Manson's Tropical Diseases

Manson's Tropical Diseases

Twentieth Edition

G. C. COOK
MD DSc FRCP FRACP FLS

President of the Royal Society of Tropical Medicine and Hygiene (1993–95)
Physician at the Hospital for Tropical Diseases, University College London Hospitals, and St Luke's
  Hospital for the Clergy
Lecturer at the London School of Hygiene and Tropical Medicine
Formerly Medical Specialist with the Royal Nigerian Army, Lecturer in Medicine at Makerere
  University College in Uganda, and Professor of Medicine in the Universities of Zambia, Riyadh
  (Saudi Arabia), and Papua New Guinea

WB Saunders Company Ltd
London   Philadelphia   Toronto   Sydney   Tokyo

W. B. Saunders Company Ltd 24–28 Oval Road
London NW1 7DX

The Curtis Center
Independence Square West
Philadelphia, PA 19106-3399, USA

Harcourt Brace & Company
55 Horner Avenue
Toronto, Ontario M8Z 4X6, Canada

Harcourt Brace & Company, Australia
30–52 Smidmore Street
Marrickville, NSW 2204, Australia

Harcourt Brace & Company, Japan
Ichibancho Central Building, 22-1 Ichibancho
Chiyoda-ku, Tokyo 102, Japan

A catalogue record for this book is available from the British Library

First published 1898
Eighteenth edition 1982
Nineteenth edition 1987
Twentieth edition 1996

ISBN 0-7020-1764-7

Typeset by Paston Press Ltd, Loddon, Norfolk

Printed and bound in Great Britain by Bath Press, Avon

CONTENTS

PREFACE TO THE TWENTIETH EDITION

Dr (later Sir) Patrick Manson produced the first edition of this text, *Tropical Diseases: a manual of the diseases of warm climates*, in 1898. Many books had previously been written on disease(s) in various tropical locations, but Manson amassed a wealth of factual material (much of it based on an increasing knowledge of protozoology and helminthology—areas in which a great deal of current research was proceeding) on diseases (mostly infectious) from all parts of the tropics. It immediately became the classic text covering *tropical medicine* and was widely used the world over. Manson saw the book through a total of six editions. Following that, his son-in-law, Dr (later Sir) Philip Manson-Bahr, became editor until the sixteenth edition, and Manson's grandson, Dr P E C Manson-Bahr, has been (jointly) editor of the last three editions.

It seems increasingly likely that *Homo sapiens* originated in a warm climate (probably in Africa); physiological studies indicate that his ability to adapt to a high ambient temperature is infinitely better than is that to a low one. Therefore, mankind has since his/her origin been surrounded (and dominated) by diseases—viral, bacterial, protozoan, and helminthic—common to warm climates. These have without doubt moulded the human genome to a greater extent than any other single factor (including environmental ones) since the species originated. As global warming becomes a likely event (in the light of mankind's gross mismanagement of the global *milieu*) the group of diseases described by Manson is likely to assume an even greater profile in the years ahead.

Manson's work was a monograph. Since then, the book has grown 'like topsy' with bits removed and others added. I decided that a radical overhaul was now required; therefore the twentieth edition includes contributions from a wide range of authors—most of them (like Manson) British in origin, but with a significant input from tropical countries themselves. I hope the balance is not too 'wide of the mark', but should there be deficiencies, these will doubtless be rectified in future editions.

'Manson' will I sincerely hope remain the 'bible' of *tropical medicine*. It will be used by physicians in temperate climes as well as those (other medical personnel included) in the developing countries of the globe. It is also my hope that as well as addressing tropical medicine it will be considered a major text covering 'medicine in the tropics'. In addition to the entities (mostly with an infective basis) originally covered by 'Manson', I have included contributions on non-infective disease in tropical countries and also ones on disciplines related to medicine—paediatrics, surgery, and obstetrics and gynaecology. Although the book is both clinically and parasitologically oriented, it should also be of use for the primary 'health care worker' without whom the pyramidal structure of health care in the developing world would collapse.

I am extremely grateful to all of those authors who (most, but not all of those invited) accepted the challenge to contribute to this edition; some contributions clearly absorbed a great deal of their time. Seón Duggan invited me to undertake this task. Dawn Mustafa provided valuable secretarial back-up. Richard Cook and Manjula Goonawardena in particular gave valuable support during the latter stages in the book's gestation.

Above all, this twentieth edition signifies a definite change in direction for 'Manson', and it is my hope that this volume will form a healthy basis for future editions of this well established British work.

G C Cook
August 1995

PREFACE TO THE FIRST EDITION (1898)

A MANUAL on the diseases of warm climates, of handy size, and yet giving adequate information, has long been a want; for the exigencies of travel and of tropical life are, as a rule, incompatible with big volumes and large libraries. This is the reason for the present work.

While it is hoped that the book may prove of practical service, it makes no pretension to being anything more than an introduction to the important department of medicine of which it treats; in no sense is it put forward as a complete treatise, or as being in this respect comparable to the more elaborate works by Davidson, Scheube, Rho, Laveran, Corre, Roux, and other systematic writers in the same field.

The author avails himself of this opportunity to acknowledge the valuable assistance he has received, in revising the text, from Dr. L. Westenra Sambon and Mr. David Rees, M.R.C.P., L.R.C.P., lately Senior House Surgeon, Seamen's Hospital, Albert Docks, London. He would also acknowledge his great obligation to Mr. Richard Muir, Pathological Laboratory, Edinburgh University, for his care and skill in preparing the illustrations.

Patrick Manson
April 1898

LIST OF CONTRIBUTORS

Dr AO Adebajo
Rheumatology Research Unit
Addenbrooke's Hospital
Cambridge CB2 2QQ
England

Dr D Adu
Queen Elizabeth Medical Centre
Queen Elizabeth Hospital
Edgbaston
Birmingham B15 2TH
England

Dr S Amor
The Rayne Institute
Neurovirology Unit
St Thomas' Hospital
London SE1 7GH
England

Dr FI Anjourin
Jos Teaching Hospital
PMB 2076
Jos
Plateau State
Nigeria

Dr OP Arya
Dept of Genito-Urinary Medicine
Royal Liverpool University Hospital
Prescott Street
Liverpool L7 8XP
England

Dr GG Baily
Regional Dept of Infectious Diseases
and Tropical Medicine
Monsall Hospital
Newton Heath
Manchester M10 8WR
England

Dr JR Baker
Royal Society for Tropical Medicine & Hygiene
Manson House
26 Portland Place
London W1N 4EY
England

Dr AH Barnett
East Birmingham Hospital
Birmingham B9 5ST
England

Dr DG Beevers
Dept of Medicine
Dudley Road Hospital
Birmingham B18 7QH
England

Dr JR Billinghurst
Rush Green Hospital
Dagenham Road
Romford
Essex RM7 0YA
England

Dr BJ Brabin
Dept of Tropical Paediatrics
& International Child Health
Liverpool School of Tropical Medicine
Pembroke Place
Liverpool L3 5QA
England

Dr MG Brook
Dept of Infectious and Tropical Diseases
Coppetts Wood Hospital
Coppetts Road, Muswell Hill
London N10 1JN
England

Dr ADM Bryceson
Hospital for Tropical Diseases
St Pancras Way
London NW1 0PE
England

Dr DA Cavan
East Birmingham Hospital
Birmingham B9 5ST
England

Dr A Cevallas
Dept of Gastroenterology
St Bartholomew's Hospital
West Smithfield
London EC1A 7BE
England

Dr PL Chiodini
Dept of Parasitology
Hospital for Tropical Diseases
St Pancras Way
London NW1 0PE
England

The late Dr WP Cockshott
Dept of Radiology
McMaster University Medical Center
Faculty of Health Sciences
1200 Main Street West
Hamilton, Ontario L8N 3Z5
Canada

Dr TJ Coleman
PHLS Leptospira Reference Laboratory
County Hospital
Hereford HR1 2ER
England

Dr GC Cook
Dept of Clinical Sciences
Hospital for Tropical Diseases
St Pancras Way
London NW1 0PE
England

Dr KJ Collins
Dept of Geriatric Medicine
St Pancras Hospital
MRC Unit
St Pancras Way
London NW1 0PE
England

Major General GO Cowan
Royal Army Medical College
Millbank
London SW1P 4RJ
England

Professor D Crawford
Dept of Microbiology
London School of Hygiene & Tropical Medicine
Keppel Street
London WC1E 7HT
England

Dr JK Cruickshank
Clinical Epidemiology Unit
Manchester University Medical School
Oxford Road
Manchester M13 9PT
England

Dr D Dance
Dept of Clinical Sciences
London School of Hygiene & Tropical Medicine
Keppel Street
London WC1E 7HT
England

Lt Col JG Dickinson
The Duchess of Kent's Military Hospital
Horne Road
Catterick Garrison
North Yorkshire DL9 4DF
England

Dr F Doua
Liverpool School of Tropical Medicine
Pembroke Place
Liverpool L3 5QA
England

Dr DB Elkins
Queensland Inst. of Medical Research
Tropical Health Programme
Branston Terrace
Herston
Queensland
Australia

Professor MJG Farthing
Dept of Gastroenterology
St Bartholomew's Hospital
West Smithfield
London EC1A 7BE
England

Professor AF Fleming
Director of Laboratory Services
University Teaching Hospital
Private Bag 12101
Lusaka
Zambia

Miss AS Garden
Dept of Obstetrics & Gynaecology
Royal Liverpool University Hospital
Prescott Street
Liverpool L7 8XP
England

Professor HM Gilles
William P Hartley Building
University of Liverpool
Brownlow Street
PO Box 147
Liverpool L69 3BX
England

Dr D Goodall
Dept of Obstetrics and Gynaecology
Queens Park Hospital
Haslingden Road
Blackburn
Lancashire BB2 3HH
England

Dr LG Goodwin
Shepperlands Farm
Park Lane
Finchampstead
Berks RG11 4QF
England

Professor Gottstein
Dept of Clinical Pharmacology
University of Berne
Murtenstrasse 35
Berne CH-3010
Switzerland

Dr TJ Harrison
Royal Free Hospital School of Medicine
Roland Hill Street
Hampstead
London NW3 2QG
England

Professor CA Hart
Dept of Medical Microbiology
and Genito-Urinary Medicine
Royal Liverpool University Hospital
Duncan Building, PO Box 147
Liverpool L69 3BX
England

Dr DB Haswell-Elkins
Queensland Inst. of Medical Research
Tropical Health Programme
Branston Terrace
Herston
Queensland
Australia

Professor JR Hay
St John's Institute for Dermatology
Guy's Hospital
St Thomas' Street
London SE1 9RT
England

Professor RG Hendrickse
Liverpool School of Tropical Medicine
Pembroke Place
Liverpool L3 5QA
England

Dr T Hien
Centre for Tropical Diseases
Cho Quan Hospital
Ho Chi Minh City
Vietnam

Mr C Holcombe
University Dept of Surgery
University of Wales College of Medicine
Heath Park
Cardiff CF4 4XW
Wales

Dr RE Holliman
Toxoplasma Reference Laboratory
St George's Hospital Medical School
Cranmer Terrace
London SW17 0RE
England

Dr N Horne
95/6 Grange Road
Edinburgh EH9 2ED
Scotland

Professor MSR Hutt
Gwernvale Cottage
Brecon Road, Crickhowell
Powys NP8 1SE
Wales

Dr P Kelly
Dept of Gastroenterology
St Bartholomew's Hospital
West Smithfield
London EC1A 7BE
England

Dr K Lam
Dept of Microbiology
London School of Hygiene & Tropical Medicine
Keppel Street
London WC1E 7HT
England

Dr HO Lobel
Malaria Branch Center for Disease Control
Atlanta
Georgia 30333
USA

Dr DCW Mabey
Dept of Clinical Sciences
London School of Hygiene & Tropical Medicine
Keppel Street
London WC1E 7HT
England

Professor C R Madeley
Dept of Clinical Virology
Medical School
University of Newcastle-upon-Tyne
Newcastle-upon-Tyne NE2 7RU
England

Dr BK Mandal
Regional Dept of Infectious Diseases
and Tropical Medicine
Monsall Hospital
Newton Heath
Manchester M10 8WR
England

Professor PD Marsden
CEP 70 849
Brasilia DF
Brazil

Dr JC Mbanya
Dept of Internal Medicine
University of Yaounde
Cameroon

Dr S Mehta
Neurovirology Unit
The Rayne Institute
St Thomas' Hospital
London SE1 7GH
England

Dr GJ Miller
MRC Epidemiology & Medical Care Unit
Northwick Park Hospital
Watford Road
Harrow HI1 3UJ
England

Dr RF Miller
Medical Unit
The Middlesex Hospital
Mortimer Street
London W1N 8AA
England

Professor DH Molyneux
Liverpool School of Tropical Medicine
Pembroke Place
Liverpool L3 5QA
England

Professor ME Molyneux
Liverpool School of Tropical Medicine
Pembroke Place
Liverpool L3 5QA
England

Mr AH Moody
Dept of Parasitology
Hospital for Tropical Diseases
St Pancras Way
London NW1 0PE
England

Dr JE McMahon
Matunda
Burrington
Avon BS18 7AA
England

Mr DDM McGavin
Dept of Preventive Ophthalmology
Institute of Ophthalmology
27–29 Cayton Street
London EC1V 9EJ
England

Dr S Nimmannitya
Children's Hospital
Ministry of Public Health
420/8 Rajvithi Road
Bangkok 10400
Thailand

Dr SK Nordeen
Chief Medical Officer
Leprosy Unit
Division of Tropical Diseases
World Health Organization
CH-1211
Geneva 27
Switzerland

Professor CLM Olweny
Manitoba Cancer Treatment and
Research Foundation
St Boniface General Hospital
409 Tache Avenue
Winnipeg R2H 2A6
Canada

Dr JH Orley
Division of Mental Health
World Health Organization
CH-1211
Geneva 27
Switzerland

Dr VK Pannikar
Leprosy Unit
Division of Tropical Diseases
World Health Organization
CH-1211
Geneva 27
Switzerland

Professor EHO Parry
Dept of Clinical Sciences
London School of Hygiene & Tropical Medicine
Keppel Street
London WC1E 7HT
England

Dr JSM Peiris
Dept of Virology
Royal Victoria Infirmary
Queen Victoria Road
Newcastle-upon-Tyne NE1 4LP
England

Dr V Pentreath
Liverpool School of Tropical Medicine
Pembroke Place
Liverpool L3 5QA
England

Dr JHS Pettit
Room 301
Bangunan Hing Yoon
42–3 Jalan Chow Yoon
50350 Kuala Lumpur
Malaysia

Dr P Piot
Dept of Microbiology
Institute of Tropical Medicine
Nationalestraat No. 155
Antwerp 2000
Belgium

Professor JHL Playfair
Medical School
Middlesex Hospital
Mortimer Street
London W1P 7PN
England

Dr J Reichen
Dept of Clinical Pharmacology
University of Berne
Murtenstrasse 35
Berne CH-3010
Switzerland

Dr J Richens
Dept of Clinical Sciences
London School of Hygiene & Tropical Medicine
Keppel Street
London WC1E 7HT
England

Dr GM Scott
Dept of Clinical Microbiology
University College Hospital
Grafton Way
London WC1E 6AU
England

Dr RA Shakir
Middlesbrough General Hospital
Ayresome Green Lane
Middlesbrough
Cleveland TS5 5AZ
England

Dr P Shears
Dept of Medical Microbiology
and Genito-Urinary Medicine
Royal Liverpool University Hospital
Duncan Building, PO Box 147
Liverpool L69 3BX
England

Dr PE Simonsen
Danish Bilharziasis Laboratory
Jaegersborg Alle 1 D
DK 2920 Charlottenlund
Denmark

Professor DIH Simpson
Dept of Microbiology & Immunology
The Queen's University Belfast
Grosvenor Road
Belfast BT12 6BN
Northern Ireland

Dr MD Smith
Oxford Tropical Medicine Research Programme
Faculty of Tropical Medicine
Wellcome Mahidol University
Rajvhi Road
Bangkok
Thailand

Dr VR Southgate
Dept of Zoology
The Natural History Museum
Cromwell Road
London SW7 5BD
England

Professor R Steffen
Inst. fur Sozial und Praventivmedizin
der Universitat Zurich
Sumatrastr. 30
Zurich CH 80006
Switzerland

Dr GM Stern
University College Hospital
Grafton Way
London WC1E 6AU
England

Dr ND Thanh
Oxford Tropical Medicine Research Programme
Faculty of Tropical Medicine
Wellcome Mahidol University
Rajvhi Road
Bangkok
Thailand

Dr EJ Threlfall
Div Enteric Pathogens
Central Public Health Laboratory
61 Colindale Avenue
London NW9 5HT
England

Dr R Thuraisingham
Queen Elizabeth Medical Centre
Queen Elizabeth Hospital
Edgbaston
Birmingham B15 2TH
England

Dr D Warhurst
Dept of Parasitology
London School of Hygiene & Tropical Medicine
Keppel Street
London WC1E 7HT
England

Professor D Warrell
Nuffield Dept of Clinical Medicine
John Radcliffe Hospital
Headington
Oxford OX3 9DU
England

Dr M Warrell
4 Larkins Lane
Old Headington
Oxford OX3 9DW
England

Dr GB White
105 Breamwater Gardens
Ham, Richmond
Surrey TW10 7SD
England

Dr NJ White
Nuffield Dept of Clinical Medicine
John Radcliffe Hospital
Headington
Oxford OX3 9DU
England

Dr SG Wright
Hospital for Tropical Diseases
St Pancras Way
London NW1 0PE
England

Professor A Zuckerman
Royal Free Hospital School of Medicine
Roland Hill Street
Hampstead
London NW3 2QG
England

Dr JN Zuckerman
Royal Free Hospital School of Medicine
Roland Hill Street
Hampstead
London NW3 2QG
England

Every effort has been made to check the drug dosages given in this book. However, as it is possible that errors have been missed or that dosage schedules have been revised, the reader is strongly urged to consult the drug companies' literature before administering any of the drugs listed.

SECTION 1
HISTORY OF DISEASE IN WARM CLIMATES

CHAPTER 1

HISTORY OF *TROPICAL MEDICINE*, AND 'MEDICINE IN THE TROPICS'

G. C. Cook

Numerous British doctors practised in tropical countries as early as the seventeenth and eighteenth centuries: in the English West Indies, India, the East Indies and later Africa—the western part of which was widely termed the 'white man's grave'.[1,2] Many also produced monographs describing their experiences, with an outline of the disease patterns at these various locations. Many infections which now fall under the 'tropical' umbrella were widely distributed in northern Europe and northern America during the seventeenth to nineteenth centuries. Shakespeare was well aware of malaria as a disease entity in England: 'he is so shak'd by the burning quotidian tertian that it is most lamentable to behold' (*Henry V*, II. i. 123). Thomas Sydenham (1624–1689) successfully used fever-tree bark (quinine) in the management of the 'intermittent fevers' during the seventeenth century.[3] Indigenous *Plasmodium vivax* infection remained present in southeast England well into the twentieth century. Plague, typhoid, cholera, typhus and smallpox were major health hazards in Britain, London included, during the Victorian era.[4] John Bunyon (1628–1688) was well aware of the consumption (tuberculosis)—now such a dominant disease in 'tropical' countries—which so often 'took him down to the grave' (*The Life and Death of Mr Badman*).

What then is tropical medicine? Balfour[2] summarized the position as he saw it, in his Presidential Address to the Royal Society of Tropical Medicine and Hygiene in 1925: 'there is in one sense no such thing as tropical medicine, and in any case many of the most erudite writings of Hippocrates are concerned with maladies which nowadays are chiefly encountered under tropical or subtropical conditions'. Some, including a number of historians, consider that 'tropical medicine' originated as a by-product of British Empire and Raj.[5] The truth of the matter is that the discipline was exploited by the Colonialists in order that the health of British personnel, both overseas and following return to the UK, could be improved (see below).[1] The specialty in fact had its origin(s) in a multidisciplinary background: major areas of progress during the nineteenth century were public health (and hygiene), travel and exploration, natural history, evolutionary theory, and a precise knowledge of the causation of disease (the 'germ theory').[6] The miasmatists and contagionists had previously held the floor! The development of clinical parasitology following the work of Manson, Ross and others, and superimposed on this complex backcloth, led to the inevitable genesis of 'tropical medicine'.[6,7]

DEVELOPMENT OF TROPICAL MEDICINE IN LONDON

THE SEAMEN'S HOSPITAL SOCIETY

In London, the Seamen's Hospital Society (SHS) (the 'foster mother of clinical tropical medicine') was formed in the winter of 1817–1818; the *raison d'être* was to provide temporary relief to distressed mariners then roaming in large numbers on London's streets.[8] The major objective was thus largely targeted at the management of illnesses (especially fevers) introduced into London from tropical and subtropical countries.[4] At a meeting held at the City of London Tavern on 8 March 1821 (William Wilberforce was amongst those present), the committee resolved to establish a permanent floating hospital on the Thames for the exclusive use of sick and distressed seamen; the venture was to be supported by voluntary contributions. A series of hulks, HMS *Grampus* (commissioned in 1821) (Figure 1.1), HMS *Dreadnought* (1831–1857) and HMS *Caledonia* (renamed *Dreadnought*, also) (1857–1870) were anchored in Greenwich Reach and used successively; they had been 48-, 98- and 120-gun vessels, respectively.[1,8] Although they served a valuable function, major practical problems arose: ventilation was poor, and nosocomial spread of disease occurred; lack of light was a major drawback during the winter months; and other problems (not least noise) associated with being situated in the midst of an extremely busy part of the river proved tiresome.[9] In 1870 the Commissioners of the Admiralty granted the SHS a 99-year lease of the Infirmary (and adjoining Somerset Ward) of the Royal Hospital, Greenwich, in lieu of the loan of the ship(s).[1,8] This move was made possible because the number of pensioners residing in the Hospital had declined rapidly during the peaceful years following the battle of Waterloo in 1815; the Infirmary was therefore no longer required by the declining institution. [In 1873 the Hospital ceased being a permanent home for Naval pensioners and became the Royal Naval College (previously based at Portsmouth).] The Greenwich Hospital had been founded in 1694 by William and Mary as the Naval equivalent of the Royal Hospital, Chelsea (founded by King Charles II), which remains in use for Army pensioners today.

EMERGENCE OF THE SPECIALTY

Following his return to London from Formosa, Amoy (where he had made his seminal discovery of the man–mosquito cycle of the nematode *Filaria sanguinis hominis* [*Wuchereria bancrofti*]—the causative agent of lymphatic filariasis) and Hong Kong, Patrick Manson (1844–1922)[10] (Figure 1.2) embarked on a series of lectures devoted to 'tropical medicine' at several London medical schools.[11] The Rt Hon Joseph Chamberlain, Secretary of State for the Colonies, was immediately impressed at the possibility of sending the Colonial medical staff on leave in Britain to these lectures, to give an update in the prevention and management of those diseases which seriously affected the servants of Empire. Regular trade, efficient administration and agricultural production were all seriously hampered by disease; furthermore, Chamberlain's concept of 'constructive imperialism' could not be adequately developed in the presence of such a great deal of morbidity and mortality. Therefore, *clinical tropical*

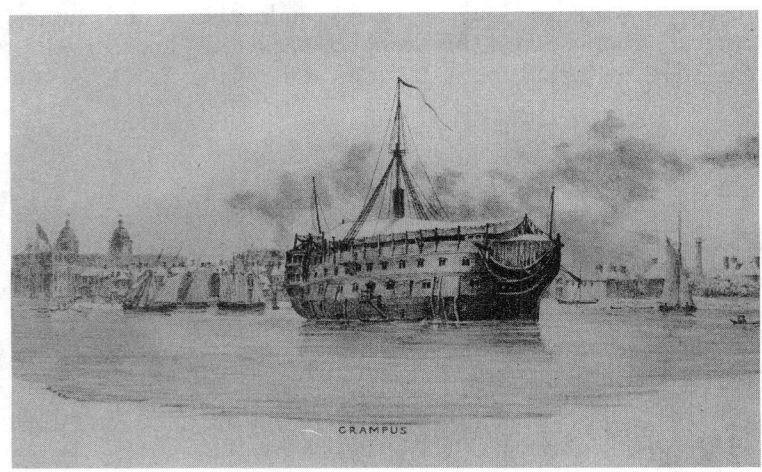

Figure 1.1 HMS *Grampus*. The first of three hospital ships sponsored by the Seamen's Hospital Society, anchored on Greenwich Reach. The disused 48-gun warship served in this capacity from October 1821 to October 1831.

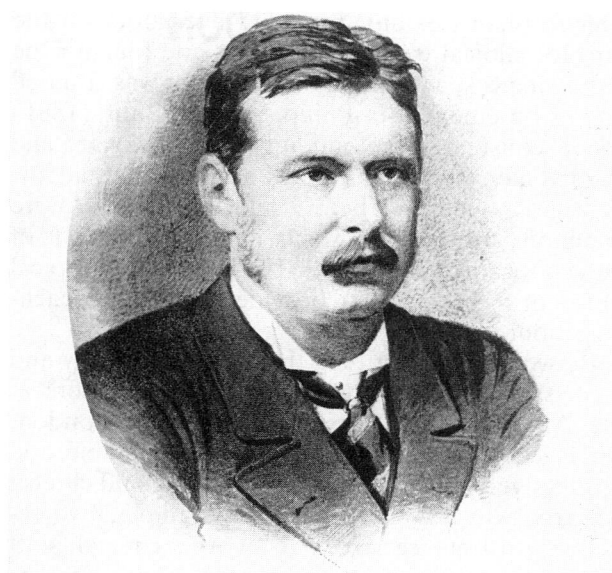

Figure 1.2 Dr (later Sir) Patrick Manson (1844–1922) aged 31 years. This photograph was probably taken whilst he was on leave in Britain from Amoy in 1875.

medicine emerged as both an important medical specialty and scientific discipline (the importance of parasites and their vector transmission in disease had recently become clear—see above); Chamberlain also considered 'tropical medicine' an essential component in the future development of British economic and social imperialism—it was, in fact, to become a 'colonial science'.[1,9] At the 1898 meeting of the British Medical Association held at Edinburgh, at which Ronald Ross' work on the role of the mosquito in avian malaria[12] was announced (his initial demonstration of *Plasmodium* spp. development in the mosquito had been published in the *British Medical Journal* the previous year), a new section devoted to Tropical Medicine was inaugurated. There were several reasons why the discipline had *not* previously emerged into the limelight. Most 'tropical diseases' had formerly existed in northern Europe (including England) and northern America (see above). There was a widespread feeling that the high mortality affecting the white man in the tropics was inevitable, and that he would never be able to live and work there successfully. The 'miasmatic theory' held sway. Furthermore, there was an understandable pessimism regarding the possibility of significant environmental improvement, most British colonies being situated on unhealthy coastlines. Also, research had until then taken a very low priority for medical staff working in the tropics; their task was to provide medical advice and clinical care to the local British community.

THE MANSON–CHAMBERLAIN COLLABORATION

In order to implement effective development of the 'new' discipline, Manson was appointed Medical Officer to the Colonial Office in 1897. Here, with Chamberlain's wholehearted support, he set about establishing a School of Tropical Medicine in London (LSTM).[1,9] A major problem related to the venue of the proposed institution. Manson favoured the Branch (Seamen's) Hospital of the Greenwich Hospital—situated near the Royal Albert Dock. However, hostility to this suggestion arose from several quarters. The War Office favoured the Royal Victoria Hospital, Netley, which, situated on Southampton Water, had been founded in 1863;[1] it had been established primarily for soldiers invalided from the Crimea and was staffed by officers of the Royal Army Medical Corps. Manson considered this option unacceptable: the atmosphere and remote situation were, in his opinion, incompatible with the teaching of clinical tropical medicine. The Royal College of Physicians was of the opinion that a new school was uncalled for! The senior medical staff of the Greenwich Hospital (led by Dr John Curnow, who was also on the editorial staff of the *Lancet*) were in opposition: they felt that removal of the 'tropical' cases to the Branch Hospital was a slight on their professional ability to manage these diseases, and was in any case undesirable because medical students from London's teaching hospitals were accustomed to visiting Greenwich for tuition in the diagnosis and management of these illnesses. The end-result was an outburst of acrimonious correspondence in the columns of the *Lancet*, the *British Medical Journal* and *The Times*, which later involved, amongst others, Sir William Broadbent, Sir William Church, Sir Jonathan Hutchinson and Sir Joseph Fayrer—the doyen of the Indian Medical Service.[1,9] However, the staunch determination of Manson and Herbert Read (Assistant Private Secretary to Chamberlain) to proceed with the project, strongly supported by Chamberlain himself, led to the rapid establishment of the proposed school at the Branch (Albert Dock) Hospital; financial assistance to the tune of £3550 came from the Colonial Office. A subcommittee was set up to 'formulate a scheme for organization and management of the LSTM in connection with the SHS'; the committee of management was composed of equal numbers of personnel from the SHS, the medical and surgical staff of the Branch Hospital, and teachers from the LSTM.

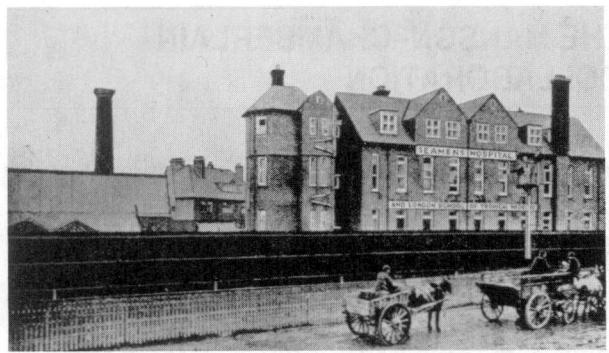

Figure 1.3 Newly opened London School of Tropical Medicine—situated on an adjoining site to the Seamen's Hospital Society's Branch (Albert Dock) Hospital—in October 1899.

SCHOOL AND HOSPITAL IN CLOSE PROXIMITY

The LSTM was officially opened on 2 October 1899. The hospital (under SHS supervision) and teaching and research facilities (LSTM) were in close proximity (Figure 1.3). With Sir Perceval Nairne (Chairman of the SHS) presiding, the inaugural address—written by Manson—was read in his absence. He later declared: 'the school strikes, and strikes effectively, at the root of the principal difficulty of most of our Colonies-disease. It will cheapen government and make it more efficient. It will encourage and cheapen commercial enterprise. It will conciliate and foster the native.'[13] Meanwhile continuous funding was necessary, and several sources of income were exploited; two charity dinners, at which Chamberlain presided, were held at the Hotel Cecil in 1899 and 1905; they raised £12000 and £11000 respectively. At the former, Chamberlain declared: 'The man who shall successfully grapple with this foe of humanity and find the cure for malaria, for the fever desolating our colonies . . . and shall make the tropics livable for white men . . . will do more for the world, more for the British Empire, than the man who adds a new province to the wide Dominions of the Queen.' A 'Tropical Diseases Research Fund' was set up, and the Dean—Sir Francis Lovell—raised funds on several overseas trips. In 1912 the school was enlarged and a new wing opened by Their Majesties King George V and Queen Mary.

In 1919 the decision was taken to relocate the school and hospital in central London; Endsleigh Palace Hotel, 23 Gordon Street, WC1, was purchased (by the SHS) for £70000 and on 11 November 1920 the Duke of York (later King George VI) opened the joint LSTM and Hospital for Tropical Diseases in this building.[1,9] The structure, which remains extant, provided five floors (at the top) for clinical tropical medicine, and four for the basic sciences; a radiology department was situated in the basement. Sir Philip Manson-Bahr (1881–1966)[9] considered the building 'dark, awkward and inconvenient, with multitudes of doors and narrow passages', but never before had there been 'more unanimity or good fellowship amongst the staffs of the school and the hospital'. The Wellcome Tropical Museum was nearby and provided invaluable teaching resources.

Between 1899 and 1929 the clinical specialty and the basic sciences were thus on the same site—first at the Albert Dock Hospital and later in London, WC1; the close proximity was both valuable and productive, and a great deal of teaching and clinical research was accomplished. For example, two research projects carried out by the clinical staff clinched the mosquito transmission of malaria saga in *Homo sapiens*.[1,9] Dr G. C. Low (1872–1952) (later largely responsible for establishing the Royal Society of Tropical Medicine and Hygiene)[14,15] and three other investigators slept between dusk and dawn—for 3 months—in a mosquito-proof hut about 7km from Rome, Italy (where *P. vivax* malaria was prevalent); by so doing they avoided a clinical *P. vivax* infection.[1] Also, in 1900, three batches of mosquitoes infected with *P. vivax* were sent from Rome to London; Manson's elder surviving son—then a medical student at Guy's Hospital, and captain of rugby football—was exposed to them, and duly acquired a clinical attack of *P. vivax* infection, which responded to quinine.[1]

FOUNDATION OF THE LONDON SCHOOL OF HYGIENE AND TROPICAL MEDICINE: CLOSE RELATIONSHIP BETWEEN TROPICAL PHYSICIANS AND BASIC SCIENTIFIC STAFF ENDS

In 1921 the Postgraduate Medical Committee recommended that an Institute of State Medicine be created in the University of London; the Rockefeller Foundation was persuaded by Professor R. T. Leiper (1881–1969) to donate $2000000 to the Ministry of Health for the development of this project.[1,9] In 1929, the London School of Hygiene and Tropical Medicine (LSHTM) was officially opened at Keppel Street (Gower Street) by the Prince of Wales (later King Edward VIII). At this point the SHS ceased managing the School, and clinical tropical medicine became detached from the basic sciences.

Clinical tropical medicine in London suffered a further temporary setback when the Ross Institute and Hospital for Tropical Diseases (Director: Sir Ronald Ross [1857–1932]—see below) was opened at Putney in 1926.[1,9,16] It was, however, clear from the outset that there was insufficient clinical material in London to justify two separate hospitals devoted to the management of tropical disease; the project therefore had no chance of becoming clinically viable! The institution ultimately became incorporated into the LSHTM, as the Ross Institute for Tropical Hygiene, in 1934; Ross had died 2 years before.

The itinerant saga of *clinical* tropical medicine in London continued unabated and the continuing survival of Manson's original concept seemed at times in serious jeopardy—not least during World War II when the specialty had to make do with a mere ten beds, with no teaching facilities, at the Dreadnought Hospital, Greenwich. For a brief period after the war a nursing home in Devonshire Street, W1, housed the discipline. The present Hospital for Tropical Diseases, situated at St Pancras, NW1, was opened on 24 May (Empire Day) 1951 by the Duchess of Kent.

Regarding the clinical discipline in London, Manson-Bahr[9] later concluded: 'In recounting the chequered history of this institution, the Hospital for Tropical Diseases, a venture one would have thought essential to the greatest of all Empires, there runs the thread of insecurity . . . the hospital became the whipping boy of medical politics . . . The Board of the SHS was always a representative body of admirals whose interest lay in the sailor, but *not* in (clinical) tropical medicine.' The saga continues: the whereabouts and date of the next removal remain anyone's guess[1,17]!

DEVELOPMENT OF TROPICAL MEDICINE IN LIVERPOOL

The Liverpool School of Tropical Medicine had opened about 6 months before that in London.[1,18] Although the concept of a School of Tropical Medicine in Liverpool developed later, the plan of action proceeded more rapidly, and the School opened to students on 21 April 1899. The initial momentum had originated in a circular from Chamberlain to the General Medical Council and leading British medical schools (11 March 1898), and a letter to the Governors of the Colonies (14 June 1898). The time-scale of the first appointments was impressive:[18,19] 20 January 1899—Dean appointed; 7 February—Demonstrator in tropical pathology (Dr H. E. Annett); 10 April—Lecturer in tropical medicine (Major Ronald Ross, IMS); 22 April—School officially opened by Lord Lister (1827–1912); May 1899—teaching started. The Liverpool School was *not* Chamberlain's 'brainchild' (unlike the LSTM), and it did not receive Government support—a source of irritation (and perhaps even anger) at the time. It owed its inception to the initiative of Mr (later Sir) Alfred Jones KCMG (1845–1909). A prominent Liverpool (like London, an important seaport) figure, and an energetic leader in the development of Liverpool's overseas trade with the West African Colonies, he controlled the Elder Dempster shipping line, which traded with the Canary Islands and West Africa (and had a thriving business in bananas, groundnuts and oil nuts). Together with several Liverpool merchants—extremely wealthy, but also generous—he provided the initiative and finance for the School's foundation. The other major personality in the foundation was Dr (later Sir) Rubert Boyce, FRS (1863–1911). In December 1898 the *Lancet*[20] reported: 'Mr Chamberlain's scheme for the teaching of tropical diseases to colonial surgeons, wherever the school may be located, has already born practical fruit. Mr. Alfred Jones of Liverpool has offered £350 annually to establish and maintain a laboratory in Liverpool for the study of tropical diseases and the scheme will be carried out by a joint committee of the Royal Southern Hospital and of University College. A laboratory for immediate investigation will be built opposite the hospital, whilst prolonged research will be carried out in the pathological laboratory of University College, under the direction of Professor Boyce. A large number of cases from the West Coast of Africa are taken into the wards of the Royal Southern Hospital, as Liverpool, being the centre of the African trade, is in constant communication with West Africa. We again have to congratulate Liverpool on the munificence of her citizens and would direct the attention of medical men about to practice in any capacity on the West Coast of Africa to the opportunity that is being afforded them for obtaining invaluable information.'

The project was supported by the Royal Society, whose Secretary wrote to the Principal of University College, Liverpool (18 November 1898):[18] 'I think the idea of starting something at Liverpool about Tropical Diseases in connection with the College, most admirable. The opportunities of studying Tropical Diseases are greater at Liverpool than anywhere else in England, excepting perhaps London. You have to arrange: 1. For teaching. 2. For investigation. No. 2 wants, I think, more support than No. 1. If you had a ward, say at the Southern Hospital, one of the physicians might take charge of it, and give lectures, clinical at the Hospital, and general say at the College—I suppose you might give him a title. For investigation you do not, I think, need a separate Laboratory at College, but a small Clinical Laboratory at the Hospital itself . . . The next point, I am in doubt about. I am inclined to think that the Pathology of Tropical Diseases should belong to the *Professor of Pathology*, who should, by virtue of this have some connection with the Tropical Diseases Ward in the Hospital, have access to the cases, &c. . . . This system of a Pathologist working with the Physician or Surgeon in Clinical charge of the sick is being very largely worked with great success in America, and in this Tropical Disease seems to offer an opportunity for it. I have talked with Lord Lister [President of the Royal Society], and he generally approves of what I have proposed, at least, thinks it most desirable that the Hospital and College should lay hold of Tropical Diseases. I myself feel very strong that it is an opportunity of *study* of these diseases. When the experts on Malaria sent out of Africa get to work on the West Coast, as they will in time do, it will be a great advantage to have an Institution for Tropical Diseases already in work at Liverpool. The experts abroad can work with the men at home.'

At a meeting convened at the offices of Messrs Elder, Dempster & Co on 23 November 1898, the following were present:[18] Alfred L. Jones; William Adamson, President of the Royal Southern Hospital; R. T. Glazebrook, Principal of University College; William Alexander, Senior Surgeon of the Royal Southern Hospital; William Carter, Physician to the Royal Southern Hospital, Professor of Therapeutics, University College; and Rubert Boyce, Professor of Pathology, University College. 'The following resolutions were unanimously passed: 1. That the gentlemen present form themselves into a Committee, with the approval of their various boards, for promoting the study of Tropical Diseases and to consider the best means of carrying out Mr. Alfred L. Jones' intentions in the munificent offer he has made to further the above object. 2. That Mr. Charles W. Jones (of Messrs Lamport and Holt) be asked to serve on this Committee. It

was decided that the above resolutions should be printed, and that Mr. Jones would hand a copy to the Rt. Hon. Joseph Chamberlain, Secretary of State for the Colonies. The Committee recommended that before the next meeting, the Professional Members should meet together to consider and suggest the best means for . . . carrying out these objects.'

At a second meeting, on 12 December 1898, a letter from Lord Ampthill (Colonial Office) to the Chairman (1 December) was read:[18] 'I have shown your letter of the 28th ult. with regard to the School of Tropical Medicine . . . to Mr. Chamberlain. He was much interested and very glad to hear of the important work you have thus commenced. You are no doubt aware of what Mr. Chamberlain has been doing himself with regard to the establishment of a School of Tropical Medicine at the Seamen's Hospital, and he considers it a great advantage that Liverpool should be co-operating on similar lines. If it would interest you, I should be very glad to send you particulars of the Colonial Office scheme and information as to what has been done already, but I dare say you have learnt all that is essential from the newspapers.'

In another letter (1 February 1899) from the Colonial Office,[18] read to a subsequent Committee meeting, it was stated that 'Chamberlain was very glad to learn that it had been decided to establish this School, but regretting that the Government could not grant any financial aid; however, in the selection of candidates for medical appointments in the Colonies, preference would be given to those who had received instruction in tropical medicine, such as that provided in the Liverpool School'. A further letter from Chamberlain (23 February) stated, however, that 'all doctors appointed to the Colonial Service must be attached to the Albert Docks' Hospital for at least 2 months'. The Committee resolved to: (1) write to the Colonial Office and express regret that Mr Chamberlain did not see his way to dispense with the latter condition in the case of students from the Liverpool School; and (2) approach the Colonial Office on the subject later. On 20 March, Professor Boyce announced that Lord Lister had written stating that he intended to approach Mr Chamberlain on behalf of the School, and it was therefore resolved to postpone further action in the matter pending receipt of information concerning the result of Lister's interview. However, Government funding was not forthcoming and there can be no doubt that this led to a significant souring of relationships (some rivalry still exists) toward Manson and the LSTM.

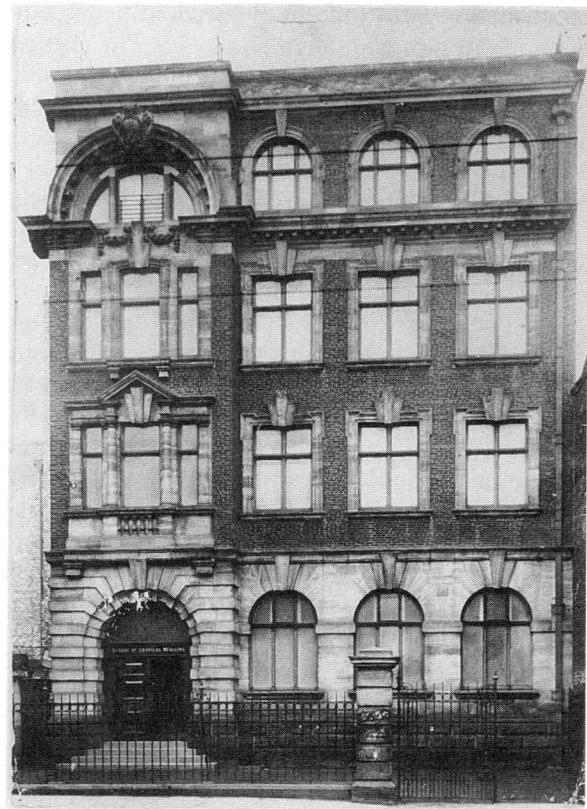

Figure 1.4 Liverpool School of Tropical Medicine—which has remained on the same site since April 1899.

FOUNDATION OF THE LIVERPOOL SCHOOL

The *Lancet*[21] summarized the inauguration of the Liverpool School (Figure 1.4): 'This School was inaugurated under fortunate auspices on April 22nd of this year by Lord Lister. "At the annual dinner of the Royal Southern Hospital on Nov. 12th, 1898, Mr. Alfred L. Jones, a prominent Liverpool citizen and West Africa merchant, made an offer of £350 a year to start a school in Liverpool for the study of tropical diseases. The offer was made in the presence of Professor Rubert Boyce of University College, Liverpool, and Dr. William Alexander of the Royal Southern Hospital". Mr. William Adamson, "the president of the Royal Southern Hospital, accepted the generous offer on condition that University College, Liverpool, and the Royal Southern Hospital should be united in the undertaking. This condition was cordially acquiesced in by Professor Glazebrook", at that time the principal of the College. "The great interest subsequently taken in the project by Mr. Alfred L. Jones, aided by the indomitable energy of Professor Boyce, resulted in subscriptions and donations coming in from all quarters towards the expenses of the proposed school. To those two gentlemen, warmly supported by the committee and medical staff of the Royal Southern Hospital, is due the establishment of the Liverpool School of Tropical Diseases. The management of the school is in the hands of a strong committee, of which Mr. Alfred L. Jones is the chairman and Mr. William Adamson . . . the vice-chairman. The committee also consists of duly appointed representatives of University College, Liverpool, the Royal Southern Hospital, the Liverpool Chamber of Commerce, the Steamship Owners' Association, and the Shipowners' Association. A sum of over £1700 has already been promised, partly in annual subscriptions and partly in donations, in support of the school", but more pecuniary support is urgently needed if the practical work already begun is to be maintained at its excellent level. "A large floor in the Royal Southern Hospital has been set apart for tropical cases. This floor includes a cheerful ward containing 12 beds, now fully occupied, also an extensive laboratory for the examination of blood, urine, faeces, &c., and furnished with the apparatus applicable to modern research". Professor Boyce superintends "the pathological department of the school, with Dr. Annett as pathological demonstrator. The committee have been fortunate in securing the services of Major Ronald Ross, IMS, as special lecturer on tropical diseases. . . . The number of malarial cases treated in Liverpool in 1898 amounted to 294. In the previous year . . . there were 242 cases of malaria, 14 of beri-beri, 30 of dysentery, and 39 of tropical anaemia. With the means of instruction in the varied forms of tropical diseases thus afforded there will be no need for Liverpool students to proceed to London to obtain that which is ready to hand at their own doors". The authorities of the Liverpool School of Tropical Medicine have lost no time in getting to real work.'

In June 1899, Ross (Figure 1.5) gave an inaugural lecture: he committed himself to the *practical* application of his malaria researches; extirpation of the mosquito, he envisaged, was the answer to the 'great malaria problem'. Ross had thus embarked on the 'sanitation' (or hygiene) tack which was to dominate much of the Liverpool School's work for the forthcoming century.

SUBSEQUENT DEVELOPMENTS IN LIVERPOOL

Shortly after its opening (in April 1899), the Liverpool School set up a series of 'expeditions': the first

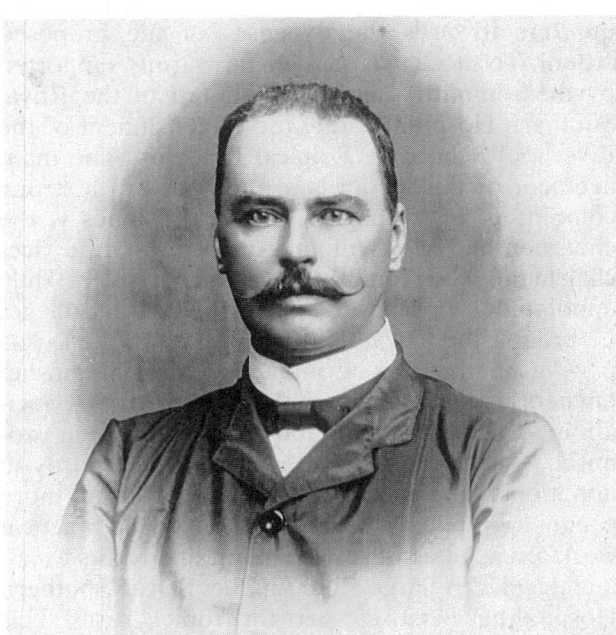

Figure 1.5 Major (later Sir) Ronald Ross (1857–1932). The photograph was probably taken around 1900.

embarked for Sierra Leone in July, and 11 more had been carried out by the end of 1903. Between its foundation and 1914, a total of 32 scientific expeditions to the tropics had taken place.[18,22] The *Annals of Tropical Medicine and Parasitology* was founded by the School's staff in 1907. The School was compelled, however, to survive by subscription; there was therefore no year-to-year stability.

At the outbreak of the Great War in 1914, teaching had been in full swing for 15 years;[23] two full courses were being given annually. An advanced practical course (1 month duration) was designed to meet the convenience of practitioners when at home on leave; those who attended this were excused the first month of the other course. Special courses on entomology designed for officers in the West African Medical Service and others were also given three times annually. Special research work was carried out at the School and the Runcorn Research Laboratories (about 16 miles from Liverpool).

The most recent historical account of the Liverpool School of Tropical Medicine is due to B. G. Maegraith;[24] in this, development of the School to the early 1970s is outlined. About this time the School had established collaborative links with some of the recently created Universities and Medical Schools of Africa, and other newly 'emergent' developing countries.

MEDICINE IN THE TROPICS

The practice of medicine in a tropical country differs in many ways from that in a temperate one—where the classical specialty (exemplified by the London and Liverpool Schools) has dominated the scenario. A major problem arises in the *definition* of 'tropical medicine'; this was addressed by Manson[7] in the preface to the first edition of his textbook in 1898: 'The title I have elected to give to this work, TROPICAL DISEASES, is more convenient than accurate. If by 'tropical diseases' be meant diseases peculiar to, and confined to, the tropics, then half a dozen pages might have sufficed for their description. . . . If . . . the expression 'tropical diseases' be held to include all diseases occurring in the tropics, then the work would require to cover almost the entire range of medicine.' The tropical practitioner (he continued): 'enjoys opportunities for original research and discovery far superior in novelty and interest to those at the command of his fellow inquirer in the well-worked field of European and American research.' Figures 1.6 and 1.7 summarize

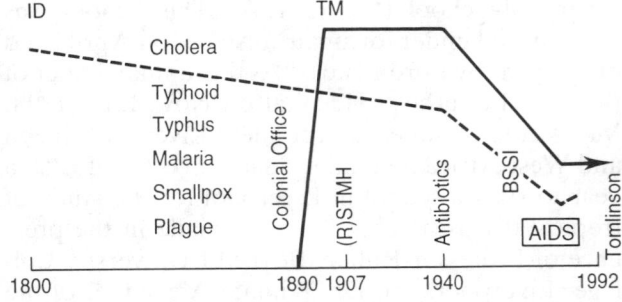

Figure 1.6 Approximate sequence of events in the foundation and development of the classical discipline: tropical medicine (TM). ID, infectious diseases; (R)STMH, (Royal) Society of Tropical Medicine and Hygiene; BSSI, British Society for the Study of Infection; AIDS, acquired immune deficiency syndrome; Tomlinson Report—published in 1992—which gave rise to sweeping changes in the British National Health Service.

some of the highlights in the development of these separate disciplines.[6]

In Britain (and other European countries) and northern America, infectious diseases dominated

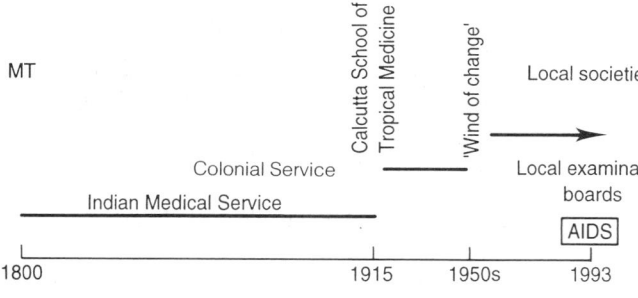

Figure 1.7 Approximate sequence of events in the progress of teaching/research in tropical (developing) countries: Medicine in the tropics (MT). AIDS, acquired immune deficiency syndrome.

the medical scene until well into the present century (see Figure 1.6); however, following the introduction of improved sanitation/hygiene in Victorian England, their prevalence slowly declined,[6] the downward trend continuing with the introduction of antibiotics in the 1940s and 1950s. Only recently has prevalence tended to move upwards—largely a result of the human immunodeficiency virus/acquired immune deficiency syndrome pandemic. *Tropical medicine*, as an organized discipline, took off in the 1890s (see above) and reached a peak during the first half of the present century. Following World War II (1939–1945) a downward trend set in; as a result, this specialty continues to decline as a specific entity. Introduction of the National Health Service 're-forms', following the Tomlinson report (published in 1992), have rendered the future of this relatively small discipline extremely vulnerable. The major priority at present is to maintain a cadre of physicians well versed in the more 'exotic' infections encountered in the UK (e.g. trypanosomiasis, leishmaniasis and schistosomiasis), a requirement which also applies to other 'temperate' countries.

In the tropical countries (Figure 1.7), the scenario is entirely different.[6] Organized medical services began with the Indian Medical Service; this was followed by the Colonial Medical Service—with a far wider influence. Although Manson had started a Medical School in Hong Kong in 1887, the first School of Tropical Medicine in a tropical country was established by Sir Leonard Rogers (1868–1962) at Calcutta in about 1920; this was a pioneering achievement. When the former British Colonies acquired 'independence' in the 1950s and later, the 'wind of change' brought in its wake many newly created indigenous universities and medical schools—e.g. Makerere University College, Kampala; Ibadan University, Nigeria; and the University (and University Teaching Hospital), Lusaka. This led to much local teaching and research, and also simultaneously the introduction of local medical societies and examining boards. These are changing times, and the future of the specialty *Tropical Medicine* is at present uncertain! But that must not be confused with 'medicine in the tropics'.

REFERENCES

1 Cook G C. *From the Greenwich Hulks to Old St Pancras: A History of Tropical Disease in London*. London: Athlone Press, 1992: 338.

2 Balfour A. Some British and American pioneers in tropical medicine and hygiene. *Trans R Soc Trop Med Hyg* 1925; 19:189–231.

3 Dewhurst K. *Dr Thomas Sydenham (1624–1689): His Life and Original Writings*. London: Wellcome Historical Medical Library, 1966: 131–139.

4 Singer C & Underwood E A. *A Short History of Medicine*, 2nd edn. Oxford: Oxford University Press, 1962: 221–223.

5 Arnold D. Introduction: diseases, medicine and empire. In Arnold D (ed.) *Imperial Medicine and Indigenous Societies*. Manchester: Manchester University Press, 1988: 1–26.

6 Cook G C. Presidential Address. Evolution: the art

of survival. *Trans R Soc Trop Med Hyg* 1994; 89: 4–18.

7 Manson P. *Tropical Diseases: A Manual of the Diseases of Warm Climates*. London: Cassell, 1898: 624.

8 McBride A G. *The History of the Dreadnought Seamens Hospital at Greenwich*. St Augustine's Hospital, Chartham: Seamen's Hospital Management Committee, 1970: 36.

9 Manson-Bahr P. *History of the School of Tropical Medicine in London: 1899–1949*. London: H K Lewis, 1956: 328.

10 Manson-Bahr P H & Alcock A. *The Life and Work of Sir Patrick Manson*. London: Cassell, 1927: 273.

11 Manson P. The necessity for special education in tropical medicine. *Lancet* 1897; ii:842–845.

12 Ross R. Report on the cultivation of proteosoma,

Labbé, in grey mosquitos. *Indian Med Gazette* 1898: 401–408, 448–452.

13 Manson P. London School of Tropical Medicine: the need for special training in tropical disease. *J Trop Med* 1899; 2:57–62.

14 Low G C. The history of the foundation of the Society of Tropical Medicine and Hygiene. *Trans R Soc Trop Med Hyg* 1928; 22:197–202.

15 Cook G C. George Carmichael Low FRCP: twelfth President of the Society and underrated pioneer of tropical medicine. *Trans R Soc Trop Med Hyg* 1993; 87:355–360.

16 Ross R. *Memoirs: With a Full Account of the Great Malaria Problem and its Solution*. London: John Murray, 1923: 547.

17 Cook G C. Future structure of clinical tropical medicine in the United Kingdom. *BMJ* 1982; 284:1460–1461.

18 *Liverpool School of Tropical Medicine: Historical Record 1898–1920*. Liverpool: University Press, 1920: 103.

19 Low G C. A retrospect of tropical medicine from 1894 to 1914. *Trans R Soc Trop Med Hyg* 1929; 23:213–232.

20 The study of tropical diseases in Liverpool. *Lancet* 1898; ii:1495.

21 The Liverpool School of Tropical Medicine. *Lancet* 1899; i:1174–1176.

22 Worboys M. Manson, Ross and colonial medical policy: tropical medicine in London and Liverpool, 1899–1914. In Macleod R & Lewis M (eds) *Disease, Medicine and Empire: Perspectives on Western Medicine and the Experience of European Expansion*. London: Routledge, 1988: 21–37.

23 Liverpool School of Tropical Medicine. *BMJ* 1914; i:324.

24 Maegraith B G. History of the Liverpool School of Tropical Medicine. *Med Hist* 1972; 16:354–368.

SECTION 2A
CLINICAL EXAMINATION

CHAPTER 2

SYMPTOMS AND SIGNS IN TROPICAL MEDICINE

M. G. Brook

In tropical medicine, perhaps more than in any other medical specialty, a carefully taken history and assiduous search for physical signs are of paramount importance. When medicine is practised in rural areas of the tropics, with little or no aid from laboratory tests, clinical acumen is the most important tool used in arriving at the correct diagnosis. Even when modern diagnostic technology is readily available, the astute practitioner can greatly benefit the patient by recognizing the multiple, often asymptomatic, pathologies that are a frequent feature of disease in a tropical context.

CLINICAL HISTORY

There are several important aspects of the history to which particular attention should be given.

TRAVEL

A precise list of places visited in chronological order, together with the extent of rural travel and exposure to water (rivers, streams, lakes) and vegetation, must be obtained, as many diseases show a marked geographical variation in incidence. For instance, in the differential diagnosis of a feverish illness, bartonellosis would only be considered in visitors to, or residents of Andean valleys in Peru, Ecuador or Colombia, whereas malaria or typhoid are so widespread as to necessitate consideration after any tropical or subtropical exposure. Some infections are common and widespread but are only acquired in certain well-defined circumstances: for example, schistosomiasis after water contact or rickettsial diseases following the bite of specific arthropod vectors in restricted ecological niches. It follows that the physician should be aware of the epidemiology of the disease(s) under consideration.

ETHNIC ORIGIN

There can be marked ethnic differences in disease incidence. Familial Mediterranean fever may present with acute fever and pain in certain Middle Eastern races, whereas a similar presentation in an African would bring sickle cell disease to mind. Similarly, tuberculosis is far more common in patients originating from the Indian subcontinent than in Europid races.

DIET

Dietary deficiencies, excess or contamination can all cause ill health. For instance, anaemia in a vegetarian (especially vegan) patient may be due to vitamin B_{12} deficiency, whilst abdominal pain in a Muslim patient during Ramadan can be caused by renal colic due to ureteric stones after self-imposed water deprivation during daylight hours. Undercooked meat may transmit a range of infections, including tapeworm, trichinellosis, salmonellosis and toxoplasmosis. Depending on the geographical location, eating fish may also cause diseases as diverse as gnathostomiasis or ciguatera poisoning.

SEXUAL CONTACTS

Sexually transmitted diseases are very common in certain parts of the tropics and frequently present with extragenital manifestations; hence, poly-arthropathy, papular rash and fever may be the presenting features of gonococcaemia; likewise, an illness that includes a generalized rash and lympha-denopathy could be caused by secondary syphilis. Human immunodeficiency virus (HIV) is spreading rapidly throughout the tropics, where it is mainly transmitted by heterosexual coitus, and should be suspected as a cause or cofactor in virtually any febrile illness.

VACCINES AND DRUGS

A history of relevant vaccination should, perhaps, never be used as a reason to exclude any condition from the differential diagnosis, although proven effective vaccination against yellow fever or hepa-titis B would virtually eliminate these diseases as a potential cause of ill health. In the same way, the appropriate use of antimalarial prophylactic drugs does not eliminate all risk for this infection but may decrease blood parasite counts to undetectable levels, thereby delaying diagnosis. Broad-spectrum antibiotics are freely available to the general public without prescription in many parts of the world and their prior use may prevent microbiological diag-nosis in bacterial disease, as well as actually causing ill-health, such as diarrhoea. Patients often try her-bal remedies and may be reluctant to admit this. There are undoubtedly many effective traditional therapies, such as the highly efficacious antimalarial qinghaosu and the Chinese herbal remedies for eczema that are as good as, if not better than, some Western medicines. However, some herbal prep-arations can also cause severe symptoms.

GENERAL INTERPRETATION

The presentation of disease is often greatly influenced by cultural factors. It can be very difficult to distinguish appropriate but exaggerated religious experiences from psychiatric disease in certain ethnic groups and a great deal of reliance may have to be placed on the opinions of others from the same culture. Words have different meanings depending on the context. A history of 'malaria' from an African patient should not necessarily be taken literally, but rather as being indicative of an acute feverish illness. This can be even more of a problem when the history is translated by a non-medical interpreter who may unintentionally change the patient's intended meaning.

SIGNIFICANCE OF SOME SPECIFIC SYMPTOMS

Physicians and health care workers practising in a rural tropical environment are often faced with a large number of patients and have to be pragmatic in their approach to the diagnosis of disease. Within a particular setting there is often only a limited range of common causes of certain symp-toms and therefore empirical therapy is offered on the basis that, if the diagnosis is correct, the patient will improve, and, if not, he or she will return unimproved. In this way the limited diagnostic re-sources available can be used in a more focused fashion. However, when investigational technology is readily to hand the practitioner will usually want to exclude a wider range of likely diseases before committing the patient to therapy. It is still possible to compile a relatively short differential diagnostic list based on the patient's presentation and travel history. The following section demonstrates the im-portant possible causes of certain symptoms, although much shorter lists can be compiled, where appropriate, according to individual patient's cir-cumstances.

FEVER (Figure 2.1)

This is one of the most common and most worrying symptoms in tropical practice. In many cases the associated symptoms and signs point to the diag-nosis. A patient with neck stiffness and generalized petechial rash, for instance, is obviously suffering from meningococcal meningitis. However, many infections can, as part of their repertoire, cause a feverish disease in which there are no associated features specific enough to allow a firm clinical diagnosis (Table 2.1). Under these circumstances it is important to give priority to the diagnosis of conditions that are rapidly progressive or associ-ated with a significant mortality, such as *Plas-modium falciparum* infection, typhoid or a viral haemorrhagic fever. In some parts of the tropics this is taken to the extreme when all such patients are given antimalarial drugs automatically, although, depending on the time of year, as few as 5% of such patients are really infected with malaria. When facilities allow, it is best to offer

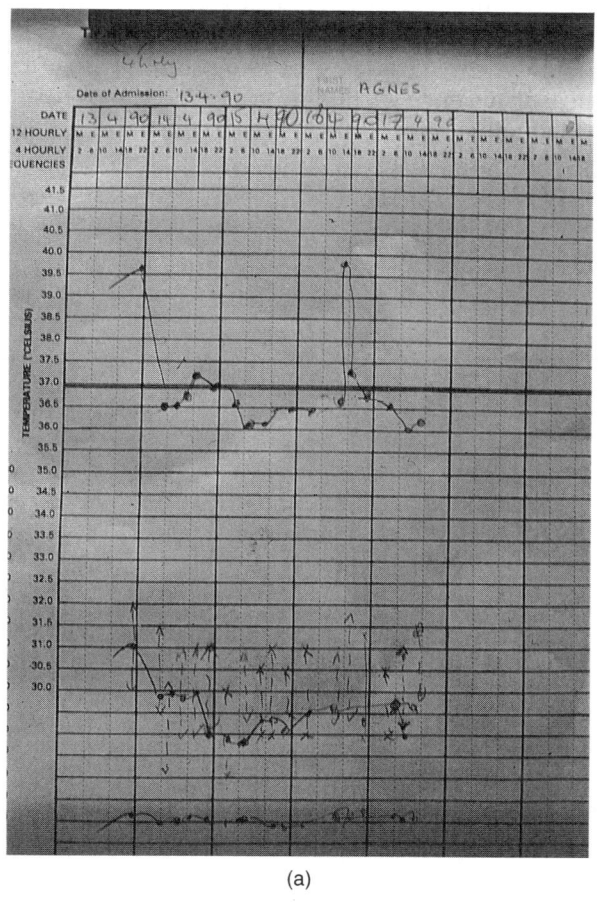
(a)

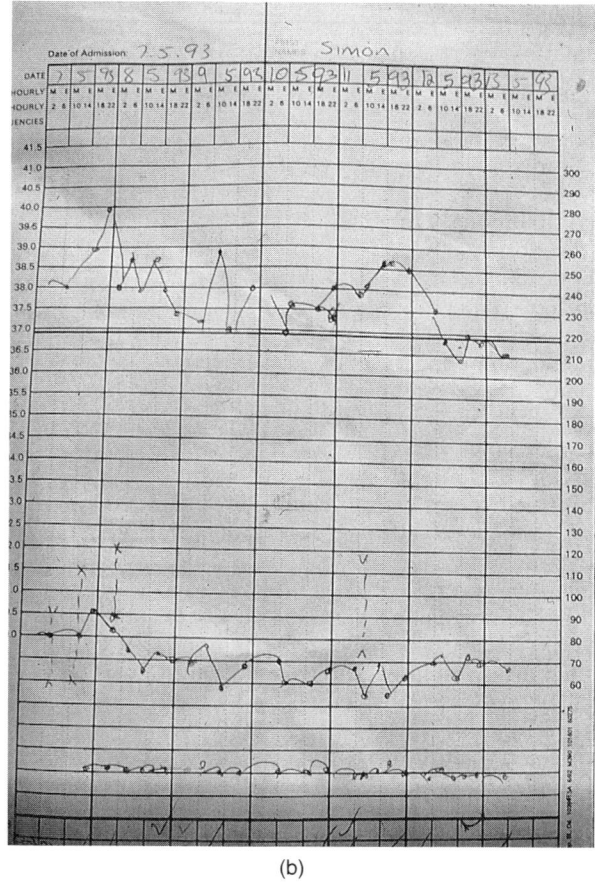
(b)

Figure 2.1   On rare occasions a fever pattern can be so characteristic as to be virtually diagnostic as in (a) the quartan (2-day gap) fever of *Plasmodium malariae* infection, or (b) the 'saddle-back' fever of dengue virus infection.

treatment only after appropriate investigation, unless the patient is in extremis.

WEIGHT LOSS, ANOREXIA AND MALAISE

These are relatively common presenting complaints and, in the most part, are readily attributable to associated disease; however, they may dominate the clinical presentation in situations where the aetiology is not obvious. Diseases to be considered in this circumstance are listed in Table 2.2.

DIARRHOEA AND VOMITING

Most symptoms in tropical practise are system specific. The physician's knowledge of clinical syndromes, disease epidemiology and geographical medicine will often lead to a rapid diagnosis. Diarrhoea is a frequent presenting complaint and in most patients will be caused by an acute primary gut infection (Table 2.3). Unfortunately, some extra-intestinal diseases, such as legionnaires' disease,

pneumococcal pneumonia or streptococcal septicaemia, can occasionally masquerade as gastroenteritis. Diarrhoea is also a frequent manifestation of certain severe diseases, including measles in malnourished children, and in the acquired immune deficiency syndrome (AIDS). Vomiting commonly accompanies diarrhoea in many gut infections but toxin-associated food poisoning (*Staphylococcus aureus*, *Bacillus cereus*), plant toxin ingestion, drugs, malaria, meningitis, renal failure, acute hypotension (septicaemia, haemorrhage), peptic ulceration and other severe systemic illnesses should also be considered.

ABDOMINAL PAIN (See also Chapter 3)

This often accompanies primary gastrointestinal infection, but there are many alternative possible causes (Table 2.4). The pain of gastroenteritis is usually spasmodic (colic), with the exception of *Campylobacter jejuni* infection—when the pain can be severe and constant, and cholera, which can

Table 2.1 Some causes of a non-specific feverish illness*.

Malaria
Typhoid fever
Influenza
Dengue fever
Prodromal viral hepatitis (A–E)
Typhus
Extrapulmonary tuberculosis
Brucellosis
Septicaemia (Gram-positive or -negative)
Epstein–Barr virus infection
Leptospirosis
Human immunodeficiency virus infection
Pneumococcal pneumonia
Legionella pneumophila infection
Hepatic amoebiasis
Visceral leishmaniasis
Parasitic hyperinfection syndromes (e.g. *Strongyloides*
hyperinfection syndrome, Katayama fever, visceral
larva migrans)
Relapsing fever
Viral haemorrhagic fevers (Lassa, Ebola, Marburg,
etc.)
Other arboviral infections (phlebotomus fever, Rift
Valley fever, etc.)
Q fever
African trypanosomiasis
Histoplasmosis
Yersiniosis
Plague
Tularaemia
Coccidioidomycosis

*In this and subsequent tables the lists are given in approximate
order of relative importance or incidence.

cause somatic muscle cramps. Most other pathologies are associated with constant pain, except that due to intestinal obstruction, which is normally colicky.

JAUNDICE

Yellow eye discoloration may be a presenting symptom, although in many cases it will be

Table 2.2 Cryptic causes of weight loss, anorexia and malaise.

Malignancy (hepatocellular carcinoma, lymphoma,
pancreatic carcinoma and others)
Extrapulmonary tuberculosis
Acquired immune deficiency syndrome
Visceral leishmaniasis
Brucellosis
Giardiasis
Hydatid disease
Schistosomiasis (malaise)
Anaemia

detected initially as a clinical sign. The physician should first of all distinguish between hepatic and haemolytic pathologies by determining the presence or absence of bile in the urine, respectively. An equally important clue lies in the patient's temperature. The primary viral hepatitides (A–E) are febrile illnesses only in the prodromal, non-icteric phase and the first 2 days of jaundice, except in the

Table 2.3 Common aetiologies of diarrhoea and vomiting.

Acute watery diarrhoea (<2 weeks)
    Vibrio cholerae
    Salmonella spp.
    Campylobacter jejuni
    Rotavirus and other enteric viruses
    Enterotoxigenic, enteropathogenic and
    enteroadherant *Escherichia coli*
    Malaria
    Shigella sonnei
    Yersinia enterocolitica
    Giardia lamblia
    Cryptosporidium parvum
    Clostridium perfringens (toxin)
    Bacillus cereus (stable toxin)
    Ciguatera fish poisoning
    Isospora belli
    Sarcocystis spp.

Bloody diarrhoea
    Shigella spp.
    Entamoeba histolytica
    Campylobacter jejuni
    Salmonella spp.
    Enteroinvasive and enterohaemorrhagic *E. coli*
    Yersinia spp.
    Clostridium difficile
    Clostridium perfringens (necrotizing enterocolitis,
        pigbel)
    Balantidium coli
    Inflammatory bowel disease (IBD)
    Schistosomiasis

Chronic diarrhoea (>2 weeks)
    Giardia lamblia
    Entamoeba histolytica
    Tropical enteropathy and 'sprue'
    Chronic pancreatitis
    Shigella spp.
    Enteroadherant *E. coli*
    Ileocaecal tuberculosis
    Disaccharide intolerance
    Postinfective irritable bowel syndrome (IBS)
    Strongyloides stercoralis
    Inflammatory bowel disease (IBD)
    Schistosomiasis
    Coeliac disease
    Trichuris trichiura
    Capillaria philippinensis

Table 2.4 Abdominal pain.

Gastroenteritis
Intestinal perforation (e.g. typhoid)
Amoebic liver abscess
Splenic rupture (e.g. malaria, Epstein–Barr virus infection)
Typhoid fever
Painful sickle cell crisis (including splenic infarction)
Peptic ulceration
Acute pancreatitis
Acute pyelonephritis
Biliary obstruction (gallstones, *Ascaris lumbricoides*, tumour)
Intestinal obstruction (volvulus, *A. lumbricoides*)
Acute salpingitis (*Neisseria gonorrhoeae*, *Chlamydia trachomatis*)
Ruptured ectopic pregnancy
Familial Mediterranean fever

rare cases of fulminant hepatic failure. Fever normally subsides with the onset of jaundice. A patient who is febrile and jaundiced concurrently is more likely to be afflicted with another, usually more severe, condition, such as falciparum malaria, typhoid, yellow fever or leptospirosis (Table 2.5). In view of the appreciable mortality of the latter conditions, their diagnosis should always be carefully considered.

HAEMATURIA AND DYSURIA

Such symptoms usually cause the patient to seek medical attention rapidly. The diagnosis is usually easy to achieve, the most common diagnostic pitfall being the failure to consider sexually transmitted diseases (Table 2.6). Where urethral discharge is the patient's primary complaint the aetiological differential diagnosis should be easy, but a significant

Table 2.5 Jaundice.

With concurrent fever	*Without concurrent fever*
Hepatic	
P. falciparum malaria	Viral hepatitis (A–E)
Typhoid	Alcoholic hepatitis
Leptospirosis (Weil's disease)	Drugs (especially antituberculous agents)
Yellow fever (and other viral haemorrhagic fevers)	Toxins (including some herbal medicines)
Epstein–Barr virus	
Septicaemia	
Pneumococcal pneumonia	
Typhus	
Brucellosis	
Mycoplasma hepatitis	
Secondary syphilis	
Miliary tuberculosis	
Posthepatic	
Ascending cholangitis	Choledocholithiasis
Amoebic liver abscess	*Clonorchis sinensis*
AIDS (cholangiopathy, drugs, cryptosporidial)	*Fasciola hepatica*
	Malignant tumours
	Pancreatitis
	A. lumbricoides
Haemolytic	
P. falciparum malaria	
Haemoglobinopathies (especially sickle cell disease)	
Glucose-6-phosphate dehydrogenase deficiency (favism, drug-induced crisis)	
Bartonella bacilliformis	
Haemolytic–uraemic syndrome (*Shigella dysenteriae*, *E. coli*)	
Drugs	

Table 2.6 Haematuria and dysuria.

Haematuria
  Bacterial urinary tract infection (*E. coli*, *Klebsiella* spp. etc.)
  Schistosoma haematobium
  Glomerulonephritis (poststreptococcal and others)
  Calculi (staghorn, ureteric or bladder)
  Renal tuberculosis
  Renal tract tumours (including bladder tumours complicating schistosomiasis)
  Gonorrhoea

Dysuria
  Haematuria of any cause
  Bacterial urinary tract infection
  Acute urethritis (*Neisseria gonorrhoeae*, *Chlamydia trachomatis*, etc.)
  Enterobius vermicularis (in female children)
  Urethral herpes simplex infection
  Genital candidiasis in the female

discharge is not always found in acute urethritis. In the male, the repertoire of symptomatic presentations of sexually transmitted disease is otherwise limited to genital ulceration and inguinal swellings, although extragenital manifestations such as gonococcal pharyngitis can be missed if an appropriate sexual history is not obtained.

SORE THROAT

The aetiology of this common complaint is very similar in both tropical and non-tropical countries (Table 2.7). Vaccination programmes in most developing countries have yet to achieve the coverage necessary to interrupt the transmission of eminently preventable conditions such as diphtheria, which should therefore always be seriously considered in this situation. An additional consideration in sub-

Table 2.7 Sore throat.

Minor viral infections
Streptococcus pyogenes
Corynebacterium diphtheriae
Epstein–Barr virus
Lassa fever
Neisseria gonorrhoeae
Secondary syphilis
Herpes simplex (especially in AIDS)
Vincent's angina

Saharan West Africa is Lassa Fever—with all the ramifications of such a diagnosis, including patient isolation and ribavirin therapy, if available.

COUGH AND DYSPNOEA

A non-productive cough presenting alone is common enough; it is most likely to be benign and caused by a minor viral throat infection. Pertussis or pleurisy due to tuberculosis are obvious exceptions. On the other hand a productive cough, or one that is non-productive with associated shortness of breath, is more ominous and should stimulate a search for signs of pneumonitis or cardiac failure, with their many possible causes (Table 2.8).

Table 2.8 Cough and dyspnoea.

Pulmonary causes
  Pneumococcal and other bacterial pneumonias
  Tuberculosis
  Typhoid (bronchitis or pneumonia)
  P. falciparum malaria (pulmonary oedema)
  Bronchiectasis (post-measles or pertussis)
  Chronic obstructive airways disease (smoke inhalation in poorly ventilated huts)
  Measles
  Amoebic lung abscess
  Pulmonary hydatid disease
  AIDS (tuberculosis, *Pneumocystis carinii*, bacterial pneumonia)
  Paragonimus spp.
  Löffler's syndrome
  Pulmonary eosinophilia
  Sarcoidosis
  Plague

Cardiac causes
  Myocarditis (enteroviral, eosinophilic, diphtheritic)
  Pericarditis (tuberculous, staphylococcal, pneumococcal)
  Cardiomyopathy (alcohol, beriberi, Chagas' disease, hypertension, endomyocardial fibrosis)
  Cardiac valve disease (rheumatic, congenital, syphilitic)
  Septicaemia

HEADACHE

Most febrile illnesses—especially malaria, typhoid and dengue fever—are accompanied by this symptom. However, primary disease of the central nervous system, including meningitis (bacterial, viral and parasitic) and space occupying lesions (abscess, tumour) should also be given due consideration.

PHYSICAL EXAMINATION

GENERAL EXAMINATION

Remembering that multiple pathology is common within the context of tropical disease, the clinician should not be surprised to find physical abnormalities additional to those expected from the primary complaint. An initial general examination should include an assessment of nutritional status. Low body mass due to malnutrition, malabsorption or the cachexia of chronic disease is a common finding. Further examination may also reveal features of vitamin deficiency. On inspection of the mouth, angular stomatitis and glossitis may suggest associated vitamin B deficiencies. Other conditions which should be actively sought include:

- *Anaemia.* Millions of children in the tropics have hookworm infection, making this the most common cause of anaemia, but there are many other possible aetiologies that should also be considered (Table 2.9).
- *Lymphadenopathy.* Residents of the tropics are frequently exposed to infectious disease and enlarged lymph nodes are a common finding which does not necessarily indicate continuing pathology. When the lymph nodes are particularly large (>2 cm) or obviously expanding then certain conditions to be considered include tuberculosis, HIV infection, lymphoma (Burkitt's type in Africa), brucellosis and African trypanosomiasis, although virtually any acute infective process may be implicated.

Table 2.10 Oedema and swelling of the limbs or face.

Extensive
  Kwashiorkor
  Nephrotic syndrome (e.g. *Plasmodium malariae*)
  Glomerulonephritis (e.g. poststreptococcal)
  Congestive cardiac failure (see Table 2.8)
  Cirrhosis (e.g. hepatitis B, alcohol, haemosiderosis)
  Hypoalbuminaemia (any chronic disease, severe diarrhoea)
  Lymphatic filariasis

Focal
  Loa loa (Calabar swelling)
  Trichinosis
  Gnathostomiasis
  Strongyloidiasis
  South American trypanosomiasis (Romaña's sign)

Table 2.9 Anaemia.

Acute
  Malaria (haemolysis)
  Haemorrhage (dysentery, typhoid, peptic ulcer, miscarriage, ectopic pregnancy)
  Bleeding diathesis (typhus, meningococcaemia, viral haemorrhagic fever)
  Sickle cell disease (haemolytic, sequestration and aplastic crises)
  Glucose-6-phosphate dehydrogenase deficiency (haemolytic crisis due to drugs or bean ingestion)

Chronic
  Helminths (hookworm, *Trichuris trichiura*, schistosomiasis)
  Pregnancy
  Menorrhagia
  Haemoglobinopathies (sickle cell disease, β-thalassaemia)
  Nutritional (e.g. B_{12} deficiency in vegans)
  Malabsorption ('sprue', giardiasis)
  Tropical splenomegaly syndrome (*Plasmodium* spp.)
  Visceral leishmaniasis
  Tuberculosis (anaemia of chronic disease)
  Malignancy
  AIDS

- *Oedema or swelling of the limbs or face.* This may be generalized or focal (Table 2.10).

SKIN (Plates 2.1 to 2.8)

The skin is frequently involved in systemic disease, e.g. the hypopigmentation and flaking appearance of kwashiorkor, and the photosensitive dermatitis of pellagra. Many problems in tropical disease practice may manifest themselves dermatologically and infections of the skin are especially common (Table 2.11). It, unfortunately, is often difficult to recognize many of the exanthemas on a black skin.

Table 2.11 Rashes.

Maculopapular
  Extensive
    Childhood exanthems (measles, chickenpox, rubella*)
    Dengue*
    Scabies
    Body lice
    Typhus*
    Secondary syphilis

  Sparse
    Gonococcaemia*
    Typhoid rose spots*
    Cutaneous myiasis
    Flea bites
    Tungiasis
    Lichen planus
    Cutaneous larva migrans
    Kaposi's sarcoma

Hypopigmentation
  Postinflammatory
  Tinea versicolor
  Leprosy
  Pityriasis alba
  Vitiligo
  Yaws
  Pinta
  Post-kala-azar dermal leishmaniasis

Ulcers
  Tropical ulcer
  Cutaneous leishmaniasis
  Desert sore (*Corynebacterium diphtheriae*)
  Typhus eschar
  Trypanosomal chancre
  Leprosy
  Yaws
  Anthrax
  Buruli ulcer (*Mycobacterium ulcerans*)

Continued

Table 2.11 Continued.

Nodules
  Onchocerciasis
  Guinea worm
  Cutaneous myiasis
  Leprosy
  Fungal infection
  Kaposi's sarcoma
  Yaws
  Subcutaneous (tuberculous abscess, pyomyositis)

Plaques/crusts
  Fungal infections
  Leprosy
  Impetigo
  Pinta
  Kaposi's sarcoma

Urticaria
  Loa loa
  Strongyloidiasis
  Schistosomiasis
  Gnathostomiasis

Petechial
  Meningococcaemia
  Typhus
  Viral haemorrhagic fevers

Vesicles
  Chickenpox/shingles
  Herpes simplex
  Orf
  Monkeypox

*May be difficult to see on a black skin.

ABDOMEN

Many of the common diseases of abdominal organs have already been considered with reference to their presenting symptoms (see Tables 2.3–2.6). Even when the primary complaint is not suggestive of abdominal disease, examination of the abdomen can be revealing.

HEPATOMEGALY AND SPLENOMEGALY

In malaria-endemic areas splenomegaly is a common finding, especially in children—where the spleen often reaches an enormous size. A wide range of other systemic diseases can also cause this sign, in addition to a frequent association with hepatomegaly (Table 2.12).

Plate 2   Infections of totally differing aetiology can produce a similar clinical presentation.

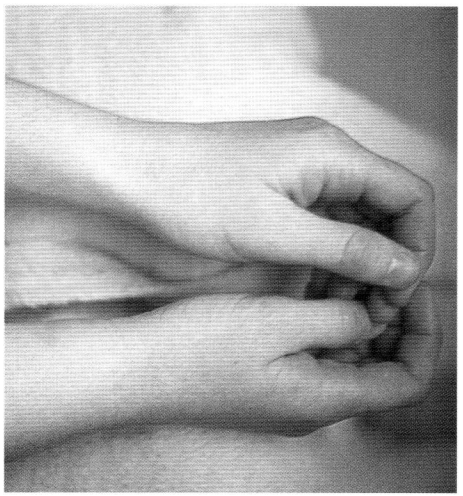

Plate 2.1   Transient swelling over the wrist in *Loa loa* infection.

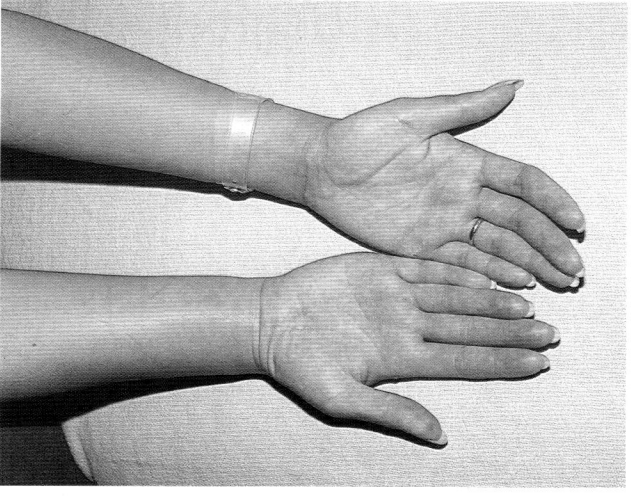

Plate 2.2   Transient swelling over the wrist in gnathostomiasis.

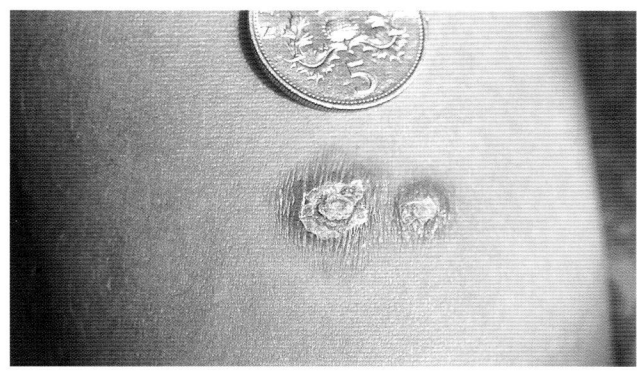

Plate 2.3   Crusted ulcers in cutaneous leishmaniasis.

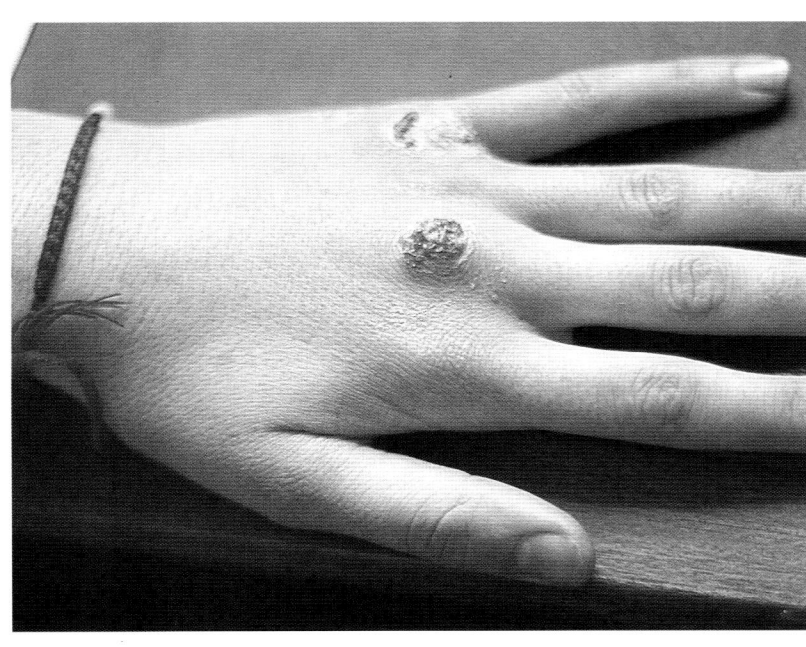

Plate 2.4   Crusted ulcers in *Staphylococcus* spp – infected insect bites.

Plate 2 Continued.

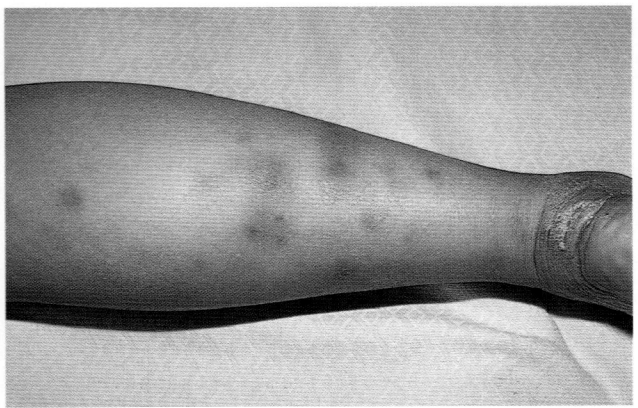

Plate 2.5 Painful nodules on the legs in erythema induratum (Bazin's disease) – related to tuberculosis.

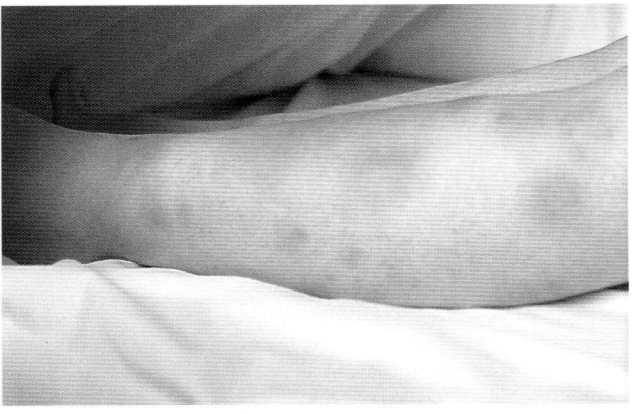

Plate 2.6 Painful nodules on the legs in erythema nodosum – related to tuberculosis.

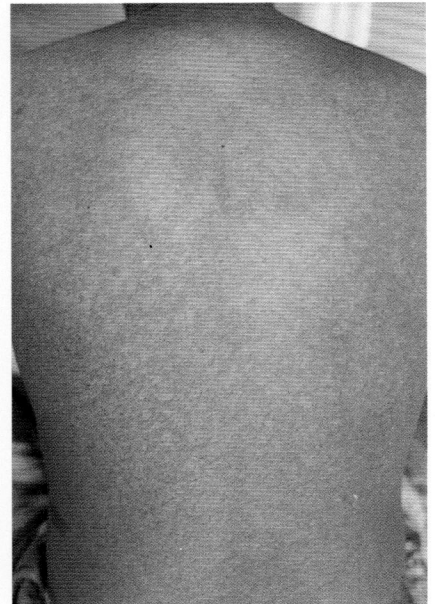

Plate 2.7 Non-confluent maculopapular rash due to dengue fever.

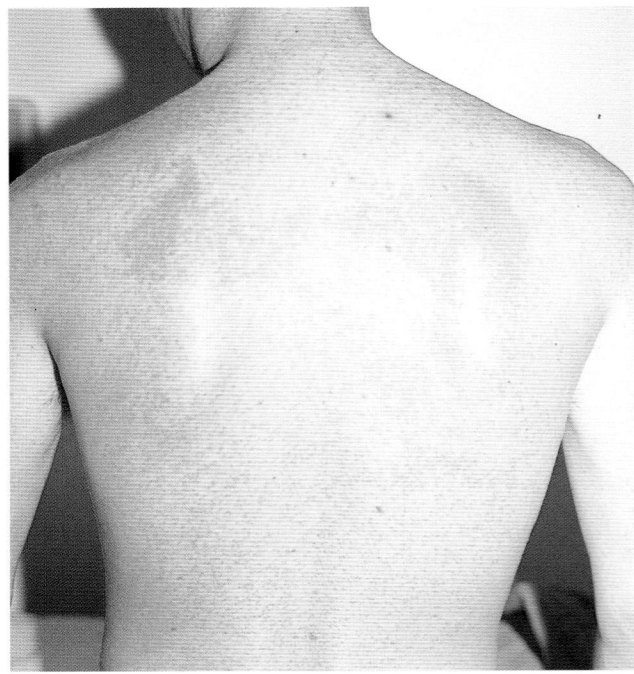

Plate 2.8 Non-confluent maculopapular rash due to rubella infection.

Table 2.12 Hepatosplenomegaly.

Predominant hepatomegaly
 Acute (usually tender)
  Viral hepatitis (A–E), Epstein–Barr virus
  Amoebic abscess
  Malaria
  Leptospirosis
  Yellow fever
  Brucellosis
  Sickle cell disease (sequestration crisis)
  Chagas' disease
  Parasitic hyperinfection syndrome (visceral larva migrans, Katayama fever)
  Veno-occlusive disease
  Beriberi

 Chronic (usually non-tender)
  Cirrhosis (hepatitis B, haemosiderosis, alcohol)
  Hepatocellular carcinoma
  Schistosomiasis
  Visceral leishmaniasis
  Hydatid disease
  Haemoglobinopathies (sickle cell, thalassaemia)
  Kwashiorkor
  Fascioliasis
  Clonorchiasis
  Trypanosomiasis
  Plague
  Bartonellosis

Predominant splenomegaly
 Malaria*
 Typhoid
 Brucellosis
 Relapsing fever
 Typhus
 Visceral leishmaniasis*
 Trypanosomiasis
 Schistosomiasis (portal hypertension)
 Haemoglobinopathies
 HIV infection
 Hydatid disease
 Lymphoma
 Leptospirosis
 Bartonellosis

*May cause massive splenomegaly.

Table 2.13 Abdominal distension.

Mass lesion(s)
 Hydatid cysts
 Amoeboma of the colorectum
 Hydronephrosis (schistosomiasis)
 Intra-abdominal malignancy
 Ovarian cyst
 Uterine fibroids

Dilated bowel
 Small-intestinal obstruction (*Ascaris lumbricoides*, intussusception, intestinal volvulus, inguinal hernia)
 Megacolon (Chagas' disease)
 Toxic megacolon (shigellosis, etc.)

Ascites
 Tuberculous peritonitis
 Hepatic cirrhosis (hepatitis B, alcohol)
 Portal hypertension (schistosomiasis, veno-occlusive disease)
 Nephrotic syndrome (*Plasmodium malariae*)
 Lymphatic filariasis (chylous ascites)
 Hypoalbuminaemia (malnutrition, chronic disease)
 Malignancy

ABDOMINAL DISTENSION

This may be due to hepatic or splenic enlargement and is also a common finding in children who are malnourished and have a high small-intestine worm load. The differential diagnosis otherwise is of mass lesions, dilated bowel or ascites (Table 2.13).

CARDIOVASCULAR SYSTEM

Cardiac failure has been discussed (see Table 2.8). Cardiomegaly has much the same range of aetiologies. Bradycardia may be a feature of Chagas' disease and diphtheritic cardiomyopathy. Relative bradycardia, a pulse slower than would be expected for a given fever, is a feature of several infections, including typhoid and yellow fever. A pulse that is disproportionately fast is a feature of myocarditis (see Table 2.8). Hypertension is an increasing problem in those who have taken to a Western life style, particularly the Afro-Caribbean races (see Chapter 26).

RESPIRATORY TRACT

Sore throat and the many likely aetiologies of lung consolidation and cavitation are discussed above (see Tables 2.7 and 2.8). Pleural effusion may complicate pneumococcal and other acute pneumonias, the former being especially common in the tropics. Tuberculosis is also a frequent cause, but other aetiologies to consider include amoebiasis and helminthic infections (*Gnathostoma spinigerum*, *Strongyloides stercoralis* and *Paragonimus* spp.).

CENTRAL NERVOUS SYSTEM

Most severe neurological diseases are also infectious in origin. The clinically important presentations are as follows.

MENINGITIS AND ENCEPHALITIS

Neck stiffness is normally a reliable sign in the early diagnosis of bacterial meningitis. The presence of a petechial rash makes a diagnosis of meningococcal disease certain, especially in the large epidemics encountered in sub-Saharan Africa in the first 6 months of the year. Although cerebral malaria may also cause severe neck stiffness, this is usually the sole alternative diagnosis to primary meningeal infection in an endemic area (Table 2.14).

Table 2.14 Meningitis and encephalitis.

Meningitis
  Neisseria meningitidis
  Streptococcus pneumoniae
  Haemophilus influenzae
  Mycobacterium tuberculosis
  Listeria monocytogenes
  Enterovirus (polio, echo, Coxsackie)
  Mumps virus
  HIV (also *Cryptococcus neoformans* in AIDS)
  Amoebae (*N. fowleri*, *Acanthamoebae*)
  Strongyloides stercoralis (hyperinfection syndrome)
  Angiostrongylus cantonensis
  Gnathostoma spp.

Encephalitis
  Acute
  Arboviruses
  Herpes simplex
  Measles
  Chickenpox
  Yellow fever
  Rabies
  Trichinella spiralis

  Subacute/chronic
  African trypanosomiasis
  Kuru

CONFUSION AND DECREASED CONSCIOUS LEVEL

Altered cerebral function may result from a variety of extracerebral conditions (Table 2.15). It may be difficult to distinguish between feverish illnesses primarily involving the central nervous system and those arising elsewhere. For example, the distinction between cerebral malarial and bacterial meningitis in children can be a difficult problem in endemic areas. Even when a firm diagnosis of malaria has been established, the child's unconsciousness may in fact be due to associated hypoglycaemia.

FITS

Although idiopathic epilepsy is well recognized in the tropics, focal or severe diffuse infections are relatively more important (Table 2.16).

NEUROPATHIES AND WEAKNESS

It is as well to remember the adage that neuropathy is due to leprosy until proven otherwise. AIDS is also becoming a relatively common cause (Table 2.17).

MUSCULOSKELETAL SYSTEM

There are relatively few infectious primary muscle conditions—although wasting is a common consequence of many severe or chronic illnesses. Tropical pyomyositis due to *Staphylococcus aureus* is particularly common in tropical Africa. Myopathy caused by the retroviruses HIV and HTLV-1 is increasingly recognized.

OSTEOMYELITIS

This condition is often caused by *S. aureus*, but tuberculosis and brucellosis are also frequently implicated, and salmonellae are a particular problem in children with sickle cell disease.

ACUTE ARTHRITIS

The degenerative and inflammatory arthritides are, in general, less important than those with an acute infective aetiology (Table 2.1).

Table 2.15 Confusion/decreased conscious level.

Infective	Non-infective
Meningitis	Drugs/alcohol/herbal medicines
Encephalitis	Dehydration
Cerebral malaria	Liver failure (acute fulminant hepatitis)
Typhoid	Hypoglycaemia (e.g. in malaria)
Dengue fever	Hypertensive stroke
Legionnaires' disease	Head injury
Leptospirosis	Psychiatric illness (hysterical conversion)
Typhus	Renal failure
Relapsing fever	
Septicaemia	
Viral haemorrhagic fevers	
Rabies	
Neurocysticercosis	
AIDS (cerebral toxoplasmosis, HIV encephalopathy, etc.)	

Table 2.16 Fits

Cerebral malaria
Meningitis/encephalitis
Cerebral tuberculoma
Neurocysticercosis
Epilepsy
AIDS (cerebral toxoplasmosis)
Schistosomiasis
Cerebral hydatid disease
Alcohol
Hypoglycaemia
Tetanus (pseudoepilepsy)

Table 2.17 Neuropathy/weakness.

Leprosy
Nutritional deficiencies (vitamin B complex)
HIV
Spinal tuberculosis
Schistosomiasis
Tropical spastic paraparesis (HTLV-1)
Lathyrism
Guillain–Barré syndrome
Diabetes mellitus
Uraemia
Toxins (e.g. ciguatera)
Drugs (e.g. isoniazid)

THE EYE

Diseases of the eye are dealt with in Chapter 10. Conjunctival injection may be caused by a primary ophthalmic condition but can also be related to systemic disease such as leptospirosis, Behçet's disease, and typhus.

FURTHER READING

Cook G C. Dealing with disease related to tropical exposure. In Toghill P J (ed.) *Examining Patients: An Introduction to Clinical Medicine*, 2nd edn. London: Edward Arnold 1995: 245–258.

SECTION 2B
SYSTEM-ORIENTED DISEASE

CHAPTER 3

TROPICAL GASTROENTEROLOGICAL PROBLEMS

G. C. Cook

The portals of entry for organisms responsible for most infections which dominate medicine in tropical countries (as elsewhere) are the skin, and respiratory and intestinal tracts. In fact a very high proportion of infections of warm climes originate from ingestion of contaminated water and foodstuffs; many resultant diseases fall into the subspecialty *tropical gastroenterology*.[1–3]

Most gastroenterological emergencies which occur in a temperate climate can also occur in tropical and subtropical countries. However, there are notable differences in prevalence.[4] Some problems are probably ethnically related (although elimination of environmental factors is often difficult), but the majority are superimposed upon an underlying communicable (infective) disease; important examples are ileal perforation or haemorrhage resulting from typhoid (enteric) fever, colonic perforation—and less often haemorrhage—in amoebic colitis and shigellosis, and hepatic abscess in invasive amoebiasis.[4]

MOUTH AND PHARYNX

The mouth and rectum are the most accessible parts of the gastrointestinal tract from a clinical viewpoint;[5] therefore, where endoscopic procedures are impossible, and that applies to many tropical and subtropical countries, as much information as possible should be derived from careful examination of these organs.

Viral, bacterial, mycotic and parasitic infections all give rise to oropharyngeal pathology, which is often most pronounced in the presence of associated malnutrition (especially in infants and children). Herpes simplex virus, Epstein–Barr virus (see Chapter 32) and many enteroviruses can produce a stomatitis; oral ulceration is a frequent manifestation in Behçet's syndrome—common in the Middle East and Japan. Lassa fever (see Chapter 30) and diphtheria (see Chapter 52) are often characterized by severe pharyngeal involvement, and in rabies (see Chapter 33) dysphagia caused by spasm of the pharyngeal muscles is an important feature of the disease. In addition to acute bacterial infections, tuberculosis, leprosy, syphilis and yaws all exert oral manifestations. Candidiasis (exceedingly common in the acquired immune deficiency syndrome (AIDS)) (see Chapter 12), histoplasmosis, South American blastomycosis and coccidioidomycosis (see Chapter 59) can also produce buccal lesions. Acute pharyngitis caused by infection with young adult *Fasciola hepatica* (ingested in raw sheep or goat liver—reported from the Middle East and India—and known locally as 'halzoun' (see Chapter 73) is caused by pentastomids.[1] Therapeutic agents such as sulphonamides (included in some antimalarial prophylactics, e.g. pyrimethamine + sulphamethoxazole (Fansidar) can give rise to the Stevens–Johnson syndrome, in which oral ulceration is common. Manifestations of specific malnutrition states (vitamin B and C deficiencies and iron deficiency anaemia) are usually obvious, whereas in kwashiorkor these are frequently combined with infective complications. Cancrum oris, a gangrenous condition involving the gums and cheeks and associated with *Borrelia vincenti* and *Fusiformis fusiformis* infection, is especially common in malnourished children,[1] especially in West Africa. Descriptions of the mouth, especially the tongue, in postinfective malabsorption (tropical sprue) (see below) were dominant in *clinical* accounts of this disease in the nineteenth century (i.e. before the advent of laboratory investigation).

Periodontal disease and dental caries are also a major problem in less developed countries.[1] Oral submucous fibrosis—a chronic disease of unknown aetiology—may affect any part of the oral cavity;[1] most reports are from the Indian subcontinent and South-East Asia. Fibroelastosis of the submucous tissues accompanied by epithelial atrophy are important sequelae and are probably premalignant.

Of malignant disease(s), buccal carcinoma is numerically pre-eminent;[5] Burkitt's lymphoma (see Chapter 32), ameloblastoma and nasopharyngeal carcinoma (see Chapter 24) are other malignancies which have important geographical distributions in tropical countries.

Hypertrophy of the salivary glands is common in malnourished children; it can also be associated with *Ascaris lumbricoides* infection and chronic calcific pancreatitis (see below).[1] Tumours of the salivary glands are probably no more common than in temperate regions.

OESOPHAGUS

The most important disease to involve this organ is oesophageal carcinoma[6] (Figure 3.1) (see Chapter 24); this malignancy possesses an enigmatic geographical distribution. It has a high prevalence in some geographical locations:[1,6] Central and East Africa (western Kenya, Malawi and eastern Zambia have the highest rates), the southern Caspian littoral (especially north-eastern Iran), and northern China (in and around the Taihand mountains). Various hypotheses have been advanced to explain the high incidence of this tumour in these areas (see Chapter 24).[1,6]

Megaoesophagus, a feature of chronic *Trypanosoma cruzi* infection (Chagas' disease) is described in Chapter 64. Table 3.1 lists some major causes of dysphagia in a tropical environment.

Oesophageal varices (Figure 3.2) usually result from advanced macronodular cirrhosis (see below); however, hepatic schistosomiasis (caused by *Schistosoma mansoni*, *Schist. japonicum*, *Schist. intercalatum*, *Schist. matthei* and *Schist. mekongi*) accounts for numerous other cases (see Chapter 72). Portal vein obstruction (see below) is also common in some parts of Africa and Asia, and probably results in most cases from umbilical sepsis in the neonatal period;[1] it is occasionally associated with hepatocellular carcinoma. The very high splenic blood flow associated with hyperreactive malarious splenomegaly (HMS) (tropical splenomegaly syndrome) can also give rise to oesophageal varices (see below).[1] Where and when available, upper gastrointestinal endoscopic sclerotherapy is of enormous value in the management of oesophageal varices, but an ideal method of dealing with bleeding varices has yet to appear; in most tropical countries, older methods (see below) remain extant.

Oesophageal trauma is a major problem in several African countries; foreign bodies (e.g. kola nuts and fish bones) and corrosive agents—which give rise to strictures—are also relatively common.[1] Achalasia, peptic oesophagitis and hiatus hernia are all encountered, but are not unduly common.

In HIV/AIDS infection, oesophageal candidiasis is a common manifestation; other systemic mycoses (see Chapter 59) can also produce an oesophagitis.

OESOPHAGUS: EMERGENCIES

The most common oesophageal lesions in tropical countries are varices (Table 3.1 summarizes the major causes) and carcinoma (see above);[4] resultant *acute* complications are upper gastrointestinal haemorrhage and obstruction, respectively. Of lesser importance, foreign bodies in the oesophagus (e.g. kola nuts) cause dysphagia, and corrosive lesions can result in stricture formation.[1]

OESOPHAGEAL VARICES

Reported prevalence rates for bleeding oesophageal varices in tropical countries are extremely unreliable.[4] Transport facilities are usually exceedingly unsatisfactory; therefore, the majority of those afflicted die before reaching primary or tertiary medical care. Also, high technology (e.g. endoscopic sclerotherapy) and blood transfusion are less often available so that outcome following medical intervention is frequently less satisfactory than in a Western country.[7] The cause of upper gastro-

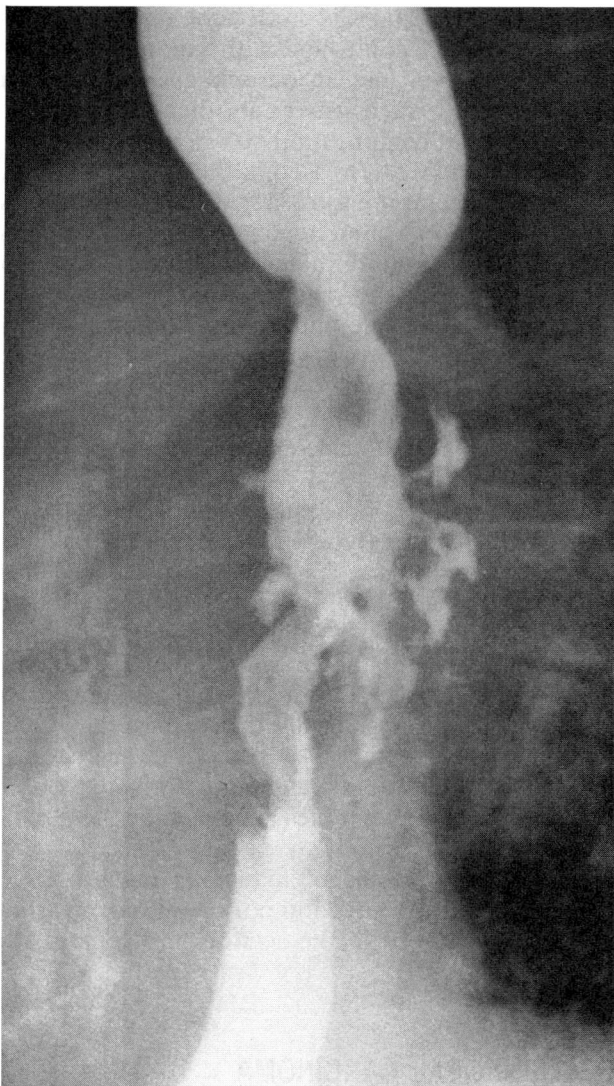

Figure 3.1 Barium swallow showing oesophageal carcinoma with gross mediastinal invasion.

Table 3.1 Some causes of dysphagia encountered in tropical countries.

Trauma	Gastritis
	Foreign bodies
	Corrosive agents
Infection	South American trypanosomiasis (Chagas' disease)
	Candidiasis (usually associated with AIDS)
	Rhizopus, Absidia (mucormycosis)
Neoplasia	Oesophageal carcinoma
Oesophageal varices	Macronodular cirrhosis (usually postviral)
	Schistosomiasis
	Portal vein thrombosis
	Hyperreactive malarious splenomegaly
Others	Achalasia
	Peptic oesophagitis
	Hiatus hernia
Extrinsic pressure	Endemic goitre

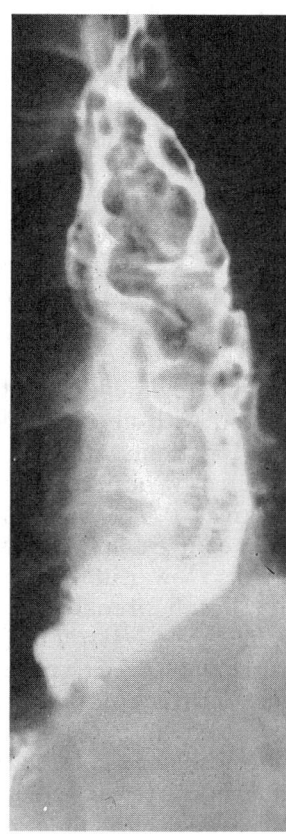

Figure 3.2 Advanced oesophageal varices in a Zambian woman with severe macronodular cirrhosis associated with HBV infection; barium swallow examination.

intestinal bleeding in 131 successive patients admitted with haematemesis or melaena to a hospital at Harare, Zimbabwe, has been analysed;[8] in 36 (27%) admissions (mean age 42 years) oesophageal varices were responsible. In 21, conservative management was followed by cessation of bleeding; however, nine suffered continuous bleeding, and six rebleeding; five patients died (four within 24 hours of admission) from haemorrhagic shock. Vasopressin infusions were used in four with the addition of oesophageal tamponade in two.

The pathophysiological mechanism(s) underlying oesophageal bleeding has been addressed on numerous occasions.[9] Both erosive and eruptive bases seem the most likely explanations; in addition, pressure and variceal size are probably important.

In Egypt, endoscopic biopsies obtained from intervariceal mucosa (within 5 cm of the cardia) in 20 individuals with, and 30 without, a history of variceal bleeding (most suffered from schistosomal liver disease) were examined histologically;[10] they showed dilated intraepithelial blood-filled channels within the squamous epithelium and lamina propria in all of the 'bleeders' and in 15 (50%) of the 'non-bleeders'. Furthermore, oesophagitis was more pronounced in the bleeders compared with the non-bleeders: 11 (55%) and 7 (23%), respectively.

The role of upper gastrointestinal endoscopy in a developing country has been studied in Kuwait;[11] 345 (4%) of 8680 patients examined successively using this technique had evidence of oesophageal varices, the usual cause being chronic schistosomal liver disease (usually in Egyptian labourers). By examining 718 successive patients who presented with upper gastrointestinal bleeding within 24 hours of admission, the exact site of the haemorrhage was delineated in 651 (91%), and the responsible lesion detected in 685 (97%). At Ibadan, Nigeria, a recent study has indicated that endoscopy gives a superior result to radiology in the diagnosis of variceal disease resulting in upper gastrointestinal haemorrhage;[12] endoscopy was successful in 64 (85%), but a barium meal correctly located the source of bleeding in only 38 (51%) of 75 patients.

Three reports from New Delhi, India, have focused on the role of endoscopic sclerotherapy in the management of bleeding oesophageal varices.[13-15] Seventy-nine patients underwent treatment (with either absolute or 50% alcohol) every 3 weeks, for oesophageal varices; active bleeding was controlled in 14 of 15 (93%) and 5 of 13 (54%) using the two fluids, respectively ($P < 0.05$); the sole disadvantage of absolute alcohol was that it produced a higher incidence of retrosternal pain. In another study, using a similar regimen, 5% ethanolamine oleate was compared with absolute alcohol in 47 randomly allocated patients; the latter solution eradicated oesophageal varices earlier (12.9 versus 8.2 weeks, respectively) ($P < 0.001$); the mean number of injection courses, and necessary amount of sclerosant were also lower in the alcohol-treated group ($P < 0.001$), but the frequency of rebleeding did not differ significantly ($P > 0.05$). Thirty-one children with variceal bleeding caused by extrahepatic portal vein obstruction (19), non-cirrhotic portal fibrosis (5) or cirrhosis (7) were treated by sclerotherapy using absolute alcohol; arrest of acute bleeding was achieved in ten by emergency sclerotherapy, and a 3-week schedule was able to achieve variceal obliteration in all of them; during a 23-month follow-up period, recurrent varices occurred in three (two with cirrhosis and one with non-cirrhotic portal fibrosis) patients; a rebleed was successfully controlled with emergency sclerotherapy in five, and an oesophageal stricture in four of them (which was easily dilated) were the only significant complications.

Although now rarely used in the Western world, oesophageal compression using a Sengstaken tube is often the only technique available. Intravenous pitressin is of limited value in acute bleeding. In long-term management, propranolol undoubtedly has a place in a developing country context.

In an attempt to provide clinical guidelines for the prediction of outcome of upper gastrointestinal bleeding in a developing country, Clamp et al[7] carried out a multicentre study based on two centres—in Sikkim and China; in the former country, 60 (69%) of the patients put into the 'high-risk' group (by applying Bayes theorem using a computer system) for rebleeding experienced this event (27 (54%) died), whereas this complication occurred in only six (2%) in the 'low-risk' group; furthermore, a simplified scoring system (little computer technology was available at Sikkim) gave almost exactly the same predictive accuracy. The authors suggest that, by using one of these systems, patients in remote areas can be categorized in order that scarce resources (which are available there) can be put to the best use.

The optimal means of managing haemorrhage resulting from extrahepatic portal venous obstruction is summarized in the section on liver disease (see below).

OESOPHAGEAL CARCINOMA

Presence of histologically diagnosed chronic oesophagitis (using upper gastrointestinal endoscopy) has been shown to be common in a high-risk population (15–26 years) in China.[16] This lesion was significantly associated with: (1) consumption of 'burning hot' beverages; (2) a family history of oesophageal carcinoma (including second degree relatives); (3) infrequent consumption of fresh fruit; and (4) infrequent consumption of dietary staples, other than maize. Associated factors which have been recorded in that population include: (1) positive cytological smears (568 individuals > 30 years of 42 190 had a positive result); and (2) a high prevalence of pharyngeal carcinoma in free-range chickens which lived off domestic scraps[17] in the local environment.

This tumour often presents late in its clinical course in the heavily affected areas; in fact, complete luminal obstruction (accompanied by inability to swallow saliva) is not uncommon at presentation.

Passage of a Celestin latex rubber tube (a palliative technique) is often the only available procedure;[6] however, blockage is a frequent problem resulting largely from the bulky African (or other) diet. Chemotherapy and radiotherapy (when available) are of very limited value.

STOMACH AND DUODENUM

Peptic ulceration was at one time considered to be an unusual cause of abdominal pain in tropical countries; it was in fact felt by many physicians to be a rare disease.[1] It is now clear, however, that this is not the case and that many difficulties facing the clinical epidemiologist in a developing country are highlighted by studies of the geographical distribution of this disease. Because sophisticated methods of diagnosis, including barium meal and upper gastrointestinal endoscopy, have not until recently been widely used in developing countries, diagnosis and attempts at establishing accurate prevalence rates have depended upon recording incidence rates of complications, especially pyloric stenosis; upper gastrointestinal haemorrhage seems an unusual presentation overall, but this probably results from the fact that such patients do not reach hospital before exsanguination occurs. Therefore, serious deficiencies exist in present knowledge regarding the true prevalence of peptic ulceration, and it is currently impossible to draw accurate conclusions on regional and rural/urban patterns, and also on variations with time, i.e. during the course of 'westernization'.

As recently as the 1950s, duodenal ulcer was considered a rare disease in Africa;[1] it is now known with certainty that this is not so, because satisfactory radiological, and more recently endoscopic, investigations have yielded accurate facts on true prevalence rate(s). Prevalence of duodenal ulcer in Africa has been reviewed using the available literature;[1,18] high prevalence areas seem to exist in parts of West Africa, Rwanda, Burundi, eastern Zaire, western Tanzania, south-western Uganda and the Ethiopian highlands. In southern India[18] (and Fijians descended from this population[19]) and Papua New Guinea the disease also seems relatively common. It has a marked male predominance; it is frequently postbulbar, and presentation with pyloric obstruction is relatively usual. Genetic factors might be important;[18] the role of diet remains difficult to assess. Whether low rates of presentation resulting from haemorrhage and/or perforation accurately reflect events, or are biased by the inability to transport a sick patient to hospital, is also impossible

to evaluate. Evidence for a causative role for *Helicobacter pylori* in chronic active gastritis, peptic ulceration and possibly gastric malignancy has escalated during the last decade;[18,20] however, Koch's postulates have not all been satisfied, and infection rate with this organism frequently approaches 100% at an early age in an affected population.

Overall, gastric ulcer is uncommon in developing countries.[1] When it occurs it usually has a male predominance, is most common in the fifth and sixth decades, and afflicts lower social strata. Pyloric obstruction is a common presentation—due frequently to the late stage of disease at presentation.

Management of a bleeding peptic ulcer has been reviewed.[1,4]

Gastritis—often resulting from alcohol and spicy foods—is a major cause of abdominal pain/discomfort[21] (Table 3.2). Infective causes (including tuberculosis) are rare overall, although they are occasionally encountered; infections which involve predominantly lower sections of the gastrointestinal tract (e.g. *Salmonella typhi* and *Shigella* spp.) occasionally produce significant gastric pathology. A heavy infection with hookworm and/or *A. lumbricoides* can also account for epigastric discomfort (see below) and must be differentiated from peptic ulceration.

When H_2-receptor antagonists (e.g. cimetidine and ranitidine) are used in developing countries, a possibility exists that they will encourage proliferation of intestinal pathogen(s)—bacterial and parasitic—for the gastric acid defence mechanism is largely removed;[22] available data are, however, presently inadequate for assessing the importance of this. Several studies of gastric acid production indicate that mean acid production probably varies little in different ethnic groups. Hypochlorhydria is relatively common in the tropics;[1] whether it is the cause or consequence of intestinal infection (of bacterial, including *S. typhi*, and/or parasitic origin) remains far from clear.

Gastric carcinoma is overall an uncommon malignancy in tropical countries (see Chapter 24).[1,23] At Sura, Fiji, gastric ulcer and carcinoma have been shown to be more common in Fijians than Indians.

Table 3.2 Some causes of *severe* abdominal pain (without features of intestinal obstruction) in relation to tropical exposure.

Site of pain	Cause
Epigastrium	Heavy nematode infection (e.g. *Ascaris lumbricoides*, hookworm) Mesenteric adenitis (helminthic eggs or tuberculosis) Acute pancreatitis (helminth-related)

Generalized	Peritonitis
	  Typhoid perforation
	  Amoebic colitis perforation (appendix, perforated peptic ulcer or diverticulitis)
	  Abdominal tuberculosis
	  Ruptured hydatid cyst
	  Sickle cell crisis
	  Recurrent familial polyserositis (familial Mediterranean fever)
	  Hyperinfective syndrome caused by *Strongyloides stercoralis*
	  Angiostrongylus costaricensis

Right upper quadrant	Helminthic infection involving biliary system
Left upper quadrant	Splenomegaly (e.g. hyperreactive malarious splenomegaly) Splenic rupture Solitary splenic abscess
Right iliac fossa	Appendicitis *Anisakis* spp. infection Ileocaecal tuberculosis

STOMACH AND DUODENUM: EMERGENCIES

Many facts remain unclear regarding upper gastrointestinal haemorrhage in tropical countries. For example, duodenal ulcer is apparently common in Indians (who are descended from southern Indians) in Fiji (see above); however, haematemesis from a chronic duodenal ulcer is more common in Fijians.

Many extant data suggest that pyloric obstruction is the most common complication of duodenal ulcer in developing countries. However, a report from Zaire, northern Nigeria, indicates that at that location perforation is by no means uncommon;[24] between 1971 and 1983, 74 (24%) of 302 patients operated for duodenal ulcer, and 29 (58%) of 50 for gastric ulcer presented with perforation; furthermore, there was a progressive incidence in the years 1971–1974 to 1979–1983 of from 16 to 45%, respectively. A rare case report from India has recorded massive haematemesis and melaena from a cholecystoduodenal fistula secondary to duodenal ulcer in a 24-year-old man;[25] he was successfully managed surgically.

Ideally, management of the complications of gastritis and peptic ulceration is exactly the same as in a Western country.

Although usually associated with oesophageal varices, gastric varices also occur alone. At New Delhi, India, 48 (16%) out of 309 patients with portal hypertension were shown to have gastric varices;[26] in six (12%) there was no evidence of associated oesophageal varices. In 11 (28%) of 40 patients who completed endoscopic sclerotherapy for oesophageal varices, gastric varices disappeared concurrently with the former, or during the following 6 months. In the light of their experience, these authors considered that 'if they persist for 6 months after eradication of oesophageal varices, a combination of paravariceal and intravariceal sclerotherapy should be attempted for their obliteration'.

ABDOMINAL PAIN

Epigastric pain/discomfort is a common presenting symptom in medical practice in tropical countries (see above);[1,27] this frequently results from heavy small-intestinal helminthic infections, especially *A. lumbricoides* and hookworm. Mesenteric adenitis as a sequel to the presence of helminthic ova, and tuberculosis, is a further cause. Helminth-related acute pancreatitis is another possibility.

Table 3.2 summarizes some causes of *severe* generalized abdominal pain. Generalized pain most commonly results from peritonitis—which has numerous aetiologies. Right upper quadrant pain is less likely to result from biliary tract disease than in a 'temperate' area of the world (see below); nevertheless, helminthic infections of the biliary system are encountered from time to time. Left upper quadrant pain can result from splenomegaly (resulting from numerous 'tropical' infections) (see below); an extreme example (HMS) occurs in most areas which are endemic for human *Plasmodium* spp. Ruptured spleen is a further cause of left hypochondrial pain; this event usually presents acu-tely. Solitary splenic abscess is by no means an uncommon event in West and Central Africa; the aetiology remains unclear.

Right iliac fossa pain is less likely to be caused by appendicitis (see below) than in most Western countries. However, an appendix-like syndrome can result from *Yersinia* spp., ileocaecal tuberculosis, and *Anisakis* spp. infection (see below). *Enterobius vermicularis* is not infrequently detected in an appendicectomy specimen; whether cause–effect related (to acute appendicitis) is frequently unclear. Less common parasites involving the appendix include *Taenia* spp., *Trichuris trichiura* and *Angiostrongylus costaricensis* (see below). A peripheral blood eosinophilia is often (but by no means always) present when a helminthiasis is causatively related to appendicitis. Ileocaecal tuberculosis can account for chronic right iliac fossa pain; an ileocaecal mass is often palpable clinically (and confirmed by ultrasonography, when this technique is available). A colonic amoeboma represents a possible source of diagnostic confusion.

SMALL INTESTINE

TROPICAL ENTEROPATHY AND SUBCLINICAL MALABSORPTION

The small-intestinal mucosa of an individual living in a developing country possesses minor structural differences compared with that in one always resident in a temperate zone.[1,28,29] Changes are not related to the clinical syndrome postinfective malabsorption (tropical sprue) (see below). Although the cause of these changes is not entirely clear, they seem to result from repeated low-grade viral and bacterial infection(s). Similarly, marginal xylose and glucose malabsorption has been demonstrated in large numbers of people indigenous to tropical countries; these abnormalities are certainly greater in lower socioeconomic groups. Subclinical malabsorption exists in many people in developing countries;[1] xylose and B_{12} malabsorption have been demonstrated in 39 and 52%, respectively, of Peace Corps workers living under rural conditions in Pakistan. Apart from repeated small-intestinal infections, other factors are probably also important. Xylose, glucose and folic acid absorption have been shown to be impaired in individuals with systemic bacterial infections, e.g. pulmonary tuberculosis and pneumococcal pneumonia. Dietary folate depletion also results in xylose malabsorption. Marginal malnutrition and pellagra have both been suggested as causing subclinical malabsorption, but evidence is contradictory.

The practical importance of subclinical malabsorption is unclear.[1,28,29] It seems likely that it significantly contributes to malnutrition in people in developing countries who subsist on a marginally adequate dietary intake consisting largely of carbohydrate. Before any rigid conclusions are drawn, however, it should be appreciated that the small intestine has a very substantial functional reserve, and that the role of the colon in absorption of carbohydrate (and other substances) (see above) remains unclear.

Diarrhoea resulting from small-intestinal disease consists of two main types:[1,29] (1) profuse watery (e.g. cholera), and (2) steatorrhoeic (exemplified by postinfective tropical malabsorption (tropical sprue)). Table 3.3 summarizes the most important causes; several of those responsible for the former type are infective and exert their pathogenic effect

Table 3.3 Small-intestinal diarrhoea.

Watery diarrhoea (large volume, fluid stool(s))
Travellers' diarrhoea (TD) (turista)
Vibrio cholerae (and other vibrios)
Escherichia coli (enterotoxigenic)
Salmonella spp.
Campylobacter jejuni
Rotavirus (and other enteric viruses)
Cryptosporidium spp.
(Food poisoning—*Staphylococcus, Clostridium perfringens*)
Hypolactasia: (1) primary—genetically determined
　　　　　　　　(2) secondary—resulting from enterocyte damage

Steatorrhoeic diarrhoea (malabsorption) (characteristically large pale, fatty, offensive stools;
microscopy often shows fat globules in faecal smear)
Postinfective tropical malabsorption ('tropical sprue')
Intestinal parasites
　　Giardia lamblia
　　Strongyloides stercoralis
　　Capillaria philippinensis
　　Coccidia: *Cryptosporidium parvum*
　　　　　　　Isospora belli
　　　　　　　Sarcocystis hominis
　　　　　　　Microsporidium spp.
　　　　　　　Cyclospora cayetanensis
HIV enteropathy
Trauma—short bowel syndrome (e.g. recovered pigbel disease)
Lymphoma—Burkitt's, Mediterranean lymphomas
Ileocaecal tuberculosis
Chronic calcific pancreatitis
Acute and chronic liver disease

(Gluten-induced enteropathy (coeliac disease) seems to be an uncommon or even rare in most
tropical populations. Occasionally it can become clinically obvious in visitors from Western
countries to the tropics)

---

via an enterotoxin (either heat stable or heat labile); invasive disease involving the enterocyte is less important. The role of intestinal hormones—especially vasoactive intestinal peptide—in the production of watery diarrhoea has become clearer.[29] The pathogenesis of diarrhoea in AIDS has a multifactorial basis, and is often by no means clear; some, but not all cases are associated with an opportunistic infection(s), especially *Cryptosporidium parvum* (see Chapter 67).[29] Other opportunistic infections in this syndrome include cytomegalovirus, *Mycobacterium avium intracellulare, Salmonella* spp., *Isospora belli, Sarcocystis hominis* and *Microsporidium* spp. infections; in addition, Kaposi's sarcoma (see Chapter 24) causes severe small-intestinal disease.

Many of the problems encountered with management, including chemoprophylaxis and chemotherapy, are exemplified by travellers' diarrhoea (see below).

TRAVELLERS' DIARRHOEA

The clinical syndrome traveller's diarrhoea (TD)[1,30–34] is arguably the world's most common disease entity; it is rarely associated with mortality (usually in the presence of debility, or at the extremes of life), but the significant morbidity with which it is associated not infrequently interferes with a crowded schedule or a leisure or sporting activity. Numerous titles have been applied, including: 'turista', 'Montezuma's revenge', 'Hong Kong dog' and 'Delhi belly'. One estimate is that 12 million individuals travel annually from an industrialized (Western) country to one in the tropics or subtropics;[35] in this group incidence of TD varies from around 20 to 50%. There is a highly significant geographical variation in prevalence; high-risk areas include[36]: North Africa, sub-Saharan Africa, the Indian subcontinent, South-East Asia, southern America, Mexico and the Middle East; intermediate ones include the north Mediterranean, Canary Islands and the Caribbean islands; low-risk ones include North America, western Europe and Australia. In a retrospective study carried out in Switzerland, a large group of travellers was asked to complete a questionnaire after travelling abroad; incidence of the disease varied greatly, the highest figure (50%) being associated with travel to Tunisia. (No detailed study exists of TD acquired in a European country.[37])

The disease tends to become less common with advancing years; it is unclear whether this is due to the fact that older travellers (≥60 years) have a more discerning life style, or whether relative immunity increases with advancing age.[30,36] Individuals resident for substantial periods in areas where TD is common, seem to experience it less frequently than those not previously exposed.[30,31]

CLINICAL FEATURES

TD is contracted by ingestion of contaminated water/food; it is characterized by acute-onset watery diarrhoea (usually of small-intestinal origin);[29–34] when colorectal involvement exists, diarrhoea may be bloody (see below). Abdominal colic, nausea and vomiting may be present; fever is unusual, being recorded in 1–10% of infected individuals. Prostration and resultant dehydration (with electrolyte imbalance) causes major problems in a *severe* case. Rarely, symptoms become chronic, and it seems likely that a small proportion of cases of TD proceed to postinfective malabsorption (see below).[28] Unfortunately for the investigator, by the time disease has become clinically overt, the initiating infection(s) has invariably been cleared. Chronic diarrhoea of lesser severity is a relatively common problem following recovery from acute disease; this can usually be attributed to: (1) *tropical enteropathy* (in which there is major derangement of enterocyte structure and function) (see above); or (2) the *irritable bowel syndrome* (see below).

On clinical grounds, an important differential diagnosis is inflammatory bowel disease— presenting for the first time during, or immediately after, tropical exposure.[38,39] In a retrospective review of UK residents presenting at the Hospital for Tropical Diseases, London, with acute onset/bloody diarrhoea, the majority had inflammatory bowel disease (usually ulcerative colitis); it was numerically more important than shigellosis and amoebic colitis.

Acute disease pursues an especially virulent course in certain high-risk groups,[30,31,36] e.g. those suffering from: achlorhydria (*Salmonella* spp. and

Vibrio spp. infections are known to be significantly more common in this group); known inflammatory bowel disease (see below); previous gastrointestinal tract surgery; a malignancy involving the gastrointestinal tract; and acquired or congenital immunodeficiency (including immunosuppressive therapy and HIV/AIDS). In addition, individuals on diuretic therapy (in whom maintenance of electrolyte balance is precarious) and others at the extremes of life also fall within the high-risk group. It is important to recognize these factors when advising chemoprophylaxis (see below).[36]

AETIOLOGY

In 1970, Rowe et al[40] recorded results of a study involving British soldiers newly arrived at Aden; in 19 (54.3%) of 33 cases in which a known pathogen was not apparent, a 'new' serotype of *Escherichia coli* was isolated in the acute phase of TD; in a further 14 (40%), several different *E. coli* serotypes were also isolated. (B. H. Keane had suggested in the 1950s (on circumstantial evidence) that bacterial pathogens were implicated.[30,31]) Sack[41] recorded the identity of *E. coli* serotypes isolated from US Peace Corps volunteers serving in various countries: Kenya 06:H16, 06:H−, 027:H7, 0159:H4 and 0159:H34; Morocco 06:H16, 0128:H12, 027:H20 and 0169:H−; Honduras 08:H9, 015:H49, 015:H− and 027:H20. Therefore, many common strains of enterotoxigenic *E. coli* (ETEC) are relevant. Many other micro-organisms can also be involved:[1,29–34] *Salmonella* spp., *Shigella* spp., *Campylobacter jejuni*, enteroadherent *E. coli* (EAEC) (see Chapter 41) and *Vibrio* spp. (see Chapter 41); rotavirus and Norwalk virus (see Chapter 35), and *Giardia lamblia*, *Coccidia* spp. (including *Cryptosporidium* spp., *I. belli* and *Blastocystis hominis*) and *Entamoeba histolytica* (see Chapter 67). Other bacteria which have been implicated include: *Aeromonas hydrophila*, *Plesiomonas shigelloides* and *Y. enterocolitica*. The causative agents vary significantly in different locations, e.g. in an affected individual in Asia, Central America or Africa the likely organism is different on probability grounds, although not relevant to a specific case. Furthermore, more than one organism is frequently present; in a study involving US Peace Corps workers in Thailand, 33% were infected by 2–4 different pathogens.[31] Although protozoan parasites are usually incorporated in the list of aetiological agents, the incubation period is usually somewhat longer than is usual in TD; this applies especially to *G. lamblia*. When the colorectum is involved predominantly, *Shigella* spp., enteroinvasive *E. coli* (EIEC), enterohaemorrhagic *E. coli* (EHEC) and *Ent. histolytica* may be responsible. Rarely, herpes simplex virus and *Chlamydia trachomatis* have been implicated. New pathogens will doubtless emerge in future years.

PATHOPHYSIOLOGY

The pathophysiology varies and depends on the site of the gastrointestinal tract involved.[1,29–34] Whereas in the small intestine toxigenic diarrhoeas predominate (see above), in the colorectum (see below) invasive disease is more common.

ETEC are characterized by both toxin production and mucosal adherence (via specific fimbriae); the latter property is required for disease production, for toxin-producing non-adherent mutants do not cause disease. Enteropathogenic *E. coli* (EPEC) (probably not a major cause of TD) adhere to intestinal mucosal cells and although they do not invade, destroy microvilli. EAEC (detected in up to 15% of patients suffering from TD) do not belong to classical serotypes of EPEC, but adhere to Hep-2 cells in culture; they neither produce a toxin nor invade.[42] EIEC behave similarly to *Shigella* spp. and account for up to 5% of cases; the main site of action is the colorectum, and the major clinical manifestation is therefore dysentery resulting from epithelial cell invasion and intracellular multiplication; there is resultant mucosal inflammation and ulceration.[42] EHEC (an uncommon cause of TD) produces disease via verotoxin production.

PROPHYLAXIS

Travellers should take maximal care to avoid water/ food likely to be contaminated; common sense is of paramount importance! Use of prophylactic agents is controversial. Wiström and Norrby[36] have summarized several studies (in different geographical locations) involving chemoprophylaxis: doxycycline, co-trimoxazole, trimethoprim, mecillinam, bicozamycin and the fluroquinolone compounds (norfloxacin and ciprofloxacin). High protection rates (≥90%) have been claimed for co-trimoxazole and the fluroquinolones; for trimethoprim a rate of around 50% has been recorded. Most cases of TD therefore possess a bacterial aetiology. The major problem with antibiotic chemoprophylaxis, however, is the risk of significant side-effects— dominated by dermatological reactions (including Stevens–Johnson syndrome) and pseudomembranous colitis (see below); using co-trimoxazole, a rate of 20% of significant skin reactions, necessitating discontinuation of prophylaxis, has been recorded.

Also, the acquisition of resistant faecal *E. coli*, during chemoprophylaxis has been recorded in several studies;[36] an increase from 21 to 100% was recorded using doxycycline in Kenya, and one of 3 to 100% with co-trimoxazole in Mexico. When chemoprophylaxis is used, either norfloxacin or ciprofloxacin seem to be most appropriate, although strains of *Campylobacter jejuni* rapidly acquire resistance.[37] In a recent study in Egypt, 2 of 105 individuals on norfloxacin developed TD, compared with 30 (26%) of 117 given a placebo.[42] (Ciprofloxacin should be avoided in children because of experimental evidence indicating cartilaginous damage in young experimental animals; there is no evidence in *Homo sapiens*.)

Should chemoprophylaxis be recommended widely in an essentially *benign* clinical syndrome? In addition to the objections so far outlined (see above), there is a possibility of inducing a false sense of security—resulting in increased exposure to other infections, e.g. viral hepatitis.[42] The following groups should be seriously considered for chemoprophylaxis (for ≤3 weeks):

- Travellers with a bad track record of TD.[29–34]
- Those in whom hypochlorhydria is a reality (or possibility).
- Individuals suffering from inflammatory bowel disease.
- HIV-infected patients.
- Those in whom electrolyte balance is precarious (e.g. those receiving diuretic therapy), and others with chronic renal failure.
- The 'elderly' (not easily defined!).
- A nebulous group in whom TD is professionally embarrassing (e.g. members of the armed services, airline pilots, athletes, politicians, businessmen and other professionals on tight schedules, etc.).

The role of prophylactic antiperistaltic agents is likewise controversial; action is unphysiological. It has been suggested that they can mask a more serious infection, e.g. *S. typhi*, although in this disease diarrhoea is an unusual presenting symptom (see Chapter 42). By delaying pathogen(s) excretion it is also possible that clinical disease is prolonged. In children, paralytic ileus is a major complication, and has occasionally precipitated mortality.[44]

Bismuth subsalicylate has a role in prophylaxis; the bismuth moiety possesses antimicrobial activity, and salicylate antisecretory properties.[31] Early studies in Mexico by DuPont et al[45] showed that, given as a suspension (the sheer bulk required precluded its use by travellers), this agent significantly reduced TD; the same group, also working in Mexico, has demonstrated that, when given in tablet form (2 four times daily for ≤3 weeks, i.e. 2.1 g daily), a 65% protection rate can be achieved;[45] at half that dose, efficacy was greatly reduced. Number(s) of pathogen-positive TD cases in a group of treated patients was seven of 29, compared with 35 of 59, in a placebo group; ETEC was present in three and 22 respectively, and *Shigella* spp. in two and eight, respectively.[45]

A B-subunit/whole-cell (BS-WC) cholera vaccine has recently been shown to produce relative protection.[46] In a study involving Finnish tourists to Morocco, BS-WC induced 52% protection against diarrhoea caused by ETEC, 65% with mixed infection, 71% when ETEC was present with another pathogen, and 82% when ETEC and *S. enterica* were present concurrently. (Sack[41] has concluded that 'any advances in prevention and treatment of diarrhoea in travellers will be directly applicable to the worldwide problem of diarrhoea in children, which is far more important on a global scale'. This statement does not apply to this BS-WC vaccine, because protection only lasts for about 3 months.) A further approach under consideration consists of oral administration of colostrum-derived antibodies against ETEC.[31]

A recent experimental investigation indicates that lactobacilli, which have the ability to adhere to the intestinal mucosa, can prevent *E. coli* colonization. In a limited clinical study, *Lactobacillus* GG reduced prevalence of TD by up to 40%.[31]

TREATMENT

Treatment (as in cholera, see below) devolves around oral rehydration (see below); all travellers should carry suitable preparations.[1,33,34] When properly constituted, Dioralyte (Rhône-Poulenc Rorer) solution contains: glucose 90, Na^+ 60, K^+ 25, Cl^- 45 and citrate 20 mmol/l. Corresponding concentrations for another proprietary preparation, Rapolyte (Janssen) are: 111, 60, 20, 50 and 10 mmol/l. WHO/UNICEF rehydration fluid contains: glucose 111, Na^+ 90, K^+ 20, Cl^- 80 and citrate 10 mmol/l. In a mild case adequate rehydration can usually be achieved using ordinary mineral water.

The role of chemotherapy in established TD remains controversial. Early work carried out by DuPont et al[45] in Mexico showed that both co-trimoxazole and trimethoprim reduced the length of symptoms. Recent trials, using antibiotics which have been given for chemoprophylaxis (see above), have also indicated that the length of symptoms can be shortened; in Mexico, ofloxacin (600 mg daily for 3 days) produced cure in 77 (95%) of 81, compared with 56 (71%) patients who received placebo ($P =$

0.0001).[47] Short-course chemotherapy can only be justified in a *severe* case; this applies at the extremes of life and in high-risk groups (see above), especially HIV-infected individuals.[32]

CHOLERA (see also Chapter 41)

This represents the archetypal disease in the context of small-intestinal secretory (watery) diarrhoea.[29,48,49]

The causative organism, *V. cholerae*, is not invasive and exerts its effect by means of an enterotoxin.[48] If untreated, the disease has a 20–80% mortality; with modern oral rehydration regimens that figure should be less then 1%. Death results from dehydration, vascular collapse and renal failure.

Historically, cholera was not confined to tropical countries and involved many temperate areas, including much of northern Europe. An epidemic in 1854 in London was traced to contaminated water supplied from the Broad Street pump in Soho. According to legend, when the handle of the pump was tied down by Dr John Snow, the London anaesthetist, a rapid decline in the incidence of new cases was recorded.[50,51]

EPIDEMIOLOGY

Cholera is endemic in India, Pakistan, Bangladesh, Afghanistan and many other countries of South-East Asia. Nosocomial transmission is reported. In recent years, epidemics have occurred in the Middle East, South America and Africa;[48] most have been localized. Cholera is endemic along the Gulf Coast of the USA. The disease is closely associated with poverty, overcrowding and low socioeconomic status.

In former times cholera was spread by population movements such as the annual hadj to Mecca; outbreaks involving air travellers have now been recorded. Overall, however, the disease is rare in British travellers.[52] It tends to affect young people more often than the elderly.

AETIOLOGY

There is probably a genetic predisposition—blood group O is associated with a higher infection rate than group A.[29]

Classical cholera is caused by *V. cholerae*, which is now localized to the Indian subcontinent, particularly the deltas of the Ganges and Brahmaputra rivers. Elsewhere, the El Tor biotype, which originated in Indonesia around 1960, and the 0139 strain have been responsible for most epidemics. *Vibrio* spp. are curved, Gram-negative, flagellated rods approximately $2\mu m$ in length. Each biotype of cholera contains three serotypes: Inaba, Ogawa and Hikojima.

The bioecology of the organism is unclear, though its habitat between epidemics might be in river estuaries.[53] A seasonal appearance has been observed in a related organism, *V. parahaemolyticus*, and this is associated with the cyclic appearance of zooplankton in the water column.

Following ingestion (often in seafood), gastric acid destroys *Vibrio* spp.; in hypochlorhydria (e.g. following gastrectomy), or after cannabis smoking, the disease is more common and often more severe.[22] The role of H_2-receptor antagonists in predisposition remains unclear. Organisms multiply within the small-intestinal lumen and do not invade the mucosa or enter the portal circulation, except in exceptional circumstances.[54]

An enterotoxin is secreted which adheres tightly to the enterocyte; this increases the activity of adenylate cyclase and subsequently the concentration of cyclic AMP. Cholera toxin has a molecular weight of 84 000, an optimal pH of 8.0 and is inactivated at 60°C. As cyclic AMP accumulates in the enterocyte, a massive net flux occurs towards the lumen. When colonic absorptive capacity (which might itself be decreased in acute cholera[49]) is overwhelmed, torrential diarrhoea results.[55]

Despite non-invasiveness, *V. cholerae* induces serum bactericidal and agglutinating antibodies, albeit at low concentration.

PATHOLOGY

Histologically, the small-intestinal mucosa is intact. Light and electron microscopical appearances are normal. Following circulatory collapse resulting from gross dehydration, renal tubular necrosis can be demonstrated.

CLINICAL FEATURES

There are no prodromal symptoms. The incubation period varies from a few hours to 5 days. The disease is similar whichever biotype is involved, but there is a wide spectrum of severity. When the El Tor biotype is responsible, a higher proportion of patients are asymptomatic. Onset is sudden, and mild diarrhoea rapidly gives way to the passage of a large volume of opalescent fluid—the classic 'rice-water' stools. Up to 30 litres of fluid, containing a high concentration of *Vibrio* spp. organisms, may be passed in 24 hours.[49] Vomiting of fluid of a similar composition is a later feature. Thirst, muscle cramps, hoarseness and anuria follow.

Clinical signs of severe dehydration may be present by 24 hours after onset in an untreated case. The body temperature is normal or mildly elevated. Circulatory failure and acute renal failure follow. Confusion, disorientation and hypoglycaemic convulsions may occur. Mortality rate is dependent on the degree of dehydration. Relative immunity is short lived. A carrier state—which lasts a few weeks—may occur, and gallbladder foci have been identified.

INVESTIGATIONS

Vibrio spp. organisms are easily identified in faecal specimens; material should be transported to the laboratory in alkaline peptone water (pH 9.0). A rapid diagnostic technique for field use has been described. For accurate serological identification of *V. cholerae*, rigid criteria are necessary. With classic cholera, organisms are present during the incubation period and for up to 5 days after an attack; in the El Tor variety, *Vibrio* spp. can persist for weeks or months.

Faecal samples are isotonic, with a protein concentration of approximately 10 g/l; pH is about 7.5; typical electrolyte concentrations are: sodium 139 mmol/l, potassium 23 mmol/l, chloride 106 mmol/l and bicarbonate 48 mmol/l. Specimens contain a high concentration of IgA. Serum IgA and IgM are elevated, the former most markedly in patients with an El Tor infection. In in vitro animal studies, cholera toxin enhances IgA secretion from crypt epithelium to ileal lumen.[56]

Serum electrolyte, urea and creatinine concentrations vary with the stage and severity of the disease. Excessive potassium loss exacerbates metabolic acidosis. Urine is concentrated and its composition also depends on the severity of the disease.

DIFFERENTIAL DIAGNOSIS

Diagnosis is usually straightforward; however, all other causes of small-intestinal diarrhoea (with and without vomiting) of acute onset (see below) should be considered. These include: travellers' diarrhoea, *E. coli*, *Staphylococcus* spp., *Clostridium perfringens*, *Cl. botulinum*, *Campylobacter jejuni* and viral causes (e.g. rotavirus, Norwalk agent). *Salmonella* spp. and *Shigella* spp. should also be considered. *V. parahaemolyticus* (conveyed by infected raw seafood) and other non-cholera *Vibrio* spp. can also produce a similar disease. Very occasionally, *P. falciparum* malaria can present with severe watery diarrhoea, particularly in infants and children. Food poisoning caused by toxic agents should be added to the list of differential diagnoses.

PREVENTION

Basic sanitation and public health procedures should be improved.[57] Sterility of water supplies is of paramount importance. Vaccination with inactivated (dead) *Vibrio* spp. organisms gives limited protection;[58] 0.5 ml and 1.0 ml vaccine should be given at an interval of 1 week, and a 0.5 ml booster every 6 months.

An inactivated oral vaccine[59,60] and a live attenuated strain (CVD 103-HgR) are likely to be available soon for adult travellers.[58,61] Important progress is being made towards an effective oral bivalent cholera–typhoid vaccine. Contacts of proven cases should be vaccinated; all faeces and bed-linen should be destroyed. The 26th Assembly of the World Health Organization recommended in 1973 that cholera vaccination should not be compulsory, due to its limited public health value. Despite this, a few countries continue to demand vaccination before entry.

Overall, vaccines have so far proved disappointing, but they offer some degree of protection to individual travellers who are at special risk, for example those living in close proximity to overcrowded, infected populations.

TREATMENT

Rehydration regimens

Treatment was revolutionized by the introduction of oral rehydration regimens.[62–65] The enterocyte sodium–glucose carrier system is not affected by cyclic AMP, and thus glucose (and glycine)-stimulated membrane transport takes place normally. Sachets of prepared glucose–electrolyte solutions[66] can be obtained commercially (for example, WHO Oral Rehydration Salts and Dioralyte (Rhône-Poulenc Rorer), see above).

It is impossible to overload the circulation by the oral route in a previously fit person. Quantity of ingested fluid should be regulated by faecal loss, best measured 2-hourly. Rehydration should be accomplished within 48 hours. In an unsophisticated situation, sucrose is often more easily obtainable than glucose; results are usually good, although if severe mucosal damage pre-exists, sucrase concen-

tration is likely to be lowered and satisfactory rehydration is less readily achieved. Cereal-based electrolyte solutions have also given satisfactory results.[65,67]

In a severe case, intravenous fluids may be necessary for initial rehydration.[65,68] A widely used fluid consists of: sodium chloride 5.0 g, sodium bicarbonate 4.0 g, potassium chloride 1.0 g, made up to 1 litre. Severity of dehydration should be assessed on clinical grounds; in a case of average severity, 5 litres should be given (the first litre within 10 minutes) to a 50 kg subject.

Drug treatment

Aspirin[69] and chlorpromazine[70] have been advocated; both inhibit prostaglandin production, and thus limit the effect of cholera toxin on enterocytes, but in practice results are not encouraging.[69] Similarly, clonidine hydrochloride (an α_2-adrenoceptor agonist)—which has also antisecretory properties—has been tested with only limited success.[71]

Analgesics may be necessary for severe muscle cramps. Intravenous calcium gluconate is of value for tetany.

Tetracycline hydrochloride, 1 g/day for 5 days, shortens duration of diarrhoea and clears the luminal content of *Vibrio* spp. organisms in the case of the El Tor biotype.[65] A single dose (1 g or 2 g) has also been shown to be effective in *V. cholerae* infection, but is associated with asymptomatic bacteriological relapse.[72,73] Tetracycline should be started several hours after rehydration therapy has begun. Single-dose doxycycline (300 mg) is probably as effective as tetracycline.[65,74] There is clear evidence that in epidemics the El Tor biotype rapidly develops resistance not only to tetracycline, but also to several other antibiotics (including trimethoprim plus sulphamethoxazole),[75] and is therefore of very limited value.

PROGNOSIS

If cholera is adequately treated, there should be no mortality and recovery complete. A suggestion has been made, however, that such patients might be predisposed to α-chain disease (see below).[76]

MALABSORPTION IN THE TROPICS

Apart from infective causes, *primary* hypolactasia (lactase deficiency)[1,77] accounts for watery small-intestinal diarrhoea in people indigenous to tropical countries. A low concentration of this enzyme in the enterocyte brush border is the normal state for adult *Homo sapiens* (as for other species within the mammalian kingdom); it is under genetic control. In a minority of the world's population, i.e. northern Europeans, Africans with a Hamitic ancestry, certain Middle-Eastern populations (e.g. Saudi Arabians), and others in northern parts of the Indian subcontinent, a high concentration is preserved into adult life. *Secondary* hypolactasia results from brush-border damage;[1,77] concentration of all disaccharidases (and other digestive enzymes) is reduced, but slow recovery occurs after the initiating insult has disappeared. Thus, whenever enterocyte destruction occurs (this includes postinfective tropical malabsorption, see below) hypolactasia develops.

Following ingestion of milk or another milk product, in which lactose is not completely hydrolysed, osmotic diarrhoea results; this is accompanied by abdominal colic, distension and flatulence ('lactose intolerance'). Yoghurt contains adequate bacterial lactase to hydrolyse the lactose component and is usually well tolerated. Lactic acid production (derived from hydrolysis of lactose by colonic bacteria) produces irritative diarrhoea—which contributes to the symptoms. The precise role of the colon in adaptation remains unclear; it is now clear that carbohydrate—in the form of free fatty acid(s) (and also nitrogen and electrolytes)—can be absorbed from this organ. Investigation of hypolactasia most often utilizes the breath hydrogen test; lactose tolerance test and lactase assay in a jejunal biopsy specimen are alternatives. In management, milk and all lactose-containing dairy products should be eliminated from the diet;[1,77] individuals in countries with *primary* hypolactasia sometimes regulate bowel function by varying lactose ingestion.

POSTINFECTIVE MALABSORPTION (PIM) (TROPICAL SPRUE)

Relatively little is known about the prevalence and severity of malabsorption in acute infective conditions of the small intestine (viral, bacterial and parasitic) and the duration for which it can continue *after* the specific organism(s) has been eliminated.

In some cases, malabsorption persists in the presence of *mixed* luminal flora, and a single infective agent cannot be detected. In others the recognizable initiating infective cause (or causes) may continue, culminating in a chronic form; a more precise term is therefore 'post*acute* infective' malabsorption. As with all infective diseases, the clinical spectrum

varies from a subclinical case to one with gross pathology (malabsorption). PIM is of particular clinical significance in tropical countries where small (and large) intestinal infections are exceedingly common.

The clinical entity *PIM related to tropical exposure* has been reviewed by Cook,[1,28,29,78,79] Tomkins,[80] Baker[81] and Mathan.[82]

HISTORY AND DEFINITION

Confusion exists between PIM and tropical sprue; however, in tropical and subtropical countries the entities seem synonymous, and much difficulty is associated with semantics.[1,28] Dr Patrick Manson first coined the term tropical sprue (derived from a word used by Dutch workers in the East Indies) in 1880.[83] It rapidly became applied to all cases of malabsorption in tropical countries—undoubtedly including some resulting from tuberculosis and various parasitoses (both protozoan and helminthic). Historically, chronic diarrhoea accompanied by wasting was recognized in India before 600 BC; although the Englishman William Hillary is often credited with the first precise description of tropical sprue at Barbados,[84] it is likely that he described either epidemic *G. lamblia* infection, or possibly strongyloidiasis. The clinical syndrome was certainly well known to British physicians in India during the eighteenth and nineteenth centuries; most descriptions were made in British expatriate populations. It was only in the early 1960s that reports of a high prevalence of epidemic PIM in indigenous Indians became available.[1,81,82] Despite early suggestions that chronic tropical diarrhoea had an insidious onset, it is clear (after careful assessment) that the vast majority of cases always presented *acutely*. Confusion has been compounded further when acute epidemic cases of small-intestinal infection, associated with gross dehydration (in addition to xylose and fat malabsorption) and acute mortality, have been designated tropical sprue, as in numerous reports from southern India.[82] It is essential therefore to include a *time factor* in the definition of this clinical *syndrome*, e.g. chronic diarrhoea and malabsorption, with weight loss, of at least 3–4 months duration. If used at all, the term tropical sprue would also be better reserved for a condition where malabsorption of nutrients is quantitatively more important than that of water and electrolytes. Although the aetiology of PIM remains conjectural (see below), it is now clear that most cases follow an *acute* small-intestinal insult by either a bacterial, viral or parasitic (or mixed) pathogen.

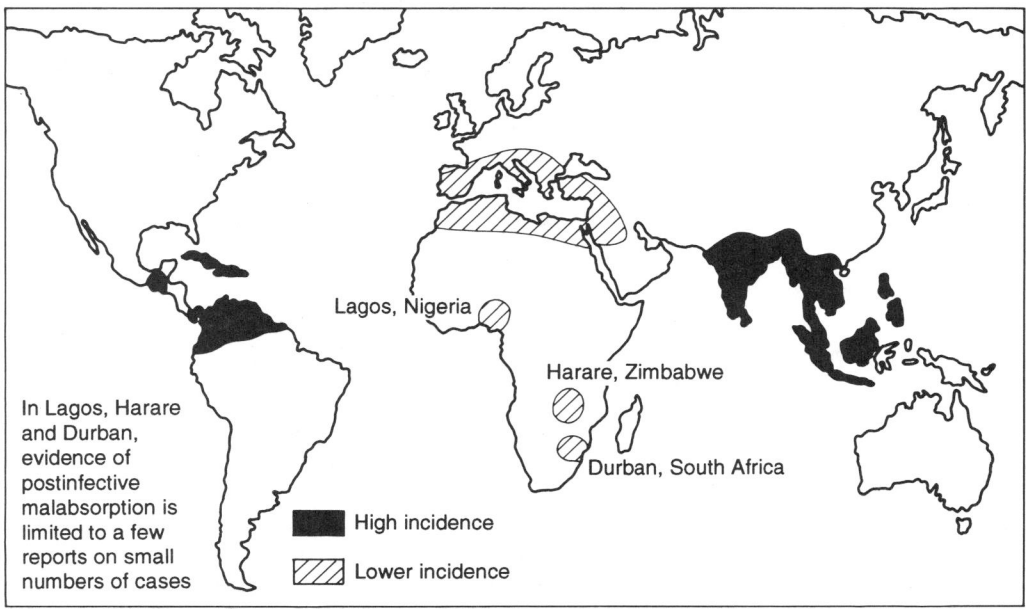

In Lagos, Harare and Durban, evidence of postinfective malabsorption is limited to a few reports on small numbers of cases

Lagos, Nigeria

Harare, Zimbabwe

Durban, South Africa

■ High incidence

▨ Lower incidence

Figure 3.3 World map showing areas where postinfective tropical malabsorption is a significant medical problem.

Overall, evidence for PIM following a small-intestinal insult is more complete for bacterial and parasitic infections. Infections of viral origin might, however, be more important numerically; lack of precise data can be largely attributed to the fact that virology remains a relatively neglected discipline in most developing countries, where infections of all types are far more common than in the Western world.

The effect of malabsorption after divergent small-intestinal insults on overall nutritional status is largely unknown (see above); children are especially at risk. The magnitude of energy loss is unclear; a deficit of 10% of dietary energy is one estimate, which is substantial in tropical populations subsisting on a marginal diet. The importance of anorexia in exacerbating associated malnutrition is also underexplored.

GEOGRAPHICAL DISTRIBUTION

Figure 3.3 summarizes the geographical localities where PIM has been reported either commonly or less frequently;[28,29] the map does *not* include areas where sporadic cases have been rarely recorded. Although the disease is common (and endemic) in Asia and the northern part of South America, it is a very unusual condition in tropical Africa. Until recently it was a common entity in overland travellers from the UK to Asia; the fact that it is now rarely seen is presumably largely a result of early antibiotic administration. In the Middle East and Mediterranean littoral, PIM is unusual, but certainly occurs.[84]

AETIOLOGY

Taking the available evidence into account, there can be no reasonable doubt that PIM has an infective basis (see above):[1,28,29,78,79] it is (1) more common in geographical areas where enteric infection abounds; (2) epidemic in some areas, including southern India; (3) the small-intestinal lumen is colonized by aerobic enterobacteria; and (4) recovery usually occurs rapidly (and dramatically) following initiation of broad-spectrum antibiotic treatment. Despite this, however, Mathan[82] is of the opinion that in southern India the primary lesion is enterocyte damage resulting from a 'persistent' lesion of the stem cell compartment occurring on a 'background of tropical enteropathy'.[85] He further considers that 'an immunity-conferring agent may be responsible for the initiating damage'. The widely used definition for this *clinical syndrome* in southern India, 'intestinal malabsorption of at least two nutrients and the exclusion of diseases that give rise to secondary malabsorption (in a tropical environment)', is inadequate; it does not exclude *tropical enteropathy* (see above), nor does it introduce a time (chronicity) clause (see above).

Genetic predisposition

All infective diseases have a genetic background. In a limited study at Puerto Rico, 25 of 27 patients with PIM (not well defined) had at least one antigen of the HLA-Aw19 series;[86] the strongest associated link was with Aw31. In India, a high frequency of HLA-B8 was documented;[87,88,99] HLA-A1, A28 and Bw35 were significantly decreased in the affected group. More data are required on genetic markers in PIM.

Infection

In severe PIM (in the absence of parasites) bacterial colonization has been demonstrated both within the jejunal lumen and in biopsy specimens.[89–91] The importance of adhesive properties of bacteria in pathogenesis in unclear; many bacteria, including *E. coli*, *S. typhimurium* and *V. cholerae*, possess adhesive properties—mediated by a transmissible plasmid. In tropical PIM, several groups have demonstrated a higher concentration of aerobic enterobacteria in relation to the enterocyte compared with luminal fluid.[91] (In the normal individual, anaerobes outnumber aerobes by about 1000-fold.) It seems likely that a variety of toxins released by these enterobacteria induce net water secretion and malabsorption.[92] In the blind-loop syndrome, enterobacteria (which are invariably obligate anaerobes) do *not produce toxins*.[93] Several months after tropical exposure the upper small-intestinal intraluminal bacterial flora (mucosal biopsy or luminal fluid) may remain abnormal;[91,94] 7 of 11 patients studied had enterobacteria in numbers ranging from 10^3 to 10^8/g or ml. The most common organisms are *Klebsiella pneumoniae*, *Enterobacter cloacae* and *E. coli*; *Citrobacter feundii*, *Serratia marcescens* and *Pseudomonas* spp. have also been detected. It seems highly likely, therefore, that these organisms had been present since the onset of disease. In southern India, a viral aetiology has been sought; there is little evidence for this. The origin of this overgrowth has not been adequately studied in tropical PIM; in patients in England with small-intestinal bacterial overgrowth, faecal flora account for most of the organisms, but salivary flora seem important in some cases.[95]

Jejunal morphology

Morphological changes are non-specific and range in severity.[96] Blunting of villi ('partial villous atrophy') with increased lymphocyte and plasma cell infiltration (not a feature of *tropical enteropathy*) are present to a variable degree; a 'flat' mucosa is exceedingly unusual. Although the number of plasma cells is increased, distribution of IgA-,

IgM- and IgG-containing cells is normal.[97] In untreated gluten-induced enteropathy, T cells expressing T-cell receptor γ/δ heterodimers are disproportionately raised; this is not so in PIM.[98] The significance of elevated jejunal surface pH (demonstrated in southern India) is unclear, but is probably merely an indicator of enterocyte damage.[99] Crypt *hyperplasia* has been demonstrated.[85,100]

Although a predisposing immunological deficit has been postulated in tropical PIM, there is no good evidence for this; immunological changes (increased IgG, IgE, C4 and orosomucoid, gastric parietal cell antibodies, and lymphopenia with a low peripheral blood T-cell count) seem to be *sequelae* of mucosal damage, and are not causally related.[85,101]

(A single case report has documented the occurrence of myeloma in a patient suffering from tropical PIM;[102] chronic immunocyte stimulation with autonomous proliferation of a malignant clone of plasma cells has been suggested.)

Small-intestine stasis

In southern India whole-gut transit time (using a radio-opaque marker technique) has been shown to be unaltered in tropical PIM, despite a striking increase in faecal weight.[103] Small-intestinal stasis has, however, been well documented in tropical PIM and might result from excessive enteroglucagon production in response to ileal (and colonic) mucosal injury (see below).[97,104] However, many patients with PIM have received diphenoxylate or loperamide for acute diarrhoea; both agents produce relative small-intestinal stasis.[105,106] They induce antiperistalsis and prevent prostaglandin-induced diarrhoea; inhibition of small-intestinal secretion also occurs.[78] This stasis is of particular interest because peristalsis is usually *increased* in the presence of intraluminal bacteria.

Gut hormones

Gut hormones have been studied in tropical PIM in the fasting state and following a standard meal.[97] Fasting and postprandial plasma enteroglucagon concentrations (produced by L cells in the distal ileum and colon) and motilin were markedly elevated; furthermore, this elevated enteroglucagon concentration shows a significant correlation with a reduction in small-intestinal transit (using the H_2 breath test). Both enteroglucagon and motilin concentrations fall after treatment.[104] Concentration of another gut hormone, plasma peptide YY (also produced by endocrine cells in the ileum and colon) has been shown to be grossly elevated in PIM;[107] it seems possible that this results from a change in peptide YY secretion, resulting from malabsorption, and is a compensatory mechanism in diarrhoea.[108] This hormone is also known to delay gastric emptying and small-intestinal transit, and to reduce gastric and pancreatic secretion. Patients with PIM have a reduced postprandial rise in gastric inhibiting polypeptide; gastrin and pancreatic polypeptide are normal.

Role of the colon

The colonic mucosa, in addition to that of the small intestine, is abnormal in tropical PIM ('tropical colonopathy').[109] Few causes of diarrhoea are strictly confined to one or other of these organs, for example shigellosis frequently involves the small intestine, and salmonellosis and *Campylobacter jejuni* infection the colon.

Recent recognition of an important role for the colon in absorption is clearly relevant. The normal colon is able to absorb 4–7 litres of water per 24 hours,[110] together with 100–160 mmol carbohydrate (as volatile fatty acid(s)). Failure of the diseased colon to salvage the increased ileal effluent increases intensity of diarrhoea.

Colonic abnormalities have been reported in tropical sprue;[111] using a colonic perfusion system, impaired water and sodium absorption was demonstrated.[112] These abnormalities might result from impaired fatty acid absorption, and the effect of free fatty acid(s) on the colonocyte.[113] Other suggested mechanisms are colonocyte damage, enterotoxin production by colonic bacteria, and the local action of bile acid(s) (unabsorbed by the small intestine). Bile acids can be converted to deconjugated, dihydroxy bile acids by colonic bacteria, and impair colonic salvage of water and salt by stimulating colonic secretion and propulsion.[114,115] Colonic bacteria are able to convert long chain fatty acid(s) to hydroxy fatty acid(s), which stimulate colonic secretion[114] and modify colonic motility, resulting in diarrhoea. A defect in sodium and water absorption from rectal mucosa has also been demonstrated using an in vivo dialysis technique;[116] Na^+, K^+-ATPase activity was significantly reduced.

Colonic function has not been investigated in PIM (contracted in a tropical environment) investigated and treated in London.

Animal model

A clinical syndrome which exhibits very close similarities to PIM has been described in the German shepherd dog.[78,117] Jejunal biopsy specimens show villous atrophy with a variable infiltration of lymphocytes and plasma cells in the lamina propria. Subcellular biochemical studies are also similar to those in the human syndrome. Xylose absorption is impaired and blood folate and serum B_{12} concentrations reduced. Aerobic bacteria are involved; both clinical and laboratory recovery take place after broad-spectrum antibiotic therapy.

CLINICAL ASPECTS

This is dominated by chronic diarrhoea with large, pale, fatty stools, and sometimes excessive flatulence, usually following an *acute* intestinal infection.[1,28,29,78,79] Weight loss may be gross and is probably related to anorexia as much as to intestinal disease. Figure 3.4 shows an affected patient before and after chemotherapy; a brief case history is appended. A wide range of clinical presentation exists, however, varying from the *acute* onset type (not strictly postinfective), described by Baker and Mathan as occurring in epidemics (with vomiting and pyrexia in up to 50%) at Vellore, India, to a far more *chronic* entity. Other clinical features, such as glossitis (aphthous ulceration was common in nineteenth century reports), megaloblastic anaemia, fluid retention, depression, apathy, amenorrhoea and infertility, occur only after several months duration.

Table 3.3 summarizes the more important differential diagnoses of chronic malabsorption in relation to tropical exposure (see below). There are also many non-infective causes of malabsorption in the tropics and subtropics; these should be excluded systematically.[1,28,29,78,79]

During, and immediately after, an acute small-intestinal infection, xylose, glucose, fat, B_{12} and folate malabsorption frequently occur (see above). After 4 months or so, moderate/severe morphological change occurs in the jejunal mucosa; serum folate and later B_{12} concentrations decline—often to very low concentrations. Hypoalbuminaemia and oedema are late signs.

Gastric acid secretion is often depressed, but whether this precedes, or is a sequel to, the initiating infection is unknown.[109,118] The role of hypochlorhydria in the production of small-intestinal infection is also unclear.[22] In a small proportion of cases in southern India, B_{12} absorption either improved or became normal with addition of intrinsic factor.[109]

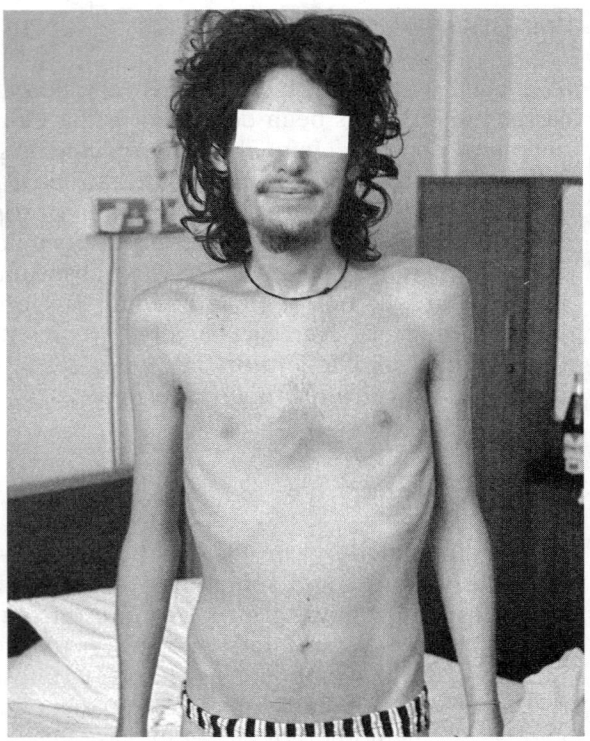
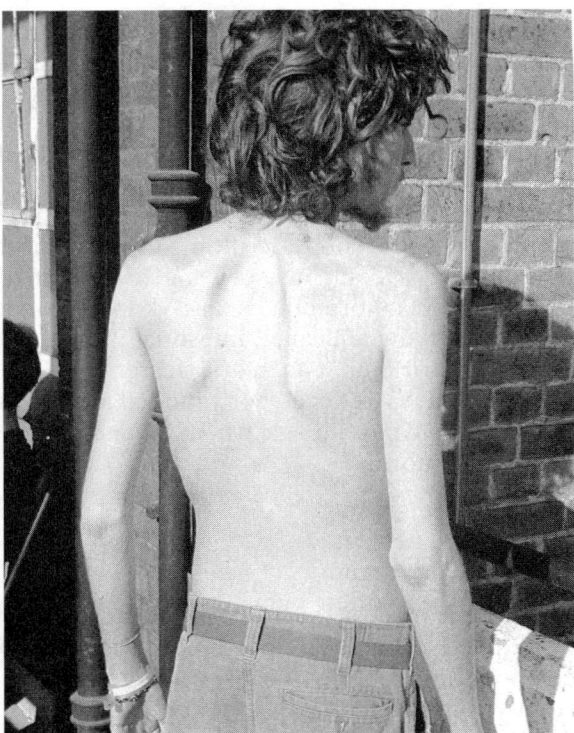

(a)

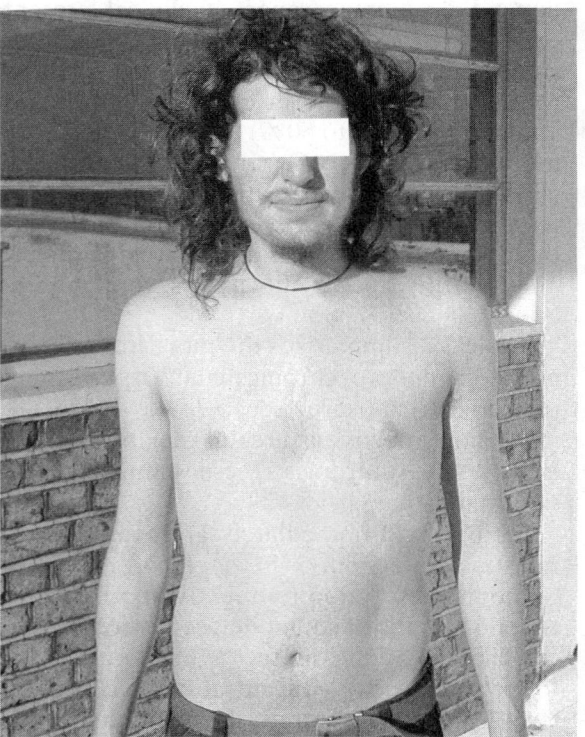
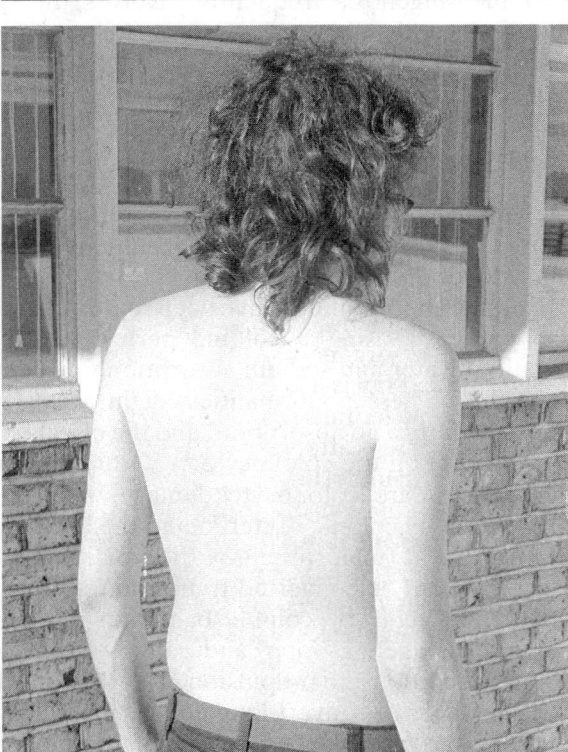

(b)

Figure 3.4   (a) A 19-year-old Englishman presented in London with postinfective tropical malabsorption (tropical sprue). Acute diarrhoea started soon after his arrival in Nepal and he lost approximately 12 kg in weight during the subsequent 2 months. The total urinary xylose excretion after a 25 g oral load was 2.5 mmol/5 hours (normal range 8.0–16.0 mmol/5 hours); the 24-hour faecal fat was 83 mmol (normal range 11–18 mmol); the Schilling test result was 0.16% urinary excretion at 24 hours (normal >10%) and the 8-hour serum concentration was 0% (normal >0.6%) of the loading dose. Jejunal biopsy histology showed marked villous blunting with increased lymphocytes in the lamina propria. Parasites were not found in several faecal samples. Serum albumin 36 g/litre; haemoglobin 13.2 g/dl; mean corpuscular volume 102.9; red blood cell folate 113 ng/l (normal >150 ng/l); serum vitamin B$_{12}$ 322 pg/l (normal >150 pg/l). The patient responded rapidly to treatment with oral tetracycline and folic acid. (b) The same man 4 weeks after initiation of treatment.

Secondary hypolactasia may be present (see above).[77]

There is no good evidence that PIM predisposes to any gastrointestinal malignancy.

INVESTIGATIONS

Investigations should include urinary D-xylose excretion after a 5 or 25 g loading dose, 72-hour faecal fat estimation, a Schilling test and jejunal biopsy; faecal parasites should be excluded. (The 1-hour blood xylose concentration is in practice probably superior to a 5-hour urinary collection in a tropical environment.[119]): serum B_{12} and red blood cell folate concentrations should be estimated; after 4 months of illness most patients have a low folate concentration. Serum albumin[120] and globulin concentrations are often depressed. Monosaccharide absorption is impaired to a greater extent than that of amino acids.[78] Barium meal and follow-through examination shows dilated loops of jejunum with clumping of barium,[120] in addition to reduced transit rate.

Jejunal mucosal changes are variable, depending on the duration of the disease. By 3 or 4 months most biopsies are ridged and/or convoluted; a flat mucosa is extremely unusual and, if present, gluten-induced enteropathy should be suspected. Submucosal invasion with lymphocytes (predominantly T cells) and plasma cells is usual

Ultrastructural changes in jejunal biopsy specimens have been studied;[121] although lysosomes, peroxisomes and mitochondrial enzymes are not depressed, the organelles are more fragile. Endoplasmic reticulum is unchanged. A significant reduction in 5-nucleotidase in the basolateral (plasma) membrane persists after recovery. The latter finding might reflect an underlying abnormality in the enterocyte of individuals susceptible to PIM.

Intestinal permeability has been investigated;[122] abnormalities in urinary excretion of lactulose and rhamnose following an oral load are similar to results obtained in gluten-induced enteropathy.

AETIOLOGY AND TREATMENT

A hypothesis to account for the aetiology of tropical PIM is summarized in Figure 3.5.[104] The 'vicious cycle' can be broken by (1) eliminating bacterial overgrowth, and (2) aiding mucosal recovery (with folic acid supplements).[123] Whilst this hypothesis has been challenged, a satisfactory alternative has not been produced. An adequate diet should be combined with tetracycline (250 mg three times a day for at least 2 weeks) and folic acid (5 mg three times a day for 1 month). Evidence of susceptibility of the responsible flora to antibiotics other than tetracycline is extremely limited.[124] Symptomatic treatment may be necessary in the *acute* stage of the disease; codeine phosphate (30 mg three times a day), diphenoxylate (2.5–5 mg four times daily), or loperamide (5–10 mg four times daily) are of value if stool frequency is excessive. Mild cases respond without treatment, but this may take several months. Recovery is usually rapid and straight-forward;[1,78,104] in the preantibiotic era a mortality rate of 10–20% was usual.

Evidence from south India suggests that response to antibiotics in that area is less satisfactory;[81,85] this is used as evidence to support a suggestion that a viral rather than a bacterial aetiology is causative in that locality.

CONCLUSIONS

The aetiology of PIM—especially that presenting in association with tropical exposure—is slowly becoming clearer.[78,104,125] It is probable that several primary insults to the enterocyte (of an infective nature) are involved. Whereas PIM resulting from most viral, bacterial and parasitic causes is usually self-limiting, the tropical sprue syndrome, when well established, is not usually so. The reason why only a minority of affected individuals who suffer acute small-intestinal infections are susceptible to PIM is unknown; a genetic (or ethnic) basis for susceptibility seems likely.

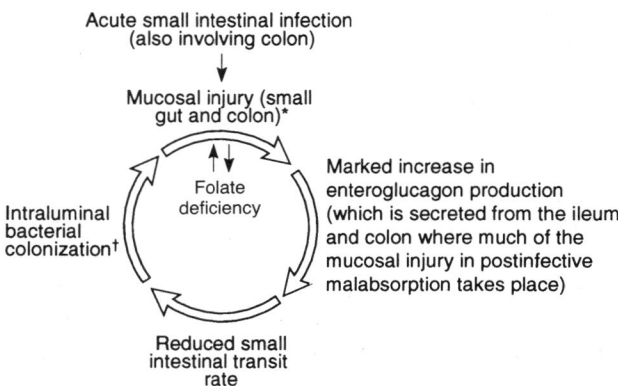

Figure 3.5 Hypothetical scheme to illustrate the pathogenesis of postinfective malabsorption. The open arrows indicate the vicious cycle which, once set in motion, is only broken by elimination of the abnormal luminal flora, and hastening of enterocyte recovery.

OTHER CAUSES OF MALABSORPTION IN THE TROPICS

Table 3.3 summarizes some of these. The role of parasitic infection has been highlighted by AIDS, in which prolonged diarrhoea accompanied by malabsorption and weight loss can be very troublesome. Incontrovertible evidence now exists that HIV infection causes chronic enteropathy with villous blunting; crypt hypoplasia results either from a direct effect of the viruses on cell replication, or by an unknown immunological reaction. This is now a very common cause of persisting malabsorption in Africa. In this context, *Cryptosporidium parvum* and *Isospora belli* have recently come to the fore and it is now also clear that these organisms can produce a self-limiting illness simulating TD in immunocompetent adults and children (see below). *G. lamblia* (see below) is undoubtedly the most common cause of parasitic malabsorption,[79] *Strongyloides stercoralis* (see below),[126] which is widespread in tropical countries, was until very recently still present in approximately 15–30% of former prisoners of war in South-East Asia during World War II; it is an underdiagnosed cause.[1]

Of all causes of malabsorption related to tropical exposure, *intestinal tuberculosis*—usually involving the ileocaecal region—is probably that with the lowest index of suspicion amongst medical personnel.[79,127,128] Abdominal tuberculosis can assume several clinical forms: apart from the hypertrophic ileocaecal form, glandular (involving the mesenteric glands), peritoneal (sometimes with ascites) and hepatic involvement (with granulomatous disease) are relatively common. With the first of these presentations, weight loss and diarrhoea are often accompanied by a low-grade febrile illness; in severe cases stools are large, pale and bulky. Examination reveals an ileocaecal mass in 35–50% of cases,[128] and occasionally enlargement of one or more lymph glands; however, there is often no clinical abnormality. Late presentation can be as adult kwashiorkor. Anaemia and hypoalbuminaemia are common.[128] Chest radiography is usually normal. Absorption tests are frequently abnormal; fat and B_{12} absorption are affected most severely. A protein-losing enteropathy may be present. Pathologically, the disease results either from miliary dissemination, or follows ileal ulceration. Malabsorption is caused by chronic bile salt loss; unabsorbed bile salts (normally reabsorbed in the terminal ileum) in turn interfere with colonic absorption. Barium meal and follow-through examination shows ileal strictures,[128] frequently multiple, in

a high percentage of cases; the ascending colon may also be shortened. The major differential diagnosis is Crohn's disease,[128] which is statistically much less common in people indigenous to the tropics. *Yersinia* spp. infection should be considered. Chest radiography is usually normal. The tuberculin test is positive in 70–90% of cases.[128] A needle liver biopsy specimen occasionally shows hepatic granulomas with caseation. Diagnostic laparotomy, or peritoneoscopy (and peritoneal biopsy), is sometimes necessary in order to obtain a tissue diagnosis, and he died with complications.[128] Treatment is with an antituberculosis regimen (see Chapter 57). Resection of stricture(s) and occasionally hemicolectomy are often necessary; chemotherapy should be initiated before surgical intervention.

A further cause of malabsorption in a tropical environment consists of the Mediterranean (α-chain) lymphoma,[29,129] which occurs sporadically in many parts of the tropics. If started early, tetracycline produces a good result.

OTHER SMALL-INTESTINAL INFECTIONS

VIRAL INFECTIONS

Significant intestinal protein loss (mean 1.7 g daily) and xylose malabsorption have been demonstrated in northern Nigerian children with measles (see Chapter 15); approximately 25% also had lactose malabsorption.[130] Other infections in children caused by enteroviruses and herpes simplex viruses are also associated with diarrhoea and weight loss; malnutrition may result;[131] the mechanism(s) (involving enterocyte damage) is probably similar to that in measles.

Volunteers infected with enteric viruses develop small-intestinal morphological lesions which are not always associated with symptoms.[132]

Jejunal mucosal changes giving rise to severe malabsorption have been well documented in viral hepatitis;[133] these may persist for a considerable time after resolution of the hepatic abnormalities. The Norwalk agent (a 27 nm picornavirus) can also produce mucosal damage and malabsorption.[134] Rotavirus infections give rise to morphological abnormalities and (especially in children) malabsorption.[135,136]

These viral infections are invasive, and the resulting diarrhoea and malabsorption are caused by enterocyte destruction. Malabsorption usually occurs after the virus has been shed into the intestinal lumen; the villi contain immature crypt-type enterocytes. In coronavirus infection(s) in piglets, which resemble human rotavirus infections, glucose absorption is significantly impaired.[137] This has practical importance in management because sodium and water secretion cannot be reversed by glucose; oral rehydration fluids, commonly used in small-intestinal (including travellers') diarrhoea (see above), contain a high glucose concentration which overwhelms the limited absorptive capacity.

Baker et al[138] have suggested that coronavirus infections are responsible for at least some cases of 'tropical sprue' in southern India (see above); this might be the case, but asymptomatic individuals often excrete these viruses and this does not therefore indicate a cause–effect relationship. Also at Vellore, a search for evidence of Berne virus infection in 'epidemic tropical sprue' proved negative.[139]

BACTERIAL INFECTIONS

Moderate to severe malabsorption is commonplace during acute intestinal infections of bacterial origin; subnormal absorptive capacity persists for variable periods after termination of the diarrhoea and apparent clinical recovery. In a study in Bangladesh, approximately 70% of patients had evidence of xylose malabsorption 1 week after the diarrhoea had ceased; this was less common after cholera than *Shigella* spp., *Salmonella* spp. and/or *Staphylococcal* spp. infections; xylose and B_{12} malabsorption persisted for up to 378 and 196 days, respectively, after the diarrhoea had cleared.[140]

Although many different infective insults to the enterocyte are probably important in PIM (see above), evidence for bacteria being responsible currently has more solid support than that involving other agents.

Escherichia coli

These organisms (with varying modes of pathogenicity) produce a spectrum of disease from TD to malabsorption by enterotoxin production and mucosal invasion—similar to that caused by *Shigella* spp. They are frequently food or water borne, and may cause outbreaks of gastroenteritis.[78] Heat-labile enterotoxins exert an effect by activating adenylcyclase by a mechanism(s) similar to *V. cholerae*. Both heat-labile and heat-stable enterotoxins are probably important in TD (see above). A large pool of resistant *E. coli* (often showing resistance to multiple antimicrobials) now exists in the community. Enterotoxin production by *E. coli* may

be transferred simultaneously with antibiotic resistance (see Chapter 43); in a study, 72 and 44% of ETEC isolated in South-East Asia were resistant to one or more, and four or more antibiotics, respectively.[141] Enterocyte adhesiveness of *E. coli* is also a property of some strains and that might be important in continuing colonization and subsequent malabsorption.[142,143] The relationship between adherence and verotoxin production remains unclear.[144] Attachment of micro-organisms to the enterocyte prevents clearance by peristaltic activity; such mucosal receptors may be determined genetically.[145] Ultrastructural studies have shown *E. coli* adherent to mucosal cells, with flattening of the microvilli, loss of the cellular terminal web and cupping of the plasma membrane around individual bacteria;[146] intracellular damage was marked in the most heavily colonized cells. Histological improvement was demonstrated following clearing of *E. coli* with neomycin and nutritional support. This mechanism can lead to protracted diarrhoea in infants. In most cases, resultant malabsorption is short lived.

Salmonellosis

Malabsorption occasionally follows infection with *Salmonella* spp. (see Chapter 42),[147,148] but the frequency is unknown.

Campylobacter jejuni

Although unusual, dysenteric disease (bloody diarrhoea) has for long been known to predispose to tropical PIM;[78] in addition to shigellosis it is clear that some cases are caused by *E. coli* (see above) and others by *Campylobacter jejuni* (see Chapter 41).

Although most cases of *Campylobacter jejuni* infection are acute, present with gastroenteritis and are self-limiting, initial symptoms can be prolonged.[149,150] The disease is a zoonosis; poultry are frequently contaminated. Many outbreaks have been traced to infected cow's milk. Dogs also constitute a reservoir of infection.[151] Although the infection is self-limiting, erythromycin probably hastens recovery when given early in a severe case. The carrier state is common.

Enteritis necroticans (pigbel disease)

Although described in Germany at the end of World War II (1939–1945), and named Darmbrand,[4,29] this

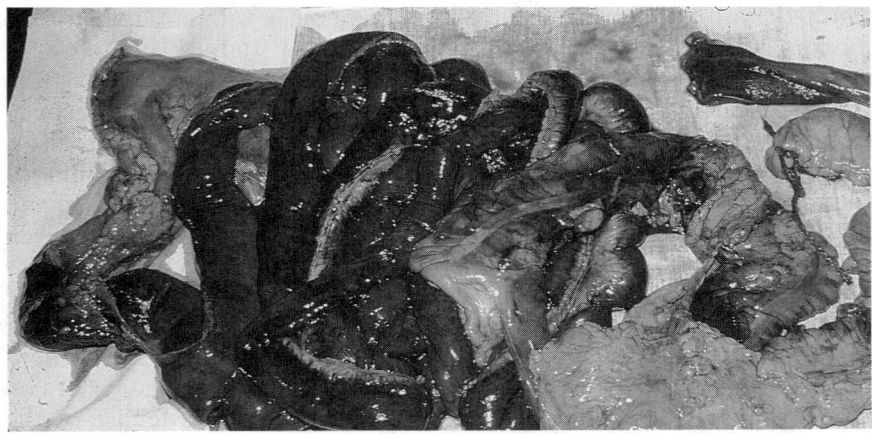

Figure 3.6 Gangrenous small intestine at post mortem in a Papua New Guinean child who had died from necrotizing enteritis (pigbel disease).

acute infection (Figure 3.6), which is more common in children than adults, occurs in several tropical countries, notably the highlands of Papua New Guinea (where it is endemic),[152] Thailand and Uganda.[1,78] Recently, enteritis necroticans has been recorded in Khmer children at an evacuation site on the Thai–Kampuchean border of Thailand; in the former report 36 (58%) out of 62 affected children (10 months–10 (mean 4) years) died.[4] It seems likely that a disease termed 'necrotizing jejunitis' in rural areas of Bihar, India—which also affects children—represents the same entity;[78] this condition ('segmental necrotizing enteritis') has also been recorded in Jaipur, India, and in Sri Lanka.[4] Scanty reports of a similar condition have also been made from northern Europe, which suggests that the disease exists worldwide, but only reaches epidemic proportions when suitable conditions exist, most importantly for the β-toxin of *Clostridium perfringens* type C (ingested in contaminated foodstuffs) to take its toll. Murrell[153] has suggested (in the light of historical evidence) that the disease was widespread in medieval Europe when 'human habitats, food hygiene, protein deficiency, and periodic meat feasting formed the basics of village life as they do in many Third World cultures today'. Enteritis necroticans is now known to be caused by the ingestion (often at pig feasts or 'mumus') of food contaminated by *Cl. perfringens* type C.[152] The pathophysiology of the disease is complex, but the presence of a low concentration of trypsin (resulting from trypsin inhibitors in foodstuffs and chronic protein–energy malnutrition) allows the β-toxin of *Cl. perfringens* to survive and produce mucosal injury.[29] It is sometimes associated with persisting structural changes in the small intestine; malabsorption may be a sequel.

Fluid and electrolyte replacement are essential (see below). Tetracycline or chloramphenicol, and type C gas gangrene antisera are of value; laparotomy is often indicated. In Papua New Guinea, immunization against *Cl. perfringens* type C has given good results;[29] in a controlled trial, marked reduction in incidence and mortality was demonstrated in the treatment group.

PARASITIC INFECTIONS

Giardiasis

The spectrum of disease caused by this flagellated protozoan is broad.[1,27,29,78] Symptoms vary from subclinical cases to those with severe malabsorption and malnutrition. The reason why some individuals are prone to symptomatic giardiasis is not clear; size of infecting dose, strain variability, genetic predisposition, acquired immunity factors, achlorhydria, a local secretory IgA deficiency, and the presence of blood group A phenotype have all been considered. An increase in IgE and IgD cell numbers has been reported in the jejunal mucosa of 20 affected patients;[154] the former reversed after treatment, when an increase in IgA cell numbers was also recorded. The actual mechanism by which the trophozoites cause an absorptive defect is also unclear. Mucosal injury, with or without invasion, bacterial overgrowth in association with parasitization, and bile salt deconjugation by bacteria and/or parasites have all been considered. The extent of jejunal morphological abnormality varies widely.[155]

Clinical presentation is usually between 1 and 3 weeks after infection; contaminated water and, less commonly, food are the usual sources of infection. Infection occurs both endemically and epidemically. The disease can probably be contracted from domestic animals.[156] It is more common in male homosexuals, but is not an opportunistic infection in AIDS sufferers. Diarrhoea of acute onset, flatus and weight loss may all be present; the stools have the characteristics of *malabsorption*. The disease is clinically indistinguishable from PIM in the absence of giardiasis; investigations also give similar results. In fact a full-blown case has all of the clinical and laboratory features of the classical (historical) reports of 'tropical sprue' (see above). Cysts may be found in a faecal specimen; trophozoites can be detected in either a jejunal biopsy or jejunal fluid, or with the string test (Enterotest). If mucosal changes and malabsorption exist, circulating antibodies to *G. lamblia* cysts can usually be detected.

Treatment is with metronidazole (2 g on 3 consecutive days); alcohol should be avoided during the treatment period. A single dose of tinidazole (2 g orally) has been used with success and there are claims that it is equally efficacious. Two 5-nitroimidazoles—ornidazole and tinidazole (as a single 1.5 g dose)—have been compared;[157] recurrence of infection during the subsequent 2 months was similar in each case (about 10%). Nimorazole has also been used. Alternatively, mepacrine (100 mg three times daily for 10 days), which is less often used, usually gives a satisfactory result.

Cryptosporidium parvum

This organism also produces a broad spectrum of disease—from a TD-like syndrome to severe PIM; however, the latter usually, but not always, occurs in the immunosuppressed (including AIDS) sufferer where the organism is opportunistic.[158] Diagnosis is similar to that for *G. lamblia* infection; oocysts are usually detectable in a faecal sample. Treatment (rarely indicated in the immunointact individual) is with spiramycin, but is usually ineffective in the immunosuppressed; although at least 70 other compounds have been tested, none, including spiramycin, has proven efficiency in vitro.[78]

Other parasites

The vast majority of small-intestinal parasitic infections do not result in signs/symptoms unless present at a very high concentration.[27] In a heavy infection, hookworm is responsible for hypochromic anaemia, and *A. lumbricoides* rarely accounts for obstruction in the small intestine and biliary and pancreatic ducts (see Chapter 71). The major clinical sequel of tapeworm infection is neurocysticercosis (*Taenia solium*) (see Chapter 76)—unrelated to the intestinal tract.

Although *A. lumbricoides*, *Ancylostoma duodenale* and *Necator americanus* have at various times been implicated in malabsorption,[159] there is no definite evidence except in rare or anecdotal case reports.[160] *Diphyllobothrium latum* infections are occasionally associated with a low serum B_{12} concentration; however, this is caused by B_{12} uptake within the small-intestinal lumen, and is not an example of true malabsorption.

Clear evidence exists that *Strongyloides stercoralis* is causally related to malabsorption.[1,29,78,79,126] This helminth can survive in the human host for several decades; some 10–20% of ex-prisoners of war in South-East Asia during World War II (1939–1945) remained infected until recently.[161] Onset of diarrhoea is less acute than with *G. lamblia*. Larvae can be demonstrated by the Enterotest, and less often by jejunal biopsy. Ova and larvae can occasionally be detected in faecal specimens. Eosinophilia may be gross; however, it is often absent. The immunofluorescent antibody test (IFAT) is positive in approximately 70% of cases; however, cross-reaction with filaria is common. The enzyme linked immunosorbent assay (ELISA) test, when available, is more specific. A negative serological result is common in the immunosuppressed patient. Treatment is with thiabendazole (1.5 g twice daily on 3 successive days); repeated courses may be required. Albendazole (400 mg daily for 3 days) is less effective. In animal experiments, cambendazole has given encouraging results; this has also been the case in limited clinical studies, but the compound has not been released for human use.[78] Other *Strongyloides* species are important, especially in children. *Strongyloides fülleborni* has been implicated in the pathogenesis of severe PIM (see above) in Zambia and Papua New Guinea, where a significant mortality rate has been recorded.[1,78]

In the northern Philippines and Thailand, *Capillaria philippinensis* has been causally associated with PIM.[1,79,159] It can occur in epidemics. Diarrhoea of acute onset is followed by malabsorption and, if untreated, infection carries a substantial mortality rate. Protein-losing enteropathy may also be present. Treatment with mebendazole, and latterly albendazole, has given good results.

The protozoa *I. belli*[1,27,79,159] and *Sarcocystis hominis* (usually conveyed by undercooked pork and beef)[161] also cause malabsorption. These organisms replicate within the enterocyte. *I. belli*, like *Cryptosporidium parvum*, causes a spectrum of disease, from TD to PIM, and is more common in the immunosuppressed individual. Pyrimethamine + sulphadiazine, and co-trimoxazole + nitrofurantoin, have been used with some success. Other protozoan parasites, such as *P. falciparum* (in an acute infection) and visceral leishmaniasis (kala-azar) can also produce significant malabsorption.

SMALL-INTESTINAL DISEASE: EMERGENCIES

Severe dehydration consequent upon secretory watery diarrhoea accounts for enormous amounts of acute morbidity and mortality throughout the tropics; this applies especially to infants and children. Intravenous replacement therapy has been in use for more than 150 years; Dr Robert Lewins MD FRCP, of Leith, recorded that he had witnessed Dr Thomas Latta inject saline intravenously to a patient suffering from cholera (see above) in 1832;[162] it is unlikely, however, that this was the first attempt at intravenous rehydration.[163] (In fact, Sir Christopher Wren, better known for his architectural achievements, had introduced the technique experimentally in 1657.) Nearly three-quarters of a century passed before Sir Leonard Rogers, working at Calcutta, demonstrated a reduction in the mortality rate in cholera patients from 70 to 20% by use of this technique.[163] Introduction of *oral* rehydration regimens had to wait much longer, in fact until the latter half of the twentieth century. Introduction of this form of management, which followed upon important basic applied physiological observations, was, in a world context, one of the most important medical advances during the present century.[1] In many acute medical conditions, gastric emptying is delayed; however, this is not the case in cholera (and presumably other acute small-intestinal infections) and does not constitute a barrier to oral rehydration, even when fluid and electrolyte loss (in the stool) is severe.[164] But oral rehydration therapy remains grossly underused,[165] and infants and children in developing countries with acute gastroenteritis continue to die unnecessarily because this simple technique is not readily applied. Those authors have concluded: 'the impediment to its wide acceptance may be that it is counterintuitive for a simpler and much less expensive treatment to be an improvement over an effective but more complicated technology'! Even the moribund can sometimes be saved.

ENTERITIS NECROTICANS (PIGBEL DISEASE)

This acute small-intestinal emergency (see above), which usually affects infants and children,[166] is characterized by gangrenous changes in the small-intestinal wall (in patchy distribution); the jejunum is most markedly affected, but the ileum is also involved. Presentation is as an acute abdominal (surgical) emergency, with abdominal pain, fever, and bloody diarrhoea (see above). A chronic stage

of the disease may ensue in which there is narrowing of the small-intestinal lumen (in one or more places) by a fibrotic stenosis or adhesion; clinical presentation is with subacute obstruction, often accompanied by malabsorption and malnutrition. Fluid and electrolyte replacement are vitally important in management; gastric suction is also required. Penicillin or another antibiotic should be given (see above). Laparotomy is frequently indicated to confirm the diagnosis and to resect the necrosed, haemorrhagic segment(s) of small intestine. Fortunately, active immunization against the β-toxin has proved effective prophylaxis in Papua New Guinea; hospital admissions for pigbel in one area of the country fell to less then one-fifth of the previous figure ($P < 0.001$) when a vaccination programme was introduced.[167] Hopefully, therefore, morbidity due to this acute abdominal emergency (with a very high mortality rate) will eventually fall in all of the seriously affected countries.

PARALYTIC ILEUS AND ACUTE OBSTRUCTION

In Pakistan, paralytic ileus has recently been recorded as a late complication of acute diarrhoeal disease in infants;[168] despite decompression and total parenteral nutrition, the mortality rate was 25%. When compared with others who did *not* develop ileus (following acute diarrhoeal disease), these infants were shown to have had significantly more antimotility agents preceding the ileus; furthermore, more had a depressed serum potassium concentration. The potential dangers associated with antiperistaltic agents, especially in infancy and childhood, are thus re-emphasized.

Acute intestinal obstruction constitutes a common surgical emergency in both children and adults in many parts of the tropics, including Africa. Strangulated hernia (usually of inguinal origin) is usually the most common cause; volvulus and intussusception are relatively common in tropical Africa; tuberculosis is a further cause—due either to stenosis or to pressure on the third part of the duodenum or jejunum. A heavy *A. lumbricoides* infection (especially in children) can also produce small-intestinal obstruction;[1,169] when diagnosed clinically, laparotomy can usually be avoided. Management consists of intravenous hydration, nasogastric suction and appropriate anthelmintic chemotherapy. Strangulated hernia, volvulus and intussusception nearly always require laparotomy.[1,169] In a recent report from southern India, 904 children presented with intestinal obstruction;[170] the most common causes in order of frequency were: necrotizing enteritis (see above), acute intussusception, band obstruction, subacute obstruction, and remnants of the vitello-intestinal duct. Rare causes of small-intestinal obstruction include: Burkitt's lymphoma, Mediterranean lymphoma (α-chain disease) (see above) and intestinal schistosomiasis. Small-intestinal trauma—caused by a road accident or knife, arrow or gunshot wound—is also important in a tropical context.

TYPHOID (ENTERIC) FEVER (see also Chapters 42 and 43)

In most areas within the developing world, typhoid (and to a lesser extent tuberculosis) accounts for much small-intestinal disease encountered in surgical practice;[171] perforation, obstruction and less often haemorrhage constitute acute surgical emergencies. This seems especially important in West Africa. *S. typhi* infection is also an increasing problem in travellers from industrialized countries to the tropics; in the USA, 2666 cases (fatality rate 1–3%) of acute enteric fever were officially notified between 1975 and 1984; 62% of them were imported, the majority of infections having originated in either Mexico or India.[172] Statistically, surgical complications are unusual and misleading emphasis emerges from several standard texts; thus in a series of 82 culture-positive cases in The Gambia there were no surgical complications;[173] this also applied in a series of 192 cases of enteric fever—most caused by *S. typhi*—in Thailand.[174]

Management of enteric fever has been reviewed.[175] Despite its relative rarity (perhaps 2–4% of cases worldwide), typhoid perforation (when it occurs) is an extremely serious event, accounting for 20–60% of deaths in this disease (a figure which is increased by late presentation, female sex, age over 40 years and the presence of multiple perforations). Late perforation is often indistinguishable from a perforated appendix, amoebic liver abscess, tuberculous peritonitis, an infected ruptured ectopic pregnancy or intestinal strangulation. The best form of management seems to be surgical, provided the patient is not too shocked to endure such a procedure (a prolonged period of preoperative resuscitation is often required). There is as yet no general agreement, however, regarding the ideal type of operative intervention;[176] simple closure, ulcer excision and closure, wedge excision and closure, ileal resection and anastomosis, resection and transverse ileotransverse colostomy, and right hemicolectomy have all found favour. When the perforation is single, simple closure (with or without excision) is the procedure of choice; an area(s) of impending perforation should never be oversewn. Closure should always be in two layers: an inner one of chromic catgut and an outer of silk. When there are three or more perforations, bowel resection is probably advisable. Peritoneal lavage with a copious amount of washing with normal saline should always be carried out. The incidence of postoperative complications is high and includes peripheral vascular failure, respiratory infections, anaemia, sepsis, abscess formation, burst abdomen and intestinal obstruction.[175,176] Reperforation or new perforation is possible. In a series of 108 consecutive cases of perforated typhoid enteritis managed in western Nigeria, 100 (93%) underwent 'debridement of the perforation and two-layer bowel closure';[177] 35 patients died, usually from overwhelming sepsis. In addition to specific chemotherapy—although chloramphenicol (1 g four times daily in an average adult, reduced to 1 g twice daily when body temperature is normal) remains the agent of choice, increasing numbers of reports of multiple-antibiotic-resistant strains of *S. typhi* are being reported (especially from India)—metronidazole, and possibly corticosteroids, seem to improve the prognosis.[175] Alternative chemotherapeutic agents include amoxycillin, co-trimoxazole, trimethoprim and ciprofloxacin; the last agent is indicated when there are serious doubts about sensitivity to the other compounds, as is frequently the case when infection has resulted in Asia.

Haemorrhage is rarely life threatening, although recorded;[175,178] whereas the majority of cases can be treated conservatively (using blood transfusion), when selective angiography, fibreoptic endoscopy and high resolution radionuclide imaging are available, localization of the bleeding site can be delineated and appropriate surgery instituted.

EMERGENCIES ASSOCIATED WITH HELMINTHIASES

Where abdominal discomfort (and pain) are common sequelae to heavy small-intestinal nematode infections (see above), especially ancylostomiasis and *A. lumbricoides* (see above), serious acute complications (see above)[179] are fortunately rare. However, they do exist. Anisakiasis for example, which is usually acquired from ingestion of undercooked or raw infected fish (sushi and sashimi), can present with an acute appendicitis-like illness.[180,181] Invasive disease caused by this organism is usually localized to the ileocaecal region; there is no satisfactory parasitological or serological test, and chemotherapy is not effective. A diagnostic laparotomy is often necessary.

Eosinophilic enteritis is a disease entity of multiple aetiology.[182] However, a recent report from Townsville, Australia, suggested that *Ancylostoma caninum* (the dog hookworm) was responsible for an epidemic (93 cases) encountered there;[183] nine were subjected to diagnostic laparotomy: eosinophilic infiltration involving a segment of ileum with indurated thickening of the distal small intestine and proximal dilatation was the usual underlying pathology. A rare case of acute mesenteric ischaemia (accompanied by segmental small-intestinal infarction and gangrene) caused by *Schist. mansoni* has been reported from Baghdad, Iraq.[184] The small intestine can also be involved in *Schist. japonicum* infection; intestinal obstruction resulting from

mesenteric ischaemia, an intussuscepting polypoid mass or fibrotic stenosis are possible sequelae. Intestinal perforation resulting from infection with the acanthocephalan worm *Macracanthorhynchus hirudinaceus*, a natural intestinal parasite of the pig, has been described at Bangkok, Thailand[185] (eight other cases are on record); this infection has also been reported from several other parts of the world, including China and southern Europe. Fatal gastrointestinal haemorrhage (associated with fluctuating jaundice, a tender liver, palpable gallbladder and an eosinophilia) has been attributed to *F. hepatica* (liver fluke) infection at Harare, Zimbabwe;[186] the site of bleeding was probably the biliary tree.

COLORECTUM

The vast majority of cases of colorectal disease occurring in a tropical environment have an infective basis (Table 3.4); they are dominated by bacterial (*Shigella* spp. (see Chapter 41) (Figure 3.7),[1,187,188] *Campylobacter jejuni* and invasive *E. coli*) and protozoan (*Ent. histolytica* (see Chapter 67)[1,189,190] and *Balantidium coli*) infections. Amoebic colitis and shigellosis present classically with

bloody diarrhoea; this should be differentiated from carcinoma, necrotizing colitis, antibiotic-associated colitis and inflammatory bowel disease (which is overall not very common in tropical countries). Whether or not amoebic colitis can proceed to inflammatory bowel disease is debatable; however, misdiagnosis of amoebic colitis as inflammatory bowel disease (with subsequent corticosteroid therapy) can result in fatality. In AIDS, cytomegalovirus colitis is common; although *Cryptosporidium* is usually a small-intestinal parasite, colonic involvement can also occur. In addition, megacolon resulting from South American trypanosomiasis (Chagas' disease) (see Chapter 64) also gives rise to colonic pathology. Of diseases localized to the anal region, lymphogranuloma is perhaps the most important, although bacterial (including donovanosis, syphilis and gonorrhoea (see Chapter 13) and parasitic (including *Ent. histolytica*, *Schistosoma* spp. and *Enterobius vermicularis*) infections enter the list of differential diagnoses.

The colorectum is the organ for which there are, *par excellence*, major differences in disease prevalence between developing and westernized populations. Overall these diseases are far less common in indigenous people in developing countries compared with individuals in industrialized ones;[1,191,192] colonic carcinoma seems, for example, to be an unusual lesion in rural communities. Moderately good evidence now exists that frequency of these diseases is increasing as urbanization advances—in Africa especially. Hypotheses to account for these differences include the greater dietary fibre consumption in most tropical countries; however, such associations rarely have a proven cause–effect relationship.

Table 3.4   Colorectal diarrhoea.*

Bacterial infection
   Shigellosis
   Campylobacter jejuni
   Escherichia coli (enteroinvasive)

Protozoan infection
   Entamoeba histolytica
   Balantidium coli

Schistosomiasis (usually *Schistosoma mansoni* and *Schist. japonicum*)

Unusual causes
   Non-specific ulcerative colitis—inflammatory bowel disease†
   Crohn's disease†
   Appendicitis
   Diverticulitis
   Haemorrhoids
   Colonic carcinoma
   Irritable bowel syndrome

---

*Characteristically, numerous small stools containing mucus, pus and blood; microscopy shows pus cells and/or red blood cells in a faecal smear.
†Although these diseases are uncommon, or even rare, in most tropical populations, they can become clinically overt for the first time in visitors from Western countries to the tropics.

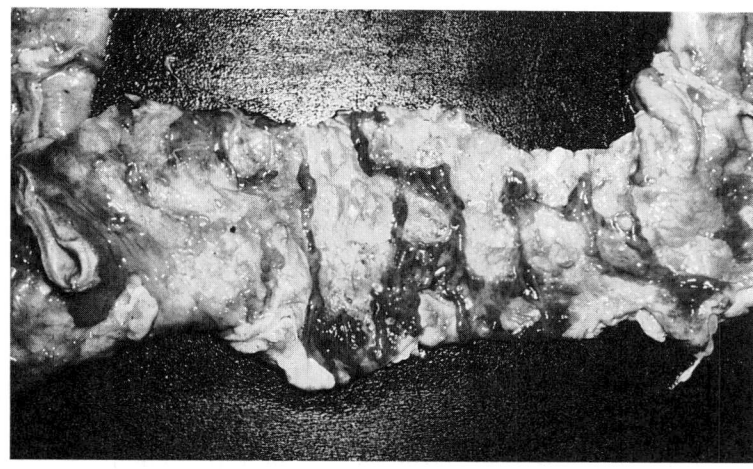

Figure 3.7 Severe amoebic colitis: operative specimen obtained from an Australian nurse misdiagnosed as having non-specific ulcerative colitis (inflammatory bowel disease) while working in Papua New Guinea.

Many data have been collected on colonic function in indigenous inhabitants of developing countries;[1] it seems likely that 24-hour faecal weight and volume is higher in Africa, and constipation unusual. Overall, intestinal transit rate also seems more rapid. Limited evidence indicates that colorectal histology is mildly different in indigenous people in developing countries, and is comparable to *tropical enteropathy* (see above). In PIM in India (see above) in vivo colonic functional abnormalities have been demonstrated. Whether colonic pathology is important in a nutritional context remains difficult to evaluate (see above); evidence now exists that this organ is important in the absorption of nitrogen and free (volatile) fatty acids.

Inflammatory bowel disease[193–195] (non-specific ulcerative colitis and Crohn's disease) is far less common overall in indigenous people in developing countries compared with the UK and other Western countries. The aetiology of these diseases is unknown,[194] although an infective basis has frequently been suggested; good evidence for a viral or bacterial (possibly mycobacterial) origin is at present lacking. Very few reports of ulcerative colitis have been made from African countries, with a few more from Asia;[193,195] in individuals in the UK from the Caribbean and Indian subcontinent the disease clearly exists. Such differences apply to Crohn's disease, probably to an even greater extent, although this disease is also well recognized in Caribbean people in the UK. Although Crohn's disease behaves very much like intestinal tuberculosis in clinical practice, response to antituberculous therapy is extremely disappointing. When inflammatory bowel disease occurs, it seems to behave similarly to that in the indigenous population of the UK. It is a common cause of bloody diarrhoea in travellers who have returned to temperate from tropical countries

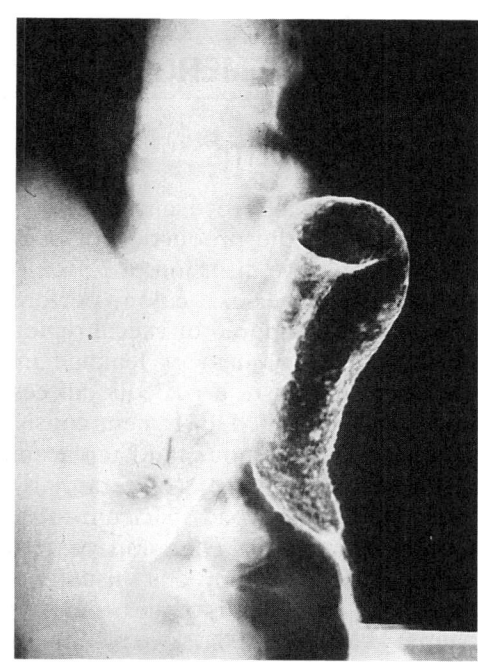

Figure 3.8 Barium enema in a 35-year-old woman who experienced bloody diarrhoea during a visit to Africa; she had not previously had significant gastrointestinal problems. Colonic biopsy specimen obtained at colonoscopy confirmed the diagnosis.

(Figure 3.8).[38,196] Similarly, appendicitis, diverticular disease and haemorrhoids are overall less common in a developing country population, and here also a high-fibre intake has been implicated; a causative association has not, however, been proved. Reasonable evidence exists that these diseases are all increasing with urbanization.

Although irritable bowel syndrome (spastic colon)[198,199] is extremely common in UK residents (and others) following an intestinal infection acquired in a tropical country, it seems to be far less significant in indigenous peoples in Africa and Asia. Whether this constitutes a genuine difference is unclear because so many of the latter have more severe symptoms of different origin(s) and these might mask symptoms resulting from irritable bowel syndrome. This syndrome does not constitute a single entity; although some cases respond to mebeverine or peppermint oil, many do not.

Enterobius vermicularis infection (see Chapter 71) is arguably the most common gastrointestinal infection in the world, overall;[200] it exists in both tropical and temperate areas.

Colonoscopy is an endoscopic technique which is now available in some, but by no means all, developing countries; frequently, it is available only at the teaching hospital and/or other (tertiary referral) centre(s) of relative excellence.

COLONIC DISEASE: EMERGENCIES

INVASIVE AMOEBIC COLITIS

Perforation—although a rare event—can complicate this disease, with the production of amoebic peritonitis;[1] there may be diffusion of *Ent. histolytica* from a blotting-paper-like colon, perforation (especially in the rectosigmoid or caecal regions or to the retroperitoneal tissues) or leakage into a confined space (resulting in a pericolic abscess or internal intestinal fistula). Management consists of gastric suction and intravenous fluid replacement; metronidazole, 500 mg 8-hourly (preferably by the intravenous route), and a broad-spectrum antibiotic should be given immediately. The colon is extremely fragile, therefore laparotomy is usually best avoided;[201] overall, mortality is of the order of 50%, and after surgery close on 100%. Two recent reports have recorded results of surgical intervention in 15 patients with fulminant amoebic colitis.[202,203] In the first, five out of six patients (four had a subtotal colectomy with ileostomy, and two a right hemicolectomy and ileostomy) subsequently died (none was diagnosed either preoperatively or during surgery);[202] in the second, three out of nine died, all of whom had exteriorization of the cut ends of the bowel following resection of the necrotic segment (four of those who died had end-to-end anastomoses, and two peritoneal drainage).[203]

SHIGELLOSIS

Perforation is less common in shigellosis compared with amoebic colitis, but haemorrhage is well docu-mented. The most recent pandemic of this disease in the western hemisphere began in Guatemala in 1969 and spread rapidly to Nicaragua, Belize, Honduras, Costa Rica, Panama and Mexico; it ended in 1973, but by then an estimated 500 000 had been affected, of whom 20 000 died.[204]

APPENDICITIS

Acute appendicitis remains a major problem in tropical countries. In Calabar, Nigeria, 603 consecutive cases were investigated prospectively during a 5-year period;[205] there were no major differences from this disease in industrialized countries, and it constituted the second most common abdominal emergency during the study period, being less common than acute intestinal obstruction. Many causative agents are involved; in a retrospective review of 2921 appendicectomies carried out at Allahabad, India, during a 25-year period,[206] 153 produced histological evidence of a specific infection: tuberculosis (70), *Ent. histolytica* (17), *A. lumbricoides* (13), *A. lumbricoides* and *Trichuris trichiura* (2), *Enterobius vermicularis* (41), and *Taenia* spp. (2). This acute disease should be differentiated from pelvic inflammatory disease, typhoid enteritis, ruptured ectopic pregnancy, psoas abscess, acute amoebic colitis, and *Schist. mansoni* colitis. Although the vast majority of cases of appendicitis in developing countries result from a bacterial cause, helminths, including *Schist. mansoni, Strongyloides stercoralis* and *Trichuris trichiura*, have also been implicated in occasional cases.[1]

VOLVULUS OF THE COLON

This is a disease with clear geographical differences; it is common in much of Central and East Africa, India and southern America;[1] many reports have been made from Uganda and Zimbabwe. Although genetic factors have been suggested for these high prevalence rates, a high-fibre diet, common in most of Africa, has also been implicated. The major complication is strangulation with gangrene of a colonic segment; this should be differentiated from primary volvulus of the small intestine, compound volvulus (usually ileosigmoid) and internal herniae. Distention can be relieved with a flatus tube; at laparotomy the precise operation, and extent of resection, depends on the length of gangrenous colon. With simple volvulus, mortality rate should be low. Zimmerman et al[207] have emphasized the value of emergency colonoscopy in the diagnosis of colonic volvulus; when the mucosa is ischaemic or necrotic, emergency laparotomy is indicated, but when appearances are normal, relief of flatus (with a flatus tube passed per rectum) together with medical management and elective surgery (resection and anastomosis), 10 days later, is recommended.

COLONIC INTUSSUSCEPTION

The common variety, especially in west Africa, is the caecocolic one; although children may be afflicted, the vast majority are in adults. Aetiology—as with that of volvulus—is conjectural; while an intestinal polyp or amoeboma accounts for some, there is no obvious clue in most cases. Gangrene is about three times more common with the ileoileal and ileocaecal varieties compared with the caecocolic type.

ACUTE COLONIC DILATATION

Several gastrointestinal infections can cause toxic megacolon. These include: *Salmonella* spp., *Campylobacter* spp., and *Y. enterocolitica* infection; recently, however, there has been a growing recognition of *Shigella* spp. in this potentially lethal condition.[208] Correct diagnosis is essential; an unnecessary laparotomy can thus usually be avoided. If the condition is misdiagnosed as ulcerative colitis, and corticosteroids administered, potentially fatal consequences can ensue. Diagnostically, the causative organism can usually be identified in a faecal sample; however, this is not always the case. Choice of an appropriate antibiotic is often difficult; in *Shigella* spp. infection, a fluoroquinolone, e.g. ciprofloxacin (200 mg intravenously 12-hourly for 10 days) seems most appropriate, and is usually indicated. Toxic dilatation of the colon has also been reported, albeit rarely, in *Ent. histolytica* infection;[209] these authors recorded a single case (in which total colectomy, and administration of metronidazole and emetine, was followed by recovery) and were able to find seven cases in the world literature.

OTHER COLORECTAL LESIONS

Anorectal infections in relation to tropical exposure have been reviewed.[210] Trauma to the colon, often resulting from road accidents, constitutes a medical emergency in most tropical countries.[1] Necrotizing colitis (the pathology is similar to that of enteritis necroticans, see above) is rarely encountered. Colonic obstruction is rarely caused by carcinoma (a rare tumour in the rural tropics) but is recorded following introduction of a foreign body per rectum.[1]

LIVER AND BILIARY SYSTEM

Liver histology in an individual indigenous to a tropical country differs from that in one who has spent his or her life in a temperate region of the world.[1] This organ is subjected to numerous systemic infections—viral, bacterial and parasitic—and it lies at the distal end of the portal circulation; it is therefore bathed with portal blood containing viruses, bacteria, parasites, ova, products of digestion and other antigens. Thus, Kupffer cell hyperplasia and periportal infiltration (with lymphocytes, plasma cells and eosinophils) are more common, and stellate fibrosis occurs more frequently. Also, hepatocyte nuclear pleomorphism and sinusoidal lymphocytosis are frequently prominent; these appearances are unusual in biopsies obtained in a temperate country. Malaria and schistosomal pigment are often also present. Granulomas are common (Figure 3.9) and a large number of differential diagnoses exist; Table 3.5 lists some of them.

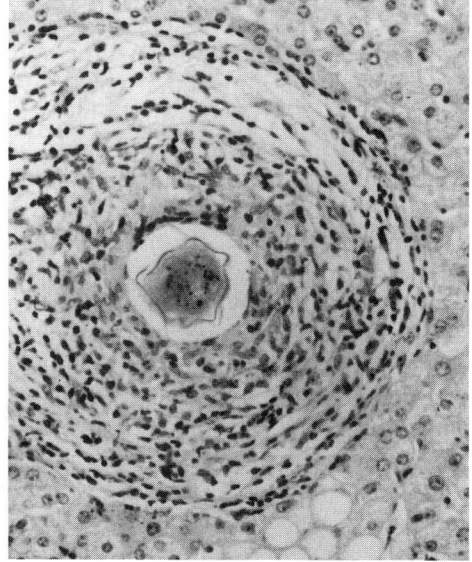

Figure 3.9 Liver biopsy specimen from a 30-year-old Zambian woman. A degenerating *Schistosoma mansoni* egg is surrounded by a well-formed granuloma.

Table 3.5 Some causes of hepatic granulomas in tropical countries.

Infection	
Viral	cytomegalovirus, Epstein–Barr virus
Bacterial	tuberculosis and atypical mycobacteria, leprosy, syphilis, Q fever, brucellosis
Parasitic	schistosomiasis, ascariasis, strongyloidiasis, toxocariasis, filariasis, enterobiasis, visceral leishmaniasis
Fungi	histoplasmosis, coccidioidomycosis, aspergillosis, actinomycosis, candidiasis
Neoplasms	lymphomas—especially intra-abdominal Hodgkin's disease
Others	(sarcoidosis) therapeutic agents—especially sulphonamides

ACUTE LIVER INFECTIONS

Jaundice in a tropical context (Table 3.6) is most commonly a result of viral hepatitis (types A, B (sometimes in a combined infection with D), C, E and F) (see Chapter 31), but other causes should also be considered;[211] Table 3.6 summarizes some of them. An important cause is the jaundice of *acute systemic bacterial infection*—most commonly caused by pneumococcal lobar pneumonia or pyomyositis.[1] The mechanism of this form of jaundice is complex and consists of hepatocellular, cholestatic and haemolytic elements; the importance of the latter depends to some extent on the underlying prevalence of glucose-6-phosphate dehydrogenase (G6PD) deficiency in the population under consideration (see Chapter 6). It is important to differentiate this form of jaundice from viral hepatitis, otherwise the appropriate antibiotic will not be administered for an underlying bacterial infection. In addition to yellow fever, several other viruses are implicated;[212] dengue fever, Kyasanur Forest disease, herpes simplex and Coxsackie virus should also be considered.

In AIDS, the liver is affected by many opportunistic organisms; these include viruses, and hepatitis B (HBV) and C (HCV) infections can be especially virulent. A liver biopsy specimen may also yield evidence of cytomegalovirus, *M. tuberculosis, M. avium intracellulare,* atypical mycobacteria, *Cryptosporidium parvum*, *Pneumocystis carinii, Crypto-*

coccus spp. and Kaposi's sarcoma. Cholestatic features are common.

In addition to septicaemia, several bacterial infections can produce jaundice;[1,213] leptospirosis is usually accompanied by renal involvement, whilst overt jaundice in typhoid fever is unusual. Melioidosis, plague, tularaemia and relapsing fever can also produce hepatitis. Of parasitic causes,[214,215] acute *P. falciparum* infection is perhaps the most important. In acute (Katayama syndrome) and *severe* chronic schistosomiasis jaundice may be present, but rarely in invasive hepatic amoebiasis. Most parasitic infections, including African trypanosomiasis (see Chapter 63) and visceral leishmaniasis (see Chapter 65), can produce significant hepatitis and deranged hepatocellular function—often in the absence of *clinical* jaundice.

Several parasites produce large duct biliary obstruction; for practical purposes, *A. lumbricoides* is probably the most important to recognize and treat.[4]

Sickle cell disease and haemoglobinopathies (see Chapter 6) are important causes of haemolytic jaundice; they possess a genetic basis. Jaundice in the presence of G6PD deficiency is frequently precipitated (or worsened) by therapeutic agents and/or toxins. In some parts of the tropics, especially Indonesia and Papua New Guinea, the Dubin–Johnson syndrome seems unusually common.

CHRONIC LIVER DISEASE

Most cases of *chronic active hepatitis* in tropical countries result from HBV and HCV infections;[216] corticosteroids should *not* be administered for they exacerbate hepatocyte viral replication; interferon-γ and adenine arabinoside have given encouraging results, but ethnic factors are probably important. There is no reliable evidence that either malnutrition (including kwashiorkor) or *Plasmodium* spp. infection are aetiologically important, although such beliefs linger.[1]

In tropical countries most cases of macronodular cirrhosis result from viral hepatitis—most commonly HBV, and to a lesser extent HCV hepatitis.[216] The sequence of events is: acute hepatitis → chronic active hepatitis → macronodular cirrhosis → and, ultimately, hepatocellular carcinoma[217] (hepatoma) (acute viral hepatitis is covered in Chapter 31 and hepatoma in Chapter 24). HBV and HCV are undoubtedly the most important aetiological factors in hepatoma, but the role of aflatoxin[1] should not be totally disregarded.

Table 3.6 Some causes of jaundice in the tropics.

Jaundice of acute bacterial infection: pneumococcal lobar pneumonia, pyomyositis

Viruses:	hepatitis (A–F) yellow fever Epstein–Barr virus cytomegalovirus Marburg and Ebola diseases Lassa fever
Bacteria:	leptospirosis typhoid fever syphilis gonococcal disease bartonellosis
Parasites:	malaria (acute *Plasmodium falciparum* and *P. vivax*) schistosomiasis amoebiasis (rarely) toxoplasmosis trichinellosis fascioliasis ⎫ clonorchiasis ⎬ predominantly large-duct obstructive jaundice opisthorchiasis ascariasis ⎭ hydatidosis (rarely)
Genetic:	sickle cell disease glucose-6-phosphate dehydrogenase deficiency Dubin-Johnson syndrome

---

Clinically, cutaneous stigmata of chronic hepatocellular disease are difficult to detect in brown or black skins;[1] similarly, other cutaneous stigmata of chronic liver disease may be absent. Diagnosis is often first suspected by abnormal liver function tests; a needle liver biopsy specimen is usually diagnostic. Peritoneoscopy is relatively simple and underused in developing countries; refined diagnostic techniques are rarely available. No treatment is of any avail in established cirrhosis. Major complications (see below) resulting from portal hypertension are: (1) haemorrhage, from oesophageal varices (see below); (2) fluid retention, including ascites; and (3) hepatic encephalopathy. Fluid retention is a major long-term problem, largely the result of a very low serum albumin concentration. This complication is often difficult to manage, largely because salt restriction is virtually impossible to impose; diuretics, e.g. frusemide (Lasix) (40–120 mg daily) and spironolactone (Aldactone) (100 mg daily), usually achieve success. Paracentesis abdominis should rarely be undertaken; this procedure depletes albumin stores further and electrolyte balance can be seriously disturbed; tapping ascitic fluid should be reserved for: (1) diagnostic purposes—to determine whether a bacterial infection, tuberculous peritonitis or hepatocellular carcinoma is present concurrently; and (2) management of *tense* ascites, accompanied by respiratory embarrassment. Hepatic encephalopathy is managed by accepted methods: oral neomycin (6 g daily) and/or lactulose (20–35 g three times daily); in the presence of hypolactasia lactose can be substituted for lactulose.

Other forms of chronic liver disease (with subsequent decompensation) (see below) include those resulting from excessive alcohol ingestion, Indian childhood cirrhosis, haemosiderosis and venoocclusive disease. Wilson's disease (hepatolenticular degeneration) and other genetically determined forms of cirrhosis are of limited importance numerically in the tropics, although they too should enter the list of differential diagnoses.

ALCOHOLIC LIVER DISEASE

Alcohol-related disease (including cirrhosis) is common in both indigenous and expatriate populations in tropical countries.[1,218] Genetic factors are undoubtedly involved; HBsAg carriers are especially vulnerable. The liver in chronic alcoholic disease is classically micronodular, but not always so; liver biopsy histology sometimes shows characteristic Mallory's hyaline deposits, and haemosiderin may be present in excess. There are no major differences from the disease in temperate climates. The quantity of daily alcohol required to produce this disease is not known with accuracy, and estimates differ widely; a wide individual variation exists, and women seem to tolerate chronic alcohol ingestion less well than men. Acute alcoholic hepatitis is underdiagnosed and possesses a high mortality rate; the role of corticosteroids continues to be disputed;[1,218] any beneficial effect is at best marginal and administration should probably be confined to severe and advanced cases.

INDIAN CHILDHOOD CIRRHOSIS

Indian childhood cirrhosis[219] is largely confined to India (especially south India, Calcutta and the Punjab) and surrounding countries; it is frequently familial. Diagnosis is usually made between 1.5 and 3 years of age; members of the upper strata of Hindu society are often affected. The disease may pursue fulminant, acute or subacute courses, and carries a high mortality rate. The clinical course therefore varies widely and is comparable to viral hepatitis (see above), with acute fulminant viral hepatitis at one extreme of the spectrum and cirrhosis (with one or all of its classic complications) (Figure 3.10) at the other. Histologically there is usually progressive fibrosis, with absence of regeneration; macronodular and micronodular cirrhosis result. Hepatocellular carcinoma is an uncommon complication. The disease is associated with a high copper intake; epidemiological evidence suggests that early weaning followed by milk-feeding from copper vessels imparts an excessive copper intake.[220] However, the possibility of an inherited defect resulting in excess copper absorption and/or metabolism has not been eliminated. There is no adequate treatment; in prevention, non-human milk for infant and childhood consumption should *not* be stored in copper-containing vessels.

HAEMOSIDEROSIS

Haemosiderosis (African or Bantu siderosis) is a disease of southern, and to a lesser extent other (tropical) parts of East and West Africa.[221] Whether it can proceed to clear-cut cirrhosis is arguable; heavy alcohol intake is commonplace in many geographical areas where the disease is common; it is

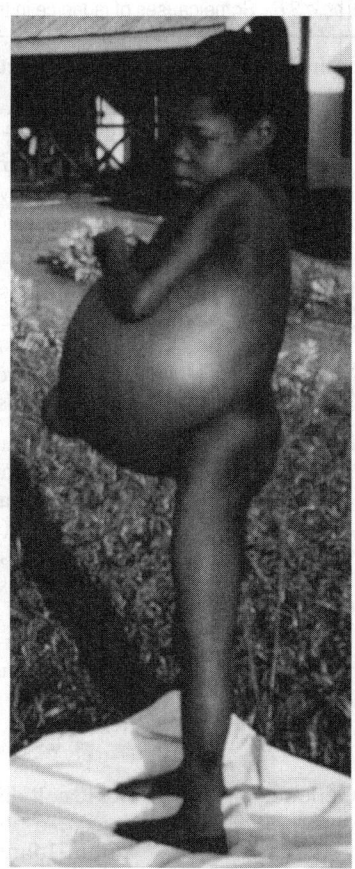

Figure 3.10   Indian child suffering from decompensated chronic liver disease—Indian childhood cirrhosis.

frequently impossible to exclude this as an aetiological factor (as with haemochromatosis). Iron-containing pots for cooking are commonly used in most areas, such as Zimbabwe, where haemosiderosis is common, but other factors also seem relevant.[222] Also, chronic pancreatitis is relatively common in these areas; evidence exists that an excess of hepatocyte iron (and fat) is common.

VENO-OCCLUSIVE DISEASE

Although first described in Jamaica, distribution of veno-occlusive disease is now known to be much wider.[223] Bush-teas, which contain pyrrolizidine alkaloids (*Heliotropium, Crotalaria* and *Senecio*) are important aetiologically. Veno-occlusive disease occurs in many localized areas of the tropics.

OTHER CHRONIC LIVER DISEASES

The liver is involved in most chronic infective diseases: tuberculosis, leprosy, syphilis, actinomycosis, visceral leishmaniasis and African histoplasmosis

Table 3.7   Causes of portal hypertension and oesophageal (and gastric) varices, showing those which are more common in developing countries.

Level of obstruction	Cause
Prehepatic	Hyperreactive malarious splenomegaly (HMS) (increased portal blood flow)* Portal vein occlusion* Splenic vein occlusion
Hepatic	Macronodular cirrhosis* Hepatosplenic schistosomiasis* Veno-occlusive disease* Congenital hepatic fibrosis
Posthepatic	Cardiac failure (secondary to chronic rheumatic disease)* Endomyocardial fibrosis* Constructive pericarditis* Inferior vena caval obstruction Hepatic vein thrombosis (Budd–Chiari syndrome)

*More common in a developing tropical country.

are examples. It is however, unusual for decompensation (and liver failure) to result. Major space occupying lesions involving the liver are: amoebic abscess (see below), pyogenic abscess and hydatid disease; tuberculomas, cysticercosis and melioidosis are of lesser importance. Of non-infective diseases, sickle cell disease, β-thalassaemia, haemoglobin-H disease, porphyria and α_1-antitrypsin deficiency produce significant hepatic pathology.

PORTAL HYPERTENSION

Portal hypertension[1,224] is a sequel to any form of chronic liver disease; Table 3.7 summarizes some causes in a tropical country. Cirrhosis and schistosomal liver disease ('pipe-stem' fibrosis) are numerically very important; however, in the latter entity hepatocellular function is preserved to a greater extent, and for longer in the course of disease than in cirrhosis; therefore, fluid retention and more importantly encephalopathy are less common. A form of non-cirrhotic chronic liver disease—sometimes associated with portal hypertension—exists in India; despite various suggestions (including arsenic poisoning), the aetiology remains unclear. Of pre-hepatic causes, HMS is the most common; portal hypertension results from an increased splenic blood flow. Portal/splenic vein obstructions, probably resulting from neonatal umbilical sepsis, are important causes throughout tropical countries, and are undoubtedly underdiagnosed; hepatocellular function is usually intact. Posthepatic causes of portal hypertension include

(Table 3.7): cardiac failure (usually resulting from chronic rheumatic cardiac disease); right-sided endomyocardial fibrosis (see Chapter 5; and constrictive pericarditis, usually but not always resulting from tuberculosis. Other causes of portal hypertension are hepatocellular carcinoma, and various dehydrating diseases, including dysentery and cholera. Splenomegaly is present whatever the cause of portal hypertension (which should be distinguished from other causes of enlargement of this organ in a tropical country). Barium swallow or upper gastrointestinal endoscopy usually confirms the presence of oesophageal varices. When available, ultrasonography is valuable in assessing portal vein patency.

BILIARY TRACT DISEASE

In tropical countries biliary pathology is largely attributable to parasites[1,214]—ascariasis (see Chapter 71), clonorchiasis and opisthorchiasis (see Chapter 73); pigment stones (often intrahepatic) occasionally complicate sickle cell disease. *A. lumbricoides* infection (see Chapter 71) is an underdiagnosed cause of large-duct obstruction. It should always be considered in this clinical situation; it may be confused with pancreatic carcinoma. Endoscopy, if available, is of value; medical treatment is usually successful. Clonorchiasis and opisthorchiasis (see Chapter 73), acquired from ingestion of raw freshwater fish, may result in cholangiohepatitis and biliary obstruction; cholangiocarcinoma is a late complication of both infections. *F. hepatica* infection (see Chapter 73) can give rise to tender hepatomegaly accompanied by jaundice; difficulty in diagnosis from viral hepatitis may be a problem; an eosinophilia is, however, common with this and all biliary trematode infections. Overall, cholesterol stones (and associated secondary infection) are uncommon in rural populations, especially in Africa. Gallbladder infection by *S. typhi* can result in the typhoid carrier state (see Chapter 42); the focus of infection is usually intrahepatic. Gallbladder carcinoma is unusual.

LIVER: EMERGENCIES

ACUTE HEPATOCELLULAR FAILURE

Acute liver failure (acute hepatic necrosis) is a major clinical problem in all developing countries (see above);[4] various hepatitis viruses (most commonly B, C, D and E, and to a lesser extent A) are involved, but some cases are caused by other viruses, bacteria or toxins. Although acute hepatocellular failure has been recorded in *severe* acute *P. falciparum* infection, this is of limited clinical importance; if it occurs (apart from a terminal event), it is of far less importance than other major organ failure.[225]

The role of the several viruses in the production of acute liver injury has been summarized.[226] Reports highlight the aetiological basis of hepatitis in tropical countries; in Egypt, HBV and hepatitis A virus (HAV) accounted for 47 and 0.7% of cases of acute hepatitis (there was serological evidence of both viral infections in a further 1.4%), whereas 14.2% of cases were HB$_s$Ag carriers, 31% 'non-A, non-B' hepatitis and 6% were drug-induced.[227] In other locations, however, hepatitis D virus (HDV) is important—especially southern America, south-eastern Asia (and probably India) and northern Africa. Thus in Thailand, HDV is frequently present in drug abusers; it is also endemic in Chandigarh, India,[228] and has been described in an epidemic of acute hepatitis in the Himalayan foothills in south Kashmir.[229] In India and South-East Asia, hepatitis E virus (HEV) is responsible for most cases of the entity previously termed 'non-A, non-B' hepatitis;[230,231] a similar situation probably pertains in Africa and southern America. This virus is transmitted by the faecal–oral route and is transmitted in contaminated drinking water; the major importance of this infection is that it produces a high incidence of hepatocellular failure in pregnant women. The 27 nm viral particles can be demonstrated in a faecal sample;[232] the way is now open for a satisfactory serological test and subsequently a vaccine for this

infection. HCV causes severe disease—including acute hepatic failure—similar to that produced by HBV.[233]

Differential diagnosis

Many other viruses present in tropical and subtropical regions may also produce acute hepatic necrosis; these include herpes simplex type 1,[234] herpes virus 6,[235] Epstein–Barr virus, cytomegalovirus, yellow fever[236] and the haemorrhagic fever viruses, which include the Lassa fever virus, the Marburg agent, Ebola virus and Rift Valley fever virus (see above).[237,238] Of bacterial causes of hepatitis, enteric fever is common, but rarely (if ever) proceeds to hepatocellular necrosis.[239] The jaundice of systemic bacterial infection[1] often follows pyomyositis, especially in Africa. *P. falciparum* malaria causes deranged liver function tests resulting from centrilobular necrosis.[225] Hepatotoxicity resulting from herbal remedies is not confined to tropical countries.[240] Alcoholic hepatitis is a significant clinical problem in both indigenous and expatriate populations.[1]

Management

Tandon et al[241] have outlined their experience of acute hepatic failure (resulting from viral hepatitis) in 145 (>12 years old) patients managed by them using a 'simple supportive therapeutic regimen' during a 5.5-year period at New Delhi, India. Criteria for inclusion were:

- Development of hepatic encephalopathy within 4 weeks of onset of symptoms and signs of acute hepatitis; and
- Absence of evidence of pre-existent liver disease.

There were 65 men and 80 women; 46 of them were pregnant and presumably infected by HEV infections.

They used a simple intensive support mechanism; this consisted of:

1 Isolation in an intensive care room.
2 Attention to general hygiene and care of a comatose patient.
3 Intravenous fluid to provide 1000–1500 calories daily using 10% dextrose, supplemented, if necessary, by 20% dextrose.
4 Nasogastric tube for aspiration of gastric contents and instillation of drugs.
5 Gut sterilization by ampicillin (1.5 g 6-hourly via nasogastric tube); bowel washes twice daily.
6 Liquid antacids (30 ml 2-hourly).
7 'Lactisyn' (1 ampoule = *Lactobacillus lactus* 490

million, *L. acidophilus* 490 million, *Streptococcus lactus* 10 million) three times daily.

8 Condom or catheter drainage of the urinary bladder.

9 Maintenance of electrolyte and fluid balance by intravenous supplementation.

Complications were managed as follows:

- Infection (diagnosis was based on clinical findings, leucocyte count $> 15 \times 10^9/l$, and/or chest radiograph abnormality): gentamicin 3.5 mg/kg body weight (as three divided doses), and/or cephalexin (2 g daily as four divided doses).

- Cerebral oedema (criteria for diagnosis were: focal or generalized seizures, abnormal reactive or unequal pupils, decerebrate posture of the body after minor stimuli, and/or sudden deterioration of vital signs): intravenous mannitol (200 ml administered during 30 minutes and repeated three or four times per 24 hours).

- Gastrointestinal bleeding (diagnosed by aspiration of fresh or altered blood via nasogastric tube): liquid antacid (30–45 ml every 2 hours), gastric lavage (with 100 ml cold saline containing 8 mg noradrenaline every 30 minutes) and occasionally cimetidine. (When the prothrombin time was >7 s compared with a control, fresh frozen plasma was administered.)

- Renal failure (the criterion used was: oliguria (urine output <400 mg/24 h, and rising blood urea) despite adequate hydration): diuretics (judiciously used!).

Overall 42 (28.9%) survived; of those ≤40 years old 41 (33%) recovered, compared with only one (4.8%) of those ≥40 years; survival was not affected by pregnancy. Indicators of poor prognosis were: grade IV coma, presence of HB_sAg, serum bilirubin concentration >20 mg/100 ml and sodium <119 mmol/l. In fatal cases the immediate complications resulting in death were: cerebral oedema (65), bleeding (31), renal failure (11) and infection (8). The authors concluded that these results were comparable with results from centres using a variety of complex therapeutic regimens (e.g. exchange blood transfusion, charcoal perfusion and haemodialysis).

CHRONIC HEPATOCELLULAR FAILURE

Cirrhosis, generally resulting from one of the hepatitis viruses (usually B or C), is a very common problem throughout tropical and subtropical countries. A recent study carried out at New Delhi, India, has addressed the problem of survival in young (<35 years old) and older patients with cirrhosis;[242] numbers in the two groups were 63 and 106,

respectively. Aetiology of cirrhosis in the young and adult groups was: HBV-related (32 and 51), alcohol-related (10 and 28), while 19 and 21, respectively, were labelled 'cryptogenic'; in the former group, one had Wilson's disease and another α_1 antitrypsin deficiency. During the surveillance period 27 and 47 deaths occurred: 40 and 64% from hepatic failure, and 52 and 26% from variceal bleeding. The 5-year survival (62 and 56%) and probability of survival within a similar grade of liver disease (Child's classification) were comparable. As anticipated, probability of survival was significantly higher in grade A and lowest in C. Aetiology of cirrhosis did not significantly influence prognosis in this study.

Hepatocellular carcinoma usually presents as a rapidly progressive malignancy; however, an acute on chronic presentation can occur due to internal necrosis and haemorrhage.[169] Such a lesion can in fact rupture into the peritoneal cavity, posing problems in differential diagnosis.

In a patient with actively bleeding oesophageal varices, differentiation of the aetiology of underlying liver disease (from postviral (or another aetiology) cirrhosis and chronic schistosomal disease) is usually impossible on clinical grounds alone. In a study carried out at Cairo, Egypt, liver ultrasonography was undertaken in 50 patients who were undergoing an operation for bleeding oesophageal varices;[243] ultrasonographic diagnosis was compared with a surgically obtained wedge biopsy specimen. The authors concluded that ultrasonography gave the more accurate diagnosis; the findings in schistosomal periportal (pipe-stem) fibrosis were characteristic and were not mimicked by other liver diseases (including cirrhosis); ultrasonography agreed with the histological diagnosis in 44 cases.

Role of ultrasonography in management

The overall value of ultrasonographic scanning and scintigraphy in the diagnosis of *chronic* liver disease in developing countries has recently been addressed;[244,245] in the former study from Durban, South Africa, 425 and 304 scans, respectively, were evaluated and the authors concluded that both techniques were superior for detection of focal (88 and 92%, respectively) compared with diffuse (27 and 54%, respectively) disease, but that their accuracy in distinguishing normal and diseased livers was low (68 and 74%). Using ultrasonography, a correct diagnosis was obtained in 81% of patients with amoebic liver abscess (see below), 29% with hepatocellular carcinoma, and 43% with metastatic carcinoma. Therefore, needle biopsy is frequently necessary to diagnose diffuse disease, but a high degree of specificity can be anticipated with a space occupying lesion.[181] A further problem surrounding ultrasonography has been highlighted:[245] in Africa and other developing countries, focal lesions 'often present so late that lesions revealed by ultrasound are huge and bizarre', and the inexperienced radiologist may therefore be baffled.

PORTAL HYPERTENSION AND ITS COMPLICATIONS

The major causes of portal hypertension (and oesophageal varices) are summarized in Table 3.7. Some geographical variations have been reviewed.[1,9] While in many parts of the world cirrhosis is the most common cause, in India non-cirrhotic portal fibrosis is relatively common.[9] Indian childhood cirrhosis (see above) also accounts for cases in the younger age group(s). Extrahepatic portal vein obstruction is common in some countries (including India);[246] however, in Egypt, Africa, the Middle East, South America, and China, *Schist. mansoni* and *Schist. japonicum*, respectively, are frequently responsible. In Jamaica, South Africa, central Asia and the south-western USA, epidemic veno-occlusive disease (see above) (caused by *Heliotropium, Crotalaria, Senecio* and other alkaloids) (see above) is important.

Pitressin (vasopressin) forms the basis of management of variceal haemorrhage; if and where available, upper gastrointestinal endoscopic sclerotherapy is of value, but this technique usually has to be repeated at 6-month intervals. The Sengstaken tube (for variceal compression) still has a place in developing countries. Haemorrhage is not a major presenting feature at most tropical hospitals (see above).

Bleeding varices resulting from extrahepatic portal obstruction

The cause of portal vein thrombosis in developing countries remains unclear; it is, however, a relatively common condition, and neonatal umbilical sepsis is usually cited as the likely aetiological factor.[1] During an 8.5-year period, 136 patients with extrahepatic portal hypertension were treated surgically at New Delhi, India;[246] in 22 it was carried out as an emergency (for variceal bleeding), and in 114 as an elective procedure (in 104 for a past haematemesis and in ten for massive splenomegaly). The emergency strategy consisted of: splenectomy and splenorenal shunt (14), transoesophageal variceal ligation (4), splenectomy and gastro-oesophageal

devascularization (3) and mesocaval shunt (1). Elective procedures were: splenectomy and splenorenal shunt (94), mesocaval shunt (8) and splenectomy and gastro-oesophageal devascularization (12). Operative mortality was 2 (9%) and 1 (1%), respectively; none of the survivors developed encephalopathy or postsplenectomy sepsis. One hundred and seventeen (86%) were followed up for 2–10 years; 17 had a further haematemesis, but 90 and 75% were alive at 5 and 10 years, respectively. Patients are often a long way from medical facilities when experiencing haematemesis in a developing country; the authors therefore considered that in this setting operative intervention was more satisfactory than endoscopic sclerotherapy or management with propranolol (variceal compression was not considered).

SPACE–OCCUPYING HEPATIC LESIONS

Invasive hepatic amoebiasis

Amoebic liver abscess is a cause of right upper quadrant pain (and hepatomegaly); this is usually accompanied by fever, and not infrequently right shoulder-tip pain. Travellers to infected areas as well as the indigenous population(s) of the tropics may be affected.[1,247] A high prevalence (16 cases of invasive disease—9 involving the liver—amongst 160 individuals) has been documented in Italian tourists to Phuket, Thailand, after their party had stayed in a 'luxury' hotel.[248] Pathogenesis is dependent on an oral infection with a potentially invasive strain (zymodeme) of *Ent. histolytica*.[249] Diagnosis is based on an appropriate serological technique (IFAT, cellulose acetate, or countercurrent immunoelectrophoresis) and hepatic ultrasonography or computerized tomography.

Clinical characteristics in a group of 52 patients suffering from amoebic liver abscesses have been recorded at Cairo, Egypt;[249] while 22 (42%) presented with an acute illness (see above), 30 (58%) had a more chronic illness with dull aching in the right hypochondria, weight loss, fatigue, moderate to low-grade pyrexia and anaemia. A right-sided pleural effusion, emphysema, ascites and jaundice was present in three (6%), four (8%), seven (13%), and seven (13%), respectively. Forty-two (81%) abscesses were solitary and in the right lobe; 29 (43%) were initially solid or heterogeneous. Response to metronidazole (750 mg three times daily for 10 days) was described as good in 50; in four aspiration was carried out on account of the large abscess size.

Whether needle aspiration of an amoebic abscess (in addition to satisfactory chemotherapy) is indicated remains controversial. A prospective, randomized controlled study carried out at New Delhi, India, has addressed this issue;[250] in 17 of 37 patients (all received appropriate chemotherapy, 2–4 g metronidazole for 10 days) who completed the study, aspiration was carried out on the day of hospital admission; clinical improvement (and cure) was similar to that in 20 controls. 'Abscess' diameter was slightly lower in those who underwent aspiration (54 versus 72 mm). However, at Benin, Nigeria, needle aspiration was considered to 'enhance clinical recovery';[251] in a non-randomized trial, 19 patients were managed by needle aspiration in addition to chemotherapy, and 17 were given chemotherapy (metronidazole, diloxanide and chloroquine) alone; 18 and 10, respectively, experienced complete resolution (as shown by ultrasonography) after 21 days ($P < 0.021$), and clinical response was also considered more rapid ($P < 0.01$), especially when the abscess was > 6 cm in diameter. Delay in ultrasonographic 'recovery' is not important, there being good evidence that a residual abnormality after a year or more is compatible with complete, uncomplicated resolution.

Although no in vitro evidence of *Ent. histolytica* resistance to the 5-nitroimidazole compounds exists, reports continue to be made from India of drug-resistant cases. The main problem with such reports is that, in few (if any) has diloxanide furoate (500 mg three times daily for 10 days) been administered; this is essential for a definitive cure because it is a far superior luminal amoebicide compared with the 5-nitroimidazole compounds—and therefore kills the cysts (which could belong to invasive zymodemes). In a prospective randomized study of 50 such resistant cases at New Delhi, four management regimens were used:[252] (1) a repeat course of conservative therapy (with 1.25 mg/kg dehydroemetine given intramuscularly daily for 10 days); (2) needle aspiration (under ultrasonographic guidance); (3) percutaneous catheter drainage (under ultrasonographic guidance); and (4) open surgical drainage with catheter insertion. The authors concluded that 'the most impressive results' were obtained with regimen 3.

To summarize, in the uncomplicated case needle aspiration (under cover of a 5-nitroimidazole compound) is indicated when: (1) the abscess(es) cavity is large and the patient seriously ill; and (2) the site of the lesion is such that perforation into a nearby viscus (most importantly the pericardium) seems probable. All cases of invasive amoebiasis should receive a course of the luminal amoebicide diloxanide furoate (500 mg three times daily for 10 days) *after* metronidazole (800 mg three times daily for 10 days) or tinidazole (2 g daily for 3 days). If this regimen is omitted, *Ent. histolytica* cysts remain in the colonic lumen and, in the event of their being of a pathogenic zymodeme, further tissue invasion (including liver abscess) might occur.

Spontaneous perforation of an amoebic liver abscess is a serious complication which is associated with high morbidity and mortality rates;[247] this applies especially when perforation takes place into the pericardial cavity. Successful percutaneous drainage (for 7–34 days) of a perforated abscess in five 'severely ill' patients (with a total of 11 lesions) under metronidazole cover has recently been recorded;[253] there were resultant abscesses in the subhepatic space, pelvis, chest, right and left paracolic gutters, lesser sac, retroperitoneum and flank, and associated fistulas were demonstrated with the bile duct, duodenum and the colon; all healed completely. No patient required a laparotomy. These authors recommend wider use of catheter drainage for this serious complication of hepatic amoebiasis.

Pyogenic liver abscess

Although in a tropical context much less common than invasive amoebiasis, pyogenic abscess is a serious disease with high morbidity and mortality—even when managed in experienced hands.[1] In most cases, a primary intra-abdominal focus of infection can be detected. Differentiation from invasive hepatic amoebiasis is usually straightforward,[254] the patient being more severely and acutely ill; jaundice, septicaemia and renal impairment are common accompaniments. Ultrasonography is usually diagnostic. At Kuala Lumpur, 25 pyogenic abscesses were encountered between 1970 and 1985;[255] during the same period, there were 90 amoebic and one tuberculous abscesses, while in 89 others the cause of the abscess was not determined. At Kingston, Jamaica, fever and abdominal pain were present in 21 (80%) out of 24 cases of pyogenic abscess encountered between 1977 and 1986;[256] the most common signs were right upper quadrant tenderness and hepatomegaly; leucocytosis, elevated alkaline phosphatase and hypoalbuminaemia were common. Reports from London[257] and California[258] have given encouraging reports of management by needle aspiration under antibiotic (usually gentamicin and metronidazole or clindamycin) cover. Another study has also recorded satisfactory results in 18 of 21 patients using this form of percutaneous drainage. Other authors have intimated, however, that this form of management should be reserved for selected patients.[259] A report from Riyadh, Saudi Arabia,[260] has provided results which were less encouraging. In Jamaica surgical drainage using a guided percutaneous technique gave comparable results.[256] Taking all reports into account, it seems wise to perform a laparotomy and to institute surgical drainage as soon as possible after diagnosis. Using ultrasonographic control, a pyogenic abscess 'resolved' significantly more rapidly than an amoebic abscess.[261] It should be appreciated, however, that this disease carries a significant mortality rate; between 1975 and 1986, these authors treated 109 children with pyogenic liver abscess; the mortality rate was 15%.[262] There is limited (suggestive) evidence that the overall prognosis is improving.[263]

Hydatid disease and schistosomiasis involving the liver

Only rarely, usually following trauma, does hydatidosis[214,264] present as an abdominal emergency.

Perforation into the peritoneal cavity may produce an anaphylactoid reaction with hypotension, and/or seeding of daughter hydatid cysts within the peritoneal cavity. Secondary bacterial infection is an unusual event.[1,260] Chemotherapy is with albendazole and/or praziquantel (see Chapter 75).[264]

Hepatic schistosomiasis[14,265] is complicated by portal hypertension and oesophageal varices in an advanced case; however, hepatocellular function is maintained late into the course of disease and hepatic encephalopathy and ascites occur as advanced (usually terminal) signs. Praziquantel is the chemotherapeutic agent of choice;[265] evidence of reversal of fibrotic changes is now available.

PANCREAS

The two major diseases involving this organ encountered in tropical countries, and which differ from those in temperate ones, are: (1) 'J-type' diabetes, first reported in Jamaica (Chapter 25); and (2) chronic calcific pancreatitis.[1,266]

Diabetes, which is not associated with pancreatic calcification in young people, is encountered throughout tropical countries; those affected are usually thin, and require high doses of insulin; however, they do not rapidly develop ketosis when insulin is discontinued. J-type diabetes might have a viral aetiology, one of the Coxsackie group of viruses being involved; a raised incidence of antibody to Coxsackie B_4 has been demonstrated in similarly affected patients in India. A suggestion has been made that these patients, especially those in Africa, are less susceptible to chronic diabetic complications than Europeans; this now seems unlikely.

A popular Indian and Chinese vegetable karela (*Momordica charantia*) possesses hypoglycaemic properties; these are enhanced by chlorpropamide, a fact that should be taken into account in the management of diabetes in a number of Asian countries.

A syndrome consisting of pancreatic calcification associated with both exocrine and endocrine impairment is common in many tropical countries (Figure 3.11);[1,266] most observations have been made in Africa (East and West), southern India and Indonesia. The aetiology of *chronic calcific pancreatitis* remains unknown. Pancreatic disruption in childhood kwashiorkor can be severe and might be relevant. Cassava (*Manihot esculenta*) has been implicated. Long-standing pancreatic damage can also follow viral hepatitis. A further hypothesis is that pancreatic ducts are blocked by secretions and inspissated mucous plugs, and later calcify; this might be more common after starvation, gastroenteritis and dehydration. Presentation is with weight loss and malabsorption (in some parts of the tropics, especially Africa, this is the most common cause of overt malabsorption); diabetes mellitus and pancre-

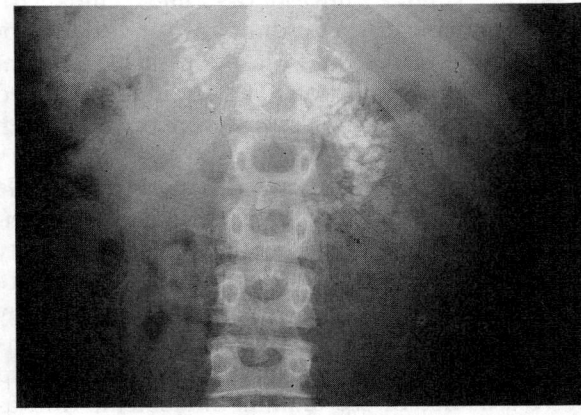

Figure 3.11 Abdominal radiograph showing calcified pancreas in the chronic calcific pancreatitis syndrome. There was no history of alcohol excess or infant malnutrition; aetiology was therefore undetermined.

atic pain are important features. Management consists of providing pancreatic supplements (e.g. pancreatin, BP, 6g orally with meals) together with diabetic control.[1] Pain is often difficult to manage and may be so severe that suicide is an unfortunate sequel.

The pancreas can also be involved in many infections including *Schist. mansoni* and *Schist. japonicum,* trichinellosis, cysticercosis and hydatid disease.

Pancreatic duct obstruction, complicated by acute pancreatitis, is most commonly a sequel to *A. lumbricoides* infection (see below); tapeworms are rarely implicated. Clonorchiasis and opisthorchiasis can involve the pancreatic duct system.

EMERGENCIES OF THE PANCREAS, AND BILIARY SYSTEM

One of the most widely distributed nematodes in tropical and subtropical countries is *A. lumbricoides*.[1,214] By entering the biliary system (from the duodenum) this parasite can cause several acute medical and surgical conditions. Reporting from Kashmir, India, Khuroo et al[267] collected 500 cases in which *A. lumbricoides* involved the liver, biliary tract and pancreas; biliary ascariasis was present in 171 cases, and in 140 there was hepatic, in eight gallbladder and in seven pancreatic involvement. These authors recognized five clinical presentations: acute cholecystitis (64), acute cholangitis (121), biliary colic (280), acute pancreatitis (31) and hepatic abscess (4). Twenty-seven had a pyogenic cholangitis which was treated by decompression and drainage—surgically in two and endoscopically in 25; removal of adult worms from the ampullary orifice (with extraction per os) led to rapid relief of biliary colic in 214, and acute pancreatitis in 16; four patients died, from acute pancreatitis (2), pyogenic cholangitis (1) and hepatic abscess (1). Worms persisted at 3 weeks in the biliary tree in 12 patients;

dead worms were removed either by surgery (5) or by using an endoscopic basket (7). *A. lumbricoides* moved out of the ductal system in 211 cases. The patients were followed up for a mean of 48 months; 76 became reinfected and had reinvasion of the biliary tree; in seven cases intrahepatic duct and bile duct calculi (superimposed on dead worms) were present.

In south-eastern Asia, the two most common biliary parasites are *Clonorchis sinensis* and *Opisthorchis* spp.[24] Although these cause chronic problems, notably secondary bacterial cholangitis[169] and adenocarcinoma of the biliary system, an acute presentation[1] is unusual. A Thai woman infected with *Opisthorchis viverrini* and *F. hepatica* who presented with abdominal pain, fever, jaundice and upper gastrointestinal bleeding of undetermined origin—which resulted from haemobilia—has been described.[268]

In most indigenous people of developing countries, gallstones are unusual; when they occur they are usually of the pigment variety, and often associated with haemolysis. A recent report from Saudi Arabia, where the average life style has rapidly become westernized (with striking changes in diet) over the last two to three decades, indicates that cholecystectomy for cholelithiasis is now one of the most common major abdominal operations to be carried out;[269] between 1977 and 1986, 2854 individuals (most of them young Saudis) underwent this operation at 14 hospitals in the Eastern Province of the country.

Acute pancreatitis is uncommon overall in developing countries, although severe abdominal pain caused by chronic calcific pancreatitis[1] can give rise to problems in differential diagnosis. The pain may be so severe that suicide is attempted. Biliary involvement by *A. lumbricoides* can result in acute pancreatitis.[1,169] Other helminths, including *Clonorchis sinensis, Opisthorchis* spp. and *Anisakis* spp. have also been associated with this condition. A rare cause is *S. typhi* infection; a single case report in a 17-year-old Guatemalan boy has been described in Mexico.[270]

SPLEEN

Table 3.8 summarizes some causes of splenomegaly in the tropics, and Figure 3.12 illustrates clinical and histological appearances in HMS.[1] Most of these causes receive attention in other chapters. The most extreme form of splenomegaly (HMS) is covered in

Chapters 6 and 61; those caused by various viral, bacterial and parasitic infections are dealt with under these respective headings.

The spleen is an extremely important defence organ against many infections, especially pneumo-

Table 3.8 Some causes of splenomegaly in the tropics.

Infections
    Viral   Epstein–Barr virus, cytomegalovirus, viral hepatitis and other virus diseases
    Bacterial   typhoid fever, brucellosis, tuberculosis
    Parasitic   malaria (especially hyperreactive malarious splenomegaly (HMS)),
                  schistosomiasis, visceral leishmaniasis, trypanosomiasis

Portal hypertension

Haemopoietic diseases
    Sickle cell disease, thalassaemia

Reticuloendothelial diseases
    Burkitt's lymphoma, leukaemia, reticuloses

Cystic lesions
    Hydatid disease

Abscess
    Amoebic; unknown aetiology

Spontaneous haemorrhage and rupture

Metabolic
    Amyloidosis

coccal and *Plasmodium* spp. infections. Splenectomized individuals in tropical countries should receive pneumococcal vaccine; prudent advice regarding malaria prophylaxis is mandatory.

Splenic abscess usually constitutes a tropical disease.[1] Aetiology is unknown; underlying viral and parasitic diseases have been suggested, but not proved. A connection with carriage of the sickle cell gene has also been suggested, but not proved. Most reports have been made in West Africa and Zimbabwe. In most, the aetiology is unknown, but some result from *S. typhi* infection. The clinical history is usually one of 2–3-weeks duration, consisting of pain/swelling in the left hypochondrium, associated with pyrexia. The splenic swelling is tender, often exquisitely so, and fluctuant. A radiograph may show gas within the abscess. Untreated, it can rupture into the peritoneal cavity; splenectomy therefore has an important role in management. Should the condition become chronic—an unusual sequel—splenectomy is the correct course in management.

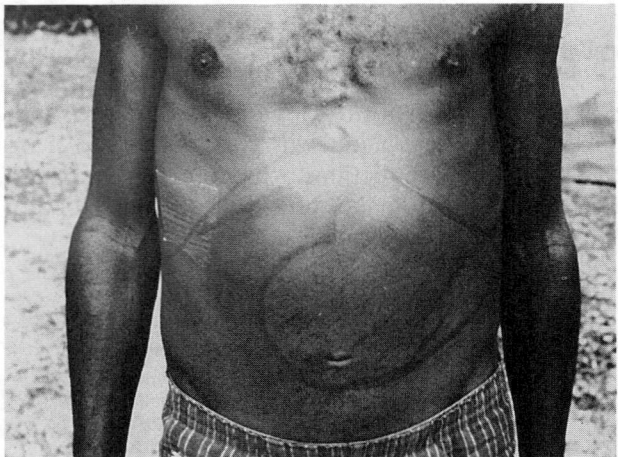

(a)

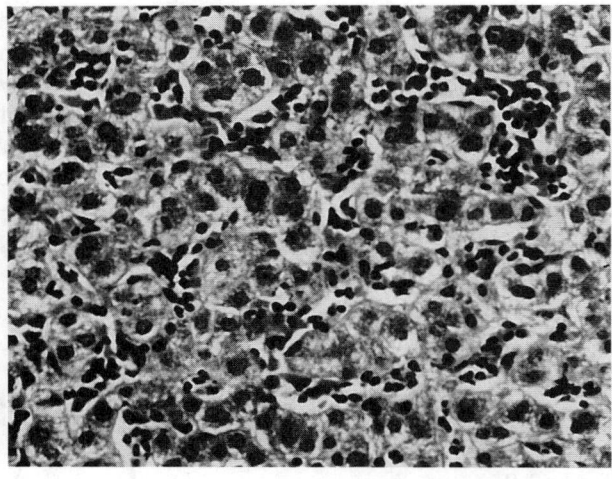

(b)

Figure 3.12 (a) Papua New Guinean man suffering from hyperreactive malarious splenomegaly (HMS); all of the features of this syndrome were present. (b) Liver biopsy specimen showing severe sinusoidal lymphocytosis, a component of the HMS syndrome.

REFERENCES

1 Cook G C. *Tropical Gastroenterology*. Oxford: Oxford University Press, 1980:484.

2 Cook G C (ed.). *Gastroenterological Problems from the Tropics*. London: BMJ Publishing Group, 1995: 146.

3 Cook G C (ed.). *Travel-Associated Disease*. London: Royal College of Physicians, 1995: 179.

4 Cook G C. Gastroenterological emergencies in the tropics. *Baillière's Clin Gastroenterol* 1991; 5:861–886.

5 Ferguson R. Diseases of the mouth. In Misiewicz J J, Pounder R E & Venables C W (eds) *Diseases of the Gut and Pancreas,* 2nd edn. Oxford: Blackwell, 1994: 93–101.

6 Watson A. Carcinoma of the oesophagus. In Misiewicz J J, Pounder R E & Venables C W (eds) *Diseases of the Gut and Pancreas,* 2nd edn. Oxford: Blackwell, 1994: 159–172.

7 Clamp S E, Morgan A G, Kotwal M R et al. Use of a multinational survey to provide clinical guidelines for upper gastrointestinal bleeding in developing countries. *Scand J Gastroenterol* 1988; 23 (supplement 144):63–66.

8 Kiire C F, Kitai I, Sigola L & Ternouth I. Upper gastrointestinal bleeding in an African setting. *J R Coll Physicians Lond* 1987; 21:107–110.

9 Okumura H, Aramaki T & Katsuta Y. Pathophysiology and epidemiology of portal hypertension. *Drugs* 1989; 37 (supplement 2):2–12.

10 El-Zayadi A, Montasser M F, Girgis F, El-Okby S, Botros B & Mohran Z. Histological changes of the esophageal mucus in bleeding versus non-bleeding varices. *Endoscopy* 1989; 21:205–207.

11 Nakib B A I, Radhakrishnan S, Liddawi H A I, Jacob G S & Ruwaih A A I. The role of gastrointestinal endoscopy in a developing country. *Endoscopy* 1986; 18:37–39.

12 Atoba M A, Ayoola E A & Olubuyide I O. Radiological and endoscopic correlation in upper gastrointestinal haemorrhage and malignancy. *Scand J Gastroenterol* 1986; 21 (supplement 124):149–151.

13 Sarin S K, Nanda R & Sachdev G. Relative efficacy and safety of absolute alcohol and 50% alcohol as variceal sclerosants. *Gastrointest Endosc* 1987; 33:362–365.

14 Sarin S K, Mishra S P, Sachdev G K, Thorat V, Dalal L & Broor S L. Ethanolamine oleate *versus* absolute alcohol as a variceal sclerosant: a prospective, randomized, controlled trial. *Am J Gastroenterol* 1988; 83:526–530.

15 Sarin S K, Misra S P, Singal A K, Thorat V & Broor S L. Endoscopic sclerotherapy for varices in children. *J Pediatr Gastroenterol Nutr* 1988; 7:662–666.

16 Wahrendorf J, Chang-Claude J, Liang Q S et al. Precursor lesions of oesophageal cancer in young people in a high-risk population in China. *Lancet* 1989; ii:1239–1241.

17 Clarke C A & Bodmer W F. Oesophageal cancer in China. *Lancet* 1989; ii:1525.

18 Langman M J S. Aetiologies of peptic ulcer. In Misiewicz J J, Pounder R E & Venables C W (eds) *Diseases of the Gut and Pancreas,* 2nd edn. Oxford: Blackwell, 1994:249–259.

19 Scobie B A, Beg F & Oldmeadows M. Peptic diseases compared endoscopically in indigenous Fijians and Indians. *N Z Med J* 1987; 100:683–684.

20 Rathbone B J & Heatley R V (eds). *Campylobacter pylori and Gastroduodenal Disease*. Oxford: Blackwell, 1989:290.

21 Tytgat G N J. Gastritis. In Misiewicz J J, Pounder R E & Venables C W (eds) *Diseases of the Gut and Pancreas,* 2nd edn. Oxford: Blackwell, 1994:221–235.

22 Cook G C. Hypochlorhydria and vulnerability to intestinal infection. *Eur J Gastroenterol Hepatol* 1994; 6:693–695.

23 Craven J L. Carcinoma of the stomach. In Misiewicz J J, Pounder R E & Venables C W (eds) *Diseases of the Gut and Pancreas,* 2nd edn. Oxford: Blackwell, 1994:335–352.

24 Mabogunje C A. Perforated duodenal and gastric ulcers in the Nigeria savannah. *Int Surg* 1985; 70:327–330.

25 Kochhar R, Krishna P R, Gupta N M & Mehta S K. Massive gastrointestinal bleeding due to cholecystoduodenal fistula. *Acta Chir Scand* 1988; 154:471–472.

26 Sarin S K, Sachdev G, Nanda R, Misra S P & Broor S L. Endoscopic sclerotherapy in the treatment of gastric varices. *Br J Surg* 1988; 75:747–750.

27 Jernigan J, Guerrant R L & Pearson R D. Parasitic infections of the small intestine. *Gut* 1994; 35:289–293.

28 Cook G C. The small intestine and its role in chronic diarrheal disease in the tropics. In Gracey M (ed.) *Diarrhea*. Boca Raton: CRC Press, 1991: 127–162.

29 Cook G C. Tropical disease and the small intestine. In Misiewicz J J, Pounder R E & Venables C W (eds) *Diseases of the Gut and Pancreas,* 2nd edn. Oxford: Blackwell, 1994:597–615.

30 DuPont H L. Travelers' diarrhea. In Gracey M (ed.) *Diarrhea*. Boca Raton: CRC Press, 1991:115–126.

31 Gorbach S L. Travelers' diarrhea. In Gorbach S L, Bartlett J G & Blacklow N R (eds) *Infectious Diseases*. Philadelphia: WB Saunders, 1992:622–628.

32 Okhuysen P C & Ericsson C D. Travelers' diarrhea. *Curr Opin Gastroenterol* 1992; 8:110–114.

33 Cook G C. Travellers' diarrhoea: slow but steady progress. *Postgrad Med J* 1993; 69:505–508.

34 Farthing M J G. Travellers' diarrhoea. *Gut* 1994; 35:1–4.

35 Black R E. Epidemiology of travelers' diarrhea and relative importance of various pathogens. *Rev Infect Dis* 1990; 12 (supplement 1):S73–S79.

36 Wiström J & Norrby R. Antibiotic prophylaxis of travellers' diarrhoea. *Scand J Infect Dis* 1990; 70:111–129.

37 Ljungh A H. Travellers' diarrhoea and the European tourist. *Eur J Gastroenterol Hepatol* 1992; 4:764–770.

38 Harries A D, Myers B & Cook G C. Inflammatory bowel disease: a common cause of bloody diarrhoea in visitors to the tropics. *BMJ* 1985; 291:1686–1687.

39 Schumacher G, Kollberg B & Ljungh Å. Inflammatory bowel disease presenting as travellers' diarrhoea. *Lancet* 1993; 341:241–242.

40 Rowe B, Taylor J & Bettelheim K A. An investigation of travellers' diarrhoea. *Lancet* 1970; i:1–4.

41 Sack R B. Travelers' diarrhea: microbiologic bases for prevention and treatment. *Rev Infect Dis* 1990; 12 (supplement 1): S59–S63.

42 Tellier R & Keystone J S. Prevention of travelers' diarrhoea. *Infect Dis Clin North Am* 1992; 6 (no. 2):333–354.

43 Scott D A, Haberberger R L, Thornton S A & Hyams K C. Norfloxacin for the prophylaxis of travelers' diarrhea in US military personnel. *Am J Trop Med Hyg* 1990; 42:160–164.

44 Bhutta T I & Tahir K I. Loperamide poisoning in children. *Lancet* 1990; 335:363.

45 DuPont H L, Ericsson C D, Johnson P C & de la Cabada F J. Use of bismuth subsalicylate for the prevention of travelers' diarrhea. *Rev Infect Dis* 1990; 12 (supplement 1):S65–S67.

46 Peltola H, Siitonen A, Kyronseppa H et al. Prevention of travellers' diarrhoea by oral B-subunit/whole cell cholera vaccine. *Lancet* 1991; 338:1285–1289.

47 DuPont H L, Ericsson C D, Matthewson J J & DuPont M W. Five versus three days of ofloxacin therapy for travelers' diarrhea: a placebo-controlled study. *Antimicrob Agents Chemother* 1992; 36:87–91.

48 Nalin D R. Cholera and severe toxigenic diarrhoeas. *Gut* 1994; 35:145–149.

49 Phillips S F. Asiatic cholera: nature's experiment? *Gastroenterology* 1986; 91:1304–1307.

50 Snow J. *On the Mode of Communication of Cholera*, 2nd edn. London: Churchill, 1855.

51 Cook G C. The Asiatic cholera: an historical determinant of human genomic and social structure. In Drasar B S (ed.) *Cholera*. London: Chapman & Hall, 1995 (in press).

52 Steffen R. Epidemiologic studies of travelers' diarrhea, severe gastrointestinal infections, and cholera. *Rev Infect Dis* 1986; 8:S122–S130.

53 Miller C J, Drasar B S & Feachem R G. Cholera and estuarine salinity in Calcutta and London. *Lancet* 1982; i:1216–1218.

54 Toeg A, Berger S A, Battat A, Hoffman M & Yust I. *Vibrio cholerae* bacteremia associated with gastrectomy. *J Clin Microbiol* 1990; 28:603–604.

55 Phillips R A. Water and electrolyte losses in cholera. *Fed Proc* 1964; 23:705–712.

56 Hamilton S K, Keren D F, Boitnott J K, Robertson S M & Yardley J H. Enhancement of cholera toxin of IgA secretion from intestinal crypt epithelium. *Gut* 1980; 21:365–369.

57 Cook G C. Preventive strategies for the avoidance of infectious diarrhoea. In Gracey M & Bouchier I A D (eds) *Infectious Diarrhoea*. London: Baillière Tindall, 1993; 7 (no. 2): 519–545.

58 Levine M M. Modern vaccines: enteric infections. *Lancet* 1990; 335:958–961.

59 Clemens J D, Harris J R, Sack D A et al. Field trial of oral cholera vaccines in Bangladesh. *Southeast Asian J Trop Med Public Health* 1988; 19:417–422.

60 Clemens J D, Sack D A, Harries J R et al. Field trial of oral cholera vaccines in Bangladesh: results from three-year follow-up. *Lancet* 1990; 335:270–273.

61 Kaper J B. *Vibrio cholerae* vaccines. *Rev Infect Dis* 1989; 11:S568–S573.

62 Avery M E & Snyder J C. Oral therapy for acute diarrhea: the underused single solution. *N Engl J Med* 1990; 323:891–894.

63 Collins B J, van Loon F P L, Molla A, Molla A M & Alam N H. Gastric emptying of oral rehydration solutions in acute cholera. *J Trop Med Hyg* 1989; 92:290–294.

64 Mahalanabis D. Oral rehydration therapy. *Crit Rev Trop Med* 1984; 2:77–91.

65 Cook G C. Management of cholera: the vital role of rehydration. In Drasar B S (ed.) *Cholera*. London: Chapman & Hall, 1995 (in press).

66 Djeddah C, Miozzo A, di Gennaro M et al. An outbreak of cholera in a refugee camp in Africa. *Eur J Epidemiol* 1988; 4:227–230.

67 Molla A M, Sarkar S A, Hossain M, Molla A & Greenough W B. Rice-powder electrolyte solution as oral therapy in diarrhoea due to *Vibrio cholerae* and *Escherichia coli*. *Lancet* 1982; i:1317–1319.

68 Cosnett J E. The origins of intravenous fluid therapy. *Lancet* 1989; ii:768–771.

69 Islam A, Bardham P K, Islam M R & Rahman M. A randomized double blind trial of aspirin versus placebo in cholera and non-cholera diarrhoea. *Trop Geogr Med* 1986; 38:221–225.

70 Rabbani G H, Greenough W B, Holmgren J & Kirkwood B. Controlled trial of chlorpromazine as antisecretory agent in patients with cholera hydrated intravenously. *BMJ* 1982; 284:1361–1364.

71 Rabbani G H, Butler T, Patte D & Abud R L. Clinical trial of clonidine hydrochloride as an antisecretory agent in cholera. *Gastroenterology* 1989; 97:321–325.

72 Islam M R. Single dose tetracycline in cholera. *Gut* 1987; 28:1029–1032.

73 Rabbani G H, Islam M R, Butler T, Shahrier M & Alam K. Single-dose treatment of cholera and furazolidone or tetracycline in a double-blind randomized trial. *Antimicrob Agents Chemother* 1989; 33:1447–1450.

74 Alam A N, Alam N H, Ahmed T & Sack D A. Randomized double blind trial of single dose doxycycline for treating cholera in adults. *BMJ* 1990; 300:1619–1621.

75 Jesudason M V & John T J. Transferable trimethoprim resistance of *Vibrio cholerae* O1 encountered in southern India. *Trans R Soc Trop Med Hyg* 1990; 84:136–137.

76 Al-Saleem T I. Evidence of acquired immune deficiencies in Mediterranean lymphoma. A possible aetiological link. *Lancet* 1978; ii:709–712.

77 Cook G C. Hypolactasia: geographical distribution, diagnosis, and practical significance. In Chandra R K (ed.) *Critical Reviews in Tropical Medicine,* vol. 2. New York: Plenum Press, 1984:117–139.

78 Cook G C. Postinfective malabsorption (including tropical sprue). In Bouchier I A D, Allan R N, Hodgson H J F & Keighley M R B (eds) *Gastroenterology: Clinical Science and Practice,* 2nd edn. London: W B Saunders, 1993: 552–537.

79 Cook G C. Persisting diarrhoea and malabsorption. *Gut* 1994; 35:582–586.

80 Tomkins A. Tropical malabsorption: recent concepts in pathogenesis and nutritional significance. *Clin Sci* 1981; 60:131–137.

81 Baker S J. Idiopathic small intestinal disease in the tropics. In Chandra R K (ed.) *Critical Reviews in Tropical Medicine,* vol. 1. New York: Plenum Press, 1982:197–245.

82 Mathan V I. Tropical sprue in southern India. *Trans R Soc Trop Med Hyg* 1988; 82:10–14.

83 Manson P. Notes on sprue. *Medical Reports for the half year ended 31 March 1880,* 19th issue. Imperial Maritime Customs 11, spec. ser. 2. Shanghai: Statistical Department of the Inspectorate General, 1880:33–37.

84 Hillary W. Of chronical diseases. In *Observations on the Changes of the Air and the Concomitant Epidemical Diseases, in the Island of Barbados,* 2nd edn. Hawes, Clarke & Collins, 1766:276–297.

85 Montgomery R D & Chesner I M. Post-infective malabsorption in the temperate zone. *Trans R Soc Trop Med Hyg* 1985; 79:322–327.

86 Mathan V I. Tropical sprue. *Springer Semin Immunopathol* 1990; 12:231–237.

87 Menendez-Corrada R, Nettleship E & Santiago-Delpin E A. HLA and tropical sprue. *Lancet* 1986; ii:1183–1185.

88 Naik S. HLA and gastrointestinal disorders. *Indian J Gastroenterol* 1986; 5:121–124.

89 Banwell J G & Gorbach S L. Tropical sprue. *Gut* 1969; 10:328–333.

90 Klipstein F A, Holdeman L V, Corcino J J & Moore W E C. Enterotoxigenic intestinal bacteria in tropical sprue. *Ann Intern Med* 1973; 79:632–641.

91 Tomkins A M, Drasar B S & James W P T. Bacterial colonisation of jejunal mucosa in acute tropical sprue. *Lancet* 1975; i:59–62.

92 Klipstein F A, Horowitz I R, Engert R F & Schenk E A. Effect of *Klebsiella pneumoniae* enterotoxin on intestinal transport in the rat. *J Clin Invest* 1975; 56:799–807.

93 Klipstein F A, Engert R F &B Short H B. Enterotoxigenicity of colonising coliform bacteria in tropical sprue and blind-loop syndrome. *Lancet* 1978; ii:342–344.

94 Tomkins A M, Wright S G & Drasar B S. Bacterial colonization of the upper intestine in mild tropical malabsorption. *Trans R Soc Trop Med Hyg* 1980; 74:752–755.

95 Hamilton I, Worsley B W, Cobden I et al. Simultaneous culture of saliva and jejunal aspirate in the investigation of small bowel bacterial overgrowth. *Gut* 1982; 23:847–853.

96 Marsh M N. Functional and structural aspects of the epithelial lymphocyte, with implications for coeliac disease and tropical sprue. *Scand J Gastroenterol* 1985; 114 (supplement):55–75.

97 Besterman H S, Cook G C, Sarson D L et al. Gut hormones in tropical malabsorption. *BMJ* 1979; ii:1252–1255.

98 Spencer J, Isaacson P G, Diss T C & MacDonald T T. Expression of disulfide-linked and non-disulfide-linked forms of the T cell receptor γ/δ heterodimer in human intestinal intraepithelial lymphocytes. *Eur J Immunol* 1989; 14:1335–1338.

99 Lucas M L & Mathan V I. Jejunal surface pH measurements in tropical sprue. *Trans R Soc Trop Med Hyg* 1989; 83:138–142.

100 Mathan M M, Ponniah J & Mathan V I. Epithelial cell renewal and turnover and relationship to morphologic abnormalities in jejunal mucosa in tropical sprue. *Dig Dis Sci* 1986; 31:586–592.

101 Ross I N & Mathan V I. Immunological changes in tropical sprue. *Q J Med* 1981; 50:435–449.

102 Levine D S, Ree H J & Crowley J P. Tropical sprue and multiple myeloma: chronic immunocyte stimulation may have led to autonomous proliferation of a malignant clone of plasma cells. *Rhode Island Med J* 1986; 69:277–279.

103 Jayanthi V, Chacko A, Gani I K & Mathan V I. Intestinal transit in healthy Southern Indian subjects and in patients with tropical sprue. *Gut* 1989; 30:36–38.

104 Cook G C. Aetiology and pathogenesis of post-infective tropical malabsorption (tropical sprue). *Lancet* 1984; i:721–723.

105 Editorial. Loperamide—what does it block? *Lancet* 1981; ii:1088–1089.

106 Sandhu B R, Tripp J H, Candy D C A & Harries J T. Loperamide: studies on its mechanism of action. *Gut* 1981; 22:658–662.

107 Adrian T E, Savage A P, Bacarese-Hamilton A J, Wolfe K, Besterman H S & Bloom S R. Peptide

YY abnormalities in gastrointestinal disease. *Gastroenterology* 1986; 90:379–384.

108 Playford R J, Domin J, Beacham J et al. Preliminary report: role of peptide YY in defence against diarrhoea. *Lancet* 1990; 335:1555–1557.

109 Mathan V I. Tropical sprue in southern India. *Trans R Soc Trop Med Hyg* 1988; 82:10–14.

110 Read N W. Diarrhoea: the failure of colonic salvage. *Lancet* 1982; ii:481–483.

111 Ramakrishna B S & Mathan V I. Water and electrolyte absorption by the colon in tropical sprue. *Gut* 1982; 23:842–846.

112 Ramakrishna B S & Mathan V I. Role of bacterial toxins, bile acids, and free fatty acids in colonic water malabsorption in tropical sprue. *Dig Dis Sci* 1987; 32:500–505.

113 Tiruppathi C, Balasubramanian K A, Hill P G & Mathan V I. Faecal free fatty acids in tropical sprue and their possible role in the production of diarrhoea by inhibition of ATPases. *Gut* 1983; 24:300–305.

114 Binder J H. Pathophysiology of bile acid and fatty acid induced diarrhoea. In Field M, Fordtran J S & Schultz S G (eds) *Secretory Diarrhea*. Bethesda: American Physiological Society, 1980: 157.

115 Snape W J, Shiff S & Cohen S. Effect of deoxycholic acid on colonic mobility in the rabbit. *Am J Physiol* 1980; 238:G321–325.

116 Ramakrishna B S & Mathan V I. Absorption of water and sodium and activity of adenosine triphosphatases in the rectal mucosa in tropical sprue. *Gut* 1988; 29:665–668.

117 Batt R M & McLean L. Comparison of the biochemical changes in the jejunal mucosa of dogs with aerobic and anaerobic bacterial overgrowth. *Gastroenterology* 1987; 93:986–993.

118 Baker S J & Mathan V I. Tropical sprue in southern India. In *Tropical Sprue and Megaloblastic Anaemia. A Wellcome Trust Collaborative Study*. London: Churchill Livingstone, 1971:189–260.

119 Gupta B, Narru N & Dhar K L. Evaluation of surface area corrected peak blood xylose as a screening test of intestinal malabsorption in the tropics. *Indian J Gastroenterol* 1987; 6:89–91.

120 McLean A M, Farthing M J G, Kurian G & Mathan V I. The relationship between hypoalbuminaemia and the radiological appearances of the jejunum in tropical sprue. *Br J Radiol* 1982; 55:725–728.

121 Peters T J, Jones P E, Wells G & Cook G C. Sequential enzyme and subcellular fractionation studies on jejunal biopsy specimens from patients with post-infective tropical malabsorption. *Clin Sci Mol Med* 1979; 56:479–486.

122 Cook G C & Menzies I S. Intestinal absorption and unmediated permeation of sugars in post-infective tropical malabsorption (tropical sprue). *Digestion* 1986; 33:109–116.

123 Haffejee I E. Effect of oral folate on duration of acute infantile diarrhoea. *Lancet* 1988; ii:334–335.

124 Albert M J, Rajan D P & Mathan V I. *In vitro* susceptibility to metronidazole of bacteria from the small intestine of tropical sprue patients. *Indian J Med Res* 1984; 79:333–336.

125 Glynn J. Tropical sprue—its aetiology and pathogenesis. *J R Soc Med* 1988; 79:599–606.

126 Grove D I. Strongyloidiasis: a conundrum for gastroenterologists. *Gut* 1994; 35:437–440.

127 Palmer K R, Patil D H, Basra N G S, Riordan J F & Silk D B A. Abdominal tuberculosis in urban Britain—a common disease. *Gut* 1985; 26:1296–1305.

128 Tandon R K. Abdominal tuberculosis. In Bouchier I A D, Allan R N, Hodgson H J F & Keighley M R B (eds). *Gastroenterology: Clinical Science and Practice,* 2nd edn. London: W B Saunders, 1993:1459–1468.

129 Rambaud J-C & Ruskoné-Fourmestraux A. Small intestinal lymphomas: immunoproliferative small intestinal disease, α-chain disease and Mediterranean lymphomas. In Bouchier I A D, Allan R N, Hodgson H J F & Keighley M R B (eds) *Gastroenterology: Clinical Science and Practice,* 2nd edn. London: W B Saunders, 1993:636–643.

130 Dossetor J F B & White H C. Protein-losing enteropathy and malabsorption in acute measles enteritis. *BMJ* 1975; 2:592–593.

131 McKenzie D, Hansen J D L & Becker W. Herpes simplex virus infection: dissemination in association with malnutrition. *Arch Dis Child* 1959; 34:250–256.

132 Agus S G, Dolin R, Wyatt R G et al. Acute infectious non-bacterial gastroenteritis: intestinal histopathology. *Ann Intern Med* 1973; 79:18–25.

133 Conrad M E, Schwartz F D & Young A A. Infectious hepatitis—a generalised disease. *Am J Med* 1964; 37:789–801.

134 Schreiber D S, Blacklow N R & Trier J S. The intestinal lesion of the proximal small intestine in acute infectious nonbacterial gastroenteritis. *N Engl J Med* 1973; 288:1318–1323.

135 McCormack J G. Clinical features of rotavirus gastroenteritis. *J Infect* 1982; 4:167–174.

136 Schoub B D. Enteric adenoviruses and rotaviruses in infantile gastroenteritis in developing countries. *Lancet* 1981; ii:925.

137 Telch J, Shephard R W, Butler D G et al. Intestinal glucose transport in acute viral enteritis in piglets. *Clin Sci* 1981; 61:29–34.

138 Baker S J, Mathan M, Mathan V I et al. Chronic enterocyte infection with cornavirus. One possible cause of the syndrome of tropical sprue? *Dig Dis Sci* 1982; 27:1039–1043.

139 Brown D W G, Selvakumar R, Daniel D J & Mathan V I. Prevalence of neutralising antibodies to Berne virus in animals and humans in Vellore, South India. *Arch Virol* 1988; 98:267–269.

140 Lindenbaum J. Malabsorption during and after recovery from acute intestinal infection. *BMJ* 1965; ii:326–329.

141 Echeverria P, Verhaert L, Ulyangco C V et al. Antimicrobial resistance and enterotoxin production among isolates of *Escherichia coli* in the Far East. *Lancet* 1978; ii:589–592.

142 Boedeker E C. Enterocyte adherence of *Escherichia coli*: its relation to diarrhoeal disease. *Gastroenterology* 1982; 83:489–492.

143 Editorial. Microbial adhesion, colonisation and virulence. *Lancet* 1981; ii:508–510.

144 Editorial. Mechanisms in enteropathogenic *Escherichia coli* diarrhoea. *Lancet* 1983; i:1254–1256.

145 Rutter J M, Burrows M R, Sellwood R & Gibbons R A. A genetic basis for resistance to enteric disease caused by *Escherichia coli*. *Nature* 1975; 257:135–136.

146 Rothbaum J C. A clinicopathologic study of enterocyte-adherent *Escherichia coli*: a cause of protracted diarrhoea in infants. *Gastroenterology* 1982; 83:441–454.

147 Iushchuk N D & Abdullaev S. Sostoianie vsasyvatel'noi funktsii tonkoi kishki pri sal'monelleze u detei. *Pediatriia* 1981; 7:23–24.

148 Mandal B K. *Salmonella typhi* and other salmonellas. *Gut* 1994; 35:726–728.

149 Blaser M J & Reller L B. Campylobacter enteritis. *N Engl J Med* 1981; 305:1444–1452.

150 Editorial. Campylobacter enteritis. *Lancet* 1982; ii:1437–1438.

151 Holt P E. Role of *Campylobacter* spp in human and animal disease: a review. *J R Soc Med* 1981; 74:437–440.

152 Murrell T G C & Walker P D. The pigbel story of Papua New Guinea. *Trans R Soc Trop Med Hyg* 1991; 85:119–122.

153 Murrell T G C. Pigbel disease in Papua New Guinea: an ancient disease rediscovered. *Int J Epidemiol* 1983; 12:211–214.

154 Gillon J, Andre C, Descos L et al. Changes in mucosal immunoglobulin-containing cells in patients with giardiasis before and after treatment. *J Infect* 1982; 5:67–72.

155 Vega-Franco L, Alvarez E L, Romo G & Bernal R M. Adsorción de proteinas en niños con giardiasis. *Bol Med Hosp Infant Mex* 1982; 39:19–22.

156 Farthing M J G. *Giardia lamblia*. In Farthing M J G & Keusch G T (eds) *Enteric Infection: Mechanisms, Manifestations and Management*. London: Chapman & Hall, 1988:397–413.

157 Jokipii L & Jokipii A M M. Treatment of giardiasis: comparative evaluation of ornidazole and tinidazole as a single oral dose. *Gastroenterology* 1982; 83:399–404.

158 Sloper K S, Dourmashkin R R, Bird R B et al. Chronic malabsorption due to cryptosporidium in a child with immunoglobulin deficiency. *Gut* 1982; 23:80–82.

159 Cook G C. Parasitic infection. In Booth C C & Neale G (eds) *Disorders of the Small Intestine*. Oxford: Blackwell, 1985:283–298.

160 Crosby W H. The deadly hookworm: why did the Puerto-Ricans die? *Arch Intern Med* 1987; 147:577–578.

161 Bunyaratvej S, Bunyawongwiroj P & Nitiyanant P. Human intestinal sarcosporidiosis: report of six cases. *Am J Trop Med Hyg* 1982; 31:36–41.

162 Cosnett J E. The origins of intravenous fluid therapy. *Lancet* 1989; i:768–771.

163 Sheehy T W. Origins of intravenous fluid therapy. *Lancet* 1989; i:1081.

164 Collins B J, van Loon F P L, Molla A et al. Gastric emptying of oral rehydration solutions in acute cholera. *J Trop Med Hyg* 1989; 92:290–294.

165 Avery M E & Snyder J D. Oral therapy for acute diarrhea: the underused simple solution. *N Engl J Med* 1990; 323:891–894.

166 Johnson S, Echeverria P, Taylor D N et al. Enteritis necroticans among Khmer children at an evacuation site in Thailand. *Lancet* 1987; ii:496–500.

167 Lawrence G W, Lehmann D, Anian G et al. Impact of active immunisation against enteritis necroticans in Papua New Guinea. *Lancet* 1990; 336:1165–1167.

168 Murtaza A, Khan S R, Butt K S, Finkel Y & Aperia A. Paralytic ileus, a serious complication in acute diarrhoeal disease among infants in developing countries. *Acta Paediatr Scand* 1989; 78:701–705.

169 Hoffman S H. Tropical medicine and the acute abdomen. *Emerg Med Clin North Am* 1989; 7:591–609.

170 Gopi V K, Joseph T P & Varma K K. Acute intestinal obstruction. *Indian Pediatr* 1989; 26:525–530.

171 Archampong E Q. Tropical diseases of the small bowel. *World J Surg* 1985; 9:887–896.

172 Ryan C A, Hargrett-Bean N T & Blake P A. *Salmonella typhi* infections in the United States, 1975–1984: increasing role of foreign travel. *Rev Infect Dis* 1989; 11:1–8.

173 Weeramanthri T S, Corrah P T, Mabey D C W & Greenwood B M. Clinical experience with enteric fever in The Gambia, West Africa 1981–1986. *J Trop Med Hyg* 1989; 92:272–275.

174 Thisyakorn U, Mansuwan P & Taylor D N. Typhoid and paratyphoid fever in 192 hospitalized children in Thailand. *Am J Dis Child* 1987; 141:862–865.

175 Cook G C. Management of typhoid. *Trop Doc* 1985; 15:154–159.

176 Gibney E J. Typhoid perforation. *Br J Surg* 1989; 76:887–889.

177 Meier D E, Imediegwu O O & Tarpley J L. Perforated typhoid enteritis: operative experience with 108 cases. *Am J Surg* 1989; 157:423–427.

178 Rubin C M E & Fairhurst J J. Life-threatening haemorrhage from typhoid fever. *Br J Radiol* 1988; 61:415–416.

179 Raj S M, Sivakumaran S & Vijayakumari S.

Morbidity due to intestinal helminthiasis. *Lancet* 1990; 336:811–812.

180 Adams A A, Beeh J L & Wekell M M. Health risks of salmon sushi. *Lancet* 1990; 336:1328.

181 Cook G C. *Parasitic Disease in Clinical Practice.* London: Springer, 1990:272.

182 Hepburn N C. Aetiology of eosinophilic enteritis. *Lancet* 1990; 336:571.

183 Prociv P & Croese J. Human eosinophilic enteritis caused by dog hookworm *Ancylostoma caninum*. *Lancet* 1990; 335:1299–1302.

184 Anayi S & Al-Nasiri N. Acute mesenteric ischaemia caused by *Schistosoma mansoni* infection. *BMJ* 1987; 294:1197.

185 Radomyos P, Chobchuanchom A & Tungtrongchitr A. Intestinal perforation due to *Macracanthorhynchus hirudinaceus* infection in Thailand. *Trop Med Parasitol* 1989; 40:476–477.

186 Bannerman C & Manzur A Y. Fluctuating jaundice and intestinal bleeding in a 6-year-old girl with fascioliasis. *Trop Geogr Med* 1986; 38:429–431.

187 Acheson D W K, Farthing M J G & Keusch G T. Shigellosis. In Bouchier I A D, Allan R N, Hodgson H J F & Keighley M R B (eds) *Gastroenterology: Clinical Science and Practice,* 2nd edn. London: W B Saunders, 1993:1358–1363.

188 Acheson D W K & Keusch G T. The shigella paradigm and colitis due to enterohaemorrhagic *Escherichia coli*. *Gut* 1994; 35:872–874.

189 Zaidman I. Intestinal amoebiasis. In Bouchier I A D, Allan R N, Hodgson H J F & Keighley M R B (eds) *Gastroenterology: Clinical Science and Practice,* 2nd edn. London: W B Saunders, 1993:1451–1459.

190 Ravdin J I. Diagnosis of invasive amoebiasis—time to end the morphology era. *Gut* 1994; 35:1018–1021.

191 Williams N S. Malignant tumours. In Bouchier I A D, Allan R N, Hodgson H J F & Keighley M R B (eds) *Gastroenterology: Clinical Science and Practice,* 2nd edn. London: W B Saunders, 1993:856–882.

192 Fielding L & Padmanabhan A. Clinical features of colorectal cancer. In Misiewicz J J, Pounder R E & Venables C W (eds) *Diseases of the Gut and Pancreas,* 2nd edn. Oxford: Blackwell, 1994:877–892.

193 Langman M J S. Inflammatory bowel disease: incidence, epidemiology and genetics. In Bouchier I A D, Allan R N, Hodgson H J F & Keighley M R B (eds) *Gastroenterology: Clinical Science and Practice,* 2nd edn. London: W B Saunders, 1993:1067–1075.

194 Rhodes J M & Tsai H H. Aetiology and pathogenesis. In Bouchier I A D, Allan R N, Hodgson H J F & Keighley M R B (eds) *Gastroenterology: Clinical Science and Practice,* 2nd edn. London: W B Saunders, 1993:1075–1091.

195 Misiewicz J J, Pounder R E & Venables C W (eds). *Disease of the Gut and Pancreas,* 2nd edn. Oxford: Blackwell, 1994:675–804.

196 Schumacher G, Kollberg B, Ljunoh Å. Inflammatory bowel disease presenting as travellers' diarrhoea. *Lancet* 1993; 345:241–242.

197 Thomson J P S & Keighley M R B. Haemorrhoids. In Bouchier I A D, Allan R N, Hodgson H J F & Keighley M R B (eds) *Gastroenterology: Clinical Science and Practice,* 2nd edn. London: W B Saunders, 1993:915–922.

198 Heaton K W. Irritable bowel syndrome. In Bouchier I A D, Allan R N, Hodgson H J F & Keighley M R B (eds) *Gastroenterology: Clinical Science and Practice,* 2nd edn. London: W B Saunders, 1993:1512–1522.

199 Holdsworth C D. Irritable bowel syndrome. In Misiewicz J J, Pounder R E & Venables C W (eds) *Diseases of the Gut and Pancreas,* 2nd edn. Oxford: Blackwell, 1994:921–930.

200 Cook G C. *Enterobius vermicularis* infection. *Gut* 1994; 35:1159–1162.

201 Ravdin J I. Intentional disease caused by *Entamoeba histolytica*. In Ravdin J I (ed.) *Amebiasis: Human Infection by Entamoeba histolytica*. New York: Churchill Livingstone, 1988:495–510.

202 Ellyson J H, Bezmalinovic Z, Parks S N & Lewis F R. Necrotizing amebic colitis: a frequently fatal complication. *Am J Surg* 1986; 152:21–26.

203 Shukla V K, Roy S K, Vaidya M P & Mehrotra M L. Fulminant amebic colitis. *Dis Colon Rectum* 1986; 29:398–401.

204 Parsonnet J, Greene K D, Gerber A R, Tauxe R V, Aguilar O J V & Blake P A. *Shigella dysenteriae* type 1 infections in US travellers to Mexico. *Lancet* 1989; ii:543–545.

205 Otu A A. Tropical surgical emergencies: acute appendicitis. *Trop Geogr Med* 1989; 41:118–122.

206 Gupta S C, Gupta A K, Keswani N K, Singh P A, Tripathy A K & Krishna V. Pathology of tropical appendicitis. *J Clin Pathol* 1989; 42:1169–1172.

207 Zimmermann J-M, de Graeve B, Coblence J-F & Colonna M-A. Attitude thèrapeutique actuelle devant le volvulus du colon pelvien en milieu tropical. *Méd Trop* 1989; 49:371–374.

208 Wilson A P R, Ridgway G L, Sarner M, Boulos P B, Brook B C & Cook G C. Toxic dilatation of the colon in shigellosis. *BMJ* 1990; 301:1325–1326.

209 Gradon J D & Lutwick L I. Toxic dilation and amebiasis. *Am J Gastroenterol* 1988; 83:206–207.

210 Cook G C. Anorectal infections in relation to tropical exposure. In Demling L & Frühmorgan P (eds) *Non-Neoplastic Diseases of the Anorectum*. Dordrecht: Kluwer, 1992:187–226.

211 McIntyre N, Benhamou J-P, Bircher J, Rizzetto M & Rodes J (eds). Viral hepatitis. In *Oxford Textbook of Hepatology*. Oxford: Oxford University Press, 1991:529–629.

212 McIntyre N, Benhamou J-P, Bircher J, Rizzetto M & Rodes J (eds). Hepatitis in other systemic viruses In *Oxford Textbook of Hepatology*. Oxford: Oxford University Press, 1991:630–655.

213 McIntyre N, Benhamou J-P, Bircher J, Rizzetto M & Rodes J (eds). Bacterial, rickettsial, and spirochaetal infections. In *Oxford Textbook of Hepatology*. Oxford: Oxford University Press, 1991:656–688.

214 Da Dilva L C, Chieffi P P & Carrilho F J. Protozoal and helminthic diseases of the liver. In Prieto J, Rodés J & Shafritz D A (eds) *Hepatobiliary Disease*. Berlin: Springer, 1992:631–664.

215 McIntyre N, Benhamou J-P, Bircher J, Rizzetto M & Rodes J (eds) Infection of the liver. In *Oxford Textbook of Hepatology*. Oxford: Oxford University Press, 1991:696–739.

216 McIntyre N, Benhamou J-P, Bircher J, Rizzetto M & Rodes J (eds). Cirrhosis and chronic active hepatitis. In *Oxford Textbook of Hepatology*. Oxford: Oxford University Press, 1991:369–390.

217 Okuda K & Okuda H. Primary liver cell carcinoma. In McIntyre N, Benhamou J-P, Bircher J, Rizzetto M & Rodes J (eds) *Oxford Textbook of Hepatology*. Oxford: Oxford University Press, 1991:1019–1053.

218 McIntyre N, Benhamou J-P, Bircher J, Rizzetto M & Rodes J (eds). Alcoholic liver disease. In *Oxford Textbook of Hepatology*. Oxford: Oxford University Press, 1991:789–862.

219 Mowat A P. Paediatric liver disease. In McIntyre N, Benhamou J-P, Bircher J, Rizzetto M & Rodes J (eds) *Oxford Textbook of Hepatology*. Oxford: Oxford University Press, 1991:1287–1301.

220 Scheinberg I H & Sternlieb I. Is non-Indian childhood cirrhosis caused by excess dietary copper? *Lancet* 1994; 344:1002–1004.

221 Brissot P & Deugnier Y. Genetic haemochromatosis. In McIntyre N, Benhamou J-P, Bircher J, Rizzetto M & Rodes J (eds) *Oxford Textbook of Hepatology*. Oxford: Oxford University Press, 1991:948–958.

222 Gordeuk V R. Bantu siderosis. *Lancet* 1986; i:1310.

223 Valla D & Benhamou J-P. Disorders of the hepatic veins and venules. In McIntyre N, Benhamou J-P, Bircher J, Rizzetto M & Rodes J (eds) *Oxford Textbook of Hepatology*. Oxford: Oxford University Press, 1991:1004–1011.

224 McIntyre N, Benhamou J-P, Bircher J, Rizzetto M & Rodes J (eds). Portal hypertension and gastrointestinal bleeding. In *Oxford Textbook of Hepatology*. Oxford: Oxford University Press, 1991:391–426.

225 Cook G C. Hepatic structure and function in experimental and human malaria. In Bianchi L, Gerok W, Maier K-P & Dienhardt F (eds) *Infectious Diseases of the Liver (Falk Symposium 54)*. Dordrecht: Kluwer, 1990:191–213.

226 Editorial. The A to F of viral hepatitis. *Lancet* 1990; 336:1158–1160.

227 Zakaria S, Goldsmith R S, Kamel M A & El-Raziky E H. The etiology of acute hepatitis in adults in Egypt. *Trop Geogr Med* 1988; 40:285–292.

228 Pal S R & Prasad S R. Delta virus infections in and around Chandigarh, Northern India: evidence for endemicity. *Trop Geogr Med* 1987; 39:123–125.

229 Khuroo M S, Zargar S A, Mahajan R, Javid G & Lai R. An epidemic of hepatitis D in the foothills of the Himalayas in South Kashmir. *J Hepatol* 1988; 7:151–156.

230 Ramalingaswami V & Purcell R H. Waterborne non-A, non-B hepatitis. *Lancet* 1988; i:571–573.

231 Zuckerman A J. Hepatitis E virus: the main cause of enterically transmitted non-A, non-B hepatitis. *BMJ* 1990; 300:1475–1476.

232 Gupta H, Joshi Y K & Tandon B N. An enzyme-linked immunoassay for the possible detection of non-A, non-B viral antigen in patients with epidemic viral hepatitis. *Liver* 1988; 8:111–115.

233 Zuckerman A J. The elusive hepatitis C virus: a cause of parenteral non-A, non-B hepatitis. *BMJ* 1989; 299:871–873.

234 Gróza S, Delić D, Žerjav S, Jovanović R & Bujko M. Recovery from herpes simplex virus type-1 hepatitis in a female adult. *Klin Wochenschr* 1988; 66:796–798.

235 Asano Y, Yoshikawa T; Suga S et al. Fatal fulminant hepatitis in an infant with human herpesvirus-6 infection. *Lancet* 1990; 335:862–863.

236 Boulos M, Segurado A A C & Shiroma M. Severe yellow fever with a 23-day survival. *Trop Geogr Med* 1988; 40:356–358.

237 Holmes G P, McCormick J B, Trock S C et al. Lassa fever in the United States: investigation of a case and new guidelines for management. *N Engl J Med* 1990; 323:1120–1123.

238 Lucia H L, Coppenhaver D H, Harrison R L & Baron S. The effect of an arenavirus infection on liver morphology and function. *Am J Trop Med Hyg* 1990; 43:93–98.

239 Khosla S N, Singh R, Singh G P & Trehan V K. The spectrum of hepatic injury in enteric fever. *Am J Gastroenterol* 1988; 83:413–416.

240 MacGregor F B, Abernethy V E, Dahabra S, Cobden I & Hayes P C. Hepatotoxicity of herbal remedies. *BMJ* 1989; 299:1156–1157.

241 Tandon B N, Joshi Y K & Tandon M. Acute liver failure: experience with 145 patients. *J Clin Gastroenterol* 1986; 8:664–668.

242 Sarin S K, Chari S, Sundaram K R, Ahuja R K, Anand B S & Broor S L. Young v adult cirrhotics: a prospective, comparative analysis of the clinical profile, natural course and survival. *Gut* 1988; 29:101–107.

243 Abdel-Wahab M F, Esmat G, Milad M, Abdel-Razek S & Strickland G T. Characteristic sonographic pattern of schistosomal hepatic fibrosis. *Am J Trop Med Hyg* 1989; 40:72–76.

244 Maharaj B, Bhoora I G, Patel A & Maharajah J. Ultrasonography and scintigraphy in liver disease in developing countries. *Lancet* 1989; ii:853–856.

245 Editorial. Clinical ultrasound in developing countries. *Lancet* 1990; 336:1225–1226.

246 Pande G K, Reddy V M, Kar P et al. Operations

for portal hypertension due to extrahepatic obstruction: results and 10 year follow-up. *BMJ* 1987; 295:1115–1117.

247 Reed S L & Braude A I. Extraintestinal disease: clinical syndromes, diagnostic profile, and therapy. In Ravdin J I (ed.) *Amebiasis: Human Infection by Entamoeba histolytica.* New York: Churchill Livingstone, 1988; 511–532.

248 Lalla F de, Rizzardini G, Cairoli G A, Rinaldi E, Santoro D & Ostinelli A. Outbreak of amoebiasis in tourists returning from Thailand. *Lancet* 1988; ii:847.

249 Sargeaunt P G. Zymodemes of *Entamoeba histolytica.* In Ravdin J I (ed.). *Amebiasis: Human Infection by Entamoeba histolytica.* New York: Churchill Livingstone, 1988; 370–387.

250 Ahmed L, Rooby A E I, Kassem M I, Salama Z A & Strickland G T. Ultrasonography in the diagnosis and management of 52 patients with amebic liver abscess in Cairo. *Rev Infect Dis* 1990; 12:330–337.

251 Sharma M P, Rai R R, Acharya S K, Ray J C S & Tandom B N. Needle aspiration of amoebic liver abscess. *BMJ* 1989; 299: 1308–1309.

252 Freeman O, Akamaguna A & Jarikre L N. Amoebic liver abscess: the effect of aspiration on the resolution or healing time. *Ann Trop Med Parasitol* 1990; 84:281–287.

253 Singh J P & Kashyap A. A comparative evaluation of percutaneous catheter drainage for resistant amebic liver abscesses. *Am J Surg* 1989; 158:58–62.

254 Ken J G, van Sonnenberg E, Casola G, Christensen R & Polanski A M. Perforated amebic liver abscesses: successful percutaneous treatment. *Radiology* 1989; 170:195–197.

255 Barnes P F, De Cock K M, Reynolds T N & Ralls P W. A comparison of amebic and pyogenic abscess of the liver. *Medicine* 1987; 66:472–483.

256 Goh K L, Wong N W, Paramsothy M, Nojeg M & Somasundaram K. Liver abscess in the tropics: experience in the University Hospital, Kuala Lumpur. *Postgrad Med J* 1987; 63:551–554.

257 Bansal A S & Prabhakar P. Clinical aspects of pyogenic liver abscess: the University Hospital of the West Indies experience. *J Trop Med Hyg* 1988; 91:87–93.

258 Berger L A & Osborne D R. Treatment of pyogenic liver abscesses by percutaneous needle aspiration. *Lancet* 1982; i:132–134.

259 Herbert D A, Fogel D A, Rothman J, Wilson S, Simmons F & Ruskin J. Pyogenic liver abscesses: successful non-surgical therapy. *Lancet* 1982; i:134–136.

260 Bowers E D, Robison D J & Doberneck R C. Pyogenic liver abscess. *World J Surg* 1990; 14:128–132.

261 McCorkell S J & Niles N L. Pyogenic liver abscesses: another look at medical management. *Lancet* 1985; i:803–806.

262 Sheen I S, Chien C S C, Lin D & & Liaw Y F. Resolution of liver abscesses: comparison of pyogenic and amebic liver abscesses. *Am J Trop Med Hyg* 1989; 40:384–389.

263 Pineiro-Carrero V M & Andres J M. Morbidity and mortality in children with pyogenic liver abscess. *Am J Dis Child* 1989; 143:1424–1427.

264 Morris D L. Echinococcus of the liver. *Gut* 1994; 35:1517–1518.

265 Strickland G T. Gastrointestinal manifestations of schistosomiasis. *Gut* 1994; 35:1334–1337.

266 Castillo C F del, Richter J M & Warshaw A L. Chronic pancreatitis. In Bouchier I A D, Allan R N, Hodgson H J F & Keighley M R B (eds) *Gastroenterology: Clinical Science and Practice,* 2nd edn. London: W B Saunders, 1993:1615–1634.

267 Khuroo M S, Zarger S A & Mahajan R. Hepatobiliary and pancreatic ascariasis in India. *Lancet* 1990; 335:1503–1506.

268 Wong R K H, Peura D A, Mutter M L, Heit H A, Birns M T & Johnson L F. Hemobilia and liver flukes in a patient from Thailand. *Gastroenterology* 1985; 88:1958–1963.

269 Tamimi T M, Wosornu L, Al-Khozaim A & Abdul-Ghani A. Increased cholecystectomy rates in Saudi Arabia. *Lancet* 1990; 336:1235–1237.

270 Hearne S E, Whigham T E & Brady C E. Pancreatitis and typhoid fever. *Am J Med* 1989; 86:471–473.

CHAPTER 4

RESPIRATORY PROBLEMS IN THE TROPICS

M. E. Molyneux

Most clinicians in the tropics have to deal with a large number of patients with chest complaints, and must do so without the armamentarium of diagnostic devices available to those working in richer nations. Fortunately a great deal can be achieved through careful history-taking and physical examination, judicious choice of which tests to do and (especially) which not to do, and a thorough knowledge of which diseases are important in the patient's environment.

In an average outpatient department, 20–40% of patients have come with respiratory complaints, and 20–30% of hospital medical admissions are for disorders predominantly affecting the lungs. Many patients are suffering from conditions such as chronic obstructive airways disease (COAD) that might occur anywhere in the world; others have diseases that are much more common in, or peculiar to, tropical areas, e.g. pulmonary schistosomiasis; and within the tropics patterns differ greatly from one region to another.

The acquired immune deficiency syndrome (AIDS) epidemic has had a major impact on the pattern of respiratory disease in the tropics, particularly in its effect on the incidence and manifestations of tuberculosis. The possibility of underlying human immunodeficiency virus (HIV) infection must influence the interpretation of symptoms and signs in patients with pulmonary problems.

Because tuberculosis is so common throughout the world, especially among HIV-infected individuals, many people with other causes of chronic cough suffer unwarranted lengthy therapeutic trials of antituberculous drugs. The therapeutic trial for 'possible tuberculosis' is sometimes sensible, but must only be embarked upon when other diagnoses have been carefully sought. Of 430 patients with 'unresponsive pulmonary tuberculosis' referred from district hospitals to a tuberculosis unit in South Africa, over half did not have tuberculosis at all (T. F. B. Collins, personal communication). The correct diagnoses in these varied, and included: non-tuberculous bronchiectasis, lung abscess, foreign body, congenital cystic lung, hydatid disease, mitral stenosis, bronchial carcinoma and sarcoidosis.

In a busy clinic a quick diagnosis may have to be made for patients with mild acute disease, but in any who are very sick or who have recurrent, chronic or unresponsive symptoms a full clinical assessment is essential.

The history may give useful clues. Look for previous events or current symptoms that might suggest HIV-related disease. Ask about previous antituberculosis treatment and the adequacy thereof: this may not be mentioned by the patient and is easily neglected by the doctor. If there is a history of tuberculosis, it would help to know whether it was proven tuberculosis or merely suspected. Look for any history of an episode of unconsciousness preceding the symptoms, e.g. general anaesthesia, epilepsy, alcoholic coma, trauma; inhalation at such a time is a common cause of localized pulmonary infection or lung abscess. Enquire about place and conditions of work, with particular emphasis on dusts and the relation of symptoms to the time of work. Work in mines, even in the distant past, may have been responsible for fibrotic lung disease. A patient who works with animals or birds may be exposed to zoonotic diseases that sometimes have a pulmonary component: tularaemia, Q fever, leptospirosis or psittacosis. Smoking has increased in many countries (see section on smoking, below) and should be carefully asked about: it may be responsible for or exacerbate the patient's illness. Remember that bronchial asthma and left ventricular failure may each give rise to cough as the major symptom, or the only one the patient mentions; other clues if sought will usually point to the diagnosis. Mitral stenosis is much more common in developing than in industrial countries. In a patient with cough, associated symptoms may help with diagnosis or management: haemoptysis, breathlessness, night sweats, weight loss. In areas where gnathostomiasis occurs, enquire about eating habits; where schistosomiasis is prevalent consider the life style and likelihood of contact with schistosomal water.

The environmental or family context may suggest important possibilities. The patient's life style may indicate a high risk of HIV infection. Pneumonic plague is contracted by inhalation from a close contact dying of septicaemic plague. Ask about contacts known to have tuberculosis, but also about any close contact known to have died recently of undiagnosed disease—tuberculosis is a strong possibility.

In the *physical examination* note the general condition. Look for features suggestive of immunosuppression: current or recent herpes zoster, oral candidiasis, and wasting. Look carefully for evidence of cardiac or abdominal abnormalities. It is easy to miss pericardial constriction or effusion, which may mimic or complicate pulmonary disease. Right ventricular hypertrophy may develop in chronic pulmonary disease; it is sometimes a feature of pulmonary schistosomiasis. Palpable lymph nodes in the axillae or supraclavicular fossae may provide a source of diagnostic material and should therefore be sought routinely and carefully. Because so many patients have advanced disease by the time they reach medical attention, a variety of physical signs are encountered that are seldom seen in industrialized countries. Abnormalities of chest movement or shape and mediastinal (tracheal) shift may indicate contraction from chronic fibrosis within the chest. A hydropneumothorax or pyopneumothorax can be identified clinically by the succussion splash and shifting dullness (percussion over the fifth intercostal space anteriorly is dull with the patient erect, and hollow when supine). Amphoric breathing and post-tussive crackles may be heard over a large cavity. Amoebic liver abscess may present as cough and haemoptysis—which may be acute or chronic; this possibility should be deliberately looked for by palpating for intercostal tenderness over the right lower chest (the liver below the costal margin may be non-tender and is sometimes not palpable, especially when an abscess has discharged some of its contents upwards). A diagnosis of lung abscess can often be made from the characteristic pungent fetor that may fill a ward. Hepatosplenomegaly in a schistosomal area or the presence of a caput medusae increase the possibility of schistosomal lung disease and cor pulmonale. COAD is common everywhere; the characteristic physical signs should indicate the diagnosis, but remember that other pulmonary disease may be difficult to detect in the presence of COAD. In particular, any evidence of tuberculosis should be searched for carefully as the two conditions commonly coexist.

A number of *tests* can contribute to diagnosis and follow-up. HIV serology helps to clarify a suspected diagnosis of AIDS; but remember that not all clinical problems are attributable to HIV infection in seropositive individuals. A peak flowmeter provides an index of airways obstruction, both for diagnosis and for observing changes and response to treatment; a small portable version such as the Wright Peak Flow Mini-meter makes a useful addition to the doctor's bag, and there should be one on every ward. The mainstay of diagnosis in tuberculosis is microscopy of the stained sputum smear, but good sputum samples may yield a lot of other information. Note the quantity and appearance; microscopy may occasionally reveal larval helminths, *Paragonimus* ova, hydatid scolices or fungal hyphae (aspergilloma). Bacterial culture is of limited value because of the plentiful commensal flora in the pharynx. Culture for tubercle bacilli yields a delayed diagnosis in a small proportion of smear-negative subjects. In HIV-infected patients, pulmonary tuberculosis is more likely to be sputum-negative than in other people[1]. The likelihood of getting useful information from the sputum is proportional to the quality of sputum sampling. Improved samples can be obtained by physiotherapy or by initiating a deep cough by spraying the vocal cords with a fine saline spray or by injecting 1 ml of sterile saline direct into the trachea through a fine needle inserted between the thyroid and cricoid cartilages.

Chest radiographs are important but expensive. (In a poor country one chest radiograph may cost as much as the entire health budget for a year for four people.) They should therefore be used with discretion, and with a clear idea of what they can and cannot do. Never use a radiograph as a short cut to the correct diagnosis as it is highly susceptible to misinterpretation and is, anyway, often rendered unnecessary by proper clinical evaluation of the patient. Toman[2] has summarized several studies indicating how commonly one expert may differ from another (or from him- or herself on different occasions) in the interpretation of chest films. There is no point in taking a chest radiograph to demonstrate what is clearly deducible from clinical features, as in lobar pneumonia, massive pleural effusion or sputum-positive tuberculosis, unless there is a definite indication that the picture may contribute to management. Follow-up radiographs in a patient clinically improving on treatment for pneumonia or tuberculosis are rarely warranted. It is better to reserve radiography for circumstances in which it can be most useful, as in the management of pneumothorax or the investigation of unresolving pneumonia.

If available, fibreoptic bronchoscopy may provide useful information towards diagnosis in a number of circumstances. The instrument is expensive, but each procedure then costs almost nothing. A physician, surgeon or radiologist may quite readily acquire the ability to use it after a period of instruction by an expert. The instrument is valuable for identifying causes of local bronchial obstruction (including small foreign bodies, tumours, etc.), for obtaining secretions from a local site by brushings or lavage (e.g. to look for acid-fast bacilli in the sputum-negative patient) and for obtaining transbronchial lung biopsies (highly effective in identifying *Pneumocystis carinii* pneumonia, but less effective for tumours distant from the hilum). The value of fibreoptic bronchoscopy is limited by the quality of laboratory facilities which can be applied to fluid or tissues obtained. The instrument must be cleaned adequately after each investigation, to eliminate the risk of HIV transmission.

ACUTE LOBAR PNEUMONIA

Lobar pneumonia is common in all tropical countries and is a major cause of death, especially in children (see section on acute respiratory infection in children, below). Evidence suggests that bacterial pneumonias are often preceded by a viral infection that presumably alters the susceptibility of the host or damages local defence mechanisms. The circumstances of an individual's illness should be noted: 'primary' pneumonia occurs in the previously healthy, 'secondary' pneumonia as a complication of another disorder (e.g. structural defect) or circumstance (e.g. period of unconsciousness with aspiration or atelectasis). Note also the immune status of the host: the HIV-infected individual, the autosplenectomized sickler, the postsplenectomy patient, the pregnant woman, the alcoholic, the diabetic and the malnourished all have an increased susceptibility to bacterial infection(s).

The symptoms and signs of lobar pneumonia are well known but sometimes confusing. In early pneumonia, the diagnosis may have to be deduced from the symptoms and presence of fever, shallow tachypnoea and reduced chest movement, in the absence of any auscultatory signs. In one study in Africa it was shown that the site of consolidation could be more reliably predicted by the 'pointing sign' than by auscultation; the patient is asked to cough and point to the place where this causes pain. When pleurisy is diaphragmatic an abdominal cause may be suspected by patient or physician. In some populations a considerable proportion of patients with lobar pneumonia develops jaundice. This may be deep but usually fades rapidly with treatment of the pneumonia (more rapidly than jaundice fades in acute viral hepatitis). This jaundice of pneumonia is of mixed type (Chapter 3) and does not seem to be associated with pre-existing chronic liver disease or hepatitis B carrier status; in one study there was a significant association with glucose-6-phosphate dehydrogenase deficiency,[3] but others have not found this. Characteristic but minor changes in liver histology have been demonstrated.

Pneumococci and *Haemophilus influenzae* have been the most common bacterial agents identified in most studies of lobar pneumonia. The organism may be identified by blood culture in about one-third of patients, or by detecting bacterial antigen in blood or urine. Direct needle aspiration from consolidated lung improves the yield but there is a small risk of pneumothorax.

Other bacterial causes of lobar consolidation may be difficult to distinguish, on the basis of the clinical features, from pneumococcal disease, but may in some circumstances be suspected. In legionella pneumonia there may be mental confusion, diarrhoea or hypotension; hyponatraemia and haematuria are common. These features, together with failure to respond to initial antibiotic treatment, should indicate the possibility of this diagnosis, for which erythromycin is the drug of choice. The incidence of legionella pneumonia in the tropics is not yet well known but the propensity of the organism to multiply in water that is perpetually above a temperature of 25°C, and the fact that about a third of UK patients have acquired the infection after travel in southern Europe, suggests that *Legionella* may be responsible for more of the pneumonia occurring in the tropics than is generally recognized.

A proportion of pneumonias in any series proves to be due to *Mycoplasma pneumoniae*, although these organisms more commonly cause a mild upper respiratory tract infection. The illness cannot be distinguished from other pneumonias by clinical features, but may be suspected in the small percentage of patients who develop extrapulmonary complications, especially arthritis or haemolytic anaemia. Tetracycline is the drug of choice but erythromycin is also effective.

A severely ill patient may have staphylococcal pneumonia, in which multiple lung cavities may develop. Many such patients are assumed to have sputum-negative tuberculosis and are given antituberculous drugs. The severity of illness and the presence of scattered, small, thin-walled cavities may alert the clinician to the correct diagnosis, when cloxacillin or a cephalosporin may be appropriate treatment. Chloramphenicol is usually as effective and a lot less expensive.

It is important, in areas where tuberculosis is common, to remember that postprimary tuberculosis may present with a clinical syndrome indistinguishable from acute bacterial pneumonia. William Osler recognized this when working in Boston in 1900, where tuberculosis was as common as it is in many tropical areas today. He taught that every patient with lobar pneumonia should be considered to have tuberculosis until clinical progress proved otherwise. This advice is much more important today when specific therapy is available.

In some areas, particularly South-East Asia, melioidosis should be considered as a possible cause of both acute and of unresolving pneumonia, especially in the debilitated or immunocompromised. Appropriate media are needed to culture the organism and to indicate the correct therapy (see Chapter 51).

Viral pneumonia cannot reliably be distinguished clinically from bacterial: the latter may complicate upper respiratory tract viral infections, so that in both there may be preceding malaise, fever and upper respiratory symptoms. In children in particular so much pneumonia is viral that many prescriptions for antibiotics are unnecessary. Careful studies in various localities are needed to provide guidelines for routine therapy (see Chapter 36).

A diagnosis that may have to be considered in patients with cough and dyspnoea, especially in the context of malnutrition or any of the conditions associated with impaired immunity, is *P. carinii* pneumonia. This appears to be much less common as a manifestation of AIDS than is the case in North America or Europe,[4] but *P. carinii* has also been recognized as the cause of a proportion of cases of acute pneumonia in otherwise healthy children and as a cause of epidemic interstitial pneumonitis. The clinical features are non-specific: dry cough, fever and dyspnoea are usual; there are characteristically few signs on auscultation. Radiographs usually show scattered reticulonodular shadows in both lungs, especially around the hila, progressing to larger areas of consolidation, but the picture is very variable. Diagnosis is most reliably made by transbronchial biopsy through a fibreoptic bronchoscope, but promising methods of detecting antigen in sputum may lead to more rapid diagnosis and a better appreciation of the role of this agent in pneumonia in tropical communities. Co-trimoxazole is the treatment of choice, as it is safer than pentamidine, which may be tried if co-trimoxazole fails.

There is no generally applicable standard treatment for pneumonia. Once the particular circumstances of an individual's illness have been carefully assessed, a policy derived from local studies of aetiological agents and drug sensitivity patterns should be applied. In some areas, particularly Papua New Guinea and South Africa, pneumococci resistant to penicillin have become common enough to alter treatment policy. In a study in Papua New Guinea, chloramphenicol was found to be effective as a routine treatment for childhood pneumonia, and it was shown to be just as valuable alone as when combined with penicillin.[5] Whatever drug treatment is given, the patient should be carefully observed for response to treatment and for the development of any complications: lung abscess, empyema, or metastatic (including cerebral) abscess.

PLEURAL EFFUSION

Patients may develop symptoms only when a pleural effusion has become massive, with no detectable resonance on the affected side, and shift of the trachea and mediastinum towards the opposite side. Such huge effusions are quite common, especially in young adults with postprimary tuberculosis. There may be a history of pleuritic pain on the affected side some days or weeks before, and breathlessness has usually ensued only recently. In addition to the classical stony dullness on percussion, bronchial breathing is usually heard over the affected hemithorax, but it is quiet and distant, heard only when the patient breathes deeply, unlike the bronchial breathing of consolidation which usually augments quiet breath sounds. A careful examination is required to search for evidence of other disease and for abnormal lymph nodes. A sample of pleural fluid should be allowed to stand for half an hour on the bench: if a coagulum or 'web' appears the fluid is likely to be an exudate. The high protein content will be confirmed in the laboratory, but if this is not possible there is a simple bedside test that can indicate the approximate the protein content of the fluid. This test depends on the fact that there is a fairly close correlation between the specific gravity and protein content of effusion fluid (or serum). Having taken the fluid sample from the patient, expel one small drop of the fluid, from a height of about 1 cm, into a solution of copper sulphate. If the drop sinks to the bottom, it has a higher specific gravity than the copper sulphate; if it floats, it is of lower specific gravity. The copper sulphate solution, which can be used several times, must be prepared in such a concentration (2.37 g of $CuSO_4 5H_2O$ dried crystals dissolved in water to a volume of 100 ml) that its specific gravity is 1.016, because this is about the same as the specific gravity of an effusion containing 3.0–3.5 g/dl of protein. If the drop of fluid sinks, it is probably an exudate; if it floats it is probably a transudate. A test of this kind can only be a rough guide, but may help guide immediate decisions concerning further investigation or management.

When drawing fluid from an exudate it is wise to take a pleural biopsy at the same time, using an Abrams' needle. If two or three specimens of pleura are taken in different directions at the same site there is a 70% chance of making a histological diagnosis, which in the young is usually tuberculosis, and in older patients may be tuberculous or malignant disease. Removing one litre of fluid will allow the lung to expand and may relieve discomfort; this can be repeated on later occasions but it is unnecessary to attempt to remove it all. A tuberculous effusion will resolve with drug treatment. Occasionally an effusion can become loculated in an unusual site—such as the anterior part of a pleural space, and may be associated with persisting fever or localized pain; the fluid should be identified by careful percussion and auscultation, with radiographic help if necessary, as removing the effusion may abolish the symptoms.

BRONCHIAL ASTHMA

Bronchial asthma is common in the tropics and there are some differences in the pattern of disease from that seen in temperate countries. In a study in Nigeria[6] most adults with asthma had first developed symptoms in adult life; a minority of patients gave a history of rhinitis, and none had suffered from eczema; most patients suffered more at night than by day; about half could relate symptoms to exposure to house dust. In most studies nearly all patients have positive skin tests to one or more allergens, most commonly house dust mites[6,7] (such tests are also positive in a large proportion of the non-asthmatic population; control groups are essential in such studies). Where staffing allows, it can be useful to hold a regular asthma clinic[8] to which patients have ready access and at which good home therapy can be taught, problems discussed and drugs dependably supplied. Another value of such a clinic is that it can be the setting for good teaching on asthma for auxiliaries, students, nurses and doctors. Each patient should be assessed for possible precipitating factors or circumstances: season, time of day, exercise, dust, drugs (e.g. salicylates—present in innumerable mixtures and tablets available from grocery stores), animals, bedding. At a clinic all patients can be taught about the need for keeping home and bedding as clean as possible, about the dangers of smoking and the possible dangers of aspirin and other drugs, and the need for early treatment of attacks. Progress can be monitored by symptom indices and measurements of the peak flow rate.

Treatment should be appropriate to the frequency and severity of attacks, with β_2-agonists (salbutamol or terbutaline) as the first line for mild attacks; cromoglycate may be assessed for prophylactic efficacy over a period of weeks for those suffering frequent attacks; severe episodes can be usefully treated with short courses of oral corticosteroids (e.g. prednisolone 60 mg daily for 3–5 days) with nebulized β_2-agonists by inhalation initially. Long-term regular steroid treatment should rarely be necessary; if embarked upon the usual dangers must be considered; antimalarial and antituberculous prophylaxis may be warranted. Although aerosol inhalers are of great value in asthma, many patients find them difficult or impossible to use; they are expensive, and should only be dispensed to those patients who demonstrate that they can inhale properly from them. This requires painstaking teaching by clinic staff.

In some areas patients with cough or wheeze may have tropical pulmonary eosinophilia, in which gross eosinophilia and lung shadows on radiography are associated with a positive filarial serological fixation test; the condition improves rapidly with antifilarial treatment (see Chapter 70). This possibility should be looked for in the asthma clinic, especially in areas where *Wuchereria bancrofti* and *Brugia malayi* are common. The condition is uncommon in Africa, but a similar combination of cough, wheeze and eosinophilia may occur due to the migrating larval stages of *Ascaris*, hookworm or strongyloides infection (see Chapter 71).

HIV AND THE LUNGS (See also Chapter 12)

Pulmonary symptoms are common in AIDS, and in many patients they are the first clinical manifestation of the disease. Organisms causing opportunist infections include: mycobacterial, bacterial, fungal and viral agents. Of these, *Mycobacterium tuberculosis* is the most common in tropical settings: the incidence of clinical tuberculosis is greatly increased in the presence of HIV infection. Pulmonary tuberculosis in HIV-infected patients is more commonly diffuse, miliary or basal in its distribution than it is in patients without HIV infection. This fact makes the confirmation of the diagnosis difficult in many patients, and presumptive treatment is commonly necessary. Drug reactions occur with increased frequency in patients with HIV-related disease. Extrapulmonary tuberculosis is more common in patients with HIV infection than in others.

P. carinii may complicate immunosuppression caused by HIV infection, but appears to be a less common opportunist than it is in temperate countries.[4] Bacterial and fungal pneumonias may be the presenting complication in patients with HIV infection.[9] Both Kaposi's sarcoma and lymphomas may present with pulmonary symptoms, or may involve the lungs as disease progresses.[10] The contribution of lymphoid interstitial pneumonitis to disease in HIV-infected children remains to be evaluated.

Although a variety of parasites causes lung problems in the tropics (see below), these infections do not appear to be increased in frequency or altered in their clinical manifestations by concomitant HIV infection or AIDS.

Pulmonary complications in HIV-infected patients are discussed in more detail in Chapter 12.

SARCOIDOSIS

In many tropical countries sarcoidosis has never been identified. Studies in some areas suggest that the apparent dearth of cases may be due to the fact that most are misdiagnosed as sputum-negative tuberculosis or another chronic infection. In temperate countries Africans, West Indians and Asians have a much higher incidence of sarcoidosis than do Caucasians living in the same vicinity. In one UK study West Indians had an incidence of sarcoidosis that was over 14 times that in Caucasians living in the same part of London.[11] Caucasians are also found to have less severe disease, with fewer systemic manifestations, than the other ethnic groups. Nevertheless the condition remains uncommon in the tropics; a special unit in Delhi has detected increasing numbers of cases in recent years,[12] but the total number identified in the entire country in the years 1957–1982 was only 90. The possibility of sarcoidosis should be considered in patients with unresolving lung disease, especially if there are accompanying extrathoracic features such as iridocyclitis, lymphadenopathy, central nervous system complications or hypercalcaemia.

PULMONARY PROBLEMS IN COMMON PARASITIC DISEASES

Those working in a tropical area, or having to deal with travellers, must be aware of pulmonary aspects of most of the common parasitic diseases; lung involvement may complicate other more usual features of those infections, or may sometimes be the major mode of presentation. In some parasitic diseases the lung is the predominant territory involved: paragonimiasis (see Chapter 73) must be considered in patients with cough, haemoptysis and cavitating lung disease, often mistaken for tuberculosis; hydatid cysts (see Chapter 75) may produce a variety of lung problems as a result of mechanical compression of intrathoracic structures. In a number of helminth infections (hookworm, *Ascaris*, *Strongyloides*) a larval stage of the parasite migrates through the lungs, when it may cause cough, fever, dyspnoea and sometimes wheeze or haemoptysis (see Chapter 71).

The severity of the illness probably depends on how many larvae are migrating at one time; the classical self-experiment of Koino[13] illustrated this. He swallowed 2000 viable *Ascaris* eggs, and within a week suffered a severe illness with high fever, dyspnoea, cyanosis, severe cough and frothy, blood-stained sputum lasting for 7 days. There was eosinophilia, and many *Ascaris* larvae were recovered from his sputum. It would be unusual for such a large number of eggs to be ingested simultaneously in natural circumstances. In schistosomia-sis, especially where portal hypertension has led to venous shunts bypassing the liver, eggs may be deposited in pulmonary capillaries and arterioles, eliciting a granulomatous reaction resulting either in pulmonary hypertension or the accumulation of large masses of granulation tissue (see Chapter 72).

Malaria may be complicated by pulmonary problems; cough is not uncommonly a symptom, even in moderately severe malaria, and in severe *P. falciparum* malaria pulmonary problems have been reported in 5–15% of cases. Although pulmonary oedema due to therapeutic fluid overload, or bronchopneumonia complicating deep coma, may occur, a more specific malarial lesion indistinguishable from adult respiratory distress syndrome has been recognized in which there is septal oedema, endothelial cell swelling and hyaline membrane formation within the alveoli (see Chapter 61). In children in endemic areas, acidosis with resultant tachypnoea is common in severe malaria, but respiratory distress syndrome is rarely seen.

SMOKING IN THE TROPICS

Over 100 developing countries have a tobacco industry that contributes to revenue, employment and trade. The end-product is, however, increasingly finding its way back to the countries of origin, where the practice of smoking has recently increased steadily. This increase has been estimated at 32% in Africa and 24% in South America between 1970 and 1980, but is much greater within certain sections of the population. In Nigeria 41% of adult men smoke. Particularly alarming are figures from secondary schools: 30–40% of pupils in some areas have been found to be regular smokers. Smoking-related diseases appear to have increased: the incidence of carcinoma of the bronchus in China increased sixfold between 1970 and 1980, and emphysema and lung cancer are rapidly becoming more common in Nigeria, India and Malaysia. Because of the delayed effects of smoking a great increase of these and other smoking-related diseases can be expected within the coming decade.

ACUTE RESPIRATORY INFECTION IN CHILDREN (See also Chapter 15)

Respiratory diseases, particularly bacterial pneumonia, tuberculosis, measles and pertussis, are major causes of death throughout the world. Children are at particular risk: at least two million and probably over five million die of respiratory infections every year. Only recently have these problems begun to receive the kind of attention that has been devoted to diarrhoeal disease, malaria and malnutrition—the other major killers in children.

The urban child, whether in the tropics or non-tropics, suffers an average of 5–8 episodes of acute respiratory infection per year. Of these, lower respiratory infections are the most lethal, particularly in the tropics where the risk of death from pneumonia in children aged 1–4 years has been recorded as 50 times as great as in comparable groups in the USA and Canada.[14] Malnourished children are at special risk; in a study in Costa Rica the mortality of acute respiratory infection was 12 times higher in malnourished infants than in those of normal weight.[15]

Upper respiratory infections are usually viral, but

the causative agent is rarely identified. Upper respiratory viral infections may progress to viral pneumonia or may be complicated by bacterial pneumonia. Of the responsible viruses, measles, respiratory syncytial virus and the influenza and parainfluenza viruses are numerically most important. The most common bacteria causing pneumonia are *Streptococcus pneumoniae* and *Haemophilus influenzae*, but staphylococci are important, especially in infants and when complicating measles or influenza. In about half of all cases of bacterial pneumonia there is clinical or serological evidence of a preceding virus infection.

Because of the enormous mortality from acute respiratory infection, the World Health Organization has urged that each nation should embark on a national programme aimed at its study and control, particularly in children.[14] The programme should include a study of aetiological agents and their relation to clinical disease pattern and prognosis—important in deciding on vaccination policies. From studies of local disease patterns, clinicians should try to draw up standard treatment and referral flow charts for the use of primary health workers and rural hospital staff, in an attempt to improve upon the currently disastrous failure to save the lives of millions of children with treatable disease. Several simple measures, in addition to clinical ones might have an important impact: the continued promotion of breast feeding, which is known to halve the risk of respiratory syncitial virus infection in infants;[16] timely vaccination in infancy against tuberculosis, measles, diphtheria, and pertussis; special vigilance for those children at greatest risk of death from respiratory infection (those with low birth weight, diarrhoeal disease and malnutrition); and insistence on continued or increased hydration and feeding during respiratory illness. Each locality will have to decide at what level staff should be allowed to give antibiotic treatment and what that treatment should be, in the light of bacterial agents and their drug sensitivities known to prevail locally.

Meanwhile there is an urgent need for new and additional vaccines, particularly against respiratory syncytial virus, pneumococci and *Haemophilus influenzae*. These too will need effective primary health and maternal child health services if they are to be deployed effectively.

REFERENCES

1 Pitchenik A E, Fertel D S & Bloch A B. Mycobacterial disease: epidemiology, diagnosis, treatment and prevention. *Clin Chest Med* 1988; 9:425–441.

2 Toman K. *Tuberculosis: Case Findings and Chemotherapy: Questions and Answers*. Geneva: WHO, 1979.

3 Tugwell P. Glucose-6-phosphate-dehydrogenase deficiency in Nigerians with jaundice associated with lobar pneumonia. *Lancet* 1973; i:968–970.

4 Elvin K M, Lumbwe C M, Luo N P et al. *Pneumocystis carinii* is not a major cause of pneumonia in HIV infected patients in Lusaka, Zambia. *Trans R Soc Trop Med Hyg* 1989; 83:553–559.

5 Shann F, Barker J & Poore P. Chloramphenicol alone versus chloramphenicol plus penicillin for severe pneumonia in children. *Lancet* 1985; ii:684–688.

6 Warrell D A, Fawcett I W, Harrison B D W et al. Bronchial asthma in the Nigerian Savanna region. *Q J Med* 1975; 174:325–347.

7 Shao J F & Shayo A. Allergen skin tests to asthmatic children screened at Muhimbili Medical Centre, Dar es Salaam, Tanzania. *East Afr Med J* 1985; 62:386–390.

8 Gill G V. An asthmatic clinic for provincial tropical hospitals. *Trop Doct* 1979; 9:155–157.

9 Blaser M J & Cohn D L. Opportunistic infections in patients with AIDS: clues to the epidemiology of AIDS and the relative virulence of pathogens. *Rev Infect Dis* 1986; 8:21–30.

10 Bayley A C. *Atypical aggressive Kaposi's sarcoma in Africa*. In Gottlieb G J & Ackermann A B (eds) *Kaposi's Sarcoma: A Text and Atlas*. Philadelphia: Lea & Febiger, 1988: 28–30.

11 McNicol M W & Luce P J. Sarcoidosis in a racially mixed community. *J R Coll Physicians Lond* 1985; 19:179–183.

12 Gupta S K, Mitra K, Chatterjee S et al. Sarcoidosis in India. *Br J Dis Chest* 1985; 79:275–280.

13 Koino R. *Jpn Med World* 1992; 2:317. quoted in Woodruff A W (ed.) *Medicine in the Tropics*. Edinburgh: Churchill Livingstone, 1974: 159.

14 World Health Organization. Memorandum. A programme for controlling acute respiratory infections in children. *Bull World Health Organ* 1984; 62:47–58.

15 James J W. Longitudinal study of the morbidity of diarrheal and respiratory infections in malnourished children. *Am J Clin Nutr* 1972; 25:690–694.

16 Pullan C R, Toms G R, Martin A J et al. Breast feeding and respiratory syncytial virus infection. *BMJ* 1980; 281:1034–1036.

CHAPTER 5

CARDIOVASCULAR DISEASE IN THE TROPICS

E. H. O. Parry and F. I. Anjorin

Any discussion of particular diseases must be seen against the background of the vast differences between tropical countries in climate, culture, environment, economic progress and health care. A form of treatment may be feasible, though costly, in some places, but unthinkable in a poor country. Investigations in tropical cardiac centres may likewise be advanced and may lead to precise anatomical and physiological diagnosis, whereas in other hospitals there may even be no radiographic film. There are also major differences within tropical countries, and it is not justifiable to write about the pattern of cardiovascular disease in a country without reference to the place and its ecology.

Traditional attitudes and practices are commonly retained in rural societies served by district hospitals, whereas the massive urban migration, so characteristic of many tropical countries, has produced new societies in which urban habits, attitudes and an informed demand for modern and expensive health care are commonplace. The vigorous physical activity of subsistence farming is replaced by the taxi ride and the search for work in the city. Against this massive change it is therefore scarcely surprising that cardiovascular disease is changing dramatically and continuously,[32,64] and so the pattern of disease described in any country describes point prevalence and no more. Good sequential or comparative studies are uncommon and their methodologies are often inconsistent, although there are reliable data from Johannesburg, South Africa[28] and some West African countries.

In Abidjan, Côte d'Ivoire, coronary arterial disease has risen as a proportion of all cases of cardiovascular disease from 1.2 to 6.5%, endomyocardial fibrosis has fallen, and pericarditis has risen (human immunodeficiency virus (HIV) infection may contribute to this) (3.5 to 8.8%), whereas rheumatic heart disease and hypertensive heart disease (36.7 to 39%) (Chapter 26) are largely unchanged.

It is not possible to extrapolate from one country to another nor to one area from another in the same country, but trends are evident. As urban life gets more influential, coronary arterial disease rises, hypertension persists and some infections decline; but HIV may lead to a rise of tuberculous and pyogenic pericarditis. When cor pulmonale is induced by smoke pollution inside small huts, housing or a change in cooking habit will reduce its prevalence. Conversely, cigarette smoking, more common in towns, will inevitably affect cor pulmonale and coronary arterial disease.

In some countries of the tropics there are distinctive cardiac diseases which depend on the local environment and its microbes:[4] Chagas' disease in Latin America, schistosomal cor pulmonale in Egypt and Sudan, cor pulmonale in parts of India and Papua New Guinea. These may affect the local prevalence of disease but the central diseases remain: rheumatic cardiac disease, dilated cardiomyopathy, hypertension, and, with urbanization, coronary arterial disease (Chapter 27).

As an individual doctor in a tropical country, the message is clear: try to establish the pattern of disease where you are and do not depend on others' data from different places in the same country. Prepare a basic protocol for your case data and do not expect everything to be the same as in the place you trained, but seek advice in establishing the criteria for diagnosis and record data very carefully. In this way knowledge of patterns of disease, local factors in pathogenesis and thus strategies for control can be developed. This chapter highlights important and/or unusual cardiovascular diseases in the tropics.

RHEUMATIC CARDIAC DISEASE

This is probably the greatest cardiovascular scourge in the tropics—it cripples and disables children,[12] adolescents and young adults, and no health service has overcome it—but the pattern is changing. As countries become richer and people have better homes, food and health care, so the disease, essentially an affliction of the overcrowded poor, is becoming less prevalent,[46] but in India, Pakistan,[26] in much of Africa,[30] and among the urban poor,[25] rheumatic fever and rheumatic heart disease account for from 12–30% of cardiovascular morbidity; there are significant differences between richer and poorer in these countries. In Hong Kong and some Latin American countries, however, the prevalence has been falling significantly[65] and in Sri Lanka lesions of the mitral valve are less severe and restenosis after surgery less common.[56] Rheumatic fever in poor communities in the tropics differs from the formerly familiar pattern in the industrialized countries:[34] it affects young children; it has different clinical features;[53] it affects the heart more commonly both in the first attack and in recurrences; and, on account of weak health services, its secondary prevention is very difficult indeed.

EPIDEMIOLOGY

Risk factors are simple: the poor, the poorly housed, the overcrowded are affected; in schools in India there is a rising prevalence from the poorest government schools to private schools. Prevalence data show that there are more cases in those parts of the tropics where rainfall is sparse and there is a harsh dry season; this is presumably due to easier transmission and/or acquisition of *Streptococcus pyogenes* in a hot dry climate. In West Africa it is the drier countries and regions, away from the west coastal belt, where the disease is more common. In all the countries where prevalence studies have been carried out as part of the major World Health Organization (WHO) programme for the prevention of rheumatic fever and rheumatic cardiac disease, a wide range in prevalence has been found (Table 5.1). The WHO studies have taken, as a baseline for the 16 collaborative project countries,[63] a mean prevalence of 10/1000 for established rheumatic heart disease and an incidence of rheumatic fever of 100/100000, but this varies greatly and available studies have not taken the same age group or used the same methods.

Table 5.1   Prevalence of rheumatic heart disease.

Area	Prevalence/1000	
	Rate	Range
Africa	4.7	3.4–12.6
East Mediterranean	4.4	0.9–10.2
The Americas	1.5	1.1–7.9
Western Pacific	0.7	0.6–1.4
South-East Asia	0.12	0.1–1.3

CRITERIA FOR DIAGNOSIS

The Duckett Jones criteria have been successively modified: chorea, subcutaneous nodules and erythema marginatum are rarely seen in the tropics and so the current criteria allow a diagnosis of rheumatic fever if carditis is the only major feature.[66] Arthralgia may occur instead of arthritis. Although much established rheumatic heart disease is seen, acute carditis is recognized much less frequently than would be expected. Rheumatic fever follows infection with *Strep. pyogenes*. For every 100 cases of sore throat, 20 are caused by *Strep. pyogenes*. For every 100 of those caused by *Strep. pyogenes*, 20 are symptomatic with fever and cervical lymph nodes. Out of the 20 symptomatic cases, two of rheumatic fever may develop, whereas only one case may develop in the 80 without symptoms, except during an epidemic, when the numbers are increased five times.

CLINICAL FEATURES

Rheumatic fever

When there is only carditis, with no other manifestations, the child may have a low grade fever and a tachycardia and so be thought to have an acute infection—or even bacterial endocarditis, but look for the dissociation between the fever and the considerable tachycardia. Look also carefully and daily for a cardiac murmur—in systole or in diastole, at the apex of the heart. This is a diagnosis which is difficult.

Rheumatic heart disease

Established disease affects (1) the mitral valve alone, resulting most commonly in mitral incompe-

Table 5.2 Comparison of streptococcal and viral sore throat.

Feature	Streptococcal	Viral
Onset	Abrupt	Gradual
Throat	Painful	Uncomfortable
Cervical nodes	Enlarged, tender	Not enlarged
Eyes and nose	Not affected	Watery eyes, runny nose
Throat/tonsils	Red, swollen, exudate	Red, vesicles, ulcers

tence, followed by mitral stenosis or mixed stenosis and incompetence; (2) combined mitral and aortic lesions; and (3) least commonly, the aortic valve alone.

Streptococcal sore throat

This may be evident before the onset of some cases of acute rheumatic fever, but it may not, and it must be recognized in the community if primary prevention is to have any hope of success. The distinction between a streptococcal and a viral infection may be difficult (Table 5.2).

PREVENTION

The fundamental aims are:

1. *Environment*: to improve homes and housing, food and health care.
2. *Primary prevention*: to detect and treat symptomatic *Strep. pyogenes* sore throat—with either benzathine penicillin 1.2 megaunits, penicillin V for 10 days, or benzyl penicillin.
3. *Secondary prophylaxis*: to establish and maintain effective secondary prophylaxis of streptococcal infection in those with known rheumatic heart disease.
   (a) *Primary health care*: a thoroughly effective system both for giving benzathine penicillin

every 3 weeks and for immediate recall of those who do not attend for their injection is essential. It is very difficult to maintain such follow-up even with dedicated community nurses.[19]
   (b) *Dose of antibiotic*: the dose of benzathine penicillin, every 3 weeks, is 600000 units for those of 30kg or less, and 1.2 megaunits for others; sulphadiazine 0.5 or 1g daily is an alternative.
   (c) *Duration*:
      (i) 5 years for those without carditis during an attack of acute rheumatic form.
      (ii) At least to age 25 for those with evidence of acute carditis; longer if wretched living conditions.
      (iii) Indefinitely for those with established rheumatic heart disease.
4. *Research*: to develop prospective studies of the relevant M types of *Strep. pyogenes* which are important in the tropics and are associated with first attacks of acute rheumatic fever or recurrences. This could lead to vaccination of those at risk.

MANAGEMENT

Acute rheumatic fever

Eradicate *Strep. pyogenes* with benzylpenicillin and establish maintenance prophylaxis with benzathine penicillin. Manage cardiac failure with bed-rest for acute carditis and give aspirin or corticosteroids, for as long as there is evidence of carditis, provided there is no evidence of cardiac failure.[9]

Chronic rheumatic heart disease

Maintain penicillin prophylaxis to prevent recurrences and infective endocarditis when necessary, and give standard treatment for valvular disease, disorders of rhythm or cardiac failure.

DILATED CARDIOMYOPATHY

Throughout the tropics patients are commonly seen who have a dilated heart without any identifiable cause. In some cases they account for about 20% of cases of cardiovascular disease.

PATHOGENESIS

There are many possible factors and this is, at best, a syndrome. Men are affected more than women, predominantly in the age group 40–49 years.

Poverty and social class

These have been identified as significant in West Africa where the condition is much more common in patients of low social class than is found with other types of heart disease.[35]

Anaemia

While severe anaemia may be associated with cardiac failure it does not appear to be a causal factor in dilated cardiomyopathy in the tropics, although it may aggravate cardiac failure.

Toxins

These are often suggested but rarely incriminated in cardiac failure. Subsistence farmers in northern Natal, South Africa, were found to store their maize very poorly, causing it to become contaminated with fungi: when they ate the maize they developed idiopathic congestive cardiomyopathy.[11] When their stores of maize were exhausted they bought well-stored maize and the incidence of cardiac failure fell. This example shows how careful clinical studies can reveal factors in the pathogenesis of cardiomyopathy that are locally important.

Alcohol

There is much evidence that alcohol,[47] often a strong traditional brew, is an important and common cause of dilated cardiomyopathy in many areas of the tropics. There may be other evidence of alcoholic dependence but many patients will not give a truthful report of the volume drunk each day, and the social climate of many is against them if they try to break their habit.

Nutrition and micronutrients

Although the less well-nourished lower social class are more commonly affected there is no evidence for a direct nutritional cause of dilated cardiomyopathy in the tropics. While some cases can be attributed to a specific deficiency, for instance the rare cases of beriberi, micronutrient deficiency (for example selenium) has not yet been proved.

Myocarditis

Damage to the myocardium from a previous viral myocarditis may prove to be more significant than is currently appreciated.

Hypertension

There is evidence to suggest that some patients may be former hypertensives: the age groups of those with hypertensive cardiac failure and dilated cardiomyopathy are similar; the aortic arch diameter in all cases of dilated cardiomyopathy is intermediate between that of hypertensive and normal individuals; in some cases the blood pressure rises as cardiac failure responds to treatment, and they may need antihypertension drugs; and in East Africa formerly-proved hypertensives presented years later with dilated cardiomyopathy but with normal blood pressure throughout.

Genetic factors

There is no certain evidence that dilated cardiomyopathy in the tropics has a genetic basis but data are very scanty and much remains to be learned.

CLINICAL FEATURES

Most patients have had some of the typical symptoms of pulmonary and/or systemic oedema for up to 2 years before they seek help. Thus the physical signs are often dominated by pulmonary oedema or dependent oedema, ascites and a large liver. The heart is large and praecordial pulsation varies, depending on the size and dilatation of the left ventricle. Atrioventricular valvular incompetence is common so the jugular pulse may show the distinctive systolic wave of tricuspid regurgitation, and panystolic murmurs are heard with a third heart sound.

Sometimes systemic embolization, for example a 'cerebrovascular accident' from an intracavitary left ventricular thrombus, is the presenting feature. Intractable heart failure despite adequate treatment may be due to a large left ventricular thrombus adding an obliterative component to the poorly contracting and dilated left ventricle.

DIAGNOSIS

In a man with normal arterial pressure and no evidence of valvular disease the diagnosis is not difficult, but if there is raised arterial pressure, retinal arterial changes and left ventricle which is thickened but dilated, the distinction from hypertensive cardiac failure may be difficult. Similarly, if there is mitral incompetence, and the patient is younger, rheumatic heart disease and even endomyocardial fibrosis may have to be considered, but the mitral valvular incompetence may be reversed by effective treatment of the cardiac failure, which is impossible when the valve or its papillary muscles are diseased, as in rheumatic carditis or in endomyocardial fibrosis.

MANAGEMENT AND PROGNOSIS

Management depends on the resources and drugs available. In district hospitals diuretics, with digoxin when there is an atrial arrhythmia, can be recommended. Other forms of treatment including vasodilators can be used at specialist hospitals. The prognosis[61] depends on the function of the left ventricle:[18] those who do worst have a high left ventricular end-diastolic pressure, end-systolic volume and end-diastolic volume with a reduced ejection fraction. If alcohol is incriminated as a causative factor then somehow the patient has to stop drinking it.

PERIPARTUM CARDIAC FAILURE

When the heart fails, the clinical manifestations are the same whatever the causes. The clinical syndrome dominates the signs, management and course, and the cause is often not obvious: peripartum cardiac failure (PPCF) is such a syndrome.

The definition varies from report to report but only in the time interval related to delivery. In Nigeria the following definition has been used: 'cardiac failure, with symptoms beginning in pregnancy or up to 6 months post partum—of up to 6 months duration, with no history of cardiac failure other than PPCF itself, and with no discernible cause for cardiac failure other than anaemia or hypertension, presumed to be acute'.[17] Others limit diagnosis of PPCF to patients whose symptoms begin during the last months of pregnancy or in the first few months after delivery. The essential issue of PPCF is cardiac failure, without a definable cause, developing in a woman who is or was recently pregnant.

DISTRIBUTION

The syndrome has been reported widely in the tropics, for example from Latin America, the Caribbean, East, West and South Africa,[39] India, China and Korea. Occasional cases are also seen in temperate countries and some important series of cases have been reported in the USA,[24] almost exclusively among black women.

FACTORS IN THE PATHOGENESIS

This is a syndrome which may conceal a number of conditions. In discussing factors in the pathogenesis, it must be emphasized that these may be important only in certain places, and they may be relevant in other places.

The syndrome is primarily one of a dilated cardiomyopathy and therefore the factors in the pathogenesis of a dilated cardiomyopathy anywhere in the world have to be considered in PPCF.

Race

The largest reported series have been in West Africans and black Americans. The syndrome is apparently also common in Korea, and cases are reported in all races.

Parity

PPCF is more common in multiparous women, and this appears to be independent of age, although increasing age is itself a risk factor.

Twin births

Data are few but the risk has been reported to be twofold in a twin pregnancy.

Blood pressure

Hypertensive disease of pregnancy has been suggested as a risk factor but data are scanty. PPCF has been called postpartum hypertensive cardiac failure in southern Nigeria. The question therefore arises as to whether PPCF patients are a potentially hypertensive cohort and whether PPCF is a form of hypertensive heart failure, as suggested in southern Nigeria, or can the hypertension is some cases be explained by some other mechanism? There is persuasive evidence from northern Nigeria that this is indeed the case in some patients.

Genetic predisposition

There are no data which establish PPCF patients as having a particular genetic predisposition, notably a distinctive human leucocyte antigen (HLA), which could affect the evolution of a viral infection.

Viral infection

Evidence of a preceding viral infection in some cases is similar to the evidence in cases of dilated cardiomyopathy. Rapidly advancing myocarditis has been described in such cases. Endomyocardial biopsy has given evidence in over 50% of cases of myocarditis, but the mechanism of this myocarditis is not known.[37,38,50]

The northern Nigerian PPCF syndrome

This is distinctive and has additional characteristic pathogenetic factors.

Cultural practices

In the area around Zaria in northern Nigeria the Hausa women after delivery traditionally take *kanwa*, a rock salt rich in sodium and potassium, in order to promote the flow of breast milk. They also traditionally lie on a heated bed for at least 40 days post partum to prevent them from becoming diseased from the cold. This is because they consider that a woman after delivery has a large area vulnerable to cold, important in the causation of many diseases, and therefore she must be protected from it. She would also take hot splashing 'baths' twice daily for the same reason. These habits are changing and so the syndrome of PPCF can be expected to become less common.

Seasonal variation

The temperature and humidity in the guinea savanna of West Africa vary greatly between the wet and dry seasons. Hospital admissions of PPCF mothers, but not of other patients, was highly significantly associated with heat and humidity, the peak of admissions following about 2 months after the hottest humid season.

The Nigerian syndrome—a possible mechanism

The factors are postpartum state, hot season and hot beds and baths, and ingestion of a sodium-rich rock salt.

The heat causes vasodilatation so that the cardiac output rises in order to maintain flow and arterial pressure, but the excessive sodium load demands a high renal arterial pressure for its excretion. This can only be at best partially achieved by a further rise of cardiac output and blood pressure.[51] Oedema therefore develops and the cycle is set for it to increase daily. The syndrome is thus established with a high output state and vasodilatation, oedema, and systemic and pulmonary venous congestion. Physiologically it is not true cardiac failure because the stroke volume can rise in response to a rise in filling pressure. This group responds rapidly with a massive diuresis, but it does not include a smaller number whose heart is dilated and who do not respond with a diuresis.

CLINICAL PICTURE

Symptoms of pulmonary and/or systemic venous congestion develop—related in time to delivery. Swelling of the whole body, even including the face, can be substantial. The physical signs are not specific: look carefully for the height of the jugular venous pressure and its wave, arterial pulsus alternans, and signs of an enlarged or hyperdynamic left ventricle with a third heart sound. These signs are useful for monitoring the effects of treatment. The blood pressure is often raised when the patient is first seen, but falls within a few days during diuretic (and digoxin) treatment. Systemic and pulmonary emboli are seen when the heart is very large.

INVESTIGATIONS

These can be used to confirm physical signs, to monitor progress, and to measure the disorders of function. The chest radiograph shows a dilated heart, pulmonary venous congestion and oedema. There is no typical pattern.

DISORDERED PHYSIOLOGY

Physiological studies in Brazil have not shown a homogeneous pattern of cardiac function. Most patients showed a raised ventricular filling pressure with low cardiac output but there was a subset with high output 'failure'.[36] This is precisely what was found in studies of the syndrome in Nigeria, where it was suggested that volume overload was responsible for the syndrome. But why? The picture in such cases is of hypervolaemia, which, when cured by diuretics, leaves a normal heart.[2] In some cases, however, and the reasons for this are not clear, there is irreversible cardiac damage.

EVOLUTION AND TREATMENT

The prognosis of this syndrome varies with its pathogenesis, from the rapidly progressive myocarditis for which cardiac transplantation alone is curative, to a syndrome of oedema and uncomplicated cardiomegaly which resolves very quickly with treatment by diuretics. Bad signs in prognosis are any arrhythmia, a persistently dilated heart, and systemic or pulmonary emboli.[3] There is no reason to take the baby off the breast, and as soon as the mother has had a major diuresis there is no reason to keep her in hospital unless she has bad prognostic signs.

In an advanced centre where endomyocardial biopsy is obtainable and a reliable histology service is available, this procedure is indicated. If myocarditis is detected, routine treatment for cardiac failure for 7 days is recommended; if this is ineffective, immunosuppressant drugs may be beneficial and must be tried. If these drugs are ineffective, the outlook is bad and little else can be done.

SUBSEQUENT PREGNANCIES

The syndrome may recur, but if the heart returns to normal after the first episode[60] there is no reason to advise against subsequent pregnancy; continuous antenatal and postnatal care are, however, imperative.

HYPERTENSION AND HYPERTENSIVE HEART DISEASE

Most people in the tropics with high blood pressure (defined by the WHO criteria) do not know that they are hypertensive, and even if they were aware and sought treatment, in many countries the public budget can not possibly stretch to supply the ideal combination of antihypertension drugs. Report after report tells the same story.

BLOOD PRESSURE IN RURAL AND URBAN SOCIETIES (See also Chapter 26)

Studies of people who live in isolated rural areas of tropical countries have shown that the prevalence of hypertension is very low and that, unlike the typical urban society, blood pressure levels remain within a remarkably narrow range throughout adult life. Although such remote people are now few, there are still many who live in simple rural communities and it is these who form the control subjects in studies of blood pressure in urban migrants.

Blood pressure in people from rural societies may rise modestly with age, but this rise is greater in people of the same ethnocultural group who now live in cities.[48] Factors in urban migrants which are important determinants of blood pressure are body weight, or indices relating weight to height, and sodium (from common salt) intake.[20] There is an associated lower intake of potassium. There are now very many such studies: some examples are given in the reference list.[8,10,23,31,45] Indeed, in Tanzania, blood pressure in normotensive urban men, who normally take a relatively low amount of salt, was

found to be peculiarly sensitive to a high salt intake.[49] Salt sensitivity has also been related to the survival of those who were transported from Africa: they survived because they could conserve sodium. Not only does the blood pressure rise with age in urban migrants but the prevalence of hypertension is greater than that among those in their original rural area. Migration apparently affects the blood pressure in women less than men. Urbanization and prosperity have to be distinguished from each other. Whereas in Hong Kong increasing prosperity has been shown to lead to a greater risk of death from ischaemic heart disease, a greater risk of death from hypertensive or cerebrovascular disease is not a sequel to increased prosperity in tropical countries.

RACE

Different origins apparently govern both the prevalence and pattern of hypertension (Chapter 26). In any society those of black African origin are most susceptible and, as discussed below, they are vulnerable to stroke; low renin hypertension is also more common.

SEQUELAE OF HYPERTENSION

Stroke is a common problem in hospital practice in the tropics and it is closely correlated with hypertension: in one study, over 27 years, stroke mortality was 11.4% in hypertensives but only 1.8% in normotensives. It is often the presenting feature of hypertension, particularly if this has not been detected previously, and so, if much hypertension goes undetected, numerous strokes can be expected.

Hypertensive cardiac failure[21] has already been discussed in relation to dilated cardiomyopathy; it is not known whether untreated hypertension leading to left ventricular hypertrophy in a population not subject to coronary arterial disease is responsible for a subsequently dilated ventricle and the syndrome of dilated cardiomyopathy. In some cases of hypertensive heart disease left ventricular hypertrophy is asymmetrical.[5] In most tropical countries hypertensive heart disease accounts for 20–35% of cases of cardiovascular admissions, and this figure remains obstinately constant. Malignant hypertension is well recognized and renal failure with severe hypertension is also often seen, but without a definite diagnosis of the underlying renal disease the cause for this remains conjectural. Retinopathy occurs in hypertension, as it does in northern countries, and must be searched for in all cases.

Coronary arterial events are much more common in Asian hypertensives than among those of black African origin.

THE PROBLEM OF MANAGEMENT

As life expectancy increases, so more and more untreated and later disabled victims of hypertension will block hospital beds and put a vast strain on resources. Severe hypertension may be detected if there is an efficient primary health care service, but, if people migrate, records of blood pressure often do not follow them and so vital data may be lost. Systems of health care will have to be modified to accommodate the identified chronic sick (hypertensive), the cost of whose care and perhaps drugs, could never be met by government alone. Can systems of community care be developed, not least to help those who have been partially disabled by stroke? Few, if any, poor tropical countries could afford to treat hypertension in all those who need drugs with an angiotensin-converting enzyme (ACE) inhibitor, a beta blocker, a calcium channel blocker and diuretic; even if they could, the problem is compounded because ACE inhibitors and beta blockers are apparently less efficacious in black people than they are in white people.

For the individual who needs drugs it is essential to establish that drug supply can be sustained indefinitely, and it is essential to ensure that treatment will be followed. The drug regimen will depend on national drug policy, whether or not there is an essential drug list and thus what drugs are available at health station, health centre, and district, regional or specialist hospital. Again, therapy will become a matter of trial to find which drugs are more effective; careful observation and good records are essential.

There is no reason why a doctor should perform the follow-up of an uncomplicated hypertensive patient: a well-trained medical assistant or clinic nurse, who works with defined criteria for referral if there is an unexpected change, should be in control in the realistic management of hypertension.

ENDOMYOCARDIAL FIBROSIS

In any discussion of tropical cardiac disease, endomyocardial fibrosis (EMF) is prominent because of its remarkable clinical and pathological features, and now its suggested pathogenesis,[40] but it is not common, and even in specialist cardiac centres in endemic areas it comprises only about 1–5% of cases. Nevertheless, there are areas in the hot and humid tropics—Kerala, Malaysia, West and Central Africa and Brazil,[22] where the disease is seen much more commonly than in other areas.

HISTORY AND EARLY STUDIES

J.N.P. Davies, pathologist at the Old Mulago Hospital, Kampala, described how at necropsy he found the left ventricle with a curious thickening of the endocardium—chiefly at the apex. He subsequently defined the pathology, and the Kampala team added more on the clinical and epidemiological and pathological features of EMF.[14,15] Meanwhile in Nigeria an Ibadan team described clinical and physiological features and the possible aetiological role of eosinophils.

WHAT IS EMF?

Endocardial thickening of the ventricle leads to physiological effects: cardiac constriction or restriction and atrioventricular valvular incompetence leading to regurgitation. The disease is understood best from the pathological changes in established—and thus possibly burnt out, cases. In the left ventricle dense fibrous tissue at the apex spreads around the cavity of the ventricle or may first appear around the papillary muscle of the posterior cusp of the mitral valve. This muscle is thus anchored so that the valve becomes incompetent. In late cases there is a curious folding over of the horizontal upper border of the endocardial thickening due to intraventricular turbulence.

Changes in the right ventricle are similar, but it loses its cavity, which is obliterated from below by the advancing fibrosis of layered mural thrombi. In late cases the papillary muscles are lost in a bed of fibrous tissue, the tricuspid valve loses its function, and the right atrium can become aneurysmal. The left, right, or both ventricles can be affected. Chronic pericardial effusion can be associated with right ventricular EMF; a pleural effusion is more common with left or biventricular disease.

The anatomical changes explain physiological dysfunction and the physical signs in established disease. Dense avascular fibrous tissue, often sharply defined from or 'dipping into' the myocardium, is characteristic of established disease. In acute disease, however, the pericardium, myocardium and endocardium are affected. There is active inflammation with lymphocytes, eosinophils which may be degranulated,[44] and many small blood vessels packed with cells. In addition, irregularly scattered throughout the myocardium, and often unrelated to overlying endocardial change, there are foci where myocardial fibres are disappearing and fibroblasts are evident.

PATHOGENESIS

The term eosinophilic endomyocardial disease has been suggested to replace endomyocardial fibrosis because the cardiac changes are explained in terms of the eosinophil and its constituents.[55] Thus EMF has changes similar to those found in the heart in patients with hypereosinophilic syndromes. The critical questions are: what is the trigger for an eosinophilia in EMF, and is it found consistently? Eosinophilia is not consistent, but that could be because the disease is often not present until its pathogenetic process is burnt out, leaving fibrotic ventricles only. There were early reports from francophone West Africa, and also more recent ones, which linked filariasis with EMF, and particularly *Loa loa*, or any other helminth which provokes an eosinophilia.[7,29] Although a clear initial illness[42] has been described, such cases are rare so that there are few investigative data.

The suggested sequence is: trigger to eosinophilia (helminthic or other infection) leads to hypereosino-

philia and liberation of eosinophilic cationic protein and major basic proteins. Eosinophilic cationic protein is toxic to a wide range of cells, including endocardial and myocardial cells: the damaged endocardium serves as a focus for mural thrombi which are themselves promoted by the release of platelet activation factor(s) from the eosinophils. Further mural thrombi are then laid down at the original and adjacent sites, and a fibrotic mass results. This is a logical and clear sequence following hypereosinophilia but the difficulty lies in reconciling it with all the data, particularly from Uganda.

So what other factors might perhaps be important in Uganda? Prevalence of EMF in Uganda was shown to differ between immigrant Rwanda and native Baganda, in a ratio of about 4–5 to 1, whereas rheumatic heart disease was just the reverse.[54] Similarly, in a kindred with the tropical splenomegaly syndrome, EMF was apparently more prevalent.[43] Causes of eosinophilia are abundant in the tropics but EMF is not. Additionally, it appears to be much less prevalent in dry grassland areas—but why? On the whole available evidence suggests that hypereosinophilia in a hot and humid environment promotes features leading to the development of endomyocardial fibrosis.

CLINICAL FEATURES

These are directly determined by the stage of the disease and the anatomical distortion of whichever ventricle is dominantly affected, together with the resultant effects on cardiac function.

Initial illness

This is the key to our future understanding. Some patients, previously quite well, have a febrile illness in which the face may swell and they become febrile, breathless and ill, and develop symptoms of pulmonary venous congestion. This may advance quickly and can be fatal within months, but little is known about this phase of the disease.[6]

Left ventricular disease

The ventricle is not enlarged and there are inevitably, in almost every case, signs of mitral valvular incompetence with a loud pulmonary closure sound, and progressive evidence of pulmonary hypertension. A third heart sound is usual—early and crisp, and it is dominant when the physiological pattern is a restricted ventricle.

Right ventricular disease

The classical picture, described from Ibadan, is of a young patient, often with delayed puberty, slight exophthalmos, central cyanosis, no peripheral oedema and massive ascites. The ascites is so dominant and the jugular pressure so very high that most cases of established right ventricular EMF are at first missed. This need not be so if the physician looks very carefully around the lobe of the ear, with the patient standing or sitting up at 90° on the bed. The jugular systolic wave, secondary to tricuspid regurgitation, can then be seen to move the ear lobe and to cause a general expansion around the neck with each ventricular systole. The high pressure jugular vein can therefore even be palpable. The stroke volume is small, therefore the arterial pulse has a small pulse pressure and atrial fibrillation is common. The heart may be impalpable either because there is a large pericardial effusion or because it is rotated by the massive right atrium which lies under the sternum, so that the left ventricle lies more posteriorly. There may be no murmur at the defunct tricuspid valve but only an abrupt third heart sound.

INVESTIGATIONS

The stage and site of disease determine findings on the chest radiograph; these vary from a massive cardiac shadow (aneurysmal right atrium or pericardial effusion) (Figure 5.1) to an almost normal heart with perhaps a prominent pulmonary artery.

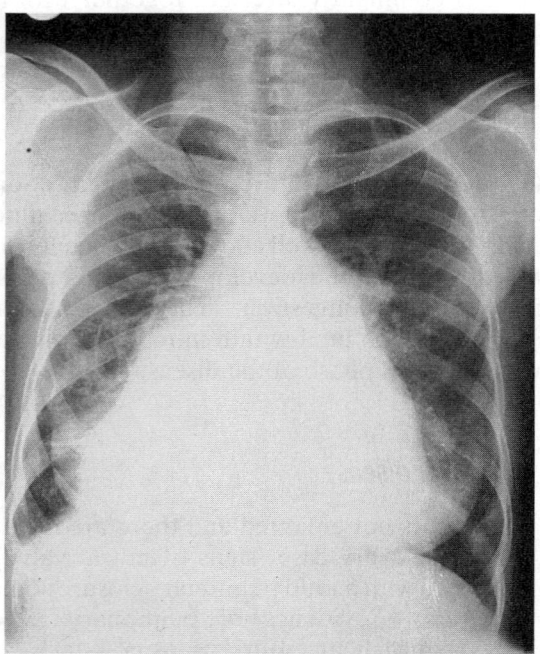

Figure 5.1 Biventricular endomyocardial fibrosis: the cardiac shadow is totally distorted with the enlarged right atrium prominent.

Echocardiography[41,62] has been found to be most valuable in making a definitive diagnosis: advanced techniques should define the anatomical changes precisely.

There is no specific diagnostic test.

DIAGNOSIS

When advanced methods including echocardiography are not available, there are three clinical problems:

1. The initial illness. This may resemble any acute myocarditis or even acute rheumatic fever: the evolution of the disease alone will probably give the diagnosis because no investigation from the limited range available can differentiate these three conclusively.
2. Established mitral incompetence. In patients with EMF there is never any evidence of mitral stenosis nor of aortic incompetence, as may be found in about 40–45% of cases of rheumatic cardiac disease; nor is the mitral lesion associated with a large hypodynamic left ventricle, as in dilated cardiomyopathy. If a clear third heart sound is audible and the heart is not large, EMF is clinically a possible diagnosis.
3. Signs of cardiac construction. Constrictive pericarditis is more common than left ventricular EMF and must be the first diagnosis when classical signs of constriction are detected. If there is any suggestion of a murmur of atrioventricular valvular incompetence, EMF is strongly suggested because valves are normal in pericardial disease.

MANAGEMENT

Established disease

Cardiac surgery has been practised in Abidjan but this is economically indefensible, although clinically appealing and logical if the disease is not active. If high protein pleural or peritoneal fluid is aspirated in large volumes the patient will lose much protein; this is therefore not advocated. Digoxin can be used to control ventricular rate in right ventricular EMF if atrial fibrillation is present. As little else can be done against the barrier of fibrous tissue it is essential to correct anaemia and any new infection.

The acute illness

If patients present with a short history and an unstable state they should be managed as for any acute myocarditis. If an eosinophilia is detected its cause should be defined and treated. The role of corticosteroids is not established. It is critically important for our understanding of EMF that any curious cases of cardiac failure in young people in endemic areas of the tropics should be observed, studied and followed up very carefully.

PERICARDIAL DISEASE

Much pericardial disease is missed in routine hospital practice because physical signs are difficult to detect, or because the primary disease demands urgent attention. In the tropics there are two important forms of pericarditis, both secondary to a major primary disease: (1) acute pyogenic pericarditis; and (2) tuberculous pericarditis. Other types of pericarditis are seen, and are also incidental to a major systemic illness or an adjacent infection—for example pericarditis complicating liver abscess due to *Entamoeba histolytica*.

PYOGENIC PERICARDITIS

The pericardium is affected as part of a bacteraemia derived from, or associated with a primary focus which may be anywhere, for example pyomyositis, lobar pneumonia or pelvic infection. In such cases local and systemic signs are dominant and pericarditis may not be recognized until it causes circulatory effects.

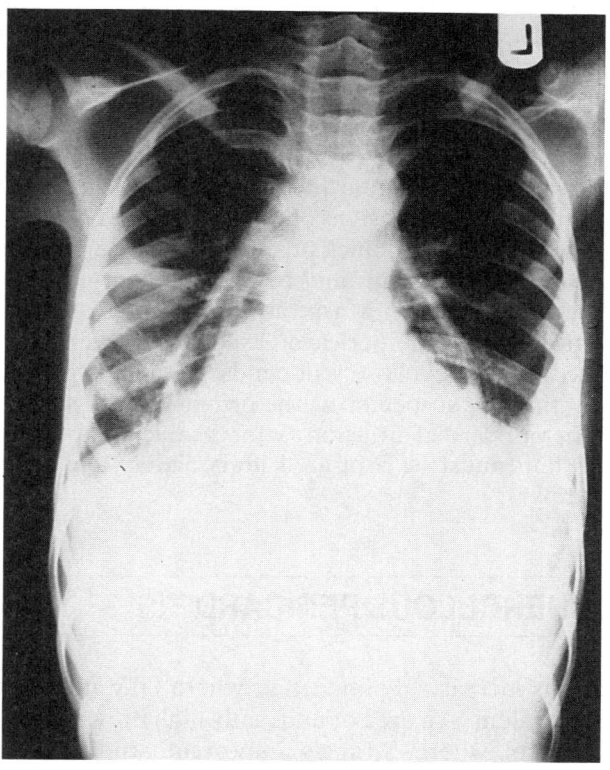

Figure 5.2 Pyogenic pericarditis: note thickness of pericardium and the associated pleural effusion and pulmonary changes.

CLINICAL FEATURES

These depend on whether or not there is a pericardial effusion and the speed at which this has formed. If the fluid forms quickly, the parietal pericardium cannot stretch adequately to accommodate it and symptoms and signs of cardiac tamponade develop. The heart is compressed and the signs therefore depend on obstruction to venous inflow and a subsequent fall in stroke output. Therefore, in any patient who has a serious systemic pyogenic illness or lobar pneumonia which is unexpectedly slow to resolve, examine the cardiovascular system carefully and monitor the jugular venous pressure and the heart rate.

The early evidence that cardiac tamponade may be developing is a slowly but steadily rising heart rate in a patient whose primary illness was considered to be getting better. There may be evidence of pericarditis—a pericardial rub, or signs of fluid,

dullness to percussion at the right border of the sternum, an impalpable cardiac impulse and very quiet heart sounds. Therefore, suspect a rapidly enlarging pericardial effusion in a patient with significant pyogenic disease who becomes restless, perhaps breathless, and who is noticed to have a rising heart rate and evidence of intense peripheral vasoconstriction: cold hands, empty veins and an arterial pulse which is rapid, of very small pulse pressure and which may diminish in amplitude during inspiration (pulsus paradoxus). The jugular venous pressure is very high with minimal pulsation; it may be so high that the observer fails to realize that it is raised. When a pyogenic pericardial effusion has developed more slowly there are not the critical signs of an acutely low cardiac output; instead, signs of effusion are dominant.

MANAGEMENT

This depends on accurate diagnosis. In an uncomplicated effusion, in a district hospital without echocardiography, a chest radiograph may reveal a large cardiac shadow but this may be difficult to interpret if there is a consolidated lobe in lobar pneumonia or a pleural effusion (Figure 5.2). Pericardial fluid (pus) confirms the diagnosis; if it is purulent, it should be aspirated totally. Aspiration by the epigastric approach with the patient sitting up in bed is the easiest, and safest in a hospital with limited resources. Use a 50ml, or 20ml, syringe with a long needle fitted with a two-way tap so that fluid can easily be expelled. Aspirate daily, but be prepared to transfer the patient to a cardiac surgical unit if there are persistent signs of fluid or cardiac compression. In such cases, thick pus sticks to the pericardial membranes and can only be removed surgically.[33] Early diagnosis with aspiration and instillation of antibiotic into the pericardial sac may prevent this. The antibiotic chosen depends on the organism identified or suspected as the primary pathogen.

In pericardial effusion with cardiac tamponade the fluid must be aspirated immediately and completely.

TUBERCULOUS PERICARDITIS

This is increasingly important where HIV infection is prevalent. An area of unusually high prevalence is Transkei where Strang's important studies have been done.[59] *Mycobacterium tuberculosis* is thought to reach the pericardium from adjacent infection in lymph nodes or possibly pleura.

CLINICAL PICTURE

This depends on the stage of the disease. Many patients present late and are thought to have liver disease because they are wasted and have tense ascites, or because the jugular venous pressure is not examined, or is very high, and thus is not recognized, hidden behind the lobe of the car. It is no longer rare to see acute tuberculous pericarditis with a friction rub alone; indeed, in contrast to cases of tuberculosis alone, those who have HIV/AIDS often show evidence of early pericardial infection. Most patients have a pericardial effusion which may be large or small, with underlying pericardial fibrosis. This is constrictive pericarditis with its distinctive signs: a small arterial pulse pressure, sometimes with pulsus paradoxus, and a venous pulse which has a high pressure and can be seen to fall sharply immediately after carotid pulsation (*y* descent).

These are the most important signs; the heart may be impalpable and, when constriction is established, a third heart sound is audible.

DIAGNOSIS

In patients with HIV/AIDS, signs of pericarditis must be assumed to be caused by tuberculosis. Aspiration of pericardial fluid is helpful: the fluid has a high protein content around 40g/l and in about 80% of cases it is bloodstained; the cells are lymphocytes. There is no characteristic chest radiograph: this depends on the volume of pericardial fluid, the presence of a pleural effusion, and whether the pericardium has calcified or not.

TREATMENT

Give antituberculosis drugs with corticosteroids—Strang showed that steroids prevent constriction.[57,58] The currently recommended initial dose is prednisolone 2mg/kg. The course of steroids is 11 weeks. This makes patients rapidly better, constriction is prevented, and pericardial fluid disappears.

OTHER INFECTIONS

VIRUSES

These are much less common. There is nothing distinctive about viral pericarditis in the tropics.

MENINGOCOCCUS

Signs of pericarditis may be detected in patients with meningococcal disease who have bacteraemia and antigenaemia. Immune complexes are formed and deposited on the pericardium. The pericarditis is transient and the prognosis is dominated by the severity of infection.

PARASITES

The only significant, but nevertheless rare, protozoan pericarditis is caused by trophozoites of *Entamoeba histolytica* which reach the pericardium from an adjacent liver abscess. The prognosis in this complication is bad because it is often not recognized early. Pericardial tamponade can develop quickly and it is therefore essential to aspirate pericardial fluid. There is no satisfactory trial of chemo- therapy: metronidazole and chloroquine orally, and metronidazole injected into the pericardial sac, have been advocated.

ARTERIAL DISEASE

AORTA AND LARGE ARTERIES

Just as EMF is more common in certain areas of tropical countries than in temperate ones, so too is idiopathic 'tropical' aortitis more common in the tropics, particularly in Asian countries: Malaysia,[16] Thailand, Singapore, Korea, China and India,[13] where some cases are named Takayasu's disease. It has also been described in many African countries, with notable studies in South Africa.[27,52] Whether this disease in Asia is the same as that seen in African countries, or whether there are distinctive tropical variants, is not known. The questions are: what are the triggers for the disease, and are they more prevalent in the tropics?

The clinical features are determined by the pathological/anatomical damage to the aorta and its large branches, so that regional ischaemia in a tissue or organ is the most common clinical presentation. Aortograms may show aneurysmally dilated or stenosed segments of aorta with an irregular lumen so that the orifices of any of its branches may be occluded.

The abdominal aorta is diseased in over 90% of cases, but pathology in the subclavian arteries in over 60%, and renal arteries in over 80% indicate where symptoms are common.

PATHOGENESIS

The cause of the arteritis is not known but certain facts may give clues. There is a systemic inflammatory phase in some patients, and the morphological changes are similar to those of temporal arteritis. Therefore, while an immune mechanism has been suggested (an associated glomerulonephritis in some patients may be suggestive evidence), there are no consistent markers of an immune reaction. The difficulty with this is that, in a disease in which there are probably phases of activity and quiescence, the absence of immune markers may merely indicate that the disease is quiescent when the samples were taken. Although it is suggested that genetic factors may be responsible, no consistent HLA patterns in series of patients from different countries have been demonstrated.

CLINICAL FEATURES

The symptoms depend on the artery affected. Most patients are young adults; in some series women predominate. Symptoms associated with hypertension are found in about one-third of cases, and visual symptoms have also been reported in about one-third of patients, as have symptoms of transient cerebral ischaemia. Physical signs depend on the vessel affected; therefore, when examining a patient, palpate all arterial pulses—in particular examine to see whether any pulses are delayed or unequal between left and right; auscultate the vessels and the abdomen, particularly around the umbilicus where a bruit from renal artery stenosis may be audible in up to 50% of cases.

INVESTIGATION

An aortogram is definitive: it will show segments of stenosis and dilatation. Selective renal angiography can be used if the abdominal aorta is obviously abnormal or if the patient has a high blood pressure.

MANAGEMENT

In many tropical hospitals the diagnosis can be suspected from symptoms and signs, and in most patients no treatment is possible. In technically advanced hospitals angioplasty or an arterial bypass may be used, but this is only reasonable for limited and symptomatic disease, for example renal arterial disease with a significantly raised blood pressure. It must be emphasized that arterial damage is widespread and treatment is unlikely to help.

CORONARY ARTERIAL DISEASE

The remarkable differences in the prevalence of coronary artery diseases between different countries in the tropics has led to many comparative studies (Chapter 27). Similarly, the pattern of disease is changing in countries which are becoming industrialized and where people's habits and diet are changing.

Clinically, coronary arterial disease causes the same symptoms, whether in tropical or temperate countries. Cardiac pain on effort, however, in a patient who is at low risk—a young adult from a rural African community—may cause a problem with diagnosis. Severe anaemia from untreated heavy hookworm infection can lead to a qualitative defect in coronary arterial flow in spite of a greatly increased cardiac output. In a patient who is not anaemic the orifices of the coronary arteries or their lumens may be occluded or stenosed. Tropical or syphilitic aortitis may involve the orifice(s); the lumen may be occluded by emboli in rheumatic cardiac disease or dilated cardiomyopathy with a left ventricular mural or cavitary thrombus. A rare curiosity which may distort a coronary artery is annular subvalvular aneurysm of the left ventricle.[1] Described in a number of tropical countries, a pouch forms and enlarges so that it may stretch the circumflex branch of the left coronary artery, appear as a rounded shadow on the left ventricle—in a chest radiograph, or grow into the septum. Mural thrombi form and may partially fill the aneurysm and lead to systemic emboli.

LEFT VENTRICULAR CAVITARY THROMBUS

Originally described at autopsy in Senegal in patients with dilated cardiomyopathy, these thrombi are now being detected by echocardiography in similar cases in West Africa and in patients with peripartum cardiac failure. In some, streptokinase has had a remarkable effect.

REFERENCES

1 Abrahams D G, Barton J, Cockshott W P et al. Annular subvalvular left ventricular aneurysms. *Q J Med* 1962; 31:345–360.

2 Adesanya C O, Anjorin F I, Sada I A et al. Atrial natriuretic peptide, aldosterone and plasma renin activity in peripartum heart failure. *Br Heart J* 1991; 65:152–154.

3 Adesanya C O, Anjorin F I, Adesoshun I O et al. Peripartum cardiac failure—a ten-year follow-up study. *Trop Geogr Med* 1989; 41:190–196.

4 Adoh A, Kouassi-Yapo F, N'Dori R et al. Etiologie des artériopathies des membres inférieurs chez les Noirs Africains à Abidjan. *Cardiol Trop* 1991; 17:59–65.

5 Ajayi A A & Akinwasi P O. Spectrum of hypertensive heart disease in Nigerians: cross-sectional study of echocardiographic indices and their correlation with treadmill exercise capacity. *J Hypertens* 1993; 11:99–102.

6 Andy J J & Bishara F F. Observations on clinical features of early disease of African endomyocardial fibrosis. *Cardiol Trop* 1982; 8:23–33.

7 Andy J J, Bishara F F & Soyinka O O. Relation of severe eosinophilia and microfilariasis to chronic African endomyocardial fibrosis. *Br Heart J* 1981; 45:672–680.

8 Astagneau P, Lang T, Delarocque E et al. Arterial hypertension in urban Africa: an epidemiological study on a representative sample of Dakar inhabitants in Senegal. *J Hypertens* 1992; 10:1095–1101.

9 Barlow J B, Marcus R H, Pocock W A et al. Mechanisms and management of heart failure in active rheumatic carditis. *S Afr Med J* 1990; 78:181–186.

10 Beevers D G & Prince J S. Some recent advances in non-communicable disease in the tropics. 1. Hypertension: an emerging problem in tropical countries. *Trans R Soc Trop Med Hyg* 1991; 85:324–326.

11 Campbell G D. Non-aflatoxin human mycotoxicosis: an experience. *Proc R Coll Physicians Edinb* 1992; 22:45–51.

12 Chauvet J, Kakou Guikahue M, Aka F et al. La gravité des cardites rheumatismales à Abidjan. A propos de 52 cas à Abidjan chez les enfants de moins de 15 ans. *Cardiol Trop* 1989; 15:77–81.

13 Chugh K S, Jain S, Sakhuja V et al. Renovascular hypertension due to Takayasu's arteritis among Indian patients. *Q J Med* 1992; 85:833–843.

14 Connor D H, Somers K, Hutt M S R et al. Endomyocardial fibrosis in Uganda (Davises' disease). *Am Heart J* 1968; 75:107–124.

15 Connor D H, Somers K, Hutt M S R et al. Endomyocardial fibrosis in Uganda (Davises' disease). *Am Heart J* 1967; 74:687–700.

16 Danaraj T J, Wong H O & Thomas M A. Primary arteritis of aorta causing renal artery stenosis and hypertension. *Br Heart J* 1963; 25:153–165.

17 Davidson N Mc D & Parry E H O. Peripartum cardiac failure. *Q J Med* 1979; 47:431–461.

18 Diaz R A, Obasohan A & Oakley C M. Prediction

of outcome in dilated cardiomyopathy. *Br Heart J* 1987; 58:393–399.

19 Edington M E & Gear J S S. Rheumatic heart disease in Soweto—a programme for secondary prevention. *S Afr Med J* 1982; 62:523–525.

20 Ekpo E B, Udofia O, Eshiet N F et al. Demographic life style and anthropometric correlates of blood pressure of Nigerian urban civil servants, factory and plantation workers. *J Hum Hypertens* 1992; 6:275–280.

21 Falase A O, Ayeni O, Sekoni G A et al. Heart failure in Nigerian hypertensives. *Afr J Med Sci* 1983; 12:7–15.

22 Guimaraes A C, Esteves J P, Filho A S et al. Clinical aspects of endomyocardial fibrosis in Bahia, Brazil. *Am Heart J* 1971; 81:7–19.

23 He J, Klag M J, Whelton P K et al. Migration, blood pressure pattern, and hypertension: the Yi migrant study. *Am J Epidemiol* 1991; 134:1085–1101.

24 Homans D C. Current concepts: peripartum cardiomyopathy. *N Engl J Med* 1985; 312:1432–1437.

25 Ibrahim Khalil S, Elhaq M, Ali E et al. An epidemiological survey of rheumatic fever and rheumatic heart disease in Sahafa Town, Sudan. *J Epidemiol Community Health* 1992; 46:477–479.

26 Ilyas M, Peracha M A, Ahmed R et al. Prevalence and pattern of rheumatic heart disease in the frontier province of Pakistan. *JPMA* 1979; 29:165–198.

27 Isaacson C A. An idiopathic aortitis in young Africans. *J Pathol Bacteriol* 1961; 81:69–79.

28 Isaacson C. The changing pattern of heart disease in South African Blacks. *S Afr Med J* 1977; 52:793–798.

29 Ive F A, Willis A J P, Ikeme A C et al. Endomyocardial fibrosis and filariasis. *Q J Med* 1967; 36:496–516.

30 Jaiyesimi F. Acquired heart disease in Nigerian children: an illustration of the influence of socio-economic factors in disease pattern. *J Trop Paediatr* 1982; 28:223–229.

31 James S A, de Almeida-Filho N & Kaufman J S. Hypertension in Brazil: a review of the epidemiological evidence. *Ethn Dis* 1991; 1:91–98.

32 Kam-sang W & Vallance-Owen J. Changing prevalence and pattern of cardiovascular diseases in Hong Kong. *Chin Med J* 1988; 101:579–586.

33 Mabogunje O A, Adesanya C O, Khwaja M S et al. Surgical management of pericarditis in Zaria, Nigeria. *Thorax* 1981; 36:590–595.

34 Majeed H A, Batnager S, Yousof A M et al. Acute rheumatic fever and the evolution of rheumatic heart disease: a prospective 12 year follow-up report. *J Clin Epidemiol* 1992; 45:871–875.

35 Malu K, Ticolat R, Renambot I et al. Enquête épidémiologique sur les myocardopathies chroniques dilatées primitives: 69 cas. *Cardiol Trop* 1991; 17:127–132.

36 Marin-Neto J A, Maciel B C, Teran Urbanetz L L et al. High output failure in patients with peripartum cardiomyopathy: a comparative study with dilated cardiomyopathy. *Am Heart J* 1991; 121:134–140.

37 Melvin K R, Richardson P J, Olsen E G J et al. Peripartum cardiomyopathy due to myocarditis. *N Engl J Med* 1982; 307:731–734.

38 Midei M G, De Ment S H, Feldman A M et al. Peripartum myocarditis and cardiomyopathy. *Circulation* 1990; 81:922–926.

39 Nkoua J L, Kimbally-Kaky G, Onkami A H et al. La myocardiopathie du postpartum: à propos de 24 cas. *Cardiol Trop* 1991; 17:105–110.

40 Olsen E G J & Richardson P J (eds). Multicentre research project on endomyocardial disease—eleven communications. *Postgrad Med J* 1983; 59:133–188.

41 Okereke O U I, Chikwendu V C, Ihenacho H N C et al. Non-invasive diagnosis of endomyocardial fibrosis in Nigeria using two dimensional echocardiography. *Cardiol Trop* 1991; 17:97–103.

42 Parry E H O & Abrahams D G. The natural history of endomyocardial fibrosis. *Q J Med* 1965; 34:383–408.

43 Patel A K, Ziegler J L, D'Arbela P G et al. Familial cases of endomyocardial fibrosis in Uganda. *BMJ* 1971; 4:331–334.

44 Po-chun Tai, Spry C J F, Obsen E G J et al. Deposits of eosinophil granule proteins in cardiac tissues of patients with endomyocardial fibrosis. *Lancet* 1987; i:643–647.

45 Poulter N R, Khaw K T, Hopwood B E C et al. The Kenya Luo migration study: observations of the initiation of a rise in blood pressure. *BMJ* 1990; 309:967–972.

46 Quinn R W. Comprehensive review of morbidity and mortality trends for rheumatic fever, streptococcal disease, and scarlet fever: the decline of rheumatic fever. *Rev Infect Dis* 1989; 11:928–953.

47 Richardson P J, Wodak A D, Atkinson L et al. Relation between alcohol intake, myocardial enzyme activity, and myocardial function in dilated cardiomyopathy: evidence for the concept of alcohol induced heart muscle disease. *Br Heart J* 1986; 56:165–170.

48 Rosenthal T, Grossman E, Knecht A et al. Levels and correlates of blood pressure in recent and earlier Ethiopian immigrants to Israel. *J Hum Hypertens* 1990; 4:425–430.

49 Mtabaji J P, Nara Y & Yamori Y. The cardiac study in Tanzania: salt intake in the causation and treatment of hypertension. *J Hum Hypertens* 1990; 4:80–81.

50 Sanderson J E, Olsen E G J & Gatei D. Peripartum heart disease: an endomyocardial biopsy study. *Br Heart J* 1986; 56:285–291.

51 Sanderson J E, Adesanya C O, Anjorin F I et al. Postpartum cardiac failure—heart failure due to volume overload? *Am Heart J* 1979; 97:613–621.

52 Schrire V & Asherson R A. Arteritis of the aorta and its major branches. *Q J Med* 1964; 33:439–463.

53 Serme D. Etude épidémiologique, clinique et évolutive de valvulopathies rheumatismales observées à Onagadongon. *Cardiol Trop* 1992; 18:93–99.

54 Shaper A G & Coles R M. The tribal distribution of endomyocardial fibrosis in Uganda. *Br Heart J* 1965; 27:121–127.

55 Spry C J F. Eosinophils in eosinophilic endomyocardial disease. *Postgrad Med J* 1987; 62:609–613.

56 Stephen S J. Changing patterns of mitral stenosis in childhood and pregnancy in Sri Lanka. *J Am Coll Cardiol* 1992; 19:1276–1284.

57 Strang J I G, Gibson D G, Nun A J et al. Controlled trial of prednisolone as adjuvant in treatment of tuberculous constrictive pericarditis in Transkei. *Lancet* 1987; i:1418–1422.

58 Strang J I G, Gibson D G, Mitchison D A et al. Controlled clinical trial of complete open surgical drainage and of prednisolone in treatment of tuberculous pericardial effusion in Transkei. *Lancet* 1988; ii:759–764.

59 Strang J I G. Tuberculous pericarditis in Transkei. *Clin Cardiol* 1984; 7:667–670.

60 Sutton M St J, Cole P & Plappert M. Effects of subsequent pregnancy on left ventricular function in peripartum cardiomyopathy. *Am Heart J* 1991; 121:1776–1778.

61 Tamburro P & Wilber D. Sudden death in idiopathic dilated cardiomyopathy. *Am Heart J* 1992; 124:1035–1045.

62 Vijayaraghavan G, Davies J, Sadanandan S et al. Echocardiographic features of tropical endomyocardial disease in South India. *Br Heart J* 1983; 50:450–459.

63 WHO Cardiovascular Diseases Unit. WHO programme for the prevention of rheumatic fever/rheumatic heart disease in 16 developing countries: report from phase I (1986–90). *Bull World Health Organ* 1992; 70:213–218.

64 Wong S L & Donnan S P. Influence of socio-economic status on cardiovascular diseases in Hong Kong. *J Epidemiol Community Health* 1992; 46:148–150.

65 Woo K S, Kong S M & Wai K H. The changing prevalence and pattern of acute rheumatic fever and rheumatic heart disease in Hong Kong (1968–1978). *Aust N Z J Med* 1983; 13:151–156.

66 Haffejee I. Rheumatic fever and rheumatic heart disease: the current status of its epidemiology, diagnostic criteria and prophylaxis. *Q J Med* 1992; 84:641–658.

CHAPTER 6

HAEMATOLOGICAL DISEASES IN THE TROPICS

Alan F. Fleming

REFERENCE RANGES

The normal values of red cell counts and indices, white cell counts, platelet counts and activities of haemostatic mechanisms vary with age, sex and pregnancy state.[1,2] There are also genetic and common environmental factors which can affect the reference ranges in certain populations.[3] It is especially important that the difference in reference ranges in all stages of life be appreciated by health workers in tropical countries, where up to half the population are aged under 15 years and women experience numerous and often complicated pregnancies.

RED CELL VALUES

Age

Full term infants

Red cell values of the fetus are almost unchanged during the last trimester of pregnancy. The full term infant is born with a high haemoglobin (Hb) concentration, red blood cell (RBC) count and mean cell volume (MCV) (Table 6.1). A rapid rate of red cell production and low splenic function are shown by the presence of nucleated RBCs, occasional Howell–Jolly bodies (red cell nuclear fragments), polychromasia, a high reticulocyte count (mean 150 $\times 10^9$/l) and target cells in the peripheral blood. In the first few hours of life, the Hb concentration of capillary blood is on average 35 g/l higher than in venous blood, due to haemoconcentration. If the blood from the placenta is allowed to transfuse into the infant, the Hb rises about 10–20 g/l.

The blood volume ranges from 50 to 100 ml (mean 85 ml) per kilogram body weight.

During the first few weeks of life, the ability of the blood to deliver oxygen is in excess of what is required, so that erythropoietin secretion is low and the bone marrow is relatively hypoplastic. Red cell survival is short, 80–100 days compared with 90–150 (mean 120) days in adults. Plasma volume increases as the infant grows. As a consequence, the Hb, packed cell volume (PCV) and RBC count decline to reach a nadir between 8 and 12 weeks of life. The large fetal red cells are replaced, and the MCV declines (Table 6.1). Fetal haemoglobin (HbF) is replaced by adult haemoglobin (HbA) (Table 6.2).[4]

Premature infants

Infants born prematurely during the third trimester have red cell values initially the same as those of full term infants. However, their basal metabolic rates, oxygen consumption, erythropoietin secretion, red cell production and red cell survival (60–80 days) are all lower. After birth, red cell values fall faster and to lower levels than in mature infants: at around 8 weeks of life the most premature but otherwise normal and well-nourished infant can have an Hb as low as 70 g/l (Table 6.3).[2]

Childhood

After the third month of life, oxygen needs exceed oxygen delivery and provide the necessary stimulus to erythropoietin secretion and red cell production: the Hb, PCV and RBC count rise steadily until puberty (Table 6.1).

Sex

The Hb continues to rise in boys but levels off in girls at puberty, so that men have on average Hb 15 g/l— higher than non-pregnant women (Table 6.1). Red

Table 6.1 Red blood cell values at various ages.

	Hb (g/l)	PCV (1/1)	RBC ($\times 10^{12}/l$)	MCV (fl)	MCH (pg)	MCHC (g/l)
Birth (cord blood)	165 ± 30	0.54 ± 0.10	6.0 ± 1.0	120 (mean)	—	300 ± 27
3 months	115 ± 20	0.38 ± 0.04	4.0 ± 0.8	95 (mean)	29 ± 5	325 ± 25
1 year	120 ± 15	—	4.4 ± 0.08	78 ± 8	27 ± 4	325 ± 25
3–6 years	130 ± 10	0.40 ± 0.04	4.8 ± 0.7	84 ± 8	27 ± 3	325 ± 25
10–12 years	130 ± 15	0.41 ± 0.04	4.7 ± 0.7	84 ± 7	27 ± 3	325 ±25
Men	155 ± 25	0.47 ± 0.07	5.5 ± 1.0	86 ± 10	29.5 ± 2.5	325 ± 25
Women	140 ± 25	0.42 ± 0.05	4.8 ± 1.0	86 ± 10	29.5 ± 2.5	325 ± 25

Values are mean ± 2 SD (95% range).
Hb, haemoglobin; MCH, mean cell haemoglobin; MCHC, mean cell haemoglobin concentration; MCV, mean cell volume; PCV, packed cell volume (haematocrit); RBC, red blood cell count.
Reproduced with permission of the authors and publishers from Dacie and Lewis.[1]

Table 6.2 Proportion of haemoglobin F found at various ages.

Age	HbF (%)
Birth	70–90
1 month	50–75
2 months	25–60
3 months	10–35
4 months	5–20
6 months	<8
9 months	<5
1 year	<2
Adults	<0.4

Reproduced with permission of the author and publishers from Huehns.[4]

Table 6.3 Haemoglobin (g/l) observed in iron-sufficient preterm infants.

	Birthweight (g)	
Age	1000–1500	1501–2000
2 weeks	163 (117–184)	148 (188–196)
1 month	109 (87–152	115 (82–150)
2 months	88 (71–115)	94 (80–114)
3 months	98 (89–112)	102 (93–118)
4 months	113 (91–131)	113 (91–131)
5 months	116 (102–143)	118 (104–130)
6 months	120 (94–138)	118 (107–126)

Values are mean (range).
Reproduced with permission of the authors and publishers from Lundström U, Siimes M A & Dallman P R. *J. Pediatr* 1977; 91:878–883.

cell volumes are 30 ± 5 ml/kg in men and 25 ± 5 ml/kg in women; plasma volume (45 ± 5 ml/kg) and total blood volume (70 ± 10 ml/kg) are the same in both sexes. Testosterone is the stimulus to additional erythropoiesis in men, whereas oestrogen depresses erythropoiesis.

Pregnancy

From the 12th week of gestation there is an increase of erythropoietin secretion, erythroid hyperplasia, reticulocytosis (2–6%) and an increase of the total red cell volume by 400–450 ml in normal and iron-sufficient pregnant women. The plasma volume increases also, by about 1250 ml in primigravidae and 1500 ml in multigravidae. As the increase in plasma volume is greater than that of the red cell volume, there is haemodilution (Figure 6.1 B,C): Hb 110 g/l and PCV 0.31 are the accepted lower limits of normal. There is a mild macrocytosis (increase of MCV) during pregnancy.[5]

Genetic and environmental differences

When large series of persons of European descent (whites) and of sub-Saharan African descent (blacks) have been matched for age, sex, pregnant state and socioeconomic status, it has been found that at all ages and in both sexes blacks have on average Hb 5–10 g/l lower than whites, and that this difference is independent of environment. A high frequency of α^+ thalassaemia, up to 50% of some black populations, explains this small genetically determined difference.

Of much greater importance are environmental factors, including malaria, other intercurrent infections and malnutrition, especially deficiencies of iron and folic acid. Apparently healthy members of

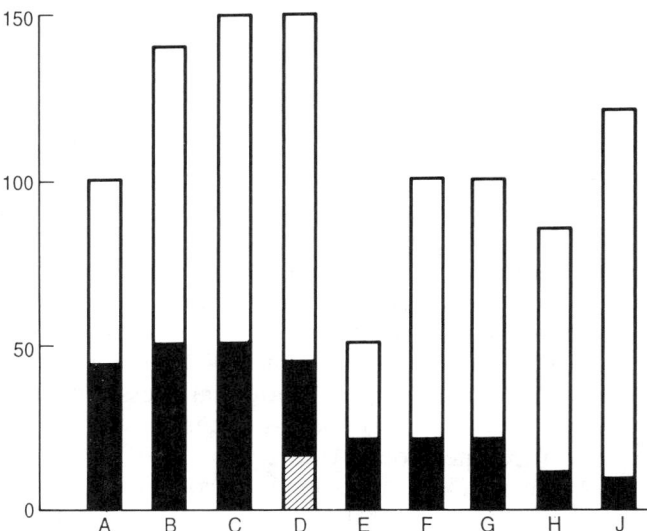

Figure 6.1 Blood volume changes in health and disease. (A) Normal (non-pregnant) adult. (B) Normal single pregnancy. (C) Normal twin pregnancy. (D) Hypersplenism, not anaemic. (E) Acute haemorrhage. (F) Acute haemorrhage, 48 hours later. (G) Moderate anaemia. (H) Severe anaemia. (J) Severe anaemia with circulatory congestion. Note that two or more of these conditions may be present in the same patient; in particular E–J are variations on A (non-pregnant), but could be shown again as variants on B (pregnant), C (multiple pregnancy) or D (hypersplenism). ▨, Red cells sequestered in the spleen; ■, red cells; □, plasma. (Reproduced with permission of the publisher from Fleming A F. In Parry E H O (ed.) *Principles of Medicine in Africa*, 2nd edn. Oxford: Oxford University Press, 1984: 706.)

communities living in the tropics frequently show an average Hb 20 g/l lower at all ages and in both sexes than the internationally accepted reference means. The control of malaria, improvements in hygiene and nutrition, and rises in social class are all associated with the range of Hb concentrations increasing towards the standard ranges.[2]

Altitude. For every 1000 m above sea level, the Hb increases on average by 2.5 g/l, due to low oxygen tension stimulating erythropoietin production.

Miscellaneous factors. The Hb rises slightly with muscular exercise and in assuming the upright posture. It is somewhat higher in the morning than the evening. It is lower in athletes in training, and is raised in tobacco-smokers.

WHITE CELL COUNTS

NEUTROPHILS

Age

There is a transiently high total white blood cell (WBC) count and a neutrophil leucocytosis at and following birth, peaking at about 12 hours of life (Table 6.4), with a high number of non-segmented neutrophils (up to $1.8 \times 10^9/l$). The number of neutrophils declines and is exceeded by the lympho-

Table 6.4 Normal leucocyte counts.

Age	Total leucocytes		Neutrophils			Lymphocytes			Monocytes		Eosinophils	
	Mean	(range)	Mean	(range)	%	Mean	range	%	Mean	%	Mean	%
Birth	18.1	(9.0–30.0)	11.0	(6.0–26.0)	61	5.5	(2.0–11.0)	31	1.1	6	0.4	2
12 hours	22.8	(13.0–38.0)	15.5	(6.0–28.0)	68	5.5	(2.0–11.0)	24	1.2	5	0.5	2
24 hours	18.9	(9.4–34.0)	11.5	(5.0–21.0)	61	5.8	(2.0–11.5)	31	1.1	6	0.5	2
1 week	12.2	(5.0–21.0)	5.5	(1.5–10.0)	45	5.0	(2.0–17.0)	41	1.1	9	0.5	4
2 weeks	11.4	(5.0–20.0)	4.5	(1.0–9.5)	40	5.5	(2.0–17.0)	48	1.0	9	0.4	3
1 month	10.8	(5.0–19.5)	3.8	(1.0–9.0)	35	6.0	(2.0–16.5)	56	0.7	7	0.3	3
6 months	11.9	(6.0–17.5)	3.8	(1.0–8.5)	32	7.3	(4.0–13.5)	61	0.6	5	0.3	3
1 year	11.4	(6.0–17.5)	3.5	(1.5–8.5)	31	7.0	(4.0–10.5)	61	0.6	5	0.3	3
2 years	10.6	(6.0–17.0)	3.5	(1.5–8.5)	33	6.3	(3.0–9.5)	59	0.5	5	0.3	3
4 years	9.1	(5.5–15.5)	3.8	(1.5–8.5)	42	4.5	(2.0–8.0)	50	0.5	5	0.3	3
6 years	8.5	(5.0–14.5)	4.3	(1.5–8.0)	51	3.5	(1.5–7.0)	42	0.4	5	0.2	3
8 years	8.3	(4.5–13.5)	4.4	(1.5–8.0)	53	3.3	(1.5–6.8)	39	0.4	4	0.2	2
10 years	8.1	(4.5–13.5)	4.4	(1.8–8.0)	54	3.1	(1.5–6.5)	38	0.4	4	0.2	2
16 years	7.8	(4.5–13.0)	4.4	(1.8–8.0)	57	2.8	(1.2–5.2)	35	0.4	5	0.2	3
21 years	7.4	(4.5–11.0)	4.4	(1.8–7.7)	59	2.5	(1.0–4.8)	34	0.3	4	0.2	3

Values are mean (95% confidence limits) $\times 10^9/l$ and mean percentage of differential counts.
Reproduced with permission of the author, the publisher and WB Saunders. From Dallman P R. In Rudolph A M (ed.) *Pediatrics*, 16th edn. New York: Appleton Century-Crofts, 1977: 1178.

cyte count after 2 weeks. From 2 years, the number of circulating neutrophils increases with age until adult life, when they contribute 40–75% of the total count of $4.0–11.0 \times 10^9$/l in caucasian adults.[2]

Sex

Women during their reproductive period of life have slightly higher WBC and neutrophil counts (average difference 0.66×10^9/l) than men, and oral contraceptives increase counts further: there are two peaks of neutrophil leucocytosis coinciding with peaks of oestrogen secretion and a fall following menstruation. Postmenopausal women have counts slightly lower than men.

Pregnancy

The WBC and neutrophil counts rise to a plateau by the second trimester (WBC mean 9.0×10^9/l, range $5.0–16.0 \times 10^9$/l; neutrophils mean 7.0×10^9/l, range $2.5–14.0 \times 10^9$/l) (Figure 6.2).[5] There is a sharp peak of neutrophil leucocytosis during obstetric delivery, when the total WBC count may reach 40×10^9/l in an uninfected patient. Neutrophil and total WBC counts fall to non-pregnant levels by the sixth day post partum. The circulating neutrophils in pregnant women are relatively young, with a shift to the left (<3% metamyelocytes and myelocytes), raised activity of neutrophil alkaline phosphatase and other enzymes and enhanced bactericidal function.

Genetic and environmental factors

A relative and absolute neutropenia has been described in children over 6 months and adults who are black Africans or of black African descent in the Americas and Europe (Table 6.5),[3] and in Palestinians, Yemeni Jews and Saudi Arabians. The total body neutrophils have been found to be the same in adults of West Indian origin living in the UK as in the white Britons, but the West Indians have a greater number of neutrophils in the bone marrow storage pool, while Europeans have more in circulation; provocation of a neutrophil response, either experimentally or by natural infection, leads to rises to the same level in both races. There is probably a genetic factor underlying this ethnic neutropenia, but environmental factors may also play a role, for example those causing splenomegaly and hypersple-

nism. The neutrophil count rises with higher socio-economic status in Africans, and declines in Europeans living in west Africa.

The WBC and neutrophil counts rise during pregnancy in African women, but remain about 3.0×10^9/l lower than in pregnant caucasians (Figure 6.2).

Miscellaneous factors. Counts are higher in the afternoon than in the morning, by about 0.5×10^9/l. Exercise mobilizes the cells marginated on the endothelium, and so raises the number of circulating cells, even up to a WBC count of 30×10^9/l with the most strenuous exertion. Emotional stress can raise counts transiently. Tobacco-smokers have persistently higher neutrophil counts.

Acute reactive neutrophil leucocytosis is seen most commonly in response to pyogenic infections (Table 6.6): immature neutrophils (metamyelocytes) are released from the bone marrow; there is an excess of deeply purple staining primary cytoplasmic granules ('toxic granulation'); occasionally oval blue staining Döhle bodies, which are RNA, are present in the cytoplasm. Neutrophil damage shows as ragged and vacuolated cytoplasm and pyknotic nuclei. With severe infections there can be a leukaemoid reaction, when the total count is above 80×10^9/l with a shift to the left as far as promyelocytes and blast cells.

EOSINOPHILS AND BASOPHILS

The eosinophil count is high at birth and declines slowly throughout childhood to less than 0.4×10^9/l in adult life (see Table 6.4).[2] There is a diurnal variation, more considerable than that of neutrophils. The eosinophil count is lower during pregnancy; the stress of obstetric delivery causes the eosinophils to vanish from the peripheral blood almost entirely, even if there was an initially high count (Figure 6.2). Symptom-free individuals living in the tropics often have high eosinophil counts due to subclinical infections by helminths (see Table 6.5); counts are higher in rural and non-elite groups than in urban and elite groups. In the tropics eosinophilia is more likely to be a response to helminthic infection than to be an indication of allergy (Table 6.6).

The basophil count is normally low (see Table 6.4); accurate electronic counting demonstrates diminished counts during stress, pregnancy, acute infections and the administration of corticosteroids. A raised count is always suggestive of leukaemia or a myeloproliferative disorder, but may be seen in some allergic conditions (Table 6.6).

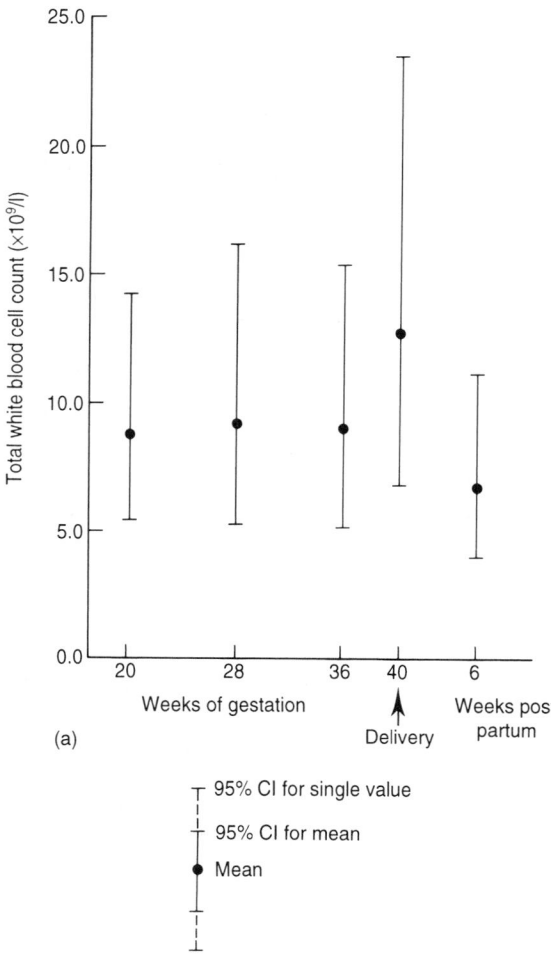

(a)

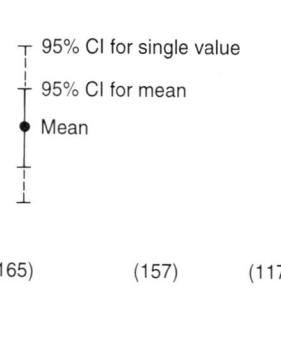

95% CI for single value

95% CI for mean

● Mean

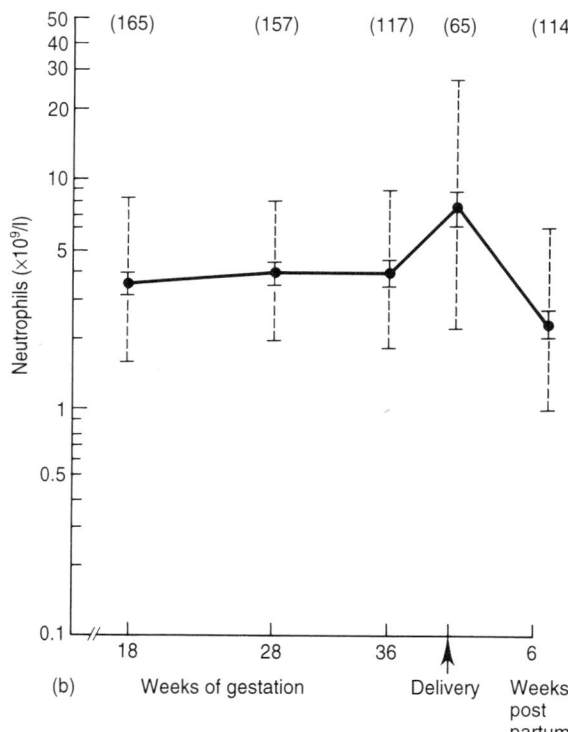

(b)

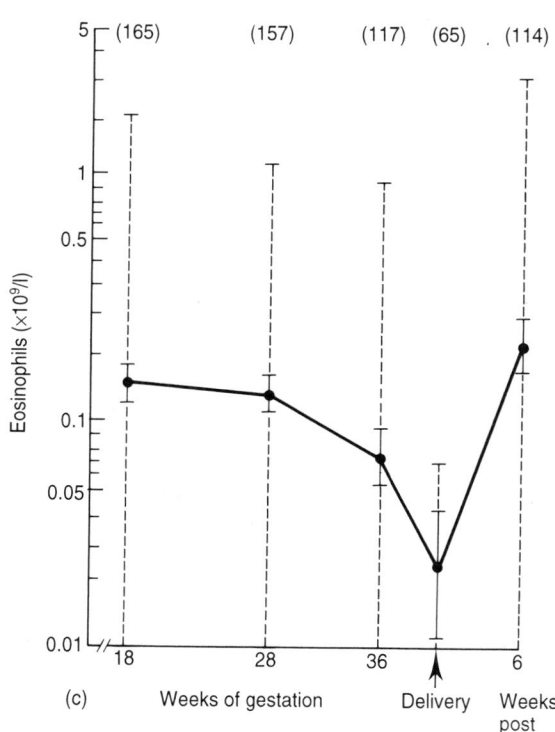

(c)

Figure 6.2 (a) Total white blood cell count (mean and 95% confidence limits for a single value) in 67 white Australian women during pregnancy. From Fleming.[5] (b) Absolute neutrophil counts and (c) absolute eosinophil counts in Nigerian primigravidae during pregnancy and the puerperium: numbers of observations are in parentheses. (Reproduced with permission from Fleming A F, Akintunde E A, Harrison K A & Dunn D. *E. Afr Med J* 1985; 62:175–184.)

Table 6.5 Leucocyte counts in 123 non-elite male Nigerian blood donors in Zaria.

	Mean	*(Range)*	*%*
Total white cells	5.1	(2.6–10.2)	—
Neutrophils	2.8	(1.1–7.1)	30–85
Eosinophils	0.11	(0–2.0)	1–30
Basophils	0.002	(0–0.02)	0–1
Lymphocytes	2.1	(0.7–3.1)	15–60
Monocytes	0.13	(0–1.3)	0–8

Values are mean (95% confidence limits) $\times 10^9$/l and range of percentage of differential counts.

Table 6.6 Some causes of reactive leucocytosis.

Leucocytosis	Causes
Neutrophilia	Acute viral infections (e.g. poliomyelitis)
	Acute bacterial infections (e.g. staphylococcal)
	Tissue damage
	Haemorrhage
	Haemolysis
	Malignancies
	Stress states
	Diabetic ketoacidosis
	Miscellaneous (drugs, corticosteroids, chemicals, renal failure, collagen diseases)
	Pregnancy and delivery
Eosinophilia	Helminthic infections of tissues
	Löffler's syndrome (larval migration of nematodes)
	Convalescence from viral or other infections
	Malignancies
	Cytotoxic therapy
	Allergic disorders
	Miscellaneous (post splenectomy, familial, lead ingestion, polyarteritis nodosa, pulmonary aspergillosis, rheumatoid arthritis)
Basophilia	Miscellaneous (hypersensitivity, myxoedema, iron deficiency, chronic haemolysis)
Lymphocytosis	Childhood infections generally
	Protozoan infections (malaria, toxoplasmosis)
	Viral infections
Monocytosis	Protozoan infections (malaria)
	Rickettsial infections
	Subacute/chronic bacterial infections (tuberculosis, brucellosis, subacute bacterial endocarditis)

LYMPHOCYTES

The lymphocyte count is normally high in the first year of life and then declines to adult levels (see Table 6.4). There are no reported differences between adult males and non-pregnant females, but the total lymphocyte count declines slightly during pregnancy; of more importance is a functional reduction of T-cell-mediated immunity during pregnancy.

A proliferation of B-cell lymphocytes is commonly seen in the tropics in response to malaria and other intercurrent infections, especially in childhood in rural and non-elite groups (Table 6.6). An absolute lymphocytosis with numerous activated lymphocytes (plasmacytoid cells) is frequently seen in children in the tropics. Atypical lymphocytes with slate-grey or blue cytoplasm are suggestive of viral infections. African adults have a relative lymphocytosis, due to neutropenia, and often an absolute lymphocytosis (see Table 6.5). Of peripheral blood lymphocytes of adults in the industrialized countries, approximately 80% are T cells, 10–15% B cells and 5–10% null cells; rural Nigerians have been reported to have higher proportions of B cells (about 30%), whereas elite Nigerians and Europeans had similar distribution of lymphocyte subsets.

MONOCYTES

The monocyte count is highest during the first 2 weeks of life (see Table 6.4); there is no other significant physiological change, except a fall during obstetric delivery. In the tropics counts may be raised in association with subclinical protozoan or other infections or lowered in subjects with splenomegaly (see Tables 6.5 and 6).

HAEMOSTASIS

Age

Platelet counts (normal $150–400 \times 10^9/l$) and function do not vary with age to any clinically significant degree.

Vitamin K is a fat-soluble vitamin, widely distributed in both vegetable and animal foods as well as being absorbed from that produced by the microbiological flora of the normal gut. Vitamin K levels of infants, especially premature infants, are critically low in the first 3 days of life because of a slow rate of transport across the placenta, low hepatic stores, the absence of an intestinal bacterial flora, and low concentrations in colostrum and breast milk. In addition, the immature liver has limited capacity for the synthesis of clotting factors. Vitamin K is essential for the synthesis by the liver of clotting factors (II, VII, IX and X) and protein C and protein S; these have low activity in umbilical cord blood, especially in preterm infants, so that the prothrombin time (PT) and partial thromboplastin time

Table 6.7 Haemostatic measurements in the newborn and adults.

	Preterm infants	Full term infants	Children over 2 months and adults
Platelets × 10^9/l	150–400	150–400	150–400
Prothrombin time (s)	13–18	12–16	11–14
Partial thromboplastin time (s)	35–50	30–45	23–35
Fibrinogen (g/l)	2–4	2–4	2–4
FDP (mg/l)	<10	<10	<10

Reproduced with permission of the author and publishers from Buchanan G R. *Clin Haematol* 1978; 7:85–109.

(PTT) are prolonged (Table 6.7).[2] Vitamin K-producing bacteria colonize the bowel and the deficiency is rectified usually by 72–120 hours. However, a few infants, especially the preterm, progress to haemorrhagic disease of the newborn. Fibrinolytic activity is essentially functional in infants.

Sex

Platelet counts are higher in women than man by about 20%, and fall following menstruation.[1]

Pregnancy

Plasma volume expansion causes the platelet count to fall about 20% during pregnancy, but function remains unchanged. The activity of the rapid extrinsic pathway is enhanced during pregnancy, with high levels of factors VII, X and fibrinogen. On the intrinsic pathway, activity of factors XII, IX and VIII are also moderately raised, but factor XI decreases. A decline of antithrombin III (AT III) adds to hypercoagulability in pregnancy, so that the thromboplastin generation time and PT are accelerated. This potential hypercoagulability is balanced by lower levels of factor XIII. Plasminogen levels are increased parallel to the rise of fibrinogen, while antiplasmin activity is unchanged. This potential for fibrinolysis is suppressed normally by the placenta producing inhibitors to plasminogen activator synthesis and release by endothelium. Fibrin/

fibrinogen degradation products (FDPs) are present in plasma low concentrations in the third trimester only.

During obstetric delivery and following separation of the placenta there is activation and consumption of platelets and coagulation factors; the fibrinolytic pathway is activated, with a transient appearance of FDPs reaching a maximum in the first 4 hours post partum. There is a return of all haemostatic factors to non-pregnant levels by the end of the second week of the puerperium.

Genetic and environmental differences

The platelet counts in the African newborns up to around 6 months of age do not differ significantly from those of European newborns and adults. Older children and adults throughout tropical Africa have a moderate thrombocytopenia, for example 70–370 × 10^9/l in symptom-free adult male Nigerians. This is probably the result of increased pooling of platelets in subclinically enlarged spleens.[1,3]

Platelets from non-elite Nigerians have been shown to be relatively resistant to aggregation by ADP, thrombin and ristocetin: aggregation can be induced either by increasing concentrations of the agonists or by resuspending the platelets in European plasma, suggesting that there are inhibitory plasma factors; these could be merely high levels of macroglobulins in response to intercurrent infections. The bleeding time and clot retraction are within standard reference ranges and there is no tendency to purpura, but the inhibition of platelet adhesion and aggregation could contribute to the low incidence of atheroma and thrombosis.[6]

Factor VIII coagulant activity of Africans is commonly greater than 150% of the activity of pooled European plasma. Levels in plasma of fibrinogen, plasminogen activators and spontaneous fibrinolysis are high in Africans and Papua New Guineans who perform heavy manual work, but levels fall with rising economic status and a more sedentary life. In Kenya and Papua New Guinea the frequency distribution of PT was shown to be skewed to the right, that is there was a subpopulation with prolonged times; subclinical hepatic disease is a probable cause, and this is likely to apply to other tropical populations.

ANAEMIA

DEFINITION

Anaemia is defined as a condition in which the Hb concentration in peripheral blood is lower than normal for age, sex and pregnancy state of the subject (Table 6.8). The Hb is usually directly related to the total red cell volume, but there are exceptional circumstances: (1) during the first hours of life, when there is haemoconcentration in the capillaries, capillary blood samples will underestimate anaemia, especially in premature, acidotic, hypotensive or hypovolaemic infants; (2) immediately following acute haemorrhage, the Hb remains unchanged until there has been compensatory expansion of the plasma volume over the following 48 hours (see Figure 6.1E, F); (3) with splenomegaly there is both an expansion of plasma volume and sequestration of red cells, so that patients with massive splenomegaly may have a Hb 80 g/l, for example, while the total red cell mass is normal (see Figure 6.1D).

AETIOLOGY

Anaemia results from three basic mechanisms: (1) blood loss (haemorrhage); (2) decreased production of red cells; and (3) increased destruction of red cells (haemolysis) (Table 6.9). Only those causes which are of major public health importance in the tropics will be discussed. These include: (1) infections such as malaria, hookworm, schistosomiasis, tuberculosis, and the human immunodeficiency viruses (HIV-1, HIV-2); (2) nutritional deficiencies of iron and

Table 6.8 Haemoglobin concentrations below which anaemia is likely to be present in populations living at sea level.

	Hb *(g/l)*
Newborn infants	140
6 months–6 years	110
6–14 years	120
Adult males	130
Adult females (non-pregnant)	120
Adult females (pregnant)	110

For each increment of 1000 m above sea level, add 2.5 g/l (2 g/l per 2500 feet). Reproduced from various sources, including the World Health Organization.[7]

Table 6.9 Aetiology of anaemia.

1 Blood loss
  (a) *Acute*
  (b) *Chronic* (e.g. hookworm) leading to iron deficiency

2 Decreased red cell production

(a) *Nutritional deficiencies*	(b) *Depressed bone marrow function*
Iron	Secondary anaemias
Folate	infections (e.g.
Vitamin B_{12}	tuberculosis)
Various	chronic hepatic disease
protein–energy,	chronic renal disease
vitamin A,	carcinomatosis
vitamin C,	HIV
vitamin E, riboflavin,	Aplastic anaemia
pyridoxine, Cu	drugs and chemicals
	infiltration
	idiopathic
	irradiation
	congenital
	Thalassaemias
	α thalassaemias
	β thalassaemias

3 Increased red cell destruction

(a) *Abnormalities of red cells*	(b) *Abnormal haemolysis*
Haemoglobin	Immune haemolysis
sickle cell disease	autoimmune
Enzymes	fetomaternal
G6PD deficiency	incompatibility
Membrane	incompatible blood
elliptocytosis	transfusion
ovalocytosis	Non-immune haemolysis
spherocytosis	infections (e.g.
	malaria)
	hypersplenism
	drugs and chemicals
	venoms
	burns
	mechanical

folate; and (3) inherited disorders of red cells, including the thalassaemias, sickle cell disease, glucose-6-phosphate dehydrogenase (G6PD) deficiency, and ovalocytosis.

EPIDEMIOLOGY

Anaemia is the most common manifestation of disease observed in the tropics (Table 6.10). Prevalence and morbidity are greatest in preschool

Table 6.10 Estimated prevalence of anaemia by geographic region and age/sex category, around 1980 (population data in millions).

	Children 0–4 years			Children 5–12 years			Men 15–59 years			Women 15–49 years Pregnant			Women 15–49 years All		
	No.	Anaemic %	No.	No.	Anaemic %	No.	No.	Anaemic %	No.	No.	Anaemic %	No.	No.	Anaemic %	No.
Region															
Africa	85.7	56	48.0	96.6	49	47.3	116.8	20	23.4	17.9	63	11.3	106.4	44	46.8
Northern America	19.6	8	1.6	27.5	13	3.6	76.3	4	3.1	3.4	—	—	64.2	8	5.1
Latin America	52.9	26	13.7	69.8	26	18.1	98.1	13	12.8	9.9	30	3.0	86.5	17	14.7
East Africa	16.1	20	3.2	25.4	22	5.6	55.8	11	6.1	2.7	20	0.5	46.9	18	8.4
South Asia	212.0	56	118.7	278.4	50	139.2	386.3	32	123.6	41.7	65	27.1	329.4	58	191.0
Europe	33.4	14	4.7	55.0	5	3.0	147.2	2	3.0	5.7	14	0.8	117.5	12	14.1
Oceania	2.3	18	0.4	3.6	15	0.5	6.9	7	0.5	0.4	25	0.1	5.5	19	0.1
Former Soviet Union	23.1	—	—	31.1	—	—	80.3	—	—	4.0	—	—	68.7	—	—
World*	445.1	43	193.5	587.6	37	217.4	967.7	18	174.2	85.8	51	43.9	825.0	35	288.4
Developed regions	86.1	12	10.3	130.7	7	9.1	346.5	3	12.0	14.8	14	2.0	285.5	11	32.7
Developing regions*	395.0	51	183.2	456.8	46	208.3	621.2	26	162.2	71.0	59	41.9	539.5	47	255.7

*Excluding China
Reproduced by permission of the World Health Organization from DeMaeyer and Adiels-Tegman.[8]

children and pregnant women, in whom it is usual to find about half to be anaemic in rural and impoverished communities. The most common causes in preschool children are iron deficiency, malaria, thalassaemias (in Asia) and sickle cell disease (in Africa). The conditions leading most frequently to an anaemia in pregnancy are iron and folate deficiencies, malaria, thalassaemia minor (in Asia) and milder forms of sickle cell disease (in Africa). Although anaemia is less common and usually less severe in school children, men and non-pregnant women, it is still a major health problem in these groups: in them, anaemia is often secondary to tuberculosis or other chronic infections. HIV-infection is now an extremely common cause of anaemia in Africa, and will be increasingly common in Asia.

PATHOPHYSIOLOGY

Anaemia reduces the oxygen-carrying capacity of the blood. The body compensates for this by: (1) increasing the release of oxygen from Hb to the tissues; (2) increasing cardiac output; (3) enhancing blood flow to vital tissues with high oxygen requirements, while reducing flow to other organs; and (4) increasing respiration. The severity of anaemia is best considered as passing through three stages: (1) compensated, (2) decompensated and (3) anaemic

cardiac failure. The severity of anaemia does not depend on the Hb concentration alone, so that cut-off points of Hb 70 g/l and 30 g/l for when decompensation and cardiac failure respectively are likely must be taken as very approximate. Older patients are more likely to progress to decompensation or heart failure than the young; infants and young children are able to tolerate extremely low Hb concentrations with few complaints. Patients who develop an anaemia acutely have less time to compensate than patients with chronic anaemias such as sickle cell disease or aplastic anaemia. Patients who are hypervolaemic as a result of pregnancy (see Figure 6.1B), especially multiple pregnancy (see Figure 6.1C), or of splenomegaly (see Figure 6.1D) are more liable to progress as far as congestive cardiac failure, as are patients with underlying cardiac, vascular or respiratory diseases. In contrast, patients with low levels of activity, including the bedridden, are less likely to become decompensated.

Compensated anaemia

The major compensatory mechanism in mild to moderate anaemia is the increase of 2,3-diphosphoglycerate (2,3-DPG) concentration in red cells: this binds to deoxyhaemoglobin, shifts the oxygen dissociation curve of Hb to the right (decreased oxygen affinity) and increases oxygen release to tissue by up to 40%.[9] Cardiac output is raised by an increase in stroke volume at rest: on exertion there is both an exaggerated tachycardia and further rise in stroke volume. Vasodilatation enhances the blood flow to the myocardium, skeletal muscle and brain, while there is vasoconstriction in the skin and kidneys. The plasma volume expands, but the total blood volume remains normal (see Figure 6.1G).

Patients complain of breathlessness on exertion only, and there are no physical signs except pallor, unless there are symptoms and signs from the underlying cause of the anaemia.

Work capacity

Maximal work capacity, as measured by the Harvard Step Test (HST), correlates directly with Hb at all levels, and is reduced by even mild anaemia: the average HST of Guatemalan labourers was 65 at Hb 130–150 g/l and 30 at Hb 70–90 g/l.[10]

Productivity and earnings of anaemic male manual workers are seriously reduced.[11,12] The earnings of anaemic women performing less strenuous factory work are also reduced.[13] Anaemia in either parent has an adverse effect on the family through low food production, low income and poor care for children; village life suffers from there being less ground under cultivation, and the national economy declines from overall low productivity.

In childhood, anaemia is associated with slow growth, delayed development and poor cognitive abilities.

Decompensated anaemia

When the Hb falls below about 70 g/l, the major mechanism for improving oxygen delivery is an increase in cardiac output.[9] Both stroke volume and the heart rate are raised at rest. The work of the ventricles is reduced by the low viscosity of anaemic blood and by peripheral vasodilatation; the circulation time is short. The blood volume is reduced in about 25% of patients (see Figure 6.1H).

Patients are breathless even at rest. There is tachycardia, arterial and capillary pulsation, a wide pulse pressure and haemic ejection systolic murmurs. It is common experience that patients who are subsistence farmers, or others wholly dependent on their own manual labour, do not seek treatment until they have reached this stage of anaemia.

About half of all maternal deaths in developing countries are associated with Hb <70 g/l, although anaemia is not the primary cause of death, and there is serious intrauterine growth retardation.

Anaemic heart failure

If anaemia progresses (Hb <30 g/l approximately), the oxygen supply to the myocardium is insufficient, no further increase of cardiac output is impossible, and high-output cardiac failure develops. The plasma volume expands (see Figure 6.1J): patients who are already hypervolaemic from pregnancy or splenomegaly are most liable to develop anaemic heart failure.

Patients are severely breathless and may complain of angina, night cramps or claudication. There is cardiomegaly, engorgement of jugular veins, pulmonary oedema, hepatomegaly, peripheral oedema and sometimes ascites. Without appropriate treatment there is a high morbidity rate: up to 20% of maternal deaths in Africa and India used to be due to anaemic heart failure, and this may still be true where obstetric and blood transfusion services have not developed. Fetal loss remains above 30% from severely anaemic pregnant women.

TREATMENT

The first principle of management is the diagnosis and treatment of the cause of the anaemia. The transfusion of concentrated red cells is required by anaemic patients in three circumstances only: (1) a patient is in danger of dying of anaemic heart failure or hypoxia before specific medication can raise the Hb; (2) a patient is about to experience stress, such as emergency major surgery, obstetric delivery or cytotoxic therapy; and (3) the anaemia is incurable, for example thalassaemia or aplastic anaemia, as will be discussed under these conditions. The inappropriate use of blood transfusion is not to be condoned, especially since the advent of HIV and the acquired immunodeficiency syndrome (AIDS).[14]

HAEMOLYTIC ANAEMIAS

This is a group of anaemias in which there is an increase of red cell turnover due to a shortening of the red cell life span from the normal range of 90–150 (mean 120) days. Haemolysis may be the consequence of an abnormal haemolytic process, or of abnormalities (usually congenital) of the red cells (see Table 6.9). Clinical and laboratory features common to all haemolytic anaemias are due to the

Table 6.11 Features of the haemolytic anaemias.

Features of extravascular and intravascular haemolysis
  Jaundice
  Hyperbilirubinaemia (unconjugated)
  Increased urinary urobilinogen
  Increased faecal urobilinogen (stercobilinogen)

Features of intravascular haemolysis
  Reduced/absent haptoglobins
  Reduced haemopexin
  Haem/methaemoglobinaemia
  Methaemalbumin (positive Schumm's test)
  Haem/methaemoglobinuria
  Haemosiderinuria

Features of increased RBC production
  Polychromasia
  Reticulocytosis
  Bone marrow erythroid hyperplasia

increased breakdown of haemoglobin and the compensatory mechanisms of increased red cell production (Table 6.11). Haemolysis may be extravascular, that is within the reticuloendothelial system (RES), when the breakdown products of haemoglobin follow the normal metabolic pathways of bilirubin. Lysis of red cells within the circulation results in the release of haemoglobin into plasma, the saturation and removal of haemoglobin- and haem-binding proteins (haptoglobins and haemopexin), and the presence of haemoglobin and its degradation products in the plasma and urine. Chronic haemolysis can lead to the formation of pigment stones in the gallbladder.

The bone marrow is capable of increasing red cell production around eight times the normal rate. Compensatory erythroid hyperplasia may be sufficient to maintain a normal or near normal Hb, but is insufficient when rates of haemolysis are most rapid. Often the haemolytic process is accompanied not by erythroid hyperplasia, but by depression of marrow activity, either as part of the pathology of the disease (e.g. malaria) or due to complicating infections, such as parvovirus B19 which precipitates the so-called aplastic crises of sickle cell disease. A rapid rate of red cell production leads to high demands for folic acid, and long-standing haemolytic anaemias are frequently complicated by folate deficiency and megaloblastic erythropoiesis, followed by more profound anaemia. Chronic erythroid hyperplasia, as in sickle cell disease and the thalassaemias, results in expansion of the bone marrow cavity, seen clinically as bossing of the vault of the skull and projection of the maxilla (gnathopathy), and on radiography of the skull—as the hair-on-end appearance (see Figure 6.7).

SPLENOMEGALY AND HYPERSPLENISM

Palpable enlargement of the spleen is a common clinical finding in the tropics, especially where malaria is endemic (Table 6.12). In many instances splenomegaly is accompanied by the syndrome of hypersplenism, when there is pancytopenia, the severity of which is usually related to the size of the spleen. The anaemia is due to: (1) increased red cell pooling in the spleen, (2) shortened red cell life span with increased destruction of the spleen, and (3) haemodilution from an increased plasma volume (see Figure 6.1D). The mechanisms of granulocytopenia and thrombocytopenia are similar: an eosinophilic response to helminthic infection may not be apparent in the peripheral blood because the eosinophils are held in the spleen, but it will be obvious in the bone marrow. The anaemia is usually normocytic and normochromic, there is a reticulocytosis and the bone marrow shows hyperplasia.

MALARIA (See also Chapter 61)

The features of malaria are described in detail in Chapter 61; here are discussed only the haematological consequences, which include anaemia, changes in the white cells and disorders of haemostasis.[15] Of the different species of parasite, *Plasmodium falciparum* is the most common and has the most profound haematological consequences; this species of malaria is implied except where stated otherwise.

Malarial anaemia

Where malaria is endemic, for example in tropical Africa, the severity and pathology (including anaemia) progress through three phases as individuals acquire partial immune protection: (1) acute malaria in non-immune children after about 6 months of age when maternally-derived immunity is lost; (2) recurrent malaria in children less than about 5 years of age; and (3) recurrent mild parasitaemia in partially immune older children and adults. Malaria in non-immune adults, such as expatriate visitors to endemic areas or inhabitants of countries where malaria is unstable, have haematological complications of acute or recurrent malaria essentially similar to those of children in the endemic areas.

Acute malaria

In non-immune individuals there is usually no anaemia within 24–48 hours of the onset of fever, but there is then a rapid fall of the Hb and haematocrit over 4–5 days, with the degree of anaemia corre-

Table 6.12 Some causes of splenomegaly (See also Chapter 3).

Generally slight (<5 cm below the costal margin)

Acute infections	— malaria, septicaemias, viraemias, hepatitis, trypanosomiasis, brucellosis, toxoplasmosis, typhus
Subacute, chronic infections	— tuberculosis, **brucellosis**, syphilis, hydatid, meningococcal septicaemia, histoplasmosis, bacterial endocarditis
Miscellaneous	— megaloblastic anaemia, iron deficiency anaemia, immune thrombocytopenia, **rheumatoid arthritis**, hyperthyroidism, myeloma, disseminated lupus erythematosus, **sarcoidosis**, amyloidosis

Generally moderate (5–10 cm below the costal margin)

Chronic haemolysis	— **recurrent malaria**, haemoglobinopathies, spherocytosis
Portal hypertension	— hepatic cirrhosis
Haematological malignancies	— **chronic lymphocytic leukaemia, lymphomas**, acute leukaemias, polycythaemia vera

Usually gross (>10 cm below the costal margin)

Hyperreactive malarial splenomegaly (HMS)

Schistosomiasis

Kala-azar

Thalassaemia major

Haematological malignancies	— chronic granulocytic leukaemia, **myelofibrosis**
Miscellaneous	— splenic cysts and tumours, lipid storage diseases

Conditions in bold print are commonly associated with hypersplenism.

sponding approximately to the intensity of parasitaemia. The anaemia is normochromic and normocytic. The reticulocyte count is low at this stage, although the bone marrow shows erythroid hyperplasia with minimal dyserythropoietic changes.[15,16] The total plasma bilirubin and unconjugated fraction are raised: increased conjugated bilirubin indicates complicating hepatic dysfunction. Haptoglobins are reduced or absent (see Table 6.11).

Malaria is immunosuppressive and is frequently complicated by secondary infections, such as bronchopneumonia, urinary tract infections and Gram-negative septicaemias; anaemia is generally more profound when there is secondary infection, especially with non-typhoid *Salmonella* septicaemia. It has been suggested that profound anaemia in some children may be the result of concurrent infection by parvovirus B19, which infects early red cell precursors preferentially and causes a transient red cell hypoplasia.[16]

The major mechanism of haemolysis is undoubtedly rupture of red cells at the time of release of merozoites, but anaemia is often more severe and more persistent than can be accounted for directly by parasitaemia. The Hb may continue to fall for between 7 and 21 days following clearing of the parasites, due apparently to both continued haemolysis and delayed release of red cells from the marrow. Survival of both autologous non-parasitized red cells and donated red cells is shortened. There is phagocytosis of the parasitized and unparasitized red cells, seen easily in the bone marrow. The direct Coombs' test (DCT) is frequently positive, associated with adsorption by red cells of immunoglobulin (Ig) G and the C3 component of complement; however, autoimmune haemolysis is not an important mechanism, although IgG-coated red cells are more rapidly removed by the RES than uncoated cells. Haemolysis of unparasitized red cells appears, therefore, to be due to a non-specific activation of the RES, hypersplenism and Fc receptor-mediated uptake.

During acute malaria there is immobilization of iron in the macrophages, and low serum iron concentrations: serum ferritin is massively increased, being an acute reactive protein. Red cell folate levels are raised above normal through mechanisms

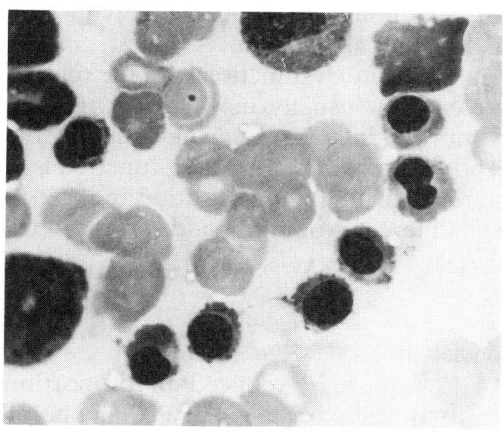
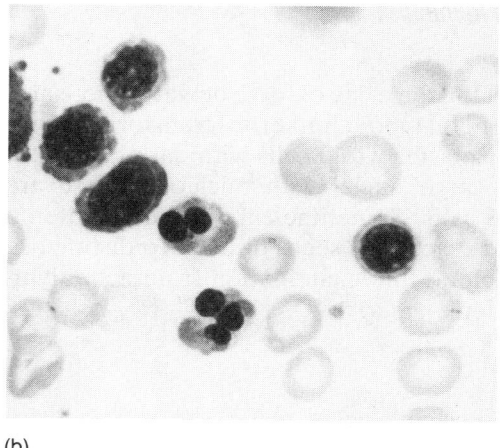

(a)   (b)

Figure 6.3 (a) and (b) Dyserythropoiesis: a term used to describe specific morphological changes in bone marrow which usually denotes ineffective erythropoiesis. These changes include cytoplasmic vacuolation, basophilic stippling, intracytoplasmic bridges, nuclear fragmentation (karyorrhexis), incomplete and unequal nuclear division and multinuclearity. Dyserythropoiesis occurs to a variable degree in many anaemias.

which are uncertain, but possible due to synthesis of folate by the parasites themselves.

Following clearance of the parasitaemia and during recovery, the peripheral blood shows a reticulocytosis, anisocytosis, macrocytosis and polychromasia (see Table 6.11).

Recurrent malaria

Children living where malaria is endemic suffer from recurrent attacks: they complain of intermittent fever and general ill health, and on examination often have moderate splenomegaly. They have a chronic normocytic, normochromic anaemia with a low reticulocyte count; anaemia may be profound during acute exacerbations but there is only a scanty parasitaemia, although gametocytes and malarial pigment may be seen in the monocytes.[15–17] The anaemia is a result of both hypersplenism and severe dyserythropoietic disturbance of the bone marrow (Figure 6.3). The mechanism of dyserythropoiesis is uncertain, but it could be secondary to hypoxia from the packing of bone marrow sinusoids with parasitized red cells, or be mediated by tumour necrosis factor (TNF).

Disturbed marrow function is reversed by successful antimalarial treatment, which is followed by a brisk reticulocytosis and rise in Hb.

Haemoglobinuria and blackwater fever

The majority of patients presenting with haemoglobinuria seen today are G6PD deficient and have been treated with oxidant drugs (see below). However, some are G6PD normal and the trigger to severe intravascular haemolysis cannot be found. In the past patients were not infrequently seen with blackwater fever. Typically such a patient was a non-immune adult expatriate who had been taking quinine irregularly as prophylaxis. The patient complained of loin pain, vomiting and diarrhoea; initially there was polyuria, but later oliguria with dark-brown or black urine. There was tender hepatosplenomegaly, jaundice and profound anaemia; malarial parasites were scanty or even absent. There was massive haemoglobinuria and all other features of intravascular haemolysis (see Table 6.11). The mechanism was probably quinine-induced immune haemolysis: blackwater fever has rarely been seen since quinine was replaced by artificial aminoquinolines, but may return with the increasing use of quinine.

Malaria in the partially immune

Where malaria is endemic, older children and adults experience recurrent malarial parasitaemia contained by acquired immunity, with moderate haemolysis and compensatory erythroid hyperplasia. This contributes largely to the mean Hb being about 20 g/l lower than accepted reference figures in both sexes in many communities.[2] There is moderate anisocytosis, macrocytosis and polychromasia. The balance between haemolysis and erythroid hyperplasia is disturbed during pregnancy (see below), after splenectomy, immune anergy—for example from malignant disease, and with hyperreactive malarial splenomegaly (HMS) (see below). Fortunately, there appears to be no interaction between malaria and HIV, except where possible during pregnancy.

Leucocytes in malaria

Lymphocytes

From about the third day of fever onwards there are, in the peripheral blood, numerous transformed lymphocytes or plasmacytoid cells with dark blue cytoplasm and large nuclei with nucleoli. These are activated B cells. Sometimes in African children a leukaemoid reaction is seen, difficult to distinguish on simple blood film examination from acute lymphoblastic leukaemia.[18]

Neutrophils

Many patients with acute malaria show a neutropenia due to margination to the endothelial surface of neutrophils in the circulation. During recovery from uncomplicated malaria there is often a leucocytosis with a shift to the left, toxic granulation, vacuolation and ragged cytoplasm. A neutrophil leucocytosis is seen often in reaction to secondary infections, and carries a poor prognosis.[15] Rarely there is a myeloid leukaemoid reaction, with an extremely high neutrophil count and shift to the left as far as myelocytes or promyelocytes and blast cells.[18]

Eosinophils

The eosinophil count is low during acute malaria, even if the initial count is high in response to helminthic infections. During recovery, there may be an eosinophilia.[18]

Monocytes

The monocyte count is raised; the cells are frequently vacuolated, and erythrophagocytosis and malarial pigment may be seen. The examination of monocytes in a thin blood film is most valuable in diagnosis as malarial pigment persists for several days after the clearance of parasitaemia; pigment remains in bone marrow macrophages for up to 20 weeks after infection.

Disorders of haemostasis in malaria

Platelets

The platelet count is reduced regularly in acute malaria; for example, in 105 Nigerian children with malaria, the mean platelet count was $132 \times 10^9/l$, as compared to $234 \times 10^9/l$ in the same subjects 12 days later after receiving treatment with chloroquine.[19] However, severe thrombocytopenia ($<50 \times 10^9/l$) was observed in only 5%. Platelet survival is reduced to 2–4 days; probable mechanisms include: reduced membrane sialic acid leading to rapid clearance, an immune mechanism involving anti-platelet IgG and hypersplenism.[15,19] There may be some megakaryocyte dysfunction with the release of giant platelets, but usually megakaryocytes are numerous, normal in appearance and actively budding in the bone marrow.[15,17] Platelet function is enhanced generally, including aggregation induced by ADP, adrenaline, thrombin and thromboxane A_2 (TXA_2).[15,19]

Coagulation

AT III levels are reduced in proportion to the severity of the parasitaemia. PT may be prolonged as a consequence of hepatic dysfunction.

In a small proportion, for example less than 10% of Thai adults, acute malaria may be complicated by disseminated intravascular coagulation (DIC).[15,18] The process is triggered by the release of thromboplastin during massive haemolysis, toxic destruction of endothelium and the activation of complement. DIC is reversed usually following active antimalarial therapy: patients may require transfusion with fresh whole blood, or even exchange transfusion; the use of heparin is controversial.[15]

Treatment of severe malarial anaemia

The management of acute malaria and its complications is discussed in Chapter 61. Malarial anaemia generally responds to antimalarial therapy, but is a major cause of morbidity and of mortality.[16] In different series between 10 and 16% of all deaths in childhood in Africa have been attributed to malarial anaemia, but these are certain to be underestimates.

In the past there has been far too great a willingness to treat malarial anaemia by blood transfusion. With the advent of HIV in Africa many thousands of children have been treated successfully for anaemia, but at the cost of developing AIDS later. Even where blood donations are screened for anti-HIV, donors may be in the window between infection and seroconversion, so that more stringent criteria for transfusion must be applied.[20] 'Red cell transfusion is required only when anaemia is associated with incipient or established cardiac failure.'[14]

Malaria in pregnancy

There is a reduction in resistance to malaria during pregnancy that has been related to a physiological suppression of cell-mediated immune responses to malarial antigen or to higher serum cortisol concentrations;[21,22] humoral immunity to malaria is un-altered. The presentation of malaria during pregnancy varies enormously according to the woman's previous exposure and level of acquired immunity.[23]

Women with no or low levels of acquired immunity to malaria, if infected during pregnancy, suffer from severe malaria, frequently complicated by cerebral malaria, renal failure, blackwater fever, profound anaemia and DIC. Women of all ages and parities are affected equally. Maternal and fetal morbidity and mortality are heavy.[23]

In women who live where malaria is stable (hyper- or holoendemic), and who have acquired high levels of immunity to *P. falciparum*, the frequency and density of parasitaemia rise to plateaux early in the second trimester, especially in primigravidae, or women in their second pregnancies to a less extent. The densities of parasitaemias do not reach levels seen in early childhood, and the women are generally asymptomatic or have mild symptoms only. However, there is haemolysis and anaemia, seen most commonly in the mid-second trimester and in primigravidae. Compensatory erythroid hyperplasia leads to high demands for folate, demands which are already increased because of pregnancy. The haemolytic process is often complicated by megaloblastic erythropoiesis, and profound anaemia follows.[23]

The frequency of palpable splenomegaly increases during pregnancy in all gravida classes, and a peak spleen rate about double that of non-pregnant women can be reached at around 16 weeks of gestation.[24] Even higher spleen rates (e.g. 70% in Nigeria) are seen in anaemic pregnant women; in Nigeria about 25% of severe anaemias in pregnancy were complicated by HMS (see below) and hypersplenism.[25] About 5% of women in the same series had a severe haemolytic process which was not controlled by antimalarials but responded to prednisolone and was presumed to be due to an immune process triggered by malaria.[23,26]

The presentation of malaria in pregnancy is intermediate between the two patterns where malaria is unstable (mesoendemic), as for example in Thailand and Zambia.

The peripheral blood picture of malarial plus folate deficiency anaemia in pregnancy is characterized by great anisocytosis, macrocytosis and polychromasia with or without nucleated red cells, but no poikilocytosis; there is a reticulocytosis; malarial parasites are usually absent or scanty. The white cell count is variable and there may be a myeloid leukaemoid reaction; the expected hypersegmentation of folate deficiency is often marked by a shift to the left. The bone marrow shows megaloblastic changes which may be gross; malarial pigment is present in the macrophages; iron stores tend to be increased unless there is concurrent iron deficiency.

Maternal and fetal morbidity and mortality are extremely high (see Anaemic Heart Failure).

Blood transfusion is indicated only if the patient is in incipient or established cardiac failure, or if the patient is approaching delivery with an Hb <70 g/l.[14] Anaemia responds rapidly in most patients following antimalarial therapy and folic acid; the haematocrit tends not to rise, but remains steady in patients with HMS;[23] in the few patients with immune haemolysis the haematocrit rises rapidly following treatment with prednisolone 60 mg/day for 1 week, 45 mg/day for 1 week and 30 mg/day maintenance in three divided doses, up to about 36 weeks of gestation.[26]

Malaria and anaemia can be effectively prevented by the administration of prophylactic antimalarials (e.g. proguanil) and folic acid supplements to pregnant women.[23] There are, however, great problems in the delivery of effective regimens to more than the few who attend antenatal clinics regularly: malaria chemoprophylaxis (Maloprim) has been given by traditional birth attendants in the Gambia, with beneficial effects on parasite rates, the haematocrit and birth weight, especially in primigravidae and also grandes multigravidae.[27]

Hyperreactive malarious splenomegaly (See also Chapters 3 and 61)

In malarious areas a varying proportion of children (and non-immune adult visitors) have splenomegaly associated with intermittent parasitaemia, and regressing with the gradual acquisition of relative immunity. In some, however, the spleen does not regress but enlarges progressively with increasing age. This condition is known as hyperreactive malarious splenomegaly (HMS), and was previously called the tropical splenomegaly syndrome (TSS). Its defining features are: (1) residence in a malarious area; (2) chronic splenomegaly, often massive; (3) serum IgM elevated to more than 2 standard deviations above the local reference mean; (4) high malarial antibody titres; (5) hepatic sinusoidal lymphocytosis; and (6) clinical and immunological response to long-term antimalarial prophylaxis.[28,29]

Pathophysiology

Central to the pathophysiology of HMS is the overproduction of IgM in response to recurrent infection by *P. falciparum*, *P. malariae* or *P. vivax*. There is familial and ethnic clustering suggesting a genetic basis. It is seen most often in groups who have migrated relatively recently to endemic malarial areas, and so are likely to lack genetic polymorphisms which confer partial protection against malaria. Such polymorphisms could include HLA-linked genetically controlled processing of malarial antigens and antibody production.[30,31] During acute malaria, there is transient production of IgM lymphocytotoxic antibodies which are specific for activated suppressor T lymphocytes (CD8+), which normally down-regulate synthesis of IgM by B cells. It has been shown in Indonesian patients with HMS that these lymphocytoxic antibodies persist, with consequent imbalance between helper T cells (CD4+) which are normal, and suppressor T cells which are greatly reduced, so that there is a lack of inhibition of B-cell activity.[32] Recurrent antigenic and mitogenic stimuli from malaria to the B cells result in gross overproduction of polyclonal IgM, of which only a small part has antimalarial specificity. The IgM forms aggregates (cryoglobulins) and immune complexes. These are phagocytosed by the RES, including the macrophages of the liver (Kupffer cells), spleen and bone marrow, stimulating macrophage hyperplasia and T-cell proliferation, seen as hepatic sinusoidal infiltration and the lymphocytosis of spleen and bone marrow. Overproduction of IgM and its complexes precedes and is the stimulus to progressive and eventual massive splenomegaly and hepatomegaly. Pancytopenia of variable severity results from hypersplenism. The apparent anaemia is caused mainly by the expansion of plasma volume (up to 130 ml/kg) and sequestration of up to one-third of the total red cells in the spleen (see Figure 6.1D). There is haemolysis of cells pooled in the spleen, and erythrophagocytosis mediated by the adsorption of immune complexes; haemolytic crises are associated with pregnancy and infection. Patients are liable to frequent and prolonged infections related to neutropenia and disturbed immune function.[33,34]

Distribution and clinical presentation

HMS has been described in Africa (Nigeria, Uganda, Kenya and Zambia), western Asia (Aden), the Indian subcontinent (Bengal, Sri Lanka), South-East Asia (Vietnam, Thailand, Indonesia), Oceania (Papua New Guinea) and South America (Amazon basin). High incidences are reported in the Fulani in northern Nigeria, Rwandan immigrants in Uganda, the Angas of Upper Watut Valley and the related Menya of Tauri Valley (Papua New Guinea), and the Yanomani in Venezuela. Prevalence rates of over 50% have been reported only in the Papua New Guinea groups and the Indonesians of the island of Flores.[28–34]

Presentation is usually in young to middle-aged adults, but can occur as early as 8 years of age and in old age. In some series women have outnumbered men, but in others there is an equal sex incidence. Patients complain most commonly of the abdominal swelling and a dragging feeling or pain from the enlarged spleen. The spleen may be huge, reaching to the left iliac fossa and across the midline. There is usually hepatomegaly. Lymphadenopathy is not a feature.[29,32]

Haematology

The anaemia is generally moderate, but may be severe during pregnancy or following acute infections; it is normocytic, but there may be macrocytosis and polychromasia with a reticulocytosis. The total WBC is generally low, with granulocytopenia. However, in west Africa in about 10% of patients there is a lymphocytosis which may mimic chronic lymphocytic leukaemia (CLL). There is a mild thrombocytopenia, but not usually sufficient to lead to haemorrhage. Malarial parasites are absent as a rule.

Sickle cell trait confers significant but partial protection against the development of HMS.

The bone marrow shows hyperactivity of erythroid, granulocyte and megakaryocyte lines. Megaloblastic changes are rare. An excess of normal lymphocytes is observed in west African patients. The frequency of depleted iron stores is not different from that of the population. Malaria pigment is not seen.[29,33]

Diagnosis

The defining feature is excessively high serum IgM. When there is a leukaemoid reaction, HMS may be distinguished from CLL by (1) the absence of lymphadenopathy, (2) the high serum IgM, whereas levels are lower than normal in CLL except when there is a monoclonal paraprotein, (3) normal lymphocyte transformation with phytohaemagglutinin (PHA), whereas transformation is reduced in CLL.[28,29,33,34]

Prognosis

The condition appears benign in most patients when seen first, but there is a high mortality without treatment; for example 46% over 15 years rising to nearly 90% in those with gross splenomegaly in the Upper Watut Valley. Death is usually from acute bacterial or other overwhelming infections.[34]

Some Nigerian patients show a haematological and immune status suggestive of transition to CLL, and in Ghana patients have been described in whom there is a clonal lymphoproliferation.[35,36] It is probable that the polyclonal expansion of B lymphocytes provides targets for somatic mutation, followed by selection of a single clone and development of CLL or lymphoma.

Treatment

The treatment of choice is the administration of antimalarial chemoprophylaxis for life. The choice of prophylactic depends on the local pattern of sensitivity of the malarial parasites: proguanil has been the most effective agent in tropical Africa. After about 3 months of treatment there is a steady decrease in splenomegaly over many months and a return of all immunological and haematological parameters to normal. Failure of treatment suggests non-compliance, malignant transformation or incorrect diagnosis.[29] Non-compliance leads to relapse, morbidity and increased mortality.

There is no place for splenectomy, despite the immediate improvement it causes, because of high operative and later mortality, the transfer of disease from splenomegaly to hepatomegaly, and the need in any case for lifelong antimalarial prophylaxis to prevent acute malaria.[29,33]

OTHER PROTOZOA

Visceral leishmaniasis (See also Chapter 65)

Infection by *Leishmania donovani* is followed by hyperplasia of macrophages and lymphocytes, massive production of IgG and progressive hepatosplenomegaly (kala-azar). The size of the spleen is related directly to the duration of infection and to the severity of pancytopenia.[18,37] Anaemia is due primarily to hypersplenism (expansion of plasma volume, haemodilution, splenic sequestration and haemolysis) (see Figure 6.1D). There are plasma cold anti-I agglutinins, the adsorption of IgG by red cells and the fixation of complement, but no convincing evidence that autoimmune haemolysis contributes to the severity of anaemia in kala-azar.[38] Dyserythropoiesis and ineffective erythropoiesis have a role in the causation of anaemia in at least some patients.[39] In India about half of patients are reported to have moderate to severe megaloblastosis, due to folate deficiency secondary to increased demands from haemolysis.[40]

In the early stages there may be leucocytosis with a shift to the left, but neutropenia becomes increasingly severe with advancing disease. Neutrophil function has been reported to be normal by some, but Italian workers have reported reduced phagocytic and bactericidal activity.[41] Neutropenia may

become profound: children in particular are liable to secondary bacterial infections, or the development of cancrum oris. The eosinophil count is reduced; lymphocyte and monocyte counts are raised and occasionally there may be leukaemoid reactions.[18]

Platelets are sequestered in the spleen and platelet survival is short: thrombocytopenia may be sufficiently severe to cause mucosal bleeding but cutaneous purpura is unusual. Hepatic dysfunction can lead to hypoprothrombinaemia with prolonged coagulation time and PT. There is increased fibrinolytic activity and reduced fibrinogen concentration in some patients with advanced disease.[18] Immune complex-mediated vasculitis and DIC have been reported from Sudan.[42]

The bone marrow is usually hyperplastic and often megaloblastic, with increased erythroid, granulocytic and megakaryocytic activity; lymphocytes and plasma cells are numerous, as are macrophages, many of which contain Leishman–Donovan bodies. In long-standing chronic kala-azar there may be bone marrow hypoplasia and fibrosis; gelatinous transformation of bone marrow has been described in one patient.[43] Pure red cell aplasia has been reported, which could have been due to coincidental infection by parvovirus B19.[44]

Successful treatment of leishmaniasis is followed by regression of the spleen and a return to haematological normality over 9 months following cure. The Hb response may be delayed due to the anaemia of chronic disorder (see below).[45,46]

Trypanosomiasis (See also Chapters 63 and 64)

African trypanosomiasis is accompanied by a haemolytic anaemia, which is usually moderate but may be severe.[18] Haemolysis has several mechanisms: (1) trypanosomes release haemolysins, which enables the parasites to utilize haem and other nutrients from the red cells; (2) there is adsorption of IgM immune complexes on to red cells with fixation of complement, and the sensitized red cells are phagocytosed throughout the RES; and (3) there is hypersplenism. There is a moderate leucocytosis, with raised lymphocyte and monocyte counts, but a neutropenia from hypersplenism. Thrombocytopenia is usual during acute infections, and may be profound due to hypersplenism. With *Trypanosoma brucei rhodesiense* infections there is, in addition, platelet aggregation and destruction, and in some patients DIC.

In infections with *T. cruzi* (American trypanosomiasis, Chagas' disease) there may be a normocytic anaemia, leucocytosis, lymphocytosis and hypoprothrombinaemia.

Toxoplasmosis

There is a high rate of transmission of *Toxoplasma gondii* in childhood in the developing countries, causing only mild disease generally; some patients may have a persistent lymphocytosis with atypical mononuclear cells like glandular fever cells and a thrombocytopenia.[18] Congenital toxoplasmosis is rare as women are almost invariably immune. Severe and congenital toxoplasmosis may be seen more commonly as a result of the AIDS pandemic.

Amoebiasis

Patients with chronic disease have a hypochromic microcytic anaemia as a result of either chronic blood loss and iron deficiency, and/or the anaemia of chronic disorders. Neutrophil leucocytosis, sometimes amounting to a leukaemoid reaction, is associated with perforation of the bowel, peritonitis, secondary bacterial infections and amoebic liver abscesses. Hepatic disease results in prolonged PT and excessively high serum vitamin B_{12} levels.

Giardiasis

Acute diarrhoea due to *Giardia lamblia* causes a malabsorption of folate, whereas about half of the patients with chronic infections have impaired absorption of vitamin B_{12} which is multifactorial, including damage to ileal receptors, utilization of the vitamin by the parasite, and bacterial overgrowth of the bowel.[18]

HAEMOGLOBINOPATHIES

The inherited disorders of haemoglobin synthesis, the haemoglobinopathies, form by far the largest group of genetically determined anaemias. They occur most frequently in Africa, Asia and the Mediterranean region, and in immigrant populations from these areas, for example Afro-Americans, but can be encountered in every ethnic group. An understanding of their pathophysiology is based on a knowledge of the genetic control and structure of normal haemoglobin(s).[47,48]

Normal human haemoglobins

Normal haemoglobin consist of two pairs of peptide chains, each made up of over 140 amino acids (Figure 6.4); each of the four peptide chains in one haemoglobin molecule is associated with one haem moiety. The earliest peptide chains to be syn-

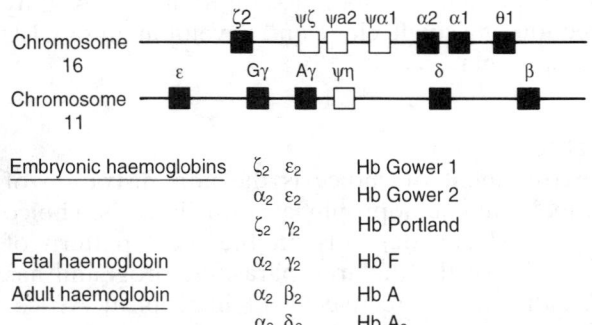

Figure 6.4 Genetic control of normal haemoglobins. Gene map of α-globin (above) and β-globin (below) gene clusters on chromosomes 16 and 11 respectively. Expressed sequences are shown as solid rectangles, pseudogenes as open rectangles. All normal haemoglobins contain one pair of globin chains produced by the α-globin gene cluster and one pair of globin chains from the β-globin gene cluster.

thesized, during the first 10–12 weeks of intrauterine life, are designated ζ, ε, α and γ: these combine to form the embryonic haemoglobins Gower 1 ($\zeta_2\varepsilon_2$), Gower 2($\alpha_2\varepsilon_2$) and Portland ($\zeta_2\gamma_2$). In the second and third trimesters of intrauterine life, HbF ($\alpha_2\gamma_2$) is predominant. During the third trimester, β-globin synthesis begins and at birth up to 30% of the total haemoglobin is HbA ($\alpha_2\beta_2$), the remainder being HbF (see Table 6.2). After birth, synthesis of γ chains falls rapidly, while that of β chains rises, so that by about 6 months of age over 95% is HbA, less than 4% is a minor fraction called HbA_2 ($\alpha_2\delta_2$) and less than 1% is HbF.

Haemoglobin chain synthesis is controlled by an α-globin gene cluster on chromosome 16 and a β-globin gene cluster on chromosome 11 (Figure 6.4). Separate pairs of allelomorphic genes control the structures of α, β, γ, δ, ε and ζ chains. Embryonic chain genes are repressed at the end of the first trimester, while α and γ genes are active during the rest of intrauterine life. Around the time of birth γ-chain genes are repressed and the β- and δ-chain genes are activated.[47,48]

Molecular basis of the haemoglobinopathies

There are two groups of inherited disorders of haemoglobin synthesis. The larger group is comprised of disorders which result from inherited defects in the *rate* of synthesis of one (or more) of the globin chains; these are referred to as the *thalassaemias*, of which β thalassaemias and α thalassaemias are clinically the most important and most common. The second group of conditions are those which result from a genetically determined alteration in the *structure* of the globin chains; of these,

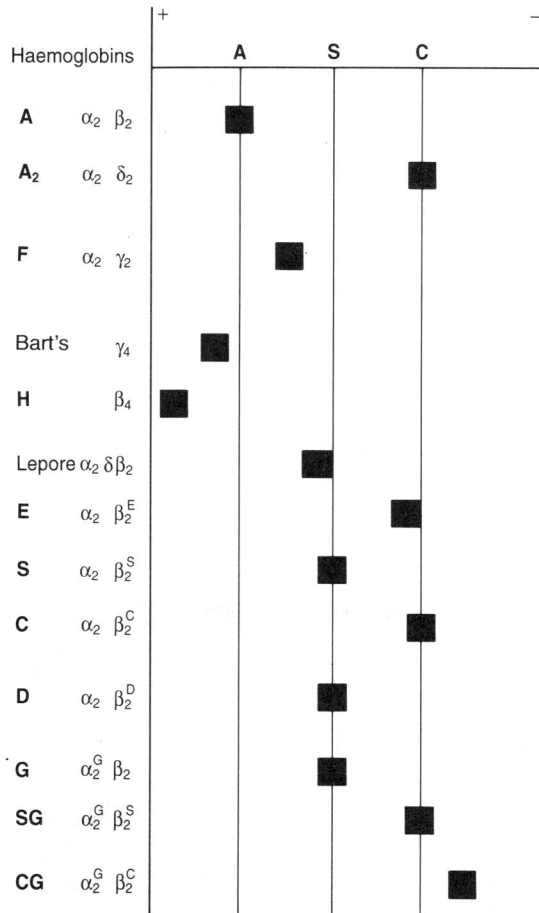

Haemoglobins		
A	α_2 β_2	
A$_2$	α_2 δ_2	
F	α_2 γ_2	
Bart's	γ_4	
H	β_4	
Lepore	α_2 $\delta\beta_2$	
E	α_2 β_2^E	
S	α_2 β_2^S	
C	α_2 β_2^C	
D	α_2 β_2^D	
G	α_2^G β_2	
SG	α_2^G β_2^S	
CG	α_2^G β_2^C	

Figure 6.5 Relative mobilities of normal and some abnormal haemoglobins on electrophoresis on cellulose acetate membrane, pH 8.9. The positions of HbA, HbS and HbC are indicated by vertical lines.

abnormalities of β and α chains only are of clinical significance, and β-chain variants are the most frequent. The most commonly applied laboratory technique for identification of normal and abnormal haemoglobins is their mobility on electrophoresis (Figure 6.5).[1]

Genes for β thalassaemia, α thalassaemia and for the β-chain variants HbS, HbC, HbD and HbE occur in certain populations at polymorphic frequencies (defined arbitrarily as being carried by 1% or more of the population). These populations all live in regions where *P. falciparum* malaria is (or was until recently) endemic. On geographical evidence, and in some instances demographic and parasitological evidence as well, it is thought that heterozygous inheritance of these abnormalities of haemoglobin synthesis renders the red cell less favourable than normal for the development of malarial parasites. Carriers enjoy, therefore, some protection against severe malaria and hence survival and genetic advantages, which balance in the popu-

lation the genetic disadvantages arising from the ill health and early deaths in the homozygotes.[31,49]

β Thalassaemias

Genetically determined reduction of β-globin synthesis, β thalassaemia, occurs in between 2 and 30% of members of populations living in a broad belt stretching from the Iberian peninsula, through the Mediterranean region, western Asia, the Indian subcontinent, southern China, South-East Asia, Indonesia to Oceania (Figure 6.6); in Africa it is found only north of the Sahara and on the Atlantic seaboard of West Africa.[50] About 3% of the world's population, or over 150 million individuals, most in Asia, carry genes for β thalassaemia.

There are known to be above 120 different β-thalassaemia mutations, but about 20 alleles account for 90% of all β-thalassaemia genes. In homogeneous populations there are as a rule only a few common alleles and some rare alleles; in heterogeneous populations there can be many alleles—for example about 40 in Israel. Most are point mutations affecting genetic control of β-globin synthesis at any level of transcription or translation, and a few are gene deletions.[50,51] All the different mutations are classified either as β^0-thalassaemia genes, when there is complete suppression of β-globin synthesis, or β^+-thalassaemia genes, where suppression is incomplete and allows for variable amounts of β globin and HbA to be formed. The β thalassaemias are classified clinically as: (1) *thalassaemia major*, when patients are chronically ill, severely anaemic and dependent on blood transfusion for survival beyond early childhood; (2) *thalassaemia intermedia*, when patients are not transfusion dependent but have a moderate degree of anaemia requiring transfusion only during intermittent crises; and (3) *thalassaemia minor*, when patients are generally symptom free and have mild anaemia only.[47,48]

β Thalassaemia major

Homozygous β^0 thalassaemia, compound heterozygous β^0/β^+ thalassaemia and most homozygous β^+ thalassaemias result in β thalassaemia major. Over 50 000 infants are born annually with this condition.[52]

Pathophysiology. Infants are normal at birth, but the disease is manifest in the early months of life as β-globin chains cannot be synthesized and HbA does not replace HbF. The excess of α chains precipitate, forming large intracytoplasmic inclusion bodies, which cause the intramedullary death of red

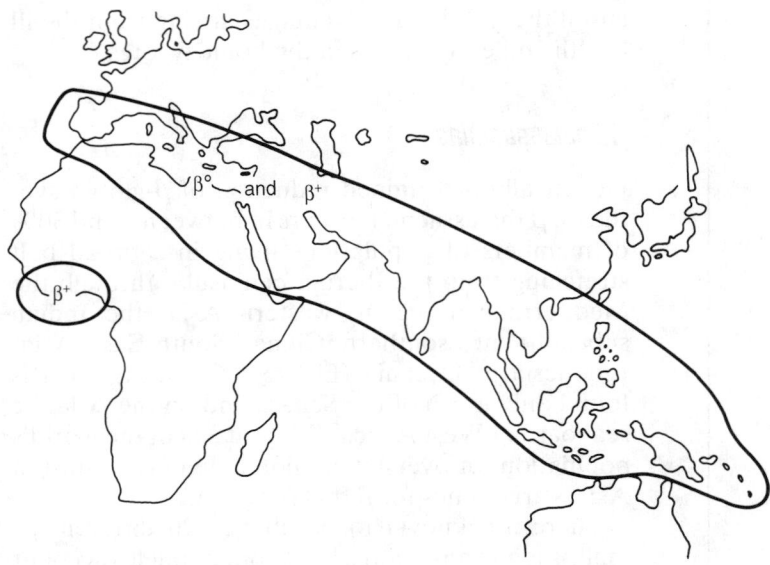

Figure 6.6 Areas of the Old World where β thalassaemias reach polymorphic frequencies. (Reproduced with permission of the publishers from Fleming A F. In Strickland G T (ed.) *Hunter's Tropical Medicine*, 7th edn. Philadelphia: WB Saunders, 1991: 36–64.)

cell precursors and ineffective erythropoiesis. The red cells which do reach the peripheral blood are also damaged by the inclusion bodies, so that there is haemolysis—especially through erythrophagocytosis in the spleen. Profound anaemia and hypoxia stimulate erythropoietin production and release, leading to chronic erythroid hyperplasia and massive expansion of the bone marrow. Demands for folate are high, deficiency is common and results in worsening of the anaemia. There is splenic hypertrophy and hypersplenism. Iron absorption is enhanced, but iron utilization in haemoglobin synthesis is poor, so that iron accumulates in tissues.[47,48]

Clinical. From about the third month of life children have pallor, suffer from intermittent fevers and fail to thrive. There is severe retardation of growth and development. Skeletal changes include gross bossing of the skull, overgrowth of the maxilla, poor dentition, blockage of sinuses and a tendency to spontaneous fractures of long bones. Radiographs of the skull show thinning of the outer table and spicules of bone in the expanded marrow cavity, giving the 'hair-on-end' appearance (Figure 6.7). The children become wasted and potbellied due to the increasing hepatosplenomegaly. Hypersplenism leads to worsening of the anaemia, a greater susceptibility to infections because of granulocytopenia, and a tendency to haemorrhage from thrombocytopenia. Progressive haemosiderosis damages tissues and organs: there is a bronze discoloration of the skin; there may be cardiac arrhythmia, pericarditis and congestive cardiac failure; endocrine dysfunctions may include diabetes mellitus, hypoparathyroidism, hypothyroidism, adrenal insufficiency and hypogonadism; there is progressive hepatic fibrosis.

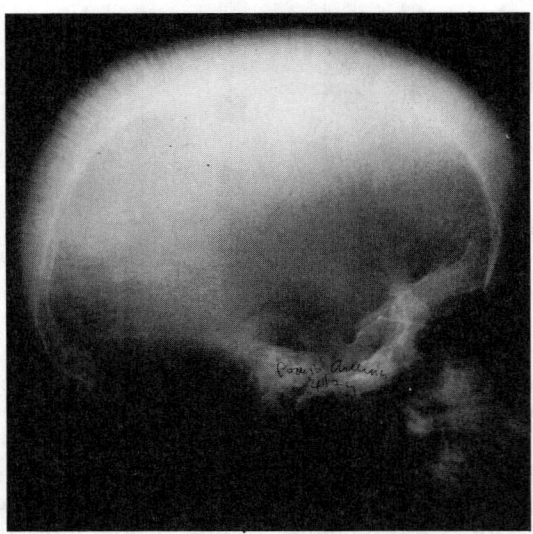

Figure 6.7 Skull radiograph in β thalassaemia major, showing hair-on-end appearance which is the result of massive expansion of the bone marrow cavity.

Where there is no appropriate treatment, children usually die from anaemic heart failure in the first 2–3 years of life. If intermittent blood transfusions are available to prevent anaemic heart failure, patients survive longer but are liable to die from overwhelming infections in later childhood. Children transfused on a regular basis to maintain an adequate Hb concentration grow and develop normally, but succumb to the complications of haemosiderosis in the late teens or early twenties.

Haematology. At first presentation the Hb is usually 20–80 g/l. The MCV and mean cell haemoglobin (MCH) are low. Red cells show anisocytosis, macrocytosis, with microcytosis, numerous target cells,

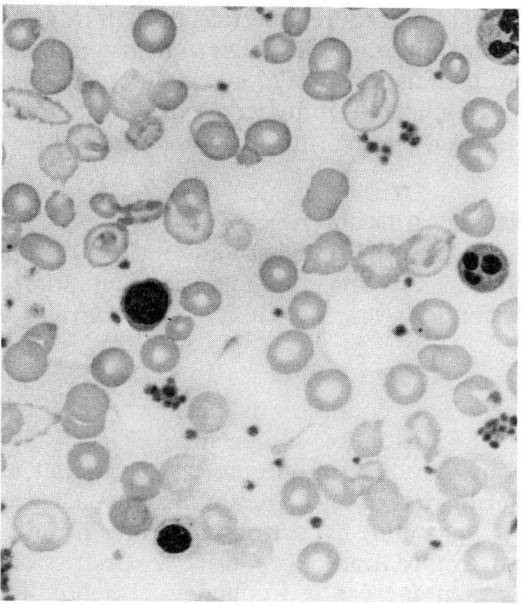

Figure 6.8 Peripheral blood film in β thalassaemia major—showing gross hypochromia, numerous target cells and nucleated red cells.

poikilocytosis, some fragmentation, gross hypochromia, numerous nucleated red cells, which may be megaloblasts, and basophilic stippling (Figure 6.8). The reticulocyte count is only moderately elevated. The white cell count may be high in response to infection, but hypersplenism can cause granulocytopenia and thrombocytopenia.

The bone marrow shows erythroid hyperplasia, which can be complicated by megaloblastosis of folate deficiency. Staining with methyl violet shows many large irregular inclusion bodies (the α chains) in the erythroid cells. Staining with the Prussian blue reaction shows a great excess of iron in the reticuloendothelial cells.

Haemoglobin electrophoresis reveals only HbF and the minor fraction of HbA_2 in patients with homozygous β^0 thalassaemia. Patients with β^+ thalassaemia have 20–90% HbF, the remainder being HbA with less than 4% HbA_2 (see Figure 6.5).

Serum iron, saturation of transferrin and ferritin levels are all high and rise progressively with age; there are the biochemical features of extravascular and intravascular haemolysis (see Table 6.11).

Treatment. The principles of management are: (1) a high blood transfusion regimen aimed at maintaining the Hb in the range 90–140 g/l and so suppressing the patient's own abnormal erythropoiesis; (2) the administration of chelating agents to reduce iron overload; (3) splenectomy when hypersplenism develops, as shown by rising transfusion needs, neutropenia and thrombocytopenia; (4) folic acid

supplements; and (5) prophylactic antimalarials in endemic areas.[53]

Transfusion is required every 6–8 weeks: concentrated red cells are rendered leucocyte and plasma free by washing or freezing, and filtering during administration, in order to avoid sensitization and reactions to serum and white cell antigens. Hb concentrations are monitored to adjust the frequency and size of transfusions.[54]

As each millilitre of red cells contains 1 mg of iron, haemosiderosis is inevitable unless a chelator is administered. Desferrioxamine (DF) therapy should be started as early as possible, in the second or third year of life or at the beginning of the high transfusion regimen. DF is administered by a slow subcutaneous infusion using a mechanical pump, through a 'butterfly' needle placed in the anterior abdominal wall: in patients without iron accumulation, DF 25–50 mg/kg is administered during 10–12 hours at night, for 5 nights a week, allowing a rest at weekends. Treatment is initiated in hospital, but parents and patients learn the technique for home care. Ascorbic acid 100–200 mg daily improves iron excretion. Urinary iron is monitored in order to adjust dosage of DF. More intensive chelation with DF is indicated for patients with established iron overload.[55]

Splenectomy should be delayed if possible until the age of 4–5 years as there is a risk of overwhelming infection in asplenic young children. Children should be vaccinated in early childhood and before splenectomy against influenza type B, pneumococcus and meningococcus. Oral prophylactic penicillin should be given after splenectomy, at least until puberty.[55]

Future developments in management may include the introduction of oral chelating agents,[56] the induction of the HbF synthesis, and the development of gene therapy. Bone marrow transplantation has been successful for selected patients, but is unlikely to be applied generally.

These regimens are extremely expensive and complex. Up to 25 units of blood are needed per patient per year and DF is costly: the total cost per patient is up to US$10 000 per annum. Compliance, especially to DF therapy, declines as patients approach puberty. The risk of transmitting HIV by blood transfusion is present, if low, in the Western world,[57] but is increasing rapidly with the progress of the pandemic in Asia; even where blood donors are screened satisfactorily, many will be in the 'window' between infection and seroconversion.

High transfusion regimens with iron chelation have been applied successfully in North America, northern Europe, Mediterranean countries and in specialist centres in Asia. However, the vast majority of patients with β thalassaemia major, mostly in Asia, still receive no appropriate management and can expect at best intermittent transfusions and palliative treatment. The major thrust of development must be towards cost-effective prevention in these communities (see below).

β Thalassaemias intermedia

Disease less severe than thalassaemia major results from the inheritance of HbE β thalassaemia in South-East Asia, HbC β thalassaemia and homozygous β^+ thalassaemia in West Africa (see Figures 6.6 and 6.12), various $\delta\beta$ thalassaemias and Hb Lepore disorders. Hb Lepore is the product of crossover between δ and β genes; $\delta\beta$ thalassaemias are less common and arise from gene deletions. Also, the coinheritance of α thalassaemia or of genes leading to enhancement of HbF production can diminish the clinical and haematological expressions of homozygous β thalassaemia.[47,48] The largest number of patients with β thalassaemia intermedia are those with HbE β thalassaemia, of whom over 40 000 are born each year in South-East Asia.[50]

Clinical. There is a wide range of severity in this heterogeneous collection of abnormalities, from moderate haemolytic anaemia (e.g. HbC β thalassaemia) to a condition close to thalassaemia major (e.g. HbE β thalassaemia), with a high rate of morbidity and mortality, especially in early childhood, splenomegaly, skeletal deformity, chronic leg ulcers, recurrent infections, a tendency to form gallstones, and iron accumulation progressing with age.[58]

Haematology. The degree of anaemia in the steady state is most variable: anaemia is worse in patients with hypersplenism, folate deficiency or intercurrent infection, and in pregnancy. Red cells are hypochromic and microcytic, with numerous target cells; osmotic fragility is reduced.

Haemoglobin electrophoresis shows characteristic features (see Figure 6.5): HbE β^0 thalassaemia, HbE and HbF only; HbE β^+ thalassaemia, HbE, HbF and HbA;[58] similarly HbC β thalassaemia, HbC and HbF or HbC, HbF plus HbA; homozygous β^+ thalassaemia, HbF with variable proportions of HbA; homozygous Hb Lepore, Hb Lepore only; homozygous $\delta\beta$ thalassaemia, HbF only.

Management. The health of patients needs continual surveillance. They require protection against infection through immunization and antimalarial prophylaxis, and folic acid supplements. They require prompt antibiotic treatment of bacterial infections. Blood transfusions are required only during anae-

mic crises, but if there is serious growth retardation or skeletal abnormalities, high transfusion regimens with iron chelation should be considered. Splenectomy is indicated if hypersplenism develops, as shown by increasing transfusion requirements.

β Thalassaemia minor

Heterozygous inheritance of either β^0 or β^+ thalassaemia genes results in β thalassaemia minor; there are probably over 150 million such carriers alive today.

Clinical. The condition is asymptomatic.[47,48] A small proportion of subjects have just palpable splenomegaly. The moderate but persistent anaemia during pregnancy causes fetal hypoxia, compensatory placental hypertrophy, mild intrauterine growth retardation, low urinary oestradiol excretion, an increased frequency of fetal distress during delivery and a high frequency, about 12%, of Apgar scores of 3 or less at 1 minute, but no significant increase of perinatal mortality.[59]

Haematology. The Hb is in the range 90–110 g/l, and during pregnancy about 20 g/l lower; the MCV and MCH are low, especially with β^0 thalassaemia, and the blood film shows moderate anisocytosis, microcytosis and hypochromia with occasional target cells and a few cells with punctate basophilia; the red cell changes are greater than expected for the mild degree of anaemia. There is mild to moderate erythroid hyperplasia in the bone marrow; there is no tendency to iron overload unless the patient has received misdirected parenteral iron therapy, and the prevalence of iron deficiency is the same as that of the general population.

The diagnosis is made by observing that the HbA$_2$ is raised to 4–6% (Figure 6.5); the HbF is also raised to about 3% in approximately half of the subjects. Osmotic fragility is reduced.

Management. It is important for the diagnosis to be made so as to avoid unnecessary treatment of the hypochromic anaemia with iron. Subjects should be reassured as to the benign nature of the condition and be offered genetic counselling (see below).

Malaria. J.B.S. Haldane was the first to hypothesize that the geographical coincidence of malaria and β thalassaemia could be due to the heterozygotes being at genetic advantage through a partial protection against *P. falciparum*.[49,50] A relative resistance to malaria was confirmed in Liberian children with thalassaemia minor.[60] Suggested mechanisms of limiting parasitaemia have included: (1) a slower than normal decline of HbF in the first two years of life;[61] (2) a greater rigidity of red cell membranes resisting parasite invasion; and (3) modified expression of parasite-induced neoantigens on red cell surfaces enhancing the development of protective cell mediated immunity.[62]

Hereditary persistence of fetal haemoglobin

Subjects are seen not infrequently in West Africa with a hereditary persistence of fetal haemoglobin (HPFH). This results from a combined deletion of the δ and β genes, but the deficit of β-globin chains is wholly compensated for by a high rate of synthesis of γ chains.[47] Heterozygotes have no clinical or haematological abnormalities except that they have HbF 20–30% of the total; acid elution and staining for HbF on a peripheral blood film shows that HbF is homogeneously distributed in all red cells, so distinguishing this from other conditions such as β^+ thalassaemia, where HbF is distributed unevenly in the erythrocytes. Homozygotes for HPFH are not anaemic, but have a thalassaemia-like appearance of the red cells and 100% HbF.

Prevention

The prohibitively high costs of treatment, the morbidity and eventual mortality even with the best available care, and the growing risk of infection with HIV through blood transfusion, make prevention of β thalassaemia major the only feasible option for the control of the disease in developing countries.[47,48,50,51] National programmes have been applied with high levels of success, that is 50–97% reduction of thalassaemia major cases, in Cyprus, Greece and Italy, and in the immigrant populations of the UK and the USA.[63–65] Strategies include the education of health professionals of all cadres, the general population, community leaders and schoolchildren, with the objectives of gaining support and compliance to screening programmes, and achieving legal and ethical acceptance of prenatal diagnosis and termination of pregnancies in which there is inheritance of β thalassaemia major.

Genetic counselling and screening for thalassaemia minor are targeted at couples before or at marriage, and at conception or early pregnancy, with the objective of identifying couples at risk of conceiving severely affected infants. Screening techniques include one tube osmotic fragility tests, and measuring red cell indices (especially MCV and MCH) using simple electronic cell counters, with HbA_2 estimations for confirmation followed by determination of the mutations in both parents. Prenatal diagnosis of major disease is possible from chorionic villus biopsy in the first trimester, followed by DNA analysis by various methods, including the use of oligonucleotide probes, Southern blotting and the polymerase chain reaction (PCR). The error rate is about 1% and the fetal loss rate following biopsy about 2%.

α Thalassaemias

Genetically determined reductions of α-globin synthesis are most often the outcomes of a variety of deletions from the α-globin gene cluster on chromosome 16 (see Figure 6.4).[47,48,50] Deletions of one or other of the two α-globin genes (denoted $-\alpha$) result in α^+ thalassaemias with partial suppression only of α-globin synthesis: these are caused by unequal cross-over events, generating at the same time triple α genes ($\alpha\alpha\alpha$) which can be observed in the normal population. Deletions of both genes (denoted $--$) result in α^0 thalassaemias with total absence of α-globin synthesis. A few α^+ thalassaemias are due to point mutations, giving rise to more severe reductions of α-globin synthesis than do the single gene deletions. The most important non-deletional α^+ thalassaemia gene is a termination codon mutation on α_2-globin gene, leading to the production of an elongated α chain which combines with β chains to form Hb Constant Spring: the abnormal mRNA is unstable so that only low levels of Hb Constant Spring are synthesized and the phenotype is a moderately severe α thalassaemia.

Pathophysiology

Three genotypes are associated with clinically asymptomatic states: (1) heterozygous α^+ thalassaemia ($-\alpha/\alpha\alpha$); (2) homozygous α^+ thalassaemia ($-\alpha/-\alpha$); and (3) heterozygous α^0 thalassaemia ($--/\alpha\alpha$).

Doubly heterozygous α^0 thalassaemia/α^+ thalassaemia ($--/-\alpha$) leaves only one active α-globin gene; the excess γ chains in fetal life combine to form tetramers γ_4 (Hb Bart's), while the excess β chains in postuterine life combine to form β_4 (HbH). Both abnormal haemoglobins have high oxygen affinity, resulting in tissue hypoxia; in addition, HbH is unstable and is precipitated as intracellular inclusion bodies, causing haemolysis and the clinical condition of HbH disease.

Homozygous α^0 thalassaemia ($--/--$) allows for only Hb Bart's to be formed in fetal life; because of its high oxygen affinity, infants are hypoxic and hydropic, inevitably dying in utero or shortly after delivery.

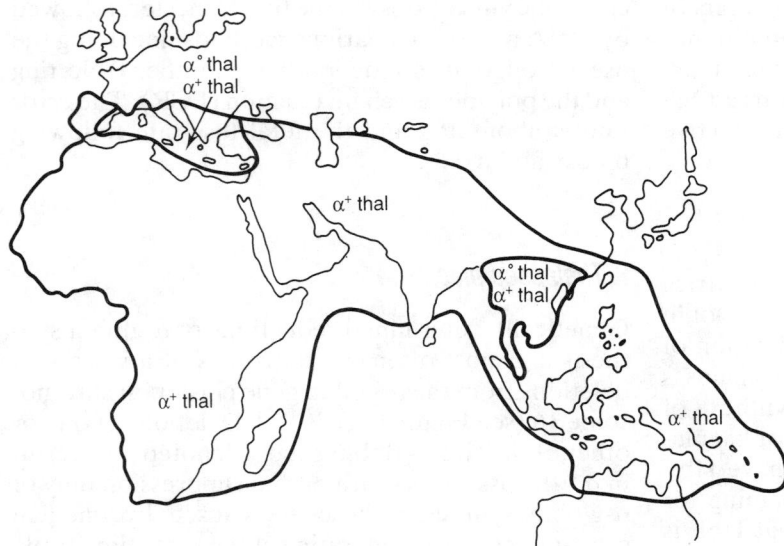

Figure 6.9   Areas of the Old World where α thalassaemias reach a polymorphic frequency.

Geographical distribution

α^0 Thalassaemia gene frequencies are highest in South-East Asia (Figure 6.9);[50] in Thailand, for example, gene frequencies for α^0 thalassaemia are 0.025, for α^+ thalassaemia 0.10–0.15 and for Hb Constant Spring 0.05–0.15. In consequence, Hb Bart's hydrops foetalis affecting about 25 000 infants each year, and HbH disease affecting about 68 000 infants each year, are major health problems.[52]

Both α^+ thalassaemia and α^0 thalassaemia deletions are seen at low frequencies in the Mediterranean region, so that HbH disease and hydrops foetalis can occur. In addition, HbH disease is seen rarely from non-deletional mutations. α^+ Thalassaemia is common in eastern Saudi Arabia (frequency 0.37); α^0 thalassaemia and hydrops foetalis do not occur but HbH disease is seen occasionally arising from the homozygous inheritance of an α_2-globin gene point mutation.[50]

On the Indian subcontinent α^+ thalassaemia gene frequencies are extremely high (above 0.70) in tribal or scheduled groups and in the Tharu of Nepal, but as α^0 thalassaemia genes are not found there is no disease.[50] Similarly, α^+ thalassaemia gene frequencies reach up to 0.70 on the coastal areas of Papua New Guinea and are high in all of Polynesia, island Melanesia and Micronesia. However, α^0 thalassaemia is not present, and HbH disease and Hb Bart's hydrops foetalis are seen only exceptionally from a non-deletional mutation.

α^+ Thalassaemia gene frequencies are in the range 0.10–0.27 throughout sub-Saharan Africa, but α^0 thalassaemia, HbH disease and Hb Bart's hydrops foetalis have never been reported (Figure 6.9).[50,66]

Haemoglobin Bart's hydrops foetalis

Infants inheriting homozygous α^0 thalassaemia $(--/--)$ are stillborn at 28–40 weeks of gestation, or they die shortly after delivery.[47,48] They are pale and grossly oedematous; the liver and spleen are enlarged massively; the placenta is large and friable.

Hb concentrations are in the range of 60–80 g/l; red cell appearances are those of thalassaemia. Haemoglobin electrophoresis shows about 80% Hb Bart's and 20% Hb Portland (see Figures 6.4 and 6.5).

Mothers of hydropic infants often exhibit during pregnancy the 'maternal syndrome' of early onset severe dependent oedema, associated rarely with albuminuria or hypertension. Maternal ill health and the psychological trauma to both parents may be prevented through screening couples for α^0 thalassaemia trait, genetic counselling, prenatal diagnosis and early termination of affected pregnancies. Prenatal diagnosis depends on chorionic villus biopsy and DNA analysis using a ζ-globin gene probe or PCR.[51,67]

Haemoglobin H disease

Doubly heterozygous α^0 thalassaemia/α^+ thalassaemia $(--/-\alpha)$, α^0 thalassaemia/Hb Constant Spring or homozygous non-deletional α^+ thalassaemias lead to a thalassaemia intermedia-like condition.[47,48] The disease may be mild, but occasionally children have retarded growth and skeletal deformities. There is a variable degree of splenomegaly

Hb concentrations are generally in the range of 70–100 g/l, but haemolytic crises may be precipitated by infections or exposure to oxidant drugs, such as sulphonamides, or during pregnancy. Red cell indices and red cell appearances are typical of thalassaemia. There is a moderate reticulocytosis, but numerous inclusion bodies of precipitated HbH are seen in the red cells after incubation with brilliant cresyl blue: prolonged incubation, up to 3 hours, is the basis of a sensitive test for HbH.[68] At birth there is up to 25% Hb Bart's, and after infancy haemoglobin electrophoresis shows HbA, normal or reduced HbA$_2$ and 5–40% HbH (see Figure 6.5).

The health of patients should be surveyed regularly, and prophylactic antimalarials and supplementary folic acid supplied. Patients should be warned against the use of oxidant drugs and advised to report if unwell or when pregnant. Progressive hypersplenism may necessitate splenectomy.

Asymptomatic α thalassaemias

At birth Hb Bart's contributes about 2.5% of the total haemoglobin in heterozygous α^0 thalassaemia ($--/\alpha\alpha$) and homozygous α^+ thalassaemia ($-\alpha/-\alpha$), and may be seen in trace amounts in about 10% of heterozygous α^+ thalassaemias ($-\alpha/\alpha\alpha$).[47,48,66] After infancy there is minimal anaemia with Hb about 5 g/l lower on average than in the reference population. The MCV is reduced to 75–80 fl, the MCH is low normal, and there is slight microcytosis and hypochromia on the thin blood film. HbH is *not* detected.

α^+ Thalassaemia is of some importance in Africa as, besides causing a slight anaemia, it ameliorates the severity of sickle cell disease and is associated with lower proportions of HbS in sickle cell trait (see below).

Malaria

The strongest evidence that α^+ thalassaemia has been selected for by malaria is epidemiological: for example, gene frequency is closely and positively correlated with endemicity of malaria in Papua New Guinea and island Melanesia.[48] As the disadvantage of α^+ thalassaemia, or even α^0 thalassaemia, is not great, only mild selective pressure would be required to achieve polymorphism. In fact, no increased fitness or control of parasitaemia has been demonstrated in heterozygotes. However, in α^+ thalassaemia increased amounts of malaria-induced neoantigens are displayed on red cell surfaces, and rapid immune clearance of parasitized cells is the probable mechanism of advantage.[50,62]

Sickle cell disease

A point mutation replaces glutamic acid with valine at position 6 on the β globin. The combination of normal α chains with the abnormal β^S chains forms sickle haemoglobin (HbS).[47,69,70] *Sickle cell disease* is defined as the condition resulting from the inheritance of two abnormal allelomorphic genes controlling β-globin formation, of which at least one is the β^S gene. Sickle cell disease includes the most common type, homozygous HbSS (referred to as *sickle cell anaemia*), and the compound heterozygous conditions of HbSC, HbS β thalassaemia, HbSD, HbSO^{Arab} and others. *Sickle cell trait* (HbAS) is the condition arising from the inheritance of one normal β-globin gene and one β^S gene.

There were about 78 million carriers of sickle cell trait in the world in 1992; of these, 65 million were in Africa south of the Sahara and north of the Zambesi river and Kalahari desert. In tropical Africa β^S gene frequencies reach to over 0.15, that is more than 30% of the adult population have HbAS (Figure 6.10).[71] The β^S gene is found at polymorphic frequencies also in the tribal (scheduled) groups of India, in the Arabian peninsula and the Mediterranean region. High gene frequencies are encountered as well in populations derived by the slave trade or voluntary emigration from Africa and the Mediterranean, such as in the Americas, the UK, other northern European countries and Australia.

DNA analysis of the β-globin gene cluster has shown that the β^S gene is linked to various β-chain haplotypes, each with a distinct geographical distribution (Figure 6.10). This implies that the sickle mutation arose independently at different times, linked to the different haplotypes. The Arab–India haplotype is found throughout the Indian tribal groups and in eastern Saudi Arabia. The Senegal haplotype is confined to the western seaboard of West Africa. The Benin haplotype is common in central West Africa, and would seem to have spread through the trans-Saharan slave trade to North Africa, the Mediterranean region and western Arabia. The Bantu haplotype (previously called Central African Republic or CAR haplotype) is found uniformly throughout the Bantu-speakers of central and southern Africa. The fourth African β^S mutation, linked to the Cameroon haplotype, is restricted to the Eton of central Cameroon.[71] These distributions are of interest not only in our understanding of selective pressures and human evolution, but because clinical expression is modified by haplotype linkages.

Each year about 156 000 infants are born with sickle cell disease, of whom 130 000 are in Africa and 33 000 in Nigeria alone. Most have sickle cell anaemia (HbSS); HbSC is also common in central West Africa (Burkina Faso, Ghana, Benin and south-western Nigeria); HbS β^+ thalassaemia is seen in West Africa, especially Liberia; HbS β^0

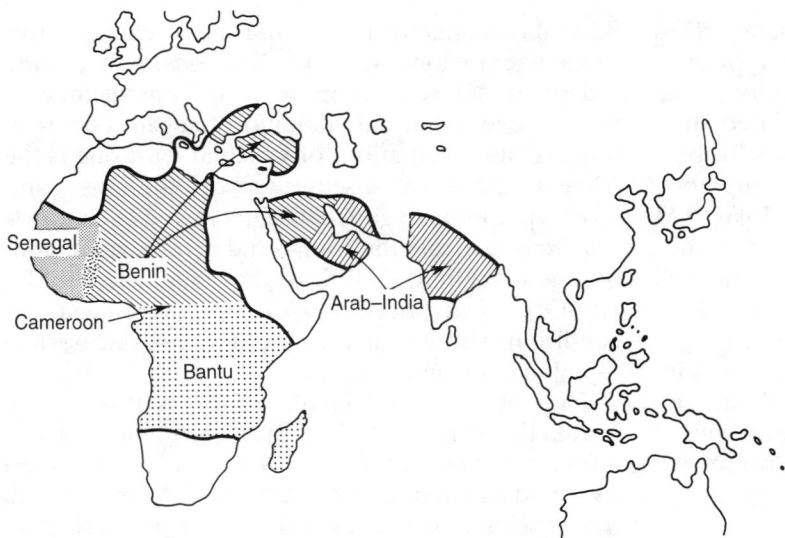

Figure 6.10   Areas of the Old World where haemoglobin S gene frequency is >0.02, and distribution of β^S haplotypes. Heavy arrows indicate probable spread of the Benin haplotype to the Mediterranean and western Asia.

thalassaemia occurs in North African, Mediterranean and mixed populations of the Americas; HbSD is seen most in the Punjab (see Figures 6.6, 6.10 and 6.12).

Pathophysiology

Valine is a hydrophobic amino acid, whereas glutamic acid is hydrophilic: as position 6 of the β globin is externally situated, the solubility of the HbS molecule is much reduced compared to HbA, especially in the deoxygenated state. Deoxy-HbS polymerizes, the contact points between molecules involving the $\beta6$ valines. The polymers form long chains of haemoglobin molecules; in cross-section, each chain consists of 14 molecules. The polymers align in parallel, and this is the probable mechanism for the distortion of the red cells into the characteristic sickle cell shape (Figure 6.11), as the polymers lie parallel with the long axis of the sickled cells. With alternating deoxygenation and oxygenation, the red cell sickles and unsickles, but eventually ill-defined losses and changes of membrane lipids and proteins lead to the membrane becoming rigid in the sickle form: the red cell is then an irreversible sickled cell, although within the membrane the haemoglobin is still capable of degelling on oxygenation. Failure of transmembrane ion exchange mechanisms leads to the loss of K^+ and water from the cell, while intracellular concentrations of Na^+ and Ca^{2+} rise, the latter by an order of one hundredfold the normal.

Sickled cells are fragile and are phagocytosed by cells of the RES, so that there is both intravascular and extravascular haemolysis. Sickled cells adhere to each other and to endothelium, so causing blockage of small blood vessels, infarction and death of tissues. Important secondary effects include an

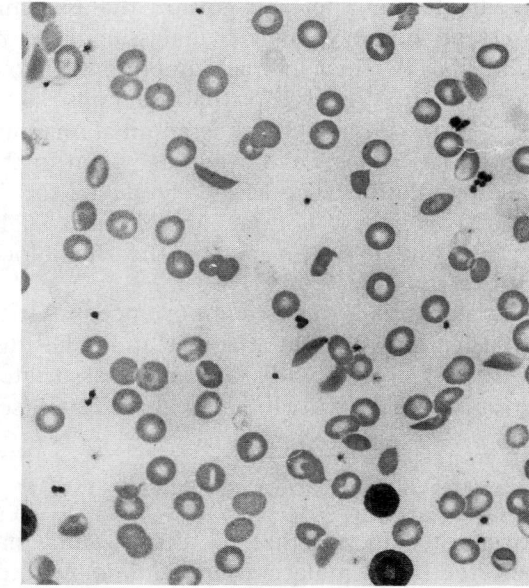

Figure 6.11   Peripheral blood film in sickle cell anaemia.

increased susceptibility to infections, which has several mechanisms: (1) mucosal and skin integrity may be breached following infarction; (2) haemoglobinaemia activates and consumes complement, so that there is a chronic defect of the alternative pathway of activation and diminished opsonization and phagocytosis of, for example, pneumococci; (3) recurrent infarction in the spleen leads to destruction of the organ (autosplenectomy) and functional hyposplenism; and (4) postinfarctive tissue necrosis provides a microenvironment favouring bacterial growth, and precedes the development of osteomyelitis and pyelonephritis. Recurrent infections and chronic ill health are associated with retardation of growth and development: chronic haemolysis creates high demands for folate, and deficiency contributes to the impaired growth and development besides leading to anaemic crisis.

Disease is worst in HbSS and HbSβ^0 thalassaemia, and is in diminishing order of severity in HbSC, HbSD, HbSO^{Arab} and HbSβ^+ thalassaemia. Sickle cell trait (HbAS) and HbS/HPFH are essentially without clinical abnormality except when under extreme stress.

Sickle cell anaemia

Infants with HbSS have complications only rarely in the early months of life while HbF concentrations remain high. The disease is manifest clinically from the third month onwards: the earliest presentation is frequently the 'hand–foot' syndrome of painful swelling of the dorsum of the hands or feet, often symmetrical, resulting from infarctions into the small bones. Due to parents coming late for advice and limited diagnostic skills at the first levels of care, the diagnosis is commonly delayed in tropical Africa (where are born about 5 out of 6 patients with sickle cell anaemia) with consequent morbidity and mortality, which could have been prevented.[72] The diagnosis is made in the first year of life in only about 10% of Nigerian children with sickle cell anaemia receiving hospital care. The most common age is 1–3 years, but up to 20% of patients are over 10 years at the time of diagnosis.

Patients suffer from chronic ill health interspersed with acute anaemic, infarctive and infective crises.

The steady state. Height and weight are below average for age throughout childhood. There is little body fat. The limbs are long and thin, and much of the loss of height is in the spinal column; there is an exaggerated lumbar lordosis and the chest is often barrel-shaped due to an increase in the anteroposterior distance. The bones of the vault of the skull and the face show bossing similar to that of β thalassaemia major (see Figure 6.7): the rounding of the forehead causes exaggeration of the supraorbital sulcus; the bridge of the nose appears sunken because of expansion of the bones around it; expansion of the maxilla causes the upper teeth to protrude. Bossing is much more pronounced in African than American patients; it is largely reversible with long-term antimalarial prophylactics, which suggests that malarial haemolysis is a contributory factor.

There is pallor and usually clinically obvious jaundice. The liver is invariably enlarged. Gallstones can be demonstrated in about 10% of African and 30% of American adult patients, but only rarely do they cause symptoms. The spleen is large in early childhood, but shrinks due to infarction, and is palpable in about 7% of patients only after puberty. In only the occasional patient is there hypersplenism. Moderate chronic cervical adenopathy is usual.

The heart is enlarged: the apex beat is displaced laterally and may be visible. The pulse rate is normal at rest but is rapid after minimal exertion or with apprehension and excitement. Mid-systolic murmurs are heard in most patients, and third heart sounds are common. Patients complain of polydipsia and polyuria, related to renal medullary infarction and loss of ability to concentrate urine: enuresis in childhood and nocturia are usual.

Most patients are remarkably well adapted psychologically, and perform their schooling well, although achievement may be poor from loss of time through ill health.

After the age of about 11 years skeletal maturation is delayed. Fusion of the epiphyses is late, and growth may continue for longer than normal, so that postpubertal HbSS subjects catch up on growth and a few go on even to reach well above average height (e.g. 190 cm). Puberty is delayed, and menarche occurs in girls on average 1 year later than in the normal population. Postadolescent patients, girls in particular, persist in a non-adult life style, so that first sexual experience and marriage is often at a relatively late age; many men are impotent following priapism (see below). Rarely, growth and development are so retarded that the patient has the appearance of a pituitary dwarf.

Haematology in the steady state. The Hb is generally in the range 60–100 g/l; patients are not in distress, even with levels constantly lower than this range, as they are compensated by high levels of erythrocyte 2,3-DPG and efficient oxygen delivery to the tissues. The red cells show great anisocytosis, macrocytosis with microcytosis, sickle cell forms, target cells, poikilocytes, polychromasia and a variable number of nucleated red cells (Figure 6.11); with hyposplenism the red cell appearance is more abnormal, and punctate basophilia and Howell–Jolly bodies may be seen. The reticulocyte count is raised up to 20%. The total white cell count is generally raised, showing a neutrophil leucocytosis with a shift to the left and toxic granulation, or a lymphocytosis with activated forms, even in the absence of obvious infection. The platelet count is high, especially when there has been autosplenectomy and following an infarctive crisis.

Haemoglobin electrophoresis shows the major fraction in the position of HbS, with a variable proportion of HbF and normal HbA$_2$ (Figure 6.5). That the major haemoglobin is HbS can be confirmed by the solubility test.[70]

The biochemical features of both intravascular and extravascular haemolysis are present (see Table 6.11); conjugated bilirubin is usually raised due to liver dysfunction.

Anaemic crises. Catastrophic declines of Hb are the result of (1) malaria, (2) acute splenic sequestration, (3) folate deficiency, and (4) aplastic crises.[72]

Acute *P. falciparum* malaria in subjects with sickle cell disease causes a severe haemolytic crisis and profound anaemia, leading often to anaemic cardiac failure, which used to be the most common observed cause of death in Africa. The most severe anaemias in acute illness are still associated with malaria, even in patients who are supposedly receiving prophylactics.

A sequestration crisis is characterized by an acutely enlarging spleen and a precipitate fall of Hb by more than 20 g/l, with a high reticulocyte count. It is most frequent in the second 6 months of life but can occur at older ages, even adulthood, in subjects who retain their spleens. Anaemic cardiac failure can develop, and it is the single most common cause of death in early life in non-malarial areas such as the West Indies.[70]

More than 10% of untreated African patients have megaloblastic erythropoiesis from folic acid deficiency when seen first. Megaloblastosis is almost inevitable during pregnancy unless prevented. Life-threatening anaemia develops rapidly.

During almost any acute infection erythropoiesis is depressed, and as patients with sickle cell anaemia are dependent on abnormally high rates of erythropoiesis the Hb drops rapidly. Of greater severity is infection by parvovirus B19 (see below).[73] 'Aplastic' crises occur in clusters in patients with sickle cell anaemia, associated with epidemic transmission of parvovirus B19 and outbreaks of erythema infectiosum in the population of normal children.

Infarctive crises. Sickling can lead to infarction in almost any organ or tissue in the body. The common sites of infarction crises are the bones, the chest and the abdomen.[72]

Up to 90% of African children seen with sickle cell anaemia between 6 months and 2 years of age have the hand–foot syndrome. If the swelling is hot, red and fluctuant, a superimposed osteomyelitis must be suspected. After about 2 years of age the sites of bone pain crises shift to the long bones. Pain is frequently localized around the joints, may be in multiple sites, be symmetrical in its distribution, and move from site to site. Onset is sudden; severity is variable, but often intense; duration is also variable, but usually there is spontaneous resolution within 5 days. Often there are no physical signs except warmth and tenderness over the affected bone, and the unwary physician is liable to underestimate the severity of the pain and overestimate the patient's reaction. Malaria, other infections, cold or damp (in the rainy season) are recognized precipitating factors, but often crises start for no apparent reason. Necrosis can lead rarely to emboli of bone marrow fat or bone to the lungs, brain, kidneys or other tissues.

Acute severe pain in the chest can be due to (1) pneumonia, (2) pulmonary infarction, (3) bone pain crisis in the thoracic cage, or rarely (4) angina pectoris. The first two conditions are serious, and often difficult to distinguish clinically or radiologically; as either one may precede and precipitate the other, the phrase 'acute pulmonary episode' is used. Lobar pneumonia and infection by the pneumococcus are more likely in early childhood, and infarction to be the primary pathology in adults.

Patients commonly complain of recurrent mild abdominal pain, but this may be severe and require admission to hospital. Pain is usually localized centrally or in the epigastrium. The patient may be vomiting. There is a history of constipation; bowel sounds are reduced and fluid levels can be seen radiologically. Aetiology is obscure, but is thought to be due to mesenteric infarcts. The condition resolves spontaneously, usually within 5 days. Other abdominal painful crises related to sickle cell disease are splenic infarction, infarction in lumbar vertebrae, duodenal ulceration, acute cholecystitis, obstruction of cystic or bile ducts, and pancreatitis. Patients may also present with abdominal crises unrelated to sickle cell disease, for example acute appendicitis.

Sickling in cerebral vessels can cause obstruction, infarction and haemorrhage. The immediate consequences of stroke include convulsions, coma, paralyses of varying extent and depth, or death. The late sequelae are contractions of limbs if no physiotherapy is available, faecal and urinary incontinence, speech defects and serious impairment of intellectual function.

Older patients can complain of blurred vision: examination reveals tortuous retinal vessels, proliferation of the retinal vessels, intraocular haemorrhages and sometimes retinal detachments. Pathology can develop until there is severe or total loss of vision.

Leg ulceration is a most common complication in the West Indies and North America, starting most often between 10 and 20 years of age. For reasons which remain obscure, ulcers are uncommon (less than 10%) in Africa even in those above 12 years of age: males are affected six times more often than females. The ulcers are usually on the lower third of the leg above the medial or lateral malleoli. They start as infarcts into the skin which show as small blisters; these develop into necrotic sloughs after 2 weeks and ulcers in about 3 weeks. Small ulcers may heal or may spread to up to 10 cm in diameter, causing serious incapacity.

Infarction in the renal pelvis leads to papillary necrosis, often complicated by haematuria and bacteriuria. Priapism is seen in adolescent or young adult males, but can occur in childhood: severity can vary from mild and transient, to moderate which resolves with 24 hours, to when the penis is hot and exquisitely tender, with pain referred to the perineum and lower abdomen. Untreated, severe priapism subsides over about 2 weeks but leads to fibrosis of the corpora cavernosa and permanent impotence.

Bacterial infections. The pneumococcus (*Streptococcus pneumoniae*) is the most common infectious cause of death in non-malarial areas; its frequency in Africa has been underestimated, and it is probably second only to malaria as a cause of morbidity and mortality.[72] Pneumococcal pneumonia, septicaemia and meningitis are seen in children between 5 months and 5 years old, and most frequently under the age of 2 years; the children have high fevers (>39.5°C) and are liable to convulsions, coma, shock and the Waterhouse–Friderichsen syndrome. Without appropriate treatment mortality is greater than 50%.

Other organisms commonly associated with acute upper or lower respiratory tract infections and bacteraemia are *Haemophilus influenzae, Staphylococci, Streptococci* and various Gram-negative bacilli. Bone infarction is complicated by acute osteomyelitis in less than 10% of all patients; invading organisms in Africa are *Salmonella* (usually *S. typhi*) in about half, other coliforms in less than half and *Staph. pyogenes* in about one-fifth.

Chronic degenerative disease. As more patients live into adult life, chronic and irreversible degenerative changes after the age of 20 years are becoming increasingly important. Irreversible organ damage leading to death includes hepatic failure, renal failure, stroke and chronic lung disease with cor pulmonale.[70,74] Major debilitation is the result of (1) avascular necrosis of bones, which can lead to loss of mobility when affecting the head of the femur or vertebral bodies, (2) retinopathy with loss of vision, and (3) leg ulcers. Men over 25 years commonly present with duodenal ulcers (over 30% in Jamaica), which have complicated clinical courses, including pyloric stenosis.[70] There can be a progressive bone marrow failure after the age of 40.[75]

Pregnancy. African women with sickle cell anaemia invariably become severely depleted of folic acid by mid-pregnancy if they are without medical supervision. About one-quarter may experience sequestration crises. Shortly before and shortly after delivery they are liable to severe bone pain crises, which may be complicated by marrow and bone embolus and systolic hypertension with albuminuria ('pseudotoxaemia'). They have high frequencies of urinary tract and other infections.

Obstetric delivery is often complicated by pelvic disproportion, the result of impaired growth during childhood. In Nigeria about half are delivered by caesarean section. During the puerperium they are liable to infection, especially wound sepsis.

Maternal mortality rates depend largely on the obstetric care available: in early series it was about 33%, but this has been reduced to nearly zero in the USA. In Nigeria mortality remains around 12%.

There is fetal growth retardation, and one-third of infants are of low birth weight. Perinatal mortality can be as high as 33% but be reduced to around 10% with good antenatal care and careful supervision of delivery and the puerperium.[76]

Prognosis. The pattern and severity of disease are governed by both environmental and genetic factors.[72] In Africa the environmental factors are of far greater importance in determining prognosis; in the USA the impact of the environment is largely controlled and the severity of disease depends more on the inherited factors.[74]

In rural tropical Africa, when there was inadequate nutrition, poor hygiene, no avoidance of mosquitoes and no practice of modern medicine, less than 2% of infants born with sickle cell anaemia survived beyond 4 years.[77] The family are all important: when they are caring, intelligent, educated and wealthy, children with HbSS do much better, even without regular medical care. The principal role of the medical profession is to support the family in the maintenance of the good health of family members with sickle cell disease (see below). Since the 1960s the provision of care has spread and improved throughout much of tropical Africa, so that it is now not unusual to see African patients with HbSS entering professional life (e.g. law, medicine, nursing) and achieving parenthood.

The expression of sickle cell disease is modified by a range of other mutations on the β-globin gene cluster, the so-called β-globin haplotypes (Figure 6.10).[71,72,74,78] The Arab–India and the Senegal haplotypes are linked to determinants of high levels of persisting HbF (means 20 and 12% respectively) in subjects with HbSS. The Benin and Bantu haplotypes are associated with lower levels of HbF (means

Table 6.13 Maintenance of health in sickle cell disease.

Early diagnosis	Laboratory techniques	— HbS solubility — Hb electrophoresis
	Screening	— pregnant women — newborn of mothers with S gene — anaemic children — siblings of patients
	Clinical awareness	
Education	Parents and patients Health professionals General public	
Sickle cell clinics	Prevent infection	— prophylactic antimalarials — immunization — prophylactic penicillin
	Nutrition	— folic acid supplements — general nutritional advice
	Advice	— avoid cold, fatigue, dehydration, excessive alcohol — no useless treatment — attend clinic regularly — report when ill — report when pregnant
Hospital	Prompt treatment of crises	
Obstetrics	Supervision of pregnancy, delivery, puerperium Family limitation to ≤ 3 viable children	

8%), but for reasons which are not yet understood, disease is more severe with the Bantu than the Benin haplotype. Sickle cell anaemia with high levels of HbF, linked to Arab–India and Senegal haplotypes, is associated with a more normal body build, more subcutaneous fat, less dactylitis, less acute chest pain, less splenic atrophy and less major organ failure in adulthood; Hb concentrations are higher, red cell survival is longer, there are fewer sickled cells, and reticulocyte and platelet counts are lower.

Coincidental inheritance of homozygous α^+ thalassaemia ($-\alpha/-\alpha$) with HbSS results in less anaemia, less haemolysis, lower MCH and MCV, fewer sickled cells and lower reticulocyte counts. Values with heterozygous α^+ thalassaemia are intermediate between those with $-\alpha/-\alpha$ and $\alpha\alpha/\alpha\alpha$. α Gene deletions do not seem to have much influence on the severity of acute complications of sickle cell disease but do decrease the risks of chronic organ damage in adults.[74]

Maintenance of health. Whenever β^S gene has high frequency, priority should be given to a system for maintaining patients in a steady state of good health through early diagnosis, supportive care at sickle cell clinics and obstetric units, easy access to appropriate care in crises, and education of the public, the patients and the health professionals (Table 6.13).[72]

To facilitate early diagnosis all pregnant women should be screened by Serjeants' HbS solubility test, with confirmation of positive results by haemoglobin electrophoresis; screening of fathers would identify couples at risk of having affected infants but it is more practical if a woman has HbS to test the newborn infant by electrophoresis (on citrate agar at pH 6–6.5). Other children at risk and to be screened are all with severe anaemia and the ill siblings of known patients with sickle cell disease. The HbS solubility test is preferable by far to the sickling test as it distinguishes heterozygotes from homozygotes and is simpler to perform: it is the test of choice in the primary health care setting. Haemoglobin electrophoresis should be set up in all hospitals of around 100 beds or more in tropical Africa and should be available for all clinicians.

Once diagnosed, sickle cell disease should be explained in detail to parents, guardians and patients in a language and phraseology they can understand. Their knowledge and comprehension must be reinforced with the aid of pamphlets and further discussions. The first essential intervention is the prevention of malaria: patients should receive a curative course of antimalarials at first attendance or following any break in attendance at the sickle cell clinic; they must be kept free from malaria through regular antimalarial prophylaxis, and proguanil is still the prophylactic of choice, being safe and effective. A regimen of once-daily folic acid supplement and once-daily proguanil is easy to remember and comply with. Prophylactic oral penicillin V potassium 125 mg twice daily up to the age of 5 years (or to adolescence) has substantially reduced the morbidity and mortality associated with pneumococcal septicaemia in the USA and the UK.[79,80] Controlled trials are needed in Africa but present problems of cost and logistics. Widespread immunization against the pneumococcus is not an option for reasons of cost, difficulties of the cold chain and the inadequate response of children under 3 years. On the other hand it is important for children with sickle cell disease to receive the expanded programme of immunization against other common infections.[72]

The coincidence of the area of Africa where the β^S gene has high frequency and where HIV is now epidemic makes it more important than ever that the health of patients with sickle cell disease be maintained so as to avoid situations where it is necessary to transfuse blood. Where there are no programmes of health care for sickle cell disease sufferers, but merely treatment of crises, which often involves transfusions of blood (appropriate and inappropriate), 20% or more of patients with sickle cell disease have been infected with HIV. In Africa 130 000 infants are born each year with sickle cell disease, and only 400 with haemophilia, who are at risk of infection by HIV through blood and blood products.[72]

Management of the patient in crisis. Prompt treatment is essential and arrangements should be made for patients in crisis to be able to report and receive attention without having to compete with the mass of sick people seen in the outpatients clinics of equatorial Africa. Regardless of the nature of the crisis it should be assumed that the patient has malaria, and treatment started without waiting for the results from a thick blood film. Prophylactic proguanil and supplementary folic acid should continue.

Anaemic crises. In the great majority of patients the haematocrit will cease to fall and will rise rapidly following treatment with antimalarials, folic acid and antibiotics if indicated. Blood transfusion is necessary only if (1) there is incipient or established anaemic heart failure, (2) there is a sequestration crisis, with Hb <60 g/l and falling rapidly, (3) obstetric delivery is imminent, with Hb <80 g/l, or (4) there are coincidental indications, such as haemorrhage or emergency surgery.[14,72]

Infarctive crises. Management is based on three principles: (1) the control of pain, (2) the restoration and maintenance of hydration and acid–base balance, and (3) the treatment of infection.[70,72,80]

The physician should assess the severity of pain and prescribe appropriate analgesics to be given at determined dosage and intervals; the physician must reassess pain at regular intervals and be prepared to increase or decrease the analgesics. Analgesic dosage should never be left to the judgements of different ward staff and the persuasive powers of the patients. Mild pain can be controlled with paracetamol, moderately severe pain with dihydrocodeine tartrate (DF118) and severe pain with opiates, such as diamorphine 10 mg at once, followed by an infusion, assessed by body size and patient's response.

Hydration is maintained by encouraging the mildly affected patient to drink; a more severely ill patient may be treated with nasogastric fluids if bowel sounds can be heard, or by intravenous fluids.

Acute infections. Antibiotics should be withheld unless there are clear indications for their use. If there are indications, antibiotics should be given promptly and in adequate dosage. Treatment must be started before results of bacteriological investigations are completed when there is (1) fever >39°C, unless due to malaria, (2) the acute pulmonary syndrome, or (3) suspected meningitis. Initial treatment could be with cefuroxime sodium 150 mg/kg per 24 hours, or alternatively ampicillin or penicillin plus chloramphenicol. Treatment of acute osteomyelitis can commence with chloramphenicol and cloxacillin.[72]

Cerebrovascular accidents. Patients should be rehydrated immediately. Some physicians advocate exchange blood transfusion but it is not possible to give general advice on this question.[80] Patients should be managed individually, taking into consideration the safety of blood transfusion in the locality.

Priapism. Treatment is aimed at relieving pain and preventing fibrosis of the corpora cavernosa.[80] Mild or 'stuttering' priapism can be relieved by micturition, walking around, avoiding sexual arousal and bathing in cold water. Moderately severe priapism will respond, usually within 24 hours, to bed-rest, sedation, analgesics, intravenous hydration, and cyproterone or stilboestrol. Initial therapy of severe

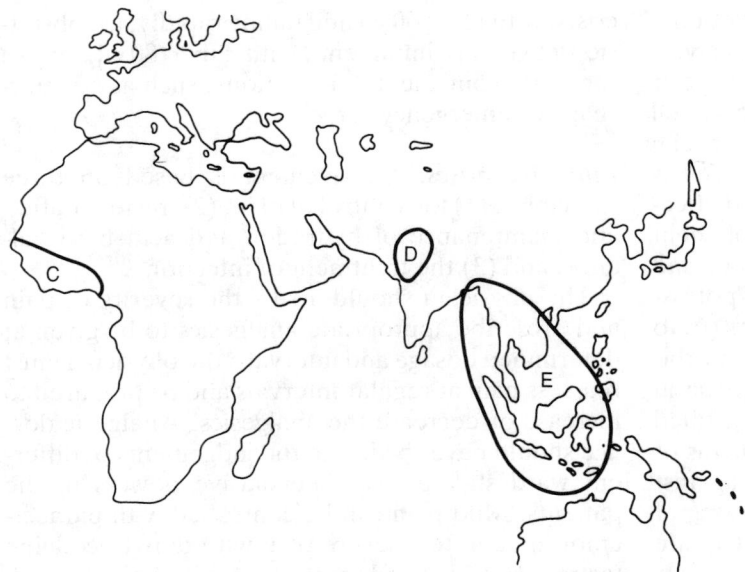

Figure 6.12   Areas of the Old World where haemoglobins C, D (Punjab or Los Angeles) and E reach polymorphic frequencies. (Reproduced with permission of the publishers from Fleming A F. In Strickland G T (ed.) *Hunter's Tropical Medicine*, 7th edn. Philadelphia: W B Saunders, 1991: 36–64.)

priapism should include opiate analgesics and rehydration; under general or spinal anaesthetic, a wide-bore needle is inserted into the lateral side of the base of the penis and the viscous blood aspirated; this is followed by repeated irrigation with saline or 10% heparin and aspiration until fresh blood only is obtained.

Leg ulceration. Small and clean ulcers are treated successfully with daily antiseptic washing and dressing. Large ulcers will heal slowly with (1) prolonged bed-rest with the affected leg raised, (2) appropriate antibiotic therapy, (3) hydrogen peroxide lotion or surgical debridement to remove the slough, and (4) antitetanus prophylaxis. Larger ulcers or those which fail to heal require skin grafts. Once healed, the legs should be protected by crepe or elastic stockings.[70]

Management during pregnancy. Health must be maintained through careful antenatal supervision and the insistence on prophylactic antimalarials and supplementary folic acid.[73] Prophylactic red cell transfusions has been advocated, but benefits are slight if any,[81] and are certainly outweighed by the risk of complications from transfusion in the tropics. Transfusion of red cells is indicated if a patient approaches obstetric delivery with Hb <80 g/l. Patients should be assessed as to the danger of pelvic disproportion, and elective caesarean delivery planned if necessary.

New treatments. There are still no specific therapies for sickle cell disease and its complications. Hydroxyurea or butyrate therapy increases the proportion of HbF and reduces the intracellular polymerization of HbS and haemolysis:[82] results of extensive and controlled trials are awaited. Selected patients have been cured by bone marrow transplantation.[83]

Prevention of sickle cell disease. Strategies for prevention of sickle cell disease include (1) screening to recognize couples at risk, (2) genetic counselling, and (3) prenatal diagnosis followed by termination of homozygous or doubly heterozygous fetuses. Postmarital screening and counselling are widely available for African couples who have had affected children already: in Nigeria in particular, there have been attempts to educate the population and to make premarital counselling available.[84]

Prenatal diagnosis is technically possible and is becoming relatively inexpensive to apply in a few centres.[85] National programmes in Africa suffer restraints of low priority from government, lack of knowledge in the whole community, lack of trained staff, lack of facilities and the illegality or ethical non-acceptance of termination of pregnancy.

Haemoglobin SC disease

The compound heterozygous inheritance of HbS and HbC occurs often in West Africa and in populations derived from West Africa (see Figures 6.10 and 6.12). The pathophysiology and clinical features are similar to those of HbSS, but the severity is much less, and some patients are nearly asymptomatic.[70] Age at presentation is generally later. Because many girls survive childhood, HbSC is the most common form of sickle cell disease to present with complications during pregnancy in West Africa.[76] Eye disease is more frequent, related to the higher Hb concentration. Because the spleen is not destroyed,

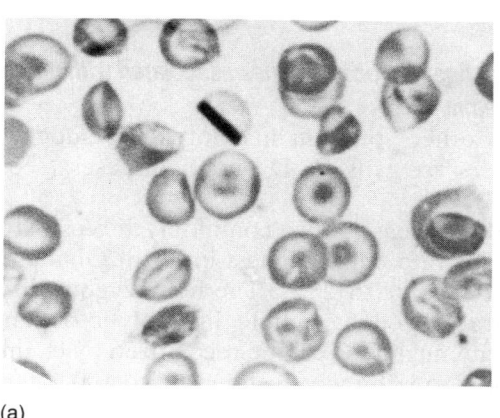

(a)

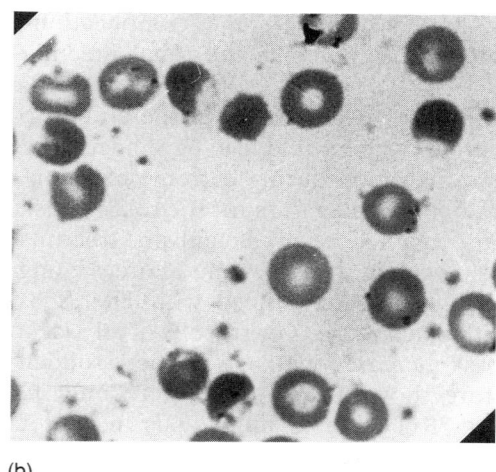

(b)

Figure 6.13   Peripheral blood films. (a) Haemoglobin C disease: there are numerous target cells and one red cell shows intracellular crystal formation. (b) G6PD deficiency: red cells showing oxidative damage. The haemoglobin seems to be separated from the membrane of the cells in certain areas and the rest of the cell looks dense. These changes occur only during a haemolytic episode.

acute sequestration crises and splenic infarcts during flight, including in pressurized aircraft, happen during adult life.

The Hb concentration is intermediate between that of HbSS and normals. The MCV is lower than in HbSS: reticulocyte counts are moderately raised. The red cell appearance is of anisocytosis, some macrocytes, some microspherocytes, numerous target cells, occasional sickle cell forms but with rounded ends, and occasional intraerythrocytic crystals of precipitated HbC (Figure 6.13). Electrophoresis shows two major fractions in the position of HbS and HbC (see Figure 6.5).

The condition of combined inheritance of HbSS plus the α-globin variant HbG^{Philadelphia} is commonly mistaken for HbSC in West Africa (see Figure 6.5). On electrophoresis the subject with HbSS + G shows HbS and the hybrid HbS/G, which moves in the position of HbC; HbS solubility easily differentiates between the two, showing the heterozygous pattern (half precipitated) with HbSC and the homozygous pattern (all haemoglobin precipitated) with HbSS + G.

Haemoglobin S β^0 thalassaemia

The inheritance of both HbS and β^0 thalassaemia occurs most often in North Africa, Sicily and in the mixed population of the Americas (see Figures 6.6 and 6.10).[70]

The clinical course is very similar to that of HbSS. Haematologically the two conditions are difficult to distinguish: the peripheral blood pictures are similar, the MCV and MCH are lower in HbS β^0 thalassaemia; HbS is the only major fraction in both, but HbA$_2$ is raised in HbS β^0 thalassaemia (see Figure 6.5). The diagnosis is made with certainty when one parent carries the β^S gene and the other has β^0 thalassaemia trait.

Haemoglobin S β^+ thalassaemia

This doubly heterozygous condition is most common in Liberia and other parts of West Africa (see Figures 6.6 and 6.10). The clinical course is mild. Anaemia is often slight, and irreversibly sickled cells are seen rarely in the blood.[70] Haemoglobin electrophoresis shows HbA 5–30%, and HbS (see Figure 6.5). It is important not to mistake HbS β^+ thalassaemia for HbAS, in which the HbS is always less than 50%.

Haemoglobin S D^{Punjab}

There are several HbDs, but only HbD^{Punjab} interacts with HbS, leading to a disease similar to HbSS, and is seen amongst Sikhs and mixed populations (see Figures 6.10 and 6.12).[70] There is moderately severe haemolytic anaemia; the peripheral blood picture resembles HbSS: electrophoresis at alkaline pH shows a single band in the position of HbS (see Figure 6.5), but the HbS solubility test yields the heterozygous pattern, and electrophoresis on agar gel separates HbS from HbD (in the position of HbA).

Sickle cell trait

The inheritance of HbAS results in what is essentially a benign condition, which is not associated with decreased life expectancy or with any haematological abnormalities except for the presence of

HbS. There are, however, some complications resulting from microinfarcts in the renal medulla and spleen.[70,86]

There is a progressive decrease in the ability to concentrate urine, which could lead to an increased tendency to dehydration during extreme exertion. This is the probable explanation for the relative risk of sudden unexplained death in enlisted recruits during basic training in the US Armed Forces being 28–40 times higher among those with HbAS as compared with black recruits or recruits of all races; the relative risk increased with age.[87] These sudden deaths are rare, however, as there were only 12 deaths among 38 600 HbAS individuals in over 2 million recruits. Other renal complications include a doubling of the expected frequency of significant bacteriuria during pregnancy, and rarely painless haematuria following renal papillary necrosis.

Incidents are reported of splenic infarcts following exertion at high altitudes. Earlier reports of splenic infarcts while flying at high altitudes in unpressurized aircraft have been largely discounted as being before haemoglobin electrophoresis and differentiation from HbS β^+ thalassaemia or even HbSC was possible.

In the absence of other causes of anaemia, the Hb, red cell indices and reticulocyte count are normal. Electrophoresis shows HbA and HbS: the proportion that is HbS has a trimodal distribution associated with the coincidental inheritance of α-thalassaemia genes; HbS is 34–38% with $\alpha\alpha/\alpha\alpha$, 28–34% with $-\alpha/\alpha\alpha$ and 20–28% with $-\alpha/-\alpha$. HbS above 45% is suggestive of HbS β^+ thalassaemia.[70]

A partial protection against *P. falciparum* malaria has been more clearly demonstrated to be associated with sickle cell trait than it has with any other inherited abnormality of the red cells.[31,49,71] In the non-immune, parasite densities, the frequency of severe malaria (e.g. cerebral malaria or malarial anaemia) and the frequency of death from severe malaria are all lower, and survival rates in childhood are higher. In areas of low endemicity female fertility is higher. In areas of stable malaria HbAS gives partial protection against HMS and severe anaemia associated with HMS during pregnancy.[23,29] There appear to be several mechanisms by which the density of parasitaemias are controlled:[31,49,71] (1) there is an increase of sickling of parasitized red cells, with subsequent removal of the parasitized and sickled cells by the spleen, so limiting the number of early parasite forms; (2) the intraerythrocyte growth during schizogony is inhibited by HbS gelling during the last 12 hours of the cycle spent in relatively hypoxic deep tissues; (3) there has been description of enhancement of cell-mediated immune responses against *P. falciparum* antigens,

possibly related to a modified expression of parasite antigens.[88]

Other haemoglobinopathies associated with haemolytic anaemia

The other common haemolytic haemoglobin disorders are Hbs C, D and E diseases (see Figure 6.12).[47]

HbC disease occurs commonly in West Africa, the carrier rate being highest in north Ghana, with an incidence of 16–28%. The homozygous disorder is characterized by a mild haemolytic anaemia and splenomegaly. It can be recognized by examination of a blood film which shows up to 100% target cell formation with intracellular crystals (Figure 6.13a). Mild microcytosis is a common but not universal feature of HbC trait and disease. Folic acid deficiency and megaloblastic erythropoiesis frequently complicate the course of pregnancy. The diagnosis can be confirmed by haemoglobin electrophoresis (see Figure 6.5).

HbD disease has been found in several racial groups. The clinical picture is that of a moderately severe haemolytic anaemia with splenomegaly. The blood film usually shows moderate numbers of target cells. There are several different types of HbD, all of which have the same rate of electrophoretic migration as HbS but do not precipitate with the HbS solubility test or result in sickling. HbD[Punjab] is the one which is associated with the most marked clinical symptoms.

HbE disease is extremely common in South-East Asia and also occurs in India, Burma and Pakistan.[50] It is occasionally associated with splenomegaly, and is characterized by a mild haemolytic anaemia with hypochromic red cells. HbE migrates in the same position as HbC and HbA_2 (see Figure 6.5).

ENZYMOPATHIES

Erythrocytes are non-nucleated but living cells dependent on several enzymatic pathways. They obtain energy from the breakdown of glucose, 95% of which is metabolized by anaerobic glycolysis to lactate and in the process adenosine triphosphate (ATP) is produced. Five per cent of glucose is metabolized via the hexose monophosphate (pentose phosphate) shunt, during which reduced nicotinamide adenine dinucleotide phosphate (NADPH) is produced. There are many enzymopathies or inherited defects of enzymes affecting the red cells, for example pyruvate kinase deficiency, but of these only deficiencies of glucose-6-phosphate dehydrogenase (G6PD), the first and rate limiting

Table 6.14 Classification of variants of G6PD.

Class	G6PD activity	Haematological manifestations	Polymorphic variants
I	Nearly absent	Congenital non-spherocytic haemolytic anaemia	—
II	Severe <10%	Intermittent haemolysis	Mediterranean, Mali, Union
III	Moderate 10–60%	Less severe intermittent haemolysis	A⁻, Canton, Mahidol
IV	Normal 60–100%	None	B, A, Gambia
V	Increased >150%	None	

enzyme of the hexose monophosphate shunt, reach polymorphic frequencies in different populations.[89,90]

G6PD deficiency

Role of the enzyme

G6PD is vital to and occurs in all cells, but in the red cell this enzyme with the hexose monophosphate pathway is the only source of NADPH. Reduced glutathione (GSH) is synthesized at high concentration in red cells, and has the function of restoring oxidized —SH groups and reducing superoxides and peroxides (through the actions of superoxide dismutase and glutathione peroxidase), but is itself oxidized to GSSG. NADPH is essential for the regeneration of GSH (with the enzyme glutathione reductase). G6PD deficiency and a reduction of synthesis of NADPH exposes the red cell to oxidation of haemoglobin with the intracellular precipitation of globin as Heinz bodies, of several enzymes and of lipids and proteins of the membrane, with consequent haemolysis.

G6PD variants

Over 400 allelic variants of G6PD have been differentiated by electrophoretic mobility, kinetic properties and spectrophotometric assay of enzymatic activity. They have been classified according to their enzymatic activity and clinical manifestations (Table 6.14). Variants of class I, causing chronic non-spherocytic haemolytic anaemias, occur sporadically in all populations. Variants of class II (e.g. Gd^{Mediterranean}) and of class III (e.g. GdA⁻) are associated with intermittent haemolytic crises triggered by oxidant stresses: all variants of major public health importance are in these two groups. Class IV includes GdB, the most common enzyme and referred to as the normal: other variants with normal activity achieve polymorphic frequency, for example GdA in Africa.

The gene controlling G6PD structure is carried on the X chromosome. Males who inherit an abnormal gene ($\overline{X}Y$) will have the variant enzyme in all their erythrocytes, as will homozygous females ($\overline{X}\overline{X}$). Heterozygous females ($\overline{X}X$) will have on average half of their red cells containing normal enzyme and half containing variant enzyme, due to the random suppression of one X chromosome in all female somatic cells. Clinically significant enzyme deficiency will be seen most often in hemizygous males; homozygous females contribute about 10% of those genetically deficient, and about 10% of female heterozygotes are also effectively deficient due to unequal inactivation of their X chromosomes. Frequency in populations is usually expressed as a percentage of males who are hemizygotes.

World distribution

About 7.5% of the world's population carry one or two genes for G6PD deficiency: the highest frequencies are in sub-Saharan Africa (e.g. 32% of males among the Luo on the shores of Lake Victoria), Saudi Arabia and South-East Asia (Figure 6.14). There are populations, for example Sardinians and Kurdish Jews, in which the frequency of G6PD deficiency in males exceeds 50%. The Old World can be divided into three zones according to which G6PD variants achieve polymorphic frequency (Figure 6.14). In zone I, covering the Mediterranean, North Africa, western Asia and the Indian subcontinent, the severely deficient (class II) Gd^{Mediterranean} is prevalent. In zone II, covering South-East Asia, China, Korea and Oceania, two class II variants (Gd^{Mediterranean} and Gd^{Union}) and two moderately severely deficient (class III) variants (Gd^{Mahidol} and Gd^{Canton}) are common. In the third zone, sub-Saharan Africa, the class III enzyme GdA⁻ is frequent, the class II Gd^{Mali} achieves local polymorphic frequency, and up to 40% carry the GdA variant with normal activity. G6PD deficiency is not found in the indigenous populations of America or Australia, but deficient variants occur com-

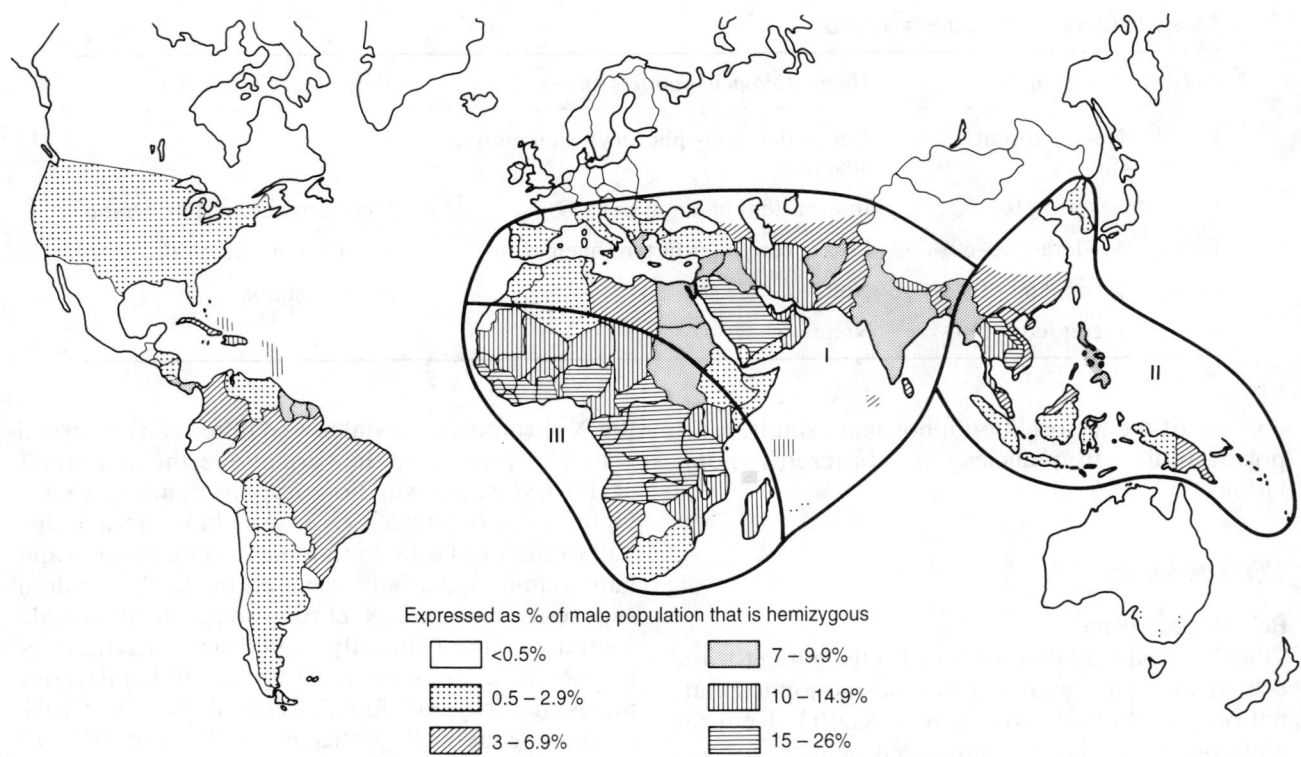

Expressed as % of male population that is hemizygous

☐	<0.5%	▦	7 – 9.9%
▦	0.5 – 2.9%	▥	10 – 14.9%
▨	3 – 6.9%	▤	15 – 26%

Figure 6.14   World distribution of G6PD deficiency. Superimposed are three zones where different G6PD variants reach polymorphic frequencies: zone I, Gd^Mediterranean; zone II, Gd^Mediterranean, Gd^Canton, Gd^Union, Gd^Mahidol; Zone III, GdA⁻. (Reproduced with permission of the World Health Organization from WHO Working Group, ref. 89).

monly in the descendants of African, Mediterranean and Asian immigrants.

About 4.5 million infants born each year are at risk for the complications of G6PD deficiency.

Clinical manifestations

Episodes of haemolysis and jaundice occur in four situations: (1) the neonatal period; (2) severe viral and bacterial infections; (3) following ingestion of certain foods; and (4) following exposure to various drugs and chemicals (Table 6.15). These intermittent episodes tend to be more severe with class II (e.g. Gd^Mediterranean) than class III (e.g. GdA⁻) variants.

Neonatal jaundice. Newborn infants are frequently jaundiced (defined as serum bilirubin >250 μmol/l (15 mg/dl)) on about the fourth day of life in all parts of the world where G6PD deficiency is common (see Figure 6.14), and neonatal jaundice is recognized as a major public health problem in Greece, Saudi Arabia, tropical Africa, the Caribbean, South-East Asia and China, although incidence figures are not often available; in Hong Kong 12% and Singapore 10% of newborns were jaundiced before the intro-

duction of successful control programmes.[91] Jaundice is often multifactorial: common causes include sepsis, prematurity, G6PD deficiency, fetomaternal ABO incompatibility, and haematomas from birth trauma. G6PD deficiency contributes in 30–80% of patients. Globally, infant mortality due to jaundice associated with G6PD deficiency is 0.7–1.6 per 1000 births, with an equal number suffering lifelong morbidity.

Identified variables which potentiate jaundice due to G6PD deficiency are: (1) the severity of the enzyme deficiency (e.g. Mediterranean versus African variants) and lower levels of G6PD in the liver; (2) prematurity; (3) genetically determined slower maturity of the liver in Asians; (4) infections, such as umbilical sepsis, septicaemia and pneumonia; (5) exposure of either the mother or the infant to oxidant drugs (Table 6.15), e.g. mothballs (in the preservation of towelling saved from an older infant), herbal medicines (e.g. Chinese *hung lian*), 'mentholated' powders applied to the umbilical cord, vitamin K analogues, sulphonamides and nitrofurantoins; and (6) breast feeding, which, however, should not be discouraged unless there are exceptional circumstances. Jaundice results from both haemolysis and poor hepatic function. Anaemia is generally moderate (e.g. Hb 130 g/l), with red

Table 6.15 Drugs and other agents commonly associated with oxidative damage to red cells.

Drugs and chemicals which cause oxidative damage to red cells in normal subjects and more severe haemolysis in G6PD-deficient subjects
>   Phenylhydrazine
>   Dapsone and other sulphones
>   Naphthalene (moth balls)
>   Phenacetin and acetanilide (in large doses only)
>   Sulphasalazine (Salazopyrin)

Drugs and chemicals which are shown to cause haemolysis in G6PD-deficient subjects
>   Acetanilide and phenacetin (therapeutic doses)
>   Methylene blue
>   Nalidixic acid
>   Niridazole (Ambilhar)
>   Nitrofurantoins
>   Orange RN (red suya food colouring)
>   Pamaquin
>   Primaquine
>   Pentaquine
>   Sulphonamides: sulphacetamide
>   sulphamethoxale/co-trimoxazole
>   sulphanilamide
>   sulphapyridine
>   Thiazosulphone
>   Toluidine blue
>   Trinitrotoluene (TNT)

Drugs and chemicals that may cause haemolysis in some types of G6PD-deficient subject but not shown to be haemolytic in GdA⁻ type
>   Aspirin (in large doses)
>   Chloroquine
>   Quinine
>   Quinidine
>   Vitamin K analogues
>   Chloramphenicol
>   Dimercaprol (BAL)
>   *Vicia faba* (broad beans)

This list is not comprehensive. In addition there are many isolated unconfirmed reports of other drugs causing haemolysis in G6PD deficiency.

cell anisocytosis, spherocytosis, polychromasia and numerous nucleated cells. Total unconjugated bilirubin levels are raised, and when above $300\,\mu$mol/l there is the danger of kernicterus and severe permanent brain damage.

While the serum bilirubin is in the range of 250–$300\,\mu$mol/l in mature and otherwise healthy infants, treatment should be with phototherapy. In the absence of designed equipment, sufficient irradiance can be obtained from a unit of at least seven 20-watt fluorescent tubes placed 40 cm above the naked infant, whose eyes are shielded.[92] Alternatively, exposure to the morning sunlight, with cooling of the body and shielding of the eyes, is effective. When the unconjugated bilirubin rises above $300\,\mu$mol/l, treatment is by exchange blood transfusion with blood from G6PD normal donors compatible with both mother and infant, at a volume twice that of the infant's blood volume (i.e. 2 × 85 ml/kg body weight), in 20 ml aliquots over 2 hours. Phototherapy and exchange transfusion are indicated at lower bilirubin levels in low weight and ill infants.[90–92]

Neonatal jaundice has been controlled and kernicterus virtually abolished in Singapore by a highly successful national campaign in which (1) G6PD activity is screened in cord blood of all infants, (2) all those deficient are observed in hospital for 2 weeks, and treated promptly if jaundice develops; (3) both the general public and health professionals are informed and educated, (4) letters are given to parents with G6PD deficiency addressed to the obstetrician who delivers the next baby, and (5) G6PD-deficient infants are issued with cards warning against potentially haemolysing drugs.[91] Other measures preventing neonatal jaundice include:

(1) adequate prenatal care, so avoiding many premature deliveries; (2) non-traumatic delivery, so avoiding extensive haematomas; and (3) hygiene in the puerperium, so avoiding sepsis.

Infection-induced jaundice. Viral infections, including hepatitis, infections of the respiratory and gastrointestinal tracts, and bacterial infections, including lobar pneumonia, typhoid, paratyphoid and septicaemia, commonly cause severe jaundice in G6PD-deficient subjects. Possible mechanisms are the generation of H_2O_2 by activated neutrophils and macrophages, triggering haemolysis of G6PD-deficient cells and liver dysfunction leading to hepatocellular jaundice. Anaemia will be more severe as a result of suppression of erythropoiesis by infection. The course may be complicated in adults, but only rarely in children, by renal failure, which can be the result of pre-existing renal disease, nephrotoxic drugs, urinary tract infection, hepatic virus infection, renal ischaemia and tubular obstruction by haemoglobin. The administration of oxidant drugs may lead to further intravascular haemolysis and life-threatening renal failure.

Management is supportive: the treatment of the primary infection, the avoidance of oxidative drugs (Table 6.15), and a regimen for renal failure.

Food-induced haemolysis. Favism is a condition of severe intravascular haemolysis precipitated by eating fava beans (*Vicia faba*) or inhalation of the pollen; it occurs commonly in G6PD-deficient inhabitants of the Mediterranean area, North Africa and western and eastern Asia. It had been thought to be associated only with Gd^Mediterranean, but has been described recently with other variants including GdA^-.[93] Favism occurs with the ingestion of fresh, dried or frozen beans, but fresh beans in the spring are the most potent. Haemolysis in breast-fed infants may follow when mothers eat fava beans. Which ingredients trigger haemolysis is not proven.

Favism affects children under 5 years most commonly. Its pathogenesis is uncertain, as some G6PD subjects are spared altogether, while others have attacks for the first time after eating beans for years without trouble. There is intravascular haemolysis of sudden onset 24–48 hours after ingestion of beans: patients show pallor and haemoglobinuria; jaundice is less pronounced than with the haemolysis triggered by infections or drugs. Anaemia may be profound and renal failure can develop.

There is no specific treatment: transfusion of G6PD normal blood may be required if there is incipient or established cardiac failure.

Haemolytic episodes are best prevented by screening of G6PD deficiency in populations with high frequency, education and avoiding eating beans.

Milder acute haemolytic episodes have followed eating red suya, a peppered kebab-like roasted meat, in Nigeria; the offending substance was Orange RN (monosodium salt of 1-phenylazo-2-naphthol-6-sulphonic acid) used as colouring. It can be predicted that other foods could have the same effect in developing countries where there is inadequate control of additives.[94]

Drug-induced haemolysis. Ingestion of a wide variety of drugs and chemicals induces haemolysis in G6PD-deficient subjects (Table 6.15). The range of precipitating substances and the severity of the crises are greater with class II (e.g. Gd^Mediterranean) than class III (e.g. GdA^-) variants. There is also considerable intrapatient variability of severity between subjects with the same G6PD variant and drug exposure.[89,90,92]

Starting from between a few hours and 3 days after exposure, there may be only transient mild anaemia, or in some there is a rapidly progressive severe anaemia reaching a nadir at 7–8 days. Patients can complain of loin and abdominal pain; there is jaundice, haemoglobinuria and transient splenomegaly. Recovery is marked by a reticulocytosis and a rise of haemoglobin after 8–9 days.

Continued exposure to the drug can lead to fatal anaemia or renal failure in the case of class II variants. However, in the milder haemolysis of GdA^- it is sometimes possible to continue with essential therapy, for example dapsone in the treatment of leprosy; patients have a transient haemolytic anaemia, followed by a state of compensated haemolysis.

Treatment is supportive and by withdrawal of the offending agent. Further attacks can be prevented by giving the patient a list of drugs to be avoided. Community strategies include screening and education.

Diagnosis

Haematology. During the steady state, subjects with the common forms of G6PD deficiency have a very mild chronic haemolysis, with a red cell life span of around 100 days. With Gd^Mediterranean the mean Hb in males is slightly decreased (141 versus 157 g/l in controls in one series). Red cell indices and appearances on blood film are normal, but there is a slight reticulocytosis (± 1.5%).

During a haemolytic crisis there are all the features of intravascular haemolysis (see Table 6.11) and a characteristic peripheral blood film appearance (see Figure 6.13B): supravital staining shows the presence of Heinz bodies.

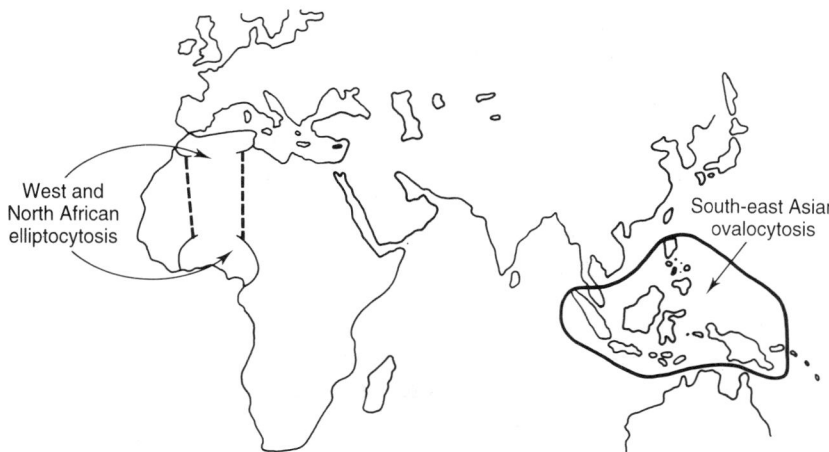

Figure 6.15 Areas of the Old World where ovalocytosis and elliptocytosis achieve (or approach) a polymorphic frequency.

G6PD screening and identification. There are several screening tests available that depend on NADPH production and its detection by direct fluorescence or by reduction of a coloured dye (e.g. methylene blue) to its colourless form.[95] These are simple, inexpensive and sensitive for the detection of hemizygous males and homozygous females when in the steady state. However, immediately following haemolytic crises, when there is a high population of young red cells, G6PD activity of whole blood may be normal, especially with class III (e.g. GdA⁻) variants; in this situation blood should be centrifuged and the older cells at the bottom of the column tested, or the test delayed for about 6 weeks.

G6PD activity can be measured quantitatively by the spectrophotometric assay of NADPH formation by red cells: this requires a basic biochemistry laboratory. Male hemizygotes, female homozygotes and more than 80% of female heterozygotes can be identified.

The different G6PD variants are identified by several techniques, including electrophoresis and enzyme kinetic studies: these investigations are performed in reference or research laboratories only.

G6PD and malaria

Evidence that G6PD deficiency may confer advantage is derived from geography, parasitology of patients and in vitro cultures of *P. falciparum*.[89,90] Globally, G6PD deficiency reaches polymorphic frequency only where *P. falciparum* is or was endemic (see Figure 6.14), suggesting that in these areas deficient subjects have a genetic advantage; this view is supported by micromapping, for example in Sardinia where deficient gene frequency declines with increasing altitude and decreasing transmission of malaria. Clinical and field studies have shown a parasitological advantage consistently only for female heterozygotes, for example Nigerian

children with GdB/GdA⁻, who had significantly lower *P. falciparum* densities than normal children with malaria; furthermore, GdB red cells were much more often parasitized than GdA⁻ red cells in the same individual. In vitro cultures of *P. falciparum* have demonstrated that parasite growth is impaired in G6PD-deficient compared with normal red cells, but in some studies additional oxidative stress was needed before the difference became apparent. The probable mechanism is through oxidative damage, to which malaria parasites are susceptible and which is more liable in G6PD-deficient than in normal red cells. Why hemizygous males apparently do not enjoy partial protection against malaria remains unresolved, but it is possible that this is related to induction of G6PD synthesis by the parasite during passage through a wholly G6PD-deficient red cell population.

MEMBRANE DEFECTS

The red cell membrane is supported by a protein skeleton consisting of a lattice of hexagons, the sides of which are spectrin tetramers: these are linked at the corners of the hexagons by actin, tropomyosin and protein 4.1, and attached to the lipid bilayer by ankyrin and protein 3 (the major transmembrane protein and anion transporter), as well as by glycoproteins such as glycophorin C. Inherited variants of either the integral or skeletal proteins of the red cell membrane may be manifest as abnormalities of shape, such as hereditary spherocytosis, elliptocytosis and ovalocytosis.[96] Membrane defects occur sporadically in all populations, hereditary spherocytosis being the most studied; only ovalocytosis in South-East Asia and Oceania achieves polymorphic frequency, but elliptocytosis is approaching polymorphic frequency in West and North Africa (see Figure 6.15).

South-East Asian ovalocytosis

The molecular basis of South-East Asian ovalocytosis is a deletion of 27 nucleotides, resulting in the deletion of nine amino acids from protein 3: the abnormal protein 3 has a higher than normal affinity for ankyrin, resulting in increased membrane rigidity and the oval shape (Figure 6.16a).[97,98] Inheritance is autosomal and dominant.

Ovalocytosis is seen at high frequency in populations of Malaysia, Indonesia, the Philippines, Papua New Guinea and the Solomon Islands, and possibly in Micronesian populations further out into

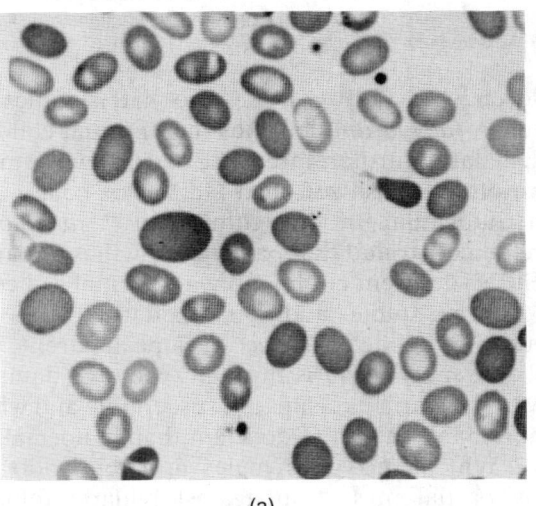

(a)

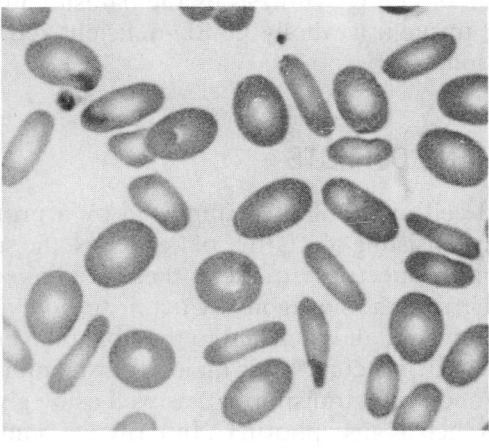

(b)

Figure 6.16 Peripheral blood films. (a) South-East Asian ovalocytosis. A high proportion of cells have a long axis which is less than twice the transverse axis (ovalocytosis). Some have two areas of central pallor (knizocytes), e.g. on the horizontal midline, towards the right edge. Some have mouth-like slits of pallor (stomatocytes), e.g. near the lower edge towards the left. (Reproduced with permission of the author and publishers from Dacie J V. *The Haemolytic Anaemias 1*, 3rd edn. Edinburgh: Churchill Livingstone, 1985.) (b) Elliptocytosis. The long axis is more than twice the transverse axis.

the Pacific (see Figure 6.15). The distribution is extremely uneven within this area, but reaches up to 50% in Sulawesi (Celebes) and 27% in coastal Papua New Guinea.

South-East Asian ovalocytosis is not associated with haemolysis or anaemia, except for the occasional report of haemolysis, possibly related to the inheritance of a second membrane defect. A high proportion of red cells are ovalocytes (with a long axis less than twice the transverse axis), stomatocytes and knizocytes (with duplicated central pallor) (Figure 6.16a). Osmotic fragility is reduced.

Malaria parasite rates are significantly lower in subjects with ovalocytosis than in those with normal red cells. Reduced invasion of ovalocytes by *P. falciparum* has been shown in vitro. The probable mechanism is through decreased mobility of membrane proteins, preventing penetration of merozoites of possibly both *P. falciparum* and *P. vivax*.

Elliptocytosis in West and North Africa

There are many mutations which result in elliptocytosis, and several have been described in West and North Africa. Two variants of spectrin are at least approaching polymorphic frequency. Spectrin αI/65 is the more common, being reported in Benin, Togo, Côte d'Ivoire and Burkina Faso in West Africa, and in the Maghreb (Tunisia, Algeria and Morocco); Tuaregs who inhabit the Sahara between these two areas have elliptocytosis, but this has not been characterized (see Figure 6.15). Spectrin αI/46 is found amongst Ewe speakers in Togo and Benin. Up to 2–3% of both northern and southern Nigerians have an uncharacterized elliptocytosis. Inheritance is dominant. The condition is usually symptomless, but there may be mild haemolysis, especially in homozygotes with the spectrin αI/65 variant. Red cells have a long axis more than twice the transverse axis (Figure 6.16b). There can be periodic episodes of slight jaundice and moderate splenomegaly following intercurrent infections; children with elliptocytosis and malaria sometimes develop profound anaemia (personal observations). Some elliptocyte variants are resistant to invasion by *P. falciparum* but there is no evidence at present as to whether there is selection for elliptocytosis in West Africa.

NUTRITIONAL ANAEMIAS

IRON

Iron is essential for the formation of haemoglobin, myoglobin and various enzymes. Its deficiency is the most common of all nutritional disorders: about 700 million individuals suffer from anaemia due to iron deficiency, out of the global total of around 1000 million anaemic persons (see Table 6.10), while an even larger number have iron depletion which has not reached the stage of anaemia.[99,100]

Dietary iron and absorption

In early postnatal life iron is derived normally from breast milk, which contains 0.3–0.5 mg/l in a readily available form (50% absorbed). Iron in all other foods is in three forms: (1) haem iron, (2) non-haem iron, and (3) contamination iron.

Haem iron is a constituent of haemoglobin and myoglobin in meat, poultry, fish and blood products; it is readily absorbed (20–30%) by the duodenal mucosal cells and utilized.

Non-haem iron is found in varying concentrations in all foods of plant origin, including cereals, tubers, vegetables and pulses. It is poorly absorbed (<5%) from common staples such as rice, maize, wheat, sorghum and millet when eaten alone. Absorption is inhibited by many vegetable ligands, including phytates in cereals, polyphenols in nuts and legumes, tannin in tea and soy protein, and by fibre; other inhibitors are egg phosphoproteins, and in those with pica, ash and clay. Absorption may be enhanced to up to 20% by consumption during the same meal of (1) fresh fruits and vegetables rich in ascorbic acid (e.g. guava, citrus, pineapple, mango, green or red peppers, cauliflower, some green leafs, potato, sweet potato, tomato and turnip), (2) amino acids from meat, poultry, fish and other seafoods, and (3) acids (e.g. lactic, citric).

Contamination iron is from two sources: dirt and iron cooking vessels. An adult male can take in 40–500 mg of contaminating iron on rice, sorghum or tef (*Eragrostis abyssinica*, a staple of the Ethiopian highlands) from the dirt picked up during threshing on earth floors and the dust of the market place; little of this absorbable. Cooking food in iron pots may increase the iron content several fold, especially with soups containing acid-rich vegetables which are simmered for a long time. Beer brewed in iron pots is rich in available iron, and nutritional iron overload can follow after years of steady consumption (see below).

Absorption is by duodenal mucosal cells and is regulated by the iron status of the individual, being more efficient in the iron depleted than in the iron replete.

Iron balance

The iron in the body is in four compartments: (1) haemoglobin iron 1.5–3.0 g, (2) storage iron 1.0–1.5 g as ferritin and haemosiderin, (3) 'essential' iron 300 mg in myoglobin and numerous enzymes, and (4) transport iron 3–4 mg as transferrin, all quantities relating to adult males. The turnover of iron is rapid, about 23 mg entering and leaving the haemoglobin compartment of an adult each day, but iron is highly conserved and basal losses by desquamation in faeces, urine and skin for adult men and postmenopausal women are only about 1 mg/day (Table 6.16). Infants have low requirements while the red cell mass diminishes during the first 4–6 months, and these are met by breast feeding. Iron needs are high relative to body size during growth in older infancy, childhood and the adolescent growth spurt. Menstruation approximately doubles the basal demand. Requirements are low during the first trimester of pregnancy but rise rapidly in the second trimester, to reach around 6–7 mg/day; approximately 1000 mg of iron is needed over the whole of one pregnancy. Lactating women secrete about 0.3 mg of iron per day in breast milk, but while they have amenorrhoea daily requirements are relatively low.

Diets with high contents of bioavailable iron are eaten by most populations in industrialized countries, and also, until recently, surviving communities of hunter–gatherers, pastoralists who eat meat and blood (e.g. Masai in Kenya) and some groups with high ascorbic acid intake (e.g. Yoruba in Nigeria); physiological demands for iron are usually met, except during pregnancy when negative balance and some depletion of stores is inevitable. The majority of the world's population eat food with intermediate, low or very low bioavailable iron, from which it is impossible to meet the basic physiological requirements for iron (Table 6.16).

Iron deficiency

Aetiology

Iron deficiency is commonly the result of *inadequate intake* of bioavailable iron not meeting physiological requirements. Ligands inhibiting iron absorption can be increased in special circumstances: food taboos applied during pregnancy; the replacement of traditional diets by convenience foods including wheat-bread and eggs; the drinking of tea (or coffee to a lesser extent) with the meal. Premature infants are a special case of nutritional deficiency as the transplacental transport of iron to the infant takes place almost wholly in the last 4 weeks of gestation.

Table 6.16 FAO/WHO recommended iron intakes (mg/day) to cover requirements of 97.5% individuals in each age/sex group for diets with different bioavailabilities (after ref. 99).

Age/sex group	Absorbed iron required	Bioavailability of dietary iron (% of iron absorbed)			
		Very low[1] (<5%)	Low[2] (5–10%)	Intermediate[3] (11–18%)	High[4] (>19%)
Children, both sexes					
0–4 months	0.5	*	*	*	*
4–12 months	0.96	24	13	6	4
13–24 months	0.61	15	8	4	3
2–5 years	0.70	17	9	5	3
6–11 years	1.17	29	16	8	5
Adolescents					
12–16 years (girls)	2.02	50	27	13	9
12–16 years (boys)	1.82	45	24	12	8
Adults					
Men	1.14	28	15	8	5
Women					
Menstruating	2.38	59	32	16	11
Pregnant: 1st trimester	0.8	—	—	—	—
3rd trimester	6.3	†	†	†	—
Lactating	1.31	33	17	9	6
Postmenopausal	0.96	24	13	6	4

* Iron from breast milk is sufficient for about the first 6 months.
† Supplementation essential.
[1] *Very low bioavailability*. Diet composed almost entirely of cereals (e.g. in India).
[2] *Low bioavailability*. Monotonous diet based on cereals, roots and tubers, with a preponderance of foods which inhibit iron absorption (maize, rice, beans, wheat, sorghum) and with negligible quantities of meat, fish or ascorbic acid.
[3] *Intermediate bioavailability diet*. Similar to above, but including some foods of animal origin and/or ascorbic acid.
[4] *High bioavailability*. A diversified diet containing generous quantities of meat, poultry, fish or foods rich in ascorbic acid: typical of most populations in industrialized countries. The regular consumption with meals of inhibitors of absorption (e.g. tea or coffee) can reduce bioavailability to the intermediate level.

Those with the greatest *physiological demands* for iron are at the highest risk of deficiency; these are preschool children, adolescents during the growth spurt, and especially menstruating girls, and pregnant women. Women who have many pregnancies, closely spaced, are especially liable to deficiency.

As normal red cells contains iron as haemoglobin 1 mg per 1 ml, *chronic blood loss* can lead easily to negative balance and depletion of iron stores. Common causes in the tropics are infection by hookworm, *Schistosoma* spp. and whipworm (*Trichuris trichiura*). Many conditions leading to chronic haemorrhage (e.g. menorrhagia, aspirin ingestion, peptic ulcers, carcinomas) occur in tropical as well as in non-tropical environments.

Hookworm. Infections with *Ancylostoma duodenale* and *Necator americanus* are widespread, and probably more than 900 million individuals, almost a quarter of the world's population, are infected (see

Chapter 71). Prevalence of 80–90% in the population in the moist tropics is not unusual.

The adult worms ingest, detach and digest the host's intestinal mucosa, causing bleeding. The daily loss of iron has been calculated as 1.2 mg and 0.8 mg per 1000 ova per gram of faeces for *A. duodenale* and *N. americanus* respectively, but as both species are now found more-or-less worldwide and mixed infections are common, the daily loss of iron of 1 mg per 1000 ova per gram of faeces regardless of species is a good working figure.

Depletion of iron stores depends on (1) the daily absorption of iron, (2) the size of the body's iron stores, and (3) the intensity of the hookworm infection. Subjects with diets poor in bioavailable iron and with low or no stores need only light infections to deplete them of iron; in contrast, adults in West Africa on traditional diets had a threshold of at least 20 000 ova per gram of faeces, equivalent to an iron loss of 20 mg/day, above which they went into negative balance. Women have lower thresholds than men. Children expose their whole body surfaces to infection when playing on the ground, and have heavy hookworm loads in relation to their body weights; the resultant *subacute hookworm anaemia* has an element of acute haemorrhage in its aetiology. *Acute hookworm anaemia* is rare but follows extremely heavy infections, usually in infants but sometimes in older children or even adults; anaemia is from acute blood loss, and shows a normochromic picture.[18]

Schistosomiasis. About 200 million people are infected by *Schistosoma*, and transmission is increasing with the spread of irrigation (see Chapter 72).

The haematuria from *S. haematobium* is short lived but can give rise to a loss of 30–40 mg of iron per day and contribute significantly to iron deficiency, especially in adolescent boys, for example in Somalia and coastal East Africa.

The mechanisms of anaemia caused by *S. mansoni* and *S. japonicum* infections are complex. Ulcers and polyps in the colon bleed and can result in a chronic loss of iron of 7–8 mg/day. Infection of the liver is followed by hepatic fibrosis and the anaemia of chronic disorders; portal hypertension leads to splenomegaly and the pancytopenia of hypersplenism; oesophageal varices may bleed acutely or intermittently, leading to iron loss.[18]

Trichuriasis. T. trichiura is one of the most prevalent helminths in the world (see Chapter 71). Blood is lost from the inflamed colonic mucosa. Heavy infections in excess of 800 worms (16 000 ova per gram of faeces) result in a blood loss of 4 ml, or iron loss of 1.5 mg, per day. Trichuriasis can contribute to iron deficiency, or be a major cause in children, as has been reported from Central America and Malaysia.[101]

Stages of iron deficiency

Iron deficiency passes through three stages. In the first stage, *iron depletion*, iron stores are reduced, but haemopoiesis remains unaffected: plasma ferritin is below normal and staining for iron in a bone marrow aspirate shows scanty (1+) or zero iron in the macrophages of a cellular fragment; plasma iron is low normal, plasma transferrin raised and its percentage saturation reduced within the normal range. In the second stage, *iron deficient erythropoiesis*, iron stores have been exhausted: plasma ferritin is reduced further, iron is absent from the bone marrow and there are no sideroblasts; plasma iron and transferrin saturation are below normal and red

cell protoporphyrin is raised; the Hb is likely to be within the normal range or there may be a slight normochromic anaemia. With further depletion, iron is not available for haemoglobin synthesis, and *iron deficiency anaemia* develops.

Iron deficiency anaemia

Clinical. Patients present with symptoms and signs of anaemia from any cause; in addition they may show angular stomatitis, koilonychia and loss of melanin skin pigmentation.

Iron is essential for many metabolic processes, and its deficiency even without anaemia has adverse effects on development during childhood, the outcome of pregnancy and work capacity. In practice it is not feasible to distinguish the results of iron deficiency *per se* from those of anaemia. The consequences of iron deficiency, and especially iron deficiency anaemia are: *in infants and children*, impaired motor development, co-ordination, language development and scholastic achievement, psychological and behavioural effects (inattention, fatigue, insecurity, etc.) and decreased physical activity; *in adults of both sexes*, decreased physical work, earning capacity and resistance to fatigue; *in pregnant women*, increased maternal and infant morbidity and mortality, premature delivery, and risk of low birth weight.[99] There is no convincing evidence that iron deficiency either enhances or significantly impairs resistance to infections, although there is some reduction of cellular immune responses.[100]

Haematology. Anaemia varies from mild to profound. The MCV, MCH and mean cell haemoglobin concentration (MCHC) are all reduced; the peripheral blood film shows microcytic hypochromic red cells and sometimes numerous target cells (Figure 6.17). In the bone marrow aspirate there are micronormoblastic red cell precursors and the total absence of storage iron. Plasma, for example in a microhaematocrit tube, is nearly colourless and water clear.

There are three considerations in confirming the diagnosis of iron deficiency anaemia: (1) limited laboratory facilities; (2) biochemical measurements of iron status giving misleading results in patients with multiple pathology; and (3) the differentiation from the microcytic hypochromic anaemias of chronic disorders and β thalassaemia minor.

With a limited laboratory the diagnosis of iron deficiency anaemia can be usually made with certainty from the blood film appearance, colourless plasma and the absence of iron in the bone marrow.

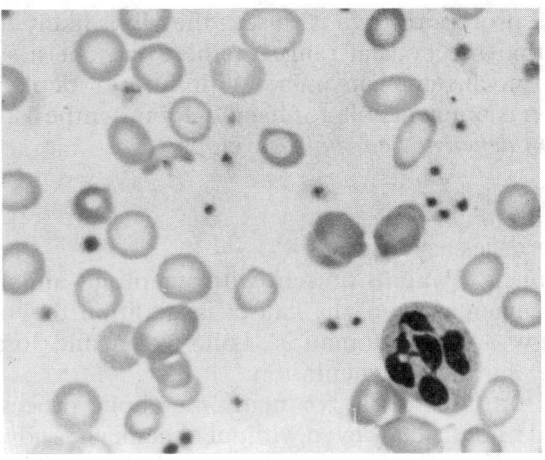

Figure 6.17 Peripheral blood film. Iron deficiency anaemia: there is variation in size of the red cells (anisocytosis) with many small cells (microcytosis), variation of shape (poikilocytosis) and hypersegmented neutrophil, suggestive but not diagnostic of folate or vitamin B_{12} deficiency; there are numerous platelets (thrombocytosis) which are likely to be a response to chronic haemorrhage.

However, iron is immobilized in the RES in the anaemia of chronic disorders, megaloblastic anaemia and protein–energy malnutrition (PEM); although iron is seen in the bone marrow and iron deficiency is not limiting erythropoiesis at the time, treatment of the primary condition can lead to the mobilization of all iron and the uncovering of iron deficiency.

Ferritin is an acute reactive protein and plasma ferritin levels are generally raised in rural populations in the tropics, and although levels correlate with the body iron stores, higher cut-off points have to be applied. Malaria, other recurrent infection and chronic hepatic disease can be accompanied by abnormally high plasma ferritins even in the face of severe iron deficiency, making the measurement of plasma ferritin of limited diagnostic value, especially in children.

In iron deficiency, the plasma iron is low and the plasma transferrin is raised, so that transferrin saturation is <16% in adults, <14% in children and <12% in infants. In contrast, in anaemia of chronic disorders and PEM, both plasma iron and plasma ferritin are reduced, and although the saturation of transferrin is decreased it remains >15%.

In β thalassaemia minor the red cell count is higher (>5.0×10^{12}/l), there is less anisocytosis (normal RBC distribution width (RDW)), greater microcytosis and less hypochromia than with iron deficiency. From these characteristics are derived several formulae to differentiate the two conditions for example the ratio MCV:RBC is >14 in iron deficiency and <14 in thalassaemia.

Treatment

Oral treatment. Tablets of ferrous salts (for example exsiccated ferrous sulphate 200 mg, containing 60 mg of elemental iron) taken orally are the cheapest effective treatment.[99] For adults and adolescents the recommended dosage is 60 mg of elemental iron per day for mild anaemia and 120 mg per day for moderate or severe anaemia. Absorption is best if the tablets are taken on an empty stomach. Treatment should continue until the Hb has reached normal limits and ceased to rise, and then for at least another 4–6 weeks in order to build up body stores.

Pregnant women should receive a combination tablet containing 250 μg of folic acid and 60 mg of iron twice a day; suitable tablets are supplied by UNICEF for \$US1 per 1000 tablets.

Infants and children may be treated with liquid preparations in divided doses to provide 5 mg of iron per kilogram body weight per day.

Oral iron can cause upper gastrointestinal side-effects (epigastric discomfort, nausea and vomiting), or lower gastrointestinal side-effects (diarrhoea or constipation). The frequency of adverse reactions is related directly to the dosage of iron and not to the ferrous compound prescribed. Oral treatment must continue if possible: dosage should be reduced and then stepped up again slowly within the patient's tolerance, or the tablets taken with meals (although this reduces absorption), or the formulation changed to a better tolerated but much more expensive slow-release preparation.

Where folate intake is poor, deficiency may develop during the response to iron therapy: folic 5 mg/day for 3 weeks should be given. Recovery may be delayed by coincidental malaria, and there is evidence that children are more susceptible to malaria during the reticulocyte response to iron therapy; an initial curative antimalarial course followed by a prophylactic for 3 weeks is recommended where malaria is endemic.

Parenteral treatment. A parenteral route is justified when (1) oral treatment has not been tolerated, (2) there is persistent non-compliance, (3) it is nearly impossible for a patient to comply because of the severity of the iron deficiency and the length of time required for oral therapy, and (4) an advanced period of gestation does not allow for full oral treatment before obstetric delivery. The extra cost of parenteral preparations is offset by savings on hospital bed occupancy and staff time, and by the rapid return of the patient to productive life.[101]

The recommended preparation is iron dextran, containing iron 50 mg/ml. The dosage required is calculated from the formula: total dose (ml) = 0.01

$\times\ W(140-Hb)$, where W is the body weight (kg) and Hb is the observed haemoglobin concentration (g/l). (Practitioners must be certain that they calculate the haemoglobin deficit in the correct units, g/l, *not* g/dl: the total dose is generally in the range of 30–50 ml in a severely anaemic adult.) Short courses of intramuscular injections, for example 2 ml daily for 10 days, are tolerated, but larger iron deficits are better managed by total dose iron infusion. This is highly effective, can be carried out as an outpatient procedure, and is safe, although it must be performed by a doctor who is prepared to treat rare anaphylactic reactions.

The patient receives promethazine hydrochloride (Phenergan) 12.5 mg (adult dose) 30 minutes before the infusion. Adrenaline 1/1000, anthisan and oxygen are to hand. The skin over the chosen vein is cleaned with soap, not an alcohol solution. The calculated total dose of iron dextran is dissolved freshly in normal saline, up to a maximum of 5% v/v (e.g. 50 ml in 1 litre). The infusion is started at less than 10 drops/min for 30 minutes, during which time the patient is observed by a doctor: if there is no reaction, the whole infusion is given over a few hours; if a serious reaction develops, the infusion is stopped and treatment for anaphylaxis is administered promptly. In addition, patients should receive folic acid 5 mg/day for 3 weeks, a curative antimalarial and a prophylactic for 3 weeks if malaria is endemic.[23]

Prevention

There are four strategies for the prevention of iron deficiency: (1) iron supplementation; (2) fortification of a staple food with iron; (3) measures to increase dietary intake of bioavailable iron; and (4) the control of hookworm and other helminthic infections.[99]

Supplementation. Supplementation with medicinal iron has the advantages of having immediate impact and of being targeted on specific groups which are known to be liable to deficiency, including pregnant women, premature infants, preschool children and adolescent girls.

Iron supplementation for pregnant women should be given the highest priority in all national programmes of prenatal care delivery.[23,99,102] A successful programme must involve policy makers, planners, managers, educators, workers, midwives, obstetricians, the pregnant women themselves and their families, in order to ensure the utilization of antenatal services, the provision of medication and compliance by pregnant women. Recommended supplementation is the UNICEF combined tablet of elemental iron 60 mg (as ferrous sulphate) and folic acid 250 μg, taken twice daily without food throughout the second half of pregnancy; if compliance is poor or if there are unacceptable side-effects, the two tablets can be taken together, or be taken with meals or be reduced to one per day. Where malaria is endemic, antimalarial prophylaxis should start from the time of first antenatal attendance. Where women are exposed to heavy hookworm infestations, albendazole 400 mg should be given orally on first attendance. Vitamin A (2.4 mg retinol/day) supplements dramatically enhanced the efficacy of iron in the prevention of anaemia in pregnancy in Indonesia.

Breast feeding for 6 months or more protects full term infants; breast-fed preterm infants require iron supplements by not later than 2 months of age. Recommended dosage is 2 mg/kg body weight, up to a maximum of 15 mg/day until iron fortified cereal foods can be introduced. Parents must be warned about the toxicity of iron overdosage. Bottle-fed infants should receive formulae containing iron 12 mg/l and vitamin E 10 iu/l;[2] unfortified brands are still being sold by the unscrupulous in developing countries.

Preschool children can be reached at child-care centres; a practical regimen is to give a 2–3 week course of iron 30 mg/day in liquid or tablet form, several times a year.[99] The administration of iron supplements to rural Gambian children at home by their mothers was successful in the treatment of iron deficiency, but led to an increased risk of severe malarial parasitaemia; it is proposed that antimalarial prophylactics should be given at the same time as iron supplementation.[103]

Food fortification. The fortification with iron of widely consumed and centrally processed staple foods is the main strategy for anaemia control in many countries.[11,99] Vehicles for fortification have included acidified milk formulae and biscuits (with added bovine haemoglobin) in Chile, sugar in Guatemala, salt in India and fish sauce in Thailand. Fortification has been followed by a slow but steady decrease of prevalence of anaemia at low cost. Fortification programmes require industrial infrastructure and organized marketing which do not exist in many countries, particularly in Africa.

Dietary modification. In the long term the ideal is for people to eat food from which they can absorb sufficient iron for normal physiological requirements.[99] Improved iron status can be achieved by increasing enhancers of iron absorption (e.g. ascorbic acid and animal protein), decreasing inhibitors (e.g. tannin and phytic acid), or by increasing total food intake so that energy needs are met fully and total iron intake improved by up to 30%. Efforts to raise the ascorbic acid content of food have the best chances of success.

However, even when the value of ascorbic acid-rich foods is understood, there are restraints of cost if purchased, and of limited water supply and expense of fencing if grown in home gardens. As ascorbic acid is destroyed by heat, encouragement should be given to eating food raw or cooked only lightly and not reheated. Germination, malting and fermentation of grains both increase ascorbic acid and decrease tannin and phytates. Attempts to increase intake of animal protein are restrained by high costs and by religious objections, for example Hinduism.

Control of helminthic infections. It has been shown, for example in Korea, that transmission of hookworm can be reduced highly effectively and cheaply by simple sanitary measures, such as pit latrines, wearing plastic sandals and abandoning human faeces as fertilizer[101] (see also Chapters 71 and Appendix III).

Iron overload

There are many congenital and acquired conditions leading to systemic iron overload, including hereditary haemochromatosis and thalassaemia.[104] In sub-Saharan Africa, dietary iron overload is associated with drinking regularly for many years beers brewed from sorghum, millet and maize (Chapter 3). The beers are fermented in iron pots or, in more recent times, steel (oil) barrels, and contain absorbable iron at a concentration of about 80 mg/l; as acid and alcohol stimulate gastric acid secretion, absorption is enhanced further. Men especially commonly drink several litres on weekends.

Dietary iron overload, as defined as hepatic iron $>360\,\mu$mol/g dry weight (normal $<17\,\mu$mol/g), was present in 26% of male and 8% of female black South Africans over 40 years of age in necropsies at Baragwanath Hospital, Soweto, in 1959–1960. The 'liberalization' of the drinking laws, allowing black South Africans to drink bottled beer, was followed by a substantial decline in prevalence of the condition. However, dietary iron overload remains common in rural areas of much of southern Africa; for example, 21% of Zimbabwean men aged 45 years or more had high serum ferritins and transferrin saturation $>70\%$ in 1986, and the condition is reported in several countries of East and West Africa. It seems probable that a high dietary intake

is not the only factor but that it is interacting with an inborn error of metabolism in the causation of iron overload in Africa.

Once the hepatic iron is above $360\,\mu$mol/g dry weight, portal fibrosis and cirrhosis develop. Other complications include pancreatic fibrosis and diabetes mellitus, cardiac fibrosis and heart failure, chronic scurvy and osteoporosis. Patients have a history of beer consumption over years, hepatomegaly with or without ascites and hyperpigmentation. The diagnosis is confirmed by finding excessively high serum iron, transferrin saturation and ferritin, and excessive iron in a liver biopsy. Benefit is described from repeated venesections; chelating agents have had no extensive trials.

FOLIC ACID

Normal metabolism

The vitamin folic acid is not found naturally in the form of the core molecule pteroylglutamic acid (PGA), but as active folates, which are reduced, conjugated and condensed forms of PGA.[105–107] The enzyme dihydrofolate reductase, found in mammalian liver cells, reduces PGA to dihydro- and tetrahydrofolates. Folates are transported and absorbed as monoglutamates, but intracellularly are often conjugated to form polyglutamates. Folates are metabolically active when condensed with one-carbon radicals (e.g. methyl, methenyl, methylene, formyl); folates function as cofactors for the transfer of these one-carbon radicals in the synthesis of purines and pyrimidines (and hence nucleic acids) and in amino acid interconversions (e.g. histidine/glutamic acid, homocysteine/methionine and glycine/serine). Folate is essential for the conversion of uridine to thymidine required for DNA synthesis; therefore, folate is necessary for normal cell division, and tissues with rapid rates of cell division, for example bone marrow and gastrointestinal mucosa, have the highest requirements.

Folates are found in a wide variety of both animal and vegetable foods. Good sources include liver, green vegetables, tubers (e.g. yams, sweet potatoes), bananas and plantains, mangoes, fresh green and red peppers, locust beans, eggs, cheese and yeast products (e.g. bread and beer). Red meat and poultry are moderately good sources. Poor sources are grains (e.g. rice, maize, sorghum, millet), roots (e.g. cassava), non-green vegetables and distilled alcohols. Folates are heat labile and water soluble, so that prolonged cooking, reheating or boiling in large volumes of water greatly reduce the available folate.

Table 6.17 Daily dietary requirements for folates and vitamin B$_{12}$ (after ref. 7).

Nutrient	Group	Daily dietary requirement (μg)
Folate	0–6 months	40–50
	7–12 months	120
	1–12 years	200
	$\geq$ 13 years	400
	Pregnant women	800
	Lactating women	600
Vitamin B$_{12}$	0–12 months	0.3
	1–3 years	0.9
	4–9 years	1.5
	$\geq$ 10 years	2.0
	Pregnant women	3.0
	Lactating women	2.5

Polyglutamates are deconjugated and folates are absorbed actively as monoglutamates in the upper jejunum. Serum transport is as *N*-5-methyltetra-hydrofolate. Storage is mainly in the liver, and is normally sufficient to meet requirements for about 3 months only. Folate is excreted in bile, but most of this is reabsorbed. There is a small loss in urine; faeces are rich in folate, but this is derived from bacterial synthesis in the colon and is extraneous to the body's metabolism. Folate is consumed in intermediary metabolism: requirements are highest during growth, pregnancy and lactation (Table 6.17).

Folate deficiency

Aetiology

Despite folates being found in a wide range of commonly eaten foods, dietary deficiency is common, often related to food shortages, destruction by cooking or eating of inappropriate foods (Table 6.18).[7,11,100,105–107] In some communities of subsistence farmers, folate deficiency is seen most frequently at the end of the dry season and in the early rainy season before the new harvest. Sometimes all the folate-rich foods are cooked in a soup or relish added to the bulky staple; this may be cooked for several hours and reheated many times before being finished, so destroying most of the folate. Individuals with highest requirements, especially pregnant women and premature infants, are the most likely to be severely deficient.[23]

Malabsorption of folate results from tropical sprue and from acute or chronic intestinal infections (e.g. giardiasis), and may also complicate systemic infections, including acute pneumonias, tuberculosis and malaria.

Haemolysis leads to erythroid hyperplasia and high demands for folate: patients with severe chronic haemolytic anaemias (e.g. sickle cell disease, thalassaemia major, spherocytosis) are almost inevitably seriously deficient if untreated. Recurrent malaria in childhood leads to dyserythropoiesis but not folate deficiency; in contrast, the main pathology of malaria in partially immune pregnant women is haemolysis and an anaemia which is normochromic at first but can progress to a profound folate deficiency megaloblastic anaemia.[23]

Dihydrofolate reductase is inactive at 39°C: high or prolonged pyrexia can lead to acute megaloblastic arrest of erythropoiesis due to this block in folate metabolism. The 2,4-diaminopyrimidines (pyrimethamine and trimethoprim) are analogues of PGA and competitive inhibitors of dihydrofolate reductase. Their affinities for the enzymes of protozoa or bacteria are high and for the enzymes of mammals low, but overdosage can lead to severe disturbance of folate metabolism and megaloblastic anaemia. This has occurred in epidemics in China following the addition of pyrimethamine to table salt. Infants are liable to be overdosed, and individuals may overtreat themselves with antimalarial prophylactics (e.g. pyrimethamine daily instead of weekly), or with therapies containing pyrimethamine (e.g. Fansidar), or with simultaneous antimalarials and co-trimoxazole in high dose.

Aetiology is often multiple. In infancy and childhood, folate deficiency commonly complicates prematurity, feeding with boiled cows' milk or with goats' milk (which contains only folate unavailable for man), poor weaning foods, diarrhoea, repeated systemic infections, and haemoglobinopathies:[107] in West Africa, for example, about one-third of children with either PEM or moderate to severe anaemia are folate deficient. Factors leading to folate deficiency during pregnancy are commonly low intake, high demands from pregnancy especially multiple pregnancy, malarial haemolysis especially in primigravidae, pyrexia and haemoglobinopathies; folate deficiency is a major aetiological factor in severe anaemias in pregnancy in around three-quarters of West African patients and two-thirds of Indian patients.[23,105] In southern Africa women present commonly about 6 months post partum with megaloblastic anaemia due to a low intake of folate from a maize-based diet not meeting the high demands of repeated pregnancies and prolonged lactation.

Clinical

Patients with folate deficiency present with the symptoms and signs of anaemia. They have an increased susceptibility to infection related to

Table 6.18 Some causes of folate and vitamin B_{12} deficiencies.

	Folate	Vitamin B_{12}
Inadequate intake	Boiling of bottle feeds	Breast feeding by B_{12} deficient women
	Goats' milk feeding of infants	
	Inappropriate weaning foods	Veganism
	Anorexia (recurrent infection, old age)	
	Seasonal shortage (end of dry season)	
	Prolonged cooking/reheating	
	Prolonged storage of food	
	Famine	
	Taboos and food fads	
	Alcoholism	
Malabsorption	Diarrhoea in infancy	Pernicious anaemia
	Acute enteric infections	Gastrectomy
	Giardia lamblia	Chronic Giardia lamblia
	Ileocaecal tuberculosis	HIV infection
	Systemic infections (pneumonia, tuberculosis)	Diphyllobothrium latum
	Coeliac disease	Stagnant loop syndrome
	Tropical sprue (acute)	Tropical sprue (chronic) (Chapter 3)
	Crohn's disease	Crohn's disease
High physiological demands	Growth (prematurity, infancy, adolescence)	
	Pregnancy	(Pregnancy)
	Lactation	
Pathologically high demands	Haemolysis (sickle cell, thalassaemia, etc.; recurrent malaria)	
	Malignant disease (Burkitt's, choriocarcinoma)	
Disturbed metabolism	Pyrexia	Nitrous oxide
	Overdosage of antagonists (pyrimethamine, trimethoprim)	Chronic cyanide intoxication (cassava)

neutropenia and immune deficiency. Rarely, there is a history of purpura or menorrhagia associated with thrombocytopenia. Mild splenomegaly is not unusual. Patients may have depression of mood and mental alertness, but not the major neurological signs of vitamin B_{12} deficiency. Long-standing folate deficiency can cause hyperpigmentation of the skin, but this is not so obvious as with vitamin B_{12} deficiency. Changes in the intestinal tract are glossitis, angular cheilosis, mild malabsorption and delayed regeneration of liver cells. Chronic deficiency causes sterility in both sexes and retarded growth and development in childhood, for example in patients with sickle cell disease. Folate deficiency in early pregnancy has an association with neural tube defects in the infants, and in later pregnancy with premature delivery.

Haematology

Anaemia varies in severity but may be profound. The MCV and MCH are raised, but the MCHC is normal. The reticulocyte count is high if the underlying cause is haemolysis, but otherwise is normal or low. The red cells show anisocytosis and macrocytosis; there is a tendency to oval forms, but poikilocytosis is unusual unless the anaemia is long-standing; cells are normochromic; there is polychromasia, punctate basophilia occasionally, nucleated cells (which may be obvious megaloblasts) and Howell–Jolly bodies (Figure 6.18a). Macrocytosis and raised MCV may not be apparent in patients who have concomitant iron deficiency or α thalassaemia. The total WBC and neutrophil counts are usually low, with hypersegmented neutrophils in the peripheral blood (Figure 6.18b); however, with complicating infections, as are common in the tropics, there may be leukaemoid reactions, with excessively high total WBC and neutrophil counts, showing a shift to the left as far as the promyelocytes or even blasts, and numerous giant metamyelocytes. The platelet count is moderately reduced commonly, but sometimes severely. Bone marrow aspirates reveal megaloblastic haemopoiesis (Figure 6.19); iron stores tend to be raised due to immobilization, but in patients with dual deficiencies, megaloblastic changes can be masked and iron absent from the marrow. Serum lactate dehydrogenase

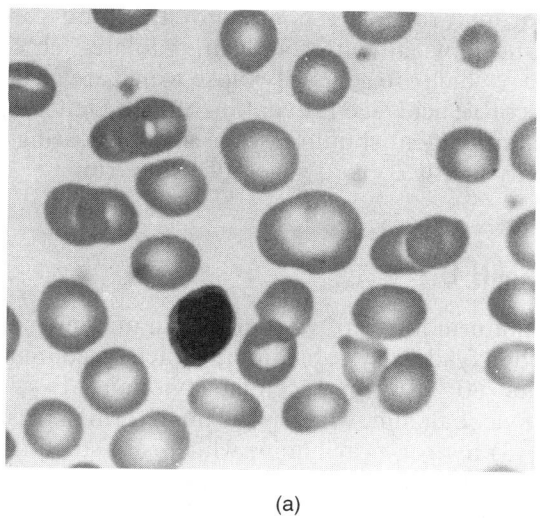

(a)

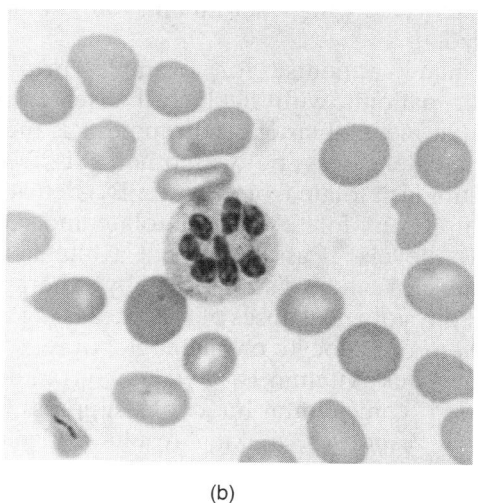

(b)

Figure 6.18 Peripheral blood films. (a) Macrocytic megaloblastic anaemia. Red cells show variation of size (anisocytosis) and large cells (macrocytes), some of which are oval. (b) Hypersegmented neutrophil of a patient with dietary vitamin B_{12} deficiency.

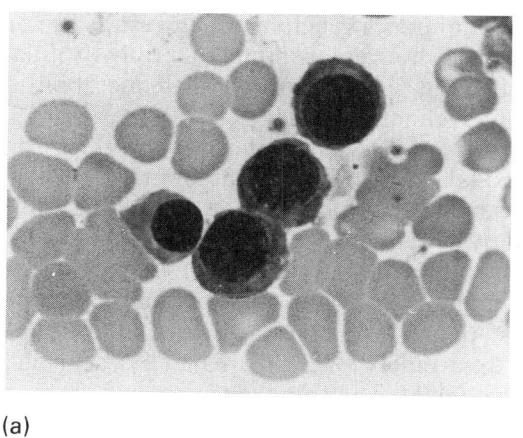

(a)

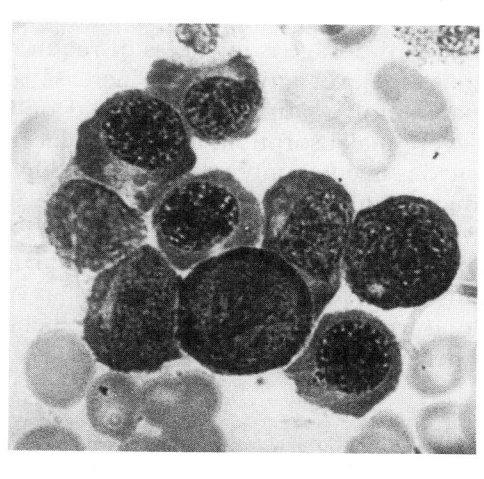

(b)

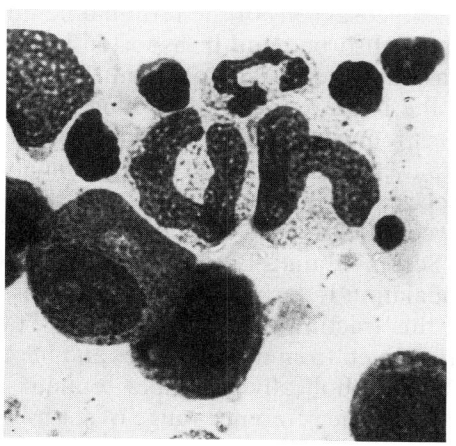

(c)

Figure 6.19 Bone marrow. (a) Normoblastic erythroid hyperplasia from a patient with haemolytic anaemia, to show the normal stages of maturation of erythroblasts. (b) Megaloblastic bone marrow: the erythroblasts are large; the nuclei are grainy (deficient in chromatin); the nuclei remain immature whereas the cytoplasm continues to develop (nuclear–cytoplasmic dissociation); there are bizarre-shaped nuclei and Howell–Jolly bodies; there is a high proportion of early forms which do not develop to late forms, but suffer intramedullary destruction. (c) Giant metamyelocytes: these are about twice the size of normal metamyelocytes and characteristic of megaloblastic bone marrows, but may be seen also with dyserythropoiesis (e.g. malaria) or following cytotoxic therapy.

levels are extremely high; serum bilirubin is moderately raised.

With many patients, for example pregnant women or patients with sickle cell disease, it is obvious that megaloblastic erythropoiesis is the result of folate deficiency, but with others it is necessary to distinguish folate from vitamin B_{12} deficiency by assaying serum folate, red cell folate and serum vitamin B_{12} levels. If assays are not available, the two deficiencies can be distinguished by a therapeutic trial of physiological doses of folic acid 50 μg/day: if there is no reticulocyte or haemoglobin response within one week, vitamin B_{12} 1 μg/day intramuscularly is tried; coincidental infections suppress haematological responses, making results difficult to interpret.

Treatment

Folic acid 5 mg/day is followed by a reticulocyte response after about 5 days, and the slow restoration of normal haematology; treatment for 3 weeks is sufficient to replace the body stores but should be continued if there are ongoing high demands or malabsorption. This dosage is in excess of requirements and there is never any need to increase to 15 mg/day; parenteral treatment is indicated only rarely with severe malabsorption, and the reduced form folinic acid is needed only to counteract dihydrofolate reductase inhibitors.

Patients with a megaloblastic anaemia can be treated initially with both folic acid and vitamin B_{12} while awaiting the results of vitamin assays, provided all blood and marrow samples have been collected for necessary investigations.

Prevention

The same three strategies of supplementation, fortification of food and dietary modification apply as in the prevention of iron deficiency.

Premature infants should be given supplements of 50 μg/day. Infants with diarrhoea should receive 50 μg in addition. Deficiency in pregnancy is prevented with the combined iron (60 mg) and folic acid (250 μg) tablets twice a day. Preconceptional supplements of folic acid are required to prevent recurrence of neural tube defects. Patients with chronic haemolytic anaemias (e.g. thalassaemia, sickle cell disease, congenital spherocytosis) are generally given folic acid 5 mg/day, this large dose being the pharmaceutical preparation usually available.

For populations with high frequencies of nutritional deficiency there is a strong case for the fortification of the staple with folic acid, for example maize flour in southern Africa; however, this has not yet been enforced.

The natural folate content of the food can be enhanced by cultivating and eating folate-rich vegetables, which are generally those which are also rich in ascorbic acid (see Prevention of Iron Deficiency). Encouragement should also be given to eating raw or only lightly cooked vegetables and fruit.

VITAMIN B_{12}

The natural forms of vitamin B_{12} in mammals are : (1) deoxyadenosylcobalamin, which accounts for about 80% of intracellular vitamin B_{12}; (2) methylcobalamin, which is the main form in plasma; and (3) hydroxycobalamin, which is in small quantities both intracellularly and extracellularly.[106,108] Cyanocobalamin occurs naturally in trace amounts only, but is stable and so finds diagnostic and therapeutic applications. There are only three biochemical reactions known to involve vitamin B_{12} in man: (1) the isomerization of methylmalonyl CoA to succinylCoA; (2) the isomerization of α-leucine to β-leucine; (3) the methylation of homocysteine to methionine, a reaction which results in conversion of methyltetrahydrofolate to tetrahydrofolate. Vitamin B_{12} is vital for normal folate metabolism and for the myelination of nerve fibres.

Vitamin B_{12} is synthesized by micro-organisms and is available to man in animal foods, especially liver, and animal products, including milk and its derivatives and eggs. Vitamin B_{12} is not found in vegetables: it is available, however, from faecally contaminated water, and this source is important in the poorest vegetarian societies.[105] Requirements are extremely low, and are met by very small intakes of animal food (Table 6.17).

Vitamin B_{12} is released from food in the stomach, and then bound to intrinsic factor (IF), a glycoprotein secreted by parietal cells. The IF–B_{12} complex is adsorbed by means of a specific receptor on to the mucosal cells of the terminal ileum; the vitamin B_{12} is absorbed and transported to the liver by the plasma protein transcobalamin II. Storage, mainly in the liver, amounts to 3–5 mg and is sufficient to meet requirements for 3–4 years. There is an enterohepatic circulation: there is a minimal loss in urine; faeces are rich in vitamin B_{12}, but this is synthesized by colonic bacteria and not absorbed.

Serum vitamin B_{12} is bound about 80% to transcobalamin I, derived from neutrophils; the function of this fraction is not understood. Transcobalamin II, derived from macrophages and hepatocytes, carries metabolically available vitamin B_{12} between tissues. The reference range of serum vitamin B_{12} is usually given as 150–900 ng/l, but higher levels are not uncommonly associated with PEM, hepatic disease, granulocytic proliferation and a genetically determined higher transcobalamin II binding capacity in Blacks.

Vitamin B₁₂ deficiency

Aetiology

Vitamin B_{12} deficiency can be the result of (1) inadequate intake, (2) malabsorption due to a failure of IF secretion by gastric parietal cells, (3) disease of the ileum, (4) competition by the fish tapeworm, *Diphyllobothrium latum*, and (5) disturbed metabolism (Table 6.18).[105,106,108] Demands are raised during pregnancy and lactation (Table 6.17), but this precipitates overt deficiency only in those whose status was marginal before pregnancy.

Dietary inadequacy. The requirements for vitamin B_{12} are so low that nutritional deficiency is rare. It is seen most commonly in infants born to and breast fed by women who are vitamin B_{12}-deficient; the disorder occurs predominantly in Indians whose mothers have tropical sprue and/or inadequate nutrition, but can result from maternal pernicious anaemia.

Strictly vegan diets, which exclude all animal products such as milk and eggs, contain inadequate vitamin B_{12} and deficiency occurs in some impoverished Indian Hindu populations and other vegans such as Rastafarians. Indian immigrants in the UK seem to be at an increased risk of deficiency, possibly because there is less bacterial contamination of water and food. Severe vitamin B_{12} deficiency has been described in long-term prisoners of oppressive governments.

Malabsorption. Classical addisonian pernicious anaemia, due to lack of IF secretion, is relatively uncommon in Africa, India and South-East Asia;[105] however, it occurs often in Blacks in non-tropical South Africa, and is being seen with increasing frequency in the tropics in elite groups, for example in Nigeria.[109]

Sprue is the most common cause of malabsorption, probably as a result of interfering with adsorption of IF–B_{12} by ileal mucosal cells. Subnormal serum vitamin B_{12} is reported in 23% of patients infected by HIV, even in the early stages of the disease.[110] The fish tapeworm is a rare cause of deficiency, even where the infestation is common.

Disturbed metabolism. The peel of the roots of cassava contains linamarin, a cyanogenic glycoside from which is released hydrocyanic acid.[111] Cassava is usually prepared by peeling, washing and drying in the sun; this destroys the source of cyanide through fermentation. Chronic cyanide intoxication can follow drought, for example in Mozambique, when the linamarin content is excessively high, or from imperfect preparation, for example in refugees during the Nigerian civil war. Patients suffer from chronic cyanide intoxication, leading to tropical amblyopia. Urinary thiocyanate excretion is high, serum cyanocobalamin is raised but total serum vitamin B_{12} is low. Tobacco amblyopia has a similar pathogenesis.

Exposure to nitrous oxide for 5–6 days or recurrent exposure induces megaloblastic anaemia through the oxidation of cobalamins to inactive forms.

Clinical

Vitamin B_{12} deficiency has the same haematological and systemic consequences as folate deficiency. In addition, the course can be complicated by peripheral neuropathy, optic atrophy, psychiatric disturbances and subacute combined degeneration of the cord, characterized by demyelination in the lateral and posterior columns. A common clinical finding is melanin hyperpigmentation, especially of palms, soles and across the small joints of the hands and feet.[105]

Neonatal deficiency, as seen in Indian infants, shows as a failure of normal development, involuntary movements, loss of muscle tone, pallor and hyperpigmentation of skin and mucous membranes; untreated the condition can progress to coma and death.[105]

Haematology

The peripheral blood and bone marrow findings are identical with those of folate deficiency, except that as vitamin B_{12} deficiency is likely to be more long standing, there tends to be more poikilocytosis and thrombocytopenia. Diagnosis is confirmed by the serum vitamin B_{12} level being well below the reference range. Malabsorption is diagnosed by measuring the absorption of radioactive vitamin B_{12} (the Schilling test): malabsorption will *not* be corrected by the addition of IF when the lesion is intestinal. The deoxyuridine (dU) suppression test is abnormal, except with nutritional deficiency of vitamin B_{12}.

Treatment

Normal stores are restored with hydroxycobalamin $1000\,\mu g$ intramuscularly, six times over 1–2 weeks: thereafter, $1000\,\mu g$ is given every 3 months to all patients with permanent malabsorption. Vegans may be treated orally, or be encouraged to eat some vitamin B_{12} containing food. Infants should receive $0.1\,\mu g$ per day orally, and the deficient mothers treated at the same time.

Cyanocobalamin is still used in some developing countries but is not as satisfactory because maintenance doses have to be given monthly, and it is useless in the treatment of cyanide intoxication.

OTHER DEFICIENCIES

Protein–energy malnutrition

PEM is a serious cause of disease, but not of anaemia. Anaemia is usually moderate (Hb 80–90 g/l), normocytic and normochromic, although the MCV may be slightly elevated.[112] The reticulocyte count is low and the marrow shows a normoblastic erythroid hypoplasia. Erythropoietin levels are increased appropriately for the degree of anaemia but there is an impaired response by erythroid precursors. Red cell survival may be moderately shortened, especially in kwashiorkor. Anaemia is more severe when there is concomitant infection related to impaired cell mediated immunity, and deficiencies of iron and folate, as occur commonly.

Vitamin C deficiency

Severe scurvy is associated with normochromic normocytic anaemia.[112] Vitamin C deficient diets are certainly deficient in folate and bioavailable iron as well, and anaemia of multiple deficiencies is usual.

Vitamin E deficiency

Premature infants bottle fed with milk rich in polyunsaturated fatty acids, deficient in vitamin E and supplemented with iron develop a haemolytic anaemia due to oxidation of the red cell membrane.

Pyridoxine deficiency

Naturally occurring pyridoxine deficiency is rare, but administration of pyridoxine antagonists, such as cycloserine and pyrazinamide, causes a failure of incorporation of iron into haemoglobin and sideroblastic anaemia.[112]

Riboflavin deficiency

Patients are reported to develop normocytic, normochromic anaemias with erythroid hypoplasia.[112]

Copper deficiency

Premature infants and infants or children with severe chronic diarrhoea and malnutrition may become deficient of copper.[112] There is anaemia and severe neutropenia. The marrow shows vacuolated erythroid cells, megaloblasts and ringed sideroblasts; myeloid cells are also vacuolated and have an arrest of maturation at the myelocyte stage.

ANAEMIAS DUE TO MARROW DEPRESSION

Acute infections

Any acute infection may result in a temporary depression of erythropoiesis, which generally goes unnoticed. Significant anaemia results if the patient is dependent on a rapid rate of erythropoiesis (e.g. sickle cell disease) or if the infection causes haemolysis as well; mechanisms of haemolysis may be: (1) specific to the infection (e.g. malaria, the lecithinases of *Clostridria*); (2) DIC and microangiopathic haemolysis following septicaemias or viraemias; (3) immune, for example complicating infection by *Mycoplasma pneumoniae*; or (4) idiosyncracies of the patient, for example G6PD deficiency.

Anaemia of chronic disorders

With chronic infections, and also malignant disease and some collagen diseases (e.g. rheumatoid arthritis), anaemia can progress over weeks to reach a constant state known as the *anaemia of chronic disorders*.[113] There are at least four mechanisms. (1) Iron is sequestrated into the RES; possibly this is mediated at sites of inflammation through the release from granulocytes of lactoferrin, a protein with a high affinity for iron and for which there is a specific receptor on macrophages. (2) There is moderate reduction of red cell life span. (3) There is a depression of production of erythropoietin. (4) There are factors which depress erythropoiesis.

The anaemia is usually moderate (Hb >80 g/l haematocrit >0.30) and normocytic, but may progress to being hypochromic and rarely microcytic. The plasma iron is reduced ($<12\,\mu mol/l$), plasma transferrin is low (unlike iron deficiency) and the saturation of transferrin is low (15–25%) but generally higher than in iron deficiency; serum ferritin is raised ($>200\,\mu g/l$) (unlike iron deficiency). In the bone marrow, iron is seen in increased quantities in the macrophages (unlike iron deficiency), but the number of siderocytic granules in normoblasts (sideroblasts) is low; erythropoiesis is normoblastic with occasional mild dyserythropoietic changes; there tends to be granulocytic hyperplasia and often an obvious increase in the number of plasma cells.

The haematological complications of three infections, tuberculosis, HIV and parvovirus B19, need to be discussed in detail because they show certain features and because of their public health importance. The anaemias of protozoal and helminthic infections have already been discussed.

Tuberculosis (See also Chapter 57)

Approximately one-third of the world's population is infected by *Mycobacterium tuberculosis*.[114] In the developing countries the majority of infected individuals are under 50 years of age. It is estimated that 8 million develop tuberculosis each year, of whom more than 4.5 million are in Asia, including China; 2.6–2.9 million die each year. The highest incidence (220/100 000 per year) was in sub-Saharan Africa, and this has now risen further by about 20% to 265/100 000 per year, due to the pandemic of HIV. It is predicted that during the next decade the incidence of tuberculosis will continue to rise in Africa, and as it seems inevitable that the incidence of HIV infections in Asia will overtake that of Africa, the impact of AIDS on tuberculosis in Asia will be catastrophic.

Tuberculosis is one of the most common causes of anaemia in adult males and non-pregnant females in the developing world, probably the most common cause amongst adults requiring hospital care, and in some communities, for example in southern Africa, the most common underlying disease leading to the need to administer blood transfusions in the management of anaemia.[115]

The major mechanism is the anaemia of chronic disorders: anaemia is more common and tends to be more severe in patients with extrapulmonary and disseminated disease. Patients, especially vegetarians, are frequently undernourished, with specific deficiencies of vitamin B_{12}, folate, iron and protein, both as predisposing factors through impairment of cell-mediated immunity and as complications of tuberculosis through anorexia and malabsorption, especially with abdominal tuberculosis. Metastatic fibrocaseous granulomas in the bone marrow give rise to a leucoerythroblastic picture and severe anaemia.

Abnormalities of the white cells are most pronounced with disseminated non-reactive miliary tuberculosis. These include: a neutrophil leucocytosis with a shift to the left and toxic granulation, and

this may amount to a leukaemoid reaction; eosinophilic reactions, which are likely to reflect coincidental helminthic infections; increased basophils, which are suggestive of an underlying myeloproliferative disease; monocytosis and lymphocytosis. Many patients have reactive thrombocytosis, sometimes exceeding $1000 \times 10^9/l$. Other patients have neutropenia, lymphopenia or thrombocytopenia due to inhibition of production related to tuberculosis, hypersplenism of tuberculous splenomegaly, or HIV infection.

The bone marrow is commonly normoblastic but may show micronormoblastic, dyserythropoietic or megaloblastic features; granulocytic and megakaryocytic hyperplasia and plasma cell excess are usual; there is an excess of iron in the macrophages unless the patient is iron deficient. Some patients may show hypoplasia of one or more cell lines, associated with severe anaemia, neutropenia and thrombocytopenia.

The various therapeutic agents used in the management of tuberculosis can lead to haematological complications. These include: (1) the sideroblastic anaemia of pyridoxine inhibitors (isoniazid, pyrazinamide, cycloserine); (2) hypoplasia or aplasia of one or more of the cell lines; (3) disturbances of folate or vitamin B_{12} metabolism; and (4) immune haemolysis.[115]

Immune deficiency states predispose to the reactivation of latent tuberculosis. For many years it has been known that tuberculosis is associated with lymphomas, leukaemias (especially chronic myeloid leukaemia), the myeloproliferative diseases and aplastic anaemia. Currently in Africa, one-third of patients presenting with AIDS have active tuberculosis; where the HIV epidemic is mature, up to 60% of all patients newly diagnosed as having pulmonary tuberculosis and a higher proportion with extrapulmonary tuberculosis are anti-HIV seropositive.

Human immunodeficiency virus (See also Chapter 12)

It is estimated that more than 18 million adults and 1.5 million children had been infected by HIV by the end of 1994.[116] Of these, 11 million were in Africa, three million in Asia, two million in the Caribbean and Latin America, one million in North America and half a million in Western Europe. It is predicted that by the year 2000, a total of at least 30–40 million men, women and children will have been infected. The greatest increase in numbers is likely to be in Asia. Up to 1995, over 4.5 million adults and children have progressed to AIDS.

Peaks of frequency of AIDS in Africa are in women aged 20–24 years, men aged 25–35 years and infancy or early childhood. AIDS must now be considered in the differential diagnosis of anaemia in these age groups. HIV-infected subjects may present with anaemia, for example in pregnancy. Anaemia becomes increasingly frequent as HIV disease progresses, until 70–95% of patients with full-blown AIDS are anaemic.[117] The major mechanism is the anaemia of chronic disorders, but other factors include direct depression of erythropoiesis by HIV, focal or diffuse fibrosis or serous fatty atrophy of the marrow cavity. Coinfections with parvovirus B19, *L. donovani* and perhaps other organisms cause severe red cell hypoplasia. Up to 23% of patients have subnormal vitamin B_{12}. Autoimmune haemolysis is rare, although up to 20% have positive direct Coombs' tests.

About half of patients with AIDS have neutropenia; lymphopenia is central to the pathology of the disease. Peripheral blood films may show hyposegmented neutrophils, activated plasmacytoid lymphocytes and vacuolated monocytes.

Thrombocytopenia increases in frequency from around 12% in the early to 70% in the later stages of disease. It is immune mediated, but there appears to be decreased production in some patients.

Bone marrows show the features of anaemia of chronic disorders. Erythropoiesis is of variable activity from hypo- to hyperplastic; dyserythropoiesis is common. Occasional patients have megaloblastic erythropoiesis, one not uncommon cause being self-medication and overdosage with trimethroprim. Erythrophagocytosis by macrophages is seen commonly. There is patchy lymphocytosis, and sometimes considerable plasmacytosis, which may be mistaken for myeloma. Iron stores may be raised, especially in African men who habitually drink home-brewed beer.

Children with AIDS have similar changes, but macrocytosis and lymphocytosis appear to be more frequent.

Parvovirus B19

Parvovirus B19 is a single stranded DNA virus which is common and distributed worldwide.[73,118] Transmission is by respiratory droplets, but also transplacentally and by exchange of blood. In tropical countries children are usually infected in the first 2 years of life, and protective antibodies are present in about 90% of adults. Between 7 and 10 days after infection there is a transient viraemia for not more than 2 weeks; this may be symptomless in up to 30%, or be accompanied by 'flu-like symptoms, or cause self-limiting erythema infectiosum (fifth disease) after 1 week, or in adults arthritis or arthralgia; vascular purpura is a rare complication.

The virus has a tropism for pronormoblasts: during viraemia there is an absence of reticulocytes, a great reduction of erythroid progenitors and the presence of giant pronormoblasts in the bone marrow. In subjects with previously normal erythropoiesis and normal immunocompetence there is only a transient depression of erythropoiesis coinciding with the viraemia, but this is tolerated and usually unnoticed. There are three situations in which parvovirus B19 has serious consequences: pregnancy, haemolytic anaemias and immune deficiency.

When parvovirus B19 infection is acquired for the first time during the first half of pregnancy, there is transplacental transmission which can cause spontaneous abortion or hydrops foetalis, increasing by 20 times the risk of fetal wastage.

Patients with a short red cell life are dependent on a compensatory rapid rate of erythropoiesis and suffer from 'aplastic crises' when infected by parvovirus B19; morbidity and mortality rates are high. This was described first with sickle cell disease but has been observed with thalassaemia, spherocytosis, enzymopathies and acquired haemolytic anaemias. It has been suggested that concomitant infection with parvovirus B19 could be a cause of severe anaemia and death in children with malaria.[119]

Parvovirus B19 viraemia can persist in patients who are immunocompromised, including those with leukaemias, lymphomas and HIV disease. There is severe chronic anaemia due to erythroid hypoplasia; occasionally there is also neutropenia and thrombocytopenia. It is certain that parvovirus B19 infections are occurring frequently in infants and young children already infected transplacentally with HIV, and it is probable that this is a common cause of profound anaemia in Africa and elsewhere.

During epidemics of parvovirus B19, susceptible subjects, such as patients with sickle cell disease and non-immune pregnant women, can be protected with intravenous normal immunoglobulin. Immunoglobulin therapy is curative of persistent viraemia and chronic anaemia in immunocompromised patients, but failures have been reported with AIDS. Vaccines are being developed.

Aplastic anaemia

Aplastic anaemia is a rare condition. The annual incidence is $2–3/10^6$ in the Western world, with peaks at 10–24 years and in old age, and a male predominance. The annual incidence is higher in young adults 15–24 years of age in Thailand (7.2 × 10^6), with a male predominance; this high incidence is probably to be found also in Japan and other Far Eastern countries, for unknown reasons.[120] No cause is found in the majority of patients, but in some exposures to antibiotics (e.g. chloramphenicol), non-steroidal anti-inflammatory drugs (e.g. indomethacin, butazones), paint, benzene and irradiation have proven aetiological associations. The easy availability of potent pharmaceuticals without prescription, and the constant exposure to benzene of unofficial vendors of petrol and sweatshop factory workers are serious, if unmeasured, risk factors in developing countries.[121] The role of hepatitis and other viruses remains unclear.

Aplastic anaemia is described fully in standard texts and recent reviews.[122]

Alcoholism

Excessive consumption of alcohol is a large and growing social and health problem in tropical communities whose traditional ways of life have been disrupted. The haematological consequences are anaemia, macrocytosis, vacuolation of the normoblasts and excess sideroblasts, as a direct result of the toxicity of alcohol on early red cell precursors (CFU-E and BFU-E). Thrombocytopenia is common, but leucopenia is unusual. Other results of alcoholism include malnutrition leading to folate deficiency and megaloblastic anaemia, and haemosiderosis (see Iron Overload). Hepatic failure can be complicated by hypoprothrombinaemia (see below).

DISORDERS OF WHITE CELLS

The peripheral blood white cell counts of healthy individuals (see Tables 6.4, 6.5 and Figure 6.2) and the causes of reactive leucocytosis (see Table 6.6) have been discussed under References Ranges.

LEUCOPENIA

The number of circulating WBCs may be abnormally low as a result of failure of production, inhibition of release, increased margination in the circulation, pooling in an enlarged spleen or excessive consumption, and there is often a combination of these factors in one patient. Both neutropenia and lymphopenia are common in the tropics, usually as the direct or indirect results of infections (Table 6.19).

LYMPHOMAS AND PARAPROTEINAEMIAS

Only the epidemiological and possible aetiological factors in the tropics will be discussed; lymphomas are described in detail in Chapter 11 and in standard texts.

Burkitt's lymphoma (See also Chapter 32)

The highest age-specific incidence of cancers (all types) in childhood has been reported from tropical Africa; there is a peak of incidence between the ages of 5 and 9 years, more marked in boys than girls and predominantly due to Burkitt's lymphoma (BL) (Figure 6.20).[123] There are three epidemiological patterns: (1) BL is *endemic* in tropical Africa and Papua New Guinea, where annual incidence is 8–12/100 000, with a peak at 4–9 years of age; (2) *intermediate* incidence of 1–2/100 000 per year is found in North Africa, western Asia and South America; (iii) BL occurs *sporadically*, <0.1/100 000 per year, in the Western world.

Table 6.19 Some causes of leucopenia in the tropics.

Neutropenia: <2.0 × 10^9/l
  Acute malaria
  Viral infections in early stages
  AIDS
  Typhoid
  Brucellosis
  Overwhelming bacterial infections
  Megaloblastosis
  Hypersplenism
  Bone marrow infiltration (e.g. leukaemia)
  Exposure to chemicals (e.g. benzene)
  Idiosyncratic reactions to drugs
  Cytotoxic therapy
  Aplastic anaemia
  Felty's syndrome
  Miscellaneous (racial, familial, cyclic, chronic,
    idiopathic)
Lymphopenia: <1.5 × 10^9/l
  Viral infections in prodromal stages
  AIDS
  Corticosteroids
  Lymphoma
  Acute leukaemias

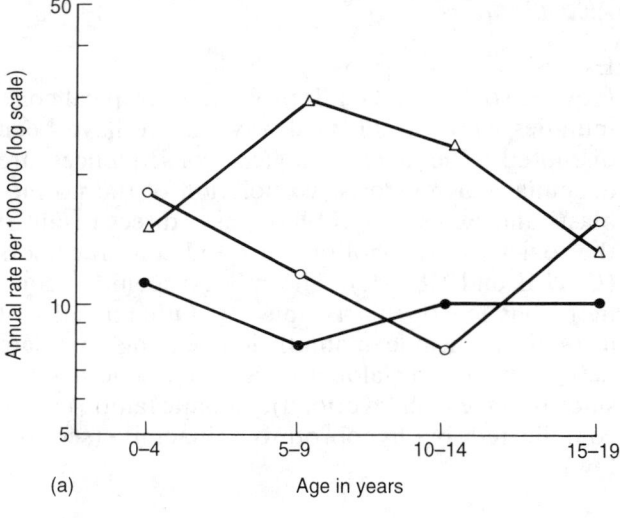

(a)

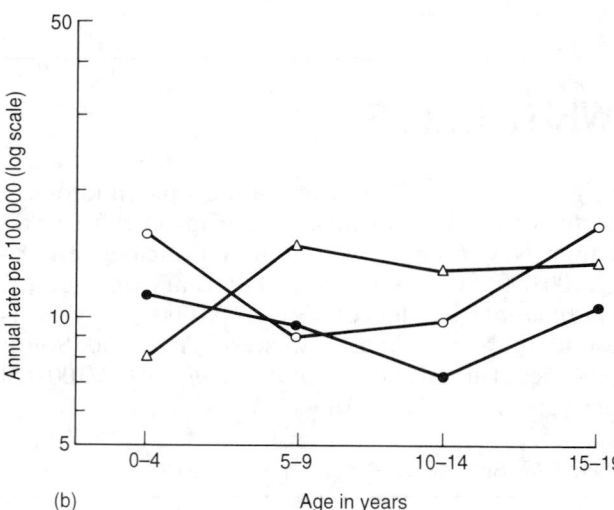

(b)

Figure 6.20   Age-specific incidence of childhood cancer (all types) in (a) males and (b) females in US whites (○) and blacks (●) (Michigan) and Nigerians (△) (Ibadan). (From data in ref. 123.)

The causation of endemic BL may be summarized: the majority of children in developing countries are infected by the Epstein–Barr virus (EBV) before the age of 1 year; infection by EBV immortalizes B cells, resulting in their proliferation; where *P. falciparum* is endemic, recurrent infections suppress T-cell regulation of B-cell proliferation, and also stimulates antigenically and mitogenically further B-cell proliferation; somatic mutations are more probable the larger is the polyclonal pool of proliferating B cells; one such mutation is a translocation involving chromosome 8 at the site of the c-*myc* proto-oncogene, with its juxtaposition to an immunoglobulin heavy chain gene sequence on chromosome 14; BL is the result of the monoclonal proliferation of cells with t8:14 in 85% of cases, or in the minority of cases the juxtaposition of the

chromosome 8 c-*myc* to immunoglobin $\varkappa$ or λ light chain sequences on chromosomes 2 and 22 respectively.[124] In areas of intermediate endemicity there are high rates of EBV transmission in early childhood, but no or low malaria transmission. Less than 20% of sporadic cases of BL are associated with EBV.

BL also results as a complication of AIDS, but this has been observed only rarely in Africa, possibly because lymphomas are late complications in long survivors, and most African patients with AIDS do not receive management which prolongs life.

Hodgkin's disease

There are four histological types of Hodgkin's disease (HD): nodular sclerosing (NS), mixed cellularity (MC), lymphocyte depleted (LD) and lymphocyte predominant (LP). The last form, LP, may be a distinct and separate entity. HD is not common, having a crude annual incidence of 2.4–3.0/100 000 in North America and Western Europe; overall, the male to female ratio is 1:1.5. There are four epidemiological patterns. Pattern I: there are high incidences (or relative frequencies) of HD in childhood in Central and South America, North Africa, western Asia and sub-Saharan Africa; there is a predominance of MC and LD, which carry poor prognoses.[125] Pattern III: in the developed countries, there is a peak of incidence in young adults (20–34 years), in whom NS is the predominant type; a second peak of HD in middle age has been described in the past, but this may have been due to overdiagnosis. Pattern II: this is intermediate between patterns I and III, and is found in rural areas of developed countries, including Eastern Europe and southern USA. Pattern IV: HD has a low incidence in eastern Asia.[126,127]

EBV genomes are expressed by the malignant Reed–Sternberg cells from a high proportion (50–70%) of HD patients aged under 15 or over 50 years, and it is most probable that EBV plays an aetiological role in these patients. In contrast, EBV genome positivity is rare in patients aged 15–34 years and with NS, suggesting a different aetiology.[126] HIV-infected persons appear to be at greater risk of developing HD.

Non-Hodgkin's, non-Burkitt's lymphomas

The remaining lymphomas, excluding BL and HD, are a heterogeneous group of tumours of B-cell and T-cell origin, the classification of which is complex and not wholly agreed. The combined incidence of all non-Hodgkin's lymphomas (NHLs) generally exceeds the incidence of HD, for example 4.9/100 000 per year for males and 4.1/100 000 per year for females in England and Wales; incidence rises with age to peak at 55–74 years.

In the developed countries, follicle centre cell lymphomas with follicular pattern are the most common NHL, with increasing incidence with age. About 75% have a translocation of chromosomes 14 and 18, juxtaposing the immunoglobulin heavy chain locus and the *bcl*-2 putative proto-oncogene. In contrast, these low or intermediate grade tumours are relatively rare in developing countries.[124] High grade NHLs have higher frequencies in Asia and Africa, and a strong association has been reported in Africa between frequency of high grade NHLs and malarial endemicity.[128,129]

Immunoproliferative small intestinal disease

This is a condition which occurs at high incidence in children and young adults in North Africa, western Asia, eastern Asia and sub-Saharan Africa. Sporadic cases have been reported in South, Central and North America, and Europe. It is associated with low socioeconomic status and recurrent or chronic enteric infections. Prolonged antigenic stimulation of intestinal lymphoid tissues and a genetic predisposition are proposed mechanisms.[124,130] In its premalignant phase, there is steatorrhoea, malabsorption and weight loss; histologically there is a lymphoproliferation and plasma cell infiltration of the small bowel mucosa and mesenteric lymph glands. The proliferating cells are IgA-producing B cells, which synthesize defective immunoglobulin α heavy chains (α heavy chain disease). The condition responds at this stage to ampicillin, metronidazole and antihelminthic agents, followed by long-term tetracycline. Untreated, the condition may progress to a high-grade malignant lymphoma of large cell immunoblastic plasmacytoid type. The annual incidence of intestinal lymphoma used to be as high as $4.8/10^6$ in Israel, but this has now dropped; the male to female ratio is around 2:1. The anaemia of chronic disorders is usual and is complicated in about 40% of patients by malabsorption of iron, folate or vitamin B_{12}.

Adult T-cell leukaemia/lymphoma

Epidemiology

The human T-cell lymphotropic virus type 1 (HTLV-1) is a type C retrovirus which is causative of adult T-cell leukaemia/lymphoma (ATL) and tropical spastic paraparesis/HTLV-1 associated myelopathy (TSP/HAM) in a small number of infected

individuals.[117] HTLV-1 is transmitted by sexual intercourse, through breast feeding and by the exchange of blood. Male to female transmission is more efficient than female to male, and is enhanced by other concomitant sexually transmitted diseases: female prostitutes have higher seroprevalence than the general population. Unidentified receptors for HTLV-1 are on surfaces of CD^{4+} T cells, CD^{8+} T cells and monocyte-derived cells. After invasion of cells and transcription, proviral DNA is integrated into the DNA of host cells.

HTLV-1 is endemic in populations of Asia, Africa, the Americas, Australasia and Oceania. Seroprevalence is high (about 10%) in south-west Japan, especially on Kyusha and Shikoku islands. HTLV-1-associated ATL is encountered sporadically in other parts of Japan and on Taiwan, and only occasionally in other Asian countries.[129] The largest pool of the virus is in sub-Saharan Africa, where there are probably about ten million infected subjects. The highest rates of seropositivity (about 10%) are reported from Gabon and southern Cameroon; prevalence declines northwards into the savanna and sahel. In West Africa seroprevalence is 3–6% in the savanna of Nigeria and Benin; rates are lower in coastal areas and further west as far as Senegal. HTLV-1 has low endemicity (about 1%) in populations of eastern and southern Africa, except in the Seychelles, where overall frequency is 6.2%. The virus is also endemic in populations of African descent in the Caribbean, Central America, southern USA and Britain (e.g. 3–6% amongst Jamaican adults). Clusters have been reported amongst Iranian Jews, Iraqis, Georgians of the Caucasus, Australian Aborigines and the inhabitants of Papua New Guinea and the Solomon Islands. Seroprevalence rises slowly with age, compatible with the slow rate of transmission in endemic areas.[117]

HTLV-1 is spreading epidemically amongst intravenous drug users and male homosexuals in North and South America and Western Europe.

The structurally similar HTLV-2 is endemic amongst groups of the aboriginal population of Central America, and is being spread epidemically amongst blood transfusion recipients and intravenous drug users in the USA and Italy. Associations with disease, such as hairy cell leukaemia, chronic neurodegenerative disease or the chronic fatigue syndrome, remain indefinite.

Pathogenesis

HTLV-1 (and HTLV-2) induces a latent infection in a small subset of cells predominantly CD^{4+} T cells. The virus does not possess oncogenes, but the regulatory gene *tax* has oncogenic potentials through inducing expression both of interleukin (IL)-2 and of IL-2 receptor. Incubation time between infection and disease is at least 15 years. The lifetime risk of developing ATL after HTLV-1 infection is about 3% in females and 7% in males, but the reason for male predominance is unknown. The pathogenesis of TSP/HAM is discussed in Chapter 8.

Clinical

Five clinical phases are recognized: (1) asymptomatic, (2) acute ATL, (3) chronic ATL, (4) smouldering ATL, and (5) lymphoma type.[117,118] Some asymptomatic patients show a preleukaemic condition, diagnosed from the incidental observation of lymphocytosis, with abnormal cells characterized by pleomorphism, multilobed nuclei ('flower' or 'clover-leaf' cells), or cytoplasmic vacuoles; pre-ATL is transient in about half of patients, but may persist and progress to ATL.

About two-thirds of patients have acute ATL. Predominant clinical findings are lymphadenopathy, hepatosplenomegaly and skin lesions, which include papules, nodules, plaques, tumours and ulcers.

Histology of the lymph nodes and of skin lesions is of a high-grade NHL. The cells originate usually from helper T cells (CD^{4+}, CD^{8-}) with functional suppressor activity. Radiology shows pulmonary infiltration and osteolytic lesions which are associated with hypercalcaemia. Anaemia and thrombocytopenia are rare. The WBC count is raised, 30–130 $\times 10^9$/l, with a predominance of the characteristic abnormal lymphocytes; the bone marrow shows infiltration, but less than would be expected from the leukaemic blood picture. The disease is generally resistant to aggressive cytotoxic therapy, and patients die within 12 months of diagnosis. Chronic ATL is associated with skin lesions, mild lymphocytosis only, and a prolonged course. Smouldering ATL shows as skin rashes and a low count of ATL cells, and remains stable for many years. The lymphoma type is clinically like NHL, without the leukaemic manifestations; prognosis is poor.

ATL (and TSP/HAM) develops amongst individuals wherever HTLV-1 is endemic: the low reported frequency, for example in tropical Africa, reflects a low rate of diagnosis.

Myeloma in black Africans

The age-adjusted incidence rates of myeloma have been reported to be 9.9/100 000 in blacks and 4.3/100 000 in whites in the USA. Similar high incidence is observed in black South Africans, and the diagnosis is made at high frequencies in the Carib-

bean and tropical Africa.[131,132] The high incidence in black Africans and those of black African descent may be genetically determined. The disease is seen in sub-Saharan Africa not infrequently in patients of 30–39 years of age, and around 65% of patients are 40–60 years old. Plasmacytomas are not uncommon.

LEUKAEMIAS

The crude incidence of all leukaemias is probably very much the same in tropical and non-tropical regions, but there are distinct differences in the age and gender distribution of the four main types: (1) acute lymphoblastic leukaemia (ALL), (2) acute myeloblastic leukaemia (AML), (3) chronic myeloid leukaemia (CML), and (4) chronic lymphocytic leukaemia (CLL). There are only a few clinical and haematological manifestations and diagnostic problems peculiar to the tropics, but there are severe limitations to their management, especially of the acute leukaemias, in the developing countries.

Acute lymphoblastic leukaemias

Immunophenotypic markers distinguish ALL according to the cells of origin of the blast cells, as precursor B-ALL (including null-ALL, common ALL (c-ALL) and pre-B-ALL), B-ALL and T-ALL. There are three epidemiological patterns of childhood ALL.[133,134] Pattern I: in countries with the poorest economic development, for example much of tropical Africa and Asia, the incidence of diagnosed ALL is low (<0.1/100 000 per year). Pattern II: in countries of intermediate economic development and where there has been the establishment of some haematological services, for example North Africa, Nigeria, Kenya and southern Africa, ALL remains uncommon (<1/100 000 per year), cALL is rare but there is a peak of T-ALL at 5–14 years of age. Pattern III: in the developed or Western countries, the incidence of ALL is 2–3/100 000 per year, with a marked peak of cALL at 2–4 years of age. ALL of all types is seen at low incidence in adults at all ages. The male to female ratio is generally 2:1. Pattern I is largely the result of the lack of medical facilities and diagnostic abilities. The rarity of cALL in pattern II is true; T-ALL has only a relatively high incidence, due to the absence of cALL, not an absolutely high incidence. The peak of incidence of cALL in early childhood in developed countries is explained by the following hypothesis: there is a putative childhood leukaemia virus, which is ubiquitous where standards of hygiene are low, and which infects children early in life, causing no or few symptoms; the mean age of first exposure rises with increasing socioeconomic status, until a significant number of women experience their first infection during pregnancy; transplacental infection by the virus is one step in the causation of cALL; within communities where primary infection in pregnancy is relatively frequent, this event and cALL are more common in first children, with high social class, in remote areas and following the mixing of populations. The children of immigrants (for example Asians and West Indians in the UK) have patterns of incidence similar to the population of their country of residence, illustrating the importance of the environment.

Several tropical countries appear to be moving from pattern II to pattern III, and cALL is being diagnosed now with increasing frequency in blacks in South Africa, in Zimbabwe, Nigeria, Saudi Arabia and South-East Asia.

Clinical

The symptoms and signs of ALL are those arising from malignant infiltration (lymphadenopathy, hepatosplenomegaly, bone pain), anaemia, haemorrhage or thrombosis, and infections from immune depression. Being uncommon in the developed countries, these symptoms and signs arouse the suspicion of leukaemia, but in the tropical world the diagnosis may be overlooked in the mass of children with anaemia, infection and hepatosplenomegaly.

Diagnosis

The total WBC count is raised in around two-thirds, but may be normal or low in one-third of patients. The leukaemic blast cells can be mistaken for activated or transformed lymphocytes in response to malaria, viral or other infections, and the diagnosis missed in the laboratory. The bone marrow is infiltrated with blasts. ALL is classified according to the French–American–British (FAB) criteria by the light microscopic appearance of the blasts: L1, the blasts are uniformly small and have little or no cytoplasm; L2, the blasts are pleomorphic with more abundant, agranular cytoplasm; L3, the blasts have dark-blue staining cytoplasm with vacuoles in both cytoplasm and nucleus. L3 corresponds to B-ALL or the leukaemic presentation of BL.

Treatment and prognosis

Supportive treatment includes red cell transfusion for anaemia, platelet transfusion for haemorrhage from thrombocytopenia, antibiotics for infection, allopurinol for hyperuricacidaemia, and antimalarial therapy and prophylaxis. Specific treatment is with complex regimens of cytotoxic agents and radiotherapy of the central nervous system: it is highly effective, especially for cALL in childhood, but cannot be undertaken except in specialized units. Regrettably, patients in most of the developing world have not benefited from the strides made in leukaemia management during the last 25 years, because of both social and biological handicaps. Patients, or parents, are not able to comply with therapeutic regimens because of their complexity, cost, distances of travel, lack of comprehension or distrust of modern medicine. Supplies of cytotoxic drugs are uncertain and radiotherapy usually wholly unavailable. Patients often show indicators of poor prognosis, including late presentation, poor nutrition, high leucocyte counts, severe thrombocytopenia, L2 blasts, T-cell markers and mediastinal masses. When all these are accounted for in multivariate analyses, black African patients still seem to have a genetically determined poor prognosis.

Acute myeloblastic leukaemias

AML is classified by FAB criteria as: M0 and M1, with malignant blast cells that have few or no granules; M2, with blasts that have granules and Auer rods; M3, promyelocytic leukaemia, of hyper- or hypogranular variants; M4, myelomonocytic leukaemia; M5, monocytic leukaemia; M6, erythroleukaemia, and M7, megakaryocytic leukaemia, which are varieties.

AML is diagnosed at equal frequency as ALL in childhood in tropical Africa, whereas in the Western world there are four cases of ALL to one of AML; this is due in part to the low incidence of cALL in Africa, but there is also a high frequency of AML in boys (male to female ratio as high as 3.8:1), associated with low socioeconomic status.[133] AML in adults has about equal gender frequency and no association with economic status. Recognized risk factors in adults include cigarette smoking, which may account for up to 20% of AML in some communities;[134] a rising incidence of AML will be one part of the large increases of cancer, mostly tobacco related, predicted for developing countries during the next few decades. Exposure to chemicals and toxic or radioactive waste at work and in the environment is increasing and is uncontrolled in the third world; factors related causatively to AML include benzene, to which are exposed informal petrol-vendors and workers in the rubber, shoe, petroleum, leather, printing and chemical industries, asbestos, chemical fertilizers, pesticides and irradiation.[121,134] As alkylating agents (e.g. cyclophosphamide) are associated causatively with AML and as they are used in the treatment of BL, NHL, HD, myeloma and CLL, all of which occur in the young or relatively young in the tropics, it may be anticipated that AML will be observed at higher than expected incidence in patients who have received cytotoxic therapy.[133]

Clinical

AML is indistinguishable from ALL clinically, except that in tropical Africa between 10 and 25% of all patients and about one-third of boys may present with a chloroma. Chloromas are solid tumours usually arising in the orbit but occurring at other sites: the freshly cut surface is characteristically green (hence the name); histologically the tumour is a myeloblastic deposit.

Diagnosis

Monocytic and myelomonocytic leukaemoid reactions from tuberculosis may be mistaken sometimes for M4 and M5 AML.[115] L2 ALL and M1 AML are differentiated by the myeloperoxidase and Sudan black reactions, which are positive with AML. The non-specific esterase reaction is strongly positive with M5 and positive with M4 AML.

Treatment and prognosis

Supportive treatment should be given as with ALL (see above). Survival without specific treatment is about 2 months. Cytotoxic therapy should be undertaken in specialist centres only: conventional chemotherapy allows for a median survival of about 9 months. Marrow ablation followed by bone marrow transplant carries much better prognosis and the possibility of cure, but needs sophisticated and expensive facilities.

In promyelocytic leukaemia (M3) there is a specific translocation which fuses the retinoic acid receptor α gene on chromosome 17 to a locus, PML on chromosome 15. All-*trans*-retinoic therapy has been followed by differentiation of M3 blasts down the neutrophil pathway,[135] a treatment which may prove possible to administer and control with limited resources.

Chronic myeloid leukaemia

Over 90% of CMLs have cells with the Philadelphia (Ph[1]) chromosome, which is a chromosome 22 that has lost much of its long arm in reciprocal translocation with chromosome 9. The translocation juxtaposes the Abelson proto-oncogene (*Abl*) from the long arm of chromosome 9 with a breakpoint cluster (*bcr*) on chromosome 22. The combination produces a chimeric mRNA, which translates a protein with tyrosine kinase activity able to confer independence from control by growth factors on several cell lines.

Annual incidence is about 1/100 000 throughout the world, with a slightly higher rate in male Blacks; males are affected more often than females. Age-specific incidence rises progressively with age from childhood: frequency peaks in the industrialized countries in the fifth decade, but in the developing countries with younger populations more patients are seen under 40 years than over. CML is the third leukaemia of childhood, and in Africa between 10 and 20% of cases occur in patients below the age of 15 years. Environmental factors associated with CML are excessive exposure to ionizing irradiation and benzene.[133,136]

Clinical

Patients complain most often of abdominal discomfort from gross hepatosplenomegaly. They may be emaciated, have generalized lymphadenopathy, and be anaemic. African patients have on average larger spleens and more severe anaemia than European patients.

Diagnosis

The WBC count is raised up to 500×10^9/l: all stages of granulocyte development are present in increasing proportions from blasts to mature granulocytes, with neutrophils predominating usually, but eosinophils and basophils are also present. Tuberculosis, meningococcal meningitis, septicaemia, megaloblastosis in pregnancy, eclampsia, acute liver necrosis, amoebic liver abscess, burns, mercury poisoning from skin-lightening ointments, and severe haemorrhages may give leukaemoid reactions resembling CML. CML and leukaemoid reactions can be distinguished by: (1) a gap in the progression of granulocyte development in CML, e.g. relatively few metamyelocytes; (2) a high basophil count in CML; (3) toxic granulation and other reactive features in leukaemoid reactions; and (4) the neutrophil leucocyte alkaline phosphatase reaction, which is strongly positive with leukaemoid reactions and negative with CML.

Treatment and prognosis

Supportive therapy should include initial antimalarial treatment and prophylaxis for life in endemic regions, and allopurinol. Cytotoxic therapy following standard regimens, for example hydroxyurea, busulphan or busulphan plus mercaptopurine, can be administered safely and be controlled in small hospitals with laboratories able to perform total and differential WBC counts. Tumour mass is reduced and the quality of life improved, but survival is not prolonged. In most patients the leukaemia undergoes blastic transformation to AML or ALL, which are generally resistant to treatment. Median survival in Ph[1] positive CML is 40–47 months from diagnosis, and is shorter in patients with large spleens or Ph[1]-negative leukaemias. Bone marrow transplant is currently the only treatment which can prolong life.

Chronic lymphocytic leukaemia

In 90–95% of CLLs the cells are of mature B-cell origin; other variants are hairy cell leukaemias (5–10%) usually of B-cell origin, T-CLL (about 1%) and B- or T-prolymphocytic leukaemias (<1%).[136] Age-adjusted incidence rates differ more than tenfold among populations, showing greater variation than any other major leukaemia type. There are three main epidemiological patterns.

Pattern I: the highest age adjusted rates (>3/100 000 per year for males) are in Canada and Scandinavia; the rest of the Western world has intermediate rates (>2/100 000 per year for males); lower rates (about 1/100 000 per year for males) are found in Central and South America. CLL is rare under 40 years of age, and thereafter incidence rises rapidly with age. The male to female ratio is about 2:1.

Pattern II: in tropical Africa, CLL occurs from the age of about 17 years, with equal numbers of men and women affected.[133,137] There is a bimodal distribution. About half the patients are aged less than 45 years; in these younger adults CLL is associated with low socioeconomic status and rural habitation: females predominate by about 2:1 in most West African series, but not in some East and Central African series; frequency rises with age in females to peak at the end of reproductive life. Over the age of 45 years the male to female ratio is 2:1, as in pattern I. It is hypothesized that the probability of somatic mutation in B cells is increased in an enlarged pool of proliferating B cells resulting from recurrent malaria and other infections; probability is greatest in individuals of low socioeconomic status and high rates of exposure to infection, and in women whose cell-mediated immunity has been depressed repeatedly during pregnancies; the probability is further enhanced in individuals with HMS (see above). A second genetic event could follow infection by a virus, whose transmission is more likely in poor communities and whose proliferation may be more rapid with depression of immunity by malaria and pregnancy.

In urban Lagos female fertility is high but malaria transmission is lower than in rural West Africa, and

CLL frequency peaks in women at 50–69 years;[138] in the Caribbean where there is no malaria there is a slight excess of women with CLL and their peak is in the seventh decade.[139]

Pattern III: CLL is rare throughout the Indian subcontinent, South-East and Far-East Asia. Genetic factors are important determinants, as Asian immigrants to Hawaii, North America and Europe have continued low incidence.

B-CLL has been reported to have an association with HTLV-1 seropositivity in Jamaica and Nigeria but this is probably not causative. CLL has some associations with solvent exposure and unidentified farming or occupational factors. About half have abnormalities of chromosomes 12 or 14.

Clinical

Onset is insidious. Patients present with hepatosplenomegaly and lymphadenopathy. Spleens tend to be larger where malaria is endemic and may reach across to the right iliac fossa.

Diagnosis

The WBC count is commonly $>40 \times 10^9/l$, with the majority of cells mature lymphocytes. Following acute malaria, cells are marginated and the count in the peripheral blood falls temporarily. It is common to see two populations of lymphocytes in the blood, one representing the malignant clone, the other reactive to recurrent malaria or other infections. The bone marrow is infiltrated with the malignant clone only.

The only condition which can give a CLL leukaemoid reaction is HMS (see above); the differentiation of the two conditions has been discussed.

Treatment and prognosis

Initial curative antimalarial therapy followed by long-term prophylaxis, for example with proguanil, is followed by a partial reduction of spleen size and peripheral lymphocyte count, supporting the view that patients with CLL have a loss of acquired immunity to malaria. In mild disease this may be the only necessary treatment. Most patients will require reduction of tumour mass by chlorambucil or chlorambucil plus prednisolone, following standard regimens. Response can be monitored and treatment controlled wherever there is a minimum of laboratory support. Median survival is about 8 years, but is dependent on the stage of disease, and is certainly shorter in tropical countries. Infections are often the terminal events.

DISORDERS OF HAEMOSTASIS

Abnormal bleeding can arise from disorders of: (1) the initiation of haemostasis, involving the vascular endothelium and platelets, and manifest as purpura and haemorrhage from or into superficial surfaces; and (2) the consolidation of haemostasis, involving the coagulation and fibrinolytic pathways, and showing clinically as uncontrolled haemorrhages from or into deeper tissues. The pathogenesis of haemorrhage is often multiple, for example a viraemia can cause damage to both endothelium and platelets, and this can lead to the consumption of platelets and coagulation factors, and the activation of fibrinolysis.

PURPURAS

Disorders of the initiation of haemostasis result from (1) abnormalities of the endothelium, (2) abnormalities of platelet function, or (3) thrombocytopenia.

VASCULAR PURPURAS

Damage to endothelium is a common cause of purpura and haemorrhage in the tropics (Table 6.20). Infections are important, leading to haemorrhage through either direct toxicity to the endothelium (the haemorrhagic fevers), or to an immune damage during convalescence from several of the common childhood diseases, or to late immune damage as in Henoch–Schönlein purpura. The viral haemorrhagic fevers include dengue, yellow fever,

Lassa fever, Rift Valley, Argentinian, Bolivian, Venezuelan, Crimea–Congo, Omsk, Kyasanur Forest, Korean, Marburg and Ebola haemorrhagic fevers. In immunocompromised individuals, herpes-viruses (simplex and varicella) and arboviruses (O'nyong-nyong, African chikungunya) can cause haemorrhages which are sometimes fatal. Dengue is the most common of the haemorrhagic fevers, being hyperendemic in South-East Asia and spreading epidemically, especially to the Americas and China: the annual incidence in Thailand was 345/100 000 in 1987.[73]

DEFECTIVE PLATELET FUNCTION

Purpura resulting from disordered platelet function (thrombopathy) can complicate the course of some of the haemorrhagic fevers (Lassa, dengue, Marburg, Ebola), alcoholism, hepatic cirrhosis, uraemia, paraproteinaemias, leukaemias and myeloproliferative disorders, or can result from ingestion of non-steroidal anti-inflammatory agents (aspirin, indomethacin) and other drugs. The bleeding tendency of patients with uraemia can be corrected temporarily by cryoprecipitate (see under Haemophilia). The thrombopathies, both acquired and congenital, are described in standard texts of haematology.

THROMBOCYTOPENIA

An abnormally low platelet count may result from defective production, destruction or consumption in the peripheral blood, splenic pooling, or a combi-

Table 6.20 Some causes of haemorrhage due to vascular endothelial disorders in the tropics.

Infections—direct toxicity:		viraemias (dengue, yellow fever, Lassa fever, other haemorrhagic fevers)
		bacteria (typhoid, Gram-negative septicaemia, meningococcal septicaemia)
	—early immune damage:	measles, scarlet fever, chickenpox, rubella, tuberculosis
	—late immune damage:	Henoch–Schönlein purpura, purpura fulminans
Drugs	—idiosyncratic reactions:	streptomycin, isoniazid, penicillin, sulphonamides, aspirin, quinine, etc.

Uraemia
Scurvy
Dysproteinaemias (e.g. myeloma)
Fat embolism (e.g. marrow embolism in sickle cell disease)
Congenital (Ehlers–Danlos, Osler–Rendu–Weber, etc.)
Miscellaneous (purpura simplex, senile purpura, factitious bleeding)

Table 6.21 Some causes of thrombocytopenia in the tropics.

Primarily low production
  Infections (e.g. typhoid, brucellosis)
  Megaloblastic anaemia
  Alcoholism
  Marrow infiltration (e.g. leukaemia)
  Aplastic anaemia
  Drugs and chemicals—cytoxic drugs
                  — overdosage (e.g.
                     pyrimethamine,
                     trimethoprim)
                  — idiosyncratic reactions
                  — occupational exposure (e.g.
                     benzene)
  Miscellaneous (cyclic, congenital)
Primarily increased consumption or destruction
  Infections (e.g. acute malaria, trypanosomiasis,
    dengue)
  Hypersplenism (see Table 6.12)
  Chronic hepatic disease
  Disseminated intravascular coagulation (see Table
    6.22)
  Immune— idiopathic thrombocytopenia (ITP)
         — acute viral infections
         — drugs (e.g. quinine, penicillin)
         — AIDS
         — onyalai
         — other autoimmune diseases
         — lymphomas, CLL

nation of these mechanisms. Many of the common causes in the tropics have been discussed already (viral, bacterial and protozoal infections, AIDS, hypersplenism, megaloblastosis, alcoholism, overdosage with pyrimethamine and trimethoprim, benzene exposure) (Table 6.21). Other conditions, such as idiopathic thrombocytopenic purpura (ITP) have no epidemiological or clinical features peculiar to the tropics, except that patients tend to have splenomegaly and anaemia.[19]

Onyalai

The work *onyalai* means blood blister in the language of the Kimbundu in western Angola.[140] It is an acquired immune thrombocytopenia which differs epidemiologically, immunologically and clinically from ITP.

Epidemiology

Onyalai has been described only in Africa south of the equator. The geographical area of distribution has shrunk over the last 60 years, due partly to the discontinuation of the habit of calling any thrombocytopenia in an African onyalai, and probably because changing life styles have removed unknown aetiological factors. Onyalai is encountered commonly in Kavango and Ovambo territories of northern Namibia and in neighbouring southern Angola. Onyalai accounts for over 1% of all hospital admissions in Kavango, where the minimum annual incidence has been calculated to be 151/100 000. There is no significant seasonal variation of frequency. Over half of all patients are aged under 20 years, which may not differ from the age structure of the whole population. The male to female ratio is 1:1.5.

Aetiology is linked clearly to some factor(s) in rural life in the Okavango valley, where millet is the main staple, and mycotoxins from fungal contamination of grain are suspected. Recently, autoantibodies to glycoprotein (GP) IIb/IIIa of platelets have been demonstrated in 12 out of 14 patients with onyalai; both IgG and IgM antibodies were present.[140] In contrast, anti-GPIIb/IIIa is found in only about one-third of patients with ITP, and it is mainly IgG.

Clinical

The clinical hallmark is the acute appearance of haemorrhagic bullae in the mucous membranes of the mouth, tongue and palate, and less frequently on the skin, including the soles of the feet. Epistaxis is often present and may be severe. Blood loss can lead to haemorrhagic shock. The median duration of haemorrhage is about 8 days, but the condition may persist for months and tends to recur.

Haematology

Patients have profound thrombocytopenia, and many are anaemic from blood loss. The bone marrow shows hyperplasia of the erythron and megakaryocytes. Platelets are morphologically normal.

Treatment and prognosis

Mortality in the acute phase used to be about 10%: patients dying of haemorrhagic shock or from cerebral haemorrhage. Treatment with transfusions of whole blood for haemorrhagic shock and of platelets, and supportive measures including oral hygiene, has reduced mortality to less than 3%. Prednisolone is not effective. Splenectomy is indicated for otherwise uncontrollable bleeding, and is followed by a return to normal platelet counts, but the condition has recurred fatally in some splenectomized patients. Intravenous immunoglobulin has been effective in four patients, but the cost is prohibitive. Vincristine may benefit some patients.

COAGULATION DISORDERS

The disorders of blood coagulation may be acquired or congenital. The acquired disorders occur more commonly in clinical practice, but have not attracted the intense medicoscientific interest given to the congenital diseases such as haemophilia.[141]

ACQUIRED COAGULOPATHIES

Hypoprothrombinaemias

Vitamin K deficiency

Haemorrhagic disease of the newborn. The newborn, especially the premature, have normally low levels of vitamin K and somewhat prolonged PTs (see Reference Ranges; Table 6.7). Classical haemorrhagic disease of the newborn (HDN) is the result of vitamin K deficiency: premature infants and infants of mothers receiving antituberculous therapy, anticonvulsants or warfarin are at increased risk; bleeding is usually into skin, mucosal surfaces, the gastrointestinal tract, or from the umbilical stump or from circumcision. Infants may present between 1 and 3 months with intracranial haemorrhage of late HDN due to vitamin K deficiency: they are exclusively breast fed and may have received antibiotics.

The incidence of HDN is not known, but is obviously high where premature infants are breast fed exclusively; late HDN has been estimated to occur in 3/1000 Thai infants. The diagnosis is confirmed by a prolonged PT. HDN is prevented by prophylactic vitamin K, 1 mg intramuscularly on the first day of life; in treatment, vitamin K should be given intravenously.

Malabsorption. Patients with biliary obstruction or small bowel disease become deficient of the fat-soluble vitamin. Gut sterilization by antibiotics can contribute to but does not cause deficiency alone. Diagnosis is based on a prolonged PT, which reverts rapidly to normal following vitamin K, 10 mg intravenously: the response will be partial only if there is liver disease.

Vitamin K antagonism

Warfarin is a competitive inhibitor of vitamin K. Haemorrhage follows inadvertent overdosage, self-administration by the psychiatrically disturbed, the simultaneous administration of medications which potentiate warfarin (e.g. co-trimoxazole, chloramphenicol), or the eating by children of warfarin laid out as rat poison. Patients remain anticoagulated for several days after warfarin has been stopped, so its effects have to be reversed by intravenous vitamin K.

Hepatic disease

Bleeding in liver disease is multifactorial. During acute infectious hepatitis, a mild disorder of haemostasis, consisting of reduced levels of V, VII and X and a prolonged PT, is not unusual. In association with liver failure, there is severe factor deficiency, afibrinogenaemia and DIC (see below). Patients with chronic hepatic disease or cirrhosis show impairment of synthesis of all vitamin K-dependent factors and fibrinogen and reduced platelet function; some patients show a reduced clearance of FDPs, which contributes to chronic DIC.

The PT is prolonged and vitamin K has little or no effect. If the PT is four times the normal or more, it is hazardous to perform a percutaneous liver biopsy. Bleeding with liver disease should be treated by transfusion of cryosupernate (residual plasma following removal of cryoprecipitate), or fresh frozen plasma or factor concentrates (if available).[14]

Disseminated intravascular coagulation

The widespread or uncontrolled deposition of fibrin in the circulation may be triggered by a large range of conditions (Table 6.22).[141] Pathogenesis starts with (1) damage to the endothelium with activation of the intrinsic pathway of the coagulation cascade, or (2) the release of thromboplastin-like materials from tissues with the activation of the extrinsic pathway, or (3) the injection of procoagulants of various snake venoms (Table 6.23) or contact with South American rubber-tappers with the caterpillar of the moth *Lonomia achelous*, which feeds on the leaves of rubber trees. During pregnancy there is normally a potential hypercoagulable and hyperfibrinolytic state (see References Ranges) and a wide range of obstetric disorders can trigger severe DIC (see Table 6.22).

The dominant feature of acute DIC is haemorrhage, which is multifactorial (Figure 6.21): there is endothelial damage, and consumption of platelets, coagulation factors and fibrinogen, rendering the blood incoagulable; plasmin is activated, both fibrin and fibrinogen are degraded, and FDPs are released into the circulation; FDPs have antithrombin activity and are incorporated into clot rendering it friable. In subacute and chronic DIC red cells are ruptured by being forced through fibrin networks in small blood vessels, resulting in microangiopathic haemolytic anaemia. The obstruction of small blood vessels can cause ischaemia, tissue necrosis and

Table 6.22 Main causes of DIC encountered in clinical practice in the tropics.

Acute	Subacute	Chronic
Infections	**Obstetric**	**Metabolic**
Viraemias	Pre-eclampsia/eclampsia	Liver disease
Septicaemias (Gram-negative, typhoid,	Retention of dead fetus	Renal disease
meningococcal)	Hydatidiform mole	
Protozoan (African trypanosomiasis, malaria rarely)	**Malignancy**	**Malignancy**
	Acute leukaemias (M3)	Prostatic carcinoma
Obstetric disorders		
Septic abortions	**Others**	
Abruptio placentae	Purpura fulminans	
Ruptured uterus		
Amniotic fluid embolus		
Shock		
Accidental trauma (birth trauma or anoxia, head injuries,		
thoracic, fractured femur)		
Surgical trauma (thoracic)		
Burns		
Heat stroke		
Envenomation		
Snake bites (see Table 6.23)		
Lonomia achelous caterpillars		
Others		
Acute hepatic necrosis		
Cytotoxic therapy		
Incompatible blood transfusion		

Table 6.23 Species of snake commonly responsible for morbidity or death from haemorrhage (after ref. 142).

Area	Latin name	Vernacular names
Africa	*Echis carinatus*	Carpet or saw-scale viper
	Bitis arietans	Puff adder
	Naja nigricollis	Spitting cobra
	Dispholidus typus	Boomslang
Asia		
Middle East	*E. carinatus*	Carpet or saw-scale viper
South-East	*Daboia russelii**	Russell's viper
	E. carinatus	Carpet or saw-scale viper
	Calloselasma rhodostoma†	Malayan pit viper
	Trimeresurus species	Green pit viper
Australia	*Notechis scutatus*	Tiger snake
	Oxyuranus scutellatus	Taipan
	Pseudonaja textilis	Eastern brown snake
America		
North	*Crotalus adamanteus*	Eastern diamond-backed rattlesnake
	C. atrox	Western diamond-backed rattlesnake
Central	*C. durissus durissus*	Central American rattlesnake
	Bothrops asper	Terciopelo, caissaca
South	*B. atrox*	Fer-de-lance, barba amirilla
	B. jararaca	Jararaca
	C. durissus terrificus	South American rattlesnake

*Formerly *Vipera russellii*.
†Formerly *Agkistrodon rhodostoma*.

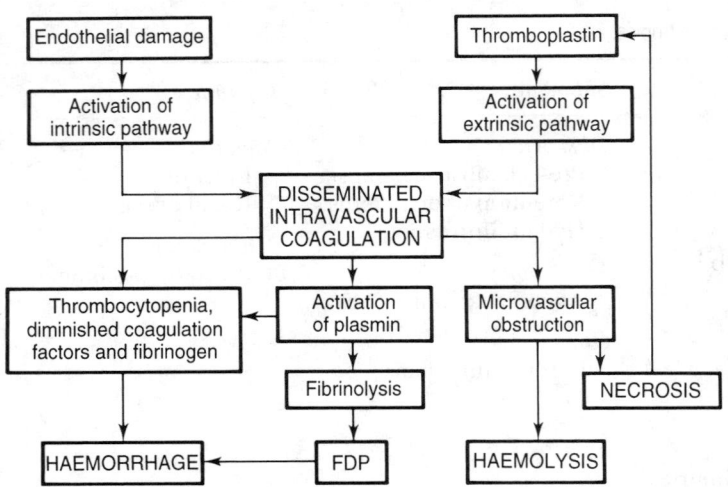

Figure 6.21 The pathogenesis of disseminated intravascular coagulation (DIC). (Reproduced with permission of the publishers from Fleming A F. In Parry E H O (ed.) *Principles of Medicine in Africa*, 2nd edn. Oxford: Oxford University Press, 1984: 733.)

renal failure; pituitary and suprarenal failure are rarer complications.

Clinical

Patients have the clinical features of their primary condition. DIC can range from a minor derangement of coagulation without bleeding to a severe haemorrhagic state. It is a dynamic condition which can progress rapidly, so that attention must be paid to minor abnormalities of clotting tests. The most usual presentation is bleeding from mucous membranes, skin, venepuncture sites or from the uterus.

Diagnosis

The platelet count is reduced, the kaolin–cephalin clotting time (KCCT), the PT and the thrombin times are prolonged, and the plasma FDPs are raised. In severe DIC the simple clotting time is prolonged or the blood may be incoagulable or nearly so, allowing for the confirmation of the diagnosis in the absence of other laboratory tests. Microangiopathic haemolytic anaemia shows the features of intravascular haemolysis (see Table 6.11); in the peripheral blood there are many small fragmented red cells with bizarre shapes (schizocytes).

Subacute or chronic DIC is confirmed when there are thrombocytopenia, raised plasma FDPs, moderate decreases in coagulation factors and evidence of microangiopathic haemolysis.

Treatment

The first principle is to treat the primary cause. If the underlying disease responds rapidly (e.g. meningococcal septicaemia to antibiotics, snake envenomation to specific antivemon, or abruptio placentae to the completion of obstetric delivery), the DIC will correct spontaneously in most instances.

Secondly, the blood volume must be restored and maintained with the transfusion of whole blood (or if not available, concentrated red cells plus saline, or saline and colloids).

Thirdly, if haemorrhage cannot be controlled, platelets, fresh frozen plasma and cryoprecipitate may have to be transfused to restore the missing factors.[14]

Fourthly, in subacute or chronic conditions in which the primary cause cannot be cured, the patient may be heparinized, with the aim of keeping the clotting time just above 15 minutes, in order to break the chain of pathogenesis.

Snake envenomation (See also Chapter 22)

Snake bites are of major public health importance in many communities as causes of haemorrhage, other morbidity and mortality, but are largely neglected in health care planning (Table 6.23).[141,142] Those at highest risk of envenomation include: (1) farmers working in paddy fields, or at the beginning of the rains in dryer climates, when small rodents and reptiles attract the snakes to the fields at the same time as farmers are digging; (2) nomadic herdsmen; (3) hunter–gatherers; (4) workers on development sites. Epidemics of snake bites follow floods, when the human and the snake populations are concentrated together. Snake venoms contain up to about 20 components with a wide range of toxicity (see Chapter 22); only snake venoms causing haemorrhage through procoagulant activities are discussed here briefly (Figure 6.22).

Africa

Echis carinatus. The carpet or saw-toothed viper is probably the most dangerous snake in the world, and is found throughout Africa north of the equator, as well as in the Middle East, the Indian subconti-

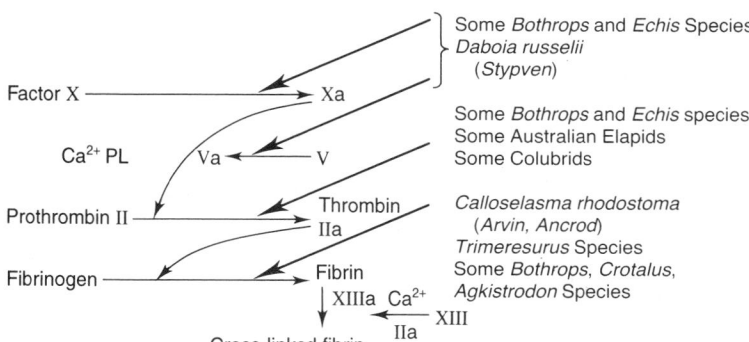

Factor X ⟶ Xa

Ca²⁺ PL Va ⟵ V

Prothrombin II ⟶ Thrombin / IIa

Fibrinogen ⟶ Fibrin

Some *Bothrops* and *Echis* Species
Daboia russelii
(*Stypven*)

Some *Bothrops* and *Echis* species
Some Australian Elapids
Some Colubrids

Calloselasma rhodostoma
(*Arvin, Ancrod*)
Trimeresurus Species
Some *Bothrops, Crotalus,
Agkistrodon* Species

| XIIIa Ca²⁺
↓ ⟵ XIII
Cross-linked fibrin IIa

Figure 6.22 Sites of action of some snake procoagulants. (Reproduced with the kind permission of D. A. Warrell.)

nent and South-East Asia. The snake is particularly prevalent in West Africa, where in rural areas during the early rains up to one-third of adult male hospital beds may be occupied by envenomed farmers. The annual incidence in the Bambur area of the Benue valley, Nigeria, has been estimated to be 600/100 000: mortality is 10–20% in those who attend hospital but do not receive appropriate attention; this has been projected to an estimated 23 000 deaths annually in West Africa.

The venom contains an activator of thrombin (Figure 6.22), causing consumption of coagulation factors, but not usually of platelets, and high levels of FDPs. The blood is incoagulable, which is diagnostic of severe *E. carinatus* envenomation where this is common. Death follows intracranial haemorrhage after 1 or 2 days, or haemorrhagic shock and renal failure after 1 week.

Therapy is with an antivenom which must be known to be effective in the locality because antigenic specificity of venoms varies, for example between East and West Africa. Both Pasteur Paris *Echis* and South African Institute for Medical Research (SAIMR) antivenoms are reliable in West Africa.

Naja nigricollis. The spitting cobra is common throughout sub-Saharan Africa, except in the central African forest and the temperate south. Besides spitting, the snakes bite, and about one-fifth of systematically envenomed victims have spontaneous haemorrhages, which may be fatal.

Procoagulant activity has been shown in vitro, but is probably not important. FDPs can be raised from about the fifth day, associated with tissue necrosis, but DIC is not a serious feature. One specific action is the destruction of platelet actin and a failure of clot retraction. In the clotting time test, clot forms normally (unlike with *E. carinatus*), but fails to retract on standing.

Polyvalent antivenoms are not effective.

Bitis arietans. The puff adder is found throughout sub-Saharan Africa except in dense forest, and occurs also up the west Atlantic seaboard to Morroco and in western Arabia. The main effects of envenomation are cytotoxic on the heart, the automatic nervous system and the kidney. Some patients have spontaneous haemorrhages, usually of gums and nose, as a result of endothelial damage, consumption of platelets and thrombocytopenia; DIC is not usual, but may occur and be complicated by microangiopathic haemolytic anaemia.

Bites by the Gaboon viper (*B. gabonica*) found throughout sub-Saharan Africa, and by the rhinoceros horned viper (*B. nasicornis*) found in a belt between West Africa and western Kenya, have similar effects.

Treatment includes specific polyvalent antivenom.

Dispholidus typus. The green African tree-snake or boomslang is widespread in wooded areas of sub-Saharan Africa, except in the dense central African forest. It is not aggressive and is inefficient in envenomation as it is back-fanged. Only those who handle snakes are liable to be bitten. Envenomation is followed after 1–2 days by spontaneous haemorrhage, due to the activation of factors II, X and XIII leading to DIC. The course may be complicated by microangiopathic haemolysis and renal failure. Mortality without treatment is high, but antivenoms are effective.

Asia

Daboia russelii. Russell's viper is widely but discontinuously distributed in South-East Asia; it is a major health problem in the rice-growing areas of the Indian subcontinent, Myanmar (Burma) and Thailand. Annual incidence of fatal snake bites in Sri Lanka is 6/100 000 and in Myanmar 3.3/100 000, of which about three-quarters is due to *D. russelii*.

Venom is cytotoxic for endothelium, platelets,

red cells, muscles, nerve cells and liver; there is vasodilatation and increased capillary permeability. Two major procoagulants activate factors X and V (Figure 6.22), causing consumption coagulopathy, DIC, deposition of fibrin in the kidneys and other organs, and fibrinolysis. With severe systemic envenomation there are widespread spontaneous haemorrhages. Causes of death include: (1) early shock from haemorrhage, vasodilatation and increased capillary permeability; (2) intracerebral and subarachnoid haemorrhages; (3) late shock from massive gastrointestinal bleeding; (4) late shock from pituitary–adrenal insufficiency following haemorrhage or infarction; and (5) acute renal failure.

Blood is usually incoagulable, FDPs are high and there is often thrombocytopenia.

Antivenom restores haemostasis but does not prevent the complications of renal failure.

Asian pit vipers. Calloselasma rhodostoma, the Malayan pit viper, is the second most important cause of envenomation in South-East Asia. There is more local swelling, pain, lymphadenopathy and tissue necrosis than with *D. russelii* bites. The proteolytic enzyme 'arvin' or 'ancrod' cleaves fibrinogen (Figure 6.22), defibrinating the victim in about half an hour: platelets are damaged, fibrinolysis is activated and the FDPs raised. Haemorrhage may be local, spread up the bitten limb or become generalized.

Many species of *Trimeresurus*, the green pit vipers, bite frequently but with less serious effects than with the Malayan pit viper.

Central and South America

About 200 deaths in Brazil and 100 in Venezuela each year are due to bites by *Crotalus* species (rattlesnakes) and *Bothrops* species (Table 6.23). Envenomation causes (1) extensive tissue necrosis, (2) defibrination from cleavage of fibrinopeptide A from fibrinogen (Figure 6.22), (3) intravascular haemolysis, (4) renal failure, and (5) neurotoxicity.

Antivenom should be administered in all cases of rattlesnake bite, even before there is evidence of systemic envenomation.

CONGENITAL DISORDERS

The prevalence of haemophilia A (congenital deficiency of factor VIII) is about 10/100 000, of von Willebrand's disease (congenital deficiency or abnormality of factor VIII-related antigen) is greater than 10/100 000, and of haemophilia B (congenital deficiency of factor IX) is about 0.1/100 000 population.[141] All other congenital disorders of coagulation are rarities. Except in consanguineous communities, there is probably little true variation of incidence between populations in the world, although the rate of diagnosis may be low in developing countries due to early death, low clinical suspicion and lack of laboratory facilities.

The clinical presentation of these disorders is much the same in the tropics as in the temperate zones. Boys present not infrequently following circumcision, and cerebral haemorrhages can result from the raised intracranial pressure of persistent coughing.

The specific treatment of choice for haemophilia A is factor VIII concentrate, but this is costly and not available in many developing countries. Cryoprecipitate, which is rich in factor VIII, can be prepared simply with a minimum of equipment. Donor blood is collected into a multipack plastic blood-collection set: the unit is centrifuged or allowed to sediment, and the plasma separated into the second pack, which is separated and frozen at $-20°C$ or colder for 24 hours; the plasma is thawed at $4°C$ and centrifuged; the cryoprecipitate is retained in the second bag and the cryosupernate separated into a third bag; both are stored at $-20°C$ until used. Because factor VIII coagulant activity is high in normal subjects in the tropics (e.g. Africans have >150% activity of pooled European plasma), cryoprecipitate of high activity can be produced with no more than a domestic deep-freezer.

During the first half of the 1980s a large number of haemophiliacs treated with factor VIII concentrates were infected with HIV through this product. Patients escaped infection when they were treated only with locally produced cryoprecipitate from donors in communities which were not yet infected by HIV, for example in Nigeria. The present situation (1995) is that factor VIII concentrates are noninfective if the virus is correctly inactivated, whereas cryoprecipitate is potentially infective. In the future, many haemophiliacs in tropical Africa, America and Asia are liable to be infected through contaminated cryoprecipitate.

Haemophilia B is best treated with virus-inactivated factor IX concentrate; cryosupernate and fresh frozen plasma can be given in the absence of the concentrate, but are potentially infectious for HIV.

Wherever possible, von Willebrand's disease should be managed with desmopressin, but cryoprecipitate may be necessary.

All blood products which are not heat inactivated are potentially infectious for HIV, hepatitis B virus (if donors are not screened for HBsAg), hepatitis C and other micro-organisms. Blood and blood products should be used appropriately: that is, only when there are definite indications for which the advantages are judged to outweigh the risks of infection.[14]

REFERENCES

1 Dacie J V & Lewis S M. *Practical Haematology*, 7th edn. Edinburgh: Churchill Livingstone, 1991: 9–17.

2 Nathan D G & Oski F A. *Hematology of Infancy and Childhood*, 3rd edn. Philadelphia: W B Saunders, 1987: 1677–1697.

3 Gilles H M. Normal haematological values in tropical areas. *Clin Haematol* 1981; 10:697–706.

4 Huehns E R. The structure and function of haemoglobin: clinical disorders due to abnormal haemoglobin structure. In Hardisty R M & Weatherall D J (eds) *Blood and its Disorders*. Oxford: Blackwell, 1974: 526–629.

5 Fleming A F. Haematological changes in pregnancy. *Clin Obstet Gynecol* 1975; 2:269–283.

6 Dupuy E, Fleming A F & Caen J P. Platelet function, factor VIII, fibrinogen, and fibrinolysis in Nigerians and Europeans, in relation to atheroma and thrombosis. *J Clin Pathol* 1978; 31:1094–1101.

7 World Health Organization. Nutritional anaemias. *WHO Tech Rep Ser* 1972; 503.

8 DeMaeyer E & Adiels-Tegman M. The prevalence of anaemia in the world. *World Health Stat Q* 1985; 38:302–316.

9 Bellingham A J. The red cell in adaption to anaemic hypoxia. *Clin Haematol* 1974; 3:577–594.

10 Viteri F E & Torún B. Anaemia and physical work capacity. *Clin Haematol* 1974; 3:609–626.

11 Baker S J & DeMaeyer E M. Nutritional anemia: its understanding and control with special reference to the work of the World Health Organization. *J Clin Nutr* 1979; 32:368–417.

12 Wolgemuth J C, Latham, M C, Hall A et al. Worker productivity and nutritional status of Kenyan road construction laborers. *Am J Clin Nutr* 1982; 32:68–78.

13 Florencio C A. Effects of iron and ascorbic acid supplementation on hemoglobin level and work efficiency of anemic women. *J Occup Med* 1981; 23:699–704.

14 World Health Organization, Global Programme on AIDS, Global Blood Safety Initiative. *Guidelines for the Appropriate Use of Blood*. WHO/GPA/Inf/89: 18. Geneva: WHO, 1989.

15 World Health Organization, Division of Tropical Diseases. Severe and complicated malaria, 2nd edition. *Trans R Soc Trop Med Hyg* 1990; 84 (supplement 2):1–65.

16 Phillips R E & Pasvol G. The anaemia of *Plasmodium falciparum* malaria. *Baillière's Clin Haematol* 1992; 5:315–330.

17 Abdalla S H. Hematopoiesis in human malaria. *Blood Cells* 1990; 16:401–406.

18 Fleming A F. Haematological manifestations of malaria and other parasitic diseases. *Clin Haematol* 1981; 10:983–1011.

19 Essien E M. Platelets and platelet disorders in Africa. *Baillière's Clin Haematol* 1992; 5:441–456.

20 Greenbury A E, Nguyen-Dinh P, Mann J M et al The association between malaria, blood transfusion, and HIV seropositivity in a pediatric population in Kinshasa, Zaire. *JAMA* 1988; 259:545–549.

21 Riley E M, Schneider G, Sambou J & Greenwood B M. Suppression of cell-mediated immune responses to malaria antigens in pregnant Gambian women. *Am J Trop Med Hyg* 1989; 40:141–144.

22 Vleugels M P H, Brabin B, Eling W M C & de Graaf F. Cortisol and *Plasmodium falciparum* infection in pregnant women in Kenya. *Trans R Soc Trop Med Hyg* 1989; 83:173–177.

23 Fleming A F. Tropical obstetrics and gynaecology. 1. Anaemia in pregnancy in tropical Africa. *Trans R Soc Trop Med Hyg* 1989; 83:441–448.

24 Brabin B J. An analysis of malaria in pregnancy in Africa. *Bull World Health Organ* 1983; 61:1005–1016.

25 Fleming A F, Allan N C & Stenhouse N S. Haemolytic anaemia in pregnancy in Nigeria: recognition by simple laboratory procedures. *West Afr Med J* 1969; 18:82–88.

26 Fleming A F & Allan N C. Severe haemolytic anaemia in pregnancy in Nigerians treated with prednisolone. *BMJ* 1969; iv:461–466.

27 Greenwood B M, Greenwood A M, Snow R W et al. The effects of malaria chemoprophylaxis given by traditional birth attendants on the course and outcome of pregnancy. *Trans R Soc Trop Med Hyg* 1989; 83:589–594.

28 Bryceson A, Fakunle Y M, Fleming A F et al. Malaria and splenomegaly. *Trans R Soc Trop Med Hyg* 1983; 77:879.

29 Bryceson A D M, Fleming A F & Edington G M. Splenomegaly in northern Nigeria. *Acta Trop* 1976; 33:185–214.

30 Crane G. The genetic basis of hyperreactive malarial splenomegaly. *Papua New Guinea Med J* 1989; 32:269–276.

31 Hill A V S. Malaria resistance genes: a natural selection. *Trans R Soc Trop Med Hyg* 1992; 86:225–226, 232.

32 Piessens W F, Hoffman S L, Wadee A A et al. Antibody-mediated killing of suppressor T lymphocytes as a possible cause of

macroglobulinemia in the tropical splenomegaly syndrome. *J Clin Invest* 1985; 75:1821–1827.

33 Fakunle Y M. Tropical splenomegaly. Part 1: tropical Africa. *Clin Haematol* 1981; 10:963–973.

34 Crane G G. Hyperreactive malarious splenomegaly (tropical splenomegaly syndrome). *Parasitol Today* 1986; 2:4–9.

35 Fakunle Y M, Greenwood B M, Fleming A F & Danon F. Tropical splenomegaly syndrome or chronic lymphatic leukaemia? *Trop Geogr Med* 1979; 31:353–358.

36 Bates I, Bedu-Addo G, Bevan D H & Rutherford T R. Use of immunoglobulin gene rearrangements to show clonal lymphoproliferation in hyper-reactive malarial splenomegaly. *Lancet* 1991; 337:505–507.

37 Cartwright G E, Chung H-L & Chang A. Studies on the pancytopenia of kala-azar. *Blood* 1948; 3:249–275.

38 Kager P A, van der Plas-van Dalen C, Rees P H et al. Red cell, white cell and platelet autoantibodies in visceral leishmaniasis. *Trop Geogr Med* 1984; 36:143–150.

39 Wickramasinghe S N, Abdalla S H & Kasili E G. Ultrastructure of bone marrow in patients with visceral leishmaniasis. *J Clin Pathol* 1987; 40:267–275.

40 Marwaha N, Sarode R, Gupta R K et al. Clinico-hematological characteristics in patients with kala azar. *Trop Geogr Med* 1991; 43:357–362.

41 Lazzarin A, Esposito R & Almaviva M. Modifications of leucocyte function in visceral leishmaniasis. *Boll Ist Sieroter Milan* 1981; 60:222–224.

42 El-Hassan A M, Ahmed M A M, Rahim A A et al. Visceral leishmaniasis in the Sudan: clinical and hematological features. *Ann Saudi Med* 1990; 10:51–56.

43 Varma N, Bhoria U, Bambery P & Dash S. Gelatinous transformation of the bone marrow and *Leishmania donovani* infection. *J Trop Med Hyg* 1991; 94:310–312.

44 Solano C, Gomez-Reino F & Fernandez-Rañada J M. Pure red cell aplasia in kala azar. *Acta Haematol* 1984; 72:205–207.

45 Kager P A & Rees P H. Haematological investigations in visceral leishmaniasis. *Trop Geogr Med* 1986; 38:371–379.

46 Pippard M J, Moir D & Weatherall D J. Mechanism of anaemia in resistant visceral leishmaniasis. *Ann Trop Med Parasitol* 1986; 80:317–323.

47 Weatherall D J. Disorders of the synthesis or function of haemoglobin. In Weatherall D J, Leddingham J G G & Warrell D A (eds) *Oxford Textbook of Medicine*, 2nd edn. Oxford: Oxford University Press, 1987: 19.108–19.130.

48 Nienhuis A W & Wolfe E. The thalassemias. In Nathan D G & Oski F A (eds) *Hematology of Infancy and Childhood*, 3rd edn. Philadelphia: W B Saunders, 1987: 699–778.

49 Luzzatto L. Genetic factors in malaria. *Bull World Health Organ* 1974; 50:195–202.

50 Hill A V S. Molecular epidemiology of the thalassaemias (including haemoglobin E). *Baillière's Clin Haematol* 1992; 5:209–238.

51 Kazazian H H. The thalassemia syndromes: molecular basis and prenatal diagnosis in 1990. *Semin Hematol* 1990; 27:209–228.

52 Fleming A F. Anaemia as a world health problem. In Weatherall D J, Ledingham J G G & Warrell D A (eds) *Oxford Textbook of Medicine*, 2nd edn. Oxford: Oxford University Press, 1987: 19.72–19.79.

53 Cao A, Gabutti V, Masera G et al. A short guide to the management of thalassaemia. Reprinted from Sirchia G & Zanella A (eds) *Thalassaemia Today — The Mediterranean Experience*. Milan: Centro Transfusional Ospedale Maggiore Policlinico di Milano, 1987. (Obtainable from the Cooley's Anaemia Foundation, USA, and the UK Thalassaemia Society.)

54 Rebulla P & Modell B for the Cooleycare Programme. Transfusion requirements and effects in patients with thalassaemia major. *Lancet* 1991; 337:277–280.

55 Fosburg M T & Nathan D G. Treatment of Cooley's anaemia. *Blood* 1990; 76:435–444.

56 Kontoghiorghes G J. Oral iron chelation is here. *BMJ* 1990; 303:1279–1280.

57 Manconi P E, Dessi C, Sanna G et al. Human immunodeficiency virus infection in multi-transfused patients with thalassaemia major. *Eur J Pediatr* 1988; 147:304–307.

58 Nguyen Cong Khanh, Le Thi Thin, Duong Ba Truc et al. Beta-thalassemia/haemoglobin E disease in Vietnam. *J Trop Pediatr* 1990; 36:43–45.

59 Fleming A F. Maternal anemia and fetal outcome in pregnancies complicated by thalassemia minor and 'stomatocytosis'. *Am J Obstet Gynecol* 1973; 116:309–319.

60 Willcox M, Björkman A & Brohult J. Falciparum malaria and β-thalassaemia trait in northern Liberia. *Ann Trop Med Parasitol* 1983; 77:335–347.

61 Metaxotou-Mavromati A D, Antonopoulou H K, Laskari S S et al. Developmental changes in hemoglobin F levels during the first two years of life in normal and heterozygous β thalassemia infants. *Pediatrics* 1982; 69:734–738.

62 Luzzi G A, Merry A H, Newbold C I et al. Surface antigen expression of *Plasmodium falciparum*-infected erythrocytes is modified in alpha- and beta-thalassemia. *J Exp Med* 1991; 173:785–791.

63 Cao A, Rosatelli C, Galanello R et al. The prevention of thalassemia in Sardinia. *Clin Genet* 1989; 36:277–285.

64 Angastiniotis M. Cyprus: thalassaemia programme. *Lancet* 1990; 336:1119–1120.

65 Old J M, Varawalla N Y & Weatherall D J. Rapid detection and prenatal diagnosis of β-thalassaemia: studies in Indian and Cypriot populations in the UK. *Lancet* 1990; 336:834–837.

66 Muklwala E C, Banda J, Siziya S et al. Alpha thalassaemia in Zambian newborn. *Clin Lab Haematol* 1989; 11:1–6.

67 Tan J A M A. An evaluation of the polymerase chain reaction for deletion of α-globin genes in the prenatal diagnosis of α^0-thalassaemia. *Ann Acad Med Singapore* 1991; 20:251–255.

68 Lin C K, Gau J P, Hsu H C & Jiang M L. Efficacy of a modified improved technique for detecting red cell haemoglobin H inclusions. *Clin Lab Haematol* 1990; 12:409–415.

69 Platt O S & Nathan D G. Sickle-cell disease. In Nathan D G & Oski F A (eds) *Hematology of Infancy and Childhood*, 3rd edn. Philadelphia: WB Saunders, 1987: 655–698.

70 Serjeant G R. *Sickle Cell Disease*, 2nd edn. Oxford: Oxford University Press, 1991.

71 Nagel R L & Fleming A F. Genetic epidemiology of the β^S gene. *Baillière's Clin Haematol* 1992; 5:331–365.

72 Fleming A F. The presentation, management and prevention of crisis in sickle cell disease in Africa. *Blood Rev* 1989; 3:18–28.

73 Hibbs J R & Young N S. Viruses and the blood. *Baillière's Clin Haematol* 1992; 5:245–271.

74 Powars D, Chan L S & Schroeder W A. The variable expression of sickle cell disease is genetically determined. *Semin Hematol* 1990; 27:360–376.

75 Morris J, Dunn D, Beckford M et al. The haematology of homozygous sickle cell disease after the age of 40 years. *Br J Haematol* 1991; 77:382–385.

76 Harrison K A. Sickle-cell disease in pregnancy. In Fleming A F (ed.) *Sickle-Cell Disease: a Handbook for the General Clinician*. Edinburgh: Churchill Livingstone, 1982: 90–99.

77 Molineaux L, Fleming A F, Cornille-Brøgger R et al. Abnormal haemoglobins in the sudan savanna of Nigeria. III. Malaria, immunoglobulins and antimalarial antibodies in sickle cell disease. *Ann Trop Med Parasitol* 1979; 73:301–310.

78 Padmos M A, Roberts G T, Sackey K et al. Two different forms of homozygous sickle cell disease occur in Saudi Arabia. *Br J Haematol* 1991; 79:93–98.

79 Gaston M H, Venter J I, Woods G et al. Prophylaxis with oral penicillin in children with sickle cell anemia. *N Engl J Med* 1986; 314:1593–1599.

80 Davis S C & Brozovic M. The presentation, management and prophylaxis of sickle cell disease. *Blood Rev* 1989; 3:29–44.

81 Koshy M, Burd L, Wallace D et al. Prophylactic red-cell transfusions in pregnant patients with sickle cell disease. *N Engl J Med* 1988; 319:1447–1452.

82 Kaufman R E. Hydroxyurea: specific therapy for sickle cell anemia. *Blood* 1992; 79:2503–2506.

83 Ferster A, De Valck C, Azzi N et al. Bone marrow transplantation for severe sickle cell anaemia. *Br J Haematol* 1990; 80:102–105.

84 Akinyanju O O & Anionwu E N. Training of counsellors in sickle-cell disorders in Africa. *Lancet* 1989; i:653–654.

85 Chehab F F & Kan Y W. Detection of sickle cell anaemia mutation by colour DNA amplification. *Lancet* 1990; 335:15–17.

86 Harkness D R. Sickle cell trait revisited. *Am J Med* 1989; 87:30–34.

87 Kark J A, Posey D M, Schumacher H R & Ruehle C J. Sickle-cell trait as a risk factor for sudden death in physical training. *N Engl J Med* 1987; 317:781–787.

88 Abu-Zeid Y A, Abdulhadi N H, Theander T G et al. Seasonal changes in cell mediated immune responses to soluble *Plasmodium falciparum* antigens in children with haemoglobin AA and haemoglobin AS. *Trans R Soc Trop Med Hyg* 1992; 86:20–22.

89 WHO Working Group. Glucose-6-phosphate dehydrogenase deficiency. *Bull World Health Organ* 1989; 67:601–611.

90 Piomelli S. G6PD deficiency and related disorders of the pentose pathway. In Nathan D G & Oski F A (eds) *Hematology of Infancy and Childhood*, 3rd edn. Philadelphia: WB Saunders, 1987: 583–612.

91 Ho N K. Neonatal jaundice in Asia. *Baillière's Clin Haematol* 1992; 5:131–142.

92 Chan M C K. Glucose-6-phosphate dehydrogenase (G6PD) deficiency. *Postgrad Doct Middle East* 1992; 15:10–15.

93 Galiano S, Gaetani G F, Barabino A et al. Favism in the African type of glucose-6-phosphate dehydrogenase deficiency (A⁻). *BMJ* 1990; 300:236.

94 Williams C K O, Osotimehim B O, Ogunmola G B & Awotedu A A. Haemolytic anaemia associated with Nigerian barbecued meat (red suya). *Afr J Med Med Sci* 1988; 17:71–75.

95 Beutler E, Blume K G, Kaplan J C et al. International Committee for Standardization in Haematology: recommended screening tests for glucose-6-phosphate dehydrogenase (G-6-PD) deficiency. *Br J Haematol* 1979; 43:465–476.

96 Palek J & Lambert S. Genetics of the red cell membrane skeleton. *Semin Hematol* 1990; 27:290–332.

97 Nurse G T, Coetzer T L & Palek J. The elliptocytoses, ovalocytosis and related disorders. *Baillière's Clin Haematol* 1992; 5:187–207.

98 Tanner M J A, Bruce L, Martin P G et al. Melanesian hereditary ovalocytes have a deletion in red cell band 3. *Blood* 1991; 78:2785–2786.

99 DeMaeyer E M, Dallman P, Gurney J M et al. *Preventing and Controlling Iron Deficiency Anaemia through Primary Health Care*. Geneva: WHO, 1989.

100 Hercberg S & Galan P. Nutritional anaemias. *Baillière's Clin Haematol* 1992; 52:143–168.

101 Fleming A F. Iron deficiency in the tropics. *Clin Haematol* 1982; 11:365–388.

102 Fleming A F. Anaemia in pregnancy: part II. *Postgrad Doct Middle East* 1991; 14:322–329.

103 Smith A W, Hendrickse R G, Harrison C et al. The effects on malaria of treatment of iron-deficiency anaemia with oral iron in Gambian children. *Ann Trop Paediatr* 1989; 9:17–23.

104 Gordeuk V. Hereditary and nutritional iron overload. *Baillière's Clin Haematol* 1992; 5:169–186.

105 Baker S J. Nutritional anaemias. Part 2. Tropical Asia. *Clin Haematol* 1981; 10:843–871.

106 Hoffbrand A V. Megaloblastic anaemia and miscellaneous deficiency anaemias. In Weatherall D J, Leddingham J G G & Warrell D A (eds) *Oxford Textbook of Medicine*, 2nd edn. Oxford: Oxford University Press, 1987: 19.93–19.108.

107 Babior B M & Lanzkowsky P. The megaloblastic anemias: folate deficiency. In Nathan D G & Oski F A (eds) *Hematology of Infancy and Childhood*, 3rd edn. Philadelphia: WB Saunders, 1987: 315–338.

108 Baboir B M & Lanzkowsky P. The megaloblastic anemias: vitamin B_{12} (cobalamin) deficiency and other congenital and acquired disorders. In Nathan D G & Oski F A (eds) *Hematology of Infancy and Childhood*, 3rd edn. Philadelphia: WB Saunders, 1987: 339–362.

109 Akinyanju O O & Okany C C. Pernicious anaemia in Africans. *Clin Lab Haematol* 1992; 14:33–40.

110 Beach R S, Mantera-Atienza E, Shor-Posner G et al. Specific nutrient abnormalities in asymptomatic HIV-1 infection. *AIDS* 1992; 6:701–708.

111 Freeman A G. Optic neuropathy and chronic cyanide intoxication: a review. *J R Soc Trop Med* 1988; 81:103–106.

112 Wickramasinghe S N. Nutritional anaemias. *Clin Lab Haematol* 1988; 10:117–134.

113 Callender S T. Normochromic, normocytic anaemias. In Weatherall D J, Leddingham J G G & Warrell D A (eds) *Oxford Textbook of Medicine*, 2nd edn. Oxford: Oxford University Press, 1987: 19.91–19.93.

114 Sudre P, ten Dam G & Kochi A. Tuberculosis: a global overview of the situation today. *Bull World Health Organ* 1992; 70:149–159.

115 Knox-Macaulay H H M. Tuberculosis and the haemopoietic system. *Baillière's Clin Haematol* 1992; 5: 101–129.

116 World Health Organization. The current global situation of the HIV/AIDS pandemic. *Weekly Epidemiol Rec* 1995; 70:7–8.

117 Weber T, Hunsmann G, Stevens W & Fleming A F. Human retroviruses. *Baillière's Clin Haematol* 5: 273–314.

118 Anderson L J & Török T J. Human parvovirus B19. *N Engl J Med* 1989; 312:536–538.

119 Jones P H, Pickett L C, Anderson M J & Pasvol G. Human parvovirus infection in children with severe anaemia seen in an area endemic for malaria. *J Trop Med Hyg* 1990; 93:67–70.

120 Gordon-Smith E C & Issaragrisil S. Epidemiology of aplastic anaemia. *Baillière's Clin Haematol* 1992; 5:475–491.

121 Niazi G A, Fleming A F & Siziya S. Blood dyscrasia in unofficial vendors of petrol and heavy oil and motor mechanics in Nigeria. *Trop Doct* 1989; 19:55–58.

122 Gordon-Smith E C. (ed.) Aplastic anaemia. *Baillière's Clin Haematol* 1989; 2:1–194.

123 Waterhouse J, Muir C, Correa P & Powell J. *Cancer Incidence in Five Continents, 3*. Lyon: International Agency for Research on Cancer, 1976.

124 Ramot B & Rechavi G. Non-Hodgkin's lymphomas and paraproteinaemias. *Baillière's Clin Haematol* 1992; 5:81–99.

125 Glaser S L. Hodgkin's disease in black populations: a review of the epidemiologic literature. *Semin Hematol* 1990; 17:643–659.

126 Jarrett R F. Hodgkins disease. *Baillière's Clin Haematol* 1992; 5:57–79.

127 Stiller C A & Parkin D M. International variations in the incidence of childhood lymphomas. *Paediatr Perinat Epidemiol* 1990; 4:303–324.

128 Schmauz R, Mugerwa J W & Wright D H. The distribution of non-Burkitt, non-Hodgkin's lymphomas in Uganda in relation to malarial endemicity. *Int J Cancer* 1990; 45:650–653.

129 Shih L-Y & Liang D-C. Non-Hodgkin's lymphomas in Asia. *Hematol Oncol Clin North Am* 1991; 5:983–1001.

130 Khojasteh A & Haghighi P. Immunoproliferative small intestinal disease: portrait of a potentially preventable cancer from the Third World. *Am J Med* 1990; 89:483–490.

131 Blattner W A, Jacobson R J & Shulman G. Multiple myeloma in South African Blacks. *Lancet* 1979; i:928–929.

132 Mukiibi J M & Mkwananzi J B. Multiple myeloma in Zimbabweans. *East Afr Med J* 1987; 64:471–481.

133 Fleming A F. Possible aetiological factors in leukaemias in Africa. *Leuk Res* 1988; 12:33–43.

134 Cartwright R A & Staines A. Acute leukaemia. *Baillière's Clin Haematol* 1992; 5:1–26.

135 Castaigne S, Chomienne C, Daniel M T et al. All-trans retinoic acid as a differentiation therapy for acute promyelocytic leukaemia. I. Clinical results. *Blood* 1990; 76:1704–1709.

136 Finch S C & Linet M S. Chronic leukaemias. *Baillière's Clin Haematol* 1992; 5:27–56.

137 Fleming A F. Chronic lymphocytic leukaemia in tropical Africa: a review. *Leuk Lymphoma* 1990; 1:169–173.

138 Okany C C & Akinyanju O O. Chronic leukaemia: an African experience. *Med Oncol Tumor Pharmacother* 1989; 6:189–194.

139 Gibbs W N, Lofters W S, Hanchard B et al. Distribution of lymphomas and leukaemias at University College Hospital of the West Indies, Jamaica. In Magrath I T, O'Conor G T & Ramot B

(eds) *Pathogenesis of Leukemias and Lymphomas: Environmental Influences*. New York: Raven Press, 1984: 99–103.

140 Hesseling P B. Onyalai. *Baillière's Clin Haematol* 1992; 5:457–473.

141 Nathwani A C & Tuddenham E G D. Epidemiology of coagulation disorders. *Baillière's Clin Haematol* 1992; 5:383–439.

142 Warrell D A. Snakes. In Strickland G T (ed.) *Hunter's Tropical Medicine* 7th edn. Philadelphia: WB Saunders, 1991: 877–888.

CHAPTER 7

RENAL DISEASE IN THE TROPICS

R. Thuraisingham and D. Adu

There are variations in the causes of renal diseases in different parts of the world and this is most marked between temperate and tropical regions. Even within tropical regions differences are seen in the pattern of renal diseases. The main factor that differentiates renal disease in the tropics from that in temperate regions of the world is the much higher frequency with an infectious aetiology. Much renal disease in the tropics is, however, idiopathic and similar to renal disease found elsewhere in the world. Whether caused by infections or not, the principles underlying the understanding of renal disease are the same in all parts of the world.

GLOMERULONEPHRITIS

Glomerulonephritis is more common in the tropics than in temperate countries. It has been calculated that the incidence of the nephrotic syndrome is 60–100 times higher in some tropical countries than it is in the USA and UK.[1] In tropical areas infections are a major cause of both acute and chronic glomerulonephritis. In most instances infection-induced acute glomerulonephritis resolves when the infection is cured, although glomerulonephritis resulting from chronic infection (e.g. malaria and schistosomiasis) is not reversed following measures that eradicate the infection.

PATHOGENESIS OF INFECTION-ASSOCIATED GLOMERULONEPHRITIS

The classical studies of Dixon et al[2] established that glomerulonephritis could be induced in experimental animals following immunization with antigen. The development of glomerulonephritis coincided with the rise in specific antibody titres and the development of circulating immune complexes. Renal tissue studied by immunofluorescence showed glomerular mesangial or capillary wall deposits of immunoglobulin (Ig), complement and antigen. These studies provided the theoretical basis for the concept of immune complex-mediated glomerulonephritis. Subsequent studies, however, showed that it was difficult to induce a glomerulonephritis by the injection of preformed antigen–antibody complexes in 'naive' animals. It therefore seems unlikely that circulating immune complexes are important in the pathogenesis of glomerulonephritis. Other factors are likely to be responsible for the development of nephritis.[3] Cationic antigen or antibody is more likely to bind to the anionic surface of glomerular basement membrane and induce a glomerulonephritis. In situ antigen–antibody complexes formed following prior fixation of antigen or antibody to glomerular structures have been shown experimentally to lead to the development of a glomerulonephritis. Finally, some antibodies formed in response to non-renal antigens have been shown to bind to glomerular structures. Only a minority of individuals with a given infection develop a glomerulonephritis, demonstrating the importance of host factors in pathogenesis. Often with a single infecting organism a variety of glomerulonephritides is seen in different individuals (Table 7.1).

CLASSIFICATION

The most helpful classification is one based on aetiology and histology. The histological changes

Table 7.1 Infection-associated glomerulonephritis.

Glomerulonephritis	Infection
Membranous nephropathy	Hepatitis B *Schistosoma mansoni* Leprosy *Loa loa* Syphilis
Mesangiocapillary glomerulonephritis	*Schistosoma mansoni* Leprosy *Loa loa* Onchocerciasis Tuberculosis Candidiasis
Focal segmental glomerulosclerosis	HIV *Schistosoma mansoni*
Proliferative glomerulonephritis	*Streptococcus* spp. *Staphylococcus* spp. *Schistosoma mansoni* Leprosy *Wuchereria bancrofti* Onchocerciasis Syphilis
Amyloid	Leprosy *Schistosoma mansoni*

may be of unknown aetiology (idiopathic), or secondary to well-defined aetiological factors. The types and clinical features of idiopathic glomerulonephritis have been reviewed elsewhere.[4]

CLINICAL PRESENTATION

The ways in which glomerulonephritis may present are fairly limited and are summarized in Table 7.2. Patients with glomerulonephritis can present with asymptomatic proteinuria and/or haematuria, with proteinuria that is heavy enough to cause a nephrotic syndrome, with an acute nephritic syndrome which may be severe enough to cause acute renal failure, or with chronic renal failure.

Table 7.2 Clinical presentation of glomerulonephritis.

Persistent microscopical haematuria
Persistent proteinuria
Nephrotic syndrome
Acute nephritic syndrome
Acute renal failure

DIAGNOSIS

Definitive diagnosis of most forms of glomerulonephritis is dependent on a renal biopsy with careful interpretation of the renal histology in the light of clinical, biochemical and immunological features of the disorder.

PATTERN OF GLOMERULAR DISEASE IN THE TROPICS

This has been reviewed by Chugh and Sakhuja.[5] In most tropical countries primary glomerular diseases are more common than secondary glomerular disease. In Jamaica, however, 54% of patients with a nephrotic syndrome have secondary glomerular disease, usually lupus nephritis.[6] In Zimbabwe, 80% of children with a nephrotic syndrome have hepatitis B or streptococcal infection,[7] and in Nigeria and Uganda quartan malarial nephropathy is a common cause of the nephrotic syndrome in children.[8] In Ghana, the Indian subcontinent and South-East Asia, however, 70–90% of adults with a nephrotic syndrome have a primary glomerular disease.[9–11]

MINIMAL CHANGE NEPHROPATHY

This is uncommon in tropical Africa, where it is found in between 4 and 30% of cases.[7,8,10] Seventy-seven per cent of children in India with a nephrotic syndrome have minimal change nephropathy, an incidence comparable with that seen in Europe and North America.[12]

MEMBRANOUS NEPHROPATHY

This is common in children in Zimbabwe[7] and also in adults in Sudan[13] and Pakistan.[14] In both Africa and Asia it is frequently a complication of hepatitis B infection.

MESANGIOCAPILLARY GLOMERULONEPHRITIS

This has been described in Indonesia, India and in Ghana and may be idiopathic but is also commonly seen in postinfectious glomerulonephritis.[5]

FOCAL SEGMENTAL GLOMERULOSCLEROSIS

This is particularly common in Ghana[10] and in Senegal.[15] Renal biopsies from the patients described in Senegal had an unusual fibrillary splitting of glomerular capillary walls with interposition of basement membrane-like material.

IgA NEPHROPATHY

This is common in Singapore, Malaysia, Hong Kong and Taiwan, and in Singapore 75% of patients with more than 1g proteinuria per 24 hours have IgA nephropathy.[9,16] IgA nephropathy is, however, uncommon in Africa.

MESANGIAL IgM PROLIFERATIVE GLOMERULONEPHRITIS

Mesangial IgM proliferative glomerulonephritis is a major cause of the nephrotic syndrome in Thailand and other parts of South-East Asia.[17] This type of glomerulonephritis can also present with asymptomatic proteinuria and haematuria.

SYSTEMIC LUPUS ERYTHEMATOSUS

Lupus nephritis is common in Malaysia and Singapore and other parts of South-East Asia, and in these areas is found mostly in people of Chinese origin.[18] Lupus nephritis is also common in Jamaica[6] and also in black Americans but is uncommon in Blacks in Africa.[10]

INFECTION-ASSOCIATED GLOMERULONEPHRITIS

ACUTE ENDOCAPILLARY PROLIFERATIVE GLOMERULONEPHRITIS

The most common cause of acute proliferative glomerulonephritis (APGN) is an infection with group A streptococci. This is common in Africa,[7] the Caribbean countries[19] and in India.[20] A similar type of glomerulonephritis has been reported with other bacteria in patients with infective endocarditis, shunt nephritis and visceral abscesses. APGN commonly develops 1–2 weeks after a streptococcal pharyngitis and 3–6 weeks after a skin infection (impetigo). With both sites of infection the risk of an ensuing glomerulonephritis is higher in children aged between 2 and 12 years. APGN has become

quite rare in Western countries but epidemic outbreaks following skin infections with streptococci still occur in tropical countries.[21]

Pathogenesis

Only certain M types (cell wall protein antigens) of Lancefield group A streptococcal infections are followed by the development of glomerulonephritis. This is an immune-mediated nephritis and would by convention be termed an immune complex nephritis. The frequent observation of hypocomplementaemia fits in with antigen–antibody-mediated nephritis. The candidate 'nephritogenic' antigen is as yet not known. Some studies have suggested that this is a soluble water-extractable antigen called endostreptosin. Other studies have suggested that M proteins or M-associated proteins may be pathogenic antigens, and in yet others a cationic streptococcal proteinase has been suggested. The sera of patients with poststreptococcal glomerulonephritis also contains rheumatoid factors and antinuclear antibodies and the role of these autoantibodies in the pathogenesis of the nephritis is unclear.

Pathology

This is the classical endocapillary proliferative glomerulonephritis. There is increased hypercellularity of glomeruli from mesangial proliferation and an influx of polymorphonuclear leucocytes, monocytes and T lymphocytes (Figure 7.1). Subepithelial humps on electron microscopy are characteristic of this disorder. Extracapillary proliferation (crescents) is infrequent. Renal biopsies show deposits of C3, IgG and sometimes IgM in the glomerular mesangium and also as large subepithelial deposits

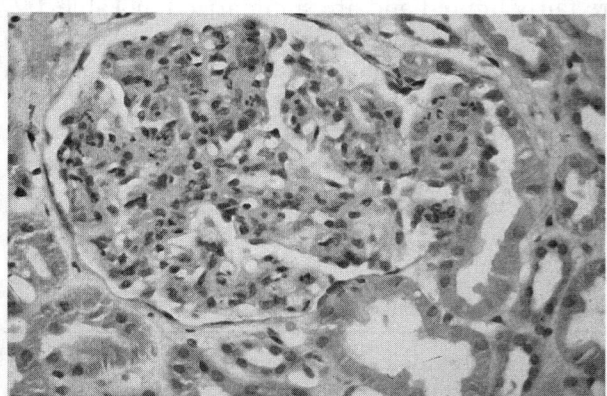

Figure 7.1 Acute postinfective glomerulonephritis. Male, 16 years, acute nephritic syndrome: solid-looking tuft filled with neutrophil polymorphs. (H & E, 250 ×.) (Courtesy of A. J. Howie.)

(humps) on immunofluorescence and electron microscopy.

Serology

Antibodies to various streptococcal antigens form the basis of diagnosis in culture-negative cases: after pharyngitis 95% of children will have an antibody response to streptolysin O, deoxyribonuclease, deoxyribonuclease B, hyaluronidase and streptokinase. After pyoderma antibody responses to deoxyribonuclease B are found, whilst responses to streptolysin O are infrequent.

Clinical

The clinical presentation ranges from asymptomatic haematuria and proteinuria, through an acute nephritic syndrome, at times accompanied by a nephrotic syndrome, and rarely a rapidly progressive glomerulonephritis. The patient with an acute nephritic syndrome presents with oliguria, reddish-brown urine due to haematuria, proteinuria, a puffy face and ankle oedema, and this is often accompanied by hypertension. Hypertension and cardiac failure are usually due to salt and water overload. Headache, vomiting and fits may complicate the rise in blood pressure. A full-blown nephrotic syndrome is infrequent and acute renal failure from extracapillary glomerulonephritis is rare, being found in less than 2% of affected children.

Management

All patients should be given a 10-day course of penicillin or erythromycin to eradicate the organism and prevent secondary spread, although this treatment has no effect on the outcome of the renal illness. The management of the acute nephritic illness is based on conventional treatment, with meticulous attention to fluid balance, together with diuretics and hypotensive drug therapy as necessary.

Outcome

The long-term prognosis of poststreptococcal glomerulonephritis is good and there are few reports of end-stage chronic renal failure as a long-term sequel. Long-term prospective studies of epidemic poststreptococcal glomerulonephritis following skin infection showed little evidence of progressive chronic renal failure or hypertension. Other studies of sporadic postpharyngitic glomerulonephritis, however, showed that up to 50% of patients have some evidence of chronic renal damage.[20]

HEPATITIS B INFECTION AND RENAL DISEASE[22]

The renal complications of hepatitis B infection are found mainly in individuals who are chronically infected. The observation by immunological techniques of hepatitis B antigen or its antibody in glomeruli strongly suggests that the renal injury is immune mediated, although the precise mechanisms are unknown. The major renal lesions of hepatitis B infection are membranous nephropathy and polyarteritis.

HEPATITIS B-ASSOCIATED MEMBRANOUS NEPHROPATHY

This is seen particularly in children who are chronic carriers of hepatitis B virus. The frequency of hepatitis B as a cause of membranous nephropathy parallels the general carrier rate of this virus in the population. Between 60 and 100% of children with membranous nephropathy in Japan, Hong Kong, South Africa and Zimbabwe have HB_sAg,[5,7,23] and by contrast this is infrequent in the USA and the UK. In children the age of onset is between 2 and 12 years, and over 80% of affected children are male. The clinical presentation is usually with a nephrotic syndrome. Most affected children have no clinical evidence of liver disease; this is more common in adults.

Serology

Sera from almost all patients with hepatitis B-associated membranous nephropathy show evidence of infection in the form of HB_sAg, HB_c antibodies, HB_eAg, and HB_e antibodies.

Pathology

The histological lesion of hepatitis B-associated membranous nephropathy differs from the idiopathic variety in that in addition to subepithelial immune deposits there are often subendothelial and mesangial deposits.

Treatment and outcome

There is no treatment of proven benefit in hepatitis B-associated membranous nephropathy. There is no evidence that corticosteroids are beneficial and indeed their use and withdrawal may lead to rebound hepatitis. The antiviral agents, interferon-α and adenosine arabinoside have been used in some patients but with no conclusive evidence of benefit. The prognosis, at least in children, is good, with reported spontaneous remissions of the nephrotic syndrome in up to two-thirds of cases.

Other glomerulonephritis

There are also reports of an increased rate of HB$_s$Ag in patients with a mesangiocapillary glomerulonephritis and mesangial proliferative glomerulonephritis, although it is unclear whether these associations are coincidental.

HEPATITIS B-ASSOCIATED POLYARTERITIS NODOSA

HB$_s$Ag has been reported in 10–40% of patients in the USA, 18–50% of patients in France and 4–8% of patients in the UK who have classical polyarteritis. This association is uncommon in tropical countries.

HUMAN IMMUNODEFICIENCY VIRUS-ASSOCIATED GLOMERULONEPHRITIS[24]

The evidence for a specific glomerulonephritis associated with human immunodeficiency virus (HIV) infection is strong, although some argue that factors such as intravenous drug abuse or opportunistic infections may be important in the development of glomerulonephritis. HIV-associated glomerulonephritis (HIV-GN) may be seen early in HIV infection and also in patients with the acquired immune deficiency syndrome (AIDS). The major clinical manifestations are proteinuria, a nephrotic syndrome and renal impairment. This complication appears to be more common in the USA than in Europe, affects Blacks predominantly and appears to be less common in white homosexuals than in Blacks and in intravenous drug abusers with AIDS.

Pathology

The characteristic histological lesion in HIV-GN is focal segmental glomerulosclerosis that resembles the idiopathic variety. There is often a marked interstitial infiltrate of lymphocytes and plasma cells. Mesangial hyperplasia has also been described in patients dying of AIDS. On immunofluorescent microscopy, mesangial and capillary wall deposits of IgM and C3 are seen. The clinical evolution in patients with HIV-associated focal segmental glomerulosclerosis once a nephrotic syndrome has developed is with rapid evolution to end-stage renal failure within weeks to months. There is no evidence of benefit from treatment with azidothymidine, although this has not been systematically studied. Patients with HIV infection and end-stage renal failure have been treated with chronic haemodialysis, although long-term survival is poor.

SCHISTOSOMIASIS (See also Chapter 72)

Schistosomiasis is widespread in the tropics. *Schistosoma haematobium* affects the urinary tract, and *S. mansoni* and *S. japonicum* the intestine(s) and liver. Significant glomerular disease has been reported only in patients with *S. mansoni* infection and hepatosplenic disease.[25,26] Overall just under 5% of patients with *S. mansoni* infection have hepatosplenic disease, and of these about 10–15% develop glomerular lesions over a period of up to 10 years. The clinical presentation is with proteinuria or nephrotic syndrome. In Egypt there is evidence that schistosomal glomerulonephritis is more common in individuals with concomitant chronic infections with *Salmonella* spp.[27]

Pathology

A mesangial proliferative glomerulonephritis is seen in mild or early cases and the most common histological change in advanced cases is a mesangiocapillary glomerulonephritis, seen in about 50% of patients. The next most frequently seen histological lesion is a focal segmental glomerulosclerosis. There are also infrequent reports of a membranous nephropathy and a proliferative glomerulonephritis. Immunofluorescent microscopy of renal biopsies shows granular deposits, predominantly of IgM but also of IgG, IgA, IgE and C3 in the mesangium and the subepithelial and subendothelial sites. Renal amyloidosis has been described in patients with *S. mansoni* infection in Sudan and in Egypt.[28]

Treatment

Treatment of schistosomal glomerulonephritis with antischistosomal drugs, prednisolone and cyclophosphamide, has been of no benefit and progression to renal failure is usual.

LEPROSY (See also Chapter 58)

The major renal lesions found in leprosy are amyloidosis and glomerulonephritis, although chronic interstitial nephritis has also been described.

Amyloidosis

Renal amyloid is a complication of long-standing leprosy and has been most often described in patients with lepromatous leprosy and rarely in patients with tuberculoid leprosy.[29,30] In earlier autopsy studies, renal amyloid was described in up to 30% of cases in North and South America, but is relatively uncommon (less than 10% of cases in India, Papua New Guinea and Africa). The amyloid fibrils in leprosy are of the AA variety that is derived from the acute phase reactant serum amyloid A (SAA). Serum levels of SAA rise in patients with erythema nodosum leprosum (ENL) reactions and there are suggestions that amyloidosis is more common in patients with recurrent ENL.[29] The clinical presentation is with proteinuria, microscopic haematuria and the nephrotic syndrome, and progression to renal failure is common.

Glomerulonephritis

Glomerulonephritis is found in up to 10% of patients with leprosy at autopsy. It tends to be more common in patients with lepromatous than with tuberculoid leprosy, and the onset of glomerulonephritis may coincide with an episode of ENL. The most common glomerular lesions are a mesangial proliferative glomerulonephritis and a focal or diffuse proliferative glomerulonephritis. Rarely a membranous nephropathy or mesangiocapillary glomerulonephritis is seen. Immunofluorescent microscopy shows granular glomerular deposits of IgG, IgM and C3 in the mesangium or on capillary walls.[30,31] The renal disease progresses to renal failure and it is unclear whether treatment for leprosy influences progression.

FILARIASIS

There are several reports of an association between filariasis and glomerulonephritis from India and Cameroon.[32,33] The clinical presentation is usually with nephrotic syndrome and rarely with an acute nephritic syndrome. Patients with *Wuchereria bancrofti* infection may develop a mesangial proliferative or a diffuse proliferative glomerulonephritis.[33] In patients with *Loa loa* infections a membranous

and a mesangiocapillary glomerulonephritis have been reported. Onchocerciasis infections have been reported to be associated with a nephrotic syndrome due to minimal-change nephropathy, mesangial proliferative glomerulonephritis and a mesangiocapillary glomerulonephritis.[32]

Pathology

On immunofluorescent microscopy glomerular deposits of IgG, IgM and C3 are seen in the mesangium and capillary walls, and in one study onchocercal antigens were identified on glomerular capillaries.

Treatment

Treatment with diethylcarbamazine probably hastens recovery in those patients with an acute nephritic presentation but has no effect in patients presenting with nephrotic syndrome.

MALARIA (See also Chapter 61)

Malaria is widespread in the tropics and is a major cause of death. In the 1930s in British Guiana Giglioli[34] established the long-suspected association between *Plasmodium malariae* infection and a nephrotic syndrome. Proteinuria, nephritis and deaths from nephritis were common in British Guiana. Patients with nephrotic syndrome in this area had a higher incidence of *P. malariae* parasitaemia than unaffected individuals, who more often had *P. vivax* and *P. falciparum* infection. In 1962 Giglioli[35] summarized his observations that following eradication of malaria from British Guiana there was a reduction in the incidence of proteinuria and nephritis and deaths from malaria.

QUARTAN MALARIAL NEPHROPATHY

The association between *P. malariae* infection and glomerulonephritis was confirmed by clinicopathological studies from Nigeria and Uganda in children with nephrotic syndrome. These children mostly had an incidence of *P. malariae* parasitaemia (up to 88% of children) that was significantly higher than in healthy controls (20%).[1,36]

Pathogenesis

Immunofluorescent microscopy of renal biopsies shows granular deposits of IgG and IgM. Further *P. malariae* antigen and antibody have been identified in the glomeruli of some children with a nephrotic syndrome in Nigeria and Uganda. Patients with malaria infections develop autoantibodies to single-stranded DNA and to IgG (rheumatoid factor) but their role in the pathogenesis of the nephritis is unclear.

Clinical features

The majority of affected individuals are children, and to a lesser extent young adults.[1,36] In children the peak age of onset is between 5 and 8 years and the sexes are equally affected. The clinical presentation is of nephrotic syndrome, often with profound hypoalbuminaemia, and ascites that is disproportionate with the degree of peripheral oedema. Microscopic haematuria is common and the proteinuria is usually poorly selective.

Pathology[36]

The glomerular lesion is a segmental glomerular capillary wall thickening with expansion of the subendothelial area, producing a double contour of the basement membrane, or a plexiform arrangement of periodic acid–Schiff-positive argyrophillic fibrils. Advanced cases show segmental and mesangial sclerosis and global glomerulosclerosis (Figure 7.2). Mesangial hypercellularity and small fibroepithelial crescents are infrequently seen. On immunofluorescent microscopy coarse granular or fine diffuse deposits of IgG, IgM and C3 are seen on the glomerular capillary walls. Electron microscopy shows that the glomerular capillary wall thickening was due to increased amounts of basement membrane material arranged in a plexiform manner in the subendo-thelial area. A characteristic feature is the demonstration of small lacunae within the glomerular basement membrane that contain material of a similar density to basement membrane.

Treatment

Treatment of quartan malarial nephropathy is unsatisfactory. Antimalarial treatment has been ineffective in inducing a remission of the nephrotic syndrome. Only a minority of children who had minor glomerular lesions responded to steroids. In most children, however, corticosteroids were ineffective and had a substantial toxicity. Azathioprine and cyclophosphamide have also not been shown to be effective therapy and in the case of azathioprine may actually worsen the prognosis.[37] Most children with quartan malarial nephropathy develop progressive renal failure.

Unanswered questions

Although *P. malariae* infection is widespread in many parts of the world, quartan malarial nephropathy has been described in only a few areas. Thus, for example, it is uncommon in Ghana and Senegal. Further glomerulonephritis that is histologically similar to quartan malarial nephropathy has been described in Senegalese children, who, however, lacked evidence of *P. malarial* infection.[15] There are several possible explanations for these discrepant observations. It is possible that only some strains of *P. malariae* are nephritogenic. It is evident that only some individuals with *P. malariae* infection develop a glomerulonephritis and this may be because of the way that their immune system reacts to this infection

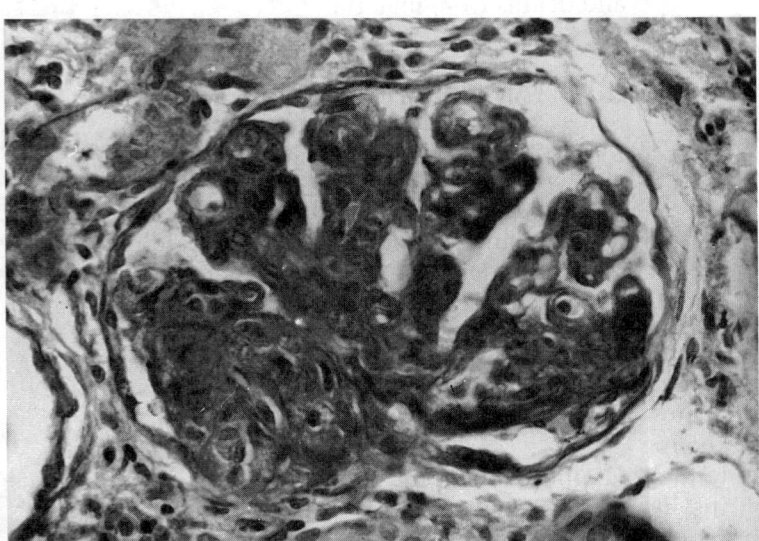

Figure 7.2 Quartan malarial nephropathy. Capillary wall thickening with double contour of capillary walls and segmental sclerosis. (PA–silver, 740 ×.) (Courtesy of R. H. R. White.)

or to environmental factors such as malnutrition or concomitant infections with other organisms.

SICKLE CELL DISEASE[38,39]

Patients with sickle cell disease often have an impaired ability to concentrate and acidify urine and to excrete a potassium load but these changes are minor and usually of no clinical significance. Glomerular filtration (GFR) and effective renal plasma flow are increased in children with sickle disease and it is suggested that the increased GFR may lead to glomerular damage in later life.

Haematuria

Microscopic haematuria is common in patients with both sickle cell disease and trait, and less commonly macroscopic haematuria that may be persistent is seen. The management is with conservative measures only. It is worthwhile screening for other causes of haematuria in these patients, e.g. schistosomiasis.

Renal papillary necrosis

This is found in both sickle cell disease and sickle cell anaemia. The clinical presentation is with haematuria that on occasion may be complicated by clot colic. Diagnosis is confirmed by intravenous pyelography, showing changes ranging from clubbing of calyces to a ring sign in which an often calcified, partly attached papilla is surrounded by a ring of contrast.

Glomerulonephritis

Focal segmental glomerulosclerosis[40]
This is the most frequently described lesion. It is found in older patients, usually aged over 30 years. The incidence of this lesion is unclear. Histologically the glomeruli are larger than normal and show segmental areas of glomerular sclerosis. Because the GFR is raised in early life in patients with sickle cell disease, it has been suggested that the segmental sclerosis is a consequence of hyperfiltration and intraglomerular hypertension. The clinical presentation is with proteinuria and the clinical course is with progressive renal impairment. The proteinuria reduces with treatment with angiotensin-converting inhibitors and it is possible that these agents, by reducing intraglomerular pressures, might reduce the rate at which renal function declines.

Mesangiocapillary glomerulonephritis[41]
The second most commonly described lesion in patients with sickle cell anaemia and proteinuria is a mesangiocapillary glomerulonephritis. The pathogenesis of this is unclear and suggestions that it is caused by the glomerular deposition of renal tubular epithelial cell antibodies and antigen await confirmation.

Acute proliferative glomerulonephritis[38]
An increased predisposition to poststreptococcal glomerulonephritis from infected leg ulcers has also been reported in older patients with sickle cell anaemia.

End-stage renal failure in sickle cell anaemia

Both continuous ambulatory peritoneal dialysis and haemodialysis have been successfully used in these patients. Anaemia is a major problem and is not helped by erythropoietin which, by increasing the levels of sickle haemoglobin, may worsen the clinical condition. Patients with sickle cell anaemia have had successful renal transplants. It is necessary to perform exchange transfusion with AA blood prior to transplantation to prevent sickling of the renal graft.

ACUTE RENAL FAILURE[42,43]

Acute renal failure complicates a wide variety of diseases. The abrupt cessation of renal function leads to uraemia, with abnormalities of fluid and electrolyte balance. The persistently high mortality in these patients leaves no room for complacency in management. Patients with acute renal failure do not necessarily present in neat diagnostic categories but more often as unexplained acute uraemic emergencies. Investigation, diagnosis and initial management must often be compressed into a few hours. The priorities in this early phase are to manage acute uraemia and electrolyte abnormalities, in particular hyperkalaemia, to establish the reversibility of the renal failure and to define its cause.

Table 7.3 Causes of acute renal failure.

Prerenal
Renal hypoperfusion (leading to acute tubular necrosis)
  Hypovolaemia
  Septicaemia
  Obstetric accidents
  Massive intravascular necrosis
  Rhabdomyolysis
Renal
  Acute tubular necrosis
  Acute interstitial nephritis
  Diffuse extracapillary glomerulonephritis
  Acute pyelonephritis
  Nephrotoxins
  Haemolytic–uraemic syndrome
Postrenal
Obstructive uropathy
Renal tubule blockage
  Myeloma (light chains)
  Uric acid, sulphadiazine
Bilateral urinary tract blockage
  Calculi
  Schistosoma haematobium
  Urethral stricture
  Prostatic hypertrophy
  Pelvic malignancy
  Posterior urethral valves

CAUSES OF ACUTE URAEMIA

The main cause of acute renal failure in the tropics is acute tubular necrosis, often as a result of infection, with glomerulonephritis presenting less commonly. Of all cases of acute renal failure in the tropics, 60% have a medical cause, 25% a surgical cause and 15% an obstetric cause.[44,45] This spectrum differs from that found in Western countries such as the UK, where 50% are medical, 47% surgical and 3% obstetric.[46] The classification of the causes of acute renal failure into prerenal, intrinsic and postrenal categories remains clinically useful in that it allows a structured approach to diagnosis and management. The major causes of acute renal failure are summarized in Table 7.3. This list is not exhaustive and is meant to emphasize the importance of seeking an aetiology in a patient with unexplained acute renal failure.

CLINICAL SYNDROMES

ACUTE TUBULAR NECROSIS

A variety of infections and hypovolaemia may lead to renal ischaemia with renal vasoconstriction and tubular cell damage with a reduction in GFR. In addition there may be tubular obstruction and back-leakage of filtrate. A similar outcome may be a result of nephrotoxic drugs, such as aminoglycosides, and also traditional herbal remedies. The clinical consequence is uraemia which is usually associated with oliguria, although some patients may be non-oliguric, producing urine volumes of 1–2 litres or higher.

RENAL PARENCHYMAL CAUSES

Acute glomerulonephritis, especially when accompanied by extracapillary proliferation (crescent formation), may lead to acute renal failure, although this is uncommon in tropical countries. Acute interstitial nephritis is seen in leptospirosis and may also be a complication of drugs such as the penicillins, sulphonamides, thiazide diuretics and frusemide and non-steroidal anti-inflammatory drugs.

OBSTRUCTIVE UROPATHY

Obstruction to the urinary tract is important because it is a common and potentially reversible cause of acute renal failure. The most common site of obstruction is at the bladder outlet due to prostatic hypertrophy or cancer, and urethral stricture. Urethral stricture is particularly common in tropical Africa.[47] Pelvic tumours in women (cervical and disseminated ovarian tumours), and in both sexes bladder cancer and less commonly retroperitoneal fibrosis or malignancy, may also obstruct the urinary tract. Obstruction at the level of the ureters or higher must be bilateral, unless there is a solitary kidney to cause acute renal failure. This is usually due to renal calculi or schistosomal-induced ureteric stenosis. Renal tubules may become blocked by uric acid crystals, particularly in patients with hyperuricaemia following chemotherapy for lymphoma, leukaemia or myeloma. Prophylactic treatment with allopurinol, hydration and alkalinization of urine in these patients now make this an infrequent cause of acute renal failure. Other causes of renal tubular obstruction include sulphadiazine therapy and high-dose methotrexate treatment.

CAUSES OF ACUTE RENAL FAILURE IN THE TROPICS

ACUTE RENAL FAILURE IN PREGNANCY

Acute renal failure from obstetric causes is common in the tropics. In the West, 3% of all causes of acute renal failure have an obstetric aetiology,[46] whereas this figure is much higher in the tropics: 25% in Ghana[45] and 15% in India.[48] The actual cause varies according to the different stages of pregnancy. In the first trimester septic abortions account for the vast majority of cases. This is common because of the lack of a legal abortion service in many tropical countries, resulting in a high prevalence of 'back street' abortions. In the third trimester the causes include pre-eclampsia and eclampsia, puerperal sepsis, haemorrhage and abruptio placentae. The most common histological lesion found is acute tubular necrosis, although cortical necrosis is found frequently in the tropics.[48] The striking decline in the incidence of acute renal failure during pregnancy in developed countries[46] can be attributed to improved obstetric care and also to liberal abortion laws.

MASSIVE INTRAVASCULAR HAEMOLYSIS

Glucose-6-phosphate dehydrogenase deficiency

Glucose-6-phosphate dehydrogenase (G6PD) deficiency is a red cell abnormality which is inherited as a sex-linked gene of partial dominance. The gene abnormality is widespread in tropical Africa, India and South-East Asia. The major clinical consequence of G6PD deficiency is haemolysis due to infections and drugs. Acute renal failure has been reported in G6PD-deficient individuals following haemolysis due to drugs[49,50] and infections such as typhoid fever.[51,52]

Malaria

Acute renal failure is a well-recognized complication of malarial infection by *P. falciparum*.[53] The prevalence of acute renal failure is of the order of 1% but in cases of severe infection can be as high as 60%.[54] The major causes of acute renal failure are severe parasitaemia and blackwater fever from massive intravascular haemolysis.[55,56] The latter may be a consequence of severe infection alone, triggered by drugs such as quinine, or caused by G6PD deficiency. The acute renal failure seen in *P. falciparum* infection usually occurs 4–7 days after the onset of fever. It can be of the oliguric or non-oliguric type and most patients are hypercatabolic. Cholestatic jaundice is often seen and there have been reports of disseminated intravascular coagulation. In severe cases multiple organ failure may develop and this signifies a poor prognosis.

The histological changes are those of acute tubular necrosis, more marked in the distal tubule, and there may be casts of haemoglobin and malarial pigment. Quinine is the drug of choice in the treatment of severe *P. falciparum* malaria in most areas and the renal failure should be treated along standard lines. Of the patients that develop acute renal failure, 60% will require dialysis and the overall mortality is less than 10%.

Diarrhoeal diseases

The acute renal failure that occurs with diarrhoeal disease is usually due to volume depletion. In one study in India 53% of cases of acute renal failure in infants and 22% in adults were due to a diarrhoeal illness.[57]

Typhoid fever

Renal complications occur in around 10% of cases of typhoid fever. Acute renal failure may be caused by massive intravascular haemolysis and this is particularly common in patients with G6PD deficiency.[51,52] There have been reports of haemolytic–uraemic syndrome in association with *Salmonella* spp. infections,[58] and also of a transient mesangial proliferative glomerulonephritis with glomerular deposits of IgM, C3 and Vi antigen.[59]

Shigella spp.

In severe *Shigella* spp. infection volume depletion and toxaemia can lead to acute renal failure from acute tubular necrosis. Acute renal failure may also occur from a haemolytic–uraemic syndrome during the diarrhoeal phase of the illness.[60] The mortality from this condition is high at 70%, with 14% of the survivors going on to develop chronic renal impairment as a result of chronic interstitial nephritis.[60]

Cholera[61]

Acute renal failure in cholera is due entirely to volume depletion. This can usually be prevented by adequate fluid replacement. Given the degree of diarrhoea in cholera, hypokalaemia is frequently present, and in addition to acute tubular necrosis there may also be evidence of vacuolation of the proximal tubular epithelium.

LEPTOSPIROSIS[62]

Leptospirosis is contracted following exposure to contaminated water, either in rivers or sewage. The clinical presentation is with myalgia, pyrexia, conjunctival congestion, headache and jaundice. There may be a bleeding diathesis with gastrointestinal and pulmonary haemorrhage. Acute renal failure occurs during the acute leptospiraemia stage in about 50% of cases and is usually accompanied by jaundice (Weil's syndrome).[17] Approximately 50% of patients develop acute renal failure and the major histological lesions are an acute interstitial nephritis with acute tubular necrosis. Minor glomerular mesangial proliferation may be seen.[63] Characteristic features of the acute renal failure are that it is hypercatabolic and that hyperuricaemia, hyperkalaemia and the rise in blood urea are disproportionate to the serum creatinine. Dark-field microscopy of urine may reveal leptospires and they may also be grown from blood culture specimens. The diagnosis may also be established by serological tests. Treatment of leptospirosis when there is renal failure is with penicillin or erythromycin. The use of penicillin may be complicated by a Jarisch–Herxheimer reaction. Patients with severe renal failure require treatment with haemodialysis or peritoneal dialysis.

HEAT STROKE[64]

Heat stroke occurs in hot climates, usually in association with exertion and poor fluid input and can lead to acute renal failure. The mechanism of the renal failure is rhabdomyolysis and disseminated intravascular coagulation. Investigations reveal evidence of haemoconcentration with a raised creatinine kinase, hyperuricaemia, myoglobinuria, hyperkalaemia, hypocalcaemia, proteinuria and often microscopic haematuria. Renal failure is treated along standard lines.

MELIOIDOSIS

This infection is caused by *Burkholeria pseudomallei*, an organism found in soil and water, and the infection is endemic in South-East Asia, Central and South America and the West Indies.[65,66] Patients with diabetes mellitus and tuberculosis have an increased susceptibility to this infection. There is a marked seasonal variation in this disease, with the majority of cases occurring in the rainy season. In northern Thailand it accounts for 20% of all community-acquired septicaemias.[66] Patients can present with a localized form of the illness with discrete foci of infection or they can present with septicaemia without any obvious site of infection. Acute renal failure is more common in patients with septicaemia (60%) than in those with the localized form of the infection (35%). In the septicaemic form

the presentation is usually one of a short history of a high temperature with diarrhoea, shock and a metabolic acidosis. There is usually radiological evidence of pneumonia, although there may be no symptoms or signs to support this. Microabscesses are sometime seen in the skin. Other features include acute renal failure, hypoglycaemia, hyponatraemia and a low white cell count. In patients with acute renal failure the mortality is high. The renal lesion is most often acute tubular necrosis but an interstitial nephritis and renal microabscesses have been seen.[66] Treatment is with doxycycline, chloramphenicol or third-generation cephalosporins. The organism is resistant to gentamicin and penicillin.

SNAKE BITE (See also Chapter 22)

Acute renal failure is a well-recognised complication of snake bites.[67] In a series from Chandrigah in India, out of 1862 patients with snake bites 3% developed acute renal failure.[68] Acute renal failure has been reported in patients bitten by snakes of the viper, colubrid and sea snake class. Following the bite of a Russell's viper between 3 and 30% of patients go on to develop renal failure.[69] The risk of developing acute renal failure depends on the venom dose and the time between the bite and the administration of antivenom. Gastrointestinal bleeding and also bleeding into the muscle, viscera and subarachnoid space may develop. Acute renal failure develops within hours to 3 days after envenomation. The mechanism for the acute renal failure differs among the various snake families. Vipers cause intravascular haemolysis and disseminated intravascular coagulation, whereas sea snake bites result in rhabdomyolysis and myoglobinuria. The most common renal histological change seen is acute tubular necrosis, but cortical necrosis may be seen in up to 3% of cases. Other renal lesions reported include proliferative glomerulonephritis (occasionally with crescents), an arteritis and renal infarcts. The main aim of treatment is adequate volume replacement and the administration of as specific an antivenom as is available as soon as possible. Treatment of renal failure is along standard lines.

NEPHROTOXINS[17] (See also Chapter 23)

A wide variety of plants used as herbal remedies in the tropics have been reported to be nephrotoxic. Renal failure has also been reported following multiple bee and wasp stings, spider bite and scorpion sting. In addition to direct nephrotoxicity the causes of acute renal failure include haemolysis and disseminated intravascular coagulation. Other causes of nephrotoxic acute renal failure include paraquat and copper sulphate poisoning.

HAEMOLYTIC–URAEMIC SYNDROME

This is a syndrome of thrombocytopenia, micro-angiopathic haemolytic anaemia with fragmented red blood cells and acute renal failure. The main cause of epidemic diarrhoea associated epidemic haemolytic–uraemic syndrome (HUS) is vero-cytotoxin-producing *Escherichia coli* (VTEC).[70] The clinical syndromes of VTEC infections include mild diarrhoea, haemorrhagic colitis and in 7–24% of patients HUS. Sporadic cases of HUS also occur and this is more common in adults. In the Indian subcontinent HUS may complicate *Shigella dysenteriae* type I infection.[71] Rare infective causes of HUS include neuraminidase-producing pneumococci and also *Salmonella typhi* infection.[58] Most cases of endemic HUS occur in infants and young children. There is usually a prodromal bloody diarrhoeal illness followed by renal failure and bleeding from the gut. Hypertension is common and focal neurological abnormalities such as fits and strokes may develop. Glomerular changes range from endothelial swelling and proliferation to thrombosis. Afferent glomerular arterioles may show fibrin deposition and may be thrombosed. In some patients a deficiency of prostacyclin-stimulating factor has been found in the plasma. The consequent defect in endothelial prostacyclin synthesis would lead to platelet aggregation and intrarenal coagulation. This provides the basis for the use of fresh plasma infusions or prostacyclin in patients with HUS. Uncontrolled studies suggest that these measures may improve the outcome in these patients.

INVESTIGATIONS[43]

These are aimed at establishing the presence and severity of acute renal failure and its aetiology, together with the history and physical examination; it is then possible to plan rational management for these patients.

Urine microscopy

Microscopic haematuria with red cell casts in the presence of proteinuria points strongly to a glomerulonephritis, whilst eosinophilluria suggests a drug-induced acute interstitial nephritis.

Haematology

A high white cell count suggests sepsis. Anaemia with thrombocytopenia, fragmented red cells and raised serum levels of fibrinogen degradation products are diagnostic of HUS or disseminated intravascular coagulation.

Radiological investigations

A chest radiograph should be performed in all patients with acute renal failure and a plain abdominal radiograph may reveal renal or ureteric calculi. An ultrasound examination of the kidneys helps to exclude obstruction and determine renal size. In patients with an obstructive uropathy, percutaneous antegrade pyelography allows visualization of the pelvis and ureter, defines the site of obstruction and allows both drainage and decompression, allowing recovery of renal function. If access to the renal pelvis is not achieved the site of the obstruction may be determined using retrograde pyelography. Radionuclide scanning with DTPA or DMSA demonstrates renal perfusion.

Renal biopsy

Renal histology is useful in all patients with unexplained acute renal failure and normal-sized unobstructed kidneys, especially if they have features suggestive of glomerulonephritis or other systemic diseases.

MANAGEMENT[43]

PREVENTION OF ACUTE TUBULAR NECROSIS

Many patients develop acute tubular necrosis after a severe infection. It is likely that many of these cases can be prevented by paying careful attention to fluid balance and avoiding nephrotoxic drugs. In this early phase acute renal failure may be potentially reversible. Oliguria, with a low urinary Na^+ (<10mmol/l), a low fractional excretion of Na^+ and a urine that is more concentrated than plasma, is indicative of incipient or prerenal acute renal failure. The ability of these urinary indices to differentiate reversible from established renal failure is imprecise and is invalidated by the loop diuretics. We and others find them of little value in practice. In patients with oliguria the first step is to correct hypovolaemia and a low cardiac output using central venous pressures or pulmonary capillary wedge pressures if necessary. A potential pitfall is that if the patient remains oliguric, pulmonary oedema may be precipitated. If oliguria persists then low dose dopamine ($0.5–3.0\mu g\,kg^{-1}\,min^{-1}$ intravenously), together with the addition of frusemide 1–2 mg/min intravenously (up to 1g), may reverse the oliguria of incipient acute tubular necrosis. Because of the possibility of inducing a massive diuresis, careful hourly monitoring of urine volume is mandatory with this regimen. At these doses dopamine is a renal vasodilator and causes an increase in glomerular filtration rate and urinary sodium excretion.

FLUID BALANCE

A daily weight chart is valuable in assessing the fluid balance of patients with acute renal failure. Clinically fluid balance can be determined by assessing the jugular venous pressure and skin turgor and looking for postural hypotension. The amount of fluids given to a patient in acute renal failure are based on: (1) measured fluid losses; (2) insensible losses minus metabolically produced water (about 600ml/day in an adult); and (3) fluid removed by dialysis.

HYPERKALAEMIA AND ACIDOSIS

Serum potassium can rise rapidly in patients who are hypercatabolic or acidotic or who have rhabdomyolysis. Hyperkalaemia is cardiotoxic and the electrocardiographic features include tall peaked T waves, prolongation of the PR interval, broadening of the QRS complex, which merges into the T wave, and ventricular arrhythmias with cardiac arrest. The serum potassium must be measured daily in patients with acute renal failure and more frequently in patients who are hypercatabolic. With milder degrees of hyperkalaemia (K^+ less than 6.0mmol/l) cation exchange resins may be used to increase faecal potassium excretion. Serum potassium levels higher than 6.0mmol/l are an indication for urgent dialysis. Intravenous glucose and soluble insulin are often helpful in reducing serum potassium pending dialysis. Most patients with acute renal failure have a metabolic acidosis and this can be severe in patients who are hypercatabolic.

DIALYSIS

There are now a variety of techniques for treating uraemia and removing fluid from patients with acute renal failure. These include haemodialysis, peritoneal dialysis, haemofiltration, continuous arteriovenous haemofiltration, continuous arteriovenous haemodialysis, and continuous venovenous haemodialysis.

Peritoneal dialysis

This has the advantage of being widely available, easy to set up and easy to run. It is effective in patients with milder degrees of renal failure who are not hypercatabolic.

Haemodialysis

As with other centres our emphasis now is on early, frequent (often daily) short (2–3-hour) haemodialyses, especially in patients who are critically ill. Other types of dialysis such as continuous arteriovenous haemodialysis are of value in the intensive care setting.

NUTRITION

Patients with acute renal failure should be given adequate nutrition in an attempt to minimize muscle catabolism and reduce malnutrition with the added risks of delayed wound healing and impaired resistance to infection.

SEPSIS

Sepsis is important both as a cause and as a complication: most studies show that sepsis is still a major cause of death in patients with acute renal failure. The major sites of sepsis are intra-abdominal and pulmonary, and septicaemia is a frequent complication.

DRUGS

Many drugs used in patients with acute renal failure are excreted by the kidneys and, unless their dose is modified, will accumulate with potentially toxic effects. It is therefore essential to know the precise pharmacokinetics of any drug before it is given to a patient with acute renal failure. Detailed guidelines to drug treatment in these patients are available.

CHRONIC RENAL FAILURE

Chronic renal failure results from the progressive and irreversible loss of renal function. The remarkable reserve in renal function means that the kidneys can support life with as little as 10% of functioning nephrons. Below that critical level death ensues unless renal function can be replaced by dialysis or renal transplantation.

AETIOLOGY

There are many causes of chronic renal failure in the tropics and these are summarized in Table 7.4. In tropical countries, glomerulonephritis, hypertension and diabetic nephropathy are major causes of chronic renal failure, as is an obstructive uropathy.[11,72,73] Early identification of the cause of chronic renal failure may help in slowing its progression to terminal uraemia.

DIABETIC NEPHROPATHY[75]

Diabetic nephropathy has been reported in tropical Africa, the Caribbean, the Indian subcontinent and South-East Asia. In most areas the prevalence of diabetic nephropathy in patients with diabetes mellitus varies between 10 and 20%. The progressive nature of diabetic nephropathy makes this likely to be a major cause of end-stage renal failure in these areas.

PATHOPHYSIOLOGY

Studies in rats who had undergone a 5/6ths nephrectomy suggested that the consequences of nephron loss, in particular glomerular hypertrophy, were responsible for progressive renal damage.[76] Glomerular hypertrophy resulting from nephron loss was accompanied by glomerular hyperperfusion, hyperfiltration and hypertension and these in turn led to progressive glomerular sclerosis, tubulointerstitial atrophy and scarring. This glomerular sclerosis occurred independently of the initial cause of the initial nephron loss. In rats reduction of intraglomerular pressures, either by a low protein diet or by an angiotensin-converting enzyme inhibitor (which reduces intraglomerular pressures by afferent arteriolar vasodilatation), slowed down the rate at which renal failure progressed.[76] These measures have been used in patients with chronic renal failure. The evidence for conclusive benefit is lacking.

BIOCHEMISTRY

Serum creatinine and urea do not rise above normal until the GFR falls below 50ml/min, i.e. until renal function is halved. This makes them inaccurate markers of renal function in mild renal impairment. Below a glomerular filtration rate of 30ml/min the serum creatinine rise is approximately linear to glomerular filtration rate. Indeed, because of tubular secretion of creatinine, serum creatinine levels become a better marker of renal function than the creatinine clearance at low levels of renal function.

HYPERKALAEMIA AND ACIDOSIS

These are not marked until the GFR falls below 20ml/min. Exceptions to this are patients with tubulointerstitial disorders.

SALT AND WATER HANDLING

In most patients, salt and water balance is maintained until the GFR falls below 15% of normal. Nevertheless some individuals with tubulointerstitial disease are salt and water losers and tend to dehydration at a higher GFR. Others with glomerular disease and hypertension, especially with hypertensive heart disease, may retain salt and water and develop heart failure.

BONE[77]

Increased blood levels of parathormone are found in mild levels of renal failure when GFR falls below 50–

Table 7.4 Causes of chronic renal failure in the tropics.

Cause	Africa[73]	India[11,72]	Malaysia[74]
Hypertensive renal disease (nephrosclerosis)	32–49	5–23	?
Glomerulonephritis	25–62	35–65	30
Pyelonephritis	2–29	7–18	2
Diabetic nephropathy	3–9	7–23	9
Obstructive uropathy	?	3–14	6
Renal calculi	12	7	?
Tuberculosis	?	1–5	?
Polycystic kidney disease	?	1–6	0.5

Values are percentages.

60 ml/min. This is probably due to inappropriately low levels of 1,25-dihydroxycholecalciferol and not to hyperphosphataemia with consequent hypocalcaemia, as previously thought. With advanced renal failure there is impaired renal synthesis of 1,25-cholecalciferol from its precursor 25-cholecalciferol. A reduction in intestinal absorption of calcium and also hyperphosphataemia increase the tendency to hypocalcaemia. This stimulates the parathyroid glands to hyperplasia and in severe cases to adenoma formation. The consequences of this are renal osteodystrophy. Vitamin D deficiency leads to osteomalacia, and hyperparathyroidism to the development of bone erosions and osteitis fibrosa.

ALUMINIUM INTOXICATION

This arises from absorption of aluminium-containing phosphate binders and dialysis against fluid containing aluminium. The bony consequences are osteomalacia. Aluminium intoxication can also cause an encephalopathy.

MANAGEMENT

The causes of chronic renal failure are varied and its clinical presentation differs between patients. Management must therefore be guided by the assessment of individual patients.

CONSERVATIVE MANAGEMENT

This is effective in individuals with a GFR of 10 ml/min or greater. The first objective is to identify and correct potentially reversible causes of progressive renal failure. Examples of this include obstructive uropathy and the use of potentially nephrotoxic drugs such as non-steroidal anti-inflammatory drugs. Good blood pressure control will probably slow down the rate of progression of renal damage. Whilst angiotensin-converting enzyme inhibitors may be particularly effective in this regard they may also impair renal function in patients with renal ischaemia, whether from large vessel disease (renal artery stenosis) or small renal vessel disease. A low-protein diet reduces the progression of renal damage in rats and possibly in humans. We arbitrarily restrict protein intake to 0.6 g/kg with a serum creatinine over $400 \mu mol/l$ and to 0.5 g/kg when the serum creatinine rises to over $600 \mu mol/l$.

The maintenance of GFR in advanced renal failure is critically dependent on salt and water balance. Salt and water overload leads to heart failure, a reduction in cardiac output and worsening of renal function. Salt and water depletion leads to volume depletion, a reduction in cardiac output and a reduction in GFR. Each patient must have careful regular assessments of their fluid status and salt and water intake and this is then optimized, if necessary, using diuretics. Once the GFR falls below 20 ml/min plasma potassium tends to rise, justifying a reduction in dietary potassium intake. Expert dietetic help adjusted to the local foods is invaluable in the management of these patients.

Renal osteodystrophy is relatively uncommon in most parts of the tropics but will undoubtedly become a problem once patients are established on maintenance dialysis programmes. Key principles in management include control of hyperphosphataemia with calcium carbonate which binds ingested phosphate and the use of 1α-hydroxycholecalciferol or 1,25-dihydroxycholecalciferol in patients who are (1) hypocalcaemic, (2) have a raised alkaline phosphatase, (3) have a raised parathormone. The dose of calcium carbonate must be adjusted to avoid hypercalcaemia.

DIALYSIS AND TRANSPLANTATION

Once the GFR falls below 10 ml/min, renal replacement with either dialysis[78] or a renal transplant is necessary if life is to be maintained. The costs of dialysis—both continuous ambulatory dialysis and haemodialysis—are substantial and this puts it out of the reach of many but not all tropical countries as a universal mode of treatment. Renal transplantation once set up is less costly in the long term. Several tropical countries have developed successful live donor transplant programmes. Organ donation from closely related and willing individuals is justified in these circumstances. Unrelated or third-party organ donors are ethically unacceptable.

OBSTRUCTIVE UROPATHY

RENAL TUBERCULOSIS[79]

Tuberculosis can affect the urinary tract in three ways. Most commonly there is parenchymal renal involvement with ureteric and bladder involvement. Parenchymal renal involvement often leads to cavitation, seen on intravenous urography as papillary ulceration or cavities in the parenchyma and these may communicate with the pelvicalyceal system. Advanced parenchymal lesions lead to a nonfunctioning kidney—so-called autonephrectomy. On plain abdominal radiographs renal calcification is often a clue to the diagnosis of tuberculosis. Bladder involvement leads to ulceration and there may be inflammation of the ureters. In advanced disease the bladder becomes obstructed and fibrosed and this, together with ureteric stricture or incompetence of the vesicoureteric junction, can lead to an obstructive uropathy. Extrarenal tuberculosis may lead to the late development of glomerular amyloid. The clinical presentation is that of renal amyloid from any other cause. Rarely tuberculosis has been associated with the development of a mesangiocapillary glomerulonephritis.

RENAL CALCULI[80]

Renal and ureteric calculi tend to be uncommon in Blacks in tropical Africa but is common in the Middle East, the Indian subcontinent and the rest of Asia. In areas with a high incidence of schistosomiasis bladder stones may be common. It is suggested that a high temperature, an inadequate fluid intake and a low urine volume predispose to stone formation in some areas. Bladder stones are common in Central Africa and parts of South-East Asia.

SCHISTOSOMA HAEMATOBIUM[81]

S. haematobium infections are widespread in the tropics. Schistosoma-mediated inflammation of the bladder and ureters can lead to fibrosis and to an obstructive uropathy. The bladder and the juxtavesical ureter are initially involved by granuloma formation. Ureteric involvement leads to ureteric dilatation, stricture and vesicoureteric reflux. Functionally these abnormalities may lead to renal failure. Diagnosis is by examining the urine for *S. haematobium* ova. A calcified bladder or ureters may be seen on abdominal radiographs (Figure 7.3). Intravenous urography shows a variety of changes including segmental dilatation of the ureter, ureteric stenosis and dilatation of the upper tracts. There is good evidence of an association between *S. haematobium* infection and the subsequent development of bladder cancer. The majority of these tumours are squamous cell carcinomas.

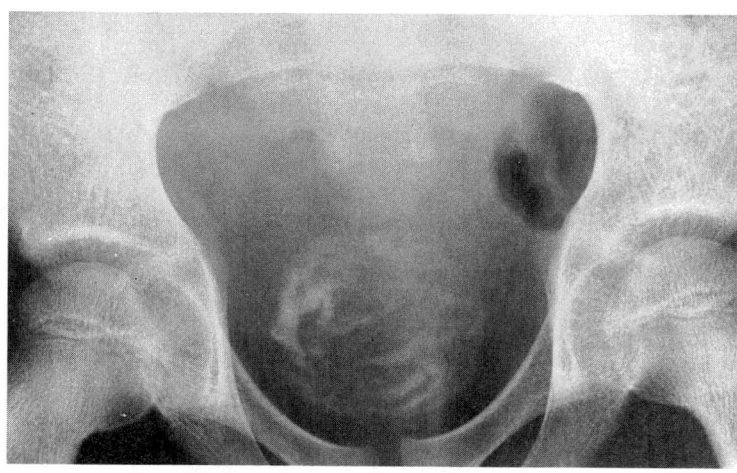

Figure 7.3 Bladder wall calcification in schistosomiasis. (Courtesy of Judy Webb, St Bartholomew's Hospital.)

REFERENCES

1 Kibukamusoke J W, Hutt M S R & Wilks N E. The nephrotic syndrome in Uganda and its association with quartan malaria. *Q J Med* 1967; 36:393–407.

2 Dixon F J, Vasquez J J, Weigle W O & Cochrane C G. Pathogenesis of serum sickness. *Arch Pathol* 1958; 65:18–28.

3 Glotz D & Druet P. Immune mechanisms of glomerular damage that affect the kidney. In Cameron J S, Davison A M, Grunfeld J-P & Ritz E (eds) *Oxford Textbook of Clinical Nephrology*. Oxford: Oxford University Press, 1992: 240–262.

4 Adu D. Idiopathic glomerulonephritis. In Weatherall D, Ledingham J G G & Warrell D A (eds) *Oxford Textbook of Medicine*, 3rd edn. Oxford: Oxford University Press, 1993: (in press).

5 Chugh K S & Sakhuja V. Glomerular disease in the tropics. In Cameron J S, Davison A M, Grunfeld J-P & Ritz E (eds) *Oxford Textbook of Clinical Nephrology*. Oxford: Oxford University Press, 1992: 486–502.

6 Morgan A G, Shah D J, Williams W & Forrester T E. Proteinuria and glomerular disease in Jamaica. *Clin Nephrol* 1984; 21:205–209.

7 Seggie J, Davies P G, Ninin D & Henry J. Pattern of glomerulonephritis in Zimbabwe. Survey of disease characterised by nephrotic proteinuria. *Q J Med* 1984; 53:109–118.

8 Seggie J L & Adu D. Nephrotic syndrome in the Tropics. In Cameron J S & Glassock R J (eds) *The Nephrotic Syndrome*. New York: Marcel Dekker, 1988: 653–695.

9 Sinniah R & Khoo O T. The pathology and immunopathology of glomerulonephritis in Singapore. *Proceedings of the 1st Asian Pacific Congress of Nephrology*, Tokyo, 1979: 114.

10 Adu D, Anim-Addo Y, Foli A K et al. The nephrotic syndrome in Ghana: clinical and pathological aspects. *Q J Med* 1981; 50:297–306.

11 Chugh K S & Sakhuja V. Renal disease in northern India. In Kibukamusoke J W (ed.) *Tropical Nephrology*. Canberra: Citforge, 1984: 428–440.

12 Srivastava R N, Mayekar G, Anand R, Choudhury V, Ghai O P & Tandon H. Nephrotic syndrome in Indian children. *Arch Dis Child* 1975; 50:626–630.

13 Musa A R M, Veress B, Kordofani A M, Asha H A, Satir A & Hassan A M E. Pattern of the nephrotic syndrome in the Sudan. *Ann Trop Med Parasitol* 1980; 74:37–42.

14 Sadiq S, Jafrey N A & Naqvi S A J. An analysis of percutaneous renal biopsies in fifty cases of nephrotic syndrome. *J Pakistan Med Assoc* 1978; 28:121–124.

15 Morel-Maroger L, Saimot A G, Sloper J C et al. 'Tropical nephropathy' and 'Tropical extramembranous glomerulonephritis' of unknown aetiology in Senegal. *BMJ* 1975; 1:541–546.

16 Levy M & Berger J. Worldwide perspective of IgA nephropathy. *Am J Kidney Dis* 1988; 12:340–347.

17 Sitprija V. The kidney in acute tropical disease. In Kibukamusoke J W (ed.) *Tropical Nephrology*. Canberra: Citforge, 1984: 148–169.

18 Prathap K & Looi L M. Morphological patterns of glomerular disease in renal biopsies from 1000 Malaysian patients. *Ann Acad Med Singapore* 1982; 11:52–56.

19 Poon-King T, Potter E V, Svartman M et al. Epidemic acute nephritis with reappearance of M-type 55 streptococci in Trinidad. *Lancet* 1973; i:475–479.

20 Chugh K S, Malhotra H S & Sakhuja V. Progression to end-stage renal disease in poststreptococcal glomerulonephritis. *Int J Artif Organs* 1987; 10:189–194.

21 Rodriguez-Iturbe B. Acute endocapillary glomerulonephritis. In Cameron J S, Davison A M, Grunfeld J-P & Ritz E (eds) *Oxford Textbook of Clinical Nephrology*. Oxford: Oxford University Press, 1992: 405–417.

22 Johnson R J & Couser W G. Hepatitis B infection and renal disease: clinical, immunopathogenetic and therapeutic considerations. *Kidney Int* 1990; 37:663–676.

23 Lai K N, Lai F M, Chan K W, Chow C B, Tong K L & Vallance-Owen J. The clinico-pathological features of hepatitis B virus-associated glomerulonephritis. *Q J Med* 1987; 240:323–333.

24 Bourgoignie J J. Renal complications of human immunodeficiency virus type 1. *Kidney Int* 1990; 37:1571–1584.

25 Andrade Z A & Rocha H. Schistosomal glomerulopathy. *Kidney Int* 1979; 16:23–29.

26 Barsoum R S. Schistosomiasis. In Cameron J S, Davison A M, Grunfeld J-P & Ritz E (eds) *Oxford Textbook of Clinical Nephrology*. Oxford: Oxford University Press, 1992: 1729–1741.

27 Barsoum R S, Bassily S, Baligh O K et al. Renal disease in hepatosplenic schistosomiasis: a clinicopathological study. *Trans R Soc Trop Med Hyg* 1977; 71:387–391.

28 Omer H O & Wahab S M A. Secondary amyloidosis due to *Schistosoma mansoni* infection. *BMJ* 1976; i:375–377.

29 McAdam K P W J, Anders R F, Smith S R, Russell D A & Price M A. Association of amyloidosis with erythema nodosum leprosum reactions and recurrent neutrophil leucocytosis in leprosy. *Lancet* 1975; ii:572–575.

30 Chugh K S, Damle P B, Kaur S et al. Renal lesions in leprosy amongst north Indian patients. *Postgrad Med J* 1983; 59:707–711.

31 Johny K V, Karat A B A, Rao P S S & Date A. Glomerulonephritis in leprosy. A percutaneous renal biopsy study. *Lepr Rev* 1975; 46:29–37.

32 Ngu J L, Chatelanat F, Leke R, Ndumbe P & Youmbissi J. Nephropathy in Cameroon: evidence for filarial derived immune complex pathogenesis in some cases. *Clin Nephrol* 1985; 24:128–134.

33 Chugh K S, Singhal P C & Tewari S C. Acute glomerulonephritis associated with filariasis. *Am J Trop Med Hyg* 1978; 27:630–631.

34 Giglioli G. Malarial nephritis: epidemiological and clinical notes on malaria. In *Blackwater Fever, Albuminuria and Nephritis in the Interior of British Guiana, Based on Seven Years' Continual Observation*. London: Churchill, 1930.

35 Giglioli G. Malaria and renal disease with special reference to British Guiana II. The effect of malaria eradication on the incidence of renal disease in British Guiana. *Ann Trop Med Parasitol* 1962; 56:225–241.

36 Hendrickse R G, Adeniyi A, Edington G M, Glasgow E F, White R H R & Houba V. Quartan malarial nephrotic syndrome: collaborative clinicopathological study in Nigerian children. *Lancet* 1972; i:1143–1149.

37 Adeniyi A, Hendrickse R G & Houba V. Selectivity of proteinuria and response to prednisolone or immunosuppressive drugs in children with malarial nephrosis. *Lancet* 1970; i:644–648.

38 Nicholson G D. Kidney in sickle cell disease. In Kibukamusoke J W (ed.) *Tropical Nephrology*. Canberra: Citforge, 1984: 272–286.

39 Statius van Eps L W. Sickle-cell disease and the kidney. In Cameron J S, Davison A M, Grunfeld J-P & Ritz E (eds) *Oxford Textbook of Clinical Nephrology*. Oxford: Oxford University Press, 1992: 700–720.

40 Falk R J, Scheinman J, Phillips G, Orringer E, Johnson A & Jennette J C. Prevalence and pathologic features of sickle cell nephropathy and response to inhibition of angiotensin-converting enzyme. *N Engl J Med* 1992; 326:910–915.

41 McCoy R C. Ultrastructural alterations in the kidney of patients with sickle cell disease and the nephrotic syndrome. *Lab Invest* 1969; 21:85–95.

42 Adu D & Kibukamusoke J W. Acute renal failure in the tropics. In Kibukamusoke J W (ed.) *Tropical Nephrology*. Canberra: Citforge, 1984: 199–215.

43 Beaman M & Adu D. Acute renal failure. In Tinker J & Zapol W M (eds) *Care of the Critically Ill Patient*. Berlin: Springer, 1992: 515–532.

44 Chugh K S & Kjellstrand C M. The changing epidemiology of acute renal failure: patterns in economically advanced and developing countries. In Andreucci V E (ed.), Fine L G, Hatano M & Kjellstrand C M (co-eds) *International Yearbook of Nephrology*. Boston: Kluwer, 1989: 207–226.

45 Adu D, Anim-Addo Y, Foli A K, Yeboah E D, Quartey J K M & Riberio B F. Acute renal failure in tropical Africa. *BMJ* 1976; i:89–91.

46 Beaman M, Turney J H, Rodger R S C, McGonigle R S, Adu D & Michael J. Changing pattern of acute renal failure. *Q J Med* 1987; 237:15–23.

47 Yeboah E D. Acute retention of urine at Korle Bu Teaching Hospital. *Ghana Med J* 1980; 19:152–155.

48 Chugh K S, Singhal P C, Sharma B K et al. Acute renal failure of obstetric origin. *Obstet Gynecol* 1976; 48:642–646.

49 Chugh K S, Singhal P C, Sharma B K et al. Acute renal failure due to intravascular hemolysis in the North Indian patients. *Am J Med Sci* 1977; 274:139–146.

50 Owosu S K, Addy J H, Foli A K et al. Acute reversible renal failure associated with glucose-6-phosphate dehydrogenase deficiency. *Lancet* 1972; i:1255–1257.

51 Lwanga D & Wing A J. Renal complications associated with typhoid fever. *East Afr Med J* 1970; 47:146–152.

52 Adu D, Anim-Addo Y, Foli A K, Yeboah E D, Quartey J K M & Ribeiro B F. Acute renal failure and typhoid fever. *Ghana Med J* 1975; 4:172.

53 Boonpucknavig V & Sitprija V. Renal disease in acute *Plasmodium falciparum* infection in man. *Kidney Int* 1979; 16:44–52.

54 Sitprija V. Nephrology forum: nephropathy in falciparum malaria. *Kidney Int* 1988; 34:867–877.

55 Dukes D C, Sealey B J & Forbes J I. Oliguric renal failure in blackwater fever. *Am J Med* 1968; 45:899–903.

56 Canfield C J, Miller L H, Bastelloni P J, Eichler P & Barry K B. Acute renal failure in *Plasmodium falciparum* malaria. *Arch Intern Med* 1968; 122:199–203.

57 Chugh K S. Etiopathogenesis of acute renal failure in the Tropics. *Ann Natl Acad Med Sci (India)* 1987; 23:89–99.

58 Baker N M, Mills A F, Rachman I & Thomas J E P. Haemolytic uraemic syndrome in typhoid fever. *BMJ* 1974; ii:84–87.

59 Musa A M, Salch S Y & Abu Asha H. Transient nephritis during typhoid fever in five Sudanese patients. *Ann Trop Med Parasitol* 1981; 75:181–184.

60 Bhuyan U N, Srivastava R N & Choudhry V P. Pathology of acute renal failure and haemolytic uraemic syndrome in acute dysentery in children. *Indian J Med Res* 1985; 81:402–408.

61 Benyajati C, Keoplung M, Beisel W R, Gangarosa E J, Spring H & Sitprija V. Acute renal failure in Asiatic cholera: clinicopathological correlations with acute tubular necrosis and hypokalemic nephropathy. *Ann Intern Med* 1960; 52:960–975.

62 Sitprija V. Renal involvement in leptospirosis. In Robinson R R (ed.) *Tropical Nephrology*. New York: Springer, 1984: 1041–1052.

63 Sitprija V, Pipatanagul V, Mertowidjojo K, Boonpucknavig V & Boonpucknavig S. Pathogenesis of renal disease in leptospirosis: clinical and experimental studies. *Kidney Int* 1980; 17:827–836.

64 Shibolet S, Coll R, Gilat T & Sohar E. Heatstroke: its clinical picture and mechanism in 36 cases. *Q J Med* 1967; 36:525–548.

65 Weber D R, Douglass L E, Brundage W G & Stelkamp T C. Acute varieties of melioidosis occurring in US soldiers in Vietnam. *Am J Med* 1969; 46:234–244.

66 Susaengrat W, Dhiensiri T, Sinavatana P & Sitprija V. Renal failure in melioidosis. *Nephron* 1987; 46:167–169.

67 Chugh K S. Nephrology forum: snake bite induced acute renal failure in India. *Kidney Int* 1989; 35:891–907.

68 Chugh K S, Aikat B K, Sharma B K, Dash K C, Mathew M T & Das K C. Acute renal failure following snakebite. *Am J Trop Med Hyg* 1975; 24:692–697.

69 Lwin M, Warrell D A, Phillips R E, Swe T N, Pe T & Lay M M. Bites of Russell's viper (*Vipera russelli siamensis*) in Burma: haemostatic, vascular and renal disturbances and response to treatment. *Lancet* 1985; ii:1259–1264.

70 Karmali M A, Petric M, Lim C, Fleming P C, Arbus G & Lior H. The association between idiopathic haemolytic uraemic syndrome and infection by verotoxin-producing *E. coli*. *J Infect Dis* 1985; 151:775–782.

71 Raghupathy P, Date A, Shastry J C, Sudarsanam A & Jadhav M. Haemolytic–uraemic syndrome complicating shigella dysentery in south Indian children. *BMJ* 1978; i:1518–1521.

72 Kirubakaran M G. Renal disease in South India. In Kibukamusoke J W (ed.) *Tropical Nephrology*. Canberra: Citforge, 1984: 448–456.

73 Matekole M, Affram K, Lee S J, Howie A J, Michael J & Adu D. Hypertension and end-stage renal failure in tropical Africa. *J. Hum Hypertens* 1993; 7(5):443–446.

74 Suleiman A B. Renal disease in South-East Asia. In Kibukamusoke J W (ed.) *Tropical Nephrology*. Canberra: Citforge, 1984: 374–382.

75 Asmal A C & D'Elia J. Diabetic glomerulosclerosis in the tropics. In Kibukamusoke J W (ed.) *Tropical Nephrology*. Canberra: Citforge, 1984: 237–256.

76 Brenner B M, Meyer T W & Hostetter T H. Dietary protein intake and the progressive nature of kidney disease: the role of haemodynamically mediated glomerular injury in the pathogenesis of progressive glomerular sclerosis in aging, renal ablation and intrinsic renal disease. *N Engl J Med* 1982; 307:652–659.

77 Reichel H, Drüeke T & Ritz E. Bony complications in chronic renal failure. In Cameron J S, Davison A M, Grunfeld J-P & Ritz E (eds) *Oxford Textbook of Clinical Nephrology*. Oxford: Oxford University Press, 1992: 1365–1389.

78 Maher J F. *Replacement of Renal Function by Dialysis: A Textbook of Dialysis*, 3rd edn. Boston: Kluwer, 1989.

79 Halim A & Gow J G. Genitourinary tuberculosis. In Husain I (ed.) *Tropical Urology and Renal Disease*. Edinburgh: Churchill Livingstone, 1984: 118–140.

80 Robertson W G. Urolithiasis: epidemiology and pathogenesis. In Husain I (ed.) *Tropical Urology and Renal Disease*. Edinburgh: Churchill Livingstone, 1984: 143–164.

81 Wallace D M & Husain I. Bilharziasis: the kidney and ureter. In Husain I (ed.) *Tropical Urology and Renal Disease*. Edinburgh: Churchill Livingstone, 1984: 237–260.

CHAPTER 8

TROPICAL NEUROLOGY

Ra'ad A. Shakir and Gerald M. Stern

Applying equally to other chapters in this book is the problem of a comprehensive yet pragmatic definition of tropical medicine—for which there appears to be no simple resolution. Even the nineteenth century rubric—those diseases which prevail between the tropics of Cancer and Capricorn—was unsatisfactory because illnesses such as cholera, typhoid, typhus and malaria occurred widely in Europe until the beginning of the twentieth century. Now, when speed and facility of travel can dramatically influence presentation of disease, definitions must be appropriately elastic. No doubt controversy will continue concerning a more suitable, precise and contemporary name for this specialty. Maurice King's term 'the medicine of poverty' is probably as succinct as can be presently contrived—to embrace afflictions arising from primitive social conditions, malnutrition, high population growths, ignorance of 'overly traditional societies', high infant mortality rates and low life expectation, all fundamentally determined by major factors beyond the powers of physicians; only the economist, engineer, agriculturalist and those who can alter the distribution of global wealth can make a significant impact.

Tropical neurology is of course not limited to bizarre manifestations of viral, bacterial and parasitic infections, but also reflects the expression of many non-infectious diseases in a particular environment where malnutrition, trauma, perinatal injury and cerebrovascular and degenerative diseases tend to show patterns of nineteenth century Western proportions; 'younger' societies may show different disease distributions. These are among the many factors that must be taken into consideration when assessing and comparing epidemiological surveys. Consider, for example, epilepsy: this is a major neurological disorder in the tropics and has important medical and social implications.[1] Attempts to determine accurately the magnitude of the problem have encountered considerable difficulties, including differences in definition and methods of case detection. It is therefore difficult to determine what significance should be attributed to the reported relatively low prevalence in India and the fact that certain regions of Africa and Latin America have a

very high prevalence, sometimes as much as ten times the average for industrialized countries. It would appear that rural prevalence is lower than in urban areas, partial seizures more common than primary generalized ones and mortality rates for epilepsy appear to be higher in tropical countries in comparison to those in industrialized areas. Known aetiological factors present a bewildering spectrum.[2] Cysticercosis accounts for about half the cases of epilepsy of late onset in several countries. Other parasitic infections known to cause epilepsy include: schistosomiasis, paragonimiasis, sparganosis, hydatid disease, toxoplasmosis, trypanosomiasis, cerebral malaria and cerebral amoebiasis. Tuberculous, pyogenic, viral and fungal infections can also cause epilepsy as a late sequel as well as being a feature of the acute illness. Poor antenatal and perinatal care resulting in perinatal brain damage probably contributes to a higher prevalence. Despite these problems there have been impressive attempts to sharpen the epidemiological profile of epilepsy. Thus a recent survey[3] of a rural Tanzanian population showed a prevalence of 11.4 per thousand in a population of 18 183. It was possible to study 203 of these in detail: 32.5% had partial seizures, 85.2% tonic–clonic ones and 8.4% had unclassifiable fits; 95% initially sought aid from outside the immediate family—a traditional healer, a priest—and 80% had consulted traditional healers. Fewer than 20% of the patients were receiving regular anticonvulsants. The authors stress the importance of improving patient attitudes, and in particular, acceptance of anticonvulsant therapy.

The crucial conditions largely determining the prevalence of this group of illnesses show no sign of improvement: most are worsening. In 1990 the population of India was 850 000 000, second only to China's 1 134 000 000, and by the year 2000 the Indian total will be 1 043 000 000, rising to 1 513 000 000 in the year 2025. Global figures are equally distressing.[4,5] Today the world population is close to 5.6 billion, and by the year 2050 is likely to exceed 10 billion. 'The growth of the earth's population has been like a long thin powder fuse that burns slowly and haltingly until it finally reaches the charge and explodes' (Kingsley Davis). To this potential explosion must be added the impact of global environmental change[6] on disease patterns.[7] Thus the effects of global warming on the distribution of parasitic and other infectious diseases– disequilibrium in physical and biological eco-systems—and the potential impact of climate changes on world food supply indicate that the developing countries are likely to bear the brunt of the problem. The disparity between developed and developing countries may become even more conspicuous. Famine is as old as humanity and 'tropical diseases' and their neurological complications are likely to increase.

NUTRITIONAL AND TOXIC FACTORS

The clinical features of the major classical nutritional disorders of the central and peripheral nervous systems are well known, as is the importance of the vitamin B complex for the development and functioning of the nervous system. Thus beriberi ('I can't, I can't', depicting profound weakness), usually due to the discarded germinal layer of polished rice, presents clinically in the wet or dry form: the salient neurological features are painful polyneuropathy with tender calves and sensitive soles. Pellagra, due to a similar dietary deficiency mainly involving the nicotinic acid obtained in white maize presents clinically—often in endemic spring attacks—with diarrhoea, a light-sensitive erythematous rash progressing to thickening and atrophy with glossitis, diplopia, dysarthria, myelopathy and neuropathy with psychological and behavioural changes. Wernicke's encephalopathy may be acute or insidious, with vomiting, nystagmus, diplopia, confusion, ophthalmoplegia, retinal haemorrhages, polyneuropathy, and a dramatic Korsakoff's syndrome with amnesia and confabulation. However, it will be appreciated that even in communities known to be thiamine deficient from the consumption of processed rice, or in maize-eating populations known to be vulnerable to pellagra from niacin deficiency, it is common to see the consequences of the lack of thiamine, pyridoxine and niacin and perhaps also pantothenic acid in combination necessitating appropriate blunderbuss therapy.

It will also be appreciated that there are numerous local and usually well-recognized (yet to appear in classical textbooks) nutritional syndromes. For example, among certain hill tribes in north-east Burma it is traditional for women to consume only polished rice while pregnant; their infants may develop an unusual pattern of beriberi with congestive heart failure, hepatosplenomegaly and aphonia due to bilateral recurrent laryngeal nerve lesions which respond promptly to parenteral pyridoxine. Strachan's syndrome (visual failure, painful neuropathy and oral, perianal and scrotal dermatitis and ulcer-ation) has been described in several parts of the world and is another probable consequence of multiple nutritional deficiencies including riboflavin, thiamine, niacin and pyridoxine. The painful burning feet described in prisoner-of-war camps was probably another example of multiple nutritional deficiency.

Clinically and epidemiologically it is often difficult to separate the consequences of nutritional deficiency from environmental toxins because they tend to occur in similar settings and the manifestations may be indistinguishable. The problem is further compounded by the increasing quantities of chemicals, often indiscriminately used in industry and agriculture as well as medicine. Toxic pesticides merit particular attention and many of the hazards arise from the lack of precautions and facilities for handling and storing these neurotoxic products safely.

The peripheral nervous system is commonly affected and has been frequently studied because it is easier to recognize clinically and to investigate electrodiagnostically and by nerve biopsy. While the pathophysiology may vary according to the putative toxin, distal axonal degeneration—so-called 'dying back' phenomenon[8]—is the most common mechanism; initially, longer or larger nerve fibres are involved, then degeneration begins in the distal regions of the nerve fibres, progressing proximally with time. However, mechanisms are probably more complex: experimental evidence suggests that many toxic agents act at the level of the axon rather than the cell body,[9] impairing axonal transport; others may disturb anabolic mechanisms in the region of the neuronal perikaryon. Whatever the precise mechanism, clinical features are similar. Early symptoms are usually sensory with paraesthesiae, suprasensitivity, hyperalgesia and pain, followed later by peripheral weakness and wasting. Impairment of tendon reflexes occurs early and all sensory modalities may be variably affected. Some have associated myelopathic disturbances with spasticity and extensor plantar responses. Involvement of the autonomic nervous system with defective sweating and vasomotor disturbances commonly occurs.

The list of known agents is legion. Heavy metals such as arsenic, lead and thallium are often found in traditional folklore medications.[10] For example, arsenical polyneuropathy (acute, or more commonly chronic) occurs very widely. Acute symptoms may include: vomiting, diarrhoea, burning discomfort in the eyes, excessive tears, photophobia, congestion and facial swelling, followed by a predominantly sensory neuropathy. Mees' lines (transverse white bands across the finger-nails) frequently occur, as does increased pigmentation of the extremities with patches of depigmentation, hyperkeratosis and descemation of palms and soles. Here the diagnosis may be confirmed, if facilities permit, by demonstrating high concentrations of arsenic in scalp hairs and nail clippings. Illicit liquor, crude arbortifacients and well water deliberately contaminated by an enemy have all been reported.[11] It will also be recalled that certain ocean fish and marine crustacea, such as the pomfret, plaice, halua and hilsa, may contain relatively high concentrations of arsenic. Another source of arsenical poisoning is said to be contaminated opium. The mechanism is thought to be direct reaction of arsenical compounds with the sulphhydryl group of proteins; electrophysiologically the signs of distal axonal degeneration and nerve biopsies show loss of myelinated fibres and degeneration of myelin into rows of myelin ovoids;[12] segmental demyelination and inflammatory changes do not occur. In the acute stages dimercaprol and/or penicillamine must be given early; when there is a delay, response may be poor.

Lead may to cause a peripheral neuropathy in adults and an encephalopathy in children. Lead neuropathy tends to be predominantly motor, more evident in the upper limbs where the extensors of the wrists and fingers are affected early and asymmetrically, tending to affect the dominant hand.[13] Proximal involvement is slow and occurs later, and sensory disturbances are minimal or absent. Associated abdominal colic and the characteristic anaemia with punctate basophilia, when present, may suggest the diagnosis. Potential sources include reconditioning of car batteries and burning lead-containing batteries for cooking, illicit liquor distillation by means of lead pipes or radiators, and contaminated water.

Thallium may be a constituent of rodenticides. The acute painful neuropathy may be associated with gastrointestinal symptoms—non-specific signs—but the occurrence of alopecia within 3 weeks should suggest the diagnosis.[14] Potassium ferro-cyanide, given orally is the present treatment of choice.

Of the many conventional medications that may provoke peripheral neuropathy brief mention will be made of those drugs widely used in the treatment of tropical bacterial and parasitic infections. Peripheral neuropathy, particularly in those genetically disposed to slow acetylation of isoniazid for the treatment of tuberculosis, is well known, as is the similar hazard of ethionamide, from sulphonamides widely used in bacillary dysentery and urinary tract infections; similarly the optic neuritis related to ethambutol. Chloroquine, a standard antimalarial agent, may produce a neuromyopathy after prolonged use, with muscle fibres showing vacuolation and peripheral nerves showing involvement of terminal axons with Schwann cell defects.[15] Clioquinol—previously widely used in the symptomatic treatment of diarrhoea and intestinal amoebiasis is now known to be the causative agent of subacute myelo-optic neuropathy;[16] unfortunately clioquinol continues to be prescribed in certain countries and the complication is still sporadically encountered. The aromatic diamidines used in the treatment of leishmaniasis and trypanosomiasis have been associated with an odd, uncommon focal disturbance of sensory function of the trigeminal nerve.

Industrial chemicals of known potential neurotoxicity rarely cause hazards in developed societies; it is where appropriate safety measures and conditions are not practised that outbreaks continue to occur. Well known is·trio-ortho-creasyl phosphate; commonly used as an industrial solvent, it has been the culprit in many reported outbreaks.[17] Accidental contamination of food, particularly edible oils, may produce not only classical peripheral mixed neuropathy, but also signs of cord involvement. Unfortunately, the damage is permanent and there is no curative or generally available protective agent. In unprotected environments, carbon disulphide and acrylamide may produce similar hazards. Insecticides widely dispensed in tropical countries are a common cause. The most common culprit is the group of organophosphorous insecticides; the defect is believed to be mainly at the postsynaptic border of the neuromuscular junction. Clinically the onset may be acute or delayed.

Particularly well documented in recent years are the toxic effects of the root crop cassava, a major crop sustaining millions of people in Africa.[18] Flour made from cassava roots may contain a high concentration of linamarin, a cyanogenic glycoside, resulting in chronic cyanide intoxication and clinically 'tropical ataxic neuropathy'. The clinical features in addition to painful neuropathy and ataxia may include blurred vision and impaired hearing of cochlear type; occasionally upper motor neurone lesions are seen. This pattern of illness is usually slowly progressive.

Konzo is a clinically distinct pattern of tropical myelopathy because of its abrupt onset and dominant upper motor neurone pattern of involvement.[19] A recent study in rural Zaire[20] was able to determine the cyanergine content of the locally used cassava flour and blood cyanide concentrations in cases and controls. This detailed study indicated that not only was there a significant sustained high blood cyanide concentration, but also that the deficient sulphur intake impaired the conversion of cyanide to thiocyanate. Even though the immediate causes are poverty and shortage of food, a relatively minor change in traditional cooking habits could prevent much disability.

Lathyrism and cycad poisoning are two other well-known examples of neurotoxic plant poisons affecting the central nervous system. Lathyrism, endemic in parts of India, Bangladesh and Ethiopia, is caused by excessive consumption of peas of the lathyrus family (chickling peas). It presents as a slowly progressive spastic paraparesis: neuropathological studies have shown selective atrophy of the pyramidal, spinocerebellar and dorsal columns of the spinal cord. The neurotoxin is an amino acid, β-N-oxalylamino-L-alanine, which is thought to act by excessive and prolonged exhaustion stimulation—a

so-called excitatory amino acid. Once damage has occurred there is no effective treatment. In a similar manner excessive consumption of the seed of the false-sago palm—either as a foodstuff or as a medicinal component—may have an excitatory neurotoxic effect and may be one of the constellation of factors responsible for the occurrence of amyotrophic lateral sclerosis and parkinsonism–dementia complex in the Pacific Mariana Islands.[21]

Rarer plant toxins include that of *Gloriosa superba* (glory lily):[22] accidental ingestion may cause alopecia, aplastic anaemia and polyneuropathy due to colchicine which impairs exoplasmic transport in peripheral nerves and also damages skeletal muscle. Podophyllin (from the dried rhizome and root of the mandrake) also has neurotoxic properties. A recent report from Hong Kong[23] described encephalopathy and sensory–motor polyneuropathy and autonomic changes after ingestion of a broth containing herbal guyjiu. Another poisonous shrub of the buckthorn family (*Karwinskia humboldtiana*), which grows freely in Mexico and Texas, may cause a progressive polyneuropathy, terminating in respiratory and bulbar paralysis.[24]

All these essentially irreversible and disabling toxic disturbances of the central autonomic and peripheral nervous systems are preventable and presumably will continue to be observed and reported in the developing world until nutritional, economic and educational disparities are resolved.

INFECTIONS

The variety of infectious agents which can damage the nervous system is vast and their clinical manifestations are protean. In addition to the general predisposing factors mentioned above—poverty, ignorance, deprivation, inadequate education—is the prevalence and persistence of insect and other vectors which thrive in humid climates and which survive throughout the seasons. In a limited review it is possible to indicate only certain salient clinical features of some of these numerous disorders which will be discussed under conventional categories.

VIRUSES (See also Chapters 12, 30, 33 and 38)

The acute exanthemas of childhood—measles, mumps and chickenpox—are still major killers, especially when epidemics occur in the presence of

severe malnutrition. The clinical scene and the therapeutic possibilities have changed considerably in recent years. Thus acute poliomyelitis (see below) is now rarely seen: an impressive example of the power of truly effective preventive medicine. Similarly subacute sclerosing panencephalitis (SSPE) is disappearing in many parts of the world where measles vaccination is available, but is still prevalent and fatal in many parts of the Middle East, Far East, India, Africa and South America; the eradication of measles should greatly diminish the incidence of SSPE. There are conflicting reports on its pathogenesis and management.[25,26] Several authors have reported the use of intraventricular interferon-α or the combined use of interferon-α plus isoprinosin.[27]

Acute viral encephalitis—due to direct invasion of the brain parenchyma—is indistinguishable clinically from the postinfectious encephalitides where perivenous demyelination is probably triggered by

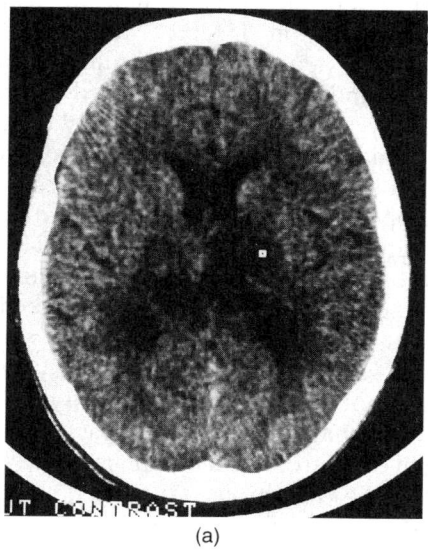
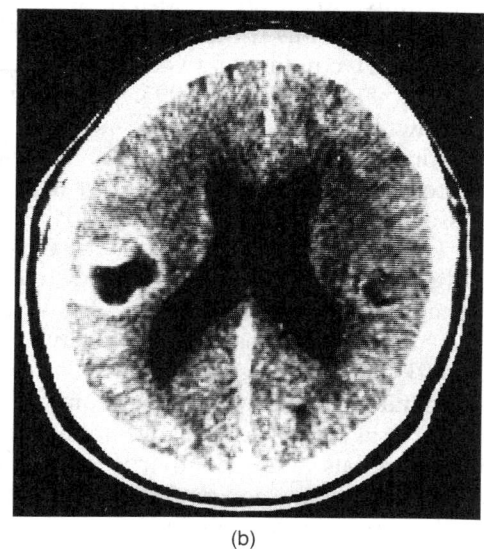

(a)   (b)

Figure 8.1   Japanese encephalitis. Brain scan (a) before and (b) after contrast showing thalamic lesions. (Courtesy of M. Gourie-Devi, National Institute of Mental Health and Neurosciences, Bangalore, India.)

allergic or immune reactions caused by a latent viral infection. Globally, viruses are by far the most common cause of encephalitis. The arboviruses cause epidemic encephalitides in many parts of the world. The majority are perpetuated by zoonoses, often inconspicuous infections obtained from birds and smaller vertebrates; transmission is by an arthropod vector such as a mosquito or tick. After replication and viraemia, encephalitis of unpredictable gravity develops. Many patients recover spontaneously after a mild attack; others may deteriorate and die within days or weeks. The clinical features are common to all: prodromal myalgia, fever and malaise, then headache, mental changes, drowsiness, with or without signs of meningeal irritation; focal neurological abnormalities such as disturbances of behaviour, mood, disorientation, deterioration of speech, level of consciousness, fits (focal or generalized), raised intracranial pressure and a deepening coma. Even when sophisticated diagnostic neuroimaging techniques such as computerized tomography (CT) or magnetic resonance imaging (MRI) are available, there may be no specific features and the EEG and cerebrospinal fluid (CSF) may not be diagnostically helpful. The demonstration of sequential changes in antibody titre in samples of serum or CSF may be the only means of establishing the true agent in sporadic cases and usually the illness has taken its course by the time the agent is confirmed.

Eastern equine encephalitis—mainly on the Atlantic and Gulf coasts of America—tends to occur in summer and autumn and the mortality may be as high as 70%;[28] *Western equine encephalitis*, which despite its name occurs throughout the USA and eastern South America, tends to be less severe.

Japanese encephalitis is a mosquito-borne arboviral infection which still claims many lives in South-East Asia. The virus is antigenically related to the flaviviruses of St Louis encephalitis and Murray Valley encephalitis and to the West Nile virus. The illness is usually severe, and fatal in about 25% of cases, with neuropsychiatric sequelae in a further 30%. It mainly affects the young, but a shift now to the elderly may be due to early immunization. CT and MRI show thalamic involvement (Figure 8.1). An inactivated Japanese encephalitis virus vaccine is now available and its use should reduce the incidence in due course.[29] Sporadic and epidemic attacks of encephalitis continue to be reported from different parts of the world and often the reasons for these fluctuations remain obscure. For example, Rift Valley fever has recently been recorded in Egypt after an absence of over 12 years. In 1993, patients began to complain of a febrile illness with headaches, retro-orbital pain, nausea, vomiting and loss of vision with or without features of a generalized encephalitis.[30] In this pattern of illness a reasonably firm clinical diagnosis can be made because of the frequent finding of macular and paramacular retinal lesions, often with haemorrhage and oedema, occurring at a time when there has been an abnormally high number of abortions in cattle and buffalo, but the true reason(s) for the recurrence remain cryptic.

Poliomyelitis. New infections are now uncommon and it is realistic to anticipate worldwide eradication by the end of the millenium. In 1992, 15 445 cases of paralytic poliomyelitis were reported, compared with 32 419 in 1988. Thus China (about 20% of the world population) conducted two national vaccination days in December of 1993, targeting all children below 4 years—the largest public health event in history. No indigenous wild poliovirus cases were reported in the USA,[31] England or Wales.[32] Vaccine-associated paralytic poliomyelitis is the prominent form of the disease not only in Western countries, but also in the developing world. In those vaccine-related cases reported in the USA there were three high-risk groups: infants receiving the first oral polio vaccine dose, unvaccinated or inadequately vaccinated adults who are in contact with receipients of oral polio vaccine, and immunocompromised individuals. Wild poliovirus causing disease is still a problem in small pockets of individuals in western Europe who for religious reasons refuse vaccination, as exemplified by the 1992 outbreak in Holland. While apparent outbreaks are still reported worldwide[33,34] it is imperative to separate paralytic poliomyelitis from other causes of paralysis in infancy.

Dengue, especially the haemorrhagic variety, still causes considerable morbidity and fatality in South-East Asia, and yellow fever similarly in Africa and South America.

Lassa fever, an acute haemorrhagic febrile illness occurring in West Africa, carries a fatality of up to 20%. It is caused by an arenavirus spread by a rodent (*Mastomys natalensis*) and causes a wide spectrum of clinical disease, from asymptomatic or trivial malaise to fatal illness, and is often associated with neurological manifestations during the acute disease or in early convalescence. Delirium, convulsions and coma occur in critically ill patients; deafness may occur towards the end of an acute illness and is believed to be the result of cochlear nerve damage. A recent paper[35] emphasizes the importance of metabolic encephalopathy, severe tremor, self-limiting encephalitis, late ataxia and subacute or chronic neuropsychiatric sequelae.

Rabies remains endemic throughout the world[36] except for the UK, Australasia, the Caribbean and Scandinavia. In Indonesia about 700 000 people are treated for exposure to the virus each year and worldwide more than one million receive rabies vaccine annually. No patient has survived the established disease. Whereas vaccines derived from cell cultures are now much safer and more effective than animal-derived preparations,[37] sadly the vast majority of human exposure to rabies occurs in developing countries, most of whom cannot afford cell culture vaccines. The majority will have access only to vaccines derived from animal neural tissue, which unfortunately may result in a disabling immune response. Reports of such neurological complications range from 1:1200[38] to 1:120.[39] Consequently many people in developing countries who are bitten and potentially exposed to rabies will deliberately avoid vaccination, fully aware of the possible hazards. Attempts to control the animal reservoir of rabies have not been successful and even in developed countries wildlife reservoirs affecting racoons and foxes still persist. The need for low-cost safe rabies vaccines equally acceptable in the developed and developing world remains a technological challenge.

Human immunodeficiency virus (HIV) infection is causing major morbidity and mortality in Africa and there is a similar trend in South-East Asia. The vast spectrum of neurological complications,[40] including opportunistic infections, tumours, neurological, manifestations attributed to HIV, from muscle disease through peripheral nerve, myelopathy, radiculopathy, meningitis and encephalopathy and other complications, cannot be adequately covered in a short review. Since the early months of 1981, when five young homosexuals in the Los Angeles area developed *Pneumocystis carinii* pneumonia, the gradual awareness of this syndrome and its complications in acquired immune deficiency states, the emergence of associated problems such as drug-resistant pulmonary tuberculosis and multiple infections such as tubercle and toxoplasmosis, have presented challenging diagnostic problems and dilemmas to physicians throughout the world, the successful management of each crisis only delaying the inevitable fatal outcome.

A recent discovery concerns the related *human T lymphotropic virus (HTLV)-I* which may be responsible for certain patterns of chronic myelopathy seen in the tropics, separating this group of illnesses from the tropical paraparesis and ataxic neuropathic group. HTLV-I-associated myelopathy was first described in the Caribbean[41] and Japan, and is also found in many parts of Africa.[42] Previously described under many guises, including tropical paraparesis and ataxic neuropathy,[43] its relation to adult T-cell leukaemia and clinical progress is now well established.[44]

HTLV-I-associated myelopathy/tropical spastic paraplegia (HAM/TSP) is a condition which appears in the fifth decade as a slowly progressive spastic paraparesis. There is usually sphincter involvement with some sensory changes. HTLV-I specific uveitis can present acutely or subacutely with vitreous opacities, mild iritis and retinal vasculitis.[45] There may be some mild pleocytosis with raised IgG and positive oligoclonal bands on a CSF study. HTLV-I specific cytotoxic T lymphocytes were isolated in the CSF of HAM/TSP patients.[46]

The transmission of HTLV-I virus is reported to be through infected T lymphocytes (this can occur sexually), through blood transfusions, or vertically from mother to infant through milk.[47]

HAM/TSP has been reported not only in the tropics but in immigrants in Europe and the USA[48] and needs to be differentiated from multiple sclerosis,[49] subacute combined degeneration, syphilis and Behçet's disease. The neuroimaging of patients with TSP/HAM shows normal myelography and periventricular low density with ventricular enlargement on brain CT; MRI shows high-intensity signals in the periventricular and subcortical white matter. Features of spinal cord atrophy have been described.[50] HTLV-II is a close relative of HTLV-I—structurally similar but molecularly distinct—and has been associated with chronic spastic paraparesis and high titres of HTLV-II antibodies in the serum and CSF.

Clearly the full spectrum of human illnesses due to this family of retroviruses is yet to be determined. All human retroviruses studied to date have been lymphotropic; whether they will all prove to cause disease of the nervous system remains to be elucidated. From the clinical point of view, presentations may be multiple; toxoplasmosis, lymphoma, progressive leucoencephalopathy and HIV encephalopathy may all overlap in the same individual. Thus multiple focal brain lesions may be due to the simultaneous development of lymphoma, toxoplasma abscesses or tuberculosis. Opportunistic infections, including parasites, fungi, bacteria as well as viruses, may cause diagnostic difficulties of unparalleled complexity.

RICKETTSIA (See also Chapter 39)

This group of illnesses,[51] which usually present as an acute meningoencephalitis, are transmitted to man by the bites of ticks or mites and occur throughout the world except in Antarctica. Mediterranean spotted fever (*Rickettsia conorii*) in Africa, Asia and the Mediterranean basin,[52] scrub typhus (*R. tsutsugamushi*) in Asia and the Pacific, typhus (*R. prowazekii*) and Q fever (*Coxiella burnetii*) are ubiquitous. Whereas the incubation period and clinical features vary between organisms, all patients manifest high fever, rash and headache, with meningoencephalitis developing during the second week of the illness.[53] Non-focal neurological features include: headache, neck stiffness and photophobia, confusion, impairment of consciousness and fits. When present, the distinctive eschar at the site of the bite may suggest the diagnosis. CSF examination is rarely helpful and treatment should be started on clinical suspicion.

The response to tetracycline or chloramphenicol is usually gratifying.

BACTERIAL INFECTIONS (See also Chapters 44, 45, 55, 57 and 58)

Bacterial meningitis in infants, children and adults remains a serious cause of morbidity and mortality.[54] Early recognition followed by prompt, appropriate and effective antibiotics is not available in many parts of the world. As vaccination is not yet comprehensively effective and not generally available this heavy burden of preventable and treatable disease will continue for the predictable future. With the exception of the neonatal period, *Haemophilus influenzae*, *Neisseria meningitidis* and *Streptococcus pneumoniae* still account for about 70% of all cases; neonatal meningitis may be caused by almost any organism and the most frequently encountered pathogens are Gram-negative bacilli, particularly *Escherichia coli* and other enteric bacilli, *Pseudomonas* and group B streptococci.[55] In the elderly, Gram-negative bacilli and *Listeria* spp. should be considered. Confirmatory CSF examination should not delay treatment. In the search for an early appropriate antibiotic in a high-incidence part of Africa, long-acting chloramphenicol injections were found to be as effective as four times a day ampicillin for 8 days.

Tuberculous involvement of the nervous system remains common, and despite the now worldwide availability of effective antituberculous therapy the classical syndromes—spinal cord compression from tuberculous osteitis, tuberculous meningitis, and intracranial tuberculomas—continue to cause significant morbidity and mortality.[56,57] As far as tuberculous osteitis is concerned it is important to appreciate that this may occur at any spinal level and is not restricted to the dorsal vertebrae; whereas in the early stages of the granulomatous process involving adjacent vertebrae and the intervening disc the cord is usually compressed anteriorly, this is not invariably so. There may be one or more posterior compressive lesions arising from tuberculous osteitis in the laminae and pedicles, and epidural tuberculomas can easily be confused with epidural tumours and other focal pathologies.

Much has been written concerning the difficulties of interpreting CSF findings in early tuberculous disease. It should be stressed that some patients with miliary tuberculosis or tuberculomas of the central nervous system may initially have an entirely normal CSF. On other occasions a marked polymorphonuclear response may be seen with a dominant eosinophilic reaction—only later changing to the more classical findings. While a significant reduction of CSF sugar content compared with a synchronous plasma level may be helpful in the diagnosis of tuberculous meningitis, the diagnosis should not be discarded because the CSF glucose remains within normal limits. Despite access to the most sophisticated diagnostic facilities it is still often necessary to embark upon antituberculous therapy on the grounds of clinical suspicion without confirmatory diagnostic support. It may be hazardous to wait until serial investigation confirms or refutes the diagnosis. Perhaps the use of polymerase chain reaction techniques will answer some of the questions.[58] The technique is more specific than CSF enzyme linked immunosorbent assay (ELISA) but false positives, in addition to the complexity of the technique, make it impractical for worldwide use.

Intracranial tuberculoma—single or multiple—remains the most common cause of a space occupying lesion in many parts of the world. CT facilities are now more widespread and the most common finding is a hypodense lesion on an unenhanced scan with a ring or disc-like enhancement with contrast and surrounding hypodensity. Where tuberculosis is common, physicians frequently promptly embark on a course of antituberculous therapy without histological verification. After 3 months of treatment a repeat brain scan will show clearing of the lesion. While there are regional differences in the optimal combination of antituberculous drugs, chemotherapy is usually given for 6–12 months, depending upon the severity of the disease and response to treatment; corticosteroids are not given routinely, but dexamethasone in high doses during the acute phase of raised pressure may be helpful in reducing cerebral oedema. Obstructive hydrocephalus may develop at any stage of the illness, sometimes acutely; it is the most likely explanation for sudden neurological deterioration and should be treated promptly by surgical drainage.

Leprosy remains by far the most common cause of chronic mononeuritis multiplex in the world.[59,60] The World Health Organization currently estimates that there are 5.5 million patients with leprosy worldwide, a fall of about 50% since the 1980s. Nevertheless, despite much publicity and public health measures, the disease is frequently overlooked or misdiagnosed, often neglected and still generally feared. Thus the extent of the illness in a community may be difficult to estimate, but all reasonable attempts to do so indicate that, despite the availability of effective treatments, prevalence throughout the world is essentially unaltered. It remains true[61] that: 'leprosy should be considered whenever confronted by a chronic and symptomless skin rash that does not correspond with a common dermatosis or which does not respond to standard treatment for similar lesions. Leprosy should be considered in all cases of transient, recurrent or persistent numbness of paraesthesiae especially when this is localized to a more or less well-defined area of skin.' Hypopigmentation, with impaired sensitivity to light touch and pinprick, and particularly focal impairment or absence of sweating, should strongly suggest the diagnosis and a careful search should be made for thickening of peripheral nerves. Most commonly palpable are the great auricular nerve in the neck, the ulnar nerve just above the medial epicondyle, the median nerve at the wrist, the lateral popliteal nerve below the head of the fibula and the sural nerve on the dorsum of the foot. Early thickening may be difficult to clinch. Trained paramedical staff often become expert in detecting and confirming the presence of leprosy in suspects. Even those with advanced disease, severe neuropathy, deformity and incapacity may be helped by skilled reconstructive surgery.

Brucellosis occurs in many tropical and subtropical areas and the nervous system may be affected in up to 5% of patients in a variety of ways.[62] It can cause an acute meningoencephalitis with papilloedema, convulsions and coma. Spinal presentation is with spastic or flaccid paraparesis due to cord compression or myeloradiculopathy, and central involvement with hemiparesis and ataxia. Diagnosis depends on blood or CSF culture of brucella, or more commonly on ELISA of the blood and CSF.[63] Treatment with rifampicin, tetracycline and streptomycin should be for 3 months in those presenting with the subacute or chronic forms.

Spirochaetes. Neurosyphilis is again on the march and is increasingly occurring in the wake of HIV infection. The old clinical adage remains true—'to know all the manifestations of syphilis is to know the whole of medicine'—but even here there are new twists to perplex even experienced physicians. When a young and apparently otherwise healthy male presents with acute onset of unilateral neural deafness, who would immediately suspect secondary syphilis? Other frequently occurring spirochaetal infections affecting the nervous system include borreliosis or relapsing fever (*Borrelia recurrentis*—louse borne; *B. duttonii*—tick borne), usually presenting as a febrile meningoencephalitis. Leptospirosis may affect any part of the nervous system, including an acute neuropathy.[64] Lyme disease (*B. burgdorferi*) is spread to man by infected ticks. While there is a very extensive literature[65] on its diverse neurological and systemic manifestations—now recognized as the leading vector-borne disease in the USA—this malady occurs mainly in temperate climates. The neural manifestations span from meningitis, encephalitis, focal cranial neuropathies, radiculitis neuropathy, encephalopathy and post-borreliosis syndromes.

PROTOZOA (See also Chapters 61, 63, 64, 67 and 68)

Plasmodium falciparum. The problems of malaria, which continues to kill 2 million children a year, with increasing death rates as the organism becomes increasingly resistant to conventional antimalarial agents,[66] are considered in detail elsewhere in this book. From the neurological aspect it remains important to stress that cerebral malaria, even when treated in research centres, still carries a mortality rate of up with to 40% with about a 10% risk of neurological sequelae[67] and all the auguries suggest that the situation will probably deteriorate further. Over 50% of deaths from cerebral malaria occur 12 hours or more after the initiation of treatment, emphasizing the importance of skilled supportive care in seizure prevention and management of raised intracranial pressure and lactic acidosis. Hypoglycaemia is an important event in cerebral malaria[68] and may well contribute to coma and neurological sequelae. The cause of the hypoglycaemia is probably multifactorial; malabsorption of glucose, parasite consumption and possibly hyperinsulinaemia resulting from the administration of quinine. Cerebral malaria continues to take its terrible toll. An effective and practical vaccine is still urgently required[69] and it is encouraging that the World Health Organization has earmarked development of potential vaccines and five *P. falciparum* antigens from different stages of the parasite life cycle. A minor but poorly recognized clinical point: *P. falciparum* can cause polymyositis[70] with muscle pain and weakness, probably due to increased blood viscosity, obstruction of capillaries with agglutinated red cells and intravascular coagulation causing muscle necrosis with myoglobinuria. Thus to the list of manifestations of 'malaria the mimic' should be added myositis.

Trypanosomiasis. African trypanosomiasis produces progressive central nervous system damage which if untreated results in death. Involvement occurs within a few weeks in the case of *Trypanosoma rhodesiense*, but usually takes much longer in the case of *T. gambiense*—months or even years. Leptomeningitis with distended ventricles, demyelination and perivascular cuffing develops and trypanosomes aggregate in the choroid plexus with an eosinophilic CSF reaction. In experimental studies trypanosomes shelter in the ependymal cells. It is also suggested that after clearing the parasite from outside the central nervous system with chemotherapy there may be an immune-mediated reaction against the intracellular parasite from outside the central nervous system and this may explain the encephalopathy noted with melarsoprol use and its prevention with steroids. Early clinical symptoms are those of an encephalopathy—with lassitude, sleepiness, walking difficulty, ataxia, tremor, dysarthria and back and neck stiffness; headaches and papilloedema may also occur. The CSF is usually under pressure, with high protein and pleocystosis and the appearance of a modified plasma cell containing a large eosinophilic inclusion of IgG (morular or Mott cells). Therapy for African trypanosomiasis has been transformed by the introduction of eflornithine,[71] which is best given intravenously and has been shown to be effective in late stages of the disease when the CNS is involved, which is not the case with pentamidine and suramin. The problems of early diagnosis and introduction of cheap, safe and effective therapy before irreversible cerebral damage occurs are immense; meanwhile the prognosis for established sleeping sickness must remain grim.

Chagas' disease (American trypanosomiasis) remains a major cause of morbidity and mortality in developing countries; the myocardium is usually heavily parasitized, frequently associated with complicated cardiac arrhythmias and presenting clinically with syncope. American trypanosomiasis caused by *T. cruzi* can involve the nervous system in the acute stage with trypanosomes in the CSF.[72] In its chronic stage enlargement of hollow organs is the diagnostic hallmark. Myositis and neuritis due to demyelination and axonal degeneration with remyelination and regeneration have been described.[73] Recent reports of the occurrence of acute Chagas' disease in patients with the acquired immune deficiency syndrome (AIDS) are usually due to reactivation of chronic or dormant infection. Fatal meningoencephalitis in patients with AIDS, as well as other causes of depressed immunity, are well recognized.[74]

Amoebiasis. Amoebic cerebral abscesses, although uncommon, have been recognized since 1849[75] and, providing the possibility of *Entamoeba histolytica* is considered early, the response to can be impressive a 5-nitroimidazole compound. *E. histolytica* can cause single or multiple cerebral abscesses which are noted on CT and may be clinically silent. Granulomatous amoebic meningoencephalitis commonly occurs in immunocompromised and debilitated individuals, including patients with AIDS. The disease has a subacute course and is generally fatal.[76] Amoebic serology is usually positive with immunofluoroescence, cellulose acetate precipitation and countercurrent immunoelectrophoresis. Brain biopsy occasionally shows *E. histolytica* trophozoites. Oral or intravenous metronidazole should be started and followed by diloxanide furoate to eliminate colonic cysts; the latter may not be successful. Surgical excision of cerebral granulomas has been reported, but the general condition of the patient should be taken into consideration carrying out invasive procedures. Most patients die despite treatment, but survival following early treatment with metronidazole supplemented with rifampicin and tetracycline has been described.

Naegleria fowleri can cause amoebic meningoencephalitis in both tropical and temperate climates. The organism prospers in moist soil and cases have been reported in children who have been swimming or playing in stagnant water. It is presumed that amoebae cross the nasal epithelium and extend to the brain through the olfactory nerves.[77] The neurological complications of meningoencephalitis may be subacute or acute. Amoebae can be isolated from the CSF, with neutrophilia and low glucose content. The changes may not be florid in patients with a subacute course due to acanthamoeba. The organisms can be identified if kept at room temperature. Treatment should start immediately with intravenous amphotericin B for 10 days; miconazole, rifampicin and tetracycline may enhance the effect of amphtericin B.

HELMINTHS (See also Chapters 70–73, 75 and 76)

The diversity and complexity of the life cycles of the numerous parasites that may affect the nervous system are considered elsewhere in this book. Here, brief consideration will be given only to the salient clinical features.

Cysticercosis. The larva of the pork tapeworm is the most common parasite to invade the central nervous system and the manifestations of neurocysticercosis may be seen worldwide. *Taenia solium* will be mainly considered in this section. Systemic infection with other adult or larval cestodes such as the dwarf tapeworm (*Hymenolepis nana*) or the beef tapeworm (*T. saginata*) are now rarely encountered. Presumably improvements in sanitation and meat inspection since the 1960s have been largely responsible. However, other cestodes such as the fish tapeworm (*Diphyllobothrium*) should not be completely forgotten because of increased consumption of sashimi and sushi from raw salmon.[78] It is believed that the fish tapeworm infects about 10% of people living in Scandanavia.[79] There, megaloblastic anaemia and its associated neurological complications may occur as a long-term consequence of infection because the adult tapeworm competes with the host for dietary vitamin B_{12}.

The larval form of *T. solium* is probably the most common cause of cystic lesions in the brain worldwide. The cysticercus, a fluid-filled bladder containing the invaginated head or scolex of the larval form, may infect all parts of the central nervous system, including the subarachnoid spaces and cisterns and, rarely, the sella turcica. Hydrocephalus is common and chronic meningitis with a lymphocytic or occasionally eosinophilic pleocytosis may be found when cysts are present in the subarachnoid space or ventricles in close proximity to the meninges.[80] CT and MRI have greatly facilitated diagnosis (Figure 8.2). The cystic lesions may be seen to contain more dense nodules, corresponding to the scolex; calcifications where cysts have died and cysts on nodules may enhance with contrast material as the cysticerci degenerate. However, there may be no radiological evidence of parasitic lesions and a negative scan does not eliminate the diagnosis if other clinical evidence is persuasive.

A less common pattern is the racemose (bunch of grapes) cluster of cysts within the cisterns.[81] The proliferating form consists of multiple interconnecting bladders of different sizes, but lacks scolices. These tend to occur in parts of the nervous system where the parasite is not closely confined by host tissue; the bladders may become large and extend into the spinal column. Careful examination may be required to reveal the degenerating scolex. It may be that racemose cysticerci are aberrant cysticerci of *T. solium* or other cestodes such as *T. multiceps* or *T. serialis* (the latter two are canine tapeworms of which the larval forms infect sheep and rabbits). Coenuri contain multiple scolices and may bud off daughter bladders; this condition is rare. To confirm the diagnosis of racemose cysticercosis requires pathological examination of the cystic lesion. When plain radiographs of soft tissues fail to reveal calcified lesions a number of available serological tests have been described. A recently introduced enzyme linked immunoelectrotransfer blot assay is sensitive and specific. Cisternal, parenchymal and intraventricular cysticerci may occur in the same patient, causing local disturbances—of which the most common is focal epilepsy. Larger cysts may produce mass effects: hydrocephalus commonly occurs and inflammation of blood vessels adjacent to

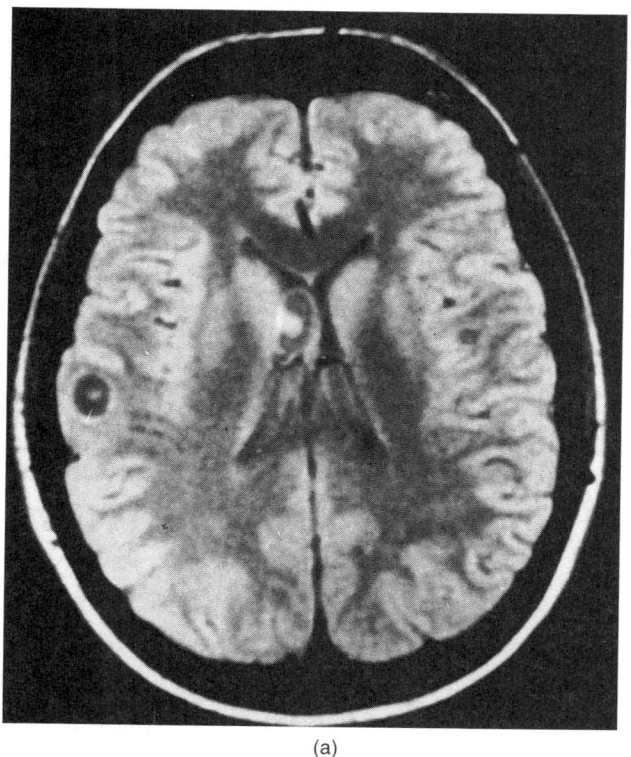

(a)

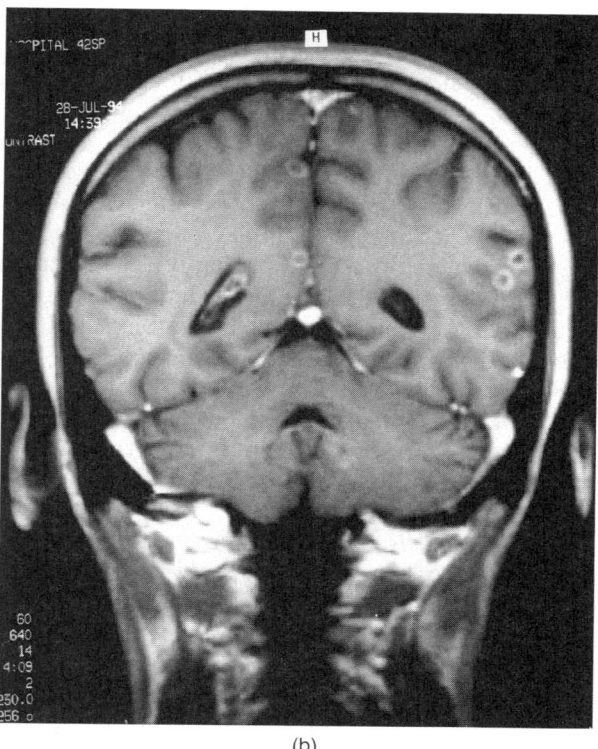

(b)

Figure 8.2 Neurocysticercosis. (a) Cysts in different stages of maturation. (b) Two cysts containing scolices.

cysts may cause brain thrombosis and infarction. Cysticercosis involving the basilar cisterns carries a poor prognosis.

Treatment of racemose and cisternal cysticercosis is difficult[82] and there are few satisfactory controlled trials to guide management. Anticysticercal drugs, corticosteroids, shunting procedures and surgical removal or decompression of cysts have been recommended. Praziquantel, an isoquinolone, and albendazole and imidazole have been used extensively in the treatment of parenchymal disease. Serial scans indicate that cysticerci are frequently eliminated or at least markedly reduced in numbers; the drugs are less effective for the cisternal and racemose manifestation. It is still not known whether albendazole is superior to praziquantel and in refractory cases both drugs are used. Praziquantel has been associated with a more adverse reaction that may be due to the host's inflammatory reaction to dying parasites, and headache, nausea and frequent seizures are common. Corticosteroids may ameliorate some of these effects and are usually prescribed, but there are few controlled trials to support this strategy.

Those with hydrocephalus due to cisternal disease and arachnoiditis will require shunting if there are symptoms and if serial scans indicate deterioration; some have recommended that a ventricular shunt

should be considered in all patients with hydrocephalus before medical therapy is attempted.[83] If racemose and cisternal cysts are focally impairing the egress of CSF, surgical removal is sometimes recommended, but such procedures may be difficult and at times hazardous.

Ischaemic cerebrovascular disease is an under-recognized and relatively common complication.[84] Inflammatory occlusion of the arteries at the base of the brain is secondary to arachnoiditis. The involved vessels are usually of small diameter provoking lacunar infarcts. However, occlusion of larger vessels such as the middle cerebral artery or even the internal carotid artery has been reported as well as transient ischaemic attacks and 'brain stem syndromes'.

While neurocysticercosis commonly seen in Latin America, Asia and Africa and in Mexico is the main cause of late-onset epilepsy, it should be borne in mind even in those whose sojourn in endemic areas has been brief and even when there is no history of possible exposure. This was clearly illustrated in a description of an outbreak of neurocysticercosis in an orthodox Jewish community residing in New York City[85] traced to a domestic employee who was found to have active parasitic infection probably acquired in her native Mexico. As man can clearly be an intermediate host through the ingestion of eggs in human faeces, it follows that the relatives of any patient with established disease should be examined—no matter how improbable the diagnosis.

Filariasis. Human filariasis may be due to *Loa loa*, *Dracunculus medinensis* or *Onchocerca volvulus*. Loiasis can cause meningoencephalitis with microfilariae in the CSF. Encephalitis with retinal haemorrhages has been described, probably as a reaction to the dying filariae with diethylcarbamazine used for treatment.[86] *D. medinensis* has been isolated from thickened peripheral nerves and can also cause paraspinal abscess by penetrating the extradural space.[87]

Wuchereria bancrofti is the cause of lymphatic filariasis. Recurrent Guillain–Barré syndrome has been reported after flare-ups of acute filariasis over a period of several years.[88]

Onchocerciasis. River blindness—endemic in large areas of Africa and Central America and caused by the filarial worm (*Onchocerca volvulus*), is transmitted by an insect vector. This breeds in fast-flowing rivers. Adult worms can survive in humans for many years, intermittently releasing microfilariae into the skin. More calamitous is migration into the anterior and posterior segments of the eye causing irreversible blindness, making onchocerciasis the most common cause of blindness in the world. The parasite occurs in both rain forests and savanna, where it is more likely to invade the eye. The anterior segment disease[89]—sclerosing keratitis and uveitis—is usually evident but the extent of posterior segment damage is more difficult to ascertain. In rain forest areas blindness is more likely to be due to posterior segment involvement with choreoretinitis and optic nerve lesions. The introduction of the antiparasitic agent ivermectin for the insect vector (*Simulium* spp.) was promising; spraying rivers with larvicide is very expensive and vector reinvasion after the discontinuation of spraying has occurred. Mass treatment with ivermectin (a semisynthetic macrocyclic lactone) is most encouraging. The drug is safe, well tolerated and effective in reducing microfilarial counts. A recent study concluded that annual ivermectin treatment may reduce the incidence of blindness by up to 80% in a savanna region. While most of the studies of onchocerciasis relate to blindness, a possible relationship with seizures has been suspected. Recent evidence[90] from western Uganda describes an improvement in seizure activity after ivermectin treatment in a community with demonstrable microfilariasis (*O. volvulus*). It may be that further studies will indicate more widespread systemic and central nervous system involvement than is currently suspected.

Nematode infections. While the adult form of *Gnathostoma spinigerum* has been known since the

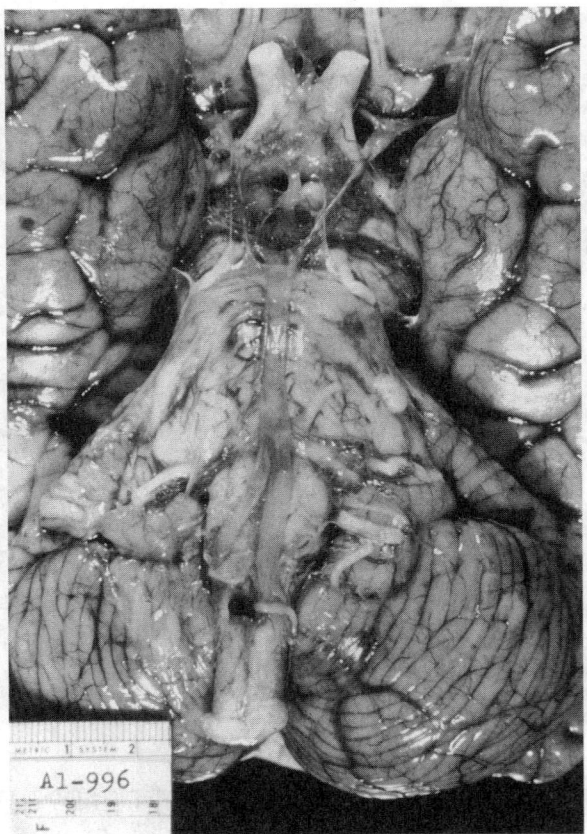

Figure 8.3 Gnathostomiasis. On the ventral surface of the lower medulla the nematodes can be seen emerging from a cavity (seen at autopsy). (Courtesy of Athasit Vejjajiva, Department of Neurology, Ramathibodi Hospital, Thailand.)

nineteenth century, when it was discovered in the stomach of a tiger in the London Zoo, the neurological manifestations of the mature parasite in man have been recognized more recently.[91] Those who prefer uncooked fish, shrimps and frogs in the tropics may acquire the larval third stage and present with a curious and sometimes fatal multifocal neurological illness (Figure 8.3). During the acute stage there may be a febrile illness with headache, neck stiffness and a rash; on occasions the parasite can be extracted from a skin lesion. A painful radiculomyelopathy may then develop with intensive girdle pain, paraparesis and eosinophilia in blood and CSF.[92] This phase may subside, but if unrecognized or untreated the parasite may then migrate through the spinal cord into the brain. Death may occur because of brain stem involvement and at autopsy the live gnathostome may be seen emerging. A patient seen recently in London had spent only a few weeks in Hong Kong on business; he had developed a complete paraplegia with a wheelchair existence and a dense hemianopia as a consequence of his preference for fresh crustacea in

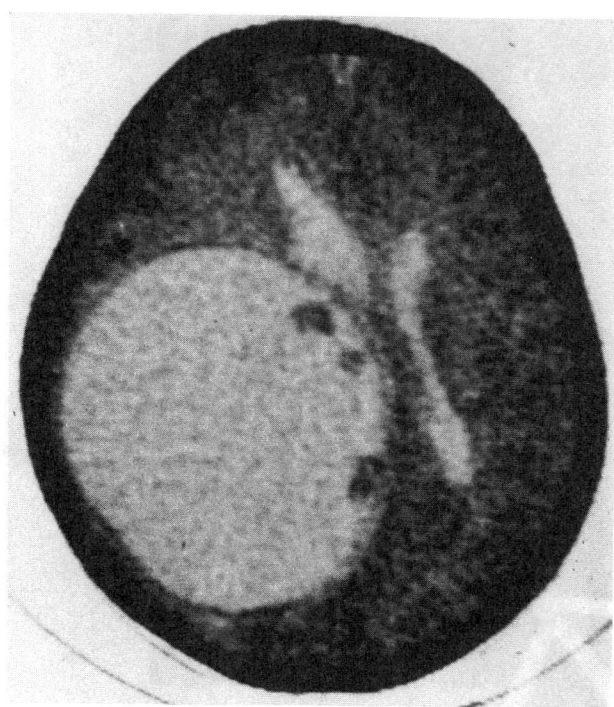

Figure 8.4 Brain scan showing large hydatid cyst with daughter cysts.

exotic restaurants. *Angiostrongylus cantonensis* (rat lungworm) similarly affects those in South-East Asia who consume poorly cooked snails, prawns and crabs. Neurological complications include meningitis, papilloedema and extraocular palsies with an eosinophilic CSF pleocytosis. Brain abscesses may occur and CT shows well-circumscribed enhancing lesions. Both these nematodes are treated with albendazole with steroid cover.

Strongyloides stercoralis, another nematode affecting the nervous system with an eosinophilic meningitis, usually occurs as part of the 'hyperinfection syndrome' with multiple cerebral infarcts, vasculitis and larval depositions.[93]

Hydatid disease. This may present as intracranial cysts, occasionally spectacularly large with the features of space occupying lesions and obstructive hydrocephalus, or with a basal arachnoiditis due to multiple smaller lesions.[94] CT and MRI (Figure 8.4) may reveal the diagnostic daughter cysts. Surgical excision and shunting are usually required. When hydatid disease affects the spine, paraplegia may result and it is usually impossible to excise all the diseased bone effectively. In consequence the prognosis is poor. Albendazole reduces cyst size and, at least in the gerbil,[95] is more effective than mebendazole and praziquantel.

Schistosomiasis. This long-known parasite of man — the earliest case known to have occurred was 5000 years ago in an Egyptian adolescent from the predy-nastic period[96]—continues to afflict mankind and it is believed that at present more than 250 million people worldwide are affected. Neuroschistosomiasis is uncommon but important because it responds well to appropriate treatment. Acute schistosomiasis (Katayama fever) presents as fever, cough, arthralgia, abdominal pain and urticaria; the neurological manifestations may be conspicuous headache, neck stiffness, evidence of raised intracranial pressure and fits. Involvement of the lower spinal cord and conus medullaris and/or cauda equina due to *Schistosoma mansoni* or *S. haematobium* has been well described,[97] but the diagnosis may be elusive even when suspected. Ova may be absent from stool and urine; available serological tests may be negative and eosinophilia absent.[98] However, eosinophilia in the CSF is usually present and the CT and MRI findings (Figure 8.5) may clinch the diagnosis. The interval of time between exposure and neurological presentation may be many years. It is recommended that all denizens where *S. mansoni* and *S. haematobium* prevail, and all travellers even with a remote history of recreational exposure to fresh water who present with a painful cauda equina or spinal syndrome, should commence praziquantel and corticosteroids without waiting for the results of laboratory or imaging tests.[99] The results may be gratifying. *S. japonicum* can also affect the cerebral hemispheres, with fits and other focal neurological presentations; this is uncommon in the West.

Toxocariasis. *Toxocara canis* transferred from dogs to humans through the eggs and the worm occasionally involves the central nervous system; unilateral retinal disease may occur in children; encephalitis and encephalomyelitis[100] have been reported in adults. Serious and persistent organic neurological and psychological deficits have been described and related to multiple brain infarcts from vasculitic lesions and eosinophilic granulomas. Myelitis with larvae in CSF and small arterial lesions may occur. Immune vasculitis should be prevented by early anthelmintic treatment, but there is a paucity of evidence of therapeutic efficacy.

Trichinosis. This parasitic disease, which develops after ingestion of undercooked meat contaminated with larvae of *Trichinella spiralis*, occurs both in tropical and temperate climates, and there have been large outbreaks in France related to the ingestion of horse meat.[101] The acute illness, with fever, headaches, myalgia, periorbital oedema, nausea and diarrhoea with a marked blood eosinophilia, increased serum muscle enzymes and specific antibodies, is well known. Less so are the neurological manifestations which are protean, making sporadic cases difficult to identify. Encephalopathy with a

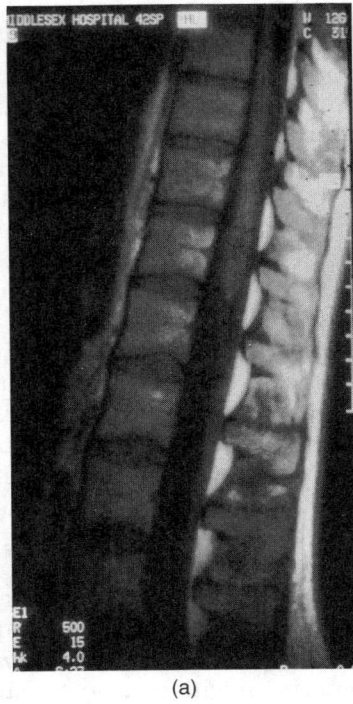

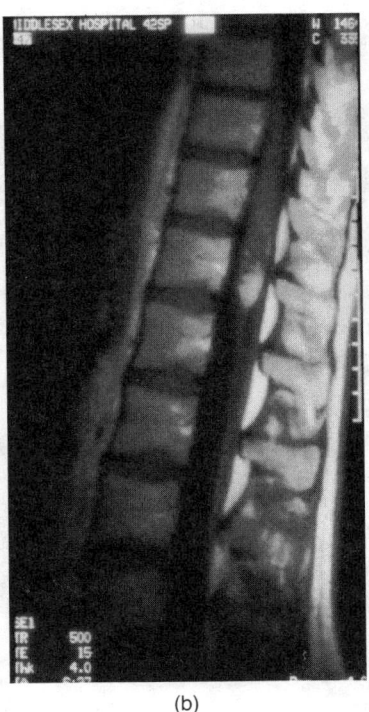

(a)   (b)

Figure 8.5   Schistosomiasis of the lower spinal cord and conus. (a) Before contrast. (b) After contrast with an irregular area of altered signal in surrounding oedema.

wide variety of focal deficits and numerous small hypodense CT changes in cortex and white matter has been clearly described.[102] The brain shows multiple small ischaemic cavities throughout the white matter and pons. Arteriolar microthrombi are present without an inflammatory infiltrate or remnants of *Trichinella* larvae. Toxaemic, allergic and larval pathogenic mechanisms have been proposed and a recent study suggests that hypereosinophilia may be implicated in the genesis of cerebral lesions. Early diagnosis and prompt treatment with anthelmintic therapy such as diffusable benzimidazole with corticosteroids is mandatory.

Paragonimiasis. This trematode causes major neurological problems in the Far East—especially Korea. It presents as an intercranial space occupying lesion. *Paragonimus westermani* is transmitted to man through ingestion of crab and crayfish; the metacercariae travel to the lungs and mature. The adult can live in the lung for several years and is usually asymptomatic. It can produce pulmonary symptoms, the most characteristic of which is cough with rusty sputum.[103] Neurological presentation is due to cerebral involvement as a result of the development of cysts in ectopic sites; various intracranial sites can be affected.[104] The diagnosis is established by demonstrating *P. westermani* eggs in sputum, faeces and pleural fluid. A monoclonal antibody assay has recently been reported. Treatment with praziquantel may be successful.[105]

CONCLUSION

To compress all the neurological manifestations of so-called 'tropical diseases' into one short chapter has necessitated brief and at times superficial accounts of an exceedingly diverse and fascinating group of illnesses. While this extent and somewhat idiosyncratic depth of coverage will not be beyond the criticism of the specialist, there should be little controversy about the need for all physicians, and particularly clinical neurologists, to be aware and reasonably well informed about this group of diseases that may affect many throughout the tropics and subtropics.

REFERENCES

1 Senanayake N & Roman G C. Epidemiology of epilepsy in the tropics. *J Trop Geogr Neurol* 1992; 2:10–19.

2 Senanayake N & Roman G C. Aetiological factors of epilepsy in the tropics. *J Trop Geogr Neurol* 1991; 1:69–80.

3 Rwiza H T, Matuja W B P & Mteza I. The past medical profile of epilepsy patients in an African rural community. *J Trop Geogr Neurol* 1992; 2:146–150.

4 Royal Society of London and US National Academy of Sciences. *Population growth resource consumption and a sustainable world: joint statement*. 1992.

5 Population Summit of the World's Scientific Academies. The statement. New Delhi, 27 October 1993.

6 Rozenzweig C & Parry M L. Potential impact of climate change on world food supply. *Nature* 1994; 367:133–137.

7 Cook G C. Effect of global warming on the distribution of parasitic and other infectious diseases: a review. *J R Soc Med* 1992; 85:688–691.

8 Cavanagh J B. The 'dying back' process: a common denominator in many naturally occurring and toxic neuropathies. *Arch Pathol Lab Med* 1979; 103:659–664.

9 Spencer P S, Sabri M I, Schaumburg H H & Moore C L. Does a defect of energy metabolism in the nerve fibre underlie axonal degeneration in polyneuropathies? *Ann Neurol* 1979; 5:501–507.

10 Senanayake N & Roman G C. Toxic neuropathies in the tropics. *J Trop Geogr Neurol* 1991; 1:3–15.

11 Senanayake N, de Silva W A S & Salgado M S L. Arsenical polyneuropathy: a clinical study. *Ceylon Med J* 1972; 17:195–203.

12 Le Quesne P M & McLeod J G. Peripheral neuropathy following a single exposure to arsenic. *J Neurol Sci* 1977; 32:437–451.

13 Windebank A J, McCall J T & Dyck P J. Metal neuropathy. In Dyck P J, Thomas P K, Lambert E H & Bunge R P (eds) *Peripheral Neuropathy*. Philadelphia:W B Saunders, 1984; 2133–2161.

14 Cavanagh J B, Fuller N H, Johnson H R M & Rudge P. The effect of thallium salts with particular reference to the nervous system. *Q J Med* 1974; 43:293–319.

15 Loftus L R. Peripheral neuropathy following chloroquine therapy. *Can Med Assoc J* 1963; 89:917–920.

16 Nakae K, Yamamoto S, Shigematsu I & Kono R. Relation between subacute myelooptic neuropathy (SMON) and clioquinol: a nationwide survey. *Lancet* 1973; i:171–174.

17 Vora D D, Dastur D K, Braganca B M et al. Toxic polyneuritis in Bombay due to ortho-cresyl phosphate poisoning. *J Neurol Neurosurg Psychiatry* 1962; 25:234–242.

18 Roman G C, Spencer P S & Schoenberg B S. Tropical myeloneuropathies: the hidden endemias. *Neurology* 1985; 35:1158–1170.

19 Howlett W P, Brubaker G, Mlingi N & Rosling H. A geographical cluster of konzo in Tanzania. *J Trop Geogr Neurol* 1992; 2:102–108.

20 Tylleskar T, Banea M, Bikangi N, Cooke R D, Poulter N H & Rosling H. Cassava cyanogens and konzo, an upper motorneurone disease found in Africa. *Lancet* 1992; 339:208–211.

21 Spencer P S, Ohta M & Palmer V S. Cycad use and motor neurone disease in Kii peninsula of Japan. *Lancet* 1987; ii:1462–1463.

22 Angunawela R M & Fernando H A. Acute ascending polyneuropathy and dermatitis following poisoning by tubers of *Gloriosa superba*. *Ceylon Med J* 1971; 16:233–235.

23 Ng T H K, Chan Y W, Yu Y L et al. Encephalopathy and neuropathy following ingestion of a Chinese herbal broth containing podophyllin. *J Neurol Sci* 1991; 101:107–115.

24 Calderon-Gonzalez R & Rizzi-Hernandez H. Buckthorn polyneuropathy. *N Engl J Med* 1967; 277:69–71.

25 Gascon G G, Crowell J, Stigsby B et al. Subacute sclerosing panencephalitis. *Neurology* 1992; 43:454–455.

26 Schoub B D, Johnson S & McAnerney J M. Observations of subacute sclerosing panencephalitis in South Africa. *Trans R Soc Trop Med Hyg* 1992; 86:550–551.

27 Steiner I, Wirguin I, Morag A et al. Intraventricular interferon treatment for subacute sclerosing panencephalitis. *J Child Neurol* 1989; 4:20–24.

28 Freier J E. Eastern equine encephalomyelitis. *Lancet* 1993; 342:1281–1286.

29 Thongchareon P. Japanese encephalitic virus encephalitis: an overview. *Southeast Asian J Trop Med Public Health* 1989; 20:559–573.

30 Arthur R R, El-Sharkawy M S, Cope S E et al. Recurrence of Rift Valley fever in Egypt. *Lancet* 1993; 342:1149–1150.

31 Strebel P M, Sutter R W, Cochi S et al. Epidemiology of poliomyelitis in the United States one decade after the last reported case of indigenous wild virus-associated disease. *Clin Infect Dis* 1992; 14:568–579.

32 Joce R, Wood D, Brown D et al. Paralytic poliomyelitis in England and Wales 1985–1991. *BMJ* 1992; 305:79–82.

33 Sutter R W, Patriarca PA, Brogan S et al. Outbreak of paralytic poliomyelitis in Oman: evidence of widespread transmission among fully vaccinated children. *Lancet* 1991; 338:715–720.

34 Otten M W, Denning M S, Jaiteh K O et al. Epidemic poliomyelitis in the Gambia following the control of poliomyelitis as an endemic disease. 1.

Descriptive findings. *Am J Epidemiol* 1992; 135:381–392.

35 Solbrig M V & McCormick J B. Lassa fever: central nervous system manifestations. *J Trop Geogr Neurol* 1991; 1:23–30.

36 Warrell D A & Warrell M J. Human rabies and its prevention: an overview. *Rev Infect Dis* 1988; 10(supplement 4):5726–5731.

37 Petricciani J C. Ongoing tragedy of rabies. *Lancet* 1993; 342:1067.

38 Nicholson K G. Rabies. *Lancet* 1990; 335:1201–1206.

39 Swaddiwuthipong W, Weniger B G, Wattanasi S & Warrell M J. A high rate of neurological complications following Semple anti-rabies vaccine. *Trans R Soc Trop Med Hyg* 1988; 82:472–475.

40 Epstein L G & Gendelman H E. Human immunodeficiency virus type 1 infection of the nervous system. Pathogenetic mechanisms. *Ann Neurol* 1993:429–436.

41 Gessain A, Barin F, Vernant J C et al. Antibodies to human T-lymphotrophic type 1 in patients with tropical spastic paraparesis. *Lancet* 1985; ii:407–409.

42 Roman G C. The neuroepidemiology of tropical spastic paraparesis. *Ann Neurol* 1988; 23(supplement):113–120.

43 Montgomery R D. The epidemiology of myelopathy associated with human T-lymphotrophic virus 1. *Trans R Soc Trop Med Hyg* 1993; 87:154–159.

44 Yamaguchi, K. Human T-lymphotropic virus type 1 in Japan. *Lancet* 1994; 343:213–216.

45 Mochizuki M, Watanabe T, Yamaguchi et al. Uveitis associated with human T-lymphotrophic virus type 1. *Am J Ophthalmol* 1992; 114:123–129.

46 Jacobson S, McFarlin D E, Robinson S et al. HTLV-1-specific cytotoxic T lymphocytes in the cerebrospinal fluid of patients with HTLV-1-associated neurological disease. *Ann Neurol* 1992; 32:651–657.

47 Hino S & Hiroshi D. Mechanisms of HTLV-1 transmission. In Roman GC, Vernant JC & Osame M (eds) *HTLV-1 and the Nervous System*. New York: Alan R Liss, 1989:495–501.

48 Cruickshank J K, Rudge P, Dalgleish A G et al. Tropical spastic paraparesis and human T cell lymphotrophic virus type 1 in the United Kingdom. *Brain* 1989; 112:1057–1090.

49 Poser C M, Roman G C & Vernant J C. Multiple sclerosis or HTLV-1 myelitis? *Neurology* 1990; 40:1020–1022.

50 Alcindor F, Valderrama R, Canaveggio M et al. Imaging of human T-lymphotrophic virus type 1-associated chronic progressive myeloneuropathies. *Neuroradiology* 1992; 35:69–74.

51 Shaked Y. Rickettsial infections of the central nervous system: the role of prompt antimicrobial therapy. *Q J Med* 1991; 79:301–306.

52 Raoult D, Zuchelli P, Weiller P J et al. Incidence, clinical observations and risk factors in the severe form of Mediterranean spotted fever among patients admitted to hospital in Marseilles 1983–1984. *J Infect* 1986; 12:111–116.

53 Kirk I J, Fine P D, Sexton J D & Muchmore G. Rocky mountain spotted fever: a clinical review based on 48 confirmed cases 1943–1986. *Medicine* 1990; 69:35–45.

54 Nosh D N. Epidemiology of bacterial meningitis: UK and USA. In Williams J D & Burnie J (eds) *Bacterial Meningitis*. London: Academic Press, 1987:93–115.

55 Ross K L, Tunkel A R & Scheld W M. Acute bacterial meningitis in children and adults. In Scheld W M, Whitley R J & Durck D T (eds) *Infections in the Central Nervous System*. New York: Raven Press, 1991:335–409.

56 Sheller J R & Des Prez R M. CNS tuberculosis. *Neurol Clin* 1988; 4:143–148.

57 Wood M & Anderson M. CNS tuberculosis. In Walton J (ed.) *Neurological Infections*. London: W B Saunders, 1988:172–196.

58 Shankar P, Manjknath N, Mohen K K et al. Rapid diagnosis of tuberculous meningitis by polymerase chain reaction. *Lancet* 1991; 337:5–7.

59 Zhang G, Li W, Yan L et al. An epidemiological survey of deformities and disabilities among 14257 leprosy patients in 11 countries. *Chin Med J* 1992; 7:216–220.

60 World Health Organization Study Group. Chemotherapy of leprosy for control programmes. *WHO Tech Rep Ser* 1982; 675.

61 Browne S G. Leprosy. *BMJ* 1968, 3:725–728.

62 Shakir R A, Al-Din A S N, Araj G F et al. Clinical categories of neurobrucellosis. *Brain* 1987; 110:213–223.

63 Araj G F, Lulu A R, Khateeb M I et al. ELISA versus routine tests in the diagnosis of patients with systemic and neurobrucellosis. *Acta Pathol Microbiol Immunol Scand* 1988; 96:171–176.

64 Turner L H. Leptospirosis. *BMJ* 1973; 1:537–540.

65 Finkel M J & Halperin J J. Nervous system borreliosis—revisited. *Arch Neurol* 1992; 49:102–107.

66 Warrell D A, Molyneux M E & Beales P F. Severe and complicated malaria. *Trans R Soc Trop Med Hyg* 1990; 84(supplement):1–65.

67 Brewster D R, Kwaitkowski D & White N J. Neurological sequelae of cerebral malaria in children. *Lancet* 1990; 336:1039–1043.

68 Phillips R E. Hypoglycaemia is an important complication of falciparum malaria. *Q J Med* 1989; 71:477–483.

69 Lockwood D N J & Pasvol G. Recent advances in tropical medicine. *BMJ* 1994; 308:1559–1562.

70 De Silva H J, Goonetilleke A K E, Senaratna N et al. Skeletal muscle necrosis in severe falciparum malaria. *BMJ* 1988; 296:1039.

71 Milord F, Pepin J, Loko L, Ethier L & Mpia B. Efficacy and toxicity of eflornithine for treatment of

Trypanosoma brucei gambiense sleeping sickness. *Lancet* 1992; 340:652–655.

72 Spina-Franca A & Mattosinho-Franca L S. American trypanosomiasis (Chagas' disease). In Vinken P J & Bruyn G W (eds) *Handbook of Clinical Neurology*, vol. 35, part III. Amsterdam: Elsevier–North Holland, 1978:85–114.

73 Woodhouse J I J. The prevalence of clinical peripheral neuropathies in human chronic Chagas disease. *J R Army Med Corps* 1993; 139:54–55.

74 Rosenberg S, Chaves C J, Higuchi N M L et al. Fatal meningoencephalitis caused by reactivation of *Trypanosoma cruzi* infection in patients with AIDS. *Neurology* 1992; 42:640–642.

75 Morehead C. Notes on the pathology and treatment of diseases of the brain, as observed in the European General Hospital at Bombay. *Trans Med Phys Soc Bombay* 1849; 9:112–115.

76 Gardner H A R, Martinez A J, Visvesvara G S et al. Granulomatous amoebic encephalitis in an AIDS patient. *Neurology* 1991; 41:1993–1995.

77 Peral I M, Visvesvara G S, Martinez A J et al. Naegleria and acanthomoeba infections: review. *Rev Infect Dis* 1990; 12:490–513.

78 Schantz P M & McAley I. Current status of food-borne parasitic zoonoses in the United States. *Southeast Asian J Trop Med Public Health* 1991; 22(supplement):65–71.

79 Salokannel J. Intrinsic factor in tapeworm anaemia. *Acta Med Scand Suppl* 1987; 517:1–51.

80 Del Brutto O H & Sotelo J. Neurocysticercosis: an update. *Rev Infect Dis* 1988; 10: 1075–1087.

81 Jung R C, Rodriguez M A, Beaver P C, Schenthal J E & Levy R W. Racemose cysticercus in human brain: a case report. *Am J Trop Med Hyg* 1981; 30:620–624.

82 Earnest M P, Reller L B, Filley C M & Grek A J. Neurocysticercosis in the United States: 35 cases and a review. *Rev Infect Dis* 1987; 9:961–979.

83 Lobato R D, Lamsa E M, Portillo J M et al. Hydrocephalus in cerebral cysticercosis: pathogenic and therapeutic considerations. *J Neurosurg* 1981; 55:786–793.

84 Del Brutto O H. Cysticercosis and cerebrovascular disease: a review. *J Neurol Neurosurg Psychiatry* 1992; 55:252–254.

85 Schantz P M, Moore A C, Munoz J L et al. Neurocysticercosis in an orthodox Jewish community in New York City. *N Engl J Med* 1992; 327:692–695.

86 Negess Y, Lanoie L O, Neafie R C et al. Loiasis: 'calabar' swellings and involvement of deep organs. *Am J Trop Med Hyg* 1985; 34:537–546.

87 Brown W J & Voge M. *Neuropathology of Parasitic Infections*. Oxford: Oxford University Press, 1982:240.

88 Bhatia B & Misra S. Recurrent Guillain–Barré syndrome following acute filiariasis. *J Neurol Neurosurg Psychiatry* 1993; 56:1133–1134.

89 Mabey D. Onchocerciasis: ivermectin and onchocercal optic nerve lesions. *Lancet* 1993; 341:153–154.

90 Kipp W, Kasoro S & Burnham G. Onchocerciasis and epilepsy in Uganda. *Lancet* 1994; 343:182–184 (letter).

91 Schmutzhard E, Boongird P & Vejjajiva A. Eosinophilic meningitis and radiculomyelitis in Thailand caused by CNS invasion of *Gnasthostoma spinigerum* and *Angiostrongylus cantonensis*. *J Neurol Neurosurg Psychiatry* 1988; 51:80–87.

92 Punyagupta S, Juttijudata P & Bunnag T. Eosinophilic meningitis in Thailand. *Am J Trop Med Hyg* 1975; 24:921–931.

93 Belani A, Leptrone D & Shands J W. Strongyloides meningitis. *South Med J* 1987; 80:916–918.

94 Cataltepe O, Colak A, Ozcan O E et al. Intracranial hydatid cyst: experience with surgical treatment in 120 patients. *Neurochirurgia* 1992; 35:108–111.

95 Taylor D H, Morris D L, Reffin D et al. Comparison of albendazole, mebendazole and praziquantel chemotherapy of *Echinococcus multilocularis* in a gerbil model. *Gut* 1989; 30:1401–1405.

96 Miller R J, Armelagos G J, Ikram S, De Jonge N, Krijger F W & Deelder A M. Palaeoepidemiology of schistomasoma infection in mummies. *BMJ* 1992; 304:555–556.

97 Haribhai H C, Bhigee A I, Bill P L A et al. Spinal cord schistosomiasis: a clinical laboratory and radiological study with a note on therapeutic aspects. *Brain* 1991; 114:709–726.

98 Blunt S B, Boulton J & Wise R. MRI in schistosomiasis of conus medullaris and lumbar spinal cord. *Lancet* 1993; 341:557.

99 Blanchard T J, Milne L M, Pollok R & Cook G C. Early chemotherapy of imported neuroschistosomiasis. *Lancet* 1993; 341:959 (letter).

100 Sommer C, Ringelstein E B, Biniek R & Glockner W M. Adult *Toxocara canis* encephalitis. *J Neurol Neurosurg Psychiatry* 1994; 57:229–231.

101 Ancelle T, Dupouy-Camet J, Bougnoux M E et al. Two outbreaks of trichinosis caused by horsemeat in France in 1985. *Am J Epidemiol* 1988; 127:1302–1311.

102 Fourestie V, Douceron H, Brugieres P, Ancelle T, Lejonc J L & Gherardi R K. Neurotrichinosis: a cerebrovascular disease associated with myocardial injury and hypereosinophilia. *Brain* 1993; 116:603–616.

103 Cook G C. Protozoan and helminthic infections. In Lambert H P (ed.) *Infections of the Central Nervous System*. New York: Marcel Decker, 1991:264–282.

104 Toyonaga S, Kurisaka M, Mori K et al. Cerebral paragonimiasis—report of five cases. *Neurol Med Chir* 1992; 32:157–162.

105 Zhang Z, Zhang Y, Shi Z et al. Diagnosis of active *Paragonimus westermani* infections with a monoclonal antibody-based antigen detection assay. *Am J Trop Med Hyg* 1993; 49:329–334.

CHAPTER 9

PSYCHIATRY

J. R. Billinghurst and J. H. Orley

Systematic psychiatry is covered in the standard textbooks on the subject. The aim of this chapter is to consider those aspects which are particularly relevant to practitioners who have to deal with psychiatric problems in the tropics but do not have the benefit of specialized training in that discipline.

In contrast to somatic diseases the pathological basis for most psychiatric disorders is obscure and confirmatory laboratory tests are lacking. Universally acceptable diagnostic criteria have, however, been hammered out in recent years—an essential prerequisite to meaningful statements about variations in prevalence and incidence between populations.

Doctors and other health workers with specialized Western-style psychiatric training are scarce in tropical lands, and in many situations psychiatrically ill patients have to be diagnosed and cared for by general medical officers and in general hospital wards and outpatient clinics. Many of those suffering from a mental disorder will never come near a Western-style doctor at all, and will stay untreated in the community, if their behaviour is not grossly disturbed. In some instances, especially in rural areas, traditional healers will be consulted and their remedies applied, since they are an integral part of the culture and can talk to the patients and their families about causes and treatments in an understandable way. It is unacceptable behaviour that will drive the family or community members to bring the mentally ill to hospitals and clinics, requesting protection for themselves and a change in behaviour by the patient. Western-style practitioners have to accept the fact that they are usually second choice helpers, only resorted to when traditional healers fail.

Since much epidemiological information has been gathered in the past from institutions whose main function was to help or provide social control, it is not surprising that this heavily biased material has led to a widespread impression that in the tropics schizophrenia and mania are relatively common, whereas the less socially disturbing conditions of depression and anxiety are rare. Standardized questionnaires and thorough case detection methods in rural communities have shown that depression and anxiety are as common there as they are in the developed world.[1] But such efforts are very laborious and time consuming and so far there are few reliably validated reports.

Whilst the number of named psychiatric diseases is small, their symptoms are protean and may be influenced by the local cultural milieu. This applies especially to delusions. If the locals believe in evil spirits, witches, sorcerers and the 'evil eye', then a patient from that locality cannot be said to be pathologically deluded if he or she too believes in such things. In addition there are culture-bound symptoms or symptom complexes, essentially neurotic, acceptable to members of one culture as a recognized way of being ill or different but very bizarre to those of other cultures. One of the best known is *running amok*, a form of violent behaviour in Malaysia and Indonesia which has given its name to the English language. Almost identical is *going berserk*, originally a Norwegian phenomenon. *Latah* is a form of imitative behaviour amongst young women in South-East Asia. *Wihtigo* afflicts certain North American tribes and is manifested by a repugnance for food of deep symbolic significance. In *koro*, Chinese men in South-East Asia believe that the penis is about to retract into the abdomen, with fatal consequences (ghosts have no genitals), and must be tied or gripped even when the afflicted person is persuaded of the anatomical impossibility of such an event. *Spirit-possession states* occur in many cultures, conferring valued status on the one possessed.

'Somatization of symptoms', the tendency to describe mental disturbances in bodily terms, is a common phenomenon in tropical practice and provides helpful insights into patients' ideas of how their bodies work and the words available in their own vernacular to describe those ideas. Symptoms commonly reported include: dizziness, palpitations, generalized or localized weakness, heat in the head or body, itching, pricking, numbness, bizarre exaggeration of pain, unclear vision, excessive belching and sexual impotence. Worms or insects seem to be biting or creeping from place to place and the patient asks for them to be expunged by purging or sneezing or another physical manoeuvre. However sure the doctor may be that the patient has got a disturbance of the mind and not the body, it is extremely difficult to convey such an unacceptable idea to the client. One has only to recall the anxiety aroused by 'palpitations' to recognize that somatization as regards the heart is a worldwide symptom, even where the scientific connection between anxiety and tachycardia is understood.

Knowing about the local culture is clearly important for health professionals in their place of work. Migrants from one culture to another take with them their own cultural ideas which may not only intensify the stress of their adjustment and determine their symptoms of mental illness if it occurs, but also affect their responses to interviews and treatment. 'Transcultural psychiatry' is a relatively new and highly relevant branch of the specialty.[2,3]

Psychotropic drugs have revolutionized both the practical care of disturbed patients and also the theoretical understanding of the likely underlying pathological chemical processes, especially at the synaptic level in schizophrenia, depression and anxiety. Significant as these are, *organic* causes of mental illness are of paramount importance in the tropics. Infections, dehydration, malnutrition, vitamin deficiencies, alcohol, toxins and drugs are all common and can all drastically affect mental functions. A 'high index of suspicion' is essential. Every patient should be as thoroughly examined and investigated for physical disease as is possible. Immediate intravenous glucose, injections of vitamins, an anti-malarial drug or a course of antibiotics, as the case may be, could prove to be dramatically beneficial if needed—and harmless if not!

TERMINOLOGY AND CLASSIFICATION

The major current international classification of mental disorders is that within the tenth edition of the International Classification of Diseases (ICD-10).[4] The major headings in the chapter on mental and behavioural disorders are:

F0 Organic, including symptomatic, mental disorders

F1 Mental and behavioural disorders due to psychoactive substance use

F2 Schizophrenia, schizotypal and delusional disorders

F3 Mood (affective) disorders

F4 Neurotic, stress-related and somatoform disorders

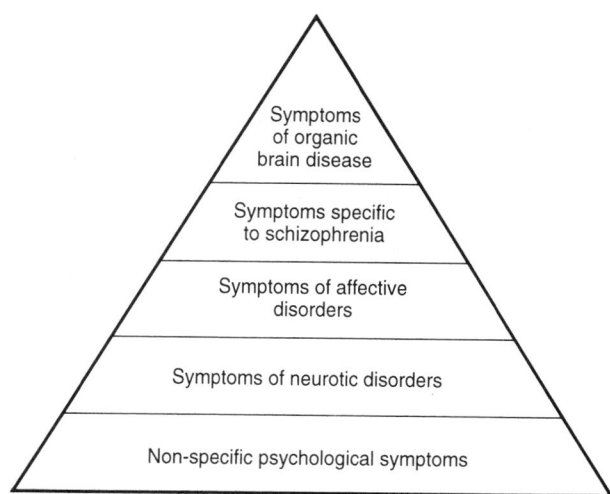

Figure 9.1 The hierarchical pyramid of symptoms.

F5 Behavioural syndromes associated with physiological disturbances and physical factors

F6 Disorders of adult personality and behaviour

F7 Mental retardation

F8 Disorders of psychological development

F9 Behavioural and emotional disorders with onset usually occurring in childhood and adolescence

This classification supersedes the older traditional division into neuroses and psychoses. Where the term 'psychosis' is still used it usually refers to the more severe mental disorders, characterized by the presence of hallucinations, delusions and abnormal behaviour.

Fould's concept of a hierarchical pyramid of symptoms, amplified by Leff,[1] provides a very helpful approach (Figure 9.1). At the bottom of the pyramid there is a large base of rather non-specific symptoms common to all mental disorders and at a level where it is difficult to say whether the patient is definitely mentally ill at all. Above the base there is another large band of neurotic symptoms, present in many mental disorders. Affective symptoms, although pointing to a diagnosis of affective disorder, may also be present in schizophrenia and organic disorders. There are, however, certain symptoms characteristic of schizophrenia (so-called 'first-rank' symptoms) which, if present, indicate that the diagnosis is schizophrenia and not affective disorder (even though affective symptoms may be present). Similarly, clouding of consciousness points strongly to the diagnosis of organic mental disorder, even if some of the symptoms of schizophrenia are present.

THE COMMON MENTAL DISORDERS IN THE TROPICS

ACUTE ORGANIC MENTAL DISORDERS (F05 and F10–19) (ACUTE CONFUSIONAL STATE, DELIRIUM, ACUTE BRAIN SYNDROME)

Acute confusional states and coma are two common presentations in patients needing hospital admission in the tropics. Since clouding of consciousness can progress rapidly to complete unconsciousness, it is helpful to consider them both under the same heading. In this context, 'acute' signifies a time interval between onset and the development of the full-blown picture of hours or days and never exceeding 1 month. From the point of view of the ICD-10, the delirium associated with drug or psychoactive drug use (through intoxication or withdrawal) is coded separately within F1, whilst that due to other extracerebral causes, intracerebral conditions, trauma or prescribed medicines is coded in F05. There may, however, be little difference between the manifestations and treatments required.

CLINICAL FEATURES

The clinical features include impairment of consciousness (all levels from inattention through rousable drowsiness to coma), disorientation (often initially in time, later in place, seldom in person), impairment of immediate recall and recent memory (difficult to assess in the presence of clouded consciousness), hallucinations (typically visual and frightening), rambling speech and abnormal even highly aggressive behaviour. Disturbances of sleep pattern and of emotions are common. Where coma is present, the Glasgow coma scale has proved to be of great practical help in assessing levels and progress.[5]

CAUSES

The organic causes to be considered are so numerous that they are divided into two tables. Table 9.1 lists likely primarily systemic disorders which disturb brain function. Table 9.2 lists diseases having pathological processes primarily within the central nervous system.

Since an acute organic psychosis is potentially reversible, the early detection and correction of the cause is of the utmost importance. More than one cause may be present, e.g. head injury or vitamin

Table 9.1   Acute organic mental disorders (acute confusional state, delirium, acute brain syndrome): likely primarily systemic (extracerebral) causes in the tropics.

Heat: high fever, heat stroke, heat exhaustion
Dehydration, electrolyte imbalance, acid–base disturbance
Infections, especially malaria, pneumonia, septicaemia, typhoid, typhus, urinary tract infection
Hypoglycaemia
Vitamin deficiency: beriberi, pellagra
Alcohol: intoxication or withdrawal
Drug of addiction: intoxication or withdrawal
Psychoactive drug
Therapeutic drug
Poisoning, herbal remedy, folk remedy
Heart failure, cardiac arrhythmias, hypotension, shock
Severe anaemia
Liver failure, portal–systemic encephalopathy
Acute renal failure
Diabetic ketoacidosis, non-ketotic hyperglycaemia

Table 9.2   Acute organic mental disorders (acute confusional state delirium, acute brain syndrome): likely primarily intracerebral causes in the tropics.

Infection: meningitis, encephalitis, brain abscess, tuberculoma, cerebral schistosomiasis, cysticercosis, hydatid disease, paragonimiasis
Epilepsy and postepileptic states
Head injury and post-traumatic states (including extracerebral haemorrhage, subdural haematoma)
Vascular disorder: haemorrhage, embolism, non-embolic infarction, sickle-cell crisis, venous thrombosis
Intracranial space occupying lesion (tumour, abscess, tuberculoma, subdural haematoma)
Raised intracranial pressure from any cause
Wernicke's encephalopathy

deficiency in alcohol intoxication. This multiplicity of causes is especially important in the tropics where one might see an infection superimposed on a vitamin deficiency, having a marked effect on brain function.

Substances causing delirium

A variety of psychoactive substances may precipitate serious mental disorder, even at relatively low doses, as may their withdrawal. This also applies to some therapeutic drugs such as antiparkinsonian drugs, isoniazid and corticosteroids. Alcohol is a frequent cause of a delirious state, due either to intoxication or to withdrawal. The intoxication may also lead to hypoglycaemia which produces further confusion or coma.

There are parts of the tropics where alcohol is a factor of major psychosocial importance. All the well-known features of intoxication and withdrawal, drink-related problems, and somatic and mental complications are seen frequently (though not always recognized initially). Fermented brews of every imaginable description are consumed, so there is a wide variation not only in the nutritional and vitamin content of the liquors but also in the presence of possible contaminants. A particularly deadly contaminant is methanol (methyl alcohol, wood spirit) which in sublethal doses may cause sudden catastrophic bilateral optic neuritis.

Social drinking is widespread. Led by the men, whole communities, even including children, may gather round communal pots and continue imbibing in a prolonged debauch. It may come as a surprise to discover that there are unsophisticated folk involved in such activities who genuinely do not recognize that there is a connection between alcohol and ill health and who not only accept this information when it is given but also act on the advice to curtail such drinking or give it up completely.[6]

Cannabis is often implicated as a cause of acute mental disorder in countries where it is grown and is used. The plant *Cannabis sativa* (Indian hemp) is easily grown in the tropics and is widely available. Popular synonyms for cannabis products include marihuana, hashish, bhang and ghanja. The active ingredient is tetrahydrocannabinol; it enters the body usually by being smoked or sometimes by being eaten, and induces in most people a pleasant, dreamy state of altered perception. Youngsters are typically introduced to its effects by groups of youths of their own age. There is a polarization of ideas about the dangers of cannabis smoking. At one extreme are those who regard it as an entirely innocuous pleasure, no more harmful than the enjoyment of alcohol in moderation, and who object to legislation against its possession and use as being liable to criminalize a section of the population rather in the same way as alcohol prohibition has been known to do. On the other hand, there are those who are convinced of its noxious effects and who also see the taking of cannabis as a prelude to involvement with 'hard' drugs (heroin, cocaine), the evil effects of which are more widely accepted. Cost and availability in the tropics, however, mean that most youngsters do not get beyond cannabis. For a minority of users the drug is not innocuous for it has been reported to precipitate anxiety and panic reactions, and manic and confusional psychoses; it may aggravate already existent schizophrenia and may even unmask a latent tendency to schizophrenia. The extensive recent literature on the chemistry, clinical effects and possible mode of action of cannabis is thoroughly reviewed by Ashton.[7] It is difficult for most practitioners in the tropics to obtain proof of the presence or recent use of cannabis but circumstantial evidence may be available and the person concerned may admit to having taken it. In the authors' experience in several parts of Africa, cannabis was a very frequently suspected cause of acute psychotic episodes, characterized by violent and highly antisocial behaviour and in most instances a complete return to normality within a few days. Control of behaviour in the meanwhile can be achieved by injections of a phenothiazine. A few individuals, however, turn out to have schizophrenia. Widespread awareness that there could be any connection at all between cannabis and violent behaviour cannot but affect public attitudes towards the drug.

DIFFERENTIAL DIAGNOSIS

In an acute functional psychosis, full consciousness tends to be preserved, but the distinction may be decidedly uncertain at first sight in a tropical setting. A patient with a low grade chronic functional psychosis may become acutely disturbed as the result of one of the causes mentioned; treatment of the latter may then unmask the hitherto unsuspected chronic disorder.

TREATMENT

Disturbed behaviour responds to neuroleptic drugs: chlorpromazine 100–400 mg and haloperidol 5–20 mg, by mouth or parenterally, are especially useful. Symptoms can also respond to the benzodiazepines. Chlormethiazole is the favoured drug for alcohol withdrawal, although its advantage over diazepam is not clear. The known or suspected underlying cause of disturbed behaviour must be treated appropriately. If there is even the faintest reason to suspect hypoglycaemia, administration of intravenous 50% glucose (dextrose) is mandatory. The treatment of the associated physical disorders is considered elsewhere in this volume and in standard textbooks.

When using the major tranquillizers it is important to remember that the *neuroleptic malignant syndrome* is a rare but potentially fatal complication of therapy by certain antipsychotic drugs and is characterized by high fever, autonomic dysfunction, disturbed consciousness and muscular rigidity simulating tetanus. The symptoms might be confused with the symptoms of the condition being treated. If suspected, the offending drug must be stopped at once. Bromocriptine and dantrolene should be tried, since they are sometimes effective in reducing symptoms.

CHRONIC ORGANIC MENTAL DISORDERS AND DEMENTIA (CHRONIC BRAIN SYNDROME)

The term chronic organic mental disorder can be applied to states in which disturbances of consciousness, orientation, memory, intellect and behaviour have persisted for longer than one month, and sometimes for years, with gradual onset and slow progress. The term is almost synonymous with dementia, but the latter suggests an even longer duration and implies irreversibility. Most of the conditions mentioned in Tables 9.1 and 9.2 as causes of acute organic mental disorder will have improved or terminated the patient's life within a month; some leave enduring sequelae; others remain active, merging into a group of diseases with a more indolent natural history. Chronic subdural haematoma is an example of a condition highly amenable to suitable treatment, and there are other conditions, mentioned in Table 9.3, the treatment of which proves rewarding. Older members of the community are the ones most likely to have vascular lesions or Alzheimer's disease. Younger patients with the symptoms of chronic organic mental disorder need careful investigation.

Table 9.3 Chronic organic mental disorders (chronic brain syndrome): likely causes in the tropics.

Prolongation or sequel of conditions mentioned in Tables 9.1 and 9.2
Chronic alcoholism, Korsakoff's psychosis
Pellograph
Chronic renal failure
Chronic subdural haematoma
Intracranial space occupying lesions
Low-grade meningitis, meningoencephalitis, encephalitis, acquired immune deficiency syndrome (AIDS), syphilis, trypanosomiasis
Uncontrolled epilepsy
Alzheimer's disease
Congenital, familial and degenerative disorders associated with dementia
Multi-infarct dementia
Sequel of brain damage at birth or in infancy

SCHIZOPHRENIA AND PARANOIA (F20–22)

CLINICAL FEATURES

The most characteristic ('first-rank') symptoms of schizophrenia are remarkably consistent all over the world, whatever the culture. They consist of the following:

- Thought disorders (echo, insertion, withdrawal, broadcasting)
- Hearing of voices giving a running commentary on the patient's behaviour or discussing the patient in the 'third person'
- Feelings of passivity, of being controlled by an outside person or agency
- Primary fixed delusions, usually persecutory, sometimes grandiose.

These symptoms are almost pathognomonic of schizophrenia. In addition, behaviour may be bizarre and inappropriate. Although most patients are socially withdrawn and slow, some become noisy, aggressive and even dangerous.

Schizophrenia can run a variety of different courses. The typical, but fortunately not most frequent, is one in which the symptoms continue unremittingly, with a progressive decline in the patient's condition. In others the symptoms remit after an initial episode but, following this, the patients may relapse periodically and some, but not all, again run a downhill course. In an appreciable number of cases, however, the patients recover and remain well. Favourable prognostic factors include a negative family history, good premorbid personality, an acute onset and a good response to treatment. Prognosis in the tropics is said to be better, perhaps because those schizophrenics who are brought for treatment are the ones whose onset was acute, and also because of a tolerant and positive attitude by the patients' families, at least in some countries.

Prevalence rates throughout the world are about 5 per 1000; annual incidence rates are much lower, a reminder of the persisting nature of the symptoms in many schizophrenics.

TREATMENT

Many phenothiazines, butyrophenones and other neuroleptics rapidly improve the symptoms, thereby also improving the patient's behaviour and social relationships. In fact, such striking amelioration of symptoms, especially the positive ones, can be achieved by antipsychotic medication that the literature is bursting with ideas and items of evidence pointing to a neurochemical basis for the disease related to brain dopamine receptors and a microanatomical abnormality.[8]

The biggest problem in the tropics is persuading the patient to continue to take the drug regularly for the many months or years required to maintain remission and prevent relapse. The co-operation of relatives or friends in this task is of the greatest importance. Compliance is made easier by using depot injections, the price of which has—for generic fluphenazine decanoate—fallen to a level which can be afforded by most. Education of the family will play an important part in preventing relapse. It is therefore worth making the most strenuous efforts to see the relatives or friends of every patient and involve them in the treatment and management as much as in the diagnosis and assessment. The follow-up of patients largely depends on whether or not it is possible to organize a community service for such a purpose. This can be achieved for diabetics and for patients on drugs to combat leprosy and tuberculosis and is therefore possible for those with schizophrenia, who are tempted to discontinue their drugs when well, like others with chronic diseases responding to treatment. In the case of schizophrenia, however, the process of relapse disturbs thinking so that the patient fails to recognize the need to resume taking the drug.

MANIA AND BIPOLAR MANIC-DEPRESSIVE AFFECTIVE DISORDERS (F30 and F31)

Clinical features, prevalence (about 2 per 1000) and treatment are similar all over the world. There is an anecdotal impression that mania is somewhat more frequent and florid in the tropics. Even without treatment manic episodes are self-limiting after a few weeks or months, and the patients are able to live normal sociable lives between the episodes. In course of time the disorder tends to become 'bipolar', with episodes of depression alternating with those of mania. Later still, episodes of depression alone may occur. This bipolar disorder has a strong genetic basis; and it can respond rewardingly to lithium. This drug, however, although inexpensive, has a narrow therapeutic range and serious side-effects when taken in excess, so that regular monitoring of serum levels is essential. The provision of such a specialized service will be beyond the means of many centres in the tropics.

DEPRESSION (F32 and F33)

Although depression in the tropics is similar to that seen elsewhere, it is harder to spot because, it is claimed, the symptoms tend to be more somatic and less psychological than in the West. Thus patients may present with disturbances of sleep and slowing, but with little emphasis on how sad they feel. Even within the psychological range of symptoms, pathological guilt and suicidal ideas and behaviour have been reported to be rarer, at least in certain parts of the tropics. Because depressive disorders tend not to lead to socially disruptive behaviour, and are not recognized as being 'diseases' curable by doctors, many sufferers do not present for treatment to Western-style physicians. Depression, however, often responds rewardingly to tricyclics or similar drugs. Monoamine oxidase inhibitors are more complicated to use and have potentially dangerous side-effects; if given at all they should be prescribed by a professional psychiatrist. Electroconvulsive therapy, when available, can often rapidly induce a complete remission from severe depression, a great advantage when drug compliance is dubious.

PUERPERAL MENTAL DISORDERS (F53)

'Postpartum blues', a relatively mild depressive state, can occur a few days after delivery, is quite common and soon passes. More severe puerperal mental disorders occur within a few weeks of childbirth and persist for weeks, even months. Depression is the most common and may be profound, the mother occasionally becoming infanticidal or suicidal. Mania and schizophrenia are also known to occur in the puerperium. Cox[9,10] has made a special study of these disorders, cultural ideas about them and management appropriate to the local setting in Uganda. It is important to detect and treat depression because it can adversely affect the care of the child and hence his/her growth and development.

ACUTE TRANSIENT PSYCHOTIC EPISODES (F23)

Sudden threatening or actual violently aggressive behaviour creates a major emergency in any society and is likely to lead to police involvement. Doctors also become involved if a 'medical' cause is suspected. Conditions to be considered include:

Acute alcoholic intoxication and withdrawal

Acute drug intoxication, especially cannabis

Other conditions listed under acute organic mental disorders

Acute mania

Acute schizophrenia

Acute stress reaction

Personality disorder.

In such confrontations, quite commonly encountered in the tropics, the harassed doctor, sometimes fumbling with language and comprehension barriers and plagued by inadequate or even misleading information, can find it remarkably difficult to be sure whether the problem is primarily organic or functional or a combination of the two; and if it is functional, whether the patient is schizophrenic or manic. A typical scenario is the dramatic entry of a couple of policemen or a posse of relatives bringing with them a young man, handcuffed or otherwise restrained, dishevelled, restless, uncooperative, rambling in speech or mute or expressing wildly extravagant or paranoid ideas. Physical examination may be difficult, even impossible. The smell of alcohol if present is a tell-tale clue but cannabis intoxication, for instance, does not produce any diagnostic physical signs.

Remaining calm and gentle in these circumstances is difficult but rewarding, and some are much better than others at knowing how to defuse such fraught situations. It is useful to have a set of 'rules' to follow, known to several members of the staff on duty. These could be based upon those set out by Essex and Gosling.[11]

Admission or detention of such patients is usually desirable, not only because they are violent and need care and treatment, but also because documented observation of their clinical course over the next few hours and days will provide essential information for diagnosis and management.

NEUROSES

Traditional societies in the tropics tend to provide a tolerant and accepting milieu for neurotics even when they cannot work, earn a living or care for their homes and families. Nowadays, however, many young adults have drifted to large cities with rootless societies, and even in the countryside things are changing under the pervasive influence of the modern 'world village'. Table 9.4 lists the contrasts in a highly polar yet helpful manner. Table 9.5 contrasts the likely location of mentally ill people in developed and developing countries, again emphasizing the paucity of neurotics in Western-style medical practice in the tropics.[1] In reviewing published material on neuroses in developing lands, Leff highlights the extremes of the range, from 0.8 per 1000 in Taiwan aborigines to 269 per 1000 in rural Uganda women. The latter study by Orley and Wing[12] used the most advanced and sophisticated methodological techniques yet applied in such research in the tropics. Comparable techniques when used in Nigeria and elsewhere are nevertheless compatible with the idea that neuroses are in fact very common.

Table 9.4 Polar attributes of traditional and modern societies.

Traditional society	Modern society
Group oriented	Individual oriented
Extended family	Nuclear family
Income-producing linked to kinship ties	Income-producing independent of kinship ties
Economic functions non-specialized	Economic functions specialized
High mortality, high fertility	Low mortality, low fertility
Status determined by age and position in family	Status achieved by own efforts
Relationships between kin obligatory	Relationships between kin permissive
Relationships determined by role and position in family	Relationships determined by individual choice
Arranged marriages	Choice of marital partner
Individuals can be replaced by others filling same roles	Individuals unique and irreplaceable
Extensive classification terminology for distant relatives	Restricted classification terminology for close relatives only
Behaviour to specific kin prescribed	Great variation in kin behaviour
Emotional relationships stereotyped	Emotional relationships differentiated

Table 9.5 Location of psychiatrically ill people in developed and developing countries.

	Developed countries	*Developing countries*
Inpatient and outpatient services	Nearly all onset psychotics; small proportion of onset neurotics	Small proportion of onset psychotics and onset neurotics
General practitioners	Most onset neurotics; tiny proportion of onset psychotics	Service not usually available
Traditional healers	No onset psychotics; small proportion of onset neurotics	Many onset neurotics and onset psychotics
Vagrants	Chronic psychotics and neurotics with previous contact with medical services	Chronic psychotics and neurotics without previous contact with medical services
Prisons	Chronic psychotics and neurotics with previous contact with medical services	Some onset psychotics
General population	Possibly a handful of onset psychotics; substantial proportion of onset neurotics	Some onset psychotics; most onset neurotics

ANXIETY, ANXIOUS DEPRESSION, PHOBIAS, ACUTE STRESS REACTIONS (F40, F41 and F43)

CLINICAL FEATURES

The symptoms of anxiety, like those of depression, are often expressed in mainly or wholly somatic terms, and when acute can merge into panic. It is essential to examine and investigate as carefully as possible for the presence of organic disease before concluding that the patient is suffering only from a mental disorder. Phobias occur but have seldom been systematically described in the tropics.

Fears for physical safety, as well as those related to the world of spirits and witches, can affect mental health profoundly. Reactions to acute stress and adjustment disorders are quite common. In addition to exceptionally severe 'life events', such as wars and disasters, long-term stressors can have psychological consequences. These can typically present as somatoform disorders.

TREATMENT

It is galling to have to face the possibility that after careful efforts to exclude organic disease, and despite the clear presence of anxiety or depression, the patient and relatives may resolutely refuse to accept a psychiatric diagnosis and may indicate their intention to seek another opinion. There can be no objection to recommending innocuous symptomatic remedies; some doctors might be unhappy with placebos, but few there must be who have not at one time or another been grateful for the availability of aspirin, ascorbic acid, magnesium trisilicate and other such simple drugs.

Benzodiazepines are the traditional anxiolytics but must be given only for a limited period, not indefinitely, because dependence is just as likely to occur in the tropics as elsewhere. Propranolol (or other β-adrenergic blocker) helpfully reduces some of the somatic manifestations of anxiety, especially 'palpitations'. Most antidepressants are also sedating and are helpful in anxiety as well as depression, provided that the patient clearly understands the need to wait for several days before the effect begins to be noticeable.

HYSTERIA (F44)

Professional psychiatrists dislike the term 'hysteria' and many are trying to drop the word altogether, despite its venerable lineage, in favour of 'dissociative (conversion) disorders'. Its psychic mechanisms may be obscure and controversial, but the non-specialist would still accept the idea that in hysteria severe psychological stress is being converted into somatic symptoms sufficiently dramatic to bring secondary benefit to the patient through him or her being labelled sick or ill—the primary benefit being the actual removal of the stress itself.[13] Hysteria is most common in, but is not exclusive to, young women and could be thought of as evidence of immaturity. The behaviour of such patients could also be considered as manipulative and, because being manipulated is strongly resented by others, hysterics tend to arouse great hostility in doctors once the 'deception' is unmasked, hostility which should be abandoned if it is accepted that the patient (unlike a malingerer) is not consciously and deliberately trying to deceive but is instead sending a cry for help. In Western society there has been a steady decline in the prevalence of hysteria throughout the twentieth century and it has now become a rare diagnosis there. In the tropics, however, hysteria is still very much alive.

CLINICAL FEATURES

The symptoms are usually neurological but do not conform to the classical descriptions of diseases of the nervous system. Instead they fit into the patient's idea of what should be wrong. The symptoms and signs can include pains, numbness, paralyses, blindness and mutism. More dramatic exhibitions include gross and bizarre involuntary movements, convulsive seizures simulating epilepsy, and apparent disturbances of consciousness ranging from overactivity to coma. In a relatively closed community, particularly a school or hostel, mass hysteria can develop, in which these manifestations, starting with one or two youngsters, quickly induce a high pitch of anxiety and are 'passed on' to many others, so as to mimic an epidemic outbreak of an infectious disease or of poisoning. Typically this outbreak of mass hysteria ceases as suddenly as it started.

TREATMENT

Organic disease can coexist with hysteria and must be treated appropriately, although such treatment may not eradicate the hysterical symptoms. Alleviating the latter by symptomatic remedies is likely to prove more rewarding than trying to explain them. Reducing the precipitating stress or modifying the behavioural response to it may be beyond the means of a busy practitioner, who can, however, take comfort that the patient will probably improve anyway in the course of time.

SOMATOFORM DISORDERS (PSYCHOGENIC SYMPTOMS AND HYPOCHONDRIASIS) (F45)

In all practices there is a large group of patients with somatic symptoms but no recognizable physical disease or obvious mental disorder. 'Psychogenic', 'psychosomatic', 'functional' or 'supratentorial' are some of the epithets applied, with innuendos only slightly less pejorative than the terms 'imaginary' or 'deliberate'. Hypochondriasis is a persistent preoccupation with fancied ill health of the body generally or of one organ in particular. Students in the tropics with imprudent work schedules are prone to worry about their brains and eyes and to develop tension headaches, inability to concentrate, various eye pains, and other visual and sleeping difficulties. This syndrome has become known as the 'brain-fag' syndrome,[14] and is considered to be a response to study stress. It has been particularly described in Africa. Advice on study methods, relaxation and discussion about the pupils' and families' expectations are the most appropriate interventions.

Malingering is definitely a derogatory term, used when deliberate deception with the intention of avoiding an uncongenial task or situation is thought to be occurring. It is familiar to those involved with the care of soldiers, schoolchildren and employees.

PERSONALITY DISORDERS (F60)

There are people who have personalities such that their behaviour is strange but who could not be said to be suffering from a named psychiatric disorder. Of major concern to human society is the person whose behaviour deviates markedly from what is acceptable or even safe. These are the 'psychopaths', often with criminal propensities, intent on instant gratification and liable to acts of violence, sexual offences, drug and alcohol abuse and arson (greatly feared where people's meagre wealth consists of clothing, wooden furniture and paper money beneath a thatched roof and where insurance schemes are non-existent). It seems that all societies contain such deviants. They pose more of a threat when the usual cohesive forces are broken down by war, disasters or the drift to cities with the relentless undermining of traditional rural values.

Neuroleptic drugs can modify behaviour but have little place in the treatment of personality disorders. There are psychotherapies with something to offer, but time, costs and cultural barriers put them far beyond the limits of practicality in most of the tropics.

MENTAL RETARDATION (F70–79)

Paediatricians are the specialists most likely to be coping with the problems created by mental retardation. Institutional care requires too many resources and is inappropriate in most cases. Most individuals are looked after at home. It is of great importance to remember that some learning, however slow, is possible for all those with mental retardation. This requires careful assessment and a degree of optimism which may at times be difficult to muster. Schemes such as the World Health Organization's community based rehabilitation programme[15] are feasible in most tropical countries.

TRADITIONAL HEALERS

All countries have their 'alternative medicines', which tend to be in competition with the government-sponsored (usually 'Western') system. Ethnocentric incomprehension and scorn have created barriers between Western-style therapists and traditional healers. 'Witch doctors', 'medicine men' and 'ju-ju', for example, are words loaded with sinister implications as regards beliefs, behaviour and even continuation of life in Afro-Caribbean settings. Respectful but not gullible inquiry into indigenous methods of healing is becoming a much more creditable area of study, along the lines pioneered by Field[16] in Ghana. It can at times be worth the effort involved in trying to find out more about what is going on locally!

REFERENCES

1 Leff J. *Psychiatry Around the Globe: A Transcultural View*. London: Gaskell Press, 1988.

2 Leff J. Transcultural psychiatry. In Weatherall D J, Ledingham J G G & Warrell D A (eds) *Oxford Textbook of Medicine*, 2nd Edn. Oxford: Oxford University Press, 1987; p. 25, 57–59.

3 Cox J L & Jorsh M S. Transcultural psychiatry. In Weller M P I & Eysenck M V (eds) *The Scientific Basis of Psychiatry*, 2nd edn. London: WB Saunders, 1992: 469–490.

4 World Health Organization. *ICD-10 Classification of Mental and Behavioural Disorders F00–F99 — Clinical Descriptions and Diagnostic Guidelines*. Geneva: WHO, 1992.

5 Teasdale G & Jennett B. Assessment of coma and impaired consciousness: a practical scale. *Lancet* 1974; ii:81–84.

6 German G A. Mental disorders. In Shaper A G, Kibukamusoke J W & Hutt M S R (eds) *Medicine in a Tropical Environment*. London: British Medical Association, 1972:329–347.

7 Ashton C H. Cannabis: dangers and possible uses (leading article). *BMJ* 1987; 294:141–142.

8 Mackay A V P & Iversen L L. Neurotransmitters and schizophrenia. In Weller M P & Eysenck M W (eds) *The Scientific Basis of Psychiatry*, 2nd edn. London: WB Saunders, 1992: 558–581.

9 Cox J L. Amakiro: a Ugandan puerperal psychosis? *Soc Psychiatry* 1979; 14:49–52.

10 Cox J L. Psychiatric morbidity and pregnancy: a controlled study of 263 semi-rural Ugandan women. *Br J Psychiatry* 1979; 134:401–405.

11 Essex B & Gosling H. *Programme for Identification and Management of Mental Health Problems*. Tropical Health Series. Edinburgh: Churchill Livingstone, 1982.

12 Orley J H & Wing J K. Psychiatric disorders in two African villages. *Arch Gen Psychiatry* 1979; 36:513–520.

13 Kendell R E. Hysteria, somatisation and the sick role. *Med Int* 1991; 95:3944–3947.

14 Prince R. Concept of culture bound syndromes: anorexia and brain fag. *Soc Sci Med* 1985; 21:197–203.

15 World Health Organization. *Training in the Community for People with Disabilities*. Geneva: World Health Organization, 1989.

16 Field M J. *Search for Security: An Ethno-psychiatric Study of Rural Ghana*. London: Faber & Faber, 1960.

CHAPTER 10

OPHTHALMOLOGY IN THE TROPICS AND SUBTROPICS

D. D. Murray McGavin

WORLD BLINDNESS

The World Health Organization (WHO) Programme for the Prevention of Blindness estimates that the number of people who will be blind by the year AD 2000 will be around 45 million, with an increase of at least one million each year in the intervening years. This is the same as the whole population of Spain, or nine times the population of Denmark. The figure does not take into account the many millions who will have only partial sight. Over 80% of blindness is in countries of the developing world and 80% of this blindness could be 'avoided', that is, either prevented or cured.

WHO CATEGORIES OF VISUAL IMPAIRMENT

Approximately 20 years ago, it was realized that there were over 70 different definitions of blindness amongst United Nations member states. Five categories of visual impairment were later defined (Table 10.1).

Table 10.1 Categories of visual impairment (adapted from the International Classification of Diseases, ninth (1975) revision).

Categories*	Visual acuity† with best possible correction	
	Maximum less than:	Minimum equal to; or better than:
1 Visual impairment	6/18 20/70 3/10 (0.3)	6/60 20/200 1/10 (0.1)
2 Severe visual impairment	6/60 20/200 1/10 (0.1)	3/60 (finger counting at 3 metres) 20/400 1/20 (0.05)
3 Blindness	3/60 (finger counting at 3 metres) 20/400 1/20 (0.05)	1/60 (finger counting at 1 metre) 5/300 (20/1200) 1/50 (0.02)
4 Blindness	1/60 (finger counting at 1 metre) 5/300 (20/1200) 1/50 (0.02)	Light perception
5 Blindness	No light perception	

*If the extent of the visual field is taken into account, patients with a visual field radius no greater than 10° but greater than 5° around central fixation should be placed in category 3. Patients with a field no greater than 5° around central fixation should be placed in category 4, even if the central acuity is not impaired.

†For the first four categories of visual impairment, the different figures in each box of the visual acuity columns represent the same level of acuity expressed according to different notations. The first line gives the notation used with the Snellen 6-metre scale (and, where applicable, the corresponding ability to count extended fingers at a set distance); the second line gives the equivalent notation used with the 20-foot scale; the third line gives the decimal notation.

Table 10.2 Major causes of blindness (after ref. 1).

	United Kingdom	*Tanzania*
Children (0–15 years)	Genetic diseases Retrolental fibroplasia Congenital anomalies	Vitamin A deficiency (measles) Congenital cataract Ophthalmia neonatorum
Adults (45 years +)	Age-related macular degeneration Chronic glaucoma Diabetic retinopathy	Cataract Trachoma Chronic glaucoma

By definition, 'blindness' is recognized in a person whose best-corrected binocular visual acuity is less than 3/60 (less than counting fingers at 3 metres) or where the central visual field is less than 10° around fixation (but greater than 5°) in the better eye. The importance of observing these guidelines cannot be overemphasized, whether using the Snellen's type, the foot-scale or the decimal notation. Agreed definitions allow comparisons between countries and regions, and between the main causes of blindness affecting different populations. It then becomes possible to consider the ophthalmic staff and equipment required to provide eye care services.

PATTERNS OF BLINDNESS

The prevalence of blindness around the world is influenced by a number of factors, including age, sex, ethnic origin, environment and geographical location.

AGE

Life expectancy is increasing in developing countries, and with the increase in the numbers of old people, there is a corresponding increase of those who are blind. In the countries of the so-called developed world, increased longevity has also resulted in more older people with chronic blinding diseases. There is, however, a contrast in the common causes of blindness between the developed and the developing world. Similarly, blinding eye disease amongst children (0–15 years) shows quite different causes of visual impairment (Table 10.2).[1] It should be remembered that in many developing countries 50% of the population is under 15 years old.

SEX

Blinding eye disease throughout the world shows some differences between males and females (Table

Table 10.3 Blinding diseases (after ref. 1).

More common in women	*More common in men*
Trachoma	Onchocerciasis
Acute glaucoma	Chronic glaucoma
Cataract	Climatic keratopathy
Diabetic retinopathy	

10.3).[1] Trachoma is 4–5 times as common amongst women compared with men, due to the recurrent cycle of reinfection affecting children and mothers (Figure 10.1). Onchocerciasis (river blindness), as a blinding disease, is more common in men who are exposed to the bites of the black biting fly (genus *Simulium*). Exposure to the fly by working in fields or by rivers where the fly breeds, greatly increases the risk of infection. In Burkina Faso, amongst the Dagara tribe, women work alongside men in the fields, and the prevalence of blinding eye disease is the same between the sexes.[2]

Closed angle glaucoma in Eskimo women is 3–4 times greater as compared with men. Conversely, open angle glaucoma amongst Africans seems to be more common in men than women.

Climatic keratopathy, due to exposure either to

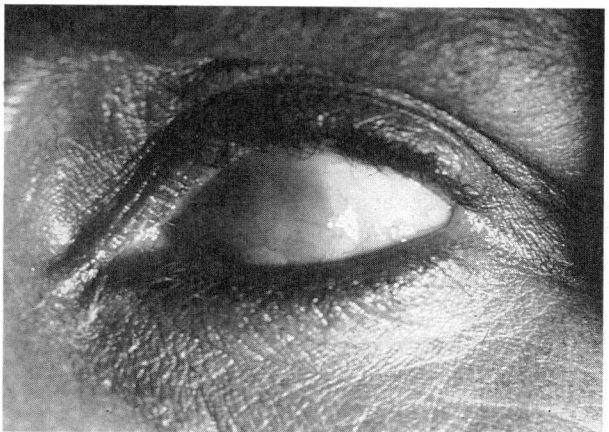

Figure 10.1 A blind eye due to trachoma in a 44-year old woman. Photo: John D C Anderson.

direct or reflected ultraviolet light, is up to five times more common amongst men than women. This relates to the exposure of men working out of doors, and is common in desert areas.

Hospital records consistently show that more men seek help for their eye problems. However, population-based surveys within communities reveal a more even pattern of disease distribution between the sexes.

ETHNIC ORIGIN

Glaucoma, in its two primary forms, shows a definite variation amongst broad ethnic regions around the world. Primary closed angle glaucoma is more common amongst Eskimos, Chinese and other races with mongoloid facial characteristics. In contrast, primary open angle glaucoma is recognized as common amongst Africans, often presenting in younger patients as compared with Caucasian races. This pattern of distribution of open angle glaucoma is also recognized amongst black Americans and in the Caribbean.

ENVIRONMENTAL FACTORS

Many environmental factors affect the prevalence of blindness in communities, and provide a huge variety of influences on eye disease. Of the common blinding diseases, both cataract and trachoma are found in populations where there are poor primary sources of water. Acute dehydration, which may have been due to acute diarrhoeal disease, is recognized as a risk factor for the later onset of cataract. The closer a community is to a good primary water source, the less likely it is that trachoma will be a major blinding scourge within that community. Tra-choma has been shown to be more common amongst cattle herders when compared with camel herders.

In a region where onchocerciasis is found, a village situated close to a river with turbulent, frothy water is more likely to have blinding eye disease due to onchocerciasis. The *Simulium* fly, which carries the microfilariae of the worm *Onchocerca volvulus,* breeds at the margins of these rivers. Thus, the name river blindness. A village which has the 'buffer' of another village situated between the river and its own community, has some degree of protection provided by the first-line village.

A poor environmental source of fruits and vegetables, or lack of basic health education where these vitamin A-rich foods may be available, place children between the ages of 1 and 6 years at risk of xerophthalmia.

GEOGRAPHICAL LOCATION

Prevalence rates of blindness in the developing countries of the world are higher when compared with those in the developed world. Estimates of the number of blind people in different regions of the world reflect population densities as well as available eye care services (Table 10.4).[3]

In the developed countries, better perinatal care allows infants to survive, but with occasional eye abnormalities such as genetic defects and retinopathy of prematurity. In countries where obstetric and neonatal care is less advanced, many premature babies do not survive.

In adult and ageing populations in the developed world, diabetic retinopathy, age-related macular degeneration and glaucoma are major causes of blindness. In the developing world, besides glaucoma, the most common eye diseases are cataract and the gross scarring effects of trachoma. In many communities, cataract is assumed to be part of the

Table 10.4 Global distribution of blindness by economic region.

Region	Reference population ($\times 10^3$)	No. of blind ($\times 10^3$)	Prevalence of blindness (%)
Established market economies	797 788	2400	0.3
Former socialist economies of Europe	346 237	1100	0.3
India	849 515	8900	1.0
China	1 133 698	6700	0.6
Other Asian and Islands	682 533	5800	0.8
Sub-Saharan Africa	510 271	7100	1.4
Latin America and Caribbean	444 297	2300	0.5
Middle-Eastern Crescent	503 075	3600	0.7
Total	5 267 414	37 900	0.7

Source: B Thylefors et al.[3]

natural process of ageing for which there is no remedy. Diabetic retinopathy is now recognized as a major cause of blindness in developing countries.

Onchocerciasis (river blindness) is found in West and Central Africa, and there are pockets of infection in Sudan, Ethiopia, Tanzania and the Yemen. It is also found in isolated foci in Central America and the northern regions of South America.

COMMON CAUSES OF WORLDWIDE BLINDNESS (Table 10.5)

We have briefly discussed the definition of blindness and some significant factors which influence blindness in the world.

In most countries of the developing world, *cataract* accounts for over 50% of those who are blind, with a worldwide total of 17–20 million. These are patients with bilateral mature or maturing cataracts and do not include the many millions who have visual impairment due to immature cataracts.

The second major cause of blindness worldwide is *trachoma*, and active infection probably affects around 150 million people. Of these, approximately 5.5 million are considered to be blind or at risk of blindness. Corneal scarring, the result of chronic and distressing infective eye disease, may ultimately lead to blindness.

Glaucoma, in its various forms, whether primary closed angle glaucoma, primary open angle glaucoma or secondary glaucoma, is found in all countries. Its onset may be acute and very painful, or chronic and insidious, without pain. About 5 million people worldwide are estimated to be blind due to glaucoma, although the actual figure may be higher.

Diabetic retinopathy is an increasing problem in the developing world, reflecting increased length of life, changing diet and improving medical services. It is estimated that approximately 2.5 million people worldwide are blind due particularly to retinopathy of diabetes.

Xerophthalmia (vitamin A deficiency affecting the eye), which is the main cause of blindness in childhood, probably affects 500 000 children each year, of whom 250 000 are irreversibly and needlessly made blind. The remainder have varying degrees of impairment of vision. An even more sobering finding is that up to 75% of blind children will die within months of the onset of their blindness. The tragedy of xerophthalmia is that remedies are readily available which would preclude any development of this avoidable eye disease.

Onchocerciasis is thought to affect about 19 million people, particularly in West and Central Africa. Perhaps 360 000 are blind by WHO definition.

In Europe, North America and other industrialized areas of the world with longer life expectancies, *age-related macular degeneration* causes sufficient reduction of central vision to place these patients within the category of blindness. It is considered that about one million people, in these countries in particular, are blind.

Eye injuries occur in all countries, and increased industrialization in the 'emerging' countries, often without adequate eye protection, results in unnecessary blindness. Up to 500 000 people are blind due to eye injuries.

In the countries of Asia, Africa and Latin America, *leprosy* is a significant cause of blindness with possibly 300 000 people blind.

EYE CARE SERVICES

There is a huge imbalance in the provision of eye care services when comparing the developed and the

Table 10.5 Causes of worldwide blindness.

Cause of blindness	No. of blind (×10⁶)	Geographical distribution
Cataract	17.0	Worldwide
Trachoma	5.5	Asia, Africa
Glaucoma (all types)	5.0	Worldwide
Diabetic retinopathy	2.5	Europe, North America
Xerophthalmia	1.0	Asia, Africa, Latin America
Age-related macular degeneration	1.0	Europe, North America
Onchocerciasis	0.5	West Africa, Latin America
Injuries	0.5	Worldwide
Leprosy	0.25	Asia, Africa, Latin America
Others	3.0	Worldwide

Source: WHO Programme for Prevention of Blindness.

developing countries of our world. In Europe and North America, there is one ophthalmologist for populations ranging from 20 000 up to 100 000. In Africa, on average, there is one ophthalmologist for one million people.

The countries of Asia reveal great variety in the provision of eye care services. India has over 100 medical schools and many trained ophthalmologists who carry out large cataract surgical lists. Eye camps may accommodate 50 or more cataract operations each day. One recent paper indicates that the incidence of blinding cataract in India in 1 year is 3.8 million.[4] Approximately 1.2 million cataract operations are carried out each year in India, and even allowing for the recognized increased mortality amongst patients with blinding cataract, compared with controls of the same age and sex, there is clearly an increasing pool of unoperated blinding cataract. The figure of 3.8 million new patients with blinding cataract each year may reflect the picture in certain parts of India.

Other countries in Asia and around the world have the same traditional method of reaching the rural populations through eye camps. However, in some countries there is little recognition of the huge numbers of patients requiring eye care who may live and die in remote areas of a country without specialist help.

A universal feature of eye care services throughout the world is the 'urbanization' of ophthalmologists—drawn to the major cities by the attractions of life style and financial reward. This gives a different picture when considering statistics for eye specialists in relation to populations, where the ratio in rural areas consistently reveals inadequate eye care facilities and expertise. Some of those who have specialized in ophthalmology do contribute generously of their time and resources in visiting distant and often impoverished communities, whether within their own native countries or by arranged visits from the more advantaged countries of the world.

If we consider that 80% of the world's blindness is in developing countries and that 80% of this blindness could be either prevented or cured, then the message of need and responsibility is clear and unequivocal.

However, there are around 100 countries in the world that have a programme for the prevention of blindness, out of the estimated 116 United Nations member states—a tribute to the considerable efforts of the team leading the WHO Programme for Prevention of Blindness.

To meet the needs of the huge numbers of cataract blind patients in Africa, surgeons are being trained who may not be medically qualified. Ophthalmic medical assistants (ophthalmic clinical officers) who have an interest and aptitude, possessing the hand skills required for eye surgery, make excellent surgeons.

The best and most effective organization of eye care services, in most developing countries, has a structure of primary health care workers, trained in the recognition of eye disease, who can provide basic treatment and advice for patients and recognize those patients who should be referred to secondary eye care units. Secondary eye care facilities will provide routine eye surgery, but should have the option of referring patients to tertiary eye care centres. These centres should be well staffed with trained ophthalmologists, ophthalmic medical assistants, optometrists, nurses and support staff, and also be equipped with necessary diagnostic and surgical instruments.

At all levels of expertise and experience, ongoing training should be given high priority. Training materials such as textbooks, manuals, teaching slide sets and posters should be made widely available. These eye health care workers can in turn develop their own programmes to provide health education for the general public.

EYE CAMPS

Eye camps may be planned and instituted in several forms. These ophthalmic outreach programmes may be described in three broad categories:

- Screening/diagnostic eye camps
- Permanent peripheral eye clinics
- Traditional surgical/operational eye camps.

The *screening/diagnostic outreach service* is being increasingly recognized following pioneer work by centres such as Aravind Eye Hospital, Madurai, India.[5] Small teams of eye care health workers visit the villages, carry out eye examinations, and refer patients to the central base hospital, often for surgery (Figure 10.2). In some situations, vehicles are provided to carry patients to the main hospital and later return them to their villages.

The *permanent peripheral eye clinic* is the establishment of a small permanent eye clinic, as a satellite to the central base hospital.[6] At regular intervals, preferably on the same day of each month, the eye team will visit the clinic and carry out eye examinations and surgery. As with all of these ophthalmic services, it is particularly important that there is local community involvement in preparation, publicity and follow-up.

The *traditional surgical eye camp* continues to be necessary where distances to the main eye hospitals or units are great or where transport is difficult,

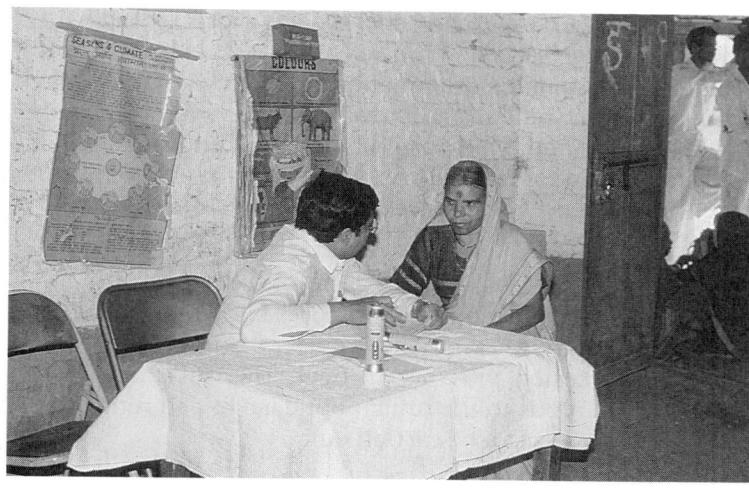

Figure 10.2 A screening/diagnostic eye camp in a school near Pune, India. Photo: Murray McGavin.

possibly with uneven and pot-holed roads. While a patient may be able to travel to the base hospital, it would be most unwise for the patient to make the return journey over a rough-surfaced road soon after cataract surgery!

EXAMINATION OF THE EYES

One of the real advantages in ophthalmology is the opportunity to visualize eye abnormalities of both the anterior and posterior segments of the eye. Thus, with a focal light and magnification, the anterior eye can be examined, and, with an ophthalmoscope, the optic nerve, retina and blood vessels can be seen.

BASIC EQUIPMENT AND DIAGNOSTIC MATERIALS

For effective examination of the eyes, only a few basic items are required.

- A test chart, e.g. Snellen's E chart
- A pin-hole disc to screen for refractive errors
- A hand torch (flashlight)
- A magnifying lens or loupe—uniocular or binocular
- A direct ophthalmoscope
- A lid speculum or retractor/s (suitably shaped paper-clips may be used)
- A Schiotz tonometer
- Eye drops: local anaesthetic drops, e.g. amethocaine 1%, benoxinate 0.4%; short-acting mydriatics (to dilate the pupil), e.g. tropicamide 1%, cyclopentolate 1%; fluorescein dye, e.g. minims (very small, disposable); paper strips. (Do not

use fluorescein eye drops from bottles as pathogenic organisms may contaminate these bottles.)

OTHER EQUIPMENT AND MEDICINES FOR TREATMENT OF EYE PATIENTS

A few basic requirements for the removal of conjunctival or corneal foreign bodies, corneal abrasions, eyelid and periorbital lacerations, infection of the eyelids, conjunctiva and cornea are as follows.

- Sterile hypodermic needles
- Fine suture material, needle-holding forceps, plain forceps
- Cotton-wool 'buds'
- Eye pads, adhesive tape, bandages
- Scissors
- Antibiotic eye drops and ointments, e.g. tetracycline 1% eye ointment, chloramphenicol 0.5% eye drops; systemic antibiotics, e.g. ampicillin 250 mg; vitamin A capsules (200 000 iu).

This chapter on eye diseases in the tropics and subtropics cannot describe the methods of examination in detail, which are always best taught by demonstration. However, a systematic approach to examination should always be followed.

1. History of the complaint

Symptoms and signs should be requested and described. What is the nature of the complaint? How long has the condition been present? Is vision affected? Is there pain, irritation, itching or discharge? What is the nature of the pain? Is the condition improving or worsening? Is there a family history of a similar complaint?

2. Measurement of visual acuity

Visual acuity should be assessed both for distance and near. Distance visual acuity should be recorded for each eye separately (Figure 10.3). If spectacles are worn for distance vision, visual acuity should be recorded with the spectacles on. If vision is reduced and there is no clear evidence of any eye disease, the pin-hole disc should be used. An improvement in vision in one or both eyes using the pin-hole indicates a likely refractive error—spectacles should improve vision.

3. Observe the general health of the patient

Is the patient, whether adult or child, healthy? Is the patient pale? What is the relationship between parent and child? Is the child distressed? A general impression of health or systemic disease is most important.

4. Examine the periorbital region of each eye

Is there swelling or inflammation—for example in the region of the lacrimal sac? Are the eyelids in the normal position, or are they everted (ectropion) or inverted (entropion)?

5. Examine both eyes together

Do the eyes appear to look straight ahead or is there any squint (strabismus)? Is there evidence of proptosis of either eye? Extraocular muscle movements can be assessed by asking the patient to gaze at an object which is moved into the various quadrants of gaze.

6. Examine the anterior eye with a focal light and magnification

Systematic examination in each eye of the conjunctiva (bulbar and tarsal), cornea, anterior chamber, iris and pupil should be carried out using the hand-held torch. To observe the upper tarsal conjunctiva, the eyelid should be everted.

7. Examination of the posterior eye

Using the ophthalmoscope and rotating different lens powers into the eyepiece, examination from the anterior vitreous through the substance of the vitreous to the retina, optic nerve and retinal blood vessels can be carried out.

8. Examination of the intraocular pressure

A crude assessment of the intraocular pressure can be effected by gently palpating the upper eyeball through the eyelid, using the two index fingers, with alternating compression. This rough method will indicate only a very hard eye with increased intraocular pressure, or a very soft eye. Much more accurate readings may be obtained using a Schiotz tonometer or an applanation tonometer. Extreme care should be observed in manipulation should there be an eye injury, particularly if perforation is a possibility. Similarly, eversion of the eyelid should not be done in the presence of a perforating injury.

These simple procedures can be carried out very quickly by a primary health care worker trained to examine the eyes. More sophisticated equipment may be available in secondary and tertiary eye care centres, for example for the measurement of central visual fields to confirm the presence of glaucoma.

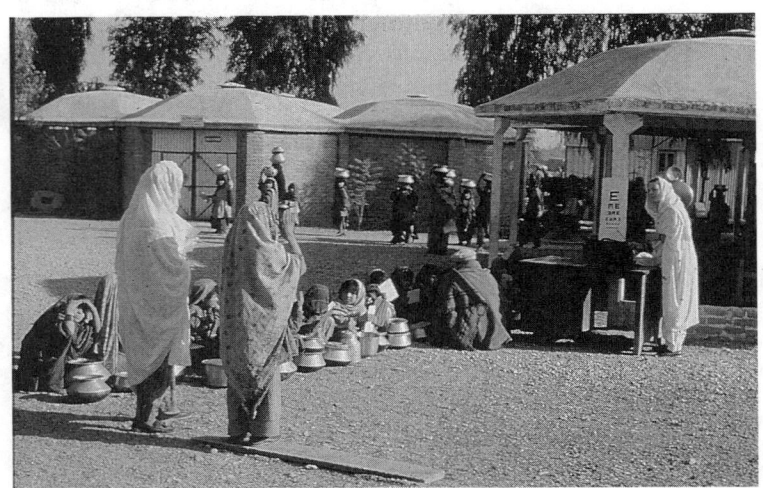

Figure 10.3 Testing the distance visual acuity of Afghan refugee children in Pakistan. Photo: Murray McGavin.

THE COMMON BLINDING DISEASES

CATARACT

Cataract is found worldwide and is the most common cause of blindness (Figure 10.4). It is estimated that 17 million people in the world are blind due to cataract. By definition, this means that the vast majority of these patients have bilateral mature or maturing cataracts. Many millions more have early or immature cataract. Most of the backlog of blind people requiring surgery is in Asia (70%), followed by Africa (20%).

Cataract may be described as congenital/developmental, traumatic, secondary or age-related. Table 10.6 gives the causes of cataract within these categories.[7]

Unfortunately, the only treatment for established cataract is the surgical removal of the lens of the eye, either as a whole (intracapsular cataract extraction) or in part (extracapsular cataract extraction). The second method is commonly used in countries with more advanced surgical techniques and this technique usually involves the insertion of an intraocular lens implant.

I have previously referred to the worldwide lack of cataract surgeons, at least within developing countries. If it should become possible to prevent or defer the onset of cataract, this would hugely contribute to easing the burden placed on inadequate eye care services, quite apart from the obvious and primary importance of alleviating much unnecessary suffering.

AETIOLOGY

Cataract is a public health problem.

Nutrition

A number of nutrients have been cited as playing a role in the development of cataract, based on animal and in vitro studies. These include: riboflavin, total protein, amino acids (especially tryptophan), vitamin C, vitamin E, selenium, calcium and zinc.[11] The question of whether malnutrition predisposes to the

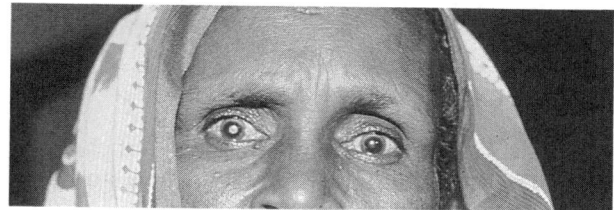

Figure 10.4   Bilateral cataract in a Somali woman. Photo: Murray McGavin.

development of cataract is difficult to elucidate. Malnutrition in developing countries is well recognized and is often associated with chronic diarrhoeal diseases, which themselves can aggravate underlying malnutrition. Chatterjee and his colleagues[12] in Punjab associated a higher prevalence of cataract with inadequate diet of proteins, including beans, lentils, milk, eggs and curd. In this study short height and low weight were also linked with the higher prevalence of cataract.

The converse of this and other studies is the question of whether the regular taking of multivitamins provides protection against the development of cataract. The Lens Opacities Case Control Study in the USA has recently indicated a decreased risk for all cataract types with regular use of multivitamins.[13] Further studies continue.

Diarrhoea/dehydrational crises

Evidence has accumulated that episodes of acute dehydration, as with severe diarrhoea or heatstroke, is a risk factor for the later onset of cataract, at least in some localities. The author was advised by a senior ophthalmologist and former professor of ophthalmology in Calcutta, India, that he recalled the 'acute' onset of cataract during epidemics of cholera. A history of severe diarrhoeal disease, sufficient to confine a patient to bed or mattress for 3 days, greatly increases the risk of the onset of cataract. It should be said that not all studies implicate acute dehydration so dramatically and, of course, a history of previous disease, when questions are specifically asked, has inevitable bias. However, the value of providing impoverished and

Table 10.6   Common causes of cataract (after ref. 7).

Developmental:	due to genetic factors, or intrauterine infection (especially rubella)
Traumatic:	due to blunt or perforating injuries
Secondary:	due to intraocular inflammation, systemic diseases or drugs
Age-related:	due to largely unknown factors associated with ageing

vulnerable communities with good water supplies is obvious. The best ophthalmologist for a community may well be the engineer who digs a deep well!

Sunlight

There are differing views as to the significance of sunlight in the aetiology of cataract. Early studies of sunlight and the prevalence of cataract in populations compared climates affecting these populations. In 1937, Wright[8] reported his study of 4000 labourers in two areas of India—one area typically with clear blue skies, and the other recognized as more cloudy. Cataract was more common in the cloudier area.

Epidemiological studies have been conducted in the USA. A cross-sectional survey of 838 watermen in Chesapeake Bay reported that lifetime sunlight exposure was associated with cortical but not nuclear cataracts. Only ultraviolet B light (295–320 nm) was associated with a weak increased risk of cortical cataract formation. After controlling for age, a doubling of cumulative exposure increased the risk by 1.60 (95% confidence interval, 1.01–2.64).[9]

A further 168 patients who required surgery for posterior subcapsular cataracts during 12 months in Maryland were compared with controls without posterior subcapsular cataracts selected from the same area and matched for age, sex and referral patterns. An association which was statistically significant was found between ultraviolet B and posterior subcapsular cataracts.[10]

Further research in this field is required. Some researchers believe that there is such significant risk associated with sunlight and the development of cataract that protective measures should be instituted. Health authorities in Australia and Canada, for example, are encouraging policies and health campaigns directed at reducing exposure to sunlight, to prevent both skin carcinoma and cataract. An environmental factor which demands our attention is the recognized thinning of the ozone layer which reduces the barrier protecting our planet from potentially harmful ultraviolet rays.

Smoking

A number of reports indicate an association between smoking and increased risk of nuclear cataracts and possibly posterior subcapsular cataracts. These studies suggest a 2–3 times increased risk of cataract with smoking. However, it is possible that smokers can reduce the risk by stopping the habit.[14]

Here is a further indictment of smoking as a highly significant risk to health.

Other risk factors for cataract

Diabetes and impaired glucose tolerance, glaucoma, hypertension, myopia and alcohol consumption are all described as increasing the risk of cataract in the developed world.[15]

SURGERY

An ongoing debate is the question of which surgical method should be used in countries of the developing world. The traditional method used for very many years to provide high volume cataract surgery is intracapsular cataract extraction (ICCE), where the entire lens is removed within its capsule. This may be effected by a variety of methods, including the use of capsule forceps and the safer procedure using the cryoprobe. The cryoprobe is applied to the surface of the lens, an ice-ball forms within the lens, and then the lens is gradually withdrawn from the eye (Figure 10.5). This method is one of the fastest methods available; magnification, which should always be used, does not need to be sophisticated, and standard, readily available instruments keep costs down. The particular disadvantage of this method is the need for aphakic correction, either with spectacles or with a contact lens. In most developing countries, a contact lens is not a realistic method of correction in view of uncertain hygiene and dusty and sandy environments, together with the difficulty older patients experience in manipulating the contact lens. Aphakic spectacles give a magnified, distorted image; in addition, they are often broken, lost or too expensive (see below).

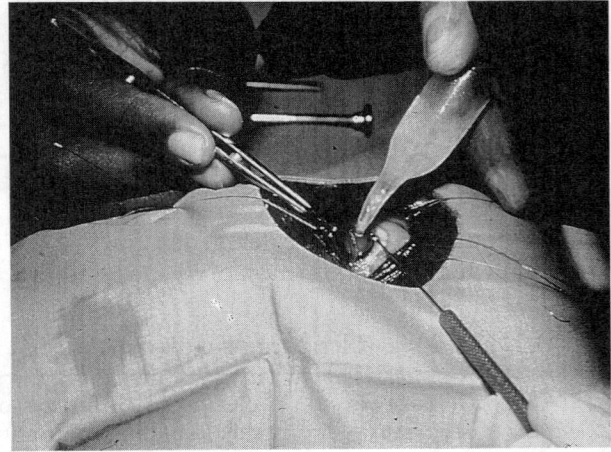

Figure 10.5 Intracapsular extraction using a cryoprobe. Photo: John D C Anderson.

The extracapsular cataract extraction (ECCE) leaves the posterior capsule of the lens in position, removing the nucleus and cortex of the lens. In the industrialized world and in much of the emerging surgical practice throughout the world, the posterior chamber intraocular lens (IOL) implant is placed within the capsular bag. Optically, this is the best method which is now being used. There should be no need postoperatively for relatively thick, convex magnifying aphakic spectacles—which may be broken or lost. Further, this type of cataract operation (ECCE + IOL) may be used for a unilateral cataract which may occur, for example, after trauma. There is no difficulty in fusing the images received by each eye, whereas aphakic spectacles worn after ICCE will magnify the image by 30%. This means that a unilateral cataract, corrected by an external aphakic lens, will result in different sizes of images seen—the patient sees double. The disadvantages of ECCE + IOL are the extra time taken to carry out surgery, the need for sophisticated magnification with coaxial illumination of the surgical field, and more expensive instrumentation.

Surgeons in developing countries are naturally keen to develop more advanced techniques and thus, in many centres throughout the world, ECCE + IOL is being routinely performed. The real problem arises when vast numbers in rural areas require routine cataract surgery, sometimes involving operating lists of up to 50 patients each day. It is also significant that surgeons training in the Western world are no longer taught the traditional ICCE, which may curtail their usefulness in visiting parts of the world where there is great need for cataract surgery to be carried out in large numbers.

Studies are being carried out to compare ICCE/aphakic spectacles and ECCE/posterior chamber IOLs (India and Thailand), and ICCE/anterior chamber IOLs and ICCE/aphakic spectacles (Nepal). Also in Nepal, the respective benefits of ICCE/anterior chamber IOLs and ECCE/posterior chamber IOLs are being studied.

Undoubtedly, techniques for the future should develop further along the lines of routine IOL surgery. The cost of IOLs is reducing—in one centre in India an excellent IOL is now produced for less than $US10. But we must be conscious of the increasing numbers of patients with cataract who may be side-lined because more advanced techniques, which are still more expensive, demand the time and energies of the ophthalmic surgeon. The great need of expertise in cataract surgery, in particular the intracapsular cataract method, is being addressed in Africa by training cataract surgeons, previously trained as ophthalmic medical assistants or ophthalmic clinical officers. This is a logical initiative which should be supported and implemented in other regions where cataract surgeons are few. Good hands and surgical skills are not confined only to those who are medically trained!

TRACHOMA

Trachoma is one of the major blinding diseases of the world. It is the most common infectious cause of blindness. Active trachoma is believed to affect around 150 million people. About 5.5 million are blind or at risk of blindness as a consequence of trachoma. This eye disease is a serious public health problem in many parts of Africa, the Middle East, central Asia, India and South-East Asia. It is also found in focal areas of Latin America and the Pacific region.

This eye disease is a recurrent, chronic eye infection. The infecting organism is *Chlamydia trachomatis*—one of a group of organisms which share characteristics of both viruses and bacteria. Of the different types of *C. trachomatis*, serotypes A, B, Ba and C cause the eye infection. Serotypes D–K mainly cause urogenital infection, where a secondary eye infection may occur, either due to infection transmitted to the newborn child during delivery (conjunctivitis of the newborn) or to a conjunctivitis occurring in association with urogenital infection in an adult. Unlike the eye-to-eye infection (serotypes A–C) which we are discussing here, chlamydial infection with serotypes D–K is a sexually transmitted disease.

Eye infection often begins in early childhood. Children a few months old may be infected with *C. trachomatis*. Recurrent episodes of reinfection, together with secondary bacterial infection, may lead on, after 10 or 20 years, to scarring of the eyelids, typically with the upper eyelid turning inwards (entropion), distortion of the eyelashes which may rub on the eyeball (trichiasis) and consequent disturbance of the corneal surface, deeper inflammation and eventually corneal scarring and blindness.

RISK FACTORS

Communities which typically have endemic trachoma are those characterized by a dry and dusty environment, with poor personal hygiene, lack of adequate sanitation, overcrowding in the homes and especially a large fly population.

Flies carry the organism *C. trachomatis*. Transmission of infection from child to child by flies has

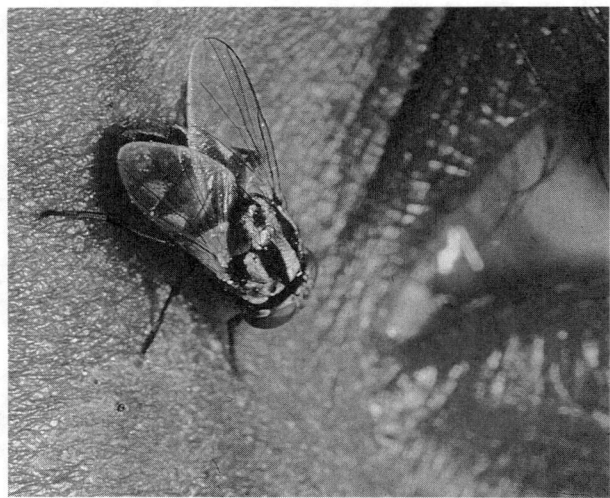

Figure 10.6   An eye-seeking fly which can carry the organism *Chlamydia trachomatis.* Photo: John D C Anderson.

been demonstrated. Eyes which have discharge attract flies (Figure 10.6). Nasal discharge attracts flies. Dirty, unwashed faces and fingers amongst children creates an environment at risk of trachoma.

The presence of faeces lying exposed, whether human or animal, will also attract flies. Well-designed ventilated pit latrines within communities, which are properly used, will reduce the prevalence of trachoma within a community. Rubbish lying in open places is a further attraction for flies.

An inadequate or far-distant primary water source is a further risk factor for trachoma. There is a direct correlation between the distance travelled to collect water and the prevalence of trachoma within a community (Figure 10.7). It is evident that a good local water supply must improve the personal hygiene of individuals within communities. The provi-

sion of a good water supply may be one of the most important interventions in reducing the prevalence of trachoma.

Lack of education, especially of mothers, is recognized as a risk factor for trachoma. Health education for parents and children should include advice about contaminated materials, for example the edge of a piece of clothing, which might be used to wipe away the discharge from a child's eyes. This can so easily be passed on to another child within the family.

One can summarize the mainly environmental risk factors for trachoma by listing the six Ds:

- Dry
- Dusty
- Dirty
- Dung
- Discharge
- Density (overcrowding in the home).

Another way of helping to remember agents of transmission of the eye disease is by listing the five Fs:

- Flies
- Faeces
- Faces
- Fingers
- Fomites (contaminated material or objects such as clothing or towels).

CLINICAL EXAMINATION

Examination of each eye should be carried out with at least 2.5× magnification, and with a good light.

1. After a brief examination of each eye for evidence of inflammation of the conjunctiva or any

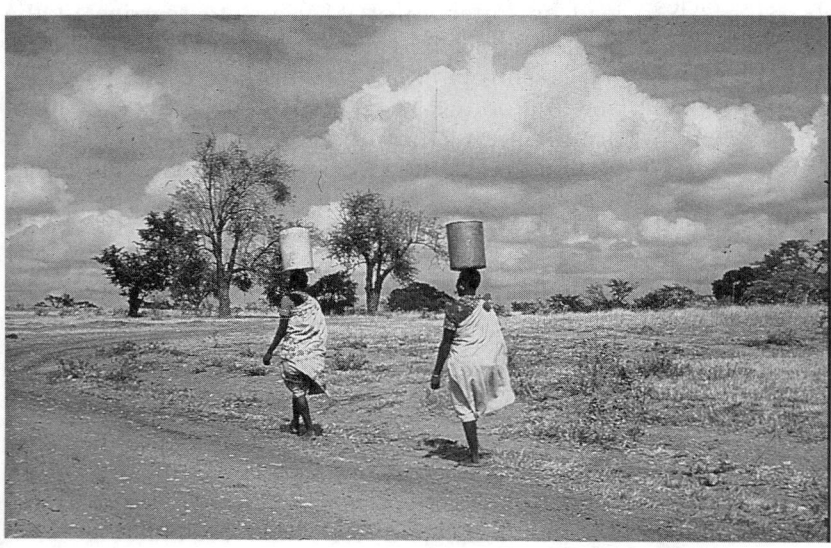

Figure 10.7   Collecting water—at a distance. Photo: Erika Sutter.

discharge, the eyelids should be carefully examined to see if any eyelashes are rubbing against the cornea.

2. It should be noted if any eyelashes have been removed (epilation).

3. The cornea is then examined for evidence of inflammation and/or corneal opacity.

4. The upper eyelid should now be turned over (everted). Ask the patient to look down, but keep the eyes open. The eyelashes are gently grasped between finger and thumb, and the other hand places a glass rod or similar object on the skin at the upper aspect of the tarsal plate of the upper eyelid, parallel to the lid margin. The upper eyelid is rotated against the slim rod and will evert. This provides a view of the upper tarsal conjunctiva.

5. The tarsal conjunctiva is examined for evidence of follicles, intense inflammation or conjunctival scarring.

SIMPLE GRADING SYSTEM (Plate 10.1)

In 1987 a new simplified grading classification for trachoma was reported in the *Bulletin of the World Health Organization*.[16] This method of assessment looks for the presence or absence of five selected signs. The order of examination for these five signs is given above.

Trachomatous inflammation—follicular (TF)

The presence of five or more follicles in the upper tarsal conjunctiva. Follicles must be at least 0.5 mm in diameter and should be situated on the flat surface of the tarsal conjunctiva. Follicles are small spots or lumps, yellowish or white and paler than the rest of the conjunctiva, which are accumulations of lymphoid cells.

Trachomatous inflammation—intense (TI)

Pronounced inflammatory thickening of the upper tarsal conjunctiva that obscures more than half of the deep tarsal vessels. In severe inflammation, the tarsal conjunctiva will appear red, rough and thickened. There is diffuse inflammatory infiltration, oedema and vascular papillary hypertrophy. There may also be many follicles present. This is an extremely infective stage of trachoma.

Trachomatous scarring (TS)

The presence of scarring in the tarsal conjunctiva. White lines in the tarsal conjunctiva show early signs of the scarring stage of trachoma. The scarring may also appear as bands or sheets and may sometimes look like the edge of a feather.

Trachomatous trichiasis (TT)

At least one eyelash rubbing on the eyeball. Evidence of removal of an eyelash/es (epilation) should also be included within this category in the grading system. Eyelashes may be removed by a patient using forceps and a mirror or some other polished or reflective surface. However, the removal of an eyelash in this way usually results in its regrowth in about 4–6 weeks.

If there is advanced conjunctival scarring and distortion of the upper eyelid, then surgery will be required for this patient.

Corneal opacity (CO)

Easily visible corneal opacity over the pupil. At least part of the pupil margin should be blurred when examining an eye with this size of corneal opacity. Thus, there should be some degree of visual impairment.

TREATMENT

Medical treatment

Treatment of active trachoma requires the application of tetracycline 1% eye ointment to both eyes. There are different regimens of treatment:

- Two times each day for 6 weeks.
- Two times each day for 5 consecutive days every month for 6 months.
- Once each day for 10 consecutive days every month for 6 months.

In practice, the first regimen of twice daily applications for 6 weeks to both eyes is usually used.

Clearly, the ointment is only effective against active trachoma, particularly follicular trachoma and intense inflammatory trachoma. However, the upper eyelid which shows conjunctival scarring may also have active inflammation as well. Whenever there is any possibility of active trachoma, a full course of tetracycline 1% eye ointment should be given.

In some patients, especially where there is intense inflammatory activity, a systemic antibiotic may be used:

- Doxycycline 100 mg, once each day for 21 days, or
- Tetracycline 250 mg, four times each day for 21 days.

  Important. These systemic antibiotics should not be given to women during pregnancy or to children under the age of 7 years.

Trials of azithromycin are taking place in the hope that this new long-acting antibiotic, taken orally, may be more effective than ointment when communities are treated.[17]

Trichiasis and epilation

When the occasional eyelash rubs against the cornea or conjunctiva causing extreme irritation, many patients remove the eyelash using forceps. They may carry a small mirror or other polished mirror-like surface to help them in this procedure. The disadvantage of this method is that the eyelash will grow again in 4–6 weeks.

A more permanent and effective method for dealing with isolated ingrowing eyelashes is to apply cautery at the base of the eyelash with the intention that the hair follicle will be destroyed. This method, of course, requires local anaesthesia by injection at the base of the eyelash.

Surgery for trachomatous entropion

There are a number of surgical procedures which have been designed to effect rotation of the eyelashes away from the eyeball by surgery to the eyelid, including the tarsal plate. In skilled hands the procedure can be most effective, and in a study carried out in Oman the most effective surgical method was bilamellar tarsal rotation.[18] Sometimes visual acuity will improve slightly following surgery for entropion, where there is some clearing of the corneal haze.

Surgery after corneal opacity

The severity of corneal scarring, which is often bilateral, usually precludes a good surgical result by corneal grafting, although this surgical procedure should not be excluded as a possible intervention in a tertiary centre.

If an area of cornea does remain clear, one possible surgical procedure is an optical iridectomy. The pupil is enlarged behind the clear cornea by removing a sector of the iris. Patients with bilateral corneal scarring may have their visual acuity improved from hand movements or doubtful counting fingers to counting fingers at 3 or 4 metres following this surgical intervention. Unfortunately, corneal scarring after trachoma is often diffuse and only occasionally allows this surgical operation.

PREVENTION

Recent studies have shown that regimens of topical treatment with tetracycline 1% eye ointment used within communities do not irradicate this eye disease. Within months the infection may return, with further inflammation and potential scarring.

Communities must be educated in the prevention of trachoma. The following advice should be suggested to the community.

- Provision of a suitable water supply.
- Regular daily face washing (and hand washing).
- Use of well-designed ventilated pit latrines.
- Rubbish lying in the open should be burned.
- Animals, especially cattle, should be housed some distance from the family home.
- Health education should be arranged for the community.

There is little anticipation at present of a vaccine that would prevent trachoma, and these measures should be communicated to communities at risk. In many countries of the world, trachoma as an eye-to-eye condition has been eradicated due to improved social, environmental and economic conditions. Foci of severe trachoma however remain. The message in preventing trachoma becomes clear: raise the standard of living and life for so many impoverished and disadvantaged communities around the world.

GLAUCOMA

Glaucoma presents in two primary forms:

- Primary open angle glaucoma (chronic simple glaucoma)
- Primary closed angle glaucoma (acute congestive glaucoma).

A congenital form of glaucoma may also occur (buphthalmos).

There are a number of secondary forms of glaucoma. Examples are:

- Glaucoma due to iridocyclitis
- Glaucoma after haemorrhage in the anterior chamber
- Phacomorphic glaucoma
- Phacolytic glaucoma
- Pigmentary glaucoma

Plate 10

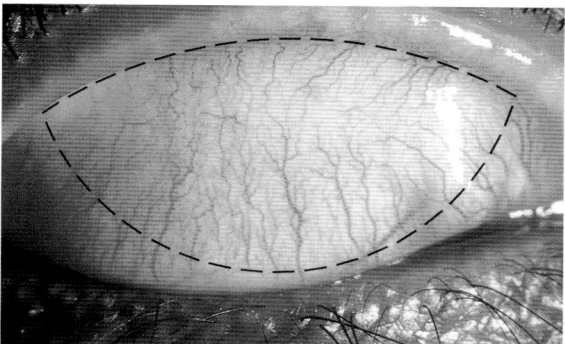

Plate 10.1   Normal upper eyelid. (The area to be examined for inflammatory changes is outlined.)

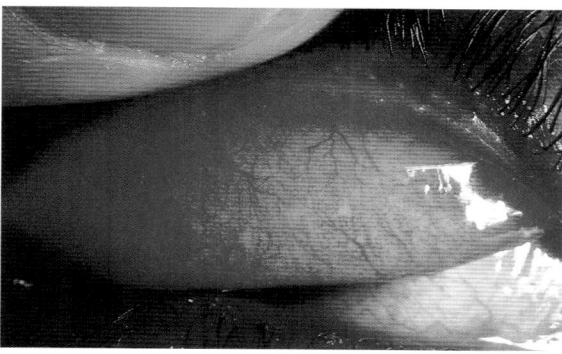

Plate 10.2   Trachomatous inflammation – follicular (TF): the presence of 5 or more follicles (each of which must be >0.5 mm diameter) on the flat surface of the upper tarsal conjunctiva.

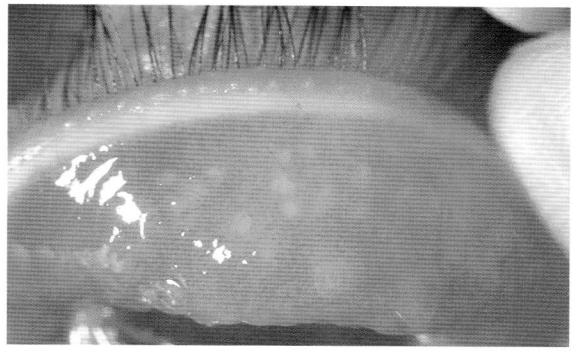

Plate 10.3   Trachomatous inflammation – intense (TI): marked inflammatory thickening of the upper tarsal conjunctiva; this obscures more than half the normal deep tarsal vessels.

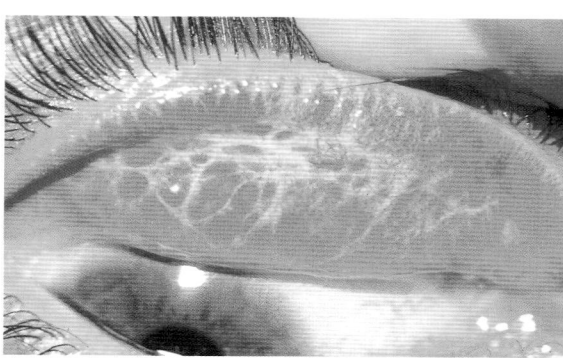

Plate 10.4   Trachomatous scarring (TS): involving the tarsal conjunctiva.

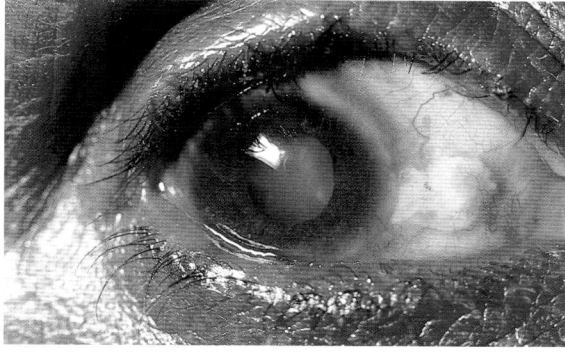

Plate 10.5   Trachomatous trichiasis (TT): evidence of one or more eyelashes rubbing on the eyeball. If one or a number of eyelashes have recently been removed, this should be graded trachomatous trichiasis.

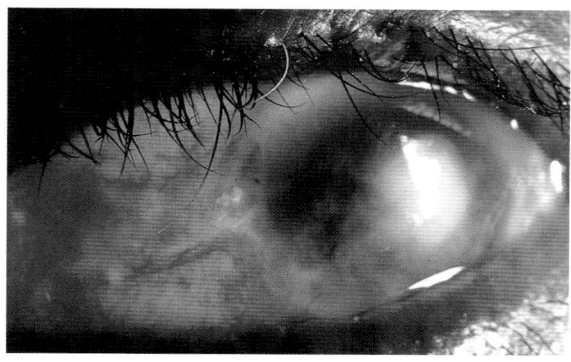

Plate 10.6   Corneal opacity (CO): corneal scarring due to trachoma where the scarring is central and sufficiently dense to obscure part of the pupil.

(Courtesy of *Journal of Community Eye Health*, International Centre for Eye Health, Institute of Ophthalmology, London.)

- Pseudoexfoliative glaucoma
- Neovascular glaucoma
- Steroid-induced glaucoma
- Epidemic dropsy.

EPIDEMIOLOGY

Glaucoma is found throughout the world. It is a blinding disease with up to 5 million blind worldwide. Estimated figures suggest 13.5 million with open angle glaucoma, 6 million with closed angle glaucoma, 2.7 million with secondary glaucoma and 300 000 children with congenital glaucoma.[19]

Open angle glaucoma is especially prevalent amongst Africans, where the disease process occurs relatively early in life, even in teenagers, with a correspondingly serious prognosis if treatment is not sought or is unavailable. However, open angle glaucoma in Africa appears to occur in clusters, with some variety in prevalence rates in different countries and regions of the African continent. The significance of this disorder amongst ethnic black races carries over to the countries of the Caribbean and also within the black populations of North America. The prevalence of open angle glaucoma amongst black Americans is 8–10 times higher than their white American compatriots. It may be that the melanin granules present in these eyes cause 'ageing' of the trabecular meshwork, in the angle of the anterior chamber, through which the aqueous fluid escapes. Open angle glaucoma is more common amongst the Caucasian populations of the industrialized world when compared with closed angle glaucoma.

The problem with open angle glaucoma is the difficulty in making an early diagnosis. The patient may be completely unaware of the condition until the visual fields are significantly reduced. Characteristic changes of the optic nerve head can be visualized by using the ophthalmoscope, but this requires expertise in the use of the instrument. The story is told of two ophthalmologists, father and son, trying out a new ophthalmoscope, with the son examining his father. On examining his father's optic nerve heads, the son realized that his father had glaucoma!

Closed angle glaucoma presents particularly amongst eastern races, such as Chinese, Vietnamese, Cambodians, Japanese and Eskimos.

It should be noted, however, that these separately described primary forms of glaucoma, in general, may occur amongst all races and there may be great variety in presentation. Thus, an intermittent closed angle form of glaucoma may occur. Clearly, the conditions described are not always absolute, falling into one category or another, but there may be some overlap in clinical presentation, still resulting in damage to the eye. Note also that patients with closed angle glaucoma have been reported in significant numbers from Nigeria, Uganda, Somalia and South Africa.

Very late diagnosis of open angle glaucoma in most of the developing countries of the world is borne out in the author's experience. In one country in central Asia, of patients examined during one calendar year in whom the diagnosis proved to be glaucoma, nearly 50% were already completely blind or nearly blind in one eye, with vision at no light perception or only slightly better, and in the second eye the vision was commonly reduced to counting fingers.

ANATOMY AND PHYSIOLOGY OF AQUEOUS FLUID CIRCULATION

The diagram of the eye in cross-section shows the production of aqueous fluid through the ciliary processes of the ciliary body. The aqueous fluid circulates around the lens of the eye and passes through the pupil, with most of the drainage of fluid being filtered through the trabecular meshwork at the angle of the anterior chamber. Any form of blockage of drainage, whether due to the root of the iris, blood, inflammatory cells, pigment, etc., can disturb the free drainage of aqueous from the eye, with a consequent rise in intraocular pressure.

OPEN ANGLE GLAUCOMA

The classical triad of ocular features which has long been taught in relation to open angle glaucoma (chronic simple glaucoma) should help us in our understanding of some of the factors which contribute to this eye abnormality:

1. Raised intraocular pressure
2. Cupped optic nerve head
3. Typical central visual field defects.

The onset of open angle glaucoma is typically insidious and may be unassociated with pain or headache. However, if a patient does complain of some headache then glaucoma must be considered in the differential diagnosis. The anterior segments of each eye are usually entirely normal in appearance. The intraocular pressure is characteristically raised and this is measured by tonometry. However, it should be noted that raised intraocular pressure alone does not necessarily mean that the patient has glaucoma. Glaucoma may be present, with visual field loss, associated with normal pressure (normal

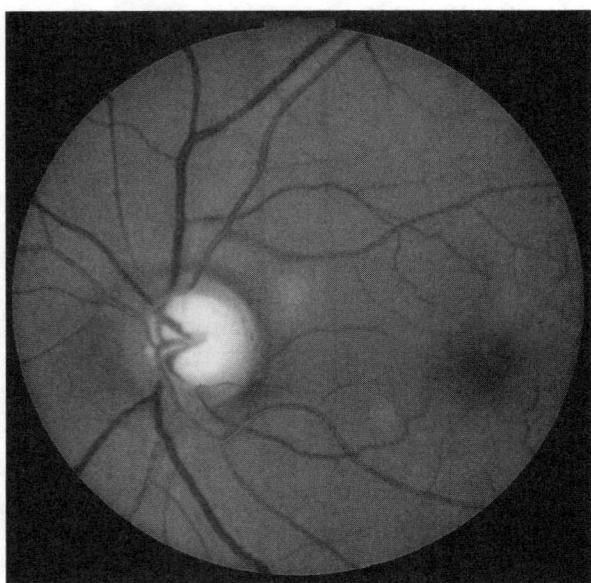

Figure 10.8 Cupping of the optic nerve head. Photo: Gordon Johnson.

tension glaucoma) and moderately raised pressures can occur in eyes that do not have classical open angle glaucoma (ocular hypertension).

Examination of the optic nerve head in each eye, using the ophthalmoscope, is of great importance in the diagnosis of glaucoma, particularly open angle glaucoma. An abnormally cupped optic nerve head can often be diagnostic of open angle glaucoma (Figure 10.8). A vertically cupped disc is more likely to be a glaucomatous cup. Borderline cupping of the optic disc, when the cup:disc ratio may be around 0.5, requires further investigation, with examination of central visual fields.

Gonioscopy is the technique used to examine the angle of the anterior chamber using a specially designed contact lens with a small mirror. Thus, the diagnosis of 'open angle', 'narrow angle', 'closed angle', 'secondary' glaucoma may be confirmed.

The central visual fields may be examined by a variety of methods from simple techniques to highly sophisticated computerized methods. Primary open angle glaucoma is typically a bilateral condition.

Treatment

The treatment of open angle glaucoma is to lower the intraocular pressure. There is a choice between surgical intervention and medical therapy. In developing countries, the approach should be surgical. This is for a number of reasons. Many patients, unfamiliar with the use of eye drops, will be confused by the instructions given, will also be very irregular in the instillation of the antiglaucoma eye drops and will not replace them when finished. This example of patient non-compliance is not confined only to developing countries. Eye drops, which generally require to be used for many years, probably for the lifetime of the patient, are costly. Also, experience in recent studies in industrialized countries have indicated that early surgery is beneficial in arresting the process of glaucoma.

If medical therapy is given, even for a short period of time, the following eye drops may be used:

- Pilocarpine 1, 2 or 4%, 3–4 times daily (alternative: carbachol 0.75 or 3%, three times daily).
- Timolol maleate (Timoptol) 0.25 or 0.5%, twice daily (alternatives: levobunolol 0.5%, twice daily; carteolol, 1 or 2%, twice daily; metipranolol 0.1, 0.3 or 0.6%, twice daily).
- Eserine 0.25 or 0.5%, 2–4 times daily.
- Adrenaline 1%, twice daily (alternative: Depivefrine, 0.1% twice daily).

Topical treatment with eye drops may be supplemented with oral acetazolamide tablets and these may be given in doses of 125 mg or 250 mg, ranging from one to four times daily. However, acetazolamide should only be used as a short-term measure; if required for a longer period of time, the patient should also be given a potassium supplement. Side-effects of acetazolamide include paraesthesiae, gastrointestinal disturbance and kidney stones.

The surgical procedure that is commonly used for open angle glaucoma is trabeculectomy. This filtering procedure allows escape of the aqueous fluid into the subconjunctival space.

Open angle glaucoma must be recognized as a condition which lasts for the remainder of the patient's life. Deterioration may continue despite treatment, but it is hoped that lowering the intraocular pressure will at least slow the progress of the disease, even if total arrest of the condition is not always achieved.

CLOSED ANGLE GLAUCOMA

Although closed angle glaucoma may occur in an intermittent form with occasional blurring of vision, the characteristic presentation of this acute eye condition is with severe pain, headache and, in extreme forms, even vomiting and disorientation. The intraocular pressure may be considerably raised, sometimes to 60 or 70 mmHg, and this must be reduced as quickly as possible.

Closed angle glaucoma is an ophthalmic emergency—delay can result in permanent loss of vision. Furthermore, without any treatment, the second eye has a greater than 50% chance of developing closed angle glaucoma within 5 years.

Clinical presentation

A typical presentation will find a patient who is distressed with severe pain and headache. The affected eye is red and congested. The cornea is often hazy due to corneal oedema and there may be awareness of coloured haloes around lights. Closer examination reveals a shallow or 'flat' anterior chamber, with the iris close against the corneal endothelium. The pupil may be dilated or semidilated and fixed, not responding to light. It may not be possible to view the posterior segment of the eye, in particular the optic nerve head, through the hazy cornea.

It should be noted that the 'closed angle' variety of glaucoma may also be 'intermittent' or even 'latent' in its presentation, always with the potential for an acute episode to occur.

The second eye, in comparison, is usually quiet and appears entirely normal. Close examination is likely to reveal a shallow anterior chamber. A shallow anterior chamber can be viewed by shining a light from the side of the eye across the anterior segment of the eye. The view of the posterior eye often shows a normal optic nerve head.

Visual acuity is usually considerably reduced in the glaucomatous eye, while often normal in the unaffected eye. Using the two index fingers, gently palpating the upper surface of the affected eye 'through' the upper eyelid, with the patient looking down, may give a sense of a hard eye when compared with the other eye. Tonometry will confirm the likely diagnosis.

Treatment

Treatment must be immediate. Acetazolamide, taken orally if possible, should be given in high doses, 250 mg four times daily. If the patient is not able to take acetazolamide orally, the drug may be given by slow intravenous infusion or by injection intramuscularly. Alternatives to acetazolamide in providing systemic treatment of markedly raised intraocular pressure are oral glycerol or intravenous mannitol. This systemic treatment is supplemented with Gutt. timolol maleate 0.5% twice daily. Pilocarpine should be given when the intraocular pressure has started to come down, and then 3–4 times daily while longer term treatment is considered.

When the eye has quietened and the intraocular pressure has returned to normal, a surgical procedure is planned. In the eye which has had the acute attack, the likely procedure is a trabeculectomy. It is of particular importance that the second eye also has surgery as a prophylactic measure. Here the procedure is an iridectomy or an iridotomy. The iridotomy can be done using the laser. This procedure creates another opening through which aqueous fluid can pass (the other opening is the pupil) and deepens the anterior chamber of the eye, drawing the root of the iris away from the trabecular meshwork and thus allowing escape of aqueous fluid which previously had been blocked.

NORMAL TENSION GLAUCOMA

It should be noted that a condition is described where typical glaucomatous field defects occur in association with a glaucomatous cup of the optic nerve head but the intraocular pressure is consistently recorded within the normal range. This is normal tension (or 'low' tension) glaucoma and indicates poor blood circulation at the optic nerve head with ischaemia, resulting in progressive optic nerve atrophy. Treatment may be difficult, but lowering the intraocular pressure further is the only approach we have at present.

CENTRAL VISUAL FIELDS AND MEDICAL TREATMENT OF GLAUCOMA

If medical therapy with eye drops is used, it is most important that the central visual fields are carefully recorded at regular intervals, often every 3–4 months. This regular attendance at the glaucoma clinic will necessarily continue for the rest of the patient's lifetime. However, surgery is usually carried out in most developing countries of the world, and now more commonly in the industrialized world.

SECONDARY GLAUCOMA

Glaucoma presents secondarily to a number of different predisposing factors. These include the following.

Iridocyclitis

Iridocyclitis can be a complication of a number of systemic disorders, including leprosy, tuberculosis, syphilis, onchocerciasis, and many others. Cells and proteins in the anterior chamber disturb the normal outflow of aqueous fluid. Using a focal light and magnification a 'flare' may be seen in the anterior chamber—like a shaft of sunlight streaming into a room full of dust. The presence of these cells and proteins in the anterior chamber may secondarily cause a rise of intraocular pressure. As a result of the inflammatory reaction within the eye there may be adhesions between the pupil margin and the anterior lens surface (posterior synechiae). The pupil will dilate irregularly if posterior synechiae are present. Occasionally the adhesions may be total, affecting the entire pupil margin, and this is described as seclusio pupillae. The iris bows forward as aqueous fluid cannot pass through the pupil and this further embarrasses the drainage angle of the anterior chamber—described as 'iris bombé'.

Haemorrhage into the anterior chamber
Degenerate red blood cells may block the trabecular meshwork at the angle of the anterior chamber and there is a secondary rise in intraocular pressure. Further, if the haemorrhage has been a result of a severe blunt injury, for example, with damage to the trabecular meshwork and the angle of the anterior chamber, later healing with fibrosis may cause a severe type of secondary raised intraocular pressure.

Phacomorphic glaucoma
The cataractous lens may become swollen (intumescent) which causes relative pupil block, the iris root is moved forward and this may result in blockage of outflow of aqueous fluid at the angle of the anterior chamber (Figure 10.9). This is a secondary form of closed angle glaucoma.

Phacolytic glaucoma
Lens material may cause blockage of outflow of the aqueous at the drainage angle and this may occur after injury (including cataract surgery) or when lens material leaks through the lens capsule or when lens material leaks through the lens capsule of a mature/hypermature lens. Macrophages, attempting to remove this abnormal material, together with the abnormal lens material may cause blockage at the angle of the anterior chamber. This is described as phacolytic glaucoma.

Pigmentary glaucoma
In certain eyes, pigment particles may circulate abnormally in the aqueous fluid, and these in turn may cause blockage at the drainage angle.

Pseudoexfoliative glaucoma
Abnormal accumulation of white particles (not unlike dandruff in appearance) may accumulate in the anterior eye. This abnormal material can cause secondary blockage of the drainage angle. Pseudo-exfoliative glaucoma is found in Sudan, Somalia, Ethiopia and Tanzania. It is less common in West Africa.

Neovascular glaucoma
A thrombosis of the central retinal vein will result in disturbance of the circulation within the eye and this may result in new vessel formation within the anterior segment of the eye. This abnormality in turn may affect the angle of the anterior chamber, where these blood vessels can be visualized, and a form of secondary glaucoma can result. Also, neovascular glaucoma may occur in diabetics where abnormal new blood vessel formation has occurred, similarly causing disturbance to the outflow of aqueous at the angle of the anterior chamber.

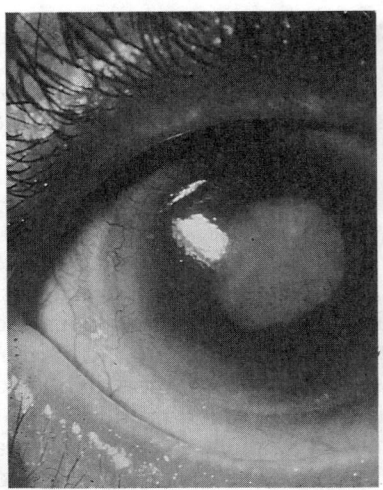
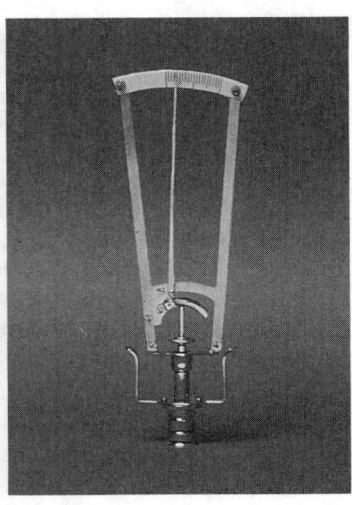

Figure 10.9 Secondary glaucoma caused by an intumescent cataract. A Schiotz tonometer is shown on the right. Photos: John D C Anderson and David's Studio.

Corticosteroid-induced glaucoma

The longer term use of topical corticosteroids can result in a rise of intraocular pressure in patients in whom there is a genetically determined susceptibility to this complication of treatment. Usually the raised intraocular pressure is reduced on discontinuing the use of topical corticosteroids.

Epidemic dropsy

This acute toxic disease is caused by the unintentional ingestion of *Argemone mexicana* oil, an adulterant of cooking oils. It has been reported in India, Mauritius, Fiji, Bangladesh and southern Africa. Rash, oedema of the lower limbs and gastrointestinal and cardiovascular disturbances may be accompanied by a secondary form of glaucoma and retinal vascular abnormalities.[20]

Treatment of the secondary glaucomas

The intraocular pressure should be reduced with acetazolamide, 125 mg or 250 mg, 2–4 times each day.

The predisposing primary condition should be treated appropriately, for example the treatment of inflammation in iridocyclitis by mydriasis and cycloplegia with atropine sulphate 1% and an anti-inflammatory agent such as a topical corticosteroid.

Blood should be removed from the anterior chamber where there is total or almost total haemorrhage (hyphaema).

An eye which has a cataractous intumescent lens should have cataract extraction. The same procedure should be followed where the diagnosis is phacolytic glaucoma.

Neovascularization within the drainage angle can be improved with panretinal photocoagulation (laser or xenon arc). This procedure will apply both to thrombotic glaucoma and where the complication is a consequence of proliferative diabetic retinopathy.

CONGENITAL GLAUCOMA (BUPHTHALMOS, OX EYE)

Congenital glaucoma occurs throughout the world. There is failure of normal development within the angle of the anterior chamber resulting in some blockage of aqueous fluid outflow. This blockage will vary according to the cause and severity of the condition. The intraocular pressure rises as a result and in these small children the eyeball, which has less rigid 'walls', can enlarge. Cupping of the optic disc may be evident.

If the condition affects only one eye, the diagnosis is usually an easy one. A larger cornea and a bigger eye is quickly recognized. However, bilateral buphthalmos may not be so immediately obvious. Other clinical features include photophoia ('fear' of light) and corneal oedema.

Treatment

Pilocarpine eye drops and acetazolamide are often given before surgery. The traditional surgical procedure is a goniotomy, in which a goniotomy knife is introduced into the anterior chamber of the eye to effect sweeping incisions along the abnormal tissue within the angle of the anterior chamber. Other surgical procedures which may be used are trabeculotomy or trabeculectomy. These are necessary if the cornea is already too cloudy to see the Ac angle for goriotomy.

DIABETES MELLITUS

Diabetes is increasing in countries of the developing world. Certain ethnic groups have a very high prevalence of diabetes. The Pima Indians of Arizona, USA, have up to one-half of the population in the age range 30–64 years with diabetes. Impaired glucose tolerance is almost 30% in Arab Omanis and also in Blacks in the USA.[21]

Earlier estimates by the WHO indicate that up to 2.5 million people worldwide are blind due to the complications of diabetes, in particular diabetic retinopathy. This estimate would make blindness due to diabetes fourth in the 'league' of causes of worldwide blindness. At least 60 million have the disease, with 40 million in developing countries.

RETINOPATHY OF DIABETES

Diabetic retinopathy is a vascular complication of both insulin-dependent and non-insulin-dependent diabetes mellitus. The prevalence of retinopathy has a recognized relationship to the duration of the systemic disease. Twenty years after the onset of diabetes, most patients with type I diabetes and more than half of those with type II diabetes have retinopathy. In industrialized countries, diabetic

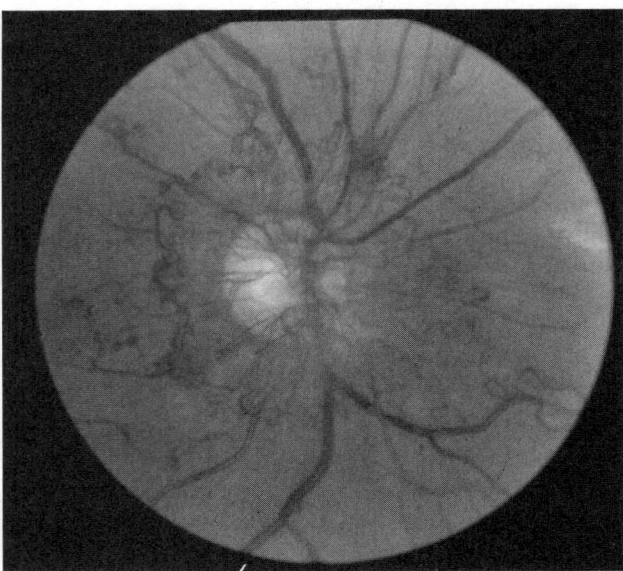

Figure 10.10 Proliferative diabetic retinopathy. Photo: Gordon Johnson.

retinopathy is a common cause of blindness amongst adults (Figure 10.10).

It is important that a patient's diabetes is well controlled, whether with or without insulin. It is a well-recognized fact that poor control is associated with retinopathy.

The progression of diabetic retinopathy is generally as follows: 'background' diabetic retinopathy → advanced non-proliferative diabetic retinopathy → proliferative diabetic retinopathy.

Retinal changes which cause visual loss are:

● Oedema of the macula.
● Proliferative diabetic retinopathy, with haemorrhage from new blood vessels, which may be retinal, preretinal or intravitreal.
● Proliferative diabetic retinopathy, with contraction of associated fibrous tissue leading to tractional retinal detachment.

Screening for diabetic retinopathy will become increasingly important in developing countries. Thus the technique of ophthalmoscopy should be taught widely and not only to those who are ophthalmologists or involved only in eye care services. (The need for good examination of the posterior eye with the ophthalmoscope has already been emphasized in the discussion of diagnosis of open angle glaucoma.)

Background diabetic retinopathy

Microaneurysms, hard exudates, cotton-wool spots and haemorrhages ('dot and blot'/flame-shaped) are typically seen on ophthalmoscopy.

Diabetic maculopathy

This is the most common cause of visual loss in diabetes mellitus. It is more common in type II disease. Exudates may be isolated or in groups or form a circinate pattern. Macular oedema will often affect vision. Fluorescein angiography shows areas of capillary non-perfusion, indicating ischaemia.

Preproliferative diabetic retinopathy

Cotton wool spots, narrowing of the arterioles, dilatation and beading of the retinal veins, large intraretinal haemorrhages and intraretinal microvascular abnormalities may be seen.

Proliferative diabetic retinopathy

This is more common in insulin-dependent diabetes.

Areas of widespread retinal capillary closure and non-perfusion occur. New vessel formation from the venous end of capillaries, with endothelial budding, respond to an angiogenesis factor recognized as a stimulant to proliferation. Fibrovascular abnormalities develop. Fragile new vessels bleed easily. Vitreous haemorrhage or detachment and contraction bands may lead to retinal detachment.

Treatment of proliferative diabetic retinopathy

● Good control of blood glucose levels.
● Reduce alcohol intake, smoking.
● Treat high blood pressure.
● Photocoagulation (laser or xenon arc).
● Avoid strenuous physical activities.

Photocoagulation

Photocoagulation, either with the laser or the xenon arc, is sight preserving in patients with severe diabetic retinopathy. With advanced new vessel formation, particularly new vessels at the optic nerve head or where neovascularization has taken place in the anterior segment of the eye, the patient is likely to require panretinal photocoagulation. With the laser, tiny focal burns may be distributed throughout the peripheral retina with 3000 or more applications. Focal laser applications in expert hands can be beneficial for clinically significant macular oedema. Also, focal laser to leaking spots associated with exudates threatening the macula may be applied. These applications should be made as far as possible before visual loss has been established.

One difficulty that will consistently require consideration, in the treatment of patients with diabetic retinopathy, is the cost of laser photocoagulators. These will necessarily require to be housed in recognized eye centres to which patients can be referred. However, the portable diode laser, attached to a slit-lamp is now being widely used for diabetic retinopathy.

As a general rule, patients with diabetes, whether type I or type II, should be examined by ophthalmoscopy once each year. This procedure is important, particularly with the passage of years since the time of onset of the disease.

VITAMIN A DEFICIENCY AND THE EYE

Vitamin A deficiency, affecting young children throughout the developing world, is an example of a condition where the simple remedy is well known but many thousands of children still become blind. Lack of public awareness of the preventive remedy, and often inadequate supplies of the vitamin where it is required result in tragic consequences.

EPIDEMIOLOGY

Vitamin A deficiency affecting the eye, which is described by the term xerophthalmia, is the most common cause of blindness in children. Seventy per cent of blindness in children is due to corneal scarring, and the vast majority of these young patients have a history of vitamin A deficiency. In many of these cases, this acute nutritional deficiency earlier in their lives has been associated with measles.

Each year about 250 000 children are irreversibly blinded due to lack of vitamin A in their diet. Perhaps another 250 000 children remain who have less profound impairment of vision but some degree of disability due to corneal damage. Further, it is recognized that 50–70% of these children will die within months of the onset of visual impairment, often due to generalized malnutrition, diarrhoeal diseases and respiratory infections.

WHO estimates report 40 million preschool children who are vitamin A deficient and, of these, 13 million have some eye damage.[22] These malnourished children are found in many countries of Asia and Africa, as well as in some areas of the Americas (Table 10.7).[23] Countries with large numbers of children and where vitamin A deficiency is widespread include: India, Bangladesh, Indonesia and the Philippines.

VITAMIN A (RETINOL)

Vitamin A plays an important part in the body's defences against infection. Deficiency of the vitamin results in an impaired immune response with a decreased resistance to infection. Squamous metaplasia of epithelial surfaces allows, for example, a greater susceptibility to lung infection.

The stores of vitamin A are mainly found in the liver, where 90% of the body's vitamin A is retained. Vitamin A undernutrition is typically associated with other nutritional deficits, which makes the young patient vulnerable to systemic disease. Of particular importance is infection with measles. The measles virus is found in the corneal epithelium and conjunctiva, respiratory tract and alimentary tract. When a child has an acute infection with measles, the poor body stores of vitamin A are quickly used up and dramatic and distressing eye changes, with corneal damage (keratomalacia), may occur.

In older children and adults, where a more accurate history may be obtained, a description of night blindness is a common presenting symptom. Vitamin A is required for the production of rhodopsin (visual purple) of the rods of the retina.

The importance of early recognition of vitamin A deficiency, particularly in the young child, is therefore not only in the preservation of sight but in many instances the saving of a young life. This recognition of vitamin A deficiency is often first appreciated by the symptoms and signs affecting the eye.

EYE CHANGES IN VITAMIN A DEFICIENCY

The following are the eye symptoms and signs (Figure 10.11) of xerophthalmia (Table 10.8).
1. *Night blindness (XN)*. Rhodopsin (visual purple) is required by the retina of the eye to allow night vision. Vitamin A is needed to replace and restore the rhodopsin of the retina. Although adults and older children may describe this symptom, it is necessary to ask the mother of a small child whether the infant bumps into objects in the evening or when it is dark.
2. *Conjunctival xerosis (X1A)*. This typically dry appearance of the conjunctival (and corneal) surfaces indicates the importance of vitamin A in maintaining healthy epithelium with adequate secretions on the surface of the eye. Damaged and unhealthy epithelium is more subject to infection and the effects of minor trauma which commonly affect the ocular surface.

This dry appearance provides the term xerophthalmia, which is commonly used to describe the condition of vitamin A deficiency affecting the eye.

Table 10.7 Countries categorized by degree of public health importance of vitamin A deficiency, by WHO region.

| WHO region | Clinical | Subclinical | | | No data: problem likely |
		Severe	Moderate	Mild	
Africa	Benin Burkina Faso Cameroon Chad Ethiopia Ghana Kenya Malawi Mali Mauritania Mozambique Niger Nigeria Rwanda Senegal Togo Uganda United Republic of Tanzania	Cape Verde Congo South Africa Zambia	Angola Guinea Namibia Sierra Leone Zaire Zimbabwe	Liberia Madagascar	Botswana Burundi Central African Republic Côte d'Ivoire Equatorial Guinea Gabon Guinea Bissau Lesotho Sao Tome & Principe Swaziland
Americas	Brazil Dominican Republic El Salvador Guatemala Haiti	Mexico Nicaragua Peru	Bolivia Ecuador Honduras	Belize Colombia Panama	Cuba
South-East Asia	Bangladesh India Myanmar Nepal	—	Bhutan Indonesia Sri Lanka Thailand	—	Maldives
Eastern Mediterranean	Afghanistan Somalia Sudan Yemen	Pakistan	Djibouti Oman	Egypt Iran Saudi Arabia	Iraq Jordan Lebanon Morocco Syria
Western Pacific	Cambodia Federal States of Micronesia Kiribati Lao People's Democatic Republic Marshall Islands Philippines Vietnam	Papua New Guinea	China Solomon Islands	Malaysia N. Mariana Islands	—

Source: WHO, May 1994.

3. *Bitot's spots (X1B)*. Bitot's spots are found on the surface of the conjunctiva—most often on the temporal bulbar conjunctiva. The typical appearance is foamy and spots may present in triangular form with the base at the corneoscleral margin.

Bitot's spots may be found in both eyes. They may occur in children under the age of 5 years, but can also persist in older children. Often the foamy spot may be removed quite easily, although it should be noted that the appearance can remain in older children beyond the period during which the child was vitamin A deficient.

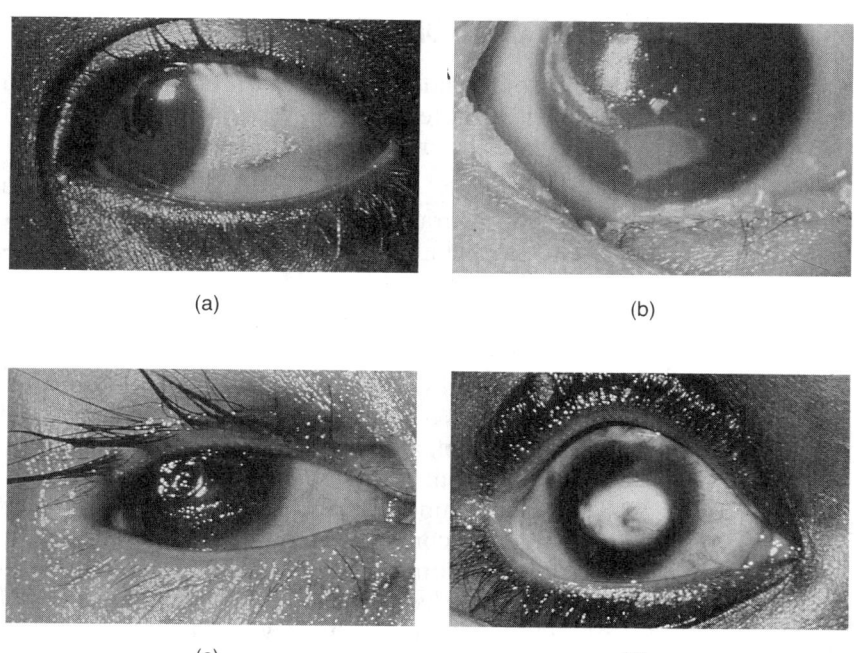

(a)

(b)

(c)

(d)

Figure 10.11 (a) Bitot's spots; (b) corneal xerosis with early ulceration; (c) corneal ulceration/keratomalacia; (d) corneal scarring. Photos: (a) Simon Franken; (b) Allen Foster; (c) Donald McLaren; (d) Gordon Johnson.

Table 10.8 Eye changes and vitamin A status.

Eye lesion	Vitamin A status*	Comments
Night blindness (XN)	Mild-moderate decrease (over 1 per 100)	Sensitive sign of low body vitamin A stores; still associated with increased illness and mortality Prevalence often increases into early school-age years Boys may be more affected than girls Cause is chemical deficiency in retina
Conjunctival xerosis (X1A)	Mild-moderate decrease (not used in WHO classification)	Dryness of conjunctiva due to decrease in goblet cells and epithelial change Difficult to diagnose reliably by clinical examination
Bitot's spots (X1B)	Mild-moderate decrease (over 5 per 1000)	White 'foamy' or 'cheese-like' spots on the conjunctiva: usually bilateral and temporal Caused by change in squamous epithelium with underlying xerosis In older children may not disappear with vitamin A treatment
Active corneal changes (X2/X3)	Severe decrease (over 1 per 10 000)	Danger signs of permanent loss of sight Cornea may 'melt' (keratomalacia) in a few hours Most common at age 2–4 years No sex differences
Corneal scars (XS)	Depends on examination timing (over 5 per 10 000)	End-stage of malnutrition eye damage Scarring (leucoma) often allows some residual vision Blinded eyes may be protuberant (anterior staphyloma) or shrunken (phthisis)

*Public Health problem criteria as defined by the WHO in children aged between 6 months and 6 years.
Source: WHO Programme for Prevention of Blindness.

Bitot's spots may take various shapes and sizes and are not always triangular in appearance. Some may contain pigment.

Bitot's spots indicate changes in the squamous epithelium of the conjunctiva overlying areas of dryness (xerosis).

As the central cornea is not involved, the vision of the child remains unaffected where Bitot's spots alone are present.

4. *Corneal xerosis (X2)*. Sharing in the overall presentation of xerophthalmia, the cornea can appear dry and lustreless. This appearance

reflects the changes in the corneal epithelium consequent upon vitamin A deficiency. It is specifically the corneal changes which will begin to affect vision in the child.

5. *Corneal ulceration with xerosis (X3A)*. The development of corneal xerosis and consequent damage to the corneal epithelium may progress to involve the deeper layers of the cornea, resulting in corneal ulceration, which can be superficial or deep. A centrally situated corneal ulcer will profoundly affect vision in the eye.

6. *Corneal ulceration/keratomalacia (X3B)*. The cornea may 'melt' dramatically (keratomalacia), with an acute onset, over a few hours. Younger children are particularly susceptible to this development, which is most often found in infants aged 1–3 years. At this stage of very severe vitamin A deficiency, treatment must be given as an emergency intervention, often to protect the other, less affected eye, thereby protecting vision. Sadly, keratomalacia may present as a bilateral condition.

7. *Corneal scarring (XS)*. The healed state following severe vitamin A deficiency with corneal ulceration and keratomalacia can result in marked corneal scarring which will often affect both eyes. Vision is severely reduced. This appearance, the result of vitamin A deficiency in a young child, with most of life ahead, is the distressing consequence of a preventable eye disease.

Many children who have this severe form of vitamin A deficiency will not survive beyond some months after the acute episode because they are particularly susceptible to intercurrent infections and diarrhoea and have poor resistance to systemic disease. For those who live through this acute phase, both their eyes, and inevitably their lives, are scarred.

Severe damage to the anterior eye may result in unsightly, bulging eyes (anterior staphylomas) or the reverse occurs and the eye begins to shrink (phthisis bulbi).

The progression of eye signs that we have described may not occur in the sequence given. For example, an individual child with an acute requirement of vitamin A, perhaps during and following measles infection, may have alarming corneal changes as the first presentation of the eye disease and the systemic deprived nutritional state.

It should be recognized that evidence of vitamin A deficiency affecting children who appear for examination indicates that others in the same family and community are likely to be vitamin A deficient, even if no signs are evident.

TREATMENT OF XEROPHTHALMIA

The recommended treatment of recognized vitamin A deficiency affecting the eye requires a schedule of three doses of oral vitamin A (Table 10.9):

- Immediately on diagnosis (first day) 200 000 iu vitamin A orally
- The following day (second day) 200 000 iu vitamin A orally
- Between 7 days and 4 weeks later 200 000 iu vitamin A orally.

It may not always be possible to see the child after 4 weeks; if this is the case, then the third dose should be given 1 week after the initial dose, or any time up to 4 weeks from the commencement of treatment.

If a child is under 1 year old or weighs less than 8 kg, half the recommended dosages should be given.

If there is vomiting which would render the oral treatment useless, an intramuscular injection of 100 000 iu of water-soluble vitamin A (not an oil-based preparation) may be used instead of the first oral dose.

Treatment should be given immediately, as soon as the diagnosis is made. Treatment is not only seeking to preserve vision but may also preserve the life of the child.

At the commencement of treatment with vitamin A, a topical antibiotic eye ointment, for example tetracycline 1% or chloramphenicol 1%, each given three times daily, is advised to prevent the complication of bacterial infection of the eye. The affected eye/s should be covered with an eye pad if the cornea is involved, making sure that the eyelid is gently closed before applying the eye pad.

The patient should be referred immediately to an eye specialist.

Table 10.9   Treatment of xerophthalmia.

Children over 1 year old
Immediately on diagnosis   200 000 iu vitamin A orally*
The following day (2nd day) 200 000 iu vitamin A orally
Four weeks later (4 weeks)   200 000 iu vitamin A orally

*If there is vomiting an intramuscular injection of 100 000 iu of water-soluble vitamin A (not an oil-based preparation) may be used instead of the first dose

Children under 1 year old or less than 8 kg in weight
Use half doses of the regimen given above

Treatment of vitamin A deficient women during the reproductive years, including pregnancy

High doses of vitamin A are contraindicated in pregnancy. There have been concerns about the effects of vitamin A on the unborn child. If a woman in this category presents with either night blindness or a Bitot's spot, she should be given a daily dose of 10 000 iu vitamin A orally for 2 weeks.

Following the birth of her child, a woman may be given three doses of vitamin A 200 000 iu on the first day, the second day and the eighth day. Vitamin A is contained within breast milk, and this will provide a protective supply for the newborn child.

PREVENTION OF XEROPHTHALMIA

Communities which have a recognized problem of vitamin A deficiency should be given well-planned instructions outlining the consequences of vitamin A deficiency, especially for their children. The advantages of prevention, very often with remedies which are readily available, should be carefully explained (Figure 10.12).

Education about nutritional needs should be emphasized:

- Encourage breast feeding.
- Mothers should be advised to supplement the feeding of infants by 6 months, with fruits such as mango or papaya. Children aged 1 year or older can be given dark green leafy vegetables, which are rich in vitamin A.
- Every effort should be made to reach health workers, mothers and children, and indeed the whole community, with instruction about foods that have a high content of vitamin A. Examples are spinach, carrots, sweet potatoes, certain fruits and green leafy vegetables. Dairy products and

eggs contain vitamin A. Red palm oil, which is used especially by populations of West Africa, has a high content of vitamin A. Vitamin A, which is mainly stored in the liver, can be found in animal liver and fish liver oils.

- Encouragement should be given to the farmers and all members of the community to plant appropriate foodstuffs, whether in small gardens or in larger plantations, so that vitamin A deficiency can be prevented.

Interventions by health workers may be necessary:

- Vitamin A capsules 200 000 iu may be given every 3–6 months to children 1–6 years of age where there is a recognized risk within communities. Note that half this dose is appropriate for children under the age of 12 months or if a child weighs less than 8 kg. This must be recognized as a short-term measure.
- Every child who has measles should be given at least one dose of vitamin A 200 000 iu orally. If there is any evidence of vitamin A changes affecting the eye or if the community is recognized to be at risk of xerophthalmia, the full treatment regimen with three doses should be given.
- Communities which have not had a programme of measles immunization should be identified, and a programme should be planned and implemented as soon as possible.
- Note the previous recommendation for women during the reproductive years or during pregnancy who present with symptoms or signs of vitamin A deficiency.

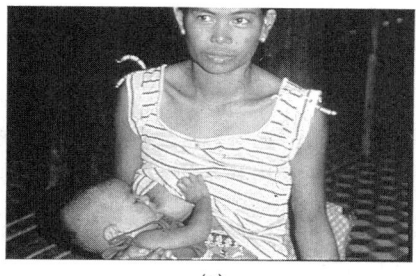 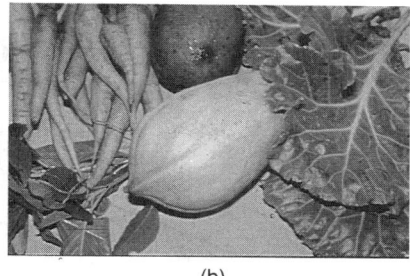

(a) (b)

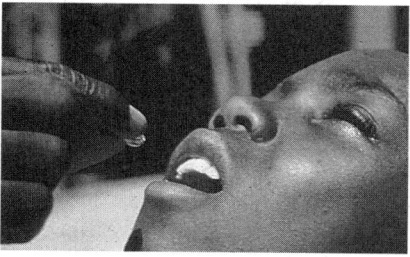 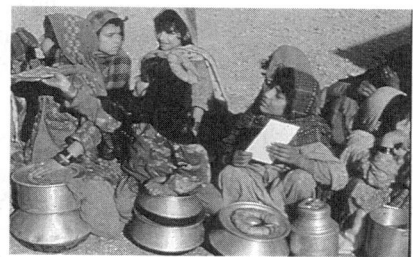

(c) (d)

Figure 10.12 (a) Breast feeding; (b) vitamin A rich fruit and vegetables; (c) vitamin A capsule; (d) milk fortified with vitamin A. Photos: (a), (b), (d) Murray McGavin; (c) Christoffel Blindenmission.

Interventions by the health authorities:

- Foods which are widely used may be fortified with vitamin A, for example sugar and milk.
- Public awareness of vitamin A deficiency and its consequences for the eye and general health should be consistently emphasized by posters, by health education at mother and child health clinics and in schools. Radio can be used to pass on information and knowledge.

MEASLES AND THE EYE

Measles is a serious infection, especially in the developing world. The WHO estimates one million deaths annually. Most of these are children. A child is 400 times more likely to die as a consequence of measles if living in a developing country.[24] Further, measles infection has often been associated with the acute onset of eye problems earlier in the life of a child or young person who presents with corneal scarring.

CLINICAL PRESENTATION

A child with measles will often have photosensitivity (sensitivity to light), watering and red eyes. There may be evidence of a punctate keratitis. Some children can develop corneal ulceration.

The measles virus is present in the superficial cornea and conjunctiva, but it is the secondary complications which can be disastrous for the eye or eyes.

- In a child with low reserves of vitamin A (mostly in the liver), where the clinical picture is characterized by poor appetite and gastroenteritis with inadequate intake of vitamin A and protein, acute vitamin A deficiency can result in corneal ulceration and keratomalacia.
- There may be depression of the immune system in association with measles infection, and a secondary infection with herpes simplex virus may complicate the picture.
- A child who is ill with measles and who is vitamin deficient and dehydrated may be listless and sufficiently ill to close the eyelids inadequately. This can result in corneal dryness due to exposure and consequent corneal ulceration. A topical antibiotic eye ointment should be used at least four times daily during the illness. Corneal exposure should be avoided.
- The situation may be complicated by a previous visit to the traditional healer which may confuse the clinical picture. Often the mother will be reluctant to admit that they have first attended the traditional healer.

TREATMENT OF MEASLES AND ITS EYE COMPLICATIONS

1. Vitamin A 200 000 iu orally should be given at least once. If there is a known risk of vitamin A deficiency in the community or if there is any symptom or sign of vitamin A deficiency affecting the eyes of the child, the full regimen of three doses of vitamin A should be prescribed.
2. A topical antibiotic should be given to each eye at least four times each day. Avoid corneal exposure.
3. Systemic treatment should be given as appropriate, for example for gastroenteritis or respiratory infection.
4. Admission to hospital may be necessary.

PREVENTION

In Africa, it is considered that about one half of childhood blindness has some relation to measles infection.

A programme of immunization should be instituted as soon as possible for the community/ies at risk. The WHO Expanded Programme on Immunization is promoting increased coverage of immunization around the world.

ONCHOCERCIASIS (See also Chapter 70)

Onchocerciasis is a parasitic disease caused by the filarial worm *Onchocerca volvulus*. The worm is transmitted by a vector, one of several species of the *Simulium* blackfly. The black biting fly breeds in rivers, with a preference for turbulent and highly oxygenated waters. Thus there is a high prevalence of disease near to rivers with turbulent streams. Both the skin and the eyes are particularly affected by the disease, which is commonly known as 'river blindness'.

EPIDEMIOLOGY

Onchocerciasis is a well recognized cause of blindness in the world. The WHO Expert Committee has estimated that the number of people infected by *O. volvulus* is about 18 million. About 75–80 million people are at risk. Around 360 000 are blind due to the disease.

About 17 million of those infected with *O. volvulus* live in West and Central Africa.[25] There are pockets of infection found in Yemen. Areas of infection are also found in Central America and northern areas of South America.

The social and economic consequences of this disease are huge, with considerable human suffering. The prevalence of blindness in villages near to fast flowing rivers may reach 15%, often affecting men of working age. The impact of this disabling infection can be such that villages have been deserted when situated close to rivers.

The development of blindness will typically affect a young man, perhaps 30–40 years old, who has lived and worked near to a fast flowing, turbulent river in West or Central Africa. During the years of childhood he will have been bitten many times by the *Simulium* fly and will have been infected and reinfected with the microfilariae of *O. volvulus*. His work may have involved daytime exposure in the fields near to his home, possibly fishing by the river, or perhaps ferrying people across the river in his boat. Gradually, over the years, the distressing symptoms and signs of onchocerciasis cause the chronic skin changes and, even more importantly, the scarring typical of the disease, affecting both the anterior and posterior eye. The condition is usually bilateral; gradually loses the visual field in each eye, vision is severely reduced leading to blindness.

The vector: the Simulium fly

The disease is spread from person to person by the blackfly of the genus *Simulium*. The female *Simulium* lays her eggs on rocks and vegetation where rivers are fast flowing and 'white' through turbulence because the eggs and larvae of the fly need oxygen for their development.

The female fly can travel up to 80 km in 1 day, although this is unusual and she is more likely to fly 5–10 km on either side of a river. During the rainy season the flies may travel to new breeding sites but when the season is dry they are more localized to permanent rivers and streams.

Around mating time, the female fly requires a blood meal to ensure development of her eggs, and as the disease is transmitted through the bite of the female fly, it is most dangerous to be living and working near to breeding sites. The female fly particularly feeds on human blood at dawn and dusk.

Life cycle of O. volvulus

When a person is already infected by the worm *O. volvulus* and is bitten by the *Simulium* fly, the small embryo worms (microfilariae) present in the skin of the infected person enter the body of the fly. There they pass through the gut wall and travel to the thoracic muscles. Further development takes place and after about 7 days the larvae move to the head of the fly, ready to be transmitted to the next human host when the fly requires another blood meal.

In this way the microfilariae of *O. volvulus* are transmitted to another person. They will take 1–3 years to develop into adult worms. One female worm can produce 0.5–1 million microfilariae in 1 year. Thus, the cycle of transmission from person to person continues.

CLINICAL PRESENTATION

The microfilariae of *O. volvulus* have a particular predilection for the skin and the eyes of the infected person but may also give rise to musculoskeletal pain interpreted as 'rheumatism'.

Skin complications

Itching is one of the first symptoms of onchocerciasis and this can be very severe, disturbing sleep. Associated with the itching there is the presence of a rash which may occur on most parts of the body but often affects the region of the buttocks. There may be very obvious scratch marks, indicating the severity of the itching.

A feature of onchocercal skin disease is depigmentation. This feature is described as 'leopard skin' and follows repeated episodes of skin inflammation associated with the death of microfilariae. There is subcutaneous fibrosis, skin atrophy and pigmentary changes. Further, the skin may look and feel like the skin of a very old person. This clinical feature has been described as 'lizard skin'.

Lymphoedema of the skin can result in chronic thickened and often blackened skin, which is the result of severe, reactive onchodermatitis. In the groin region, lymph node enlargement in the inguinal areas can disturb lymphatic drainage and the skin of the region is greatly enlarged. These folds of skin may not retract to the original, more normal situation and remain as the 'hanging groin' of onchocerciasis.

Subcutaneous nodules are found in different regions of the body, often around the hips or on the head. They are firm, discrete and painless. A nodule is formed by a fibrous reaction around coiled adult

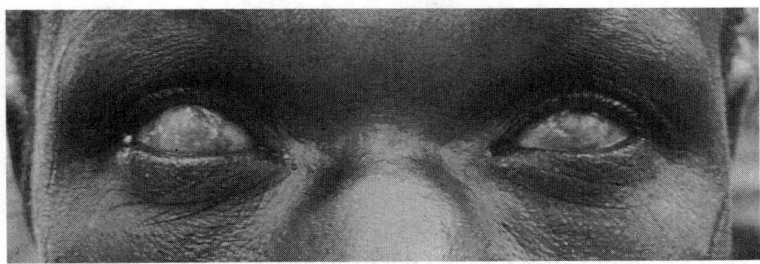

Figure 10.13   Sclerosing keratitis in onchocerciasis.
Photo: Pak Sang Lee

worms. Surgical removal of nodules (nodulectomy) may be considered, particularly where nodules are situated in the region of the head or shoulders.

Eye complications

Most of the symptoms and signs characteristic of onchocerciasis, including those affecting the eyes, are caused by the microfilariae of *O. volvulus*. Typically both eyes will be involved. As with the skin changes, it is the dead microfilariae which cause the inflammatory reaction within the eye. Microfilariae may be seen circulating in the aqueous fluid behind the cornea if sufficient magnification is available for close observation.

Eye inflammation can affect both the anterior and the posterior eye.

'Snowflake' and punctate keratitis

White-grey spots may be seen in the superficial cornea and these indicate a reaction to dead microfilariae within the cornea. Inflammatory cells accumulate around the dead microfilariae, resulting in opacities. There may be a red eye with photosensitivity and watering. A good response in treatment is usually obtained with topical corticosteroids, but these must only be given by the eye specialist as corticosteroids have their own complications for which follow-up is required.

Sclerosing keratitis

Sclerosing keratitis is one of the common inflammatory features of onchocerciasis which can cause blindness (Figure 10.13). Typically the clinical presentation is seen at the nasal and temporal aspects of the cornea, and the opacity then extends throughout the lower part of the cornea. Advanced sclerosing keratitis can result in a total corneal scar. There is no specific treatment for sclerosing keratitis but a patient with this condition should be referred for specialist advice.

Iridocyclitis

Inflammation of the iris (iritis) and of the ciliary body (cyclitis) can contribute to reduced vision. The pupil of the eye affected by onchocerciasis may be drawn down in its lower aspect due to inflammatory reaction affecting the lower iris, where accumulated dead microfilariae may be found. In association with iridocyclitis, or incidental to it, a cataract can occur, resulting in a grey-white pupil and profoundly reduced vision. These patients should also be referred to the eye specialist for treatment. Iridocyclitis will be treated with a topical mydriatic and cycloplegic, often using atropine sulphate 1% eye drops and anti-inflammatory agents. A cataract will need to be removed, preferably in an eye which is quiet without active inflammation.

Optic neuritis and choroidoretinitis

Onchocerciasis affecting the posterior eye is a recognized cause of visual loss, where a patient may first be aware of loss of visual field. The clinical picture may show optic nerve atrophy and choroidoretinal atrophy. In severe optic atrophy, the optic nerve head is abnormally pale and white, whereas the normal optic disc is a faint pink colour, although slightly paler in its central part. Areas of the retina may be pale with scattered clumps of pigmentation. This appearance of choroidoretinal atrophy follows inflammation of the choroid and retina with consequent damage to the choroid, retinal pigment epithelium and the retina itself (Figure 10.14). Experience in the use of the ophthalmoscope is important in diagnosing posterior segment eye disease, although this will only be possible if the cornea and the lens in each eye are clear. There is no treatment for optic atrophy and choroidoretinal atrophy.

DIAGNOSIS

Clinical features

The symptoms and signs of onchocerciasis are often sufficient to make a certain diagnosis: onchodermatitis, signs of scratching, depigmentation of the skin, 'lizard' skin and subcutaneous nodules. Further, the presence of microfilariae in the anterior chamber or in the cornea may be seen using the slit-lamp microscope.

The skin snip

A small piece of superficial skin may be removed, often from the region of the iliac crest or from the shoulder, using a sterile needle with a razor blade. Alternatively, a purpose-designed skin punch may remove the superficial skin. The tiny piece of skin is placed on a dry microscope slide and a drop of saline is added. After at least 30 minutes, and if possible sometime later, the skin and saline are visualized through the microscope. Mobile microfilariae can be seen moving in the fluid when using 40× magnification (see also Appendix V).

CONTROL

Onchocerciasis control can be effected in four ways:

1. By inhibiting the development of the *Simulium* flies.
   (a) Vector control to stop breeding.
   (b) Removal of obstacles which cause white, turbulent water. This may include removing rocks or even structures made by man.
2. By reducing the number of bites by the *Simulium* fly on man:
   (a) Wearing clothing which covers most of the skin surface.
   (b) Communities removing from sites near to the breeding areas for the *Simulium* fly.
3. By killing the microfilariae: chemotherapy with microfilaricides.
4. By killing the adult worms:
   (a) Removal of the subcutaneous nodules (nodulectomy).
   (b) Chemotherapy with macrofilaricides.

Vector control

Vector control is by spraying larvicides to kill the larvae of the *Simulium* fly and this has been most effectively carried out in West Africa by the huge Onchocerciasis Control Project. This project has had good results over the last 20 years in West Africa, but it is impossible effectively to control breeding at all sites. Also, flies invade from the regions and countries which have not had a programme of larvicide spraying. *Simulium* larvae have developed some resistance to the larvicides used. The OCP has organized this programme in 11 countries of West Africa, with vector control and more recently ivermectin distribution.

Nodulectomy

Removal of a coiled mass of adult worms within the fibrous nodule which forms the subcutaneous lump, often in the region of the head or the hips, is thought to be beneficial, particularly where nodules are situated near to the eyes. The rationale for this procedure is that it will reduce the number of microfilariae which are produced.

Macrofilaricides

In the past suramin has been used, given in weekly intravenous injections. However, suramin is toxic and can cause serious systemic and ocular reactions. It is not routinely recommended, although new regimens of administration are being tested.

New macrofilaricides are also being field tested at the present time.

Microfilaricides

Formerly, the established treatment by the oral route was with diethylcarbamizine which kills microfilariae. However, diethylcarbamazine can also pro-

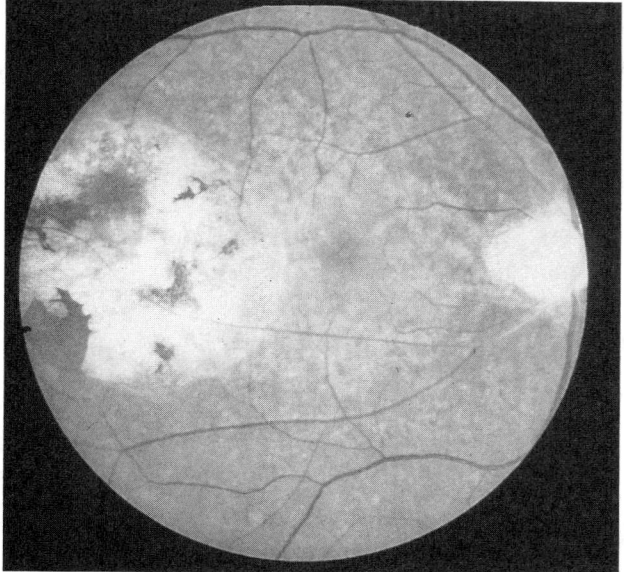

Figure 10.14 Choroidoretinal atrophy and optic nerve atrophy after onchocerciasis. Photo: Ian Murdoch.

duce a severe systemic and ocular reaction with intense itching, a rash with skin eruption, fever, headache and joint pains. This is described as the Mazzotti reaction. The effective killing of microfilariae within the eye, while ultimately producing systemic benefit, has resulted in further ocular damage and loss of sight. Diethylcarbamazine is no longer routinely used.

Ivermectin ('Mectizan')

Ivermectin kills the microfilariae of the worm *O. volvulus* but typically with only mild reactions, unlike diethylcarbamizine. Of particular significance is the knowledge that ocular damage does not routinely occur. Ivermectin is providing real hope for the future in the treatment of onchocerciasis.

Ivermectin has the following advantages:

- It kills microfilariae.
- It has been shown to prevent blindness due to optic nerve disease by 50%.
- The production of microfilariae by the adult female worm is inhibited for some months.
- The tablet or tablets need only to be taken every 6–12 months.
- There is no severe ocular reaction.
- The oral route provides easy delivery of the drug.
- Ivermectin has been donated free of charge by Merck, Sharp and Dohme.

The main logistical problem in treating populations with Ivermectin is the provision of manpower and facilities to effectively provide the drug to communities in need.

The drug is given every 6–12 months by mouth. The dose is 150 µg per kg by weight. It should not be given to the following groups of patients:

- Children under 5 years old or weighing less than 15 kg.
- Women who are pregnant.
- Women who are breast feeding a child under 1 month old.
- Patients who are severely ill, particularly with meningitis or trypanosomiasis.

Side-effects of Ivermectin include mild itching, fever, rash, headache, oedema, lymphadenopathy, myalgia and generalized body aches. More severe reactions, which are uncommon, include hypotension, asthma attacks in known asthmatics and bullous skin lesions after 1–2 weeks (Table 10.10). Most reactions occur within the first 2 or 3 days. Aspirin or an antihistamine may be given.

Table 10.10 Adverse reactions to ivermectin ('Mectizan') therapy (Mazzotti).

Mild	Severe
Pruritus	Hypotension
Fever	Asthma attacks (in known
Rash	patients)
Headache	Bullous skin lesions (after 1–2
Oedema	weeks)
Lymphadenopathy	
Myalgia	
Generalized body aches	

AGE-RELATED MACULAR DEGENERATION

Age-related macular degeneration is a common cause of bilateral blindness in the developed world (Figure 10.15). The main risk factor, as the name suggests, is age, and the condition becomes more common with advancing years. By definition the patient with bilateral macular degeneration may be registered as blind, but the great reassurance that may be given to the patient who has these changes of the central retina is that 'total' blindness will not occur. The patient will be able to see to move around, because peripheral vision is retained, although central vision can be severely affected.

Age-related macular degeneration occurs more

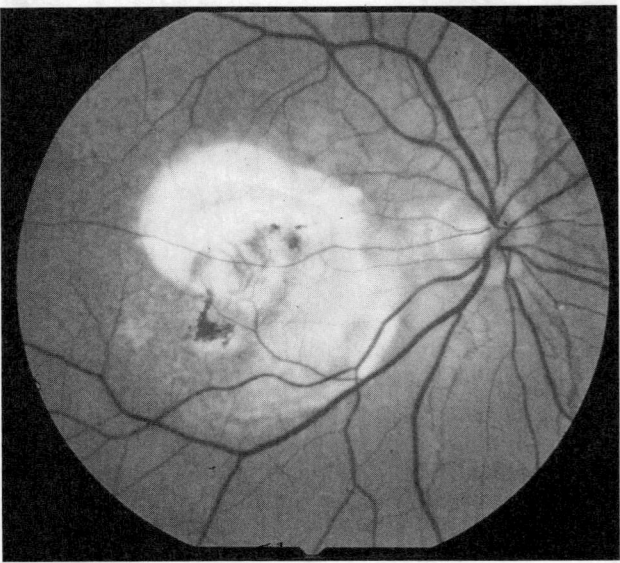

Figure 10.15 Age-related macular degeneration. Photo: Gordon Johnson.

often in caucasians, in females, where there is a family history of the eye disease, and is associated with cigarette smoking.

Two broad groups are described. Non-exudative ('dry') and exudative ('wet') macular disease. Most cases of blindness are due to the exudative form.

Exudates, in the 'wet' form of the disease, relate to the presence of subretinal neovascularization. Fluorescein angiography, where the injected fluorescein dye reveals new vessel formation, will indicate the possibility of treatment with laser photocoagulation. The neovascular membrane must be extrafoveal for the applications of laser burns to be possible.

In general, however, age-related maculopathy is a bilateral and progressive eye disease. Low-vision aids may benefit these patients.

LEPROSY AND THE EYE (See also Chapter 58)

In 1989, ffytche described leprosy, and particularly its ocular complications, as one of the great challenges for preventive medicine.[26]

EPIDEMIOLOGY

It is estimated that around 250 000 leprosy patients are blind due to the disease. Leprosy, which is sometimes called Hansen's disease, affects an estimated total of 5.5 million people worldwide.[23] The distribution of leprosy is shown in the table on p. 1017. It should also be recognized that many thousands of leprosy patients, who may be receiving little medical advice and care, are blind due to non-leprosy-associated eye disease.

CLINICAL PRESENTATION

Leprosy is a chronic bacterial disease caused by an *Mycobacterium leprae*, which has acid-fast bacillus low-grade infectivity, and a preference for cooler temperatures. Thus, the slightly cooler anterior segment of the eye is particularly affected by the presence of the organism. Two alternative subdivisions of clinical leprosy are recognized:

1. Tuberculoid (TT)
   Borderline tuberculoid (BT)
   Borderline borderline (BB)
   Borderline lepromatous (BL)
   Lepromatous leprosy (LL).

and

2. Paucibacillary leprosy (PB)—equivalent to TT and BT leprosy.
   Multibacillary leprosy (MB)—equivalent to BB, BL and LL leprosy.

The different forms of clinical presentation of leprosy reflect the immune reaction of the patient to the presence of *Mycobacterium leprae*. The spectrum of immune reaction shows high cellular immunity with a correspondingly low bacterial count in patients with tuberculoid leprosy, to very low cellular immunity with a high bacterial count in patients with lepromatous leprosy.

The clinical presentation of leprosy reflects either an acute immunological response or is the result of huge bacterial infection causing atrophy of the tissues involved. These different responses are reflected in the eye involvement of leprosy.

TYPE I REACTION (REVERSAL REACTION)
(Table 10.11)[27]

Acute redness and thickening in the skin and certain peripheral nerves can cause both motor and sensory nerve loss. Involvement of both the fifth and seventh cranial nerves can result in corneal anaesthesia (fifth nerve) and lagophthalmos (seventh nerve), where the patient is unable to close the eyelids. Type I reactions may occur with all types of borderline leprosy (BT, BB, BL).

Eye complications associated with a type I reaction

Lagophthalmos (seventh cranial nerve)
Lagophthalmos is the most common eye complication found in leprosy and may be associated with all forms of the disease (Figure 10.16). However, lagophthalmos and corneal anaesthesia are the expected complications found in association with a type I reaction. Lagophthalmos is diagnosed when there is inability to close the eyelids, which can be found with both gentle and attempted forced closure of the eyelids.

Corneal anaesthesia (fifth cranial nerve)
Corneal anaesthesia may occur in association with lagophthalmos, and the combined effect of inadequate lid closure and corneal insensitivity provides considerable danger to the eye through exposure and the effects of minor (or more severe) trauma.

Treatment of eye complications associated with type I reaction

1. Treatment of an acute type I reaction requires systemic corticosteroids for 4–6 months (e.g. prednisolone 30 mg per day decreasing over 6 months).
2. Treatment of lagophthalmos and corneal anaesthesia is recorded in Table 10.12.[27] The patient must be taught to 'think blink'—that is, the regular and deliberate blinking of both eyes many times each day.
3. Protective spectacles may be worn during the day.
4. Any possibility of exposure, particularly involving the cornea, requires an antibiotic eye ointment as a protective measure at night.
5. A tarsorrhaphy, often a lateral tarsorrhaphy, where the upper and lower eyelids are permanently sutured together, must be considered. Other surgical methods which are used include correction of ectropion (the lower eyelid turning out and drooping), which may involve a 'sling' procedure which will support the lax lower eyelid.

TYPE II REACTION (Table 10.11)[27]

The clinical presentation of a type II reaction, which occurs commonly in association with lepromatous leprosy, is with fever, subcutaneous nodules, swelling of nerves and inflammatory foci. A type II reaction affecting the eye can cause acute iridocyclitis, episcleritis and scleritis.

Eye complications associated with a type II reaction

Acute iridocyclitis

Treatment of acute iridocyclitis is similar to treatment of this inflammation due to many other causes. Atropine sulphate 1% eye drops together with corticosteroid eye drops should be given. Systemic corticosteroids should not be required.

Episcleritis and scleritis

An episcleritis will respond quickly to topical corticosteroids. The deeper inflammation of scleritis, particularly severe bilateral scleritis, which is often associated with an anterior iridocyclitis (anterior uveitis), is a well-recognized complication of severe type II reactions. Topical treatment should be given as described above, with atropine sulphate 1% and corticosteroids, but short courses of systemic corticosteroids—together with clofazimine—will be required. There is always the danger of scleral staphyloma formation (bulging of the inflamed sclera with adherent choroid and ciliary body behind), sometimes associated with scleral thinning.

Chronic iridocyclitis

This less acute form of iridocyclitis presents with some haziness of the aqueous fluid within the anterior chamber of the eye due to the presence of cells and protein (Figure 10.17). While posterior synechiae formation (adherence of the pupil margin to the anterior lens face) is not common, the pupils may become small (miosis) and resist dilatation with mydriatics. Keratic precipitates may be found on the corneal endothelium. These are foci of cells adherent to the back of the cornea. In treating chronic

Table 10.11 Eye complications in leprosy, related to classification* (after ref. 27).

Cause of complications	Complications	Paucibacillary	Multibacillary
Type I reaction	Lagophthalmos	+	+
	Corneal anaesthesia	+	+
Type II reaction	Acute iritis	−	+
	Scleritis	−	+
?	Chronic iritis	−	+
Bacilli in high numbers	Madarosis	−	+
	Blepharochalasis	−	+
	Blocked lacrimal sac	−	+
	Limbal leproma	−	+
	Leprous keratitis	−	+
	Iris pearls	−	+
	Neuroparalytic iritis	−	+
	Iris atrophy	−	+

*Exceptions may occur due to variations in the grading of patients.

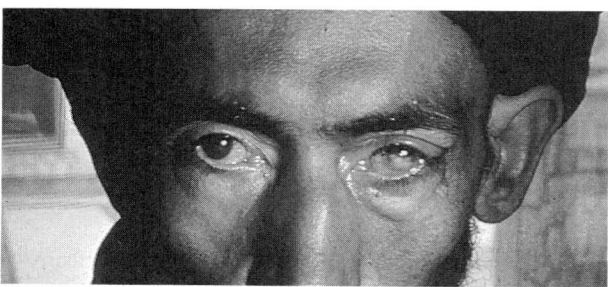

Figure 10.16   Bilateral facial paralysis due to leprosy. Temporal tarsorrhaphies have been carried out, but the left eye has severe corneal ulceration. Photo: John D C Anderson.

iridocyclitis it is important to keep the pupil as dilated and active as possible using phenylephrine 2.5–5% eye drops.

GENERAL TREATMENT

In treating the eye complications of leprosy it is vital to confirm that the patient is receiving adequate and careful systemic treatment. (See Chapter 58.) Tuberculoid leprosy requires a combination of dapsone (DDS) 100 mg per day together with rifampicin for a minimum of 6 months. Lepromatous leprosy requires a combination of dapsone, rifampicin and clofazimine for a minimum of 2 years.

It should be kept in mind that, after treatment for leprosy, eye disease will often remain and perhaps worsen.

OTHER EYE SIGNS

Thus far we have discussed the eye complications of leprosy which can result in visual loss and blindness. We shall now look briefly at other features which present clinically and can confirm the diagnosis of systemic leprosy with eye complications.

Madarosis

There is loss of eyebrow hair which may be associated with loss of eyelashes. A hair-bearing skin graft may be used to provide a 'new' eyebrow. Alternatively a dark pencil may be used.

Blepharochalasis

Excessive folds of the skin of the upper eyelid can occur after inflammatory reactions deep to the eyelid skin have disappeared. The treatment is surgical.

Lacrimal duct obstruction

This usually results in excessive watering of the affected eye (epiphora) and may occur following inflammation of the nasal mucosa and sometimes collapse of the nasal cartilage. Removal of the tear sac (dacryocystectomy) may be required.

Limbal leproma

A painless pinkish or yellowish nodule may present at the corneoscleral margin (limbus). This should resolve slowly with supervised multiple systemic drug treatment.

Leprous keratitis

Corneal deposits which are chalk-like in appearance may occur, often in both eyes and at the upper aspect or outer quadrant of the cornea. These usually do not affect visual acuity and are evidence of corneal invasion by *M. leprae*.

Iris atrophy

In long-standing lepromatous leprosy the iris stroma may become thin and atrophic, with the dilator muscle of the iris affected. The result is that the pupils become miotic and 'pin-point' in appearance. Irregular atrophy of the iris may result in pupil distortion. Before this appearance develops attempts should be made to maintain pupil dilatation using phenylephrine 2.5–5%.

Iris pearls

Small white nodules may appear on the surface of the iris. These are pathognomonic for leprosy and are formed by calcified foci of dead leprosy bacillae.

Age-related cataract in leprosy patients

Age-related (senile) cataract is a most important cause of blindness amongst leprosy patients. Often these patients do not receive the attention given to others with age-related cataract who do not have leprosy. It is a sensible precaution to require that a patient has had 6 months of systemic antileprosy treatment, without any recognized reaction, prior to intraocular surgery.

Leprosy and the intraocular pressure

Raised intraocular pressure may occur in association with iridocyclitis. However, the intraocular pressure is often slightly lower than average (ocular hypotension) where atrophy of the ciliary body has occurred.

Table 10.12   Treatment of lagophthalmos (after ref. 27).

Duration	Treatment
<6 months	Prednisolone (30 mg/day), decreasing over 6 months Blinking exercises Protective spectacles
>6 months	Eye health education
No exposure keratitis	Protective spectacles and other protective measures
Normal corneal sensation	'Think-blink-habit'
With exposure keratitis/ectropion and/or corneal sensation reduced	Permanent tarsorrhaphy Ectropion correction or tarsal sling procedure

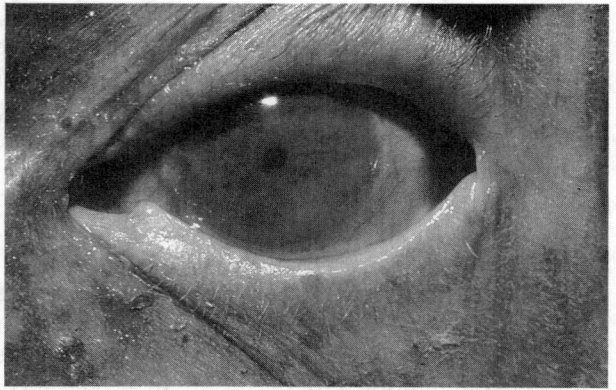

Figure 10.17   Chronic iridocyclitis in leprosy. Photo: Hans Limburg.

SUMMARY: EXAMINATION OF THE EYES IN LEPROSY AND EYE HEALTH EDUCATION

1. Record the visual acuity in each eye. Where visual acuity is reduced below 6/12 in either eye, refer to the eye specialist.
2. Note if the patient blinks regularly. Ask the patient to gently close the eyes. If necessary, ask the patient to close the eyelids forcibly. Record any evidence of lagophthalmos.
3. The patient with lagophthalmos or corneal anaesthesia should be taught to think-blink—many times each day. This patient requires referral to the eye surgeon.
4. Note any redness of either eye. Particularly examine the corneoscleral margin (limbus) for redness, which can indicate acute iridocyclitis. Any patient who has a red eye should be referred to the eye specialist.
5. Test the corneal sensation with a fine tip of 'rolled' cotton wool.
6. Examine, with magnification, the anterior chamber of the eye for evidence of any haziness suggesting circulating cells and proteins.
7. Note any evidence of a grey-white pupil which

can suggest the presence of cataract. This can be confirmed if an ophthalmoscope is available.

8. Dilate the pupil with a short-acting mydriatic (e.g. cyclopentolate 1% eye drops). The pupil's response to the mydriatic, together with evidence of haziness of the aqueous fluid behind the cornea, may suggest acute or chronic iridocyclitis. Evidence of posterior synechiae or a miotic pupil which fails to dilate will indicate the presence of active or previous iridocyclitis.
9. It should be confirmed with each patient that they are on the correct systemic treatment for their leprosy.

SUPPURATIVE KERATITIS

Corneal ulceration, due to either bacteria or fungi, is a common and often difficult problem in many countries (Figure 10.18). The cornea has been described as the 'battleground for sight', and central ulceration, when healing does occur, will usually

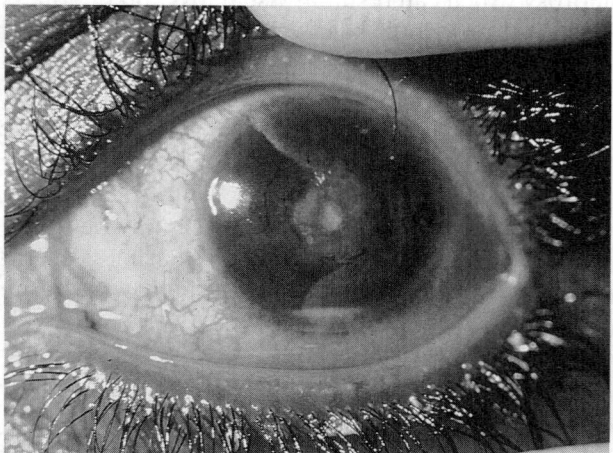

Figure 10.18   Corneal ulceration with hypopyon formation. Photo: Allen Foster.

leave a central corneal scar with marked reduction of vision. The clinical treatment of this problem can often be made difficult by lack of antibiotics and particularly antifungal agents.

Damage to the corneal epithelium alone, without corneal stromal involvement, can result in healing without scarring. However, damaged epithelium may allow entry of a great variety of organisms, with consequent deep ulceration and later scarring. Further, if the infection penetrates within the eye, pus cells may accumulate and settle at the lower aspect of the anterior chamber (hypopyon), and more severe involvement can result in endophthalmitis with irreversible damage and eventual shrinkage of the eyeball (phthisis).

Many organisms may cause suppurative keratitis. Bacterial keratitis can often be caused by *Streptococcus pneumoniae*, *Pseudomonas* spp. and *Staphylococcus aureus*. Fungi which commonly may cause a suppurative keratitis most commonly are *Aspergillus*, *Fusarium* and *Candida albicans*. Fungi are often found in humid tropical areas such as coastal West Africa and South-East Asia. Agricultural accidents and injuries with vegetable matter predispose to fungal infection.

CLINICAL APPEARANCE

It is not possible, clinically, to be certain whether a corneal ulcer is due to bacterial or fungal infection. However, a demarcated or multifocal ulceration with central and satellite foci may suggest infection due to a fungus.

LABORATORY DIAGNOSIS

Gram staining and microscope examination are possible within half an hour. The procedure for obtaining and examining material from a corneal scrape is shown in Table 10.13.[28] This procedure will demonstrate the presence of bacteria or fungi. Bacteria will be shown as Gram positive or Gram negative, as rods or cocci, under a 100× oil emersion objective. Fungal hyphae are seen under a 40× objective.

TREATMENT

The treatment of suppurative keratitis/corneal ulceration is urgent. Initial treatment may be given according to Gram stain results. Treatment can be changed if culture and sensitivity tests are available, although at least 24 hours will be required to obtain results.

Different regimens of treatment are given in Tables 10.14 and 10.15.[28]

Enriched tetracycline 1% ointment, which contains polymyxin, is a suitable antibiotic to use when treatment is given topically, before results of a Gram stain are available (or if this facility is not available).

Chloramphenicol is active against most Gram-

Table 10.13 Materials and procedure for a corneal scrape (after ref. 28).

Materials
Topical anaesthetic (ideally preservative-free if culture is to be performed)
Scalpel blades, needles or platinum spatula
Alcohol or gas burner
Matches or lighter
Clean glass microscope slides (labelled)
Wax or diamond marker
Culture media (labelled)

Procedure
Put nothing in the eye except anaesthetic until the specimen is taken
Explain the procedure to the patient
Children require sedation
Apply topical anaesthetic if required
Use sterile, cooled blade or needle to sample representative areas of ulcer (a spirit lamp may be used for sterilization)
Avoid touching lids and lashes
Use each scrape to prepare one smear or culture
Spread material thinly on to microscope slides
Resterilize and cool instrument between scrapes
Fix slides for microscopy with gentle heat (or alcohol)
Label slides and cultures with name and date

Table 10.14   Topical treatment of suppurative keratitis according to results of Gram stain (after ref. 28).

	Ideal circumstances	*Practical alternatives*
Gram-positive cocci	Cefuroxime 50 mg/ml *or* Cefaxolin 33 mg/ml	Gentamicin 14 mg/ml *or* Chloramphenicol 0.5% *or* Enriched tetracycline 1% (with polymyxin)
Gram-negative rods	Gentamicin 14 mg/ml	Gentamicin 14 mg/ml *or* Chloramphenicol 0.5% *or* Enriched tetracycline 1% (with polymyxin)
Gram-negative cocci	Penicillin G 10 000 u/ml *or* Cefuroxime 50 mg/ml	Enriched tetracycline 1% (with polymyxin)
Fungal elements	Econazole 1% *or* Miconazole 1%	Natamycin 5%

Table 10.15   Treatment of suppurative keratitis of unknown aetiology (after ref. 28).

Gentamicin drops (14 mg/ml) + cefaxolin drops (33 mg/ml)
  or
Gentamicin drops (14 mg/ml) + chloramphenicol drops 0.5%
  or
Gentamicin drops (14 mg/ml) + enriched tetracycline 1%
  or
Gentamicin 40 mg s.c. + benzyl penicillin 500 000 iu

If there is no response to therapy in 48 hours then an antifungal agent should be added:

Miconazole 1% or econazole 1% drops
  or
Natamycin 5%

positive and Gram-negative organisms, but gentamicin should be used where the infection is recognized as due to *Pseudomonas* spp. Many strains of *Neisseria gonorrhoeae* and *Staph. aureus* are resistant to penicillin G.

Topical treatment may be supplemented with subconjunctival injections. Examples are gentamicin 40 mg or penicillin G 500 000 units.

Antifungal agents include the imidazoles: miconazole, clotrimazole, econazole and ketoconazole. Amphotericin B may be tried, but it is toxic to the cornea and natamycin has poor corneal penetration. Flucytosine is active against *Candida albicans* but should be used in conjunction with an imidazole to prevent acquired resistance.

An alternative is treatment with topical silver sulphadiazine 1% ointment.

Any eye with corneal ulceration should also be given a mydriatic/cycloplegic, such as atropine sulphate 1%, used at least once daily.

For treatment of ophthalmia neonatorum, see p. 257.

EYE INJURIES

In many countries of the world, ocular trauma results in a great deal of eye pathology and human distress. Mine blasts often cause damage to limbs and eyes, in many cases involving young people and children.

Injuries to the eye may be superficial or deep. They may be due to penetrating injury or blunt injury. Burns, which may be chemical or due to excessive heat, may affect one or both eyes.

CORNEAL ABRASION

Superficial injury to the cornea can have many causes. It may be due to the scraping of the nail of a child against the mother's cornea, catching the eye on a twig, or injury with a contact lens. If the corneal epithelium only is involved, this can heal without any scarring.

Treatment

Instil antibiotic drops or ointment for at least 5 days. Give a mydriatic/cycloplegic drop, e.g. cyclopentolate 1% once. Pad and bandage the eye with the eyelid carefully closed, until the epithelium heals, but at least for 24 hours. Larger abrasions may require rebandaging for a further 24 hours following repeat instillation of the antibiotic. If vegetable matter is involved in causing the injury, remember the possibility of fungal infection complicating the injury.

SUPERFICIAL RETAINED FOREIGN BODY

A great variety of foreign bodies may cause superficial injury. These are often metallic but may also be stone, wood, an eyelash, etc. The foreign body may be situated on the tarsal conjunctiva and be revealed by everting the eyelid.

Treatment

Instil local anaesthetic drops, e.g. amethocaine 1% or benoxinate 0.4%. Remove the foreign body with a cotton-wool bud or a sterile hypodermic needle. If the foreign body is metallic, there may be some surrounding rust present. Do not be energetic in removing this as the central cornea is only about 0.5mm in depth. Give antibiotic drops or ointment for at least 5 days. Give a mydriatic/cycloplegic drop, e.g. cyclopentolate 1% once. Pad and bandage for at least 24 hours.

PENETRATING INJURIES

A penetrating injury may be due to a retained intraocular foreign body or any sharp object, such as a thorn, which penetrates the eye.

The evidence of injury may not, at first sight, be obvious. In some instances only careful examination will reveal the track of a retained intraocular foreign body. Very occasionally the patient may be quite unaware that a foreign body has entered the eye.

Clinical examination

There is no substitute for careful examination of the disturbed eye, using magnification. A retained foreign body which is radio-opaque should be shown on X-ray. However, the localization of a foreign body prior to surgery requires exact localizing methods.

Treatment

Where a penetrating injury is evident, or suspected, the patient should be given antibiotic cover, both topically and systemically, and referred to the eye specialist. The damaged eye should be protected with a shield, either a Cartella shield or an improvised shield using radiographic film.

BLUNT INJURY

A blunt injury, or non-penetrating injury, can cause considerable damage to an eye. Injuries may be caused by objects such as a stone or a fist.

It is good clinical practice to examine the eye from the front through to the back of the eye, beginning with the periorbital region and eyelids. Fractures may occur at the orbital margin and the bony floor of the orbit may fracture (a blow-out fracture), which in turn may cause adherence of the inferior extraocular muscles. Bruising may occur affecting the eyelids and the conjunctiva and there may be bleeding into the anterior chamber of the eye (hyphaema). The cornea can be damaged, resulting in oedema. Intraocular tissues may be torn, such as a tear of the root of the iris (iridodialysis). A cataract may form. The lens itself may be dislocated. Bleeding in the posterior segment of the eye may result in vitreous haemorrhage and there can be isolated or associated retinal haemorrhages. Retinal oedema may be apparent on ophthalmoscopy.

Treatment

In most instances the correct treatment of a blunt injury is rest until the condition resolves. Should there be a total, or near total hyphaema in the anterior chamber of the eye, the intraocular pressure must be carefully monitored. A pressure rise in the presence of a hyphaema may result in blood elements entering the corneal stroma, with consequent corneal blood staining. Any suggestion of a rise in intraocular pressure in the presence of a large hyphaema is a clear indication for a paracentesis, with release of the blood from the anterior chamber.

As rest is indicated in these patients, it will not be

sensible to ask a patient to travel any distance, perhaps over uneven roads, for further assessment. It is advisable to provide topical antibiotic eye drops and possibly a systemic antibiotic. A mydriatic/cyclopegic such as cyclopentolate 1% may be given. In the presence of bleeding from the iris, movement of the iris should be avoided. Any moderate intra-ocular pressure rise can be controlled by oral aceta-zolamide.

BURNS OF THE EYE

Burns of the eye may be due to chemicals or fire. In the case of chemical injury, both acid or alkali may be involved, with alkali burns generally being more serious.

Treatment

Where a burn of the eye(s) has occurred, *immediately* begin thorough irrigation of the eye(s) with water. Keep washing for 10–15 minutes until you feel all the substance which has caused the burn has been washed out. Remember to irrigate under the eyelids as well. Any fragments of chemical or ash, or other material, may be picked off with plain forceps. Antibiotic drops and ointment should be applied frequently, at least hourly, during the first day or two. Eyelids should be kept mobile with deliberate movement of the lids a number of times each day. If there is any question of possible permanent damage, such as corneal haze or adhesions between the eyelids and the eyeball, the patient should be urgently referred to the eye specialist.

SNAKE VENOM CONJUNCTIVITIS

In regions of the world where the spitting cobra is found snake venom can cause a conjunctivitis.

SOLAR BURN (ECLIPSE RETINOPATHY)

Our natural and sensible precaution is to avoid the direct glare of the sun's rays, but in certain situations this does not happen. An eclipse of the sun should only be viewed, if at all, with appropriate and adequate filters, otherwise a macular burn will follow because sunlight will focus on the retina.

In at least one central Asian country children play a 'game', competing with each other to see who can gaze longest at the sun! A macular burn may occur resulting in a permanent central scotoma. This may also be found in young people who sun-gaze while under the influence of drugs.

CATERPILLAR HAIR CONJUNCTIVITIS (OPHTHALMIA NODOSUM)

The conjunctival reaction to an unusual foreign body, a caterpillar hair, is recognized as an entity in ophthalmology, also described as *ophthalmia nodosum*. A granuloma or granulomas may form, each of which contains a foreign body. Treatment requires removal of the hair, otherwise deeper invasion may occur.

CLIMATIC DROPLET KERATOPATHY

Climatic droplet keratopathy is a degenerative condition in which translucent droplets accumulate in the superficial stroma of the cornea (Figure 10.19). It has been described in many countries and regions including Eritrea, southern Africa, India, New Guinea, Australia, Labrador, Greenland, Iceland,[29] Somalia[30] and Mongolia.[31]

It is considered that high exposure to ultraviolet sunlight is the main aetiological factor in the pathogenesis of this corneal disease, which can cause significant visual impairment.

Treatment, where necessary, can involve sector iridectomy, debridement (scraping) of the central cornea, lamellar or penetrating keratoplasty and more recently ablation by excimer laser.

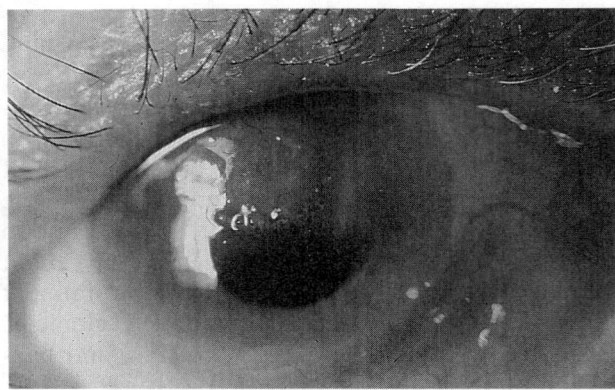

Figure 10.19 Climatic droplet keratopathy. Photo: Gordon Johnson.

TOXINS AND THE OPTIC NERVE

In patients with nutritional deficiency, particularly of the vitamin B complex, the optic nerve is susceptible to toxic damage.

Tobacco smoking in excess, often with considerable *alcohol* consumption and relatively poor nutrition can result in a toxic optic neuropathy. Pipe smokers have long been recognized to be at risk of this condition. Methyl alcohol is sometimes drunk with disastrous effects, including optic neuropathy and subsequent blindness. The author was called to examine a senior official in an Asian country because of the possibility of eye damage after drinking methyl alcohol. The patient did not survive the toxic effects of this bout of drinking.

Cassava is eaten in many tropical countries. Inadequately prepared cassava can cause optic neuropathy and peripheral nerve abnormalities due to cyanide toxicity. The cyanide content of the foodstuff, which is found particularly in the roots, may accumulate in the nervous system, causing toxic damage. Water used for soaking cassava must be discarded, together with any fermenting cassava; then the cassava must be dried before grinding into flour.

Drugs which may cause a toxic optic neuropathy include ethambutol, quinine and isoniazid.

Treatment of these conditions requires avoidance or moderation in the use of the agents which may have toxic effects.

OPTIC NERVE DISEASE OF UNKNOWN AETIOLOGY

OPTIC NERVE DISEASE AND MACULAR ABNORMALITIES IN TANZANIA[32]

A recent report describes a form of macular degeneration accompanied by optic atrophy which has appeared in the coastal regions of Tanzania. Africans of both sexes, mainly aged 10–25 years, described the subacute onset of painless bilateral loss of central vision. Visual acuity was usually 6/36 or 6/60 at the time of presentation. A few patients had some recovery of vision during the following months.

The pigment beneath the macula was dispersed and clumped, sometimes forming a small ring. Thus far this eye disease has been noted only in indigenous Africans, but of 35 different tribes. There is as yet no clear evidence as to the cause, although the history and clinical appearance suggest some unidentified toxic agent.

OPTIC NERVE DISEASE IN CUBA[33]

It is appropriate to include here reference to an epidemic of general neuropathy in Cuba during 1992–1994. More than 50 000 cases have been reported, with the epidemic moving from west to east. Most patients have been middle-aged and males are slightly more often affected (3:2). Painful paraesthesiae, mainly in the legs, with ataxia were reported. The number of patients with optic nerve involvement is uncertain, but some estimates suggest nearly 50% of cases. The aetiology is obscure but factors considered are poor nutrition, toxic influences such as tobacco or alcohol, or a virus. Patients do seem to benefit by receiving B complex vitamins and the number of new cases has declined dramatically.

EYE DISEASE IN CHILDREN

Although the exact number of blind children in the world is not known, it is estimated that the figure is approximately 1.5 million, with up to 500 000 new cases every year. Approximately 85% of these children live in Africa and Asia.[34] Many children die during the months after blindness occurs. Seventy per cent of blindness in childhood (0–15 years) is due to corneal scarring. Most of these patients with corneal scarring have had acute episodes of vitamin A deficiency, often associated with measles infection. Other causes of corneal scarring include newborn conjunctivitis (ophthalmia neonatorum), herpes simplex keratitis and the use of harmful traditional eye medicines.

In certain countries, rubella infection in mothers during pregnancy can result in the congenital rubella syndrome which, amongst other abnormalities, may result in blinding bilateral cataract. Inherited genetic factors may also result in congenital cataract and some retinal dystrophies may cause visual loss. Premature babies are at risk of retinopathy of prematurity.

VITAMIN A DEFICIENCY AND THE EYE

See pp. 239–244, and Chapter 21.

NEWBORN CONJUNCTIVITIS (OPHTHALMIA NEONATORUM)

Newborn conjunctivitis, where infection of the child's eyes occurs during the birth of the child, is a very serious problem in many parts of the developing world. Infection involving the conjunctiva is usually the first evidence, sometimes with a purulent discharge, and danger to the cornea with subsequent perforation or scarring and blindness is our first concern.

By definition, newborn conjunctivitis occurs in a child within the first 30 days of life. Two organisms commonly cause newborn conjunctivitis: *Neisseria gonorrhoeae* and *Chlamydia trachomatis* (Table 10.16).[35]

The World Health Organization has estimated a yearly adult incidence of 25 million cases of gonorrhoea and 50 million of genital chlamydial infection.

Gonococcal newborn conjunctivitis due to *N. gonorrhoeae* typically has a dramatic onset with bilateral purulent conjunctivitis and profuse discharge of pus, associated with tense and swollen eyelids (Figure 10.20). The condition usually presents within the first few days of birth. This is an eye emergency and treatment must be started immediately. For treatment of newborn conjunctivitis due to *N. gonorrhoeae*, see Table 10.17.[35]

Newborn conjunctivitis due to *C. trachomatis* is less dramatic in onset, presenting as irritable, red eyes but without purulent discharge unless secondary bacterial infection occurs. Often the infection presents some days later than with the gonococcal infection. Treatment for newborn conjunctivitis due to *C. trachomatis* is given in Table 10.17.

It is important to remember that treatment for these infective conditions should include systemic therapy because the infection is not confined to the eyes alone. Systemic treatment must also be given for both parents.

Other bacteria which may cause newborn conjunctivitis include *Haemophilus*, *Str. pneumoniae*, *Staphylococcus* and *Pseudomonas*.

Prevention of newborn conjunctivitis requires prophylactic treatment of the newborn child (Table 10.18).[35] The eyelids of both eyes should be carefully swabbed with sterile saline *as soon as each child is born*. A single application of tetracycline 1% eye ointment is given to each eye. Alternatively, silver nitrate 1% eye drops may be used, but the silver

Table 10.16 Causes of newborn conjunctivitis (after ref. 35).

Microbial
Sexually transmitted diseases (STD)
    Chlamydia trachomatis
    Neisseria gonorrhoeae

Other micro-organisms, often mixed
    Haemophilus spp.
    Staphylococcus spp.
    Streptococcus pneumoniae
    Streptococcus group D
    Escherichia coli
    Pseudomonas spp.

Chemical
Silver nitrate

Table 10.17 Management of newborn conjunctivitis (after ref. 35).

Gonococcal
A. Admission to hospital
    Penicillin i.m. or i.v.
    Topical antimicrobial therapy, e.g. tetracycline 1% ointment, intensively at first (hourly) then reducing to three times a day for 14 days

B. *If PPNG* prevalence more than 1%*
    Single i.m. injection of cefotaxime 100 mg/kg or kanamycin 25 mg/kg plus tetracycline 1% ointment or erythromycin 0.5% ointment as indicated in (A)

Chlamydial: systemic treatment
Erythromycin estolate orally (syrup) 5 mg/kg per day for 14 days

Non-gonococcal, non-chlamydial
Tetracycline 1% ointment or erythromycin 0.5% ointment four times a day for 14 days

Treatment of parents

_____

* Penicillinase-producing *N. gonorrhoeae*.

Table 10.18 Prevention of newborn conjunctivitis (after ref. 35).

Detection and treatment of infected pregnant women
Screening of all pregnant women is difficult in most countries and expensive
May be possible to screen high-risk groups

Eye prophylaxis in the neonate at birth
Mechanical cleaning of the eyelids immediately at birth, plus tetracycline 1% ointment or silver nitrate 1% drops

Treatment of the neonate as an index case
Only applicable where:
• prevalence of gonococcal infection low
• main sexually transmitted disease causing newborn conjunctivitis is *Chlamydia trachomatis*
• all infected infants can be detected and treated
• facilities exist for diagnosis of *C. trachomatis*

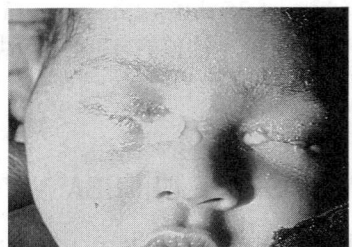

Figure 10.20 Newborn conjunctivitis due to *Neisseria gonorrhoeae*. Photo: John D C Anderson.

nitrate must be well preserved, avoiding any exposure to light or evaporation.

RETINITIS PIGMENTOSA

The hereditary degenerations of the retina can be autosomal recessive, autosomal dominant or X-linked recessive in inheritance.

Symptoms include night blindness (nyctalopia) and gradual loss of vision due to field defects. Dark adaption is affected, a typical ring scotoma is the recognized visual field abnormality, and progressive disease causes characteristic 'bone corpuscle' pigmentary disturbance of the peripheral and equatorial retina. The blood vessels become attenuated and the optic nerve head has a pale appearance. The condition may be associated with a number of other disorders or syndromes. It may also present with atypical forms.

There is no specific treatment. Close intermarriage (consanguinity) in many countries increases the risk of this disorder and genetic counselling should be offered to affected families.

SICKLE CELL DISEASE

Hereditary abnormalities affecting haemoglobin is found in Blacks, with red blood cells developing a sickle shape in conditions where low oxygen tension exists. Eye changes include conjunctival vascular abnormalities, focal iris ischaemia, peripheral retinal vascular disturbance with new blood vessel formation, haemorrhages, fibrosis and sometimes a detached retina.

Argon laser photocoagulation should be used to 'treat' any peripheral neovascularization. Late stage disease may require surgical removal of the vitreous (vitrectomy). Retinal detachment surgery may also be necessary.

See Chapter 6.

THALASSAEMIA

Also a hereditary disorder of haemoglobin, thalassaemia is found mainly in the Mediterranean region, Middle East, India and South-East Asia.

CONGENITAL CATARACT

It is important to recognize congenital cataract as early as possible so that treatment can be given, thus avoiding the danger of amblyopia or 'lazy' eye.

Congenital cataract may be the result of inherited genetic factors so that brothers and sisters may also be born with cataract. Rubella during the early

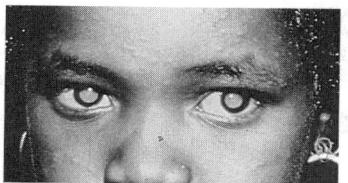

Figure 10.21   Bilateral congenital cataract after rubella infection during the mother's pregnancy. Photo: John D C Anderson.

months of the mother's pregnancy can result in cataract which is evident at birth (Figure 10.21). Chickenpox and toxoplasmosis affecting the mother may also cause cataract in the unborn child. Down's syndrome (mongolism) may be associated with congenital cataract.

Other causes of cataract include metabolic disorders with abnormal biochemical functions, for example, galactosaemia.

Prevention of congenital cataract can especially be effected by immunization against rubella. Vaccination may be given to all babies in infancy, often together with immunization against mumps and measles. Alternatively, young girls can be vaccinated at puberty.

Treatment of congenital cataract requires surgery. A child with congenital cataract, whether unilateral or bilateral, should be referred to the eye surgeon as soon as the diagnosis is made. If surgery is delayed, the eye or eyes will become amblyopic or 'lazy', with the retina lacking the necessary stimulation to develop fine and detailed vision. If both eyes are involved, the surgeon will operate on each eye, as early as possible, with the second operation sometimes within a few days of the first.

In most developing countries the child will be provided with aphakic spectacles. Refraction should be carried out every 6 months to maintain accuracy in the lenses provided. Methods which may also be considered are contact lenses, intraocular lens implants and epikeratophakia (onlay lamellar corneal graft).

RETINOPATHY OF PREMATURITY

There is evidence that retinopathy of prematurity is again becoming a cause of childhood blindness in the USA and Europe. Increasingly sophisticated neonatal care has resulted in the survival of tiny, premature babies who can develop the condition. In moderately developed countries, with improving neonatal care, babies who now survive premature birth are also at risk of retinopathy of prematurity.

Retinopathy of prematurity is a proliferative retinopathy in premature babies with immature retinal blood vessels. There is often a history of exposure to

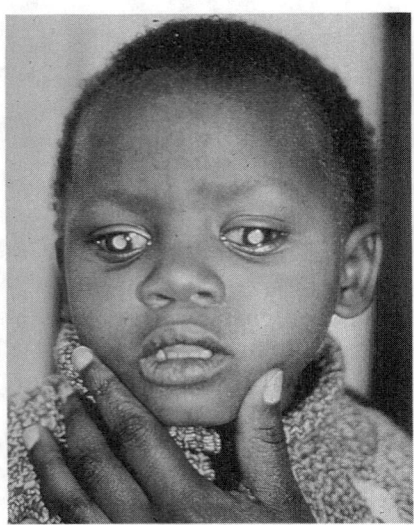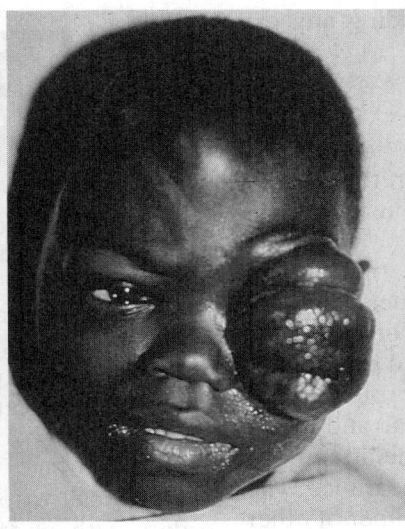

Figure 10.22 Bilateral retinoblastoma (left) Advanced retinoblastoma (right). Photos: Volker Klauss.

high oxygen concentration. Spasm of the retinal vessels is followed by dilated vessels, new vessel formation, vitreous haemorrhage, vitreous traction, retinal folds and retinal detachment.

Treatment in expert hands, using cryotherapy or the laser, can prevent progression of the disease when applied in the early stages.

RETINOBLASTOMA[36]

Retinoblastoma is the most common malignant eye tumour of childhood. The tumour arises in the retinal cells.

Most children in developing countries present for examination and treatment too late, with the tumour far advanced, commonly extraocular and often extraorbital (Figure 10.22). The tumour extends along the optic nerve to the brain. In the later stages, metastases occur to other parts of the body.

Retinoblastoma will usually first be noticed because of the presentation of a white pupil. Tumour tissue in this presentation is situated behind the lens in the eye. Other eye abnormalities which may lead to a discovery of retinoblastoma include a squint, glaucoma, visual loss, a painful red eye and orbital cellulitis. The tumour may present at any time during the first 5 years of life.

In the child a developing retinal cell can lose both of a pair of 'antioncogenes' or tumour suppressing genes. These are situated on the long arm of chromosome 13. Two-thirds of children with retinoblastoma develop the tumour because of random somatic mutations. This is uncommon and so these children present with a single, unilateral tumour, typically at a relatively older age than other children

with retinoblastoma. If they survive, these children do not pass on a genetic defect to their offspring.

The remaining one-third of children who develop retinoblastoma have lost one of each antioncogene pair in every cell in the body. Either the defect is inherited or this abnormality occurs at the time of conception. A random mutation will then occur affecting the second antioncogene, often in more than one retinal cell. Thus, foci of retinoblastoma are multiple, normally bilateral and occur at a relatively younger age.

Multiple or bilateral tumours can be considered to be genetically determined.

It is most important, following the discovery of a single tumour, that both eyes are examined very carefully. Examinations must continue regularly, every 3–6 months, until at least the age of 5 years.

Adults who have had multiple retinoblastoma, and survived, must be advised that there is a one in two chance of their children being affected.

Occasionally a tumour regresses spontaneously; thus the parents of a child with retinoblastoma should be examined, together with each of the siblings.

The differential diagnosis of this whitish, raised tumour (when still intraocular) includes infestations such as toxocariasis, retinopathy of prematurity and other causes of a 'white' pupil. Investigations should involve ultrasonography or computerized tomography, if available.

Effective treatment of retinoblastoma is largely dependent on early recognition of the tumour while it is still contained within the eye. The patient must be referred immediately to the specialist. In most eye centres in developing countries the correct treatment requires surgical excision of the eye (enucleation), removing as much of the attached optic nerve as possible. Some specialist centres will be able to provide chemotherapy and radiotherapy for these children. Chemotherapy uses vincristine, carboplatin and etopopside. Cyclophosphamide and doxorubicin are alternatives in appropriate regimens in experienced hands.

For smaller intraocular tumours, where the tumour does not extend to the ora serrata, or where there is no vitreous seeding, lens-sparing radiotherapy may be used. Focal radiotherapy can use surgically inserted scleral plaques, such as cobalt-60 or iodine-125. Cryotherapy can also be applied directly to a small tumour, and indirect xenon arc photocoagulation can be placed *around* a tumour less than 5 mm in diameter and situated away from the optic disc. It should be noted that an eye which has the original tumour can often be retained, and after expert treatment for more than one focus of retinoblastoma the first affected eye may have better vision than the other affected eye.

CONGENITAL GLAUCOMA (BUPHTHALMOS)

Glaucoma in childhood may be present at birth or can develop during the first few years of life. Increased intraocular pressure in a young child causes the more elastic tissues of the eyeball to stretch and so the eye enlarges. For this reason the description of buphthalmos, or 'ox eye', is used. Congenital glaucoma may be unilateral or bilateral. The unilateral enlarged eye is usually more quickly recognized.

The condition may cause discomfort, with photosensitivity (avoidance of bright light), and reduced vision may also be evident. On examination it may be obvious that the cornea is larger than it should be and in some instances the cornea may be hazy. On examination under anaesthesia, the optic nerve head may be cupped.

Treatment requires surgery to allow the aqueous fluid to drain out of the eye. Often persistent congenital remnants in the drainage angle of the anterior chamber of the eye have caused some degree of obstruction to the outflow of aqueous.

HARMFUL (TRADITIONAL) EYE MEDICINES

Many patients will attend the local traditional healer before considering a visit to the health worker trained in what we consider to be standard medical practice. It should be recognized that traditional healing can provide considerable benefit to patients and some centres, for example in India, have traditional healer at the local health centres. However, some applications to the eyes used by these local healers can cause severe adverse reactions.

The clinical picture which does not provide a clear diagnosis when seen by the health worker may have been confused by the superimposed application of harmful eye medicines into an eye already suffering the original disease. In these situations the history of the eye problem will be important. It should be kept in mind that the patient, or the parent who has brought a child, may be very hesitant to admit that a traditional eye medicine has been used.

A variety of harmful medications may be used: the juice of squeezed plant leaves, lime juice, kerosene, toothpaste, breast milk and urine (both animal or human). A chemical or caustic keratoconjunctivitis may occur, or infection, such as with *N. gonorrhoea* from human urine, may be introduced. In Zimbabwe, tomato juice may be given for mild conjunctivitis and lemon peel juice for discharging eyes. Powdered herbs can be blown into a diseased eye.[37] The constructive approach of discussion with traditional healers and herbalists has been encouraged in Zimbabwe.

Treatment is often difficult. Topical therapy with an antibiotic 3–4 times each day, and a mydriatic/cycloplegic such as atropine sulphate 0.5% or 1%, once daily, may be used. The original eye disease, if identified, should be treated accordingly.

REFRACTIVE ERRORS

It is beyond the scope of this chapter to discuss refractive errors. However, the recognition of refractive needs and the provision of spectacles is vital to most populations during the various stages and ages of life. Myopia, hypermetropia and/or astigmatism can severely affect the performance of a child in school. Successful school screening programmes have been implemented, for example in India. For screening purposes a pin-hole disc can indicate if poor vision is due to a refractive error. Middle and old age brings the need for presbyopic correction—for reading, for sewing, or for picking stones out of rice! Aphakic spectacle corrections are required after intracapsular cataract surgery. Correctly prescribed spectacles can transform the quality of life for many around the world. Further, it has been increasingly appreciated that the provision of low-vision optical aids must be energetically pursued so that patients who are visually impaired can have the opportunity of considerably improved visual capacity.

DIFFERENTIAL DIAGNOSIS OF THE RED EYE

INFLAMMATION OF THE EYELIDS

Blepharitis

Inflammation of the eyelids is a common complaint which is typically chronic in character. Chronic seborrhoeic blepharitis presents with redness of the lid margins with crusts on and at the base of eyelashes. *Staph. aureus* may be involved. Treatment of this chronic condition can be difficult and the inflammation will often recur. Crusts should be removed with moist cotton wool (warm water) and antibiotic eye ointment should be applied to the lid margins. If there is a severe infective blepharitis a systemic antibiotic, such as tetracycline 250 mg orally for a minimum of 3 months, may be considered.

Inflammation of the eyelid skin or eyelid margins may also be due to a virus or be allergic in origin. Viruses associated with this type of inflammation include the common wart, herpes simplex, herpes zoster ophthalmicus and molluscum contagiosum.

Stye (hordeolum)

A localized abscess at or near the base of an eyelash follicle requires treatment with heat and antibiotic eye ointment. A wooden spoon wrapped in cotton wool and a bandage, dipped in boiling water, can then be held close to the eyelid (not against the eyelid), so that the steam can 'bathe' the lesion.

Ectropion and entropion

Abnormal positions of the eyelids, such as an eyelid which turns out (ectropion) or turns in (entropion), may result in considerable discomfort and inflammation.

Ectropion, which usually involves the lower eyelid, results in exposure of the tarsal conjunctiva. Epiphora (overflow of tears) usually occurs. Ectropion can follow weakness of the orbicularis oculi or facial nerve paralysis. Injury or infection with associated scarring can cause a cicatricial ectropion.

Entropion can commonly affect both upper and lower eyelids. The scarring of trachoma is often associated with upper eyelid entropion. Injuries may cause entropion. In older age, a spastic lower eyelid may turn in, causing considerable irritation due to eyelashes rubbing on the cornea.

Chalazion (meibomian cyst, tarsal cyst, lipogranuloma)

The meibomian glands, which are situated in the tarsal plates of each eyelid, open along the lid margins. Ducts may become blocked, resulting in a retention cyst with ensuing inflammatory reaction. Often a chalazion will require incision. Following local anaesthetic injection beside the cyst and eversion of the eyelid with a chalazion clamp, an incision is made into the cyst vertically, away from the lid margin. The contents of the cyst are curetted out. A topical antibiotic eye ointment is given for some days.

Eyelid tumours

Both basal cell carcinoma and squamous cell carcinoma may result in nodular or ulcerating lesions on the eyelids.

Other eyelid inflammations

Considerable inflammation and scarring of the eyelids may be caused by conditions such as anthrax, actinomycosis, leishmaniasis and yaws.

ORBITAL CELLULITIS

Inflammation within the bony orbit of the eye can result in swelling of the eyelids, with associated proptosis of the eye. Conjunctival chemosis (oedema of the conjunctiva) is usually present. The patient may have a fever and be very unwell.

Complications of acute orbital cellulitis include corneal ulceration, endophthalmitis, septicaemia and cavernous sinus thrombosis.

Treatment is with high doses of a systemic antibiotic. A topical antibiotic eye ointment may be given, mainly to protect the eye. Supportive therapy should include adequate intake of fluids and control of the associated fever.

A characteristic presentation of orbital cellulitis is described with infection by *Loa Loa*, also described as Calabar swelling.

DACRYOCYSTITIS

Inflammation of the tear sac can result in swelling at the side of the nose near to the inner canthus of the eye. This can progress to an acutely inflamed abscess or may become chronic in nature.

Blockage of the tear ducts, which often occurs in the nasolacrimal duct running from the tear sac to below the inferior turbinate of the nose, may be a precursor of this type of inflammation. Blockage may also occur in the superior or inferior canaliculi and also the common canaliculus, which run from the inner canthus of the eye into the tear sac.

Treatment is with topical and systemic antibiotics and subsequent syringing of the tear ducts with normal saline. Failure to open the tear ducts by this method will subsequently require surgery. Blockage of the nasolacrimal duct will require a dacryocysto-rhinostomy.

INFLAMMATION OF THE CONJUNCTIVA AND CORNEA

A large variety of organisms may cause inflammation of the conjunctiva (conjunctivitis) and/or of the cornea (keratitis).

Bacterial or fungal infections typically present with a red eye and discharge. Both bacteria and fungi may cause suppurative conjunctivitis and keratitis. Infection with viruses more usually present with a red eye and watering, although secondary infection with bacteria is not uncommon, causing subsequent discharge with pus.

Allergic conjunctivitis is characterized by a red eye and extreme itching. This may be associated with conditions such as hay fever.

VERNAL KERATOCONJUNCTIVITIS (SPRING CATARRH)

This common disorder, which often affects children and teenagers, has a typical presentation affecting both the tarsal conjunctivae and the limbal region (corneoscleral margin). The eyes are red, irritable and may show strands of mucus. Severe itching is typical. Papillae may be pronounced and often have an appearance like 'cobblestones'. The exact cause is unknown and it is difficult to treat.

Treatment of vernal keratoconjunctivitis is most effective using topical corticosteroids. However, a word of warning regarding the use of topical corticosteroids: this treatment must be continued under strict specialist ophthalmic supervision. It must be recognized that topical corticosteroids have dangerous side-effects. A *steroid-induced glaucoma* can result in damage to the optic nerve due to raised intraocular pressure. The author vividly recalls a young man of 18 years presenting at the eye hospital in Kabul, Afghanistan, blind due to bilaterally cupped optic nerve heads. This young man had been troubled with vernal keratoconjunctivitis and had been treated intermittently with topical corticosteroids. A vigorous, healthy young Afghan, he was blind at the very beginning of manhood. Further, it should be noted that topical corticosteroids can be a disaster where a red eye is caused by infective

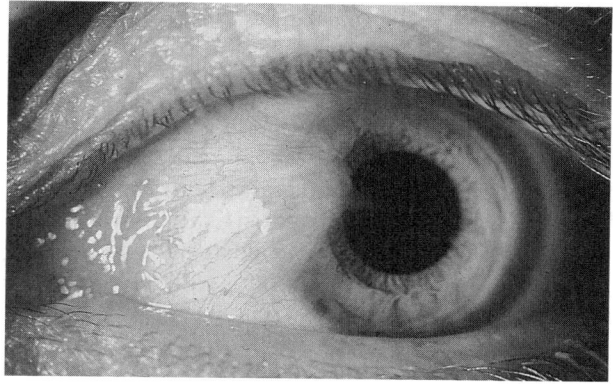

Figure 10.23   Nasal pterygium. Photo: Murray McGavin.

agents. Thus, a herpes simplex keratitis, treated with topical corticosteroids, can cause great harm to the eye, with consequent severe visual loss.

Other forms of treatment for vernal conjunctivitis are topical antihistamines or sometimes a systemic antihistamine in the late evening. If available, topical disodium chromoglycate 2% (Opticrom, Aarane, Intal) may be used four times or more each day. Symptomatic relief may be obtained to some extent with eye drops such as zinc sulphate. Cold compresses may be of some benefit.

If trachoma is present as well this should be treated before topical corticosteroids are given.

PINGUECULA

The accumulation of fatty deposits at the nasal or temporal conjunctival limbus is a common finding in middle or older age. Occasionally the pinguecula may become inflamed, when a topical anti-inflammatory agent may be used. The best form of treatment is to leave them alone.

PTERYGIUM

A pterygium is a 'wing' of conjunctival and subconjunctival tissue which grows across the cornea from either the temporal or the nasal side (Figure 10.23). Its presence in the interpalpebral area suggests several external factors which influence its growth. Although poorly understood, these may relate to ultraviolet light and to irritation in different climates, especially hot, dry and dusty conditions. Some pterygia are pale and flat and cause few problems. Others are fleshy, more often inflamed and, if surgery is required, tend to recur. Anti-inflammatory agents may be used topically if required. Surgery should be avoided if at all possible but may become necessary if the pterygium begins to approach the visual axis.

PHLYCTENULOSIS

A phlycten appears most commonly at or near to the limbus and is evidence of bacterial allergy, particularly associated with the tubercle bacillus. A phlycten is a microabscess which appears as a raised, pinkish nodule. It responds quickly to topical corticosteroids. Again, the diagnosis should be certain and any use of topical corticosteroids should be carefully monitored. Any patient with a phlycten be examined for systemic disease.

KERATOCONJUNCTIVITIS SICCA (THE DRY EYE, XEROSIS)

Keratoconjunctivitis sicca is a common condition where dryness of the eyes causes symptoms of irritation, with grittiness (like sand in the eye) and redness. It is more common with advancing years but may also occur in younger persons where damage has occurred to the lubricating glands, both lacrimal, in the upper outer region of the orbit, and conjunctival. There is a recognized association with rheumatoid arthritis. In tropical countries dry eyes can follow trachoma, in which conjunctival glands are damaged.

The diagnosis may be confirmed using a Schirmer's tear test in which strips of filter paper are hooked over the lower eyelid and the length of wetting of the strip is measured after 5 minutes. A drop of rose bengal 1% eye drops will reveal punctate staining of the cornea and conjunctiva and filaments of epithelium on the cornea (filamentary keratitis). In an eye with severe dryness, rose bengal will cause considerable discomfort.

Treatment is with artificial tear preparations such as hypromellose 0.3% eye drops.

TRACHOMA

See pp. 229–232.

CORNEAL ULCERS AND CORNEAL SCARRING

See pp. 254–256.

VITAMIN A DEFICIENCY (XEROPHTHALMIA, KERATOMALACIA)

Although xerophthalmia is often apparent in a quiet eye, a devitalized anterior eye may be subject to other influences, such as infection, which will result in a red eye.

INFLAMMATION OF THE EPISCLERA AND SCLERA

Episcleritis

Episcleritis is essentially a self-limiting condition in which the aetiology can be uncertain. It is a recognized complication of leprosy and has been associated with herpes zoster ophthalmicus, gout and rheumatoid arthritis. Treatment can be most effective, using topical corticosteroids when required.

Scleritis

Inflammation of the sclera is often associated with uveal tract inflammation, resulting in a sclerouveitis. Scleritis is most commonly associated with rheumatoid arthritis and 30% of patients presenting with scleritis are found to have rheumatoid disease. Infective conditions associated with a scleritis are leprosy, tuberculosis and herpes zoster ophthalmicus.

Scleritis requires systemic treatment, either with non-steroidal anti-inflammatory agents or systemic corticosteroids. Other immunosuppressive agents may also be used. Topical treatment will be with atropine sulphate 1%, at least once daily, and topical corticosteroids. Subconjunctival injections of corticosteroids should *not* be used because focal necrosis can occur.

INFLAMMATION OF THE ANTERIOR UVEA (ANTERIOR UVEITIS, IRIDOCYCLITIS)

Inflammation of the iris (iritis) and of the ciliary body (cyclitis) may be described as iridocyclitis or anterior uveitis.

Iridocyclitis presents typically with pain, redness, photophobia and blurred vision. The condition may be unilateral or bilateral. Examination with magnification will reveal a haziness of the aqueous fluid in the anterior chamber of the eye due to the presence of circulating proteins and inflammatory cells. Deposits of cells may be found on the endothelium of the cornea and these are described as keratic precipitates. Inflammation of the iris and its pupil margin may result in adherence of parts of the pupil to the anterior lens face. These are described as posterior synechiae. Synechiae may also occur at the base of the iris, across the angle of the anterior chamber to the base of the cornea, described as peripheral anterior synechiae.

Secondary effects of inflammation can result in secondary glaucoma and, in some instances, secondary cataract formation.

The causes of iridocyclitis are many. Systemic disease which presents with a classical granulomatous type of iridocyclitis with large keratic precipitates includes sarcoidosis, tuberculosis and leprosy.

Injury to an eye can occasionally result in a 'sympathetic' inflammation of the second eye. It is said that this may occur days, months or even years after the original injury. The originally injured eye, described as the 'exciting' eye, may induce inflammation of the second eye, the 'sympathizing' eye. This can result in difficulties in management. Topical corticosteroid therapy is required, and also systemic corticosteroids. Other immunosuppressive drugs may be considered.

There are a variety of factors influencing the onset of iridocyclitis which may relate to genetic characteristics, sex and race. For example, the presence of the HLA-B27 antigen is often associated with ankylosing spondylitis and uveitis. Males are more likely to develop ankylosing spondylitis or Reiter's syndrome. Reiter's syndrome is characterized by nonspecific urethritis, polyarthritis, conjunctivitis or possibly iridocyclitis. Certain racial factors influence uveitis in conditions such as Behçet's syndrome, which is more common in eastern Mediterranean people and the Japanese. Behçet's syndrome typically presents with recurrent ulcers of the mouth and genitalia associated with a severe uveitis. The iridocyclitis of sarcoidosis is more common in the black population of North America.

ACUTE CLOSED ANGLE GLAUCOMA

See pp. 234–235.

EYE INJURIES

See pp. 254–256.

INFLAMMATION OF THE EYEBALL

Endophthalmitis

Infection which develops in the interior of the eye, for example when a bacterial or fungal corneal ulcer perforates or when a penetrating foreign body enters the eye, especially stone, wood or coal, may result in a severe intraocular inflammatory reaction. Usually this is disastrous for the eye. Vigorous treatment is required with systemic and local antibiotics and often systemic corticosteroids. Subconjunctival and intravitreal antibiotic injections may be required.

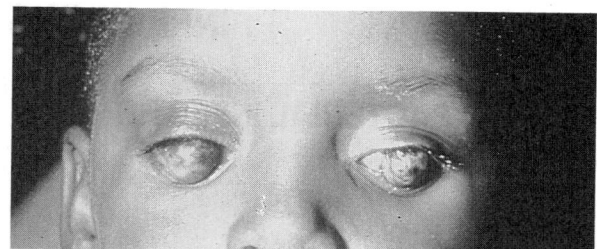

Figure 10.24   Gross staphylomata after measles and vitamin A deficiency. A blind unsightly eye will usually be enucleated. Photo: Simon Franken.

Staphyloma

A staphyloma is a bulging of the eye where, by definition, uveal tissue is adherent behind the bulging wall of the eye; thus a staphyloma may be a corneal staphyloma or a scleral staphyloma. In its initial stages the eye is usually severely inflamed with a weakened cornea or sclera. This appearance may be associated with vitamin A deficiency (Figure 10.24), in which inflammation will be minimal, or possibly follow severe injury.

Phthisis bulbi

A shrunken eye may follow severe inflammation, such as endophthalmitis or panophthalmitis, and injury from a variety of causes. The intraocular pressure is low (hypotony). The resulting shrunken eye can be quiet but during the damaging process, of whatever origin, the eye is usually inflamed.

If the patient is not complaining, nothing need to done. However, an artificial eye may be inserted either on top of the phthisical eye or after the eye has been removed surgically. The appearance can be greatly improved.

ANTERIOR SEGMENT BLEEDING WITHOUT INJURY

A *subconjunctival haemorrhage* may occur spontaneously and is shown as a dramatic red area over the white sclera. This will resolve in 2–3 weeks. Unless the patient has similar haemorrhages elsewhere, it is likely to be an isolated episode of no consequence. If in any doubt, however, the blood pressure and blood picture should be determined.

Spontaneous bleeding in the anterior chamber of the eye causing a hyphaema indicates intraocular pathology, such as new vessel formation on the iris, which may occur, for example, in diabetes.

INFECTIONS AND THE EYE

SYSTEMIC BACTERIAL INFECTIONS AND THE EYE

BRUCELLOSIS (UNDULANT FEVER; MEDITERRANEAN FEVER) (See Chapter 45)

Brucellosis is caused by infection with organisms which are Gram-negative bacilli: *Brucella abortus*, *B. melitensis* or *B. suis*. Other organisms within the same family include *B. ovis*, *B. canis neotomae,* but these cause infections in animals, with *B. canis* once reported in human beings. The disease is widespread throughout the world and can include eye changes. The systemic disease is described in Chapter 45. There has been an increase in the number of cases in eastern Mediterranean countries since 1985 (WHO).[22]

Eye complications

A uveitis which is chronic and granulomatous in character is described. Keratitic precipitates with cells and circulating proteins in the anterior chamber indicate an iridocyclitis. A posterior uveitis may occur also. However, as with anterior uveitis, the appearance of any posterior uveitis is similar in presentation to a number of other causes of posterior eye inflammation.

Keratitis may occur with some epithelial opacities. An optic neuritis is rare. Extraocular muscle abnormalities can appear, either due to local inflammation or sixth cranial nerve paralysis due to a basal meningoencephalitis.

The diagnosis of brucellosis is based on the isolation of the organism from blood, urine or pus, or serological tests.

Treatment

Treatment of the eye disease is that given for an anterior uveitis, with topical mydriasis/cycloplegia using eye drops such as atropine sulphate 1% and topical corticosteroids.

Treatment of the systemic disease with tetracycline and intramuscular streptomycin is described in Chapter 45. Trimethoprim–sulphamethoxazole may also be given.

TULARAEMIA (See Chapter 48)

Tularaemia is caused by a small Gram-negative bacillus, *Francisella tularensis (Pasteurella tularensis)*. The human infection is found in Europe, Japan and North America.

The systemic disease and its transmission from animals such as rabbits and other rodents, is described in Chapter 48.

Eye complications

The eye changes associated with tularaemia occur when the organism penetrates the conjunctiva. After a period of up to 2 weeks, symptoms and signs, such as itching, photosensitivity and pain, together with redness and conjunctival oedema (chemosis), appear. Granulomas may appear and the regional lymph nodes become enlarged. This clinical picture is one of the characteristic descriptions of Parinaud's oculoglandular syndrome. Dacryocystitis has been described.

Treatment

Treatment is with streptomycin and the tetracyclines. Details of systemic treatment are given in Chapter 48.

TUBERCULOSIS (See Chapter 57)

Tuberculosis is widespread and there is evidence that there is an increase in the infection worldwide. The WHO estimates over 8 million new cases each year, with more than 3 million deaths.[22] In countries where HIV/AIDS is endemic, tuberculosis is showing a disturbing increase. The causative organism is an acid-fast bacillus *Mycobacterium tuberculosis*.

Eye complications

The disease may affect all systems of the body, including the eyes. Infection of the skin (lupus vulgaris) can result in eyelid scarring and secondary corneal involvement due to exposure. External eye involvement can include small miliary tubercles, which are grey or yellow nodules. A papillary conjunctivitis can occur. Phlyctenular keratoconjunctivitis is a hypersensitivity reaction to the tuberculoprotein, presenting as small yellow/white nodules, often situated on the corneoscleral margin but also on the conjunctiva, associated with an inflammatory response. This nodule is a microabscess and any patient, often a child, presenting with this allergic response should have a systemic examination for tuberculosis. A keratitis is described which is typically an 'interstitial' keratitis. Scleritis, inflammation of the sclera, may be either anterior or posterior. The latter, posterior scleritis, may be associated with considerable thickening of the sclera due to granuloma formation.

An anterior uveitis (iridocyclitis) is typically granulomatous in type with large keratitic precipitates, described as 'mutton fat' because of their appearance. Examination with magnification may reveal small white nodules at the pupil margin or on the iris stroma (Koeppe nodules). Posterior uveitis (choroiditis), and a panuveitis can result in considerable disturbance to the eye. Both optic neuritis and consequent atrophy are described.

The systemic disease is described in Chapter 57.

Treatment

The systemic treatment of tuberculosis with isoniazid, together with rifampicin or ethambutol and other medications, in a variety of regimens, is described in Chapter 57.

The treatment of eye disease should be appropriate to the local condition diagnosed. A phlycten responds quickly to topical corticosteroid therapy as the nature of the lesion is a hypersensitivity reaction. It should be noted that corticosteroids should only be used when the diagnosis is certain and where specialist advice has been sought.

Periphlebitis retinae

It is considered that periphlebitis retinae is most commonly associated with systemic tuberculosis in developing countries. The vascular disturbance may vary, from mild retinal vasculitis, evident on examination of the retinal periphery, to new vessel formation and gross bilateral vitreous haemorrhages. The condition is also described as Eales's disease, which is now recognized as a group of diseases with different aetiologies. The author has seen both forms of the disease and in one central Asian country (Afghanistan) Eales's disease is found in the more florid form. It does seem significant that tuberculosis in this same country, both in its pulmonary and particularly in its extrapulmonary form, was a well-recognized and common medical problem. How-

ever, other causes of retinal neovascularization and vitreous haemorrhage must be excluded.

A variety of causes of retinal vasculitis include sarcoidosis, Behçet's disease, systemic lupus erythematosus and multiple sclerosis.

MENINGOCOCCAL MENINGITIS (See Chapter 44)

Epidemics of meningococcal meningitis (cerebrospinal meningitis) occur particularly in tropical countries, although the disease is found worldwide. Apart from 'epidemic' years, 300 000 cases will occur each year and 10% of patients will die. A 'meningitis belt' has been described across the savanna of sub-Saharan Africa, from Sudan to The Gambia. The organism is the Gram-negative *N. meningitidis* which typically is shown on microscopy as pairs of cocci or as a single coccus.

The systemic disease is described in Chapter 44.

Eye complications

Extraocular muscle imbalance can occur due to involvement of the cranial nerves, in particular the sixth nerve, although a partial third nerve paralysis is not uncommon. The patient may present with an unblinking appearance with open palpebral apertures. Encephalitis with optic neuritis may result in postneuritic atrophy. These features are associated with basal meningitis and the chronic meningitis can cause a secondary hydrocephalus.

The pupils react in a variety of ways according to the particular site of inflammation intracranially. In the early stages there may be miosis but mydriasis will occur with the onset of coma.

A conjunctivitis and also an anterior uveitis can occur associated with meningococcaemia. A panophthalmitis is uncommon.

Involvement of the visual cortex can result in loss of vision with entirely normal ocular features and reactions. This visual disturbance or blindness may sometimes remain for days or even weeks with some recovery of sight in time, following treatment.

Treatment

The treatment of the systemic disease with penicillin or chloramphenicol is described in Chapter 44.

Local inflammation involving the eye or eyes should be treated appropriately with an antibiotic for external infection, and with mydriasis/

cycloplegia and topical corticosteroids for anterior ureitis.

DIPHTHERIA (See Chapter 52)

Diphtheria is caused by infection with a Gram-positive bacillus *Corynebacterium diphtheriae*.

The disease is a public health problem in some developing countries, for example Sudan and India. Due to immunization, diphtheria has been reduced in distribution and effects worldwide, although recent reports in Russia bring news of a disturbing number of patients with the disease.

Eye complications

Local involvement of the eyes can present with a membranous conjunctivitis and eyelid oedema, discharge and local lymph node enlargement. Corneal ulceration can occur.

The classical sign of the infection with the bacillus is a 'dirty' grey membrane which forms where infection has occurred. The discharge can be blood-stained. On removal of the membrane the surface uncovered is raw and often has petechial haemorrhages. The exotoxins formed by the organisms are particularly damaging to the heart, kidneys and central nervous system. Cranial nerve paralysis can occur, affecting the extraocular muscles, particularly the sixth cranial nerve but with the fourth and third nerves sometimes also affected.

It should be noted that a membrane may form with other infections, such as with *Streptococcus* or *Pneumococcus*.

The systemic disease is described in Chapter 52.

Treatment

Diphtheria antitoxin should be used and then treatment with penicillin or erythromycin. Treatment of the disease is given in Chapter 52.

ANTHRAX (See Chapter 49)

Cutaneous anthrax can involve the eyelids and periorbital regions. Infection is by direct contact with contaminated skins and other animal products, most often amongst those who work with live or dead animals. The organism can also be transmitted by flies. A red papule forms at the site of inoculation with the organism, *B. anthracis*. The area of inoculation becomes black (eschar). The woman from

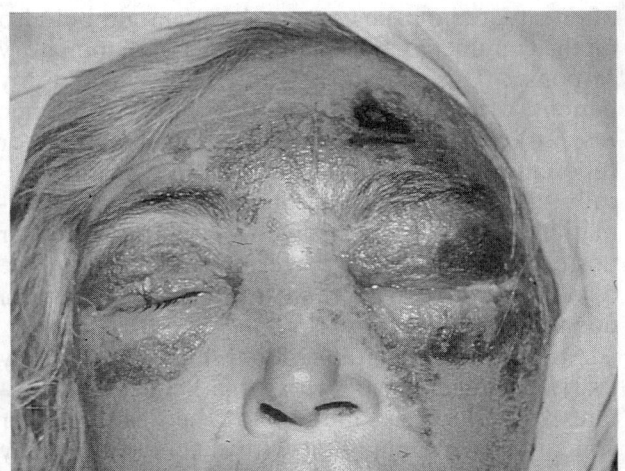

Figure 10.25   Anthrax in Central Asia. Notice the black eschar on the forehead. Photo: Murray McGavin.

central Asia, shown in Figure 10.25, related that an insect had bitten her forehead and a dark eschar can be seen at the site.

Eye complications

Eschar formation affecting the eyelids can progress to considerable scarring, resulting in dramatic cicatricial ectropion—the eyelid can turn 'inside out'.

Treatment

Systemic treatment with the penicillins is described in Chapter 49.

Eyelid surgery requires horizontal division of the scar tissue externally—to allow the eyelid to resume its original position—with a full-thickness skin graft in the region of divided scar tissue.

CHOLERA (See Chapters 3 and 41)

Cholera is a gastrointestinal disease caused by the bacillus *Vibrio cholerae*. The disease is widespread in tropical countries and has occurred in devastating epidemics. Profuse watery diarrhoea and vomiting results in acute dehydration.

A cholera pandemic, beginning in the East, has gradually spread in the last 30 years, reaching Latin America by 1991. The disease is described in Chapters 3 and 41.

Eye complications

The severely dehydrated patient will present with 'sunken' eyes. Conjunctivitis, corneal ulceration and corneal oedema have been reported. The great danger to the eyes is in the severely ill patient where poor eye care allows the patient to leave the eyelids open, with consequent dehydration, exposure keratoconjunctivitis and ulceration.

Of particular importance in the context of cholera is the increased risk of cataract due to acute dehydration. The author has discussed with Professor Indra Sekhar Roy, of Calcutta, the acute onset of cataract which he has described during cholera epidemics in India.

Treatment

Treatment is with fluid and electrolyte replacement and antibiotics. Tetracycline or furazolidone or erythromycin may be used. In the individual case, trimethoprim–sulphamethoxazole or chloramphenicol are effective (see Chapters 3 and 41).

TYPHOID FEVER (See Chapter 42)

Infection with the bacterial organism S*almonella typhi* causes fever, abdominal pain and prostration. The bacilli may be harboured by a carrier of the infection and the organism is also found in water, milk, ice-cream and other foodstuffs. This infective disease is widespread throughout the world and is particularly common in the tropics.

For a full description of the disease and its clinical features see Chapter 42.

Eye complications

Classically, rose spots may be described on the conjunctiva of patients with typhoid fever. They are found in association with similar rose spots distributed on the trunk and limbs, which may amount to only a few lesions or a considerable number on the body surface. During epidemics, cataract may form, possibly related, at least in part, to the associated dehydration. Involvement of the nervous system may result in a variety of complications, including extraocular muscle involvement and pupillary abnormalities. A meningitis is not common and S. *typhi* is recovered only occasionally from the cerebrospinal fluid.

Treatment

The treatment of choice remains chloramphenicol. For a full description of treatment options in typhoid fever see Chapter 42.

SPIROCHAETAL DISEASES AND THE EYE

SYPHILIS (See Chapter 13)

Syphilis is caused by the spirochaete *Treponema pallidum* which may be transmitted by venereal contact or, in the congenital form of the disease, from the mother to the unborn child. An annual incidence of 3.5 million is reported by the WHO.[22]

Congenital syphilis

A great variety of clinical symptoms and signs may occur in congenital syphilis and the disease may be sufficiently severe to cause abortion. The distinctly ocular changes of congenital syphilis can be relatively mild, although this is not always so, and severe ocular defects are well recognized. These include inflamed eyelids, dacryocystitis, conjunctivitis, extraocular muscle paresis, interstitial keratitis, iridocyclitis, pupil abnormalities (an Argyll Robertson pupil may be seen occasionally), choroidoretinitis with the classic appearance of pigment granules and yellow/red spots (the 'salt and pepper' fundus), and optic neuritis and optic atrophy. Typically congenital syphilis becomes latent and then reactivates, often during the teenage years, and often manifests as an interstitial keratitis. The patient then complains of severe discomfort or pain with photosensitivity and a red eye or eyes. The area of the cornea so affected may attract fine new blood vessels and the oedematous and inflamed area appears pink, which has been described as a 'salmon patch' appearance. Associated inflammation will include an iridocyclitis. Corneal scarring may also be a consequence. Later, tiny, empty blood vessels in the cornea are described as 'ghost vessels'.

Adult acquired syphilis

In acquired syphilis the primary stage of the disease is manifest as a painless, ulcerated 'chancre', where the spirochaete has gained entry, and this may be associated with a local lymphadenopathy. The chancre will heal and some time later second stage syphilis develops. Eye changes associated with this stage of syphilis can include iridocyclitis, retinal vasculitis and optic neuritis. Inflammation of the iris (iritis) may be obviously hyperaemic (roseolae). Tertiary stage syphilis may ensue after a variable period of time and can have similar clinical features. Also, the classical Argyll Robertson pupil may occur. Bilateral involvement of the pupils usually causes irregular pupils, and the affected pupil does not react to either direct or consensual light stimulation but will constrict on accommodation. Optic atrophy may be found. These eye findings are usually associated with systemic disease.

A description of the systemic disease in its different stages and the diagnostic tests for syphilis are given in Chapter 13.

Treatment

Treatment of the inflammatory disease of the anterior eye will require mydriasis and cycloplegia using eye drops such as atropine sulphate 1% together with topical corticosteroids.

A description of the general treatment of syphilis, using penicillin, is given in Chapter 13.

LEPTOSPIROSIS (See Chapter 56)

Leptospirosis is caused by a number of spirochaetes of the genus *Leptospira*. The organisms are found worldwide. Man is infected by contact with a variety of domestic and wild animals, including rats, pigs, dogs and cattle, mostly due to contact with urine-contaminated water and soil. After an incubation period of 8–12 days, the patient develops fever and chills with general malaise and photosensitivity. The conjunctival vessels may be dilated and there may be subconjunctival haemorrhages.

The systemic disease is described in full in Chapter 56.

Eye complications

An iridocyclitis can occur, although the onset of the intraocular inflammation may be weeks or some months after the initial infective phase has passed. In its severe systemic form leptospirosis has been described as Weil's disease, with jaundice and an enlarged liver and severe kidney disease.

See Chapter 56 for details of appropriate treatment. Antibiotics in high doses are indicated.

RELAPSING FEVER (See Chapter 55)

Relapsing fever is caused by the spirochaetes *Borrelia recurrentis* and *Borrelia duttoni*, which may be louse borne or tick borne, respectively. Humans harbour the body louse, and rodents and other animals can be infested with ticks. The disease is widespread and is found in all the warmer continents of the world.

The patient has a dramatic fever with severe headache, photosensitivity, muscle and joint pains, upper respiratory tract inflammation, nausea and vomiting. A rash is common. After the initial episode, which subsides spontaneously, the patient may feel well for a few days but a recurrence of the symptoms and signs may follow. This cycle may recur.

Eye complications

Eye complications of relapsing fever include anterior uveitis, which may be acute or chronic in character. Haemorrhages and exudates of the retina have been described. A meningitis may result in ptosis and extraocular muscle abnormalities due to cranial nerve paralysis.

Treatment

Both tetracycline and penicillin may be used, with tetracycline preferred except in children under 7 years and pregnant women. The patient needs total nursing and supportive care.

A full description of the systemic disease, diagnostic tests and treatment is given in Chapter 55.

YAWS (See Chapter 54)

Yaws is caused by the spirochaete *Treponema pertenue*, which is found in many geographical locations including Asia, Africa, South America and the Caribbean. An ulcerating papilloma forms the primary lesion.

As the disease progresses there may be the appearance of papules at a variety of sites. During the later stages the characteristic lesion is an ulcerating granuloma (gumma) which heals with scarring. This lesion, affecting the nose or orbit, can destroy bone and cartilage in the region (gangosa).

Eye complications (See Chapter 54)

Eye changes particularly involving the eyelids are due to scarring. Consequent deformities may cause the lower eyelid to turn out due to scar tissue formation (cicatricial ectropion). However, there can be considerable destruction in the region of the eye and orbit.

PINTA

Pinta is caused by the spirochaete *T. carateum*, which is found in the Central Americas and the

Caribbean. The disease process can result in scarring involving the eyelids which may cause eyelid deformities.

CHLAMYDIAL INFECTIONS AND THE EYE

TRACHOMA

Infection with *Chlamydia trachomatis* is described on pp. 229–232.

LYMPHOGRANULOMA VENEREUM

Lymphogranuloma venereum is caused by an organism of the *Chlamydia* (or *Bedsonia*) group of infective agents. It is a venereal disease, transmitted by sexual contact. The organism is widespread geographically.

The initial lesion, the primary sore, is usually in the genital region and within days there follows a regional lymphadenitis, with fever, headache, malaise, nausea and skin changes. A description of the systemic disease is given in Chapter 13.

Eye complications

Eye changes associated with lymphogranuloma venereum include a follicular conjunctivitis with a lymphadenopathy, particularly of the preauricular lymph node. This is also the clinical picture of Parinaud's oculoglandular syndrome. A keratitis may be associated with corneal infiltration and new vessel formation. An iridocyclitis has been described. Posterior eye changes include dilatation of the retinal veins, some retinal haemorrhages and oedema at the optic nerve head.

Treatment

Tetracyclines are the drugs of choice. A description of the treatment of lymphogranuloma venereum is given in Chapter 13.

RICKETTSIAL INFECTIONS AND THE EYE

TYPHUS

Typhus fever may be louse borne, where the infecting organism is *Rickettsia prowazeki*, or tick, mite or flea borne. The characteristic systemic diseases associated with these infections, together with details of the vectors and the rodents and other animal hosts involved are described in Chapter 39. Vasculitis is a significant feature in the systemic manifestations of these diseases.

Eye complications

Eye complications associated with typhus fever can include conjunctivitis with photosensitivity. Subconjunctival haemorrhages may occur. Other complications include: iridocyclitis, retinal changes with haemorrhages, and optic nerve oedema. Optic atrophy may ensue.

Treatment

Chloramphenicol and the tetracyclines are the drugs of choice.

ROCKY MOUNTAIN SPOTTED FEVER

This rickettsial disease is caused by *R. rickettsii* and is found in the Western hemisphere. The vector is the tick—carried by wild rodents and dogs.

A conjunctivitis with photosensivity and petechial haemorrhages of the bulbar and tarsal conjunctivae are described.

Treatment is with chloramphenicol and the tetracyclines.

VIRAL INFECTIONS AND THE EYE

MEASLES

Measles and the eye and its association with vitamin A deficiency is discussed on p. 244.

RUBELLA

The disease is caused by an RNA virus of the arbovirus group. It is most often diagnosed when it appears in epidemics. The disease presents with a maculopapular rash, which is pink/red, on the face, trunk and extremities.

Rubella infection in susceptible mothers during the first 3 months of a pregnancy has an 80% chance of affecting the unborn child. The expanded rubella syndrome can have both minimal and severe effects. Apart from eye complications, the child may be deaf or mentally retarded and there may be cardiovascu-

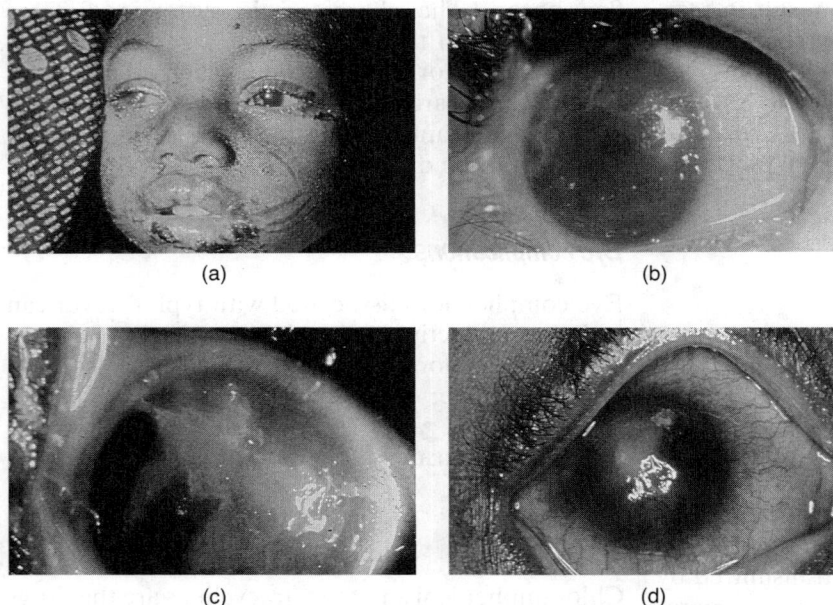

(a)

(b)

(c)

(d)

Figure 10.26 Herpes simplex keratitis.
Photos: (a), (c) John Sandford-Smith; (b) Allen
Foster; (d) David Yorston.

lar abnormalities. Growth of the fetus may be inhibited, and in the most severe form the fetus may be aborted or the child stillborn.

Eye complications

Cataract may occur in around half of all children affected by rubella in utero. This form of congenital cataract may be unilateral or bilateral. The virus may remain in the lens for some years after birth and surgical removal of the cataract may result in a uveitis. Other eye defects include congenital glaucoma (buphthalmos), rubella retinopathy, which can have a 'salt and pepper' appearance, optic atrophy, squint, nystagmus and microphthalmos.

Treatment

The treatment of rubella is preventive. Young females should be immunized; immunization may be carried out at 1 year of age or before puberty. This provides lasting immunity.

HERPES SIMPLEX AND THE EYE[38]

The herpes simplex virus (HSV) is distributed worldwide and can have severe effects on the eye. The virus contains a DNA core and this insinuates itself into the cell and the cell nucleus, where it is able to reproduce itself. Most individuals will have experienced a 'cold sore' on our face, but the effect

on the cornea is clearly much more significant. In many countries a lack of recognition of the infection, which causes a herpes simplex keratitis and the consequent use of topical corticosteroids, which are contraindicated in this infection unless used by the experienced eye specialist, can be disastrous for the eye. Most herpes simplex keratitis is caused by type I infections, although occasionally type II infections occur, particularly in the newborn—when infection occurs in the mother's birth canal.

It appears that the virus can remain latent for a long time within the nervous system, particularly the ganglion of the fifth cranial nerve (trigeminal). It should be noted that herpes simplex infection is more severe in immunocompromised individuals and may, for example, complicate the picture of measles keratitis and vitamin A deficiency.

In one study in Tanzania, HSV was responsible for 36% of corneal ulcers found in children (1981–1985)[39] and for 59% of corneal ulcers in patients of all ages (1988–1989).[38]

Although herpes simplex keratitis may be immediately obvious due to the presence of the classical dendritic figure, confusion may occur as the ulcer often presents in developing countries with an atypical appearance. The ulcer may be larger and can be described as geographic or amoeboid in appearance (Figure 10.26). These presentations may relate to the length of time before treatment is sought, but may also be the result of wrong diagnosis and wrong treatment, particularly with corticosteroids, or the consequence of treatment with inappropriate traditional eye medicines.

Table 10.19 Distinguishing signs of herpetic corneal ulcers.

Typical, narrow branching dendritic ulcer
Large, irregular geographic ulcer
Intense corneal vascularization
Dense stromal infiltrate
Stromal necrosis and/or facetting
Reduced corneal sensation
Scarring/facetting/vascularization from previous attacks
Central corneal oedema, with keratitic precipitates (disciform)

Reproduced from Yorston D. Measles and childhood blindness. *J Community Eye Health* 1991; 4 (Issue No. 8): 2–4.

Eye complications

Herpes simplex ulceration of the cornea has a tendency to recur and, should the infection and inflammation spread deeper than the corneal epithelium, corneal scarring is likely to result in reduced vision. Recurrence may be stimulated by a number of factors, including fever, exposure to ultraviolet light, minor trauma, measles and psychological factors. Thus, herpes simplex keratitis is consistently found in association with malaria and other causes of high fever.

Symptoms of HSV keratitis include pain and photosensitivity. Signs (Table 10.19) include watering (lacrimation), a red eye with circumcorneal injection, and in the classic presentation, a branching dendritic figure. This appearance of the superficial cornea is well delineated by instilling fluorescein dye. The same dye will, of course, also outline a larger ulcer, such as the geographic ulcer previously noted. A severe host immune reaction to the presence of the virus in the stroma of the cornea can result in considerable inflammation. Neovascularization is likely to develop, particularly with ulcers close to the limbus. When healing occurs a scar remains and it can also result in an irregular corneal surface. Deep inflammation of the cornea due to HSV infection provides a complicated problem in treatment. A uveitis may develop and sometimes the evidence of previous corneal epithelial infection can only be found with careful examination under magnification.

Treatment

Previously, treatment of superficial HSV keratitis affecting only the corneal epithelium was mechanical removal of the infected cells of the epithelium.

Idoxuridine (IDU) was the first antiviral agent used. IDU 0.1% drops should be given intensively each hour until epithelial healing takes place and then the dosage can be reduced to four times daily for a few days. Alternatively, IDU 0.5% eye ointment should be given five times each day. Unfortunately, IDU may itself result in corneal ulceration if used excessively and long-term use can result in occlusion of the lacrimal puncta.

Other forms of treatment are now more commonly used and these include acyclovir 3% eye ointment, which should be given five times daily, or vidarabine eye ointment, five times daily, or trifluorothymidine 1% solution, five times daily.

In experienced hands it may be necessary to use topical corticosteroids in a patient in whom there has been an immune response resulting in a deep disciform keratitis. The weakest effective dose of steroid should be used and (only) after treatment with an antiviral agent has been started and probably continued. The antiviral agent can be discontinued when a very weak corticosteroid is used, e.g. when prednisolone is reduced to 0.1%.

The eye health worker should refer any patient with herpes simplex keratitis to an experienced colleague after beginning treatment with a topical antiviral agent only, if this is available.

In the longer term, an unhealed HSV ulcer may require a conjunctival flap or a tarsorrhaphy to effect healing. (A tarsorrhaphy is a surgical procedure, which is usually temporary, in which the eyelids are partially sutured together.) Many years ago the author's father required this latter form of surgical intervention after intermittent treatment with IDU eye drops which also caused lacrimal punctal occlusion. The result was a healed cornea but with scarring.

Fortunately, most herpes simplex infections of the eye are unilateral, although this is not always the case. Scarring may require a later corneal graft which can be highly successful, although recurrence of the HSV infection can occur within the graft itself.

HERPES ZOSTER OPHTHALMICUS

The virus of herpes zoster is a DNA virus which lies dormant in sensory nerve root ganglia after a previous infection with chickenpox (varicella). A variety of stimuli may cause the development of herpes zoster (shingles) but, most commonly, herpes zoster affects the older age group and the immunocompromised individual. The development of shingles may be the first evidence of infection with the HIV/AIDS virus and this has become particularly apparent in African countries. Most often shingles affects the trunk but herpes zoster ophthalmicus, affecting the periorbital region and eye, occurs in less than 10% of patients who develop shingles. In these patients the ophthalmic division of the fifth cranial nerve is affected.

The clinical features of herpes zoster ophthalmicus include the classic rash, which is red and vesicular, develops crusts and later resolves with multiple tiny scars. The rash is typically 'one sided' in the region of the eyelids, supraorbital region and to a variable extent backwards above the hair line. The patient is generally unwell with headache and often depression. A distressing characteristic of the infection is postherpetic neuralgia which can persist for a year or two or more.

Eye complications

Eye complications occur in around 50% of patients and these can be expected if the nasociliary branch of the ophthalmic division of the fifth nerve is affected, with vesicles on the side of the nose. There may be lid scarring, a conjunctivitis, episcleritis, scleritis, keratitis, anterior uveitis, secondary glaucoma, extraocular nerve and muscle involvement and optic neuritis. Herpes zoster keratitis may take a variety of forms, including punctate epithelial erosions, filamentary keratitis and disciform keratitis.

Treatment

The patient requires rest, adequate fluids and analgesia to allow relief of the often severe pain. Antiviral drugs should be applied topically, both to the skin and to the eye. Acyclovir is most commonly used as a cream to the skin and as an ointment for the eye. Acyclovir may also be given systemically, especially if a patient is immunocompromised. A topical cycloplegic, such as atropine sulphate 1% eye drops, should be given to prevent posterior synechiae and to reduce spasm of the intraocular muscles. A topical corticosteroid may also be given if there is deep inflammation of the cornea or an iridocyclitis, but this must be under supervision of an eye specialist.

CHICKENPOX (VARICELLA)

This common virus infection of childhood is characterized by fever, malaise and rash, which appears 12–16 days after infection has occurred. The rash is erythematous with vesicles occurring in groups which are widespread over the body surface. It may, however, occur at any age and can be a complicated and serious disease. The virus is a DNA virus identical to the herpes virus group. The patient has immunity to varicella following infection.

Eye complications

Vesicles may occur on the eyelids, conjunctiva and at the corneoscleral margin(s). Superficial punctate keratitis, deeper inflammation of the corneal stroma (interstitial keratitis) and iridocyclitis have been described. Occasionally, extraocular muscle involvement, pupil abnormalities and optic neuritis have occurred. The retina can be involved in immunocompromised individuals.

Treatment

Antibiotic ointment can prevent secondary bacterial infection of skin lesions. Any systemic complication, such as a pneumonia, will require suitable antibiotic cover for secondary bacterial infection.

VARIOLA AND VACCINIA

It is excusable to mention these viruses if only to provide encouragement that a previously devastating disease has been effectively eradicated worldwide.

Variola (smallpox)

This virus infection has been eradicated due to a campaign of universal vaccination. Variola was a disease characterized by high fever, malaise, generalized aches and pains, followed by a typical rash, which was papular and vesicular, progressing to a pustular phase. Eye complications involved the eyelids, conjunctiva and the cornea. Corneal ulceration progressed to often gross scarring and loss of vision. Scars can still be seen in older patients in some countries. Deeper involvement sometimes occurred with choroiditis, optic neuritis and extraocular muscle involvement.

Vaccinia

A similar virus to the smallpox virus, vaccinia was used for immunization to prevent smallpox. Vaccination could be followed by systemic complications, including eczema and vaccinia necrosum. The author has seen a child with the latter condition in whom, following vaccination, it was discovered that there was hypogammaglobulinaemia. Sometimes vaccinia was transferred from the vaccination site to the eye, usually by the patient's fingers, resulting in vesicles on the lids, conjunctiva or cornea. This could occur in a child, or sometimes a mother transferred the virus to her own eye from the child's vaccination site.

MUMPS

An acute fever associated with a parotitis, sometimes involving other organs, causing orchitis, oophoritis and pancreatitis, is due to a virus which, following infection, provides long-term immunity.

Eye complications include dacryoadenitis, conjunctivitis, keratitis, scleritis, iridocyclitis, retinitis and optic neuritis. Treatment is supportive with analgesics and appropriate treatment of any eye complications.

MOLLUSCUM CONTAGIOSUM

Molluscum contagiosum is caused by a DNA virus which usually infects children. Infection in adults, especially in Africa, may be a sentinel lesion for HIV infection. A small papule with a central umbilicus is the typical lesion. There may be an isolated lesion or groups of papules. When situated on the eyelid, or possibly the conjunctiva, a conjunctivitis or sometimes a keratitis may occur. Curetting of the lesions, after local anaesthesia, with the application of chemical cautery using tincture of iodine or carbolic acid is usually successful. When working in Asia, the author recalls dealing with approximately 70 lesions on the face and chest of a child, with encouraging results. In this case a general anaesthetic was necessary.

CYTOMEGALOVIRUS

Infection with this virus has been particularly associated in recent years with the HIV/AIDS epidemic. Thus, it is a relatively common infection in the immunocompromised host. HIV/AIDS is discussed in Chapter 12.

Eye complications

Eye changes associated with the infection include an anterior uveitis, retinal oedema and necrosis, retinitis with widespread haemorrhages and sometimes retinal detachment. The optic nerve may be involved, with progressive optic atrophy. Opacities may occur in the vitreous and a posterior uveitis may also occur.

Infection affecting a woman who is pregnant can result in general and ocular abnormalities in the fetus. General features include a low birth weight, purpura, deafness, mental retardation, pneumonitis, and an enlarged liver and spleen. Eye changes include a cataract, uveitis, optic nerve atrophy, choriodoretinitis and microphthalmos.

BURKITT'S LYMPHOMA

The Epstein–Barr virus has been implicated as the casusative factor in this form of lymphoma. The tumour is found especially in sub-Saharan, middle Africa, but also in South America, Papua New Guinea and sporadically elsewhere.

Most commonly found in children under 10 years old, the maxillary region and orbit are often involved. The abdomen is often affected and also the central nervous system. A cranial nerve palsy can occur. The considerable upper jaw swelling can involve the eyelids and the anterior eye surfaces.

Treatment is by surgery, radiotherapy and chemotherapy (see Chapters 24 and 32).

HIV/AIDS AND THE EYE (See also Chapter 12)

HIV infection is most often a sexually transmitted disease caused by the human immunodeficiency virus. It can also be transmitted by transfusion of contaminated blood and by unsterile needles associated with drug abuse.

While HIV infection in developed countries occurs particularly in homosexual populations and amongst drug users, in Africa it is mainly transmitted by heterosexual activity. Seropositivity is significantly linked with a history of sexually transmitted disease, genital ulcer disease, contact with prostitutes and lack of male circumcision. Age-specific peaks of HIV infection are found amongst children under the age of 5 and amongst young adults.[40]

The WHO has estimated that by early 1992 there were 10–12 million people infected with HIV. Around 90% of these were in sub-Saharan Africa; child mortality rates may reach 50% in some countries of the region. The projected figures for the year 2000 are: HIV infection, 30–40 million; AIDS, approaching 10 million.[23]

It does seem that the rate of progression from HIV seropositivity to clinical AIDS and death advances more quickly in Africans than in Americans.

HIV has been isolated from most body fluids, with semen, vaginal secretions and blood of most importance in transmission of the disease.

HIV has been found in the tears, conjunctiva, the cornea, the aqueous humour and the vascular endothelium of the retinal vessels. These findings, in relation to potential transmission of the infection, are important, for example when examining patients with an applanation tonometer. However, there is no report of transmission occurring through tears. Isopropyl alcohol swabbing of the tonometer tip is an adequate means of sterilization. The possible transmission of HIV as a result of corneal transplant surgery is an obvious concern.

Retinopathy has fluffy white 'cotton-wool' spots as the most common sign of systemic infection, seen in 25–50% of AIDS patients. Typically they are not found in HIV infected children. These spots are an indication of severe disease and also indicate ischaemic injury of the nerve fibre layer of the retina. Retinal haemorrhages indicate a progressive vascular abnormality and can be associated with microaneurysms and focal areas of vasculitis.

Opportunistic infections include infection with *cytomegalovirus* (CMV), which is the most common infection found, occurring in up to 30% of patients with AIDS, in 50% of whom the condition is bilateral. The overall incidence is less in developing countries, around 5–10%. Yellow-white necrotic areas with irregular margins are found at the posterior pole and along the distribution of the main blood vessels. CMV infection can severely damage the retina within months. Ganciclovir, given intravenously, may be prescribed for CMV retinitis, but not at the same time as treatment of AIDS with zidovudine. Patients are treated initially with ganiclovir 5 mg/kg intravenously twice daily for 2 weeks, followed by 6 mg/kg i.v. on 5 days each week (or 5 mg/kg i.v. each day). Side-effects of ganciclovir include bone marrow depression with reduction of white cells. Foscarnet may also be used for CMV retinitis. CMV retinitis appears to be less common in heterosexuals than in homosexuals and is correspondingly less common amongst African patients.

Other infective agents which may take advantage of the depressed immune state in AIDS include *Cryptococcus neoformans*, *Pneumocystis carinii*, *Mycobacterium avium-intracellullare*, *Toxplasma gondii*, *Histoplasma capsulatum* and *Candida albicans*.

Herpes zoster ophthalmicus is a marker for HIV infection in Africa. The course of this disease is more severe in HIV-positive patients, with more subjective discomfort. It also occurs in a younger age group. Intravenous or oral acyclovir is the preferred treatment, but the drug is expensive. Retinal necrosis may occur in association with herpes zoster and this can present in two clinical forms. The typical form has necrotic areas in the peripheral fundus, with vasculitis, haemorrhages and vitreous and anterior chamber involvement. The other presentation, more often found with HIV seropositivity, shows many yellowish lesions scattered throughout

the fundus and less often vitreous and anterior chamber inflammation. Treatment is with high doses of acyclovir or foscarnet intravenously. Prognosis is very poor.

The eyelids may have multiple warts or the umbilicated papules of molluscum contagiosum, both suggestive of HIV/AIDS infection.

Some of the rarer ophthalmological abnormalities associated with HIV infection may be associated with cryptococcal meningitis or toxoplasmosis. These include motor nerve palsies, pupil abnormalities and optic nerve inflammation and atrophy.

Herpes simplex keratitis is more often recurrent in AIDS patients and is often less responsive to treatment.

Syphilis, not unexpectedly, is more common amongst HIV seropositive patients. All patients with syphilis should be tested for HIV. The converse is also necessary. Eye disease includes uveitis, optic neuritis and retinal vasculitis.

Tuberculosis is similarly more common amongst HIV seropositive patients, and this may progress to miliary disease, foci of infection in the choroid or widespread choroidal and retinal invasion, with a poor prognosis for vision and life.

Tumours described in association with HIV/AIDS are: Kaposi's sarcoma, B-cell lymphomas and conjunctival squamous cell carcinoma. Kaposi's sarcomas may appear on the eyelid or conjunctiva, and rarely within the orbit.

FUNGAL INFECTIONS AND THE EYE

Over 100 fungal species, whether filamentous fungi, yeasts or dimorphic organisms, have been associated with eye infections. Difficulties in management of the oculomycoses relate to problems in diagnosis and often an inadequate resource of antifungal agents. A suppurative keratitis, for example, may be due to either bacteria or fungi but this cannot be firmly decided on clinical grounds alone. A simple measure for determining the type of organism involved is to carry out a Gram stain (see Chapter 59). Although many antifungal medications have been developed, their ready availability has been limited, partly because the financial return for pharmaceutical companies producing these eye medicines has been uncertain.

PATHOGENIC FUNGI AND EYE INFECTION (OCULOMYCOSES)

Fungi causing eye infections are most commonly filamantous fungi and yeasts.

- *Filamentous fungi*. These are multicellular organisms with projections known as hyphae. Hyphae may have divisions or be non-septate. Septate filamentous fungi include important organisms causing eye infections: *Fusarium*, *Aspergillus* and *Penicillium*. Non-septate filamentous fungi, for example *Rhizopus* and *Phycomycetes*, less commonly involve the eye.
- *Yeasts*. *Candida albicans* and *Cryptococcus neoformans* are species of yeasts that may be involved in eye infections. They are distinguished by the fact that they are unicellular organisms that reproduce by budding.
- *Dimorphic fungi*. These fungi, such as *Blastomyces dermatitidis*, may be responsible for ocular and orbital disease following blood and lymphatic spread.

Oculomycoses are found worldwide but particularly in countries with hot and humid climates. The geographical pattern of these infections worldwide is gradually emerging as the literature on mycotic infections of the eye increases. In some parts of the tropics, between a third and a half of adult corneal ulcers are caused by fungi. The filamentous fungi *Aspergillus* and *Fusarium* are most commonly found affecting the eye. *Candida albicans* is also found worldwide.

In terms of the treatment of fungal eye infections, the most significant anatomical site is the cornea where suppurative keratitis, ulceration, hypopyon formation and possible corneal perforation mean that early recognition of the infection and prompt treatment is vital.

A fungal corneal ulcer is suggested by a dry, slowly worsening, necrotic ulcer with stromal infiltrate and multifocal lesions, particularly if the ulcer fails to respond to antibiotic treatment. However, these signs are not consistently present.

Fungi are associated with vegetable matter, so injuries, such as abrasions of the cornea with twigs, thorns and husks, must always be examined with an awareness of the possibility of fungal infection.

Fungi may also involve the canaliculi of the lacrimal duct system.

ASPERGILLOSIS

The genus *Aspergillus* contains over 300 identified species and is common in warm and humid climates. The nose and paranasal sinuses are often infected, which can lead on to ocular involvement with extraocular muscle palsies. Intracerebral abscess formation can cause eye complications due to a space occupying lesion.

Keratitis with corneal ulceration and an endophthalmitis are well recognized in aspergillosis.

Aspergilli may infect the lacrimal canaliculi and an associated conjunctivitis may be present.

FUSARIOSIS

Fusarium spp. may cause a suppurative keratitis, with or without hypopyon formation. As with any suppurative keratitis, corneal scarring is likely when the area of infection and inflammation heals. At a later time corneal grafting may be indicated.

CANDIDIASIS (MONILIASIS)

Candida albicans is an organism commonly found in the mouth, throat and vulva.

The fungus may affect the eyelids, lacrimal system, conjunctiva and cornea. Often infection will follow injury to the eye, whether accidental or (sometimes) surgical.

The fungal organism can also spread by the endogenous route, especially in patients whose immune system is compromised, such as drug addicts and those on immunosuppressants. Intraocular infection may occur, with anterior uveitis, choroidoretinitis and vitreous abscess formation.

CRYPTOCOCCOSIS

Cryptococcosis neoformans is a yeast-like fungus which may have systemic effects involving the skin, lungs and meninges. It may cause a mycotic corneal ulceration and hypopyon may form. Endogenous spread through the bloodstream results in involvement of either the anterior or posterior uveal tract. Infection of the meninges may cause raised intracerebral pressure with the ocular sign of papilloedema and subsequent optic atrophy. Cranial nerve abnormalities also occur.

BLASTOMYCOSIS

Blastomycosis dermatitidis is found in the Americas and Africa and affects the skin, lungs and various other organs. The infection is characterized by suppurative granulomas which may be found in the mouth, nose and also sometimes involving the eyelids. The orbit, lacrimal canaliculi, conjunctiva and cornea may be affected.

COCCIDIOIDOMYCOSIS

Infection with *Coccidioides immitis* usually begins with inhalation of the organism causing a pneumonitis. The disease may also involve skin, subcutaneous tissues, bone and meninges. Eye involvement can include a hypersensitivity response manifest as a phlyctenular conjunctivitis. The eyelids may be affected, and intraocular involvement has been recorded, causing a posterior uveitis. As with many fungi an endophthalmitis can occur.

RHINOSPORIDOSIS

Rhinosporidium seeberi, mostly reported in India and Sri Lanka, commonly affects the nasal mucosa but eye involvement of the conjunctiva causes watering and photosensitivity. The lacrimal passages may become infected.

HISTOPLASMOSIS

Infection by the fungus *Histoplasma capsulatum* is widespread. The organism is found in the soil and is inhaled.

The eye changes associated with this infection are described as 'presumed ocular histoplasmosis syndrome' (POHS), and based on evidence of infection elsewhere, but no organism has been isolated from the eye. It is presumed that histoplasmosis has a predilection for the posterior uvea and the characteristic lesions are multifocal atrophic choroidal and disciform macular changes.

If subretinal neovascular membranes form, treatment is with argon laser photocoagulation.

TREATMENT OF FUNGAL INFECTIONS

The imidazoles (miconazole 1%, clotrimazole 1%, ketoconazole 1% and econazole 1%) are the preferred antifungal agents. They are unfortunately not always freely available. Other antifungals have a number of limiting factors in their use: amphotericin B can be toxic to the cornea; natamycin 5% has poor corneal penetration; flucytosine 1% is only effective against yeasts and must be used in conjunction with an imidazole to avoid the development of resistance.

Silver sulphadiazine 1% eye ointment has been used effectively as an antifungal agent and povidone iodine (5% or less) is being advocated as a topical antiinfective eye drop also effective against the common fungi.

If possible, immediate empirical antifungal treatment should be avoided and a Gram stain of a corneal scrape carried out. If a mycotic corneal ulcer is suspected, when antibacterial therapy has been unresponsive after 48 hours, an antifungal agent should be used.

Natamycin 5% eye drops are most effective against filamentous fungi, including *Aspergillus* and *Fusarium*, but may not always achieve good results. Dosage is one drop half-hourly, then 6–8 times per day after 3–4 days.

Amphotericin B is most effective against yeasts, particularly *Candida* and *Cryptococcus*. It may be given intravenously and topically.

Flucytosine 1% is effective against yeasts, including *Candida* and *Cryptococcus*, although some strains are resistant. It must therefore be given with an imidazole. It may be given in oral form and topically.

The imidazoles have a broad spectrum of antifungal activity. All are used topically. Clotrimazole 1%, miconazole 1%, ketoconazole 1% and econazole 1% are often used in treatment of the keratomycoses caused by filamentous fungi and yeasts. They do not invariably achieve a good result.

Silver sulphadiazine 1% eye ointment has proved beneficial in treating *Aspergillus* and *Fusarium*.[41]

Systemic antifungal treatment will be necessary in endogenous infections, such as with *Candida*, where flucytosine 150 mg/kg per day and ketoconazole 200 mg/kg per day for 3 weeks may be given. Alternatively, amphotericin B in 5% dextrose can be administered intravenously over several days until a total of 200 mg is given.

DISEASES CAUSED BY PROTOZOA

TOXOPLASMOSIS (See Chapter 66)

Toxoplasmosis is caused by *Toxoplasma gondii*. The distribution of toxoplasmosis is worldwide, with as many as one-third of adults infected. There is some geographical variation which mainly relates to the dietary habits of populations, particularly consumption of uncooked or raw meat, and the presence of cats, often domestic pets, which are the recognized hosts of the organism. A description of the systemic disease is given in Chapter 66.

Eye complications

Toxoplasmic retinochoroiditis is the common manifestation of the disease affecting the eyes. Typically the condition is seen in a quiescent form, with

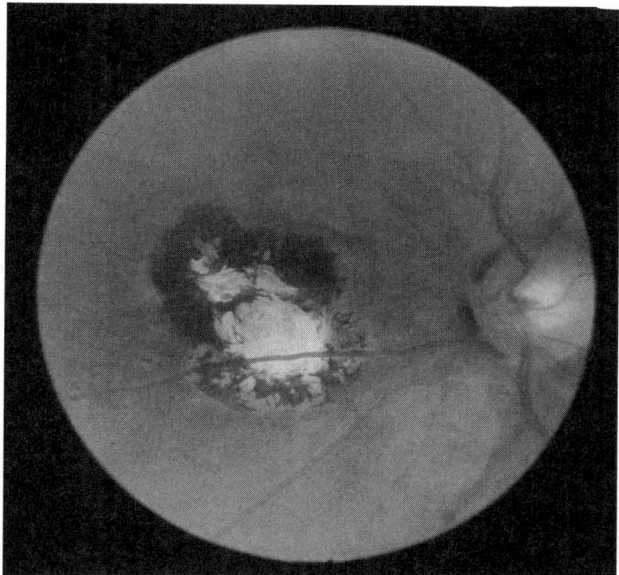

Figure 10.27 Old toxoplasmic retinochoroidal atrophy. Photo: Gordon Johnson.

scarring affecting the posterior segment of the eye. By far the most common presentation is the result of congenital toxoplasmosis, with infection of the fetus during pregnancy. Descriptions of acquired toxoplasmic retinochoroiditis have been reported but these are uncommon. Eye disease due to toxoplasmosis is found more commonly in patients with AIDS.[42]

Congenital toxoplasmosis which has caused a retinochoroiditis may present with a squint or nystagmus. The typical scarring of old retinochoroidal atrophy is often found during routine eye examinations in teenage or adult life where vision has not been significantly affected and the patient is unaware of any eye abnormality. However, most eye changes affecting the retina and choroid are situated at the posterior pole of the eye, often in the region of the macula, and the patient may complain of poor vision (Figure 10.27). This is one form of infective posterior uveitis.

The acute, 'acquired' infection is characterized by focal, necrotizing retinitis. The patient may complain of blurred vision, floaters and photosensitivity. The lesions may be multifocal, although the final 'punched-out' scar may be seen as an isolated lesion, often situated at the posterior pole of the eye or in the area around the optic nerve head. In the acute phase the foci of inflammation are 'fluffy' white with hazy margins. Later the scar is clearly demarcated, white-grey in colour, often with pigment at its margins. Vitritis and iridocyclitis may be associated. Cystoid macular oedema can develop.

Treatment

If treatment is necessary during the acute or chronic infective stage, pyrimethamine is given at 25 mg/day for 3–4 weeks. Children should be given 2 mg/kg per day for 3 days, followed by 1 mg/kg per day for 4 weeks. Folinic acid should also be given, 5–10 mg daily, to inhibit any toxic effects of pyrimethamine on the blood. Together with the pyrimethamine, trisulphapyrimidine, 2–6 g/day for 3–4 weeks, is prescribed for adults, or 100–200 mg/kg per day for 3–4 weeks for children.

Pyrimethamine should not be given to pregnant women. Periocular corticosteroid injections are contraindicated.

It may be necessary to give systemic corticosteroids where active retinochoroiditis is present. Corticosteroids should be given in conjunction with pyrimethamine and trisulphapyrimidine. An alternative therapy is with clindamycin, an antibiotic which can cause antibiotic-associated colitis.

LEISHMANIASIS (See also Chapter 65)

Leishmaniasis is a protozoan disease caused by parasites of the genus *Leishmania*. The insect vector which transmits the parasite is the sandfly. It is found in many developing countries, with up to 12 million cases estimated.

A description of the systemic disease in its various forms worldwide is given in Chapter 65.

Eye complications (visceral leishmaniasis)

The visceral form of leishmaniasis is known as kala-azar and eye disease is uncommon with this condition. Retinal haemorrhages have been described, typically bilateral and multiple in distribution.[43] Iridocyclitis has been reported, with occasional descriptions of keratitis.

Eye complications (cutaneous leishmaniasis)

Cutaneous leishmaniasis has been described as tropical sore (oriental sore), mucocutaneous leishmaniasis (espundia) and disseminated anergic cutaneous leishmaniasis.

Eye changes commonly affect the eyelids, with occasional involvement of the lacrimal ducts or conjunctiva. The cutaneous lesion has a variety of appearances, with ulcer formation after the initial appearance of nodules or papules, often situated on the face, sometimes affecting the eyelids. Skin involvement leaves a characteristic scar.

Treatment

Sodium stibogluconate or meglumine antimonate may be given, 20 mg/kg per day either intramuscularly or intravenously, for up to 20 days. The maximum daily dose should be 850 mg. An alternative treatment is with amphotericin B, 0.25–1 mg/kg in 500 ml of 5% dextrose, given intravenously, either daily or every second day. The daily dose should not exceed 50 mg. Care must be observed in initiating and continuing the use of amphotericin B in view of its toxicity.

AMOEBIASIS (See Chapter 67)

Amoebiasis is the intestinal protozoal disease due to the organism *Entamoeba histolytica*.

The disease is found worldwide, with 500 million infected (1984 estimate, WHO). It is found in deprived communities, being associated with poverty and inadequate sanitation. It is a major health problem in parts of Africa, Asia and Latin America, where highly virulent strains may exist. Over 50 000 deaths probably occur each year.

A description of the systemic disease is given in Chapter 67.

Eye complications

In many populations where infection with *Ent. histolytica* is endemic, or even epidemic, it is difficult to determine whether eye changes are specifically associated with the systemic infection. Much of the literature suggesting an association lacks proof, in that the organism was not demonstrated within the eye. However, a relatively uncommon but well-recognized complication of amoebiasis is a cerebral focus of infection, and reports of improvement in eye lesions, for example keratitis, associated with systemic treatment of amoebiasis do suggest an occasional association. Braley and Hamilton[44] described cysts in the region of the macula with associated small retinal haemorrhages and disturbance of the retinal pigment epithelium. King and his colleagues[45] described five patients with a similar appearance, three of whom also had opaque, yellow foci within the cysts described.

Treatment

Treatment should be with a combination of metronidazole, 800 mg three times a day for 10 days followed by diloxanide furoate, 500 mg three times daily for 10 days.

Alternatively, instead of metronidazole, paromomycin 500 mg three times a day may be given for 7 days.

GIARDIASIS (See Chapter 67)

Giardiasis is an infective condition of the intestine caused by the protozoan organism, *Giardia lamblia*. Giardiasis is found in populations worldwide and typically results in gastroenteritis following ingestion of contaminated food or water, particularly water where contamination with faecal matter has occurred. It is believed that around 200 million people are infected.

Eye complications

Presumed giardiasis affecting the eyes has most commonly involved anterior and posterior uveitis with iridocyclitis, choroiditis, retinal and subretinal haemorrhages and macular disturbance. However, it should be noted that these descriptions of giardiasis affecting the eyes have no definite evidence. Patients responded to systemic treatment for the disease with improvement in the eye abnormalities.[46]

Treatment

Systemic treatment may be given with metronidazole 2 g three times daily for 3 days.

Alternatively mepacrine 100 mg three times daily for 5 days or furazolidone 100 mg four times daily for 7 days may be used. These dosages are for adult patients. For children the dose of metronidazole is 5 mg/kg, for mepacrine 2 mg/kg and for furazolidone a paediatric liquid is given at 1.25 mg/kg. Each regimen is similar to those for adults.

AFRICAN TRYPANOSOMIASIS (See Chapter 63)

Trypanosomiasis in Africa is caused by two protozoa, *Trypanosoma brucei gambiense* and *T. b. rhodesiense*. The insect vector for the disease is the tsetse fly of the genus *Glossina*.

The distribution of the disease, commonly known as 'sleeping sickness', is in Africa, between latitudes 15°N and 15°S. As many as 50 million people are at risk.

A description of the clinical disease is given in Chapter 63.

Eye complications

A variety of clinical eye abnormalities have been reported. Eyelid oedema with conjunctival redness and photosensitivity may occur. Interstitial keratitis and iridocyclitis are reported. In the severe form of the disease, with the onset of meningoencephalopathy, there may be widespread neurological changes, ptosis, extraocular muscle involvement, optic neuritis and papilloedema.[47]

Treatment

A description of the treatment African trypanosomiasis is given in Chapter 63. Suramin or pentamidine may be given by intramuscular injection. If the central nervous system is affected, intravenous melarsoprol is prescribed. An alternative is eflornithine.

AMERICAN TRYPANOSOMIASIS (See Chapter 64)

Also known as Chagas' disease, American trypanosomiasis is caused by a protozoan parasite, *T. cruzi*. The insect vectors transmitting the organism are the blood-sucking reduviid bugs of the genera *Triatoma*, *Rhodnius* and *Panstrongylus*.

Geographically the disease is found in Central and South America, extending from Mexico to Argentina. Up to 15–18 million people are estimated to be infected, with 90 million at risk.

Eye complications

Characteristic evidence of Chagas' disease, where the inoculation site is in the region of the eye, is oedema of the eyelids, which is typically unilateral (Romana's sign). The lacrimal gland can be involved in the inflammation. A single report in 1981 described granulomatous uveitis in a premature child.[48]

Treatment

Nifurtimox is the drug of choice. An alternative drug is benznidazole.

MALARIA (See Chapter 61)

Malaria is caused by protozoan infection with organisms of the *Plasmodium* species, the cause of the severe form of the disease in the tropics,

P. falciparum. Other species are: *P. vivax*, *P. ovale* and *P. malariae*. It remains a devastating disease in tropical countries and just under 300 million are believed to be infected worldwide.

Eye complications

Retinal haemorrhages are seen in association with malaria. In some patients the retinal haemorrhages may have associated retinal exudates.

In severe cerebral malaria there may be extraocular muscle pareses, optic neuritis, and cortical blindness due to brain damage.

An important eye abnormality associated with the treatment of malaria is the rare complication chloroquine retinopathy.[49] Chloroquine is used routinely in the treatment of malaria, but in a number of countries individuals who are unwell for a variety of different reasons will regularly take chloroquine as a general form of treatment. Chloroquine can damage the central retina, disturbing the macula and producing a pathognomonic 'bull's eye' maculopathy. The disturbed retinal pigment epithelium forms a ring or oval which provides the reason for the descriptive term. Central vision is affected.

A well-recognized eye complication associated with malaria is herpes simplex keratitis.

Treatment

The treatment of malaria is described in Chapter 61).

PNEUMOCYSTOSIS (See Chapter 60)

Pneumocystosis is caused by the organism *Pneumocystis carinii*. There is some debate as to whether the organism should have a protozoan classification or be associated with fungi.

In recent years *Pn. carinii* has caused infection, particularly a pneumonia, in immunodeficient individuals. It has been associated with an interstitial pneumonia in nutritionally deficient infants. Those with AIDS are particularly susceptible. Thus it has been found amongst homosexuals, drug addicts and haemophiliacs.

Eye complications

It is accepted that at least some of the retinal changes found in patients with AIDS during recent years are associated with *Pn. carinii* infection. These appearances are described as cotton-wool spots, which appear as fluffy, whitish foci in the retina. A choroiditis due to *Pn. carinii* is recognized.[50]

Treatment

A combination of trimethoprim and sulphamethoxazole is recommended. An alternative is pentamidine isethionate.

A description of systemic treatment is given in Chapter 60.

DISEASES CAUSED BY NEMATODES

ONCHOCERCIASIS

By far the most common cause of blindness within this group of infections, onchocerciasis and its effects on the eye are discussed in detail in Chapter 70.

TOXOCARIASIS (See Chapter 71)

Toxocariasis is caused mainly by the organism *Toxocara canis*; it results from contact with the host, especially puppies. Occasionally toxocariasis is caused by *Toxocara cati*, where the host is the cat.

Toxocariasis is distributed worldwide, and is found in both developing and industrialized countries.

The systemic disease is described as *visceral larva migrans*, which is described in Chapter 71.

Eye complications

Ocular larva migrans may present with an eye problem such as squint or a white pupil (leucocoria). The typical abnormality is a single isolated granuloma at the posterior pole of the eye, although the lesion may occur peripherally and more than one focus may be evident. Intraretinal tracks of 'wandering' larvae may be seen on ophthalmoscopic examination. The presence of granulomatous inflammation may result in a variety of other clinical features, including keratitis, iridocyclitis, chronic endophthalmitis, detached retina and optic neuritis. In the 'quiet state' the retina and choroid may show atrophic scarring.[51]

It is important to differentiate ocular toxocariasis from the malignant intraocular tumour of childhood, retinoblastoma. Both of these eye abnormalities may present with leucocoria. It should be noted that ocular larva migrans may occur as a congenital infection.

Treatment

Most eye lesions are quiescent and no therapy is indicated. Treatment with diethylcarbamazine, thiabendazole or mebendazole is generally ineffective and may worsen inflammation while killing the organism. The granulomatous inflammation affecting the posterior segment of the eye has a variety of cell types, including eosinophils and epithelioid and giant cells; occasionally evidence of destroyed larvae may be found. If severe intraocular inflammation is present, systemic or periocular corticosteroids may be required. Intraocular inflammation can result in endophthalmitis, membrane formation or traction on the retina and retinal detachment. Expert surgical intervention will involve vitrectomy, division of membranes and retinal detachment surgery, as each intervention is appropriate.

LOIASIS (See Chapter 70)

Loiasis is found in West and Central Africa and is caused by the filarial helminth *Loa loa*. The insect vector of the worm is the fly of the genus *Chrysops*.

Eye complications

The most typical evidence of infection with *L. loa* is the presence of the worm under the conjunctiva of the eyeball.[52] There may be conjunctival redness and some discomfort. The more dramatic presentation shows considerable swelling due to oedema of the eyelids (Calabar swelling), caused by the presence of the worm subcutaneously. Usually this swelling will settle in a few days.

Other eye features described include: the presence of worms in the anterior chamber, a uveitis and a retinopathy.

Treatment

Diethylcarbamazine should be used and the regimen of treatment is described in Chapter 70.

The presence of a subconjunctival worm first requires topical anaesthesia. A suture is passed under the worm and tied tightly and the worm is dissected out. Alternatively a cryoprobe may immobilize the worm before surgical removal.

THELAZIASIS

The oriental eye worm, *Thelazia callipaeda*, has principally been reported in patients from Japan and other countries in the Far East. Transmission is possibly by flies.

A description of the systemic disease is given in Appendix III.

Eye complications

Typically the patient complains of irritation and watering with a congested eye, often associated with pain. The worm may be seen within the conjunctival sac. An intraocular infection was described in an 8-year-old Pakistani girl in whom the worm was found on the endothelial surface of the cornea.[53] Following instillation of cocaine drops the worm was removed surgically.

Treatment

Any worm present on the surface of the eye can be removed after the application of a local anaesthetic.

BANCROFTIAN AND BRUGIAN FILARIASIS

Filariasis caused by *Wuchereria bancrofti* has a widespread distribution in Africa, Asia and Latin America, with 70–75 million infected (WHO). *Brugia malayi* occurs principally in South-East Asia, while *Brugia timori* is found in Indonesia; about 6 million are infected with these worms. These lymphatic filariases have a wide variety of clinical presentations (Chapter 70).

Transmission is by mosquitoes.

Eye complications

Adult worms have been isolated in the conjunctiva, with associated pain and redness. A subretinal adult worm has been found and larvae can infiltrate the anterior chamber, iris,[54] lens capsule, retina and choroid. Worms have been found in the eyelid and also the lacrimal gland.

Treatment

An adult worm may be removed from beneath the conjunctiva after the application of topical anaesthetic to the bulbar conjunctiva.

The preferred treatment is with diethylcarbamazine and the regimen used is described in Chapter 70.

DRACUNCULIASIS

Dracontiasis (dracunculosis) due to the guinea worm, *Dracunculus medinensis*, is widely distributed, mainly in sub-Saharan Africa but it is also found in southern Asia. It is estimated by the WHO that the number of people infected is now less than 3 million. Few die of the disease. Water which is contaminated with the smaller crustacean, *Cyclops*, is ingested and the patient becomes infected. After an incubation period of up to 1 year a worm will often emerge through the skin.

The systemic features of the infection are described in Chapter 70.

Eye complications

In one 12-year-old girl from India, who had an irritable, watering eye and swelling of the conjunctiva, an adult female guinea worm was removed surgically.[55] The older literature has reported involvement of the orbit in association with dracunculiasis.

Treatment

Niridazole, metronidazole and thiabendazole have been used and may help to reduce inflammation, allowing easier removal of emerging worms.

A description of treatment is given in Chapter 70.

TRICHINOSIS

Trichinosis is caused by infection with the larvae of *Trichinella spiralis*.

Trichinosis is commonly the result of eating infected, uncooked meat, most often pork. A great variety of other animals are also infected, including dogs, rodents, bears and jackals. The disease is found worldwide, including both Europe and America, where raw meat may be eaten.

A description of the systemic disease is given in Chapters 5, 14 and 71.

Eye complications

The most common sign which may present to an eye specialist is bilateral eyelid oedema. This may be a consequence of invasion of the extraocular muscles with the organism, and pain on eye movement can be a feature. There may be associated oedema of the conjunctiva (chemosis).[47]

Photosensitivity and blurring of vision can occur. Small haemorrhages may occur. These may present subconjunctivally and also within the eye, for example as a retinal haemorrhage. There may be an optic neuritis and optic nerve oedema.

Treatment

Treatment of the eyes is with a cycloplegic, such as atropine sulphate 1%, and topical corticosteroids. Swelling may be reduced with the application of cold compresses.

The systemic treatment of trichinosis with thiabendazole is described in Chapter 71.

GNATHOSTOMIASIS

Most reports of gnathostomiasis have been from Thailand and Japan, although other reports have been recorded from a number of countries, principally in Asia.

Infection is caused by eating uncooked fish, chicken or pork.

The human disease has been mainly due to infection with *Gnathostoma spinigerum*, the inflammatory consequences being caused by the larvae, with hypersensitivity reactions within the tissues. Central nervous system involvement may present with pain in the limbs followed by permanent paraplegia.

Both cutaneous and visceral forms of infection occur; a full description of the systemic disease is given in Chapter 8.

Eye complications

A great variety of eye complications may occur in association with the systemic disease. The eyelids, the anterior surface of the eye and intraocular tissues may be involved, and there may be an orbital cellulitis. Corneal ulceration, uveitis, worms in the anterior or posterior chambers, cataract and secondary glaucoma are described.[56] The worm may cause retinal disturbance and inflammatory changes can occur along the track made by the moving worm.

Treatment

The only well-recognized form of treatment is the removal of the worm after anaesthesia. It has been suggested that cryotherapy could be used to immobilize the worm before surgery.

ANGIOSTRONGYLIASIS

The form of angiostrongyliasis which causes eye disease is caused by the worm *Angiostrongylus can-*

tonensis. Also described as eosinophilic meningitis, the transmission of the disease to humans follows the ingestion of snails, prawns, crabs or vegetables which are uncooked. Areas for preparing food should be kept clean. Angiostrongyliasis is a disease of rodents and is found mainly in Asia and the Pacific region. The parasite has been identified in Egypt and Cuba (Chapter 8).

Eye complications

The adult worm has been found in the anterior chamber of the eye and reports have identified a worm under the retina.[57] The third stage larva has been found in the vitreous in two patients.

Symptoms and signs have included visual loss, pain, blepharospasm and evidence of iridocyclitis. Posterior segment inflammatory consequences, including retinal pigment disturbance or retinal detachment, can occur.

Optic neuritis occurs in association with eosinophilic meningitis and the sixth cranial nerve can be affected.

Treatment

Surgical removal of the worm is indicated. One method of removing the worm from the posterior segment is to use a cryoprobe to immobilize the worm before incision and removal. Considerable care is necessary in preparing the site of entry in order to avoid retinal detachment.

Anterior segment inflammation will require treatment with topical atropine sulphate 1% and topical corticosteroids.

DISEASES CAUSED BY CESTODES

CYSTICERCOSIS (See Chapter 76)

Cysticercosis is associated with the encysted form of the larvae of the tapeworm *Taenia solium*, and only occasionally by *T. saginata*. Faecal contamination of food and water is the most common cause of the acquired form of the disease, although the consumption of raw pork or beef means that the infection is widespread throughout the world. Muslims and Jews do not eat pork and therefore the disease is less common in these communities.

T. solium cysticerci have been found in many tissues, including brain, spinal cord, muscles, lungs, subcutaneous tissues and eyes.

The systemic disease is described in Chapter 76.

Eye complications

Cysticercosis affecting the eye is commonly intra-ocular and is particularly found in the posterior segment of the eye, either subretinally or within the vitreous.[58] *T. solium* cysticerci may also occur in the anterior chamber and other eye tissues. The typical form of the intraocular cyst may show movement and the protoscolex may move 'in or out' of the cyst.[59]

Symptoms and signs include pain, double vision, blurring of vision and sometimes flashes of light.

Treatment

The systemic treatment of cystisercosis with praziquantel is described in Chapter 76. Corticosteroids may be used in association with praziquantel.

It is necessary to attempt removal of the intra-ocular cyst surgically.

ECHINOCOCCOSIS (See Chapter 75)

Also described as hydatid disease, this infection is most often due to the larvae of the tapeworm *Echinococcus granulosus*. The disease is widespread and other species are found in particular geographical locations. Most cysts are found in the liver and lungs. The systemic disease is described in Chapter 75.

Eye complications

Typically ocular echinococcosis is found within the bony orbit.[60] The most common sign is proptosis. There may be associated conjunctival chemosis, congestion and exposure keratitis.

The author operated on two patients with these orbital cysts while working in Central Asia.

Treatment

Treatment of the orbital cyst is by surgical removal.

The treatment of the systemic disease is described in Chapter 75.

COENURIASIS

Coenuriasis can involve the central nervous system and the eyes; the larvae of *Taenia multiceps* are particularly implicated.

The disease is relatively rare but has been reported worldwide.

Eye complications

The infection may involve the orbit and also be found inside the eye.[61] Extraocular involvement can affect the eyelids or extraocular muscles. Intra-ocular infection is typically at the posterior segment of the eye. Reaction to the presence of the cyst may cause pain, and intraocular inflammation can result in severe ocular damage.

Treatment

Surgical removal of the cyst should be attempted before inflammatory consequences occur.

Treatment of the systemic disease is given in Chapter 77.

SPARGANOSIS

Sparganosis, due to infection with larvae of the cestode of the genus *Spirometra*, is found worldwide, but particularly in the Far East.

Humans can develop sparganosis by drinking contaminated water or eating infected snakes, birds or mammals. The flesh of an infected frog may be placed on ulcers and eye problems are usually caused by direct contact. For example, in China raw flesh may be applied to the eyes of patients who have fever.

Eye complications

The application of the flesh of a frog to inflamed or painful eyes can result in infection with the parasite, and eyelid oedema, watering and extreme irritation may develop. A worm may be found subconjunctivally and retrobulbar invasion can occur. The larva has been identified in the anterior chamber of the eye.[62]

Treatment

The worm or nodule should be removed surgically.

DISEASES CAUSED BY TREMATODES

PARAGONIMIASIS (See Chapter 73)

A number of lung flukes of the genus *Paragonimus* have been implicated in this infection, which is particularly prevalent in the Far East but is also found in Africa and Latin America. The organism is carried by many animals and human infection may follow the consumption of uncooked meats, including crab and other crustaceans.

The systemic disease is described in Chapter 73.

Eye complications

Typically the onset of eye inflammation is characterized by severe pain which is intermittent in nature. There is a uveitis leading to considerable intraocular inflammation. The immature worm may cause anterior segment inflammation with hypopyon formation. There may be vitreous and retinal haemorrhages.[47]

Treatment

In ocular paragonimiasis the helminth should be removed surgically.

Treatment of the systemic disease is described in Chapter 73.

SCHISTOSOMIASIS (See Chapter 72)

Schistosomiasis (bilharziasis) probably affects around 200 million people, with as many as 600 million at risk. This helminthic infection is mainly caused by *Schistosoma japonicum*, *S. mansoni* and *S. haematobium*. Dams and irrigation canals have increased the spread of schistosomiasis because these waters contain the snail which is the intermediate host for the worm.

A description of the systemic disease is given in Chapter 72.

Eye complications

Egg granulomas are found on the conjunctiva but also in the choroid[63,64] and in the lacrimal gland. The most frequent infecting agent is *S. haematobium*.

An *S. mansoni* adult has been found in the anterior chamber of an eye.

There are records of uveitis and retinal haemorrhages that have been observed in patients with schistosomiasis.

Treatment

The drug of choice in the systemic treatment of schistosomiasis is praziquantel. The regimens for treatment and alternative therapies are given in Chapter 72.

DISEASE CAUSED BY ARTHROPODS

MYIASIS (See Chapter 79)

The larvae (maggots) of certain flies may cause ocular myiasis. These infestations are found in the Mediterranean region, Central America and Africa but also in temperate regions. Orbital involvement has been reported in many countries around the world.

Eye complications

External ocular myiasis can affect the eyelids, nasolacrimal ducts, lacrimal sac and conjunctiva.[65] There is acute redness with irritation and discharge. This extremely unpleasant infection requires surgical removal of the larvae.

Internal ocular myiasis may result in uveitis, which can be severe. Usually the inflammation is due to a single larva and the prognosis is relatively good.[66]

Orbital myiasis is often found in patients with poor personal hygiene; maggots invade the periorbital regions.

Treatment

External ocular myiasis requires the careful removal of the larvae after applying local anaesthetic eye drops.

Internal ocular myiasis requires treatment of any inflammation with topical therapy, including corticosteroids. Occasionally it may be necessary to remove the larvae surgically.

Orbital myiasis requires removal of the maggots with the application of antiseptic solutions and the likely need of systemic antibiotics to deal with secondary bacterial infection.

ESSENTIAL EYE DRUGS

Table 10.20 gives details of medications routinely used in ophthalmic practice. Many of these drugs can be manufactured from ready-prepared materials.[67]

Table 10.20 Essential eye drugs* (after ref. 67).

Topical antimicrobial agents	Antibiotic† Antiherpetic† Pan antiinfective†	0.5% Chloramphenicol eye drops 0.1% Idoxuridine eye drops 5% Povidone-iodine 1% Tetracycline eye ointment (enriched with polymyxin B) This last, being an ointment, has to be purchased in bulk
Local anaesthetic	Topical†	0.5% Amethocaine hydrochloride eye drops
Mydriatic	Diagnostic† Therapeutic†	1% Cyclopentolate hydrochloride 1% Atropine sulphate
Topical steroids	Weak† Normal† Strong†	0.1% Prednisolone 0.5% Prednisolone 1.0% Prednisolone
Corneal stain	†	Fluorescein paper strips
Subconjunctival drugs	Antibiotic Steroid Mydriatics	Gentamycin 40 mg/ml Hydrocortisone succinate 100 mg ampoule Methyl prednisolone 40 mg/ml (Depo-prep) Atropine sulphate 1 mg/ml Adrenaline hydrochloride 1/1000
Oral agents		Tab. Acetazolamide 250 mg Tab. Prednisolone 5 mg Tab./Amp. Vitamin A 200 000 iu Tab. Ivermectin (in areas where onchocerciasis occurs)

*Many of these can be locally made and are already in use by some National Prevention of Blindness programmes.
†These drops can be locally prepared from raw materials.

GLOSSARY

Abrasion: injury to the cells lining the surface of the anterior eye, often describing superficial injury of the corneal epithelium.

Amblyopia ex anopsia: also described as a 'lazy' eye; the result of inadequate stimulus to the retina in the child, often in an eye that squints.

Anterior uveitis: inflammation of the anterior uveal tract.

Aphakia: an eye in which the lens has been removed or has dislocated.

Band keratopathy: deposition of calcium between the epithelium and Bowman's membrane across the middle and lower part of the cornea.

Bitot's spot: an often triangular foam-like plaque on the bulbar conjunctiva associated with vitamin A deficiency.

Blepharitis: inflammation of the eyelids.

Blepharospasm: tonic contraction of the eyelids.

Bowman's membrane: the interface between the corneal epithelium and the corneal stroma.

Buphthalmos: congenital glaucoma ('ox eye').

Cataract: opacity in the lens of the eye.

Chalazion: a cyst in the region of the meibomian glands of the eyelid.

Chemosis: oedema of the conjunctiva.

Chlamydia: the genus of micro-organisms that includes those causing trachoma.

Choroiditis: inflammation of the choroid.

Choroidoretinitis: inflammation of the choroid and retina.

Climatic keratopathy (solar keratopathy, Labrador keratopathy): corneal changes and opacities caused by excessive exposure to ultraviolet light.

Cobblestones: a descriptive term used for the papillae of the tarsal conjunctiva found in vernal (spring) catarrh.

Conjunctivitis: inflammation of the conjunctiva.

Corneal anaesthesia: loss of corneal sensitivity.

Corneal grafting: the surgical technique used to replace a centrally scarred cornea with a donor graft.

Corneal stroma: the main thickness of the cornea (9/10) between Bowman's and Descemet's membranes.

Cryotherapy: treatment by freezing.

Cycloplegia: paralysis of the ciliary muscle of the eye.

Dacryocystectomy: surgical removal of the lacrimal sac.

Dacryocystitis: inflammation of the lacrimal sac.

Dacryocystorhinostomy (DCR): surgery to create a new opening from the lacrimal sac into the nose to allow tears to drain into the nose.

Dendritic ulcer: the typical appearance of a primary corneal ulcer caused by the herpes simplex virus.

Descemet's membrane: the membrane in the cornea between the stroma and the corneal endothelium.

Ectasia: outward bulge of thinned tissue.

Ectropion: outward turning of the eyelid.

Endophthalmitis: extensive inflammation inside the eye.

Entropion: inward turning of the eyelid.

Enucleation: removal of the eyeball, most often as a surgical procedure.

Epilation: removal of an eyelash.

Epiphora: overflow of tears.

Episcleritis: inflammation of the episclera.

Evert: turning inside out; for example, turning the upper eyelid to examine the tarsal conjunctiva.

Evisceration: removal of the contents of the eye by curettage, leaving the sclera, optic nerve and extraocular muscles.

Extraocular: outside the eye.

Facial nerve palsy: paralysis of the facial (sixth cranial) nerve.

Filtration angle: the region between the base of the iris and the cornea where aqueous fluid drains through the trabecular meshwork.

Fluorescein: a dye used topically on the surface of the eye to stain an area of corneal ulceration. The dye is also used by injection to view vascular and other abnormalities of the retina and choroid (fluorescein angiography).

Follicles: small yellow/white lumps on the conjunctiva which vary from 0.2 to 2 mm in diameter. Histologically they consist of lymphoid tissue.

Foreign body: usually a tiny fragment causing eye injury, it may be metal, dust, wood, stone, etc.

Gonioscopy: examination of the filtration angle of the anterior chamber of the eye with a contact lens (gonioscope).

Goniotomy: a surgical procedure with a goniotomy knife used in congenital glaucoma.

Gram's stain: a stain used to identify organisms both bacteria and fungi, microscopically.

Halo: a diffuse circle of rainbow-like colours around a light when corneal oedema is present.

Hypermetropia: long sight.

Hyphaema: blood in the anterior chamber of the eye.

Hypopyon: pus in the anterior chamber of the eye.

Hypotony: low intraocular pressure.

Intumescent: swollen; often used to describe an enlarged hypermature cataractous lens.

Iridocyclitis: inflammation of the iris and the ciliary body.

Keratic precipitates (KP): clumps of cells and/or pigment on the corneal endothelium due to inflammation of the iris and possibly ciliary body.

Keratitis: inflammation of the cornea.

Keratoconjunctivitis: inflammation of the cornea and the conjunctiva.

Keratoconjunctivitis sicca: dry eyes due to a reduced and abnormal precorneal tear film.

Keratomalacia: destructive melting of the cornea associated with vitamin A deficiency.

Keratomycosis: fungal infection of the cornea.

Lacrimation: secretion and flow of tears.

Lagophthalmos: inability to close the eyelids; may be associated with facial nerve paralysis, e.g. in leprosy.

Laser iridotomy: the creation of a hole in the iris using the laser.

Lens-induced uveitis: inflammation of the uvea due to leakage of protein through the lens capsule.

Leucoma: a white scar of the cornea.

Madarosis: loss of eyebrow hair and/or eyelashes.

Mazzotti reaction: systemic reaction following the use of diethylcarbamazine and suramin for onchocerciasis.

Miosis: constriction of the pupil.

Molluscum contagiosum: a virus-induced small papilloma.

Mydriasis: dilatation of the pupil.

Myopia: short sight.

Night blindness: poor vision at night.

Nodulectomy: surgical removal of nodules (onchocercomas) in onchocerciasis.

Onchocercomas: nodules formed by the encapsulated mass of adult worms in onchocerciasis.

Ophthalmia neonatorum: infection of a newborn child's eyes within 30 days of birth.

Optical iridectomy: surgical enlargement of the pupil to improve vision.

Optic neuritis: inflammation of the optic nerve.

Orbit: the bony skeleton (part of the skull) which contains the eye and extraocular muscles, nerves, blood vessels and fat.

Pannus: a superficial fibrovascular membrane of the upper cornea, associated with trachoma.

Panretinal photocoagulation: multiple small burns of the retina either with laser or xenon arc photocoagulators; commonly used for proliferative diabetic retinopathy.

Papilloedema: oedema of the optic nerve head.

Peripheral anterior synechiae (PAS): inflammatory adhesions in the angle of the anterior chamber of the eye.

Peripheral iridectomy: the surgical removal of a small piece of peripheral iris.

Phacolytic glaucoma: raised intraocular pressure due to macrophages and lens protein blocking the filtration angle, often associated with hypermature cataract.

Phlycten: a microabscess, usually at the corneoscleral margin, often associated with an allergic reaction to the tubercle bacillus.

Photophobia: fear (dislike) of light.

Phthisis bulbi: shrunken eye.

Pinguecula: fatty deposit on the bulbar conjunctiva.

Pinhole disc: a tiny aperture or multiple apertures in a card or plastic disc; used to assess visual acuity.

Posterior synechiae: inflammatory adhesions between the pupil margin and the anterior surface of the lens.

Proptosis: forward displacement of the eye.

Pseudoexfoliation: the accumulation of white particles within the anterior segment of the eye, collecting on the anterior lens capsule, pupillary margin, ciliary body and zonule.

Pterygium: fleshy growth which grows across the cornea from the conjunctiva and subconjunctiva.

Ptosis: drooping of the eyelid.

Refractive error: a variation from the accepted normal optics of an eye, usually corrected by suitable spectacles.

Retinoblastoma: a malignant tumour of the retina found in young children.

Rhodopsin (visual purple): a substance required by the rods of the retina to allow some vision at night.

Schiotz tonometer: an instrument designed to measure intraocular pressure.

Scleritis: inflammation of the sclera.

Sclerosing keratitis: scarring of the peripheral cornea in association with inflammation.

Snellen's 'E' chart: a standard chart to measure visual acuity.

Staphyloma: outward bulge of the cornea or the sclera with the uvea adherent behind.

Stye: infection at or near an eyelash follicle.

Subconjunctival haemorrhage: bleeding under the conjunctiva.

Subluxated: partial dislocation, usually describing a lens which is out of position.

Tarsal conjunctiva: conjunctiva lining the under surface of the eyelids.

Tarsorrhaphy: stitching together of the eyelids, usually partial and a temporary measure.

Trabecular meshwork: a connective tissue network in the angle of the anterior chamber through which the aqueous fluid drains out of the eye.

Trabeculectomy: a surgical filtering procedure, usually for open angle glaucoma.

Trabeculotomy: a surgical procedure for congenital glaucoma.

Trachoma: eye infection caused by the micro-organism *Chlamydia trachomatis*.

Traditional eye medicines (TEM): medicines used by traditional healers in developing countries.

Trichiasis: eyelashes turning inwards and scratching the external surface of the eyeball.

Vernal catarrh (spring catarrh): a type of allergic conjunctivitis.

Visual acuity: the measurement of vision.

Xerophthalmia: 'dry eye'; used to describe the eye changes associated with vitamin A deficiency.

Xerosis: dryness of the surface of the eye, often associated with vitamin A deficiency.

ACKNOWLEDGEMENTS

The author is very grateful to Professor Gordon Johnson and Ms Susan Stevens who reviewed the manuscript. Review articles from the *Journal of Community Eye Health*, for which publication the author is editor, have provided abundant material and resource—which have been very much appreciated (please see references). An authorative source on parasites and the eye, *Ophthalmic Parasitology* by B. H. Kean, Tsieh Sun and Robert M. Ellsworth (Igaku-Shoin), is the standard text in the field to which the author constantly referred for that section of the chapter.

Thanks are also due to Ms Faith Wakeford, Ms Keren Fisher and Ms Sarah Stubbs who typed the script and coped admirably with many rethinks and changes.

The references were compiled by Ms Susan M. Stevens RGN RM OND FETC, Ophthalmic Resource Coordinator, International Resource Centre, International Centre for Eye Health, Insti-tute of Ophthalmology, Bath Street, London, EC1V 9EL, UK.

REFERENCES

1 Foster A. World Distribution of Blindness. *J Community Eye Health* 1988; 1 (Issue No. 1): 2–3.

2 World Health Organization. *10 Years of Onchocerciasis Control in West Africa. Review of the Work of the Onchocerciasis Control Programme in the Volta River Basin Area from 1974–84.* WHO/OCP/GVA/85.1B. Geneva: WHO, 1985.

3 Thyelfors B, Negrel A-D, Pararajasegaram R & Dadzie K Y. *Global Data on Blindness—An Update.* WHO/PBL/94.40. Geneva: WHO, 1994: 12.

4 Minassian D C & Mehra V. 3.8 Million blinded by cataract each year: projections from the first epidemiological study of incidence of cataract blind-ness in India. *Br J Ophthalmol* 1990; 74:341–343.

5 Venkataswamy G. Cataract Surgery—Eye Camps—Alternative Delivery System. *J Community Eye Health* 1989; 2 (Issue No. 4): 9.

6 Johnson G J. Audit of results of cataract surgery. *J Community Eye Health* 1992; 5 (Issue No. 10): 1–2.

7 Foster A & Johnson GJ. Treatable blindness. *Trop Doc* 1988; 18: 112–115.

8 Wright R E. The possible influence of solar radiation on the production of cataract in certain districts of Southern India: a preliminary investigation. *Indian J Med Res* 1937; 24: 917–920.

9 Taylor H R, West S K, Rosenthal F S et al. Effect of ultraviolet radiation on cataract formation. *N Engl J Med* 1988; 319: 1429–1433.

10 Bochow T W, West S K, Azar A, Munoz B, Sommer A & Taylor H R. Ultraviolet light exposure and risk of posterior subcapsular cataracts. *Arch Ophthalmol* 1989; 107: 369–372.

11 Bunce G E, Kinoshita J & Horwitz J. Nutritional factors in cataract. *Ann Rev Nutr* 1990; 10: 233–254.

12 Chatterjee A, Milton R C & Thyle S. Prevalence and aetiology of cataract in Punjab. *Br J Ophthalmol* 1982; 66: 35–42.

13 Leske M C, Chylack L T & Wu S Y. The Lens Opacities Case–Control Study Group. The lens opacities case–control study: risk factors for cataract. *Arch Ophthalmol* 1991; 109: 244–251.

14 West S K. Cataract: a challenge for public health ophthalmology. *J Community Eye Health* 1992; 5 (Issue No. 9): 1–2.

15 Harding J J. *Cataract: Biochemistry, Epidemiology and Pharmacology.* London: Chapman & Hall, 1991.

16 Thyelfors B, Dawson C R, Jones B R, West S K & Taylor H R. A simple system for the assessment of trachoma and its complications. *Bull World Health Organ* 1987; 65 (4): 477–483.

17 Bailey R L, Arullendran P, Whittle H C & Mabey DCW. Randomised controlled trial of single-dose azithromycin in treatment of trachoma. *Lancet* 1993; 342: 453–456.

18 Reacher M H, Huber M J E, Camarearatnam R & Alehassany A. A trial of surgery for trichiasis of the upper lid from trachoma. *Br J Ophthalmol* 1990; 74: 109–113.

19 Thylefors B & Negrel A-D. The global impact of glaucoma. *Bull World Health Organ* 1994; 72: 323–326.

20 Sachdev M S, Sood N N, Verma L K, Gupta S K & Jaffrey N F. Pathogenesis of epidemic dropsy glaucoma. *Arch Ophthalmol* 1988; 106: 1221–1223.

21 King H & Rewers M. Diabetes in adults is now a third world problem. *Bull World Heath Organ* 1991; 69: 643–648.

22 World Health Organization. *Global Health Situation and Projections.* WHO/HST/92.1. Geneva: WHO, 1992.

23 Cohen N. Vitamin A deficiency and the eye. *J Community Eye Health* 1988; 1 (Issue No. 1): 4–5.

24 Morley D. Severe measles. *J Community Eye Health* 1991; 4 (Issue No. 8) 1–2.

25 WHO Expert Committee on Onchocerciasis. Third Report. *WHO Tech Rep Ser* 1987; 752.

26 ffytche T. Ocular leprosy. *J Community Eye Health* 1989; 2 (Issue No. 3): 1.

27 Hogeweg M. Leprosy and the eye. *J Community Eye Health* 1989; 2 (Issue No. 3): 2–5.

28 Wright E & Foster A. Suppurative keratitis: a blinding corneal infection. *J Community Eye Health* 1988; 2 (Issue No. 2): 5–7.

29 Gray R H, Johnson G J & Freedman A. Climatic droplet keratopathy. *Surv Ophthalmol* 1992; 36: 241–253.

30 Johnson G J, Minassian D C & Franken S. Alterations of the anterior lens capsule associated with climatic keratopathy. *Br J Ophthalmol* 1989; 73: 229–234.

31 Minassian D C, Baasanhu J & Johnson G J. The relationship between cataract and climatic droplet keratopathy in Mongolia. *Acta Ophthalmol* 1994; 72: 490–495.

32 Johnson G J, Mtanda A T, Kinabo N N, Sangawe J L F, Masesa D E & Negrel A-D. Optic nerve and macular atrophy of unknown origin in Tanzania. *Arch Public Health* 1993; 51: 561–571.

33 Thomas P K, Plant G, Baxter P & Santiago Luis R. An epidemic of optic neuropathy and painful sensory neuropathy in Cuba: clinical aspects. 1994 (unpublished).

34 Gilbert C. Childhood blindness: major causes and

strategies for prevention. *J Community Eye Health* 1993; 6 (Issue No. 11): 3–6.

35 Klauss V. Newborn conjunctivitis (ophthalmia neonatorum). *J Community Eye Health* 1988; 1 (Issue No. 2): 2–4.

36 Hungerford J. Retinoblastoma. *J Community Eye Health* 1990; 3 (Issue No. 5): 2–6.

37 Chana H S. Traditional eye medicine in Zimbabwe. *J Community Eye Health* 1989; 2 (Issue No. 4): 10.

38 Yorston D. Herpes simplex disease of the eye. *J Community Eye Health* 1990; 3 (Issue No. 6): 2–4.

39 Foster A & Sommer A. Corneal ulceration, measles, and childhood blindness in Tanzania. *Br J Ophthalmol* 1987; 71: 331–343.

40 Kestelyn P. Ocular problems in AIDS. *Int Ophthalmol* 1990; 14: 165–172.

41 Mohan M, Gupta S K, Kalra V K, Vajpayee R B & Sachdev M S. Topical silver sulphadiazine: a new drive for ocular keratomycosis. *Br J Ophthalmol* 1988; 72: 192–195.

42 Weiss A, Margo C E, Ledford D K et al. Toxoplasmic retinochoroiditis as an initial manifestation of the acquired immune deficiency syndrome. *Am J Ophthalmol* 1986; 101: 248–249.

43 DeCock K M, Rees P H, Klauss V et al. Retinal hemorrhages in kala-azar. *Am J Trop Med Hyg* 1982; 31: 927–930.

44 Braley A E & Hamilton H E. Central serous choroidosis associated with amebiasis. A record of 9 cases. *Arch Ophthalmol* 1957; 58: 1–14.

45 King R E, Praeger D L & Hallett J W. Amebic choroidosis. *Arch Ophthalmol* 1964; 72: 16–22.

46 Anderson M L & Griffith D G. Intestinal giardiasis associated with ocular inflammation. *J Clin Gastroenterol* 1987; 7: 169–172.

47 Kean B H, Sun T & Ellsworth R M. *Ophthalmic Parasitology*. New York: Igaku-Shoin, 1991.

48 Rodger F C. *Eye Diseases in the Tropics*. Edinburgh: Churchill Livingstone, 1981: 84–85.

49 Sassani J W, Brucker A J, Cobbs W et al. Progressive chloroquine retinopathy. *Am J Ophthalmol* 1983; 15: 19–22.

50 Rao N A, Zimmerman P L, Boyer D et al. A clinical, histopathologic, and electron microscopic study of *Pneumocystis carinii* choroiditis. *Am J Ophthalmol* 1989; 107: 218–228.

51 Molk R. Ocular toxocariasis: a review of the literature. *Ann Ophthalmol* 1983; 15: 216–231.

52 Lee B Y P & McMillian R. *Loa loa*: Ocular filariasis in an African student in Missouri. *Ann Ophthalmol* 1984; 16: 456–458.

53 Choudry A R. Thelaziasis. *Am J Ophthalmol* 1969; 67: 773–774.

54 Joseph A & Raju N S D. Immature stage of *Wuchereria bancrofti* in the human eye. *Indian J Ophthalmol* 1980; 28: 89–90.

55 Verma A K. Ocular dracontiasis. *Int Surg* 1968; 50: 508–509.

56 Kittiponghansa S, Prabriputaloong A, Pariyanonda S et al. Intracameral gnathostomiasis: a cause of anterior uveitis and secondary glaucoma. *Br J Ophthalmol* 1987; 71: 618–622.

57 Kanchanaranya C, Prechanond A & Punyagupta S. Removal of living worm in retinal *Angiostrongylus cantonensis*. *Am J Ophthalmol* 1972; 74: 456–458.

58 Topilow H W, Yimoyines D J, Freeman H M et al. Bilateral multifocal intraocular cysticercosis. *Ophthalmology* 1981; 88: 1166–1172.

59 Kruger-Leite E, Jalkh A E, Quiroz H et al. Intraocular cysticercosis. *Am J Ophthalmol* 1985; 99: 252–257.

60 Chana H S, Klauss V & Shah A. Orbital hydatid disease in Kenya. *Am J Trop Med Hyg* 1986; 35: 991–994.

61 Manschot W A. Coenurus infection of eye and orbit. *Arch Ophthalmol* 1976; 94: 961–964.

62 Sen D K, Muller R, Gupta V P et al. Cestode larva (sparganum) in the anterior chamber of the eye. *Trop Geogr Med* 1989; 41: 270–273.

63 Orefice F, Jimal C R & Pittella J E H. Schistosomatic choroiditis. I. Funduscopic changes and differential diagnosis. *Br J Ophthalmol* 1985; 69: 294–299.

64 Pittella J E H & Orefice F. Schistosomatic choroiditis. II. Report of first case. *Br J Ophthalmol* 1985; 69: 300–302.

65 Masseo V, Ercolani D, Trombetti D et al. External ophthalmomyiasis: report of four cases. *Int Ophthalmol* 1987; 11: 73–76.

66 Syndalen P, Nitter T & Mehl R P. Ophthalmomyiasis interna posterior. Report of case caused by the reindeer warble fly larva and review of previous reported cases. *Br J Ophthalmol* 1982; 66: 589–593.

67 Taylor J. Appropriate eye drugs for developing countries. *J Community Eye Health* 1991; 4 (Issue No. 7): 2–6.

CHAPTER 11

DERMATOLOGICAL PROBLEMS

J. H. S. Pettit

Most doctors working in tropical areas are consulted by patients who demand treatment for their skin ailments. The diseases for which these patients seek attention fall into three groups.

1. Common dermatoses of worldwide incidence of the presentation and treatment of which do not vary according to geography (e.g. warts, molluscum contagiosum, scleroderma, dermatitis herpetiformis, mycosis fungoides).
2. Diseases also of worldwide distribution which have a different presentation or require a different approach to treatment (e.g. acne vulgaris, lupus vulgaris, psoriasis).
3. Dermatoses, the acquisition of which is dependent on residence, permanent or temporary, in tropical areas (e.g. Buruli ulcer, leishmaniasis, rhinoscleroma, Brazilian pemphigus).

Attempts are not made here to cover diseases falling in the first group; many suitable textbooks are available to advise on the diagnosis and treatment of such cases. Diseases discussed in this chapter will fall into one of the two other groups mentioned above.

REGIONAL VARIANTS OF WORLDWIDE DERMATOSES

ACNE VULGARIS

This common disease of adolescence usually presents as a combination of a greasy skin with comedones and pustules most frequently on the face but, in more severe cases, also affecting the chest and upper back. The condition may vary from a mild scattering of a few blackheads on the temples or forehead to a severe eruption in which the face is covered with pustulocystic lesions which leave deforming crateriform scars when the patient finally (with the doctor's assistance) manages to shake off the disease (Plate 11.1). It is mainly because of these cosmetic deformities that it is worthwhile undertaking treatment to prevent patients being scarred for life.

TROPICAL VARIANTS OF PRESENTATION

Greasiness is a feature of acne; when patients move from a temperate to a tropical zone they will not only perspire more but will produce more sebum. This means that those whose acne starts in a temperate climate may find on transfer to the tropics that they get worse—some authorities have used such phrases as 'tropical acne' or 'summer acne' for such a situation. It is also possible that young people who have been fortunate enough to avoid the development of acne when living in a cool climate will find that a holiday in a warmer country will precipitate the eruption.

A high proportion of ethnic groups in the tropics (e.g. those of the Amazon valley and South-East Asia) are relatively less hirsute than their Caucasian counterparts and consequently have less sebaceous glands and show a tendency for their acne to be less severe.

TREATMENT IN THE TROPICS

Routine therapy consists of degreasing the skin either with 1% cetrimide lotion or a suitably medicated soap; the application of a keratolytic—sulphur 6% in calamine lotion, 5% benzoyl peroxide lotion or 0.05% retinoic acid lotion—will usually be sufficient for the comedone type of acne. Patients with a predominance of pustules will need tetracycline (500 mg once or twice daily for several months) to suppress formation of pustules and so reduce the number of resultant scars.

13-*cis*-retinoic acid has recently become popular for severe pustular acne. It is only rarely needed for patients living in the tropics. Preferably it should not

Plate 11

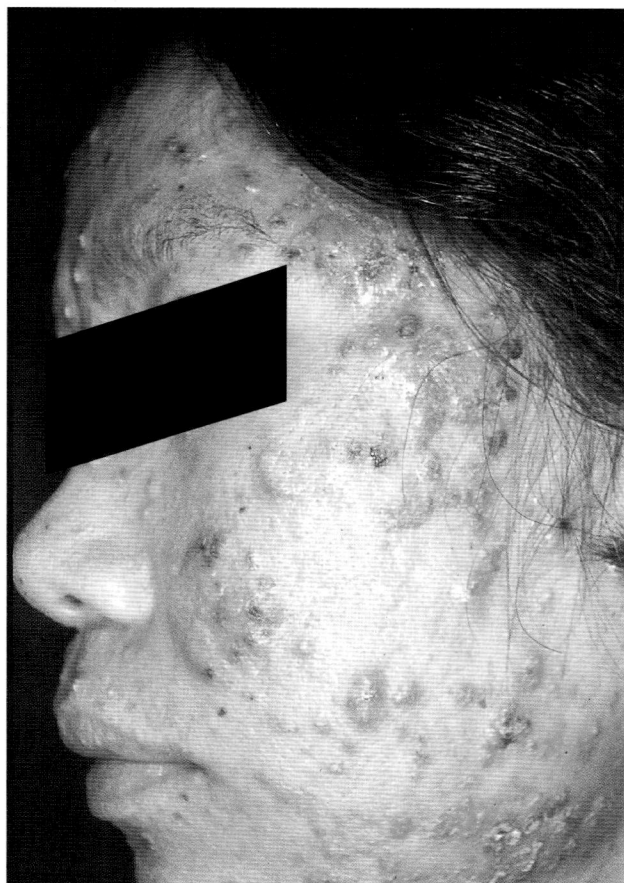

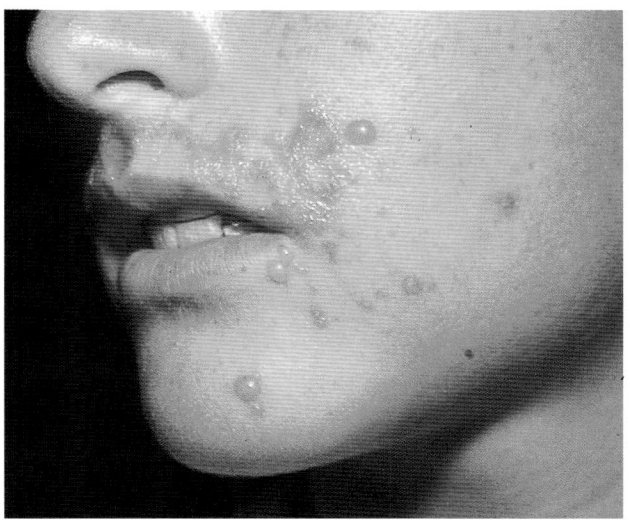

Plate 11.2 Impetigo. Lesions usually start as bullae which break down to form crusts.

Plate 11.1 Acne vulgaris. Severe nodulocystic pustular acne; in such cases the back is often affected.

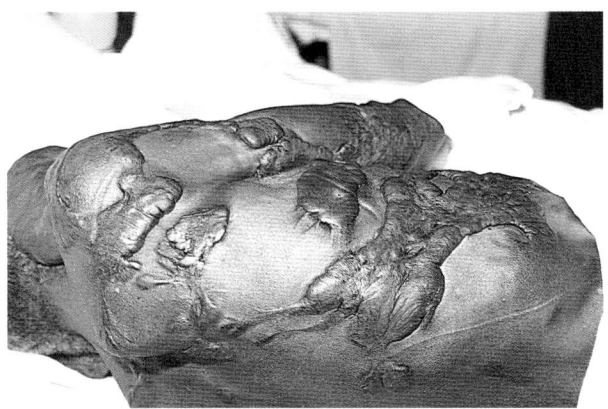

Plate 11.3 Keloid – following extensive burns.

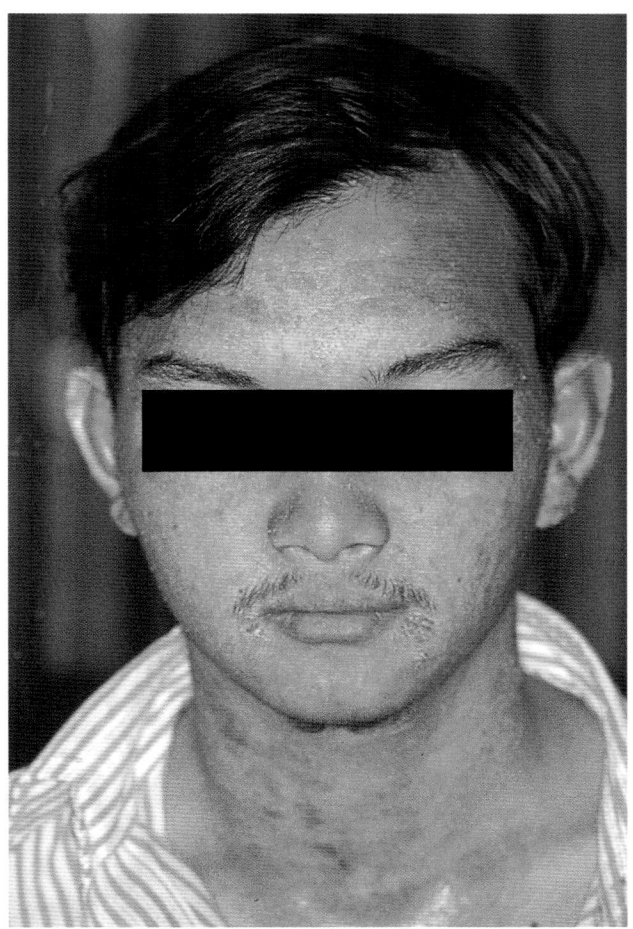

Plate 11.4 Photodermatitis. Red pruritic skin of exposed areas in a patient undergoing treatment with chlorothiazide. (Courtesy of Radzi bin Jaafar.)

Plate 11 Continued.

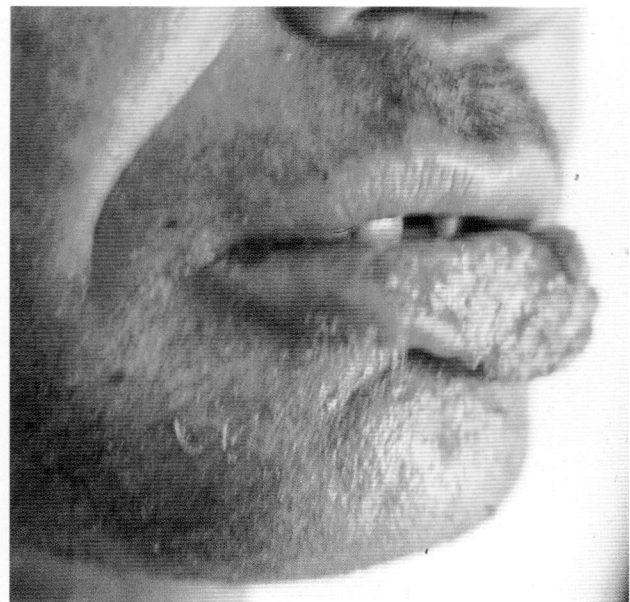

Plate 11.5 Squamous cell carcinoma. Proliferating and ulcerating tumour on the lower lip of a man in an Iranian village.

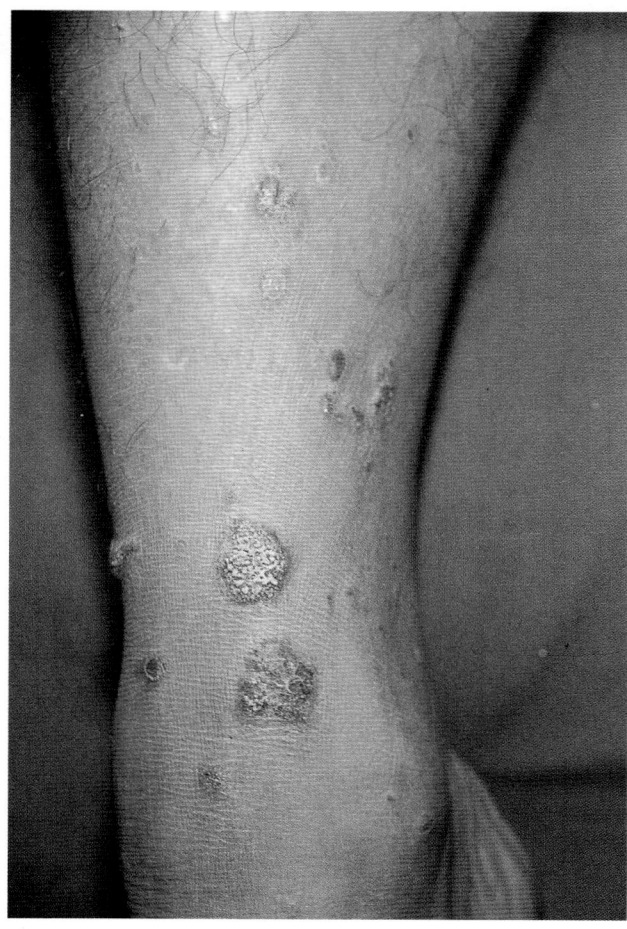

Plate 11.6 Lichen planus (hypertrophic). Numerous dark warty patches on the anterior tibial borders with lichen planus involving the mouth.

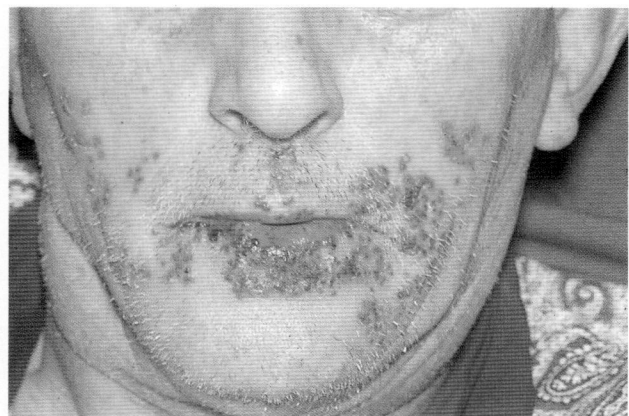

Plate 11.7 Herpes simplex associated with a *Plasmodium falciparum* infection. (See Chapter 61.)

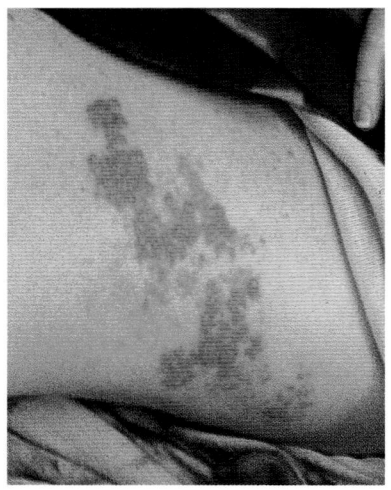

Plate 11.8 Herpes zoster in an otherwise fit individual (See Chapter 11.)

Plate 11 Continued.

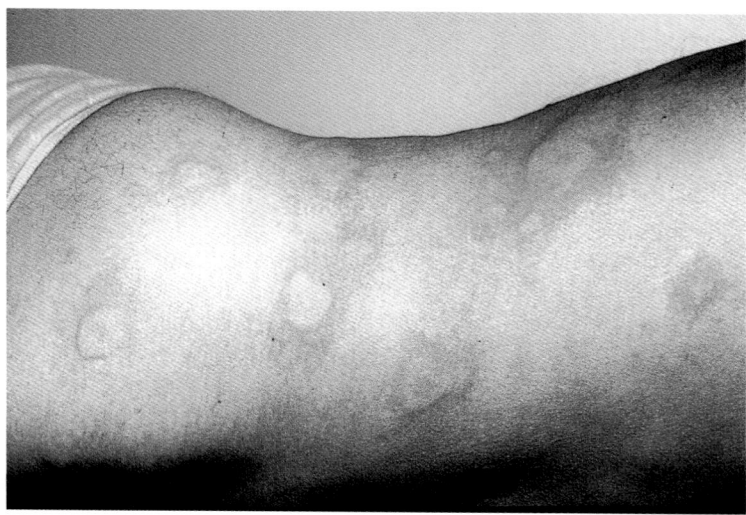

Plate 11.9 Giant urticaria in a patient suffering from acute schistosomiasis (Katayama fever). (See Chapter 72.)

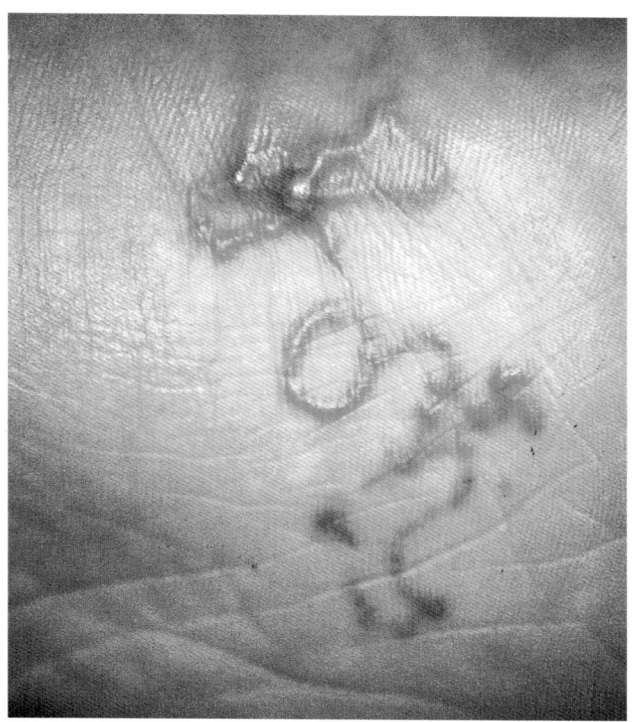

Plate 11.10 Larva migrans – caused by *Ancylostoma brasilliense* – acquired whilst walking barefooted on a beach in the Caribbean.

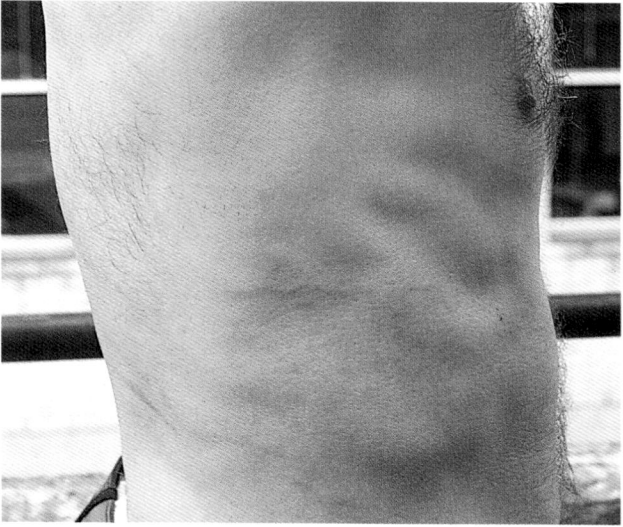

Plate 11.11 Larva currens in an elderly man infected with *Strongyloides stercoralis* for many years.

be prescribed for women in the reproductive period of life.

PYOCOCCAL INFECTIONS

Impetigo contagiosa and ecthyma are the most common forms of pyococcal infections of the skin. Impetigo is classically described as consisting of bullous or crusted lesions on exposed areas usually caused by staphylococci or streptococci (Plate 11.2); studies from various parts of the world seem unable to agree as to which form of disease is caused by which organism.

Ecthyma is a rather deeper crusted infection often penetrating the basal layer and leaving a scar after healing, a finding which is not characteristic of impetigo.

ROPICAL VARIANTS OF PRESENTATION

arefoot or barelegged children in the fields or rdens of rural areas are exposed to all sorts of ditional superficial lesions of the skin (boils, tches, grazes, bites, etc.) which when second- infected by pyococcal organisms produce a trum of infection which is best called pyoderma. untreated these infections result in the devel- nt of hypopigmented scars which stay visible shins for many years.

MENT IN THE TROPICS

ses of pyoderma usually respond well to twice daily with warm water and soap by the local application of an antibiotic h as neosporin or sodium fusidate; but in re such sophisticated products are either ive or not available a satisfactory substi- made by mixing the contents of a 250 mg etracycline with 25 g of a simple cream. extensive cases will respond more stemic antibiotic therapy but it should ed that penicillin is often unsuccessful. bacteriological studies are frequently and in such cases erythromycin or re usually helpful. ities hold that all cases of pyoderma d systemically because of the possi- ren may develop acute glomerulo- a nephritogenic *Streptococcus* spp. rapy has not been convincingly nt acute glomerulonephritis[1] it is h treatment should only be given

for extensive cases of pyoderma and not used for milder infection(s).

ECZEMA–DERMATITIS

Throughout the world about half the people who seek treatment for a skin condition are suffering from various infections—bacterial, fungal, viral, parasitic, etc. The eczema–dermatitis complex makes up about 30% of all the other dermatoses put together. In the past the words 'eczema' and 'dermatitis' have been used interchangeably for a group of physical signs which start with a mildly pruritic erythema and soon develop a scattering of vesicles throughout the lesion associated with an increasing pruritus. Later the vesicles rupture, often as a result of scratching, and the consequent combination of oozing and scaliness produces a sticky crusted patch which can become secondarily infected. More recently it has become the custom in many centres to use the word 'eczema' to describe those cases that have an endogenous cause and the word 'dermatitis' to describe a similar clinical picture produced as a reaction to some extrinsic irritant or sensitizing application to the skin.

ENDOGENOUS ECZEMA

Most often eczema presents in a discoid or nummular form mainly affecting young people in their late teens or early twenties. Scattered on the arms and legs are well-defined circular mixtures of erythemas, vesicles and crusts, usually less than 2 cm in diameter which are often mistaken for small patches of tinea corporis—potassium hydroxide preparations will show that no fungus is present. This is an exceedingly chronic condition and at any one time the patient has a combination of newly erupting and slowly healing circular patches which may continue for several years. No one has any idea as to the cause of this troublesome condition which may need small (5–15 mg) doses of prednisolone daily to keep the patient comfortable. This manifestation of eczema is found rather more frequently in the tropics than in temperate zones, and as patients in warm countries do not take kindly to persistent use of creams and ointments the best treatment may be a combination of systemic corticosteroids and 1% hydrocortisone lotion. In Hawaii it has been found that a single deep intramuscular injection of 40 units of triamcinolone acetonide every 4–6 weeks is both effective and acceptable.

POMPHOLYX

When a potentially vesicular eruption affects the hands and the fingers the thickness of the keratin layer effectively modifies the clinical appearance, and patients complain less of redness and crusting and more of itching and deeply sited vesicles. The condition often starts along the sides of the fingers and is particularly common in hot weather, being therefore usually limited to the summer months in temperate zones but occurring all year round in the tropics.

Some patients develop this clinical picture as a sensitization phenomenon associated with badly treated athlete's foot but in most cases the cause is unknown; the not infrequent association of pompholyx with discoid eczema leads some dermatologists to suspect that the same unknown aetiology may precipitate either clinical condition. Increased perspiration exacerbates pompholyx but is not the cause.

Local applications of corticosteroids are not very helpful unless the affected part is occluded by a plastic glove or finger-stall; such dressings should be kept airtight and need be changed only once a day.

CONTACT DERMATITIS

Certain materials (soaps, strong acids or alkalis, etc.) will irritate any skin to produce reddening, vesiculation, exudation and scaliness. Persistent use of such irritants will cause a condition often called 'housewife's dermatitis' or 'dish-pan hands'.

Other, more unfortunate individuals develop a similar group of symptoms as an allergic reaction to a material to which they have become sensitized. The list of these sensitizers is pretty well unending: medicaments, preservatives, fragrances, metals and chemicals may all cause sensitization.[2]

In the less developed parts of the world where industrialization has not yet attained unwelcome proportions, contact dermatitis is inexorably spreading and industrial medical officers should learn not only to recognize the arrival of these allergic industrial dermatoses but also how to investigate them by the use of suitable patch-testing equipment.[3]

It must also be remembered that various foods, fruits and plants are potential sensitizers but in such cases the patient (frequently a housewife or shop assistant) will usually be aware of the cause and take necessary avoiding action.

A short course of oral prednisolone combined with local application of a corticosteroid will satis-factorily relieve the patients of their symptoms but it must be emphasized that *all* sources of the sensitizer should be eliminated from the patient's environment before a cure can be expected.

ATOPIC ECZEMA

This unpleasant condition, frequently found in association with asthma and hay fever, is not true eczema and vesicles are rarely seen in any of the dermatological presentations: the skin is abnormally pruritic and reacts to scratching by the development of thick patches of the skin, variously called lichenification or neurodermatitis.

In the tropics patients or their parents often blam various forms of fish, crustacea, eggs or dairy pro ucts for the exacerbations of this condition dermatologists seem to be slowly recognizing atopic patients may indeed be sensitive to ing allergens. Despite this, relatively few childre cured by modifications of their diet. Stresses teething, illness, school, and family or wor lems often seem to play an important part in tating periods of exacerbation of th diathesis.

Long-term use of a weak steroid crea ary and this can sometimes be useful with 2–3% liquor picis carbonis or 2 acid. Oral corticosteroids should much as possible as it is often diffic medication once it has begun.

FUNGUS DISEASES OF T

Many fungi infect the skin, us following superficial or de ditions are described in Ch

KAPOSI'S SARCO

First described by F name of 'idiopathic condition was initi ope and norther nodules varying bean occurring enlarged to fo extended alo marked boar puric lesion lesions we involved and although Kaposi originally said the disease was fatal in 2–3 years, it was often found to take a longer course.

It was not until the 1930s that the disease was recognized in central Africa, at which time it was said to occur almost always in men.

ACQUIRED IMMUNE DEFICIENCY SYNDROME (AIDS) (See Chapter 12)

The unhappy explosion of this frightening disease has drawn worldwide attention to Kaposi's sarcoma. Initially recognized in the homosexual communities in North America[4] it is now realized that AIDS is common in central and East Africa where it now affects men and women in about equal numbers. Kaposi's sarcoma affects about half the American cases of AIDS but it occurs less frequently (15–20%) in Africans.

Nowadays the presentation varies somewhat from the original description, the initial lesions, frequently symmetrical, being somewhat paler and more widely scattered and even appearing behind the ears and on the mucosae and gingivae, and later spreading to the internal organs (Chapter 24).

KELOIDS

Surgeons, physicians and even dermatologists seem to be easily confused by the strange spontaneously developing lesions which are seen far more commonly in central Africa than in other parts of the world. The not infrequent development of hypertrophic scars of the skin, usually following trauma, surgery or even inoculations (particularly BCG) are mistaken for keloids but, although keloids may be triggered off by trauma, the classical keloid lesion appears spontaneously, often occurring on the chest wall over the sternomanubrial area, which is probably one of the least frequently damaged parts of the body (Plate 11.3).

Starting as a small, hard nodule which extends peripherally to give a firm, very pruritic plaque it can be differentiated from an ordinary hypertrophic scar (which does not spread) by the characteristic pseudopodial extensions typical of a true keloid.

Differentiation is important as a hypertrophic scar in a non-keloidal patient can be excised with little danger of recurrence, while a true keloid, whether starting spontaneously or following trauma, reacts badly to surgical excision in the scar and a larger lesion will return.

Many patients with true keloids seek treatment, sometimes because of the intractable pruritus but at others for cosmetic reasons. The best form of treatment is to inject a corticosteroid into the lesion but this procedure is extremely painful and local anaesthetic must be injected under the keloid prior to actual treatment. It is best to use a corticosteroid which has been formulated for intra-articular use.

Although not easily available in the tropics, superficial X-irradiation is sometimes effective, with or without simultaneous surgical excision; the dosage should be left in the hands of the radiotherapist.

PSORIASIS

There was a time when European dermatologists taught that psoriasis was less common in the warmer parts of the world; they were wrong. Reports from various parts of the tropics show that some 3–5% of all patients seen in skin clinics are suffering from psoriasis. It is, however, true that most patients (of whatever race) are less severely affected than those who live in cooler areas, probably because they have a much greater exposure to sunlight and are less affected because of this accidental therapeutic irradiation.

These well-demarcated erythematosquamous lesions can easily be recognized by an average medical student and are seen anywhere on the body. They occur in small guttate lesions in children while in adults psoriasis occurs in larger plaques on the trunk, limbs and scalp. When it appears in the groins or other relatively moist flexures the appearance will be modified—well demarcated and erythematous but not scaly.

TREATMENT IN THE TROPICS

The wide range of medications and applications used throughout the world is ample evidence that a cure is not possible. Details of routine therapy can be obtained from a more specialized dermatological textbook but certain features should be mentioned here. Guttate psoriasis has been treated with success, particularly in South America and Malaysia by the use of dapsone 100 mg orally each day; smaller doses should be given to children. It is now recognized that haemolysis of red blood cells is dose related and this rarely occurs in adults taking less than 200 mg daily.

It is obvious that in the tropics those who have widespread psoriasis will be unwilling to cover large areas of their bodies with sticky or malodorous applications and, ideally, treatment should be administered systemically rather than locally, but the considerable value of dithranol ointment (anthralin in the USA) should not be overlooked.

A recent acceptable change in approach has led to the use of 0.5% dithranol in Lassar's paste being applied to the patches for no more than an hour each evening. This treatment does not stain the skin to anything like the extent caused by longer application and will often be accepted by patients who will otherwise reject dithranol.

In some of the more sophisticated parts of the world the use of oral psoralens associated with ultraviolet A light (PUVA therapy) has attained a high degree of popularity. This time-consuming and expensive therapy is rarely necessary in the tropics but patients who wish to spend the money may take two capsules of methoxsalen at 11 a.m. and spend their lunch-time from 1 to 2 p.m. sitting in the sun as completely unclothed as local tradition permits.

When patients are severely affected it may be necessary to resort to the oral administration of etretinate (1 mg/kg daily) for 3–6 months but this is not only expensive but has a number of side-effects which diminish the enthusiasm of many of its users.

The use of antimetabolites—methotrexate, hydroxyurea, etc.—should not be attempted by the non-specialist.

SCABIES (See Chapter 81)

This infestation by *Acarus scabiei* is found throughout the world, being readily spread from person to person; consequently more than one member of the family is usually affected at the same time. Pruritic papules first appear on the finger-webs and fronts of the wrists and spread from there to the axillae, areola and around the umbilicus, later involving the genitalia, particularly the scrotum. It is seen more frequently in children where the itching is often so badly scratched that patients become secondarily infected and complain of a pyoderma.

In addition to having infected papules it is not unknown for patients to become sensitized to the presence of acari and consequently to develop a widespread papular urticaria looking somewhat like chickenpox. This may cause diagnostic confusion as the urticarial papules do not contain acari and scrapings will be negative. In any case, and contrary to the classical teaching, presence of the acarus is usually difficult to demonstrate in the tropics and diagnosis will often have to depend on the classical distribution of the lesions, combined with a history of nocturnal pruritus affecting several members of the family at the same time.

It is often not realized that patients who have been infected for the first time do not itch for the first 3–4 weeks and, because of this, some members of the patient's household may not know they have the disease: despite their protests *all* the members of the household (including the servants) should be treated at the same time. According to availability, treatment can be benzyl benzoate emulsion 25%, malathion lotion 0.5% or monosulfiram 25% diluted with 2 or 3 parts of water. Any one of these lotions should be applied all over the body (omitting the head and neck which are rarely affected in adults), left on for 24 hours and then washed off. The treatment should be repeated on two or three consecutive nights. For children the same routine should be used although the lotion should be diluted to half-strength for those between 8 and 12 years of age and a quarter-strength for those between 4 and 8 years. Children under 4 should not be treated with these lotions; instead 6% sulphur ointment or 10% crotamiton can be used twice daily.

CRUSTED SCABIES

Although it was first recognized in Norway more than 100 years ago the condition now known as crusted scabies is still seen intermittently in the tropics, being found particularly in leprosaria or children's homes. It seems that patients with lepromatous leprosy or Down's syndrome are particularly susceptible to invasion by the *A. scabiei* and do not react to such infections in the usual way. A massive proliferation of the acari stimulates an enormous non-pruritic scaliness of the skin which may be taken for an erythroderma. Not infrequently the presence of such cases in a ward is only recognized when an epidemic of scabies affects other patients, nurses, doctors, ward attendants and laundry assistants. All contacts must be treated with routine antiscabies treatment but the index case often needs several weeks of daily treatment carefully applied.

SOLAR DERMATOSES AND EPIDERMAL MALIGNANCIES

Although Africans, Indians and other deeply pigmented groups are usually careful to protect themselves from the sun's rays as much as possible, Caucasians often seem to imagine that despite their lack of protective pigmentation they can expose themselves to the dangers of solar irradiation with impunity. Because of this there is a high incidence of abnormalities of the skin caused by sunlight in Australia, the southern parts of the USA, and other areas where a white population lives in an unsuitable geographical situation.

PHOTODERMATITIS

While it is obvious that excessive exposure to the sun may be expected to damage the cells of the epidermis to give various degrees of sunburn it is often forgotten that certain individuals, hypersensitive to the sun's rays, may develop skin lesions from no more than ordinary exposure. Such patients show a diffuse eczematous reaction limited to the exposed areas of the skin: forehead, nose, cheeks, V of the neck, forearms and hands (Plate 11.4).

Drugs that produce this clinical picture include tetracyclines, phenothiazines, thiazides and the sulpha drugs, while among local applications that may sensitize the patient are buclosamide, topical antihistamines and the halogenated salicylanilides which have all been easily available to the public at various times and in various places.

Treatment is primarily directed at recognizing the cause of solar sensitivity but, unfortunately, the elimination of the cause is not always followed by an amelioration of the dermatitis, in which case not only are systemic steroids necessary in small doses but a sun-barrier lotion or cream should be used on the exposed parts of the skin in the daylight hours. A large number of barriers are available, the simplest and cheapest being made with 10% *p*-aminobenzoic acid in 60% alcohol.

THE PORPHYRIAS

Sometimes patients (either in childhood or adult life) develop a bullous sun sensitivity associated with scarring of the skin. If there is no evidence of the use of either local or systemic sun sensitizers it may be suspected that the patient has a form of porphyria that affects the skin.[5] Expert biochemical assistance should be obtained.

EPIDERMAL MALIGNANCIES

Actinic keratoses

Long-term exposure to sunlight is now recognized as being the most frequent cause of epidermal cancer. Paler-skinned individuals are much more prone to these malignancies, which are therefore most common in Caucasians who spend long hours in direct sunlight in oil fields, tin mines, rubber plantations, farms, golf courses, etc. The first sign of trouble is an increased dryness and wrinkling of the skin associated with histological evidence of damage to the elastic tissue in the dermis (solar elastosis) and this is later followed by the appearance on the exposed areas of small scaly lesions with a bright erythematous base which show histologically that cells in the epidermis are undergoing malignant change. These actinic keratoses are potentially premalignant and, although patients report that some keratoses fall off, others ultimately change into one of the forms of cancer mentioned below. It is advisable to treat the keratoses before transformation occurs.

In locations where liquid nitrogen or other forms of cryotherapy are available dermatologists often freeze individual lesions; other forms of direct destruction are not recommended. The best method of treatment is to use 5-fluorouracil; a 5% cream is usually needed for keratoses on the dorsum of the hands, the arms and legs but this is often too strong for the face and a 1% lotion can be used which is made by adding the contents of a 5 ml ampoule of 5-fluorouracil (containing 250 mg) to 20 ml of propylene glycol. This lotion should be applied all over the face, the ears and the neck twice daily for 3 weeks, by which time there will be a strong reaction in all visible lesions, perhaps even some erosions. The reaction will not only affect the previously visible keratoses but will also appear in unexpected sites where presumably subclinical lesions are in the early stages of development. Patients find this an uncomfortable treatment and may need to spend most of the daylight hours indoors during the last half of the 3-week course but, after that, the use of 1% hydrocortisone lotion will clear the irritated skin and with any luck there will be no recurrences for at least 4 years.

Basal cell carcinoma (See Chapter 24)

Most doctors can recognize these skin-coloured papules which slowly enlarge producing a pearly rolled edge. Later the centre breaks down to form a typical rodent ulcer, a locally malignant tumour which extends remorselessly but almost never metastasizes. These lesions need to be taken seriously (especially if they are close to the eye) but there are various schools of thought concerning the best method(s) of therapy. Many dermatologists curette the lesions extensively under local anaesthesia and cauterize the base; others use liquid nitrogen or radiotherapy. All treatments seem to be successful 80–90% of the time, but it is recommended here that management should consist of a thorough curettage under a local anaesthetic with the subsequent application of 5% 5-fluorouracil ointment to the residual ulceration; this will satisfactorily kill off any malignant cells which have escaped the curette. Such therapy takes longer than the others but may be expected to produce a higher percentage of cures.

Squamous cell carcinoma

This condition also appears in light-exposed areas, the tumour being particularly common on the lip. Starting as a rapidly growing fleshy nodule it soon breaks down to give a mixture of crusting, ulceration and proliferation (Plate 11.5). Lesions are truly malignant and must always be treated seriously.

Similar malignancy may occur in any chronic ulcer of the skin seen in the tropics (tropical ulcer (Chapter 2), Buruli ulcer (Chapter 57), leprosy, etc.); sometimes it is difficult to decide whether the proliferating tissue at the edge of an ulcer is truly malignant or whether the patient simply has pseudo-epitheliomatous hyperplasia.

All cases of squamous cell carcinoma should be treated by the combined attention of a surgeon and radiotherapist.

Malignant melanoma (See Chapter 24)

These highly invasive malignancies arise from melanocytes which normally live in the basal layer producing melanin and injecting it into nearby basal cells, thereby helping to protect the epidermal cells against solar damage. In Australia the incidence of melanoma rises in direct relationship to nearness to the equator, and the risk of melanoma has been shown to increase with accumulated sun exposure throughout life.[6]

Any new growth showing varied colours—black, brown, red or even blue—should be viewed with suspicion and, although melanomas do not always develop in a previously existing cellular naevus, patients with numerous moles should be warned to seek medical attention if such lesions change their shape or their colour or if they start to bleed spontaneously.

Malignancies in achromic skin lesions

Most skin malignancies occur in Caucasians, Japanese and the paler Chinese skins but Asians and Africans, whose normal skin colour provides a reasonably effective protection against the depreda-

tions of ultraviolet light, may have trouble if they suffer from any form of dermatosis which takes the form of a hypopigmented or achromic patch. Patients with long-standing vitiligo or albinism will find that after 10 or more years actinic keratoses and other forms of superficial skin malignancies may develop in the unprotected areas; consequently they should always use sun-barrier lotions during the daytime. When they occur epidermal malignancies should be treated in the ordinary way.

TUBERCULOSIS OF THE SKIN

Whether due to improved treatment or to the widespread use of BCG tuberculous infections are much less of a problem in temperate zones than they used to be. The varied clinical manifestations that used to be easily recognized are now less often seen in Europe and North America. These different presentations are usually caused by the patient's past exposure to tuberculosis and the consequent underlying immunity.

Those who have never previously been infected by *Mycobacterium tuberculosis* will produce a primary chancre if the organism is inoculated into the skin. A small, slowly growing nodule breaks down to form a painless ulcer not infrequently associated with similarly painless regional lymphadenopathy. This often takes a long time to heal and if the patient cannot develop a high resistance one of the other forms of skin tuberculosis may appear at the site of the initial infection.

All other forms of skin tuberculosis are associated with some deeper form of infection. Scrofuloderma overlies colliquative necrosis of tuberculous glands (usually in the neck) and shows a combination of fluctuant nodules and discharging sinuses; tuberculous osteitis (knee, wrist, rib, etc.) sometimes spreads to the overlying skin to cause a tuberculous ulcer in which the chronic granulation tissue on the floor of the ulcer is surrounded by a delicate bluish-white edge.

Lupus vulgaris occurs when an organism lodges in the skin of a patient who already has a positive Mantoux reaction. It causes tuberculoid granulomas in the dermis which manifests itself initially as small brownish-red nodules which on vitropression are supposed to appear as translucent greenish-yellow 'apple-jelly' nodules. They extend centrifugally leaving in the centre an atrophic epidermis which may ulcerate or ultimately even become malignant. In the past, lupus vulgaris was particularly common round the face and nose.

TROPICAL VARIANTS IN PRESENTATION

In those parts of the world where individuals are exempted from the need to wear thick, or indeed any clothing superficial skin trauma is more easily experienced. In such areas pulmonary tuberculosis is by no means uncommon and it follows that previously uninfected children may develop a primary tuberculous chancre anywhere on the body where trauma has been associated with penetration by tubercle bacilli. A high 'index of suspicion' must be maintained as otherwise these small painless ulcers may be treated lightly and the disease not diagnosed until one of the more extensive forms of tuberculosis has appeared.

Tuberculosis verrucosa cutis is the most common form of tuberculosis in many parts of the less developed world. It is somewhat similar to lupus vulgaris, with a chronic tuberculoid granuloma appearing in the dermis after traumatic inoculation in a patient with high immunity but, in addition to the granuloma in the dermis, a reactive hyperplasia of the epidermis causes the lesion(s) to be markedly warty. They will usually produce roughly concentric rings on the buttocks, elbows or ankles; these sites are probably due to the fact that in some parts of the world people sitting on a wooden floor may be damaged by a splinter that has been contaminated by infected sputum from another member of the family.

A further problem has recently been recognized in those parts of the world where the incidence of AIDS is high. Tuberculosis occurs far more frequently than expected in such communities. Leprosy workers fear that Hansen's disease may be finding a foothold in such areas, but evidence is presently lacking.

TREATMENT IN THE TROPICS

In those parts of the world where there is a continuing high incidence of pulmonary tuberculosis of the lung it is not surprising that skin tuberculosis is seen more often than in the more affluent regions. It has, however, been pointed out from Kenya that skin manifestations are less common than might have been expected. It must be remembered that before the discovery of specific antituberculous drugs in the late 1940s various forms of ultraviolet light and vitamin D (calciferol) were used for the treatment of skin tuberculosis and it is possible that numerous patients with a fairly high resistance do not develop an infection following inoculation because they are exposed for hours a day to preventive doses of sunshine.

Such treatment cannot, however, be relied on and some form of antituberculous therapy must be used. Care should always be taken to investigate the probability of tuberculosis simultaneously infecting other sites and, even if such complications remain undiscovered, it is wise to treat the patient as though there is a hidden infection. The initial treatment should consist of isoniazid 200–300 mg daily and two other first-line drugs (rifampicin, streptomycin or ethambutol) in suitable doses followed by a period of 6–12 months when the patient continues isoniazid with one of the other drugs (see Chapter 57).

In many parts of the tropics, skin tuberculosis is often treated with isoniazid alone; this treatment is often dermatologically effective but should only be undertaken if it is certain there is no other active manifestation of tuberculosis in the body. Isoniazid resistance may develop.

URTICARIA

Every adult at one time or another experiences an attack of acute urticaria. This usually starts as a sudden eruption of raised white oedematous wheals on an erythematous base which are usually pruritic enough to prevent sleep. Most cases of acute urticaria are manifestations of food sensitivity (shellfish, fish, dairy products, etc.). In the tropics urticaria is seen in all countries but the causes vary according to local habits of eating.

CHRONIC URTICARIA

This is usually defined as the persistence of urticarial attacks for more than 2 months. It is rarely due to food allergens for even the least observant individual will slowly recognize the association between an item of diet and a further attack and take suitable steps to avoid recurrence. Ingested drugs, particularly aspirin and other salicylates, and benzoates and the yellow colouring known as tartrazine, are often unrecognized causes of chronic urticaria.[7]

In the tropics all the usual causes of chronic urticaria may be recognized but it must not be forgotten that many patients are reacting to parasitic infestations. All long-standing cases should have their stools examined for hookworm, tapeworms, and roundworms and the patient should be carefully examined for evidence of trichinosis (Chapter 71), onchocerciasis, dracunculosis and lymphatic filariasis (Chapter 70) and strongyloidiasis (Chapter 71).

Treatment is aimed at removing any recognized cause but it should be remembered that a dermatosis as common as urticaria may exist coincidentally with some parasitoses without there necessarily being an aetiological connection.

A single daily tablet of astemizole (a non-sedating antihistamine) will usually be sufficient to suppress the symptoms.

DERMATOSES LIMITED MAINLY TO THE TROPICS

Residents of countries in or adjacent to the tropics not only develop the diseases that are found uniformly throughout the world but are also liable to acquire other conditions, usually infective, the causative organisms of which can only exist in warmer or moister zones. Such diseases may be bacterial (e.g. anthrax, Buruli ulcer, leprosy and yaws), superficial and deep fungus infections (e.g. blastomycosis, paracoccidioidomycosis and rhinosporidiosis) and parasitic (e.g. amoebiasis, dracunculosis, filiariasis, leishmaniasis, onchocerciasis, schistosomiasis). They are all discussed in the appropriate chapters.

There are, however, a number of other dermatoses, not of infective origin, whose incidence is much higher in the tropics; some of the more frequently occurring are discussed below.

ARSENISM

In the first half of the twentieth century the medical profession gradually and apparently somewhat reluctantly abandoned the habit of prescribing arsenic but there remain a number of other ways in which individuals may be poisoned by arsenic.

In some countries such as Argentina and the USA certain rivers are known to contain a higher than usual amount of arsenic and in several parts of the world communities living in the neighbourhood of tin mines have been poisoned by arsenic seeping into nearby wells to give a concentration of more than 0.1 mg/l, the level which is usually considered dangerous. Another source, recognized in Iran, was the contamination of wells by a leaking drainpipe which led from the local public baths in which bathers had used an arsenical paste as a depilatory during bathing. In Thailand and Malaysia capsules containing up to 25% of arsenious trioxide have been sold in rural communities as an all-purpose tonic.

Dermatological manifestations due to arsenic are always slow to appear—acute arsenical poisoning does not have any time to produce skin lesions. After some years of persistent low-grade ingestion changes appear, starting with an abnormality of

pigmentation particularly affecting the trunk; there is a diffuse hyperpigmentation of a rather slaty-grey colour, scattered throughout which are small areas of normal skin which have in the past been described as 'raindrop hypopigmentation'. This is often the only manifestation of chronic arsenical poisoning but sometimes—usually a few years later—small hard callus-like keratoses appear, particularly on the palms and soles. These protrude from the surface and so do not particularly resemble plantar warts but may be mistaken for verruca vulgaris, although usually they are more numerous. Patients seek treatment if walking is painful but the recognized therapies for warts or actinic keratoses do not usually succeed and patients often resort to the use of pumice stone or a similar dermabrasive.

Despite a reputation to the contrary, arsenical keratoses rarely, if ever, turn malignant but the concomitant development of skin malignancies (especially Bowen's disease) is not uncommon.[8] Bowen's disease is a form of intraepidermal premalignancy looking somewhat like a patch of psoriasis; it often occurs in association with internal malignancies, particularly of the lungs and the stomach. As it is known that chronic arsenism is frequently associated with such neoplasms it is not clear whether the bowenoid lesions are a direct result of arsenical poisoning or a manifestation of an arsenically caused internal malignancy. All patients should be regularly examined for evidence of neoplasia and any recognized lesion must be treated in the normal way. At the same time tests should be made to ensure that the water supply is safe. It is wise to remind communities whose water is contaminated that boiling it does not make it safe.

BRAZILIAN PEMPHIGUS FOLIACEUS

The group of bullous eruptions which jointly shares the name of pemphigus are autoimmune diseases characterized by the histological presence of acantholysis in which disruption of intercellular bridges permits separation of epidermal cells. Consequent development of intraepidermal bullae develop, the type of pemphigus being determined by the site of the blister. If the intercellular split is low down in the epidermis or just above the basal layer the disease is called pemphigus vulgaris, while if it is higher (at or near the granular layer) a diagnosis of pemphigus erythematosus or pemphigus foliaceus is made. In these cases the blister roof will be more easily rubbed off and the patients will have less intact bullae and more erosions. These pemphigus diseases occur worldwide and, until recent improvements in therapy, were usually fatal. All such diseases occur in middle or later life and their aetiology is unknown.

A strange variant of pemphigus is apparently limited to certain areas in Brazil (particularly the state of Goiás). This is in many ways indistinguishable from true pemphigus foliaceus but there are some features that are startlingly different. Almost half the cases start before the age of 21 and in many there is a family history. Clinically, however, the appearance is much the same, the eruption usually starting on the face and scalp and then spreading to the presternal regions as a scaly crusted redness in which only a few intact bullae are visible at any one time. The condition may persist for years but sometimes resolves spontaneously. In most cases the skin is increasingly involved by a scaly oozing erythema, the scalp hair becomes matted and this is followed by widespread diffuse alopecia, while a combination of blistering and papillomatous lesions may affect the flexures.[9,10]

It is not unusual for the bullae to be particularly sited around the edges of the erythematous patches. The disease is often complicated by bacterial superinfection and sometimes viral contamination will cause a widespread varicelliform eruption of the type originally described by Kaposi.

TREATMENT

Whether the Brazilian disease is the same as ordinary pemphigus foliaceus remains uncertain but usually the same treatment is successful. Initial high doses of oral corticosteroids (up to 250 mg of prednisolone daily) rapidly suppress the appearance of new bullae and the dosage can quickly be reduced until further bullae erupt. The addition of small doses of methotrexate or azathioprine may permit the further reduction of corticosteroids until only one or two 5 mg tablets are necessary each day. Mepacrine 0.3–0.6 g daily or dapsone 100 mg daily are also useful as supplementary medications.

As many cases of Brazilian pemphigus foliaceus suffer from pulmonary tuberculosis it may be necessary to avoid the use of corticosteroids until the tuberculosis is under control; in this case mepacrine and dapsone may be particularly helpful.

LICHEN AMYLOIDOSUS

The systemic forms of amyloidosis, whether primary or secondary, occur rarely but widely throughout the world. Primary systemic amyloidosis usually shows cutaneous, subcutaneous and systemic masses of amyloid deposited widely to produce cutaneous plaques, alopecia, macroglossia, etc. Sometimes found in a family distribution, other cases are associated with plasma cell myeloma but in most patients there is no recognizable cause. Secondary systemic disease which rarely, if ever, involves the skin is usually the manifestation of some underlying chronic disease such as ulcerative colitis, tuberculosis or erythema nodosum leprosum (Chapter 58).

A third form of amyloidosis is localized to the skin and is called lichen amyloidosus. This has a worldwide distribution but is seen much more commonly in Asia, being particularly frequent in Indonesia, Malaysia and south India. It is not associated with the forms of systemic disease mentioned above. Starting as a pruritus of the shins it occurs less commonly on the arms and rarely on the trunk. The area slowly becomes hyperpigmented and rows of small maculopapules appear which gradually become darker, more raised and dome shaped and finally appear somewhat like the ripples seen on a sandy shore at the sea's edge. Histologically amyloid can be found deposited in the dermal papillae.

In severe cases the papular lichenoid eruption of the shins is associated with macular hyperpigmentation on the back of the shoulders and between the scapulae but, although this discoloration is often quite extensive, it rarely changes into the dome-shaped papules that are diagnostic on the shins. Macular amyloidosis is usually not pruritic.

TREATMENT

Patients are often more distressed by the itching than the appearance, and local use of corticosteroid ointment (applied once a day and occluded by a plastic sheet) will often help the pruritus but prolonged use of this or of intralesional corticosteroid injections leads to atrophy of the skin and an increasingly unpleasant mottled appearance of the shins.

Triamcinolone A intramuscularly every 6 weeks

often markedly diminishes the itching but produces relatively little change in appearance. Patients with only mild pruritus sometimes respond to one of the more sedative antihistamines: chlorpheniramine maleate in the daytime or promethazine hydrochloride at night.

Retinoic acid cream or lotion (0.05%) applied locally may soften the keratotic papules.

LICHEN PLANUS AND LICHENOID ERUPTIONS

Lichen planus is a relatively uncommon disease, the typical lesions being flat-topped, shiny, pruritic papules which often have a violaceous colouring in Caucasians. Although seen most frequently on the fronts of the wrists they can also be found scattered across the body, on the genitalia and even on the buccal mucosa where the condition takes the form of bluish-white streaks inside the cheeks or on the tongue or palate. Histology shows the epidermis to have a thickening of the granular and keratin layers as well as liquefaction degeneration of the basal layer, while a heavy infiltrate of T lymphocytes is present in the upper part of the dermis.

During the Second World War Caucasians fighting in the tropics not infrequently developed a papular pruritic eruption which was called 'tropical lichen planus'. As time went on it was realized that this was a drug eruption following the use of mepacrine as an antimalarial. Routine treatment was changed to chloroquine; this drug did not produce a skin reaction and tropical lichen planus disappeared.

HYPERTROPHIC LICHEN PLANUS

Although lichen planus occasionally shows hypertrophic lesions, inhabitants of southern Indian and Sri Lanka often develop an eruption in which hypertrophic lesions are the only ones seen. Most common around the lower leg and the ankle, thick warty deeply pigmented and highly pruritic nodules may last for years (Plate 11.6). Frequent intralesional injections of corticosteroids are liable to cause atrophy of the skin and it is better to give intramuscular injections of triamcinolone acetonide once every 4–6 weeks, or ACTH 40 units weekly for 6–8 weeks. Some workers have recently claimed that griseofulvin 500mg twice daily for 3 months is effective but this should be tried only as a last resort.

ACTINIC LICHEN PLANUS

This condition has sometimes, rather confusingly, been called 'lichen planus tropicus' but the name 'actinic lichen planus' is preferred for this peculiar lichenoid eruption[11] which occurs particularly on the face and forehead and is probably due to excess exposure to the sun. Itching, mildly hyperpigmented papules gradually extend and take on an annular appearance with a central depression; as they enlarge they may coalesce.

It seems to occur particularly along the north coast of Africa, in Egypt and the Near East. It is highly pruritic and takes 2–3 weeks to resolve, responding slowly, if at all, to the usual therapies given for lichen planus.

A slightly different condition described in Kenya as lichenoid melanodermatitis seems much the same as other forms of actinic lichen planus but it apparently runs a more rapid and less pruritic course.[12]

PIGMENTARY PROBLEMS

VITILIGO

It is not known why so many people develop this cosmetically disquieting abnormality in which areas of skin in any part of the body suddenly lose all their colour and become not simply hypopigmented but totally achromic; if it occurs on the scalp, hairs in the affected area usually lose their pigment. The darker-skinned races are more particularly alarmed by this condition, especially if it appears on the face or other uncovered areas of the body, and seem to seek attention more frequently than Caucasians. Whether this is because the disease is cosmetically less acceptable in pigmented peoples or whether such communities have a higher incidence of vitiligo is not certain. Patients, dreading the possibility of vitiligo, often consult their doctors urgently for hypopigmented lesions such as pityriasis alba, pityriasis versicolor or the early stages of leprosy.

Treatment

It is very difficult to know what advice to give to dark-skinned patients who have vitiligo. A few fortunates find the condition resolves, particularly if it has only been present for a few weeks, but the longer the condition lasts the less likelihood there will be of satisfactory treatment. Repigmentation appears initially around hair follicles, and patients are frequently cheered by the appearance of these dark dots on the skin of the shins or trunk. Unfortunately, the repigmentation only rarely extends fully across the lesions and, after a year or so of expensive treatment, vitiligo often remains visible. It must be realized that pigmentation, returning as it does from the depths of the hair follicles, will not occur on the lips, areola, glans penis, palms or soles and patients must never be allowed to believe that colour will return to these sites.

It is necessary, therefore, to tell patients that treatment is successful in 25% of cases at most but many are so distressed by the condition that they press for treatment even if little success is anticipated. It is unfair to allow patients to pay large sums of money for medications the success of which is not guaranteed, and therapy should not be continued for more than 3 months, unless greater than usual success is being obtained.

Various psoralens are the most frequently prescribed medications, sensitizing the skin to sunlight and, theoretically, encouraging the achromic areas to repigment. It is usually suggested that two 10mg tablets of ammoidin or two 10mg capsules of methoxsalen should be taken 2 hours before exposure to natural sunlight; the treatment known as PUVA is a combination of psoralens and carefully graded doses of UVA light. It should be remembered that vitiliginous patches which were previously heavily pigmented will be exceedingly susceptible to the side-effects of these treatments (elastosis, increased risk of 'non-fatal' cancer) and the long-term use of PUVA therapy is unwise unless it is producing dramatic results.

In some of the more sophisticated parts of the world it is possible to obtain various waterproof camouflaging preparations; Covermark, Dermocover and Keromask are proprietary products which all have various shades of masking and toning creams and finishing powders which can in experienced hands be very effective in covering areas of discoloration and so alleviating the patient's embarrassment. Where these preparations are not obtainable, potassium permanganate 0.1% or even walnut juice may be used to mask the patches. In any case all patients should be advised to cover the achromic areas with a sun-barrier preparation as it is not unknown for actinic keratoses or lupus erythematosus to develop in these unprotected areas.

MELASMA

The appearance of a brownish-black macular pigmentation over the cheek bones, the nose, the upper lip and the forehead has for many years been attributed to the combination of multiple pregnancies and exposure to the sun, the disease attaining its highest incidence in the Middle East, North Africa, India and Central America. In the past the condition was called 'chloasma uterinum' but, as it is now considered that it may also be due to a combination of sunlight and the prolonged use of oral contraceptive pills, it is better known as 'melasma'.

Monobenzyl ether of hydroquinone is available in various strengths from 2 to 10% and when applied to the pigmented areas will slowly lighten the skin; a similarly effective application consists of p-methyloxyphenol 10% in a water-soluble base. The best prophylaxis is for the patient or her partner to use a non-hormonal form of contraception.

PHRYNODERMA

In 1933 two papers were published associating the appearance of dome shaped follicular hyperkeratotic papules with deficiency of vitamin A. At that time numerous associated symptoms were described, including severe or fatal diarrhoea, peripheral neuritis and extensive oedema. It is now realized that these patients had multiple dietary deficiencies—the condition being most frequently found in severely malnourished prisoners or indentured labourers. This symptom complex is nowadays rarely seen except under famine conditions.

The skin lesions now known as phrynoderma (toad skin) continue unabated in children and adolescents, being rare over the age of 18. Scattered raised papules with a hyperkeratotic punctum are grouped in areas 5–6cm in diameter, most often over the knees and elbows and often having a clearly visible hypopigmented background.[13]

TREATMENT

Despite occasional claims to the contrary, vitamin supplements do not have much effect on this condition which responds best to emollient soap and various keratolytic creams. Retinoic acid 0.5% is often quite helpful, while if younger children (6–10 years old) find this to be too irritating, it may be advisable to mix the retinoic acid cream with an equal amount of hydrocortisone ointment.

The condition rarely, if ever, persists into adult life and should be considered as a follicular disorder of keratin formation and not as a vitamin deficiency.

REFERENCES

1 Dillon H C Jr. *Int J Derm* 1980; 19:443.
2 Cronin E. *Contact Dermatitis*. New York: Churchill Livingstone, 1981.
3 American Academy of Dermatology. *Patch-testing in Allergic Contact Dermatitis*, 7th edn. Evanston, IL: AAD, 1984.
4 Jaffe H W, Choi K, Thomas P A et al. *Ann Intern Med* 1983; 99:145.
5 Bhutani L K & Kumar A S. *Int J Dermatol* 1981; 20:380.
6 Green A. *Aust J Dermatol* 1984; 25:99.
7 Warin R P & Smith R J. *Br J Dermatol* 1975; 93 (supplement II):19.
8 Reymann F, Moller R & Nielson A. *Arch Dermatol* 1978; 114:378.
9 Azulay R D. *Int J Dermatol* 1982; 21:122.
10 Beutner E H, Prigenzi L S, Hale E W et al. *Proc Soc Exp Biol Med* 1968; 127:81.
11 Zanca A & Zanca A. *Int J Dermatol* 1978; 17:506.
12 Verhagen A R H B & Koten J W. *Br J Dermatol* 1979; 101:651.
13 Pettit J H S. *Int J Dermatol* 1983; 22:117.

CHAPTER 12

HIV/AIDS—WITH AN EMPHASIS ON AFRICA

Peter Piot

The acquired immune deficiency syndrome (AIDS) was first described in the USA in 1981.[1] Over 10 years later, by mid-1993, over 700 000 cases of AIDS had been reported from nearly all countries to the World Health Organization (WHO).[2] However, WHO estimates that well over 2.2 million cases had cumulatively occurred in adults.[2] Perhaps more importantly, it is (conservatively) estimated that over 14 million adults and children were infected in 1993 with the human immunodeficiency virus (HIV), the cause of AIDS.

For surveillance purposes AIDS is defined as an illness characterized by the presence of a reliably diagnosed disease at least moderately predictive of cellular immunodeficiency, and by the absence of an underlying cause for immunodeficiency or any defined cause for reduced resistance to the disease. Diseases at least moderately predictive of cellular immunodeficiency are listed in Table 12.1. In addition to AIDS, HIV causes a broad spectrum of clinical diseases, as described below. In many developing countries, AIDS is now a major public health problem, which is most likely to grow in the near future. To quote the *World Development Report 1993*:[3] 'Historians will look back on the latter half of this century as having had one great medical triumph, the eradication of smallpox, and one great medical tragedy, AIDS'.

GEOGRAPHICAL DISTRIBUTION

Infection with HIV is occurring in all continents, but the major foci are in North America, sub-Saharan Africa, Latin America and the Caribbean, and South and South-East Asia. Figure 12.1 shows the distribution of HIV infection in the world, illustrating that the overwhelming majority of cases occur in the developing world.

Sub-Saharan Africa is by far the most affected region, with the highest HIV prevalence rates occurring in the eastern and southern parts of the continent, and a second epidemic focus around Ivory Coast in West Africa (Figure 12.2).

In the major cities of East and Central Africa, and in Abidjan, AIDS patients make up at least 50% of patients hospitalized in medical services. In the same areas AIDS has also become the leading cause of death among hospitalized adults, and in a city such as Abidjan or a rural area such as Masaka District in Uganda, even the major cause of adult death among men, and second only to pregnancy and abortion-related death among women.[4–6] Thus, in Masaka district, the mortality attributable to HIV infection was 44% for adult males, 50% for adult females, and as much as 89% for adults aged 25–34 years.[6] These figures demonstrate the profound impact that the HIV epidemic has on adult mortality in sub-Saharan Africa, even in some rural populations.

It is estimated that by mid-1993 over 1.5 million AIDS adult cases had occurred in this region, making up two-thirds of the global total (Table 12.2). Another half million children with AIDS should be added to this figure.[2]

In general there are an equal number of men and women among AIDS cases and among people with HIV infection. However, in countries such as Uganda and Zaïre women outnumber men by a factor of 1.2, whereas in West Africa there are more men than women among AIDS cases.

HIV seroprevalence rates among the general population in Africa vary widely, from well below 1% in many rural areas or in a country like Madagascar, to over 30% among adults in cities such as Kigali, Rwanda, and Kampala, Uganda.[7,8] Seroprevalence rates usually peak between 16 and 29 years,

Table 12.1 Diseases (at least) moderately predictive of cellular immunodeficiency.

Candidiasis of the oesophagus, trachea, bronchi or lungs
Cryptococcosis, extrapulmonary
Cryptosporidiosis and isosporiasis
Cytomegalovirus diseases of an organ other than liver, spleen or lymph nodes in a patient >1 month of age
Herpes simplex virus infection causing a mucocutaneous ulcer persisting for longer than 1 month, or oesophagitis
Disseminated *Mycobacterium avium-intracellulare* infections
Pneumocystis carinii pneumonia
Cerebral toxoplasmosis
Extrapulmonary tuberculosis
Recurrent *Salmonella* spp. septicaemia
Kaposi's sarcoma (epidemic type, see Table 12.7)
Primary lymphoma of the brain
Non-Hodgkin's lymphoma
Progressive multifocal leucoencephalopathy
Lymphoid interstitial pneumonia
HIV wasting syndrome (emaciation)
HIV encephalopathy
In children <13 years of age: multiple or recurrent bacterial infections (septicaemia, pneumonia, meningitis, bone or joint infection, abscess of an internal organ or body cavity)

with the peak often occurring at a lower age for women than for men. Another indication of the importance of sexual activity in the spread of HIV infection is the very high prevalence rates of HIV documented among female prostitutes and patients with other sexually transmitted diseases. It is not unusual to find HIV seroprevalence rates over 80% in prostitutes and over 50% among patients with sexually transmitted diseases in sub-Saharan Africa, and even in areas where HIV infection is still uncommon infection rates exceeding 10% are often found in these two populations.[7,8]

Whereas a rapid spread of HIV in sexually highly exposed populations has been observed from the early 1980s in Africa,[9] there is now increasing evidence that, particularly in women, HIV infection is not confined any longer to people with high-risk sexual behaviour. This is supported by studies in pregnant women in Kenya, Malawi and Rwanda,[10–12] suggesting that the sexual behaviour of the partner is also an important risk factor of HIV infection.

HIV incidence rates are usually below 1% per year, but may be as high as 5% in the general population.[7] In contrast, such annual incidence rates may reach a staggering 50% among female prostitutes.[13] In some populations the HIV incidence appears to roughly equal the mortality from

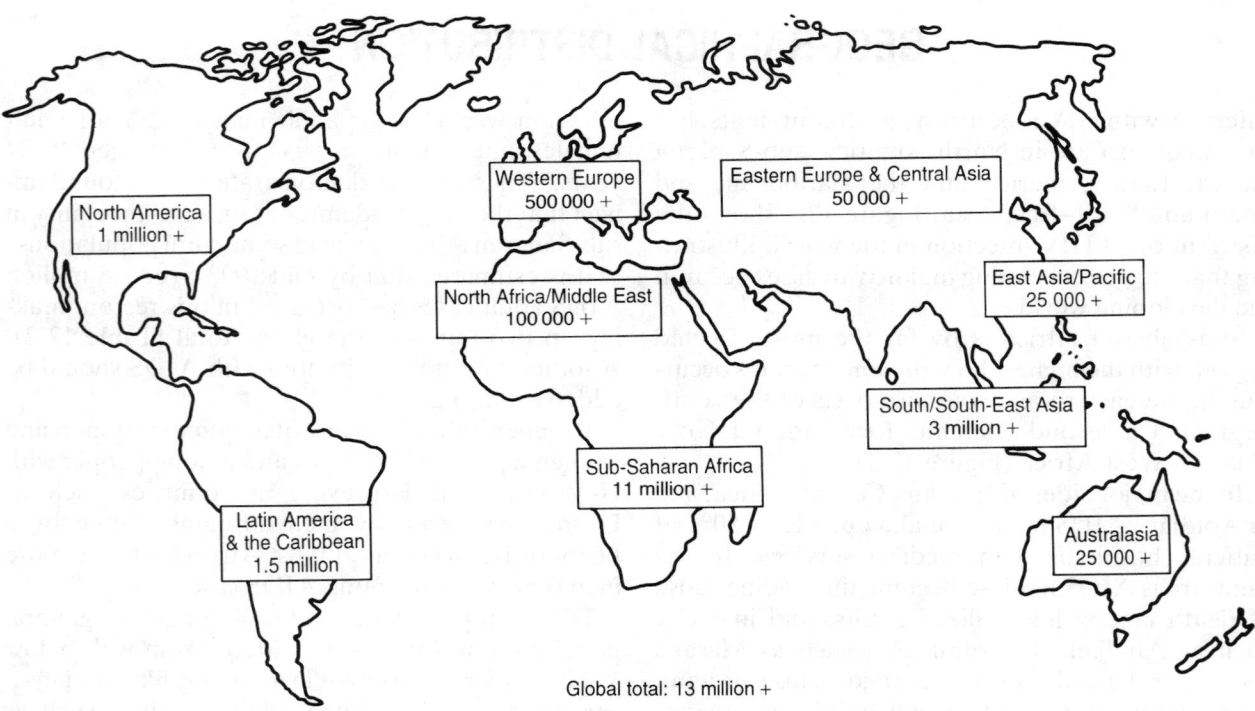

Global total: 13 million +

Figure 12.1 Estimated global distribution of cumulative HIV infections in adults, by continent or region at the end of 1994. (Source: Global Programme on AIDS, World Health Organization.)

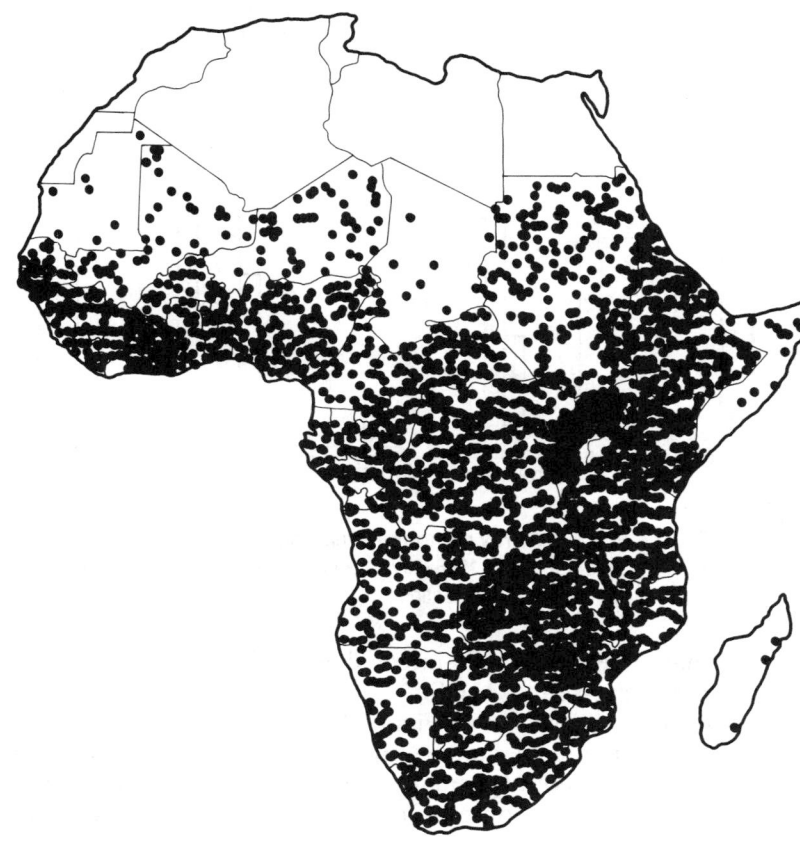

Figure 12.2 Distribution of estimated cumulative HIV infections in adults in sub-Saharan Africa, 1992. (Source: Global Programme on AIDS, World Health Organization.)

Table 12.2. Estimated and projected HIV prevalence in adults by 'macro' region.

'Macro' region	End of 1994		2000	
	*Estimated HIV prevalence**	*Estimated population aged 15–49 years (1990)*	*Projected HIV prevalence*	*Projected population aged 15–49 years*
Australasia, Europe and North America	>1.2 million	646 million	1 million	675 million
Latin America and Caribbean	>1.5 million	227 million	>2 million	282 million
Africa	>8 million	289 million	>9 million	397 million
Asia	2.5 million	1527 million	8 million	1843 million
Global total	>13 million	2689 million	>20 million	3197 million

*Total number of HIV-infected people currently alive.

HIV infection, resulting in a stable or very slowly rising seroprevalence.[14]

HIV-2 is a closely related human immunodeficiency virus which circulates mainly in West Africa, and to a limited extent in Angola, Mozambique and India.[15] Whereas in Guinea-Bissau it is the predominant HIV (with 10% of the adult population being infected), HIV-1 is far more common than HIV-2 in other West African countries, where HIV-1 is spreading fast, but prevalence levels of HIV-2 remain stable. As for HIV-1, the most sexually active populations have the highest infection rates with HIV-2. Both sexual and mother-to-child transmission of HIV-2 are less efficient than is the case for HIV-1.

AIDS is also an increasing public health problem in Latin America and the Caribbean, where some islands have among the highest cumulative incidence rates of AIDS in the world. By mid-1993 over 250 000 cases of AIDS had occurred in this region.[2]

Figure 12.3 shows HIV-1 seroprevalence rates among patients with sexually transmitted diseases in

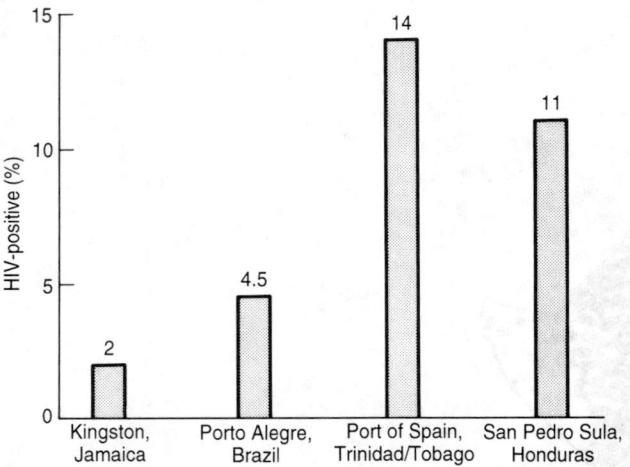

Figure 12.3 HIV prevalence in sexually transmitted disease clinic attenders in Latin America and the Caribbean, 1991–1992. (Source: Global Programme on AIDS, World Health Organization.)

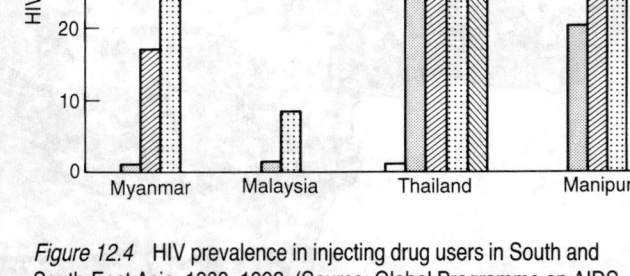

Figure 12.4 HIV prevalence in injecting drug users in South and South-East Asia, 1988–1992. (Source: Global Programme on AIDS, World Health Organization.)

Latin America and the Caribbean, showing that between 2 and 14% of such patients are infected. Prevalence rates among antenatal clinic attenders in the region range from 1 to 3% in Sao Paulo, Santo Domingo and the Bahamas, to around 10% in certain communities in Haiti.[3]

Whereas homosexual and bisexual contacts have been the main mode of spread of HIV, heterosexual intercourse and injecting drug use have become the main routes of transmission in many countries.[16,17] As a result, the male-to-female ratio among AIDS cases is declining in most countries in the region.

In South and South-East Asia, HIV has recently been spreading extensively, with over 1.5 million people infected by mid-1993. However, less than 4000 cases of AIDS were reported from Asia by that time, though the actual number is probably closer to 30 000. The full impact of HIV infection in Asia will only be seen after the year 2000 when many of the currently HIV-infected individuals will have progressed to AIDS.[18]

As shown in Figure 12.4 the spread of HIV was fulminant among injecting drug users in selected areas of Myanmar, north-east India, and Thailand, where seroprevalence rates of 50% are not uncommon.[8] Simultaneously the virus has been spreading heterosexually, which is now the major mode of transmission of HIV in Asia. Both in Thailand and several Indian cities, such spread occurred most dramatically in female prostitutes.[19] At least in Thailand HIV has now spread well beyond the groups at highest risk for HIV. Thus, nearly 7% of young military recruits in Thailand in 1991 were HIV positive, with 15.3% of men from the upper north region of the country being infected with HIV.[20] Prostitution, sex with prostitutes, and sexually transmitted diseases are the main risk factors for HIV infection in Thailand.

EPIDEMIOLOGY

HIV is transmitted by sexual contact (heterosexual or homosexual), administration of infected blood or blood products, contaminated injections, and from infected mothers to their infants. In contrast to North America and Europe, where the overwhelming majority of AIDS patients acquired the disease by homosexual contact or were intravenous drug addicts, bidirectional heterosexual transmission is the major mode of infection in the developing world.

In the absence of amplifying factors, the efficiency of penile–vaginal intercourse is low for HIV transmission (well below 1%). Factors which enhance the risk of heterosexual transmission of HIV include higher viraemia (during acute infection and more advanced stages of the disease) in the infecting partner, sex during menstruation, receptive anal intercourse, the presence of other sexually transmitted diseases, and possibly lack of circumcision in men, cervical ectopy and the use of desiccating vaginal agents.[21]

In particular, genital ulcers such as chancroid, syphilis, and genital herpes, and to a lesser extent, gonorrhoea and chlamydial infection, enhance the risk of sexual transmission of HIV.[22,23] This has been studied extensively in Kenya and Zaïre, where relative risks of up to 10 for genital ulcers for HIV transmission were found and of 3–5 for non-ulcerative sexually transmitted disease.[24,25] However, as non-ulcerative sexually transmitted diseases are much more common in most countries, their contribution to the heterosexual spread of HIV may be greater.

Mother-to-child transmission during pregnancy, during delivery or through breast feeding is the second most common mode of spread of HIV-1 in the developing world. It is striking that the observed rates of mother-to-child transmission of HIV-1 have been consistently higher in Africa than in Europe or North America (30–40% as compared with 15–20%, respectively).[26] Factors playing a role in this higher risk of transmission include transmission through breast feeding, more frequent advanced immuno-deficiency (associated with higher HIV viraemia) and more common occurrence of chorioamnionitis as a result of genital infection.

In several, but not all, studies maternal HIV-1 infection was associated with adverse pregnancy outcome, including stillbirth, premature delivery and low birth weight.[27,28]

Blood transfusions continue to be a source of HIV infection in many parts of the developing world, particularly in sub-Saharan Africa.[29] This clearly demonstrates that the existence of a fairly simple technology—HIV antibody tests—is not enough for assuring safe blood transfusions.

Finally, nosocomial transmission of HIV by syringes and needles undoubtedly occurs, but its role in the spread of HIV is poorly documented—although it is probably very low.[30] However, outbreaks of infection-associated nosocomial infection in eastern Europe demonstrate that infections for medical purposes can be a source of HIV infection in the community.

There is much heterogeneity in the epidemiology of HIV throughout the world. The HIV/AIDS epidemic is still in an expanding phase in most parts of the world, with continuing geographical spread and changing epidemiological patterns.[31]

Numerous variables may influence the spread of HIV, either directly (i.e. sexual behaviour) or indirectly (i.e. demography, poverty). These include sexual behaviour, rate of condom use, the age structure and sex ratio of urban and rural populations, migration patterns, levels of sexually transmitted diseases, the quality and accessibility of health services, women's status, and in general the public response to the epidemic.

The impact of AIDS on the most severely affected countries is already considerable but the situation will become worse as the number of people with HIV-induced illness continues to increase. AIDS not only affects infected individuals and their relatives and friends, but also communities at large with a long-term impact on households, on the health sector, on demography and on the economic and social system.[3]

The health sector is directly affected by a growing demand for health care, as illustrated by the large numbers of men and women with AIDS occupying often over 50% of all medical beds in the hospitals of many African cities.[4,5] Absorbing this growing burden of patients is a major challenge for health care systems in the developing world. Moreover, as a results of AIDS the incidence of tuberculosis is rising in many countries (see below).[32,33]

The long-term demographic impact of AIDS is uncertain, and will probably differ from one country to another.[34] However, AIDS is already the leading cause of death in adults in many African cities, and is also increasing the under-5 child mortality, reversing the achievements of child survival programmes in high HIV prevalence areas. In addition, the number of orphans from parents who died from AIDS is rapidly growing, with over one million AIDS orphans projected for 1998 in Uganda alone.[35]

Economically, AIDS is now among the top five leading causes of loss of healthy life in urban sub-Saharan Africa, accounting for 15% of the total disease burden.[36] As HIV infection occurs mainly in young adults in their most productive years, it increasingly affects many economic and social sectors as well.

AETIOLOGY AND PATHOGENESIS

AIDS is caused by HIV, which belongs to the lentiviruses, of which two distinct viruses have been identified in man: HIV-1 and HIV-2.[37,38]

Important biological properties of HIV include the presence of a reverse transcriptase, an enzyme enabling this RNA virus to make a DNA copy of its genome, the integration of viral DNA into the genome of the host cell, and the preferential infection of T lymphocytes with the helper phenotype (CD4+). HIV infection of helper T lymphocytes may result in cell destruction, but the virus may also remain in a state of latency in the lymphocytes or replicate without causing any obvious cell damage or clinical disease. Infected individuals carry the virus for life.

HIV has been isolated from lymphocytes, cell-free blood, semen, cervicovaginal secretions, brain tissue, cerebrospinal fluid, saliva, tears, breast milk, urine and bone marrow, and can be isolated from other tissues, body fluids, secretions and excretions.

By nucleic acid analysis of the complete *gag* genes at least seven distinct HIV-1 genotypes can be identified (designated types A–G).[39] An even higher degree of genetic variation exists in the envelope region, which contains hypervariable regions interspersed with highly conserved sequences.[40] In addition, HIV isolates differ in their biological properties such as replication rate, syncytium-inducing capacity and host range.

Whereas HIV-1 isolates from patients in the developing world are similar to those found in the industrialized world, African isolates generally exhibit more genetic heterogeneity.

A second human lentivirus, occurring mostly in West Africa, shares approximately 40% nucleic acid homology. Simian immunodeficiency viruses (SIVs) are non-human primate lentiviruses which are more or less related to the HIVs. They closely parallel HIVs in genomic organization and biological properties. Figure 12.5 shows the genetic relationship between HIV-1 and HIV-2, and SIVs from sooty mangabeys (SIV$_{sm}$), African green monkeys (SIV$_{agm}$), mandrills (SIV$_{mnd}$), rhesus macaques (SIV$_{mac}$) and chimpanzees (SIV$_{cpz}$).[41]

The pathogenesis of HIV infection and AIDS is not fully understood.[42–44] A typical course of HIV infection is shown in Figure 12.6.[44] During the early period after primary infection there is widespread dissemination of virus and a sharp decrease in the number of CD4 T cells in peripheral blood. An immune response to HIV ensues, with a decrease in detectable viraemia followed by a prolonged period of clinical latency. The CD4 T-cell count continues to decrease during the following years, until it reaches a critical level below which there is a substantial risk of opportunistic diseases.[44]

The basic clinical features of AIDS originate from the critical injury of the immune system, due to the selective infection of helper T lymphocytes. As a result of this, the host becomes susceptible to life-threatening opportunistic infections and malignancies. Functional defects can be identified in almost every part of the immune system, including cellular and humoral immunity. Thus, the main immunological disorders include lymphopenia, a decrease in helper T lymphocytes, T-cell dysfunction, defective monocyte cytotoxic function, polyclonal B-cell activation, non-specific antilymphocyte antibodies, increased levels of β_2-microglobulin and defective delayed hypersensitivity (cutaneous anergy).

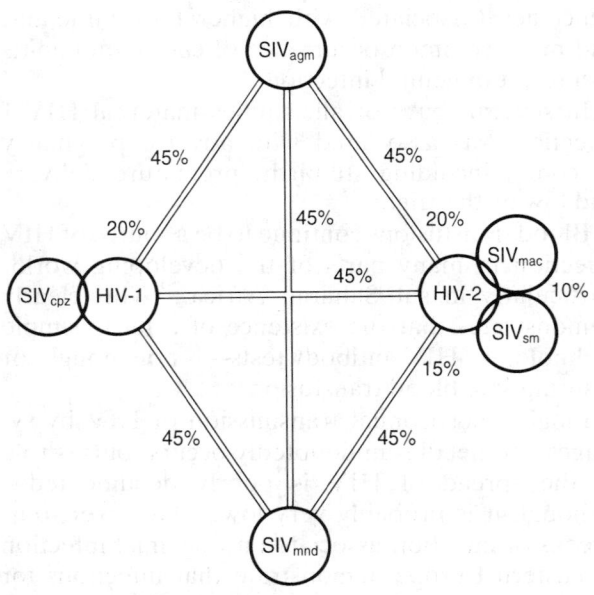

Figure 12.5 Relationship between human and non-human primate lentiviruses on the basis of amino acid homologues. Percentages in the lines are approximate values of amino acid divergences in the *pol* gene product. (Reproduced with permission from Peeters *et al.*[41])

CLINICAL FEATURES

The clinical expression of HIV infection is very diverse, varying from a healthy carrier state to potentially fatal opportunistic diseases. The clinical manifestations associated with HIV infection also vary in different populations, possibly due to the relative frequency of endemic infections. This brief review will focus on the particular aspects of the disease as occurring in Africa, where tuberculosis,

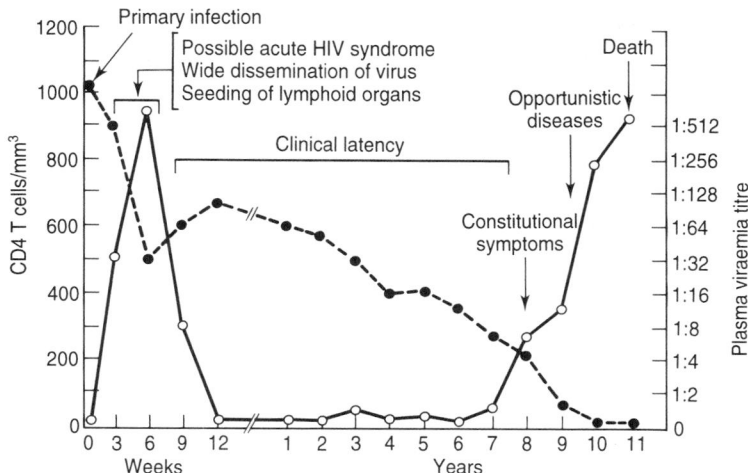

Figure 12.6 Typical course of HIV infection. ●--●, CD4 T-cell count; ○——○, plasma viraemia titre. (Reproduced with permission from G. Pantaleo *et al.*[44])

gastrointestinal and dermatological manifestations are more common than in Europeans and Americans with AIDS.[45–47]

ACUTE ILLNESS

Early in the infection with HIV an acute illness may occur characterized by a mononucleosis-like syndrome, including fatigue, diarrhoea, fever, cough, pruritus, pallor, candidiasis, lymphadenopathy, hepatosplenomegaly and rhinorrhoea.[48] Occasionally patients may develop a transitory aseptic meningoencephalitis, mononeuritis or polyneuritis.

ASYMPTOMATIC HIV INFECTIONS

Latent virus infection may last for at least 10 years after the acquisition of infection. Whereas the median time of progression to disease among individuals with HIV infection is 10–12 years in the industrialized world, this clinical evaluation may be more rapid in Africa.[49–51] Thus, in a well-documented rural cohort in Uganda, the rate of disease progression was as high as 12.4% per year.[51] This may be due to a lack of medical care and prophylaxis for opportunistic infections, as well as to a higher occurrence of other endemic diseases, such as parasitoses and tuberculosis, which may cause immune depletion. This is supported by a study in Haiti in which prophylaxis with isoniazid in patients with both HIV and *Mycobacterium tuberculosis* infections considerably prolonged life expectancy.[52]

During this latent period, the patient is infective and HIV can be detected in various body fluids and in lymph nodes. Antibody to HIV can be demonstrated in serum.

SYMPTOMATIC HIV INFECTION

Weight loss and weakness (asthenia) are the most common clinical manifestations in patients with HIV infection in Africa. Table 12.3 summarizes clinical findings in three series of patients.[53–55] These signs and symptoms are often intermittent and can disappear spontaneously during variable periods.

Lymphadenopathy involving two or more extra-inguinal sites is found in a majority of HIV-positive patients. Lymphadenopathy occurs most frequently in the cervical and axillary regions. Lymph nodes are firm, mobile, non-tender and generally do not exceed 6cm in diameter. Lymph nodes larger than 6cm in diameter in HIV-infected patients are often of tuberculous origin. They can regress during progression of the disease.

Mucocutaneous manifestations are common in patients with HIV infection. A characteristic generalized papular pruritic eruption is found in approximately 20–60% of African and Haitian patients with HIV infection.[56,57] It is often seen in the early stages of illness but is generally found intermittently throughout the course of the disease. Its aetiology is unknown. The initial lesion is a small firm and very pruritic papule which releases a small drop of fluid when scratched. The papules become hyperpigmented macules. They are symmetrically distributed over the body, but are most frequently found on the extremities. Histological features are nonspecific and include perivascular infiltration of the skin and subcutaneous tissue with mononuclear cells with a variable number of eosinophils.

Recurrent mucocutaneous herpes simplex infections are found in 5–10% of African patients with HIV infection. Over 10% of patients with HIV infection experience a varicella zoster infection, which is recurrent in one-quarter of the cases. The

Table 12.3. Clinical manifestations in patients with AIDS in Africa.

Sign or symptom	Percentage of AIDS patients		
	Uganda[53] (N = 5142)	Tanzania[54] (N = 2000)	Zaire[55] (N = 196)
Weight loss (>10% of body weight)	82	91.5	99
Asthenia (weakness)	NA	97.5	91
Fever (>1 month)	79	79	54
Diarrhoea (>1 month)	60	75	41
Cough	41	42.5	37
Pruritus	NA	31	30
Dysphagia	NA	23.5	35
Headache (>1 month)	NA	NA	33
Dyspnoea	21	NA	23
Amenorrhoea	NA	77	42
Oral candidiasis (thrush)	36	56.5	47
Pruriginous papular eruption	36	70.5	20
Generalized lymphadenopathy	20	36.5	9
History of shingles (zoster)	10	6.5	9
Neurological abnormalities	NA	72	20
Focal neurological disorder	NA	10.5	NA

NA, not available.

initial episodes of varicella zoster infection are often the first manifestation of HIV-associated illness.

Oral candidiasis in the absence of antimicrobial immunosuppressive therapy or an immunosuppressive illness is highly associated with HIV infection. Its occurrence in an HIV-positive patient is often a bad prognostic sign and an indication of progression towards 'full-blown' AIDS.

Cutaneous hypersensitivity reactions occur with an increased frequency in individuals with HIV infection. They are particularly common during high-dose co-trimoxazole, sulphadiazine or thiacetazone treatment.[58,59]

The predominant clinical presentation of AIDS in adults in the tropics is a diarrhoea–wasting syndrome.[47,60,61] Patients may lose several litres of liquid stool a day, sometimes leading to severe dehydration. The cause of this secretory diarrhoea is not known, and established intestinal pathogens can be detected in only a minority of patients. Thus, *Cryptosporidium parvum*, microsporidia and *Isospora belli* are found in variable proportions of patients with HIV/AIDS. Fever is a very common symptom in African patients with HIV infection. It is often of unknown origin, and may be due to endemic infections unrelated to underlying HIV infection, such as malaria.

Non-opportunistic bacterial infections are an important cause of morbidity and mortality in adults with HIV infection in Africa.[62,63] *Salmonella typhimurium* and *Streptococcus pneumoniae* are the major conventional pathogens in HIV-infected patients, but other bacteria such as *Staphylococcus aureus*, *Haemophilus influenzae*, *Escherichia coli* and *Shigella* spp. also occur.

Neurological syndromes such as chronic and acute meningitis, myelopathy, encephalopathy with dementia, and peripheral neuropathy complicate the clinical course of a majority of AIDS cases. The most common neurological disorder is a progressive change in behaviour associated with dementia, which usually progresses towards severe dementia.

Cough in AIDS patients with *Pneumocystis carinii* pneumonia or with lymphoid interstitial pneumonitis is usually non-productive and frequently associated with dyspnoea. Haemoptyses and pleural effusion are mainly caused by tuberculosis or Kaposi's sarcoma. However, *P. carinii* pneumonia is relatively rare in African patients and the most common cause of pulmonary disease in the developing world is tuberculosis (see below).

HIV INFECTION IN CHILDREN

Clinical disorders in infants and children with AIDS include failure to thrive, persistent oral candidiasis, fever, persistent pulmonary infiltrates, hepatosplenomegaly, chronic parotitis, generalized lymphadenopathy and recurrent diarrhoea.[64] The rate of progression from HIV-1 infection to AIDS is faster in children than in adults. Among children with

Table 12.4. Differences between AIDS in children and adults (after ref. 64).

- Lymphoid interstitial pneumonitis and chronic parotitis are more common in children
- Severe and/or recurrent bacterial infections are a major problem in children
- Tuberculosis seems less prevalent in children
- Central nervous system opportunistic infections (*Cryptococcus neoformans* meningitis and toxoplasmosis) are uncommon in children
- Kaposi's sarcoma and central nervous system lymphomas are rare in children
- HIV encephalopathy seems more frequent in children
- Lymphopenia is rare in children
- Hypergammaglobulinaemia is more pronounced in children

symptomatic HIV-related disease seen in Kigali, 40% were diagnosed before 12 months of age, and 70% before 24 months.[64] However, children with HIV-1 infection may remain asymptomatic for many years, though only 39% of perinatally infected children followed in Rwanda remained symptom free after 18 months of age.[63]

The mortality rate in children with HIV infection has been much higher in Africa than elsewhere, varying between 14 and 39% during the first year of life.[64–66]

Some clinical differences between AIDS in children and adults are listed in Table 12.4.

OPPORTUNISTIC INFECTIONS AND TUMOURS

An opportunistic infection is defined as an infection with an organism that usually does not cause disease in a healthy person, but that may cause a severe and life-threatening illness in the presence of immunodeficiency. Opportunistic infections in AIDS generally result from reactivation rather than from primary infection.

Though all opportunistic diseases may occur in AIDS patients throughout the world, the relative importance of specific diseases may be different. For instance, major opportunistic diseases in Europe, the Americas and Asia, such as *P. carinii* pneumonia, atypical mycobacteriosis and Kaposi's sarcoma, are less frequent in African AIDS patients than elsewhere.[67–69] In contrast, tuberculosis, chronic diarrhoea, cerebral toxoplasmosis and bacteraemia due to non-opportunistic pathogens, such as *Salmonella typhimurium* and *Streptococcus pneumoniae*, are all very common.[33,62,70] In South-East Asia systemic infection with *Penicillium marneffei* is a common opportunistic mycosis in patients with HIV infection. Thus, in Chiang Mai, northern Thai-

land, penicillinosis was diagnosed in 140 (35%) of 400 consecutive AIDS cases.[71]

The most commonly identified opportunistic diseases in African patients with AIDS are listed in Table 12.5.

Patients with cryptococcal meningitis often present with mild headache, low-grade fever and weight loss. In Kinshasa a generally mild neck stiffness occurred in only 60% of cases during the course of the disease. Lumbar puncture is therefore always indicated whenever an HIV-infected patient develops headache.

P. carinii pneumonia is less frequent among Africans with AIDS than among European or American patients, in whom it is the most common presenting opportunistic infection.

Toxoplasma encephalitis was diagnosed by biopsy or at autopsy in 21% of patients in Ivory Coast,[72] indicating that this is a significantly more common opportunistic infection than among American AIDS cases. It is characterized by headache, confusion, focal neurological signs, fever and grand mal seizures. Serum antibody titres against *Toxoplasma gondii* are of little use for diagnosis, and difficult to interpret.

Tuberculosis is not only the leading opportunistic infection among adult AIDS patients in Africa, but is itself greatly affected by the HIV epidemic, with rising incidence rates wherever HIV has become endemic.[32,32,73] Thus, in several African countries with a reasonably well-functioning tuberculosis control programme, the annual incidence of tuberculosis doubled between 1985 and 1990. This rise in incidence is probably entirely attributable to the spread of HIV infection in populations where 50–80% of all adults are infected with *M. tuberculosis*.

In Africa and Haiti around 30–50% of tuberculosis patients are now infected with HIV (Table 12.6). In other developing countries the HIV prevalence is still low among tuberculosis patients, but is usually higher than in the general population. However, as pulmonary tuberculosis may develop across a broad spectrum of HIV-associated immunodeficiency in tuberculosis endemic populations, it is of limited use as an AIDS-defining illness.[74]

Additional consequences of dual HIV/*M. tuberculosis* infection include a high mortality among tuberculosis patients with HIV infection (mostly due to HIV-related illness), a growing rate of multidrug resistance of *M. tuberculosis*, and an up to tenfold increase in severe skin reactions—including Stevens–Johnson syndrome, during antituberculous therapy in HIV-positive patients.[59,75,76]

Extrapulmonary tuberculosis has been diagnosed in 10–20% of HIV-positive patients with tuberculosis in Africa.[32,33,75] Radiological features of pulmon-

Table 12.5. Frequency of opportunistic diseases in four groups of African patients with AIDS (after refs 46, 53–55).

	% of AIDS patients with opportunistic disease			
	Uganda	*Tanzania*	*Zaire*	*Africans in Europe*
Candidal oesophagitis	NA	23.5	27	23
P. carinii pneumonia*	NA	NA	17	25
Diarrhoea >1 month:				
with *Cryptosporidium*	NA	NA	6	9
with *Isospora belli*	NA	NA	1	4
Cryptococcosis	NA	NA	5	30
Herpetic ulceration for >1 month	5	7.5	3	25
Cerebral toxoplasmosis	NA	NA	NA	18
Tuberculosis	11	11	13	12
Atypical mycobacterial infection	NA	NA	NA	8
Generalized cytomegalovirus infection	NA	NA	NA	25
Progressive multifocal leucoencephalitis	NA	NA	NA	2
Kaposi's sarcoma	4	13.5	4	21
Lymphoma	NA	0.5	NA	0

NA, not available.
*Bilateral pneumonia of unknown aetiology.

Table 12.6 HIV seroprevalence among patients with tuberculosis.

Country	*Year*	*No. patients studied*	*HIV positive (%)*
Africa			
Burundi	1985–1986	328	55
Ivory Coast	1989–1990	2043	40
Kenya	1990	NA	27
Zaire	1990	1011	20
Zambia	1988–1990	346	60
Asia			
Hong Kong	1985–1991	1548	0
Tamil Nadu, India	1991–1992	278	1
Latin America/Caribbean			
Brazil	1991	1398	3
Haiti	1990	NA	57
Mexico	1991	NA	5

NA, not available.
Source: US Bureau of the Census, 1992.

ary tuberculosis in Africans with HIV infection are usually typical (upper lobe infiltration and/or cavitation or miliary pattern), although atypical patterns are more common in advanced stages of HIV infection. Tuberculous lymph nodes in AIDS patients frequently show no granulomas, due to an inadequate cellular response. Cutaneous anergy to tuberculin has been reported in a wide range of patients with both HIV infection and tuberculosis (20–93%).[32]

In 'standard' 12-month chemotherapy regimens not including rifampicin, both the therapy failure rate and relapse rate are higher in HIV-positive patients than in HIV-negative patients with tuberculosis.[76,77]

Kaposi's sarcoma, an angioproliferative disorder of endothelial origin, is found in 4–15% of African patients with AIDS, as compared with nearly half of American and European homosexual men with AIDS. In contrast to the 'classic' endemic form of Kaposi's sarcoma in Central Africa (see Chapter 24), which is not associated with HIV infection or

Table 12.7. Criteria for epidemic Kaposi's sarcoma, Uganda Cancer Institute (after ref. 69).

1. Oral Kaposi's sarcoma
2. Genital Kaposi's sarcoma
3. Diffuse lymphadenopathy*
4. Disseminated cutaneous Kaposi's sarcoma†
5. Gastrointestinal Kaposi's sarcoma
6. Pulmonary Kaposi's sarcoma

*Enlargement >2 cm at ≥2 extrainguinal sites.
†Involvement of face, trunk, upper and lower extremities.

immunosuppression, it presents as a generalized aggressive disease, with involvement of the skin, lymph nodes and various organs, particularly the pulmonary and gastrointestinal systems. In general, lesions appear as hyperpigmented black plaques on the black skin, and as purple plaques on the white skin. Some lesions may be infiltrative or present as nodules or tumours (ulcerated or not). Lesions may be surrounded by oedema, as in the classical type of Kaposi's sarcoma. They appear on all parts of the body. In the mouth, lesions are mainly found on the hard palate.[69]

Table 12.7 lists locations of Kaposi's sarcoma typical of the HIV-associated epidemic form.

CAUSE OF DEATH

The cause of death in patients with HIV infection in the developing world is not well documented.[68] In a

Table 12.8 Prime cause of death and pathology prevalence among 247 hospitalized patients with HIV infection at Abidjan, Ivory Coast.[72]

Disease	Prime cause of death (%)	Pathology prevalence (%)
Tuberculosis	32	38
Bacteraemia	11	16
Cytomegalovirus	2	18
Cerebral toxoplasmosis	10	15
Pyogenic pneumonia	8	30
Pneumocystis pneumonia	2	3
Kaposi's sarcoma	2	9
Purulent meningitis	5	5
Cryptococcosis	2	3
Non-specific enteritis	3	10
Other causes and undetermined	15	45

large study on a representative sample of patients who died during hospitalization in Abidjan, Ivory Coast, tuberculosis, bacteraemia due to Gram-negative rods and cerebral toxoplasmosis caused 53% of deaths.[72] Tuberculosis was found in half of the cadavers with an AIDS-defining pathology, as compared with only 4% for *P. carinii* pneumonia (Table 12.8). Interestingly, in this population where both HIV-1 and HIV-2 occur, patients with HIV-2 infection had severe cytomegalovirus infection and HIV-associated encephalitis more often than patients with HIV-1 infection, which is compatible with a more prolonged course of disease.

DIAGNOSIS

The diagnosis of AIDS is initially a clinical one, and is based on the identification of an opportunistic infection or a malignancy listed in Table 12.1. Whenever possible the presence of serum antibody to HIV should be demonstrated by a well-evaluated serological test. However, in many developing countries, diagnostic and laboratory facilities may be insufficient to diagnose reliably most opportunistic diseases associated with AIDS. Therefore a clinical case definition of AIDS was developed by WHO (Table 12.9).[78] The specificity and sensitivity of this definition for the diagnosis of HIV infection vary widely, but are generally between 60 and 90% among hospitalized patients.[79–81] Tuberculosis represents one of the major problems in the differential diagnosis using this definition. It should be stressed that criteria were developed as a surveillance tool.

However, the diseases listed in Table 12.1 are often impossible to diagnose in the absence of sophisticated laboratory support, and therefore the clinical definition for surveillance can be a useful tool in many areas.

HIV antibody detection offers the most satisfactory approach to the laboratory diagnosis of HIV infection. Serological tests are used for confirming a clinical diagnosis, for screening blood and for epidemiologic surveys.

An enzyme linked immunosorbent assay (ELISA) is most commonly used as an initial test for the demonstration of HIV antibody, but more rapid and simpler tests are also used, including gelatin particle agglutination, passive haemagglutination and dot immunoassays. The sensitivity and specificity of most commercially available tests are over

Table 12.9 WHO clinical case definition of AIDS where diagnostic resources are limited.[78] (Definition developed at WHO Workshop on AIDS at Bangui, Central African Republic.)

Adults
AIDS in an adult is defined by the existence of at least two of the major signs associated with at least one minor sign, in the absence of known causes of immunosuppression such as cancer or severe malnutrition or other recognized aetiologies.
1. Major signs
   (a) Weight loss >10% of body weight
   (b) Chronic diarrhoea >1 month
   (c) Prolonged fever >1 month (intermittent or constant).
2. Minor signs
   (a) Persistent cough for >1 month
   (b) Generalized pruritic dermatitis
   (c) Recurrent varicella zoster
   (d) Oropharyngeal candidiasis
   (e) Chronic progressive and disseminated herpes simplex infection
   (f) Generalized lymphadenopathy.
The presence of generalized Kaposi's sarcoma or cryptococcal meningitis are sufficient by themselves for the diagnosis of AIDS.

Children
Paediatric AIDS is suspected in an infant or child presenting with at least two major signs associated with at least two minor signs in the absence of known causes of immunosuppression.
1. Major signs
   (a) Weight loss or abnormally slow growth
   (b) Chronic diarrhoea >1 month
   (c) Prolonged fever >1 month.
2. Minor signs
   (a) Generalized lymphadenopathy
   (b) Oropharyngeal candidiasis
   (c) Repeated common infection(s) (otitis, pharyngitis, etc.)
   (d) Persistent cough
   (e) Generalized dermatitis
   (f) Confirmed maternal HIV infection.

98%. WHO regularly publishes operational characteristics of available serological tests.[82]

WHO RECOMMENDATIONS FOR HIV TESTING STRATEGIES

WHO[83] recommends three testing strategies to maximize accuracy while minimizing cost. Which strategy is most appropriate will depend on the objective of the test and the prevalence of HIV in the population, as shown in Table 12.10. Selected tests can be purchased at reduced prices through WHO.

STRATEGY I

All serum samples are tested with one ELISA or rapid/simple assay. Serum that is reactive is considered HIV antibody positive. Serum that is non-reactive is considered HIV antibody negative.

STRATEGY II

All serum samples are first tested with one ELISA or rapid/simple assay. Any serum found reactive on the first assay is retested with a second ELISA or rapid/simple assay based on a different antigen preparation and/or different test principle (e.g. indirect versus competitive). Serum that is reactive on both tests is considered HIV antibody positive. Serum that is non-reactive on the first test is considered HIV antibody negative. Any serum that is reactive on the first test but non-reactive on the second test is also considered antibody negative.

STRATEGY III

As in strategy II, all samples are first tested with one ELISA or rapid/simple assay, and any reactive samples are retested using a different assay. Strategy III, however, requires a third test if serum is found reactive on the second assay. The three tests in this strategy should be based on different antigen preparations and/or different test principles. Serum reactive at all three tests is considered HIV antibody positive; serum that is non-reactive on the first test is considered HIV antibody negative, as is serum that is reactive in the first test but non-reactive in the second. Serum that is reactive in the first and second tests but non-reactive in the third test is considered to be equivocal (see Equivocal (Borderline) Test Results below for further details).

In the selection of the HIV antibody test for use in strategies II and III, the first test should have the highest sensitivity, whereas the second and third tests should have higher specificities than the first.

When diagnosis is the objective, an additional blood sample should be obtained and tested from all persons newly diagnosed as seropositive on the basis of the first sample. This will help eliminate any possible laboratory or clerical error.

For all three strategies, it is most important that quality assurance procedures be stringently complied with so as to maximize the accuracy of the

Table 12.10 WHO recommendations for HIV testing strategies according to test objective and prevalence of infection in the population.

Objective of testing	Prevalence of infection	Testing strategy
Transfusion/donation safety	All prevalences	I
Surveillance	>10%	I
	≤10%	II
Diagnosis		
Clinical signs/symptoms of HIV infection/AIDS	All prevalences	II
Asymptomatic patients	>10%	II
	≤10%	III

Strategy I: All samples are tested with one ELISA or rapid/simple test (hereafter referred to as test).

Strategy II: All samples are first tested with one test. Any reactive samples are subjected to a second test based on a different principle and/or a different antigen preparation.

Strategy III: All samples are first tested with one test. Any reactive samples are retested with a different test. Samples found reactive by the second test are subjected to a third and different test.

laboratory results. Procedures for detecting both laboratory and clerical errors must be included in all protocols. For example, procedures that guarantee the correct identification of initially reactive units of donated blood—which must be discarded, are essential to the maintenance of a safe blood supply.

Any positive test results obtained with testing strategy I must not be used for purposes of diagnosis of HIV infection in an individual. If a blood or tissue donor is to be notified of test results, the testing strategies for diagnosis must be used (Table 12.10). Guidelines for counselling persons regarding HIV testing, infection and disease are available from WHO.

Users should note that differentiation between HIV-1 and HIV-2 infections cannot always be achieved with the currently available antibody tests, even when the two types (HIV-1 and HIV-2) of Western blot are used. WHO is currently undertaking studies aimed at the development of evaluation of testing strategies for differentiation using ELISA and/or rapid/simple assays.

EQUIVOCAL (BORDERLINE) TEST RESULTS

Serum from persons being tested for the purpose of diagnosis should be retested if the results are equivocal, that is neither clearly positive nor clearly negative. If the serum again produces equivocal results, testing with western blot may be considered, especially for persons from low-prevalence (<1%) populations. A second blood sample should be obtained after a minimum of 2 weeks following the first sample and both should be retested using the appropriate strategy. If the second serum sample also produces an equivocal result, the person is considered to be HIV antibody negative.

Equivocal results obtained for surveillance should be reported and analysed separately.

Units of donated blood yielding equivocal test results must be discarded, as must units found reactive.

MANAGEMENT

The management of patients with HIV infection and AIDS represents one of the most complex issues that health care workers have to deal with. In addition to complicated diagnostic and therapeutic problems, clinicians and relatives and friends have to assure psychological and social support. It is essential that clinical follow-up is organized in collaboration with community-based initiatives.

WHO and many countries have published guidelines for standardized case management.[84] These are usually based on a syndromic approach using flow charts.

As specific antiretroviral therapy with zidovudine or other nucleoside analogues is rarely available or is too expensive, and as several opportunistic diseases are difficult to diagnose (e.g. cerebral toxoplasmosis) or not treatable with essential drugs (e.g. cytomegalovirus infection), the major aim of man-

Table 12.11 Therapy for opportunistic infections in AIDS patients.

Infection	Drug	Usual daily adult dose	No. of doses	Route	Minimum duration*
Pneumocystis pneumonia	Trimethoprim–sulphamethoxazole	15–20 mg/kg trimethoprim *with* 75–100 mg/kg sulphamethoxazole	3 times a day	Intravenous	21 days
	or pentamidine isethionate	4 mg/kg	Once a day	Intravenous	21 days
Maintenance therapy	Trimethoprim–sulphamethoxazole	160 mg trimethoprim *with* 800 mg sulphamethoxazole	Once a day	Oral	For life
	or Dapsone	100 mg	Twice a week	Oral	For life
	or Pentamidine	300 mg	Every 4 weeks	Aerosol	For life
Toxoplasmosis	Pyrimethamine	75 mg once, then 25–50 mg	Once a day	Oral	28 days
	and Sulphadiazine	4–6 g	Once a day	Oral	28 days
	and Calcium folinate	15 mg	3 times a week	Oral Intravenous	
Maintenance therapy	Pyrimethamine	25 mg		Oral	For life
	and Sulphadiazine	2 g	3–5 times a week	Oral	For life
Cryptosporidiosis	No drug known to be effective				
Isospora belli	Trimethoprim–sulphamethoxazole	160 mg trimethoprim	4 times a day *then*	Oral	10 days
		800 mg sulphamethoxazole	twice a day		21 days
Oral candidiasis	Gentian violet (1% aqueous solution)		4 times a day	Local application	7–10 days
	or Nystatin	500 000 units	4 times a day	Oral	7–10 days
	or Ketoconazole	200–400 mg	Once a day	Oral	7–10 days
Candida oesophagitis	Ketoconazole	400 mg	Once a day	Oral	7–10 days
Cryptococcosis	Amphotericin B	0.3 mg/kg	Once a day	Intravenous	42 days
	and Flucytosine	150 mg/kg	4 times a day	Oral	42 days
	or Amphotericin B	0.5–0.6 mg/kg	Once a day	Intravenous	
Maintenance therapy†	Amphotericin B	1 mg/kg	Once a week	Intravenous	For life
	or Fluconazole	200 mg	Once a day	Oral	For life
Herpesvirus infection	Acyclovir	5–10 mg/kg	3 times a day	Intravenous	7 days
		200 mg	5 times a day	Oral	7 days
Zoster	Acyclovir	10 mg/kg	3 times a day	Intravenous	7 days
		800 mg	3 times a day	Oral	7 days
Cytomegalovirus infection	Acyclovir	5 mg/kg	Twice a day	Intravenous	14–21 days
Maintenance therapy	Acyclovir	5 mg/kg	Once a day	Intravenous	For life
Atypical mycobacterial infection	No drug known to be effective				
Tuberculosis	Standard antituberculosis treatment (avoiding thiacetazone)				

*Optimal duration of therapy in AIDS patients is not well established.
†For at least 6 months after culture conversion.

agement of AIDS patients is to reduce suffering from conditions caused by HIV infection itself and by common opportunistic diseases.

Table 12.11 lists therapeutic regimens for infectious diseases in AIDS patients in case such drugs are available. Primary chemoprophylaxis of tuberculosis is a promising preventive intervention but requires operational evaluation as to its feasibility and cost-effectiveness.

The management of patients with AIDS requires no special facilities or quarantine, except for patients with tuberculosis, who may be highly contagious. However, contact with mucosal surfaces, blood and other secretions and excretions of such patients should be avoided by wearing gloves when drawing blood or examining mucous membranes. In general, gloves should always be used when assisting in delivery or performing invasive procedures because in some populations a considerable proportion of women are infected with HIV. Finally, taking care of AIDS patients may be a heavy psychological burden for health workers, as well as for their families. Hospital personnel should be thoroughly informed on HIV infection and patient management.

PREVENTION

Since no effective therapy or vaccine is available, control of AIDS is of necessity based on prevention. The latter is complicated by social, economic and political constraints in many developing countries. The prevention of sexual transmission of HIV infection is based on a reduction in the number of sex partners, the use of condoms and the early treatment of bacterial sexually transmitted diseases.

Transmission through blood transfusions can be drastically reduced by screening blood donors for HIV antibody. Disposable or properly sterilized needles and syringes should be used (and the number of injections given should be reduced). Interruption of perinatal transmission may be achieved by the prevention of HIV infection in girls and in women of childbearing age and counselling on contraception for HIV-seropositive women. All these measures require a substantial financial and organizational effort, which is increasingly being taken up by national AIDS control programmes.

AIDS and HIV infection now clearly represent one of the most dramatic challenges to the public health system in many developing countries. Unless control programmes are successful, HIV infection will have a growing negative impact on health and health care services in Africa and other areas of the developing world.

REFERENCES

1 Gottlieb M S, Schroff R, Schanker H M et al. *Pneumocystis carinii* pneumonia and mucosal candidiasis in previously healthy homosexual men. *N Engl J Med* 1981; 305:1425–1431.

2 World Health Organization. *The HIV/AIDS Pandemic: 1993 Overview*. WHO/GPA/CNP/EV A/93.1. Geneva: WHO, 1993.

3 World Bank. *World Development Report 1993. Investing in Health*. New York: Oxford University Press, 1993.

4 De Cock K M, Barrere B, Diaby L et al. AIDS: the leading cause of adult death in the West African city of Abidjan, Ivory Coast. *Science* 1990; 249:793–796.

5 Hassig S E, Perriëns J, Baende E et al. An analysis of the economic impact of HIV infection among patients at Mama Yemo Hospital, Kinshasa, Zaire. *AIDS* 1990; 4:883–887.

6 Mulder D W, Nunn A J, Wagner H-U, Kamali A & Kengeya-Kayondo J F. HIV-1 incidence and HIV-1 associated mortality in a rural Ugandan population cohort. *AIDS* 1994; 8:87–92.

7 Nkowane B M. Prevalence and incidence of HIV infection in Africa: a review of data published in 1990. *AIDS* 1991; 5 (supplement 1): S7–S16.

8 United States Bureau of the Census, Center for International Research. *AIDS/HIV Surveillance Database*. Washington, DC: Bureau of the Census, 1993.

9 Piot P, Plummer F A, Rey M-A et al. Retrospective epidemiology of AIDS virus infection in Nairobi populations. *J Infect Dis* 1987; 155:1108–1112.

10 Temmerman M, Mohammed Ali F, Ndinya-Achola J O, Moses S, Plummer F A & Piot P. Rapid increase of both HIV infection and syphilis among pregnant women in Nairobi, Kenya. *AIDS* 1992; 6:1181–1185.

11 Dallabetta G A, Miotti P G, Chiphangur J D et al. High socio-economic status is a risk factor for human immunodeficiency virus type 1 (HIV-1) infection but not for sexually transmitted diseases in women in Malawi: implications for HIV-1 control. *J Infect Dis* 1993; 167:36–42.

12 Allen S, Lindan C, Serufila A et al. Human immunodeficiency virus infection in urban Rwanda: demographic and behavioural correlates in a representative sample of child bearing women. *JAMA* 1991; 226:1657–1663.

13 Ngugi E N, Plummer F A, Simonsen J N et al. Prevention of HIV transmission in Africa: the effectiveness of condom promotion and health

education among high-risk prostitutes. *Lancet* 1988; ii:887–890.

14 Anderson R M, May R M, Boily M C, Garnett G P & Rowley J T. The spread of HIV-1 in Africa: sexual contact patterns and the predicted demographic impact of AIDS. *Nature* 1991; 352:581–589.

15 De Cock K M, Brun-Vézinet F & Soro B. HIV-1 and HIV-2 infections and AIDS in West Africa. *AIDS* 1991; 5 (supplement 1): S21–S28.

16 Hospedales J, White F, Gayle C, Newton E, Francis C & Poumerol G. Epidemiology of HIV/AIDS in the Caribbean. In Lamptey P, White F, Figueroa J P & Gingle R (eds) *The Handbook for AIDS Prevention in the Caribbean*. Research Triangle Park, NC: Family Health International, 1992: 1–23.

17 Pan American Health Organization/World Health Organization. *1990 AIDS/HIV/STD Annual Surveillance Report*. Washington, DC: PAHO/WHO, 1991.

18 Li P C K & Yeoh E K. Current epidemiological trends of HIV infection in Asia. In Volberding P & Jacobson M A (eds) *AIDS Clinical Review 1992*. New York: Marcel Dekker, 1992: 1–24.

19 Weniger B G, Limpakarnjanarat K, Ungchusok K et al. The epidemiology of HIV infection and AIDS in Thailand. *AIDS* 1991; 5 (supplement 2): S71–S85.

20 Nopkesorn T, Mastro T D, Sangkharomya S et al. HIV-1 infection in young men in Northern Thailand. *AIDS* 1993; 7:1233–1240.

21 Johnson A M & Laga M. Heterosexual transmission of HIV. *AIDS* 1988; 2 (supplement 1): S49–S56.

22 Wasserheit J N. Epidemiological synergy: inter-relationships between HIV infection and other STDs. *Sex Transm Dis* 1992; 19:61–77.

23 Laga M, Nzila N & Goeman J. The interrelationship of sexually transmitted diseases and HIV infection: implications for the control of both epidemics in Africa. *AIDS* 1991; 5 (supplement 1): S55–S64.

24 Cameron D W, Simonsen J D, D'Costa L J et al. Female-to-male transmission of human immunodeficiency virus type 1: risk factors for seroconversion in men. *Lancet* 1989; ii:401–407.

25 Laga M, Manoka A T, Kivuvu M et al. Non-ulcerative sexually transmitted diseases as risk factors for HIV-1 transmission in women: results from a cohort study. *AIDS* 1993; 7:95–102.

26 Dunn D T, Newell M L, Ades A E & Peckham C S. Risk of human immunodeficiency virus type 1 transmission through breast feeding. *Lancet* 1992; 340:585–587.

27 Newell M L, Peckham C S & Lepage P. HIV infection in pregnancy: implications for women and children. *AIDS* 1990; 4(supplement:)S111–S117.

28 Ryder R W & Temmerman M. The effect of HIV-1 infections during pregnancy and the perinatal period on maternal and child health in Africa. *AIDS* 1991; 5 (supplement 1): S75–S86.

29 Jäger H, Jersild C & Emmanuel J C. Safe blood transfusions in Africa. *AIDS* 1991; 5 (supplement 1): S163–S169.

30 Berkley S. Parenteral transmission of HIV in Africa. *AIDS* 1991; 5 (supplement 1): S87–S92.

31 Piot P, Laga M, Ryder R W et al. The global epidemiology of HIV infection: continuity, heterogeneity, and change. *J Acquir Immune Defic Syndr* 1990; 3:403–412.

32 Perriëns J H, Mukadi Y & Nunn P. Tuberculosis and HIV infection: implications for Africa. *AIDS* 1991; 5 (supplement 1): S127–S133.

33 De Cock K M, Soro B, Coulibaly I M & Lucas S B. Tuberculosis and HIV infection in sub-Saharan Africa. *JAMA* 1992; 268:1581–1587.

34 Anderson R M, May R & McLean A R. Possible demographic consequences of AIDS in developing countries. *Nature* 1988; 332:228–234.

35 Barnett T & Blaikie P. *AIDS in Africa: its present and future impact*. London: Bellhaven Press, 1992.

36 Over M & Piot P. *HIV Infection and Sexually Transmitted Diseases*. Washington, DC: World Bank, 1991.

37 Barré-Sinoussi F, Chermann J C, Rey F et al. Isolation of a T-lymphotropic retrovirus from a patient at risk for acquired immunodeficiency syndrome (AIDS). *Science* 1983; 220:868–871.

38 Popovic M, Sarngadharan M G, Read E & Gallo R C. Detection, isolation and continuous production of cytopathic viruses (HTLV-III) from patients with AIDS and pre-AIDS. *Science* 1984; 224:497–500.

39 Louwagie J, McCutchan F E, Peeters M et al. Phylogenetic analysis of 70 international HIV-1 isolates provides evidence for multiple genetic subgroups. *AIDS* 1993; 7:769–780.

40 Meyers G, Korber B, Berzofsky J A, Smith T F & Pavlakis G N (eds). *Human Retroviruses and AIDS*. Los Alamos: Los Alamos National Laboratory, 1992.

41 Peeters M, Piot P & van der Groen G. Variability among HIV and SIV strains of African origin. *AIDS* 1991; 5 (supplement 1): S29–S36.

42 Levy J A. Pathogenesis of human immunodeficiency virus infection. *Microbiol Rev* 1993; 57:183–289.

43 Weiss R A. How does HIV cause AIDS? *Science* 1993; 260:1273–1278.

44 Pantaleo G, Graziosi C & Fauci A S. The immunopathogenesis of human immunodeficiency virus infection. *N Engl J Med* 1993; 328:327–335.

45 Piot P, Kapita B M, Ngugi E N, Mann J M, Colebunders R & Wabitsch R. *AIDS in Africa. A Manual for Physicians*. Geneva: W H Organization, 1992.

46 Colebunders R L & Latif A S. Natural history and clinical presentation of HIV-1 infection in adults. *AIDS* 1991; 5 (supplement 1): S103–S112.

47 Goodgame R W. AIDS in Uganda: clinical and social features. *N Engl J Med* 1990; 323:383–389.

48 Colebunders R L, Ryder R W, Francis H et al. Seroconversion rate, mortality and clinical manifestations associated with the receipt of an human immunodeficiency virus infected blood transfusion. *J Infect Dis* 1991; 164:450–456.

49 N'Galy B, Ryder R W, Kapita B et al. Human

immunodeficiency virus infection among employees in an African hospital. *N Engl J Med* 1988; 319:1123–1127.

50 Anzala A, Wambugu P, Plummer F A et al. Incubation time to symptomatic disease and AIDS in women with known duration of infection. *VII International Conference on AIDS*, Florence, June 1991. Abstract TUC 103.

51 Mulder D, Kamali A, Nakyinge J, Nunn A J, Wagner H V & Kengeya-Kayondo J F. HIV-1 associated mortality in a rural Ugandan cohort: result at two year follow-up (14193 person years). *IX International Conference on AIDS*, Berlin, June 1993. Abstract WS-CO3-6.

52 Pape J W, Jean S S, Ho J L, Hagner A & Johnson W D Jr. Effect of isoniazid prophylaxis on incidence of active tuberculosis and progression of HIV infection. *Lancet* 1993; 342:268–272.

53 Berkley S F, Okware S & Namaara W. Surveillance for AIDS in Uganda. *AIDS* 1989; 3:79–85.

54 Howlett W P, Nkya W M, Mmuni K A & Missalek W R. Neurologic disorders in AIDS and HIV disease in the northern zone of Tanzania. *AIDS* 1989; 3:289–296.

55 Colebunders R, Mann J, Francis H et al. La clinique du SIDA en Afrique. *Méd Mal Infect* 1986; 15:350–355.

56 Colebunders R, Mann J M, Francis H et al. Generalized papular pruritic eruption in African patients with human immunodeficiency virus infection. *AIDS* 1987; 1:117–121.

57 Hira S K, Wadhawan D, Kamanga J et al. Cutaneous manifestations of human immunodeficiency virus in Lusaka, Zambia. *J Am Acad Dermatol* 1988; 19:451–457.

58 Colebunders R, Ryder R W, Nzila N et al. HIV infection in patients with tuberculosis in Kinshasa, Zaïre. *Am Rev Respir Dis* 1989; 139:1082–1085.

59 Nunn P, Kibuga D, Gathua S et al. Cutaneous hyper-sensitivity reactions due to thiacetazone in HIV-1-seropositive patients treated for tuberculosis. *Lancet* 1991; 337:627–630.

60 Serwadda D, Mugerwa R D, Sewankambo N K et al. Skin disease: a new disease in Uganda and its association with HTLV-III infection. *Lancet* 1985; ii:849–852.

61 Colebunders R, Lusakumunu K, Nelson A M et al. Persistent diarrhoea in Zairian AIDS patients: an endoscopic and histological study. *Gut* 1988; 29:1687–1691.

62 Gilks C F, Ojoo S A & Brindle R J. Non-opportunistic bacterial infections in HIV-seropositive adults in Nairobi, Kenya. *AIDS* 1993; 5 (supplement 1): S113–S116.

63 Gilks C F, Brindle R J, Otieno L S et al. Life-threatening bacteraemia in HIV-1 seropositive adults admitted to hospital in Nairobi, Kenya. *Lancet* 1990; 336:545–549.

64 Lepage P & Hitimana D-G. Natural history and clinical presentation of HIV-1 infection in children. *AIDS* 1991; 5 (supplement 1): S117–S125.

65 Ryder R W, Nsa W, Hassig S E et al. Perinatal transmission of the human immunodeficiency virus type 1 to infants of seropositive women in Zaire. *N Engl J Med* 1989; 320:1637–1642.

66 Lallemant M, Lallemant-Le Coeur S, Cheynier D et al. Mother–child transmission of HIV-1 and infant survival in Brazzaville, Congo. *AIDS* 1989; 3:643–646.

67 Mbaga J M, Pallangyo K J, Bakari M & Aris E A. Survival time of patients with acquired immunodeficiency syndrome: experience with 274 patients in Dar-es-Salaam. *East Afr Med J* 1990; 3:55–61.

68 Lucas S B, Odida M & Wabinga H. The pathology of severe morbidity and mortality due to HIV infection in Africa. *AIDS* 1991; 5 (supplement 1): S143–S148.

69 Desmond-Hellmann S D & Katongole-Mbidde E. Kaposi's sarcoma: recent developments. *AIDS* 1991; 5 (supplement 1): S135–S142.

70 Taelman H, Bogaerts J, Batungwanayo J et al. Community acquired bacteraemia, fungaemia and parasitaemia in febrile adults infected with HIV in Central Africa. *V International Conference on AIDS in Africa*, Kinshasa, October 1990. Abstract FOD1.

71 Sirisanthana F. Mycotic infections in patients infected with HIV. *IX International Conference on AIDS*, Berlin, June 1993. Abstract PS-07-2.

72 Lucas S B, Hounnou A, Peacock C et al. The mortality and pathology of HIV infection in a West African city. *AIDS* 1994; 7:1569–1579.

73 Murray C J L, Styblo K & Rouillon A. Tuberculosis in developing countries: burden, intervention and cost. *Bull Int Union Tuberc Lung Dis* 1990; 65:6–24.

74 Mukadi Y, Perriëns J H, St Louis M E et al. Spectrum of immunodeficiency in HIV-1 infected patients with pulmonary tuberculosis in Zaire. *Lancet* 1993; 342:143–146.

75 Elliott A M, Luo M, Tembo G et al. Impact of HIV on tuberculosis in Africa: a cross-sectional study. *BMJ* 1990; 301:412–415.

76 Perriëns J H, Colebunders R L, Karahunga C et al. Increased mortality and tuberculosis treatment failure rate among HIV-seropositive compared with HIV-seronegative patients with pulmonary tuberculosis treated with 'standard' chemotherapy in Kinshasa, Zaïre. *Am Rev Respir Dis* 1991; 144:750–755.

77 Hawken M, Nunn P, Gathua S et al. Increased recurrence of tuberculosis in HIV-1 infected patients. *Lancet* 1993; 342:332–336.

78 World Health Organization. Provisional WHO clinical case definition for AIDS. *Weekly Epidemiol Rec* 1986; 61:69–73.

79 Colebunders R, Mann J M, Francis H et al. Evaluation of a clinical case definition of acquired immunodeficiency syndrome in Africa. *Lancet* 1987; i:492–494.

80 Widy-Wirsky R, Berkley S, Downing R et al. Evaluation of the WHO clinical case definition for AIDS in Uganda. *JAMA* 1988; 260:3286–3289.

81 Katabira E T & Wabitsch R. Management issues for patients with HIV infection in Africa. *AIDS* 1991; 5 (supplement 1): S149–S155.

82 World Health Organization. *Operational Characteristics of Commercially Available Assays to Determine Antibodies to HIV-1 and/or HIV-2 in Human Sera*. Geneva: WHO, 1992.

83 World Health Organization. Global programme on AIDS—Recommendations for the selection and use of HIV antibody tests. *Weekly Epidemiol Rec* 1992; 20:145–149.

84 World Health Organization. *Guidelines for the Clinical Management of HIV Infection in Adults*. WHO/GPA/IDS/HCS/91.6. Geneva: WHO, 1991.

CHAPTER 13

SEXUALLY TRANSMITTED DISEASES (EXCLUDING HIV)

David Mabey and John Richens

Sexually transmitted diseases (STDs) are among the most common reasons for seeking medical care in developing countries, accounting for 10% or more of medical consultations in some parts of Africa.[1] Nevertheless, and in spite of their serious consequences (particularly for women and children), and increasing evidence that they may facilitate the transmission of human immunodeficiency virus (HIV) through heterosexual contact, they have often been accorded low priority by medical professionals and health planners. The consequent lack of good facilities for their management has led many patients with these conditions to seek treatment outside the formal health sector, with inadequate treatment regimens leading to increasing antimicrobial resistance among sexually transmitted pathogens. Because no statistics are available for patients treated outside the formal health sector, the extent of the problem continues to be underestimated.

EPIDEMIOLOGY

Certain broad generalizations can be made about the epidemiology of STDs. Clearly they are diseases of the sexually active, although mother-to-child transmission also occurs. None of the sexually transmitted agents described in this chapter has an epidemiologically significant non-human reservoir. They are more common among young adults, among single people of both sexes, and among those who travel. Although no sexually active individual is immune, certain groups can be identified whose behaviour places them at higher risk than others. Such groups include commercial sex workers and their clients, bar workers, the military, truck drivers and sailors.

Accurate STD prevalence figures are not available for any developing country, but studies in Swaziland and Uganda have estimated the incidence of gonorrhoea to be 3000 and 15 000 respectively per 100 000 total population per annum.[2] For comparison, the annual incidence of gonorrhoea in England and Wales is less than 100 per 100 000.

The prevalence of certain STDs among antenatal clinic attenders in a variety of developing countries is shown in Table 13.1. This group is considered to

Table 13.1 Prevalence of STDs among antenatal clinic attenders in developing countries.

Country	Neisseria gonorrhoeae (%)	Chlamydia trachomatis (%)	Treponema pallidum (%)	Trichomonas vaginalis (%)
Gambia[3]	6.7	6.9	1	32
Kenya[4]	6.6	10.0	—	—
Swaziland[5]	3.9	—	14	23
Zambia[6]	11.2	—	12.5	38
Nigeria[7]	3.4	—	0.5	21
Ghana[8]	3.4	7.7	—	—

Table 13.2 Factors contributing to the high incidence of STDs in developing countries.

1. Demographic factors (high proportion of population are young adults)
2. Rural–urban migration with breakdown of traditional customs
3. Prostitution
4. Lack of adequate medical services
5. High prevalence of antibiotic-resistant strains of *Neisseria gonorrhoeae*, *Haemophilus ducreyi*.
6. Polygamy

be representative of the general sexually active population, although there is a paucity of studies among rural populations, and gives an estimate of the likely public health importance of congenitally acquired STDs. Table 13.2 shows a number of factors which may explain the higher incidence and prevalence of STDs in developing compared with industrialized countries. Females who sell sex are a major reservoir of infection in developing countries.[9]

The relative importance of certain STDs is much greater in developing countries. For example chancroid remains the most common cause of genital ulceration in many African countries but has almost disappeared from Europe. Sporadic outbreaks among impoverished communities in North America in the 1980s suggest that this has more to do with socioeconomic factors than with climate. Donovanosis (granuloma inguinale) is highly prevalent in certain parts of Papua New Guinea, south-east India and South Africa but appears to be rare outside these areas. The lack of reliable and cheap diagnostic tests for the three classical 'tropical STDs', chancroid, donovanosis and lymphogranuloma venereum (LGV) has hindered attempts to study their epidemiology.

Because of the lack of adequate diagnostic and treatment facilities for STDs in many developing countries, complications are commonly seen, particularly among women and children. Pelvic inflammatory disease (PID), due in the majority of cases to gonorrhoea or chlamydial infection, is the most common cause of admission to gynaecology wards in Africa.[10] Ectopic pregnancy as a sequela of PID is up to three times as common in Africa as in Europe, and tubal infertility, another common sequela, is widespread, with up to 20% of women affected in some regions of Africa.[3,11] The incidence of carcinoma of the cervix is extremely high in many developing countries. Of infants born in many African cities, 2–3% develop gonococcal ophthalmia neonatorum, and congenital syphilis is the major cause of hospital admission among infants aged less than 3 months in Lusaka, Zambia.[12,13]

Table 13.3 lists organisms transmissible by sexual contact and the diseases they cause. In this chapter only those responsible for major morbidity in developing countries will be considered further.

HISTORY-TAKING AND EXAMINATION IN THE STD CLINIC

It is not possible to provide a good clinical service for STDs unless one gains the confidence of the patient(s). This requires *privacy* and the *avoidance of a moralistic attitude*.

It is usually possible to take a history and examine a patient with an STD in 10 minutes. When taking a *history*, the following information should be collected, in addition to name, occupation, address and date of birth.

1. The nature and duration of the symptoms.
2. The nature of any treatment already taken for this condition.
3. A sexual history, which should include marital status and the nature and frequency of recent sexual contacts with regular or casual partners.

This information is essential in order to attempt contact tracing and/or partner notification.
4. Past medical history.
5. In female patients a menstrual and obstetric history should be taken.

During any interview with an STD patient it is the duty of the clinician to advise the patient of the dangers implicit in recent sexual behaviour, in particular the risk of acquiring HIV infection, and to counsel the patient concerning the reduction of high-risk sexual activity.

The *examination* should be carried out in private in a good light. After examination of the mouth and palms, patients should be stripped from the umbilicus to the knees. The skin of the abdomen, groins and perineum should be examined in particular for

Table 13.3 Sexually transmitted diseases in humans.

	Agent	Disease
STDs producing genital lesions		
Viruses	Herpes simplex virus	Genital herpes, disseminated and neonatal herpes infection
	Human papilloma virus	Genital warts, juvenile laryngeal papillomatosis, squamous carcinoma in anogenital area
	Molluscum contagiosum virus	Molluscum contagiosum
Bacteria	*Neisseria gonorrhoeae*	Gonococcal infections of urethritis, epididymis, pharynx, rectum, conjunctiva, upper genital tract of women, disseminated gonorrhoeal infection
	Chlamydia trachomatis, serotypes D–K	As for gonorrhoea, except for disseminated infection; also infantile pneumonia and reactive arthritis
	Chlamydia trachomatis, L1,2,3 serotypes	Lymphogranuloma venereum
	Ureaplasma urealyticum	Non-gonococcal urethritis
	Mycoplasma hominis	Salpingitis, postpartum fever
	Haemophilus ducreyi	Chancroid
	Treponema pallidum	Syphilis
	Gardnerella vaginalis and anaerobes	Bacterial vaginosis
	Calymmatobacterium granulomatis	Donovanosis (granuloma inguinale)
Fungi	*Candida albicans*	Genital candidiasis
Protozoa	*Trichomonas vaginalis*	Trichomoniasis
Arthropods	*Phthirus pubis*	Pediculosis
	Sarcoptes scabiei	Scabies
Infections which can be sexually transmitted but which do not generally produce genital lesions		
Viruses	Hepatitis viruses	Hepatitis A–D
	Cytomegalovirus (CMV)	CMV infections of newborn and immunosuppressed
	HIV	Acquired immune deficiency syndrome
	HTLV-1	Tropical spastic paraparesis, T-cell leukaemia/ lymphoma
Bacteria	*Shigella* spp.	Shigellosis
	Campylobacter spp.	Campylobacter enteritis
	Salmonella spp.	Salmonellosis
	Group B streptococcus	Neonatal sepsis
Protozoa	*Giardia lamblia*	Giardiasis
	Cryptosporidium spp.	Cryptosporidiosis
	Entamoeba histolytica	Amoebiasis*
Helminths	*Enterobius vermicularis*	Enterobiasis
	Strongyloides stercoralis	Strongyloidiasis
	Trichuris trichiura	Trichuriasis

* Occasionally produces anogenital ulceration in tropical countries.

evidence of scabies and pediculosis, and the inguinal glands palpated. In males the penis should be inspected, after retraction of the foreskin in uncircumcised patients. If a urethral discharge is not apparent, evidence of urethritis can be sought by milking the urethra forward and examining the meatus for discharge. The scrotum should be palpated for evidence of epididymitis. Female patients should be examined in the lithotomy position. The lower abdomen should be palpated for evidence of PID (masses and/or tenderness) and, after inspection of the vulva, a vaginal speculum should be passed. The cervix should be examined and the speculum then slowly withdrawn while the walls of the vagina are examined. Bimanual examination should then be performed to identify pelvic masses and/or tenderness. The presence of pain on moving the cervix (cervical excitation tenderness) suggests the presence of PID. In both sexes the perianal skin should also be inspected and if receptive anal intercourse is suspected, proctoscopy should be performed.

The *laboratory investigations* requested will depend on the facilities available. In general they should be selected on the principle that a patient with one STD is also at increased risk of other STDs; that is, they should not be limited to tests designed to identify the cause of the present symptoms. All patients with an STD should be screened for syphilis. Whether they should also be screened for HIV depends on the availability of counselling and of treatment for those found to be positive.

DISEASES CAUSING A GENITAL DISCHARGE

URETHRAL DISCHARGE IN MALES

Urethritis in males is either gonococcal, non-gonococcal or of mixed aetiology; the presence of gonococci is easily demonstrated by Gram stain. In most developing countries the majority of cases presenting to hospital are gonococcal. Up to 50% of cases of non-gonococcal urethritis are due to *Chlamydia trachomatis*; a proportion of the remaining cases are associated with *Ureaplasma* or *Mycoplasma* species, and a small percentage may harbour *Trichomonas vaginalis*. Because coinfections with *Neisseria gonorrhoeae* and *C. trachomatis* are common, it is generally advisable to treat cases of gonorrhoea for both gonorrhoea and chlamydial infection when follow-up cannot be guaranteed.

GONORRHOEA

Gonorrhoea is the most prevalent bacterial STD in the tropics. The causative organism, *N. gonorrhoeae*, a Gram-negative oval diplococcus found only in man, is especially adept at colonizing the epithelial surfaces of the male and female urogenital tract, conjunctiva, pharynx, rectum and synovium.

Pathogenesis

Virulence is conferred by the presence of pili which mediate adherence, sufficient to withstand hydrodynamic forces within the urethra, and which also inhibit uptake by phagocytes. Invasion and multiplication has been demonstrated in mucus-secreting non-ciliated cells of the fallopian tubes. No specific toxins produced by *N. gonorrhoeae* have been identified but the lipo-oligosaccharide and peptidoglycan components have been implicated in inhibition of ciliary function and the genesis of synovitis respectively. *N. gonorrhoeae* is highly adept at avoiding the host immune response. The pilus antigens, the protein designated P.II and the lipo-oligosaccharide are all capable of antigenic variation sufficient to permit repeated reinfection of the same host within a short period. In recent studies from Nairobi it was shown that the mean time to reinfection among a group of prostitutes was 12 days.[9] Antibodies to the P.III protein do not fix complement and can block bactericidal, complement-fixing antibodies to the lipo-oligosaccharide. The bacteria produce an IgA_1 protease which may impair the host mucosal immune response. The mucosal immune response to infection is characterized by the production of IgA, IgM and IgE which can inhibit adherence and facilitates opsonization. These responses have been demonstrated in both infected and non-infected, exposed contacts of infected individuals. Strains responsible for disseminated gonococcal infection have been shown to be less susceptible to killing by human serum, are less chemotactic to neutrophils and elicit greater amounts of blocking antibody.

Clinical features

The risk of contracting gonorrhoea after a single exposure is about 20% for males and probably much higher for females. Most men develop symptoms after a 2–5-day incubation period and 90% will experience symptoms within 14 days. Asymptomatic infections are much more frequent in women—up to 80% of infections detected in contacts of symptomatic partners.

Symptomatic uncomplicated infections in males manifest typically a thick, yellow urethral discharge. In females vaginal discharge or dysuria are the major symptoms. Accompanying symptoms include a variable degree of meatal itching, burning, dysuria, frequency and oedema. Infections of the pharynx and rectum (mostly asymptomatic) can result from orogenital and genitoanal sexual contact in males, but in females the rectum is easily infected by contamination from an infected vaginal discharge. Gonococcal infection may present as vulvovaginitis in children infected by sexual abuse or by infected fomites.[14]

Complications in men

In males, spread of the infection to the epididymis, usually unilaterally, is the most common complication (20% of patients not receiving antibiotics). Acute epididymitis has initially to be distinguished from acute torsion. Because it is often difficult to establish an aetiological diagnosis, sexually active males should be given treatment that is effective for gonorrhoea and chlamydia. Some cases will be due to mumps virus infection, and in older men Gram-negative bacilli may be responsible.

The older literature on gonorrhoea describes a number of complications seldom encountered in industrialized countries but which may still be seen in the tropics.[15] These include abscess and fistula formation resulting from spread of infection to various glands associated with the genitourinary tract (prostate, glands of Tyson, Littré, Cowper). Ultimately these may lead to urethral stricture, a difficult complication to manage, which appears to show marked geographical variation in the tropics.[16,17]

Complications in women

In women, common local complications are infections of the paraurethral (Skene's) glands and Bartholin's glands (Figure 13.1). Much more serious

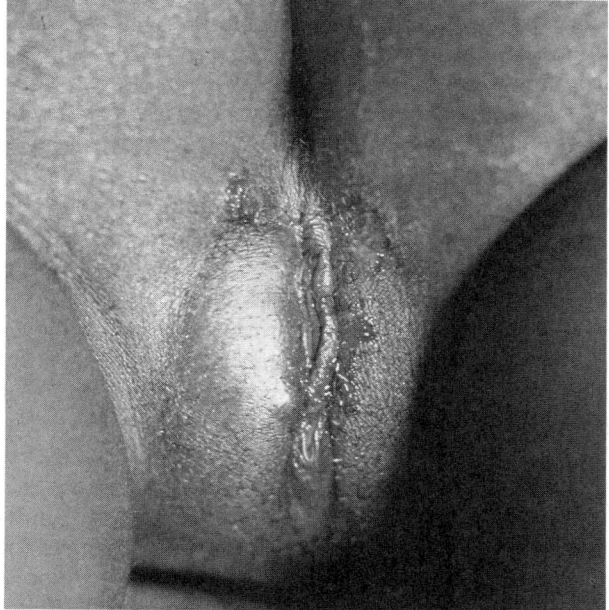

Figure 13.1   Acute bartholinitis due to gonorrhoea (posterior view).

complications may ensue when infection spreads into the uterus and fallopian tubes. Abortion, delivery and insertion of intrauterine devices are risk factors for ascending infection. Unusual uterine bleeding in sexually active women should prompt consideration of a possible gonococcal endometritis. Further spread may lead to acute complications such as acute salpingitis and abscess formation or long-term problems of chronic PID, and increased risk of ectopic pregnancy (increased tenfold after one episode of salpingitis). Acute salpingitis has to be differentiated clinically from ectopic pregnancy (pregnancy test, ultrasonography) and acute appendicitis (laparoscopy).

Sterility may complicate both overt and silent infection in either sex. In a recent study from Central Africa fallopian tube occlusion was present in 83% of infertile women.[18] Acute salpingitis has been estimated to produce sterility in 17% of patients, the risk rising with multiple episodes of infection, in older patients and with more severe inflammation. Gonorrhoea in pregnancy has been associated with low birth weight,[19] premature rupture of membranes, chorioamnionitis and postpartum upper genital tract infection.[20] There is also a higher risk of disseminated gonococcal infection.

Disseminated infection

Disseminated gonococcal infection may arise in about 2% of patients with gonorrhoea overall. The local infection from which it originates is often asymptomatic. It manifests most often as an asymmetric oligoarthritis with a predilection for knees, ankles, and large and small joints of the upper limb. Tenosynovitis occurs frequently. The skin lesions (classically the tender necrotic pustule, but many other forms also occur) often noted in white skins are rare in dark-skinned patients. Gonococcal arthritis accounts for as much as 20% of acute arthritis in young adults in the tropics.[21] It has to be differentiated from other septic arthritides, and in particular from reactive arthritis which is also often sexually acquired. Rarer manifestations of disseminated gonococcal infection include endocarditis and meningitis. Disseminated infections can no longer be expected to respond to penicillin as in the past. Treatment effective against penicillinase-producing strains may be required. Seven days therapy is recommended.

Ocular gonococcal infections

Ocular gonococcal infection in adults, which is presumed to follow autoinoculation with a contaminated finger in most cases, is a common and potentially blinding complication in developing

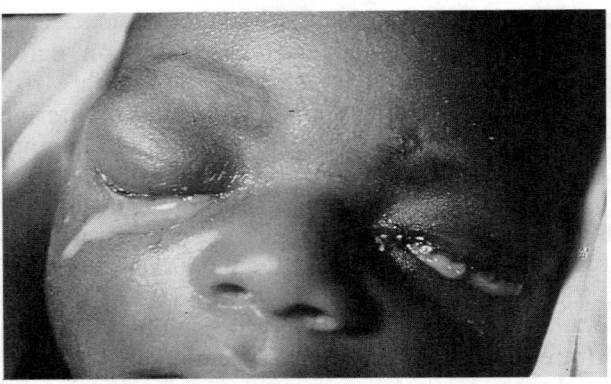

Figure 13.2 Gonococcal ophthalmia in a 7-day-old neonate.

countries.[22] It presents as an acute purulent conjunctivitis which may progress rapidly to corneal perforation in the absence of adequate systemic and topical antimicrobial treatment.

Ophthalmia neonatorum

Ophthalmia neonatorum is defined as an acute conjunctivitis occurring in the first month of life. The high incidence of infection with *N. gonorrhoea* and *C. trachomatis* among pregnant women in many tropical countries is reflected in a correspondingly high incidence of ophthalmia neonatorum which occurs in 30–50% of children born to infected mothers if prophylaxis is not administered.

Ophthalmia neonatorum usually presents as an acute bilateral purulent conjunctivitis (Figure 13.2). Gonococcal infections frequently present in the first week and can lead to blindness. The diagnosis can often be made by microscopy (Gram stain for gonorrhoea, Giemsa stain for chlamydial inclusions). Cultures should be made when possible. Systemic and topical treatment (Tables 13.4 and 13.5) should be administered to the neonate, and the mother and her sexual partner(s) should also be treated.

The use of ocular prophylaxis in countries where the prevalence of gonorrhoea in antenatal women exceeds 1% is highly cost-effective. A recent trial from Kenya showed that the instillation of 1% silver nitrate or 1% tetracycline ointment into the eyes of infants at delivery was equally effective in preventing gonococcal ophthalmia neonatorum.[24]

Laboratory diagnosis

The definitive diagnosis of gonorrhoea rests on the isolation of *N. gonorrhoeae*. In many parts of the tropics this is not feasible. The demonstration of Gram-negative diplococci in urethral smears (Figure 13.3) has a sensitivity and specificity of >95% for the diagnosis of gonorrhoea in males, but both sensitivity and specificity are considerably lower in females, where culture is the method of choice. In disseminated infection specimens from joints, blood or skin lesions give a rather poor yield and the organism may be isolated more readily from the genital tract.

When cultures are to be made, the sites for swabbing should be determined by the history and examination findings. In males it is best to obtain a urethral specimen by insertion and rotation of a swab in the urethra for 5 seconds. For women the ectocervix should be wiped clean and a swab should be inserted into the cervical os and rotated for 10 seconds. Rectal swabs are best obtained through a proctoscope. *N. gonorrhoeae* is a delicate organism, highly susceptible to drying, and prompt inoculation of media and careful adherence to recommended laboratory technique is important to maximize isolation rates. Of newer reported methods for the diagnosis of gonorrhoea (e.g. antigen detection by immunofluorescence or enzyme immunassay, serology, detection of gonococcal DNA), none has so far been shown to be superior to traditional methods.[25]

Treatment (Tables 13.4 and 13.5)

Gonorrhoea is treated ideally with a single dose of supervised oral treatment. The dose administered should give a serum level of at least three times the minimum inhibitory concentration for 8 or more hours. Throughout the tropics an increasing proportion of isolates of *N. gonorrhoea* show both plasmid and chromosomally-mediated resistance to penicillin and other cheap antibiotics such as tetracycline and co-trimoxazole.[26] Penicillinase-producing *N. gonorrhoeae* (PPNG) account for 30–50% of isolates in many tropical countries. In developed countries new antibiotics such as ceftriaxone, cefixime or fluorinated quinolones such as ciprofloxacin are now widely used to ensure that PPNG strains will be effectively treated.[27] In the tropics these drugs are rarely available outside the private sector. The cheapest drugs which show some efficacy against PPNG are co-trimoxazole and tetracycline, but in many areas this efficacy is unacceptably low. Other drugs widely used in the treatment of gonorrhoea due to PPNG in the tropics are listed in Table 13.4. Test of cure 3–5 days after treatment is undertaken where resources permit.

Treatment of contacts should extend to all individuals exposed within 2 weeks of the onset of symptoms in the index case and within 4 weeks of diagnosis of asymptomatic infected individuals. The issue of whether to give blind treatment for

Table 13.4 Recommended treatment for STDs.

Disease	Recommended treatment	Schedule*	Alternatives	Schedule	Notes
Gonorrhoea[1]	Ceftriaxone[2]	1	Kanamycin	1	[1]Concurrent chlamydial therapy is often recommended [2] Equivalent third generation cephalosporin, e.g. cefixime, may be used [3]Equivalent quinolone may be used [4]These regimens may be effective against PPNG when combined with clavulanic acid in areas where chromosomal resistance to penicillin is not too high
	Ciprofloxacin[3]	—	Thiamphenicol	1	
	Spectinomycin	—	Co-trimoxazole	1	
			Amoxycillin[4] + probenecid 1 g orally	—	
			Procaine penicillin[4] + probenecid 1 g orally	1	
			Doxycycline	1	
			Tetracycline hydrochloride	1	
Ophthalmia neonatorum (gonococcal)	Ceftriaxone	2	Kanamycin i.m. + tetracycline ointment	2	Special precautions need to be taken to avoid nosocomial spread of the infection
Chlamydial infection	Doxycycline	1	Erythromycin	1 or 5	—
	Tetracycline hydrochloride	1	Sulphafurazole	—	
Chlamydial ophthalmia	Erythromycin syrup	—	—	—	Not helped by topical therapy
Early syphilis (i.e. primary, secondary or latent <2 years duration)	Benzathine penicillin	1	Doxycycline[1]	4	[1]Suitable for non-pregnant penicillin-allergic individuals [2]Efficacy questionable. Can be used for pregnant women allergic to penicillin
	Procaine penicillin	2	Tetracycline hydrochloride[1]	4	
			Erythromycin[2]	4	
Congenital syphilis	Crystalline penicillin	—	—	—	[1]For cases with abnormal CSF [2]For cases with normal CSF
	Procaine penicillin[1]	3	—	—	
	Benzathine penicillin[2]	2	—	—	
Chancroid	Ceftriaxone	1	Ciprofloxacin	—	More data required on efficacy of ciprofloxacin. These regimens may be ineffective in patients with HIV infection
	Erythromycin	1	—	—	
	Co-trimoxazole	2	—	—	
Lymphogranuloma venereum	Doxycycline	3	Erythromycin	3	Repeated courses of antibiotics may help in difficult cases
	Tetracycline hydrochloride	3	Sulphadiazine	—	Equivalent sulphonamide may be used
Donovanosis	Co-trimoxazole	3	Erythromycin	3	Combination therapy recommended for difficult cases, e.g. patients with AIDS. Lincomycin and erythromycin useful in pregnancy. [1]Can be combined with streptomycin 1 g i.m. daily

continued

Table 13.4 Continued

Disease	Recommended treatment	Schedule*	Alternatives	Schedule	Notes
	Doxycycline	3	Norfloxacin	—	
	Tetracycline hydrochloride[1]	3	Thiamphenicol	2	
			Lincomycin	—	
Trichomoniasis	Metronidazole	1	Clotrimazole[1]	1	[1]Much less effective than metronidazole
Bacterial vaginosis	Metronidazole	2 or 3	—	—	—
Candidiasis	Nystatin		—	—	—
	Miconazole or clotrimazole	1 or 2	—	—	Other imidazoles may be used
Primary genital herpes	Acyclovir	1	—	—	—
Complicated genital herpes	Acyclovir	2	—	—	—
Recurrent herpes	Acyclovir	3 or 4	—	—	Gives marginal benefit only
Pelvic inflammatory disease	1. Treatment for gonorrhoea +		Thiamphenicol	2	Intrauterine device removal recommended
	2. tetracycline or doxycycline +	2 2			
	3. metronidazole	4			
Epididymitis	1. Treatment for gonorrhoea +		1. Treatment for gonorrhoea +		—
	2. tetracycline or doxycycline	2 2	2. erythromycin	2	

*Details of dosage schedules are given in Table 5.
Source: World Health Organization.[23]

chlamydial infection to all patients with gonorrhoea is controversial but certainly worth serious consideration. This practice has been officially recommended in some developed countries. Drawbacks include a substantial amount of unnecessary treatment, cost, risks of adverse effects, masking of other infections and promoting tetracycline resistance.

Prevention

The major obstacle to the control of gonorrhoea is the large reservoir of asymptomatic or clinically non-specific infections in women and the difficulty of establishing the diagnosis in women. The greatly increased cost of effective treatment for PPNG is an added burden for tropical countries. Given these constraints it is more appropriate to direct resources to condom promotion and other safe sex messages rather than costly strategies to increase case-finding and treatment. The development of vaccines for gonorrhoea has been hindered by the antigenic variation manifest by the organism. It is hoped that a vaccine to the relatively invariant P.I protein may prove useful in the future.

CHLAMYDIAL INFECTIONS

The demonstration in 1909 of chlamydial inclusions in cervical scrapings from the mother of an infant with inclusion conjunctivitis and in urethral scrapings from her male partner laid the basis for our understanding of genital chlamydial infections, but it was not until it became possible to isolate *C. trachomatis* in tissue culture in 1965 that the extent of the morbidity due to this organism became clear.

Epidemiology

C. trachomatis is the most prevalent sexually transmitted bacterial pathogen in industrialized countries,[28] and appears to be at least equally prevalent in developing countries (see Table 13.1). Studies in industrialized countries have shown that genital chlamydial infection is more prevalent in younger age groups, even after taking account of differences in sexual activity, implying that some degree of protective immunity may develop after natural infection.

Aetiology

C. trachomatis is a Gram-negative bacterium which is an obligate parasite of eucaryotic cells, since it lacks enzymes of the cytochrome oxidase pathway. The genus *Chlamydia* has a unique life cycle. The metabolically inert infectious elementary body has a rigid cell wall and is adapted for extracellular sur-

Table 13.5 Dosage schedules for drug treatment of STDs.

Drug	Route	Dose		Duration	Notes
Acyclovir	Oral	Schedule 1	200 mg 5 times daily	7 days	—
	i.v.	Schedule 2	5 mg/kg 8-hourly	5–7 days	—
	Oral	Schedule 3	200 mg 5 times daily	5 days	—
	Oral	Schedule 4	800 mg twice daily	5 days	—
Amoxycillin	Oral	3 g		1 dose	—
Benzathine penicillin	i.m.	Schedule 1	2.4 million iu, split between 2 injection sites	1 dose	Further doses after 1 and 2 weeks may be given to patients with latent and secondary syphilis. HIV-positive individuals may require higher dosage
		Schedule 2	50 000 iu/kg	1 dose	
Ceftriaxone	i.m.	Schedule 1	250 mg	1 dose	For gonorrhoea 125 mg may be sufficient
		Schedule 2	50 mg/kg (max. 125 mg)	1 dose	
Ciprofloxacin	Oral	500 mg		1 dose	Equivalent quinolones may be used
Co-trimoxazole (tablets of trimethoprim 80 mg, sulphamethoxazole 400 mg)	Oral	Schedule 1	10 tablets	Daily for 3 days	—
		Schedule 2	2 tablets twice daily	7 days	Contraindicated in pregnancy
		Schedule 3	2 tablets twice daily	14 days	—
Crystalline benzylpenicillin	i.m.	50 000 iu/kg in 2 divided doses		10 days	—
Doxycycline	Oral	100 mg twice daily	Schedule 1	7 days	—
			Schedule 2	10 days	—
			Schedule 3	14 days	—
			Schedule 4	15 days	—
Erythromycin	Oral	Schedule 1	500 mg 4 times daily	7 days	—
		Schedule 2	500 mg 4 times daily	10 days	—
	Oral	Schedule 3	500 mg 4 times daily	14 days	—
	Oral	Schedule 4	500 mg 4 times daily	15 days	—
		Schedule 5	250 mg 4 times daily	7 days	For patients unable to tolerate 500 mg 4 times daily
Erythromycin syrup	Oral	50 mg/kg per day in 4 divided doses		2 weeks	—
Kanamycin	i.m.	Schedule 1	2 g	1 dose	—
		Schedule 2	25 mg/kg (max. 75 mg)		
Lincomycin	Oral		500 mg 4 times daily	14 days	—
Metronidazole	Oral	Schedule 1	2 g	1 dose[1]	Contraindicated in first trimester of pregnancy. Patients should avoid alcohol. [1] Nursing mothers should suspend breast feeding for 24 hours
		Schedule 2	2 g	1 dose repeated after 48 hours	—
		Schedule 3	500 mg twice daily or 250 mg three times daily	7 days	—
		Schedule 4	1 g twice daily	10 days	—
Miconazole or clotrimazole	Intravaginal	Schedule 1	100 mg daily	7 days	—
		Schedule 2	200 mg daily	3 days	—
Norfloxacin	Oral	400 mg twice daily		2–11 days	—
Nystatin	Intravaginal	100 000– 1 000 000 iu daily		14 days	—
Procaine penicillin	i.m.	Schedule 1	4.8 million iu	1 dose	—
		Schedule 2	1.2 million iu daily	10 days	15 days is sometimes recommended for secondary or latent syphilis
		Schedule 3	50 000 iu/kg	10 days	—

continued

Table 13.5 Continued

Drug	Route	Dose			Duration	Notes
Spectinomycin	i.m.	2 g			1 dose	—
Sulphadiazine	Oral	1 g 4 times daily			14 days	—
Sulphafurazole	Oral	500 mg 4 times daily			7 days	—
Thiamphenicol	Oral	Schedule 1	2.5 g		Daily for 2 days	—
		Schedule 2	2.5 g followed by 500 mg 4 times daily		10 days	—
Tetracycline hydrochloride	Oral	500 mg 4 times daily	Schedule 1		7 days	Contraindicated in pregnancy
			Schedule 2		10 days	—
			Schedule 3		14 days	—
			Schedule 4		15 days	—
Tetracycline eye ointment	Topical	Hourly for 24 hours, then 8 hourly			10 days	—

Source: World Health Organization.[23]

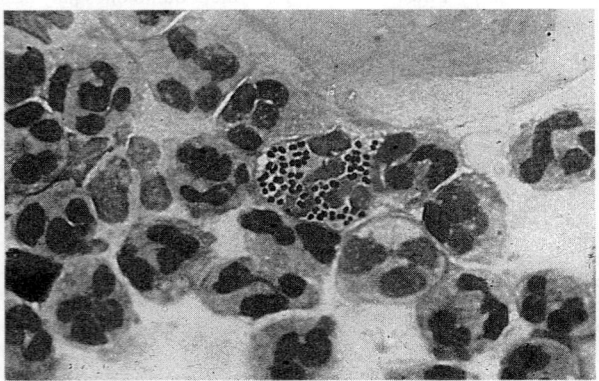

Figure 13.3 Appearance of *N. gonorrhoeae* in a Gram-stained smear of urethral discharge.

vival. It appears to infect preferentially columnar epithelial cells, by which it is actively taken up. After entering the host cell it differentiates over a number of hours to the metabolically active reticulate body, which divides by binary fission until an intracellular inclusion is formed which may contain several thousand organisms. The life cycle is completed when reticulate bodies condense to form elementary bodies, which are released from the inclusion after lysis of the host cell.

A number of serotypes of *C. trachomatis* have been identified by the microimmunofluorescence test of Wang and Grayston. Serotypes A–C cause ocular infection in trachoma endemic areas, whereas serotypes D–K cause genital tract infections worldwide. Serotypes L1, L2 and L3 are more invasive both in vitro and in vivo, and cause LGV.

Pathology

The pathological hallmarks of infection with *C. trachomatis* are: (1) the subepithelial lymphoid follicle; and (2) fibrosis and scarring. The latter may

progress for months and years even in the absence of chlamydial organisms demonstrable by conventional means. The host immune system is believed to play an important part in the pathogenesis of chlamydial infections, and a chlamydial heat shock protein of 57 kDa which has been shown to elicit a delayed hypersensitivity reaction in previously infected animals may also be a determinant of immunopathology in humans.[29]

Clinical features

The clinical spectrum of disease due to chlamydial infection is similar to that seen in gonococcal infection. Although in general chlamydial infections are less likely than gonococcal to cause severe symptoms, they are more likely to cause serious sequelae, particularly in women.[30]

In males, chlamydial infection causes urethritis and, in a proportion of cases, epididymo-orchitis. It is possible that urethral stricture is a late sequela of chlamydial urethritis.

In females, chlamydial cervicitis is often asymptomatic. Sometimes patients will complain of vaginal discharge, and the finding of a mucopurulent discharge at the cervical os is suggestive of chlamydial or gonococcal cervicitis. Ascending infection of the female genital tract may lead to endometritis, salpingitis or PID and this is facilitated by trauma to the cervix, for example during childbirth, insertion of an intrauterine device or termination of pregnancy. Because the symptoms of chlamydial PID are often mild, patients may present only when the sequelae of irreversible damage to the fallopian tubes (infertility, ectopic pregnancy) become apparent. Infection may track to the right upper quadrant, giving rise to a perihepatitis with characteristic adhesions between the liver capsule and peritoneum (the Curtis–FitzHugh syndrome).

Some 30% of infants born to infected mothers become infected. In the majority of cases the only consequence of this is a self-limiting conjunctivitis presenting within the first 2 weeks of life, but occasionally chlamydial ophthalmia is more severe and if it persists it may give rise to conjunctival scarring. A small proportion of infected infants develop chlamydial pneumonitis, presenting usually between the ages of 6 weeks and 3 months with a paroxysmal cough and tachypnoea in the absence of fever. Rales may be heard on clinical examination, and a chest radiograph often reveals extensive bilateral pulmonary infiltrates with hyperinflation. There is characteristically a raised serum total IgG and IgM, and a mild eosinophilia.[31]

Diagnosis

While isolation in tissue culture remains the gold standard for the diagnosis of chlamydial infection, and is the only test which is 100% specific, several antigen detection tests are now commercially available which are almost equally sensitive and specific as well as being cheaper and more widely available. Most diagnostic laboratories now use an antigen detection enzyme immunoassay, confirming positive results either by direct immunofluorescence or by the blocking reaction which is now incorporated in some commercially available tests.[32]

Whichever of these tests is used, specimen collection is of paramount importance. Swabs from females should be collected from the endocervix and urethra. Urethral swabs from males should be inserted at least 2 cm beyond the meatus. A first catch urine specimen appears to be as good as a urethral swab for diagnosing chlamydial infection in males, and is less invasive.[33]

Serology has no place in the diagnosis of uncomplicated chlamydial infections with the exception of the more invasive LGV, but may be helpful in the diagnosis of suspected PID and is the method of choice for the diagnosis of neonatal chlamydial pneumonia.

Management

C. trachomatis remains sensitive to tetracyclines and erythromycin, and these are the treatments of choice (see Tables 13.4 and 13.5). The new macrolide antibiotic azithromycin shows promise as an effective single dose therapy for genital chlamydial infection.[34]

VAGINAL DISCHARGE IN WOMEN

The three most prevalent causes of vaginal discharge are *Candida albicans*, *Trichomonas vaginalis* and bacterial vaginosis. *N. gonorrhoeae* and *C. trachomatis*, which infect the endocervix rather than the vagina, are less commonly associated with symptomatic discharge. Unfortunately it is not possible clinically to distinguish reliably between these infections, although the presence of mucopurulent discharge at the cervical os has been proposed as a marker of gonococcal or chlamydial infection. A wet preparation, examined with a phase contrast microscope, can usually distinguish between candidiasis, trichomoniasis and bacterial vaginosis.

VULVOVAGINAL CANDIDIASIS

Candida albicans can be isolated from the vagina of up to 50% of sexually active women, the majority of whom are asymptomatic. Although sexual transmission may occur, the gastrointestinal tract has also been implicated as a source of infection. Symptomatic disease is associated with an increase in the number of yeasts present in the vagina; factors which predispose to this are pregnancy, antimicrobial therapy, oral contraceptive use, immunosuppression (e.g. HIV related) and glycosuria. It has also been suggested that tight, poorly ventilated nylon underclothing, by increasing perineal moisture, may predispose to symptomatic disease in warm climates.

The cardinal clinical features of vulvovaginal candidiasis are pruritus vulvae and vaginal discharge. The discharge is typically whitish, with curd-like plaques adhering to the vaginal wall, and does not smell. There may be erythema and/or oedema of the vulva and vaginal walls.

The diagnosis can be made on a wet preparation made from the vaginal discharge, the sensitivity of which can be increased by adding 10% potassium hydroxide. Typical mycelia and yeast cells are seen. For the treatment of vulvovaginal candidiasis, see Table 13.4.

TRICHOMONIASIS (Chapter 69)

T. vaginalis has been found in the vagina of up to 30% of antenatal clinic attenders in certain African centres (see Table 13.1). Studies in the USA have shown that its prevalence is higher among women with many partners, and that it can be isolated from a high proportion of male contacts of infected women, suggesting that transmission is primarily through sexual contact. In males most infections are believed to be asymptomatic and self-limiting, although occasionally it may give rise to urethritis.

Up to 75% of women attending STD clinics with *T. vaginalis* infection complain of vaginal discharge. Pruritus vulvae, dyspareunia and dysuria are also common symptoms. On examination a profuse yellow-green frothy discharge, which is not malodorous, is typically noted. The vulva and vaginal walls may be excoriated and erythematous in severe cases, and punctate haemorrhages may be seen on the cervix.[35]

The diagnosis can be made on a wet preparation collected from the posterior fornix. Under phase contrast, increased numbers of polymorphonuclear leucocytes are usually seen, and motile flagellated parasites, slightly larger than polymorphonuclear leucocytes are present. Compared with culture, direct microscopy is less than 80% sensitive, so that culture should also be performed when available. For the treatment of trichomoniasis, see Table 13.4.

BACTERIAL VAGINOSIS

Bacterial vaginosis is a syndrome in which a malodorous vaginal discharge is associated with charac-teristic changes in the vaginal bacterial flora. There is an increase in numbers of anaerobes, *Gardnerella vaginalis* and *Mycoplasma hominis*, such that lactobacilli are no longer predominant. Bacterial vaginosis appears to be more prevalent among women with many sexual partners, but since it has been found in sexually inexperienced women it is not clear that it is a sexually transmitted condition.

The discharge of bacterial vaginosis is typically homogeneous and white, and associated with increased vaginal pH (>4.5). The characteristic fishy smell is more easily detectable after the addition of a drop of 10% potassium hydroxide to a drop of discharge on a slide. Bacterial vaginosis has been shown to be associated with adverse pregnancy outcome (premature labour, chorioamnionitis, postpartum endometritis).[36]

The diagnosis of bacterial vaginosis depends on the identification of clue cells in a wet preparation or Gram stain made from the vaginal discharge. These are squamous epithelial cells which are covered with many adherent bacteria, giving them a granular appearance. For the treatment of bacterial vaginosis, see Table 13.4.

DISEASES CAUSING GENITAL ULCERATION

CHANCROID

Chancroid, or soft sore, was first distinguished from the hard chancre of syphilis by Ricord in 1838. In 1889 Ducrey, in Naples, showed that the inoculation of material from chancroidal ulcers into the skin of the forearm caused ulceration which could be serially passaged, and identified the causative organism which now bears his name. The development of defined solid media for the isolation of *Haemophilus ducreyi* in the 1970s enabled detailed epidemiological studies of chancroid to be carried out for the first time.[37]

Epidemiology

Chancroid is the most common cause of genital ulceration in Africa, where it accounts for more than 60% of genital ulcers seen, and probably also in other areas of the developing world.[38] Although generally rare in industrialized countries, there have been several well-documented outbreaks in North America since the 1970s. Characteristic features of these outbreaks have been a high male-to-female case ratio, the involvement of prostitutes and the low socioeconomic status of the populations affected. A study in Nairobi investigated the role of asymptomatic females in the transmission of the disease and concluded that they were of little importance.[39] Studies among Australian solders during the Vietnam war suggest that chancroid is more common among uncircumcised than circumcised males.[40]

The prevalence of chancroid is high among commercial sex workers in the cities of Africa (Figure 13.4), as is the prevalence of HIV infection.[41] Prospective studies among both males and females at high risk of HIV infection in Nairobi have suggested that chancroid significantly increases the risk of transmission of HIV via heterosexual contact, either by increasing infectivity, susceptibility or both.[42]

Aetiology

Chancroid is caused by *H. ducreyi*, a small facultatively anaerobic Gram-negative bacillus which requires haemin (X factor), reduces nitrate to nitrite and forms typical streptobacillary chains on Gram stain. It is a fastidious organism which will only grow on enriched media and grows best at 30–33°C in an atmosphere of 5% carbon dioxide.

Pathogenesis

Histopathologically, chancroidal ulcers contain three distinct zones: a superficial zone consisting of necrotic tissue, fibrin and numerous bacteria; an intermediate zone showing oedema and new vessel formation; and a deep zone containing a dense infiltrate of neutrophils and plasma cells with fibroblastic proliferation.

The pathogenesis of chancroid is not well understood. The application of *H. ducreyi* to the human forearm does not produce a lesion unless the skin is traumatized. Certain strains are avirulent in the human and in a rabbit model, but lack of virulence in the rabbit does not necessarily imply a strain is avirulent in the human. There is some evidence that virulent strains are relatively resistant to phagocytosis by human polymorphonuclear leucocytes and to complement-mediated killing by normal human and rabbit serum. The suppurating lymphadenopathy of chancroid is notable for the large number of neutrophils and small one of bacilli present.

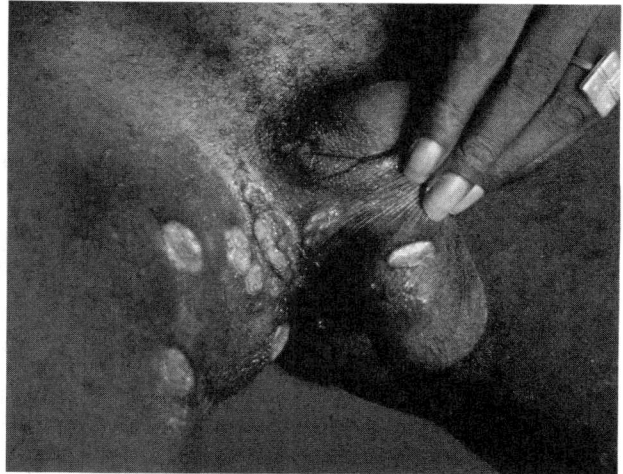

Figure 13.5 Chancroid: multiple soft painful ulcers.

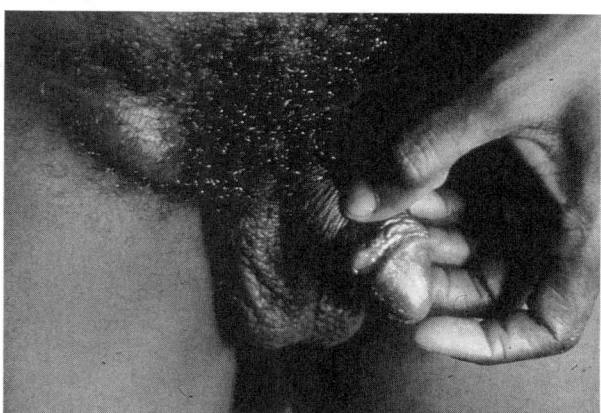

Figure 13.6 Chancroid: ulcer of corona accompanied by a painful bubo.

Clinical features

After an incubation period of 3–7 days, a papule appears at the site of inoculation which soon ulcerates. The typical ulcer of chancroid (Figure 13.5) is painful and soft, has a purulent base with an undermined edge, and bleeds on contact. Multiple ulcers are commonly present, and there is painful inguinal lymphadenopathy (Figure 13.6) in some 50% of cases, often unilateral. Atypical presentations are, however, common, and even in experienced hands chancroid cannot reliably be distinguished from primary syphilis on clinical grounds.[43] Herpes simplex, LGV and donovanosis must also be considered in the differential diagnosis of chancroid.

Chancroid may cause extensive local destruction

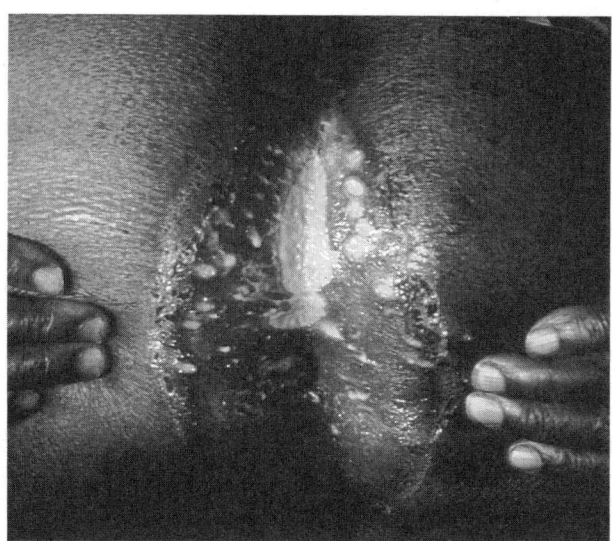

Figure 13.4 Extensive perianal ulceration resulting from an *H. ducreyi* infection in a prostitute.

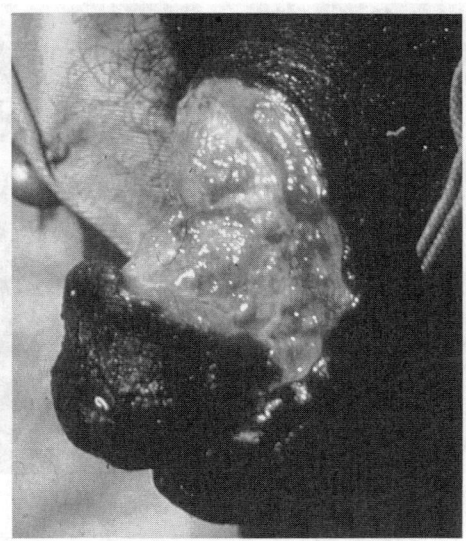

Figure 13.7 Phagaedenic chancroid: destructive ulcer of penile shaft.

(Figure 13.7), particularly in HIV-infected individuals who may fail to respond to antimicrobial treatment, but the infection does not disseminate.

Diagnosis

Gram stain of smears obtained from ulcers has been advocated in the past for the diagnosis of chancroid, but this lacks both sensitivity and specificity. The laboratory diagnosis of chancroid depends on the isolation of *H. ducreyi* from the ulcer. Swabs should be taken from the ulcer base or its undermined edge and plated directly on appropriate blood-containing media enriched with fetal calf serum and Vitox and made selective with vancomycin. For optimal rates of isolation media made up from both GC agar and Mueller–Hinton agar base should be inoculated. Plates should be incubated for at least 72 hours in an atmosphere of 5% carbon dioxide at 33°C. *H. ducreyi* is identified by its typical colonial morphology (colonies are difficult to break up and can be moved intact across the surface of the agar), Gram stain and inability to ferment sugars.

An enzyme immunoassay has been described for the serological diagnosis of chancroid, but it has not been fully evaluated and is not yet commercially available.[44]

Management (Tables 13.4 and 13.5)

Chancroidal ulcers should be kept clean and dry, with regular washing in soapy water. The mainstay of antimicrobial treatment has for a number of years been co-trimoxazole or erythromycin in standard dosage given by mouth for 7 days. However, an increasing proportion of strains worldwide are now resistant to sulphonamides, and many trimethoprim-resistant strains have been isolated in Thailand and Kenya. Ciprofloxacin 500 mg daily for 3 days by mouth and ceftriaxone 500 mg as a single intramuscular dose appear to be effective alternatives, although in HIV-infected patients much longer courses of treatment may be required.

SYPHILIS

History

Syphilis, a young shepherd boy, was the eponymous hero of a Latin poem written in 1530 by the Italian G. Fracastorio. He succumbed to an apparently new disease which had swept across Europe a few years earlier in the wake of the French army's retreat from Naples. The timing of this epidemic led to the suggestion that syphilis had been brought back from the New World by Columbus and his men in 1493. An alternative hypothesis put forward by E.H. Hudson, a physician working in the 1930s in Mesopotamia (now Iraq), was that syphilis originated as an endemic infection of childhood (yaws) in the hot humid tropics, and that venereal transmission only became important when living standards improved sufficiently to prevent transmission in childhood giving rise to long-lasting immunity. This so called unitarian hypothesis is supported by recent evidence of very close DNA homology between *Treponema pallidum* and *T. pertenue* (recently reclassified as *T. pallidum* subsp. *pertenue*).[45]

Although syphilis in all its clinical aspects had been described in detail by nineteenth century physicians, notably Hutchinson in Britain, and Fournier in France, it was not until 1905 that the causative organism, *T. pallidum*, was first identified by Schaudin and Hoffman; in 1906 Wasserman described the first serological test for the diagnosis of syphilis.

Epidemiology

The incidence of syphilis has declined steadily for most of the twentieth century in Western Europe and North America, with the exception of a brief rise during and immediately after each world war, although in the late 1980s an increased incidence was observed in certain American inner city populations.

There are no reliable incidence figures for developing countries. Seroprevalence surveys have shown high rates of positivity among urban antenatal clinic attenders in many African countries (see Table 13.1), but in the absence of supportive clinical information such studies should be interpreted with caution. For example, while there is no doubt that venereal syphilis poses a major threat to the health of neonates in Lusaka, Zambia, follow-up of a rural antenatal population in The Gambia with a similar seroprevalence (12%) found no difference in pregnancy outcome between seropositive and seronegative women.[46] The relative rarity of late syphilis in parts of Africa where early syphilis is common has led to speculation that the disease has become more common in recent years, perhaps reflecting loss of herd immunity following the mass treatment campaigns against endemic treponemal disease in the 1950s and 1960s.

Transmission by sexual contact requires exposure to moist mucosal or cutaneous lesions; experiments in the rabbit suggest that an inoculum of some 50 organisms is sufficient to initiate infection. The rate of transmission from an infected partner is approximately 30%.

Aetiology

Syphilis is caused by *T. pallidum*, one of a small group of treponemas (of the order Spirochaetales) pathogenic to man. It cannot be distinguished in the laboratory from the agents responsible for yaws and pinta (*T. pallidum* subsp. *pertenue* and *T. carateum* respectively). It is a spiral organism 6–15 μm in length and 0.15 μm in width, visible by light microscopy only under conditions of dark-field illumination, and cannot be grown on artificial media. In tissue culture and in animal models it divides slowly, with a replication time of approximately 30 hours. It is highly susceptible to drying.

Pathogenesis

T. pallidum has not been shown to produce either exotoxins or endotoxins. Following experimental infection in the rabbit, *T. pallidum* begins to replicate once it has passed through the epithelium. An initial polymorphonuclear leucocyte response at the lesion is soon replaced by an infiltrate of T and B lymphocytes. The primary chancre also contains mucoid material, mainly hyaluronic acid and chondroitin sulphate, which may modulate the host immune response. Both circulating *T. pallidum* specific T cells and specific antibody can be found in the majority of cases of primary syphilis. At the same time as these are first noted, the number of organisms in the lesion decreases and the ulcer

begins to heal, suggesting that the immune system is controlling the infection.

The appearance of secondary lesions some weeks later, due to the dissemination of organisms and circulating immune complexes, indicates that this is not the case, although the mechanism by which such a slow growing organism evades the host immune response is not clear. Much of the pathology of secondary syphilis may be immune complex mediated. High levels of antitreponemal antibody are present in the circulation, but cell-mediated immune responses are depressed.

Eventually cell-mediated immune responses to *T. pallidum* are restored as the lesions are brought under control, leading to the latent stage. Follow-up studies in the prepenicillin era showed that relapse of infectious secondary lesions occurred in up to 25% of cases. The organism can survive in the body for many years thereafter, causing tertiary lesions characterized by the presence of a small number of organisms and a lymphocytic host response giving rise to an endarteritis.

Clinical features

After an incubation period of 10–70 days (median 21 days), a *primary chancre* (Figure 13.8) develops at the site of inoculation. The chancre is typically painless, indurated, with a clean base and a raised edge, and does not bleed on contact. There is usually only a single lesion; in the male it is most commonly on the glans, the foreskin, the coronal sulcus or the shaft of the penis, and in the female on the cervix or vulva. The primary chancre is often accompanied by inguinal lymphadenopathy; the glands are charac-

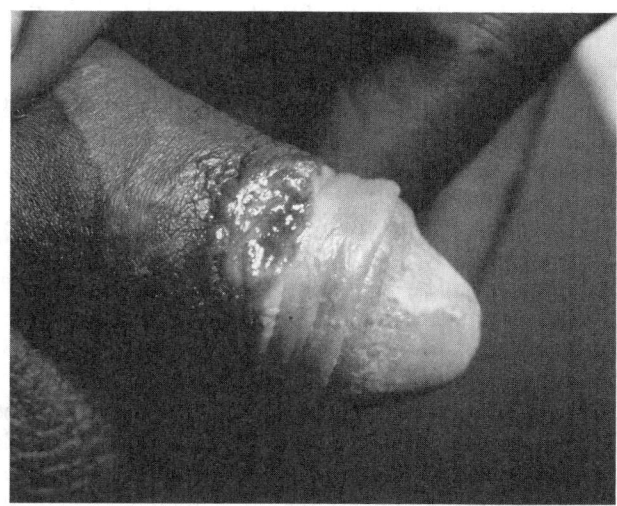

Figure 13.8 Syphilis: primary chancre.

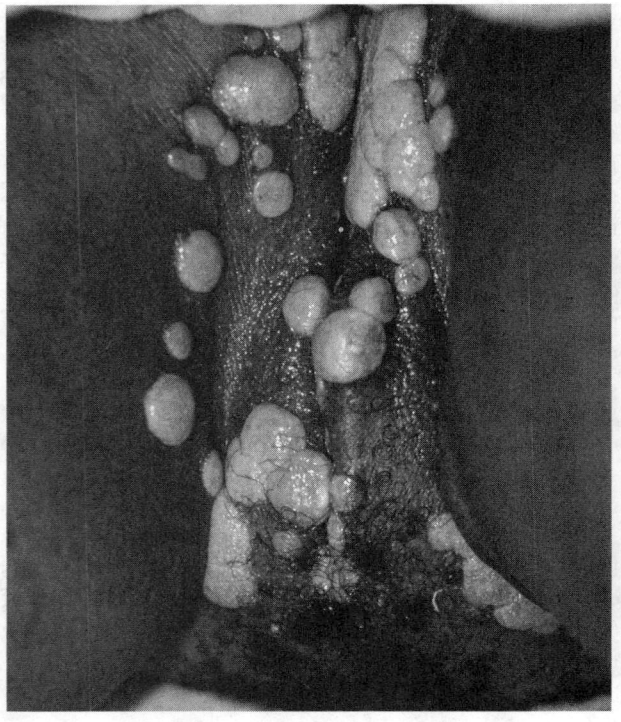

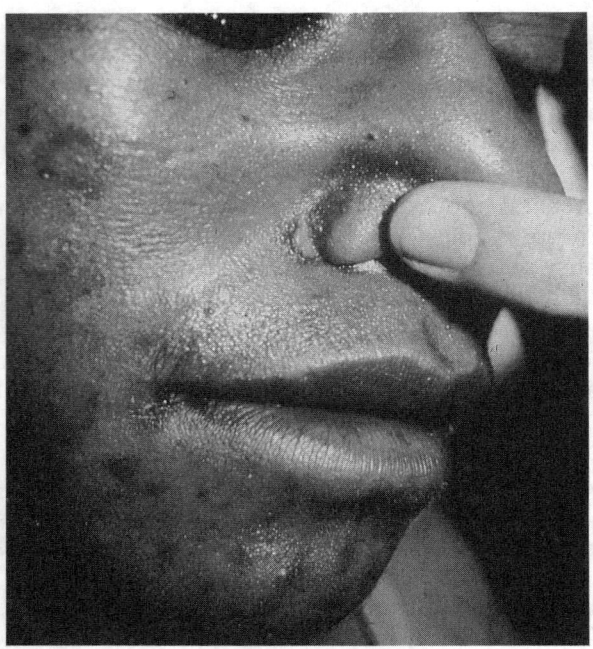

Figure 13.10   Secondary syphilis: condyloma abutting on ala nasi.

Figure 13.9   Secondary syphilis: condylomata lata.

teristically hard (the 'bullet bubo' of Hutchinson) and painless.

The primary chancre generally resolves spontaneously over several weeks. Between 3 and 6 weeks after its first appearance the features of *secondary syphilis* appear. The rash of secondary syphilis may take many forms: papular, macular or pustular; annular lesions are not uncommon. It often desquamates, but in moist areas of the body (e.g. perineum, axilla) soft raised condylomata lata may be seen (Figures 13.9 and 13.10). It generally affects the palms (Figure 13.11) and soles, and does not itch. The mucous membranes may be involved, with mucous patches or oral ulceration sometimes in the form of the characteristic 'snail track' ulcer. In addition to its cutaneous manifestations secondary syphilis may cause systemic illness (fever, malaise), generalized lymphadenopathy, nephritis, hepatitis, meningitis or uveitis.

The lesions of secondary syphilis generally resolve after several weeks, although relapses commonly occurred in the preantibiotic era. In the absence of adequate treatment the patient then enters the latent stage of the disease, and is liable to develop *tertiary syphilis* at some time in the future.

The lesions of tertiary syphilis fall into three categories: the gumma, cardiovascular disease and central nervous system disease. The classic Oslo study of untreated syphilis, in which some 1400 patients were followed for up to 50 years, found that

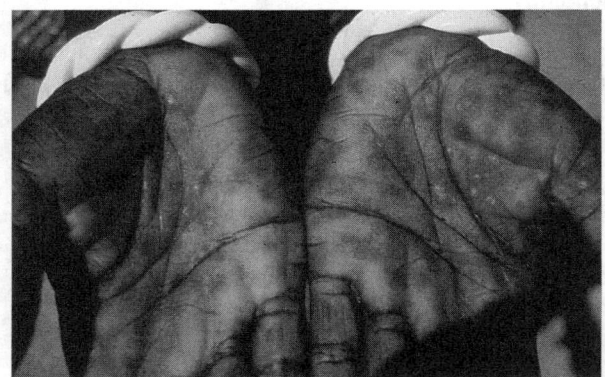

Figure 13.11   Secondary syphilis: typical palmar rash.

the most common manifestation was the gumma, a painless 'punched out' ulcer with little or no inflammatory reaction, which developed in 15%: 70% were cutaneous, 10% involved bone and rarely the viscera were involved. Most cases occurred in the first 15 years following infection. Cardiovascular lesions (aortitis, aortic valve disease or coronary ostial occlusion) were seen in 15% of males and 8% of females, with onset typically 30–40 years after infection. Neurological manifestations were seen in 9% of males and 5% of females, with meningovascular disease typically occurring after 15–20 years and tabes dorsalis or general paresis after 20–30 years.[47] The Tuskegee study of untreated black Americans showed similar results. It is therefore surprising that tertiary syphilis, and in particular neurosyphilis, appears rather uncommon in Africa in spite of the high incidence of early syphilis.

CONGENITAL SYPHILIS

Early congenital syphilis

Pregnant women with untreated early or latent syphilis are liable to give birth to congenitally infected infants. The risk is highest among those with primary or secondary syphilis during pregnancy, and diminishes as the duration of latent syphilis increases. Studies conducted in the preantibiotic era found that untreated early syphilis in the mother led to stillbirth in 25% of cases, neonatal death in some 15% of cases and a syphilitic infant in about 40% of cases. Corresponding figures for untreated late syphilis were 12, 9 and 2%.[48]

Signs of congenital syphilis in the neonate include a bullous rash (Figure 13.12), anaemia, jaundice and hepatosplenomegaly. The infant is often small for dates and may have feeding difficulties. The prognosis is poor in infants with signs of congenital syphilis at birth. More commonly, the syphilitic infant appears normal at birth, and presents in the first 3 months of life with: failure to thrive; a rash which resembles that of secondary syphilis, with desquamation usually involving the palms (Figure 13.13) and soles; persistent nasal discharge (sometimes bloodstained); and anaemia or hepatosplenomegaly (Figure 13.14). Periostitis of the long bones, with or without metaphyseal abnormalities, is radiologically evident in more than 90% of cases, and may present clinically as pseudoparalysis of one or more limbs. The prognosis is very much better in those presenting in the postneonatal period.[49]

Late congenital syphilis

Late congenital syphilis in the child or adolescent corresponds to tertiary syphilis in the adult,

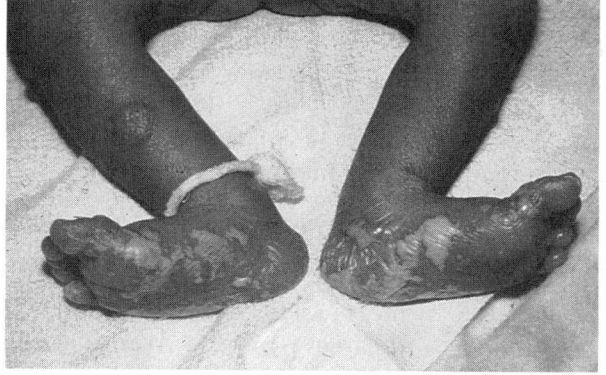

Figure 13.12 Congenital syphilis in a neonate: bullous lesions of feet.

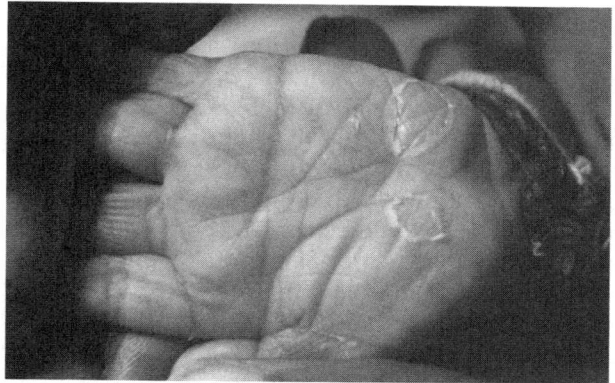

Figure 13.13 Congenital syphilis in a 3-month-old infant: desquamating lesion of palm.

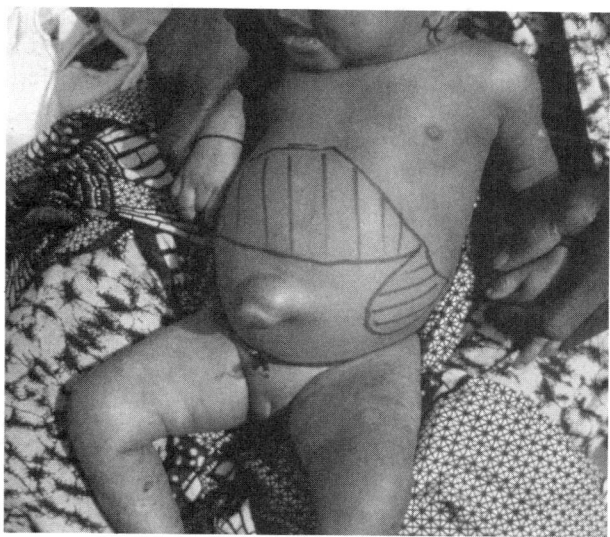

Figure 13.14 Congenital syphilis in a 3-month-old infant: hepatosplenomegaly.

although the cardiovascular system is seldom involved. Manifestations include bony and dental abnormalities (skull bossing, Hutchinson's teeth) and inflammatory lesions of the cornea (interstitial keratitis) and joints (Clutton's joints). Eighth nerve deafness is commonly seen, and symptomatic neurosyphilis may occur, corresponding to tabes dorsalis or general paresis in the adult. In view of the high incidence of early congenital syphilis in many African cities, late manifestations of the disease are surprisingly rare in Africa.

Diagnosis

Clinically it may not be possible to distinguish a syphilitic primary chancre from other causes of genital ulceration. In most parts of Africa chancroid is the most important differential diagnosis, but in areas where donovanosis is prevalent this should also be considered. The primary chancre should also be distinguished from LGV, herpes and non-venereal causes of genital ulceration. Secondary syphilis may resemble a variety of other skin conditions, but rashes which do not itch and affect the palms and soles should be considered syphilitic until proved otherwise. Early congenital syphilis in the neonatal period may be confused with perinatally acquired herpes simplex on account of the bullous rash, or with other intrauterine infections causing hepatosplenomegaly, anaemia and jaundice (e.g. cytomegalovirus, toxoplasmosis, rubella).

Dark-field microscopy

T. pallidum may be demonstrated by dark-field microscopy in fluid from ulcerated or moist lesions of early syphilis, or in bulla fluid from lesions of early congenital syphilis. It can be distinguished from other spirochaetes which may be present under the foreskin by its characteristic shape and motility. Dark-field microscopy is likely to be negative in patients who have applied antiseptics to the lesion or taken antibiotics.

Serological diagnosis

Two categories of test are available for the serological diagnosis of syphilis: non-specific or reagin tests (e.g. Venereal Disease Research Laboratory (VDRL), rapid plasma reagin (RPR)) and treponemal tests (*T. pallidum* haemagglutination (TPHA), fluorescent treponemal antibody (FTA)). The reagin tests are useful for monitoring the response to treatment because they exhibit a falling titre after successful therapy, but they may give false-positive reactions in subjects with other chronic infections. The treponemal tests generally remain positive for life, and cannot therefore distinguish between a current and a past infection. They are more specific than the reagin tests but cannot distinguish between sexually acquired and endemic treponemal infections. The RPR and TPHA tests are simple to perform and do not require sophisticated laboratory equipment. In the neonate it is necessary to demonstrate IgM antibodies by the FTA test in order to distinguish between true infection and passively acquired maternal antibody; however, in an infant with signs of congenital syphilis, a positive maternal reagin test is sufficient grounds for treatment.

Management (Tables 13.4 and 13.5)

T. pallidum remains fully sensitive to penicillin. Because it is a slowly dividing organism it is necessary to ensure adequate circulating penicillin levels for at least 10 days. Recommended treatment regimens are shown in Table 13.4. It has been suggested that single dose benzathine penicillin does not ensure adequate levels in the cerebrospinal fluid, and recent anecdotal evidence suggests that it may be ineffective in HIV-infected patients. If it is possible to ensure compliance, ten daily doses of aqueous procaine penicillin 1.2 million units is preferable. Epidemiological treatment is recommended for sexual contacts.

Early congenital syphilis should be treated with procaine penicillin 50 000 units/kg i.m. daily for 10 days. If compliance is considered unlikely, benzathine penicillin 50 000 units/kg i.m. as a single dose may be given, although this does not give therapeutic levels in the cerebrospinal fluid. The mother and her sexual partner(s) should be investigated and treated appropriately. If possible, infants should be followed up after 6 months to ensure that the RPR or VDRL test has reverted to negative.

Prevention

Congenital syphilis can be prevented by serological screening of pregnant women at antenatal clinics. Experience in Lusaka, Zambia, has shown that in a developing country setting this is only successful if serological tests are performed in the clinic and treatment given immediately.

LYMPHOGRANULOMA VENEREUM

Lymphogranuloma venereum (LGV) is also known as lymphogranuloma inguinale, lymphopathia venereum, tropical or climatic bubo and Durand–Nicolas–Favre disease.

Epidemiology

It is an STD largely confined to the tropics. In most places it accounts for only a small proportion of patients, although its prevalence in parts of Ethiopia and Nigeria reaches up to 20% of patients with STDs. The disease is seen five times more often in men than women, though the late anorectal complications are more prevalent in women.

Aetiology

LGV is caused by the invasive L1, L2 and L3 strains of *C. trachomatis* which show enhanced resistance to phagocytosis compared with other serotypes of *C. trachomatis*.

Pathology

The characteristic pathological features are a thrombolymphangitis and perilymphangitis with proliferation of the endothelial cells of the lymphatics. In the lymph nodes prominent migration of neutrophils leads to characteristic stellate abscess formation.

Clinical features

The disease is important chiefly as a cause of bubo. When a sexually active adult presents with an inguinal bubo not associated with genital ulcer, LGV is an important diagnosis to consider. The initial event in infection, occurring 3–30 days after exposure, is typically a small, painless, usually herpetiform ulcer of the genitalia which may pass unrecognized and resolves spontaneously. It is thought likely that some patients develop asymptomatic infections of the urethra and cervix. The second phase of the illness is the development of increasingly painful lymphangitis and lymphadenitis, accompanied by fever and malaise. The infected nodes (bilateral in a third of cases) coalesce into a matted mass which may project outwards below or above the inguinal ligament to give the classical 'groove sign'. The nodes are liable to rupture, forming multiple sinuses. Untreated, the disease may cause extensive lymphatic damage resulting in elephantiasis of the genitalia (Figure 13.15). The combination of elephantiasis with skin breakdown sometimes seen in late cases is referred to as esthiomène. An additional characteristic feature in long-standing cases is the development of fenestrations in the labia. In women and homosexual men the disease may present as an acute proctocolitis which, in a proportion of cases, leads much later to abscess formation, fibrosis, fistula and rectal stricture. In the Caribbean a high incidence of vulval carcinoma has been recorded among premenopausal women with scars of either LGV or donovanosis.[50] A substantial proportion of cases of rectal stricture may also develop carcinoma.

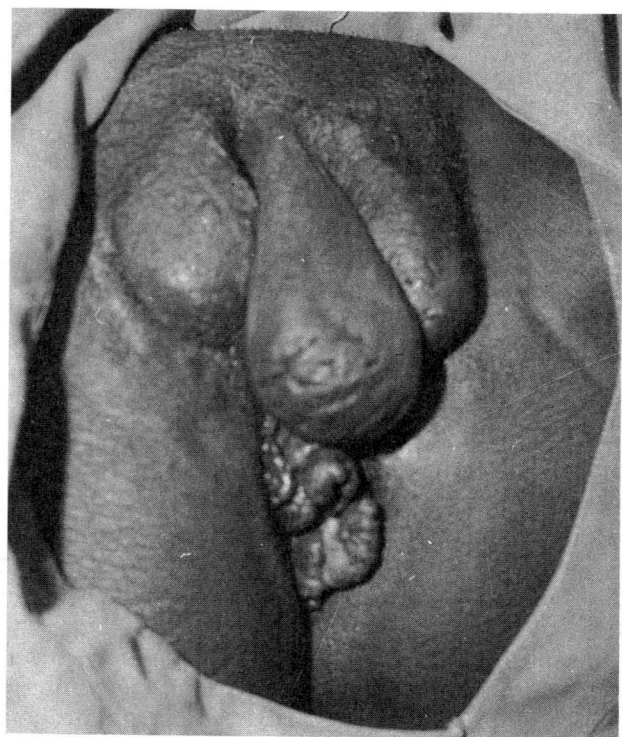

Figure 13.15 Lymphogranuloma venereum: elephantiasis in long-standing case. (Reproduced with permission of the publishers from Arya O P, Osoba A O & Bennett F J. *Tropical Venereology*. Edinburgh: Churchill Livingstone, 1980.)

1925, is no longer available. It was abandoned because of lack of sensitivity and specificity, particularly early in the disease. The presence of stellate abscesses in biopsy material is suggestive of LGV. Immunofluorescence may be used to demonstrate chlamydial elementary bodies in tissue or discharge from buboes. Additional laboratory findings include leucocytosis, an elevated erythrocyte sedimentation rate and increases in IgG and cryoglobulins. The rectal stricture of LGV tends to be more long and tubular than a malignant lesion.

Diagnosis

The diagnosis of LGV can only be confirmed in specialist centres with facilities for the isolation and identification of *C. trachomatis* L1–3 strains, or equipped to carry out either the complement fixation or microimmunofluorescent test.[51] Serological tests lack sensitivity and show cross-reaction with other serovars of *C. trachomatis*. Accepted criteria for a positive diagnosis are a complement fixation test titre of 1:64 or a microimmunofluorescence titre of 1:512. The Frei test, a skin test introduced in

Treatment (Tables 13.4 and 13.5)

The drugs recommended for treatment of acute cases are of the tetracycline group or erythromycin as for other chlamydial infections. Benefit in late cases, e.g. with rectal stricture, is slight. Plastic surgical operations may be of benefit in cases with extensive elephantiasis or deformity.[52] Suspicious areas in healed scars should be biopsied for malignant change. Aspiration of buboes through adjacent healthy skin is usually advised.

DONOVANOSIS

Synonyms: granuloma inguinale, granuloma venereum. It is important not to confuse this disease with *lympho*granuloma venereum (see above) or to confuse Donovan bodies (see below) with Leishman–Donovan bodies (leishmaniasis). The disease was first recognized in India, where Donovan observed the bodies that bear his name in an oral lesion of the disease. Sir Patrick Manson did much to promote awareness of the disease by devoting a chapter to 'ulcerating granuloma of the pudenda' in the first edition of this textbook. Endemic areas are localized to a few specific areas of the tropics. The most important of these are currently south-east India, Papua New Guinea (PNG), Brazil, The Guianas, and eastern parts of South Africa. The disease is strongly associated with prostitution and low socio-economic status. Major epidemics of donovanosis have been reported from PNG but are unlikely to be seen again. Outside PNG the highest recently reported incidence of donovanosis has been from Durban, South Africa, where a recent study found 16% of genital ulcers in men to be due to donovanosis.[53] There is strong evidence that the disease is sexually transmitted in most patients, although some authors have put forward arguments for a non-sexual mode of transmission.[54] The risks of transmission to partners appears to be lower than for other STDs. Perinatal transmission is the subject of a single case report.[55] Recent work in South Africa has shown that a history of donovanosis is a risk factor for acquisition of HIV.

Aetiology

The disease is caused by a poorly characterized, encapsulated, Gram-negative coccobacillus called *Calymmatobacterium granulomatis* which lives intracellularly. Successful culture has only exceptionally been reported. Growth has been obtained in the yolk sac of fertile chick eggs and liquid or semi-liquid media containing yolk, soya or lactalbumin.[56]

Pathology

The disease primarily attacks the skin. The bacteria are carried to inguinal nodes where they occasionally cause a suppurating periadenitis ('pseudobubo') but more often they escape to produce ulcers in the overlying skin. The key histological features are (1) epithelial hyperplasia, (2) a dense dermal infiltrate of plasma cells, and (3) scattered large macrophages containing clusters of Donovan bodies. Donovan bodies stain poorly with haematoxylin and eosin but with Giemsa they typically display a capsule and bipolar densities which give a characteristic closed safety-pin appearance.

Clinical features

The first manifestation, appearing after a 3–40-day incubation period, is usually a small papule which ruptures to form a granulomatous lesion which is characteristically pain free, 'beefy-red' in colour, bleeds readily on contact and is often elevated above the level of the surrounding skin. The lesion has to be differentiated from other forms of genital ulcer. Most likely to cause confusion are chancroid,[57] condylomata lata, ulcerated warts and squamous carcinoma. Untreated, the ulcers slowly extend (Figure 13.16), particularly along skin folds towards the groins (Figure 13.17) and anus. Special features are extragenital lesions (mostly neck and mouth), cervical lesions (resemble carcinoma or tuberculous cervicitis), involvement of uterus, tubes and ovaries (hard masses, abscesses, 'frozen pelvis', hydronephrosis) and rare cases of haematogenous dissemination to lung, liver, spleen and bone. Complications include rapid extension of lesions secondarily infected with fusospirochaetal organisms, scarring (in some populations very prominent), elephantia-

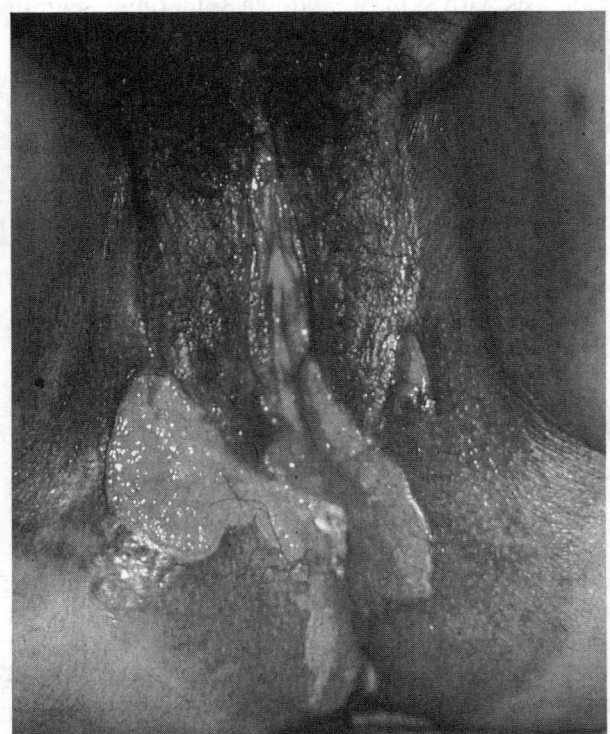

Figure 13.16 Donovanosis: slowly extending painless ulceration.

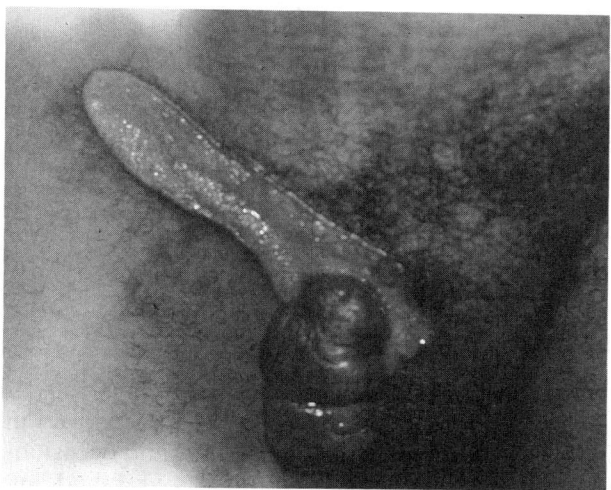

Figure 13.17 Donovanosis: lesion extending along inguinal fold.

sis, and the development of squamous carcinoma. Deaths from the disease are now rare.

Diagnosis

The diagnosis requires the demonstration of *intracellular* Donovan bodies (Figure 13.18) in either biopsy material (best stained with silver stains or Giemsa) or smears taken from active areas which can be stained by Giemsa or Leishman stains. For collection of specimens, a recommended technique is to thoroughly clean the lesions of surface debris, detach a small piece of tissue by any suitable means (local anaesthetic is not always necessary) and then,

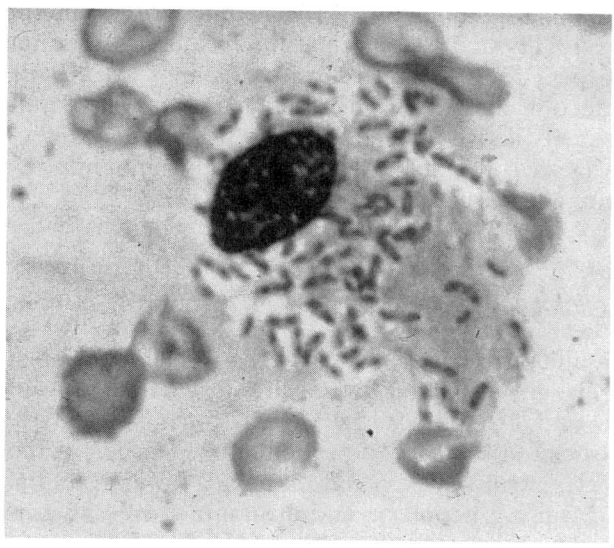

Figure 13.18 Donovan bodies: Giemsa-stained smear from genital ulcer demonstrating intracellular organisms with bipolar densities.

between two glass slides, crush and spread for staining.[58]

Treatment (Tables 13.4 and 13.5)

The bacteria respond to many broad-spectrum antibiotics active against Gram-negative bacilli.[56] The most widely used in recent years have been: tetracylines, chloramphenicol, co-trimoxazole and erythromycin. Thiamphenicol, lincomycin and norfloxacin[59] have recently been shown to be of value. Treatment should be continued until lesions have resolved and, if possible, a little longer to reduce the risk of relapse. Combined therapy, e.g. lincomycin and erythromycin, should be considered in high-risk or difficult cases, e.g. pregnant women who show accelerated disease and are at risk of haematogenous dissemination, patients with the acquired immune deficiency syndrome (AIDS) and patients with extensive disease. Plastic surgical procedures are required in some patients. Treatment of contacts without lesions is not thought necessary.

GENITAL HERPES

Genital herpes is an ulcerative STD caused principally by herpes simplex virus type 2 (HSV-2) and to a lesser extent by herpes simplex virus type 1 (HSV-1), the usual cause of oral herpes. Genital herpes accounts for a much lower proportion of patients with genital ulcer in the tropics than it does in developed countries. It has been suggested that the higher frequency of HSV-1 infection in the tropics gives some degree of protective cross-immunity to HSV-2.

Clinical features

The clinical picture is highly characteristic in many cases with its localized clusters of vesicles which break down to form ulcers (Figure 13.19), crust over and then resolve. Sites of involvement include the external genitalia, neighbouring skin, the urethra and cervix (both endocervix and ectocervix), pharynx and rectum. Tender lymphadenopathy may occur. During the primary attack the virus ascends the peripheral nerves to local ganglia where a latency is established which is liable to be interrupted by periodic recurrences for the remainder of the patient's life. The primary attack is notably more severe than subsequent episodes, with lesions covering a wider and more symmetric area. It is notorious for causing an excruciating urethritis in some women. The complications of genital herpes include

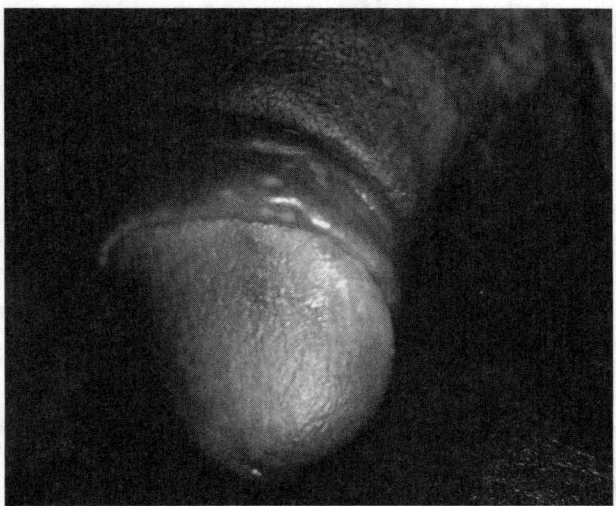

Figure 13.19 Recurrent genital herpes: cluster of small painful ulcers of corona.

a sacral radiculomyelopathy which may manifest with constipation and retention of urine as well as shooting pains down the legs. The latter neuritic pains may be a particularly troublesome feature of recurrent disease. Other complications include aseptic meningitis, extragenital lesions, yeast vaginitis and disseminated herpes. In pregnant women recurrences and dissemination are more frequent and premature delivery may complicate primary attacks. Severe and intractable infections occur in patients with AIDS.

Diagnosis

Clinical diagnosis alone is often sufficient. Genital herpes has to be distinguished from other STDs that cause painful genital ulcer and from non-infectious conditions such as Behçet's syndrome and Crohn's disease. The definitive diagnosis rests on viral isolation. Kits for antigen detection are available. Serological diagnosis is only of value in a primary attack. In less sophisticated settings the diagnosis can be made by looking for characteristic mononucleated giant cells with eosinophilic intranuclear inclusions (Cowdry type A bodies) in smears from lesions (Tzanck test).[60]

Treatment (Tables 13.4 and 13.5)

Specific treatment can rarely be offered in the tropics, none the less patients require explanation, reassurance and advice, just as elsewhere. Patients need to be instructed to keep the lesions clean and dry. They should be told that the disease is likely to recur and that they will transmit the infection to others if they have sexual intercourse while they have lesions. Acyclovir has been shown to be of value in ameliorating symptoms of the primary attack, treatment of infected neonates and adults with immunosuppression or disseminated disease. Continuous prophylactic therapy has been found useful in ameliorating and preventing recurrences in patients particularly troubled by recurrent disease.

Herpes in pregnancy

Transmission from mother to child occurs in 50% of cases with a primary attack at term, is much lower in patients with recurrences (about 1%) and occasionally occurs as a result of asymptomatic viral shedding by the mother at term. Neonatal herpes carries a 60% mortality which has changed little with the introduction of acyclovir. The presence of active herpetic lesions of the cervix at term is an indication for caesarean section, though this operation does not fully protect against infection developing in the neonate. Antenatal cultures for HSV in at-risk women are no longer recommended as they fail to identify neonates at risk. The use of acyclovir in late pregnancy is being investigated and it has been suggested that pregnant women at risk should be screened with specific HSV-2 serology.[61]

GENITAL WARTS

Epidemiology

In developed countries genital infection with the human papillomavirus (HPV) is the most common viral STD and is four times as frequent as genital herpes. Using the most sensitive diagnostic methods infection can be demonstrated in as many as 40% of sexually active women.[62] In the tropics HPV infections are common but are of relatively minor importance compared with the bacterial STDs.

Aetiology

Genital warts are caused by HPVs. The types most prevalent in genital lesions are designated HPV-6, -11 and -16. Of these HPV-16 has been particularly associated with the development of cancer of the cervix, whilst HPV-6 and -11 have a lower potential for causing neoplasia and are more closely associated with exophytic (as opposed to flat) lesions and with the development of respiratory papillomas in children born to infected mothers.

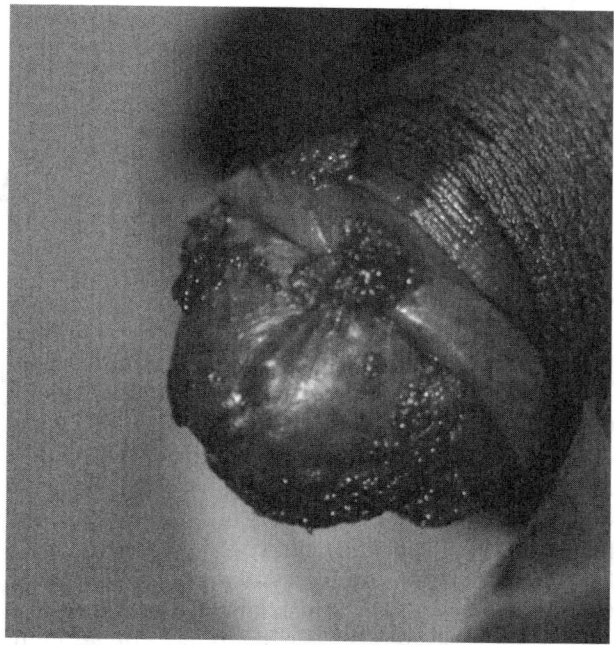

Figure 13.20 Genital warts: condylomata acuminata caused by human papilloma virus.

Pathology

The virus infects the basal layer of differentiating squamous epithelium and produces a pathognomonic large, clear, perinuclear zone known as koilocytotic atypia. Full assembly of viral particles is confined to the more superficial layers of the epithelium. HPV is implicated in the causation of cancer of the cervix,[63] a cancer with a very high incidence in many parts of the tropics.

Clinical

The lesions produced by HPV vary from the well-known soft, fleshy, vascular condylomata acuminata with their frond-like appearance (Figure 13.20) to papular warts which resemble those seen on other parts of the body, pigmented and non-pigmented papules and leucoplakia. Warts may sometimes grow in the urethra. Recent research has shown that many patients have subclinical HPV infections that can only be visualized by colposcopy after application of 5% acetic acid or detected in tissue specimens by techniques such as the polymerase chain reaction. In pregnancy, in immunosuppressed patients and in the presence of genital discharges there is a tendency for warts to grow rapidly. The lesions showing the greatest similarity to genital warts are condylomata lata of secondary syphilis and, occasionally, verrucose forms of donovanosis.

Diagnosis and treatment

Biopsy confirmation of the diagnosis of condylomata acuminata warts is optional but cervical cytology, where available, is recommended for female patients and female contacts in order to detect progression of lesions to cervical intraepithelial neoplasia. Treatment is generally reserved for macroscopic lesions because subclinical infections show high spontaneous regression rates and also show a strong tendency to relapse with currently available forms of treatment. Specific treatment for warts[64] includes treatment with trichloroacetic acid and the traditional application of 20% podophyllin (maximum 0.5 ml) once or twice weekly. Cure rates with podophyllin, at <50%, are not very satisfactory. Care is needed to avoid burning normal skin, which can be protected with glycerine. Podophyllin should be washed off after 4 hours and is contraindicated in pregnant women. Larger warts can be removed with cryotherapy or diathermy. More modern treatments include the application of 5-fluorouracil ointment, self-treatment with podophyllotoxin, and carbon dioxide laser treatment.

CONTROL AND PREVENTION OF STDs

The important components of an STD control programme are: (1) gathering of information, e.g. STD morbidity surveillance, special surveys on the aetiology of genital ulcer in a particular area, data on antibiotic sensitivities of local strains of *N. gonorrhoeae* and *H. ducreyi*; (2) provision of management guidelines; (3) training programmes; (4) provision of health care to patients with STDs wherever they may present; (5) co-ordinated programmes of education about STDs for patients and the general public; and (6) management and supervision of the programme. Each of these will be discussed in more detail.

INFORMATION GATHERING

Morbidity surveillance in the tropics is often incomplete and unreliable. Given the rudimentary facilities available in many centres, it is often best to record numbers of patients with ulcer, discharge, etc., rather than specific diagnoses. Good reporting from a few representative sentinel sites may be more useful than unreliable reports collated from the whole country. When possible, special surveys should be undertaken periodically, such as studies of the prevalence of gonorrhoea, chlamydial infection and syphilis in antenatal mothers. Statistics on ophthalmia neonatorum, congenital syphilis, PID, ectopic pregnancy and infertility may be useful for impressing upon health planners the full extent of STD morbidity.

STANDARD MANAGEMENT GUIDELINES FOR STDs

When a reasonable amount of information is available about the picture of STDs in a country and the antibiotic sensitivity patterns of local isolates, it is possible to draw up rational guidelines for the management of patients presenting with the common STD syndromes such as discharge, genital ulcer, bubo, epididymitis and PID. These guidelines can be tailored to different levels of the health system according to the availability of supporting laboratory tests and drugs. Such guidelines can be conveniently set out as flow charts or algorithms in pocket manuals which are supplied to all health workers who need to manage STDs. Examples of such algorithms are given in a recent publication from the World Health Organization.[23] In view of the constantly changing pattern of antibiotic sensitivities of *N. gonorrhoea* and *H. ducreyi*, it is important that guidelines are reviewed and revised at 3–4-yearly intervals.

TRAINING

The high incidence of STDs in tropical populations makes it important for all health workers to acquire the basic skills to manage patients appropriately according to standard guidelines, to prevent ophthalmia neonatorum and congenital syphilis, and to promote the following health education messages which are important in STD prevention.

- Reduction of the number of sexual partners.
- Avoidance of sex with high-risk partners.
- Use of condoms for protection against STDs.
- Knowledge of the symptoms, sequelae and transmissibility of STDs.
- Avoidance of sexual contact when symptoms are present.

- Knowledge of what AIDS is and how HIV is transmitted.
- Obtaining proper treatment promptly for STD symptoms.
- Ensuring that the patients' contacts are treated whether they have symptoms or not.

PROVISION OF SERVICES FOR PATIENTS WITH STDs

The aim should be to maximize coverage and access of STD services for men and women and to have a way of referring problem cases. Costs to patients should be kept as low as possible and confidentiality safeguarded. Specialist STD clinics are valuable where the volume of patients is high, but in general the provision of specialist clinics for the treatment of STDs, which has been successful in controlling these diseases in certain industrialized countries, is neither appropriate nor feasible in most developing countries where patients with STDs should be managed at the primary health care level. Family planning and antenatal clinics provide opportunities for STD control activities which tend to be underutilized at present.

EDUCATION PROGRAMMES

The appropriate content for education messages has been described above. These messages must be expressed in a sensitive manner after widespread consultation and careful pretesting before they are disseminated by health workers, through posters and by the media. It is particularly important to target schoolchildren, commercial sex workers and patients attending for treatment of STDs. Interest has recently focused on the use of peer educators to encourage people to listen to health messages. Condom promotion is of particular importance and the social marketing of condoms recently introduced into many African countries shows promise.

SUPERVISION AND MANAGEMENT OF STD CONTROL

It is important for programmes of STD and AIDS control to be fully integrated because of their many shared objectives. The delegation of much routine STD treatment and control to the primary health care level is unlikely to succeed unless the morale and commitment of health care workers responsible for treating patients with STDs is maintained by regular supportive visits by programme managers.

REFERENCES

1 Piot P & Hira S. Control and prevention of sexually transmitted diseases. In Lamptey P & Piot P (eds) *The Handbook for AIDS Prevention in Africa*. Durham, NC: Family Health International, 1990: 83–104.

2 Meheus A & Piot P. Epidémiologie des maladies sexuellement transmissibles dans les pays en train de développement. *Ann Soc Belg Méd Trop* 1983; 63:281–311.

3 Mabey D C W, Lloyd-Evans N, Conteh S & Forsey T. Sexually transmitted diseases among randomly selected attenders at an antenatal clinic in The Gambia. *Br J Vener Dis* 1984; 60:331–336.

4 Laga M, Plummer F, Nsanze H et al. Epidemiology of ophthalmia neonatorum in Kenya. *Lancet* 1986; ii:1145–1148.

5 Meheus A, Friedman F, van Dyck E & Guyver T. Genital infections in prenatal and family planning attendants in Swaziland. *East Afr Med J* 1979; 57:212–217.

6 Hira S K. Sexually transmitted disease—a menace to mother and children. *World Health Forum* 1986; 7:243–247.

7 Osoba A O & Onifade A. Venereal diseases among pregnant women in Nigeria. *West Afr Med J* 1973; 22:23–25.

8 Bentsi C, Klufio C A, Perine P L et al. Genital infections with *Chlamydia trachomatis* and *Neisseria gonorrhoeae* in Ghanaian women. *Genitourin Med* 1985; 61:48–50.

9 D'Costa L J, Plummer F A, Bowmer I et al. Prostitutes are a major reservoir of sexually transmitted diseases in Nairobi, Kenya. *Sex Transm Dis* 1985; 12:64–67.

10 Muir D G & Belsey M A. Pelvic inflammatory disease and its consequences in the developing world. *Am J Obstet Gynecol* 1980; 138:913–928.

11 Cates W, Farley T M M & Rowe P J. Worldwide patterns of infertility: is Africa different? *Lancet* 1985; ii:596–598.

12 Mabey D, Hanlon P, Hanlon L, Marsh V & Forsey T. Chlamydial and gonococcal ophthalmia neonatorum in The Gambia. *Ann Trop Paediatr* 1987; 7:177–180.

13 Hira S K, Ratnam A V, Sehgal D, Bhat G J, Chintu C & Mulenga R C. Congenital syphilis in Lusaka. Incidence in a general nursery ward. *East Afr Med J* 1982; 59:241–246.

14 Osoba A O & Alausa K O. Vulvovaginitis in Nigerian children. *Niger J Paediatr* 1974; 1:26.

15 Pelouze P S. *Gonorrhoea in the Male and Female*. Philadelphia: W B Saunders, 1941.

16 Bewes P C. Urethral stricture. *Trop Doct* 1973; 3:77–81.

17 Osegbe D N & Amaku E O. Gonococcal strictures in young patients. *Urology* 1981; 18:37–41.

18 Collet M, Reniers S, Frost E et al. Infertility in Central Africa: infection is the cause. *Int J Gynaecol Obstet* 1988; 26:423–428.

19 Elliot B, Brunham R C, Laga M et al. Maternal gonococcal infection as a preventable risk factor for low birth weight. *J Infect Dis* 1990; 161:532–536.

20 Plummer F A, Laga M, Brunham R D et al. Postpartum upper genital tract infections in Nairobi, Kenya: epidemiology, etiology, and risk factors. *J Infect Dis* 1987; 156:92–98.

21 Stein C M & Hanly M G. Acute tropical polyarthritis in Zimbabwe: a prospective search for a gonococcal aetiology. *Ann Rheum Dis* 1987; 46:912–914.

22 Kestelyn P, Bogaerts J & Meheus A. Gonorrhoeal keratoconjunctivitis in African adults. *Sex Transm Dis* 1987; 14:191–194.

23 World Health Organization. Management of patients with sexually transmitted diseases. Report of a WHO Study Group. *WHO Tech Rep Ser* 1991; 810.

24 Laga M, Plummer F A, Piot P et al. Prophylaxis of gonococcal and chlamydial ophthalmia neonatorum; a comparison of silver nitrate and tetracycline. *N Engl J Med* 1988; 318:653–657.

25 Ison C A. Laboratory methods in genitourinary medicine. Methods of diagnosing *gonorrhoea*. *Genitourin Med* 1990; 66:433–439.

26 Lind I. Epidemiology of antibiotic resistant *Neisseria gonorrhoeae* in industrialized and developing countries. *Scand J Infect Dis Suppl* 1990; 69:77–82.

27 Moran J S & Zenilman J M. Therapy for gonococcal infections: options in 1989. *Rev Infect Dis* 1990; 12(supplement 6): S663–S644.

28 Thompson S E & Washington A E. Epidemiology of sexually transmitted *Chlamydia trachomatis* infections. *Epidemiol Rev* 1983; 5:96–123.

29 Morrison R P, Lyng K & Caldwell H D. Chlamydial disease pathogenesis. Ocular hypersensitivity elicited by a genus-specific 57 kD protein. *J Exp Med* 1989; 169:663–675.

30 Westrom L & Mårdh P-A. Chlamydial salpingitis. *Br Med Bull* 1983; 39:145–150.

31 Beem M O & Saxon E M. Respiratory tract colonisation and a distinctive pneumonia syndrome in infants infected with *Chlamydia trachomatis*. *N Engl J Med* 1977; 296:306–310.

32 Ridgway G L & Taylor Robinson D. Current problems in microbiology. Chlamydial infections: which laboratory test? *J Clin Pathol* 1991; 44:1–5.

33 Sellors J, Mahony J, Jang D et al. Rapid, on-site diagnosis of chlamydial urethritis in men by detection of antigens in urethral swabs and urine. *J Clin Microbiol* 1991; 29:407–409.

34 Steingrimsson O, Olaffson J H, Thorarinsson H et al. Azithromycin in the treatment of sexually transmitted disease. *J Antimicrob Chemother* 1990; 25(supplement A):109–114.

35 Wolner-Hanssen P, Krieger J N, Stevens C E et al. Clinical manifestations of vaginal trichomoniasis. *JAMA* 1989; 261:571–576.

36 Gravett M G, Preston Nelson H, DeRouen T, Critchlow C, Eschenbach D A & Holmes K K. Independent association of bacterial vaginosis and *Chlamydia trachomatis* infection with adverse pregnancy outcome. *JAMA* 1986; 256:1899–1903.

37 Hammond G W, Slutchuk M, Scatliff J et al. Clinical epidemiological, laboratory and therapeutic features of an urban outbreak of chancroid in North America. *Rev Infect Dis* 1980; 2:867–879.

38 Morse S A. Chancroid and *Haemophilus ducreyi*. *Clin Microbiol Rev* 1989; 2:137–157.

39 Plummer F A, D'Costa L J, Nsanze H et al. Epidemiology of chancroid and *Haemophilus ducreyi* in Nairobi. *Lancet* 1983; ii:1293–1295.

40 Hart G. Venereal disease in a war environment. Incidence and management. *Med J Aust* 1975; 1:808–810.

41 Cameron D W, D'Costa L J, Gregory M M et al. Female to male transmission of human immunodeficiency virus type 1: risk factors for seroconversion in men. *Lancet* 1989; ii:403–407.

42 Plummer F A, Simonsen J N, Cameron D W et al. Co-factors in male to female transmission of HIV. *J Infect Dis* 1991; 163:233–239.

43 Fast M V, D'Costa L J, Nsanze H et al. The clinical diagnosis of genital ulcer disease in men in the tropics. *Sex Transm Dis* 1984; 11:72–76.

44 Museyi K, Van Dyck E, Vervoort T, Taylor D, Hoge C & Piot P. Use of an enzyme immunoassay to detect serum IgG antibodies to *Haemophilus ducreyi*. *J Infect Dis* 1988; 157:1039–1043.

45 Hudson E H. *Non-venereal Syphilis*. Baltimore, MD: Williams & Wilkins, 1958.

46 Greenwood A, D'Alessandro U, Sisay F & Greenwood B. Treponemal infection and the outcome of pregnancy in a rural area of the Gambia, West Africa. *J Infect Dis* 1992; 166:842–846.

47 Gjestland T. The Oslo study of untreated syphilis. *Acta Derm Venereol Suppl (Stockh)* 1955; 35:1.

48 Ingraham N R. The value of penicillin alone in the prevention and treatment of congenital syphilis. *Acta Derm Venereol* 1951; 31 (supplement 24): 60.

49 Hira S K, Bhat G J, Patel J B et al. Early congenital syphilis: clinicoradiologic features in 202 patients. *Sex Transm Dis* 1985; 12:177–183.

50 Sengupta B S. Vulval cancer following or co-existing with chronic granulomatous diseases of the vulva. *Trop Doct* 1981; 11:110–114.

51 Perine P L, Andersen A J, Krause D W et al. Diagnosis and treatment of lymphogranuloma venereum in Ethiopia. In Nelson J D & Grassi C (eds) *Current Chemotherapy and Infectious Disease*. Washington, DC: American Society for Microbiology, 1980: 1280–1282.

52 Parkash S & Radhakrishna K. Problematic ulcerative lesions in sexually transmitted diseases: surgical management. *Sex Transm Dis* 1986; 13:127–133.

53 O'Farrell N, Hoosen A A, Coetzee K D & Van den Ende J. Genital ulcer disease in men in Durban, South Africa. *Genitourin Med* 1991; 67:327–330.

54 Goldberg J. Studies on granuloma inguinale. VII. Some epidemiological considerations of the disease. *Br J Vener Dis* 1964; 40:140–145.

55 Scott C W, Harper D M, Jason R S & Helwig E B. Neonatal granuloma venereum. *Am J Dis Child* 1952; 85:308–315.

56 Richens J. The diagnosis and treatment of donovanosis (granuloma inguinale). *Genitourin Med* 1991; 67:441–452.

57 Verdich J. *Haemophilus ducreyi* infection resembling granuloma inguinale. *Arch Derm Venereol* 1984; 64:452–455.

58 Cannefax G R. The technic of the tissue spread method for demonstrating Donovan bodies. *J Vener Dis Inf* 1948; 29:210–214.

59 Ramanan C, Sarma P S A, Ghorpade A & Das M. Treatment of donovanosis with norfloxacin. *Int J Dermatol* 1990; 29:298–299.

60 Folkers E, Orange A P, Dun ven Voorden J N, Van der Veen J P W, Rijlaarsdam J U & Emsbroek J A. Tzanck smear in diagnosing genital herpes. *Genitourin Med* 1988; 64:249–254.

61 Mercey D E & Mindel A. Preventing neonatal herpes? *Genitourin Med* 1991; 67:1–2.

62 Rando R F. Human papillomavirus: implications for clinical medicine. *Ann Intern Med* 1988; 108:628–631.

63 Munoz N, Bosch X & Kaldor J M. Does human papillomavirus cause cervical cancer? The state of the epidemiologic evidence. *Br J Cancer* 1988; 57:1–5.

64 Eskelinen A & Mashkilleyson N. Optimum treatment of genital warts. *Drugs* 1987; 34:599–603.

FURTHER READING

1 Arya O P, Osoba A O & Bennett F J. *Tropical Venereology*, 2nd edn. Edinburgh: Churchill Livingstone, 1988.

2 Holmes K K, Mårdh P A, Sparling P F et al. (eds) *Sexually Transmitted Diseases*, 2nd edn. New York: McGraw-Hill, 1990.

3 Osoba A O (ed.). Baillière's clinical tropical medicine and communicable diseases. *Sexually transmitted*

diseases in the tropics. London: Baillière Tindall, 1987.

4 Schulz K F, Cates W Jr & O'Mara P R. Pregnancy loss, infant death, and suffering: legacy of syphilis and gonorrhoea in Africa. *Genitourin Med* 1987; 63:320–325.

5 Sexually Transmitted Diseases Treatment Guidelines. *Rev Infect Dis* 1990; 12 (supplement): S577–S690.

CHAPTER 14

MUSCULOSKELETAL DISEASES

A. O. Adebajo

Musculoskeletal disorders are increasingly being recognized as an important and growing cause of morbidity in the tropics. In addition it is believed that the study of these conditions in the tropics may provide useful aetiopathogenetic clues.[1] For too long, these disorders have been neglected in the tropics, with the earliest reports almost all dating back little more than half a century ago.

As the term implies, musculoskeletal diseases are those which affect muscles, tendons, ligaments, joints, the connective tissues and even bone. Not surprisingly many of these disorders in the tropics are of infectious origin (Table 14.1).

Table 14.1 Infectious agents particularly associated with rheumatic disorders in the tropics.

Viruses
  O'nyong-nyong
  Dengue
  Chikungunya
  Hepatitis B
  Yellow fever
  Human immunodeficiency virus (HIV)
  Sandbis
  Ross river

Spirochaetes
  Yaws
  Syphilis

Bacteria
  Staphylococcus spp.
  Salmonella spp.
  Neisseria gonorrhoeae
  Brucella spp.

Parasites
  Malaria
  Schistosomiasis
  Dracontiasis
  Filariasis
  Amoebiasis

Fungi
  Histoplasmosis
  Madura foot

DISEASES OF SKELETAL MUSCLE, TENDONS AND LIGAMENTS

Primary diseases of skeletal muscle are uncommon in the tropics. Muscle disorders are more commonly seen in association with another pathology, such as prolonged corticosteroids given therapeutically, endocrine disorders such as thyrotoxicosis, and in association with neoplasms such as hepatoma. The apparent absence of polymyalgia rheumatica in the tropics is of interest and remains unexplained.

POLYMYOSITIS

Although this inflammatory disorder is uncommon in the tropics it does occur.[2,3] Classical acute phase proteins, electromyographic and muscle biopsy changes are found. However, elevated serum creatinine kinase levels may occur in healthy black males[4] and must be interpreted with caution.

INFECTIVE PYOMYOSITIS

Pyomyositis is an acute inflammation of skeletal muscle mainly confined to the subtropics and tropics.[5–7] It occurs at any age but most frequently in children and young male adults. The initiating lesion may be a penetrating injury or crush injury or it may be secondary to a staphylococcal arthritis. *Staphylococcus pyogenes* is the usual infecting organism. It is possible that the disorder may arise when the staphylococcus reaches a muscle recently damaged by a viral myositis, but malnutrition and various parasitic infections have also been postulated.

Muscular pain is usually the first symptom, followed within the next week by fever, localized induration and oedema. Any muscle group may be affected but most commonly the proximal limb muscles (gluteal and quadriceps) are involved. The erector spinae and shoulder girdle muscles can also be affected. The clinical features are those of a localized abscess with mild to moderate systemic features. If untreated the condition will progress over the next 4 weeks until there is extensive muscle destruction. Pus can often be aspirated from 10 days onwards. Occasionally the systemic picture predominates and multiple muscle abscesses occur as a late finding. There is often a minor degree of polymorphonuclear leucocytosis, and a moderate eosinophilia of about 10% is common. Treatment involves the administration of an adequate dose of an appropriate antibiotic effective against penicillinase-producing organisms, given parenterally at least initially. Treatment for several weeks is often required and surgical drainage of fluctuant abscesses should be carried out. Despite the destruction of a large muscle bulk, functional and cosmetic recovery is usually remarkably good.

PARASITIC PYOMYOSITIS

Several parasites can give rise to a myositis. Trypanosomiasis causes an acute myositis, often with encephalomyelitis and myocarditis. The same appears to be true of filariasis.

SOFT TISSUE DISORDERS

Diseases involving the musculoskeletal soft tissues (tendons and ligaments) present clinically in a man-

ner identical to that found in temperate countries. Patients with these problems do not usually seek medical attention, as observed with shoulder lesions.[8] Similarly back pain is very prevalent in the tropics, often in association with manual work. The fact that health insurance schemes and compensation claims for injuries are uncommon in many tropical countries may be one reason why only a proportion of back pain sufferers seeks medical attention.

HYPERMOBILITY

Hypermobility is due to laxity of the ligaments surrounding a joint as a result of genetic and/or environmental causes (Figure 14.1). Studies on hypermobility indicate that African populations have a higher prevalence of hypermobility than Caucasians, although this prevalence may be lower than amongst populations from the Indian subcontinent.[9–11]

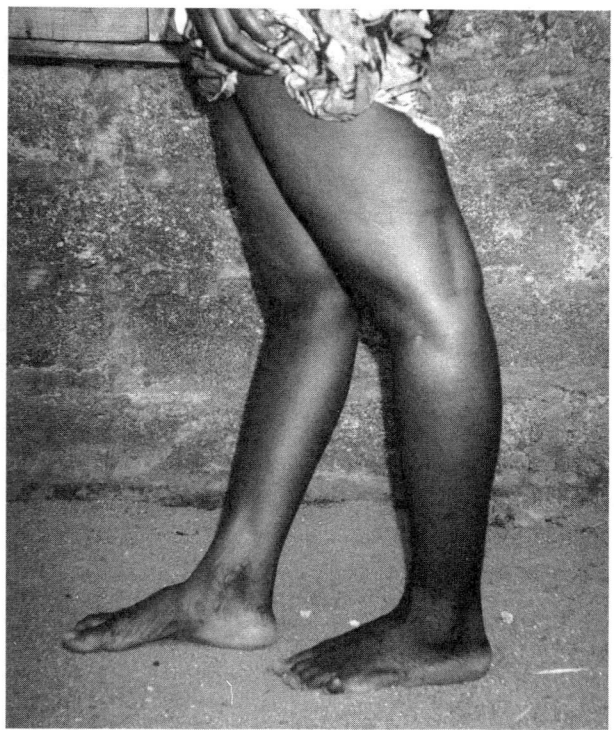

Figure 14.1 Hyperextensibility (hypermobility) of the knee in an African woman.

DISEASES OF JOINTS

Diseases of joints form the bulk of the musculoskeletal disorders and particularly those seen in hospital. Arthralgia refers to significant joint pain occurring in the total or virtual absence of any physical signs. Arthritis, on the other hand, refers to an inflammatory process of the joint lining, with the classical features of redness, warmth, swelling and limitation of function in addition to joint pain. Arthralgia occurs commonly in association with infectious diseases such as those due to arboviruses. Arthritis can be involved in a number of infective, immunological and metabolic conditions. Although treatment usually involves the use of analgesics, non-steroidal anti-inflammatory drugs, disease-modifying drugs and physiotherapy there are certain problems peculiar to the tropics. These include the question of the use of antimalarial drugs for inflammatory joint problems in regions with endemic malaria, as well as the of sulphasalazine where glucose-6-phosphate dehydrogenase deficiency is common.

RHEUMATOID ARTHRITIS

Rheumatoid arthritis is the most studied rheumatic disorder in the tropics. The disorder is a chronic inflammatory deforming and destructive polyarthritis usually affecting joints, often in a peripheral and symmetrical manner (Figure 14.2). In addition it is a systemic disease affecting various organs and body systems. The disorder is a relatively recent condition on the African continent.[12] The cause of this disease is unknown but there is a strong genetic association with the DR4 haplotype. Environmental factors may also be important.[13,14] There is some evidence to suggest that the disease is more prevalent in urban than rural areas.[15,16] In India the disease is infrequent and mild, with systemic manifestations and subcutaneous nodules occurring rarely.[17] In Jamaica there is a high prevalence of the disease but it is mainly mild and rheumatoid factor seronegative.[18] In East Africa and among urban but not rural black South Africans rheumatoid arthritis has a similar pattern to that in Caucasian populations[15,16,19,20] In West Africa, however, the disease is uncommon and mild.[21,22] A similar pattern has been found in some studies conducted in China.[23,24] In Malaysia rheumatoid nodules and other extra-articular features are uncommon.[25]

SPONDYLOARTHROPATHIES

Spondyloarthropathies such as ankylosing spondylitis are uncommon in Africans[26] and in the Middle East,[27] in keeping with the low prevalence of HLA-B27 in these areas. Ankylosing spondylitis is less common in the Chinese than in white populations[28] but its prevalence may be higher in rural parts of China.[23] Ankylosing spondylitis is characterized by limited spinal movement, squaring of the vertebral bodies and ossification of the disc margins and longitudinal spinal ligaments resulting in a 'bamboo' spine.

Reiter's syndrome, comprising the triad of urethritis, conjunctivitis and arthritis, occurs predominantly after venereal disease in Africa and in Papua New Guinea.[29–31] Other seronegative arthropathies are uncommon in the tropics.

OSTEOARTHRITIS

Osteoarthritis is a progressive joint disease characterized by destruction of articular cartilage and the generation of osteophytes. Osteoarthritis may be mono-, oligo- or polyarticular in joint distribution. Polyarticular disease is uncommon in many parts of the tropics.[32–34] Heberden's nodes (osteophytes involving the distal interphalangeal joints) are uncommon in Africans and Jamaicans.[35,36] Osteoarthritis of the hip joint is uncommon, in contrast with

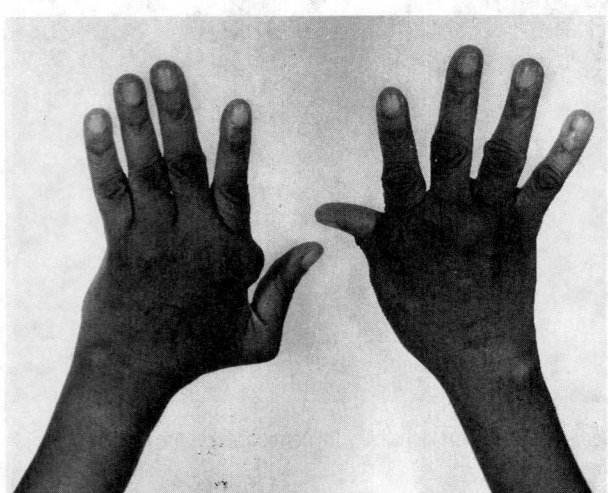

Figure 14.2 Hand deformity in an African woman with rheumatoid arthritis.

Table 14.2 Hip and knee joint involvement in Nigerian and British patients with osteoarthritis.

Patients	Hip (%)	Knee (%)
Nigerian (Adebajo, 1991)[34]	1.4	47.0
British (Cushnaghan and Dieppe, 1991)[82]	19.0	41.2

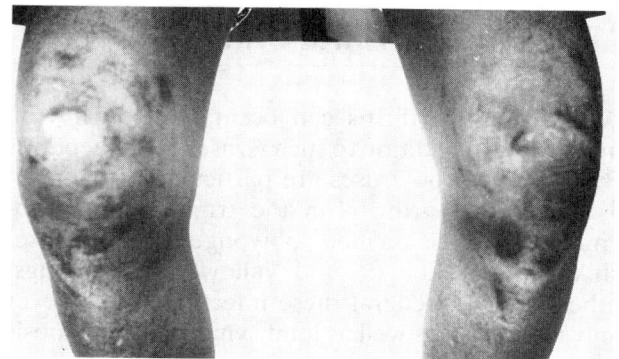

Figure 14.4 Right knee swelling in a young man with Reiter's syndrome.

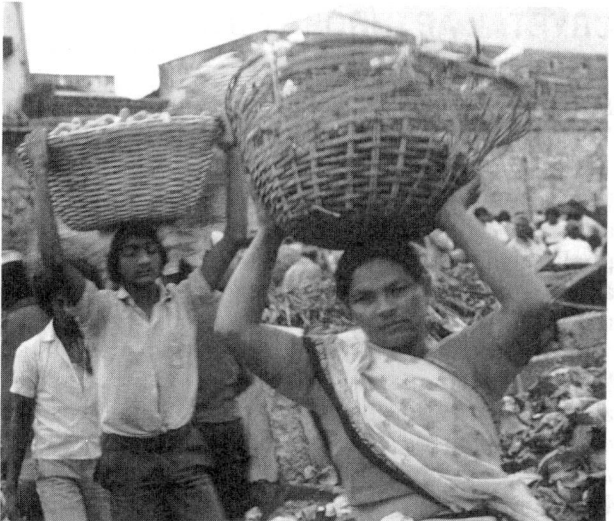

Figure 14.3 Carrying loads on the head is common in the tropics but is not associated with cervical spondylosis in the general population.

osteoarthritis of the knee (Table 14.2), among Chinese,[37,38] Africans,[39,40] Indians[41] and in the Middle East.[27] Various sociocultural activities including squatting and kneeling, either in prayer or as a form of greeting, have been suggested as influencing this distribution of osteoarthritis. Developmental knee abnormalities from rickets, trauma or parasitic infections and a low prevalence of congenital hip abnormalities in many parts of the tropics may also determine the joint distribution. Interestingly, the habit of carrying loads on the head by some populations does not seem to predispose to cervical spondylosis (Figure 14.3).

An interesting degenerative arthropathy known as Mseleni disease has been observed in southern Africa.[42] It is believed to be an unusual form of bone dysplasia, commonly affecting females before the age of 40 years and most frequently involving the hip joint, although other joints—particularly the knees and ankles, can be affected. The clinical course is

that of a slowly progressive disability and the treatment is as for osteoarthritis.

ARTHRITIS OF BACTERIAL ORIGIN (SEPTIC ARTHRITIS)

Various organisms can give rise to septic arthritis. An acute pyogenic joint infection is one of the most common causes of joint disease in the tropics. It is commonly due to Staph. aureus. The hip joints are most commonly affected in infants and the knee joint in older children and adults.[43]

Salmonella joint infections are also common, particularly in those with sickle cell disease. Meningococcal arthritis can occur either as a localized suppurative arthritis or as generalized polyarthritis. The synovial fluid of affected joints may be sterile, indicating that immune complexes could play a large part in the pathogenesis of the disease.[44] In children, acute rheumatic fever causes migratory joint involvement involving predominantly the large joints.

Gonococcal arthritis can occur following spread of Neisseria gonorrhoeae from the urogenital tract. It may mimic Reiter's syndrome (Figure 14.4) but, unlike the latter, the organism may be isolated from the synovial fluid and responds to penicillin.

Tuberculosis may affect any joint, particularly the hip or the knee, but is usually monoarticular. There may also be other evidence of tuberculosis but diagnosis is often difficult and may require synovial biopsy. Brucellosis occurs either as a local suppurative arthritis or a generalized non-suppurative polyarthritis in many parts of the tropics. Pastoral and nomadic populations are at particular risk.[45,46]

In all suspected cases of septic arthritis the affected joint should be aspirated and appropriate antibiotics given.

ARTHRITIS OF VIRAL ORIGIN

Arthralgia or arthritis can occur with most viral infections. In addition to such viruses as the hepatitis B virus, the arboviruses are particularly important as a cause of arthritis in the tropics. The arboviral infections include o'nyong-nyong disease, chikungunya, dengue and yellow fever amongst others.[47–50] In general these infections cause fever and a skin rash as well as joint symptoms. Diagnosis is usually made by identifying raised viral titres. Although in a few cases chronic arthralgia or arthritis may persist, the prognosis is usually good and analgesics are the mainstay of treatment.

ARTHRITIS OF PARASITIC AND FUNGAL ORIGIN

Various parasitic infections may be associated with arthritis, or more commonly arthralgia. Malaria is one of the most common causes of polyarthralgia in the tropics. Arthralgia and backache may occur as an extraintestinal symptom of amoebic dysentery and may even be a predominant symptom. Dracontiasis, schistosomiasis and filariasis have all been associated with joint problems. Usually there is arthralgia; however synovitis may occur and the adult worm or larval form may be recovered from the joint fluid. Onchocerciasis in particular may be associated with disabling back pain.

Fungal infection due to *Histoplasma duboisii* as well as madura foot may be associated with a periarthritis and even erosive changes.

ACUTE TROPICAL POLYARTHRITIS

Acute or idiopathic tropical polyarthritis is a condition which has generated considerable interest as it is still uncertain as to whether it is a homogeneous entity or a diagnostic waste-paper basket for acute arthritis associated with unknown or undiagnosed tropical infections.[51–53] The condition affects young adults of both sexes and usually involves large joints. Constitutional features including fever may be present and the erythrocyte sedimentation rate is raised. The white cell count, joint radiographs and synovial fluid analysis are normal. Spontaneous resolution of the condition commonly occurs and treatment is symptomatic.

CRYSTAL ARTHROPATHIES

Hyperuricaemia and gout are common in some Polynesian islands.[54] There is evidence that in some tropical countries gout is associated with urbanization, although both rich and poor may be affected.[55–57] Gout commonly affects the metatarsophalangeal joint of the large toe. Affected joints are acutely inflamed and very tender. Acute attacks may be precipitated by trauma or heavy drinking and thus may recur. Urate deposition into tissues leads to subcutaneous tophi, and renal stones may also occur. In addition to these clinical features, the diagnosis is made by a raised serum uric acid level and evidence of uric acid crystals in synovial fluid. Radiographs may show areas of bone destruction around affected joints. Colchicine or non-steroidal anti-inflammatory drugs are useful for acute attacks, while xanthine oxidase inhibitors which reduce uric acid synthesis, such as allopurinol, are used to lower the serum uric acid level.

Chondrocalcinosis or pseudo-gout differs from gout in that calcium pyrophosphate crystals rather than uric acid crystals are deposited in the synovium and tissues. Pseudo-gout has been reported from the tropics.[58]

CONNECTIVE TISSUE DISORDERS

Connective tissue disorders such as systemic lupus erythematosus (a syndrome characterized by vasculitis, photosensitive skin rash, fever, nephritis and neuropsychiatric disturbances, in association with antinuclear antibodies) are uncommon in Africa.[59,60] Systemic lupus erythematosus is, however, common in China,[28] Malaysia,[61] India,[62] Puerto Rico[63] and the West Indies.[64] In Malaysia those of Chinese ethnic origin seem to be more vulnerable to systemic lupus erythematosus than Malays or those of Indian origin.[63,65] It has been suggested that tropical infections such as malaria may protect Africans against connective tissue diseases,[66] perhaps mediated through tumour necrosis factor.[6] Alternatively systemic lupus erythematosus and other connective tissue diseases may be under-diagnosed in many parts of the tropics as a result of the immunodiagnostic tests required. Diseases like tuberculosis may also mimic some of these connective tissue disorders.[59] Another problem is that autoantibodies that are usually found in patients with systemic lupus erythematosus may also occur in association with various tropical infections.[67]

Other connective tissue disorders such as scleroderma, systemic sclerosis and polyarteritis nodosa have all been reported from the tropics.[19,68–79]

DISEASES OF BONE

Infections are the most common form of bone disease in the tropics but bone tumours, particularly Burkitt's lymphoma, are also found. Sickle cell disease can be complicated by bone lesions in those parts of the tropics where the disease occurs (mainly West Africa and the Caribbean). Rickets is still common in many parts of the tropics, but other metabolic bone diseases are less frequently seen. Congenital lesions of bone are rare.

INFECTIVE DISEASE OF BONE

As with infective diseases of joints, many different organisms may be responsible. Acute osteomyelitis is commonly seen with or without any obvious focus of infection such as skin sepsis. In patients with sickle cell disease *Salmonella* organisms are common pathogens.[55] A chronic infection may develop with the formation of a sequestrum of dead bone which can act as a nidus for the systemic spread of organisms. Acute infections are treated with antibiotics and drainage, while chronic infections often require prolonged antibiotics and excision of dead bone.

Tuberculosis can affect virtually any bone of the body. Tuberculosis of the vertebrae (Pott's disease) is a common problem in the tropics. The infection occurs most commonly in the thoracic spine, leading to vertebral collapse with a kyphosis. The spinal cord may be affected as a result of direct pressure of inflammatory tissue, or more commonly by occlusion of nutrient arteries. A paravertebral abscess may track around the abdominal or thoracic wall or in front of the psoas muscle to point in the groin as a psoas abscess. Spinal tuberculosis can be treated on an outpatient basis with antituberculous chemotherapy.

Brucella infection occurs most frequently in the lumbar spine but spinal cord damage is uncommon. Radiographs show osteolytic lesions with new bone formation. Diagnosis is difficult but brucellosis should be considered in a patient with severe backache and radiological signs of bone destruction.[71] Treatment is with appropriate antibiotics.

BONE TUMOURS

Primary tumours of bone are uncommon, although osteogenic sarcomas may mimic acute osteomyelitis. Secondary deposits often arise from lymphomas or hepatocellular carcinomas.

METABOLIC BONE DISEASE

Rickets remains a common problem in the tropics and is sometimes related to a poor diet as well as the wearing of purdah by mothers which may lead to calcium deficiency in their babies (Figures 14.5–14.7).

Blount's disease occurs in parts of the tropics, mainly amongst Blacks,[72] and is an osteochondrosis affecting the medial tibial physis, causing tibia vara. Treatment is by tibial osteotomy.

Osteoporosis is uncommon in many parts of the tropics;[73,74] this may be due to protection by socio-cultural factors—in particular exercise.

Other metabolic bone diseases such as marble bone disease and Paget's disease appear to be uncommon in most parts of the tropics.

HAEMOGLOBINOPATHIES

Apart from osteomyelitis, bone lesions associated with haemoglobinopathies include bone crises as a result of infarction of bone(s), as well as bossing of the skull, biconcave vertebrae and dactylitis. Avascular necrosis of the femoral, or less commonly

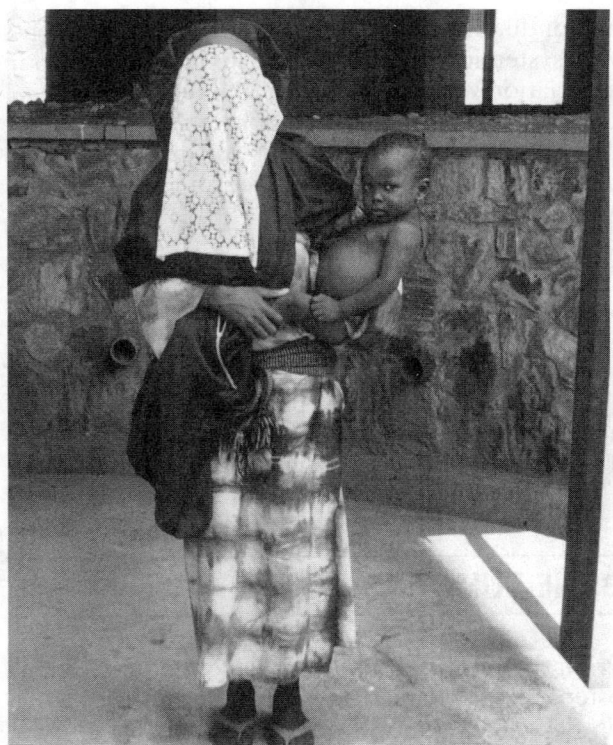

Figure 14.5   A mother in purdah; her child has rickets.

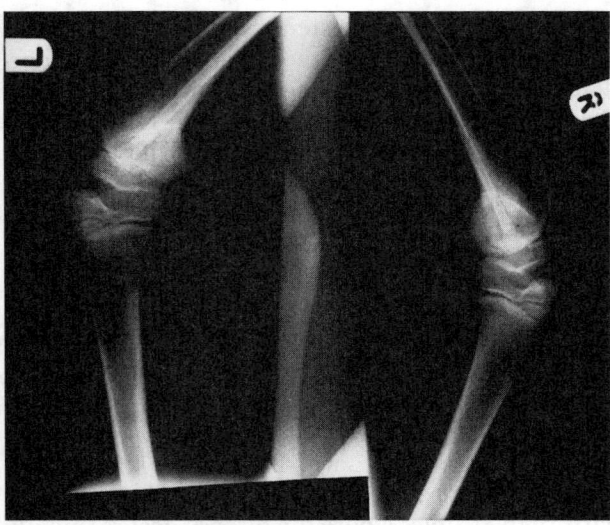

Figure 14.7   Radiograph of a child with rickets.

humeral, head is seen in patients with haemoglobin SC or SS disease.

OTHER BONY LESIONS

Ainhum is a condition in which a stricture slowly develops between the fifth toe and the foot, leading

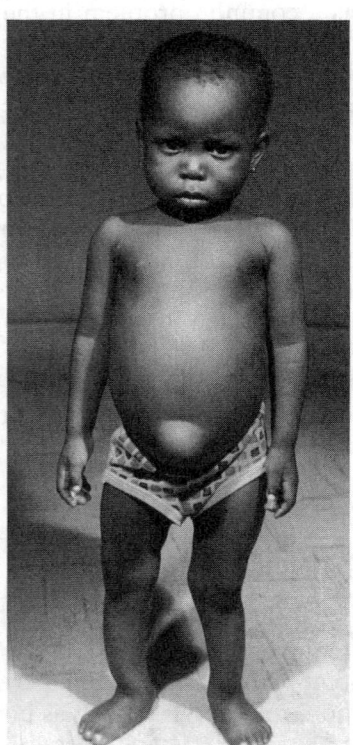

Figure 14.6   Child with rickets showing limb deformities.

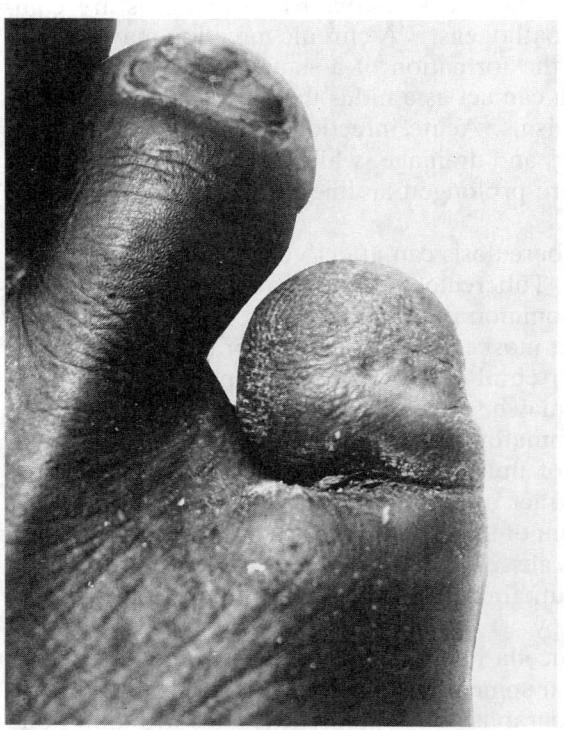

Figure 14.8   Ainhum at its height. (Courtesy of W. M. Meyers.)

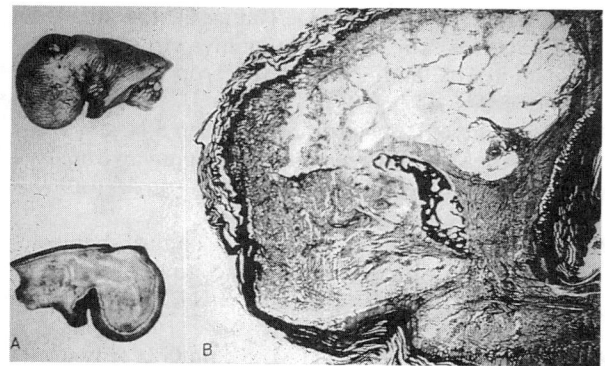

Figure 14.9   An amputated toe from a patient suffering from ainhum, showing constriction at the base. (Courtesy of B. H. Kean.)

to spontaneous amputation. It has its highest incidence in Africa, especially amongst women of the Transkei in South Africa,[75] but also occurs in people of African descent in the New World,[76] Polyne-sians[77] and Indians.[78] The aetiology is obscure and is considered as being due to abnormal fibrogenesis,[79] angiodysplasia[80] or a common toxic cause (possibly of plant origin) for both ainhum and phocomelia.[75] It is most common in people who walk barefoot. Clinically, there is a slow development of a constriction encircling the little toe at the level of the metatarsophalangeal joint(s). Pain may occur and the distal portion of the toe may swell. After some years the toe may remain attached to the foot by a fragile cutaneous pedicle only, and at this stage spontaneous or deliberate amputation usually occurs (Figures 14.8 and 14.9). There is no proven treatment for the condition but when troublesome the affected toe should be amputated.

Transkei foot is a disorder consisting of marked lateral deviation of the fifth toe; it has been described in the Xhosa population of the Transkei and is possibly of genetic origin.[81]

REFERENCES

1 Muirden K D. What can be learned from Third World rheumatism. *Br J Rheumatol* 1987; 26: 1–2.

2 Stein M & Davis P. Rheumatic disorders in Zimbabwe: a prospective analysis of patients attending a rheumatic diseases clinic. *Ann Rheum Dis* 1990; 40:400–402.

3 Gelfand M & Taube F. Polymoysitis in the African. *J Trop Med Hyg* 1966; 69:232–235.

4 Worrall J G, Phongsathorn V, Hooper R J L & Paice E W. Racial variation in serum creatinine kinase unrelated to lean body mass. *Br J Rheumatol* 1990; 29:371–373.

5 Horn C V & Master S. Pyomyositis tropicans in Uganda. *East Afr Med J* 1968; 45:463–471.

6 Levin M J, Gardner P & Waldevogel F A. Tropical pyomyositis. *N Engl J Med* 1971; 284:196–198.

7 Chiedozi L C. Polymyositis. Review of 205 cases in 112 patients. *Am J Surg* 1979; 137:255.

8 Adebajo A O & Hazleman B L. Soft tissue shoulder lesions in the African. *Br J Rheumatol* 1992; 31:275–276.

9 Beighton P, Solomon L & Seskilne C L. Articular mobility in an African population. *Ann Rheum Dis* 1973; 32:413–418.

10 Adebajo A O & Eastmond C J. Racial variation in lumbar spine flexion. *Br J Rheumatol* 1989; 28:13.

11 Birrell F, Adebajo A O, Hazleman B L & Silman A J. *Br J Rheumatol* 1994; 33:56–59.

12 Adebajo A O. Rheumatoid arthritis: A twentieth century disease in Africa. *Arthritis Rheum* 1991; 34:248.

13 Silman A J. Is rheumatoid arthritis an infectious disease? *BMJ* 1991; 303:200–201.

14 Adebajo A O. Is rheumatoid arthritis an infectious disease? *BMJ* 1991; 303:786.

15 Solomon L, Robin G & Valkenburg H A. Rheumatoid arthritis in an urban South African negro population. *Ann Rheum Dis* 1975; 34:128–135.

16 Beighton P, Solomon L & Valkenburg H A. Rheumatoid arthritis in a rural South African negro population. *Ann Rheum Dis* 1975; 34:136–141.

17 Chopra A, Raghunath D, Singh A & Subramain A R. The pattern of rheumatoid arthritis in the Indian population: a prospective study. *Br J Rheumatol* 1988; 27: 454–456.

18 Lawrence J S, Brenner J M, Bull J A & Burch T. Rheumatoid arthritis in a subtropical population. *Ann Rheum Dis* 1966; 25:59–66.

19 Lutalo S K. Chronic inflammatory rheumatic diseases in black Zimbabweans. *Ann Rheum Dis* 1985; 44:121–125.

20 Bagg L R, Hansen D P, Mutibuko I K et al. Chronic polyarthritis at the Kenyatta National Hospital. *East Afr Med J* 1976; 53:567–572.

21 Greenwood B M. Polyarthritis in Western Nigeria. I. Rheumatoid arthritis. *Ann Rheum Dis* 1969; 28:488–496.

22 Adebajo A O & Reid D M. The pattern of rheumatoid arthritis in West Africa and comparison with a cohort of British patients. *Q J Med* 1991; 292:633–640.

23 Beasley P, Bennett P H & Lin C C. Low prevalence of rheumatoid arthritis in Chinese. *J Rheumatol* 1983; 10 (supplement): 11–15.

24 Moran H, Chen Shun-le, Muirden K D et al. A comparison of rheumatoid arthritis in Australia and China. *Ann Rheum Dis* 1986; 45:572–578.

25 Toy B H, Sengupta S, Ang A H, White J C & Lav K S. Pattern of rheumatoid arthritis in West Malaysia. *Ann Rheum Dis* 1973; 32:151–156.

26 Chalmers I M. Ankylosing spondylitis in African blacks. *Arthritis Rheum* 1980; 23:1366–1370.

27 Rajapakse C N. The spectrum of rheumatic diseases in Saudi Arabia. *Br J Rheumatol* 1987; 26:22–23.

28 Chang N C. Rheumatic diseases in China. *J Rheumatol* 1983; 10 (supplement): 41–45.

29 Maddocks I. Reiter's syndrome in Port Moresby Papua. *Br J Vener Dis* 1967; 43:280–283.

30 Hall L. Polyarthritis in Kenya. *East Afr Med J* 1966; 43:161–170.

31 Csonka G W. The course of Reiter's syndrome. *BMJ* 1958; i:1088–1090.

32 Bremner J M, Lawrence J S & Miall W E. Degenerative joint disease in a Jamaican rural population. *Ann Rheum Dis* 1968; 27:326–332.

33 Brighton S W, de la Harper A L & van Staden D A. The prevalence of osteoarthrosis in a rural African community. *Br J Rheumatol* 1985; 24:321–325.

34 Adebajo A O. The pattern of osteoarthritis in a West African teaching hospital. *Ann Rheum Dis* 1991; 50:20–22.

35 Lawrence J S & Molyneux M. Degenerative joint disease among populations in Wensleydale, England and Jamaica. *Int J Biometeorol* 1968; 12:163–175.

36 Solomon L, Beighton P & Lawrence J S. Osteoarthrosis in a rural South African population. *Ann Rheum Dis* 1976; 35:274–278.

37 Hoagkund F T, Yau A & Wong W L. Osteoarthritis of the hip and other joints in Southern Chinese in Hong Kong: incidence and related factors. *J Bone Joint Surg [Am]* 1973; 55:545–547.

38 Gunn D R. Don't sit—squat! *Clin Orthop* 1974; 103:104–105.

39 Ebong W W & Lawson E A L. Pattern of osteoarthritis of the hip in Nigerians. *East Afr Med J* 1978; 55:81–84.

40 Solomon L. Pathogenesis of osteoarthritis. *Lancet* 1972; i:1072.

41 Mukhopadhaya B & Barooak B. Osteoarthritis of the hip in Indians: an anatomical and clinical study. *Indian J Orthop* 1967; 1:55–63.

42 Yach D & Botha J L. Mseleni joint disease in 1981: decreased prevalence rates, wider geographical location than before, and socioeconomic impact of an endemic osteoarthrosis in an underdeveloped community in South Africa. *Int J Epidemiol* 1985; 14:276–284.

43 Onyemelukwe G & Sturrock R D. Septic arthritis in Northern Nigeria. *Rheumatol Rehabil* 1979; 18:13–17.

44 Greenwood B M, Mohammed I & Whittle H C. Immune complexes and the pathogenesis of meningococcal arthritis. *Clin Exp Immunol* 1985; 59:513–519.

45 Manson-Bahr P E C. Clinical aspects of brucellosis in East Africa. *J Trop Med Hyg* 1955; 59:103–106.

46 Ali-Rawi Z S, Al-Khateeb N & Khalifa S J. Brucella arthritis among Iraqi patients. *Br J Rheumatol* 1987; 26:24–27.

47 Carey D E, Myers R M, De Ranitz C M, Jodhar M & Reuben R. The 1964 chikungunya virus infection in man in Thailand. *Trans R Soc Trop Med Hyg* 1969; 63:434–445.

48 Nimmannitya S, Halstead S B, Cohen S N & Margiotta M R. Dengue and chikungunya virus infection in man in Thailand. *Am J Trop Med* 1969; 17:107–111.

49 Haddow A J & Ellice J M. Studies on bush-babies (*Galago* spp) with special reference to the epidemiology of yellow fever. *Trans R Soc Trop Med Hyg* 1964; 58:521–538.

50 Causey O R, Madbouly H M, Kemp G E & Lee V H. Arbovirus surveillance in Nigeria, 1964–1967. *Bull Soc Pathol Exot* 1969; 62:249–259.

51 Editorial. Acute tropical polyarthropathy: homogeneous entity or diagnostic scrap heap? *Lancet* 1988; i:627–628.

52 Adebajo A O. Tropical polyarthritis. *Lancet* 1988; i:1103–1104.

53 Stein C M. Tropical polyarthritis. *Lancet* 1988; i:1103.

54 Prior I A M, Rose B S, Harvey H P B & Davidson F. Hyperuricaemia, gout and diabetic abnormality in polynesian people. *Lancet* 1966; i:333–338.

55 Mongola E N & Odeny J W. Gouty arthritis. *Nairobi J Med* 1972; 5:6.

56 Fleischmann V & Adadevoh B K. Hyperuricaemia and gout in Nigerians. *Trop Geogr Med* 1973; 25:255–261.

57 Mody G M & Naidoo P D. Gout in South African Blacks. *Ann Rheum Dis* 1984; 43:394–397.

58 Ducloux M & Lartigau J. Un cas de chondrocalcinose articulaire diffuse chez le noir d'Afrique de l'Ouest. *Bull Soc Med Afr Noire* 1969; 14:451–456.

59 Taylor H G & Stein C M. Systemic lupus erythematosus in Zimbabwe. *Ann Rheum Dis* 1986; 45:645–648.

60 Adebajo A O. Does tumour necrosis factor protect against lupus in West Africans? *Arthritis Rheum* 1992; 35:839–840.

61 Frank A O. Apparent predisposition to systemic lupus erythematosus in Chinese patients in West Malaysia. *Ann Rheum Dis* 1980; 39:266–269.

62 Malaviya A, Misra R, Banerjee S et al. Systemic lupus erythematosus in Indian Asians: a prospective analysis of clinical and immunological features. *Rheumatol Int* 1986; 6:97–101.

63 Mendez-Bryan R, Gonsalez-Alcover R & Roger L. Rheumatoid arthritis: prevalence in a tropical area. *Arthritis Rheum* 1964; 7:171–176.

64 Harris E N, Williams E, Shah D J & De Ceular K. Mortality of Jamaican patients with systemic lupus erythematosus. *Br J Rheumatol* 1989; 28:113–117.

65 Veerapen K, Wong F, Bosco J & Manivasagar M. Systemic lupus erythematosus (SLE): a profile of 419 patients from Malaysia. *Br J Rheumatol* 1988; 27:40.

66 Greenwood B M, Herrick E M & Voller A. Can parasitic infection suppress autoimmune disease? *Proc Soc Med* 1970; 63:19–20.

67 Adebajo A O, Charles P, Maini R N & Hazleman B L. Autoantibodies in Malaria, tuberculosis and hepatitis B in a West African population. *Clin Exp Immunol* 1993; 92:73–76.

68 Buchanan W M & Gelfand M. Polyarteritis nodosa in the African. *Cent Afr J Med* 1970; 16:274–275.

69 Greenwood B M. Autoimmune disease and parasitic infections in Nigerians. *Lancet* 1968; ii:380–381.

70 Davis P, Stein M, Ley H & Johnston C. Serological profiles in connective tissue diseases in Zimbabwean patients. *Ann Rheum Dis* 1989; 48:73–76.

71 Rajapakse C N A, Al-Aska A K, Al Orainey I, Halim K & Arabi K. Spinal brucellosis. *Br J Rheumatol* 1987; 26:28–31.

72 Golding J S R & McNeil-Smith J D G. Observations on the etiology of tibia vara. *J Bone Joint Surg [Br]* 1963; 45:320–325.

73 Adebajo A O, Cooper C & Grimley Evans J. Fractures of the hip and distal forearm in West Africa and the United Kingdom. *Age Ageing* 1991; 20:435–438.

74 Solomon L. Osteoporosis and fracture of the femoral neck in the South African Bantu. *J Bone Joint Surg [Br]* 1968; 50:2–13.

75 Daynes W E S. Ainhum: its possible causation by ingestion of plants. *S Afr Med J* 1973; 47:320–321.

76 Kean B H, Tucker H A & Miller W C. Ainhum: clinical summary of 45 cases on Isthmus of Panama. *Trans R Soc Trop Med Hyg* 1946; 39:331–334.

77 Browne S G. Ainhum. A Clinical and etiological study of 83 cases. *Ann Trop Med Parasitol* 1961; 55:314–320.

78 Aggarwal N D & Singh H. Ainhum. Report of an atypical case. *J Bone Joint Surg [Br]* 1963; 45:376–378.

79 Browne S G. True ainhum: its distinctive and differentiating features. *J Bone Joint Surg [Br]* 1965; 47:52–55.

80 Dent D M, Fataar S & Rose A G. Ainhum and antiodysplasia. *Lancet* 1981; ii:396–397.

81 Schwartz P A, Shlugman D, Daynes G et al. Transkei foot. *S Afr Med J* 1974; 48:961–962.

82 Cushnaghan J & Dieppe P. Study of 500 patients with limb joint osteoarthritis. I. Analysis by age, sex and distribution of symptomatic joint sites. *Ann Rheum Dis* 1991; 50:8–13.

SECTION 3
RELATED SPECIALTIES IN THE TROPICS

Tropical medicine has traditionally focused strictly on *medical* entities. However, 'medicine in the tropics' encompasses a far wider scenario; special problems arise in certain groups. A high proportion of the population of a developing country consists of infants and children; therefore, it is important that some of the major diseases affecting this group are emphasized and brought to the fore. Surgical conditions are also common, and all too frequently first-class care is not available; in consequence, many cases are not dealt with until the disease under consideration has reached an advanced stage; additionally, inadequate training and inept surgical practice all too frequently result in unfortunate consequences following an operative procedure. Obstetric and gynaecological problems abound; these too are frequently subject to all manner of complications which are often exceedingly difficult to manage with the limited facilities available.

This section seeks to highlight some of the special problems posed by infants and children and the pregnant woman in a tropical environment; major surgical and gynaecological problems are also covered, albeit somewhat cursorily. It is essential, however, that the reader takes this section in conjunction with other components within the book where greater in-depth coverage of relevant disease entities—especially those with an infective basis—is to be found.

CHAPTER 15

PAEDIATRICS IN THE TROPICS

R. G. Hendrickse and B. J. Brabin

This chapter aims to summarize various specific paediatric problems associated with a tropical environment. Many of the diseases covered in other sections also have paediatric implications.

OVERVIEW

Children constitute 40–50% of the population of developing countries which are situated mainly in the tropics and subtropics. Adults indigenous to these countries have considerable immunity to endemic diseases that may be life-threatening to non-immune, recent arrivals. It was long overlooked (perhaps ignored), and is frequently still forgotten, that babies born in these countries constitute the majority of 'non-immune recent arrivals'; they are highly susceptible to endemic diseases which cause greater morbidity and mortality in children than in adults and whose clinical manifestations may differ remarkably, not only from adult experience, but also between the infant, toddler and adolescent.

Most 'statistics' concerning children in developing countries are based on sample surveys and other techniques for estimating vital statistics when reliable records are missing. Such estimates are subject to bias and inaccuracies. Reservations about the quality of the data should, however, *not* obscure the scale of the inequity that characterizes childhood survival (or death) when comparisons are made between the least and most developed countries in the world. Infant mortality rates (i.e. deaths per 1000 livebirths in the first year of life) are on average five times higher in the lesser developed than the more developed countries, while comparison between the worst of the former (e.g. Afghanistan) and the best of the latter (e.g. Sweden) reveals a difference of about 30:1. The risk of dying is expected to diminish rapidly after the hazards of infancy, but the mean difference in the 1–4 year death rate between the more and less developed countries is about 20:1; between extremely disadvantaged countries like Guinea and Sierra Leone and affluent countries like Sweden and Finland the rate rises to 50:<1 in this age group.[1]

The causes of this enormous mortality in the tropical developing countries differ at different ages. At the start of life they are greatly influenced by events during pregnancy and labour and the underlying status of maternal health. Perinatal mortality rates (i.e. stillbirths and all deaths per 1000 births in the first week of life per 1000 total births) are very high, especially in areas where pregnant women have no antenatal care and their deliveries are unsupervised. Maternal ill health, including malaria in pregnancy, other parasitic, bacterial and viral infections, severe anaemia, rheumatic heart disease, diabetes mellitus, haemoglobinopathies, severe malnutrition and so forth, contribute to stillbirths, low birth weight and prematurity; poor obstetrics exposes mother and baby to trauma, including neonatal asphyxia, and to infections including tetanus of the newborn and sometimes of the mother as well.

Paediatric interventions have very limited potential for reducing perinatal mortality. Improved survival in late fetal and early neonatal life requires determined efforts to improve maternal health, on which fetal and neonatal health depend. Unfortunately a very high proportion of girls enter motherhood under-aged, undernourished, undersized, underprivileged, uneducated and unwell and may be denied access to medical services for cultural, religious or economic reasons. It is certain that unless and until there is significant improvement in womens' health and social status and access to medical services, perinatal mortality in the tropics is unlikely to show significant improvement.

Neonatal jaundice has in recent years emerged as a serious 'new' problem in hospital based paediatrics in the tropics. In countries like Nigeria it has now reached the proportions of a serious issue in public health.[2] The causes of this alarming increase in the incidence and severity of neonatal jaundice, which kills many and causes cerebral palsy due to kernicterus in many more, remain obscure. Glucose-6-phosphate dehydrogenase (G6PD) deficiency and ABO blood group incompatibility have been incriminated in several studies, but these genetic factors have long been stabilized in the community and cannot be the direct cause of the current problem, which seems more likely to be due to some unidentified environmental factor. Facilities for exchange transfusion and phototherapy, which are essential for effective management of severe neonatal jaundice, are often lacking in hospitals in the tropics. Where exchange transfusions can be done there now lurks the spectre of transmitting human immunodeficiency virus (HIV) infection, especially in countries where a significant proportion of 'healthy' blood donors are HIV positive.

Neonatal tetanus continues to be an important cause of neonatal death throughout the tropics. Evidence is accumulating that giving two doses of tetanus toxoid during pregnancy, as has been recommended for the prevention of neonatal tetanus, may not be a reliable way of preventing the disease in everyone. Infants born in circumstances which risk exposure to tetanus can be provided with absolute protection from the disease by a small dose (e.g. 500–750 units) of anti-tetanus serum if given before the onset of any symptoms of tetanus.

Excluding malaria, the principal killers in late childhood in the tropics are essentially the same as those that decimated the child population in Europe and North America during and following the industrial revolution. These include diarrhoeal diseases, respiratory tract infections, acute infectious diseases like measles, pertussis, diphtheria and typhoid, and chronic infections like tuberculosis, all occurring against a background of malnutrition, overcrowding and poor environmental sanitation.

The death rate from malaria in childhood is unquestionably high but actual rates quoted differ widely by region and within regions from time-to-time. In areas holoendemic for *Plasmodium falciparum* malaria, children and pregnant women are the primary targets for severe disease. Cerebral malaria is a disease of early childhood and is rare in the indigenous adult population, including pregnant women who tend to develop severe anaemia when assailed by *P. falciparum*.

The nature of paediatrics in the tropics is changing quite rapidly in countries where urbanization of rural communities is proceeding apace. It is predicted that by the year 2000 the majority of the world's population will be urban-based. Disruption of rural family life, abandoning of traditional child rearing practices like breast feeding, the need for women to go out to work to augment family income to survive in a city's 'cash' economy rather than rural 'subsistence' economy, have all contributed to rapid escalation of neglect, abuse, exploitation and abandonment of children in urban areas. The enormous scale of these problems can be gauged by the fact that in the cities of South and Central America alone there are currently estimated to be in excess of 20 million 'abandoned' children among whom morbidity and mortality from violence, drugs and physical neglect now exceed sickness and death from tropical diseases.

NUTRITIONAL DISORDERS (See also Chapter 21)

PROTEIN–ENERGY MALNUTRITION

In the cool temperate parts of the world where kwashiorkor does not occur a spectrum of nutritional states which grade smoothly from obesity, to normal, to underweight, to marasmus can be traced, permitting a rational classification of protein–energy malnutrition (PEM) on the basis of weight for age or, preferably, weight for height, which can discriminate between acute and chronic PEM (Table 15.1). In the tropics where kwashiorkor occurs, correlations between severity of kwashiorkor and severity of malnutrition assessed by anthropometric

Table 15.1 Determination of nutritional status (after ref. 7).

Height for age (%)	Weight for height (%)		
	<80	80–120	>120
<90	(1) Chronic malnutrition	(2) Stunted but no malnutrition	(3) Stunted and obese
>90	(4) Acute malnutrition	(5) Normal	(6) Obese

Action required: (1) Long-term socioeconomic development; (3) and (6) nutrition education; (2) and (5) nil; (4) emergency measures to relieve an acute situation.

criteria like weight and height are very variable and inconstant. Fatal kwashiorkor can occur in children who, by anthropometric criteria, are normally nourished! This implies that the aetiology of kwashiorkor involves factors other than food deprivation and the nutrient composition of diet.

MARASMUS

Persistent undernutrition in childhood leads sequentially to arrested linear growth, stationary weight, then progressive weight loss as subcutaneous and other fat depots are depleted and muscles waste away to provide energy and other requirements needed to maintain vital functions. This ultimately leads to the clinical state known as marasmus which in its worse form fits the description 'skin and bones' (Figure 15.1). There are many causes of nutritional failure in childhood, but the overwhelming majority of marasmic children seen in the developing countries become malnourished simply because they do not get enough to eat. Unfortunately nutritional failure, once initiated, may be complicated by diarrhoea which aggravates the situation and may establish a vicious cycle of malnutrition–diarrhoea–malnutrition.

The combination of natural disasters like recurrent droughts and man-made disasters like civil wars, associated with a precipitous decline in the economic fortunes of developing countries in the tropics in recent years, has determined that food deprivation, amounting to actual starvation in many areas, is now rife in many countries, where childhood marasmus now occurs on an epidemic scale.

There is little that direct medical intervention can achieve in these circumstances. The practice of regular weight monitoring is regarded as an essential activity to promote nutrition and child health. But when nothing can be offered or done for starving sick children, routine, regular weighing only monitors childrens' misery and is otherwise a purposeless exercise.

Marasmic children are usually unhappy and irritable but respond to attention, are usually eager to feed, and speedily gain weight if offered sufficient food to satisfy their needs. Failure of an adequate diet to promote weight gain in a child diagnosed as suffering from nutritional marasmus indicates some underlying condition of which primary tuberculosis is the most common. In some areas Kala-azar might need to be considered and acquired immune deficiency syndrome (AIDS) has now emerged as a problem in parts of Africa. There are no confirmatory laboratory tests for nutritional marasmus. Even when wasting is extreme, except for fluctuations in serum electrolyte levels that may occur following diarrhoea, there are no biochemical or haematological abnormalities that characterize marasmus.

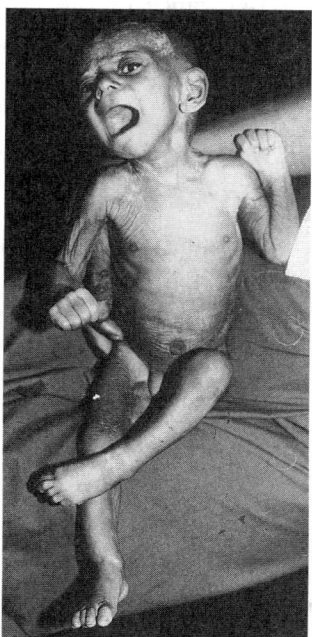

Figure 15.1 Marasmus. The child has an alert look but shows marked wasting and lax skin with an appearance of prominent bony protuberances.

KWASHIORKOR

It is now generally acknowledged that the aetiology of kwashiorkor remains obscure and that the long held concept that the condition results from protein deficiency is no longer tenable. Kwashiorkor impinges on and interacts with underweight and marasmus but seems not to be an integral part of the spectrum of disorders directly attributable to nutritional inadequacy of protein and/or energy that justifies the designation PEM.

During the past decade associations have been established between kwashiorkor and aflatoxins.[3,4] The hypothesis that implicates aflatoxins in the aetiology and pathogenesis of kwashiorkor[5] is attractive because it is reconcilable with all the known facts about the epidemiology and clinical behaviour of the disease; it also demystifies all the 'mysteries' about the disease, first enumerated by Trowell, Davies and Dean in their original classical account of the disease.[6] If the aflatoxin hypothesis is validated the prevention and management of kwashiorkor will require radical review. Table 15.2 compares marasmus, kwashiorkor and problems attributable to aflatoxins and demonstrates the

Table 15.2 Comparing marasmus, kwashiorkor and aflatoxin, ingestion.

Feature	Marasmus	Kwashiorkor	Aflatoxins
Geography	Worldwide	Mainly tropics	Mainly tropics
Climate	Any	Hot and humid	Hot and humid
Seasonality	No	Yes: rainy > dry	Yes: rainy > dry
Biochemical derangements	Nil specific	Depression of: protein synthesis, glucose metabolism, enzyme induction, lipid metabolism	Depression of: protein synthesis, glucose metabolism, enzyme induction, lipid metabolism
Liver pathology	Normal or fatty	Fatty $+ \rightarrow +++$	Fatty $+ \rightarrow +++$
Immunosuppression	$0 \rightarrow + \rightarrow ++$	Always $+++$	$+++ \rightarrow ++++$

remarkable similarities between the latter two entities.

Main clinical features of kwashiorkor

The syndrome occurs mainly in children who have recently been weaned. The age incidence tends therefore to reflect differences in weaning practices. The disease may rarely occur in fully breast-fed babies. Onset is usually insidious over a period of weeks but may be more acute. Oedema associated with hypoproteinaemia occurs in all cases but varies greatly in severity from case to case. The mental state of these children is characteristically a combi-

nation of apathetic misery and peevish irritability when approached or handled. Most cases show dermatoses of variable extent and character and hair tends to lose its colour and normal texture and to become sparse and easily pluckable (Figure 15.2). Complicating infections are common as these children are invariably immunosuppressed. Hypothermia and hypoglycaemia occur frequently, and hypokalaemia and hypomagnesaemia can be assumed in almost every case.

Further consideration of kwashiorkor will be confined to some recommendations on management of the disease that reflect accumulated clinical experience and take cognizance of the possible role of aflatoxins in aetiology.

Management of kwashiorkor

Acute resuscitation
Correct any fluid and electrolyte imbalance and shock if present or impending; correct *severe* anaemia; check for and correct hypothermia and hypoglycaemia; vigorously treat any infection present or suspected. In malarious areas give curative dose of antimalarials; leave uninfected skin lesions exposed; keep mother with child and involve her in care.

Establishing feeding
Commence frequent small oral feeds as soon as possible with a mixture of equal parts 10% dextrose and WHO oral rehydration solution or Darrow's solution. Use a nasogastric tube if oral fluids are stubbornly refused. Aim to restore normal calorie intake as soon as possible but avoid sudden intro-

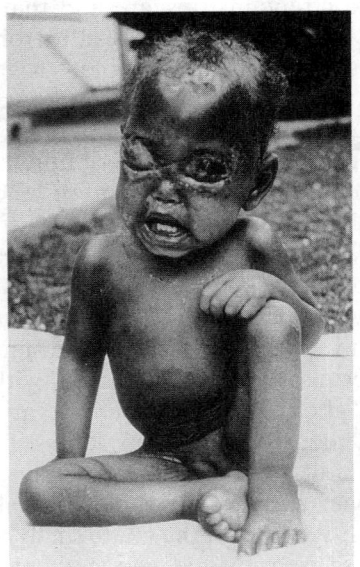

Figure 15.2 Kwashiorkor in a young child. Note the miserable appearance, facial oedema with periorbital infection, hair changes and peripheral oedema.

duction of large milk intake. Establish full mixed feeding based on local foods as soon as possible, ensuring that all ingredients are *fresh and of good quality*.

The quality of food, particularly cereals, must be carefully monitored. 'Spoiled' foods are likely to contain aflatoxins and, irrespective of whether aflatoxins cause kwashiorkor, eating aflatoxin-contaminated food would be expected to compromise recovery.

Supplements to diet

Give folic acid 5 mg daily plus a general vitamin supplement, with large amounts of vitamin A in areas where this vitamin is deficient. These children have a large deficit in total body potassium; oral potassium supplements as well as magnesium should be given during the first weeks of treatment. Zinc supplementation may also be beneficial and is recommended.

VITAMIN A AND D, AND ZINC DEFICIENCIES

VITAMIN A

Deficiency of vitamin A is now widely recognized as a risk factor for child mortality in areas where xerophthalmia is a problem. This conclusion is based on the results of several intervention trials in which vitamin A was administered prophylactically to young children. Child deaths were reduced by as much as 54% in one of these studies in South India,[8] which used a weekly vitamin A dosage of 8333 iu). Other studies have used 200 000 iu every 4 or 6 months. The severity of illness episodes, especially diarrhoeal disease, is reduced following such supplementation. In severe measles there is good evidence for a protective effect as children who received 400 000 iu recovered more rapidly from pneumonia and diarrhoea. These benefits are also reported in children with measles who have subclinical deficiency of vitamin A.

Vitamin A supplementation is effective in preventing xerophthalmia. Xerophthalmia pre-eminently affects the young child (1–5 years), and not so much the infant, who may be protected by prolonged breast feeding. The clinical classification of xerophthalmia is shown in Table 15.3 and a pigmented Bitot's spot and xerotic patch in Figure 15.3.

Table 15.3 Clinical classification of xerophthalmia.

Ocular sign	Classification
Night blindness	XN
Conjunctival xerosis	X1A
Bitot spot	X1B
Corneal xerosis	X2
Corneal ulcer/keratomalacia	X3
Corneal scar	XS
Xerophthalmia fundus	XF

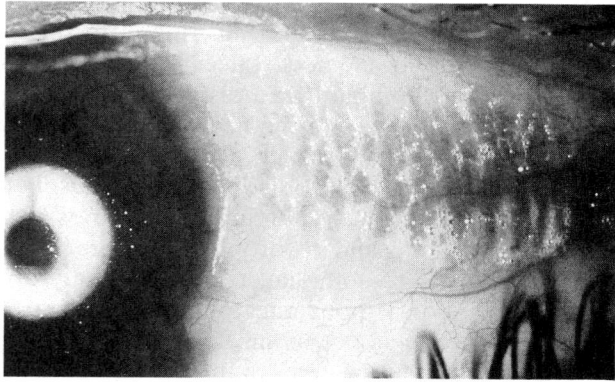

Figure 15.3 Pigmented Bitot's spot and xerotic patch (Courtesy of the late H A P C Oomen).

The treatment of xerophthalmia recommended by the World Health Organization (WHO)[9] is vitamin A, in the form of retinyl palmitate or acetate in an oily solution, 200 000 iu orally immediately on diagnosis, repeated a day later and again 4 weeks later, or sooner if there is clinical deterioration. If there is vomiting or severe diarrhoea, 100 000 iu water-miscible vitamin A by intramuscular injection is preferred. In babies under 8 kg weight and/or less than 1 year old, half of these doses should be given.

In discussing the prevention of nutritional blindness we have to be aware that the affection is easily curable without ophthalmological skills, that the survivor of the corneal stages, if untreated or if treated too late, will be blind and that the medicinal cure is cheap. Promotional measures should encourage the use of green leafy vegetables which are an excellent, underutilized, inexpensive source of vitamin A in food.

RICKETS

Nutritional rickets occurs primarily in countries where for religious and/or social reasons women and children are not exposed to the sun. It is quite common in Pakistan, Egypt, Ethiopia, the Middle

East and West Africa, but is considered rare in East Africa.

It commonly presents between 6 and 18 months of age and is increasingly recognized in very low birth-weight babies. Rickets is a disease of growth and is infrequent therefore in severe PEM. Diagnosis is straightforward. The child may appear well nourished but restless and pale and a history of diarrhoea or respiratory infection may be given. Head sweating is common. Motor development is delayed, with poor linear growth. Infantile tetany may occur. Characteristic bony lesions in infancy include craniotabes, delayed closure of the fontanelles, delayed dentition, and epiphyseal enlargement best seen in the wrists and costochondral junctions. Bossing of the head, bow legs, knock knees and other limb deformities are common features in older children. Clinical diagnosis is confirmed by wrist radiographs and serum chemistry, which always shows raised alkaline phosphatase and depressed phosphate levels. The therapeutic vitamin D dose varies from 1500 to 5000 iu/day and the prophylactic dose is 400–600 iu/day. Where compliance with the long-term daily medication is poor and follow-up difficult, a single massive dose of vitamin D may be given by injection. This practice is quite common in the Middle East where the danger now exists that 'shopping around' for treatment may result in children receiving multiple doses of 100 000–200 000 iu vitamin D. Breast milk may contain sufficient vitamin D to protect infants but supplementation is required in high-risk infants and for those whose mothers keep them up out of the sun.

ZINC DEFICIENCY

This is now recognized as having a role in PEM, especially during nutritional rehabilitation. Studies have demonstrated the requirement of zinc for growth and have led to recommendations to include zinc supplements during rehabilitation. Diets rich in fibre and phytate may contribute to a reduced zinc status in many rural tropical populations.

NUTRITIONAL ANAEMIAS

IRON-DEFICIENCY ANAEMIA

Prevalence of these anaemias in young children in low socioeconomic groups is frequently 50–70% of those examined. Iron-deficiency anaemia continues to be the most common nutrient deficiency in the world, with peak prevalence at 6–24 months. The main causes for this relate to poor dietary intake and low bioavailability of iron, blood loss caused by intestinal parasites and high requirements for iron in growing infants. Healthy breast-fed babies are unlikely to become iron-deficient before 6 months of age. Iron stores at birth are reduced in premature babies and, because of their high growth rate, anaemia usually occurs as early as 2–3 months of age. Fetal anaemia is also reported by several authors in studies of maternal and cord haemoglobin values from developing countries.[10] Infants fed cow's milk from an early age are prone to anaemia as this is a poor source of iron and increases intestinal blood loss. Iron-deficiency in the first year of life delays psychomotor development and these deficits have been shown to persist into childhood.[11] These findings are of importance because they indicate that behavioural deficit in children may relate to the early onset of iron-deficiency in infants.

It is important to treat iron-deficiency anaemia in children. The dose required is 5 mg/kg/day of elemental iron and this must be given over 2–3 months in order to replenish stores. Clinical and dietary history and examination of the child, blood film and red cell indices should provide the diagnosis. If there is doubt, a therapeutic trial of iron should be given, together with dietary advice.

FOLATE DEFICIENCY

Folate deficiency occurs much more frequently in children in tropical countries than elsewhere. It is a well recognized complication of kwashiorkor, sickle cell anaemia and other inherited haemolytic anaemias, goat's milk feeding in infancy, and malabsorption from many causes. Low birth weight babies are very susceptible to folate deficiency, which should be suspected when these infants become anaemic and fail to thrive. Folate deficiency can cause persistent diarrhoea in infancy. Routine administration of folic acid, 2.5–5 mg daily, is recommended for the following conditions in childhood: sickle cell anaemia, thalassaemia and other inherited haemolytic anaemias; kwashiorkor; low birth weight babies; and children receiving long-term medication with drugs that have significant antifolate activity. Folate deficiency usually responds rapidly to treatment but megaloblastic anaemia in kwashiorkor may prove an exception.

IMPORTANT CONGENITAL MICROBIAL INFECTIONS

Since the original description of the TORCH agents (Toxoplasmosis, Rubella, Cytomegalovirus and *Herpes simplex* virus) several more agents have been linked with congenital infection, e.g. HIV, hepatitis B virus (HBV), parvovirus, *Varicella zoster* virus, Epstein–Barr virus and *Listeria monocytogenes*. To these must, of course, be added syphilis and malaria, both of which have long been recognized as important causes of congenital infections in the tropics. Tuberculosis, trypanosomiasis and leishmaniasis should be borne in mind when confronted by neonatal illness of obscure cause in the tropics as these infections may, rarely, be transplacentally transmitted. A few of the more prevalent, well-recognized and important congenital infections in the tropics are discussed below.

HUMAN IMMUNODEFICIENCY VIRUS (See also Chapter 12)

HIV-1 infection in African children is acquired largely from the mother, either in utero or at birth. The risk of vertical transmission has been estimated to be between 15 and 40%. A positive maternal viral culture in advanced maternal disease is associated with increased infant morbidity and mortality. Studies from Europe in children with perinatal HIV-1 infection have reported HIV-1-associated signs in 82% of seropositive children at a median age of 5 months.[12] The median survival time was 96 months. In a study of infants with positive cord cultures, 45% were dead by 1 year.

In parts of East and Southern Africa, where up to 30% of women attending antenatal clinics are infected and perinatal transmission rates are 30–40%, HIV has become one of the major paediatric problems. Reasons for the higher vertical transmission rate in Africa are not clear; the stage of symptomatic disease during pregnancy and in some cases acquisition of infection during pregnancy or around the time of delivery may be important.

Recommendations that breast feeding be discouraged when the mother is HIV-1 seropositive is based upon isolation of the virus from breast milk as well as documented postnatal transmission in a small number of infants. The frequency of breast milk transmission is unknown. In view of the importance of breast feeding in maintaining child health in developing countries it should still be encouraged as the risks associated with bottle feeding far exceed the risks of acquiring HIV by breast feeding.

The diagnosis in a symptomatic child over 15 months of age is confirmed by a repeatedly positive HIV-specific IgG antibody test, e.g. the enzyme-linked immunosorbent assay (ELISA), with a confirmatory Western blot test. Under 15 months a positive ELISA and Western blot must have additional clinical evidence to support the diagnosis, unless HIV culture, antigen capture methods or polymerase chain reaction techniques are available.

Clinical manifestations frequently show in the first months of life. The most common features include failure to thrive, respiratory infections, chronic diarrhoea, recalcitrant thrush, recurrent bacterial infections and interstitial pulmonary disease. Developmental delay may result from chronic debility or involvement of the central nervous system. Other findings include diffuse lymphadenopathy, hepatosplenomegaly and parotid gland enlargement. A rising number of children are being orphaned by AIDS and in East and Southern Africa there is growing concern about their present and future care.

HEPATITIS B VIRUS (See also Chapter 31)

Vertical transmission can result from acute maternal hepatitis B virus (HBV) infection or from the chronic maternal asymptomatic carrier state. Between 70 and 90% of mothers with evidence of high infectivity, i.e. high hepatitis B surface antigen (HBsAg) titre or e antigen (HBeAg) positivity, can be expected to transmit HBV to their infants; 85–90% of them will become chronic carriers. It has been estimated that more than 25% of these individuals will die in later life, either of hepatocellular carcinoma or cirrhosis of the liver. In the neonatal period these babies may remain asymptomatic or present with late onset neonatal hepatitis. Horizontal spread amongst children is thought to occur via cuts and abrasions in skin, or via saliva when in very close contact.

Children can be protected by immunization. In areas where many carrier mothers are HBeAg positive, e.g. in South-East Asia, infants should be vaccinated at birth. Indeed, mass vaccination of all infants during their first year of life is recommended in endemic areas where the majority of mothers are HBeAg positive. The HBV vaccine can be incorporated into the WHO Expanded Programme of Immunization (EPI) schedule of vaccination.

For babies born to carrier mothers the most effective protection is provided by a combination of hyperimmune globulin (HBIg) and HBV vaccine given by intramuscular injection at birth, with repeat of the HBV vaccine at 1 and 6 months. This schedule reduces the risk of infants becoming carriers from 90% to about 5%.[13] The use of vaccine alone only reduces the risk of carrier status to about 25%.

HBsAg has been detected in breast milk in a few carriers and it is plausible that breast feeding may provide an oral route of infection. However, there is insufficient evidence to consider withholding breast feeding in babies born to carriers.

CONGENITAL SYPHILIS (See also Chapter 54)

This is a resurgent problem in tropical countries. Suspicion may arise in high-risk pregnancies (e.g. drug abusers). Other clues include an unexplained large placenta, unexpected previous abortions and/or stillbirths, and ill-defined rashes or ulcerating lesions at unusual sites (mouth, anus or breast). Most infants present at between 1 and 3 months with pallor due to haemolysis, hepatosplenomegaly and skin lesions. Such lesions include peeling and involvement of the palms and soles, condylomata lata, and perianal rashes which may resemble a persistent nappy rash. Other features are persistent nasal discharge ('snuffles'), failure to thrive, pseudoparesis of one or more limbs secondary to syphilitic epiphysitis, delayed closure of fontanelles and frontal bossing. Symptomatic newborns are often jaundiced.

The diagnosis of overt disease should not present a real diagnostic difficulty if syphilis is borne in mind. Positive serology in the presence of any of the classical clinical manifestations of congenital syphilis is diagnostic. X-ray examination of the knees and legs will often reveal distinctive syphilitic pathology in children with indefinite clinical signs or who may be suspected on other grounds of having syphilis. This is particularly helpful when reliable serology is not easily or quickly available.

Where facilities permit, diagnosis should be firmly established by appropriate serological tests, but when diagnostic laboratory facilities are lacking, as is often the case in the tropics, proof of diagnosis relies on response to treatment. Definitive serological diagnosis is usually based on a positive Venereal Disease Research Laboratory (VDRL) test with persistently high or rising titres or a persistent positive fluorescent antibody absorption test (FTA-ABS).

Penicillin is the drug of choice and is recommended in a dose of 50 000 units/kg of aqueous procaine penicillin, by intramuscular injection, daily for 7–10 days. A large dose of a long-acting benzathine penicillin (at least 100 000 units/kg) given once, or preferably twice, a week apart, is recommended when daily treatment is not feasible or patient compliance is suspect. All children with syphilis should be followed up to ensure control of all symptoms and to monitor serology. Persistence of positive serology 6 months after treatment is an indication for a further course of treatment.

PARASITIC DISEASES

MALARIA (See also Chapter 61)

The estimated one to two million malaria deaths each year are mainly due to *P. falciparum* infections in children under 5 years of age. The clinical picture of malaria in children varies with the endemicity of the disease. Where malaria transmission is low or markedly seasonal, severe disease may occur at any age. Under conditions of persistent year-round transmission (stable or holoendemic malaria), severe disease occurs almost exclusively in very young children who, if they survive, develop a high degree of acquired immunity by 5–6 years of age which is sufficient to protect them thereafter from life-threatening malaria. In early infancy transplacentally-acquired maternal malarial antibody provides passive immunity which suppresses, but does not prevent, malarial infection in the infant. Exclusive breast feeding is believed to protect in a similar way, i.e. not by preventing infection but by reducing parasite density.

In some areas, *P. falciparum* prevalence approaches 100% by 12 months of age. There seems to be a persistent misapprehension that in such areas clinical manifestations of malaria tend to occur *after* 6 months of age. This is not true. There is abundant evidence that life-threatening malaria occurs in infants under 6 months. Cases may present as early as 6 weeks, the incidence increasing gradually thereafter to reach a peak sometime after 6 months. Fever (usually without rigors), cough, vomiting, pallor and convulsions are the well-known presenting symptoms in childhood. Acute haemolytic episodes causing jaundice are unusual. The serious complications seen when severe infections present late include coma, cardiac failure from severe anaemia, haemoglobinuria and its associated renal problems, circulatory collapse, hypoglycaemia and rarely spontaneous bleeding.

CEREBRAL MALARIA

The definition of cerebral malaria in children is the same as in adults: unrousable coma in *P. falciparum* malaria in the absence of an alternative or additional cause for altered consciousness. Peak prevalence occurs at 2–3 years and well-nourished children are more frequently and severely affected than malnourished ones. The condition is exceptionally rare in kwashiorkor. Clinical history is usually short, 1–2 days; convulsions preceded by alteration of consciousness and followed by coma is the most common mode of presentation. Headache and fever are common preceding complaints. The age incidence of 'febrile convulsions', which is 6 months to 5 years, overlaps precisely with the age incidence of cerebral malaria in holoendemic malarious areas and this causes diagnostic difficulties in practice. Rapid recovery of full consciousness within half an hour of a convulsion virtually excludes cerebral malaria in childhood.

A common clinical finding is hepatosplenomegaly but not infrequently neither organ is enlarged. Opisthotonos may occur and suggests the diagnosis of meningitis or tetanus. Hypoglycaemia occurs quite commonly in young children and may aggravate and prolong coma if unrecognized and uncorrected. In West Africa a popular traditional remedy for convulsions; causes hypoglycaemia this is frequently given to children with cerebral malaria. The immediate administration of intravenous glucose is recommended for any child so treated who shows alteration of consciousness.

Case fatality is high (between 10 and 40%), with most deaths occurring within 24 hours. Time from starting of treatment to resolution of coma in children is short (1–2 days). If the child recovers neurological sequelae are few.

MALARIA AND ANAEMIA

Anaemia is a very frequent and often serious complication of *P. falciparum* malaria in early childhood. There appears to be an inverse correlation between degree of anaemia and cerebral involvement, i.e. the greater the degree of anaemia the less the likelihood of cerebral malaria. The main cause of the anaemia appears to be dyserythropoeisis with a maturation arrest at the normoblast stage in bone marrow. Malarial anaemia responds very well to effective antimalarial treatment but there is a lag period of 4–5 days before reticulocytosis occurs as a prelude to a rapid steady rise in haemoglobin concentration.

CONGENITAL MALARIA

This may be either symptomatic or asymptomatic and in a proportion of cases only cord parasitaemia occurs. The risk of congenital symptomatic malaria is low (<1%) in babies born to women living under holoendemic conditions. If symptomatic at birth these babies present with anaemia, jaundice and splenomegaly. The diagnosis is frequently missed. Those with asymptomatic parasitaemia at birth may either suppress this spontaneously, or present with clinical symptoms in the late neonatal period.

QUARTAN MALARIA

In terms of acute sickness *P. malariae* quartan malaria is the most benign species of human malaria but it has the ability to compromise immune function(s). Quartan malarial nephrotic syndrome is the clinical expression of an immune complex nephritis caused by *P. malariae* which is arguably the most common cause of chronic parenchymatous renal disease in childhood in the tropics. Patients present with classical signs of nephrotic syndrome such as oedema, massive albuminuria, hypoproteinaemia and hypercholesterolaemia but, with few exceptions, do not show a satisfactory response to any form of treatment and eventually die from hypertension and renal failure.[14] The use of corticosteroids in these cases is fraught with danger and is only very rarely beneficial. A decision to try prednisolone in the management of this condition is only justified if the patient is under tight clinical control that enables early detection of adverse effects and withdrawal of treatment if it is harmful.

MANAGEMENT OF SEVERE MALARIA

The management is similar to that in adults. If a child has a convulsion this is usually controlled with paraldehyde, 0.1–0.2 ml/kg body weight i.m. (given in a glass syringe), or a slow intravenous injection of diazepam, 0.15 mg/kg to a maximum of 10 mg.

Diazepam, 0.5–1.0 mg/kg, can be given intrarectally if injection is not possible. The choice of antimalarial is the same as for adult malaria but weighing of children is mandatory and the dose of antimalarial should be calculated on a body-weight basis.

If hypoglycaemia occurs it should be treated with an intravenous bolus injection of 50% glucose (up to 1.0 ml/kg body weight), followed by a slow intravenous infusion of 10% glucose to prevent recurrence of hypoglycaemia.

In children presenting with oliguria and dehydration careful rehydration with isotonic saline is mandatory, with frequent re-examination of the jugular venous pressure and blood pressure.

TRYPANOSOMIASIS (See also Chapters 63 and 64)

Congenital infection with African trypanosomiasis has been described in 15 cases.[15] There is evidence from areas endemic for *Trypanosomal gambiense* infection that infected women can carry apparently normal pregnancies through to full term delivery. Two of these infants remained asymptomatic until the second year of life, when they presented with neurological sequelae and illness. Children with unexplained neurological problems in the first few years of life who live in endemic areas should be investigated for possible trypanosomiasis.

Congenital infection with South American trypanosomosis is not infrequent, the incidence ranging from 2 to 10% in some areas.

KALA-AZAR (See also Chapter 65)

The clinical picture varies depending on the immune competence to *Leishmania donovani* of the population. In recent epidemics in India and Sudan, children and adolescents constituted the majority of cases. Case fatality was about 6% in the Indian epidemic. Kala-azar may occur as early as 4 months of age in an endemic area, where any infant who presents with high irregular fever, vomiting, toxaemia, hepatosplenomegaly and lymphadenopathy should be suspected of having infantile Kala-azar. Rare cases of congenital kala-azar have been reported following maternal infection in pregnancy. In the acute form the condition may resemble malaria, acute tuberculosis, or typhoid and it may also be confused with infectious mononucleosis. Usually the disease presents insidiously with vague symptoms and progressive development of splenomegaly. The presenting complaint often relates to secondary infections which frequently occur as a consequence of the immunocompromised state.

Haematological abnormalities include moderate to severe anaemia, leucopenia and thrombocytopenia or agranulocytosis. Polyclonal hypergammaglobulinaemia is invariably present. Bilateral pneumonia and tuberculosis are well-known complications. In childhood a bone marrow examination for amastigotes is the preferred diagnostic method. Pentavalent antimonials are the treatment of choice.

PARASITIC CAUSES OF CHILDHOOD FITS

The main causes of childhood fits, other than malaria, are neurocysticercosis and toxoplasmosis. Cysticercosis prevalence is probably grossly underestimated in children with epilepsy living in areas with a high pork consumption. Among 88 epileptic patients (>15 years of age) in northern Togo (West Africa), 27 suffered from cysticercosis.

Convulsions, intracranial calcification and hydrocephalus in the newborn point to the diagnosis of toxoplasmosis. In later childhood, epilepsy, mental retardation, microcephalus and cranial nerve palsies are other sequelae.

Other parasitic causes of seizures include echinococcosis, cerebral paragonimiasis and African trypanosomiasis.

DISEASES POTENTIALLY PREVENTABLE BY VACCINATION

The WHO EPI (see above) was established in 1974 to protect the world's children against six common vaccine-preventable diseases: pertussis, tetanus, poliomyelitis, diphtheria, measles and tuberculosis. An EPI recommended vaccine schedule to achieve protection as early in life as possible is shown in Table 15.4.

Table 15.4 Recommended immunization schedule for achieving protection as early in life as possible.

Contact	Age of child	Vaccines
1	At birth	BCG and OPV
2	6 weeks	DPT and OPV
3	10 weeks	DPT and OPV
4	14 weeks	DPT and OPV
5	9 months	Measles

DPT, diphtheria, pertussis, tetanus; OPV, oral poliomyelitis vaccine.

TUBERCULOSIS (See also Chapter 57)

Infants, adolescents and pregnant women have heightened susceptibility to tuberculosis. These facts, plus the debilitating influence of endemic malnutrition in childhood, determine that tuberculosis remains one of the most serious and intractable problems in paediatrics in the tropics; is now being aggravated by the increasing incidence of AIDS.

Tuberculosis is discussed in detail elsewhere. The focus here is on some specific aspects of tuberculosis in childhood that have special relevance in clinical practice.

Interpretation of tuberculin test results

A positive tuberculin test is the rule in postprimary infections but a negative result does not exclude active disease. The test may be negative if:

- It is carried out in the preallergic phase, i.e. too early.
- The child is immunosuppressed by drugs (most commonly prednisolone); malnutrition (mainly kwashiorkor); or diseases like measles, Kala-azar, pertussis, malignancy, etc.
- It may be a false-negative test because the tuberculin used was denatured or the technique used for the test was faulty.

Problems associated with BCG vaccination

Widespread routine BCG administration in infancy has created some difficulties in interpreting the results of tuberculin tests in childhood. The following points reduce these difficulties:

- BCG tuberculin sensitivity is rarely demonstrable using Mantoux 1/10 000.
- Induration caused by Mantoux 1/1000 after BCG is usually <10 mm and almost never exceeds 15 mm.

- There is a persistent response to tuberculin following tuberculosis but the response always wanes after BCG.

Use of BCG as a diagnostic test/protective measure

Some children who show no sensitivity to the strongest concentrations of purified protein derivative (PPD) or old tuberculin (OT) may show a cellular immune response to BCG in the form of an accelerated BCG reaction in which local induration occurs within 48 hours, followed by ulceration, scab formation and healing by scarring within 2–3 weeks. BCG vaccination may therefore be employed as the final test for tuberculin sensitivity in children suspected of having the disease.

Diagnosis of tuberculosis by therapeutic trial

In desperately ill children suspected of having severe tuberculosis (pulmonary, miliary, or meningitic) and in whom the diagnosis cannot be established by other means, a therapeutic/diagnostic trial of antituberculous drugs is justified. Streptomycin and rifampicin should be avoided as they can be active against non-tuberculous organisms. Isoniazid in high dose, 20 mg/kg/day, + para-aminosalicylic acid + pyrazinamide are in theory the best drugs for a therapeutic trial, but where choice is limited the most powerful combination of antituberculous drugs available should be used for desperately ill children suspected of having tuberculosis.

Tuberculosis in pregnancy and after delivery

Avoid streptomycin in pregnancy because it can cross the placenta and cause eighth nerve damage in the baby. Active pulmonary tuberculosis in the mother does not call for separation from her infant and cessation of breast feeding. She should be given full chemotherapy for her disease, and her baby should receive prophylactic isoniazid, 5–10 mg/kg, in a single dose daily for 6 months or until the mother is sputum-negative for acid-fast bacilli. The infant must also be given BCG, preferably the isoniazid resistant form if this is locally available.

Tuberculous meningitis

Once believed to be rare in the tropics, tuberculous meningitis is now recognized as one of the most common types of meningitis seen in hospital practice. It is associated with high mortality and serious, chronic sequelae and disability; these mainly reflect delay in starting treatment, usually caused by a combination of late presentation and delay in establishing the diagnosis. Early diagnosis relies above all on a 'high index of suspicion'. A good working rule that is firmly recommended in paediatric practice in the tropics is to regard lymphocytosis associated with reduced sugar in any specimen of CSF as indicative of tuberculous meningitis and treat accordingly until proved otherwise. In recent years results of treatment of tuberculous meningitis have been greatly improved by early insertion of valve drainage to relieve intraventricular pressure.

BCG vaccine in young children gives good protection against miliary tuberculosis and tuberculous meningitis. Adverse reactions are uncommon and not more than 1% of children should show suppurative lymphadenitis. BCG is also sufficiently effective against leprosy (vaccine efficacy about 50%) in East and Central Africa to be considered an important element of leprosy control in that region. BCG should not be given to children with symptomatic HIV infection.

MEASLES

Measles is now seldom seen in the Western world, where most children have now received measles vaccination, but it is still widespread in the tropics where vaccine coverage has been patchy and vaccine failures common. It is a disease of the under fives, with many cases in the first year of life and a peak incidence in 2–3-year-old children. The early phases of the disease are as is classically described but the rash is not easy to see in dark skins, especially in bad light. A haemorrhagic rash occasionally occurs. Misdiagnosed patients with measles are often admitted to general wards where the disease then spreads to non-immune children with other serious diseases.

In malnourished children, skin desquamation following the exanthem is usually extensive, severe and prolonged for several weeks. This is a period of debility and immunosuppression, with many infectious complications and when most deaths occur. Multiple complications are the rule rather than the exception; bronchopneumonia is the most frequent. Stomatitis and other oral lesions, including cancrum oris (noma), and chronic diarrhoea with fluid and electrolyte disturbances are frequent complications. Acute measles encephalitis occurs not infrequently and subacute sclerosing panencephalitis occasionally. Activation of primary tuberculosis and miliary or bronchogenic spread are constant risks following measles. Otitis media and skin sepsis are very common, but rarely fatal complications. Chronic otitis

may lead to a hearing impairment. Measles vaccination remains the only safeguard against the disease. Megadose vitamin A should be given to children with measles on admission to hospital, in areas where vitamin A deficiency occurs, as this significantly reduces mortality.

PERTUSSIS

This epidemic disease, which follows cycles from a few to several years, is still a serious health problem. Cough, 'whoop' and vomiting are the characteristic signs. Young infants often do not whoop, although the cough is still spasmodic and followed by vomiting. After a bout of coughing, apnoea may occur, leading to unconsciousness. Attacks may last several weeks and be complicated by pneumonia, malnutrition, conjunctival haemorrhages and rectal prolapse. Death may result from an encephalopathy or in infants from respiratory complications. Current interest is in the development of an acellular pertussis vaccine containing purified identifiable antigens.

DIPHTHERIA

Diphtheria can be mild or life threatening. Before vaccination was available the disease showed epidemic cycles with 2–4 year intervals. Epidemics still occur in parts of Africa.[16] A child may not appear ill with early tonsillar diphtheria but within a few days will become very toxic with extensive membrane formation. The membrane may be difficult to see if there is tonsillar oedema. Bull-neck diphtheria results from extensive buccal and pharyngeal swelling and has been mistaken for mumps. Acute airways obstruction may resemble viral 'croup' in infants. If death does not occur from the toxic effects to the myocardium or from respiratory or pharyngeal paralysis then recovery is complete. Neurological complications which generally appear after a variable latent period are predominantly bilateral and usually motor. Cutaneous diphtheria is not uncommon in the tropics and this can lead to a high level of immunity in children. Diphtheria from the skin of one child may cause faucial diphtheria in another.

Antibiotics are not a substitute for treatment with antitoxin but are needed to prevent the production of diphtheria toxin. Penicillin and erythromycin are effective against most strains. Antitoxin must be administered by the intravenous route as early as possible. Tests for sensitivity to horse serum must be performed before administration. The occurrence of a recent epidemic in Africa illustrates that a sporadic case of diphtheria in a partially immunized community warrants serious efforts to curb the spread of the disease.

POLIOMYELITIS (See also Chapter 38)

Poliomyelitis is a disease of early life in indigenous populations in the tropics: its maximal impact is in the first 3 years of life. It represents 'infantile paralysis', as poliomyelitis was originally called. A very high proportion of patients have established paralysis when first seen. It is virtually impossible to recognize poliomyelitis by the early prodromal symptoms. Children seen in the preparalytic phase of the disease may have severe limb pain that simulates osteomyelitis, painful sickle cell crises, etc. Gentle passive movement of the limbs will differentiate poliomyelitis as it is the only condition in which pain is not aggravated, and may even be relieved, by these manoeuvres. Meningeal irritation in poliomyelitis needs to be differentiated from pyogenic or tuberculous meningitis. Polymorphs may be present in significant numbers early in poliomyelitis before lymphocytes become dominant. The glucose content of the CSF is normal in poliomyelitis, whereas it is reduced in meningitis.

Typically, poliomyelitis paralysis occurs 1–3 days after onset of symptoms, often preceded by meningism, restlessness and apprehension. Paralysis is rapid in onset and may continue to spread over a period of 2 to 3 days. Large muscles are affected more frequently than small and legs more frequently than arms. Paralysis is flaccid and tendon reflexes are lost in affected muscles, which waste rapidly. Severe paralysis of trunk muscles, including intercostals, may lead to respiratory failure and/or pulmonary complications. Bulbar involvement can lead to drowning in secretions that cannot be swallowed, which collect in the throat and are aspirated into the respiratory passages. Once the active phase of poliomyelitis has passed, usually within 1 or 2 weeks, paralysed muscles start showing some improvement and may continue to do so for up to a year or more with appropriate physiotherapy.

The severity of poliomyelitis is influenced by:

- *Age*: more severe in older than younger patients and in prepubertal boys than girls.
- *Injections*: if given during or just prior to onset cause 'provocation paralysis'.

Muscle fatigue before or during the illness increases risk of paralysis. Corticosteroid administration and immune deficiency increase risk of severe disease. Removal of tonsils, adenoids and teeth in non-immunes exposed to poliomyelitis greatly increases the risk of bulbar involvement and severe disease. These procedures must be avoided during outbreaks of poliomyelitis.

Pregnancy adversely affects the outcome of poliomyelitis but this is not a problem in indigenous populations who are immune long before they can become pregnant.

Death in poliomyelitis is usually from respiratory failure, to which many factors may contribute: bulbar paralysis; respiratory muscle paralysis; cardio-respiratory failure from vital centre involvement which can also cause hyperpyrexia; pulmonary pathology such as atalectasis, oedema and pneumonia; and technical mishaps related to tracheostomy tubes, breathing apparatus, etc. Injudicious over-sedation, and conversely extreme anxiety, and gastric dilatation are factors that can aggravate respiratory problems.

MENINGITIS, RESPIRATORY INFECTION AND POLYSACCHARIDE VACCINES

The meningococcal A and C vaccines are safe and effective in terminating outbreaks and large epidemics. They are least protective for children under 2 years, who are at greatest risk. These vaccines do not prevent group B meningococcal disease. The new *Haemophilus influenzae* conjugate vaccines are immunogenic in younger children. As a higher proportion of children under 2 years of age may have severe *H. influenzae* infections (meningitis and cellulitis) in developing countries, vaccines with an improved vaccine efficacy in young children and infants are required. A pneumococcal polyvalent vaccine has shown a 59% efficacy in reducing mortality in children under 5 years in the Papua New Guinea highlands.[17]

RESPIRATORY INFECTIONS (See also Chapters 4 and 36)

Of all infant deaths from respiratory infections, 98% occur in developing countries. One estimate suggests that 2.5 million infants and 1.5 million children aged 1–4 years die from respiratory infection each year. Acute respiratory infections can be classified as upper or lower respiratory tract and case management guidelines have been developed by the WHO to be used by health care workers to determine the necessity for antibiotic treatment or referral to secondary care. The system uses respiratory rate thresholds (>50 breaths per minute) and chest indrawing to diagnose and classify severity. Children with chest indrawing require hospital referral, children with fast breathing but no indrawing require outpatient antibiotics, and those without fast breathing or chest indrawing do not need antibiotics and can be managed at home. Penicillin and co-trimoxazole are highly effective antibiotics.

STREPTOCOCCAL DISEASE

The Lancefield group A, β-haemolytic streptococci tend to be underrated villains in the spectrum of pathogens that cause acute, recurrent and chronic illness in childhood in the tropics. They are one of the most common causes of respiratory tract infections which include nasopharyngitis with low grade fever, cervical adenitis and purulent nasal discharge in the under 3 year group that might persist for weeks or months and be associated with weight loss, otitis media and sinusitis. In older children group A streptococci cause follicular tonsillitis and pharyngitis the immediate complications of which include parapharyngeal and retropharyngeal abscess, and whose late sequelae include glomerulonephritis and rheumatic fever, both the initial and the recurrent attacks. Rheumatic heart disease is the most common type of acquired heart disease in childhood worldwide, it causes much suffering and disability and makes heavy demands on medical services.

Other clinical problems attributable to streptococci include impetigo, erysipelas and secondary infection of scabies, which in the tropics is more frequently the cause of acute nephritis than is pharyngitis. Scarlet fever, pneumonia, wound and puerperal infections were much feared streptococcal infections in preantibiotic days. They retain their threat to health and life in communities remote from modern medical care.

Streptococci have remained sensitive to penicillin, which is the drug of choice for treatment—preferably given by the intramuscular route.

DENGUE HAEMORRHAGIC FEVER AND DENGUE SHOCK SYNDROME
(See also Chapter 34)

Dengue haemorrhagic fever (DHF) and dengue shock syndrome (DSS) occur mainly in children and are most common in South-East Asia and Oceania, where they annually account for hundreds of thousands of paediatric admissions and thousands of deaths. The pathological features that distinguish DHF/DSS from dengue are vascular permeability, contraction of plasma volume, hypotension, thrombocytopenia and a haemorrhagic diathesis.

There are four types of dengue viruses which are transmitted by mosquitoes of the genus *Aedes*, mainly *A. aegypti*. These mosquitoes also transmit the Chikungunya virus which also can cause DHF. The *A. aegypti* mosquito is well adapted to urban existence and occurs in high density in DHF endemic areas, which generally have high population density and poor sanitation.

Four grades of severity of DHF/DSS are recognized. Grade I: febrile with non-specific constitutional symptoms and a positive tourniquet test. Grade II: in addition to the foregoing there is haemorrhage in skin, gastrointestinal tract and other sites. Grade III: circulatory failure with rapid weak pulse, small pulse pressure, cold clammy extremities and hypotension. Grade IV: profound shock and moribund clinical state with undetectable pulse and blood pressure.

The syndrome may occur at any age from infancy but most cases occur between 5 and 10 years. Fever is usually continuous and a moderate enlargement of the liver occurs with all grades of the disease. There may be a maculopapular eruption. As the disease progresses bleeding occurs, mainly as petechial haemorrhages in grade II and gastrointestinal bleeding in grades III and IV, when increasing haemoconcentration and thrombocytopenia occur. The onset of hypovolaemic shock may be associated with restlessness and clouding of consciousness and evidence of peripheral circulatory failure, abdominal pain and effusions in serous cavities, notably the right pleura. CNS symptoms, including convulsions, meningism and opisthotonos, extensor plantar responses and raised intracranial pressure may occur but the CSF shows no abnormality. Slight lymphadenopathy may occur with mild splenomegaly.

In dengue-endemic areas any febrile illness of unspecified cause in childhood, of less than 7 days duration, especially during the rainy season, should be suspected to be DHF and a tourniquet test performed. If the test proves positive, DHF is likely. Febrile illness presenting after 7 days duration virtually excludes the diagnosis of DHF/DSS.

The diagnosis of DHF/DSS is clinical. Confirmation of diagnosis relies on detecting a fourfold or greater rise of HI antibody titre in convalescent sera or HI antibody of ≥1:640 in both acute or convalescent sera.

The clinician walks a tightrope in managing DHF/DSS. On the one hand, inadequate administration of intravenous fluids will increase the risk of hypovolaemia and shock, while on the other hand, giving too much fluid may overload the circulation. Constant careful monitoring of vital signs, and other important parameters like the haematocrit and platelet count, and constant careful supervision of therapy are mandatory. Corticosteroids may be helpful in severe shock but are not routinely used. Antibiotics may be needed for associated or complicating illness. Large fluid collections in body cavities are best aspirated to ease respiratory embarrassment. Adequate treatment of DHF/DSS is often dramatically rewarded and recovery is almost always complete. Vector control is the only preventive measure in the absence of an effective polyvalent dengue virus vaccine.

REFERENCES

1 Grant J P. In *UNICEF. The State of the World's Children*. Oxford: Oxford University Press, 1989.

2 Effiong C E, Aimaku V E, Bienzle U, Oyedeji G A, Ibezi G & Ikpe D E. Neonatal jaundice in Ibadan: incidence and aetiological factors in babies born in hospital. *J Natl Med Assoc* 1975; 67:208–213.

3 Hendrickse R G, Coulter J B S, Lamplugh S M et al. Aflatoxins and kwashiorkor: a study of Sudanese children. *BMJ* 1982; 285:843–846.

4 Ramjee G, Berjazk M, Adhikani M & Dutton M F. Aflatoxins and kwashiorkor in Durban, South Africa. *Ann Trop Paediatr* 1992; 12:241–247.

5 Hendrickse R G. Kwashiorkor: the hypothesis that incriminates aflatoxins. *Pediatrics* 1991; 88:376–379.

6 Trowell H C, Davies J N & Dean R F A. *Kwashiorkor*. London: Edward Arnold, 1954.

7 Waterlow J C. Notes on the assessment and classification of protein-energy malnutrition in children. *Lancet* 1973; ii:87–89.

8 Mavalanker D V & Clemens J. Vitamin A and childhood mortality. *Lancet* 1991; 337:1409–1410.

9 World Health Organization. *Vitamin A Supplements. A Guide to their Use in the Treatment and Prevention of Vitamin A Deficiency and Xerophthalmia*. Geneva: WHO, 1988.

10 Brabin B. Fetal anaemia in developing countries: its causes and significance. *Ann Trop Paediatr* 1992; 3:1–8.

11 Walter T, Andraca I & Chadud P. Iron deficiency anaemia: adverse effects on infant psychomotor development. *Pediatrics* 1989; 84:7–17.

12 Tovo P A, de Martino M, Gabiano C et al. Prognostic factors and survival with perinatal HIV-1 infection. *Lancet* 1991; 339:1249–1253.

13 Ip H M, Lelie P N, Wong V C W et al. Prevention of hepatitis B virus carrier state in infants according to maternal serum levels of HBV DNA. *Lancet* 1989; i:406–410.

14 Hendrickse R G & Adeniye A. Quartan malarial nephrotic syndrome. *Kidney Int* 1979; 16:64–74.

15 Brabin L & Brabin B J. Parasitic infections in women and their consequences. *Adv Parasitol* 1992; 31:1–81.

16 Van Geldermalsen A A & Wenning U. A diphtheria epidemic in Lesotho, 1989. Did vaccination increase the population's susceptibility? *Ann Trop Paediatr* 1993; 13:13–19.

17 Riley I, Lehmann D, Alpers M P et al. Pneumococcal vaccine prevents death rate from acute lower-respiratory-tract infections in Papua New Guinean children. *Lancet* 1986; ii:877–881.

CHAPTER 16

SURGERY IN THE TROPICS

C. Holcombe

Any doctor who has worked in a developing country will not easily forget the widespread and pathetic evidence of surgical neglect in the villages; huge hernias and hydroceles, unsightly lumps on the faces of women and children, and the failure of so many countries to provide even a basic level of surgical care for their people.

Samiran Nundy,
All India Institute of Medical Sciences

Tropical surgery involves the management of trop- ical surgical pathological entities, and also the treat- ment of many who present late and must inevitably be managed with minimal resources.

There is a huge unmet surgical need in the tropics. Nordberg[1] in Kenya estimated that only 10% of operations needed were actually performed. Health care must involve the whole person, and the primary health care physician must be able to refer a patient with a surgical problem to a surgeon who will deal with it both competently and efficiently.

SURGICAL PRINCIPLES IN THE TROPICS

THE BALANCE OF RISK: WHEN TO OPERATE

Surgery is practical, management is all important and the decision whether or not to operate is vital. For many patients the difficulties of referral are insurmountable. Those in dire need who will die without surgery should be operated upon, even if facilities and skill are not ideal. On the other hand someone with a chronic problem which causes inconvenience but allows life to continue should only be operated upon if a good outcome is assured. The tendency for the 'non-surgeon' is to wait too long before operating. Repeated careful examin- ation with hourly measurement of the pulse, tem- perature, blood pressure and urine output are the keys to decision-making.

WHO SHOULD OPERATE

There is a shortage of trained surgeons throughout the tropics, and those who are trained are concen- trated in the large cities. Watters and Bayley,[2] in a study in Zambia of over 21 000 operations, found that 18 000 (86%) were not complex and could be taught to non-surgeons. They concluded that gen- eral doctors must be taught and encouraged to perform surgery in district hospitals. They argued cogently that teaching hospital trained surgeons should concentrate their time on more difficult oper- ations, teaching surgical trainees and supporting district hospital doctors.

IMPROVISATION

Resources are limited and without the will to impro- vise the tropical surgeon is lost. Improvisation does not mean poor surgery. At the heart of improvisa- tion is a concern for the patient. There is often a choice between no operation, or an operation with less than perfect facilities. For the majority, espe- cially the acutely ill, the latter is almost always preferable.

SURGERY OF SEPSIS

The Western doctor visiting a hospital ward in the tropics for the first time cannot fail to be impressed by the quantity, severity and variety of infective complications: infected compound fractures, large abscesses, empyema of the chest, chronic ulcers and gas gangrene are all common. Management principles are the same for all: *debridement to healthy bleeding tissue and adequate dependent drainage* (Figure 16.1).

ABSCESSES

The management of pus is surgical. Abscesses show the classical signs of redness (replaced by shininess in dark-skinned people), increased temperature and pain. The pus must be drained, generally by a wide

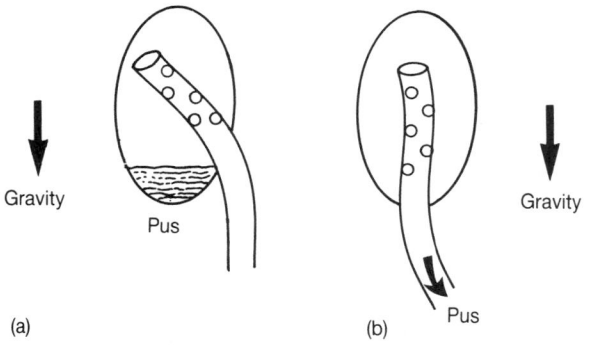

Figure 16.1 Dependent drainage must be achieved: (a) correct; (b) incorrect.

and adequate incision with excision of the skin edges, to allow dependent drainage, packing, daily dressing and granulation.

TROPICAL PYOMYOSITIS

Tropical pyomyositis is characterized by the apparently spontaneous appearance of bacterial abscesses within the fascial boundaries of skeletal muscles, usually muscles with large bulk. *Staphylococcus aureus* is the organism isolated in the majority of cases. Pyomyositis accounts for 3–4% of surgical admissions in Uganda[3] and 2% of surgical admissions in tropical Ecuador.[4]

AETIOLOGY

Taylor et al[5] have documented virus-like particles on electron microscopy of skeletal muscle adjacent to areas of tropical pyomyositis and suggest that these (arena) viruses cause an initial injury which becomes secondarily infected with *Staph. aureus*.

MANAGEMENT

Without treatment the prognosis is grave with a gradual deterioration in health; the patient eventually takes to the bed and dies. Treatment is adequate drainage of all abscess cavities under antibiotic cover.

HUMAN IMMUNODEFICIENCY VIRUS INFECTION AND THE ACQUIRED IMMUNE DEFICIENCY SYNDROME (See also Chapter 12)

The human immunodeficiency virus (HIV) has made an enormous impact on tropical surgical practice.

RISK TO THE SURGEON

Between 11 and 24% of surgical patients in Zambia are HIV positive.[6] The surgeon is at risk from 'sharps' injuries, with a seroconversion rate estimated at 1 in 200.

CHANGES IN SURGICAL PRESENTATION AND MANAGEMENT

Surgery may be required as a result of conditions related to HIV positivity, e.g. intussusception of the bowel in Kaposi's sarcoma in a patient with acquired immune deficiency syndrome (AIDS) or because of indirect complications of HIV infection, e.g. postoperative infection. There is an increased risk of sepsis in the HIV-positive patient. Pyogenic infection may or may not be a result of reduced immunocompetence, but appendicitis, wound infection or perianal sepsis will be worse and more difficult to manage in those with reduced immunocompetence. Reconstruction needs to be regarded in a different light: implants should be avoided and flaps and skin grafts used only if there is no alternative as they are less likely to take.

Intervention for pyogenic sepsis should be earlier and more aggressive. The difficulty is that in those who are immunocompromised the classic signs of infection are reduced, making for delay when one should be expediting surgical intervention. At the time of surgery the differentiation between dead and live tissue is more difficult, and surgery should err on the side of being more rather than less aggressive in debridement.[7]

AIDS-RELATED PATHOLOGY

In 1983 Bayley,[8] working in Zambia noted the emergence of a new and aggressive form of Kaposi's sarcoma. Patients with this aggressive form of Kaposi's sarcoma, characterized by symmetrical lymphadenopathy, respiratory distress, weight loss and poor response to chemotherapy, were found to have positive serology for human T lymphotropic virus I (HTLV-III) in contrast to endemic Kaposi's sarcoma.[9] Non-specific cystitis, chronic osteitis and peripheral vascular disease have been noted in HIV-positive patients with no other known pathologies, so that in areas where there is a high prevalence of HIV infection, HIV-related pathology makes up a significant proportion of the surgical workload.

THE ACUTE ABDOMEN (See also Chapter 3)

The common causes are obstruction, peritonitis, appendicitis, duodenal ulcer and trauma (Table 16.1). Peritonitis secondary to infection of the female genital tract is relatively common compared with the West. Peritonitis carries significant mortality, recorded as 25% in a series of 55 patients from Zambia.[12] In the tropics patients tend to be young and fit, without other medical problems, which improves prognosis, although this is offset by the fact that they often present late.

MANAGEMENT

The initial management priority is resuscitation with intravenous fluids. Fluid replacement can be monitored simply and effectively by hourly urine measurement. Intravenous antibiotics should also be given. In most cases laparotomy is indicated with the aim of stopping further soiling of the peritoneum and washing out the peritoneal cavity. Peritoneal lavage with several litres of warm fluid is vital. Conservative management of peritonitis may

occasionally be attempted if the patient's peritonitis is of some days duration, there is evidence that the source of contamination has sealed and that the peritoneal cavity is coping with the infection. Where there is diagnostic difficulty laparoscopy is a useful adjunct; this reduced the unnecessary laparotomy rate from 14 to 6% when introduced in Jos, Nigeria.[14]

TYPHOID PERFORATION (Chapter 42)

The major surgical complication of typhoid fever is intestinal perforation.

PATHOLOGY

Salmonella typhi is transmitted by the orofaecal route, gaining entry through the intestinal mucosa in the region of the Peyer's patches. Initially there is hyperplasia of the Peyer's patches, followed by

Table 16.1 Reasons for emergency laparotomy in East and Central Africa.

			Percentage due to:				
Place	Year(s)	Total	Obstruction	Peritonitis	Appendix	Duodenal ulcer	Trauma
Rwanda[10]	1977–81	204	44	8	8	11	16
Zambia[11]	1975–76	77	49	5	17	0	13
Zambia[12]	1985–87	150	21	26	17	3	35
Uganda[13]	1983–86	100	37	24	ns	ns	12

necrosis and ulceration, usually within 45 cm of the ileocaecal valve, on the antimesenteric border.

FREQUENCY

The incidence of typhoid perforation varies widely and is highest in West Africa at 8–18%.[15] A perforation rate of 3.5% has been reported in Cairo,[16] 1–5% in South Africa,[17] 0.5% in Nepal[18] and 11% in India.[19]

MANAGEMENT

The primary objective of management is early and aggressive resuscitation in preparation for swift simple surgery and this can be achieved with a mortality of only 5%.[20] A combination of chloramphenicol and metronidazole should be given and the peritoneal cavity thoroughly washed out. In 15% there are up to five separate perforations. Perforation occurs within 45 cm of the ileocaecal valve in 95%. Resection is rarely necessary (only 1% in the series from Ghana) and multiple perforations can be sutured.

AETIOLOGY OF HIGH PERFORATION RATE IN WEST AFRICA

Late arrival of patients to hospital, an unusually virulent strain of *S. typhi*, diminished host resistance and local tissue allergy have all been suggested.

APPENDICITIS

INCIDENCE

Appendicitis was rare in the tropics and remains uncommon. This is graphically illustrated by Osman[21] in a study from Khartoum. He analysed all operations done in the Khartoum Hospital from 1929 and showed a rapid rise in the incidence of appendicectomy from 1957. In the Melanesian population the annual incidence of appendicectomy is 29 per 100 000[22] compared with 210 per 100 000 in Australia.[23]

Katzen[24] and Onuigbo[25] have noticed seasonal variations in incidence in Africa, suggesting the possible involvement of an infective agent, and Barker and Morris[26] have recently published data suggesting an infective aetiology for appendicitis. Infection acquired at a young age causes little harm. However, as hygiene in the community improves, infection is acquired by the older child or adult,

and this results in appendicitis; if hygiene improves further, infection is never acquired, so leading to a reduction in the incidence of appendicitis, as is now occurring in the West.

APPENDICITIS IN THE TROPICS

Presentation is similar, although the perforation rate is higher, reaching 18% in Malaysia.[27] Schistosomal ova are occasionally found but are of doubtful significance.[28]

DIVERTICULOSIS

Diverticulosis occurs in up to one-third of patients over 60 years old in the West,[29] yet in a series of 216 adult barium enemas in southern Nigeria (mean age 40 years) only three (1%) had diverticula,[30] while Archampong et al[31] found 16 cases (4%) of diverticulosis in 362 barium enemas. In India 2% of 969 barium enemas showed diverticula (mean age 58 years), and the authors suggested that an increasingly urbanized and Westernized life style may be responsible for this increase.[32] Diverticulosis is likely to become more common as dietary fibre intake is reduced and the age of the population increases.

GALLSTONES

INCIDENCE

Overall, gallstones are rare in the tropics.[33] In a postmortem study in Uganda Owor[34] found an incidence of only 0.87%. In the 1980s only 7–8 cases of gallstones were being treated each year at University Hospital, Ibadan, Nigeria.[35] Even in the 1990s in East Africa a series of 20 patients with gallstones was considered worthy of publication.[36] There has, however, been a recent increase and Adedji et al[37] have suggested that this may be due to an increasingly 'Western' diet and better access to hospital care.

AETIOLOGY

Burkitt and Walker[38] have related the low incidence of gallstones in the tropics to increased fibre in the tropical diet. Gallstones are more common in patients with sickle cell disease,[39] but the incidence is less than in patients with sickle cell disease in the

USA, suggesting that the protective effect of diet is still active.[40] In a proportion of patients biliary infection by *Ascaris lumbricoides* is important, particularly where there are intrahepatic calculi.[41]

CLINICAL PRESENTATION AND MANAGEMENT

The complications of gallstone disease tend to present later in the tropics than in the West: the diagnosis is often not considered in the tropics, and patients present late. In Zimbabwe 25% presented with a right upper quadrant mass, 30% with obstructive jaundice and 6% with peritonitis.[42] Delayed surgery, after acute cholecystitis has settled, is wise. Ajao et al[43] have reported an 18% incidence of common bile duct injury in those operated on acutely.

INTESTINAL OBSTRUCTION

INTRODUCTION

In a typical series of 103 African cases with intestinal gangrene,[44] strangulated hernias accounted for 63%, intussusception 20%, adhesions 12% and volvulus 3%. This pattern changes markedly with improved health care, as shown by Lee and Ong[45] and Ti and Yong.[46] As health care improves the age of patients increases, adhesions replace hernias as the most common cause of obstruction, and the incidence of obstruction due to tuberculosis decreases. The cause of obstruction is different in children, where Gopi et al[47] found necrotizing enteritis to be the most common cause of obstruction in India.

PRESENTATION AND MANAGEMENT

The four cardinal signs of intestinal obstruction are colicky abdominal pain, abdominal distension, vomiting and absolute constipation. Patients in the tropics present late and are severely fluid and electrolyte depleted, requiring up to 6–7 litres of fluid. The patient should have a urinary catheter passed and the urine output measured hourly. An hourly output of at least 30 ml is desirable.

Operation is urgent if there is evidence of a gangrenous segment and/or perforation of intestine. This is suggested by signs of local or generalized peritonitis, a raised peripheral white cell count and toxic shock. Operation should also be carried out soon if there is a closed loop obstruction.

HERNIAS

Hernias are common in Africa. Inguinal hernias predominate: of 2011 hernias operated upon in northern Nigeria, 92% were inguinal.[48] Nordberg[1] has estimated that only 10% of operations needed for strangulated hernias are carried out. This unmet surgical need leads to many of the features of this disease in the tropics.

Strangulation is relatively common, accounting for 75% of cases of intestinal obstruction in Accra.[44]

Faecal fistula from a hernia is rare in the West but occurs in the tropics, either from neglect of a strangulated hernia or from the intervention of the 'native healer' with a red-hot piece of metal.

Giant hernias are defined as those larger than the average human head which on occasion become so large that they drag on the ground and develop callosities. Surgical repair is problematic as return of the abdominal contents to the abdomen can cause respiratory distress. Induction of a progressively increasing pneumoperitoneum preoperatively can be helpful.

Umbilical hernia is very common in African children; it is self-limiting and does not usually need surgical repair. However, those with a neck greater than 5 cm may persist and irreducibility, strangulation, and increase in size with age are indications for operation.

INTUSSUSCEPTION

Ninety-five per cent of cases of intussusception occurs in infants under 5 years of age.[49] Ileocaecal intussusception is common throughout Africa, and in southern Nigeria caecocolic intussusception is common.[50] It has been suggested that this is initiated by contraction of the caecal wall opposite the ileocaecal valve, which may be caused by 5-hydroxytryptamine which is common in plantain and bananas,[51] or by excretion products of *A. lumbricoides* which can also cause marked bowel contraction. Parasites, fasting and feasting, enlarged ileocaecal lymph nodes, intestinal polyps and a mobile caecum have all been implicated in the aetiology of intussusception.[52]

PRESENTATION

The key presenting features are colicky abdominal pain, vomiting, a palpable tumour, diarrhoea and the passage of blood and mucus per rectum.

DIAGNOSIS

Plain abdominal radiography provides the diagnosis, with confirmation by barium enema if necessary. A barium enema can also be therapeutic in reducing the intussusceptum; however this should be used with extreme care in the tropics where patients present late and the incidence of gangrene is high.

TREATMENT

Management is by operation at which the intussusceptum gently is squeezed back, rather than pulled out. In the presence of gangrene or an irreducible intussusception a hemicolectomy with ileocolic anastomosis may be necessary.

VOLVULUS

Sigmoid volvulus is common in East Africa, and small intestinal volvulus more common in West and South Africa. In a series from Zimbabwe there were 81 cases of large bowel volvulus (sigmoid in 78), 72 cases of small intestinal volvulus, and 30 cases of ileosigmoid knotting.[53]

SIGMOID VOLVULUS

Sigmoid volvulus is the most common cause of intestinal obstruction in Addis Ababa[54]; it is common in Sudan, accounting for 18% of all cases of acute intestinal obstruction.[55]

Aetiology

High residue diet has been suggested but does not account for the male predominance.

Native enemas contain ginger, pepper, and herbal extracts and may cause excess bowel motility and volvulus.

Anatomy: the sigmoid has to have a long mesentery for volvulus to occur and this has been demonstrated radiologically and at autopsy.[53] The sigmoid loop is longer in men and those with a history of constipation.

Presentation

Gross abdominal distension is the most striking feature and the diagnosis can be confirmed on a plain abdominal radiograph which shows a huge inverted U outlining the distended loop from pelvis to diaphragm and frequently surmounting two fluid levels.

Treatment

Distension can usually be relieved using the sigmoidoscope, which untwists the bowel and is accompanied by an explosive, but satisfying, emission of liquid faeces and flatus. A flatus tube is then passed through the sigmoidoscope to maintain decompression. This conservative method is contraindicated if there is a compound volvulus or signs of gangrene and peritonitis, in which case laparotomy is needed. Decompression is safe but recurrence is likely in over 50%. The best method of treatment is unclear. Elective resection is possible but it may be difficult to persuade patients to have an operation when they are well. Laparotomy and primary anastomosis may be ideal in very good hands[56] but cannot be advocated for most parts of the tropics. Operative detorsion with temporary 'Foley catheter colostomy' may be both safe and effective at preventing recurrence.[57]

SMALL INTESTINAL VOLVULUS

Small intestinal volvulus accounted for 20% of all cases of intestinal obstruction in Nairobi,[58] and is also common in Ethiopia.[59] In addition to the signs of intestinal obstruction circulatory collapse is often a marked feature. Active resuscitation and laparotomy is required.

ASCARIASIS (See also Chapter 71)

Ascaris lumbricoides has been reported to infect up to 70% of children in tropical countries[60] and causes obstruction of the terminal ileum. Over 80% of patients can be treated conservatively[61] with nasogastric suction and intravenous infusion. When the patient has passed flatus or faeces a vermifuge, either piperazine or a benzimidazole compound should be given. These patients must be closely observed and if there are signs of volvulus or perforation, laparotomy is mandatory.

TRAUMA

In the Third World, trauma is an epidemic of staggering proportions.

Imre Loefler, 1992[62]

Introduction: In a multicentre study from Nigeria[63] trauma accounted for 10% of all admissions; the majority of these (75%) were due to road traffic accidents. In Dar-es-Salaam nearly half of all paediatric surgical admissions were due to trauma, which was the leading cause of death,[64] and in Nigeria there are over 8000 recorded deaths annually[65] due to road traffic accidents.

BLUNT TRAUMA TO THE ABDOMEN

Of 195 children with abdominal injuries in Nigeria almost 80% were brought in dead or died shortly after admission.[66] The major priority of management is resuscitation, and urgent laparotomy in those who are shocked. Resuscitation should be with blood or colloid but can utilise any intravenous fluid available. Laparotomy can be life saving and should be combined with autotransfusion of the free blood in the peritoneum which can be strained through sterile gauze and then transfused.[67] Although splenic preservation following trauma has been practised in the tropics,[68] the spleen, if damaged, is probably best removed, particularly if the operator is inexpert. Ihekwaba[69] found no increased rate of infection in 94 patients who had undergone splenectomy.

HEAD INJURIES

No head injury is so severe as to be despaired of, nor so trivial as to be lightly ignored.

Hippocrates

Head injuries are common in the tropics; few wear seat belts or crash helmets and road traffic accidents account for 60–80% of injuries. In a review of head injuries in Zaria there was a mortality rate of 30%, and 50% in Zambia.[70,71]

In initial management of the unconscious patient, preservation of the airway is all important and the patient should be put in the recovery position, due attention being given to the neck in case this has also been injured. Following hospital admission each patient should have his/her grade on the Glasgow coma scale recorded. The most useful guide to management is a change in this, particularly if the patient was initially lucid but becomes rapidly unconscious, suggesting a possible extradural haematoma, for which urgent burr holes are needed.

PENETRATING ABDOMINAL INJURIES

The incidence and nature of penetrating injury is dependent on the degree of urbanization and civil conflict in the country concerned. A distinction needs to be made between high- and low-velocity injuries. The amount of energy release, and consequently the amount of tissue damage is much greater with a high-velocity injury, making exploration and debridement mandatory,[72] whereas low-velocity injuries can be treated safely by an expectant 'watch and wait policy'. Norris and Sugrue[73] have pointed out that it can be difficult to distinguish these and each wound must be treated on its merits.

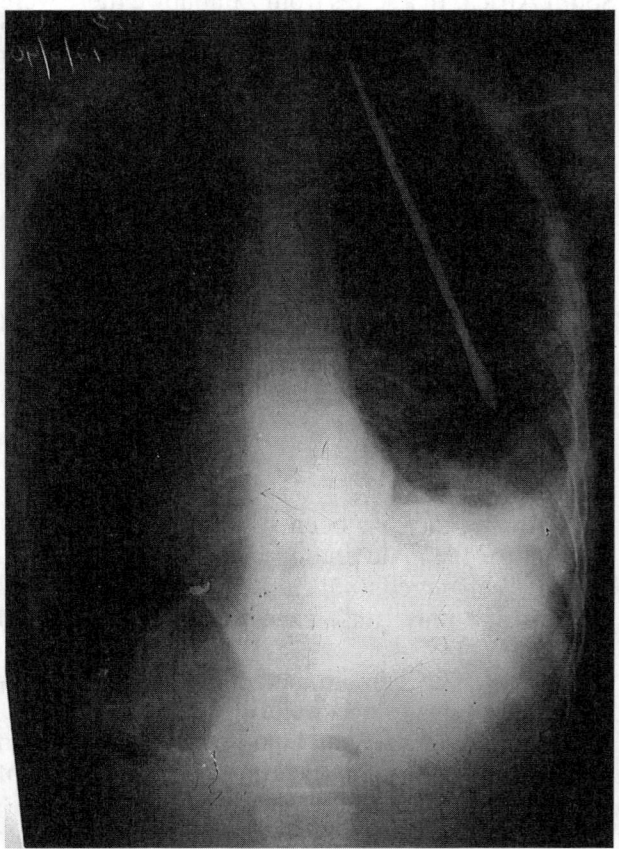

Figure 16.2   The bow and arrow remains an effective weapon.

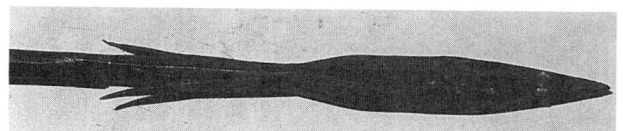

Figure 16.3 The barbs on this arrowhead are clearly seen.

Up to 30% of penetrating abdominal wounds can be managed conservatively.[74] Frequent observation is vital,[75] and if this is not possible laparotomy is safer. Similar conservative management of penetrating injuries of the neck is also safe.[76] Controversy remains regarding the management of colonic injuries. In the tropics, where the facilities for treatment are frequently not ideal, the provision of a temporary covering colostomy seems prudent. In some areas of the tropics the bow and arrow are still commonly used. Victims who are stable and reach hospital need formal laparotomy or thoracotomy as

the barbs prevent simple removal (Figures 16.2 and 16.3).

INJURIES OF THE LIMBS

In Canada there are 700 orthopaedic surgeons for a population of 22 million; in East and Central Africa there are 25 orthopaedic surgeons for a population of over 75 million.[77] Treatment must be appropriate:[78] the use of Western techniques, particularly internal fixation, is often inappropriate (Figure 16.4). Very often injuries present late after the traditional bone setter has failed. Initial management must concentrate on soft tissues, drainage of infection, debridement, and closed treatment of fractures whenever possible.

PLASTIC AND RECONSTRUCTIVE SURGERY

Plastic and reconstructive surgery makes up a fifth of the surgical workload in the tropics[79] and the basic principles should be known by all health personnel. Open fires are still used for cooking and heating and burns are common, particularly amongst children;[80] initial management is often not ideal and post-burn contractures are common (Figure 16.5). Trauma is common and often neglected. Tumours present late and need reconstructive surgery even for palliation (Figure 16.6). Finally, specific tropical problems such as cancrum oris, lymphoedema and keloids also need a plastic surgery input.

PRINCIPLES OF PLASTIC SURGERY

A sound application of the principles of plastic surgery and wound care is important.[81] The key to eliminating wound breakdown, with all its attendant debility, is adequate debridement, good blood supply, and suture lines without tension. If either of these cannot be achieved the wound should be left to granulate and heal by secondary intention. Be bold in debridement, be timid in suturing: even very large defects will heal by secondary intention.

CANCRUM ORIS (NOMA)

Dzo-ma-ga (running horse gangrene) is a disease that spreads rapidly . . . foul black gangrene appears

next to the teeth. Then the dead tissues fall away and expose the underlying roots. A few days later the cheek may perforate and the lip necrose.

Chinese Surgeon, 1617

AETIOLOGY

Eighty per cent of cases occur in 2–6-year-old children.[82] Three factors are necessary: a predisposing debilitated state, ulcerative gingivitis, and a precipitating general illness, often measles or malaria.[83]

CLINICAL FEATURES

The first sign is Vincent's gingivitis, with a sore mouth and mucosal ulceration. The overlying cheek then becomes gangrenous and secondary infection heralds the onset of systemic upset. Following demarcation the slough separates and healthy granulation tissue forms. The disfigurement is extreme (Figure 16.7). Trismus is caused by mucosal contracture and can progress to ankylosis of the lower jaw, with inability even to eat.[84]

TREATMENT

Acute management addresses the cause, with attention to general nutrition and local desloughing. The

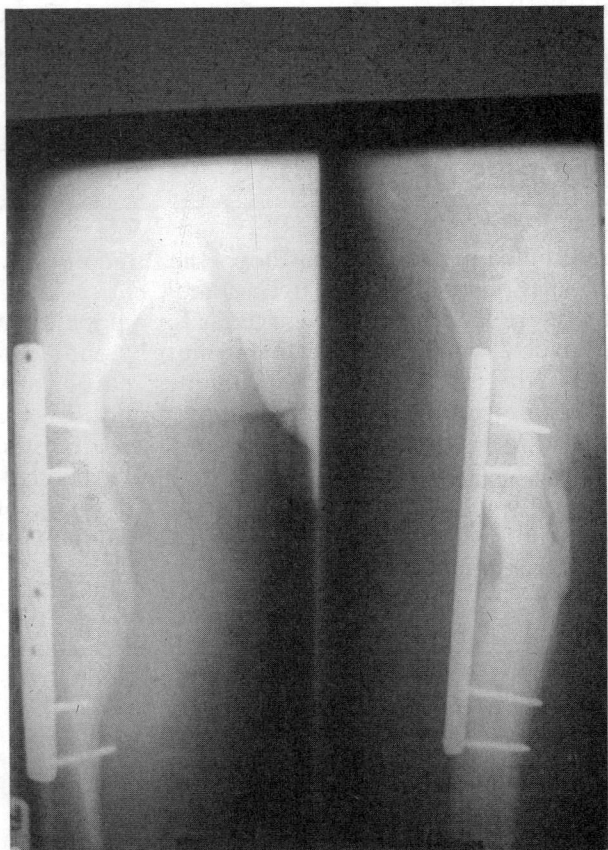

Figure 16.4   Chronic osteomyelitis following internal fixation of the femur.

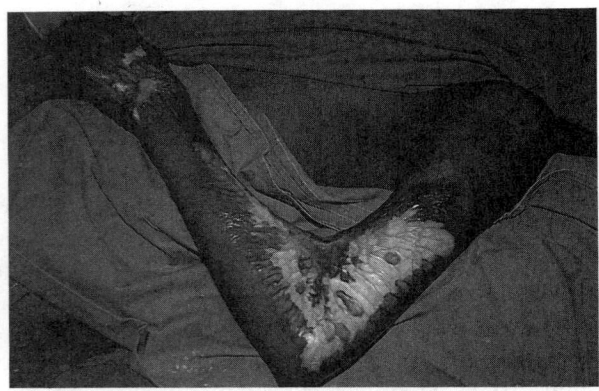

Figure 16.5   Burn contracture of the elbow.

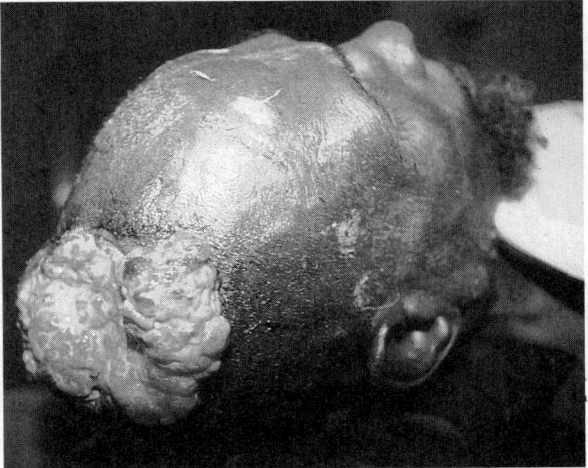

Figure 16.6   A large squamous cell carcinoma of the scalp.

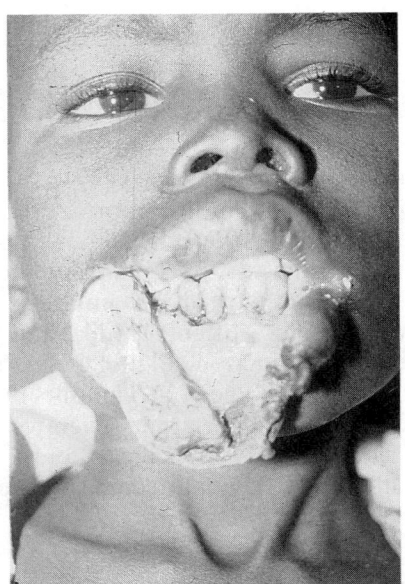

Figure 16.7   Cancrum oris.

An average of seven operations per patient was required by Durrani.[85]

TROPICAL ULCERS (See also Chapter 11)

ACUTE PHAGEDENIC ULCER

Clinical features

three pillars of treatment are iron, penicillin and antimalarials.

Reconstruction presents a formidable problem, involving release of trismus, the replacement of lost cheek lining and replacement of lost cheek cover.

The disease is limited to tropical and subtropical areas of the world and has decreased markedly with improvement in standards of living. Ninety-five per

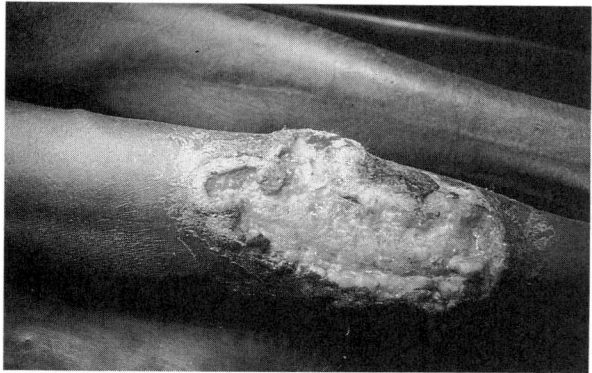

Figure 16.8 Squamous cell carcinoma developing in a long-standing tropical ulcer.

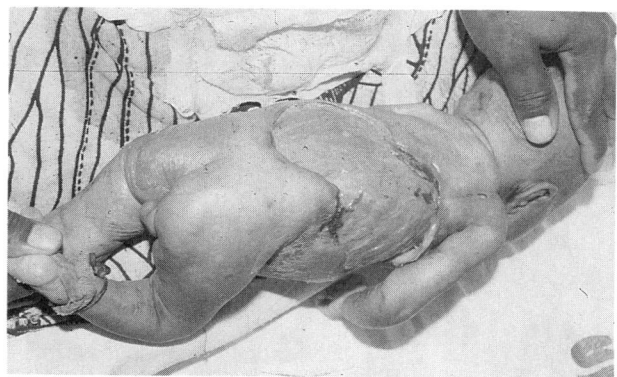

Figure 16.9 Buruli ulcer involving most of the trunk.

cent occur around the ankle and lower third of the leg. Initially there is constitutional disturbance, fever, pain and restlessness. The lesion is preceded by minor trauma and presents with a tender indurated area which forms a round or oval ulcer. These early lesions have been experimentally produced by the inoculation of *Bacillus fusiformis* and spirochaetes into volunteers.[86]

There is rapid spread and tissue destruction. The underlying muscles and tendons may be exposed and the ulcer is painful at this stage. After about 4 weeks the ulcer becomes stationary and painless; it either heals or becomes a chronic non-specific ulcer.

Chronicity

Neglected ulcers become chronic, form a fibrous avascular base and may persist for 30 years or more. In about 2% of these ulcers a squamous cell carcinoma will develop. This is a common tumour in northern Nigeria[87] and is the reason for 20% of all lower limb amputations[88] (Figure 16.8).

Treatment

Prevention can be achieved by wearing shoes and long trousers and the early lesion responds dramatically to penicillin. If the ulcer is less than 2.5 cm antibiotics and daily dressing will lead to rapid healing. Ulcers larger than 2.5 cm require daily dressing(s) and antibiotics for 5–7 days followed by split-skin grafting. Chronic ulcers need excision and grafting.

BURULI ULCER

Buruli ulcer is a chronic necrotizing skin ulcer with undermined edges caused by *Mycobacterium ulcer-*

ans; it may involve a large part of the trunk or limb (Figure 16.9). The ulcer may penetrate deep fascia, exposing bone and tendons which usually slough, resulting in severe deformity.[89] Treatment is surgical with wide excision and primary closure or grafting.

CHRONIC LYMPHOEDEMA

FREQUENCY

In East Africa over a quarter of a million people have elephantiasis,[90] while in Ethiopia endemic elephantiasis of the lower leg has an incidence of 87 per 1000.[91]

AETIOLOGY

Filariasis (Chapter 70) is the best known cause of elephantiasis, but primary chronic lymphoedema is due to absorption of aluminosilicate and silicon (Chapter 28). This initially causes peripheral and then more proximal lymphatic obstruction.[92] It is, however, more common in certain families, and this is probably due to an hereditary hypoplasia of the lymphatics.

Treatment

Early treatment may arrest the disease process and should be aimed at the underlying cause. If lymphoedema is established, prolonged standing must be avoided, the foot elevated whenever possible and elastic stockings fitted. Kager et al[93] found encouraging results with intermittent pneumatic pressure in Kenya. Hygiene is also important as the majority of exacerbations are associated with infection.

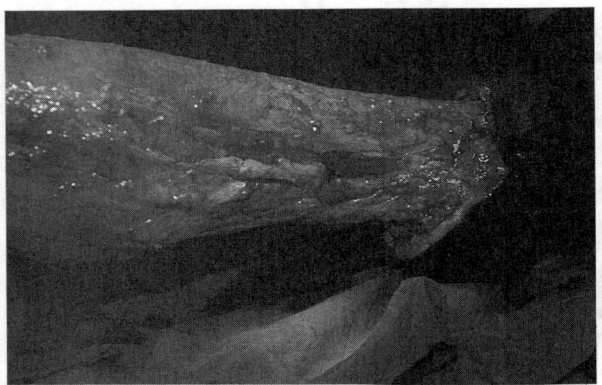

Figure 16.10   Charles' procedure for chronic lymphoedema.

The mainstay of surgery is Charles' operation, first described in 1912. This involves excision of all subcutaneous fat down to the deep fascia, on to which split skin is applied.[94] This is a reasonably major surgical procedure and should be done under tourniquet to avoid excessive blood loss (Figure 16.10).

KELOID

Keloid is a benign, proliferative non-neoplastic connective tissue overgrowth localized to the dermis; it occurs in response to cutaneous trauma and grows beyond the confines of the original scar. Keloid formation is more common over the sternum, back, shoulders and face and thickens preferentially along lines of tissue tension. Keloids are much more common in coloured people, with a ratio of about 3.5:1.[95] Oluwasanmi[96] found a high concentration of immunoglobulin (IgG) in keloid tissue in Nigerians and an immunological basis for the disease has been suggested.

TREATMENT

Tempest[95] has recommended masterly inactivity, particularly for chest keloids, and this is perhaps good advice for all keloids. Complete excision is followed by recurrence in 70%, and as the scar is now longer the keloid is bigger.

Partial excision within the lesion, with or without skin grafting, has some success and surgery can be combined with radiotherapy and has been claimed to give a good result.[97] Intralesional injection of steroids, most commonly triamcinolone, can also be successful and has been combined with surgery to prevent a recurrence. Pressure has been used in keloid therapy since 1894,[98] and has recently given good results in East Africa.[99] The results are best if pressure is applied early; it needs to be applied for several months.

REFERENCES

1 Nordberg E M. Incidence and estimated need of caesarian section, inguinal hernia repair and operation for strangulated inguinal hernia in rural Africa. *BMJ* 1984; 289:71–72.

2 Watters D A K & Bayley A C. Training doctors and surgeons to meet the surgical needs of Africa. *BMJ* 1987; 295: 761–763.

3 Horn C V & Master S. Pyomyositis tropicans in Uganda. *East Afr Med J* 1968; 45:463–471.

4 Kerrigan K R & Nelson J. Tropical pyomyositis in eastern Ecuador. *Trans R Soc Trop Med Hyg* 1992; 86:90–91.

5 Taylor J F, Fluck D & Fluck D. Tropical myositis: ultrastructural studies. *J Clin Path* 1976; 29:1081–1084.

6 Bayley A C. Surgical pathology of HIV infection: lessons from Africa. *Br J Surg* 1990; 863–686.

7 Loefler I J P. Surgeons and AIDS in Africa. *Surgery* (*add on*) 1992; 10:95–96.

8 Bayley A C. Aggressive Kaposi's sarcoma in Zambia, 1983. *Lancet* 1984; i:1318.

9 Bayley A C, Downing R G, Cheingsong-Popov R et al. HTLV-III serology distinguishes atypical and endemic Kaposi's sarcoma in Africa. *Lancet* 1985; i:359–361.

10 Dewulf E. Abdominal emergencies: a four year experience in Central Africa. *Trop Doct* 1986; 16:129–131.

11 Umerah B C & Obadike G O. Acute abdomen in the Zambian African. *East Afr Med J* 1978; 55:77–80.

12 Watters D A K. Severe peritoneal sepsis. *Baillière's Clin Trop Med Commun Dis* 1988; 3:275–300.

13 Ecookit S J, Omaswa F G & Upolei A L. Operations at Ngora Hospital. *Proc Assoc Surg East Afr* 1987; 10.

14 Ogbonna B C, Obekpa P O, Nomoh J T, Obafunwa J O & Nwana E J C. Laparoscopy in developing countries in the management of patients with an acute abdomen. *Br J Surg* 1992; 79:964–966.

15 Archampong E Q. Surgical complications of enteric fever. *Baillière's Clin Trop Med Commun Dis* 1988; 3:301–309.

16 El Ramli A H. Chloramphenicol in typhoid fever. *Lancet* 1950; i:618–620.

17 Keenn J P & Hadley G P. The surgical management of typhoid perforation in children. *Br J Surg* 1984; 71:928–929.

18 Kurlberg G & Frisk B. Factors reducing mortality in typhoid ileal perforation. *Trans R Soc Trop Med Hyg* 1991; 85:793–795.

19 Khosla S N. Typhoid perforation. *J Trop Med Hyg* 1977; 80:83–87.

20 Archampong E Q. Tropical diseases of the small bowel. *World J Surg* 1985; 9:887–896.

21 Osman A A. Epidemiological study of appendicitis in Khartoum. *Int Surg* 1974; 59:218–221.

22 Foster H McA & Webb S J. Appendicitis and appendicectomy in a Melanesian population. *Br J Surg* 1989; 76:368–369.

23 *Hospital Inpatient Statistics: Most Common Principal Procedures*. New South Wales Department of Health, Sydney: 1986.

24 Katzen M. Some observations on the acute abdomen in children. *S Afr Med J* 1966; 40:566–569.

25 Onuigbo W I B. Acute appendicitis in Nigerian Igbos—review of 182 cases. *Am J Proctol Gastroenterol Colon Rectal Surg* 1981; 32:6–7.

26 Barker D J P & Morris J. Acute appendicitis, bathrooms and diet in Britain and Ireland. *BMJ* 1988; 296:953–955.

27 Lee C M & Teoh M K. Perforated appendicitis—the Malaysian experience. *J R Coll Surg Edinb* 1990; 35:83–87.

28 Adebamowo C A, Akang E E U, Ladipa J K & Ajao O G. Schistosomiasis of the appendix. *Br J Surg* 1991; 78:1219–1221.

29 Burkitt D P. Non-infective disease of the large bowel. *Br Med Bull* 1984; 40:387–389.

30 Bohrer S P & Lewis E A. Diverticula of the colon in Ibadan, Nigeria. *Trop Geogr Med* 1974; 26:9–14.

31 Archampong E Q, Christian F & Badoe E A. Diverticular disease in an indigenous African community. *Ann R Coll Surg Engl* 1978; 60:464–470.

32 Kochhar R, Goenka M K, Nagi G, Bhasin D K & Mehta S K. The emergence of colonic diverticulosis in urbanised Indians. A report of 23 cases. *Trop Geogr Med* 1989; 41:254–256.

33 Burkitt D P & Tunstall M. Gall-stones: geographical and chronological features. *J Trop Med Hyg* 1975; 78:140–144.

34 Owor R. Gallstones in the autopsy population at Mulago Hospital, Kanpala. *East Afr Med J* 1964; 41:251.

35 Akute O O & Adekunle O O. Cholelithiasis in Ibadan, Nigeria. *East Afr Med J* 1984; 61:45.

36 Ogutu E O, Orinda D A O, Nusau B M & Lule G N. Cholelithiasis in the Kenyan African. *East Afr Med J* 1990; 67:656–660.

37 Adedji A, Akande B & Olumide F. The changing pattern of cholelithiasis in Lagos. *Scand J Gastroenterol* Suppl 1986; 124:63–66.

38 Burkitt D P & Walker A R. Saint's triad: confirmation and explanation. *S Afr Med J* 1976; 50:2136–2138.

39 Durosinmi M A, Ogunseyinde A O. Olatunji P O & Esan G J. Prevalence of cholelithiasis in Nigerians with sickle cell disease. *Afr J Med Med Sci* 1989; 18:223–229.

40 Adekile A D. Experience with cholelithiasis in patients with sickle cell disease in Nigeria. *Am J Pediatr Hematol Oncol* 1985; 7:261–264.

41 Schulman A. Non-western patterns of biliary stones and the role of ascariasis. *Radiology* 1987; 162:425–430.

42 Faranisi C T & Chimuka D. Gall bladder disease in Zimbabwe. *East Afr Med J* 1989; 66:115–121.

43 Ajao O G, Al-Saigh A A, Malatani T & Ladips J K. Timing of surgery in acute cholecystitis. *East Afr Med J* 1991; 68:490–494.

44 Fashakin E. O. Experience with 103 cases of intestinal gangrene in Ife-Ife, Nigeria. *Trop Doct* 1989; 19:25–27.

45 Lee S H & Ong E T L. Changing pattern of intestinal obstruction in Malaysia: a review of 100 consecutive cases. *Br J Surg* 1991; 78:181–182.

46 Ti T K & Yong N K. The pattern of intestinal obstruction in Malaysia. *Br J Surg* 1976; 63:963–965.

47 Gopi V K, Joseph, T P & Varma K K. Acute intestinal obstruction. *Indian Pediatr* 1989; 26:525–530.

48 Okukak E E, Grundy D J & Lawrie J H. Hernia in northern Nigeria. *J R Coll Surg Edinb* 1983; 28:147.

49 Kark A E & Rundle W J. The pattern of intussusception in Africans in Natal. *Br J Surg* 1960; 48:296–309.

50 Adekunle O O. Acute intestinal obstruction: a review of 300 cases treated at University College Hospital, Ibadan. *Niger Med J* 1977; 7:37–40.

51 Foy J M & Parratt J R. A note on the presence of noradrenaline and 5-hydroxytryptamine in plantain. *J Pharm Pharmacol* 1960; 12:360.

52 Awojobi Q A. Intussusception. In Adeloye A (ed.) *Davey's Companion to Surgery in Africa*. Edinburgh: Churchill Livingstone, 1987:328.

53 Wapnick S, Mufundi F & Musengesi L. Aetiological factors related to intestinal obstruction. *Cent Afr J Med* 1975; 21:53–57.

54 Gurovsky A. Survey of patients with volvulus of the sigmoid colon in Eritrea. *Ethiop Med J* 1969; 7:111–116.

55 El Masri S H & Khalil T. Volvulus of the sigmoid colon in Eritrea. *Trop Geogr Med* 1976; 28:297–302.

56 Loefler I J P. Bantu volvulus. *Surgery (add on)* 1990; 84:1996–1198.

57 Mout P. Temporary colostomy as a permanent treatment for sigmoid volvulus: a simple and safe one-stage procedure. *Trop Doct* 1989; 19:20–30.

58 Warambo M W. Acute volvulus of the small intestine. *East Afr Med J* 1971; 48: 209–212.

59 Lindtjorn B, Breivik K & Lende S. Intestinal volvulus in Sidamo, Ethiopia. *East Afr Med J* 1981; 58:208–211.

60 Louw J H. Abdominal complications of *Ascaris lumbricoides* infestation in children. *Br. J. Surg* 1966; 53:510–521.

61 Mokoena T & Luvuno F M. Conservative management of intestinal obstruction due to *Ascaris* worms in adult patients: a preliminary report. *J R Coll Surg Edinb* 1988; 33:318–321.

62 Loefler I J P. Trauma in the Third World: a Third World perspective. *Surgery* (*add on*) 1992; 10:64a.

63 Odelowo B O O. The problem of trauma in Nigeria. *Trop Geogr Med* 1991; 43:80–84.

64 Shija J K & Omar O S. Trauma as a major paediatric surgical problem in Dar-es-Salaam. *Proc Assoc Surg East Afr* 1985; 3:169–170.

65 Obeme A & Fagbayi A. Road traffic accidents in Kaduna metropolis: a three month survey. *East Afr Med J* 1988; 65:572–577.

66 Adejuyigbe O, Aderounmu A O & Adelusola K A. Abdominal injuries in Nigerian children. *J R Coll Surg Edinb* 1992; 37:29–33.

67 Moran B J. Traumatic rupture of the spleen in the rural tropics. *Trop Doct* 1988; 18:110–111.

68 Mabogunje O A. Splenic studies: II. Preservation of the ruptured spleen. *East Afr Med J* 1985; 62:597–601.

69 Ihekwaba F N. Splenectomy for trauma. *Trop Doct* 1988; 18:62–64.

70 Watters D A K & Sinclair J R. Outcome of severe head injuries in Central Africa. *J R Coll Surg Edinb* 1988; 33:35–38.

71 Muhammad I. Management of head injuries at the ABU hospital, Zaria. *East Afr Med J* 1990; 67:447–451.

72 Coupland R M. Technical aspects of war wound excision. *Br J Surg* 1989; 76:663–667.

73 Morris D S & Sugrue W J. Abdominal injuries in the war wounded of Afghanistan: a report from the International Committee of the Red Cross Hospital in Kabul. *Br J Surg* 1991; 78:1301–1304.

74 Demetriades D, Charalambides D, Lakhoo M & Pantanowitz D. Gunshot wound of the abdomen: role of selective conservative management. *Br J Surg* 1991; 78:220–322.

75 Stein A. Stab wounds of the abdomen. *S Afr Med J* 1973; 47:551.

76 Ngakane H, Muckart D J J & Luvuno F M. Penetrating visceral injuries of the neck: results of a conservative management policy. *Br J Surg* 1990; 77:908–910.

77 Fullard H, Darby H C, Willet B M & Gayland D. *The University Atlas*, 21st edn. London: George Philip, 1981.

78 Jellis J E. Taking orthopaedics to the people. *Baillière's Clin Trop Med Commun Dis* 1988; 3:257–274.

79 Goodacre T E E. Plastic surgery in a rural African hospital: spectrum and implications. *Ann R Coll Surg Engl* 1986; 68:42–44.

80 Onuba O. Pattern of burns injury in Nigerian children. *Trop Doct* 1988; 18:106–108.

81 McGregor I A. *Fundamental Techniques of Plastic Surgery and their Surgical Applications*. Edinburgh: Churchill Livingstone, 1989, 8th edition.

82 Tempest M N. Cancrum oris. *Br J Surg* 1966; 53:949–969.

83 Adeloye A. Cancrum oris. In Adeloye A (ed.) *Davey's Companion to Surgery in Africa*. Edinburgh: Churchill Livingstone, 1987:147–159.

84 Oluwasanmi J O, Sulaman, B L & Akinyemi O O. Ankylosis of the mandible from cancrum oris. *Plast Reconstr Surg* 1976; 57:342–350.

85 Durrani K M. Surgical repair of defects from noma (cancrum oris). *Plast Reconstr Surg* 1973; 52:629–634.

86 McAdam I W J. Tropical phagedenic ulcers in Uganda. *J R Coll Surg Edinb* 1966; 11:196–205.

87 Holcombe C & Babayo U. The pattern of malignant disease in north east Nigeria. *Trop Geogr Med* 1991; 43:189–192.

88 Holcombe C & Hassan S. Major limb amputation in northern Nigeria. *Br J Surg* 1991; 78:885–886.

89 Okoro A. *Mycobacterium ulcerans* infection. *Postgrad Doct Afr* 1980; 2:41.

90 Price E W. Endemic elephantiasis of the lower legs: natural history and clinical study. *Trans R Soc Trop Med Hyg* 1974; 68: 44–52.

91 Price E W. The site of lymphatic blockade in endemic (non-filarial) elephantiasis of the lower legs. *J Trop Med Hyg* 1977; 80:230–237.

92 Editorial. Non-filarial elephantiasis. *Lancet* 1980; i:349.

93 Kager P A, Rees P H & Bhatt K M. Non-filarial elephantiasis. *Lancet* 1980; i:1419.

94 Dellon A L & Hoopes J E. The Charles procedure in primary lymphoedema. Long term clinical results. *Plast Reconstr Surg* 1977; 60:589–595.

95 Tempest M N. Wound healing in the Tropics. In Schwartz S I, Adesola A O, Elebute E A & Rob C G (eds) *Tropical Surgery*. New York: McGraw-Hill, 1971; 66–87.

96 Oluwasanmi J O. Keloids in Ibadan. *Trop Geogr Med* 1974; 26:231–241.

97 Ramakrishnan K M, Thomas K P & Sundararajan C R. Study of 1000 patients with keloids in South India. *Plast Reconstr Surg* 1974; 53:276–280.

98 Ketchum D, Cohen I K & Masters R W. Hypertrophic scars and keloids. A collective review. *Plast Reconstr Surg* 1974; 53:140–154.

99 Haq M A & Haq A. Pressure therapy in treatment of hypertrophic scar, burn contracture and keloid: the Kenyan experience. *East Afr Med J* 1990; 67:785–793.

CHAPTER 17

OBSTETRICS AND GYNAECOLOGY IN THE TROPICS

A. S. Garden and D. Goodall

OBSTETRICS

MATERNAL MORTALITY: MAJOR CAUSES AND MANAGEMENT

The World Health Organization (WHO) estimates that 500 000 maternal deaths occur each year, 99% of them in developing countries (Figure 17.1). Over half the maternal deaths in the world occur in Asia and, of these, three-quarters are in India, Pakistan and Bangladesh.[1]

A maternal death is defined as a death of a woman while pregnant or within 42 days of the termination of a pregnancy, irrespective of the duration or the site of the pregnancy. The maternal mortality rate is expressed as the number of maternal deaths per 100 000 total deliveries. While the definition is succinct and accurate, the information obtained is less so because of the problems in data collection.[2] In many countries the death of a woman is not notified. Pregnancies may be registered late, if at all, so that deaths may not be reported as pregnancy related. In addition, there may be cultural or religious pressures not to attribute pregnancy as a factor in the cause of death, for instance if the woman was unmarried. In other situations pregnancy may not be recognized as the triggering factor in a death by the attending medical personnel. Despite these recognized shortcomings in the registration system, maternal mortality statistics make sobering reading. In areas of rural Gambia, rates as high as 2000 per 100 000 are reported, while a study in one region of India reports rates of 874 per 100 000 in rural areas and 545 per 100 000 in urban areas.[1] This compares with rates of around 4–8 per 100 000 in Western Europe. The levels of morbidity associated with pregnancy are even more difficult to calculate, although it has been estimated that 50 million women per year suffer complications of pregnancy, which may produce long-term debilitating symptoms such as vesicovaginal fistula, infertility and chronic pelvic pain.

The causes of maternal death are multifactorial and related to the status of women in the society, the level of nutrition, female literacy rates and availability of transport, as well as to the standard of medical and obstetric care. The main obstetric causes of maternal death in developing countries, however, are hypertensive disorders of pregnancy,

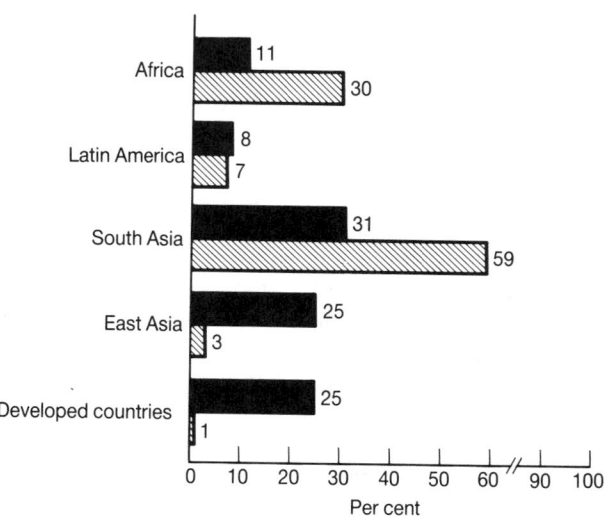

Figure 17.1 Percentage of women of reproductive age (▨) and maternal deaths (■) by geographic region, 1980s. Reproduced with permission from Maine D *Safe Motherhood Programs: Options and Issues*, New York: Center for Population and Public Health, Colombia University.

Table 17.1 Main causes of maternal deaths in hospitals in selected developing countries.

	India	Pakistan	Malaysia	Vietnam	Indonesia	Islamic Republic of Iran	Fiji	Nigeria	Ghana	Malawi	Zimbabwe	Kenya	United Republic of Tanzania	Egypt
Haemorrhage	+	+	+	+	+	+	+	+	+	+	+	+	+	+
Sepsis	+	+			+	+		+	+	+	+	+	+	+
Toxaemia	+	+	+	+	+	+	+	+	+	+			+	+
Abortion							+	+			+			+
Obstructed labour/ ruptured uterus		+		+				+	+	+	+	+	+	
Hepatitis	+					+	+				+			
Anaemia	+	+		+			+	+					+	
Abnormal haemoglobin														
Cardiac disease				+		+	+							

Reproduced with permission from Royston R and Armstrong S (eds) *Preventing Maternal Deaths*, Geneva: WHO, 1989.

infection and sepsis, haemorrhage, obstructed labour, anaemia and abortion (Table 17.1). Medical and obstetric inputs to reduce maternal mortality and morbidity must therefore focus on these problems.[3]

HYPERTENSIVE DISORDERS OF PREGNANCY (See also Chapter 26)

Pregnancy-induced hypertension is a multisystem disease characterized by increased blood pressure, non-dependent oedema and proteinuria. The disease occurs more commonly in primigravidae and in poorly nourished women in the late second and third trimesters of pregnancy. It is also more common in young (under 16 years of age) and in older mothers (over 35 years of age). In severe cases the condition progresses to eclampsia which is characterized by epileptiform seizures and coma. Prior to the onset of fits the woman may complain of frontal headaches, visual disturbances (particularly flashing lights), epigastric pain and vomiting. Examination shows her reflexes to be exaggerated. Urinary output decreases. These symptoms and signs must not be ignored.

Pregnancy-induced hypertension is classified as being mild, moderate or severe depending on the level(s) of blood pressure and the degree of proteinuria. The progress of the disease is extremely unpredictable, some patients having only mild disease throughout the latter part of their pregnancy whilst others progress rapidly within 24 hours from apparently mild disease to fulminating pre-eclampsia and eclampsia. Treatment is by delivery of the fetus and placenta. In the mild or moderate forms, especially before 36 weeks gestation, treatment with antihypertensives under supervision may allow the pregnancy to be prolonged for a few weeks. It must be remembered, however, that hypertension is just one symptom of a multisystem disorder and control of the blood pressure does not imply cure of the disease.

MANAGEMENT

Mild and moderate forms of the disease can only be detected by antenatal care, as the disease is symptomless at this stage other than perhaps for the appearance of non-dependent oedema. The treatment of these patients is expectant. Labour can usually be induced without risk to the fetus after 37 weeks gestation. The objective of management prior to this time is to control blood pressure and monitor the maternal and fetal condition to ensure that deterioration does not occur. Control of blood pressure can be achieved with any of the standard antihypertensive agents such as methyldopa, hydralazine, nifedipine or labetalol (Chapter 26). The earlier betablockers such as propranolol should be avoided if possible as they tend to cause fetal bradycardia and hypoglycaemia in neonates.

In areas with inadequate antenatal care provision or utilization, most women will present with severe forms of the disease or with eclampsia. Management in these circumstances is based on stabilizing the maternal condition and delivery of the fetus irrespective of gestation. Vaginal delivery is usually possible by rupturing the membranes and the judicious use of oxytocin, if available. Careful monitoring of fluid intake and output is essential during this time as these patients are frequently oliguric and may develop pulmonary oedema. If the patient does not progress in labour, delivery by caesarean section may be necessary. Control of blood pressure is by the use of intravenous antihypertensives. Intravenous anticonvulsants should also be used. The most commonly used are diazepam, phenytoin and magnesium sulphate, which can also be given intramuscularly. Diazepam may cause maternal respiratory depression and may also affect the fetus. Magnesium sulphate may also cause respiratory and cardiac arrest if serum magnesium levels become too high. Care must be taken, therefore, when using magnesium sulphate to check renal output and the presence of reflexes before giving a further dose. Suppression of the reflexes always occurs prior to respiratory or cardiac arrest. Phenytoin is less reliable in its action, is more expensive and requires close monitoring of the patient.

Patients are at risk of eclamptic fits up to 48 hours after delivery. During this time they should therefore receive intensive nursing in a semiprone position in a quiet room. Antihypertensive and anticonvulsant therapy should be continued.

COMPLICATIONS

Complications of the hypertensive disorders of pregnancy may be due to the disease itself, secondary to seizures or to the side-effects of drugs or other treatment given. Complications directly due to the disease process include renal failure, hepatic failure, disseminated intravascular coagulation and adult respiratory distress syndrome. Complications secondary to seizures include intracranial haemorrhage and retinal detachment. The main complications of treatment are related to respiratory depression and fluid overload.

INFECTION AND SEPSIS

SEPSIS

Following delivery or abortion, whether spontaneous or induced, the presence of a large denuded area of the uterus predisposes to the development of puerperal sepsis. Sepsis may also occur secondary to laceration of the genital tract and in the presence of retained products of conception. Poor hygiene on the part of the birth attendant and poor sterilization of instruments inserted into the genital tract during delivery or abortion are a particular risk. The presence of a genital tract infection is suspected by the presence of foul-smelling lochia or discharge. Less specific symptoms include abdominal pain, vomit-

ing, headache and loss of appetite. Examination reveals pyrexia and a tender bulky uterus. In more advanced stages of the disease tender masses in the adnexa or in the posterior fornix may be found, suggesting the presence of tubo-ovarian or Pouch of Douglas abscesses. Septicaemia may also occur.

Treatment in the early stages is by the use of broad-spectrum antibiotics followed by evacuation of the uterus after approximately 24 hours if retained products of conception are suspected. In more advanced cases, following the administration of intravenous antibiotics, laparotomy to drain the tubo-ovarian abscesses is necessary, and in extreme cases hysterectomy and pelvic clearance may be required. Laparotomy should not be delayed more than 12 hours after the administration of antibiotics as this is associated with a higher mortality. Abscesses in the Pouch of Douglas may be drained by colpotomy but a significant proportion of such patients will subsequently require laparotomy.

VIRAL HEPATITIS (See also Chapter 31)

Viral hepatitis [hepatitis A (HAV), B (HBV) and C (HCV), and E (HEV)] is a major cause of maternal mortality. Pregnant mothers in developing countries are both at greater risk of contracting hepatitis and have a higher mortality associated with the disease related to their poor nutritional status. Fulminating hepatitis usually occurs during the third trimester. The early symptoms include nausea, malaise, fever, headache and joint pains. Later symptoms include epigastric pain and jaundice, with hepatic coma being the cause of death. Premature labour and postpartum haemorrhage are the common obstetric complications.

Treatment is supportive with bed-rest being extremely important. A high carbohydrate diet is required, with intravenous glucose infusion in labour. Fresh blood should be transfused if a postpartum haemorrhage occurs. The newborn child should be given vitamin K.

MALARIA (See also Chapter 61)

Malaria in general, and particularly infection with *Plasmodium falciparum*, is a problem in pregnancy. Pregnant women living in endemic areas tend to lose their immunity to malaria, particularly during the second trimester, and are at increased risk of infection which tends to be more severe. Women in the second trimester of their first pregnancy are at greatest risk. The most serious effect of malaria in pregnancy is the development of haemolytic anaemia which, if severe enough, may lead to hypoxia of both the mother and fetus. Hepatorenal syndrome and/or cerebral malaria is often the cause of death.

The presentation of malaria in pregnancy, however, may be atypical and its presence should be suspected in any pregnant woman in endemic areas with fever or jaundice. Risks specific to pregnancy are abortion or premature labour and intrauterine growth retardation secondary to the presence of trophozoites in the placenta.

Treatment is dependent on the geographical area and the local pattern of drug resistance. Chloroquine is the treatment of choice in chloroquine-sensitive areas. Neonatal deafness has been reported but not from the doses used in the prophylaxis of malaria.[4] Pyrimethamine and proguanil are folic antagonists and therefore have a theoretical risk to the fetus; supplementary folate should be given. In endemic areas all pregnant women should have prophylaxis with chloroquine (in the absence of resistance) from 20 weeks gestation.

TETANUS (See also Chapter 48)

Maternal tetanus infection may result from abortion with improperly sterilized instruments or from delivery in unclean surroundings. Neonatal tetanus may result from traditions such as the application of cow dung to the umbilical cord. Treatment is described in Chapter 48, but mortality figures remain high.

Prevention therefore must be the main aim. Training of birth attendants, particularly in the use of a clean delivery technique, will reduce the risk of infection. Two doses of tetanus toxoid should be given to all pregnant women in the antenatal period.

ACQUIRED IMMUNE DEFICIENCY SYNDROME

(See also Chapter 12)

The number of maternal deaths due to acquired immune deficiency syndrome (AIDS) will undoubtedly increase in the future. WHO figures suggest that 1 in 40 women in sub-Saharan Africa are affected with the virus.[5] Although the evidence suggests that the infection has been more recently introduced to South-East Asia, the epidemic mirrors that of the early stages in Africa with the rapid spread of the virus among urban prostitutes.

Maternal death in women with AIDS in pregnancy is usually the result of *Pneumocystis carinii* pneumonia. Treatment is with trimethoprim–sulphamethoxazole and other supportive measures. Other maternal risks include anaemia, toxoplasmosis infection and tuberculosis. Fetal risks of AIDS include an increased incidence of spontaneous abor-

tion, preterm labour, intrauterine growth retardation and stillbirth.

The risk of perinatal spread of HIV human immunodeficiency virus (HIV) to the fetus has been estimated variously as between 13 and 60%.[6] Recent studies have shown that HIV may be spread by breast feeding,[7] and bottle feeding is advised for HIV-infected mothers in developed countries. In developing countries, however, this advice has to be balanced against the risk of gastroenteritis in the infant and the fact that bottle feeding may be seen as indicative of HIV infection in areas which traditionally breast feed. The advice to mothers in areas where the risk of gastrointestinal infections is high must be to breast feed their infants.[8]

Obviously, appropriate care to prevent spread of infection to health care workers is a priority.

HAEMORRHAGE

This is a major cause of maternal morbidity and mortality and of perinatal death.[9] Anaemia will be discussed later in this chapter and is an important contributory problem. Many women will be at substantial risk, even from a relatively small volume of blood loss before, during or after delivery.

Antepartum haemorrhage is defined as that occurring after 28 weeks gestation (although in the developed world 24 weeks is a more realistic figure). The two common causes are abruptio placentae and placenta praevia. The former may be associated with pre-eclampsia. If the retroplacental haemorrhage is large it will lead to immediate fetal death and place the mother at risk due to hypotension, shock and possible disseminated intravascular coagulation. If the haemorrhage is concealed (i.e. completely contained between the placenta and the myometrium with no visible vaginal loss) the condition may be recognized by the signs of a tense, tender uterus, with the fetal parts difficult or impossible to palpate and the fetal heart silent. Prompt action to perform an artificial rupture of the membranes and replace fluids with plasma expanders or substitutes (if blood is not available) will expedite delivery and reduce subsequent risks of disseminated intravascular coagulation. Intervention by caesarean section, whilst now common in developed countries, should be considered with extreme caution. The priority is the survival of the mother.

In patients with placenta praevia the maternal and fetal condition may remain satisfactory until haemorrhage is considerable. Recognition of the likely diagnosis, through the signs of a high presenting part, unstable or transverse lie, will ensure prompt intervention by caesarean section.

The third member of the 'haemorrhage triad' is postpartum haemorrhage. The risks of postpartum haemorrhage are higher in mothers who have had an antepartum haemorrhage and those of high parity, multiple pregnancy and a previous history of postpartum haemorrhage. Prevention through active management of the third stage of labour is appropriate. Intramuscular or intravenous ergometrine, 0.5 mg, or ergometrine maleate with oxytocin ('Syntometrine') or intravenous oxytocin, 10 units, should be given at the birth of the anterior shoulder. The placenta should be delivered by controlled cord traction once it is evident that the uterus has contracted and signs of separation of the placenta are evident.

When postpartum haemorrhage occurs, prompt resuscitation with intravenous fluids, plasma substitutes and blood, if available, will decrease the risk to the mother. It is important to remember that it may also be due to vaginal or cervical lacerations, especially following an instrumental delivery.

OBSTRUCTED LABOUR

The majority of labours and deliveries in developing countries are conducted by untrained persons and, whilst the outcome may be a vaginal delivery, if the labour is prolonged then the likelihood of fetal hypoxia is high and the consequence may frequently be stillbirth or neonatal death.

If there are serious complications associated with the prolonged labour, such as cephalopelvic disproportion, or malpresentation, such as a transverse lie brow, or shoulder presentation, then this will result in obstructed labour. In some cases vaginal delivery may still occur but at a cost not only of fetal death but also serious maternal morbidity such as vesicovaginal fistula due to pressure necrosis. In more extreme cases uterine rupture and subsequent maternal death will be the outcome.[10]

The aim of antenatal care in the high-risk approach (see below) will be to identify those mothers prior to labour who may be considered to be at real risk of obstructed labour and endeavour to ensure that they are referred to appropriate centres where facilities are available to provide safe delivery. However, it will not be possible to clearly identify a proportion of these mothers until labour is established. The use of the partograph in the conduct and management of all labours therefore becomes essential.[11] The fundamental purpose is to recognize when labour is not progressing normally,

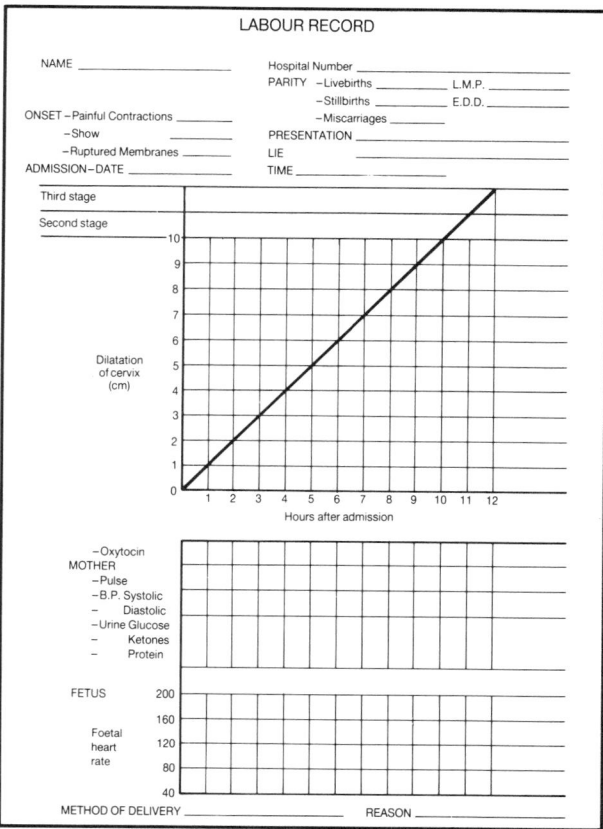

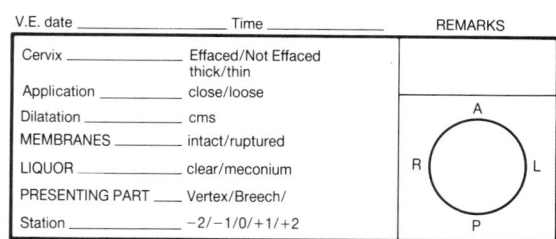

Figure 17.2 Simple partograph.

allowing for appropriate action to be taken by the attendant concerned.[12] Since a large number of deliveries are conducted by traditional birth attendants, attempts have been made to evolve simple systems which will enable them to recognize the signs which precede obstructed labour and thereby enable the mother to be referred to an appropriate centre where medical staff and facilities are available.[13,14]

A large number of mothers are cared for and delivered within the primary health care systems of different countries either at village subcentres or primary health centres. It is essential that those health care professionals involved (auxiliary nurses, midwives, doctors) should use the partograph.[15] This will enable them to identify when there is failure of progress and to take action to correct this by the judicious use of oxytocin to improve uterine

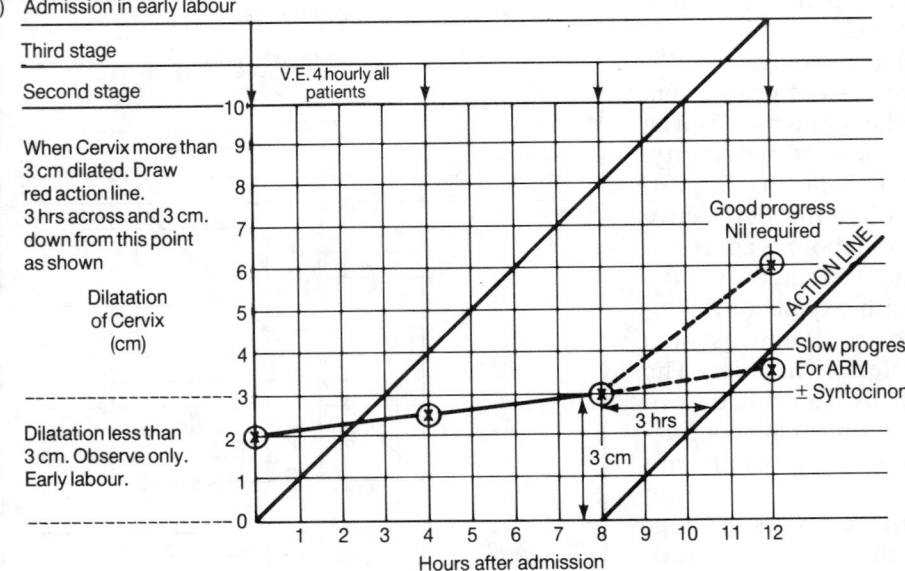

a) Admission in early labour

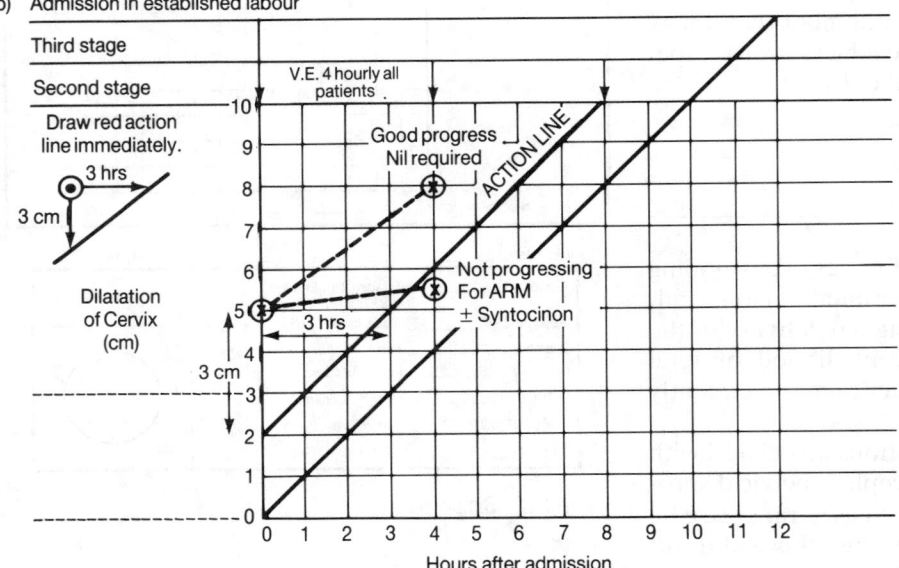

b) Admission in established labour

Figure 17.3 Use of partograph shown in Figure 17.2.

contractions, providing cephalopelvic disproportion and malpresentation have been excluded.[16–18] Further lack of progress requires intervention by caesarean section which can be performed early to ensure fetal survival and prevent maternal mortality and morbidity.

One of the simplest forms of partograph which can be used is shown in Figure 17.2. When labour is established and the cervix is more than 3 cm dilated an action line is drawn at 3 hours along and 3 cm down, as illustrated in Figure 17.3. Subsequent vaginal examination in 4 hours will indicate whether progress is normal or action such as performing artificial rupture of the membranes or commencing oxytocin infusion is necessary. Trained staff will subsequently be alerted as to the need for medical intervention.

ANAEMIA

The official definition of anaemia is a haemoglobin concentration <11 g/dl. However, in many communities it is not uncommon for women to have a haemoglobin level <7 g/dl. As a consequence, this is both a direct cause of maternal death and contributes to the problems of haemorrhage and infection.

Anaemia is the end-result of many factors in a woman's life. Poor nutrition in childhood may result in her starting her first pregnancy with low iron stores; repeated pregnancies too close together will deplete her iron, B_{12} and folate levels further; dietary traditions in pregnancy together with common infections such as hookworm and malaria compound the problem. Heavy periods prior to conceiving or blood loss during pregnancy may also be factors.

Investigation can be limited to measuring the haemoglobin with exclusion of an underlying cause. Field workers should be trained to recognize the clinical signs of anaemia by examination of the mucous membranes. Haemoglobin levels should be measured in pregnancy at booking, 30 weeks and 36 weeks gestation.

In order for treatment to be effective, women need to be registered for antenatal care at an early gestation and their haemoglobin level checked at follow-up visits. Along with nutritional advice, a daily dose of 30–60 mg of elemental iron for women with a normal iron store and 120–240 mg for those women with low iron stores, accompanied by 0.8 mg of folate, is usually sufficient. A rise in the level of haemoglobin should be seen within a month of commencing treatment. If there is no response it may be due to an underlying disorder such as sickle cell disease or haemoglobinopathy, failure to comply with treatment or failure to absorb the oral therapy.

The problem of absorption may be overcome by the use of parenteral iron such as iron dextran given by a series of intramuscular injections or by total dose intravenous infusion. The dose of parenteral iron required is calculated by the formula:

Amount required = 0.66 × patient's weight (kg) × haemoglobin deficiency

If given intramuscularly, a test dose of 25 mg is given on the first day and, if no adverse reaction is encountered, a daily dose of 250 mg thereafter until the total dose has been given. If given intravenously it is essential that the staff are trained to recognize and treat anaphylactic reactions. These usually occur within the first few millilitres of the infusion. Between 0.5 and 1.0 ml of adrenaline 1:1000 should be given subcutaneously should an anaphylactic reaction occur. It must be emphasized that parenteral iron does not increase the haemoglobin level any more quickly than oral therapy and should be reserved for those who cannot tolerate or absorb oral therapy.

For those patients who present in late pregnancy or in labour with a very low haemoglobin level, blood transfusion may be necessary, although in areas with endemic HIV infection this is an option that will be employed only as a last resort. Care must be taken to prevent cardiac failure when transfusing women with very low haemoglobin levels as the anaemia may lead to inefficient cardiac action and fluid overload. Exchange transfusion may be employed where facilities exist or the transfusion may be accompanied by intravenous diuretic therapy.

Death due to cardiac failure may occur with haemoglobin levels below 4 g/dl. Women whose haemoglobin level is between 4 and 7 g/dl are also at greater risk of dying from infection due to poor resistance or from haemorrhage. Blood losses as low as 500 ml, easily tolerated by a woman with a normal haemoglobin level, may be fatal. Other effects of anaemia in pregnancy include stillbirth, intrauterine growth retardation and premature labour.

Prevention of anaemia is of the utmost importance. Much can be done by health workers in promotion of a good diet, the composition of which will vary depending on the region but which should include green vegetables, staples, cereals and meat. Encouraging the use of iron cooking pots will also improve iron consumption. Promotion of family planning programmes to encourage family spacing is essential.

ABORTION AND ECTOPIC PREGNANCY

Spontaneous abortion is a common problem in developing countries as in developed countries. The major risk to the mother is the delay in reaching a centre with appropriate facilities, thereby allowing the complications of infection and haemorrhage to occur. Where abortion is complete these risks are minimal and further intervention is unnecessary. However, incomplete abortion frequently leads to continued vaginal bleeding and consequent anaemia. The retained products may also give rise to uterine sepsis. Prompt evacuation of the uterus will minimize these problems. Whilst in developed countries termination of unwanted pregnancies is readily available, this is not so in developing countries. Consequently, a high proportion of women presenting with incomplete abortion have associated sepsis due to the abortion originally being performed by unskilled or untrained personnel. In such cases treatment of the infection or septicaemia is the wiser course of action before evacuation of the uterus. An additional complication may be that of postabortal tetanus which has a very poor prognosis.

With more effective family planning programmes and education it may be hoped that unwanted pregnancies can be kept to a minimum and that centres for the medical termination of pregnancy, if more widely available, can reduce the maternal risks. However, experience in developed countries is that the incidence of unwanted pregnancies remains high, placing a burden on these services and causing problems of morbidity among women.

Ectopic pregnancy can be a major life-threatening condition. The incidence has been reported as varying between 1 per 43 and 1 per 175 births and is increasing. The main risk factors include age, previous pelvic inflammatory disease, use of an intrauterine contraceptive device, pelvic surgery, and induced abortion. Rupture of the ectopic pregnancy leads to the classical signs of acute lower abdominal pain and hypotension with signs of haemoperitoneum. Immediate intervention is by laparotomy with partial salpingectomy to control the bleeding. In many areas where there are no blood transfusion facilities, it is appropriate to carry out intraoperative autotransfusion, with aspiration of blood from the peritoneal cavity into a sterile bottle containing 50 ml of citrate phosphate dextrose. The collected blood should then be filtered and transfused back into the patient. This can be done before dealing with the ectopic pregnancy and will reduce the risk(s) to the patient.[19]

In some cases the condition is chronic with slow leakage of blood into the peritoneal cavity, causing intermittent lower abdominal pain and pelvic tenderness or a pelvic mass. Anaemia will develop. Laparoscopy, if available, will allow a positive diagnosis and appropriate intervention.

ORGANIZATION AND IMPLEMENTATION OF ANTENATAL CARE

Although the knowledge and skills to deal with the obstetric problems outlined above are essential for any member of the health team caring for pregnant women, it is equally important for the health care scheme to provide comprehensive antenatal care. It is a sad fact that most of the 500 000 maternal deaths occurring each year, principally in developing countries, could have been prevented with adequate antenatal care.

The aim of comprehensive antenatal care for large populations, both in rural areas and in urban situations, is to identify pregnant women as early as possible and arrange appropriate referral for those at high risk. It is essential in such a programme to have good communication and to make maximum use of each member of the health care team.[20] The involvement of the local community is also necessary.

HIGH-RISK APPROACH STRATEGY

While no screening programme in obstetrics can predict or prevent every obstetric emergency, problems such as obstructed labour, particularly in parous women, can be identified by screening programmes and the woman referred to the appropriate primary, secondary or tertiary level of care. Suitable screening programmes must be developed for use by workers at all levels.[21] Those used by traditional birth attendants may be no more than 'too early, too close, too many, too late', whereas medical, nursing and midwifery staff can be trained to use the guidelines shown in Tables 17.2 and 17.3.

A major factor in the success of a high-risk approach is the early identification of all pregnant

Table 17.2 Risk factors at booking.

Older (>yr 30) or young (<yr 16) primigravida
Grand multipara (>five deliveries)
History of vaginal bleeding
History of infertility
Family history of:
   diabetes
   hypertension
   multiple pregnancy
   congenital abnormalities
Past obstetric history of:
   small/large for dates
   fetal abnormality
   three or more spontaneous miscarriages
   pre-eclampsia or eclampsia
   stillbirth or neonatal death
   preterm labour
   caesarean section
   problems in third stage
Short stature (actual height varies with population)

Table 17.3 Risk factors arising during pregnancy.

Haemoglobin <8.5 g/dl
Poor weight gain
Proteinuria
Glycosuria
Cardiac disease
Diabetes mellitus
Blood pressure >140/90
Rhesus negative
Polyhydramnios
Oligohydramnios
Vaginal bleeding
Reduced fetal movements
Malpresentation
Multiple pregnancy
Abnormal fundal height

women. Village health workers are extremely important in ensuring and arranging for antenatal registration, as are health workers who have no direct connection with maternal health, such as those involved in leprosy programmes. In addition to allowing appropriate screening and care, early identification of pregnant women is essential for collecting statistics about trends in maternal mortality.

COMMUNICATION

For a high-risk strategy to work, it is essential that there is good communication at all levels so that women so identified may be referred to the appropriate level of care. Ideally, the person identifying the problem should accompany the woman to the referral centre, which has the additional advantage that the health care workers can receive training. In practice this is rarely possible due to the volume of work and distances to be travelled. An alternative strategy is that personnel from the referral centre, usually a midwife or doctor, should regularly visit each centre for which they are responsible at intervals of not less than 2 months. At this visit, all women who have been referred can be discussed, the progress of their pregnancy reviewed and plans made for further management. Also at this time the opportunity can be taken to discuss any maternal deaths which may have occurred since the last visit and avoidable factors and improvements in management considered. This should be done in a constructive and helpful way and not seen to be merely a means of apportioning blame. Such a strategy requires considerable input from more senior levels of staff. Adequate training and supervision are essential if a comprehensive antenatal care scheme is to be successful and permit each member of the health care team to work to his or her maximum potential.

For effective communication, information should be passed both ways between referral and referring centres. The use of simple patient-held records is one solution to the problem. In labour the partograph (see above) provides all the essential information.

USE OF PERSONNEL

Each member of the health care team must be enabled to work to his or her maximum potential. Village health workers and traditional birth attendants can and should be trained to carry out routine antenatal care.[22] Midwives can and should be trained to perform simple forceps and ventouse deliveries and manual removal of placenta. Doctors at first referral level can and should have the facilities to perform caesarean section and administer anaesthetics and blood transfusions. Obstetricians at district hospital level and above should provide a consultant role, evaluating high-risk women, managing the difficult obstetric complications and training and supervising other members of staff. Using doctors to perform normal vaginal deliveries is a waste of midwifery skills and prevents doctors from improving the services for which they are responsible.

INVOLVEMENT OF THE COMMUNITY

The community can be involved at every level of maternity care. Community education programmes about warning signs in pregnancy, nutrition and family spacing methods will help the message to be received by the individual pregnant woman, and often, more importantly, her husband or mother-in-law. The local community can also help by the provision of a clinic room and in taking responsibility for the village health care worker. The involvement of the community is also essential for providing transport, both for referral visits and in an emergency.

PROBLEMS WITH THE HIGH-RISK APPROACH

There are three main problems with the high-risk approach. The first is providing the appropriate training of all levels of staff, as previously mentioned. The second problem is acceptance of the advice by the women. Many women do not wish to deliver outside their community or in a hospital. Some problems of acceptance are due to local tradition and require considerable efforts on behalf of the health care team to overcome them. In addition, nursing and medical personnel in the referral centre must provide a welcoming and caring atmosphere.

The greatest difficulty to be overcome, however, is the transport of pregnant women. Many live a considerable distance from roads and may take days to reach the referral centre. It is often difficult to persuade owners to lend or hire any form of transport. This problem has been overcome in some communities by the provision of a maternity home or village which will allow pregnant women to await the onset of labour close to the level of required care. In other communities, families pay into a fund which can then be used to hire transport for women as required. There is no doubt that a lack of transport is the greatest problem to be overcome in providing comprehensive maternity care in any rural area in the developing countries.

GYNAECOLOGY

FAMILY PLANNING

The objective of maternity services is to ensure a healthy outcome for the mother and baby. In order to achieve this objective, maternity care should extend beyond the period of pregnancy and childbirth. In the first instance the mother-to-be should be helped to plan her pregnancy at the optimum time to reduce risks to her health. After delivery a subsequent pregnancy should be postponed until she has regained her health and the need for breast feeding is over. Family planning services should, therefore, be an integral part of any maternity service.

The proper planning of pregnancy will help reduce the hazards of childbirth. 'Too early, too close, too many and too late' presents considerable risks to mother and child. Such an unfavourable pattern is all too common in developing countries. It has been estimated that if women were able to plan their pregnancies for an optimal time, about 200 000 maternal deaths (out of the 500 000 annual deaths— see above) and about 560 000 infant deaths (out of more than 12 million) could be averted.

Although obstetric and contraceptive services may be provided separately, there are advantages if they are integrated. Information and education about family planning can be provided as part of postpartum care. Pregnancy may be the first point of contact with the health services.

Breast feeding is critical for child survival by providing high quality, no cost, clean nutrients. It is also a natural method of child spacing as return of fertility is delayed through lactational amenorrhoea.[23] The duration of this is extremely variable and can range from 4 to 24 months. It should be remembered that a lactating woman may become pregnant in her first ovulatory cycle before her periods recommence. It is important therefore for women to consider other contraceptive measures after the first 6 months, which do not interfere with the continuation of breast feeding.

There is a wide range of contraceptive methods available which allows for a choice to suit the different needs and circumstances of the users. Barrier methods such as condoms with spermicides can be used with safety after delivery and may be adequate to supplement the contraceptive effect of lactational amenorrhoea. The intrauterine contraceptive device (IUCD) is a convenient method since it does not interfere with lactation and is a 'once only' insertion with no further action required by the user.

The ideal time for insertion is 6 weeks after delivery when the uterus has involuted. Under these circumstances the expulsion rate is 5–20 per 100 woman years. It may not be practicable to delay insertion, however, particularly if the woman lives some distance from family planning services or if there is concern that she may not reattend. In these circumstances, an IUCD can be inserted within a few days of delivery, although the expulsion rate may be higher. Careful insertion into the fundus of the uterus with a sponge forceps will reduce the risk of expulsion in this situation.[24] The original inert devices such as the Lippes' loop are now being replaced by copper-bearing devices such as the 'copper T', the addition of copper increasing the effectiveness and the smaller size reducing the blood loss at menstruation and the risk of expulsion. If complications of bleeding or pain persist, then the IUCD should be removed. Despite the IUCD, pregnancy may occur, with an increased incidence of ectopic implantation.

With regard to oral contraceptives, the 'minipill', containing only a progestogen, which does not affect lactation, can be safely used, although good compliance is required. The oestrogen content in the combined oral contraceptive pill does affect lactation and should not therefore be used in the first 6 months after delivery.

If injectables such as medroxyprogesterone acetate ('Depo-Provera') or norethisterone acetate ('Noristerat') are approved for use in a particular country, they can be safely used in breast-feeding women as they do not affect lactation.

Surgical methods of contraception have an important place in postpartum decisions about contraception. Providing the couple are certain that their family is complete, postpartum tubal occlusion is a relatively straightforward procedure. This can be performed under a local or general anaesthetic. Vasectomy may be an acceptable alternative.

PELVIC INFLAMMATORY DISEASE AND SEXUALLY TRANSMITTED DISEASES

The increasing incidence of pelvic inflammatory disease, and sexually transmitted disease(s) is a major worldwide health problem for women but particularly in developing countries. While the exact figures are not known, one recent survey reported that 24% of the women in an area of rural India had symptoms suggestive of pelvic inflammatory disease.[25]

Within communities, differences in social, sexual and contraceptive behaviour influence the prevalence of pelvic inflammatory disease and sexually transmitted diseases. The factors of greatest influence are the age of onset of sexual activity, the number of partners and the frequency of intercourse. The use of barrier methods of contraception decreases the incidence of infection.

PELVIC INFLAMMATORY DISEASE

The main organisms involved in pelvic inflammatory disease are *Neisseria gonorrhoeae* and *Chlamydia trachomatis*. There is frequently a secondary infection with Gram-negative or anaerobic bacteria.

The symptoms of pelvic inflammatory disease are lower abdominal pain, which is usually low suprapubic and bilateral, accompanied by purulent, often foul-smelling, vaginal discharge, dyspareunia and fever. In addition the woman may experience irregular vaginal bleeding, urinary symptoms of frequency or dysuria, and nausea, vomiting and diarrhoea. Abdominal examination reveals tenderness, particularly suprapubically and in both iliac fossae; bimanual pelvic examination reveals tenderness of the uterus and adnexa. Movement of the cervix produces extreme pain on the adnexal side under tension (cervical excitation tenderness). Many cases, however, are silent and only diagnosed when the woman presents with some of the sequelae of pelvic infection such as ectopic pregnancy or tubal infertility. Although accurate figures are not available the incidence of both these conditions is rising, suggesting an increase in the number of silent infections. There is some evidence that pelvic inflammatory disease associated with chlamydia, as opposed to gonorrhoea, presents in a less acute fashion and so may be more difficult to diagnose.

If facilities exist, investigations should be carried out before antibiotic therapy is started. Bacteriological swabs should be taken from the upper vagina, cervix and urethra. Endocervical swabs containing endothelial cells are essential for the isolation of *C. trachomatis*. Additional baseline investigations include white cell count and ESR, which may be performed serially to assess the response to therapy.

Antibiotics should be started after taking the bacteriology swabs—without waiting for the results. Treatment in areas where *C. trachomatis* is the most common organism should be with a 2 week course of tetracycline or erythromycin, combined with a broad-spectrum antibiotic effective such as gentamicin, against Gram-negative organisms, and metronidazole to treat any anaerobic infection. If it is more likely that gonorrhoea is the basic infection, ampicillin should be used unless there is a high chance that ampicillin resistance has developed.

Response to treatment, as judged by the patient's well-being, resolution of pyrexia and a reduction in white cell count and ESR, should be seen in 24–48 hours. If there is no improvement laparotomy should be considered. Surgical intervention is required earlier when a pelvic mass is felt, particularly if there is no reduction in size following antibiotic therapy. Surgical intervention includes drainage of the abscess and removal of all infected and necrotic tissue.

SEXUALLY TRANSMITTED DISEASES

The treatment of the more common sexually transmitted diseases will be outlined below. It must be remembered, however, that treatment of the woman's partner and contact tracing is mandatory for complete eradication of all these infections.

Syphilis (See also Chapters 12 and 13)

The incidence of syphilis is increasing in areas where HIV infection is endemic. Initial lesions or chancres are seen most commonly on the labia, fourchette and cervix and appear as painless papules which progress to red, round, firm ulcers with a granulating base. They are accompanied by regional lymphadenopathy. Confirmation of the diagnosis is by darkfield microscopy of a wet swab preparation from the chancre. Chancres heal within around 3 to 8 weeks and, if untreated, are followed by the disseminated symptoms of secondary syphilis which appear within 4 to 10 weeks of the primary lesion. They include the classical dermatological lesions—genital condylomata lata and systemic lesions—fever, malaise, anorexia and headache. CNS involvement may also be present. If untreated at this stage the disease will progress through a latent phase, reappearing in 20–30% of patients in the tertiary form—characterized by granulomatous gummas of the skin, bone or viscera, by cardiovascular lesions—particularly involving the aorta, and by neurosyphilis.

Treatment is with benzylpenicillin, 2.4 million units intramuscularly, as a single dose for early lesions and in the treatment of partners. Treatment is given weekly over 3 weeks for those with longstanding infection.

Gonorrhoea (See also Chapter 13)

Gonorrhoea is probably the most common sexually transmitted disease worldwide. The causative organism is *N. gonorrhoeae*, a Gram-negative intracellular diplococcus, which may be identified from cervical or urethral secretions.

The infection is usually localized to the site of primary infection, although pelvic inflammatory disease may occur (see above). Symptoms are usually purulent vaginal discharge, urinary frequency and dysuria. Infection of Skene's glands or the Bartholin's gland duct opening may also be present. Treatment is with penicillin or ampicillin, except in areas where resistance is common; here, the cephalosporins should be used.

Chlamydia (See also Chapter 13)

Infections with *C. trachomatis* are becoming increasingly common in the West and are the most common sexually transmitted disease in the USA. The problems associated with laboratory detection and the relative frequency of asymptomatic infections mean that very few studies have been performed in developing countries to ascertain the prevalence.

Chlamydia are small intracellular Gram-negative bacteria. Diagnosis is made by the detection of inclusion bodies within the cytoplasm of cells obtained from swabs from the urethra or endocervix. The success of culture depends largely on the adequacy of sampling and the laboratory technique.

Chlamydia infections cause mucopurulent cervicitis which, if untreated, may progress to cause an ascending genital tract infection with endometritis and salpingitis. These conditions may result in infertility or ectopic pregnancy from damaged fallopian tubes. If present at the time of delivery, a *C. trachomatis* infection of the fetus may result in severe conjunctivitis, which presents about a week after birth, or pneumonia, which may not present until several months later. Chlamydial infection in the genital tract may also cause premature labour.

Treatment is with tetracycline, 500 mg four times daily, or erythromycin, 500 mg four times daily. Both regimens should be continued for a minimum of 7 to 14 days.

REFERENCES

1 Royston E & Armstrong S. The dimensions of the problem. In Royston E & Armstrong S (eds) *Preventing Maternal Deaths*. Geneva: WHO, 1989: 30–44.

2 Walker G J, McCaw-Binns A, Ashley D E et al. Identifying maternal deaths in developing countries: experience in Jamaica. *Int J Epidemiol* 1990; 19:599–605.

3 Sai F T & Measham D M. Safe Motherhood Initiative: getting our priorities straight. *Lancet* 1992; 339:478–480.

4 Bruce-Chwatt L J. Malaria and pregnancy. *BMJ* 1983; 286:1457–1458.

5 Johnson A M. Epidemiology of HIV infection. *Baillière's Clin Obstet Gynaecol* 1992; 6:13–31.

6 Mok J Y Q. Vertical transmission. *Baillière's Clin Obstet Gynaecol* 1992; 6:85–100.

7 Van de Perre P, Simonson A, Msellati P et al. Postnatal transmission of human immuno-deficiency virus type 1 from mother to infant. *N Engl J Med* 1991; 325:593–598.

8 Cutting W A M. Breast feeding and HIV infection. *BMJ* 1992; 305:788–789.

9 Lennox C E. Assessment of obstetric high risk factors in a developing country. *Trop Doct* 1984; 14:125–129.

10 Lawson J B. Sequelae of obstructed labour. In Lawson J B & Stewart D B (eds) *Obstetrics and Gynaecology in the Tropics and Developing Countries*. London: Edward Arnold, 1974: chap. 12.

11 World Health Organization. *The Partograph: A Managerial Tool for the Prevention of Prolonged Labour*. Section I: the principle and the strategy. WHO/MCH/88.3. Section II: a user's manual. WHO/MCH/88.4. Section III: facilitator's guide. WHO/MCH/89.1. Section IV: guidelines for operations research on the application of the partograph. WHO/MCH/89.2. Geneva: WHO, 1988.

12 Dujardin B, De Schampheleire I, Sene H & Ndiaye F. Value of the alert and action lines on the partogram. *Lancet* 1992; 339:1336–1338.

13 Thouw J. Delegation of obstetric care in Indonesia. *Int J Gynaecol Obstet* 1992; 38(supplement): S45–S47.

14 Daly C & Pollard A J. Traditional birth attendants in the Gambia. *Midwives Chron* 1990; 103:104–105.

15 Urrio T F. Maternal deaths at Songea Regional Hospital, southern Tanzania. *East Afr Med J* 1991; 68:81–87.

16 O'Driscoll K & Meagher D. *Active Management of Labour*, 2nd edn. London: Baillière Tindall, 1986.

17 Mola G & Rageau O. Augmentation of labour by a standard protocol in Papua New Guinea. *Asia Oceania J Obstet Gynaecol* 1990; 16:219–224.

18 Bood T. Experience with active labour management

protocol and reduction of caesarean section rate in Nicaragua. *Trop Doct* 1990; 20:115–118.

19 Laskey J & Wood P B. Ectopic pregnancies and intraoperative autotransfusion. *Trop Doct* 1991; 21:116–118.

20 Fauveau V, Steward K, Khan S A & Chakraborty J. Effect on mortality of community-based maternity-care programme in rural Bangladesh. *Lancet* 1991; 388:1183–1186.

21 Chabot H T & Rutten A M. Use of antenatal cards for literate health personnel and illiterate traditional birth attendants: an overview. *Trop Doct* 1990; 20: 21–24.

22 Begum J A, Kabir I A & Mollah A Y. The impact of traditional birth attendants in improving MCH care in rural Bangladesh. *Asia Pac J Public Health* 1990; 4: 142–144.

23 Perez A, Labbok M H & Queenan J T. Clinical study of the lactational amenorrhoea for family planning. *Lancet* 1992; 339:968–970.

24 Filshie M & Guillebaud J. *Contraception, Science and Practice*. London: Butterworth, 1989.

25 Bang R A, Bang T A, Baitule M, Choudhary Y, Sarmakaddam S & Tale O. High prevalence of gynaecological diseases in rural Indian women. *Lancet* 1989; i:85–88.

SECTION 4
ENVIRONMENTAL/GENETIC DISORDERS

Classical 'tropical medicine' has been centred on a variety of 'exotic' infections—dominated by those of parasitic origin. In recent years a far greater emphasis has, rightly, been placed on disease entities that do not have an infective basis. Although these can be roughly divided into those with a predominantly environmental *or* genetic background, the majority (as with most disease entities in a non-tropical environment) fall somewhere within a grey area between these two poles; in fact in many of them both genetic and environmental factors operate in conjunction. This section therefore focuses on a miscellaneous group of disorders, most of which were not given due recognition in previous editions of this text.

Travellers' diseases, heat illness and altitude sickness all have obvious associations with environmental phenomena. Nutrition-associated diseases—dominated by those precipitated by a deficiency of major and/or specific dietary ingredients, and 'toxicity' of animal and vegetable origin—are also clearly related to local environmental factors.

Areas of 'medicine in the tropics' that have hitherto been grossly underplayed in *Manson's Tropical Diseases* are malignant disease and three major diseases commonly associated with an affluent environment: diabetes mellitus, hypertension, and lipid disorders and ischaemic cardiac disease. These already account for large numbers of cases in many of the more urbanized tropical areas. In each of them any attempt at dissecting genetic from environmental predisposing factors poses problems which are often seemingly insuperable.

The two other diseases covered in this section are podoconiosis and recurrent familial polyserositis (familial Mediterranean fever). The former has a relatively well delineated geographical distribution and is confined to those areas where silica abounds and particles enter the lymphatics of the lower limbs via bare feet; the resultant clinical abnormality is barely distinguishable from lymphatic filariasis (elephantiasis). The latter is an underrecognized disease which usually (but not always) affects members of certain clearly defined ethnic groups; here, genetic factors are clearly involved but they are not yet very well delineated.

Doubtless other disease entities falling into the non-infective category will emerge and attain full and detailed coverage in subsequent editions of this text. For the present, the major purpose of this section is to highlight several of the more important entities which have hitherto received far less attention than seems justified in the light of present knowledge.

CHAPTER 18

TRAVEL MEDICINE

R. Steffen and H. O. Lobel

Travel, especially to tropical and subtropical countries, is associated with an increased risk of morbidity and mortality. The purpose of travel medicine is to reduce these risks by increasing travellers awareness of them and by promoting the use of preventive measures. The choice of preventive measures is guided by balancing the risk of illness or death against the risks, costs and benefits of prevention. Pretravel advice is based on modifying behaviour; prevention by immunization, chemoprophylaxis and personal protective measures; and medication for self-treatment. Travel medicine is interdisciplinary and includes many specialities other than tropical medicine or infectious diseases, such as accident prevention, psychiatry, high altitude pathophysiology (Chapter 20) and behavioural sciences.

Travel medicine has become increasingly import-

ant for the 30–35 million residents of industrialized nations who travel annually to developing countries.[1] Between 80 and 95% of these are short-term travellers. Some who work abroad may either make repeated short visits (airline crews or business persons) or reside there for prolonged periods (missionaries, volunteer workers). Health risks differ between these groups and, depending on the environment and their behaviour, may vary within a single group.

In this chapter the data on risks of morbidity and mortality associated with travel will be reviewed and related to available preventive and self-therapy measures (Figure 18.1). Only frequent health risks for which epidemiological data are available will be considered. Various other exotic infections rarely occur in travellers.

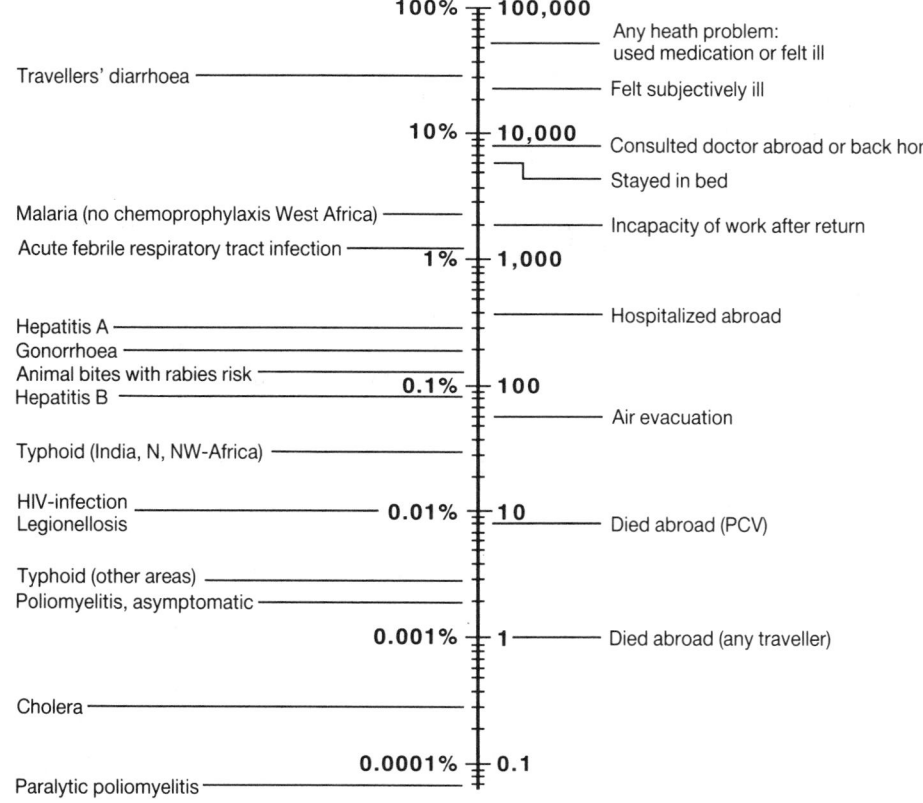

Figure 18.1 Morbidity and mortality in travellers to developing countries: incidence rates per month of stay abroad.

DEATHS

Accidents are a leading cause of death for intercontinental travellers. Of Swiss travellers who died overseas, 44% were killed by accidents, 15% by cardiovascular diseases, 9% by other illnesses and 3% by infections; for 29% the cause of death remained unknown.[2] Among US travellers, cardiovascular diseases were the number one cause of death (49%), followed by intentional and unintentional injuries.[3] Of almost 8000 United Nations military and civilian personnel stationed for 12 months in Namibia, 16 died; 14 of these deaths were due to motor vehicle crashes.[4] Deaths abroad due to injuries are two to threefold higher in 15–44-year-old travellers than in the same age group in industrialized countries.[2] Fatal accidents are mostly due to motor vehicle injuries, with motorcycles and a lack of seat belts in rental cars as important risk factors. Drowning is also an important cause of death and accounted for 16% of all deaths due to injuries among US travellers.[3] It is often due to swimming while under the influence of alcohol or by being swept away by sea currents. Assaults or terrorism are infrequent causes of death. Trauma was also the main reason for aeromedical evacuation from Africa, Asia and Latin America, especially following traffic accidents.[5]

The following strategies have been proposed to prevent accidents (adapted from Hargarten et al.):[2]

1. Host/traveller factors
   (a) Avoid alcohol and driving, alcohol and food before swimming.
   (b) Use available safety equipment (seat belts, helmets, etc.).
2. Vehicle factors
   (a) Select safe cars, check availability of seat belts, good tyres and brakes.
   (b) Rent larger vehicles when possible.
   (c) Avoid using motorcycles and riding on the back of open trucks.
   (d) Avoid small, non-scheduled aircraft.
3. Environmental factors
   (a) Avoid travel at night.
   (b) Employ a local driver who knows traffic and pedestrian patterns.
   (c) Carefully select swimming areas.
   (d) Know the local emergency medical system.

ILLNESS

Surveys among Swiss travellers returning from intercontinental travels found that up to 75% of short-term travellers experience some health impairment.[6] Few of these self-reported health problems are severe: 21–43% feel sick, but only 5% require medical attention, and less than 1% warrant hospitalization, usually for only a few days. The most common health impairment is due to travellers' diarrhoea, while malaria and human immunodeficiency virus (HIV) are among the most serious infectious hazards to which travellers may be exposed.

TRAVELLERS' DIARRHOEA (See also Chapter 3)

EPIDEMIOLOGY

Travellers' diarrhoea is the most frequent illness of travellers to developing countries (Figure 18.1). The incidence rates per 2 week stay vary between destinations (Figure 18.2). Most of these data were obtained in the late 1970s,[7] but data for destinations in the southern and eastern Mediterranean were obtained again in 1989[8] and the rates had decreased by less than 1% per year. Consistent incidence rates have also been observed among travellers to Mexico (H. L. DuPont, personal communication). There are three levels of risk: (i) travellers from industrialized countries and staying for 2 weeks in Canada or the USA, northern and central Europe, Australia and New Zealand have a low incidence rate, up to 8%; (ii) intermediate incidence rates (8–20%) are experienced by travellers to most destinations in the Caribbean, in southern Europe, Israel, Japan and South Africa; (iii) the incidence rates of travellers' diarrhoea among those travelling to developing countries varies between 20 and 50% during the first 2 weeks of stay.

The incidence rate is especially high among infants and young adults. Travellers' diarrhoea often has a particularly severe and long-lasting course in small children.[9] The risk increases when food is consumed from street vendors, native families or other places with low sanitary conditions.[10–12]

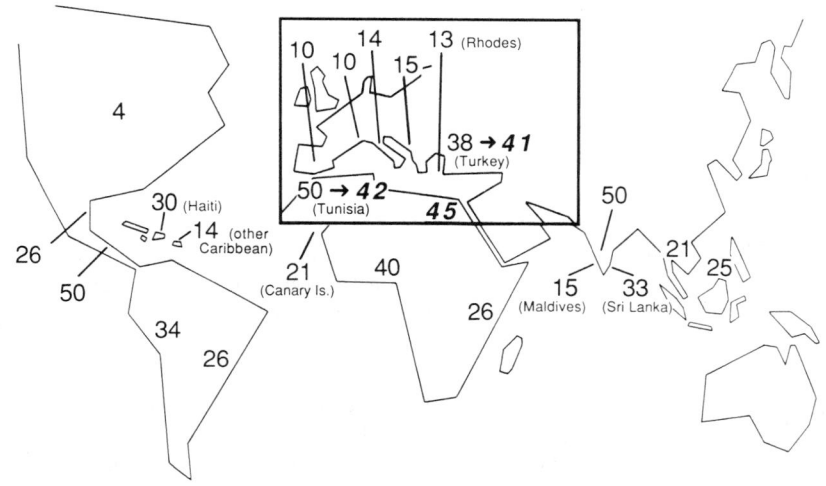

Figure 18.2 Incidence of travellers' diarrhoea per 14 days of stay in 20 645 European tourists at various destinations. **(7)**, data from 1975–1981; **(8)**, data from 1989.

Table 18.1 Aetiology of travellers' diarrhoea: range of isolation rates (%) in various studies.[14–16]

	Asia	Central America	North-East Africa	West Africa
ETEC*	20–34	28–72	31–75	42
Salmonella spp.	11–15	0–16	0	4
Shigella spp.	4–7	0–30	0–15	7
Campylobacter jejuni	2–11	Few	Few	1
Aeromonas hydrophila	1–57	NA	NA	0
Vibrio parahaemolyticus	1–16	Few	Few	NA
Giardia lamblia	<5	0–9	NA	0
Entamoeba histolytica	<5	0–9	NA	2
Rotavirus	NA	?–36	0	NA
Various	0–10	0–5	0–8	14
Multiple	9–22	NA	NA	10
No pathogen	33–53	15–30	15–55	40
Number of studies	8	15	3	1

*Enterotoxigenic *Escherichia coli*.
NA, no data available.

Persons with an impaired gastric acid barrier may be at higher risk of gastroenterological infection.[13]

Travellers' diarrhoea is usually caused by faecal contamination of food and beverages. Bacterial agents predominate, especially enterotoxigenic *Escherichia coli* (ETEC) which are responsible for about 40% of cases[14–16] (Table 18.1). *Salmonella* spp., *Shigella* spp., *Campylobacter jejuni* and other species of bacterial pathogens, as well as *Giardia lamblia* and *Entamoeba histolytica,* each cause fewer than 5% of the cases. Despite extensive microbiological assessment 20–40% of all cases remain of undetermined aetiology. Bacterial agents probably cause most of these cases because the disease can be diminished by use of antimicrobial agents.[17]

The symptoms of travellers' diarrhoea in tourists frequently start on the third day of the stay abroad, with a second episode beginning about a week after arrival in 20% of cases. Untreated, the mean duration is 4 days (median 2 days), and the symptoms may persist for over a month in 1%.[7] It is usually a mild disease with fewer than six bowel movements per 24 hours, but the accompanying symptoms may be disturbing (Figure 18.3). Twenty-two per cent of patients show signs of mucosal invasive disease with fever and/or blood in the stool(s).

PREVENTION

There are various options for preventing travellers' diarrhoea. Dietary restrictions using the rule of 'boil

18%
23%
1-2
6+
3-5
59%
(a)
Cramps
66%
Nausea
46%
Fever
18%
Blood
15%
Vomiting
12%
Dysentery
(Blood and/ or fever)
22%
0 10 20 30 40 50 60 70
Per cent
(b)

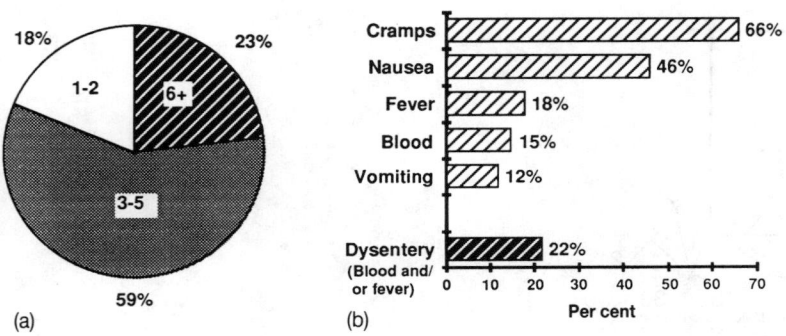

Figure 18.3 Severity and symptoms of travellers' diarrhoea: (a) bowel movements per 24 hours; (b) concomitant symptoms.

it, cook it, peel it or forget it' will reduce the incidence. These precautions are rarely adhered to: during the first 3 days of a stay in Kenya or Sri Lanka, 98% of Swiss tourists ate salads, puddings and sandwiches with mixed fillings, used ice cubes in their drinks or even chose raw oysters or steak tartare.[18] Many drugs have been proposed for the prevention of travellers' diarrhoea but only antimicrobial agents are at least 80% effective.[17] They are not indicated for every traveller because of possible adverse reactions but they may be considered under special circumstances (Figure 18.4). Drugs of choice include quinolones and co-trimoxazole, although resistance against the latter agent is increasing in the Far East. Quinolones have been associated with neuropsychiatric adverse events[19] and potential interactions with drugs such as chloroquine and mefloquine must be considered.

Effective polyvalent immunization against traveller's diarrhoea is not yet available.[20] Currently available vaccines against typhoid or cholera do not prevent it. Parents with infants who intend to travel to developing countries for pleasure are advised to postpone their travel.

SELF-THERAPY

Because of the inadequate efficacy of prophylaxis against travellers' diarrhoea, self-therapy abroad is

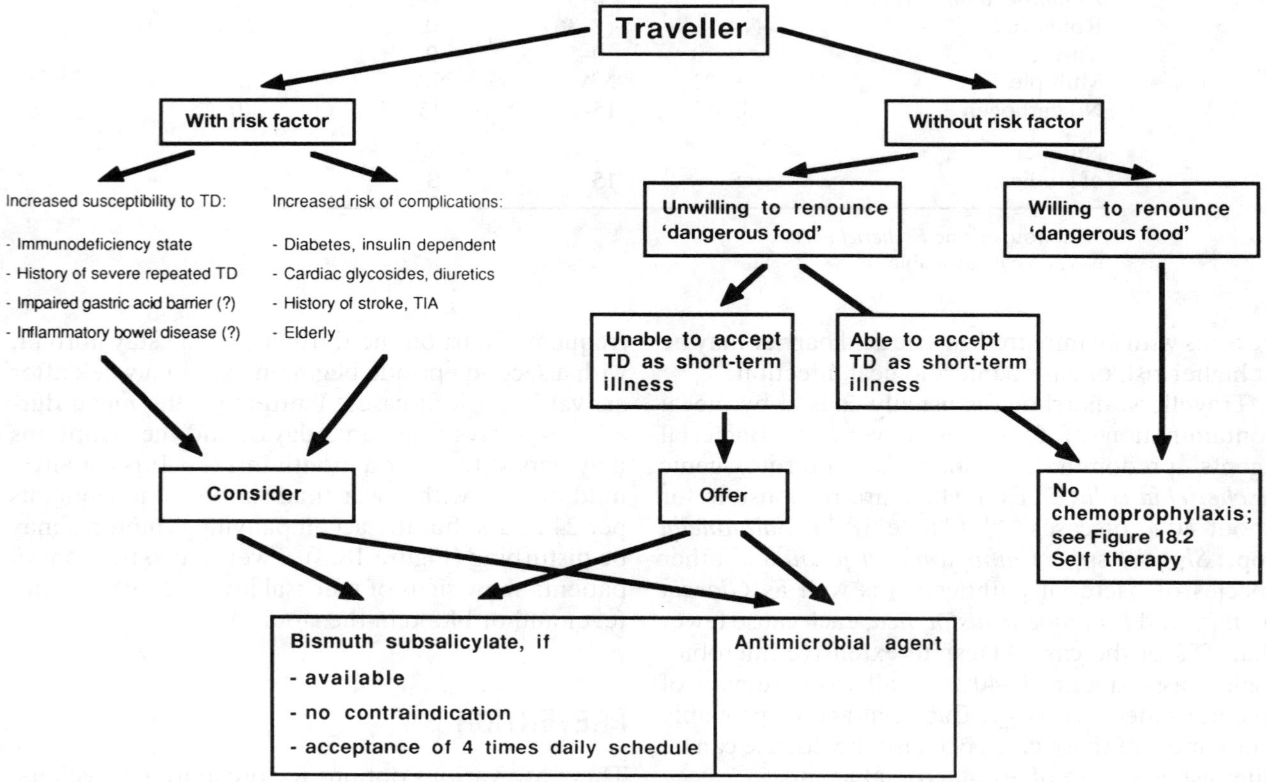

Traveller
With risk factor
Without risk factor
Increased susceptibility to TD:
- Immunodeficiency state
- History of severe repeated TD
- Impaired gastric acid barrier (?)
- Inflammatory bowel disease (?)
Increased risk of complications:
- Diabetes, insulin dependent
- Cardiac glycosides, diuretics
- History of stroke, TIA
- Elderly
Unwilling to renounce 'dangerous food'
Willing to renounce 'dangerous food'
Unable to accept TD as short-term illness
Able to accept TD as short-term illness
Consider
Offer
No chemoprophylaxis; see Figure 18.2 Self therapy
Bismuth subsalicylate, if
- available
- no contraindication
- acceptance of 4 times daily schedule
Antimicrobial agent

Figure 18.4 Chemoprophylaxis of travellers' diarrhoea (TD), duration limited to 3 weeks. TIA, transient ischaemic attack.

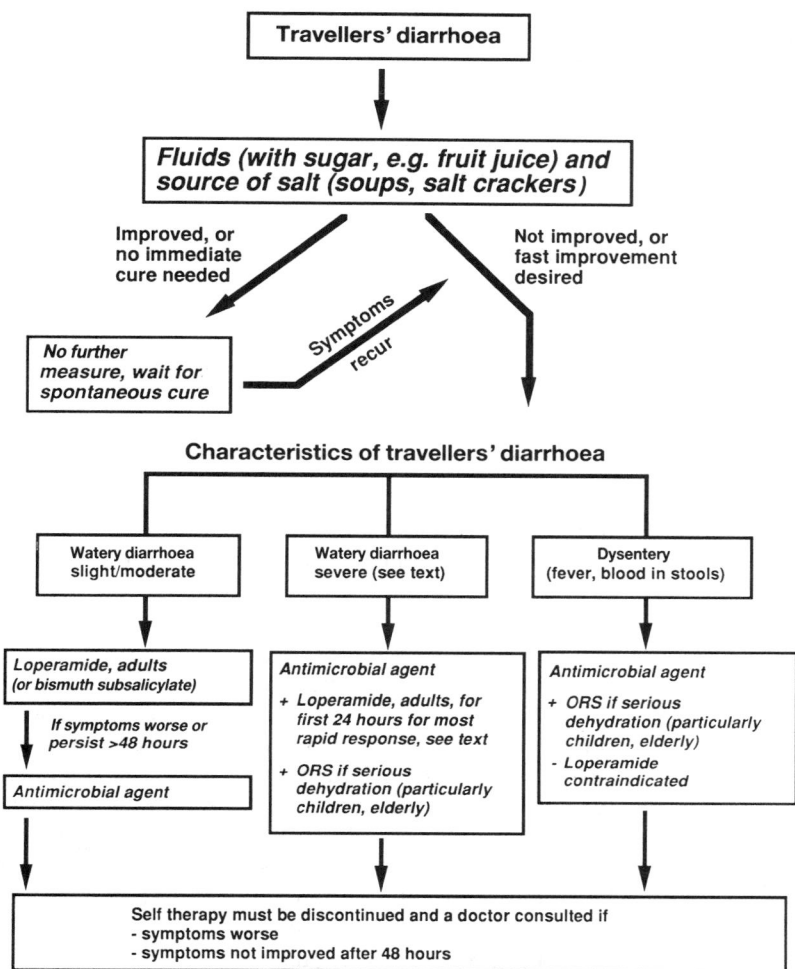

Travellers' diarrhoea

↓

Fluids (with sugar, e.g. fruit juice) and source of salt (soups, salt crackers)

Improved, or no immediate cure needed

Not improved, or fast improvement desired

Symptoms recur

No further measure, wait for spontaneous cure

Characteristics of travellers' diarrhoea

| Watery diarrhoea slight/moderate | Watery diarrhoea severe (see text) | Dysentery (fever, blood in stools) |

Loperamide, adults (or bismuth subsalicylate)

If symptoms worse or persist >48 hours

Antimicrobial agent

Antimicrobial agent
+ *Loperamide, adults, for first 24 hours for most rapid response, see text*
+ *ORS if serious dehydration (particularly children, elderly)*

Antimicrobial agent
+ *ORS if serious dehydration (particularly children, elderly)*
- *Loperamide contraindicated*

Self therapy must be discontinued and a doctor consulted if
- symptoms worse
- symptoms not improved after 48 hours

Figure 18.5 Self-therapy of travellers' diarrhoea in adults. ORS, oral rehydration solution.

important. In most cases it would be reasonable to wait until the symptoms of the self-limited illness subside and to replace fluid and electrolyte losses. Oral rehydration solution is the correct strategy for children and elderly patients, in whom dangerous dehydration may occur. However, adult travellers often want an immediate cure which is not provided by oral rehydration solutions.[21] Loperamide is the fastest acting agent for the treatment of non-invasive travellers' diarrhoea.[22] This is the treatment of choice in mild to moderate, non-invasive illness (Figure 18.5). It should not be used on its own in invasive illness characterized by fever and/or blood in the stools because it may lead to an aggravation of symptoms in patients with dysentery.[23,24] In such cases only antimicrobial agents can be recommended. Treatment with a combination of loperamide and an antimicrobial agent results in rapid disappearance of symptoms with a mean duration of illness of 1 hour.[22] Thus, two drugs can be recommended for inclusion in the travel kit: loperamide and an antimicrobial agent, usually a quinolone. Drugs which are neither antimotility agents nor antibiotics have shown no significant effect, with the exception of bismuth subsalicylate.[25]

MALARIA (See also Chapter 61)

EPIDEMIOLOGY

Malaria is present in most tropical and subtropical countries. Using surveillance data and the numbers of travellers to the respective destinations, we can roughly estimate the risk of malaria in travellers visiting different countries. The risk of infection, particularly with *Plasmodium falciparum,* is much higher in Africa than in Asia or Latin America (Table 18.2), especially in most of the frequently visited tourist centres. However, foci with high transmission rates are present in Asia and Latin America. One study[26] estimated the monthly incidence rate of *P. falciparum* malaria in travellers to West Africa to be 24 cases per 1000 travellers if no chemoprophylaxis was used. Assuming a case fatal-

Table 18.2 Estimated monthly incidence rate of malaria without chemoprophylaxis per 100 000 travellers.

	Morbidity			
		Plasmodium falciparum		Mortality (2% case fatality rate)
Destination	All cases (n)	(%)	(n)	
East Africa	1500	90	1350	27
West Africa	2400	90	2160	43
Indian subcontinent	350	20	70	1
Far East	100	30	30	0.6
Central America and Mexico	<10	10	1	0.02
South America	50	16	8	0.2

ity rate of 2%,[27] 0.4 deaths per 1000 travellers would be expected.

PREVENTION

Prevention of malaria is based on protection against *Anopheles* mosquito bites between dawn and dusk and on taking chemoprophylaxis.

Anti-mosquito measures

Contact with mosquitoes can be reduced by remaining in well-screened areas, using mosquito nets and wearing clothes that cover most of the body. The protective effect of such clothing is enhanced when it is impregnated or sprayed with a repellent or an insecticide.[28] Topical repellents with diethyltoluamide are effective, but they need to be applied every 2–3 hours. The concentration of DEET should be between 25 and 30%. Higher concentrations should be avoided in infants and children. Insecticides and coils are effective; in non-air-conditioned and inadequately screened rooms the mosquito net remains by far the most effective tool. Impregnation with permethrin increases the usefulness of nets.[29] Unfortunately, few travellers use antimosquito measures adequately.[26,30]

Chemoprophylaxis

Use of effective drugs can prevent clinical malaria. For several decades chloroquine was an effective and well-tolerated drug for prevention of malaria. Because of widespread resistance to this drug, it can now be recommended only for those at risk of malaria infection travelling to Central America, Haiti, the Dominican Republic and the Near East.

Several drugs may be considered for travellers to areas with chloroquine-resistant malaria: mefloquine, doxycycline, or chloroquine + proguanil. The tolerance and effectiveness of different chemoprophylactic regimens have recently been investigated in 140 000 short-term travellers to East Africa[26] and in a longitudinal cohort study of Peace Corps volunteers in Africa.[31] In East Africa, mefloquine appears to be the most effective agent, with more than 90% protection, whereas the protection provided by chloroquine at a dosage of 300 mg base/week was not significantly better than that achieved with no prophylaxis[26] (Table 18.3). Among Peace Corps volunteers in West Africa mefloquine was 94% more effective than chloroquine alone and 86% more effective than the combination of weekly chloroquine + daily proguanil.[31]

The rate of serious neuropsychiatric events (convulsions, psychosis) attributed to malaria chemoprophylaxis was identical (1 per 10 000) among 40 000 users of chloroquine with or without proguanil and among 53 000 users of mefloquine; no such events have been observed during 3 years of use of mefloquine for prophylaxis in Peace Corps volunteers. Questionnaire surveys among the European travellers indicated that self-reported subjective mild adverse events were experienced by 11–23% of the travellers and were not clearly associated with any particular drug used for prophylaxis (Figure 18.6). Also among Peace Corps volunteers subjective mild adverse events were reported with equal frequency by users of mefloquine as by users of chloroquine. In addition, the frequency of these events declined with prolonged use of mefloquine. These studies suggest that mefloquine, when used in prophylactic dosage, is tolerated as well as other agents currently recommended. The drug is contraindicated for persons with hypersensitivity to mefloquine. The use in pregnant women in the first trimester and, in children under 5 kg must be justified by an unavoidable high risk of infection.

Doxycycline is an effective alternative for persons

Table 18.3 Synopsis of vaccines and immune globulin (IG) for use by travellers.

Indication	Route	Regimen (days)	Efficacy (%)	Effective from day*	Duration of protection
Cholera (WC inactiv.)	ID/SC/IM	0/(−28 optional)	30–60	P6,R1	O:6mo,E:3–4 mo
(WC-BS)	PO	0/7–14	80	P6	O/E. 6 months
(CVD-103HgR)	PO	0	80	P6,R1	O/E: 6 months
Diphtheria	IM	0 (B)	80	15	5(−10) years
Yellow fever	SC	0	>99	P10,R1	O: 10y, E: >15 years
Hepatitis A (active)	IM	0/(−14–30§)/180–365	98	<14	10–25 years
(IG)	IM	0	85	2	3–5 months
Hepatitis B	IM	0/14–30/180–365	90	30	3–8 years
Japanese encephalitis	IM	0/7–14/(14–28)/365	90	7	1–4 years
Measles	SC	0	90	30	Usually >20 years
Meningococcal meningitis	IM	0	70–90	7	1–3 years
Poliomyelitis	PO	0 (B)	>99	30	10 years
	IM		>99	30	5(−10) years
Rabies	IM/ID	0/7/21–28	>99	7	2–3 years
Tetanus	IM	0 (B)	>99	15	10 years
Tuberculosis	ID	0	50	60	10 (?) years
Typhoid fever (Ty21a)	PO	0/2/4	70	15	1(−7) years
(TAB)	IM	0/28	70	15	2–7 years
(Vi CPS)	IM	0	70	<28	>3 years

P, primary; R, revaccination; O, officially; E, effectively. B if only booster needed.
*If more than one dose is necessary, number of days after completion of series.
§If Havrix® 720 EL.U., unnecessary if 1440 EL.U. used.

who cannot use mefloquine.[32–34] This drug is contraindicated for pregnant women and children under 8 years of age. Side-effects of doxycycline include monilial vaginitis, gastrointestinal symptoms (nausea or vomiting) in 3–7% of users, and phototoxicity after intense sun exposure.[35]

If neither mefloquine nor doxycycline can be used, travellers may use chloroquine plus proguanil, but they need to be aware that this regimen has only limited effectiveness.

Emergency stand-by medication

Some experts suggest that travellers to areas with a very low risk of infection carry a stand-by medication instead of using chemoprophylaxis (Figure 18.7).[36] The rationale for such a strategy is that in such areas the risk of adverse events may well exceed the benefit of avoided infection. Travellers with stand-by medication are instructed that, should malaria symptoms occur, they should first seek medical care. The stand-by medication can be used by the local doctor, or for self-treatment if no medical care can be obtained within 12–24 hours after the onset of illness. Persons using mefloquine or doxycycline for prophylaxis do not need to carry stand-by medication. Only persons not using chemoprophylaxis or using chloroquine with or without proguanil in areas with chloroquine-resistant *P. falciparum* should carry medication with them.

There are various concerns about advocating such stand-by medication. First, malaria symptoms are difficult to explain to untrained persons: even doctors often find it difficult to diagnose this infection. Second, travellers may decide to change their

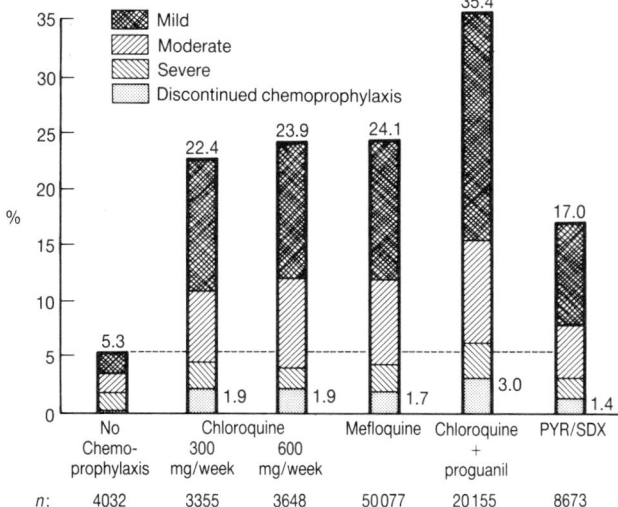

Figure 18.6 Adverse events of malaria chemoprophylaxis. PYR/SDX, pyrimethamine + sulfadoxine ('Fansidar').

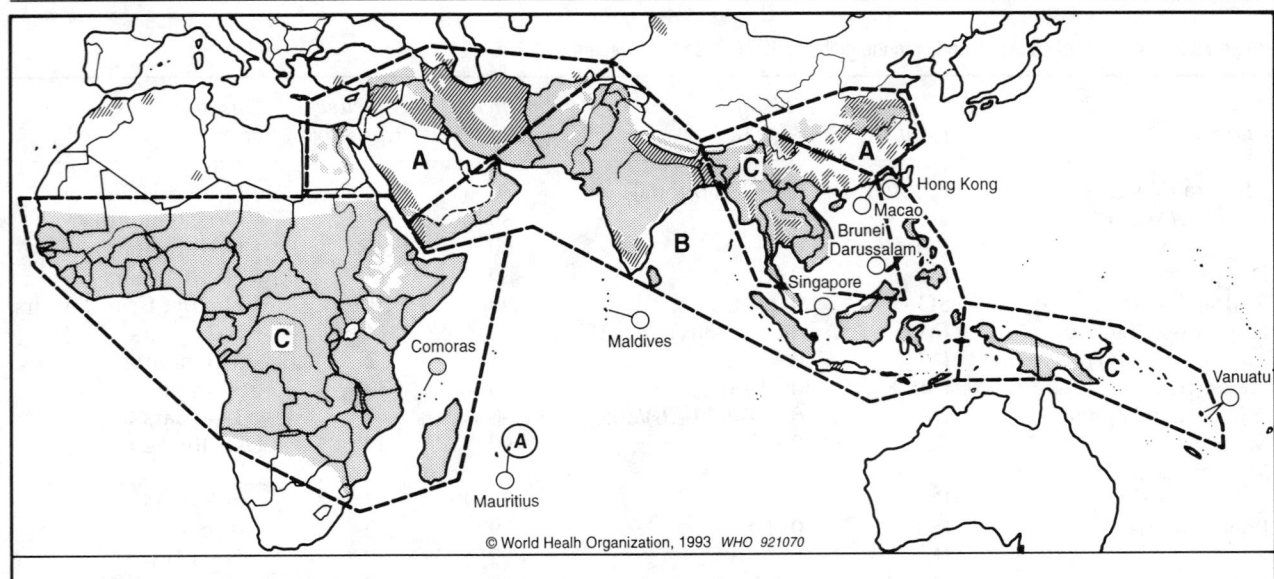

A	In zone A, risk generally low and seasonal; no risk in many areas (for example urban areas). *P. falciparum* absent or sensitive to chloroquine.	*either:* chloroquine prophylaxis *or:* (in case of very low risk): no prophylaxis
B	Low risk in most of the areas of zone B. Chloroquine alone will protect against *P. vivax*. Chloroquine with proguanil will give some protection against *P. falciparum* and may alleviate the disease if it occurs despite prophylaxis.	**prophylaxis:** chloroquine + proguanil *or:* chloroquine alone (if proguanil is not available) *or:* (in case of very low risk): no prophylaxis
C	In Africa, risk high in most areas of zone C, except in some high-altitude areas. Risk low in most areas of this zone in Asia and America, but high in parts of the Amazon basin (colonization and mining areas). Resistance to sulfadoxine–pyrimethamine common in zone C in Asia, variable in zone C in Africa and America.	**prophylaxis:** chloroquine + proguanil (for certain countries of Africa only) *or:* doxycycline *or:* mefloquine *or:* (in case of very low risk): no prophylaxis

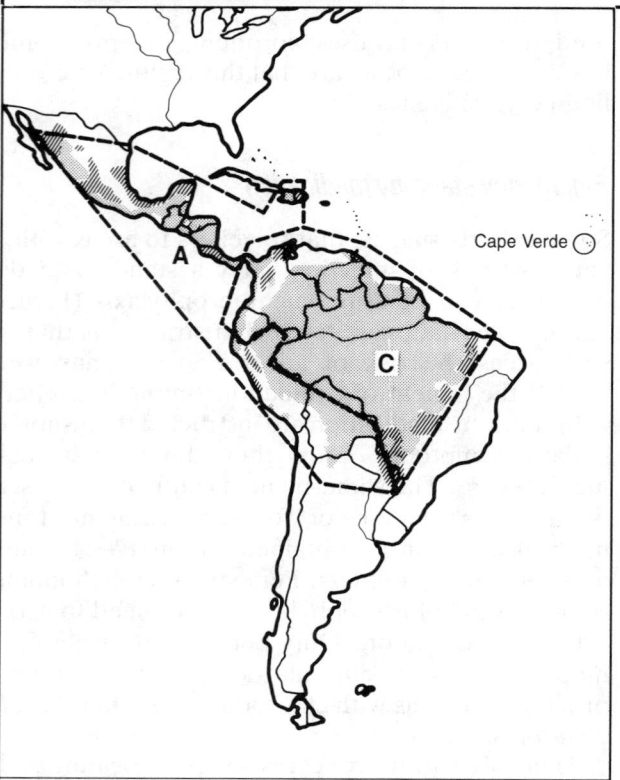

○ Areas in which malaria has disappeared, been eradicated or never existed

◩ Areas with limited risk

◓ Areas where malaria transmission occurs

Figure 18.7 WHO recommendations for malaria chemoprophylaxis.

itinerary and visit high-risk malaria areas for which they should have received chemoprophylaxis.

Among the drugs recommended for use as stand-by medication, 'Fansidar' appears to be effective outside South-east Asia and South America, and it is well tolerated when used for treatment. Halofantrine also appears to be effective outside limited areas in Thailand but since incidents of sudden death have been associated with QT_c prolongation attributed to this drug it is no longer recommended for self-treatment. Mefloquine, 25 mg base/kg (maximum 1500 mg in 2 doses) often results in severe dizziness and in approximately 0.2% in psychosis or seizures.

HUMAN IMMUNODEFICIENCY VIRUS
(See also Chapter 12)

Casual sexual contacts abroad play an important role in the transmission of human immunodeficiency virus (HIV) infection.[37] Other sources of HIV include contaminated blood and use of contaminated needles and syringes. Available data on sexual behaviour of short-term tourists and of long-term overseas workers is of concern because of the worldwide epidemic of HIV and sexually transmitted diseases.[38] Seventeen (4.8%) of 354 British respondents who had been abroad and 31 (6.4%) of 484 Swiss short-term travellers had had casual sex. Among Belgian men working in Central Africa, who were tested HIV-negative, 51% and 31% reported casual sex with a local woman or prostitute, respectively.[39] A more recent study of 1968 Dutch expatriates working in sub-Saharan Africa showed that 31% of males and 13% of females had casual sexual contacts with African partners, and 'always' condom use was reported by less than 25% of the study participants.[40] Among short-term vacationers, 5% had casual sexual contacts, half of these unprotected by condoms.[41,42]

The World Health Organization (WHO) estimates that 75% of all HIV infections worldwide are sexually transmitted and that the efficiency of transmission per sexual contact ranges from 0.1 to 1%. This efficiency can be greatly increased by the presence of other sexually transmitted diseases and genital lesions.[43] In populations with a high prevalence of HIV and other sexually transmitted diseases, as is often the case in female prostitutes in developing countries, the transmission probability of HIV is greatly enhanced.[43,44] Studies indicate that the prevalence of HIV ranged from 0.4% in Dutch expatriates to 1.1% in Belgians and 8.6% in Danish volunteers. These rates are 100 to 500 times higher when compared with the general population of these countries.[39]

Because of the risk of acquiring incurable viral sexually transmitted diseases such as HIV, the emphasis should be on safe sex, such as always using a condom, for all those who travel and engage in casual sex. Other preventive measures include avoidance of unscreened or inadequately screened blood (the chance of needing a blood transfusion during travel is small) and use of sterile needles and syringes which should be included in the travel kit.

VACCINE-PREVENTABLE DISEASES

EPIDEMIOLOGY

The morbidity and mortality of the most frequent vaccine-preventable diseases has been estimated (Figure 18.8). Among these, hepatitis A and B infections are the most important ones. Hepatitis A may infect anyone, even those residing in luxury tourist hotels, and the monthly incidence rate is high (3 cases per 1000 travellers). Persons eating and drinking under poor hygienic conditions have a monthly incidence rate of 20 per 1000 travellers. The average duration of incapacity to work is 33 days, and the case fatality rate 0.1%.[45] Hepatitis A is responsible for about 60% of hepatitis cases in travellers returning from developing countries. Hepatitis B and hepatitis non-A non-B (HCV and HEV) were each diagnosed in about 15% of the cases, while about 10% remained unclassified.

Hepatitis B is mostly diagnosed in expatriates in highly endemic areas such as Asia but tourists are rarely infected.[46] Risk factors include casual sexual contacts, tattooing, acupuncture, and occasionally medical and dental treatment in developing countries. Persons living in close contact with the indigenous population may be infected by minor injuries. Future studies need to determine the role of hepatitis C and E (HCV and HEV) in travellers.

Typhoid fever may cause infections in foreigners, especially on the Indian subcontinent, and in many parts of North and West Africa, excluding Tunisia, as well as in travellers eating and drinking under poor hygienic conditions. Otherwise the incidence rate per month is lower;[47–50] the case fatality rate did not exceed 1% in these surveys of travellers. At most tourist destinations the risk of typhoid fever is 100 times lower than the risk of hepatitis A.

Many cases of rabies in travellers have been reported. The rate of exposure to animal bites is estimated to be 0.2–0.4% per month; in the majority of these incidents there was some concern about rabies infection.[51]

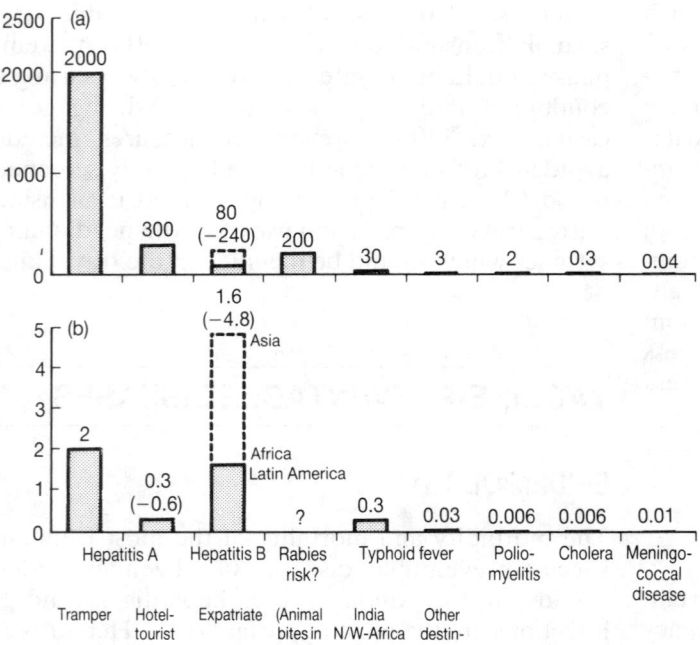

Figure 18.8 (a) Morbidity and (b) mortality of vaccine-preventable diseases per 100 000 non-immune travellers.

Yellow fever is extremely rare in travellers. Only five cases in travellers (four unvaccinated) have been published since the early 1980s, due to the fact that immunization is required in most countries where this infection occurs.[52]

The risk of poliomyelitis is probably underestimated: 47 cases of imported poliomyelitis in residents of Europe, Canada or the USA, who had often been in a developing country for less than a week, were reviewed.[53] In the UK imported poliomyelitis accounts for an important proportion of all diagnosed cases.[54] Because asymptomatic infections occur more frequently than symptomatic ones, we must assume that the incidence of asymptomatic infection in unvaccinated travellers is at least 20 per 1 000 000. Only 18 contact cases in industrialized nations have been recorded.

There are various other vaccine-preventable diseases about which little epidemiological data in travellers exist, as only anecdotal cases have been reported. The incidence rate is probably less than 1 per million travellers per month. Outbreaks of meningococcal disease have occurred in situations in which travellers lived in crowded conditions, such as after trekking or after the Hadj to Mecca.[55] Although an increased endemicity of Japanese encephalitis has lately been observed in the indigenous population in an area including all Asian countries east and north-east of India, fewer than thirty cases of Japanese encephalitis in civilian visitors have been recorded in the literature.[56,57] Only two cases of plague were reported in international travellers

between 1966 and 1990.[58] No plague infection has been confirmed in a traveller in the 1994 epidemic in India. It is often difficult to decide whether tuberculosis has been imported from abroad or has been acquired locally. Except for a few reports of in-flight transmission, infection apparently occurs almost exclusively when there is prolonged and intense contact with patients. There are few published data on diphtheria, tetanus and pneumococcal infections in travellers.[59]

Travellers are rarely infected with cholera. This infection is usually limited to the low-income groups within the autochthonous population. Typically, the recent epidemic in South America has led to infection of a relatively few visitors who had not adhered to fundamental hygienic rules, such as eating improperly cooked fish after having it imported illegally into the USA. Of the 96 travel-associated cholera cases in the USA since 1 January 1992, 75 were associated with an outbreak on board an aeroplane from Argentina.[60] Between 1975 and 1981 only 129 imported cases of cholera were reported to WHO. Detailed analysis showed an attack rate of two cases per 1 000 000 travellers.[60–62] Many of these infections were imported from North Africa and Turkey to Europe (mainly by foreign workers) and their families returning from home leave. Some of the countries which they had visited had reported no cholera cases to WHO for fear of endangering tourism. All infected patients had a short stay in hospital and the case fatality rate in travellers was below 2%. Cases are rarely treated abroad and asymptomatic infections do not cause epidemics in temperate regions.

PREVENTION

According to the International Health Regulations only yellow fever immunization is mandatory. There is no valid indication for cholera vaccination and even remote border posts have gradually realized that this can no longer be required. Saudi Arabia often requires pilgrims to be immunized against meningococcal disease. Up-to-date information on required immunizations can be obtained from airlines. Their information regarding recommended immunizations is often unreliable!

The main regimens for malaria chemoprophylaxis are summarized in Table 18.4.

The International Health Regulations indicate that yellow fever vaccination is required for entry into most countries of tropical Africa or northern South America, where the infection is endemic. Additionally some countries in Asia and in the Pacific require passengers who have travelled through infected or endemic areas within the previous 10 days to show proof of vaccination. Since the yellow fever epidemic in Kenya in 1992 most experts recommend yellow fever vaccination for any stay in an endemic area even if no cases of the infection have been detected for decades, since the vector is present and epidemics may theoretically occur anytime. Yellow fever vaccination must be performed in centres which are approved by the national authorities and it must be documented in the international vaccination certificate.

Immunization for hepatitis A (HAV) has a high priority. An active vaccine was introduced in several countries in 1992. The very low prevalence rates of anti-hepatitis A virus antibodies in persons up to the age of 50 years, according to recent European and North American studies, makes prevaccination testing useless unless the future traveller is over 50 years old or has stayed in a developing country for longer than a year or has a history of jaundice[63] (and V. Ansdell, personal communication). Hepatitis A immunization may be recommended to any traveller visiting the developing countries but it is unnecessary for visits to the Caribbean (except Hispaniola) or to southern Europe. In countries where the active vaccine is available it should be preferred to immune globulin because of the higher efficacy and longer duration of protection. In countries where active hepatitis A vaccine is not yet available, immune globulin may be injected at a dose of 2 ml for visits of less than 3 months duration, and 0.06 ml/kg body weight for a protection of up to 5 months. Regular booster doses are necessary for longer exposure.

For long-term residents, hepatitis B vaccination is indicated, and it may also be considered for short-term visitors who intend to engage in high-risk sex (although this still leaves them unprotected for HIV infection!).

Vaccination against typhoid fever seems indicated for persons who may eat and drink under poor hygienic conditions, and those who will stay for over one month in developing countries or who visit the Indian subcontinent, Peru or North or West Africa, excluding Tunisia.

Rabies vaccination should be considered for all long-term residents, particularly for those who will live in close contact with the autochthonous population.

Other special risk vaccinations are those against meningococcal disease, which may be recommended to trekkers in Nepal and to visitors in areas where the infection is epidemic or highly endemic, such as for stays in the Sahel zone, particularly

Table 18.4 Prophylactic effectiveness of various regimens of malarial chemoprophylaxis in East Africa.

Regimen	Cases	Pers-Mo*	Effectiveness† (±95% C.I.)
No chemoprophylaxis	39	3137	0
Chloroquine 300 mg/wk	43‡	3827	(-43) 10 43
Chloroquine 600 mg/wk	35	4897	6 42 64
Chloroquine + proguanil	41	11912	56 72 82
Mefloquine	35	31412	85 91 94
Pyrimethamine + sulfadoxine ('Fansidar')	36	16206	71 82 89

*Person-months of exposure.
†With good and bad compliance.
‡Four deaths.

involving close contact with natives. Japanese encephalitis vaccine may be recommended for persons staying for at least 2 weeks in rural areas in endemic countries. There is a decreasing trend in the recommendation immunization against tuberculosis to long-term residents abroad because one wishes to be able to diagnose infection from seroconversion to tuberculin.

For reasons unrelated to travel, persons living in industrialized countries should be immunized against poliomyelitis, tetanus and diphtheria, as well as measles, mumps and rubella. As this applies even more for visits to the developing world, a medical consultation prior to departure makes it possible to administer necessary booster doses, or sometimes to initiate vaccination against these infections.

Unless primary vaccination is needed (which requires several doses) most vaccines may be given simultaneously.

CONCLUSIONS

Every physician or nurse who counsels intending travellers must tailor specific recommendations based on a balance between the health risks to be expected during travel and the benefits and tolerance of protective measures.[64] One should not protect or advise travellers against rare risks while failing to protect them against more likely or severe diseases.[64]

Four strategies are available to reduce the health risks of foreign travel: (1) appropriate behaviour can prevent sexually transmitted diseases, and reduce the risks of malaria and diarrhoea and the danger of injuries; (2) prophylactic drug use can prevent malaria; (3) drug therapy for travellers' diarrhoea can reduce duration and morbidity; and (4) immunizations can prevent some diseases without requiring compliance from the traveller.

REFERENCES

1 Handszuh H. Tourism trends and patterns. In Lobel H O, Steffen R & Kozarsky P E (eds) *Travel Medicine 2*. Proceedings of the Second Conference on International Travel Medicine. Atlanta, GA: International Society of Travel Medicine, 1992: 8–9.

2 Hargarten S W, Baker T D & Guptill K. Overseas fatalities of United States citizen travellers: an analysis of deaths related to international travel. *Ann Emerg Med* 1991; 20:622–626.

3 Lustenberger I. *Todesfälle von Schweizern im Ausland*. Thesis, University of Zurich, 1990.

4 Steffen R, Desaules M, Nagel J et al. Epidemiological experience in the mission of the United Nations Transition Assistance Group (UNTAG) in Namibia. *Bull World Health Organ* 1992; 70:129–133.

5 Wenker O. *Repatriierungsflüge der REGA 1983*. Thesis, University of Zurich, 1990.

6 Steffen R & Lobel H O. Epidemologic basis for the practice of travel medicine. *J. Wilderness Med* 1994; 5:56–66.

7 Steffen R & Boppart I. Travellers' diarrhoea. *Baillière's Clin Gastroenterol* 1987; 1:361–376.

8 Brenner D, Steffen R & Schorr D. Travellers' diarrhea in Egypt, Tunisia and Turkey 1989. *Trav Med Int* 991; 9:68–71.

9 Pitzinger B, Steffen R & Tschopp A. Epidemiology of travellers' diarrhea in infants and children. *J Pediatr Infect Dis* 1991; 10:719–723.

10 Ericsson C D, Pickering L K, Sullivan P & DuPont H L. The role of location of food consumption in the prevention of travellers' diarrhea in Mexico. *Gastroenterology* 1980; 79:812–816.

11 Tjoa W S, DuPont H L, Sullivan P et al. Location of food consumption and travellers' diarrhea. *Am J Epidemiol* 1977; 106:61–66.

12 Dickens D L, DuPont H L, Johnson P C. Survival of bacterial enteropathogens in the ice of popular drinks. *JAMA* 1985; 253:3141–3143.

13 Farthing M J G, DuPont H L, Guandalini S, Keusch G T & Steffen R. Prevention and treatment of travellers' diarrhoea. *Gastroenterol Int* 1992; 5:162–175.

14 Black R E. Pathogens that cause travellers' diarrhea in Latin America and Africa. *Rev Infect Dis* 1986; 8:S131–135.

15 Taylor D N & Echeverria P. Etiology and epidemiology of travellers' diarrhea in Asia. *Rev Infect Dis* 1986; 8:S136–141.

16 Steffen R, Mathewson J, Ericsson C D et al. Travellers' diarrhea in West Africa and Mexico: fecal transport systems and liquid bismuth

subsalicylate for self-therapy. *J Infect Dis* 1988; 157:1008.

17 DuPont H L, Ericsson C D, Johnson P C & Cabada F J. Antimicrobial agents in the prevention of travelers' diarrhea. *Rev Infect Dis* 1986; 8:S167–171.

18 Kozicki M, Steffen R & Schar M. 'Boil it, cook it, peel it or forget it': does this rule prevent travellers' diarrhoea? *Int J Epidemiol* 1985; 14:169–172.

19 Norrby S R. Side effects of quinolones: comparisons between quinolones and other antibiotics. *Eur J Clin Microbiol Infect Dis* 1991; 10:378–383.

20 Peltola H, Siitonen A, Kyronseppa H et al. Prevention of travellers' diarrhoea by oral B subunit/whole-cell cholera vaccine. *Lancet* 1991; 338:1285–1289.

21 World Health Organization. *Diarrhoeal Diseases Control Programme Drugs in the Management of Acute Diarrhoea in Infants and Young Children.* WHO/CDD/CMT/86.1 Rev. 1. Geneva: WHO, 1988.

22 Ericsson C D, DuPont H L, Mathewson J J, Stewart West M, Johnson P C & Bitsura J A M. Treatment of traveler's diarrhea with sulfamethoxazole and trimethoprim and loperamide. *JAMA* 1990; 263:257–261.

23 Murphy G S, Bodhidatta L, Echeverria P et al. Ciprofloxacin and Loperamide in the treatment of bacillary dysentery. *Ann Int Med* 1993; 118:582–586.

24 DuPont H L & Hornick R B. Adverse effect of lomotil therapy in shigellosis. *JAMA* 1973; 226:24–31.

25 Steffen R. Worldwide efficacy of bismuth subsalicylate in the treatment of traveler's diarrhea. *Rev Infect Dis* 1990; 12:S80–86.

26 Steffen R, Fuchs E, Schildknecht J et al. Mefloquine compared with other malaria chemoprophylactic agents in tourists visiting East Africa. *Lancet* 1993; 341:1299–1303.

27 Steffen R & Behrens R. Travellers' malaria. *Parasitol Today* 1982; 8:61–66.

28 Christophers R. Mosquito repellents. *J Hyg* 1947; 45:176–231.

29 Schmid R A. *Personal protection against malaria, excluding chemoprophylaxis.* Thesis, University of Zurich, 1992.

30 Lobel H O, Phillips-Howard P A, Brandling-Bennet A D et al. Malaria incidence and prevention among European and North American travellers to Kenya. *Bull World Health Organ* 1990; 68:209–215.

31 Lobel H O, Miani M, Eng T, Bernard K W, Hightower A W, Campbell C C. Long-term malaria prophylaxis with mefloquine. *Lancet* 1993; 341:848–851.

32 Pang L W, Boudreau E F, Limsomwong N & Singharaj P. Doxycycline prophylaxis for falciparum malaria. *Lancet* 1987; ii:1161–1164.

33 Watanasook C, Singharaj P, Suriyamongkol V et al. Malaria prophylaxis with doxycycline in soldiers deployed to the Thai–Kampuchean border.

Southeast Asian J Trop Med Public Health 1989; 20:61–64.

34 Singharaj P, Eamsila C, Bhothisuwan A et al. Efficacy of doxycycline as malaria prophylaxis in the soldiers deployed to the Thai-Kampuchean border. *R Thai Army Med J* 1987; 40:165–170.

35 Frost P, Weinsteain G D & Gomez E. Phototoxic potential of minocycline and doxycycline. *Arch Dermatol* 1972; 105:681–683.

36 World Health Organization. *International Travel and Health.* Geneva: WHO, 1992.

37 De Schrijver A & Meheus A. International travel and sexually transmitted diseases. *World Health Stat Q* 1989; 42:90–99.

38 Laga M. Risk of HIV infection and other sexually transmitted diseases for travellers. In Lobel H O, Steffen R & Kozarsky P E (eds) *Travel Medicine 2.* Proceedings of the Second Conference on International Travel Medicine. Atlanta, GA: *International Society of Travel Medicine,* 1992; 201–203.

39 Bonneux L, van der Stuyft P, Taelman H et al. Risk factors for HIV infections among European expatriates in Africa. *BMJ* 1988; 297:581–584.

40 Houweling H, De Grave A, Smits S P et al. Prevalence of HIV infections and risk factors among Dutch expatriates in sub-Saharan Africa. In Lobel H O, Steffen R & Kozarsky P E (eds) *Travel Medicine 2.* Proceedings of the Second Conference on International Travel Medicine. Atlanta, GA: *International Society of Travel Medicine,* 1992; 204–206.

41 Hawkes S, Hart G J, Johnson A M et al. Risk behaviour and HIV prevalence in international travellers. *AIDS* 1994; 8:247–252.

42 Stricker M, Steffen R, Hornung R, Gutzwiler F, Eichmann A & Wittasek F. Flüchtige sexuelle Kontakte von Schweizer Touristen in den Tropen. *Munch Med Wochenschr* 1990; 132:175–177.

43 Laga M, Nzila N & Goeman J. The interrelationship of sexually transmitted diseases and HIV infection: implications for the control of both epidemics in Africa. *AIDS* 1991; 5(supplement):SS55–63.

44 Piot P & Tezzo R. The epidemiology of HIV and other STD in the developing world. *Scand J Infect Dis Suppl* 1990; 69:839–897.

45 Steffen R, Kane M A, Shapiro C N et al. Risk of hepatitis A in travelers. *JAMA* 1994; 272:885–889.

46 Steffen R. Risks of hepatitis B for travelers. *Vaccine* 1990; 8:S31–32.

47 Public Health Laboratory Service. Communicable disease report. *Community Med* 1984; 6:72–75.

48 Steffen R. Typhoid vaccine, for whom? *Lancet* 1982; i:625–626.

49 Taylor D N, Pollard R A & Blake P A. Typhoid in the United States and the risk to the international traveler. *J Infect Dis* 1983; 148:599–602.

50 Ryan C A, Hagrett-Bean N T & Blake P A. *Salmonella typhi* infections in the United States, 1975–84. *Rev Infect Dis* 1989; 11:1–8.

51 Bernard K W & Fishbein D B. Pre-exposure rabies

prophylaxis for travellers: are the benefits worth the cost? *Vaccine* 1991; 9:833–836.

52 Anonymous. Yellow fever. *Weekly Epidemiol Rec* 1986; 61:59–60.

53 Kubli D, Steffen R & Schar M. Importation of poliomyelitis to industrialized nations between 1975 and 1984: evaluation and conclusions for vaccination recommendations. *BMJ* 1987; 295:169–171.

54 Joce R, Wood D, Brown D & Begg N. Paralytic poliomyelitis in England and Wales, 1985–91. *BMJ* 1992; 305:79–82.

55 Koch S & Steffen R. Meningococcal disease in travellers. Vaccination recommendations. *J Travel Med* 1994; 1:4–7.

56 Centers for Disease Control. Inactivated Japanese encephalitis virus vaccine. *MMWR* 1993; 42:RR1, 1–15.

57 Macdonald W B G, Tink A R & Ouvrier R A. Japanese encephalitis after a two-week holiday in Bali. *Med J Aust* 1989; 150:334–339.

58 Centers for Disease Control. Imported bubonic plague. *MMWR* 1990; 39:895–901.

59 Editorial. Pneumococcal vaccination for travel to Spain? *Lancet* 1992; 340:84–85.

60 Weber J T, Levine W C, Hopkins D P, Tauxe R V. Cholera in the United States, 1965–1991. *Arch Intern Med* 1994; 154:551–556.

61 Snyder J D & Blake P A. Is cholera a problem for US travelers? *JAMA* 1982; 247:2268–2269.

62 Morger H, Steffen R & Schär M. Epidemiology of cholera in travellers and conclusions for vaccination recommendations. *BMJ* 1983; 286:184–186.

63 Studer S, Joller H, Steffen R & Grob P J. Prevalence of hepatitis A antibodies in Swiss travellers. *Eur J Epidemiol* 1993; 9:50–54.

64 Steffen R & DuPont H L. Travel Medicine. What's That? *J Travel Med* 1994; 1:1–3.

FURTHER READING

Cook G C (ed). *Travel-associated Disease*. London: Royal College of Physicians of London, pp. 179, 1995.

CHAPTER 19

HEAT STRESS AND ASSOCIATED DISORDERS

K. J. Collins

Constant internal body temperature is achieved by processes of heat exchange adjusting heat loss to heat gain. Heat balance is usually expressed in the form of an equation:

$$M \pm w = \pm R \pm C \pm k - E$$

where M = the rate of metabolic heat production,
w = the external work performed by or on the body,
R = the loss or gain of radiant heat
C = the loss or gain of heat by convection
k = the conductive loss or gain of heat through body contact with solids or fluids
E = the evaporative heat loss from the body surface by sweating and respiration.

If the body temperature is not kept in a steady state, a heat storage component ($\pm S$) must be introduced into the equation to account for a rising or falling temperature.

In health, heat balance is maintained by an efficient thermoregulatory system despite considerable heat loads imposed by high ambient temperatures and/or physical work. The system allows body temperature fluctuations, normally about $\pm 0.3°C$ diurnal change at rest in a neutral environment, extending to $\pm 2.0°C$ in more extreme ambient conditions and physical activity. Should the accumulation of environmental and metabolic heat exceed the capacity of the thermoregulatory system to dissipate heat (positive heat storage), body temperature will rise and a spectrum of symptom complexes, known collectively as heat disorders, may occur. At one end of this spectrum is heat stroke, a life-threatening condition with severe complications resulting from heat damage to tissues.

THERMOREGULATION

An immediate response to hot conditions is a rise in skin temperature and vasodilatation by (1) autonomic vasomotor reflexes acting through the neural centres controlling heat loss, and (2) direct warming of the skin. Much of the large increase in skin blood flow due to heat exposure comes from opening of arteriovenous anastomoses deep to the skin capillaries.[1] Dilatation of the large cutaneous vascular network causes a redistribution of blood from the body core to the skin and concomitant reduction in splanchnic blood flow. The compensatory fall in renal and hepatic blood flow produces oliguria in the heat and a reduced hepatic metabolic clearance. If the heat stress is great, the skin temperature rises and approaches 35°C over the whole of the body surface. At or near this point the deep body temperature is stabilized by the secretion of sweat, which increases with body temperature drive. Sweat that is not evaporated but drips from the body surface (as occurs in hot humid environments) is useless for cooling. Fully evaporated sweat may, on the other hand, contribute to large heat losses, of the order of 670 watts for every litre of sweat evaporated. Up to 10 litres of hypotonic fluid per day may be lost by profuse sweating in hot environments. Serious dehydration is therefore a possible outcome of this physiological process and is a primary concern, especially when water supplies are low. With the fluid loss by sweating there is also a loss of salt, which may pose another potential problem. Salt concentration in sweat may vary from 1 g per litre in heat-acclimatized personnel to 3 g per litre in those who are not acclimatized. The rate of sweating and dietary intake of salt are other variables that determine sweat salt concentration. Immediate and long-term endocrine regulations are brought into play when water and salt imbalance occurs in hot environments.[2]

Cardiovascular strain develops from the increasing demand for a cardiac output to transfer heat and water to vasodilated vascular beds in the skin for heat loss. In resting conditions, extensive shunting of blood to the skin induces a fall in blood pressure and an increase in heart rate. With an adequate venous pressure, stroke volume is maintained and cardiac output increased. Dehydration with excessive sweating leads to a marked decrease in circulating blood volume, a reduction in stroke volume and an increased heart rate. With exercise in hot conditions blood is shunted to working muscles as well as to the skin for thermoregulation. In unacclimatized humans there is an initial period of cardiovascular instability characterized by increasing body temperature, heart rate and plasma volume with a decrease in stroke volume. Stability returns with acclimatization when plasma volume and stroke volume increase and heart rate decreases.[3] Several standard works describe these and other general thermoregulatory responses to heat in greater detail.[4-6]

CENTRAL NERVOUS CONTROL

Temperature regulation is integrated by a controlling system in the central nervous system which responds to the heat content of tissues. Receptors sensitive to thermal information from the skin, deep tissues and the central nervous system itself provide feedback signals to a central controller with a principal centre in the hypothalamus. The temperature of blood perfusing the hypothalamus is a major drive in temperature control. An essential role in processing thermal signals has been ascribed to the preoptic region of the anterior hypothalamus (heat-loss centre) and posterior hypothalamic heat-gain centre. An analysis of human thermoregulation by means of direct human calorimetry has suggested that control is mainly through warm sensors in the preoptic area of the hypothalamus and cold sensors in the skin.[7] These and other related hypotheses on the functional organization of thermoregulatory centres in the brain have been the focus of enquiry for more than a century. Ideas on the need for a hypothalamic 'set-point' have been developed in order to explain how body temperature is maintained at predetermined constant levels.[8] How the central nervous system interprets the information received from thermosensors also remains a controversial issue, with central 'set-point' or 'gain' determinants providing plausible models.[9]

Excessive increases in brain temperature affecting the integrative function of central nervous structures is likely to have profound deleterious consequences on the controlling system. It has been postulated that some protection of the brain against hyperthermia may be afforded by the anatomy of the blood circulatory system of the head which permits selective cooling of the brain.[10]

HEAT ACCLIMATIZATION

Writing more than 200 years ago on the heat hazard to newcomers to the tropics, Lind[11] pointed out that habituation to hot climates reduced the danger to health. The process of heat acclimatization was originally associated with improved ability to perform work in the heat.[12] In fact a useful degree of acclimatization to heat can be attained simply by hard physical training in a cool environment. Marked physiological changes occur after a few days of work in hot conditions. Heart rate and deep body temperature do not rise so high and the sweating mechanism becomes more efficient. A total sweat rate of 0.5–1 litre per hour may increase to 2 litres or occasionally 3 litres per hour in a fully acclimatized man, though such high rates cannot be maintained for longer than an hour or so. A major part of the improvement in sweat output is due to increased cellular secretory capacity of the sweat glands brought about by sweat gland training,[13] although there is also likely to be a central nervous component with a lowered threshold for the onset of

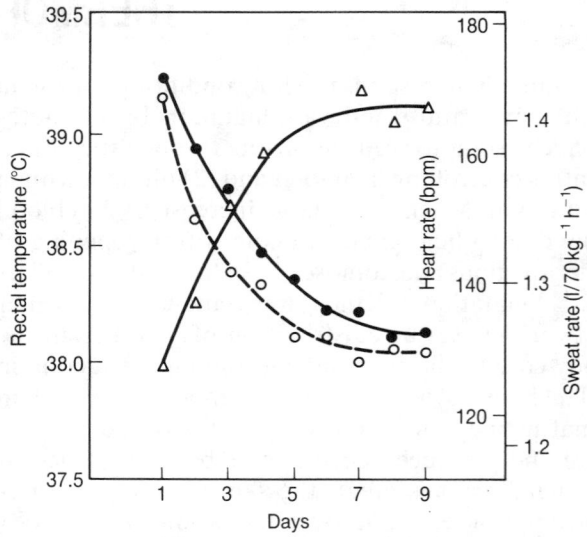

Figure 19.1 Typical average rectal temperatures (●), pulse rates (○) and sweat losses (△) of a group of men during the development of acclimatization to heat. (Adapted from Lind and Bass.)[16]

sweating. With initial acclimatization, the salt content of sweat is reduced in response to a salt deficit and reduced plasma volume.[2] Concentration may increase again during prolonged daily heat exposure.[14] Acclimatization to heat is associated with increments in blood volume, plasma volume, extracellular fluid volume and total body water content.[15]

Heat tolerance can be achieved artificially by daily sessions of controlled hyperthermia or work–rest routines for 3–4 hours in a climatic chamber (acclimation) or naturally by normal daily physical work in the tropics (acclimatization). The adaptive process develops rapidly over the first 3 or 4 days and is virtually complete by 9 or 10 days (Figure 19.1). When exposure to heat ceases, the physiological adaptations are retained for up to 2 weeks but thereafter the benefits are rapidly lost.[4] Part of the longer-term process of heat adaptation involves behavioural adjustments, such as resting during the hottest part of the day. This is intuitive to tropical indigenes who normally seek to avoid the stresses of hyperthermia and in consequence they are often not fully heat acclimatized.

For healthy young adults, such as men in the armed forces, acclimation to heat has been shown to greatly reduce the incidence of heat disorders. In the gold mines in South Africa, heat acclimation chambers, in which recruits are initially trained by graded work in the heat, have proved to be very effective in achieving the same goal.[17]

HEAT STRESS

The heat stress of a given working situation is defined as the sum of all those factors that contribute to the heat gain of the body. It is necessary to consider both climatic factors, such as ambient temperature, humidity and air movement, as well as non-climatic factors such as physical work and clothing. Heat stress indices[1] provide the equivalence of various environmental heat factors, usually with physical activity and clothing insulation as independent variables.

Various heat stress indices have been proposed, divided broadly into: (1) those which have been empirically derived by assessing the physiological effects on a test group of people under varying climatic conditions, e.g. the effective temperature scale, the wet bulb globe temperature (WBGT) index;[18] and (2) those derived by theoretical consideration of the effects of environmental heat, physical activity and clothing on the body's heat balance, e.g. the heat stress index,[19] the predicted 4 hour sweat rate,[20] ISO 7933.[21] No index or standard is universally applicable to all situations since all are affected to differing degrees by the environmental and human variables. The WBGT index calculated from 0.7 wet bulb (WB) + 0.3 globe temperature (GT) indoors, or 0.7 WB + 0.2 GT + 0.1 dry bulb (DB) outdoors is probably the most widely used. It was originally devised for use outdoors where there is a solar radiation component to the heat stress, and was effectively employed to reduce the incidence of heat casualties in unacclimatized marine recruits.[22] Safe physical activity schedules may be set according to the predicted environmental heat loads for the day, e.g. WBGT < 18°C (low risk), WBGT > 28°C (very high risk).[23] Heat stress indices are often used in industry to predict average tolerance times for various work/heat situations.[4,24] The increase in knowledge and understanding of human thermoregulation and the processes of heat exchange have led to the development of mathematical models of human responses to hot environments[25] and to the rapid assessment of heat stress.

HEAT DISORDERS

The pathological conditions associated with the effects of heat arise from four main aetiologies:

1. Circulatory instability
   (a) Heat syncope
   (b) Heat oedema

2. Heat-induced skin disorders
   (a) Hidromeiosis
   (b) Prickly heat (miliaria rubra)
   (c) Anhidrotic heat exhaustion
3. Water and electrolyte imbalance
   (a) Heat cramps

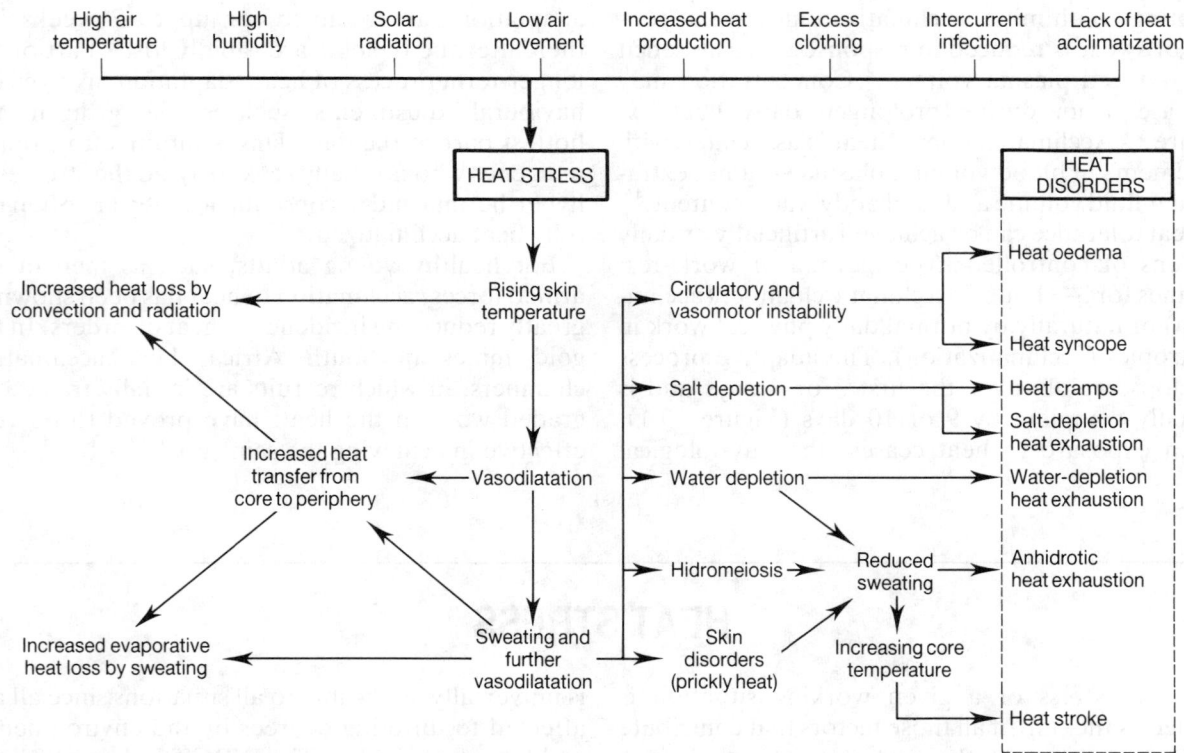

Figure 19.2 Heat stress and heat disorders.

  (b) Water-depletion heat exhaustion
  (c) Salt-depletion heat exhaustion
4. Hyperthermic failure of thermoregulation
  (a) Heat stroke.

The various factors contributing to heat stress and the development of heat disorders are summarized in Figure 19.2.

Another category of heat disorder is sometimes described under the general heading of psychological effects of heat.[26] The predominant psychological heat effects are characterized by deterioration in performance and loss of efficiency presenting as 'acute heat neurasthenia', or 'tropical fatigue' as a chronic form of heat neurotic reaction. The syndromes are ill-defined and may not be attributable solely to the effects of heat.

Predisposing factors

Severely hot conditions, particularly when high humidity or intense solar radiation is combined with heavy physical work and lack of acclimatization, provide the background to most heat disorders. Any factor that compromises the normal processes of thermoregulation is implicated in the aetiology. Personnel most at risk often have a history of heat intolerance or skin disorder, are overweight or physically unfit. Another factor of major importance is failure on the part of the supervising authority, or

the individuals concerned, to appreciate the potential dangers involved in exposure to severe heat stress.

Heat exposure aggravates underlying pathology, especially cardiovascular disease, and in this respect the elderly are particularly at risk. Occult infections have been observed to cause transient anhidrosis[27] and the influence of endogenous pyrogens is thought to raise the 'set-point' around which body temperature is regulated.[28] Many heat stroke victims present with a previous history of infection or fever. Heat intolerance can be extreme in cases of thyrotoxicosis, mucoviscidosis and congenital absence of sweat glands in ectodermal dysplasia. It should also be borne in mind that many pharmacological agents interfere with body heat balance or the processes of temperature regulation.[29] Special care is required in high-temperature conditions with patients who have been prescribed diuretics, anticholinergics or central nervous stimulants and depressants or other drugs that may influence thermoregulation.

MINOR HEAT DISORDERS

HEAT OEDEMA

Unacclimatized people arriving in the tropics may at first experience mild swelling of the feet and ankles which usually resolves within a few days.[4] There is uncertainty about the precise aetiology of this disorder but it is likely to be due to cutaneous vasodilatation and venous stasis in the legs. Mild oedema may also be a manifestation of an expansion of the extracellular fluid space, influenced by aldosterone and antidiuretic hormone activity.[2] Some newcomers to hot climates show their apprehension of the heat by overloading themselves with salt and water.

HEAT SYNCOPE

Fainting is common in unacclimatized people exposed to heat and it is usually precipitated by prolonged standing, sudden cessation of exercise or change in posture. Heat syncope occurs because of peripheral vascular pooling and collapse of venomotor tone leading to cerebral anoxia. The patient is pale with a slow pulse and slow sighing breathing. Consciousness is usually lost for a minute or so, but returns as cerebral circulation is restored when the patient is placed in a head-low position. Other causes of loss of consciousness must be excluded. Syncope may also be the prelude to more serious disorders due to heat.

HEAT CRAMPS

These painful cramps are probably due to mild water intoxication in the heat, or to salt depletion (q.v.), and occur in people who are sweating profusely while at the same time drinking large amounts of unsalted fluids.[4] Cramps may be experienced more frequently by those who exercise regularly and adhere to a low-salt diet. Spasms usually last less than 1 minute, occasionally for 2 or 3, but they may recur every few minutes for several hours. Heat cramps must be distinguished from tetany, observed in some normal individuals with raised body temperature in the heat who may hyperventilate sufficiently to develop acute respiratory alkalosis.[30,31]

For severe cramps, intravenous normal saline (0.5–1 litre) can be given, or even a small quantity of 5% hypertonic saline. This should be followed by liberal quantities of salt in drinks (disguised by citrus flavouring) until the urine contains at least 2–3 g chloride per litre. Marked hyperthermia and other systemic manifestations of heat exposure are not part of the heat cramp syndrome as currently defined. Prevention entails the provision of salted drinks at the place of work.

SKIN DISORDERS WITH SWEAT SUPPRESSION

HIDROMEIOSIS

With sustained wetting of the skin in hot humid climates where sweat evaporation is prevented, sweat production may diminish because of a physical process termed hidromeiosis (described previously as 'sweat gland fatigue'). In this case, suppression of sweating is caused by obstruction of sweat glands by swelling of the keratin layer of the skin when water is absorbed at high skin temperatures.[1,32] The process can be readily reversed by moving the patient into a hot dry environment. Hyperthermia develops more readily in hot humid environments because of lack of effective evaporative cooling and hidromeiosis.

PRICKLY HEAT

This is a common problem in hot climates, causing considerable irritation and discomfort. It appears to occur more frequently in Caucasians with a fair complexion but is by no means restricted to this group. The condition arises from acute (miliaria rubra) or chronic (miliaria profunda) blockage of the sweat ducts, usually as a result of maceration of the stratum corneum. The pathogenesis therefore resembles that of hidromeiosis, but the sweat ducts become more permanently blocked by plugs of mucopolysaccharide debris and there is distension of the ducts by secreted sweat.[33] The rash of miliaria rubra is an erythematous epidermal vesicular eruption that is pruritic, and it is accompanied by a prickling or tingling sensation when sweating is provoked. Subsequently miliaria profunda may develop, characterized by dermal vesicles without erythema or pruritus. Secondary bacterial and fungal infections may occur.

Treatment consists of removing the patient to cool quarters if possible, to avoid sweating, and removing tight-fitting clothing. Prickling can be relieved by a cool shower, thorough drying of the skin and application of calamine lotion or zinc oxide powder. Mildly astringent lotions such as those containing mercuric chloride are useful, as are topical antimicrobial agents.

ANHIDROTIC HEAT EXHAUSTION

Impairment of sweating by miliaria profunda or other skin disorders may lead to a state of heat exhaustion affecting personnel exposed for several months to a hot climate. The condition may occur in humid heat or in desert climates. Dyshidrosis is probably a more accurate term to describe the sweat suppression since complete absence of sweating does not usually occur. Skin pathologies such as exfoliative dermatitis and other atrophic skin disorders are sometimes involved. Patients are unable to perform even small amounts of work without suffering undue fatigue and discomfort in the heat. Attempts to do so may precipitate other heat disorders, including heat stroke.

BODY FLUID IMBALANCE

WATER-DEPLETION HEAT EXHAUSTION

People working in hot conditions frequently do not completely replace the volume of water lost by sweating (voluntary dehydration) and usually maintain a slight negative water balance averaging 1 or 2% of total body weight. This minor degree of dehydration is sufficient to impair maximum physical performance. More serious degrees of dehydration may develop when water supplies are restricted, and yet though water depletion is thought to cause mild reductions in thermal sweating[4] high sweat rates appear to be maintained during the most extreme dehydration produced experimentally.[34] The classic situations producing water-depletion heat exhaustion have been described among castaways at sea in the tropics, travellers stranded in the desert and labourers and service personnel working hard in extreme heat when water supplies are inadequate. An accessory factor is often the additional loss of fluid by vomiting and diarrhoea.

Dehydration due predominantly to water depletion is characterized symptomatically by intense thirst, fatigue, weakness, anxiety and impaired judgement. Irritability and faintness appear as water loss approaches 6% of body weight.[4] Urine is scanty and concentrated. Extracellular fluid volume is diminished, with increasing osmolality, and water moves from the cells into the extracellular compartment. Haemoconcentration is marked and serum protein and sodium levels elevated. It is important to decide whether heat exhaustion is due mainly to water or salt depletion. The circumstances of onset are usually quite different. Sweat is hypotonic and a relatively far greater amount of water than salt is lost so that progressive water-depletion heat exhaustion is always more rapid in development than salt-depletion heat exhaustion. Differential diagnosis may be established by the symptoms and signs set out in Table 19.1.[4] In its severest form when heat exhaustion occurs in hot dehydrating desert conditions in individuals stranded without water, the situation may become rapidly fatal within a day. Studies by Adolph[34] of dehydration in the desert suggest that death is ultimately due to oligaemic shock and to heat stroke due to loss of thermoregulatory control.

Treatment consists of rest in cool surroundings with carefully controlled rehydration sufficient to ensure a net gain of 2–3 litres over the first 24 hours and 0.5–1 litre per day subsequently. Excessively rapid correction of hypernatraemia may cause cerebral oedema, convulsive seizures and death due to uncal herniation. Unconscious patients will require intravenous fluid replacement and if there is doubt

Table 19.1 Differential diagnosis of salt- and water-depletion heat exhaustion.

	Predominant salt depletion	Predominant water depletion
Duration of symptoms	3–5 days	Often much shorter
Thirst	Not prominent	Prominent
Fatigue	Marked	Less marked
Giddiness	Prominent	Less prominent
Muscle cramps	In most cases	Absent
Vomiting	In most cases	Usually absent
Thermal sweating	Probably unchanged	Diminished
Haemoconcentration	Early and marked	Slight until late
Urine chloride	Negligible amount	Normal
Urine concentration	Moderate	Pronounced
Blood sodium	Below average	Above average
Mode of death	Oligaemic shock	Oligaemic shock; heat stroke

whether the patient is predominantly water depleted or salt depleted, isotonic saline should be given; otherwise the fluid of choice is 5% glucose solution. Recovery is indicated by increased urine output but it is essential to avoid fluid overload if renal damage has occurred.

Salt-depletion heat exhaustion

Without extra salt unacclimatized people who have a naturally high salt content in sweat may lose enough salt to cause a negative balance during the first few days of heat exposure. Supplementation over and above a normal daily dietary intake of about 10 g sodium chloride is required if daily losses of 5 litres of sweat contain 3 g per litre. This is usually unnecessary in heat-acclimatized individuals since balance is gradually restored by the salt-conserving action of aldosterone on sweat glands[35] and salt concentration may reduce to about 1 g per litre. More severe salt depletion can occur in the absence of any salt replacement when water intake is high.[4]

The classical clinical and laboratory findings in human salt deficiency have been described by McCance.[36] Plasma volume is reduced, with haemoconcentration and a high blood urea. The concentration of sodium and chloride in urine is very low. Extracellular fluid osmolality is reduced, causing hypovolaemia and a shift of water into the intracellular compartment. Plasma sodium may sometimes be deceptively normal but the sodium and chloride content of whole blood is reduced. Fatigue, giddiness, nausea and muscle cramps are common clinical features. Anorexia, diarrhoea and vomiting reduce the already inadequate intake of salt and establish a vicious circle of events.[4] Thirst is not a feature, unlike water depletion. In contrast to predominant water depletion, salt depletion does not generally predispose rapidly to heat stroke.

Treatment is usually easier than for water depletion and consists of bed-rest in cool conditions with a high salt intake in the form of salted drinks. Salt should be added to cool fruit drinks (7 g per litre) and salty food encouraged to achieve an intake of up to 20 g daily. Complete clinical recovery occurs usually only after 5–7 days of rest and treatment and is accompanied by the consistent appearance of significant amounts of chloride in urine. For comatose patients, isotonic saline may be given intravenously at the rate of 2–4 litres during 12–24 hours. When extreme hyponatraemia causes symptoms of water intoxication, rarely is hypertonic saline indicated. It is important to examine neck veins and lung bases during treatment for signs of circulatory overloading.

HEAT STROKE

Heat stroke is a condition caused by excessive rise in body temperature brought about by overloading or failure of the thermoregulatory system. It is characterized primarily by hyperthermia with core temperature above 40.6°C, central nervous system dysfunction resulting from tissue damage, and by metabolic derangement and coma. It is the least common but most serious of heat disorders and it carries a high mortality rate if effective treatment is not given immediately.

Epidemiology

Heat stroke occurs during heat waves even in temperate regions. It is found that infants, the elderly and heart disease patients are most at risk in hot weather.[37–40] Heat stroke also occurs in physically active people, e.g. service personnel, marathon runners during prolonged exercise or those doing unaccustomed hard work in hot conditions.[41,42] Each year, a mass of people, currently about two million, gathers at Mecca to make the traditional seven day Hadj pilgrimage. There is high radiant heat and high ambient temperature, aggravated by many people assembled in a very restricted area. Many of the pilgrims suffer from heat disorders during the Hadj: over 1000 may be treated for heat stroke and some hundreds may die before reaching treatment centres.[43]

Precise statistics for morbidity and mortality are not available because of poor certification of the condition and the difficulty in defining the size and composition of the population at risk. In the South African gold mines, where the working population is homogeneous in its social background, heat stroke cases are reported at rates of 0.3 per 1000 per year in environments of 32°C WB and 4.0 per 1000 per year at 34.4°C WB.[17] During the Hadj in 1961 there was an incidence of 1.8 per 1000 in 0.27 million foreign pilgrims. Reported mortality ratios vary considerably, from 0 to 80%, but it is not always clear whether treated cases have been included.

Aetiology

Two types of heat stroke have been described:[44,45] (1) 'classical' heat stroke is associated with intolerably hot conditions or heat waves, without significant physical exertion, particularly in sick or elderly people; (2) 'exertional' heat stroke is generally observed in younger individuals generating high metabolic loads by exercise or physical work in the heat.

Table 19.2 Presentation of 'classical' and 'exertional' heat stroke.[46]

Feature	'Classical'	'Exertional'
Age group	Infants, elderly	15–65-years-old
Health status	Chronic illness	Usually healthy
History of febrile illness	Occasionally	Common
Activity	Sedentary	Usually highly active
Drug use	Diuretics, haloperidol, phenothiazines	Amphetamines, cocaine
Sweating	Usually absent	Usually present
Respiratory alkalosis	Dominant	Mild
Lactic acidosis	Absent or mild	Often marked
Rhabdomyolysis	Seldom severe	Severe
Hyperuricaemia	Modest	Severe
Creatinine phosphokinase/ aldolase	Mildly elevated	Markedly elevated
DIC	Mild	Marked
Hypoglycaemia	Uncommon	Common

Some differences between the two categories are given in Table 19.2, but there are common characteristics, e.g. hyperthermia, lack of acclimatization, dehydration, skin mottling and flushing, psychotic behaviour, convulsions, shock and coma.

Malignant hyperthermia leading to heat stroke is a rare and often fatal complication of general anaesthesia. In susceptible patients with familial myopathy, halothane anaesthesia typically produces sustained muscle contraction resulting in a rapid rise in body temperature. The biochemical basis appears to involve an abnormally large release of calcium into the myoplasm.[47]

Pathology

At about 42°C deep body temperature, hyperthermia causes denaturation of enzymes, liquefaction of membrane lipids, mitochondrial damage and destabilization of lipoproteins. The high temperature is primarily responsible for tissue damage, but cellular hypoxia, congestion, endotoxaemia and disseminated intravascular coagulation (DIC) are contributory.

Malamud and others[48] classically described the anatomical and histological changes found at autopsy. The meninges and brain are oedematous with petechial haemorrhages. Neuronal degeneration is particularly marked in the cerebellum. The predominance of alterations in cerebellar structures corresponds to the clinical picture of central nervous system damage in patients who survive severe heat stroke. These patients often show cerebellar ataxia with marked dysarthria, polyneuropathy or dysmetria.[49] Haemorrhages are also observed in serous cavities and in the heart, kidneys, liver and gastrointestinal mucosa. Mycocardial damage is common[50] and, characteristically, subendocardial haemorrhages occur beneath the left interventricular septum. Skeletal muscle may show necrosis if rhabdomyolysis has accompanied heat stroke. Liver damage is one of the most prominent features, with centrilobular fatty changes, congestion and degenerating hepatocytes resembling Councilman bodies. The kidneys are damaged and show hyperaemia and petechial haemorrhages. Deleterious effects in the blood include haemolysis, megakaryocyte damage, DIC with bleeding diatheses and widespread fibrin deposition. DIC contributes to both the bleeding manifestations and shock syndrome.[51]

Clinical features

In most cases of heat stroke the onset of delirium or coma is sudden but, in some, several days ill health precede the onset of coma and severe hyperthermia. With acute onset heat stroke, prodromal symptoms lasting minutes or hours include headache, disorientation, stupor, emotional outbursts, dizziness, excessive thirst and locomotor changes.

Central nervous system disturbances are typical presenting features. Often the patient is in coma with a rectal temperature of 40.6°C or more and there may be involuntary movements closely resembling epilepsy with tonic and clonic convulsions, and frequently urinary and faecal incontinence. Hyperpnoea with tetany is commonly observed.[30] Sweating is often present at the stage of collapse, particularly in young active heat stroke casualties.[52] Anhidrosis with a hot dry skin, contrary to some

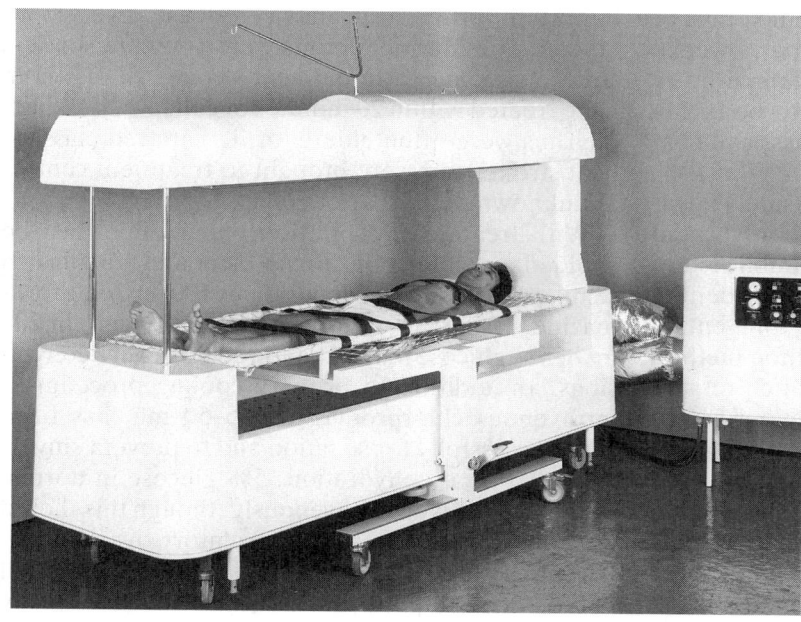

Figure 19.3 Body Cooling Unit for treatment of hyperthermia and heat stroke. (Photograph by courtesy of Guardian Medical Products.)

earlier accounts, cannot therefore be regarded as pathognomonic. On admission the patient's pulse is thready and the face flushed or cyanotic. In some cases, blood pressure and pulse pressure may be increased, whereas in others there is profound hypotension and shock. The electrocardiogram often shows flattened or inverted T waves, transient conduction abnormalities and myocardial damage.[4] Gastrointestinal haemorrhage with haematemesis or melaena can sometimes occur as manifestations of coagulopathy.

Diagnosis

Heat stroke can be suspected in any patient who loses consciousness under conditions of heat stress. The diagnosis is highly probable if body temperature is 40°C or above in the presence of clinical features described previously. Measurement of rectal temperature is crucial but is often difficult in a struggling patient. High-reading, metal-cased thermometers or electronic probes should be made available where heat stroke is a known risk.

Cooling measures are urgently required, leaving little time for exploring alternative diagnoses. The possibility of high fevers from other causes must, however, be kept under consideration. In the tropics, malaria is the most important differential diagnosis, for which appropriate treatment is urgently needed. High fevers from other causes such as meningitis, typhoid and arbovirus infection, encephalitis, bacterial pneumonia, septicaemia, tetanus and cerebral (pontine) haemorrhage are also to be considered. It is important to examine the skull

for signs of injury which may have occurred during convulsions.

Laboratory findings include leucocytosis and thrombocytopenia. Changes in the plasma concentration of sodium, chloride and potassium are not consistent, though hypokalaemia has been frequently observed in acute heat stroke.[46,53] Serum glutamic oxaloacetic transaminase, serum glutamic pyruvic transaminase, lactic dehydrogenase and creatine phosphokinase are usually elevated within 24 hours of admission. The levels continue to rise for about 2 days and remain elevated for 12–14 days. Serum enzyme changes are of diagnostic and prognostic significance.[54] Severe renal involvement with rising urea nitrogen is evident in many fatal cases.

Treatment

In the field situation, the patient should be placed in the shade, clothing removed and the skin kept wet and fanned. An effective degree of conductive cooling can be obtained simply by immersing the patient in a bath of cold water or water and ice, and the body and limbs massaged vigorously to promote skin circulation. In hospital, the patient may be placed on a slatted trolley, exposing the skin to good air movement from an electric fan and a fine spray of water. Alternatively, the patient can be cooled by tepid water sponging or by wrapping in a wet sheet and fanning.

The need to avoid vasoconstriction during cooling and yet enable the management of a violent, delirious, incontinent and vomiting patient has led to the development of a Body Cooling Unit (BCU) to treat heat stroke[55,56] (Figure 19.3). This method utilizes evaporative and convective cooling from sprays of atomized water at 20°C combined with a powerful flow of air at 50°C to maintain skin temperature above 31–32°C. The BCU has proved to be highly satisfactory in the management of classical heat stroke patients among the hadj pilgrims.[43]

Ice water immersion is a simple and usually available form of treatment which has been advocated since the first edition of textbook was published in 1898.[57] The method, however, appears to deny a critical principle of heat dissipation by preventing cutaneous vasodilatation. In defence of the method it has been suggested that the hydrostatic pressure of water during immersion increases venous return to the heart in hypotensive patients and that pathological, rather than physiological vasomotor responses occur, such that the body–shell insulative barrier may not be significant at the onset of heat stroke.[58] Furthermore, it is reported that there have been no deaths during the treatment by ice water immersion of 252 heat stroke cases in Marine Corps recruits in the last 15 years. Though a mean mortality of 12.1% using the BCU was observed in Hadj pilgrims in 1982,[43] there are obviously

important differences between these two populations. The Marine recruits were young fit soldiers suffering from exertional heat stroke, all of whom were treated within 20 minutes of collapse. The hadj pilgrims were often elderly or ill, suffered classical heat stroke, and were brought to treatment centres at unknown periods after collapse.

With treatment, aspiration pneumonia must be avoided by keeping the airway clear and nursing in a semilateral position. Meperidine, 100 mg, chlorpromazine, 100 mg, and promethazine, 100 mg, in 200 ml of 5% glucose may be required for severe convulsions. In addition to primary cooling procedures, intravenous chlorpromazine, 25–50 mg, has been used successfully for sedation and to prevent shivering.[43] To treat dehydration, 5% glucose in normal saline can be given intravenously, though this should be done with care to avoid circulatory overloading. Oxygen should be given while danger to the central nervous system persists. DIC has been successfully treated with heparin,[59] though fresh plasma provides a safer alternative. Dextran should be avoided since it may impair platelet function.

PREVENTION OF HEAT DISORDERS

Prevention of the ill effects of heat stress entails, for doctors working in the tropics, in industry, ships and other places where the risk occurs, knowledge of the technique for measuring heat stress (e.g. the use of the WBGT index for assessing heat stress and heat tolerance times),[24] and the factors relating to work or rest in these conditions. The predictions concerning global environmental changes warn that the temperate regions of the world may come to experience the health hazards of environmental heat stress more frequently.[60] Migrants and individuals moving into hot regions or those working in hot industries require supervision and advice on the effects of high temperatures. Prevention of the ill effects broadly involves the control of human activities in outdoor heat and reduction of indoor heat loads by control measures so that temperatures are brought within recognized safety limits. It is essential to have a

prepared treatment centre where cooling can be given at once to any patient in need.

Special care is required when conditions are hostile, when escape from hot conditions is difficult or when water is in short supply. Due attention must therefore be paid to the provision of adequate potable water supplies, suitable clothing and thermally comfortable living quarters. Supplemental salt may be necessary, particularly for unacclimatized persons. Large, heavy meals and excess alcohol, especially during the hottest part of the day, are to be avoided. Successful prevention is often the result of careful selection and continuous medical screening of heat-exposed personnel and, if possible, artificial acclimatization to heat beforehand. Regular exercise helps to provide a degree of heat acclimatization.

REFERENCES

1 Kerslake D McK. *The Stress of Hot Environments.* Cambridge: Cambridge University Press, 1972.

2 Collins K J & Weiner J S. Endocrinological aspects of exposure to high environmental temperatures. *Physiol Rev* 1968; 48:785–839.

3 Rowell L B. Cardiovascular aspects of human thermoregulation. *Circ Res* 1983; 52:367–379.

4 Leithead C S & Lind A R. *Heat Stress and Heat Disorders.* London: Cassell, 1964.

5 Clark R P & Edholm O G. *Man and his Thermal Environment.* London: Edward Arnold, 1985.

6 Collins K J. Regulation of body temperature. In Tinker J & Zapol W M (eds) *Care of the Critically Ill Patient,* 2nd edn. Berlin: Springer, 1992:155–173.

7 Benzinger T H. Mechanisms of human thermoregulation. In Khogali M & Hales J R S (eds) *Heat Stroke and Temperature Regulation.* New York: Academic Press, 1983:53–64.

8 Hensel H. *Thermoreception and Temperature Regulation.* New York: Academic Press, 1981.

9 Bligh J. Basic concepts and applied aspects of body temperature regulation. In Khogali M & Hales J R S (eds) *Heat Stroke and Temperature Regulation.* New York: Academic Press, 1983:41–52.

10 Cabanac M & Caputa M. Natural selective cooling of the human brain: evidence of its occurrence and magnitude. *J Physiol (Lond)* 1979; 286:255–264.

11 Lind J. *An Essay on Diseases Incidental to Europeans in Hot Climates.* London: T. Becket, 1768.

12 Bass D E, Kleeman C R, Quinn M, Henschel A & Hegnauer A H. Mechanisms of acclimatization to heat in man. *Medicine* 1955; 34:323–380.

13 Collins K J, Crockford G W & Weiner J S. Sweat-gland training by drugs and thermal stress. *Arch Environ Health* 1965; 11:407–422.

14 Streeten D H P, Conn J W, Louis L W et al. Secondary aldosteronism: metabolic and adrenocortical responses of normal men to high environmental temperatures. *Metabolism* 1960; 9:1071–1092.

15 Bass, D E & Henschel A. Responses of body fluid compartments to heat and cold. *Physiol Rev* 1956; 36:128–144.

16 Lind A R & Bass D E. The optimal exposure time for the development of acclimatization to heat. *Fed Proc* 1963; 22:704–706.

17 Wyndham C H. A survey of the causal factors in heat stroke and of their prevention in the gold mining industry. *J S Afr Inst Min Metall* 1965; 66:125–155.

18 International Standards Organization. *Hot Environments: Estimation of the Heat Stress on Working Man, Based on the WBGT Index (Wet Bulb Globe Temperature),* ISO 7243. Geneva: ISO, 1989.

19 Belding H S. *Engineering Approach to Analysis and Control of Heat Exposure.* New York: Academic Press, 1972.

20 Macpherson R K. *Physiological Responses to Hot Environments,* MRC Special Report No. 298. London: HMSO, 1960.

21 International Standards Organization. *Hot Environments: Analytical Determination and Interpretation of Thermal Stress using Calculation of Required Sweat Rate,* ISO 7933 . Geneva: ISO, 1989.

22 Minard D, Belding H S & Kingston J R. Prevention of heat casualties. *JAMA* 1957; 165:1813–1818.

23 Shapiro Y & Seidman D S. Field and clinical observations of exertional heat stroke patients. *Med Sci Sports Exerc* 1990; 22:6–14.

24 British Occupational Hygiene Society. *The Thermal Environment,* Technical Guide No. 8. Leeds: Science Reviews, 1990.

25 Wissler E H. A review of human thermal models. In Mekjavic I B, Bannister E W & Morrison J B (eds) *Environmental Ergonomics.* London: Taylor & Francis, 1988: 267–285.

26 Pepler R D. Psychological effects of heat. In Leithead C S & Lind A R (eds) *Heat Stress and Heat Disorders.* London: Cassell, 1964: 237–253.

27 Bannister R G. Anhidrosis following bacterial pyrogen. *Lancet* 1960; ii:118–122.

28 Veale W L, Ruwe W & Cooper K E. Mechanism of fever and antipyresis. In Khogali M & Hales J R S (eds) *Heat Stroke and Temperature Regulation.* New York: Academic Press, 1983: 79–97.

29 Lomax P & Schonbaum E. *Body Temperature Regulation: Drug Effects and Therapeutic Implications.* New York: Marcel Dekker, 1979.

30 Iampietro P F. Heat-induced tetany. *Fed Proc* 1963; 22:884–886.

31 Sprung C L, Portocarrero C J, Fernanine A V et al. The metabolic and respiratory alterations of heat stroke. *Arch Intern Med* 1980; 140:665–669.

32 Collins K J & Weiner J S. Observations on arm-bag suppression of sweating and its relationship to thermal sweat-gland 'fatigue'. *J Physiol* (Lond) 1962; 161:538–556.

33 O'Brien J P. A study of miliaria rubra, tropical anhidrosis and anhidrotic asthenia. *Br J Dermatol* 1947; 59:125–158.

34 Adolph E F. *Physiology of Man in the Desert.* New York: Interscience, 1947.

35 Collins K J. The action of exogenous aldosterone on the secretion and composition of drug-induced sweat. *Clin Sci* 1966; 30:207–221.

36 McCance R A. Experimental sodium chloride deficiency in man. *Proc R Soc* Lond [Biol] 1936; 119:245–268.

37 Ellis F P. Heat Illness. I. Epidemiology. *Trans R Soc Trop Med Hyg* 1976; 70:402–411.

38 Ellis F P. Heat illness. II. Pathogenesis. *Trans R Soc Trop Med Hyg* 1976; 70:412–418.

39 Ellis F P. Heat illness. III. Acclimatization. *Trans R Soc Trop Med Hyg* 1976; 70:419–425.

40 Kilbourne E M, Choi K, Jones S & Thacker S B. Risk factors for heat stroke. *JAMA* 1982; 247:332–336.

41 Sutton J R & Bar-Or O. Thermal illness in fun running. *Am Heart J* 1980; 100:778–781.

42 Jardon O. Physiologic stress, heat stroke and malignant hyperthermia: a perspective. *Milit Med* 1982; 147:8–14.

43 Khogali M & Hales J R S. *Heat Stroke and Temperature Regulation.* New York: Academic Press, 1983.

44 Knochel J P. Environmental heat illness. *Arch Intern Med* 1974; 133:841–864.

45 Shibolet S, Lancaster M C & Danon Y. Heat stroke: a review. *Aviat Space Environ Med* 1976; 47:280–301.

46 Knochel J P. Heat stroke and related heat disorders. *Dis Mon* 1989; 35:301–377.

47 Moulds R F W & Denborough M A. Biochemical basis of malignant hyperpyrexia. *BMJ* 1974; ii:241–244.

48 Malamud N, Haymaker W & Cluster R P. Heatstroke: a clinico-pathologic study of 125 fatal cases. *Milit Surg* 1946; 99:397–449.

49 Mehta A C & Baker R N. Persistent neurological deficits in heat stroke. *Neurology* (*NY*) 1970; 20:336–340.

50 Kew M C, Tucker B K, Bersohn I & Seftel H C. The heart in heat stroke. *Am Heart J* 1969; 77:324–335.

51 Mustafa M K Y, Khogali M, Gumaa K & Al Nasr N M A. Disseminated intravascular coagulation among heat stroke cases. In Khogali M & Hales J R S (eds) *Heat Stroke and Temperature Regulation*. New York: Academic Press, 1983: 109–117.

52 Hubbard R W. The role of exercise in the etiology of exertional heat stroke. *Med Sci Sports Exerc* 1990; 22:2–5.

53 Austin M G & Berry J W. Observations on one hundred cases of heat stroke. *JAMA* 1956; 101:1525–1529.

54 Kew M, Bersohn H & Seftel H. The diagnostic and prognostic significance of the serum enzyme changes in heat stroke. *Trans R Soc Trop Med Hyg* 1971; 65:325–330.

55 Weiner J S & Khogali M. A physiological body cooling unit for treatment of heat stroke. *Lancet* 1980; i:507–508.

56 Khogali M & Weiner J S. Heat stroke: report on 19 cases. *Lancet* 1980; ii:276–278.

57 Manson P. *Tropical Diseases*. London: Cassell, 1898: 211–213.

58 Costrini A. Emergency treatment of exertional heat stroke and comparison with whole body cooling techniques. *Med Sci Sports Exerc* 1990; 22:15–18.

59 Weber M B & Blakely J A. The haemorrhagic diathesis of heat stroke: a consumptive coagulopathy successfully treated with heparin. *Lancet* 1969; i: 1190–1192.

60 World Health Organization. *Potential Health Effects of Climatic Change,* Report of a WHO Task Group. Geneva: WHO, 1989.

CHAPTER 20

HIGH ALTITUDE PROBLEMS

J. G. Dickinson

Although problems of high altitude were traditionally considered in terms of mountaineering (Figures 20.1 and 20.2) and exploration, they are now of importance in a wide variety of leisure pursuits, including skiing, mountain marathon running, canoeing on high-altitude rivers, mountain cycling, hang gliding, ballooning and diving into high-altitude lakes. They are also of military importance: in 1963 Indian Army troops were rushed by air to a high airfield in Ladakh where they were to face well-acclimatized Chinese troops who had crossed the Tibetan plateau on foot. This generated the largest series of cases of acute mountain sickness (AMS) in one paper: 1925 cases reported by Singh et al[1] in 1969. More recently, the US Marine Corps was involved in a training exercise at only 2000–2600 m and found that nine out of 624 soldiers were affected.[2] In addition to acute problems, chronic mountain sickness has long been known and subacute forms have recently been described. Extra precautions at high altitude may be necessary for patients with a number of general medical conditions.

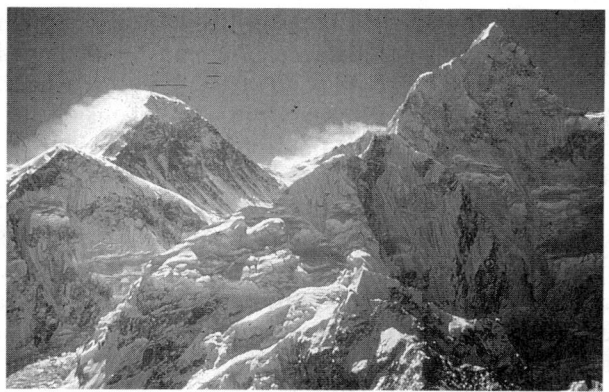

Figure 20.1 Mount Everest (left of centre) attracts thousands of trekkers every year, as well as mountaineers.

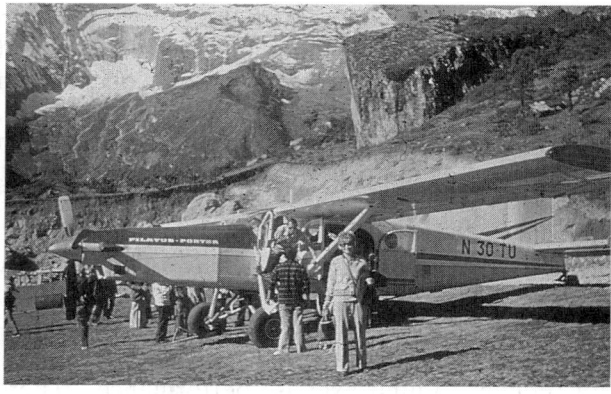

Figure 20.2 The 'vector of acute mountain sickness' can take unacclimatized visitors to over 4000 m.

PHYSIOLOGY OF HIGH ALTITUDE

Ascent to high altitude gives exposure to reducing levels of barometric pressure. Though the *percentage* of oxygen is constant throughout the atmosphere, the *partial pressure* falls in proportion to barometric pressure. As Po_2 falls to levels corresponding to the steep part of the oxygen dissociation curve of haemoglobin, desaturation occurs. This stimulates ventilation which is then driven by hypoxaemia in place of the normal stimulus, hypercapnia. However, the increased ventilation modifies itself by an additional negative feedback mechanism: it leads to low Pco_2 levels, which provide a brake that limits the ventilatory response in the first few days. During this time the kidneys partially correct the respiratory alkalosis, gradually reducing the inhibitory effect on ventilation, which can then increase

Table 20.1 Some measurements on the summit of Everest (after ref. 4).

| | Summit, 8848 m | | Sea level | |
	mmHg	kPa	mmHg	kPa
Barometric pressure	253	33.7	760	101.3
Alveolar Po_2	35	4.7	149	19.9
Arterial Po_2	28	3.7	95	12.7
Arterial Pco_2	7.5	1.0	40	5.3
pH	>7.7	—	7.4	—
Base excess (mmol/l)	−7.2	—	—	—
Haemoglobin (g/dl)	18.4	—	15	—

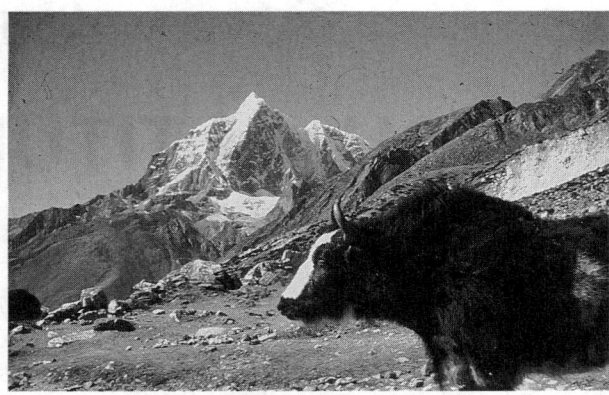

Figure 20.3 The yak: adapted to high altitude in having no pulmonary arteriolar constriction in response to hypoxia.[6]

further.[3] This process is known as ventilatory acclimatization. The degree to which these changes may occur is illustrated by measurements[4] carried out on a single subject at the summit of Mount Everest, 8848 m (Table 20.1). These findings would be alarming at sea level.

Changes take place in the red cells, producing an increased level of 2,3-diphosphoglycerate which shifts the oxygen dissociation curve for haemoglobin to the right. This counteracts the left shift due to alkalosis and low Pco_2 but, as it favours unloading of oxygen in the tissues only at the expense of uptake in the lungs, it is of doubtful benefit.[5]

In the lungs, pulmonary arteriolar constriction takes place, leading to pulmonary hypertension. This response, which at sea level assists in the matching of ventilation and perfusion, is inappropriate at high altitude, where all alveoli are equally hypoxic. It does not occur in animals adapted to high altitude, such as the yak (Figure 20.3).[6] The circulation generally performs well at high altitude and is not thought to limit exercise performance.[7] There are changes in the distribution of body fluids.[8,9] Diuresis, shift of water from the vascular to the extravascular space and a further shift from the

extracellular to the intracellular space combine to produce haemoconcentration. The packed cell volume of blood therefore rises early, even though the marrow response takes much longer. There is an advantage in that more oxygen is carried per unit of blood, but increased blood viscosity leads to an increase in cardiac work and increased risk of thrombosis. In the case of long-term exposure to high altitude, erythropoietin secretion leads to increased bone marrow activity and true polycythaemia. When combined with pulmonary hypertension this can lead to the cardiac failure of chronic mountain sickness.

Hormonal changes at altitude have been extensively studied and some will be mentioned later. It is difficult to know the extent to which results are compounded by other physiological stresses, such as cold and exercise, and to distinguish physiological from pathological responses.

Sleep at high altitude shows characteristic changes.[10] Periodic respiration is usual, leading to marked swings of arterial Po_2. Sleep is then disturbed and unrefreshing.

ACUTE MOUNTAIN SICKNESS (AMS)

A complex of clinical conditions occurs in the first few days of exposure to high altitude. Table 20.2 compares three different systems of classification and terminology. That of Ravenhill (1913)[11] was the result of remarkably accurate observations on Peruvian miners. The one that the author proposed in 1982[12] was an attempt to improve one then in common use in order to help non-medical climbers to recognize serious diseases and to open medical

minds to pathophysiological processes other than oedema. However, a version of the older system has now been accepted by the Lake Louise Consensus,[13] which is certainly the body best fitted to make judgements.

All these conditions are more likely to occur in those who ascend fast, especially by vehicle or plane, and in general the prevalence is proportional to the altitude reached. A recent prevalence study[14]

Table 20.2 Systems of classification and terminology.

Ravenhill[11] *1913*	*Dickinson*[12] *1982*	*Lake Louise* *Consensus*[13] *1992*
Normal puna*	Benign acute mountain sickness. Malignant acute mountain sickness	Acute mountain sickness (AMS)
Cardiac puna	(a) Pulmonary acute mountain sickness	High altitude pulmonary oedema (HAPO, HAPE)
Nervous puna	(b) Cerebral acute mountain sickness	High altitude cerebral oedema (HACO, HACE)
	(c) Mixed pulmonary and cerebral forms	

'Puna' is the local Peruvian name for mountain sickness.
High-altitude retinal haemorrhage and high-altitude subcutaneous oedema are features that may occur with or without other signs and symptoms.

has shown, for example, benign AMS features in 9% at 2850 m, 13% at 3050 m, 34% at 3650 m and 53% at 4599 m. Several other studies have given similar results. It is important to realize that severe, even fatal, AMS can occur at altitudes between 2000 and 3000 m, that is below 9000 feet. Although benign AMS may precede malignant AMS, and provide a useful warning, malignant AMS may occur without such warning.

BENIGN AMS

Symptoms include headache, anorexia, nausea, vomiting, disturbed sleep and a feeling of discomfort in the chest. Findings that may be associated are retinal haemorrhages (Figure 20.4), which can be seen in asymptomatic people at high altitude and are of no significance unless they lie over the macula,

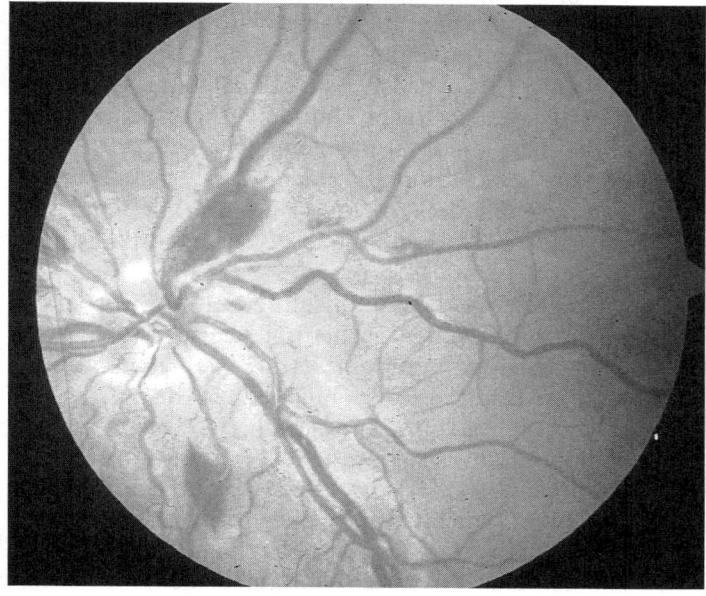

Figure 20.4   Retinal haemorrhages: not necessarily associated with other features of mountain sickness.

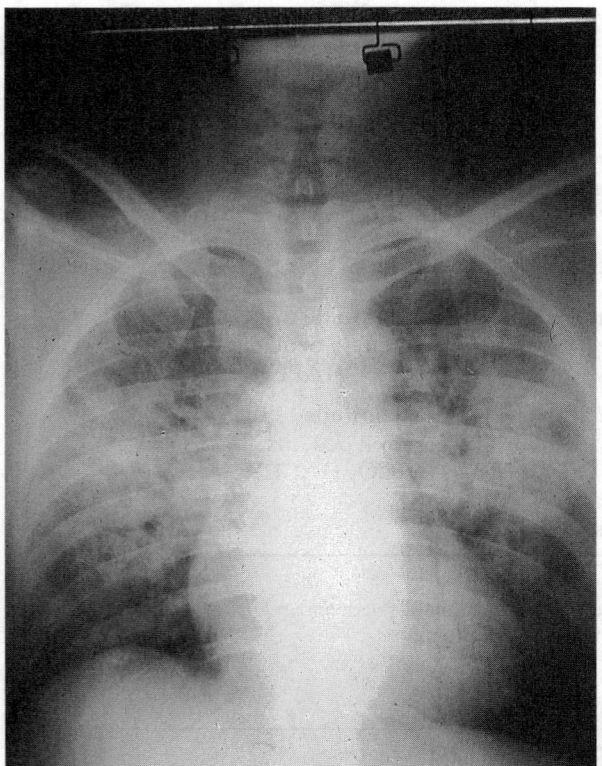

Figure 20.5   Bilateral shadowing in pulmonary AMS.

and subcutaneous oedema, which seems more common in women and is harmless in itself.

Symptoms usually resolve after a few hours or days of rest and treatment is not essential. There has been demonstrable improvement since treatment was with acetazolamide or dexamethasone, and climbers may continue to ascend cautiously after they have recovered.

PULMONARY AMS

The main symptom is breathlessness at rest and there may be a cough. Basal crepitations, tachycardia and increased cyanosis may be found. A chest radiograph shows pulmonary oedema (Figure 20.5), which may be unilateral; oedema is confirmed at autopsy.[15] This is often associated with thrombosis in pulmonary vessels and sometimes with an inflammatory exudate which may represent secondary infection.[16,17]

Studies have failed to demonstrate any elevation of left atrial or pulmonary wedge pressure[18] and bronchopulmonary lavage has shown the fluid to have a low protein content, suggesting that the oedema is due to increased capillary permeability.[19]

CEREBRAL AMS

The onset of this is frequently at night, when arterial desaturation is most severe. Common presentations are ataxia, headache, abnormal behaviour and drowsiness, which may slip rapidly into coma. Papilloedema is often, but not always, present and there may be a variety of other neurological signs, including paresis.[17,20] At autopsy, brain oedema is usual and there are frequently both haemorrhages and thromboses.[16,17]

MIXED PULMONARY AND CEREBRAL AMS

This is the most common clinical pattern in the 'malignant' group, occurring for example in 33 of 50 victims (66%).[17] Pure cerebral AMS occurred in 22% and pure pulmonary AMS in only 12%. However, this was a series studied following evacuation; pulmonary AMS responds more rapidly to evacuation to lower altitude and may have been underrepresented. It seems likely that the additional desaturation caused by pulmonary oedema predisposes to the development of added cerebral AMS.

TREATMENT

Victims of benign AMS may remain at the altitude of onset in the expectation of likely recovery and may then continue to ascend with caution. If they show no improvement, or deteriorate, they must descend. However, all cases of malignant AMS must be evacuated to lower altitude without delay, overcoming all logistical problems (Figure 20.6). Helicopter evacuation is ideal but may involve unacceptable delay. If drugs are used they must be regarded only as an adjunct to the essential step of urgent descent.

Oxygen may be administered but rarely produces much improvement. This is because it is hard to provide, in a mountain setting, sufficient flow to increase inspired Po_2 significantly in the presence of a very high level of ventilation. Use of a pressure chamber to restore the ambient barometric pressure towards normal is an effective but cumbersome treatment which is rarely available on a mountain. The Gamow bag is a portable chamber that can be supplemented by a self-contained life support sys-

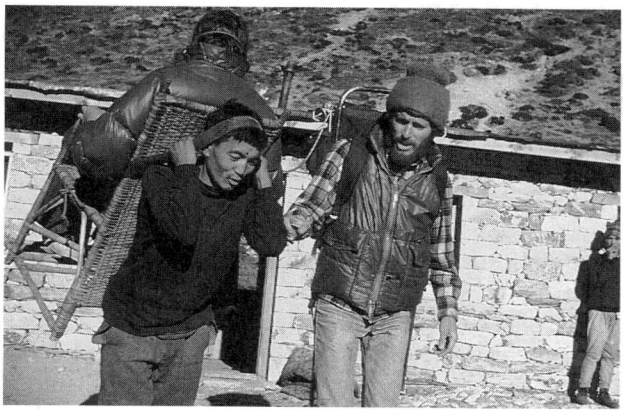

Figure 20.6 Early evacuation is the essence of management of malignant AMS; oxygen is less important.

tem[21] and can provide emergency care on remote expeditions. It is quite costly.

Acetazolamide can relieve symptoms in benign AMS.[22] It probably acts by correcting alkalosis and therefore stimulating ventilation, but it is not clear if this is entirely as a result of its effect on renal carbonic anhydrase or whether it also has an effect on the brain. There is some evidence that benzolamide, a selective renal carbonic anhydrase inhibitor, has an equivalent effect.[23]

Dexamethasone may also be useful in the treatment of benign AMS and mild cerebral AMS.[24–26] Its action may be to impair prostaglandin synthesis, reducing mediators of inflammation and thus reducing capillary permeability.[27]

Nifedipine, a calcium antagonist, seems to benefit victims of pulmonary AMS,[28] possibly by reducing pulmonary artery pressure, but it may also act on mediator release in the lungs.[29]

Although rebreathing of carbon dioxide was thought to be beneficial in one study,[30] this has since been refuted.[31] This demonstrates the difficulty of therapeutic trials in these conditions.

PREVENTION

It is not possible to identify susceptible individuals accurately before exposure to high altitude, though climbers who have previously suffered from AMS are more likely to suffer on future ascents. To prevent sickness and fatality it is therefore necessary to plan all ascents to high altitude with care. Those involved, and especially those in charge, should be familiar with the risk(s) and should plan

accordingly. Exact rates of ascent will depend on the terrain and facilities, but, in general, overall daily altitude gain above 3000 m should be no more than 300–350 m, and above 5000 m it should be no more than 200 m. This appears restrictive to many expeditions but is mitigated by the fact that higher altitudes may be reached during the daytime if the climbers return to lower altitudes to sleep, and adopt the 'climb high, sleep low' policy. So called 'rest days' also assist acclimatization; during these days, climbers go as high as they wish, but must return to the previous night's altitude to sleep. In order to minimize the risk of malignant mountain sickness, climbers who are experiencing symptoms of benign AMS should not climb any higher until they have recovered, as already mentioned. As this may require dividing a party, such a contingency must be considered in planning. Because of the variation in susceptibility even these precautions will not prevent certain individuals from developing malignant AMS, so evacuation routes and methods must always be considered in the planning of an ascent.

On the subject of drug prophylaxis, agreement is far from complete.[32] Acetazolamide has been known for some years to reduce or prevent benign AMS symptoms.[33,34] Because it reduces periodic respiration, it improves sleep quality. The small diuretic effect is probably of no value, and although the drug increases cerebral blood flow this is probably not a therapeutic action.[35] A dose of 250 mg 8-hourly seems to be sufficient, but even this may cause troublesome paraesthesiae which may themselves cause disturbance of sleep. There are no firm grounds for believing that the drug prevents malignant AMS and, indeed, there have been severe cases including death in climbers taking it.[36,37]

Studies of prophylaxis with dexamethasone,[38,39] using 4 mg 8- or 12-hourly, have also shown a reduction of symptoms with few side-effects in the short term other than mild hyperglycaemia. It may be that mild degrees of cerebral mountain sickness are also prevented, but, as with acetazolamide, cerebral and pulmonary AMS may occur.[37] Theoretically either drug may increase the risk of malignant AMS by suppressing warning symptoms.

Although there is considerable pressure to prescribe one or other of these drugs for groups and individuals going to high altitudes, the author's personal preference is not to do so routinely, but to concentrate on sensible rates of ascent and good planning. Drug prophylaxis can then be used for essential high-risk ascents such as rescue missions.

PATHOPHYSIOLOGY

Many basic details of the causation of AMS remain to be elucidated. Hypoxia and to a lesser extent hypobaria are the probable root causes, but individual idiosyncracy seems important, at least in determining which people will suffer at relatively low altitudes. It seems likely that susceptible individuals are either limited in their physiological response to hypoxia, or produce a response that is harmful in itself. There is reasonable evidence that they retain more water at high altitude,[1,40] and attempts have been made to correlate this with hormone changes, especially aldosterone and atrial natriuretic peptide.[40-42]

Those who are susceptible probably have a blunted ventilatory response to hypoxia which, although it makes physiological sense, is curious because studies have shown that Sherpas and elite mountaineers also have blunted responses, whereas they might be expected to respond briskly.[43]

Many ingenious theories have been developed to explain pulmonary oedema at high altitude. The final explanation may turn out to be a combination of high pulmonary artery pressure, patchy flow, and increased permeability due to mediator release.[29]

Cerebral oedema is certainly present in most cases of cerebral AMS that come to autopsy but, as we have seen, thromboses and haemorrhages are also common. They could result from the effects of haemoconcentration due to hypoxia and dehydration, but it is also possible that thrombus forms in relation to microbubbles of inert gas released as a result of decompression due to hypobaria. There is some evidence that neurotransmitter release might be impaired by hypoxia, interfering with neural function.[44,45]

The cause of cerebral oedema is not clear. It does not appear to be a function of cerebral blood flow, though the latter does increase markedly at altitude. It is tempting to ascribe it to a depression of the sodium–potassium pump at the neural cell surface, but there is no proof of this. Another interesting hypothesis[46] resembles one of the possible mechanisms for lung oedema: the fully dilated cerebral capillaries may be exposed to surges of blood pressure, especially at night when transient hypertension occurs in response to arterial desaturation. This could lead to fluid exudation. Mediators of inflammation may also play a part.

It is commonly believed, but not proven, that benign AMS simply represents early cerebral oedema, and the beneficial effects of dexamethasone are adduced to support this. However, it seems best to keep an open mind on this matter.

CHRONIC MOUNTAIN SICKNESS

First described by Professor Carlos Monge in Peru in 1928,[47] this condition occurs in long-term residents at high altitude in the Andes. It is almost unknown in Nepal, but has recently been described in Tibet, affecting the immigrant Han population rather than the indigenous Tibetans. Features include neuro-psychiatric symptoms, marked polycythaemia, cyanosis, finger clubbing, pulmonary hypertension, and cardiac failure. These features improve dramatically during a period of residence at low altitude, only to reappear when the patient returns to the mountain(s).

SUBACUTE MOUNTAIN SICKNESS

The influx of Han people to Lhasa in Tibet revealed a subacute infantile form of AMS in babies born at high altitude[48] which is frequently fatal. This appears much closer than Monge's disease to the so-called brisket disease of cattle taken to high altitude. A rather similar condition has since been described in adults by an Indian group studying soldiers evacuated after residence at over 6000 m for up to 6 months.[49]

The epidemiology of these conditions raises fascinating questions as to the physiological characteristics of ethnic groups such as the Sherpas and Tibetans that seem resistant to them, showing adaptation to high altitude rather than mere acclimatiz ation. The absence of pulmonary arteriolar reac-

tivity and muscularization may be important factors.[50]

OTHER CONDITIONS

Doctors are sometimes asked to advise patients with pre-existing medical conditions who wish to go to high altitude. It is important to consider how high they intend to go, the rate and means of getting there and the degree of exertion that will be required. Clearly exertion at high altitude creates greater demands on the oxygen delivery systems, lungs, heart and circulation, than does equivalent activity at sea level. Patients with chronic respiratory or cardiac failure are best advised to remain below 3000 m and to limit physical activity even above 2000 m. Hypoxaemia clearly increases the severity of angina and could lead to cardiac failure in persons with ischaemic or other myocardial disease. Anaemia combined with hypoxaemia may lead to tissue hypoxia.

Asthmatics generally perform reasonably well at high altitude as air pollution is minimal and allergens few, though attacks can be precipitated by exertion or cold. An asthmatic who is able to be physically active at sea level is probably fit for high altitude, whereas one with exercise limitation all the time at sea level might be at risk.

Black people with sickle cell disease or trait, or with haemoglobin SC disease are at risk of crises as a result of deformity of the red cells due to hypoxia at high altitude. Whereas homozygotes are generally well informed about such risks, such crises may come as an unpleasant surprise to heterozygotes.

Much remains to be learned about the mechanisms of human response to high altitude, but the message to the average traveller[51] is simple: 'Be well informed, plan carefully, do not go too high too fast and be prepared to come down if you feel unwell.'

REFERENCES

1 Singh I, Khanna P L, Srivastava M C et al. Acute mountain sickness. *N Engl Med J* 1969; 280:175–184.
2 Pigman E C & Karakla D W. Acute mountain sickness at intermediate altitudes: military mountainous training. *Am J Emerg Med* 1990; 8:7–10.
3 Rahn O & Otis A B. Man's respiratory response during and after acclimatization to high altitude. *Am J Physiol* 1949; 157:445–462.
4 West J B. Climbing Everest without oxygen: an analysis of maximal exercise during excessive hypoxia. *Respir Physiol* 1983; 52:265–279.
5 Winslow R M, Samaja M & West J B. Red cell function at extreme altitude on Mount Everest. *J Appl Physiol* 1984; 56:109–116.
6 Heath D, Williams D R & Dickinson J G. The pulmonary arteries of the yak. *Cardiovasc Res* 1984; 18:133–139.
7 Reeves J T, Groves B M, Sutton J R et al. Operation Everest II: preservation of cardiac function at extreme altitude. *J Appl Physiol* 1987; 63:137–142.
8 Hannon J P, Chinn K S K & Shields J L. Alterations in serum and extracellular electrolytes during high altitude exposure. *J Appl Physiol* 1971; 31:266–273.
9 Hannon J P, Chinn K S K & Shields J L. Effect of acute high altitude exposure on body fluids. *Fed Proc* 1969; 28:1178–1184.
10 Weil J V, Kryger M H & Scoggin C H. Sleep and breathing at high altitude. In Guilleminault C & Dement W C (eds) *Sleep Apnea Syndromes*. New York: Alan R Liss, 1978: 119–136.
11 Ravenhill T H. Some experiences of acute mountain sickness in the Andes. *J Trop Med Hyg* 1913; 20:313–320.
12 Dickinson J G. Terminology of acute mountain sickness. *BMJ* 1982; 2:720–721.
13 Sutton J R, Coates G & Houston C S (eds). Lake Louise Consensus. In *Hypoxia and Mountain Medicine*. Burlington, VT: Queen City Press, 1992.
14 Maggiorini M, Buhler B, Walter M et al. Prevalence of acute mountain sickness in the Swiss Alps. *BMJ* 1990; 301:853–855.
15 Nayak N C, Roy S & Narayanan T K. Pathologic features of altitude sickness. *Am J Pathol* 1974; 45:381–391.

16 Dickinson J G, Heath D, Williams D R & Gosney J. Altitude-related deaths in seven trekkers in the Himalayas. *Thorax* 1983; 38:646–656.

17 Dickinson J G. *Acute mountain sickness*. DM Thesis, University of Oxford, 1981: 22.

18 Peneloza D & Sime F. Circulatory dynamics during high altitude pulmonary oedema. *Am J Cardiol* 1969; 23:369.

19 Schoene R B, Hackett P H, Henderson W R et al. High altitude pulmonary oedema. Characteristics of lung lavage fluid. *JAMA* 1986; 256:63–69.

20 Houston C S & Dickinson J G. High altitude illness: a cerebral form. *Lancet* 1975; 2:758–761.

21 Kasic J F, Smith H M & Gamow R I. A self-contained life support system designed for use with a portable hyperbaric chamber. *Biomed Sci Instrum* 1989; 25:79–81.

22 Bradwell A R, Winterborn M, Wright A D et al. Acetazolamide treatment of acute mountain sickness. *Clin Sci* 1988; 74(supplement 18): 62P.

23 Swenson E R, Leatham K L, Roach R C et al. Renal carbonic anhydrase inhibition reduces high altitude sleep periodic breathing. *Resp Physiol* 1991; 86:333–343.

24 Ferrazini M, Maggiorini M, Kriemler S et al. Successful treatment of acute mountain sickness with dexamethasone. *BMJ* 1987; 294:1380–1382.

25 Hackett P H, Roach R C, Wood R A et al. Dexamethasone for prevention and treatment of acute mountain sickness. *Aviat Space Environ Med* 1988; 59:950–954.

26 Levine B D, Yoshimura K, Kobayashi T et al. Dexamethasone in the treatment of acute mountain sickness. *N Engl J Med* 1989; 321:1707–1713.

27 Coote J H. Pharmacological control of altitude sickness. *Trends Pharmacol Sci* 1991; 12:450–455.

28 Oelz O, Ritter M & Henni R. Nifedipine for high altitude pulmonary oedema. *Lancet* 1989; ii:1241–1244.

29 Reeves J T & Schoene R B. When lungs on mountains leak. *N Engl J Med* 1991; 325:1306–1307.

30 Harvey T C, Winterborn M, Lassen N A et al. Effect of carbon dioxide in acute mountain sickness: a rediscovery. *Lancet* 1988; ii:639–641.

31 Bartsch P, Baumgartner R W, Waber U et al. Comparison of carbon dioxide-enriched, oxygen-enriched and normal air in treatment of acute mountain sickness. *Lancet* 1990; 336:772–775.

32 Dickinson J G. Acetazolamide in acute mountain sickness. *BMJ* 1987; 295:1161–1162.

33 Forwand S A, Landowne N, Follansbee J N et al. Effect of acetazolamide on acute mountain sickness. *N Engl J Med* 1968; 279:839–845.

34 Birmingham Medical Research Expeditionary Society Mountain Sickness Study Group. Acetazolamide in control of acute mountain sickness. *Lancet* 1981; i:180–183.

35 Jensen J B, Wright A D, Lassen N A et al. Cerebral blood flow in acute mountain sickness. *J Appl Physiol* 1990; 69:430–433.

36 Greene N K, Kerr A M, McIntosh I B et al. Acetazolamide in the prevention of acute mountain sickness: a double blind crossover study. *BMJ* 1981; 283:811–813.

37 Naije R & Melot C. Acute pulmonary oedema on the Ruwenzori mountain range. *Br Heart J* 1990; 64:400–402.

38 Rock P B, Johnson T S, Cymerman A et al. Effect of dexamethasone on symptoms of acute mountain sickness at Pike's Peak Colorado (4300 m). *Aviat Space Environ Med* 1987; 58:668–672.

39 Ellsworth A J, Meyer E F & Larson E B. Acetazolamide or dexamethasone versus placebo to prevent acute mountain sickness on Mount Rainier. *West Med J* 1991; 154:289.

40 Bartsch P, Pfluger N, Audetat M et al. Effects of ascent to 4559 m on fluid homeostasis. *Aviat Space Environ Med* 1991; 62:105–110.

41 Milledge J S, Catley D M, Blume D et al. Renin, angiotensin converting enzyme and aldosterone in humans on Mt Everest. *J Appl Physiol* 1983; 55:1109–1112.

42 Milledge J S, Beeley J M, McArthur S et al. Atrial natriuretic peptide, altitude and acute mountain sickness. *Clin Sci* 1989; 77:509–514.

43 Milledge J S. The ventilatory response to hypoxia: how much is good for a mountaineer? *Postgrad Med J* 1987; 63:169–172.

44 Lipton P & Whittingham T S. Cerebral neuronal transmission. *Semin Resp Med* 1981; 3:68–69.

45 Dickinson J G. High altitude cerebral oedema: acute cerebral mountain sickness. *Semin Respir Med* 1983; 3:151–158.

46 Sutton J R & Lassen N A. Pathophysiology of acute mountain sickness and high altitude pulmonary oedema: an hypothesis. *Bull Eur Physiopathol Respir* 1979; 15:1045–1052.

47 Monge M C. La enfermedad de los Andes, sindromes eritremicos. *Ann Fac Med Lima* 1928; 11:314.

48 Sui G L, Liu Y H, Cheng X S et al. Subacute infantile mountain sickness. *J Pathol* 1988; 155:161–170.

49 Anand I S, Malhotra R M, Chandrashekhar Y et al. Adult subacute mountain sickness: a syndrome of congestive heart failure in man at very high altitude. *Lancet* 1990; 335:561–565.

50 Heath D. Missing link from Tibet. *Thorax* 1989; 44:981–983.

51 Dickinson J G. High Altitude. In Dawood R M (ed.) *Travellers' Health,* 3rd edn. Oxford: Oxford University Press, 1992: 224–231.

FURTHER READING

Heath D & Williams D R. *High Altitude Medicine and Pathology*. London: Butterworth, 1989 (3rd edition of *Man at High Altitude*)

Houston C S. *Going High. The Story of Man and Altitude*. New York: American Alpine Club, 1980.

Sutton J R (ed.). Man at altitude. *Semin Respir Med* 1983; 5(2).

Ueda G, Kusama S & Voelkel N F (eds). *High Altitude Medical Science*. Matsumoto: Shinshu University, 1988.

Ward M P, Milledge J S & West J B. *High Altitude Medicine and Physiology*. London: Chapman & Hall, 1989.

CHAPTER 21

NUTRITION-ASSOCIATED DISEASE

G. C. Cook

NUTRITIONAL REQUIREMENTS IN THE TROPICS

Energy requirement for an adult man of 25 years working an 8-hour day is estimated at 3200 calories (13 000 kJ) per 24 hours in the temperate zone. The effect of a hot climate on these requirements is not more than a 10–20% decrease at most. It has been estimated that some villagers consume only 2040 calories (8500 kJ) per day and are permanently hungry.

Pregnancy and breast feeding increase the energy requirement and a baby during the first 6 months at the breast will require an extra 600 calories (2500 kJ) daily via the mother's food intake. Growing children require extra, so that pregnant women and nursing mothers, as well as growing children, are the most vulnerable to nutritional deficiencies. This is shown by the average lower weight of children from under-developed countries as compared with well-fed children from temperate ones. Diets in the tropics are unbalanced as well as being deficient in calories. In the UK, of the 3200 calories (13 000 kJ) daily intake, 88 g consist of protein, of which 54 g are animal protein. In India, of the 2040 calories (8500 kJ) daily intake, 53 g consist of protein, of which only 6 g are animal protein.

In addition to the energy-deficient, unbalanced diet available to tropical people there is the added effect of bacterial and parasitic infections which are very prevalent. Social and cultural customs and breakdown of society from the impact of towns and industrial development have all played a major part in producing these nutritional deficiencies which are so common in many tropical areas.[1–5]

NUTRITION AND INFECTION

The relationship between infection and nutrition had been reviewed.[6] Infection may have an effect on nutritional status, and nutritional status may affect the resistance to infection in the individual.

In protein nutrition, infection has its most serious effect on the nitrogen balance. Intestinal infections may cause some decrease in nitrogen absorption from the gastrointestinal tract but the most important effects are from increased excretion of urinary nitrogen, and diminished intake from anorexia.[6] An outstanding feature of kwashiorkor is the frequency with which it is precipitated by an attack of acute diarrhoeal disease. The increased excretion of nitrogen and decreased intake of food associated with active tuberculosis is of importance in regions where protein malnutrition is common. All viral diseases exert a detectable adverse effect on nitrogen balance and measles, of all communicable diseases, imposes an unusually severe nutritional stress. Measles probably precipitates kwashiorkor in West Africa more frequently than any other infectious disease. It is an important contributory cause of kwashiorkor in many tropical areas and there is a strong association between failure to thrive, diarrhoeal disease and bacterial colonization of the small intestine. Heavy *Ascaris lumbricoides* infections may divert protein from the host, since an adult worm contains a lot of protein. An unusually heavy infection with an intestinal helminth can probably induce protein malnutrition in persons whose diet is otherwise adequate; some observers believe that infection with helminths may precipitate kwashiorkor. The consequence of moderate and light helminthic infection is more debatable and adequate epidemiological studies to determine their effect are not available.

Infection may have an effect on vitamin deficiencies. There is evidence that blindness caused by onchocerciasis is less common in areas where red palm oil, which is high in vitamin A content, is used.

Infectious diseases can precipitate clinical beri-beri in individuals on a diet deficient in vitamin B_1.

Systemic infections can induce anaemia when folic acid is deficient, and fish tapeworm may cause anaemia because of its high requirement of vitamin B_{12}.

Hookworm disease is responsible for iron deficiency anaemia, due to iron loss from small-intestinal mucosal haemorrhage. Chronic infections of bacterial or viral origin produce an 'anaemia of infection' by interfering with iron binding capacity and red cell life span.

Heavy infections with *Giardia lamblia* or *Strongyloides stercoralis* may interfere with absorption; unless the infection is heavy, intestinal helminths as a rule do not interfere with absorption.

IMMUNOCOMPETENCE MALNUTRITION

It is now well recognized that immunocompetence is severely affected in malnutrition. Both T-cell and B-cell-dependent immune systems are depressed but this deficiency is reversible with nutritional repletion. Defects in cellular immunity have been found in 75% of children with protein–energy malnutrition and malnourished children show thymic atrophy and depressed cell-mediated immunity, possibly, as has been suggested, a result of zinc deficiency.[7] The effect on humoral immunity is less clear. Low IgG, albumin and secretory IgA levels have been found in malnutrition, but the production of antibodies was shown not to be inhibited and it is probable that it is the quality of antibody formed which is important; this limits ability to remove antigen. Immunosuppression from infections such as malaria plays an important role in susceptibility to infections in malnutrition.

MALNUTRITION AND RESISTANCE TO INFECTION(S)

When malnutrition impairs immunity to infection the effect is termed synergic; when malnutrition affects the infectious agent more than the host it is termed antagonistic. Many observations have shown that tuberculosis is more common in malnourished individuals and that diarrhoeal diseases and upper respiratory illnesses occur more frequently and last longer in malnourished compared with well-nourished children. There is some evidence, especially in Africa, that amoebic dysentery is more severe in individuals on a deficient diet. Synergism is usual and antagonism rare. From experimental studies on animals synergism is the characteristic reaction with bacteria, rickettsiae, intestinal protozoa and helminths. Antagonism is relatively common with viruses.

The results of several studies support a general view that moderate to severe nutritional deficiencies increase the severity of infection in man.

MALNUTRITION

Malnutrition is extremely common throughout the developing countries.[8–12] Estimates of incidence:

	Africa	Asia	South America
Severe malnutrition	3 million	6 million	1 million
Moderate malnutrition	16 million	64 million	10 million

worldwide indicate that 10 million children are at risk of death and one-third will die even if treated. Certain well-defined syndromes exist:

- Protein–energy malnutrition (kwashiorkor, marasmus)[11,13]
- Vitamin deficiencies
- Nutritional neuropathies.

PROTEIN–ENERGY MALNUTRITION (KWASHIORKOR) (PEM) (See also
Chapter 15)

Kwashiorkor has many other names, including: Mehlnährschaden (Germany), obwosi (Uganda), diboba, m'buaki (Zaire), culebulla (Mexico), bouffisure d'Annam (Indo-China), depigmentation oedema syndrome, pellagroide beri-berico (Cuba). The disease is similar to Mehlnährschaden, a starch or flour dystrophy described by Czerny and Keller in Vienna in 1906. The first clinical description in the tropics was given in Kenya. In Ghana, Cicely Williams first gave it its distinctive name, kwashiorkor or 'deprived child', and described its pathology.[14]

GEOGRAPHICAL DISTRIBUTION

PEM is found in many countries including: Africa,[2,11] India, Papua New Guinea, Indonesia, China,[10,15] Japan, Malaysia, Mexico and many South American countries. Cases have been found in Hungary, Italy and in Puerto Rican families living in New York.

AETIOLOGY

The cause of PEM is multifactorial, although dietary intake is dominant; infection and psychosocial factors are also important.

Diet

The primary cause of PEM is the diet in infancy, low in protein but containing some calories derived from carbohydrate when protein needs are much greater than in adult life.[16] For the first 6 months the breast-fed infant gains weight and is protected from infections by antibody transfer across the placenta. In the second 6 months breast milk decreases, supplementary foods which consist largely of carbohydrate are insufficient and, at the same time, passive immunity declines. In the second year of life breast feeding may cease or if it continues is insufficient and supplementary foods consist mainly of carbohydrate. At this time the non-immune child is exposed to infection, with its nutritional consequences. The child's weight remains constant or it may decline and PEM develops (Figure 21.1).

In the third and fourth years weight gain resumes its upward trend but at a lower level than would be regarded as normal. The diet is then deficient in protein and calorie intake may also be reduced due to the low quality of staple food. In addition, there may be mineral and vitamin deficiencies. Cultural habits, ignorance and poverty all contribute to this poor diet.[17]

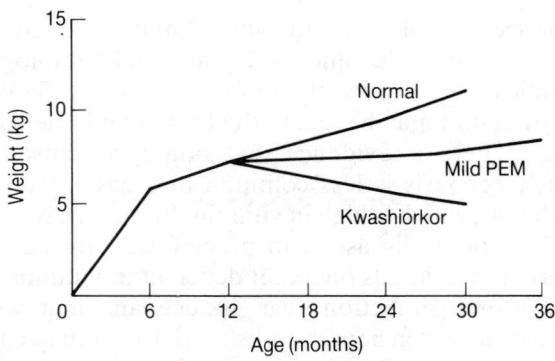

Figure 21.1   Weight gain in mild malnutrition and kwashiorkor.

Infections

Infection is an important aetiological factor in kwashiorkor (Figure 21.2). One line of defence against invading organisms is to produce free radicals (lipid peroxides and toxic carbonyls) to kill them. There are a number of protective pathways against free radicals which require micronutrients (zinc, selenium) for their efficient function. A recent hypothesis postulates that a deficiency of any of these micronutrients will lead to a loss of protection, resulting in cellular damage which gives rise to the oedema, fatty liver, pigmentary changes, diarrhoea, immuno-incompetence and mental changes typical of kwashiorkor.

Psychosocial factors[18–20]

Weaning and the arrival of another child cause feelings of deprivation which result in anorexia and a decrease in food intake.

Toxins

Aflatoxin has been incriminated as a factor in the cause of kwashiorkor (Chapter 15)[21] but as a major factor it is probably not to blame.[22] The finding of high levels of aflatoxin in kwashiorkor might well be due to the inability of the fatty liver to eliminate the toxin.

PATHOLOGY

Protein deficiency exerts a severe nutritional effect by interfering with carbohydrate, fat and protein metabolism. Changes occur in enzyme-secreting organs, but *all* tissues are affected. Bones become osteoporotic and skeletal muscles flabby.

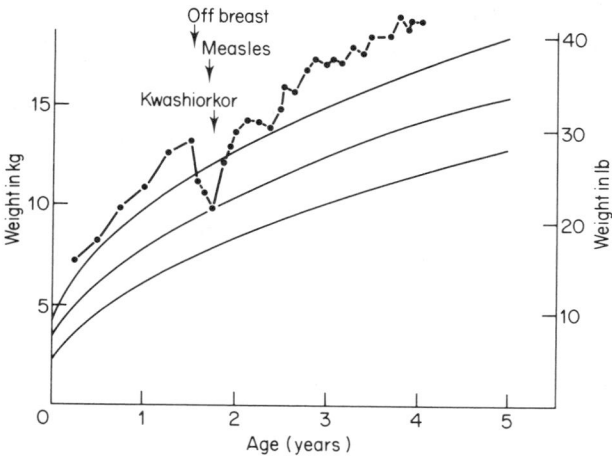

Figure 21.2 Effect of measles on weight gain. Recovery occurred after a stay in hospital. (After Morley.[17])

Liver

Macroscopically the liver is fatty and greasy.[23] Fat first appears in the periphery of the lobules and later involves the centre as small droplets which coalesce to form large fat globules fill practically the whole cell (Figure 21.3). There is a fibrous stellate pattern round each portal tract and, although there is an increase in lymphocytes and plasma cells in the sinusoids during recovery, there is no evidence that cirrhosis is a late sequel.[24] With adequate treatment the fat disappears in reverse order and the fatty changes are totally reversible.[24] Liver function is usually well preserved and, when in advanced cases the serum bilirubin and transaminase concentrations are raised, prognosis is bad and sudden death may occur—possibly from liver failure.

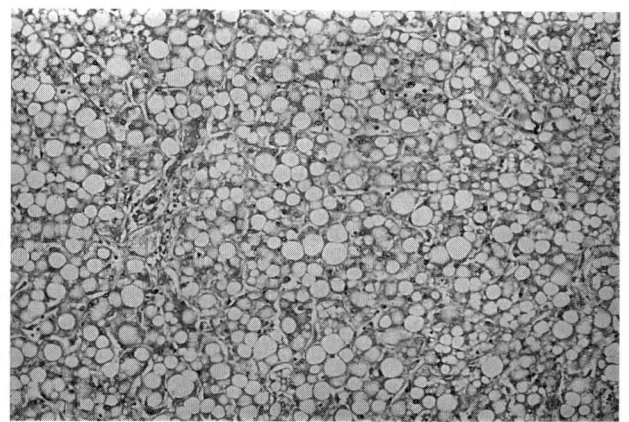

Figure 21.3 Histology of liver of a child with kwashiorkor, showing severe fatty vacuolation of hepatocytes.

Pancreas

The pancreas is pale and atrophic.[16] Microscopically there is atrophy, vacuolation and loss of zymogen granules from the acinar cells, with dilatation of ducts and interstitial fibrosis. Calcification can occur and there is some evidence that chronic calcific pancreatitis in later life is a sequel to kwashiorkor in infancy (see Chapter 3).[25] The salivary glands show marked atrophy with loss of acinar cells.

Gastrointestinal tract

The enzyme-secreting cells of the mucosa are atrophied and there is blunting and broadening of villi with an increase of cells in the lamina propria.[26] This results in loss of disaccharidases (and impaired monosaccharide adsorption), which results in lactose and glucose intolerance after recovery from PEM; lactose and glucose cause diarrhoea. Bacterial contamination of the small intestine causes malabsorption and protein loss; diarrhoeal disease(s) and measles further worsen the position.

Heart

The heart is small and atrophied with histological and biochemical evidence of myocardial dysfunction.[27] A rise in cardiac enzymes and return to normal following recovery suggests dead or dying myocardial cells. Cardiac output is reduced to one-half to one-third of normal with serious danger of circulatory overload during treatment.

Thymus

The thymus is atrophied; this is related to the immunodepression evident in PEM.

Brain and central nervous system[28]

The weight of the brain is decreased. Atrophy, vacuolation and chromatolysis with neurofibrillary disorganization is present in the central nervous system of experimental animals. The anterior horn cells of the spinal cord show similar changes. There are degenerative and atrophic changes in the central ganglia, with a reduction in the size of cortical neurones.

Skin

The skin shows hyperpigmentation with subsequent exfoliation, atrophy, hypopigmentation and a combination of ulcers, fissures and hyperkeratosis. The nails are thin and soft. Microscopically the horny layer is thickened—with basophilia and atrophy of the cells of the granular layer, and vacuolation and atrophy of the cells of the malpighian layer. The dermis is congested and oedematous and the collagen bundles swollen and fragmented. Hair bulbs are atrophic, with loss of pigment from the shafts.

Kidneys

Hyalinization of the glomeruli and fatty degeneration of convoluted tubules have been observed. Albuminuria indicates reduced glomerular flow and tubular activity, which combined with reduced cardiac output leads to electrolyte and water imbalance.

Hormone changes

Hormone changes represent an adaptation to nutritional stress. The plasma cortisol concentration is raised with an increase in growth hormone (sometimes this is reduced, leading to nutritional dwarfism) and the level of insulin is reduced. With recovery growth hormone and cortisol levels return to normal but the insulin level remains low, resulting in reduced ability to handle glucose.[25]

Anaemia (see also Chapter 6)

Some degree of anaemia is always found in children with PEM. There is usually moderate but occasionally severe normocytic normochromic anaemia.

B₁₂ and folate

Macrocytosis and megaloblastic marrow changes have been described in some individuals and giant metamyelocytes have been reported in the marrow. However, there is no demonstrable deficiency of vitamin B_{12} or folate in serum and the defect may be due to a failure to convert folic acid.

Iron

Iron deficiency is not a consistent feature of the anaemia of PEM, although on refeeding stores become depleted, and iron deficiency anaemia may result.

Erythropoietin

An appropriate erythropoietin response to the degree of anaemia has been demonstrated.

The anaemia of PEM usually responds to refeeding and treatment of infection(s); with restoration of marrow function iron deficiency limits haematological recovery, but due to the possibility of an exacerbation of *Plasmodium* spp. and other infections on recovery iron supplements should be postponed until after refeeding.[29]

Oedema

Oedema is a constant feature of PEM. Its causation is a matter of controversy. The classical view is that it is due to hypoalbuminaemia; other factors can also contribute. Cardiac output is reduced and there are decreases in renal blood flow and glomerular infiltration, with an inability to concentrate urine and handle sodium. There are also electrolyte deficiencies: potassium, magnesium and phosphorus depletion can all contribute to oedema formation. All these factors may operate but a low serum albumin is probably the overriding factor.[30]

Carbohydrate metabolism

Hypoglycaemia is frequently observed; this may be due to hepatic failure and is one cause of death. Glucose absorption and the handling of intravenous glucose and galactose loads are abnormal. Enzymatic abnormalities of glucose oxidation have been described.

Lipid metabolism

An intestinal mucosal defect is responsible for a marked reduction in the absorption of different lipid fractions; this persists for many weeks after clinical recovery. Intolerance to milk lipid(s) has been described. Abnormalities in lipid transport are probably related to a deficiency of protein 'carriers'.

Protein and amino acid metabolism

There is a severe disturbance of protein metabolism in kwashiorkor; serum protein concentration is invariably reduced. The serum albumin is reduced owing to decreased synthesis. The α_1- and α_2-globulins are relatively increased and β-globulin frequently decreased. The γ-globulin is also elevated and the albumin/globulin (A/G) ratio reversed. As a result of impaired hepatic circulation and altered serum protein concentration, liver function tests are abnormal and there is a high bromsulphthalein retention in kwashiorkor. Nitrogen balance studies have demonstrated retention of a larger proportion of dietary protein than in normal children and there is increased recycling of body amino acids.

Blood urea and urinary urea excretion are reduced. Urinary creatinine is reduced but amino acid nitrogen, purine derivatives and protein amino acid metabolites are elevated.

Serum activity of various enzymes (amylase, pseudocholinesterase and alkaline phosphatase) is constantly reduced but concentrations of other enzymes associated with destruction of parenchymatous organs are raised.

IMMUNITY

Immunocompetence is severely affected in PEM; both T-cell and B-cell-dependent systems are depressed but recover with nutritional repletion (see Appendix I). Infections such as measles[7,31] and malaria further depress immunity, and secondary infections are common. Tuberculosis is a major problem, and bronchitis and bronchopneumonia frequently result in death.

CLINICAL FEATURES

The main clinical features of kwashiorkor are failure to grow, oedema, skin and hair changes, diarrhoea and mental changes. The *onset* during the second year of life is often quite abrupt and is triggered by an attack of diarrhoea, measles[17,31] or removal from the mother (displacement by a new infant). Kwashiorkor has been recorded in breast-fed infants who are fed an excess of sugar and starch in addition to small amounts of breast milk; they are known as 'sugar babies' in the Caribbean.

Failure to grow

Of all the indices which have been used to forecast PEM, weight records are the most valuable[17,32] and the effect of removal of a child from the mother and/or an attack of measles are well shown in Figure 21.2. In prolonged PEM growth becomes stunted and ossification of bone is delayed.

Oedema

Pitting oedema is of variable degree—from slight pitting of the legs to generalized oedema in which the child is blown up, with massive swelling of the

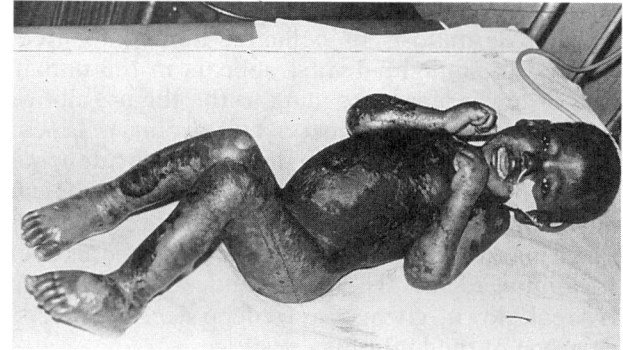

Figure 21.4 Oedema and dermatological lesions in kwashiorkor. (Courtesy of Jelliffe and Barber.)

eyelids blocking the eyes (Figure 21.4). The oedema may be deceptive and the child looks fat and plump so that when recovery begins and excess fluid is lost he or she changes into a wizened little creature with sunken cheeks, pot-belly and spindly legs. In 'sugar babies' (who receive adequate calories but an excess of carbohydrate) body tissue(s) beneath the oedema are not wasted.

Dermatological lesions

Skin lesions, which may be slight or absent, are characteristic of kwashiorkor (Figure 21.5). The skin always shows some degree of atrophy and, the typical dermatosis is present with varying degrees of frequency and severity. It starts as large areas of erythema resembling second-degree burns which become progressively dry, hyperkeratotic and hyperpigmented. In other cases lesions begin as small areas of hyperkeratosis and hyperpigmentation; they grow and become confluent. The epidermis peels off, leaving a depigmented, often tender and reddish oozing surface referred to as 'crazy pavement', 'alligator' or 'mosaic' skin. The

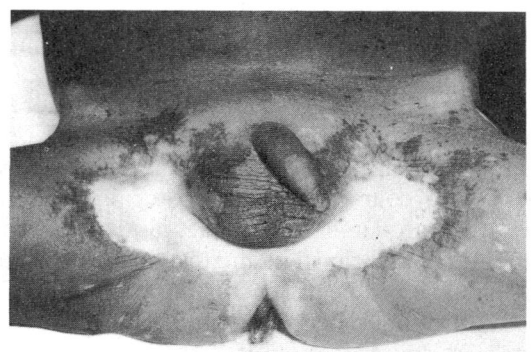

Figure 21.5 Kwashiorkor in a Fijian boy aged 2 years, showing characteristic dermatological lesions—depigmentation and hyperpigmentation.

dermatosis mainly affects pressure areas and is not, like the dermatosis of pellagra, limited to areas exposed to sunlight. It first appears in the napkin area or lower legs, spreading to the thighs, elbows and flexures of the knee(s) and groin(s). Linear flexural fissures extending into the subcutaneous tissues may be present around the pinna of the ear and behind the knee. In severer cases the dermatosis is well marked over the legs, and in milder cases over the lumbar region. There is a tendency for the skin to break down, giving rise to deep necrotic ulcers; gangrene of the limbs may ensue.

Hair changes (achromotrichia)

Hair changes are a virtually constant feature, but are variable. The hair becomes dry and thin, loses its normal sheen and can easily be pulled out. Hair grown during periods of malnutrition loses its colour; black hair becomes brown, reddish yellow or even white, and periods of depigmented growth alternating with periods of more pigmented growth are responsible for the 'flag sign' ('signale la bandera'). Similar but less marked changes may be present in the eyelashes and nails.

Diarrhoea

A recent history of diarrhoea is almost always present. The diarrhoea is non-specific; undigested food may be present in faeces. A large faecal volume indicates malabsorption. Vomiting is common, especially if the child is made to eat more than he or she is accustomed to. Dehydration and electrolyte imbalance resulting from diarrhoea allows hypovolaemia to coexist with oedema.

Mental changes

The kwashiorkor child is dull, apathetic and miserable. He or she rarely screams or cries but produces a low and miserable whimper and resists examination. An urge to fight or scream is absent. There is a great falling off in expression and comprehension. A syndrome resembling encephalitis has been described, with coarse tremors, postural abnormalities, exaggerated tendon reflexes and myoclonus; these features are transient and disappear with treatment. Transient electroencephalographic (EEG) abnormalities have been reported. Brain weight(s) of children dying of malnutrition are significantly lower when compared with control 'non-malnourished' children. EEG and histological evidence of brain damage has been found in protein-

deficient animals but there is as yet no evidence that these findings are applicable to the progress of children recovering from protein–energy malnutrition.[33]

Cardiovascular changes

The heart is small and atrophied pathologically; therefore, some disturbance of cardiovascular function is to be expected and anaemia and fluid retention are important causes of heart failure. The heart appears small on a chest radiograph and there is a low cardiac output. The extremities are frequently cold and cyanotic, and blood pressure is low with reduced pulse pressure. Low serum potassium and magnesium affect myocardial excitability and the heart is extremely sensitive to digitalis. During recovery there may be marked cardiovascular changes with an increase in cardiac diameter and gallop rhythm; cardiac failure may occur after blood or plasma infusion(s).

The electrocardiogram shows non-specific changes: dwarfing of all complexes and an abnormally short or long P–R interval with flat or inverted T waves over the left praecordium. During recovery bizarre ST and T patterns have been noted—often with asymmetrical peaking of the T wave.

Associated nutritional deficiencies

Associated vitamin deficiencies are frequently present but are inconstant and vary geographically. Vitamin A deficiency is potentially the most important since its absorption, transport and utilization are impaired in kwashiorkor, and there is a high frequency of severe ocular lesions due to vitamin A deficiency in children with protein–energy malnutrition in areas where vitamin A deficiency is endemic (see Chapter 10).

Trace metals

Deficiency of trace metals, particularly copper and zinc, may be important.[34,35] Zinc deficiency is now assuming an important role (see Chapter 15).

Associated infections

Associated infections are common.[36–39] Bronchitis and pneumonia may occur in a patient with kwashiorkor who may die quite suddenly of respiratory failure due to bronchopneumonia without previous evidence of fever or dyspnoea. Paradoxically, malaria may flare up during recovery due to the improved nutritional status of the patient; other infections may also relapse.

TREATMENT

Treatment is based primarily upon the administration of a diet high in protein and of good biological value, which contains sufficient energy.[40-44] Dehydration and electrolyte imbalance must be corrected and since there is usually severe potassium deficiency replacement must be achieved. Since the cardiac reserve is diminished intravenous fluids must be given cautiously.

The basis of treatment is skimmed milk powder (50 g) which can be used with calcium caseinate (50 g), sucrose (20 g), and cottonseed oil (30 g) in water to 1 litre. The milk powder is made to a paste with cold water, hot water is added and brought to the boil and the whole is blended and made up to 1 litre. Total intake of 3–5 g/kg body weight of protein of high biological value should be maintained and the total energy intake should be about 120–140 calories (500–600 kJ)/kg body weight daily. Small frequent feeds are necessary from the start. Specific supplements are needed only if there is a particular deficiency, such as vitamin A; this should be corrected intramuscularly. Potassium chloride (1 g daily) is also recommended; rapid clinical and electrocardiographical improvement is achieved by adding magnesium. Blood transfusion may be needed. Iron should be given in the case of iron-deficiency anaemia, and folic acid for megaloblastic anaemia. The weight curve and consistency of the stool(s) form important guides and weight may be lost at first due to loss of oedema. In some infants diarrhoea may develop owing to carbohydrate intolerance, especially involving lactose. Lactose-free nutrient made from groundnuts 150 g, wheat flour 50 g, maize flour 100 g, cottonseed oil 25 g, and sucrose 75 g, made into biscuit, has been used successfully.

Recovery takes place in two stages.[45,46] During the first stage oedema disappears and the major biochemical and physiological abnormalities return to normal values. This stage lasts 2–3 weeks and weight is lost. During the second stage the child recovers the lost weight and reaches the normal weight for height. This takes 2–3 months.

PREVENTION

Various aid programmes exist.[47] Prevention depends on educating mothers to avoid artificial feeding in the absence of correct knowledge of how to handle it, and on adopting satisfactory weaning habits using local products containing readily available protein. Malnutrition in a developing country is a highly complex matter; 'overall' solutions are not readily available.[48-55]

'Incaparina' prepared by the Institute of Central America and Panama is an economic, easily cooked mixture of ground maize, whole ground sorghum, cottonseed flour, yeast and calcium carbonate, enriched with vitamin A. This protein supplement is widely used in Central America to prevent the development of protein–energy malnutrition.

MILD TO MODERATE PEM

This is clinically manifest by inadequate physical growth.[55] The child is small and less active. Bone maturation is retarded and mental development slowed; whether this is irreversible or not is debatable (see above).

MARASMUS

The most common form of marasmus in the developing world has a primary origin and results from starvation of small children.[55]

Children are fed a diet which is adequate qualitatively, but grossly deficient in energy for the requirements of the rapidly growing child. Energy is the limiting factor and the child 'lives on its own tissues'. The disease develops in infants fed on mother's milk, which in malnourished mothers is deficient in amount, or by prolonged breast feeding, with inadequate supplementation or inadequate artificial feeding with overdiluted cow's milk or starchy gruels. Social changes and urbanization are forcing mothers to wean early and the adoption of artificial feeding precipitates infective diarrhoea. An important cause of marasmus is malabsorption caused by bacterial colonization of the small intestine brought about by a constant intake of infected water and food, from an insanitary environment.

There is marked atrophy of all organs and tissues. Anaemia is not a feature unless a superimposed cause is present. Intestinal absorptive mechanisms are adequate. Small intestinal enzymes are normal in marasmus, in contrast to kwashiorkor.

Serum proteins are normal and serum enzymes, e.g. amylase and pseudocholinesterase, are not affected.

Marasmus is more frequent in infants than older children because they are growing more rapidly and are more likely to be subject to a marasmus-producing type of diet. With restriction of food intake, growth almost ceases and the infant utilizes subcutaneous fat followed by muscle. The infant is hungry and cries continuously. There may be constipation due to diminished food intake. Infectious diseases act as precipitating and aggravating factors. The child is extremely emaciated; the muscles are atrophic. Skin is thin, flaccid and wrinkled. Hair is not altered. The mind is alert, but the typical face of the marasmic child resembles that of a little very old man. Often there is added dehydration from infective vomiting and diarrhoea.

Practically all cases recover after adequate dietary treatment unless severe complications, such as dehydration, electrolyte imbalance or infection, are present concurrently. The diet should be complete, balanced and adequate for the apparent biological age, and higher in energy than would be required for a normal child; 200 calories (850 kJ)/kg body weight daily are required. Progress should be monitored by regular weighing.

FAMINE OEDEMA

True famine oedema is due to a deficiency of protein and usually occurs in adults. It occurs during war and other social disturbances, and was common in central Europe during the First World War (1914–1918). Famine oedema was common in Japanese prison camps during the Second World War (1939–1945) and was confused with beriberi. The Dutch 'hungeroedem' was synonymous with the wet beriberi of the British medical staff.

The condition is due to lack of fat and protein in the diet. The primary effect is a reduction in serum protein concentration—below 40–50 g/l. Generalized oedema develops without albuminuria or evidence of cardiac failure or peripheral neuropathy. Serum albumin is greatly reduced. Recovery takes place when patients are placed on a diet containing sufficient protein of high biological value. Many cases of so-called adult kwashiorkor are in reality famine oedema. Epidemic dropsy caused by the consumption of contaminated cottonseed or mustard oil can also produce a similar picture.

ENDEMIC GOITRE

Goitre consists of slowly developing enlargement of the thyroid gland—caused by a deficiency of iodine in the diet, or the influence of goitrogens.

GEOGRAPHICAL DISTRIBUTION

Worldwide endemic goitre is distributed in certain restricted localities, away from the sea, at the head of rivers, and in isolated valleys with poor soil and high rainfall. In the tropics it is found in Africa, Central and South America and in Asia. Papua New Guinea has been the focus of much research.[56]

In *Africa* it is a problem in the Atlas mountains, the Nile valley, and highland areas of Kenya, Tanzania, Rwanda, Burundi, Cameroon, Gambia, Congo basin and Nigeria.

It is present in large areas of *Central* and *South America*.

In *Asia* it is found in the Himalayas—from the Pamirs to Kashmir, Nepal, Myanmar and China (Yunnan) and also in Thailand, Vietnam and Malaysia.

AETIOLOGY

The cause of endemic goitre is a failure of the thyroid gland to obtain adequate iodine to maintain its normal structure and function. This failure may be brought about by a deficiency of iodine in the diet—which results from a deficiency in the environment, thus accounting for the geographical distribution of endemic goitre. It may also be caused by goitrogens, substances which impose an abnormal physiological demand on the thyroid or interfere metabolically with the utilization of iodine by that gland. Goitrogens include: cyanide containing compounds (cassava) and fluoride, which interfere with the ability of the gland to trap iodine from the circulation; and antimony and cobalt, which interfere with the production of thyroid hormone(s). Goitrogens are also found in vegetables of the *Brassica* (cabbage) family.

Endemic cretinism

Endemic cretinism is the most serious effect of endemic goitre and is found where urinary iodine excretion is <20 μg daily. In parts of Papua New Guinea the prevalence of cretinism approaches 15%. There are two forms: the 'neurological', which predominates and is characterized by mental retardation, deaf mutism, spastic diplegia and strabismus; and the 'myxoedematous', with signs of congenital hypothyroidism. The latter presentation predominates in central Africa, where dietary goitrogens may also play a part.

Cretinism can be prevented by iodine supplements; these should be given before conception—since iodine deficiency causes neurological damage in early fetal life, and by iodized oil prophylaxis to the general population.

PATHOLOGY

The thyroid enlarges in response to secretion of pituitary thyroid stimulating hormone (TSH) In the early stages follicular hyperplasia occurs and colloid is reduced. In the later chronic stages, when the iodine stores have been exhausted, the gland becomes soft and enlarged with large amounts of colloid in the follicles. Nodular formation takes place and haemorrhage and calcification may occur. The gland does not become 'toxic' and there is no evidence that malignancy ensues.

Severe iodine depletion may interfere with corneal neuronal dendrites and is the major factor in the pathogenesis of endemic cretinism.

CLINICAL FEATURES

Large goitres are easily recognized. Moderate degrees of thyroid enlargement are diagnosed on goitre surveys and graded by inspection, palpation and neck measurement. Presence of thyroid enlargement in a significant number of persons living in an area is sufficiently strong evidence for the diagnosis of endemic goitre. Tracheal pressure may produce interference with the recurrent laryngeal nerve and hoarseness. The patient is almost always euthyroid.

DIAGNOSIS

Urinary excretion of iodine may be as low as 10 μg daily. The uptake of radioactive ^{131}I is increased. Thyroid hormones are normal. Rarely, hormone concentrations are depressed and the patient is hypothyroid.

TREATMENT

If treated early the goitre may disappear completely following the administration of iodine—30 mg potassium iodide made up to 20 ml distilled water, and administered as 4–6 drops daily in a glass of water. Beneficial results will be observed in 4–6 weeks, and the patient should then be maintained on a daily regimen. Advanced goitres must be treated surgically if they are causing symptoms.

EPIDEMIOLOGY

Areas of iodine deficiency are those, far away from the sea, in which there are isolated areas of poor soil because the rainfall has leached the soil, and there is no natural supply of iodine. Areas of endemicity can be found by surveys and measurement of the size of thyroid glands in the population. Serum protein-bound iodine concentrations are low and uptake of ^{131}I is also low in these areas.

PREVENTION

Goitre can be prevented by the addition of iodized salt; 100 μg iodine added to the daily diet is sufficient. A more practical solution is to give a deep intramuscular injection of 5 ml of iodized oil containing about 400 mg iodine per ml; this is effective for several years.[56,57]

SCURVY

GEOGRAPHICAL DISTRIBUTION

Scurvy is found worldwide especially in hot, dry desert areas where fresh vegetables and fruit are sparse.

AETIOLOGY

The disease is due to a lack of vitamin C (ascorbic acid) which catalyses oxidation by the introduction of hydroxyl groups, and is essential for the formation of collagen.

PATHOLOGY

Inadequate formation of collagen leads to extravasation of blood, loosening of the teeth and easily fractured bones with subperiosteal haemorrhages. Autopsy shows extensive haemorrhage in internal organs.

CLINICAL FEATURES

Scurvy occurs both in adults and infants.

Adult scurvy

Onset is insidious with loss of weight, progressive weakness and, characteristically, stiffness in the leg muscles and any other muscle groups in extensive use. Haematomas in the calf muscles may be the first sign. The acute symptoms are brought on by physical exertion. The gums soon become affected with swelling and sponginess of the alveolar margin(s) and fungating masses projecting beyond the teeth—which loosen and fall out. Subcutaneous petechiae form on the limbs and trunk producing scorbutic purpura; wounds fail to heal. The anaemia is characteristically microcytic and hypochromic and responds only to ascorbic acid.

Infantile scurvy

The majority of cases present in the second half of the first year—especially in premature and artificially fed infants. There is a triad of irritability, tenderness of the legs, and failure to use them (pseudoparalysis). Bleeding manifestations are confined to the site(s) of erupting teeth. The infant lies in a characteristic position with legs flexed at the knees and hips partially flexed and internally rotated due to pain from subperiosteal haemorrhages, which may be palpable at the distal end of the femur and proximal end of the tibia. Costochondral beading (scorbutic rosary) is also usually palpable. Anaemia is microcytic and hypochromic but may be megaloblastic due to accompanying folate deficiency resulting from lack of folate coenzymes associated with vitamin C.

Bone radiographs show characteristic epiphyseal changes with a line of rarefaction at the point of epiphyseal growth and a ground glass appearance of the shafts.

DIAGNOSIS

The main differential diagnosis is from rickets which may coexist as 'scurvy rickets'. In rickets there is a dense line at the epiphyseal junction(s). The capillary permeability test (Hess) is performed using a sphygmomanometer to occlude venous return to the arm; petechiae appear in scorbutic cases. The vitamin C saturation test is performed by saturating the body with ascorbic acid and measuring excretion in the urine; if any ascorbic acid is retained there is vitamin C deficiency.

TREATMENT

Ascorbic acid (50 mg four times daily) should be given for 1 week in infantile scurvy—followed by 50 mg twice daily for 1 month. Vitamin C may also be given as 100–200 ml fresh orange juice daily. Adult scurvy should be treated with 250 mg four times daily until all signs have disappeared.

EPIDEMIOLOGY

Scurvy is not common in most tropical areas since vitamin C is abundant. The disease can occur in infants who are fed on dried cereal and boiled milk and soldiers, prisoners and refugees in camps in dry desert areas who are not provided with fresh fruit and vegetables.

PREVENTION

Vitamin C is destroyed by heat—especially prolonged cooking—and the presence of alkalis. Foods which are steamed and cooked rapidly retain much of their vitamin C content. The recommended intake of vitamin C is 30 mg daily for infants, 40–45 mg for children, and 70 mg for adults. Scurvy may be prevented in camps and groups of men living on dry rations by giving 100 mg of ascorbic acid daily in tablet form. Artificially fed infants should receive supplements in the form of fresh orange juice daily, or as ascorbic acid supplement.

RICKETS AND OSTEOMALACIA

GEOGRAPHICAL DISTRIBUTION

Rickets is now rare in temperate countries but still occurs sporadically in many parts of the world where custom deprives infants and/or women of sunlight due to social or religious custom.[58]

AETIOLOGY

Rickets and osteomalacia are caused by vitamin D deficiency. Vitamin D is a sterol; vitamin D_1 (calciferol) results from the action of ultraviolet light on ergosterols in plants, and vitamin D_2 (cholecalciferol) from the action of sunlight on 7-dehydrocholesterol in mammalian skin. Vitamin D has a direct effect on bone calcification where it increases the rate of secretion and resorption of minerals. A high dietary phytate content may impair the absorption of calcium and phosphorus.

PATHOLOGY

Defective calcification of developing long bones results in slowing of calcium and phosphorus precipitation in the newly formed matrix; a mass of osteoid tissue which fails to calcify—causes enlargement at the growing ends of the bone—in rickets at the costochondral junction (rickety rosary), and a softening of all the bones in both rickets and osteomalacia.

CLINICAL FEATURES

Rickets

Onset during the first 2 years of life is later than that in scurvy. The child becomes ill, pale, flabby and irritable, prone to tetany and laryngeal stridor. There is general physical and mental retardation and deformity of ribs, spine, pelvis and limbs (Figure 21.6). The skull shows bossing (craniotabes). Both liver and spleen may be palpable. As the child grows, the skeletal changes heal but marked deformities may remain, such as pigeon-chest, spinal curvature, knock-knees and bow-legs.

Osteomalacia

Osteomalacia occurs in women of childbearing years—usually in the first pregnancy. The bones, especially those of the pelvic girdle, ribs and femora,

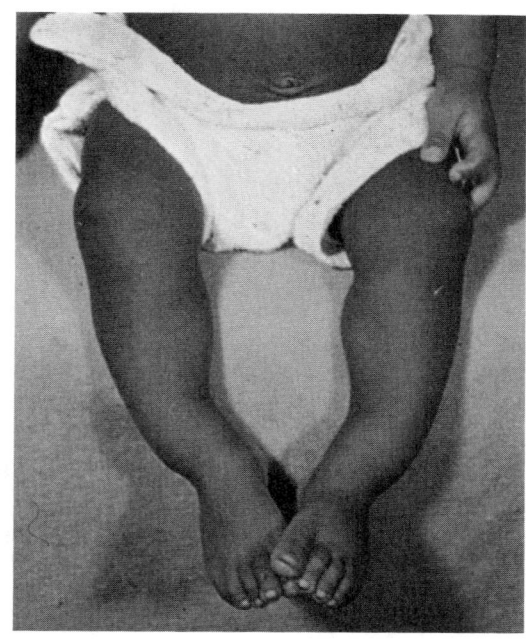

Figure 21.6 Curvature of the legs resulting from rickets.

become soft, painful and deformed. The gait is characteristic, the patient swaying the leg outward before putting the foot to the ground. Tetany is common. Anaemia is present and spontaneous fracture(s) may occur. Fetal bones show no signs of rickets.

DIFFERENTIAL DIAGNOSIS

The differential diagnosis of rickets from infantile scurvy may be difficult but rickets usually occurs in older infants and there are no subperiosteal haemorrhages; other possibilities are congenital syphilis, achondroplasia and osteogenesis imperfecta. Renal rickets in chronic renal disease does not respond to vitamin D.

DIAGNOSIS

Radiographs of the wrist may show characteristic changes in the epiphyses. The line of osteochondral calcification is broadened and rarefied (Figure 21.7). Serum calcium is low (6–7 mg/dl); clinical rickets can occur with normal calcium and phosphorus levels.

TREATMENT

Treatment is based on providing an adequate calcium and vitamin D intake. Vitamin D should be

Figure 21.7 Radiograph of the hand in rickets (right), compared with a normal radiograph (left).

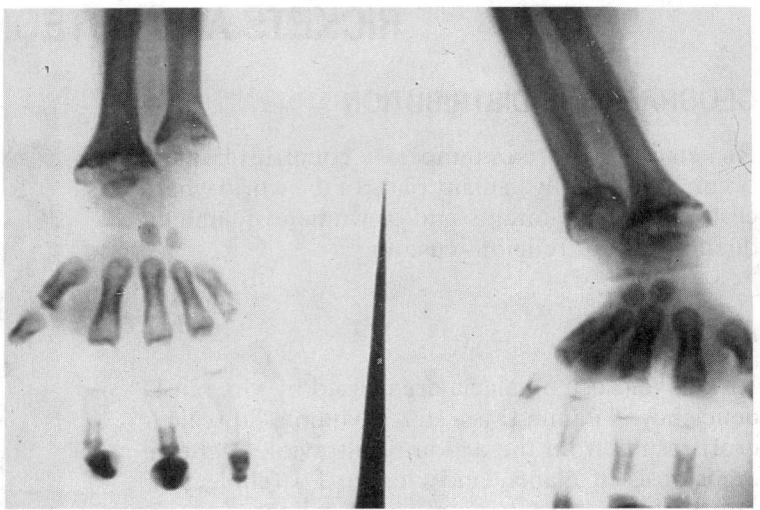

given, 2000–5000 iu daily and calcium as milk 500 ml daily.

EPIDEMIOLOGY

Rickets

In the tropics rickets may occur where sunlight is reduced by high rise buildings; in Asia it is a disease of cities. The San Blas Indians of Panama protect their children from the sun because of the high incidence of albinism. In Guatemala cases have been found in sunny rural areas where toddlers are kept in houses because the mothers have to go out to work. It has been suggested that rural rickets in Iran and Kashmir might be due not to a high phytate content but to an 'anticalcifying' factor present in high extraction flour (chupatty).[59]

Osteomalacia

In India, osteomalacia is widespread in women whose diets are inadequate in calcium and vitamin D and who are kept in 'purdah'; this prevents the sunlight reaching the skin. In northern China a similar cause for osteomalacia as for rickets has been suggested—namely, an 'anticalcifying' factor in chupatty flour; biochemical healing has been obtained with a chupatty-free diet.

PREVENTION

An adequate intake of milk, clearance of slums and action against atmospheric pollution should be undertaken, as well as health education for children and women. They should obtain adequate sunlight and receive a daily intake of 400 iu of vitamin D as cod-liver oil or bread fortified with calcium and vegetable fats with calciferol.

VITAMIN A DEFICIENCY (NIGHT BLINDNESS, XEROPHTHALMIA, KERATOMALACIA)

GEOGRAPHICAL DISTRIBUTION

Vitamin A deficiency is common in parts of South and South-East Asia, the Middle East, Africa and Latin America where it usually accompanies PEM.[60–62]

AETIOLOGY

Vitamin A (retinol) is utilized by epithelial cells throughout the body. When deficient, they undergo squamous metaplasia; the cells becoming flattened and heaped upon each other. The sweat glands become blocked with secretion and sweat diminishes. The lack of tears and the change(s) in the conjunctiva leads to *xerophthalmia* and, in the cornea, *keratomalacia*; the diminished supply to the rod cells of the retina leads to failure of dark adaptation and *night blindness*. Similar changes in the skin lead to *follicular keratosis*.

The pathology, clinical features, treatment and prevention of these conditions are dealt with in Chapters 10 and 15.

VITAMIN B₁ DEFICIENCY (BERIBERI)

GEOGRAPHICAL DISTRIBUTION

Until relatively recently beriberi was common in many tropical and subtropical areas and was formerly the scourge of mines and plantations in Malaysia, China, Indonesia and other parts of the Far East, wherever rice was the staple diet; it was the cause of enormous mortality and morbidity. It was common among workers in the tropics on such major engineering projects as the Panama Canal and Congo (Zaire) Railway. Outbreaks have occurred in institutions such as mental homes in Ireland, the USA and France and in fishermen in Newfoundland, the North American coast and Iceland. Beriberi was formerly a major problem in the Japanese Navy and was almost universal in prisoner-of-war and internment camps in the Far East in the Second World War (1939–1945). Beriberi was formerly prevalent in the crews of ships. From 1894 to 1920 the disease was common in crews of Swedish and Norwegian ships and yet was comparatively rare in British ones. The explanation was that during these years bread baked from white flour or a mixture of wheat and rye was used in the Scandinavian ships so that the diet was inadequate in B vitamins.

AETIOLOGY

Vitamin B₁ deficiency, or beriberi, is due to a deficiency of vitamin B₁ or thiamine. Vitamin B₁ is present in the tissues in the phosphorylated form (diphosphothiamine) which acts as a coenzyme for the metabolism of carbohydrate in the Krebs citric acid cycle and exerts a role in the oxidative breakdown of pyruvic acid. Since the brain and nervous tissue and heart muscle use glucose in large amounts as a primary source of energy, it is these tissues in which carbohydrate metabolism is especially deranged in vitamin B₁ deficiency. Pyruvic acid accumulates in blood and the central nervous system and is excreted in excess in the urine. Vitamin B₁ is also involved in the synthesis of acetylcholine and in neural transmission. Another factor resulting from breakdown in the Krebs cycle is a metabolic acidosis resulting from the accumulation of blood lactic acid; this is important in alcoholic beriberi.[63]

Vitamin B₁ is widely distributed in raw foodstuffs, the richest sources being whole cereals—especially rice, in which it is found in the pericarp of the aleurone layer and in the grain embryo. The rice grain in its natural condition is enclosed in a husk. In 'husking' the husk is removed but the pericarp is retained; this is termed 'unpolished' rice. In milling and polishing both the embryo and pericarp are removed and the grains are polished by rubbing with talc between sheepskins. This product is known as polished or white rice. Vitamin B₁ is also found in yeast which is an exceptionally potent source and can be used as a dietary supplement.

Vitamin B₁ is a colourless, water-soluble, crystalline substance melting at 248–250°C which is stable at 100°C for 24 hours in dry conditions. Rate of destruction is increased by the presence of water and alkali but ordinary cooking in the absence of soda does not destroy the vitamin; it is, however, denatured by pressure cooking and autoclaving—when yeast and liver are subjected to heat and pressure. Most vitamin B₁ is stored in the liver, kidneys and muscles and it is abundant in normal heart muscle. Vitamin B₁ is excreted in urine in which the kidney concentrates it from the plasma, but only a small part of the vitamin given by the mouth is excreted, the remainder being destroyed in the body. It is also excreted in milk but not faeces. An excretion of less than 12.1 iu/day in the urine is evidence of vitamin B₁ deficiency. The international unit is the antineuritic activity of $3\,\mu$g of pure vitamin B₁. Minimum daily requirement for an adult of 70 kg on 3000 calories (12 600 kJ)/day would be 300 iu or 1 mg, but 500–700 iu (1.75–2.3 mg) is desirable. A larger amount is required when metabolic rates are increased in pregnancy, lactation, infancy and childhood; there is a high incidence of beriberi among pregnant women and mothers. Hard physical work also increases the requirement; thus beriberi was more prevalent among stokers than sailors. Since the metabolic rate rises during fever there is an association of beriberi with *Plasmodium* spp. and other pyrexias illnesses.

Secondary (alcoholic) beriberi

Alcoholic cardiomyopathy causes low output cardiac failure; it has a complex aetiology and is not a direct result of beriberi.

True alcoholic beriberi is a form of oedematous cardiac disease with high output failure occurring in certain severe alcoholics; it responds rapidly to vitamin B_1. It is not common in the West but has been described as 'palm-wine tapper's heart' in Gambia, which develops in palm tappers whose work is arduous and involves the climbing of numerous palm trees and consumption of the fermenting sap.

Drug-induced beriberi has been reported from East Africa resulting from use of nitrofurazone in the treatment of trypanosomiasis—which interferes with pyruvate metabolism.

PATHOLOGY

As a result of a breakdown in carbohydrate metabolism those systems of the body which utilize glucose most rapidly are affected; these are the central and peripheral nervous system and cardiac muscle. Degenerative nerve changes may be detected in the neurones in the anterior and posterior horn cells and sympathetic ganglia. The vagus is involved—with degenerative changes in its nucleus in the floor of the fourth ventricle. Microscopically the nerve trunks show changes ranging from slight medullary degeneration to complete neural destruction (Wallerian degeneration). Regenerative processes can occur side by side with the degenerative. Some fibres of the vagus and sympathetic nerves escape and the bronchial and oesophageal twigs are usually unaffected. In Wernicke's encephalopathy foci of congestion and haemorrhage are scattered symmetrically in the grey matter of the brain stem and hypothalamic regions. The mamillary bodies are virtually always affected. The lesions show specific selectivity for the vegetative centres, being most severe in the lateral horns and Clarke's nuclei at the thoracic level. There are also numerous perivascular haemorrhages and widespread degenerative changes throughout the brain.

In the heart the primary lesion is a loss of contractility of the heart muscle due to water retention. Microscopic examination of cardiac muscle shows intracellular oedema, sarcolysis and hydropic degeneration—probably due primarily to an excess of lactic acid brought about by defective oxygenation. These changes cause 'beriberi heart' (Chapter 5), the essential features of which are: a hyperkinetic circulation, peripheral vasodilatation, enlargement of the right side of the heart and dilatation of the pulmonary artery with increased circulation time—causing high output failure. The cause of the hyperkinetic circulation is low peripheral arterial resistance resulting from vasodilatation, in spite of increased plasma catecholamines, due to a loss of control of muscular arteriolar tone. It may be a compensatory mechanism which is brought into play to counteract tissue anoxia, which is simulated by a failure of carbohydrate metabolism, or vasodilatation in the muscles may be responsible by causing arteriovenous shunting. Post-mortem appearances are those of severe right heart failure. The right side of the heart is dilated, especially the atrium, the walls of which may be paper thin. There is gross congestion of the venous return and right atrium and ventricle. Serous effusions are present in the pleural and peritoneal cavities and cellular tissues. There is oedema of the lungs and severe central congestion of the liver with 'nutmegging'.

CLINICAL FEATURES

Beriberi assumes varyious clinical forms according to the extent and degree of cardiac involvement. There are two main forms of the disease: neurological or 'dry' beriberi and oedematous or 'wet' beriberi. However, both constitute the same disease and a mixture of the two forms is usual.

The period of development of beriberi in man after being placed on a vitamin B_1-deficient diet has been determined at 80–90 days. The onset is usually insidious but may occasionally be ushered in by an acute onset, ending fatally within a few hours without any symptoms referable to the central nervous system.

Paraplegic or dry beriberi (See also Chapter 8)

The signs and symptoms are those of a peripheral neuropathy of mixed motor and sensory type. There is a gradual onset of weakness of the lower limbs followed by ataxia; there may be paraesthesiae with burning and tingling in the limbs.

Motor signs

Flaccid weakness with wasting, develops at first in the muscles of the lower limbs. The extensors of the foot and toes are involved with foot and toe drop and the gastrocnemii become weak and wasted. This weakness gradually spreads to involve the extensors of the legs and later the extensors and flexors of the thigh. At this stage the patient is not able to rise from the squatting position with the hands held above the head. This constitutes the 'jongck' or 'squatting

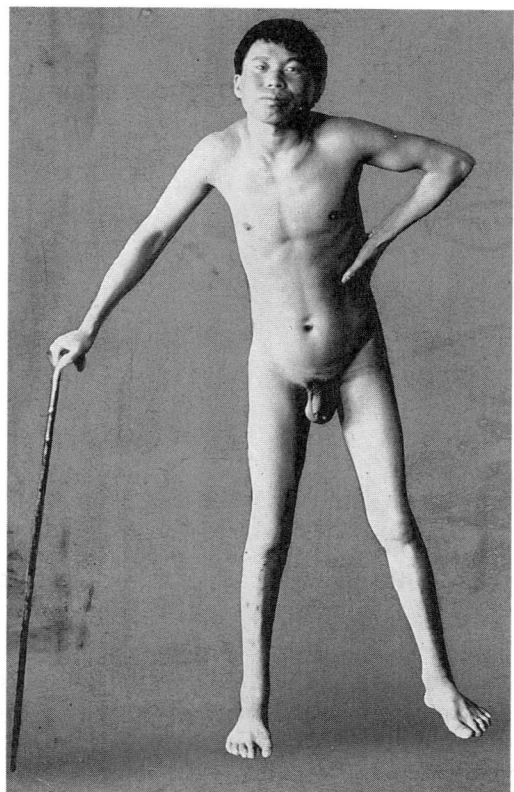

Figure 21.8 Ataxic or paraplegic beriberi—showing the characteristic gait.

test'. The upper limbs are eventually affected—with weakness and wasting of the thenar, hypothenar, plantar and arm muscles, which may show fibrillary twitchings. There may be marked wrist drop. There is also loss of the deep reflexes. The knee jerks, ankle jerks and arm reflexes are all lost. The fibres of the affected muscles show myoedema and contract painfully when struck with the patella hammer. Electrical reactions reveal the 'pattern of degeneration'.

Sensory changes

Sensory changes are marked. There is a sensory neuropathy of peripheral type with glove and stocking anaesthesia spreading up from the feet over the tibiae to the thighs. A similar loss of sensation spreads up from the tips of the fingers. There is loss of sensation to pain, light touch and heat and cold; deep sensibility elicited by compression of the Achilles tendon is lost.

A severe ataxia develops owing to the marked loss of postural sensation and the patient is unable to button his jacket or pick up a pin. The gait becomes ataxic and he/she walks with a high-stepping gait on a broad base, requiring the use of a stick (Figure 21.8). The cranial nerves are not involved and there

are no tremors. The bladder and rectal sphincters are only involved in the terminal stages.

Cardiac or wet beriberi (see also Chapter 5)

Cardiac beriberi consists of high output right heart failure in which the circulation time is increased.

Oedema

There is generalized oedema of the arms, legs, hands and trunk and the face is puffy. The urine is scanty, of high specific gravity; there is no albuminuria.

Circulatory changes

In the early stages the extremities are warm and the pulse rapid. Blood pressure is low with a high pulse pressure. In the later stages when heart failure appears the hands may become cold. 'Pistol shot' sounds may be heard over the larger arteries and occasionally heart block may supervene. The jugular venous pressure is greatly raised with marked venous pulsation in the neck due to tricuspid incompetence. The heart is enlarged to the right and the heart sounds are evenly spread, causing a 'tic-tac rhythm' with reduplication of the second heart sound. A loud pansystolic murmur is heard over the entire praecordium including the tricuspid area. Paralysis of the recurrent laryngeal nerve by a grossly distended atrium has been recorded. The liver is enlarged and tender and may pulsate. There is usually uni- or bilateral hydrothorax, and ascites.

Radiography of the heart shows a typically globular enlargement affecting the right and left ventricles (Figure 21.9). Pericardial effusion is rare at this stage. The electrocardiogram shows distinct changes: low voltage, inverted or flattened T waves in all leads, a decreased P–R interval and prolongation of the Q–T interval. Changes indicating right ventricular strain are also present.

Progress

Most patients die from paralysis and right heart failure complicated and aggravated by pulmonary oedema, diaphragmatic paralysis, hydrothorax or hydropericardium. Sudden cardiac failure is common (shoshin, as described by Japanese workers).

Infantile beriberi

Infantile beriberi occurs in breast-fed infants of vitamin B₁-deficient mothers—especially if they are taking a high carbohydrate diet. It can also occur in

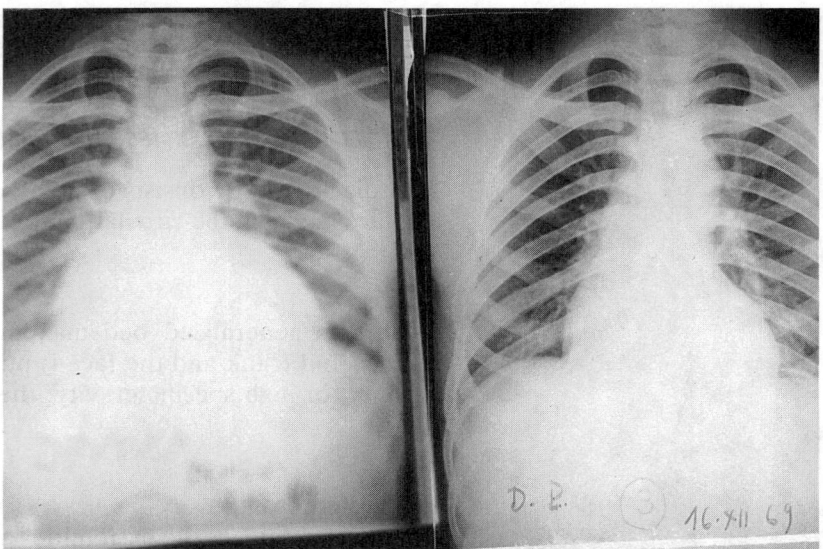

Figure 21.9 Beriberi heart. Left, before treatment; right, after treatment. Transverse cardiac diameter is significantly decreased 11 days after vitamin B$_1$ treatment.

artificially fed infants if the feed is deficient in vitamin B$_1$ or the carbohydrate level is too high.

It is probable that vitamin B$_1$ deficiency is not the sole cause of infantile beriberi; some of the features are probably caused by certain toxic products in breast milk. It is considered that breakdown products from incomplete metabolism of carbohydrate, especially methyl glyoxal, are toxic to the infant.

Characteristically, onset is during the second and third months of life especially the ninth, tenth and eleventh weeks. The baby is rather fat and flabby. The onset is with restlessness, attacks of crying, oliguria and minor puffiness of the body. This may be followed by vomiting of milk (Figure 21.10).

The cardiorespiratory phase is the most dramatic and rapidly fatal form of the disease. There is a fairly sudden onset of peripheral and central circulatory failure. The lungs become moist, the heart enlarges with 'tic-tac' rhythm and the pulse becomes rapid and thready. There is venous engorgement of the neck veins with tender enlargement of the liver.

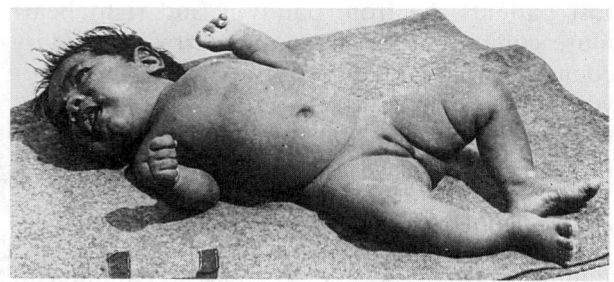

Figure 21.10 A child in the convulsions of infantile beriberi. Note the generalized fluid retention.

Oedema collects and the child may die within 36–48 hours from cardiorespiratory failure.

A chronic phase occurs in slightly older infants. There is anorexia, loss of weight and constipation. Dysphonia and aphonia—ascribed to paralysis of the left recurrent laryngeal nerve by pressure to the left atrium—are common and give rise to a characteristic cry. There is oedema and oliguria. Paralysis of muscles and loss of tendon reflexes are also found (polyneuritic phase).

Thiamine concentration in milk can be estimated. The critical level is probably 6–7 μg/100 ml.

Wernicke's encephalopathy

A combination of ataxia, clouding of consciousness and ophthalmoplegia was described by Wernicke in 1881. Subsequently this syndrome was associated with chronic alcoholism. From 1933 onwards its connection with vitamin B$_1$ deficiency was suspected and a similar condition was described in a nutritional disease of silver foxes in America. Outbreaks of this disease occurred in prisoner-of-war camps in the Far East in the Second World War (1939–1945). Diagnosis was established at autopsy by demonstration of haemorrhage(s) in the mamillary bodies (see above). The cause of the syndrome was established to be vitamin B$_1$ deficiency by the rapidity with which it responded to vitamin B$_1$ injections. Predisposing causes are dysentery, diarrhoea, failure to adapt to a rice diet and febrile conditions such as sepsis and malaria.

In 90% of cases of the B$_1$ deficiency type other forms of beriberi are associated. There are signs of severe disturbance(s) of the midbrain with oculomotor signs and cranial nerve lesions with general clouding of consciousness. The first symptom is persisting anorexia followed by evidence of cranial nerve lesions.

General signs include clouding of consciousness, insomnia, disorientation and semi-coma.

Oculomotor signs and symptoms include wavering of the visual fields on looking sideways, diplopia and photophobia. Horizontal nystagmus is the earliest sign. In a quarter of cases there is an external rectus palsy, sometimes with complete disconjugate wandering of the eyes. Loss of visual acuity, ptosis and retinal haemorrhage(s) are also present.

Other cranial nerve lesions occur in the trigeminal, facial, auditory and glossopharyngeal nerves.

Symptoms and signs are promptly relieved by vitamin B₁ injections, 50–100 mg daily.

DIFFERENTIAL DIAGNOSIS

Dry beriberi must be distinguished from: alcoholic peripheral neuropathy—in which there are associated tremors and mental changes including Korsakoff's psychosis; tabes dorsalis in which there are Argyll Robertson pupils and posterior column changes; arsenical neuropathy in which there are pigmentation of the skin and hyperkeratosis of the palms and soles of the feet; chronic lead poisoning in which there is a blue line on the gums and the neuropathy is purely motor; lathyrism—in which there is a pyramidal lesion with spasticity of the legs, increased tendon reflexes and extensor plantar responses; triorthocresyl phosphate (ginger or jake) paralysis in which there is a pure motor flaccid paralysis; other nutritional neuropathies such as 'burning feet' and combined degeneration of the cord when both posterior columns and pyramidal tracts are involved. In the rapidly ascending paralysis of the Guillain-Barré syndrome cerebrospinal fluid usually contains a raised protein content.

Wet beriberi must be distinguished from other causes of right cardiac failure with a high output: anaemic heart failure, hookworm disease, and chronic nephritis. In famine oedema and epidemic dropsy signs of peripheral neuropathy are absent.

DIAGNOSIS

Laboratory tests
Pyruvic acid concentration in the blood is raised and is of diagnostic value. In acute beriberi the pyruvic acid level approximate to 2 mg/dl and in untreated

chronic beriberi 1.5 mg/dl. After thiamine administration the level falls to about 0.5 mg/dl.

Red blood cell transketolase (RBC-TK) levels are reduced and blood lactic acid levels raised.

Meyer's test
There is an increase in audible sounds in the antecubital fossa after subcutaneous injection of adrenaline.

Volhard's diuresis test
In a normal fasting person after drinking 1 litre of water all the fluid is excreted in 4 hours. In beriberi water retention is present which disappears after treatment with thiamine.

Acute cardiac beriberi responds dramatically within a few hours to an intravenous vitamin B₁ injection of 50–100 mg.

SEQUELAE

It was formerly considered that there were no long-term sequelae to wet beriberi. However, a case of gradually progressive congestive cardiomyopathy following severe wet beriberi acquired in a Far Eastern prisoner-of-war camp apparently proved fatal 30 years later.

TREATMENT

Wet beriberi

Specific treatment is with thiamine. Dramatic effects are observed in acute cardiac cases when large doses are given intravenously. Intravenous injections of 50 mg of thiamine should be repeated two or three times in 24 hours until serial radiographs show that the heart has been reduced to normal size. In moribund patients the injection has been made into the jugular vein. In severe cases venesection, taking 250–300 ml of blood from the arm, is of great value. In a straightforward case the patient should be confined to bed and given a high protein diet with restriction of salt and fluids, with the addition of thiamine to the diet in the form of tablets or by intramuscular injection.

Dry beriberi

Treatment with thiamine injections relieves the pain and subjective dysthesiae. Signs of peripheral neuropathy take some time to disappear but results are disappointing in some parts of the world where the patients will inevitably relapse after returning home and resuming a diet of polished rice.

Infantile beriberi

After a thiamine injection improvement will be noted in a few hours; sometimes it is dramatic. In acutely ill children thiamine 25 mg should be injected intravenously and a further 25 mg intramuscularly once or twice daily until the symptoms have subsided, when an oral dose of 10 mg should be given daily for several weeks. The child should be removed from the breast and given artificial feeds for 24 hours while the mother is given thiamine. Breast milk should be drawn off and discarded so that after 24 hours the mother is ready to feed her baby again.

PREVENTION

Beriberi can be eradicated by the prohibition of polished rice. This has been attempted in some countries but to legislate against the use of white rice in countries where rice is the staple food results in the appearance of a black market in this product. Unpolished (red) rice and parboiled rice—in which the vitamin is retained—are satisfactory foods. Beriberi can also be prevented by using mixed diets containing other sources of thiamine, such as pulses, groundnuts, whole wheat, vegetables, fruit and milk.

Health education and the development of methods of milling rice, in which the germ is retained, have led to the disappearance of beriberi from most eastern communities.

PELLAGRA

GEOGRAPHICAL DISTRIBUTION

Pellagra has been reported from most parts of the world where maize is consumed as a staple diet. Since the Second World War (1939–1945) pellagra has vanished from most parts of the world where it was formerly present and is now confined to parts of Kenya, Malawi, Zambia, Lesotho and South Africa. Its presence often follows social disturbances and the establishment of large camps for internment or refugees.

AETIOLOGY

Pellagra is a syndrome caused by a deficiency of a variety of specific factors, nicotinic acid (nicotinamide, niacin) being the most important. The amino acid tryptophan is a precursor of nicotinic acid in man; therefore, a diet with a high tryptophan but low nicotinic acid content is not pellagrogenic.

The richest sources of nicotinic acid are liver, kidney and yeast; others are wholemeal flour and green vegetables. Of staple foods maize contains the least available nicotinic acid, possibly because a large proportion of the nicotinic acid is in a bound form which can be liberated by alkaline hydrolysis; this is achieved by treatment of maize with lime as practised in Central America. The daily nicotinic acid requirement is about 10–15 mg but can be replaced by excess dietary tryptophan. Nicotinic acid is found in the tissues as a nucleotide, diphosphopyridine nucleotide (DPN) usually designated coenzyme I, formed by the combination of adenine ribose phosphate and nicotinamide. There is also a corresponding coenzyme II, triphosphopyridine nucleotide.

Coenzymes I and II are the coenzymes responsible for the oxidative enzyme dehydrogenases; they act as intermediate carriers for the hydrogen released from various substrates by the dehydrogenase enzymes. The enzymes containing nicotinamide are concerned with many important energy producing metabolic reactions. Nicotinic acid deficiency leads to metabolic disturbances in many tissues; the nervous system is seriously involved. There is also an impairment of pyruvic acid metabolism in pellagra which is more marked in pellagrins with neurological manifestations than in those without. Following administration of nicotinic acid alone for 15 days a group of pellagrins, pyruvic acid concentration returned to normal, suggesting that nicotinic acid deficiency was the cause of deranged pyruvate metabolism; there was also a significant improvement in neurological status after nicotinic acid therapy alone.

Pellagra appeared soon after the introduction of maize to Europe and advanced with the extension of maize cultivation. Epidemics of pellagra occur among maize (or sorghum) eaters. Pellagra is also present in non-maize-eating countries, such as India, Cuba and Brazil. In Central America where maize is also the staple, pellagra is rare. This may be due to the treatment of maize with lime which releases more tryptophan, or to coffee consumption, which is rich in niacin. The cause of pellagra is more complicated than a simple deficiency and is due to the disturbance of a delicate chemical balance between certain toxins present in relatively large amounts in maize and some essential dietary factors, of which nicotinic acid and tryptophan are the most important. Leucine, for instance, which is plentiful in sorghum, affects tryptophan and nicotinic acid metabolism in man. Analogues of nicotinic acid can produce pellagra-like effects in animals but it is not certain whether these result from poisonous substances present in maize. The main problem of pellagra is one of biochemical imbalance.

Secondary pellagra is due to non-absorption of the necessary vitamin(s) by a 'non-functioning' intestinal mucosa. It also occurs after prolonged treatment with large doses of isoniazid (used in chemotherapy of tuberculosis—Chapter 57) which replaces the nicotinic acid in the oxidative reduction coenzyme DPN.

PATHOLOGY

There is an increased excretion of coproporphyrin in the urine which has been regarded either as indicating faulty metabolism or abnormal absorption. It occurs especially in alcoholic pellagra but it has been demonstrated that the amount of coproporphyrin in the urine is inversely proportional to the nicotinic acid intake. Since oral gastrointestinal and neurological manifestations of pellagra can be evoked by exposure to sunlight it has been suggested that porphyrin metabolism in pellagra is abnormal. There is marked emaciation of the body. The viscera show fatty degeneration and a characteristic deep pigmentation. The intestinal mucosa and the liver and spleen are atrophied. The suprarenal capsules may be atrophied and the cortex appears black; the medulla may be the seat of haemorrhage(s). The heart shows 'brown atrophy'.

Central nervous system

Central nervous system manifestations have been summarized.[64] In the brain the main alterations are found in the Betz cells of the motor cortex and to a lesser extent the Purkinje cells, periventricular cell groups, and the nuclei of the cranial motor nerves. Chromatolysis, poor staining of nuclei and nucleoli

and an increase in intracellular pigment are the most constant findings. The frontal lobes are most affected but the basal ganglia may also show some degree of change. There is some endothelial thickening and hyaline degeneration of the walls of capillary blood vessels. In advanced cases gliosis may be present.

The spinal cord shows more or less symmetrical degeneration of the dorsal columns with scattered demyelination. The spinocerebellar and pyramidical tracts are involved to a lesser extent. The cells of Clarke's column show chromatolysis and pigmentary degeneration, the column of Goll being most affected. Myelin degeneration of the peripheral nerves is common. The myelin sheaths become irregular due to swelling and atrophy, and may present a honeycombed appearance.

CLINICAL FEATURES

The cardinal signs of pellagra constitute the well-known triad: 'diarrhoea, dermatitis and dementia'.

Prepellagrinous state

The initial symptoms consist of vague 'functional' digestive disturbances which recur during repeated exacerbations with periods of quiescence for years without the appearance of skin eruptions. The patient appears pale, has a peculiar lifeless staring look with dilated pupils and complains of non-specific symptoms, giddiness and vague but often severe pains in the back and joints. The complexion is 'muddy' with bluish leaden-coloured sclerae. The character changes, becoming irritable and at the same time stupid and morose. The earliest signs are difficult to define and a great many people suffering from chronic ill-health in an endemic pellagra area may really suffer from the prepellagrous state.

Other early vitamin B deficiencies may be associated with the prepellagrous state: angular stomatitis, an atrophic condition of the lips (perlèche), and cheilosis—associated with ariboflavinosis.

The disease may not advance beyond this point but it may progress to the fully developed syndrome.

Gastrointestinal symptoms and signs

The gums become swollen and bleed easily (alpine scurvy). The tongue may be scarlet, raw and fissured and the lingual papillae atrophied. A characteristic symptom is pyrosis—a burning sensation in the oesophagus causing dysphagia. The appetite is variable. There is tenderness in the epigastrium and over the lower abdomen. Although there may be constipation, diarrhoea is common and the stools are often pale and fermenting, resembling those of 'tropical sprue' (Chapter 3).

Dermatological lesions

Dermatological lesions appear on sites exposed to the sun and/or pressure. At first an erythema—not unlike severe sunburn—is observed on the parts of the body which are as a rule unclothed and exposed to the sun. The eruption is symmetrical and characteristic. It appears suddenly first on the back of the hands and feet, then on the forearms, legs, chest, neck, face and sometimes on the scrotum and female genitalia, anus and other regions subject to mechanical pressure and irritation. Patches of erythema are irregular in outline and intensity. Very characteristic is a symmetrical eruption behind the mastoid process, or a ring and collar around the neck (Casal's necklace) (Figure 21.11). The affected area is swollen and tense and the seat of burning or itching sensations—which become acute on exposure to the sun.

Congestion disappears completely but temporarily on pressure. Petechiae are common on the affected parts; blebs with clear opaque or blood-stained contents of feebly alkaline reaction may form. The eruption usually lasts about a fortnight and is followed by hyperkeratosis and desquamation, leaving the skin rough, thickened and stained a light sepia. This is especially marked on the backs of the hands and elbows. There may be malar or supraorbital pigmentation. Hyperkeratosis may follow and involve the whole body. Linear haemorrhagic strips of purpura may occur after exposure to the sun and after trauma, caused by increased permeability of the blood vessels; this was observed in prisoners in Indonesia.

Pellagra differs in individuals with a black or brown skin; erythema becomes a blackish or purplish patch on black skin. In olive-skinned races these appear sepia.

After the eruption has subsided atrophic patches of skin remain in the interdigital clefts and these, combined with wasting, produce the appearance of 'washerwoman's fingers'. The hands become aged and the nails atrophic and brittle.

Nervous system

The brain, spinal cord and peripheral nervous system may all be involved.

Central nervous system

The time of appearance of mental symptoms varies widely. They may be present from the start or occur during convalescence. The patient suffers from obstinate insomnia but occasionally from sleepiness. In general there is an anxiety neurosis with depressive features; depression is common. Psychosensory disturbances are common with intolerance of bright light, colours and noises; the affected individual becomes fidgety, quarrelsome and irritable. General deterioration of mental and physical health may antedate continued manifestations of disease or acute mania; confusion may herald death.

Encephalopathy and nicotinic acid deficiency

Acute encephalopathic states associated with a nicotinic acid deficiency are accompanied by an acute metabolic disturbance of a reversible nature. Certain stuporose and psychotic states in malnourished individuals have been found to respond to nicotinic acid. A clinical picture has been described consisting of clouding of consciousness, cogwheel rigidity of the extremities, and uncontrollable gasping and sucking reflexes. This syndrome has been observed in association with pellagra, alcoholism, polyneuropathy, Wernicke's encephalopathy and scurvy. No response was obtained with thiamine, but after nicotinic acid 1000 mg daily in divided doses parenterally, recovery occurred between the third and fifth days of treatment. Stupor, delirium and acute psychotic symptoms are sometimes present in association with a mild pellagrinous rash, and may respond dramatically to intravenous nicotinic acid.

Psychoses and pellagra

It has been estimated that 4–10% of patients with pellagra become permanently insane; in the USA pellagrins were formerly numerous in lunatic asy-

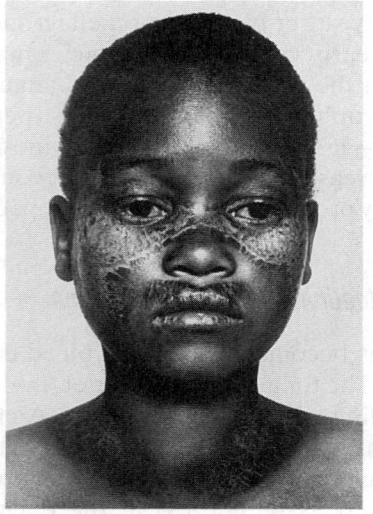

Figure 21.11 Butterfly skin lesions and Casal's necklace in pellagra.

lums. Not only may pellagra lead to insanity but those insane from other causes were formerly liable to pellagra. It was found that in certain mental institutions in the USA the number of mentally insane developing pellagra was a constant proportion of the total. In a review of pellagra in asylums in England it was found that, at the time of onset, pellagrins had been resident from 6 months to several years. The form of psychosis is a profound melancholia with suicidal tendencies preceded by restlessness and insomnia; it may closely resemble general paralysis of the insane. The mental aberration may be characterized by profound dementia, hallucinations and catatonia.

Spinal cord and peripheral nerve disturbances

Spinal cord or peripheral nerve involvement may precede, accompany or follow the cutaneous, oral and alimentary lesions of pellagra. In the early stages neurological manifestations are commonly those of a psychoneurotic kind, but later peripheral neuropathy or paraplegia of the ataxic or spastic type, or a combination of both may develop. Cord changes are more common than those of a neuropathy. Tremors and rigidity—possibly of extrapyramidal origin, may occur. Burning, tingling and aching feet suggest neuropathy; exaggerated knee jerks and extensor plantar responses suggest a pyramidal lesion, and ataxic paraplegia is not uncommon in the late stages of the disease. The cranial nerves may be involved and eighth nerve deafness, retrobulbar neuritis and central scotomas have been recorded.

The variable incidence of these neurological complications in different pellagrous communities, together with the fact that they sometimes appear after recovery from pellagra and are resistant to treatment with nicotinic acid, suggest that they are caused by associated vitamin B deficiencies and are not features of pellagra *per se*. They are considered more fully in Chapter 8.

Associated vitamin B deficiencies

Ariboflavinosis with angular stomatitis and cheilosis may occur in the early stages of pellagra. 'Burning feet' is a common symptom and is probably associated with pantothenic acid deficiency.

Ocular changes

The eyes may be affected, with oedema of the conjunctivae, corneal dystrophy and lens opacities of three types—powder-like, multiple, irregular and tongue-like—extending from the peripheral zone towards the centre.

Course

The symptoms may abate 2–3 months after onset and although the affected skin remains dark and rough, the disease appears to be arrested. The following spring, however, if the diet similar, it recurs in a more severe form. The eruption assumes a darker colour and the depression of spirits deepens into melancholia which may have maniacal interludes and a peculiar tendency to suicide. The general feeling of weakness increases, the affected individual loses weight and is unable to work, and the gait becomes uncertain and of the spastic paraplegic type. The tongue is tremulous. Pains in the back become acute and there may be lightning pains, cramps, twitching, tremors and even epileptiform convulsions of cortical type. Diarrhoea becomes troublesome. Symptoms may persist for years unless the diet is improved.

Secondary pellagra

Pellagra due to voluntary dietary restriction has been recognized for several years; slimming, ketogenic and faddist diets have all been held responsible. It is also considered that hyperthyroidism predisposes to pellagra.

Surgical pellagra

Pellagra may follow major surgical operations on the gastrointestinal tract, such as partial colectomy or total or partial gastrectomy. It may also be associated with an organic lesion of the gastrointestinal tract, such as oesophageal stricture, gastric carcinoma, pyloric stenosis, carcinoma of the colon, stricture of the rectum, rectal polyposis, Crohn's disease, chronic intestinal amoebiasis and malabsorption syndromes such as coeliac disease and 'tropical sprue'. Failure of biosynthesis of vitamins is a possible cause in such cases.

Alcoholic pellagra

Alcoholic pellagra occurs especially in those who drink methyl alcohol; it is possible that chronic gastritis interferes with the production of intrinsic factor and absorption of nicotinic acid.

Drug-induced pellagra

Isoniazid, used in the treatment of tuberculosis (Chapter 57), may cause pellagra when administered in doses >300 mg daily, by displacing nicotinic acid in the oxidative reduction coenzyme DPN. In these cases nicotinic acid supplements must be given along with the isoniazid. Sulphonamides interfere with the action of nicotinic acid and can also cause pellagrous rashes.

DIAGNOSIS

In acute pellagra, blood nicotinic acid concentration is <0.31 mg/dl; on treatment this rises to >0.55 mg/dl. A combination of localized erythema of seasonal recurrence with neurological, particularly mental, disturbance in a person from an endemic pellagrous area is not likely to be confused with any other disease.

The rash may be mistaken for: acrodynia, erythema multiforme, dermatitis venenata, lupus erythematosus or eczema solare. The combination of mental and neurological signs must be distinguished from: hysteria, cerebrovascular syphilis, general paresis of the insane, ergotism, lathyrism and other nutritional neuropathies.

TREATMENT

The most important aspect of management of pellagra is to provide an ample balanced diet and most pellagrins will improve as rapidly on a good hospital diet as on any other treatment. There is evidence that rapidly increasing the intake of one vitamin may precipitate imbalance and produce deficiency in another. A high energy diet—3000–4000 calories (12 600–16 800 kJ) is necessary with good supplies of fresh meat, liver, milk, eggs and in addition a source of vitamin B complex, such as yeast 25–30 g daily.

Nicotinic acid

Nicotinic acid should be given at 50 mg three times daily for 10–14 days; this dose should be doubled in a severe case. There is usually a pharmacological reaction with tingling and warmth over the malar regions and neck, caused by vasodilatation. Overdosage may cause tingling and numbness of the tongue and lower jaw.

In acute mania, or encephalopathy associated with pellagra, intravenous nicotinic acid at high dose (1000 mg daily in divided doses) may produce a dramatic recovery. The spinal symptoms of pellagra are largely resistant to treatment and nicotinic acid has limited value in chronic psychotic pellagrins.

Maize and sorghum—both associated with pellagra—contain large amounts of leucine, which affects the metabolism of tryptophan and nicotinic

acid. Isoleucine counteracts this metabolic effect and pellagrous patients (sorghum eaters) have been treated with 5 g of isoleucine daily; cure occurs in about 15 days. Controls kept on the sorghum diet without isoleucine did not improve.

Riboflavin

Since ariboflavinosis (see below) frequently accompanies pellagra, treatment should be reinforced with riboflavin 1–3 mg daily.

Parentrovite

'Parentrovite' is a proprietary multivitamin preparation which is of great value in the treatment of pellagra.

EPIDEMIOLOGY

Seasonal incidence

In Europe pellagra appeared formerly during the spring and autumn, being most severe in the spring. In Egypt the incidence was similar. In Malawi, pellagra was prevalent during August, September and October, the 'southern spring'. In the northern USA the disease exhibited the usual double incidence, the spring outbreak occurring during May/June and the autumnal one in September/October. In the Deep South the disease used to appear as early as January. This clear seasonal periodicity indicated that climatic factors have an important though indirect effect and it is likely that exposure to sunlight, which exacerbates all the manifestations of pellagra, is responsible.

Sex

Both sexes are liable to the disease but in different geographical locations the disease exhibits a different predilection for one or other sex in accordance with occupation and habit. In the USA it was more prevalent in women of childbearing age because of the debilitating effect(s) of menstruation, pregnancy and lactation. Elderly people living alone are especially liable, owing to their monotonous diet.

Age

Pellagra is a disease of middle age, the majority of cases occurring between 20 and 50 years. So-called 'infantile pellagra' is now known to be synonymous with protein–energy malnutrition (see above), and is not a pellagrinous condition.

Occupation

Pellagra is most prevalent amongst field labourers undertaking hard manual work. It is very prevalent amongst prison population. Epidemics of pellagra commonly occur when an apparently healthy prison or camp population is suddenly exposed to unaccustomed hard physical labour, such as building an airfield or road.

Diet

The dietary factor is all-important. In the southern USA, pellagra was common when the main diet consisted of molasses and corn (maize). With improved social and economic conditions and the development of supermarkets, pellagra-preventing foods such as milk and eggs became freely available, and pellagra has vanished from the community. Pellagra is a disease of poverty, backwardness and subsistence agriculture—affecting large populations involved in plantation labour.

PREVENTION

Pellagra may be prevented by a change in the economic and social conditions that cause it. In institutions and prisons the diet must not be confined to maize meal, but must include fresh fruit and vegetables and foods containing B vitamins. Hard physical work should be avoided when the diet is inadequate.

ARIBOFLAVINOSIS

GEOGRAPHICAL DISTRIBUTION

Ariboflavinosis is present worldwide and is associated with other deficiency syndromes such as pellagra and PEM; it was common in prisoner-of-war camps in the South-east Asia in the Second World War (1939–1945).

AETIOLOGY

Ariboflavinosis is caused by deficiency of riboflavin (vitamin B_2). Riboflavin (vitamin B_2) is present in tissues as a dinucleotide, flavinadenine dinucleotide (FADN) or flavine, which occupies a key position in reactions leading to the oxidation of hydrogen to water. The main sources are meat, legumes, milk and wholemeal flour. Riboflavin is destroyed on exposure to light, and signs of riboflavin deficiency occur when the daily intake is <0.2–0.3 mg. Daily intake of 0.35–0.5 mg is adequate, but daily intake of 2 mg riboflavin is considered ideal for an adult.

PATHOLOGY

Lack of tone in small blood vessels is believed to be the cause of the lesions at the junction of skin with mucous membranes and epithelial surfaces.

CLINICAL FEATURES

Sore red lips (cheilosis), a marked increase in vertical fissuring of the lips (perlèche), fissured angles of the mouth (angular stomatitis) and a purplish raw tongue covered with enlarged granular papillae are among the most constant signs of ariboflavinosis. Other signs are facial lesions consisting of seborrhoeic excrescences (dyssebacea), varying in length—up to 1 mm—and sparsely scattered over the face. The mouths of sebaceous glands are plugged with inspissated sebum giving the skin a roughened appearance which, when it occurs on the shoulders, arms and legs, is known as follicular hyperkeratosis, phrynoderma or 'toad's skin'. This may, however, be a manifestation of vitamin A deficiency (see above) and is not caused by ariboflavinosis. Scrotal dermatitis, an eczematous condition of the scrotum, is due to ariboflavinosis. Ariboflavinosis frequently complicates other deficiency syndromes such as pellagra and PEM, and was frequently associated with the deficiency syndromes occurring in prisoner-of-war camps in South-east Asia during the Second World War (1939–1945).

TREATMENT

Ariboflavinosis is rapidly cured by administration of 2–5 mg of riboflavin daily. Measures designed to improve the diet in a general manner with an increased intake of legumes, roots and animal proteins will prevent deficiency.

REFERENCES

1 Carpenter K J. Nutritional science and the Third World. *Am J Clin Nutr* 1993; 57:86–87.

2 Igbedioh S O. Undernutrition in Nigeria: dimension, causes and remedies for alleviation in a changing socio-economic environment. *Nutr Health* 1993; 9:1–14.

3 Magnani R J, Mock N B, Bertrand W E & Clay D C. Breast-feeding, water and sanitation, and childhood malnutrition in the Philippines. *J Biosoc Sci* 1993; 25:195–211.

4 Malnutrition and diet-related death rates remain rampant in some nations. *Soz Praventivmed* 1993; 38:104–105.

5 International Conference on Nutrition (news). *World Health Forum* 1993; 14:207–209.

6 Scrimshaw N S, Taylor C E & Gordon J E (eds). Interactions of nutrition and infection. *WHO Monogr* 1968; 57:1–329.

7 Golden M H N, Golden B E, Holland P S E G & Jackson A A. Zinc and immunocompetence in protein–energy malnutrition. *Lancet* 1978; i:1226–1228.

8 Brown K H & Begin F. Malnutrition among weanlings of developing countries: still a problem begging for solutions. *J Pediatr Gastroenterol Nutr* 1993; 17:132–138.

9 Onis M de, Monteiro C, Akré J & Glugston G. The worldwide magnitude of protein–energy malnutrition: an overview from the WHO Global Database on Child Growth. *Bull World Health Organ* 1993; 71:703–712.

10 Popkin B M, Keyou G, Zhai F, Guo X, Haijiang M & Zohoori N. The nutrition transition in China: a cross-sectional analysis. *Eur J Clin Nutr* 1993; 47:333–346.

11 Shimeles D & Lulseged S. Clinical profile and pattern of infection in Ethiopian children with severe protein–energy malnutrition. *East Afr Med J* 1994; 71:264–267.

12 Wandel M. Nutrition-related diseases and dietary change among Third World immigrants in northern Europe. *Nutr Health* 1993; 9:117–133.

13 Pryer J A. Body mass index and work-disabling morbidity: results from a Bangladeshi case study. *Eur J Clin Nutr* 1993; 47:653–657.

14 Williams C D. Nutritional disease of childhood associated with maize diet. *Arch Dis Child* 1933; 8:423–433.

15 Liu L S. Nutrition in China. *Acta Cardiol* 1993; 48:469–470.

16 Trowell H C, Davies J N P & Dean R F A. *Kwashiorkor*. London: Edward Arnold, 1954: 308.

17 Morley D. Prevention of protein–calorie deficiency syndromes. *Trans R Soc Trop Med Hyg* 1968; 62:200–208.

18 Gardner J M M & Grantham-McGregor S M. Physical activity, undernutrition and child development. *Proc Nutr Soc* 1994; 53:241–248.

19 Jain S & Choudhry M. Mother surrogate and nutritional status of preschool children. *Indian J Pediatr* 1993; 60:429–433.

20 Kusin J A, Kardjati S & Renqvist U H. Chronic undernutrition in pregnancy and lactation. *Proc Nutr Soc* 1993; 52:19–28.

21 Hendrickse R G. The influence of aflatoxins on child health in the tropics with particular reference of kwashiorkor. *Trans R Soc Trop Med Hyg* 1984; 78:427–435.

22 Leading article. Aflatoxins and kwashiorkor. *Lancet* 1984; ii:1133–1134.

23 Brooks S E H, Doherty J F & Golden M H N. Peroxisomes and the hepatic pathology of childhood malnutrition. *West Indian Med J* 1994; 43:15–17.

24 Cook G C & Hutt M S R. The liver after kwashiorkor. *BMJ* 1967; iii:454–457.

25 Cook G C. Glucose tolerance after kwashiorkor. *Nature* 1967; 215:1295–1296.

26 Cook G C & Lee F D. The jejunum after kwashiorkor. *Lancet* 1966; ii:1263–1267.

27 Gupta S, Singh B & Minocha S K. Fulminant right sided endocarditis in a malnourished patient. *J Assoc Physicians India* 1993; 41:740–741.

28 Gyárfás I. Nutrition and chronic disease – the viewpoint of WHO. *Acta Cardiol* 1993; 48:477–479.

29 Murray M J, Murray A B, Murray M B & Murray C J. The adverse effect of iron repletion on the course of certain infections. *BMJ* 1978; ii:1113–1115.

30 Waterlow J C. Kwashiorkor revisited: the pathogenesis of oedema in kwashiorkor and its significance. *Trans R Soc Trop Med Hyg* 1984; 78:436–441.

31 Arya S C. Ideal age for measles vaccination with persisting maternal antibody, human immunodeficiency virus infection and protein–calorie malnutrition. *Infection* 1993; 21:256–257.

32 Bani I A. The problems and challenges in growth monitoring. *East Afr Med J* 1993; 70:743–745.

33 Stanfield J P. Some aspects of the long-term effects of malnutrition on the behaviour of children in the Third World. *Proc Nutr Soc* 1993; 52:201–210.

34 Allen L H. Nutritional influences on linear growth: a general review. *Eur J Clin Nutr* 1994; 48 (supplement 1):S75–S89.

35 Tomkins A, Behrens R & Roy S. The role of zinc and vitamin A deficiency in diarrhoeal syndromes in developing countries. *Proc Nutr Soc* 1993; 52:131–142.

36 Hlaing T. Ascariasis and childhood malnutrition. *Parasitology* 1993; 107 (supplement):S125–S136.

37 Lunn P G & Northrop-Clewes C A. The impact of gastrointestinal parasites on protein–energy malnutrition in man. *Proc Nutr Soc* 1993; 52:101–111.

38 Murrell K D. Presidential address. Dr Stoll's wormy world revisited: the neglected animal diseases. *J Parasitol* 1994; 80:173–188.

39 Stephenson L S. Helminth parasites, a major factor in malnutrition. *World Health Forum* 1994; 15:169–172.

40 Berg A. Sliding toward nutrition malpractice: time to reconsider and redeploy. *Annu Rev Nutr* 1993; 57:3–7.

41 Berg A. Sliding toward nutrition malpractice: time to reconsider and redeploy. Martin J. Forman Memorial Lecture. Presented at the annual meeting of the National Center for International Health, Washington, DC, June 24, 1991.

42 Berg A. Malnutrition and 'nutrition engineering' in low-income countries: a rejoinder. *Int J Health Serv* 1993; 23:615–619, 621–623.

43 Brewster D R. Nutritional malpractice: a pediatric perspective. *Am J Clin Nutr* 1993; 58:575–576 & 580–581.

44 Csete J. Malnutrition and 'nutrition engineering' in low-income countries: a comment on Alan Berg's vision of the nutrition track record. *Int J Health Serv* 1993; 23:607–614.

45 Golden M H. Is complete catch-up possible for stunted malnourished children? *Eur J Clin Nutr* 1994; 48 (supplement 1):S58, S71.

46 Grantham-McGregor S, Powell C, Walker S, Chang S & Fletcher P. The long-term follow-up of severely malnourished children who participated in an intervention program. *Child Dev* 1994; 65:428–439.

47 Seaman J. Aid programmes for malnutrition and the role of the nutritionist. *Proc Nutr Soc* 1993; 52:175–182.

48 Carriere R C. Ending malnutrition: whose responsibility? *Am J Clin Nutr* 1993; 58:577–578, 580–581.

49 The Children's Health Care Collaborative Study Group. The causes of children's institutionalization in Romania. *Child Care Health Dev* 1994; 20:77–88.

50 Choudhury A Y & Bhuiya A. Effects of biosocial variables on changes in nutritional status of rural Bangladeshi children, pre- and post-monsoon flooding. *J Biosoc Sci* 1993; 25: 351–357.

51 Ghebremeskel K & Crawford M A. Nutrition and health in relation to food production and processing. *Nutr Health* 1994; 9:237–253.

52 Herrick J B. The gentle cow as scapegoat for world hunger? *J Am Vet Med Assoc* 1993; 202:882–883.

53 Mo-suwan L, Junjana C & Peutpaiboon A. Increasing obesity in school children in a transitional society and the effect of the weight control program. *Southeast Asian J Trop Med Public Health* 1993; 24:590–594.

54 Uauy-Dagach R. The practice of clinical nutrition in a developing nation. *J Nutr* 1994; 124 (supplement 8):1449S–1454S.

55 Waterlow J. Malnutrition of children in developing countries: what can we do? *Med War* 1993; 9:108–115.

56 Buttfield I H & Hetzel B S. Endemic goitre in Eastern New Guinea with special reference to the use of iodized oil in prophylaxis and treatment. *Bull World Health Organ* 1967; 36:243–262.

57 Trowbridge F L, Harris S S, Cook J et al. Coordinated strategies for controlling micronutrient malnutrition: a technical workshop. *J Nutr* 1993; 123:775–787.

58 Prentice A & Bates C J. Adequacy of dietary mineral supply for human bone growth and mineralisation. *Eur J Clin Nutr* 1994; 48 (supplement 1):S161, S177.

59 Dunnigan M G, McIntosh W B & Ford J A. Rickets in Asian immigrants. *Lancet* 1976; i:1346.

60 Bellagio brief: vitamin A deficiency and childhood mortality. *Bull Pan Am Health Organ* 1993; 27:192–197.

61 Olson J A. Hypovitaminosis A: contemporary scientific issues. *J Nutr* 1994; 124 (supplement 8):1461S–1466S.

62 Underwood B A. Hypovitaminosis A: international programmatic issues. *J Nutr* 1994; 124 (supplement 8):1467S–1472S.

63 Campbell C H. The severe lacticacidosis of thiamine deficiency: acute pernicious or fulminating beriberi. *Lancet* 1984; ii:446–449.

64 Spillane J D (ed.). *Tropical Neurology*. London: Oxford University Press, 1973:448.

CHAPTER 22

ANIMAL TOXINS

D. A. Warrell

VENOMOUS BITES AND STINGS

Venoms are complex mixtures of compounds with toxic, irritant or allergic properties which are secreted by some groups of animals to be injected into their prey or squirted at their enemies. Possession of venom by an easily recognizable and often highly coloured reptile, amphibian or bird may confer protection on its species and the harmless species which mimic its appearance or behaviour. The venoms secreted on to the skin of some amphibians may protect their moist integument against infection as well as being distasteful, poisonous and therefore deterrent to predators. Animals have evolved various methods of injecting venom into their prey or aggressors. Mammals (Insectivora and vampire bats), snakes, lizards, spiders, centipedes, ticks, leeches and octopuses inject their venoms by biting with teeth, fangs, venom jaws, beak or other hardened mouth parts; duck-billed platypuses, fish, coelenterates, echinoderms, insects and scorpions do so by stinging. Some snakes, toads, scorpions and other arthropods squirt their venom at enemies. Poisoning which results from the ingestion of the flesh and viscera of aquatic animals is discussed in the second part of this chapter (see p. 509). Allergic reactions to injected venoms and ingested poisons are in some cases far more dangerous than their direct toxic effects. This is a large subject in its own right; here it will be referred to only briefly.

VENOMOUS MAMMALS

The duck-billed platypus (*Ornithorhynchus anatinus*) is an aquatic egg-laying mammal of eastern Australia. Males have sharp spurs on their hindlimbs connected by a duct to crural venom glands. This venom apparatus is used defensively and in fights between males during the breeding season. Each year, at least one human is stung by a platypus in Victoria.[1] However, fewer than 20 cases have been reported.[1,2] The venom can cause agonizing local pain, persistent local swelling and inflammation with regional lymphadenopathy, but no cases of life-threatening envenoming has been reported. Experimentally, the venom is weakly haemolytic, coagulant and causes local haemorrhage, oedema and fatal hypotension in animals.

Several species of Insectivora produce a venomous secretion from enlarged and granular submaxillary salivary glands which discharge at the base of the lower incisors, which may be grooved. Venom is conducted along the concave surfaces of these teeth and probably serves to immobilize amphibian and rodent prey.[3] Venomous species include the Haitian solenodon (*Solenodon paradoxus*) and possibly the Cuban solenodon (*Aoptogale cubanus*), the European water shrew (*Neomys fodiens*), Mediterranean shrew (*N. anomalous*) and the short-tailed shrew of the eastern USA and Canada (*Blarina brevicauda*). The venom of the last of these species is the most toxic and is probably a protein. It produces fatal cardiorespiratory and neurotoxic effects in rodents and lagomorphs. In humans, bites by these species occasionally result in local pain, swelling and inflammation. The saliva of vampire bats (Desmodontinae) increases capillary permeability, inhibits platelet aggregation, inhibits activation of factor XI by factor XII and activates plasminogen (desmokinase) causing fibrinolysis.[4] These effects presumably promote the flow of blood from the animal on which the bats are feeding.

VENOMOUS SNAKES

TAXONOMY, IDENTIFICATION AND DISTRIBUTION

Of the 2500–3000 species of snakes, about 500 belong to the four families of venomous snakes, Atractaspididae, Elapidae, Hydrophiidae and Viperidae. Only about 200 species have caused death or permanent disability by biting humans. More than 30 species of another family, the Colubridae, once considered harmless, have produced signs of envenoming in man and five species have caused fatal bites.[5] Among non-venomous snakes, only the giant constrictors (family Boidae) are potentially dangerous to man. There have been a number of fatal attacks by these snakes reported from Africa (rock python, *Python sebae*), South-East Asia (especially Indonesia) (reticulated python, *Python reticulatus*) and South America (anaconda, *Eunectes murinus*). Some of the victims, even adults, were swallowed.

Snakes are classified on morphological grounds, from the arrangement of their scales (lepidosis), dentition, osteology, myology, sensory organs, the form of the hemipenes, and more recently by immunological studies of their venoms and serum proteins and sequence analysis of DNA encoding important mitochondrial and other enzymes.[6]

Legless lizards, such as slow worms, glass lizards (Anguidae), worm-like geckos (Pygopodidae) (Figure 22.1) and legless skinks, may be distinguished from snakes by the presence of eyelids, external ears, friable tails and by the lack of enlarged ventral scales. Some have vestigial limbs. Amphisbaenids have worm-like annular grooves along the length of their bodies and caecilians (legless amphibians) lack obvious eyes and scales. Eels and pipe-shaped fish are distinguished from snakes by their gills and fins.

All medically important species of snakes have one or more pairs of enlarged teeth with grooves or venom channels, the fangs, in the upper jaw, by which venom is introduced through the skin of a human victim. Approximately 400 of the 2500 species of Colubridae have short, immobile fangs or enlarged solid teeth at the posterior end of the maxilla (Figure 22.2). The African and Middle Eastern burrowing asps or stiletto snakes (genus Atractaspis, family Atractaspididae), also known as burrowing or mole vipers or adders, false vipers or side-stabbing snakes, have very long front fangs on which they impale their victims by a side-swiping motion, the fang protruding from the corner of the partially closed mouth (Figure 22.3). The Natal black snake (*Macrelaps microlepidotus*), now included in Atractaspididae, possesses two very large grooved fangs at the posterior ends of its maxillae. The Elapidae (cobras—*Naja*; kraits—*Bungarus*; mambas—*Dendroaspis*; shield-nosed snakes—*Aspidelaps*; Asian and American coral snakes—*Calliophis*, *Maticora*, *Micrurus*; African garter snakes—*Elapsoidea*; terrestrial venomous Australasian snakes, etc.) have relatively short, fixed front fangs (Figure 22.4). The Hydrophiidae, sea snakes (Figure 22.5), have short, fixed fangs like elapids (Figure 22.6). The Viperidae (vipers, adders, rattlesnakes, moccasins, lance-headed vipers and pit vipers) have highly developed long, curved, hinged, front fangs which have a closed venom channel, giving them a structure like a hypodermic needle (Figure 22.7). The subfamily Crotalinae (pit vipers) includes the rattlesnakes (genera *Crotalus* and *Sistrurus*), moccasins (*Agkistrodon*) and lance-headed vipers (genera *Bothrops*, *Bothriechis*, *Porthidium*,

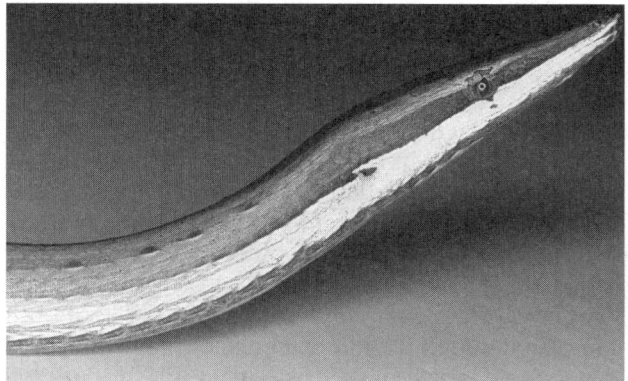

Figure 22.1   A legless lizard, Burton's snake-lizard (*Lialis burtonis*: family Pygopodidae) from Papua New Guinea. Note external ear. (Copyright D.A. Warrell.)

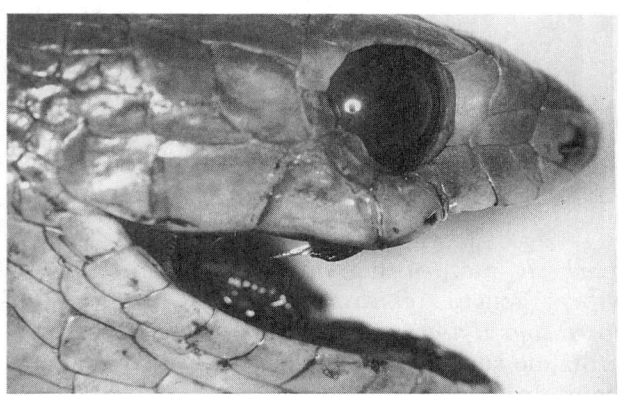

Figure 22.2   Rear fangs of the boomslang (*Dispholidus typus*), a dangerous African colubrid. (Copyright D.A. Warrell.)

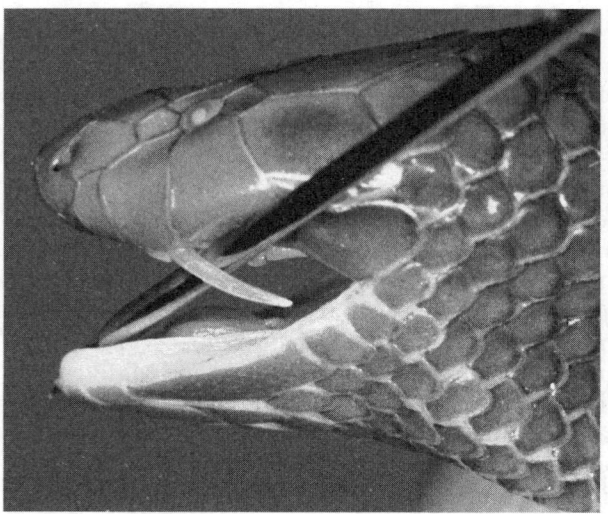

Figure 22.3   Very long front fang of a West African burrowing asp (*Atractaspis aterrima*: family Atractaspididae).

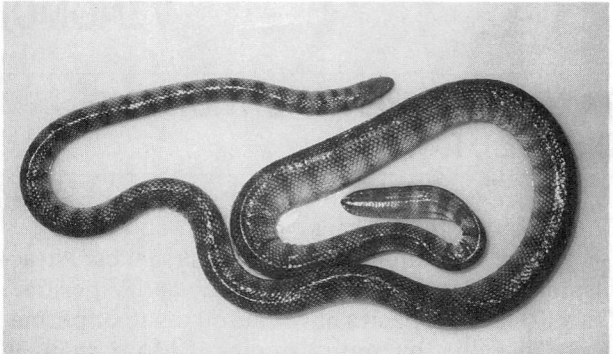

Figure 22.5   A common sea snake of South-East Asia (*Hydrophis cyanocinctus*: family Hydrophiidae). Note flattened tail. Specimen 1.4 metres long, from the Gulf of Siam. (Copyright D.A. Warrell.)

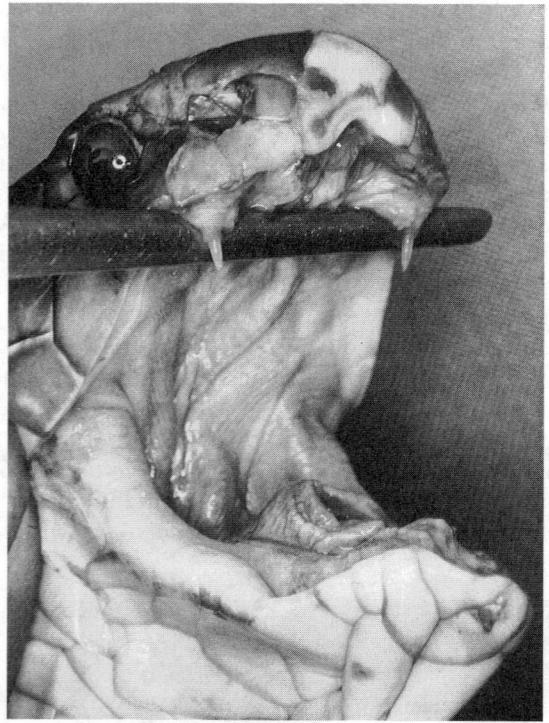

Figure 22.4   Short front fangs of the monocellate Thai cobra (*Naja kaouthia*: family Elapidae).

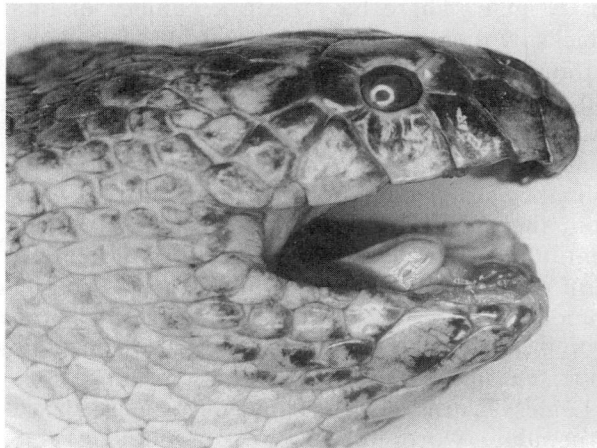

Figure 22.6   Short front fang of the sea snake (*Lapemis hardwickii*). (Copyright D.A. Warrell.)

Lachesis, etc.) of the Americas and the Asian pit vipers (genera *Agkistrodon*, *Deinagkistrodon*, *Calloselasma*, *Trimeresurus*, *Hypnale*, etc.). The pit of crotaline snakes is a heat-sensitive organ, situated between the eye and nostril, which detects warm-blooded prey (Figure 22.8). Snakes of the subfamily Viperinae, the Old World vipers and adders, have

no pit organ. The English words viper and adder have not been strictly applied to distinguish those species which produce live young (ovoviviparous) and those which lay eggs.

None of the care and skill lavished on the identification of parasites and their vectors is devoted by medical staff to the identification of venomous snakes. In some cases, however, a precise diagnosis can be life-saving. For example, the two common South-East Asian kraits, *Bungarus fasciatus* and *B. candidus*, are superficially similar in appearance, but monospecific *B. fasciatus* antivenom is ineffective in patients envenomed by *B. candidus*.[7] There is no simple and reliable method of distinguishing venomous from non-venomous snakes. The mouth can be examined for the presence of fangs but these may be very small in the case of elapids, and folded back inside a sheath in vipers. However, the most dangerous species are usually well known in the areas where they occur. The characteristic hood of

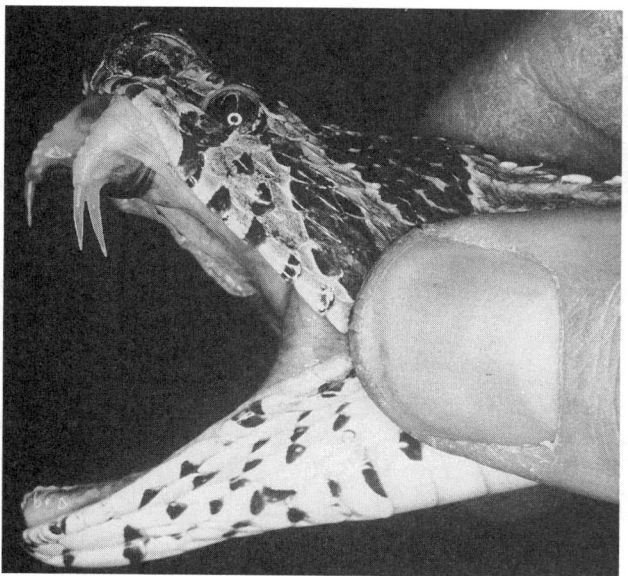

Figure 22.7   Long hinged front fangs, with reserve fang on its left side, enclosed in dental sheath, in a Thai Russell's viper (*Daboia russelii siamensis*: family Viperidae; subfamily Viperinae). (Copyright D.A. Warrell.)

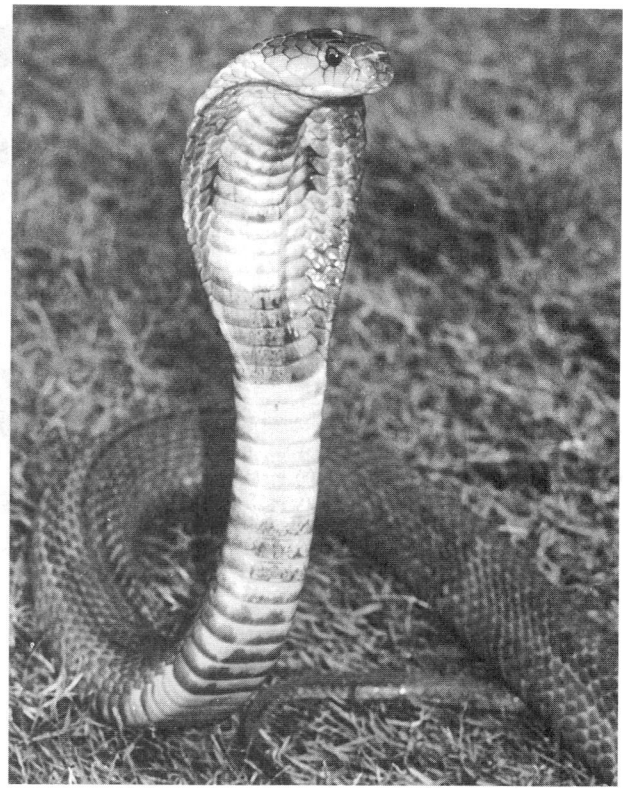

Figure 22.9   Thai spitting cobra, brown phase (*Naja siamensis*: family Elapidae) showing spread hood in threatening/defensive attitude. Specimen 1.3 metres long from central Thailand. (Copyright D.A. Warrell.)

cobras and some other elapids is evident only when the snake is rearing up in a defensive attitude (Figure 22.9). Vipers are often identifiable by their repeated and sometimes colourful dorsal pattern (Figure 22.10). Russell's viper (*Daboia russelii*) and puff adders (*Bitis arietans*) make a loud hissing sound by expelling air through their large nostrils, the saw-scaled or carpet vipers (genus *Echis*) produce a characteristic rasping sound by rubbing their coils together (Figure 22.11), rattlesnakes produce an unmistakeable sound and king cobras (*Ophio-*

phagus hannah) 'growl'. Some harmless species are readily confused with the venomous ones which they mimic: for example *Telescopus* (cat snake) and *Dasypeltis* (egg-eating snake) with *Echis* (saw-scaled viper) species in Africa; *Boiga multomaculata* with *Daboia russelii* in Thailand; various species of *Dryocalamus* and *Lycodon* with *Bungarus candidus* and *B. caeruleus* and *Xenodon severus* with *Bothrops brazili* and similar species. Table 22.1 lists the species which, in each continent, are responsible for most snake bite deaths and severe morbidity. Some species, although notorious for the potency of their venom (e.g. many species of sea snakes and Australasian elapids), or their great size (e.g. king cobra, *Ophiophagus hannah* and Gaboon viper *Bitis gabonica*), have not been included because they rarely bite humans. The African night adders (genus *Causus*), Asian green pit vipers (genus *Trimeresurus*) and Latin American hog-nosed vipers (e.g. *Porthidium nasutum*) bite many people but rarely cause severe envenoming. Illustrated books, papers and keys have been published for the identification of venomous snakes in most parts of the world, but most are out of print

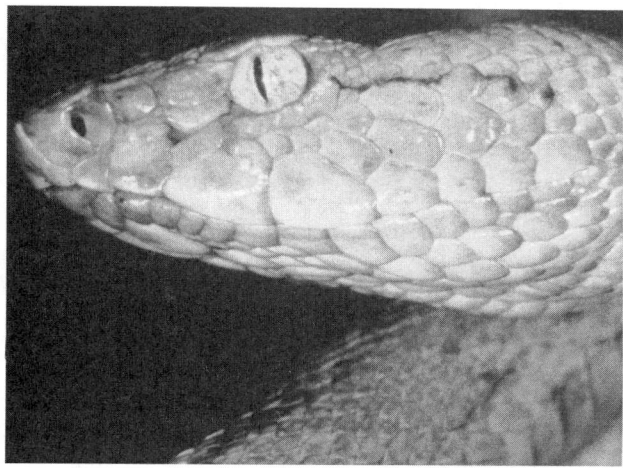

Figure 22.8   Japanese Tokara habu (*Trimeresurus tokarensis*: family Viperidae; subfamily Crotalinae) showing heat-sensitive pit organ between eye and nostril. (Copyright D.A. Warrell.)

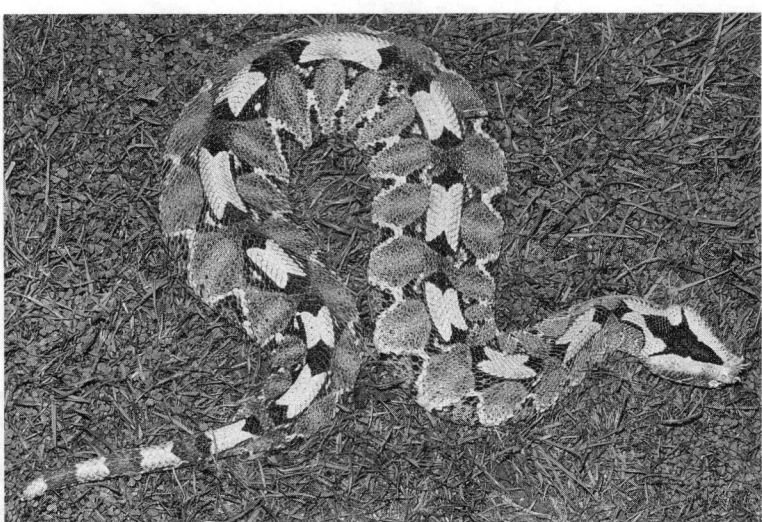

Figure 22.10 Rhinoceros or nose-horned viper of the African rain forest (*Bitis nasicornis*) showing distinctive repeated dorsal pattern. Specimen 90 cm long from Cameroon. (Copyright D.A. Warrell.)

and available only in libraries or through antiquarian booksellers.

Venomous snakes are widely distributed, up to altitudes of 4000 metres (*Agkistrodon himalayanus*), especially in tropical countries. One species (*Vipera berus*) just enters the Arctic Circle. There are no other venomous species in the Arctic, Antarctic, in North America, north of about latitude 51°N, Newfoundland, Nova Scotia, in most of the islands of the western Mediterranean, Atlantic and Caribbean (except in Martinique, Santa Lucia, Margarita, Trinidad and Aruba), in Madagascar and Chile (where there are mildly venomous colubrid snakes), New Caledonia, New Zealand, Hawaii and some other Pacific Islands, Crete, Ireland and Iceland. Sea snakes exist in the Indian and Pacific Oceans between latitudes 30°N and 30°S as far north as Siberia (*Pelamis platurus*), in estuaries, rivers and in some freshwater lakes (e.g. *Hydrophis semperi* in Lake Taal, Philippines; *Enhydrina schistosa* in Ton Ley Sap, Cambodia).

EPIDEMIOLOGY

The determinants of incidence and severity of snake bite are summarized in Table 22.2. The incidence of snake bite and its related morbidity and mortality has been determined most precisely in industrialized countries such as the USA[8] and Australia.[1] In the tropical countries where snake bite is a serious problem there are few reliable data. Records of patients treated by traditional methods are lost to the official statistics. Hospital records, the sole source of most snake bite reporting, are likely to

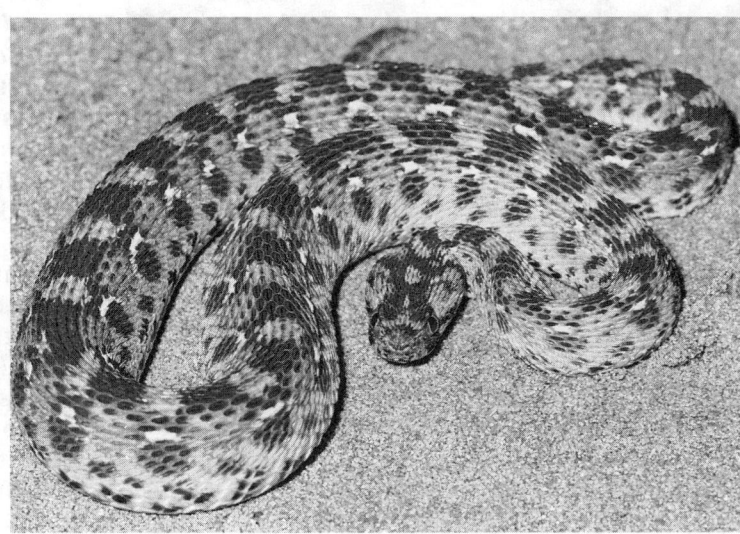

Figure 22.11 Saw-scaled or carpet viper (*Echis ocellatus*). Specimen 55 cm long from north-eastern Nigeria. (Copyright D.A. Warrell.)

Table 22.1 Species of snake probably responsible for most deaths and morbidity.

Area	Scientific name	English name
North America	*Crotalus adamanteus*	Eastern diamondback rattlesnake
	Crotalus atrox	Western diamondback rattlesnake
	Crotalus viridis subspecies	Western rattlesnakes
Central America	*Crotalus durissus durissus*	Central American rattlesnake
	Bothrops asper	Terciopelo, caissaca
South America	*Bothrops atrox, B. asper*	Fer-de-lance, barba amarilla
	Bothrops jararaca	Jararaca
	Crotalus durissus terrificus	South American rattlesnake, cascabel
	Lachesis muta	Bushmaster
Europe	*Vipera berus*	Viper, adder
	Vipera ammodytes	Long-nosed viper
Africa	*Echis* species	Saw-scaled or carpet vipers
	Bitis arietans	Puff adder
	Naja nigricollis, N. mossambica, etc.	African spitting cobras
	Naja haje	Egyptian cobra
	Dendroaspis species	Mambas
Asia, Middle East	*Echis* species	Saw-scaled or carpet vipers
	Vipera (Macrovipera) lebetina	Levantine viper
	Vipera palaestinae	Palestine viper
Indian subcontinent and South-East Asia	*Naja naja, N. kaouthia*, etc.	Asian cobras
	Bungarus species	Kraits
	Daboia russelii subspecies	Russell's vipers
	Calloselasma rhodostoma	Malayan pit viper
	Trimeresurus species	Green pit vipers
	Echis carinatus, E. sochureki	Saw-scaled or carpet vipers
Far East	*Naja atra*, etc.	Asian cobras
	Bungarus multicinctus	Chinese krait
	Trimeresurus flavoviridis	Japanese habu
	Trimeresurus mucrosquamatus	Chinese habu
	Agkistrodon blomhoffii	Mamushi
Australasia	*Acanthophis* species	Death adder
	Pseudonaja textilis	Eastern brown snake
	Notechis scutatus	Tiger snake
	Oxyuranus scutellatus	Taipan

Table 22.2 Determinants of snake bite incidence and severity of envenoming.

Incidence of bites	Severity of envenoming

1. Frequency of contact between snakes and humans, depends on:
  (a) Population densities
  (b) Diurnal and seasonal variations in activity
  (c) Types of behaviour (e.g. human agricultural activities)
2. Snakes' 'irritability'—readiness to strike when alarmed or provoked—varies with species
	1. Dose of venom injected—depends on mechanical efficiency of bite and species and size of snake
	2. Composition and hence potency of venom—depends on species and, within a species, the geographical location, season and age of the snake
	3. Health, age, size and (?) specific immunity of human victim
	4. Nature and timing of first aid and medical treatment

overrepresent the more seriously envenomed patients, and depend on the enthusiasm and workload of the hospital superintendent. Population surveys[9] give a more accurate picture of the incidence of snake bite. Certain hunter–gatherer tribes are at greatest risk from snake bite. Snakes were responsible for 2% of adult deaths in the Yanomamo of Venezuela, 5% in the Waorani of Ecuador and 24% in the Cashinaua of Acré, Brazil. Snake bite appeared to be the most important cause of death in some villages in the kuru-endemic area of the Papua New Guinea highlands. The Phi Tong Luang of the Thailand–Laos border, the Hadza of Tanzania and the Aborigines of central Australia have also suffered a high mortality from snake bite. An estimated 15 000–20 000 people die each year from snake bite in India. In the 1930s the annual snake bite mortality reported in Burma exceeded 2000 (15.4 per 100 000 population).[10] Thirty years later it was still estimated to exceed 1000 (3.3 per 100 000) per year and has been as high as the fifth most important cause of all deaths.[11] In 1984, about 900 snake bite deaths were recorded in Sri Lanka, an incidence of six per 100 000 per year. In the Amami and Okinawa Islands of Japan, there were 5488 bites by the habu (*Trimeresurus flavoviridis*) with 50 deaths during the 9 years from 1962 to 1970. The highest incidence of bites on one of the islands was 4.6 per 1000 population per year.[12] In the Benue Valley of northeastern Nigeria the incidence of snake bites was found to be 497 per 100 000 population per year with a mortality of 12.2%.[13] Snake bite is also common in Latin America. In Brazil, the case fatality of snake bites in the preantivenom era was thought to be about 25%, and the total number of bites 19 200 each year. By 1970, the estimated incidence was 51 026 bites and 1153 deaths per year, but recent figures indicate an average of 20 170 bites and 122 deaths per year. In the USA there are 7000 bites by venomous snakes each year with 12 to 15 deaths, and in Australia 1000–2000 bites per year with an average of two deaths per year. In Britain, there are more than 200 adder bites (*Vipera berus*) each year but there have been only 14 deaths during the last hundred years. There were 44 deaths caused by this species in Sweden between 1911 and 1978, and in Finland 21 deaths in 25 years with an annual incidence of almost 200 bites.

In tropical countries, snake bite is an occupational disease of farmers, herders and hunters. Rice farmers in Burma, Sri Lanka and central Thailand tread on Russell's vipers or inadvertently pick them up in a handful of paddy during the harvest[11] (Figure 22.12). In the savannah of West Africa farmers are bitten by *Echis* species as they dig the fields at the start of the rainy season.[13] Rubber-tappers in South-East Asia tread on Malayan pit vipers in the dark and are bitten as they make their early morning rounds of the rubber trees, and in the jungles of western Brazil the collectors of natural rubber ('seringueiros') are bitten by *Bothrops atrox*.

Sea snake bites have been an occupational hazard of fishermen in those parts of South-East Asia where hand nets were used. Records of 144 sea snake bites were collected in north-west Malaya in 1955–1956.[14] Mechanization of fishing methods in this region has

resulted in a dramatic decrease in sea snake bites, but they still occur along the coast of south Vietnam.[15] The beaked sea snake (*Enhydrina schistosa*) has caused most bites and deaths. Other common and medically important species are *Hydrophis cyanocinctus* (see Figure 22.5), *H. spiralis* and *Lapemis hardwickii* (see Figure 22.6).

In the more industrialized countries venomous snakes are increasingly popular as pets. Most bites are inflicted on the hands when the snakes are picked up and in the USA 25% of bites resulted from snakes being attacked or handled. Stories of unprovoked attacks by such species as mambas and king cobras can be discounted, but snakes will bite if they are cornered or feel threatened. Some species, notably *Bungarus caeruleus* in India and Sri Lanka, *B. candidus* in South-East Asia and *Naja nigricollis* in West Africa, enter human dwellings at night in pursuit of their prey (rodents, lizards, toads) and may strike at a sleeping person if startled. Epidemics of snake bite have resulted from a sudden increase in snake population density, for example after flooding in Colombia, Pakistan, India and Bangladesh, but in the case of *Echis ocellatus* in Togo in the 1950s a dramatic increase in snakes and bites was unexplained.[13] Invasion of the snake's habitat by large numbers of people may also be followed by an increased incidence of snake bite. This has happened during the building of new roads through jungles in South America and moving farmers to newly irrigated areas in the former dry zone of Sri Lanka.

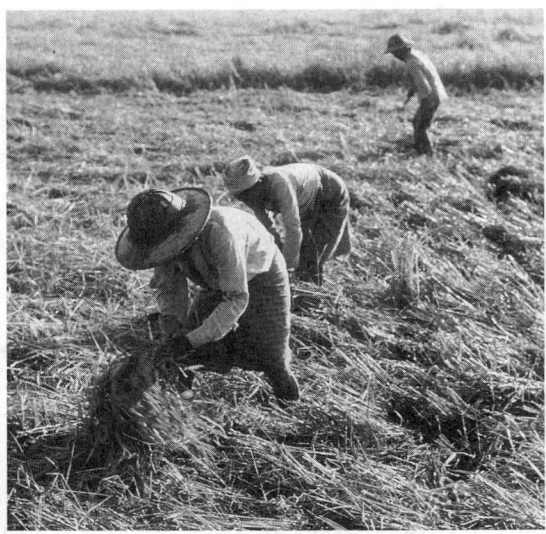

Figure 22.12 Burmese rice farmers harvesting the paddy, an occupation with a high risk of Russell's viper bite. (Copyright D.A. Warrell.)

VENOM APPARATUS[16]

COLUBRIDAE

The most primitive method for injecting venom is found in the back-fanged Colubridae. The posterior part of the superior labial gland (Duvernoy's gland) drains into a periodontal fold of buccal mucosa. The venom tracks down grooves in the anterior surfaces of the several enlarged posteriorly situated fangs (see Figure 22.2). This arrangement is effective for envenoming the natural prey, for example a chameleon in the case of the boomslang, which is held in the snake's mouth until it is dead. Human envenoming is a very rare accident. The snake must seize and chew at the finger of its victim, usually a herpetologist.

ATRACTASPIDIDAE

The venom apparatus of Atractaspididae differs from all other venomous snakes in many respects and the homology of the venom glands is uncertain.[16] In *Atractaspis engaddensis* and *A. microlepidota*, as in some species of Elapidae (*Maticora*) and Viperidae (*Causus*), the venom glands are very long—perhaps one-sixth of the snake's total length. The fangs of Atractaspididae and their method of striking are also distinctive (see p. 318).

ELAPIDAE, HYDROPHIIDAE AND VIPERIDAE

In these families, the venom glands lie behind the eye. Compressor muscles, principally the adductor superficialis in Elapidae and Hydrophiidae, and the compressor glandulae in Viperidae, squeeze venom out of the gland through the venom duct to the base of the fang. Venom is transmitted to the tip of the fang through a partially closed groove in its anterior surface or through a closed canal in the case of the Viperidae (Solenoglypha). In several species of elapid, the African spitting cobras *Naja nigricollis*, *N. katiensis*, *N. pallida* and *N. mossambica*, the South African ringhals or rinkals (*Hemachatus haemachatus*) and Asian spitting cobras (*N. sumatrana*, *N. siamensis*, *N. sputatrix*, etc.), the fang is modified to allow the snake to eject a spray of venom into the eyes of an aggressor. Instead of opening downwards at the tip of the fang, the venom channel is angled forward at its point of exit in the anterior surface of the fang, a few millimetres above its tip.[17]

The performance of the venom apparatus has been studied in very few species. The Palestine viper (*Vipera palaestinae*) can inject doses of venom lethal to its natural prey at each of ten or more consecutive strikes. When snakes have bitten two or more humans in rapid succession the second or third victims were sometimes more severely envenomed than the first. However, Russell's viper appears to inject most of its available venom at the first strike. More than half the people bitten by some venomous species (e.g. Malayan pit viper) show little or no envenoming. This has suggested to some that snakes might be capable of biting defensively without injecting venom. However, there is little evidence that snakes can control their injection of venom or vary the amount according to the size of the prey: the strike is essentially a reflex action. The snake's venom apparatus has been evolved to deliver a mechanically effective bite with injection of a supra-lethal dose of venom into its natural prey. When the snake lashes and strikes at a human foot or ankle after it has been trodden upon it is far less likely, for purely anatomical reasons, that an adequate injection of venom will be achieved.

VENOM COMPOSITION

The most complex of all poisons, snake venoms may contain 20 or more components. More than 90% of the dry weight is protein, comprising a rich variety of enzymes, non-enzymatic polypeptide toxins and non-toxic proteins. Non-protein ingredients of venom include carbohydrate and metals (often in the form of glycoprotein metalloprotein enzymes), lipids, free amino acids, nucleotides and biogenic amines. The precise role of most venom enzymes in the process of natural envenoming and digestion of the snake's prey is unknown. Enzyme function and pathophysiological disturbances are most clearly related in case of venom procoagulants. For example, Russell's viper venom contains at least two proteases which activate the mammalian blood clotting cascade. RVV-X, a glycoprotein, activates factor X by a calcium-dependent reaction and also acts on factor IX and protein C. RVV-V, an arginine ester hydrolase, activates factor V. *Echis* venoms contain a zinc metalloprotein, 'Ecarin', which activates prothrombin. Malayan pit viper venom contains a glycoprotein serine protease, ancrod (Arvin), which cleaves fibrinopeptide A from the fibrinogen molecule. Phospholipase A_2 is the most widespread and extensively studied of all venom enzymes. Under experimental conditions it damages mitochondria, red blood cells, leucocytes, platelets, skeletal muscle, vascular endothelium and other membranes, produces presynaptic neurotoxic activity, opiate-like sedative effects and the autopharmacological release of histamine. Few, if any, of these properties can be linked with certainty to pathophysiological disturbances in man. The acetylcholinesterase found in most elapid venoms is no longer thought to contribute to their neurotoxicity. Hyaluronidase may serve to promote the spread of venom through tissues; proteolytic enzymes (hydrolases) may be responsible for local changes in vascular permeability leading to oedema, blistering and bruising, and to necrosis. L-amino acid oxidase, which gives yellow viper venoms their colour, may have a digestive function.

The polypeptide toxins, often called neurotoxins, are low molecular weight, non-enzymatic proteins found almost exclusively in elapid and hydrophiid venoms. Postsynaptic (α) neurotoxins such as α-bungarotoxin and cobrotoxin, contain about 60–70 amino acid residues and bind to acetylocholine receptors on the motor end-plate. Presynaptic (β) neurotoxins such as β-bungarotoxin, crotoxin and taipoxin, contain about 120–140 amino acid residues and a phospholipase A subunit and prevent release of acetylcholine at the neuromuscular junction. Biogenic amines such as histamine and 5-hydroxytryptamine, found particularly in viper venoms, may contribute to the local pain and permeability changes at the site of a snake bite.

Clearly, snake venom cannot be regarded as a single toxin. The variation of venom composition from species to species explains the clinical diversity of snake bite. There is also considerable variation in the relative proportions of different venom constituents within a single species throughout its geographical distribution, at different seasons of the year, and as a result of ageing.

CLINICAL FEATURES OF ENVENOMING

In patients bitten by snakes, the symptoms and signs are explained by fear, the direct action of the various venom components on tissues, indirect effects such as complement activation and autopharmacological release of endogenous vasoactive substances, effects of treatment and complications such as secondary infections.

LOCAL SWELLING

In the bitten limb, increased vascular permeability leads to swelling and bruising. The factors responsible include proteases, phospholipases, membrane-damaging polypeptide toxins, hyaluronidase and endogenous autacoids released by the venom, such as histamine, 5-hydroxytryptamine and kinins. Venoms of some Viperidae, such as *D. russelii*, *V. berus* and *Crotalus* species, can produce a diffuse increase in vascular permeability resulting in pulmonary oedema, serous effusions, conjunctival and facial oedema and haemoconcentration.

Local tissue necrosis results from the direct action of myotoxic and cytolytic factors, possibly polypeptide toxins, and ischaemia caused by thrombosis, external compression by a tight tourniquet, or compression of arteries by swollen muscle within a tight fascial compartment.

HYPOTENSION AND SHOCK

Profound hypotension is part of the autopharmacological syndrome which may occur within minutes of bites by *Vipera palaestinae*, *V. berus*, *D. russelii* and *Actractaspis engaddensis*. Presumably this is caused by release of vasodilating autacoids. Oligopeptides in Viperidae venoms (e.g. *Bothrops* species) inhibit bradykinin-deactivating enzymes and angiotensin-converting enzymes (ACEs) and were the models for synthetic ACE inhibitors used to treat hypertension.[18] Some people, such as snake handlers, may become sensitized to snake venoms and can suffer life-threatening anaphylactic reactions within minutes of being bitten. Leakage of plasma or blood into the bitten limb and elsewhere or massive gastrointestinal haemorrhage may cause hypovolaemia after viper bites. Vasodilatation, especially of splanchnic vessels, and a direct myocardial action may contribute to hypotension after viper and rattlesnake bites.

BLEEDING AND CLOTTING DISTURBANCES[19]

These are seen after bites by some vipers, pit vipers, Australasian elapids and the few dangerously venomous colubrids. Snake venoms can cause haemostatic defects in a number of different ways: venom procoagulants can activate intravascular coagulation and produce consumption coagulopathy leading to incoagulable blood. For example, procoagulants in the venom of Colubridae, *Echis* species and *Notechis scutatus* activate prothrombin, *Daboia russelii* venom has procoagulants activating factors V and X, and many Crotalinae venoms have a direct thrombin-like action on fibrinogen. Some venoms, such as those of the rattlesnakes *Crotalus atrox*[20] and *C. adamanteus*,[21] cause defibrinogenation by activating the endogenous fibrinolytic system. Anticoagulant activity, sometimes identifiable with phospholipase, does not seem to be clinically significant. Thrombocytopenia is a common accompaniment of systemic envenoming and many venoms affect platelet function in vitro. Few studies of platelet function in envenomed humans have been attempted. In patients bitten by Malayan pit vipers and green pit vipers (*Trimeresurus albolabris*) there was initially inhibition of platelet agglutination followed by activation and the appearance of circulating clumps of platelets.[22] In the absence of trauma, defibrination induced by venom coagulants such as ancrod (Arvin) from *C. rhodostoma* venom is a relatively benign state. Spontaneous systemic bleeding is attributable to distinct venom components, haemorrhagins, which damage vascular endothelium. The combination of defibrination, thrombocytopenia and vessel wall damage will result in massive bleeding, a common cause of deaths from viper bites. This group of venom activities is often referred to, inappropriately, as 'vasculotoxic'. 'haematotoxic' or even 'haemolytic'.

INTRAVASCULAR HAEMOLYSIS

Although most snake venoms are haemolytic in vitro, this effect is rarely of clinical significance. However, envenoming by some *Bothrops* species, Russell's viper (in India and Sri Lanka), some Australasian elapids and members of the colubrid genera *Dispholidus*, *Thelotornis* and *Rhabdophis* may be associated with massive intravascular haemolysis contributing to renal failure. Evidence of mild microangiopathic haemolysis is sometimes found in patients with severe bleeding and clotting disturbances.

COMPLEMENT ACTIVATION[23]

Elapid and some colubrid venoms activate complement via the alternative pathway (e.g. 'cobra venom factor' may be the cobra's C3b), whereas some viperid venoms activate the classical pathway. The role of complement activation in the pathogenesis of envenoming is unknown, but there are many possible interactions with the clotting system and other humoral mediators.[24]

RENAL FAILURE

Renal failure is a rare complication of severe envenoming by almost any species of snake, even those which usually cause only mild envenoming such as *Trimeresurus albolabris*, the hump-nosed viper (*Hypnale hypnale*) and *Vipera berus*. However, it is a common event following bites by Russell's vipers,[11] the tropical rattlesnake (*Crotalus durissus*

terrificus) and sea snakes; in these cases it is the major cause of death. Possible mechanisms of acute tubular necrosis are prolonged hypotension, disseminated intravascular coagulation, a direct toxic effect of the venom on the renal tubule, haemoglobinuria, myoglobinuria and hyperkalaemia. Russell's viper venom produces hypotension, disseminated intravascular coagulation, direct nephrotoxicity[25] and, in Sri Lanka and India, intense intravascular haemolysis.[26] The mechanisms in victims of *C. d. terrificus* is most likely to be generalized rhabdomyolysis, combined with hypotension in some cases.[27] A large variety of renal histological changes have been described after snake bite. Pre-existing chronic renal disease and the effects of antivenom (serum sickness) may confuse interpretation.

NEUROTOXICITY

The neurotoxic polypeptides and phospholipases of snake venoms cause paralysis by blocking transmission at the neuromuscular junction. Paralytic symptoms are characteristic of most elapids, such as kraits, coral snakes, mambas and cobras, but not of the African spitting cobras (*Naja nigricollis*, *N. pallida*, *N. mossambica*, etc.).[24] Venoms of terrestrial Australasian snakes, sea snakes and a few species of Viperidae, notably *C. d. terrificus*, Pallas' pit viper (*Agkistrodon blomhoffii brevicaudus*), Sri Lankan and possibly South Indian *D. russelii* and the berg adder (*Bitis atropos*) are also neurotoxic in humans. Patients with paralysis of the bulbar muscles may die of upper airway obstruction or aspiration but the most common mode of death after neurotoxic envenoming is respiratory paralysis. Anticholinesterases, by prolonging the life of the neurotransmitter, may lead to a dramatic improvement in paralytic symptoms in patients bitten by snakes whose neurotoxins are predominantly postsynaptic in their action (e.g. Asian cobras). Some patients bitten by elapids or vipers are unphysiologically drowsy in the absence of respiratory or circulatory failure. This is unlikely to be an effect of neurotoxic polypeptides as these do not cross the blood–brain barrier. An intriguing possibility is the release of endogenous opiates by a venom component or binding to an opiate receptor. For example, intracerebral injection of β-RTX (receptor-active protein) from *D. russelii* venom produced sedation in rats.[28]

RHABDOMYOLYSIS

Generalized rhabdomyolysis with release of myoglobin, muscle enzymes and potassium is an effect in man of presynaptic neurotoxins of most species of true sea snakes, many of the terrestrial Australasian elapids such as tiger snake (*Notechis scutatus* and *N. ater*), king brown or mulga snake (*Pseudechis australis*), taipan (*Oxyuranus scutellatus*), rough-scaled snake (*Tropidechis carinatus*) and small-eyed snake (*Cryptophis nigrescens*) and several species of Viperidae, the tropical rattlesnake (*C. d. terrificus*),[27] canebrake rattlesnake (*C. horridus atricaudatus*),[29] Mojave rattlesnake (*C. scutulatus*) and Sri Lankan Russell's viper (*D. r. pulchella*).[26] Patients may die of bulbar and respiratory muscle weakness, from acute hyperkalaemia or later renal failure.

VENOM OPHTHALMIA[30]

Venoms of the spitting cobras and ringhals are intensely irritant and even destructive on contact with mucous membranes such as the conjunctivae and nasal cavity. Corneal erosions, anterior uveitis and secondary infections may result.

ENVENOMING BY DIFFERENT FAMILIES OF VENOMOUS SNAKES

COLUBRIDAE (back-fanged snakes)[5]

Severe or fatal envenoming is reliably reported in patients bitten by five species of back-fanged colubrid snake: boomslang (*Dispholidus typus*) (see Figure 22.2), vine, twig or bird snake (*Thelotornis kirtlandi* and *T. capensis*) of central and southern Africa, yamakagashi (*Rhabdophis tigrinus*) of Japan, the red-necked keelback (*R. subminiatus*) of South-East Asia and *Philodryas olphersii* of Brazil. Snakes of this family claimed the lives of two outstanding herpetologists, K. P. Schmidt (*Dispholidus typus*) and R. Mertens (*Thelotornis kirtlandi*). Severe envenoming is possible only if the snake is able to retain its grip and chew for 15 seconds or longer. All the species give rise to similar symptoms. Nausea with repeated vomiting, colicky abdominal pain and headache develop hours after the bite. There is bleeding from old and recent wounds such as venepunctures, and spontaneous gingival bleeding, epistaxis, haematemesis, melaena, subarachnoid haemorrhage, haematuria and extensive ecchymoses. Intravascular haemolysis and microangiopathic haemolysis have been described. Most of the fatal cases died of renal failure from acute tubular necrosis many days after the bite. Local effects of the venom are usually trivial but several patients showed some local swelling and one bitten

by *Dispholidus typus* had massive swelling with blood-filled bullae. Investigations reveal incoagulable blood, defibrination, elevated fibrin(ogen) degradation products (FDPs), severe thrombocytopenia and anaemia. These clinical features are explained by disseminated intravascular coagulation triggered by a venom procoagulant which activates prothrombin.

ATRACTASPIDIDAE (burrowing asps and Natal black snake)

Sixteen species of the genus *Atractaspis* and one species of *Macrelaps* have been described in Africa and the Middle East. All are venomous, but fatal or near fatal envenoming has been described in only three species: *A. microlepidota*, *A. irregularis* and *A. engaddensis*. Local effects include pain, swelling, blistering, necrosis, tender enlargement of local lymph nodes and in some cases local numbness or paraesthesiae in areas conforming to the distribution of a cutaneous nerve. The most common systemic symptom is fever. Most of the fatal cases died within 45 minutes of the bite after vomiting, producing profuse saliva and lapsing into coma.[31] Severe envenoming by *A. engaddensis* may produce violent autonomic symptoms (nausea, vomiting, abdominal pain, diarrhoea, sweating and profuse salivation) within minutes of the bite. One patient developed severe dyspnoea with acute respiratory failure and two showed abnormal electrocardiograms (ST–T changes and prolonged PR interval). Rarely, mild abnormalities of blood coagulation and liver function have also been described. *Atractaspis* venom has very high lethal toxicity. Recently, the venom of *A. engaddensis* was shown to contain three 21 amino acid peptides—sarafotoxins which show remarkable (60%) sequence homology with endogenous endothelins and cause coronary vasoconstriction and atrioventricular block.[32] The venom also contains haemorrhagic and necrotic factors but no true neurotoxins.[33] Bites by *Macrelaps microlepidotus* are said to have resulted in collapse and loss of consciousness.

ELAPIDAE (cobras, kraits, mambas and coral snakes)

Elapid venoms are best known for their neurotoxic effects. In the case of kraits, mambas, coral snakes, most of the Australian elapids (see below) and some of the cobras (e.g. Egyptian cobra, *Naja haje*; Cape cobra, *Naja nivea*), local effects are minimal. However, patients bitten by African spitting cobras (*N.*

nigricollis, *N. pallida*, *N. katiensis* and *N. mossam-bica*) and Asian cobras (*N. naja*, *N. kaouthia*, *N. siamensis*, *N. sumatrana*, *N. sputatrix*, *N. atra*, etc.) commonly develop tender local swelling, which may be extensive (Figure 22.13), and regional lympha-denopathy. Blistering may appear within 24 hours, often at the edge of a demarcated pale or blackened anaesthetic area of skin (Figure 22.14). The lesion smells putrid and eventually breaks down with loss of skin and subcutaneous tissue, which may be extensive (Figure 22.15). Prolonged morbidity may result and some patients may lose a digit or the affected limb if there is secondary infection. Severe envenoming by the king cobra (*Ophiophagus han-nah*) results in swelling of the whole limb and forma-tion of bullae at the site of the bite but there is minimal local necrosis.[34] However, rapidly develop-

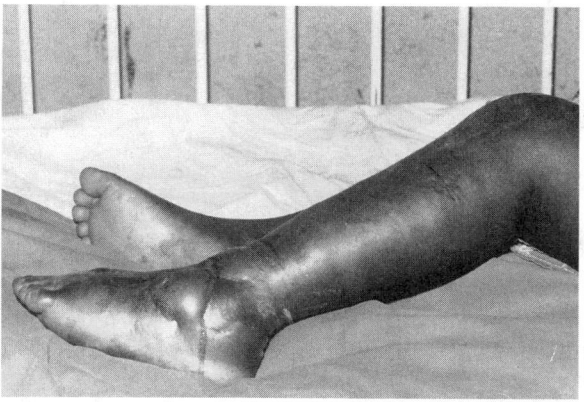

Figure 22.13 Nigerian girl with swelling of the whole limb, blistering and early signs of necrosis 48 hours after being bitten on the dorsum of the left foot by a black-necked or spitting cobra (*Naja nigricollis*). (Copyright D.A. Warrell.)

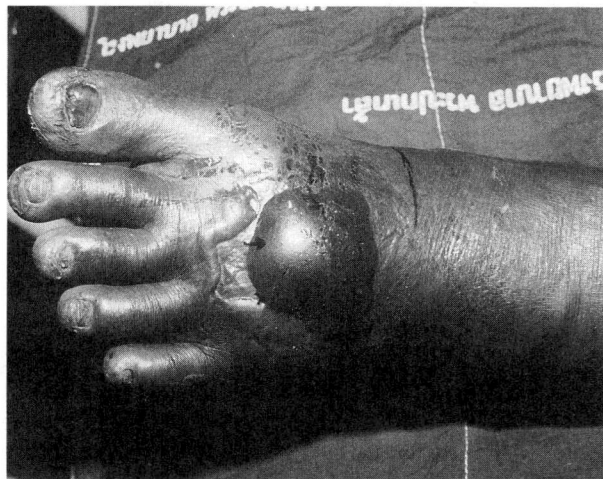

Figure 22.14 Blistering which appeared 36 hours after a bite by a monocellate Thai cobra (*Naja kaouthia*). (Copyright D.A. Warrell.)

ing neurotoxicity is the dominant clinical feature of patients envenomed by this species. Neurotoxic effects are also seen in patients envenomed by Asian cobras (it is the predominant feature in victims of *N. philippinensis*) and other elapids, but have yet to be documented adequately in victims of African spit-ting cobras. The earliest symptom of systemic enve-noming is repeated vomiting, but the use of emetic herbal medicines may confuse the interpretation of this symptom. Other early preparalytic symptoms include contraction of the frontalis (before there is demonstrable ptosis), blurred vision, paraesthesiae especially around the mouth, hyperacusis, head-ache, dizziness, vertigo and signs of autonomic ner-vous stimulation such as hypersalivation, congested conjunctivae (Figure 22.16) and 'goose-flesh'. Paral-ysis is first detectable as ptosis and external ophthal-moplegia, as ocular muscles are most sensitive to neuromuscular blockade (Figure 22.17). These signs may appear as early as 15 minutes after the bite (cobras or mambas) but may be delayed for 10 hours or more following krait bites. Later, the facial muscles, palate, jaws, tongue, vocal cords, neck muscles and muscles of deglutition may become paralysed (Figure 22.18). Many patients are unable to open their mouths, but this can be overcome by force. In a minority the jaw is said to hang open. Respiratory arrest may be precipitated by obstruc-tion of the upper airway by the paralysed tongue or inhaled vomitus. Intercostal muscles are affected before the limbs, diaphragm and superficial muscles and, even in patients with generalized flaccid paral-ysis, slight movements of the digits may be possible, allowing the patients to signal that they are con-scious. Loss of consciousness and generalized con-vulsions are usually explained by hypoxaemia in patients who have respiratory paralysis. However, drowsiness, before the development of significant paralysis, has often been described but remains unexplained. In patients whose eyelids are drooping as a result of physiological tiredness, ptosis may be inferred incorrectly, unless the extent of lid retrac-tion with upward gaze is formally assessed. Patients with systemic envenoming suffer from headache, malaise and generalized myalgia. Intractable hypo-tension can occur in patients envenomed by Asian cobras, despite adequate respiratory support. Neurotoxic effects are completely reversible, either acutely in response to antivenom or (for example in Asian cobra bites) to anticholinesterases,[35] or they may slowly wear off spontaneously. In the absence of specific antivenom, patients supported by mech-anical ventilators recover sufficient diaphragmatic movement to breathe adequately in 1–4 days. Ocu-lar muscles recover in 2–4 days and there is usually full recovery of motor function in 3–7 days.

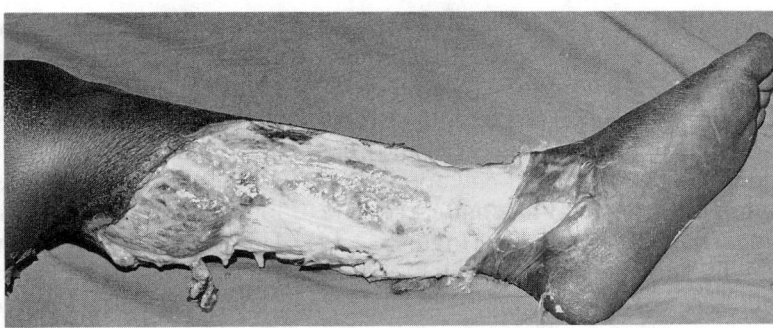

Figure 22.15 Extensive necrosis of skin and subcutaneous tissues in a Nigerian woman bitten 10 days earlier by a black-necked or spitting cobra (*Naja nigricollis*). (Copyright D.A. Warrell.)

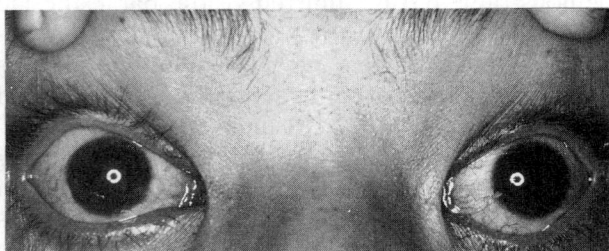

Figure 22.16 Bilateral ptosis, complete external ophthalmoplegia and conjunctival congestion in a Burmese man bitten 24 hours earlier by a king cobra (*Ophiophagus hannah*). (Copyright D.A. Warrell.)

Bites by Australasian elapids[1,36]

Venoms of these snakes result in three main groups of symptoms: neurotoxicity similar to that seen with other elapid bites (Figure 22.19), generalized rhabdomyolysis and haemostatic disturbances (Figure 22.20). Local signs are usually mild, but extensive local swelling and bruising with localized necrosis has been reported, especially after bites by the king brown or mulga snake (*Pseudechis australis*). Painful and tender local lymph nodes are a common feature in patients developing systemic envenoming. Early symptoms include vomiting, headache and syncopal attacks similar to those experienced after some viper bites (see below).

Persistent bleeding from wounds and spontaneous systemic bleeding from gums and gastrointestinal tract is found in association with incoagulable blood following bites by many Australasian species (Figure 22.20). Venoms of 15 out of 19 species exhibited procoagulant activity in vitro.[1,37] Some venoms (e.g. *Pseudonaja*, *Pseudechis* and *Micropechis ikaheka*, the New Guinean small-eyed snake) are anticoagulant. Haemostatic abnormalities are particularly frequent and serious in patients bitten by tiger snakes (*Notechis* species), taipans (*Oxyuranus* species) and brown snakes (*Pseudonaja* species), uncommonly with bites by black snakes (*Pseudechis* species) and never with bites by death adders (*Acanthophis* species).

In the past, there has been some confusion between haemoglobinuria and myoglobinuria in

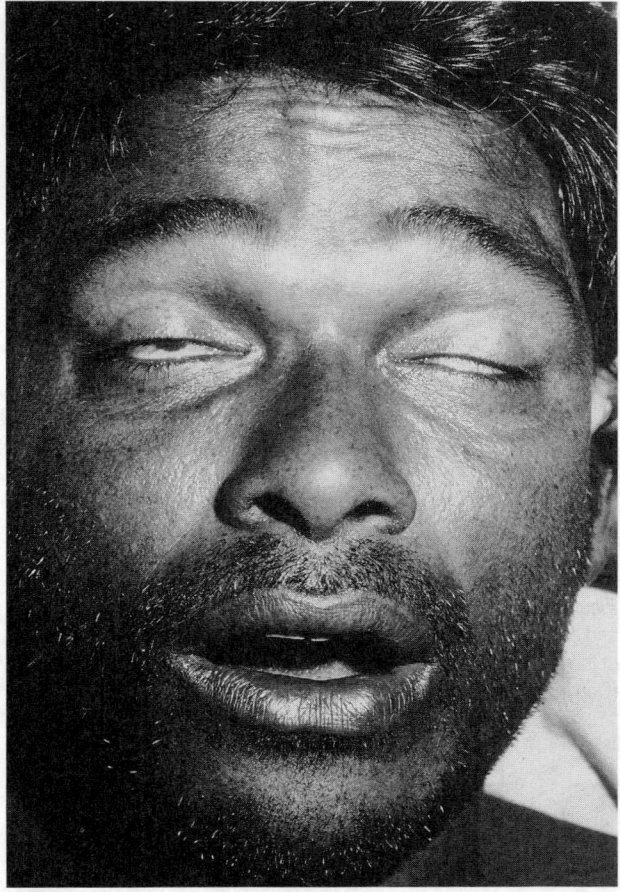

Figure 22.17 Severe ptosis, external ophthalmoplegia and inability to open the mouth, protrude the tongue or swallow in a Sri Lankan patient bitten by a common krait (*Bungarus caeruleus*). (Copyright D.A. Warrell.)

patients passing dark urine. It is now clear, however, that haemoglobinaemia and haemoglobinuria can occur as a result of intravascular haemolysis (e.g. with envenoming by *Pseudechis australis*) but that myoglobinuria caused by generalized rhabdomyolysis (see below) is also a feature of envenoming by some species (e.g. *Notechis*, *Oxyuranus* and *Pseudechis australis*, etc.). Renal failure may result from haemoglobinuria or myoglobinuria.

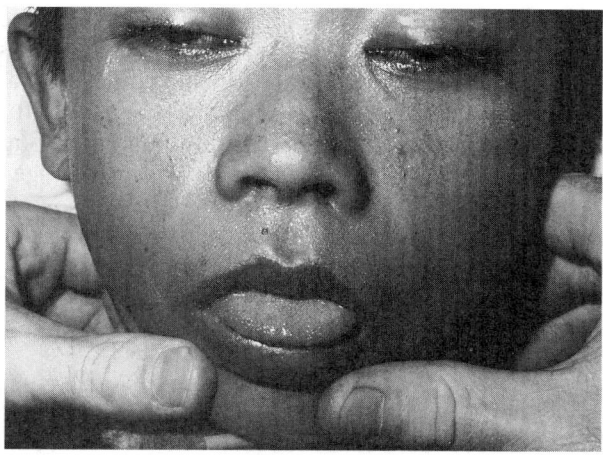

Figure 22.18 Ptosis and inability to open the mouth or protrude the tongue in a Thai patient bitten by a Malayan krait (*Bungarus candidus*). (Copyright D.A. Warrell.)

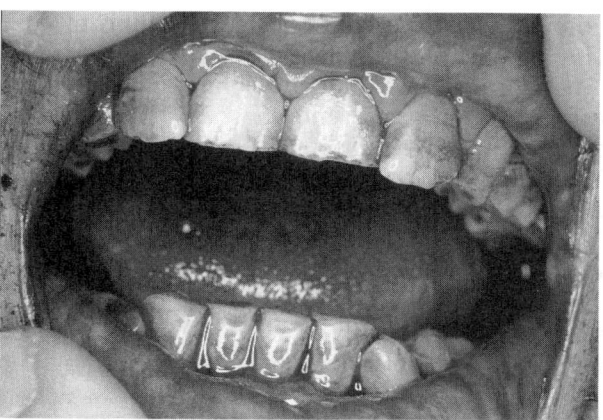

Figure 22.20 Bleeding from the gingival sulci in a Papua New Guinean man bitten 6 hours previously by a taipan (*Oxyuranus scutellatus canni*). (Copyright D.A. Warrell.)

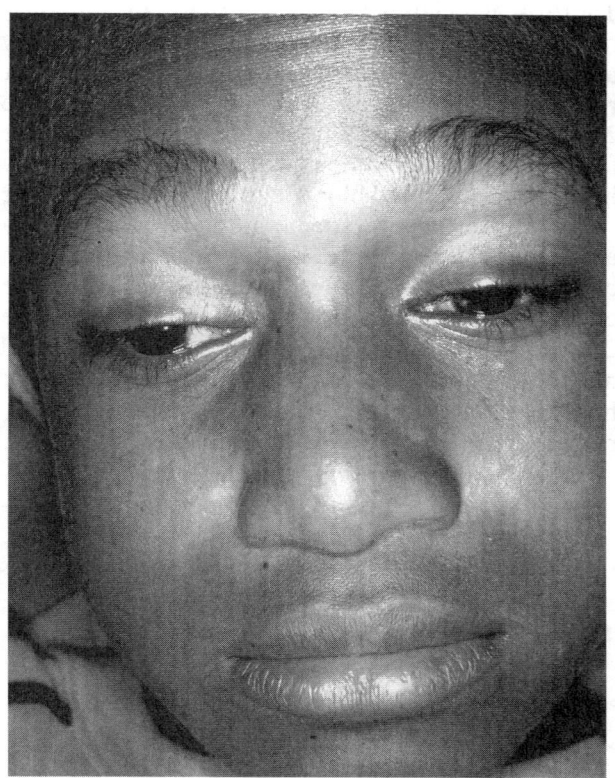

Figure 22.19 Ptosis, external ophthalmoplegia and facial paralysis in a Papua New Guinean boy bitten 24 hours previously by a taipan (*Oxyuranus scutellatus canni*). (Copyright D.A. Warrell.)

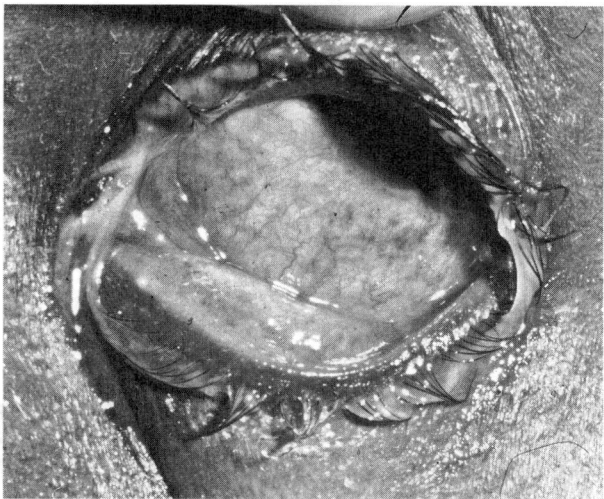

Figure 22.21 Intense conjunctivitis with leucorrhoea (and corneal erosions) in a patient 'spat' at 3 hours previously by an African black-necked or spitting cobra (*Naja nigricollis*). (Copyright D.A. Warrell.)

or fluorescein examination reveals corneal erosions in more than half the patients spat at by *N. nigricollis*.[30] Secondary infection of the corneal lesions may result in permanent opacities causing blindness or panophthalmitis with loss of the eye. Rarely venom is absorbed into the anterior chamber causing hypopyon and anterior uveitis.

HYDROPHIIDAE (sea snakes)[15,38]

The bite is usually painless and may not be noticed by the wader or swimmer, but teeth are frequently left in the wound. There is no local swelling or involvement of local lymph nodes. Generalized rhabdomyolysis is the dominant feature of enve-

Snake venom ophthalmia

Venom ophthalmia may result when venom of the spitting elapids (see above) enters the eye. There is intense local pain, blepharospasm, palpebral oedema and leucorrhoea (Figure 22.21). Slit-lamp

noming by these snakes. Early symptoms of envenoming include headache, a thick feeling of the tongue, thirst, sweating and vomiting. Generalized aching, stiffness and tenderness of the muscles becomes noticeable between 30 minutes and $3\frac{1}{2}$ hours after the bite. Trismus is a common feature (Figure 22.22). Passive stretching of the muscles is resisted. Later, there is progressive flaccid paralysis starting with ptosis, as in elapid envenoming (Figure 22.23). The patient remains conscious until the respiratory muscles are sufficiently affected to cause respiratory failure. Myoglobinaemia and myoglobinuria de-

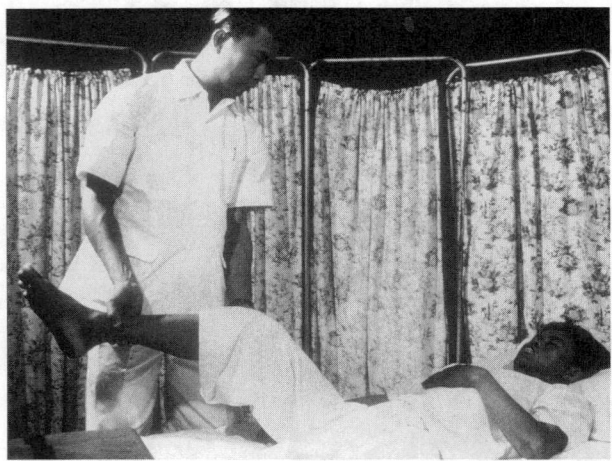

Figure 22.22 Malayan patient showing trismus and muscle stiffness and tenderness (on passive stretching) after a bite by a sea snake. (Courtesy of the late H.A. Reid.)

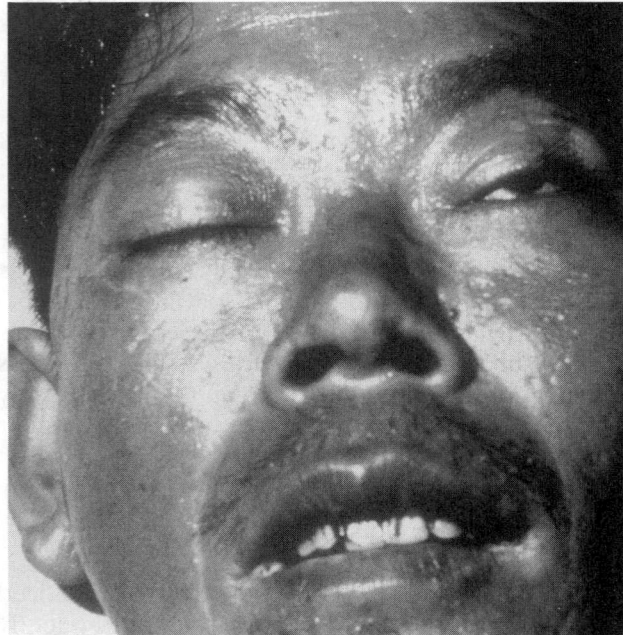

Figure 22.23 Bilateral ptosis and external ophthalmoplegia in a Malayan fisherman envenomed by a sea snake. (Courtesy of the late H.A. Reid.)

velop 3–8 hours after the bite (Figure 22.24). These are suspected when the serum/plasma appears brownish and the urine dark reddish brown ('Coca-Cola-coloured'). 'Stix' tests will appear positive for haemoglobin/blood in urine containing myoglobin. Myoglobin and potassium released from damaged skeletal muscles may cause renal failure, while hyperkalaemia may develop within 6–12 hours of the bite and lead to cardiac arrest.

VIPERIDAE (Old World pitless vipers and adders, New World rattlesnakes, moccasins and lance-headed vipers, Asian pit vipers)

Venoms of vipers and pit vipers usually produce more local effects than other snake venoms. Swelling may appear within 15 minutes, but rarely is delayed for several hours. It spreads rapidly, sometimes involving the whole limb and adjacent trunk. There is associated pain, tenderness and enlargement of regional lymph nodes. Bruising, especially along the path of superficial lymphatics and over regional lymph nodes, is commonly seen (Figure 22.25) and there may be persistent bleeding from the fang marks. Swollen limbs can accommodate many litres of extravasated blood leading to hypovolaemic shock. Blistering may appear at the bite site as early as 12 hours after the bite. Blisters may be filled with clear or bloodstained fluid and, in cases of severe envenoming, extend up the bitten limb (Figure 22.26). Necrosis of skin, subcutaneous tissue and muscle (Figure 22.27) may develop in up to 10% of hospitalized cases, especially following bites by rattlesnakes (e.g. *Crotalus adamanteus*, *C. atrox*, *C. horridus* and *C. viridis*), South American lance-headed vipers (genus *Bothrops*) and the bushmasters (*Lachesis muta*) and Asian pit vipers (e.g. *Calloselasma rhodostoma*, *Deinagkistrodon acutus*

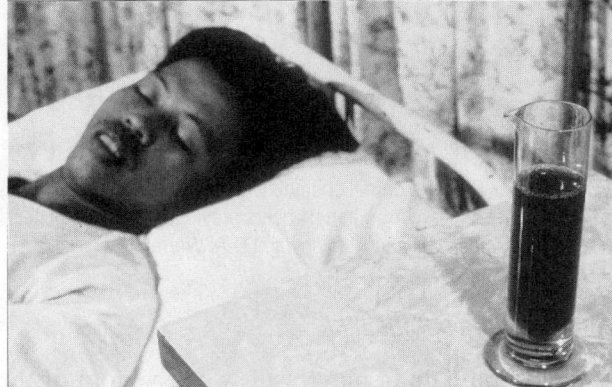

Figure 22.24 Myoglobinuria resulting from generalized rhabdomyolysis in a Malayan fisherman envenomed by a sea snake. (Courtesy of the late H.A. Reid.)

and *Trimeresurus flavoviridis*), African vipers (genus *Bitis*), saw-scaled vipers (genus *Echis*) and Palestine viper (*V. palaestinae*). Bites on the digits and in areas draining into the tight fascial compartments, such as the anterior tibial compartment, are particularly likely to cause necrosis. In these cases high intracompartmental pressure may add ischaemic necrosis to the direct necrotic effects of the venom.[39] Severe pain associated with tense swelling, subcutaneous anaesthesia and pain on stretching the intracompartmental muscles (e.g. dorsiflexion of the foot in the case of the anterior tibial compartment) should raise the possibility of raised intracompartmental pressure. Sudden severe pain, absence of arterial pulses and a demarcated cold segment of limb suggests thrombosis of a major artery. The absence of detectable local swelling 2 hours after a viper bite usually means that no venom was injected. However, there are important exceptions to this rule: fatal systemic envenoming by the tropical rattlesnake (*Crotalus durissus terrificus*), Mojave rattlesnake (*Crotalus scutulatus*) and Bur-

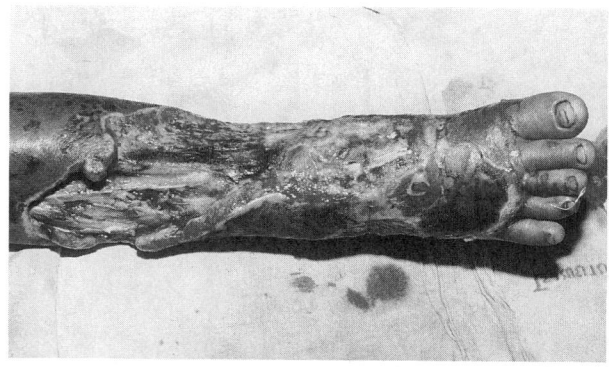

Figure 22.27 Extensive necrosis of the skin and muscle in a 5-year-old Thai child 10 days after being bitten by a Malayan pit viper (*Calloselasma rhodostoma*). (Courtesy of Sornchai Looareesuwan, Bangkok.)

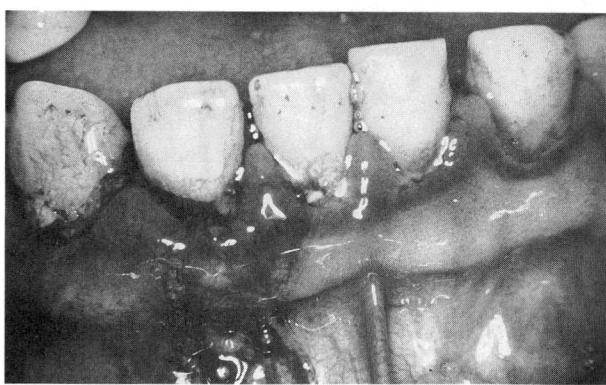

Figure 22.28 Bleeding from gingival sulci in a Nigerian patient bitten by a saw-scaled or carpet viper (*Echis ocellatus*). (Copyright D.A. Warrell.)

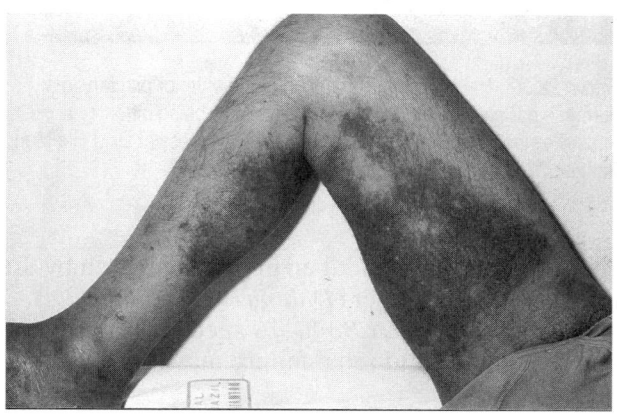

Figure 22.25 Extensive bruising in a Brazilian patient 36 hours after being bitten on the ankle by a jararaca (*Bothrops jararaca*). (Copyright D.A. Warrell.)

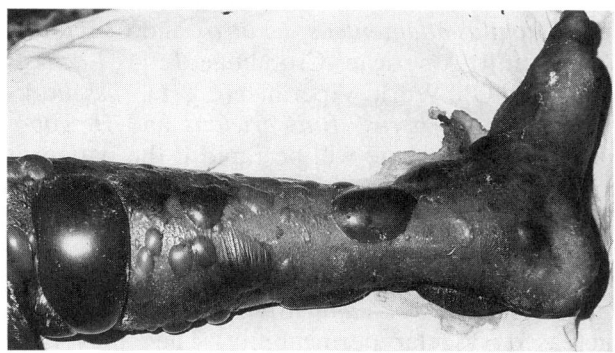

Figure 22.26 Massive swelling and bulla formation in a Thai patient 36 hours after being bitten by a Malayan pit viper (*Calloselasma rhodostoma*). (Copyright D.A. Warrell.)

mese Russell's viper (*D. r. siamensis*) may occur in the absence of local signs. In fact, patients bitten by *C. d. terrificus* rarely show any local swelling.

Haemostatic abnormalities are characteristic of envenoming by Viperidae, but are usually completely absent in patients bitten by the smaller European vipers (*V. berus*, *V. aspis*, *V. ammodytes*, etc.) and some species of rattlesnakes. Persistent bleeding from the fang puncture wounds and from new injuries such as venepuncture sites and from old partially healed wounds may be the first clinical evidence of a bleeding diathesis. Spontaneous systemic haemorrhage is most often detected in the gingival sulci (Figure 22.28). Saliva and sputum may contain blood which usually derives from bleeding gums or epistaxis. True haemoptysis is rare. Haematuria may be detected a few hours after the bite. Ecchymoses, intracranial and subconjunctival haemorrhages, and bleeding into the floor of the mouth, tympanic membrane, and gastrointestinal and genitourinary tracts also occur. Discoid ecchy-

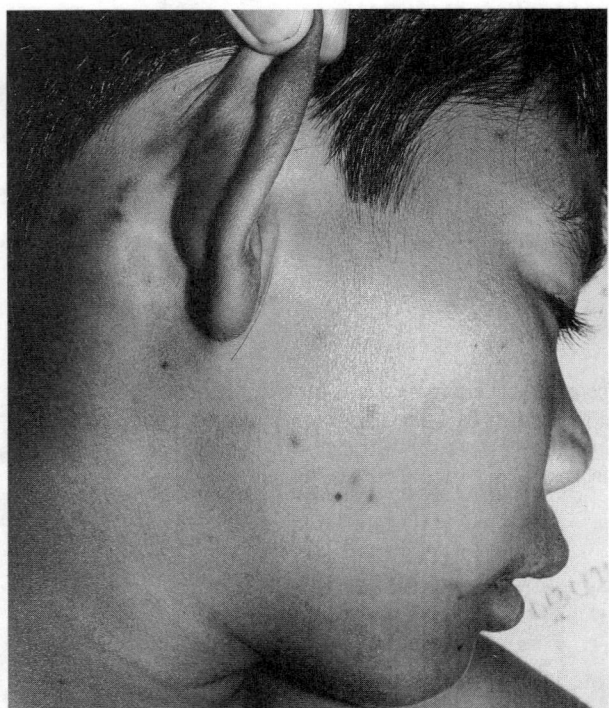

Figure 22.29   Discoid haemorrhages in a Thai boy 6 hours after being bitten by a Malayan pit viper (*Calloselasma rhodostoma*). (Copyright D.A. Warrell.)

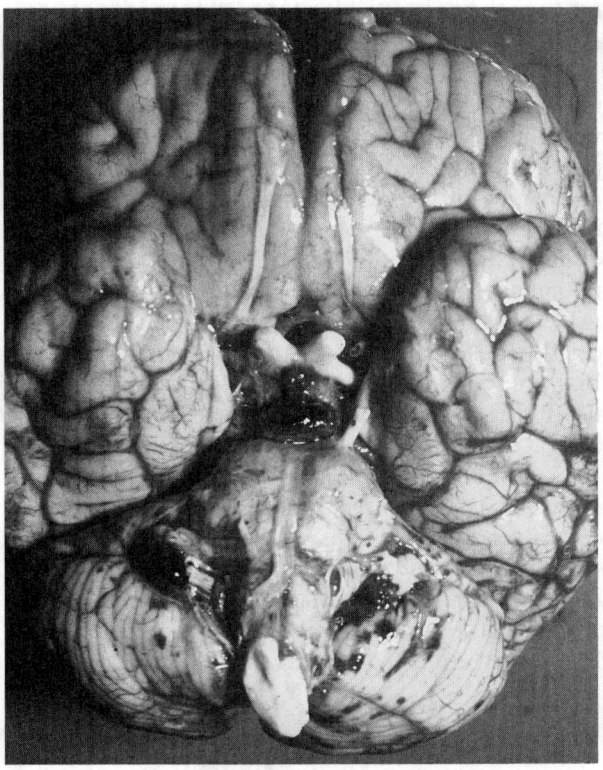

Figure 22.30   Haemorrhagic infarction of the anterior pituitary in a Burmese patient who died in shock 5 days after being bitten by a Russell's viper (*Daboia russelii siamensis*). (Courtesy of Dr U Hla Mon, Rangoon.)

moses, especially of the face and trunk, are seen in patients bitten by Russell's vipers, *Bothrops* species and *Calloselasma rhodostoma* (Figure 22.29). Bleeding into the anterior pituitary (resembling Sheehan's syndrome) has been described in patients bitten by Burmese and Indian Russell's vipers (Figure 22.30) and by *Bothrops jararacussu*. Menorrhagia and antepartum and postpartum haemorrhage have been described in women envenomed by vipers. Severe headache and meningism suggest subarachnoid haemorrhage, evidence of a developing central nervous system lesion (e.g. hemiplegia), irritability, loss of consciousness and convulsions suggest (in the absence of cardiorespiratory failure) an intracranial haemorrhage. Abdominal distension, tenderness and peritonism with signs of haemorrhagic shock but no external blood loss (haematemesis or melaena) suggest retroperitoneal or intraperitoneal haemorrhage. Incoagulable blood resulting from defibrination is a common and important finding in patients systemically envenomed by members of the following genera: *Atheris*, *Daboia*, *Vipera*, *Echis*, *Lachesis*, *Agkistrodon*, *Gloydius*, *Bothrops*, *Calloselasma*, *Crotalus*, *Deinagkistrodon* and *Trimeresurus*.

Intravascular haemolysis, causing haemoglobinaemia (pinkish plasma) and black or greyish urine (haemoglobinuria or methaemoglobinuria), has

been convincingly described in patients bitten by Sri Lankan Russell's viper (*Daboia russelii pulchella*),[26] and South American *Bothrops* species. Progressive severe anaemia and renal failure may result.

Circulatory shock (hypotensive) syndromes

A fall in blood pressure is a common and serious event in patients bitten by vipers, especially in the case of some of the North American rattlesnakes (e.g. *Crotalus adamanteus*, *C. atrox* and *C. scutulatus*), South American Crotalinae (e.g. *Lachesis muta*) and Old World Viperinae (e.g. *D. russelii*, *V. palaestinae*, *V. berus*, *Bitis arietans* and *B. gabonica*). The pulse rate will be rapid if the patient is compensating for hypovolaemia resulting from external haemorrhage, blood loss into the tissues or local or generalized increase in capillary permeability. Patients envenomed by Burmese Russell's viper (*D. r. siamensis*) show evidence of increased vascular permeability. They may have conjunctival oedema (Figure 22.31), serous effusions (Figure 22.32), pulmonary oedema (Figure 22.33), haemoconcentration and a fall in serum

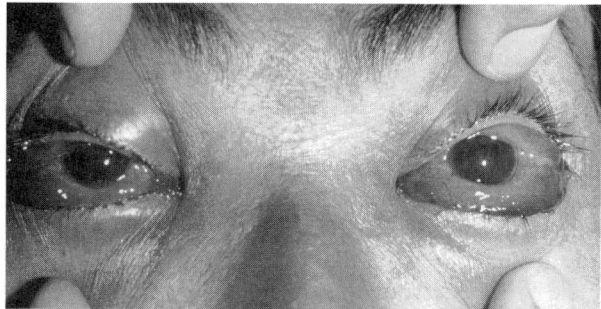

Figure 22.31 Intense bilateral conjunctival oedema (chemosis) in a Burmese man bitten 24 hours previously by a Russell's viper (*Daboia russelii siamensis*). (Copyright D.A. Warrell.)

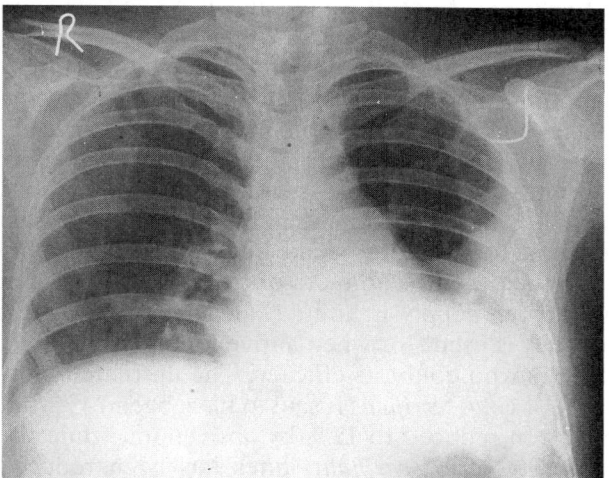

Figure 22.32 Chest radiograph showing a pleural effusion in a Burmese woman bitten by a Russell's viper (*Daboia russelii siamensis*). (Copyright D.A. Warrell.)

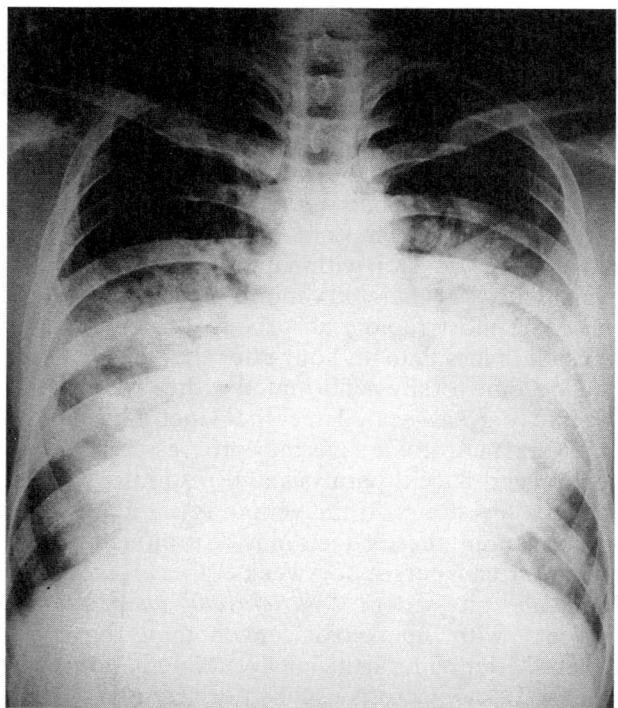

Figure 22.33 Chest radiograph of a Burmese man who developed pulmonary oedema after being bitten by a Russell's viper (*Daboia russelii siamensis*). (Copyright D.A. Warrell.)

albumin concentration.[11] The pulse rate may be slow or irregular if the venom is affecting the heart directly or reflexly (e.g. *Vipera berus*, *Bitis arietans*, *Calloselasma rhodostoma*). Vasovagal syncope may be precipitated by anxiety in certain individuals. Early repeated and usually transient syncopal attacks associated with features of an autopharmacological or anaphylactoid reaction are seen in patients bitten by some members of the genus *Vipera* (e.g. *V. palaestinae*, *V. berus*, *V. aspis* and *D. russelii*). Vomiting, sweating, colic, diarrhoea (with incontinence), shock and angioneurotic oedema of the face, lips, gums, tongue and throat may appear as early as 5 minutes or as late as many hours after the bite. These symptoms may resolve spontaneously or recur and persist, leading to death. Hypotension is also an important feature of the systemic anaphylaxis which may complicate antivenom therapy (see below). *Renal failure* is a rare complication of severe envenoming by any species of snake, but it is a regular occurrence and the most frequent cause of death in victims of Russell's viper throughout its range, tropical rattlesnake (*Crotalus durissus terrificus*), some species of *Bothrops*, Merrem's hump-nosed viper (*Hypnale hypnale*) and the bushmaster (*Lachesis muta*). Patients bitten by Russell's viper may become oliguric within a few hours of the bite. Loin pain and tenderness may be experienced within the first 24 hours and, in 3 or 4 days, the patient may become irritable, comatose or convulsing, with hypertension and evidence of metabolic acidosis. Neurotoxicity, attributable to venom phospholipases A_2, is a feature of envenoming by a few species of *Viperidae* (e.g. *C. d. terrificus*, *Agkistrodon blomhoffii*, *Bitis atropos* and Sri Lankan *D. r. pulchella*). The clinical features are the same as with elapid envenoming (Figure 22.34) but progression to respiratory or generalized paralysis rarely if ever occurs. Associated myalgia suggests the possibility of rhabdomyolysis.

CLINICAL COURSE AND PROGNOSIS

Local swelling is usually evident within 2–4 hours of bites by vipers and cytotoxic cobras and may develop even more rapidly following bites by some rattlesnakes. Swelling is maximal and most extensive on the second or third day after the bite. Resolution of swelling and restoration of normal function in the bitten limb may be delayed for months, especially in the older age group (e.g. after bites by the European adder (*Vipera berus*). The earliest systemic symptoms such as vomiting and syncope may develop within minutes of the bite, but even in the case of elapid venoms, which are thought to be the most rapidly absorbed, deaths are most unusual in less than an hour after the bite. Patients may become totally defibrinated within 1–2 hours of the bite (e.g. saw-scaled or carpet viper *Echis ocellatus*)[40] and neurotoxic signs may progress to a state of generalized flaccid paralysis and respiratory arrest within a few hours. If the venom is not neutralized by antivenom, these effects may be prolonged. Defibrination can persist for weeks (*E. carinatus* and Malayan pit viper *Calloselasma rhodostoma*). Patients with neurotoxic envenoming have recovered after being artificially ventilated for up to 10 weeks. Tissue necrosis usually declares itself within

a week of the bite. Sloughing of necrotic tissue and secondary infections including osteomyelitis may occur during subsequent weeks or months. Early deaths from neurotoxic envenoming are caused by airways obstruction or respiratory paralysis, whereas later deaths may result from technical complications of mechanical ventilation or intractable hypotension. Late deaths, more than 5 days after the bite, are usually the result of renal failure. Delayed shock with recurrent spontaneous haemorrhage has been described in Burmese victims of Russell's viper: pituitary and other intracranial haemorrhages have been found at autopsy.

Even when the fangs of a venomous snake have pierced the skin, envenoming is not inevitable. About 20% of patients bitten by North American rattlesnakes, Central American lance-headed vipers (mainly *Bothrops*), *Calloselasma rhodostoma* and *Daboia russelii* show absolutely no evidence of envenoming, and as many as 80% of those bitten by sea snakes and 50% by *C. rhodostoma* or *D. russelii* have trivial or no envenoming. Untreated snake bite mortality is hard to assess, for hospital admissions include a disproportionate number of severe cases, and data for untreated snake bites are available only from the preantivenom era or from occasions when antivenom supply is limited, an antivenom of low potency is used[13] or when antivenom is withheld by doctors who doubt its efficacy. The untreated mortality of *C. d. terrificus* is said to have been 74%, but has been reduced to 12% by antivenom, while the mortality of *E. carinatus* bites has been reduced from about 20 to 3% with antivenom. Prognosis appears to be worst in infants and in the elderly, but there is no convincing evidence that children have a worse prognosis than young adults, despite the larger dose of venom relative to their body weight.

INTERVAL BETWEEN BITE AND DEATH

Death after snake bite may occur as rapidly as 'a few minutes' (reputedly after a bite by the king cobra *Ophiophagus hannah*) or as long as 41 days after a bite by the saw-scaled or carpet viper (*Echis carinatus*). However, the rapidity of death after snake bite has generally been exaggerated. Most elapid deaths occur several hours after the bite, most sea snake bites between 12 and 24 hours after the bite, and viper bites within days of the bite.

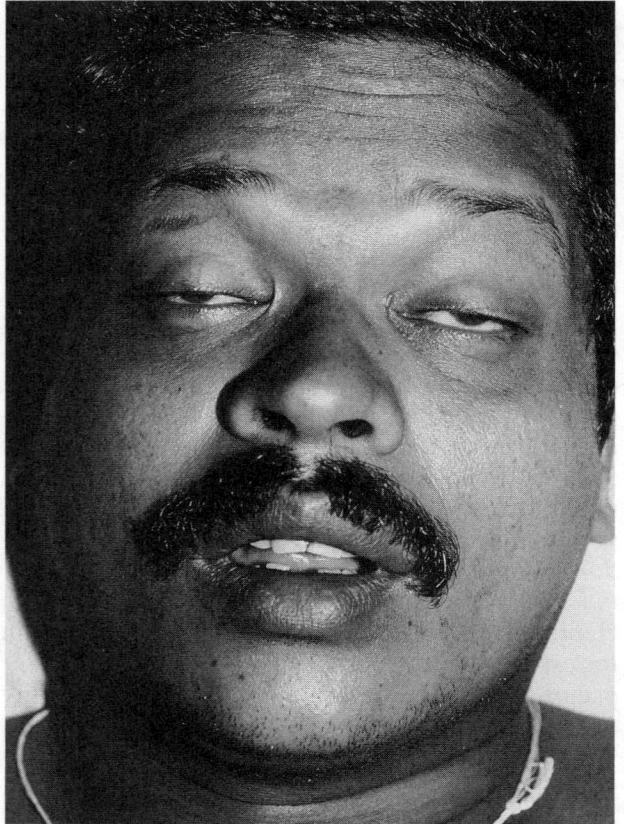

Figure 22.34 Sri Lankan man with neurotoxic envenoming by Russell's viper (*Daboia russelii pulchella*). There is ptosis, ophthalmoplegia and inability to open the mouth and protrude the tongue. (Copyright D.A. Warrell.)

LABORATORY INVESTIGATIONS

Systemic envenoming by most species excites a neutrophil leucocytosis: counts above 20 000 cells/μl indicate severe envenoming. Haematocrit may be high initially because of haemoconcentration when there is generalized increase in capillary permeability (e.g. *Crotalus* species, Burmese *V. russelii*). A subsequent fall in haematocrit is usual: the causes include bleeding into the bitten limb and elsewhere and, uncommonly, from intravascular haemolysis, especially from microangiopathic haemolysis in patients with disseminated intravascular coagulation. In these cases, the blood film will show fragmented erythrocytes (schistocytes or helmet cells). Thrombocytopenia is commonly associated with snake venom coagulopathies (e.g. *D. russelii, Calloselasma rhodostoma* and *Crotalus viridis helleri*) and is also a feature of bites by the puff adder (*Bitis arietans*), although there are no other disturbances of haemostasis in humans bitten by this species.

Incoagulable blood is a cardinal sign of systemic envenoming by the majority of Viperidae, many of the Australasian elapids and the medically important Colubridae. For clinical purposes, a simple all-or-nothing test of blood coagulability is adequate. A few millilitres of blood taken by venepuncture are placed in a new, clean, dry glass test tube, left undisturbed at room temperature for 20 minutes, then tipped to see if there is clotting or not (Figure 22.35). More sensitive tests which are reasonably simple to perform are whole blood or plasma prothrombin times and detection of an unequivocally elevated FDP concentration (e.g. 80 μg/ml) by agglutination of sensitized latex particles (Thrombo-Wellcotest). Serum concentrations of creatine phosphokinase and aspartate aminotransferase and blood urea are commonly raised in patients with severe envenoming, probably because of muscle damage. In patients with generalized rhabdomyolysis caused by venoms of sea snakes and Australasian snakes there is a steep rise in serum creatine phosphokinase, myoglobin and potassium concentrations. Plasma appears brownish in the presence of gross myoglobinaemia, but is stained pink when there is intravascular haemolysis. Heparinized blood should be allowed to sediment spontaneously (without centrifugation) for detection of haemoglobinaemia. The urine of patients with intravascular haemolysis is black (as in 'blackwater fever') but brownish, pinkish or reddish in those with haematuria or myoglobinuria. Blood urea and serum creatinine and potassium concentrations should be measured in patients who become oliguric, especially in cases with a high risk of renal failure (e.g. *D. russelli, C. d. terrificus, Bothrops* species, terrestrial Australasian snakes, Hydrophiidae and Colubridae). Severely sick, hypotensive and shocked patients will develop lactic acidosis (increased anion

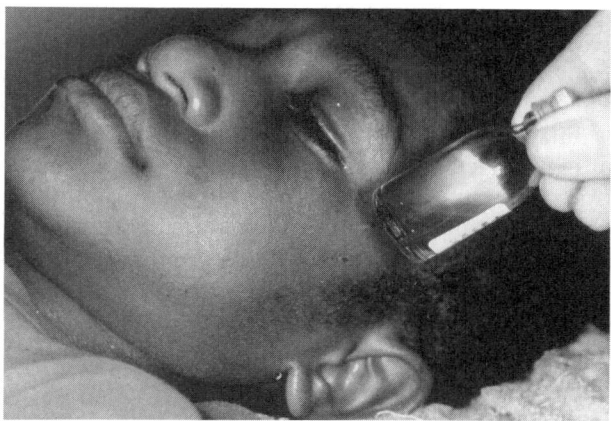

Figure 22.35 Simple whole blood clotting test. In this Papua New Guinean patient envenomed by a taipan (*Oxyuranus scutellatus canni*) a few millilitres of venous blood was placed in the new, clean, dry, glass bottle and was left to stand at room temperature for 20 minutes. At the end of this time the blood is still liquid, indicating defibrinogenation. (Copyright D.A. Warrell.)

gap), those with renal failure will also develop a metabolic acidosis (decreased plasma pH and bicarbonate concentration, reduced arterial $P\text{CO}_2$), and patients with respiratory paralysis will develop respiratory acidosis (low pH, high arterial $P\text{CO}_2$, decreased $P\text{O}_2$) or respiratory alkalosis if they are overventilated.

All snake-bitten patients should be encouraged to empty their bladder on admission. Urine should be examined for blood/haemoglobin and protein ('stix' test) and for microscopic haematuria and red cell casts.

Electrocardiographic abnormalities are unusual but important. Sinus bradycardia, ST–T changes, various degrees of atrioventricular block and evidence of hyperkalaemia have been described, especially in patients envenomed by Viperidae, Australasian elapids and Atractaspididae.

Chest radiographs are useful for detecting pulmonary oedema (e.g. European *Vipera* and *D. russelii* (see Figure 22.33), intrapulmonary haemorrhages and pleural effusions (*D. russelii*) (see Figure 22.32).

IMMUNODIAGNOSIS

The immunological detection of venom antigens in body fluids of snake bite victims has improved diagnosis, understanding of pathophysiological mechanisms, assessment of first aid methods and control of antivenom treatment.[41] Enzyme immunoassays (EIA) have been the most widely used[41,42] but immunodiagnostic test kits are generally available only in Australia (from the Commonwealth

Serum Laboratories). These tests are highly sensitive but their specificity may be inadequate to distinguish between different species and false-positive reactions are common, especially in the sera of rural populations in the tropics. Relatively high venom antigen concentrations (e.g. from wound swabs or aspirates) can be detected within 15–30 minutes, which is just fast enough to allow the selection of the appropriate monospecific antivenom. For retrospective diagnosis, including forensic cases, tissue around the fang punctures, wound and blister aspirate, serum and urine should be stored for EIA immunodiagnosis.

MANAGEMENT OF SNAKE BITE

FIRST AID

First aid can be carried out only by the person who is bitten or by others who happen to be nearby at the time, using materials which are readily available, close at hand.

1. Reassure the victim, who will almost certainly be terrified.
2. Do not tamper with the bite wound in any way, but immobilize the bitten limb using a splint or sling. If available, firm binding of the splint with a crepe bandage is an effective form of immobilization.
3. Take the patient as quickly as possible to the nearest health clinic, dispensary or hospital where medical treatment can be given. Muscular contraction in the bitten limb will promote spread of venom, so this should be avoided as far as possible. Ideally, the patient should be transported by motor vehicle, bicycle (as a passenger), boat or on a stretcher.
4. Avoid harmful and time-wasting treatments (see below).
5. Since species diagnosis is critically important, the snake should be taken along to hospital if it has already been killed. However, if the snake is still at large, do not risk further bites and waste time by searching for it. Even snakes which appear to be dead should not be touched with the bare hands but carried in a bag or dangling across a stick. Some species (e.g. *Hemachatus haemachatus* sham death, and even a severed head can inject venom!

Rejected or controversial first aid methods

Procedures which inflict further trauma or other interference to the bite site are potentially harmful and should not be used. These include cauterization, incision or excision, amputation of the bitten digit, suction by mouth, vacuum pumps or 'venom-ex' apparatus, instillation of chemical compounds such as potassium permanganate, cooling with ice (cryotherapy) and electric shocks.[43] Incisions will lead to uncontrolled bleeding in patients with incoagulable blood, may damage nerves, blood vessels or tendons and introduce infection. Suction, chemicals and cryotherapy may cause necrosis of tissues. None of these methods aimed at removing venom from the site of the bite has received consistent support from the results of animal experiments. No clinical studies have been attempted. The use of tourniquets, compression pads and bandages, in an attempt to impede the systemic uptake of venom, remains controversial. In animals, tight (arterial) tourniquets have been shown to prevent the absorption of venom and to prolong survival after the injection of venoms of elapids and vipers. The splinting and crepe bandaging method ('pressure immobilization') advocated by Sutherland in Australia also proved effective in limiting the absorption of venom in restrained monkeys.[44] In the original experiments, crepe bandaging was thought to exert a pressure of about 55 mmHg, that of a venous tourniquet. The splint and crepe bandage is certainly an effective way of immobilizing the bitten limb, and is a less painful way of applying an obstructive pressure than is the arterial tourniquet. However, in practice, it is difficult to judge how tightly to apply the crepe bandage, difficult for the patient to apply unaided and might accentuate the locally necrotic effects of some snake venoms.[45] Dangers of tourniquets and other occlusive methods include ischaemia and gangrene, if they are applied for more than about 2 hours, damage to peripheral nerves (especially the lateral popliteal nerve), increased fibrinolytic activity, congestion, swelling, increased bleeding, increased local effects of venom and shock or rapid development of life-threatening systemic envenoming after their release. Few convincing clinical data are available, but in Thai patients bitten by *Calloselasma rhodostoma*, and Burmese patients bitten by *D. russelii*, systemic venom antigen concentrations did not increase after the tourniquets applied by country people had been released.[46,47] Tourniquets/constricting bands are the most widely used first aid method in most countries but, because of the danger, their use should be *strongly discouraged*. However, if a patient is bitten by a dangerous neurotoxic elapid (such as a mamba, king cobra or taipan) or by a sea snake, and medical attention is likely to be delayed for 1–2 hours, there is a risk that respiratory paralysis might develop en route to hospital. *In these cases alone* it seems reasonable to apply a firm crepe bandage and splint (if available), or a tight tourniquet (upper arm or thigh) in the hope of delaying the onset of life-threatening neurotoxicity until the patients reach a place where they can be resuscitated.

TREATMENT OF EARLY SYMPTOMS

Distressing and dangerous manifestations of envenoming may appear before the patient reaches hospital.

Local pain may be intense. Oral paracetamol is preferable to aspirin, which commonly causes gastric erosions and could lead to persistent gastric bleeding in patients with incoagulable blood. *Severe pain* can be treated with pethidine or pentazocine.

Vomiting is a common early symptom of systemic envenoming. Patients should lie on their side with the head down to avoid aspiration. Persistent vomiting can be treated with intravenous chlorpromazine (25–50 mg in adults, 1 mg/kg in children).*

Syncopal attacks and anaphylactic shock

Patients may collapse within minutes of the bite and show features either of a vasovagal attack or of an autopharmacological reaction with angioneurotic oedema, abdominal colic and diarrhoea. An antihistamine such as chlorpheniramine maleate (10 mg in adults, 0.2 mg/kg in children) can be given by intravenous or intramuscular* injection. Hypotension or bronchoconstriction can be treated with adrenaline 0.1% (1 in 1000) (0.5 ml in adults, 0.01 ml/kg in children) by *subcutaneous injection*.

Respiratory distress

This may result from upper airway obstruction if the jaw and tongue are paralysed or from paralysis of the respiratory muscles. Patients should be laid on the side, the airway cleared, if possible using a suction pump, an oral airway inserted and the jaw elevated. If the patient is cyanosed, or respiratory movements are very weak, oxygen should be given by any available means. If clearing the airway does not produce immediate relief, artificial ventilation must be given. In the absence of any equipment, mouth-to-mouth or mouth-to-nose ventilation can be lifesaving. Manual ventilation by Ambu bag and anaesthetic mask is rarely effective. Ideally, the patient should have a cuffed endotracheal tube inserted,

using a laryngoscope, or a cuffed tracheostomy tube inserted. The patient can then be ventilated by Ambu bag. If no femoral or carotid pulse can be felt, external cardiac massage should be instituted.

TREATMENT AT HEALTH CLINIC, DISPENSARY OR HOSPITAL BY MEDICALLY TRAINED STAFF

Clinical assessment

Snake bite is a medical emergency. The history, symptoms and signs must be assessed rapidly so that appropriate treatment can be started without delay. The three most important preliminary questions are: Where (in which part of your body) were you bitten? How long ago were you bitten? Have you brought the snake or, if not, did you see what kind of snake it was? If the snake has been killed but not brought, one of the accompanying friends or relatives should be despatched to collect it posthaste. If the snake can be diagnosed confidently as non-venomous, the patient can be discharged immediately after receiving a booster dose of tetanus toxoid. Patients should be asked whether they have taken any herbal or other treatment, whether they have vomited, fainted, or have noticed any bleeding or other ill-effects of the bite and whether they have passed urine since being bitten. Physical signs should be assessed before any tourniquet is removed. Fang marks are sometimes invisible and rarely help the diagnosis, although the discovery of two or three discrete puncture marks does suggest fangs of a venomous snake. Local swelling, tenderness and lymph node involvement are early signs of envenoming. The gingival sulci should be examined carefully as these are usually the earliest site where spontaneous bleeding is detectable. Bleeding from venepuncture sites, recent wounds and skin lesions suggests that the blood is incoagulable. If the patient is shocked (collapsed, sweating, cold, cyanosed extremities, low blood pressure, tachycardia) the foot of the bed should be raised, and an intravenous infusion of a plasma expander such as fresh frozen plasma, dextran, Haemaccel or fresh blood started immediately. The jugular venous pressure or, preferably, the central venous pressure should be observed. The earliest symptom of neurotoxicity after elapid bites is often blurred vision, a feeling of heaviness in the eyelids and drowsiness. The earliest sign is contraction of the frontalis muscle (raised eyebrows and puckered forehead) even before true ptosis can be demonstrated. Signs of respiratory muscle paralysis (dyspnoea, exaggerated

---

*In patients with incoagulable blood, intramuscular and subcutaneous injections can lead to haematoma formation. Pressure dressings should be applied to venepuncture sites to prevent oozing.

abdominal respiration and contraction of intercostal muscles and cyanosis) must be detected and the blood pressure measured. Patients with generalized rhabdomyolysis have trismus and stiff and tender muscles which resist passive stretching. Urine output may dwindle very early in the course of Russell's viper bite. Dark urine suggests myoglobinuria or haemoglobinuria.

It may be obvious from this preliminary assessment that antivenom should be given, but even if there is no evidence of significant envenoming patients should be admitted to a ward where they can be observed closely for at least 24 hours. Every hour, ptosis should be looked for and symptoms, level of consciousness, pulse rate and rhythm, blood pressure, respiratory rate, extent of local swelling and other new signs should be recorded. If there is any evidence of neurotoxicity, the ventilatory capacity or expiratory pressure should also be recorded every hour. Useful investigations include the simple whole blood clotting test (or more sensitive tests of haemostasis, FDP estimation, etc. if available), peripheral leucocyte count, haematocrit, urine microscopy and 'stix' testing and electrocardiography.

ANTIVENOM (ANTIVENIN, ANTIVENENE, ANTI-SNAKE BITE SERUM)

Antivenom is the whole serum or enzyme-refined immunoglobulin of animals, usually horses or sheep, which have been immunized with venom. It is the only specific treatment available and has proved effective against many of the lethal and damaging effects of venoms. In the management of snake bite the most important clinical decision is whether or not to give antivenom, for only a minority of snake-bitten patients need it, it may produce severe reactions, and it is expensive and often in short supply.

INDICATIONS FOR ANTIVENOM

Systemic envenoming

1. Haemostatic abnormalities: spontaneous systemic bleeding, incoagulable blood or prolonged clotting time, elevated FDP, thrombocytopenia.
2. Cardiovascular abnormalities: hypotension, shock, abnormal electrocardiogram, cardiac arrhythmia, cardiac failure, pulmonary oedema.
3. Neurotoxicity.
4. Generalized rhabdomyolysis.
5. Impaired consciousness.

6. In patients with definite signs of local envenoming, the following indicate significant systemic envenoming: neutrophil leucocytosis, elevated serum enzymes such as creatine phosphokinase and aminotransferases, haemoconcentration, uraemia, hypercreatininaemia, oliguria, hypoxaemia, acidosis and vomiting in the absence of a history of ingesting emetic agents.

Severe local envenoming

The development at any stage of local swelling involving more than half the bitten limb or extensive blistering or bruising, especially in patients showing the abnormalities listed above under (6) and in patients bitten by species known to cause local necrosis (e.g. Viperidae, Asian cobras, African spitting cobras, *Naja nigricollis*, *N. pallida* and *N. mossambica*). Bites on the digits by these species carry a high risk of necrosis and so antivenom is also indicated in such cases.

Some wealthy countries can afford a wider range of indications for the use of antivenom. The following *additional* indications have been suggested.

- *United States and Canada*. Following bites by the most dangerous rattlesnakes (*Crotalus atrox*, *C. adamanteus*, *C. viridis*, *C. horridus* and *C. scutulatus*) antivenom therapy has been recommended if there is rapid spread of local swelling, even without evidence of systemic envenoming, and after bites by coral snakes (*Micruroides euryxanthus* and *Micrurus fulvius*) if there is immediate pain or any other symptom or sign of envenoming.
- *Australia*. Antivenom is recommended in any proved or suspected case of snake bite if there is any evidence of systemic spread of venom, including tender regional lymph nodes, and if there has been an effective bite by any identified highly venomous species.[1]
- *Europe*. To improve the rate of recovery of local swelling after bites by *Vipera berus*, antivenom has been recommended in adults with swelling extending up the forearm or leg within 2 hours of the bite.[48]

Contraindications

Atopic patients and those who have had reactions to equine antiserum on previous occasions have an increased risk of developing severe antivenom reactions. In such cases antivenom should not be given unless there are definite signs of severe (potentially life-threatening) systemic envenoming. Reactions may be ameliorated by pretreatment with adrenaline, antihistamine and corticosteroid (doses given below). Rapid desensitization is not recommended.

PREDICTION OF ANTIVENOM REACTIONS

Hypersensitivity testing by intradermal or subcutaneous injection or intraconjunctival instillation of diluted antivenom has been widely practised in the past. However, these tests delay the start of antivenom treatment, are not without risk, and have recently been proved to have no predictive value for early (anaphylactic) or late (serum sickness type) antivenom reactions.[49]

ADMINISTRATION OF ANTIVENOM

The range of venoms neutralized by an antivenom is usually stated in the package insert and is to be found in compendia of antivenoms.[50] If the biting species is known or can reliably be deduced, the appropriate monospecific antivenom should be used. In parts of the world where several species produce identical signs, patients who fail to bring the dead snake must be treated with polyspecific antivenom, which will contain a lower concentration of specific antibody to each species than the monospecific antivenom.

Manufacturers' expiry dates are often extremely conservative. Liquid lyophilized antivenoms stored at below 8°C usually retain most of their activity for 5 years or more.[51] Opaque solutions should not be given as precipitation of protein indicates loss of activity and an increased risk of reactions. Antivenom should be given as soon as it is indicated, but it is almost never too late to give it as long as signs of systemic envenoming persist (e.g. up to 2 days after a sea snake bite and many days or even weeks for prolonged defibrination following bites by Viperidae). In contrast, local effects of venoms are probably not reversible by antivenom delayed more than 1–2 hours after the bite. The intravenous route is the most effective. An infusion over 30–60 minutes of antivenom diluted in isotonic fluid may be easier to control than an intravenous 'push' injection of reconstituted but undiluted antivenom given over 10–20 minutes. There is no difference in the incidence of severity of antivenom reactions in patients treated by these two methods.[49] In the rural tropics, the intravenous push method has the advantage that it involves less expensive equipment, is quicker to initiate and compels someone to remain with the patient at least while the injection is being given.

In the absence of anyone capable of giving an intravenous injection, antivenom may be given by deep intramuscular injection (e.g. into the anterior thighs but not into the gluteal region) followed by massage to promote absorption. However, the volumes of antivenom normally required would make this route impracticable, as would the risk of haematoma formation in patients with incoagulable blood. Local injection of antivenom, for example into the fang marks, seems rational but is difficult, painful and hazardous (especially when the bite is on a digit or other tight compartment) and has not proved effective in animal studies.

The average initial dose of antivenom required should be based on results of clinical studies, but these are rarely available. Most manufacturers base their recommendations on the mouse assay which may not correlate with clinical findings.[52] Initial doses of some important antivenoms are given in Table 22.3. The apparent serum half-lives of antivenoms in envenomed patients range from 26 to 95 hours, depending on how they are prepared.[53–55] Systemic envenoming may recur several days after an initial good response to antivenom.[45] This is probably the result of continuing absorption of venom from the injection site after antivenom has been largely cleared from the circulation. The implication is that an initial dose of antivenom, however large, may not prevent late or recurrent envenoming. *Children must be given the same or larger doses of antivenom than adults*. The response to antivenom will determine whether further doses should be given. Neurotoxic signs may improve within 30 minutes of antivenom treatment but usually take several hours. Hypotension, sinus bradycardia and spontaneous systemic bleeding may respond within 10–20 minutes and blood coagulability is usually restored between 1 and 6 hours, provided sufficient antivenom has been given. A second dose of antivenom should be given if severe cardiorespiratory symptoms persist for more than about 30 minutes, and incoagulable blood persists for more than 6 hours, after the start of the first dose. Enormous doses of antivenom may be required to treat patients bitten by species capable of injecting very large amounts of venom or extremely potent venom. Thus a patient bitten by the king cobra (*Ophiophagus hannah*) was given 1150 ml of specific antivenom and prolonged artificial ventilation.[34] Other exceptionally large species include the bushmaster (*Lachesis muta*), diamondback rattlesnakes (*C. adamanteus* and *C. atrox*), Gaboon viper (*Bitis gabonica*) and black mamba (*Dendroaspis polylepis*).

ANTIVENOM REACTIONS

Antivenom treatment may be complicated by three types of reaction: early (anaphylactic), pyrogenic

Table 22.3 Guide to initial dosage of some important antivenoms.

| Species | | Manufacturer, antivenom | Approximate initial dose |
Latin name	English name		
Acanthophis species	Death adder	CSL,* monospecific	3000–6000 units
Bitis arietans	Puff adder	Behringwerke, North/Central Africa; SAIMR;† polyspecific	80 ml
Bothrops jararaca	Jararaca	Brazilian manufacturers, *Bothrops* polyspecific	20 ml
Bungarus caeruleus	Common krait	Haffkine polyspecific	100 ml
Calloselasma (Agkistrodon) rhodostoma	Malayan pit viper	Thai Red Cross (Saovabha), Bangkok, monospecific	100 ml
		Thai Government Pharmaceutical Organization, monospecific	50 ml
Crotalus adamanteus	Eastern diamondback rattlesnakes		
Crotalus atrox	Western diamondback rattlesnakes	Wyeth, (Crotalidae) polyspecific	30–100 ml
Crotalus viridis subspecies	Western rattlesnakes		
Daboia (Vipera) russelii	Russell's vipers	Burma Pharmaceutical Industry, monospecific	40 ml
		Haffkine polyspecific	100 ml
		Thai manufacturers, monospecific	50 ml
Echis species	Saw-scaled or carpet vipers	SAIMR, *Echis*, monospecific	20 ml
		Behringwerke, North Africa/Near and Middle East, polyspecific	100 ml
Hydrophiidae	Sea snakes	CSL, sea snake/tiger snake	1000 units
Naja kaouthia	Monocellate Thai cobra	Thai Red Cross, monospecific	100 ml
Naja naja	Indian cobra	Haffkine; Central Research Institute, Kasauli; Serum Institute of India, polyspecific	100 ml
Notechis scutatus	Tiger snake	CSL, monospecific	3000–6000 units
Pseudechis textilis	Eastern brown snake		
Oxyuranus scutellatus	Taipan	CSL, monospecific	12000 units
Trimeresurus albolabris	Green pit viper	Thai Red Cross, monospecific	100 ml
Vipera berus	European adder	Immunoloski Zavod-Zagreb Vipera polyspecific	10 ml
		Therapeutic Antibodies (Inc), Fab monospecific BeriTAB	100–200 mg
Vipera palaestinae	Palestine viper	Rogoff Medical Research Institute, Tel Aviv, Palestine viper monospecific	50–80 ml

*Commonwealth Serum Laboratories, Australia.
†South African Institute for Medical Research.

and late (serum sickness-type). Pretreatment with antihistamine, corticosteroid and subcutaneous 0.1% adrenaline reduces the incidence of early and late reactions.

Early antivenom reactions are not usually type I IgE-mediated hypersensitivity reactions to equine serum proteins for they are not predicted by hypersensitivity tests.[49] Antivenoms activate complement in vitro,[56] while the clinically similar reactions to homologous serum are associated with complement activation and immune complex formation in vivo. The complement system is probably activated by aggregates of IgG. Reactions usually develop within 10 to 180 minutes of starting antivenom. There is itching, urticaria (Figure 22.36), fever, tachycardia, palpitations, cough, nausea and vomiting. The reported incidence, which varies from 3 to 54%, appears to increase with the dose and to decrease when refined antivenom is used and administration is by intramuscular rather than intravenous injection. Unless patients are watched carefully for 3 hours after treatment, mild reactions may be missed and deaths may be misattributed to the envenoming itself. Up to 40% of patients with early reactions show features of severe systemic anaphylaxis: bronchospasm, hypotension or angio oedema, but deaths are rare. Early reactions respond readily to adrenaline given by a subcutaneous injection of between 0.5 and 1.0 ml of 0.1% (1:1000, 1 mg/ml) in adults (children 0.01 ml/kg) at the first sign of trouble. Antihistamines such as chlorpheniramine maleate (adult dose 10 mg, children 0.2 mg/kg) should be given by intravenous injection to combat the effects of histamine released during the reaction.

Pyrogenic reactions result from contamination of the antivenom by endotoxin-like compounds. High fever develops 1–2 hours after treatment and is associated with rigors, followed by vasodilatation and a fall in blood pressure. Febrile convulsions may be precipitated in children. Patients should be cooled and given antipyretic drugs such as paracetamol, by mouth, powdered and washed down a nasogastric tube (15 mg/kg) or in the form of a suppository.

Late (serum sickness-type) reactions develop 5–24 (mean 7) days after treatment. The higher the dose of antivenom the higher the incidence of these reactions and the speed of their development. Symptoms include fever, itching, urticaria, arthralgia, including the temporomandibular joint, lymphadenopathy, periarticular swellings, mononeuritis multiplex, albuminuria and rarely encephalopathy. This is an immune complex disease which responds to an antihistamine such as chlorpheniramine (adults 2 mg four times a day, children 0.25 mg/kg per day in divided doses), or, in more severe cases, to corticosteroid (prednisolone 5 mg four times a day for 5 days in adults, 0.7 mg/kg per day in divided doses for 5 days for children).

SUPPORTIVE TREATMENT (ASSUMING THAT ADEQUATE DOSES OF ANTIVENOM HAVE BEEN GIVEN)

Artificial ventilation was first suggested for neurotoxic envenoming more than one hundred years ago but patients continue to die for lack of this simple procedure. Neurotoxic effects are fully reversible with time: a patient bitten by *Bungarus multicinctus* in Canton recovered completely after being ventilated manually for 30 days, and a patient probably envenomed by *Tropidechis carinatus* recovered after 10 weeks mechanical ventilation in Queensland, Australia. Endotracheal intubation or tracheostomy, using cuffed tubes, is needed. The patient can be ventilated manually with an anaesthetic or Ambu bag or, preferably, with a mechanical ventilator (Figure 22.37).

Anticholinesterase drugs may produce a rapid useful improvement in neuromuscular transmission in some patients envenomed by some species of

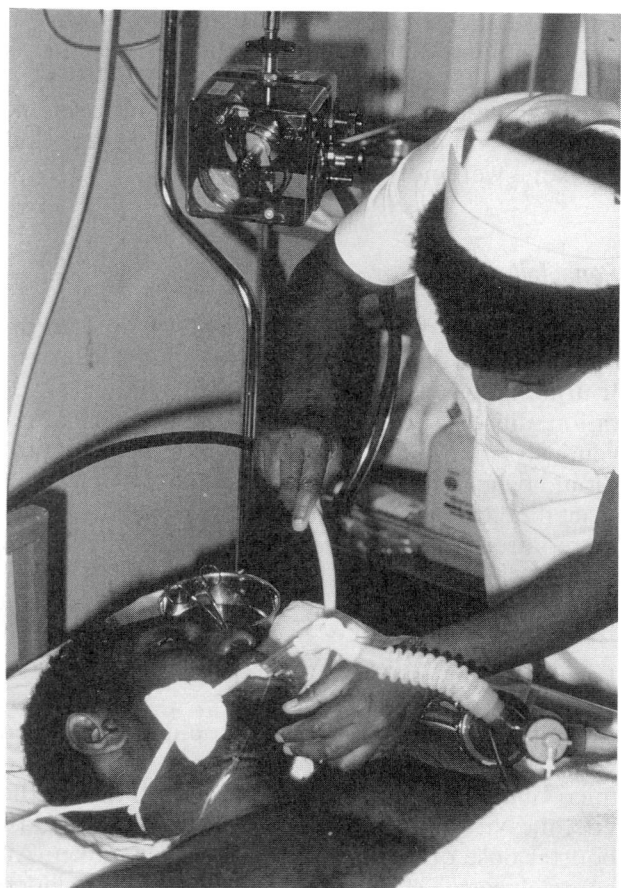

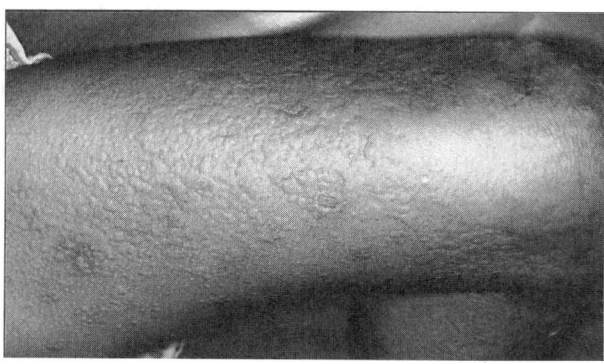

Figure 22.36 Urticaria of the thigh, coalescent over the knee, in a patient experiencing an early antivenom reaction 15 minutes after the start of treatment. (Copyright D.A. Warrell.)

Figure 22.37 Artificial ventilation by Bird ventilator in a patient with complete flaccid paralysis following a bite by a taipan (*Oxyuranus scutellatus canni*) in Central Province, Papua New Guinea. (Copyright D.A. Warrell.)

Asian and African cobras, mambas, death adders (*Acanthophis* species), coral snakes (*Micrurus* species) and kraits.[35] It is worth trying the 'Tensilon test' in all cases of severe neurotoxic envenoming, as with suspected myasthenia gravis. Atropine sulphate (adults 0.6 mg, children 50 μg/kg) is given first by intravenous injection to block unpleasant muscarinic effects of acetylcholine (increased secretions, abdominal colic). Edrophonimum chloride (Tensilon) is then given by slow intravenous injection in an adult dose of 10 mg, or 0.25 mg/kg for children. Patients who respond convincingly can be maintained on neostigmine methylsulphate, 50–100 μg/kg and atropine 4-hourly or by continuous infusion.

Hypotension and shock

These usually result from hypovolaemia and should be treated by infusing a plasma expander, preferably fresh whole blood or, failing that, fresh frozen plasma. Central venous pressure or pulmonary arterial catheter monitoring is the safest way to control volume replacement. Hypotensive patients envenomed by Burmese Russell's viper responded to dopamine, 2.5 μg/kg per minute by intravenous infusion; but methylprednisolone, 30 mg/kg, and naloxone were not effective.[11]

Renal failure

If urine output drops below 400 ml/24 hours, urethral and central venous catheters should be inserted. If urine flow fails to increase after cautious rehydration, diuretics (e.g. frusemide up to 1000 mg intravenously) and dopamine (2.5 μg/kg per minute) should be given and the patient should be placed on strict fluid balance. Peritoneal or haemodialysis will be required in most patients with established renal failure.

Local infection

Infection at the site of the bite should be prevented with penicillin or erythromycin (or by an antimicrobial effective against the bacterial flora of the buccal cavity and venoms of local snakes)[57,58] and a booster dose of tetanus toxoid should be given. An aminoglycoside such as gentamicin should be added if the wound has been tampered with or there is evidence of local necrosis. Bullae are best left alone. Snake-bitten limbs should be nursed in the most comfortable position. *Necrotic tissue* should be excised as soon as possible and the denuded area covered with split-skin grafts.

Intracompartmental syndromes

Swelling of muscles within tight fascial compartments may raise the tissue pressure to such an extent that perfusion is impaired and ischaemic damage is added to the effects of the venom. The signs of an intracompartmental syndrome include excessive pain, weakness of the compartmental muscles and pain when they are passively stretched, hypoaesthesia of areas of skin supplied by nerves running through the compartment and obvious tenseness of the compartment.[39] Palpation of peripheral pulses or their detection by Doppler ultrasound does not exclude intracompartmental ischaemia. An intracompartmental pressure of more than 45 mmHg indicates a high risk of ischaemic necrosis.[39] In these circumstances, fasciotomy may be justified to relieve the pressure in the compartment, but this treatment did not prove effective in saving envenomed muscle in animal experiments.[59] Necrosis occurs most frequently after digital bites. Fasciotomy must not be attempted before blood coagulability has been restored by adequate doses of specific antivenom, accelerated if possible by the transfusion of fresh whole blood or clotting factors.

Corticosteroids, heparin, antifibrinolytic agents such as aprotinin (Trasylol) and ε-aminocaproic acid, antihistamine, trypsin and a variety of traditional herbal remedies have been used and advocated for snake bite. Most are potentially harmful and none has been proved to be effective.

SNAKE VENOM OPHTHALMIA

The 'spat' venom should be washed from the eye or mucous membrane as soon as possible using large volumes of water or other bland fluid. Unless a corneal abrasion can be excluded by fluorescein staining or slit-lamp examination, treatment should be the same as for any corneal injury: a topical antimicrobial agent such as tetracycline or chloramphenicol and closure of the eye with a dressing pad.[30] 0.1% adrenaline eyedrops relieve the pair.

PREVENTION

The incidence of snake bite can be greatly reduced by taking simple precautions. Unfortunately, these methods are impracticable for those, such as farmers, who have to do hard physical work in hot snake-infested areas. Snakes should never be disturbed, attacked or handled unnecessarily even if they are thought to be harmless species or appear to be dead. Venomous species should never be kept as pets or as performing animals. Protective clothing— boots, socks, long trousers—should be worn when walking in undergrowth or deep sand and a light should always be carried at night. Particular care should be taken while collecting firewood, moving logs, boulders, boxes or debris likely to conceal a snake, and climbing rocks and trees covered with dense foliage or swimming in overgrown lakes and rivers. Wading in the sea, especially in sand or near coral reefs, is a dangerous pastime (see below, fish stings) and should be avoided if possible. Shuffling is safer than a high stepping gait. Divers should keep clear of sea snakes. Fishermen who catch sea snakes in nets or on lines should return them to their element without touching them.

Domestic animals such as chickens and rodent pests attract snakes into human dwellings. Snakes can be discouraged by rodent-proofing, by removing unnecessary junk and litter and by using solid building materials. Various toxic chemicals such as naphthalene, sulphur, insecticides (e.g. DDT, dieldrin and pyrethrins) and fumigants (e.g. methyl bromide, formaldehyde, tetrachloroethane) are lethal or repellent to snakes.

PROPHYLACTIC IMMUNIZATION AGAINST SNAKE VENOMS

Venom toxoids (venoids) have been used to immunize farmers at high risk of habu bite (*Trimeresurus flavoviridis* in the Ryukyu and Amami Islands in Japan.[60] Elsewhere, there has been some progress in producing venoids to protect against Russell's viper bite. In this case, the rapid development of renal damage, irreversible by antivenom, is a strong argument for pre-exposure prophylaxis.[11] The production and modification of venom antigens by genetic engineering is an exciting new development which could lead to the production of snake venom vaccines.[61]

VENOMOUS LIZARDS[62]

Two species of venomous lizard (genus *Heloderma*) are capable of envenoming humans. The venom glands are in the lower jaw. The Gila monster (*H. suspectum*) is striped, with a short, thick tail, and grows up to 60 cm in length (Figure 22.38). It occurs in the south-western USA and the adjacent areas of Mexico. The Mexican beaded lizard or escorpión (*H. horridum*) is spotted, with a relatively long, thin tail, and reaches 80 cm in length. It is found in western Mexico and Central America. Bites are rare. The lizard hangs on with its powerful jaws and is difficulty to disengage. There is immediate severe local pain with tender swelling and regional lymphadenopathy. Symptoms include weakness, dizziness, hypotension, syncope, sweating, rigors, tinnitus, nausea and vomiting. There may be leucocytosis, coagulopathy and electrocardiographic changes.[63] No fatal cases have reliably been reported. Specific antivenom is not generally available. A powerful

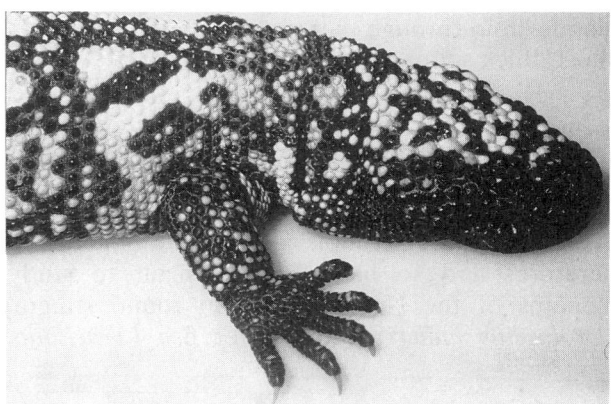

Figure 22.38 Gila monster (*Heloderma suspectum*), one of the two species of venomous lizards. (Copyright D.A. Warrell.)

analgesic may be required. Hypotension should be treated with plasma expanders and perhaps adrenaline or a pressor agent such as dopamine.

VENOMOUS FISH[64]

TAXONOMY

More than 100 species of fish, inhabiting temperate and tropical seas, possess a defensive venom-injecting apparatus which can inflict dangerous stings. Fatal stings from members of the groups have been reported: order Chondrichthyes (cartilagenous fish); order Squaliformes (sharks and dogfish); order Rajiformes (stingrays and mantas); order Osteichthyes (bony fish); suborder Siluroidei (catfish); family Trachinidae (weever fish); family Scorpaenidae (scorpion fish, stonefish) (Figure 22.39) and family Uranoscopidae (stargazers or stone-lifters).

VENOM APPARATUS

Venom is secreted around spines or barbs in front of the dorsal, anal or pectoral fins and tail and opercular spines in the gill covers. The venom gland in stingrays lies in a groove beneath a membrane covering the barbed precaudal spine up to 30 cm long. The most advanced venom apparatus is found in the genus *Synanceja* (stonefish): bulky venom glands drain through paired ducts to the tips of the short, thick spines.

VENOM COMPOSITION

Fish venoms are unstable at normal ambient temperatures and so have been difficult to study. Venoms of the North American round stingray (*Urolophus halleri*) and weever fish (*Trachinus*) were found to contain peptides, protein, enzymes and a variety of vasoactive compounds (kinins, 5-hydroxytryptamine, histamine, adrenaline and nor-adrenaline). Pharmacological effects include local necrosis, direct actions on cardiac, skeletal and smooth muscle, causing electrocardiographic changes, hypotension and paralysis, and central nervous system depression.

INCIDENCE AND EPIDEMIOLOGY OF FISH STINGS

There are hundreds of weever fish stings around the British coast each year, especially in Cornwall. The peak incidence is in August and September. Fifty-eight cases were seen at a hospital in Pula on the Adriatic over 13 years. In the USA, 1500 stings by rays and 300 stings by scorpion fish are thought to occur each year. Eighty-one cases of stonefish sting were seen over a 4 year period at a hospital in Pulau Bukom, an island near Singapore. Ornate but highly venomous and aggressive members of the genera *Pterois* and *Dendrochirus* (zebra, lion, tiger, turkey or red fire fish or coral or fire cod) are popular aquarium pets. Fatal fish stings are very rarely reported. Stings usually occur when people wading near the shore tread on fish which are lying in the sand or shallow water. Most victims are stung on the sole of the foot, but stingrays lash their tails and usually impale the ankle. Fishermen, scuba divers and aquarium enthusiasts are often stung on the fingers while carelessly handling or attempting to touch the fish.

SYMPTOMS OF ENVENOMING

Immediate, sharp, agonizing pain is the dominant symptom. Even stoical adults may collapse screaming with pain and are thought to be hysterical. Bleeding may be seen from single or multiple puncture sites. Hot, erythematous swelling extends rapidly up the stung limb.

STINGRAYS[65]

These fish are widely distributed in oceans and rivers.[66] The large barbed spine may cause severe lacerating injuries, usually to the lower part of the

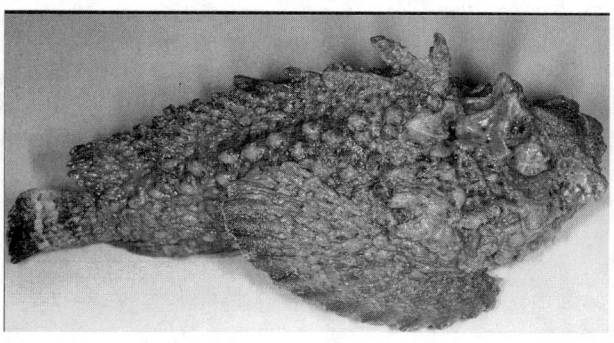

Figure 22.39 Stonefish (*Synanceja horrida*) from Papua New Guinea. (Copyright D.A. Warrell.)

legs but occasionally penetrating the body cavities, heart and viscera when the swimmer falls or lies on the fish. Deaths from this mechanical trauma have been reported from Mexico and New Zealand. The spine and fragments of its integument may remain in the wound. The venom produces local swelling and sometimes necrosis (Figure 22.40), with a high risk of secondary infection unless the broken spine and other foreign material are removed from the wound. Systemic effects include hypotension, cardiac arrhythmias, muscle spasms, generalized convulsions, vomiting, diarrhoea, sweating and hypersalivation.

WEEVERS[67]

Stings by Trachinidae produce intense local pain with slight swelling. Systemic symptoms are rare but some patients develop severe chest pain simulating myocardial ischaemia, cardiac arrhythmias and hypotension.

SCORPION FISH AND STONEFISH

The family Scorpaenidae comprises more than 350 species which are widely distributed in some temper-

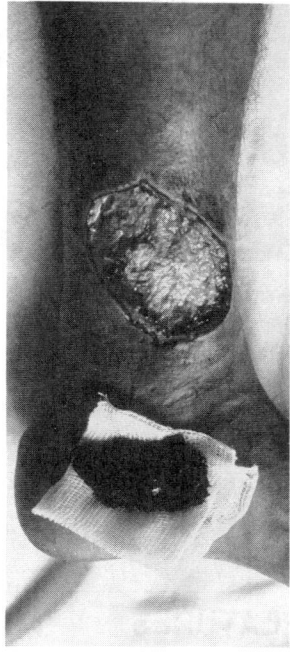

Figure 22.40   Sloughing of necrotic tissue 20 days after a sting by a freshwater ray (*Potamotrygon hystrix*) in the Amazon region of Brazil. (Courtesy of João Luiz Costa Cardoso, São Paulo.)

ate and all tropical seas and are especially abundant around the coral reefs of the Indo-Pacific region. The stonefish (genus *Synanceja*) (see Figure 22.39) are the most dangerous of venomous fish. They occur from East Africa, across the Indian Ocean, to the Pacific. Stings are excruciatingly painful, as are all fish stings, but symptoms may persist for 2 days or more. There is local swelling, discoloration, sweating and paraesthesia and sometimes local lymphadenopathy. Systemic symptoms are more common than with other fish stings. They include nausea, vomiting, hypotension, cardiac arrhythmias, respiratory distress, neurological signs, convulsions and evidence of autonomic nervous system stimulation. People have died within an hour of being stung by *S. verrucosa*.

TREATMENT

The most effective treatment for pain is to immerse the stung limb in water that is uncomfortably hot but not scalding (i.e. just under 45°C). Temperature can be assessed with the unstung limb. It is not necessary to add magnesium sulphate to the water. Injection of local anaesthetic such as 1% lignocaine, for example as a ring block in the case of stung digits, is less effective. The spine, membrane and other foreign material must be removed from the wound. Prophylactic antibiotics and tetanus toxoid should be given to patients stung by rays or scorpion fish because of the size of wound and risk of necrosis, but these measures are not justified for weever fish stings. Local injection of potassium permanganate solution or acidifying solutions such as emetine hydrochloride were said to cure local pain, but they may promote local necrosis and are less effective than immersion in hot water. In patients with severe systemic envenoming, an adequate airway should be established and cardiorespiratory resuscitation instituted when necessary. Severe hypotension can be treated with adrenaline and bradycardia with atropine. The only antivenom now available commercially is manufactured by the Commonwealth Serum Laboratories in Australia. It neutralizes the venoms of *S. trachynis*, *S. verrucosa* and *S. horrida* and has paraspecific activity against venoms of the North American scorpion fish (*Scorpaena guttata*) and other members of the Scorpaenidae family. Two millilitres (2000 units), one ampoule, is given intravenously for each two puncture marks found at the site of the sting. The dose is increased in patients with severe symptoms.[1]

PREVENTION (See p. 494–495)

Bathers and waders should adopt a shuffling gait to reduce the risk of stepping on a venomous fish skulking in sand or mud. Footwear protects against most species except stingrays.

VENOMOUS MARINE INVERTEBRATES[64]
COELENTERATES (HYDROIDS, STINGING CORALS, MEDUSAE, PORTUGUESE MEN-O'-WAR OR BLUEBOTTLES, JELLYFISH, BLUBBERS, BOX-JELLIES, STINGING ALGAE, SEA ANEMONES AND SEA PANSIES)

The venom apparatus of the coelenterates is the stinging capsule or nematocyst which, when triggered by physical contact or chemicals, everts a thread-like tubule with sharpened tip which can penetrate the skin and inject toxin. The tentacles of coelenterates are armed with myriads of these nematocysts which produce lines of painful irritant wheals on the skin of swimmers unlucky enough to make contact with them. Coelenterate venoms contain peptides together with vasoactive compounds such as 5-hydroxytryptamine, histamine, prostaglandins and kinins which cause immediate severe pain, inflammation and urticaria.

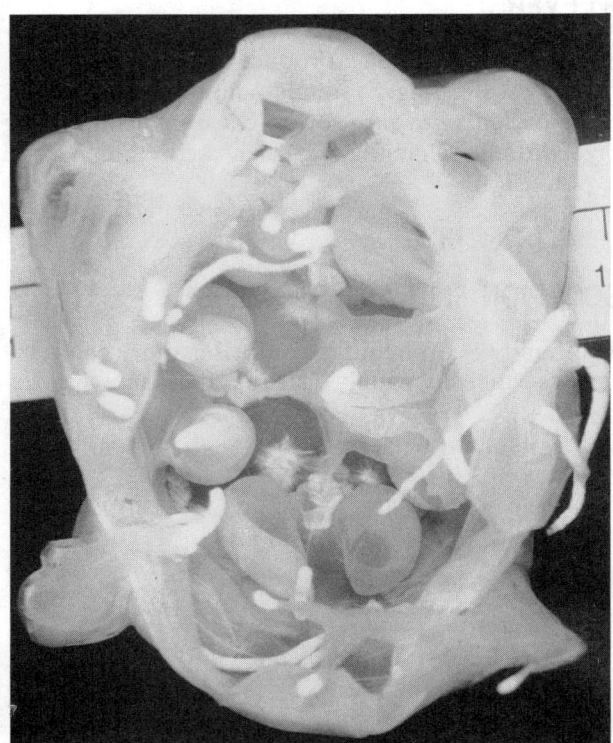

Figure 22.41 Underside of a box jellyfish from Sri Lanka (*Chiropsalmus buitendijki*). The bell is approximately 12 cm in diameter. (Copyright D.A. Warrell.)

EPIDEMIOLOGY

The most dangerous coelenterate to man, the box-jellyfish (*Chironex fleckeri*) has been found along the northern coast of Australia from Darwin to Port Curtis and has been responsible for 63 deaths since 1883. Most stings occur in December and January. Fatal jellyfish stings have also been reported from Bougainville Island in the east to the west coast of India and north to the Philippines where a similar species *Chiropsalmus quadrigatus* is common (Figure 22.41). During a three-and-a-half year period, 116 cases of marine stings were seen in Cairns, north Queensland.[68] Forty per cent of the patients had clinical features of 'Irukandji sting' caused by *Carukia barnesi*. Prodigious swarms of the scyphomedusa *Pelagia noctiluca* appeared along the northern Adriatic coast during the summers of 1977–1979. In 1978 it was estimated that 250 000 swimmers had been stung. At Pula on the Adriatic coast, 55 patients stung by a sea anemone (*Anemonia sulcata*) were seen from 1965 to 1980.[69] This coelenterate is widely distributed in the eastern Atlantic and Mediterranean. Coelenterate stings are common in most parts of the world but few reliable statistics are available.

CLINICAL FEATURES

The imprint of nematocyst stings on the skin may have a diagnostic pattern. *Chironex fleckeri* produces immediate brownish or purplish wheals 8–10 mm wide with cross-striations. More extensive swelling, erythema and vesiculation develops, with areas of necrosis and eventual healing with scar formation. *Carukia barnesi* produces an oval erythematous area about 7 cm in diameter and then transient papules with surrounding hyperhidrosis. Portuguese man-o'-war (*Physalia*) stings produce chains of oval wheals surrounded by erythema. These lesions persist for only about 24 hours. Histological sections of the skin lesions may reveal identifiable nematocysts, allowing differentiation between stings by different genera.

The dominant symptom of the coelenterate sting is immediate severe pain coming in waves and sometimes becoming incapacitating in its intensity. Systemic symptoms are most severe following stings by cubomedusae (box-jellyfish), genera *Chironex* and *Chiropsalmus* (Figure 22.41). The victim, usually a child swimming in shallow water, suddenly screams with pain and within minutes becomes cyanosed, suffers generalized convulsions and is found to be pulseless. The whole jellyfish or a length of tentacles may still be adherent to the patient's skin. Autopsies reveal pulmonary oedema. Patients envenomed by *Carukia barnesi* develop severe systemic effects minutes to hours after the sting but with little or no local effect. Systemic effects of coelenterate stings include cough, nausea, vomiting, abdominal colic, diarrhoea, rigors, severe musculoskeletal pains, syncope and signs of autonomic nervous system stimulation such as profuse sweating. The Portuguese man-o'-war (*Physalia*) occasionally causes systemic symptoms and has been known to produce intravascular haemolysis leading to haemoglobinuria and renal failure. Rare fatalities have been attributed to *Physalia*. The sea anemone *Anemonia sulcata* produces painful local papules, erythema, oedema and vesiculation. Systemic symptoms such as sleepiness, dizziness, nausea, vomiting, myalgia and periorbital oedema are occasionally produced.

TREATMENT

First aid is all important as patients may die within minutes of the sting. Lifeguards and others working on coelenterate infested beaches should be trained to deal with jellyfish stings. The patient must be taken out of the water. The nematocysts in fragments of tentacles stuck to the skin must be inactivated to prevent further discharge and envenoming. For *Chironex* and *Physalia*, commercial vinegar or 3–10% aqueous acetic acid is effective;[70] but for *Chrysaora*, a widely distributed Atlantic genus, baking soda and water (50% w/v) proved effective. Alcoholic solutions (methylated spirits, suntan lotion, aftershave, etc.) were advocated until recently when it was shown that they cause massive discharge of nematocysts. Pressure immobilization is recommended. Mouth-to-mouth artificial ventilation has proved life saving in several patients who developed severe respiratory depression with cyanosis, coma and pulselessness. If no pulse can be detected, external cardiac massage should be started. Experimentally, the venom of *Chironex* affects the heart directly and the central nervous system. Clinically, respiratory depression appears to be more important than cardiotoxicity but recent work suggests that verapamil might reverse this effect.

A specific 'sea wasp' antivenom is manufactured by the Commonwealth Serum Laboratories in Australia for *Chironex fleckeri* stings. The antivenom should be administered intravenously (or in the absence of a medically qualified person intramuscularly) if symptoms of systemic envenoming persist after first aid treatment.

PREVENTION

People, and especially children, should keep out of the sea at times of the year when dangerous coelenterates are most prevalent and especially when they have been sighted and warning notices have been displayed. Wet suits and other clothing will protect against the stings.

ECHINODERMS (STARFISH AND SEA URCHINS)[64]

Echinoderms have hard protective exoskeletons. Starfish (Asteroidea) sprout numerous sharp spines which can penetrate human skin, releasing a violet-coloured liquid. *Acanthaster planci* of the Red Sea and Indian and Pacific Oceans is up to 60 cm in diameter and possesses venomous spines 6 cm long. The venom causes severe pain, redness, swelling, muscle weakness, hyper/hypoaesthesia, facial oedema, cardiac arrhythmias, vomiting and paralysis. Sea urchins (Echinoidea) (Figure 22.42), especially of the tropical families Diadematidae and Echinothuridae, have brittle, articulated spines (30 cm long in *Diadema*) and grapples (globiferous pedicellariae) (Figure 22.43). Both contain venom which is released when they are embedded in the skin. Severe pain, syncope, numbness, generalized paralysis, aphonia, respiratory distress and even death may result. The fragments of spines embedded in the skin may cause secondary infection, and granuloma formation several months later. Penetration of bones and joints may cause destructive changes.

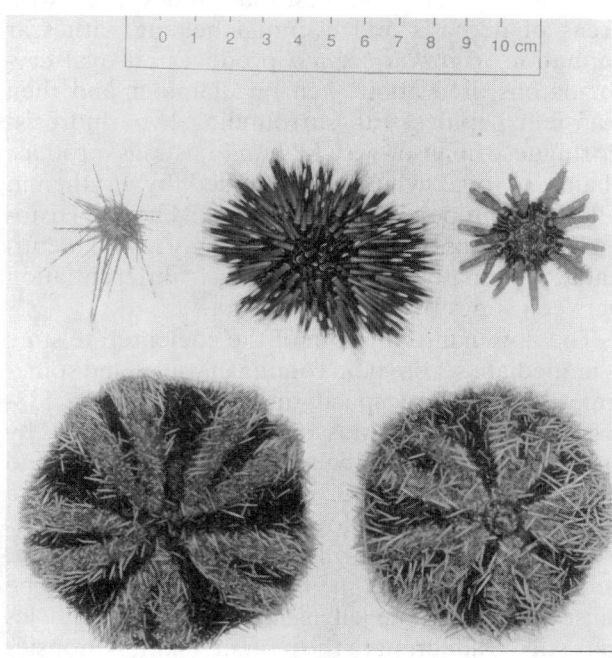

Figure 22.42 Sea urchins (Echinodermata) from Papua New Guinea. Above (left to right): *Diadema setorum*, *Echinometra methiae*, *Prioncidaris verticillata*. Below: *Tripeneuster gradua*, *T. gratilla*. (Copyright D.A. Warrell.)

TREATMENT

Spines and pedicellariae must be removed as soon as possible as they may continue to inject venom and give rise to later complications. The sites of penetration are usually on the soles of the feet. The superficial layer of thickened epidermis should be pared down and 2% salicylic acid ointment applied for 24–48 hours to soften the skin. Most spines can then be extruded, but deeply embedded ones may require surgical removal under local anaesthetic.[71]

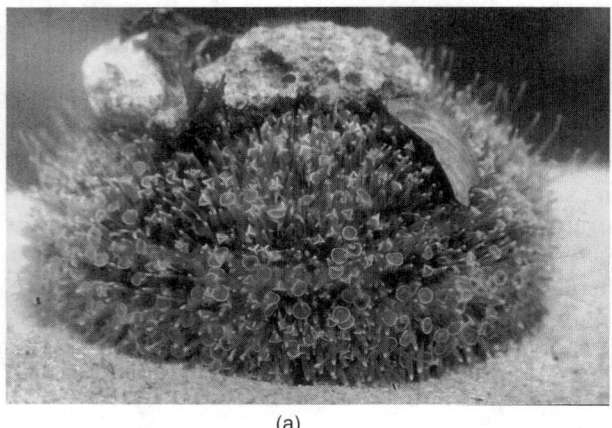

(a)

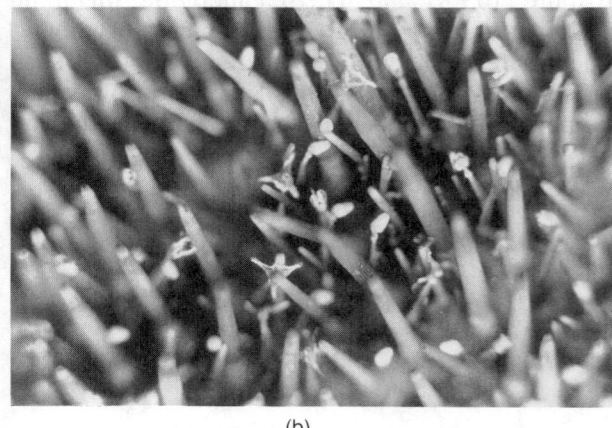

(b)

Figure 22.43 Flower or felt cap sea urchin (*Toxopneustes pileolus*) from Sri Lanka. (a) Whole animal. (b) Venom apparatus—pedecellariae. (Courtesy of Malik Fernando, Colombo, Sri Lanka.)

MOLLUSCS (CONE SHELLS AND OCTOPUSES)[64]

Cone shells (family Conidae) (Figure 22.44), up to 20 cm in length, are found in the Pacific and Indian Oceans. They kill their prey of small fish and other marine animals by harpooning them with a venom-filled radular tooth or dart. In humans, the venom produces local paraesthesiae and numbness and paralysis which progressed to fatal respiratory paralysis in eight out of the 30 reported cases. The venom of *Conus geographus* was found to contain several neurotoxic peptides including one that produced irreversible inhibition of the release of transmitter at neuromuscular junctions by preventing calcium entry.[72] No specific treatment is available. If respiratory paralysis develops, mouth-to-mouth respiration may be needed, followed by prolonged mechanical ventilation. An arterial tourniquet or crepe bandage and splint might delay absorption of the venom until the patient had reached hospital.

Cephalopods (cuttlefish, squids and octopuses) secrete toxic saliva which is inoculated by the sharp and powerful beak. The venom contains tetrodotoxin-like activity (see p. 350), other toxins, vasoactive amines and hyaluronidase. Cephalopod bites are usually painful and produce bleeding, swelling, redness, heat and irritation. Systemic

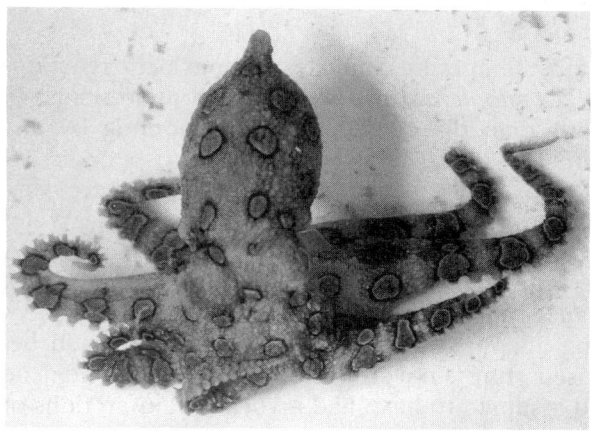

Figure 22.45 Spotted or blue-ringed octopus (*Octopus lunulatus*) from Madang, Papua New Guinea. (Copyright D.A. Warrell.)

symptoms include numbness of the mouth and tongue, blurring of vision, dysphonia, dysphagia and paralysis of the legs and arms. A number of severe cases including two fatalities have been reported from Australia; they were caused by small (20 cm long) octopuses, the common blue-ringed or banded octopus (*Octopus maculosus*, also known as *Hapalochlaena maculosa*) and the blue-ringed or spotted octopus (*O. lunulatus*) (Figure 22.45). *O. maculosus* is abundant around the coast of Australia, especially in the south and frequents shallow water and rock pools. The two patients who died had handled octopuses while they were out of the water. They vomited soon after the bite, then developed respiratory paralysis and died 90 and 120 minutes later.

There is no specific treatment for octopus bites; the effects resemble rapidly developing tetrodotoxin poisoning. Mouth-to-mouth respiration combined with external cardiac massage (if the patient is pulseless) may be life-saving. An arterial tourniquet or crepe bandage and splint should be applied to delay absorption of the venom until the patient has reached hospital. Mechanical ventilation and other intensive care may be needed. It would be worth testing the response to anticholinesterase (see Tensilon test, p. 333) and treating bradycardia with atropine.

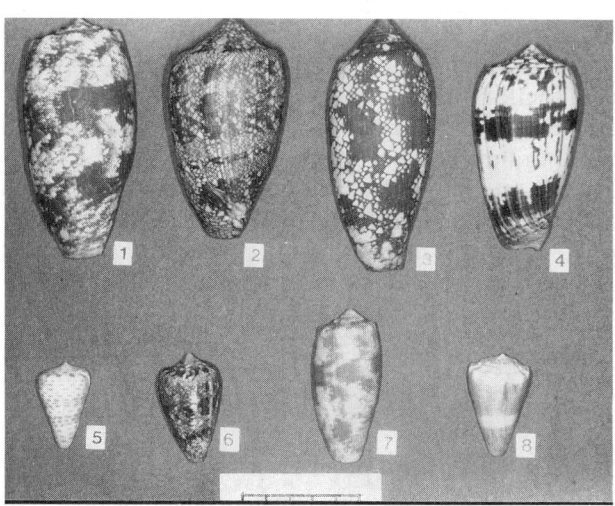

Figure 22.44 Venomous cone shells, family Conidae, from Sri Lanka. 1, *Conus geographus*; 2, *C. textile*; 3, *C. aulicus*; 4, *C. striatus*; 5, *C. tessulatus*; 6, *C. abbas*; 7, *C. tulipa*; 8, *C. lividus*. (Scale in centimetres.) (Copyright D.A. Warrell.)

INSECT STINGS
HYMENOPTERA STINGS (BEES, WASPS, YELLOW JACKETS, HORNETS, FIRE ANTS)

In most temperate countries, anaphylactic reactions to *Hymenoptera* stings are a more common cause of death than direct effects of envenoming by any animal.[73]

For example, between 1959 and 1972 there were 61 deaths from insect stings in England and Wales but only one death from adder bite. In the USA there are between 40 and 50 deaths a year from *Hymenoptera* stings. Deaths from *Hymenoptera* sting anaphylaxis are probably underreported because a sting is not suspected in patients found dead and assumed to have had myocardial infarctions or cerebrovascular accidents. *Hymenoptera* venoms also have direct toxic effects but these are not seen in man unless there have been many, usually hundreds of, stings, as in the case of mass attacks by Africanized honey-bees (*Apis mellifera scutellata*) in Middle and South America. Since the accidental release of swarms of these aggressive bees in Brazil, in 1957, they have spread throughout Latin America and have reached the USA. An average of 30 deaths have been reported each year from mass attacks by these insects.[74]

In other countries, *Hymenoptera* stings are usually caused by members of the Apidae (e.g. *Apis mellifera*, the honey-bee) and Vespidae (e.g. wasps such as *Paravespula vulgaris*), American yellow jackets, genus *Dolichovespula*, and hornets, genus *Vespa*, including the enormous East Asian *V. mandarinia* which can reach a length of almost 4 cm and a weight of 3 g. In North America millions of stings each year are caused by imported fire ants (*Solenopsis*), hypersensitivity is common and there have been cases of fatal anaphylaxis.

VENOM APPARATUS AND COMPOSITION[75,76]

Venoms are injected through a barbed sting. Bees inject approximately $50\,\mu g$ of venom, the total capacity of the venom sac, and leave the stings embedded in the skin, but wasps and hornets can sting repeatedly. The venoms contain biogenic amines (histamine, 5-hydroxytryptamine and acetylcholine), enzymes such as phospholipase A and hyaluronidase and toxic peptides; kinins in the case of Vespidae; apamin, melittin and anti-inflammatory compounds such as mast cell degranulating peptide in Apidae.

CLINICAL FEATURES

Direct toxic effects in non-allergic subjects

In people who are not allergic to the venom, single stings usually produce only local effects attributable to the injected biogenic amines, particularly 5-hydroxytryptamine. Pain, and an area of heat, redness, swelling and wealing develop rapidly but rarely exceed 2–3 cm in diameter or last more than a few hours. Local effects are dangerous only if the airway is obstructed, for example following stings on the tongue.

In non-allergic subjects, fatal systemic toxicity can result from as few as 30 stings in children, while adults have survived more than 2000 stings by *Apis mellifera*. In some patients the clinical effects of massive envenoming resemble histamine overdose: vasodilatation, hypotension, vomiting, diarrhoea, throbbing headache and coma.[77] However, mass attacks by Africanized bees in Latin America can cause intravascular haemolysis, generalized rhabdomyolysis (causing grossly elevated serum creatine phosphokinase, aminopeptidases and myoglobin), hypercatecholinaemia (hypertension, pulmonary oedema, myocardial damage), bleeding, hepatic dysfunction and acute renal failure (Figure 22.46). Rhabdomyolysis followed by myoglobinuria and renal failure can occur after multiple hornet stings (*Vespa affinis*). Intravascular haemolysis with haemoglobinuria (*Vespa orientalis*), thrombocytopenic purpura, myasthenia gravis (*Polistes* species) and various renal lesions, including nephrotic syndrome, have also been described.

Allergic effects

Three to 4% of the population may be hypersensitive to *Hymenoptera* venoms. Clinical suspicion of venom hypersensitivity arises when reactions to successive stings are increasingly severe, or when systemic symptoms follow a sting. In England, sensitization to bee venom appears to require more stings (average 81 on 23 occasions) than sensitization to wasp venom (average four stings).[78] Most patients allergic to bee venom are bee-keepers or their relatives. Systemic symptoms include tingling scalp, flushing, dizziness, visual disturbances, syncope, wheezing, abdominal colic, diarrhoea and tachycardia developing within a few minutes of the sting.

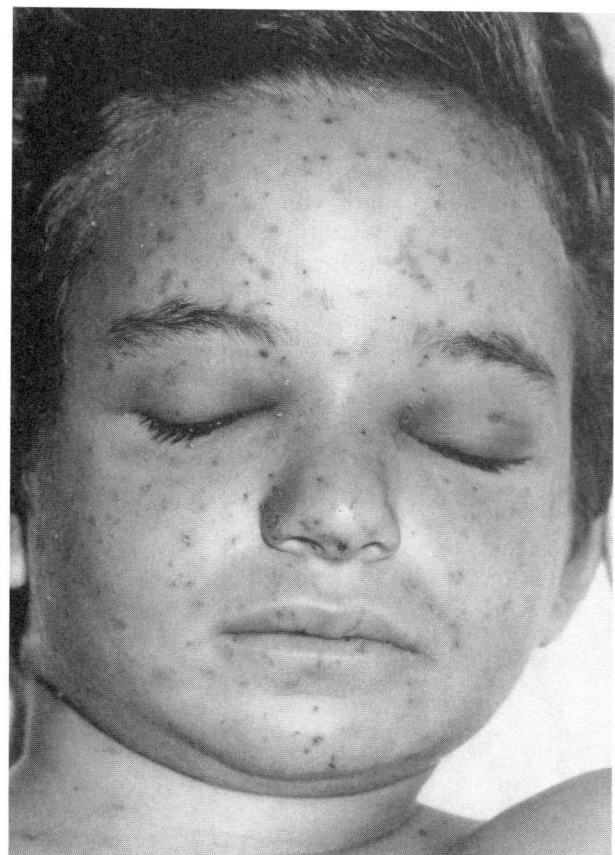

Figure 22.46 Multiple bee stings by Africanized honey-bees (*Apis mellifera scutellata*) causing severe envenoming in a 14-year-old Brazilian boy. (Copyright D.A. Warrell.)

Over the next 15–20 minutes urticaria, angio-oedema, oedema of the glottis, profound hypotension and coma may develop. Patients may die within minutes of the sting. In a few cases, serum sickness develops a week or more after the sting. Atopy does not predispose to sting allergy but asthmatics who are allergic to venom are likely to suffer severe reactions. Reactions are enhanced by beta blockers and non-steroidal anti-inflammatory agents. The diagnosis of venom hypersensitivity can be confirmed by intradermal skin testing with dialysed specific venoms in concentrations of $0.01–1\,\mu g/ml$, or by detecting specific IgE antibodies in serum by the radioallergosorbent test (RAST). Whole body extracts of bees and wasps, traditionally used for skin testing, do not discriminate between hypersensitive patients and controls. A postmortem diagnosis of insect sting anaphylaxis can be supported by detecting specific IgE in the victim's serum. Pathological findings in cases of fatal systemic anaphylaxis include acute pulmonary hyperinflation, laryngeal oedema, pulmonary oedema and intra-alveolar haemorrhage.

TREATMENT

The embedded bee sting should be removed as quickly as possible, without squeezing, which will inject more venom. It can be scraped out with a blade or fingernail. Domestic meat tenderizer (papain), diluted roughly 1 in 5 with tap water, is said to produce immediate relief of pain. Aspirin is an effective analgesic favoured from long experience by bee-keepers. Local antiseptics are acceptable but topical antihistamines should not be used as they promote sensitization.

TOXIC EFFECTS

In cases of severe systemic envenoming, large doses of parenteral antihistamines and corticosteroids should be given and, if needed, bronchodilators and adrenaline. No specific antivenoms are available. As in crush syndrome, renal damage by myoglobinuria or haemoglobinuria may be prevented by correcting hypovolaemia and giving mannitol and bicarbonate. Acute tubular necrosis will require treatment with haemofiltration or renal dialysis.

ALLERGIC EFFECTS

The most effective treatment for sting anaphylaxis is 0.1% adrenaline in an adult dose of 0.5–1 ml, children 0.01 ml/kg, given by subcutaneous or intramuscular injection. Patients known to be hypersensitive should wear an identifying tag (such as provided by Medic-Alert in Britain) as they may be discovered unconscious after a sting. They should be trained to give themselves adrenaline subcutaneously and should always carry a pre-loaded syringe of adrenaline for this purpose. Adrenaline delivered by a pressurized inhaler (Medihaler-epi delivering $200\,\mu g$ of adrenaline acid tartrate per puff) will relieve bronchospasm, but insufficient is absorbed to combat other effects of anaphylaxis. Injection of an antihistamine (e.g. chlorpheniramine maleate, 10 mg intravenously or intramuscularly) will alleviate the mild urticarial symptoms, and antihistamine should be given for the next 24–48 hours to combat the effects of histamine released during the reaction. Severe reactions may require cardiorespiratory resuscitation. Salbutamol is an effective bronchodilator and large doses of hydrocortisone may help the resolution of massive oedema. Respiratory tract obstruction is the main cause of death. Stings in the mouth may cause serious airway obstruction even in people who are not hypersensitive to venom.

PREVENTION OF *HYMENOPTERA* STING ANAPHYLAXIS

In 1978, a controlled trial proved that hyposensitization using pure venom was effective in protecting allergic patients against anaphylactic reactions to sting challenge.[79] However, immunotherapy is probably only necessary in adult patients with histories of severe reactions and demonstrable venom-specific IgE. Most people are stung when they inadvertently crush the bee or wasp or interfere with their nests (i.e. bee-keepers). Wasps congregate where sweet things are manufactured or consumed and in orchards and vineyards. Vespidae are attracted by brightly-coloured floral patterns and perfumes. Some of the largest hornets (*V. veluntina* and *V. mandarinia*) are so aggressive that their territory cannot be cultivated until the nests have been destroyed.

SCORPION STINGS

Scorpions (order Scorpionida) capable of inflicting fatal stings in humans are all members of the families Buthidae and Scorpionidae.[75] Examples of the most deadly species are: *Androctonus australis* (North Africa and Middle East), *A. crassicauda* (Turkey, Middle East and North Africa), *Buthus occitanus* (countries bordering the Mediterranean and Middle East), *Leiurus quinquestriatus* (North Africa and Middle East), *Parabuthus* (South Africa), *Tityus trinitatis* (Trinidad and Venezuela), *T. serrulatus* (Figure 22.47) and *T. bahiensis* (Brazil, Argentina), *Centruroides sculpturatus* (California, New Mexico, Arizona and Baha California), *C. limpidus* and *C. suffusus* (Mexico) and *Mesobuthus tamulus* (India).

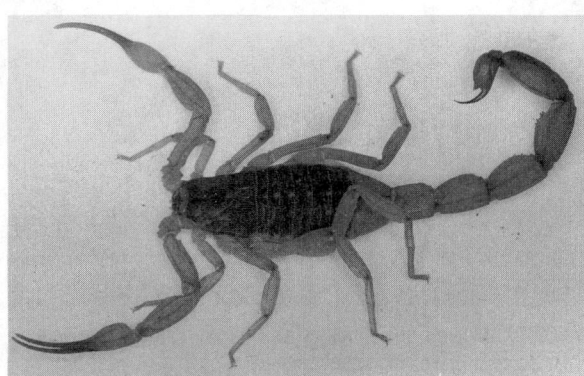

Figure 22.47 Brazilian scorpion (*Tityus serrulatus*; family Buthidae). (Scale in centimetres.) (Copyright D.A. Warrell.)

EPIDEMIOLOGY

Painful scorpion stings are a common event throughout the tropics; however, fatal envenoming is frequent only in parts of Latin America, North Africa, the Middle East and India. In southern Libya there were 900 stings with seven deaths per 100 000 population in 1979.[51] There has been no death from scorpion sting in the USA since 1968, but in Mexico there are between one and two thousand deaths each year, with an incidence of 84 deaths per 100 000 per year in Colima state and a mere three deaths per 100 000 per year in the infamous Durango state. Case mortality is about 50% in children up to 4 years old.[80] In Brazil, mortality increases from around 1% in adults to 15–25% in children less than 6 years old. In Algeria there was an average of 1260 stings and 24 deaths per year. In India there are many cases of stings by the red scorpion (*Mesobuthus tamulus*), with fatalities in adults and children.

CLINICAL FEATURES

Rapidly developing, very intense local pain is the most common symptom. Local signs such as swelling, redness, heat and regional lymph node involvement are never extensive. Local necrosis is most unusual except following stings by *Hemiscorpius lepturus* in Iraq and Iran. Systemic symptoms may develop within minutes, but may be delayed for as much as 24 hours. Features of autonomic nervous system excitation are initially cholinergic and later adrenergic. There is hypersalivation, profuse sweating, hyperthermia, vomiting, diarrhoea, abdominal distension, loss of sphincter control, and priapism. Release of catecholamines, as in phaeochromocytoma, produces hypertension and toxic myocarditis with arrhythmias (most commonly sinus bradycardia), cardiac failure and pulmonary oedema.[81] These cardiovascular effects are particularly prominent following stings by *Leiurus quinquestriatus* and *Mesobuthus tamulus*. Neurotoxic effects such as fasciculation, spasms and respiratory paralysis are a particular feature of stings by *Centruroides sculpturatus*.

Hemiplegia and other neurological lesions have been attributed to fibrin deposition resulting from disseminated intravascular coagulation. Hypercatecholaminaemia could explain hyperglycaemia and glycosuria in patients stung by scorpions, but in the case of stings by the black scorpion on Trinidad (*Tityus trinitatis*), acute pancreatitis may be the mechanism. Fifteen to 120 minutes after the initial searing pain of the sting, patients stung by this scorpion begin to salivate, feel nauseated and vomit persistently, producing coffee-grounds or frank haematemesis. Hyperglycaemia, glycosuria and sometimes albuminuria can be detected a few hours after the sting. There is abdominal pain with distension and rigidity. Electrocardiographic abnormalities (T wave inversion, QRS segment abnormalities and QTC prolongation) are common and may last for 3–6 days. Other features include pyrexia, sweating, bradycardia, cardiac arrhythmias, hypotension and neuromuscular irritability. Acute oedematous or haemorrhagic pancreatitis with development of pancreatic pseudocysts has been demonstrated at autopsy or laparotomy.

TREATMENT

Pain may respond to local infiltration or ring block with local anaesthetic. Local injection of emetine is said to relieve the pain but may cause necrosis. Parenteral opiate analgesics such as pethidine and morphine may be required but are said to be dangerous in victims of *Centruroides sculpturatus*.

The use of antivenom is controversial, but is advocated by doctors in Middle and South America, North Africa and parts of the Middle East. Antivenoms are manufactured in many countries.[50]

Many accessory treatments have been suggested. There is some clinical evidence to support the use of the following treatments:

1. For patients with cardiovascular symptoms (hypertension, bradycardia and early pulmonary oedema) vasodilators are recommended.[82] The use of atropine (except in cases of life-threatening sinus bradycardia), cardiac glycosides and beta blockers is controversial.
2. Anticonvulsants such as phenobarbitone for neurotoxic symptoms (*Centruroides sculputratus*).

No antivenom is commercially available for the treatment of *Mesobuthus tamulus* stings in India. In this case, patients who develop priapism, dilated pupils, sweating and bradycardia are at high risk of progressing to pulmonary oedema. Early energetic treatment with vasodilators may prevent this.

Prophylactic immunization with scorpion venom toxoid has been considered in Mexico.

SPIDER BITES[83]

The spiders (Araneae) are an enormous group containing more than 30 000 known species. A single family, containing less than 1% of these species, is non-venomous. Only 12 species of spider are known to cause dangerous envenoming in humans, while another 24 are suspected of doing so. Spiders bite with a pair of fangs, the chelicerae (Figure 22.48), to which the venom glands are connected.[75] A central venom duct opens near the tip of the fang.

CLINICAL FEATURES

Two main clinical syndromes, 'necrotic' and 'neurotoxic', are caused by spider bite.

NECROTIC ARANEISM

Skin lesions, varying in severity from mild localized erythema and blistering to quite extensive tissue necrosis, have been attributed to a variety of species of spiders. The members of the genus *Loxosceles* are the most important causes of the syndrome. Many of these spiders are extending their geographical ranges. *L. laeta* is widely distributed in Central and South America, especially in Chile. *L. reclusa*, the brown recluse spider, has caused at least 200 bites with six deaths in the USA this century. More than 60 cases were reported in Texas between 1959 and 1962. *L. rufescens* occurs in the Mediterranean region, North Africa, Israel and elswhere.

Eighty per cent of patients are bitten indoors, usually in their bedrooms while asleep or dressing,

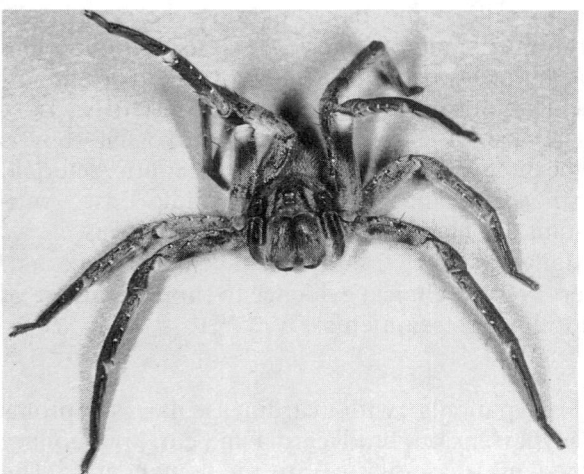

Figure 22.48   Threatening posture of a female Brazilian 'banana spider' (*Phoneutria keiserlingi*). Note venom jaws. (Copyright D.A. Warrell.)

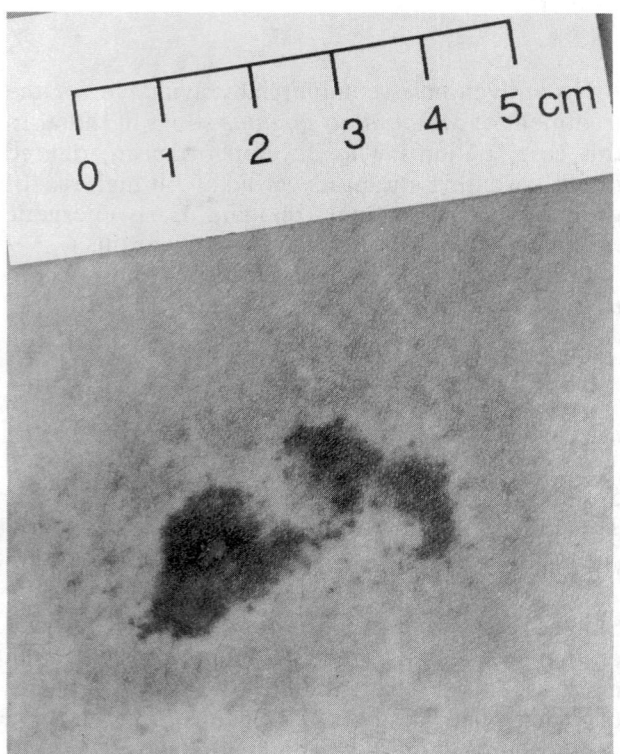

Figure 22.49   Early ischaemic lesion at the site of the bite of a Brazilian spider (*Loxosceles gaucho*). (Copyright D.A. Warrell.)

and in the USA a number of men were bitten on their genitals while they sat on outdoor lavatories in which the spiders had spun their webs. There is burning pain at the site of the bite, oedema and development of a violaceous plaque (Figure 22.49) which, over the course of a few days, becomes a black eschar (Figure 22.50) which sloughs in a few

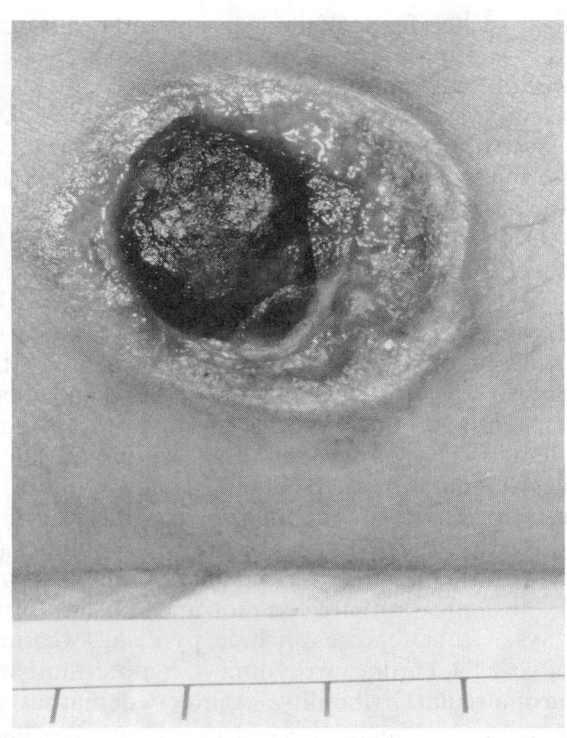

Figure 22.50   Necrotic eschar or slough at the site of a bite by a Brazilian spider (*Loxosceles gaucho*). (Scale in centimetres.) (Copyright D.A. Warrell.

weeks, sometimes leaving a necrotic ulcer. Rarely, the necrotic area may cover an entire limb. In 12% of cases there are systemic effects including haemo-globinuria and jaundice resulting from haemolytic anaemia, fever, scarlatiniform rash (Figure 22.51), respiratory distress and collapse. The average mortality among all reported cases is 6% and about 30% in those with systemic envenoming.

NEUROTOXIC ARANEISM

Members of the genus *Latrodectus* (widow, hour-glass, button or red-back spiders) are the most widespread and numerous of all venomous animals dangerous to man. *L. mactans* (black widow spider) (Figure 22.52) occurs in the Americas. Sixty-three deaths were attributed to this species in the USA from 1950 to 1959. *L. tredecimguttatus*, widely but incorrectly known as 'tarantula', lives in fields in the Mediterranean countries where it has been responsible for epidemics of bites. Nine hundred and forty-six cases were reported in Italy between 1946 and 1951. *L. hasselti*, the Australian and New Zealand 'red-back spider' or 'katipo' causes up to 340 reported bites each year in Australia.[1] Twenty deaths are known to have occurred. *L. mactans* and a related species *L. geometricus* also cause some

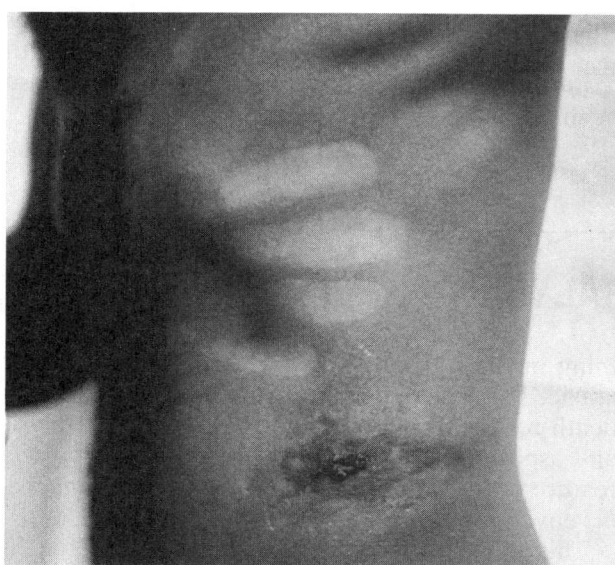

Figure 22.51 Scarlatiniform rash, blanching on pressure, associated with fever in a Brazilian patient bitten above the iliac crest 18 hours previously. (Courtesy of João Luiz Costa Cardoso, São Paulo.)

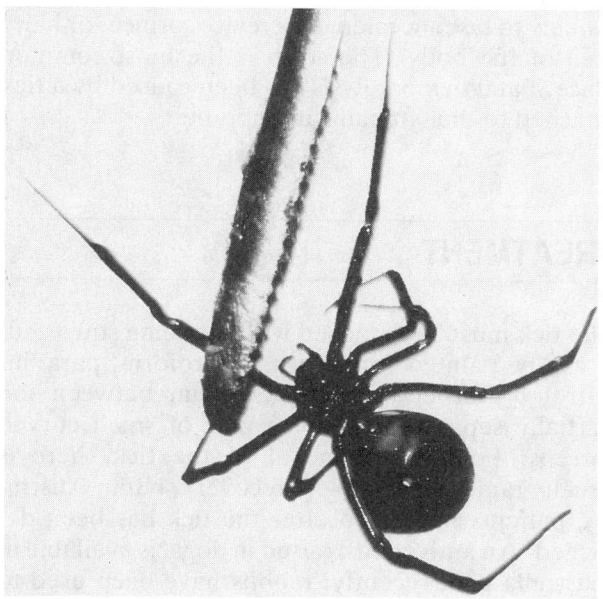

Figure 22.52 'Black widow' spider (*Latrodectus mactans*). Note 'hourglass' pattern on ventral surface of abdomen. (Copyright D.A. Warrell.)

muscle tremors and spasms which may be severe enough to demand artificial ventilation.

L. mactans bites produce minimal local changes. Local dull aching or numbness may develop after 30–40 minutes. Painful muscle spasms and lymphadenopathy spread and increase in intensity during the next few hours until the trunk, abdomen and limbs are involved and respiration may be embarrassed. Other features include tachycardia, hypertension, irritability, psychosis, vomiting and priapism. Similar effects are produced by the Brazilian 'banana spider', *Phoneutria nigriventer* (see Figure 22.48), which causes bites and deaths in South American countries. These spiders may be exported in bunches of bananas to temperate countries where they have been responsible for a few bites and deaths.

Funnel web spiders, genus *Atrax*, are confined to south-eastern Australia and eastern Tasmania.[1] *A. robustus*, the famous Sydney funnel-web spider, occurs within a 160 mile radius of Sydney. Unusually amongst spiders, the aggressive male is more dangerous to man than the larger female. The powerful chelicerae of this large spider produce a painful bite but with minimal local changes. Numbness around the mouth and spasm of the tongue may develop within 10 minutes, followed by nausea and vomiting, abdominal colic, profuse sweating, salivation and lacrimation, dyspnoea and coma. There are local or generalized muscle fasciculations and spasms, hypertension and in some of the fatal cases, pulmonary oedema, thought to be neurogenic in origin. Thirteen deaths, occurring between 15 minutes and 6 days after the bite, were reported between 1927 and 1980.

TREATMENT

FIRST AID TREATMENT

In the case of bites by spiders with rapidly active potent venom such as *A. robustus*, firm crepe bandaging and splinting of the bitten limb or a tight tourniquet may delay venom spread until the patient reaches hospital.

SPECIFIC TREATMENT

Antivenoms are manufactured in several countries.[50] Neurotoxic araneism seems more responsive to antivenom than does the necrotic type. Oral dapsone (100 mg twice a day) is said to reduce the extent of necrotic lesions.

bites in South and eastern Africa. *L. hasselti* bites produce local heat, swelling and redness, which is rarely extensive. Intense local pain develops in about 5 minutes; after 30 minutes there is pain in local lymph nodes and after about an hour headache, nausea, vomiting and sweating occur. Tachycardia and hypertension may follow and there are

SUPPORTIVE TREATMENT

Calcium gluconate (10 ml of a 10% solution given by slow intravenous injection) relieves the pain of muscle spasms caused by *Latrodectus* venom rapidly and more effectively than muscle relaxants such as diazepam or methocarbamol. Antihistamines, corticosteroids, beta blockers and atropine have also been advocated.

TICK BITE PARALYSIS[84,85]

TAXONOMY AND EPIDEMIOLOGY

Ticks, with mites, form the order of Acari of the class Arachnida. Adult females of about 30 species of hard tick (family Ixodidae) and immature specimens of six species of soft tick (family Argasidae) have been implicated in human tick paralysis.[86] The tick's saliva contains a neurotoxin which causes presynaptic neuromuscular block and decreased nerve conduction velocity. The tick embeds itself in the skin with its barbed hypostome introducing the salivary toxin while it engorges with blood.

Although tick paralysis has been reported from all continents, most cases occur in western North America (*Dermacentor andersoni*), eastern USA (*D. variabilis*) and eastern Australia from north Queensland to Victoria (*Ixodes holocyclus*, known as the bush, scrub, paralysis or dog tick). In British Columbia there were 305 cases with 10% mortality between 1900 and 1968. About 120 cases have been reported in the USA, and in New South Wales there were at least 20 deaths between 1900 and 1945.

CLINICAL FEATURES

Ticks are picked up in the countryside or from domestic animals, particularly dogs, in the home. A majority of patients and almost all fatal cases are children. After the tick has been attached for about 5 or 6 days a progressive ascending, lower motor neurone paralysis develops with paraesthesiae. Often a child, who may have been irritable for the previous 24 hours, falls on getting out of bed first thing in the morning, and is found to be weak or ataxic. Paralysis increases over the next few days: death results from bulbar and respiratory paralysis and aspiration of stomach contents. Vomiting is a feature of the more acute course of *Ixodes holocyclus* envenoming.

This clinical picture is often misinterpreted as poliomyelitis, although in North America the peak incidence of tick paralysis is earlier in the year than the epidemic season for poliomyelitis. Other neurological conditions, including Guillain–Barré syndrome, paralytic rabies, Eaton–Lambert syndrome, myasthenia gravis or botulism, may also be suspected. Diagnosis depends on finding the tick, which is likely to be concealed in a crevice, orifice, or hairy area of the body. The scalp is the most common place. Fatal tick paralysis has been caused by a tick attached to the tympanic membrane.

TREATMENT

The tick must be detached without being squeezed. It can be painted with ether, chloroform, paraffin, petrol or turpentine, or prised out between the partially separated tips of a pair of small curved forceps. Following removal of the tick there is usually rapid and complete recovery, but in Australia, patients have died after the tick has been detached. An antivenom, raised in dogs, is available in Australia and, recently, rabbits have been used to produce an antitoxin against *I. holocyclus* saliva.[50] This is recommended for severely affected or very young patients; 20–30 ml are given intravenously.

CENTIPEDE AND MILLIPEDE BITES[75]

CENTIPEDES

Many species of centipede (Chilopoda) can inflict painful bites, producing local pain, swelling, inflammation and lymphangitis. Systemic effects such as vomiting, headache, cardiac arrhythmias and convulsions are extremely rare and the risk of mortality was probably greatly exaggerated in the older literature. The most important genus is *Scolopendra* which is distributed throughout tropical countries. Local treatment is the same as for scorpion stings. No antivenom is available.

MILLIPEDES (DIPLOPODA)[87]

Most species possess glands in each of their body segments which secrete, and in some cases squirt out, irritant liquids for defensive purposes. These contain hydrogen cyanide and a variety of aldehydes, esters, phenols and quinonoids. Members of at least eight genera of millipedes have proved injurious to man. Important genera are *Rhinocricus* (Caribbean), *Spirobolus* (Tanzania), *Spirostreptus* and *Iulus* (Indonesia), and *Polyceroconas* (Papua New Guinea). Children are particularly at risk when they handle or try to eat these large arthropods. When venom is squirted into the eye, intense conjunctivitis results and there may be corneal ulceration and even blindness. Skin lesions are initially stained brown or purple, blister after a few days, and then peel. First aid is generous irrigation with water. Eye injuries should be treated as for snake venom ophthalmia (see p. 494).

POISONING BY INGESTION OF MARINE ANIMALS[64]

A variety of illnesses, usually categorized as 'food poisoning', are caused by eating seafood. The most common are attributable to bacterial or viral infections. These include *Vibrio parahaemolyticus* (after eating crustaceans, especially shrimps), *V. cholerae* (crabs and molluscs), non-O1 *V. cholerae* (oysters), *V. vulnificus* (oysters), *Aeromonas hydrophila* (frozen oysters), *Plesiomonas shigelloides* (oysters, mussels, mackerel, cuttlefish), *Salmonella typhi* (molluscs), *Campylobacter jejuni* (clams), *Shigella* species (molluscs), hepatitis A virus (molluscs, especially clams and oysters), Norwalk agent (oysters and other molluscs) and 'small round viruses' (cockles and other molluscs). Botulism has been reported in people eating smoked fish and canned salmon. Since 1953, approximately 100 000 Japanese are thought to have been affected by methyl mercury poisoning (Minamata disease) after eating fish and molluscs contaminated with methyl mercury derived from industrial waste dumped in Minamata Bay and at the mouth of the Agano River in Japan. The victims developed severe central nervous system damage, with a mortality of 33% in the initial outbreak. Pregnant women exposed to methyl mercury gave birth to infants who were mentally retarded and had cerebral palsy and convulsions.

A number of clinical syndromes have been recognized which are related to the presence in the ingested flesh or viscera of marine animals of toxins either derived ultimately from dinoflagellates (e.g. ciguatera, tetrodotoxic or paralytic shellfish poisoning) or resulting from the decomposition of fish during storage (scombrotoxic fish poisoning).[88,89]

GASTROINTESTINAL AND NEUROTOXIC SYNDROMES

Nausea, vomiting, abdominal colic, tenesmus and watery diarrhoea may precede the development of neurotoxic symptoms. Paraesthesiae of the lips, buccal cavity and extremities are early symptoms. Other neurotoxic manifestations include a peculiar distortion of temperature perception so that cold objects feel hot (like dry ice) and vice versa, dizziness, myalgia, weakness starting with muscles of phonation and deglutition and progressing to respiratory paralysis and flaccid quadriplegia in some cases, ataxia, involuntary movements, convulsions, visual disturbances, hallucinations and psychoses, cranial nerve lesions and pupillary abnormalities.

Cardiovascular abnormalities include hypotension and bradycardia and some patients develop florid cutaneous lesions.

Distinguishable within this general pattern of symptoms are a number of conditions related to the ingestion of a particular taxonomic group of animals. Some of the more important syndromes are described below.

CIGUATERA FISH POISONING

The word ciguatera seems to derive from the Cuban word 'cigua' for a poisonous marine snail (*Livona pica*, the west Indian top shell) which was coined by early Spanish settlers.[64] Ciguatera is now applied to an illness resulting from the ingestion of more than 400 species of warm-water, shore or reef fish. The highest incidence of ciguatera seems to be in the Pacific region. Three thousand and nine cases with 0.1% mortality were reported during a 14-year period from New Caledonia, where it is known as 'la gratte' ('the itch'),[90] and more than 400 cases a year occur in Vanuatu. In Guadeloupe (Antilles) there were an average of 30 cases of ciguatera poisoning per 10 000 inhabitants each year. The fish most often associated with ciguatera are from the families Serranidae (groupers), Lutjanidae (snappers), Scaridae (parrot fish) and Scombridae (mackerel). Other important groups are moray eels (Muraenidae), barracudas (Sphyraenidae) and jacks (Carangidae).

It is now known that the toxins responsible for ciguatera fish poisoning originate from benthic dinoflagellates. *Gambierdiscus toxicus* has been implicated. It settles on algae such as *Spysidia filamentosa* in the neighbourhood of tropical reefs and is ingested by herbivorous fish. These in turn are the prey of the carnivorous fish which, when eaten by humans, may give rise to severe gastrointestinal, neurotoxic and cardiovascular symptoms. Ciguatoxins are concentrated in the intestine, gonads and viscera. The acquisition of toxin by fish cannot be predicted; there is no seasonal variation in its prevalence but the risk of poisoning is greater with some species, e.g. Moray eels, and definitely increases as the fish gets larger.

Three toxins, ciguatoxin, maitotoxin and scaritoxin (from the parrot fish *Scarus sordidus*) have been identified but their molecular structures are not yet known. Until recently there was no better method of deciding whether a fish contained toxin than by feeding part of it to an animal and waiting for clinical symptoms to develop. One recent method is to measure the LD_{50} of fish extract injected intrathoracically in *Aedes aegypti* mosquitoes, but an even more promising method consists of piercing the suspect fish with a bamboo stick and detecting ciguatoxin using a monoclonal antibody EIA method.

The effect of ciguatoxin was thought to resemble anticholinesterase, but more recent work suggests a direct effect on excitable membranes by competing with calcium ions. In animals the venom produces respiratory failure followed by hypotension, bradycardia and cardiac arrhythmias.

Clinical features

Exceptionally, symptoms first appear as early as minutes or as long as 30 hours after eating the poisoned fish; however, the usual interval is 1–6 hours. The earliest symptom is numbness or tingling of the lips, tongue, throat and extremities, a metallic taste and a dry mouth or hypersalivation. Reversed perception of heat and cold is a distinctive symptom. In many cases, especially with milder poisoning, the earliest symptoms are gastrointestinal: sudden abdominal colic, nausea, vomiting and watery diarrhoea. Myalgia, ataxia, vertigo, visual disturbances and pruritic skin eruptions develop later. In severely neurotoxic cases flaccid paralysis and respiratory arrest may develop. Gastrointestinal symptoms resolve within a few hours but paraesthesiae may persist for a week or longer.

Ciguatera poisoning from eating moray eels (*Gymnothorax* species) is particularly rapid and severe because of the high concentration of toxin in these animals.

Chelonitoxication results from the ingestion of marine turtles (Chelonia). Its clinical features resemble ciguatera poisoning. Most outbreaks have been in the Indo-Pacific area. The species usually implicated are green hawksbill and leathery turtles. The mortality rate among reported cases is 28%.

TETRODOTOXIC (PUFFER FISH) POISONING

More than 50 species of tropical scaleless fish of the order Tetraodonitiformes have proved poisonous. They include porcupine fish (*Chilomycterus*), molas or sunfish (*Mola*) and puffer fish or toadfish (Tetraodontidae—genera *Arothron*, *Fugu*, *Lagocephalus*, etc). The flesh of the puffer fish (Japanese fugu) is particularly relished in Japan where, despite the stringent regulations and skilful fugu cooks, there are 250 cases of tetrodotoxin poisoning reported each year with a 60% mortality. The peak mortality was probably 470 in 1947. Cases have been reported in Thailand and many other Indo-Pacific countries. Tetrodotoxin is an aminoperhydroquinazoline which has been synthesized. It is one of the most potent non-protein toxins known. It is found mainly in the ovaries, viscera and skin. There is a definite seasonal variation in the toxin concentration which reaches a peak during the spawning season (May to June in Japan). Tetrodotoxin impairs nervous conduction by blocking the sodium ion flux without affecting potassium, producing neurotoxic and cardiotoxic effects. The origin of this toxin is unknown. It may, like ciguatoxin, be acquired through the food chain. An identical toxin has been found in the skin of newts (genus *Taricha*), frogs (genus *Atelopus*) and salamanders and the saliva of octopuses (genus *Octopus*) (see p. 341), in the digestive glands of several species of gastropod mollusc, a star fish, flat worm (*Planorbis*) and nemertine worms in Japan, and is produced by some bacteria.

Clinical features

Paraesthesia, dizziness and ataxia become noticeable within 10–45 minutes of eating the fish. Generalized numbness, hypersalivation, sweating and hypotension may develop. Some patients remain aware of their surroundings despite appearing comatose. Gastrointestinal symptoms may be completely absent. Death from respiratory paralysis usually occurs within the first 6 hours and is unusual more than 2 hours after eating the fish. Erythema, petechiae, blistering and desquamation may appear.

PARLYTIC SHELLFISH AND CRUSTACEAN POISONING

Bivalve molluscs, such as mussels, clams (*Saxidomus*), oysters, cockles and scallops, xanthid crabs, coconut crabs (*Birgus*), and the eggs of horseshoe crabs (*Carcinoscorpius*), may acquire neurotoxins such as saxitoxin from the dinoflagellates *Alexandrie* (formerly *Gonyaulax*) *catenella*, *A. tamarensum* and *A. excavatum* which occur between latitudes 30°N and 30°S. The dinoflagellates may be sufficiently abundant during the warmer months of May to October to produce a 'red tide'. The dangerous season is announced by the discovery of unusual numbers of dead fish and sea birds. Symptoms develop within 30 minutes of ingestion. They include perioral paraesthesia, gastrointestinal symptoms, ataxia, visual disturbances and pareses (progressing to respiratory paralysis within 12 hours) in 8% of cases. Milder gastrointestinal and neurotoxic symptoms without paralysis have been associated with ingestion of molluscs contaminated by neurotoxins from *Gymnodinium breve* (formerly *Ptychodiscus brevis*), which also causes a 'red tide'.

HISTAMINE SYNDROME (SCOMBROTOXIC POISONING)

The red flesh of scombroid fish such as tuna, mackerel, bonito and skipjack, and of canned non-scombroid fish like sardines and pilchards, may be decomposed by the action of bacteria such as *Proteus morgani*, converting muscle histidine into saurine, histamine and unidentified toxins. Toxic fish may produce a tingling or smarting sensation in the mouth when eaten. Between minutes and a few hours after ingestion, flushing, burning, urticaria and pruritus of the skin, headache, abdominal colic, nausea, vomiting, diarrhoea and bronchial asthma may develop. Identical symptoms have been described in Sri Lankan patients who ate a histamine-rich fish, the skipjack, while taking isoniazid, a histamine inhibitor, for tuberculosis.

POISONING BY INGESTION OF CARP'S GALLBLADDER

In parts of the Far East, the raw bile and gallbladder of various species of freshwater carp (e.g. the grass carp *Ctenopharyngodon idellus*; 'plaa yeesok' *Probarbus jullienii*) are believed to have medicinal properties. Patients in China, Taiwan, Hong Kong, Thailand and elsewhere have developed acute abdominal pain, vomiting and watery diarrhoea 2–18 hours after drinking the raw bile or eating the raw gallbladder of these fish. One patient developed flushing and dizziness. Hepatic and renal damage may develop, progressing to oliguric or non-oliguric acute renal failure (acute tubular necrosis). The hepatonephrotoxin has not been identified, but is heat stable and may be derived from the carp's diet.

TREATMENT

The differential diagnosis includes bacterial and viral food poisoning and allergic reactions. No specific treatments or antidotes are available. Gastrointestinal contents should be eliminated by emetics and purges. Activated charcoal absorbs saxitoxin and other shellfish toxins. Atropine is said to improve gastrointestinal symptoms and sinus bradycardia in patients with gastrointestinal and neurotoxic poisoning. Oximes, such as pralidoxime and 2-pyridine aldoxime, have been claimed to benefit the anticholinesterase features of ciguatera poisoning but the evidence is not convincing. Calcium gluconate may relieve mild neuromuscular symptoms. In scombroid poisoning, antihistamines and bronchodilators should be used. In cases of respiratory paralysis, endotracheal intubation and mechanical ventilation have proved life saving. Cardiac resuscitation may also be required. There is some evidence supporting the use of 20% mannitol intravenously in ciguatera poisoning.

PREVENTION

Ciguatera, tetrodotoxin and the other toxins responsible are heat-stable, so cooking does not prevent poisoning. In tropical areas the flesh of fish should be separated, as soon as possible, from the head, skin, intestines, gonads and other viscera which may have high concentrations of toxin. All scaleless fish should be regarded as potentially tetrodotoxic, while very large fish carry an increased risk of being ciguateratoxic. Moray eels should never be eaten. Some toxins are fairly water-soluble and may be leeched out, so water in which fish are cooked should be thrown away. Scombroid poisoning can be prevented by prompt freezing or by eating the fish fresh. Shellfish should not be eaten during the dangerous season and when there are red tides.

REFERENCES

1 Sutherland S K. *Australian Animal Toxins. The Creatures, their Toxins and Care of the Poisoned Patient*. Melbourne: Oxford University Press, 1983: 199.

2 Fenner P J, Williamson J A & Myers D. Platypus envenomation: a painful learning experience. *Med J Aust* 1992; 157:829–832.

3 Dufton M J. Venomous mammals. *Pharmacol Ther* 1992; 53:199–215.

4 Hawkey C M. Salivary antihemostatic factors. In Greenhall A M & Schmidt U (eds) *Natural History of Vampire Bats*. Boca Raton: CRC Press, 1988: 133–141.

5 Minton S A. Venomous bites by non-venomous snakes: an annotated bibliography of colubrid envenomation. *J Wilderness Med* 1990; 1:119–127.

6 Knight A, Densmore L D & Rael E D. Molecular systematics of the Agkistrodon complex. In Campbell J A & Brodie E D (eds) *Biology of the Pit Vipers*. Tyler, TX: Selva, 1992: 49–69.

7 Warrell D A, Looareesuwan S, White N J et al. Severe neurotoxic envenoming by the Malayan krait *Bungarus candidus* (*Linnaeus*): response to antivenom and anticholinesterase. *BMJ* 1983; 286:678–680.

8 Parrish H M. *Poisonous Snakebites in the United States*. New York: Vantage Press, 1980.

9 Pugh R N H, Theakston R D G, Reid H A & Briar I S. Malumfashi endemic diseases research project. XIII. Epidemiology of human encounters with the spitting cobra, *Naja nigricollis*, in the Malumfashi area of northern Nigeria. *Ann Trop Med Parasitol* 1980; 74:523–530.

10 Swaroop S & Grab B. Snakebite mortality in the world. *Bull World Health Organ* 1954; 10:35–76.

11 Myint-Lwin, Warrell D A, Phillips R E, Tin-Nu-Swe, Tun-Pe & Maung-Maung Lay. Bites by Russell's viper (*Vipera russelli siamensis*) in Burma: haemostatic, vascular and renal disturbances and response to treatment. *Lancet* 1985; ii:1259–1264.

12 Sawai Y, Makino M, Kawa-Mura Y et al. Epidemiological study of habu bites on the Amami and Okinawa Islands of Japan. In Ohsaka A, Hayashi K & Sawai Y (eds) *Plant, Animal and Microbial Toxins*, vol. 2. New York: Plenum Press, 1976: 439–450.

13 Warrell D A & Arnett C. The importance of bites by the saw-scaled or carpet viper (*Echis carinatus*). Epidemiological studies in Nigeria and a review of the world literature. *Acta Trop (Basel)* 1976; 33:307–341.

14 Reid H A & Lim K J. Sea-snake bite. A survey of fishing villages in northwest Malaya. *BMJ* 1957; ii:1266–1272.

15 Warrell D A. Sea snake bites in the Asia-Pacific region. In Gopalkrishnakone P (ed.) *Sea Snake Toxinology*. Singapore University Press (in press).

16 Kochva E. Oral glands of the reptilia. In Gans C & Gans K A (eds) *Biology of the Reptilia*. London: Academic Press, 1978: 43–161.

17 Bogert C M. Dentitional phenomena in cobras and other Elapids with notes on adaptive modifications of fangs. *Bull Am Mus Nat Hist* 1943; 81:285–360.

18 Douglas W W. Polypeptides: angiotensin, plasma kinins and others. In Goodman A G, Gilman L S, Rall T W & Murad F (eds) *The Pharmacological Basis of Therapeutics*. New York: Macmillan, 1985: 639–659.

19 Hutton R A & Warrell D A. Action of snake venom components on the haemostatic system. *Blood Rev* 1993; 7:176–189.

20 Budzynski A Z, Pandya B V, Rubin R N, Brizuela B S, Soszka T & Stewart G J. Fibrinogenolytic afibrinogenaemia after envenomation by western diamondback rattlesnake (*Crotalus atrox*). *Blood* 1984; 63:1–14.

21 Kitchens C S & Van Mierop L H S. Mechanism of defibrination in humans after envenomation by the eastern diamondback rattlesnake. *Am J Hematol* 1983; 14:345–353.

22 Hutton R A, Looareesuwan S, Ho M et al. Arboreal pit vipers (genus Trimeresurus) of Southeast Asia: bites by *T. albolabris* and *T. macrops* in Thailand and a review of the literature. *Trans R Soc Trop Med Hyg* 1990; 84:866–874.

23 Vogt W. Snake venom constituents affecting the complement system. In Stocker K F (ed.) *Medical Use of Snake Venom Proteins*. Boca Raton: CRC Press, 1990: 79–96.

24 Warrell D A, Greenwood B M, Davidson N McD, Ormerod L D & Prentice C R M. Necrosis, haemorrhage and complement depletion following bites by the spitting cobra (*Naja nigricollis*). *Q J Med* 1976; 45:1–22.

25 Ratcliffe P J, Pukrittayakamee S, Ledingham J G G & Warrell D A. Direct nephrotoxicity of Russell's viper venom demonstrated in the isolated perfused rat kidney. *Am J Trop Med Hyg* 1989; 40:312–319.

26 Phillips R E, Theakston R D G, Warrell D A et al. Paralysis, rhabdomyolysis and haemolysis caused by bites of Russell's viper (*Vipera russelli pulchella*) in Sri Lanka: failure of Indian (Haffkine) antivenom. *Q J Med* 1988; 68:691–716.

27 Azevedo-Marques M M, Hering S E & Cupo P. Evidence that *Crotalus durissus terrificus* (South American rattlesnake) envenomation in humans causes myolysis rather than hemolysis. *Toxicon* 1987; 25:1163–1168.

28 Bevan P & Hiestand P. β-RTX. A receptor-active protein from Russell's viper (*Vipera russelli russelli*) venom. *J Biol Chem* 1983; 258:5319–5326.

29 Kitchens C S, Hunter S & Van Mierop L H S. Severe myonecrosis in a fatal case of envenomation by the canebrake rattlesnake (*Crotalus horridus atricaudatus*). *Toxicon* 1987; 25:455–458.

30 Warrell D A & Ormerod L D. Snake venom ophthalmia and blindness caused by the spitting cobra (*Naja nigricollis*) in Nigeria. *Am J Trop Med Hyg* 1976; 25:525–529.

31 Warrell D A, Ormerod L D & Davidson N McD. Bites by the night adder (*Causus maculatus*) and burrowing vipers (genus Atractaspis) in Nigeria. *Am J Trop Med Hyg* 1976; 25:517–524.

32 Sokolovsky M. Structure–function relationships of endothelins, sarafotoxins and their receptor subtypes. *J Neurochem* 1992; 59:809–821.

33 Weiser E, Wollberg Z, Kochva E & Lee S Y. Cardiotoxic effects of the venom of the burrowing asp, *Atractaspis engaddensis* (Atractaspididae, Ophidia). *Toxicon* 1984; 22:767–774.

34 Tin-Myint, Rai-Mra, Maung-Chit, Tun-Pe & Warrell D A. Bites by the king cobra (*Ophiophagus hannah*) in Myanmar: successful treatment of severe neurotoxic envenoming. *Q J Med* 1991; 80:751–762.

35 Watt G, Theakston R D G, Hayes C G et al. Positive response to edrophonium in patients with neurotoxic envenoming by cobras (*Naja naja philippinensis*). A placebo-controlled study. *N Engl J Med* 1986; 315:1444–1448.

36 Campbell C H. Symptomatology, pathology and treatment of the bites of elapid snakes. In Lee C Y (ed.) *Snake Venoms. Handbook of Experimental Pharmacology*. Berlin: Springer, 1979: 898–921.

37 Marshall L R & Herrmann R P. Coagulant and anticoagulant actions of Australian snake venoms. *Thromb Haemost* 1983; 50:707–711.

38 Reid H A. Symptomatology, pathology and treatment of the bites of sea snakes. In Lee C Y (ed.) *Snake Venoms. Handbook of Experimental Pharmacology*. Berlin: Springer, 1979: 922–955.

39 Matsen F A. *Compartmental Syndromes*. New York: Grune & Stratton, 1980: 162.

40 Warrell D A, Davidson N McD, Greenwood B M et al. Poisoning by bites of the saw-scaled or carpet viper (*Echis carinatus*) in Nigeria. *Q J Med* 1977; 46:33–62.

41 Ho M, Warrell M J, Warrell D A, Bidwell D & Voller A. A critical reappraisal of the use of enzyme-lined immunosorbent assays in the study of snake bite. *Toxicon* 1986; 24:211–221.

42 Theakston R D G, Lloyd-Jones M J & Reid H A. Micro-ELISA for detecting and assaying snake venom and venom-antibody. *Lancet* 1977; ii:639–641.

43 Hardy D L. A review of first aid measures for pit viper bite in North America with an appraisal of Extractor™ suction and stun gun electroshock. In Campbell J A & Brodie E D (eds) *Biology of the Pit Vipers*. Tyler, TX: Selva, 1992: 405–414.

44 Sutherland S K, Coulter A R & Harris R D. Rationalisation of first-aid measures for elapid snake bite. *Lancet* 1979; i:183–186.

45 Warrell D A. The global problem of snake bite: its prevention and treatment. In Gopalakrishnakone P & Tan C K (eds) *Recent Advances in Toxinology Research*, vol. 1. National University of Singapore, 1992: 121–153.

46 Ho M, Warrell D A, Looareesuwan S et al. Clinical significance of venom antigen levels in patients envenomed by the Malayan pit viper (*Calloselasms rhodostoma*). *Am J Trop Med Hyg* 1986; 35:579–587.

47 Tun-Pe, Tin-Nu-Swe, Myint-Lwin, Warrell D A & Than-Win. The efficacy of tourniquets as a first aid measure for Russell's viper bites in Burma. *Trans R Soc Trop Med Hyg* 1987; 81:403–405.

48 Reid H A. Adder bites in Britain. *BMJ* 1976; ii:153–156.

49 Malasit P, Warrell D A, Chanthavanich P et al. Prediction, prevention and mechanism of early (anaphylactic) antivenom reactions in victims of snake bites. *BMJ* 1986; 292:17–20.

50 Theakston R D G & Warrell D A. Antivenoms: a list of hyperimmune sera currently available for the treatment of envenoming by bites and stings. *Toxicon* 1991; 29:1419–1470.

51 World Health Organization. Progress in the characterization of venoms and standardization of antivenoms. *WHO Offset Publ* 1981; No. 58.

52 Warrell D A, Warrell M J, Edgar W, Prentice C R M, Mathison J H & Mathison J. Comparison of Pasteur and Behringwerke antivenoms in

envenoming by the carpet viper (*Echis carinatus*). *BMJ* 1980; 280:607–609.

53 Thein-Than, Kyi-Thein & Mg-Mg-Thwin. Plasma clearance time of Russell's viper (*Vipera russelli*) antivenom in human snake bite victims. *Trans R Soc Trop Med Hyg* 1985; 79:262–263.

54 Ho M, Silamut K, White N J et al. Pharmacokinetics of three commercial antivenoms in patients envenomed by the Malayan pit viper (*Calloselasma rhodostoma*) in Thailand. *Am J Trop Med Hyg* 1990; 42:260–266.

55 Theakston R D G, Fan H W, Warrell D A, Da Silva W D, Ward S A, Higashi H G & BIASG. Use of enzyme immunoassays to compare the efficacy and assess dosage regimens of three Brazilian *Bothrops* antivenoms. *Am J Trop Med Hyg* 1992; 47:593–604.

56 Sutherland S K. Serum reactions. An analysis of commercial antivenoms and the possible role of anticomplementary activity in de-novo reactions to antivenoms and antitoxins. *Med J Aust* 1977; 1:613–615.

57 Theakston R D G, Phillips R E, Looareesuwan S, Echeverria P, Makin T & Warrell D A. Bacteriological studies of the venom and mouth cavities of wild Malayan pit vipers (*Calloselasma rhodostoma*) in southern Thailand. *Trans R Soc Trop Med Hyg* 1990; 84:875–879.

58 Jorge M T, de Mendonça J S, Ribeiro L A, da Silva M L R, Kusano E J U & Cordeiro C L dos S. Flora bacteriana da vacidade oral, presas e veneno de *Bothrops jararaca*: possível fonte de infecção no local da picada. *Rev Inst Med Trop São Paulo* 1990; 32:6–10.

59 Garfin S R, Castilonia R R, Mubarak S J, Hargens A R, Russell F E & Akeson W H. Rattlesnake bites and surgical decompression: results using a laboratory model. *Toxicon* 1984; 22:177–182.

60 Sawai Y. Vaccination against snake bite poisoning. In Lee C Y (ed.) *Snake Venoms. Handbook of Experimental Pharmacology*. Berlin: Springer, 1979: 881–897.

61 Ménez A. Immunology of snake toxins. In Harvey A L (ed.) *Snake Toxins: International Encyclopedia of Pharmacology and Therapeutics*, sect. 134. New York: Pergamon Press, 1991: 35–90.

62 Russell F E & Bogert C M. Gila monster, venom and bite: a review. *Toxicon* 1981; 19:341–359.

63 Preston C A. Hypotension, myocardial infarction and coagulopathy following Gila monster bite. *J Emerg Med* 1989; 7:37–40.

64 Halstead B W. *Poisonous and Venomous Marine Animals of the World*, 2nd edn. New Jersey: Darwin Press, 1988.

65 Russell F E, Panos T C, Kang L W, Warner A M & Colket T C. Studies on the mechanism of death from stingray venom: a report on two fatal cases. *Am J Med Sci* 1958; 235:566–584.

66 Castex M N. Freshwater venomous rays. In Russell F E & Saunders P R (eds) *Animal Toxins*. Oxford: Pergamon Press, 1967: 167–176.

67 Maretić Z. Some epidemiological, clinical and therapeutic aspects of envenomation by weeverfish sting. In De Vries A & Kochva E (eds) *Toxins of Animals and Plant Origin*, vol. 3. New York: Gordon & Breach, 1973: 1055–1065.

68 Barnes J H. Observations on jellyfish stingings in North Queensland. *Med J Aust* 1960; 2:993–999.

69 Maretić Z, Russell F E & Ladavać J. Epidemic of stings by the jellyfish *Pelagia noctiluca* in the Adriatic. In Eaker D & Wadström T (eds) *Natural Toxins*. Oxford: Pergamon Press, 1980: 77–82.

70 Williamson J & Exton D. *The Marine Stinger Book*. Brisbane: Surf Life Saving Association of Australia, 1985.

71 Alender C B & Russell F E. Pharmacology. In Boolootian R A (ed.) *Physiology of Echinodermata*. New York: Interscience, 1966: 529–543.

72 Olivera B M, Rivier J, Scott J K, Hillyard D R & Cruz L J. Conotoxins. *J Biol Chem* 1991; 266:22067–22070.

73 Mueller U R. *Insect Sting Allergy. Clinical Picture, Diagnosis and Treatment*. Stuttgart: Gustav Fischer, 1990.

74 Winston M L. *Killer Bees. The Africanized Honey Bee in the Americas*. Cambridge, MA: Harvard University Press, 1992.

75 Bettini S. (ed.) *Arthropod Venoms. Handbook of Experimental Pharmacology*, vol. 48. Berlin: Springer, 1978.

76 Piek T. *Venoms of the Hymenoptera. Biochemical, Pharmacological and Behavioural Aspects*. London: Academic Press, 1986.

77 Murray J A. A case of multiple bee stings. *Cent Afr J Med* 1964; 10:249–251.

78 Ewan P W. Allergy to insect stings: a review. *J R Soc Med* 1984; 78:234–239.

79 Hunt K J, Valentine M D, Sobotka A K, Benton A W, Amodio F J & Lichtenstein L M. A controlled trial of immunotherapy in insect hypersensitivity. *N Engl J Med* 1978; 299:157–161.

80 Mazzotti L & Bravo-Becherelle M A. Scorpionism in the Mexican Republic. In Keegan H L & Macfarlane W V (eds) *Venomous and Poisonous Animals and Noxious Plants of the Pacific Region*. Oxford: Pergamon Press, 1963: 111–131.

81 Bawaskar H S. Diagnostic cardiac premonitory signs and symptoms of red scorpion sting. *Lancet* 1982; i:552–554.

82 Gueron M, Ilia R & Sofer S. The cardiovascular system after scorpion envenomation. A review. *Clin Toxicol* 1992; 30:245–248.

83 Maretić Z & Lebez D. *Araneism*. Pula: Novit, 1979.

84 Pearn J. The clinical features of tick bite. *Med J Aust* 1977; 2:313.

85 Murnaghan M F & O'Rourke F J. Tick paralysis. In Bettini S (ed.) *Handbook of Experimental Pharmacology*, vol. 48. Berlin: Springer, 1978: 419–464.

86 Gothe R, Kunze K & Hoogstraal H. The mechanism of pathogenicity in the tick paralyses. *J Med Entomol* 1979; 16:357–369.

87 Radford A J. Millipede burns in man. *Trop Geogr Med* 1975; 27:279–287.

88 Hughes J M, Merson M H & Gangarosa E J. When friends or patients ask about . . . the safety of eating shellfish. *JAMA* 1977; 237:1980–1981.

89 World Health Organization. Aquatic (marine and freshwater) biotoxins. *Environmental Health Criteria* 37. Geneva: WHO, 1984.

90 Bagnis R, Kuberski T & Laugier S. Clinical observations on 3009 cases of ciguatera (fish poisoning) in the South Pacific. *Am J Trop Med Hyg* 1979; 28:1067–1073.

CHAPTER 23

PLANT POISONS

L. G. Goodwin

Most people in tropical countries depend for their food upon small farms and gardens and in times of political unrest, military action or climatic disaster their livelihood may be threatened or destroyed. Drought, flood and warfare create famine; food shortages often lead to poisoning. Hungry people will eat badly stored, rotting, contaminated or adulterated foodstuffs even if they know them to be harmful; migrants will eat unfamiliar plants and fruits—anything that looks edible—and poisoning occurs. Seeds, including many used as human food, contain a great range of toxic substances and must be suitably prepared before they are eaten.[1] Harmful effects are also caused by contact with plants that have stinging hairs or irritant latex, resulting in toxic or allergic dermatitis. People in the tropics rely heavily for advice and treatment on traditional herbalists; many patients admitted to hospital have already received herbal medicines or enemas administered by local practitioners. These remedies, although they may have been in use for generations, are not necessarily safe; many contain pharmacologically potent or toxic substances with effects that may be immediate, or may be slow or cumulative poisons with hepatotoxic, carcinogenic or mutagenic activity. Very few traditional remedies have been submitted to the rigorous tests now demanded before a new synthetic medicine can be registered and used. When given together with synthetic medicines, herbal remedies can be especially dangerous, the pharmacological effects of the combinations often being unpredictable.

Paradoxically, the use of traditional herbal preparations by ethnic minority groups, and because of their reputed stimulant, aphrodisiac or health-giving properties, is increasing in the West as 'alternative medicine'; their toxic effects arebeing seen more frequently in Europe and North America. In addition, the active principles of plants used in their countries of origin for their psychotropic effects—notably cannabis, the opium alkaloids and cocaine—have become serious addictive drug problems in the West. Plant poisons have also been used throughout history for criminal purposes.

The treatment of poisoning often presents difficulty unless there is clear evidence of the cause, as in the case of a child who has been observed to consume something known to be toxic. It is important to prevent continued absorption from the alimentary tract by giving an emetic or gently washing out the stomach and, unless there is diarrhoea already, making sure that the rest of the gut is emptied. The patient needs to be closely observed and appropriate supportive treatment given as symptoms develop. It is always important to correct and maintain fluid and electrolyte balance and to check the levels of glucose and other blood constituents. In serious cases, dialysis or life support systems may be needed. In some institutions it is now possible to screen the urine and serum for the presence of known drugs and poisons and this facility should be used, if available, to help track down the source of poisoning.

Plant poisoning may therefore occur as a result of:

- Accidental poisoning from:
  toxic or contaminated foodstuffs;
  toxic seeds and fruits
  contact with irritant plants.
- The use of traditional medicines.
- The use of plants for their psychotropic properties.
- The use of plant poisons for criminal purposes.

ACCIDENTAL POISONING

TOXIC OR CONTAMINATED FOODS

CASSAVA AND YAMS

Manihot utilissima (Euphorbiaceae) is a native of Brazil and is widely grown in the tropics for the production of flour and tapioca. It occurs in 'sweet' and 'bitter' varieties but both contain cyanogenetic glycosides. The grated roots must be thoroughly washed to remove the toxic material; badly prepared cassava causes signs of hydrocyanic acid poisoning: nausea, vomiting, abdominal distension and respiratory difficulty. Diets that rely predominantly on cassava have also been shown to cause goitre,[2] parotid hypertrophy, pancreatitis, diabetes and ataxic neuropathy.

Yams are the tubers of *Dioscorea* (Dioscoreaceae); there are many palatable, cultivated varieties. There are also bitter, toxic species, such as *D. dumetorum* and *D. hirsuta*, that contain the alkaloid dioscorine. They may be eaten if sliced, steeped and washed in water but if badly prepared are toxic. Bitter yams are sometimes interplanted with edible varieties in order to deter theft by strangers, and deaths have occurred from the consumption of bitter yams during food shortages.[3]

CYCADS

In some countries the root stocks of cycads (*Cycas* and *Zamia*) are used to produce edible flour. This must be carefully washed to remove the toxic glycoside cycasin, which causes lesions of the central nervous system and hepato-cellular cancer.

The seeds of *Cycas circinalis* eaten by the Chamorro people of Guam and neighbouring islands, contain a neurotoxic amino acid, β-N-methylamino-L-alanine, which is possibly the cause of amyotrophic lateral sclerosis, Parkinsonism and dementia that occur in that area.[4,5]

PEAS AND BEANS (LEGUMINOSEAE)

Leguminous plants provide valuable foods but there are many toxic species that must be avoided.

Lathyrism is caused by *Lathyrus sativus*, the grass pea, which is nutritious, high yielding, resistant to drought, flooding and weed growth—qualities that should make it an ideal food plant for the tropics. Unfortunately it contains β-N-oxalylamino-L-alanine, which mimics the depolarizing action of the neurotransmitters, glutamate and aspartate. If used as a major dietary ingredient for 2–6 months it causes spastic paralysis of the legs, ranging in severity from limping to crawling on all fours. Grass pea consumption follows food shortages in India and Africa, and its use is increasing. It is a profitable cash crop that is used as a cheap adulterant in flour from other pulses; lathyrism is therefore likely to appear in places remote from grass pea cultivation. Attempts are now being made to select strains with a low content of the toxic principle.[6,7]

Favism is a haemolytic condition associated with the consumption of beans (*Vicia faba*) by individuals with glucose 6-phosphate dehydrogenase (G6PD) deficiency. The deficient erythrocytes are damaged by substances such as divicine and isouramil from the beans because their proteolytic enzyme systems are impaired.[8] The condition is common in the Middle East[9] but rare in Thailand, probably because the G6PD mutants that occur there are different.[10]

Many species of beans contain lectins that, if not destroyed by cooking, may cause serious toxic effects. Lectins recognize and bind selectively to carbohydrate receptors on cell surfaces. They act as information molecules that promote efficient symbiosis between the plant and nitrogen-fixing bacteria in the root nodules, and they also provide powerful protection against fungi and predatory insects.[11] As part of the human diet, lectins act as growth factors for the small intestine and influence health, digestive function and the bacterial ecology of the alimentary tract. In excess, they disturb intestinal structure and function and cause loss of body weight; large doses cause severe vomiting and bloody diarrhoea, followed by damage to the central nervous, and cardiovascular systems and kidneys.

CONTAMINATION WITH WEED SEEDS

Crops grown with weeds, when harvested, produce contaminated foods, and some weeds have poisonous seeds. The Mexican poppy, *Argemone mexicana* is a common weed in countries as far apart as India and Australia; it contains the toxic benzphenanthridine alkaloid sanguinarine and its effects have been known for many years. As a contaminant of a widely used cooking oil derived from mustard seed, it has led to outbreaks of 'epidemic dropsy' in many tropical countries.[12,13] The small, black oily seeds resemble those of mustard and become mixed with them accidentally or by deliberate adulteration. Village lads in India, while grazing cattle, can collect

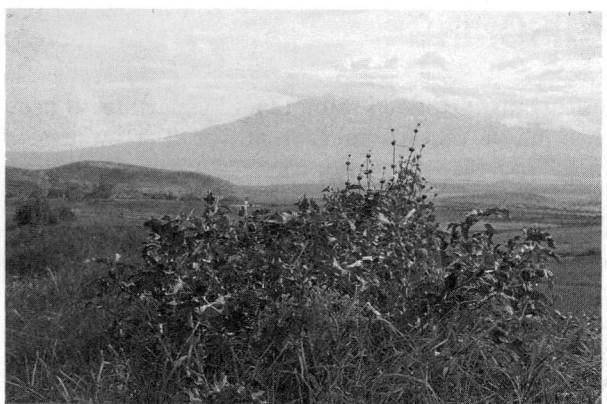

Figure 23.1   Datura stramonium. (Reproduced with permission from *Trans R Soc Trop Med Hyg* 1992; 86: cover.)

up to 8 kg of *Argemone* seeds a day in summer, and may sell them to unscrupulous dealers. Sanguinarine is absorbed from the intestinal tract, and also through the skin if oil containing it is used for massage.[14] It causes capillary dilatation and increased permeability, resulting in oedema, beginning in the legs and spreading, sometimes to the whole body. Fever, diarrhoea, vomiting, glaucoma and an erythematous skin rash are sometimes observed. Anaemia, wasting and weakness occur and pleural and pericardial effusions cause respiratory and cardiac dysfunction. Sanguinarine is also car-

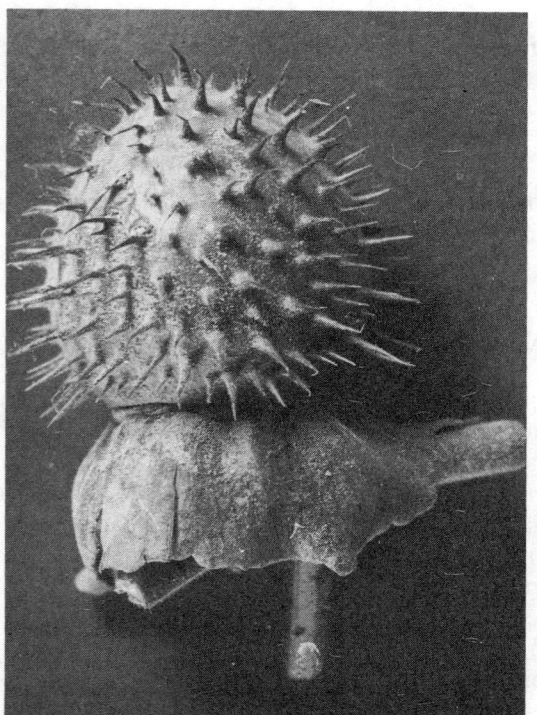

Figure 23.2   The poisonous fruit of Datura stramonium. (Reproduced with permission from *Trans R Soc Trop Med Hyg* 1984; 78: 134.)

cinogenic. It can be detected in oil by means of a sensitive test based on paper chromatography and an orange fluorescence under ultraviolet light that changes to brilliant blue in the presence of alkali.[15]

The thorn apple or Jimson weed, *Datura stramonium* (Figures 23.1 and 23.2), also grows in most parts of the world and is a frequent cause of poisoning in cereal crops. The seeds contain alkaloids of the tropane series, notably hyoscyamine, which causes psychosis with hallucinations, tachycardia and dilated pupils. Outbreaks are common; one example in Tanzania involved the consumption of porridge made from millet distributed by a local branch of the National Milling Corporation.[16]

Contamination of a local cereal, 'gondli', with the seeds of *Crotalaria* has caused veno-occlusive disease of the liver (see below) in central India,[17] and the weed *Heliotropium popovii* has been responsible for recurrent outbreaks of the same disease, with a high incidence and mortality, in villages in northwestern Afghanistan.[18]

CONTAMINATION WITH FUNGI

Ergot (*Claviceps purpurea*) is the classical example of a fungal food poison. The sclerotia, containing ergotoxine and related alkaloids that stimulate smooth muscle, are harvested with the ears of rye and other grasses. The flour causes uterine and vascular contraction, with abortion, arterial occlusion and painful gangrene—the St Anthony's fire of the Middle Ages. Ergot poisoning, although easy to prevent, still occurs from careless harvesting in times of food shortage. Vasodilator drugs ease ischaemic pain and help to prevent gangrene.

Wheat harvested in Ethiopia has sometimes contained seeds of the grass *Lolium temelentum*, itself contaminated with a fungus, probably *Endoconidium*. When ingested it leads to epidemics of 'miscara' (tipsy), with dizziness, headache, slurred speech, tremors and staggering gait.[19]

Consumption of mouldy grains infected with *Fusarium* or *Stachybotris* leads to alimentary toxic aleukia, probably caused by toxic tricothecenes. *Aspergillus flavus* and *A. parasiticus* produce aflatoxins that are toxic to the liver and are carcinogenic; the consumption of contaminated groundnuts has been linked with the common occurrence of hepatic carcinoma in Africa and Asia.[20] Other moulds are associated with chronic renal disease(s), and the inhalation of fungal spores may cause respiratory disease from direct invasion (histoplasmosis and actinomycosis), the effect of toxic metabolites (stachybotryosis) or allergic reactions.[21,22]

Accidental fungal poisoning also occurs when

toxic mushrooms, such as *Amanita phalloides*, are eaten in mistake for harmless species.

TOXIC SEEDS AND FRUITS

Jequirity beans (*Abrus*) and castor oil seeds (*Ricinus*) are bright and attractive to children and are sometimes made into necklaces. They contain poisons that, after a delay of 1–48 hours, can cause fatal gastroenteritis; the toxic principle of castor oil seeds, ricin, is one of the most poisonous substances known. Acute poisoning is treated by gastric lavage, demulcents and adjustment of fluid and electrolyte balance; diarrhoea empties the lower part of the gut. Abdominal pain may require analgesics, and for serious cases, respiratory support or haemodialysis may be needed.

Jenghol, or djenkol, beans (*Pithecolobium*) cause poisoning in Malaysia and Java. Blood, casts and crystals of djenkolic acid appear in the urine, and the renal tract may be blocked, causing dysuria and anuria. Diagnosis is obvious from the strong sulphurous odour of the breath and the urine. Treatment is to render the urine strongly alkaline (pH 8) by giving sodium bicarbonate by intravenous infusion (250 ml of 3.5% solution four times in a single day for a 70 kg adult). Continued blockage may need gentle catheterization under general anaesthesia.[23]

The broken kernels of *Prunus* spp. (plums, peaches, cherries, apricots, almonds) and those of loquats (*Eriobotrya*) contain a cyanogenetic glycoside that causes vomiting, weakness, ataxia, dyspnoea and coma.[24] The active principle, amygdalin (Laetrile) has been given to patients with cancer, and side-effects have not been uncommon. Treatment is to wash out the stomach and fill it with 5% sodium thiosulphate solution. Dicobalt edetate (20 ml of 1.5% solution) is given intravenously followed immediately by 50 ml of 50% dextrose through the same needle. Oxygen and respiratory support should be available.

The ackee, *Blighia sapida* (named after Captain Bligh of the Bounty) is a native of West Africa but is common in the West Indies and South America. The fruit has a large, fleshy aril with a pleasant taste and, when ripe, is good to eat; but when eaten unripe, before the fruit has opened on the tree, it is poisonous and has claimed the lives of many children in Jamaica and other islands, where circumscribed epidemics of 'vomiting sickness' were once common in rural areas. Unripe ackee fruits contain toxic hypoglycins, polypeptides that block gluconeogenesis in the liver and cause acute hypoglycaemia.[25]

A previously healthy child complains of abdominal discomfort and after vomiting several times,

recovers and may fall asleep. A few hours later severe vomiting returns, with convulsions and coma. The temperature is usually normal or subnormal, the pulse rate 90–100 and the respiratory rate 26–30—sometimes, as death approaches, of the Cheyne–Stokes type. Extreme hypoglycaemia with blood sugar levels as low as 22 mg/dl are found, and unless glucose is given promptly, death usually occurs within 12 hours of the initial vomiting.[26,27] The liver shows fatty changes, with almost complete absence of glycogen. Treatment is to wash out the stomach and to give glucose by intravenous infusion. Large doses of glycine may also be of value.[28] For those who recover, convalescence is usually complete in 24 hours.

Coral plants, *Jatropha curcas*, *J. glandulifera* and *J. multifida* (Euphorbiaceae), grow rapidly and are used in Africa and the West Indies as hedging plants. The fruits, 'physic nuts', taste like sweet almonds but have been reported to cause colic, cramps and thirst, with a subnormal temperature. Another species, *J. gossypifolia* is known in the West Indies as the 'bellyache bush' and its seeds contain an intestinal irritant like croton oil.

CONTACT WITH IRRITANT PLANTS

Many tropical plants cause toxic or allergic dermatitis that may appear as erythema, vesiculation or urticaria. A further species of *Jatropha, J. urens*, has leaves provided with stinging hairs that cause itching, smarting, flushing of the face, swelling of the lips and fainting.

Contact with the leaves of poison ivy (*Rhus toxicodendron* and *R. juglandifolia*) or poison sumach (*R. vernix*) causes intense irritation and inflammation. In Japan severe dermatitis may follow contact with lacquer made from *R. vermicifera*. Repeated attacks do not lead to immunity. Treatment consists of thorough washing of the skin with soap and water and removal of the poison from clothes by soaking in 1% hypochlorite solution.

Pyrethrum (*Chrysanthemum cinereriaefolium*) dermatitis occurs in Kenya where the plant is grown on a commercial scale for the production of insecticide. Exposure to the leaves and flowers causes itching, usually beginning at the corners of the eyes with lacrimation, followed by an irritating vesicular rash, peeling of the skin and the formation of painful fissures. Sweating and exposure to sunlight exacerbate the lesions.

The manichneel, *Hippomane mancinella*, like many other members of the family Euphorbiaceae, produces a highly irritant latex. It is a small tree, common along the coastline of South and Central America, the West Indies and India. There are two varieties, one with leaves like holly and the other like laurel; both are equally poisonous. The fruit resembles a crab-apple and sensitive people who touch it are likely to suffer from a skin eruption with erythema, bullae and vesiculation. The wood and even the sawdust are irritant and cause dermatitis, frequently of the genitalia and anus, with a vesiculo-pustular eruption sometimes confined to the glans penis. In the eye, the latex causes conjunctivitis with pain, photophobia and blepharospasm. If the fruit is eaten, by children or unwary strangers, it causes vesiculation of the buccal mucosa, bloody diarrhoea and sometimes death.

Latex on the skin should be washed off at once in the sea; blisters should be protected against infection and, if extensive, treated like second-degree burns. Emesis should be induced if the fruit has been eaten.

In China, a light sensitive dermatosis known as 'atriplicism' results from eating the spinach plant *Atriplex littoralis*. Itching of the hands is followed by oedema and the appearance of bullae; there may be gangrene of the fingertips, cutaneous haemorrhages and cyanosis and oedema of the face and eyelids. The condition resembles Raynaud's disease. A similar syndrome has been reported after consumption of *A. serrata* or *Chenopodium hybridum*.

Many plants and flowers, such as the euphorbias, orchids, primulas, lillies and mangoes, are capable of causing allergic dermatitis in sensitive people. The juice of some of the umbelliferae contains photosensitizing furanocoumarin derivatives that on contact with the skin cause erythema and vesication after exposure to light. Seaweed dermatitis has been reported from Hawaii, probably as a result of contact with a blue-green alga, *Lyngbya majuscula*, which produces a toxic rash in persons bathing in the sea off windward beaches. It responds to local treatment with antihistamine.

Idiosyncrasy to wood dust is not uncommon. Iroko (African teak) is the trade name for *Chlorophora exelsa*, a tree used for furniture; the sawdust produces the usual signs of allergy, with skin irritation, facial oedema, blepharospasm, acute coryza and pharyngitis. Other woods—mahogany, teak, satin wood and obeche—may produce similar symptoms.

TRADITIONAL MEDICINES

Herbal medicines are widely used and are still a source of new and useful remedies. The Chinese 'qinghaosu' (*Artemisia annua*) has been used for the treatment of fever for centuries and is now proving of value in the control of strains of malaria parasites that have developed resistance to the synthetic anti-malarial compounds (Chapter 61). But traditional medicines exist in many forms, lack standardization, and very few have been rigorously tested for toxicity, especially for their long-term effects. They are prescribed by herbalists, usually as complex mixtures with an uncertain pharmacology, or are prepared and taken by the patients themselves. Poisoning occurs because the herb contains toxins, because it has been mixed accidentally or deliberately with other, poisonous, plants and medicines, or because, as in the Asian 'kushtays', it has been mixed with appreciable amounts of the oxides of arsenic, mercury, tin, zinc or lead.[29] Synthetic drugs are now also being used to reinforce herbal medicines and the often unpredictable effects of such combinations is adding to the hazards.[30]

It is also dangerous to use herbal medicines as adjuncts to normal drug therapy. Thus, heart remedies containing cardioactive glycosides (*Strophanthus, Convallaria, Cytisus, Scilla*) seriously interfere with the control of digitalized patients, and hypotensive herbs (*Rauwolfia, Crataegus, Viscum*) affect the control of blood pressure if given during treatment with synthetic anti-hypertensive drugs. Karela, the fruit of *Momordica charantia* (Cucurbitaceae) is used in curries and is a traditional Indian remedy for diabetes; it has a hypoglycaemic action that interferes with the control of diabetes in patients receiving orthodox treatment.

'BUSH TEAS'

The most common herbal remedies are bush teas, infusions made from fresh or dried flowers, fruits, leaves, bark or roots by steeping in hot or cold water. Some of them are undoubtedly toxic.

Veno-occlusive disease (Chapter 3), which occurs in the West Indies, East and West Africa and India, is an acute, subacute or chronic condition affecting the central and sublobular hepatic veins. In the West Indies it is related to the consumption of bush tea made from *Crotalaria fulva* which contains toxic pyrrolizidine alkaloids. These compounds, which occur in *Crotalaria, Senecio, Heliotropium* and other composite plants, may also enter the human diet through the contamination of cereals with weed seeds. They are well-known poisons of farm animals in many parts of the world and produce similar lesions in the livers of laboratory animals.

The primary pathological change is subendo-thelial oedema followed by intimal overgrowth of connective tissue, with narrowing and occlusion of the central and sublobular hepatic veins. Atrophy or necrosis of liver cells, with consequent fibrosis, leads to gross changes similar to those seen in cardiac cirrhosis.[31] It has been estimated that veno-occlusive disease accounts for about one-third of all cases of liver cirrhosis in the West Indies.[32] The symptoms and signs are due to portal hypertension and its associated complications; the patient is usually a child with tender hepatomegaly and ascites. About half of those affected recover and 20% die in the acute stage. The remainder pass into a subacute or chronic stage, with continuing portal hypertension.[33]

GINSENG

The root of *Panax ginseng* (Araliaceae) has been used in China, Korea and Japan for centuries in the belief that it counters fatigue and stress and confers health, virility and longevity. The pharmacological basis for its reputation is slender, but ginseng is now in fashion worldwide. Several species are cultivated, but they are all expensive and the drug is therefore frequently found adulterated with *Eleutherococcus* (Russian ginseng), *Mandragora, Rauwolfia* and other roots of similar appearance. Ginseng contains a complex mixture of steroids and saponins; it can cause nervous excitation, tremor, hypertension and oestrogen-like effects.

COTTON ROOT BARK

The bark of *Gossypium* (Malvaceae) contains a compound that depresses spermatogenesis and has been used as a male contraceptive. It may cause an increased loss of potassium through the kidney.

MAKLUA

The fruit of *Diospyros mollis* (Ebenaceae) contains a derivative of hydroxynaphthalene and is used in Thailand for the expulsion of intestinal worms. It has been reported to cause optic neuritis in children.

TOBACCO

The leaves and flowers of *Nicotiana* spp. have been universally smoked, snuffed or chewed for their stimulant effect(s); they are also a well-known irritant and carcinogen and a danger to health. Preparations of the leaves applied to the chest to relieve respiratory complaints have sometimes given rise to toxic effects by percutaneous absorption of nicotine. An unusual nostrum made by the Yoruba people of Nigeria is 'cow's urine mixture', consisting of green tobacco leaves, rock salt, citron (*Citrus medica*), the leaves of the bush basil, *Ocimum viride*, and cow's urine. The remedy is given by mouth or rubbed into the skin for the prevention and treatment of epileptic or eclamptic fits; the toxic effects are those of nicotine—central nervous excitation, with vomiting, diarrhoea, dehydration and hypoglycaemia, followed by depression and coma, sometimes with permanent neurological lesions or death.[34]

Convulsions must be controlled and glucose given intravenously. The poison is removed by gastric lavage or cleansing of the skin, and blood glucose, electrolytes and fluid balance monitored.

PSYCHOTROPIC DRUGS

Herbal remedies that relieve mental tension, stress, and anxiety, or otherwise give relief from the troubles of life, have been discovered and prepared in all countries. Some of them have become dangerous drugs of addiction.

ALCOHOL

Addiction to alcohol occurs in tropical countries, with the same effects as in temperate ones. Rum (65–72% alcohol) is distilled from fermented molasses in the West Indies and South America; arrack or sake (50–60%) is manufactured in India, China, Java and Japan from fermented rice. Toddy, made from the sweet sap of various palms, is drunk in India, Sri Lanka and West Africa. A potent drink, pulque, is made in South America from the juice of agaves.

OPIUM

The opium habit, both eating and smoking, is common in the tropics, especially in the East, where the opium poppy, *Papaver somniferum* is grown. Refined alkaloids of the morphine series are illegally exported to Western Europe and North America to supply addicts.

COCA

Erythroxylon coca is widely grown in South America and India and is used as a stimulant and intoxicant. The leaves, first dried in the sun, are chewed with lime or, as in India, with betel. There is loss of sensation in the tongue and lips, followed by acceleration of the pulse and a period of hilarity, exaltation and the ability to do without food. The drug addict soon becomes emaciated and cachectic. Cocaine is a major illegal drug traffic problem in Europe and America.

INDIAN HEMP (HASHEESH)

Cannabis indica is grown in India and the Middle East; it is a variety of the common hemp, *C. sativa*, used for making ropes. The leaves are dried and powdered and chewed or smoked ('bhang'). An extract of the resinous flowers is known as 'ganja'. Both preparations cause intense nervous excitement. If used persistently they can lead to insanity, with illusions and hallucinations. Hasheesh, in various preparations, often with the addition of solanaceous plants such as *Datura*, is habitually taken by millions in Africa and Asia. It has become a serious drug of addiction in Western countries.

KAVA

The powdered root of *Piper methysticum*, prepared as a beverage, is drunk on festive occasions throughout Polynesia. Formerly the root was prepared by mastication by specially selected girls, a practice which caused the spread of tuberculosis. Overindulgence in kava induces a state of hyperexcitement, with loss of power in the legs. Chronic intoxication leads to debility with ataxia, visual and auditory defects and coarse, roughened skin.

BETEL

Chewing betel, the leaves of *Piper betel*, together with lime and areca nuts (*Areca catechu*) is a common practice in India, Sri Lanka and other Eastern countries. The mouth, lips and cheeks are stained bright red. The drug produces flushing of the face and it has mild stimulant and possibly anthelmintic properties. In Central and West Africa, the nuts of the kola tree (*Cola acuminata* and *C. nitida*) are habitually chewed and act as a sialagogue and stimulant, without obvious detrimental effects.

KHAT

Khat (cafta, miraa, muiragi) is derived from a small tree, *Catha edulis*, indigenous to North Africa. The leaves and twigs are chewed, infused or smoked and are reputed to produce a happy, mellow sense of friendliness. The leaves contain cathinone, a phenylalkylamine derivative with effects similar to those of amphetamine; cases of mental disturbance in addicts have been reported.

CRIMINAL POISONING

Many species of plants are used in the tropics for suicide and murder. They are often those that grow in the locality, and have been used traditionally as arrow poisons for hunting and warfare, or for ceremonies such as trial by ordeal. Many potent substances—the cardiac glycosides, tropane alkaloids, strychnine, eserine and curare—now important drugs in Western medicine, have been derived from these sources. For criminal purposes, plant products are frequently supplemented with another available poison such as arsenic, and introduced into foods such as flour, seeds or sweets.

Plants containing cardioactive glycosides are commonly used. In Madras and Bombay a potent extract is made from the roots of the white oleander, *Nerium odorum* (Apocynaceae), and in the West Indies *Urechites suberecta* exerts similar effects—a cumulative cardiac poison that eventually results in sudden death and is not easily detected. Other members of the Apocynaceae, such as *Cerbera odollum*, *Thevetia neriifolia* and *Strophanthus* spp., contain rapidly acting substances that cause death from cardiac failure within hours. In Zaire, all of the traditional arrow poisons contained extracts of

Strophanthus, often supplemented with haemolytic saponins.

A decoction of the bulbs of the lily, *Gloriosa superba*, allied to squill, also contains cardioactive glycosides and is used for criminal and suicidal purposes in Southern India, Sri Lanka, Burma and parts of Africa. The active principles, superbine and colchicine, cause gastrointestinal irritation and death from cardiac failure in about 4 hours.

By far the most frequently encountered criminal poisons in India, Sri Lanka and other tropical countries are the seeds of various species of *Datura* (Solanaceae). They contain atropine, hyoscyamine and scopolamine and cause mental excitation followed by coma. Preparations of the seeds have relatively little taste and are easily introduced into food or drink. *D. fastuosa* was a favourite poison of the Thugs in India, *D. sanguinea* is used in Colombia and Peru, *D. ferox* and *D. arborea* in Brazil, and the leaves of the related *Hyoscyamus fahezlez* by the Tuareg in the Sahara. The seeds of *D. stramonium* with *D. metel*, a common cause of poisoning through the contamination of cereal crops, are used in East Africa for criminal purposes, as an inebriant to facilitate robbery or to elicit confessions of witchcraft.[16] Poisoning with tropane alkaloids is effectively treated by injections of physostigmine.

The juice of the milkweed, *Asclepias*, is used in India as an infanticide; the symptoms—vomiting, salivation and cramps—are not easy to distinguish from those resulting from other causes. The roots of various species of aconite, such as *Aconitum ferox* are employed for the same purpose; they usually kill the infant in a few hours.

In Indonesia an extract of the roots of *Milleria sericea*, a leguminous plant allied to *Wisteria*, is used as a fish poison and also for criminal purposes. It produces debility, headache and diarrhoea, followed by collapse and death.

In China, opium is the most commonly used poison for suicide, especially by women.

Curare, the arrow poison of the South American forest tribes, was derived from the giant vines of the Amazon and the Orinoco; the main source was *Chondodendron tomentosum*. The drug blocks neuromuscular transmission; the muscles relax and the victim collapses. It has revolutionized anaesthesia in modern medicine and synthetic substitutes for natural D-tubocurarine have been prepared and are widely used.

Other South American poisons are derived from *Paullinia pinnata* and *Thevetia ahonai*, both of which cause vomiting and respiratory failure.

In West Africa, one of the most common criminal poisons is 'red water' or 'sassy' bark, from the tree *Erythrophleum guineense*. In contains the alkaloid erythrophleine, which causes vomiting, difficulty in breathing, convulsions and a cardiac effect resembling that of digitalis. It also has some local anaesthetic activity and, like the 'ordeal bean', *Physostigma venenosum*, was once widely used in trial by ordeal, in which the poison was given and the suspect observed to see if recovery occurred; if it did, the individual was not guilty.

The latex of the common African hedge cactus (*Euphorbia*), as well as causing dermatitis, is escharotic and cathartic, and has been used as an ingredient of arrow poison and as an unpleasant murder weapon.

Toxic species of mushrooms are found in all countries and have also been used for criminal purposes.

In cases of criminal poisoning the cause is seldom known and treatment usually has to depend on emptying the gastrointestinal tract and dealing with signs and symptoms as they arise. A toxicology screen, if available, may help to identify the poison and indicate appropriate life-saving measures.

REFERENCES

1 Bell E A. Toxic compounds in seeds. In Murray D R (ed.) *Seed Physiology*, vol. 1. London: Academic Press, 1984: 245–264.

2 Ekpechi O L. Pathogenesis of endemic goitre in Eastern Nigeria. *Br J Nutr* 1967; 21:537–545.

3 Dalziel J M. *The Useful Plants of West Tropical Africa*. London: Crown Agents for the Colonies, 1948: 491.

4 Spencer P S, Nunn P B, Hugon J, Ludolph A C, Ross S M, Roy D N, Robertson R C. Guam amyotrophic lateral sclerosis – Parkinsonism – dementia linked to a plant excitant neurotoxin. *Science* 1987; 237:517–522.

5 Bell E A & Nunn P B. Neurological disease in man: are plants to blame? *Biologist* 1988; 35:39–43.

6 Haimanot R T, Kidane Y, Wahib E, Kalissa A, Alemu T, Zlin Z A, Spencer P S. Lathyrism in rural Northwestern Ethiopia: a highly prevalent neurotoxic disorder. *Int J Epidemiol* 1990; 19:664–672.

7 Roy D. The neurotoxic disease lathyrism. *Natl Med J India* 1988; 1:70–80.

8 Morelli A, Grasso M, Meloni T, Forteleoni G, Zocchi E & de Flora A. Favism. Impairment of proteolytic systems in red blood cells. *Blood* 1987; 69:1753–1758.

9 Hedayat S H, Farhud D D, Mentazami K & Ghadrian P. The pattern of bean consumption, laboratory findings in patients with favism, G6PD deficiency and a control group. *J Trop Paediatr* 1981; 27:110–113.

10 Kitayaporn D, Charoenlarp P, Pataroarechachai J & Pholpoti T. G6PD deficiency and fava bean consumption do not produce haemolysis in Thailand. *Southeast Asian J Trop Med Public Health* 1991; 22:176–181.

11 Pusztai A J. *Plant Lectins*. Cambridge: Cambridge University Press, 1991.

12 Steyn D G. Poisoning with the seeds of *Argemone mexicana* (Mexican poppy) in human beings. Indian epidemic dropsy in South Africa. *S Afr Med J* 1950; 24:333–339.

13 Tandon R K, Tandon H D, Nayak N C & Tandon B N. Liver in epidemic dropsy. *Indian J Med Res* 1976; 64:1064–1069.

14 Sood N N, Sachdev M S, Mohan M, Gupta S K & Sachdev H P S. Epidemic dropsy following transcutaneous absorption of *Argemone mexicana* oil. *Trans R Soc Trop Med Hyg* 1985; 79:510–512.

15 Hakim S A E. Death, cardio-myopathy, symptomless glaucoma and cancer from edible oils containing argemone. *Maharashtra Med J* 1970; 17:109–130.

16 Rwiza H T. Jimson weed poisoning; an epidemic at Usangi rural government hospital. *Trop Geogr Med* 1991; 43:85–89.

17 Tandon B N, Tandon R K, Tandon H D, Narndranathan M & Joshi Y K. An epidemic of veno-occlusive disease of liver in Central India. *Lancet* 1976; i:271–272.

18 Mohabat O, Srivastava R N, Younos M S, Mozad A A, Sediq G G & Aram G N. An outbreak of hepatic veno-occlusive disease in Northwestern Afghanistan. *Lancet* 1976; ii:269–271.

19 Brinton D. An unusual form of epidemic food poisoning with neurological symptoms. *Proc R Soc Med* 1946; 39:173–175.

20 Krishnamachari K A V R, Bhat R V, Nagarajan V & Tilak T B G. Hepatitis due to aflatoxicosis. An outbreak in Western India. *Lancet* 1975; i:1061–1063.

21 Ellenhorn M J & Barceloux D G (eds). Plants, mycotoxins and mushrooms. In *Medical Toxicology*. Amsterdam, Elsevier, 1988: 1209–1349.

22 World Health Organization. Mycotoxins. *Environmental Health Criteria*. Geneva: WHO, 1970.

23 West C E, Perrin D D, Shaw D C, Heap G J & Soemanto. Djenkol bean poisoning (djenkolism): proposals for treatment and prevention. *Southeast Asian J Trop Med Public Health* 1973; 4:564–570.

24 Rubino M J & Davidoff F. Cyanide poisoning from apricot seeds. *JAMA* 1979; 241:359.

25 Hassall C H & Reyle K. The toxicity of the ackee (*Blighia sapida*) and its relationship to the vomiting sickness of Jamaica. *West Indian Med J* 1955; 4:85–90.

26 Jelliffe D B & Stuart K L. Acute toxic hypoglycaemia in the vomiting sickness of Jamaica. *BMJ* 1954; 1:75–77.

27 Stuart K L, Jellife D B & Hill R R. Acute toxic hypoglycaemia occurring in the vomiting sickness of Jamaica. *J Trop Paediatr* 1955; 1:69–87.

28 Sherratt H S A & Al-Bassam S S. Glycine in ackee poisoning. *Lancet* 1976; ii:1243.

29 Aslam M, Davis S S & Henly M A. Heavy metals in some Asian medicines and cosmetics. *Public Health* 1979; 93:274–284.

30 Penn R G. Adverse reactions to herbal and other unorthodox medicines. In D'Arcy P F & Griffin J P (eds) *Iatrogenic Diseases*, 3rd edn. Oxford: Oxford University Press, 1985: 898–918.

31 Edington G M & Gilles H M. *Pathology in the Tropics*. London: Edward Arnold, 1969; 488–490.

32 Bras G, Brooks S E H & Watler D C. Cirrhosis of the liver in Jamaica. *J Pathol Bacteriol* 1961; 82:503–512.

33 Stuart K L & Bras G. Veno-occlusive disease of the liver. *Q J Med* 1957; 26:291–316.

34 Elegbe R A & Oyebola D D O. Cow's urine poisoning in Nigeria: cardiorespiratory effects of cow's urine in dogs. *Trans R Soc Trop Med Hyg* 1977; 71:127–132.

FURTHER READING

Chopra R N. *Poisonous Plants of India*. Calcutta: Government of India Press, 1940.

Chopra R N. *Indigenous Drugs of India,* 2nd edn. Calcutta: Dhat, 1958.

Dalziel J M. *The Useful Plants of West Tropical Africa*. London: Crown Agents for the Colonies, 1948.

Lampe K F & Fagerstrom R. *Plant Toxicity and Dermatitis*. Baltimore, MD: Williams & Wilkins, 1968.

Lampe K F & McCann M A. *AMA Handbook of Poisonous and Injurious Plants*. Chicago: American Medical Association, 1985.

Watt J M & Breyer-Brandwijk M G. *Medicinal and Poisonous Plants of Southern and Eastern Africa*. Edinburgh: Livingstone, 1962.

CHAPTER 24

MALIGNANT DISEASE

C. L. M. Olweny and M. S. R. Hutt

Any account of the problem of cancer must take into consideration several accepted generalizations. The term cancer is used to describe a group of conditions which are characterized by an abnormal proliferation of particular cells. Each tumour is classified according to its cell of origin, anatomical site and biological behaviour, and each is due to a specific factor or constellation of factors, the majority of which are determined by geographical, social, economic or cultural factors, acting through physical, chemical or biological agents. Tumours due to direct genetic mechanisms are very rare, though genetic factors may render individuals or groups of people susceptible to particular environmental influences. The majority of tumours show an age-related incidence which reflects length of exposure to carcinogenic factors in the environment.

Contrary to the common belief associating cancer with industrialization and urban life style, cancer occurs very frequently in the developing world. Numerically, there are more cancer victims in developing countries than in the developed countries: of the estimated 5.9 million new cases of cancer diagnosed globally every year, 3 million come from the former; of the 4.3 million estimated annual cancer deaths, 2.3 million occur in the developing countries.

GLOBAL VARIATIONS

There are global cancer incidence variations due to the fact that political boundaries rarely, if ever, comprise a population that is genetically, culturally and socioeconomically homogeneous.[1] There is thus considerable variation of cancers observed in different regions of the world. Cancer of the cervix for instance, the most common cancer in the developing countries, is the tenth most common in the developed countries. On the other hand colorectal cancer, second only to lung cancer in the developed countries, is number eight in the developing countries (Table 24.1).[2] These differences underscore the variations in health care priorities.

Table 24.1 The ten most common cancers globally.[2]

Developing countries	Developed countries
1. Uterine cervix	1. Lung
2. Stomach	2. Colorectal
3. Oropharynx	3. Breast
4. Oesophagus	4. Stomach
5. Breast	5. Prostate
6. Lung	6. Bladder
7. Liver	7. Lymphoma
8. Colorectal	8. Oropharynx
9. Lymphoma	9. Uterine body
10. Leukemia	10. Uterine cervix

CANCER IN THE TROPICS

During the first half of this century little was known or published about cancer in tropical countries and it was thought by many to be rare in the 'native' populations of these regions. However, a few individuals recognized not only that cancer occurred but also that the incidence and behaviour of some tumours was quite different from that seen in temperate climates. By the 1930s it was known that there was a high incidence of squamous cell carcinoma of the bladder in regions with a high prevalence of *Schistosoma haematobium* infection, of oral cancer in the Indian subcontinent and of nasopharyngeal carcinoma in the Far East. The first large series of histologically proven malignant tumours in Africans, published in 1934, showed several peculiar features, including descriptions of lymphosarcomas of the jaw, almost certainly Burkitt's lymphoma.

Although the incidence of stomach cancer is decreasing in many parts of the world it remains an important cause of mortality in most Western countries and particularly in Japan. This tumour is relatively uncommon in most tropical regions such as Africa, the Indian subcontinent and much of the Far East. However, there are focal areas of high incidence such as that found around Mount Kilimanjaro in Tanzania and in the adjacent part of Kenya, near Lake Kivu in Zaire and in the countries of

Rwanda and Burundi. High rates are also found in the mountainous regions of Colombia and in Chile. Carcinoma of the pancreas, which is increasing in frequency in Western populations, is uncommon in most tropical countries.

SMOKING AND LUNG CANCER

Unfortunately with the increasing adoption of a Western life style, especially smoking, lung cancer incidence is expected to rise sharply in the developing countries. Such an increase has already been observed in Shanghai, China's largest city, in India and in Zimbabwe. The male lung cancer incidence recorded in Bulawayo, Zimbabwe in 1968–1972 was 70.6/100 000 population. Such phenomenal increase calls for an urgent need to counteract the ruthless and sophisticated smoking campaign launched by the tobacco companies. It is not enough to merely persuade individuals to give up smoking or for governments to legislate against tobacco. There are powerful economic interests served by the production, promotion and sale of tobacco products which seek to maximize consumption at all cost.[3] Tobacco is the major source of foreign exchange earnings in some countries. The most prominent cancer risk factor is cigarette smoking, associated primarily with lung cancer but contributing considerably to cancers of the oro-pharynx, oesophagus and urinary bladder. It has been suggested that tobacco smoking is the most deadly form of drug addiction, and that it is exacting a heavier toll in lives and dollars than cocaine, heroin, the acquired immune deficiency syndrome (AIDS), traffic accidents, murder and terrorist attacks combined.[4] Lung cancer epidemic is threatening most developing countries. If we are to win the war against cancer, we must first win the battle against tobacco.[5]

OTHER CAUSES OF CANCER

Although genetic factors are known to play some role in the causation of certain cancers, notably increased incidence of skin cancers in individuals with defective capacity to repair DNA damage caused by ultraviolet light (xeroderma pigmentosa),[6,7] it is now recognized that most cancers are due to factors in the environment (Table 24.2). These factors are physical, chemical, biological and, most importantly, life style related.

CANCER REGISTRATION

The establishment of medical schools in many former colonial countries of the tropics after the

Table 24.2 Cancers associated with environmental factors.

Factors	Examples	Cancers
Physical	Ultraviolet light	Skin cancers,
	Ionizing radiation	e.g. melanoma
Chemicals	Aflatoxin	Liver
	Asbestosis	Mesothelioma
	Vinyl chloride	Liver
Biological: viruses	Hepatitis B virus	Liver
	Human papilloma virus	Uterine cervix
	Epstein–Barr virus	Nasopharynx
		Burkitt's lymphoma
Biological: parasites	*Schistosoma haematobium*	Bladder
	Clonorchis sinensis	Liver
Life style	Smoking	Lung
		Oropharynx
		Bladder
		Oesophagus
	Diet	Colorectal
		Breast
	Alcohol	Liver
		Oesophagus

Second World War coincided with the extension of epidemiological interests and techniques in the field of non-infectious diseases, including cancer. During this period cancer registries were established in many tropical countries throughout the world and these were able to obtain for the first time age-specific cancer rates in several localized areas, usually around teaching hospitals where diagnostic facilities were of a high order and where there was an accurate census of the populations served. These incidence rate surveys were supplemented by proportional frequency studies (the frequency of individual tumours as a percentage of the whole) from different areas and tribal or ethnic groups in countries or regions.

These studies have shown not only that there are marked differences between the cancer pattern of tropical and of temperate countries, but also that there are large variations in frequency of specific cancers within regions and countries of the tropics. Some of the most important aetiological discoveries in the cancer field have stemmed from these geographical studies.

There are, however, few reliable estimates of cancer incidences in the tropics, especially in Africa. Some cancer registries e.g. Kyadondo county in Uganda, record only histologically confirmed cases.[8] For others, though population based, e.g. Bamako in Mali,[9] the proportion of histologically confirmed cases is rather low by the accepted standards of developed countries. There are several reasons to account for this shortfall. First, the autopsy rates are low in some countries for religious and cultural reasons. Second, histopathological facilities are inadequate and are often located only in university teaching hospitals. Third, because of the costs incurred, most clinicians opt for simpler diagnostic techniques, e.g. α-fetoprotein (AFP) estimation for liver cancer. Fourth, most patients in the tropics present at an advanced stage of their illness when therapeutic intervention is less important and histological diagnosis becomes an academic exercise.

CANCER CONTROL AND PREVENTION

Cancer control is the application of existing knowledge covering the whole spectrum of approaches designed to actively prevent, cure or manage cancer. The aim of a national cancer control programme is to reduce morbidity and mortality due to cancer and to improve the quality of life of cancer patients. Treating cancer is an expensive, high technology process that few tropical countries can afford.[3] Prevention must therefore be their primary focus. Fortunately in the tropics, a number of cancers are amenable to primary and secondary prevention. Liver cancer is mostly due to hepatitis B virus. An effective and affordable vaccine is available and is currently undergoing clinical trial in the Gambia to assess its efficacy in preventing chronic liver disease and hopefully primary liver cancer.[10] Given the fact that cancer of the uterine cervix is the most common cancer in the tropics, consideration must be given to prevention of this cancer by screening. The principles of screening are outlined on Table 24.3. Cancer of the cervix meets most of the required guidelines.

The rest of this chapter will discuss only some of the common tumours encountered in the tropics. The choice for inclusion is based on the frequency, whether it is preventable and whether there is a lesson to learn from the tumour in question.

Table 24.3 Principles of screening.

1. The disease should be an important health problem
2. Its natural history should be well understood
3. It should be recognizable at an early stage
4. Early stage treatment must be more beneficial than late stage treatment
5. A suitable test exists to detect the disease at an early stage
6. The test should be acceptable to the general population
7. Adequate facilities must exist for diagnosis and treatment of cases identified.
8. Benefit from screening must outweigh any possible physical or psychological harm
9. The benefits must clearly outweigh the costs involved

CANCER OF THE UTERINE CERVIX (See also Chapter 17)

Cancer of the cervix is the most common cancer affecting women in the tropics. About 80% of the 500 000 cases diagnosed globally every year are in the developing countries.[11] In Latin America and the Caribbean, cancer of the cervix is considered to be the leading cause of death among women. It is estimated that approximately 1 in every 1000 women aged 30–55 years will develop cervical cancer every year. The rates are particularly high in Brazil, Columbia, Chile, Costa Rica and the Indian subcontinent, with rates ranging from 35.1 to 48.2/100 000.[12] In Africa the situation has been described as tragic.[13] The disease affects young premenopausal women in over 50% of cases. More often than not there is considerable delay in diagnosis and most centres lack appropriate treatment facilities. Recent studies in Kenya,[14] Nigeria,[15] Tanzania,[16] and Zimbabwe[17] all confirm these observations.

AETIOLOGY

The relationship between cancer of the cervix and sexual behaviour is well established.[18] The most important factors are age at first intercourse and the number of sexual partners. Many studies show a 2–3-fold increased risk in women with more than one partner.[19] Cancer of the cervix is far more common in married than unmarried women, and multiple live births seem to increase the risk. The role of the male partner is increasingly being recognized.[20,21] In addition, there are some non-sexual factors, notably smoking and oral contraceptive pill use, that seem to play an important role. The relative risk increases up to 13-fold in smokers when compared to non-smokers, even after correcting for sexual characteristics.[22] The exact role of smoking and oral contraceptives is still debatable[23,24] and this is particularly so in the tropics[25] where female smoking and oral contraceptive use are recent introductions in life style and behaviour.

Exposure to sexually transmitted agent or agents has been in the limelight for over two decades. Initial interest in the 1970s focused on herpes simplex virus type 2 (HSV-2). It was suggested that HSV-2 might be the initiating agent.[26] More recently human papilloma virus (HPV) (especially HPV types 16 and 18) has emerged as the putative transmissible factor for cancer of the cervix.[27,28] HPV is a double-stranded DNA virus and is found in 95% of cervical condylomata acuminata. The evidence for incriminating HPV is based on clinical observations and molecular biological investigations.[29] Numerous studies have found HPV-DNA in cervical cancer tissues. HPV is capable of transforming rodent cells in vitro. The relative risk for cancer of the cervix in the presence of HPV-DNA increases from twofold to almost tenfold with increasing intensity of the hybridization reaction and this increase persists even after adjusting for other major risk factors. HPV-16/18 infection rates appear

to be higher in Latin America (32%) than in Germany (2–13%) or Denmark (6–13%). Latin America has the highest recorded incidence rates for cancer of the cervix. These and other observations provide circumstantial evidence for the hypothesis that HPV is an aetiological agent in cancer of the cervix.

Certain histological variants seem to be associated with specific HPV type. HPV-16 appears commonly in squamous cell carcinoma while HPV-18 is seen frequently in adenocarcinomas.

Using Southern blot hybridization or the more sensitive polymerase chain reaction (PCR) techniques HPV-DNA was detected in almost 85% of tumours. PCR is an in vitro DNA amplification technique capable of 100 000-fold amplification of specific DNA sequences using heat-stable DNA polymerase. In about 15% of cervical cancer cases HPV-DNA sequences cannot be detected. There are several possible explanations. First, HPV may only play a role in the early intraepithelial stages of tumour development and the viral DNA sequences may get lost at later stages of disease progression.[30] Second, metastatic disease spread may also lead to loss of viral DNA sequences.[30,31] Third, it is possible some cervical cancers are associated with HPV types only remotely related to the known genital HPVs and are undetected by the currently available diagnostic methods. Lastly, a proportion of cancers may indeed develop independently of any HPV infection.

STAGING

The staging system in wide use is the one recommended by the International Federation of Gynecology and Obstetrics (FIGO) (Table 24.4).

Pretreatment evaluation and assignment of stage, in addition to history and physical examination, must include pelvic examination under anaesthesia, chest X-ray, intravenous pyelography, barium enema, cystoscopy and/or sigmoidoscopy. A recent study using computerized tomography (CT) and magnetic resonance imaging (MRI) to determine the utility of these imaging techniques in detecting local or regional metastasis concluded that the 60% accuracy was too low to warrant routine use of these tests for staging.[32] The majority of patients present with advanced disease stage with 80–90% being stages III and IV as observed in a number of African studies.[14–17] The full prestaging protocol proposed tends to be time consuming and expensive. A cost-effective protocol which omits some investigations

Table 24.4 FIGO staging of carcinoma of the uterine cervix: 1988 update.

Stage	Characteristics
0	*Carcinoma in situ, intraepithelial carcinoma* (cases of stage 0 should be included in statistics for invasive carcinoma)
I	*Carcinoma strictly confined to the cervix*
I-A1	Minimal, microscopically-evident carcinoma of the cervix
I-A2	Lesion detected microscopically that can be measured. The lesion must invade less than 5 mm below the base of the surface or glandular epithelium and extend to no more than 7 mm in the horizontal plane
I-B	Lesions larger than stage I-A2. Preformed space involvement should not alter the staging but should be recorded
II	*Carcinoma extends beyond the cervix* but does not reach the pelvic wall. The carcinoma involves the vagina, but not the lower third
II-A	No obvious parametrical involvement
II-B	Obvious parametrical involvement
III	*Carcinoma extends to the pelvic wall.* On rectal examination there is no cancer-free space between the tumour and the pelvic wall. The tumour involves the lower third of the vagina. All cases with hydronephrosis or non-functional kidney should be included unless known to be due to other causes
III-A	No extension to the pelvic wall
III-B	Extension to the pelvic wall
IV	*Carcinoma extending beyond the true pelvis* or clinically involving the mucosa of the bladder or rectum
IV-A	Spread to adjacent organs
IV-B	Spread to distant organs

without harming patients has been proposed for developing countries.[33]

PROGNOSTIC FACTORS

The most reliable prognostic factors are stage at diagnosis, nodal status and size and grade of differentiation of primary tumour.[30] In addition HPV-negative tumours have a significantly worse overall recurrence rate (2.6× higher risk of recurrence) than HPV-positive patients. Relapse-free survival at 24 months is of the order of 77% for HPV-positive patients and only 40% for the HPV-negative group. HPV-negative tumours have significantly (4.5×) higher risk of distant metastases than HPV-positive

tumours. It would thus appear that HPV-negative cancers may represent a biologically distinct subset of tumours that are more aggressive and carry poorer prognosis than HPV-positive cancers.[30,34,35]

PREVENTION

The process of carcinogenesis from induction to development of invasive cancer is approximately 10 years. Precancerous changes can be detected several years before the development of invasive cancer by a simple test, the Papanicolaou (Pap) test, named after its developer Dr George N. Papanicolaou. Early detection by Pap test (screening) if properly organized and executed has been shown to save lives.[36–38] The test is reasonably sensitive but does occasionally produce abnormal results (false positive) in the absence of disease and normal findings (false negative) in women who subsequently are found to have disease. Furthermore, screening programmes tend to attract married healthy women, particularly those in the higher socioeconomic groups, while the women most at risk are habitually missed. There is, in addition, lack of international agreement on the age range for screening and the frequency for such screening. Considerable disquiet is growing in some circles about the possibility that cervical screening may actually cause psychological harm by engendering anxiety.[39]

It has also been suggested by others that cervical screening is not cost 'effective'.[40] Most of these observations do reflect Western culture where cancer of the cervix is not common and it would therefore cost exorbitant sums of money to identify one case. The situation in the tropics is clearly different, and although cost–benefit analyses have not been systematically undertaken the sheer numbers of victims would suggest that screening should be advocated. What is needed is proper education of the population in question and the installation of appropriate treatment facilities to handle the cases identified. It is, however, disheartening to observe that many cytological screening programmes set up in Africa have either collapsed or do not function properly. It is therefore imperative that any projected schemes undertake very careful study and analysis of current failures.

TREATMENT

Cervical screening, if successfully carried out, will reduce the incidence of clinically invasive squamous cell carcinoma and thus lower morbidity and mortality.[37]

Cancer in situ (stage 0) is best treated by abdominal hysterectomy, with or without vaginal cuff. If the patient wishes to retain fertility and she can be relied upon to return for regular review, then a cone biopsy may be adequate. The outcome for stage 0 is excellent, with less than 2% of patients developing recurrent cancer in situ or invasive carcinoma.[41] The treatment of stage I-A with minimal invasion is similar to that for stage 0. For stages I-B and II-A the treatment is either surgery (radical hysterectomy and pelvic lymphadenectomy) or radiotherapy, which consists of external beam irradiation and brachytherapy (temporary insertion of intrauterine and vaginal colpostats loaded with isotope, usually caesium-137). Surgery is the preferred approach for younger women who wish to retain ovarian function and avoid vaginal irradiation. Radiotherapy is to be recommended for patients who are elderly and/or have surgical contraindications. The survival for the two approaches (radiation and surgery) is about equivalent, with survival at 5 years ranging from 60 to 80% under ideal conditions. Stages II-B and III patients are to be considered for radical hysterec-tomy and pelvic lymphadenectomy or external beam irradiation (4500–5500 cGy) followed by intracavitary brachytherapy. Patients with locally invasive stage IV-A or recurrence after radiotherapy may be considered for pelvic exenteration. Down-staging for patients with locally advanced disease is being advocated, especially in tropical areas, and clinical trials are to be activated.

The role of chemotherapy for cancer of the cervix is less well defined and the results less impressive. Single agent therapy with cisplatin may give responses in about 30% of cases. Combination chemotherapy may slightly improve on this, to 50%.

The situation in Africa and most developing countries is such that the recommendations highlighted above may be inappropriate. Most patients present with disease at very advanced stage when even pelvic exenteration may not be done. In many situations neither radiotherapy nor chemotherapy is available. Survival is difficult to ascertain as default rate is high. Most patients request for discharge to try alternative forms of therapy.[15] Such pathetic situations underscore the need to develop comprehensive palliative care services, including pain control.

HEPATOCELLULAR CARCINOMA (See also Chapters 3 and 31)

Primary liver cancer includes hepatocellular carcinoma (HCC), which is very common, cholangiocellular carcinoma, which is rare, and angiosarcoma of the liver, which is very rare. This discussion will concentrate on HCC only. HCC is among the ten most common cancers worldwide.[2] It is estimated that there are at least 260 000 new cases every year; the majority of these are to be found in sub-Saharan Africa, South-East Asia and the western Pacific. In Shanghai the incidence rate is 34.4/100 000 males and 11.6/100 000 females. In the Philippines the figures quoted are 17.5/100 000 males and 7.1/100 000 females.[12] In sub-Saharan Africa, primary liver cancer is the most common cancer affecting men. The highest recorded incidence rate is in Mozambique, with an incidence rate of over 100/100 000 population.[42] A more recent survey in Mozambique recorded incidence rates ranging from 9.3 to 60.7/100 000 males and from 3.7 to 13.0/100 000 females.[43] The striking feature was the high rates in the very young, with estimated crude rates for those aged 20–29 years being 82.2/100 000 and for those aged 30–39 being 85.8/100 000. The incidence rates for other African countries are shown in Table 24.5.[9]

Table 24.5 Incidence rates of liver cancer in several African countries.[9]

Country	Years	Incidence per 100 000	
		Male	*Female*
Gambia	1986–88	33.1	12.6
Mali (Bamako)	1987–88	48.6	15.3
Nigeria (Ibadan)	1960–69	10.4	3.9
Senegal (Dakar)	1969–74	25.6	9.0
Swaziland	1979–83	10.5	3.0
Zimbabwe (Bulawayo)	1968–72	64.6	25.4

By contrast, HCC is uncommon in northern India (1.4/100 000 annually in Bombay), although proportional frequencies suggest the tumour is more common in the southern part of the subcontinent. Rates intermediate between those of the Far East and those of Europe and North America are reported in countries of the Middle East, the Caribbean and parts of South America.

AETIOLOGY

HCC is multifactorial in aetiology and causal factors differ in different parts of the world. Hepatitis B virus (HBV) is believed to play a causal role in about 80% of patients with HCC worldwide.[44] In low-risk populations about one-half of HCC cases in men and one-third in women can be attributed to a viral aetiology.[45] The non-viral aetiological factors associated with HCC are aflatoxin, cigarette smoking, oral contraceptives and alcohol ingestion.

HEPATITIS B VIRUS

About 80% of HCCs result from infection with HBV, a virus which causes other liver ailments as well and is second only to tobacco as a known single cause of cancer. The evidence for its causal role in HCC is derived from epidemiological case–control and cohort studies, clinical data and laboratory investigations. Follow-up of patients with chronic liver disease associated with HBV markers indicate that hepatitis B surface antigen (HBsAg)-positive individuals with chronic hepatitis and/or cirrhosis have a greater risk of developing HCC. Retrospective investigations of HBV serum markers show a substantially higher rate in patients who subsequently develop HCC than in controls. The most convincing epidemiological evidence, however, comes from the prospective case–control surveillance of 22 000 middle-aged Chinese males in Taiwan observed for 75 000 man-years of follow-up. In the 15% who were HBsAg carriers there was a 223-fold excess risk of HCC over the non-carriers.[46] Molecular biology studies show HBV-DNA integration in tissues of patients with chronic hepatitis and HCC. The process of integration makes the elimination of HBV-DNA in chronic carriers impossible. Integration of HBV-DNA into human hepatocytes was first detected in a continuous cell line expressing HBsAg derived from a male HBV carrier with HCC. HBV-DNA is now known to be incorporated into the host genome of HCC patients whether they have evidence of viral infection or not.[47,48] However, the existence of low incidence regions of HCC despite a high prevalence of HVB infection may indicate that HBV infection acting alone may have little carcinogenic effect and that it may need to be potentiated by another factor or factors.

Although HCC and HBV are closely associated, some patients with HCC have no serological evidence of past or active HBV infection. Tissue from 75–100% of patients with HCC who have no sero-

logical marker of HBV have no HBV-DNA detected by hybridization studies and 50–90% have no HBV-DNA detectable by PCR. In Japan and in Europe 54–69% of patients with HCC without serological markers for HBV have antibodies to hepatitis C virus (HCV). Seven well-documented cases have been reported in which chronic non-A, non-B hepatitis (HCV) had been prospectively followed and had progressed to HCC.[49] Cirrhosis is found in 86–100% of anti-HCV positive HCC patients. The mechanism of oncogenesis for HCV is not clear as available data indicate lack of HCV integration in the host cell. Although it was previously felt that blood transfusion was the major mode of transmission, available evidence currently indicates that over 90% of anti-HCV-positive blood donors have no history of having received transfusions. It is currently estimated that over 50% of HCC diagnosed annually in Japan is probably HCV-related.[48] The role of HCV in the tropics is entirely unknown but probably minimal.

AFLATOXIN

Aflatoxin was first isolated in 1961 following an outbreak of fatal jaundice in turkeys. The 'turkey-X' disease was traced to poultry feed containing peanuts contaminated with *Aspergillus flavus* imported from Brazil. Subsequently aflatoxin B (so called because of its blue fluorescence) was found to be potently hepatotoxic and carcinogenic in a variety of animal species. Aflatoxins are a group of compounds produced by the mould *A. flavus* which grows readily in warm, humid conditions. Although groundnuts are the substrate of choice for the mould, it can grow on other cereals, notably maize, millet, peas and sorghum.

People in some areas of the tropical world are frequently exposed to food contaminated with aflatoxin. In Mozambique 8% of prepared meal samples contain measurable aflatoxin. The average contamination level is 38.1 μg/kg wet food. The aflatoxin levels in food samples observed in Mozambique are the highest in the world.[43] In the Transkei the frequency of food sample contamination is much higher (25%) but the level of contamination is much lower than that in Mozambique.

The carcinogenic risk of aflatoxin has been evaluated and reported.[50] Laboratory research has demonstrated the hepatocarcinogenic properties of aflatoxin.[51,52] There is a clear correlation between HCC and the rate of aflatoxin ingestion[43,53,54] (Table 24.6). Further confirmation of an aetiological role for aflatoxin in HCC has come from a case–control study in the Philippines where the mean

Table 24.6   Aflatoxin ingestion and hepatocellular carcinoma in different countries (after ref. 43).

Country	Location	Aflatoxin B_1 ingestion (μg/kg)	HCC rate/100 000 per year
Kenya	High altitude	3.5	1.2
	Middle altitude	5.9	2.5
	Low altitude	10.0	4.0
Swaziland	High veld	5.1	2.2
	Middle veld	8.9	3.8
	Low veld	43.1	9.2
Mozambique	Inhambene	77.7	12.1
	Homoine-Maxixe	131.4	17.7
	Zavala	183.7	14.0

contamination level of different dietary items was established and individual levels of consumption determined retrospectively.[55] Studies in Kenya[56] and Thailand have more or less found similar results. In Egypt, a country with a very low level of aflatoxin contamination because the climate is hot and dry, the incidence of HCC is relatively low. In Botswana, which is very dry, and Greenland, which is very cold, the incidence of HCC is low and presumably *A. flavus* growth in such unfavourable climates is inhibited.

The mechanism of carcinogenesis is not well understood, but several plausible explanations have been suggested. Aflatoxin B is metabolized by a microsomal mixed function oxidase system to produce aflatoxin B-2,3-epoxide which is believed to be the carcinogen.[57] It has also been suggested that aflatoxin may suppress cell-mediated immunity and facilitate persistent HBV infection and eventually HCC.[58] There is a suggestion that aflatoxin only accumulates in the liver after the liver's ability to degrade aflatoxin has been impaired by persistent HBV infection.[59]

CIGARETTE SMOKING

Cigarette smoking has only recently permeated rural developing countries. Its impact on HCC must therefore be minimal. Where studies have been done, as in South African Blacks, the evidence supports the conclusion that cigarette smoking plays no aetiological role in HCC in South Africa.[60] In low-risk areas of the world, cigarette smoking is a significant risk factor with a relative risk ratio of greater than 2.[61]

ALCOHOL

It is estimated that heavy alcohol consumption is another risk factor, especially in the low incidence areas. HCC is almost fivefold as common in men who imbibe more than 80 g of ethanol per day than in non-drinkers.[61] However, in tropical countries most HCCs are associated with macronodular posthepatitic rather than micronodular alcoholic cirrhosis.[62] There is very little evidence to implicate alcohol as playing a role in high incidence areas of HCC. A case–control study in South Africa gave no indication that alcohol could be incriminated as a risk factor.[63]

ORAL CONTRACEPTIVE USE

The use of oral contraceptive pills has been shown to be significantly related to HCC in women, with a 5.5-fold increase in relative risk[61] in those women using it for over 5 years. Like cigarette smoking, the use of oral contraceptives is only beginning to take root in rural tropical areas and their impact on the incidence of HCC, though largely undetermined, must be minimal. Earlier reports suggested that oral contraceptives mostly caused liver adenomas, although some have transformed into carcinomas. The mechanism whereby oestrogens, including those used in oral contraceptive pills, cause cancer is not clearly understood, although it has been suggested that they may be powerful promoters of hepatocarcinogenesis in laboratory animals.[64]

CLINICAL FEATURES

HCC presents with right upper quadrant pain or discomfort, abdominal mass and distension. Physical examination reveals hepatomegaly in 90% of cases, wasting and ascites in 50%. Abdominal venous collaterals, if looked for, occur in 30% and icterus in 25%. A few patients may present with pathological fractures due to bone metastases. In Uganda, bone is the second most common site of metastases in HCC. Some patients have marked itching due to obstructive jaundice and about 10% may present with haematemesis and melaena following rupture of oesophageal varices in cases of advanced cirrhosis. Elevated alkaline phosphatase is detected in 75% of cases and AFP is above the normal level in 60%.

HCC affects young individuals, with remarkably high rates in the 10–29 year age group in Mozambique.[43] In Uganda the peak incidence is observed during the third and fourth decades. The male: female ratio is 2–4:1. The clinical diagnosis of HCC in the tropics is relatively simple. This is because other tumours likely to metastasize to the liver are relatively rare. Thus in the tropics any young adult male presenting with abdominal pain and mass and found to have hepatomegaly has HCC until otherwise proven. If alkaline phosphatase is elevated this raises the suspicion even further. A positive AFP almost certainly confirms the diagnosis. However, if an intervention is contemplated a needle biopsy is recommended. The most common differential diagnosis in the tropics is an amoebic liver abscess.

PROGNOSIS

HCC in the tropics runs a fulminant downhill course. The mean interval from onset to death in South African patients was 11 weeks.[65] In a study which included Algerian and French patients, the mean survival time of untreated patients was 73 days, suggesting the natural history of French patients may be similar to African and Asian patients with HCC.[66] Most patients present with a very advanced single massive tumour when first seen (Figure 24.1).

The fibrolamellar variant of HCC,[67] which occurs primarily in the young (peak in second to third decade), affects both male and female patients with non-cirrhotic livers and is rarely associated with positive AFP but has a good prognosis (average survival 44 months), is extremely rare in the tropics. No case of fibrolamellar HCC has been seen in South African Blacks.[68]

Signs of poor prognosis include wasting, abdominal venous collaterals, ascites, elevated bilirubin and encephalopathy.[66,69–71]

TREATMENT

The treatment of HCC remains unsatisfactory. Surgical resection provides the only prospect for cure. However, less than 2% present at a stage when this approach is feasible. Even apparently early cases have advanced cirrhosis and recurrence in the remaining lobe after apparently curative resection is the rule rather than the exception.

The goal of treating most patients with HCC is palliation. Hepatic artery ligation is an effective way of relieving symptoms, especially pain and in individuals who have had spontaneous intraperitoneal rupture, a common complication.[72] The rationale is based on the observation that liver tumours (primary and secondary) derive their blood supply from the hepatic artery, while normal liver is supplied from both the hepatic artery and the portal vein. Before hepatic artery ligation can be recommended the patency of the portal vein must be established.

Radiation therapy is rarely recommended because liver tissue is extremely sensitive even to low-dose radiation. However, ^{90}Y-labelled microspheres are undergoing clinical trials.

Chemotherapy appears to be an effective form of palliation. The best single agent seems to be the anthracycline doxorubicin.[71,73] The overall response rate is of the order of about 40%. A recent multicentre study conducted under the auspices of the African Organization for Research and Training in Cancer (AORTIC) showed that epirubicin and doxorubicin were equally efficacious, although the latter was more toxic (C.F. Kiire, personal communications).

Several drug combinations have been tried, with disappointing results.[73,74] The combination of doxorubicin and cisplatin has been reported to result in a dramatic response, although it was complicated by the reactivation of hepatitis B infection.[75]

It should be stressed that in tropical areas the goal of treatment of HCC is to relieve symptoms and therefore the patient's quality of life is paramount.

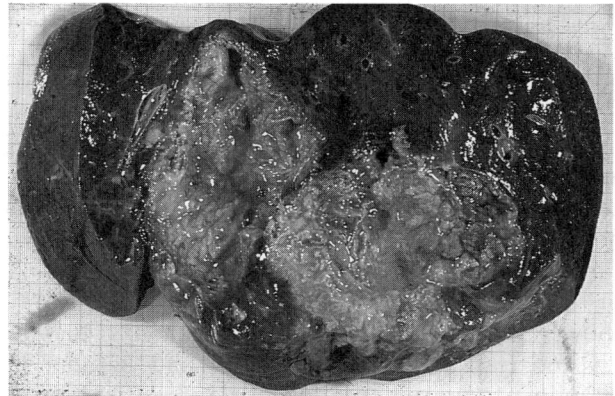

Figure 24.1 Hepatocellular carcinoma. Mass in liver.

PREVENTION

Since 80% of HCC is attributed to HBV infection and an effective vaccine against the virus is now available, the prospect for cancer prevention is now in sight.[76] A vaccination trial sponsored by the World Health Organization is underway in the Gambia, West Africa to determine its efficacy in preventing chronic liver disease and HCC in particular.[8] As HBV transmission in Africa occurs by horizontal spread, with a second wave of infection occurring at the time of school entry, it is possible to include HBV vaccine in the expanded programme of immunization.

Screening using modern imaging techniques, CT and ultrasonography, as well as serial AFP testing has been tried[77] but this approach is clearly not cost effective in many tropical countries.

CANCER OF THE OESOPHAGUS (See also Chapter 3)

Apart from the French provinces of Brittany and Normandy, which have incidence rates in excess of 80/100 000 population, cancer of the oesophagus is relatively rare in most of Europe. Outside Europe, high rates are recorded in Linxian in Northern China, in the province of Mazandarin in Iran on the Caspian sea, in East, Central and Southern Africa, India and Central America. In Linxian province of the Peoples' Republic of China the incidence rate is 130/100 000 population and oesophageal cancer is second only to stomach cancer as the leading cause of cancer deaths in China according to the 1974–1976 statistics.

In most tropical areas, cancer of the oesophagus has an uneven geographical distribution. Both rural and urban dwellers appear to be equally affected. In South Africa cancer of the oesophagus was a curiosity in the 1920s but it has now become one of the most common cancers affecting black males.[78,79] The highest rates are recorded in the Transkei: up to 63/100 000 males and 65/100 000 females. More recently, high rates have been recorded in Zimbabwe, Zambia, Malawi, parts of Tanzania and in the region around Kisumu in Kenya. By contrast oesophageal carcinoma appears to be rare in south-west Uganda, Zaire and in West Africa. In all high incidence areas there is a strong male dominance but in recent years the tumour has been increasing in frequency in women in South Africa.[80]

AETIOLOGY

Alcohol and tobacco acting together have been established as the major cause of oesophageal cancer in the industrialized world. Epidemiological studies in France show that those who smoke or drink heavily run a 44 times greater risk of oeso-phageal cancer than the light drinkers and smokers. It has been postulated that alcohol might act as a solvent facilitating the passage of carcinogens into the inner layers of the oesophagus. The role of alcohol in the causation of cancer of the oesophagus in developing countries is not clearly documented. In Iran, for instance, it is not the custom of Turkoman people to drink and very few of the oesophageal victims smoke. In China, of 527 patients 83% reported that they did not drink alcohol, and those who drank did so only on a few special occasions. In his study in South Africa, Oettle[81] concluded that smoking and alcohol use did not contribute as aetiological agents, and that the major factor appeared to be fortuitous, connected with a common African habit but not fundamental to it. In a more recent study, multiple logistic regression models identified four parameters which best discriminated cases from controls.[82] These were: smoking commercial cigarettes, smoking a pipe, eating bought (commercial) maize and eating butter or margarine. Earlier studies had indicated that 20–30% of oesophageal cancer patients had never smoked.[83] Even more at variance with the usual pattern of risk factors in the West is the apparent lack of appreciable effects of alcohol usage on the disease in Zulus. Observations in South Africa appear to lend support to nutritional predisposing factors to cancer of the oesophagus. Dietary staples appear to be low in vitamins and minerals.[84] In China and Iran oesophageal cancer may also be related to nutritional factors. It has been demonstrated that victims of oesophageal cancer are malnourished and get neither vitamin A or C nor riboflavine requirements. One study showed over 40% consumed less than 10% in winter and less than 20% in spring and autumn of vitamin A requirements. A deficiency of vitamin A has been shown to lead to carcinogenesis, while an adequate intake of vitamin C has been shown to have an anticarcinogenic effect. In China death from oesophageal cancer has been closely linked with ingestion of pickled vegetables.

In areas of Iran and China at high risk of oesophageal cancer precursor lesions of cancer of the oesophagus have been described as occurring prior to the development of invasive squamous cell carcinoma.[85,86] Unfortunately the addition of riboflavine, retinol and zinc had no effect on the high prevalence of precancerous oesophageal lesions.[87] There are several possible explanations for this negative result. First, the treatment may not have been given for a period long enough or the dosages were not large enough to effect change. Second, the precancerous oesophageal lesions, like gastritis, may be irreversible. Third, the hypothesis linking riboflavine/retinol deficiency with precancerous oesophageal lesions may not be correct.

CLINICAL FEATURES

In high incidence areas cancer of the oesophagus may be seen in the fourth and fifth decades of life. Men are 2–3 times more commonly affected, except in northern Iran, where women predominate, and in South Africa, where the frequency in women is on the increase. The disease often becomes symptomatic with progressive dysphagia and severe weight loss and wasting.

STAGING

Pretreatment evaluation for accurate staging should include history, physical examination, barium swallow, upper gastrointestinal endoscopy and biopsy and a CT scan of the thorax and upper abdomen if available. Direct laryngoscopy and bronchoscopy is advisable. Staging recommended by the American Joint Committee on Cancer (AJCC), as shown in Table 24.7, applies the tumour, node and metastasis (TNM) system. A simplified staging with its TNM equivalent is shown in Table 24.8. The following clinical, radiographic and endoscopic evidence may suggest extension of the cancer outside the oesophagus: (1) recurrent laryngeal, phrenic or sympathetic nerve involvement; (2) fistula formation; (3) tracheal or bronchial tree involvement; (4) vena caval or azygos vein obstruction; and (5) malignant effusion.

Table 24.7 AJCC staging system for cancer of the oesophagus.

Stage	Description
T_x	Minimum requirement to assess primary tumour not met
T_0	No evidence of primary tumour
T_{is}	Cancer in situ
T_1	Involves 5 cm or less of oesophageal length, producing no obstruction and no circumferential involvement and no extraoesophageal spread
T_2	Greater than 5 cm of oesophageal length without extraoesophageal spread or tumour of any size that produces obstruction
T_3	Any tumour with extraoesophageal spread
N_x	Minimum requirement for nodal assessment not met
N_0	No clinically palpable or radiological evidence of nodal involvement
N_1	Movable unilateral palpable nodes or radiological evidence of <1 cm diameter nodes
N_2	Movable bilateral palpable or radiological evidence of >1 cm, <3 cm diameter nodes
N_3	Fixed palpable nodes >3 cm on radiology
M_x	Minimum requirement to assess metastases not met
M_0	No evidence of distant metastases
M_1	Distant metastases present

Table 24.8 Simplified staging for oesophageal cancer.

Stage	TNM component	Description
0	$T_{is} N_0 M_0$	Carcinoma in situ with no invasion or spread
I	T_1, N_0, M_0	Involves <5 cm of oesophageal length with no spread or obstruction
II	$T_1, N_1; N_2; M_0$ $T_2 N_0–N_2 M_0$	Tumour causing obstruction or >5 cm in length; unilateral or bilateral palpable movable nodes
III	T_3 and N; M_0 Any T, N_3, M_0	Extraoesophageal spread, fixed palpable nodes, no distant metastases
IV	Any T, and N, M_1	Distant metastases

TREATMENT

Squamous cell carcinoma of the oesophagus is a devastating disease with long-term survival rates from unselected series of about 5%. The goal of treatment is palliation. There are several possible approaches: surgery, radiotherapy, laser therapy, intubation and combined chemoradiotherapy. Surgical mortality has dramatically improved[88–90] with most series reporting 1–2% mortality. Following 'curative' resection, the 5-year survival ranges from 8 to 22%.[91,92] Improved outlook for surgically-treated patients is the result of better preoperative and postoperative care, especially nutritional and respiratory support.

Improvements in the results of radiotherapy have been less impressive. Pearson's[93] results, with survival at 5 years of 25% for cervical, 16% for mid and 12% for lower oesophagus, remain unchallenged in Western countries. Controlled trials comparing radiotherapy with surgery are rare. Radiotherapy on its own or in addition to surgery has not altered prognosis.[94–96] Radiotherapy is frequently chosen as a means of palliation but its effectiveness may be marred by serious complications. These include fistula formation, if the tumour is adherent to the bronchus, and postirradiation stricture.

It is clear that late presentation is the limiting factor in improving results. Intubation should be reserved for patients with advanced disease and limited prognosis. Intubation provides poor palliation. Blockage of the tube is not infrequent and swallowing is far from normal.

Given the limited usefulness of both surgery[94] and radiotherapy[94] and since systemic disease is a major factor in the failure pattern, there is growing interest in neoadjuvant trials (giving chemotherapy before definitive primary surgery).[97] Animal models have suggested the superiority of giving systemic therapy prior to surgery. In addition, preoperative chemotherapy allows an in vivo assessment of tumour sensitivity to the drugs.

More recently concurrent chemoradiotherapy is being advocated. This was based on promising observations of a similar approach for anal canal and rectal cancers. Preliminary observations reported greatly improved palliation as well as improved 12- and 24-month survival rates using preoperative chemoradiotherapy.[98] At Wayne State University the approach utilized 5-fluorouracil and mitomycin-C, later changed to 5-fluorouracil and cisplatin (because of the unpredictable toxicity of mitomycin-C), concurrently with radiotherapy.[99,100] The choice of 5-fluorouracil and cisplatin is based on their known antitumour activity in oesophageal cancer and because they are established radiation sensitizers.[101–103] Apart from possible radiosensitization of hypoxic cells, other mechanisms postulated include inhibition of repair of sublethal or potentially lethal damage, increased induction of chromosomal aberrations and binding to thiols. The pathological complete response is about 25–30%. Such combined chemoradiotherapy appears to provide excellent palliation but no studies have been done to assess the quality of life of patients undergoing such treatment. The toxicity encountered includes nausea, vomiting, oesophagitis, mucositis, stomatitis, leucopenia and thrombocytopenia.

MALIGNANT TUMOURS OF THE SKIN (See also Chapter 11)

The skin is sometimes referred to as the window of human biology and pathology because many processes of life are reflected on the body surface. In addition, the skin is the largest organ of the body.

In light-pigmented people, i.e. inhabitants of Europe and North America, exposure to solar ultraviolet light is responsible for the very high incidence of skin cancers such as basal cell and squamous cell cancers and melanomas. Other factors which may influence the frequency and distribution of skin cancers include occupation, clothing, hairstyles and leisure habits, all of which determine the degree of exposure to the ultraviolet component of the sun.

Dark-skinned individuals appear to be well adjusted to the hot tropical environments. The protective and adaptive elements include the increased melanin and the large number of sweat glands. The dark pigment absorbs heat readily, such that 'sun bathing' is not a comfortable activity for dark-skinned people, contrary to the general belief that dark-skinned people enjoy heat! In any case, more suntan is not needed and not prized. Ultraviolet-related skin cancers are commonly observed in individuals with certain genetic abnormalities such as albinism, a group of inherited conditions in which there is a defect in melanin production and metabolism. Decreased pigmentation is particularly noticeable in the skin, hair and eyes. The skin becomes dry and wrinkled on exposure to sunlight. Albinos develop multiple skin tumours (basal cell and squamous cell), usually in the exposed areas of the body (head, neck, ears, conjunctiva and limbs). It is estimated that albinos are one thousand times more likely to develop basal cell cancers than pigmented people. Another genetic disorder associated with skin cancers is xeroderma pigmentosum, an inherited defect of DNA repair following ultraviolet-induced damage.[6,7]

SQUAMOUS CELL CANCER

Squamous cell cancer of the skin is common in some tropical populations, especially in poverty-stricken rural areas. In the tropics squamous cell cancers are clinically and aetiologically distinct from those seen in Europe. The majority arise in areas of damaged skin, most frequently in scars of long-standing tropical ulcers (Figure 24.2), old burns or epithelialized sinuses. In Uganda the annual incidence of squamous cell cancer is 1.70 men and 1.33 women per 100 000 population; it accounts for 12% of all malignancies. This relative frequency is similar to what has been observed in other tropical areas as far apart as Nigeria in West Africa and the Solomon Islands in the South Pacific. Squamous cell cancer may also occur as a result of certain cultural practices, such as the Kangri cancer of India.

Since about 80% of these cancers are superimposed upon or complicate long-standing tropical ulcers, the increased availability of clean water, soap and to a lesser extent antibiotics may lead to marked decline of these tumours in the tropics. However, once the tumour is established wide surgical excision of the localized lesion remains the treatment of choice. The role of radiotherapy and chemotherapy in the management of these tumours is not well documented.

MALIGNANT MELANOMA

Malignant melanomas arise from the cells that produce skin pigmentation. Malignant melanomas of the skin occur most commonly in those areas of the world where light-skinned people by default live in an environment of abundant sunshine, e.g. Australia, Israel and South Africa. Sunbathing is a popular summer relaxation with light-skinned people. In dark-skinned persons the primary site of malignant melanoma is on the non-pigmented sole of the foot (Figure 24.3) or less commonly on the palmar side of the hands or fingers. It is extremely rare for dark-skinned people to develop melanoma in a pigmented site. If they do there is often preceding vitiligo. Vitiligous patches, if looked for, can often be found concurrently at other sites in dark-skinned patients with malignant melanoma.

It is probable that melanomas arise from preexisting naevi, but because of the generally dark skin colour, changes that predict malignant change may be difficult to observe and overlooked, especially if the primary lesion is located on the sole of the foot. Thus malignant melanoma tends to present at a very advanced stage as an exophytic fungating lesion with or without regional adenopathy. It has been suggested that trauma (physical, chemical or thermal) may play a role in the aetiology of these tumours in the tropics. There has, however, been no reduction of incidence observed among shoe-wearing urban dwellers in the tropics.

There is a clear relationship between thickness of the tumour and survival.[104] Early melanoma is potentially curable by wide excision. In the past the accepted surgical approach was a wide excision with a 5 cm margin. The current trend is towards a narrower margin tailoring to tumour thickness.[105] In general for tumours less than 1 mm thickness, a 1 cm

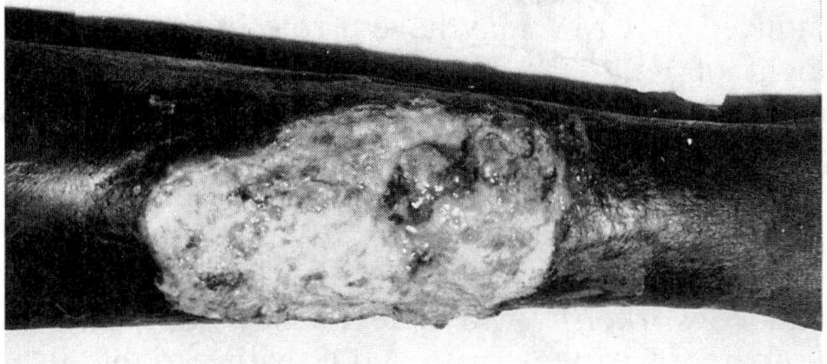

Figure 24.2 Squamous cell carcinoma in long-standing tropical ulcer. (Courtesy of E.H. Williams).

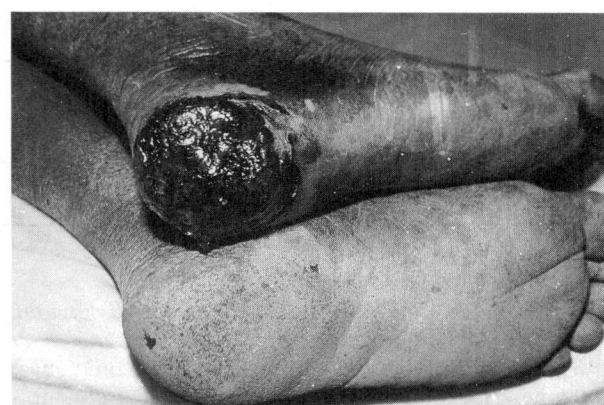

Figure 24.3 Malignant melanoma on sole of foot. (Courtesy of E.H. Williams.)

margin is adequate, while 2–3 cm margins are recommended for thicker tumours. The role of elec-tive node dissection, radiotherapy, chemotherapy and immunotherapy remains to be defined.

KAPOSI'S SARCOMA (See also Chapter 12)

Kaposi's sarcoma (KS) is a tumour that commonly presents with skin involvement, although visceral and bone tumours are frequently observed. Epidemiologically KS can be classified into sporadic, endemic and epidemic forms (Table 24.9). The sporadic (classic) form represents what was originally described in 1872 by Moritz Kaposi. It is commonly seen in elderly males of Jewish, South European and Mediterranean origin. The endemic form was described in sub-Saharan Africa, especially Eastern Zaire and Western Uganda, with decreasing incidence from this 'epicentre'. The epidemic form was first described in the large North American cities of New York and Los Angeles and is associated with human immunodeficiency virus (HIV) infection.

Aggressive forms of KS were observed in Uganda and Zambia at about the same time as the epidemic variety was described in North America. The distribution of AIDS in Africa corresponds closely to that of the endemic pre-epidemic KS. There is often confusion as to the nature of a particular case. There are no reliable figures for incidence of epidemic AIDS-related KS in the tropics. In the USA the incidence of KS complicating AIDS is actually on the decline.[106] At the beginning of the epidemic 35–40% of reported AIDS cases had KS. The incidence appears to have dropped and currently about 14% of AIDS cases have KS. This may be due to early mortality from opportunistic infections. In the Ivory Coast 9.3% of AIDS patients have KS and only 1.1% of AIDS deaths are due to it.

All forms of KS (sporadic, endemic and epidemic) share similar histological features, including lymphatic and vascular proliferations, spindle cell formation and mononuclear cell infiltration.

Table 24.9 Clinicoepidemiological correlation of Kaposi's sarcoma.

Epidemiology	Clinical Form	Behaviour
Sporadic	Nodular	Indolent
Endemic	Nodular, plaque	Indolent
	Florid	Aggressive
Epidemic	Generalized	Aggressive

AETIOLOGY AND PATHOGENESIS

Kaposi's sarcoma is one of the tumours that is known to develop in iatrogenically immunosuppressed renal transplant recipients.[107] Anecdotal reports of spontaneous regression of KS in such patients upon discontinuation of immunosuppressive therapy supports the relationship between the integrity of the immune system and the development of KS.[108,109] However, there have been cases of AIDS-related KS with no clinical or laboratory evidence of impaired immunity. Available data do suggest that activation of the immune system may play a role in the pathogenesis of AIDS-related KS.[110] In case of endemic African KS, multiple parasitic infestations, including malaria and bacterial and viral infections, could be the source of continuous activation. In classic KS high levels of anti-cytomegalovirus (CMV) antibodies have been reported.

The multiple and disseminated nature of KS suggests a role of unique circulating transforming growth factors locally produced.[111] HIV-infected T cells, monocytes and transformed cells produce growth factors and viral regulatory protein (Tat protein) that result in autocrine and paracrine stimulation of host cell proliferation and viral expression.[112] Most of these cytokines (as growth factors are generally called) are angiogenesis factors which stimulate vascular endothelial cell proliferation and new blood vessel formation. Cytochemical and phenotypic marker studies have demonstrated KS cells to have features of vascular channel and endothelial cell lineage.[113]

It has been suggested that cell transformation induced by CMV may have a role in the development of KS.[114,115] However, DNA hybridization experiments indicate that only a small subset of KS samples (15–20%) contain CMV-DNA sequences, which in some cases may have been derived from productively infected cells.[116,117] In vitro DNA amplification techniques (PCR), described by Saiki and co-workers,[118] to detect CMV footprints in tumours of patients with AIDS with variable incidence of KS led to the conclusion that CMV infection is probably unrelated to the development of KS in patients with AIDS. HIV genome appears to be absent in AIDS-related KS tissue. Other factors may play a cofactor role in tumorigenesis, e.g. CMV in KS and Epstein–Barr virus (EBV) in lymphomas.[119] However, irrespective of the underlying aetiology the final common pathway appears similar to all, hence the uniform morphological features.

CLINICAL FEATURES

There are features which distinguish epidemic AIDS-related KS from endemic African KS. These include peak age at presentation, sex distribution, clinical course and response to therapy (Table 24.10). In addition, opportunistic infections are commonly observed in epidemic KS. In the tropics tuberculosis is the most common infection related to HIV, while *Pneumocystis carinii* is rare.[120] 'Slim disease', a clinical syndrome dominated by chronic diarrhoea and weight loss, is a common presentation.[121] In some parts of Africa enteropathic AIDS (slim disease) accounts for over 70% of AIDS cases. The cause is as yet unknown, but the protozoa *Cryptosporidium parvum*, *Isospora belli* and *Enterozoa* are likely to be involved. In the tropics there are no real high-risk groups for HIV infection, as is the case in Europe and North America where homosexuality and intravenous drug abuse are high-risk factors. In the tropics HIV is spread by heterosexual contact. Blood screening is not universally practised and non-screened blood may be a common mechanism of spread as well.

Endemic KS presents mostly with unilateral limb oedema and skin nodules (Figure 24.4). Nodules may arise in the subcutaneous tissue (nodular form) (Figure 24.5) or from deeper than the deep fascia and may resemble granuloma pyogenicum (florid form). Visceral involvement is frequent. The lymphadenopathic form of KS is rare in endemic form except in children[122] but is common in epidemic AIDS-related KS. Complications reported include haematemesis,[123] intestinal obstruction,[124] perfo-

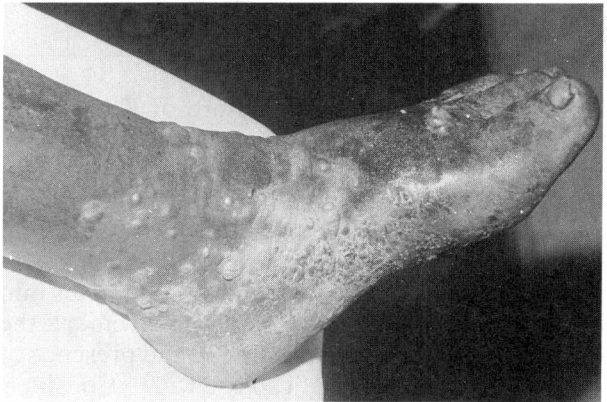

Figure 24.4 Endemic Kaposi's sarcoma. Tumour nodule on foot with oedema. (Courtesy of E.H. Williams.)

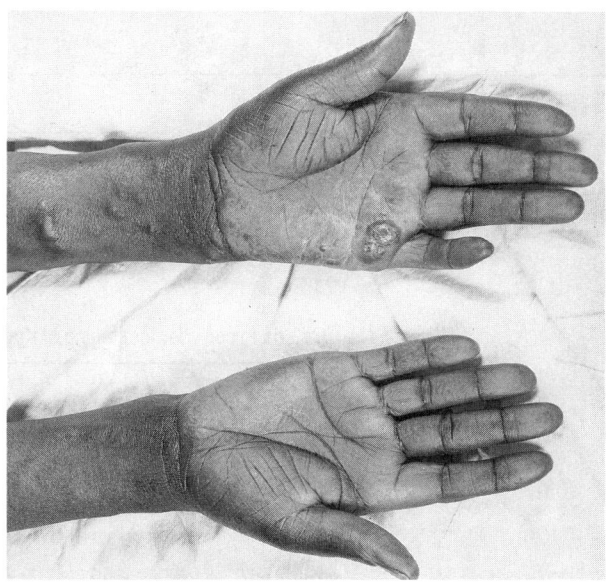

Figure 24.5 Endemic Kaposi's sarcoma of the hands showing tumour nodules. (Courtesy of E.H. Williams.)

ration,[125] diarrhoea with protein-losing enteropathy[126] and intussusception.[127] Studies from East Africa have suggested that visceral involvement may occur frequently, despite a lack of abdominal or pulmonary symptoms and signs.[128,129] The epidemic AIDS-related KS presents with a combination of marked cachexia, skin hyperpigmentation and oropharyngeal involvement. The oropharynx may either exhibit purple KS nodules or ulcerations and plaques due to tumour or secondary fungal infections. Visceral involvement, especially pulmonary, is common. Systemic symptoms of fever, diaphoresis and weight loss are of prognostic significance.

Table 24.10 Clinical features of Kaposi's sarcoma.

Feature	Endemic	Epidemic
Age (years)	40–50	20–30
Gender M:F	12:1	2–3:1
Clinical course	Indolent Aggressive	Always aggressive
Treatment response	Excellent	Poor
Prognosis	Good–excellent	Poor

STAGING

Because of the multicentric nature of KS, staging has been difficult. The four-stage classification originally described by Krigel and co-workers[130] included epidemic as well as non-epidemic forms of disease. The staging system of Mitsuyasu and Groopman[131] was designed especially for classification of epidemic AIDS-related KS and takes into consideration the extent of tumour involvement, the presence of systemic symptoms and the presence of opportunistic infections (Table 24.11). Considerable data also support the use of immunological staging as a predictor of both survival and response to therapy. Patients with systemic symptoms are likely to have a low number of CD^4 cells and low $CD^4:CD^8$ ratios. The poor prognosis of such patients is related to the presence of opportunistic infections.[132]

TREATMENT

Studies from Uganda indicated that nodular and plaque forms of endemic KS respond to simple therapies, including oral alkylating agents.[133,134] The more aggressive endemic forms responded well to combination chemotherapy consisting of actinomycin D, vincristine and imidazole carboximide.[135] Localized endemic forms respond well to radiotherapy. Aggressive multiagent chemotherapy exacerbates the existing immune impairment of patients with epidemic AIDS-related KS and such combination chemotherapy not only worsens the prognosis but may increase mortality. Studies are underway to ascertain whether hemibody radiation or oral single agents may improve the quality of life of these patients.

AIDS-ASSOCIATED TUMOURS

The coexistence of classic KS and endemic KS with other malignancies, especially of the lymphoreticular system, has previously been documented.[136,137] KS is the most common malignancy complicating AIDS. Initial Centers for Disease Control (CDC) criteria for diagnosis of AIDS included occurrence of opportunistic infections and KS with unexplained immunosuppression.

Table 24.11a   Criteria to consider for staging of Kaposi's sarcoma.

Feature	Good risk (all of following)	Poor risk (any of following)
Tumour (T)	Confined to skin and/or lymph nodes and/or minimal oral disease	Tumour-associated oedema or ulceration
		Extensive oral KS Gastrointestinal or visceral KS
Immune system (I)	CD^4 cells $\geq 300/\mu$l	CD^4 cells $< 300/\mu$l
Systemic illness (S)	No history of opportunistic infection or thrush No systemic symptoms	History of opportunistic infection or thrush Systemic symptoms

Table 24.11b   Suggested staging for epidemic Kaposi's sarcoma.

Stage	Characteristics
I	No prior or coexisting opportunistic infection. No systemic symptoms, CD^4 $>300/\mu$l
II	No prior or coexisting opportunistic infection. No systemic symptoms, CD^4 $<300/\mu$l
III	No prior or coexisting opportunistic infection. Systemic symptoms
IV	Prior or coexisting opportunistic infection

Table 24.12 HIV-associated conditions.

HIV-associated malignancies
Kaposi's sarcoma*
Non-Hodgkin's lymphoma
  Intermediate grade
  High grade*
Primary CNS lymphoma*
Hodgkin's disease

Possible HIV-associated diseases
Cervical dysplasia
Paediatric smooth muscle tumours
T-cell non-Hodgkin's lymphoma

*AIDS-defining disease.

Other AIDS-related tumours include malignant lymphomas, cloagenic cancer of the anorectum, squamous cell cancer of the tongue, cervical dysplasia and soft tissue sarcomas of children (Table 24.12). CDC indicate that 2.9% of AIDS patients had non-Hodgkin's lymphomas, a rate of 60 times greater than the general population.[138] Lymphomas are predominantly high-grade B-cell non-Hodgkin's lymphomas, usually immunoblastic, and Burkitt's lymphomas with dismal prognosis; response to chemotherapy does not translate to improved survival. Age appears to be an important factor in the lymphoma subtype. The incidence of the immunoblastic type increases steadily with age, while Burkitt's lymphoma occurs mostly in the 10–19 year age group. Usually at diagnosis 75% of AIDS lymphomas have stage III/IV disease, often with extranodal involvement including the central nervous system and marrow.

Cervical dysplasia has been found with greater frequency in women with HIV infection.[139] In one study cervical dysplasia was found in 41% of females with HIV infection versus 9% for HIV-negative intravenous drug users and 4% in the general population.[140] Anorectal (cloagenic) tumours, and in particular those associated with certain strains of HPV, have a notably aggressive course in both men and women with HIV.[141,142]

Children infected with HIV may have an increased risk of developing a variety of smooth muscle tumours that do not commonly arise in the setting of other immunodeficiency diseases.[143] Leiomyosarcoma is particularly common[144] and, given the low incidence of this tumour in the paediatric age group, its association with HIV is unlikely to be due to chance.

BURKITT'S LYMPHOMA (See also Chapter 32)

Burkitt's lymphoma (BL) is a malignant lymphoma of B-cell origin. Dr Burkitt,[145] a British surgeon working in Kampala, Uganda, drew attention to the fact that some features of this disease occurred with certain repetitiveness. Other observers had noted similar tumours presenting at separate sites like jaws, orbits, ovaries, kidneys, adrenals, thyroid, testes and breasts and had concluded that they were all separate entities. Dr Burkitt felt that although the involved sites varied from patient to patient, a pattern emerged that suggested a unitary process. He then undertook a journey around Africa (the famous 'tumour safari') and was able to map out the geographical distribution of this tumour within Africa. He further observed that the distribution was very similar to the malaria map and suggested that the tumour might be caused by an arthropod (mosquito)-borne virus. Subsequently, at a conference on lymphoreticular tumours held in Paris in 1963, it was unanimously agreed to give the tumour the eponym Burkitt's lymphoma in recognition of his pioneering work. Soon after, Dalldorf (1964) reaffirmed that the distribution of BL was related to that of holo- or hyperendemic malaria.

EPIDEMIOLOGY

Burkitt's lymphoma is restricted to the geographical latitudes 10–15° north and south of the equator and to altitudes below 1500 metres. It is rare in places where the diurnal temperature drops to below 16°C frequently and in places where the rainfall is less than 50 cm per annum. Outside tropical Africa BL is found in those areas of the tropical belt with the above climatic conditions, namely Papua New Guinea. In these endemic regions BL accounts for more than 50% of childhood tumours.

The highest incidence of BL is in the West Nile district of Uganda where the number recorded approaches 13/100 000 population. It is in the same area where time–space clustering has been recorded.[146] A time trend has also been observed and over the last decade there has been a noticeable

Table 24.13 Comparison between endemic and sporadic Burkitt's lymphoma.

Features	*Endemic*	*Sporadic*
Epidemiology	Related to climate	Unrelated
	Very common in children	Rare in children
EBV association	>95% are associated with EBV	Rarely associated with EBV
Chromosomal translocations	Invariably found	Invariably found
Clinical features	Presents commonly with jaw tumour; nodal disease rare	Presents commonly with abdominal, nodal, marrow disease
	Long-term survival with simple therapy	Long-term survival only after aggressive therapy

downward trend in the number of cases diagnosed both in Uganda and Tanzania. In Ibadan, Nigeria it is estimated that the incidence is 15/100 000 children aged 5–9 years. Outside this endemic belt, sporadic cases of BL have been observed in the USA, Europe and the Middle East. More recently several cases have been noted in association with the AIDS epidemic.[147] The clinical features of these non-endemic cases differ from those of the endemic forms (Table 24.13).

AETIOLOGY

Burkitt's lymphoma has provoked extensive tumour investigations because of its possible aetiological association with EBV, the influence of malaria, the specific chromosomal abnormality, the role of oncogenes in lymphomagenesis, and the role of growth factors in tumourigenesis.

EPSTEIN-BARR VIRUS

EBV was initially discovered in 1964 in cells from endemic BL.[148] For a long time it has been a forerunner as a candidate for an oncogenic virus. For a virus to be considered oncogenic it has to fulfil certain criteria. These criteria (Henle–Koch's postulates) include:

- The ability of the candidate virus to transform in vitro.
- The finding of significant immune response to viral products in patients compared with controls.
- The detection of viral tumour markers, e.g. viral genomes, and viral products, e.g. antigens, in the tumour.
- The ability of the candidate virus to cause malignant tumours in vivo.

EBV is known to transform human B lymphocytes in vitro; patients with BL have a significantly higher EBV serological response (viral capsid antigen, VCA; early antigen, EA; EB-determined nuclear antigen, EBNA) than controls and Burkitt's tumours carry footprints of the virus (EBV genome), detected either as EBV-DNA or EBNA.[149] In addition, EBV can transform B lymphocytes of some simian hosts, and these transformed cells can grow progressively, and kill, after reimplantation into the original autochthonous host. In marmoset and owl monkeys EBV has direct oncogenic activity: it can induce lymphomas and these tumours carry the EBV genome.

In the large seroepidemiologic study carried out in the West Nile district of Uganda, more than 40 000 children were bled and followed up for several years to determine the features of those that developed BL.[150] The hypotheses tested were that BL was due to delayed EBV infection, as in infectious mononucleosis; that EBV is a passenger virus and that BL developed in children heavily and chronically infected with EBV. During the follow-up period 14 children with previously stored sera developed BL. This and other studies led to the conclusion that BL was not due to delayed infection as patients developing BL seroconverted 6–24 months prior to BL becoming manifest. High VCA titre was not protective; on the contrary it favoured the development of BL. The failure to detect EBV genome in non-BL tumours, although these tumours came from individuals with positive EBV serology, negated the passenger hypothesis.[151]

Although EBV has more or less fulfilled the Henle–Koch's postulates, there are still a number of features that do not fit. For instance, EBV is ubiquitous and yet BL is only found in restricted areas of the world. Even in the so-called endemic belt very few patients succumb to the disease. EBV-DNA is only associated with endemic BL. The non-endemic, e.g. American, BL only very rarely contains EBV-DNA. Even in Africa only 90% of BL tumours are EBV genome positive. Thus EBV is not absolutely necessary in the development of BL. The role of malaria in endemic BL may be to facilitate the development of lymphoma through either polyclonal B-cell proliferation and/or T-cell immuno-suppression. Malaria prophylaxis was started in the North Mara province of Tanzania and this appeared to coincide with a downward trend. However, the curious geographical distribution of endemic BL in sub-Saharan Africa and in Papua New Guinea is best explained on the basis of malaria endemicity. In addition, recent studies in Uganda have suggested that other non-Burkitt, non-Hodgkin's lymphomas may also be related to malaria endemicity.[152]

CHROMOSOMAL ABNORMALITIES

Manolov and Manolova first reported a characteristic chromosome abnormality in BL in 1972. Part of the long arm of chromosome 8 was translocated to the long arm of chromosome 14.[153] Ninety per cent of BL tumours have this translocation, which always involved the same bands of the two chromosomes, namely band q24 of chromosome 8 and band q32 of chromosome 14. The remaining 10% of BL tumours exhibited two variant translocations: a reciprocal translocation involving q24 of 8 with either band p11 of chromosome 2 or band q11 of chromosome 22. These translocations were observed in all BL tumours irrespective of EBV genome status and whether they were endemic or non-endemic.

HUMAN IMMUNOGLOBULINS

It was later discovered that the genes for human immunoglobulin heavy chains are located on band q32 of chromosome 14, whereas the genes for the κ and λ light chains are on band p11 of chromosome 2 and band q11 of chromosome 22 respectively. George Klein predicted that chromosome 8 probably carried an oncogene and the translocation was transferring this oncogene close to the immuno-globulin gene. His predictions have been borne out. The c-*myc* oncogene has been identified on band q24 of chromosome 8. It is believed they may have an immortalization function. In other words, while the translocation of the c-*myc* oncogene close to an immunoglobulin constant region is a constant feature, this, though necessary, is not sufficient to cause tumour. A second oncogene, B-*lym* of N-*ras*, appears to be needed to complete the neoplastic transformation.

CLINICAL FEATURES

BL presents usually with jaw swelling (75%), abdominal swelling (60%) and central nervous system involvement (30%). Patients with jaw swellings generally present with maxillary involvement more commonly than mandibular tumour. Maxillary tumour often spreads upwards to involve the orbit (Figure 24.6). Bilateral maxillary tumour is common. Bilateral mandibular disease is rare unless all four quadrants are involved. Patients present complaining of loose teeth, and a lateral oblique radiograph of the jaw reveals loss of lamina dura. Abdominal swelling is a presenting feature in about 60% of patients, usually more so in females than in males. Almost any organ within the abdomen can and does get involved in the tumorous process and often malignant ascites is an accompanying feature. Central nervous system involvement is seen in about 30% of patients at presentation. This may be either as cranial nerve palsy (III, VI, VII commonly) or paraplegia or just malignant CSF pleocytosis alone. The peak age at presentation is 4–9 years. The tumour is unseen below 1 year, less than 1% under 2 years and peaks from 4 to 9 years, and then falls off such that less than 5% of patients are under 15 years of age.

The diagnosis of BL is often evident because of the clinical presentation in a child from an endemic area. However, histological confirmation must always be sought as other tumours, notably

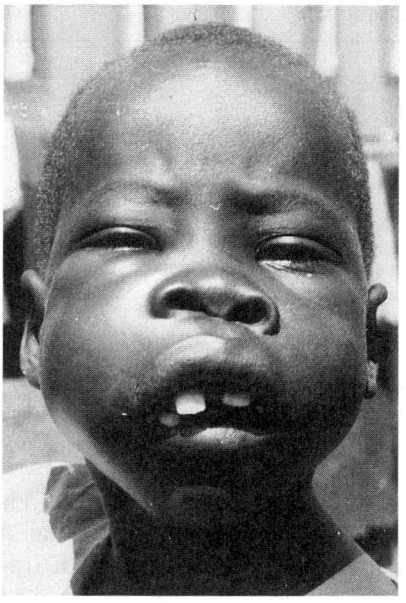

Figure 24.6 Burkitt's lymphoma. Jaw tumour.

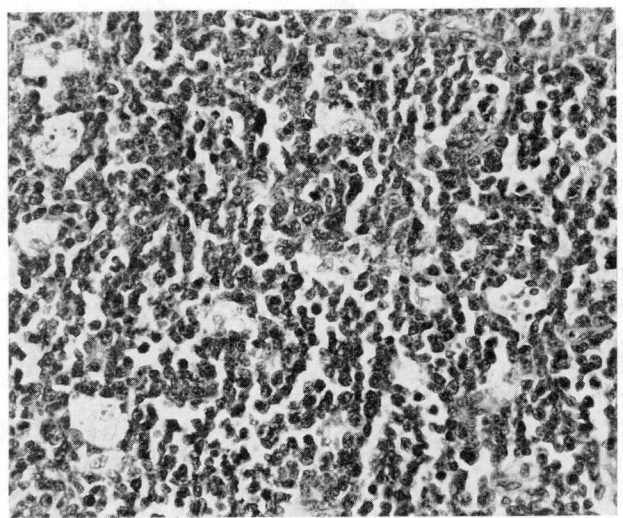

Figure 24.7   Burkitt's lymphoma. 'Starry sky' picture.

embryonal rhabdomyosarcoma, neuroblastoma, lymphoblastic lymphoma and Wilms' tumour, may all mimic BL. Histologically the classical 'starry sky' picture (Figure 24.7) is suggestive of BL and is due to the presence of large numbers of phagocytic macrophages among tumour cells.

STAGING

The staging system commonly applied to endemic BL was suggested by Ziegler and Magrath. It is based on the volume of tumour and reflects prognosis (Table 24.14).

Table 24.14   Staging of Burkitt's lymphoma

Stage	Feature
A	Solitary extra-abdominal site
AR	Resected intra-abdominal tumour
B	Multiple extra-abdominal sites
C	Intra-abdominal tumour
D	Abdominal tumour with sites of tumour other than facial

CELL KINETICS

Burkitt's lymphoma is a very rapidly growing tumour. It is the fastest growing tumour in man and has been referred to as the human equivalent of the L1210 mouse model. BL has a growth fraction of 100%, mean cell cycle time of 26 hours and observed volume doubling time of 2.8 days.

TREATMENT

Because of the peculiar cell kinetics BL is extremely responsive to drug therapy and is one of the early tumours noted to be curable by drugs alone. However, the management of this tumour requires a multidisciplinary approach. The role of surgery includes biopsy for diagnosis, spinal cord decompression and insertion of an Ommaya reservoir, but, most importantly, debulking. BL is one of the tumours where debulk surgery has been clearly shown to be beneficial.[154] An attempt should be made by the surgeon to remove as much tumour (>90%) as possible. In case of bilateral ovarian involvement this means bilateral oophorectomy. Patients who have had more than 90% of their tumour taken out surgically have a survival advantage equal to those with early stage I or A disease. If the surgeon cannot remove sufficient tumour, removal of less tumour does not influence prognosis. BL is a radiosensitive tumour but because of its peculiar rapid growth conventional radiotherapy is ineffective as the tumour regrows between each day's therapy. This problem is circumvented by superfractionation of each day's dose of irradiation into three treatments given 4 hours apart. However, prophylactic craniospinal irradiation failed to show any value in preventing or delaying central nervous system relapse.[155]

The treatment of choice for BL is chemotherapy. The single most effective agent is cyclophosphamide. Although single-agent cyclophosphamide is as effective as a three-drug combination consisting of cyclophosphamide, vincristine and methotrexate (COM), the combination is superior in preventing systemic relapse.[156] All in all about 80% of patients achieve complete tumour regression, 10% partial response. About 50% will relapse: those who relapse early, within 3 months, do poorly, while those who relapse late, after 3 months, respond well even to initial induction agents.[157] Patients remaining relapse-free after 1 year can be considered cured and the overall relapse-free survival at 10 years is 35–50%.[158]

PREVENTION

Dr Epstein[159,160] and his colleagues have developed an EB vaccine using the high molecular weight glycoprotein component of EBV membrane antigen. This vaccine conferred 100% protection against a lymphomagenic dose of EBV in the cotton-top tamarine (a South American marmoset). Preliminary safety studies are under way. It will be necessary to ascertain its efficacy in preventing infectious

mononucleosis, and then BL and nasopharyngeal carcinoma.

NASOPHARYNGEAL CARCINOMA (See also Chapter 32)

INCIDENCE AND GEOGRAPHICAL DISTRIBUTION

Nasopharyngeal carcinoma (NPC) is an uncommon tumour in the white populations of Europe and North America but has long been recognized as an important problem in parts of the Far East, particularly southern China. In regions which have a high incidence the tumours are poorly differentiated, non-keratinizing squamous cell carcinomas and often show a heavy infiltration with lymphocytes and other inflammatory cells. This feature gave rise to the old term lymphoepithelioma. These tumours appear to be aetiologically distinct from the well-differentiated squamous cell carcinomas that may occur anywhere in old people. The highest incidence rates are found in the southern provinces of China, particularly around Guandong, and in Hong Kong and Singapore, where rates of between 12 and 20/ 100 000 are recorded. There is also a high incidence in the Chinese population of Malaysia, Thailand, Indonesia and Hawaii. NPC is some 20 times more common in the Chinese population of Malaysia than in Indians living there. The incidence of NPC in south-east Asia is directly related to the degree of inbreeding with immigrant populations from southern China.

Regions of intermediate frequency (from 1.5 to 9/ 100 000 a year) are found in several parts of Africa; these include the highland areas of Kenya, parts of the Sudan, Tunisia, Morocco and Algeria. In some of these countries the age distribution of the tumour shows two peaks with the first occurring between 10 and 20 years.

AETIOLOGY

The high incidence of NPC in peoples of southern Chinese descent who live in different environments, often contrasting with a low incidence in neighbouring ethnic groups, is suggestive of a genetic factor. HLA-typing has shown that Cantonese Chinese with A2, B17, BW46 haplotypes have an increased risk of developing NPC.

EPSTEIN-BARR VIRUS

Clinical disorders associated with EBV include infectious mononucleosis, endemic BL and NPC. In infectious mononucleosis both IgG and IgM antibodies directed at the VCA are detected. Nuclear antigen antibodies are absent as these develop 2–6 months after initial infection. The relationship between NPC and EBV was postulated on the basis of the finding of antibodies to EBV in the serum and the identification of viral genomes by in situ hybridization of epithelial tumour cells.[161] In NPC IgG specific to EBV EA is often present as well as the IgA directed against VCA. There is a correlation with the histological classification (Table 24.15), with the keratinizing squamous cell type (type I) having a much lower incidence of positive antibodies than the non-keratinizing or undifferentiated types.

Until recently EBV was considered to be exclusively a B-lymphotropic herpes virus and the observed presence of EBV in epithelial cells in NPC was difficult to explain. However, EBV receptors have now been demonstrated on, and virus binding to, the surface of epithelial cells.

Table 24.15 World Health Organization classification of nasopharyngeal carcinoma and EBV antibodies.

Classification	Description	EBV antibodies	
		IgG-EA (%)	*IgA-VCA (%)*
Type I	Keratinizing squamous cell	35	16
Type II	Non-keratinizing squamous cell	94	84
Type III	Undifferentiated carcinoma	83	89

DIETARY FACTORS

It has been observed that ethnic differences in similar geographical regions (e.g. Southern China) are associated with marked variations in the frequency of NPC and that these differences may be related to dietary habits. Evidence of the causative role of salted fish, especially if it is consumed early in life, has been postulated. Relatively high levels of nitrosamines have been identified in Cantonese salted fish and extracts have been shown to activate EBV in Raji cells (a BL cell line) in vitro.[162]

CLINICAL FEATURES

The diagnosis of NPC is often difficult because the nasopharynx is hard to visualize and the primary lesion tends to infiltrate submucosally and can easily be missed in a superficial biopsy.

Many cases of NPC are diagnosed late or remain undiagnosed until they present with clinical nodes without an obvious primary site.[163] The majority of patients seen with NPC in East Africa present with enlarged, often massive, cervical lymph nodes which may be mistaken for tuberculosis or malignant lymphoma (Figure 24.8). In some instances lymphadenopathy is a late phenomenon and such patients have, in addition, multiple cranial nerve palsies and

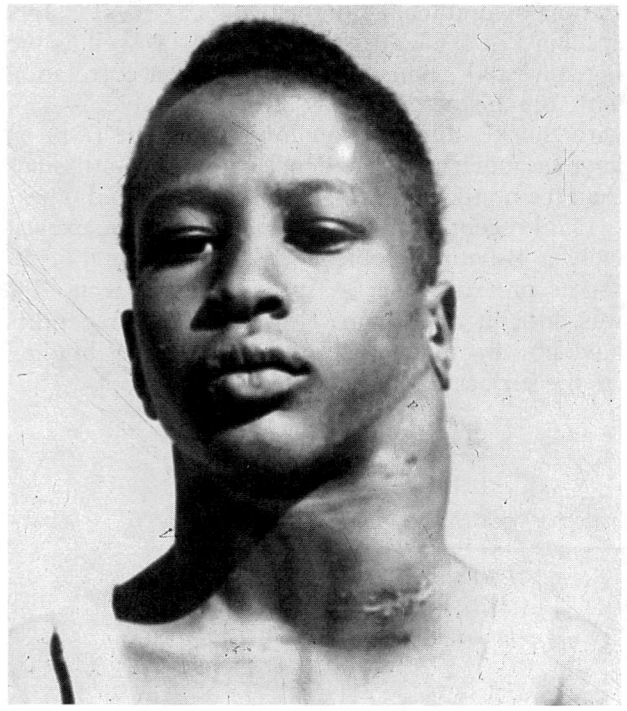

Figure 24.8 Nasopharyngeal carcinoma with massive cervical lymphadenopathy. (Courtesy of M.A.O. Malik.)

pain due to tumour extension through the base of the skull. A small percentage (about 5%) present only with cranial nerve palsies. Because of the location of the primary tumour patients may present with blockage of the eustachian tube causing otitis media. Thus any adult with persistent or recurrent otitis media should be suspected of having NPC. Less frequently patients may present with nasal blockage or epistaxis.

TREATMENT

Radiotherapy is the primary treatment of NPC regardless of the stage. The recommended dose is 6500–7000 cGy delivered to a port encompassing the nasopharynx as well as the base of the skull. Often a boost to the nasopharynx is considered, using intracavitary implants.[164] Surgery plays a limited role and is usually reserved for salvage therapy of residual cervical nodal disease. Several cytotoxic agents show activity in NPC. These include methotrexate, bleomycin, 5-fluorouracil, doxorubicin, cisplatin and vinblastine. Combination chemotherapy has often been given in sequential fashion with radiotherapy.[165] Concurrent chemoradiotherapy applying radiosensitizers, notably cisplatin, is undergoing clinical trial.

In most tropical areas mortality from NPC is high because patients present at a very advanced disease stage and most do not have access to radiotherapy facilities. Whenever possible focus should be placed on prevention.

PREVENTION

Because 10–20% of healthy donors may have false-positive EBV antibodies, these may not be very useful for screening. However, some success using serological tests for EBV have been demonstrated in China.[166] In a study involving 67 891 healthy subjects, 9% were found to have elevation of IgA-VCA ($\geq$1:10). Of the 6102 with high titres, 48 (0.8%) were found on mirror examination to have obvious NPC. Endoscopic examination and blind biopsy of 130 randomly selected from the remaining 6054 individuals detected NPC in 5.4%.[166] Thus serological screening should be considered for high-risk populations.

Prevention should also focus on dietary education. The prospect for vaccination is in sight (see section on Burkitt's lymphoma, above). Such vaccines may be of value for high-risk groups.

ORAL AND OROPHARYNGEAL CARCINOMA

INCIDENCE AND GEOGRAPHICAL DISTRIBUTION

Mouth cancer is the most common cancer in South-East Asia, home of one-fifth of the world's population. Squamous cell carcinoma of the mucosa of the oral cavity and oropharynx is a tumour whose incidence is closely related to particular cultural habits. There is a high incidence in most of the populations of the Indian subcontinent and in peoples of Indian extraction living in other countries of the Far East such as Singapore, Sri Lanka, Thailand and Vietnam. These types of cancer account for nearly 50% of cancer patients registered at the Tata Memorial Hospital in Bombay, and incidence rates of over 20/100 000 have been recorded in some districts of India. In Malaysia these tumours account for 30% of all malignancies, and in Sri Lanka and India approximately 35–40% of all cancers occur in the oral cavity, compared with only 2–3% in the UK and USA.[167,168] Low rates are observed in Chinese and an intermediate pattern in Malaysia.

AETIOLOGY

A high incidence of oropharyngeal tumour is related to the cultural practice of chewing betel quid and, less frequently to smoking locally made cheroots called bidi. Betel quid consists of the young leaf of betel vine (*Piper betel*) mixed with slices of areca nut and varying quantities of slaked lime. Tobacco and spices are often added to this mixture. The resultant quid is held for long periods of time in the buccal sulcus. The development of squamous cell carcinoma is usually preceded by the development of precancerous leucoplasic changes in the oral epithelium. A high alcohol intake, vitamin A deficiency, dental caries and sepsis may be contributory factors in some patients. There is conflicting evidence as to the relative roles of tobacco and other constituents of the quid in the development of cancer.

PREVENTION AND MANAGEMENT

Up to 15 years may lapse before lesions in the mouth turn cancerous. Various studies in India have indicated a high prevalence of oral premalignant lesions.[169] These are leucoplakia and oral submucous fibrosis. If these lesions, which are the first signs of danger, are detected in sufficient time for treatment, the disease is curable through surgery and radiotherapy. Unfortunately, most patients seek medical attention only when they are in pain, which is a late symptom, and therefore too late for any therapy but pain relief.

In a study using primary health care workers in Sri Lanka it was demonstrated that the precancerous lesions can be detected by this category of workers.[170] This approach has been found to be reliable and pragmatic, and since these primary health care workers outnumber dentists by a ratio of 10 to 1, they may give a lead on how to approach other cancers in remote populous tropical environments. Any improvement in general nutrition, particularly an adequate intake of vitamins, trace elements and animal protein, is likely to reduce the incidence in high-risk populations. Reduction of alcohol intake, and particularly tobacco consumption, should also be encouraged.

CARCINOMA OF THE BLADDER (See also Chapter 7)

INCIDENCE AND GEOGRAPHICAL DISTRIBUTION

Bladder cancer is the sixth most common form of cancer in the developed world (see Table 24.1) with an age-standardized rate of approximately 25/ 100 000. The majority of tumours are transitional in histological type and over 75% occur in elderly men. Within most of the tropics the rates are low but in parts of East, Central and Southern Africa, Egypt and the Sudan and some regions of the Middle East rates are high. In Bulawayo, Zimbabwe, for example, they are 28.7 and 7.0/100 000 in men and women respectively, and at the Cairo Cancer Institute bladder cancer accounts for 38.5% of all cancers in men and 11.3% in women. The tumours in these high-incidence regions are predominantly squamous in histological type.

AETIOLOGY

The geographical distribution of high-incidence bladder cancer in the tropics parallels that of *S. haematobium*, an association that was first noted by Fergusson[171] in Egypt in 1911. Case–control studies in Zimbabwe, using bladder calcification as an index of infection, have shown a significantly higher rate of infection in patients than controls.[172] Estimated incidence rates in different districts and regions of East and Central Africa show a close relationship between the prevalence and intensity of *S. haematobium* infection and high rates of bladder cancer.

The mechanisms of carcinogenesis are uncertain. Heavy, chronic infection with *S. haematobium* leads to inflammation, fibrosis and calcification of the bladder with impairment of function and inadequate emptying. This predisposes to recurrent, mixed bacterial infections. In such patients carcinogenic nitrosamines which are formed from excreted nitrates and nitrites have been detected.[173,174] It is thought that these substances acting on hyperplastic and metaplastic epithelium give rise to the characteristic squamous cell carcinomas.

CLINICAL FEATURES

Schistosomal bladder cancer occurs mostly in young individuals. It is commonly a well-differentiated squamous cell carcinoma and has less tendency to spread via the bloodstream and lymphatics. The mean age at presentation is about 45 years and in Egypt about 75% of the victims are under 50 years of age. It is rarely observed in the under 20 age group. This is in contradiction to non-schistosomal bladder cancer where the mean age is about 65 years and less than 10% are under 50 years of age. The male: female ratio for schistosomal bladder cancer is 4–5:1. The male preponderance may be related to increased male exposure to schistosomal infection. Unfortunately the cardinal early sign of bladder cancer (painless haematuria) is often ignored in schistosomal endemic areas as most of the populace will have had haematuria since childhood. For this and other reasons the great majority of the cases present very late with symptoms of cystitis and obstructive uropathy. A plain radiograph of the

Table 24.16   TNM staging of bladder carcinoma: UICC classification.

Stage	Description
T_{is}	Carcinoma in situ, 'flat tumour'
T_a	Non-invasive papillary carcinoma
T_1	Tumour invades subepithelial connective tissue
T_2	Tumour invades superficial muscle
T_3	Tumour invades deep muscle or perivesical fat
T_4	Tumour invades prostate, uterus, vagina, pelvic wall or abdominal wall
N_1	Metastasis in a single lymph node 2 cm or less in greatest dimension
N_2	Metastasis in a single lymph node, 2–5 cm in greatest dimension or multiple nodes ≤5 cm
N_3	Metastasis in node >5 cm in greatest dimension
M_0	No distant metastasis
M_1	Distant metastasis

abdomen may reveal a calcified outline of the urinary bladder. Cystoscopy and biopsy establishes the diagnosis. In centres such as the Cairo Cancer Institute, where investigators are experienced, urine cytology provides a fairly accurate diagnosis.[175] Biopsy is still necessary to confirm the diagnosis, although 'aggressive biopsy' to determine the depth of tumour muscle invasion may cause perforation because of the advanced nature of most cases. Pre-staging work-up should include history and physical examination, urinalysis for cytology, looking for schistosomal eggs and for malignant cells, and a plain radiograph of the abdomen. Urography should be followed by an examination under anaesthesia. Cystoscopy to map out the location of bladder tumour and biopsy are essential. The currently recommended staging system is the TNM staging advocated by the International Union Against Cancer (UICC) (Table 24.16).

TREATMENT

Radical surgery is the only curative treatment modality. However, radical cystectomy is associated with postoperative morbidity and mortality as high as 15–30% in some series. Adjuvant radiotherapy has been used postoperatively to prevent or delay recurrence. Preoperative radiotherapy has been tried in Cairo and the preliminary results are encouraging.[176] Radiotherapy as the sole treatment modality has been disappointing. This may be due to the massive tumour bulk associated with fibrosis and bacterial infection. Effective single cytotoxic agents include cisplatin, bleomycin and methotrexate. The efficacy of combination chemotherapy or concurrent chemoradiotherapy has yet to be demonstrated.

PREVENTION

The prevention of bladder cancer in those regions where schistosomiasis is endemic is dependent on effective schistosomal control (see Chapter 72). There is a minimum of 20 years lag period between infection and the development of bladder cancer. Schistosomal bladder cancer should therefore be amenable to screening. Screening has been advocated for high-risk populations in Egypt. Before such a practice is embarked upon on a wide scale, its cost-effectiveness needs to be carefully evaluated.

REFERENCES

1 Tomatis L. Environmental cancer risk factors: a review. *Acta Oncol* 1988; 27:465–472.

2 Parkin D M, Laara E & Muir C S. Estimates of the world wide frequency of sixteen major cancers in 1980. *Int J Cancer* 1988; 41:184–197.

3 Olweny C L M. Global inequalities in cancer care. *Trans R Soc Trop Med Hyg* 1991; 85:709–710.

4 Bailey B J. Tobaccoism is the disease—cancer is the sequela (editorial). *JAMA* 1986; 255:1923.

5 Olweny C L M. Goals and rationale of cancer treatment. *Med J Aust* 1991; 155:187–192.

6 Cleaver J R. Defective repair replication of DNA in xeroderma pigmentosum. *Nature* 1968; 218:652–656.

7 Takebe H, Nishigori C & Satoh Y. Genetics and skin cancer of xeroderma pigmentosum in Japan. *Jpn J Cancer Res* 1987; 78:1135–1143.

8 Templeton A C, Buxton E & Bianchi A. Cancer in Kyadondo County, Uganda 1968–1970. *J Natl Cancer Inst* 1972; 48:865–874.

9 Bayo S, Parkin D M, Koumare A K et al. Cancer in Mali. *Int J Cancer* 1990; 45:679–684.

10 Whittle H C, Inskip H, Hall A J, Mendy M, Downer R & Hoare S. Vaccination against hepatitis B and protection against chronic viral carriage in the Gambia. *Lancet* 1991; 337:747–750.

11 Parkin D M, Stjernsward J & Muir C. Estimates of worldwide frequency of 12 major cancers. *Bull World Health Organ* 1984; 62:163–182.

12 Whelan S L, Parkin D M & Masuyer E (eds). Patterns of cancer in five continents. *IARC Sci Publ* 1990; 102.

13 Grant M C. Cancer of the cervix: a tragic disease in South Africa. *S Afr Med J* 1982; 61:819–822.

14 Rogo K O, Omany J, Onyango J N, Ojwang S B & Stendahl U. Carcinoma of the cervix in the African setting. In *Human Papilloma Virus and Human Immunodeficiency Virus Infection in Relation to Cervical Cancer*. Umea University Medical Dissertations No. 293, part I, 1990; 1–22.

15 Briggs N D & Katchy K C. Pattern of primary gynaecological malignancies as seen in a tertiary hospital situated in the River State of Nigeria. *Int J Gynaecol Obstet* 1990; 31:157–161.

16 Mgaya H N & Mbura J S. The pattern of cervical cancer at Muhimbili Medical Centre, Dar-es-Salaam, Tanzania. *Tanzania Med J* 1985; 2:11–17.

17 Kasule J. The pattern of gynaecological malignancy in Zimbabwe. *East Afr Med J* 1989; 66:393–399.

18 Brinton L A & Fraumeni J F Jr. Epidemiology of uterine cervical cancer. *J Chronic Dis* 1986; 39:1051–1065.

19 Brinton L A, Hamman R F, Huggins G R et al. Sexual and reproductive risk factors for invasive squamous cell cervical cancer. *J Natl Cancer Inst* 1987; 79:23–30.

20 Skegg D C G, Corwin P A, Panel C & Doll R. Importance of the male factor in cancer of the cervix. *Lancet* 1982; ii:581–583.

21 Brinton L A, Reeves W C, Brenes M M et al. The male factor in the etiology of cervical cancer among sexually monogamous women. *Int J Cancer* 1989; 44:199–203.

22 Brinton L A, Schairer C, Haenzel W et al. Smoking and invasive cervical cancer. *JAMA* 1986; 255:3265–3269.

23 Layde P M. Smoking and cervical cancer: cause or coincidence? *JAMA* 1989; 261:1631–1632.

24 Piper J M. Oral contraceptives and cervical cancer. *Gynecol Oncol* 1985; 22:1–14.

25 Yach D & Townsend G S. Smoking and health in South Africa. *S Afr Med J* 1988; 73:391–399.

26 Zur Hausen H. Condylomata acumunata and human genital cancer. *Cancer Res* 1976; 36:794.

27 Meanwell C A, Cox M F, Blackledge G & Maitland N J. Human papilloma virus 16 DNA in normal and malignant cervical epithelium: implications for aetiology and behaviour of cervical neoplasia. *Lancet* 1987; i:703–707.

28 Wright T C Jr & Richart R M. Role of human papilloma virus in the pathogenesis of genital tract warts and cancer. *Gynecol Oncol* 1990; 37:151–164.

29 Reeves W C, Brinton L A, Garcia M et al. Human papilloma virus infection and cervical cancer in Latin America. *N Engl J Med* 1989; 320:1437–1441.

30 Riou G, Favre M, Jeannel D, Bourhis J, Le Dousaal V & Orth G. Association between poor prognosis in early-stage invasive cervical carcinoma

and non-detection of HPV DNA. *Lancet* 1990; 335:1171–1174.

31 Fuchs P G, Girardi F & Pfister H. Human papilloma virus 16 DNA in cervical cancer and in lymph nodes of cervical cancer patients: a diagnostic marker for early metastases. *Int J Cancer* 1989; 43:41–44.

32 Brodman M, Friedman F, Dottino P et al. A comparative study of computerized tomography, magnetic resonance imaging and clinical staging for detection of early cervix cancer. *Gynecol Oncol* 1990; 36:409–412.

33 Du-Toit J P. A cost effective but safe protocol for the staging of invasive cervical cancer in a Third World country. *Int J Gynaecol Obstet* 1988; 26:261–264.

34 Kurman R J, Schiffman M H, Lancaster W D et al. Analysis of individual human papilloma virus types in cervical neoplasia: a possible role of type 18 in rapid progression. *Am J Obstet Gynecol* 1988; 159:293–296.

35 Barnes W, Delgado G, Kurman R J et al. Possible prognostic significance of human papilloma virus type in cervical cancer. *Gynecol Oncol* 1988; 29:267–273.

36 Day N E. Screening for cancer of the cervix. *J Epidemiol Community Health* 1989; 43:103–106.

37 Anderson G H, Boyes D A, Benedet J L et al. Organization and results of the cervical cytology screening programme in British Columbia. *BMJ* 1988; 296:975–978.

38 International Agency for Research on Cancer, Working Group on Evaluation of Cervical Cancer Screening Programmes. Screening for squamous cervical cancer; duration of risk after negative results of cervical cytology and implication for screening policies. *BMJ* 1990; 293:659–664.

39 Marteau T M. Ethics of clinical research. *BMJ* 1989; 299:513–514.

40 Raffle A E, Aldar B & MacKenzie E F D. Six years audit of laboratory workload and rates of referral for colposcopy in cervical screening programme in three districts. *BMJ* 1990; 301:907–911.

41 Van Nagell J R Jr, Hanson M B, Donaldson E S & Gallion H H. Treatment of cervical intraepithelial neoplasma III by hysterectomy without intervening conization in patients with adequate colposcopy. *Cancer* 1985; 56:2737–2739.

42 Prates M D & Torres F O. A cancer survey in Lourenco Marques, Portuguese East Africa. *J Natl Cancer Inst* 1965; 35:729–757.

43 Van Rensburg S J, Cook-Mozaffari P, Van Schalkwyk D J, Van Der Watt J J, Vincent T J & Purchase I F. Hepatocellular carcinoma and dietary aflatoxin in Mozambique and Transkei. *Br J Cancer* 1985; 51:713–726.

44 Kew M C. The hepatitis B virus and hepatocellular carcinoma. *Semin Liver Dis* 1981; 1:59–67.

45 Yu M C, Tong M J, Coursaget P et al. Prevalence of hepatitis B and hepatitis C viral markers in black and white patients with hepatocellular carcinoma in the United States. *J Natl Cancer Inst* 1990; 82:1038–1041.

46 Beasley R P, Hwang L Y, Lin C C & Chien C S. Hepatocellular carcinoma and hepatitis B virus. *Lancet* 1981; ii:1129–1133.

47 Shafritz D A, Shouval D, Sherman N I, Hadziyannis S J & Kew M C. Integration of hepatitis B virus DNA into the genome of liver cells in chronic liver disease and hepatocellular carcinoma. *N Engl J Med* 1981; 305:1067–1073.

48 Brechot C, Nalpas B & Courouce A et al. Evidence that hepatitis B virus has a role in liver-cell carcinoma in alcoholic liver disease. *N Engl J Med* 1982; 306:1384–1387.

49 Hepatitis C virus, a causative infectious agent of non-A, non-B hepatitis: prevalence and structure. Summary of a conference of hepatitis C virus as a cause of hepatocellular carcinoma. *J Natl Cancer Inst* 1992; 84:86–90.

50 International Agency for Research on Cancer. Evaluation of carcinogenic risk of chemicals to man. *IARC Monogr* 1976; 10.

51 Newberne P M & Butler W H. Acute and chronic effects of aflatoxin on the liver of domestic and laboratory animals: a review. *Cancer Res* 1969; 29:230–235.

52 Carnaghan R B A. Hepatic tumurs and chronic liver changes in rats following administration of aflatoxin. *Br J Cancer* 1967; 21:811–814.

53 Peers F, Bosch X, Kaldor J, Linsell A & Pluijmen M. Aflatoxin exposure, hepatitis B virus infection and liver cancer in Swaziland. *Int J Cancer* 1987; 39:545–553.

54 Peers F G, Gilman G A & Linsell C A. Dietary aflatoxin and human liver cancer. A study in Swaziland. *Int J Cancer* 1976; 17:167–176.

55 Bulatao J, Almero E M, Castro Jardeleza Ma T R & Salamat L A. A case-control dietary study of primary liver cancer from aflatoxin exposure. *Int J Epidemiol* 1982; 11:112–119.

56 Linsell C. Aflatoxin and liver cancer. *Trans R Soc Trop Med Hyg* 1977; 7:471–473.

57 Campbell T & Hayes J. Role of aflatoxin metabolism in its toxic lesion. *Toxicol Appl Pharmacol* 1976; 35:195–222.

58 Lutwik L. Relations between aflatoxin, hepatitis B virus and hepatocellular carcinoma. *Lancet* 1979; i:755–757.

59 Coady A. The aflatoxin–hepatoma hepatitis B surface antigen story. *BMJ* 1975; 3:592–593.

60 Kew M C, Dibisceglie A M & Paterson A. Smoking as a risk-factor in hepatocellular carcinoma. A case-control study in Southern African blacks. *Cancer* 1985; 56:2315–2317.

61 Yu M C & Tong M J. Non viral risk factors for hepatocellular carcinoma in low-risk population, the non-Asians of Los Angeles County, California. *J Natl Cancer Inst* 1991; 83:1820–1826.

62 Maynard E P, Sedikali F, Anthony P P & Barker L F. Hepatitis-associated antigen and cirrhosis in Uganda. *Lancet* 1970; ii:1326–1328.

63 Higginson J & Oettle A G. Cancer incidence in Bantu and 'Cape Colored' races of South Africa: report of a cancer survey in the Transvaal (1953–1955). *J Natl Cancer Inst* 1960; 24:589–671.

64 Li J J & Li S A. High incidence of hepatocellular carcinoma after synthetic oestrogen administration in Syrian golden hamsters fed alpha-naphthoflavine: a new tumour model. *J Natl Cancer Inst* 1984; 73:543–547.

65 Kew M C, Kassianides C, Hodkinson J, Coppon A & Paterson A C. Hepatocellular carcinoma in urban born blacks: frequency and relation to hepatitis B virus infection. *BMJ* 1986; 293:1339–1341.

66 Attali P, Prod'homme S, Pelletier G et al. Prognostic factors in patients with hepatocellular carcinoma. *Cancer* 1987; 59:2108–2111.

67 Sowl S H, Titelbaum D S, Gansler T S et al. The fibrolamellar variant of hepatocellular carcinoma. Its association with focal nodular hyperplasia. *Cancer* 1987; 60:3049–3055.

68 Van Tonder S, Kew M C, Hodkinson J & Fernandes-Costa F. Serum vitamin B_{12} binders in Southern African blacks with hepatocellular carcinoma. *Cancer* 1985; 56:789–792.

69 Vogel C L & Linsell C A. International Symposium on hepatocellular carcinoma, Kampala, Uganda. *J Natl Cancer Inst* 1972; 48:567–571.

70 Primack A, Vogel C L, Kyalwazi S K et al. A staging system for hepatocellular carcinoma: prognostic factors in Ugandan patients. *Cancer* 1975; 35:1357–1364.

71 Olweny C L M, Toya T, Katongole-Mbidde E, Mugerwa J, Kyalwazi S K & Cohen H. Treatment of hepatocellular carcinoma with adriamycin: preliminary communication. *Cancer* 1975; 36:1250–1257.

72 Chen M, Hwang T, Jeng L, Jan Y & Wang C. Surgical treatment for spontaneous rupture of hepatocellular carcinoma. *Surg Gynecol Obstet* 1988; 167:99–102.

73 Olweny C L M, Katongole-Mbidde E, Bahendeka S, Otim D, Mugerwa J & Kyalwazi S K. Further experience in treating patients with hepatocellular carcinoma in Uganda. *Cancer* 1980; 46:2717–2722.

74 Bezwoda W R, Weaving A, Kew M & Derman D P. Combination chemotherapy of hepatocellular cancer. *Oncology* 1987; 44:207–209.

75 Olweny C L M & Johnson R. Rapid response to cisplatin and doxorubicin in hepatitis B virus reactivation. *J Gastroenterol Hepatol* 1987; 2:533–537.

76 Prevention of hepatocellular carcinoma by immunization. *Bull World Health Organ* 1983; 61:731–744.

77 Kobayashi K, Sugimoto T, Makino H et al. Screening methods for early detection of hepatocellular carcinoma. *Hepatology* 1985; 5:1100–1105.

78 Rose E F. Oesophageal cancer in the Transkei: 1955–1969. *J Natl Cancer Inst* 1973; 51:7–16.

79 Cook P. Cancer of the oesophagus in Africa. *Br J Cancer* 1971; 25:853.

80 Van Rensburg S J, Benade A S, Rose E F & du Plessis J P. Nutritional status of African populations predisposed to oesophageal cancer. *Nutr Cancer* 1983; 4:206–216.

81 Oettle A G. *Cancer Research in Africa.* Johannesburg: Witwatersrand University Press, 1967.

82 Van Rensburg S J, Bradshaw E S, Bradshaw D & Rose E F. Oesophageal cancer in Zulu men, South Africa: A case-control study. *Br J Cancer* 1985; 51:399–405.

83 Bradshaw E & Schonland M. Smoking, drinking and oesophageal cancer in African males of Johannesburg, South Africa. *Br J Cancer* 1974; 30:157–163.

84 Van Rensburg S J. Epidemiologic and dietary evidence for a specific nutritional predisposition to esophageal cancer. *J Natl Cancer Inst* 1981; 67:243–251.

85 Crespi M, Munoz N, Grassi A et al. Oesophageal lesions in Northern Iran: a premalignant condition. *Lancet* 1979; i:217–221.

86 Munoz N, Crespi M, Grassi A et al. Precursor lesions of oesophageal cancer in high risk population in Iran and China. *Lancet* 1982; i:876–879.

87 Munoz N, Wanrendorf J, Bang L J et al. No effect of riboflavin, retinol and zinc on prevalence of precancerous lesions of oesophagus. *Lancet* 1985; ii:111–114.

88 Ropp M B, Hawley D, Reising J et al. Improved survival in squamous oesophageal cancer, preoperative chemotherapy and irradiation. *Arch Surg* 1986; 121:1330–1335.

89 Ellis F H & Maggs P R. Surgery for carcinoma of the lower oesophagus and cardia. *World J Surg* 1981; 5:527–533.

90 Orringer M B. Technical aids in performing transhiatal esophagectomy without thoracotomy. *Ann Thorac Surg* 1984; 38:128–132.

91 Hennessy T P J. Choice of treatment in carcinoma of the oesophagus. *Br J Surg* 1988; 75:193–194.

92 Skinner D B. Surgical treatments for oesophageal carcinoma. *Semin Oncol* 1984; 11:135–143.

93 Pearson J G. The present and future potential of radiotherapy in the management of esophageal cancer. *Cancer* 1977; 39:882–890.

94 Earlam R & Cunha-Melo J R. Oesophageal squamous cell carcinoma: I. A critical review of surgery. *Br J Surg* 1980; 67:381–390.

95 Earlam R & Cunha-Melo J R. Oesophageal squamous cell carcinoma: II. A critical review of radiotherapy. *Br J Surg* 1980; 67:457–461.

96 Launois B, Delarne D, Campion J P et al. Preoperative radiotherapy for carcinoma of the oesophagus. *Surg Gynecol Obstet* 1981; 153:690–692.

97 Kelsen D. Multimodality therapy of oesophageal

carcinoma: still an experimental approach. *J Clin Oncol* 1987; 5:530–531.

98 Steiger Z, Franklin R, Wilson R F et al. Complete eradication of squamous cell carcinoma of the oesophagus with combined chemoradiotherapy and radiotherapy. *Am J Surg* 1981; 47:95–98.

99 Leichman L, Steiger Z, Seydel H G et al. Combined preoperative chemotherapy and radiation therapy for cancer of the oesophagus. *Semin Oncol* 1984; 11:178–185.

100 Poplon E, Fleming T, Leichman L et al. Combined therapies for squamous cell carcinoma of the esophagus: a Southwest Oncology Group Study (SOGS-8037). *J Clin Oncol* 1987; 5:622–628.

101 Forastieve A A, Orringer M B, Perez-Tamayo C et al. Concurrent chemotherapy and radiotherapy followed by transhiatal esophagectomy for local regional cancer of the oesophagus. *J Clin Oncol* 1990; 8:119–127.

102 Dewit L. Combined treatment of radiation and cisdiamine dichlonoplatinum (II): a review of experimental and clinical data. *Int J Radiat Oncol Biol Phys* 1987; 13:402–426.

103 Pfeffer M R, Teicher B A, Holder S A, al-Achi A & Herman T S. The interaction of cisplatin plus etoposide with radiation +/− hyperthermia. *Int J Radiat Oncol Biol Phys* 1990; 19:1439–1447.

104 Ho V C & Sober A J. Therapy of cutaneous melanoma: an update. *J Am Acad Dermatol* 1990; 22:159–176.

105 Balch C M. Excising melanoma: how wide is enough? And how to reconstruct? *J Surg Oncol* 1990; 44:135–138.

106 Friedman-Kien A E & Saltzman B R. Clinical manifestations of classical, endemic African and epidemic AIDS-associated Kaposi's sarcoma. *J Am Acad Dermatol* 1990; 22:1237–1250.

107 Harwood A R, Osoba P, Hostader S W et al. Kaposi's sarcoma in recipients of renal transplants. *Am J Med* 1979; 67:759–765.

108 Stribling J, Weitzner S & Smith G U. Kaposi's sarcoma in renal allograft patients. *Cancer* 1978; 42:442–446.

109 Penn I. Kaposi's sarcoma in organ transplant recipients. Report of 20 cases. *Transplantation* 1979; 27:8–11.

110 Safai B, Sarngadharan M G, Koziner B et al. Spectrum of Kaposi's sarcoma in the epidemic of acquired immunodeficiency syndrome. *Cancer Res* 1985; 45:4646–4648.

111 Ensoli B, Nakamura S, Salahuddin S Z et al. Acquired immunodeficiency syndrome Kaposi's sarcoma derived cells express cytokines with autocrine and paracrine growth effects. *Science* 1989; 243:223–226.

112 Ensoli B, Barillari G, Salahuddin S Z et al. Tat protein of HIV-1 stimulates growth of cells from Kaposi's sarcoma lesions of AIDS patients. *Nature* 1990; 345:84–86.

113 Salahuddin S Z, Nakamura S, Biberfield P et al. Angiogenic properties of Kaposi's sarcoma derived cells after long-term culture in vitro. *Science* 1988; 242:430–433.

114 Drew W L, Miner R C, Ziegler J L et al. Cytomegalovirus and Kaposi's sarcoma in young homosexual men. *Lancet* 1982; ii:125–127.

115 Giraldo G, Beth E & Huang E S. Kaposi's sarcoma and its relationship to cytomegalovirus (CMV) III, CMV-DNA and CMV early antigen in Kaposi's sarcoma. *Int J Cancer* 1980; 26:23–29.

116 Delli Bovi P, Donti E, Knoules II D M et al. Presence of chromosomal abnormalities and lack of acquired immunodeficiency syndrome retrovirus DNA sequences in AIDS-associated Kaposi's sarcoma. *Cancer Res* 1986; 46:6333–6338.

117 Grody W W, Lewis K J & Naeim F. Detection of cytomegalovirus DNA in classic and epidemic Kaposi's sarcoma by in situ hybridization. *Hum Pathol* 1988; 19:524–528.

118 Saiki R K, Gelfand D H, Stoffel S et al. Primer-directed enzymatic amplification of DNA with a thermostable DNA polymerase. *Science* 1988; 239:487–491.

119 Neri A, Barriga F, Inghirami F et al. Epstein–Barr virus infection preceeds clonal expansion in Burkitt's and acquired immunodeficiency syndrome-associated lymphoma. *Blood* 1991; 77:1092–1095.

120 Reeve P A. HIV infection in patients admitted to a general hospital in Malawi. *BMJ* 1989; 298:1567–1568.

121 Serwadda D, Mugerwa R D, Sewankambo N K et al. Slim disease: a new disease in Uganda and its association with HTLV III infection. *Lancet* 1985; ii:359–361.

122 Olweny C L M, Kaddu-Mukasa A, Atine I, Owor R, Magrath I & Ziegler J. Childhood Kaposi's sarcoma: clinical features and therapy. *Br J Cancer* 1976; 33:555–560.

123 Grore J H. Kaposi's disease: report of an unusual case. *Radiology* 1955; 65:236–239.

124 Coetzee T & LeRoux C G J. Kaposi's sarcoma presentation with intestinal obstruction. *S Afr Med J* 1967; 41:442–445.

125 Mitchell N & Feder A. Kaposi's sarcoma with secondary involvement of the jejunum, perforation and peritonitis. *Ann Intern Med* 1949; 31:324–329.

126 Novis B H, King N & Banks N. Kaposi's sarcoma presenting with diarrhoea and protein-losing enteropathy. *Gastroenterology* 1974; 67:996.

127 Khorshid K A, Erzingatsian K, Watters D A K & Bailey A C. Intussusception due to Kaposi's sarcoma. *J R Coll Surg Edinb* 1987; 32:339–341.

128 Cook J. The clinical features of Kaposi's sarcoma in the East African Bantu. *Acta Un Int Cancr* 1962; 18:388–398.

129 Slavin G, Cameron H McD, Forbes C et al. Kaposi's sarcoma in East African children: a report of 51 cases. *Pathology* 1970; 100:189–199.

130 Krigel R L, Laubenstein L J & Muggia F M. Kaposi's sarcoma: a new staging classification. *Cancer Treat Rep* 1983; 67:531–534.

131 Mitsuyasu R T & Groopman J E. Biology and therapy of Kaposi's sarcoma. *Semin Oncol* 1984; 11:53–59.

132 Taylor J, Afrasiabi R, Fahey J L et al. A prognostically significant classification of immune changes in AIDS with Kaposi's sarcoma. *Blood* 1986; 67:666–671.

133 Kyalwazi S K. Chemotherapy of Kaposi's sarcoma: experience with Trenimon. *East Afr Med J* 1968; 45:17–26.

134 Olweny C L M, Sikyewunda W & Otim D. Further experience with Razoxane (ICRF 159—NSC 129943) in treating Kaposi's sarcoma. *Oncology* 1980; 37:174–176.

135 Olweny C L M, Toya T, Katongole-Mbidde E et al. Treatment of Kaposi's sarcoma combination of actinomycin-D, vincristine and imidazole carboxamide (NSC 45388): results of a randomized clinical trial. *Int J Cancer* 1974; 14:649–656.

136 Safai B, Mike V, Giraldo G, Beth E & Good R A. Association of Kaposi's sarcoma with secondary primary malignancies: possible etiopathogenic implications. *Cancer* 1980; 45:1472–1479.

137 Olweny C L M, Hutt M S R & Owor R (eds). Kaposi's sarcoma. In *Antibiotics and Chemotherapy*, vol. 29. Basel: Karger, 1981:30.

138 Beral V, Peterman T, Berkelman R & Jaffe H. AIDS-associated non-Hodgkin's lymphoma. *Lancet* 1991; 337:805–809.

139 Spurrett B, Jones D S & Stewart G. Cervical dysplasia and HIV infection. *Lancet* 1988; i:232–238.

140 Schafer A, Friedman W, Mielke M et al. The increased frequency of cervical dysplasia–neoplasia in women infected with the human immunodeficiency virus related to the degree of immunosuppression. *Am J Obstet Gynecol* 1991; 164:593–599.

141 Kiviat N, Rompalo A, Bowden R et al. Anal human papilloma-virus infection among HIV-seropositive and seronegative men. *J Infect Dis* 1990; 162:358–361.

142 Maiman M, Fruchler R G, Serur E et al. HIV infection and cervical neoplasia. *Gynecol Oncol* 1990; 38:377–382.

143 Chadwick E G, Connor E J, Hanson C G et al. Tumours of smooth muscle origin in HIV-infected children. *JAMA* 1990; 263:3182–3184.

144 McLoughlin L C, Nord K S, Joshi V V et al. Disseminated leiomyosarcoma in a child with AIDS. *Cancer* 1991; 67:2618–2621.

145 Burkitt D P. A sarcoma involving the jaws in African children. *Br J Surg* 1958; 197:218–223.

146 Pike M C, Williams E H & Wright D. Burkitt's tumour in the West Nile district of Uganda. *BMJ* 1967; ii:395–399.

147 Ziegler J L, Drew W L, Miner R C et al. Outbreak of Burkitt's-like lymphoma in homosexual men. *Lancet* 1982; ii:631–633.

148 Epstein M A, Achong B G & Barr Y M. Virus particles in cultured lymphoblasts from Burkitt's lymphoma. *Lancet* 1964; i:702–703.

149 Nonoyama M & Ragano J S. Homology between Epstein–Barr virus DNA and viral-DNA from Burkitt's lymphoma and nasopharyngeal carcinoma determined by DNA–DNA reassociation kinetics. *Nature* 1973; 242:44–47.

150 de-The G, Geser A, Day N E et al. Epidemiological evidence for a causal relationship between Epstein–Barr virus and Burkitt's lymphoma: results of the Ugandan prospective study. *Nature* 1978; 274:756–761.

151 Olweny C L M, Atine I, Kaddu-Mukasa A et al. Epstein–Barr virus genome studies in Burkitt and non-Burkitt lymphomas in Uganda. *J Natl Cancer Inst* 1977; 58:1191–1196.

152 Schmauz R, Mugerwa J W & Wright D H. The distribution on non-Burkitt, non-Hodgkin's lymphomas in Uganda in relation to malaria endemicity. *Int J Cancer* 1990; 45:650–653.

153 Zech L, Haglund U, Nilsson K et al. Characteristic chromosomal abnormalities in biopsies and lymphoid cell lines from patients with Burkitt and non-Burkitt lymphomas. *Int J Cancer* 1976; 17:47–56.

154 Magrath I T, Lwanga S, Carswell W & Harrison N. Surgical reduction of tumour bulk in the management of abdominal Burkitt's lymphoma. *BMJ* 1974; ii:308–312.

155 Olweny C L M, Atine I, Kaddu-Mukasa A et al. Cerebrospinal irradiation of Burkitt's lymphoma. Failure in preventing central nervous system relapse. *Acta Radiol Ther Phys Biol* 1977; 16:225–231.

156 Olweny C L M, Katongole-Mbidde E, Kaddu-Mukasa A et al. Treatment of Burkitt's lymphoma: randomized clinical trial of single versus combination chemotherapy. *Int J Cancer* 1976; 17:436–440.

157 Ziegler J L, Bluming A Z, Fass L & Morrow R H. Relapse patterns in Burkitt's lymphoma. *Cancer Res* 1972; 32:1267–1272.

158 Olweny C L M, Katongole-Mbidde E, Otim D, Lwanga S K, Magrath I & Ziegler J L. Long-term experience with Burkitt's lymphoma in Uganda. *Int J Cancer* 1980; 26:261–266.

159 Epstein M A. Vaccination against Epstein–Barr virus: current progress and future strategies. *Lancet* 1986; i:1425–1427.

160 Epstein M A. Recent studies on a vaccine to prevent Epstein–Barr virus-associated cancers. *Br J Cancer* 1986; 54:1–5.

161 Wolf H, zur Hausen H & Becker V. Epstein–Barr virus genomes in epithelial nasopharyngeal cancer cells. *Nature [New Biol]* 1973; 244:245–247.

162 Shao Y M, Poirier S, Ohshima H et al. Epstein–Barr virus activation in Raji cells by extracts of preserved food from high risk areas for nasopharyngeal carcinoma. *Carcinogenesis* 1988; 9:1455–1457.

163 Jesse R H, Perez C A & Fletcher G H. Cervical lymph node metastasis: unknown primary cancer. *Cancer* 1973; 31:854–859.

164 Ho J H. Nasopharyngeal carcinoma. *West J Med* 1985; 143:70–73.

165 Holoye P Y, Byers R M & Gard D A. Combination chemotherapy of head and neck cancer. *Cancer* 1978; 42:1661–1669.

166 Wei W I, Sham J S, Zong Y-S, Choy D & Ng M H. The efficacy of fibreoptic endoscopic examination and biopsy in the detection of early nasopharyngeal cancer. *Cancer* 1991; 67:3127–3130.

167 Binnie W H. Oral cancer. In Dolby A E (ed.) *Oral Mucosa in Health and Disease*. Oxford: Blackwell, 1975: 301–333.

168 Pindborg J J. Epidemiological studies of oral cancer. *Int Dent J* 1977; 27:172–178.

169 Mehta F S et al. *Oral Cancer and Precancerous Conditions in India*. Copenhagen: Munksgaard, 1971.

170 Warnakulasuriya K A A S, Ekanayake A N I, Sivayoham J et al. Utilization of primary health care workers for early detection of oral cancer and precancer cases in Sri Lanka. *Bull World Health Organ* 1984; 62:243–250.

171 Fergusson D R. Associated bilharziasis and primary malignant disease of the urinary bladder. *J Pathol Bacteriol* 1911; 16:76–79.

172 Gelfand M, Weinberg R W & Castle V M. Relation between carcinoma of the bladder and infestation with *Schistosoma haematobium*. *Lancet* 1967; i:1249–1251.

173 Hicks R M, Walters C L, el Sebai I et al. Demonstration of nitrosamines in human urine. Preliminary observations on a possible etiology for bladder cancer associated with chronic urinary infection. *Proc R Soc Med* 1977; 70:413–417.

174 el Aaser A A & el Merzabani M M. Etiology of bladder cancer. In el-Sebai I & Hoogstraten B (eds) *Bladder Cancer*, vol. I (CRC Series on Experiences in Clinical Oncology). Boca Raton: CRC Press, 1983; 39–58.

175 el-Bolkainy M N, Ghoneim M A, el-Morsey B A & Nasrs M. Cancer of bilharzial bladder: diagnostic value of urine cytology. *Urology* 1974; 3:319.

176 Awward H K, Abdel Baki H, el-Bolkainy M N et al. Preoperative irradiation of T$_3$ carcinoma in bilharzial bladder: a comparison between hyperfractionation and conventional fractionation. *Int J Radiat Oncol Biol Phys* 1979; 5:787.

CHAPTER 25

DIABETES MELLITUS IN THE TROPICS

David A. Cavan and Anthony H. Barnett

Diabetes mellitus is a worldwide disease but varies greatly in prevalence. In temperate regions there are two common types, type I (insulin dependent) and type II (non-insulin dependent), accounting for about 15 and 85% of cases respectively. These diseases also occur in the tropics and, while the prevalence of type I diabetes is generally low, some discrete populations have very high incidences of type II diabetes.

A third type of disease is seen in tropical countries. This has been termed variously as J-type, Z-type, type III or tropical pancreatic diabetes. Such cases are often associated with malnutrition and, for the purposes of this account, the general term malnutrition-related diabetes mellitus (MRDM) will be used. As discussed below, this shares features of both type I and type II diabetes.

The epidemiology and pathogenesis of each type of diabetes will be discussed separately, with particular emphasis on regional variations and the pattern of disease in tropical countries.

TYPE I DIABETES MELLITUS

Type I diabetes is predominantly a Caucasoid disease[1] and the highest prevalence rates occur in northern European countries. Although only scanty data are available in some cases, evidence suggests that the prevalence is low in most other races, including Asian Indians,[2] Chinese,[3] Japanese[1] and black Africans[1] (Table 25.1). The prevalence of the disease in black Americans and Afro-Caribbeans is, however, intermediate between that seen in white Caucasians and black Africans.[4] This may result from admixture of Caucasian genes in the negroid genome (estimated to be around 21% in black Americans). Within Europe there is a North–South gradient of prevalence rates, which range from 2.2 per 1000 population in Finland[5] to 0.24 per 1000 in France.[6] Both genetic and environmental factors have been implicated to explain these differences.

Type I diabetes is characterized by T-cell-dependent destruction of pancreatic β cells.[7] This depends on activation of $CD4^+$ T cells following presentation of antigen bound to the human leucocyte antigen (HLA) molecule on the surface of antigen-presenting cells. Type I diabetes is associated with certain HLA types and antigen presentation, and hence disease susceptibility may

Table 25.1 Worldwide prevalence of type I diabetes.

Country	Prevalence per 1000
Finland	2.2
USA	1.0
UK	0.7
France	0.24
India	0.06–0.7*
China	0.09
Japan	0.03
Tropical Africa	0.03†

*The range given reflects regional differences in prevalence rates in India.
†Accurate prevalence figures not yet available for Tropical Africa; the figure given is a realistic estimate based on available data.

therefore be partly influenced by the nature of the HLA molecule(s). In Caucasians, 95% of affected subjects possess either HLA-DR3 or DR4[8] or both,

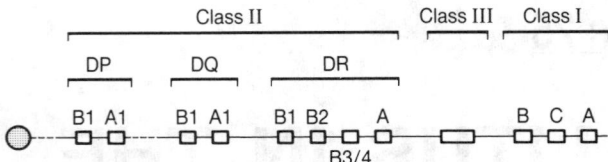

Figure 25.1 Simplified diagram of the HLA system on chromosome 6.

while DR2 and DRw6 appear to be protective.[9] These antigens are encoded by the *DRB1* gene of the major histocompatibility complex (MHC) on chromosome 6 (Figure 25.1). The MHC genes exhibit much variation or polymorphism and there is strong linkage disequilibrium between specific variants (alleles) of the *DRB1* gene and those of the *DQA1* and *DQB1* genes. This implies that certain alleles will occur together at a frequency greater than expected by chance. Analysis of *DQA1* and *DQB1* genes in different ethnic groups has demonstrated that particular alleles show consistent disease associations in many races and may represent primary susceptibility determinants.[8] Furthermore, those races with low disease incidences have a reduced frequency of these susceptibility alleles (the DR4-related allele *DQA1*0301* is rare in Asians[10] and the DR3-related allele *DQB1*0201* is rare in Japanese[11]). Absence of these alleles in a particular ethnic group may directly influence the prevalence of type I diabetes in that race.

Despite the strong evidence for inherited susceptibility, studies of identical twins suggest that this accounts for only 30–40% of disease susceptibility.[12] Environmental factors must also play an important role. Seasonal variation in the onset of disease has been reported in many different populations, indicating a possible viral aetiology.[13] Migrants from low-risk to high-risk areas assume the higher risk of their host country, e.g. Japanese migrants to Hawaii and French migrants to Canada, suggesting that disease susceptibility may be influenced by the host environment.[14] Temporal changes in disease incidence have also occurred, with a doubling in incidence in 3 years in an area of western Poland.[15] These observations could be explained by viral infection triggering autoimmune β-cell destruction. The nature of such infection remains elusive.

In summary, type I diabetes appears to be rare in the tropics. This may be due to the lack of one or more susceptibility genes or the absence of a disease-inducing environmental agent. The increased mortality from the disease in poor countries with limited health resources may also play a part in reducing the prevalence rates in these countries compared with developed nations. When it occurs, the disease is clinically indistinguishable from that seen in Caucasians.[1]

TYPE II DIABETES MELLITUS

Type II diabetes is by far the more common of the two main types of the disease. It is characterized by the presence of residual endogenous insulin secretion and peripheral insulin resistance.[16] The latter has been suggested as the primary pathogenetic abnormality in type II diabetes as well as obesity and hypertension, with which it is often associated.[17] Insulitis does not occur but abnormal islet amyloid peptides have been demonstrated in some subjects, although their role, if any, in pathogenesis is unclear.[18]

Like type I diabetes it shows a marked ethnic variation in prevalence (Table 25.2). In general, prevalence in developed nations lies between 1 and 4%, but is as high as 6% in Asian Indians, both in India[19] and in migrants to Africa,[20] whereas the prevalence in black Africans is low.[21] Asian migrants to South Africa[22] and the UK,[23] however, show a marked increase in disease prevalence. There are also discrete populations with very high disease rates, around 50% in Pima Indians in the United States[24] and in the Micronesians of Naura.[25] These ethnic variations suggest a genetic basis for type II diabetes. This is supported by the 90% disease concordance in identical twins.[12] Unlike type I diabetes, however, there has been little success in identifying possible susceptibility genes.

Apart from differences in prevalence, other racial differences also occur. Whereas onset is rare below the age of 40 years in Caucasians, the disease quite commonly appears in the third decade in Asian and, to a lesser extent, Black subjects.[23] Such cases may need to be carefully evaluated to avoid unnecessary treatment with insulin: absence of ketosis, duration of presenting symptoms and the detection of plasma C peptide may help to distinguish this entity from type I diabetes.

Asian Indians with type II diabetes have a high prevalence of hypertension and coronary heart disease. One study demonstrated higher fasting insulin

Table 25.2 Prevalence of type II diabetes in different populations.

Population	Prevalence (%)
White Caucasian	
Europe	2
USA	4
Asian	
South India	6
North India	1.2
UK	12
South Africa	20
Tanzania	7
Afro-Caribbean	
Tanzania	1.1
Nigeria	1.4
USA	5
Others	
Mauritius	10
Pima Indians (USA)	50
Micronesians (Naura)	50

and triglyceride levels and higher blood pressure in Asian compared with European type II diabetic subjects.[26] This may indicate a greater role for insulin resistance in the disease in this race, which together with the early age of onset may account for the high prevalence of coronary heart disease.

Within the Asian Indian population, the prevalence amongst urban dwellers is up to four times that of rural communities.[27,28] This suggests that environmental, as well as genetic, factors are important in disease pathogenesis. Obesity is the most important nutritional factor in the aetiology of type II diabetes[29] and its rarity in rural workers may help explain their low prevalence of disease. Obesity is common, however, in the relatively wealthy urban dwellers who have access to plentiful food and who may take less exercise. This would explain the relative increase in prevalence in Asians in the UK compared with those in Tanzania, for example.

Indeed many of the populations with very high incidences of type II diabetes have experienced a sudden increase in wealth over the last few decades associated with increasing urbanization and obesity. As well as the Pima Indians and Micronesians cited above, similar trends have been observed in black Americans[30] and some Arab populations.[31]

The high frequency in Asians compared with, for example, white Europeans, cannot, however, be explained by increased wealth and urbanization in the former. Available evidence points to a genetic predisposition to the disease in these populations, mostly within the tropics, which is manifest as type II diabetes with the adoption of a more 'Western' life style. These observations led to the 'thrifty genotype' hypothesis first put forward nearly 30 years ago.[32] It was suggested that, in populations where famine alternated with periods of food abundance, individuals with a predisposition to type II diabetes used the limited food supply more efficiently and therefore had a selective advantage during famine. The 'progress' which has abolished famine in these populations has resulted in the expression of this genotype as type II diabetes and obesity.

This is supported by data from Tanzania which showed a low prevalence of type II diabetes (0.87%) in black Africans.[21] The prevalence of impaired glucose tolerance (defined as glucose tolerance between normal value(s) and frank diabetes, and may be associated with later development of type II diabetes), however, was similar to that of North Americans. This suggests that disease expression in rural Africans is inhibited by the absence of those environmental factors present in the US population.

This is an attractive hypothesis but cannot account for all cases of type II diabetes in tropical countries. Although rare, the disease does occur in rural Africans, many of whom (43% in one study) are underweight.[21] Another study of urban Kenyans showed a lower body mass index in diabetic than in control subjects.[33]

In summary, type II diabetes is very common in some Asian and other races but is relatively rare in much of tropical Africa. An urban life style and increased wealth and availability of food correlate with increasing disease prevalence.

MALNUTRITION-RELATED DIABETES MELLITUS

In 1955 the term J-type diabetes was used to describe those patients in Jamaica (around 6%) who could not be classified as having either type I or type II diabetes.[34] Despite an early age of onset, low body weight and the requirement for high doses of insulin, they were ketosis-resistant. A condition termed

Z-type or tropical pancreatic diabetes was reported from Indonesia in 1959.[35] In addition to the above features, this was characterized by a history of childhood malnutrition and pancreatic calcification and fibrosis. Both types have since been reported in most tropical countries, including India, Ethiopia, Nigeria, Uganda, Ghana, Tanzania, Malawi, Kenya, Zaire, Cameroon, Pakistan, India, Sri Lanka, Brazil, Madagascar, Zimbabwe, Singapore, Brunei and Papua New Guinea.[36]

The World Health Organization (WHO) proposed the term malnutrition-related diabetes mellitus (MRDM) to incorporate the above types of tropical diabetes and others which had been described since the early twentieth century.[37] It was thus implied that they constituted a single entity but this is doubted by some authors, as is the relationship with malnutrition: indeed in some cases malnutrition may result from the disease rather than be causative.

Under the WHO classification, MRDM is subdivided into protein-deficient pancreatic diabetes (PDPD) and fibrocalculous pancreatic diabetes (FCPD), which largely correspond to the J- and Z-types respectively. FCPD implies the presence of pancreatic calcification and fibrosis, which result from a form of chronic pancreatitis known as tropical calcific pancreatitis (TCP).[36]

The diagnostic criteria for PDPD are: blood glucose greater than 11.1 mmol/l, disease onset under the age of 30 years, body mass index less than 19 kg/m^2, absence of ketosis, poor socioeconomic status or history of childhood malnutrition and insulin requirement of more than 60 units per day.[38] Additional criteria for the diagnosis of FCPD include a history of recurrent abdominal pain from an early age and radiographic or ultrasonographic evidence of pancreatic calculi in the absence of alcoholism, gallstones or hyperthyroidism.[39]

An alternative series of criteria which emphasize the presence of malnutrition has also been proposed: the two major criteria required for diagnosis are residence between the tropics of Cancer and Capricorn, and chronic low protein and calorie intake; in addition there are three supportive minor criteria (the presence of exocrine pancreatic disease, a requirement for insulin and early age of onset).[40]

Disease prevalence is often difficult to establish for the same logical reasons as with the other types of diabetes. These difficulties are compounded by a lack of consensus regarding diagnostic criteria and possible overlap with types I and II diabetes, especially in view of the young age of onset of the latter in many tropical countries. Thus one study from India which found that MRDM accounted for 23% of cases of diabetes[41] probably included cases of type II diabetes. Up to 80% of cases in Indonesia[35] and 50% of those under 20 years of age in Nigeria[42] are reported to have MRDM. Other reports, however, suggest much lower rates. FCPD was present in only 0.4% of 3100 cases in Madras, India;[43] a recent study from Nigeria found that only 6% of young patients could be classified as having MRDM[44] and it is absent from parts of Ethiopia.[45]

PATHOLOGY AND PATHOGENESIS

Available information on the pathological changes in MRDM is incomplete and largely confined to the FCPD variant. The hallmark is pancreatic fibrosis, which is much more marked in FCPD than PDPD. Pancreatic calcification and damage to exocrine tissue occur mainly in FCPD.[36] Islet tissue is affected to varying degrees but evidence of autoimmune damage has not been reported. In some cases the liver is involved and may show cirrhosis, fatty change or glycogen infiltration.[36]

The original concept of MRDM was that it resulted from malnutrition *per se*. Severe protein–energy malnutrition is associated with a diminished insulin response to oral glucose[46] and raised basal serum growth hormone: both factors may contribute to glucose intolerance. Resistance to ketosis may reflect impaired hepatic function and lack of non-esterified fatty acids in such patients.[36] Thus severe protein malnutrition could account for the typical findings, including absence of ketosis, in MRDM. Signs of malnutrition, hepatic dysfunction and fat malabsorption in the PDPD subtype of MRDM improved with insulin treatment and a nutritional diet in one study.[47] Subsequent withdrawal of insulin did not, however, correct the underlying glucose intolerance: all remained hyperglycaemic and some went on to become ketotic. Furthermore, a diminished glycaemic response to insulin has been demonstrated in several studies of MRDM, indicating insulin resistance.[36,41] It appears, therefore, that factors other than protein malnutrition may be involved in the aetiology of MRDM (Figure 25.2). Severe protein–calorie malnutrition occurs in many parts of the world where MRDM is unknown; conversely, many subjects with the disease show no signs of malnutrition.[40]

It has been suggested that cassava (tapioca) ingestion may trigger pancreatic dysfunction.[48] Cassava is the staple food in many areas where MRDM occurs,

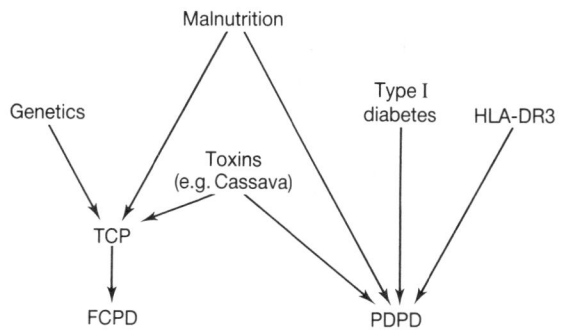

Figure 25.2 Possible factors in the aetiology of MRDM.

supplying perhaps up to three-quarters of total carbohydrate and one-half of protein intake. It contains the cyanogenic glycoside, linamarin, which on hydrolysis releases hydrocyanic acid. This toxin is normally inactivated by conjugation with sulphydryl groups derived from the amino acids methionine, cystine and cysteine to form thiocyanate. Deficiency of these amino acids in protein–calorie malnutrition may lead to accumulation of hydrocyanic acid which may directly damage the pancreas.[36] This is an attractive, albeit unproven, hypothesis but cassava consumption itself does not adequately explain the distribution of MRDM. It is not consumed in two areas of India where MRDM is recognized (although another cyanide-containing food, ragi, is in regular use in these areas).[40] In addition, MRDM is not endemic in all cassava-consuming areas, although this may reflect differences in cooking habits.

A variant of the disease (previously termed K-type) is related to alcohol consumption.[49] This occurs in men aged over 30 years in Kenya, Uganda and South Africa. Kaffir beers in these areas are thought to be responsible and it has been suggested that these also contain small amounts of cyanide.[36,40]

The similarity of the clinical features of PDPD to type I diabetes has led to speculation that it is in fact a form of the latter, and that the observed weight loss is secondary to untreated diabetes.[50] There is some genetic data from Ethiopia in support of this hypothesis where HLA-DR3 was significantly positively associated and DR2 negatively associated both with PDPD and type I diabetes compared with controls.[51] Interestingly, however, DR4 was not associated with PDPD, although it was associated with type I diabetes. It has been suggested that DR3 is associated with a milder form of type I diabetes than DR4,[52] and PDPD may represent a variant of DR3-associated type I diabetes. This is an interest-

ing observation and further genetic and histological evidence is required to substantiate it.

TROPICAL CALCIFIC PANCREATITIS AND FIBROCALCULOUS PANCREATIC DIABETES (See also Chapter 3)

Although FCPD is thought to be secondary to TCP, not all cases of TCP develop frank diabetes: in some glucose tolerance is impaired while in others it remains normal.[53] The latter tend to be younger, however, and longitudinal studies are required to ascertain whether all cases of TCP eventually become diabetic. The exocrine pancreatic dysfunction in FCPD has been shown to correlate directly with the extent of β-cell loss: in one study plasma C-peptide concentration (which reflects β-cell function) was severely diminished (but detectable) in 75% and immunoreactive trypsin (a marker of exocrine function) almost undetectable in 66% of subjects with FCPD.[53] There was a significant correlation between these two parameters in all subjects with TCP, regardless of their glucose tolerance, indicating that both exocrine and endocrine function decrease occur concomitantly, presumably as a result of the same pancreatic lesion. Most studies report residual insulin secretion, which would prevent the development of ketosis.[39,54]

The pancreatic lesion in TCP reflects chronic pancreatitis: the pancreas becomes shrunken, firm and fibrosed with multiple stones in the major ducts.[36] The cause of pancreatitis is unclear and, while originally thought to result from malnutrition, other possibilities include toxic effects, particularly from cassava consumption, and genetic predisposition. Although most patients are underweight, evidence of malnutrition may be present in only 25%.[39] Plasma albumin has been shown to be normal in cases of TCP without diabetes and low only in those who had developed FCPD.[53] This suggests that protein malnutrition does not precede TCP and may result from it. Given the associated impairment of exocrine function (a third of one study group had steatorrhoea[39]), it could be expected that TCP itself may lead to malabsorption and weight loss.

Support for a genetic component to susceptibility in FCPD comes from the occurrence of familial aggregation of FCPD in south India.[55] Ten per cent of patients had a family member with pancreatic calculi or exocrine pancreatic pathology and there was a high prevalence of abnormalities of glucose tolerance.[56] Molecular genetic studies have shown associations of FCPD with a DQB restriction fragment length polymorphism (RFLP) similar to that found in type I diabetes, and a stronger association with the class 3 allele of the hypervariable region of the 5' flanking region of the insulin gene, which was also associated with type II diabetes.[57]

In summary, MRDM is a geographically widespread condition which is still poorly understood.

The FCPD subtype probably results from TCP which is of unknown aetiology and leads to pancreatic calcification and both endocrine and exocrine dysfunction. In PDPD only the endocrine pancreas is affected. The relative importance of malnutrition, toxin ingestion and genetic predisposition in the aetiology of both conditions remains to be elucidated.

CONCLUSIONS

Although the clinical picture of each type of disease is similar wherever it occurs, there is a wide geographical diversity in the rates of the different types of diabetes mellitus within the tropics. Increased awareness of the differences between the types of disease should result in more accurate diagnosis and better epidemiological data, which will be invaluable in further studies of the pathogenesis of this important and common condition.

ACKNOWLEDGEMENTS

D.A.C. was supported by the Medical Research Council (UK).

REFERENCES

1 Odugbesan O & Barnett A H. Racial differences. In Barnett A H (ed.) *Immunogenetics of Insulin Dependent Diabetes.* Lancaster: MTP Press, 1987: 91–101.

2 Vaishnava H, Bashin R C & Galati P O. Diabetes mellitus with onset under 40 years in North India. *J Assoc Physicians India* 1974; 22:879–888.

3 Shanghai Diabetes Research Cooperative Group. Diabetes mellitus survey in Shanghai. *Chin Med J* 1980; 93:663–667.

4 Lorenzi M, Cagliero E & Schmidt J J. Racial differences in incidence of juvenile onset type I diabetes: epidemiologic studies in southern California. *Diabetologia* 1985; 28:734–738.

5 Koivisto V A, Åkerblom H K & Wasz-Höckert O. The epidemiology of juvenile diabetes mellitus in Northern Finland. *Nord Counc Arct Med Res* 1976; 15:58–65.

6 Lestradet H & Besse J. Prevalence and incidence of juvenile insulin-dependent diabetes in France. *Diabete Metab* 1977; 3:229–234.

7 Todd J A. Genetic control of autoimmunity in Type I diabetes. *Immunol Today* 1990; 11:122–129.

8 Jenkins D, Mijovic C, Fletcher J A, Jacobs K H, Bradwell A R & Barnett A H. Identification of susceptibility loci for type I (insulin-dependent) diabetes by trans-racial gene mapping. *Diabetologia* 1990; 33:387–395.

9 Cavan D A, Penny M A Jacobs K H, et al. Both DQA1 and DQB1 genes are implicated in HLA-associated protection from Type 1 diabetes in a British Caucasian population. *Diabetologia* 1993; 36:252–257.

10 Jenkins D, Mijovic C, Jacobs K H, Penny M A, Fletcher J & Barnett A H. Allele-specific gene probing supports the DQ molecule as a determinant of inherited susceptibility to type I (insulin-dependent) diabetes mellitus. *Diabetologia* 1991; 34:109–113.

11 Jacobs K H, Jenkins D, Mijovic C H et al. An investigation of Japanese subjects maps susceptibility to type I (insulin-dependent) diabetes mellitus close to the DQA1 gene. *Hum Immunol* 1992; 33:24–28.

12 Barnett A H, Eff C, Leslie R D G & Pyke D A. Diabetes in identical twins: a study of 200 pairs. *Diabetologia* 1981; 20:87–93.

13 Gamble D R & Taylor K W. Seasonal incidence of diabetes mellitus. *BMJ* 1969; iii:631–633.

14 Diabetes Epidemiology Research International. Preventing insulin-dependent diabetes mellitus: the environmental challenge. *BMJ* 1987; 295:479–481.

15 Rewers M, LaPorte R E, Walczak M, Dmochowski K & Bogaczynska E. An apparent 'epidemic' of youth onset insulin-dependent diabetes mellitus in Western Poland. *Diabetes* 1987; 36:106–113.

16 Flier J S. Insulin receptors and insulin resistance. *Ann Rev Med* 1983; 34:145–160.

17 Reaven G M. Role of insulin resistance in human disease. *Diabetes* 1988; 37:1595–1607.

18 Cooper G J S, Willis A C, Clark A, Turner R C, Sim R B & Reid K B M. Purification and characterisation of a peptide from amyloid-rich pancreases of type 2 diabetic patients. *Proc Natl Acad Sci USA* 1987; 84:8628–8632.

19 Rao P V, Ushabala P, Seshiah V et al. The Eluru survey: prevalence of known diabetes in a rural Indian population. *Diabetes Res Clin Pract* 1989; 7:29–31.

20 Swai A B M, McLarty D G, Sherriff F et al. Diabetes and impaired glucose tolerance in an Asian community in Tanzania. *Diabetes Res Clin Pract* 1990; 8:227–234.

21 McLarty D G, Swai A B M, Kitange H M et al. The prevalence of diabetes and impaired glucose tolerance in rural Tanzania. *Lancet* 1989; i:871–875.

22 Jackson W P U. Epidemiology of diabetes in South Africa. *Adv Metab Disord* 1978; 9:111–146.

23 Mather H M & Keen H. The Southall diabetes survey: prevalence of known diabetes in Asians and Europeans. *BMJ* 1985; 291:1081–1084.

24 Knowler W C, Bennett P H, Hamman R F & Miller M. Diabetes incidence and prevalence in Pima Indians. *Am J Epidemiol* 1978; 108:497–505.

25 Zimmet P, Pinkstone G, Whitehouse S & Thomas K. The high incidence of diabetes mellitus in the Micronesian population of Naura. *Acta Diabetol Lat* 1982; 19:75–79.

26 McKeigue P M, Shah B & Marmot M G. Diabetes, insulin resistance and central obesity in South Asians and Europeans. *Diabetic Med* 1989; 6 (supplement 1):A41–42.

27 Tripathy B B, Panda N C, Tej S C, Sahoo G N & Kar B K. Survey for detection of glycosuria, hyperglycaemia and diabetes mellitus in urban and rural areas of Cuttack district. *J Assoc Physicians India* 1971; 19:681–692.

28 Gupta O P, Joshi M H & Dave S K. Prevalence of diabetes in India. *Adv Metab Disord* 1978; 9:147–165.

29 World Health Organization Expert Committee on Diabetes Mellitus. Second Report. *WHO Tech Rep Ser* 1980; 646:1–80.

30 Bonham G S & Brock D B. *The Relationship of Diabetes with Race, Sex and Obesity.* America Statistical Association, Proceedings of the Social Statistics Section, 1982; 397–402.

31 Bacchus R A, Bell J L, MadKour M & Kilshaw B. The prevalence of diabetes mellitus in male Saudi Arabs. *Diabetologia* 1982; 20:87–93.

32 Neel J V. Diabetes Mellitus: a 'thrifty' genotype rendered detrimental by 'progress'? *Am J Hum Genet* 1962; 14:353–362.

33 Obel A O K. Body mass index in non-insulin dependent diabetics in Kenya. *Trop Geogr Med* 1988; 40:93–96.

34 Hugh-Jones P. Diabetes in Jamaica. *Lancet* 1955; ii:891–897.

35 Zuidema P J. Cirrhosis and disseminated calcification of the pancreas in patients with malnutrition. *Trop Geogr Med* 1959; 11:70–74.

36 Abu-Bakare A, Taylor R, Gill G V & Alberti K G M M. Tropical or malnutrition-related diabetes: a real syndrome? *Lancet* 1986; i:1135–1138.

37 World Health Organization Study Group on Diabetes Mellitus. *WHO Tech Rep Ser* 1985; 727.

38 Ahuja M M. Diabetes: special problems in developing countries. *Bull Deliv Health Care Diabet Devel Countries* 1980; 1:5–6.

39 Mohan V, Mohan R, Sushjeela L et al. Tropical pancreatic diabetes in South India: heterogeneity in clinical and biochemical profile. *Diabetologia* 1985; 28:229–232.

40 McMillan D E. Tropical malnutrition diabetes. *Diabetologia* 1986; 29:127–128.

41 Tripathy B B & Kar B C. Observations on clincal patterns of diabetes mellitus in India. *Diabetes* 1965; 14:404–412.

42 Osuntokun B O, Akinkugbe F M, Francis T I, Reddy S, Osuntokun O & Taylor G O L. Diabetes mellitus in Nigerians: a study of 832 patients. *West Afr Med J* 1971; 20: 295–312.

43 Viswanathan M, Mohamud U, Krishnamoorthy M & Balachandran P K. Diabetes in the young: a study of 166 cases. *Antiseptic* 1966; 63:741–745.

44 Akanji A O. Malnutrition-related diabetes mellitus in young adult diabetic patients attending a Nigerian diabetic clinic. *J Trop Med Hyg* 1990; 93:35–38.

45 Lester F T. A search for malnutrition diabetes in an Ethiopian diabetic clinic. *IDF Bull* 1984; 29:14–16.

46 Garg S K, Marwaha R K, Ganapathi V et al. Serum growth hormone, insulin and blood sugar responses to oral glucose in protein energy malnutrition. *Trop Geogr Med* 1989; 41:9–13.

47 Abdulkadir J, Mengesha B, Gebriel W et al. The clinical and hormonal (C-peptide and glucagon) profile and liability to ketoacidosis during nutritional rehabilitation in Ethiopian patients with malnutrition-related diabetes mellitus. *Diabetologia* 1990; 33:222–227.

48 McMillan D E & Geevarghese P J. Dietary cyanide and tropical malnutrition diabetes. *Diabetes Care* 1979; 2:202–208.

49 Mngola E N. Diabetes mellitus in the African environment: the dilemma. In Mngola E N (ed.) *Diabetes 1982*, Excerpta Med Int Congr Ser no. 600. Amsterdam: Excerpta Medica, 1983:3–9.

50 Lester F T. Nutritional status of young adult Ethiopians before onset and after treatment of diabetes mellitus. *Ethiop Med J* 1990; 28:1–7.

51 Abdulkadir J, Worku Y, Schreuder G M T, D'Amaro J, de Vries R R P & Ottenhoff T M H. HLA-DR and DQ antigens in malnutrition-related diabetes mellitus in Ethiopians: a clue to its aetiology? *Tissue Antigens* 1989; 34:284–289.

52 Ludvigsson J, Samuelsson U, Baeufort C et al. HLA DR3 is associated with a more slowly progressive form of type I (insulin-dependent) diabetes. *Diabetologia* 1986; 29:207–210.

53 Yajnik C S, Shelgikar K M, Sahasrabudhe R A et al.

The spectrum of pancreatic exocrine and endocrine (beta-cell) function in tropical calcific pancreatitis. *Diabetologia* 1990; 33:417–421.

54 Mohan V, Snehalatha C, Ramachandran A, Jayashree R & Viswanathan M. Pancreatic B-cell function in tropical pancreatic diabetes. *Metabolism* 1983; 32:1091–1092.

55 Pitchumoni C S. Familial pancreatitis. In Pai K N,

Suman C R & Varghese R (eds) *Pancreatic Diabetes.* Trivandrum: Geo-Printers, 1980:46–48.

56 Mohan V, Chari S, Hitman G A et al. Familial aggregation in tropical fibrocalculous pancreatic diabetes. *Pancreas* 1989; 4:690–693.

57 Kambo P K, Hitman G A, Mohan V et al. The genetic predisposition to fibrocalculous pancreatic diabetes. *Diabetologia* 1989; 32:45–51.

CHAPTER 26

HYPERTENSION IN THE TROPICS

J. C. Mbanya, J. K. Cruickshank and D. G. Beevers

High blood pressure has only recently been regarded as an important health problem in the developing and developed countries of the tropics (see also Chapter 5). The quickening pace of change and increasing mass communication have put more Western life styles within the immediate reach of people in developing countries so that cardiovascular diseases, and particularly hypertension, now have a sharply rising incidence, morbidity and mortality. As the main risk factors for cardiovascular disease are themselves treatable, it is to be hoped that they will not reach the epidemic proportions that have been seen in the West. However, if cardiovascular disease prevention is to be achieved in tropical countries, major changes will be necessary in the methods of administering medical care.

Hypertension is one of three major risk factors for the development of heart attack and stroke, renal failure, cardiac failure and peripheral vascular disease. The other factors, cigarette smoking and raised plasma lipid levels, should also be preventable.[1] These three risk factors themselves have a synergistic or multiplicative effect on each other in causing cardiovascular disease (Figure 26.1).

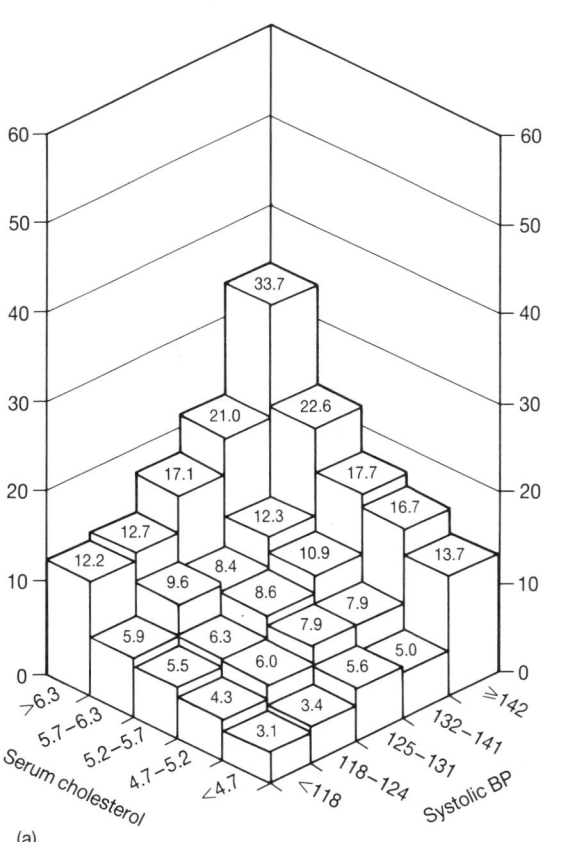

(a)

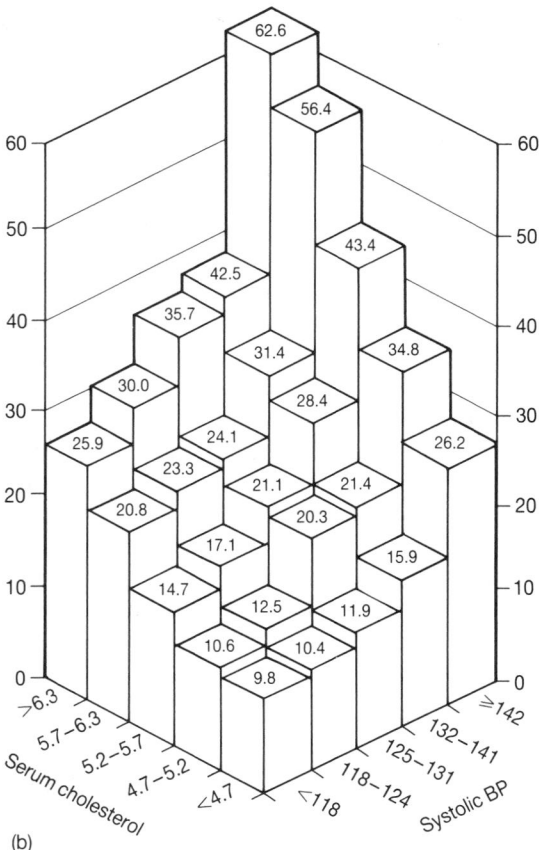

(b)

Figure 26.1 Coronary heart disease mortality per 10 000 person-years. (a) Non-smokers; (b) smokers. (Adapted from Multiple Risk Factor Intervention Trial (MRFIT) examinees.[1])

Programmes to implement the control of high blood pressure are now on the agenda of such bodies as the Pan American Health Organization, and the governments of countries in South-East Asia, India and many Pacific islands. In South America, major initiatives have been taking place in Brazil. In tropical Africa, the Pan African Society of Cardiology is actively promoting initiatives to deal with hypertension even though funding remains limited. An important factor that has encouraged these bodies is that programmes directed towards high blood pressure control are applicable to other chronic conditions including diabetes mellitus and coronary heart disease.[2]

In the field of adult medicine, hypertensive disease is having a major impact in clinical practice. In urban Brazil and in the West Indies, as well as many parts of urban Africa, up to one-third of all outpatients and acute medical admissions can be related to high blood pressure. In West Africa, hypertensive cardiac failure is now more common than rheumatic or other heart diseases. In parts of South Asia, diabetes mellitus and hypertension commonly coexist and predispose to the developing epidemic of coronary heart disease which has also struck migrant Indian origin people wherever they have settled. In South-East Asia, vascular diseases are now routine diagnoses, even if myocardial infarction remains relatively uncommon. In the West Indies and sub-Saharan Africa, hypertension, renal failure and stroke are common but again coronary heart disease remains relatively less common. A similar pattern is seen amongst the African-origin black communities in the UK and the USA.[3]

High blood pressure is also a major risk factor for perinatal and maternal mortality. Throughout the tropical world, eclampsia—which has many features akin to hypertensive encephalopathy, is thought to be killing over 50 000 women per year.

Much of our knowledge of hypertension and its consequences in tropical settings has come from studies of African or Indian subcontinental settlers in the West Indies, Britain and the USA, as well as studies of migrants in Africa from rural subsistence farming areas to the expanding cities and their associated shanty towns. These studies can assist our understanding of the relative roles of genetic versus environmental factors in the pathogenesis of hypertension.

THE EPIDEMIOLOGICAL TRANSITION

The transitions outlined above from traditional infective to chronic cardiovascular disease lead to the inescapable conclusion that attaining or struggling towards typical Westernized life styles, with all the social, financial, dietary and stress-related influences, as well as increasing tobacco and alcohol consumption, have profound long-term blood pressure elevating effects. The observation that hypertension and its consequences are almost unheard of in remote tribal areas whilst reaching epidemic proportions in the cities, implies that environmental factors are primarily responsible for the aetiology of hypertension (Figure 26.2). The emergence of the same problems in widely differing populations makes a major genetic basis for hypertension much less likely.[4–6] It follows, therefore, that hypertension and its sequelae are generally preventable or reversible.

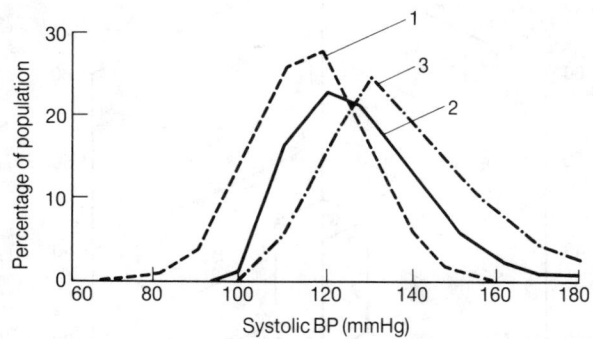

Figure 26.2 Blood pressure distribution in three different populations: 1, Kenyan nomads; 2, London civil servants; 3, Japanese railwaymen. Although mean blood pressures were higher in the Japanese railwaymen, the shape of the distribution curve is preserved, indicating a difference throughout the population. (Adapted from Swales J D, Sever P S & Peart W S. *Clinical Atlas of Hypertension.* London: Gower, 1991).

DEFINITIONS OF HYPERTENSION

Blood pressure in any population is distributed in a 'normal' or gaussian curve so that any definition of hypertension depends on arbitrary levels of blood pressure, above which individuals can be labelled as hypertensive and below which they are considered to be either borderline or normotensive (Figure

26.2). Those populations with a high prevalence of hypertension are also the populations with higher average blood pressures. Thus, in a sense, the whole population could be regarded as hypertensive when compared with societies where hypertension is rare. The preventive solution to hypertension would, therefore, require a whole population strategy. From a clinical standpoint, the definition of hypertension must rely on the available evidence of the value of blood pressure reduction. Thus, a pragmatic definition of hypertension, taking into account the epidemiological principles and the current state of knowledge of the benefits of blood pressure reduction, is 'that level of blood pressure above which treatment does more good than harm'.[7] This blood pressure level now approximates to the dividing line for the definition of hypertension originally provided by the World Health Organization (WHO). The WHO guidelines are based on three blood pressure measurements on two successive visits to a clinic, using diastolic phase V (final disappearance of sounds). Irrespective of age, the level chosen was 160 mmHg for systolic and 95 mmHg diastolic blood pressure (Table 26.1).

The updated guidelines from the United States

Table 26.1 Definition of hypertension by WHO criteria.

	Systolic blood pressure (mmHg)		*Diastolic blood pressure (mmHg)*
Normal	<140	with	<90
Borderline	140–159	and/or	90–94
Definite	≥160	and/or	≥95
Mild hypertension	160–179	and/or	95–104

It is important to note that these take no account of the age of the patient, the number of blood pressure readings or the presence of pre-existing vascular complications of hypertension.

Joint National Committee on Blood Pressure and the British Hypertension Society were published in 1993.[8,9] Both take into account the results of the recent therapeutic trials of the management of hypertension. These guidelines are therefore relevant for clinicians in all parts of the world, although because of problems of feasibility and expense, they have not been tested in tropical settings.

MEASUREMENT

Important clinical decisions are made on the basis of the height of blood pressure but sadly this measurement is often inaccurate. The standard mercury manometer, when used properly, is still the gold standard. Electronic automatic machinery should be treated with suspicion. The main problem with mercury manometers are related to their incorrect use, and medical and related staff should ideally be retrained. The British Hypertension Society[10] has provided simple guidelines on the measurement of blood pressure and these are briefly outlined here. The manometer should be well maintained with the mercury column vertical and at rest the mercury should be at 0 mmHg. If the manometer is sloping away from the vertical, due to damaged hinges, this leads to overestimation of the pressure. The rubber bladder inside the arm cuff should encircle at least 80% of the upper arm. In order to achieve this, it is strongly recommended that the old 'adult cuff' with a bladder measuring 12.5 × 23 cm should be replaced by the 'alternative adult cuff' with a bladder measuring 12.5 × 33 cm. This cuff is applicable for individuals with arm circumferences of up to 43 cm.

The use of too small a cuff leads to overestimation of blood pressure.

Blood pressures should normally be measured with the subject seated with the cuff level with the heart. The arm should be slightly externally rotated and supported to avoid the isometric exercise required to hold the arm raised, as this causes false elevations of blood pressure. The manometer cuff should be inflated to about 15 mmHg above the level needed to occlude the brachial pulse and the diaphragm of the stethoscope should be placed where the pulse was felt, slightly to the medial side of the antecubital fossa. The column of mercury should be deflated slowly (2 mm/s). The systolic blood pressure is taken at the first appearance of Korotkoff sounds (phase I) and diastolic pressure at the final disappearance of sounds (phase V). Measurement of diastolic blood pressure at the phase of muffling of sounds (phase IV) is now obsolete. Blood pressures are measured to the nearest 2 mmHg.

On all occasions, blood pressure should be measured twice and decisions made on the basis of the second reading. In patients with mild hypertension, decisions on starting drug therapy should only be made after two readings on four separate occasions.

Failure to follow these simple guidelines will lead to overestimation of blood pressure and needless or excessive use of antihypertensive agents. Many people have blood pressures which are mildly elevated on first measurement but which settle on rechecking. These 'white coat hypertensives' may receive unnecessary drug therapy.

The careful training of observers, possibly with audiovisual aids, is important as the accurate assessment of hypertensive patients will differentiate between those requiring drug therapy, those requiring careful observation only, and those who can be reassured. Whilst many hypertensive patients remain undiagnosed, many are overtreated because of unreliable measurement techniques.

EPIDEMIOLOGY

In developing countries where many populations do not have easy access to health care facilities, the diagnosis of hypertension is often made only after complications have set in. Hypertension is not being diagnosed at the milder and presymptomatic stage when drug treatment is of proven value. The underdiagnosis of hypertension is a major problem in all countries and can only be solved when the routine screening of all apparently fit symptomless adults becomes an accepted part of medical care.

In most black populations, except those few remaining unexposed to 'development', hypertension is generally more common than in white or Indo-European communities. Hence, if health care facilities are limited, hypertension may appear to be more severe in blacks by giving rise to higher mortality rates at a younger age. However, the small number of follow-up studies of blacks do not support this view. For a given level of blood pressure, an individual black person has virtually the same prognosis as a white or Asian subject. This trend was found in studies in the USA, Jamaica and Trinidad.[11] The contention that black hypertensive patients have more severe hypertension than whites arises from the clinical fallacy of more people being at risk and thus being seen with the complications.

An important factor in the epidemiology of hypertension is that in all non-tribal societies average blood pressure rises with advancing age. Thus at the age of 70, about one-half of the population will have hypertension using WHO criteria. This rise in blood pressure with age is primarily due to environmental factors as it is not seen in genetically similar rural populations. There is evidence that the blood pressure age gradient is steeper in urban Africans than in the white communities of Europe and the USA. The consequences of raised blood pressure, and particularly stroke, thus become more common with advancing age in tropical countries. African-origin black communities of Europe and the USA also show a steeper rise of blood pressure with age than the white communities in the same cities.

PREVALENCE

Blood pressures requiring drug therapy are seen in 5–10% of adult white populations in Europe and the USA, depending on the age distribution of the population, and are substantially more common in blacks. There is good evidence that these levels of blood pressure are also common in Africa where the prevalence of hypertension may reach 20%—the highest figures being seen in the cities. In some regions, hypertension accounts for 10 and 5% of adult hospital morbidity and mortality, respectively.

In some areas of Africa, between 4 and 6% of children aged 5–15 years have elevated blood pressure. There are few reliable data comparing blood pressures of black and white populations in Africa. Comparisons of studies in Africa with those done in Europe or the USA tend to be confounded by lack of standardization of methods and failure to take into account the effects of obesity and alcohol as well as the age distribution of the population(s). Another important consideration is the effect of ambient temperature (for a 1°C increase in temperature blood pressure falls by 1 mmHg). There is, however, evidence that hypertension is more common in black South Africans than in whites.[12] Urban/rural comparisons in several parts of Africa, including Cameroon, Gambia, Ghana, Ivory Coast, Nigeria, South

Africa and Kenya, report consistently higher rates (5–10%) in urban areas. In Western countries, hypertension is more common in men until the age of about 50 years. At this stage, the difference between the genders lessens and hypertension eventually becomes more common in women, possibly in part because of the impact of premature death in the men with higher blood pressures.

RISK FACTORS FOR HYPERTENSION

SOCIAL GRADIENT

An emerging phenomenon in tropical countries is that people of middle and upper socioeconomic class tend to have higher rates of hypertension than poorer groups. This excess is partly due to greater body mass but other factors, including physical inactivity and nutritional influences such as alcohol consumption and a high-salt diet with a low intake of potassium-rich foods, may also be involved.[13] Social status incongruity and the stress associated with social betterment and rapid changes in the structure of societies may also be important. Studies in developed societies show the opposite phenomenon, with an inverse relationship between social class and blood pressure. As urbanization and development in the tropics settles down, this trend for hypertension and its complications to be more common in people of higher social class may reverse, as it did in the West about 50 years ago. Until then, hypertension is selectively killing off economically active members of the community.

ALCOHOL

Excess alcohol intake is a well-established risk factor for hypertension. Its pressor effects may be more important in tropical settings where other cardiovascular risk factors are few, but we know of no studies addressing this point. It is of interest that the second ever study reporting the relationship between alcohol and blood pressure was conducted in Bombay.[14] Whilst earlier reports suggest that the risk of hypertension appeared at the level of about five drinks per day, recent data suggest that there is a relationship even at lower alcohol levels.[13] Epidemiological and clinical studies strongly suggest that the alcohol–blood pressure relationship is rapidly reversible with moderation or cessation of drinking.

CATIONS

There is evidence from well-designed cross-sectional and longitudinal studies that a difference in mean sodium intake of 100 mmol/day is associated with a 7–10 mmHg difference in systolic blood pressure rise over 30 years. Furthermore, lower dietary potassium intakes are associated with an increased risk of hypertension. Both salt restriction and potassium supplementation effectively reduce blood pressure. Current evidence emerging from the INTERSALT study, which was the largest ever international comparative study of hypertension in 30 countries, demonstrates that hypertension is most common in populations with the lowest potassium consumption and the highest 24-hour urinary sodium excretion.[13] The role of these dietary factors in hypertension needs further investigation in urban and rural tropical areas. Clinical studies conducted in the USA suggest that black people are more sensitive to a given dietary salt load, exhibiting a greater rise in blood pressure and a delayed natriuresis when compared with white people.[15] Thus, black people may be more salt-sensitive even though they may consume similar amounts of salt.

Some of the electrolyte differences may be related to socioeconomic factors. Potassium-rich foods, generally considered to be beneficial—by reducing blood pressure and hence strokes, are expensive and there is evidence, mainly from the USA, that their consumption in poor urban black communities is lower than in the rural populations and also lower than in white people.

CATION TRANSPORT

Electrolyte membrane abnormalities may be associated with essential hypertension in man. Hypertensives have significantly higher intracellular sodium levels compared with normotensives and the ouabain sensitive sodium pump, responsible for extruding sodium from cells, is depressed and there is also raised intracellular calcium. A difference in sodium–potassium countertransport across cell membranes may be genetically determined, predisposing black more than white people to hypertension.[16] Higher intrasodium concentrations are found in both normotensive and hypertensive black people when compared with whites.

THE RENIN–ANGIOTENSIN SYSTEM

Studies in North America, the UK and South Africa have consistently shown that adult black subjects have lower plasma renin and angiotensin II levels than whites.[17] Since this difference is not immediately related to a higher salt intake, these low renin levels may be genetically determined. It is possible, however, that genetic factors were originally less important as people living in tropical hunter–gatherer societies tended to die prematurely if they had higher renin levels and lacked the capacity to retain sodium. The low-renin/sodium-retaining people tended to survive. In the high-salt-consuming societies today, the capacity to retain sodium has become disadvantageous as it causes a rise in blood pressure.

INSULIN METABOLISM

A series of abnormalities associated with resistance to insulin-stimulated glucose uptake, including hyperinsulinaemia, impaired glucose tolerance, increased plasma triglyceride concentration(s), decreased high-density lipoprotein concentration(s) and high blood pressure, have been reported in studies in Britain and the USA. All of these factors are independently related to the development of ischaemic cardiac disease. Based on these considerations, it has been suggested that insulin resistance and hyperinsulinaemia may be involved in the aetiology of hypertension.[18] However, there is inconsistent evidence of a relationship between insulin resistance and hypertension in non-European populations. Since there is still a low incidence of ischaemic heart disease in hypertensive patients in Africa, it could be argued that insulin-resistance and its effects on lipid metabolism are less important.

Animal fat intake in Africa is lower than in the West and this may explain the relative rarity of coronary heart disease, whilst hypertension-related strokes and renal failure are common. As in all populations, there is an excess of hypertension associated with diabetes mellitus. Community studies carried out in Cameroon and Madagascar put the association at between 20 and 30%. The association of raised blood pressure with non-insulin dependent diabetes mellitus is associated with increased mortality rate(s) from cardiovascular disease. Both risk factors are closely related to life style so their rising prevalence should be preventable.

UNDERLYING CAUSES OF HYPERTENSION

In a tiny minority of hypertensive patients, a treatable underlying disease may be found which is the cause of raised blood pressure[19] and the reader is referred to the standard textbooks of hypertension. Intrinsic renal diseases (glomerulonephritis, polycystic renal disease, pyelonephritis), renal artery stenosis, endocrine diseases (Cushing's syndrome, primary aldosteronism, phaeochromocytoma and acromegaly) and coarctation of the aorta do not seem to occur with greater frequency in the tropics than in Europe or North America. There does, however, appear to be an excess incidence of systemic lupus erythematosus which can be an important cause of high blood pressure, especially in young women. Estimations of the prevalence of secondary hypertension are influenced by the availability of modern diagnostic facilities and this presents problems for most tropical countries. Extensive investigation reveals that between 10 and 20% of patients with hypertension presenting to hospital in some African countries have evidence of renal impairment but this kidney damage is a consequence rather than a cause of the hypertension. It is possible that glomerulonephritis is more common in West Africa than in Europe but this point can only be proved by extensive use of renal biopsies, which would be of doubtful feasibility or value.

HYPERTENSION IN PREGNANCY (See also Chapter 17)

This is an important problem in the tropics and is associated with increased maternal and fetal mortality. Perinatal and maternal mortality rates are high in developing countries and about one-third of these deaths may be due to hypertension. The diagnosis of pre-eclampsia is made on the presence of proteinuria and there is usually elevation of blood pressure. The drug treatment of severer grades of hypertension at this stage of pregnancy is worthwhile. Patients who have pre-existing or chronic hypertension may sustain a fall in pressure in early pregnancy. If the diastolic blood pressure remains consistently below 100 mmHg, drug treatment should not be given. Many mothers develop gestational or pregnancy-induced hypertension in which blood pressure rises in pregnancy and falls after pregnancy is over. Where this elevation of blood pressure is mild, and not associated with proteinuria, drug treatment should not be given.

It is probable that raised blood pressure in pregnancy is associated with the development of established hypertension in later life, and also that this problem runs in families. There is now evidence that low birth weight babies, resulting from maternal hypertension, may be more prone to hypertension in adulthood.

HYPERCHOLESTEROLAEMIA AND CIGARETTE SMOKING

The presence of hypercholesterolaemia or cigarette smoking exerts a major influence on prognosis amongst hypertensive patients. Hypercholesterolaemia is not common in Blacks in Africa or the Caribbean. By contrast, it has become a major problem in the Indian subcontinent and the Pacific Islands and amongst Asians living the Caribbean.[20] The promotion of tobacco in the developing countries constitutes an international scandal. Neither of these risk factors themselves cause hypertension.

SYMPTOMS AND SIGNS

Patients with mild-to-moderate hypertension rarely complain of symptoms. Dizziness, fatigue, headache and palpitations are more often due to anxiety or the side-effects of antihypertensive drugs. Severely hypertensive patients may present for the first time, with stroke or evidence of renal impairment or heart disease.

Clinical examination may reveal evidence of left ventricular enlargement. For a given level of blood pressure, if left ventricular hypertrophy is present, the mortality is four times greater. Malignant hypertension is diagnosed if there are retinal haemorrhages and or exudates with or without papilloedema. In such cases, the diastolic blood pressure is usually more than 120 mmHg.

In the Indian subcontinent and in Asian populations resident in the West, coronary heart disease is a common complication of hypertension. Examination may reveal evidence of other arterial disease with absent peripheral pulses, as well as xanthelasmas, xanthomas, corneal arcus and femoral or carotid bruits. Clinical signs of heart failure may be due to coronary heart disease but severe hypertension alone can also cause heart failure. Alternatively, heart failure may be due to congestive cardiomyopathy or concurrent rheumatic cardiac disease.

INVESTIGATIONS

Investigation depends on the severity of the hypertension and availability of facilities. All patients receiving antihypertensive drug therapy should ideally have routine urine testing, and full biochemical haematological profiling together with an ECG.

Urine testing should be regarded as routine in all patients. Haematuria, where present, may be due to malignant hypertension and proteinuria may be due to hypertension itself or to underlying renal disease. For a given level of pressure, if there is proteinuria, mortality is approximately doubled. The presence of proteinuria is a better predictor of mortality than estimations of serum creatinine or urea levels. The measurement of microproteinuria (urine albumin below 300 mg/l) is of value in diabetic hypertensives but its significance in other hypertensives is uncertain.

All patients should undergo at least one blood test to estimate plasma sodium and potassium levels. Serum potassium levels are low in both primary and secondary hyperaldosteronism, and if hypokalaemia is encountered this needs detailed investigation. The most common cause of hypokalaemia is diuretic therapy, which must be discontinued at least 4 weeks prior to testing. Serum urea or creatinine levels should be measured to obtain an estimate of renal function. The estimation of creatinine clearance is not valuable unless there is severe renal failure. Serum cholesterol levels should be measured in the non-fasting state in populations where hypercholesterolaemia is common. If the ECG shows evidence of left ventricular hypertrophy, with the sum of the R wave in leads V_5 or V_6 and the S wave in V_1 or V_2 amounting to more than 35 mm, then the prognosis is bad. Because left ventricular hypertrophy is such an important prognostic factor, a routine ECG in hypertensive patients is desirable.

Haematological profiling with estimations of plasma viscosity or ESR may provide evidence of connective tissue diseases which may cause high blood pressure. In such cases, proteinuria may also be present.

If renal impairment is present or there is unexplained hypokalaemia, more detailed investigation with renal ultrasound scanning or intravenous urography is necessary. If the kidneys are found to be small but with a smooth outline, then the possibility of correctable renal artery stenosis should be borne in mind and renal angiography is worth considering. If the kidneys are small with an irregular outline, pyelonephritis is more likely and investigations should be conducted to exclude obstructive uropathy with vesicoureteric reflux. If hypokalaemia is present, patients should undergo estimation of plasma renin and aldosterone levels. In primary hyperaldosteronism, plasma renin is low, whilst concurrent plasma aldosterone levels are high. If these features are found, patients should proceed to computerized tomography to detect an adrenal adenoma. In Conn's syndrome, removal of the aldosterone-secreting adenoma may lead to cure of hypertension.

Patients with symptoms of a paroxysmal nature with sweating, flushing, blanching, tachycardia, weight loss, constipation and panic attacks should be investigated to exclude phaeochromocytoma. This requires a 24-hour urine test for catecholamines, metanephrines or 4-hydroxy-3-methoxymandelic acid.

MANAGEMENT

The effective management of hypertension can reduce mortality and morbidity from stroke, and to a lesser extent heart attack.[21] In developing countries, socioeconomic considerations dictate that costs should be kept to a minimum. For this reason, non-pharmacological methods of reducing blood pressure need to be applied even more rigorously. Dietary recommendations should emphasize the importance of the reduction of salt intake. Patients should be counselled on the avoidance of salty foods and told they should never add salt to food when cooking or at the table. An increase in potassium-rich foods, which can be achieved by increasing the consumption of fresh fruit and vegetables, will also help to lower blood pressure. Supplementation with potassium chloride tablets is not recommended.

All cigarette smokers should be instructed to stop. Smoking is an independent risk factor for heart attack and stroke but is not itself associated with hypertension.

A high alcohol intake is an established factor in hypertension, requiring action by the part of the clinician. Males should consume no more than 21 units of alcohol per week and females no more than 14 units per week (one unit of alcohol is equivalent to half a pint (300 ml) of beer, or a single measure of spirits or a glass of wine). Enquiries about the amount of alcohol consumed is important but must be conducted with discretion.

Weight reduction in obese patients is important and where this can be achieved there will be a significant fall in both systolic and diastolic blood pressure.

There is good evidence that regular physical exercise lowers blood pressure on a long-term basis, even though at the time of exercise pressures may rise acutely. A structured exercise programme should be encouraged, although in urban areas with limited facilities this may be difficult to achieve.

These recommendations are relevant to all people and not just those with raised blood pressure. Advice on achieving dietary goals should be administered by trained paramedical or nursing staff, who may be more aware of local food prices and availability. There is evidence that well-trained nurses can achieve better results when treating mild hyper-

tension than their medical colleagues. Training programmes are necessary to provide nurses with the appropriate skills to manage chronic diseases like hypertension. Non-pharmacological methods of treating mild hypertension should be continued for at least 6 months. In severer cases, drug therapy will need to be initiated at an earlier stage but there is evidence that alcohol and salt restriction are additive to most antihypertensive drugs.

DRUG THERAPY

In many hypertensive patients, unfortunately, non-pharmacological methods are insufficient to reduce diastolic blood pressure below 90 mmHg. In such patients, antihypertensive drugs will be required (Figure 26.3) and there is a wide choice but many of the newer drugs are expensive.[6] Once drug treatment has been started, it is usually necessary to continue indefinitely or at least until the age of 80. Compliance with long-term antihypertensive medication is often difficult to achieve and this problem

may be compounded by limited or intermittent availability of antihypertensive drugs in some countries. Once-daily tablet regimens should be used routinely. Careful, sympathetic and systematic follow-up is necessary, preferably by suitably trained nurses or paramedical staff.

Antihypertensive drugs were first introduced in the 1950s and there are now seven different classes acting by various mechanisms. The drug treatment of hypertension can bring about approximately a

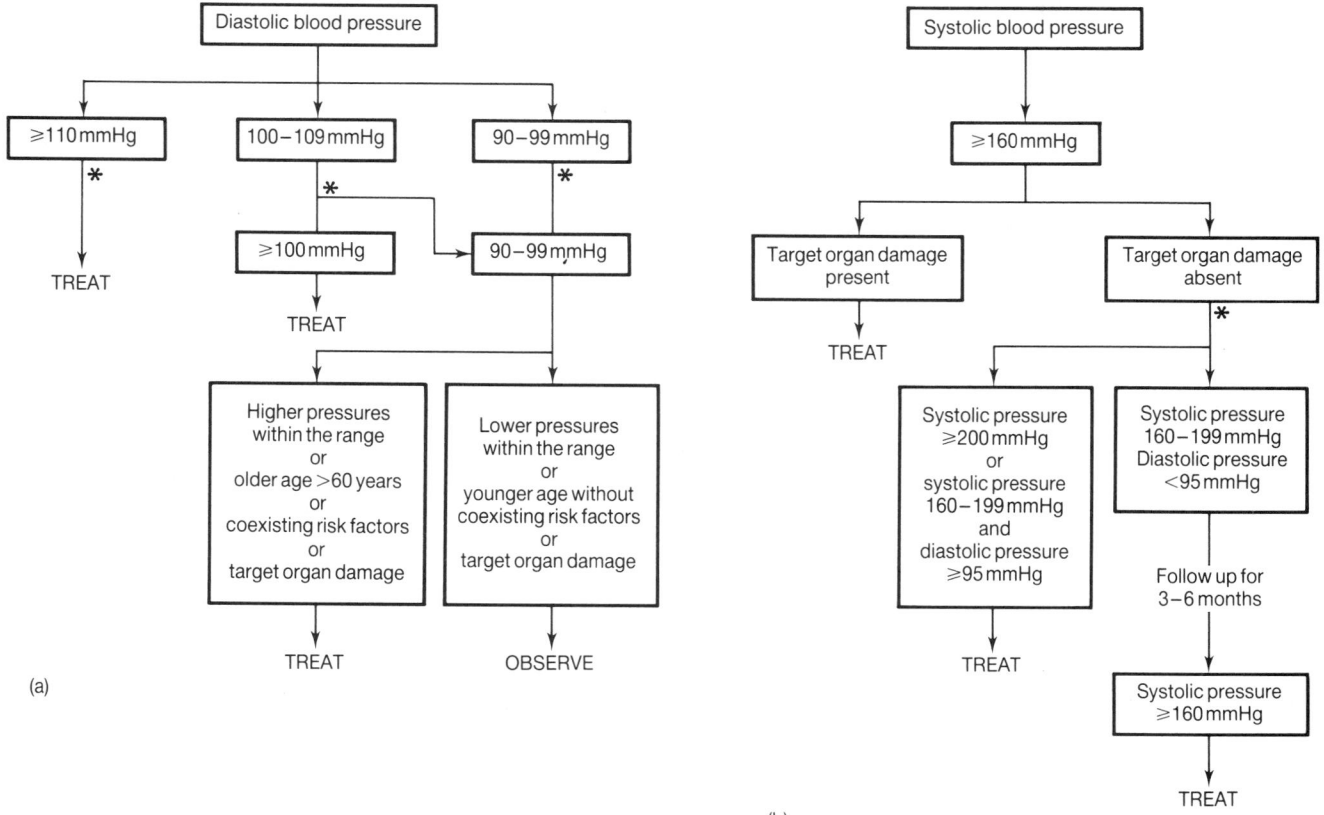

Figure 26.3 Thresholds for drug treatment of hypertension with reference to (a) diastolic blood pressure (all patients given non-pharmacological advice) and (b) systolic blood pressure ≥ 160 mmHg. *Repeated measurements. British Hypertension Society Guideline, 1993.

Table 26.2 Limitations on use of hypotensive drugs in patients with a second condition. (Drugs not listed in ranking order.)

Coexisting disease	Thiazide diuretic	Beta blocker	ACE inhibitor	Calcium antagonist	Alpha-1 blocker
Diabetes	Care needed*	Care needed†	Yes	Yes	Yes
Gout	No	Yes	Yes	Yes	Yes
Dyslipidaemia	Controversial§	Controversial§	Yes	Yes	Yes
Ischaemic heart disease	Yes	Yes	Yes	Yes	Yes
Heart failure	Yes	No	Yes	Care needed‡	Yes
Asthma	Yes	No	Yes	Yes	Yes
Peripheral vascular disease	Yes	Care needed‡	Care needed‡	Yes	Yes
Renal artery stenosis	Yes	Yes	No	Yes	Yes

*Diuretics may exacerbate diabetes.
†Beta blockers should be used with care in diabetes because awareness of insulin hypoglycaemia may be dulled. In non-insulin dependent disease beta blockers may worsen glucose tolerance and exacerbate the deranged lipid profile.
‡Care needed when using calcium antagonists, particularly verapamil and diltiazem, in heart failure and when using angiotensin converting enzyme inhibitors and beta blockers in peripheral vascular disease, because of an association with renal artery stenosis a condition in which extreme care should be taken.
§Choice of beta blockers and diuretics in patients with dyslipidaemia is controversial.

Table 26.3 Known and common or important side-effects with different classes of drug. (Side-effects not listed in ranking order for different classes of drugs.)

Common side-effects	Thiazide diuretic	Beta blocker	ACE inhibitor	Calcium antagonist	Alpha-1 blocker
Headache	−	−	−	+	−
Flushing	−	−	−	+	−
Dyspnoea	−	+	−	−	−
Lethargy	−	+	−	−	−
Impotence	+	+	−	−	−
Cough	−	−	+	−	−
Gout	+	−	−	−	−
Oedema	−	−	−	+	−
Postural hypotension	+	−	−	−	+
Cold hands and feet	−	+	−	−	−

40% reduction in the incidence of stroke and a 20% reduction in coronary heart disease. The aim of treatment is to reduce the systolic blood pressure to below 160 mmHg and the diastolic blood pressure to below 90 mmHg. Side-effects can be kept to a minimum by employing the lowest possible doses in the first instance.

Tranquillizers and sedatives have no place in antihypertensive regimens and they should be reserved exclusively for patients with primary psychiatric ailments. There is no convincing evidence that any of the traditional or herbal remedies available in some countries have any useful effects on blood pressure and some of them may even be dangerous.

The choice of antihypertensive drugs depends on availability and cost as well as efficacy and side-effects (Tables 26.2 and 26.3). Broadly speaking, all antihypertensive regimens are about equally effective. The central acting alpha-agonists and the beta blockers have the most side-effects (sedation, lethargy, cold extremities, bradycardia and wheeze). Of the seven classes of blood pressure-lowering drugs only methyldopa, the thiazide diuretics and the beta blockers have been demonstrated to prevent heart attacks or strokes and no agent has been shown convincingly to prevent renal failure. The newer classes of drugs have fewer side-effects and are more theoretically attractive but as yet no trials have been conducted to prove that they prolong life. The angiotensin converting enzymes (ACE inhibitors) are a particularly useful class of drug as they may be the most effective agent(s) in reversing left ventricular hypertrophy, delaying renal failure in diabetic as well as non-diabetic hypertensives.

1. CENTRALLY-ACTING ALPHA AGONISTS

This class includes methyldopa, clonidine and the reserpine group of drugs. Clonidine is generally regarded as being unacceptable due to side-effects. The main problem with these drugs is that they cause lethargy and sometimes depression, and reserpine, when used in high doses, has been associated with suicide. In very low doses, these centrally acting drugs are effective and tolerable in mild hypertension and they are useful because they have the major advantage of being very cheap.

2. THIAZIDE DIURETICS

These agents, which are also cheap, are still the mainstay of antihypertensive therapy for older patients. They should be prescribed only at the lowest possible dose, e.g. bendrofluazide, 2.5 mg daily. Increased doses provide no further reduction of blood pressure but cause increased adverse side-effects, including erectile impotence, glucose intolerance, elevation of plasma lipid levels, hyperuricaemia and hypokalaemia. Thiazides are best avoided in younger patients and particularly in sexually active men.

3. THE BETA-BLOCKERS

These drugs, introduced in 1965, were rapidly shown to be effective, not only in treating hypertension but also in the management of angina and the secondary prevention of myocardial infarction. Their impact on primary coronary prevention has been disappointing. The hydrophilic beta blockers (e.g. atenolol) cause fewer central nervous system side-effects (lethargy, sleep disturbance) than the lipophilic drugs like propranolol.

4. THE ALPHA-BLOCKERS

The early alpha blockers, indoramin, phenoxybenzamine and prazosin, have now largely fallen from use because of side-effects and complexity of dosage. The recent introduction of doxazosin and terazosin has largely overcome these problems. These newer alpha blockers are very safe and may have beneficial effects on sexual function in men and also relieve prostatic symptoms. They also reduce plasma lipid levels slightly.

5. THE DIRECT-ACTING VASODILATORS

Hydralazine has been used mainly as an additive drug to control blood pressure where the thiazides and the beta blockers together have proved ineffective. Side-effects include the drug-induced lupus phenomenon. Because hydralazine has to be given twice or thrice daily it has largely fallen from use. Minoxidil is a very powerful vasodilator which should only be used in the most resistant hypertensive patients in conjunction with beta blockers and a loop diuretic.

6. ACE INHIBITORS

These expensive drugs can cause overrapid and dangerous falls in blood pressure if used in high doses in patients with renal impairment or those already receiving diuretic therapy. They are contraindicated in patients with renal artery stenosis. The ACE inhibitors are the only class of drug which has been convincingly shown to prolong life in patients with heart failure and should probably now be used in all such cases. They may also be specifically indicated in diabetic hypertensives as they have no adverse effects on insulin sensitivity or plasma lipid levels and they do preserve renal function in patients with hypertensive or diabetic nephrosclerosis. The main side-effect is a dry, persistent, irritating cough in about 10% of patients. Life-threatening angioneurotic oedema is occasionally encountered.

7. THE CALCIUM CHANNEL BLOCKERS

This group can be subdivided into the dihydropyridines and the non-dihydropyridines (diltiazem and verapamil). The last two agents are effective at reducing blood pressure and are antianginal but, due to negative chronotropism and ionotropism, they are absolutely contraindicated in patients with heart failure and should not be used in conjunction with beta blockers. The dihydropyridines are very safe but cause headache, flushing and ankle oedema. They appear to be the least effective drugs in reducing left ventricular hypertrophy and are contraindicated after a myocardial infarction.

INDIVIDUAL VARIATIONS OF DRUG RESPONSE

In general, if one antihypertensive drug is ineffective at its usual dose, it is best to change to a different class rather than to increase the dose. There are, however, some reasonably predictable differences in drug response or suitability which may influence the choice of first-line drug therapy.

SPECIFIC GROUPS

BLACK HYPERTENSIVES

Patients of black African origin, as stated earlier, have consistently lower plasma renin and angiotensin II levels than other ethnic groups. It is not surprising, therefore, that these drugs which partly act by blocking renin release (i.e. the beta blockers) or by inhibiting the generation of angiotensin II (i.e. the ACE inhibitors) are less effective in black patients.[22] By contrast, the thiazide diuretics, the centrally acting drugs, the calcium channel blockers and the alpha blockers are effective (Figure 26.4). Salt restriction is effective in black patients and this manoeuvre as well as the thiazide diuretics may potentiate ACE inhibitors or the beta blockers.

SOUTH ASIANS

The response of antihypertensive drugs in South Asians is broadly similar to that in whites. However, the high incidence of diabetes mellitus, glucose intolerance and hyperlipidaemia means that the thiazide diuretics are frequently contraindicated.

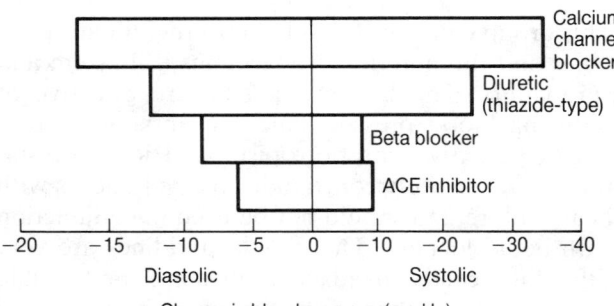

Figure 26.4 Average reduction in systolic and diastolic BP in large clinical trials of monotherapy with four different classes of antihypertensive drug used for the treatment of mild-to-moderate essential hypertension in black men and women. (Reproduced from Hall.[16]).

There is a very high incidence of coronary heart disease in people of Indian subcontinental origin and coronary preventative manoeuvres are particularly necessary.

ORIENTAL PATIENTS

Hypertension is particularly common in people of oriental origin, especially the Japanese. This may, in part, be related to the very high salt intake in the North-West Pacific rim. Salt restriction is effective in reducing the very high incidence of strokes in this area. Coronary heart disease is relatively uncommon but its incidence may be rising as dietary fat intake rises.

PACIFIC ISLANDERS

This group has a high incidence of extreme obesity, diabetes mellitus, hypertension, hyperuricaemia and alcohol excess. Non-pharmacological and pharmacological approaches to these problems are mandatory and the choice of antihypertensive drugs depends on the individual patient and the concurrent risk factors.

THE ELDERLY

Antihypertensive drug therapy has been shown to be particularly useful in the elderly and is now indicated in hypertensive patients up to the age of about 80 years.

Stroke and coronary prevention has been achieved with the use of the thiazide diuretics in low doses. Beta blockers and ACE inhibitors are slightly less effective in reducing blood pressure in the elderly compared with younger patients, but the dihydropyridines can be used safely.

RESISTANT HYPERTENSION

Approximately 10% of patients have blood pressures which cannot be reduced despite the use of

three concurrent antihypertensive drugs. Some of these patients may be found to have a history of chronic alcohol abuse; many will give a history of long-standing hypertension with long interruptions of dietary and drug treatment. There are usually ECG changes of left ventricular hypertrophy.

All resistant hypertensives should undergo more detailed investigation to exclude any underlying cause for their high blood pressure. There are some antihypertensive regimens which are particularly effective and should be considered in such patients. These are the ACE inhibitors with the dihydropyridine calcium channel blockers, minoxidil with a beta blocker and a loop diuretic, and an ACE inhibitor with frusemide in high dosage.

Many apparently resistant hypertensives are, in fact, known not to comply with drug therapy. Compliance of therapy can be improved if drug regimens are simplified. Preferably, no antihypertensive regimen should require drugs to be taken more often than once daily.

CONCLUSIONS

Antihypertensive therapy has been validated. It prevents heart attacks and strokes and prolongs life by reducing death rates from these diseases. The dramatic decline in malignant hypertension and hypertensive cardiac failure in the Western world is closely related to the mass treatment of millions of hypertensive patients. The prognosis in hypertensive patients is more closely related to the accuracy of long-term blood pressure control than the severity of the hypertension when first diagnosed.

Much of the rising prevalence of hypertension in tropical countries is related to potentially reversible environmental factors and dietary habits. There is still time to bring about preventive measures in order to avoid a coronary 'epidemic', which has afflicted Western countries over the last 50 years. The principles of managing hypertension are similar in all communities, and intervention at an early, mild, presymptomatic stage is worthwhile. However, the health care facilities of many countries should be amended to take on this major but preventable hazard to health.

REFERENCES

1 Stamler J, Wentworth D & Neaton J D. Is relationship between serum cholesterol and risk of premature death from coronary heart disease continuous or graded? *JAMA* 1986; 256:2823–2828.

2 Pobee J O M. Should hypertension control be considered a public health imperative in black Africa? *J. Human Hypertens* 1990; 4:199.

3 Cruickshank J K, Beevers D G, Osbourne V L, Haynes R A, Corlett J C K & Selby S. Heart attack, stroke, diabetes and hypertension in West Indian, Asians and Whites in Birmingham, England. *BMJ* 1980; 281:1108.

4 Sever P S, Gordon D, Peart W S & Beighton P. Blood pressure and its correlates in urban and tribal Africa. *Lancet* 1980; ii: 60–64.

5 Akinkugbe O O. World epidemiology of hypertension in blacks. In Hall W D, Saunders E & Shulman N B (eds) *Hypertension in Blacks*. Chicago: Year Book Medical Publishers Inc,1985:3–16.

6 Shaper A G & Saxton G A. Blood pressure and body build in a rural community in Uganda. *East African Med J* 1969; 46:228–235.

7 Evans J G & Rose G. Epidemiology of non-communicable disease hypertension. *Br Med Bull* 1971; 23:37–42.

8 Joint National Committee on Detection, Evaluation and Treatment of High Blood Pressure. The Fifth Report of the Joint National Committee on Detection, Evaluation and Treatment of High Blood Pressure (JNC-V). *Arch Intern Med* 1993; 153:154–183.

9 Sever P, Beevers D G, Bulpitt C et al. Management guidelines in essential hypertension: report of the Second Working Party of the British Hypertension Society. *BMJ* 1993; 306:983–987.

10 British Hypertension Society. Recommendations on blood pressure measurement. *BMJ* 1986; 293:611.

11 Ashcroft M T & Desai P. Blood pressure and mortality in a rural Jamaican community. *Lancet* 1978; i:1167–1170.

12 Seedat Y K, Seedat M A & Hackland D B T. Prevalence of hypertension in the urban and rural Zulu. *J Epidemiol Community Health* 1982; 36:256–261.

13 INTERSALT Cooperative Research Group. Intersalt: an international study of electrolyte

excretion and blood pressure: results of 29 hour urinary sodium and potassium excretion. *BMJ* 1988; 297:319–328.

14 Shah W W & Kunjannam P V. The incidence of hypertension in liquor permit holders and teetotallers. *J Assoc Physicians India* 1959; 7:243–267.

15 Luft F C, Rankin L I, Bloch R et al. Cardiovascular and humoral responses to extremes of sodium intake in normal white and black men. *Circulation* 1979; 60:697–706.

16 Weissberg P L, Woods K L, West M J & Beevers D G. Genetic and ethnic influences on the distribution of sodium and potassium in normotensive and hypertensive subjects. *J Clin Hypertens* 1987; 3:20–25.

17 Freis E D, Materson B J & Flamenbaum V. Comparison of propranolol or hydrochlorothiazide alone for treatment of hypertension: III. Evaluation of the renin–angiotensin system. *Am J Med* 1983; 74:1029–1041.

18 Reaven G M. Role of insulin resistance in human disease. *Diabetes* 1988; 37:1595–1607.

19 Kaplan N M. *Clinical Hypertension*, 5th edn. Baltimore, M D: Williams & Wilkins, 1990.

20 Millar G J, Beckles G L A & Byam N T A. Serum lipoprotein concentrations in relation to ethnic composition and urbanisation in men and women in Trinidad, West Indies. *Int J Epidemiol* 1984; 13:413–421.

21 Collins R, Peto R, MacMahon S et al. Blood pressure, stroke and coronary heart disease. Part 2: Short-term reductions in blood pressure: overview of randomised drug trials in their epidemiological context. *Lancet* 1990; 335:827–838.

22 Hall W D. Pathophysiology of hypertension in blacks. *Am J Hypertens* 1990; 3: 366S-371S.

CHAPTER 27

ISCHAEMIC HEART DISEASE AND LIPID DISORDERS

G. J. Miller

ISCHAEMIC HEART DISEASE

Ischaemic heart disease (IHD) is the collective term for disorders arising from occlusion of the coronary arteries. Nineteenth century physicians associated narrowing of the coronary vasculature with angina pectoris, aneurysmal dilatation of the heart and cardiac failure, but believed that complete occlusion of a major coronary artery invariably caused sudden death. The diagnosis of non-fatal myocardial infarction had to await the cogent account by Herrick,[1] published in 1912. Improvements in the interpretation of the electrocardiogram between 1920 and 1935, linking abnormal Q waves and certain RS–T changes with myocardial infarction, played a considerable part in the emergence of the disorder from obscurity. However, increased awareness and diagnostic ability could not have accounted for IHD to become the leading cause of death in the industrialized nations after 1945. By 1963, IHD accounted for about 30% of deaths in the USA. The realization that the developed world was suffering a massive epidemic of premature death due to this disease spurred a research effort into its causes, prevention and treatment that continues to this day.

RECENT EPIDEMIOLOGY

The global epidemiology of IHD during the 1980s is summarized in Figures 27.1 and 27.2, derived from World Health Organization statistics.[2] Much of the world population remains economically undeveloped and retains its historical pattern of disease. In such communities birth rates and infant mortality rates are high, there is a heavy burden of communicable diseases and a relatively short life expectancy, and mortality from the non-communicable diseases is low. Health surveillance systems are rudimentary

and vital statistics not generally available. Any IHD is essentially confined to the elite, whose socio-economic status is way above that of the general community. Such territories are not represented in Figures 27.1 and 27.2.

In countries in the transitional phases of development, improvements in nutrition and environmental hygiene first appear in the urban centres and progress gradually into the rural areas. The communicable diseases are brought under control and life expectancy increases. Increasing numbers of patients with non-communicable disorders are seen in hospitals serving the urban centres. Physicians are aware of the changing pattern of disease, but what health statistics are available may be unreliable at first. Children of the more well-to-do in the urban centres begin to show signs of the changes in life style, with increasing adiposity, a reduction in physical activity and rising blood cholesterol levels[4,5] which augur ill for cardiovascular health. Jamaica exemplifies such territories (Figure 27.2).

Only in the later stages of transition towards full development do populations acquire the disease patterns of the older industrialized world in which infant mortality and communicable disease rates are low, life expectancy is relatively high, and IHD and cancers are the leading causes of death. Territories shown in Figures 27.1 and 27.2 which typify such countries include Singapore, Cuba and Trinidad and Tobago. Their current mortality from IHD can be seen to be similar to, or even higher than that of Great Britain and the USA. While IHD is declining in some of the older industrialized regions it is increasing in many of the newly industrialized territories.[6]

The reasons for the downward trend in IHD mortality in the older industrialized countries (see Figure 27.1) have not been delineated clearly. First

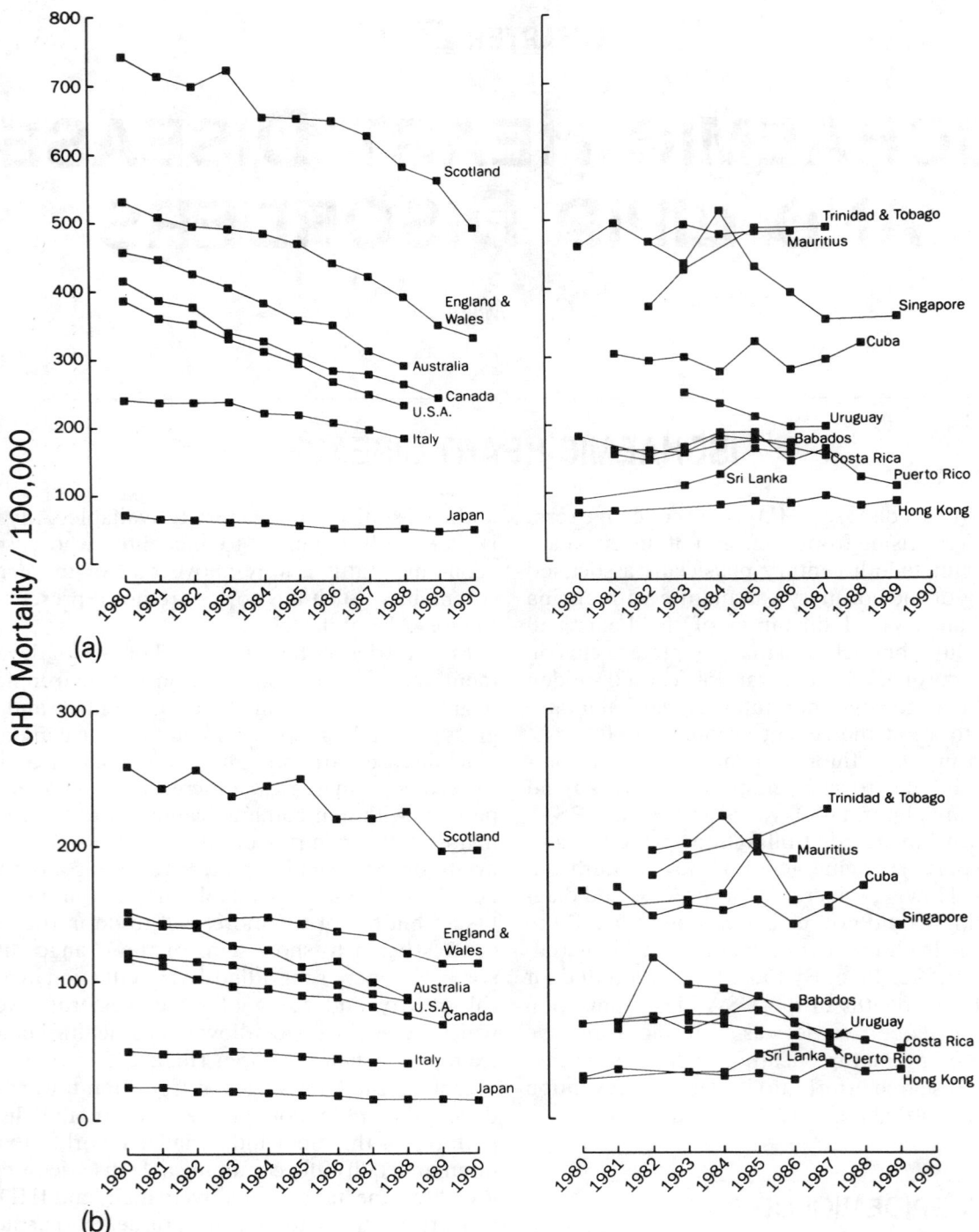

Figure 27.1 Annual mortality rates from ischaemic heart disease (ICD-9, basic tabulation list, code 270) for (a) men and (b) women aged 55 to 64 years in seven older-developed and 10 newly developing nations between 1980 and 1990. (Reproduced from World Health Organization[2]).

observed in California and Utah in the mid-1960s,[7] it is likely to have been partly a response to preventive measures and partly a result of earlier diagnosis and advances in management leading to a reduction in case fatality.[8] This experience in the developed world has prompted calls for 'primordial' prevention of IHD in the developing nations.[9] Through public health initiatives with political support, the develop-ing territories are to be discouraged from acquiring those aspects of a 'Western' life style causally linked to IHD. Rather they are to be encouraged to retain certain features of their traditional way of life that are consistent with cardiovascular health. Thus the campaign against IHD is shifting into the global arena.

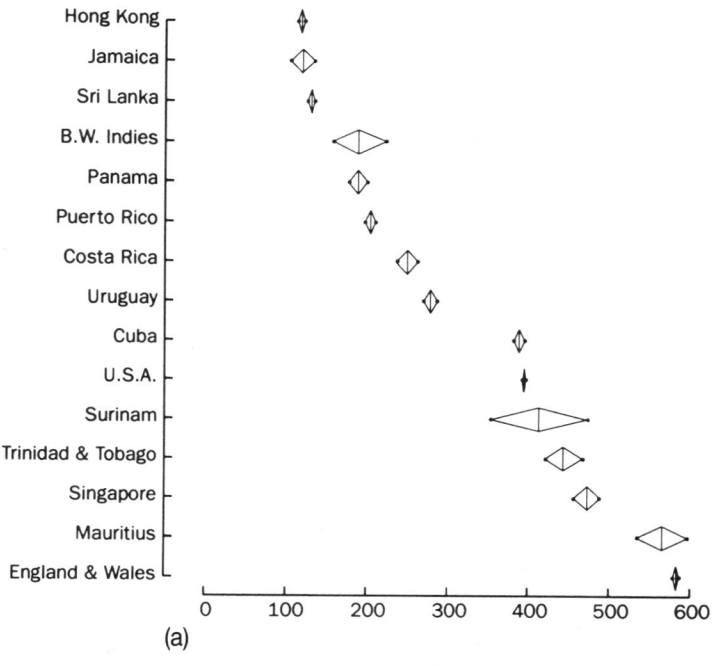

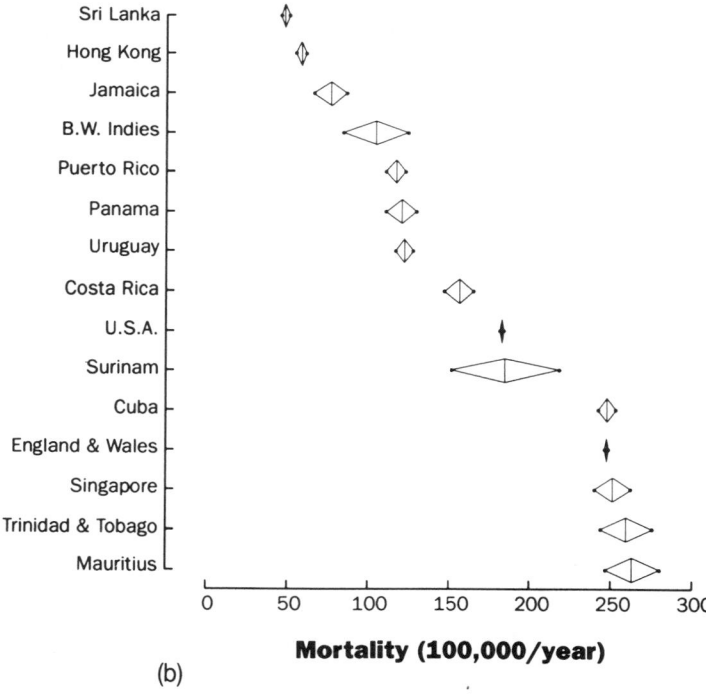

Figure 27.2 Age-standardized annual mortality rates from ischaemic heart disease (ICD-9, basic tabulation list, code 270) for (a) men and (b) women aged 45 years or more in 15 territories. Best estimates are given as vertical bars flanked by their 5th and 95th percent confidence intervals. Rates are averages across 1983–1985 except for: Hong Kong, 1984–1986; Jamaica, 1984; British West Indies (Bahamas, Barbados, Belize, St Vincent), all data available for 1982–1985; Surinam, 1984–1985; Trinidad and Tobago, 1983, 1984, 1986. (Reproduced from World Health Organization[2]. Rates have been standardized see Segi.[3]

PATHOLOGY

The IHD emerging in the developing world differs in no important respect from that on the wane in the older industrialized world. However, the relative contributions made by the multiple factors underlying the pathology of this complex disease, coronary atheroma and thrombosis, will differ somewhat between societies owing to distinctions in genetic composition and life style.

THE ATHEROMATOUS LESION

Atheromas are discrete and often eccentric intimal lesions of large arteries. They are characterized by a proliferation of smooth muscle cells, infiltration by monocytes and macrophages, an accumulation of

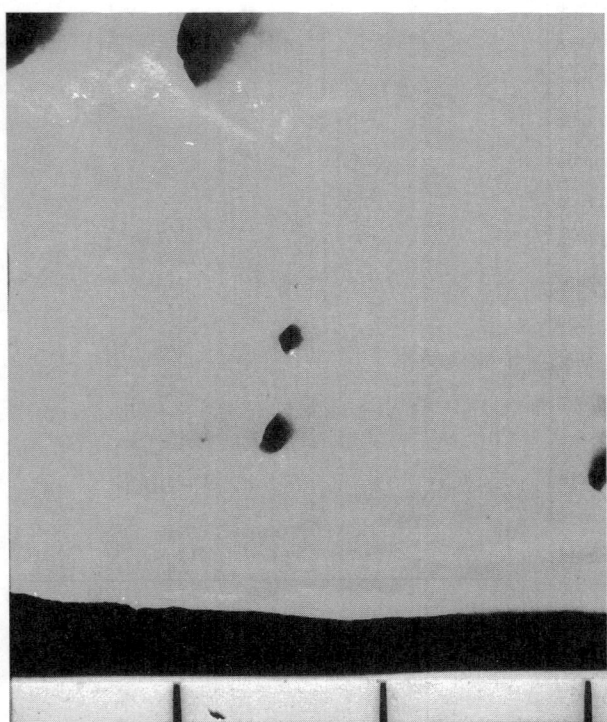

Figure 27.3 A surface view of the endothelium of the aorta, showing fatty streaks that are especially prominent around the ostia of branch vessels.

collagen, elastic fibres and proteoglycans, and deposition of intracellular and extracellular lipid (mainly cholesterol ester). Fibrin is often present as a meshwork on the surface of the lesion, and in large amounts more deeply within advanced lesions.[10] The precursor of the atheromatous lesion is believed to be the fatty streak (Figure 27.3). More advanced lesions are termed fibrous plaques.

The fatty streak

The arterial wall is subjected continuously to wear and tear, for which there has evolved a complex system of repair. Microscopic injury to the vascular endothelium induces the synthesis of several regulatory peptides including platelet-derived growth factor (now known to be produced also by endothelial cells and macrophages). The cellular responses to these peptides include:

- Migration of circulating monocytes into the intima and their phenotypic transformation to scavenger cells or macrophages.
- Proliferation and migration of contractile smooth muscle cells from the media into the intima with

subsequent transformation to the synthesizing phenotype.
- Secretion of collagen and other components of the extracellular matrix by transformed smooth muscle cells.
- Activation of vascular endothelial cells at the site of injury with transformation of their normally anticoagulant surface to one with procoagulant properties.
- Fibroblast proliferation and other neutrophil responses.

This co-ordinated response normally leads to the restoration of the vascular endothelium and intima. None of these responses would in itself lead to the deposition of lipid at the site of injury.

However, even under normal circumstances, many plasma constituents traverse the intima and such fluxes are probably increased at times of injury. The internal elastic lamina at the intima–media junction is thought to behave as a 'molecular sieve', trapping macromolecular structures such as the larger plasma lipoproteins within the intima. The uptake of trapped and modified lipoprotein particles by cells at sites of injury is believed to be the origin of the fatty streak.

Fatty streaks are found frequently in childhood in all populations, irrespective of the background mortality from IHD.[11,12] Each consists of smooth muscle cells and lipid-laden macrophages within the intima, lying beneath an endothelium of normal microscopic appearance. Fatty streaks commonly develop at the same anatomical sites as fibrous plaques found at older ages, which suggests a potential precursor–product relation.[13] However, the existence of fatty streaks in the coronary arteries of children and adults in societies with a very low mortality from IHD implies that this lesion is innocuous *per se* and does not necessarily lead to plaque formation.

The fibrous plaque

The conditions which convert a fatty streak to a fibrous plaque (Figure 27.4) have not been fully elucidated, but seem to involve:

- Recurrent and excessive damage to the endothelium, evoking the cellular responses that produce fatty streaks.
- Raised plasma concentrations of atherogenic lipoproteins,[14] with increased flux into the arterial wall. First among these are the cholesterol-rich low-density lipoproteins (LDLs), particularly the small, dense subclass. Intermediate-density lipo-

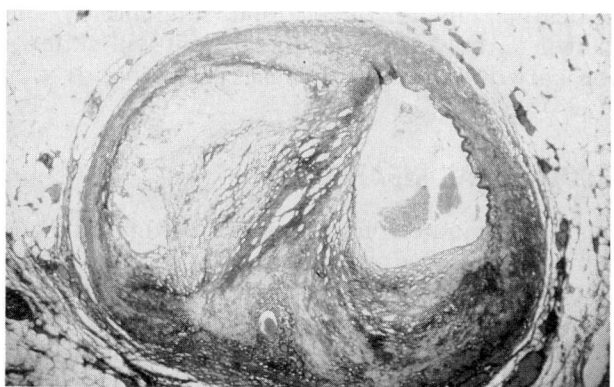

Figure 27.4 Transverse section of a coronary artery in a patient with ischaemic heart disease, showing an eccentric and advanced atheromatous plaque. The spaces at the base of the lesion were filled with a cholesterol-rich pool of tissue debris. Overlying this pool is a cellular-rich region, the whole being covered with a fibrous cap. The remainder of the lumen is patent.

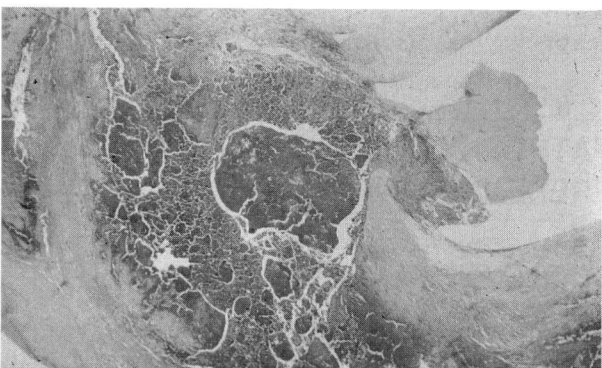

Figure 27.5 Section through an atheromatous plaque that has fissured, showing a haemostatic plug within the body of the lesion, and some extension of thrombus into the vessel's lumen.

proteins (IDLs), and probably also the smaller subclass of the very-low-density lipoproteins (VLDLs) are likely to play a similar role to LDL.

- Oxidative damage to trapped lipoproteins leading to intracellular and extracellular lipid accumulation.
- Impaired cholesterol clearance from macrophages and other peripheral tissue cells, owing to disturbances to the metabolism of high-density lipoprotein (HDLs).
- Necrosis of the deeper layers of the plaque, creating a cholesterol-rich pool of tissue debris.
- Fibrin deposition on the lesion and its incorporation into the plaque.

These factors are discussed in detail below. In the coronary arteries, fibrous plaques are found most commonly in the first 3 cm of the left coronary vessel and the proximal segment of its anterior descending branch. Their distribution is patchy and often eccentric. At the base of the plaque is a variable amount of necrotic debris with cholesterol crystals and some calcification. Overlying this is a highly cellular region, rich in smooth muscle cells, macrophages, intracellular and extracellular lipid, and connective tissue. The whole is covered by a fibrous cap with smooth muscle cells embedded in dense connective tissue. Large amounts of fibrin are frequently found in more advanced lesions, especially the gelatinous type of plaque with a prominent lipid-rich region.[10] Fibrin is present on the surface of the cap and in bands interspersed between collagen. These raised lesions gradually occlude the vessel's lumen and are liable to fissuring or rupture (Figure 27.5).

CORONARY THROMBOSIS

Several factors appear to be involved in the generation of an occlusive clot or thrombus within a coronary artery:

- Plaque fissuring or rupture
- The coagulability of the plasma
- The adhesiveness and aggregability of platelets
- Disturbances of local blood flow
- Loss of the natural anticoagulant properties of the vascular endothelium
- Hyperviscosity of blood
- Impaired fibrinolysis.

Fibrous plaques fissure under mechanical stress (Figure 27.5), frequently at the junction of the fibrous cap with healthy intima, although at times in the centre of the cap. In eccentric plaques with a large pool of cholesterol and debris, the fibrous cap can tear completely. In about 25% of cases the injury is more superficial, with partial tearing of a cap containing large numbers of lipid-laden macrophages.[15] Exposure of subendothelial collagen and cells which express tissue factor (the cofactor for factor VII) on their surfaces leads to thrombin formation, fibrin deposition, platelet adhesion and platelet aggregation (see below, Haemostatic Factors). Tears range from the microscopic to those demonstrable by coronary angiography. A haemostatic plug forms in the fissure and may encroach upon the lumen (Figure 27.5), sometimes producing complete occlusion with extension distally. Coronary angiography has revealed the high frequency of thrombus formation at sites of fissuring in patients with unstable angina pectoris and acute myocardial infarction;[16] hence the rationale for thrombolytic therapy. Some degree of coronary thrombosis is nearly always found following sudden cardiac death.[17]

PATHOPHYSIOLOGY AND CLINICAL PRESENTATION

STABLE ANGINA PECTORIS

Obstruction of the coronary artery reduces the maximum rate of blood flow through the vessel. Ischaemia occurs when the demand of the myocardium supplied by the obstructed artery exceeds its metabolic reserve of oxygen, as dictated by maximal coronary flow and maximal oxygen extraction. The myocardial oxygen demand is a function of the cardiac frequency and the tension in the ventricular wall, the latter being a function of ventricular pressures during systole. Cardiac metabolism is almost entirely aerobic, so that a rapid deterioration in myocardial contractility occurs with ischaemia. Left ventricular end-diastolic pressures rise and stroke volume falls. Regional disturbances of myocardial metabolism and electrophysiological processes are manifested respectively as an increased production of lactate and ST segment depression on the electrocardiogram (ECG). If ischaemia persists, characteristic pain develops. This symptom is usually precipitated by exertion or emotion, commencing retrosternally and radiating to the left arm, throat and back. The pain is classically described as 'gripping' or 'tight', but sometimes only a mild ache or discomfort is noticed, there may be no radiation, or pain spreads to an unusual site. Pain induced by physical exercise is relieved promptly by rest. At times, ischaemic pain can be induced at rest simply by an increase in cardiac frequency (increasing myocardial oxygen requirement) or by spasm of the coronary arteries.

UNSTABLE ANGINA PECTORIS

A previously asymptomatic patient, or a patient with stable angina pectoris, may suddenly notice bouts of chest pain of unpredictable onset, often when at rest and relaxed. The underlying lesion appears to be plaque fissuring with intermittent superimposition of thrombotic material which transiently increases the severity of occlusion of the affected coronary artery. Such changes have been observed in unstable angina by fibreoptic angioscopy. There is frequently biochemical evidence of activation of platelets and the haemostatic system (see below) but no evidence of necrosis of the myocardial tissue (myocardial infarction). The danger is, however, that the patient will suffer a coronary thrombosis that causes infarction.

MYOCARDIAL INFARCTION

About 20 minutes of cessation of coronary flow is sufficient to cause myocardial necrosis. In patients who survive several hours, there will often (but not always) be diagnostic changes in the plasma and on the ECG. Severe disruption of cell membrane permeability allows macromolecules such as cardiac enzymes to leak from cells into the extracellular space and thence into the circulation. Serum aspartate transaminase concentrations are generally elevated within 12–24 hours, returning to normal 48–72 hours later. This enzyme is not cardiospecific, however, and is released following pulmonary or hepatic cell damage. Lactic dehydrogenase (LDH) is released from damaged myocardium more slowly, rising to a peak at 72–84 hours and remaining raised for up to 10 days. Its isoenzyme, LDH_1, is relatively cardiospecific and is usually assayed in terms of its α-hydroxybutyrate dehydrogenase activity. The most specific cardiac enzyme is the MB isoenzyme of creatine phosphokinase (MB-CPK). Its plasma level rises within 12 hours of the onset of the clinical attack, peaks at about 24 hours, and returns to normal after 48–72 hours. Thus repeated MB-CPK measurement aids the early diagnosis of myocardial infarction, whereas LDH_1 is more useful when investigation has been delayed. Laboratories should establish their own 'upper normal' limits for the communities they serve. Men generally have higher normal levels of total serum creatine phosphokinase than women, and black adults considerably higher normal levels than other ethnic groups.[18,19] In one study, the increased levels of creatine phosphokinase in Blacks were confined to the MM (skeletal muscle) isoenzyme.[20] Ischaemic injury to the myocardium can also induce incomplete repolarization of the cell membrane during diastole, creating a 'current of injury' between the ischaemic zone and neighbouring healthy tissue. The result is depression of the TQ segment of the ECG. Since this part of the electrocardiographic cycle is taken as the baseline when the record is read, the appearance given is that of ST segment elevation. When infarction extends as far as the epicardial surface, the full thickness of the ventricular wall becomes electrically inert. An electrode overlying this region records the cardiac cavity potential as a pathological QS complex (i.e. no positive R wave deflection) or a pathological Q wave. Infarction can also injure the cardiac conducting tissue, producing various forms of heart block.

Myocardial infarction may cause left ventricular failure and orthopnoea. Systemic hypotension may be apparent. Ventricular fibrillation is another serious complication, but in the absence of hypotension and cardiac failure it is usually amenable to modern techniques of resuscitation. Supraventricular tachycardias are also common, including atrial fibrillation. Late complications include cardiac aneurysm, rupture of the interventricular septum, papillary muscle necrosis with mitral incompetence, and cardiac rupture.

SUDDEN CARDIAC DEATH

This term is usually applied when an acute coronary occlusion causes death within 1 hour. Frequently there is a history of angina or previous myocardial infarction. The realization that an appreciable proportion of patients die before they reach hospital has led to intensive efforts to take treatment and resuscitation facilities to the patient, and to speed admission for intensive care. In an appreciable number of patients plaque fissuring and thrombosis trigger a lethal arrhythmia, possibly by provoking vasospasm or embolism into the vessels supplying the conduction system. Recent myocardial necrosis may or may not be found at autopsy. In other patients, there is advanced coronary stenosis without significant thrombus formation, often with old myocardial scarring and ventricular hypertrophy. The poorly functioning ventricle is susceptible to re-entrant arrhythmias and ventricular fibrillation. Sudden ischaemic cardiac deaths have to be differentiated from those due to cardiomyopathy, right ventricular dysplasia, valvular disease with prolapse, myocarditis and the Wolff–Parkinson–White syndrome.

AETIOLOGICAL AND PATHOGENIC FACTORS

Individuals at increased risk for IHD have certain physicochemical characteristics of predictive value, referred to as risk factors. This term also includes aspects of the individual's environment and way of life. Of course, a characteristic of predictive value may be either causally or non-causally associated with the disease process, and much research has been undertaken to distinguish one from the other. Those with a role in the aetiology of IHD can be conceived of as forming a web of causation (Table 27.1). First (group 1) are those characteristics inti-

Table 27.1   Risk factors for ischaemic heart disease.

Group 1

Plasma lipoproteins

Low-density lipoproteins		↑
High-density lipoproteins		↓
Intermediate-density lipoproteins		↑
Very-low-density lipoproteins		↑
Postprandial chylomicronaemia		↑
Lipoprotein (a)		↑
Total cholesterol		↑
Total triglyceride		↑

Plasma apolipoproteins

Apolipoproteins B-100 and B-48		↑
Apolipoprotein E; E_2 isoform		↑
Apolipoprotein A-I		↓

Haemostatic and platelet characteristics

Factor VII coagulant activity		↑
Fibrinogen concentration		↑
Platelet aggregability	?	↑

Fibrinolytic factors

Plasminogen activator inhibitor type 1		↑
Dilute clot lysis time		↑

Causes of and responses to endothelial cell injury

Antioxidant status		↓
Blood pressure		↑
Blood viscosity		↑
Plasma homocysteine concentration		↑
White cell count		↑
Plasma Von Willebrand factor concentration		↑
Urine albumin		↑
Plasma endothelin concentration		↑

Group 2

Obesity		↑
Insulin resistance; diabetes mellitus		↑
Ageing		↑
Physical fitness		↓

Group 3

Dietary energy		↑
Dietary fat intake (and composition)		↑
Vitamins A, C, E	?	↓
Dietary marine/fish oils	?	↓
Habitual level of physical activity		↓
Smoking tobacco, especially as cigarettes		↑
Alcohol consumption (inverse association)	↓↓ or ↑	↑
Psychosocial stress		↑
Social supports and coping mechanisms		↓
Certain industrial exposures		
Carbon disulphide		↑
Carbon monoxide		↑
Organic nitrates		↑

Arrows indicate direction of change associated with increased risk; ? signifies that more supportive data are needed.

Table 27.2 Lipoprotein class.

	Chylomicron*	VLDL	IDL	LDL	HDL
Hydrated density (g/ml)	<0.95	0.95–1.006	1.006–1.1019	1.019–1.063	1.063–1.210
Source	Intestine	Mainly liver; some intestine	A metabolic 'remnant' of VLDL	A catabolic product of IDL	Complex assembly in peripheral circulation
Function	Transport of dietary triglyceride	Transport of endogenous triglyceride	—	Major transporter of lipoprotein cholesterol	Reverse cholesterol transport
Lipid composition (%)					
Triglyceride	90	60	40	10	5
Cholesterol	5	12	30	50	20
Phospholipid	3	18	20	15	25
Protein	2	10	10	25	50
Apolipoproteins					
A	A-I, A-II, A-IV	—	—	—	A-I, A-II
B	B-48	B-100	B-100	B-100	—
C	C-I, C-II, C-III	C-I, C-II, C-III	—	—	C-I, C-II, C-III
E	E	E	E	—	—

*The chylomicron remnant is a particle of density >0.95 g/ml which contains apo-B48. It is normally cleared rapidly and, like the chylomicron is not present in fasting plasma.

mately related to the atherogenic and thrombogenic processes at the vascular endothelial surface, for example the plasma lipoproteins, certain haemostatic and fibrinolytic factors, and markers of endothelial cell injury. Second (group 2) are those metabolic, physiological and genetic changes that have a direct influence on group 1. Lastly are those environmental, behavioural and life style factors that influence the disease by their effects on factors in group 1 and group 2.

PLASMA LIPIDS, LIPOPROTEINS AND APOLIPOPROTEINS

Plasma lipoproteins are complex macromolecular structures which transport triglyceride and cholesterol from the splanchnic region to peripheral tissues, and cholesterol from peripheral cells to the liver (reverse cholesterol transport). Their metabolic processing is directed by their specific proteins (apolipoproteins) which act as ligands for cell surface receptors, cofactors for enzymes, and structural components. Each particle consists of a core of lipid enveloped in a surface layer of apolipoproteins and phospholipid. Particles range in diameter from 5 nm to greater than 500 nm, and the larger they are, the greater their lipid content and the lower their density. These differences in density and apolipoprotein content permit separation of the lipoproteins into many classes and subclasses (Table 27.2).

The chylomicron

These, the largest of the lipoproteins, are synthesized in the small intestinal mucosa for transport of dietary lipids. Apolipoproteins (apo) B-48, A-I, A-II and A-IV are among their surface components. They are secreted into the intestinal lymph where they acquire the apo C proteins and apo E from HDLs. Apo B-48 is so named because it is about 48% of the size of apo B-100 present in VLDLs and their metabolic products, and contains the aminoterminal 2152 amino acids of apo B-100. Lacking the carboxy-terminal of apo B-100, apo B-48 is not recognized by the B/E receptor (the so-called LDL receptor). In the circulation, chylomicrons are rapidly sequestered in the capillaries where most of their triglyceride is hydrolysed to glycerol and unesterified fatty acid by the surface-bound enzyme, lipoprotein lipase. Apo C-II is an activating cofactor for lipoprotein lipase. With transfer of fatty acids to the tissue cells and to albumin, the chylomicron shrinks in size and its redundant surface materials are lost, to reappear in HDL. Within 5–10 minutes, the chylomicron is reduced to a remnant which is then probably metabolized further by hepatic lipase and eventually bound to a remnant receptor which recognizes apo E, to be taken up by the hepatocyte. Plasma apo B-48 levels in fasting plasma are normally extremely low, perhaps only 0.1% of those for apo B-100. Nevertheless, the ratio of apo B-48 to apo B-100 in fasting plasma is increased in patients with clinical IHD,[21] possibly because of an overproduction of endogenous triglyceride in VLDLs by the liver and increased competition between chylomicron and VLDL remnants for the apo E receptor.

Very-low-density lipoproteins

Plasma VLDL particles are secreted by the liver and small intestine and transport endogenous lipid to peripheral tissues. Like the chylomicron, they are sequestered in capillaries and their lipid core is hydrolysed by lipoprotein lipase. They can be removed by the liver at any stage of their catabolism by way of the apo B/E receptor, for which apo B-100 and apo E serve as ligands. Particles whose core triglyceride is almost completely hydrolysed are ultimately transformed to smaller IDLs. In healthy persons, a proportion of IDL is cleared directly by the liver through the binding of apo E, and the remainder is hydrolysed further by hepatic lipase to LDL, with loss of apo E.

Low-density lipoproteins

These are the end-products of VLDL catabolism, each particle retaining the single molecule of apo B-100 that belonged to its progenitor. The concentration of LDL in plasma is a function of the rate of secretion of VLDL, the partitioning of IDL between hepatic clearance and further catabolism to LDL, and the rate of uptake of LDL by the B/E receptor. About 50–75% of LDL is normally cleared through the liver. After binding to B/E receptors, the particles are endocytosed and undergo lysosomal degradation with release of cholesterol.

Plasma LDL particles lack apo E and are therefore cleared relatively slowly. Prolonged residence in the circulation can induce further modifications in their composition, especially in the presence of hypertriglyceridaemia. It appears that there is transfer of triglyceride and cholesterol between VLDL and LDL, involving cholesterol ester transfer protein, with subsequent metabolic processing of the triglyceride-enriched LDL particle by hepatic lipase. The product of these transfer processes is a small dense LDL particle (LDL-III),[22] thought to be particularly atherogenic. However, small dense LDL is also seen in populations with low dietary intakes of cholesterol and saturated fat, raising the possibility that LDL particle size may not be as good a predictor of IHD risk as is LDL cholesterol concentration across communities.

High-density lipoproteins

Plasma HDL particles are heterogeneous, and can be divided into subclasses, either on the basis of

Table 27.3 Approximate mean lipoprotein cholesterol concentrations (mmol/l) in middle-age according to population risk of IHD.

IHD risk	Men			Women		
	Total	LDL	HDL	Total	LDL	HDL
0	3.0	1.8	0.9	3.0	1.8	0.9
Very low	3.5	2.2	1.0	3.5	2.2	1.0
Low	4.5	2.7	1.0	4.5	2.7	1.1
Moderate	5.0	3.1	1.1	5.1	3.2	1.2
High	5.5	3.5	1.1	5.7	3.7	1.4
Very high	6.0	3.8	1.2	6.4	4.0	1.6

their density into HDL_2 (1.063–1.112 g/ml) and HDL_3 (1.112–1.210 g/ml), or according to their apolipoprotein composition (e.g. particles containing apo A-I alone, apo A-I plus apo A-II, etc.). The importance of HDL appears to relate to its function in the transport of cholesterol from peripheral tissues to the liver, the only organ that can catabolize this molecule in substantial amounts.[23]

There are at least four sources of nascent HDL particles:

1. Redundant surface of triglyceride-rich lipoproteins generated during lipolysis.
2. The intestine: particles containing apo A-I predominantly.
3. The liver: particles containing mostly apo E.
4. Macrophages: particles rich in apo E.

These nascent particles are discoid and consist of apolipoproteins, phospholipids and unesterified cholesterol. They acquire cholesterol from peripheral cells, which is then esterified by the enzyme lecithin–cholesterol acyltransferase. In this way a lipid core is created and the particle becomes spherical. Esterified cholesterol appears to be returned to the liver by several routes:

- Initial transfer to chylomicrons and VLDL with subsequent hepatic clearance as a component of their remnant particles. This process involves cholesterol ester transfer protein.
- Direct uptake of whole HDL particles in the liver, possibly involving an HDL receptor.
- Temporary 'docking' of HDL on the surface of the hepatocyte while the particle's cholesterol ester content is released to the cell interior.

PLASMA CHOLESTEROL AND POPULATION MORTALITY DUE TO IHD

Plasma total cholesterol (the sum of its concentrations in the several lipoprotein classes) differs widely between populations (Table 27.3). The lowest levels are found in aboriginal societies, where mean values in adults average about 3 mmol/l(1 mmol/l = 38.7 mg/dl). The standard deviation about this mean is about 0.5 mmol/l, and levels differ negligibly with age and sex. Plasma LDL and HDL cholesterol average about 1.8 and 0.9 mmol/l respectively. In such communities, IHD is rare.

Plasma total cholesterol concentrations are somewhat higher in agricultural communities of the developing world, being in the region of 3.5 mmol/l, with average LDL and HDL cholesterol levels of around 2.2 and 1.0 mmol/l respectively. Total and LDL cholesterol concentrations increase with increasing obesity (an association found even in aboriginal societies such as the Yanomamo of Brazil).[24] The incidence of IHD is very low in such communities; for example, the annual mortality from IHD for men aged 55–64 years is reported to be less then 1.0/1000 in parts of rural China,[2] where plasma cholesterol averages about 3.3 mmol/l.[25]

In populations reporting annual mortality rates from IHD in middle-aged men of between 1.0 and 2.4/1000, mean cholesterol levels for such men are generally between 4 and 5 mmol/l, with levels of LDL and HDL cholesterol of about 3.0 and 1.0 mmol/l respectively. For example, in Costa Rica, with an IHD mortality of 1.4/1000 men aged 55–64 years in 1987,[2] mean cholesterol values in adults under 65 years were reported to be 4.5 and 4.7 mmol/l in rural and urban men, and 4.6 and 4.9 mmol/l in rural and urban women.[26]

In the Seychelles, with an annual IHD death rate of 1.9/1000 men aged 55–64 years in 1985–1987,[2] cholesterol levels for men and women aged 25–64 years were about 5.0 and 5.3 mmol/l respectively.[27] Precise comparison of lipid concentrations between populations is unreliable unless care is taken to standardize the method of analysis.

Completing the biological range of blood cholesterol are those communities with high rates of IHD. In the USA, the IHD mortality in middle-aged men was about 3/1000 per year in the late 1980s. Their average serum cholesterol concentration was about 5.5 mmol/l, with a mean LDL and HDL cholesterol of about 3.5 and 1.1 mmol/l respectively. Middle-aged men in England and Wales have a mean cholesterol of the order of 6.0 mmol/l, LDL cholesterol being about 3.8 mmol/l and HDL cholesterol about 1.2 mmol/l on average. In Scotland, which has an extremely high IHD mortality (see Figure 27.1), about 11% of the adult population has a serum cholesterol of 7.8 mmol/l or more, with a smaller percentage having values in excess of 8.5 mmol/l.[28]

Figures 27.1 and 27.2 show that the newly-industrialized countries Trinidad and Tobago, Mauritius and Singapore have mortality rates from IHD that are similar to the highest rates now found in the developed world. Mean plasma cholesterol levels in their men and women of middle age are 5.7 mmol/l (220 mg/dl) or above, while LDL cholesterol concentrations are at least 4.0 mmol/l (155 mg/dl) and frequently higher ([29–31]). However, a high proportion of their populations is of Indian (South Asian) descent. The particular susceptibility of South Asian people to IHD is discussed below (Ethnicity and IHD).

Thus population average blood cholesterol levels range from about 3 to 6 mmol/l in adults, while individual concentrations can be as low as 2.5 mmol/l or higher than 8.5 mmol/l, due mainly to variation in LDL cholesterol. The time lapse between the development of a raised blood cholesterol concentration and the onset of clinical IHD can be several decades. By contrast, changes in life style can alter the lipid profile within weeks. Consequently, in some communities that have acquired a Westernized diet only in the very recent past, plasma cholesterol concentrations may be high while IHD rates remain low. This appears to be the situation among the Inuit people of Greenland, for example. The people of Nanortalik in south-west Greenland have total cholesterol levels averaging more than 6.0 mmol/l,[32] and ultrasonography has revealed a similar degree of atherosclerosis among them as in Danish adults.[33] So far, however, IHD mortality in Greenland Inuit remains low.

PLASMA CHOLESTEROL AND INDIVIDUAL RISK OF IHD

In affluent and industrialized societies a continuous, positive and curvilinear relation exists between blood total cholesterol and an individual's risk of IHD.[34] This association, the population comparisons outlined above, and evidence from clinical trials for a reduction in risk when high blood cholesterol levels are lowered by drug therapy, have led to programmes aimed at the reduction of cholesterol levels on a national basis. The largest of these, the National Cholesterol Education Program of the USA,[35] aims to reduce the average American's blood cholesterol concentration by 10% or more, and has selected levels below 5.17 mmol/l (200 mg/dl) as 'desirable' for adults. This strategy, combined with more aggressive management of the 'high-risk' patient, is expected to reduce the burden of IHD on the community substantially. 'Desirable' and 'high' LDL cholesterol levels have been set at less than 3.36 mmol/l (130 mg/dl) and 4.13 mmol/l (160 mg/dl) or more respectively.[35] As a rule of thumb, a 1% reduction in a raised blood cholesterol concentration is accompanied by a 2% reduction in individual risk of IHD.[36] The hypercholesterolaemic states are discussed below (Lipid Disorders).

PLASMA TRIGLYCERIDE CONCENTRATION AND POPULATION MORTALITY FROM IHD

Triglyceride in plasma is of dietary and hepatic origin. In fasting plasma, the vast majority of triglyceride is normally found only in VLDL and IDL, while in the postprandial state it is also found in chylomicrons. On their traditional diets, low in total fat, saturated fatty acids and cholesterol, the fasting triglyceride concentrations of aboriginal and agricultural societies average about 1.0–1.2 mmol/l (1 mmol/l = 88.5 mg/dl). In some individuals, fasting levels are as low as 0.5 mmol/l. With increasing intake of saturated fatty acid there is a gradual increase in fasting triglyceride, which falls slowly on return to a low-fat diet.[37] In communities with a high mortality from IHD, mean fasting triglyceride concentrations range between 1.4 and 2.0 mmol/l in men, and somewhat less in women. In neither sex, however, does the population mean concentrations correlate with national mortality rates from IHD.[38]

PLASMA TRIGLYCERIDE AND INDIVIDUAL RISK OF IHD

In most prospective surveys, individuals with a high fasting triglyceride concentration have an increased risk of IHD, possibly reflecting disorders of lipid metabolism witH both atherogenic and thrombogenic consequences. Triglyceride *per se* appears to be neither directly atherogenic nor thrombogenic; rather high triglyceride levels are an indicator of an increased risk of IHD when they signify increases in VLDL and IDL particle concentrations. Simple enrichment of VLDL particles with triglyceride (as for example on a high carbohydrate diet), without an increase in particle concentration, is thought unlikely to be of pathogenic significance for IHD.

Delayed clearance of chylomicron and VLDL remnants may encourage their uptake by macrophages with the development of foam cells.[39] Furthermore, their delayed clearance may promote the transfer of cholesterol into remnant particles from LDLs and HDLs via the cholesterol ester transfer protein. This may interfere with hepatic uptake of cholesterol and lead to the generation of particularly atherogenic small, dense LDL particles. Hypertriglyceridaemia is also associated with a reduced HDL cholesterol concentration, itself strongly associated with IHD. In many patients with a dietary-induced increase in triglyceride, or a genetic hypertriglyceridaemia, LDL cholesterol levels are also raised. Finally, hypertriglyceridaemia is accompanied by increases in factor VII coagulant activity and plasminogen activator inhibitor type I (PAI-1) concentration, markers of thrombogenic risk.

A single measurement of fasting triglyceride generally carries little additional statistical information about an individual's risk of IHD when other factors such as LDL and HDL cholesterol concentrations and factor VII activity have been taken into account. This lack of independent predictive power has led some to argue that there is insufficient epidemiological evidence to warrant screening for and treatment of high triglyceride concentrations.[40] Others have emphasized the difficulty in interpretation of multivariate statistical analyses such as these, in which the predictive variables are strongly correlated and measurement errors can be large.[41] A single measurement of fasting triglyceride is a relatively poor estimate of an individual's 'usual' fasting concentration, and is even worse as an estimate of the 'usual' daily average concentration. This problem is compounded by the lack of certainty as to whether fasting or postprandial levels are more important for pathogenesis.

Faced with these statistical problems the argument has been advanced for giving increased weight to the metabolic evidence for a role of VLDL in IHD, and to treat a raised plasma triglyceride level accordingly.[42] Fasting levels exceeding 2.26 mmol/l (200 mg/dl) are thought to merit attention,[43] especially when the ratio of LDL cholesterol to HDL cholesterol concentration is above 5.0.[44] Patients with hypertriglyceridaemia commonly present with fasting concentrations of more than 4.5 mmol/l, and in familial lipoprotein lipase deficiency, concentrations may exceed 12 mmol/l, owing to fasting chylomicronaemia. In this latter condition, however, in which LDL cholesterol levels can be very low and factor VII coagulant activity is normal, risk relates to pancreatitis rather than IHD.

HIGH-DENSITY LIPOPROTEIN AS A MARKER OF RISK OF IHD

Plasma HDL cholesterol concentration is inversely related to the risk of IHD in both sexes, an increase in concentration of 0.1 mmol/l being associated with a reduction in risk of about 10%[45] in populations with a high mortality from IHD. Yet at the same time, a low HDL cholesterol (about 0.8 mmol/l) is a common finding in communities where IHD is rare. The probable explanation for this apparent paradox is related to the effects of dietary fat on HDL.

Most populations with a low IHD mortality consume little saturated fatty acid and cholesterol and have relatively low levels of LDL and HDL cholesterol. Change to a diet rich in these constituents produces a variable increase in the plasma concentrations of both particles,[46,47] which revert upon return to the traditional diet. The concentration of HDL cholesterol on a high-fat diet is influenced by sex (women having higher values, as shown in Table 27.3), smoking habit (reduced concentrations in smokers), physical activity (lower in sedentary people) and alcohol consumption (increased in a dose–response manner). Plasma HDL cholesterol levels are also related inversely to obesity and fasting triglyceride concentrations.

The epidemiological evidence therefore suggests that individual risk of IHD is strongly and inversely related to the concentration of HDL cholesterol that can be sustained when on a high saturated-fat diet. By contrast, national mortality rates are poorly related to the population averages of HDL cholesterol concentration.

The principal apolipoprotein of HDL, apo A-I, is a cofactor for the enzyme lecithin–cholesterol acyltransferase. Apo A-I synthesis is stimulated by oestrogens. A familial disorder characterized by isolated reductions in apo A-I and HDL cholesterol concentration carries a high risk of premature IHD.[48,49]

LIPOPROTEIN (a)

Lipoprotein (a) (Lp(a)) is a circulating complex consisting of an LDL particle coupled to a highly glycosylated protein called apolipoprotein (a) (apo(a)). The striking feature of apo(a) is its close sequence homology with plasminogen, the zymogen of the fibrinolytic enzyme plasmin. Plasminogen's structure contains a serine protease domain and a finger-like extension of five ring structures known as kringles. Apo(a) possesses a closely homologous protease and kringle 5 domain, but kringle 4 of plasminogen is repeated in tandem for a variable number of times in apo(a). This variation in the number of kringle 4 coding sequences in the apo(a) gene on chromosome 6 results in more than 20 alleles for isoforms of different size. Large isoforms of apo(a) tend to be associated with low plasma concentrations of Lp(a), and small isoforms with high Lp(a) levels.

Considerable differences exist in the distribution of Lp(1) concentration between populations. High Lp(a) levels have been reported in Sudanese and Nigerian adults and low levels in Singapore Chinese and Tibetans.[50,51] European and Indian populations tend to have intermediate values. The frequency of alleles coding for the large isoforms of apo(a) appears to be higher in Chinese, Indians and Sudanese, whereas the smaller isoforms are more prevalent in Western groups. In all populations an inverse relation exists between isoform size and Lp(a) concentration. However, for any isoform, large differences in Lp(a) concentration exist between populations, indicating that apo(a) size is not the only determinant of Lp(a) level.

The high level of Lp(a) in the black Sudanese, despite their tendency to a higher frequency of the larger isoforms, accords with experience among Blacks elsewhere. At birth, black and white infants of both sexes have similarly low Lp(a) concentrations.[52] In all groups, concentrations reach adult levels by 2 years of age. In both sexes, black children have considerably higher levels of Lp(a) than white children,[53] a difference which persists into adulthood, as shown by studies in the USA,[54] Congo,[55] Sudan,[50] Nigeria,[51] and the Seychelles.[27]

A positive association between Lp(a) concentration and risk of IHD has been described in some populations.[56] The sequence homology between the apo(a) and plasminogen genes has suggested that Lp(a) may be a risk factor for IHD because apo(a) couples to the plasminogen receptor on the vascular endothelium, thereby binding an LDL particle to the vessel wall and competitively inhibiting the activation of plasminogen. In all ethnic groups, Lp(a) concentration and the frequency of the small isoforms of apolipoprotein(a) are higher in patients with IHD than in healthy individuals.[57] The lower IHD rates in Blacks than in Whites in many communities, despite the higher Lp(a) levels of the former, emphasize the multifactorial nature of the disease.

Increased Lp(a) levels are resistant to dietary changes and lipid-lowering drugs, apart from nicotinic acid. Raised concentrations in postmenopausal women may be reduced by hormone replacement therapy. High levels in diabetic patients and those with chronic renal failure may also fall when these conditions are controlled.

HAEMOSTATIC FACTORS

The size and composition of thrombus forming on a plaque fissure is most probably determined by the thrombogenic potency of exposed subendothelial tissues, and by the responsiveness of the haemostatic system. Hypercoagulable plasma and hyperaggregable platelets may therefore convert an otherwise minor complication of atherosclerosis into a life-threatening event.

Hypercoagulability

The coagulation component of haemostasis consists of an interdependent series of reactions in which at each stage the enzyme generated acts upon its zymogen substrate to generate the enzyme that catalyses the subsequent step. Each stage is regulated by circulating serine protease inhibitors (serpins) including antithrombin III, antitrypsin and C1 inhibitor. Hypercoagulability is conceived of as a procoagulant imbalance between the generation of a coagulant enzyme and the activity of its inhibitors at one or more steps of the haemostatic pathway, causing an overresponsiveness to thrombogenic stimuli. One marker of hypercoagulability is thought to be a high factor VII coagulant activity (VIIc), which has been found in British men at high risk of IHD.[58] Low VIIc levels have been reported in Bantu men,[59] Westernized black South Africans[60] and rural Gambians.[61] Plasma VIIc is associated positively with dietary fat intake[62] and plasma triglyceride concentration,[63] thereby providing a link between dietary, lipid and haemostatic factors in IHD (see below, Dietary Factors).

The latent coagulant activity of factor VII will depend upon the plasma concentration of the protein, and upon the proportion circulating as the fully active enzyme (VIIa). Coagulant activity is expressed only when factor VIIa forms a complex with tissue factor, its cofactor on the surface of subendothelial cells and activated endothelial cells. The greater is VIIc, then the greater is likely to be the potential for thrombin generation following vascular injury.

Hyperaggregability

Circulating platelets scan the endothelial surface with a system of surface membrane receptors which facilitate their adhesion and aggregation at points of vascular damage. The first set of receptors are adhesive glycoproteins, many belonging to the integrin family, which recognize collagen and other adhesive proteins of the subendothelium such as von Willebrand factor, fibronectin and thrombospondin. Ligand–receptor coupling triggers changes in platelet shape, the generation of eicosanoids, including the proaggregatory molecule thromboxane, and the release of stored ADP and serotonin from platelet-

dense granules and adhesive proteins and coagulation factors from the α granules. The whole process is augmented by exposure of the platelets to thrombin which initiates aggregation by coupling to and cleaving its own receptor on the platelet membrane. Activation of platelets by ADP and thrombin induces surface expression of the fibrinogen receptor (glycoprotein IIb-IIIa). Receptors on adjacent activated platelets bind to shared fibrinogen molecules, thereby inducing aggregation.

Platelet behaviour appears to depend upon the composition of the lipid membrane in which its receptor systems are embedded. Enrichment of platelet membranes with cholesterol reduces their fluidity, which may help to explain reports of increased platelet aggregability ex vivo in hyperlipidaemic patients. On the other hand, in an epidemiological study no associations were found between plasma cholesterol or triglyceride levels and platelet responsiveness to ADP.[64] The enrichment of platelet membrane phospholipid with very long chain polyunsaturated fatty acids of the n-3 series (eicosapentaenoic acid and docosahexaenoic acid) by consumption of large amounts of marine mammal and fatty fish oils will reduce platelet aggregability by displacing arachidonic acid of the n-6 series. This diverts platelet eicosanoid metabolism from the production of thromboxane of the diene series (TXA_2) to that of the triene series (TXA_3), a much weaker platelet aggregating agent. Whether dietary manipulation of platelet membrane composition influences risk of IHD remains to be established. In one study of patients who had recovered from a myocardial infarction survival was significantly reduced in those whose platelets aggregated spontaneously and rapidly ex vivo.[65] In another study, a 29% reduction in mortality was reported in survivors of a myocardial infarction following advice to eat fatty fish at least twice weekly.[66]

There have been few ethnic comparisons of platelet function. In Uganda, platelet adhesiveness to glass beads did not differ between African and Indian men, despite large differences in risk of IHD.[67] In London, platelet responsiveness to ADP was less in West Indians than in Europeans.[64]

Plasma fibrinogen

Plasma fibrinogen concentration and risk of IHD are strongly and positively associated in both sexes where the disease is common.[58,68] Fibrinogen may influence risk through effects on blood viscosity (itself a marker of risk), platelet aggregation, or the rate of accumulation of fibrin in the atheromatous plaque. A strong, dose–response relationship exists between fibrinogen and smoking, and plasma concentrations fall rapidly when the habit is stopped (though not returning to non-smoking levels for several years). Fibrinogen levels tend to be higher in women than in men, and to increase after the menopause. There appears to be no effect of diet on fibrinogen, except perhaps a tendency for levels to fall with increased consumption of fish oils. Obesity and glucose intolerance are associated with increased concentrations, while alcohol consumption and physical activity are inversely related to plasma fibrinogen levels.

International and ethnic contrasts in fibrinogen levels do not fully accord with contrasts in IHD mortality. For example, high concentrations have been reported from rural parts of the Gambia.[61]

Fibrinolytic factors

The fibrinolytic system dissolves thrombi, thereby maintaining a patent vascular system. The serine protease plasmin degrades fibrin to soluble fragments. Plasmin is generated from plasminogen by tissue-type plasminogen activator (t-PA) or urokinase-type plasminogen activator (u-PA). Plasma t-PA is the more important of the two activators, and is normally present at concentrations of about 1 nmol/l. An important property of t-PA is its strong binding affinity to fibrin, being adsorbed together with its substrate plasminogen. The plasmin produced remains fibrin-bound and resistant to inactivation by α_2-antiplasmin. These properties explain the success of t-PA as a thrombolytic agent in coronary thrombosis.

Plasma t-PA is inhibited by a protein with very high binding affinity called plasminogen activator inhibitor type 1 (PAI-1), present in plasma, platelets, endothelial cells and smooth muscle cells. Most t-PA circulates as a complex with PAI-1, leaving excess PAI-1 in reserve. Various forms of stress can provoke release of t-PA, for example physical exercise, thereby generating a brief period of fibrinolytic activity.

Interest in PAI-1 has been stimulated by the discovery that its levels are increased in men who have survived a first myocardial infarction.[69] Plasma PAI-1 levels are also raised with obesity, hypertriglyceridaemia[70] and diabetes mellitus. Dilute clot lysis time, a crude measure of fibrinolytic activity, is weakly associated with IHD.[58] Times are reported to be shorter (i.e. lytic activity is greater) in the Bantu of South Africa[59] and in the rural Gambia[61] than in Europeans.

MARKERS OF ENDOTHELIAL CELL DYSFUNCTION

Endothelial dysfunction arising from injury is believed to predispose to both atherogenesis and thrombosis. Several markers of endothelial damage have been proposed, for example Von Willebrand factor, a glycoprotein secreted by the endothelium which circulates as a complex with factor VIII. Raised levels of Von Willebrand factor have been reported to be a risk factor for recurrent myocardial infarction.[71] Microalbuminuria, which may reflect a renal component of a more generalized endothelial dysfunction, has also been found to be an independent predictor of IHD.[72] Another putative marker is the plasma concentration of the peptide endothelin, a powerful vasoconstrictor and vascular smooth muscle mitogen secreted by vascular endothelium, which is increased in patients with myocardial infarction.[73] These and other candidate markers are under intensive study at present.

DIETARY FACTORS

Dietary fat and cholesterol

Most aboriginal peoples subsist on a diet that contains very little fat and cholesterol although nutritionally adequate, apart from periods of famine. Their blood cholesterol levels are very low. When such people forgo their traditional diet for one more typical of affluent, industrialized and sedentary societies (that is, rich in total fat, saturated fatty acids and energy) there is a prompt increase in blood total, LDL and HDL cholesterol levels, and in plasma triglyceride concentration.[74] When there is positive energy balance, rapid gains in weight are observed[74] which, if persistent, can be accompanied by high rates of non-insulin dependent (type II) diabetes mellitus.[75,76] These changes are corrected by reversion to the traditional diet. Educational programmes aimed at discouragement of those aspects of the Western diet with adverse effects on cardiovascular health form a major component of 'primordial' prevention.

The dietary saturated fatty acids responsible for the increase in blood cholesterol are of chain length C-12 (lauric acid), C-14 (myristic acid) and C-16 (palmitic acid). How these fatty acids exert their effects on blood cholesterol is uncertain, but experiments in non-human primates suggest that they suppress the activity of the B/E (LDL) receptor, thereby impeding the clearance of cholesterol-rich lipoproteins from the blood.[77]

Large amounts of dietary cholesterol will also

increase the plasma total and LDL cholesterol concentrations of aboriginal peoples,[46], although the effect is less marked than that of saturated fatty acid. The action of dietary cholesterol on blood cholesterol tends to be more obvious when taken in a diet rich in saturated fatty acid.

These effects of dietary fat on blood lipids are believed to explain their strong relations with mortality rates from IHD at an international level.[78] However, the relations are not straightforward. In the South-west Pacific region, the traditional diet of some Polynesian peoples had a high content of saturated fat obtained from coconut oil, rich in lauric acid and myristic acid. In other respects the diet was typical of aboriginal peoples, with sufficient calories only for energy balance and little protein. Although this high consumption of coconut oil was associated with a high plasma cholesterol concentration, a study of Polynesian men aged 40 years or more yielded no evidence of IHD.[79] Conceivably, other aspects of an aboriginal life style may protect the vascular system even when saturated fat is a major source of dietary energy.

The recommended diet

A palatable and nutritionally adequate diet cannot be constructed with a saturated fat content of less than about 7% of energy. Intakes close to this minimum are, however, compatible with health. The recommended diet proposed for the USA and Europe has a saturated fat content of 10% of total energy. Communities with a high mortality from IHD consume about 15–20% of energy as saturated fat. Whereas saturated fat tends to increase blood cholesterol, increases in polyunsaturated fat tend to have the opposite effect, while changes in monounsaturated fat have no significant influence on blood cholesterol *per se*.[80,81] No natural diet contains more than about 8% of energy in the form of polyunsaturated fatty acids. Higher intakes may predispose to malignancy and immune suppression and the generation of oxidized lipids in vivo (see below). Monounsaturated fat (mainly oleic acid) generally supplies about 10–15% of energy in an affluent diet (though it can be higher in the Mediterranean diet). Thus the optimal diet is envisaged as containing about 10% saturated fat, 8% polyunsaturated fat and 12% monounsaturated fat (making a total of 30% of energy as fat),[82] though some authorities would accept a greater proportion of energy as monounsaturated fat if needed for palatability. In Puerto Rico, a starch-rich (and hence reduced-fat) diet was associated with a relatively low incidence of IHD.[83] Dietary cholesterol intake is positively associated with risk of IHD, possibly because of adverse effects on the ratio of LDL cholesterol to HDL cholesterol, particularly in the non-obese.[84] On this account, a daily cholesterol intake of under 300 mg is generally recommended.[82]

Fish oils and eicosanoid metabolism

Activation of platelets and endothelial cells triggers the release of arachidonic acid (C20:4, n-6) from membrane phospholipids for immediate eicosanoid synthesis. The principal end-product of this pathway in the platelet is TXA_2, a potent platelet aggregating agent and vasoconstrictor, while in the endothelial cell it is prostacyclin (PGI_2), an inhibitor of platelet aggregation and a vasodilator. Arachidonic acid can be displaced from phospholipid by eicosapentaenoic acid (C20:5, n-3) and docosahexaenoic acid (C22:6, n-3), derived from fatty fish and marine mammals. Entry of these very long chain polyunsaturated fatty acids into the eicosanoid pathway leads to the production of thromboxane and prostacyclin of the triene series (TXA_3 and PGI_3), the former product lacking the platelet aggregatory effect of TXA_2 and the latter having a similar potency to PGI_2. These effects are thought to explain the prolonged bleeding time and diminished platelet aggregation ex vivo in the traditional Inuit, and raise the possibility that a diet rich in fatty fish may protect against IHD.[66]

Micronutrients, fatty acids and oxidative attack

Free radicals such as superoxide are continuously generated as intermediate products of normal cell metabolism. If released, these highly reactive species attack other molecules, particularly polyunsaturated fatty acids, with potentially very serious consequences. A series of protective mechanisms has evolved which minimize such untoward reactions. Firstly, the active centres of enzymes that generate free radicals are structured so as to prevent their escape before further processing. Secondly, a system of enzymes (superoxide dismutase, catalase, glutathione reductase) reduces superoxide to hydrogen peroxide, which subsequently decomposes to water. The third line of defence comprises the antioxidant vitamins which neutralize highly reactive species that have evaded the first two systems. Lipids are protected by vitamin E and the carotenoids. Vitamin C appears to function in the regeneration of vitamin E that has reacted with free radicals. Thus the risk of oxidative damage to lipoprotein lipid depends upon the rate of production of free radicals, the susceptibility of the lipoprotein lipid to oxidative attack (i.e. the proportion as polyunsaturated fatty acid), the effectiveness of the defensive enzymes such as superoxide dismutase, and the reserve of antioxidant vitamins. Peroxidation of polyunsaturated fatty acids by hydroxyl radicals generates aldehyde species which attack covalent bonds in apo-B100, the principal protein component of VLDL, IDL and LDL, causing its fragmentation. The existence of circulating auto-antibodies to oxidized LDL in human plasma is strong evidence for the occurrence of these processes in vivo[85] and the recognition of denatured lipoproteins as antigenic by the immunological system.

Monocytes and macrophages cannot be converted to foam cells (the typical cell of the fatty streak and fibrous plaque) simply by prolonged exposure to normal LDL, but only by contact with damaged LDL. Oxidized material that is endocytosed cannot be degraded within the cell, and is probably toxic for the macrophage. Thus the final outcome is macrophage degeneration with leakage of lipid and cell debris into the extracellular space[86] to produce the basal pool of the atheromatous plaque.

The susceptibility of polyunsaturated fatty acids to oxidative damage has caused concern about dietary enrichment with these species. The possibility that antioxidant vitamins retard the advancement of atheromatous lesions is supported by reported associations between low dietary, blood and tissue levels of vitamins E and C and increased risk of IHD.[87,88]

OBESITY, HYPERGLYCAEMIA AND INSULIN RESISTANCE

Obese adults are at increased risk of IHD. The accumulation of body fat during adulthood is associated with many other characteristics associated with IHD, particularly when this is deposited abdominally (the so-called male-type obesity, with an increased ratio of waist circumference to hip circumference). These characteristics include raised LDL cholesterol and VLDL triglyceride concentrations, a reduced HDL cholesterol concentration, an increased blood pressure, a raised factor VII coagulant activity and plasma fibrinogen concentration, glucose intolerance and hyperinsulinaemia. Hyperinsulinaemia is related to a high risk of IHD, but the metabolic disturbances linking this state with cardiovascular disease are not well understood. There is evidence (but not proof) to suggest that an increased abdominal fat mass releases excessive unesterified fatty acid into the portal system, which is then converted to glucose or assembled as triglyceride in hepatocytes. Subsequent release of these products

raises peripheral glucose and VLDL concentrations. Excess hepatic triglyceride may suppress the processing of insulin by the liver, allowing its escape into the systemic circulation. The resultant peripheral hyperinsulinaemia provokes a compensatory down-regulation of peripheral insulin receptors, giving rise to impaired glucose tolerance on oral glucose challenge. Glycosylation of proteins exposed to raised glucose concentrations, such as albumin, may generate products that are injurious to the vascular endothelium. Insulin resistance and non-insulin dependent diabetes mellitus are associated with raised levels of several suspected markers of endothelial damage, including PAI-1, urine albumin excretion and plasma endothelin. Further research is needed to substantiate this chain of events, or reveal in what ways it requires modification.

Adipocytes in the gluteal region, the hips and thighs appear metabolically distinctive from those in the abdominal region, and in women subserve functions relating to pregnancy and lactation. Obesity of this female type is probably not necessarily related to a positive energy balance or other changes that increase the risk of IHD. Women in many tropical communities essentially free of IHD are noted for their striking obesity of this type, for example in parts of Polynesia,[89] the Caribbean[90] and South Africa.[91] However, some women will have a more generalized obesity with associated increases in blood pressure and non-insulin dependent diabetes mellitus. In Britain, women of Afro-Caribbean descent are heavier than European women for their height, and have a larger waist:hip ratio, yet they have the lower mortality from IHD, presumably because of advantageous differences in other risk factors.

Central obesity appears to be an early response to urbanization and affluence in societies in transition, though of course fat is also deposited elsewhere, such as over the triceps muscles.[74] This development may well presage an increase in IHD mortality in years to come, as appears to have happened, for example, in many South Asian (Indian) communities that have migrated overseas (see below, Ethnicity and IHD). Reaven[92] has referred to the clustering of glucose intolerance, hyperinsulinaemia, hypertriglyceridaemia, a low plasma HDL cholesterol concentration and increased blood pressure as syndrome X.

PHYSICAL INACTIVITY

In aboriginal and agricultural underdeveloped societies, physical exertion is a necessity. By contrast, in industrialized and mechanized society, physical exertion is regarded as a leisure activity, the prerogative of the young. The motivation to expend muscular energy is no longer survival, but rather the same health-conscious attitude which encourages an avoidance of obesity, control of the diet, and refrainment from cigarette smoking. Physical activity appears to be not only a marker of an attitude conducive to health, but also cardioprotective in its own right. Strenuous physical exertion is followed by a transient increase in plasma fibrinolytic activity due to release of tissue plasminogen activator. An increase in habitual physical activity is accompanied by an improved lipoprotein profile (reduced VLDL triglyceride and increased HDL cholesterol).[93] Regular vigorous exercise is also associated with reductions in plasma fibrinogen concentration and factor VII coagulant activity, and improvements in insulin sensitivity and blood pressure levels. Sustained brisk walking is sufficient to improve exercise endurance in sedentary people, and the associated metabolic responses may explain the reduced risk of IHD in those taking regular physical exercise.

CIGARETTE SMOKING

In societies with a low mortality from IHD and low plasma cholesterol concentrations, cigarette smoking shows little association with the extent of coronary atherosclerosis or risk of clinical IHD.[94,95] By contrast, in communities in which IHD is common, a dose–response association exists between smoking and risk of the disorder, with those who inhale having a higher risk than non-inhalers. Ex-smokers are at lower risk than current smokers, but whether they ever reacquire the risk of non-smokers is debatable.

Chronic smokers seem to suffer vascular endothelial cell injury. They have a relative leucocytosis, and some studies have suggested that this is accompanied by white cell activation with increased generation of free radicals. The plasma LDL particles of smokers may have an increased susceptibility to peroxidative damage, owing perhaps in part to a reduced content of antioxidants, a consequence of dietary deficiency. Tissue injury and a chronic inflammatory response may help explain the raised plasma fibrinogen level of the cigarette smoker, an acute-phase protein. The association between smoking and fibrinogen has dose–response characteristics, and fibrinogen levels fall when the habit is given up. Platelet survival is shortened in smokers, and the raised urinary excretion of the products of eicosanoid metabolism in the smoker may indicate increased platelet activation.

Smokers have changes in lipid metabolism that may contribute to their high risk of IHD. Plasma HDL cholesterol concentrations are reduced and chylomicron remnant clearance is impaired.

BLOOD PRESSURE

Hypertension can be common in communities that experience little IHD. For example, in parts of the Caribbean, prevalence rates of hypertension exceeding 20% have been recognized in middle-aged adults for at least 50 years, whereas IHD has remained rare until relatively recently.[96] When IHD emerges as a major cause of morbidity and mortality, whether in tropical[97] or temperate[98] countries, both systolic and diastolic blood pressure become strong predictors of individual risk of IHD. There is no threshold to this relation, the positive gradient extending across the full range of blood pressure. Drug therapy sufficient to lower diastolic pressure by 5 mmHg or more can lead to an appreciable decrease in the risk of IHD.[98]

PSYCHOLOGICAL FACTORS

Individuals in all societies face the unpredictability of life and the psychological stress of adverse economic and social circumstances. Societies differ, however, in the supports given to the individual within the family, neighbourhood and workplace to lessen the strains of adverse circumstances. Japan is frequently cited as exemplifying those societies which emphasize loyalty to the social group, while North American culture places a high premium on individualism. Although both nations are highly affluent and industrialized, Japan has the longer life expectancy and a much lower mortality from IHD, which is falling.[99] While the traditional Japanese diet, very low in fat, probably makes a major contribution to this disparity in IHD, certain supportive characteristics of Japanese culture may also have a role. When Japanese men living in California were classified according to their degree of social assimilation into the host American community, those holding most to traditional Japanese culture had much the lower prevalence of IHD, an association not explained by differences in diet, smoking habits, blood cholesterol or blood pressure.[100] Psychological stresses imposed by social and economic pressures in an unsupportive society have been proposed as one explanation for the social class gradient in IHD mortality in many industrialized countries including Britain.[101] What the pathophysiological responses to psychosocial stress that promote IHD might be are unclear at present, and constitute an area in need of further research.

ETHNICITY AND IHD

Ethnic differences in sociocultural factors and gene pools are important for IHD insofar as they are responsible for ethnic contrasts in the risk factor profile for IHD. Ethnic contrasts in mortality from IHD are discerned most clearly in societies containing both indigenous and immigrant groups, as in England.

SOUTH ASIANS

Many millions of people around the world trace their origins to the Indian subcontinent. Their migration dates essentially from the mid-nineteenth century, and many communities resettled in their new homeland more than 100 years ago. Such populations are found in Guyana, Trinidad, Mauritius, Natal, Fiji, Singapore and East Africa, while more recent resettlement has occurred in England and North America. Despite their very considerable cultural diversity, their differences in geographical origin across the Indian subcontinent, and the varying extent to which they have assimilated into the general culture of their new homeland, people of South Asian (Indian) ancestry have a considerably higher mortality from IHD than their neighbours of other ethnic origins.[102] This contrast is particularly striking in the long-established urban community of Indian descent in Trinidad, where cultural assimilation has been extensive.[97] The remarkable predisposition of these people to non-insulin dependent diabetes mellitus, and failure of this characteristic or any other standard risk factor to account for their high IHD mortality, has led to suggestions that both disorders are the outcome of a common underlying trait, such as a distinctive pattern of insulin metabolism akin to syndrome X.[103] Diabetes mellitus has been recognized for centuries among the affluent and obese in India, and IHD is seen throughout the subcontinent, especially in large urban centres.[104]

Whether IHD is more a public health problem in Indian communities overseas than in cities in the subcontinent is uncertain. Population-based mortality data for IHD are not available for India or Pakistan. In Britain, where the IHD death rate among adults of Indian, Pakistani or Bangladeshi origin is high,[105] the prevalence of electrocardiographic major Q waves in middle-aged men of these ethnic groups (about 4%) is similar to that reported in the major urban centres of India.[104,106] These comparisons suggest that IHD is common in urban India, in agreement with the experience of physicians with urban practices.[107] The prevalence of major Q waves appears to be much lower in rural parts of India.[108]

AFRICANS

The belief that the descendants of Africans in the USA and elsewhere are resistant to IHD despite their high prevalence rates of hypertension, hypercholesterolaemia and cigarette smoking is not supported by epidemiology. In the USA for example, higher age-adjusted IHD mortality rates were reported for black males than white males in 23 of 34 eastern states in which the comparison could be made.[109] While part of the mortality difference may reflect ethnic differences in health care, the figures should dispel any misconception about ethnic immunity. Black males are often found to have a higher HDL cholesterol and a lower triglyceride concentration than white males, but there is no evidence for any genetic basis for this difference. National mortality rates for IHD in Britain's community of Afro-Caribbean descent are currently intermediate between rates in the West Indies and the overall rate for Britain. Many West Indian territories are witnessing increases in hospital admission rates for IHD as their populations forgo their traditional life styles for habits held responsible for the high mortality from IHD in Europe and North America.

While IHD is the leading cause of mortality in black adults in the USA,[110] the disease is much less common in black populations of Africa, Latin America and territories bounding the Indian Ocean. In some of these territories data are restricted to hospital experience. For example, in Abidjan (Ivory Coast), myocardial infarction accounts for 3% of patient admissions.[111] Almost all are men, many being less than 50 years of age, and they not uncommonly have a normal coronary arteriogram with few coronary risk factors. In Ouagadougou (Burkina Faso), fewer than 2% of admissions for cardiac disorders are due to IHD.[112] In Northern Nigeria, hospital admission for IHD is a rarity.[113,114] In the Mamprobi (Ghana) survey, electrocardiographic Q–QS abnormalities were found in 2% of men and women aged 35 to 69 years.[115] Similarly low prevalence rates apply to much of East Africa and South Africa. For example, one analysis of deaths among black South Africans in selected districts concluded that, at ages 36–64 years, IHD accounted for about 7% of deaths in men and 4% in females. These percentages were much less than those for white South Africans.[116] In large samples of urban and rural black South African adults aged over 60 years, far fewer than 1% had electrocardiographic changes suggestive of IHD.[117,118]

The electrocardiogram in black populations

In epidemiology it is standard practice to describe the electrocardiographic findings in terms of the Minnesota code.[119] This classification focuses on Q and QS patterns, R wave amplitudes, ST segment and T wave items which in white populations indicate an increased probability of underlying cardiac disease. This system has confirmed that the age-specific prevalence of high-amplitude R waves in left ventricular leads and deep S waves in right ventricular leads is higher in Blacks than in other ethnic groups,[120–122] even when allowance is made for blood pressure.

In parts of the USA and South Africa increased QRS voltages, major and minor ST segment and T wave patterns, and prolonged PR intervals are more common in Blacks than in Whites, but are associated with risk of clinical IHD only in Whites.[123,124]

NATIVE AMERICANS

Data on IHD in native Americans are relatively sparse, partly because for statistical purposes they have in the past been pooled with other ethnic minorities in the USA. There are several hundred native American tribes which together comprise about 0.6% of the American population. The largest of these tribes is the Navajo, numbering approximately 200 000. This diversity makes any consideration of native Americans as a single entity questionable, particularly when it is recalled that while some still strive to pursue their traditional life style, a large number now live in urban centres.

Much of the information for native Americans pertains to Pima and Papago Indians of the south-western USA, who have extremely high prevalence rates for non-insulin dependent diabetes mellitus.[125] Around 1980, diseases of the heart accounted for 21% of deaths in native Americans and Alaskans, as compared with 38% for the total population of the USA,[126] figures to be interpreted bearing in mind the young age structure of native American communities and their high rates of competing causes of premature death.

In the 1960s, IHD rates appeared to be low among the Pima, Navajo and Apache peoples of the south-western USA.[127,128] However, between then and the late 1970s, the disease became increasingly common.[129] Whereas formerly, serum cholesterol levels in Navajo people were low, nowadays those in men under 55 years exceed those of the general USA population, although cholesterol concentrations in Navajo women are still relatively low.[130] High IHD mortality rates have been reported in the Chippawa[131] and Sioux.[132] The overall impression is that IHD nowadays affects urbanized Indians similarly to the general population. In the more isolated south-western American tribes, IHD rates are increasing but are still lower than in Whites. The risk factors for IHD, documented for the white population, appear to behave similarly in native Americans, among whom increases in LDL cholesterol levels, obesity, dietary saturated fat, glucose intolerance and high blood pressure are causes for concern.

CHINESE

In China, Hong Kong and Taiwan the prevalence of IHD has been estimated to be approximately 4–8 times lower than in Western populations.[133] Within China, mortality rates from IHD are higher in the north than south, even in urban centres, and higher in urban than rural areas.[134] Rates are highest in urban Beijing, where in the mid-1980s IHD mortality was reported to be respectively 33 and 65% of that of men and women in the USA.[134] The impression is that IHD has become more common in these territories during the past 30 years, although some of this may have been due to ageing of their populations. In Singapore, age-standardized death rates from IHD among its Indian and Malay communities exceeded those for the USA and England and Wales in the early 1980s, whereas they remained low in the Chinese community, although not as low as in Japan.[135]

The clinical presentation, pattern of complications and short-term prognosis of IHD in the Chinese conform to those in Western populations.[136] Chinese patients who have recovered from an acute myocardial infarction have significantly higher concentrations of plasma triglyceride, cholesterol and apo B, and a lower concentration of apo A-I than control patients.[137] In a comparison of cardiovascular mortality rates and IHD risk factor levels by county in China, however, LDL cholesterol levels did not correlate with IHD mortality, whereas plasma triglyceride concentration did so (positively).[25] In Singapore, ethnic differences in cigarette smoking rates, blood pressure levels, serum cholesterol and serum triglyceride did not explain the relatively low IHD mortality in the Chinese sector of the population, but HDL cholesterol levels were higher in the Chinese than in other ethnic groups.[135]

CONTROL AND PREVENTION

The high mortality outside hospital following coronary thrombosis is well recognized, and has led to intensive efforts to improve the immediate care of such emergencies. Defibrillation and management of other complications of the acute attack, together with more rapid admission for intensive care, have reduced the case fatality in communities where IHD rates have reached epidemic levels. Incidence rates and fatality rates remain so high, however, that prevention remains the only long-term solution.

In developing countries that are witnessing the emergence of IHD as a significant health problem, authorities are being urged to embark upon health promotion through risk factor intervention.[6,9] The decline in IHD mortality in Europe and North America, some of which is due to improvements in risk factor status,[138] testifies to the effectiveness of this approach. Principal among these measures would appear to be the prevention of male-type (central) obesity by control of energy balance, control of blood lipid levels by limitation of saturated fat intake, discouragement of tobacco smoking, and prompt management of raised blood pressures. Such a strategy may well control both the atherogenic and thrombogenic components of the disease. Families in whom IHD emerges first may well be genetically predisposed to the deterioration in risk factors that follows in the wake of life style changes, and family members of all patients presenting with IHD should be examined and counselled accordingly. Control programmes are likely to be more effective when they combine advocacy of the health aspects of the traditional life style with education about the negative health consequences of the Western life style to which many aspire.

LIPID DISORDERS

HYPERCHOLESTEROLAEMIC STATES

FAMILIAL HYPERCHOLESTEROLAEMIAS

Many mutations of the B/E (LDL) receptor gene are recognized, leading to defective synthesis or function of the LDL receptor, causing a diminished clearance of LDL particles from the circulation. In many European populations, the frequency of the heterozygotic state is about 1 in 400, while in certain more closed communities, where there is evidence for a founder effect, this can rise to 1 in 80 (e.g. Lebanese, Quebecois French-Canadian, Afrikaaners). The disorder affects Asian, Arabian and black African peoples.[139]

In the heterozygote, blood cholesterol ranges between 7 and 15 mmol/l due to the high LDL cholesterol, while HDL cholesterol tends to be reduced. Xanthomas appear by early adulthood, typically in the Achilles tendon and the tendons of the extensors as they run over the heads of the metacarpal bones. Xanthelasmas, in or close to the eyelids, and premature corneal arcus may be present. Premature atherosclerosis often culminates in clinical IHD before 50 years of age. In the very rare homozygote or double heterozygote, cholesterol levels may be as high as 25 mmol/l and IHD can present in the first decade of life.

FAMILIAL COMBINED HYPERLIPIDAEMIA

This is an imprecisely defined inherited disorder which probably consists of several genetic and molecular defects presenting with a similar phenotype. There is a strong familial tendency to increased plasma cholesterol and triglyceride concentrations. Different members of a single family may have elevations in either lipid alone, and the lipid profile is sometimes inconstant in affected individuals. The LDL particles tend to be small and dense, with a high ratio of apo B-100 to cholesterol. Plasma HDL cholesterol is often low, and there appears to be an increased synthesis of VLDL. In many European communities, the disorder affects 1–2% of families and is present in 10–15% of patients with IHD. Xanthelasmas are not a feature of this disorder.

Presumably the genetic characteristics underlying this disorder are present in all populations, but phenotypic expression may require the presence of certain acquired factors such as a high-fat diet and obesity. Conceivably, families with these genotypes will be among the first to manifest hyperlipidaemia and atherosclerosis when societies shift from traditional 'low-risk' life styles and acquire Western patterns of behaviour.

REMNANT HYPERLIPOPROTEINAEMIAS

Clearance of chylomicron remnants and VLDL remnants (i.e. IDL) is by way of a receptor which binds to apo E but not to Apo B-100. Three common alleles are present for the apo E gene, designated E_2, E_3 and E_4. The respective isoforms of the apolipoprotein have different binding affinities for the receptor, which in the case of E_2 is defective and predisposes to impaired remnant removal from the circulation. Poor clearance of remnant particles leads to a combined hyperlipidaemia. A marker of this disorder is the presence of VLDL particles with β mobility rather than pre-β or α_2 mobility on electrophoresis, a high ratio of cholesterol to triglyceride, and an abnormally high content of apo E.

In the apo E_2 heterozygote (E_2/E_3 or E_2/E_4), a mild elevation in remnant particles is associated with a reduction in LDL cholesterol concentration. The apo E_2 homozygote state accounts for nearly all cases of remnant (type III) hyperlipoproteinaemia, the remainder being due to rarer variants of apo E. However, only about 2% of E_2 homozygotes express the phenotype, other conditions needing to be present for remnants to accumulate (e.g. hypothyroidism, diabetes mellitus, other genetic disorders of lipid metabolism, renal disease). Phenotypic expression is associated with characteristic orange planar xanthomas in the palmar creases, tuberous xanthomas at the elbow and other sites, and an increased risk of IHD and peripheral vascular disease.

The frequency of the E_2 allele differs significantly between populations. For example, reported frequencies are 12% in New Zealand, 8% in Germany, 4% in Finland and Japan and 3% in Nigeria,[140] and as low as 1.5% in the Greenland Inuit people.[32]

HYPERTRIGLYCERIDAEMIC STATES

DIETARY HYPERTRIGLYCERIDAEMIA

As with hypercholesterolaemia, dietary factors are the most common causes of a raised fasting triglyceride concentration. Among the important dietary characteristics are its energy content, fat composition, its carbohydrate component and the amount of alcohol consumed.

Hypercaloric diets stimulate hepatic production and secretion of VLDL particles, and ultimately lead to obesity, which itself is a frequent cause of hypertriglyceridaemia. Saturated fatty acids may also increase triglyceride levels when taken in large amounts, possibly by affecting VLDL metabolism. Substitution of monounsaturated or polyunsaturated fatty acids for saturated fat will sometimes lower plasma fasting triglyceride levels. This is particularly the case when the diet is enriched with very long chain polyunsaturated fatty acids of marine mammal or fish origin, which reduce hepatic synthesis of VLDL triglyceride.

A shift from a high-fat, low-carbohydrate diet to a low-fat, high-carbohydrate diet may induce a temporary increase in VLDL triglyceride, due mainly to increased loading of VLDL particles. This is of little if any clinical relevance for IHD.

GENETIC HYPERTRIGLYCERIDAEMIAS

The increased plasma triglyceride levels in familial combined hyperlipidaemia and remnant (type III) hyperlipoproteinaemia have been described above. Familial hypertriglyceridaemia is a condition in which isolated high triglyceride levels are present in several family members. There appears to be overproduction of large triglyceride-enriched VLDL particles. The condition is inherited in an autosomal dominant manner, and does not respond to restriction of dietary fat intake. Other rare inherited conditions associated with high fasting triglyceride concentrations are familial lipoprotein lipase deficiency, hepatic triglyceride lipase deficiency and lecithin–cholesterol acyltransferase deficiency.

REFERENCES

1 Herrick J B. Clinical features of sudden obstruction of the coronary arteries. *JAMA* 1912; 59:2015–2020.

2 World Health Organization. *World Health Statistics Annual*. Geneva: WHO, 1980–1992.

3 Segi M. *Cancer Mortality for Selected Sites in 24*

Countries (1950–1957). Sendai, Japan: Department of Public Health, Tokohu University School of Medicine. 1960.

4 Miller G J, Saunders M J, Gilson R J C & Ashcroft M T. Lung function of healthy boys and girls in relation to ethnic composition, test exercise performance, and habitual physical activity. *Thorax* 1977; 32:486–496.

5 Badruddin S H, Khurshid M, Molla A, Manser W W T, Lalani R & Vellani C W. Factors associated with elevated serum cholesterol levels in well-to-do Pakistani schoolchildren. *J Trop Med Hyg* 1991; 94:123–129.

6 Dodu SRA. Emergence of cardiovascular disease in developing countries. *Cardiology* 1988; 75:56–64.

7 Hechter H H & Borhani N O. Mortality and geographic distribution of arteriosclerotic heart disease. *Public Health Rep* 1965; 80(1), 11 January.

8 Goldman L & Cook E F. The decline in ischemic heart disease mortality rates: an analysis of the comparative effects of medical interventions and changes in lifestyle. *Ann Intern Med* 1984; 101: 825–836.

9 Litvak J, Ruiz L, Restrepo H E & McAlister A. The growing noncommunicable disease burden, a challenge for the countries of the Americas. *Bull Pan Am Health Organ* 1987; 21:156–171.

10 Smith E P. Fibrinogen, fibrin and fibrin degradation products in relation to atherosclerosis. *Clin Haematol* 1986; 15:355–370.

11 McGill H C. Fatty streaks in the coronary arteries and aorta. *Lab Invest* 1968; 18:100–104.

12 Freedman D S, Newman W P, Tracy R E, Voors A E & Srinivasan S. Black–white differences in aortic fatty streaks in adolescence and early adulthood: The Bogalusa Heart Study. *Circulation* 1988; 77:856–864.

13 Leary T. The genesis of atherosclerosis. *Arch Pathol* 1941; 32:507–555.

14 PDAY Research Group. Relationship of atherosclerosis in young men to serum lipoprotein cholesterol concentrations and smoking. A preliminary report. *JAMA* 1990; 264:3018–3024.

15 Davies M J. Morphology and natural history of atherosclerotic lesions in the human arterial tree. In Woolf N. & Davies M J (eds) *Atherosclerosis in Ischaemic Heart Disease: The Mechanisms*, vol. 1. London: Science Press, 1990: 2:1–2:52.

16 Davies M J. Thrombosis in acute myocardial infarction and sudden death. In Mehta J L, ContiC R and Brest A N (eds) *Thrombosis and Platelets in Myocardial Ischemia*. Philadelphia: F A Davis, 1987: 151–159.

17 Davies M J & Thomas A. Thrombosis and acute coronary-artery lesions in sudden cardiac ischaemic death. *N Engl J Med* 1984; 310:1137–1140.

18 Wong E T, Cobb C, Umehara M K et al. Heterogeneity of serum creatine kinase activity among racial and gender groups of the population. *Am J Clin Pathol* 1983; 79:582–586.

19 Hooper R J L, Worrall J G, Phongsathorn V & Paice E W. Effect of racial variation in serum creatine kinase on interpretation: a case report. *Ann Clin Biochem* 1992; 29:229–230.

20 Black H R, Quallich H. & Gareleck C B. Racial differences in serum creatine kinase levels. *Am J Med* 1986; 81:479–487.

21 Simons L A, Dwyer T, Simons J et al. Chylomicrons and chylomicron remnants in coronary artery disease: a case-control study. *Atherosclerosis* 1987; 65:181–189.

22 Kraus R M. Relationship of intermediate and low-density lipoprotein subspecies to risk of coronary artery disease. *Am Heart J* 1987; 113:578–582.

23 Reichl D & Miller N E. Pathophysiology of reverse cholesterol transport. Insights from inherited disorders of lipoprotein metabolism. *Arteriosclerosis* 1989; 9:785–797.

24 Mancilha-Carvalho J J & Crews D E. Lipid profiles of Yanomamo Indians of Brazil. *Prev Med* 1990; 19:66–75.

25 Wenxun F, Parker R, Parpia B et al. Erythrocyte fatty acids, plasma lipids, and cardiovascular disease in rural China. *Am J Clin Nutr* 1990; 52:1027–1036.

26 Campos H, Bailey S M, Gussak L S, Siles X, Ordovas J M & Schaefer E J. Relations of body habitus, fitness level, and cardiovascular risk factors including lipoproteins and apolipoproteins in a rural and urban Costa Rican population. *Arterioscler Thromb* 1991; 11:1077–1088.

27 Bovet P, Shamlaye C, Kitua A, Riesen W F, Paccaud F & Darioli R. High prevalence of cardiovascular risk factors in the Seychelles (Indian Ocean). *Arterioscler Thromb* 1991; 11:1730–1736.

28 Tunstall-Pedoe H, Smith W C S & Tavendale R. How-often-that-high graphs of serum cholesterol. Findings from the Scottish Heart Health and Scottish Monica Studies. *Lancet* 1989; i:540–542.

29 Miller G J, Beckles G L A, Byam N T A et al. Serum lipoprotein concentrations in relation to ethnic composition and urbanization in men and women of Trinidad, West Indies. *Int J Epidemiol* 1984; 13:413–421.

30 Hughes K, Yeo P B, Lun K C et al. Cardiovascular diseases in Chinese, Malays, and Indians in Singapore. II. Differences in risk factor levels. *J Epidemiol Community Health* 1990; 44:29–35.

31 Tuomilehto J, Li N, Dowse G et al. The prevalence of coronary heart disease in the multi-ethnic and high diabetes population of Mauritius. *J Intern Med* 1993; 233:187–194.

32 de Knijff P, Johansen L G, Rosseneu M, Frants R R, Jespersen J & Havekes L M. Lipoprotein profile of a Greenland Inuit population. Influence of anthropometric variables, apo E and A4 polymorphism, and lifestyle. *Arterioscler Thromb* 1992; 12:1371–1379.

33 Hart Hansen J P, Hancke S & Moller Petersen J. Atherosclerosis in native Greenlanders: an ultrasonographic investigation. *Arch Med Res* 1990; 49:151–156.

34 Stamler J, Wentworth D, Neaton J D for the MRFIT Research Group. Is the relationship between serum cholesterol and risk of premature death from coronary disease continuous and graded? Findings in 356 222 primary screenees of the Multiple Risk Factor Intervention Trial (MRFIT). *JAMA* 1986; 256:2823–2828.

35 Expert Panel on Population Strategies for Blood Cholesterol Reduction: executive summary. National Cholesterol Education Program. *Arch Intern Med* 1991; 151:1074–1084.

36 Lipid Research Clinics Program: The Lipid Research Clinics Coronary Primary Prevention Trial: II. The relationship of reduction in incidence of coronary heart disease to cholesterol lowering. *JAMA* 1984; 251:365–374.

37 Antonis A & Bersohn I. The influence of diet on serum triglyceride in South African white and Bantu prisoners. *Lancet* 1961; i:3–9.

38 Simons L A. Interrelations of lipids and lipoproteins with coronary artery mortality in 19 countries. *Am J Cardiol* 1986; 57:5G–10G.

39 Van Lenten B J, Fogelman A M, Jackson R J, Shapiro S, Haberland M E & Edwards P A. Receptor-mediated uptake of remnant lipoproteins by cholesterol-laden human monocyte-macrophages. *J Biol Chem* 1985; 260:8783–8788.

40 Avins A L, Haber R J & Hulley S B. The status of hypertriglyceridemia as a risk factor for coronary heart disease. *Clin Lab Med* 1989; 9:153–168.

41 Phillips A N & Davey Smith G. How independent are 'independent' effects? Relative risk estimation when correlated exposures are measured imprecisely. *J Clin Epidemiol* 1991; 44:1223–1231.

42 Hamsten A. Hypertriglyceridaemia, triglyceride-rich lipoproteins and coronary heart disease. *Baillière's Clin Endocrinol Metab* 1990; 4:895–922.

43 Assmann G, Gotto A M & Paoletti R. The hypertriglyceridemias: risk and management. Introduction. *Am J Cardiol* 1991; 68:1A–4A.

44 Assmann G & Schulte H. Relation of high-density lipoprotein cholesterol and triglycerides to incidence of atherosclerotic coronary artery disease (the PROCAM experience). *Am J Cardiol* 1992; 70:733–737.

45 Gordon D J, Probsfield J L, Garrison R J et al. High-density lipoprotein cholesterol and cardiovascular disease. Four prospective American studies. *Circulation* 1989; 79:8–15.

46 McMurray M P, Connor W E, Lin D S, Cerqueira M T & Connor S L. The absorption of cholesterol and the sterol balance in the Tarahumara Indian of Mexico fed cholesterol-free and high cholesterol diets. *Am J Clin Nutr* 1985; 41:1289–1298.

47 Brunner D, Weissbort J, Fischer M et al. Serum lipid response to a high caloric, high fat diet in agricultural workers during 12 months. *Am J Clin Nutr* 1979; 32:1342–1349.

48 Third J L H C, Montag J, Flynn M, Freidel J, Laskarzewski P & Glueck C J. Primary and familial hypoalphalipoproteinemia. *Metabolism* 1984; 33:136–146.

49 Ordovas J M, Cassidy D K, Civeira F, Bisgaier C L & Schaefer E J. Familial apolipoprotein A-I, C-III, and A-IV deficiency and premature atherosclerosis due to deletion of a gene complex on chromosome 11. *J Biol Chem* 1989; 264:16339–16342.

50 Sandholzer C, Hallman D M, Saha N et al. Effects of the apolipoprotein (a) size polymorphism on the lipoprotein (a) concentration in 7 ethnic groups. *Hum Genet* 1991; 86:607–614.

51 Cobbaert C & Kesteloot H. Serum lipoprotein (a) levels in racially different populations. *Am J Epidemiol* 1992; 136:441–449.

52 Rifai N, Heiss G & Doetsch K. Lipoprotein (a) at birth, in blacks and whites. *Atherosclerosis* 1992; 92:123–129.

53 Srinivasan S R, Dahlen, G H, Jarpa R A, Webber L S & Berenson G S. Racial (black–white) differences in serum lipoprotein (a) distribution and its relation to parental myocardial infarction in children. Bogalusa Heart Study. *Circulation* 1991; 84:160–167.

54 Guyton J R, Dahlen G H, Patsch W, Kautz J A & Gotto A M. Relationship of plasma lipoprotein Lp (a) levels to race and to apolipoprotein B. *Arteriosclerosis* 1985; 5:265–272.

55 Parra H-J, Luyeye I, Bouramore C, Demerquilly C & Fruchart J-C. Black–white differences in serum Lp(a) lipoprotein levels. *Clin Chim Acta* 1987; 167:27–31.

56 Dahlen G, Berg K, Gillnas T & Ericson C. Lp(a): pre-beta-lipoprotein in Swedish middle-aged males and in patients with coronary heart disease. *Clin Chem* 1975; 7:334–341.

57 Sandholzer C, Saha N, Kark J D et al. Apo(a) isoforms predict risk for coronary heart disease. A study in six populations. *Arterioscler Thromb* 1992; 12:1214–1226.

58 Meade T W, Mellows S, Brozovic M et al. Haemostatic function and ischaemic heart disease: principal results of the Northwick Park Heart Study. *Lancet* 1986; ii:533–537.

59 Merskey C, Gordon H & Lachner H. Blood coagulation and fibrinolysis in relation to coronary disease. A comparative study of normal white men, white men with overt coronary heart disease, and normal Bantu men. *BMJ* 1960; i:219–227.

60 Vermaak W J H, Ubbink J B, Delport R, Becher P J, Bissbort S H & Ungerer J P J. Ethnic immunity to coronary heart disease? *Atherosclerosis* 1991; 89:155–162.

61 Meade T W, Stirling Y, Thompson S G et al. An international and interregional comparison of haemostatic variables in the study of ischaemic heart disease. *Int J Epidemiol* 1986; 15:331–336.

62 Miller G J, Cruickshank J K, Ellis L J et al. Fat consumption and factor VII coagulant activity in middle-aged men. *Atherosclerosis* 1989; 78:19–24.

63 Mitropoulos K A, Miller G J, Reeves B E A, Wilkes H C & Cruickshank J K. Factor VII

coagulant activity is strongly associated with the plasma concentration of large lipoprotein particles in middle-aged men. *Atherosclerosis* 1989; 76:203–208.

64 Meade T W, Vickers M V, Thompson S G, Stirling Y, Haines A P & Miller G J. Epidemiological characteristics of platelet aggregability. *BMJ* 1985; 290:428–432.

65 Trip M D, Cats V M, van Capelle F J L & Vreeken J. Platelet hyperreactivity and prognosis in survivors of myocardial infarction. *N Engl J Med* 1990; 322:1549–1554.

66 Burr M L, Fehily A M, Gilbert J F et al. Effects of changes in fat, fish, and fibre intakes on death and myocardial reinfarction: diet and reinfarction trial (DART). *Lancet* 1989; ii:757–761.

67 Shaper A G, Jones K W, Kyobe J & Jones M. Fibrinolysis in relation to body fatness, serum lipids and coronary heart disease in African and Asian men in Uganda. *J Atheroscler Res* 1966; 6:313–327.

68 Kannel W B, D'Agostino R B & Belanger A J. Fibrinogen, cigarette smoking, and risk of cardiovascular disease: insights from the Framingham Study. *Am Heart J* 1987; 113:1006–1010.

69 Hamsten A, de Faire U, Walldius G et al. Plasminogen activator inhibitor in plasma: risk factor for recurrent myocardial infarction. *Lancet* 1987; ii:3–9.

70 Crutchley D J, McPhee G V, Terris M F & Canossa-Terris M A. Levels of three hemostatic factors in relation to serum lipids. Monocyte procoagulant activity, tissue plasminogen activator, and type-1 plasminogen activator inhibitor. *Arteriosclerosis* 1989; 9:934–939.

71 Jansson J H, Nilsson T K & Johnson O. Von Willebrand factor in plasma: a novel risk factor for recurrent myocardial infarction and death. *Br Heart J* 1991; 66:351–355.

72 Yudkin J S, Forrest R D & Jackson C A. Microalbuminuria as predictor of vascular disease in non-diabetic subjects. Islington Diabetes Survey. *Lancet* 1988; ii:530–533.

73 Miyauchi T, Yanagisawa M, Tomizawa T et al. Increased plasma concentrations of endothelin-1 and big endothelin-1 in acute myocardial infarction. *Lancet* 1989; ii:53–54.

74 McMurray M P, Cerqueira M T, Connor S L & Connor W E. Changes in lipid and lipoprotein levels and body weight in Tarahumara Indians after consumption of an affluent diet. *N Engl J Med* 1991; 325:1704–1708.

75 Saad M F, Knowler W C, Pettitt D J, Nelson R G, Mott D M & Bennett P H. The natural history of impaired glucose tolerance in the Pima Indians. *N Engl J Med* 1988; 319:1500–1506.

76 Knowler W C, Bennett P H, Hamman R F & Miller M. Diabetes incidence and prevalence in Pima Indians: a 19-fold greater incidence than in Rochester, Minnesota. *Am J Epidemiol* 1978; 108:497–505.

77 Nicolosi R J, Stucchi A F, Kowala M C, Hennessy L K, Hegsted D M & Schaefer E J. Effect of dietary fat saturation and cholesterol on LDL composition and metabolism. *Arteriosclerosis* 1990; 10:119–128.

78 Keys A, Aravanis C, van Buchem F S P et al. The diet and all-causes death rate in the Seven Countries study. *Lancet* 1981; ii:58–61.

79 Hunter J D. Diet, body build, blood pressure, and serum cholesterol levels in coconut-eating Polynesians. *Fed Proc* 1962; 21:36–43.

80 Keys A, Anderson J & Grande F. Serum cholesterol response to changes in the diet. *Metabolism* 1965; 14:747–787.

81 Mensink R P & Katan M B. Effect of dietary fatty acids on serum lipids and lipoproteins. A meta-analysis of 27 trials. *Arterioscler Thromb* 1992; 12:911–919.

82 Expert Panel. Report of the National Cholesterol Education Program Expert Panel on detection, evaluation and treatment of high blood cholesterol in adults. *Arch Intern Med* 1988; 148:36–69.

83 Gordon T, Kagan A, Garcia-Palmieri M et al. Diet and its relation to coronary heart disease and death in three populations. *Circulation* 1981; 63:500–515.

84 Goff D C, Shekelle R B, Katan M B, Gotto A M & Stamler J. Does body fatness modify the association between dietary cholesterol and risk of death? Results from the Chicago Western Electric Study. *Arterioscler Thromb* 1992; 12:755–761.

85 Palinski W, Rosenfeld M E, Yla-Herttuala S et al. Low density lipoprotein undergoes oxidative modification in vivo. *Proc Natl Acad Sci USA* 1989; 86:1372–1376.

86 Luc G & Fruchart J-C. Oxidation of lipoproteins and atherosclerosis. *Am J Clin Nutr* 1991; 53:2065–2095.

87 Gey K F, Puska P, Jordan P & Moser U K. Inverse correlation between plasma vitamin E and mortality from ischemic heart disease in cross-cultural epidemiology. *Am J Clin Nutr* 1991; 53:326S–334S.

88 Riemersma R A, Wood D A, MacIntyre C C A, Elton R A, Gey K F & Oliver M F. Risk of angina pectoris and plasma concentrations of vitamins A, C and E and carotene. *Lancet* 1991; 337:1–5.

89 Prior I A M, Rose B S, Harvey H P B & Davidson F. Hyperuricaemia, gout and diabetic abnormality in Polynesian people. *Lancet* 1966; i:333–338.

90 Beckles G L A, Miller G J, Alexis S D et al. Obesity in women in an urban Trinidadian community. Prevalence and associated characteristics. *Int J Obes* 1985; 9:127–135.

91 Seftel H C. The rarity of coronary heart disease in South African blacks. *S Afr Med J* 1978; 54:99–105.

92 Reaven G M. role of insulin resistance in human disease. *Diabetes* 1988; 37:1595–1607.

93 Lakka T A & Salonen J T. Physical activity and serum lipids: a cross-sectional population study in Eastern Finnish men. *Am J Epidemiol* 1992; 136:806–818.

94 Robertson T L, Kato H, Gordon T et al. Epidemiologic studies of coronary heart disease and stroke in Japanese men living in Japan, Hawaii and California. *Am J Cardiol* 1977; 39:244–249.

95 Viel B, Donoso S & Salcedo D. Coronary atherosclerosis in persons dying violently. *Arch Intern Med* 1968; 122:97–103.

96 Kean B H. Blood pressure studies on West Indians and Panamanians living on the isthmus of Panama. *Arch Intern Med* 1941; 68:466–475.

97 Miller G J, Beckles G L A, Maude G H et al. Ethnicity and other characteristics predictive of coronary heart disease in a developing community: principal results of the St James Survey, Trinidad. *Int J Epidemiol* 1989; 18:808–817.

98 MacMahon S, Peto R, Cutler J et al. Blood pressure, stroke and coronary heart disease. *Lancet* 1990; 335:765–774, 827–838.

99 Marmot M G & Smith G D. Why are the Japanese living longer? *BMJ* 1989; 299:1547–1551.

100 Marmot M G & Syme S L. Acculturation and coronary heart disease in Japanese Americans. *Am J Epidemiol* 1976; 104:225–247.

101 Marmot M G, Adelstein A M, Robinson N & Rose G A. Changing social class distribution of heart disease. *BMJ* 1978; ii:1109–1112.

102 McKeigue P M, Miller G J & Marmot M G. Coronary heart disease in South Asians overseas: a review. *J Clin Epidemiol* 1989; 42:597–609.

103 McKeigue P M, Shah B & Marmot M G. Relation of central obesity and insulin resistance with high diabetes prevalence and cardiovascular risk in South Asians. *Lancet* 1991; 337:382–386.

104 Chadha S L, Radhakrishnan S, Ramachandran K, Kaul U & Gopinath N. Epidemiological study of coronary heart disease in urban population of Delhi. *Indian J Med Res* 1990; 92:424–430.

105 Marmot M G, Adelstein A M & Bulusu L. *Immigrant Mortality in England and Wales 1970–78*, OPCS Studies of Medical and Population Subjects No. 47. London: HMSO, 1984.

106 Sarvotham S G & Berry J N. Prevalence of coronary heart disease in an urban population in northern India. *Circulation* 1968; 37:939–953.

107 Agarwal B H. A reappraisal of pattern of cardiovascular disorders in India. *J Indian Med Assoc* 1975; 65:125–129.

108 Dewan B D, Malhotra K C & Gupta S P. Epidemiological study of coronary heart disease in a rural community in Haryana. *Indian Heart J* 1974; 26:68–78.

109 Leaverton P E, Feinleib M & Thom T. Coronary heart disease mortality rates in United States blacks, 1968–1978: interstate variation. *Am Heart J* 1984; 108:732–737.

110 Gillum R F. Coronary heart disease in black populations. I. Mortality and morbidity. *Am Heart J* 1982; 104:839–851.

111 Chauvet J, Renambot J, Ehra A et al. Study of 35 cases of myocardial infarction with coronarography and ventriculography in Black Africans in Abidjan. *Trop Cardiol* 1991; 17(supplement 1):21–27.

112 Serme D, Lengani A & Ouandaogo B J. Heart diseases among hospitalized patients in the medical department of the Ouagadougou Hospital. *Trop Cardiol* 1991; 17:24–30.

113 Abengowe C U. Cardiovascular disease in Northern Nigeria. *Trop Geogr Med* 1979; 31:553–560.

114 Idahosa P E. Coronary heart disease in blacks. *Lancet* 1985; i:634.

115 Pole D, Ikeme A C, Pobee J O M, Larbi E, Williams H & Blankson J. The Mamprobi Survey: a screening survey for cardiovascular disease and risk factors in Africa: methodology and validity. *Bull World Health Organ* 1979; 57:81–87.

116 Wyndham C H. Mortality from cardiovascular diseases in the various population groups in the Republic of South Africa. *S Afr Med J* 1979; 56:1023–1030.

117 Walker A R P. The epidemiology of ischaemic heart disease in the different ethnic populations in Johannesburg. *S Afr Med J* 1980; 57:748–752.

118 Walker A R P. Coronary heart disease in blacks: is it increasing? *S Afr Med J* 1981; 60:763–764.

119 Prineas R J, Crow R S & Blackburn H. *The Minnesota Code Manual of Electrocardiographic Findings. Standards and Procedures for Measurement and Classification*. Boston: Wright, 1982.

120 Ashcroft M T, Miller G J, Beadnell H M S G & Swan A V. A comparison of T-wave inversion, S–T elevation and R S amplitudes in precordial leads of Africans and Indians in Guyana. *Am Heart J* 1971; 81:467–475.

121 Miall W E. Myocardial disorders in a Jamaican community. *Postgrad Med J* 1972; 48:770–774.

122 Beaglehole R, Tyroler H A, Cassel J C, Deubner D C, Bartel A & Hames C G. An epidemiological study of left ventricular hypertrophy in the biracial population of Evans County, Georgia. *J Chronic Dis* 1975; 28:554–559.

123 Bartel A, Heyden S, Tyroler H A, Tabesh E, Cassel J C & Hames C G. Electrocardiographic predictors of coronary heart disease. *Arch Intern Med* 1971; 128:929–937.

124 Walker A R P & Walker B F. The bearing of race, sex, age, and nutritional status on the precordial electrocardiograms of young South African Bantu and Caucasian subjects. *Am Heart J* 1969; 77:441–459.

125 Nagulesparan M, Savage P J, Mott D M, Johnson G J, Ungar R H & Bennett P H. Increased insulin resistance in obese, glucose-intolerant Southwestern American Indians. Evidence for a defect not explained by obesity. *J Clin Endocrinol Metab* 1980; 51:739–742.

126 Kumanyika S K & Savage D D. Ischemic heart disease risk factors in American Indians and Alaska Natives. In *Report of the Secretary's Task Force on Black and Minority Health*, vol. IV, part 2.

Washington: US Department of Health and Human Services, 1986: 445–473.

127 Fulmer H S & Roberts R W. Coronary heart disease among the Navajo Indians. *Ann Intern Med* 1963; 59:740–764.

128 Sievers M L. Myocardial infarction among Southwestern American Indians. *Ann Intern Med* 1967; 67:800–807.

129 Sievers M L & Fisher J R. Disease of North American Indians. In Rothschild H R (ed.) *Biocultural Aspects of Disease*. New York: Academic Press, 1981:191–252.

130 Sugarman J R, Gilbert T J, Percy C A & Peter D G. Serum cholesterol concentrations among Navajo Indians. *US Public Health Rep* 1992; 107:92–99.

131 Gillum R F, Gillum B S & Smith N. Cardiovascular risk factors among urban American Indians. Blood pressure, serum lipids, smoking, diabetes, health knowledge and behaviour. *Am Heart J* 1984; 107:756–776.

132 Welty T K. Cholesterol levels among the Sioux. *Indian Health Serv Provider* 1989; 14:35–38.

133 Woo K S & Donnan S P B. Epidemiology of coronary arterial disease in the Chinese. *Int J Cardiol* 1989; 24:83–93.

134 Tao S, Huang Z, Wu X et al. CHD and its risk factors in the People's Republic of China. *Int J Epidemiol* 1989; 18(supplement 1):S159–S163.

135 Hughes K, Yeo P P B, Lun K C et al. Ischaemic heart disease and its risk factors in Singapore in comparison with other countries. *Ann Acad Med Singapore* 1989; 18:245–249.

136 Woo K S. Pathology of fatal acute myocardial infarction in the Chinese. *Aust N Z J Med* 1990; 20:20–25.

137 Schwartzkopff W, Schleicher J, Pottins I, Yu S-B, Han C Z & Du D-Y. Lipids, lipoproteins, apolipoproteins, and other risk factors in Chinese men and women with and without myocardial infarction. *Atherosclerosis* 1990; 82:253–259.

138 Sytkowski P A, Kannel W B & D'Agostino R B. Changes in risk factors and the decline in mortality from cardiovascular disease. The Framingham Heart Study. *N Engl J Med* 1990; 322:1635–1641.

139 Marais A D, Firth J C, Rose A G & Berger G M B. Fatal outcome of homozygous familial hypercholesterolaemia in a black patient. A case report. *S Afr Med J* 1990; 77:588–590.

140 Sepehrnia B, Kamboh M I, Adams-Campbell L L, Nwankwro M & Farrell R E. Genetic studies of human apolipoproteins. VII. Population distribution of polymorphisms of apolipoproteins A-I, A-II, A-IV, C-II, E and H in Nigeria. *Am J Hum Genet* 1988; 43:847–853.

CHAPTER 28

PODOCONIOSIS (NON-FILARIAL ELEPHANTIASIS)

G. C. Cook

Much confusion has existed between elephantiasis caused by the lymphatic filariases (*Wuchereria bancrofti* and *Brugia malayi*) (Chapter 70) and endemic elephantiasis — which is not helminth-related. This latter disease is caused by microparticles of silica and aluminosilicates which enter the lymphatics of the lower limbs through the soles of the feet; it is a disease of rural communities and affects individuals who do not use footwear. The term podoconiosis (Greek: *podos*, of the foot; *konion*, dust) has recently gained acceptance to describe the disease.[1] It is often known locally as 'big foot disease'.

HISTORY

Podoconiosis was probably described by the Latin philosopher Pliny, Augustine of Hippo (now Tunisia) and Isidore of Seville in Spain.[1] It was recognized as a 'specific' disease by the Persian physician Muhammad Ibn Zakariya (El Razi) in the tenth century AD; his original description in Arabic is (or was) housed at the Baghdad Medical School. He considered that 'if the disease is attended to at its onset and treated appropriately it can be cured or stopped and will not increase'; this differentiated it from filarial elephantiasis. Amongst early illustrations which probably depict podoconiosis is one in the thirteenth century *Mappa Mundi* (map of the world) preserved at Hereford Cathedral,[2] a carved oak pew-end in the church at Dennington, Suffolk, and in the sixteenth century *Cosmographia Universalis* of Munster.[1] Realization in the late nineteenth century that most cases of elephantiasis are associated with *W. bancrofti* (and later *B. malayi*) infection[3,4] led to confusion regarding the aetiology of the disease, especially in parts of Africa where this helminthiasis seemed to be absent. In Guatemala there was confusion with lepromatous leprosy.[1]

EPIDEMIOLOGY

In Africa, where most cases of the disease have been described, podoconiosis is most common in highland areas in east and central parts of the continent.[1,5] Here the red clays are related to volcanism in prehistory.[6,7] In West Africa, highland areas are very limited—involving only Cameroon,[8,9] part of Nigeria and the Island of Malabo, Gabon;[10] although *Onchocerca volvulus* is present in some highland areas, *W. bancrofti* is invariably absent. The disease has also been recorded in several volcanic oceanic islands: the Cape Verde Islands, Canary Islands, and Malabo Island (formerly Fernando Po).[10] It has also been recorded in Central America, from Mexico to Colombia and Ecuador. Other descriptions are from Guatemala, Costa Rica, Puerto Rico, Surinam, French Guiana and Brazil. Reports also exist from north-west India[11] and Sri Lanka.

Most affected individuals are from families of barefooted agriculturalists; the disease is less common in pastoral areas.[1] The altitudes, climates and soil composition in areas endemic for podoconiosis have been studied extensively.[12] The soil is invariably volcanic and of red clay, which becomes extremely slippery after rain.[1,11,13] Electron diffraction analysis shows this to consist of alumino-silicate kaolinite, with ultrafine particles of amorphous silica and iron oxides. Thermoluminescence and exoemission studies indicate that the dynamic surface properties of endemic soils are important criteria in cytotoxicity.

In summary, characteristics of an endemic area are:[1] (1) a temperate or near-temperate climate situated within the tropics at an altitude >1500 m;

(2) reddish-brown soil, of which approximately half (by weight) consists of microparticles <10 μm in diameter and one-third <2 μm; (3) microparticles with a predominance of silica in the 2–10 μm portion (silts), and of the aluminosilicate kaolinite in the <2 μm portion (clay); (4) approximately half of the clay portion is <0.4 μm and often 0.1 μm; and (5) the local population is agrarian and walks barefooted.

PATHOGENESIS

Podoconiosis consists of a slowly progressive obstructive lymphopathy caused by particles of optimal size (in suitable soil) having penetrated the soles of the feet; this has been confirmed by analysis of biopsy specimens from the dermis, lymphatic vessels, lymph glands (by elemental analysis of incinerated residues) and by electron microscopic microanalysis of particles in thin tissue sections.[14]

The initial pathogenetic event is, therefore, entry of toxic mineral microparticles into the dermis of the foot; the pathological consequences are dependent on particle size.[15] This takes place to a greater extent in the soft thin skin of young people, and by the age of 10–15 years a sufficient load of toxic material is present in the foot to produce clinical evidence of tissue damage.[1] The lymphatic vessels leading from the dermis become fibrosed and in some cases completely obstructed. Regional lymph node involvement (in the groin) occurs subsequently. These event are followed by fibrotic changes.

PATHOLOGY

Changes result from lymphatic obstruction and fibrosis; the anatomy and physiology of the lower limb lymphatics have been studied extensively. Associated lesions are 'pillowy' oedema, fibrous nodulation, hyperkeratosis, interdigital bacterial and fungal infection, tuberculous adenitis, and other changes consequent upon 'traditional' management.[1]

CLINICAL FEATURES

Podoconiosis commonly begins between the ages of 10 and 19 years—in both sexes—but has been recorded as early as 5 and as late as 60 years.[1] A burning sensation of the sole following a long walk often heralds the disease; it may become worse in bed—at night, after excessive alcohol intake, after prolonged exertion, while standing in front of a fire, and during menstruation. A local swelling of the foot, usually on the dorsum near the first toe cleft, slowly diminishes in size but recurs after further exertion. The lower part of the affected leg is progressively involved over a few months to several years, but the thigh is rarely affected. Although both legs are in fact always affected, the disease develops asymmetrically, so that the swelling of one leg usually increases whilst the other remains constant. Femoral lymphadenitis is common and a cluster of nodes may reach 5 cm in length and weigh 5–6 g. Recurrent acute febrile episodes are a usual, but inconstant feature, and these lead progressively to lymphatic obstruction. The acute episodes may be mistaken for a localized bacterial infection and in consequence an antibiotic prescribed. After a varying period of time, lymphoedema (elephantiasis) becomes firmly established.

In an endemic area, early disease should be suspected in any young person complaining of discomfort in the lower legs and feet, especially in bed at night and after excessive exertion. Price[1] has summarized early signs indicating oedema of the dorsal tissues of the foot and the plantar region: (1) increased skin markings and indentation on pressure; (2) a large second toe; (3) a splayed forefoot; (4) lymph dampness of the forefoot skin; (5) hyperkeratosis ('mossy foot'); (6) 'block toes' (early oedema of the forefoot causes the toes to appear rigid, as if they were wooden and were nailed to the forefoot); (7) plantar oedema; and (8) persistent itching of a lower part of one or other leg.

In a fully developed case, appearances vary from lymphoedema, at one end of a spectrum, to thickened, rough and leathery skin of the foot, i.e. traditional elephantiasis, at the other.[1] In most cases both features are present. In the oedematous form ('water bag' leg) the skin pits on pressure and can be pinched up with the fingers; it is smooth with little hyperkeratotic change. There may be slight oozing of lymph, and skin hairs are usually lost. Secondary infection may supervene. *Streptococcus* spp. lymphangitis may be a complication. In the fibrotic ('leathery' leg) form, the fibrotic dermis may be 3 cm or more in thickness and become fixed to the deep tissues; it does not pit and cannot be pinched up between the fingers. Hyperkeratosis is common and hyperpigmentation is present. Nodulation is common at the base of the toes or in front of the ankle. Inguinal nodes are usually prominent and tender, and abdominal nodes (sometimes tender) may be palpable on abdominal examination. In a small minority of cases, the affected area may extend above the knee(s). Several conditions associated with prolonged lymphatic blockage (including tuberculous adenitis) have been summarized (see above).

MANAGEMENT

Rhazes, writing in the ninth century AD, considered that 'This malady, if it takes hold, is incurable', but he continued 'if it is treated at the beginning it can be stopped with no further advances'.[1] Those observations remain valid today because the pathogenic effect of silica and aluminosilicate penetration into the tissues of the foot causes slowly progressive but irreversible pathological changes. Individuals living in endemic areas have for many centuries recognized an association with the soil, and have also been aware that migration away from an area of high prevalence to one free of the disease arrests its progress, and vice versa. Sections of the community afflicted by this disorder usually originate in the lower strata of society in which financial resources for footwear, etc., are very limited. Underlying principles of management are as follows:[1] (1) the treatment of symptoms caused by early or established disease; (2) reduction to a minimum of any additional load of silica particles in the dermis; and (3) either elevation of a limb and/or elastic stockings may help to assist in reducing the oedema. Obviously, use of footwear prevents further absorption of the responsible mineral particles. The use of matting to cover the bare ground within residential huts should be encouraged; this not only controls the progress of early disease but prevents the mineral load reaching pathogenetic proportions in other (usually younger) members of the family. If possible, a young individual with early signs of the disease should be encouraged to take up residence in a non-endemic area, and may return to the location of high prevalence when footwear is available and is being widely used. A change of occupation, which reduces contact between the bare foot and soil, will clearly be beneficial; home industries such as weaving and dressmaking may be encouraged. Oedema and fibrogenesis are interrelated; prolonged oedema produces fibrosis, and similarly prolonged fibrosis predisposes to oedema. Oedema can be reduced by elevation of the limb or by compression with bandaging or a stocking. A variety of drugs has been used with the object of reversing established fibrosis; in Africa various traditional plant derivatives have been used, but to no avail.

Surgical procedures are unlikely to provide satisfactory results, even when the uptake of mineral microparticles has been arrested. No method is available by which particles can be removed from the dermis, lymphatic tissues of the lower leg and regional lymph nodes. Surgery is indicated in the following situations:[1] (1) excision of 'nodules' on the foot; (2) removal of a femoral node which is subject to repeated attacks of adenitis; and (3) removal of superfluous skin, after the use of compression methods, in the lymphoedematous type of swelling.

PREVENTION

Podoconiosis is certainly a preventable disease; with greater future recognition of its prevalence geographically, exposure to pathogenic particles can be avoided.[1] However, prevention is also heavily dependent on the raising of socioeconomic standards, and provision of footwear, etc.

REFERENCES

1 Price E W. *Podoconiosis: Non-Filarial Elephantiasis*. Oxford: Oxford University Press, 1990: 131.

2 Chancey M. *Mappa Mundi*. Hereford: Hereford Cathedral Publications, 1987.

3 Price E W. The elephantiasis story. *Trop Dis Bull* 1984; 81:R1–R12.

4 Cook G C. *From the Greenwich Hulks to Old St Pancras: A History of Tropical Disease in London*. London: Athlone Press, 1992: 332.

5 Price E W. Endemic elephantiasis of the lower legs in Rwanda and Burundi. *Trop Geogr Med* 1976; 28:283–290.

6 Oomen A P. Studies on elephantiasis of the legs in Ethiopia. *Trop Geogr Med* 1969; 21:236–253.

7 Price E W. Endemic elephantiasis of the lower legs in Ethiopia: an epidemiological survey. *Ethiop Med J* 1974; 12:77–90.

8 Price E W & Henderson W J. Endemic elephantiasis of the lower legs in the United Cameroon Republic. *Trop Geogr Med* 1981; 33:23–29.

9 Price E W, McHardy W J & Pooley F D. Endemic elephantiasis of the lower legs as a health hazard of barefooted agriculturalists in Cameroon, West Africa. *Ann Occup Hyg* 1981; 24:1–8.

10 Corachan M, Tura J W, Campo E, Solely M & Traveria A. Podoconiosis in Aequatorial Guinea: report of two cases from different geological environments. *Trop Geogr Med* 1988; 40:359–364.

11 Kalra N L. Non-filarial elephantiasis in Bikaner, Rajasthan. *J Commun Dis* 1976; 8:337–340.

12 Hirsch A. *Handbook of Geographical and Historical Pathology*. London: New Sydenham Society, 1886; 3:712.

13 Price E W. The association of endemic filariasis of the lower legs in East Africa with soil derived from volcanic rocks. *Trans R Soc Trop Med Hyg* 1976; 70:288–295.

14 Heather C J & Price E W. Non-filarial elephantiasis in Ethiopia: analytical study of inorganic material in lymph nodes. *Trans R Soc Trop Med Hyg* 1972; 66:450–458.

15 Spooner N T & Davies J E. Possible role of soil particles in the aetiology of non-filarial (endemic) elephantiasis: a macrophage cytotoxicity assay. *Trans R Soc Trop Med Hyg* 1986; 80:222–225.

CHAPTER 29

FAMILIAL MEDITERRANEAN FEVER (RECURRENT HEREDITARY POLYSEROSITIS)

G. C. Cook

A clinical syndrome with a probable genetic basis which gives rise to recurrent febrile episodes associated with systemic manifestations, notably abdominal pain, pleurisy and arthropathy, affects members of certain groups with an ethnic origin usually on the Mediterranean littoral or the Middle East.[1] The major importance of this disease is that it forms an important differential diagnosis from other febrile illnesses; in addition, it gives rise to substantial morbidity but not mortality in those affected,.

HISTORY

The first description of a familial condition comprising 'recurring attacks of a peculiar nature' was made by Janeway and Mosenthal[2] in 1908: a 16-year-old Jewish schoolgirl 'without special neurotic inheritance' had suffered febrile bouts associated with abdominal pain, which consisted of prodromal, crescendo and recovery phases, since the age of 2 weeks. Several subsequent reports originated in the USA and were dominated by those from individuals with a Jewish origin.[3–5] More recently, large series of cases have been recorded involving Jewish residents of Israel,[6] Turks,[7] Armenians (most of them in the USA)[8,9] and 'fair-skinned' Arabs.[10] Many names have been applied to the syndrome, including:[1] benign paroxysmal peritonitis, periodic disease, periodic fever, periodic peritonitis, maladie dite périodique, épanalepsie méditerranéenne, familial paroxysmal polyserositis, recurrent polyserositis, paroxysmal peritonitis, familial Mediterranean fever (FMF), familial paroxysmal polyserositis, familial recurrent polyserositis and recurrent hereditary polyserositis. Renal amyloidosis was first demonstrated in this condition by Mamou and Cattan[11] in 1952 (see below). Colchicine was first used successfully in FMF by Goldfinger[12] in 1972, and the first clear evidence that its administration prevents renal amyloid deposition was provided by Zemer and her coworkers[13] in Jerusalem in 1986.

EPIDEMIOLOGY

One estimate is that 2 million people suffer, or have suffered from FMF, although the precise magnitude of the problem worldwide is impossible to ascertain. The major ethnic groups affected are Jews (both Sephardic and Ashkenazi), Arabs, Armenians and Turks. In Sephardic and Iraqi Jews an estimated gene frequency of 1:45 with a prevalence of 1:2000 homozygous individuals has been calculated.[1] Corresponding figures for Armenians in Lebanon are 1:32 and 1:1000. Gene frequencies varying between 1:52 and 0.032, in non-Ashkenazi Jews and Armenians respectively, have been suggested.[9] Sporadic cases (without a clear family history of the disorder) have been recorded from many countries, including the UK, Ireland, France, Germany, Sweden, the former USSR, Japan and India.[1] Occasional reports of a comparable syndrome have recently been made in Maoris. In virtually all of the reported series a significant male predominance has been recorded,[6,10] the mean ratio being of the order of 1.7:1. Most studies have indicated mendelian recessive transmission,[1,9] although a dominant mode of inheritance has been claimed by some. Prevalence rates around 18% have been recorded when both parents are healthy, and 36% when one is affected. If there were full penetrance, the anticipated figures would be 25% and 50%, respectively. In one study, the number of offspring affected was significantly lower than that expected.[14] Incomplete penetrance might be more common in females; late appearance of the syndrome in some children has been suggested as an explanation for this inequality.

AETIOLOGY AND PATHOGENESIS

Table 29.1 summarizes some of the numerous aetiological and pathogenic bases for FMF.[1,4] Many investigators have concentrated on the likelihood of an immunological defect; suppressor T-cell activity and chemotaxis are decreased in the untreated disease, and these abnormalities are corrected after colchicine administration. A C5a-inhibitor deficiency in joint and peritoneal fluids suggests that this defect might be causatively related to the acute inflammatory attacks.[15,16] A genetically determined enzyme defect with recessive mendelian inheritance remains a possibility. Other suggested metabolic abnormalities include: a defect in one of the lipocortin proteins, a defect in the formation and elimination of circulating monohydroxy and dihydroxy fatty acids, and an inherited enzymatic error in catecholamine metabolism. There is no known relationship with a genetic marker; neither an ABO nor HLA association has been recorded. There is a notable absence of descriptions of this syndrome in historical texts involving affected groups (including the Bible and the Koran);[1] this, therefore, leaves the possibility open that a relatively recently introduced environmental factor (possibly dietary) might trigger the onset of the overt clinical syndrome.

Table 29.1 Some suggested aetiological and pathogenic bases for FMF, together with some known precipitating factors.[1]

Possible aetiological factor(s)
Infective agent of unknown identity
'Immune defect'
'Allergen'
Dietary 'allergy'
Angioneurotic oedema
'Autoimmune'
C5a-inhibitor deficiency (joint/peritoneal fluid)
Inborn error of metabolism
Lipocortin-protein defect
Abnormal catecholamine metabolism
Endocrine

Some known precipitating factors
Stress/anxiety
Cold
Physical exercise
Menstruation

PATHOLOGY

FMF is characterized by serosal inflammation and hyperaemic manifestations involving small blood vessels, venules and arterioles;[6] ultrastructural changes in the latter consist of basement membrane thickening, concentric layers being separated by ground substance. Serous membranes exhibit both hyperaemia and an acute inflammatory exudate containing neutrophils, lymphocytes, monocytes, plasma cells and eosinophils. When present, adhesions are thin. Synovia are also affected. When present (see below), dermatological changes consist of mild acanthosis and hyperkeratosis with infiltration by neutrophils, lymphocytes and histiocytes around smaller blood vessels.

CLINICAL FEATURES

Approximately 50% of cases have an onset during the first decade of life; most present by the end of the second, and only about 1% at >40 years.[10] Table 29.2 summarizes the major clinical features of FMF. Vomiting in association with abdominal pain is common, but diarrhoea is unusual. A high percentage of affected individuals have undergone a previous abdominal operation (usually an appendicectomy). Prevalence of symptoms and signs varies in different series, but arthropathy seems to be more severe in Sephardic Jews. Dermatological lesions consist most commonly of erysipelas-like lesions involving the legs, ankles and dorsum of the feet. Schönlein–Henoch purpura, urticaria, bullous lesions and vasculitis have also been recorded. Symptoms are frequently alleviated during pregnancy.[5,8] A classical presentation is as follows:

> A 46-year-old Arab man, who had been born in Jerusalem, was referred to a London hospital on account of irregular bouts (usually at intervals of about 2 months) of abdominal pain since age 18 years. A clinical diagnosis of Crohn's disease had been made and sulphasalazine was prescribed. Fifteen years earlier he had been subjected to appendicectomy on account of abdominal pain. His mother's sister's son had experienced similar attacks. Extensive investigation between attacks proved negative; ESR 18 mm/h. Following initiation of colchicine chemotherapy (see below) he became completely asymptomatic.

Table 29.3 summarizes some less common clinical features of FMF, and Table 29.4 gives some clinical differential diagnoses.[1]

Precise criteria for a clinical diagnosis of FMF are difficult to establish, but the following have been suggested: (1) >4 attacks (24–72 hours duration) of peritonitis and/or pleurisy in the presence of fever, and in many cases, arthropathy also; (2) absence of

Table 29.2 Clinical features of uncomplicated FMF.[1]

Abdominal pain (24–48 h) + pyrexia (38–40°C) + tachycardia
Acute peritonitis (constipation common; diarrhoea unusual)
Pleurisy (+ effusion) (approx 50%)
Arthropathy (large joints; symmetrical; usually non-destructive) (approx 50%)
Dermatological lesions (usually resembling erysipelas) (10–70%)
Immune complex nephropathy

Table 29.3 Some less common clinical features of FMF.[1]

Severe headaches
Pharyngitis
Pericarditis
Myocarditis
Myalgia
Panniculitis
Ophthalmic problems: colloid bodies, episcleritis
Acute orchitis—infertility
Mollaret's meningitis
Childhood growth retardation

Table 29.4 Some clinical differential diagnoses of FMF.[1]

Pyrexia of undetermined origin
Abdominal infection
    Appendicitis
    Cholecystitis
    Perforated peptic ulcer
    Diverticulitis
Relapsing pancreatitis
Acute intermittent porphyria
Pulmonary embolism/atelectasis
Septic arthropathy
Juvenile rheumatoid arthritis
Tuberculous arthritis
Systemic lupus erythematosus
Other causes of amyloidosis

symptoms between attacks; and (3) a lack of known underlying aetiological and/or pathological factors.

Clinically, the most important complication of FMF is amyloid AA formation, the compound being deposited in many tissues, including the kidneys (renal glomerulae),[11,17] spleen, lung, heart, liver and intestine. This complication is significantly more common in Sephardic Jews and Turks;[18] Ashkenazi Jews, Armenians and Arabs are largely 'immune' from this complication. It seems possible that genetic mechanisms (so far undefined) also protect some ethnic groups from amyloid formation.[18] It is however possible, though by no means established, that FMF in Sephardic Jews, Ashkenazi Jews and Armenians results from different (separate) recessive disorders, expressing mutations at different gene loci, but affecting the same metabolic pathway.

INVESTIGATIONS

Acute phase reactants and ESR are elevated during an acute episode. However, this does not distinguish the syndrome from other conditions with an underlying inflammatory basis. The polymorph leucocyte count is elevated, there may be transient haematuria, and abnormalities can occur in both the electrocardiogram and electroencephalogram. Although initially considered to be of value, a metaraminol provocation test[19] and dopamine-β-hydroxylase concentration[20] have not stood the test of time. In affected individuals, rectal/gum biopsy shows amyloid deposition. This can be confirmed in a renal biopsy specimen; however, renal biopsy is not without a complication rate, haemorrhage being a significant possibility in the presence of amyloid deposition.

MANAGEMENT

Numerous therapeutic agents have been used in the management of FMF and these have included: *para*-aminobenzoic acid, chloroquine, corticosteroids, adrenaline, ephedrine, atropine, reserpine, nicotinic acid and tuberculin desensitization. In addition, numerous analgesics, narcotics, antiemetics and non-steroidal anti-inflammatory compounds have been tried, with limited degrees of success. In some studies a low-fat diet has been claimed to be effective, and one low in tyrosine has also been advocated. Successful management dates back to the introduction of colchicine in 1972 (see above).

The mode of action of colchicine is unknown, but 0.5–1.5 mg daily is usually adequate to prevent attacks.[12,21,22] Unfortunately, this agent has been associated with male infertility, but this problem probably does not apply to women. Following the widespread use of colchicine in the prevention of acute episodes, clear evidence later emerged that this form of management also prevents onset of the amyloid nephropathy.[13] Therefore in the high-risk groups it is of paramount importance that regular colchicine administration be continued indefinitely.

PROGNOSIS

This is dependent on the presence or absence of amyloid AA deposition. Those in a low-risk group for this complication (Ashkenazi Jews and Armenians), and others successfully treated with colchicine should have a normal life expectancy.

REFERENCES

1 Cook G C. Recurrent hereditary polyserositis or familial Mediterranean fever: an overview. *Ann Saudi Med* 1991; 11:576–584.

2 Janeway T C & Mosenthal H O. An unusual paroxysmal syndrome, probably allied to recurrent vomiting, with a study of the nitrogen metabolism. *Trans Assoc Am Physicians* 1908; 23:504–518.

3 Alt H L & Barker M H. Fever of unknown origin. *JAMA* 1930; 94:1459–1461.

4 Reimann H A. Periodic disease: periodic fever, periodic abdominalgia, cyclic neutropenia, intermittent arthralgia, angioneurotic edema, anaphylactoid purpura and periodic paralysis. *JAMA* 1949; 141:175–178.

5 Siegal S. Familial paroxysmal polyserositis: analysis of fifty cases. *Am J Med* 1964; 36:893–918.

6 Sohar E, Gafni J, Pras M & Heller H. Familial Mediterranean fever: a survey of 470 cases and review of the literature. *Am J Med* 1967; 43:227–253.

7 Ozedmir A I & Sokmen C. Familial Mediterranean fever among the Turkish people. *Am J Gastroenterol* 1969; 51:311–316.

8 Schwabe A D & Peters R S. Familial Mediterranean

fever in Armenians: analysis of 100 cases. *Medicine (Baltimore)* 1974; 53:453–462.

9 Rogers D B, Shohat M, Petersen G M et al. Familial Mediterranean fever in Armenians: autosomal recessive inheritance with high gene frequency. *Am J Med Genet* 1989; 34:168–172.

10 Barakat M H, Karnik A M, Majeed H W A et al. Familial Mediterranean fever (recurrent hereditary polyserositis) in Arabs: a study of 175 patients and review of the literature. *Q J Med* 1986; 60: 837–847.

11 Mamou H & Cattan R. La maladie périodique (sur 14 cas personnels dont 8 compliqués de néphropathies). *Sem Hôp Paris* 1952; 28:1062–1070.

12 Goldfinger S E. Colchicine for familial Mediterranean fever. *N Engl J Med* 1972; 287:1302.

13 Zemer D, Pras M, Sohar E et al. Colchicine in the prevention and treatment of the amyloidosis of familial Mediterranean fever. *N Engl J Med* 1986; 314:1001–1005.

14 Armenian H K. Genetic and environmental factors in the aetiology of familial paroxysmal polyserositis: an analysis of 150 cases from Lebanon. *Trop Geogr Med* 1982; 34:183–187.

15 Matzner Y & Brzezinski A. C5a-inhibitor deficiency in peritoneal fluids from patients with familial Mediterranean fever. *N Engl J Med* 1984; 311:287–290.

16 Schwabe A D & Lehman T J A. C5a-inhibitor deficiency: a role in familial Mediterranean fever? *N Engl J Med* 1984; 311:325–326.

17 Mamou H. Maladie périodique amylogène. *Sem Hôp Paris* 1955; 31:388–391.

18 Pras M, Bronshpigel N, Zemer D & Gafni J. Variable incidence of amyloidosis in familial Mediterranean fever among different ethnic groups. *Johns Hopkins Med J* 1982; 150:22–26.

19 Barakat M H, El-Khawad A O, Gumaa K A et al. Metaraminol provocative test: a specific diagnostic test for familial Mediterranean fever. *Lancet* 1984; i:656–657.

20 Barakat M H, Gumaa K A, Malhas L N et al. Plasma dopamine beta-hydroxylase: rapid diagnostic test for recurrent hereditary polyserositis. *Lancet* 1988; ii:1280–1283.

21 Dinarello C A, Wolff S M, Goldfinger S E, Dale D C & Alling D W. Colchicine therapy for familial Mediterranean fever: a double-blind trial. *N Engl J Med* 1974; 291:934–937.

22 Zemer D, Revach M, Pras M et al. A controlled trial of colchicine in preventing attacks of familial Mediterranean fever. *N Engl J Med* 1974; 291:932–934.

SECTION 5A
VIRAL INFECTIONS

When the first edition of this text was written (in 1898), the discipline *virology* was as yet unborn; the vast range of tropical 'fevers' (after *Plasmodium* spp. had been excluded) remained without a delineated aetiological agent. Since then, viruses—some commonplace and widely distributed, and others rare and with a localized geographical distribution—have been implicated in a high proportion of febrile illnesses in many tropical countries; although not exhaustive, this section covers many of them.

Dengue accounts for much morbidity, but rarely mortality, in tropical countries, whilst its major clinical manifestation *dengue haemorrhagic fever* is the cause of serious illness and mortality in children—especially in south-east Asia. The cosmopolitan Epstein–Barr virus (EBV) causes an acute illness (infectious mononucleosis) the world over, but its role in the causation of Burkitt's lymphoma and nasopharyngeal carcinoma in several tropical locations is rapidly becoming clearer and is the subject of a great deal of current research. Of the more exotic viruses, some of those causally related to the viral haemorrhagic fevers periodically hit the media headlines—for example, Lassa fever and Ebola disease—an outbreak of which in Zaire in 1995 attracted widespread attention. But there can be no doubt that the 'tropical' virus (most likely derived from a sub-human primate arising in Africa) which has really shaken the world (medicine and politics included) is the human immunodeficiency virus (HIV).

Viral hepatitis accounts for a vast amount of morbidity and mortality in tropical countries. Previous editions of Manson have paid less attention to the pathogens responsible for this group of infections than they clearly warranted; hopefully this deficiency has been rectified in this twentieth edition. The role of gastrointestinal viruses—for example, rotavirus—in tropical paediatrics rapidly becomes clearer. Also, the viruses responsible for respiratory tract disease, and those causing measles and other childhood maladies are gaining their rightful place in 'medicine in the tropics'. A short time ago the mere mention of rabies caused alarm and denoted a death sentence. Research into preventive strategies for this disease has progressed at a remarkable pace, and the spectacular advances surrounding this viral infection are summarized in this section.

It is perhaps of interest that the first human infection to have been swept from the face of the globe—varicella (smallpox)—was caused by a virus. Whilst 'tropical medicine' was, in its formative years dominated by advances in protozoology and helminthology—with virology a distant 'dream'—this might seem surprising. But, it should be recalled that almost two centuries before, Edward Jenner—a Gloucestershire general practitioner—had introduced the appropriate preventive strategy which ultimately dealt a lethal blow (as Jenner envisaged) to this devastating worldwide disease, the last naturally occurring case of which arose in October 1977.

CHAPTER 30

ARBOVIRUS INFECTIONS

D. I. H. Simpson

Most diseases caused by arboviruses (*ar*thropod-*bo*rne *viruses*) are zoonoses; that is, they are primarily infections of vertebrates other than man, and of the arthropod vectors, and can be transmitted to man. Two apparent exceptions are o'nyong-nyong fever (ONN) and dengue (DEN), of which the only known vertebrate host is man, although a monkey host has been suggested for dengue in rural settings. These viruses are usually spread by the bites of arthropods, but some can also be transmitted by other means (through milk, excreta or aerosols). The arbovirus infections 'are maintained in nature principally, or to an important extent, through biological transmission between susceptible vertebrate hosts by blood-sucking insects; they multiply to produce viraemia in the vertebrates, multiply in the tissues of the insects and are passed on to new vertebrates by the bites of insects after a period of extrinsic incubation'.[1] In the same publication, however, Chumakov prefers the following definition: 'Arboviruses are zoonotic viral agents which, when circulating in the natural foci of infection, are transmitted in a more or less regular manner by arthropods, but in certain circumstances may be transmitted in other ways than by arthropods.'

Smith[2] suggests that the safest definition is that arboviruses are 'potential zoonotic viruses which cannot be otherwise classified'.

The names by which these viruses are known are of mixed origin. Some are dialect names for the illnesses they cause (chikungunya, o'nyong-nyong), some are place names (West Nile, Bwamba) and some derive from clinical characteristics (Western equine encephalitis, yellow fever).

AETIOLOGY

Most arboviruses are spherical, measuring 17–150 nm or more, a few are rod-shaped, measuring 70 × 200 nm.[1] All are RNA viruses. Many circulate in a natural environment and do not infect man. Some infect man only occasionally or cause only a mild illness; others are of great clinical importance,

causing large epidemics and many deaths. The arboviruses of clinical importance belong to the Togaviridae, the alphaviruses, flaviviruses, the Bunyaviridae, nairoviruses, phleboviruses and other subgroups (Table 30.1).

Alphaviruses are all transmitted by mosquitoes in nature, but in experimental work the range of mosquito species capable of transmission is larger than the known range of vectors in nature. Flaviviruses are transmitted by mosquitoes and ticks and many have been isolated worldwide from the salivary glands of bats, but only one has caused a laboratory infection in man. Some phleboviruses are transmitted by sandflies and mosquitoes.

EPIDEMIOLOGY

VERTEBRATE HOSTS

The vertebrate hosts have been differentiated as maintenance, incidental, link and amplifier hosts.

Maintenance hosts

These 'are essential for the continued existence of the virus'.[3] They usually live in symbiosis with the viruses, without causing actual disease, but they develop antibody.

The maintenance hosts provisionally recognized include the following, though some have only been incriminated experimentally[4] (see footnote for list of abbreviations).

Abbreviations: EEE, Eastern equine encephalitis; WEE, Western equine encephalitis; VEE, Venezuelan equine encephalitis; SLE, St Louis encephalitis; JE, Japanese encephalitis; MVE, Murray Valley encephalitis; TBE, tick-borne encephalitis; RSSE, Russian spring–summer encephalitis; KFD, Kyasanur Forest disease; LGT, Langat virus; JUN, Junin virus; MAC, Machupo virus; LI, louping ill; POW, Powassan virus; YF, yellow fever; DEN, dengue fever; CE, California encephalitis; TAH, Tahyna virus; RB, Rio Bravo virus; CTF, Colorado tick fever; ONN, o'nyong-nyong virus.

Table 30.1 Arboviruses.

Virus	Geographical distribution	Transmission	Fever	Clinical form	Rash
TOGAVIRIDAE					
Alphaviruses					
*Chikungunya (CHIK)	Africa, India, South-East Asia	Mosquito	+	H	+
*Mayaro (Uruma)(MAY)	South America	Mosquito	+		+
*O'nyong-nyong (ONN)	Africa	Mosquito	+		+
*Ross River (RR)	Australia, South Pacific	Mosquito	+	Arthritis	+
*Sindbis (SIN)	Africa, Saudi Arabia, India, South-East Asia, Australia, Sweden	Mosquito	+		+ (Africa only)
Mucambo (MUC)	Brazil	Mosquito	+		
Semliki Forest (SF)	South Africa, East Africa	Mosquito	+		
Ockelbo	Sweden	Mosquito	+		+
*Eastern equine encephalitis (EEE)	North America	Mosquito	+	E	
*Western equine encephalitis (WEE)	North and South America	Mosquito	+	E	
*Venezuelan equine encephalitis (VEE)	North and South America	Mosquito	+	E	
Flaviviruses					
Mosquito-borne					
*Dengue-type 1 (DEN1)	Africa, Pacific, Far East, Caribbean	Mosquito	+	H	+
*Dengue-type 2 (DEN2)	Far East, Trinidad, Belize	Mosquito	+	H	+
*Dengue-type 3 (DEN3)	Philippines, India	Mosquito	+	H	+
*Dengue-type 4 (DEN4)	Philippines	Mosquito	+	H	+
Ilhéus (ILH)	South and Central America	Mosquito	+	E	
*Japanese encephalitis (JE)	Japan, Far East	Mosquito	+	E	
Banzi (BAN)	Africa	Mosquito	+		
Bussuquarra (BSQ)	South America	Mosquito	+		
*Murray River encephalitis (MVE)	Australia, New Guinea	Mosquito	+	E	+
*West Nile (WN)	Africa, India, Europe	Mosquito	+	E	+
Kunjin (KUN)	Australia, Sarawak	Mosquito	+		+
*St Louis encephalitis (SLE)	Americas	Mosquito	+	E	
Wesselsbron (WSL)	South Africa	Mosquito	+		+
*Yellow fever	Africa, South and Central America	Mosquito	+	H	
Zika (ZIKA)	Africa, South-East Asia	Mosquito	+	Lab	+
Spondweni (SPO)	South Africa	Mosquito	+		
Sepik (SE)	Australia	Mosquito	+		
*Rocio (ROC)	Brazil	Mosquito	+	E	
Tick-borne					
*Kyasanur Forest disease (KFD)	India	Ixodid tick	+	H	+
Kumlinge (KUM)	Finland	Tick	+	E	+
Langat (LAN)	Malaysia	Ixodid tick	+	E	
Louping ill	Britain	Ixodid tick	+	E	
*Omsk haemorrhagic fever (OHF)	Former USSR	Ixodid tick	+	H	+
*Powassan (POW)	Canada, USA	Ixodid tick	+	E	
*Tick-borne encephalitis (TBE)					
Far Eastern (Russian spring–summer encephalitis (RSSE)	Former USSR, Asia	Ixodid tick	+	E	
Central European	Europe and Scandinavia	Ixodid tick	+	E	
Negishi (NEG)	Japan	? Tick	+	E	
Other vectors					
Rio Bravo (RB)	USA, Trinidad	? Bat saliva	+	E, meningitis	

Table 30.1 Arboviruses (Continued).

Virus	Geographical distribution	Transmission	Fever	Clinical form	Rash
BUNYAVIRIDAE					
Bunyamwera group					
Bunyamwera (BUN)	Africa	Mosquito	+		
Calovo (CUO)	Europe	Mosquito	+		
Germiston (GER)	Africa	Mosquito	+		
Guaroa (GRO)	South and Central America	Mosquito	+		
Ilesha	Africa	Mosquito	+		
Tensaw	North America	Mosquito	+	E	
Wyeomyia	Central and South America	Mosquito	+		
Maguari	South America	Mosquito	+		
Bwamba group					
Bwamba (BWA)	Africa	Mosquito	+		
C Group					
Apeu (APEU)	South America	Mosquito	+		
Caraparu (CAR)	South America	Mosquito	+		
Itaqui (ITQ)	South America	Mosquito	+		
Marituba (MTB)	South America	Mosquito	+		
Murutuca (MUR)	South America	Mosquito	+		
Madrid (MAD)	Panama	Mosquito	+		
Oriboca (ORI)	South America	Mosquito	+		
Ossa (OSSA)	Panama	Mosquito	+		
Restan (RES)	Trinidad	Mosquito	+		
Nepuyo (NEP)	Central America	Mosquito	+		
Tataguine (TAT)	Nigeria	Mosquito	+		
California group					
*California encephalitis (CE)	USA, Canada	Mosquito	+	E	
Inkoo	Finland	Mosquito	+	Meningism	
*La Crosse (LAC)	USA, Canada	Mosquito	+	E	
*Tahyna (Lumbo) (TAH)	Europe, Africa	Mosquito	+		
Trivattatus	USA	Mosquito	+		
Simbu group					
*Oropouche (ORO)	South America	Mosquito	+	E	
Shuni	Africa	Mosquito	+		
Guama group					
Guama (GMA)	South America	Mosquito	+		
Catu (CATU)	South America	Mosquito	+		
Other Bunyaviridae					
Bhanja	India, southern Europe	Tick	+		
Thogoto (THO)	Africa, Mediterranean	Tick	+	E	
Nairoviruses					
Crimean–Congo group					
*Crimean–Congo haemorrhagic fever (C–CHF)	Europe, Africa, Middle East, central Asia, Pakistan	Ixodid tick	+	H	+
Hazara	Pakistan	Ixodid tick		H	
Nairobi sheep disease group					
Dugbe	Africa	Ixodid tick	+		
Ganjam	Africa, India	Ixodid tick	+		
Nairobi sheep disease	Africa, India	Ixodid tick	÷		
Phleboviruses					
*Phlebotomus fever (sandfly fever) Neapolitan (SFN) Sicilian (SFS)	Africa, Asia	Phlebotomine sandflies	+		
*Rift Valley fever (RVF) (Zinga)	Africa	Mosquito	+	H	
Candiru (CDU)	Brazil	?	+		
Chagres (CHG)	Panama	*Phlebotomus*	+		

Table 30.1 Arboviruses (Continued).

Virus	Geographical distribution	Transmission	Fever	Clinical form	Rash
Uukuviruses					
Uukuniemi	Finland, Norway, Eastern Europe	Tick	+		
*Hantaan virus, Puumala virus (murine virus nephropathy, MVN). Haemorrhagic fever with renal syndrome (HFRS)	China, Korea, European Russia, Scandinavia, Balkans, Europe	Contamination from rodent urine or rodent bite	+	H	
ORBIVIRIDAE					
Changuinola group					
Changuinola	Central America	*Phlebotomus*	+		
Kemerovo group					
Kemerovo (KEM)	Europe	Tick	+		
Tribec	Europe	Tick	+		
*Coltivirus					
Colorado tick fever (CTF)	North America	Tick	+	HE (in children)	+
Ungrouped					
Orungo (ORU)	Central Africa and Cameroon	Mosquito	+		
RHABDOVIRIDAE					
Vesicular stomatitis group					
Vesicular stomatitis (Indiana and New Jersey)	North and Central America	*Phlebotomus*	+		
Chandipura	India, Africa	Mosquito	+		
Piry	South America	Mosquito	+		

H, haemorrhagic; E, encephalitis.
* Of clinical importance.
For a complete list of mosquito vectors and the arboviruses they transmit (Appendix IV).

Birds
Prairie chicken, red-winged blackbird, blue jay, pheasant, pigeon, cardinal, sparrow, wren, grackle, wood thrush, catbird (EEE, WEE, SLE), heron, egret (JE). Migrating birds can carry viruses over long distances (MVE, EEE, WEE, SLE).

Hantaviruses
Hantaan virus, Pumala virus, Seoul virus, Prospect Hill virus (murine virus arthropathy, haemorrhagic fever with renal syndrome (HFRF), nephropothica epidemica, hantavirus pulmonary syndrome.

Rodents and insectivores (VEE, KFD, LGT, JUN, MAC)
Vole, shrew, rat, *Arvicanthis*, field mouse, hedgehog, squirrel, lemming, chipmunk (European TBE, RSSE, LI), groundhog (POW), deer mouse, porcupine (CTF), sloth, small marsupials, voles, deer, mice, rats.

Primates
Monkey (YF, ?DEN).

Leporidae
Rabbit, hare (CE, ?TAH).

Ungulates (cattle, deer)
(?European TBE, LI).

Bats
(?RB).

Marsupials, reptiles and amphibia
Kangaroo, snake (?EEE, WEE), lizard, alligator, turtle (?EEE).

Incidental hosts

These become infected, but transmission from them does not occur with sufficient regularity for stable maintenance. Man is usually an incidental host, often, but not always being a dead end in the chain. Incidental hosts may or may not show symptoms. They may be necessary for the maintenance of transmission as they are the main hosts of ticks, keeping these arthropods alive in sufficient numbers to be effective carriers.

Link hosts

These bridge a gap between maintenance hosts and man (e.g. between small mammals and man by goats (via milk) in tick-borne encephalitis, and between wild birds and man by sparrows in SLE).

Amplifier hosts

These increase the weight of infection to which man is exposed, for instance pigs, which act between wild birds (especially herons) and man in JE. Dogs may also be involved.

The mode of transmission between maintenance hosts may differ from that responsible for infection of incidental hosts, including man.

The populations and characters of the vertebrate hosts and their threshold levels of viraemia are important. Small rodents multiply rapidly and have short lives, thus providing a constant supply of susceptible individuals, especially to the tick-borne viruses. On the other hand, monkeys and pigs multiply slowly, and once they have recovered from an infection with YF and JE respectively, they remain immune for life. Immunity also affects pigs in the early months of life, having been transmitted via the placenta from immune mothers, and this no doubt is a feature in other animals. African monkeys are relatively resistant to YF, but Asian and American monkeys are susceptible, probably because, unlike the African monkeys, they have not been exposed continuously for centuries to the infection. It is also possible that infection with other related arboviruses may partly immunize African monkeys (and man) against YF.

So far as is known, the only vertebrate host of ONN is man and the conditions for the spread of this infection seem to depend on the human populations involved, and the multiplicity of vector mosquitoes. In urban conditions, with a concentrated human population and prolific breeding of *Aedes aegypti*, the cycle of yellow fever and dengue is also usually man–mosquito–man.

INVERTEBRATE HOSTS

These include mosquitoes, sandflies and ticks and also *Culicoides* (involved in some animal viruses).

After these vectors have imbibed virus from a vertebrate in a state of viraemia, the virus undergoes an incubation period within the arthropod, known as the extrinsic incubation period. In mosquitoes this period is short: 10 days at 30°C ambient temperature and longer at lower temperatures. Mosquitoes remain infective for life without any apparent ill-effects. Their infectivity appears to increase with time after infection and their effectiveness as transmitters depends upon the frequency with which they bite.

It is also possible that arthropods, whose mouth parts are contaminated by virus in the act of feeding, could transmit the virus mechanically if they feed on another animal. For instance, chikungunya virus can be transmitted mechanically by *Ae. aegypti* for 8 hours after infection.

Most arboviruses have been recovered from mosquitoes and a list of the vectors is given in Table 30.1 (p. 616) and Appendix IV.

Ixodid ticks are involved in a closely interrelated subgroup of group B arboviruses and also in some of the other groups. Genera of ticks involved include *Haemaphysalis*, *Ixodes* and *Dermacentor* (see also Appendix IV).

In general, mosquitoes are refractory to tick-borne viruses and ticks to mosquito-borne viruses but there may be exceptions in some conditions.[1]

TRANSMISSION

Transmissions by arthropods involves several processes:

- Ingestion by the arthropods of virus in the blood (usually) or tissue fluids of the vertebrate hosts.
- Penetration of the viruses into the tissue of the arthropods, in the gut wall, or elsewhere after passing through the gut wall ('gut barrier').
- Multiplication of the viruses in the arthropod cells, including those of the salivary glands.[1]

Stage 2 and part of stage 3 represent the extrinsic incubation period of the disease.

The quantity of blood, and therefore the amount of virus ingested, seems to be important; each arthropod species must ingest a minimum quantity of a given virus before multiplication can take place. The same mosquito species can have two different thresholds for two different viruses and if one species has a low threshold, other species may have high thresholds or be completely resistant. This threshold phenomenon is extremely important in determining the efficiency of a vector and may also vitally affect the course of an epidemic.

The viruses persist in ixodid ticks for months or years and in mosquitoes for practically their whole lives, though there may be a gradual decrease of concentration of the virus with time. Viruses have been reported to persist in overwintering mosquitoes and this could be important, for instance in *Culex tritaeniorhynchus* infected with JE, and *C. tarsalis* infected with WEE (infective by bite up to 8 months).

Trans-stadial persistence of virus is normal in ticks and transovarial passage has been observed in some species; both are of great epidemiological importance. Transovarial passage in mosquitoes does not occur although evidence for transovarial passage of YF virus in *Ae. furcifer-taylori* has been given. Arthropods do not appear to be harmed by these infections.

IMPORTANT FACTORS IN TRANSMISSION BY ARTHROPODS

- Susceptibility of the arthropods to infection and ability to transmit it. There is wide variation in this.
- Breeding habits of the arthropods and preferred habitats, whether near man and other hosts of the virus.
- Biting habits of the arthropods; in mosquitoes whether they are anthropophilic or zoophilic, exophilic or endophilic.
- Longevity of the arthropods, which depends to a great extent on temperature, humidity and (especially in ticks) the availability of hosts to feed on. Overwintering mosquitoes can carry virus from one year to the next—*C. tarsalis* can carry WEE for 8 months.
- Abundance of the arthropods; for mosquitoes the availability of suitable breeding places (and therefore the rainfall) is a major factor. An efficient vector may have a wide range of animals on which to feed, but if the arthropod species is abundant, and even if it bites man only infrequently in the presence of other (and preferred) animals, the large numbers enable it to maintain transmission to man. For instance, *C. tritaeniorhynchus*, which mostly bites birds, Bovidae, dogs and especially porcines, and only to a limited extent man, can maintain transmission of JE from pigs to man by sheer numbers. *C. tarsalis* feeds indiscriminately on mammals in summer, when WEE and SLE tend to occur in man and horses, but at other times it feeds on birds which carry the virus.
- Migratory birds can help by spreading virus which is circulating in their blood or by carrying infected ticks.
- Ecological systems are of primary importance in

transmission and biocenosis determines the formation of natural foci of infection. A case in point is the circulation of YF virus among forest monkeys and tree-living mosquitoes, occasionally reaching mosquitoes haunting banana plantations raided by the monkeys, and thence reaching man and perhaps spreading from man to man by peridomestic mosquitoes. Similarly, man becomes infected with KFD when he enters the domain of infected monkeys and picks up infected ticks. Other mosquito-borne and tick-borne infections are variations on the same theme.

The mosquito-borne and tick-borne infections differ in that ticks attach themselves to vertebrates for relatively long periods and can therefore overlap a viraemic phase. In the case of KFD the populations of ticks are maintained at high levels by domestic cattle, on which they feed, and the cattle are close enough to the sources of viraemia (monkeys, and possibly birds and small rodents) to maintain enough ticks to carry on the cycle in animals. Man is an intruder and though he becomes infected he is not a link in the chain. The subject is discussed in more detail in the section on KFD, p. 643.

Transmission may be represented diagrammatically, as in Figure 30.1.

OTHER FACTORS IN TRANSMISSION

Although transmission of arboviruses usually takes place through the bites of arthropods, it is important to remember that some of the viruses can, exceptionally, be transmitted in other ways. European TBE can be acquired by drinking the milk of infected goats, Junin and Lassa viruses through contact with excreta of infective rodents, VEE (in cotton rats) apparently via urine or faeces infecting the nasopharynx, WEE possibly through aerosol from a patient and EEE (in pheasants) by one bird pecking another. Laboratory infections have been reported with Kunjin virus in Australia, and others. Muroid virus nephropathy can be transmitted by aerosol from infected rodents. CTF virus is reported to have been transmitted by blood transfusion.

Many human activities encourage transmission of these animal viruses to man. Irrigation often promotes the breeding of enormous numbers of mosquitoes. For instance, the development of rice fields encourages *C. tritaeniorhynchus* in Sarawak, spreading JE, and *Mansonia uniformis* and *Anopheles gambiae* in Kenya spreading chikungunya, ONN, possibly West Nile and Sindbis, and malaria. The seasonal cutting of old vegetation in Sarawak

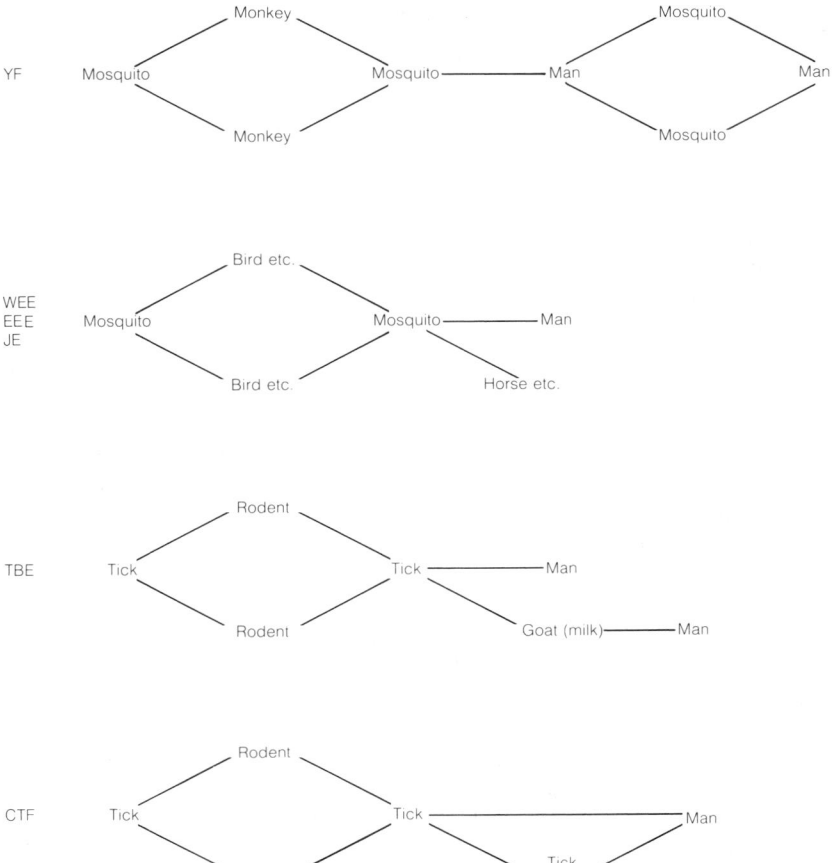

Figure 30.1 Transmission of some arboviruses.
For abbreviations, see p. 615.

produces heavily polluted pools which support massive populations of culicines. The keeping of cattle driven into marginal forest areas in India, promotes the growth and transport of ticks and the intrusion of man into forest areas lays him open to infection with yellow fever and the tick-borne diseases.

For a fuller discussion of these points the paper on epidemiology by Smith et al[5] should be consulted.

IMMUNITY

After a vertebrate has been infected by an arbovirus the virus probably multiplies first in the regional lymph glands where the earliest formation of antibodies also probably takes place. The antibodies are immunofluorescent (IFA), haemagglutination-inhibiting (HI), complement fixing (CF) and neutralizing (N). In general HI antibodies appear early and may be long lasting; CF antibodies appear later and may last 2–5 years; and N antibodies appear early and are long lasting. But there are differences; some arboviruses do not produce high titres of antibodies in man and some antibodies are short-lived or appear late.

Of these antibodies, HI and CF are important in diagnosis, but the only protective antibody is N, which is also the most specific antibody.

Arboviruses are grouped according to antigenic characters, but after inoculation of one virus into a fresh animal, not only the homologous antibodies, but also heterologous antibodies reacting with other viruses of the same group tend to appear. Recovery from an infection by a member of one group of arboviruses may provide some degree of resistance to a subsequent infection by another member of the same group; for instance, infection with West Nile virus may have modified the Ethiopian epidemic of YF in 1962.[6] Again, the effect of prior infection with Zika, Uganda S and other related viruses in the forest belt of Nigeria, leading to a high incidence of related antibodies, is suggested as the explanation of the absence of epidemic YF in man in that area. These related infections probably modify the disease rather than prevent infection.[7]

ACTIVE IMMUNITY IN GENERAL

A person who recovers from an attack of YF possesses a solid immunity against reinfection. Neutralizing antibodies can be found as early as a few days after the beginning of the disease and are found constantly for many years in the sera of such persons. This persistence of immunity does not depend upon exogenous reinfection and the mechanism by which the antibodies are produced is not clear. It has been commented[8] that a mosquito infected with YF is not harmed by it, but continues to excrete the virus throughout life. This means a continuous release of virus, probably from epithelial cells of the salivary glands. The virus enters man (or other animals) and gains the liver and other epithelium, provoking the early antibodies in the blood, which neutralize circulating viruses. But antibodies which can be detected for so many years in man must stem from a continuing stimulus, and the sensitive cells and their progeny probably have a prophase equivalent of the virus incorporated into their genetic structure, with occasional reversion to productive development which provides the stimulus for further antibody formation. The solid and fundamental immunity probably lies at the genetic level. A degree of immunity of this kind may possibly be provided when a related virus invades epithelial cells.

Epidemics of MVE, JE and West Nile are not reported in the endemic areas of dengue, possibly because of cross-protection. There seems to be an analogy with the protective effect in schistosomiasis of infection with heterologous schistosomes.

The immunology of arbovirus infections is in line with the immunological principles of virus infections in general.

PASSIVE IMMUNITY IN GENERAL

Infant rhesus monkeys and human infants born of mothers immune to YF have protective antibodies in their sera at birth which persist for several months. These immune bodies are probably transmitted by the placenta rather than in the mothers' milk, because antibodies may disappear from infant sera while they are still suckling. This passive immunity is transient. Passive immunity induced by injection of homologous immune serum, however, has been used for protection against TBE in circumstances of special risk and similar sera could be used against other infections, particularly after laboratory accidents.

CLINICAL FEATURES IN GENERAL

After the virus enters the body it reaches the lymphatic system where it multiples and from which it is released into the blood (viraemic phase) and thence to the organs affected.

Most arbovirus infections are inapparent (producing no symptoms) or mild (producing some fever and occasionally a rash), diagnosable retrospectively by serological methods. For instance, in an epidemic of JE it was estimated that for each case of apparent disease there were 500–1000 inapparent infections. The proportions no doubt vary with circumstances.

If clinical manifestations arise after infection they do so after an intrinsic incubation period lasting from a few days to a week or more. Some arboviruses damage the endothelial lining of the capillaries, increasing permeability, which allows the virus to pass the blood–brain barrier, causing meningoencephalitis (encephalitides). Others damage the parenchymatous organs by direct damage to the cells in which they are situated, while with others damage is caused by the immune system of the host from the formation of antigen–antibody complexes and disordered complement formation which damage the renal tubules and alter the coagulation and fibrinolytic systems of the body, causing haemorrhage (viral haemorrhagic fevers). There is a general pattern of biphasic illness, the first phase associated with viraemia, ending when antibodies appear in the blood, and the second phase when the virus is located in organs, such as the liver or brain.

The onset of clinical manifestations is nearly always abrupt, generally occurring after the onset of viraemia. *Fever* is usual and is sometimes the only sign. In many cases the clinical manifestations last only while the virus is disseminated, recovery following without sequelae, but in other cases there is *remission*, short or long. If long, the disease is biphasic. After this *fever returns*, with signs indicating localization of the virus in certain organs: albuminuria, jaundice, meningeal signs, encephalitis and myelitis. If the period of viraemia has been without symptoms and the virus becomes localized in the central nervous system, encephalitis appears late and may seem to be primary. In haemorrhagic cases there is a special risk of shock, which can rapidly become irreversible unless treated promptly.

All degrees of involvement may be observed in a single epidemic, but some arboviruses cause generally mild disease, others tend to severity.

The syndromes may be grouped as follows:

1 Systemic febrile disease (see Table 30.2; p. 623)
2 Viral haemorrhagic fever (VHF) (see Table 30.3; p. 628)
3 Encephalitides (see Table 30.4; p. 655).

SYSTEMIC FEBRILE ILLNESSES

This is the largest group and the mild forms of all arbovirus diseases are of this kind (Table 30.2). The course may be biphasic and the infection may go on to the more serious haemorrhagic or encephalitic forms.

In addition to fever, which may suggest influenza, the following symptoms may occur:

- *Anorexia,* with nausea and vomiting (phlebotomus fevers), or respiratory symptoms may predominate (Tahyna).
- A *rash*, erythematous or itchy maculopapular, with congestion of the face and neck (phlebotomus), inflammation of the palate, vesicles on the feet (Sindbis), or even petechiae of more extensive haemorrhages.
- *Conjunctivitis*, with photophobia and orbital pain (phlebotomus) or even central retinitis and chorioretinitis (Rift Valley).
- *Epidemic polyarthritis* (Ross River in Australia).
- *Arthralgia* (o'nyong-nyong, chikungunya) or myalgia (especially in dengue), which can be responsible for excruciating pain, sometimes so severe as to render the patient incapable of movement ('break-bone fever'); lumbar pain is also common (phlebotomus).
- *Inflammation* and enlargement of the lymphatic glands (o'nyong-nyong, chikungunya, West Nile).
- *Leucopenia*, which is common, and thrombocytopenia (Colorado).

Table 30.2 Systemic febrile diseases.

Chikungunya	Tahyna
O'nyong-nyong	Oropouche
Ross River fever	Rocio virus
Mayaro	Sandfly fever
Sindbis	

DIAGNOSIS

VIROLOGICAL DIAGNOSIS

Blood should be taken as soon as possible after the onset of the disease, part being reserved for isolation of the virus (only useful in the first few days), and part for serological tests. Suckling mice, hamsters, guinea-pigs and tissue culture techniques are used for isolation of the virus.

If there are meningeal signs the cerebrospinal fluid (CSF) may be used for isolation and is occasionally positive in TBE, CTF, JE, WEE, SLE and YF. Cells may be sedimented and examined by the fluorescent antibody technique.

After death, specimens of tissue should be taken as soon as possible, emulsified and quickly inoculated into suckling mice 1–3 days old, or adult mice, newborn hamsters, chick embryos or even guinea-pigs (Junin virus). The material to be inoculated is usually treated with antibiotics, and part is kept frozen for confirmation by reisolation of the virus.

SEROLOGICAL DIAGNOSIS

After infection the virus probably first multiplies in the regional lymph glands, where the earliest antibody formation also probably starts. Serological diagnosis is based on the detection of IFA, HI, CF and N antibodies and on the variations in titre found in paired sera at various stages. IFA and HI antibodies are cross-reactive within the arbovirus groups, and may need confirmation by tests for N antibodies. CF antibodies are separate and distinct from N antibodies. N antibodies are usually the most specific.

If the patient has been exposed to an arbovirus of the same group as the one responsible for the illness, serological diagnosis is difficult because group antibodies are at high titre—even to some extent the N antibodies.

The gel precipitin test has been used successfully with antigens produced in cell cultures, for tests on paired sera. It has also been used to differentiate various viruses, though consistently satisfactory antisera for this purpose may be difficult to obtain.

The fluorescent antibody test has been used as a reliable test for antigen in acute-phase blood clots in CTE and on postmortem material, for instance in JE.

Some of the reagents—antigens and immune fluids—used for tests are described in a World Health Organization publication.[1]

CHIKUNGUNYA (CHIK)

GEOGRAPHICAL DISTRIBUTION

Antibody studies have shown that this virus is widespread in Africa and is also present in Saudi Arabia, Borneo, Malaysia and the Philippines, and clinical outbreaks have occurred in many parts of Africa as

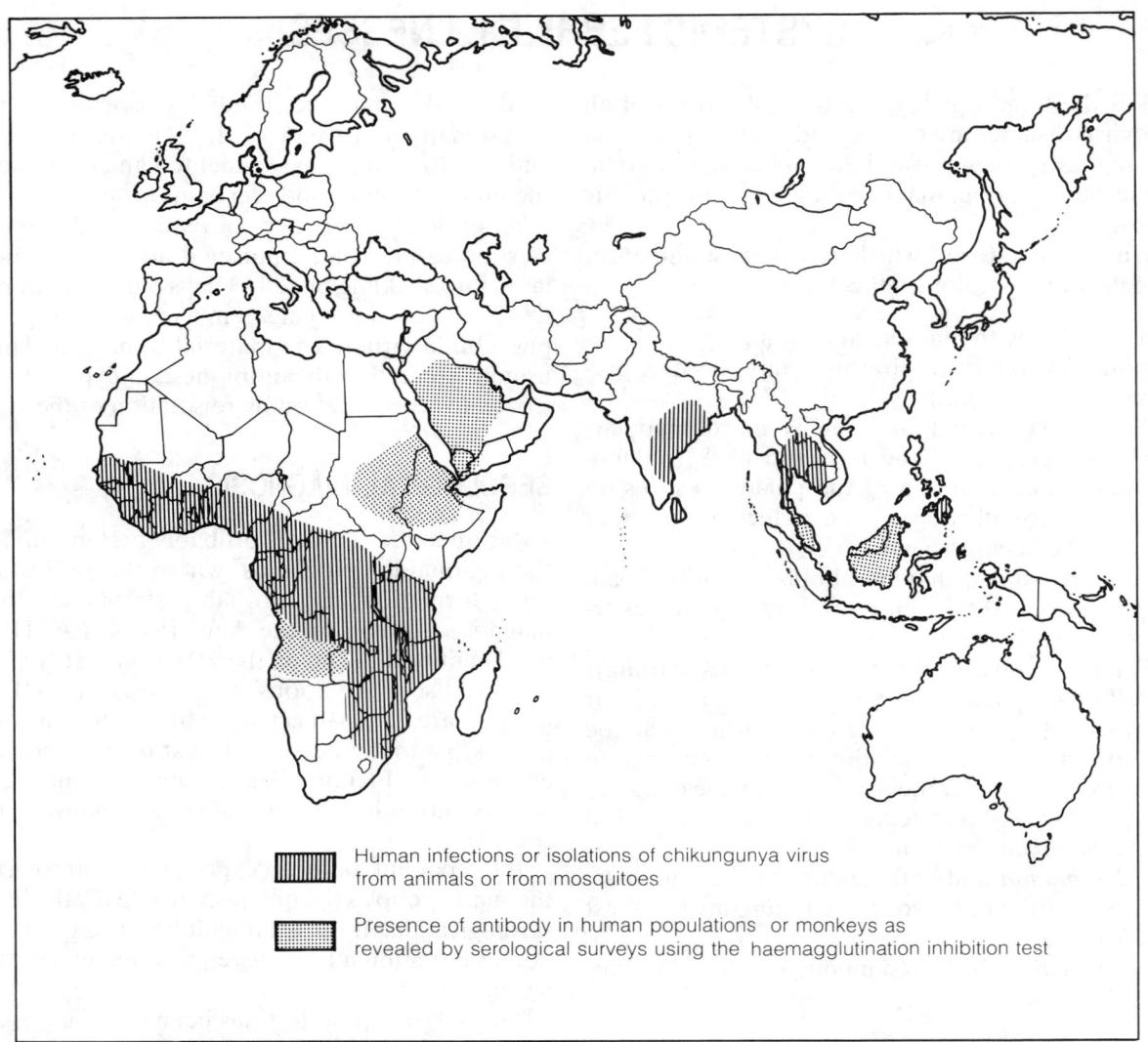

Figure 30.2 Geographical distribution of chikungunya virus (courtesy of the Department of Entomology, London School of Hygiene and Tropical Medicine).

well as Thailand, Cambodia, Burma, Sri Lanka and India (Calcutta, Madras, Vellore) (Figure 30.2).

AETIOLOGY

Chikungunya virus is an alphavirus closely related to o'nyong-nyong.

TRANSMISSION

In Africa the main vector to man is *Ae. aegypti* but a forest cycle is maintained by *Ae. africanus* and several species of *Mansonia*. In Asia the main vectors are *C. fatigans* (*quinquefasciatus*), *C. tritaeniorhynchus* and *C. gelidus* (see Table 30.1 (p. 616) and Appendix IV).

PATHOLOGY

The pathology is not known but is probably the same as dengue.

SYMPTOMS AND SIGNS

Natural history

Chikungunya is an acute self-limiting febrile disease with a forest and human cycle and no haemorrhagic or central nervous system complications (although in Thailand it has been associated with haemorrhagic dengue).

The *incubation period* is 2–4 days. The disease is biphasic. Onset is abrupt with severe pain in the joints and the patient prostrated. After 1–4 days the

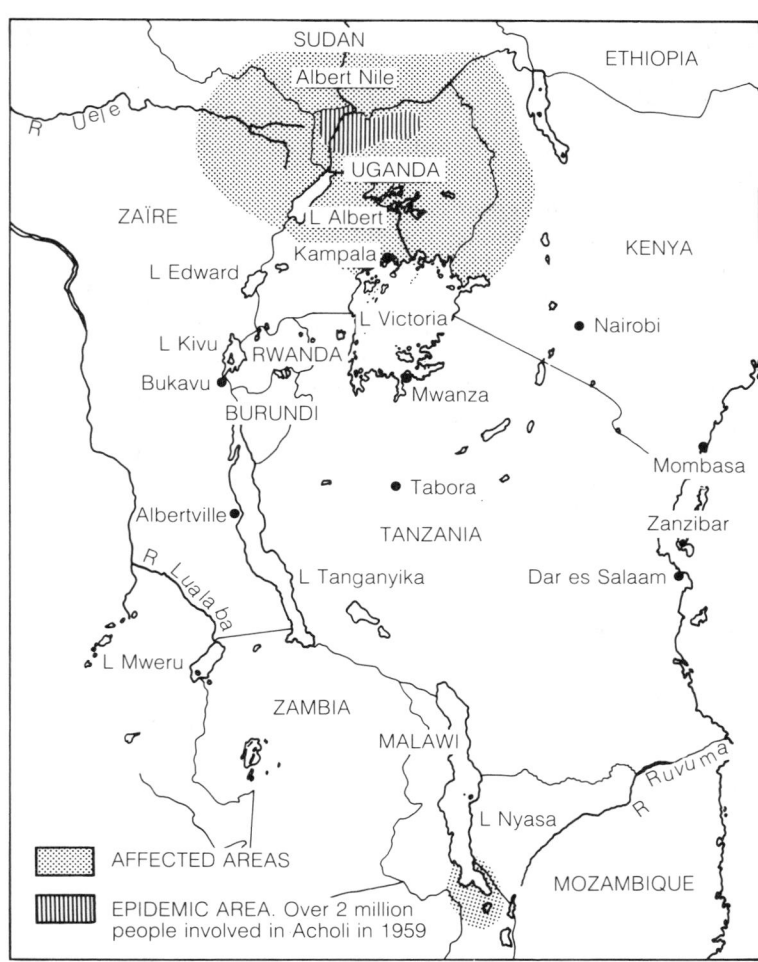

Figure 30.3 Geographical distribution of o'nyong-nyong fever (courtesy of the Department of Entomology, London School of Hygiene and Tropical Medicine).

fever subsides and there is an afebrile period of 3 days when the fever returns with an itching maculo-papular rash on the trunk and extensor surfaces of the limbs. After another 3–6 days the fever subsides and there is complete recovery. In Asia it is associated with mild haemorrhagic features but no shock. There are no chronic sequelae but a crippling arthralgia may occur intermittently for up to 4 months.

DIAGNOSIS

Diagnosis is by paired sera for HI and N antibodies but there are cross-reactions with other alpha-viruses, Semliki Forest and o'nyong-nyong.

EPIDEMIOLOGY

There is a forest cycle involving monkeys (vervets and baboons) transmitted by *Ae. africanus* and other mosquitoes. Rodents may also be hosts since they show a transient viraemia on being inoculated with virus, while monkeys show a high viraemia.

O'NYONG-NYONG (ONN)

GEOGRAPHICAL DISTRIBUTION

ONN is present in Uganda, Kenya, Tanzania and southern Sudan (Figure 30.3).

AETIOLOGY

ONN virus is an alphavirus closely related to CHIK.

TRANSMISSION

Anopheles funestus is the major vector but *Anopheles gambiae* is also involved (see Appendix IV).

SYMPTOMS AND SIGNS

Natural history

ONN is an acute, self-limiting disease which is a purely human infection.

The *incubation period* is 8 days. Onset is abrupt with rigor and epistaxis; the fever settles rapidly (one-third afebrile). There is severe arthralgia involving the knees, elbows, wrists and ankles symmetrically and suffusion of the conjunctivae. On the fourth day an irritant pink maculopapular rash appears, beginning on the face and spreading to the limbs and trunk, which fades in a week. The cervical lymph glands are enlarged and the axillary and inguinal glands may also be affected. Recovery takes place within a week but joint pains may persist. There is a leucopenia with relative lymphocytosis.

EPIDEMIOLOGY

There is no animal reservoir and the cycle is purely man to man. Large epidemics occur when there are enough susceptible subjects, in which 70% of the population may be attacked with all the age groups affected.

CONTROL

Wearing of mosquito nets and anti-*Anopheles funestus* measures will control the epidemics.

ROSS RIVER FEVER (EPIDEMIC POLYARTHRITIS)[9]

GEOGRAPHICAL DISTRIBUTION

Ross River fever occurs annually in epidemics in northern and eastern Australia, and epidemically in Fiji, American Samoa, Cook Islands and New Caledonia. Antibody studies have shown infection to be present in New Guinea, Solomon Islands, the Moluccas and Vietnam.

TRANSMISSION

Transmission is by *Ae. vigilax* and *C. annulirostris* in Australia and *Ae. polynesiensis* in the Cook Islands. *Ae. aegypti* and *Ae. albopictus* are efficient experimental vectors (see Table 30.1 (p. 616) and Appendix IV).

PATHOLOGY

Observation based on examinations of joint fluids suggests that the virus multiplies in synovial cells.

CLINICAL FEATURES

Natural history

It is an acute self-limiting infection with arthritis lasting a week, mainly a human infection.

The *incubation period* is 3–9 days. Onset is abrupt with fever, myalgia and arthralgia. In 20% of cases there is an irritant maculopapular rash on the extremities and trunk. Knees, ankles and wrists are painful and swollen with joint effusions. Recovery occurs within a week but persistent arthritic pains may occur up to one year.

DIAGNOSIS

HI antibodies appear in blood and joint fluid.

EPIDEMIOLOGY

The reservoir vertebrate hosts are unknown but wallabies are suspected. In epidemics the virus is spread from man to man and in Australia cases occur annually between summer and autumn. Explosive epidemics have occurred in Fiji, Samoa and the Cook Islands when the disease encountered a fresh non-immune population. Infection rates were 90%, with 40% of the population showing clinical attacks.

MAYARO[10]

Mayaro virus causes an acute self-limiting dengue-like disease in South America. It is transmitted by *Haemagogus* mosquitoes and wild vertebrates maintain the virus in nature and amplify it. Epidemics have occurred in north and eastern South America, affecting settlers along the Trans-Amazon Highway. There is a great potential for outbreaks among new immigrants and settlers opening up forested country (see Table 30.1 (p. 616) and Appendix IV).

SINDBIS[11]

Sindbis virus causes a self-limiting disease in South Africa, with fever, diffuse papular rash and, in severer cases, vesicles on the feet, from which virus has been recovered. It is transmitted by *C. univittatus*, *C. antennatus* and *C. perexiguus*. Migratory birds are involved in the spread of infection (see Table 30.1 (p. 616) and Appendix IV).

TAHYNA (LUMBO)

Tahyna virus causes a respiratory disease in the Czech Republic and Slovakia and has been found in southern France. It is transmitted by mosquitoes (see Table 30.1 (p. 616) and Appendix IV).

OROPOUCHE VIRUS (ORO)[10]

GEOGRAPHICAL DISTRIBUTION

Oropouche virus is a major cause of disease in the Amazon region of Brazil.

AETIOLOGY

Oropouche virus is a member of the Simbu group of bunyaviruses (see Table 30.1).

TRANSMISSION

The virus is transmitted to man as a zoonosis and thus from man to man by culicine mosquitoes, *Ae. serratus* and *C. quinquefasciatus*. The reservoir is sylvatic animals and ORO virus has been isolated from the three-toed sloth (*Bradypus tridactylus*) (see Table 30.1 (p. 616) and Appendix IV).

CLINICAL FEATURES

Natural history

The infection is short lived with severe disease and aseptic meningitis in some cases[12] but no fatalities. There are a large number of inapparent infections.

Symptoms and signs

The onset is sudden, with chills, headache, myalgia, arthralgia and photophobia being most common. There is a high fever which subsides rapidly, although some of the patients suffer a relapse.

DIAGNOSIS

A high level of antibody develops in the blood.

EPIDEMIOLOGY

The attack rate is twice as high in females as in males. The ORO virus circulates predominantly as a zoonosis in sylvatic animals but periodically is capable of causing severe urban epidemics when it is transmitted from man to man with *C. paraensis*, the primary vector in these epidemics.

ROCIO VIRUS (ROC)

Rocio virus caused an outbreak in 1975 and 1976 in coastal areas of São Paulo state in Brazil. There were 825 cases with 95 deaths. It caused an illness with fever, headache and vomiting, with signs of meningitis and encephalitis. The source of virus was wild birds, and *Psorophora ferox* the vector (see Table 30.1 (p. 616)).

SANDFLY FEVER (PHLEBOTOMUS FEVER, PAPPATACI FEVER)

GEOGRAPHICAL DISTRIBUTION

Sandfly fever is widespread throughout the Mediterranean and Middle East, Malta, Aegean Islands, Egypt and Iran, North Africa, Red Sea and Arabian Gulf; in Asia in the Caucasus and Himalayas up to 4000 feet (Figure 30.4).

AETIOLOGY

The virus causing sandfly fever is a phlebovirus with eight antigenically distinct strains, only two of which, Sicilian and Neapolitan, cause human disease. The others have been isolated from insects and animals.[13]

TRANSMISSION

The sandfly responsible for transmission, *Phlebotomus papatasii*, becomes infective 6 days after feed-

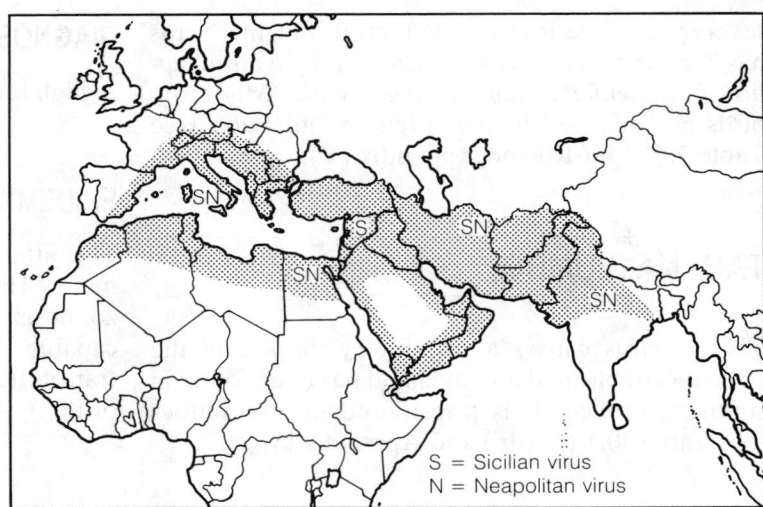

Figure 30.4 Endemic areas of sandfly fever viruses (courtesy of the Wellcome Tropical Institute).

S = Sicilian virus
N = Neapolitan virus

Table 30.3 Viral haemorrhagic fevers.

Arbovirus	Name of disease	Animal hosts	Transmission	Geographical area
Dengue virus	Dengue haemorrhagic (DHF)	Monkeys	Mosquitoes	Africa, Asia, America
Rift Valley fever virus	Rift Valley fever (RVF)	Various mammals	Mosquitoes	Africa
Yellow fever virus	Yellow fever (YF)	Monkeys	Mosquitoes	Africa, America
Omsk haemorrhagic fever virus	Omsk haemorrhagic fever (OHF)	Small mammals	Ticks	Asia, Siberia
Kyasanur Forest virus	Kyasanur Forest disease (KFD)	? rodents, monkeys	Ticks	Asia, India
Crimean–Congo haemorrhagic fever virus	Crimean–Congo haemorrhagic fever (C–CHF)	Small mammals	Ticks	Africa, Asia
Hantaan virus	Muroid virus nephropathy (MVN)	Small rodents	Rodent saliva and urine	Asia, Europe, Africa
Puumala virus	(Haemorrhagic fever with renal syndrome) (HFRS)			
Arenaviruses				
Junin virus	Argentinian haemorrhagic fever	Rodents	Rodent urine	South America
Machupo virus	Bolivian haemorrhagic fever	Rodents	Rodent urine	South America
Lassa virus	Lassa fever	Rodents	Rodent urine	West Africa
Guanarito	Venezuelan haemorrhagic fever	Rodents	Rodent urine	South America
Filoviruses				
Marburg virus	Marburg virus disease	Unknown	Nosocomial	Africa
Ebola virus	Ebola virus disease	Unknown	Nosocomial	Africa

ing and remains infective for life. Transovarial transmission occurs so that newly emerged sandflies are capable of transmitting infection. It is possible that a parasitic mite of the sandflies acts as a reservoir.

CLINICAL FEATURES

Natural history

It is an acute self-limiting disease lasting 2–4 days, with complete recovery and immunity to further attacks, and no mortality.

The *incubation period* is 3–6 days.

Symptoms and signs

The onset is abrupt, with high fever, congested face and neck stiffness. Ocular symptoms are marked, with intense supraorbital pain and injected conjunctivae (papilloedema has been described). There is stiffness of limbs. After 3 (range 2–8) days the fever settles. Occasionally there is a recrudescence (saddle back fever) lasting for a day or two. There is a leucopenia. The CSF pressure is increased and there is a pleocytosis with raised protein.

DIAGNOSIS

Paired sera for HI and N antibody tests are required. There is no specific treatment

EPIDEMIOLOGY

There are no animal reservoirs. In endemic areas transmission lasts from April to October. Epidemics occur among non-immune entrants to the community, especially military forces.

VIRAL HAEMORRHAGIC FEVERS (VHF)

Viral haemorrhagic fevers are caused by a number of different viruses which may be arboviruses, arenaviruses or filoviruses. A list is given in Table 30.3. In the main these viruses cause mostly mild infections but all of them can cause severe and fatal disease with haemorrhagic manifestations, and some have caused devastating epidemics in South America and the Far East.

The pathogenesis of these haemorrhagic features has been the subject of much research and may be caused by one or a combination of a number of factors. These factors are vascular damage, disorders of coagulation, immunopathology and direct damage to organs.

The viruses have a special affinity for the endothelium of capillaries and small vessels which are severely affected directly by the virus, resulting in an increased permeability. Complement activation with the formation of immune complexes which are deposited in the walls of small vessels further damages them, leading to capillary fragility (positive tourniquet test) and haemorrhage with bleeding from the mucous membranes, and even cerebral haemorrhage. Widespread haemorrhage produces hyperconcentration of the blood, hypovolaemia, hypoxia of the tissues, acidosis and hyperkalaemia which, with vomiting and dehydration, may lead to irreversible shock. Other factors involved may be maturation arrest of megakaryocytes in the bone marrow, with platelet abnormalities and disseminated intravascular coagulation leading to fibrinogen depletion. Some viruses directly damage the cells of organs (e.g. hepatic necrosis in YF).

The management and immunology of viral haemorrhagic fevers is considered in general before describing each one in detail.

MANAGEMENT OF VIRAL HAEMORRHAGIC FEVERS[14]

A case of possible VHF must be approached correctly from the start.

HISTORY

An accurate history must establish the symptoms, exact location of travel (cf. areas endemic for various VHFs) and, most important, specific contact with ill persons or their tissues and secretions and direct or indirect contact with local animals (except in the case of mosquito-borne VHF). An interval of 3 weeks between the last possible exposure and onset of illness rules out the diagnosis of VHF.

SYMPTOMS

Many symptoms are non-specific but certain specific symptoms will suggest VHF: pharyngitis, conjunctivitis, vomiting, diarrhoea, abdominal pain and, most important, haemorrhagic manifestations and shock.

DIAGNOSIS

Rapid diagnosis is most important because it affects management of the case. Other febrile illnesses associated with shock and haemorrhage must be excluded: falciparum malaria, meningococcaemia, leptospirosis, typhus, septicaemia, plague, *Escherichia coli* septicaemia.

Extreme care must be taken in obtaining blood specimens because blood is highly infective in the first few days of viraemia. Specimens must be specially labelled so that their infectivity is clear.

ISOLATION

Care must be taken not to alarm the public. Although people in direct contact with patients, such as doctors, nurses, pathologists and technicians are at risk, further spread outside to the community at large does not occur except with mosquito-borne viruses.

Strict isolation, preferably under negative pressure or under a sealed tent with an anteroom where staff can don protective clothing, is necessary to protect the staff. Protective clothing includes masks and goggles. The patient should use a chemical toilet. In the case of possible mosquito-borne VHF, isolation under a mosquito net or in a mosquito-proof room is all that is necessary. Those working in the tropics will realize that much of the foregoing is impracticable. Experience has shown that *normal* barrier nursing techniques are sufficient to prevent transmission of these diseases in hospital.

VERIFICATION OF DIAGNOSIS

Verification of diagnosis must first exclude other possible non-VHF causes. Specimens to be collected immediately are:

- A throat swab
- A clean mid-stream urine specimen
- Venous blood for antibody studies and virus isolation using a disposable needle and syringe which must be discarded in disinfectant immediately. A blood smear for malaria parasites is absolutely necessary but once fixed is safe to be examined (see Appendix V).

Convalescence

Most cases of VHF are over the infectious stage quite quickly but with arenaviruses virus can be excreted in the urine for a period of months following an attack.

TREATMENT

The careful management of fluid and electrolyte balance from the onset of disease is the most important facet of treatment.

Shock

Shock is a feature of many haemorrhagic fevers and the following treatment has been used for haemor-

rhagic dengue, and may be appropriate for other diseases leading to shock.[15] Treatment is supportive and good nursing is essential. Oxygen is useful at first. Water balance must be maintained at as near normal as possible. To restore fluids and electrolytes, infusion of 5% dextrose in half-strength normal saline, at the rate of 100 ml/kg body weight daily, is recommended. Or 10–15 ml of Ringer lactate solution/kg body weight (see below) may be infused intravenously for 1 hour, followed by a less concentrated electrolyte replacement fluid. Plasma or a substitute may be given to combat shock. Blood transfusion is not recommended in the hypotensive phase but may be given after recovery from shock if the patient shows signs of having had severe haemorrhage.

Hypovolaemia is usual and packed cell volume should therefore be watched; if it remains the same, or increases during replacement indicating loss of fluid to extracellular spaces, plasma should be given to maintain an adequate circulating blood volume, at the rate of 10–20 ml/kg per hour until the packed cell volume begins to decline.

In the hypotensive phase, hydrocortisone 50–100 mg daily, or aldosterone 0.1 mg/kg daily, in conjunction with the infusion fluid, may reduce mortality and sometimes has a dramatic effect. (Aldosterone raises blood pressure, conserves sodium and causes potassium to be excreted in the urine; it is therefore a rational treatment. The dose quoted is high.)

During recovery, when vascular fluid returns to the circulation, infusion of fluid should cease.

Ringer lactate solution contains approximately 131 mmol sodium, 5 mmol potassium, 4 mmol calcium, 29 mmol bicarbonate (as lactate) and 111 mmol chloride in each litre.

Some children with metabolic acidosis do not easily metabolize lactate and should therefore receive 1–2 ml/kg of 3.75% sodium bicarbonate solution intravenously every 10–15 minutes until improvement is noted.[16]

To control thrombocytopenic bleeding, transfusion of fresh human platelet concentrates is valuable. One unit of platelet concentrate is obtained from one pint of blood; the dose used in Thai children ranged from 0.2 unit to 10 units/kg body weight.

Curative treatment

Immune plasma

Although the efficacy of immune plasma obtained from a patient who has recovered has not yet been scientifically established, it appears to have benefited some. The immune plasma must be administered early in the illness, preferably in the first week. Later the presence of virus and naturally occurring antibody may cause the deposition of antigen–antibody complexes, which in themselves cause pathological changes.

Antiviral drugs

Ribavirin if administered during the first week of illness has been of benefit in Lassa fever (see p. 648) and Rift Valley fever (see p. 635). Other possible antiviral drugs include interferon inducers.

CONTROL

VECTOR CONTROL

Vector control has been successful in some circumstances, for instance, during the construction of the Panama Canal when by strict discipline all collections of water capable of breeding *Ae. aegypti* (and vectors of malaria) were eliminated from the area. Similar methods were applied to cities and towns in South America under the threat of YF. When DDT was introduced, extensive use in Guyana and elsewhere soon eradicated *Ae. aegypti* and with it the threat of urban YF. In Africa, however, *Ae. aegypti* has recently shown resistance to DDT, and in some areas it is exophilic in habit, so that spraying dwellings with insecticide is ineffective. Forest mosquitoes, of course, are not susceptible to ordinary methods of spraying. Tick control by residual insecticides has, however, achieved some success in the former USSR. However, the problems of vector control, especially in rural areas, are formidable.

IMMUNIZATION

Vaccines which have been developed for VHF are highly effective but are available only for YF, Rift Valley fever and Omsk haemorrhage fever. For most other arbovirus diseases they are either experimental or can be used only in restricted groups of people, such as laboratory workers, in face of threatened outbreaks or in reservoir animals (e.g. pigs for JE), or are not yet available. The multiplicity of the viruses creates a difficulty, which may to some extent be reduced by the development of group vaccines, where these give some cross-protection.

Many vaccines have been developed for YF since Hindle and Aragão independently first used emulsions of organs from infected animals for that purpose. Hindle used a phenol–glycerin emulsion and later an emulsion treated with formalin after reduction of virulence by freezing.

Active immunity in YF is now provoked by vaccines consisting of virus selected by serial intracerebral passage in mice. Early vaccines were given along with specific immune human serum with the intention of preventing severe reactions, but some branches of the immune serum were found to carry the virus of hepatitis, and to cause that disease in the recipients; the method was therefore discontinued.

A more successful vaccine was derived from a highly virulent strain of YF virus isolated from an African named Asibi, in Ghana, and cultivated in vitro in mouse embryonic tissue. This procedure greatly reduced the viscerotropism of the strain without altering its neurotropism. The virus was then grown in tissue culture of minced chick embryos from which the central nervous system had been removed before mincing; after prolonged propagation in this medium it was found that neurotropism and viscerotropism were both greatly reduced, but the virus retained its antigenic properties. This was the famous vaccine 17D, still widely used and highly effective, giving protection for at least 10 years, and only very rarely causing any untoward reaction. In 120 000 persons, mostly under 12 years old, vaccinated with 17D, only two developed meningoencephalitis. 17D is a live vaccine but it cannot be passed from person to person by mosquitoes.

Infants should preferably not be given YF vaccine before the age of 9 months because of the somewhat greater risk of encephalitis below that age.

The French Dakar vaccine is a neurotropic virus. Of 1 880 000 persons vaccinated with this, 246 developed meningoencephalitis and 23 died.

These live vaccines all provoke active immunity, not so persistent as the immunity developed after natural infection, but nevertheless extremely effective for several years.

Immunization against YF is required by law before travellers are allowed into certain countries either for their protection or to prevent the importation of the disease to areas where *Ae. aegypti* is present.

Apart from YF, vaccines have been produced against several arbovirus diseases, for use in animals (for instance horses) as well as in man.

Attenuated strains of VEE, Langat, West Nile and WEE viruses (some grown on chick embryo) have been developed, and the Langat vaccine may protect against Powassan, KFD and RSSE too. Strains of chikungunya, TBE, SLE, KFD, Rift Valley and CTF have been inactivated, some by formalin, and tested experimentally. For TBE the early brain vaccines gave meningoencephalitis, and were

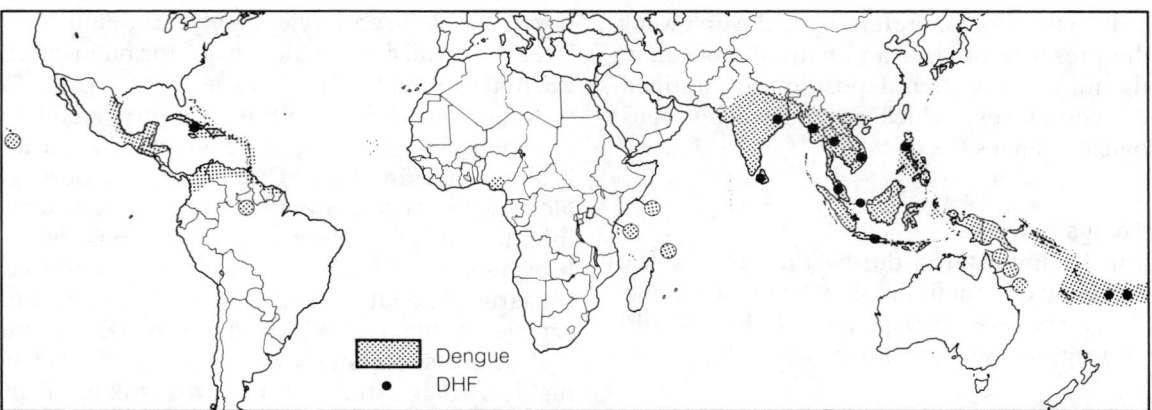

Figure 30.5   Geographical distribution of dengue and dengue haemorrhagic fever (DHF) (courtesy of the Department of Entomology, London School of Hygiene and Tropical Medicine).

superseded by cell culture vaccines. Dengue and JE vaccines have also been devised. For various reasons these vaccines are not widely used.[17]

After vaccination against SLE, HI antibody appears in the first weeks, to a peak in the third week. CF antibody, which is more specific, appears in the second week to a peak in the second month. CF antibody was at a low titre at 18–22 months in one Florida outbreak, but neutralizing antibodies persisted; they tend to appear early.

Immunological phenomena may play a part in the pathogenesis of haemorrhagic fever and encephalitis, and this risk needs to be carefully considered in vaccinating against some arbovirus infections. Allergic encephalitis is one such risk.

DENGUE (See also Chapter 34)

GEOGRAPHICAL DISTRIBUTION

Dengue has a worldwide tropical and subtropical distribution between 30° north and 40° south (Figure 30.5). It is endemic in South-East Asia (types 1, 2, 3 and 4), the Pacific (type 2), West Africa (types 1 and 2), East Africa (type 2), Caribbean (types 1 and 4) and the Americas (types 2 and 3).

AETIOLOGY

The dengue virus, a member of the flavivirus group, is an RNA virus, 17–25 mm in diameter, which can be grown in a variety of mosquitoes and tissue cultures. It possesses antigens which overlap with YF, JE and West Nile viruses and there are four serotypes (1, 2, 3 and 4), all of which can be involved in both classical dengue and dengue haemorrhagic

fever. It can survive at 4°C for several weeks and −70°C for years. Dengue virus can be passed vertically in *Aedes* experimentally but the epidemiological significance of this is uncertain.

TRANSMISSION

Dengue is transmitted by mosquitoes (see Table 30.1 and Appendix IV). The classical type is transmitted worldwide by *Ae. aegypti* and by *Ae. albopictus* (Asia, Philippines and Japan); *Ae. polynesiensis*, *Ae. scutellaris* and *Ae. pseudoscutellaris* (Pacific Islands and New Guinea); *Ae. polynesiensis* (Society Islands) and *Ae. niveus* (Philippines) (see also Appendix IV). Mosquitoes can be infected from the onset until the fourth day of illness and become infective from 8 to 11 days after feeding, remaining infective for life. Transovarial transmission of all four dengue viruses by *Ae. albopictus* has been demonstrated.[18]

PATHOLOGY

After inoculation the virus reaches the regional lymph glands and disseminates to the reticulo-endothelial system, in which it multiplies and from which it seeds the blood. In classical dengue changes can be seen in the skin, where there is swelling of the endothelium of small blood vessels and perivascular infiltration with mononuclear cells.

IMMUNITY

Immunity is antibody mediated and after recovery there is a long-standing immunity to the homologous strain but none to other serotypes or other flaviviruses, although some common antigens are possessed.

CLINICAL FEATURES

The *incubation period* is 2–7 days.

Natural history

Classical dengue is a short-lived infection with complete recovery and is not usually fatal but under certain circumstances it can cause a severe haemorrhagic fever which can be fatal.

Symptoms and signs

The onset is sudden with high fever (40°C) which is biphasic. Severe muscle pains ('break bone fever'), headache and prostration are characteristic. After an early erythematous rash, a few days later a morbilliform or scarlatiniform rash appears, beginning on the extremities, accompanied by generalized lymphadenopathy. The liver is moderately enlarged and there is a profound leucopenia. The second febrile phase lasts 2–3 days and the rash then desquamates. Convalescence is long and may be accompanied by tachycardia, general debility and often severe mental depression. Classical dengue is seldom fatal.

DIAGNOSIS

Virus isolation in the early stages is achieved by inoculation of cell cultures: LLC-MK2 or Vero cells, cells of *Ae. albopictus, Ae. pseudoscutellaris*, or live mosquitoes (*Ae. aegypti*), inoculated intrathoracically and examined after 7–14 days by immunofluorescence. The type can be identified by CF or N tests or immunofluorescence with type-specific monoclonal antibodies. The early stages must be distinguished from malaria and hepatitis. Chikungunya, sandfly fever and Rift Valley fever closely resemble dengue, but without the rash.

Serological diagnosis

The HI test performed on acute stage serum taken in the first 4 days and convalescent serum taken 2–3 weeks later will show a fourfold increase to one or more of the four serotype antigens. Neutralization tests will distinguish clearly between the four serotypes.

TREATMENT

The treatment is symptomatic only.

COMPLICATIONS

Encephalopathies have been associated with proven dengue in Indonesia.[19] Dengue haemorrhagic fever is considered later.

EPIDEMIOLOGY

A jungle cycle of dengue involving forest mosquitoes and wild monkeys has been postulated in Malaya and West Africa where antibodies have been found in monkeys, the significance of which is not yet clear.

Dengue fever epidemics involve many thousands of cases, with attack rates of 75–80%, completely disrupting the life of communities. These epidemics result from the introduction of a new serotype or the availability of a susceptible population (immigrants and young persons born since the last epidemic). These epidemics have swept up the Caribbean and eastern seaboard of the Americas and up the eastern shores of East Africa, involving the islands. More recently dengue has caused vast epidemics in South-East Asia.

CONTROL

Control of dengue rests upon vector control, mainly the domestic breeding of *Ae. aegypti* in domestic water containers. The *Aedes* index can be used to monitor the population of mosquitoes and hence foresee outbreaks and institute proper vector control. A satisfactory vaccine has yet to be developed, but, for dangers, see below in section on dengue haemorrhage fever.

DENGUE HAEMORRHAGIC FEVER (DHF)

GEOGRAPHICAL DISTRIBUTION

DHF is a perennial problem in South-East Asia where it is a major cause of child morbidity and mortality. DHF has also appeared in Cuba, the Caribbean[19] and in the Pacific (Fiji). So far DHF has not been documented from Africa.

AETIOLOGY

The cause is still not clear. Halstead[20] proposed the concept of two sequential infections with different dengue serotypes, the first infection sensitizing the patient to the second, producing a severe response which has been shown to be immunologically mediated and involving the complement system. A critical period of about 6 months between the two infections has been thought to be necessary. This view is supported by experience in Fiji, which suffered outbreaks of dengue in 1971 and 1972, with the occurrence of haemorrhagic fever in people of all ages and in expatriates. There had been no dengue in Fiji for 30 years.[21–23] (Rosen[24] has suggested that an abnormally virulent strain of virus might be responsible.)

PATHOLOGY

The basic pathological change responsible for DHF is increased capillary permeability leading to rapid shifts of extracellular fluid, allied to fluid depletion from decreased intake and increased loss resulting in haemoconcentration, hypovolaemia, reduced tissue perfusion and oxygenation, acidosis and widespread cellular damage leading to shock. The capillary leakage is most likely to be caused immunologically by the activation of complement by dengue antigen–antibody complexes, which may also initiate disseminated intravascular coagulation. The *liver* shows mid-zonal hyaline or acidophilic necrosis of parenchymal liver cells and Kupffer's cells, with the appearance of Councilman lesions. The *kidneys* rarely show glomerulonephritis, probably due to immune complexes. There is a *reticuloendothelial* reaction (proliferation of lymphocytes, plasmacytoid cells and increase in phagocytosis), maturation arrest of *megakaryocytes* and hypocellularity of the bone marrow. Capillary damage results in leakage of fluid, plasma and erythrocytes into interstitial spaces and serous cavities causing pleural and peritoneal effusions, and retroperitoneal oedema. Haemorrhages are not generally severe but major gastrointestinal bleeding may appear in adolescents and adults.

IMMUNITY

The immune status of the host is the important component which determines the development of DHF. The presence of non-neutralizing antibodies to a heterologous serotype can cause 'immune enhancement' of dengue virus growth in lymphoid cells with the release of factors increasing capillary permeability. There is a strong association of this process with a second infection on a prior exposure to another serotype or, in the case of infants, to the presence of maternal antibody to suggest that this is a cause, but it is possible that a more virulent strain might do it on its own (see section on aetiology, above).

CLINICAL FEATURES

On the second to fifth days of classical dengue illness at the end of the first phase the patient deteriorates rapidly, with development of the shock syndrome. Restlessness, sweating and hypotension appear, coincident with a positive tourniquet test, petechiae, ecchymoses and spontaneous haemorrhages. There is tender enlargement of the liver in some cases, with hypoproteinaemia, hyponatraemia, mild elevation of the liver enzymes and some nitrogen retention. The presence of disseminated intravascular coagulation is shown by the alteration in clotting factors and reduced fibrinogen. Without treatment, 50% of the patients die, but with treatment the mortality is reduced to 5% and recovery is usually rapid.

DIAGNOSIS

A positive tourniquet test or spontaneous haemorrhages, thrombocytopenia and evidence of haemoconcentration (plus 20% or more) are the diagnostic criteria for DHF.

SEROLOGY

The CF and HI tests will be positive to all strains of dengue but neutralizing antibodies to both the primary and secondary infection will be raised, whereas to the other serotypes will be negative; thus each of the causative serotypes of dengue can be identified.[25]

TREATMENT

This is discussed in the section on management of VHF (see p. 630). Isolation of the patient is not necessary except that mosquitoes should be excluded by mosquito nets or screens. Care, however, must be taken to prevent contamination with blood in the few days of the illness during the period of viraemia.

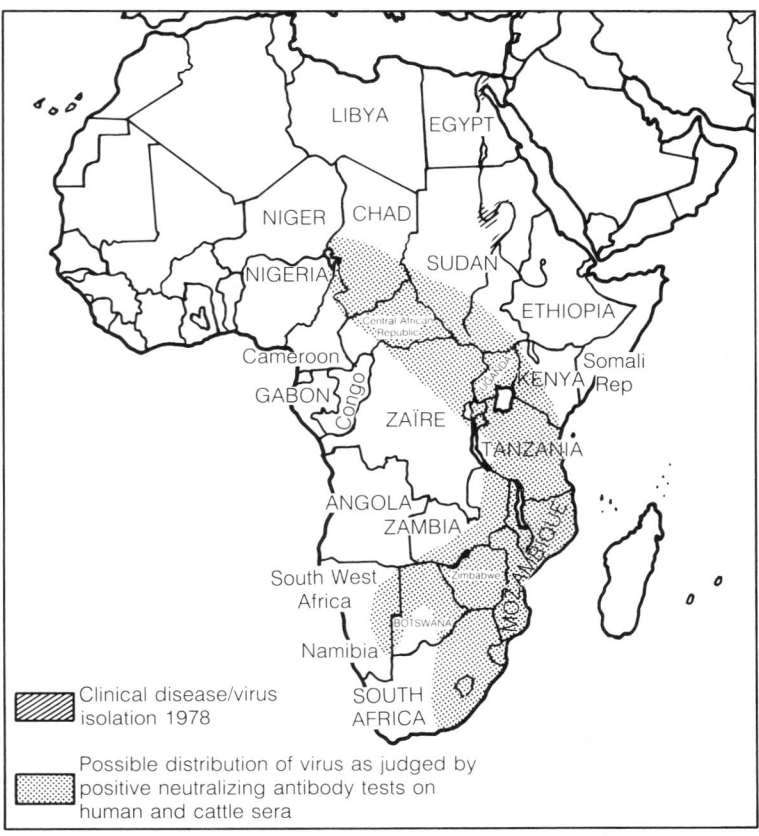

Figure 30.6 Geographical distribution of Rift Valley fever (courtesy of the Department of Entomology, London School of Hygiene and Tropical Medicine).

EPIDEMIOLOGY

DHF in South-East Asia affects mainly indigenous young children. Adults and expatriates will develop classical dengue but escape DHF. Foreign residents living in good conditions in Bangkok with piped water tend to escape. An outbreak of DHF which started in Manila in 1963 then invaded Thailand (150000–200000 cases) and South Vietnam.

CONTROL

Control measures are those applied to classical dengue fever. Immunization with vaccines presents a problem because an individual with antibodies to one serotype runs the danger of developing DHF when infected with another serotype.

RIFT VALLEY FEVER (RVF)

GEOGRAPHICAL DISTRIBUTION

Rift Valley fever was first recognized in Kenya in 1931 as causing disease in sheep and man. Until 1977 it was restricted to man and domestic animals in sub-

Saharan Africa, with epizootics in Kenya, South Africa, Zimbabwe, Sudan, Egypt, Uganda, Tanzania and Zambia. A similar virus (Zinga virus) was found to be present in West Africa (Mali, Nigeria and Zaire) and in Botswana and Mozambique but without epizootics. In 1977 RVF spread to Egypt where it caused massive epidemics and epizootics and showed a capability to spread beyond sub-Saharan Africa (Figure 30.6). The Egyptian episode was largely centred in the Nile delta where approximately 600 human deaths are thought to have occurred. This was probably preceded by a massive epizootic along the Nile bank from Aswan in the south to Cairo in the north. Rift Valley fever occurred again in Aswan in 1993 and several cases with ophthalmic complications have been seen in the Nile delta.

AETIOLOGY

RVF is a member of the genus *Phlebovirus* of the family Bunyaviridae (see Table 30.1). The virus is spherical, 90–110 nm in diameter, with a lipid envelope from which glycoprotein spikes protrude, and can be found in host membrane systems. Two strains of the virus have been found, RVF and Zinga virus, which have been shown to be the same virus by the neutralization test.[26]

PATHOLOGY

The pathogenesis of RVF is still not clear but is thought to be a direct effect of the virus of increased virulence on cells, or a sensitization phenomenon similar to that seen in dengue, or some form of synergism between the virus and endemic schistoso-miasis.

The pathology closely resembles that of YF. The liver is the main organ affected, with mid-zonal hyaline changes leading to necrosis and bodies re-sembling the Councilman bodies of YF. The kidney tubules and spleen show toxic changes and there are haemorrhages in all the viscera. The causes of these changes are a vasculitis from viral infection of endo-thelial cells and antigen–antibody immune com-plexes. Encephalitis and extensive retinal changes may also be found.

TRANSMISSION

Transmission between the zoonotic hosts is by mos-quitoes of the *Eretmapodites, Coquillettidiae, Man-sonia, Aedes* and *Culex* groups (see Table 30.1 and Appendix 4). and possibly to man by *A. caballus* and *C. theileri* in South Africa and *C. pipiens* in Egypt. Direct transmission, especially during epidemics, is by the aerosol route from infected animal tissues. Person-to-person transmission does not occur but acute phase blood as well as infected animals are highly infectious, especially in abattoirs.

IMMUNITY

Active immunity

Immunity is antibody mediated and there is pro-longed immunity to reinfection with the homolo-gous strains after recovery. Antibodies formed are of the usual viral response (HI, CF and N). HI and CF antibodies are used in diagnosis whereas N antibodies give specificity.

Passive immunity

A passive immunity can be transferred via the pla-centa to the child and lasts for several months; the possession of antibodies, especially N antibodies, can be used in treatment using convalescent sera.

CLINICAL FEATURES

Natural history

RVF is a self-limiting disease in the great majority of infections, with a short, acute febrile phase with complete recovery but, in less than 5% of cases, complications—haemorrhagic and encephalitic—can occur with fatal results.

Symptoms and signs[27]

The *incubation period* is 3–7 days. The onset is abrupt with fever, headache, joint and muscle pains and photophobia. In the majority of cases this is followed by complete recovery. In a few cases there may be recrudescence of symptoms after the initial short illness and convalescence may be prolonged. In a small proportion (less than 5% in the Egyptian epidemic) the illness is much more severe, with the onset of haemorrhagic manifestations (purpura, haematemesis and melaena) and liver failure (jaun-dice). Other complications include meningoen-cephalitis, ocular involvement with retinitis, retinal haemorrhages and blindness due to retinal vasculitis and retinal detachment (South Africa,[28] Zim-babwe,[29] and Egypt[30]).

DIAGNOSIS

When cases of fever present in numbers and the three complications—haemorrhage, encephalitis and blindness—occur then there is a strong indi-cation that these are cases of RVF, especially if associated with an epizootic in sheep and cattle. Isolation of virus within the first 7 days from the blood can be done by intracerebral inoculation into baby mice, and most kinds of cell culture. Serolo-gical diagnosis is by the HI test on paired sera, using a standard antigen from the World Health Organiz-ation.[31] Other tests are CF, agar gel diffusion, immunofluorescence and enzyme linked immuno-sorbent assay (ELISA). The detection of N anti-bodies are diagnostic for RVF because there is no cross-reaction between these antibodies and other phleboviruses.

TREATMENT

Cases should be managed as in all VHFs. Isolation from mosquitoes must be enforced and attendants should be protected from infected blood in the early stages. Symptomatic treatment is that of other VHFs (see p. 630). There is as yet no curative drug

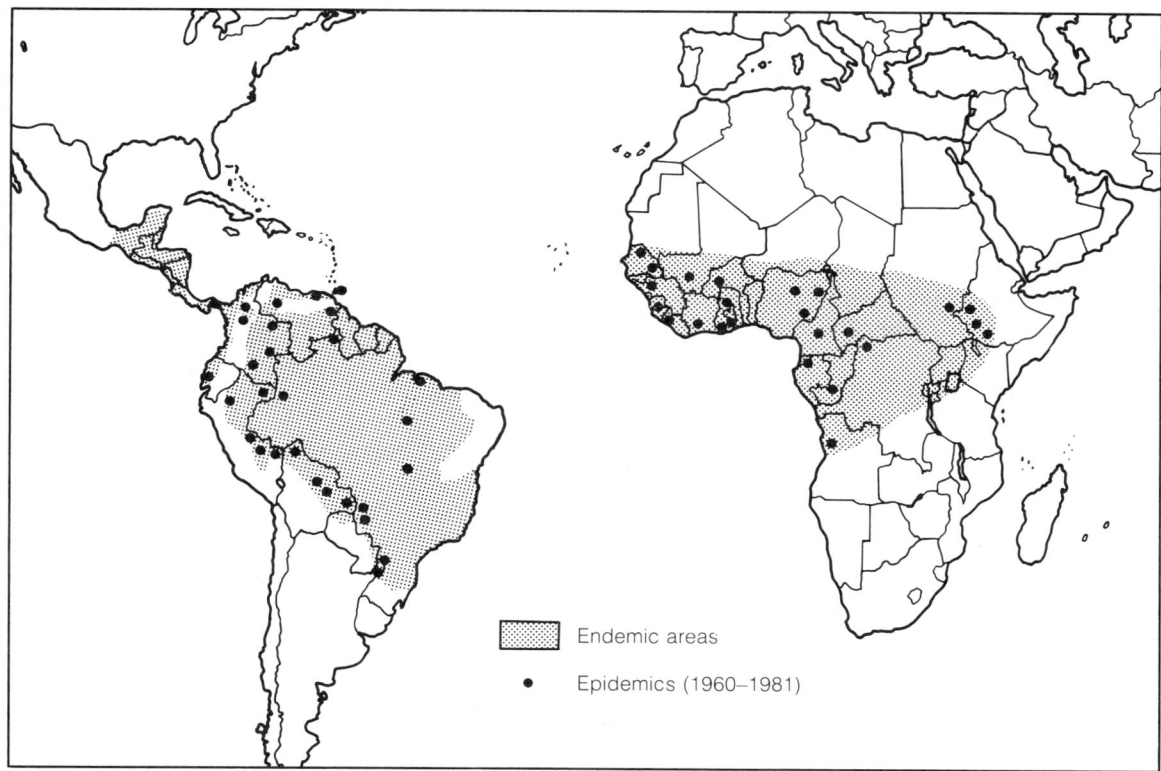

Figure 30.7 Geographical distribution of yellow fever.

but laboratory experiments suggest that interferon inducers, antiviral drugs (ribavirin) or immune serum could be useful, and convalescent serum from cases of RVF who have recovered should certainly be used in severe cases.

EPIDEMIOLOGY

RVF is maintained in the forest in an enzootic fashion in an as yet poorly understood maintenance cycle. Rodents have been thought to be responsible but no viral isolations, only antibodies, have been found. Spectacular epizootics in domestic animals are the result of large numbers of susceptible (European) breeds of cattle and sheep, high arthropod densities and spillover from the forest cycle. Originally restricted to domestic animals and man in sub-Saharan Africa it has, since 1977, spread to Egypt, causing explosive epidemics in man and domestic animals. The spread was possibly by camels from the Sudan carrying infection or arthropods establishing new enzootic foci in the changing arthropod and vertebrate population after the construction of the High Aswan Dam. Spread can occur to other areas in North Africa and South-West Asia with the construction of new dams and irrigation schemes.[32,33]

CONTROL

Quarantine is not effective but movements of animals should be controlled and sick animals should be allowed to die or recover and not be slaughtered, to avoid spreading the infection in abattoirs. Control of abattoirs and vaccination of workers should be enforced.

IMMUNIZATION

Vaccination of exposed laboratory workers and veterinary staff using a formalin-inactivated cell culture vaccine (expensive) should be performed.

Veterinary vaccines are the first line of defence against the spread of RVF. Both live and inactivated vaccines have been used to control the spread in animals with some success.[34]

YELLOW FEVER (YF) (See also Chapter 3)

GEOGRAPHICAL DISTRIBUTION

Yellow fever is found in the tropical forest areas of Africa and South America (Figure 30.7) and until early in this century caused large epidemics in the Caribbean and the subtropical and temperate regions of North American as far north as Baltimore and Philadelphia. 'Jungle' YF still occurs in Brazil and there was an outbreak in Trinidad in 1978–1979, with 18 cases and eight deaths. Many other epidemics have occurred in South America, and a large epidemic in Ethiopia was responsible for many deaths in 1960–1962, and in Senegal in 1965–1966. YF has caused fatalities in tourists, especially in West Africa, who have not been vaccinated.

West Africa was probably the original home of YF, which may have been transported to the Americas by ships carrying infected mosquitoes in the post-Columbian period. YF has never been established in Europe, Asia or Australasia although potential vectors (*Ae. aegypti* in South-East Asia) abound, so that if it were introduced into Asia catastrophic epidemics could occur.

AETIOLOGY

Yellow fever is a flavivirus (see Table 30.1), 25–65 nm in size, which can survive at 4°C for a month and freeze dried for many years. It can be grown on a variety of vertebrate cell cultures, chick or mouse embryo, KB or HeLa cell cultures with a cytopathic effect. There are seven strains which can infect man. Freshly isolated strains which are pantropic lose viscerotropism in the chick embryo. African strains of yellow fever possess an antigen absent from American strains and the 17D strain, which is so successfully used as a live vaccine, has acquired an antigen absent from the original 'Asibi' strain from which it was developed.[2]

TRANSMISSION

Mosquitoes (See Table 30.1 and Appendix IV)

In nature YF is transmitted by mosquitoes of several genera. In the Americas the forest cycle is maintained by *Haemagogus spegazzinii* as the principal vector, with *H. leucocelaenus*, *H. janthinomys* (= *falco*) and *Sabethes chloropterus* also involved. *Ae. aegypti* is responsible for urban outbreaks. Virus has also been isolated from *Ae. fulvus* in Brazil. In Africa *Ae. africanus* maintains the monkey–mosquito–monkey cycle in the forest, while *Ae. simpsoni,* which breeds close to man in the axils of plants (bananas), becomes infected from monkeys raiding the plantations, and transmits YF to man. Other *Aedes* involved in the forest cycle are *Ae. vittatus, Ae. luteocephalus, Ae. metallicus* and *Ae. taylori,* from which evidence of transovarial trans-

mission has been obtained under natural conditions in Senegal, suggesting an ideal vector for transmission among monkeys.[35] The urban cycle is maintained by *Ae. aegypti* (see Appendix IV).

Mosquitoes become infected from the first to third day of fever. The intrinsic cycle in the mosquito is 4 days at 37°C and 18 days at 18°C. Mosquitoes remain infected for life, about 2–4 months. The possibility of transovarial transmission has already been mentioned.

Ticks

YF virus has been isolated from *Amblyomma variegatum* in Brazil and trans-stadial transmission was demonstrated by infecting nymphs and passing on the infection to uninfected monkeys at the adult stage. The epidemiological significance of this is not clear.[36]

Other methods of transmission

Human blood is infective in the first 3 days of illness and handling of infected monkeys in the early stages of viraemia could cause infection. Interhuman transmission is unimportant but laboratory work with infected monkeys and mosquitoes can be dangerous.

PATHOLOGY

There is no evidence of any immune reactions influencing the pathogenesis of YF. The virus affects highly specialized epithelial or myocardial cells only; stroma cells are not involved. The changes are toxic, beginning with cloudy swelling and going on to degenerative fatty changes and coagulative necrosis. There is no inflammatory response.

Liver

Typical lesions may not be found in biopsy specimens from patients who later recover and serological evidence is necessary for diagnosis in such cases. In fatal cases, however, the liver is not shrunken; it may be reddish-yellow and feels greasy. The typical lesions form a characteristic triad: microglobular fatty degeneration of epithelial liver cells throughout the hepatic lobule; dissociation of the hepatic lobule, most marked in the mid-zone (but some normal liver cells always remain around the central zone); and coagulative necrosis of the epithelial liver

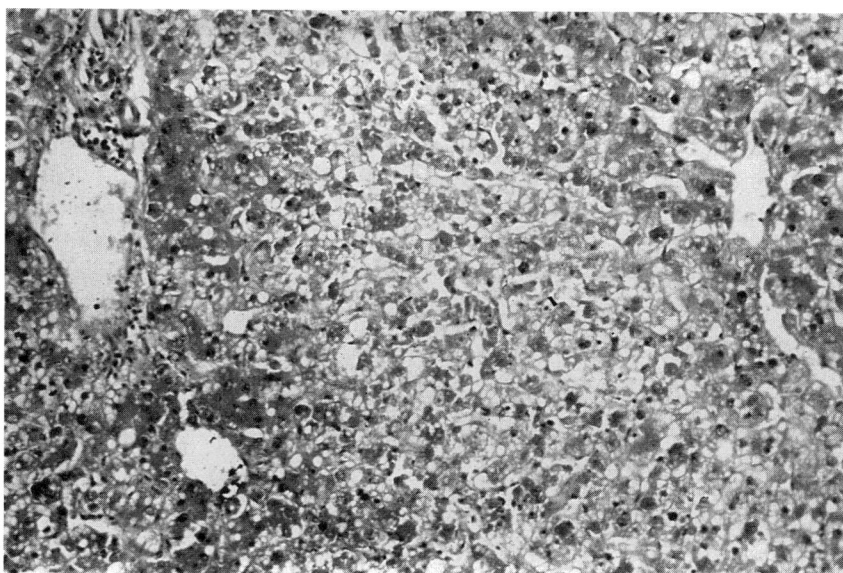

Figure 30.8 Postmortem appearance of the liver of a rhesus monkey with yellow fever, showing well-marked mid-zonal necrosis and minimal inflammatory changes.

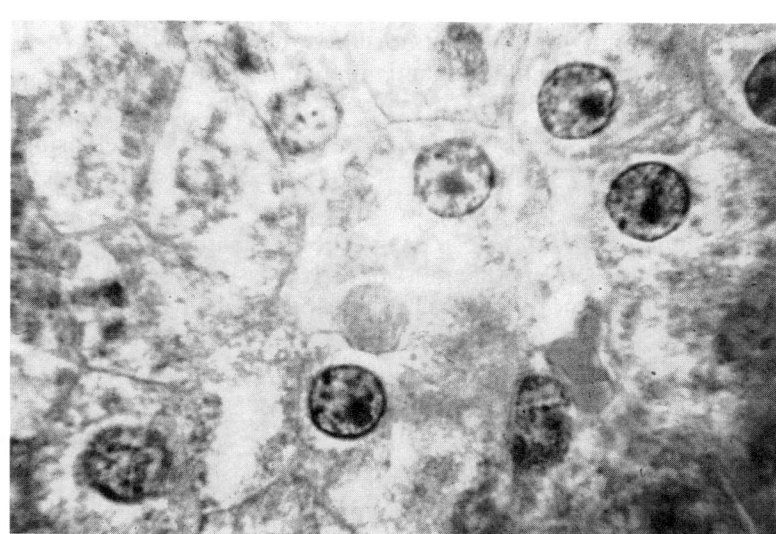

Figure 30.9 Councilman body in the liver cell of a rhesus monkey affected with yellow fever.

cells, mainly affecting the mid-zone (Figure 30.8). The nuclei of the liver cells are pyknotic and the coagulated contents of the cells stain deeply with eosin, the Councilman bodies resulting from this degeneration taking on a salmon-pink colour (Figure 30.9). Under low power a stained section looks as if red pepper has been scattered on it.

Other organs

The lesions are variable: some degree of nephritis or nephrosis (with transient proteinuria in mild cases), adrenal lesions, lesions of the heart (fatty changes, even in the sinoatrial node and the bundle of His, corresponding with the clinical bradycardia) and lesions of the brain (perivascular haemorrhages). In the kidneys there are fatty changes with necrosis of

tubular epithelium and casts in both cortex and medulla. Encephalitis was not formerly thought to be part of the picture of naturally occurring YF, but meningoencephalitis was a dominant feature of the epidemic of 1960 in the Sudan and Ethiopia. Severe haemorrhages may take place in the digestive system, the internal cavities, the lungs (common), liver, spleen and kidneys. Death results from failure of the liver or kidneys or both, though cardiac damage may contribute. Patients who recover show complete replacement of lost tissue by direct regeneration and hypertrophy of surviving cells.

IMMUNITY

Immunity is antibody mediated and lifelong immunity follows infection with YF virus. In many endemic areas where contact with virus-carrying mosquitoes is constant, i.e. near the forest, infection is common in childhood, leading to a solid immunity. The immunity is antibody mediated, HF and N antibodies being found from the end of the first week of infection.

CLINICAL FEATURES

Natural history

In the majority of cases the infection is short and sharp with full recovery. Inapparent infections, especially in endemic areas, are common, leading to the apparent freedom from infection of the indigenous inhabitants, in contrast to new arrivals, immigrants or armies. In a minority of cases and in epidemics the infection is severe, with biphasic fever, jaundice and severe haemorrhages leading to the 'black vomit' with a high mortality. This illness was known in the eighteenth and nineteenth centuries as the 'yellow jack'.

Symptoms and signs

The *incubation period* is 3–6 days. The spectrum of infection varies from the mild abortive case (the majority) to the more severe classic case of YF (only 10–20% of cases).

Mild case

An acute febrile illness with sudden onset of fever and headache without other symptoms lasting 48 hours or less. In some other patients the headache is more severe, accompanied by myalgia and slight proteinuria. The characteristic bradycardia in relation to the temperature (Faget's sign) is present and the illness may last several days with recovery.

Haemorrhagic fever

Period of infection

This is the period of viraemia and lasts 3 days. There is an abrupt onset, with fever up to 40°C, chills, severe headache, nausea, vomiting, abdominal pain and distressing pain in the back, loins and limbs. The patient is dehydrated with a dry tongue and foul breath. There is a yellow tint in the conjunctivae which deepens with the appearance of jaundice in the skin. Minor gingival haemorrhages or epistaxis may occur. Despite a rising temperature the pulse may decrease and Faget's sign, a falling pulse with a constant temperature or a constant pulse with a rising temperature, is present.

Period of calm

A short period of calm follows the initial fever and in milder cases recovery may take place. This period lasts several hours to a day.

Period of recrudescence

Viraemia is now absent and antibodies appear. The fever returns and the patient's condition deteriorates rapidly. Hepatorenal failure develops. The abdominal pain continues and the patient vomits altered blood ('coffee-ground' or 'black vomit') or fresh blood. There is melaena and diarrhoea may be present with fresh blood in the stools. Bleeding may take place from eyes, nose, mouth, bladder, rectum and other organs.

Hepatic involvement

Jaundice becomes evident (but is never so deep as in relapsing fever or hepatitis) and the liver function tests deteriorate. There is no splenic enlargement.

Renal involvement

There is a heavy proteinuria with a tendency to suppression of urine and granular casts and haemoglobin can be found in the urine with azotaemia.

Myocardial involvement

There can be hypotension and hypokinetic heart failure, and ST segmental changes are commonly seen in the electrocardiogram. The patient may recover rapidly after a period of 3–4 days, or recovery may take over 2 weeks. Death occurs on the seventh to tenth day of illness. Bad prognostic signs are increasing proteinuria, haemorrhages, a rising pulse, hypotension, oliguria and azotaemia.

CNS involvement

Signs that the CNS is affected suggest meningitis or encephalitis and include slurred speech, nystagmus, incoordination of movements with tremor of hands and limbs, and brisk tendon reflexes. There may be convulsions and sudden death. If the patient recovers from a severe attack convalescence tends to be long but usually without sequelae. Late deaths after convalescence are very rare and are related to myocardial damage, cardiac arrhythmia or cardiac failure. Suppurative parotitis and bacterial pneumonia may complicate the disease.

Laboratory findings

There is a leucopenia with thrombocytopenia and prolonged clotting and prothrombin times.

Liver. Liver enzymes (SGOT, SGPT) are elevated in jaundiced patients (but not in non-jaundiced patients) and peak between the fifth and tenth day, returning to normal by the tenth to twentieth day. There may be hypoglycaemia associated with severe liver damage.

Renal. At first the urine contains a small amount of albumin, which increases on the fourth or fifth day reaching levels of 3–5 g/litre. There is biliuria.

CNS. The CSF is clear without cells but may be under increased pressure with slightly elevated protein.

DIAGNOSIS

The diagnosis has to be made from other haemorrhagic fevers without jaundice (Lassa, Ebola, Marburg, Junin, Machupo) and with jaundice from Rift Valley fever. Other conditions which must be distinguished are falciparum malaria, louse-borne relapsing fever, infectious hepatitis and leptospirosis. A dictum worth remembering is that an epidemic of a fatal disease in which jaundice is so noteworthy as to be remarked upon is *not* one of YF but is more likely to be relapsing fever or infectious hepatitis. Fever and heavy proteinuria is suggestive. Virus can be isolated from the blood in the first 3 days, with detection of virus by ELISA.

Serological diagnosis

IFA, HI and N antibodies appear within 1 week of onset and CF antibodies later. Paired acute and convalescent sera showing a rising titre are diagnostic. There are cross-reactions with other flaviviruses but N antibodies are specific. Background immunity in tropical populations can render serodiagnosis difficult.

Liver biopsy

Formerly, the presence of Councilman bodies in a liver biopsy was considered specific for YF but their presence in other VHFs, such as Rift Valley fever, makes this no longer certain.

MANAGEMENT AND TREATMENT

The only isolation necessary is from mosquito bites and the patients should be nursed in a screened environment. Blood is infectious in the first 3 days. Treatment is as for other VHFs (see p. 630).

EPIDEMIOLOGY

There are two cycles: the forest cycle (jungle yellow fever) and the urban cycle (urban yellow fever) (see Table 30.1 and Appendix IV).

Forest cycle (jungle yellow fever)

America

YF virus is maintained probably in rodents (experimental infections have been recorded in the spiny rat *Proechimys dimidiatus* and *Heteromys* with persistent viraemia), maintained by *Haemagogus* mosquitoes as the principal vector. Recurrent epizootics occur in howler (*Alouatta*) monkeys who die in large numbers, starting in Panama and spreading up the east coast of Central America to Guatemala, confirming the belief recorded by Balfour in 1914 that a 'silent forest' where all the howler monkeys had died denoted the presence of YF.

Africa

In the forests of West, Central and East Africa a jungle cycle exists as an inapparent infection in monkeys, mainly *Cercopithecus* (vervet) monkeys. Other susceptible primates with inapparent infections include colobus (important in Ethiopia), mangabeys (*Cercocebus*) and baboons (*Papio*). In East Africa some species of bushbaby (*Galago*) which are susceptible to the virus have been shown to possess antibodies in nature, suggesting that the virus may circulate in these nocturnal animals transmitted by other ectoparasites, and passed on to susceptible primates and thence to man.[37]

Human infection

Human infection occurs because of ecological changes created by man: in Africa, by cutting down the forest and planting banana plantations, bringing monkeys into contact with *Ae. simpsoni*, a plant axil breeder which passes the infection on to man. In the Americas humans contract the disease by engaging in woodcutting, and *Haemagogus* mosquitoes bite in and around houses in forest clearings. *Sabethes* (a drought-resistant mosquito) transmits infection during the dry season (see Appendix IV).

An endemic area population will show a rising percentage of positive antibody tests with age, whereas an epidemic situation will be shown by antibodies in the older age and none in the younger age groups.

Urban cycle (urban yellow fever)

When there is a high population of *Ae. aegypti*, intense transmission among humans occurs, with large epidemics where there are enough non-immunes in the population, which can be brought about by immigration, or a rising number of people born since the last epidemic. Up the early years of this century huge epidemics of this nature frequently spread throughout the Caribbean and up the east coast of North America. These epidemics of 'yellow jack' terrified the inhabitants. Similar epidemics occurred in the 'White Man's Grave' in West Africa. Once *Ae. aegypti* was controlled these epidemics became a thing of the past and no urban cases of YF have been described from the Americas for the past 40 years.

However, *Ae. simpsoni* spreading up wooded valleys in an otherwise deforested environment can come into contact with man, with resulting epidemics. In the Nuba mountains of southern Sudan in 1940 there was an epidemic (17 000 cases, 10% mortality rate) and in south-western Ethiopia along the Omo river in 1960–1962 (15 000–30 000 deaths, mortality rate up to 85%). In 1965–1966 in Senegal there was an epidemic mainly affecting children under 10 years with a mortality rate of 15%. Mass vaccination had been suspended in 1960.

CONTROL

Urban cycle (urban yellow fever)

Eradication and control of *Ae. aegypti* is the key to the prevention of urban YF. This includes an attack on the breeding sites in water containers and tanks and an *Aedes* monitoring system which gives an *Aedes* index of the numbers of *Aedes* mosquitoes. When this reaches a certain height an epidemic can result. In the presence of an epidemic, adult control by 'fogging' of towns and cities with insecticide will bring the epidemic to a halt. *Ae. aegypti* had been eradicated from the USA but has now returned to Louisiana, once a hotbed of YF, in its previous numbers.

VACCINATION

Yellow fever 17D is a safe, live, attenuated vaccine providing a long-lasting immunity. For purposes of certificates 10 years is considered the limit but immunity after 40 years has been documented and it may be lifelong. Vaccination to YF is imperative for travellers to endemic areas and certificates are demanded for travellers from endemic areas to non-infected tropical areas. Immunity develops within 10 days after vaccination. No serious complications have been found. No consequences for the fetus have been recorded but pregnant women should avoid vaccination unless the risk from YF is considered great. Infants under 1 year of age should not be vaccinated unless this is unavoidable because they have a slight risk of developing encephalitis. The vaccine is prepared in chick embryos and persons sensitive to egg protein may have reactions. The French neurotropic vaccine produced in mouse brain, used in parts of Africa, has caused allergic encephalomyelitis among children. A general decline in the incidence of 'jungle' YF has resulted from the mass vaccination programme in Brazil using 17D vaccine.

OMSK HAEMORRHAGIC FEVER (OHF)

GEOGRAPHICAL DISTRIBUTION

OHF occurs in the Omsk area of Siberia.

AETIOLOGY

The virus of OHF is a flavivirus (see Table 30.1) separable into two subgroups: (1) isolated from human blood, and (2) isolated from *Dermacentor marginatus*. The virus can be grown on HeLa cells or chick embryos.

TRANSMISSION

The virus is harboured by ticks—*D. pictus* (*reticulatus*) and *D. marginatus*—with trans-stadial and transovarial transmission. The ticks transmit the infection to man from rodents, mainly musk-rats (see Table 30.1 and Appendix IV). The mechanism of interrodent transmission in nature is not known but mites may transmit the infection between musk-rats and other rodents. Infection by direct contact with musk-rat carcasses and pelts is common, and interhuman transmission occurs. There is some evidence of infection by the respiratory route.

PATHOLOGY

The pathology of fatal cases is that of VHF with haemorrhage in tissues and necrotic areas in the liver. Immunity is antibody mediated; little is known about second attacks.

CLINICAL FEATURES

OHF is essentially a self-limiting acute infection in the majority of cases. Little is known about the occurrence of inapparent infections.

The *incubation period* is 3–7 days.

Symptoms and signs

The onset is abrupt with fever and a papulovesicular eruption on the soft palate followed by haemorrhagic features, epistaxis, melaena and uterine haemorrhage. The fever lasts 5 days and then remits with recovery and there is a leucopenia. Sometimes the fever is biphasic, recurring for 2–3 days. Complete recovery is usual with a fatality of 1–3%. There is no CNS involvement.

DIAGNOSIS

Virus can be isolated from the blood in the febrile period. Serological diagnosis is made by the CF and HI tests.

EPIDEMIOLOGY AND CONTROL

The reservoir of infection is the musk-rat and ticks. Human infection depends upon musk-rat–human contact, which may be via tick or the handling of musk-rat carcasses and pelts. When there is a great mortality of musk-rats then contact is greater and outbreaks occur.

VACCINATION

A formalized mouse brain vaccine has been developed and should be used to protect those at risk, such as trappers and water course workers.

KYASANUR FOREST DISEASE (KFD)

Local synonym: 'Monkey disease'

GEOGRAPHICAL DISTRIBUTION (See Figure 30.14)

KFD was first described in 1957 in the Kyasanur Forest of Mysore (now Karnataka).[38] Small outbreaks occurred in the Shimoga district in 1958–1971 and since 1972 there have been small local outbreaks now invading North Kanara district.

AETIOLOGY

KFD virus is a flavivirus (see Table 30.1) antigenically related to TBE, Langat, OHF and West Nile viruses but there is no cross-immunity. The virus can be grown in suckling mice, hamster or monkey kidney cells or HeLa cells with cytopathic effect.

TRANSMISSION

KFD virus is transmitted by the nymphal stages of ticks which have been infected in the larval stage from a rodent or monkey. The ticks are *Haemaphysalis spinigera*, *H. turturis* and *H. papuana* (*kinneari*). KFD virus is also carried by *Ixodes petauristae* and *I. ceylonensis* and has been recovered from *Dermacentor* nymphs. KFD is not normally transmitted from person to person but the blood is potentially infective up until the twelfth day (see Table 30.1 and Appendix IV).

PATHOLOGY

There are degenerative changes in the large organs. The spleen shows reduction of malpighian corpuscles and erythrophagocytosis. There is focal haemorrhagic bronchopneumonia with focal necrosis of the liver and gastrointestinal tract. The kidneys show acute degeneration of the proximal and collecting tubules. There is no encephalitis (monkeys show encephalitis and anterior horn cell damage).

IMMUNITY

Immunity is antibody mediated. Little is known about immunity to second attacks but monkeys who recover are immune. There is no cross-immunity to other flaviviruses.

CLINICAL FEATURES

Natural history

KFD is a fever with a vesicular eruption on the palate with, in some cases, meningoencephalitis and haemorrhagic manifestations. Complete recovery after a long convalescence is usual in all except the 5% of cases who die. Little is known about inapparent infection but antibodies to KFD virus have been found in man and domestic animals in Kutch in north-west India.

Symptoms and signs

The *incubation period* is from 3 to 8 days after the infective tick bite. In about 20% of cases the disease is biphasic.

First phase

The onset is sudden with malaise and fever up to 40°C by the third or fourth day. Severe conjunctivitis is a feature, with a papular or vesicular eruption on the palate. There is vomiting, diarrhoea and dehydration. Myalgia in the back and calf muscles is severe. There is a general lymphadenopathy in most cases, with cervical, axillary and, more rarely, epitrochlear in others. The liver may be enlarged with raised SGOT and SGPT levels but jaundice does not occur. In the majority of cases there are no haemorrhages but gastrointestinal bleeding and haemoptysis may occur. Hypotension and bradycardia are found from the ninth day, lasting a week, and after 10 days the illness subsides.

Second phase

In 20% of cases, 1–2 weeks after the first phase the fever returns, lasting 1–7 days. There may now be symptoms of meningoencephalitis, with neck stiffness, mental disturbance, tremors and giddiness, lasting until the fever subsides. After recovery there is a prolonged convalescence, the patient remaining weak for some time. There is a marked leucopenia and a heavy albuminuria with casts in the urine. The CSF is normal in the first phase but shows increased protein but without cells in the second phase.

DIAGNOSIS

KFD most closely resembles YF, from which it can be distinguished by the geographical distribution (see Figure 30.14) (although at first KFD was thought to be YF) so an accurate travel history is important. Virus can be isolated from the blood up until the 12th day in suckling mice or tissue culture, with rising antibody (IFA, HI and N) titres in acute and convalescent sera.

TREATMENT

Patients must be cared for in a tick-free environment and care taken in the first 12 days to avoid contamination of medical and nursing staff with blood. The treatment is as for other VHFs (see p. 630).

EPIDEMIOLOGY

KFD virus circulates in forest rodents, especially the shrew (*Suncus murinus*) but also *Rattus wroughtoni*, *R. blandfordi* and a squirrel (*Funambulus tristriatus*), maintained by larval ticks of *Haemaphysalis spinigera*, *H. turturis* and *H. papuana* (*kinneari*).

Monkeys (langur) (*Presbytes entellus*) and bonnet macaque (*Macaca radiata*) pick up larval ticks when foraging on the ground and become infected. Many die but some recover and are immune for life. When infected the monkeys show a heavy viraemia. The larvae emerge from the ground as nymphs and come into contact with man, to whom they transmit the infection as a dead-end infection.

Birds (grey jungle fowl and golden-backed woodpecker) are important because they carry adult ticks around and spread the infection; although antibodies have been found in some, they are not thought to play any role in maintaining the infection in nature.

Amplifying mechanism[38]

Under natural conditions the contact of man and monkey with ticks is low and to raise the number of ticks to epizootic levels it is necessary to increase their numbers and the rate of infection. Monkeys provide an efficient source of infection because of their heavy viraemia, and the number of ticks is increased by man's activity in bringing cattle into the forest where they provide a good source of food for *Haemaphysalis* ticks, thus increasing their numbers. The monkeys move around the forest forming foci of infection. KFD has spread since man invaded the forest for rice cultivation, timber extraction and cattle ranching. The cut-down forest forms an interface of lantana thicket in which many species of birds nest and which is crossed by innumerable trails used by cattle, deer, ground birds and small mammals. Infection of man is basically an occupational disease contracted by males who enter the forest, and is preceded by illness and death in langur and macaque monkeys.

CONTROL

Control is essentially a breaking of the tick–man contact. Alteration of the environment and keeping cattle out of the forest are important. Personal protection involves regular (daily) deticking of the body and repellents. A formalized vaccine has shown promising results.

Special care must be taken in undertaking post-mortems on dead monkeys found in the forest.

CRIMEAN–CONGO HAEMORRHAGIC FEVER (C–CHF)

GEOGRAPHICAL DISTRIBUTION

C–CHF is found widely in Africa, Asia, the former USSR, eastern Europe, the Middle East, Iran and Pakistan.

AETIOLOGY

The virus causing C–CHF is in the Crimean–Congo group of bunyaviruses (see Table 30.1).

TRANSMISSION

Transmission is by ixodid ticks of the genus *Hyalomma*, in which the virus survives by trans-stadial and transovarian transmission (see Table 30.1 and Appendix IV). Transmission is also possible by infected blood in a hospital setting or as an epidemic in an endemic area, when the exact method is not known but may be by aerosol spread.

PATHOLOGY

The pathology is that of a VHF with haemorrhagic and liver lesions.

In the *liver* there is a mid-zonal necrosis with Councilman bodies, and in the *spleen*, lymphocyte depletion, necrosis of pulp, haemorrhage in kidney and other organs.

IMMUNITY

Immunity is antibody mediated. Little is known about second attacks.

CLINICAL FEATURES

The disease is an acute, self-limiting infection except under epidemic conditions, when the mortality may be high (30–50%). Mild and inapparent infections occur.

Symptoms and signs

The *incubation period* is 3–6 days, followed by sudden onset of fever, headache, chills, myalgia and vomiting. There is a fine petechial rash and haemorrhage on the soft palate. In more than 25% of cases severe haemorrhage on the fourth or fifth day is a feature and collapse is common. The fatality rate varies from 15% in sporadic cases to 70% in epidemics. There is a leucopenia and thrombocytopenia and occasional liver involvement. CNS complications do not occur. In Africa the haemorrhagic syndrome and death are rare.

DIAGNOSIS

The virus can be isolated from the blood during the febrile period and antibodies measured by serological methods—CF, IH and IFAT. Failure to isolate virus from the blood in 7 days or detect antibody by the 20th day rules out the diagnosis of C–CHF.

TREATMENT

Patients must be nursed in strict isolation (see p. 630) under negative pressure or in a sealed tent isolator because medical and nursing staff are susceptible to aerosol spread and blood is infectious during the febrile period. When facilities do not allow this, strict barrier nursing should be enforced and staff should wear gloves and masks.

EPIDEMIOLOGY AND CONTROL

The C–CHF virus circulates between symptomatic wild and domestic animals (sheep, goats, cattle, hares) and is transmitted to man by a *Hyalomma* tick bite. Sporadic cases occur in animal herds and small epidemics occur with interhuman spread. Secondary cases in hospital workers occur from contact with infected blood and tissues. No vaccine is yet available.

MUROID VIRUS NEPHROPATHY (MVN)[39]

Synonyms. Korean haemorrhagic fever (HFRS), epidemic haemorrhagic fever with renal symptoms (HFRS), haemorrhagic nephrosonephritis (HNN). In 1993 a new syndrome, Hantavirus pulmonary syndrome, was recognized in the south-western USA.

AETIOLOGY

The MVN virus is a member of the Uukuvirus group of bunyaviruses (see Table 30.1).[40] It is 80–115 nm in diameter. There are four antigenically distinct groups,[41] each associated with a different rodent species: *Apodemus* (field mouse) (Hantaan virus),

Clethrionomys (vole) (Puumala virus), rats from Korea, Japan and the USA, and *Microtus* from the USA.

GEOGRAPHICAL DISTRIBUTION

The four antigenically distinct viruses have a world-wide distribution in China, Kenya, Japan (Hantaan virus), north-eastern Asia, Scandinavia, the Balkans, Belgium and France (Puumala virus) and *Microtus*-derived virus in Alaska, eastern USA, Bolivia and India.

TRANSMISSION

No case-to-case spread has yet been recorded in man and transmission of the virus is from chronically infected rodents, which excrete virus in saliva and faeces for a month and in urine for at least 2 years, to man. The greatest concentration is in rodent lungs and human infection is probably contracted by the aerosol route, or an environment contaminated with rodent urine, and occasionally by rodent bite.[42]

PATHOLOGY[43]

The pathogenesis of MVN is of immunological origin rather than a direct viral destructive process. Viral antigen combines with viral antibody to form complexes which trigger the classic complement pathway, with destruction of platelets, activation of the coagulation and fibrinolytic systems with severe renal damage (tubular and glomerular necrosis). The vascular endothelium is a primary target of the virus and there is severe vascular damage with capillary engorgement, leakage of red cells and interstitial and retroperitoneal oedema with little or no cellular response.

The kidney shows severe renal damage with homogeneous eosinophilic tubular deposits.

IMMUNITY

Immunity is antibody mediated and the majority of infections recover with complete immunity to reinfection. Most infections are mild or inapparent.

CLINICAL FEATURES

Natural history

The majority of cases develop a mild fever without nephropathy or haemorrhagic symptoms, with complete recovery. Most cases of infection are inappar-

ent. In some cases, especially the Far Eastern form, there is severe illness with haemorrhagic and renal symptoms with a 5–20% mortality.

Incubation period

The incubation period is about 14–20 days, as measured from a rodent bite.[42]

Symptoms and signs

The illness may be so mild as to make diagnosis difficult but all patients have proteinuria and azotaemia and there is an erythematous rash which sometimes becomes petechial. One-fifth of the Far Eastern cases show severe features with shock, haemorrhage and gross fluid and electrolyte imbalance. The course of the disease may be divided into five phases.

1 *Febrile phase (days 1–4)*. The onset is abrupt with retro-orbital headache, eye pain, photophobia and mild myalgia. Gastrointestinal symptoms (abdominal pain, nausea and vomiting) are common. There is typically an erythematous rash which may become petechial on the face, neck, shoulders and upper thorax.
2 *Hypotensive phase (days 5–8)*. This starts about the fifth day of illness with marked proteinuria, haemoconcentration, hypotension and occasionally shock.
3 *Oliguric phase (days 9–11)*. This starts about the ninth day with decreased urinary output and signs of renal failure. Haemorrhagic manifestations appear with haematuria. Serious haemorrhage is unusual, but may take the form of haematemesis, melaena and cerebrovascular complications.
4 *Diuretic phase (days 12–14)*. The patient improves with diuresis.
5 *Convalescent phase (15th day onwards)*. This phase is protracted, lasting up to 4 months. Sequelae are rare, except those resulting from CNS complications.

DIFFERENTIAL DIAGNOSIS

This includes leptospirosis (more severe muscle pain and jaundice), typhus, relapsing fever, acute nephritis, JE, TBE, other haemorrhagic fevers (Crimean–Congo and Omsk), plague and scurvy.

DIAGNOSIS

There is an initial leucocytosis followed in the haemorrhagic phase by leucopenia and thrombocytopenia.

Serodiagnosis is the diagnostic tool.

Immunofluorescent IgM antibodies appear very early by the fifth to seventh day of illness, specific titres rising to 1/64, to fall after 6–8 weeks. Other fluorescent IgG and neutralizing antibodies persist at high titre for more than three decades.

TREATMENT

The patient must be nursed in strict isolation (see p. 000) until convalescence. Aerosol and blood contamination of medical attendants must be avoided. In the first stages acute shock requires careful fluid balance and albumin infusions; during the haemorrhagic phase sedation and replacement of blood products; and during the renal phase careful fluid balance and electrolyte adjustment with dialysis in the most severe cases.

EPIDEMIOLOGY

There are three epidemiological types of infection, rural, urban and laboratory acquired, which are determined by the host species of the virus concerned.

Rural

The rural disease is widespread and patchy in the northern hemisphere. There are two types: the severe Far Eastern (Hantaan virus) associated with *Apodemus* (field mouse), and the mild northeastern European (Puumala virus) associated with *Clethrionomys* (vole). The reservoir rodents live in fields but invade houses at the beginning of winter, causing peaks of disease in spring and autumn. Epidemics arise during war (especially trench warfare) and many outbreaks have occurred in the past. In the Far East endemic disease is considerable in poor countries.

Urban

The urban form, which is caused by house rats, is a mild disease of major importance in China.

Laboratory

Infections are acquired from laboratory rat colonies and are usually mild.

CONTROL

Prevention of contact between the human population and rodents depends on improvement in living conditions. No vaccine is yet available but vaccination of targeted populations such as agricultural workers could achieve some control.

ALTAMIRA HAEMORRHAGIC FEVER

In January 1972, 22 cases of a haemorrhagic syndrome involving the skin and in some cases the mucous membranes, with melaena and bleeding from the gums and nose, occurred among some 7000 recent settlers in the Altamira region on the Trans-Amazon highway in Brazil (Altamira haemorrhagic syndrome). A further 70 cases were identified later in a larger population. Several deaths were attributed to the disease. The condition was first diagnosed as thrombocytopenic purpura; the platelet counts were very low. Attempts to isolate bacteria or a virus failed and the cause remains unknown, but it appears to have affected only recent immigrants and to be related to the abundance of black flies (Simuliidae) in the rainy season. It has been suggested that the syndrome is a hypersensitivity reaction to the bites of these flies.[44]

ARENAVIRUSES[45]

Arenaviruses are a group, numbering 14 at present, of single-stranded RNA viruses 50–500 nm (110–130 nm mean) in diameter with a lipid membranous envelope, with projections on the surface and granules (arenaceus = sandy) inside the virion, all sharing certain antigenic components. They all can cause acute or persistent infections of rodents. Only five—lymphocytic choriomeningitis (LCM), Lassa, Junin, Machupo and Guanarito—are human pathogens. The remaining nine are Mozambique (Mopeia) and Acar from the Old World, and Tacaribe, Amapari, Flexal, Pichende, Latino, Parana and Tamiami from the New World. Tacaribe virus has been isolated from bats and mosquitoes in Trinidad; Pichiende has

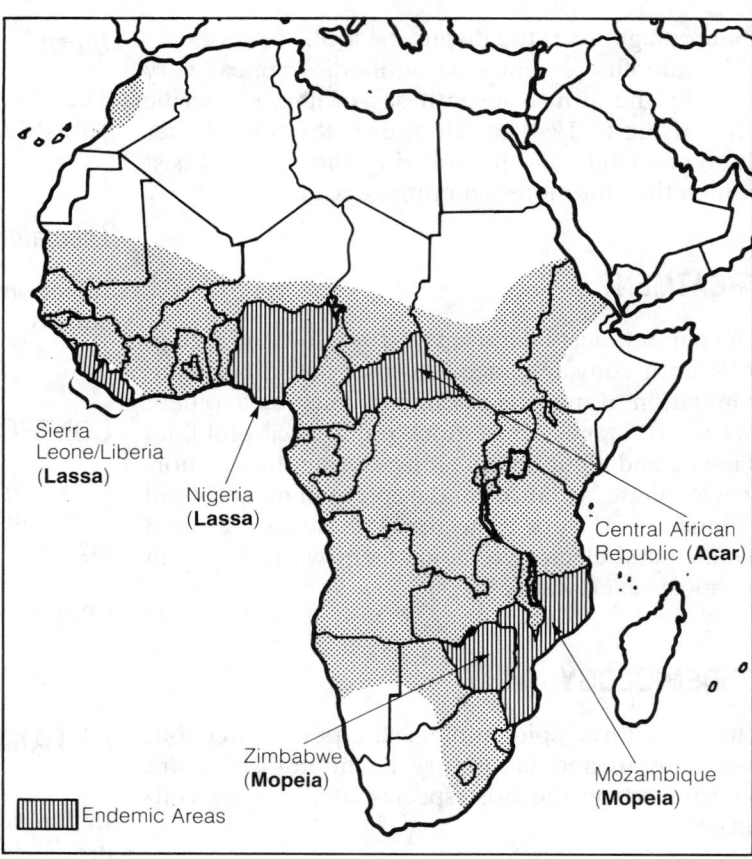

Figure 30.10 Geographical locations of Lassa and related viruses from Africa. The stippled area represents the distribution of the single major rodent host (*Mastomys* (*Praomys*) *natalensis*) in this continent. (Reproduced from Howard and Young.[38])

been isolated from haemolytic anuric disease in children and healthy adults in Brazil. Lassa, Junin, Machupo and Guanarito are conveyed to man by contact with rodent excreta (see Figures 30.10 and 30.11).

LASSA FEVER[46] (See also Chapter 38)

GEOGRAPHICAL DISTRIBUTION (Figure 30.10)

Lassa fever is confined to West Africa, from where it was first described in Lassa, northern Nigeria, and Central Africa. Small outbreaks have occurred in Zorzor, Liberia, Panguma Tongo in Sierra Leone, and cases have occurred in various parts of Nigeria.

Serological evidence of human infection has been found in Guinea, Senegal, Mali and Zaire. It has been shown[47,48] in Sierra Leone and Nigeria that the infection occurs widely in communities as a minor illness or inapparent infection. Recent estimates suggest that there are 100 000 cases annually with 5000 fatalities.[49]

AETIOLOGY

Lassa fever is an arenavirus which grows readily on Vero cells with cytopathic effect. Strains of virus from Sierra Leone, Liberia, Nigeria, the Central African Republic, Mozambique and Zimbabwe are serologically distinct.[50]

TRANSMISSION

Lassa fever virus is basically an inapparent infection of the multimammate mouse (rat) (*Mastomys natalensis*), from which infection spreads to man by direct contact in households, or indirect contact via food or water contaminated by rodent urine. The virus is not transmissible by aerosol in the hospital or laboratory. Nosocomial transmission occurs in a hospital setting by direct and indirect contact via blood and fomites. There is no evidence of transmission by ectoparasites or any insect.

PATHOLOGY[51]

The mechanism of the pathological changes is the same as that of other VHFs, with formation of antigen–antibody complexes as well as a direct effect of the virus on capillaries causing an increase in permeability. In the *liver* there is a widespread parenchymal focal eosinophilic necrosis of hepatic cells with the presence of eosinophilic bodies resembling Councilman bodies but there is no zonal pattern of necrosis (unlike YF and RVF). The *spleen* shows lymphoid depletion with areas of eosinophilic necrosis; the *lungs* show pleural and peritoneal effusions and focal patches of pneumonitis; and the *kidneys* focal necrosis of renal tubules. There are interstitial haemorrhages in other organs, heart and renal medulla. The *CNS* shows meningoencephalitis with oedema, congestion, neuronophagia and perivascular cuffing.[52]

IMMUNITY

Immunity is antibody mediated and little is known about second attacks. Inapparent infections are the rule and may protect against severe infections.

CLINICAL FEATURES[53]

Natural history

The majority of infections take their natural course with complete recovery without sequelae. In others, a minority, there is a severe deterioration in condition after the first week, with death from haemorrhagic shock. In these cases mortality rates vary from 30% in Nigeria, 20% in Sierra Leone to 14% in Liberia.

The *incubation period* is 3–16 days, generally 7–10 days.

Symptoms and signs

The *onset* is insidious with fever which lasts 7–17 days, and malaise and pain in limb muscles. On the seventh day in severe cases there is a sudden deterioration with a severe fall in blood pressure. There is vomiting, sore throat, continuous troublesome cough with chest pains, headache and diarrhoea. The pharynx is inflamed with characteristic white or yellow patches on the tonsils and there may be ulcers, with characteristic oedema of eyelids and face (an important physical sign, caused by increased capillary permeability). Occasionally there is a maculopapular rash. The blood pressure is low with a bradycardia. There is a leucopenia with albuminuria and casts in the urine. Death occurs from shock, hypotension, peripheral vasoconstriction, hypovolaemia and anuria. There are no clinical signs of meningoencephalitis.

Convalescence is from the second to fourth week with extreme weakness for several weeks and alopecia, which recovers. Deafness (20% of cases) is usually reversible but may be permanent.

DIFFERENTIAL DIAGNOSIS

At onset, Lassa fever is almost indistinguishable from other acute fevers: falciparum malaria, other VHFs, meningococcaemia and septicaemia.

The characteristic pharyngitis with white tonsillar patches and facial oedema are important distinguishing features.

DIAGNOSIS[54]

A detailed travel history is all important. Laboratory diagnosis must be undertaken with precautions as for dangerous category 4 pathogens (see p. 000). Viraemia persists well into the second week and in the urine in convalescence (up to 63 days). Isolation from the blood on Vero cell cultures can give a diagnosis within 72 hours. The IFAT test will show antibodies by the second week, and an ELISA test is now available for the detection of both antigen and antibody allowing for early diagnosis before the development of antibody.[55] Isolation from pharyngeal secretions and from urine is also possible.

TREATMENT[56]

Treatment is as for VHF (see p. 630): in isolation with strict barrier nursing and with special care taken about fomites and blood and urine specimens.

Immune convalescent serum with high antibody content has been used and should be given on or before the tenth day, when the treatment is very successful.[57] Possible dangers, such as infection of non-Lassa patients with the serum, and the formation of antigen–antibody complexes are not met with in practice.[55] It is important that convalescent serum is obtained late in convalescence, 90–180 days after onset of illness, and it should match the strain of the virus.

Chemotherapy

Effective therapy with ribavirin has now been demonstrated.[58]

EPIDEMIOLOGY

The virus has been repeatedly isolated from the multimammate mouse (rat) (*Mastomys natalensis*), which is spread throughout the whole of Africa south of the Sahara. In this rodent the virus causes a chronic inapparent infection with persistent viraemia and viruria. With increasing man–rodent contact from grain stores in houses, direct and indirect infection of man occurs from food contaminated by rodent excreta or aerosol inhalation from rodent urine. Direct man-to-man spread is only found in a hospital environment where, although secondary cases are common, tertiary cases are very rare. One case of Lassa fever entering a non-endemic area should not arouse the fear of an epidemic.

CONTROL

Rodent control and decreasing man–rodent contact are the methods used. A vaccine is not yet available but the possibilities have been discussed by Clegg.[49] Surveillance of case contacts should be carried out for 21 days and any contacts developing fever isolated. Special care must be undertaken with laboratory specimens.

JUNIN VIRUS (ARGENTINIAN HAEMORRHAGIC FEVER—AHF)

GEOGRAPHICAL DISTRIBUTION

The endemic–epidemic area is 100 000 km² in the pampas north-west of Buenos Aires which has a population of one million people (Figure 30.11).

AETIOLOGY

Junin virus can be grown on HeLa cells with a cytopathic effect or in suckling mice, and cross-reacts with Machupo virus.

TRANSMISSION

Junin virus causes a chronic infection of the rodents *Calomys musculinus* and *Calomys laucha*, in which it maintains persistent viraemia and viruria with virus in the saliva. The virus is transmitted to man by direct contact with rodents or indirectly from contaminated food. Direct person-to-person transmission is very rare.

PATHOLOGY

There is no evidence of any immunopathological process playing a part in the pathology. The virus enters the body by the alimentary or respiratory tract and collects in local lymph glands, where it multiplies, invading the reticuloendothelial system including immunocompetent cells, thus impairing the host's immune response. The virus causes capillary damage with haemorrhagic and hypovolaemic shock. There is lymphadenopathy and focal haemorrhages in many organs, especially the brain, endothelial swelling in capillaries and arterioles, focal non-zonal necrosis of the liver and renal tubular necrosis. There is some evidence of disseminated intravascular coagulation.

IMMUNITY

Immunity is antibody mediated and little is known about second attacks.

CLINICAL FEATURES[59]

Natural history

Infection of man causes severe disease, with a high mortality and death between the eighth and tenth day in many infections. Inapparent infection does not occur.

Symptoms and signs

The *incubation period* is 8–12 days.

There is a slow, insidious onset with chills, headache, myalgia, retro-orbital pain and nausea. This is followed by fever, conjunctival injection, oedema of face, neck and upper thorax with a petechial rash in the axilla and generalized lymphadenopathy. On the sixth to eighth day there is a sudden deterioration, with haemorrhage, haematemesis, melaena, haematuria and oliguria proceeding to anuria. Pronounced *neurological* disturbances occur, with tremors, psychic changes and coma. Death is caused by hypovolaemic shock. There is a heavy albuminuria with leucopenia, thrombocytopenia and altered clotting factors. Patients who recover do so when the fever falls, and there is a prolonged convalescence with alopecia. Relapse may occur.

DIAGNOSIS

Virus can be isolated from the blood during the acute febrile period. Viral antigen can be identified

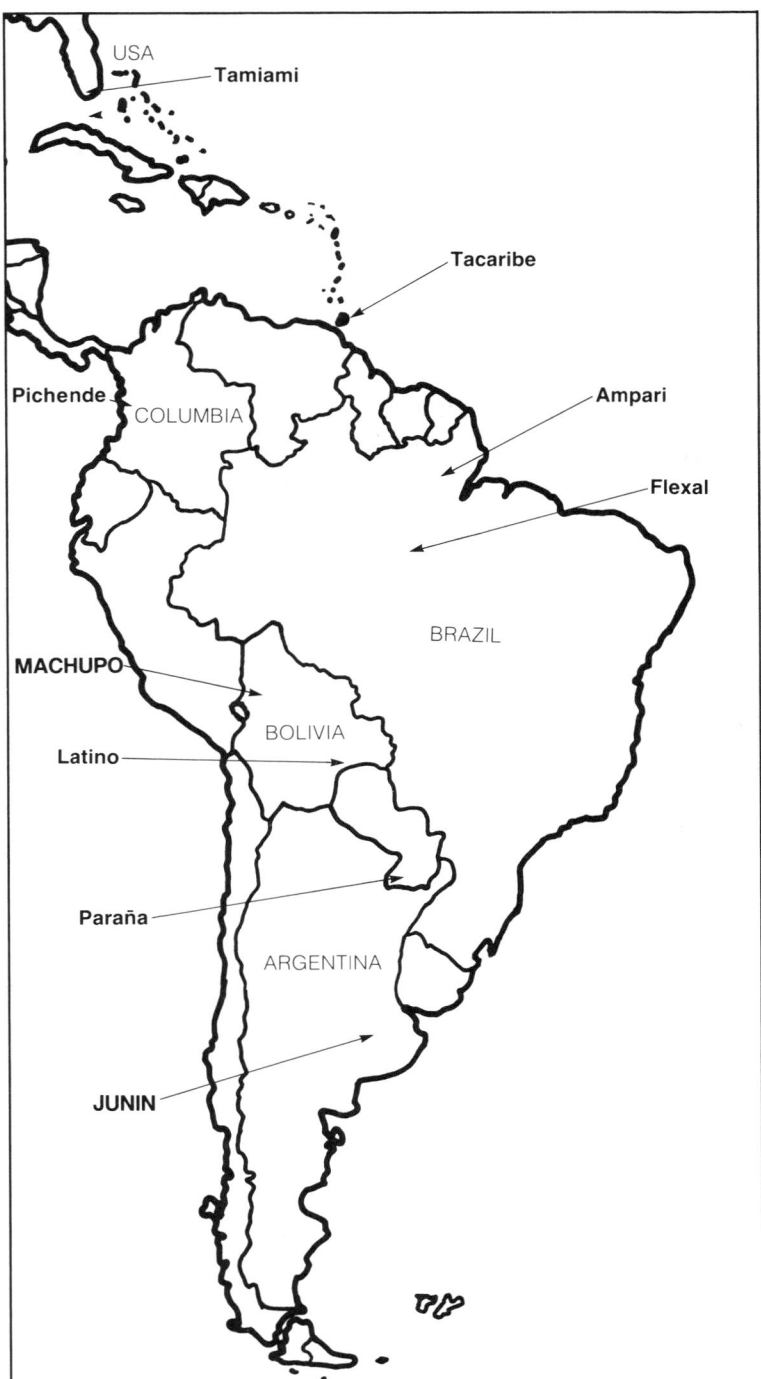

Figure 30.11 Geographical locations of arenavirus isolates in the New World that are serologically defined as being members of the Tacaribe complex. (Reproduced from Howard and Young.[38])

in cells with specific immune serum. IFA tests on acute and convalescent sera can clinch the diagnosis.

TREATMENT (see p. 630)

Immune plasma, provided it is given within 8 days of onset, is helpful. A complication is a benign febrile encephalitis 4–6 weeks after the onset of infection.

EPIDEMIOLOGY

The two main reservoir hosts *Calomys laucha* and *Calomys musculinus* live and breed in maize fields and the surrounding banks. The disease is occupational and is prevalent in rural workers (four males to one female). It occurs mainly in May when the maize is being harvested, at which time there is a great increase in rodents and male harvesters. AHF has occurred in quite large epidemics and between 1958 and 1974 there were 16 000 cases notified.

CONTROL

The methods are control of rodents by trapping and rodenticides and reducing man–rodent contact by mechanization of harvesting. Two types of vaccine are under trial—a formalized mouse brain vaccine and an attenuated (live) vaccine.

MACHUPO VIRUS (BOLIVIAN HAEMORRHAGIC FEVER)

GEOGRAPHICAL DISTRIBUTION

Rural area in north-east Bolivia (Figure 30.11).

AETIOLOGY

Machupo virus is similar to Junin and Lassa fever viruses.

TRANSMISSION

The natural reservoir is the rodent *Calomys callosus*, in which it causes a chronic infection with persistent viraemia and viruria. Transmission to man is by contamination of food and water by direct contact through skin abrasions. Man-to-man transmission is almost unknown, except on one occasion in a non-endemic area where the index case caused five secondary cases, with four deaths.

PATHOLOGY

These is congestion and interstitial haemorrhages in the gastrointestinal tract and CNS. Eosinophilic inclusion bodies are found in the Kupffer's cells of the liver. There is an interstitial pneumonia in all cases.

SYMPTOMS AND SIGNS[60]

There are almost identical to AHF.

The *incubation period* is 7–14 days.

The onset is insidious, with fever, conjunctival injection and flushing of the face and neck. The disease is not so severe as AHF and many recover. In those who do not, on the sixth to tenth day there is a sudden deterioration with collapse and hypovolaemia. Haemorrhagic manifestations (30%) and neurological disturbances (50%) may occur. There is leucopenia and thrombocytopenia. This stage lasts 2–4 days and may be followed by recovery. The acute phase, which lasts 2–3 weeks, is followed by a prolonged convalescence with generalized weakness and alopecia. Inapparent infection is very rare. Relapses may occur.

EPIDEMIOLOGY

First recognized in 1959 in the Beni region of north-east Bolivia, it is an urban disease. The first epidemic devastated and caused the abandonment of a village. The natural reservoir, *Calomys callosus*, is found throughout the grasslands but invades houses in small towns and comes into intimate contact with man, infecting him indirectly from a chronic viraemia and viruria. The disease reaches its maximum during the dry season, April to September; adult males are the most affected.

CONTROL

Rodent control (cats and traps) in town can stop the epidemics but can do nothing about the rural rodents, which are extending the endemic–epidemic area.

FILOVIRUSES (MARBURG AND EBOLA VIRUSES) (See also Chapter 3)

Marburg and Ebola viruses are very similar in morphology but are antigenically distinct. They share no antigens with any other viruses and are classified separately as filoviruses. Virus particles are pleomorphic and appear as long filamentous U- or S-shaped particles, 2 nm long × 70–80 nm in diameter, or as circular bodies composed of an internal structure and a surface layer with numerous spikes. Multiplication is by budding from this structure. For virological studies see Johnson et al,[61] Bowen et al[62] and Pattyn et al.[63]

EBOLA VIRUS DISEASE[64]

GEOGRAPHICAL DISTRIBUTION

The disease first appeared in 1976 in the equatorial provinces of southern Sudan and northern Zaire. Epidemics have occurred and sporadic cases and serological surveys show that Ebola virus is still active in northern Zaire. Considerable alarm was raised in the USA in 1989 when cynomolgus monkeys imported from the Philippines were found to be infected with a strain (Reston) of Ebola. No clinically obvious infections were recorded in man.

AETIOLOGY

Ebola virus, of which there are two biotypes, is the cause. It is closely related but antigenically distinct from Marburg virus.

TRANSMISSION

Transmission is person-to-person by contact with a patient in the acute stage of the disease and by direct contact with blood-contaminated syringes, needles and other fomites. There is no evidence of any animal reservoir or insect vectors.

PATHOLOGY

There is no evidence of any immunological mechanisms at work in the causation of the pathology. The virus is pantropic and invades cells producing necrotic lesions in all organs. The *liver* shows necrosis of single hepatocytes with fatty degeneration and necrosis at the periphery of the lobules. Eosinophilic cytoplasmic inclusions are common. The *spleen* shows atrophy and lymphocyte depletion with plasma cell infiltration. The *kidneys* show glomerular changes and focal tubular necrosis. The *heart* shows interstitial oedema and lymphocytic infiltration, and bone marrow shows degeneration of granulocyte but no change in the red cell precursors.

IMMUNITY

Immunity is antibody mediated and there is no evidence of second attacks. Convalescent serum may help recovery.

CLINICAL FEATURES

Natural history

Most cases who show symptoms proceed inevitably to death but inapparent infection can occur, as shown by serological surveys.

The *incubation period* is 7–14 days.

The onset is sudden, with fever, severe headache, myalgia, abdominal pain and sore throat, with herpetic lesions on the mouth and pharynx. There is severe conjunctival injection and gingival haemorrhages. Diarrhoea, which is a prominent feature, continues until the tenth day and measures the severity of the disease. Bleeding occurs in the majority of cases, appearing towards the end of the fifth day with haematemesis and bloody diarrhoea. On the fifth to seventh day a morbilliform rash (never haemorrhagic) is visible on white but not African skins. Neurological manifestations (hemiplegia and psychosis) are common. Death occurs most commonly on the ninth day, but between the second and twenty-first day. Mortality rates vary from 50–60% in the Sudan to 80% in Zaire. There is a prolonged convalescence. There is a leucopenia at first, with later an increase in granulocytes and the appearance of large cells with dark cytoplasm (virocytes) which are activated lymphocytes and lymphoblasts. Hypoproteinaemia and a raised transaminase level are present with heavy albuminuria.

DIAGNOSIS

Diagnosis is from YF, LF and Marburg as well as other haemorrhagic fevers and a travel history is imperative. Virus can be isolated from blood by inoculation of weanling mice or guinea-pigs and then subinoculated into Vero cells. IFA tests on paired sera show antibodies and distinguish from Marburg disease.

TREATMENT

The cases must be nursed under full VHF precautions (see p. 630). Anti-Ebola convalescent serum may be of help.

EPIDEMIOLOGY

So far there has been no evidence of an animal reservoir. The infection is conveyed from an index case to other persons by communal syringes in Zaire, and is mainly caused by nursing infected cases in a rural hospital environment in Sudan. Droplet infection is not a feature. There is evidence of continuing transmission in northern Zaire.

CONTROL

Cases must be strictly isolated and nursed under conditions for class 4 pathogens. All contact with blood, urine and other excreta must be avoided.

MARBURG VIRUS DISEASE[65]

GEOGRAPHICAL DISTRIBUTION

The original cases came from workers who had handled monkeys from the Kyoga region of Uganda and serological evidence of infection has been found in monkeys in Uganda, baboons in Kenya and three monkey trappers.

AETIOLOGY

Marburg virus is closely related but antigenically distinct from Ebola

TRANSMISSION

The primary infections were infected by handling monkey organs and tissue cultures from vervet monkeys (*Cercopithecus aethiops*), through the intact skin by contact with infected blood. Secondary cases involved medical staff exposed to the index case, from blood and in one case semen (up to 11 weeks later).

CLINICAL FEATURES

These are almost identical to Ebola virus disease. Relapses occur and Marburg virus has been isolated from semen 83 days in one and 60 days in another case after the onset of illness. Uveitis complicated one case[66] and virus was isolated from the anterior chamber of the eye 80 days after onset. In one laboratory infection, recorded by Emond et al,[67] the illness was mild and recovery complete after a long convalescence.

DIAGNOSIS

Diagnosis is by IFA test from Ebola virus.

EPIDEMIOLOGY AND CONTROL

There have been three outbreaks so far: the first in a West German laboratory from handling infected monkeys; a second from a visitor to the Wankie park in Zimbabwe; and a third in a sugar worker in Kenya who infected the doctor who intubated him.[68] There have been 32 cases, with eight deaths. Monkeys are clearly not maintenance hosts since they have fatal infections. No primary host has yet been identified but insect bites have been suggested as a factor.

ARTHROPOD-BORNE ENCEPHALITIDES

Almost all arboviruses are neurotropic in mice and are able to cause encephalitis (Table 30.4) in man, although only a few do so in nature.

Transmission is by mosquito or tick bite, although droplet spread can occur (VEE).

The pathological changes are mostly in the grey matter of the midbrain, basal ganglia, brain stem and cerebellum, where histology shows meningo-encephalitis with mononuclear cell infiltration and perivascular cuffing.

PATHOLOGY IN GENERAL

The virus enters the bloodstream from the insect vector bite and settles in the cells of the reticuloendothelial system where it replicates, causing a fever and a systemic reaction. In the majority of cases the antibody defences of the host eradicate the infection and recovery ensues after a short febrile illness. In some cases the virus enters the nervous system and invades the cells, causing irreversible destruction.

CLINICAL MANIFESTATIONS

The majority of people infected develop a short, sharp febrile attack with complete recovery and immunity to reinfection. In many endemic areas a number of inapparent infections are revealed by serological surveys. In some cases the infection is biphasic and after a short period of recovery the symptoms return and signs of meningoencephalitis appear (excitability, somnolence, coma, delirium,

Table 30.4 Arthropod-borne encephalitis of clinical importance.

Virus	Disease	Hosts	Geographical distribution
Mosquito-borne			
Equine encephalitides			
Alphavirus	Eastern equine encephalitis (EEE)	Wild and domestic birds, spillover to man and equines	USA, Central and South America
	Western equine encephalitis (WEE)	Wild and domestic birds, spillover to equines and man	Western North America
	Venezuelan equine encephalitis (VEE)	Wild forest rodents, spillover to equines and man	South America
Japanese–West Nile complex			
Flavivirus	Japanese encephalitis (JE)	Wild birds and pigs, spillover to man	Asia, Japan, Korea, Taiwan, China, Indo-China, Philippines, Thailand, Bangladesh, eastern and southern India
	St Louis encephalitis (SLE)	Passerine birds, possibly bats, spillover to equines and man	Temperate areas North America, Argentina, Brazil, Surinam, Panama, Trinidad, Jamaica
	Murray Valley encephalitis (MVE)	Birds	Australia, New Guinea
	West Nile virus	Wild birds, spillover to man	Widely distributed in Old World, South Africa and Israel
Bunyaviruses	California encephalitis (CE)		
	La Crosse (LAC)	Wild birds	North America, Canada
Tick-borne			
Flavivirus	Russian spring–summer (RSSE)	Rodents	Eastern Siberia
	European tick-borne encephalitis (TBE)	Rodents, spillover to goats and man	Eastern Europe, Scandinavia
	Powassan		Canada

hyperthermia and epileptiform convulsions). In some cases, especially children, the flaccid paralyses, which may be permanent, develop.

DIAGNOSIS

Virus can be cultivated from the blood in the acute phase and antibody titres are shown to be raised in convalescent sera taken 10–30 days later. A specimen of clotted blood sent on ice to the appropriate laboratory for culture and serology is necessary.

EQUINE ENCEPHALITIDES (ALPHAVIRUS)

Equines (horses and donkeys) are affected in an epizootic preceding an epidemic in man and act as amplifier hosts between the reservoir hosts (birds, rodents) and man.

WESTERN EQUINE ENCEPHALITIS (WEE)

GEOGRAPHICAL DISTRIBUTION (Figure 30.12)

WEE is found in Texas, Colorado, Saskatchewan and in Argentina, Brazil, Mexico and Guyana, where human infections are unknown but equine epizootics occur.

AETIOLOGY

WEE is an RNA virus, 55 nm in diameter, that can be cultured in tissue cultures with a cytopathic effect. Chick embryo fibroblasts are favoured.

TRANSMISSION

Transmission is by mosquitoes. *Culex tarsalis*, which feeds readily on birds, transmits the infection in the western USA, and *Culiseta melanura* in areas where *Culex tarsalis* does not occur (eastern USA) (see Appendix IV).

IMMUNITY

Immunity is antibody mediated and protects against second attacks. Serological surveys show inapparent infections and children are most affected in epidemics.

PATHOLOGY

Pathology in fatal cases is that of a meningoencephalitis.

CLINICAL FEATURES

The majority of infections are inapparent and most overt cases in adults recover without any sequelae but 50% of young children develop neurological complications with some permanent neurological changes. Mortality rate is 10%.

Symptoms and signs

The *incubation period* is 5–10 days.

The onset is gradual, with mild fever, malaise, headache, stiff neck and drowsiness. In the minority of severe cases the fever increases, with signs of CNS involvement, somnolence, coma, flaccid and spastic paralyses which recover. There is a leucocytosis in the early stages and the CSF shows a pleocytosis with increased protein in those with CNS involvement.

DIAGNOSIS

Viral isolation in acute phase, with CF and HI tests on convalescent sera.

EPIDEMIOLOGY

WEE virus circulates in more than 75 species of wild birds and some domestic ones. The basic transmission cycle is between *Culex tarsalis* and birds in the summer. Over-wintering of the virus may be in hibernating mammals but more likely in overwintering mosquitoes. Epizootics in horses acting as amplifying hosts precede human epidemics. In man the highest attack rates are in infants and young males in a rural environment.

CONTROL

Antimosquito measures are difficult in rural areas but where small towns are involved 'fogging' from the air with insecticide may terminate an epidemic. A non-neurotropic strain of virus isolated from birds has been used successfully as a vaccine but only experimentally.

EASTERN EQUINE ENCEPHALITIS (EEE)

GEOGRAPHICAL DISTRIBUTION (Figure 30.12)

EEE is found in the eastern USA (where epizootics occur in horses but human cases are rare), Mexico, Panama, Brazil, Argentina and Guyana. Two small human outbreaks have occurred in Dominica and Jamaica, and in 1962 there was a major epidemic of 6762 cases in Venezuela; 0.6% were fatal.

AETIOLOGY

EEE virus is 50 nm in diameter and can be cultured in many tissue culture systems. There are two antigenic types, North and South American.

TRANSMISSION

Transmission is by mosquitoes; *Culiseta melanura* and *Culiseta morsitans, Ae. sollicitans* and *Ae. taeniorhynchus* are the main vectors but isolations of

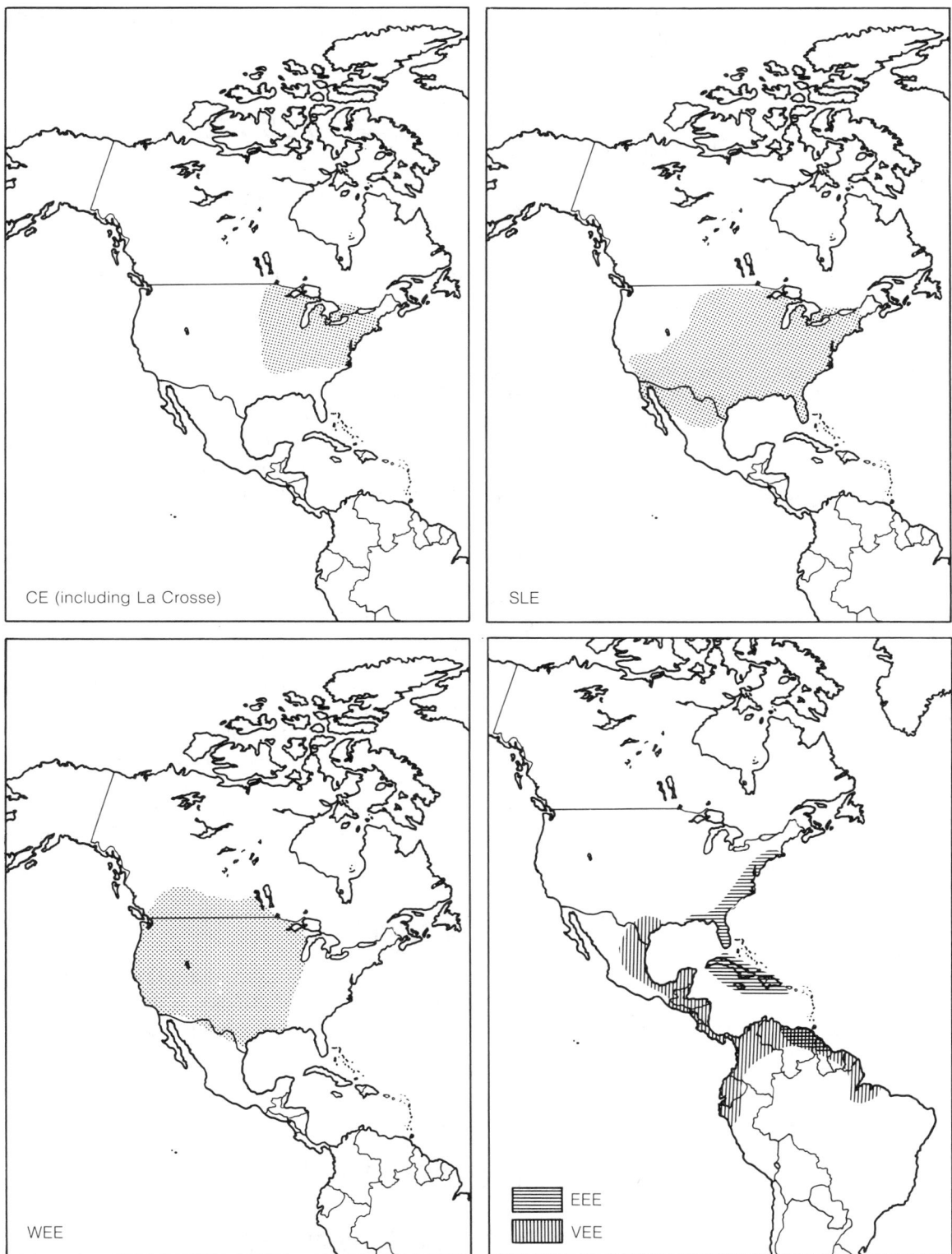

Figure 30.12 Distribution of mosquito-borne encephalitis in the New World. CE, California encephalitis; SLE, St Louis encephalitis; WEE, Western equine encephalitis; EEE, Eastern equine encephalitis; VEE, Venezuelan equine encephalitis. (Courtesy of the Department of Entomology, London School of Hygiene and Tropical Medicine.)

virus have been made from other mosquitoes in the field (see Table 30.1 and Appendix IV).

IMMUNITY

Immunity is antibody mediated and affords protection against second attacks.

SYMPTOMS AND SIGNS

Natural history

EEE is more severe than WEE in both horses and man. Many cases recover after a short febrile attack but in others, chiefly children and young infants, the disease is biphasic and symptoms return with CNS involvement.

The *incubation period* is 7–10 days.

The onset is gradual with fever and meningism which may resolve. However, in young children and infants the disease is biphasic and symptoms return after 1–2 days with the onset of symptoms of encephalitis. There is a leucocytosis with pleocytosis and increased protein in the CSF. Neurological sequelae occur.

EPIDEMIOLOGY

Transmission is maintained by birds and mosquitoes in an extensive geographical area. Infection of horses and man is accidental and in the centre of the area serological evidence of inapparent human infection can be found. EEE may cause a high mortality in birds, both wild and domestic. Infection in horses is severe, most dying within a few days.

CONTROL

Mosquito control is the only method. Vaccination is not yet available

VENEZUELAN EQUINE ENCEPHALITIS (VEE)

GEOGRAPHICAL DISTRIBUTION (Figure 30.12)

Extensive outbreaks with human cases have occurred in Venezuela (100 000 cases in 1962, almost wiping out the equine population), Trinidad, Colombia, Brazil and Panama. The virus is now extending its area and evidence of human infection has been found in Florida.

AETIOLOGY

VEE virus is a round particle 65–80 nm in diameter. It grows in many different cell cultures with cytopathic effect. There are a number of antigenic subtypes.

TRANSMISSION

The main vectors are *Ae. serratus* and *Ae. taeniorhynchus* and culicine species including *Culex fatigans*. Isolations have been made from about 40 other species (see Table 30.1 and Appendix IV). *Simulium* may transmit infections and there is a possibility of man-to-man spread by droplet infection, and spread among horses can occur without an insect vector.

IMMUNITY

Immunity is antibody mediated and provides protection against second attacks. It therefore takes about 10 years to build up a susceptible population of man and equines to sustain a new epidemic.

JAPANESE–WEST NILE VIRUS COMPLEX

These are all diseases caused by flaviviruses and transmitted by mosquitoes from birds, which are the main reservoir hosts.

SYMPTOMS AND SIGNS

Natural history

Most infections are inapparent and the majority of the overt infections are mild and transient, though virulence may vary in epidemics.

The *incubation period* is 2–5 days.

The onset is sudden, with rigor, fever and myalgia. A sore throat and upper respiratory symptoms are a feature and diarrhoea is common (first phase lasting 1–5 days). After a short illness recovery is complete. In some cases, and in about 4% of children under 15, the disease is biphasic and symptoms return, with involvement of the CNS. Convulsions and coma and long-term sequelae, flaccid and spastic paralyses and mental depression, are common. There is a leucopenia, with pleocytosis and raised protein in the CSF.

DIAGNOSIS

Virus may be isolated from the blood in the acute phase and also from the throat, suggesting droplet spread. Antibody titres on paired sera are diagnostic.

EPIDEMIOLOGY

VEE virus circulates silently in small mammals and with a high rainfall and an increase in the number of mosquitoes and their biting, horses become infected acting as amplifying hosts. Equine cases precede human cases, most commonly children in whom the disease is more severe. A high proportion of equines develop immunity so that 10 years is necessary to build up another susceptible population.

CONTROL

Mosquito control is difficult in rural conditions and a vaccine has not yet been developed.

ST LOUIS ENCEPHALITIS (SLE)

GEOGRAPHICAL DISTRIBUTION (Figure 30.12)

This is the most important arbovirus in the USA. It is widespread throughout North America but has also occurred in Jamaica and evidence of infection in birds is found in Central America, Brazil and Argentina.

AETIOLOGY

The SLE virus is 30–40 nm in diameter and is best grown in newborn white mice but also grows on hamster and chicken kidney cell cultures. It shares antigens with Japanese and West Nile viruses.

TRANSMISSION

The basic transmission cycle is between birds and several culicine mosquitoes. After the winter the virus is introduced by migrant birds or long-term infection of bats. The main vector to man is *Culex quinquefasciatus* in the eastern and *C. tarsalis* in the western USA. Transovarial transmission is usual (see Table 30.1 and Appendix IV).

SYMPTOMS AND SIGNS

Natural history

Most infections are inapparent, in a ratio of 100:1. Overt infections usually last a few days with fever and complete recovery. In a very few cases, chiefly elderly persons, CNS signs develop, usually recovering rapidly with no permanent sequelae.

The *incubation period* is a few days.

Onset is sudden, with fever and severe headache, followed after a few days by recovery. CNS involvement is shown by drowsiness, tremor, dysarthria and photophobia with convulsions. This lasts 10 days, with complete recovery. Lymphocytosis is common. The CSF shows pleocytosis and a raised protein.

EPIDEMIOLOGY

C. quinquefasciatus, being an urban mosquito, is responsible for urban outbreaks, while *C. tarsalis* in the western USA is responsible for rural outbreaks. In urban areas both are affected equally but elderly people are most affected. In rural areas males are affected more than females. Epidemics occur in the late summer and early autumn.

CONTROL

Environmental sanitation to control *C. quinquefasciatus* in urban areas is essential. 'Fogging' with insecticides may be necessary.

JAPANESE ENCEPHALITIS (JE)

GEOGRAPHICAL DISTRIBUTION

JE is found in eastern Asia from Siberia to southeast India, Japan, Okinawa, Guam, Philippines and Indonesia.

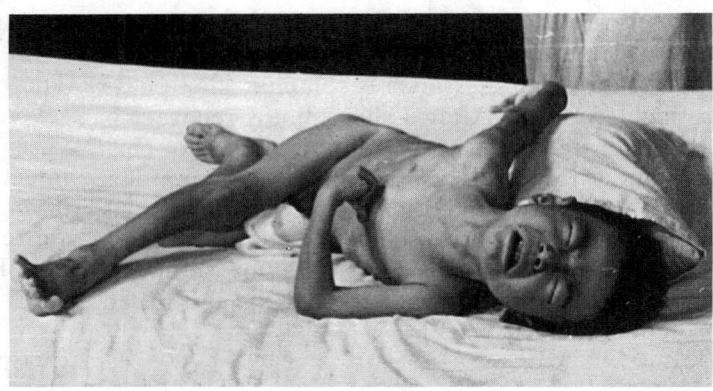

Figure 30.13   A 5-year-old boy with Japanese encephalitis.

AETIOLOGY

JE virus is 50 nm in diameter and shares antigens with SLE and MVE. It grows well on hamster and pig kidney cells and in animals and certain donkeys after intracerebral inoculation.

TRANSMISSION

Culex tritaeniorhynchus, a rice-field breeder, is the main vector in north Asia and Japan, *C. pipiens* in the eastern USSR, *C. annulirostris* in Guam, *C. gelidus* in Malaysia, and *C. vishnui* in India (see Table 30.1 and Appendix IV).

PATHOLOGY

In the brain there are areas of necrosis with small haemorrhages and perivascular cuffing in the grey matter, most marked in the thalamus and substantia nigra. Fine calcareous particles may be seen.

IMMUNITY

An antibody-mediated immunity protects against second attacks and builds up resistance in the population.

SYMPTOMS AND SIGNS

Natural history

Many infections are inapparent but in about 0.2% the infection is overt and severe, reaching a mortality rate in elderly persons of up to 50%. This is the most severe of the viral encephalitides.

The *incubation period* is 4–14 days.

The onset is sudden and within 24 hours there are signs of an acute meningoencephalitis. The face and conjunctivae are suffused. There is a characteristic

attitude with head retracted, arms and knees bent and shoulders pressed to the chest (Figure 30.13). After 3 days stupor, delirium, coma and decerebrate rigidity follow. The temperature fluctuates widely. If the acute stage is survived then recovery is slow. Upper motor neurone paralyses and extrapyramidal lesions are common. Death may occur suddenly in convalescence. Permanent sequelae, mental impairment, emotional instability, motor neurone lesions and aphasia are common. There is a leucopenia in the early stages. The CSF remains normal in half the cases, and shows a pleocytosis with increased protein in the other half.

DIAGNOSIS

HI and CF tests become positive from the third to seventh, maximum at the fortieth day. N test is positive later and remains positive for years. There are cross-reactions with other flaviviral antigens. Virus can be isolated from the brain at post mortem.

TREATMENT

Convalescent serum, 20 ml daily, during the first week is thought to help but is of no use when the CNS is involved.

EPIDEMIOLOGY

The main source of infection is the rice fields where the vector *C. tritaeniorhynchus* breeds, becoming infected from pigs or birds. Three weeks after mosquito breeding begins in the spring, virus can be found in birds and pigs but man is not involved until there is a high density of mosquitoes. The infection is amplified by pigs and conveyed to man. Birds (night heron and egrets) carry the infection from rural to urban areas. There is a seasonal summer incidence, with epidemics every year in Japan where children are affected more than adults. Most cases are in children and old people but visitors of any age are affected.

CONTROL

A formalized mouse brain vaccine is available and is given in three injections 2 months before the epidemic season.

MURRAY VALLEY ENCEPHALITIS (MVE)

GEOGRAPHICAL DISTRIBUTION

MVE is found in Australia and New Guinea.

AETIOLOGY

MVE is spherical, 25–35 nm in diameter. It is antigenically related to JE. It can be cultured in hamster kidney cells, KB cells and in chick embryos with cytopathic effect.

PATHOLOGY

MVE closely resembles JE.

NATURAL HISTORY

The majority of infections are inapparent, in the ratio of 700:1.

The *incubation period* is 1–2 weeks.

The signs and symptoms are the same as JE and the overt disease is very severe, with a mortality rate as high as 35%. Serious sequelae are common (residual paralyses and mental impairment).

DIAGNOSIS

The serological diagnosis is difficult because of the presence of dengue and other flaviviruses in these areas.

EPIDEMIOLOGY

The virus is maintained in a cycle involving wild birds and mosquitoes. The vector *C. annulirostris* is infected from birds who carry the infection widely by migration (see Table 30.1 and Appendix IV).

WEST NILE FEVER

GEOGRAPHICAL DISTRIBUTION

Serological surveys indicate that the virus is widely spread from South Africa to Egypt and Israel, southern Europe, the Middle East and south India.

AETIOLOGY

West Nile virus is 20–40 nm in diameter. It is constructed of a nucleocapsid enclosed in a lipid-containing envelope.

TRANSMISSION

The main vectors are: in Egypt, South Africa and Israel *C. univittatus* and *C. pipiens*; in Israel and France *C. modestus*; and in India *C. vishnui*. Virus has been isolated from ticks: *Ornithodorus* spp., *Dermacentor* spp., *Rhipicephalus* spp. and *Hyalomma* spp. in the former USSR (Table 30.1 and Appendix IV).

PATHOLOGY

Little is known because although deaths have occurred from meningoencephalitis, no post mortems have been recorded. In monkeys encephalitic changes are present in the cerebral grey matter and the cerebellum.

SYMPTOMS AND SIGNS

Natural history

In the great majority of cases West Nile fever is an inapparent infection; in others there is an acute dengue-like fever (for which it has often been mistaken) followed by recovery, but a few cases develop meningoencephalitis.

The *incubation period* is 3–6 days.

The onset is sudden, with nausea, fever, photophobia, congested eyes and face. After 5–6 days the fever falls by lysis and there is complete recovery. In children the fever may be saddle back. There is a generalized lymphadenopathy and a maculopapular rash on the chest, shoulders, upper arms and back. In elderly patients the first phase may be followed by the development of a meningoencephalitis.

DIAGNOSIS

The virus can be isolated from the blood in the first 6 days into suckling mice or embryonated eggs. Retrospective diagnosis with paired serum can be difficult because there is cross-reaction with persons inoculated with 17D virus against yellow fever.

EPIDEMIOLOGY

Virus circulates widely in birds (pigeons, crows), especially in the nesting season, and the young become infected with a high viraemia. The infection is spread widely by migration. *C. univittatus* is an avid feeder on birds and *C. pipiens* transmits the infection in the cooler season. Eighty per cent of the residents of Egypt show evidence of past infection. There have been epidemics of West Nile fever in South Africa and Israel.

CALIFORNIA ENCEPHALITIS (CE)

The California serogroup of viruses cause illness in the USA (see Figure 30.12). CE was the first to be isolated; it frequently infects man but rarely causes clinical illness. La Crosse (LAC) virus, on the other hand, is an important pathogen of man. LAC virus circulates in chipmunks, tree squirrels and cottontail rabbits in a rural forest environment and is transmitted by *Aedes, Culex, Anopheles* and *Psorophora* mosquitoes (see Table 30.1 and Appendix IV). The principal vector is *Ae. triseriatus,* in which there is transovarial transmission. It causes an acute fever with encephalitis involvement, mainly in children. The incubation period is 5–10 days, the onset gradual with fever, headache, neck rigidity, convulsions and coma. Permanent CNS changes are rare and the mortality less then 1%.

TICK-BORNE ENCEPHALITIS (TBE)

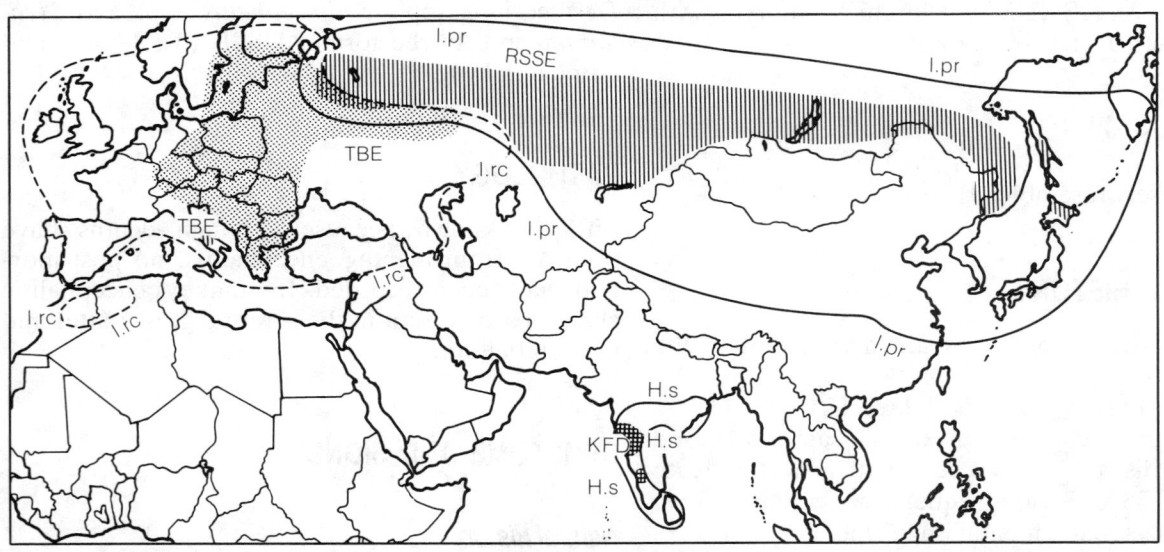

Figure 30.14 Geographical distribution of tick-borne encephalitis—Russian spring–summer encephalitis (RSSE), European tick-borne encephalitis (TBE) and Kyasanur Forest disease (KFD)—and the main vectors. I.pr, *Ixodes persulcatus*; I.rc, *Ixodes ricinus*; H.s, *Haemophysalis spinigera*. (Courtesy of the Department of Entomology, London School of Hygiene and Tropical Medicine.)

RUSSIAN SPRING–SUMMER ENCEPHALITIS (RSSE) AND EUROPEAN TICK-BORNE ENCEPHALITIS

GEOGRAPHICAL DISTRIBUTION (Figure 30.14)

TBE is seasonally epidemic in scattered foci in the far eastern part of the former USSR (RSSE) and in European Russia, Austria, Hungary, the Balkans, Czech Republic, Slovakia and Scandinavia (European TBE). The Powassan type is found in Canada and western Ontario.

AETIOLOGY

The virus is spherical, 20–30 nm in diameter, with a dense centre and surface membrane. It shares antigens with the viruses causing louping ill, Omsk haemorrhagic fever, and Kyasanur Forest disease, but not Japanese encephalitis.

TRANSMISSION (See also Table 30.1 and Appendix IV)

The vectors are *Ixodes persulcatus* in the eastern part of the former USSR and *I. ricinus* in the West. Viral infection is maintained by transovarial transmission. People may also become infected from drinking infected goat's milk.

PATHOLOGY

The virus multiplies in the liver before circulating in the blood, where it alters the vascular permeability and enters the brain, especially the basal ganglia and anterior horn cells of the cervical region. Histologically there is severe neuronal damage, with softening and death of cells, glial proliferation, neuronophagia and lymphoid proliferation around vessels. The cervical segments of the cord, medulla, midbrain and pons are affected.

SYMPTOMS AND SIGNS

Natural history

The infection is often inapparent but when overt is severe, the Eastern (RSSE) form (30% mortality) being more severe than the European form (TBE) (3% mortality).

The *incubation period* is 8–14 days.

Onset is sudden, with severe headache, fever, nausea and photophobia. In non-fatal cases the fever subsides after a week. In others the disease is biphasic and, after a period of several days recovery, the second phase develops with signs of a meningoencephalitis, which in the Eastern form is severe but in the European form mainly benign. Death comes from ascending paralysis and respiratory failure within a week of onset of the second phase. The mortality rate is higher in children. There is a leucopenia at the start, with a leucocytosis at the end. The CSF shows a pleocytosis with raised protein. Residual paralyses are common, involving the upper extremities and shoulder girdle.

DIAGNOSIS

Virus can be isolated from the blood in the first week. The CF test is not so reliable as the HI and N tests.

TREATMENT

Hyperimmune serum used in the first week has been helpful but is of no use when meningoencephalitis has set in.

EPIDEMIOLOGY

The virus circulates in small wild animals, chiefly rodents, and is transmitted by larval and nymphal ticks who, when they mature, feed on larger mammals, including man. The incidence of the disease is seasonal—spring and early summer—occurring in small epidemics in the eastern part of the former USSR, where it is a disease of the forest and the taiga. In Europe it is a forest disease and occurs from late spring until early autumn, and outbreaks often follow a period when voles are numerous.

CONTROL

In some areas of the far eastern part of the former USSR, forests are closed to all visitors because of this infection. Tick repellents may be of help. A formalized mouse brain vaccine is available and is used to protect laboratory workers but there are side-reactions. A safe and effective vaccine is available. It is recommended for holiday makers and sportsmen in the forested areas of Europe. It is given in two doses 4–6 weeks apart, followed by a booster after 12 months.[69]

COLORADO TICK FEVER (CTF)

Colorado tick fever is found in the Rocky Mountain area especially in Colorado. Fever is usually biphasic and mild, sometimes with a maculopapular rash or petechiae, and sometimes causing haemorrhages and encephalitis in children, who mostly recover without sequelae. The most important hosts are the chipmunk and the golden-mantled ground squirrel, which infect immature ticks (*Dermacentor andersoni*). Other species of rodents may act as alternative secondary hosts for the virus.

REFERENCES

1 World Health Organization. Arboviruses and human disease. Report of a WHO Scientific Group. *Wld Hlth Org Tech Rep Ser* 1967; 369:1–84.

2 Smith C E G. *Abstr Hyg* 1968; 43:1397.

3 Smith C E G. *Scient Basis Med Ann Rev* 1964; 125.

4 Simpson D I H. Arboviruses and free-living wild animals. *Symp Zool Soc London* 1968; 24:13–28.

5 Smith C E G. Studies on arbovirus epidemiology associated with established and developing rice culture. Introduction. *Trans R Soc Trop Med Hyg* 1970; 64:481–2.

6 Pinto M R. *Kongressbericht über die III Tagung der Deutschen Tropenmedizinischen Gesellschaft e V. 1967; 22–22 April.* Munich: Urban Schwarzenberg, 1967:153.

7 MacNamara F N, Horn D W & Porterfield J S. Yellow fever and other arthropod-borne viruses. A consideration of two serological surveys made in South Western Nigeria. *Trans R Soc Trop Med Hyg* 1959; 53:202–212.

8 Boyd J S K. *12th Annual Conference of the Indian Association of Pathologists* 1961; 118.

9 Rosen L, Shroyer D A, Tesh R B et al. Transovarial transmission of dengue viruses by mosquitoes: *Aedes albopictus* and *Aëdes aegypti. Am J Trop Med Hyg* 1983; 32:1108–1109.

10 Pinheiro F P, Freitas R B, Travassos Da Rosa J F et al. An outbreak of Mayaro virus disease in Belterra, Brazil. I. Clinical and virological findings. *Am J Trop Med Hyg* 1981; 30:674–681.

11 McIntosh B M, McGillivray G M, Dickson D B et al. Illness caused by Sindbis and West Nile viruses in South Africa. *S Afr Med J* 1964; 38:291–294.

12 Pinheiro F P, Rocha A G, Freitas R B et al. Meningite associada às infecções por vírus Oropouche. (Engl. Abstr.) *Rev Inst Med Trop São Paulo* 1982; 24:246–251.

13 Tesh R B, Saidi S, Gajdamovič S J et al. Serological studies on the epidemiology of sandfly fever in the old world. *Bull Wld Hlth Org* 1976; 54:663–673.

14 Center for Disease Control. *Morbidity and Mortality Weekly Report* (Supplement) 1983; 32:2S.

15 World Health Organization. Mosquito-borne haemorrhagic fevers of South-east Asia and the western Pacific. *Bull Wld Hlth Org* 1966; 35:17–33. Prasong T. Therapy and therapeutic studies of Thai Haemorrhagic fever. *Bull Wld Hlth Org* 1966; 35:74.

16 Bukkavesa S. Physiological disturbance in Thai Haemorrhagic fever. *Bull Wld Hlth Org* 1966; 35:51. Balankura M, Valyasevi A, Kampanart-Sanyakorn C et al. Treatment of the Dengue Shock Syndrome. *Bull Wld Hlth Org* 1966; 35:75.

17 World Health Organization. Human Viral and Rickettsial vaccines. Report of a WHO Scientific Group. *Wld Hlth Org Tech Rep Ser* 1966; 325:1–79.

18 Fraser H S, Wilson W A, Thomas E J et al. Dengue shock syndrome in Jamaica. *Br med J* 1978; i:893–894.

19 Sumaro W H, Jahja E, Gubler D J et al. Encephalopathy associated with dengue infection. [Letter]. *Lancet* 1978; i:449–450.

20 Halstead S B. Observations related to pathogenesis of dengue hemorrhagic fever. VI. Hypotheses and discussion. *Yale J Biol Med* 1970; 42:350–62.

21 Editorial. Dengue. *Lancet* 1976; ii:239–340.

22 Editorial. Dengue. *Br Med J* 1977; ii:1175–1176.

23 Editorial. *Asian J Inf Dis* 1978; 2:112.

24 Rosen L. The Emperor's New Clothes revisited, or reflections on the pathogenesis of dengue hemorrhagic fever. *Am J Trop Med Hyg* 1977; 26:337–343.

25 Van Tongeren H A E. Dengue haemorrhagic fever—case report. *Trans R Soc Trop Med Hyg* 1983; 77:198–200.

26 Meegan J M, Digoutte J P, Peters C J et al. Monoclinal antibodies to identify Zinga virus at Rift Valley fever virus. [Letter.] *Lancet* 1983; i:641.

27 Peters C J & Meegan J M. In Beran G W (ed.) *Viral Zoonoses*, vol 1. Boca Raton, Florida: CRC, 1981:403–420.

28 Van Velden D J J, Meyer J D, Oliver J et al. Rift Valley fever affecting humans in South Africa: a clinicopathological study. *S Afr Med J* 1977; 51:867–871.

29 Swanepoel R, Manning B & Watt J A. Fatal Rift Valley fever of man in Rhodesia. *Cent Afr J Med* 1979; 25:1–8.

30 Laughlin L W, Meegan J M, Stausbaugh L J et al. Epidemic Rift Valley fever in Egypt: Observations of the spectrum of human illness. *Trans R Soc Trop Med Hyg* 1979; 73:630–633.

31 Shope R E, Peters C J & Davies F G. The spread of Rift Valley fever and approaches to its control. *Bull Wld Hlth Org* 1982; 60:299–304.

32 Meegan JM. The Rift Valley fever epizootic in Egypt 1977–78. 1. Description of the epizootic and virological studies. *Trans R Soc Trop Med Hyg* 1979; 73:618–623.

33 Hoogstraal H, Meegan J M, Khalid G M et al. The Rift Valley fever epizootic in Egypt 1977–78. 2. Ecological and entomological studies. *Trans R Soc Trop Med Hyg* 1979; 73:624–629.

34 World Health Organization. The use of veterinary vaccines for prevention and control of Rift Valley fever: Memorandum from a WHO/FAO meeting. *Bull Wld Hlth Org* 1983; 61:261–268.

35 *Weekly Epidemiological Record* 1978; 4:305.

36 Cornet J P, Juard M, Camicas J L et al. Transmission expérimentale du virs de la fièvre jaune par la tique *Aroblyomma variegatum* (fabr.) (Acarida: Ixodida). *Bull Soc Path Exot Fil* 1982; 75:136–140. (Engl. Abstr.).

37 Haddow A J & Ellice J M. Studies on bush-babies (galago spp.) with special reference to the epidemiology of yellow fever. *Trans R Soc Trop Med Hyg* 1964; 58:521–538.

38 Boshell J. Kyasanur forest disease: ecologic considerations. *Am J Trop Med Hyg* 1969; 18:67–80.

39 Fisher-Hock S P & McCormick J B. *Abstr Hyg Comm Dis* 1985; 60:R2–R20.

40 McCormick J B, Palmer E L, Sasso D R et al. Morphological identification of the agent of Korean haemorrhagic fever (Hantaan virus) as a member of the bunyaviridae. *Lancet* 1982; i:765–771.

41 Schmaljohn C S, Hasty S E, Harrison S A. et al. Characterization of Hantaan virions, the prototype virus of hemorrhagic fever with renal syndrome. *J Inf Dis* 1983; 148:1005–1012.

42 Dournon E, Moriniere B, Matheron S et al. HFRS after a wild rodent bite in the Haute-Savoie—and risk of exposure to Hantaan-like virus in a Paris laboratory. [Letter]. *Lancet* 1984; i:676–677.

43 Yang S H, Gu X S, Wang D Q et al. Studies on immunopathogenesis in epidemic hemorrhagic fever: role of classical complement pathway activation in pathogenesis. *Chin Med J* 1981; 94:789–798.

44 Pinheiro F P, Bensabath G, Costa D Jun et al. Haemorrhagic syndrome of Altamira. *Lancet* 1974; i:639–642.

45 Howard C R & Young P R. Variation among New and Old World arenaviruses. *Trans R Soc Trop Med Hyg* 1984; 78:299–306.

46 Monath T P & Casal J. Diagnosis of Lassa fever and the isolation and management of patients. *Bull Wld Hlth Org* 1975; 52:707–715.

47 Fraser D M, Campbell C C, Monath T P et al. Lassa fever in the Eastern Province of Sierra Leone, 1970–1972. I. Epidemiologic studies. *Am J Trop Med Hyg* 1974; 23:1131.

48 Arnold R B & Gary G M. A neutralization test survey for Lassa fever activity in Lassa, Nigeria. *Trans R Soc Trop Med Hyg* 1977; 71:152–154.

49 Clegg J C S. Possible approaches to a vaccine against Lassa fever. *Trans R Soc Trop Med Hyg* 1984; 78:307–310.

50 Jahrling P B. Protection of Lassa virus-infected guinea pigs with Lassa-immune plasma of guinea pig, primate, and human origin. *J Med Virol* 1983; 12:93–102.

51 Buckley S M & Casals J. Pathobiology of Lassa fever. *Int Rev Exp Path* 1978; 18:97–136.

52 Sato K, Ikerionun S E & Katchy K C. *Jap J Trop Med Hyg* 1982; 10:23–31.

53 Emond R T D, Bannister B, Lloyd G et al. A case of Lassa fever: clinical and virological findings. *Br Med J* 1982; ii:1001–1002.

54 World Health Organization. *Wkly Epidem Rec* 1974; 41:341.

55 Jahrling P B, Niklasson B S & McCormick J B. Early diagnosis of human Lassa fever by ELISA detection of antigen and antibody. *Lancet* 1985; i:250–252.

56 Monath T P. Lassa fever: review of epidemiology and epizootiology. *Bull Wld Hlth Org* 1975; 52:577–92.

57 Frame J D, Verbrugge G P, Gill R G et al. The use of Lassa fever convalescent plasma in Nigeria. *Trans R Soc Trop Med Hyg* 1984; 78:319–324
Frame J D, Jahrling PB, Yalley-Ogunro J E et al. Endemic Lassa fever in Liberia. II. Serological and virological findings in hospital patients. *Trans R Soc Trop Med Hyg* 1984; 78:656–660
Frame J D, Yalley-Ogubro J E, Hanson A P. Endemic Lassa fever in Liberia. V. Distribution of Lassa virus activity in Liberia: hospital staff surveys. *Trans R Soc Trop Med Hyg* 1984; 78:761–763

58 McCormick J B, King I J, Webb P A et al. Lassa fever. Effective therapy with ribavirin. *N Engl J Med* 1986; 314:20–26.

59 Elsner B, Schwarz F, Mando O G et al. Pathology of 12 fatal cases of Argentine hemorrhagic fever. *Am J Trop Med Hyg* 1973; 22:229–236.

60 Child P L, Mackenzie R B, Velverde L et al. Bolivian hemorrhagic fever. A pathologic description. *Arch Path* 1967; 83:434–435.

61 Johnson K M, Webb P A, Lance J V et al. Isolaton and partial characterization of a new virus causing acute haemorrhagic fever in Zaire. *Lancet* 1977; i:569–571.

62 Bowen E T M, Platt G S, Lloyd G et al. Viral haemorrhagic fever in southern Sudan and northern Zaire. Preliminary studies on the aetiological agent. *Lancet* 1977; i:571–573.

63 Pattyn S, Jacob W, van der Groen G et al. Isolation of Marburg-like virus from a case of haemorrhagic fever in Zaire. *Lancet* 1977; i:573–574.

64 World Health Organization. Brès P. The epidemic of Ebola haemorrhagic fever in Sudan and Zaire, 1976: introductory note. *Bull Wld Hlth Org* 1978; 56:247–271.

65 Transactions Royal Society of Tropical Medicine and Hygiene. *Symposium on Marburg Virus Disease* 1969; 63:295.

66 Gear J J S, Cassel G A, Gear A J et al. Outbreak of Marburg virus disease in Johannesburg. *Br Med J* 1975; 4:489–493.

67 Emond R T D, Evans B, Bowen E T W et al. A case of Ebola virus infection. *Br Med J* 1977; ii:541–544.

68 Smith D H, Johnson B K, Isaacson M et al. Marburg-virus disease in Kenya. *Lancet* 1982; i:816–820.

69 Simpson D I H & Varma M G R. Vaccination against tick-borne encephalitis. (Letter]. *Br Med J* 1982; 284:1787–1788.

CHAPTER 31

VIRAL HEPATITIS

Arie J. Zuckerman, Tim J. Harrison and Jane N. Zuckerman

Since the 1970s there has been an explosion in knowledge of viral hepatitis, a major public health problem throughout the world affecting several hundreds of millions of people. Viral hepatitis is a cause of considerable morbidity and mortality in the human population, both from acute infection and chronic sequelae which include, with hepatitis B and hepatitis C infection, chronic active hepatitis, cirrhosis and primary liver cancer (see also Chapter 3).

The hepatitis viruses include a range of unrelated and often unusual human pathogens:

- *Hepatitis A virus (HAV)*: a small unenveloped symmetrical RNA virus which shares many of the characteristics of the picornavirus family. This virus has been classified in the hepatovirus genus, and is the cause of infectious or epidemic hepatitis transmitted by the faecal–oral route.
- *Hepatitis B virus (HBV)*: a member of the hepadnavirus group double-stranded DNA viruses which replicate by reverse transcription. Hepatitis B virus is endemic in the human population and hyperendemic in many parts of the world.
- *Hepatitis C virus (HVC)*: an enveloped single-stranded RNA virus which appears to be distantly related (possibly in its evolution) to flaviviruses, although hepatitis C is not transmitted by arthropod vectors. Infection with this virus is common in many countries, and it is associated with chronic liver disease and also with primary liver cancer, at least in some countries.
- *Hepatitis D virus (HDV)*: an unusual single-stranded circular RNA virus with a number of similarities to certain plant viral satellites and viroids. This virus requires hepadnavirus helper functions for propagation in hepatocytes, and is an important cause of acute and severe chronic liver damage in some regions of the world.
- *Hepatitis E virus (HEV)*: an enterically transmitted non-enveloped, single-stranded RNA virus which shares many biophysical and biochemical features with caliciviruses. Hepatitis E virus is an important cause of large epidemics of acute hepatitis in the subcontinent of India, Central and South-East Asia, the Middle East, parts of Africa and elsewhere; this virus is responsible for high mortality during pregnancy.

HEPATITIS A (See also Chapter 3)

Outbreaks of jaundice have been described for many centuries and the term 'infectious hepatitis' was coined in 1912 to describe the epidemic form of the disease. Hepatitis A virus (HAV) is spread by the faecal–oral route and is endemic throughout the world and hyperendemic in areas with poor standards of sanitation and hygiene. The seroprevalence of antibodies to HAV has declined since World War II in many industrialized countries.

The incubation period of hepatitis A is about 28 days. The virus replicates in the liver. Very large amounts of virus are shed in the faeces during the incubation period, before the onset of clinical symptoms and a brief period of viraemia occurs (Figure 31.1). The severity of illness ranges from asymptomatic to anicteric or icteric hepatitis and rarely fulminant hepatitis. The virus is non-cytopathic when grown in cell culture. Its pathogenicity in vivo, which involves necrosis of parenchymal cells and histiocytic periportal inflammation, may be mediated via the cellular immune response. By the time of onset of symptoms, excretion of virus in the faeces has declined and may have ceased and anti-HAV IgM, which is diagnostic of acute infection and appears late during the incubation period, increases in titre. Anti-HAV IgG may be detected 1–2 weeks later and persists for years.

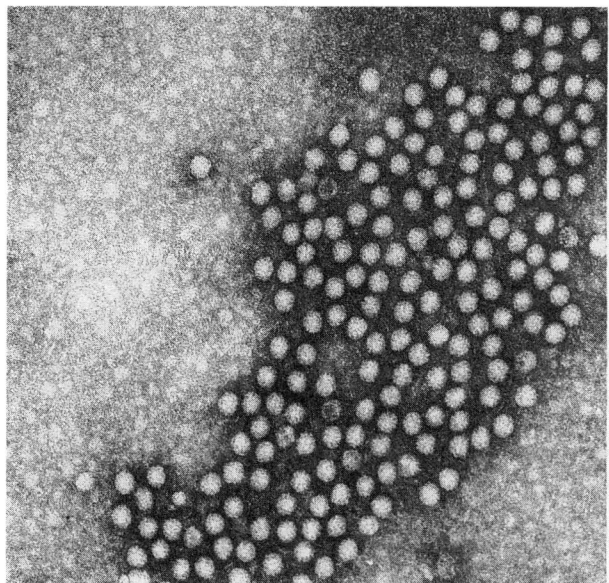

Figure 31.1 Electron micrograph showing the large number of hepatitis A virus particles in faeces during the incubation period of the infection. (Reduced from 120000×; From a series by Anthea Thornton and A.J. Zuckerman.)

CLASSIFICATION

Examination by electron microscopy of concentrates of filtered faecal extracts from patients during the incubation period reveals 27 nm unenveloped spherical particles typical of the Picornaviridae. HAV was classified in 1983 in the genus *Enterovirus* (as enterovirus 72) of the family Picornaviridae on the basis of its biophysical and biochemical characteristics, including stability at low pH. However, this classification preceded the isolation and analysis of complementary DNA (cDNA) clones leading to the determination of the entire nucleotide sequence of the viral genome.[1] Comparison with other picornavirus sequences revealed limited homology to the enteroviruses or, indeed, the rhinoviruses; however, the structure and genome organization is typical of the Picornaviridae. HAV is now considered as a separate genus (*Hepatovirus*) within the Picornaviridae as are the cardioviruses (of mice) and apthoviruses (foot and mouth disease viruses).

ORGANIZATION OF THE HAV GENOME

The HAV genome comprises about 7500 nucleotides (nt) of positive sense RNA which is polyadenylated at the 3′ end and has a polypeptide (VPg) attached to the 5′ end. A single, large open reading

Table 31.1 Passive immunization with normal immunoglobulin for travellers to highly endemic areas.

Body weight (kg)	Dose (iu anti-HAV (ml)/L)	
	<3 months stay	>3 months stay
<25	50 (0.5)	100 (1.0)
25–30	100 (1.0)	250 (2.5)
<50	200 (2.0)	500 (5.0)

frame (ORF) occupies most of the genome and encodes a large polyprotein.

The viral polyprotein is processed to yield the structural (located at the amino-terminal end) and non-structural viral polypeptides. Many of the features of replication of the picornaviruses have been deduced from studies of prototype enteroviruses and rhinoviruses, in particular poliovirus type 1.

PREVENTION AND CONTROL OF HEPATITIS A

PASSIVE IMMUNIZATION

Control of hepatitis A infection is difficult. Since faecal shedding of the virus is at its highest during the late incubation period and the prodromal phase of the illness, strict isolation of cases is not a useful control measure. Spread of hepatitis A is reduced by simple hygienic measures and the sanitary disposal of excreta.

Normal human immunoglobulin, containing at least 100 iu/ml of anti-hepatitis A antibody, given intramuscularly before exposure to the virus or early during the incubation period will prevent or attenuate a clinical illness. The dosage should be at least 2 iu anti-hepatitis A antibody/kg body weight, but in special cases, such as pregnancy or in patients with liver disease, that dosage may be doubled (Table 31.1). Immunoglobulin does not always prevent infection and excretion of HAV, and inapparent or subclinical hepatitis may develop. The efficacy of passive immunization is based on the presence of hepatitis A antibody in the immunoglobulin, but the minimum titre of antibody required for protection has not yet been established. Immunoglobulin is used most commonly for close personal contacts of patients with hepatitis A and for those exposed to contaminated food. Immunoglobulin has also been used effectively for controlling outbreaks in institutions such as homes for the mentally handicapped and in nursery schools. Prophylaxis with immuno-globulin is recommended for persons without hepa-titis A antibody visiting highly endemic areas. After a period of 6 months the administration of immuno-globulin for travellers should be repeated, unless it has been demonstrated that the recipient has devel-oped his or her own hepatitis A antibodies.

HEPATITIS A VACCINES

In areas of high prevalence most children have antibodies to HAV by the age of 3 years and such infections are generally asymptomatic. Infections acquired later in life are of increasing clinical sever-ity. Less than 10% of cases of acute hepatitis A in children up to the age of 6 years are icteric but this increases to 40–50% in the 6–14 age group and to 70–80% in adults. Of 115 551 cases of hepatitis A in the USA between 1983 and 1987, only 9% of the cases, but more than 70% of the fatalities, were in those aged over 49. It is important, therefore, to protect those at risk because of personal contact with infected individuals or because of travel to highly endemic areas. Other groups at risk of hepatitis A infection include staff and residents of institutions for the mentally handicapped, day care centres for children, sexually active male homosexuals, intra-venous narcotic drug abusers, sewage workers, health care workers, military personnel and mem-bers of certain low socioeconomic groups in defined community settings. It is also recommended that food handlers should be immunized. In some devel-oping countries the incidence of clinical hepatitis A is increasing as improvements in socioeconomic con-ditions result in infection later in life and strategies for immunization are yet to be agreed.

KILLED HEPATITIS A VACCINES

The foundations for a hepatitis A vaccine were laid in 1975 by the demonstration that formalin-inactivated virus extracted from the liver of experi-mentally infected marmosets induced protective antibodies in susceptible marmosets on challenge with live virus. Subsequently HAV was cultivated, after serial passage in marmosets, in a cloned line of fetal rhesus monkey kidney cells (FRhK6), thereby opening the way to the production of hepatitis A vaccines. Later it was demonstrated that prior adap-tation in marmosets was not a prerequisite to growth of the virus in cell cultures and various strains of virus have been isolated directly from clinical material using several cell lines, including human diploid fibroblasts, and various techniques have been employed to increase the yield of virus in cell culture. Safety and immunogenicity studies of formalin-inactivated hepatitis A vaccines with an adjuvant have been completed and the vaccine had been licensed in several countries by the end of 1992. Other preparations of killed hepatitis A vaccines are under clinical trial.

LIVE ATTENUATED HEPATITIS A VACCINES

The major advantages of live attenuated vaccines, such as the Sabin type of oral poliomyelitis vaccines, include the ease of administration on a large scale by the oral route, relatively low cost, and the fact that, since the virus vaccine strain replicates in the gut, the production of both local immunity in the gut and humoral immunity thereby mimicking natural infec-tion, antibodies tend to persist longer. Disadvan-tages include the potential of reversion towards virulence, interference with the vaccine strain by other viruses in the gut, relative instability of the vaccine and shedding of the virus strain in the faeces for prolonged periods and the potential of spread to contacts.

The most extensively studied live attenuated hepatitis A vaccines are based on the CR326 and HM175 strains of the virus attenuated by prolonged passage in cell culture.

Two variants of the CR326 strain have been investigated after passage in marmoset liver in FRhK6, MRC5 and WI-38 cells. Inoculation of susceptible marmosets demonstrated seroconver-sion, and protection on challenge. Biochemical evi-dence of liver damage did not occur in susceptible chimpanzees, although a number had histological evidence of mild hepatitis with the F variant and the vaccine virus was shed in the faeces for about 12 weeks prior to seroconversion. There was no evi-dence of reversion towards virulence. Studies in human volunteers indicated incomplete attenuation of the F variant, but better results were obtained with the F^1 variant without elevation of liver enzymes.

Studies with the HM175 strain, which was isolated and passaged in African green monkey kidney cells, showed that this strain was not fully attenuated for marmosets, although it did not induce liver damage on challenge. Further passages and adaptation of HM175 revealed some evidence of virus replication in the liver of chimpanzees and minimal shedding of the virus into faeces. Other studies are in progress in non-human primates.

Markers of attenuation of HAV have not been identified and reversion to virulence may occur. On the other hand, there is also concern that 'over-attenuated' viruses may not be sufficiently immunogenic. Current candidate live attenuated hepatitis A vaccines require administration by injection. Prep- arations which may be suitable for oral adminis- tration are not presently available.

HEPATITIS E

Retrospective testing of serum samples from patients involved in various epidemics of hepatitis associated with contamination of water supplies with human faeces led to the conclusion that an agent other than hepatitis A or hepatitis B was involved. Epidemics of enterically transmitted non-A, non-B hepatitis in the Indian subcontinent were the first to be reported, in 1980, but outbreaks involving tens of thousands of cases have also been documented in the former USSR, South-East Asia, northern Africa and Mexico. The average incu- bation period is longer than that for hepatitis A, with a mean of 6 weeks. The highest attack rates are found in young adults, and high mortality rates (up to 20%) have been reported in women in the third trimester of pregnancy.

Virus-like particles measuring 28–34 nm in diam- eter have been detected in faecal extracts of infected individuals by immune electron microscopy using convalescent serum. However, such studies have often proved inconclusive because a large pro- portion of the excreted virus may be degraded during passage through the gut. Cross-reaction studies between sera and virus in faeces associated with a variety of epidemics in several different countries suggest that a single serotype of virus is involved.

Studies on hepatitis E virus (HEV) have pro- gressed following transmission to susceptible non-human primates. HEV was first transmitted to cynomolgous macaques, and a number of other species of monkey, including chimpanzees, have also been infected. Reports of transmission to pigs and rodents await confirmation. Reports on repli- cation of the virus in cell culture have thus far not been confirmed.

The problem of degradation of HEV in the gut was circumvented when the bile of infected monkeys was found to be a rich source of virus. This material permitted the molecular cloning of DNA comp- lementary to the HEV (RNA) genome and the entire 7.5 kb sequence was determined. The organ- ization of the genome is distinct from the Picornavir- idae and the non-structural and structural polypeptides are encoded respectively at the 5′ and 3′ ends. HEV resembles the caliciviruses in the size and organization of its genome as well as in the size and morphology of the virion.

LABORATORY TESTS

Sequencing of the HEV genome has resulted in the development of a number of specific diagnostic tests. For example, HEV RNA was detected, using the polymerase chain reaction (PCR), in faecal samples. An enzyme linked immunosorbent assay (ELISA), which detects both IgG and IgM anti-HEV, has been developed using a recombinant HEV–glutathione-S-transferase fusion protein and used to detect antibodies in sporadic cases of infec- tion in children and adults and during a number of epidemics.

HEPATITIS B (See also Chapter 3)

Hepatitis B virus (HBV) was originally recognized as the cause of 'serum hepatitis', the most common form of parenterally transmitted viral hepatitis, and an important cause of acute and chronic infection of the liver. The incubation period of hepatitis B is variable, with a range of between 1 and 6 months. The clinical features of acute infection resemble those of the other viral hepatitides. Frequently, acute hepatitis B is anicteric and asymptomatic, although a severe illness with jaundice can occur and acute liver failure may develop. The virus persists in about 10% of infected immunocompetent adults and in as many as 90% of infants infected perina- tally, depending on the ethnic group of the mother. About 350 million people worldwide are persistent carriers of hepatitis B. Liver damage is mediated by the responses of the cellular immune response of the host to the infected hepatocytes. Approximately

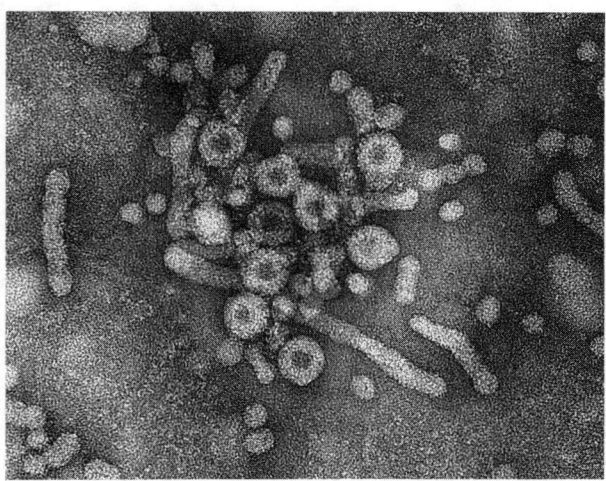

Figure 31.2   Hepatitis B virus. (Reduced from 250000×; From a series by A.J. Zuckerman et al.)

25% of all patients with chronic hepatitis will progress to cirrhosis and about 20% of those with cirrhosis will develop hepatocellular carcinoma. Hepatocellular carcinoma is one of the most common cancers worldwide.

During the first phase of chronicity, virus replication continues in the liver and replicative intermediates of the viral genome may be detected in DNA extracted from liver biopsies. Markers of virus replication in serum include HBV DNA, the pre-S1 proteins (see below) and a soluble antigen, hepatitis B e antigen (HBeAg), which is secreted by productively infected hepatocytes. In those infected at a very young age this phase may persist for life but, more usually, virus levels decline over time. Eventually in most individuals there is immune clearance of infected hepatocytes associated with seroconversion from HBeAg to anti-HBe. During the period of replication the viral genome may integrate into the chromosomal DNA of some hepatocytes and these cells may persist and expand clonally. Rarely, seroconversion to anti-HBs follows clearance of virus replication but, more frequently, the surface antigen (HBsAg) persists during a second phase of chronicity as a result of the expression of integrated viral DNA.

STRUCTURE OF THE VIRUS

The hepatitis B virion is a 42 nm particle comprising an electron-dense nucleocapsid or core, 27 nm in diameter, surrounded by an outer envelope of the surface protein (HBsAg) embedded in membraneous lipoprotein derived from the host cell (Figure 31.2). The surface antigen is produced in

excess by the infected hepatocytes and is secreted in the form of 22 nm particles (initially referred to as Australia antigen) and tubular structures with the same diameter.

The 22 nm particles are composed of the major surface protein in both non-glycosylated (p24) and glycosylated (gp27) form in approximately equimolar amounts, together with a minority component of the so-called middle proteins (gp33 and gp36) which contain the pre-S2 domain, a glycosylated 55 amino acid N-terminal extension. The surface of the virion has a similar composition but also contains the large surface proteins (p39 and gp42) which include both the pre-S1 and pre-S2 regions. These large surface proteins are not found in the 22 nm spherical particles (but may be present in the tubular forms in highly viraemic individuals) and their detection in serum correlates with viraemia. The domain which binds to the specific HBV receptor on the hepatocyte resides within the pre-S1 region.

The nucleocapsid of the virion consists of the viral genome surrounded by the core antigen (HBcAg). The carboxyterminus of the core protein is arginine rich and this highly basic domain is believed to interact with the genome. The genome, which is approximately 3.2 kb in length, has an unusual structure and is composed of two linear strands of DNA held in a circular configuration by base pairing at the 5′ end. One of the strands is incomplete and the 3′ end is associated with a DNA polymerase molecule which is able to complete that strand when supplied with deoxynucleoside triphosphates. In the past, this endogenous DNA polymerase reaction was used as a serological assay for the hepatitis B virion but this has now been superseded by DNA–DNA hybridization and the PCR. The 5′ ends of both strands of the genome are modified. The 5′ end of the complete strand is covalently linked to a protein and the 5′ end of the incomplete strand is an oligoribonucleotide. In both cases these moieties seem to be primers for the synthesis of the respective strands during the genome replication. A motif of 12 base pairs is directly repeated in the genome near to the 5′ ends of the two strands (DR1 and DR2 respectively) and these sequences play an important role in replication.

ORGANIZATION OF THE HBV GENOME

To date, the genomes of more than a dozen isolates of HBV have been cloned and the complete nucleotide sequences determined. Analysis of the coding potential of the genome reveals four ORFs which are conserved between all of these isolates (Figure

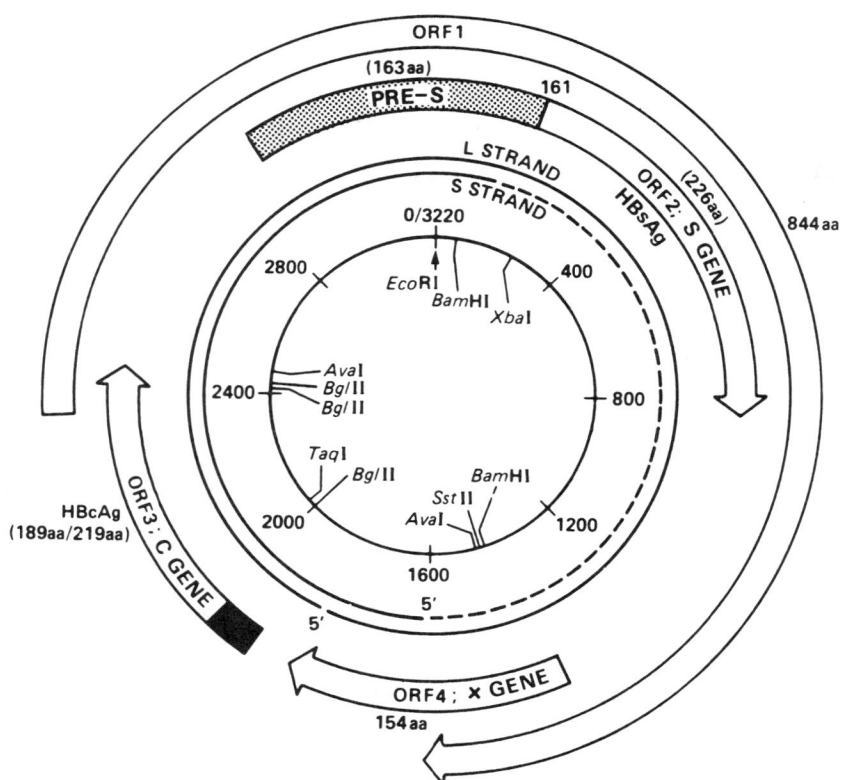

Figure 31.3 Organization of the genome of hepatitis B virus.

31.3). These have the same polarity as the incomplete strand of genomic DNA, which therefore has been designated the plus strand.

The first ORF encodes the various forms of the surface protein and contains three in-frame methionine codons which are used for initiation of translation. Both the middle (gp33 and gp36) and major (p24 and gp27) proteins are translated from a family of 2.1 kb mRNAs transcribed from a promoter located in the pre-S1 region and polyadenylated in response to a signal sequence located just downstream from the start of the core ORF.

A second promoter is located upstream of the pre-S1 initiation codon. This directs the synthesis of a 2.4 kb mRNA which is coterminal with the other surface messages and is translated to yield the large (pre-S1) surface proteins. This promoter seems to be weak (or may be down-regulated) so that the message is of low abundance and relatively little of the large surface proteins is synthesized. Unlike the middle and major surface proteins, the large surface protein is not secreted from the cell. In fact its synthesis inhibits the secretion of the smaller proteins and may be a signal for virus assembly.

The core ORF also has two in-phase initiation codons. The 'precore' region is highly conserved, has the properties of a signal sequence, and is responsible for the secretion of HBeAg.

The third ORF, which is the largest and overlaps the other three, encodes the viral polymerase. The fourth ORF was designated 'x', identified recently as a transcriptional transactivator, and may be an 'early' gene product which functions to up-regulate the viral promoters.

REPLICATION OF THE HBV GENOME

Following infection of a hepatocyte the single-stranded region of the virion DNA is repaired by the endogenous polymerase and the genome appears on a covalently closed, circular form in the nucleus. This DNA is the template for the transcription of all of the viral RNAs. Synthesis of minus strand DNA is primed by a protein, now believed to be the amino-terminal domain of the polymerase, and proceeds with the concomitant degradation of the RNA template by the RNAase H activity. There is no semi-conservative replication of the covalently closed circular DNA in the nucleus and a pool of up to 30 copies of template DNA initially is built up by transfer of some of the progeny DNA from the cytoplasm to the nucleus. The mode of replication of the viral genome resembles those of the phylogenetically related retroviruses and, and more closely, a family of plant viruses (the caulimoviruses).

PREVENTION AND CONTROL OF HEPATITIS B

The discovery of variation in the epitopes presented on the surface of the virions and subviral particles identified subtypes of HBV which differ in their geographical distribution. All isolates of the virus share a common epitope, *a*, which is a domain of the major surface protein and seems to protrude as a double loop from the surface of the particles. Two other pairs of mutually exclusive antigenic determinants, *d* or *y* and *w* or *r*, are also present on the major surface protein. These variations have been correlated with single nucleotide changes in the surface ORF which lead to variation in single amino acids in the protein. Four principal subtypes of HBV are recognized: *adw*, *adr*, *ayw* and *ayr*. Subtype *adw* predominates in northern Europe, the Americas and Australasia and is also found in Africa and Asia. Subtype *ayw* is found in the Mediterranean region, eastern Europe, northern and western Africa, the Near East and the Indian subcontinent. In the Far East, *adr* predominates but the rarer *ayr* may occasionally be found in Japan and Papua New Guinea.

The major response to immunization with the current hepatitis B vaccines is to the common *a* epitope with consequent protection against all subtypes of the virus.

PASSIVE IMMUNIZATION

Hepatitis B immunoglobulin (HBIG) is prepared from pooled plasma with high titre of hepatitis B surface antibody (anti-HBs) and may confer temporary passive immunity under certain defined conditions. The major indication for the administration of HBIG is a single acute exposure to HBV, such as occurs when blood containing surface antigen is inoculated, ingested or splashed on to mucous membranes and conjunctivae. The optimal dose has not been established but doses in the range of 250–500 iu have been used effectively. It should be administered as early as possible after exposure and preferably within 48 hours, usually 3 ml (containing 200 iu of anti-HBs per ml) in adults. It should not be administered 7 days following exposure. It is generally recommended that two doses of HBIG should be given 30 days apart.

Results with the use of HBIG for prophylaxis in babies at risk of infection with HBV are encouraging if the immunoglobulin is given as soon as possible after birth or within 12 hours of birth, and the chance of the baby developing the persistent carrier state is reduced by about 70%. More recent studies using combined passive and active immunization indicate an efficacy approaching 90%. The dose of HBIG recommended in the newborn is 1–2 ml (200 iu of anti-HBs per ml).

ACTIVE IMMUNIZATION

Immunization against hepatitis B is required for groups which are at an increased risk of acquiring this infection. These groups include individuals requiring repeated transfusions of blood or blood products, prolonged inpatient treatment, patients who require frequent tissue penetration or need repeated access to the circulation, patients with natural or acquired immune deficiency and patients with malignant diseases. Viral hepatitis is an occupational hazard among health care personnel and the staff of institutions for the mentally handicapped and in some semiclosed institutions. High rates of infection with hepatitis B occur in narcotic drug addicts and drug abusers, male homosexuals who change partners frequently and prostitutes. Individuals working in high endemic areas are also at increased risk of infection. Women in areas of the world where the carrier state in that group is high are another segment of the population requiring immunization in view of the increased risk of transmission of the infections to their offspring. Young infants, children and susceptible persons living in certain tropical and subtropical areas where present socioeconomic conditions are poor and the prevalence of hepatitis B is high should also be immunized.

The failure to grow HBV in tissue culture has directed attention to the use of other preparations for active immunization. Since immunization with HBsAg leads to the production of protective surface antibody, purified 22 mm spherical surface antigen particles have been developed as vaccines. These vaccines have been prepared from the plasma of symptomless carriers. Trials on protective efficacy in high-risk groups have demonstrated the value of the vaccines and their safety. There is no risk of transmission of the acquired immune deficiency syndrome (AIDS) or any other infection by vaccines derived from plasma which meet the World Health Organization requirements of 1981, 1983 and 1987. Local reactions reported after immunization have been minor, occurring in less than 20% of immunized individuals, and consist of slight swelling and reddening at the site of inoculation. Temperature elevations of up to 38°C were observed in only a few individuals.

SITE OF INJECTION FOR VACCINATION

Hepatitis B vaccination should be given intramuscularly in the upper arm or the anterolateral aspect of the thigh and *not* in the buttock. There are over 100 reports of unexpectedly low antibody seroconversion rates after hepatitis B vaccination using injection into the buttock. In one centre in the USA a low antibody response was noted in 54% of healthy adult health care personnel. Many studies have since shown that the antibody response rate was significantly higher in centres using deltoid injection than centres using the buttock. On the basis of antibody tests after vaccination, the Advisory Committee on Immunization Practices of the Centers of Disease Control, USA, recommended that the arm be used as the site for hepatitis B vaccination in adults, as have the Departments of Health in the United Kingdom.

A comprehensive study in the USA by Shaw et al [2] showed that participants who received the vaccine in the deltoid had antibody titres that were up to 17 times higher than those of subjects who received the injections into the buttock. Furthermore, those who were injected in the buttock were two to four times more likely to fail to reach a minimum antibody level of 10 miu/ml after vaccination. (Recent reports have also implicated buttock injection as a possible factor in a failure of rabies postexposure prophylaxis using a human diploid cell rabies vaccine.)

The injection of vaccine into deep fat in the buttocks is likely with needles shorter than 5 cm, and there is a lack of phagocytic or antigen presenting cells in layers of fat. Another factor may involve the rapidity with which antigen becomes available to the circulation from deposition in fat, leading to delay in processing by macrophages and eventually presentation to T and B cells. An additional factor may be denaturation by enzymes of antigen which has remained in fat for hours or days. The importance of these factors is supported by a finding at the Royal Free Hospital, London, and elsewhere that thicker skin fold was associated with a lowered antibody response.[3]

These observations have important public health implications, well illustrated by the estimate that about 20% of subjects immunized against hepatitis B via the buttock in the USA by March 1985 (about 60 000 people) failed to attain a minimum level of antibody of 10 miu/ml and were therefore not protected.

Hepatitis B surface antibody titres should be measured in all individuals who have been immunized against hepatitis B by injection into the buttocks, and when this is not possible a complete course of three injections of vaccine should be administered into the deltoid muscle or the anterolateral aspect of the thigh—the only acceptable sites for hepatitis B immunization.[4].

INTRADERMAL IMMUNIZATION

The high cost of hepatitis B vaccines is a serious economic obstacle to extensive immunization against hepatitis B, which is needed in many countries in Africa and Asia. The possibility of reducing the amount of antigen required for immunization by reducing the dose of vaccine or by using the intradermal route has been explored. Presentation of antigen to the immune system intradermally results in a macrophage-dependent T-lymphocyte response via specific epidermal cells, and the intradermal route has been used for immunization against tuberculosis, diphtheria, typhoid, cholera, influenza, rabies and other infections. A second reason for attempting to use hepatitis B vaccine intradermally is to accelerate the immune response in persons who suddenly experience a high risk of infection—for example, after accidental exposure to hepatitis B or infants born to carrier mothers.

A review of reports on the intradermal administration of hepatitis B vaccines[5] raises several important and unresolved issues.

1. The immunogenicity of the plasma-derived vaccine given intradermally in doses of 0.1 ml (2.0 μg of antigen protein) has been clearly demonstrated. However, although the antibody titres after two intradermal or intramuscular doses given 1 month apart were similar, the booster injection at 6 months resulted in anti-HBs levels which were ten times higher after intramuscular than intradermal inoculation.

2. Multisite intradermal inoculation of a single reduced dose of rabies vaccine resulted in rapid seroconversion and antibody levels similar to those obtained with the extended intramuscular immunization route. However, after multisite intradermal inoculation of a single reduced dose of hepatitis B vaccine, seroconversion was slower than that with intramuscular injection, and the antibody titres after the booster injection were also lower after intradermal than after intramuscular injections.

3. Intradermal inoculation requires skill, and subcutaneous injection into fat will result in a poor immune response.

4. Although adverse reactions after intradermal injection were not marked, local reactions at the site of administration of the vaccine (which contains aluminium hydroxide as adjuvant) frequently included the development of an erythematous macule 5–10 mm in diameter after 24–48 hours; the lesion would subside after days or weeks, leaving a small pigmented macule, occasionally overlying a small palpable nodule.

5. The use of jet injectors for inoculation of hepatitis B vaccine has been considered. Current advice is that until further studies clarify the risk of transmission of infection (such as hepatitis B and the human immunodeficiency virus) by different types of jet injectors their use should be restricted to special situations where large numbers of persons need to be immunized within a short time. The use of jet injectors in the UK has been generally discouraged (although this does not apply to the use of jet injectors by individuals for self-administration of insulin or low-dose heparin).

Trials of intradermal hepatitis B vaccines in Gambian children illustrate many of the problems reviewed above. In the first trial 1 μg of a plasma-derived vaccine was given to neonates intradermally in the same syringe with BCG followed by two further doses of 1 μg of intradermal HBV vaccine. The trial was considered a failure because 19 of 32 neonates (59.4%) had a low response of less than 10 miu/ml of anti-HBs compared with two of the 33 neonates who received the vaccine intramuscularly ($P < 0.01$). In the second trial in young children, two different regimens were used: two doses of 2 μg of the vaccine were given intradermally after a 20 μg intramuscular dose or three doses of 2 μg were given intradermally. In both cases the geometric mean antibody responses were significantly lower than in the control group who were given 20 μg intramuscularly followed by two 10 μg doses intramuscularly. Vaccine failures, defined as the presence of surface antigen or core antibody or the absence of surface antibody, were also significantly higher in the intradermal groups. In the third trial, 4 μg of vaccine were given intradermally with a multiple orifice puncture gun to 20 young children and all had a good surface antibody response. It was pointed out, however, that this was a large dose, 40% of the recommended intramuscular dose, and might have been just as successful if it had been given intramuscularly. It was concluded that in an endemic area people soon become infected with hepatitis B virus and that at present the conventional intramuscular regimens using relatively large doses of vaccine are to be preferred, despite their considerable costs.[6]

The overriding consideration is efficacy of protection. In most of the studies reported to date, those who received hepatitis B vaccine intradermally were young healthy subjects, in whom the antibody response is known to be good, and the vaccine was given by experienced staff under ideal conditions. There are no data on the longer term duration of anti-HBs, on the subclass(es) of the antibody induced, or on antibody specificity and affinity. Furthermore, protective efficacy studies of intradermal immunization against hepatitis B have not been reported so far.

International and national requirements for vaccine manufacture and licence require assurance on safety, immunogenicity and protective efficacy of the recommended dosage and schedule of administration. It seems imprudent to ignore these requirements and recommendations. Careful evaluation and review of the intradermal route (and indeed of low-dose schedules) are essential, especially in countries where circumstances are not ideal either for storage or for accurate intradermal administration of a vaccine.

INDICATIONS FOR IMMUNIZATION AGAINST HEPATITIS B

The current indications for the use of hepatitis B vaccines in low prevalence areas are summarized below, although these recommendations are under review. The recommendation for immunization against this infection in intermediate and high prevalence regions also include universal immunization of infants.[7,8] Many countries, including the USA and Italy, introduced universal immunization for infants in 1992 and it is expected that most countries will implement this policy by 1996.

Current policy in the UK

1. All health care personnel in frequent contact with blood or needles; groups at the highest risk in this category include:
   (a) Personnel, including teaching and training staff, directly involved over a period of time in patient care in residential institutions for the mentally handicapped where there is a known high risk of hepatitis.
   (b) Personnel directly involved in patient care over a period of time, working in units giving treatment to persons known to be at high risk of hepatitis B infection.
   (c) Personnel directly involved in patient care working in haemodialysis, haemophilia and

other centres regularly performing maintenance treatment of patients with blood or blood products.

(d) Laboratory workers regularly exposed to increased risk from infected material.

(e) Health care personnel on secondment to work in areas of the world where there is a high prevalence of hepatitis B infection, if they are to be directly involved in patient care.

(f) Dentists and ancillary dental personnel with direct patient contact.

2. Patients:

(a) Patients on first entry into those residential institutions for the mentally handicapped where there is a known high incidence of hepatitis B.

(b) Patients treated by maintenance haemodialysis.

(c) Patients for major surgery who are likely to require a large number of blood transfusions and/or treatment with blood products.

3. Contacts of patients with hepatitis B: the spouses and other sexual contacts of patients with acute hepatitis B or carriers of HBV, and other family members in close contact.

4. Other indications for immunization:

(a) Infants born to mothers who are persistent carriers of HBsAg or are HBsAg positive as a result of recent infection, particularly if HBeAg is detectable, or HBV-positive mothers without antibody to e antigen (anti-HBe). The optimum timing for immunoglobulin to be given at a contralateral site is immediately at birth or within 12 hours.

(b) Health care workers who are accidentally pricked with needles used for patients with hepatitis B. The vaccine may be used alone or in combination with hepatitis B immunoglobulin as an alternative to passive immunization with hepatitis B immunoglobulin only. Studies on the efficacy of these different schedules of immunization are nearing completion.

5. Immediate protection: infants born to carrier mothers. Whenever immediate protection is required, as, for example, for infants born to HBsAg-positive mothers (see 4(a) above) or following transfer of an individual into a 'high-risk' setting or after accidental inoculation, active immunization with the vaccine should be combined with simultaneous administration of hepatitis B immunoglobulin at a different site. It has been shown that passive immunization with up to 3 ml (200 iu anti-HBs per ml) of hepatitis B immunoglobulin does not interfere with an active immune response. A single dose of hepatitis B immunoglobulin (usually 3 ml for adults; 1–2 ml for the newborn) is sufficient for healthy individuals. If infection has already occurred at the time of the first immunization, virus multiplication is unlikely to be inhibited completely, but severe illness and, most importantly, the development of the HBV carrier state may be prevented in many individuals, particularly in infants born to carrier mothers.

6. The immune response to the current hepatitis B vaccines is poorer in immunocompromised patients and in the elderly. For example, only about 60% of patients undergoing treatment by maintenance haemodialysis develop anti-HBs. It is suggested therefore that patients with chronic renal damage be immunized as soon as it appears likely that they will ultimately require treatment by maintenance haemodialysis or renal transplant. Consideration should be given to the use of blood from healthy immunized donors with high titres of anti-HBs for the routine haemodialysis of such patients who respond poorly to immunization against hepatitis B.

7. Other groups at risk of hepatitis B include the following:

(a) Individuals who frequently change sexual partners, particularly promiscuous male homosexuals and prostitutes.

(b) Intravenous drug abusers.

(c) Staff at reception centres for refugees and immigrants from areas of the world where hepatitis B is very common, such as South-East Asia.

(d) Although they are at 'lower risk', consideration should also be given to long-term prisoners and staff of custodial institutions, ambulance and rescue services, and selected police personnel.

(e) Military personnel are included in some countries.

DEVELOPING NEW HEPATITIS B IMMUNIZATION STRATEGIES

There is now strong support for the introduction of universal antenatal screening to identify hepatitis B carrier mothers and the vaccination of their babies. It is important that any other strategies do not interfere with the delivery of vaccine to this group. Immunization of this group will have the greatest impact in reducing the number of new hepatitis B carriers. For children outside this group it is difficult to estimate the lifetime risk of acquiring a hepatitis B infection.

There are four main approaches:

1. To continue vaccination of the 'high risk' babies, as defined above.
2. Universal infant immunization.
3. Universal adolescent immunization.
4. Vaccinate everybody.

VACCINATION OF ADOLESCENTS

This approach delivers vaccination at a time close to that when 'risk behaviour' would expose adolescents to infection. Vaccination could be delivered as part of a wider package on health education in general, to include sex education, risk of AIDS, dangers of drug abuse, smoking and the benefits of a healthy diet and life style.

The problems with this approach are as follows:

- Persuading parents to accept vaccination of children against a sexually transmitted disease—a problem they may not wish to address at that time.
- Ensuring that a full course of three doses is given.
- Difficulty in evaluating and monitoring vaccine cover. The systems for monitoring uptake of vaccine in this age group may not operate efficiently.

VACCINATION OF INFANTS

The advantages of this approach are:

- It is known that vaccination can be delivered to babies.
- Parents would accept vaccination against hepatitis B along with other childhood vaccinations without reference to sexual behaviour.

The disadvantages of this approach are:

- The question of whether immunity would last until exposure occurred in later life. This was however to become less of a problem as more people were vaccinated because the chance of exposure to infection was reduced.
- That the introduction of further childhood vaccination would reduce the uptake of other childhood vaccinations. This problem would be avoided if hepatitis B vaccine could be delivered in combination with diphtheria, pertussis and tetanus (DPT) vaccine and this proposal may have to await the production and evaluation of a suitable vaccine.

Vaccination of infants is preferable to vaccination of adolescents as there are sufficient mechanisms to ensure, monitor and evaluate cover. A booster dose could be given in early adolescence, combined with a health education package. A rolling programme could be introduced, giving priority to urban areas.

POLYPEPTIDE VACCINES

Hepatitis B polypeptide vaccines containing specific hepatitis B antigenic determinants of the major non-glycosylated peptide I of the surface antigen with a molecular weight of 22 000–24 000 and its glycosylated form, a polypeptide with a molecular weight in the range of 22 000–24 000 have been prepared in micellar form.[9] The individual polypeptides of the surface antigen are immunogenic, and the purified 24 000 (designated as p24) and 27 000 (gp27) molecular weight polypeptides are effective antigens. Clinical trials of the polypeptide micelle vaccine have been conducted.[10]

PRODUCTION OF HEPATITIS B VACCINES BY RECOMBINANT DNA TECHNIQUES

Recombinant DNA techniques have been used for expressing HBsAg and HBcAg in prokaryotic cells (*Escherichia coli* and *Bacillus subtilis*) and in eukaryotic cells, such as mutant mouse LM cells, HeLa cells, COS cells, CHO cells and yeast cells (*Saccharomyces cerevisiae*).

Recombinant yeast hepatitis B vaccines have undergone extensive evaluation in clinical trials. The results have indicated that this vaccine is safe, antigenic and free from side-effects (apart from minor local reactions in a proportion of recipients). The immunogenicity is similar, in general terms, to that of the plasma-derived vaccine. Recombinant yeast hepatitis B vaccines are now being used in many countries. A vaccine based on HBsAg expressed in mammalian (CHO) cells is in use in the People's Republic of China.

HEPATITIS B VACCINES CONTAINING PRE-S EPITOPES

A disadvantage of plasma-derived and recombinant hepatitis B vaccines containing only the major protein of HBsAg (without pre-S sequences) is the lack of immune responsiveness of a minority of vaccinees. The identification of an immunodominant domain in the pre-S2 region of HBsAg and the observation that mice which were immunologically non-responsive to the major protein of HBsAg made antibodies to a synthetic peptide corresponding to this epitope stimulated interest in incorporation of pre-S sequences in hepatitis B vaccines. Itoh et al[11] demonstrated that a synthetic peptide encompassing 19 amino acids from the pre-S2 region, when coupled to keyhole limpet haemocyanin, elicited a protective antibody response when administered to chimpanzees. The middle (pre-S2 + S) and large (pre-S1 + pre-S2 + S) forms of HBsAg have been expressed in yeast using constitutive and inducible promoters, respectively. The former preparation has been evaluated for safety and immunogenicity. A vaccine containing all three (large, middle and major) forms of HBsAg, synthesized in Chinese hamster ovary cells, has been tested in Singapore. The preparation proved safe and immunogenic with a rapid antibody response in 96% of the recipients.[12]

HYBRID VIRUS VACCINES

Potential live vaccines using recombinant vaccinia viruses have been constructed for hepatitis B, and also for herpes simplex, rabies and other viruses. Foreign viral DNA is introduced into the vaccinia virus genome by construction of chimaeric genes and homologous recombination in cells because the large size of the genome of vaccinia virus (185 000 base pairs) precludes gene insertion in vitro. A chimaeric gene consisting of vaccinia virus promoter sequences ligated to the coding sequence for the desired foreign protein is flanked by vaccinia virus DNA in a plasmid vector.

Recloned vaccinia virus containing hepatitis B surface antigen sequences has been used successfully for 'priming' experimental animals. At present, however, there is no accepted laboratory marker of attenuation or virulence of vaccinia virus for man, either in the host directly inoculated with the virus or after several passages in the same species. Alterations in the genome of vaccinia virus which are concomitant with the selection of recombinants may alter the virulence of the virus. Changes in host range or tissue tropism of vaccinia viruses may occur as a result of their genetic modification and these could be caused by changes in the virus envelope as a result of the incorporation of gene products of the foreign viral genes inserted into the vaccinia virus.

The advantages of a vaccinia virus recombinant as a vaccine include low cost, ease of administration by multiple pressure or by the scratch technique, vaccine stability, long shelf-life and the possible use of polyvalent antigens. The known adverse reactions with vaccinia virus vaccines are well documented and their incidence and severity must be carefully weighed against the adverse reactions associated with existing vaccines which a new recombinant vaccine might replace. There are also reports of spread of current strains of vaccinia virus to contacts and this may present difficulties. Other recombinant viruses as vectors are being explored, and in particular the oral adenovirus vaccines which have been in use for some 20 years (reviewed by Zuckerman[13]).

NOVEL HEPATITIS B VACCINES USING HYBRID PARTICLES

Other developments include the use of the envelope proteins of HBV (HBsAg) in a particulate form by expressing the proteins in mammalian cells. In-phase insertions of variable length and sequence of another virus (poliomyelitis virus type I) were made in different regions of the S gene of HBV. The envelope proteins carrying the surface antigen and the insert are assembled with cellular lipids in the cultured mammalian cells after transfection. The inserted polio neutralization peptide was found to be exposed on the surface of the hybrid envelope particles and induced neutralizing antibodies against poliovirus in mice immunized experimentally. This approach may also be useful for studying the biological activity of other peptides incorporated into the surface of an organized multimolecular complex. The expression and secretion of hybrid envelope particles by established cell lines may thus provide an efficient system for the production of potential new vaccines.

Another potentially excellent carrier vehicle for human and veterinary vaccines in addition to hepatitis B is the use of the core particles of HBV. The advantage of the core structure as a particle includes its ability to induce antibody with approximately 100-fold greater efficiency than the surface antigen particle, and an ability to augment T-helper cell function. The feasibility of this approach was recently demonstrated with synthetic and biosynthetic peptides of foot and mouth disease virus after fusion to hepatitis B core.

CHEMICALLY SYNTHESIZED HEPATITIS B VACCINES

The development of chemically synthesized polypeptide vaccines offers many advantages in attaining the ultimate goal of producing chemically uniform, safe and cheap viral immunogens to replace many current vaccines, which often contain large quantities of irrelevant microbial antigenic determinants, proteins and other material additional to the essential immunogen required for the induction of a protective antibody.[13,14] The preparation of antibodies against viral proteins using fragments of chemically synthesized peptides mimicking viral amino acid sequences is now a possible and attractive alternative approach in immunoprophylaxis.

Successful mimicking of determinants of HBsAg using chemically synthesized peptides in linear and cyclical forms has been reported by several groups of investigators. Peptides have been synthesized which retain biological function and appropriate secondary structure, even though they have a limited sequence homology with the natural peptide or are much smaller.

Enhancement in the immunogenicity of the pre-S region of HBsAg has been demonstrated in mice, using chemically synthesized amino acid residues. The immune response to the pre-S2 region was shown to be regulated by H-2 linked genes which are distinct from those which regulate the response to the S region. It was also demonstrated that immunization of a 'non-responder' murine strain with particles which contain both S and pre-S2 can circumvent non-responsiveness. More recently a protein sequence which mediates the attachment of HBV virus to human hepatoma cells was identified. A synthetic peptide analogue, which is recognized by both cell receptors and viral antibodies, elicited antibodies reacting with the virus. Such a preparation may elicit protective antibodies by blocking the attachment of virus to the cells.

However, designing proteins with the correct tertiary structure and with functional activities is exceedingly difficult because it is not possible to predict the tertiary structure of a protein from its amino acid sequence alone. X-ray crystallography and interactive computer graphics are essential and available tools. The first step is to obtain a highly purified protein which can be crystallized to diffraction quality. The electron density of the crystal can then be calculated and since crystallography provides information on the non-hydrogen atoms in proteins it is possible to build a scaffold model for fitting the known amino acid sequence into this structure. The model can then be refined by using sets to test co-ordinates to improve the density map. More recent techniques using synchrotron X-ray sources may allow the collection of structural information from protein in solution. However, there are no proven principles yet for *de novo* protein design, although it is equally clear that significant advances are being made in the construction of secondary patterns of proteins.

Nevertheless, there are several reports which show that the modification of peptides based on secondary structure predictions and model building is now feasible. Peptides have been synthesized which retain biological function and appropriate secondary structure, even though they have a limited sequence homology with the natural peptide or are much smaller. For example, studies with hormones have shown that it is possible to stabilize a turn by cyclization of the molecule, either by introducing a disulphide bond or by designing a cyclic peptide.

Synthetic peptides may therefore be employed in due course as vaccines, although mixtures of more than one of the peptides may be required. Of the many questions which remain to be answered, the critical issues are whether antibodies induced by synthetic immunogens will be protective and whether protective immunity will persist. Some of the carrier proteins and some of the adjuvants which had been linked to the synthetic molecules cannot be used in man, and it is therefore essential to find acceptable and safe material for covalent linkage, or to synthesize sequences which do not require linkage.

HEPATITIS B ANTIBODY ESCAPE MUTANTS

The emergence of mutants of HBV resistant to vaccine-induced antibody has been reported in Italy[15] and in Singapore[16] and more recently elsewhere. In most cases in Italy, and all in Singapore, the neonate of an infectious carrier mother became chronically infected despite circulating anti-surface antibody (anti-HBs) following combined immunoprophylaxis with HBIG and vaccine. Nucleotide sequence analysis of the region of the HBV genome encoding the major antigenic domain of the surface protein revealed a point mutation (guanosine to adenosine) which specifies a coding change from glycine to arginine in the surface antigen. The amino acid residue involved is located in the second loop of the *a* determinant. Although it has not been possible to detect the variant in the mothers' sera, it is likely that their infecting dose of virus may have included the variant. It is possible then that the anti-HBs antibody present in HBIG neutralized wild-type virus, leaving the variant to become established in the neonate despite vaccination. This hypothesis is supported by a report from the USA[17] of the identical mutation in an HBV variant isolated from an adult following transplantation for HBV-related liver disease. The human monoclonal anti-HBs which was given in an unsuccessful attempt to prevent reinfection of the graft seems to have selected the mutant. Identical mutants have been reported from Japan, and preliminary studies suggest a similar mutant in Brazil.

HBV PRECORE MUTANTS

When DNA–DNA hybridization replaced the less sensitive assay of the endogenous DNA polymerase activity as a method for detecting hepatitis B virions in serum, it became clear that some patients with anti-HBe were seropositive for virus.[18,19] These and other early reports suggested that this finding was more common in Greece and other Mediterranean regions than elsewhere, raising the possibility of the involvement of a variant form(s) of HBV.

Vaudin et al[20] reported the nucleotide sequence of the genome of a strain of HBV cloned from the serum of a naturally infected chimpanzee. A surprising feature was a point mutation in the penultimate codon of the precore region which changed the tryptophan codon (TGG) to an amber termination codon (TAG). The nucleotide sequence of the HBV precore region from a number of anti-HBe-positive Greek patients was investigated by direct sequencing PCR-amplified HBV DNA from serum (Carman et al).[21] An identical mutation of the penultimate codon of the precore region to a termination codon was found in seven of eight anti-HBe-positive patients who were positive for HBV DNA in serum by hybridization. In most cases there was an additional mutation in the preceding codon. Similar variants were found in an Italian study by amplification of HBV DNA from serum from a further seven anti-HBe-positive patients, one of whom seemed to be coinfected with wild-type virus. These variants are not confined to the Mediterranean region; the same nonsense mutation (without a second mutation in the adjacent codon) has been observed in patients from Japan and elsewhere, as well as rarer examples of defective precore regions caused by frameshifts or loss of the initiation codon for the precore region.

Patients without HBeAg with high levels of HBV replication from various geographical areas may be infected frequently by viruses with variant precore regions. Presumably these can replicate without secretion of HBeAg. The majority of patients who are infected with these variants are anti-HBe-positive, implying past infection with non-defective HBV. It is not clear whether these patients were infected originally with a mixture of wild-type and mutant viruses or whether the variants arose throughout the course of natural infection. The process of seroconversion from HBeAg to anti-HBe seems to select the variant viruses and this may be related to the expression of HBeAg on the surface of hepatocytes infected by the wild-type virus.

In many cases precore variants have been described in patients with severe chronic liver disease and who may have failed to respond to therapy with interferon. This observation raises the question of whether they are more pathogenic than the wild-type virus. For example, a nosocomial outbreak of fatal fulminant hepatitis B in Israel was associated with transmission of mutant HBV from a common source to five individuals; and in a study of British patients with fulminant hepatitis B, precore mutants were found in eight of nine HBeAg-negative patients but in none of six who were HBeAg, positive on presentation.

HBV AND HEPATOCELLULAR CARCINOMA (See also Chapters 3 and 24)

Regions of the world where persistent carriage of HBV is common have been found to coincide with a high prevalence of primary liver cancer. Furthermore, in these areas patients with the tumour are almost invariably seropositive for HBsAg. In a prospective study in Taiwan, 184 cases of hepatocellular carcinoma occurred in 3454 carriers of HBsAg at the start of the study, but only ten such tumours occurred in 19 253 control males who were HBsAg negative.[22]

Southern hybridization of tumour DNA yields evidence of chromosomal integration of viral sequences in at least 80% of hepatocellular carcinomas from HBsAg carriers. There is no similarity in the pattern of integration between different tumours, and variation is seen both in the integration site(s) and in the number of copies or partial copies of the viral genome. Sequence analysis of the integrants reveals that the direct repeats in the viral genome often lie close to the virus–cell junctions, suggesting that sequences around the ends of the viral genome may be involved in recombination with host DNA. Integration seems to involve microdeletion of host sequences, and rearrangements and deletions of part of the viral genome may also occur. When an intact surface gene is present, the tumour cells may produce and secrete HBsAg in the form of 22 nm particles. Production of HBcAg by tumours is rare, however, and the core ORF is often incomplete and modifications such as methylation may also modulate its expression. Cytotoxic T cells targeted against core gene products on the hepatocyte surface seem to be the major mechanism of clearance of infected cells from the liver, and cells with integrated viral DNA which are capable of expressing these proteins may also be lysed. Thus there may be immune selection of cells with integrated viral DNA which are incapable of expressing HBcAg.

The mechanism(s) of oncogenesis by HBV remains obscure. HBV may act non-specifically by stimulating active regeneration and cirrhosis, which may be associated with long-term chronicity. However, HBV-associated tumours occur occasionally in the absence of cirrhosis and it is difficult to explain the frequent finding of integrated viral DNA in tumours. In rare instances the viral genome has been found to be integrated into cellular genes such as cyclin A and a retinoic acid receptor. Translocations and other chromosomal rearrangements also have been observed. Although insertional mutagenesis of HBV remains an attractive explanation for oncogenicity, supportive evidence is lacking. In contrast with these findings in human hepatocellular carcinoma, liver cancer in woodchucks associated with persistent infection with the woodchuck hepatitis virus frequently involves integration of the viral genome in or near to cellular *myc* genes.

An alternative possibility is that tumour forma-tion is associated with a viral gene product. The product of the x gene is known to be a transactivator of transcription and so may cause inappropriate up-regulation of cellular genes. Truncated forms of HBsAg, which may be produced from incomplete surface ORFs integrated in tumour cells, can also have transactivating activity, perhaps through interaction with receptors in the cell membrane. Like many other cancers, the development of hepato-cellular carcinoma is likely to be a multifactorial process. The clonal expansion of cells with integrated viral DNA seems to be an early stage in this process and such clones may accumulate in the liver throughout the period of active viral replication. In areas where the prevalence of primary liver cancer is high, virus infection usually occurs at an early age and virus replication may be prolonged, although the peak incidence of tumour is many years after the initial infection.

HEPATITIS D

STRUCTURE AND REPLICATION OF HDV

Delta hepatitis was first recognized following the detection of a novel protein, delta antigen (HDAg), by immunofluorescent staining in the nuclei of hepatocytes from patients with chronic active hepatitis B. Hepatitis delta virus (HDV) requires a helper function of HBV for its replication. HDV is coated with HBsAg which is needed for release from the host hepatocyte and for entry in the next round of infection.

Two forms of delta hepatitis infection are known. In the first, a susceptible individual is coinfected with HBV and HDV, often leading to a more severe form of acute hepatitis caused by HBV. Vaccination against HBV also prevents coinfection. In the second, an individual chronically infected with HBV becomes superinfected with HDV. This may accelerate the course of the chronic liver disease and cause overt disease in asymptomatic HBsAg carriers. HDV itself appears to be cytopathic and HDAg may be directly cytotoxic.

Delta hepatitis is common in some areas of the world with a high prevalence of hepatitis B infection, particularly the Mediterranean region, parts of eastern Europe, the Middle East, Africa and South America. It has been estimated that 5% of HBsAg carriers worldwide (approximately 15 million people) are infected with HDV. In areas of low prevalence for hepatitis B, those at risk of hepatitis B infection—particularly intravenous drug abusers—are also at risk of HDV infection.

The HDV particle is approximately 36 nm in diameter and is composed of an RNA genome associated with HDAg, surrounded by an envelope of HBsAg. The virus reaches higher concentrations in the circulation than HBV—up to 10^{12} particles per millilitre have been recorded. The HDV genome is a closed circular RNA molecule of 1679 nucleotides with extensive sequence complementarity that permits pairing of approximately 70% of the bases to form an unbranched rod structure. The genome thus resembles those of the satellite viroids and virusoids of plants, and similarly seems to be replicated by the host RNA polymerase II with autocatalytic cleavage and circularization of the progeny genomes via *trans*-esterification reactions (ribozyme activity). Consensus sequences of viroids which are believed to be involved in these processes are also conserved in the delta virus.

Unlike the plant viroids, however, HDV codes for a protein, HDAg. This antigen, which contains a nuclear localization signal, was originally detected in the nuclei of infected hepatocytes and may be detected in serum only after removing the outer envelope of the virus with detergent.

HEPATITIS C

Before the identification of hepatitis C virus (HCV), transmission studies in chimpanzees established that the main agent of parenterally acquired non-A, non-B hepatitis was likely to be an enveloped virus some 30–60 nm in diameter.[23,24] The studies by Bradley et al[23] provided a pool of plasma that contained a relatively high titre of the agent. In order to clone the genome, the virus was pelleted from the plasma. Because it was not known whether the genome was DNA or RNA, a denaturation step was included prior to the synthesis of cDNA so that either DNA or RNA could serve as a template. The resultant cDNA was then inserted into the bacteriophage expression vector λ gt11 and the libraries screened using serum from a patient with chronic non-A, non-B hepatitis.[25] This approach led to the detection of a clone (designated 5-1-1) which was found to bind to antibodies present in the sera of several patients with non-A, non-B hepatitis. This clone was used as a probe to detect a larger, overlapping clone in the same library. It was possible to demonstrate that these sequences hybridized to a positive-sense RNA molecule of around 10 000 nt which was present in the livers of infected chimpanzees but not in uninfected controls. By employing a 'walking' technique it was possible to use newly detected overlapping clones as hybridization probes in turn to detect further virus-specific clones in the library. Thus clones covering the entire viral genome were assembled and the complete nucleotide sequence determined. The organization of the genome closely resembles those of the pestiviruses and flaviviruses.

DETECTION OF HCV INFECTION

Since the 5-1-1 antigen was originally detected by antibodies in the serum of an infected patient it was an obvious antigen for the basis of an ELISA to detect anti-HCV antibodies. A larger clone, C100, was assembled from a number of overlapping clones and expressed in yeast as a fusion protein using human superoxide dismutase sequences to facilitate expression. This fusion protein formed the basis of first generation tests for HCV infection. The 5-1-1 antigen comprises amino acid sequences from the non-structural, NS4, region of the genome and C100 contains both NS3 and NS4 sequences. It is now known that antibodies to C100 are detected relatively late following an acute infection. Furthermore, the first generation ELISAs were associated with a high rate of false positivity when applied to

low incidence populations and there were further problems with some retrospective studies on stored sera. Data based on this test alone should, therefore, be interpreted with caution.

Second generation tests include antigens from the nucleocapsid and further non-structural regions of the genome. The former (C22) is particularly useful, and antibodies to the HCV core protein seem to appear relatively early in infection. These second generation tests confirmed that HCV is the major cause of parenterally transmitted non-A, non-B hepatitis. Routine testing of blood donations is now in place in many countries and prevalence rates vary from 0.2–0.5% in northern Europe, to 1.2–1.5% in southern Europe and Japan. Most of those with antibody have a history of parenteral risk, such as a history of transfusion or administration of blood products or of intravenous drug abuse. There is little evidence for sexual or perinatal transmission of HCV and the natural routes of transmission have yet to be identified.

The availability of the nucleotide sequence of HCV made the use of the PCR possible as a direct test for the genome of the virus itself. The first step is the synthesis of a cDNA copy of the target region of the RNA genome using reverse transcriptase (primed by the antigenomic PCR primer or, better, by random hexamers) and the product of this reaction is then a suitable target for amplification. The concentration of virus in serum samples is often very low so that the mass of product(s) from the PCR reaction is insufficient for visualization on a stained gel. Thus either a second round of amplification (with nested primers) or detection of the primary product by southern hybridization is required. There is considerable variation in nucleotide sequences among different isolates of HCV, and the 5' non-coding region, which seems to be highly conserved, is the preferred target for the PCR.

Current data suggest that about 50% of infections with HCV progress to chronicity. Histological examination of liver biopsy-specimens from asymptomatic HCV carriers reveals that none has normal histology, and that up to 70% have chronic active hepatitis and/or cirrhosis. Whether the virus is cytopathic or whether there is an immunopathological element remains unclear. HCV infection is also associated with progression to hepatocellular carcinoma, at least in some countries. For example, in Japan, where the incidence of hepatocellular carcinoma has been increasing despite a decrease in the prevalence of HBsAg, HCV is now the major risk factor. There is no DNA intermediate in the repli-

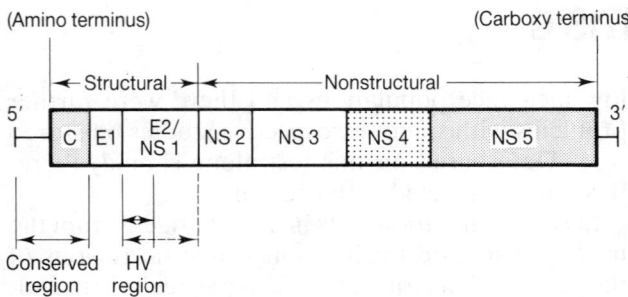

(Amino terminus)   (Carboxy terminus)

Figure 31.4 Hepatitis C viral genome. HV, hypervariable region.

cation of the HCV genome or integration of viral nucleic acid, and viral pathology may contribute to oncogenesis as a result of cirrhosis and regeneration of liver cells.

ORGANIZATION OF THE HCV GENOME

The genome of HCV (Figure 31.4) resembles those of the pestiviruses and flaviviruses in that it comprises around 10 000 nt of positive-sense RNA, lacks a 3′ polyA tract and has a similar gene organization. It has been proposed that HCV should be the prototype of a third genus in the family Flaviviridae. All of these genomes contain a single large ORF which is translated to yield a polyprotein from which the viral proteins are derived by posttranslational cleavage and other modifications.

There is a short, untranslated region at the 5′ end of the genomic RNA and a further untranslated region at the 3′ end, the large ORF accounting for over 95% of the sequence. The structural proteins are located towards the 5′ end and the non-structural proteins towards the 3′ end. The first product of the polyprotein is the non-glycosylated capsid protein, C, which complexes with the genomic RNA to form the nucleocapsid. As with the flaviviruses, a hydrophobic domain may anchor the growing polypeptide in the endoplasmic reticulum and facilitate cleavage by a cellular signalase, releasing the nucleocapsid precursor (anchored C). The amino-acid sequence of the nucleocapsid protein seems to be highly conserved among different isolates of HCV.

The next domain in the polyprotein also has a signal sequence at its carboxy-terminus and may be processed in a similar fashion. The product is a glycoprotein which is probably found in the viral envelope and is referred to as E1/S or gp35. The third domain may be cleaved by a protease within the viral polyprotein to yield what is probably a second surface glycoprotein, E2/NS1 or gp70. These proteins are of considerable interest because of their potential use in tests for the direct detection of viral proteins and for HCV vaccines. Nucleotide sequencing studies reveal that both domains contain hypervariable regions. It is possible that this divergence has been driven by antibody pressure and that these regions specify important immunogenic epitopes.

The non-structural region of the HCV genome is divided into regions NS2–NS5. In the flaviviruses, NS3 has two functional domains, a protease which is involved in cleavage of the non-structural region of the polyprotein and a helicase which is presumably involved in RNA replication. Motifs within this region of the HCV genome have homology to the appropriate consensus sequences, suggesting similar functions. NS5 seems to be the replicase and contains the gly-asp-asp motif common to viral RNA-dependent RNA polymerases.

OTHER HEPATITIS VIRUSES

It is likely that there are other human hepatitis viruses. Whilst HCV is clearly the major cause of parenterally transmitted non-A, non-B hepatitis, data from some of the original and other transmission experiments suggest that at least one other agent might be involved. A number of candidates are already emerging. Togavirus-like particles have been observed in the livers of patients with fulminant, sporadic (community acquired) non-A, non-B hepatitis.[26] A number of these patients proceeded to transplantation, with apparent reinfection of the graft with haemorrhagic manifestations. A severe form of sporadic hepatitis, characterized histologically by large syncytial giant hepatocytes and perhaps caused by a paramyxovirus, has also been described,[27] and other viruses may well await discovery.

TREATMENT OF ACUTE VIRAL HEPATITIS

There is no specific treatment (see also Chapter 3). General measures include bed-rest and a generally nutritious diet. Patients should be encouraged to exercise regularly if they feel well. Consumption of alcohol should be avoided during the acute phase and continue to be modest after convalescence.

Corticosteroids and non-steroidal anti-inflammatory drugs are *not* indicated and should not be used.

TREATMENT OF CHRONIC HEPATITIS B INFECTION

Specific treatment is now available following the demonstration that interferon-α inhibits replication of HBV, and that prolonged treatment can lead to remission of the disease (reviewed by Dusheiko and Zuckerman[28]).

Antiviral therapy is aimed at patients with active disease and viral replication, preferably at a stage before signs and symptoms of cirrhosis or significant injury have occurred. Eradication of the disease is possible in only a minority of patients. Permanent loss of HBV DNA and HBeAg results in an improvement in necroinflammatory change(s), and reduced infectivity. It is possible that the accompanying histological improvement reduces the risk of cirrhosis and hepatocellular carcinoma.

Unfortunately, treatment of chronic hepatitis with interferon is effective in less than half of those treated. It is relatively expensive, requires administration by injection, is often confusing in its effects, and is not free of side-effects. None the less, recombinant interferon-α has been licensed for treatment of chronic hepatitis B in the UK and several European countries.

The interferons act by interaction with specific membrane receptors, thereby inducing a number of enzymes and proteins, the best characterized of which are the $2',5'$-oligoadenylate synthetases ($2',5'$- A synthetases) and protein kinases. The expression of the class I major histocompatibility antigen (MHC) genes are activated by all interferons, and those of class II by interferon-γ, to increase the expression of MHC at the cell surface, and thereby amplify viral antigen recognition and display. Interferons also modify the cellular and humoral immune response.

Three preparations of interferon-α are currently available, two of which are recombinant preparations and one of which is prepared from a lymphoblastoid cell line. Approximately 40% of patients respond. Highest response rates are usually seen in carriers with higher baseline serum aminotransferase levels, lower levels of HBV DNA and without AIDS. Although these factors provide some predictive information, none of these criteria is absolute, and individual carriers, for example ethnic Chinese, with active disease, or those patients with anti-HIV antibodies but normal CD^4 lymphocyte counts, may respond, making the prediction of treatment outcome somewhat difficult. The appropriate dose of interferon is not yet established, but 5–10 mu three times weekly for 3–4 months is currently prescribed.

The subclinical exacerbation of the hepatitis frequently seen in responders suggests that interferon acts by augmenting the immune response to HBV, perhaps triggered by the inhibition of viral replication as well as the effects of interferon on cytotoxic T cells. Although residual HBV DNA can be detected by PCR, the disease appears to be ameliorated. Approximately 20% of patients who respond to treatment with clearance of HBeAg will also clear HBsAg within a year of treatment, and up to 65% may later clear HBsAg after 6 years of follow-up.

Patients who do not respond to interferon-α represent a difficult management problem. Lower doses given for a longer period are currently being studied.

Pulsed corticosteroid treatment and interferon may also be of benefit in patients without elevated serum aminotransferases. This treatment regimen should be used with caution in those patients with decompensated hepatitis B because of the risk of inducing severe hepatic necrosis.

The major early side-effects of interferon include an influenza-like illness. Later side-effects include: malaise, muscle aches, headaches, poor appetite, weight-loss, increased need for sleep, irritability, anxiety and depression, hair loss, thrombocytopenia and leucopenia. Unusual or severe side-effects include: seizures, acute psychosis, bacterial infections, autoimmune reactions, thyroid disease, proteinuria, cardiomyopathy, skin rashes and interferon antibodies.

OTHER ANTIVIRAL DRUGS

A number of other agents have been used for the treatment of hepatitis B. These include interferon-γ, acyclovir (acycloguanosine), 6-deoxyacyclovir, ganciclovir, foscarnet (tri-sodium phosphonoformate), azido-3'-deoxythymidine triphosphate, 2',3'-dideoxycytidine and 2',3'-dideoxyinosine, adenine arabinoside 5'-monophosphate (ara-AMP), phyllanthrus amarus, interleukin-2, isoprinosine, thymosin, tumour necrosis factor, transfer factor, adenine arabinoside 5'-monophosphate conjugated with lactosaminated albumin, interferon-γ and -α, interferon-γ and -β, acyclovir and interferon, and levamisole. Few of these agents are useful clinically, but ganciclovir, ara-AMP and foscarnet may suppress HBV in some patients.

Several newer nucleoside analogues suppress hepatitis B in vitro, and these drugs are at present undergoing clinical trial in humans.

TREATMENT OF CHRONIC HEPATITIS C INFECTIONS

Interferon-α treatment is indicated for patients with well-documented chronic hepatitis C in whom other causes of chronic hepatitis have been excluded, and who have at least a twofold elevation of serum alanine aminotransferase. Interferon-α ameliorates disease activity in approximately 50% of patients with hepatitis C after short courses (6 months) of treatment. Liver biopsy histology provides useful information regarding the extent of liver damage. Treatment should be started at a dose of 3×10^6 units, three times weekly, and administered subcutaneously for 6 months. Treatment can be discontinued after 3 months if no response has occurred. However, approximately 50% of responders relapse when treatment is stopped. Almost all of these relapses tend to re-respond to retreatment.

Ribavirin, a nucleoside analogue which is taken orally, has also been shown to inhibit HCV. This drug may be a better choice for patients with cirrhosis, who respond poorly to interferon. The major side-effect of ribavirin is haemolysis, and the drug is still under study.

REFERENCES

1 Cohen J L, Ticehurst J R, Purcell R M et al. Complete nucleotide sequence of wild-type hepatitis A virus: comparison with different strains of hepatitis A virus and other picornaviruses. *J Virol* 1987; 61:51–59.

2 Shaw F E Jr, Guess I J A, Roets J M et al. Effect of anatomic site, age and smoking on the immune response to hepatitis B vaccination. *Vaccine* 1989; 7:425–430.

3 Cockcroft A, Soper P, Insail C et al. Antibody response after hepatitis B immunisation in health care workers. *Br J Ind Med* 1990; 47:199–202.

4 Zuckerman J N, Cockcroft A & Zuckerman A J. Site of injection for vaccination. *BMJ* 1992; 305:1158.

5 Zuckerman A J. Appraisal of intradermal immunisation against hepatitis B. *Lancet* 1987; i:435–436.

6 Whittle H C, Lamb W H & Ryder R W. Trials of intradermal hepatitis B vaccines in Gambian children. *Ann Trop Paediatr* 1987; 7:6–9.

7 Zuckerman A J. Who should be immunised against hepatitis B? *BMJ* 1984; 289:1243–1244.

8 Deinhardt F D & Zuckerman A J. Immunization against hepatitis B: report on a WHO meeting on viral hepatitis in Europe. *J Med Virol* 1985; 17:209–217.

9 Skelly J, Howard C R & Zuckerman A J. Hepatitis B polypeptide vaccine in micelle form. *Nature* 1981; 290:51–54.

10 Hollinger F B, Trois C, Heiberg D, Sanchez V, Dreesman G R & Melnick J L. Response to hepatitis B polypeptide vaccine in micelle form in a young adult population. *J Med Virol* 1986; 19:229–240.

11 Itoh Y, Takai E, Ohnuma H et al. A synthetic peptide vaccine involving the product of the pre-S(2) region of hepatitis B virus DNA; protective efficacy in chimpanzees. *Proc Natl Acad Sci USA* 1986; 83:9174–9178.

12 Yap L, Guan R & Chan S H. Recombinant DNA hepatitis B vaccine containing pre-S components of the HBV coat protein: a preliminary study on immunogenicity. *Vaccine* 1992; 10:439–442.

13 Zuckerman A J. Immunization against hepatitis B. *Br Med Bull* 1990; 46:383–398.

14 Zuckerman A J. Synthetic hepatitis B vaccine. *Nature* 1973; 241:499.

15 Carman W F, Zanetti A R, Karayiannis P et al. Vaccine-induced escape mutant of hepatitis B virus. *Lancet* 1990; 336:325–329.

16 Harrison T J, Hopes E A, Oon C J, Zanetti A R & Zuckerman A J. Independent emergence of a vaccine-induced escape mutant of hepatitis B virus. *J Hepatol* 1991; 13(supplement 4):S105–S107.

17 McMahon G, Ehrlich, P H & Moustafa Z A. Genetic alterations in the gene encoding the major HBs-DNA and immunological analysis of recurrent HBsAg derived from monoclonal antibody-treated liver transplant patients. *Hepatology* 1992; 15:757–766.

18 Lieberman H M, LaBrecque D R, Kew M C, Hadziyannis S J & Shafritz D A. Detection of hepatitis B virus DNA directly in human serum by a simplified molecular hybridization test: comparison to HBE-Ag/anti-HBe status in HBsAg carriers. *Hepatology* 1983; 3:285–291.

19 Hadziyannis S J, Lieberman H M, Karvountzis G G & Shafritz D A. Analysis of liver disease, nuclear HBcAg, viral replication, and hepatitis B virus DNA in liver and serum of HBeAg vs. anti-HBe positive carriers of hepatitis B virus. *Hepatology* 1983; 3:656–662.

20 Vaudin M, Wolstenholme A J, Tsiquaye K N, Zuckerman A J & Harrison T J. The complete nucleotide sequence of the genome of a hepatitis B virus isolated from a naturally infected chimpanzee. *J Gen Virol* 1988; 69:1383–1389.

21 Carman W F, Jacyna M R, Hadziyannis S, Karayiannis P & Thomas H. Mutation preventing formation of e antigen in patients with chronic hepatitis B. *Lancet* 1989; 2:588–591.

22 Beasley R P & Hwang L-Y. Overview on the epidemiology of hepatocellular carcinoma. In Hollinger F B, Lemon S M & Margolis H S (eds) *Viral Hepatitis and Liver Disease*. Baltimore, MD: Williams & Wilkins, 1991: 532–535.

23 Bradley D W, McCaustland K A, Cook E H, Schable C A, Ebert J W & Maynard J E. Posttransfusion non-A, non-B hepatitis in chimpanzees. Physicochemical evidence that the tubule-forming agent is a small, enveloped virus. *Gastroenterology* 1985; 88:773–779.

24 He L F, Alling D, Popkin T, Shapiro M, Alter H J & Purcell R H. Determining the size of non-A, non-B hepatitis virus by filtration. *J Infect Dis* 1987; 156:636–640.

25 Choo Q L, Kuo G, Weiner A J, Overby L R, Bradley D W & Houghton M. Isolation of a cDNA clone derived from a blood-borne non-A, non-B viral hepatitis genome. *Science* 1989; 244:359–362.

26 Fagan E A, Ellis D S, Tovey G M et al. Toga virus-like particles in acute liver failure attributed to sporadic non-A, non-B hepatitis and recurrence after liver transplantation. *J Med Virol* 1992; 38:71–77.

27 Phillips M J, Blendis L M, Pourcell S et al. Syncytial giant-cell hepatitis. Sporadic hepatitis with distinctive pathological features, a severe clinical course, and paramyxoviral features. *N Engl J Med* 1991; 324:455–460.

28 Dusheiko G M & Zuckerman A J. Therapy for hepatitis B. *Curr Opin Infect Dis* 1991; 4:785–794.

CHAPTER 32

EPSTEIN–BARR VIRUS AND ASSOCIATED DISEASES

Kitty Lam and Dorothy H. Crawford

Epstein–Barr (EB) virus was first isolated from cultures of Burkitt's lymphoma (BL) biopsy-material and was rapidly shown to be a unique herpesvirus.[1] Subsequent studies have shown the virus to be worldwide in distribution, infecting most individuals. EB virus is the established aetiological agent of infectious mononucleosis (IM)[2] and is also associated with certain types of human cancer, namely BL[3], anaplastic nasopharyngeal carcinoma (NPC),[4] lymphoproliferative disorders and lymphoma in the immunocompromised (including non-Hodgkin's lymphoma (NML)),[5] and, most recently, a subset of Hodgkin's disease. In addition, oral hairy leucoplakia, a recently described non-malignant lesion of epithelial cells, is also caused by EB virus.[6]

BIOLOGICAL PROPERTIES

EB virus is a human herpesvirus which is known to infect B lymphocytes[7] and squamous epithelial cells.[8] Infection of B cells occurs via a specific cellular receptor—the CD21 molecule—which also functions as the CR2 receptor for the C3d component of complement.[9] A similar molecule has now been identified on a subset of squamous epithelial cells.[10] In vitro infection of squamous epithelial cells results in a lytic infection with release of new virus particles and cell death. In contrast, infection of B cells results in immortalization of the cells, giving rise to continuously proliferating lymphoblastoid cell lines.[11] This type of infection is termed 'latent' and is associated with a restricted pattern of viral gene expression. At present only nine virus-coded latent proteins have been identified in lympho-blastoid cell lines. These comprise the EB virus nuclear antigen (EBNA) complex of six proteins (EBNA1–6); latent membrane proteins (LMP)1 and LMP2A and LMP2B. The function of these proteins are for the most part unknown, but EBNA1 is necessary for maintenance of the viral genome as multiple plasmids in the host cell nucleus. EBNA2 and LMP act as viral oncogenes, and are essential in the immortalization process. In contrast to the small number of latent proteins, many lytic cycle proteins are expressed. Three major complexes can be identi-fied: the membrane antigen (MA) complex of three glycoproteins, early antigen (EA) complex com-posed of a restricted EA(R) and diffuse EA(D) form and the viral capsid antigen (VCA) complex.[12]

INFECTION IN HEALTHY INDIVIDUALS

Primary infection with EB virus is commonly sub-clinical, occurs predominately in childhood and gives rise to a lifelong carrier state. Seropositivity increases with age, and 90% of adults are seroposi-tive in most populations. However, the rate of seroconversion varies according to economic status, such that up to 90% of children over the age of 2 years in developing countries have evidence of past infection, whereas seroconversion may be delayed until adolescence in high socioeconomic groups of developed countries.[13]

Virus infection usually occurs through the mouth

by close contact with a seropositive individual. Lytic infection of squamous epithelial cells in the oropharynx occurs with production of infectious virus particles into the pharyngeal cavity. Recently the squamous epithelium of the uterine cervix has been identified as a second site of virus replication, suggesting the possibility of sexual transmission in some cases.[14] Peripheral blood B lymphocytes become infected as they pass through sites of virus replication and then enter the general circulation. This type of dual infection persists for life.[15]

Viral replication in squamous epithelium and persistence in peripheral blood B lymphocytes is controlled by EB virus-specific humoral and cellular immunosurveillance mechanisms. Humoral activity is mediated by neutralizing antibody directed to the MA complex of the virus envelope which inhibits virus binding to the CR2 receptor on susceptible cells.[16] In addition, antibodies to VCA and EBNA persist for life at easily detectable levels. Cellular immunity is provided by EB virus-specific, CD8[+] cytotoxic T lymphocytes which can be detected in the circulation in all normal seropositive individuals.[17] To date, all the EB virus latent proteins expressed on infected B cells with the exception of EBNA 1 have been recognized as target antigens by EB virus specific CTL which are killed in an MHC class I restricted manner.[18–20] Thus in the carrier state a balance exists between virus replication and host immune mechanisms which successfully control the infection at a subclinical level. However, in the immunocompromised host this balance may be tipped in favour of virus replication and may lead to EB virus-associated disease.[21]

INFECTIOUS MONONUCLEOSIS

HISTORY

Infectious mononucleosis (IM) was first documented as a clinical entity by Sprunt and Evans (1920)[22] and the association between EB virus and IM was first suggested when a laboratory technician acquired serum antibodies to EB virus during the course of IM.[23] This suggestive observation was later confirmed in a prospective study of university students[13] where it was convincingly shown that students with antibodies to EB virus prior to the study did not suffer from IM; students leaving university with no antibody to EB virus did not develop IM during the study period; and the acquisition of EB virus antibody was coincident with the development of clinical IM in 50% of cases. In the other 50% of students, seroconversion occurred with no clinical illness.

EPIDEMIOLOGY

EB virus infects all known population groups, though IM is commonly seen in Western societies and is rare in non-industrial countries. In addition, IM is more common in high than low socioeconomic groups in the USA and UK. This is because IM usually occurs when a primary infection is delayed until 15–25 years, an age at which most individuals of low socioeconomic status in developing countries have already seroconverted[24] (see above).

TRANSMISSION

The mode of transmission of EB virus is by the oral route and infectious virus can be isolated from saliva and throat washings of most seropositive adults.[25] EB virus has also been detected in squamous epithelial cells of the uterine cervix and in semen from seropositive individuals, suggesting that virus transmission may occur by sexual contact.[26] These sites of virus replication may account for the peak age incidence of IM in adolescents and young adults, when new social contacts are being formed. IM has also been acquired through blood transfusions to seronegative individuals.[27]

PATHOGENESIS

EB virus entering the host via the mouth establishes a productive infection in the squamous epithelial cells of the oropharynx. Secondary infection of B lymphocytes at this site allows spread throughout the body via the peripheral blood circulation. The host immune response to EB virus is rapid and vigorous so that by the time of onset of clinical symptoms both humoral and cellular mechanisms are detectable. Humoral immune mechanisms

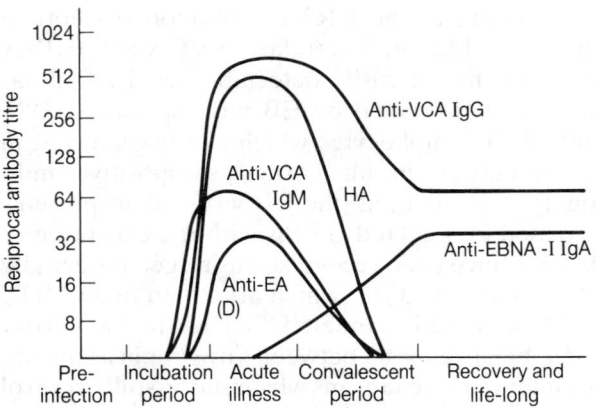

Figure 32.1 Profile of serum antibodies to EB virus-associated antigens before, during and after primary infection. EA(D), diffuse form of early antigen; VCA, viral capsid antigen; HA, heterophile antigen; EBNA, EB virus nuclear antigen.

characterize the course of infection, with IgM, IgA and IgG antibodies to VCA reaching a peak titre coincidentally with clinically overt disease (Figure 32.1). Simultaneously, IgG antibodies to EA(D) and MA are produced, with the latter functioning as a neutralizing antibody preventing further virus infection and spread. Heterophile antibodies are clearly detectable during acute IM and are characteristic of an active infection. These antibodies are directed against antigens unrelated to the virus, such as sheep and horse red cells, and, although their relationship in the virus infection remains unclear, they are a useful diagnostic marker of IM. During convalescence, some 6–12 weeks after onset, titres of IgM and IgA antibodies to VCA and IgG antibodies to EA(D) fall to undetectable levels. IgG antibody to VCA and MA decline and maintain plateau levels throughout life. IgG antibody to EBNA1 only becomes detectable in convalescence, rises to a plateau level and then persists for life. Antibodies to the other EBNA proteins (2–6) are not consistently detectable during or after primary infection. Heterophile antibodies disappear within 2–6 months but occasionally persist for as long as 2 years.[28] Cell-mediated immune functions are depressed during early infection, with anergic responses to various mitogens and antigens. A distinctive feature of IM is a lymphocytosis with the appearance of atypical lymphocytes in the peripheral blood which are predominately CD8 positive. These lymphocytes have been shown to have suppressor cell function and also cytotoxic activity against virus-infected cells and act in a non-MHC restricted manner. Their precise function still remains unclear but they are probably important in controlling and confining the virus infection.[29]

HISTOPATHOLOGICAL FINDINGS

Excision biopsy is rarely performed for a diagnosis of IM but may be required in cases of unusual or complicated infection. Histological appearances in lymph node, liver and spleen typically show a mononuclear cell infiltrate with immunoblastic appearance. These are mainly CD8$^+$ T cells, interspersed with occasional EBNA-positive B cells. Lymph nodes are generally enlarged, with developed lymphoid follicles and germinal centres. Infiltrates are found in widely dilated sinuses and intersinusoidal cords. Cellular infiltration in hepatic portal areas and splenic white pulp have also been reported. These histological changes are not pathogenic for IM and may mimic B cell lymphoma.

CLINICAL MANIFESTATIONS

SYMPTOMS AND SIGNS

After an incubation period estimated at 30–50 days, the onset of IM is often abrupt, although a prodromal period characterized by chills, sweats and feverish sensations may occur.[30] Most cases present with fever, neck swelling and sore throat accompanied by a number of non-specific symptoms, including malaise, headache, abdominal pain, anorexia and myalgia. Tonsillar enlargement, lymphadenopathy and splenomegaly are the most frequent clinical signs and may be accompanied by hepatomegaly and jaundice in some cases. Skin rashes can occur, most commonly induced by the administration of ampicillin.

COMPLICATIONS

In a vast majority of cases IM is a benign and self-limiting disease lasting 6–8 weeks and resulting in full recovery. In some cases, however, relapses may occur within the 6-month period following the acute disease. Fatalities rarely occur and are usually the result of one of the following complications of IM: acute liver necrosis; splenic rupture (which may be spontaneous or follow mild trauma); pharyngeal or tracheal obstruction; neurological complications and haematological disorders, including autoimmune thrombocytopenia and haemolytic anaemia.[31] A rare familial condition, X-linked lymphoproliferative syndrome, is associated with invariably fatal primary EB virus infection in 50% of the male offspring of carrier females. The precise abnormality associated with this genetic defect is unknown.[32]

LABORATORY DIAGNOSIS

The central finding in IM is the 'atypical' mononuclear cell in peripheral blood, accounting for 30% of the mononuclear lymphocytosis.[30] However, the presence of these cells is not diagnostic of IM because they are also found to a lesser extent in other infections, including cytomegalovirus infection, viral hepatitis, toxoplasmosis, rubella, mumps and roseola.[33] A firm diagnosis of IM relies on the detection of serum IgM anti-VCA antibodies, with or without anti-EA(D) antibodies.[28,34] Additionally, the presence of heterophil antibody which causes haemagglutination of red cells from species other than humans is characteristic of infection.[35] A commercial kit is available (Monospot test) which is rapid and reliable, detecting over 90% of acute IM cases and rarely giving false-positive results.[36] This test is generally used as a first-line diagnostic test for IM, although negative results, particularly in children, should be checked with the IgM anti-VCA test.

MANAGEMENT AND TREATMENT

Treatment of IM is largely supportive since more than 95% of patients recover without specific therapy. Sore throats and fever can be alleviated with analgesics, and strenuous exercise should be avoided. Corticosteroids are often advocated and offer some relief for acute symptoms, although their use remains controversial in uncomplicated illness and is probably best reserved for the treatment of tracheal obstruction, autoimmune phenomena and neurological symptoms.[37] Antiviral chemotherapy has been used in a limited number of cases, with little beneficial effect.[38]

BURKITT'S LYMPHOMA (See also Chapter 24)

HISTORY

BL was first described in African children by Denis Burkitt in 1958 as a malignant tumour which principally affected the jaw and represented a new clinical and pathological entity[39] (Figure 32.2).

EPIDEMIOLOGY

Endemic BL represents the most common childhood cancer in parts of equatorial Africa and Papua New Guinea, with an annual incidence in Africa of 15–20 cases per 100000 population annually[40] (Figure 32.3a). The tumour also occurs worldwide but at a 20–200-fold lower incidence than in Africa, and these sporadic BL cases show some epidemiological, clinical and cellular differences to endemic BL. This review concentrates on African BL. Endemic BL occurs between the ages of 3–15 years with a peak incidence at 5–7 years and with a male predominance. The tumour is found in geographically restricted regions of equatorial Africa, occurring only at an altitude of less than 1200m where rainfall is greater than 60cm/year and temperatures are above

16°C. These observations led Denis Burkitt to suggest the involvement of the mosquito vector and a virus in the development of BL. It is now recognized that intense malaria transmission and high levels of persistent EB virus infection predispose the individual to tumour development[41] (see later).

SEROEPIDEMIOLOGY

The geographical restriction of endemic BL suggested an infectious cofactor in tumour development and this was identified when a new herpesvirus, later named as Epstein–Barr (EB) virus, was detected in cell lines grown from endemic BL biopsy-material.[1] These observations, in conjunction with the discovery of EB virus as the aetiological agent of IM, raised the question of whether BL represented a malignant form of IM. Consequently, a prospective study aimed at identifying individuals who may be predisposed to BL development was conducted in which serum antibody titres to EB viral antigens VCA and EA were determined. Of the 42000 children studied, aged 0–8 years and residing in four counties of the Western Nile district of Uganda, 16 new cases of BL were reported over a 2-year period. Examination of their serum antibodies to EB virus

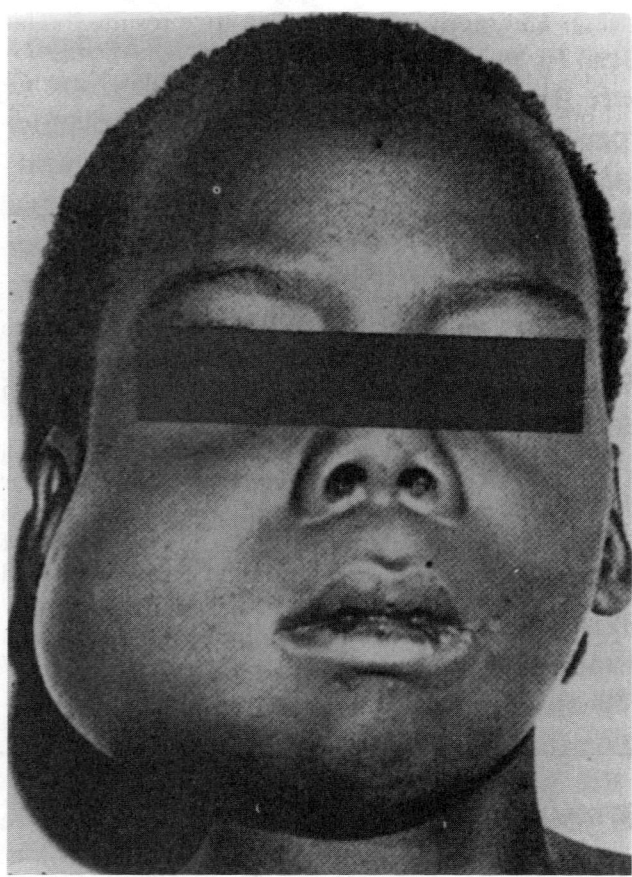

Figure 32.2   An African male child with Burkitt's lymphoma of the jaw.

prior to tumour development showed that all had been seropositive for several years although they exhibited ten times higher anti-VCA geometric mean titres than age/sex/locality-matched controls. It was calculated that the increased risk of developing BL was approximately 30 times higher for children who had VCA titres two dilutions or more above the geometric mean titre. The VCA titre did not increase at tumour onset, though antibodies to EA developed in some cases. These data showed that BL, unlike IM, was not the result of a primary EB virus infection, but suggested that EB virus was an important factor in the development of the disease.[42]

PATHOGENESIS

ASSOCIATION WITH EB VIRUS

No single finding has provided evidence that EB virus is the direct causative agent of BL, but a number of observations imply that it is involved in the malignant process. Firstly, seroepidemiological data suggest a unique pattern of EB virus serum antibody levels before the onset of BL[3] (see above). Secondly, examination of BL biopsy-material identified multiple copies of EB virus DNA and EB virus coded proteins in 96% of BL biopsies originating from endemic areas.[43] Thirdly, EB virus has an immortalizing capacity for B lymphocytes in vitro, resulting in a continuously proliferating lymphoblastoid cell line; in addition BL cells containing EB virus readily grow as cell lines in vitro. Finally, the virus can cause lymphoid tumours in certain non-human primates[44] (see later).

CHROMOSOMAL ABNORMALITIES

All BL tumour cells and their derived cell lines show a characteristic chromosomal translocation between the immunoglobulin gene loci on chromosomes 14, 2 or 22 and the c-*myc* oncogene on chromosome 8.[45] In a normal cell, the c-myc protein is involved in control of the cell cycle, such that it is functional in actively proliferating cells and inactive in quiescent cells. Deregulation of this gene in BL, due to its translocation, probably accounts for the continued proliferative capacity of the BL cell as well as the inability to differentiate.[46] These specific translocations occur in both endemic and sporadic BL cells but can be distinguished by the site of their breakpoints in the Ig gene loci.[47]

HOLOENDEMIC MALARIA

Since EB virus is found worldwide and endemic BL is geographically restricted, other cofactors must be involved in the disease process. Holoendemic *Plasmodium falciparum* malaria has been suggested because the geographical distribution of the two diseases is strikingly similar and subsequent observations have confirmed this association. Thus the incidence of BL has been reduced in areas where malaria-carrying mosquitoes have been eradicated; in urban areas where malaria transmission is lower than in rural areas and in individuals who are carriers of the sickle cell anaemia trait and are thereby protected from severe malaria.[48] These observations led to the proposal of a multistep scenario in the development of endemic BL incorporating the various associated factors. This proposes that chronic malaria infection, which results in polyclonal activation of B cells, increases the chance(s) of an aberrant chromosomal translocation involving the c-*myc* oncogene. EB virus infection of such a cell would release it into autonomous cell growth. This process is enhanced by malaria-induced immunosuppression decreasing the efficiency of EB virus-

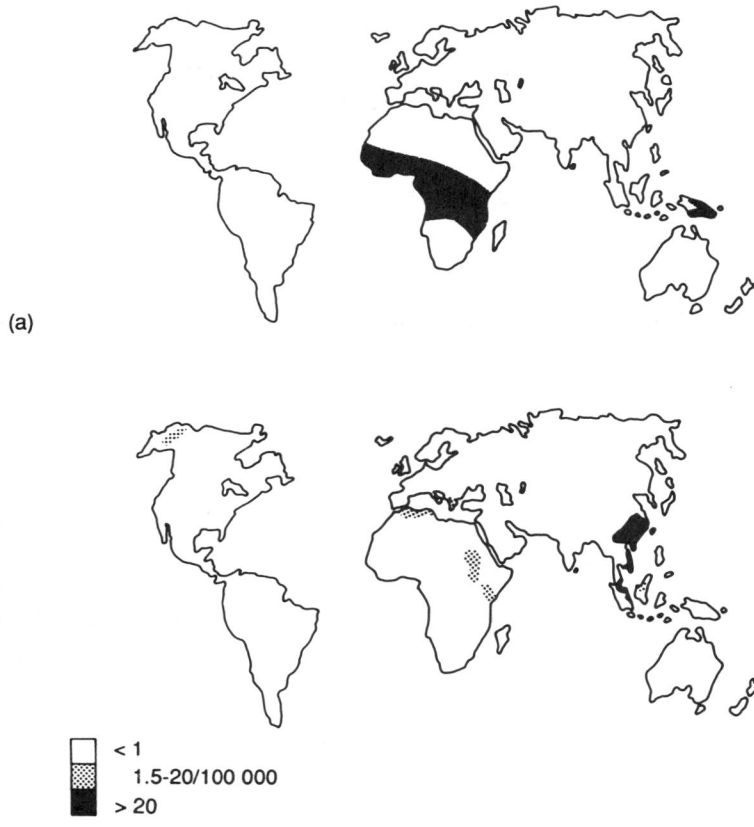

(a)

(b)

☐ < 1
▨ 1.5-20/100 000
■ > 20

Figure 32.3 Worldwide distribution of incidence to EB virus-associated tumours: (a) Burkitt's lymphoma, and (b) nasopharyngeal carcinoma.

specific immune mechanisms.[49] Aspects of this hypothesis have been substantiated by the observations that children with acute malaria have a reduced EB virus-specific cytotoxic T-cell activity and a correspondingly higher number of EB virus-carrying B cells which return to normal levels in convalescence.[50,51]

HISTOPATHOLOGY

Original histopathological observations made by O'Connor and Davis (1960)[52] identified the tumour described by Burkitt to be a lymphoma. The malignant tumour consists of lymphoid cells which are undifferentiated and monomorphic, possessing amphophilic cytoplasm with clear vacuoles and non-cleaved nuclei with 2–5 basophilic nucleoli. A large number of histiocytes infiltrate the tissue, giving it a characteristic 'starry sky' appearance (Figure 32.4). There still remains some controversy over the histological classification of BL and in the present working formulation of non-Hodgkin's lymphoma (NHL); BL belongs to the high-grade, malignant lymphoma, small non-cleaved cell group.[53]

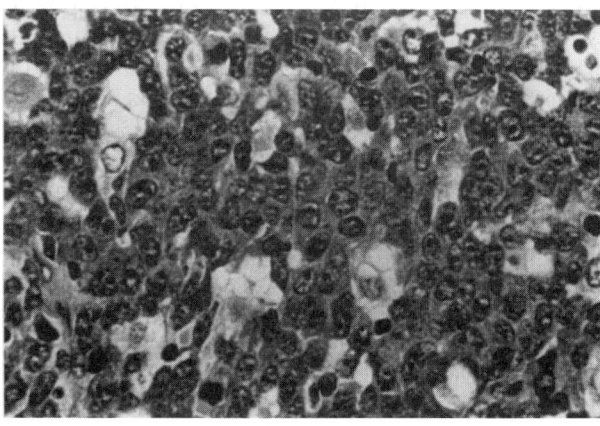

Figure 32.4 Histological section of Burkitt's lymphoma showing monomorphic lymphoid cells with histiocytic infiltration. (H & E, 800×.) (Courtesy of P. Isaacson, University College Hospital, London.)

CLINICAL FEATURES

Sixty per cent of cases of BL present with a tumour of the jaw, with or without orbital or mandibular invasion.[54] However, at presentation, the tumour is usually found to be multifocal, with other common sites being the testis, ovaries, breast (in pubertal girls), liver, stomach and intestine. Lymph nodes and spleen are rarely involved and bone-marrow invasion only occurs during the terminal phase of the disease. Intracranial invasion is common at a late stage, with lymphomatous deposits in extradural spaces which may lead to partial or complete paralysis.

LABORATORY DIAGNOSIS AND TREATMENT

The diagnosis of BL in endemic areas is made on clinical and histological evidence. Initially, treatment of the tumour centred on radiation and surgery, though later cyclophosphamide was found to be successful, giving an excellent remission rate.[55] Chemotherapy now generally includes cyclophosphamide, vincristine, methotrexate, cytosine arabinoside and BCG. If clinical relapse occurs within the first 9 months, survival does not usually exceed 2.5 years.[56] Titres of serum antibodies can be used as prognostic markers, with high titres of anti-EA(R) heralding a relapse. Remission and long-term survival is accompanied by low or undetectable levels of anti-EA(R), and high levels of antibody to MA.[57]

LYMPHOMA IN HUMAN IMMUNODEFICIENCY VIRUS-INFECTED INDIVIDUALS (See also Chapter 12)

HISTORY AND EPIDEMIOLOGY

The World Health Organization estimates that nine million individuals worldwide are infected with the human immunodeficiency virus (HIV)—who additionally have an increased incidence of opportunistic infections, Kaposi's sarcoma, squamous cell carcinoma and malignant lymphomas.[58] In the USA, the incidence of NHL has increased in parallel with the acquired immune deficiency syndrome (AIDS) epidemic, and this clinical association led to the inclusion of it as a diagnostic criterion for AIDS.[59] A recent study shows a 5% overall incidence of AIDS-NHL, which is approximately 60 times the frequency of NHL arising spontaneously in the general population.[60] In addition, with increasing longevity resulting from successful antiretroviral therapy, a cumulative rate of 28.6% at 30 months has been calculated for those on long-term azidothymidine therapy.[61] Attempts to identify risk factors in the development of AIDS-NHL in the USA have identified the following parameters: it occurs twice as commonly in men as in women; it occurs in white more than black populations; it is more common in haemophiliac patients; and it is less common in patients of African or Caribbean origin or in patients acquiring HIV through heterosexual contact. No difference in incidence was seen between intravenous drug users and homosexual men with regard to NHL histological cell type, grade or disease progression.[60] Statistical data of AIDS-NHL in Africa has been difficult to obtain without accurate information on the size of groups at risk. Data on common disease associations with AIDS patients in Africa are slowly being defined, though much of the evaluation has been derived from patients examined in Europe where resources permit expensive procedures. Initial data show a similar range of diseases encountered in Western countries, although the relative prevalences differ. Such data as exist suggest that AIDS-NHL is rare in Africa, perhaps due to the high rate of heterosexual transmission and early death from opportunistic infection(s).[62]

HISTOPATHOLOGY AND PATHOGENESIS

The aetiology of AIDS-NHL is unknown but reactive lymphoid hyperplasia, progressive HIV-induced immunosuppression, and EB virus infection are thought to be important contributing factors. The majority are of B lymphocyte origin, but recently T cell lymphomas have also been recognized in the AIDS setting. A wide spectrum of histological types have been observed, from which two major categories can be identified.[63] The first group are large cell lymphomas of immunoblastic/plasmacytoid type which account for 60–80% of

AIDS-NHL and occur more commonly in the older (>40 years) age groups with severe immunosuppression. These tumours are similar to those arising in immunosuppressed patients, particularly organ transplant recipients in that they usually arise at extranodal sites, in particular the gastrointestinal tract or central nervous system (CNS) and usually contain EB viral DNA and express viral proteins.[64] There is a suggestion that mutations of the tumour suppressor gene p53 is an event involved in the tumorigenic process. The EB virus association is particularly marked in primary CNS lymphoma, where virus involvement may even be as high as 100%.[65] This tumour is several thousand times more likely to occur in HIV-seropositive individuals than in the general population.

The second category of AIDS-NHLs, which constitutes about 20% of all NHL reported in the USA, are undifferentiated tumours of small, non-cleaved cells. This tumour is BL-like and is around 1000 times more common in HIV-positive individuals than in normal ones. The tumours occur relatively early in HIV-infection when immune function is relatively unimpaired. All tumour cells show a chromosomal translocation normally of either t8:22 or t2:8 variant type involving the c-*myc* oncogene, with the majority showing a chromosomal break point analogous to that found in sporadic BL.[66] The intense stimulation of B cells seen in early HIV infection is thought to predispose the cell towards this translocation.[66,67] Only in a minority of AIDS-associated BL tumours are EB virus-associated.[68]

Hodgkin's Disease (HD) in AIDS patients shows histological features that are compatible with a mixed cellularity subtype. The polymorphous infiltrate is composed of small lymphocytes, plasma cells, histiocytes, occasional eosinophils and frequent Reed-Sternberg cells. The aggressive and atypical behaviour of HD in AIDS patients is probably attributable to the severe immune deficiency. EB virus is found in around 80% of cases.

CLINICAL FEATURES

AIDS-NHL exhibits an aggressive clinical pattern with rapid progression and a fatal outcome. Clinically , AIDS-NHLs are characterized by the extent of disease at presentation involving extranodal sites and the high frequency of accompanying systemic symptoms.[69] The most common sites of tumour presentation are: gastrointestinal tract (27%), CNS (25%), bone marrow, liver and lung. Other more unusual sites, such as oral mucosa, cardiac muscle, large bowel including anus and rectum, have been reported. Systemic symptoms are present in up to 82% of patients and typically include fever, drenching night sweats and severe weight loss in excess of 10% of normal body weight. In addition, a common presenting feature is rapidly enlarging lymph nodes which have to be distinguished from persistent generalized lymphadenopathy.[70,71]

TREATMENT

Patients with AIDS-NHL have been treated with a similar combination of chemotherapy regimens known to be effective against aggressive lymphomas in non-AIDS patients. However complete response rates range from 30–50% and are lower than the corresponding rates seen in non-HIV infected individuals, presumably due to the underlying disease.[70] The median survival time of treated patients ranges from 4 to 6 months and relapses occur rapidly. Radiation therapy has been used as treatment for CNS tumours. This method, in conjunction with partial tumour resection and systemic chemotherapy, has resulted in complete responses in only a few patients. A median survival time of 5.5 months is quoted in one study—with death usually due to recurrent lymphoma or opportunistic infection(s).[72]

NASOPHARYNGEAL CARCINOMA (See also Chapter 24)

HISTORY

Nasopharyngeal carcinoma (NPC) is a tumour of the nasopharyngeal squamous epithelium. The original clinical description of NPC was formulated by Durand-Fardel (1837)[73] and the histopathological documentation was by Michaux (1944).[74] The association between EB virus and undifferentiated (u)NPC was made in 1966 by Old from the observation that all uNPC patients had high serum antibodies to EB virus VCA.[4,75] More recently the differentiated forms of the tumour also have been shown to be EB virus-associated.[76]

EPIDEMIOLOGY

The incidence of NPC shows great geographical variation with the highest incidences (12–20 cases/100000 per year) found in southern China, Hong Kong and Singapore, where it is the most common tumour in men and the second most common in women[77] (see Figure 32.3b). Areas of intermediate incidence (1.5–9 cases/100000 per year) include Alaska, Iceland and North and East Africa, where it accounts for 7% of all cancers in males. In the rest of the world NPC is a rare tumour accounting for approximately 0.25% of all cancers (1–10 cases/100000 per year).[78] Further studies within the southern provinces of China have identified tumour prevalence amongst distinct ethnic groups, with the highest incidence of uNPC occurring among the Han Chinese and Cantonese Chinese populations. Males have a higher incidence than females (2.7:1), irrespective of race and geographical location. The age distribution for tumour development varies slightly according to the different geographical areas and is characterized by two peaks. In the high incidence areas there is an initial peak at 20–24 years and a larger, second peak at 50–55 years, with a sharp fall thereafter.[79]

SEROEPIDEMIOLOGY

The association between EB virus and NPC was first suggested when sera from uNPC patients were shown to contain high titre antibodies to EB viral antigens. In particular, elevated levels of anti-VCA antibodies were found in NPC sera, with 8–10-fold differences in geometric mean titres between patients with tumour compared with matched controls.[80] This is similar to that documented for BL.[75] IgG and IgA antibodies to EA(D) are most frequently seen, and rising titres correlate with increasing tumour burden. IgA antibodies to EA(D) are also found in saliva from uNPC patients and are thought to be diagnostic of the disease.[81,82]

PATHOGENESIS

ASSOCIATION WITH EB VIRUS

No single fact provides sufficient evidence for direct aetiological involvement of EB virus in NPC. However, the following findings suggest that EB virus plays more than a mere casual role. Firstly, EB virus DNA can be detected in the malignant epithelial cells in all cases studied as well as EBNA1 and LMP in the majority of uNPC biopsy specimens from different countries.[43,83] Secondly, seroepidemiology has convincingly shown that high titre antibodies to EB viral antigens correlate with the development and progression of uNPC.[84] Finally, uNPC biopsy cells can be induced to produce infectious EB virus which are indistinguishable from EB virus derived from BL or IM.[85]

COFACTORS

Genetic factors involved in tumour development have been suggested by familial clustering found in high incidence areas. This has been substantiated by HLA typing of Chinese patients with NPC and normal controls which shows that individuals who expressed A2BW46 have a relative risk of 1.96 for tumour development, and the AW19BW17 haplotype occurs more frequently in patients with NPC than in controls.[86,87] In addition, long-term survivors show a significant decrease in frequency of the BW17 marker, suggesting its association with a poor prognosis.[88] The decline in uNPC after several generations of Chinese who migrate from a high to a low incidence area is thought to be due to intermarriage with non-Chinese races. However, these NPC-associated haplotypes have not been observed in patients with NPC from intermediate incidence areas.

Environmental carcinogens are another suggested cofactor for NPC. Studies on Chinese patients have shown an association between NPC and prior nasal illness, the use of chinese herbal medicines, exposure to smoke and consumption of certain preserved foodstuffs.[89] A consistent factor found with all these associations is the presence of carcinogens used in the preservation of food and sources of traditional Chinese medicines such as extracts from the Euphorbiaceae.[90]

HISTOPATHOLOGY

The World Health Organization has devised a classification recognizing three types of NPC.[91]

1. Keratinizing squamous cell carcinoma.
2. Non-keratinizing squamous carcinoma showing evidence of keratinocyte differentiation but in which squamous maturation is not obvious. These cells have well-defined cell margins and exhibit a stratified or pavement arrangement.
3. Undifferentiated squamous carcinoma where

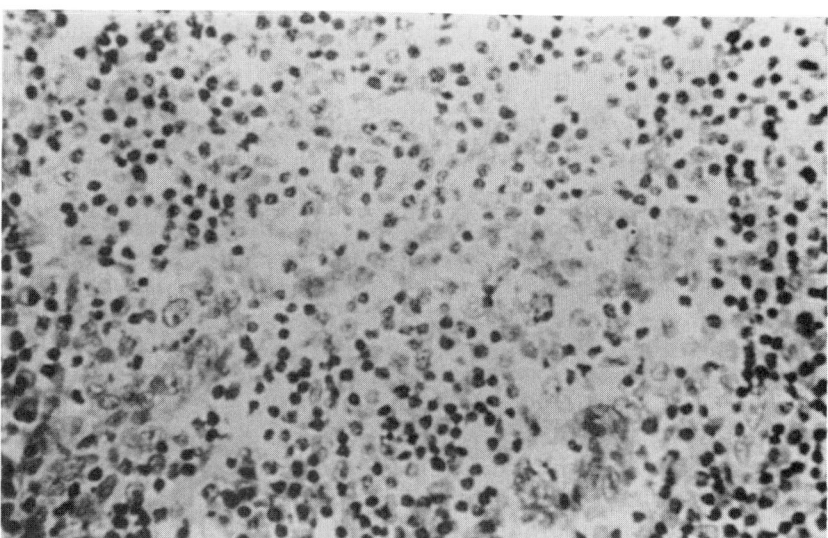

Figure 32.5 Histological section of undifferentiated nasopharyngeal carcinoma showing scattered malignant epithelial cells with heavy infiltrate of small lymphocytes. (H & E, 400×.)

cells exhibit syncytial qualities rather than a pavement appearance, and tumour cells appear as strands of loosely connected cells within a lymphoid stroma. The latter is composed of a heavy infiltrate of lymphocytes, predominantly T cells, which are non-malignant and which may be remnants of the abundant lymphoid tissue in the nasopharyngeal walls (Figure 32.5). This observation led to the earlier classification of the tumour as lymphoepithelioma and it is this form of NPC which is regularly associated with EB virus.

The frequency of these histopathological types varies according to age and geography. Differentiated squamous cell carcinomas are commonly found in older patients and constitute a greater proportion of cases in low-risk populations. Conversely, uNPC is common in younger patients in the high-risk areas.

CLINICAL FEATURES

The clinical symptoms of NPC are determined by the site of tumour presentation: it commonly arises in the fossa of Rosenmüller on the posterior wall of the nasopharynx. From this site it metastasizes early to draining lymph nodes, resulting in bilateral upper cervical lymph node enlargement, the most frequent presenting symptom. Less frequent symptoms are nasal obstruction, postnasal discharge, epistaxis, partial deafness and cranial nerve palsies. Three modes of clinical progression have been described by Ho.[92]

1. A metastatic type (43% of cases in high-risk areas) characterized by rapid invasion of cervical lymph nodes with limited extension of the primary tumour and distant metastases involving the lung, liver and spinal cord.
2. An invasive type (10% of cases) with direct spread of the primary tumour to adjacent muscles, bone, cranial nerves, sinuses, orbits, veins and base of skull with little involvement of cervical lymph nodes.
3. A combined type involving direct spread from the primary tumour and metastatic spread to regional lymph nodes and distant sites. This represents the most common type in high-risk areas.

LABORATORY DIAGNOSIS

Diagnosis of NPC is made on histological examination of an excision biopsy. EB virus serology has been found to be increasingly useful for confirming uNPC as well as in monitoring disease progression because IgA anti-VCA and anti-EA(D) are raised in serum and saliva prior to therapy. After successful therapy, antibody titres decline to become undetectable.[82] Patients who relapse with metastatic spread after therapy show rising antibody titres. The characteristic high levels of IgA anti-VCA and anti-EA(D) in the saliva have allowed the early detection of tumours before metastasis, resulting in more successful treatment.[84]

MANAGEMENT AND TREATMENT

If left untreated, NPC is rapidly fatal, with death commonly due to laryngeal or pharyngeal obstruction. Surgical treatment of the tumour is usually unsatisfactory because of the site and the early spread to regional lymph nodes. Various chemotherapeutic agents have been tried with little success; radiotherapy continues to be the preferred treatment for both primary and secondary metastatic sites. The prognosis for the metastatic type is 5–8 years, even after adequate radiotherapy.

EB VIRUS VACCINE PRODUCTION AND THERAPEUTIC IMPLICATIONS

A vaccine against EB virus was first proposed with the aim of preventing two human malignancies associated with EB virus, namely BL and uNPC.[93] Such a vaccine would also be advantageous to individuals at risk of developing severe IM, especially male children of X-linked lymphoproliferative syndrome carriers. Furthermore, the vaccine would benefit organ transplant recipients who are EB virus negative and therefore at risk of developing B-cell lymphoproliferations and lymphomas after primary infection.

EB virus-coded MA (gp340) has been chosen as a candidate vaccine antigen because antibodies directed to this antigen are neutralizing—preventing virus infection and spread. MA (gp340) preparations have been shown to produce high levels of specific antibodies in an animal model (cotton-top tamarins) and to protect against subsequent challenge with a 100% tumourigenic dose of EB virus.[94] Three recombinant virus vectors based in vaccinia, varicella and adenoviruses have been constructed which express gp340.[95–97] Successful results in animals offer considerable hope for testing the vaccine in clinical trials in humans in the near future, ultimately with a view to developing international vaccination programmes.

REFERENCES

1 Epstein M A, Achong B G & Barr Y M. Virus particles in cultured lymphoblasts from Burkitt's lymphoma. *Lancet* 1964; i:702–703.

2 Henle G, Henle W & Diehl V. Relation of Burkitt's tumor associated herpes-type virus to infectious mononucleosis. *Proc Natl Acad Sci USA* 1968; 59:94–101.

3 Klein G, Clifford P, Klein E & Stjernsward J. Search for tumor-specific immune reactions in Burkitt lymphoma patients by the membrane immunofluorescence reaction. *Proc Natl Acad Sci USA* 1966; 55:1628–1635.

4 Old L J, Boyse E A, Oettgen H F et al. Precipitating antibody in human serum to an antigen present in cultured Burkitt's lymphoma cells. *Proc Natl Acad Sci USA* 1966; 56:1699–1704.

5 Crawford D H, Thomas J A, Janossay G et al. Epstein–Barr virus nuclear antigen-positive lymphoma after cyclosporin. A treatment in patients with renal allograft. *Lancet* 1980; i:1355–1356.

6 Greenspan J S, Greenspan D, Lennette E et al. Replication of Epstein–Barr virus within the epithelial cells of oral 'hairy' leukoplakia, an AIDS-associated lesion. *N Engl J Med* 1985; 313:1564–1571.

7 Pattengale P L, Smith R W & Gerber P. Selective transformation of B lymphocytes by EB virus. *Lancet* 1973; ii:93–94.

8 Sixbey J W, Vesterinen E H, Nedrud J G, Raab-Traub N, Walton L A & Pagano J S. Replication of Epstein–Barr virus in human epithelial cells infected in vitro. *Nature* 1983; 306:480–489.

9 Fingeroth J D, Weis J J, Tedder T F, Strominger J L, Biro P A & Fearon D T. Epstein–Barr virus receptor of human B lymphocytes is the C3d receptor. *Proc Natl Acad Sci USA* 1984; 81:4510–4516.

10 Young L S, Clarke D, Sixbey J W & Rickinson A B. Epstein–Barr virus receptors on human pharyngeal epithelia. *Lancet* 1986; i:240–242.

11 Pope J H, Horne M K & Scott W. Transformation of foetal human leucocytes in vitro by filtrates of a human leukaemic cell line containing herpes-like virus. *Int J Cancer* 1968; 3:857–866.

12 Kieff E & Lieboweitz D. Epstein–Barr virus and its replication. In Fields B N & Knipe M S (eds) *Virology*. New York: Raven Press, 1990: 1889–1920.

13 Niederman J C, Evans A S, Subrahmanyan L & McCollum R W. Prevalence, incidence and persistence of EB virus antibody in young adults. *N Engl J Med* 1970; 283:361–365.

14 Sixbey J W, Lemon S M & Pagano J S. A second site for Epstein–Barr virus shedding: the uterine cervix. *Lancet* 1986; ii:1122–1124.

15 Allday M J & Crawford D H. Role of epithelium in EB virus persistence and pathogenesis of B-cell tumours. *Lancet* 1988; i:855–857.

16 Pearson G R, Dewey F, Klein G & Henle W.

Relation between neutralization of Epstein–Barr virus and antibodies to cell membrane antigens induced by the virus. *J Natl Cancer Inst* 1970; 45:989–995.

17 Moss D J, Rickinson A B & Pope J H. Long-term T cell-mediated immunity to Epstein–Barr virus in man I. Complete regression of virus-induced transformation in cultures of seropositive donor leukocytes. *Int J Cancer* 1978; 22:662–668.

18 Moss D J, Misko I S, Burrows S R, Burman K, McCarthy R & Sculley T B. Cytotoxic T-cell clones discriminate between A- and B-type Epstein–Barr virus transformants. *Nature* 1988; 331:719–721.

19 Burrows S R, Sculley T B, Misko I S, Schmidt C & Moss D J. An Epstein–Barr virus-specific cytotoxic T cell epitope in EBV nuclear antigen 3 (EBNA 3). *J Exp Med* 1990; 171:345–349.

20 Murray R J, Kurilla M G, Brooks J M et al. Identification of target antigens for the human cytotoxic T cell response to Epstein–Barr virus (EBV): implications for the immune control of EBV-positive malignancies. *J Exp Med* 1992; 176:157–168.

21 Crawford D H, Edwards J M B, Sweny P, Janossy G & Hoffbrand A V. Long-term T-cell mediated immunity to Epstein–Barr virus in renal allograft recipients receiving cyclosporin A. *Lancet* 1981; i:10–13.

22 Sprunt T P & Evans F A. Mononuclear leucocytosis in reaction to acute infections (in infectious mononucleosis). *Bull Johns Hopkins Hosp* 1920; 31:410–417.

23 Henle G & Henle W. Immunofluorescence in cells derived from Burkitt's lymphoma. *J Bacteriol* 1966; 91:1248–1256.

24 Diehl V, Raylor J, Parlin J A, Henle G & Henle W. Infectious mononucleosis in East Africa. *East Afr Med J* 1969; 46:407–413.

25 Gerber R, Goldstein L I, Lucas S, Nonoyama M & Perlin E. Oral excretion of Epstein–Barr viruses by healthy subjects and patients with infectious mononucleosis. *Lancet* 1972; ii:988–989.

26 Israelson V, Shirley P & Sixbey J W. Excretion of the Epstein–Barr virus from the genital tract of men. *J Infect Dis* 1991; 163:1341–1343.

27 Wising P J. A study of infectious mononucleosis (Pfeiffer's disease) from the etiological point of view. *Acta Med Scand Suppl* 1942; 133:1–102.

28 Henle W, Henle G & Horowitz C A. Epstein–Barr virus-specific diagnostic tests in infectious mononucleosis. *Hum Pathol* 1974; 5:551–565.

29 Rickinson A B. *The Epstein–Barr Virus: Recent Advances*. London: Heinemann, 1986: 75–125.

30 Hoagland R J. The transmission of infectious mononucleosis. *Am J Med Sci* 1955; 229:262–272.

31 Smith J N. Complications of infectious mononucleosis. *Ann Intern Med* 1956; 44:861–864.

32 Purtilo D T, Cassel C, Yang J P S et al. X-linked recessive progressive combined variable immunodeficiency (Duncan's disease). *Lancet* 1975; i:935–941.

33 Wood T A & Frenkel E P. The atypical lymphocytes. *Am J Med* 1967; 42:923–926.

34 Henle W, Henle G, Niederman J C, Klemola E & Haltra K. Antibodies to early antigens induced by Epstein–Barr virus in infectious mononucleosis. *J Infect Dis* 1971; 124:58–67.

35 Davidsohn I & Lee C L. Serologic diagnosis of infectious mononucleosis. A comparative study of five tests. *Am J Clin Pathol* 1964; 41:115–125.

36 Basson V & Sharp A A. Monospot: a differential slide test for infectious mononucleosis. *J Clin Pathol* 1969; 22:324–325.

37 Bender C E. The value of corticosteroids in the treatment of infectious mononucleosis. *JAMA* 1967; 199:529–531.

38 Andersson J, Britton S, Ernberg I et al. Effect of acyclovir on infectious mononucleosis: a double-blind, placebo-controlled study. *J Infect Dis* 1986; 153:283–290.

39 Burkitt D P. A sarcoma involving the jaw in African children. *Br J Surg* 1958; 46:218–223.

40 Williams E H, Smith P G, Day N E, Geser A, Ellice J & Tukei P. Space–time clustering of Burkitt's lymphoma in the West Nile district of Uganda: 1961–1975. *Br J Cancer* 1978; 37:109–122.

41 Burkitt D. A children's cancer dependent on climatic factors. *Nature* 1962; 194:232–234.

42 de-Thé G, Geser A, Day N E et al. Epidemiological evidence for causal relationship between Epstein–Barr virus and Burkitt's lymphoma: results of the Ugandan prospective study. *Nature* 1978; 274:756–761.

43 Nonoyama M & Pagano J S. Homology between Epstein–Barr virus DNA and viral DNA from Burkitt's lymphoma and nasopharyngeal carcinoma determined by DNA–DNA reassociation kinetics. *Nature* 1973; 242:44–47.

44 Miller G, Shope T, Cooper D et al. Lymphoma in cotton-top marmosets after inoculations with Epstein–Barr virus: tumour incidence, histologic spectrum, antibody responses, demonstration of viral DNA and characterisation of viruses. *J Exp Med* 1977; 145:948–967.

45 Manolova Y, Manolov G, Kieler J, Levan A & Klein G. Genesis of the 14q+ marker in Burkitt's lymphoma. *Hereditas* 1979; 90:5–10.

46 Bentley D L & Groudine M. Novel promoter upstream of the human c-*myc* gene and regulation of c-*myc* expression in B-cell lymphomas. *Mol Cell Biol* 1986; 6:3481–3489.

47 Neri A, Barriga F, Knowles D M, Magrath I T & Dalla-Favera R. Different regions of the immunoglobulin heavy chain locus are involved in chromosome translocations in distinct pathogenic forms of Burkitt's lymphoma. *Proc Natl Acad Sci USA* 1988; 85:2748–2752.

48 Kafuko G W & Burkitt D P. Burkitt's lymphoma and malaria. *Int J Cancer* 1970; 6:1–9.

49 Lenoir G M & Bornkamm G W. Burkitt's lymphoma—a human cancer model for the study of

the multistep development of cancer. Proposal for a new scenario. *Adv Virol Oncol* 1987; 6:173–206.

50 Whittle H, Brown J, Marsh K et al. T cell control of EB virus infected B cells is lost during *P. falciparum* malaria. *Nature* 1986; 312:449–450.

51 Lam K M C, Syed N, Whittle H & Crawford D H. Circulating Epstein–Barr virus-carrying B cells in acute malaria. *Lancet* 1991; 337:876–878.

52 O'Connor G T & Davies J N P. Malignant tumours in African children with special reference to malignant lymphoma. *J Pediatr* 1960; 56:526–535.

53 Rosenberg S A. National Cancer Institute sponsored study of classification of non-Hodgkin's lymphomas. Summary and description of a working formulation for clinical usage. *Cancer* 1982; 49:2112–2135.

54 Burkitt D & O'Connor G T. Malignant lymphoma in African children I. A clinical syndrome. *Cancer* 1961; 14:258–269.

55 Nkrumah F K & Biggar B J. Combination chemotherapy in abdominal Burkitt's lymphoma. *Cancer* 1977; 46:1410–1416.

56 Ziegler J L, Morrow J H, Templeton A C, Bluming A Z, Fass L & Kyalwazi S K. Clinical features and treatment of childhood malignant lymphoma in Uganda. *Int J Cancer* 1970; 5:415–425.

57 Henle W, Henle G, Gunven P, Klein G, Clifford P & Singh S. Patterns of antibodies to Epstein–Barr virus-induced early antigens in fatal cases of Burkitt's lymphoma and long term survivors. *J Natl Cancer Inst* 1973; 50:1163–1173.

58 Centers for Disease Control. Diffuse, undifferentiated non-Hodgkin's lymphomas among homosexual males: United States. *MMWR* 1982; 31:277–279.

59 Centers for Disease Control. Revision of the case definition of acquired immunodeficiency syndrome for national reporting: United States. *MMWR* 1985; 31:373–375.

60 Beral V, Peterman T, Berkelman R & Jaffe H. Non-Hodgkin's lymphoma in persons with AIDS. *Lancet* 1991; 337:805–809.

61 Pluda J M, Yarchaon R, Jaffe E S et al. Development of non-Hodgkin's lymphoma in an antiretroviral therapy. *Ann Intern Med* 1990; 113:276–282.

62 Lucas S B, Odida M & Wabinga H. The pathology of severe morbidity and mortality caused by HIV infection in Africa. *AIDS* 1991; 5(supplement):S143–S148.

63 Levine A M. Lymphoma in acquired immunodeficiency syndrome. *Semin Oncol* 1990; 17:104–112.

64 Thomas J A & Crawford D H. EBV associated B cell lymphoma in AIDS and after organ transplantation. *Lancet* 1989; i:1075–1076.

65 MacMahon E, Glass J D, Hayward S D et al. Epstein–Barr virus in AIDS-related primary central nervous system lymphoma. *Lancet* 1991; 338:969–973.

66 Pelicci P G, Knowles D M, Magrath I T & Dalla-Favera R. Chromosomal breakpoints and structural alterations of the c-*myc* locus differ in endemic and sporadic forms of Burkitt's lymphoma. *Proc Natl Acad Sci USA* 1986; 83:2984–2988.

67 Subar M, Neri A, Inghirami G, Knowles D M & Dalla-Favera R. Frequent c-*myc* oncogene activation and infrequent presence of Epstein–Barr virus genome in AIDS-associated lymphoma. *Blood* 1988; 72:667–671.

68 Haluska F G, Russo G, Kant J, Andreef M & Croce C M. Molecular resemblance of an AIDS-associated lymphoma and endemic Burkitt's lymphoma: implications for their pathogenesis. *Proc Natl Acad Sci USA* 1989; 86:8907–8911.

69 Zeigler J L, Beckstead J A, Volberding P A et al. Non-Hodgkin's lymphoma in 90 homosexual men: relation to generalized lymphadenopathy and the acquired immunodeficiency syndrome. *N Engl J Med* 1984; 311:565–570.

70 Knowles D M, Chamulak G A, Subar M et al. Lymphoid neoplasia associated with the acquired immunodeficiency syndrome (AIDS). *Ann Intern Med* 1988; 108:744–754.

71 Lowenthal D A, Straus D J, Campbell S, Gold J W M, Clarkson B D & Koziner B. AIDS-related lymphoid neoplasia: the Memorial Hospital experience. *Cancer* 1988; 61:2325–2337.

72 Kaplan L D, Abrams D I, Feigal E et al. AIDS-associated non-Hodgkin's lymphoma in San Francisco. *JAMA* 1989; 261:719–724.

73 Dirand-Fardel. Cancer du pharynx–ossification dans la substance musculaire du coeur. *Bull Soc Anat (Paris)* 1837; 12:73–80.

74 Michaux L. Ophthalmologic and neuralogic symptoms at malignant nasopharyngeal tumors: clinical study comprising 454 cases, with special reference to histopathology and possibility of earlier recognition. *Acta Psychiatr Scand Suppl* 1944; 31:1–323.

75 Henle W, Henle G, Ho H C et al. Antibodies to EB virus in nasopharyngeal carcinoma, other head and neck neoplasms and control groups. *J Natl Cancer Inst* 1970; 44:225–231.

76 Raab-Traab N, Flynn K, Pearson G et al. The differentiated form of nasopharyngeal carcinoma contains Epstein–Barr virus DNA. *Int J Cancer* 1987; 39:25–29.

77 Hiryama T. Descriptive and analytical epidemiology of nasopharyngeal cancer. In de Thé G & Ito Y (eds) *Nasopharyngeal Carcinoma: Etiology and Control.* Lyon: IARC, 1978: 167–190.

78 de Thé G. Role of Epstein–Barr virus in human diseases: infectious mononucleosis, Burkitt's lymphoma and nasopharyngeal carcinoma. In Klein G (ed.) *Viral Oncology.* New York: Raven Press, 1980: 769–797.

79 Shanmugaratnam K. Variations in nasopharyngeal cancer incidence among specific Chinese communities (dialect groups) in Singapore. In de Thé G & Ito Y (eds) *Nasopharyngeal Carcinomas: Etiology and Control.* Lyon: IARC, 1978: 191–198.

80 De Schryver A, Friberg S Jr, Klein G et al. Epstein–Barr virus-associated antibody patterns in carcinoma of the post-nasal space. *Clin Exp Immunol* 1969; 5:443–459.

81 Henle W, Ho H C, Henle G & Kwan H C. Antibodies to Epstein–Barr virus-related antigens in nasopharyngeal carcinoma. Comparison of active cases with long term survivors. *J Natl Cancer Inst* 1973; 51:363–369.

82 Henle G & Henle W. Epstein–Barr virus-specific IgA serum antibodies as an outstanding feature of nasopharyngeal carcinoma. *Int J Cancer* 1976; 17:1–7.

83 zur Hausen H, Schulte-Holthausen H, Klein G et al. EBV DNA in biopsies of Burkitt tumours and anaplastic carcinomas of the nasopharynx. *Nature* 1970; 228:1056–1058.

84 Henle W, Ho J H C, Henle G, Chau J C W & Kwan H C. Nasopharyngeal carcinoma: significance of changes in Epstein–Barr virus related antibody patterns following therapy. *Int J Cancer* 1977; 20:663–672.

85 Trumper P A, Epstein M A, Giovanella B C & Finerty S. Isolation of infectious EB virus from the epithelial tumour cells of nasopharyngeal carcinoma. *Int J Cancer* 1977; 20:655–662.

86 Simons M J, Wee G B, Day N E, de-Thé G, Morris P J & Shanmugaratnam K. Immunogenetic aspects of nasopharyngeal carcinoma. I. Difference in HLA antigen profiles between patients and comparison groups. *Int J Cancer* 1974; 13:122–134.

87 Simons M J, Wee G B, Goh E H et al. Immunogenetic aspects of nasopharyngeal carcinoma. IV. Increased risk in Chinese of nasopharyngeal carcinoma associated with a Chinese-related HLA profile (A2, Singapore 2). *J Natl Cancer Inst* 1976; 57:977–980.

88 Simons M J, Chan S H, Wee G B et al. Nasopharyngeal carcinoma and histocompatibility antigens. In de-Thé G & Ito Y (eds) *Nasopharyngeal Carcinoma: Etiology and Control*. Lyon: IARC, 1978:271–282.

89 Ho J H C. An epidemiologic and clinical study of nasopharyngeal carcinoma. *Int J Radiol Oncol Biol Phys* 1978; 4:181–198.

90 Ito Y, Kawanishi M, Hirayama T & Takabaysashi S. Combined effect of the extracts from *Croton tiglium*, *Euphorbia lathyris* or *Euphorbia tizcalli* and *N*-butyrate on Epstein–Barr virus expression in human lymphoblastoid P3HR-1 and Raji cells. *Cancer Lett* 1981; 12:175–180.

91 Shanmugaratnam K & Sobin L H. Histological typing of upper respiratory tract tumors. In *International Histological Classification of Tumors*, No. 19. Geneva: WHO, 1978.

92 Ho J H C. The natural history and treatment of nasopharyngeal carcinoma. In Lee Clarke R, Cumley J E, McCay J E & Copeland M (eds) *Oncology*. Medical Publishers, 1970: 1–14.

93 Epstein M A. Epstein–Barr virus—is it time to develop a vaccine program? *J Natl Cancer Inst* 1976; 56:697–700.

94 Epstein M A, Morgan A J, Finerty S, Randle B J & Kirkwood J K. Protection of cottontop tamarins against Epstein–Barr virus-induced malignant lymphoma by a prototype subunit vaccine. *Nature* 1985; 318:287–289.

95 Morgan A J, Mackett M, Finerty S, Arrand J R, Scullion F T & Epstein M A. Recombinant vaccinia virus expressing Epstein–Barr virus glycoprotein gp340 protects cottontop tamarins against EBV-induced malignant lymphomas. *J Med Virol* 1988; 25:189–195.

96 Lowe R, Keller P, Davison A, Kieff E, Morgan A & Ellis R. Varicella zoster virus as a live vector for the expression of foreign genes. *Proc Natl Acad Sci USA* 1987; 84:3896–3900.

97 Ragot T, Tosoni-Pittoni E, Finerty S, Morgan A J & Perricaudet M. Recombinant adenoviruses which express the Epstein–Barr virus membrane antigen gp340/220, gp220 only or a secreted form of gp340 induce persistent virus-neutralizing antibodies in rabbits. In Ablashi DV (ed.) *Epstein–Barr Virus and Human Disease*. Humana Press, 1991: 231–236.

CHAPTER 33

RABIES

M. J. Warrell

Rabies is a widespread infection of certain animal species which is occasionally transmitted to man. Other names for rabies include hydrophobia, la rage (in French), la rabbia in Italian, la rabia (in Spanish), and in German, die Tollwut.

HISTORY

Transmission of the infection from dogs' saliva was known to the Egyptians at the time of the Pharaohs, and suggested methods of treatment are found in Chinese manuscripts from the fifth century BC.[1] Animal rabies was described by Aristotle in the fourth century BC, and the Roman, Celsus, wrote of the human illness in the first century AD, when knowledge and fear of the disease was widespread. A sixteenth century Italian physician, Fracastoro, described the clinical features of rabies.[2]

John Hunter initiated a scientific approach to rabies in 1793 and experiments on transmission of the infection were carried out in Germany by Zinke, and in France by Magendie early in the nineteenth century. Louis Pasteur's work in the 1880s demonstrated that rabies was an infection of the central nervous system. He repeatedly passaged virulent 'street' virus in rabbits, attenuating it to a 'fixed' laboratory strain, used to make the first rabies vaccine.[2]

Growth of the virus in tissue culture was achieved in the 1930s and the virus was first visualized by electron microscopy in the early 1960s.[3]

VIRUS

Rabies virus is the prototype of the genus *Lyssavirus* (Gk *lyssa* rage/frenzy) of the large family of Rhabdoviridae (Gk *rhabdos* rod). Eleven of the recognized lyssaviruses are antigenically related and form the rabies serogroup.[4] They are found in arthropods and mammals and include three rabies-related viruses known to infect man: Mokola, Duvenhage and European bat lyssavirus (see p. 703). Other rhabdoviruses which occasionally cause disease in humans are: the vesicular stomatitis viruses, Chandipura, Piry and Le Dantec viruses.[5]

The bullet-shaped rabies virion (Figure 33.1) measures 180×75 nm approximately, and contains a single strand of negative-sense RNA, which, combined with a nucleoprotein, forms a helical coil. Two more viral proteins, a phosphoprotein and RNA polymerase (needed to transcribe mRNA) are associated with the coil. This whole structure is the ribonucleoprotein complex. It is covered by a matrix protein and then by a glycoprotein bearing club-shaped spikes (Figure 33.1b) which project outward through a host cell-derived lipid layer.[6]

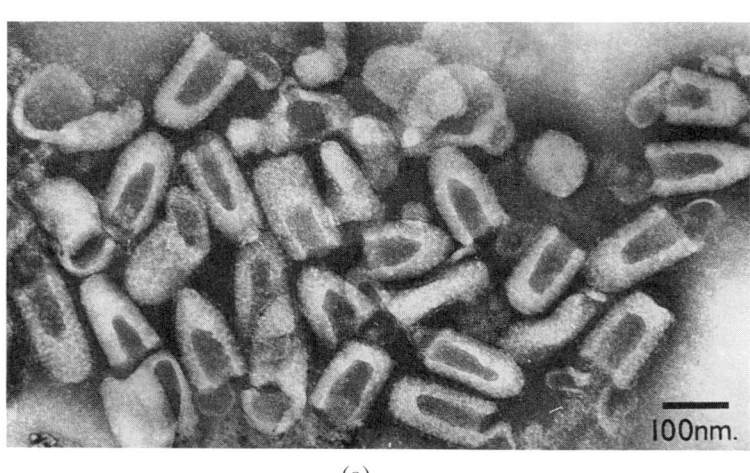

(a)

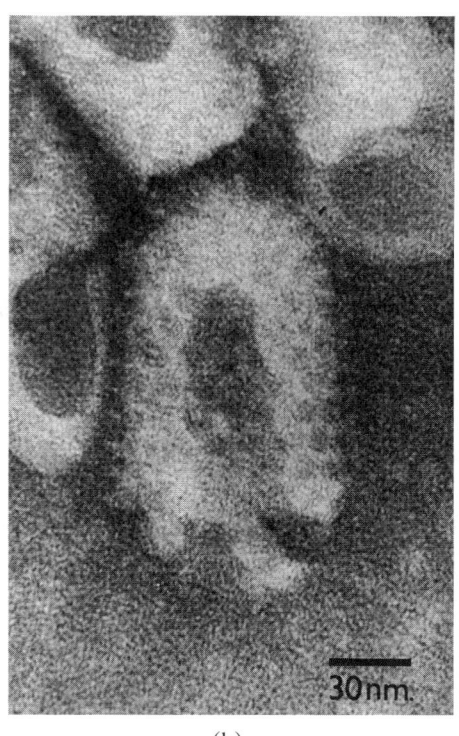

(b)

Figure 33.1(a) and (b)   Negatively stained electron micrographs of bullet-shaped rabies virions; (b) shows projections on the surface of the glycoprotein coat, covering all but the blunt end of the virion. (Courtesy of C.J. Smale and Joan Crick.)

INACTIVATION

Rabies virus is rapidly inactivated by heat. At 56°C the half-life is less than a minute, but at 37°C it is prolonged to several hours in moist conditions. At 4°C there is little loss after 2 weeks.[7]

The lipid coat is disrupted by detergents or a simple 1% soap solution. Other viricidal agents include 45% ethanol, iodine solutions (1:10 000 available iodine) and 1% benzalkonium chloride,[8] but phenol is not so effective.[9]

GEOGRAPHICAL DISTRIBUTION

Rabies is a widespread zoonosis, occurring in separate cycles within dogs and wild mammal vector species. Strains of virus from different groups can be identified by typing viral antigens using a panel of monoclonal antibodies. The infection sometimes spills over to non-vector species such as humans. The *urban* enzootic in domestic dogs is of most importance to man, and is the cause of more than 90% of human rabies cases (Figure 33.2).[10] Dogs also frequently infect cats and other domestic species. The pattern of *sylvatic* (wildlife) rabies shows great geographical variation, and knowledge of local current epizootics is important in the prevention of human rabies fatalities. The distribution of dominant vector species is summarized in Table 33.1.

Areas of the world which have recently been

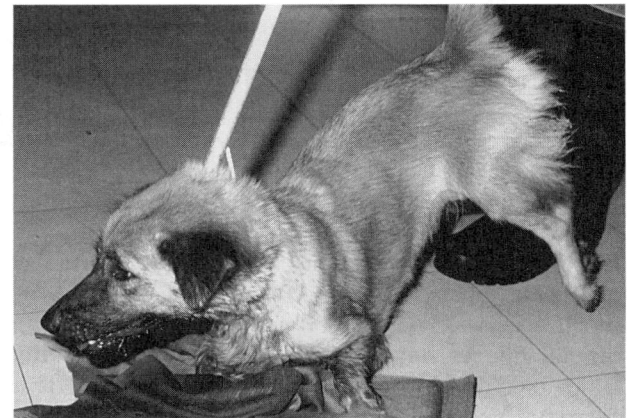

Figure 33.2   Domestic dog with paralytic rabies in Bangkok, Thailand. Note paralysis of limbs and drooling of saliva. (Courtesy of D.A. Warrell.)

Table 33.1   Distribution of important rabies vector species.

Species	Distribution
Africa[11]	
Domestic dog	Widespread dominant vector
Black-backed jackals (*Canis mesomelas*)	Zambia, Zimbabwe, Namibia
Yellow mongoose (*Cynictis penicillata*)	South Africa
Americas	
Arctic fox[12] (*Alopex lagopus*)	North-west Canada, Alaska
Striped skunk[12] (*Mephitis mephitis*)	Central Canada and USA, California
Racoon[13] (*Procyon lotor*)	Mid-Atlantic states and south-east USA
Fox[12]	Arizona, Texas and north-eastern USA
Insectivorous bats[12]	USA and South America
Domestic dog	Widespread Mexico, Central and South America
Vampire bat[14] (Desmodontidae)	Southern Texas, Mexico, Central and South America south to Argentina and Chile; Trinidad and Tobago
Mongoose[15] (*Herpestes* species)	Puerto Rico, Grenada, Cuba, Dominican Republic
Asia[11]	
Domestic dog	Widespread dominant vector
Wolf	Iran, Iraq, Afghanistan
Europe	
Fox	Widespread from France east to Russia
Arctic fox[11] (*Alopex lagopus*)	Northern Russia
Racoon dog[16] (*Nycterentes procyonoides*)	Baltic states, Russia, Poland, Ukraine
Wolf[16]	Russia
Dog	Turkey, southern Russian states
Insectivorous bats[17]	Germany, Denmark, Netherlands, Russia, Poland, Spain, France, Czech Republic, Switzerland

reported to be free of rabies include: Australia; New Zealand; Papua New Guinea; Japan; Taiwan; Hong Kong Islands; Singapore; some islands of Indonesia (e.g. Bali), and in the Indian Ocean; many Pacific islands, e.g. Solomon Islands, Fiji, Samoa and Cook Islands; UK; Ireland; Iceland; Finland; Sweden; mainland Norway; the Iberian peninsula; Mediterranean islands; some Caribbean islands (e.g. Barbados, Bahamas, Jamaica and Antigua); and Antarctica.

Although some countries have no urban or sylvatic rabies, infected wild animals cross land borders (e.g. Greece, Italy, Malaysia and Hong Kong Northern Territories). Imported rabies is a universal risk.

INCIDENCE

In endemic tropical areas, especially where dogs are the dominant vector, the true incidence of human rabies is unknown because of underreporting or lack of published figures.[18] In India estimates of mortality are 25000–50000 per year,[19] although the official figures have been less than 100! In China 5000–7000 deaths per year occurred 10 years ago but there has been a dramatic fall to about 1000 per year ($0.09/10^5$ population). In 1992 in Bangladesh the estimate was 2000 cases ($1.8/10^5$ population); in Sri Lanka 112 were reported ($0.64/10^5$ population); and in Nepal 200 ($1.1/10^5$ population). Other countries with a high incidence include Ethiopia, Nepal, Brazil, Mexico, Colombia, Ecuador and El Salvador.[18,20,21]

There has been an impressive reduction in the number of local human cases following vector control campaigns, for example after dog vaccination and population control in Latin America,[10] and rabies was eliminated from areas such as Taiwan, Japan and peninsular Malaysia by these means. Despite this there has been no evidence of a significant change in the overall incidence of human rabies in tropical endemic areas for decades.

Only 0.01% of human rabies cases occur in temperate zones.[18] In the USA, where sylvatic rabies is endemic, there have been an average of 1.6 rabies deaths per year over 30 years, and 37% of these were infected abroad.[22]

RABIES-RELATED VIRUS INFECTIONS (Table 33.2)

Rabies and rabies-related viruses are now classified as six genotypes (Table 33.2). Rabies is genotype 1, and four others, genotype 3, Mokola, genotype 4 Duvenhage and genotypes 5 and 6 European bat lyssaviruses, are known to have infected at least six people. Mokola virus caused fatal encephalitis in a Nigerian child, while another recovered from pharyngitis and probably a febrile convulsion.[23,24] A laboratory worker recovered from an accidental infection.[29] Duvenhage virus is named after a patient who had rabies-like encephalitis.[25]

Rabid bats have been found occasionally in Europe since 1954. When a woman was bitten by a rabid *Eptesicus serotinus* insectivorous bat in Denmark in 1985,[30] an extensive search revealed many rabid bats also in Germany and the Netherlands, a few in Russia, Poland, Spain,[17] France[31] and Czech Republic. These bat viruses are similar to but antigenically distinct from Duvenhage virus and form the European bat lyssavirus group (genotype 5).[26] Two Russian girls died of rabies following bat bites, and at least one virus was a European bat lyssavirus strain.[27] In Finland in 1985, a zoologist bitten by a bat from an unknown source died of furious rabies-like encephalitis.[28] The virus isolated can be distinguished from the other European bat viruses but is similar to two isolates from Dutch *Myotis* bats, and together these form a second biotype of European bat lyssavirus (genotype 6).[26,31]

Table 33.2 Rabies-related viruses known to have infected humans.

Genotype	Virus	Source	Known geographical area	Human disease
3	Mokola	Shrews (*Crocidura* sp.)	Nigeria, Cameroon	—
		Harsh furred mouse (*Lophuromys sikapusi*)	Central African Republic	—
		Cat	South Africa	—
		Cat, dog, rodents	Zimbabwe	—
		Human	Nigeria	Pharyngitis and recovery Fatal encephalitis (no hydrophobia)
4	Duvenhage	Insectivorous bat	South Africa, Zimbabwe	—
		Human	South Africa	Furious rabies-like encephalitis
5	European bat lyssavirus (biotype 1)	Insectivorous bat (esp. *Eptesichus serotinus*)	Germany, Denmark, Netherlands, Russia, Poland, Spain, France	—
6	European bat lyssavirus (biotype 2)	Human	Russia	Furious rabies-like encephalitis
		Insectivorous bat (*Myotis dasyncneme*)	Netherlands	
	Finland virus	Human	Unknown	Rabies-like encephalitis

See text for references.
Genotype 2, Lagos bat virus has not been found in humans.

TRANSMISSION OF INFECTION

ANIMAL CONTACT

Inoculation of rabies virus into a wound or on to a mucous membrane may result in infection. This includes contamination of an unhealed lesion. Intact skin is a barrier against viral entry. Humans are usually infected by virus-laden saliva, inoculated during the bite of a rabid dog. The chance of developing rabies following exposure is revealed by data from the prevaccine era (see below, Efficacy of Postexposure Prophylaxis).

HUMAN-TO-HUMAN

Transmission via infected secretions has never been documented virologically,[32] even from patients producing copious saliva and nursed at home. Viraemia has not been detected.[32]

Transmission has occurred through *grafting of infected corneas*. Four virologically proven cases followed transplants from donors with unsuspected rabies.[32] Another patient who received a cornea from an infected donor survived following treatment with high-dose postexposure therapy including interferon.[33]

Transplacental infection occurs in animals and recently a Turkish woman and her 2-day-old infant died of virologically confirmed rabies.[34] This is exceptional. Many mothers with rabies have been delivered of healthy babies.

There are old anecdotal reports of infections from contact with human saliva, kissing, biting, sexual intercourse, breast feeding and eating infected meat, but these routes remain unproven in man.

INHALATION

Inhalation of rabies virus in aerosols infected two people in bat-infested caves.[35] Two more inhaled aerosols of 'fixed' virus in laboratory accidents.[36,37]

RABIES VACCINES

Vaccines for human use no longer contain live rabies virus, but *live attenuated vaccines* are available for animals. These have not caused human disease following accidental inoculation and no postexposure treatment is recommended by the American authorities.[38]

PATHOGENESIS

The extraordinary journey of rabies virions along nerves up to the brain, and then outward to many organs, is poorly understood. It usually begins with the bite of a rabid animal inoculating virus-laden saliva through the skin, often into muscle. Experiments show viral replication occurring locally in striated muscle or mucous membrane,[39] or directly invading a nerve cell.[40] The virus can probably attach to several types of cell receptors.[41] One important site of attachment is the nicotinic acetylcholine receptor at neuromuscular junctions, where binding is competitive, not only with cholinergic ligands, but also with a snake venom neurotoxin, α-bungarotoxin, which has homologous sequences with rabies glycoprotein.[42]

Once inside a neurone the virus is carried centripetally in an incomplete form, perhaps as naked nucleocapsids.[43] The flow of axoplasm transports it towards the brain, at a rate of 3 mm/h experimentally.[44] Its progress can be halted by sectioning nerves[45] or by metabolic inhibitors, such as colchicine.[41] Rabies spreads across synapses, through ganglia, eventually reaching the brain, where intraneuronal replication occurs on a massive scale.[41,46] Infection of the limbic system causes aggressive behaviour and enables transmission from a vector species to another host.

The rabies virus remains virtually confined to neurones as centrifugal dissemination then progresses via autonomic and peripheral nerves.[46] Virus has been isolated from human skeletal and cardiac muscle, skin, lung, kidney, adrenal, lacrimal and, of course, salivary glands.[47,32]

In contrast to events in neurones, virus replication in acinar cells of the salivary glands produces large amounts of extracellular virus.[46] Although there is no evidence of viraemia, rabies virus is shed in human lacrimal and respiratory tract secretions, occasionally in urine[32] and possibly in milk.

A striking difference in behaviour of virulent street viruses and attenuated rabies strains has been linked to the presence of a particular amino acid component (arginine in position 333) of the glycoprotein molecule.[48] Substitution of this marker of virulence by another amino acid results in attenuation.[46] The mechanism is unknown and other molecular sites may also influence virulence.

Rabies virus evades recognition by the immune system until a late stage of the disease. At the site of inoculation, some virus is briefly exposed, but once within the CNS, virions and their antigens are hidden from immune surveillance. During the final centrifugal phase of infection, when rabies antigens are eventually expressed on cell membranes and extracellular virus is produced, the immune response is too late to combat the overwhelming infection.

PATHOLOGY

Cerebral congestion and a few petechial haemorrhages are usual findings in rabies encephalitis, but not gross cerebral oedema.[49,50] A lymphocytic perivenous infiltrate is common, and neutrophils are occasionally seen, perhaps only early in the disease. Eosinophilic cytoplasmic inclusions (Negri bodies) are found in 75% of cases, most frequently in large neurones of the hippocampus, Purkinje cells of the cerebellum and medulla.[51] Neuronophagia, microglial reaction, foci of demyelination and perineural infiltration (Babès' nodules) also occur.[51] The brain stem and spinal cord are predominantly affected, but changes are often widespread. A meningeal reaction is common in children, and in paralytic disease the spinal cord is most severely affected. The extent of the histopathological change varies from complete disruption of neuronal structure and axonal degeneration of peripheral nerves following intensive care,[52] to an absence of any inflammation or degeneration.[49,50,53]

Negri bodies consist of eosinophilic rabies nucleoprotein matrix and occasional virions. They contain small basophilic masses, probably fragments of host cell organelles, mechanically trapped during fusion of smaller inclusions.[3]

Extraneural pathology consists of focal degeneration of salivary glands, liver, pancreas, adrenal medulla and lymph nodes;[54] there is also interstitial myocarditis.[55]

IMMUNITY

RESPONSE TO INFECTION

Following a rabid bite, no immune response is detectable in unvaccinated subjects before encephalitis has developed. Rabies antibody is first found in serum, then in CSF about a week after the onset.[56,57] Neutralizing antibody may rise to a high level if life is prolonged. Specific rabies IgM antibody is occasionally found, but it is not helpful in diagnosis as it does not appear very early and can also be present in postvaccinal encephalitis.[58]

There is little evidence of lymphocyte-mediated responses to encephalitis in man. Pleocytosis is observed in only 60% of patients, with a mean leucocyte count of 75/mm^3.[56] Peripheral blood lymphocyte transformation has been shown in a few cases of furious rabies.[59] Experimentally, rabies infection suppresses the lymphocyte-mediated response to other antigens.[60] Only very low levels of interferon have been found in the serum and CSF of about 30% of patients with rabies encephalitis.[61]

RESPONSE TO VACCINE

The best available simple measure of immunity after vaccine treatment is the level of neutralizing antibody,[62] which usually appears 7–14 days after starting a primary vaccine course. The amount of antibody needed for protection against rabies in man cannot be determined, but the World Health Organization (WHO) recommends that a minimum neutralizing antibody level of 0.5 u/ml should be attained to demonstrate unequivocal seroconversion.[63]

The degree of protection from vaccine and the production of antibody in animals are genetically controlled, although unlinked traits.[64] In man there is an apparent genetic link with production of neutralizing antibody following rabies vaccine. A relatively delayed, lower level of response occurred in about 10% of vaccinees.[65] Increasing age (over 50 years) also impairs antibody production.[66]

The induction of antibody can be accelerated by increasing the dose of antigen,[67] or dividing the vaccine between multiple sites over the body.[68]

An injection of rabies vaccine induces a wide range of antibodies, both to viral antigens and to non-viral vaccine components which may be associated with side-effects (see below). The spiky glycoprotein coat of the virion bears the only antigens capable of stimulating the protective neutralizing antibody,[69] and so the glycoprotein is thought to be the most important component of a rabies vaccine.

In animals, injections of purified core ribonucleoprotein also induce protective immunity, in association with non-neutralizing antibody, helper T-lymphocyte activity and interferon-γ induction.[69] This protection is effective against a variety of rabies and rabies-related strains,[70] unlike the glycoprotein-mediated immunity. The glycoprotein does, however, bear epitopes which stimulate T lymphocytes,[71] and specific transformation of human peripheral blood lymphocytes can be demonstrated in vitro following vaccine treatment. The role of these helper T lymphocytes,[72] and the cytotoxic T-cell response,[70] in protection against disease is not clear.

A small amount of interferon may be induced briefly following a first dose of rabies vaccine,[73] but it is very unlikely to afford significant protection in man.[62]

CLINICAL FEATURES

INCUBATION PERIOD

The interval between inoculation and the onset of symptoms is between 20 and 90 days in at least 60% of cases, but it has varied from 4 days to 19 years.[74,75] Short incubation periods have recently been reported from Thailand, where 42% of patients develop symptoms after 10–20 days.[76] In general, the nearer the bite is to the head, the shorter the incubation period,[77] but this is a loose correlation and cannot be relied upon in individual cases.

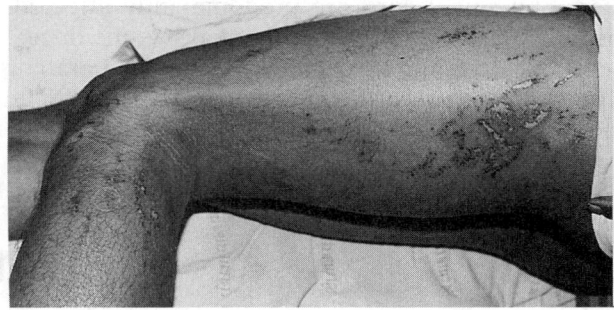

Figure 33.3 Intense itching of the bitten limb provoking scratching and excoriation, a common prodromal symptom of rabies encephalitis. (Courtesy of Sornchai Looareesuwan.)

PRODROMAL SYMPTOMS

Itching or paraesthesiae at the site of the healed bite wound are the only specific prodromal symptoms, occurring in about 40% of patients (Figure 33.3).[78] The wide range of non-specific features include: fever, headache, myalgia, fatigue, sore throat, gastrointestinal symptoms, irritability, anxiety and insomnia. The disease progresses to either furious or paralytic rabies encephalitis, usually within a week.[79]

FURIOUS RABIES

This well-known form is probably the more common. Malfunction of the brain stem, limbic system and higher centres results in the characteristic hydrophobic spasms. This is a reflex contraction of inspiratory muscles provoked by attempts to drink water, and later even the sound or mention of water, and also sometimes by draughts of air (aerophobia), touching the palate, bright lights or loud noises.

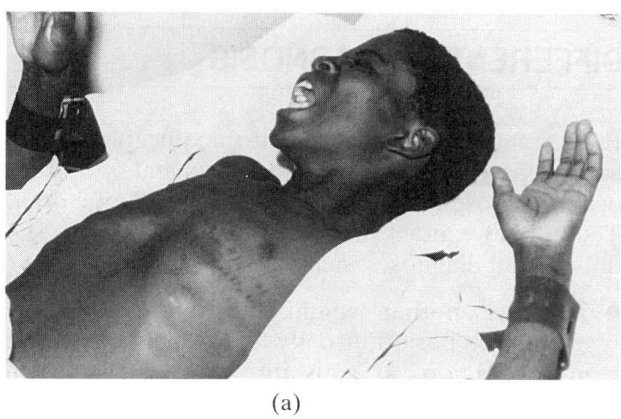
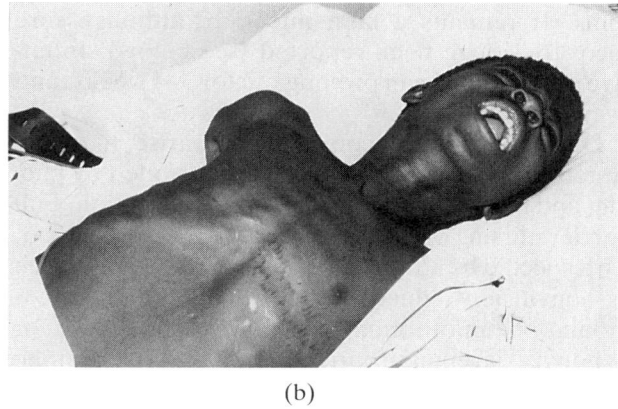

(a)   (b)

Figure 33.4   Progression of a hydrophobic spasm associated with terror in a Nigerian boy with furious rabies. (a) Note the powerful contraction of the diaphragm (depressing the xiphisternum) and sternocleidomastoid muscles. (b) The episode terminates in opisthotonos. (Courtesy of D.A. Warrell.)

Intense thirst forces patients to try to drink. They may have a tight feeling in the throat, the arm trembles, and jerky spasms of the sternomastoids, diaphragm and other inspiratory muscles lead to a generalized extension, sometimes with convulsions and opisthotonos (Figure 33.4).[79] There is an associated inexplicable feeling of terror which occurs during the first episode, which is not a learned response.[80] Respiratory or cardiac arrest following a hydrophobic spasm is fatal in one-third of cases.

Excitation, aggression, anxiety or hallucinations occur between calm, lucid intervals, when no neurological abnormality may be detectable. Other features include cardiac arrhythmias, myocarditis, labile blood pressure and temperature, respiratory disturbances (e.g. Cheyne–Stokes respiration, cluster breathing), meningism, lesions of cranial nerves III, VII and IX, abnormal pupillary function, muscle fasciculation,[79] autonomic stimulation with lacrimation and salivation and rarely increased libido, priapism and spontaneous orgasms.[81,82] Coma eventually ensues, with flaccid paralysis (Figure 33.5), and the agonizing illness rarely lasts more than a week without intensive care.

PARALYTIC RABIES

Less common than furious rabies, paralytic or 'dumb' rabies may be missed unless there is a high level of suspicion. Paralytic disease is characteristic of vampire bat-transmitted rabies[14,83] and it is more common following infections by attenuated viruses,[36,37,84] and perhaps after postexposure vaccination.[57]

Prodromal symptoms are followed by paraesthesiae or hypotonic weakness, commonly starting near the site of the bite and spreading cranially. Fasciculation, myoedema or piloerection may be seen. The ascending paralysis results in constipation, urinary retention, respiratory failure and inability to swallow. Flaccid paralysis, especially of proximal muscles, is associated with loss of tendon and plantar reflexes, but sensation is often normal. Hydrophobic spasms may occur in the terminal phase and death ensues after 1–3 weeks.[79]

TREATMENT AND COMPLICATIONS

All rabies patients should be admitted to hospital and sedated heavily to relieve their agonizing symp-

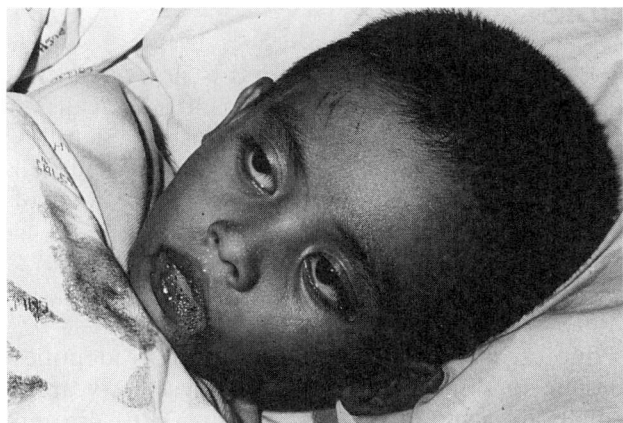

Figure 33.5   Hypersalivation, sweating and haematemesis in a 5-year-old Thai boy with furious rabies. (Courtesy of D.A. Warrell.)

toms. It remains a fatal infection, although rare recoveries have been reported (see below). Intensive care therapy can prolong life for 3–4 weeks, and even up to 133 days.[85]

During this time complications arise in every system. Cardiac arrhythmias are controlled by pacing, and respiratory failure requires ventilation. Full barrier nursing of the unconscious patient is needed, with specific treatment for likely complications such as convulsions, fluctuating blood pressure, pneumonia, pneumothorax, cerebral oedema, hyper- or hypopyrexia, inappropriate antidiuretic hormone secretion, diabetes insipidus and haematemesis from stress ulceration.[79]

Treatment with hyperimmune serum and several antiviral agents—including intrathecal tribavirin (ribavirin) and interferon-α have not been effective.[5,61,86]

RECOVERY FROM RABIES

Four individuals are claimed to have survived rabies encephalitis. Two patients, who had been given postexposure prophylaxis and then intensive care, recovered completely,[87,88] and another recent case has neurological sequelae. The diagnoses were based on high rabies neutralizing antibody levels in the serum and CSF. No virus or antigen was identified.

The fourth patient was a previously vaccinated microbiologist who inhaled fixed rabies virus. The diagnosis was again made serologically,[37] and he has residual neurological impairment.

DIFFERENTIAL DIAGNOSIS

Rabies should be suspected if inexplicable neurological, psychiatric or laryngopharyngeal symptoms occur in those who have been to an endemic area. The animal contact may have been forgotten. The differential diagnoses include the following.[79]

- *Tetanus*, another wound infection, has a short incubation period, usually less than 15 days. The muscle rigidity is constant, without relaxation between spasms. The CSF is always normal.
- *Intoxications* with drugs acting on the CNS, poisons and even delirium tremens could be confused with rabies.
- *Rabies phobia* is a hysterical response, usually very soon after a bite, with aggressive behaviour and an excellent prognosis.
- *Guillain–Barré syndrome* may present as paralytic rabies, and very rarely follows rabies tissue culture vaccine treatment (see p. 714).
- *Postvaccinal encephalitis*, an allergic response to nervous tissue-containing rabies vaccine, can be clinically indistinguishable from paralytic rabies (see p. 714).
- *Other viral encephalitides* including Japanese encephalitis, poliomyelitis and treatable herpes simiae B, from a monkey bite, should be considered.

DIAGNOSIS

INTRAVITAM DIAGNOSIS OF HUMAN RABIES ENCEPHALITIS

The diagnosis of rabies can be confirmed by virus isolation, rapid identification of antigen or, in unvaccinated people, antibody detection.

ISOLATION OF RABIES VIRUS

Culture of the virus is most successful during the first week of illness—from saliva, throat, tracheal or eye swabs, brain biopsy samples, CSF and occasionally urine.[56] The method of inoculation of suckling mice[9] yields results in 1–3 weeks, and is now being replaced by tissue culture techniques in BHK cells or the more sensitive murine neuroblastoma cells. A microculture technique takes up to 4 days,[89] but cell cultures are more sensitive to the toxic effects of contaminated inocula.

ANTIGEN DETECTION

A fluorescent antibody test (FAT) rapidly identifies antigen in skin biopsies taken from a hairy area, usually the nape of the neck (Figure 33.6). Frozen sections of punch biopsies reveal rabies antigen in nerve twiglets around the base of hair follicles (Figure 33.7).[90] Careful controls of specificity are

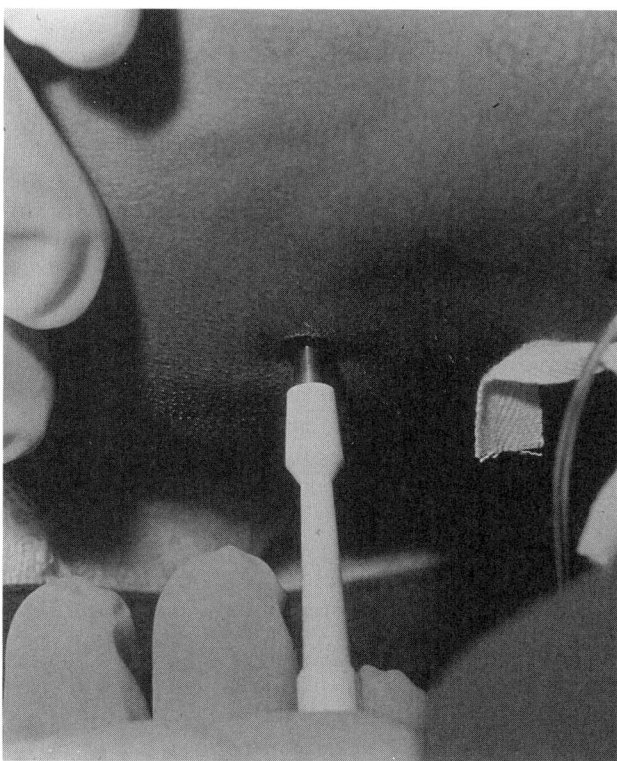

Figure 33.6 Punch biopsy of skin in the hairy nuchal region for rabies antigen detection in a patient with suspected rabies encephalitis. (Courtesy of D.A. Warrell.)

needed, but this method is 60–100% sensitive.[58,91] False positives have not been reported.

The corneal smear test is too insensitive to be useful[56,58] and false positives have occurred.

ANTIBODY DETECTION

In unvaccinated patients, rabies seroconversion often occurs during the second week of illness and is diagnostic,[56] but absence of antibody up to 24 days after the onset of symptoms has been observed, possibly related to interferon therapy.[92]

In vaccinated people, very high levels of antibody in the serum, and especially in the CSF, are needed to make the diagnosis.[88] CSF antibody is produced later than in serum and is between two and four times lower in titre.[56]

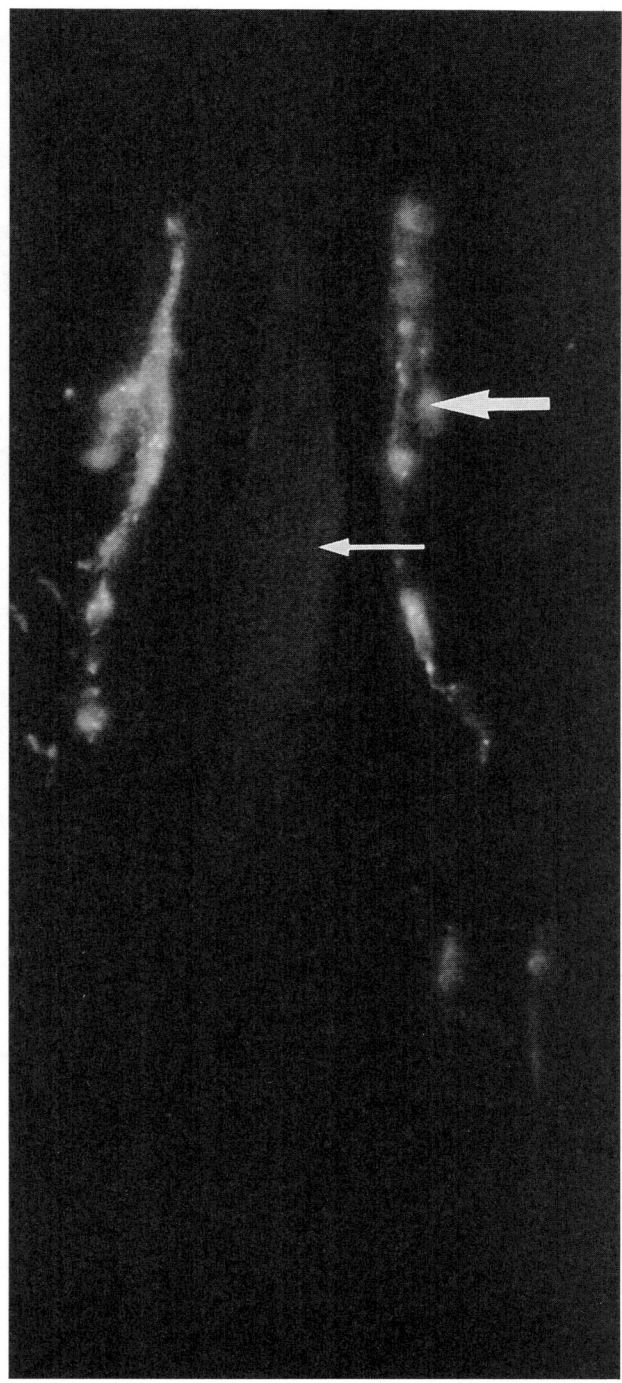

Figure 33.7 Diagnosis of rabies during life from a skin biopsy. Vertical section through a hair follicle. The small arrow shows the hair shaft. The bright fluorescence (large arrow) indicates rabies antigen in nerve cells around the follicle.

POSTMORTEM DIAGNOSIS IN HUMANS

Although virus isolation from secretions is usually unsuccessful after 2 weeks of illness, culture of brain tissue should be possible post mortem, even if the FAT antigen test is negative. Samples can be obtained without a full postmortem examination. Brain necropsies are taken with a Vim–Silverman needle via the medial canthus of the eye—through the superior orbital fissure or an occipital approach through the foramen magnum.

Retrospective diagnosis using formalin-fixed brain specimens is possible by trypsin digestion and labelled antibody staining with immunofluorescent[93] or enzymatic[94] techniques.

DIAGNOSIS IN THE BITING MAMMAL

If laboratory facilities are available, suspect rabid animals should be killed without delay and their brains tested for rabies infection.[95] Observation in captivity is potentially dangerous and uncertain.[75] Ideally, samples of hippocampus, brain stem and cerebellum should be tested, but brain specimens can be obtained from dogs without craniotomy via the occipital foramen.[96] FAT staining of acetone-fixed impression smears takes a few hours[97] and is the usual method of diagnosis. It is about 98% sensitive compared with viral culture by the mouse

inoculation test[97] and has replaced the classical Sellers' stain for Negri bodies. The FAT is unreliable in detecting rabies-related viruses.[17]

An epi-illumination adaptor for standard light microscopes has been produced,[98] but if fluorescence microscopy is not available, a rapid enzyme immunodiagnostic kit will test for antigen in brain tissue suspensions. This is 3% less sensitive than the FAT.[99]

No single test should be relied upon to make this important diagnosis. Ideally, virus isolation is attempted on all FAT-negative samples, by inoculation of suckling mice or tissue culture (see above, Postmortem Diagnosis in Humans).

Strains of street rabies, or rabies-related viruses from different vector species or geographical areas, can be differentiated by antigenic typing. Virus isolates are identified by observing their reaction pattern with a panel of monoclonal antibodies,[12,17,31] or more precisely by sequence analysis of the nucleoprotein gene.[100]

CONTROL OF ANIMAL RABIES

The optimum method of protecting man from rabies infection or economic loss due to rabies varies greatly in different endemic areas. The species of vector, its prevalence and interaction with man dictate whether elimination or vaccination of animals is appropriate and economically feasible.

URBAN RABIES

The control of endemic rabies in urban areas, where dogs are the dominant vectors, requires: epidemiological surveillance; laboratory diagnostic facilities; education to avoid unnecessary contact with animals, especially stray dogs; and vaccination of dogs, cats and humans.[95]

The size of a population of stray dogs depends on available food and shelter. Attempts at control by killing dogs results in an increased reproduction rate and rapid restoration of numbers. Elimination of urban rabies by reducing the stray population and vaccinating can be successful, as in peninsular Malaysia and Japan.[11] Mass vaccination campaigns—aimed at immunizing 80% of dogs—have eliminated canine rabies in densely populated urban areas of Argentina, Brazil and Peru.[10]

Efficient postexposure vaccine treatment of dog-bite victims should be ensured. This includes a rapid diagnostic service and adequate supplies of vaccine and immune serum.

SYLVATIC (WILDLIFE) RABIES

For some vector species active control is not attempted, but simple measures prevent contact with man. Insectivorous bats in North America and Europe are examples, due to the low rate of transmission to other species and lack of effective methods. In contrast, where infection of domestic animals and humans is likely, as with fox rabies in Europe, campaigns for population control and vaccination have been mounted.

Trapping, gassing, poisoning and hunting are generally inefficient means of population reduction. Only Denmark has succeeded in eliminating rabies by these methods.[101]

Two types of oral fox vaccine have been used to great effect. Live attenuated rabies virus vaccine, disguised in chicken head or sausage-like baits, has been distributed by aircraft over areas of Canada and many European countries including Germany,

Belgium, Switzerland, Austria, France, Italy and the former Czechoslovakia. As a result, virtually all of Switzerland and large parts of other countries are now free of rabies.[102] A live vaccinia recombinant vaccine expressing rabies glycoprotein[103] is effective experimentally in foxes, racoons[104] and skunks,[105] and also against fox rabies in the field in Belgium.[106]

In Latin America vampire bat rabies is a major cause of death in cattle,[14] with disastrous economic consequences. Specific control methods include treatment with anticoagulants, diphenadione or warfarin, to which bats but not cattle are highly sensitive. Genetically engineered vaccines such as the vaccinia–rabies glycoprotein recombinant vaccine may in future be used for cattle.[107]

POSTEXPOSURE PROPHYLAXIS

This treatment is aimed at killing or neutralizing rabies virus in a wound before any virions enter a nerve ending. Once within the nervous system, the immune response is thought to be incapable of preventing disease. Postexposure treatment is needed after possible contact with rabies virus through an open wound or mucous membrane (Figure 33.8). Intact skin is a barrier against infection.

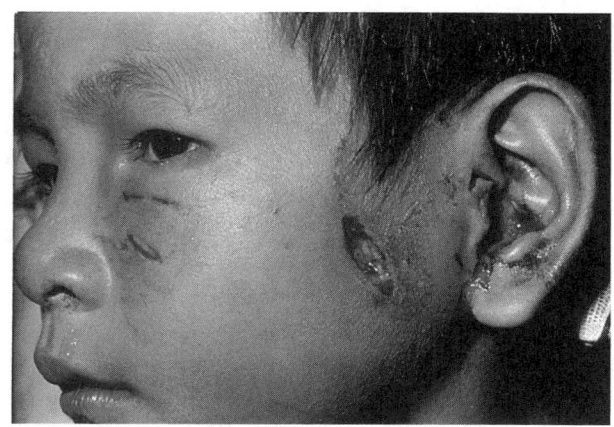

Figure 33.8 Facial bites inflicted by a rabid dog in Thailand. (Courtesy of D.A. Warrell.)

ASSESSING THE RISK OF RABIES INFECTION

In rabies endemic areas strenuous efforts should be made to have the biting animal put down and its brain examined for rabies.[95] An unprovoked attack by an unvaccinated animal with abnormal behaviour (for example excitable or partially paralysed) indicates a high risk of rabies. Nevertheless, vaccinated animals have transmitted rabies.[108]

If the biting animal has escaped or there is any doubt, postexposure prophylaxis should be given, irrespective of the length of time since the bite. The official WHO recommendations are summarized in Table 33.3.

Postexposure treatment has three components: wound treatment, active immunization and passive immunization with rabies immune globulin.

Table 33.3 Specific postexposure prophylaxis for use in a rabies endemic area (following contact with a domestic or wild rabies vector species, whether or not the animal is available for observation or diagnostic tests)*.

Exposure	Treatment
Minor (including licks of broken skin, scratches or abrasions without bleeding)	• Start vaccine administration immediately • Stop treatment if animal remains healthy for 10 days • Stop treatment if animal's brain proves negative for rabies by appropriate laboratory tests
Major (including licks of mucosa, minor bites or major bites—multiple or on face, head, fingers or neck)	• Immediate rabies immune globulin and vaccine • Stop treatment if domestic cat or dog remains healthy for 10 days • Stop treatment if animal's brain proves negative for rabies by appropriate laboratory tests

*This scheme is a simplification of the recommendations of the WHO Expert Committee on Rabies (1992).[95]

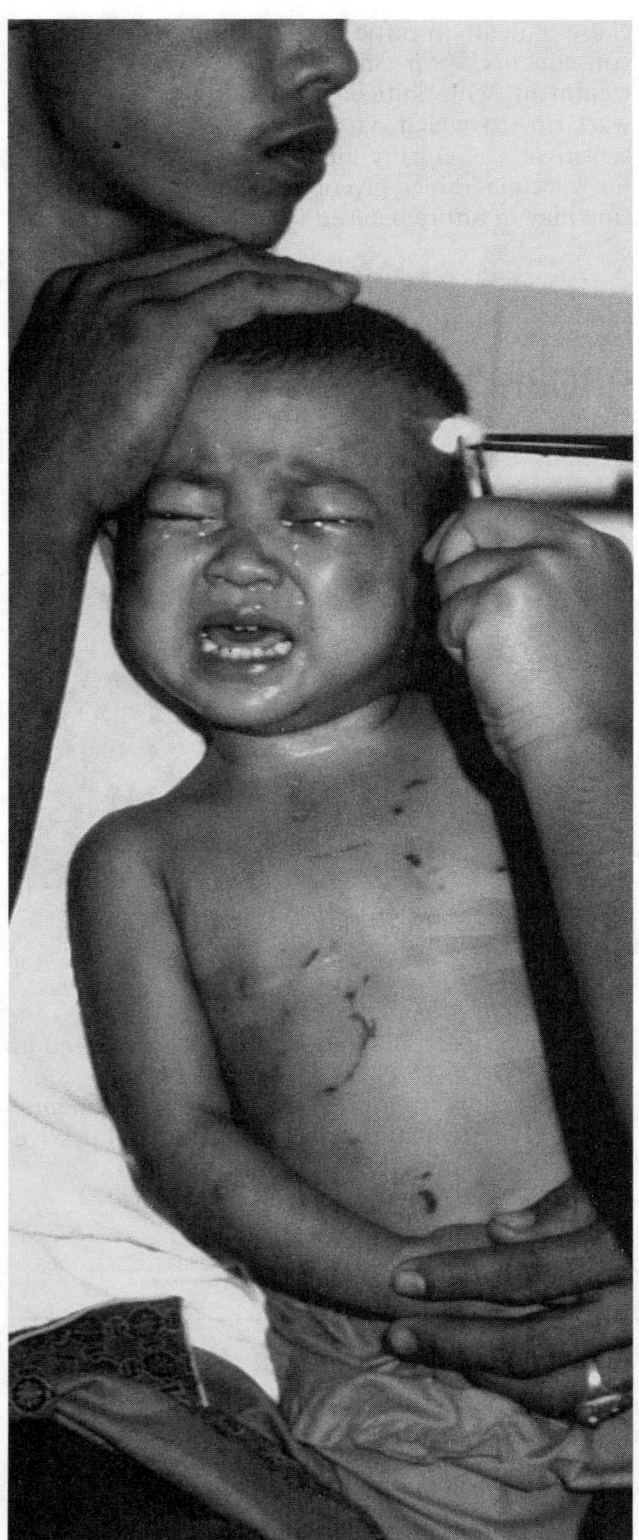

Figure 33.9 Thorough wound cleaning following an attack by a rabid dog (as for this Thai boy) is an essential part of postexposure prophylaxis. (Courtesy of D.A. Warrell.)

WOUND TREATMENT

Immediate cleaning of the wound or site of contact with a rabid animal is imperative for rabies protection (Figure 33.9). Thorough scrubbing with concentrated (20%) soap solution or detergent and debridement should be followed by rinsing under running water. If possible, swab with a virucidal agent: iodine solutions or 40–70% alcohol.[109] Quaternary ammonium compounds are neutralized by soap and are not generally recommended.[110] Energetic wound cleaning may require local or even general anaesthesia. Suturing should be delayed or avoided to prevent inoculation of virus deeper into the tissues.[95]

Tetanus prophylaxis may be required, and other bacterial infections associated with mammal bites may be treated with antibiotics; for example, *Pasteurella multocida* is usually sensitive to ampicillin, tetracycline and co-trimoxazole.

ACTIVE IMMUNIZATION

RABIES VACCINES

All human rabies vaccines currently produced contain killed whole virus which has been grown on a variety of substrates.

Nervous tissue vaccines

These are inactivated homogenates of infected sheep, goat or suckling mouse brains. Fourteen or 21 daily injections are given subcutaneously over the anterior abdominal wall because it is a large area of lax tissue able to accommodate the large volume of vaccine. Nervous tissue vaccines are still produced in 24 countries, and it is likely that most recipients of postexposure treatment today have these.

Semple vaccine was first produced in 1911 and is still widely used in India, where there are an estimated 3 million recipients annually.[21] Fuenzalida's suckling mouse brain vaccine is used in South America and parts of Asia. The potency of Semple vaccine is variable, and 7% of 707 Thai patients with rabies had had a full course of vaccine.[76] Although postvaccinal encephalitis is a serious complication (see p. 714), postexposure treatment is urgent so, if it is the only vaccine available, treatment should be started and a change to modern tissue culture vaccine can be made at any time.

Vaccine produced on embryonated eggs

An American duck embryo vaccine was withdrawn 15 years ago but a highly purified inactivated rabies duck embryo vaccine is now manufactured in Switzerland. It is claimed to be free of all myelin and other neural proteins and is used according to the regimens for tissue culture vaccines.[111]

Vaccines produced in tissue culture

A change to the use of tissue culture vaccine occurred about 15 years ago in Europe and North America, and since then increasingly in other countries including China, Japan, Thailand and Russia.

The original French human diploid cell vaccine (HDCV) is produced in slow-growing fibroblast monolayer cultures. An HDCV is also made in Germany and Canada. Although effective, it is too expensive for widespread use so many other cell lines are now used to make cheaper products. Two vaccines which are exported to tropical endemic areas are a German purified chick embryo cell (PCEC) vaccine and a French purified vero cell vaccine (PVRV) (Table 33.4). PVRV is made in cells on the surface of dextran particles in a suspension culture, permitting economical large-scale production. Tissue culture vaccines are also made, mainly for local use, in China, Japan, Russia, the Netherlands and the USA.[112,113]

TISSUE CULTURE VACCINE REGIMENS

The standard WHO recommended regimen for all these vaccines is a 1.0 ml dose intramuscularly into the deltoid (or anterolateral thigh in children, but never the buttock) on days 0, 3, 7, 14 and 30.[38,95] At $US124 per course for HDCV, this is too expensive for widespread use,[76] and it is relatively slow at inducing measurable immunity, so other schemes have been devised to decrease the amount of vaccine while accelerating the immune response.

One such regimen has been tested in patients bitten by proven rabid animals, and only those with severe bites (see below) also received immune globulin, as is common in tropical areas. This multiple-site intradermal method for HDCV has a wide margin of safety, and consists of:[114]

Day 0   0.1 ml intradermally at eight sites (right and left deltoid, suprascapular, thigh and lower abdominal areas) using up the whole 1.0 ml ampoule.

Day 7   0.1 ml intradermally at four sites (deltoids and thighs).

Days 28 and 91 0.1 ml intradermally at one site (deltoids).

The distribution of sites is designed to stimulate many different groups of lymph nodes. A *separate syringe and needle* must be used for every patient to prevent viral cross-infection.[115] Neutralizing antibody induction is fast, 88% are positive by day 7, and antibody is detectable a year later, whether or not immune globulin was also given.[114] Less than two ampoules of vaccine are needed—a 60% reduction of the intramuscular regimen. Only four visits to the clinic are required, instead of up to 17 for nervous tissue vaccines, which considerably reduces the cost of travel and time off work for patients.

Other multisite postexposure regimens suggested include a two-site intramuscular method, using four doses of HDCV within 21 days. This induces short-lived antibody[116] and is not economical. An intradermal regimen using PVRV has been tested postexposure, with immune globulin in every case.[117] The manufacturer's instructions should be followed for all other vaccines.

Postexposure treatment for those who have had previous vaccination

Wound care and booster doses of vaccine are still vital and urgent. Provided that a full pre- or postexposure course of HDCV or other established tissue

Table 33.4 Widely-used rabies tissue culture vaccines for humans.

Vaccine*	Abbreviation	Cell line	Virus	Origin	Licensed
Human diploid cell vaccine	HDCV	Human fibroblast MRC-5	PM1503	France	1974
Purified vero cell rabies vaccine	PVRV	Vero cell	PM1503	France	1985
Purified chick embryo cell	PCEC	Primary chick embryo cell	LEP	Germany	1985

*All three are inactivated with β-propiolactone.

culture vaccine has been given, or if at least 0.5 iu/ml of rabies neutralizing antibody has been documented following any other treatment, a boosting course of two or three doses of tissue culture vaccine intramuscularly on days 0 and 3 are recommended, and passive immunization is not required. Otherwise a full course of vaccine and rabies immune globulin are needed.

VACCINE COMPLICATIONS

Side-effects of tissue culture vaccines

Minor local reactions occur in about 15% of vaccinees, and include pain, erythema, swelling, aching and paraesthesia.[118] Multiple-site intradermal injections cause local itching in 35%.[114] Mild systemic reactions, reported by 7% of vaccinees, consist of influenza-like symptoms, headache, fever, malaise, myalgia, nausea, dizziness or a rash.[118]

Booster doses of HDCV, usually about a year after previous treatment, have caused systemic allergic reactions in 6% of American vaccinees. After 3–13 days, urticaria, rash, angio-oedema and arthralgia appear, but always respond promptly to symptomatic treatment.[119] This is an IgE-mediated response to non-viral vaccine constituents. β-Propiolactone, which inactivates the virus in most tissue culture vaccines, reacts with and alters human serum albumin and other proteins in the vaccine, rendering them immunogenic.[120] Highly purified vaccines may not have this complication.[121]

Extremely rare neurological illness following HDCV are either Guillain–Barré-like (in four patients) or local limb weakness (in two patients).[118] Recovery is usually rapid, and none have been fatal.

Rabies vaccines can be safely given in pregnancy.

Postvaccinal neuroparalytic reactions to nervous tissue vaccines

These are inflammatory, demyelinating, autoimmune responses to myelin and other neural antigens contained in the vaccine.[122] Estimates of their incidence vary with different products, but if complications are sought by active surveillance, the frequency is up to 1:220 recipients of Semple vaccine, with a mortality rate of 3%.[123] Symptoms usually appear within 2 weeks of starting the course, but may not appear until 2 months later.[5] A wide variety of meningoencephalitic or localized neurological signs are seen.[122]

Suckling mouse brain vaccines have a lower complication rate (1:8000[124] to 1:27000[125]) but periph-eral nervous system signs, such as Guillain–Barré syndrome, frequently predominate and are fatal in 22% of cases.[124]

Postvaccinial encephalitis can be clinically identical to paralytic rabies, and the diagnosis must be made by exclusion. The skin biopsy technique of rabies antigen detection has proved a useful rapid method.[58]

No further nervous tissue vaccine must be given, but the course completed with a tissue culture vaccine. High-dose corticosteroid therapy is conventional, and cyclophosphamide in addition has been suggested.[126]

PASSIVE IMMUNIZATION

Rabies immune globulin (RIG) provides passive protection during the first 7–10 days of a primary postexposure course of vaccine, when no neutralizing antibody is detectable. This not only neutralizes virus in the wound, but also enhances the presentation of vaccine antigens to T lymphocytes.[127]

The efficacy of RIG treatment combined with rabies vaccine has been proved by many animal studies and natural experiments when wolves have bitten large numbers of people in Iran[128] and China.[129] The mortality from head wounds was reduced fivefold by the addition of immune serum to vaccine treatment.[130]

A dose of 40 iu/kg of equine RIG or 20 iu/kg of human RIG should ideally accompany every primary postexposure vaccine course, but it is essential following severe bites: that is, on the head, neck or fingers and multiple or deep bites.[95] RIG is infiltrated around the wound if anatomically possible, and any remaining injected intramuscularly at a site remote from the vaccine. RIG given days or even hours before the vaccine is started impairs the immune response.[131] The dose must not be exceeded because RIG may reduce the immunogenicity of the vaccine.

Human RIG is prohibitively expensive ($US296 per person) for third world use, and even equine RIG ($US28 per person)[76] is available and affordable by less than 5% of Thai patients.[132]

The incidence of serum sickness following equine RIG varies between 1 and 6%, depending on which product is used.[132] An intradermal skin test does not predict reactions and should be abandoned.[133] Adrenaline should always be at hand in case of anaphylaxis. Human RIG has not been associated with serum sickness.

EFFICACY OF POSTEXPOSURE PROPHYLAXIS

The untreated mortality from rabid animal bites depends on the part of the body affected and the severity of the bite. Data from the prevaccine era give an estimate of the chance of infection from suspect rabid dogs. The mortality from multiple bites on the head was 60–80%, from a single facial bite 30%, and from bites on the hand 15–67%.[134,135] In India the overall mortality from proven rabid dog bites was 35–57%.[136,137] Regretably, no information on wound treatment is given in these studies.

If wound treatment, HDCV and RIG, are given on the day of the bite in the correct manner, prophylaxis is 100% effective.[138] This also applies to reports of other tissue culture vaccines to date. Nevertheless, more than 60 patients are known to have died of rabies after receiving some of these vaccines. This mortality can be attributed to human or circumstantial failure to deliver optimum treatment, and not to reduced antigen content or other failure of the vaccine.

There are four known causes of these rabies deaths:

1. Any delay in starting vaccine increases the chance of rabies virus entering neurones before the immune response is generated. The mortality following head wounds from Iranian rabid wolves doubled if vaccine was delayed beyond 8 days.[130] Treatment is urgent, and it is never too late to begin. Vaccine and RIG should both be used even if the bite occurred months before.
2. Rabies immune globulin is frequently not available in areas where it is most needed,[132] and infiltration of the wound is sometimes omitted.
3. Injecting vaccine into the buttock instead of the deltoid impairs antibody production.[139]
4. Inability of the patient to mount an immune response may be due to chronic disease (e.g. cirrhosis) or immunosuppressive drugs (e.g. steroids).[138]

Street rabies virus strains show a high degree of homology with the strains used in vaccine production, but there is great antigenic diversity among the rabies-related viruses. Whether tissue culture vaccines will protect against European bat lyssavirus infection is debatable.[140] It is likely that the protection afforded against rabies-related viruses is less efficient than that against street rabies virus strains.

A reduced or delayed immune response to postexposure prophylaxis can sometimes be predicted:[141] if treatment is late (e.g. more than 2 days after exposure); if no RIG is available for severely bitten patients; if there is underlying disease or immune deficiency; if potentially immunosuppressive drugs are being taken; if the contact was a rabid bat in Europe; or in other circumstances suggesting a rabies-related virus infection. In any of these instances the immune stimulus can be increased, either by doubling the initial dose of vaccine (one intramuscular dose in each deltoid) or by dividing the first dose between eight sites intradermally, as for the economical HDCV regimen (see above).[114]

PRE-EXPOSURE PROPHYLAXIS

This is advisable for anyone likely to be in contact with a rabid animal. This may include veterinarians, animal handlers, laboratory staff, zoologists, wildlife enthusiasts, health workers, travellers and residents in endemic areas where dogs are the dominant vector species.

A pre-exposure course consists of three doses of tissue culture vaccine, given intramuscularly on days 0, 3 and 28 (or 21).[38,95] An economical alternative for HDCV,[38] PCEC[142] and PURV vaccines is intradermal injections of 0.1 ml at the same intervals. A separate syringe must be used for each patient.[115]

Chloroquine taken as malaria prophylaxis, and other unidentified factors in Americans vaccinated in tropical countries, can suppress the antibody response to intradermal primary pre-exposure treatment.[143,144] In these circumstances, the full dose of vaccine must be given intramuscularly.

Confirmation of seroconversion is generally unnecessary.[38] Booster doses may be given intradermally or intramuscularly at intervals of 6 months to 3 years, depending on the risk of infection. Laboratory staff handling rabies virus should either check that their neutralizing antibody level is at least 0.5 iu/ml, or have a booster injection every 6 months.[38,95] A booster dose 6 months to 2 years after the primary course prolongs the presence of antibody, which is regularly detectable for 5 years and even up to 8 years.[145] Although the titre of antibody falls more rapidly after intradermal than intramuscular inoculation, the response to a booster dose is dramatic whatever the original route.[146]

Repeated booster injections should only be given when necessary because of the risk of hypersensitivity reactions (see p. 714).[119]

REFERENCES

1 Théordoidès J. *Histoire de la Rage, Cave canem.* Paris: Masson, 1986.

2 Wilkinson L. The development of the virus concept as reflected in corpora of studies on individual pathogens. 4. Rabies—two millennia of ideas and conjecture on the aetiology of a virus disease. *Med Hist* 1977; 21:15–31.

3 Matsumoto S. Rabies virus. *Adv Virus Res* 1970; 16:257–301.

4 Calisher C H. Antigenic relationships among Rhabdoviruses from vertebrates and hematophagous arthropods. *Intervirology* 1989; 30:241–257.

5 Warrell M J & Warrell D A. Rhabdovirus infections of man. In Porterfield J S & Tyrell D A J (eds) *Handbook of Infectious Diseases*, vol. 3. Exotic viral infections. London, Chapman and Hall: 1995.

6 Wunner W H, Larson J K, Dietzschold B & Smith C L. The molecular biology of rabies viruses. *Rev Infect Dis* 1988; 10:S771–S784.

7 Michalski F, Parks N F, Soko F & Clark H. F. Thermal inactivation of rabies and other rhabdoviruses: stabilization by the chelating agent EDTA at physiological temperatures. *Infect Immun* 1976; 14:135–143.

8 Kaplan M M, Wiktor T & Koprowski H. An intracerebral assay procedure in mice for chemical inactivation of rabies virus. *Bull World Health Organ* 1966; 34:293–297.

9 Koprowski H. The mouse inoculation test. In Kaplan M M & Koprowski H (eds) *Laboratory Techniques in Rabies*, 3rd edn. Geneva: WHO, 1973: 85–93.

10 Larghi O P, Arrosi J C, Nakajata-a J & Villa-Nova A. Control of urban rabies. In Campbell J B & Charlton K M (eds) *Rabies*. Boston: Kluwer, 1988: 407–422.

11 Blancou J. Epizootiology of rabies: Eurasia and Africa. In Campbell J B & Charlton K M (eds) *Rabies*. Boston: Kluwer, 1988: 243–265.

12 Smith J S. Rabies virus ectopic variation: use in ecologic studies. *Adv Virus Res* 1989; 36:215–253.

13 Jenkins S R, Perry B D & Winkler W G. Ecology and epidemiology of raccoon rabies. *Rev Infect Dis* 1988; 10:S620–S628.

14 Baer G M. Vampire bat and bovine paralytic rabies. In Baer G M (ed.) *The Natural History of Rabies*, 2nd edn. Boca Raton: CRC Press, 1991: 389–403.

15 Everard C O R & Everard J D. Mongoose rabies. *Rev Inf Dis* 1988; 10:S610–S614.

16 Cherkasskiy B L. Roles of the wolf and the raccoon dog in the ecology and epidemiology of rabies in the USSR. *Rev Infect Dis* 1988; 10:S634–S636.

17 King A & Crick J. Rabies-related viruses. In Campbell J B & Charlton K M (eds) *Rabies*. Boston: Kluwer, 1988: 177–199.

18 Acha P N & Arambulo P V. Rabies in the tropics— history and current status. In Kuwert E, Merieux C, Koprowski H & Bogel K (eds) *Rabies in the Tropics*. Berlin: Springer, 1985: 343–359.

19 Sehgal S & Bhatia R. Rabies. Current status and proposed control programmes in India. *Proceedings of a Workshop on Rabies Surveillance and Control, NICD Delhi*. Delhi: National Institute for Communicable Diseases, 1985.

20 Bahnemann H G. Rabies in South East Asia. In Kuwert E, Merieux C, Koprowski H & Bogel K (eds) *Rabies in the Tropics*. Berlin: Springer, 1985: 541–544.

21 Bögel K & Motschwiller E. Incidence of rabies and post-exposure treatment in developing countries. *Bull World Health Organ* 1986; 64:883–887.

22 Fishbein D B. Rabies in humans. In Baer G M (ed.) *The Natural History of Rabies*. Boca Raton: CRC Press, 1991: 519–549.

23 Familusi J B & Moore D L. Isolation of a rabies related virus from the CSF of a child with 'aseptic meningitis'. *Afr J Med Sci* 1972; 3:93–96.

24 Familusi J B, Osunkoya B O, Moore D L et al. A fatal human infection with Mokola virus. *Am J Trop Med Hyg* 1972; 21:959–963.

25 Meredith C D, Rossouw A P & van Praag Koch H. An unusual case of human rabies thought to be of chiropteran origin. *S Afr Med J* 1971; 45:767–769.

26 King A, Davies P & Lawrie A. The rabies viruses of bats. *Vet Microbiol* 1990; 23:165–174.

27 Selimov M A, Tatarov A G, Botvinkin A D et al. Rabies related Yulivirus: identification with a panel of monoclonal antibodies. *Acta Virol (Praha)* 1989; 33:542–546.

28 Lumio J, Hillbom M, Roine R et al. Human rabies of bat origin in Europe. *Lancet* 1986; i:378.

29 Crick J. Rabies. In Gibbs E P J (ed.) *Virus Diseases of Food Animals*, vol. II. London: Academic Press, 1981: 469–516.

30 Bitsch V, Westergaard J & Valle M. Bat virus— Europe. *MMWR* 1986; 35:430–432.

31 Hirose J A, Bourhy H & Lafon M. A reduced

panel of anti-nucleocapsid monoclonal antibodies for bat rabies virus identification in Europe. *Res Virol* 1990; 141:571–581.

32 Helmick C G, Tauxe R V & Vernon A A. Is there a risk to contacts of patients with rabies? *Rev Infect Dis* 1987; 9:511–518.

33 Sureau P, Portnoi D, Rollin P et al. Prévention de la transmission inter-humaine de la rage après greffe de cornée. *C R Acad Sci* 1981; 293:689–692.

34 Sipahioglu U & Alpaut S. Transplacental rabies in humans. *Mikrobiyol Bül* 1985; 19:95–99.

35 Winkler W G. Airborne rabies. In Baer G M (ed.) *The Natural History of Rabies*, vol. II. New York: Academic Press, 1975: 115–121.

36 Winkler W G, Fashinell T R, Leffingwell L et al. Airborne rabies transmission in a laboratory worker. *JAMA* 1973; 226:1219–1221.

37 Centers for Disease Control. Rabies in a laboratory worker—New York. *MMWR* 1977; 26:183–184.

38 Centers for Disease Control. Rabies prevention— United States, 1991: recommendations of the Immunization Practices Advisory Committee (ACIP). *MMWR* 1991; 40:RR-3.

39 Murphy F A. Rabies pathogenesis, brief review. *Arch Virol* 1977; 54:279–297.

40 Coulon P, Derbin C, Kucera P et al. Invasion of the peripheral nervous systems of adult mice by the CVS strain of rabies virus and its avirulent derivative AV01. *J Virol* 1989; 63:3550–3554.

41 Tsiang H. Pathophysiology of rabies virus infection of the nervous system. *Adv Virus Res* 1993; 42:375–412.

42 Lentz T L. Rabies virus binding to an acetylcholine receptor alpha-subunit peptide. *J Mol Recognit* 1990; 3:82–88.

43 Gosztonyi G, Dietzschold B, Kao M et al. Rabies and Borna disease: a comparative pathogenetic study of two neurovirulent agents. *Lab Invest* 1993; 68:285–295.

44 Tsiang H, Ceccaldi P E & Lycke E. Rabies virus infection and transport in human sensory dorsal root ganglia neurons. *J Gen Virol* 1991; 72:1191–1194.

45 Baer G M. Animal models in the pathogenesis and treatment of rabies. *Rev Infect Dis* 1988; 10:S739–S750.

46 Wunner W H. Rabies viruses—pathogenesis and immunity. In Wagner R R (ed.) *The Rhabdoviruses*. New York: Plenum Press, 1987: 361–426.

47 Dueñas A, Belsey M A, Escobar J et al. Isolation of rabies virus outside the human central nervous system. *J Infect Dis* 1973; 127:702–704.

48 Dietzschold B, Wunner W H, Wiktor T J et al. Characterization of an antigenic determinant of the glycoprotein that correlates with pathogenicity of rabies virus. *Proc Natl Acad Sci USA* 1983; 80:70–74.

49 Tangchai P, Yenbutr D & Vejjajiva A. Central nervous system lesions in human rabies. A study of

twenty-four cases. *J Med Assoc Thai* 1970; 53:471–486.

50 Dupont J R & Earle K M. Human rabies encephalitis. A study of forty-nine fatal cases with a review of the literature. *Neurology* 1966; 15:1023–1034.

51 Perl D P. The pathology of rabies in the central nervous system. In Baer G M (ed.) *The Natural History of Rabies*, vol. I. New York: Academic Press, 1975; 235–272.

52 Maton P N, Pollard J D & Newsom-Davies J. Human rabies encephalomyelitis. *BMJ* 1976; i:1038–1040.

53 Iwasaki Y, Liu D-S, Yamamoto T & Konno H. On the replication and spread of rabies virus in the human central nervous system. *J Neuropathol Exp Neurol* 1985; 44:185–195.

54 Sandhyamani S, Roy S, Gode G R & Kalla G N. Pathology of rabies: a light and electronmicroscopical study with particular reference to the changes in cases with prolonged survival. *Acta Neuropathol (Berl)* 1981; 54:247–251.

55 Metze K & Feiden W. Rabies ribonucleoprotein in the heart. *N Engl J Med* 1991; 324:1814–1815.

56 Anderson L J, Nicholson K G, Tauxe R V & Winkler W G. Human rabies in the United States, 1960 to 1979: epidemiology, diagnosis and prevention. *Ann Intern Med* 1984; 100:728–735.

57 Hattwick M A W. Human rabies. *Public Health Rev* 1974; 3:229–274.

58 Warrell M J, Looareesuwan S, Manatsathit S et al. Rapid diagnosis of rabies and post-vaccinal encephalitides. *Clin Exp Immunol* 1988; 71:229–234.

59 Hemachudha T, Phanuphak P, Sriwanthana B et al. Immunologic study of human encephalitic and paralytic rabies. Preliminary report of 16 patients. *Am J Med* 1988; 84:673–677.

60 Wiktor T J, Doherty P C & Koprowski H. Suppression of cell-mediated immunity by street rabies virus. *J Exp Med* 1977; 145:1617–1622.

61 Merigan T C, Baer G M, Winkler W G et al. Human leucocyte interferon administration to patients with symptomatic and suspected rabies. *Ann Neurol* 1984; 16:82–87.

62 Turner G S. Immune response after rabies vaccination: basic aspects. *Ann Inst Pasteur Virol* 1985; 126E:453–460.

63 World Health Organization, Working Group II. Vaccine potency requirements for reduced immunization schedules and pre-exposure treatment. *Dev Biol Stand* 1978; 40:268–270.

64 Templeton J W, Holmberg C, Garber T & Sharp R M. Genetic control of serum neutralizing-antibody response to rabies vaccination and survival after a rabies challenge infection in mice. *J Virol* 1986; 59:98–102.

65 Kuwert E K, Barsenbach C, Werner J et al. Early/ high and late/low responders among HDCS vaccinees? In Kuwert E K, Wiktor T J &

Koprowski H (eds) *Cell Culture Rabies Vaccines and their Protective Effect in Man.* Geneva: International Green Cross, 1981: 160–167.

66 Anderson L J, Winkler W G, Smith J S et al. Post-exposure rabies prophylaxis with 5 doses of a tri-*N*-butyl phosphate inactivated human diploid cell vaccine. In Kuwert E K, Wiktor T J & Koprowski H (eds) *Cell Culture Rabies Vaccines and their Protective Effect in Man.* Geneva: International Green Cross, 1981: 300–306.

67 Anderson L J, Baer G M, Smith J S, Winkler W G & Holman R C. Rapid antibody response to human diploid rabies vaccine. *Am J Epidemiol* 1981; 113:270–275.

68 Turner G S, Aoki F Y, Nicholson K G et al. Human diploid cell strain rabies vaccine. Rapid prophylactic immunisation of volunteers with small doses. *Lancet* 1976; i:1379–1381.

69 Dietzschold B & Ertl H C J. New developments in the pre- and post-exposure treatment of rabies. *Immunology* 1991; 10:427–439.

70 Celis E, Ou D, Dietzschold B & Koprowski H. Recognition of rabies and rabies-related viruses by T-cells derived from human vaccine recipients. *J Virol* 1988; 62:3128–3134.

71 Macfarlan R I, Dietzschold B, Wiktor T J et al. T cell responses to cleaved rabies virus glycoprotein and to synthetic peptides. *J Immunol* 1984; 135:2748–2752.

72 Celis E, Miller R W, Wiktor T J et al. Isolation and characterization of human T-cell lines and clones reactive to rabies virus: antigen specificity and production of interferon-γ. *J Immunol* 1986; 136:692–697.

73 Nicholson K G, Kuwert E K, Werner J & Harrison P. Interferon response to human diploid cell strain rabies vaccines in man. *Arch Virol* 1979; 61:35–39.

74 Smith J S, Fishbein D B, Rupprecht C E & Clark K. Unexplained rabies in three immigrants in the United States. A virological investigation. *N Engl J Med* 1991; 324:205–211.

75 Editorial. Human rabies: strain identification reveals lengthy incubation. *Lancet* 1991; 337:822–823.

76 Wilde H, Chutivongse S, Tepsumethanon W et al. Rabies in Thailand: 1990. *Rev Infect Dis* 1991; 13:644–652.

77 Wang S P. Statistical studies of human rabies in Taiwan. *J Formosan Med Assoc* 1956; 55:548–555.

78 Kaplan C, Turner G S & Warrell D A. *Rabies. The Facts,* 2nd edn. Oxford: Oxford University Press, 1986: 21–67.

79 Warrell D A. The clinical picture of rabies in man. *Trans R Soc Trop Med Hyg* 1976; 70:188–195.

80 Warrell D A, Davidson N Mc D, Pope H M et al. Pathophysiologic studies in human rabies. *Am J Med* 1976; 60:180–190.

81 Talaulicar P M. Persistent priapism in rabies. *Br J Urol* 1977; 49:462.

82 Udwadia Z F, Udwadia F E, Rao P P & Kapadia F.

Penile hyperexcitability with recurrent ejaculations as the presenting manifestation of a case of rabies. *Postgrad Med J* 1988; 64:85–86.

83 Hurst E W & Pawan J L. An outbreak of rabies in Trinidad, without history of bites, and with the symptoms of acute ascending myelitis. *Lancet* 1931; ii:622–628.

84 Pará M. An outbreak of post-vaccinal rabies (rage de laboratoire) in Fortaleza, Brazil in 1960. Resistant fixed virus as the etiological agent. *Bull World Health Organ* 1965; 33:172–182.

85 Emmons R W, Leonard L L, De Genaro F et al. A case of human rabies with prolonged survival. *Intervirology* 1973; 1:60–72.

86 Warrell M J, White N J, Looareesuwan S et al. Failure of interferon alfa and tribavirin in rabies encephalitis. *BMJ* 1989; 299:830–833.

87 Porras C, Barboza J J, Fuenzalida E et al. Recovery from rabies in man. *Ann Intern Med* 1976; 85:44–48.

88 Hattwick M A W, Weis T T, Stechschulte C J, Baer G M & Gregg M B. Recovery from rabies: a case report. *Ann Intern Med* 1972; 76:931–942.

89 Rudd R J & Trimarchi C V. Development and evaluation of an in vitro virus isolation procedure as a replacement for the mouse inoculation test in rabies diagnosis. *J Clin Microbiol* 1989; 27:2522–2528.

90 Bryceson A D M, Greenwood B M, Warrell D A et al. Demonstration during life of rabies antigen in humans. *J Infect Dis* 1975; 131:71–74.

91 Blenden D C, Creech W & Torres-Anjel M J. Use of immunofluorescence examination to detect rabies virus antigen in the skin of humans with clinical encephalitis. *J Infect Dis* 1986; 154:698–701.

92 Centers for Disease Control. Human rabies acquired outside the United States from a dog bite. *MMWR* 1981; 30:537–540.

93 Swoveland P T & Johnson K P. Identification of rabies antigens in human and animal tissues. *Ann NY Acad Sci* 1983; 420:185–191.

94 Fekadu M, Greer P W, Chandler F W & Sanderlin D W. Use of the avidin–biotin peroxidase system to detect rabies antigen in formalin-fixed paraffin-embedded tissues. *J Virol Methods* 1988; 19:91–96.

95 World Health Organization. Expert Committee on Rabies Eighth Report. *WHO Tech Rep Ser* 824. 1992 Geneva: WHO.

96 Hirose J A, Bourhy H & Sureau P. Retro-orbital route for brain specimen collection for rabies diagnosis. *Vet Rec* 1991; 129:291–292.

97 Trimarchi C V & Debbie J G. The fluorescent antibody in rabies. In Baer G M (ed.) *The Natural History of Rabies,* 2nd edn. Boca Raton: CRC Press 1991: 219–233.

98 Polsuwan C, Lumlertdaecha B, Tepsumethanon W & Wilde H. Using the UV Paralens adaptor on a standard laboratory microscope for fluorescent rabies antibody detection. *Trans R Soc Trop Med Hyg* 1992; 86:107.

99 Perrin P & Sureau P. A collaborative study of an experimental kit for rapid rabies enzyme immunodiagnosis (RREID). *Bull World Health Organ* 1987; 65:489–493.

100 Smith J S, Orciari L A, Yager P A, Seidel H D & Warner C K. Epidemiologic and historical relationships among 87 rabies virus isolates as determined by limited sequence analysis. *J Infect Dis* 1992; 166:296–307.

101 Wandeler A I. Control of wildlife rabies: Europe. In Campbell J B & Charlton K M (eds) *Rabies*. Boston: Kluwer, 1988: 365–380.

102 Wandeler A I. Oral immunization of wild life. In Baer G M (ed.) *The Natural History of Rabies*, 2nd edn. Boca Raton: CRC Press, 1991:485–503.

103 Kieny M P, Blancou J, Lathe R et al. Development of animal recombinant DNA vaccine and its efficacy in foxes. *Rev Inf Dis* 1988; 10:S799–S802.

104 Rupprecht C E, Hamir A N, Johnston D H & Koprowski H. Efficacy of a vaccinia–rabies glycoprotein recombinant virus vaccine in raccoons (*Procyon lotor*). *Rev Infect Dis* 1988; 10:S803–S809.

105 Tolson N D, Charlton K M, Stewart R B et al. Immune response in skunks to a vaccinia virus recombinant expressing the rabies virus glycoprotein. *Can J Vet Res* 1987; 51:363–366.

106 Brochier B, Kieny M P, Costy F et el. Large-scale eradication of rabies using recombinant vaccinia–rabies vaccine. *Nature* 1991; 354:520–522.

107 Koprowski H. Glimpses into the future of rabies research. *Rev Infect Dis* 1988; 10:S810–S813.

108 Wilde H, Choomkasien P, Hemachudha T et al. Failure of rabies post exposure treatment in Thailand. *Vaccine* 1989; 7:49–52.

109 Kaplan M M & Cohen D. Studies on the local treatment of wounds for the prevention of rabies. *Bull World Health Organ* 1962; 26:765–775.

110 Anderson L J & Winkler W G. Aqueous quaternary ammonium compounds and rabies treatment. *J Infect Dis* 1979; 139:494–495.

111 Glück R, Wegmann A, Germanier R et al. A new highly immunogenic duck embryo rabies vaccine. *Lancet* 1984; i:844–845.

112 Roumiantzeff M, Ajjan N, Montagnon B & Vincent-Falquet J C. Rabies vaccines produced in cell culture. *Ann Inst Pasteur Virol* 1985; 136E:413–424.

113 Centers for Disease Control. Rabies vaccine, adsorbed: a new rabies vaccine for use in humans. *MMWR* 1988; 37:217–218, 223.

114 Warrell M J, Nicholson K G, Warrell D A et al. Economical multiple site intradermal immunisation with human diploid-cell-strain vaccine is effective for post-exposure rabies prophylaxis. *Lancet* 1985; i:1059–1062.

115 Koepke J W, Reller L B, Masters H A & Selner J C. Viral contamination of intradermal syringes. *Ann Allergy* 1985; 55:776–778.

116 Chutivongse S, Wilde H, Fishbein D B et al. One-year study of the 2-1-1 intramuscular post exposure rabies vaccine regimen in 100 severely exposed Thai patients using rabies immune globulin and Vero cell rabies vaccine. *Vaccine* 1991; 9:573–576.

117 Chutivongse S, Wilde H, Supich C et al. Post-exposure prophylaxis for rabies with antiserum and intradermal vaccination. *Lancet* 1990; 335:896–898.

118 Gardner S D. Prevention of rabies in man in England and Wales. In Pattison J R (ed.) *Rabies: A Growing Threat*. Wokingham: Van Nostrand Reinhold, 1983: 39–49.

119 Dreesen D W, Bernard K W, Parker R A et al. Immune complex-like disease in 23 persons following a booster dose of rabies human diploid cell vaccine. *Vaccine* 1986; 4:45–49.

120 Swanson M C, Rosanoff E, Gurwith M et al. IgE and IgG antibodies to β-propiolactone and human serum albumin associated with urticarial reactions to rabies vaccine. *J Infect Dis* 1987; 155:909–913.

121 Fishbein D B, Dreesen D W, Homes D E et al. Human diploid cell rabies vaccine purified by zonal centrifugation: a controlled study of antibody response and side effects following primary and booster pre-exposure immunizations. *Vaccine* 1989; 7:437–442.

122 Hemachudha T, Griffin D E, Giffels J J et al. Myelin basic protein as an encephalitogen in encephalomyelitis and polyneuritis following rabies vaccination. *N Engl J Med* 1987: 316:369–374.

123 Swaddiwuthipong W, Prayoonwiwat N, Kunasol P & Choomkasien P. A high incidence of neurological complications following Semple anti-rabies vaccine. *Southeast Asian J Trop Med Public Health* 1987; 18:526–531.

124 Held J R & Lopez Adaros H. Neurological disease in man following administration of suckling mouse brain antirabies vaccine. *Bull World Health Organ* 1972; 46:321–327.

125 Larghi O P. Improvement of post- and pre-exposure immunization in Latin America. In Kuwert E K, Wiktor T J & Koprowski H (eds) *Cell Culture Rabies Vaccines and their Protective Effect in Man*. Geneva: International Green Cross, 1981: 283–287.

126 Swamy H S, Shankar S K, Chandra P S et al. Neurological complications due to beta-propiolactone (BPL)-inactivated antirabies vaccination. *J Neurol Sci* 1984; 63:111–128.

127 Celis E, Wiktor T J, Dietzschold B & Koprowski H. Amplification of rabies-virus induced stimulation of human T-cell lines and clones by antigen-specific antibodies. *J Virol* 1985; 56:426–433.

128 Baltazard M & Bahmanyar M. Practical trial of antirabies serum in people bitten by rabid wolves. *Bull World Health Organ* 1955; 13:747–772.

129 Fang-tao L, Shu-beng C, Guan-Fu W et al. Study of the protective effect of the primary hamster kidney cell rabies vaccine. *J Infect Dis* 1986; 154:1047–1048.

130 Fathi M, Sabeti A & Bahmanyar M.

Séroprophylaxie antirabique chez les sujets mordus par loups enragés en Iran. *Acta Med Iran* 1970; 13:5–9.

131 Wiktor T J, Lerner R A & Koprowski H. Inhibitory effect of passive antibody on active immunity induced against rabies by vaccination. *Bull World Health Organ* 1971; 45:747–753.

132 Wilde H, Chomchey P, Prakongsri S et al. Adverse effects of equine rabies immune globulin. *Vaccine* 1989; 7:10–11.

133 Wilde H, Chomchey P, Prakongsri S & Punyaratabandhu P. Safety of equine rabies immune globulin. *Lancet* 1987; ii:1275.

134 Babès V. *Traité de la Rage*. Paris: Baillière, 1912.

135 Suzor R. *Hydrophobia*. An account of M Pasteur's system containing a translation of all his communications on the subject, the techniques of his method, and the latest statistical results. London: Chatto & Windrush, 1887.

136 Cornwall J W. Statistics of antirabic inoculations in India. *BMJ* 1923; 298.

137 Veeraraghavan N. Annual report of the Director 1969 and scientific report 1970. Coonoor: Pasteur Institute of Southern India, 1971.

138 Editorial. Rabies vaccine failures. *Lancet* 1988; i:917–918.

139 Fishbein D B & Weir E H. Administration of human diploid-cell rabies vaccine in the gluteal area. *N Engl J Med* 1988; 318:214–215.

140 King A & Davies P. Bat rabies. *State Vet J* 1988; 42:140–148.

141 World Health Organization. Rabies treatment. *Weekly Epidemiol Rec* 1989; 64:112–114.

142 Nicholson K G, Farrow P R, Bijok U & Barth R. Pre-exposure studies with purified chick embryo cell culture rabies vaccine and human diploid cell vaccine: serological and clinical responses in man. *Vaccine* 1987; 5:208–210.

143 Pappaioanou M, Fishbein D B, Dreesen D W et al. Antibody response to pre-exposure human diploid-cell rabies vaccine given concurrently with chloroquine. *N Engl J Med* 1986; 314:280–284.

144 Bernard K W, Fishbein D B, Miller K D et al. Pre-exposure rabies immunization with human diploid cell vaccine: decreased antibody responses in persons immunized in developing countries. *Am J Trop Med Hyg* 1985; 34:633–647.

145 Roumiantzeff M, Ajjan N & Vincent-Falquet J C. Experience with pre-exposure rabies vaccination. *Rev Infect Dis* 1988; 10:S751–S757.

146 Turner G S, Nicholson K G, Tyrrell D A J & Aoki F Y. Evaluation of a HDCS rabies vaccine: final report of a 3 year study of pre-exposure immunization. *J Hyg (Camb)* 1982; 89:101–110.

CHAPTER 34

DENGUE AND DENGUE HAEMORRHAGIC FEVER

S. Nimmannitya

Dengue infections caused by the four antigenically distinct dengue virus serotypes (DEN1, DEN2, DEN3, DEN4) of the family Flaviviridae are the most important arbovirus diseases in humans, both in terms of morbidity and mortality. The infection is transmitted from person to person by *Aedes* mosquitoes. Dengue infections may be asymptomatic or may lead to an undifferentiated fever (or viral syndrome), dengue fever or dengue haemorrhagic fever (DHF).[1]

DENGUE FEVER

GEOGRAPHICAL DISTRIBUTION

Dengue is a worldwide condition spread throughout the tropical and subtropical zones between 30°N and 40°S, where environmental conditions are optimal for dengue virus transmission by *Aedes* mosquitoes. It is endemic in South-East Asia (types 1–4), the Pacific (types 1–3), East and West Africa (types 1–4), the Caribbean (types 1–4) and the Americas (types 1–4).[2]

AETIOLOGY

The dengue virus, a member of the flavivirus group in the family *Flaviviridae*, is a single-stranded enveloped RNA virus, 30 nm in diameter, which can grow in a variety of mosquitoes and tissue cultures. There are four distinct but closely related serotypes (DEN1–4). They possess antigens that cross-react with yellow fever, Japanese encephalitis and West Nile viruses. Although the four dengue serotypes are antigenically distinct, there is some evidence that serological subcomplexes may exist within the group. DEN1 and DEN3 have been shown to share some antigenic determinants by neutralization tests and by immunofluorescence using monoclonal antibodies. A close genetic relationship has been demonstrated between DEN1 and DEN4 using cDNA hybridization probes. DEN2 appears to be quite distinct from the others as it shows low sequence homology with all other serotypes.[3]

There is evidence from field and laboratory studies to suggest that there are distinct strain differences between dengue viruses. Recent developments in molecular virology provided further proof for strain variation. Multiple genetic topotypes have been identified by RNA oligonucleotide fingerprinting for DEN1, DEN2 and DEN3 serotypes. The data suggest that most dengue viruses circulating in a particular geographic area are similar to each other, while viruses from different geographic areas show some biological and antigenic differences.[4,5] However, this is not always the case; in the Caribbean basin countries two topotypes of DEN2 have been documented.[2] Marked differences were also observed between DEN2 viruses isolated from forest mosquitoes and those isolated from human or from *Ae. aegypti* mosquitoes in an urban setting in West Africa, suggesting that enzootic strains of dengue virus in West Africa are genetically distinct from epidemic or endemic strains.[5]

The role that strain variation plays in the distribution and spread of epidemic dengue and in the determination of disease severity is not yet known. It is noteworthy that there are still no known biological or biochemical markers that can be used to identify virulent strains of dengue virus.

TRANSMISSION

Dengue virus is transmitted from human to human by mosquito bites. Man is the main reservoir of the virus, though studies have shown that the monkey is the jungle reservoir in Malaysia and Africa.[2]

Ae. aegypti is the most efficient of the mosquito vectors because of its domestic habit. The female mosquito bites humans during the day. After feeding on a person whose blood contains the virus, the female *Ae. aegypti* can transmit dengue, either immediately by a change of host when its feeding is interrupted, or after an incubation period of 8–10 days during which time the virus multiplies in the salivary glands. Once infected, the host remains infective for life.

Other *Aedes* mosquitoes capable of transmitting dengue include *Ae. albopictus*, *Ae. polynesiensis* and several species of the *Ae. scutellaris* complex. Each of these species has its own particular geographic distribution and they are in general less efficient vectors than *Ae. aegypti*.

Transovarian transmission of dengue viruses has been documented but its epidemiological importance has not been established.[2]

PATHOLOGY

From experimental studies in rhesus monkeys after inoculation the virus reaches the regional lymph nodes and disseminates to the reticuloendothelial system in which it multiplies and from which it enters the blood.[6] Skin lesions in non-fatal, uncomplicated dengue fever seen in human volunteers were studied by biopsy. The chief abnormality occurred in and around small blood vessels and consisted of endothelial swelling, perivascular oedema and infiltration with mononuclear cells. Extensive extravasation of blood without appreciable inflammatory reaction was observed in the petechial lesions.[7]

IMMUNITY

Immunity is antibody mediated. After an acute phase of infection by a particular dengue serotype there is an antibody response to all four dengue serotypes. There is a long-lasting immunity to the homologous serotype of the infecting strain. A cross-reactive heterotypic immunity has been reported by Sabin[7] to last for about 2 months in experimental human volunteers, while another community study reported a period of up to 1 year.[8] After infection by one serotype, the individual concerned will be immune to other serotypes for 2–12 months and become susceptible thereafter. A second attack of dengue has been reported.[9] The waning cross-reactive heterotypic antibody is implicated in the occurrence of DHF.[10]

CLINICAL FEATURES

The clinical features of dengue fever are age dependent: infants and children infected with dengue virus for the first time (i.e. primary dengue infection) usually develop a simple fever or undifferentiated febrile illness; dengue fever is most common in adults and older children and may be benign or may be a classical incapacitating disease with severe muscle and joint pain (break bone fever).[1]

Typically, after an incubation period of 5–8 days following an infective mosquito bite, the disease in adults begins with a sudden onset of fever with severe headache, and any of the following: chilliness, pain behind the eyes—particularly on eye movement or eye pressure, photophobia, backache, and pain in the muscles and joints of the extremities.

The temperature is usually high (39–40°C); the fever may be sustained for 5–6 days and may occasionally have a biphasic course. As the disease progresses the patient becomes anorexic and may show marked weakness and prostration. Other common symptoms include sore throat, altered taste sensation, colicky pain and abdominal tenderness, constipation, dragging pain in the inguinal region and general depression. A relative bradycardia is common during the febrile phase. Symptoms vary in severity and usually persist for several days.

Several types of skin rash have been described. Initially, diffuse flushing, mottling or fleeting pinpoint eruptions may be observed on the face, neck and chest. These are transient in nature. A second type of skin rash is a conspicuous rash that may be maculopapular or scarlatiniform and appears on approximately the third or fourth day. This rash starts on the chest and trunk and spreads to the extremities and face and may be accompanied by itching and dermal hyperaesthesia.

There is generalized enlargement of the lymph nodes but the liver and spleen are not usually palpable. A positive tourniquet test and petechiae on extremities are not uncommon.

Towards the end of the febrile period or immediately after defervescence the generalized rash fades and localized clusters of petechiae may appear over the dorsum of the feet and on the legs, hands and

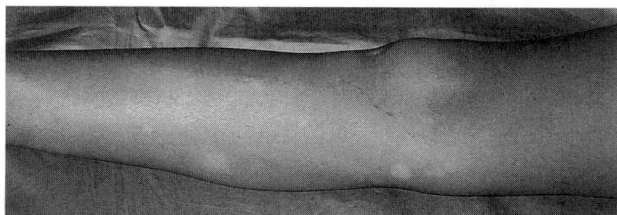

Figure 34.1   Dengue fever: convalescent rash.

arms. This confluent petechial rash is characterized by a scattered pale round area of normal skin (Figure 34.1).

Convalescence may be abrupt and uneventful but is often prolonged, sometimes taking several weeks, and may be accompanied by pronounced asthenia and depression. Bradycardia is common during this period. Loss of hair has been reported during convalescence.

Haemorrhagic complications such as epistaxis, gum bleeding, gastrointestinal haemorrhage, haematuria and hypermenorrhoea have been reported in many epidemics of dengue fever, and on rare occasions severe bleeding has caused deaths in some epidemics.[7,9]

Dengue fever with encephalitic signs but with normal cerebrospinal fluid has been reported in some epidemics.[9] Reye's syndrome associated with dengue infection is not uncommon.[11]

DIAGNOSIS

It is not possible to make a diagnosis of mild dengue or classical dengue fever from the clinical features as they resemble those of many other diseases, particularly chikungunya infection. Differential diagnosis includes malaria and other viral, bacterial and rickettsial diseases. The diagnosis is best accomplished by serological tests for antibodies and virus isolation.

VIROLOGICAL DIAGNOSIS

See DHF below.

TREATMENT

This is entirely symptomatic and supportive.

EPIDEMIOLOGY

The first reported epidemics of dengue or dengue-like disease occurred in 1779 and 1780 in Egypt and Indonesia and in 1780 in the USA (Philadelphia).[9] It is clear that dengue and other arboviruses with similar ecology had a widespread distribution in the tropics as long as 200 years ago. Historically, Asia has been the area of highest endemicity, with all four dengue serotypes circulating in the large urban centres in most countries.[2]

During and after World War II, *Ae. aegypti* became more widespread in Asia and with anincreased facility of communication and travel of susceptible foreigners into the endemic areas, together with the subsequent urbanization that occurred in most countries, the incidence of dengue infection increased dramatically. These changes coincided with the emergence of a newly described DHF in the 1950s. The advent of commercial jet air transport in the 1960s promoted the ideal mechanism for the carriage of dengue virus by persons who had visited endemic areas and were travelling during the incubation period. A trend of increased spread of dengue throughout the world has since developed. Increased epidemic activity was observed in the Pacific Islands and the Caribbean basin in the 1970s and epidemics of all four dengue serotypes were documented in both regions. In the American region, all four viruses are probably now endemic.[2]

In the 1980s increased dengue activity was observed in Africa, and all four dengue serotypes have now been documented in Africa.[2]

The incidence of dengue infection has increased markedly since the 1960s, first in Asia then in the Pacific and Americas and finally in Africa. It appears that most of the tropical world, with an estimated population of 1.5 billion, is at risk of infection with dengue.

Dengue transmission occurs throughout the year in endemic tropical areas; however in most countries there is a distinct cyclical pattern, with increased transmission usually associated with the rainy season. While in some areas increases in dengue transmission coincide with periods of increased rainfall, the interactions between temperature and rainfall or variation in daily microclimates may be important determinants of dengue transmission.[2]

In dengue endemic areas with multiple serotypes children become infected early in childhood. Classical dengue fever is rare among indigenous people as most of adults are immune. In these areas both mild dengue illness and DHF occur mainly in children.

CONTROL

See DHF below.

DENGUE HAEMORRHAGIC FEVER (See also Chapters 15 and 30)

GEOGRAPHICAL DISTRIBUTION

DHF is widespread in the South-East Asian and Western Pacific regions. It is now occurring in all countries in tropical Asia, with the exception of Bangladesh and Pakistan. DHF has also appeared in Cuba, the Caribbean, the Pacific islands, Venezuela and Brazil. So far it has not been reported from Africa.

AETIOLOGY

All four dengue serotypes are capable of causing dengue fever or DHF, depending on the immune status and probably age of the host as DHF occurs almost exclusively in children under the age of 16 years and is associated with secondary dengue infection. A strong association between DHF and secondary dengue infection has led to the proposed concept of two sequential infections by Halstead. Based on his in vitro and monkey studies, an antibody-dependent immune enhancement theory has been hypothesized by Halstead:[10] it is suggested that during the second infection with a heterotypic dengue virus which differs from the first one, pre-existing antibody from the first infection fails to neutralize and may instead enhance viral uptake and replication in the mononuclear phagocytes. Such infected cells may then become the target of an immune elimination mechanism which can trigger the production of mediators with activation of complement and the clotting cascade and eventually produce DHF.[10]

In Thailand, studies over the last 30 years have demonstrated transmission of all four dengue serotypes, with dengue type 2 as the predominating serotype.[12] The studies and experience in Thailand, as well as in Cuba, led to a suggestion that the interval between the two dengue infections (probably 1–5 years) and the sequences of infecting dengue serotypes may be important factors in determining the occurrence and severity of DHF.[10,13]

Other theories involving a virulent strain of dengue virus[14] and the genetic difference in the hosts[15,16] have been proposed. The biological and antigenically distinct strains in different geographic areas have been noted; but so far a virulent strain has not been identified.[2]

PATHOPHYSIOLOGY AND PATHOLOGY

The pathophysiological hallmarks of DHF are leakage of plasma and abnormal haemostasis. Evidence supporting plasma leakage includes a rapid rise in haematocrit, pleural effusion and ascites, hypoproteinaemia and reduced plasma volume. A critical/hypoalbuminaemia loss of plasma leads to hypovolaemic shock and death. The acute onset of shock and the rapid and often dramatic clinical recovery when the patient is treated properly, together with the absence of inflammatory vascular lesions, suggest a transient functional increase in vascular permeability that results in plasma leakage.

A disorder in haemostasis involves all three major factors: vascular change(s), thrombocytopenia and coagulopathy. Acute-type disseminated intravascular clotting is documented and is responsible for the severe bleeding. Bone marrow studies show depression of marrow elements, with maturation arrest of megakaryocytes during the early phase of the illness, which is readily reversed when the fever subsides and during the stage of shock.[18]

Kidney studies in non-fatal cases show changes similar to glomerulonephritis but these are usually mild and transient.[1]

Postmortem studies show that serous effusions with high protein content and widespread petechial haemorrhages in many organs are constant findings.

HISTOLOGICAL CHANGES[1,16]

Significant changes are found in three major organ systems.[17,18]

- Vascular changes include vasodilatation, congestion, perivascular haemorrhage and oedema of arterial walls.
- Proliferation of reticuloendothelial cells with accelerated phagocytic activity is observed frequently.
- The lymphoid tissues show increasing activity of the B-lymphocyte system with active proliferation of plasma cells and lymphoblastoid cells.
- In the liver there is focal necrosis of the hepatic and Kupffer cells, with formation of Councilman-like bodies.

Dengue virus antigen is found predominantly in cells of the spleen, thymus and lymph nodes, in Kupffer cells and in the sinusoidal lining cells of liver and alveolar lining cells of the lung.

The pathogenetic mechanism of DHF is presumed to be immunological, involving both humoral and cell-mediated immune modulation. A constant finding in DHF is activation of the complement system with profound depression of C3 and C5 levels.[1] Immune complexes have been described in DHF cases associated with secondary infection, and they may contribute to complement activation. The C3a and C5a anaphylatoxins are released and their association with the time of leakage, shock and disease severity have been demonstrated.[18] They are the most likely vascular permeability increasing mediators among the other yet unidentified agents.

IMMUNITY

The immune status of the host appears to be the important component that determines the development of DHF as the disease occurs with high frequency in two immunologically defined groups: (1) children who have experienced a previous dengue infection; and (2) infants with waning levels of maternal dengue antibody. The acute phase of infection by a particular dengue serotype is believed to provoke long-lasting homotypic immunity. A cross-reactive heterotypic immunity has been reported to last about 2 months in one study of experimental infection,[7,9] while another community study presented epidemiological data suggesting that this cross-reactive heterotypic immunity might last up to 1 year.[8] It is hypothesized that this cross heterotypic antibody, when weak and failing to neutralize the infecting dengue virus during the second infection, can enhance virus multiplication in the mononuclear phagocyte and trigger immune modulation and eventually produce DHF. Passive IgG dengue antibody from the mothers of infants under the age of one year has been shown to be capable of enhancing

virus replication when falling to below the neutralization level and produce DHF during primary infection.[10,20]

A study of the cell-mediated immune response revealed that during a secondary dengue infection serotype cross-reactive dengue-specific T lymphocytes are activated and proliferate with production of lymphokines and monokines. It is suggested that this response, while contributing to recovery from infection, may also in some circumstances play a role in the immunopathogenesis of DHF.[21]

A second attack of DHF is very rare: it has been shown to occur in about 0.5% of cases in a study over a 16-year period at the Children's Hospital in Bangkok.[22]

CLINICAL FEATURES (Figure 34.2)

DHF is a severe form of dengue infection that is accompanied by haemorrhage and a tendency to

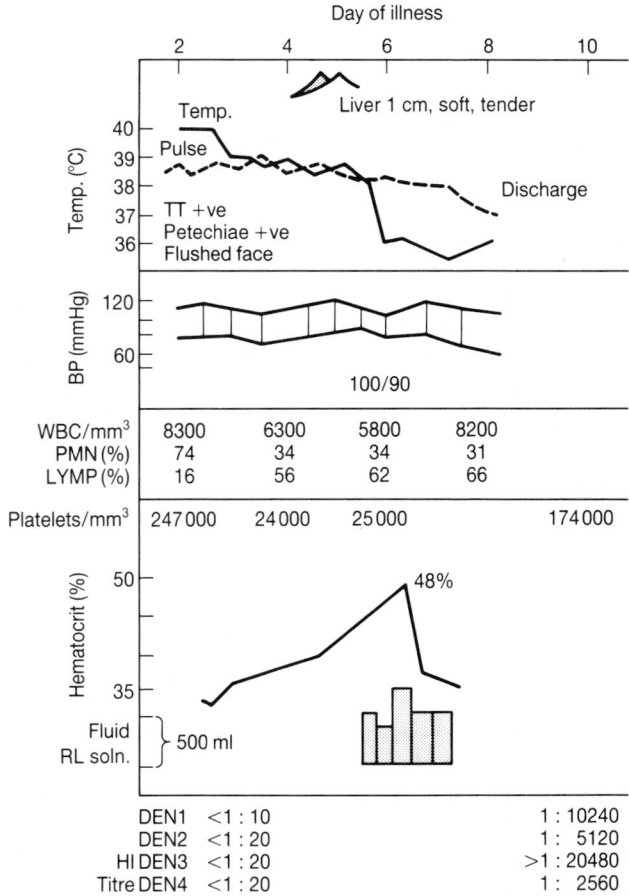

Figure 34.2 Dengue haemorrhagic fever: typical clinical course in a 9-year-old girl (with secondary dengue infection). TT, tourniquet test; PMN, polymorphonuclear leucocytes; LYMP, lymphocyte; RL, Ringer's lactate; HI, haemagglutination inhibition (antibody test by HI-titres).

develop fatal shock (dengue shock syndrome) as a consequence of plasma leakage.

Typically the disease begins with an abrupt onset of high fever accompanied by facial flush and head-ache. Some patients with an infected pharynx may complain of sore throat but rarely have rhinitis or cough. Anorexia, vomiting and abdominal pain are common. During the first few days of the febrile phase, which usually lasts for 2–7 days, the illness resembles dengue fever in many respects but a maculopapular rash and myalgia are less common. Occasionally the body temperature may be as high as 40–41°C and febrile convulsions may occur.

A haemorrhagic diathesis commonly presents as scattered petechiae on extremities, axillae, trunk and face. A positive tourniquet test and tendency to bruise at venepuncture sites are invariably present. Bleeding from the nose, gums and gastrointestinal tract are less common. Haematuria is extremely rare.

The liver is often enlarged, soft and tender but jaundice is not observed. Splenomegaly is rarely observed in small infants. Generalized lymphadeno-pathy is noted in about half of the cases.

The critical stage is reached by the time the fever subsides. Accompanying, or shortly after, a rapid drop in the temperature there are varying degrees of circulatory disturbance. The child is often sweating and restless and has cool extremities. In less severe cases the changes in vital signs are minimal and transient; the patient recovers spontaneously or after a brief period of therapy. In more severe cases shock ensues. The skin is cold and clammy and the pulse pressure is narrow (≤20 mmHg). The course of shock is brief and stormy. If no treatment is given the patient deteriorates rapidly into the stage of profound shock with an imperceptible pulse and blood pressure and dies within 12–24 hours. Pro-longed shock is often complicated by metabolic acidosis and severe bleeding—which indicates a poor prognosis. However, if the patient is properly treated before irreversible shock has developed, rapid, often dramatic recovery is the rule. In-frequently encephalitic signs associated with meta-bolic disturbances, intracranial haemorrhage or hepatic failure (a form of Reye's-like syndrome) occur and give rise to a more complicated course and grave prognosis.[11]

Convalescence is usually short and uneventful. Sinus bradycardia is common. A characteristic con-fluent petechial rash with scattered round areas of pale skin, as described in dengue fever, is frequently observed on the lower extremities. The course of the illness is about 7–10 days in most cases.

A normal white blood count or leucopenia is common and neutrophils may predominate initially.

Lymphocytosis with more than 15% of atypical lymphocytes is usually observed towards the end of the febrile period. Thrombocytopenia and haemo-concentration are constant findings. The platelet count drops shortly before or simultaneously with the haematocrit rise and both changes occur before the subsidence of fever and before onset of shock. Clotting abnormalities are usually found. Other changes include hypoproteinaemia, hypoalbumi-naemia, hyponatraemia and mildly elevated alanine aminotransferase/aspartate aminotransferase levels.

Disease severity is arbitrarily classified as 'non-shock' cases (grades I and II—grade II is more severe than grade I with the presence of spon-taneous haemorrhage) and 'shock' cases (grades III and IV—the latter is a profound shock with imper-ceptible pulse and/or blood pressure).[1,23]

DIAGNOSIS

The clinical features of DHF are rather stereotyped; thus it is possible to make a correct clinical diagnosis based on the major characteristic manifestations as described. The World Health Organization estab-lished criteria for clinical diagnosis:[1] high continu-ous fever for 2–7 days; a haemorrhagic diathesis; hepatomegaly and shock; together with two labora-tory changes—thrombocytopenia ($\leq 100\,000/mm^3$) and concurrent haemoconcentration (haematocrit elevation of 20% or more). The time–course re-lationship between the drop in platelet count and a rapid rise in haematocrit appears to be unique in DHF. These changes, which represent the major pathophysiological hallmarks of DHF, i.e. abnor-mal haemostasis and plasma leakage, clearly dis-tinguish DHF from dengue fever and other diseases.

VIROLOGICAL DIAGNOSIS

Aetiological diagnosis can be confirmed by serologi-cal testing and virus isolation from the blood during the early febrile phase. Antibodies to dengue virus antigens increase rapidly in patients with secondary dengue infection. A diagnostic (fourfold) increase in dengue antibody by the haemagglutination inhi-bition test can usually be demonstrated from paired sera obtained early in the febrile phase or on ad-mission, and 3–5 days later. A third specimen 2–3 weeks after onset is, however, required to confirm diagnosis of primary dengue infection.

Serological diagnosis by detection of anti-dengue IgM and IgG by enzyme linked immunosorbent assay (ELISA) is now widely used to document primary and secondary infection. The IgM antibody capture (MAC)-ELISA is a relatively new test. It is specific in distinguishing dengue from other flavivirus infections and has the advantage over the haemagglutination test in that a definite diagnosis can be made from an acute blood specimen alone, with a sensitivity of about 78%; when convalescent sera are tested the sensitivity is >97%.[24]

TREATMENT

The management of DHF is entirely symptomatic and supportive and is principally aimed towards replacement of plasma loss during the period of active leakage of about 24–48 hours. Prognosis depends on early clinical recognition and frequent monitoring for a drop in platelet count and rise in haematocrit. Early volume replacement when the haematocrit rises sharply as plasma leaks out can modify severity and prevent shock.

The management of DHF during the febrile phase is similar to that of dengue fever. Antipyretics may be needed to control the high fever; aspirin must not be used (to avoid gastric irritation and bleeding and as a precaution to prevent Reye's syndrome associated with dengue). Oral fluid and electrolyte therapy is recommended for patients who have anorexia and vomiting.

The critical period when plasma leakage and shock may develop is at the transition from the febrile to the afebrile phase, which is from the third day. A drop in the platelet count to $100\,000/mm^3$ or less usually precedes a rise in haematocrit. A rise in haematocrit of 20% (e.g. from 35 to 42% or more) indicates significant plasma loss and intravenous fluid therapy is indicated. In mild to moderately severe cases (grades I and II) fluid therapy can be given for a period of 12–24 hours at an outpatient clinic. Patients who are restless and have cool extremities, acute abdominal pain and oliguria should be admitted to hospital.

The fluid used for volume replacement in DHF should be an isotonic solution that has an electrolyte composition similar to plasma. The total volume needed is usually approximately maintenance plus 5–6% deficit (similar to mild or moderate dehydration). The rate of intravenous fluid infusion must be adjusted according to the rate of plasma leakage, which is more rapid during the first 6 hours of the critical phase. The need for intravenous therapy usually lasts for no more than 48 hours in uncomplicated cases.

When shock has developed, satisfactory results have been obtained with the following regimen:

1. Immediately and rapidly correct hypovolaemia from plasma loss with isotonic salt solution (5% dextrose in saline, Ringer lactate or acetate solution) and colloid (plasma or plasma expander) in cases of profound shock until improvement in vital signs is apparent.
2. Continue to replace further plasma losses to maintain effective circulation for a period of 24–48 hours.
3. Correct metabolic and electrolyte disturbances (acidosis and hyponatraemia).
4. Give fresh blood transfusions and occasionally platelet-rich plasma in cases of significant bleeding.

It is important to adjust the rate of intravenous infusion according to the extent of leakage, as guided by the haematocrit level, vital signs and urine output, to avoid excessive fluid replacement. Fluid replacement must be stopped when haematocrit and vital signs return to normal and become stable and a diuresis ensues. If further fluid replacement is given at this stage it can cause cardiac failure and/or acute pulmonary oedema when extravasated plasma is reabsorbed.

With this regimen the fatality rate of shock cases at the Children's Hospital in Bangkok has fallen to below 1%. There is no evidence that corticosteroids are of benefit in reducing the fatality rate or reducing the disease severity.[25,26] The efficacy of heparin in the treatment of cases with severe bleeding from disseminated intravascular coagulation has not been proved.

Good nursing care with close observation 24 hours a day is essential for management of patients with DHF.

EPIDEMIOLOGY

Since it was first recognized in the Philippines in 1954, DHF has occurred in Thailand, Malaysia, Singapore, Sri Lanka, Vietnam, India, Burma, Myanmar and Malaysia, several Pacific islands, China, Laos and Kampuchea. Between 1956 and 1990, there were 3 071 245 cases with 51 087 deaths reported from 12 Asian countries, the Pacific Islands, Cuba and Venezuela. The first outbreak of DHF to occur outside the South-East Asian and Western Pacific regions was in Cuba in 1981. Since then sporadic cases of DHF have been reported from the Caribbean and small outbreaks occurred in Venezuela in 1989 and Rio de Janeiro in 1991.[27]

Outbreaks occur most frequently in areas where most environmental conditions are optimal for dengue transmission and multiple types of dengue virus are simultaneously endemic or sequentially epidemic, and infections with heterologous types are frequent. In endemic areas where dengue infection is frequently asymptomatic and occurs in early childhood, classical dengue fever is rarely a recognizable disease among indigenous people. DHF occurs most frequently in children aged between 2 and 15 years. Older and many of the younger inhabitants are usually immune and escape DHF. However, cases in infants as young as 2 months and in young adults have been reported. DHF is usually associated with secondary dengue infection but can appear during a primary infection, especially in infants under the age of 1 year, all of whom possess maternal IgG dengue antibody.[10,23]

A seasonal incidence pattern usually coincides with the rainy season in many countries in tropical zones.

PREVENTION AND CONTROL

The control of dengue depends on control of the vector, particularly *Ae. aegypti*, an anthropophilic domestic mosquito which lives intimately with its human host(s). These mosquitoes breed primarily in man-made containers such as those used for water storage, flower vases, old jars, tin cans and used tyres in and around human dwellings. Elimination of these breeding sites is an effective and definitive method of controlling the vector and preventing dengue transmission. The use of larvicides and insecticides during the outbreaks has some limitations. Efforts are now focusing on health education and community participation in an attempt to control the vector(s) by eliminating or reducing the breeding sites.

There is no dengue vaccine available for public health use at present. Research is in progress to develop an effective and safe tetravalent dengue vaccine. Recently, a live attenuated tetravalent dengue vaccine prepared by serial passages through primary dog kidney cells has been developed and is currently undergoing phase 2 studies in children.[28] In the absence of a dengue vaccine for public health use at present, prevention and containment of dengue outbreaks will require an effective long-term vector control and aggressive epidemiological surveillance.

REFERENCES

1 World Health Organization. *Dengue Hemorrhagic Fever: Diagnosis, Treatment and Control*. Geneva: WHO, 1986.

2 Gubler D I. Dengue. In Monath T P. (ed.) *The Arboviruses: Epidemiology and Ecology*. Boca Raton: CRC Press, 1988: 223–260.

3 Henchal E A & Putrak J R. The dengue viruses. *Clin Microbiol Rev* 1990; 3:376–396.

4 Trent D W, Grant J A, Rosen L & Monath T P. Genetic variation among dengue 2 virus of different geographic areas. *Virology* 1983; 128:271.

5 Kerschner J H, Vorndam A V, Monath T P & Trent D W. Genetic and epidemiologic studies of dengue type 2 virus by hybridization using synthetic deoxyoligonucleotides as probe. *J Gen Virol* 1986; 67:2645.

6 Marchette N J, Halstead S B, Falker W A Jr, Stenhouse A & Nash D. Studies on the pathogenesis of dengue infection in monkeys III: sequential distribution of virus in primary and heterologous infections. *J Infect Dis* 1973; 128:28–30.

7 Sabin A B. Dengue. In Rivers T M & Horsfall F L (eds) *Viral and Rickettsial Infections of Man*. Philadelphia: Lippincott, 1959: 361–373.

8 Winter P E, Nantapanich S & Nisalak A. Recurrence of epidemic dengue hemorrhagic fever in an insular setting. *Am J Trop Med Hyg* 1969; 18:573–579.

9 Schlesinger R W. *Dengue Viruses*. New York: Springer, 1977: 90–91.

10 Halstead S B. The pathogenesis of dengue: the Alexander D Langmuir Lecture. *Am J Trop Med Hyg* 1981; 114:632–648.

11 Nimmannitya S, Thisyakon U & Hemserchart V. Dengue hemorrhagic fever with unusual manifestation. *Southeast Asian J Trop Med Public Health* 1987; 18:398–406.

12 Hoke C H, Nimmannitya S, Nisalak A & Burke D S. Studies on dengue hemorrrhagic fever at Bangkok Childrens Hospital 1962–1984. Pang T & Pathmanathan R (eds). *Proc Int Conf Dengue/DHF.* University of Malaysia Press, 1984.

13 Sangkawibha N, Rojanasuphots S, Ahandrik S et al. Risk factors in dengue shock syndrome: a prospective epidemiological study in Rayong, Thailand. *Am J Epidemiol* 1984; 120:653–669.

14 Rosen L. The Emperor's New Clothes revisited, or reflections on the pathogenesis of dengue hemorrhagic fever. *Am J Trop Med Hyg* 1977; 26:337–343.

15 Chiewsilp P, Scott R M, Bhamarapravati N et al. Histocompatibility antigens and dengue hemorrhagic fever. *Am J Trop Med Hyg* 1981; 30:1100–1105.

16 Guzman M G, Kouri G P, Bravo J, Soler M, Vazquez S & Morier L. Dengue hemorrhagic fever in Cuba, 1981; a retrospective seroepidemiologic study. *Am J Trop Med Hyg* 1990; 42:179–184.

17 Bhamarapravati N, Tuchinda P & Boonyapaknavik V. Pathology of Thai haemorrhagic fever: a study of 100 autopsy cases. *Ann Trop Med Parasitol* 1967; 61:500–510.

18 Bhamarapravati N. Hemostatic defects in dengue hemorrhagic fever. *Rev Infect Dis* 1989; 11(suppl): 826–829.

19 Malasit P. Complement and dengue hemorrhagic fever/shock syndrome. *Southeast Asian J Trop Med Public Health* 1987; 18:316–320.

20 Klick S C, Nimmannitya S, Nisalak A & Burke D S. Evidence that maternal dengue antibodies are important in the development of dengue hemorrhagic fever in infants. *Am J Trop Med Hyg* 1988; 38:411–419.

21 Kurane I, Innis B L, Nimmannitya S et al. Activation of T lymphocytes in dengue virus infections: high levels of soluble interleukin 2 receptor, soluble CD4, soluble CD8, interleukin 2, and interferon γ in sera of children with dengue. *J Clin Invest* 1991; 88:1473–1480.

22 Nimmannitya S, Kalayanarooj S, Nisalak A & Innis B L. Second attack of dengue hemorrhagic fever. *Proceedings of the International Symposium on dengue and DHF.* 1–3 October 1990, Bangkok.

23 Nimmannitya S, Halstead S B, Cohen S N & Margiotta M R. Dengue and chikungunya virus infection in man in Thailand 1962–1964. *Am J Trop Med Hyg* 1969; 18:954–971.

24 Innis B L, Nisalak A, Nimmannitya S et al. An enzyme linked immunosorbent assay to characterize dengue infections where dengue and Japanese encephalitis co-circulate. *Am J Trop Med Hyg* 1989; 40:418–427.

25 Sumarmo M D, Talogo W, Asrin A, Isnuhandojo B & Sahudi A. Failure of hydrocortisone to affect outcome in dengue shock syndrome. *Pediatrics* 1982; 69:45–49.

26 Nimmannitya S. Clinical spectrum and management of dengue hemorrhagic fever. *Southeast Asian J Trop Med Public Health* 1987; 18:392–397.

27 Dengue Newsletter. Vol 17, WHO, 1992.

28 Bhamarapravati, N. Dengue vaccine Development. In Thongcharoen, P (ed.) *Monograph on Dengue/ Dengue Hemorrhagic Fever*, WHO/SEARO No. 22. New Delhi, 1993.

CHAPTER 35

DIARRHOEA CAUSED BY VIRUSES

C. A. Hart

Enteropathogenic viruses and in particular rotaviruses are a major cause of infantile diarrhoea (see also Chapter 40). All affect the upper small intestine and produce a non-inflammatory diarrhoea. The relative importance of each is shown in Table 35.1.

ROTAVIRUS

Rotavirus (HRV) was first described as a human pathogen in 1973 on thin-section electron microscopy of duodenal biopsies. The same investigators subsequently demonstrated that the virus was shed in large numbers in faeces and could be detected by direct negative-stain electron microscopy.[1]

GEOGRAPHICAL DISTRIBUTION

Rotavirus infection is found as frequently in developed as in developing countries. It is, however, more likely to produce life-threatening diarrhoea in developing countries.[2]

Table 35.1 Relative importance of the various viral enteropathogens in children.*

Pathogen	No of cases	(%)†
Rotavirus	342	(35)
Adenovirus	78	(8)
Astrovirus	98	(10)
Calicivirus	59	(6)
Small round structureless virus (including Norwalk agent)	59	(6)
Coronavirus	2	(0.2)
Breda virus	1	(0.1)
Mixed‡	20	2

*Data from 980 cases of infantile diarrhoea at Alder Hey Children's Hospital, Liverpool over 2 years.
†Percentage of cases of diarrhoea.
‡Mixed viral or viral and bacterial diarrhoea.

EPIDEMIOLOGY

HRV is the major cause of infantile gastroenteritis. In hospital-based surveys it is found to be responsible for 25–65% of cases and in community-based surveys from 5 to 15% of cases. The peak of infection in most parts of the world occurs from 4 months to 3 years of age, although most will have been infected by 2 years. Adults can be infected and epidemics of infection can occur when antigenically different strains of rotavirus emerge.[3]

In temperate countries infections peak in the winter months, with low numbers of cases at other times. In tropical countries, although more cases of infection occur in cooler drier months, infection is highly prevalent throughout the year.[4]

VIROLOGY

Rotavirus is one of the six genera of the family Reoviridae. It has a double-shelled capsid and is approximately 70nm in diameter, with a characteristic wheel-like (L. *rota* wheel) morphology (Figure 35.1). It has an 11-segmented double-stranded RNA (dsRNA) genome and each segment encodes a single polypeptide (Table 35.2). The functions have been ascribed to some of the virus proteins (VPs). VP6 is the major inner capsid protein comprising 80% of its mass and carries the major group and subgroup antigens. VP4 is a haemagglutinin and

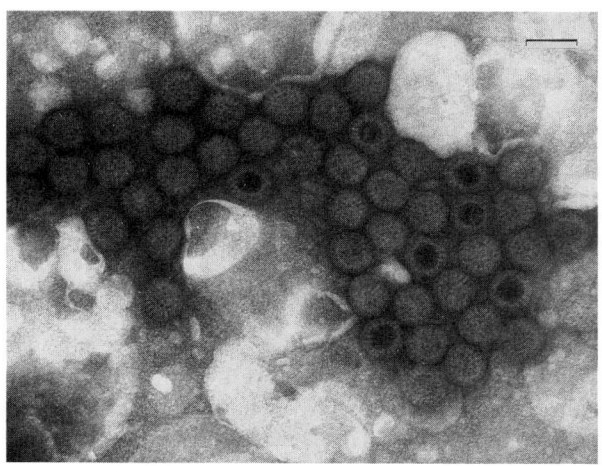

Figure 35.1 Negative-stain electron micrograph of rotavirus in faeces. (Bar = 1 μm.)

presumably mediates attachment of the virus to enterocytes. VP4 is cleaved by intestinal trypsin to produce VP5 and VP8 which are necessary for enhanced infectivity. Rotavirus can be grown in tissue culture but requires trypsin to be present in the culture medium.

Rotaviruses are classified into group, subgroup and serotype. Group (A–G) and subgroup specificities are located on VP6. Group A encompasses most of the rotaviruses infecting man. There are two major subgroups of A (I and II) as determined by enzyme linked immunosorbent assay (ELISA). Serotype specificity is determined by neutralization assays or PCR and 11 serotypes have been delineated according to epitopes on VP7. Most human infections are due to serotypes 1–4.[5] Group B rotaviruses are found in rats and pigs but also cause large outbreaks in children and adults.[3] Group C rotaviruses cause occasional human outbreaks, and groups D and E are associated with birds and pigs. Rotaviruses can also be subdivided into two main patterns (long and short) and a large number of lesser variants according to the mobility of their dsRNA segments (Figure 35.2). However, genotypes and serotypes come and go with perplexing rapidity.[6]

PATHOGENESIS

Rotavirus is excreted in large amounts (up to 10^{11} particles/ml) in the faeces of infected individuals. Although person-to-person faecal–oral transmission is the most likely route it is possible that the respiratory route may also be taken. In addition water-borne outbreaks do occur. The infective dose for rotavirus is low (10^2–10^4 particles), and the incubation period usually 1–3 days. Most of the information on the replication of rotavirus is derived by analogy from animal infection.

The enterocyte receptor for rotavirus appears to be acetylated sialic acid.[7] Rotavirus infects the villous enterocytes of the small intestine, with no evidence of infection of the stomach or colon. Within 12–24 hours of infection levels of brush-border enzymes (disaccharidases) are markedly depressed with no evidence of structural damage to the brushs border or enterocyte.[8] Subsequently the infected enterocytes die, resulting in blunting of the

Table 35.2 Genes and polypeptides of rotavirus.

RNA segment	MW ($\times 10^6$)	Gene product	MW ($\times 10^5$)	Location	Function
1	2.2	VP1	125	Inner capsid	?
2	1.68	VP2	94	Inner capsid	?
3	1.60	—	—	—	—
4	1.60	VP4	88	Outer capsid	Haemagglutinin, cleaved to VP5 and VP8 for infectivity by trypsin
5	0.98	NS53	53	Non-structural	?
6	0.81	VP6	41	Inner capsid	Group and subgroup specific antigens
7	0.5	NS34	34	Non-structural	?
8	0.5	NS35	35	Non-structural	?
9	0.5	VP7	34	Outer capsid	Glycoprotein, major neutralization antigen
10	0.3	NS29	29	Non-structural	Role in capsid assembly
11	0.2	VP9	26	Outer capsid	?

VP, virus protein; NS, non-structural.

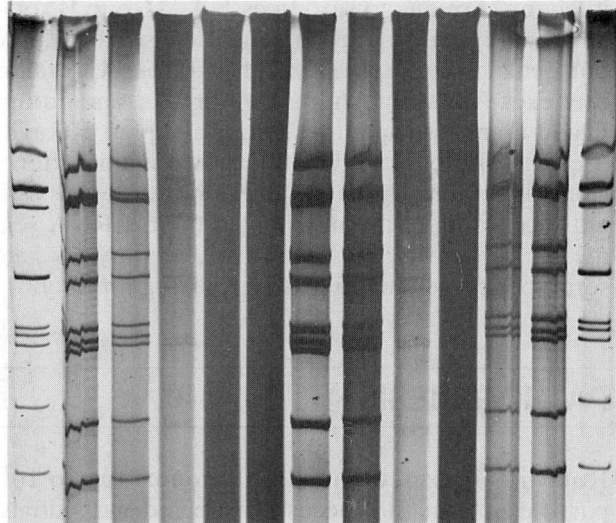

Figure 35.2 Polyacrylamide gel electrophoresis of rotavirus RNA from faeces showing 11 double-stranded segments of RNA.

villi. The virus cannot infect the immature villous crypt cells and this limits the infection.

IMMUNITY

The role of the various arms of the immune system in immunity to rotavirus infection are incompletely understood. Infection with rotavirus elicits both serum and mucosal antibody production.[9,10] IgM anti-HRV first appears in the 8–12-month age group and prevalence is high thereafter. The percentage of sera containing neutralizing antibodies to only one HRV serotype is high in young infants (8–12 months) but with age, activity against multiple serotypes occurs, indicating sequential infection with different serotypes.[11] The role of such antibodies is unclear. In challenge experiments only serum IgG but not serum neutralizing antibody correlated with protection from infection and only jejunal neutralizing antibody and not serum IgG was associated with protection from clinical infection.[9] The role of cell-mediated immunity in rotavirus infection is even less clear.

Human breast milk contains both HRV antibodies and trypsin inhibitors which protect against infection.[12] However, HRV infection in neonates rarely produces diarrhoea (10–20% of infections). Interestingly, neonatal HRV infection produces immunity to subsequent HRV gastroenteritis.[13] Neonatal rotavirus isolates have recently been shown to have similarities in the sequence of dsRNA segment 4 which encodes VP4[14] and which is different from infant isolates. VP4 must be cleaved by trypsin to produce a fully virulent virus and it is possible that the neonatal HRV VP4 is less susceptible to trypsin digestion.

CLINICAL FEATURES

HRV infection can vary from mild short-lived watery diarrhoea to an overwhelming gastroenteritis with dehydration, leading to death. The latter presentation is more common in children who are already malnourished or have measles. Vomiting is often part of HRV gastroenteritis and usually precedes diarrhoea. Infantile gastroenteritis due to HRV tends to be more severe than that due to other enteropathogens.[15] Respiratory tract signs are often noted during HRV gastroenteritis but the role of HRV in this is unclear since the virus has not been demonstrated in the respiratory mucosa. Infection at other sites has been described but is extremely rare. For example HRV has been detected in an hepatic abscess and in a child with a ventriculoperitoneal shunt infection.

It is not possible to distinguish HRV gastroenteritis from other viral causes or other noninflammatory diarrhoeas on clinical grounds. The stools are usually pale and watery or loose and are said to have a characteristic milky odour. In hospitalized patients the duration of diarrhoea is from 2 to 23 with a mean of 6 days. Patients continue to excrete virus for extended periods of time[16] and may thus be a reservoir for infecting others.

Dehydration, which can be hyponatraemic or hypernatraemic, is often associated with a metabolic acidosis.

DIAGNOSIS

Rotavirus was first discovered using negative-stain electron microscopy of faeces.[1] This is still a valuable diagnostic tool since it is a 'catch all' technique that will also detect other potential viral enteropathogens. However, the equipment is expensive to buy and maintain and requires a skilled operator. A variety of simpler, cheaper diagnostic tests are available which will only detect rotavirus.

Antigen detection tests include ELISA and latex particle agglutination (LPA).[17] The sensitivity and specificity of these tests is generally high (90–95%) but can be relatively costly. LPA is useful for a 'one off' test and ELISA for batches of samples. Surprisingly, rotavirus can also be detected by polyacrylamide gel electrophoresis of RNA extracted directly from faeces (Figure 35.2). This technique is relatively simple with good specificity (100%) and sensitivity (80–90%), and can be performed in tropical countries relatively cheaply.[17,18] It has the added advantage of providing epidemiological information because the electrophoretic pattern of the 11 dsRNA segments varies between HRV strains. Detection of viral genome by the reverse transcriptase polymerase chain reaction is a research tool which provides information on the epidemiology and duration of shedding of HRV.[5,16]

Although HRV can be cultured this is not a useful diagnostic test. Similarly, antibody detection can be undertaken but this is of little value diagnostically.

In addition to the specific diagnostic tests, measurement of serum electrolytes, urea and bicarbonate will help greatly in the management of dehydration.

TREATMENT

The mainstay of management is assessment and replacement of fluid loss. In the majority of cases this can be accomplished using oral rehydration therapy. The major limiting factors are severe dehydration with shock or the high rate of vomiting that can occur early in HRV infection. In such circumstances intravenous rehydration will be needed.

There is no specific antiviral chemotherapy for rotavirus but human or bovine colostrum and hyperimmune serum immunoglobulin have been used to manage chronic rotavirus infection.

PREVENTION AND CONTROL

Rotavirus infection is highly prevalent in both developed and developing countries so it would seem unlikely that improving public and family hygiene could prevent infection. The infective dose of HRV is low (approximately 10^2 particles) and infected individuals excrete virus in massive quantities (approximately 10^{11} particles).

To prevent HRV infection by immunization would be a major advance. A variety of live attenuated vaccines have been developed, including animal (bovine and simian) rotaviruses, reassortant strains and temperature-sensitive HRV mutants.[15,18] Although most vaccines provide some protection, none is completely effective and nonreactive. The use of 'neonatal strains' to immunize neonates is being evaluated.[13,14,18]

ADENOVIRUS

Adenoviruses are unenveloped DNA viruses of from 60 to 90 nm in diameter. Although several different adenoviruses are excreted in faeces it is only adenoviruses types 40 and 41 that cause diarrhoea. These are only artificially cultivable in the presence of rotaviruses or deficient adenoviruses. The incubation period is longer (8–10 days) than for other viral pathogens.

Enteric adenoviruses appear to be associated with 4–8% of cases of infantile gastroenteritis, although in one survey in Thailand they were associated with only 2.6%.[19]

The clinical features associated with adenovirus 40/41 do not differ from those due to other viral enteropathogens.

Specific diagnosis is either by immunoelectron microscopy or by ELISA.[20] There is no vaccine for prevention of infection.

ASTROVIRUS

Astroviruses are small (about 28 nm) unenveloped RNA viruses with a characteristic five or six-pointed star 'stamped' on their surface (Figure 35.3). In most surveys they are the second most common viral cause of gastroenteritis in young children. In temperate countries infection tends to peak in winter months. There is no information on seasonal variation in the tropics. In Thailand astroviruses were responsible for almost 9% of cases of infantile diarrhoea[19] and were second only to rotavirus (19% of cases). Astrovirus has also been described as a cause of infantile diarrhoea in Malawi.[21] The gastroenteritis caused by astrovirus is similar to that due to other viruses but rotavirus is more likely to cause dehy-dration.[19] Diagnosis is by electron microscopy or ELISA.[19]

CALICIVIRUS

Caliciviruses are small (38nm) non-enveloped RNA viruses with cup-shaped (Gk *kalux* cup) depressions around their periphery (Figure 35.4). Calicivirus is a less frequent (3.6%) cause of infantile gastroenteri-tis. Serological evidence of calicivirus infection has been found in South-East Asia and Africa.[22,23] Diagnosis is by electron microscopy or ELISA.[24]

NORWALK AGENT

The agent of 'winter-vomiting disease' is a small (32nm) unenveloped RNA virus, named after the town in the USA where it was first described. It is closely related to calicivirus. Serological surveys have shown that most children in developing countries such as Ecuador or Bangladesh have acquired antibody by 5 years of age and acquisition of antibody is usually related to an episode of diar-rhoea.[25] Vomiting is a major feature of infection.

Virus tends to be excreted in large amounts only during the first or second days of infection; thus the value of electron microscopy in specific diagnosis is limited. Antigen detection by ELISA is a useful alternative.[26]

OTHER VIRUSES

A variety of other viruses including small round structureless viruses, coronaviruses, Breda viruses or picobirnaviruses have been associated with a minority of cases of gastroenteritis in developed countries. Their role in tropical countries is un-known.

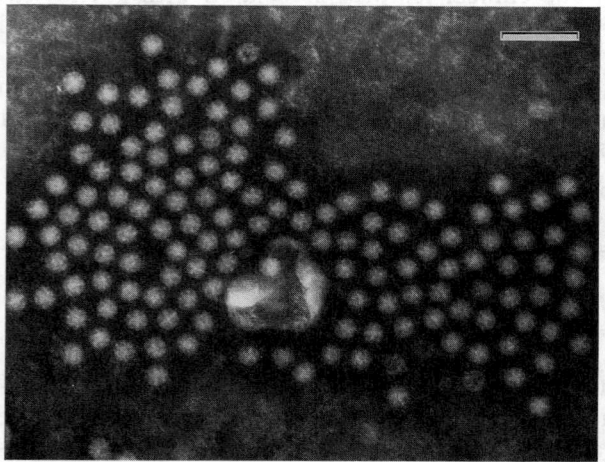

Figure 35.3   Negative-stain electron micrograph of astrovirus. (Bar = 1 μm.)

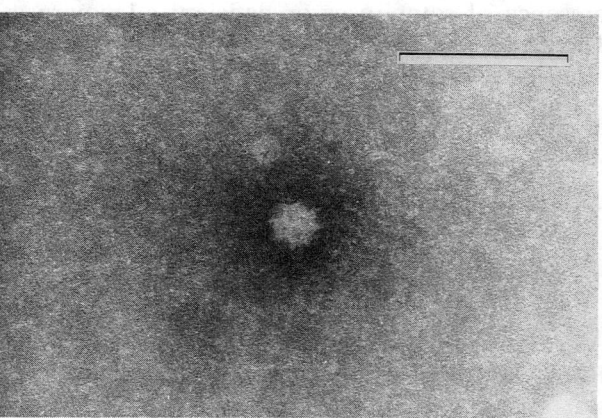

Figure 35.4   Negative-stain electron micrograph of calicivirus. (Bar = 1 μm.)

REFERENCES

1 Bishop R F, Davidson G P, Holmes I H & Ruck B J. Detection of a new virus by electronmicroscopy of faecal extracts from children with acute gastroenteritis. *Lancet* 1974; i:149–151.

2 Hart C A & Ibrahim O S. Rotavirus and gastroenteritis. *Postgrad Doct* 1989; 12:252–260.

3 Hung T, Chen G, Zhaoying F et al. Waterborne outbreak of rotavirus diarrhoea in adults in China caused by a novel rotavirus. *Lancet* 1984; i:1139–1142.

4 Bingnan F, Unicomb L, Rahim Z et al. Rotavirus-associated diarrhoea in rural Bangladesh: two year study of incidence and serotype distribution. *J Clin Microbiol* 1991; 29:1359–1363.

5 Tabassum S, Shears P & Hart C A. Genomic characterization of rotavirus strains obtained from hospitalized children with diarrhoea in Bangladesh. *J Med Virol* 1994; 43:50–56.

6 Editorial. Puzzling diversity of rotavirus. *Lancet* 1990; 335:573–575.

7 Willoughby R E & Yolken R H. SA11 rotavirus is specifically inhibited by an acetylated sialic acid. *J Infect Dis* 1990; 161:116–119.

8 Batt R M, Embaye H, Van der Waal S, Burgess D, Edwards G B & Hart C A. Application of organ culture of small intestine to the investigation of enterocyte damage by equine rotavirus infection in foals. *J Ped Gastroenterol Nutr* 1995; 20: 326–332.

9 Ward R C, Bernstein D I, Shukla R et al. Effects of antibody to rotavirus on protection of adults challenged with a human rotavirus. *J Infect Dis* 1989; 159:79–88.

10 Aiyar J, Bhan M K, Bhandari N, Kumar R, Raj P & Sazawal S. Rotavirus-specific antibody response in saliva of infants with rotavirus diarrhoea. *J Infect Dis* 1990; 162:1383–1384.

11 Brussow H, Werchan H, Liedtke W et al. Prevalence of antibodies to rotavirus in different age groups of infants in Bochum, West Germany. *J Infect Dis* 1988; 157:1014–1022.

12 Jayashree S, Bhan M K, Kumar R et al. Protection against neonatal rotavirus infection by breast milk antibodies and trypsin inhibitors. *J Med Virol* 1988; 26:333–338.

13 Bishop R F, Barnes G L, Cipriani F & Lund J J. Clinical immunity after neonatal rotavirus infection. *N Engl J Med* 1983; 309:72–76.

14 Flores J, Midthun K, Hoshino Y et al. Conservation of the fourth gene among rotaviruses recovered from asymptomatic newborn infants and its possible role in attenuation. *J Virol* 1986; 60:972–979.

15 Perez-Schael I, Garcia D, Gonzalez M et al. Prospective study of diarrhoeal diseases in Venezuelan children to evaluate the efficacy of rhesus rotavirus vaccine. *J Med Virol* 1990; 30:219–229.

16 Wilde J, Yolken R, Willoughby R & Eiden J. Improved detection of rotavirus shedding by polymerase chain reaction. *Lancet* 1991; 337:323–326.

17 Ibrahim O S, Sunderland D & Hart C A. Comparison of four methods for detection of rotavirus in faeces. *Trop Doct* 1990; 20:30–32.

18 Kapikian A Z, Flores J, Hoshino Y et al. Prospects for development of a rotavirus vaccine against rotavirus diarrhea in infants and young children. *Rev Infect Dis* 1989; 11(supplement 3):S539–S546.

19 Herrmann J E, Taylor D N, Escheverria P & Blacklow N R. Astroviruses as a cause of gastroenteritis in children. *N Engl J Med* 1991; 324:1757–1760.

20 Wood D J, Bijlsma K, de Jong J C & Tonkin C. Evaluation of a commercial monoclonal antibody-based enzyme immunoassay for detection of adenovirus types 40 and 41 in stool specimens. *J Clin Microbiol* 1989; 27:1155–1158.

21 Pavone R, Schinaia N, Hart C A, Getty B, Molyneux M & Borgstein A. Viral gastroenteritis in children in Malawi. *Ann Trop Paediatr* 1990; 10:15–20.

22 Nakata S, Chiba S, Terashima H & Nakao T. Prevalence of antibody to human calicivirus in Japan and South-East Asia determined by radio-immunoassay. *J Clin Microbiol* 1985; 22:519–521.

23 Cubitt W D & McSwiggan D A. Seroepidemiological survey of the prevalence of antibodies to a strain of human calicivirus. *J Med Virol* 1987; 21:361–368.

24 Nakata S, Estes M K & Chiba S. Detection of human calicivirus antigen and antibody by enzyme-linked immunosorbent assay. *J Clin Microbiol* 1988; 26:2001–2005.

25 Blacklow N R, Herrmann J E & Cubitt W D. Immunobiology of Norwalk virus. *Ciba Found Symp* 1987; 128:144–161.

26 Herrmann J E, Nowak N A & Blacklow N R. Detection of Norwalk virus in stools by enzyme-immunoassay. *J Med Virol* 1985; 17:127–133.

CHAPTER 36

RESPIRATORY VIRUSES

C. R. Madeley and J. S. M. Peiris

No individual can survive without a functioning respiratory tract. It is frequently invaded by infective agents of all kinds, including viruses, bacteria and other agents. The consequences depend not only on the particular agent but also on the individual patient. Pre-existing impairment of the tract by congenital malformations or damage from previous episodes of infection, as well as the circumstances of the individual as a whole (malnutrition, poverty, overcrowding, sanitation, etc.), will profoundly affect the outcome. This chapter primarily concerns viruses but other micro-organisms may be involved, alone or in combination. The respiratory tract may also be involved in part of a more extensive disease process which may itself be due to a virus. Infection of one part of the respiratory tract should therefore not be seen in isolation; the wider implications must be considered.

Acute respiratory infections are estimated to cause 4.5 million childhood deaths annually. The overwhelming majority occur in developing countries and they account for one-third of all deaths in childhood. Bacterial infections in general have a higher case fatality than acute viral infections, but viruses are far more common causes of acute respiratory infection. Overall they contribute to at least one-third of the deaths caused by acute respiratory infection in the developing world.

CLINICAL PICTURE (See also Chapter 4)

The respiratory tract can be divided into an upper and a lower part, with the boundary at the lower end of the larynx. Viral infections confined to the upper part (upper respiratory tract infection, URTI) are rarely life threatening, with the exception of croup in the tropics. They can be uncomfortable but do not usually call the individual's future into question. Such infections do not automatically spread to the lower respiratory tract, but where the lower respiratory tract is involved the process is extensive and rarely confined to one lobe or even one lung. This is in contrast to pneumococcal pneumonia which is typically confined to one lobe of one lung. Although widespread, the process of viral infection is usually less intense than that seen in bacterial pneumoni; otherwise such infections would be much more lethal. The most common manifestations of a lower respiratory tract infection (LRTI) are bronchiolitis (in infants) or an atypical pneumonia. When an LRTI occurs, the upper tract is also involved and the causative virus can usually be isolated from it. The main exception is cytomegalovirus pneumonitis in the immunocompromised patient, where the virus may not be readily recovered from the upper respiratory tract.

There are no clear-cut differences between the clinical presentation(s) of any viruses in the respiratory tract. For example, although respiratory syncytial virus (RSV) is the most common cause of bronchiolitis worldwide, this clinical condition may be caused by parainfluenzaviruses, influenzaviruses, adenoviruses or rhinoviruses. Consequently, it is unsafe to assume that two patients with similar clinical illnesses will be infected by the same virus. This is particularly so in babies and young children.

THE VIRUSES

Table 36.1 lists those viruses generally associated with the respiratory tract. Nevertheless, other viruses may be present as part of a generalized process in which the respiratory component is only a (small) part.

Table 36.1 is divided into two sections. Section A lists those viruses usually associated with respiratory tract disease. Identifying their presence will usually confirm the cause of the illness, although dual and even triple infections occasionally occur, particularly in the compromised host. They are listed in approximately descending order of importance in terms of numbers of cases annually and potential severity. By almost any criterion RSV would head the list but the others could be ranked in various order, depending on the age, time of year and geographic location of the population. This is discussed further under Epidemiology, below.

Section B lists three viruses which may be found in the respiratory tract of clinically normal individuals. Herpes simplex virus may cause no overt lesions in the respiratory tract, although its presence indicates a potential to cause damage if the opportunity occurs—particularly in compromised patients. Enteroviruses and reoviruses are not proven pathogens in the respiratory tract, although the former are frequently isolated from the throats of children.

Important features of each virus are discussed below.

RESPIRATORY SYNCYTIAL VIRUS

This virus is distributed worldwide and is found wherever it has been sought. It is frequently associated with bronchiolitis in babies under 2 years of age—with a peak incidence at about 6 months—and

Table 36.1 Viruses infecting the respiratory tract.

Virus	No. of serotypes	Group antigen?	Common disease presentation[a]
A. Usually pathogenic in the respiratory tract			
RSV	1 (2 subtypes: A and B)	Yes[b]	Bronchiolitis in <2 years (also URTI, failure to thrive, febrile fits)
Influenza A	Genetically unstable→ sequential variants[c]	Yes	URTI, influenza
Influenza B	Genetically unstable→ sequential variants[c]	Yes	URTI, influenza, may include abdominal pain
Parainfluenza	1–4a,b	No	URTI, croup, bronchiolitis
Adenovirus	47[d]	Yes	URTI, acute respiratory disease
Rhinovirus	>100	No	URTI ('common cold')
Coronavirus	Several[e]	No	URTI ('common cold')
Epstein–Barr virus	1	Yes[b]	Glandular fever
Cytomegalovirus	1	Yes[b]	Various (in the immunocompromised only)[f]
Measles	1	Yes[b]	Measles[g]
B. May be recovered from the respiratory tract but role in respiratory disease uncertain			
Herpes simplex (hominis)	1	Yes[b]	—[h]
Enteroviruses	68	No	—
Reovirus	3	No	—[i]

[a] Although this column lists the more common presentations, there is considerable overlap in clinical signs and symptoms between respiratory viruses.
[b] There is only one serotype. This is used as a group antigen for diagnostic purposes.
[c] The RNA of influenza A and B viruses is constantly undergoing mutation which is reflected antigenically, causing 'drift' in both influenza A and B and 'shift' in influenza A.
[d] Most respiratory infections are due to types 1–7.
[e] The total is not known.
[f] Usually no overt illness in the immunocompetent, except congenital damage and for some examples of glandular fever.
[g] Rash may be absent in the immunocompromised.
[h] Causes stomatitis and may be a cause of pneumonitis in compromised patients.
[i] No identified disease in man.

is the most common virus detected, especially in children under 1 year of age (see below). Large epidemics occur annually at the same season. The starting date and extent of the epidemic may vary a little but the annual epidemic can be relied on. For diagnostic purposes there is only one serotype. Two subtypes (A and B) have been described but distinguishing them requires the use of appropriate monoclonal antibodies.

INFLUENZA A AND B VIRUSES

Genetically, these are the most unstable respiratory viruses. Both exhibit antigenic *drift*, in which the surface antigens of the virus change gradually in the face of immunological pressure from the host species. One or two variants predominate at a given time. In this evolving change, they are unique among respiratory viruses. Influenza A also shows occasional major antigenic *shift* changes as a result of genetic reassortment with animal strains, effectively making a completely new virus. The time, extent and direction of *drift* or *shift* have so far been completely unpredictable. However, when viruses with antigenic shift appear in the human population, a worldwide pandemic of influenza A is a possibility, with memorable examples in 1918 ('Spanish flu') and 1957 ('Asian flu'). With no animal reservoirs to provide new strains, shift does not occur in influenza B.

PARAINFLUENZAVIRUS

There are four serotypes of parainfluenza; type 4 possesses two subtypes 4a and 4b. Types 1 and 2 typically cause croup, a high-pitched barking cough in children which is profoundly irritating to their parents. Type 3 can cause bronchiolitis or pneumonia and, less often, croup. In temperate countries types 1 and 2 (together with RSV) are more prevalent in the winter months, whereas type 3 is unusual (amongst respiratory viruses) in occurring more often in spring and early summer. This dissociation between the peaks of activity of parainfluenza type 3 and RSV has also been observed in tropical regions.[1,2]

ADENOVIRUS

There are 47 different serotypes but the majority of respiratory infections involve types 1–7. Types 1, 2,

5 and 6 are usually associated with endemic disease in temperate regions, and types 3, 4 and 7 with epidemics. The higher-numbered serotypes appear in the respiratory tract from time to time but a considerable proportion of them have been found only in the gut.

Adenoviruses are unusual in that prolonged carriage (up to 2 years in some cases) may occur in the tonsils of children, often with no continuing illness. The clinical significance of adenoviruses isolated from the throat of children must therefore be interpreted cautiously. However, they may cause a primary and severe pneumonia in debilitated children, in whom it may be rapidly fatal.

RHINOVIRUS

These are frequent causes of the common cold, itself a common winter and summer illness in temperate countries. Information on the seasonality of rhinoviruses in the tropics is scanty. They can be difficult to grow in culture (the only practical way to diagnose infection) and are very underreported, mainly because diagnosis is not attempted. Although the infection is usually uncomfortable, it is not severe. Nevertheless, rhinoviruses have occasionally been the sole pathogens present in the lungs of immunocompromised patients dying with respiratory signs and symptoms.

CORONAVIRUS

These viruses are the second main cause of the common cold. Little is known about them, other than their existence and that there may be over 30 serotypes. They require specialist techniques for diagnosis that are not widely available, and most laboratories (even in research studies) do not attempt to document their role.

MEASLES (See also Chapters 15 and 37)

Measles is often not recognized as a major cause of LRTI morbidity or mortality, and there are a number of factors that may contribute to this underassessment of the true disease burden.[3] Children with measles may not always be admitted to a general paediatric ward, the aetiology may be attributed to a superinfecting pathogen rather than to measles, and some patients with measles (especially when immunocompromised as a result of malnutrition, cytotoxic drug treatment or for other reasons) will fail to develop the typical rash. In patients who do not manifest typical clinical features, laboratory diagnosis of measles is difficult, even in the developed world, because the virus is not isolated readily and good antisera for reliable immunofluorescence are not commercially available. Where the diagnosis has been actively sought in developing countries, measles is found to be a major cause of LRTI, accounting for 6–21% of morbidity and 8–50% of the mortality attributed to LRTI. The effects of the virus on the respiratory tract can be direct (giant cell pneumonitis) or indirect. The latter includes the depressive effects of the virus on the host immune system, stores of vitamin A and overall nutritional status. All of these can lead to an increased risk of superinfection with other viral or bacterial pathogens.

CYTOMEGALOVIRUS

This is an opportunist pathogen in immunocompromised patients, in whom it can cause respiratory complications. Perinatal cytomegalovirus infection may occasionally present as pneumonitis in the newborn and (together with chlamydiae) must be considered in the differential diagnosis.

Apart than such occasional illnesses most cytomegalovirus infections are clinically silent, although serological surveys have shown positivity rates approaching 100% in some overcrowded populations.

OTHER AGENTS

The diagnosis of several other agents has been undertaken in virus laboratories because these agents cause respiratory infections which overlap clinically with those due to viruses, and they are diagnosed serologically (see below). They include psittacosis, Q fever and mycoplasmosis, and isolation of the causative organism is either difficult or dangerous. They also include *Chlamydia pneumoniae* (TWAR), which is now becoming recognized as a cause of community-acquired pneumonia although there is currently no widely available diagnostic test.

The activities of these agents are underdocumented in most parts of the world. Since they are amenable to antibiotic therapy, it is important that they are diagnosed.

EPIDEMIOLOGY

The aetiology and epidemiology of acute respiratory infections have been intensively studied in the temperate areas of the world. Information from tropical regions is more scanty, but what evidence there is does not suggest major differences in the epidemiological patterns.[4-8] Although there are a large number of viruses indigenous to the tropics (most notably a large number of insect-transmitted viruses), there is no evidence that they contribute significantly to respiratory tract disease. The viruses responsible for respiratory disease in the tropics are no different from those found in temperate countries. However, the severity of illness and its consequences may be markedly different in the developing world.

Even where high-quality, competent diagnostic services are available, not every clinical respiratory disease yields unequivocal evidence of infection by a virus or other micro-organism. The proportion in whom a positive diagnosis is made varies from a quarter to a half, depending on laboratory, area, population and time of year.

In temperate regions, respiratory infections have generally been shown to increase in the autumn and winter, although the exact mechanisms are unknown. Similar periodicity is shown in tropical regions but this may be related to fluctuations of rainfall rather than temperature. It is not clear how these variations in climatic conditions translate into changes in virus activity.

The data on respiratory infections obtained by Jacob John and his colleagues[2] in Vellore, India, and shown in Tables 36.2 and 36.3, confirm a pattern of activity familiar to workers elsewhere. RSV is the predominant virus in young children under 2 years of age and accounts for 163 out of 367 (44%) of the viruses detected. Parainfluenza type 3 was the second most common virus and, other than RSV, is probably more predictable in its epidemiology than any of the others listed. The activities of

Table 36.2 Frequency of virus detection, by age, in 809 subjects with acute respiratory infection.*

	No. of children of indicated age in whom virus was detected				
Virus	<1 year (*n* = 359)	1 year (*n* = 226)	2 years (*n* = 92)	3 years (*n* = 74)	≥4 years (*n* = 58)
RSV	108	32	16	6	1
Influenza A	6	3	2	4	1
Influenza B	3	2	3	2	4
Parainfluenza 1	9	7	4	3	2
Parainfluenza 2	1	4	0	2	0
Parainfluenza 3	29	18	7	4	4
Adenovirus	9	13	1	6	2
Other viruses positive†	23	10	12	3	1
Total no. (%)	177 (49)	79 (35)	42 (46)	29 (39)	15 (26)

*Reproduced with permission from Jacob John et al.[2]
†Two different viruses were isolated in 11, 10, 3 and 1 children of <1, 1, 2 and 3 years of age, respectively.

Table 36.3 Frequency of virus detection, by syndrome, in 331 children with lower respiratory tract infection (LRTI).*

Type of LRTI	No. of children	No. (%) positive for virus	No. in whom virus was detected:				
			RSV	Influenza	Parainfluenza	Adenovirus	Other†
Pneumonia	178	65 (37)	34	3	15	6	11
Bronchiolitis	116	83 (72)	67	1	13	4	3
Tracheobronchitis	14	7 (50)	2	1	2	2	0
Croup	8	4 (50)	0	0	5	0	1
Other†	15	4 (27)	3	0	1	0	0
Total	331	163 (49)	106	5	36	12	15

*Reproduced with permission from Jacob John et al.[2]
Two viruses were detected in four children with pneumonia, five with bronchiolitis, two with croup.
†Enterovirus (21 children), herpes simplex (13), measles virus (7), mumps virus(1), unidentified virus (7).
†Acute exacerbation of bronchial asthma (8), tropical pulmonary eosinophilia (2), tuberculosis (2), foreign body aspiration (2) and membranous tracheitis (1).

influenza A and B remain impossible to predict and can fluctuate greatly from year to year. The appearance of a 'new' strain of either A or B can be associated with an epidemic the size of which will be greater as the size of the antigenic change increases. With no shift changes in influenza B, major epidemics are less common.

HOSPITALIZED VERSUS COMMUNITY PATIENTS

Berman[9] has summarized the data from developing countries and found that the percentage of hospitalized patients who were virus positive was about twice the figure found in those attending as out-patients. This difference is not surprising and probably reflects both the greater opportunity to make a specific diagnosis in the hospitalized patient and the severity of their disease. The majority of trivial episodes (head colds and increased nasal secretions) are not subjected to virus diagnosis and the causative viruses are unconfirmed.

It could be argued that infections too trivial to require hospital admission can be mostly ignored—a dismissal even more appropriate for those remaining at home. This argument, however, is flawed for two reasons. First, human viruses are caught from other humans, although the severity varies. Hence most respiratory viral transmission occurs within the community. Second, patients may become too ill to attend a hospital, a situation exacerbated by other contributing factors such as poverty and lack of facilities.

OTHER FACTORS

As with most other diseases, respiratory infections are made worse by other components of the patient's environment. Poverty, malnutrition and overcrowding (common in urban environments everywhere in the world) are well recognized to contribute to the frequency and severity of respiratory illness. The effects may be direct or indirect through the presence of other disease, poor sanitation and poor personal hygiene (Figure 36.1).

Nevertheless, although a poor, malnourished child in a densely populated inner city slum will have many respiratory illnesses, viruses are no respecters of persons and his or her better-off cousin in a wealthy environment may also have a considerable number of infections. Where the difference lies is that the latter will cope with them better and have fewer longer-term sequelae. These will include: chronic respiratory impairment, wheezing, asthma, bronchitis and bronchiectasis.

LABORATORY DIAGNOSIS

There are three main reasons for providing a laboratory diagnosis of viral respiratory infections: to tell the clinician what is causing the illness (individual diagnosis); to monitor routine virus activity in the community (epidemiology); or to do a special investigation.

Individual diagnosis may help the clinician decide not to use antibiotics and very occasionally, in selected high-risk patients (see below), whether to use antiviral agents. In addition, control of hospital cross-infection is assisted by precise aetiological diagnoses. For example, patients with RSV can be cohorted and nursed away from other vulnerable patients. It is self-evident that individual diagnosis must be quick if it is to influence clinical management. Rapidity of diagnosis is also important in epidemiological studies because the clinician is likely to lose interest in sending specimens if there is not a rapid feed-back on the cause of the patient's illness. It is not surprising that the epidemiological data are patchy, but they can reflect year-by-year variations if the proportion of patients on whom studies are performed remains sufficiently constant.

Rapid viral diagnosis of respiratory infection is achievable (within 2–3 hours) using techniques such as antigen detection[10] (see below). However, these techniques are not universally available, even in hospitals of the developed world, mainly because they are labour intensive and are perceived as being expensive. In the developing world this is compounded by a shortage of staff experienced in the use of such techniques. While availability of viral diagnosis is not likely to be widespread in the tropics, there is a sound argument for ensuring availability of competent diagnostic facilities in a few centres, at least, to provide continuing epidemiological data and to underpin clinical training.

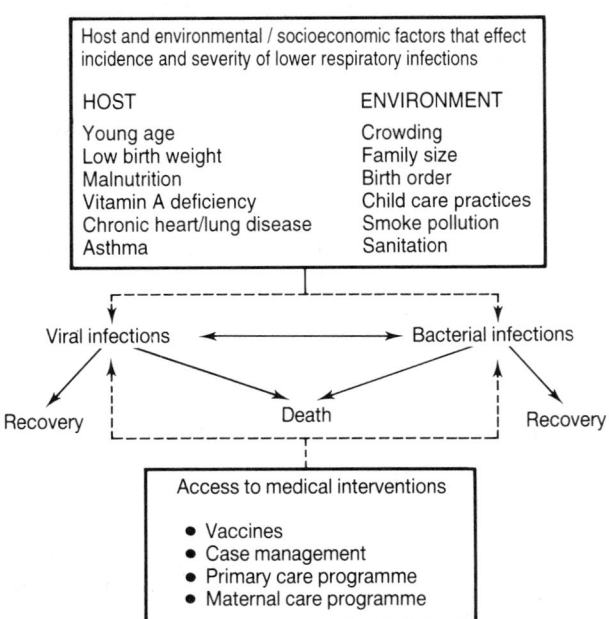

Figure 36.1 Aetiology and epidemiology of lower respiratory tract infections in developing countries. (Reproduced with permission from Berman.[9])

METHODS OF VIRAL DIAGNOSIS

Laboratory diagnosis of respiratory virus infections depends on the demonstration of *either* virus or viral components in the patient at the acute stage of the illness, *or* subsequently an immune (serological) response to the virus.

Table 36.4 Advantages and disadvantages of various techniques of virus diagnosis.

Technique	Advantages	Disadvantages
Immunofluorescence	• Rapid, i.e. same day • Allows assessment of specimen quality • Sensitive and specific in experienced hands	• Labour intensive • Requires experienced observer(s) • Requires high quality reagents • Obtaining good specimens requires skill and determination
Enzyme immunoassay	• Relatively rapid • Suitable for large numbers • Can be semiautomated • Detects incomplete virus particles	• No feedback on specimen quality • Requires high-quality reagents • Automated equipment expensive • Difficult to assess results at threshold of positivity
Culture	• Provides more virus for further analysis • Confirms presence of infective virus • Generally regarded as the gold standard • Only currently feasible method for some viruses (e.g. rhinoviruses and enteroviruses)	• Expensive and a continuing expense • Labour intensive • Some viruses difficult to isolate • Mixed infections pose problems • Requires high-quality reagents to identify isolates
Detection of nucleic acid by polymerase chain reaction (PCR)	• Can be made both very sensitive and specific • Can detect virus in the presence of antibody	• Expensive • Requires constant vigilance against cross-contamination • Unsuitable for large numbers • Labour and skill intensive

DEMONSTRATION OF VIRUS

There are several approaches to this. They include demonstration of: (1) viral antigens by immunofluorescence[11,12] or enzyme immunoassays;[10] (2) viral infectivity by growth in cell culture; or (3) viral nucleic acid by various techniques. Details of the techniques are not given in this account, but the advantages and disadvantages of each are indicated in Table 36.4. Before setting up a diagnostic laboratory the aims of the operation should be clearly thought out. If the catchment population is very large, the number of specimens may also be large and the advantages of automation (e.g. in machine-based enzyme immunoassays) may be worth having. However, this is rare and the number of available specimens may be fewer. Automation may then be less advantageous and is often minimal except in serology (see below). Except for special studies, most of the specimens will come from hospitalized patients because of the practical difficulties of collecting specimens in the community. In any case, virology specimens are perishable and must be delivered to the laboratory without delay.

DEMONSTRATION OF IMMUNE RESPONSE

This, at present, means demonstrating a serum antibody response to the stimulus provided by the virus. If current trends continue, this will be eventually replaced by assays of salivary antibody.

For a valid diagnosis, a convalescent specimen of serum (taken after a response has occurred) is needed but may be difficult to collect 2 weeks after onset from patients who may by then be totally recovered and unwilling to oblige the investigator's interest! This is particularly true of children. Nevertheless, unless an antibody response can be demonstrated (seroconversion or a rising titre) some uncertainty over the validity of the result will remain. The alternative is demonstration of an IgM-class response but this suffers from the two disadvantages that such tests are not available for all viruses and the sample (to be reliably positive) may have to be taken after the illness, with the problem(s) already mentioned.

Serology remains the routine choice for some respiratory agents which, although not viral in nature, are traditionally diagnosed by virus laboratories. These include: psittacosis, Q fever and *Mycoplasma pneumoniae* infection. All cause an illness with an insidious onset and are difficult and/or dangerous to isolate. Since all, therefore, are susceptible to antibiotics, a diagnosis is important and can be life saving. The role of *Chlamydia pneumoniae* is poorly documented at present in the absence of an easily used test.

INFECTIONS IN THE IMMUNOCOMPROMISED HOST (See also Chapter 12)

A detailed analysis of the respiratory complications of the immunocompromised patient (oncology, leukaemia, transplantation) is outside the compass of this book but some mention is necessary of opportunistic infections in patients infected with the human immunodeficiency virus (HIV) or who have the acquired immune deficiency syndrome (AIDS). They are likely to contract any of the viruses already mentioned and may have difficulty in eradicating them. However, viral respiratory infections are not in themselves a life-threatening problem in patients with AIDS, with three exceptions: measles, varicella-zoster and cytomegalovirus.

Giant cell pneumonitis due to measles can be fatal, and may occur even in patients who have past immunity (naturally-derived or vaccine induced). Chickenpox may be severe and include respiratory complications. Cytomegalovirus pneumonitis (although less commonly seen than in other groups of immunocompromised patients) can also be fatal.

The diagnosis of chickenpox is usually clinically obvious, but measles may present problems because the skin rash is often absent in the immunocompromised patient. Immunofluorescent examination of nasopharyngeal secretions for measles-infected cells provides a rapid diagnosis, but this facility is unlikely to be widely available. Cytomegalovirus can be cultured from the sputum (conventional or induced) or detected in bronchoalveolar lavage/lung biopsy specimens, if available.

NOSOCOMIAL INFECTION

RSV and influenza viruses are particularly highly infectious, and are notorious causes of cross-infection in hospitals. This may pose particular hazards to patients at higher risk, such as those with underlying heart or lung disease (e.g. congenital heart damage or bronchopulmonary dysplasia). Transmission of RSV (as with most other respiratory viruses) is by direct contact or via infected surfaces or fomites. Influenza A, on the other hand, is efficiently spread by aerosols.

Precautions that may help reduce the risk of cross-infection include the isolation or cohort nursing of infected patients and scrupulous care in hand-washing between patients. It is essential to remember that viruses can also infect medical and other hospital staff (RSV may be asymptomatic or cause a 'cold' in adults) and be transmitted by and through them.

PREVENTION AND TREATMENT

With the cells of the target organ immediately accessible to viruses, it is proving difficult to produce an effective vaccine to respiratory tract virus(es). Other than in measles, which has a systemic phase, vaccines have had only limited success. In the tropics, even the measles vaccine has limitations because much of the impact of this virus on morbidity and mortality is during infancy, and existing measles vaccines are not effective at inducing immunity in the face of passive maternal antibody. Newer vaccines, including one using canarypox virus as a vector, are presently being evaluated. A second dose of vaccine has also been suggested but cost may make this impractical in many countries.

Influenza vaccine is used for persons at high risk (e.g. patients with underlying heart, respiratory or immunocompromising diseases, patients on dialysis, the elderly) and contains components of both influenza A and B. The constituents are modified as the prevalent strains alter but inevitably will always lag behind wild strains. In addition, it is not yet known how to induce the long-term secretory IgA mucosal antibody which is probably necessary for protection. Within these limitations the vaccine, usually formalin-killed egg-grown virus, has provided useful protection, particularly in the elderly and those with pre-existing lung damage in whom even minimal protection may be enough to prevent death. An alternative approach to a live attenuated vaccine by cold-adapting influenza strains has been used widely in Russia, particularly in schools, but has yet to be introduced elsewhere to any great extent.

An experimental enteric coated vaccine to adenovirus 14 was developed for use in the US Army to combat epidemics in recruit camps but has found no application elsewhere.

Prevention of severe measles and varicella in susceptible (immunocompromised or severely malnourished) contacts may be achieved by passive immunization. Normal human γ-globulin is effective in preventing/attenuating measles if administered within 3 days of contact. For the prophylaxis of varicella, high titre varicella-zoster human immune globulin (ZIG) must be used. Maximum protection (from severe disease, not from infection) follows administration within 48 hours of contact, but some benefit may accrue if given within 10 days.

Amantadine, and its alternative rimantadine, have been shown to provide protection against influenza A (but *not* influenza B) but to be of little use in treatment. Its main use has been to give short-term passive protection to limit spread of influenza A in closed communities or in vulnerable patients (see above).

The management of viral respiratory infections is essentially symptomatic and is dealt with elsewhere (Chapter 4). Antibiotics are not routinely indicated for viral respiratory infections unless secondary bacterial superinfection occurs. The 'atypical' bacterial infections mentioned above (Q fever, mycoplasmosis and chlamydiosis) are amenable to antibiotic therapy. (T)ribavirin given as an aerosol inhalation is claimed to reduce the severity of RSV infection in infants, but this remains controversial. It is a very expensive drug, but may be life-saving in those with congenital heart and/or lung damage for whom RSV infection may be the final insult which pushes them into heart or lung failure. (T)ribavirin may have some effect in influenza but the evidence is minimal.

Acyclovir (given intravenously) is effective in the treatment of varicella or herpes simplex infections in the immunocompromised patient. It should also be used in an immunocompetent patient (usually an adult) with varicella pneumonia. Ganciclovir and foscarnet are useful in cytomegalovirus infection in the immunosuppressed, but this problem is beyond the scope of this book.

SUMMARY

Respiratory infections are very common throughout the world and are worse where social conditions are inadequate. Much childhood respiratory tract disease is either totally due to viruses or is virus initiated and the same viruses appear to be involved in all regions, tropical or temperate. Epidemiological data are incomplete everywhere (but more so for the poorer parts of the world) and originate mostly from hospitalized patients. Nevertheless, RSV is a universal childhood pathogen, found everywhere it has been sought. In Newcastle upon Tyne and the Tyneside conurbation (population approximately 1 million) there are regularly between 500 and 600 *virologically confirmed* cases a year. There are likely to be many more in the crowded cities of India, China, the Philippines and Brazil. The effects of RSV (and other viruses) are exacerbated by: overcrowding, malnutrition, deficient medical care, poor sanitation, air pollution, etc. Respiratory disease, like diarrhoea, results in significant morbidity and mortality in the developing world and will require an enormous commitment of resources to abate. Both viruses and bacteria are involved and there are few effective vaccines at present.

REFERENCES

1 Suwanjutha S, Chantarojanasiri T, Watthana-Kasetr S et al. A study of nonbacterial agents of acute lower respiratory tract infection in Thai children. *Rev Infect Dis* 1990; 12 (supplement 8):S923–S928.

2 Jacob John T, Cherian T, Steinhoff M C, Simoes E A F & John M. Etiology of acute respiratory infections in children in tropical Southern India. *Rev Infect Dis* 1991; 13 (supplement 6):S463–S469.

3 Markowitz L E & Nieburg P. The burden of acute respiratory infection due to measles in developing countries and the potential impact of measles vaccine. *Rev Infect Dis* 1991; 13 (supplement 6):S555–S561.

4 Bale J R (ed.). Symposium on Etiology and Epidemiology of Acute Respiratory Tract Infection in Children in Developing Countries. *Rev Infect Dis* 1990; 12 (supplement 8):S861–S1083.

5 Steinhoff M C (ed.). Bellagio Conference on The Pathogenesis and Prevention of Pneumonia in Children in Developing Regions. *Rev Infect Dis* 1991; 13 (supplement 6):S451–S580.

6 Assaad F & Cockburn W C. A seven year study of WHO virus laboratory reports on respiratory viruses. *Bull World Health Organ* 1974; 51:437–445.

7 Forgie I M, Campbell H, Lloyd-Evans N et al. Etiology of acute lower respiratory tract infections in children in a rural community in The Gambia. *Paediatr Infect Dis J* 1992; 11:466–473.

8 McIntosh K, Halonen P & Ruuskanen O. Report of a workshop on respiratory viral infections: epidemiology, diagnosis, treatment and preventions. *Clin Infect Dis* 1993; 16:151–164.

9 Berman S. Epidemiology of acute respiratory infections in children of developing countries *Rev Infect Dis* 1991; 13 (supplement 6):S454–S462.

10 Arstila P P & Halonen P. Direct antigen detection. In Lennette E H, Halonen P & Murphy F A (eds) *Laboratory Diagnosis of Infectious Diseases. Principles and Practice*, vol. II. New York: Springer, 1988:60–75.

11 Gardner P S & McQuillin J. *Rapid Virus Diagnosis. Application of Immunofluorescence*, 2nd edn. London: Butterworth, 1980.

12 Madeley C R. Respiratory Viruses. In *Immunofluorescence Antigen Detection Techniques in Diagnostic Microbiology*. London: Public Health Laboratory Service, 1992:33–48.

CHAPTER 37

CUTANEOUS VIRAL DISEASES

G. C. Cook

MEASLES

GEOGRAPHICAL DISTRIBUTION

Measles has a worldwide distribution.[1] It is one of the most prevalent infectious diseases of the tropics, and certainly the most serious of the acute childhood communicable illnesses.[2] Its introduction to many countries—which had previously been free—such as Fiji, Tasmania, Greenland, and many tropical areas where there were isolated people without previous contact with the disease, frequently had disastrous results.

AETIOLOGY

The causative agent, which is closely related to rinderpest and canine distemper, is a single-stranded RNA virus with a pleomorphic appearance on electron microscopy (120–250 nm in size); it consists of two components, an outer envelope with short projections and an inner nucleocapsid of RNA and a glycoprotein. There is only one strain and no known antigenic variation; alterations in virulence worldwide is due to underlying host and environmental factors. The virus grows slowly in human and monkey cell cultures. Viraemia occurs 4–5 days before the appearance of the rash, and abates within 24–48 hours. The virus can also be isolated from the throat in the coryzal stage.

TRANSMISSION

Measles is one of the most contagious of infections; approximately 90% of susceptible individuals will contract the disease after contact with a case. Transmission is direct—from secretions from the respiratory tract—by droplet spread. Cases are infectious only in the early stages, when virus can be isolated from the throat. Transplacental spread does not seem to occur, and although it is possible that fetal damage may follow measles contracted during pregnancy, this is not proven.

PATHOLOGY

Infection begins in the nose and throat from which, following limited multiplication, the virus spreads (via leucocytes) to the cells of the reticuloendothelial system; here it attacks the lymphocytes of the immune system. Further multiplication precedes the viraemic phase; epithelial cells are affected and the clinical signs and symptoms of measles develop after an incubation period of 10–14 days. Virus multiplication occurs in the reticuloendothelial system, in which it produces the appearance of large multi-nucleate giant cells. Target organs affected are the skin, conjunctivae, mouth, larynx, bronchial tree, and gastrointestinal tract. The essential lesion is 'catarrhal' inflammation of the respiratory and gastrointestinal tracts, the initial inflammation of epithelial cells being rapidly followed by fatty degeneration and exfoliation of dead cells. Complete resolution with recovery is the rule, although widespread denudation of epithelium in the gastro-cutestinal tract may result in significant enteropathy (see Chapter 3).

IMMUNITY

Immunity to measles is both antibody- and cell-mediated; following an acute attack this is lifelong. Antibodies appear simultaneously with the rash and IgM concentration peaks at 10 days—disappearing after 1 month; a resulting elevated IgG concentration decreases slowly over 6 months. Passive immunity (transferred from mother to infant trans-

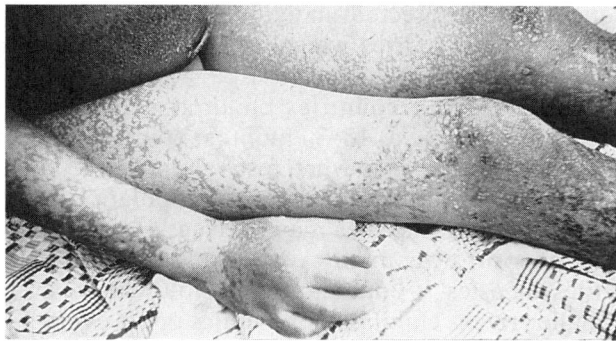

Figure 37.1 Measles rash near the knee in an African child. In a dark skin the rash has a deep bluish colour. (Courtesy of David Morley.)

placentally) lasts for the first few months of life and evidence of inapparent infection during months of declining maternal antibody can be found in one–quarter of older children. Cell-mediated immunity plays an important role in virus elimination. Resultant on its action on the cells of the reticuloendothelial system, measles depresses cell-mediated immunity, which can also be reduced simultaneously by malnutrition. This accounts for the severity of the disease in many tropical countries. Depressed cell-mediated immunity also reactivates tuberculosis and allows secondary infections, which are common in measles, to develop.

CLINICAL FEATURES

NATURAL HISTORY

Measles consists of an acute self–limiting infection; recovery occurs in the majority of cases; in tropical populations it can be complicated by severe bronchopneumonia, diarrhoea, malabsorption, malnutrition, severe conjunctivitis and blindness, gangrene of limbs and death.[1,2] Case mortality in the tropics is estimated to be about 5% (sometimes reaching 10% in rural areas).[3,4] In some village epidemics, 40% of children have died as a result of measles; a combination of pertussis and measles is particularly dangerous.

SYMPTOMS AND SIGNS

Incubation period is 10–14 days. Onset is gradual; fever and coryzal symptoms appear within 24 hours. Severe conjunctivitis and cough follow; this prodromal phase lasts for 3–4 days. Within 3 days of onset (and 24 hours before the rash) Koplik's spots can be visualized as blobs of bright red with a small bluish-white centre on the buccal mucous membrane. The exanthem (Figure 37.1) appears 24 hours later, first on the forehead and neck—spreading to invade the trunk over 3–4 days. The lesions are at first reddish maculopapular, later becoming brown, and in dark skin appearing totally different to lesions in pale skins, with a diffuse deep-red or purple rash followed by severe desquamation 2–4 days later. This may lead to patchy depigmentation and, occasionally, boils.

Haemorrhagic measles with a purpuric rash and accompanied by bleeding from mucous membranes is rare; it carries a high mortality rate.

Other systems

The mouth becomes sore, interfering with sucking and eating; this leads to malnutrition and cancrum oris. Laryngitis is common; this is followed by bronchopneumonia—which carries a high mortality rate. Diarrhoea sometimes accompanied by tenesmus and blood and mucus in the stool, leads to dehydration; parenteral replacement may be necessary to prevent death.

Central nervous system

The most common manifestation is a short, generalized convulsion early in the course of infection, from which recovery is complete.

Encephalitis

Measles encephalitis is associated with generalized convulsions—the risk increasing with age; the course is variable. Onset is usually 4–7 days after appearance of the rash (48 hours to 2 weeks after onset) and is characterized by fever, irritability, meningism and coma. The cerebrospinal fluid shows moderate pleocytosis and an increase in protein concentration. Mortality rate can be as high as 10–15%, and one-quarter of affected children are left with a permanent neurological deficit. This phenomenon probably has an immunological basis, as shown by the histological changes, perivascular cuffing, demyelination and gliosis.

Subacute sclerosing panencephalitis

This complication is caused by a persistent viral infection within the brain. It usually manifests 5–10 years after infection, and pursues a slow degenerative course, starting with personality change(s) and deterioration of intellect (with signs of mental deterioration), and progressing to a state of decerebrate rigidity. Very high levels of antibody to measles virus are present in cerebrospinal fluid.

COMPLICATIONS

Depression of cell-mediated immunity can give rise to giant cell pneumonia, also seen in patients with defective cell-mediated immunity. Severe ulcerative herpes of the mouth and eye result from cell-mediated immune depression. Severe conjunctivitis, often associated with vitamin A deficiency,[5–7] causes corneal perforation and blindness. Measles is one of the most common causes of blindness in the tropics (see Chapter 10). Gangrene of the extremities may develop. Malnutrition associated with measles can precipitate kwashiorkor and marasmus. Otitis media leads to mastoiditis and a hearing deficit. Measles exerts a major impact on infant/child development.

DIAGNOSIS

The association of cough, conjunctivitis, coryza and a morbilliform rash is usually diagnostic, but other conditions with dermatological manifestations have often been mistaken for measles; tick-borne and louse-borne typhus, meningococcaemia, scarlet fever and infectious mononucleosis are also associated with morbilliform rashes. There is a leucocytosis in the early stage(s), followed by an increase in lymphocytes—some of the Turk type.

During the prodromal phase large multinucleate (giant) cells can be visualized in stained smears of sputum/urine. Serological tests on acute and convalescent sera reveal haemaglutination-inhibiting (HI) and neutralizing (N) antibodies, with a fourfold rise in titre following the initial infection.

TREATMENT

No chemotherapeutic agent influences the course of the viraemia. Food and fluid intake should be maintained, and rehydration undertaken.[8] Antibiotics are essential when otitis media, bacterial pneumonia and skin infections are present.

EPIDEMIOLOGY

Man is the sole reservoir of infection. The incidence of measles worldwide is diminishing in developed countries, where the mean age of onset is now over 5 years. As infant immunization becomes more widely practised, the mean age of infection rises; consequently, unprotected individuals and visitors to developing countries which have no immunization programme are at increased risk.

In developing countries children generally develop the disease at 18–30 months; epidemics occur during the dry season when festivals and concourses of people take place. In isolated populations, e.g. nomadic ones, measles may occur at any age if the last exposure was many years previously. In large cities measles is endemic throughout the year; in smaller towns childhood epidemics occur every 2–3 years and infection spreads to the villages.

CONTROL

Both passive immunization with human immunoglobulin and active immunization with a live attenuated vaccine are highly successful.[9–13]

PASSIVE IMMUNIZATION

Passive immunization (human gammaglobulin 0.25 mg/kg) is effective if given within 5 days of exposure. In one study, passive immunization of children on admission to hospital gave complete protection—which was immediate.

ACTIVE IMMUNIZATION

A live attenuated strain of the virus is used; this gives a 98% seroconversion rate under ideal conditions. Fever of moderate severity and a mild rash occur rarely. Encephalitis is a rare complication.

Immunization can be combined with that for diphtheria, tetanus toxoid and pertussis (DPT) without loss of immunogenicity. Maternal antibody is transferred transplacentally and this inhibits vaccine efficacy up to the age of 6 months. Normally, vaccination is aimed at children of 9 months of age,[14] but vaccination at 6 months despite a lower seroconversion rate, is used in areas of high risk, sometimes in conjunction with a booster dose 1 year later. In order to eradicate the disease immunization uptake rates of 90–95% are required.[15]

A 49% reduction in mortality in African children hospitalized with pneumonia and gastroenteritis has been recorded when measles vaccine was given as a routine admission procedure. Human immunoglobulin should be combined with measles vaccine in malnourished children.

Live vaccines are rapidly inactivated at room temperature and the difficulty of maintaining the 'cold chain' is a major handicap to its use in most tropical countries. Monitoring of seroconversion rates should be a feature of all antimeasles campaigns.

An aerosol-administered vaccine has been successfully developed; it can be administered by anyone (with minimum qualifications) by hand pump, and should prove a great advance compared with previous methods of mass immunization. A heat-stable vaccine is under development.

A major problem is that measles vaccination campaigns have to be repeated regularly; it is essential that measles vaccine is incorporated into the regular health care system for rural areas, together with other immunizations.

POXVIRAL DISEASES

ORTHOPOX VIRUSES

The orthopox viruses are DNA double-stranded viruses, brick or ovoid-shaped, and 200–250 nm in size; they are all antigenically related and include cowpox, ectromelia (mice), monkeypox, Turkmenia rodent pox, and vaccinia. The only members of the group that have infected man are variola (smallpox), vaccinia (see Chapters 2 and 15), monkeypox and cowpox. Tanapox, although not an orthopox virus, is closely related.

MONKEYPOX

GEOGRAPHICAL DISTRIBUTION

The disease is confined to tropical Africa (Figure 37.2). Although monkeypox has been recorded since 1958 in captive monkeys, the first human case was recognized in Zaire in 1970;[16,17] since then more than 200 cases have been reported, mainly in Zaire, but also Liberia, Nigeria, Ivory Coast, Cameroon and Sierra Leone. It has only rarely been reported outside these areas of tropical rainforest.

AETIOLOGY

Monkeypox is a 'brick–shaped' orthopox virus (200–250 nm in size) which forms cytoplasmic inclusions and is morphologically indistinguishable from variola. It can be readily distinguished in culture because the pocks on chick chorioallantoic membrane are slightly larger and more haemorrhagic than those caused by variola. Unlike variola, monkeypox virus is pathological in rabbits, and has a higher temperature ceiling for growth. It grows readily in the green monkey and rodent cell cultures. Four strains of poxviruses have been isolated from monkey kidney cells and rodents; these differ from monkey-pox, but are closely related to variola, from which they can be distinguished by DNA analysis. These are known as 'white-pox' viruses; their relation to human infection is unknown.

TRANSMISSION

The usual mode of transmission from monkey to man is unclear, but infection is sometimes direct, resulting from handling dead monkeys for eating, or by droplet spread via the respiratory tract.[16] Transmission by a chimpanzee bite has also been recorded. The disease is not readily transmitted from man to man, but secondary cases have been recorded. Little tertiary spread occurs and epidemic spread is not a feature.

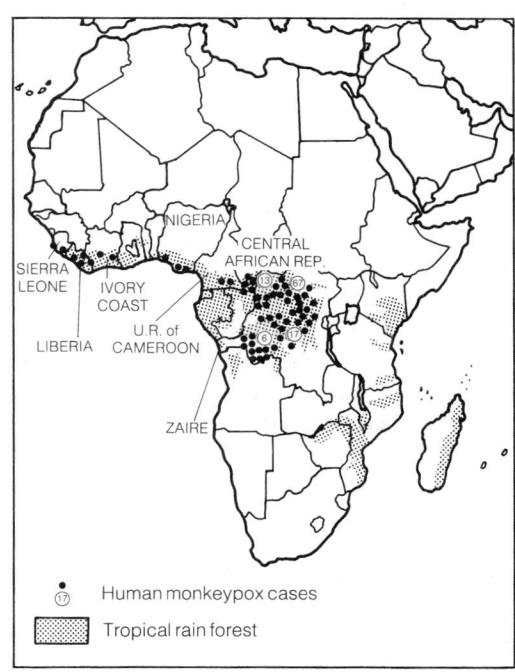

Figure 37.2 Geographical distribution of human monkeypox showing number of cases reported from 1970 to 1984. (Courtesy of the World Health Organization.)

PATHOLOGY

Few individuals are known to have died from monkeypox; no post mortems have been performed, and therefore no histopathological information is available. It seems likely that pathological changes resemble those previously attributable to smallpox.

IMMUNITY

There is well-defined immunity to reinfection, and complete cross-immunity with variola and vaccinia. Monkeypox has never been recorded in an individual vaccinated for smallpox[16].

CLINICAL FEATURES

Natural history

Monkeypox infection in man is a dead-end infection, manifesting itself as a typical smallpox-like illness. It possesses a 2–3-day prodromal period, and the smallpox-like rash evolves over 2–4 days. The illness is usually mild, and followed by complete recovery. When deaths have occurred they have usually been in children.

Symptoms and signs

The incubation period is 5–17 days. The onset is abrupt with fever and a prodromal illness lasting 2–3 days.[16] On the third day a rash appears; this consists of a single crop of discrete papules, more abundant on the face and extremities than on the trunk. The soles of the feet and palms are involved. The papules form pustules which become umbilicated and are covered with crusts which separate after about 10 days, leaving small scars. Marked lymphadenopathy may occur (Figure 37.3). Mild atypical cases occur in which there may be fewer than ten lesions, separation of the crusts occurring by the fifth day. There are no recorded complications.

DIAGNOSIS

The differential diagnosis was formerly from smallpox; diagnosis is based on epidemiology and a history of contact with monkeys.[16] Lymphadenopathy was an important distinguishing feature. Isolation of the virus, together with its cultural characteristics and antigenic structure provide the definitive diagnosis.

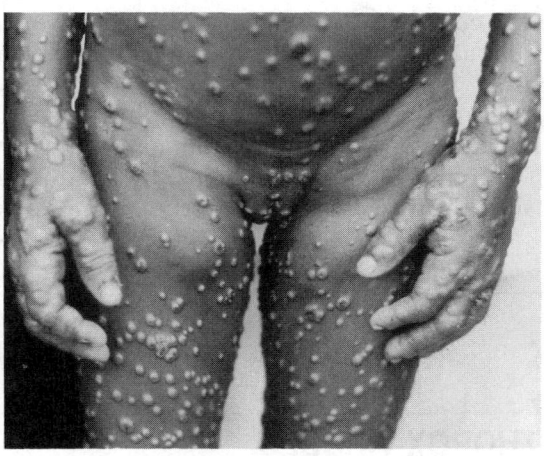

Figure 37.3 Monkeypox showing characteristic inguinal and femoral lymphadenopathy. (Reproduced with permission from Breman J G, Kalisa–Ruti, Steniowski M V et al. *Bull World Health Organ* 1980; 58: 849–868.)

TREATMENT

Treatment is symptomatic/supportive.

EPIDEMIOLOGY

Whether the primary maintenance hosts are chimpanzees, other primates, or small mammals is unknown. Most patients give a clear account of contact with monkeys which they have caught and/or eaten.[16] Most cases occur during the dry season. Children are affected more than adults. The attack rate is 10% in susceptible individuals in close contact with a primary case, in contrast to smallpox infection in which it was 20%. Secondary spread occurs amongst families, but tertiary transmission is rare and epidemics are not a feature. Now that vaccination level in communities has fallen dramatically, human monkeypox may become far more common.

TANAPOX

Tanapox was first described in 1957 and 1962 in epidemics in the lower Tana river of Kenya. Serological surveys have shown continuing transmission along the lower Tana river. Human infections have since been recorded in the forest area of Zaire. A closely related virus has been isolated from outbreaks in primate colonies in the USA, and in contacts of human cases.

AETIOLOGY

Tanapox virus is not an orthopox virus; with the Yabapox virus it forms a distinct subgroup of poxviruses. It cannot be cultured on chick chorioallantoic membrane, but grows well on green monkey kidney cell and Vero cell cultures.

TRANSMISSION

Epidemiological features suggest that the virus is transmitted from monkeys to man by mosquitoes; outbreaks in man have occurred in low-lying country near the Tana river after floods isolated wild animals, humans and their domestic animals on islands in the flood water, on which *Mansonia uniformis* and *M. africanus* had proliferated in immense numbers. There is no evidence of direct person-to-person spread.

PATHOLOGY

Pathology is limited to the epidermis—where the pock forms. There are few or no destructive changes. Hypertrophied epidermal cells containing acidophilic inclusion bodies predominate; cellular infiltration is mild and the dermis escapes intact.

IMMUNITY

Virtually nothing is known about second attacks. Antibodies which develop in infected individuals and monkeys persist for some years. There is no cross-immunity with vaccinia; recently-vaccinated people can develop the disease.

CLINICAL FEATURES

Natural history

The infection is usually mild: fever heralds the appearance of one or two pock-like lesions. Complete recovery follows.

Symptoms and signs

The incubation period is unknown. Onset is abrupt with fever lasting 3–4 days, accompanied in some cases by severe headache and prostration. Severity is open to doubt because histories have usually been recorded retrospectively, long after the event—in the major published studies. During the febrile episode one or two (but never more) pock-like lesions

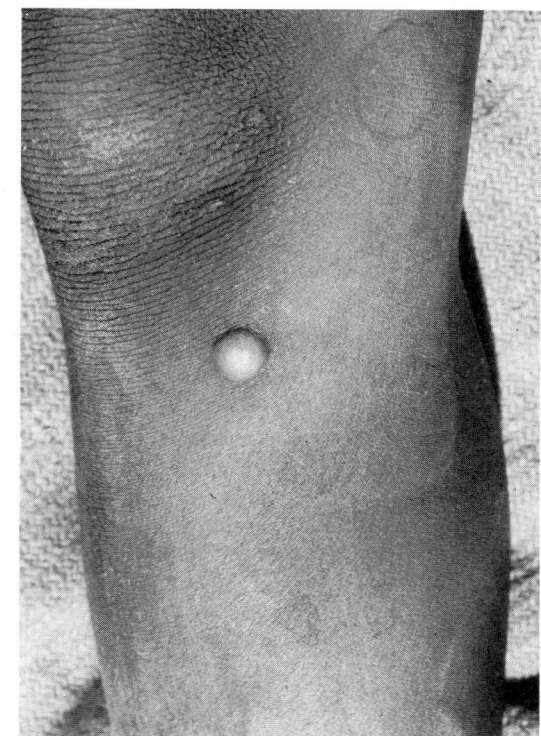

Figure 37.4 Tanapox. Solid pock containing firm cheesy material.

appear on the skin, resembling those formerly caused by smallpox. Lesions become umbilicated; they never proceed to pustule formation, but form firm cheesy centres instead (Figure 37.4). The pocks occur mainly on the exposed surfaces: upper arms, face, neck and trunk, but never on the hands, legs or feet. Recovery takes place rapidly; no scars are left and there are no residual complications.

DIAGNOSIS

Tanapox had formerly to be distinguished from modified smallpox in a vaccinated person; the character of the pock (which at first looks like smallpox) differs in its larger size, firm, solid nature and absence of pustulation. Electron microscopical appearances are similar to those previously associated with smallpox. Virus can be isolated by culture in green monkey kidney or Vero cells, and is clearly distinguished by antigenic structure from orthopox viruses. Serum antibodies develop slowly, but complement fixation and neutralizing tests on both human and monkey sera show antibody at low titre; this persists for some years and can be used for a retrospective diagnosis.

TREATMENT

Treatment is unnecessary.

EPIDEMIOLOGY

The epidemiology is poorly documented. The primary maintenance hosts are unknown; many monkeys, especially vervet (*Cercopithecus aethiops*) are susceptible, and are common in the endemic area(s). Small outbreaks have occured after flooding, but transmission was shown to be continuing along the lower Tana river in serological surveys carried out in 1971 and 1976; infection persisted since 1962. Antibodies were detected in 9.2% of the population, and in children between the ages of 2 and 12. There is no evidence of direct person-to-person transmission.

REFERENCES

1 Katz S L & Gellin B G (eds) Measles control—resetting the agenda: a report of the Children's Vaccine Initiative ad hoc Committee on an investment strategy for measles control. *J Infect Dis* 1994; 170 (Supplement 1): S1–S66. 2 Egunjobi L. Spatial distribution of mortality from leading notifiable diseases in Nigeria. *Soc Sci Med* 1993; 36:1267–1272.

3 Aaby P, Andersen M & Knudsen K. Excess mortality after early exposure to measles. *Int J Epidemiol* 1993; 22:156–162.

4 Uyirwoth G P. Measles in Mashonaland Central Province: Zimbabwe. *East Afr Med J* 1993; 70:455–459.

5 Hussey G D & Klein M. Routine high-dose vitamin A therapy for children hospitalized with measles. *J Trop Pediatr* 1993; 9:342–345.

6 Latham M C. Vitamin A and childhood mortality. *Lancet* 1993; 342:549.

7 Ross D A. Vitamin A and childhood mortality. Ghana Vitamin A Supplementation Trials Study Team. *Lancet* 1993; 342:861.

8 Foster S O, Spiegel R A & Mokdad A. Immunization, oral rehydration therapy and malaria chemotherapy among children under 5 in Bomi and Grand Cape Mount counties, Liberia, 1984 and 1988. *Int J Epidemiol* 1993; 22 (supplement 1):S50–S55.

9 Garenne M, Leroy O, Beau J P & Sene I. Efficacy of measles vaccine after controlling for exposure. *Am J Epidemiol* 1993; 138:182–195.

10 Longini I M Jr, Halloran M E, Haber M & Chen R T. Measuring vaccine efficacy from epidemics of acute infectious agents. *Stat Med* 1993; 12:249–263.

11 Nokes D J & Cutts F T. Immunization in the developing world: strategic challenges. *Trans R Soc Trop Med Hyg* 1993; 87:353–354, 398.

12 Tulchinsky T H, Ginsberg G M, Abed Y, Angeles M T, Akukwe C & Bonn J. Measles control in developing and developed countries: the case for a two-dose policy. *Bull World Health Organ* 1993; 71:93–103.

13 Orenstein W A, Markowits L E, Atkinson W L & Hinman A R. Worldwide measles prevention. *Isr J Med Sci* 1994; 30:469–481.

14 Aaby P, Andersen M, Sodemann M, Jakobsen M, Gomes J & Fernandes M. Reduced childhood mortality after standard measles vaccination at 4–8 months compared with 9–11 months of age. *BMJ* 1993; 307:1308–1311.

15 Burstrom B, Aaby P & Mutie D M. Child mortality impact of a measles outbreak in a partially vaccinated rural African community. *Scand J Infect Dis* 1993; 25:763–769.

16 Cook G C. Human monkeypox: a viral disease with an uncertain future in Africa. *Trop Dis Bull* 1988; 85:R1–R16.

17 Cook G C. Monkeypox in Africa. *Lancet* 1987; i:369.

CHAPTER 38

VIRUS INFECTIONS OF THE CENTRAL NERVOUS SYSTEM

Sandra Amor and Surekha Mehta

Although virus infections of the central nervous system are rare they are responsible for some of the most devastating and diverse effects of disease in man and animals. The hydrophobia following rabies virus infection or the chronic debilitating effects of herpes virus infection are two such examples.

Central nervous system (CNS) viral infections were first reported in Babylonian times and trepanning in early times was possibly the earliest treatment for such diseases. However, with the explosion in advances in the fields of virus isolation techniques, immunology and pharmacology, many CNS infections may be controlled by prophylactics such as immunisation and vector control, or following pharmacological intervention.

The broad spectrum of clinical manifestations of CNS infections poses the clinician not only the problem of prompt diagnosis but also that of treatment and aggressive management to allow recovery with little chance of sequelae. The major clinical manifestations are outlined in Table 38.1.

VIRAL SPREAD TO THE CENTRAL NERVOUS SYSTEM

Consideration of how viruses may enter the CNS is paramount in determining the methods by which

Table 38.1 Clinical manifestations of viral infections of the CNS.

Disease	Duration	Clinical signs	Examples
Acute meningitis	Days	Rapid onset of high fever, stiff neck, altered mental state, photophobia, raised intracranial pressure	Viral meningitis
Chronic meningitis	Months	Gradual onset of signs associated with the above	Enteroviruses
Acute encephalitis	Days	Association with systemic illness, nausea, vomiting, seizures. Specific signs associated with tropism of virus, e.g. temporal lobe lesions following HSV infection	Measles, herpes simplex
Chronic encephalitis	Months to years	Gradual onset of signs as above, progressing to severe disability and death. General debility and dementia may develop	SSPE, HIV encephalitis
Postinfectious	Days to weeks	Onset of signs following recovery from viral infection. Such signs include the development of chronic fatigue syndrome or Guillain–Barré syndrome	Postinfectious encephalomyelitis
Slow viruses	Months to years	Progressive signs of neuronal destruction. Observed following immunosuppressive therapy	PML
Prion diseases	Months to years	Progressive signs of neurological dysfunction. Not associated with conventional virus	Creutzfeldt–Jakob, Kuru

HSV, herpes simplex virus; SSPE, subacute panencephalitis; HIV, human immunodeficiency virus; PML, progressive multifocal leucoencephalopathy.

Table 38.2 Routes of entry of neurotropic viruses.

Route of entry		Example
Inoculation:	arthropod bite	Arboviruses
	animal bite	Rabies
	blood transfusion	Cytomegalovirus
	transplantation	Creutzfeldt–Jakob
Respiratory		Influenza
Enteric		Polio
Venereal		HIV
Transplacental		Cytomegalovirus

such potential infections may be avoided or controlled. Space does not allow detail on entry of viruses and the reader is referred to Johnson[1] and Fields et al.[2] Although the skin is the most extensive barrier to the entry of viruses, once this barrier is broached by some form of inoculation viruses may then rapidly invade. Likewise the respiratory, gut and genitourinary tracts, which form the most formidable barrier due to mucous film and secretory immunoglobulin, may nevertheless be permeable to acid-resistant viruses such as the enteroviruses. The major portals of entry of viruses causing human CNS infections are summarized in Table 38.2.

Following entry into the host the virus must disseminate and enter the CNS either through the neural route and be transported via axonal transport, the olfactory route, or via the blood and cross the blood–brain barrier.

NEURAL ROUTE

Viral spread along peripheral nerves is well known for rabies since the time for onset of clinical disease is relative to the site of the inoculation. Furthermore, rabies may be detected in the peripheral nerve and experimental disease prevented if the infected nerve is severed.[3] Likewise, neural spread of poliomyelitis, varicella zoster and herpes simplex virus (HSV) has also been shown experimentally.[4]

OLFACTORY ROUTE

Experimental intranasal infection with HSV and some togaviruses show that virus is spread to the CNS via the olfactory route, resulting in an early infection of the CNS with histological changes in the olfactory tracts.

HAEMATOGENOUS ROUTE

The majority of viruses inducing CNS infections are acquired from the blood. The presence of a 'blood–

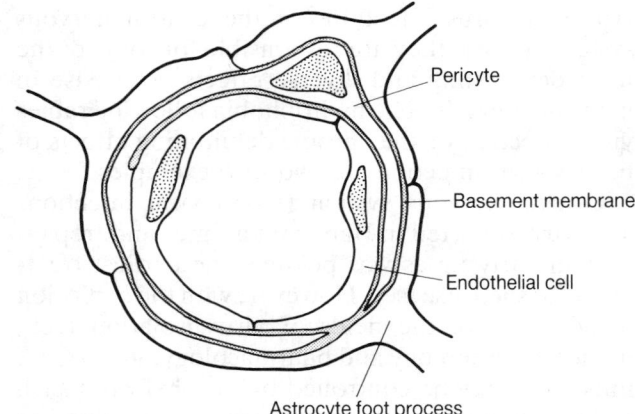

Figure 38.1 The blood–brain barrier.

brain barrier' (BBB) was based on the finding that following peripheral dye injections in small animals it was noticed that all tissues were stained with the exception of the brain.[5] Conversely, injection of dye into the cerebrospinal fluid (CSF) stained the brain but not peripheral tissues. The morphological BBB is represented by the cerebral endothelial cells, which lack fenestrations but are joined by tight junctions, pericytes which form a discontinuous layer round the endothelial cells with which they share a common basement membrane. Discontinuities in the basement membrane allow the endothelial cells direct contact with the pericytes.[6] Astrocytic foot processes surround the pericytes. A diagrammatic representation of the BBB is shown in Figure 38.1.

In general the physical and chemical nature of the molecule determines its ability to cross the BBB and thus, whereas lipid-soluble molecules are readily transferred across the BBB, charged non-lipid soluble molecules are less effective. The BBB also forms a barrier for the entry of viruses, nevertheless most viruses invade the CNS. Transfer of viruses across the BBB may take place either following infection of leucocytes, as is observed for measles and mumps virus, or adherence of virus to erthro-

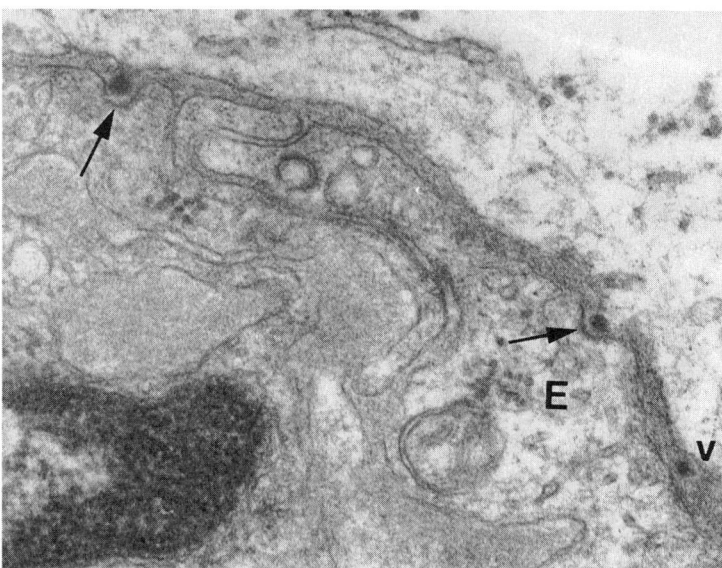

Figure 38.2 Brain capillary endothelial cell (E) showing the formation of coated vesicle containing mature virus (arrows). Mature virus (V) also present in the basement membrane. Semliki Forest × 60,000. (Kindly provided by L Pathak, St Thomas' Hospital.)

cytes, as is seen with toga- and paramyxoviruses. The infected cells may then migrate across the BBB during infection due to the upregulation of cellular adhesion molecules.[7] Such traffic is limited in the normal situation, although it may be extensive during injury or infection. Alternatively viruses may be taken up by receptors, induce the formation of pynocytotic vesicles on the endothelial cells and are actively transported, as Pathak and Webb[8] have described for Semliki Forest virus infection (Figure 38.2).

SPREAD WITHIN THE NERVOUS SYSTEM

Whether viruses reach the CNS via the haematogeneous, olfactory or neural route the progression of clinical signs is dependent on the subsequent spread of virus within the tissue. Additionally the tropism of viruses for different cells determines the characteristic clinical signs and manifestation of disease associated with specific viruses (see Table 38.1). For example the spread of herpes simplex virus within the temporal lobes leads to temporal lobe seizures, whereas infection of oligodendrocytes by JC papovavirus induces lesions of demyelination.

Attachment of viruses to cells prior to entry is obviously important in the development of disease and binding domains or receptors for numerous viruses have been identified, such as the β-adrenergic receptor for reoviruses.[9] The utilization of neurotransmitter receptors by viruses and interference in the functioning of specific neurones may

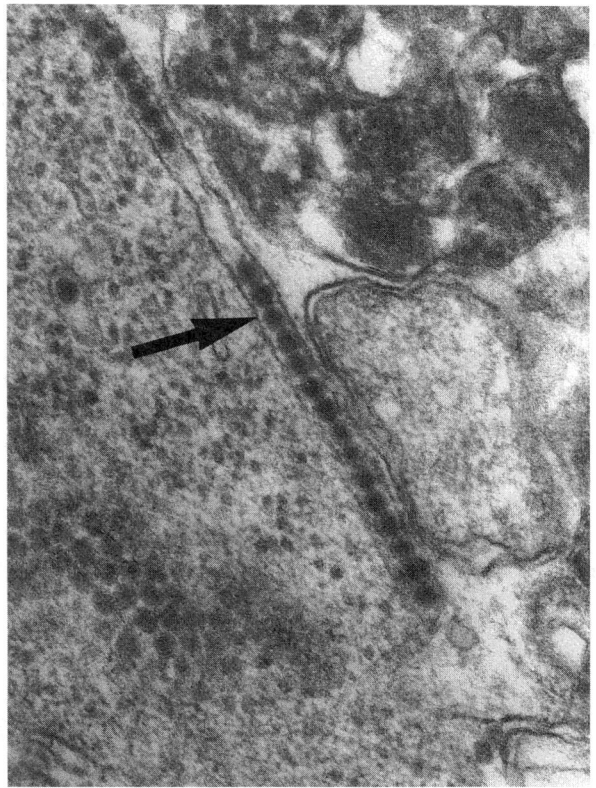

Figure 38.3 Langat virus (family *Flaviviridae*) (arrow) within the extracellular space of CNS tissue.

Table 38.3 Arthropod-borne viruses responsible for CNS diseases.

Arbovirus	Genus	Family
California encephalitis	Bunyavirus	Bunyaviridae
La Crosse	Bunyavirus	Bunyaviridae
Crimean haemorrhagic fever	*Nairovirus*	Bunyaviridae
Tensaw	Bunyamwera group	Bunyaviridae
Rift Valley fever	*Phlebovirus*	Bunyaviridae
Dengue		Flaviviridae
Ilheus		Flaviviridae
Japanese B		Flaviviridae
Kumlinge		Flaviviridae
Murray Valley encephalitis		Flaviviridae
Negishi		Flaviviridae
Powassan		Flaviviridae
Russian spring–summer encephalitis		Flaviviridae
Rocio		Flaviviridae
St Louis encephalitis		Flaviviridae
West Nile		Flaviviridae
Yellow fever		Flaviviridae
Colorado tick fever	*Orbivirus*	Reoviridae
Chikungunya	*Alphavirus*	Togaviridae
Eastern equine encephalitis	*Alphavirus*	Togaviridae
O'Nyong-Nyong	*Alphavirus*	Togaviridae
Semliki Forest	*Alphavirus*	Togaviridae
Venezuelan equine encephalitis	*Alphavirus*	Togaviridae
Western equine encephalitis	*Alphavirus*	Togaviridae
Thogoto	Ungrouped	

explain why viruses have been implicated in chronic fatigue syndrome.[10] Other receptors include the CD^4 receptor for the human immunodeficiency virus (HIV),[11] acetylcholine receptor for rabies[12] and fibroblast growth factor receptor for HSV-1.[13]

Once the virus has gained entry into the cell replication and dissemination are necessary for progression of disease. Although cell-to-cell spread is the most obvious there is little evidence for any virus that this occurs. Viruses have been observed in the extracellular spaces (Figure 38.3) and reduction of togavirus titres by specific antibody[14] suggests that extracellular movement must occur. Alternatively transport via glial cells and axons has been suggested.[15]

As with entry of viruses into the CNS the infiltrating leucocytes may be important in the spread of virus within the tissue. Additionally the role of the immune response in the progression of the disease must be considered since autoimmune responses initiated by viruses are an important phenomenon.[16]

ARBOVIRUSES (See also Chapter 30)

The vast majority of CNS infections are due to viruses transmitted by arthropod vectors, such as mosquitoes or ticks, and are termed arboviruses (*ar*thropod-*bo*rne viruses). The arbovirus group, which includes approximately 500 viruses, spans several families, i.e. Bunya-, Toga-, Flavi-, Reo- and Rhabdoviridae (Table 38.3). These arboviruses and viruses of other families implicated in CNS disorders are discussed under the virus family heading(s).

ARENAVIRIDAE

The name is derived from the Latin for 'arena', meaning sand, to describe the granules observed inside the virions. The two major groups that make up the Arenaviridae family, the lymphocytic choriomeningitis (LCM) group and the Tacaribe complex, are distinguished on the basis of antigenic reactivity.

These viruses are single-stranded RNA viruses of various sizes.

LCM complex is comprised of LCM and Lassa in which aseptic meningitis, encephalomyelitis and meningoencephalomyelitis have been described. LCM virus (LCMV) was the first virus isolated from aseptic meningitis in man. The other members of this complex, namely Ippy, Mopeia and Mobala, are not associated with human disease.

Epidemiology

LCMV, although now rarely identified in humans, is transmitted by rodents to humans via exposure of open wounds or contamination of food by infected animal excrement. Human-to-human contact has not been reported and, due to the nature of transmission, animal handlers or those living in impoverished conditions are at higher risk. Although LCMV infections of humans have not been documented for several years the seroprevalence is thought to be less than 0.1%.[17] LCMV infection in humans ranges from asymptomatic infection, mild systemic illness to CNS involvement. The severity of the illness may depend on dose, route of infection and host immunogenetic background.

Early fetal or transovarian infection in mice does not induce a sufficient immunological response to clear the virus and gives rise to a persistent infection in which virus is secreted in respiratory droplets, faeces and urine. Infection of adult mice induces a severe encephalitis and is an example of the pathological effect of the immunological response to a neurotropic virus.

Clinical features

The typical disease begins with fever, malaise, weakness, headache and myalgia, which is most severe in the lumbar region. The incubation period is 6–13 days and in some cases haematological disturbances such as leucopenia are observed. Anorexia, nausea and dizziness are also common. As many as 50% of patients may have any combination of sore throat, vomiting and arthralgias, with chest pain and pneumonitis. Neurological complications signified by headaches, stiff neck and typical signs of encephalitis have been reported in approximately 15% of infections, of which some are severe encephalitis. Fatal cases have also been reported.[18]

The white blood cell count is often 3000/mm³ or less with a mild thrombocytopenia. CSF from patients with meningeal signs contains several hundred white cells, predominantly lymphocytes (>80%), with increased protein and occasionally low sugar levels. Virus is often found in the spinal fluid during acute disease.[19] Convalescence is prolonged, with persistent fatigue and dizziness.

LASSA FEVER

Epidemiology

Lassa fever was first described in West Africa in the 1950s, although the virus was not isolated until 1969. The only known reservoir of Lassa fever virus in West Africa is *Mastomys natalensis*, one of the most commonly occurring rodents in Africa. The virus is rapidly spread from man to man giving rise to 30–66% mortality; consequently knowledge of the pathological features is limited. Rates of seroconversion to Lassa virus range from 5 to 20% in populations of Sierra Leone villages.[20] The highest rates are in crowded, highly mobile populations. Clinically, infection gives rise to haemorrhage, nephropathy, myocarditis and encephalitis.

Clinical diagnosis

Lassa fever begins 7–18 days following primary infection leading to onset of fever, headache and malaise.[21,22] Patients with Lassa fever show features of anxiety and there is an elevated respiratory rate. In 15–20% of patients bleeding occurs from gums and nose. Oedema of the face and neck are commonly seen in severe cases. Important clinical events in fatal disease are intractable hypovolaemic shock and/or severe CNS involvement, bleeding and oedema of the face. There is also endothelial and platelet dysfunction. The white blood cell count is often 3000/mm³ or less with a mild thrombocytopenia.

Pathogenesis and pathology

The most common and consistently observed lesions in fatal human Lassa fever are focal necroses of the liver, adrenal glands and spleen.[23–25] Although high virus titres occur in other organs, such as the brain, ovary, pancreas, uterus and placenta, no significant lesions have been found.

Prevention and control

The ideal method of prevention is to prevent contact between rodents and humans. This can be achieved by improving the housing and food storage which might reduce the domestic rodent population.

Vaccination

There are two vaccines for arenaviral diseases. A live attenuated vaccine has been extensively used. A second vaccine has been made by cloning and expressing the Lassa virus glycoprotein gene into vaccine virus.[26] This vaccine has proven highly suc-

cessful in preventing severe disease and death in challenged monkeys.[27]

Treatment

Ribavirin can prevent death in Lassa fever when given at any point in the illness but it is more effective when given early and administered intravenously.[28]

BUNYAVIRIDAE

The Bunyaviridae family is divided into five genera (*Bunyavirus*, *Nairovirus*, *Phlebovirus*, *Uukuvirus*, *Hantavirus*) and comprises over 250 members (Table 38.4). The viruses are between 80 and 120 nm in size and have a lipid envelope derived from the host cell membranes during maturation. The structure and replication of bunyaviruses are excellently covered in Fields' *Virology*.[29]

This section will concentrate on those viruses within the genera that are important with respect to causing significant human diseases. Other reviews may be referred to for more detailed study of the Bunyaviridae.[30–33]

BUNYAVIRUSES

The most important serogroup with respect to induction of human diseases is the California (CAL) group which include California encephalitis and La Crosse (LAC) viruses. This group of viruses has 14 serotypes, the prototype virus being La Crosse virus first isolated from a child in La Crosse, Wisconsin in 1960.[34]

Epidemiology

Members of the California encephalitis virus serogroup have been isolated in Canada, the USA, Trinidad, Europe, Africa and Finland,[35,36] although each has a very narrow host range and geographical distribution. Animals such as chipmunks and squirrels are commonly involved. La Cross virus, the prototype virus, is transmitted by the mosquito *Aedes triseriatus* which is the most important vector in California, although other Aedes species may be involved. Children and young adults aged 1–19 years are at greatest risk of exposure to this vector, which is a woodland mosquito, during activities such as camping and hiking.

La Crosse infection is the second most prevalent mosquito-borne viral infection in the USA and accounts for approximately 75 definite cases a year, although seroprevalence may reach 20% in older persons. La Crosse virus is transmitted mainly by *Ae. triseriatus*, a treehole-breeding woodland mosquito that frequently feeds on small mammals, particularly chipmunks and squirrels.[37] An alternative mosquito habitat is provided by discarded tyres, which hold rainwater on which egg rafts may be laid. This virus produces an acute encephalitis in chil-

Table 38.4   Genera and serogroups within the family Bunyaviridae.

Genus	Serogroups
Bunyavirus	Anopheles A, Anopheles B, Bunyamwera, Bwamba, California, Capim, Gamboa, Guama, Koongol, Olifantsvlei, Patois, Simbu, Teteu, Turlock
Nairovirus	Crimean–Congo, Dera Gharzi Khan, Hughes, Nairobi SD, Qalyub, Sakhalin
Phlebovirus	Phlebotomus, Rift Valley fever
Uukuvirus	Uukuniemi
Hantavirus	Hantaan

dren.[38] The acute illness lasts 10 days or fewer in most cases. The first symptoms are non-specific and last for 1–3 days, followed by the involvement of the CNS. The symptoms include stiff neck, lethargy and seizures. Earlier examination shows high counts of both polymorphonuclear neutrophil leucocytes and mononuclear cells in about 65% of patients. The most important sequelae of La Crosse encephalitis is epilepsy, which occurs in about 10% of the children. A few patients (2%) have persistent paresis. Learning disabilities and other objective cognitive deficits have been reported in a small proportion of patients. Tahyna virus, a bunyavirus related to California virus, has been associated with mild encephalitis in Slovakia.

Pathology

The lesions induced by bunyaviruses are typical of acute viral encephalitis. Examination of the CNS reveals perivascular cuffing of mononuclear cells and, in severe cases, necrotic areas. Histopathologically the lesions, which consist of scattered glial nodules, perivascular cuffs, mild leptomeningitis and occasional areas of focal necrosis, are more often found in the cerebral cortex and to a lesser extent the brain stem and medulla.

Clinical features

Following an incubation period of 3–7 days features associated with acute encephalitis are observed. Brief 'flu-like' symptoms and primary viraemia, which follows the arthropod bite, are observed. The secondary phase is marked by fever and a secondary viraemia coinciding with CNS involvement. Clinical expression includes headache, fever and meningo-encephalitis, with upper motor neuronal signs and occasionally chorea. Neurological sequelae may occur, in which persistent seizures are observed. Onset of seizures may be rapid with no other signs of disease. Acute arthritis is observed with Tahyna virus, whereas respiratory system involvement is more commonly seen in Jamestown Canyon virus infections.

Diagnosis

Clinical diagnosis of La Crosse virus may be made as a result of localization of neurological lesions. Specific diagnosis is based on complement fixation (CF) or haemagglutination inhibition (HI) assays, although neutralization tests (NT) are also used. Artsob[39] has described an enzyme linked immunosorbent assay (ELISA) for serotyping. Isolations in suckling mice and Vero cells have been used for virus typing.

Prevention and control

To date no specific treatment for the California serogroup virus infections is available. Anticonvulsants are used to control seizures.

PHLEBOVIRUSES

RIFT VALLEY FEVER

History and epidemiology

Rift valley fever (RVF) virus is the most notable virus in the genus *Phlebovirus*. An epidemic outbreak of fever chills and myalgia in which a few people developed encephalitis was reported in Egypt in 1979.[40] Additional outbreaks have been observed throughout Africa, including Nigeria, Egypt, Sudan and Kenya. Over 20 species of mosquitoes have been implicated as possible vectors. *Culex pipiens*, *Cx. theileri*, *Ae. caballus* and other mosquitoes of the *Culex* and *Aedes* group may be involved. The major sources of reservoirs are animals such as sheep, cattle and goats, although camels and antelopes can be infected. Transmission of the virus from animal to animal during epidemics may result from biting flies.

Clinical features

RVF illness is biphasic. The primary phase is associated with fever, back and joint pains, and headaches that last about 1 week. After 1–2 days remission, the second phase consists of similar symptoms for 1–2 days, with nausea and sometimes a haemorrhagic diathesis with evidence of liver and renal damage. Occasionally disturbed vision, with evidence of a retinitis and cotton-wool exudates in the region of the macula, is observed. Altered levels of consciousness are observed with, in some cases, persistent fever. Meningeal irritation occurs, with focal motor signs and hallucination(s).[41]

Diagnosis

Identification of increasing levels of IgM specific antibodies in the CSF is used for the specific diagnosis.

Management

No specific treatment for Rift Valley fever exists, although a formalin-inactivated vaccine may be of use for laboratory workers.

CORONAVIRIDAE

Members of the Coronaviridae family are pleomorphic RNA viruses of 80–130 nm diameter which replicate within the cytoplasm. The family includes several animal viruses, including murine hepatitis virus known to induce demyelination in the CNS of infected mice and several human serotypes implicated in chronic bronchitis in adults.

History and epidemiology

The neurotropic strain of mouse hepatitis virus, JHM, was first isolated from a spontaneously paralysed mouse. The virus induces lesions of acute demyelination in the brain and spinal cord.[42] Virions are observed within the neurones. The relevance of this infection to human disease is the finding of coronaviruses in the brains of patients with multiple sclerosis.[43] Thus coronaviruses may be involved in the pathogenesis and aetiology of this human demyelinating disease.

FLAVIVIRIDAE

Formerly classified as Group B arboviruses the Flaviviridae were reclassified as an independent family by Westaway et al.[44] This family comprises the largest group of viruses known to induce CNS diseases and contains the yellow fever virus which, although not implicated in CNS disease, is the prototype virus, (*L. flavus* yellow). Flaviviruses are small icosahedral enveloped viruses which replicate and mature cytoplasmically, deriving the lipid envelope from the internal membrane of the host cell. Flaviviruses may be subdivided depending on the mode of transmission, i.e. mosquitoes or ticks (Table 38.5) and consist of approximately 66 viruses. Further serological subgroups may be distinguished on the basis of reactivity in HI and neutralization assays.[45]

JAPANESE ENCEPHALITIS

History

A disease resembling Japanese encephalitis (JE) was recorded as early as 1871. In 1935, an infectious

Table 38.5 Insect vector and examples of viruses in the family Flaviviridae.

Insect vector	Virus
Mosquito	Japanese B encephalitis (JE)
	West Nile (WN)
	St Louis encephalitis (SLE)
	Murray Valley encephalitis (MVE)
	Rocio virus
Tick	Tick-borne encephalitis (TBE), e.g. Russian spring–summer encephalitis (RSSE)
	Powassan encephalitis
	Louping ill
	Negishi

agent was recovered from the brain of a human in Tokyo and was virologically and serologically established as the prototype (Nakayama) strain. JE virus is the prototype of the JE antigenic complex. The complete nucleotide sequence of the JE viral genome has been determined.[46] Antigenic variations have been shown by antibody adsorption HI, CF, kinetic neutralization, agar gel diffusion and monoclonal antibody analysis.[47] At least two immunotypes have been identified: Nakayama and JaGAr01 (isolated from *Culex* mosquitoes). The virus replicates in a number of primary and continuous cell cultures of hamster, porcine, monkey, Vero and mosquito. JE virus produces a lethal encephalitis in infant mice by any route, whereas weanling mice succumb to intracerebral virus inoculation. Hamsters and monkeys die after intracerebral inoculation but develop asymptomatic viraemia after intraperitoneal inoculation. JE virus does not produce mortality in rabbits and guinea-pigs after inoculation by any route.

Epidemiology

JE continues to be the major type of encephalitis in eastern, south-eastern and southern Asia including Japan, Far East, Guam, the former USSR, Malaysia, India and Western Pacific Island areas.[48] In endemic areas, children are affected most, with attack rates in the 3–15-year age group 5–10 times higher than in older people because of the higher incidence of protective immunity in older age groups. Among factors which influence mortality are age, different virus strains and crossprotective immunity to other flaviviruses, especially dengue. The *Cx. tritaeniorhynchus* and *Cx. vishnui* mosquitoes are the most important vectors.[49] Other species of *Culex*, *Aedes*, *Anopheles* and *Mansonia* have been implicated. Pigs and many birds, including herons and egrets, may be the chief source of virus. Other domestic animals can get infected and humans may play a part in epidemics.

Clinical illness

Clinical illness is characterized by headache, fever and other signs of meningitis. Convulsions occur in children. Upper motor neurone involvement with extrapyramidal disturbances is a feature of this disease. Mortality rate of those with meningoencephalitis is around 20% in children and up to 50% in those over 50 years old. Motor and psychological disturbances are common sequelae.[50]

Pathogenesis and pathology

Pathogenicity in mice varies with different strains of JE virus. During the acute stage oedema and small haemorrhages are found in the brain. Destruction of cerebellar Purkinje cells may occur. Lesions include neuronal degeneration and necrosis, glial nodules and perivascular inflammation. These changes occur mainly in grey matter and predominantly affect diencephalic, mesencephalic and brain stem structures. In the extraneural tissue a variety of pathological features, including hyperplasia of germinal centres of lymph nodes, enlargement of malpighian bodies in spleen, interstitial myocarditis and focal haemorrhages in the kidneys, are seen. Transplacental infection in swine results in abortion and stillbirth. Pregnant mice inoculated intraperitoneally also transmit JE virus to the fetus, with subsequent abortion.[51]

Diagnosis

The IgM-capture ELISA is especially well suited for diagnosis by detection of locally synthesized antibody in the CSF.[52] The HI, CF assays and NT are applicable.

Prevention and control

Vaccination

Formalin-inactivated vaccines for use in humans are prepared from infected adult mouse brains or infected primary hamster kidney cell cultures in Japan and China, respectively.[53,54] Primary immunization requires two doses at a 7–14-day interval. Booster vaccinations are given during the first year after primary immunization and then at 3–4-year intervals. A bivalent vaccine has been developed incorporating Nakayama and JaGAr-01 (the two subtypes of JE virus). This vaccine has also proved to be effective. Vaccination of horses with formalin-inactivated vaccines has been successful.

Vector control

Use of pesticides in rice growing areas have reduced populations of *Cx. tritaeniorhynchus*. Spraying of residual insecticides in livestock pens have reduced the case incidence in China.[55]

Treatment consists of good general management and nursing care, especially in the semicomatose and comatose patient. Hyponaetremia secondary to inappropriate antidiuretic hormone secretion is managed with water restriction. Elevations in intracranial pressure should be considered in severely ill patients with deepening coma and loss of brain stem reflexes. Anticonvulsant therapy may be required.

WEST NILE VIRUS

Epidemiology

This virus is distributed in Africa, Europe and Asia.[56] It has a mosquito as a vector. *Culex* species and other ornithophilic mosquitoes are involved. Birds, including domestic poultry, are the reservoirs.

Clinical illness

The symptoms presenting include: fever, headaches, retrobulbar and muscular pain, sore throat, nausea and vomiting. Development of maculopapular rash on the trunk, face and limbs may be seen. Occasionally arthralgia may occur. The disease is usually mild in the young but in older age groups a second phase with mild meningoencephalitis can develop with no sequelae.

ST LOUIS ENCEPHALITIS VIRUS

History

St Louis encephalitis (SLE) virus was first identified in Illinois in 1932 and associated with human disease. The virus was later isolated from monkeys previously infected with human brain tissue. SLE virus is transmitted by the mosquitoes *Cx. tarsalis* and *Cx. pipiens*, giving rise to one of the most common and important epidemic arbovirus infections in the USA. Since the 1930s numerous outbreaks have been described in Texas,[57] Ohio and Florida.[58]

Epidemiology

SLE in central USA is commonly dependent on *Cx. pipiens* and *Cx. quinquefasciatus* whereas in Florida *Cx. nigripalpus* is the principal vector. In western USA *Cx. tarsalis* is the major vector. Epidemic outbreaks appear every 10 years and appear to be dependent on the breeding of *Cx. pipiens*. Disease occurs in late summer and early autumn and the number of affected humans ranges from 0.1 to 8%.

Clinical illness

SLE induces febrile headache, aseptic meningitis and encephalitis. Although persons of all ages are affected, morbidity and mortality is seen more commonly in the elderly. Following a 3–4-day incubation a generalized illness is observed, with malaise, fever, myalgia, headache and vomiting.[59] After a similar period the symptoms may resolve or progress to clinical findings indicative of neurological involvement. Of those patients with neurological signs 50% die within 7 days of exhibiting signs and a further 30% succumb in the second week. Many patients surviving neurological involvement have persistent headaches and memory loss and others have overt neurological sequelae such as speech or sensory disturbances.

Diagnosis

Patients exhibiting signs of encephalitis in SLE endemic areas, particularly in late summer and early autumn, should be investigated for SLE. Virus isolation from biological specimens such as blood and urine may be difficult, although virus has been isolated from brain tissue. Confirmation of SLE infection is made by HI or CF tests. IgM-capture ELISA is useful for diagnosis.

Prevention and control

There is no specific treatment or vaccine for SLE. Education of individuals within infected areas and vector control has been shown to be useful following detection of SLE virus activity.

MURRAY VALLEY ENCEPHALITIS

History

In 1917 and 1918 an infectious agent was isolated following inoculation of monkeys.[60] In 1951 Murray Valley encephalitis (MVE) virus was first isolated from human brain following an outbreak of disease and referred to Australian X disease. MVE virus is a member of the JE antigenic complex.

This virus can be propagated in various cell lines, including primary chick embryo and continuous lines of pig kidney, monkey kidney and hamster kidney cells. Immune enhancement of virus growth has been shown in primary chick embryo fibroblast cultures mediated by a subpopulation of macrophages having Fc receptors.[61]

The host range of MVE is wide. Monkeys, horses,

sheep and some birds develop encephalitis after intracerebral (i.c.) inoculation. Pigeons and chickens infected subcutaneously develop viraemic infections without clinical illness.

Epidemiology

MVE virus is found in Australia and Papua New Guinea.[62] *Cx. annulirostris* is the major mosquito vector. *Ae. normanensis* may be involved. Birds, including herons, cormorants and other water birds, are the major reservoir of this virus.

Clinical illness

Onset is sudden with headaches, fever and symptoms of a meningoencephalitis. Paresis of both upper and lower motor neurones may occur and breathing and swallowing may become impaired. With modern intensive care the fatalities are reduced dramatically to 20%. However, as a result of increased survivors, the number of people with both upper and lower motor neurone and psychiatric sequelae has increased.[63]

Prevention and control

No specific treatment for MVE exists. Vector control is as with other members of this family and massive insecticide programmes are deployed when vector breeding is increased.

ROCIO ENCEPHALITIS

Rocio (ROC) virus is typical of flaviviruses, being spherically shaped with a diameter of 43 nm and crossreacting with other members of the group, i.e. SLE, Ilheus, JE and MVE virus. Infection of mice, either intraperitoneally (i.c.) or i.c. in hamsters induces encephalitis and death.

History

In March 1975 an outbreak of encephalitis was recorded in São Paulo, south-east Brazil, from which an epidemic spread; between March and June 1975 465 cases with 61 deaths were recorded.[64] The majority of those affected were workers who frequented the forest areas; this was thus suggestive of an arbovirus infection. In 1975 an unknown arbovirus was isolated from the cerebellum and spinal cord of a 39-year-old farmer and referred to as Rocio virus.[65] Further analysis identified 47 arbovirus isolates in an area previously unknown for arbovirus infections.

Epidemiology

Outbreaks in neighbouring areas followed the 1975–1976 epidemic which affected 18 counties. The disease spread south in 1977. The epidemic peaks followed seasonal parameters which favoured the increased population of mosquitoes.

Pathogenesis

The pathology has been detailed by Rosenberg.[66] Interstitial mononuclear infiltration, microglial proliferation and perivascular cuffing are observed. In acute disease neuronophagia is evident with a distinctive topographical pattern in which the dentate nucleus is more susceptible and the brain stem less so.

Clinical diagnosis

In humans the incubation period is between 7 and 14 days. The clinical features include headache, fever, vomiting, anorexia, nausea, hyperaemia of the oropharynx and conjunctivae and photophobia. Involvement of the CNS has been detailed by Tiriba et al.[67] These include meningeal irritation, alteration in consciousness, motor abnormalities and abnormalities in cranial nerve functions.

Diagnosis

Epidemiological background and clinical history is paramount. Diagnosis is by cytochemical analysis of the CSF and isolation of the virus in 2-day-old mice from infected tissue. Haemagglutination, CF and plaque reduction techniques in Vero cells, IgM antibody-capture ELISA and ultimately histological examination confirm infection.

Prevention and control

The use of larvicides in ditches and flooded areas and sanitary measures to drain stagnant waters have decreased the incidence of infection. Formalin-treated extract of infected mouse brain is used as a vaccine.

TICK-BORNE ENCEPHALITIS

The tick-borne encephalitis (TBE) virus complex consists of 14 antigenically closely related viruses, eight of which cause human disease. Russian spring–summer encephalitis (RSSE) and Central European encephalitis virus (CEE) are very closely related antigenically and are considered to be subtypes of the same virus. They are separated on the basis of kinetic HI and CF tests and at the molecular level.[68] Peptide maps of both the E and the largest non-structural protein (NS5) of the two subtypes show some differences.

TBE complex viruses grow in a variety of cell cultures, including pig, bovine and chick embryo, HeLa, human amnion, Hep 2, Vero and primary reptilian and amphibian cells.[69] Cytopathic effect and plaquing are variable. TBE viruses cause encephalitis in rats, guinea-pigs, sheep, monkeys and swine after i.c. inoculation. Infant and weanling mice develop fatal encephalitis by all routes of inoculations. Experimental inoculation of wild vertebrate species, including rodents, foxes, birds, hares and bats, results in viraemia and antibody formation. Cows, goats and sheep infected by inoculation or tick bite develop viraemia and secrete virus in their milk. The Far Eastern virus type (RSSE) is more virulent for sheep and monkeys inoculated intracerebrally than the Western (CEE) virus.[70]

Epidemiology

TBE encompasses a wide area including Siberia across to Scandinavia, through Vienna into Belgium, to Scotland and Northern Ireland, across Canada, the USA and Japan. The disease occurs in areas which are favourable for ticks. The virus is maintained in nature in a cycle involving ticks and wild vertebrate hosts. Small rodents such as shrews, moles and hedgehogs are believed to be important reservoirs. Large mammals, such as goats, sheep and cattle, serve as host for adult *Ixodes* ticks. *I. ricinus* and *I. persulcatus* are responsible for transmission in Europe and the former Soviet Union, respectively.[71] Other tick species, of the genera *Dermacentor* and *Haemaphysalis*, have been implicated in transmission, especially in areas that do not support *Ixodes* ticks.

Transmission to humans occurs mainly in adults over 20 years old who come in contact with infected animals. The disease occurs in two peaks (May–June and September–October) coinciding with the activity of adult *Ixodes* ticks. Small outbreaks involving all age groups result from consumption of raw sheep or goat's milk or cheese.

Pathology and pathogenesis

In monkeys the anterior horn cells of the spinal cord and cerebellar cortex appear to be more affected than other neuronal cells. Members of the TBE complex cause persistent infection in experimental animals. For instance, CEE virus has been isolated from monkey tissues by cocultivation and explant techniques long after infection. Mice infected with Kyasanur Forest virus are shown to survive for months, with paralysis, low titres of virus in the brain and absence of detectable neutralizing antibodies.[72] Monkeys infected with TBE complex develop a chronic encephalitis with degenerative spongiform lesions and astrocytic proliferation.[73] Chronic progressive human encephalitis and seizure disorders have been associated with RSSE virus.[74]

Histopathology consists of meningeal and perivascular inflammation, neuronal degeneration and necrosis and glial nodule formation in areas such as cerebellar cortex, brain stem, basal ganglia, cerebrum and spinal cord. The anterior horn cells of the cervical cord are especially vulnerable, which may result in the lower motor neurone paralysis seen in many cases.

Clinical features

The clinical characteristics of TBE infection in humans has been described by Radsel-Medvescek et al.[75] Most of the tick-borne viruses have been associated with human diseases but there is a gradation of virulence. The Far Eastern (Siberian) strains (formerly called Russian spring–summer encephalitis virus) cause severe encephalitis, often with bulbar and cervical cord involvement, a high fatality rate and frequent sequelae. The disease seen in Central Europe is frequently biphasic, with influenza-like symptoms and signs of mild encephalitis. The strains found in Scotland and Northern Ireland cause a sheep disease called louping ill, which is characterized by cerebellar ataxia.

Diagnosis and investigation

Definitive diagnosis depends on virus isolation or serology. The virus may be isolated from the blood during the first phase of illness and from brain tissue of patients dying early in the infection. Suckling mice, embryonated eggs and chick embryo cell cultures (with detection of virus by interference assay or immunofluorescence) have been used for virus isolation. Serological diagnosis including HI, CF, single radial haemolysis and NT have been used. Diagnosis by estimation of IgM antibodies is valuable for rapid diagnosis and is applicable to both serum and CSF.

Prevention and control

In the former USSR, formalin-inactivated mouse brain vaccines were used before World War II (1939–45). Recently vaccines have been produced in embryonated eggs or chick embryo cell cultures. However, the most effective vaccine is derived from chick embryo cell culture-grown virus which is highly purified and inactivated by formalin.[76] The vaccine produces serological conversions in over 95% of recipients and has provided 99% protection in field trials. Preventative measures include pasteurization or boiling of raw milk, avoidance of tick bite by use of repellents and protective clothing.

HERPETOVIRIDAE

Herpesviruses are double-stranded DNA viruses approximately 100–110nm in diameter and are able to establish latency and reactivation. Of the nearly 100 herpesviruses that have been at least partially characterized, the following have been isolated from humans:

- Herpes simplex virus 1 (HSV-1)
- Herpes simplex virus 2 (HSV-2)
- Human cytomegalovirus (HCMV)
- Varicella-zoster virus (VZV)
- Epstein–Barr virus (EBV)
- Human herpesvirus 6 (HHV6)
- Human herpesvirus 7 (HHV7)

The simian herpesvirus, B virus (*Crypotetia crypta*), is also known to result in CNS disturbances in humans.

For further details the reader is referred to Roizman[77] and Whitley and Schlitt.[78]

HERPES SIMPLEX VIRUS

History

Infections caused by HSV have been known since the time of ancient Greece where the name herpes was used to mean 'creep' or 'crawl' and probably described the spreading nature of some of the skin lesions resulting from infections. Mouth ulcers and lip vesicles associated with fever were referred to as *herpes febralis* by the Roman scholar Herodotus. It was only later that herpetic lesions and genital infections were associated and by the late nineteenth century the vesicular nature of the lesions were characterized. Histological descriptions of herpes infections were identified in the early twentieth century. The infectious nature of herpesvirus was shown by Lowenstein in 1919: lesions on the rabbit cornea were induced by extracts obtained from a human with herpes simplex.[79] Furthermore such experiments also showed that material from the lesions of herpes induced encephalitis.[80] The recurrent nature of HSV was first described in the 1930s and Nahmias and Dowdle[81] identified two antigenic types of HSV, which were later referred to as HSV-1, pertaining to infections 'above the belt', and HSV-2 to those 'below the belt', i.e. genital infections. Major advances in antiviral therapy and molecular biology have allowed the rapid elucidation of the replication of these viruses and the subsequent control of infection.

Epidemiology

Herpes simplex viruses are distributed worldwide and since animal vectors have not been described humans are deemed to be the sole reservoir for transmission from individuals to susceptible hosts during close personal contact. There is no seasonal variation in infections and because of the nature of infection it is estimated that over one-third of the world population is infected. Antibody prevalence studies have demonstrated that geographical location, socioeconomic status and age influence the frequency of infections.

Pathogenesis

The pathogenesis of both HSV types is unclear, although it is apparent that both primary and recurrent HSV infection may result in CNS disease. Experiment has shown that HSV gains entry to the CNS via the olfactory and trigeminal nerves,[82] although whether this occurs in humans is unknown. Whether HSV is reactivated within the CNS to result in recurrent disease episodes is also unknown.

Pathology

Acute necrotizing encephalitis is the most common type of acute encephalitis and is observed in all age groups, with the exception of young children. The gross appearance of the brain in adults shows acute inflammation, congestion and softening of the brain. The necrosis is widespread and asymmetrical, predominantly associated with the temporal lobes. The necrotic tissue is sometimes haemorrhagic. In patients who survive for more than several weeks the tissue starts to disintegrate. Severe microglial reactivity is observed and in cases of disseminated HSV infection mononuclear infiltrates and perivascular cuffing are observed. Viral inclusion bodies may be detected in the nuclei of neurones and to a lesser extent the oligodendrocytes and astrocytes.

Clinical features

The effects of herpes simplex encephalitis on the CNS vary with the type of infection. Patients present with the sudden onset of an acute febrile encephalitic illness characterized by headaches, confusion and meningeal irritation. This is rapidly followed by a deterioration in consciousness and may include focal epilepsy and focal motor neurological signs. Disseminated HSV infection is commonly observed in neonates and related to HSV-2.

Diagnosis

Patients presenting with neurological involvement and suspected herpes simplex encephalitis may be evaluated by scanning procedures such as computerized tomography or magnetic resonance imaging, together with CSF analysis. Imaging often shows evidence of oedema and midline shift in cortical structures. However virus isolation remains the definitive diagnosis for HSV and allows for typing of the virus. In cases of encephalitis a brain biopsy is necessary to establish diagnosis and eliminate conditions that mimic HSV encephalitis. The most commonly used tests are CF, NT and ELISA.[82] The development of DNA amplification assays will be of value in that non-invasive diagnostic procedures may be carried out on CSF samples to avoid biopsy.

Management

Due to the high risk of infection during birth in women with active genital HSV, infants born to such mothers should be isolated and cultures obtained after birth and repeated at intervals to exclude infection, otherwise therapy should be administered.

Prevention and control

HSV infections may be controlled by avoidance of infectious secretions, vaccination or antiviral therapy. Patients thus presenting with obvious HSV sores should avoid contact with persons at risk, particularly neonates.

The antiviral agents vidarabine and acyclovir have proved useful in the therapy of HSV encephalitis, although the outcome is dependent on factors of age, level of consciousness and disease duration. Such agents have also been suggested to be of use prophylactically for the newborn and for women at the onset of labour.[82]

Vaccination remains the preferred method for the prevention of virus infection, although recurrent episodes of infection occur in the presence of antibody and this introduces problems. However protection from life-threatening infections has been achieved in experimental animal models.[83]

VARICELLA-ZOSTER VIRUS

History

VZV causes two distinct diseases: chickenpox and 'shingles'. Chickenpox (varicella) is the primary disease, generally of children, that results in a highly contagious, generalized exanthem which occurs in epidemics. (The disease should not be confused with smallpox (variola) with which there is no relation.) The name 'chickenpox' is thought to be derived from the French *chich* (chickpea), referring to the appearance of the vesicle or pox. Shingles (herpes zoster) is a less common disease that occurs in immunocompromised or older individuals and is characterized by dermatomal vesicular rashes. *Herpes zoster* is regarded as a secondary infection associated with the reactivation of VZV that has remained latent since an earlier attack of varicella. The name 'shingles' is derived from the Latin *cingulum*, meaning girdle, which is the appearance of the lesions on the dermatome.

The association between varicella and zoster was described in 1888 by von Bókay[84] who noted the appearance of chickenpox in a family after exposure to zoster. Furthermore, serological testing could not distinguish between the viruses and the ultimate confirmation came from studies by Weller and Stoddard[85] who isolated virus from varicella lesions and zoster lesions and determined that the recovered viruses were identical.

Epidemiology

Varicella is endemic in the population and becomes epidemic during late winter and early spring. The disease affects 90% of children under the age of 10. Intimate contact is necessary for infection. In contrast zoster infections are a consequence of reactivation of VZV. Patients at greatest risk are those with Hodgkin's and non-Hodgkin's lymphoma and immunosuppressive conditions such as the acquired immune deficiency syndrome (AIDS). The incidence of CNS complications following varicella is unknown but has been reported at between 0.1 and 0.75%.[86] In contrast, the incidence of encephalitis following zoster is much higher, particularly in immunosuppressed patients.

Pathogenesis

Primary infection with VZV results from respiratory droplet transmission. The virus enters the mucosa of the upper respiratory tract, and to a lesser extent the conjunctiva, and disseminates via the blood. Cycles of replication occur, giving rise to a secondary viraemia from which the virus becomes widespread before the formation of cutaneous lesions. The complications of neurological involvement following varicella infection are classified into (1) cerebellar ataxia, (2) generalized meningoencephalitis, (3) transverse myelitis, and (4) aseptic meningitis. The pathogenesis of these conditions is unknown, although immunological mechanisms of tissue damage, as a result of infection, have been suggested.[87]

In general the CNS involvement following zoster infections is associated with higher mortality than varicella. Complications following infection include encephalitis, ophthalmic zoster, myelitis, multifocal leucoencephalopathy, Guillain–Barré syndrome and cranial and peripheral nerve palsies. VZV has been isolated from several patients with zoster encephalitis, and inclusions have been found in the glial cells and neurones. Antiviral antibodies have been demonstrated in the CSF of such patients.[88]

Pathology

The neuropathological changes observed in varicella or zoster virus infections depend on the complication induced. In fatal varicella encephalitis mononuclear infiltration and demyelination have been reported.[89] A more detailed pathology has been reported for zoster complications due to the higher incidence of mortality. Zoster meningoencephalitis includes mononuclear infiltration of the meninges, necrosis and axonal degeneration. Degeneration may also involve the posterior columns where neurophagia is observed.

Clinical features

Varicella

The incubation period in children is between 14 and 15 days and is associated with malaise and mild fever. Anorexia and a sore throat are additional clinical features of adult varicella infection. The rash proceeds to the characteristic vesicles which crust. CNS involvement occurs more often in children who present with cerebellar ataxia a few days after the onset of the rash.[86]

Zoster

The rash of zoster is preceded with pain in the dermatome affected. The lesions, which resemble varicella, appear unilaterally and generally do not cross the midline. Crusts appear up to a week after eruption and last for approximately 2 weeks. Neurological complications of zoster may precede the appearance of the rash or appear as late as 10 months afterwards.[90] Further complications are observed in immunosuppressed patients as a result of persistence of virus within the CNS.

Diagnosis

The onset of neurological signs concomitant with the appearance of varicella or zoster rash would suggest such infection of the CNS. However infection is not usually verified by virus isolation from the brain tissue, the exception being at necropsy. Serological assessment utilizes CF, immunofluorescence, ELISA and radioimmunoassays.[91]

Prevention and control

There is generally no specific treatment, aside from antipyretics (not aspirin), for varicella in the immunocompetent host. Neurological complications of varicella, particularly in the immunocompromised host, are important because of the high morbidity and mortality. Although α-interferon is effective, two nucleoside analogues, vidarabine and acyclovir, are also employed, although side-effects have been reported. The possibility that immune-mediated reactions contribute to the CNS manifestations has given rise to the use of corticosteroids as a treatment of CNS involvement. In contrast, since evidence suggests active viral replication within the CNS, it would appear that antiviral agents should be employed.

EPSTEIN–BARR VIRUS (See also Chapter 32)

EBV infections are known to give rise to several CNS complications, such as meningoencephalomyelitis, encephalitis and neuropsychiatric syndromes,[92] however the frequency of such manifestations is extremely low. The more usual association is that of Guillian–Barré syndrome. The CSF of patients with CNS disorders following EBV infection shows an increased protein level.

In patients dying from EBV infection the CNS is more often affected and shows perivascular cuffing, oedema and demyelination.

CERCOPITHECINE HERPESVIRUS 1 (B VIRUS)

The non-human primate cercopithecine herpesvirus 1 (B virus) is highly pathogenic to humans. Originally transmitted by the bite of rhesus or macaque monkeys the virus is now thought to be transmitted from person to person.

History

In 1932, following the bite from a monkey, a physician developed a localized reaction, lymphangitis, lymphadenitis and transverse myelitis and died.[93] The virus was subsequently recovered from the CNS of the patient[94] and found to be lethal to rabbits following injection.

Epidemiology

The B virus is indigenous to Old World monkeys. Although B virus has only been reported in 22 human cases and is generally transmitted via a bite, individuals in Florida have been affected (two fatally), suggesting person-to-person spread of the virus.[95] Virus is secreted in the saliva and stools of infected animals and these must therefore be considered as potential sources of infection for humans.

Pathogenesis

After the bite a local reaction occurs, followed by lymph node involvement. The course of the disease is dependent on the route of inoculation (as deter-

mined from animal studies), although transverse myelitis is a prominent neurological finding before invasion of the CNS. As with other herpesviruses the B virus becomes latent and may be reactivated under certain conditions.[96] Virus spread to the brain is suggested to occur via the neural routes, as with HSV.

Pathology

All regions of the brain may be infected by B virus and show haemorrhagic foci, necrosis and inflammation in the form of perivascular cuffing of mononuclear cells.[97] Motor neurones are affected and show degeneration. Astrocytosis is observed, with gliosis.

Clinical features

Incubation of B virus varies from 2–3 to 24 days. The neurological involvement is observed after 3–7 days of the appearance of the vesicular rash. Death may ensue within 10–14 days, although the progression of the disease depends on the age, site of bite and immunological status of the patient. Clinically the patients present with a localized inflammatory reaction at the site of the bite, or with a respiratory illness, as has been described in two individuals.

Diagnosis

Although serological tests demonstrate the presence of B virus a significant problem is the crossreactivity with HSV antigens. Diagnosis must thus be dependent on the isolation of virus, particularly from the CSF of humans suspected of being infected, and the use of cell lines susceptible to B virus. These include rabbit kidney cells or cell lines such as BSC or LLC-RK1. Definitive diagnosis may be made using molecular methods[98] and neutralization of isolates in serological assays.

Prevention and treatment

Procedures which limit the transmission of the virus should be adhered to. These include limited contact with Macaque monkeys and the routine screening of such animals. The use of hyperimmune serum has not proved effective in controlling human infection, although some success has been achieved in experimental infections.[99]

Antiviral therapy has concentrated on the nucleoside analogues: vidarabine, acyclovir and ganciclovir. The use of acyclovir in humans has been reported to slow the infection.[100]

ORTHOMYXOVIRIDAE

Orthomyxoviruses are large enveloped RNA viruses and consist of the influenza viruses which infect swine, horses, seals and a large variety of birds as well as humans.[101] Genetic reassortment produces subtypes which give rise to epidemics of highly contagious, acute respiratory illness afflicting humans.

Epidemiology

Influenza viruses are unique among the respiratory tract viruses in that they undergo significant antigenic variation. Antigenic drift involves minor antigenic changes in haemagglutinin and neuraminidase.

Pathogenesis and pathology

A wide spectrum of CNS involvement has been shown during influenza A virus infection in humans,[102–105] ranging from irritability, drowsiness and confusion to more serious manifestations of psychosis and coma. There are two specific CNS syndromes: influenza encephalopathy and post-influenza encephalitis.

Encephalopathy occurs at the height of the influenza illness and may progress to death.[106,107] Histological changes are minimal. The CSF is usually normal and the brain shows severe congestion at autopsy. The postencephalitis syndrome is extremely rare and occurs from 2 to 3 weeks after recovery from influenza. The CSF findings suggest that inflammatory changes have occurred. Influenza A virus has only rarely been isolated from the brain or CSF.[104,108] It has been suggested that the syndrome of encephalitis lethargica followed by postencephalitic Parkinson's disease was associated with the influenza epidemics of 1918.[109]

Febrile convulsion may occur in children with and without underlying CNS abnormalities. Pregnant women in the second or third trimester have an increased risk of developing fatal influenza disease,[110,111] and increases in congenital abnormalities and haematological malignancies have been reported following influenza virus infection in pregnancy.[112,113] Toxic shock syndrome has been seen during influenza virus infection in humans and is believed to be the consequence of bacterial exotoxin secreted by a colonizing *Staphylococcus aureus* strain.[114]

Clinical features

Influenza A virus infections in avian species vary with the strain of the virus. Infection with most strains of influenza virus are asymptomatic. However some strains cause chronic respiratory infections and a minority lead to a rapidly fatal infection accompanied by CNS involvement, with death occurring within 1 week.

Prevention and control

Antiviral drugs

There are several antiviral drugs that are effective against influenza virus. Amantadine hydrochloride, which has a tricyclic structure, has antiviral properties against all subtypes of influenza A virus but not against influenza B or C viruses.[115,116] The antiviral activity of this drug is exerted after adsorption of the virus to cells but before primary transcription.[117,118] Amantadine and rimantadine, an analogue of amantadine, are useful for prophylaxis against H1N1, H2N2, and H3N2 influenza A virus infections in adults and children.[119] Ribavirin has an antiviral activity against influenza A and B viruses in tissue cultures and in mice but not in humans.[120,121] The antiviral activity is exerted after adsorption, penetration and uncoating have taken place.[122] Interferon induces resistance to influenza infection in mice but has no effect in humans. Preliminary studies with recombinant α-interferon indicate slight protection against illness and virus shedding.[123]

Vaccines

Inactivated influenza A and B virus vaccines are commonly used. The vaccines are either designated whole virus (WV) or split product (SP). The WV vaccines contain intact formalin-treated virus, while SP vaccines contain purified formalin-treated virus disrupted with chemicals that solubilize the lipid-containing viral envelope. In addition, experimental vaccines containing the isolated haemagglutinin (HA) and neuraminidase (NA) surface proteins are called subunit vaccines. Other types of vaccine are those which contain a monovalent influenza A H1N1 virus of a mixture of H1N1, H3N2 and B viruses.

PAPOVAVIRIDAE

The family Papovaviridae is divided into the two subfamilies: polyomaviruses and papillomaviruses which, although they share several properties, are not related immunologically or genetically.

POLYOMAVIRUSES

History

The first human disease associated with a polyoma-virus was a rare demyelinating disease of the CNS called progressive multifocal leucoencephalopathy (PML). The disease is observed in immunodeficient individuals and was suggested, in 1961, to be due to a common virus which in the immunocompromised host runs an atypical course of infection.[124] In 1971 two viruses implicated in PML were isolated from the brain (JC virus) of a patient with PML and the urine (BK virus) of a renal transplant patient.[125] JC and BK viruses are contracted in early childhood, persist in the host and are reactivated in cases of immunocompromise, such as in AIDS.

Epidemiology

Polyomaviruses are widely distributed in many species of animals, although they are generally species specific. BK and JC viruses do not naturally infect species other than man. Antibody titres to BK virus are acquired by 50% of children by 3 years of age and against JC virus by 50% at 6 years of age.[126] PML is worldwide in distribution and occurs as a complication in lymphoproliferative disorders, chronic disease such as sarcoidosis, in immunodeficiency diseases and in patients on long-term immunosuppressive therapy. Reactivation of both JC and BK viruses are also known to occur in pregnancy, diabetes, chronic disorders and old age. Approximately 20% of patients with PML have AIDS, whereas PML is reported to occur in as many as 3.8% of AIDS patients presenting with neurological disorders.[127]

Pathogenesis

Primary JC infections of healthy individuals are not associated with illness, although BK virus has been linked with mild respiratory illness. The mode of transmission of BK and JC viruses is unknown, although the rapid acquisition of antibodies has been suggested to be consistent with respiratory disorders. Following primary infection the virus remains latent in the kidney and is reactivated under immunosuppression.

Pathology

The PML brain is characterized by foci of demyeli-nation[128] that are widespread and vary in size. In advanced cases the areas may be necrotic. The lesions occur in the absence of inflammatory cells and are more frequent in the white matter of the cerebrum. Nuclear changes in the oligodendrocytes at the edge of the demyelinated plaques are associated with the presence of JC. The lesions are also marked with bizarre giant astrocytes and oligodendrocytes with enlarged nuclei which, at light microscopical level, are deeply basophilic and may contain inclusion bodies. Neurones are unaffected.

Clinical features

Symptoms of a multifocal brain disease without signs of raised intracranial pressure in an immunocompromised host suggest the diagnosis of PML.

Diagnosis

Computerized tomography or magnetic resonance imaging of the brain will detect lesions of demyelination. Verification of PML may be carried out following examination of brain tissue in which JC virus may be identified by electronmicroscopy, immunohistological identification in CNS sections, cultivation of the virus in fetal glial cells and characterization of viral DNA by in situ hybridization and PCR.[129]

Treatment and control

There is no certain treatment for PML, although the accepted regimen is to discontinue the immuno-suppressive therapy in combination with the use of antiviral drugs. Attempts at treatment with nucleic acid-based analogues have been attempted.

PARAMYXOVIRIDAE

The Paramyxoviridae family consists of negative-stranded enveloped RNA viruses. These viruses are classified into the three genera *Paramyxovirus*, *Morbillivirus* and *Pneumovirus* and include four important human pathogens: measles, mumps, para-influenza (types 1–4) and respiratory syncytial viruses.

MORBILLIVIRUSES

The *Morbillivirus* genus is important in that it contains the human neurotropic virus measles and the canine distemper virus.

MEASLES (See also Chapter 37)

History

Measles as a disease was first described by Sydenham in the early seventeenth century and the implication that this was a virus infection was established in the 1920s. The disease is generally a childhood illness and is not lethal, although it may be serious in the very young or elderly. Great epidemics of measles have been described, such as the 'black measles' of the eighteenth century. Waves of measles infection are occasionally observed, with the greatest incidence between November and March.

Epidemiology

In the less developed countries measles is the most important cause of death between the ages 1 and 5 years.[130] Death occurs predominantly from respiratory and CNS complications. Measles does not have animal reservoirs and no vectors are involved. The principal mode of transmission is via droplets of infected respiratory tract secretions inhaled as a consequence of face-to-face exposure.[131–133] However, air-borne transmission may be important in certain settings, including school, hospitals and other institutions.

Virus is present in respiratory secretions and in the conjunctivae during the latter part of the incubation period. Viraemia is also present during this time. Virus is present in the urine for 4 or more days after the onset of rash. Patients are considered infectious from the onset of symptoms through the fourth day of rash.[132,134] Maternal antibodies provide protection during the first 6 months of life and often longer. Cell-mediated immunity is required to clear measles virus infection, however both humoral and cell-mediated immunity appear to be capable of preventing infection in normal individuals infected with the virus. The slow infection of measles in humans, i.e. subacute sclerosing panencephalitis (SSPE) is a rare disease in which virus persists in the CNS. The incidence of SSPE is more common in males than females and it is more prevalent in rural areas. The average age of onset is between 5 and 15 years and infection with measles before the age of 15 increases the risk of developing SSPE. In the USA the mean annual incidence rate of SSPE was estimated at 0.06 cases per million (under age 20) in 1980.

Clinical features

Measles begins, after an incubation period of 8–12 days, with fever, malaise and anorexia followed by conjunctivitis and cough. The infection then spreads to the epithelial surfaces of the mouth, vasopharynx, respiratory tract and gastrointestinal tract.

Two to three days before the onset of the rash, Koplik's spots appear on the buccal mucosa.[135] Koplik's spots are small (1–3mm) irregular bright red spots, each of which has a minute bluish-white speck at its centre. The temperature reaches 39.4–40.6°C at the height of the eruption on the fifth day of the illness. The rash starts around day 3 or 4 of prodromal symptoms and spreads downward over the face, neck and trunk and continues downward until it reaches the feet by the third day. Cough and coryza follow as a result of an intense inflammatory reaction that involves the mucosa throughout the respiratory tract. The most common complications involve the middle ear, CNS, eyes and the skin.[136,137]

There are three forms of measles encephalitis. Acute postinfectious measles encephalitis is the most common neurological complication of measles. Children under the age of 2 are rarely affected but it occurs in older children in the ratio of 1 in 1000. It appears a short time after the rash. Between 10 and 20% die and the majority of the survivors have some neurological sequelae. Histopathology shows perivascular inflammatory changes and demyelination.

A second form of measles encephalitis, acute progressive infectious encephalitis, occurs in immunosuppressed patients following exposure to measles.[138,139] Seizures, motor and sensory deficits and lethargy occur. In the absence of normal cell-bound immunity, unrestricted cytolytic replication of the virus occurs.

The third form of measles encephalitis is a rare late complication of measles. The symptoms develop over months, reflecting loss of cerebral cortical function.[140,141] In the early stage subtle mental changes and diminishing intellectual capacity are seen. Later, myoclonic jerks occur and progress to chorioathetosis, ataxia and finally coma. Focal retinitis occurs in the majority of the cases leading to blindness.

Pathogenesis and pathology

Measles virus replicates initially in the respiratory mucosa and spreads, perhaps carried intracellularly in pulmonary macrophages and other cells, to draining lymph nodes where further replication occurs. Virus then enters the bloodstream and from here dissemination of the virus throughout the reticuloendothelial system takes place. This results in a secondary viraemia that disseminates the infection to tissues throughout the body.

The most striking feature of measles virus infection in vivo and in vitro is the formation of multinucleated giant cells which result from the fusion of infected cells with the adjacent cells.[142,143] In tissue culture these giant cells contain eosinophilic cytoplasmic inclusion bodies and their nuclei show condensation of chromatin at the nuclear membrane.

The CNS of patients with SSPE shows inflammation of meninges and perivascular cuffing in both grey and white matter. In the later stages of disease demyelination and gliosis are observed. Although the mechanisms of myelin damage are unknown it may be a result of either neural damage or the involvement of an autoimmune response since T lymphocyte reactivity to the myelin constituent, myelin basic protein, has been observed.[144]

Diagnosis

Most measles infections are easily recognizable by the distinctive Koplik's spots, rash and catarrhal symptoms. Effective tests for laboratory diagnosis are available and include virus isolation in primary human or monkey cells and antibody determination by simple HI test and by ELISA.[145,146] Serological tests are effective in identifying cases of SSPE. Patients with this disease have increased serum antibody titres which are 10–100 times higher than those seen in late convalescent-phase sera. There is also a pronounced local production of oligoclonal measles virus antibodies in the CNS.[147] Viral antigen can be identified by immunofluorescence.

Treatment

No effective treatment is available although in vitro measles virus replication is sensitive to interferon and ribavirin treatment.

Prevention and control

No treatment is presently available but pooled immunoglobulin can be administered for postexposure prophylaxis up to 5 days after exposure.

Live attenuated vaccines are widely used. The rate of seroconversion after vaccination exceeds 90%. Vaccine complications are very rare. Encephalitis occurs at the same rate as in non-vaccinated individuals and the frequency of occurrence of SSPE is reduced by a factor of at least 10 in vaccinated persons.[148,149]

CANINE DISTEMPER VIRUS

Canine distemper virus (CDV) deserves mention in this chapter because of its relationship with measles virus and implication in the human neurological disease multiple sclerosis. This virus gives rise to a chronic relapsing disease of dogs in which demyelination lesions are observed.[150] Furthermore several studies have suggested associations between the incidence of multiple sclerosis and canine distemper in the dog population.[151]

PARAMYXOVIRUSES

MUMPS

History

Mumps has been recognized from the fifth century BC when Hippocrates described the disease as one of swellings behind the ears accompanied by swelling of the testes. However the first description of neurological involvement was that by Hamilton[152] in the eighteenth century. Transfer of disease from filtered secretions of an affected patient into experimental animals suggested the disease had a viral aetiology.

Epidemiology

Mumps infection increases in the winter months. Immunity to mumps is usually acquired between the ages of 5 and 14, with maximal humoral antibody occurring between 4 and 7 years of age.[153,154] Mortality from mumps is related primarily to the complications of meningitis/encephalitis and orchitis. These occur as age- and sex-specific hazards, with a peak risk in postpubertal males. The incidence of CSF pleocytosis is reported in 30% of patients with mumps parotitis, whereas encephalitis occurs in as many as 35% cases.[155]

Clinical features

The most characteristic feature of mumps is the swelling of the salivary glands which occurs in up to 95% of all symptomatic cases. The parotid glands are often involved. A moderate febrile response is present at the time of the disease onset. A wide variety of other organs have been involved and include the testes, CNS, epididymis, prostate, ovaries, liver, pancreas, spleen, thyroid, kidneys, eyes, thymus, heart and joints.

The onset of mumps meningitis is marked by fever, with vomiting, neck stiffness, headache and lethargy.[156] Seizures occur in 21–30% of patients with CNS symptoms. In cases of CNS involvement about one-third of all patients have evidence of intrathecal IgG synthesis and the presence of oligoclonal immunoglobulins during the first week of CNS symptoms.

Examination of the CSF shows abnormalities in the vast majority of the cases. The protein content in the CSF is markedly elevated in 60–70% of all the cases. This may be due to a damaged BBB, as indicated by high albumin indices that do not normalize for several weeks to months after the onset of the CNS symptoms. The CSF glucose content is depressed to 17–41% of the serum value in 6–29% of all cases.[157]

Pathogenesis and pathology

It has been suggested that the natural infection is initiated by droplet spread with primary viral replication in nasal mucosa or upper respiratory mucosal epithelium. The incubation period from exposure to first clinical symptoms is about 18 days. Virus is actively shed in saliva for as long as 6 days before the onset of symptoms. During this time it is likely that the virus multiplies in the upper respiratory mucosa and spreads to draining lymph nodes with subsequent transient plasma viraemia. Plasma viraemia is terminated by the developing humoral antibodies as early as 11 days after experimental infections of humans.[158]

Mumps virus has been shown to infect human lymphocytes in vitro and appears to preferentially infect activated cells of the T-lymphocyte subset. This could imply that cell-associated viraemia may be another mode of virus dissemination.

Viral replication in the parotid glands is accompanied by periductal interstitial oedema and a local inflammatory reaction involving lymphocytes and macrophages.[159] Once within neurones, virus is then able to distribute widely along neuronal pathways.

Viral invasion of the CNS occurs across the choroid plexus, although rarely is mumps meningoencephalitis fatal. CNS pathology is restricted to perivascular infiltration with mononuclear cells, scattered foci of neuronophagia and microglial rod cell proliferation.[160] Perivascular demyelination also occurs; this may be the result of an autoimmune attack on the brain tissue. Persistence of mumps virus has been suggested within the CNS of humans. Deafness is probably the result of direct damage to the cochlea and, to a lesser extent, cochlear neurones.[161] Most cases of mumps meningitis resolve without sequelae. However, ataxia and behavioural disturbances may be slow to resolve following mumps meningoencephalitis.[162–164]

Diagnosis

The clinical diagnosis of mumps is seldom problematic in the presence of parotitis. Laboratory diagnosis includes determination of virus-specific IgM and IgG levels. Mumps meningitis can be confirmed on the basis of elevated CSF serum antibody ratio.

Treatment and control

Hyperimmune γ-globulin to modify the course of mumps is used in selected cases. Two general types of vaccines have been used. The most widely used are the live attenuated mumps virus preparations; killed mumps virus antigens have a more restricted use.[165] Vaccination of susceptible children with a single subcutaneous inoculation of Jeryl Lynn B vaccine does not produce clinical symptoms, and vaccine virus cannot be isolated from blood, urine or saliva. Neutralizing antibody is usually measurable within 2 weeks of vaccination.[166]

PARVOVIRIDAE

To date parvoviruses have not been implicated in human CNS disease although infections of experimental animals with parvoviruses are known to induce cerebellar ataxia[167] and affect the development of the cerebellum during the perinatal period.

PICORNAVIRIDAE

The Picronaviridae family consists of small RNA viruses and comprises four genera: *Enterovirus*, *Rhinovirus*, *Aphthovirus* and *Cardiovirus*. Those involved in neurological disease are listed in Table 38.6.

ENTEROVIRUSES

Enteroviruses multiply throughout the alimentary tract and tend to be resistant to known antibiotics and chemotherapeutic agents. The host range of the enteroviruses is varied and may be readily induced to yield variants, which has led to the development of attenuated polio vaccine strains. The viruses of this genus, which are important CNS pathogens of humans, are the polio- and coxsackieviruses. For more detailed studies on enteroviruses the reader is referred to Melnick.[168]

POLIOVIRUS (See also Chapter 8)

History

The disease poliomyelitis has existed since ancient times although the fact that the causative agent was a virus was only first demonstrated in 1909 by Landsteiner and Popper[169] Studies in monkeys and the adaptation to tissue culture resulted in the development of methods of purification and the production of reliable vaccines through which infection can now be controlled. Poliomyelitis may be caused by one of three strains of virus: polio types 1, 2 or 3. Three forms of clinical disease have been recognized: paralysis, aseptic meningitis and minor febrile illness.

Epidemiology

Poliovirus was, until very recently, endemic worldwide, infecting susceptible infants and producing paralytic poliomyelitis in those that were not protected by maternal antibody. In 1916 80% of cases were in those under 5 years of age.[170] The change in sanitation and hygiene in the late nineteenth century, with industrialization in the north of Britain, decreased the incidence in infants but resulted in a higher incidence of paralytic poliomyelitis in later childhood due to delay in exposure to the virus. In the epidemics of 1950 the peak age was 5–9 years, although about one-third of cases and two-thirds of deaths were in those over 15 years.[168] Since 1985 most of the cases of polio worldwide have been in developing countries, although the number of

Table 38.6 Picornaviruses implicated in human neurological disease.

Genus	Virus	Disease
Enterovirus	Human polio	Paralysis, aseptic meningitis, febrile illness aseptic meningitis, paralysis
	Human coxsackie (groups A and B)	Aseptic meningitis, paralysis, meningoencephalomyelitis
	Echoviruses	Aseptic meningitis, paralysis, encephalitis, ataxia, or Guillain–Barré syndrome
	Enterovirus (types 70, 71)	Paralysis, meningoencephalitis
Cardiovirus	Encephalomyocarditis	

deaths due to other diseases may mask the true incidence of infantile paralysis.

Pathogenesis

Following ingestion poliovirus replicates in the pharynx and intestines, from which it is excreted. Transmission is by the faecal–oral route and thus the necessity for hygiene is paramount. After initial replication in the lymphoid tissue of the pharynx and gut, which leads to viraemia, the virus infects the CNS via the blood. Neural spread has been demonstrated in children following tonsillectomy.[168]

Pathology

The anterior horn cells of the spinal cord are susceptible to infection with poliovirus and are damaged or, in severe cases, completely destroyed.[171] The lesions observed in the CNS may extend to the hypothalamus and thalamus. Neuronophagia is commonly observed, with inflammation being secondary to neuronal attack. In less severe cases oedema, which results in temporary disturbance of neural functions, subsides and the cells recover completely.

Clinical features

Following infection approximately 1% of patients present with clinical disease. Abortive poliomyelitis is the most common form of the disease in which fever, malaise, drowsiness, headache and sore throat are experienced to varying degrees. The signs abate within a few days. Stiffness and pain in the back of the neck may also be experienced, in which case non-paralytic poliomyelitis, or aseptic meningitis, is diagnosed. The disease may become biphasic, whereby a minor illness is followed by a remission, but which subsequently develops into a major severe illness.

Diagnosis

Antibodies are usually present by the time paralysis occurs and a viraemia may be detected and used to determine the subtype using serological techniques.[172] More recently molecular biological techniques have been used to demonstrate poliovirus in CSF.

Prevention

In the early 1950s Jonas Salk calculated the inactivation kinetics of formalin on poliovirus grown in monkey kidney cells.[173] A vaccine was developed which was licensed in the USA in 1955, the aim of which was to induce protection by way of stimulating antibody production. Using the formalin-inactivated vaccine it was necessary to reimmunize at 1 and 6 months with successive boosters. The advance of cell culture techniques has enabled the production of large batches of virus and more effective vaccines. In contrast oral polio vaccines were developed using live attenuated virus which today consists of a mixture of three strains. The oral vaccine protects by producing both systemic antibody and local secretory IgA which would block virulent virus, preventing spread from the gut. These vaccines have the advantages over killed preparations of ease of administration and long-lasting immunity, although they have the 'disadvantage' of being excreted and thus have the potential to spread to non-vaccinated persons.[174]

COXSACKIE AND ECHOVIRUSES

Of the non-polio enterovirus infections echovirus 9 is the most frequent cause of enterovirus disease and the most common virus to be isolated in epidemics.

The chief viruses implicated in CNS disease are Coxsackie B1-6, A7 and A9, although many echoviruses have been associated with meningitis, as has enterovirus type 70. Severe CNS disease has been observed in enterovirus 71 infections, particularly in the severe epidemic of 1975 in Bulgaria.[175] Many polio encephalitic cases with meningitis were recorded, in which 21% developed paralysis. Antibodies to enterovirus 71 were detected in 72% of patients presenting with paralysis and virus isolations were made from numerous tissues including the CNS. Of the seven reported epidemics with enterovirus 71 all reported evidence of CNS involvement.[176]

POXVIRIDAE

Neurological complications of poxvirus infections are generally associated with vaccination, namely *postvaccinial encephalitis*. The pathogenesis and pathology resemble other postinfectious encephalitides and include perivascular cuffing, mononuclear infiltration and demyelination.

PRION DISEASES

Several so-called 'slow virus infections' of the CNS that are not a result of conventional virus infection, although transmissible, are classified as prion diseases or subacute spongiform encephalopathies. They are listed in Table 38.7.

These transmissible agents are thought to have a unique characteristic in being devoid of nucleic acid and yet able to transfer disease. Transmission of disease does not occur if the agents are treated with proteases. Additionally, attempts at molecular cloning are negative and nucleic acid antagonists have been shown to be ineffective. The name of the so called infectious agents, termed *prions*, is derived from *pro*tein and infec*tion*, meaning that the infectious agent is protein devoid of nucleic acid. This 'protein only' hypothesis is still under debate.

Of particular importance is the presence of a normal form of the protein found on all cells, particularly neurones. The two forms of prion proteins (PrP) (normal and infectious) are identical in terms of amino acid sequences but differ in their conformations. Furthermore the normal protein is broken down by enzymes, whereas the abnormal prion protein (PrP^{sc}) is resistant to attack by enzymes and only found in the CNS during disease where the protein accumulates in the cell.

KURU

Kuru was restricted to the population of villages in the highland of Papua New Guinea. The disease, which means shaking or shivering in the Fore language, is characterized by tremors which progress to lack of motor control and complete cerebellar ataxia. The clinical course of the disease generally results in death within 1 year of onset, although prolonged disease has been reported. Kuru was described by Gajdusek.[177] The disease was more common in children and females than males and thought to be due to the practice of certain tribal rituals. The changes in ritual cannibalism and treatment of corpses has halted the contact of persons with infected brain tissue, resulting in a vistual cessation in the incidence of disease.

The pathological picture is restricted to the CNS and is characterized by diffuse neuronal degeneration and astrocytic hypertrophy.[178] The term 'spongiform encephalopathy' is derived from the large vacuolation of the large neurones of the striatum. In many cases amyloid-containing plaques are observed and electronmicroscopy reveals scrapie-associated fibrils common to other diseases in this group.

CREUTZFELDT–JAKOB DISEASE AND GERSTMANN–STRÄUSSLER–SCHEINKER SYNDROME

Patients with Creutzfeldt–Jakob disease (CJD) present with rapidly progressive dementia and motor dysfunction; like Kuru, it is usually fatal within 1–2 years following onset. The incidence of CJD is low (prevalence of 1 per million) and is generally sporadic, although there is evidence for a familial trait in 10% of all cases. Furthermore rare mutations in the natural PrP segregate with disease which may be linked with genetic predisposition.[179] The disease is transmissible experimentally, as

Table 38.7 Prion diseases of man and animals.

Host	Disease
Man	Kuru
	Creutzfeldt–Jakob disease
	Gerstmann–Sträussler–Scheinker syndrome
Animals	Scrapie
	Transmissible mink encephalopathy
	Chronic wasting disease of mule deer and elk
	Bovine spongiform encephalopathy

shown in laboratory animals,[180] or as a result of 'accidental transmission' to man following surgery.[181] Although the average age of CJD onset is in middle to late life the disease has been described in young (4–19-year-old) patients undergoing growth hormone therapy. In these transmissions the disease resembled Kuru rather than typical CJD and suggests that Kuru may have originated in New Guinea as a result of contamination of tissue from a patient with CJD.

Gerstmann–Sträussler–Scheinker syndrome (GSS) is a variant of CJD in which patients present with progressive cerebellar ataxia, giving rise to a longer period from onset to death compared with CJD. Again several mutations in the PrP have been described and the disease is transmissible to laboratory animals.

Prevention and control

The resistance of the CJD/GSS prion to common sterilization procedures, such as boiling or the use of ultraviolet light, has resulted in a change in operating procedures and the use of hypochlorate and sodium hydroxide for sterilization.[182] To date no treatment for the human diseases has been effective. Future therapeutic regimens will possibly include drugs that interfere with the PrP^{sc}, preventing it from accumulating in the cell, or gene therapy to switch off production of the protein.

ANIMAL PRION DISEASES

Scrapie was observed in the 1930s following the use of louping ill virus vaccine produced in scrapie-contaminated brain tissue, although the disease has been recognized in sheep breeders for over two centuries.[183] The disease is a chronic disease in which affected animals present with progressive ataxia tremor and wasting. The name 'scrapie' is derived from the necessity of animals to rub or scrape themselves as a result of the disease. Susceptibility to scrapie is dependent on the strain of sheep and is linked to polymorphisms in ovine PrP.

The disease, like the human prion infections, is characterized histologically by the presence of vacuolated neurones and spongiform changes and may be experimentally induced in laboratory mice and guinea-pigs. The use of transgenic mice, in which mutations in the PrP are deliberately introduced with resulting neurological defect, supports the role of this protein in initiating disease. Furthermore transgenic mice lacking the gene coding for the natural PrP are resistant to infection with the scrapie PrP.[184] The use of experimental prion disease has allowed the investigation of potential therapies and although no effective treatment is available the use of amphotericin B has been shown to reduce concentration of scrapie PrP during the preclinical phase and prolong the incubation period of the disease.[185]

Transmissible mink encephalopathy, which is very similar to scrapie, is spread through mink colonies as a result of fighting and cannibalism and is thought to have originated from contaminated food derived from cattle. Infected tissue can transfer disease. Likewise bovine spongiform encephalopathy, first described in England in 1986, is possibly a result of feeding scrapie-contaminated food.[186]

REOVIRIDAE

The family Reoviridae contains the three genera *Reovirus*, *Rotavirus* and *Orbivirus*. To date the first two are not known to be implicated in human neurological diseases.

ORBIVIRUSES

Many of the viruses of this genus are important in veterinary disease and produce illness in a wide variety of animals, including horse sickness and bluetongue disease.[187] The exception is the dengue-like illness of humans, Colorado tick fever.

COLORADO TICK FEVER

History

Colorado tick fever (CTF) was first described in the mid-nineteenth century in the Rocky Mountain states. Florio et al[188] isolated the virus from human blood and later demonstrated that CTF virus could be isolated from the tick *Dermacentor andersoni*.[189]

Epidemiology

This disease is confined to the geographical distribution of the adult *Dermacentor andersoni* tick[190] in the Rocky Mountain states and in parts of north-western Canada; it is a common infection in hikers and foresters during May and June.

Pathogenesis

Infection with CTF virus gives rise to little or no disease in the natural host and induces a prolonged or persistent viraemia in vertebrate hosts such as ground squirrels and chipmunks that serve as amplificatory rodents. CTF virus is involved in bone marrow precursor cells and its presence in erythrocyte precursors renders the host susceptible to haemorrhagic disorders.[191] The onset of disease occurs 3–6 days after the tick bite.

Pathology

CTF virus infections do not generally result in death and thus pathological features are not well described. However following experimental infections of mice the cerebellum shows widespread necrosis and cellular infiltration.

Clinical features

A febrile illness develops, with headache and myalgia. A macular papular rash is seen in about 50% of patients. Colorado tick fever is a benign disease but in very rare cases a bleeding diathesis may develop[192] and, particularly in children, there may be a typical meningoencephalitic illness. Resolution of the acute phase may last 5–10 days. Infection in the CNS may be observed as a mild meningeal reaction to severe encephalitis. The frequency of CNS involvement ranges from 1 to 10%.[193]

Diagnosis

Abnormalities include leucopenia and thrombocytopenia; virus may be isolated from the blood due to its persistence in the erythrocytes. Some time after disease onset CF and neutralizing antibodies may be detected in the blood. CSF findings are typical of encephalitis.

Prevention

At present there is no treatment for CTF, although health awareness when hiking in the affected areas may help to limit exposure to tick bites.

RETROVIRIDAE

Several features of retroviruses, such as their unique replication cycle, oncogenic ability and the wide variety of interactions with the host, including their ability to remain latent, have led to the intense scientific attention these viruses have received. Retroviruses are classified into the three subfamilies: Oncovirinae, Lentivirinae (lentiviruses, e.g. maedi-visna, which results in chronic inflammation of the CNS, and human immunodeficiency viruses which result neurologically in AIDS dementia and demyelination) and Spumavirinae.

uses in which neurological damage has been recognized.

MAEDI-VISNA

Maedi-visna (*maedi* laboured breathing; *visna* wasting and paralysis (Icelandic translations)) is the prototype lentivirus in which the slow onset of clinical disease resulting from prolonged incubation of the virus is very similar to the prion disease of sheep, i.e. scrapie.[194]

Epidemiology

The disease was first recognized in Iceland[195] but is observed in most countries with large sheep populations. Early transmission studies in Iceland showed that the disease could be transmitted from infected sheep to naive sheep by intracerebral inoculation. Many strains of visna have been obtained

LENTIVIRUSES

In contrast to those viruses which cause acute disease and where virus is finally eliminated, the lentiviruses include those which are able to escape such elimination and persist in the host. These include the maedi-visna of sheep that give rise to chronic neurological disorders, and human immunodeficiency vir-

which vary in their ability to, for example, be propagated in tissue culture.[196]

Pathogenesis

Virus is isolated from many tissues, particularly the lymphatics, spleen and peripheral blood leucocytes.[197] Higher titres are isolated from the brain and lung. Conversion of the maedi illness to visna may occur as a result of infected peripheral blood leucocytes crossing the BBB and subsequently infecting the CNS.

Pathology

Following experimental infection severe meningitis and encephalitis is observed, coinciding with perivascular lesions of inflammatory cells. The inflammatory cells observed in the CNS consist of monocytes/macrophages, plasma cells and T lymphocytes. Depending on the duration of the disease the brain may show large areas of focal demyelination. Additionally, inflammatory lesions and/or demyelination may occur in the presence of areas of necrosis and gliosis.[198,199]

Clinical features

Clinical disease is observed as lymphadenopathy, pneumonia and CNS involvement. The sheep appear dyspnoeic with loss of flesh. The appearance of clinical disease is dependent on the strain of animal and dose of inoculation.[200]

Prevention and control

Due to the expense of developing vaccines for animals very few studies on controlling infection have been attempted. However, sheep hyperimmunized with disrupted virus are known to develop neutralizing antibodies which were able to confer some protection against homologous virus infection.[200]

HUMAN IMMUNODEFICIENCY VIRUS (See also Chapter 12)

The human immunodeficiency viruses consist of HIV-1 and HIV-2 and are typical lentiviruses (Chapter 12). This chapter will only concentrate on the CNS disease in HIV infections. Details of other features are to be found elsewhere in this book and in other comprehensive articles.[201,202]

CNS disorders associated with HIV infections are important because they are commonly seen during all stages of the disease and contribute to the outcome of the disease. The variations in clinical manifestation are dependent on both the stage of HIV disease and opportunistic infections, whether viral, such as JC infection giving rise to PML, or bacterial, e.g. *Listeria monocytogenes* meningitis.

The gross clinical features observed in neurological complications of HIV infections have been outlined by Price et al[201] and are classified by the neuroanatomical localization, i.e. whether the brain or cord is involved and whether the lesions are focal or non-focal. With regard to the neurological complications, these may be categorized depending on the stage of the disease: (1) during acute HIV infection of the CNS; (2) asymptomatic infection; (3) aseptic meningitis and headache; and (4) AIDS dementia complex. CNS syndromes of children give rise to a fifth syndrome resulting in abnormal neurological development and arrested intellectual and motor function.

HIV-infection of the CNS

HIV may enter the brain across the BBB or by infecting monocytes (macrophages and microglia) which are productively infected by virtue of having surface CD^4 molecules. Such macrophages may then cross the BBB, thus allowing the HIV access to the CNS. During the asymptomatic phase CNS involvement is common and at least 40% of all persons with HIV have abnormal CSF, with increased cell counts and protein levels.[202] Anti-HIV antibodies are detectable in the CSF and in some patients oligoclonal bands are observed. It has been suggested that aseptic meningitis and headache, AIDS dementia complex and progressive encephalopathy of children are due to the direct effects of HIV infection.[203]

Aseptic meningitis

The common neurological symptoms of early or primary HIV-1 infection are headaches and photophobia, which may be either acute or chronic.[204] Although the cause of such clinical symptoms is not known in all patients, headaches have been related to systemic disease such as *Pneumocystis carinii*. Such features may subside or progress to encephalitis, meningitis or ataxia. Aseptic meningitis affects 5–10% of HIV-infected patients; HIV may be diagnosed by positive virus culture or p24 antigen in the serum or CSF.

AIDS dementia complex

AIDS dementia complex (ADC) is commonly observed in the later stages of HIV-1 infection in relation to major systemic infections, although in a small group of patients ADC occurs in the absence of opportunistic infections and may be related to HIV-1 infection of the brain. Infection and disease are not synonymous. ADC may be classified into five major stages ranging from stage 0, which encompasses normal mental and motor functions, to stage 4, in which the patient demonstrates rudimentary levels of intellectual and social comprehension and is paraparetic or paraplegic.[201]

Epidemiology

The progression of HIV-1 infection to ADC is related, in general, to the level of immunosuppression in the patient. In the early disease with opportunistic infections approximately 10–30% of patients exhibit ADC stage 1 while 5–15% exhibit severe neurological disturbances (stage 2–3). In contrast, in the late stages of infection the majority of AIDS patients show severe disability (stage 4).[201]

Pathology

Pathological changes in the CNS of patients with ADC are most prominent in the subcortical regions correlating with the observed subcortical clinical abnormalities. The most common changes include: (1) pallor of the white matter and demyelination; (2) gliosis, necrosis and mild neuronal loss; (3) multinucleated giant cells, which may be observed in the later stages of disease; and (4) spongiform changes, which are related to severity of dementia.[201]

Clinical features

Patients with ADC show distinct cognitive changes associated with subcortical, as opposed to cortical, changes. There is general mental slowing, including apathy, impaired concentration and features associated more with depression than CNS infection. Confusion, hallucinations, impaired memory and problem-solving deficiencies are common prior to obvious dementia. ADC may progress in steps or with sudden deterioration associated with systemic infection.

Diagnosis

In patients with ADC computerized tomography and magnetic resonance imaging show cerebral atrophy, although such a finding is non-specific. The CSF of ADC patients contains HIV-specific cytotoxic T cells, increased protein, oligoclonal bands and soluble intercellular adhesion molecule 1 (ICAM-1), which may serve as a marker for disease.[205]

Prevention and control

Zidovudine (formerly AZT) has been shown to improve neuropsychological performance[206] and reduce the incidence of the AIDS dementia complex.[207] Psychiatric disorders such as mania may be treated using lithium, as in non-infected patients.

CNS syndromes in children

Mother-to-child transmission accounts for 80% of HIV infections in children.[208] Infected children present with encephalopathy, either progressive or static, and may be seen from the age of 2 months. The children with progressive encephalopathy become inactive and may develop paralysis and, if untreated, die within 1 year. The CSF may show increased protein and high levels of HIV-specific antibodies. Antibody levels in the serum (as a means of diagnosis) may be difficult to interpret due to the presence of transplacental maternal antibodies. The brains of HIV-infected children are atrophic and contain perivascular inflammation, and the small vessels show calcification.

Opportunistic viral infections of the CNS

Although a variety of opportunistic CNS infections occur with HIV infection, only viral infections will be considered in this section. The major infections are observed with JC virus that gives rise to PML (see under Papoviruses) and cytomegalovirus (CMV). PML occurs in 2–5% of AIDS patients; its effects are observed as dementia and/or focal neurological signs. Herpesvirus infections, in the form of CMV, VZV and HSV-1 and -2, give rise to 'secondary viral encephalomeningitides'. CMV may result in encephalitis and retinal infiltration, which is observed in approximately 20% of AIDS patients. As a result of immunosuppression VZV may be reactivated, giving rise to neurological syndromes such as hydrocephalus or ventriculitis.

RHABDOVIRIDAE

The family Rhabdoviridae is divided into the genera *Lyssavirus*, which contains rabies virus, and *Vesiculovirus*, containing vesicular virus (VSV). The name Rhabdoviridae is derived from the Greek '*rhabdos*', meaning rod. The viruses in this family are rod- or bullet-shaped and infect a wide variety of species.

LYSSAVIRUSES (See also Chapter 33)

The name of this genus is derived from the Greek '*lyssa*', meaning rage or frenzy, and includes rabies virus. The Duvenhage and Mokola viruses of this genus are also associated with human disease.

The rabies virus is a 180×75 nm helical nucleocapsid with a lipid bilayer from which protrude 10 nm protein spikes. Of the five proteins identified, those designated G and N have been most extensively characterized. The G protein is the only viral protein that induces virus neutralizing antibody and is also a target for T-helper and T-cytotoxic lymphocyte reactivity. The importance of such antigenic determination offers an approach for the development of vaccines. For further literature on rabies virus the reader is referred to the excellent reviews of Whitley and Middlebrooks[209] and Fields' *Virology*.[210]

History

Literary references to rabies infections have been recorded since before 2000 BC and they have been mentioned in a number of historical documents, including those of Democritis, Aristaeus and Artemis. There have been six important events in the history of rabies since the 1880s including the application of the human rabies vaccine (1885) and the finding of the pathognomonic Negri bodies for diagnosis (1903).[211] In the 1940s a mass application of potent rabies vaccine for dogs was introduced which greatly diminished the spread of disease. More recently the introduction of oral vaccination of foxes has resulted in virtual elimination of rabies from Switzerland.[212] Rabies hyperimmune antiserum was used in addition to the human vaccine regimen (1954) and the adaptation of rabies virus to cell culture and the development of a fluorescent antibody test for diagnosing infected animal brains (1958) has resulted in a dramatic improvement in the control of the disease.[213]

Epidemiology

Rabies virus is capable of infecting all warm-blooded animals, but there is a hierarchy for susceptibility.[214] Most susceptible are foxes, coyotes, jackals and wolves. The opossum is the least susceptible species. Moderately susceptible animals include dogs, the most frequent vector for transmission to humans,[215] as well as cats, racoons and skunks. An increasing source of rabies is observed in the bat population(s)[216,217] and accounts for approximately 10% of rabies-infected animals in the USA. The epidemiology of human rabies parallels that in the animal population. A higher incidence is observed in areas where public health programmes are not implemented, such as in India and Mexico where the incidence is 3.3 cases per 100 000.

Pathogenesis

The major route of infection is invariably via the bite from a rabid animal, although transmission by aerosols and as a result of corneal grafts must be taken into account. Once introduced, rabies virus is quickly sequestered. It was thought that the virus stayed in the nervous tissue close to the wound site, although studies by Murphy et al[218] indicated that the virus replicates in muscle tissue before progressing to the peripheral nervous tissue via the neuromuscular connections. That rabies virus travels to the central nervous tissue via the nerves has been demonstrated experimentally by DiVestea and Zagari,[219] who showed that severing the sciatic nerve prior to injection of rabies virus in the foot of an animal prevented disease. The incubation period of the disease varies and may be as short as 2 weeks but is more commonly 1–3 months, and in a few cases more than 1 year. Although it is widely accepted that the incubation period is related to the distance between the site of the bite and proximity to the CNS, a study by Dupont and Earle[220] did not support this view.

Pathology

Human rabies pathology, apart from the pathognomonic Negri body, consists of perivascular cuffing, some neuronophagia and limited neuronal necrosis. The limited pathology does not match the marked symptoms of hydrophobia, aerophobia, excitation and coma. There is pathology in other organs, and

Negri bodies have been found in corneas and adrenal glands.

Clinical features

Development of infection depends on the severity of the exposure, the site of the bite and possibly other factors. Neurological findings may be classified as either 'furious' or 'paralytic' and are not exclusive. Furious rabies is far more common and is characterized by spasms in response to tactile, auditory, visual and olfactory stimuli, e.g. aerophobia and hydrophobia. Such symptoms alternate with periods of lucidity, agitation, confusion and autonomic dysfunction. The alternative form of paralytic rabies ranges from paralysis of one limb to quadriplegia. Disease progresses to coma with neurological complications associated with abnormal hormonal homeostasis, alterations in temperature and inability to control blood pressure.

Diagnosis

Clinical diagnosis of rabies may be difficult in patients presenting with a paralytic or Guillain–Barré-like syndrome and the World Health Organization (WHO) Committee on Rabies[221] has emphasized that rabies must be included in the differential diagnosis of all persons presenting with neurological involvement.

The laboratory diagnosis of rabies may be performed by fluorescent antibody techniques, on smears or frozen sections and by the use of ELISA. A rapid rabies enzyme immunodiagnosis assay allows the antigen to be visualized by the naked eye and is thus a test that can be carried out in the field (with a special test kit). Molecular tests, such as the polymerized chain reaction, are available. Virus isolation can be performed using a murine neuroblastoma cell line (NAC1300), which reduces the diagnosis time by 2 days.

Prevention and control

Rabies mortality can be reduced by preventing exposure to the virus, aborting infection and thereby preventing illness, or curing clinical disease.

The WHO committee has stressed the importance of the adoption and establishment of international and regional surveillance systems in combination with dog control. In over 80 countries rabies is prevalent in dogs, which appear to be the most dangerous reservoir. Each year approximately 4 million people in these areas receive treatment after exposure to rabies and in 99% of all human cases the virus is transmitted by dogs. Furthermore 90% of people who receive postexposure treatment live in areas of canine rabies.

Vaccination

The control of rabies is through oral immunization of domestic, and more recently, wild animals. Recombinant vaccines making use of poxvirus, baculovirus and adenoviruses are possible. The vaccines available for human immunization are: (1) brain tissue vaccine (possible side-effects of autoreactivity to brain tissue); (2) purified duck embryo vaccine inactivated with β-propriolactone; and (3) tissue culture vaccines. For animal vaccination nervous tissue-derived virus has been shown to be effective in mass vaccination of the canine population in North Africa. In contrast cell culture-derived virus (either inactivated or modified live virus) for canine rabies has been used in a combined vaccination programme with distemper, hepatitis, parvo and leptospirosis vaccines. Combined vaccines with foot and mouth vaccine are used for cattle, sheep and goats. For feline control the rabies vaccine is combined with panleucopenia virus, feline calicivirus and feline parvovirus vaccines.

The WHO report (1992) describes the use of postexposure treatment. This makes use of three vaccine doses applied in the deltoid muscle of the right and left arm at day 0 and a further dose on day 7. The results show an increase in both the cellular and humoral response. Such treatment has also been combined with antirabies immunoglobulin.

Monoclonal antibodies

Postexposure treatment with murine monoclonal antibodies, and more recently murine–human chimeric antibodies and humanization of monoclonal antibodies, offers a more specific treatment regimen.

Interferon and interferon inducers

Recombinant α-interferon administration with vaccines decrease rabies virus in subhuman primates. Exogenous interferon has already been shown to be effective in a patient given a corneal transplant from a patient with rabies.

TOGAVIRIDAE

The family Togaviridae originally contained the genera of alphaviruses, flaviviruses and rubiviruses, based on various characteristics such as size, mode of replication and transmission by mosquitoes. The name is derived from the structure of the virus which consists of a ribonucleic acid within a lipid envelope (L. *toga* coat). With advances in virology the structure of the genomes and replication strategies of the genera have become more distinct and the flaviviruses are now classified as a separate family. Detailed studies of togaviruses and flaviviruses may be found in an excellent review by Schlesinger and Schlesinger.[222]

The togaviruses are now divided into the alphaviruses, rubiviruses and pestiviruses.

ALPHAVIRUSES (See also Chapter 30)

The knowledge of the structure and replication of alphaviruses has been based on Sindbis (SIN) and Semliki Forest viruses (SFV), which provide valuable models for study. Of the alphaviruses that are important encephalitogenic agents, eastern equine encephalitis (EEE), Venezuelan equine encephalitis (VEE) and western equine encephalitis (WEE) viruses are the most important, although chikungunya virus infection is also known to induce neurological complications.

CHIKUNGUNYA

History

The word *chikungunya*, meaning 'to contort or bend', was used by a tribe in Tanzania to describe the clinical manifestations of a virus epidemic of 1952–1953. Since this virus invariably results in crippling arthritis, chikungunya virus (CHIK) infection was probably responsible for the epidemic in 1779 in Indonesia.[223]

Epidemiology

CHIK is found in Africa, including Tanzania, Zimbabwe, Transvaal, Zambia and the Congo, and India, Sri Lanka and South-East Asia, including Vietnam and Thailand.[224–226] The disease is transmissible by mosquitoes. *Ae. aegypti* and various *Culex* species are the vectors in urban epidemics in Asia. In Africa, the vector involved in forest areas is *Ae. africanus* and in Sudan *Ae. leuteocephalus*.

Clinical illness

The disease is biphasic. In the first phase, symptoms include fever and severe joint, limb, and spine pains. This phase can last 6–10 days. The second phase occurs after a febrile period of 2–3 days and is associated with an irritating maculopapular rash over the body, particularly on the extensor surface of the limbs. Joint pains may persist occasionally, without fever, for up to 4 months. In some cases myocarditis and peripheral circulatory failure have been seen.[227] In this second phase, encephalitis and manifestations of neurological involvement are occasionally observed.[228] Mortality is estimated at 0.4% but in patients under 1 year old it may be as high as 2.8% and similarly over the age of 50 years the death rate may increase.

Diagnosis

Definitive diagnosis is by specific serological analysis such as HI, CF and ELISA, although the combination of febrile illness and rheumatic manifestations in a patient returning from sub-Saharan Africa or parts of Asia are characteristic features of CHIK infection.

Treatment and control

Supportive care for patients with CHIK infections are important with respect to the arthralgia. In severe cases chlorquine phosphate may be administered.

Inactivated virus vaccines have been shown to be effective but vaccination is restricted to laboratory workers, although a live attenuated virus is undergoing trials in experimental animals.

EASTERN EQUINE ENCEPHALITIS

History

Eastern equine encephalitis (EEE) was first isolated in 1933[229] and retrospective studies of epidemics are suggestive of EEE as early as 1931.

Epidemiology

EEE virus is endemic along the eastern coast of the USA, Canada, Trinidad, Guyana, Mexico, Panama, Brazil, Peru, Columbia and Argentina.[230]

In most areas the virus is transmitted between marsh birds and *Culiseta melanura* mosquitoes, which do not feed on large vertebrates. With alterations in the conditions of the marshes or swamps, the virus is transmitted to other host mosquitoes that feed on small rodents, reptiles and amphibians. *Culex* species are considered to be the vectors for transmission of EEE virus in South America.[231] Human and equine cases are seen only when the spread becomes endemic.

Pathogenesis and pathology

Viraemia occurs soon after infection and may be accompanied by a febrile prodrome. Virus gains access to the nervous system and results in severe encephalitis. HI and neutralizing antibody is present in samples taken during the first 3–5 days of encephalitis.[232] However this effective humoral immune response does not eradicate the virus from the brain and neural destruction continues through direct cytopathic effect, inflammatory damage and vasculitis. The primary pathological features of EEE are confined to the CNS.[233,234] Lesions are scattered throughout the cortex and are particularly severe in basal ganglia and the brain stem; the cerebellum and spinal cord are minimally involved. There is extensive neuronal damage as well as thrombosis of arterioles and venules. Inflammatory cells are widespread in lesions, perivascular areas and meninges. The cells are predominantly polymorphonuclear in the first week, but later mononuclear cells may predominate. Virions are present in oligodendrocytes.

Clinical illness

Human infections are rare but when they occur the ratio of inapparent to apparent infection is remarkably low. In children, the ratio is estimated to be from 2:1 to 8:1; in adults, from 4:1 to 50:1. In severe cases the onset is abrupt, with high fever followed by all the features of meningitis, including coma, convulsions and neurological damage. Age is not a major factor in mortality but severe sequelae are more pronounced in children under 10 years of age.[234,235]

Diagnosis and investigation

The abrupt onset of a severe febrile CNS illness is suggestive of this disease, and mortality in horses, associated with hot, wet summers and the proximity of salt marshes, gives further credence to EEE infection.

The virus may be isolated from serum during the initial infection but most cases are diagnosed by testing paired sera in conventional HI or NT.[235] Very high CF titres occur in most convalescing EEE cases. IgM antibodies are readily detected in acute sera by ELISA.[236] Virus may be isolated at post mortem.

Prevention and control

A vaccine inactivated by formalin treatment is available for use in laboratory workers or others at high risk of exposure.[237] The same vaccine is used to protect endangered whooping cranes, which are susceptible to lethal visceral infection.

VENEZUELAN EQUINE ENCEPHALITIS (VEE)

This virus was first isolated by Beck and Wyckoff[238] from equine encephalitis epizootics in Venezuela. Viral strains belonging to the VEE IABC group are pathogenic for horses and have been involved in human infections. In contrast, other VEE strains (ID-F, II, III, IV, V, VI) are not known to be virulent in horses.

Epidemiology

VEE is endemic in Central and South America and parts of North America, and has occurred particularly in Venezuela, Colombia, Equador, Panama, Brazil, Mexico, Florida, Texas and Trinidad. Mosquitoes of both the *Aedes* and *Culex* genera are involved. *Cx. melanoconion* and *Deinocereites* species are the main vectors in rodent-to-rodent transmission. Horses are a major reservoir of infection and transmission of the virus can occur from horse to horse as well as transplacentally. Over 150 different animal species, including domestic and wild dogs and pigs, have been found to be infected with this virus. Birds have low viraemias but could infect mosquitoes which may spread the disease and cause new epidemics.[239]

Pathogenesis

Conventional serological methods show that the viruses grouped into the VEE complex are all closely related. The viruses in this group were further divided into subtypes and variants by Young et al[240] using the HI test, and it seems that these minor distinctions are responsible for the fundamental differences in pathogenicity and biochemical significance.

The earliest humoral immune response appears around day 5 in hamsters and is directed to virion surface component.[241,242] An epitope on E2 is shown to produce the most dominant protective neutralizing antibodies. In the mouse model, cell transfer experiments suggest that T-helper lymphocyte activity is important in protection.

Clinical illness

The clinical disease in man resembles an influenza-like syndrome, with fever lasting for 1–4 days. Occasionally this is complicated by shock and coma, in which case there appears to be widespread destruction of lymphoid tissues. Meningoencephalitis can occur particularly in children but is much less common in adults. Mortality can occur in undernourished populations and in the absence of medical care.

Diagnosis

VEE should be suspected in any person suffering from febrile myalgic illness 6 days after being exposed to an enzootic biotope.

WESTERN EQUINE ENCEPHALITIS

Epidemiology

Western equine encephalitis (WEE) virus is found in the USA but human infections are limited to the western two-thirds of the country. It is also found in Canada, particularly Manitoba, Saskatchewan, Alberta and British Columbia, and South America.[229] The disease is transmitted by various species of mosquito vectors. These include *Cx. tarsalis*, *Culiseta melanura* and other mosquitoes of these two genera. *Aedes* and *Anopheles* species may be slightly involved. The natural cycle is between *Cx. tarsalis* mosquitoes and wild birds. *Culex* mosquitoes readily feed on large vertebrates, so equine and human cases occur annually. The number of cases is dependent on rainfall because mosquito breeding is largely in ground pools.

Pathogenesis and pathology

The pathogenesis of WEE in humans resembles that of EEE. However, WEE is less neuroinvasive and neurovirulent, both in humans and laboratory animals. In the CNS the pathology consists of multiple foci of necrosis, often without cellular infiltrate, found predominantly in areas such as the striatum, globus pallidus, cerebral cortex, thalamus and pons. In some areas polymorphonuclear infiltrates occur. There is widespread perivascular cuffing and meningeal reaction. The pathogenesis in rodents is similar to that of other alphaviruses.[243]

Clinical illness

WEE is characterized by sudden onset of fever, headache and general symptoms of meningoencephalitis that can be clinically severe but rarely fatal. Neurological and psychological sequelae are seen primarily in children under 2 years of age. The ratio of inapparent to apparent clinical infection is estimated at 50:1–8:1 in children and over 1000:1 in adults.

Prevention and control

Social activities such as screening of windows and doors and avoiding external pursuits are necessary to avoid infection. An inactivated vaccine is available for workers at risk from infection.

SEMLIKI FOREST VIRUS

Although Semliki Forest virus (SFV) has been assumed not to infect humans, the death of a scientist from whom SFV was isolated may suggest otherwise. More recently mild febrile illness has been reported in humans in Africa and was suggested to be due to SFV. The fact that SFV is known to induce neurological disease in experimental animals, with perivascular infiltrates and demyelination (Figure 38.4), warrants mention of this virus in this chapter.

SFV was originally isolated in Uganda in 1944. Experimentally the virus induces encephalitis in a variety of laboratory rodents. Infection of mice with the A7 or M9 strains of SFV gives rise to lesions of demyelination in the CNS.[16]

RUBIVIRUSES

History

The sole member of the rubivirus genus, rubella virus, was initially described in the early 1800s.[244] Although it is primarily a childhood illness the

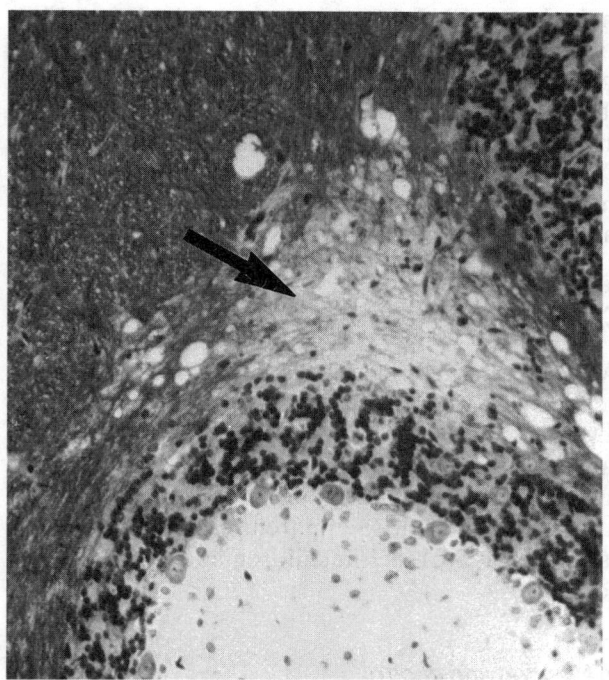

Figure 38.4   Demyelination (arrow) within the cerebellum of a mouse infected with Semliki Forest virus.

disease is endemic worldwide and serious complications such as encephalomyelitis and postinfectious encephalopathy have been reported in adults and children. The large number of studies by German scientists have given rubella virus the synonym 'German measles', although the organism is unrelated to measles virus.

Epidemiology

Unlike most other togaviruses, rubella has no known vertebrate host and the only natural reservoir is man.

Rubella virus infections are found worldwide and in the temperate regions the epidemics occur in late winter and early spring. Periods of increased incidence every 6–9 years occur, with major epidemics every 10–30 years.[245] Such epidemics are related to the susceptibility of individuals and factors which increase the transmission. Infection is generally acquired in childhood and approximately 60% of the population have antibodies by the age of 14. With the introduction of the rubella vaccine in 1969[246] the incidence of rubella has decreased, although the seroprevalence rates approach 90–95%. The incidence of infection is higher in the tropics. Postinfectious encephalopathy or encephalomyelitis is estimated to occur in 1 in 6000 cases of natural rubella.

Pathology and pathogenesis

The pathology resulting from rubella infection is dependent on the mode of infection, i.e. whether it is due to maternal–fetal transmission or is acquired postnatally. The effect on the fetus depends on the gestation period. In the first trimester there is a high risk of infection and developmental growth is arrested, although the mechanism of damage is unknown. Maternal infection after the first trimester does not appear to damage the fetus, although the risk of congenital disease is known to increase before birth. Delayed neurological disease has been reported following late-onset rubella infection and may be associated with either congenital rubella or a rare complication of natural rubella acquired in childhood.

The pathological features of CNS involvement, particularly in the adult, include perivascular lesions of mononuclear cells and demyelination. In childhood encephalopathy neural degeneration is more apparent than in the adult, whereas perivascular infiltrates and demyelination are less common. The suggestion that autoreactivity may play a role in the pathology of late-onset rubella encephalitis, often referred to as progressive rubella panencephalitis, chronic progressive panencephalitis or non-congenital rubella, comes from studies in which lymphocytes proliferate in response to CNS proteins such as myelin basic protein.[247]

Clinical features

Rubella infection in early childhood or adult life is usually mild and asymptomatic. Symptoms of postinfectious rubella encephalopathy are observed shortly after the onset of the rash of typical rubella. The clinical features of encephalitis are similar to other forms of encephalitis, including headache, vomiting, stiff neck, fevers, convulsions and altered levels of consciousness. The mortality is approximately 20%, with death occurring within a few days of the onset of symptoms.

The late-onset rubella encephalitis is similar to other slow virus infections of the CNS. Following a prolonged asymptomatic period neural degeneration is observed, usually in the second decade of life. Symptoms include behavioural changes, ataxia and seizures. Death usually results within 8 years of onset.

Diagnosis

The common symptoms of rubella, such as low-grade fever and maculopapular rash, should not be confused with other such infections. Confirmation of rubella may be made following isolation of the virus or by specific serological assays such as ELISA. The CSF cell count of patients with rubella encephalitis is high ($50/mm^3$); the majority of the cells are lymphocytes. The electroencephalogram is abnormal, oligoclonal bands are observed in the CSF[248] and rubella virus may be isolated.[249]

Treatment and prevention

Treatment of rubella encephalitis with corticosteroids has been reported.[250] Rubella vaccines, developed in the 1960s, have been used to vaccinate both school-aged children (USA) and women of child-bearing age (UK) in an attempt to decrease the incidence of congenital rubella infection. The attenuated viruses used are capable of infecting the fetus and thus vaccination of pregnant women is not recommended. More recently the policy of including the combined measles–mumps–rubella (MMR) vaccination procedure for all preschool children has been implemented in the UK. Future development of subviral vaccines may be necessary to counter the side-effects of vaccination using attenuated virus.

REFERENCES

1 Johnson R T. *Viral Infections of the Nervous System.* New York: Raven Press, 1982.

2 Fields B N, Knipe D M, Chanock R M et al. *Virology,* 2nd edn. New York: Raven Press, 1990.

3 Nicolau S & Meteiesco E. Septinvrites à virus rabique des rues. Préuves de la marche centrifuge du virus dans les nerfs périphérique des lapins. *C R Acad Sci* 1928; 186:1072–1074.

4 Cook M L & Stevens J G. Pathogenesis of herpetic neuritis and ganglionitis in mice: evidence of intra-axonal transport of infection. *Infect Immun* 1973; 7:272–278.

5 Goldmann E E. Vitalfarbung am Zentralnervensystem. *Abh Preuss Akad Wiss, Phys-Math* 1913; 1(1):1–60.

6 Dodge A B, Hechtman H B & Shepro D. Microvascular endothelial-derived autocoids regulate pericyte contractibility. *Cell Motil Cytoskeleton* 1991; 18:180–188.

7 Springer T A. Adhesion molecules of the immune system. *Nature* 1990; 346:425–434.

8 Pathak S & Webb H E. The entry and the transport of Arboviruses into and throughout mouse brain: an electronmicroscopic study. *Electronmicroscopy* 1980; 2:492–493.

9 Co M S, Gaulton G N, Tominaga A, Homcy C J, Fields B N & Green M I. Structural similarities between mammalian β-adrenergic and reovirus type 3 receptors. *Proc Natl Acad Sci USA* 1985; 82:5315–5318.

10 Webb H E & Parsons L M. Treatment of the post-viral fatigue syndrome—rationale for the use of antidepressants. In Jenkins R & Mowbray J (eds) *Post Viral Fatigue Syndrome.* New York: Wiley, 1991:297–303.

11 Sattenau Q J & Weiss R A. The CD4 antigen: physiological ligand and HIV receptor. *Cell* 1988; 52:631–633.

12 Lentz T L, Burrage T G, Smith A L, Crick J & Tignor G. Is acetylcholine receptor a rabies virus receptor? *Science* 1982; 215:182–184.

13 Kaner R J, Baird A, Mansukhani A et al. Fibroblast growth factor receptor is a portal of cellular entry for herpes simplex virus type 1. *Science* 1990; 248:1410–1413.

14 Levine B, Hardwick J M, Trapp B D, Crawford T O, Bollinger R C & Griffin D E. Antibody-mediated clearance of alphavirus infection from neurons. *Science* 1991; 254:856–860.

15 Griffin J W & Watson D F. Axonal transport in neurological disease. *Ann Neurol* 1988; 23:3–13.

16 Fazakerley J K, Amor S & Webb H E. Reconstitution of Semliki Forest virus infected mice induces immune mediated pathological changes in the CNS. *Clin Exp Immunol* 1983; 52:115–120.

17 McCormick J B & Johnson K M. Lassa fever: historical review and contemporary investigation. In Pattyn S R (ed.) *Ebola Virus Haemorrhagic Fever.* Amsterdam: Elsevier–North Holland, 1978:279–292.

18 Warkel R L, Rinaldi D F, Bancroft W H, Cardiff R D, Holmes G E & Wilsnack R E. Fatal acute meningoencephalitis due to lymphocytic choriomeningitis virus. *Neurology* 1973; 23:198–203.

19 Vanzee B E, Douglas R G Jr, Betts R F, Bauman A W, Frazer D W & Hinman A R. Lymphocytic choriomeningitis virus in university hospital personnel. Clinical features. *Am J Med* 1975; 58:803–809.

20 McCormick J B, Webb P A, Krebbs J W, Johnson K M & Smith E S. A prospective study of the epidemiology and ecology of Lassa fever. *J Infect Dis* 1987; 155:437–444.

21 McCormick J B, King I J, Webb P A et al. Lassa fever: a case-control study of the clinical diagnosis and course. *J Infect Dis* 1987; 155:445–455.

22 Monath T P & Casals J. Diagnosis of Lassa fever and the isolation and management of patients. *Bull World Health Organ* 1975; 52:707–715.

23 Edington G M & White H A. The pathology of

Lassa fever. *Trans R Soc Trop Med Hyg* 1972; 66:381–389.

24 Frame J D, Baldwin J M, Gocke D J & Troup J M. Lassa fever, a new virus disease of man from West Africa. 1. Clinical description and pathological findings. *Am J Trop Med Hyg* 1970; 73:219–224.

25 Walker D H, McCormick J B, Johnson K M et al. Pathologic and virologic study of fatal Lassa fever in man. *Am J Pathol* 1982; 107:349–356.

26 Auperin D D, Espositi J J, Lange J V, Bauer S P, Knight J & Sasso D R. Construction of a recombinant vaccinia virus expressing the Lassa virus glycoprotein gene and protection of guinea pigs from a lethal Lassa virus infection. *Virus Res* 1988; 9:233–248.

27 Fisher-Hoch S P, McCormick J B, Auperin D et al. Protection of rhesus monkeys from fatal Lassa fever by vaccination with a recombinant vaccinia virus containing the Lassa virus glycoprotein gene. *Proc Natl Acad Sci USA* 1989; 86:317–321.

28 McCormick J B, King I J, Webb P A et al. Lassa fever. Effective therapy with ribavirin. *N Engl J Med* 1986; 314:20–26.

29 Gonzalez-Scarano F & Nathanson N. Bunyaviruses. In Fields B N, Knipe D M, Chanock R M et al (eds) *Virology*, 2nd edn. New York: Raven Press, 1990:1195–1228.

30 Obijeski J F & Murphy F A. Bunyaviruses: recent biochemical developments. *J Gen Virol* 1977; 37:1–14.

31 Porterfield J S, Casals J, Chumakov M P, Gaidamovich S V & Hannoun C. Bunyaviruses and Bunyaviridae. *Intervirology* 1976; 6:13–24.

32 Murphy F A, Harrison A K & Whitfield S G. Bunyaviruses: morphologic and morphogenetic similarities of Bunyamwera serologic supergroup viruses and several other arthropod-borne viruses. *Intervirology* 1973; 1:297–316.

33 Horzinek M C. The structure of togaviruses and bunyaviruses. *Med Biol* 1975; 53:406–411.

34 Thompson W H, Kalfayan B & Anslow R O. Isolation of Californian encephalitis group virus from a fatal human illness. *Am J Epidemiol* 1965; 81:245–253.

35 Hammon W Mc D & Reeves W C. California encephalitis virus—a newly described agent. 1. Evidence of a natural infection in man and other animals. *Calif Med* 1952; 77:303–309.

36 Calisher C H. Toxonomy, classification and geographical distribution of Californian serogroup bunyaviruses. In Calisher C H & Thompson W H (eds) *Californian Serogroup Viruses*. New York: Alan R Liss, 1983:1–16.

37 Grimstad P R, Craig G B, Ross Q E & Yuill T M. *Aedes triseriatus* and La Crosse virus: geographical variation in vector susceptibility and ability to transmit. *Am J Trop Med Hyg* 1977; 26:990–996.

38 Sabatino D A & Cramblett H G. Behavioural sequelae of California encephalitis virus infection in children. *Dev Med Neurol* 1968; 10:331–337.

39 Artsob H. Distribution of California serogroups and virus infection in Canada. In Calisher C H & Thompson W H (eds) *California Serogroup Viruses*. New York: Alan R Liss, 1983:277–292.

40 Meegan J M. The Rift Valley fever epizootic in Egypt 1977–1978. 1. Description of the epizootic and virological studies. *Trans R Soc Trop Med Hyg* 1979; 73:618–623.

41 Maar S A, Swanepoel R & Gelfand M. Rift Valley fever encephalitis. A description of a case. *Cent Afr J Med* 1979; 25:8–11.

42 Lampert P W, Sims J K & Kniazeff A J. Mechanism of demyelination in JHM virus encephalomyelitis. Electron microscopic studies. *Acta Neuropathol (Berl)* 1973; 24:76–85.

43 Burks J S, De Vald L D, Jankcvsky L D & Gerdes J C. Two coronaviruses isolated from the central nervous system tissue of two multiple sclerosis patients. *Science* 1980; 209:933–934.

44 Westaway E G, Brinton M A, Gaidamovich S Y et al. Flaviviridae. *Intervirology* 1985; 24:183–192.

45 De Madrid A T & Porterfield J S. The Flaviviruses (group B arboviruses): a cross-neutralization study. *J Gen Virol* 1974; 23:91–96.

46 Sumiyoski H, Mori C, Fuke I et al. Complete nucleotide sequence of the Japanese encephalitis virus genome RNA. *Virology* 1987; 161:497–510.

47 Kobayashi Y, Hasegawa H, Oyama T, Tamai T, Shiroguchi T & Kusaba T. Antigenic analysis of Japanese B encephalitis virus using monoclonal antibodies. *Infect Immun* 1984; 44:117–123.

48 Umenai T, Krzysko R, Bektimirov T A & Assaad F A. Japanese encephalitis: current worldwide status. *Bull World Health Organ* 1985; 63:625–631.

49 Gressler I, Hardy J L, Hu S M K & Scherer W F. Factors influencing transmission of Japanese B encephalitis virus by a colonized strain of *Culex tritaeniorhynchus* Giles, from infected pigs and chicks to susceptible pigs and birds. *Am J Trop Med Hyg* 1958; 7:365–370.

50 Weaver O M, Haymaker W, Pieper S & Kurland R. Sequelae of the arthropod-borne encephalitides. V. Japanese encephalitis. *Neurology* 1958; 8:887–890.

51 Mathur A, Arora K L & Chaturvedi U C. Transplacental Japanese encephalitis virus (JEV) infection in mice during consecutive pregnancies. *J Gen Virol* 1982; 59:213–217.

52 Burke D S, Nisalak A, Lorsomrudee W, Ussery M A & Laorpongse T. Virus specific antibody-producing cells in blood and cerebrospinal fluid in acute Japanese encephalitis. *J Med Virol* 1985; 17:283–292.

53 Hsu T C & Hsu S T. Supplementary report. Effectiveness of Japanese encephalitis vaccine. Study in the second year following immunisation. In Hammon W Mc D, Kitaoka M & Downs W G (eds) *Immunisation for Japanese Encephalitis*. Baltimore, M D: Williams & Williams, 1971:266–267.

54 Oya A. Japanese encephalitis vaccine. In Fukumi

M (ed.) *The Vaccination*. Tokyo: International Medical Foundation of Japan, 1975.

55 Huang C H. Studies of Japanese encephalitis in China. *Adv Virus Res* 1982; 27:71–101.

56 Chamberlain R W. Epidemiology of arthropod-borne togaviruses: the role of arthropods as hosts and vectors and of vertebrate hosts in natural transmission cycles. In Schlesinger R W (ed.) *The Togaviruses: Biology, Structure, Replication*. New York: Academic Press, 1980:175–227.

57 Henderson B E, Pigford C A, Work T & Wende R D. Serological survey for St Louis encephalitis and other group B arbovirus antibodies in residents of Houston, Texas. *Am J Epidemiol* 1970; 91:87–98.

58 Quick D J, Thompson J M & Bond J O. The 1962 epidemic of St Louis encephalitis in Florida. IV. Clinical features of cases in the Tampa Bay area. *Am J Epidemiol* 1965; 81:415–427.

59 Finley K & Riggs N. Convalescence and sequelae. In Monath T P (ed.) *St Louis Encephalitis*. Washington, DC: APHA, 1980: 535–550.

60 French E L. Murray valley encephalitis: isolation and characterization of the aetiological agent. *Med J Aust* 1952; 1:100–103.

61 Kliks S C & Halstead S B. An explanation for enhanced virus plaque formation in chick embryo cells. *Nature* 1980; 285:504–505.

62 Doherty R L, Carley J G, Fillippich C, White J & Gust I D. Murray valley encephalitis in Australia, 1974: antibody response in cases and community. *Aust NZ J Med* 1976; 6:446–453.

63 Bennett N Mc K. Murray Valley encephalitis, 1974: clinical features. *Med J Aust* 1976; 2:446–450.

64 de Souza Lopes O, de Abreu Sacchetta L, Coimbra T L, Pinto G H & Glasser C M. Emergence of a new arbovirus disease in Brasil. II. Epidemiological studies on 1975 epidemic. *Am J Epidemiol* 1978; 108:394–401.

65 de Souza Lopes O, Coimbra T L, de Abreu Sacchetta L & Calisher C H. Emergence of a new arbovirus disease in Brasil. I. Isolation and characterisation of the etiological agent, Rocio virus. *Am J Epidemiol* 1978; 107:444–449.

66 Rosenberg S. Neuropathology of Sao Paulo south coast epidemic encephalitis (Rocio encephalitis). *J Neurol Sci* 1980; 45:1–12.

67 Tiriba A C, Miziara A M, Lorenco R, da Costa C B, Costa C S & Pinto G H. Primary human epidemic encephalitis induced by Arbovirus found at the sea shore south of the State of Sao Paulo. Clinical study in an emergency hospital. *Rev Assoc Med Bras* 1976; 22:415–420.

68 Porterfield J S. Antigenic characteristics and classification of Togaviruses. In Schlesinger R W (ed.) *The Togaviruses: Biology, Structure, Replication*. New York: Academic Press, 1980:13–46.

69 Pudney M & Varma M G R. The growth of some tick-borne arboviruses in cell cultures derived from tadpoles of the common frog, *Rana temporaria*. *J Gen Virol* 1971; 10:131–138.

70 Zilber L A. Pathogenicity of Far Eastern and Western (European) tick-borne encephalitis viruses in sheep and monkeys. In Libikova H (ed.) *Biology of Viruses of the Tick-Borne Encephalitis Complex*. New York: Academic Press, 1960:260–265.

71 Shope R E. Medical significance of togaviruses: an overview of diseases caused by togaviruses in man and in domestic and wild vertebrate animals. In Schlesinger R W (ed.) *The Togaviruses: Biology, Structure, Replication*. New York: Academic Press, 1980:47–82.

72 Price W H. Chronic disease and virus persistence in mice inoculated with Kyasanur forest disease. *Virology* 1966; 29:679–681.

73 Zlotnik I, Grant D P & Carter G B. Experimental infection of monkeys with viruses of the tick-borne encephalitis complex: degenerative cerebellar lesions following inapparent forms by the disease or recovery from clinical encephalitis. *Br J Exp Pathol* 1976; 57:200–210.

74 Ogawa M, Okubo H, Tsuji Y, Yasui N & Someda K. Chronic progressive encephalitis occurring 13 years after Russian spring–summer encephalitis. *J Neurol Sci* 1973; 19:363–373.

75 Radsel-Medvescek A, Marolt-Gomiscek M & Gajsek-Zima M. Clinical characteristics of patients with TBE treated at the University medical centre hospital for infectious diseases in Ljubljana during the years 1974–1977. *Zentralbl Bakteriol (Suppl)* 1980; 9:277–280.

76 Kunz C, Heinz F X & Hofmann H. Immunoreactivity and reactigenicity of a highly purified vaccine against tick-borne encephalitis. *J Med Virol* 1980; 6:103–109.

77 Roizman B. Herpesviridae: a brief introduction. In Fields B N, Knipe D M, Chanock R M et al (eds) *Virology*, 2nd edn. New York: Raven Press, 1990:1787–1793.

78 Whitley R J & Schlitt M. Encephalitis caused by herpesviruses, including B virus. In Scheld W M, Whitley R J & Durack J T (eds) *Infections of the CNS*. New York: Raven Press, 1991:41–46.

79 Lowenstein A. Aetiologische Untersuchungen uber den Fieber haften Herpes. *Munch Med Wochenschr* 1919; 66:769.

80 Goodpasture E W. Herpetic infections with special reference to involvement of the nervous system. *Medicine* 1929; 8:843.

81 Nahmais A J & Dowdle B. Infection with herpes simplex viruses 1 and 2. *N Engl J Med* 1973; 289:667–781.

82 Whitley R J. Herpes simplex viruses. In Fields B N, Knipe D M, Chanock R M et al (eds) *Virology*, 2nd edn. New York: Raven Press, 1990:1843–1887.

83 Meignier B. Vaccination against herpes simplex virus infections. In Roizman B & Lopez C (eds) *The Herpesviruses. Immunobiology and Prophylaxis of Human Herpes Virus Infections*, vol. 4. New York: Plenum Press, 1985:265.

84 von Bókay J. Über den ätiologischen Zusammangenhamg der Varizellen mit gewissen

Fällen von herpes Zoster. *Wien Klin Wochenschr* 1888; 22:1323–1326.

85 Weller T H & Stoddard M B. Intranuclear inclusion bodies in cultures of human tissue inoculated with varicella vesicle fluid. *J Immunol* 1952; 68:311–319.

86 Johnson R & Milborne P E. Central nervous system manifestations of chickenpox. *Can Med Assoc J* 1970; 102:831–834.

87 Applebaum E, Rachelson M H & Dolgopol V B. Varicella encephalitis. *Am J Med* 1953; 15:223–230.

88 Gershon A, Steinberg S, Greenberg S & Taber L. Varicella-zoster-associated encephalitis: detection of specific antibodies in cerebrospinal fluid. *J Clin Microbiol* 1980; 12:764–767.

89 Heppleston J D, Paerch K M & Yates P O. Varicellar encephalitis. *Arch Dis Child* 1959; 34:318–321.

90 Gelb L D. Varicella-zoster virus. In Fields B N, Knipe D M, Chanock R M et al (eds) *Virology*, 2nd edn. New York: Raven Press, 1990:2011–2054.

91 Uen W C, Luka J & Pearson G R. Development of an enzyme-linked immunosorbent assay (ELISA) for detecting IgA antibodies to the Epstein–Barr virus. *Int J Cancer* 1988; 41:479–482.

92 Schiff J, Schaefer J & Robinson J. Cell-associated Epstein–Barr virus in the cerebrospinal fluid of a patient with meningoencephalomyelitis complicating infectious mononucleosis. *Yale J Biol Med* 1982; 55:59–63.

93 Sabin A B. Fatal B virus encephalomyelitis in a physician working with monkeys. *J Clin Invest* 1949; 28:808.

94 Gay F P & Holden M. The herpes encephalitis problem. II. *J Infect Dis* 1933; 53:287–303.

95 Centers for Disease Control. Herpes B encephalitis—California. *MMWR* 1973; 22(40):333–334.

96 Vizoso A D. Latency of herpes simiae (B virus) in rabbits. *Br J Exp Pathol* 1975; 56:489–494.

97 Hummeler K, Davidson W L, Henle W, LaBoccetta A C & Rush H G. Encephalomyelitis due to infection with herpevirus simiae (herpes B virus): a report of two fatal, laboratory acquired cases. *N Engl J Med* 1959; 261:64–68.

98 Hilliard J K & Kalter S S. Development of molecular probes for simian herpesvirus detection. *Dev Biol Stand* 1985; 59:79–86.

99 Buthala D A. Hyperimmunised horse anti-B virus globulin: preparation and effectiveness. *J Infect Dis* 1962; 111:101–106.

100 Boulter E A, Thornton B, Bauer E J & Bye A. Successful treatment of experimental B virus (herpesvirus simiae) infection with acyclovir. *BMJ* 1980; 280:681–683.

101 Easterday B C. Animal influenza. In Kilbourne E D (ed.) *The Influenza Viruses and Influenza*. Orlando: Academic Press, 1975:449–481.

102 Dubowitz V. Influenzal encephalitis. *Lancet* 1958; i:140–141.

103 Louria D B, Blumenfeld H L, Ellis J T, Kilbourne E D & Rogers D E. Studies on influenza in the pandemic of 1957–1958. II. Pulmonary complications of influenza. *J Clin Invest* 1959; 38:213–265.

104 Price D A, Postlethwaite R J & Longson M. Influenza virus A2 infections presenting with febrile convulsions and gastrointestinal symptoms in young children. *Clin Pathol* 1976; 15:361–367.

105 Flewett T H & Hoult J G. Influenzal encephalopathy and post-influenzal encephalitis. *Lancet* 1958; ii:11–15.

106 Delorme L & Middleton P J. Influenza A virus associated with acute encephalopathy. *Am J Dis Child* 1979; 133:822–824.

107 Hoult J G & Flewett T H. Influenzal encephalopathy and postinfluenzal encephalitis. Histological and other observations. *BMJ* 1958; 1:1847–1850.

108 Forbes J A. Severe effects of influenza virus infection. *Med J Aust* 1958; 2:75–79.

109 Ravenholt R T & Foege W H. Before our time. 1918 influenza, encephalitis lethargica, parkinsonism. *Lancet* 1982; ii:860–864.

110 Martin C M, Kunin C M, Gottlieb L S, Barnes M W, Liu C & Finland M. Asian influenza A in Boston, 1957–1958. *Arch Intern Med* 1959; 35:71–76.

111 Soto P J Jr, Broun G O & Wyatt J P. Asian influenzal pneumonitis. 1959. A structural and virologic analysis. *Am J Med* 1959; 27:18–25.

112 Hakosalo J & Saxen L. Influenza epidemic and congenital defects. *Lancet* 1971; ii:1346–1347.

113 Randolph V L & Heath C W Jr. Influenza during pregnancy in relation to subsequent childhood leukemia and lymphoma. *Am J Epidemiol* 1974; 100:399–409.

114 MacDonald K L, Osterholm M T, Hedberg C W, Schrock C G & Peterson G F. Toxic shock syndrome: a newly recognised complication of influenza and influenza-like illness. *JAMA* 1987; 257:1053–1058.

115 Consensus Development Conference at National Institutes of Health. Amantidine: does it have a role in the prevention and treatment of influenza? *Ann Intern Med* 1980; 92:256–258.

116 Zlydnikov D M, Kubar O I, Kovaleva T P & Kamforin L E. Study of rimantadine in the USSR: A review of the literature. *Rev Infect Dis* 1981; 3:408–421.

117 Kato N & Eggers H J. Inhibition of uncoating of fowl plague virus by 1-adamantanamine hydrochloride. *Virology* 1969; 37:632–641.

118 Rickman D D, Hostetler K Y, Yazaki P J & Clark S. Fate of influenza A virion proteins after entry into subcellular fractions of LLC cells and the effect of amantadine. *Virology* 1986; 151:200–210.

119 Dolin R, Reichman R C, Madore H P, Maynard R, Linton P N & Webber-Jones J. A controlled trial of amantadine and rimantadine in the prophylaxis of influenza A infection. *N Engl J Med* 1982; 307:580–584.

120 Gilbert B E, Wilson S Z, Knight V et al. Ribavirin

small-particle aerosol treatment of infections caused by influenza virus strains A/Victoria/7/83 (H1N1) and B/Texas/1/84. *Antimicrob Agents Chemother* 1985; 27:309–313.

121 Gilbert B E & Knight V. Biochemistry and clinical applications of ribavirin. *Antimicrob Agents Chemother* 1986; 30:201–201.

122 Oxford J S. Inhibition of the replication of influenza A and B viruses by a nucleoside analogue (ribavirin). *J Gen Virol* 1975; 28:409–414.

123 Treanor J J, Betts R F, Erb S M, Roth F K & Dolin R. Intranasally administered interferon as prophylaxis against experimentally induced influenza A infection in humans. *J Infect Dis* 1987; 156:379–383.

124 Richardson E. Progressive multifocal leukoencephalopathy. *N Engl J Med* 1961; 265:815–823.

125 Gardner S. The new human papovaviruses: their nature and significance. In Waterson A P (ed.) *Recent Advances in Clinical Virology*. New York: Livingstone, 1977:93–115.

126 Taguchi F, Kajioka J & Miyamura T. Prevalence rate and age of acquisition of antibodies against JC and BK virus in human sera. *Microbiol Immunol* 1982; 26:1057–1064.

127 Berger J R, Kaszovita B, Donavan Post J & Dickinson G. Progressive multifocal leukoencephalopathy associated with human immunodeficiency virus infection. *Ann Intern Med* 1987; 107:78–87.

128 Shah K V. Polyomaviruses. In Fields B N, Knipe D M, Chanock R M et al. (eds) *Virology*, 2nd edn. New York: Raven Press, 1990:1609–1623.

129 Flaegstad T, Sundsfjord A, Arthur A A, Pedersen M, Traavik T & Subraman S. Amplification and sequencing of the control regions of BK and JC virus from human urine by polymerase chain reaction. *Virology* 1991; 180:553–560.

130 Preblud S R & Katz S L. Measles vaccine. In Plotkin S A & Mortimer E A Jr (eds) *Vaccines*. Philadelphia: W B Saunders, 1988: 182–222.

131 Babbott F L & Gordon J E. Modern measles. *Prog Med Sci* 1954; 228:334–361.

132 Black F L. Measles. In Evans A S (ed.) *Viral Infections of Humans. Epidemiology and Control*, 3rd edn. New York: Plenum Press, 1989:451–469.

133 Littauer J & Sorensen K. The measles epidemic at Umanak in Greenland in 1962. *Dan Med Bull* 1965; 12:43–50.

134 Christensen P E, Schmidt H, Jensen O, Bang H O, Andersen V & Jordal B. An epidemic of measles in Southern Greenland 1951: Measles in virgin soil. II. The epidemic proper. *Act Med Scand* 1952; 144:430–449.

135 Koplik H. The diagnosis of the invasion of measles from a study of the exanthema as it appears on the buccal mucous membrane. *Arch Pediatr* 1896; 13:91.

136 Krugman S, Katz S L, Gershon A A & Wilfert C M. Measles (rubeola). In Mosby C V (ed.) *Infectious Diseases of Children*. St Louis: 1985:152–166.

137 Morgan E M & Rapp F. Measles virus and its associated diseases. *Bacteriol Rev* 1977; 41:636–666.

138 Markowitz L E, Chandler F W, Roldan E O et al. Fatal measles pneumonia without rash in a child with AIDS. *J Infect Dis* 1988; 158:480–483.

139 Wolinsky J S, Swoveland P, Johnson K P & Baringer J R. Subacute measles encephalitis complicating Hodgkin's disease in an adult. *Ann Neurol* 1977; 1:452–457.

140 Jabbour J T, Carcia J H, Lemmi H, Ragland J, Duenas D A & Sever J L. Subacute sclerosing panencephalitis: a multidisciplinary study of eight cases. *JAMA* 1969; 207:2254–2258.

141 Font R L, Jenis E H & Tuck K D. Measles maculopathy associated with subacute sclerosing panencephalitis. *Arch Pathol* 1973; 96:168–174.

142 Milles G. Measles pneumonia with a note on the giant cell of measles. *Am J Clin Pathol* 1945; 15:334–338.

143 Pinkerton H, Smiley W L & Anderson W A D. Giant cell pneumonia with inclusions: lesion common to Hecht's disease, distemper and measles. *Am J Pathol* 1945; 21:1–23.

144 Fleischer B & Kreth H W. Clonal expansion and functional analysis of virus-specific T lymphocytes from cerebrospinal fluid in measles encephalitis. *Hum Immunol* 1983; 7:239.

145 Norrby E & Gollmar Y. Identification of measles virus-specific hemolysis inhibiting antibodies separate from hemagglutinating-inhibiting antibodies. *Infect Immun* 1975; 11:231–239.

146 Kleiman B M, Blackburn L K, Zimmerman E S & French V L M. Comparison of enzyme linked immunosorbent assay for acute measles with hemagglutination inhibition, complement fixation and fluorescent antibody methods. *J Clin Microbiol* 1981; 14:147–152.

147 Vandvik B & Norrby E. Oligoclonal IgG antibody response in the central nervous system to different measles virus antigens in subacute sclerosing panencephalitis. *Proc Natl Acad Sci USA* 1973; 70:1060–1063.

148 Landrigan P J & Wittle J J. Neurologic disorders following live measles-virus vaccination. *JAMA* 1973; 223:1459–1462.

149 Modlin J F, Jabbour J T, Witte J J & Halsey N A. Epidemiologic studies of measles vaccine and subacute sclerosing panencephalitis. *Pediatrics* 1977; 59:505–513.

150 Raine C S. On the development of CNS lesions in natural canine distemper encephalomyelitis. *J Neurol Sci* 1976; 30:13–28.

151 Cook S D, Dowling P C & Russell W C. Neutralising antibody to canine distemper and measles virus in multiple sclerosis. *J Neurol Sci* 1979; 41:61–70.

152 Hamilton R. An account of a distemper, by the common people in England, vulgarly called the mumps. *London Med J* 1790; 11:190–211.

153 Anderson R M, Cromble J A & Grenfell B T. The epidemiology of mumps in the UK: a preliminary study of virus transmission, herd immunity and the potential impact of immunization. *Epidemiol Infect* 1987; 99:65–84.

154 Philip R N, Reinhard K R & Lachman D B. Observation on a mumps epidemic in a 'virgin' population. *Am J Hyg* 1959; 69:91–111.

155 Murray H G S, Feild C M B & McLeod W J. Mumps meningoencephalitis. *BMJ* 1960; 1:1850–1853.

156 Scheid W. Mumps virus and central nervous system. *World Neurol* 1961; 2:117–130.

157 Wilfert C M. Mumps meningoencephalomyelitis with low cerebrospinal-fluid glucose, prolonged pleocytosis and elevation of protein. *N Engl J Med* 1969; 280:855–859.

158 Weller T G & Craig J R. Isolation of mumps virus at autopsy. *Am J Pathol* 1949; 25:1105–1115.

159 Bruyn H B, Sexton H M & Brainerd H D. Mumps meningoencephalitis. A clinical review of 119 cases with one death. *Calif Med* 1957; 86:153–160.

160 Taylor F B & Toreson W E. Primary mumps meningoencephalitis. *Arch Intern Med* 1963; 112:114–119.

161 Lindsay J R, Davey P R & Ward P H. Inner ear pathology in deafness due to mumps. *Ann Otol Rhinol Laryngol* 1960; 69:918–935.

162 Oldfelt V. Sequela of mumps-meningoencephalitis. *Acta Med Scand* 1949; 134:405–414.

163 Spataro R F, Lin S R, Horner F A, Hall C B & McDonald J V. Aqueductal stenosis and hydrocephalus: rare sequelae of mumps virus infection. *Neuroradiology* 1976; 12:11–13.

164 Thompson J A. Mumps: a case of acquired aqueductal stenosis. *J Paediatr* 1979; 94:923–924.

165 Brunell P A, Brickman A & Steinberg S. Evaluation of a live attenuated mumps vaccine Jeryl Lynn: with observations on the optimal tissue for testing serologic responses. *Am J Dis Child* 1969; 118:435–440.

166 Hilleman M R, Weibel R E, Buynak E B, Stokes J & Whiteman J E. Live attenuated mumps virus vaccine. 4. Protective efficacy measured in field evaluation. *N Engl J Med* 1967; 276:252–258.

167 Kilham L & Margolis G. Cerebellar ataxia in hamsters inoculated with rat virus. *Science* 1964; 143:1047–1048.

168 Melnick J L. Enteroviruses: polioviruses, coxsackieviruses, echoviruses and newer enteroviruses. In Fields B N, Knipe D M, Chanock R M et al (eds) *Virology* 2nd edn. New York: Raven Press, 1990:549–605.

169 Landsteiner K & Popper E. Ubertragung der Poliomyelitis acuta auf Affen. *Z Immunitatsforsch Orig* 1909; 2:377–390.

170 Lavinder C H, Freeman A W & Frost W H. Epidemiological studies of poliomyelitis in New York City and northeastern United States during the year of 1916. *Public Health Bull* 1918; 91:1–309.

171 Bodian D. Poliomyelitis: pathogenesis and histopathology. In Rivers T M & Horsfall F L Jr (eds) *Viral and Rickettsial Infections of Man*, 3rd edn. Philadelphia: Lippincott 1965:479–518.

172 van Wezel A L & Hazendonk A G. Intratypic serodifferentiation of poliomyelitis virus strains by strain specific antisera. *Intervirology* 1979; 11:2–8.

173 Salk J & Salk D. Control of influenza and poliomyelitis with killed virus vaccines. *Science* 1977; 195:834–837.

174 Benyesh-Melnick M, Melnick J L, Rawls W E et al. Studies on the immunogenicity, communicability and genetic stability of oral poliovaccine administered during the winter. *Am J Epidemiol* 1967; 86:112–136.

175 Shindarov L M, Chumakov M P, Voroshilova M K et al. Epidemiological, clinical and pathomorphological characteristics of epidemic poliomyelitis-like disease caused by enterovirus 71. *J Hyg Epidemiol Microbiol Immunol* 1979; 23:284–295.

176 Melnick J L. Enterovirus type 71 infections: a varied clinical pattern sometimes mimicking paralytic poliomyelitis. *Rev Infect Dis* 1984; 6:387–390.

177 Gajdusek D C. Kuru. *Trans R Soc Trop Med Hyg* 1963; 57:151–169.

178 Klatzo I, Gajdusek D C & Zigas V. Pathology of kuru. *Lab Invest* 1959; 8:799–847.

179 Goldgaber D, Goldfarb L G, Brown P et al. Mutations in familial Creutzfeldt–Jakob disease and Gerstmann–Sträussler's syndrome. *Exp Neurol* 1989; 106:204–206.

180 Gajdusek D C & Gibbs C J Jr. Transmission of two subacute spongiform encephalopathies of man (kuru and Creuzfeldt–Jakob disease) to new World monkeys. *Nature* 1971; 230:588–591.

181 Anonymous. Rapidly progressive dementia in a patient who received cadavaric dura mater graft. *MMWR* 1987; 36:49–50.

182 Brown P, Rohwer R G & Gajdusek D C. Sodium hydroxide decontamination of Creutzfeldt–Jakob disease virus. *N Engl J Med* 1984; 310:727.

183 Stockman S. An obscure disease of sheep. *J Comp Pathol* 1913; 26:317–327.

184 Weissmann C, Bueler H, Fischer M, Sauer A & Aguet M. Susceptibility to scrapie in mice is dependent on PrPC. *Philos Trans R Soc Lond [Biol]* 1994; 343: 431–433.

185 Amor S & Mehta S. Prions, viruses and antiviral drugs. *Lancet* 1993; 342:545.

186 Morgan K L. Bovine spongiform encephalopathy: time to take scrapie seriously. *Vet Res* 1988; 122:445–446.

187 Howell P G & Verweord D W. Bluetongue virus. In Gard S, Hallauer C & Meyer K F (eds) *Virology Monographs*, vol. 9. New York: Springer, 1971:37–74.

188 Bowen G S, McLean R G, Shriner R B et al. The ecology of Colorado tick fever in Rocky Mountain National Park in 1974. II. Infection in small mammals. *Am J Trop Med Hyg* 1981; 30:490–496.

189 Florio L, Miller M S & Mugrege E R. Colorado tick fever. Isolation of the virus from *Dermacentor andersoni* in nature and a laboratory study of the transmission of the virus in the tick. *J Immunol* 1950; 64:257–263.

190 Florio L & Miller M S. Epidemiology of Colorado tick fever. *Am J Public Health* 1948; 38:211–216.

191 Ater J L, Overall J, Yeh T & O'Brien A. Circulating interferon and clinical symptoms in Colorado tick fever. *J Infect Dis* 1985; 151:966–968.

192 Ekland C M, Kohls G M, Jellison W L, Burgdorfer W, Kennedy R C & Thomas L. The clinical and ecological aspects of Colorado tick fever. In *Proceedings of the Sixth International Congress on Tropical Medicine and Malaria*, vol. V, September 5–13. Lisbon: Institute of Tropical Medicine, 1958:197–203.

193 Fraaer C H & Scheff D W. Colorado tick fever encephalitis. Report of a case. *Pediatrics* 1962; 29:187–190.

194 Prusiner S B. Novel proteinaceous infectious particles cause scrapie. *Science* 1982; 216:136–144.

195 Sigurdsson B. Observations on three slow infections of sheep, maedi, paratuberculosis, rida, a slow encephalitis of sheep with general remarks on infections which develop slowly and some of their special characteristics. *Br Vet J* 1954; 110:255–270.

196 Querat G, Barban V, Sauze N et al. Highly lytic and persistent lentiviruses naturally present in sheep with progressive pneumonia are genetically distinct. *J Virol* 1984; 52:672–679.

197 Petursson G L, Nathanson N, Georgsson G, Panitch H & Palsson P A. Pathogenesis of visna. I. Sequential virologic, serologic, and pathologic studies. *Lab Invest* 1976; 35:402–412.

198 Georgsson G, Martin J R, Klein J, Palsson P A, Nathanson N & Petursson G L. Primary demyelination in visna. An ultrastructural study of Icelandic sheep with clinical signs following experimental infection. *Acta Neuropathol (Berl)* 1982; 57:171–178.

199 Nathanson N, Georgsson G, Lutley R, Palsson P A & Petursson G L. Pathogenesis of visna in Icelandic sheep: demyelinating lesions and antigenic drift. In Mims C A, Cuzner M L & Kelly R E (eds) *Viruses and Demyelinating Diseases*. London: Academic Press, 1983:111–124.

200 Narayan O & Clements J E. Lentiviruses. Bunyaviruses. In Fields B N, Knipe D M, Chanock R M et al. (eds) *Virology*, 2nd edn. New York: Raven Press, 1990:1571–1589.

201 Price R W, Brew B J & Roke M. Central and peripheral nervous system complications of HIV-1 infection and AIDS. In Devita V, Hellman S & Rosenberg S (eds) *AIDS: Etiology, Diagnosis, Treatment and Prevention*. Philadephia: J B Lippincott Company, 1992: chap. 14.

202 Appelman M E, Marshall D W, Brey R L, Houk R W, Beatty G P & Winn R E. Cerebrospinal fluid abnormalities in patients without AIDS who are seropositive for human immunodeficiency virus. *J Infect Dis* 1988; 158:193–199.

203 Evans B K, Donley D K & Whitaker J N. Neurological manifestations of infection with the human immunodeficiency viruses. In Scheld W M, Whitley R J & Durak D T (eds) *Infections of the Central Nervous System*. New York: Raven Press, 1991:201–232.

204 Carne C A, Tedder R S, Smith A et al. Acute encephalopathy coincident with seroconversion for anti-HTLV-III. *Lancet* 1985; ii:1206–1208.

205 Heidenrich F, Arendt G, Jander S, Jablonowski H & Stoll G. Serum and cerebrospinal fluid levels of soluble intercellular adhesion molecule 1 (sICAM) in patients with HIV associated neurological diseases. *J Neuroimmunol* 1994; 52:117–126.

206 Schmitt F A, Bigley J W, McKinnis R, Logue P E, Evans R W & Drucker J L. Neuropsychological outcome of zidovudine (AZT) treatment with AIDS and AIDS-related complex. *N Engl J Med* 1988; 319:1573–1578.

207 Portegies P, de Gans J, Lange J M et al. Declining incidence of AIDS dementia complex after introduction of zidovudine treatment. *BMJ* 1989; 299:819–821.

208 American Academy of Pediatrics Task Force on Pediatric AIDS. Perinatal human immunodeficiency virus infection. *Pediatrics* 1988; 82:941–944.

209 Whitley R J & Middlebrooks M. Rabies. In Scheld W M, Whitley R J & Durack D T (eds) *Infections of the Central Nervous System*. New York: Raven Press, 1991:127–144.

210 Baer G M, Bellini W J & Fishbein D B. Rhabdoviruses. In Fields B N, Knipe D M, Chanock R M et al (eds) *Virology*, 2nd edn. New York: Raven Press, 1990:883–930.

211 Negri A. Beitrag zum Studium der Aetiologie der Tollwuth. *Z Hyg Infektionskr* 1903; 43:507–528.

212 Wandeler A I, Capt S, Kappeler A & Hauser R. Oral immunisation of wildlife against rabies: concept and first field experiments. *Rev Infect Dis* 1988; 10:649–653.

213 Goldwasser R A & Kissling R E. Fluorescent antibody staining of street and fixed rabies virus antigens. *Proc Soc Exp Biol Med* 1958; 98:219–233.

214 World Health Organization. Sixth report of the expert committee on rabies. *WHO Tech Rep Ser* 1973:523.

215 Tierkel E S. Control of urban rabies. In Baer G M (ed.) *The Natural History of Rabies*, vol. II. Orlando: Academic Press, 1975:189–201.

216 Graubelle P C, Baagoe H J, Fekadu M, Westergaard J & Zoffman N. Bat rabies in Denmark. *Lancet* 1987; 1:379–380.

217 Centers for Disease Control. Bat rabies—Europe. *MMWR* 1986; 35:430.

218 Murphy F A, Harrison A K, Winn W C & Bauer S P. Comparative pathogenesis of rabies and rabies-like viruses. Infection of the CNS and centrifugal

spread of virus to peripheral tissues. *Lab Invest* 1973; 28:361–376.

219 DiVeistea A & Zagari G. La transmission de la rage par voie nerveuse. *Pasteur Ann* 1889:237–248.

220 Dupont J R & Earle K M. Human rabies encephalitis: a study of forty-nine cases with a review of the literature. *Neurology* 1966; 15:1023–1034.

221 WHO Expert Committee on Rabies. *WHO Tech Rep Ser* 1992; 824:1–84.

222 Schlesinger S & Schlesinger M J. *The Togaviridae and Flaviviridae*. New York: Plenum Press, 1986.

223 Peters C J & Dalrymple J M. Alphaviruses. In Fields B N, Knipe D M, Chanock R M et al (eds) *Virology*, 2nd edn. New York: Raven Press, 1990:713–761.

224 Thiruvengadam K V, Kalyanasundaram V & Rajgopal J. Clinical and pathological studies on chickunguya fever in Madras City. *Indian J Med Res* 1965; 53:720.

225 Deller J J Jr & Russell P K. Fever of unknown origin in American soldiers in Vietnam. *Ann Intern Med* 1967; 66:1129.

226 Halstead S B, Nimmannitya S & Margiotta M R. Dengue and chickungunya virus infection in man in Thailand 1962–1964. Observations on disease in out-patients. *Am J Trop Med Hyg* 1969; 18:972–978.

227 Weinbren M P, Haddow A J & Williams M C. The occurrence of chikungunya virus in Uganda. I. Isolation from mosquitoes, II. The occurrence of chikungunya virus in man on the Entebbe peninsula, and III. Identification of the agents. *Trans R Soc Trop Med Hyg* 1958; 52:253–262.

228 Halstead S B. Dengue and haemorrhagic fevers in Southeast Asia. *Yale J Biol Med* 1965; 37:434–437.

229 Hayes R O. Eastern and western encephalitis. In Steele J H & Beran G W (eds) *Handbook Series in Zoonoses*, *Section B: Viral Zoonoses*, vol. 1. Boca Raton, FL: CRC Press, 1981:29–57.

230 Monath T P, Lee V H, Wilson D C, Fagbami A & Tomori O. Arbovirus studies in Nupeko Forest, a possible natural focus of yellow fever virus in Nigeria. I. Description of the area and serological survey of humans and other vertebrate hosts. *Trans R Soc Trop Med Hyg* 1974; 68:30–38.

231 Downs W G, Aitkin T H G & Spence L. Eastern equine encephalitis virus isolated from *Culex nigripalpus* in Trinidad. *Science* 1959;130:1471.

232 Goldfield M, Taylor B F & Welsh J N. The 1959 outbreak of eastern encephalitis in New Jersey. 3. Serological studies of clinical cases. *Am J Epidemiol* 1968; 87:18–22.

233 Bastain F O, Wende R D, Singer D B & Zeller R S. Eastern equine encephalitis. Histopathological and ultrastructural changes with isolation of the virus in a human case. *Am J Clin Pathol* 1975; 64:10–13.

234 Farber S, Hill A, Connerly M I & Dingle J H. Encephalitis in infants and children caused by the virus of the eastern variety of equine encephalitis. *JAMA* 1940; 114:1725–1731.

235 Goldfield M, Taylor B F & Welsh J N. The 1959 outbreak of eastern encephalitis in New Jersey. 6. The frequency of prior infection. *Am J Epidemiol* 1968; 87:39–49.

236 Calisher C H, El-Kafrawi A O, Al-Deen Mahmud M I & Travassos da Rosa A P. Complex-specific immunoglobulin M antibody patterns in humans infected with alphaviruses. *J Clin Microbiol* 1986; 23:155–159.

237 Cole F E Jr. Inactivated eastern equine encephalomyelitis vaccine propagated in rolling-bottle cultures of chick embryo cells. *Appl Microbiol* 1971; 22:842–845.

238 Beck C E & Wyckoff R W G. Venezuelan equine encephalomyelitis. *Science* 1938; 88:530.

239 McConnell S & Spertzel R O. Venezuelan equine encephalomyelitis. In Steele J H & Beran G W (eds) *CRC Handbook Series in Zoonoses*, *Section B: Viral Zoonoses*. Boca Raton, CRC Press, 1981:59.

240 Young N A, Johnson K M & Gauld L W. Viruses of the Venezuelan equine encephalomyelitis complex. *Am J Trop Med Hyg* 1969; 18:290–296.

241 Jahrling P B, Hesse R A & Metzger J F. Radioimmunoassay for quantitation of antibodies to alphaviruses with staphylococcal protein A. *J Clin Microbiol* 1978; 8:54–60.

242 Jahrling P B, Hesse R A, Anderson A O & Gangemi J D. Opsonization of alphaviruses in hamsters. *J Med Virol* 1983; 12:1–16.

243 Griffin D E. Alphavirus pathogenesis and immunity. In Schlesinger S & Schlesinger M J (eds) *The Togaviridae and Flaviviridae*. New York: Plenum Press, 1986:209–249.

244 Wesselhoeft C. Rubella (German measles). *N Engl J Med* 1947; 236:943–950.

245 Witte J J, Karchmer A W, Case G et al. Epidemiology of rubella. *Am J Dis Child* 1969; 118:107–111.

246 Polk B F, Modlin J F & White J A. A controlled comparison of joint reactions among women receiving one of two rubella vaccines. *Am J Epidemiol* 1982; 115:19–25.

247 Johnson R T, Griffin D E, Hirsch R L et al. Measles encephalomyelitis—clinical and immunological studies. *N Engl J Med* 1984; 310:137–141.

248 Vandvik B, Weil M L, Grandien M & Norrby E. Progressive rubella panencephalitis: synthesis of oligoclonal virus-specific IgC antibodies and homogenous free light chains in the central nervous system. *Acta Neurol Scand* 1978; 57:53–64.

249 Squadrini F, Taparelli F, DeRienzo B, Giovannini G & Pagani C. Rubella virus isolation from cerebrospinal fluid in postnatal rubella encephalitis. *BMJ* 1977; 2:1329–1330.

250 Neveh Y & Friedman A. Rubella panencephalitis successfully treated with corticosteroids. *Clin Pediatr* 1975; 22:143–148.

SECTION 5B
RICKETTSIAL INFECTIONS

SECTION 5B
RICKETTSIAL INFECTIONS

CHAPTER 39

RICKETTSIAL INFECTIONS

G. O. Cowan

The typhus and 'spotted' fevers are caused by bacteria of the family Rickettsiaceae, which are obligate intracellular, Gram-negative, non-flagellate small pleomorphic coccobacilli (0.3–0.6 × 0.8–2.0 μm), which are often carried to man by insects from reservoirs in animals or in the insects themselves, in which they may be maintained transovarially.

The species of the genus *Rickettsia* are divided into:

- The *typhus group*, containing *R. prowazekii*, the agent of classical epidemic typhus, transmitted by the human body louse, and *R. typhi* (*mooseri*), the cause of endemic murine typhus, carried by the rat flea.
- The '*spotted fever*' *group*, containing a large number of species (*R. rickettsii*, *R. conorii*, etc.) transmitted from rodents and other animals by ticks (except *R. akari*).
- *Scrub typhus*, caused by *R. tsutsugamushi*, transmitted by larval trombiculid mites.

The genus *Rochalimaea* contains two closely related species, *Rochalimaea quintana*, the cause of *trench fever* in man, and *Rochalimaea vinsoni*, which occurs in voles.

Coxiella burnetii, the only species of its genus, causes *Q fever*.

The tribe Ehrlichieae comprises *Ehrlichia sennetsu* and *E. canis*, which can both cause fever in man, and several equine species, *Cowdria ruminantium*, the cause of 'heartwater' in cattle and other domestic animals in Africa, and *Neorickettsia helminthoeca*, which causes illness in North American canines eating salmonid fish infected with flukes containing the bacterium.

HISTORY

'*Typhus*' is derived from *τυφος*, the ancient Greek word for 'fever with stupor' or 'smoke' cognate with the Sanskrit word for 'smoke', *dhupa*.

The earliest reference to epidemic typhus is in the account by Thucydides of the Great Plague of Athens in 430 BC in the second year of the Pelopennesian war. The historical centres of the disease were in the Middle East, North Africa and the eastern shores of the Mediterranean Sea. In the eleventh century AD, epidemics occurred in Sicily and Bohemia, but it was not until siege warfare on a large scale became common in the late fifteenth century that epidemics spread through armies to the civilian population (e.g. Granada 1459, Naples 1528, and Metz 1552).

The earliest medical accounts of typhus were written by Cardano (1536)[1] and Fracastoro[2] (1546) from Venice. Coyttarus (1578)[3] first suggested that typhoid and typhus were different diseases, a distinction which took three centuries to resolve. Cober (1685)[4] proposed that the body louse was involved in the spread of typhus.

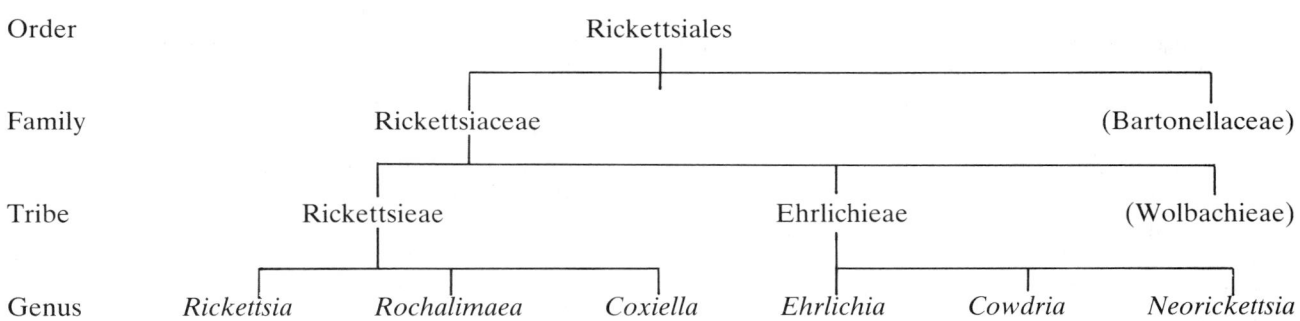

Order		Rickettsiales			
Family		Rickettsiaceae			(Bartonellaceae)
Tribe	Rickettsieae		Ehrlichieae		(Wolbachieae)
Genus	*Rickettsia* *Rochalimaea* *Coxiella*		*Ehrlichia* *Cowdria* *Neorickettsia*		

Epidemics were common in the latter half of the sixteenth century in the Italian cities, Hungary, Germany, the Netherlands, and in England, and flourished in the armies of the Thirty Years War (1618–1648) and the English Civil War. In the eighteenth century fevers were classified as 'continued', 'putrid', 'malignant' or 'spotted'; physicians recognized that armies, ships and prisons were fertile sources of 'spotted'·fever.

Damaging outbreaks of typhus occurred in the British Government army in Scotland in 1746,[5] on both sides in the American War of Independence in 1776, in the British army after the retreat from Corunna in 1809, and in Napoleon's Grand Army in Russia in 1812. The first modern clinical description was given by Von Hildenbrand from Vienna in 1810[6] and led to the eponymous title of the disease. Typhus was common in the tenements of Edinburgh in the early nineteenth century, and epidemics occurred in Ireland in the potato blight famines of 1816–1817 and 1846–1847, with migration carrying the disease to Liverpool, Glasgow and the USA. The Reverend Patrick Brontë's two oldest daughters, Maria and Elizabeth, died of typhus in an epidemic of 45 cases at their boarding school in west Lancashire in 1826, an episode described by Charlotte in her novel *Jane Eyre*.

Gerhard in 1832 in Philadelphia first described the pathological differences between typhus and typhoid fevers, and was soon followed by Perry (1836), Stewart (1840) and Ritchie (1846), who first coined the phrase 'enteric fever'. Sir William Jenner expanded on the differences in his Gulstonian Lectures of 1853 but the Registrar-General of England and Wales did not separate the two diseases statistically until 1869. To this day in Germany typhoid fever is known as *typhus abdominalis* and typhus as *typhus exanthematicus*.

Nicolle[7] in 1910 in Algeria proved that typhus is carried by the body louse; da Rocha Lima (1916)[8] described the organism and proposed the name *Rickettsia prowazekii* to honour Howard Taylor Ricketts and Stanislaus von Prowazek who had both recently died of typhus acquired in the research laboratory.

Louse-borne typhus caused large epidemics in the First World War in Serbia, Poland, eastern Germany and Mesopotamia, and in the Second World War in the Balkans, Naples, Russia and Germany, especially in the concentration camps at Belsen, Auschwitz and Buchenwald.

Flea-borne (murine) typhus had been described in Mexico in 1570 by Bravo,[9] and the complicating myocarditis was to kill Ricketts there in 1910. It was described clinically in grain silo workers in South Australia by Hone in 1923, but the final bacteriologi-

cal separation from *R. prowazekii* did not occur until studies by Maxcy (1926)[10] and Mooser (1928)[11], the organism being named *R. mooseri* or *R. typhi*.

Earlier work by Ricketts was on Rocky Mountain spotted fever (RMSF), which had been first described in 1872 in the Bitter Root Valley of western Montana and on the Snake River in Idaho in the USA.[12] He identified the causative organism in 1906, and demonstrated that ticks were its vector,[13] the first bacterial disease proved to be transmitted by an insect. The organism was named *R. rickettsii*.

Old world tick-borne typhus was not described until 1910 by Conor and Bruch in Tunisia[14] as *fièvre éruptive*—transmitted by ticks, and by Megaw in 1916 in the Himalayan foothills. The species was named *R. conorii*.

Scrub typhus, or Japanese river fever, was known in Japanese folklore to be associated with the jungle mite or chigger which was named 'dangerous bug' (*tsutsu ga mushi*). The illness was described by Hashimoto in 1810 and again in 1878 by Palm, a missionary at Nagaoka, and in 1879 by Baelz and Kawakami.[15] Dowden (1915) and Fletcher and Lesslar in 1925[16] reported the disease in Malaya, and Ogata in 1931[17] isolated the organism and named it *R. tsutsugamushi*.

Trench fever was first described by Graham[18] and Hunt and Rankin[19] in 1915 in soldiers on the Western Front, and by His[20] in 1916 in the Volhynia region of Poland. Töpfer[21] (1916) isolated the organism from body lice. It was named *Rochalimaea quintana*.

Rickettsial pox was described in the Kew Gardens district of the borough of Queens, New York by Sussman in 1946[22] and the organism was named *R. akari*.

Q fever (query fever) was reported by Derrick in abattoir workers in Brisbane, Australia in 1937[23] and the organism subsequently named *Coxiella burnetti*.

The earliest crude vaccine was made by Weigl in 1924 and widely used until a purified version devised by Cox and Bell in 1940[24] superseded it for use against epidemic and endemic typhus. Fulton and Joyner in 1945[25] developed a vaccine for scrub typhus from the lungs of infected cotton rats, but the vaccines were largely superseded in 1947 by the introduction of chloramphenicol for treatment and prophylaxis, initially for scrub typhus in Malaya by Smadel et al,[26] and soon for all types of typhus with the tetracyclines, which remain in use today.

Serological diagnosis was pioneered by Weil and Felix in 1916,[27] who described heterophile antibody agglutination of the OX-2 and OX-19 strains of *Proteus mirabilis* by typhus sera; this was extended to scrub typhus by Fletcher and Lesslar in 1926,[28] who named an agglutinated variant strain OX-K in honour of their colleague Kingsbury.

Rickettsiae grow in guinea-pigs injected with infected human blood; *R. tsutsugamushi* and *R. akari* also grow in mice. Only *C. burnetii* and *Rochalimaea quintana* can be cultured in vitro.

PATHOGENESIS

The rickettsial diseases consist of acute fevers accompanied by general constitutional symptoms and especially by headache and, in severe cases, neurological disturbances, and often by a skin rash, either macular or haemorrhagic. In some types of typhus fever the site of inoculation may form a characteristic skin ulcer with a black crust (eschar).

The early part of the febrile illness represents a period of proliferation of rickettsiae in the blood and on the endothelial surface of small blood vessels. Toxins are produced which damage endothelial cell integrity, leading to leakage of fluid into tissues and to platelet aggregation and proliferation of polymorphonuclear leucocytes and monocytes within the vessel wall and in the perivascular spaces. This results in a focal occlusive endangiitis of small venules and arterioles leading to microinfarction, producing the characteristic histological appear-

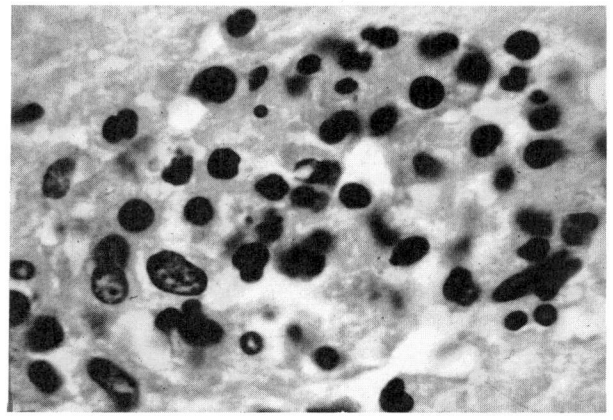

Figure 39.1   Typhus, or Wohlbach's nodule.

ances of the 'typhus nodule' described by Fränkel and Wohlbach[29] (Figure 39.1).

All body tissues may be involved in this process, with important effects especially in the brain, cardiac and skeletal muscles, the skin, lungs, and kidneys; in severe cases the endangiitis causes venous thromboses and peripheral gangrene. In the latter part of the fever, if significant rickettsaemia persists, excessive immune-complex deposition may occur within the skin, kidneys and other tissues. Convalescent patients exhibit delayed hypersensitivity reactions to injected rickettsial antigens which may perpetuate the endangiitis.

EPIDEMIC LOUSE-BORNE TYPHUS

EPIDEMIOLOGY

R. prowazekii is transmitted by the human body or clothing louse *Pediculus humanus* from person to person. Rickettsiae from the blood of a human case are ingested by the biting louse and multiply in the gut of the insect so that its faeces are heavily infected. Scratching of a subsequent bite inoculates the organisms, which can also enter the body through rubbing into the conjunctival membrane. Infected lice may die of the disease but can transmit the rickettsiae to other lice through ingestion of faeces. Transovarial vertical transmission does not occur in lice. Air-borne infection can occur in crowded conditions by the inhalation of dried louse faeces. Blood transfusion has rarely transmitted the disease. Laboratory infection is a major risk. Specimens suspected of containing rickettsiae must be

treated as for a 'dangerous pathogen'. In the USA *R. prowazekii* has also been isolated from flying squirrels (*Glaucomys volans*), and is transmitted between them by their lice and fleas; the significance of this finding in transmission to humans is uncertain.

Foci of endemic human infection from which epidemic spread can occur in times of famine, war, migration and overcrowding exist mainly in the cooler mountainous regions of tropical countries, e.g. Rwanda, Burundi, Uganda, Ethiopia, Lesotho, Transkei, Ciskei, Transvaal, Namibia, Nigeria, Kurdistan, Northern India and Pakistan, China, Papua New Guinea, the Andes mountains, Guatemala, Mexico, and Serbia and Greece (Figure 39.2). Chronic human carriage of *R. prowazekii* may result in later relapses of typhus fever, a phenomenon first described by Brill in 1910[30] in Jewish migrants from the Balkans to New York, and subsequently con-

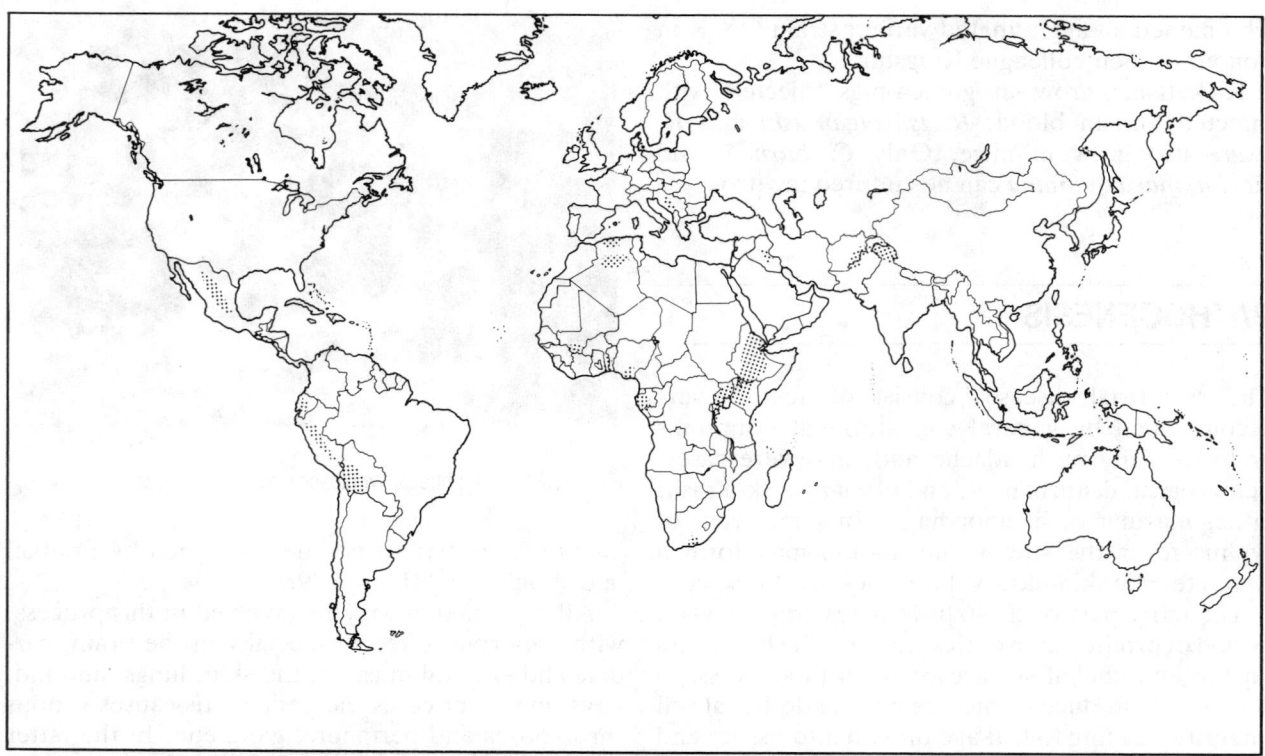

Figure 39.2 Present-day endemic foci of louse-borne typhus (*R. prowazekii*). (Courtesy of the Department of Entomology, London School of Hygiene and Tropical Medicine.)

firmed by Zinsser[31] (Brill–Zinsser disease). Such patients are thought to form a source of potential infection if louse infestation becomes common in prisons and refugee camps or in insanitary crowded conditions.

CLINICAL DESCRIPTION

In the populations at risk of epidemic typhus fever, nutrition and general immunity to infection are inadequate, so that the illness is often severe, with a mortality rate up to 20% overall, and over 50% in the weak and aged. The incubation period averages 12 days. There is an abrupt onset of fever, prostration and severe headache, with pain in the limbs, especially the shins, and nausea and vomiting. Fever rises rapidly to 39–40°C, and remains high until death or resolution by 'crisis' towards the end of the second week, if untreated. The conjunctivae are suffused, the face congested, and the patient looks vacant and depressed as if drugged or drunk (Figure 39.3). Delirium may ensue and a mid-brain ischaemic syndrome of akinetic mutism is described. There is foetor oris, and epistaxis and a dry cough are common. Splenomegaly is usual. The typhus rash appears on the second to fourth day of fever,

mainly on the trunk and proximal limbs (Figure 39.4). It consists of small irregular pink macules which rapidly darken to a mulberry or purple colour, and may become frankly petechial (Figure 39.5). Coalescence to a generalized patchy purple mottling under the skin may occur a few days later. There is *no* eschar at the site of inoculation. Patients are said to smell of mice, boot polish, or rifle-barrel washings. Constipation is usual, and paralytic ileus may occur.

In up to 50% of severe cases a meningoencephalitis ensues with meningism, tinnitus and hyperacusis followed by deafness, dysphagia, dysphoria, agitated delirium and coma. Survivors may suffer transverse myelitis, hemiparesis, peripheral neuropathy with hyperaesthesia, and prolonged psychiatric disturbances.

Other possible complications include secondary infection leading to bronchopneumonia, suppurative parotitis or otitis media, and peripheral blood vessel occlusion resulting in leg vein thrombosis and peripheral gangrene, e.g. of digits. An important further complication is myocarditis, which can occur during recovery with or without specific treatment. This presents with hypotension, tachycardia and low-output cardiac failure or sudden arrhythmic collapse.

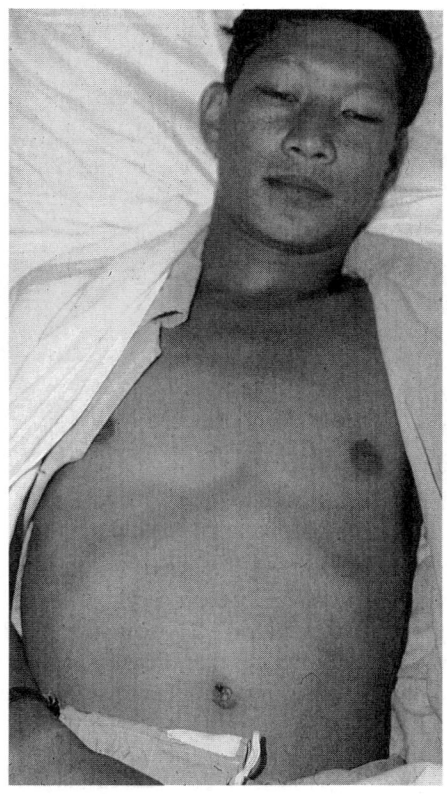

Figure 39.3 A patient with mild typhus eacephalitis.

DIFFERENTIAL DIAGNOSIS

The differential diagnosis of epidemic typhus includes:

- Typhoid fever. This may be clinically very similar and should be excluded by blood or bone marrow culture(s) for *Salmonella typhi*.
- Measles, especially if haemorrhagic. The rash of measles affects the face severely, unlike that of typhus.
- Viral haemorrhagic fevers, e.g. dengue, Rift Valley fever, Congo–Crimea haemorrhagic fever, and yellow fever. These may require to be excluded serologically.
- Meningococcal septicaemia, which can be excluded by culture of blood or cerebrospinal fluid (CSF).
- Louse-borne relapsing fever. This may be very similar clinically, with a haemorrhagic rash. Blood cultures should be performed.
- Leptospirosis. This may be clinically similar in the early stages of the illness. Distinguishing features include marked skeletal muscle tenderness and peripheral blood polymorphonuclear leucocytosis.
- *Plasmodium falciparum* malaria, especially if cerebral involvement has occurred. Blood films

should be stained to exclude this, although rashes and skin haemorrhage are rare in malaria.

DIAGNOSIS

Routine blood investigations in typhus are unhelpful, with a normal total and relative white blood cell count. More severe cases have reduced serum levels of sodium, chloride and albumin, and features diagnostic of diffuse intravascular coagulation. CSF may be at increased pressure, with modest rises in protein and monocyte count, but normal glucose content.

Specific diagnosis may be made:

- On clinical grounds, in an epidemic situation, confirmed by rapid response to specific treatment.
- Serologically by the demonstration of heterophile antibodies to *Proteus mirabilis* OX-19 and OX-2 strains, in the Weil–Felix test.

It may also be made, in specialized laboratories only:

- By isolation of rickettsiae by inoculation of blood into guinea-pigs or fertile duck eggs.
- Serologically by a group-specific microagglutination test (MAT) or species-specific immunofluorescence antibody test (IFAT), or enzyme linked immunosorbent assay (ELISA). IFAT can be modified for use without a fluorescent microscope in the indirect immunoperoxidase reaction, and the ELISA test can also be modified for field use by application to filter paper.
- By detection of the organism by polymerase chain reaction (PCR),[32] by gas–liquid chromatography of acute serum, and by antigen detection by immunofluorescence on, skin biopsy.

TREATMENT

General medical and nursing care is important, with attention to fluid balance, mouth toilet, avoidance of bed sores, adequate analgesia, treatment of agitation with judicious doses of diazepam, appropriate antibiotics (e.g. amoxycillin) for secondary lung and middle ear infection and, in severe cases, the prescription of oral prednisolone 40 mg initially and 20 mg daily for several days, followed by reducing doses. Oliguria and anuria may require peritoneal or haemodialysis.

Specific chemotherapy should be with:

- *Chloramphenicol* in an adult dose of 500 mg, 6-hourly, orally or intravenously for 7 days, or in

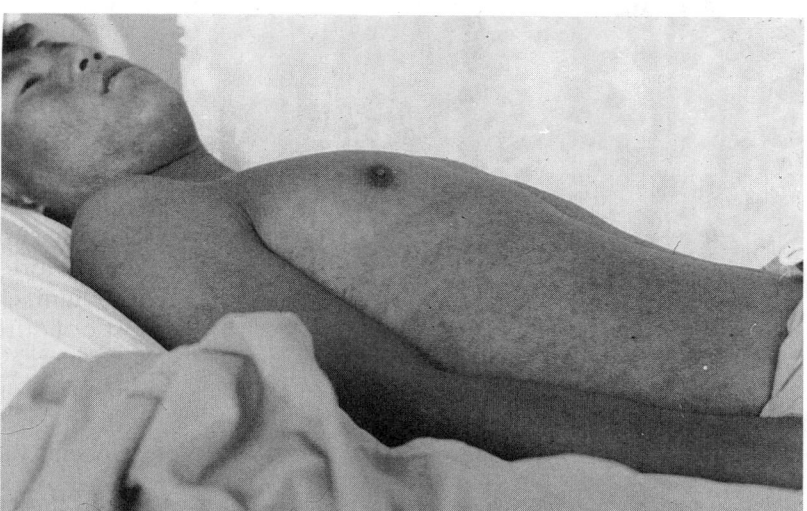

Figure 39.4   The rash of typhus fever. (Courtesy of G. W. Brown.)

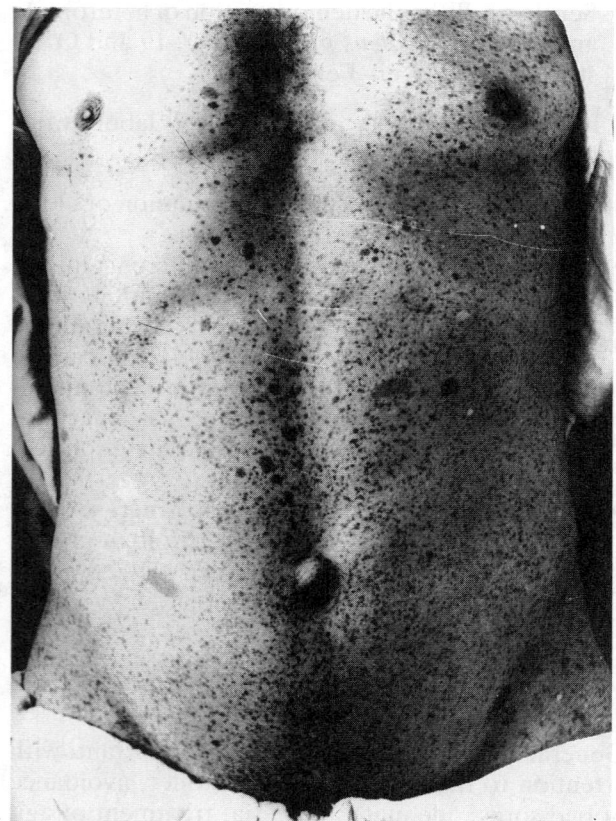

Figure 39.5   Typhus rash in the second week showing the typical distribution. The dark-coloured areas are petechial; the lighter-coloured, discrete areas disappear on pressure.

children at 75 mg/kg per day, divided 6-hourly, for 7 days; or

- *Tetracycline* at an adult dose of 500 mg, 6-hourly, orally or intravenously for 7 days, or in children at 50 mg/kg per day, divided 6-hourly for 7 days; or
- *Doxycycline* (Vibramycin) in a single oral dose of 200 mg for adults or 100 mg for children, repeated once later if necessary.[33]

Rickettsiae are also sensitive to rifampicin and quinolones but these agents are expensive and unnecessary.

Rapid defervescence should be anticipated within 48 hours if the diagnosis is correct.

Measures directed against the louse vector are essential. On admission, patients should be stripped of clothing and washed thoroughly with soap and water. Clothing should be incinerated or autoclaved. Delousing powder (1% malathion) can be applied to hospital clothing and bed sheets. Treatment of medical and nursing attendants with delousing powder once weekly is also desirable.

PREVENTION AND CONTROL

Epidemic typhus should be controlled by:

1. Delousing of patients and all members of closed communities (e.g. refugee camps, prisons) where infection occurs—using 1% malathion powder.
2. Consideration of doxycycline single-dose treatment of all contacts and residents of infected areas, and medical and nursing attendants.
3. Use of a formalinized purified vaccine from chick embryo culture, made by the Swiss Serum and Vaccine Institute. This is not widely available and is normally given only to workers in laboratories handling infected specimens.

MURINE, ENDEMIC, 'SHOP' TYPHUS

EPIDEMIOLOGY

Murine typhus is caused by *R. typhi* (*R. mooseri*) which is transmitted to man by *Xenopsylla cheopis* fleas living on *Rattus rattus* (the black rat) *Rattus norvegicus* (the brown rat), and various species of mouse, and between rats by the louse *Polyplax spinulosa* and the mite *Liponyssus bacoti*. Flea faeces infected with rickettsiae contaminate the flea bite, which is then scratched, so inoculating the infection, or may be inhaled when dried or rubbed into the conjunctival membrane. Rodents with rickettsaemia of this type do not suffer serious illness and so act as a reservoir of infection. Humans are infected by close contact with rodents and their fleas in granaries, breweries, shops and food stores, and domestically in developing countries. Garbage workers are at special risk. Human disease is known to occur in the USA, Mexico, the north of South America, Israel, Pakistan, India, South-East Asia, China and Australia (Figure 39.6). It is an important cause of fever in Khmer refugees in Thailand.[34]

CLINICAL DESCRIPTION

The incubation period is similar to that of louse-borne typhus, and the illness is also similar, but generally much less severe, with a mortality rate of only 1–2%. Headache and muscular pains are the predominant symptoms. There is *no* eschar at the site of inoculation, and the rash of fine red macules is less extensive than in epidemic typhus. Serious neurological, renal and other complications are very ususual.

DIFFERENTIAL DIAGNOSIS

The differential diagnosis of murine typhus includes:

- Typhoid fever—excluded by blood or bone marrow culture.
- Louse-borne and scrub typhus—distinguished only by specific serological tests, and treated identically.
- Arbovirus infections with a macular rash, e.g. dengue and chikungunya—distinguished serologically.

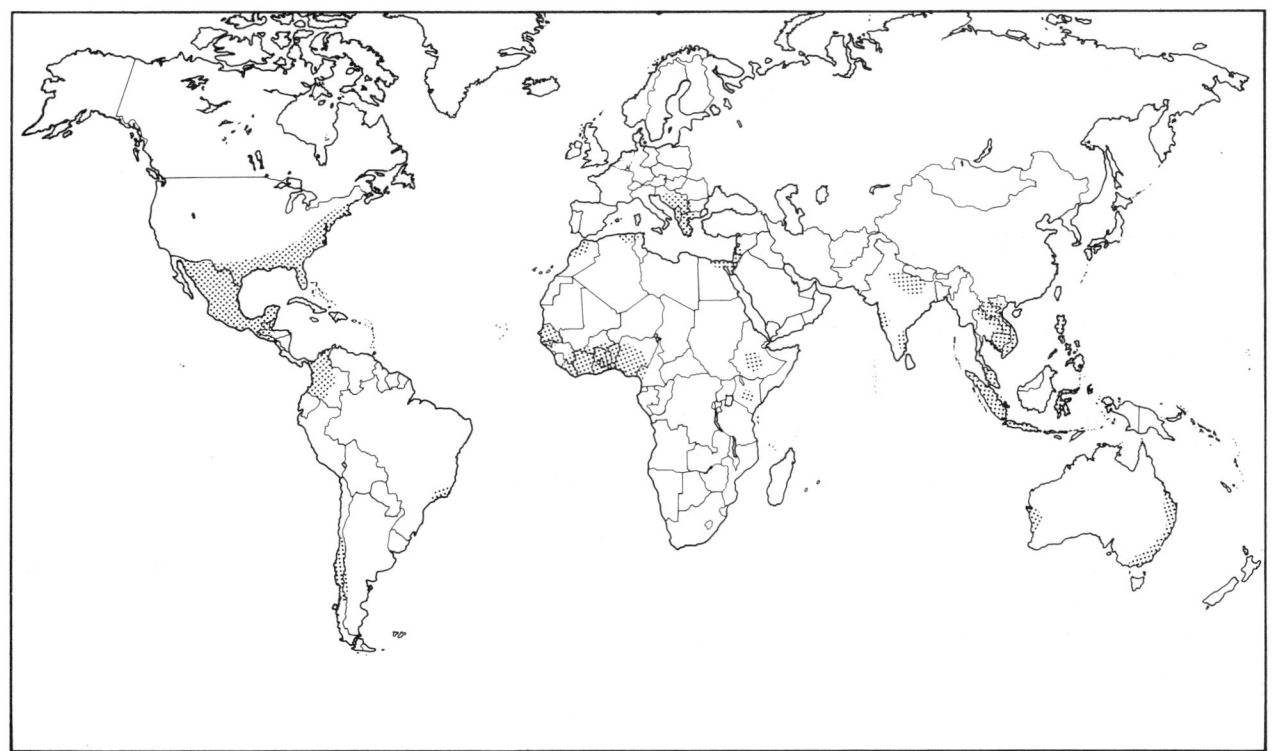

Figure 39.6 Geographical distribution of flea-borne (murine) typhus (*R. mooseri*). (Courtesy of the Department of Entomology, London School of Hygiene and Tropical Medicine.)

- Relapsing fever, transmitted by lice or ticks distinguished by blood culture.
- Leptospirosis—distinguished by exquisite muscle tenderness and polymorphonuclear leucocytosis.
- Malaria—excluded by stained blood films.
- Other causes of fever with macular rash, e.g. Epstein–Barr virus, human immunodeficiency virus (HIV) seroconversion illness—distinguished serologically.

DIAGNOSIS

The diagnosis is made by the same method(s) as in louse-borne typhus. The Weil–Felix reaction may be positive to OX-19 and OX-2 strains, but less strongly. Group-specific serology is not helpful in differentiation from *R. prowazekii* but a specific ELISA will distinguish *R. mooseri* antibodies.

TREATMENT

The general and specific treatment of murine typhus is the same as for louse-borne typhus. Steroid treatment is needed only exceptionally.

PREVENTION AND CONTROL

The prevention of murine typhus has to depend on reducing human contact with rodents and their fleas by:

1. Urban and domestic rodent control using warfarin.
2. Proofing of grain and other food stores against rodents.
3. Residual insecticide spraying of rat runs in stores and breweries.
4. The wearing of protective clothing by garbage workers.

RICKETTSIAL SPOTTED FEVERS

These infections are caused by a large number of rickettsial species, all of which, except *R. akari*, are transmitted to humans by the bite of animal ticks (Table 39.1), or by inoculation of tick faeces or body fluids if the attached tick is crushed. Many other species of tick-borne rickettsiae exist (in animal reservoirs) which have yet to be characterized or identified.

ROCKY MOUNTAIN SPOTTED FEVER

Rocky Mountain spotted fever (RMSF), due to *R. rickettsii*, is a potentially life-threatening infection. Following its original description in the mountain states of north-west USA in the late nineteenth century and the demonstration of the organism in its tick vector by Ricketts in 1906, it has since been recognized as an important cause of illness throughout the USA, especially now in the south-eastern states and on the eastern seaboard. In all, some 700 cases are reported annually in the USA (Figure 39.7). It also occurs in Canada, Mexico, Colombia and Brazil, especially in the area of São Paulo.

The ixodid tick vectors are:

- *Dermacentor andersoni* (wood tick)—western USA.
- *Dermacentor variabilis* (dog tick)—western USA.

- *Amblyomma americanum* (lone-star tick)—south and south-eastern USA.
- *Amblyomma cajennense*—Brazil and Colombia.
- *Haemaphysalis leporispalustris*—this rabbit tick does not bite humans but transmits the infection between rabbits, which act as a reservoir for transmission to man-biting ticks (Figure 39.8).

Transovarial transmission of rickettsiae occurs in ixodid hard ticks, which are thus the main reservoir of infection.

Dermacentor andersoni ticks normally live on goats, sheep, badgers, lynx and black bears, and their larvae on squirrels. *Dermacentor variabilis* and *Amblyomma* ticks live on domestic dogs, rabbits, foxes, opossums, gophers, and racoons, and their larvae on field mice.

CLINICAL DESCRIPTION

Surprisingly, in RMSF there is rarely an eschar at the site of the tick bite. After an inoculation period of 6–10 days there is an abrupt onset of fever with severe headaches and muscle pains, and a dry cough. After 2–3 days the typhus rash of fine pink macules develops (Figure 39.9), which in this disease is most marked on the soles of the feet, wrists and forearms. In more severe infections the rash quickly spreads and becomes petechial with large ecchymoses and the potential for gangrene of digits

Table 39.1 Rickettsial spotted fevers.

Disease	Agent	Vector Reservoir	Mammals also involved	Geography
Rocky Mountain spotted fever (RMSF) (Brazilian spotted fever)	*R. rickettsii*	Ticks	Rodents Dogs Rabbits Opossums	USA South America Canada
Boutonneuse fever (tick typhus)	*R. conorii*	Ticks	Dogs	Africa Mediterranean Middle East India
South African tick typhus	*R. conorii*(?)	Ticks	Cattle	Zimbabwe South Africa
Israeli tick typhus	*R. sharoni*	Ticks	Rodents Deer Cattle Horses	Israel
Siberian tick typhus	*R. sibirica*	Ticks	Rodents	Armenia Kazakhstan Kirghizia East Asia Czechoslovakia
Japanese tick typhus	*R. japonica*	Ticks	Rodents Dogs	Japan
Queensland tick typhus	*R. australis*	Ticks	Rodents	Australia South East Asia

Other rickettsiae in ticks and animals not proved to cause human disease:

	R. montana	Ticks	Rodents, birds	North America
	R. parkeri	Ticks	Rodents, birds	North America
	R. rhipicephalus	Ticks	Dogs	North America
	R. helvetica	Ticks	Rodents	Europe
	R. heilongjangi	Ticks	Rodents	China
	R. belli	Ticks	Rodents, dogs	North America
	R. canada	Ticks	Rabbits, hares	Ontario California

and others as yet untyped in Thailand, Brunei, Sicily, Pakistan, etc.

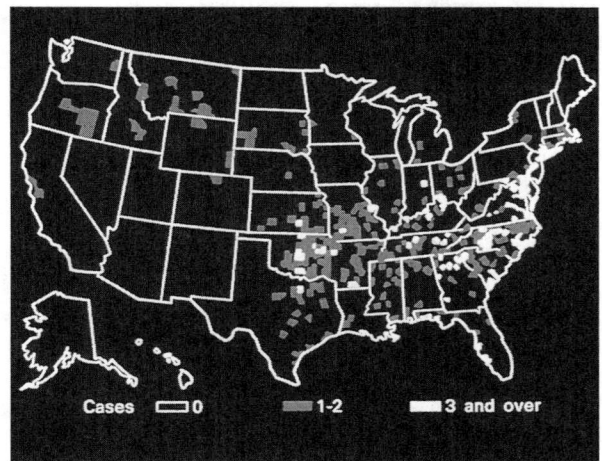

Figure 39.7 Typhus fever—tick borne (Rocky Mountain spotted fever). Reported cases by county—USA, 1988.

and pressure areas. The overall mortality rate is 7–10%, and in young children and elderly adults up to 25%. Meningoencephalitis is common in severe cases, and, as the illness progresses, the stuporose or comatose patient will become hypotensive, oliguric or anuric, and uraemic. Other complications are similar to those seen in severe louse-borne typhus and include bronchopneumonia, otitis media, parotitis and intestinal ileus. In severe cases disseminated intravascular coagulation is a common accompaniment.

DIFFERENTIAL DIAGNOSIS

RMSF should be distinguished from:

● Meningococcal septicaemia—by blood and CSF culture.

- Tick-borne relapsing fever—by blood culture.
- Haemorrhagic measles—by serological methods.
- Tularaemia—by blood culture.
- Lyme disease—by serological methods.

DIAGNOSIS

The diagnosis of RMSF is based on similar methods to those used in epidemic typhus. The Weil–Felix reaction may be positive for OX-19 antibodies but specific IFAT or immunoperoxidase methods should be used if available.

TREATMENT

Treatment with chloramphenicol, tetracycline or doxycycline is the same as for louse-borne typhus. Intensive supportive management may be needed for uraemia and diffuse intravascular coagulation—as appropriate, and severe cases should receive large doses of corticosteroid(s) initially.

PREVENTION AND CONTROL

It is not possible to eradicate the infection in ticks and animals, but the number of human cases can be reduced by:

1. The wearing of stout boots and outer garments during hunting and rambling expeditions in forests; clothing may be impregnated, e.g. with permethrin, to reduce tick bites.
2. Surveillance for tick attachment after episodes of exposure to animal contact and forest habitats; ticks still attached should be treated with absolute alcohol and then removed gently with tweezers, taking care to remove the head.
3. Residual insecticide spraying of established woodland tracks.
4. Surveillance of domestic dogs for ticks, with use of insecticide powders and impregnated collars.

There is no useful vaccine available for the prevention of RMSF.

Brazilian spotted fever is caused by *R. rickettsii* with *Amblyomma cajennense* as the vector tick. An eschar at the site of the tick bite is usual; the illness is otherwise similar to RMSF.

Mediterranean tick typhus (*fièvre boutonneuse*) occurs throughout the coastal countries of the Mediterranean and is increasingly recognized in France and Spain.[35] *R. conorii* is transmitted by the dog tick *Rhipicephalus sanguineus*, and the main reservoir of infection is in domestic dogs, rabbits, and rodents. The illness is similar to RMSF, with the possibility of

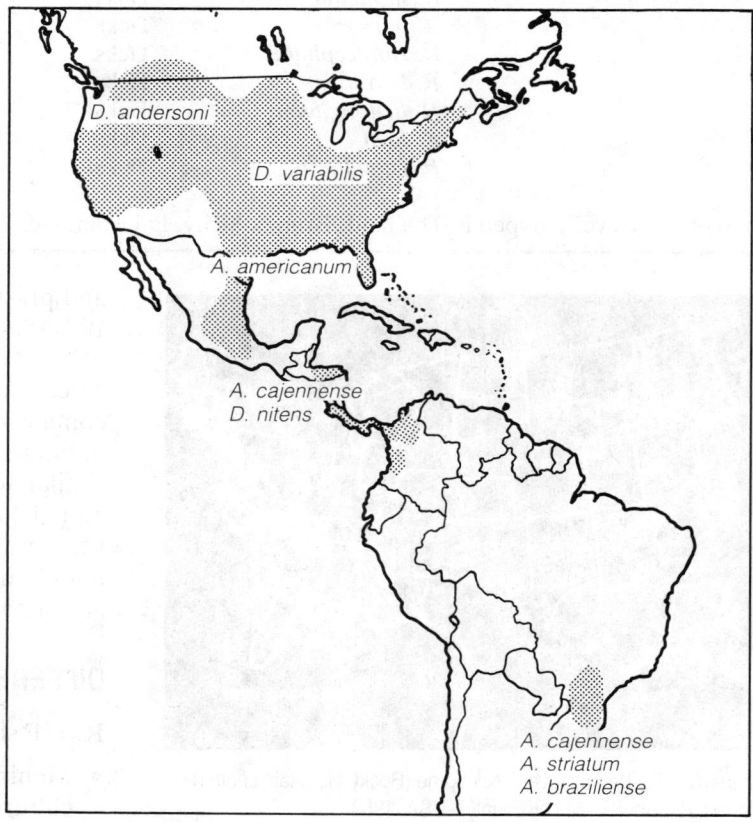

Figure 39.8 Geographical distribution of Rocky Mountain spotted fever (*R. rickettsii*). (Courtesy of the Department of Entomology, London School of Hygiene and Tropical Medicine.)

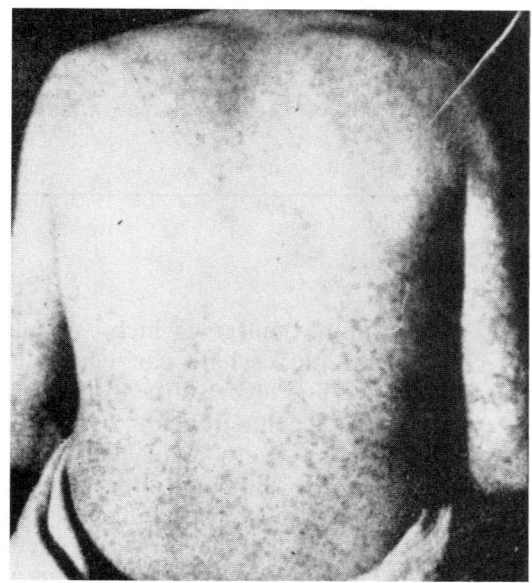

Figure 39.9 The rash of Rocky Mountain spotted fever.

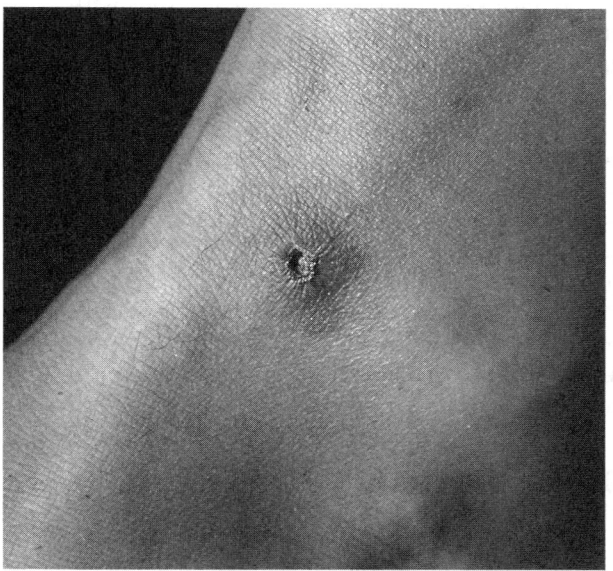

Figure 39.10 A primary eschar of African tick typhus.

a haemorrhagic rash and renal and cerebral involvement, but in most cases it is less severe.

There is almost always an eschar (*tache noire*) at the site of the tick bite, with regional adenitis (Figure 39.10).

The differential diagnoses include typhoid, meningococcal septicaemia and measles. Specific serological tests are similar to those for other forms of typhus. The Weil–Felix reaction produces positive results at low titres for OX-19 and OX-K. Treatment is as for other forms of typhus. Prevention depends on methods similar to those for RMSF to reduce tick bites. There is no vaccine.

Israeli tick typhus, which is caused by a variant organism, *R. sharoni*, is transmitted by *Rhipicephalus* dog ticks, but eschar formation is unusual.

African tick typhus, due to *R. conorii*, is reported from most African countries, including South Africa. Various dog and other animal ticks act as vectors and main reservoirs. Savanna and veld are the main areas of risk, travellers being exposed on safari holidays. The illness closely resembles Mediterranean tick typhus. A variant form in Zimbabwe is probably due to a separate rickettsial species with a reservoir in domestic cattle.[36] The differential diagnoses in Africa included tick-borne relapsing fever, typhoid, meningococcal septicaemia, measles and viral haemorrhagic fevers. Treatment is as for other forms of typhus.

OTHER FORMS OF TICK TYPHUS

Tick-borne typhus occurs in the mountainous northern fringes of the Indian subcontinent, and as far west as Astrakhan, where it is caused by *R. conorii*. The Siberian form is due to a separate type, *R. sibirica*, which also infects birds and domestic animals, and occurs in Siberia, Kirghizia, Kazakhstan, Armenia and Eastern Europe.

Separate species have also been found in Japan (*R. japonica*)[37] and Australia (*R. australis*), and suspected in Thailand. As yet untyped rickettsial species probably exist in nature for potential transmission to humans by ticks. In general these illnesses resemble Mediterranean tick typhus, and there is an eschar in over 75% of cases. Specific serological diagnosis should be attempted if possible. Antibiotic treatment is as for other forms of typhus.

Rickettsial pox is a spotted fever which produces a distinctive rash and is caused by *R. akari* which is transmitted by *Allodermanyssus sanguineus*, a mite which lives on house and field mice. Foci of this infection are known to exist in the eastern USA, including New York City, Central and South Africa, Crimea, Korea and Costa Rica. *R. akari* is serologically more akin to *R. australis* than to *R. conorii* and *R. rickettsii*. After an incubation period of 7–10 days an eschar is present at the inoculation site in 90% of cases. Fever and general symptoms are as in other forms of typhus. The rash appears rapidly and consists of sparse macules and papules which become vesicular before crusting and fading. The differential diagnoses include chickenpox, monkeypox and secondary syphilis.

The Weil–Felix reaction is negative in rickettsial pox. It can be distinguished from other rickettsial infections by specific agglutination but not by group antigen serology. Treatment is as for other forms of typhus. Preventive measures should be directed at rodent control and efficient garbage clearance.

SCRUB TYPHUS

EPIDEMIOLOGY

Scrub typhus is a significant and widespread disease in Asia. It is due to *R. tsutsugamushi*, also known as *R. orientalis*, of which at least six distinct serological strains (Gilliam, Karp, Kato, Shimokoshi, Kawasaki, Kuroki) can be detected by immunoperoxidase reactions.[38] It occurs in Japan (some 900 cases annually), South Korea, Taiwan, the Philippines, southern China (including Hong Kong and Hainan), East and West Malaysia, Thailand, Cambodia, Vietnam, Laos, Myanmar, Sri Lanka, India, Nepal, northern Pakistan, the islands of the Indian Ocean, Indonesia, Papua New Guinea and its neighbouring islands, Queensland and northern New South Wales (Figure 39.11).

The vector insect to humans is the larva of a number of trombiculid mites in which transovarial transmission maintains the infection in nature. There is also a wild rodent reservoir, and the infection characteristically occurs in discrete foci ('mite islands') where infected mites live on the jungle grass *Imperata cylindrica*, known as *lalang* (Malaysia, Indonesia), *illuk* (Philippines) or *kunai* (Papua New Guinea, Australia), which grows only where primary jungle has been cleared for cultivation or to build villages (Figure 39.12). Human cases occur when workers in oil palm and rubber estates, and policemen and soldiers traverse this habitat, brushing against the sharp stiff blades of waist-high *Imperata* grass, allowing the larval mites access. It is an important military disease, many thousands of cases having occurred in the Far East theatre in the Second World War.[39]

CLINICAL DESCRIPTION

The incubation period is 5–10 days. The mite bite has usually passed unnoticed, but the patient may be aware, as the febrile illness begins, of painful axillary or inguinal lymph nodes. Careful examination will reveal an adjacent eschar, especially on the scrotum (Figure 39.13) or in the axilla, in 50–80% of cases. This is a firm adherent black scab, 3–6 mm in diameter, with a fine red margin, which is painless (Figure 39.14). Multiple eschars can occur, e.g. under a trouser belt. The fever starts abruptly and has the usual typhus accompaniments of suffused conjunctivae and face, severe headache, drowsiness, apathy, pain in the shins and other muscles, and, more characteristically, generalized lymphadenopathy and hepatosplenomegaly. Other symptoms may include nausea and vomiting, tinnitus and hyperacusis followed by deafness, constipation, epistaxis and a dry cough.

The rash is similar to that of louse-borne typhus and occurs mainly on the arms, thighs and trunk. In severe cases, meningoencephalitis ensues with neck stiffness, delirium, focal signs, papilloedema and coma. Myocarditis may complicate this phase, and oliguria with uraemia is common in severe cases.

Indigenous peoples of areas endemic for scrub typhus commonly have a less severe illness, often without any rash or eschar. This is one of the most common causes of 'pyrexia of unknown origin' in such areas,[40] after malaria is excluded, but severe pneumonia has also been described.[41]

Immunity to scrub typhus following an attack is remarkably short-lived, lasting only a few months, and is specific to each strain of the organism, so that further attacks are common.

DIFFERENTIAL DIAGNOSIS

Scrub typhus should be distinguished from:

- Malaria—by stained blood films.
- Arbovirus infections—e.g. dengue, by serological methods.
- Leptospirosis—by blood cultures and serology.
- Meningococcal disease—by blood and CSF cultures.
- Typhoid—by blood and bone marrow cultures.
- Infectious mononucleosis and HIV seroconversion illness—by serological methods.

DIAGNOSIS

As in other forms of typhus, routine blood examinations are unhelpful. The Weil–Felix reaction of

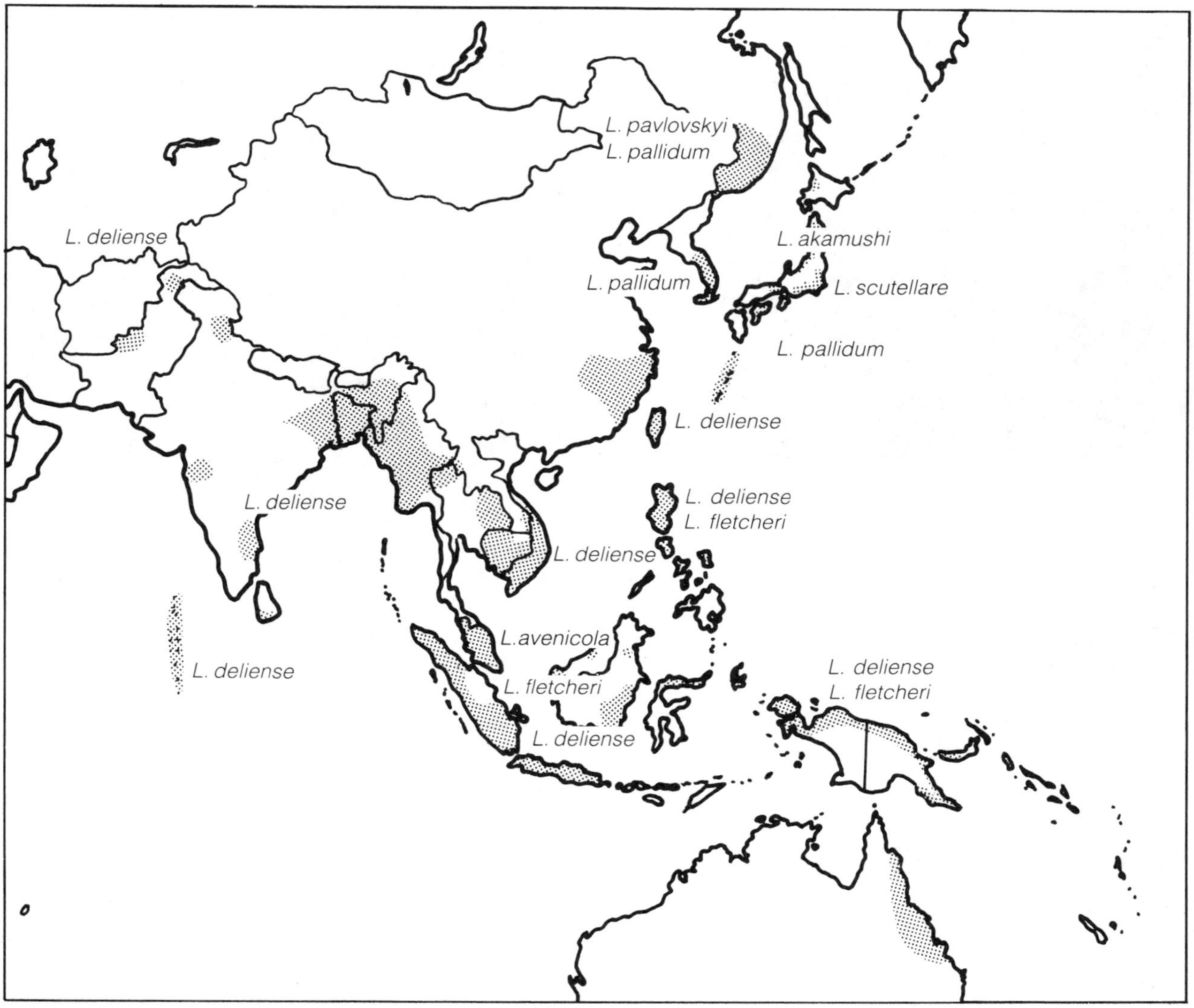

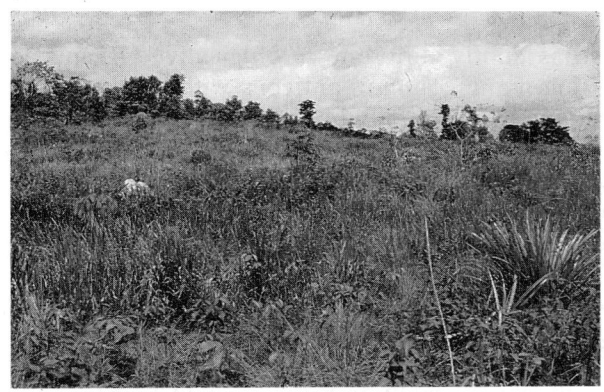

Figure 39.11 Geographical distribution of scrub (mite-borne) typhus (*R. tsutsugamushi* (*orientalis*)). (Courtesy of the Department of Entomology, London School of Hygiene and Tropical Medicine.)

Figure 39.12 Typical scrub typhus country. (Courtesy of G. W. Brown.)

specific agglutination of *Proteus* OX-K is positive in only 50% of cases, and positive titres may be delayed for up to 3 weeks. Specific immunoperoxidase or PCR serology should be sought where available. Commonly, the clinical diagnosis is based on the geographical history and physical signs and confirmed by the rapid response to specific chemotherapy. The occurrence of a Jarisch–Herxheimer reaction after the institution of treatment with tetracycline suggests that leptospirosis was either the primary diagnosis, or coexisted.

TREATMENT

The treatment of scrub typhus is now most commonly with a single oral 200 mg dose of doxycycline for adults, and 100 mg for children. In the small

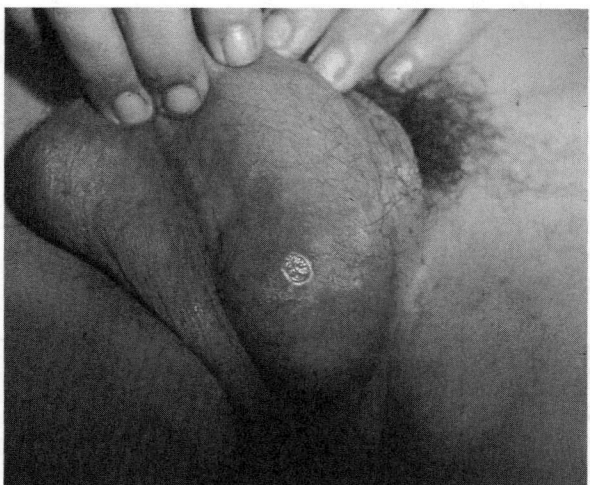

Figure 39.13   The eschar of scrub typhus. (Courtesy of G. W. Brown.)

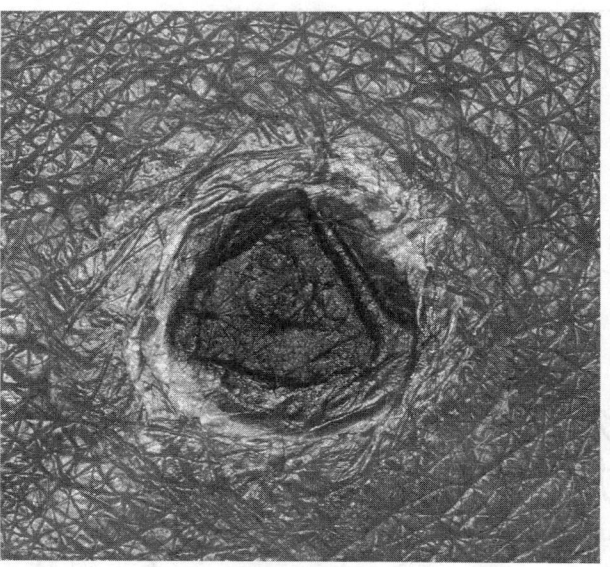

Figure 39.14   The eschar of scrub typhus, close-up view. (Courtesy of G. W. Brown.)

proportion of cases in which the usual rapid defervescence is followed by a relapse of fever 5–7 days later, an identical second dose is given. Continuous chloramphenicol or tetracycline therapy can be given for 7 days, as in louse-borne typhus, but in all forms of typhus tetracycline should not be given to oliguric or anuric patients; doxycycline is safe in such circumstances.

PREVENTION AND CONTROL

Scrub typhus can be partly prevented or controlled by:

1. The wearing of stout boots with trousers well tucked in or strapped at the ankle with gaiters or puttees in those likely to be occupationally exposed to infection.
2. Impregnation of clothing with permethrin in those at occupational risk.
3. Avoidance of cleared jungle areas known to contain infected 'mite islands'.
4. Clearance by burning of *lalang* grass in peridomestic settings, e.g. refugee camps, *kampongs*, military camps.
5. Consideration of use of chemoprophylaxis with doxycycline 200 mg weekly by those at high occupational risk, e.g. soldiers on field operations.
6. Use of cotton-rat lung vaccine; this is not now generally available.

TRENCH FEVER

EPIDEMIOLOGY

Trench fever (His–Werner disease, Wolhynia fever) was first described as an epidemic disease in the First World War—in 1915 on the Western Front and in 1916 in Poland. It is still known to occur in Mexico, Canada, Ethiopia, Burundi, China and Japan. The causative organism, *Rochalimaea quintana*, is closely related to the Rickettsiae but is not an obligate intracellular parasite and can thus be cultured on blood agar. It is transmitted by the human body louse, *Pediculus humanus*. It is thought that wild voles and other rodents may act as a reservoir, although the organism in voles, *Rochalimaea vin-*

soni, is subtly different serologically. Organisms sharing many common antigens with *Rochalimaea quintana* have recently been found in HIV-positive patients with fever, with peliosis hepatis, and with bacillary angiomatosis,[42] but there is no evidence implicating such an infection in the aetiology of Kaposi's sarcoma.

CLINICAL DESCRIPTION

The illness is usually fairly mild, with fever, headache, lumbar muscle pains, dizziness, nausea and vomiting. There is usually a sparse macular rash, but no eschar. The patient may have a single episode of fever lasting a few days, or suffer recurrent fever at intervals of about 5 days (quintan fever), or a more prolonged 'typhoidal' fever. Full recovery is usual and mortality negligible, although some patients suffer prolonged debility with dyspnoea on exertion, but without objective evidence of myocarditis.

DIFFERENTIAL DIAGNOSIS

Trench fever should be distinguished from:

- Louse-borne typhus, although the treatment is identical.
- Louse-borne relapsing fever—by blood cultures and serology.
- Typhoid—by blood and bone marrow cultures.
- Brucellosis—by serological methods.
- Q fever—by serological methods.

DIAGNOSIS

Rochalimaea quintana can be isolated from blood by culture on blood agar in a CO_2-enriched environment. A specific serological agglutination test is also possible.

TREATMENT

Trench fever is treated with doxycycline or other tetracyclines—as for scrub typhus.

PREVENTION AND CONTROL

Outbreaks of trench fever require that cases should be treated, and patients and attendants deloused—as in epidemic typhus.

Q FEVER

EPIDEMIOLOGY

Q fever was so named by Derrick in 1937 as 'query fever' before the causative organism was discovered, and not after Queensland where he discovered it. The strange name has persisted, despite the naming of the causative agent as *Coxiella burnetii*. The disease has also been known as 'Balkan grippe', 'Red River fever' (Zaire) and 'Nine Mile fever' (from a creek in the Rocky Mountains). *C. burnetii* is a very small ($0.2 \times 1.5\,\mu$m) rickettsia-like organism which is particularly resistant to heat and drying. It can be cultured in yolk sacs or minced chicken embryo cell cultures. It exists in nature as a zoonosis of rodents, rabbits and birds; it is transmitted to domestic goats and cattle by ticks and thence to humans, not usually by insects but by direct infection through milk, placental products and dried faeces in dust, although rarely sheep and cattle ticks transmit it to humans. It has a worldwide geographical distribution (Figure 39.15) and is an important cause of abortion in domestic goats and cattle.

C. burnetii produces is an intracytoplasmic infection in which the organism multiplies especially in splenic histiocytes and the Kupffer cells of the liver, where it elicits a granulomatous response.[43]

CLINICAL DESCRIPTION

The clinical course of Q fever may vary from an inapparent infection with seroconversion through a mild brief fever, or a chronic debilitating febrile illness with hepatitis, pneumonitis, pericarditis and a later risk of destructive valvular endocarditis.[44] The initial illness may resemble the typhus fevers, but without rash, although many patients present with 'atypical pneumonia' with clinical and radiological evidence of patchy pneumonitis. Hepatomegaly with biochemical evidence of hepatitis occurs in up to 30% of cases, but marked jaundice is unusual. Splenomegaly and generalized lymphadenopathy may resemble that present in Epstein–Barr virus infection. The acute illness may subside spontaneously and complicating endocarditis may not be apparent from the usual clinical features, until many months have elapsed. Cardiac involvement may occur in up to 10% of cases. The destruction of a previously healthy or congenitally abnormal valve usually involves the aortic valve, and often necessitates operative valve replacement; subsequent reinfection of a prosthetic valve can occur, indicating that infection is difficult to eradicate.

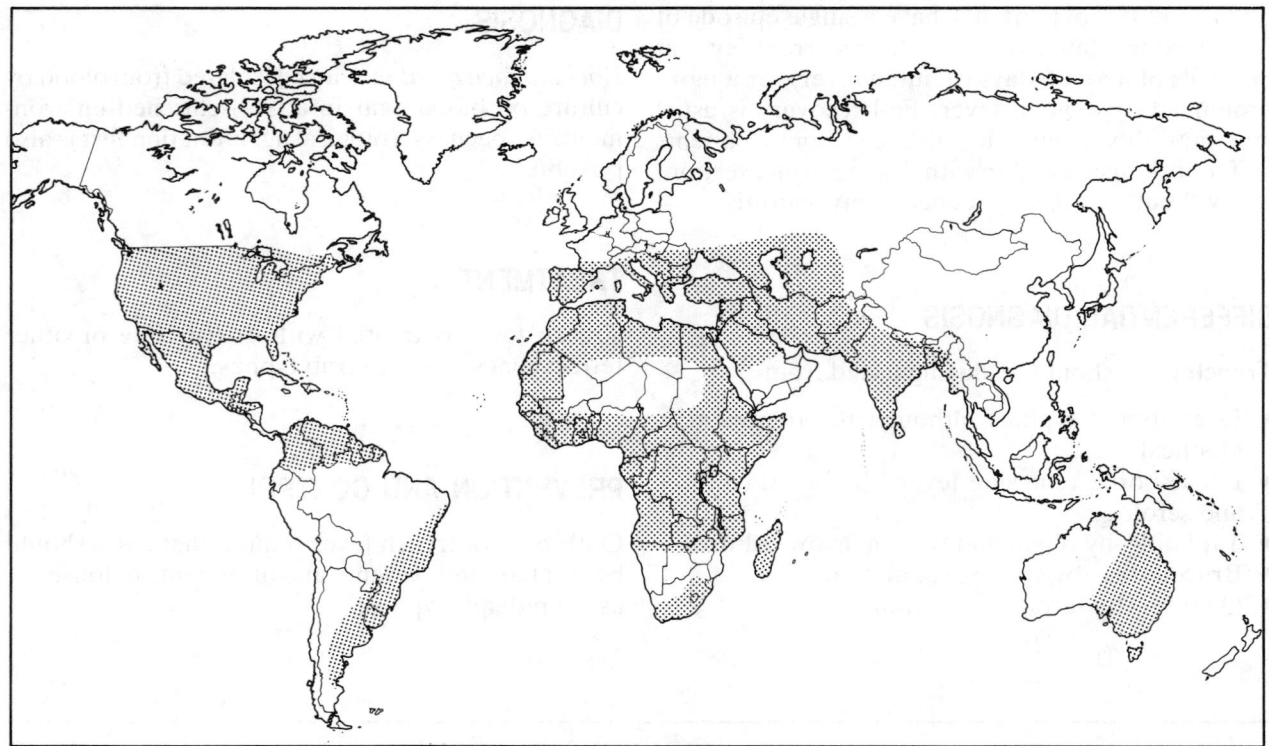

Figure 39.15   Geographical distribution of Q fever.

DIFFERENTIAL DIAGNOSIS

Q fever should be distinguished from:

- Typhoid—by blood and bone marrow culture.
- Other causes of atypical pneumonia, e.g. viruses, mycoplasma pneumoniae, ornithosis—by appropriate serological methods.
- Toxoplasmosis—by serology.
- Virus infections such as Epstein–Barr, HIV, cytomegalovirus—by appropriate serology.
- Viral hepatitis—by serology.
- Miliary tuberculosis—by chest radiography and tuberculin testing.
- Syphilis—by serology.
- Other causes of bacterial endocarditis—by blood cultures, and Lyme disease—by serology.

DIAGNOSIS

The diagnosis of Q fever is best made serologically by a fourfold-rise in antibody titre on complement fixation tests separated by 10–14 days.

ELISA and IFAT serological tests are also available. Liver biopsy shows a granulomatous hepatitis but this has many other possible causes.

TREATMENT

The treatment for early uncomplicated Q fever is as for other forms of typhus fever—with tetracycline, doxycycline or chloramphenicol.

In endocarditis, combination chemotherapy for many months is required with rifampicin and co-trimoxazole, or tetracycline and co-trimoxazole. Quinolone antibiotics may also be effective. Cardiac surgical treatment may be required.

PREVENTION AND CONTROL

Aerosol dissemination of *C. burnetii* is very difficult to prevent as control of the disease in domestic animals is difficult. Milk should be pasteurized, and slightly higher temperatures may be needed for milk from herds known to be infected.

A formalinized vaccine is available for the protection of abattoir workers, farmers and herdsmen, and laboratory workers; this is widely used in Australia.

EHRLICHIOSIS

Ehrlichia sennetsu, an intraleucocytic bacterium closely related to the Rickettsiae, was first isolated in Japan in 1954 from a patient with an illness similar to infectious mononucleosis,[45] and named accordingly—*sennetsu* being the Japanese name for glandular fever. Similar cases have been reported in Japan, Malaysia and the Philippines. No insect vector has yet been implicated in its transmission. Tetracyclines are successful in treatment.

E. canis has been known since 1935 to be the cause of tropical canine pancytopenia, transmitted by *Rhipicephalus sanguineus*, the brown dog tick.

Dogs suffer an initial acute illness with fever, lymphadenopathy and thrombocytopenia, which passes into a chronic phase with bone-marrow hypoplasia, which may prove fatal.[46] This disease is known to occur in the USA and South-East Asia and probably exists worldwide.

Human infection with *E. canis*, transmitted by dog ticks, was not reported until 1986 in the USA,[47] where cases were described of a febrile illness following a tick bite similar to RMSF, but without a rash. Intraleucocytic organisms were detected, and antibodies against *E. canis* found at high titre. Features of the illness included a macular rash, encephalopathy, renal insufficiency, joint pains and thrombocytopenia. The response to treatment with chloramphenicol, doxycycline and corticosteroids, with haemodialysis, was satisfactory. A few patients with acquired immune deficiency syndrome (AIDS) have also been reported as having *E. canis* infection.

The human infection has recently been separately characterized as *E. chaffeensis*.[48,49]

In Hong Kong an illness very similar to scrub typhus, but with negative specific serological tests for *R. tsutsugamushi*, has recently been seen, and named 'Lion Rock fever' after a geographical feature overlooking the area where cases have been reported.[50] It is possible that this is also a form of ehrlichiosis, although an unknown Rickettsia could be responsible. The illness responds dramatically to doxycycline.

REFERENCES

1 Cardano G. *De malo recentiorum medicorum medendi usu libellus*. Venetiis, apud O. Scotum, 1536.

2 Fracastoro G. *De sympathia et antipathia rerum liber unus. De contagione et contagiosis morbis et curatione*. Venetiis, apud heredes L. Iuntae, 1546.

3 Coyttarus J. *De febre purpura epidemiali et contagiosa libri duo*. Parisiis, apud M. Juevenem, 1578.

4 Cober T. *Observationum medicorum Castrensium Hungaricarum Helmstadii*, F. Linderwald, 1685.

5 Pringle J. *Observations on the Nature and Cure of Hospital and Jayl-Fevers*. London: Millar & Wilson, 1750.

6 von Hildenbrand J V. *Ueber den Ansteckenden Typhus*. Wein, 1810.

7 Nicolle C J H. Recherches experimentales sur le typhus exanthematique. *Ann Inst Pasteur* 1910; 24:243–275; 1911; 25:97–144; 1912; 26:250–280, 332–350.

8 da Rocha-Lima H. Zür Aetiologie des Fleckfiebers. *Berl Klin Wochenschr* 1916; 53:567–569.

9 Bravo F. *Opera Medicinalia*. Mexico: Ocharte, 1570, 1–90.

10 Maxcy K F. Clinical observations on endemic typhus in Southern United States. *Public Health Rep* 1926; 41:1213–1220, 2967–2995.

11 Mooser H. Experiments relating to the pathology and etiology of Mexican typhus (tabardillo). *J Infect Dis* 1928; 43:241–272.

12 Maxey E E. Some observations on the so-called spotted fever of Idaho. *Med Sentinel* (Portland, OR) 1899; 7:433–438.

13 Ricketts H T. The transmission of Rocky Mountain spotted fever by the bite of the wood tick (*Dermacentor occidentalis*). *JAMA* 1906; 47:358.

14 Conor A L J & Bruch A. Un fièvre éruptive. *Bull Soc Pathol Exot* 1910; 3:45–96.

15 Baelz E & Kawakami. Das japanische Fluss-oder-Ueberschwemmungs-Fieber, eine acute Infections-Krankheit. *Virchows Arch [Pathol Anat]* 1879; 78:373–420, 528–530.

16 Fletcher W & Lesslar J E. *Tropical Typhus in the Federated Malay States, with a Compilation on Epidemic Typhus*. London: John Bale, 1925.

17 Ogata N. Aetiologie der Tsutsugamushi-Krankheit; Rickettsia tsutsugamushi. *Zentralbl Bakteriol* (Abt Orig) 1931; 122:249–253.

18 Graham J H P. A note on a relapsing febrile illness of unknown origin. *Lancet* 1915; ii:703–704.

19 Hunt G H & Rankin A C. Intermittent fever of obscure origin occurring among British soldiers in France. *Lancet* 1915; ii:1133–1136.

20 His W. Ueber eine neue periodische Fieberkrankung (Febris Wolhynica). *Berl Klin Wochenschr* 1916; 53:322–323.

21 Töpfer H W. Zür Ursache und Uebertragung des Wolhynischen Fiebers. *Munch Med Wochenschr* 1916; 63: 1495–1496.

22 Sussman L N. Kew Gardens spotted fever. *N Y Med* 1946; 2(15):27–28.

23 Derrick E H. Q Fever, a new fever entity; clinical features and laboratory investigations. *Med J Aust* 1937; 2:281–299.

24 Cox H R & Bell E J. Epidemic and endemic typhus. Protective value for guinea-pigs of vaccines prepared from infected tissues of the developing chick embryo. *Public Health Rep* 1940; 55:110–115.

25 Fulton F & Joyner L. Cultivation of Rickettsia tsutsugamushi in lungs of rodents. Preparation of a scrub typhus vaccine. *Lancet* 1945; ii:729–734.

26 Smadel, J E, Woodward T E, Ley H L et al. Chloramphenicol (chloromycetin) in the treatment of tsutsugamushi disease (scrub typhus). *J Clin Invest* 1949; 28:1196–1215.

27 Weil E & Felix A. Zür seroligischen Diagnose des Fleckfiebers. *Wein Klin Wochenschr* 1916; 29:33–35.

28 Fletcher W & Lesslar J E. *The Weil–Felix Reaction in Sporadic Tropical Typhus.* London: John Bale, 1926.

29 Wohlbach S B. *The Aetiology and Pathology of Typhus.* Cambridge, MA; Harvard University Press, 1922.

30 Brill N E. An acute infectious disease of unknown origin. A clinical study based on 221 cases. *Am J Med Sci* 1910; 139:484–502.

31 Zinsser H. Varieties of typhus vaccine and the epidemiology of the American form of European typhus fever (Brill's disease). *Am J Hyg* 1934; 20:513–532.

32 Carl M, Tibbs C W, Dobson M E et al. Diagnosis of acute typhus infection using the polymerase chain reaction. *J Infect Dis* 1990; 161:791–793.

33 Huys J, Freyens P, Kahiyigi J & Van den Berghe G. Treatment of epidemic typhus. *Trans R Soc Trop Med Hyg* 1973; 67:718–721.

34 Duffy P E, Le Guillozic H, Gass R F & Innis B L. Murine typhus identified as a major cause of febrile illness in a camp for displaced Khmers in Thailand. *Am J Trop Med Hyg* 1990; 43:520–526.

35 Rauolt D, Weiller P J, Chagnon A et al. Mediterranean spotted fever: clinical, laboratory and epidemiological features of 199 cases. *Am J Trop Med Hyg* 1986; 35:845–850.

36 Kelly P J, Mason H R, Matthewman L A & Rauolt D. Sero-epidemiology of spotted fever group rickettsial infections in humans in Zimbabwe. *J Trop Med Hyg* 1991; 94:304–309.

37 Uchida T, Yu X, Uchiyama T & Walker D M. Identification of a unique spotted fever group rickettsia from humans in Japan. *J Infect Dis* 1989; 159:1122–1125.

38 Tange Y, Kanemitsu N & Kobayashi Y. Analysis of immunological characteristics of newly isolated strains of *Rickettsia tsutsugamushi* using monoclonal antibodies. *Am J Trop Med Hyg* 1991; 44:371–381.

39 Sayers M H P & Hill I G W. The occurrence and identification of the typhus group of fevers in South East Asia Command. *J R Army Med Corps* 1948; 90:6–22.

40 Brown G W, Shirai A, Jegathesan M et al. Febrile illness in Malaysia—an analysis of 1629 hospitalised patients. *Am J Trop Med Hyg* 1984; 33:311–315.

41 Chayakul P, Panich V & Silpapojakul K. Scrub typhus pneumonitis: an entity which is frequently missed. *Q J Med* 1988; 68:595–602.

42 Relman D A, Loutit J S, Schmidt T M et al. The agent of bacillary angiomatosis. *N Engl J Med* 1990; 323:1573–1580.

43 Whittick J W. Necropsy findings in a case of Q fever in Britain. *BMJ* 1950; i:979–980.

44 Turck W P G, Howitt G, Turnberg L A et al. Chronic Q fever. *Q J Med* 1976; 45:193–217.

45 Misao T & Kobayashi Y. Studies on infectious mononucleosis (glandular fever). I. Isolation of etiologic agent from blood, bone marrow and lymph nodes from a patient with infectious mononucleosis by using mice. *Kyūshū J Med Sci* 1955; 6:146–152.

46 Huxsoll D L, Bildebrandt P K, Nims R M & Walker J S. Tropical canine pancytopenia. *J Am Vet Med Assoc* 1970; 157:1627–1632.

47 Maeda K, Markowitz N, Hawley R C et al. Human infection with *Ehrlichia canis*, a leukocytic rickettsia. *N Engl J Med* 1987; 316:853–856.

48 Taylor J P, Betz T G, Fishbein D B et al. Serological evidence of possible human infection with *Ehrlichia* in Texas. *J Infect Dis* 1988; 158:217–220.

49 Dawson J E, Anderson B, Fishbein D B *et al*. Isolation and characterization of an *Ehrlichia* sp. from a patient diagnosed with human ehrlichiosis. *J Clin Microbiol* 1991; 29:2741–2745.

50 Cohen M A H, Li P K T, Cheng A F B et al. A fatal case of rickettsial spotted fever in Hong Kong—Lion Rock Fever. *J HK Med Assoc* 1989; 41:185–186.

SECTION 5C
BACTERIAL INFECTIONS

The emergence of successive generations of antibiotics during the last few decades has engendered much false optimism regarding control of bacterial disease in tropical and subtropical countries. However, the present situation gives cause for a great deal of pessimism, and indeed alarm. Tuberculosis remains a problem of enormous significance; in fact in 1995 this disease probably accounts for a greater degree of morbidity and mortality than any other single bacterial infection, despite the fact that streptomycin was first introduced into clinical medicine in 1944! A further problem of vast magnitude has resulted from the fact that *Mycobacterium* spp. infections are of major significance as opportunistic infections in the context of the human immunodeficiency virus (HIV) and the acquired immune deficiency syndrome—a problem which will inevitably escalate during the years ahead. Resistance to antituberculous agents is now also of major importance.

Intestinal infections are also rapidly becoming exceedingly difficult to treat: bacterial resistance has, for example, become a major problem in *Salmonella* spp. and *Shigella* spp. infections. Numerically, the archetypal small-intestinal infection *Vibrio cholerae* has, far from being brought under control, expanded its boundaries to much of southern America and also Africa. A further prob-lem of great topicality is that the non-O1 variant (to which classical *V. cholerae* renders no immunological protection) is becoming commonplace in southern Asia.

Of the more exotic infections, plague is again proving a major problem in many developing countries; this 'historical' disease has been responsible for many of the pestilences of the past and has exerted a major influence on human civilization, probably for many millennia.

Many of these infections are especially lethal in those under 5 years old. This applies especially to intestinal infections—in which a vicious cycle with malnutrition results in failure to thrive and a great deal of mortality.

Although in many cases appropriate antibacterial agents are available, the cost to the health budgets of developing countries is frequently insuperably high, putting them quite out of reach. Thus, to most of the world's populations, such agents might just as well not exist!

Overall, therefore, although the antibiotic era has led to a sharp decline in bacterial infections in the developed world, this certainly does not apply to those vast areas of the globe situated in the tropics and subtropics. Many of these infections are reviewed in this section.

CHAPTER 40

INTRODUCTION TO ACUTE INFECTIVE DIARRHOEA

C. A. Hart

Diarrhoeal disease is a major cause of mortality throughout the world. It is estimated that there are approximately 5–6 million deaths worldwide each year due to gastroenteritis,[1] and that gastroenteritis is second only to acute respiratory tract infection as the major cause of death due to infection.

Gastroenteritis exerts its greatest toll in children under 5 years old (see Chapter 35). In developing countries estimates of the annual incidence of diarrhoea vary from 3.3 episodes,[2] to 7.9 episodes,[3] to 10 episodes in a periurban area in Lima.[4] In contrast the incidence is much less in children in developed countries; for example, children in Winnipeg were reported to experience 0.8 diarrhoeal episodes per year.[5] The contrast between paediatric diarrhoea in developing and developed countries is shown in Table 40.1. In addition to the morbidity and mortality associated with diarrhoeal disease, it is also a major drain on health resources in developing countries. For example, it has been estimated that in Indonesia the per capita health budget is $5.41 per annum and that $2.50 per annum is spent per child on management of diarrhoeal disease.

Although it is not possible to diagnose the aetiological agents causing gastroenteritis clinically, it is convenient to subdivide diarrhoeal disease into inflammatory and non-inflammatory diarrhoea. There is some overlap between the two but this classification does provide a basis for discussing diarrhoeal disease (Table 40.2). In addition to the above there are pathogens that produce a disease that is predominantly vomiting with little or no diarrhoea. This is usually due to contamination of food by either *Staphylococcus aureus* or *Bacillus cereus* which liberate emetic toxins.

Table 40.1 Paediatric diarrhoea in developed and developing countries (after ref 6).

Feature	Developed countries	Developing countries
Episodes per annum	<1	3–10
Seasonality	Winter	None
Severe dehydration	Rare	Frequent
Nutritional sequelae	Rare	Usual
Measles associated	Non-existent	15–63%
Epidemic	Rare	Frequent
Polymicrobial	Unusual	>20%
Case:fatality rate	<0.01%	0.6%

Table 40.2 Clinical features of inflammatory and non-inflammatory diarrhoea.

	Non-inflammatory	Inflammatory
Symptoms	Nausea, vomiting; abdominal pain and fever not major features	Abdominal pain, tenesmus, fever
Stool	Voluminous, Watery	Frequent, small volume; blood-stained, pus cells present, mucus
Site	Proximal small intestine	Distal small intestine, colon
Mechanism	Osmotic or secretory	Invasion of enterocytes leading to mucosal cell death and inflammatory response

NON-INFLAMMATORY DIARRHOEA

The pathogens causing non-inflammatory diarrhoea are shown in Table 40.3. For the majority of these their principal site of action is the upper small intestine. Since the transit time is so rapid through the small intestine an important pathogenetic factor is the ability to adhere to the small intestinal mucosa. The mechanisms most commonly employed in producing diarrhoea are osmotic and secretory. In the former there is an inability to degrade, for example disaccharides to monosaccharides. Since only monosaccharides can be absorbed by enterocytes the disaccharides pass down the intestine taking water with them. In secretory diarrhoea the enterocyte is stimulated to secrete fluid into the gut lumen.

Table 40.3 Pathogens in inflammatory and non-inflammatory diarrhoea.

	Inflammatory	*Non-inflammatory*
Viruses (see Chapter 35)	Nil	Rotavirus Adenovirus 40/41 Astrovirus Norwalk agent Calicivirus Small round structureless virus Coronavirus Bredavirus Picobirnavirus
Bacteria (see Chapter 41)	Enteroinvasive *E.coli* (EIEC) Enterohaemorrhagic *E.coli* (EHEC) Enteroaggregative *E.coli* (EAggEC) *Aeromonas hydrophila* *Campylobacter* spp. *Salmonella* spp. *Shigella* spp. *Yersinia enterocolitica* *Clostridium difficile*	Enterotoxigenic *E.coli* (ETEC) Enteropathogenic *E.coli* (EPEC) *Vibrio cholerae* *Vibrio parahaemolyticus* *Campylobacter* spp. *Salmonella* spp. *Bacillus cereus* *Clostridium perfringens*
Protozoa (see Chapter 67)	*Entamoeba histolytica*	*Cryptosporidium parvum* *Giardia intestinalis (lamblia)* *Blastocystis hominis* *Isospora belli* *Enterocytozoon bieneusi*

INFLAMMATORY DIARRHOEA

Although there is some overlap (e.g. *Salmonella* spp. and *Campylobacter* spp. can cause non-inflammatory diarrhoea), the pathogens causing inflammatory diarrhoea form a distinct group (Table 40.3). Their site of action is usually the colon and distal ileum and they produce disease by destroying parts of the enteric mucous membranes, leading to an inflammatory response. This in turn leads to the excretion of neutrophils and erythrocytes in faeces which can be detected by simple wet film microscopy.

EPIDEMIOLOGICAL ASPECTS

The prevalence of different enteropathogens varies with the age of the individual, how the diarrhoea is acquired (e.g. food poisoning or traveller's diarrhoea), between acute and chronic diarrhoea, and with the state of the host's immunity.

AGE

In general, paediatric diarrhoea is most often due to viral enteropathogens (see Chapter 35). Approximately 60% of cases in most hospital-based surveys are due to viruses, with rotavirus accounting for a large proportion of cases, followed by adenovirus 40/41 and then astrovirus. Bacterial enteropathogens such as enteropathogenic *Escherichia coli* (EPEC), enterotoxigenic *E.coli* (ETEC), enteroaggregative *E.coli* (EAggEC), salmonellae, *Campylobacter jejuni* and shigellae and the protozoan *Cryptosporidium parvum* are responsible for the majority of the remaining cases where a pathogen is found.

In adults bacteria assume greater importance, although viral gastroenteritis does occur. For example it is estimated that *C. jejuni* is responsible for 17–20% of episodes of adult diarrhoea.

FOOD POISONING

Diarrhoeal disease following ingestion of food or water contaminated by bacteria, toxins or protozoa is still an important problem in both developed and developing countries. Although high intensity animal rearing is important in the maintenance of human enteropathogens in developed countries, in developing countries human enteric pathogens such as *Salmonella* spp. and *C. jejuni* and enterohaemorrhagic *E.coli* (EHEC) may still be implicated in outbreaks of food poisoning. Recently, water-borne outbreaks or *C. parvum* have been assuming greater importance.

TRAVELLERS' DIARRHOEA (turista, Aztec two-step, Delhi belly, etc.)

It is estimated that approximately 16 million people will travel from their domicile in industrialized

Table 40.4 Enteropathogens in travellers' diarrhoea.

Pathogen	Prevalence (%)
Enterotoxigenic *E.coli*	30–80
Campylobacter jejuni	*c.* 20
Shigella spp.	5–15
Salmonella spp.	3–15
Giardia lamblia	0–3
Cryptosporidium parvum	?
Entamoeba histolytica	0–3
Rotavirus	?
Astrovirus	?
Norwalk Agent	?
Unknown	15–20

?, Described, but imprecise or regionally restricted figures.

countries to less-developed countries. Approximately one-third of these will develop diarrhoeal disease and in the majority of cases this will be due to an infective agent.[7] A large number of different enteropathogens have been implicated but in most surveys ETEC are the predominant pathogens (Table 40.4) followed by *C. jejuni* and *Salmonella* spp. The aetiological agents vary considerably according to the countries visited, for example *C. parvum* has recently been shown to be important in visitors to the Caribbean[8] and Africa.[9] Viral enteropathogens can cause travellers' diarrhoea but have, for example, been more frequently associated with shipboard epidemics in which astrovirus and calicivirus have been implicated.

IMMUNOCOMPROMISED HOST

In tropical countries the immune compromise due to malnutrition and human immunodeficiency virus (HIV) are of major importance; both affect the frequency and severity of diarrhoeal disease. With the appearance of the acquired immune deficiency syndrome, diarrhoeal disease due to previously unrecognized pathogens, such as *C. parvum*, *Isospora belli*, *Enterocytozoon bieneusi* and *Mycobacterium avium-intracellulare*, has assumed increasing importance, albeit more often causing chronic diarrhoea.[10] Interestingly there is little information on the role of rotavirus—the major cause of infantile gastroenteritis, in HIV-infected children.

MANAGEMENT OF ACUTE DIARRHOEA

The mainstay of management of diarrhoeal disease is the assessment of dehydration and the appropriate replacement of fluid and electrolytes.[11] Although diarrhoeal disease can produce dehydration at any age, its impact is greatest in those under 5 years old. This is because, as a result of their relatively greater surface area and thus greater fluid loss through skin, infants require 2.5 times more water per kilogram body weight than older individuals. Fluid and electrolyte loss is also greatly exacerbated by vomiting. Both the initial degree of dehydration and the response to rehydration therapy should be monitored clinically (Table 40.5).

Table 40.5 Clinical assessment of rehydration.

Severity	Body weight loss	Clinical state	Signs
Mild	<5	Not unwell	Thirsty, mucous membranes dry
Moderate	5–10	Apathetic	Sunken eyes, sunken fontanelle, tachypnoea, oliguria, loss of skin turgor
Severe	10–15	Shocked	Hypotensive, peripheral circulatory failure
Critical	>15	Moribund	Severely shocked, comatose

Originally, rehydration was exclusively intravenous. This resulted in a tremendous drop in fatality rates, for example in cholera from 40% to less than 1% when properly administered. A major advance was made when an effective oral rehydration regimen was devised.

ORAL REHYDRATION THERAPY

Early oral rehydration solutions (ORS) contained only electrolytes and water and it was not until it was realized that glucose or sucrose were required to enhance sodium absorption that effective oral rehydration therapy became available. Glucose and sodium transport into enterocytes are coupled. Sucrose, a dimer of glucose and fructose, must be cleaved by brush-border sucrase for it to be ab-

sorbed. Nevertheless glucose and sucrose seem to be equally effective in ORS,[12] although there may be minor advantages with glucose.[13]

There is also some debate over the use of bicarbonate or citrate to correct acidosis. Both are equally effective but citrate is more stable, and has replaced bicarbonate in World Health Organization solutions. A further modification has been the incorporation of glycine which is taken into the enterocyte by a specific amino acid transport system. Glycine, when present in ORS at a concentration of 111 mmol/l, was found to decrease both duration of diarrhoea and stool volume.[14] The composition of various ORS is shown in Table 40.6. ORS can be obtained in packets from UNICEF or can be made up locally. They should contain sodium chloride (3.5 g), potassium chloride (1.5 g), glucose monohydrate (22 g) made up to 1 litre with potable water (sucrose, 40 g, may replace glucose, and trisodium citrate dehydrate, 2.9 g, sodium bicarbonate). To be fully effective ORS should be available at the village level so therapy can be initiated as rapidly as possible. This will require the solution(s) to be available either prepacked or in bulk, with appropriate measuring spoons, a method of providing the correct volume of potable water, and instructions on use as well as to discard unused solution within 24 h. Studies have shown that when properly instructed 98% of mothers can prepare ORS with a sodium range of 30–110 mmol/l.[15] Recently, rice powder-based ORS have been investigated, since these are more readily available. Rice powder at 30–50 g/l is an effective substitute for glucose. It tastes better than simple electrolyte–glucose ORS and is thus more acceptable to children. A recent meta-analysis of 13 randomized trials of rice-based versus glucose-

Table 40.6 Composition of oral rehydration solutions.

| Component | Concentration (mmol/l water) | | |
	Citrate ORS	Bicarbonate ORS	Glycine ORS*
Sodium	90	90	90
Potassium	20	20	20
Chloride	80	80	80
Citrate	10	—	—
Bicarbonate	—	30	30
Glucose	111	111	111
Glycine	—	—	111

*May contain either bicarbonate or citrate.

Table 40.7 Guidelines for rehydration.

Degree	Age group	Type of fluid	Volume (ml/kg body weight)	Timing
Mild	All	ORS	50	Every 4 hours
Moderate	All	ORS	100	Every 4 hours
Severe	Infants	i.v. (Hartman's)	70	Every 3 hours
Severe and shock	All	i.v. (Hartman's)	70–100	Every 4 hours

based oral rehydration therapy demonstrated the superiority of the rice-based solution in cholera diarrhoea, although the benefit was considerably smaller for children with acute non-cholera diarrhoea.[16] During the initial phase of oral rehydration therapy, while the patient is dehydrated, adults can consume 750 ml/h and children up to 300 ml/h. Maintenance therapy of 20 ml solution per kg body weight should be started as soon as signs of dehydration have gone. ORS are suitable for rehydration of all except severely dehydrated infants and those with shock (Table 40.7).

INTRAVENOUS REHYDRATION

Approximately 98% of children will respond to oral rehydration therapy. The remainder are generally infants with severe dehydration or those with profuse vomiting or a high purging rate. These will require rehydration by the intravenous route. Suitable solutions include: Ringer's lactate (Hartman's), consisting of NaCl 6.2 g, KCl 0.4 g, Na lactate 2.3 g and 2 ml 50% glucose in one litre of solution; Dacca solution (NaCl 5 g, NaHCO$_3$ 4 g, KCl 1 g and 50% glucose per litre); or acetate solution (NaCl 5 g, KCl 1 g, Na acetate 6.5 g and 2 ml 50% glucose per litre of solution). Oral rehydration therapy should be started as soon as possible following institution of intravenous rehydration, but if signs of severe dehydration persist it may be necessary to continue using Ringer's lactate at 100 ml/kg body weight per 4 hours.

ADJUNCT THERAPY

Other potential therapeutic interventions include antimicrobial agents, antimotility drugs and antisecretory drugs. They have varying degrees of efficacy and some are absolutely contraindicated for certain conditions.

ANTIMICROBIAL DRUGS

In general, infants with acute watery diarrhoea are best managed without recourse to antibiotics. However, if there is evidence of systemic spread, cholera or dysentery then antimicrobials will shorten the course of diarrhoea and ameliorate its effects. With the advent of the fluroquinolones such as ciprofloxacin and ofloxacin the debate on the use of antimicrobials has been reopened. Firstly, there is no doubt that the widespread indiscriminate use of antimicrobials, often in subtherapeutic regimens, encourages resistance in both pathogens and normal enteric flora.[17] On the other hand, even with ETEC early treatment with co-trimoxazole[18] or ciprofloxacin can decrease the severity of diarrhoea. This is preferred to the widespread prophylactic use of these antimicrobials which will certainly produce resistant bacteria.

In cholera, tetracycline or ciprofloxacin decrease the duration of diarrhoea and shedding of bacteria. In countries where *Shigella* spp. dysentery is endemic or when epidemics occur, antimicrobials are of benefit but development of resistance during the course of epidemics occurs with monotonous regularity.[17] Metronidazole (or tinidazole) is valuable in the treatment of giardiasis or amoebic dysentery.

ANTIMOTILITY DRUGS

These should be avoided.

ANTISECRETORY DRUGS

These will of course only be effective if there is a secretory component to the diarrhoea. The value of loperamide as an adjunct in treating diarrhoea in well-nourished children has been demonstrated[19] but these authors warned against its use in malnourished children.

Compounds such as kaolin or charcoal which, it is postulated, act by absorbing toxins have had little effect in controlled trials.

CONTROL OF DIARRHOEAL DISEASE

In industrialized countries it has been the separation of human and animal excreta from potable water and foodstuffs that has contributed to the great decline in the incidence of diarrhoeal disease. In addition, improvement in facilities for personal hygiene within the home have decreased the intrafamilial spread of enteropathogens. To implement these measures in developing countries will need a massive input from industrialized countries. There is little doubt that measles and malnutrition increase the morbidity and mortality of diarrhoeal disease, and control of measles by immunization should be possible.

Finally, it is unlikely that spread of some enteric pathogens, such as rotavirus, can be prevented completely by public health and good hygiene. A safe and effective vaccine against rotavirus would be of major benefit.

CONCLUSIONS

CONCLUSIONS

Diarrhoeal disease is still a major cause of mortality even though it has been shown that introduction of oral rehydration therapy can decrease mortality to less than 0.5% in defined study areas.

MORBIDITY

Malnutrition greatly affects immunity[20,21] and the incidence and severity of diarrhoeal disease. Similarly, diarrhoeal disease will greatly exacerbate malnutrition, thus creating an inexorable downward spiral. Acute diarrhoeal disease can become chronic, and chronic diarrhoea, for example that due to *C. parvum*, can become greatly prolonged.[22] Disaccharide (principally lactose) intolerance following certain types of diarrhoea has been a source of great controversy. Certain pathogens such as rotavirus or EPEC produce a great decrease in small-intestinal disaccharidase levels. Some consider that infants should not be given their normal diet because of the problem of disaccharide intolerance. Most evidence now suggests that infants should return to their normal diet within 24 hours of onset of diarrhoea unless there are specific contraindications.[23]

REFERENCES

1 Snyder J D & Merson M H. The magnitude of the global problem of acute diarrheal disease: a review of active surveillance data. *Bull World Health Organ* 1982; 60: 605–613.

2 WHO/CDD/VID/84.4 Diarrhoeal Disease Control Programme. *Report of the Third Meeting of the Scientific Working Group on Viral Diarrhoeas. Microbiology, Epidemiology, Immunology and Vaccine Development.* Geneva: WHO, 1984:8–14.

3 Mata L, Simhon A, Urrutia J, Kronmal R, Fernandez R & Crareia B. Epidemiology of rotavirus in a cohort of 45 Guatemalan Mayan Indian children from birth to age 3 years. *J Infect Dis* 1983; 148:452–461.

4 Black R C, Lopez de Romana G, Brown K H, Bravo N, Bazalar O G & Kanashiro H C. Incidence and etiology of infantile diarrhea and major routes of transmission in Huascar, Peru. *Am J Epidemiol* 1989; 129:785–799.

5 Gurwith M, Wenman W, Hinde D, Feltham S & Greenberg H. A prospective study of rotavirus infection in infants and young children. *J Infect Dis* 1981; 144:218–224.

6 Kumate J & Isibasi A. Pediatric diarrheal diseases: a global perspective. *Pediatr Infect Dis J* 1986; S1:21–28.

7 Steffan R, van der Linde F, Gyr K & Schar M. Epidemiology of diarrhea in travellers. *JAMA* 1983; 249:1176–1180.

8 Ma P, Kaufman D C, Helmick C G, D'Souza A J & Navin T R. Cryptosporidium in tourists returning from the Caribbean. *N Engl J Med* 1985; 312:647–648.

9 Soave R & Ma P. Cryptosporidium: traveller's

diarrhea in two families. *Arch Intern Med* 1985; 145:70–72.

10 Smith P D. Gastrointestinal infections in AIDS. *Ann Intern Med* 1992; 116:63–77.

11 Cash R A. Oral rehydration therapy. In Farthing M J G & Keusch G T (eds) *Enteric Infection*. London: Chapman & Hall, 1989:441–451.

12 Sack D A, Chowdhury A M A K, Eusof A et al. Oral rehydration in rotavirus diarrhoea: a double blind comparison of sucrose with glucose electrolyte solution. *Lancet* 1978; ii:280–283.

13 Nalin D R, Levine M M, Mata L et al. Comparison of sucrose with glucose in oral therapy of infant diarrhoea. *Lancet* 1978; ii:277–279.

14 Mahalanabis D & Patra F C. In search of a super oral rehydration solution: can optimum use of organic solute medicated transport lead to the development of an absorption promoting drug? *J Diarrhoeal Dis Res* 1982; 2:76:81.

15 Bhatia S, Cash R A & Cornaz I. Evaluation of the oral therapy expansion program (OTEP) of the Bangladesh rural advancement committee (BRAC). Swiss Development Cooperation and Humanitarian Aid. January 24–February 12 1983.

16 Gore S M, Fontaine O & Pierce N F. Impact of rice based oral rehydration solution on stool output and duration of diarrhoea: meta-analysis of 13 clinical trials. *BMJ* 1992; 304:287–291.

17 Shears P. A review of bacterial resistance to antimicrobial agents in the tropics. *Ann Trop Paed* 1993; 13:219–226.

18 DuPont H R, Randall R R, Galindo E, Sullivan P S, Wood L V & Mendiola J G. Treatment of traveller's diarrhea with trimethoprim/sulfamethoxazole and with trimethoprim alone. *N Engl J Med* 1982; 307:841–844.

19 Diarrhoeal Diseases Study Group (UK). Loperamide in acute diarrhoea in childhood: results of a double blind placebo controlled multicentre clinical trial. *BMJ* 1984; 289:1263–1267.

20 Chandra R K. Nutrition, immunity, and infection: present knowledge and future directions. *Lancet* 1983; i:688–691.

21 Dowd P & Heatly R. The influence of undernutrition on immunity. *Clin Sci* 1984; 66:241–248.

22 Sallon S, Deckelbaum R J, Schmid II, Harlap S, Baras M & Spira D T. *Cryptosporidium*, malnutrition and chronic diarrhea in children. *Am J Dis Child* 1988; 142:312–315.

23 Committee on Nutrition. Use of oral fluid therapy and posttreatment feeding following enteritis in children in a developed country. *Pediatrics* 1985; 75:358–361.

CHAPTER 41

GASTROINTESTINAL BACTERIA

P. Shears and C. A. Hart

The adult human comprises 10^{14} cells but only 10% of these are mammalian. The remaining 9×10^{13} consist of the bacteria and fungi that make up normal flora. The gastrointestinal tract is the major reservoir for these flora. Although bacteria can be found in the stomach and small intestine they are present in low numbers (10^2–10^4 cfu/ml) and are usually transient(s). In contrast the lower ileum and colon contain large numbers of bacteria (c. 10^{12} cfu/ml) and half the weight of faeces is made up of bacteria. To detect small numbers of pathogens in this mass of normal flora can therefore be problematic.

HELICOBACTER PYLORI

Since the beginning of this century histopathologists have described spiral bacteria in the stomach. It was not until 1983 that a bacterium was grown, rather serendipitously.[1] This micro-organism was originally named *Campylobacter pyloridis* renamed *C. pylori* for grammatical reasons, and was finally designated *Helicobacter pylori*.[2,3] It is now accepted that *H. pylori* causes acute and chronic non-autoimmune gastritis. Its role in peptic ulcer disease is less well established, and it may play a role in the development of gastric carcinoma.

EPIDEMIOLOGY

Infection with *H. pylori* is present in all areas of the world surveyed.[2,3] In developed countries approximately 10% of healthy individuals under 30 years of age have serological evidence of infection and this rises to 60% in those over 60. In developing countries infection is highly prevalent and develops at a younger age. For example in the Gambia 15% of infants under 20 months, and 46% of those under 5 years had antibodies to *H. pylori*[4]; in Peru 48% of children aged 2 months to 12 years had evidence of infection.[5] In most developing countries virtually 100% of individuals are seropositive by early childhood.[6] Humans appear to be the major reservoir for the bacterium but how it is transmitted is unclear. Person-to-person spread via endoscopes, pH electrodes or nasogastric feeding tubes[3] has been documented but this is unlikely to be a major mode of transmission. Close contact promotes spread; for example, families of infected children have a higher incidence of infection, as have gastroenterologists who are endoscopists.[7] The faecal–oral route is the most likely mode of spread but *H. pylori* has not yet been detected in faeces. Others have suggested that interoral spread is most important.[7] Water-borne spread has also been suggested as a major factor in developing countries.[5] Finally, some animal species, including the macaque and pig, have been shown to harbour *H. pylori* and might act as reservoirs.

MICROBIOLOGY

H. pylori is a sinusoidal Gram-negative bacterium approximately 3.5 μm long by 0.5–1 μm in diameter. It has a smooth surface and 4–6 sheathed flagellae with terminal bulbs (unlike *Campylobacter* spp.). The bacterium produces a powerful urease and seems well adapted to living beneath the mucous layer attached to the surface of gastric enterocytes. *H. pylori* is fastidious and slow growing. It requires enriched selective media for isolation from clinical sites. Growth is optimal at 37°C under humidified microaerophilic conditions in 10% carbon dioxide and takes 4–6 days.

PATHOGENESIS

Koch's postulates have been largely accepted for an association of *H. pylori* with antral non-

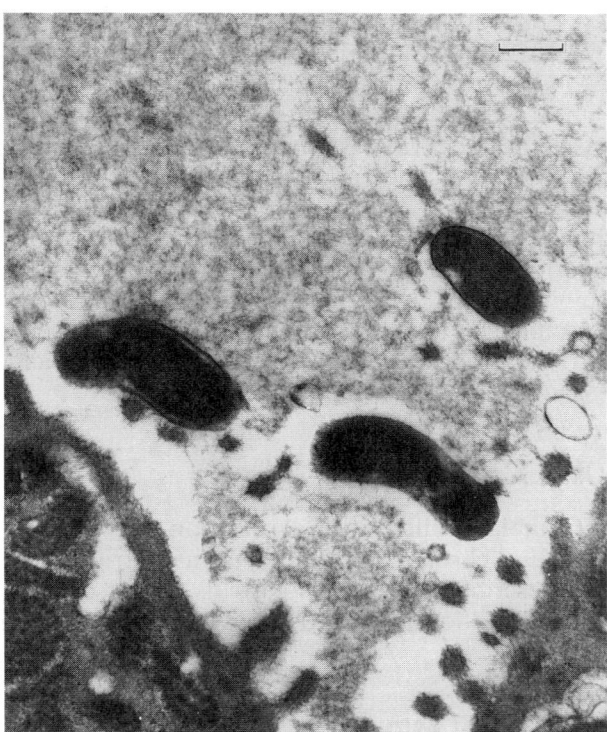

Figure 41.1 H. pylori overlaying gastric enterocytes beneath the mucin layer (bar = 1 μm).

autoimmune (type B) gastritis both in adults and children.[2,3,8,9] There is also a strong association between *H. pylori* and peptic ulceration but it may or may not be causative.[2] In feeding experiments doses of between 10^5 and 10^9 cfu have established infection but the minimum dose has not been determined. *H. pylori* appears to be able to survive an acidic gastric pH to penetrate the mucus covering the gastric epithelial cells. It has been postulated that the bacterium's spiral morphology and flagellae are important in this aspect of pathogenesis.[8] The bacteria can exist free in the mucous layer (Figure 41.1) or firmly attached to the epithelial cells. *H. pylori* then elaborates a powerful urease which helps to neutralize the acidic pH, a cytotoxin which causes vacuolation, a protease which hydrolyses mucus, and other factors which stimulate gastric acid secretion. The role of these factors in the pathogenesis of disease is not clear. Infected individuals mount a systemic and local humoral immune response. *H. pylori*-specific secretory IgA can be detected both in saliva and gastric juice. What role this plays in immunity is unclear since antibody is detectable in patients who are colonized or infected.

PATHOLOGY

H. pylori is strongly associated with chronic antral gastritis and with its active phase. Although macro-

scopic inflammation is usually not present examination of biopsies reveals *H. pylori* in close apposition to the gastric mucosa which shows an infiltrate with mono- and polymorphonuclear leucocytes. *H. pylori* and evidence of inflammation may also be found in areas of gastric metaplasia in the oesophagus (Barrett's oesophagus) or duodenum.

CLINICAL FEATURES

Chronic epigastric pain is very common in the populations of many developing and developed countries. In sub-Saharan Africa non-ulcerous dyspepsia and duodenal ulcer are the most common causes of epigastric pain.[10,11] Infection with *H. pylori* was found in 141 (88%) of adult Malawians undergoing gastroscopy for chronic epigastric pain.[11] Other features associated with *H. pylori* gastritis include nausea, vomiting and flatulence. Similar features may also be seen in children with *H. pylori* infection.[9] The clinical features of gastritis relapse and remit, thus it is possible to detect *H. pylori* infection in individuals who have histological evidence of gastritis but no signs or symptoms.

Duodenal ulceration is associated with chronic antral gastritis. *H. pylori* can be detected in both antrum and duodenal ulcer tissue, but it will not colonize the duodenum except in areas of duodenal metaplasia.[12]

DIAGNOSIS

Specific diagnosis may be reached by invasive or non-invasive techniques.

Invasive techniques

These have a higher sensitivity and specificity than the non-invasive techniques. Gastroscopic biopsies from the antrum, duodenal ulcer(s) or other areas of potential colonization are examined by culture and histology and for urease activity. Two biopsy specimens from the antrum are sufficient to detect *H. pylori*.[11] Histological samples may be stained by Giemsa, silver impregnation or acridine orange for detection of *H. pylori*. This is more sensitive than culture in most surveys.

For culture, biopsy specimens are either rolled on the surface of an appropriate culture medium (e.g. brain–heart infusion-enriched Columbia blood agar incorporating Skirrow's antibiotics) or homogenized and similarly applied. In tropical countries it is advisable to incorporate an antifungal such as amphotericin B into the medium. A '1 minute' urease test in which the biopsy is immersed in a urea (10% in deionized water) solution containing a pH indicator (phenol red) has proved highly sensitive and specific.[11]

Non-invasive techniques

Detection of antibody to *H. pylori* in serum or saliva is possible using an enzyme linked immunosorbent assay (ELISA). Such tests have proved highly sensitive[8,9] but the specificity is variable since it is possible to detect antibody in those who are no longer infected.[11]

Breath tests which involve administering [^{13}C] urea and measuring the release of the isotope in the patient's breath have proved useful in developed and developing countries.[5] They depend upon the presence of *H. pylori* urease which hydrolyses the urea with release of $^{13}CO_2$.

MANAGEMENT AND TREATMENT

Often non-ulcer dyspepsia is not treated other than by symptomatic management. *H. pylori* is susceptible in vitro to a wide range of antimicrobials, including ampicillin, quinolones, cephalosporins, nitroimidazoles and macrolides, but all fail in vivo. Combination of tripotassium dicitratobismuthate and ampicillin or metronidazole achieve 40% and 80% eradication rates, respectively[13] but require 2–4 weeks administration. Unfortunately resistance of *H. pylori* to metronidazole is high in African countries.[11]

Whether *H. pylori* is an epiphenomenon associated with peptic ulceration or plays a role in ulceration is not yet determined. Although treatment with H_2 blockers heals most duodenal ulcers, the majority (70–80%) relapse within 12 months. A combination of bismuth salts with amoxicillin and metronidazole with or without H_2 blockers is associated with ulcer healing, eradication of *H. pylori* and a greatly decreased relapse rate.[13,14]

COMPLICATIONS

In Gambian children an association between *H. pylori* and chronic diarrhoea and malnutrition has been described.[4] *H. pylori* gastritis was associated with protein-losing enteropathy in South African children.[15]

PREVENTION AND CONTROL

Infection with *H. pylori* is ubiquitous throughout the world but highly localized in individuals. Until more is known about the mode of spread, pathogenesis and immunity, prevention and control are impossible.

ESCHERICHIA COLI (See also Chapter 3)

Escherichia coli is the major aerobic component of the normal intestinal flora (*c.* 10^7 c fu/ml) but is also a major cause of diarrhoeal disease. In some surveys it is estimated that *E. coli* is responsible for up to 30% of cases of gastroenteritis.[16] The strains of *E. coli* causing diarrhoea were originally termed enteropathogenic *E. coli* (EPEC) but as the different mechanisms of pathogenicity were determined EPEC became used to describe one particular mechanism. To date, five different mechanisms have been described: EPEC, enterotoxigenic *E.coli* (ETEC), enteroinvasive *E. coli* (EIEC), enterohaemorrhagic *E. coli* (EHEC) and enteroaggregative *E. coli* (EAggEC).

E.coli was first described as a cause of gastroenteritis by its association with outbreaks of diarrhoea in infants.[17,18] This was done by showing that all infants were excreting strains of *E. coli* with the same O or somatic antigen. Different O antigens were associated with the different enteropathic mechanisms of *E. coli* (Table 41.1). However, these are associations, and to test for O serogroup is not sufficiently specific to ascribe pathogenicity to a particular strain of *E. coli*. To do this the specific pathogenicity genes, or their gene products must be sought.

ENTEROTOXIGENIC *E. COLI*

EPIDEMIOLOGY

ETEC have a worldwide distribution and are a major health hazard in adults and children in developing countries. In addition, they are a major cause of travellers' diarrhoea. In community-based studies in developing countries ETEC are responsible for 15–20% of cases of diarrhoea.[19,20] In most hospital-based studies ETEC are second only to rotavirus as a

Table 41.1 *Escherichia coli* and gastroenteritis.

Bacterium	Associated O antigens	Disease association(s)
Enterotoxigenic *E. coli*	O6, O8, O15, O20, O25 O128, O139, O148, O153, O159	Secretory diarrhoea in adults and children; travellers' diarrhoea
Enteroinvasive *E. coli*	O28, O29, O124, O136, O143, O144, O152, O164, O167	Dysentery in adults and children
Enteropathogenic *E. coli*	O55, O86, O111, O119, O125, O126, O127, O128, O142	Non-inflammatory diarrhoea in infants; travellers' diarrhoea
Enterohaemorrhagic *E. coli*	O26, O111, O157	Haemorrhagic colitis, haemolytic–uraemic syndrome in children
Enteroaggregative *E. coli*	O44, O111, O126	Chronic inflammatory diarrhoea in children

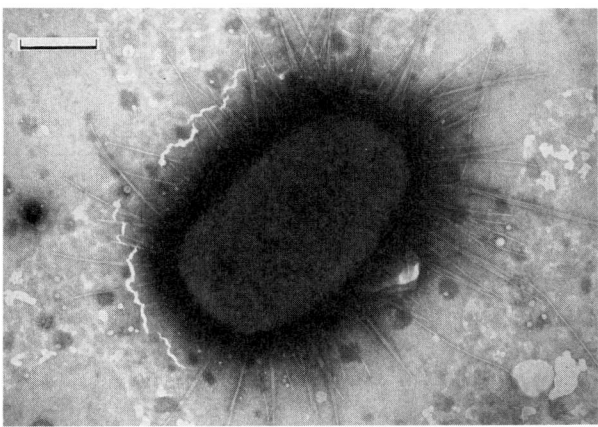

Figure 41.2 Enterotoxigenic *E. coli* showing numerous fimbriae (pili) (bar = 0.5 μm).

cause of gastroenteritis. ETEC infections occur throughout the year but are most common in the wet season.[20] Spread is by the faecal–oral route either directly or indirectly via food or water. Infants are at particular risk at weaning. The infective dose is high in the normal host (10^6–10^{10} cfu).

PATHOGENESIS

In order to produce disease, ETEC must be able to colonize the small intestine and elaborate one or both of heat-labile toxin (LT) and heat-stable toxin (ST). ETEC colonize the small intestine by means of protein spikes, called fimbriae or pili (Figure 41.2), that bind to specific receptors on the enterocyte surface. The bacteria then release their toxins. LT is a subunit toxin with a structure and mode of action similar to cholera toxin. Subunit B, the toxophore, binds to GM_1 ganglioside on the enterocyte surface and allows subunit A to activate adenylate cyclase inside the enterocyte. The raised intracellular cyclic AMP concentrations cause an efflux of Cl^-, Na^+ and water from villous crypt cells and have an antiabsorptive effect on villous tip cells. The net effect is that a large fluid load enters the colon and a voluminous watery stool is produced. ST is a low-molecular weight protein which activates guanylate cyclase. This results in secretion of fluid and electrolytes into the intestinal lumen. There are no specific histopathological changes to be seen in the small-intestinal mucosa, and no evidence of inflammation. The genes encoding pili, LT and antibiotic resistance can be carried on plasmids in ETEC.

CLINICAL FEATURES

The incubation period is 1–2 days with anorexia, vomiting and abdominal cramps in 25% of patients. The diarrhoea is explosive, voluminous and watery, up to 10 times a day. The illness is self-limiting and usually lasts 1–5 days in well nourished, but up to 3 weeks in malnourished children. Dehydration is the major complication which, in a study in Bangladesh, was seen in 46% of adults and 16% of children.[20]

DIAGNOSIS

Specific diagnosis depends upon culture of *E. coli* from faeces and detection of pathogenicity genes (fimbriae, LT, ST) by DNA hybridization, or their gene products by ELISA, immunoprecipitation or bioassay. To rely on O serogrouping is not sufficiently sensitive or specific.

TREATMENT

The mainstay of treatment is the assessment of dehydration and replacement of fluid and electrolytes. Administration of antibiotics has been shown to shorten the course of illness and duration of excretion of ETEC in adults in endemic areas[21] and in traveller's diarrhoea.[22] The antibiotic used depends upon susceptibility patterns in the particular geographic region. Currently trimethoprim or fluorinated quinolones such as ciprofloxacin are most likely to be effective.

PREVENTION

Although a B-subunit/whole-cell cholera vaccine provided 86% protection in Bangladeshi mothers and children, it was short lived (<3 months). A similar preparation was 52% effective in preventing ETEC diarrhoea in tourists.[23]

ENTEROINVASIVE E. COLI

This is a small group of E. coli that produce inflammatory diarrhoea by invading and killing colonic enterocytes (Figure 41.3). They resemble Shigella in O antigens and in being non-motile and have similar

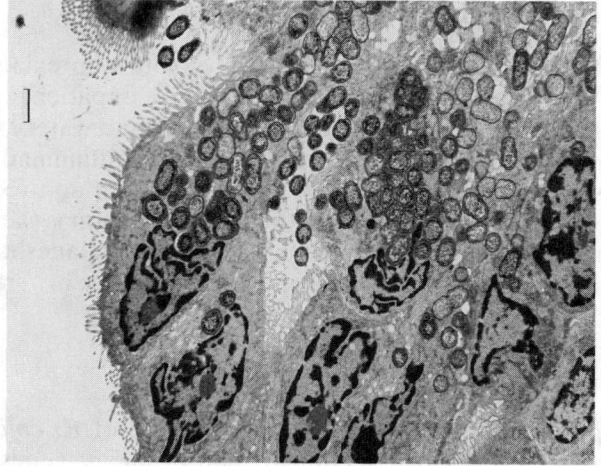

Figure 41.3 Enteroinvasive E. coli within colonic enterocytes (bar = 2 μm).

pathogenicity genes on a large plasmid that encodes surface proteins mediating invasion into cells. Infection is less common than that due to shigellae. For example, EIEC were responsible for 4.2% episodes of endemic diarrhoea in children in Thailand and shigellae for 23%.[24] Infection is uncommon in children under 1 year old but can be a cause of travellers' diarrhoea. The clinical features of EIEC infection are similar to those of shigellae but the latter may produce more severe diarrhoea. Diagnosis is by stool culture and detection of EIEC pathogenicity genes by DNA hybridization,[24] or gene products by ELISA.[25]

No vaccine is currently available for prevention.

ENTEROPATHOGENIC E. COLI

In the early 1970s when the pathogenesis of ETEC and EIEC had been defined it became apparent that a large number of the classical O serogroup did not elaborate LT or ST, nor were they invasive. However, they were able to produce diarrhoea in volunteers.[26] Since these were the original classical O serogroups that caused outbreaks of infantile diarrhoea they were termed enteropathogenic E. coli.

EPIDEMIOLOGY

The first infections with EPEC were described in the UK and the USA in the 1940s and 1950s in epidemics of infantile diarrhoea.[17,18] Nowadays they are a cause of sporadic disease. In developing countries EPEC are still a major cause of infantile diarrhoea.[27–29] In Thailand 11% of children under 1 year old with diarrhoea in a refugee camp were infected with EPEC,[28] and in an outbreak in preterm neonates in Kenya, 13 of 30 were infected with EPEC, three of whom died.[29] EPEC has also been associated with travellers' diarrhoea. Transmission is by the faecal–oral route either directly or in food or water.

PATHOGENESIS

The ingested EPEC adhere to the mucus overlying the small-intestinal enterocytes using fimbriae. They then penetrate between the microvilli of the brush border to become intimately attached to the enterocyte surface.[30] This then causes the brush border to be lost by a process of vesiculation.[31] This process is

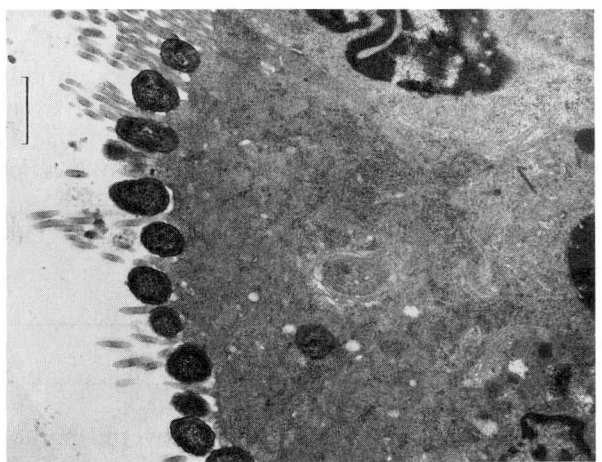

Figure 41.4 Enteropathogenic *E. coli* producing attaching effacement on duodenal enterocytes (bar = 1 μm).

termed 'attaching effacement' (Figure 41.4). Although the process is maximal in the small intestine it can occur throughout the gastrointestinal tract.[30] The net result is that large areas for absorption of nutrients are lost. In addition because the disaccharidase enzymes are integral proteins in the microvillous membrane, levels of these enzymes are markedly depressed.[32] The disaccharides sucrose, lactose and maltose in the diet must be hydrolysed to monosaccharides to be absorbed. Because of loss of the brush border the disaccharides cannot be cleaved and are thus not absorbed. They pass to the colon and cause a non-inflammatory osmotic diarrhoea, although in some cases there also appears to be a secretory component.[26]

CLINICAL FEATURES

EPEC tend to produce more severe and prolonged diarrhoea which may remit and relapse. There is initially vomiting, with fever and profuse diarrhoea with mucus but no blood. Fatality rates in epidemics range from 30 to 50% but with oral rehydration and antibiotic therapy mortality rates have decreased to less than 8%.[33]

DIAGNOSIS

This depends upon culture of *E. coli* from faeces or duodenal aspirate. Specific diagnosis involves detection of *E. coli* carrying *eae* (EPEC attaching effacement) genes by DNA hybridization.[34]

TREATMENT AND PREVENTION

The initial treatment should be to rehydrate. Because the diarrhoea can be prolonged, enteral or parenteral nutrition and antibiotics may be indicated. Ampicillin is unlikely to be effective even if the EPEC are sensitive. Administration of oral non-absorbable antibiotics such as neomycin or polymyxin B is effective. Oral absorbable antibiotics such as fluorinated quinolones or trimethoprim may also be of benefit. However, antibiotic resistance to most antibiotics has been observed in EPEC.

A vaccine is not available for prevention of infection.

ENTEROHAEMORRHAGIC *E. COLI*

EHEC were first described in Canada in 1983 when they were linked to cases of haemorrhagic colitis[35] and haemolytic–uraemic syndrome.[36]

EPIDEMIOLOGY

Infections with EHEC have been described largely in industrialized countries. Here they tend to cause outbreaks of infection, usually as the result of the consumption of incompletely cooked beef or pork.[37] EHEC can be part of the normal enteric flora of cattle and pigs.

An initial survey of adults in Thailand with diarrhoea showed that 2% of 458 patients were infected by EHEC.[38] There have recently been large outbreaks of haemorrhagic colitis in southern Africa[39] apparently associated with cooked market foods and due to EHEC.

PATHOGENESIS

EHEC produce attaching effacement, limited to the terminal ileum and colon. In addition they release one or both of the toxins verocytotoxin (VT) 1 or 2. VT-1 is also called shiga-like toxin 1. These toxins inhibit protein synthesis and are cytotoxic. In the colon they kill enterocytes, leading to an inflammatory haemorrhagic colitis. If they enter the systemic circulation they can damage endothelial cells and precipitate the haemolytic–uraemic syndrome.[37]

CLINICAL FEATURES

Haemorrhagic colitis presents with abdominal cramps and watery diarrhoea that is followed by a haemorrhagic discharge resembling a colonic bleed. There is rarely an accompanying fever. Haemolytic–uraemic syndrome is one, if not the most common cause of acute renal failure in childhood in industrialized countries. In an Indian study, EHEC were implicated in 19 of 28 cases of haemolytic–uraemic syndrome and *Shigella* spp. in only six.[40] Haemolytic–uraemic syndrome presents with acute renal failure, thrombocytopenia, coagulopathy and evidence of a microangiopathic haemolytic anaemia. With peritoneal dialysis the outlook is good, with the fatality rate falling from 50% to less than 10%.

DIAGNOSIS

The first strains of *E. coli* associated with haemorrhagic colitis and haemolytic–uraemic syndrome were of serogroup O157; they were sorbitol non-fermenters. Thus serogrouping and sorbitol MacConkey agar are used to diagnose infections. However, other serogroups (Table 41.1) are also implicated and these are sorbitol fermenters. Thus specific diagnosis depends upon detection of VT or its genes (by DNA hybridization) or of EHEC fimbrial adhesin genes.[38] Excretion of EHEC beyond the period of diarrhoea is short lived. For retrospective diagnosis it is possible to detect serum antibody to VT.[41]

TREATMENT AND PREVENTION

The treatment of haemorrhagic colitis is essentially treatment of dehydration. Antibiotics have no role and in some cases (as with *Sh. dysenteriae* 1) may increase the risk of complications.[37] For haemolytic–uraemic syndrome peritoneal dialysis is the most important intervention. No vaccine is currently available.

ENTEROAGGREGATIVE *E. COLI*

EAggEC are the most recently discovered pathogenic group. They are named for their characteristic pattern of adherence to tissue culture cells: in large aggregates.

EAggEC are particularly associated with persistent diarrhoea. In a survey of EAggEC infection in India the most notable clinical features were fever, vomiting, overt blood in the stool and a mean duration of diarrhoea of 17 days.[42] How diarrhoea is produced is not known but in a rat model, villous tip enterocytes were destroyed and villi were blunted.

Diagnosis is by culture of *E. coli* that produce a distinctive aggregative pattern on cultured cells and that hybridize with the EAggEC DNA probe.[43]

CAMPYLOBACTER JEJUNI

The genus *Campylobacter* is a major cause of gastroenteritis in both developed and developing countries. Although *C. fetus* was recognized as an opportunist pathogen as early as 1947, the full role of *Campylobacter* spp. as major enteric pathogens was not realized until appropriate selective media were devised.[44,45]

EPIDEMIOLOGY

The major enteric pathogens in the genus are *C. jejuni* (I and II), *C. coli* and *C. laridis*. Of these, *C. jejuni* is the most common cause of gastroenteritis. All can be normally present in the gastrointestinal tract of domestic and wild animals, which act as the major reservoir for infection. *C. laridis* in particular can be part of the normal intestinal flora of birds. Campylobacters can survive for 2–5 weeks in cow's milk or water kept at 4°C but they do not multiply. Infection is spread faeco-orally, human-to-human or animal-to-human (there have even been cases of

human-to-animal spread), either directly or indirectly in food and water.

Animal-to-human. Close contact with animals such as that in villages in developing countries where poultry, goats, cattle and dogs roam freely increases the risk of infection.

Human-to-human. Transmission may occur from infected individuals or from convalescent carriers, especially young children. Epidemics of infection can occur in nurseries or paediatric wards.

Food. Contamination can occur during preparation of food from the animal's intestinal content(s) or by incomplete cooking.

Milk. Consumption of raw unpasteurized milk is strongly associated with illness[46,47] as is contamination of bottled milk following attack by birds.[48]

Water. Excreta from wild and domesticated animals can contaminate surface water, and water-borne transmission is important in developing countries.

The incubation period is 2–5 days[47] with an infective dose of 500 organisms. The median duration of excretion of *C. jejuni* following cessation of diarrhoea is 2–3 weeks.

Infection is most common in those under 1 year old, with a decrease in attack rate with increasing age. *C. jejuni* is isolated in from 5 to 10% of children with gastroenteritis in developing countries,[24] but it may be isolated as frequently from children without diarrhoea.[49]

BACTERIOLOGY

Campylobacters are Gram-negative bacteria with single polar flagellae (Figure 41.5). They are spiral or bent rods 0.2–0.5 μm in diameter and 1.5–3.5 μm long. They are thermophilic and will grow at 42°C but prefer a microaerophilic atmosphere. *C. jejuni* can hydrolyse hippurate, which distinguishes it from *C. coli* and *C. laridis*. *C. coli* is sensitive to nalidixic acid but *C. laridis* is resistant. All can be cultivated on simple media.

PATHOGENESIS

Campylobacters can produce both an inflammatory diarrhoea and a non-inflammatory diarrhoea. In the latter, patients suffer a voluminous watery diarrhoea and this is due to the release by *C. jejuni* of an enterotoxin and cytotoxin following attachment to the enterocyte surface via non-fimbrial adhesins. The enterotoxin is similar in structure and mode of action to *E. coli* LT and cholera toxin.[50] The role and mode of action of the cytotoxin is unclear but it may play a role in the inflammatory diarrhoea. The dysentery-like diarrhoea is considered to be due to penetration of terminal ileal and colonic entero-

cytes, leading to cell death and an inflammatory response.

Immunity to infection is acquired following one or more infective episodes but duration of immunity is unknown. Following infection, serum and secretory antibodies to *Campylobacter* flagellae, enterotoxin, lipopolysaccharide and other surface antigens that are involved in attachment are produced. In developing countries antibodies are acquired in early life[51,52]—perhaps because of continuous exposure from animals. This may account for the lower prevalence of infection in adults in developing countries compared with developed countries, and the higher prevalence of asymptomatic infection in the former. It is probable that the presence of secretory IgA against *Campylobacter* spp. is the main determinant of immunity.

In a small proportion of those infected, usually the immunoincompetent, bacteria translocate from the intestinal lumen, causing bacteraemia.

PATHOLOGY

In the dysentery-like illness, inflammatory infiltrates into the lamina propria and crypt abscesses can be seen in the rectal, colonic and terminal ileal mucosa. This is a similar finding to that seen in *Shigella* spp. or *Salmonella* spp. infections, Crohn's disease or ulcerative colitis.

CLINICAL FEATURES

In developing countries *Campylobacter* spp. enteritis is generally less severe than that in developed countries. It is more likely to be of the non-inflammatory type, without fever or bloody diarrhoea.[51] However, severe bloody diarrhoea resembling bacillary dysentery can occur and will also occur in travellers acquiring infection in developing countries. In general diarrhoea is self-limiting and resolves in 2–7 days.

Disseminated infection can occur and predisposing factors include: malnutrition, hepatic dysfunction, malignancy, diabetes mellitus, renal failure and immunosuppression. Extraintestinal and rare forms of infection include: asymptomatic bacteraemia, meningitis, deep abscesses and cholecystitis. Reactive arthritis may follow *Campylobacter* spp. enteritis in genetically susceptible individuals (HLA-B27).

DIAGNOSIS

The features of *Campylobacter* infection are not sufficiently distinct to make a clinical diagnosis.

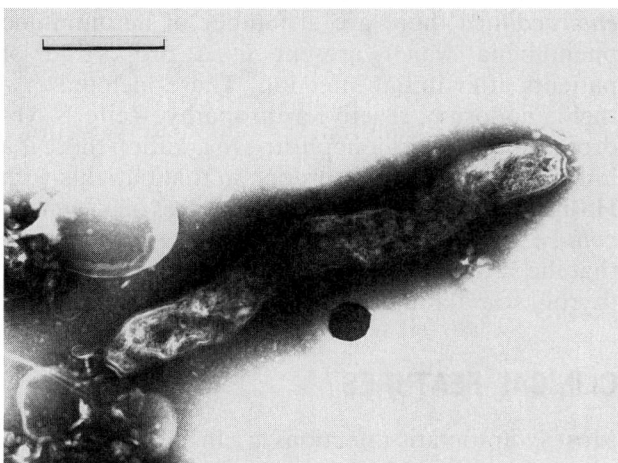

Figure 41.5 *C. jejuni* showing terminal flagellae (bar = 1 μm).

Examination of faecal smears by Gram stain or dark field microscopy can provide a rapid presumptive diagnosis. Where laboratory facilities are not optimal this may be the best diagnostic tool. However, the basis of specific diagnosis is isolation of the bacteria from faeces. *Campylobacter* spp. will grow on most basal media, especially if lysed blood is incorporated. In order to make the media selective, antibiotics such as trimethoprim are incorporated.[53] Culture is usually at 42°C (to inhibit gut commensals) and in a microaerophilic atmosphere. Culture plates and swabs should be kept out of the light prior to use since *Campylobacter* spp. are rapidly killed by free radicals generated by ultraviolet irradiation.

TREATMENT

Severe watery diarrhoea will need adequate rehydration. Cases of severe dysentery or disseminated infection will require antimicrobial chemotherapy. *C. jejuni* is usually sensitive to erythromycin, but *C. coli* may occasionally be resistant. Nevertheless, erythromycin remains the best choice.

PREVENTION AND CONTROL

There is no vaccine for prevention of infection; thus non-specific methods for prevention such as improvements in sanitation and provision of clean potable water are important.

YERSINIA ENTEROCOLITICA

The genus *Yersinia* spp. comprises *Y. pestis*, the cause of plague, *Y. pseudotuberculosis* and *Y. enterocolitica*. Of these, *Y. enterocolitica* is the only important cause of diarrhoea.[54,55]

EPIDEMIOLOGY

Although *Yersinia* spp. infection is said to have a world-wide distribution, it is found much more commonly in temperate zones than in the tropics. Even in temperate countries infection is more prevalent in colder climates and is more common in winter.[54] In most surveys of acute diarrhoeal disease where *Y. enterocolitica* was sought, it was either absent, or present in less than 1% of cases.[56] However, cases of generalized infection have been recorded in South Africa[57] and serological evidence of infection has been found in Nigeria.[58]

The reservoir for *Y. enterocolitica* is a variety of animal species, including birds, frogs, fish, snails, oysters and most mammals. The organism is excreted in faeces from pigs and cattle and can persist in lakes, streams, soil and vegetables. Patient-to-patient spread is rare except by blood transfusion. The incubation period is 1–11 days and bacteria are excreted for 14–97 (mean 42) days.

BACTERIOLOGY

Y. enterocolitica is a small Gram-negative rod with peritrichous flagellae. It will grow on simple media and is lactose non-fermenting on MacConkey agar. It is psychrophilic, and isolation from clinical samples often involves a cold enrichment step. O serogrouping is used to subdivide strains.

PATHOGENESIS

Pathogenic strains of *Y. enterocolitica* carry a large plasmid which encodes surface proteins and lipopolysaccharides mediating cell attachment, resistance to phagocytosis and serum resistance. Chromosomal genes encode the ability to invade epithelial cells. Although *Y. enterocolitica* produces a toxin similar to LT, its role in pathogenesis is unclear. *Y. enterocolitica* invades ileal enterocytes and passes to Peyer's patches, where it multiplies. This produces inflammatory diarrhoea. Bacteria may pass to local lymph nodes, thence to produce systemic disease.

In addition to disease produced directly by *Y. enterocolitica* there are a number of autoimmune phenomena which present in a proportion of patients after initial infection. These include: erythema nodosum, reactive arthropathy, Reiter's syndrome and glomerulonephritis. In addition there is a linkage with thyroid disorders, in that patients with Hashimoto's thyroiditis have high titres of *Y. enterocolitica* agglutinating antibodies. It is noteworthy that the surface of *Y. enterocolitica* has receptors for thyroid stimulating hormone.

CLINICAL FEATURES

Most symptomatic infections are in children under 5 years of age.[54,55] Characteristically, clinical features consist of diarrhoea, low-grade fever and abdominal pain. The diarrhoeic stool will be frankly blood-stained in a quarter of cases. Nausea, vomiting, headache and pharyngitis are minority presentations. The abdominal pain may be present alone or with mild diarrhoea and is often termed the pseudoappendicular syndrome. Infection may spread elsewhere to produce bacteraemia, peritonitis, hepatic, renal and splenic abscesses, pyomyositis and osteomyelitis.[54,55,57] These are more likely to occur in patients who are immunocompromised or who have iron overload—as in haemochromatosis.[57] The extraintestinal manifestations are more likely to occur in adults, as are the autoimmune phenomena. Of those with reactive arthritis, 80% are of HLA-B27 histoincompatibility type.

DIAGNOSIS

Y. enterocolitica can be isolated from stool, appendix, mesenteric lymph nodes, blood and other focal sites of infection using simple media. Strategies for isolation include MacConkey agar incubated at 25–30°C for 48 hours or selective media such as cefsulodin–irgasan–novobiocin (CIN) agar at 37°C. For isolation from food or water, cold enrichment in phosphate-buffered saline for up to 4 weeks at 4°C prior to plating on to CIN agar greatly increases the yield of both pathogenic and non-pathogenic *Yersinia* spp. Speciation is obtained by biochemical tests and it is noteworthy that all non-pathogenic *Y. enterocolitica* have pyrizinamidase activity. Pathogenic *Y. enterocolitica* all possess the virulence plasmid. For retrospective diagnosis, serology using ELISA, whole cell agglutination, or compliment fixation tests can be performed. They can be difficult to interpret and cross-reactions, for example *Y. enterocolitica* 0:9 with *Brucella abortus*, *E. coli*, *Morganella morganii* and *Salmonella* spp., do occur. The specificity of the test can be improved by detecting a greater than fourfold increase in titre between acute and convalescent sera.

TREATMENT AND CONTROL

In children with uncomplicated diarrhoea, antimicrobial treatment is of little benefit.[59] In complicated infection co-trimoxazole, tetracycline or chloramphenicol should be effective. Although natural infection with *Y. enterocolitica* produces immunity no vaccine is available.

CLOSTRIDIUM SPP.

Clostridia are anaerobic sporing Gram-positive rods. Two species *Cl. perfringens* and *Cl. difficile* are associated with diarrhoeal disease.

CLOSTRIDIUM PERFRINGENS

Two forms of diarrhoeal disease are associated with *Cl. perfringens* (formerly *welchii*). The first is a food poisoning illness due to ingestion of *Cl. perfringens* type A or the α toxin (enterotoxin) it produces. Although this is a common cause of food poisoning in industrialized countries it produces mild, short-lived disease and is extremely uncommon in the tropics.

Cl. perfringens type C, in contrast, is common in certain areas of the tropics and produces a severe necrotic enteritis.

EPIDEMIOLOGY

Cl. perfringens type C has been implicated in enteritis necroticans (Darmbrand) seen in malnourished individuals in Northern Europe after World War II[60] and 'pigbel' in the highlands of Papua New Guinea.[61]. A similar disease has been described in Uganda,[62] Malaysia, Thailand, Indonesia and China.[63] (See also Chapter 3.)

Infection can occur sporadically[62,63] but also in epidemics.[60,61] It occurs at any age but is more likely to present as acute toxic or acute surgical problems in children under 10 years old.[61,63] In Papua New Guinea pigbel is associated with large 'pig feasts' that occur every 3–10 years. Infection is more common in males than females; whether this represents a true difference in susceptibility or male greed is unclear. *Cl. perfringens* type C can be found in the human normal intestinal flora, in pig excreta and in soil.

MICROBIOLOGY

Cl. perfringens type C produces both α and β toxins which, it is presumed, are responsible for disease manifestations.

PATHOGENESIS

Since *Cl. perfringens* type C can be found as part of the normal intestinal flora, it is considered that host-dependent factors are also involved. Firstly, the bulk of the normal anaerobic flora is found in the large bowel and one hypothesis is that overgrowth of *Cl. perfringens* type C in the jejunum might be related to development of disease. A more attractive hypothesis links malnutrition and type of diet with disease. β Toxin is readily inactivated by intestinal proteases. Protein deficiency decreases intestinal protease levels; in addition, the sweet potato, which is a staple diet in highland Papua New Guinea, contains heat-stable trypsin inhibitors. Thus consumption of meat contaminated by *Cl. perfringens* type C or its β toxin in an individual with low intestinal protease activity due to malnutrition or dietary protease inhibitors would allow the toxin to produce intestinal damage.[63,64]

PATHOLOGY

Gross pathology shows patchy segmental acute ulcerative necrosis of the jejunum, and to a lesser extent the ileum, caecum and colon. This may rapidly progress to segmental gangrene with gas in the mucosa, mesentery or lymph nodes. Microscopically the intestinal wall shows separation of the mucosa from the submucosa, with large denuded areas covered with a pseudomembrane of dead enterocytes and infiltrating neutrophils and red blood cells. Healing occurs with fibrosis, and strictures and adhesions may form later.

CLINICAL FEATURES

Pigbel varies in severity from mild diarrhoea to a rapidly fatal necrotizing enteritis, with high mortality (up to 85%). The incubation period is approximately 48 hours after the feast but can vary from 24 hours to up to a week.

Disease has been classified into four main presentations.[60,61] Type I (acute toxic) presents with fulminant toxaemia and shock. Type II (acute surgical) presents as mechanical and paralytic ileus, acute strangulation, perforation and peritonitis. Type III (subacute surgical) presents later with complications of mild type II. Finally, type IV (mild or trivial) presents with mild diarrhoea but may rarely progress to type III. Type I disease occurs most commonly in young children and has the highest mortality (85%). Type II disease has a 42% mortality, type III 44% mortality, and type IV is never fatal. In type II and type III disease a palpable segment of thickened intestine may be found. The stool will contain blood and pus cells and there is a neutrophil leucocytosis in peripheral blood. The differential diagnosis includes: acute causes of inflammatory diarrhoea, peritonitis, acute abdominal obstruction, acute pancreatitis, acute amoebic colitis, and sickle cell crises.

DIAGNOSIS

Cl. perfringens can be cultured from faeces, peritoneal fluid or other infected sites by plating on to neomycin blood agar and incubating anaerobically. *Cl. perfringens* type C is differentiated from other *Cl. perfringens* by serological techniques, including immunofluorescence and type C antibody-coated silica beads.[65] Interpretation of results can be difficult since *Cl. perfringens* type C is also found in normal individuals. Detection of antibodies to the β toxin can be useful in reaching a diagnosis in survivors.[61]

TREATMENT

Acute resuscitation is by fluid and electrolytes intravenously, together with bowel decompression by restricting oral intake and nasogastric intubation. Antibiotics will be needed if there is extraintestinal spread of the organism (e.g. peritonitis) and metronidazole, ampicillin, chloramphenicol or penicillin should be of value. A *Cl. perfringens* type C antiserum is also beneficial.[61] Surgical intervention will be necessary if there is persisting obstruction, increasing signs of toxaemia, or signs of peritonitis or of strangulation. There is some evidence that early surgical intervention can decrease mortality.[61]

PREVENTION

Active immunization with a toxoid prepared from *Cl. perfringens* type C toxins has decreased the incidence of pigbel in children.[66]

CLOSTRIDIUM DIFFICILE

Cl. difficile is the cause of antibiotic-associated colitis, and of pseudomembranous colitis. The organism and toxin can be detected in asymptomatic infants but their finding in older individuals is related to disease. Although the bacterium can be found worldwide it is probably an unusual cause of diarrhoeal disease in developing countries.[67]

AEROMONAS AND *PLESIOMONAS*

These two genera within the Vibrionaceae family are both aquatic micro-organisms and can be readily isolated from fresh and salt water, fish, soil and food.

AEROMONAS HYDROPHILA

EPIDEMIOLOGY

A. hydrophila has been associated with gastroenteritis in many countries throughout the world.[68] In tropical countries, it can be isolated from healthy as well as diarrhoeic individuals. In Thailand, *Aeromonas* spp. were isolated from 9% of cases of gastroenteritis and was second in importance only to ETEC.[69]

MICROBIOLOGY

The genus *Aeromonas* encompasses three motile species A. hydrophila, A. caviae and A. sobria. A fourth non-motile species A. salmonicida is a fish pathogen and will not grow above 30°C. They are oxidase positive and will grow on most simple media. Aeromonas produces a wide range of extracellular factors including: proteases, elastases, esterases, DNase, haemolysins, cytotoxins and enterotoxins.

PATHOGENESIS

Aeromonas is associated with both inflammatory and non-inflammatory diarrhoea. It possesses both fimbrial and non-fimbrial adhesins for attachment to the intestinal mucosa. It produces an enterotoxin which has a similar mode of action to *E. coli* LT but uses a different receptor. The haemolysins of aeromonas are also cytotoxic for cultured cells. Finally, aeromonas can invade cells in vitro and in vivo and this property might be related to production of inflammatory diarrhoea.

CLINICAL FEATURES

Gastroenteritis associated with *Aeromonas* spp. can vary from acute watery diarrhoea with fever, to chronic dysentery with fever and abdominal cramps.

DIAGNOSIS

Aeromonas can be isolated from faeces using selective media such as ampicillin blood agar. Prior enrichment in alkaline peptone water increases the sensitivity of isolation. Since *Aeromonas* spp. can be isolated from normal individuals, isolation does not prove causation. For the future it may be necessary to detect pathogenicity factors (toxins, adhesins or invasiveness) to link isolation with the disease in a particular patient.

TREATMENT

Rehydration is usually the only intervention needed. If infection becomes disseminated or there is chronic dysentery, antimicrobials such as fluorinated quinolones might be of benefit.

PLESIOMONAS SHIGELLOIDES

This micro-organism has been isolated with food-borne (usually fish) gastroenteritis in Mali and India,[70,71] and there has even been a case of snake-to-human transmission.[72]

SHIGELLOSIS (BACILLARY DYSENTERY) (See also Chapter 3)

Dysentery has been a disease of poor and crowded communities throughout history, and continues to be a major cause of morbidity and mortality in the tropics. Dysentery bacilli were first demonstrated by Shiga in 1898, and subsequent studies showed that four species (serogroups) *Shigella dysenteriae, Sh.* *flexneri, Sh. boydii* and *Sh. sonnei* were responsible for the disease described as bacillary dysentery.[73] *Sh. dysenteriae* and *Sh. flexneri* are responsible for most infections in the tropics, with case fatality rates up to 20%.[74] Shigellosis occurs both endemically and as epidemics. In many tropical countries,

Table 41.2   Epidemics of *Shigella dysenteriae* 1 since 1970.

Date	Area	Attack rate (%)	Mortality rate (%)
1969–1970	Central America	2–16	3–7
1980	Zaire/Rwanda	6	2–6
1984	India/Bangladesh	5–10	2–14
1984–1987	Burma/Thailand	10–70*	NA

NA, not available.
* The higher attack rates represent data from individual affected villages.

Table 41.3   Classification of *Shigella* serotypes.

Species	No. of serotypes	Glucose	Mannitol (fermentation)	Lactose
Sh. dysenteriae	10	+	–	–
Sh. flexneri	6	+	+	–
Sh. boydii	15	+	+	–
Sh. sonnei	1	+	+	Late

endemic infection is largely due to *Sh. flexneri* and is more commonly a disease of children. Studies in Thailand[75] and Bangladesh[76] have shown *Shigella* spp. to be isolated from 50% of children presenting with bloody diarrhoea. In children admitted to hospital with shigellosis in Bangladesh, fatality rates have ranged from 6 to 20%.[76] Since 1970 major epidemics of *Sh.dysenteriae* 1 have occurred in Central America,[77] Central Africa,[78] the Indian subcontinent[79] and South-East Asia[80] (Table 41.2).

BACTERIOLOGY

Shigella spp. are members of the Enterobacteriaceae, and are aerobic, Gram-negative, non-motile bacilli. They are typically non-lactose fermenting, lysine-decarboxylase-negative and do not produce gas from glucose. The exceptions are *Sh. sonnei* which ferments lactose slowly, and *Sh. flexneri* 6 and *Sh. boydii* 13 which produce gas from glucose. *Sh. dysenteriae*, *Sh. flexneri* and *Sh. boydii* are each divided into a number of serotypes (Table 41.3).

Serotype (O) antigens comprise the outer polysaccharide chains of the lipopolysaccharide component of the cell wall. Being non-motile, *Shigella* spp. do not possess H antigens.

For epidemiological studies, serotypes may be subdivided by molecular methods such as plasmid and chromosomal DNA restriction endonuclease digests.[81]

In pure growth, *Shigella* spp. are readily cultured on non-selective media, but for isolation from clinical specimens, selective media such as MacConkey and xylose lysine deoxycholate are necessary.

Shigella spp. are sensitive to heat and are killed in 1 hour at 55°C. Survival on inanimate objects is longer at low temperatures, ranging from up to 1 month at 15°C to less than 1 day at 45°C.[82] *Shigella* spp. are sensitive to most disinfectants, being killed in 15–30 minutes by 1% phenol.

PATHOGENESIS

Shigella dysentery is characterized by invasion of the colonic mucosa, local spread of the infecting organism and death of intestinal epithelial cells. In a proportion of cases, extraintestinal complications occur, including seizures, hyponatraemia and hypoglycaemia, septicaemia, Reiter's syndrome, encephalopathy, and the haemolytic–uraemic syndrome. A number of pathogenic factors and their genetic determinants have been described. Invasion is associated with specific outer membrane proteins that are coded by plasmid (extrachromosomal) DNA of size 220 kb. Strains not containing these plasmids have been shown to be non-virulent. The lipopolysaccharide component of the cell membrane, which includes the polysaccharide sidechains specific to different O antigenic types, is a further virulence factor.[83] The lipid A component has endotoxic activity and contributes to the systemic effects of infection. The O antigen polysaccharides provide the bacteria with resistance to host defence mechanisms including opsonization, phagocytosis and intracellular killing. O polysaccharide genes are generally chromosomally encoded. However, in *Sh. sonnei* the genes are present on a 180 kb plasmid, and in *Sh. dysenteriae* 1, a 9 kb plasmid, in conjunction with chromosomal genes, is associated with O antigen synthesis. In addition to these virulence factors, *Sh. dysenteriae* 1 strains produce a toxin. Early animal studies suggested that this was primarily a neurotoxin. Subsequent work has shown that it has cytotoxic and enterotoxic properties, and is similar to the verotoxin produced by *E. coli* O157 that is associated with haemorrhagic colitis and haemolytic–uraemic syndrome.[84]

PATHOLOGY AND IMMUNOLOGY

Invasion of the colonic mucosa leads to distortion of the crypts, the formation of microabscesses, and areas of haemorrhage. Sigmoidoscopy reveals a red, bleeding, mucosa with patches of necrotic membrane, which may separate to leave ulcerated areas. The inflammatory process may extend through the submucosa to the muscle layer. In severe cases, complete healing may not occur, resulting in fibrous tissue formation and persistent ulceration. Bacteraemia is uncommon in shigella infection, but is a probable risk factor for increased mortality. In a study in Bangladesh, *Shigella* spp. bacteraemia occurred in 4% of 2018 shigella cases, but bacteraemia (including other Enterobacteriaceae) occurred in 29% of 239 patients with shigellosis who died.[85] Circulating endotoxin is likely to play an important role in the systemic manifestations of shigella infection. In *Sh. dysenteriae* 1 infections, the shiga toxin exerts both enterotoxic effects, through specific glycolipid binding sites, and as described earlier, is responsible for the haemolytic–uraemic syndrome. Infection with *Shigella* spp. leads to both local (gut) immunity and the production of circulating antibodies. Circulating antibodies are directed against the O (lipopolysaccharide) antigens and have been shown to be serotype specific.[86] Serological studies in Vietnam have shown persistent levels of antibody following infection with *Sh. flexneri*, and epidemiological studies suggest that such antibodies are protective against reinfection by the same serotype.

EPIDEMIOLOGY

Man is the only natural host for infection by *Shigella* spp. Infection is by ingestion, the infective dose being as low as 10–100 bacteria for *Sh. dysenteriae*. The incubation period is 1–5 days. Shigellosis occurs as an endemic disease in conditions of crowding, poor sanitation and inadequate water supply, and is primarily a disease of poor disadvantaged communities in the tropics.

Endemic shigellosis is largely a paediatric disease, most cases occurring in children below 10 years of age. Routes of infection include direct person-to-person transmission (from cases of asymptomatic excreters), and transmission via contaminated water or food. The evidence for person-to-person transmission in endemic areas of the tropics comes from a number of community studies that show a high frequency of secondary household cases in the family of an index case, but no differences between families with cases, and control families in relation to water or food supply.[87] In epidemics of *Sh. dysenteriae* 1, person-to-person transmission is also more common than point-source food or water outbreaks.[75] Occasional water-borne epidemics have been described in the tropics.[88]

There is some evidence that flies may act as mechanical vectors, though most studies have been unable to separate the possible role of flies from direct routes in areas of poor hygiene. A seasonal pattern of shigellosis is seen in most endemic areas. In Bangladesh, peak transmission rate occurs at the beginning of the monsoon season, with a second, lower peak, in the winter season.[89]

The epidemiology of shigella infections in endemic areas of the tropics is complicated by the wide range of serotypes isolated. In Ethiopia, 22 different serotypes were isolated from patients in Addis Ababa. In a community study in Bangladesh, up to four different serotypes were isolated from household contacts of a given index case. These findings suggest that in endemic areas there are multiple strains and numerous routes of transmission.

In epidemics of *Sh. dysenteriae* 1 a single strain most commonly is responsible. Subtyping of outbreak strains by plasmid profiling in Bangladesh demonstrated a common plasmid profile in all isolates in an epidemic in 1983, and different profiles in *Sh. dysenteriae* 1 isolates obtained from sporadic cases in the previous year. Attack rates in epidemics of *Sh. dysenteriae* 1 have ranged from 6% in the 1980–1982 epidemic in central Africa to 70% in an epidemic affecting an island in the Bay of Bengal. Crude case fatality rates have ranged from 2 to 6% in documented epidemics, but much higher rates may occur in malnourished children.[90]

CLINICAL FEATURES

Shigellosis may vary from relatively mild watery diarrhoea to severe dysentery with intestinal and extraintestinal complications. In severe cases, the onset is abrupt, with tenesmus, fever and frequent

Table 41.4 Complications of *Shigella* spp. infection associated with increased risk of mortality.

Complication	Presentation
Intestinal	
Intestinal perforation	Peritonitis leading to sepsis, fluid shifts and shock
Toxic megacolon	Intestinal perforation; metabolic abnormalities; development of haemolytic–uraemic syndrome
Dehydration	Hypovolaemic shock
Systemic	
Septicaemia	Septicaemic shock
Hyponatraemia	Obtundation, coma and seizures leading to aspiration; with prolonged seizures, anoxia
Hypoglycaemia	Prolonged seizures leading to cerebral anoxia
Seizures	Prolonged seizures leading to cerebral anoxia
Haemolytic–uraemic syndrome	Renal failure leading to hyperkalaemia and fluid overload; severe anaemia and forward failure
Pneumonia	Tachypnoea, hypoxaemia

passage of bloody, mucoid stools. The degree of dehydration may be considerably less than in other diarrhoeas, though stool frequency may be as many as 100 times per day. Intestinal complications include toxic megacolon, perforation and a protein-losing enteropathy. Electrolyte imbalance may arise, in particular prolonged hyponatraemia. *Sh. dysenteriae* and *Sh. flexneri* infections may result in a number of extraintestinal complications. Haemolytic–uraemic syndrome occurs particularly with *Sh. dysenteriae* 1 and can develop 7–10 days after the onset of disease.

Convulsions may occur with infections caused by all species of *Shigella*, particularly in children. They may occur before diarrhoea begins, and are usually accompanied by a rising fever. They rarely result in permanent sequelae.

Table 41.4 summarizes the complications of shigellosis that are associated with an increased risk of mortality. Management of each complication in widespread epidemic in areas with limited health resources presents one of the major challenges in shigella infections.

DIAGNOSIS

In many parts of the tropical world, the diagnosis and subsequent management of shigella infections occur in the absence of laboratory facilities. Clinical algorithms (Figure 41.6) have been used to aid the differential diagnosis of dysentery symptoms.

While such an approach may be inevitable in peripheral areas, laboratory confirmation of diagnosis is necessary for epidemiological investigations, and to enable antimicrobial sensitivities to de determined.

The clinical distinction between invasive and watery diarrhoea, and between bacillary and amoebic dysentery, is often unclear. In a study in a rural area of Bangladesh, 16% of children presenting with watery diarrhoea were shown to have a *Shigella* spp. infection.

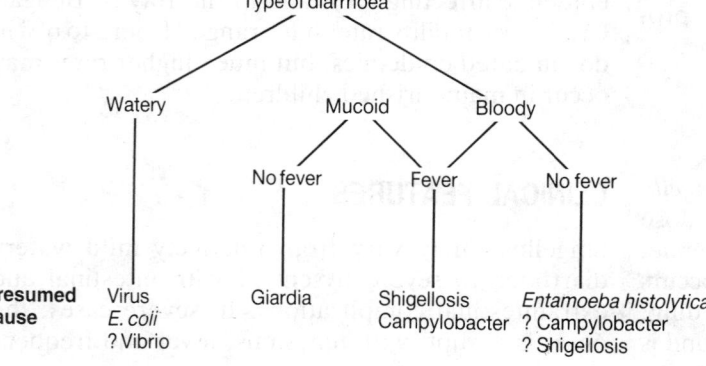

Figure 41.6 Clinical algorithm in the differential diagnosis of diarrhoea.

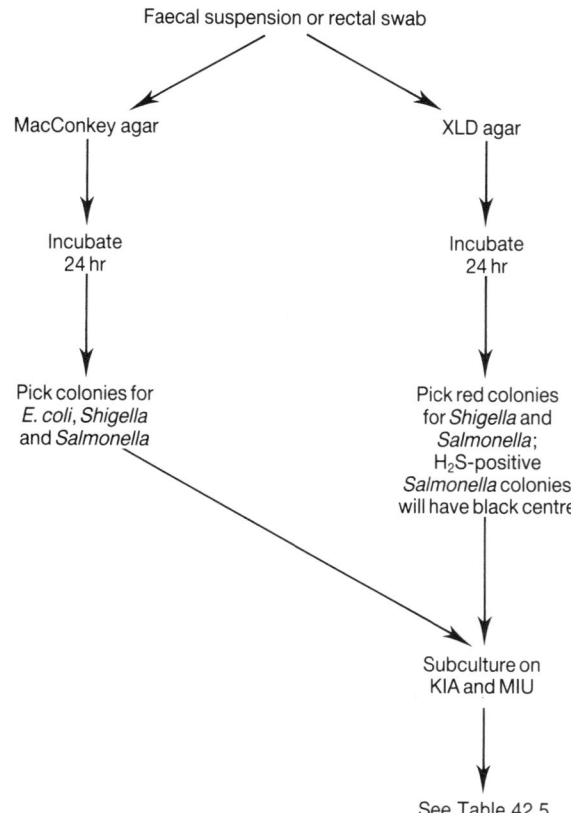

Faecal suspension or rectal swab

MacConkey agar → Incubate 24 hr → Pick colonies for *E. coli*, *Shigella* and *Salmonella*

XLD agar → Incubate 24 hr → Pick red colonies for *Shigella* and *Salmonella*; H₂S-positive *Salmonella* colonies will have black centre

Subculture on KIA and MIU

See Table 42.5

Figure 41.7 Culture protocol for isolation of *Shigella* spp.

Stool microscopy demonstrating the presence of leucocytes with associated clinical features may enable a presumptive diagnosis of shigella infection to be made.

A confirmed diagnosis of shigellosis requires culture and identification from faecal specimens or rectal swabs. Shigellae survive poorly in ambient temperatures in the tropics, and specimens should be transported in Cary–Blair medium or buffered glucose saline if there is more than a few hours delay before culture. Figure 41.7 shows the World Health Organization guidelines for the culture of specimens for isolation and identification of *Shigella* spp.

Faecal specimens or rectal swabs should be cultured overnight on MacConkey medium and a more selective medium such as xylose–lysine–deoxycholate agar (XLD). Shigellae appear as pale, non-lactose-fermenting colonies on MacConkey medium, and as pink colonies on XLD. Suspect colonies are incubated overnight on Kligler iron agar and motility indole urea medium. Table 41.5 shows the typical reactions of *Shigella* spp. in these composite media. Positive isolates may be typed by slide agglutination using the appropriate shigella antisera. Antimicrobial sensitivities should be determined using a disc diffusion method.

Where detailed epidemiological information is required, strains can be further typed by plasmid profiling and restriction endonuclease digests of chromosomal DNA.

Serology is of limited value in the diagnosis of acute cases but has been used to determine the prevalence of infection in epidemiological studies.[86]

MANAGEMENT

The management of shigella cases requires appropriate rehydration and electrolyte therapy, antimicrobial treatment, and the management of complications. Dehydration is rarely severe: oral rehydration is usually sufficient to restore water and electrolyte imbalances. Effective antimicrobial therapy will shorten the duration of illness and is particularly necessary in severe cases. Resistance of *Shigella* spp. to commonly used antimicrobial agents is an increasing problem in many tropical countries (see Chapter 43) and data on local sensitivities are essential if effective treatment is to be implemented.

Multiple antimicrobial resistance has been demonstrated in *Sh. dysenteriae* and *Sh. flexneri* throughout the tropics. Resistance patterns of epidemic strains of *Sh. dysenteriae* have included TcSuSmC in central America in 1970, ApTcSuTmC in Zaire and Rwanda in 1978 and TcSmCTm in South Asia, Burma and Thailand in 1978 (see Table 41.6 for an explanation of abbreviations). In Bangladesh, *Sh. dysenteriae* strains have been isolated with resistance to all commonly available oral antimicrobial agents including nalidixic acid.

Genetic studies have shown that multiple resistance in *Shigella* spp. is primarily plasmid mediated, and that multiple resistance plasmids may be transferred both within and between species. Endemic *Sh. flexneri* strains may be sensitive to a wider range of antimicrobial agents than epidemic strains of *Sh. dysenteriae*.

Table 41.6 shows the results of recent studies on sensitivity patterns of strains isolated in the tropics. In most areas, for the treatment of *Sh. flexneri*, ampicillin or co-trimoxazole continue to be suitable first line agents. In outbreaks of *Sh. dysenteriae* 1, monitoring of antimicrobial sensitivities is essential. In some cases, quinolones such as ciprofloxacin may be the most appropriate treatment, but the use of such drugs should be reserved only for cases where strains are known to be resistant to other antimicrobials.

PREVENTION AND CONTROL

Shigellosis is primarily a disease of crowded and usually poor communities, living in an environment

Table 41.5 Reactions of *Shigella* spp. on Kligler iron agar (KIA) and motility indole urea (MIU) medium.

Bacterium	Urea	Slant	Butt	H_2S	Gas	Motility	Indole
E. coli	−	A	A	−	+	(+)	d
Sh. dysenteriae	−	K	A	−	−	−	d
Sh. flexneri	−	K	A	−	−*	−	d
Sh. boydii	−	K	A	−	−†	−	d
Sh. sonnei	−	K	A	−	−	−	−

K, alkaline (red) reaction; A, acid (yellow) reaction; +, positive reaction; −, negative reaction; d, different biochemical types.
*Some *Sh. flexneri* serotype 6 gas (+).
†Serotypes 13 and 14 gas (+).

Table 41.6 Resistance patterns of *Shigella* spp. isolated in different tropical countries.

Date	Country	Serotype	Resistance pattern
1970	Central America	Sh. dysenteriae 1	C Tc Su Sm
1980	Zaire	Sh. dysenteriae 1	Ap Tc C Tm Sm Su
1984	India	Sh. dysenteriae 1	Ap Sm Tc C
1985	Burma	Sh. dysenteriae 1	C Tc Su Sm
1988	Bangladesh	Sh. dysenteriae 1	Ap Tc Sm Tm C Nal
1988	Ethiopia	Sh. dysenteriae 3	Ap C Tc Su
1988	Ethiopia	Sh. flexneri 2	Ap C Tc Su Sm

Ap, ampicillin; Tc, tetracycline; Su, sulphonamide; Sm, streptomycin; Tm, trimethoprim; C, chloramphenicol; Nal, nalidixic acid.

characterized by inadequate sanitation and often polluted water. In the long term, the incidence of shigellosis will be reduced only by improved public health and the alleviation of poverty.

Since most transmission is from person to person, improvements in water supply quality alone may have little impact.[91] Most studies show that increased water quantity, and allowing general improvement in the level of hygiene, does reduce the incidence of diarrhoeal disease. Improvement in hygiene at the household level, particularly through the provision of soap for hand washing, has been shown to reduce the transmission of shigellosis.[92]

In epidemics of shigellosis co-ordinated action will be necessary at the local and regional level in diagnosis, local public health intervention and possibly restrictions on population movements, markets, religious gatherings, etc.

No effective vaccines for shigellosis are currently available. Research is in progress to develop oral vaccines, which may be attenuated living organisms, with deletion of virulence genes, or recombinant vaccines where genes for protective shigella antigens are inserted into *E. coli*.[93]

CHOLERA (See also Chapter 3)

Cholera occurs endemically in many areas of the tropics, particularly in South and South-East Asia and Africa. In 1991, cholera appeared in Latin America for the first time in the twentieth century. A cholera-like disease was described by early Indian, Greek and Chinese writers, but it is uncertain whether the disease spread beyond the Indian subcontinent before the nineteenth century. How-

ever, there is at least one report of a cholera-like illness in Africa in the seventeenth century.[94] From 1817 to 1923 there were six pandemics of cholera, spreading extensively from its natural home in the Ganges plain and delta (Table 41.7). The devastating effect of the 1817 epidemic on both city and rural populations in India has been well described[95]—the vernacular term 'murri', meaning death, being aptly

Table 41.7 The first six cholera pandemics.

Pandemic	Date	Indian subcontinent	South-East Asia	Middle East	Europe	North Africa	East Africa	America
First	1817–1823	+	+	+	—	—	+	—
Second	1826–1837	+	+	+	+	+	+	+
Third	1842–1862	+	+	+	+	+	+	+
Fourth	1865–1875	+	+	+	+	+	+	+
Fifth	1881–1896	+	+	+	+	+	+	+
Sixth	1899–1923	+	+	+	+	—	+	—

Table 41.8 Differentiating properties of classical and El-Tor biotypes of *Vibrio cholerae* O1.

	Classical	El Tor
Chicken cell haemagglutination	−	+
Voges–Proskauer test	−	+
Polymyxin B sensitivity	Sensitive	Resistant

Table 41.9 Viability of *Vibrio cholerae*: survival in food.

	Survival at 30–31°C (days)	Survival at 5–10°C (days)
Cooked food	2–5	3–5
Fresh vegetables	1–7	7–10
Fish and seafood	2–5	7–14
Fruits	1–3	3–5
Milk and milk products	7–14	>14
Cereal	1–3	3–5

used to describe the impact of the disease. In each pandemic, transportation routes, commercial centres and pilgrimages mapped out the spread of the disease. The seventh pandemic of cholera, which began in 1961, is described under epidemiology (see below).

BACTERIOLOGY

In 1883, Koch demonstrated the bacterial cause of cholera during a visit to Egypt, and subsequent work defined the species *Vibrio cholerae*.[96] Vibrios are comma-shaped, aerobic Gram-negative bacteria which have a characteristic darting movement. They are oxidase positive, and ferment sucrose and glucose but not lactose. Vibrios possess both flagellar and somatic antigens. The species *V. cholerae* is divided into several serovars according to somatic antigens. *V. cholerae* O1 is the causative agent for cholera. Other serovars may cause a cholera-like illness, and are described below. There are two biotypes of *V. cholerae* O1: classical and El Tor. Table 41.8 summarizes their characteristic properties. *V. cholerae* El Tor was first isolated from pilgrims at the El Tor quarantine station in Sinai in 1906.[97] Until 1961, the El Tor biotype was isolated only in Sulawesi, Indonesia, causing four localized epidemics between 1937 and 1958. The classical and El Tor biotypes are each divided into three serotypes: Ogawa, Inaba and Hikojima.

V. cholerae does not form spores, is killed by heating at 55°C for 15 minutes and by phenolic and hypochlorite disinfectants. It can survive in saline conditions at low temperatures for up to 60 days,

and from 10 to 13 days at ambient temperature. Excluding seafoods, *V. cholerae* survives for only a limited time on foodstuffs (Table 41.9), although contaminated food may act as a vehicle for transmission. In fish and shellfish, *V. cholerae* may survive from 2 to 5 days at ambient temperatures, and 7 to 14 days in refrigeration.

PATHOGENESIS AND IMMUNITY

Cholera is characterized by severe watery diarrhoea leading to dehydration, electrolyte imbalance and hypovolaemia, with a mortality ranging from 3 to 40%.

There is a wide spectrum of severity, and mild and asymptomatic cases may occur. *V. cholerae* O1 is non-invasive; pathogenesis is due to an enterotoxin that causes excessive fluid and electrolyte loss. The initial step in pathogenesis is adherence of the vibrios to the outer mucosa of the small intestine. Adherence is due to both outer membrane protein and flagellar adhesins.[98] Cholera toxin comprises two subunits: B (binding) and A (active). The binding subunit comprises five polypeptides, each of molecular weight 11 500 and binds to a specific monosialyl ganglioside, GM_1, on small gut epithelial cells. The A subunit is then able to migrate through the epithelial cell membrane.[99] This subunit has ADP ribosyl transferase activity and causes the transfer of ADP ribose from NAD to a GTP binding protein that regulates adenylate cyclase activity. There is a resulting increase in cyclic AMP activity which, by inhibiting sodium chloride absorption and stimulating chloride excretion, results in a net loss of water, sodium chloride, potassium and bicarbonate.

Infection with *V. cholerae* results in the production of antibodies to the enterotoxin, and to O-antigenic components. Serum vibriocidal antibodies have been demonstrated in volunteers following experimental infection, and in community studies in endemic areas.[100] While they are an indication of past exposure, protective immunity is dependent on the immune response within the gut, where both locally-produced IgA and serum-derived IgG and IgM may be present. Vibriocidal antibodies within the gut inhibit adherence and are serotype specific. Antitoxin antibodies are produced to both the A and B subunits of the enterotoxin.

EPIDEMIOLOGY

Man is the only known natural host of *V. cholerae*. Transmission is by ingestion, through contaminated water or food. The infective dose is high, up to 10^{11} bacteria being required. The incubation period ranges from a few hours to 5 days.

Serological studies have shown that, in both endemic areas and during outbreaks, for each symptomatic case there may be from 5 to 40 infected but asymptomatic or mildly symptomatic cases. Contamination of water or food may thus occur from symptomatic cases or asymptomatic, transient carriers. Most are free from infection within 2–3 weeks, and there have been few examples of persistent carriage. In a study in the Philippines infection rates were 13, 8 and 0.3% in household contacts, neighbours and the general community, respectively.[101] *V. cholerae* has been shown to survive for several months in saline environments in association with certain aquatic plants and crustaceans.[102]

It is uncertain whether such natural reservoirs are important in maintaining infection in the absence of human cases. There are important epidemiological differences between classical and El Tor *V. cholerae*. For El Tor, the ratio of carriers to cases may range from 30:1 to 50:1, compared with 5:1 for classical. El Tor can also survive for longer periods in the environment.[103] These factors give El Tor an epidemiological advantage in the spread of the disease, which has occurred in the seventh pandemic and has contributed to the displacement of the classical type by El Tor. Only in Bangladesh has the classical biotype persisted.[104]

In 1961 the seventh pandemic of cholera began,

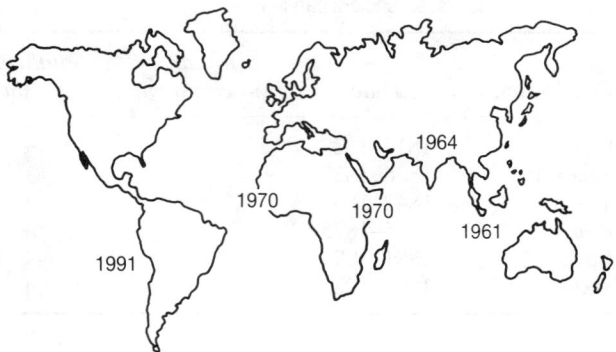

Figure 41.8   Global spread of the seventh cholera pandemic.

and continues to the present time (Figure 41.8). The pandemic, due to *V. cholerae* O1 El Tor, originated in Sulawesi and spread initially to South-East Asia. In 1963, the first El Tor strains were isolated in the Indian subcontinent and by 1966 had replaced classical strains except in East Bengal, where the two biotypes coexisted. In 1970 the pandemic had reached North and West Africa, and by the end of that decade had spread to most countries in Africa.[105] In January 1991, cholera reappeared in South America for the first time in the twentieth century. The strain is *V. cholerae* O1, biotype El Tor, serotype Inaba, and was first isolated from cases on the Pacific coast of Peru. By mid-1991 a total of 260 000 cases had been reported from six countries in South and Central America.[106]

Epidemiological studies in two cities of Peru concluded that the principal routes of transmission were via municipal drinking water, with potential points of contamination in wells, distribution systems and houses.[107] The study also implicated contaminated ice and beverages, locally grown vegetables and raw shellfish. Molecular studies have shown a similarity between strains isolated in South America and Asia.[108]

In endemic areas there are often seasonal peaks of cholera infection. In Bangladesh this occurs in the winter months after the monsoon; in South America most cases have been in the early summer. Seasonality in Bangladesh is thought to be partly related to the increased growth of algae in saline, estuarine areas after the monsoon period, improving the viability of vibrios.

In any region where cholera is endemic, natural disasters and political upheaval may lead to cholera outbreaks, and refugee movements may spread the disease to new areas. Cholera is frequently associated with cyclones and floods in Bangladesh.[109] Scarcity of clean water, crowding, and population movements have resulted in cholera outbreaks in drought and refugee-affected areas of Africa.[110,111]

Both contaminated water sources and partially cooked foodstuffs left at ambient temperatures were implicated in the spread of the disease. Where hospitals are overcrowded, and the population is undernourished, hospital outbreaks have occurred, possibly due to person-to-person spread as well as contamination of water or food.[112]

CLINICAL FEATURES

The clinical picture of infection with *V. cholerae* O1 may range from mild diarrhoea to severe dehydration with death occurring within hours. In most cases there is progress from the onset of diarrhoea to shock in 4–12 hours, with death following in several days if adequate management is not instituted. The symptoms are a reflection of the severe dehydration, electrolyte loss and metabolic acidosis. Hypovolaemia and hypotension lead to impaired consciousness and to renal failure. Hypoglycaemia may occur, particularly in children. Electrolyte loss leads to hyponatraemia and hypokalaemia. The latter may result in ileus, muscle weakness and cardiac arrhythmias.

A rapidly fatal picture has been described as 'cholera sicca'. In these cases there may be little diarrhoea or vomiting but rapid collapse and high mortality rate.

DIAGNOSIS

In epidemics the diagnosis of cholera may presumptively be made on clinical and epidemiological grounds. Laboratory diagnosis may be required when sporadic cases occur, and when an extensive outbreak requires confirmation and typing of the aetiological agent. Dark-field microscopy of faecal specimens may show the characteristic darting movement of the vibrios. Inhibition of movement by addition of diluted O1 antisera to the slide will provide strong evidence that *V. cholerae* O1 is the causative agent.[113] To confirm the diagnosis, specimens need to be cultured on a selective medium, such as thiosulphate citrate bile salts sucrose (TCBS) agar. Specimens should be transported from the field in alkaline peptone water or Cary–Blair transport medium and kept cool. *V. cholerae* O1 yields yellow, oxidase-positive colonies after overnight incubation on TCBS, which may be confirmed by slide agglutination with antiserum. In outbreak investigations, isolates should be sent to a reference laboratory for biotyping and serotyping. Sensitivity to tetracycline and other antimicrobial agents should be performed on a selected number of isolates. Where detailed epidemiological data are required, molecular methods have been used to distinguish different strains.[114]

CASE MANAGEMENT

The successful management of cholera cases relies on adequate and appropriate rehydration and restoration of electrolyte balance. Except in the most severe cases, oral replacement solutions may be used. Oral solutions are based on the role of glucose enhancing the active uptake of sodium and water.[115] As glucose is rarely available in rural areas, sucrose and rice-water-based solutions have been used with success.[116] The volume of replacement will depend on the degree of dehydration and the rate of continuing fluid loss. Considerable success has been achieved in the community level management of cholera cases in epidemics using 'home made' rehydration solutions. In refugee camps on the India–Bangladesh border during the 1971 war of independence, mortality rates were kept below 5% by the use of locally produced oral rehydration fluids.[117] When dehydration is severe or the patient is in shock, intravenous rehydration will be required. Replacement should be monitored by simple but supervised clinical assessment of the patient(s). In the severely ill child, hypoglycaemia may be anticipated and may require intravenous glucose.

Antimicrobial agents have been shown to shorten the period of diarrhoea and the amount of fluid loss. Tetracycline or doxycycline are the drugs of choice in adults where strains are sensitive, but the increasing occurrence of resistant strains limits their usefulness. Co-trimoxazole and furazolidone have been used, but antibiotics are secondary to the importance of early rehydration. Antisecretory agents have been studied in the management of cholera, but at the present time, none is of adequately proven value.

ANTIMICROBIAL RESISTANCE

Prior to 1977 only sporadic isolates of *V. cholerae* had been reported to be tetracycline resistant (Chapter 43). During an epidemic in Tanzania in 1977 the development of tetracycline resistance following its mass use in chemoprophylaxis was demonstrated.[118] In Bangladesh strains have been isolated resistant to ampicillin and co-trimoxazole in addition to tetracycline. In a given location the pattern of resistance varies in different years and surveillance of resistance patterns is necessary. Antimicrobial resistance in *V. cholerae* is usually plasmid mediated, and resistance genes may be transferred from multiply-resistant Enterobacteriaceae in the gut.

PREVENTION AND CONTROL

Cholera is transmitted by the faecal–oral route through the contamination of water or food. Hence public health measures to improve water and sanitation are essential for long-term control. The management of outbreaks is based on interrupting transmission, appropriate control and management of cases and contacts, and effective surveillance. In most cholera outbreaks the source and routes of transmission are not obvious and general sanitary measures will need to be imposed. These may include chlorination of water supplies, boiling of water at household level, and construction and maintenance of temporary latrines. Action will need to be taken to control the cleanliness of markets, and the postponement of festivals and gatherings. Adequate, though basic, sanitation facilities must be made for disposal of faeces from cases during treatment.[119]

The most appropriate group for chemoprophylaxis are household contacts of cases. The relatively high carriage of *V. cholerae* in this group has been described previously. Assuming strains are sensitive, tetracycline or doxycycline may be used in adults.[120] For doxycycline a single oral dose of 300 mg is adequate.

The currently available killed whole cell vaccines, given parentally, have no useful role to play in the management or prevention of cholera outbreaks: individual protection does not exceed 50–60%; vaccination does not reduce excretion of vibrios and is likely to give a false sense of security to both the affected population and the authorities.

Effective surveillance is an essential component of cholera control. Active reporting of suspected cases in areas previously uninfected, with appropriate bacteriological confirmation, will allow the early introduction of the control measures described above.[121] At the international level, systematic reporting of cases to the World Health Organization and its collaborative bodies will help to co-ordinate the international response and limit spread between countries.

Cholera vaccines

While the currently available killed whole cell, parenterally-administered vaccine is of limited value, new vaccines are being developed on an improved understanding of the pathophysiology of cholera, and using genetic engineering techniques. Both antibacterial and antitoxin immunity within the gut is necessary for protection. Toxoid vaccines using inactivated toxin have been shown to be ineffective. Promotion of antitoxin activity is based on the understanding of the activity of the A and B subunits. Either purified B subunit combined with killed bacteria may be given, or genetically engineered vaccine strains deficient in the genes for the A subunit may be produced. Such vaccines will give B-subunit immunity, and antibacterial immunity, but being deficient in the A subunit will be non-pathogenic. Two candidate vaccines are currently undergoing field testing. In Bangladesh, extensive studies have been made with a whole cell/B subunit (WC/B) vaccine comprising a mixture of killed classical and El Tor biotypes, of both Inaba and Ogawa serotypes, plus the purified B subunit protein.[122] Preliminary results, using three doses, have shown 85% protective efficacy in the first 6 months following administration. A second candidate vaccine is CVD-103, a live oral vaccine in which the A subunit genes have been deleted. The vaccine has been shown to produce an adequate immune response without side-effects.

The spread of the current cholera pandemic throughout South America is an indication that cholera is likely to remain a disease of considerable importance in the tropics; the development of effective vaccines may contribute to improved control.

V. CHOLERAE O139

Vibrio cholerae O139 is a new serotype which first appeared in southern India towards the end of 1992. Unlike disease caused by other non-O1 strains, this serotype has both the epidemiological and clinical characteristics of cholera. The first outbreak was reported in October 1992 in Madras, and in January 1993 further outbreaks occurred in other parts of Tamilnadu State. In December 1992, an outbreak of cholera occurred in southern Bangladesh and *V. cholerae* 0139 was isolated from 65% of cases examined.[123] By the end of March 1993, 12 southern districts were affected by outbreaks caused by O139. These outbreaks differed from *V. cholerae* O1 outbreaks in Bangladesh in that most of the cases were adults, and they occurred outside of the usual cholera season. The high attack rate in adults suggests that previous exposure to the O1 serotype does not confer protection. This finding will have major implications for the current candidate vaccines, which rely partly on immunity to the O1 somatic antigen of classical and El-Tor. Environmental studies in Bangladesh have shown O139 to be present in ponds, lakes and rivers and so the new serotype appears to have rapidly found an ecological niche. In April 1993, *V. cholerae* O139 strains were isolated from cholera cases in Thailand, indicating that the serotype has the potential for extensive geographical spread.[124]

NON-CHOLERA VIBRIOS

Vibrio species other than *V. cholerae* O1 and O139 may cause diarrhoeal diseases in the tropics but are rarely associated with extensive outbreaks. Five species have been associated with diarrhoeal diseases: *V. cholerae* non-O1, *V. parahaemolyticus*, *V. fluvialis*, *V. hollisae* and *V. minicus*. Among *V. cholerae* O1 strains, some have been isolated that are non-toxigenic but cause diarrhoea. They have been isolated from 1–3% of patients admitted to the cholera hospital in Dhaka.[125] *V. parahaemolyticus* is principally associated with seafoods. *V. fluvialis* has been implicated in an outbreak of diarrhoeal disease in Bangladesh.[126] Few data are currently available on the prevalence of these vibrios in most tropical countries.

REFERENCES

1 Marshall B J, Royce, H & Annear D I. Original isolation of *Campylobacter pyloridis* from human gastric mucosa. *Microbiol Lett* 1985; 25:83–88.

2 Peterson W I. *Helicobacter pylori* and peptic ulcer disease. *N Engl J Med* 1991; 321:1043–1048.

3 Hart C A, Murray A E & Walker S J. *Helicobacter pylori* and gastritis. *Postgrad Doct* 1990; 6:60–66.

4 Sullivan P B, Thomas J E, Wight D G D et al. *Helicobacter pylori* in Gambian children with chronic diarrhoea and malnutrition. *Arch Dis Child* 1990; 65:189–191.

5 Klein P D, Graham D Y, Gaillour A, Opekun A R & O'Brien Smith E. Water source as risk factor for *Helicobacter pylori* infection in Peruvian children. *Lancet* 1991; 337:1503–1506.

6 Megraud F, Brassen-Rabbe M P, Denis F, Belbouri A & Hoa D Q. Seroepidemiology of *Campylobacter pylori* infections in various populations. *J Clin Microbiol* 1989; 27:1870–1873.

7 Lee A, Fox J G, Otto G, Hegedus Dick E & Krakowa S. Transmission of *Helicobacter* spp. A challenge to the dogma of faecal–oral spread. *Epidemiol Infect* 1991; 107:99–109.

8 Blaser M J. *Helicobacter pylori* and the pathogenesis of gastroduodenal inflammation. *J Infect Dis* 1990; 161:626–633.

9 Drumm B. *Helicobacter pylori*. *Arch Dis Child* 1990; 65:1278–1282.

10 Rouvroy D, Bogaerts J, Nsengiumwa O et al. *Campylobacter pylori* gastritis and peptic ulcer disease in central Africa. *BMJ* 1987; 295:1174.

11 Harries A D, Stewart M, Deegan K M et al. *Helicobacter pylori* in Malawi, Central Africa. *J Infect* 1992; 24:269–276.

12 Wyatt J I, Rathbone B J, Sobala G M et al. Gastric epithelium in the duodenum. Its association with *Helicobacter pylori* and inflammation. *J Clin Pathol* 1990; 43:981–986.

13 McKinlay A W. Antibiotics in the treatment of peptic ulcer disease. *J Antimicrob Chemother* 1992; 29:92–96.

14 Rauws E A J & Tytgat G N J. Care of duodenal ulcer associated with eradication of *Helicobacter pylori*. *Lancet* 1990; 335:1233–1335.

15 Hill I D, Sinclair-Smith C, Lastovica A J, Bowie M D & Emms M. Transient protein-losing enteropathy associated with acute gastritis and *Campylobacter pylori*. *Arch Dis Child* 1987; 62:1215–1219.

16 Moyenuddin M, Rahman K M & Sack D A. The aetiology of diarrhoea in children at an urban hospital in Bangladesh. *Trans R Soc Trop Med Hyg* 1987; 81:299–302.

17 Bray J & Beavan T E D. Slide agglutination of *Bact. coli* neapolitanum in summer diarrhoea. *J Pathol* 1948; 60:395–401.

18 Neter E. Enteritis due to enteropathogenic *Escherichia coli*. Present day status and unsolved problems. *J Pediatr* 1959; 55:223–239.

19 Guerrant R C, Kirchhoff L V, Nations M K et al. Prospective study of diarrhoeal illness in north eastern Brazil. *J Infect Dis* 1983; 148:986–987.

20 Black R E, Merson M H, Rahman A S M M et al. A two year study of bacterial viral and parasitic agents associated with diarrhoea in rural Bangladesh. *J Infect Dis* 1980; 142:660–665.

21 Merson M H, Sack R B, Islam S et al. Disease due to enterotoxigenic *E. coli* in Bangladesh adults. Clinical aspects and a controlled trial of tetracycline. *J Infect Dis* 1980; 141:702–711.

22 DuPont H L, Reves R R, Galindo E et al. Treatment of traveller's diarrhoea with trimethoprim/sulfamethoxazole and trimethoprim alone. *N Engl J Med* 1982; 307:841–844.

23 Peltola H, Siitonen A, Kyronseppa H et al. Prevention of traveller's diarrhoea by oral B-subunit/whole cell cholera vaccine. *Lancet* 1991; 338:1285–1289.

24 Taylor D N, Echeverria P, Sethabutr O et al. Clinical and microbiologic features of *Shigella* and enteroinvasive *Escherichia coli* infections detected

by DNA hybridization. *J Clin Pathol* 1988; 26:1362–1366.

25 Pal T, Pasca S, Emody L & Voros S. Antigenic relationship among virulent enteroinvasive *Escherichia coli*, *Shigella flexneri* and *Shigella sonnei* detected by ELISA. *Lancet* 1983; ii:102.

26 Levine M M, Berquist E J, Nalin D R et al. *Escherichia coli* strains that cause diarrhoea but do not produce heat-labile or heat-stable enterotoxins and are non-invasive. *Lancet* 1978; i:1119–1122.

27 Edelman R & Levine M M. Summary of a workshop on enteropathogenic *Escherichia coli*. *J Infect Dis* 1983; 147:1108–1118.

28 Echeverria P, Taylor D N, Bettelheim K A et al. HeLa cell-adherent enteropathogenic *Escherichia coli* in children under 1 year of age in Thailand. *J Clin Microbiol* 1987; 25:1472–1475.

29 Senerwa D, Olsvik O, Mutanda L N et al. Enteropathogenic *Escherichia coli* serotype O111:HNT isolated from preterm neonates in Nairobi Kenya. *J Clin Microbiol* 1989; 27:1307–1311.

30 Embaye H, Batt R M, Saunders J R, Getty B & Hart C A. Interaction of enteropathogenic *Escherichia coli*: O111 with rabbit intestinal mucosa in vitro. *Gastroenterology* 1989; 96:1079–1086.

31 Embaye H, Hart C A, Getty B et al. Effects of enteropathogenic *Escherichia coli* on microvillar membrane proteins during organ culture of rabbit intestinal mucosa. *Gut* 1992; 33:1184–1189.

32 Taylor C J, Hart C A, Batt R M, McDougall C & McLean L. Ultrastructural and biochemical changes in human jejunal mucosa associated with enteropathogenic *Escherichia coli* (O111) infection. *J Pediatr Gastroenterol Nutr* 1986; 5:70–73.

33 Rothbaum R, McAdams A J, Giannella R & Partin J C. A clinicopathologic study of enterocyte-adherent *Escherichia coli*: a cause of protracted diarrhoea in infants. *Gastroenterology* 1982; 83:441–454.

34 Jerse A E, Yu J, Tall B D & Kaper J B. A genetic locus of enteropathogenic *Escherichia coli* necessary for the production of attaching and effacing lesions on tissue culture cells. *Proc Natl Acad Sci USA* 1990; 87:7839–7843.

35 Riley L W, Remis R J, Helgerson S D et al. Haemorrhagic colitis associated with a rare *Escherichia coli* serotype. *N Engl J Med* 1983; 308:681–685.

36 Karmali M A, Steele B T, Petric M & Lim C. Sporadic cases of haemolytic uraemic syndrome associated with faecal cytoxin-producing *Escherichia coli*. *Lancet*; i:619–620.

37 Karmali M A. Infection by Verocytoxin-producing *Escherichia coli*. *Clin Microbiol Rev* 1989; 2:15–38.

38 Bettelheim K A, Brown J E, Lolekha S & Echeverria P. Serotype of *Escherichia coli* that hybridized with DNA probes for genes encoding Shiga-like toxin I, Shiga-like toxin II and serogroup O157 enterohaemorrhagic *E. coli* fimbriae isolated

from adults with diarrhoea in Thailand. *J Clin Microbiol* 1990; 28:293–295.

39 Isaacson M, Canter P H, Effler et al. Haemorrhagic colitis epidemic in Africa. *Lancet* 1993; 341:961.

40 Kishore K, Rattan A, Bagga et al. Serum antibodies to verotoxin-producing *Escherichia coli* (VTEC) strains in patients with haemolytic uraemic syndrome. *J Med Microbiol* 1993; 37:364–367.

41 Chart H, Smith H R, Scotland S M et al. Serological identification of *Escherichia coli* O157:H7 infection in haemolytic uraemic syndrome. *Lancet* 1991; 337:138–140.

42 Bhan M K, Raj P, Levine M M et al. Enteroaggregative *Escherichia coli* associated with persistent diarrhoea in a cohort of rural children in India. *J Infect Dis* 1989; 159:1061–1064.

43 Baudry B, Savarino S J, Vial P, Kaper J B & Levine M M. A sensitive and specific DNA probe to identify enteroaggregative *Escherichia coli*, a recently discovered diarrhoeal pathogen. *J Infect Dis* 1990; 161:1249–1251.

44 Butzler J P, Dekeyser P, Detrain M & Dehaen F. Related vibrio in stools. *J Pediatr* 1973; 82:493–496.

45 Skirrow M B. Campylobacter enteritis: a 'new' disease. *BMJ* 1977; 2:9–11.

46 Potter M E, Blaser M J, Sikes R K, Kaufmann A F & Wells J G. Human campylobacter infection associated with certified raw milk. *Am J Epidemiol* 1983; 117:475–483.

47 Korlath J A, Osterholm M T, Judy L A, Forgang J C & Robinson R A. A point source outbreak of campylobacteriosis associated with consumption of raw milk. *J Infect Dis* 1985; 152:592–596.

48 Southern J P, Smith R M M & Palmer S R. Bird attack on milk bottles: possible mode of transmission of *Campylobacter jejuni* to man. *Lancet* 1990; 336:1425–1427.

49 Rajan D P & Mathan V I. Prevalence of *Campylobacter fetus* subsp. *jejuni* in healthy populations in India. *J Clin Microbiol* 1982; 15:749–751.

50 Walker R I, Caldwell M D, Lee E C et al. Pathophysiology of *Campylobacter* enteritis. *Microbiol Rev* 1986; 50:81–94.

51 Glass R I, Stoll B J, Huq M I et al. Epidemiologic and clinical features of endemic *Campylobacter jejuni* infection in Bangladesh. *J Infect Dis* 1983; 148:292–296.

52 Black R F, Levine M M, Brown K H, Clements M L & Lopez de Romana G. Immunity to *Campylobacter jejuni* in man. In Pearson D A, Skirrow M B, Lior H & Rowe B (eds) *Campylobacter III*. London: Public Health Laboratory Service, 1985: 129.

53 Butzler J P & Skirrow M B. Campylobacter enteritis. *Clin Gastroenterol* 1979; 8:737–765.

54 Cover T L & Aber RC. *Yersinia enterocolitica*. *N Engl J Med* 1989; 321:16–24.

55 Bottone E J. *Yersinia enterocolitica*: a panoramic view of a charismatic microorganism. *Crit Rev Microbiol* 1977; 5:211–241.

56 Gomes T A T, Rassi V, MacDonald K C et al. Enteropathogens associated with acute diarrhoeal disease in urban infants in Sao Paulo, Brazil. *J Infect Dis* 1991; 164:331–337.

57 Rabson A R, Hallett A F & Koornhof H J. Generalized *Yersinia enterocolitica* infection. *J Infect Dis* 1975; 131:447–451.

58 Awunor-Renner C & Lawande R V. Yersinia and chronic glomerulopathy in the savannah region of Nigeria. *BMJ* 1982; 285:1464–1465.

59 Pai C H, Gillis F, Tuomanen E & Marks M I. Placebo-controlled double-blind evaluation of trimethoprim sulfamethoxazole treatment of *Yersinia enterocolitica* gastroenteritis. *J Pediatr* 1984; 104:308–311.

60 Jeckeln E. Uber 'Darmbrand': das pathologisch antatomische Bild des Darmbrandes. *Dtsch Med Wochenschr* 1947; 11:105.

61 Murrell T G C, Roth L, Egerton J, Samels J & Walker P D. Pigbel:enteritis necroticans. A study in diagnosis and management. *Lancet* 1966; i:217–222.

62 Foster W D. The bacteriology of necrotising jejunitis in Uganda. *East Afr Med J* 1966; 45:550.

63 Shann F, Lawrence G & Jun-Bi P. Enteritis necroticans in China. *Lancet* 1979; i:1083–1084.

64 Lawrence G & Walker P D. Pathogenesis of enteritis necroticans in Papua New Guinea. *Lancet* 1976; i:125–126.

65 Lawrence G, Brown R, Baters J et al. An affinity technique for isolation of *Clostridium perfringens* type C from man and pigs in Papua New Guinea. *J Appl Bacteriol* 1984; 57:333–338.

66 Lawrence G, Shann F, Freestone D S & Walker P D. Prevention of necrotising enteritis in Papua New Guinea by active immunization. *Lancet* 1979; i:227–230.

67 Griffin GE. *Clostridium difficile*. In Farthing M J G & Keusch G T (eds) *Enteric Infections*. London:Chapman & Hall, 1989: 327–336.

68 Ljungh A & Wadstron T. Aeromonas and Plesiomonas. In Farthing M J G & Keusch G (eds) *Enteric Infections*. London: Chapman &Hall, 1989:169–181.

69 Echeverria P, Seriwatana J, Taylor D N, Yanggratoke S & Tirapat C. A comparative study of enterotoxigenic *Escherichia coli*, *Shigella*, *Aeromonas* and *Vibrios* as etiologies of diarrhoea in north eastern Thailand. *Am J Trop Med Hyg* 1985; 34:547–554.

70 Vandepitte J, VanDamme L, Fofana Y & Desmyter J. *Edwardsiella tarda* et *Plesiomonas shigelloides*: leur rôle comme agents de diarrhées et leur épidémiologie. *Bull Soc Pathol Exot* 1980; 73:139–149.

71 Sakazaki R, Tamura K, Prescott L M et al. Bacteriological examination of diarrhoeal stools in Calcutta. *Indian J Med Res* 1971; 59:1025–1034.

72 Davis W A, Chretien J H, Gargarusi V F & Goldstein MA. Snake to human transmission of *Aeromonas (Pl.) shigelloides* resulting in gastroenteritis. *South Med J* 1978; 71:474–476.

73 Topley W W C & Wilson G S. *Principles of Bacteriology and Immunology*. London: Edward Arnold, 1964.

74 Bennish M L. Potentially lethal complications of shigellosis. *Rev Infect Dis* 1991; 13 (supplement 4):S319–324.

75 Taylor D N, Bodhidatta L & Echeverria P. Epidemiological aspects of shigellosis and other causes of dysentery in Thailand. *Rev Infect Dis* 1991; 13 (supplement 4):S231–237.

76 Ronsmans C, Bennish M L & Wierzeba T. Diagnosis and management of dysentery by community health workers. *Lancet* 1988; ii:552–555.

77 Gangarosa E J, Perera D R, Mata L J, Morris M C, Cuzma G & Reller L B. Epidemic shiga bacillus dysentery in central America II. Epidemiological studies. *J Infect Dis* 1970; 122:181–190.

78 Frost J A, Rowe B, Vandepitte J & Threlfall E J. Plasmid characterization in the investigation of an epidemic caused by multiply resistant *Shigella dysenteriae* in central Africa. *Lancet* 1981; ii:1074–1075.

79 Pal S C. Epidemic bacillary dysentery in West Bengal, India 1984. *Lancet* 1984; i:1462.

80 Taylor D N, Bodhidatta L, Brown J E et al. Introduction and spread of multi-resistant *Sh. dysenteriae* 1 in Thailand. *Am J Trop Med Hyg* 1989; 40:77–85.

81 Litwin C M, Stom A L, Chipowsky S & Ryan K J. Molecular epidemiology of Shigella infections: plasmid profiles, serotype correlation, and restriction endonuclease analysis. *J Clin Microbiol* 1991; 29:104–108.

82 Nakamura M. The survival of *Shigella sonnei* on cotton, glass, wood, paper and metal at various temperatures. *J Hyg (Camb)* 1962; 30:35.

83 Lindberg AA, Karnell A & Weibtraub A. The lipopolysaccharide of Shigella bacteria as a virulence factor. *Rev Infect Dis* 1991; 13 (supplement 4):S279–284.

84 Brown J E, Griffin D E, Rothman S W and Doctor B. Purification and characterization of shiga toxin for *Shigella dysenteriae* 1. *Infect Immun* 1982; 36:996–1005.

85 Streulens M J, Patte D, Kabir I, Salam A, Nath S K & Butler T. Shigella septicaemia: prevalence, prevention, risk factors and outcome. *J Infect Dis* 1985; 152:784–790.

86 Lindberg A A, Cam P D, Chan N et al. Shigellosis in Vietnam: Sero-epidemiologic studies with use of lipopolysaccharide antigens in enzyme immunoassays. *Rev Infect Dis* 1992; 13 (supplement 4):S231–237.

87 Boye J M, Hughes J M, Alim A R et al. Patterns of Shigella infection in families in rural Bangladesh. *Am J Trop Med Hyg* 1982; 31:1015–1020.

88 Matham V I, Bhat P, Kapadia C R, Ponniah J & Baker S J. Epidemic dysentery caused by the Shiga

bacillus in a south Indian village. *J Diarrhoeal Dis Res* 1984; 2:27–32.

89 Hassain M A, Albert J M & Hasan K Z. Epidemiology of shigellosis in Teknaf, a coastal area of Bangladesh: a 10 year survey. *Epidemiol Infect* 1990; 105:41–49.

90 Keusch G T & Bennish M L. Shigellosis: recent progress, persisting problems and research issues. *Paediatr Infect Dis* 1989; 8:713–719.

91 Levine R J, Khan M R, D'Souza S & Nahn D R. Failure of sanitary wells to protect against cholera and other diarrhoeas in Bangladesh. *Lancet* 1976; ii:86–89.

92 Khan M U. Interruption of shigellosis by hand washing. *Trans R Soc Trop Med Hyg* 1982; 76:164–168.

93 WHO Research priorities for diarrhoeal disease vaccines: memorandum from a WHO meeting. *Bull World Health Organ* 1991; 69:667–676.

94 Pankhurst R. The history of cholera in Ethiopia. *Med Hist* 1966; 12:262–269.

95 Tod J. *Annals and Antiquities of Rajasthan*, vol. 2. New Delhi:India NDB Publishers, 1978:552.

96 Pollitzer R. *Cholera*, Monograph No.43. Geneva:WHO, 1959.

97 Khan M, Bart K J & Huq Z. The changing pattern of cholera in East Pakistan: the appearance of El-Tor *Vibrio Cholerae*. *JPMA* 1970; 20:43–48.

98 Aldridge S R & Rowley D. The role of the flagellum in the adherence of *V. cholerae*. *J Infect Dis* 1983; 147:864–872.

99 Holmgren J. Actions of cholera toxin and the prevention and treatment of cholera. *Nature* 1981; 292:413–417.

100 Bart K J, Huq Z, Khan M U, Mosley W H, Nuruzzman M & Kibriya A K. Seroepidemiologic studies during a simultaneous epidemic of infection with El-Tor Ogawa and classical Inaba *Vibrio cholerae*. *J Infect Dis* 1970; 121 (supplement):S17–24.

101 World Health Organization Expert Committee on Cholera. *WHO Tech Rep Ser* 1967; 3520.

102 Feacham R G. Environmental aspects of cholera epidemiology II. Occurrence and survival of *Vibrio cholerae*. *Trop Dis Bull* 1981; 78:865–880.

103 Woodward W E & Mosley W H. The spectrum of cholera in rural Bangladesh: comparison of El-Tor Ogawa and classical Inaba infection. *Am J Epidemiol* 1972; 96:342–351.

104 Siddique A K, Baqui A H, Eusof A et al. Survival of classic cholera in Bangladesh. *Lancet* 1991; i:1125–1127.

105 Stock R F. *Cholera in Africa*, African Environment Special Report 3. London: International African Institute, 1976.

106 Pan American Health Organization. Cholera situation in the Americas: an update. *Epidemiol Bull* 1991; 12:1–4.

107 Pan American Health Organization. Environmental health conditions and cholera vulnerability in Latin America and the Caribbean. *Epidemiol Bull* 1991; 12:5–10.

108 Faruque S M & Albert J. Genetic relation between *Vibrio cholerae* O1 strains in Ecuador and Bangladesh. *Lancet* 1992; 339:740–741.

109 Siddique AK, Islam Q & Akram K. Cholera epidemic and natural disasters: where is the link. *Trop Geog Med*. 1989; 41:377–382.

110 Tauxe R V, Holmberg S D, Dodin A, Wells J V & Blake PA. Epidemic cholera in Mali: high mortality and routes of transmission in a famine area. *Epidemiol Infect* 1988; 100:279–289.

111 Mulholland K. Cholera in Sudan: an account of an epidemic in a refugee camp. *Disasters* 1985; 9:247–258.

112 Cliff J L, Zinkin P & Martelli A. A hospital outbreak of cholera in Maputo, Mozambique. *Trans R Soc Trop Med Hyg* 1986; 80:473–476.

113 Benenson A S, Islam M R & Greenough W B. Rapid identification of *Vibrio cholerae* by darkfield microscopy. *Bull World Health Organ* 1964; 30:827–831.

114 Kaper J B, Bradford H B, Roberts N C & Falkow S. Molecular epidemiology of *Vibrio cholerae* in the US Gulf Coast. *J Clin Microbiol* 1982; 16:129–134.

115 Hirschom N. Decrease in net stool output in cholera during intestinal perfusion with glucose containing solutions. *N Engl J Med* 1968; 279:176–181.

116 Patra F C, Mahalanbis D, Jalan KV et al. Is oral rice-water electrolyte solution superior to glucose electrolyte solution in infantile diarrhoea? *Arch Dis Child* 1982; 57:910–912.

117 Mahalanbis D, Sack R B, Jacobs B et al. Oral fluid therapy of cholera among Bangladesh refugees. *Johns Hopkins Med J* 1975; 132:197–205.

118 Mhalu F S, Mmar P W & Ijumba J. Rapid emergence of El-Tor *Vibrio cholerae* resistant to antimicrobial agents in Tanzania. *Lancet* 1979; i:345–347.

119 World Health Organization. *Guidelines for Cholera Control*, 1993 WHO/CDD/SER/80.4. Geneva:WHO.

120 MacCormack W M, Chowdhury A M, Jahangir N et al. Tetracycline prophylaxis of families of cholera patients. *Bull World Health Organ* 1986; 38:787–792.

121 Vugia D C, Koehler J E & Ries A A. Surveillance for epidemic cholera in the Americas. *MMWR* 1992; 41:27–34.

122 Sack R B. Prospects for control of cholera with oral vaccines. *J Diarrhoeal Dis Res* 1992; 10:1–3.

123 Albert M J, Siddique A K, Islam M S et al. Large outbreak of clinical cholera due to *Vibrio cholerae* non-O1 in Bangladesh. *Lancet* 1993; (1) 704.

124 Shears P. Cholera – a review. *Ann Trop Med Parasitol* 1994; 88:109–122.

125 Stoll B J, Glass R I, Banu H et al. Surveillance of patients attending a diarrhoeal disease hospital in Bangladesh. *BMJ* 1982; 285:1185–1188.

126 Huq M I, Alim A R, Brenner D J & Morris G K. Isolation of vibrio like group EF-6 from patients with diarrhoea. *J. Clin Microbiol* 1980; 11:621–624.

CHAPTER 42

SALMONELLA INFECTIONS

Bibhat K. Mandal

BACTERIOLOGY

Salmonellae are flagellated non-spore-bearing Gram-negative bacilli belonging to the family Enterobacteriaceae (see also Chapter 3). Ability to ferment glucose but not lactose differentiates most salmonellae from other members of the Enterobacteriaceae. The genus *Salmonella* consists of only one species which has been named *Salmonella enterica*. Within this single species there are seven subspecies, *enterica*, *salamae*, *arizonae*, *diarizonae*, *houtenae*, *bongori* and *indica*, based on DNA structure or biochemical properties.[1] The subspecies members can be divided into serotypes (serovars) based on their somatic (O) and flagellar (H) antigens and more than 2100 are known. The serotypes of *enterica* subspecies account for most human and warm-blooded animal infections. These serotypes are grouped on the basis of sharing of a common O antigen (Kaufmann–White scheme).[2] Examples of commonly occurring groups of *enterica* subspecies serotypes are given in Table 42.1.

S. typhi also possesses a cell wall lipopolysaccharide virulence antigen (Vi), so named because Vi antigen-positive strains are highly pathogenic to mice. The antigen is also sometimes found in *S. paratyphi* C and some other enterobacterial organisms.

Further differentiation of strains within individual serotypes by bacteriophage typing and DNA fingerprinting helps epidemiological investigations.

On the basis of host preference and disease manifestations in man, the salmonellae can be conveniently placed into two broad categories:

- *S. typhi*, *S. paratyphi A*, *S. paratyphi B* and *S. paratyphi C*. These serotypes are primarily host-adapted to man and cause typhoid and paratyphoid fevers which are prolonged bacteraemic illnesses with minimal diarrhoea—at least initially.
- Other serotypes. These are host-adapted to animals, and infection in man is usually confined to the bowel and presents as acute diarrhoea.

Table 42.1 Some examples of commonly occurring salmonella serotypes and the groups to which they belong.

Group	Serotype
A	*S. paratyphi A*
B	*S. paratyphi B*
	S. stanley
	S. saintpaul
	S. agona
	S. typhimurium
C	*S. paratyphi C*
	S. cholerae-suis
	S. virchow
	S. thompson
D	*S. typhi*
	S. enteritidis
	S. dublin
	S. gallinarum

TYPHOID AND PARATYPHOID FEVERS (SYNONYMS: ENTERIC FEVER, EBERTH DISEASE)

Typhoid fever got its name from typhus because it was so like this disease. The confusion between the two was resolved only with the publication in 1850 of William Jenner's book *On the Identity and Non-Identity of Typhoid and Typhus Fevers*.[3]

The terms 'enteric fever' and 'Eberth disease' have been applied both to typhoid fever, and collectively to typhoid and paratyphoid fevers.

EPIDEMIOLOGY

Typhoid and paratyphoid fevers are endemic in the Indian subcontinent, South-East and Far-East Asia, the Middle East, Africa, Central and South America. A low level of endemicity also exists for paratyphoid B infections in the southern and eastern parts of Europe. In the rest of Europe, North America and Australasia enteric fevers occur almost exclusively as imported infections. Paratyphoid C is rare, with occasional cases in Guyana and eastern Europe.

TRANSMISSION

The ultimate source is almost always human. Transmission is through food or water contaminated with faeces or urine of a patient or carrier. Paratyphoid infections are less often water-borne because they need a higher infective dose which is unlikely to be found in water as multiplication does not occur. Raw fruit and vegetables are important vehicles in some countries where human faeces is used as manure. Shellfish harvested in coastal water polluted by raw sewage, may cause outbreaks.[4] Canned meat is generally safe but outbreaks have occurred through faulty canning processes.[5]

PATHOGENESIS

Natural infection in enteric fever is by ingestion, followed by penetration through the intestinal mucosa. Disease production is dependent on several factors: number of organisms swallowed; state of gastric acidity; and possession of Vi antigen by the organisms. The infecting dose of *S. typhi* needs to be large to produce illness in healthy individuals. In volunteers, a dose of 10^9 organisms induced disease in most (95%) but a dose of 10^3 rarely did so. Twenty-five per cent of the volunteers became ill after ingesting 10^5 organisms.[6] Possession of Vi antigen is linked with increased pathogenicity: Vi antigen-positive strains caused illness more commonly than non-Vi variants in healthy volunteers.[6] Gastric acidity is important defencively against enteric infections, and gastric hypoacidity from any cause will allow a greater number of organisms to enter the small intestine.[7] Once in the small intestine, the organisms penetrate rapidly through the intestinal mucosa,[8] although at which site is uncertain. Jejunal biopsy in experimental human infec-

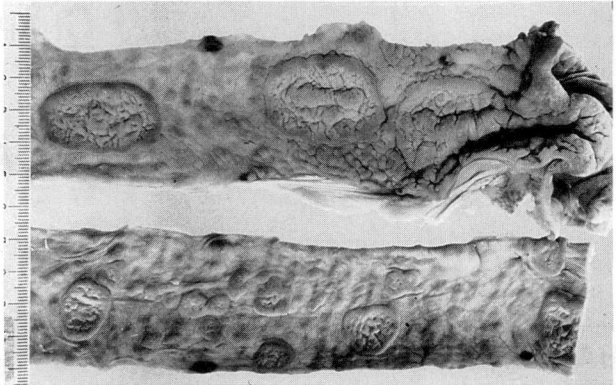

Figure 42.1   Typhoid ulceration of the small intestine. (Courtesy of the Wellcome Tropical Institute Museum (WTIM).)

tions has shown inflammatory changes suggesting local penetration.[9] Organisms also multiply in the lumen for a short period, as indicated by frequently-positive stool cultures during the first 4 days of the incubation period.[6]

From the submucosa the organisms travel to mesenteric lymph nodes. After a brief period of multiplication here the organisms enter the bloodstream via the thoracic duct (transient primary bacteraemia) and are transported to liver, spleen and other reticuloendothelial tissues. After a period of further multiplication at these sites huge numbers of organisms enter the bloodstream, marking the onset of clinical illness (secondary bacteraemia). During this secondary bacteraemia, which continues for the greater part of the illness, very few organs escape invasion but the involvement of the gallbladder and Peyer's patches in the lower small intestine have important clinical significance. The gallbladder is probably infected via the liver and the resultant cholecystitis is usually subclinical. The infected bile renders stool cultures positive. Pre-existing gallbladder disease predisposes to chronic biliary infection, leading to chronic faecal carriage.

Invasion of the Peyer's patches occurs either during the primary intestinal infection or during the secondary bacteraemia, and further seeding occurs through infected bile.[10] The Peyer's patches become hyperplastic, with infiltration of chronic inflammatory cells. Later, necrosis of the superficial layer leads to formation of irregular, ovoid ulcers along the long axis of the gut, so that stricture formation does not occur after healing (Figure 42.1). When an ulcer erodes into a blood vessel, severe haemorrhage results and transmural perforation leads to peritonitis.

The pathogenesis of the prolonged fever and toxaemia of enteric fever are poorly understood. A major role for continuing endotoxaemia has been discounted on the following grounds: (1) volunteers rendered endotoxin-tolerant still developed the typical fever of typhoid infection when challenged with experimental infection;[6] (2) it has not been possible to produce a state of prolonged fever by continuous infusion of endotoxin;[6] and (3) failure to demonstrate endotoxaemia in natural typhoid fever.[11] Pyrogens and mediators produced at the sites of inflammation have been postulated as factors responsible for the prolonged fever.[12,13]

MECHANISM OF IMMUNITY

Production of humoral antibody appears to play little role in recovery from acute infection as the patient often continues to deteriorate despite the appearance of O, H and Vi antibodies. Cell-mediated immunity is probably the key factor in recovery and its existence has been documented[14,15] The ability of Vi antibody to prevent infection is demonstrated by the efficiency of Vi antigen vaccine.[16] However, protection afforded by phenolized killed vaccine, which does not contain Vi antigen, indicates a role for other antibodies. Local gut immunity is probably important in preventing re-infection. Specific secretory IgG and IgA antibodies have been demonstrated in gut.[15]

In the endemic countries, enteric fevers have the highest prevalence in the young, adults having acquired substantial immunity through previous exposure(s).

CLINICAL MANIFESTATIONS

The incubation period of typhoid fever varies with the size of the infecting dose[6] and averages from 10 to 20 (range 3–56) days. In paratyphoid fever it ranges from 1 to 10 days.

The duration of illness in untreated cases of average severity is usually 4 weeks. In the *first* week the features are non-specific, with headache, malaise and a rising remittent fever. Constipation and a mild non-productive cough are common. During the *second* week the patient looks toxic and apathetic with sustained high temperature. The abdomen is slightly distended and splenomegaly is common. In about 50% of cases, crops of 2–4 mm diameter pink papules (rose spots), which fade on pressure, develop on the upper abdomen and lower chest, between the 7th and 12th days. They are difficult to detect in dark-skinned individuals. Rose spots may also occur in invasive salmonellosis[17] and shigellosis.[18] The spots are caused by bacterial embolization

and rose spot cultures may be positive. Relative bradycardia is common during the first 2 weeks and the pulse may have a characteristic notch (dicrotic pulse).

With the onset of the *third week* the patient becomes more toxic and ill. Continuous high fever persists and a delirious confusional state sets in (typhoid state). Abdominal distension becomes pronounced, with scanty bowel sounds. Diarrhoea is common, with liquid, foul green-yellow stools (pea soup diarrhoea). The patient is weak with a feeble pulse and rapid breathing; crackles may develop over the lung bases. Death may occur at this stage from overwhelming toxaemia, myocarditis, intestinal haemorrhage or perforation. Considerable weight loss is common. In patients who survive into the *fourth week*, the fever, mental state and abdominal distension slowly improve over a few days but intestinal complications may still occur. Convalescence is prolonged.

Variation in the clinical picture is common. Mild and inapparent infections are frequent. Diarrhoea may occur even during the first week,[19] and children may present with a high fever and febrile convulsion(s). Chronic or recurrent fever with bacteraemia may occur in association with concurrent schistosomiasis, as salmonellae are able to survive within the parasites protected from the body's defences.[20,21]

RELAPSE

Between 10 and 20% of patients treated with antibiotics suffer a relapse after initial recovery, whereas in the preantibiotic era the incidence used to be somewhat lower (8–12%). A relapse typically occurs a week or so after stoppage of therapy but occurrence after 70 days has been reported.[3] The blood culture is again positive, even in the presence of high serum levels of H, O and Vi antibodies, and rose spots may reappear. A relapse is generally milder and shorter than the initial illness.

Rarely, second or even third relapses may occur. It is noteworthy that the relapse rate is much lower following treatment with the new quinolone drugs which have effective intracellular penetration.[22]

COMPLICATIONS

Intestinal

The two most dreaded complications of enteric fever are intestinal haemorrhage and perforation, which usually occur when the sloughs overlying the Peyer's patches separate during the late second or early third week of the illness. Signs of *haemorrhage* are a sharp fall in body temperature and blood pressure, and sudden tachycardia. The blood passed per rectum is usually bright red but may be altered if intestinal stasis is present. Sometimes there may not be any passage of blood—when frank ileus is present.

Management of haemorrhage is conservative, with sedation and transfusion unless there is evidence of perforation, when surgery is indicated.

Unlike other causes of intestinal perforation, typhoid *perforation* occurs in a patient who already had a vaguely tender distended abdomen with scanty bowel sounds. Therefore, recognition of perforation can be difficult.[23,24] Usually pain and tenderness worsen, the pulse rises and the temperature falls suddenly. However, abdominal rigidity may not be prominent and bowel sounds may not disappear altogether. Frequently the discovery of free fluid in the abdomen is the only sign of perforation. Demonstration of gas under the diaphragm is a valuable aid to diagnosis.

Conservative management with nasogastric suction, antibiotic therapy and general supportive care will reduce the mortality to 30%,[25] but nowadays consensus favours surgery.[26] Most surgeons prefer simple closure of perforation with drainage of the peritoneum, and reserve small bowel resection for patients with multiple perforations. Early diagnosis, energetic resuscitation and rapid, simple surgery are the key to lower mortality. The prognosis is clearly related to the time elapsed between perforation and surgery.

Liver, gallbladder and pancreas

Mild jaundice may occur in enteric fever and may be due to hepatitis, cholangitis, cholecystitis or haemolysis. Biochemical changes indicative of hepatitis are common during the acute stage.[27] Liver biopsy in such cases often shows cloudy swelling, balloon degeneration with vacuolation of hepatocytes, moderate fatty change and focal collection of mononuclear cells—'typhoid nodules' (Figure 42.2). Intact typhoid bacilli can be seen at these sites.[28] Pancreatitis has also been reported.[29]

Cardiorespiratory

Toxic myocarditis is a significant cause of death in endemic countries.[30] It occurs in severely ill toxaemic patients and is characterized by tachycardia, weak pulse and heart sounds, hypotension and electrocardiographic abnormalities. Mild bronchitis is

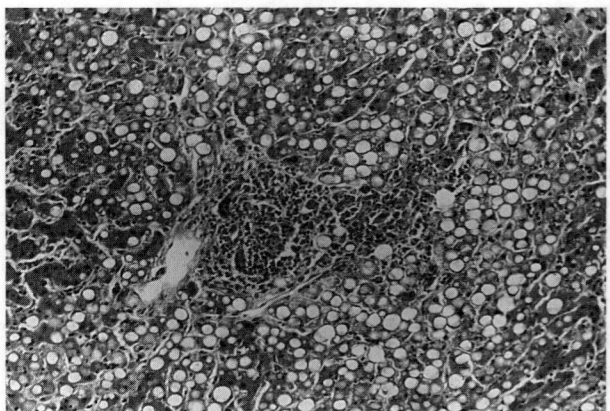

Figure 42.2 Typhoid nodule in portal tract of liver. (Courtesy of WTIM.)

common and bronchopneumonia or lobar consolidation may develop rarely.

Nervous system

A toxic confusional state, characterized by disorientation, delirium and restlessness, is characteristic of late-stage typhoid but occasionally these and other neuropsychiatric features may dominate the clinical picture from an early stage.[31] Facial twitching or convulsion(s) may be the presenting features; sometimes paranoid psychosis or catatonia may develop during convalescence.[32] Meningism is not uncommon but meningitis is rare. Encephalomyelitis may develop and the underlying pathology may be that of demyelinating leucoencephalopathy.[33] Rarely, transverse myelitis, polyneuropathy or cranial mononeuropathy may develop.

Haematological and renal

Subclinical disseminated intravascular coagulation occurs commonly in typhoid fever;[10] this rarely manifests as haemolytic–uraemic syndrome.[34] Haemolysis may also be associated with glucose 6-phosphate dehydrogenase (G6PD) deficiency. Immune complex glomerulitis has been reported and IgM immunoglobulin, C3 and *S. typhi* antigen can be demonstrated in the glomerular capillary wall.[35] Nephrotic syndrome may complicate chronic *S. typhi* bacteraemia associated with urinary schistosomiasis.[36]

Musculoskeletal and other systems

Skeletal muscle characteristically shows Zenker's degeneration (a hyaline degeneration of muscle fibres), particularly affecting the abdominal wall and thigh muscles; clinically evident polymyositis may occur.[37]

Localization may occur in almost any organ/system and involvement of bones, joints, meninges, endocardium, spleen and ovary have all been reported but such cases are rare.[38]

DIFFERENCE(S) BETWEEN TYPHOID FEVER AND PARATYPHOID FEVER

In general illness in paratyphoid B infection is milder and of shorter duration than in typhoid fever and complications are less frequent.[39] It can also present as acute gastroenteritis. Paratyphoid A and C fall between typhoid and paratyphoid B fevers in severity.

LABORATORY FINDINGS

Mild leucocytosis may develop initially but, with disease progression, leucopenia and neutropenia commonly develop. Even in uncomplicated cases, low grade normocytic anaemia, mild thrombocytopenia, modestly elevated serum transaminases and mild proteinuria are common.

DIAGNOSIS

The definitive diagnosis of enteric fever requires isolation of the organism from blood or bone marrow. Isolation from stool or urine provides strong presumptive evidence only in the presence of a characteristic clinical picture.

BLOOD AND BONE MARROW CULTURE

In the untreated, blood cultures are usually positive in about 80% during the first week, declining to 20–30% later in the course of the disease.[40] A success rate of about 90% is obtained from bone-marrow culture.[41] Prior antibiotic therapy makes positive blood culture less likely but the bone-marrow culture often remains positive.[41] A high yield (60%) has also been reported from rose spot cultures in such a situation.[41]

FAECAL AND URINE CULTURES

With modern techniques faecal cultures are often positive even during the first week, though the percentage positivity rises steadily thereafter. Urine cultures are positive less often.

SEROLOGY

The traditional Widal test measures antibodies against flagellar (H) and somatic (O) antigens of the causative organism. In acute infection, 'O' antibody appears first, rising progressively, later falling and often disappearing within a few months. H antibody appears a little later but persists for longer. Rising or high O antibody titre generally indicates acute infection, whereas raised H antibody helps to identify the type of enteric fever. However, the Widal test has many limitations.[42–44] Raised antibodies may have resulted from previous typhoid immunization or earlier infection(s) with salmonellae sharing common O antigens with S. typhi or S. paratyphi. In endemic countries, patients have higher H antibody titres. Some patients show a poor or negligible antibody response to active infection.[42] Vi antibody is often raised during acute infection and persists afterwards during chronic carriage. However, its use as a screening test for the carrier state is limited because of the frequency of false positives and false negatives.[42,43]

NEWER DIAGNOSTIC METHODS

Currently, several newer methods of serodiagnosis of typhoid fever are under evaluation, e.g. indirect haemagglutination, indirect fluorescent Vi antibody, enzyme linked immunosorbent assay (ELISA); all perform better than the Widal test in terms of sensitivity and specificity.[45,46] An indirect ELISA for IgM and IgG antibodies to S. typhi polysaccharide is also promising.[47]

The use of monoclonal antibodies against S. typhi flagellin[48] and DNA probes[49] for detection of S. typhi in blood are other promising developments.

CARRIER STATE IN ENTERIC FEVER

FAECAL CARRIER

After clinical recovery, faecal cultures remain positive in a high proportion of patients during the immediate convalescent period but the frequency of positivity declines rapidly and up to 3% will remain positive by the end of the third month. Between 1 and 3% will continue to excrete organisms in their stools for more than a year and will be designated as chronic carriers—they are likely to remain so for the rest of their lives. The incidence of chronic carriage is higher in women and in the elderly.[50] A similar situation exists with paratyphoid infections. Treatment with chloramphenicol or co-trimoxazole does not affect postconvalescence faecal carriage but amoxycillin may lessen it.[51] Carriage rate is distinctly lower following treatment with newer quinolones.[22]

URINARY CARRIER

In the absence of urinary tract pathology, persisting urinary carriage is rare after the third month, but it is common in countries where urinary schistosomiasis is endemic.

TREATMENT

Patients should be managed under strict enteric precautions, with attention to adequate hand washing and safe disposal of faeces and urine. Antibiotic therapy is essential and should begin empirically if the clinical suspicion is strong.

CHOICE OF ANTIMICROBIAL AGENTS IN ENTERIC FEVER

Chloramphenicol

Since its introduction in 1948, chloramphenicol has proved to be remarkably effective in the treatment of enteric fever worldwide. It produces a rapid improvement in the patient's general condition, followed by defervescence in 3–5 days. The recommended adult dose is 500 mg every 4 hours till defervescence, then 6-hourly for a total course of 14 days. The drug is given orally unless the patient is nauseous or having diarrhoea, when the intravenous route should be used initially. The intramuscular route should be avoided as this gives unsatisfactory blood levels and may delay defervescence. The disadvantages of chloramphenicol are: rare marrow toxicity and aplastic anaemia, higher relapse rate following its use; and emergence of resistant strains of *S. typhi*. *S. typhi* strains with plasmid-mediated resistance to chloramphenicol began to appear in the 1960s[52] and later became widespread in many of the endemic countries of the Americas and South-

East Asia, highlighting the need for alternative agents.

Ampicillin and amoxycillin

Although ampicillin is distinctly inferior to chloramphenicol, its close relative amoxycillin is at least as effective as chloramphenicol in respect of defervescence and relapse rate, and convalescence carriage occurs perhaps less commonly.[51] It is usually given orally four times daily for 14 days.

Co-trimoxazole

This combination of trimethoprim and a sulphonamide is also as effective as chloramphenicol in terms of defervescence and relapse rate,[53] and is given orally 960 mg twice daily but can be given parenterally if necessary.

'Toxic crisis'—an exacerbation of toxaemia and other symptoms, which may sometimes complicate chloramphenicol treatment[54]—appears to be rare with co-trimoxazole. Rare side-effects: are neutropenia and thrombocytopenia.

Emergence of multiresistant typhoid fever

Since 1989 there has been a rapid emergence and spread of *S. typhi* strains with simultaneous plasmid-mediated resistance to chloramphenicol, ampicillin and co-trimoxazole in the Indian subcontinent and parts of South-East Asia.[52,55] (See also Chapter 43.)

Ciprofloxacin and other 4-quinolone drugs

Ciprofloxacin has proved to be highly effective in thetreatment of typhoid and paratyphoid fevers. Defervescence occurs in 3–5 days; convalescent carriage and relapses are rare.[22] Other 4-quinolone drugs such as ofloxacin, norfloxacin and pefloxacin are equally effective.[52] Ciprofloxacin is usually given orally 500 mg twice daily for 14 days, but shorter courses may be adequate. If vomiting or diarrhoea is present, the drug should be given intravenously, 200–400 mg twice daily. The 4-quinolone drugs are highly effective against multiresistant strains.[55]

The 4-quinolone drugs are not currently recommended for use in children and pregnant women because of their observed potential for causing cartilage damage in growing animals. However, arthropathy has not been reported in children following the use of nalidixic acid—an earlier quinolone known to produce similar joint damage in young animals,[56] or in children with cystic fibrosis despite high-dose ciprofloxacin treatment.[57]

Third generation cephalosporins

Cefotaxime, ceftriaxone and cefoperazone have excellent in vitro activity against *S. typhi* and other salmonellae and have acceptable efficacy in the treatment of typhoid fever.[58] Only intravenous formulations are available. Cefotaxime is given 1 g three times daily (in children: 200 mg/kg daily in divided doses) for 14 days.

Furazolidone

This nitrofurantoin derivative has been used mainly in the Indian subcontinent. It has the advantage of being cheap but appears to be somewhat less effective than chloramphenicol.[53] It is less well tolerated and can precipitate haemolysis in G6PD deficient individuals. Its role in the treatment of multiresistant typhoid remains to be established.

CURRENT THERAPEUTIC STRATEGY

Because of the efficacy and low relapse and carrier rates associated with their use, the 4-quinolone drugs are now the drugs of choice in the treatment of adult typhoid, certainly in areas where multiresistant typhoid fever has been reported. However, because of its cheapness, choramphenicol will continue to be used in other areas where the local strains are sensitive.

In children with possible multiresistant typhoid, a third generation cephalosporin, e.g. cefotaxime will be the preferred drug if 4-quinolone drugs are to be avoided. However, their cost and the need for intravenous administration are significant disadvantages, particularly in the developing countries and ciprofloxacin is being used increasingly in children with typhoid.[59]

Corticosteroid therapy

High-dose dexamethasone (initially 3 mg/kg body weight, followed by eight doses of 1 mg/kg 6-hourly) reduces mortality in severely ill patients with depressed levels of consciousness or shock.[60]

In the non-endemic countries, patients should be kept under bacteriological surveillance after clinical recovery until six consecutive negative faecal and urine cultures are obtained.

MANAGEMENT OF CHRONIC CARRIERS

Prolonged courses of amoxycillin or co-trimoxazole may be effective, but the failure rate is high if there is chronic gallbladder disease. Ciprofloxacin (750 mg twice daily)[61] and norfloxacin (400 mg twice daily)[62] have been much more effective, with cure rates of 78 and 83% respectively.

Cholecystectomy is not always successful because of persisting hepatic infection. It is a major operation which should be performed only if strictly indicated for the patient's gallbladder disease, but not for the sole purpose of eradicating the carrier state.

Chronic urinary carriers should be investigated for urinary tract abnormalities, including schistosomiasis.

PROGNOSIS

Early antibiotic therapy has transformed a previously life-threatening illness of several weeks duration with a mortality rate approaching 20% into a short-lasting febrile illness with negligible mortality. The high mortality rates which continue to be reported from some endemic countries are undoubtedly related to delayed diagnosis and/or inappropriate treatment.

PREVENTION

In the endemic countries the most cost-effective strategy for reducing the incidence of enteric fever is the institution of public health measures to ensure safe drinking water and sanitary disposal of excreta. The effects of these measures are long lasting and will also reduce the incidence of other enteric infections which are a major cause of morbidity and mortality in those areas. In the absence of such a strategy, mass immunization with typhoid vaccines at regular intervals will also reduce the incidence of infections considerably.[63]

No effective paratyphoid vaccines are available.

Three types of typhoid vaccine are currently in use.

1. Heat-killed phenolized vaccine

Two 0.5 ml doses of this 'whole cell' vaccine given subcutaneously or intramuscularly 4–6 weeks apart give about 70% protection against water-borne infections but a higher infecting dose, which may occur in contaminated food, may break through this partial immunity. Local and systemic reactions are common. Booster doses are necessary every 3 years. An intradermal injection of 0.1 ml is suitable for this purpose as side-effects are much less.

2. Vi capsular polysaccharide antigen vaccine

This is a newly introduced single parenteral dose vaccine from the Merieux Institute. Observed overall protection rates of 75% in Nepal[64] and 64% in South Africa[16] compare favourably with the efficacy of the killed vaccine and it has the advantage of minimal side-effects. Booster doses are necessary every 3 years to maintain protection. It is not suitable for children under 18 months of age as polysaccharide antigens evoke a weak antibody response.

3. Live attenuated oral vaccines

An oral vaccine containing live attenuated *S. typhi* Ty21a strains in an enteric-coated capsule is now commercially available and has given a 67% protection rate in Chile[65] lasting for 3 years after three doses given on alternate days. A four-dose schedule, which appears to give better protection,[66] is preferred in the USA. However, only 42% efficacy was recorded in Indonesia, suggesting that the vaccine may not be as effective in areas where exposure is intense.[67]

Typhoid vaccination is recommended for travellers to highly endemic areas in Asia, Africa and the Americas. However, as the protection is at best partial, close attention to personal, and food and water hygiene should be maintained.

OTHER *SALMONELLA* INFECTIONS (SALMONELLOSIS)

Although human salmonellosis occurs worldwide, it has become a major public health problem in the developed countries over the second half of the twentieth century. Individual cases and outbreaks in community and institutions are common. Of the large number of salmonella serotypes, only a few account for the vast majority of human infections. Worldwide, examples of common human isolates are: *S. enteritidis*, *S. typhimurium*, *S. virchow*, *S. newport*, *S. hadar*, *S. heidelberg*, *S. agona* and *S. indiana*, the order of prevalence is variable according to geography and time. For years, the dominant strain throughout the world was *S. typhimurium* but in recent years *S. enteritidis* has become the most prevalent serotype in many Western countries.[68]

EPIDEMIOLOGY

The organisms are widely distributed in the animal kingdom. Domestic animals, notably cattle, pigs and poultry are frequent excretors and many wild animals are also infected. Household pets such as dogs, cats, birds and turtles are all potential sources of human infection. Human cases and convalescent carriers are also important sources. Transmission is faecal–oral, usually through ingestion of contaminated foods such as improperly prepared poultry, meat and egg. The carcass of an animal harbouring salmonella in its gut becomes contaminated during evisceration and infection spreads to other non-infected carcasses during large-scale storage. Thus, inadequately cooked meat or precooked food contaminated from raw meat in the kitchen are important vehicles of transmission. Salmonella survives deep freezing, and adequate thawing is essential before cooking. In recent years, fresh shell hen eggs infected through vertical transmission have emerged as an important source of *S. enteritidis* infection in both Europe and the USA.[68]

The factors that are responsible for the dramatic rise of salmonella infections in the West since the 1950s are the adoption of large-scale intensive farming methods for rearing food animals and the use of bulk-imported infected animal feeds, both of which create conditions suitable for rapid spread of infection among the animals. The rising incidence of drug-resistant salmonellae has been linked to the extensive and poorly controlled use of antimicrobials in farm animals.[69] Transmission from a human source is infrequent; convalescent excretors with adequate standards of personal hygiene rarely transmit infection once their stools are formed. However, infected asymptomatic food-handlers have caused a number of restaurant-associated outbreaks. Institutional outbreaks are usually food related but outbreaks in maternity, neonatal and geriatric units have followed admission of patients with an undiagnosed salmonella infection.

Unpasteurized milk is a recognized source in some countries. Unusual sources include pharmaceutical or diagnostic products of animal origin.[70] In the developing countries, the epidemiological pattern is different as large-scale rearing of food animals is not common and methods of cooking are different. Salmonellosis is uncommon in adults. However, it is an important cause of childhood infection, often contracted in hospitals through cross-infection, and there is some evidence that the hospitals are acting as a reservoir for maintaining infection in the community.[71]

PATHOGENESIS

SITE OF INVASION

Most of our understanding about the mechanisms of disease production by salmonella infection in man have come from work in animals. After evading the hostile environment(s) of the stomach and upper small intestine the organisms attach themselves to the epithelial cells of the ileum and to a lesser extent of the colon. They then penetrate and migrate to the lamina propria[72] causing inflammation, characterized by local leucocyte infiltration, congestion and oedema. Similar changes in colonic mucosa have been shown in humans with salmonella diarrhoea.[73,74] Bloodstream invasion may occur from these sites.

MECHANISM OF DIARRHOEA PRODUCTION

The exact mechanisms responsible for diarrhoea are unclear. Mucosal invasion and inflammation are clearly important, at least accounting for the bloody, mucoid type of stools which occur commonly, but do not explain the copious watery stools in the early stages. Observations in experimental animals of an enteropathy with water and electrolyte transport defects suggests the existence of secretory mechanisms.[75] Production of prostaglandin-like secretagogues and other mediators by the inflammatory tissues[76,77] and toxin production by the organisms[78] have been suggested. Salmonellae produce an enterotoxin and a cytotoxin. The enterotoxin activates adenylate cyclase and has some physicochemical characteristics in common with cholera toxin but limited antigenic homology.

INFECTING DOSE

The size of the infecting dose is important to the outcome of a salmonella infection. The rarity of water-borne outbreaks of salmonellosis suggests the necessity of a large infecting dose that can usually be found only in food following multiplication. Limited experimental evidence in volunteers suggests an infecting dose of 10^5 in the production of clinical illness.[79] However, very small infecting doses, possibly as low as 17 organisms, have caused outbreaks.[68] The size of the infecting dose is clearly influenced by the virulence of the organism and host factors such as age, immune status, underlying debilitating disease or stress factors, and the physiological state of the stomach and upper small intestine at the precise time of intake of the organism. Gastric acidity is a significant barrier to enteric infection, and hypoacidity or increased transit time increase the susceptibility to infection.[7]

VIRULENCE OF THE ORGANISM

The serotypes vary greatly in their potential to produce invasive illness outside the gastrointestinal tract. Although any serotype can cause invasive disease, some are more invasive than others. *S. cholerae-suis* regularly produces septicaemic or metastatic illnesses, and less commonly gastroenteritis.[80] Other serotypes with increased invasiveness are *S. virchow* and *S. dublin*.[81] The multiresistant *S. typhimurium* strains which have caused large outbreaks in Africa, India and the Middle East produce a high incidence of septicaemia and metastatic organ involvement.[71] What governs this virulence potential is unclear, but in animal models serotypes bearing high molecular weight plasmids (virulence plasmids) have the ability to spread beyond the initial site of infection in the intestine.[82] Virulence plasmids may be important in the pathogenesis of bacteraemia in humans.[83]

CLINICAL MANIFESTATIONS

There is wide variation in both the severity and the nature of manifestations of salmonellosis. Two often overlapping clinical syndromes are seen: acute enterocolitis (most common) and invasive salmonellosis with septicaemia or metastatic extraintestinal localization of infection. The incubation period is usually between 12 and 48 hours but longer incubation periods of up to 72 days have been reported.[84]

ACUTE ENTEROCOLITIS

This is the preferred term to describe the acute diarrhoea of salmonellosis because both small and large intestines are involved in the disease process.

The illness begins with nausea and vomiting, often

associated with malaise, headache and fever. Very soon, cramp-like abdominal pains and diarrhoea supervene. Initially the stools are of large volume and watery without visible blood or mucus; later, the volume may decrease as blood and mucus appear, indicating development of colitis. This may be associated with localization of pain over the left iliac fossa and some degree of rebound tenderness may develop. The severity of diarrhoea is quite variable, from a mild attack of several loose stools for a day to voluminious watery stools every half-hour or so over several days—leading to dehydration. The elderly, particularly those with debilitating illnesses, and individuals with gastric hypoacidity are prone to develop severe diarrhoea; this may have a cholera-like intensity in patients with a partial gastrectomy.

Occasionally, *colitis* may dominate the clinical picture with the passage of frankly bloodstained stools containing pus. Toxic dilatation may complicate the picture.[73,85] Sigmoidoscopy shows mucosal oedema, hyperaemia, petechial haemorrhages and, in severe cases, friable mucosa with ulcerations.[73] Histological features include dilatation and congestion of capillaries in the mucosa and submucosa with focal collections of polymorphonuclear leucocytes in the lamina propria (Figure 42.3a). In others there may also be a diffuse increase in chronic inflammatory cells in the lamina propria (Figure 42.3b). Crypt abscesses may be seen, but crypt architecture is usually normal with a normal goblet cell population; however, but in severe cases crypt distortion with mucus depletion may occur and distinction from inflammatory bowel disease is difficult (Figure 42.3c). Barium enema usually shows features of diffuse colitis but segmental involvement may occur, mimicking Crohn's disease.

Alternatively, ileal involvement may be the predominant feature, with pain and tenderness localized over the right lower abdomen; this may be misdiagnosed as appendicitis.

INVASIVE SALMONELLOSIS

Bacteraemia is not uncommon in salmonella infection, even in previously healthy invidivuals, and its frequency depends on the serotype of the organism and host factors. Overall, bacteraemia rates of 8% have been observed, with higher rates for some serotypes, e.g. *S. cholerae-suis*, *S. virchow* and *S. dublin*.[81] The incidence of bacteraemia is higher in the elderly[81] and in the very young.[86] Apart from age, other host factors are: immune suppression, malignancy, gastric hypoacidity, debilitating disease, bartonellosis and sickle cell disease.

In previously healthy individuals, bacteraemia is usually a transient event but in a minority of patients, particularly those with the risk factors outlined, bacteraemia may be significant and characterized by either a septicaemic illness (swinging fever, rigors and general toxicity complicating the diarrhoeal illness) or a typhoid-like illness (sustained fever, splenomegaly and even rose spots but minimal diarrhoea[16]) or evidence of metastatic localization in the meninges, bone and joints, lungs, endocardium and arteries, liver, spleen, ovary and kidneys.[38] Soft tissue localization can also occur. Metastatic infections may be unassociated with a diarrhoeal illness, as in *S. cholerae-suis* infections.[80] Meningitis occurs almost exclusively in neonates and children under 2 years of age and reports of high incidence have come from a number of the developing countries.[71] Salmonella infection accounts for most cases of aortic and other vascular infections in the elderly. Atherosclerotic aneurysms of the abdominal aorta or iliac vessels, or prosthetic valves and grafts may all be infected. Normal arteries are affected very rarely. Children with sickle cell disease are particularly prone to developing osteomyelitis. Patients with chronic schistosomiasis are prone to suffer from recurrent bacteraemia from salmonella organisms living within the helminther.[87]

REACTIVE ARTHRITIS

Sterile synovitis may follow salmonella infection, particularly in HLA-B27-positive individuals. The symptoms usually develop 1–2 weeks after the acute infection. Any joint may be affected, although the knees and ankles are most frequently involved. Occasionally, there is migratory polyarthritis, resembling acute rheumatic fever, or bilateral proximal interphalangeal joint involvement, as in rheumatoid arthritis. Acute iridocyclitis may complicate the picture. Deposition of salmonella polysaccharide in the synovial cells may be an important factor in the pathogenesis of reactive arthropathy.[88]

CARRIER STATE

Adults recovering from salmonellosis usually continue to excrete the organism(s) for 4–8 weeks; infants and the elderly excrete for longer periods. Chronic carriage beyond 1 year occurs in far fewer than 1% of cases.[89]

DIAGNOSIS

Definitive diagnosis of salmonella enterocolitis requires positive faecal isolation. Blood cultures

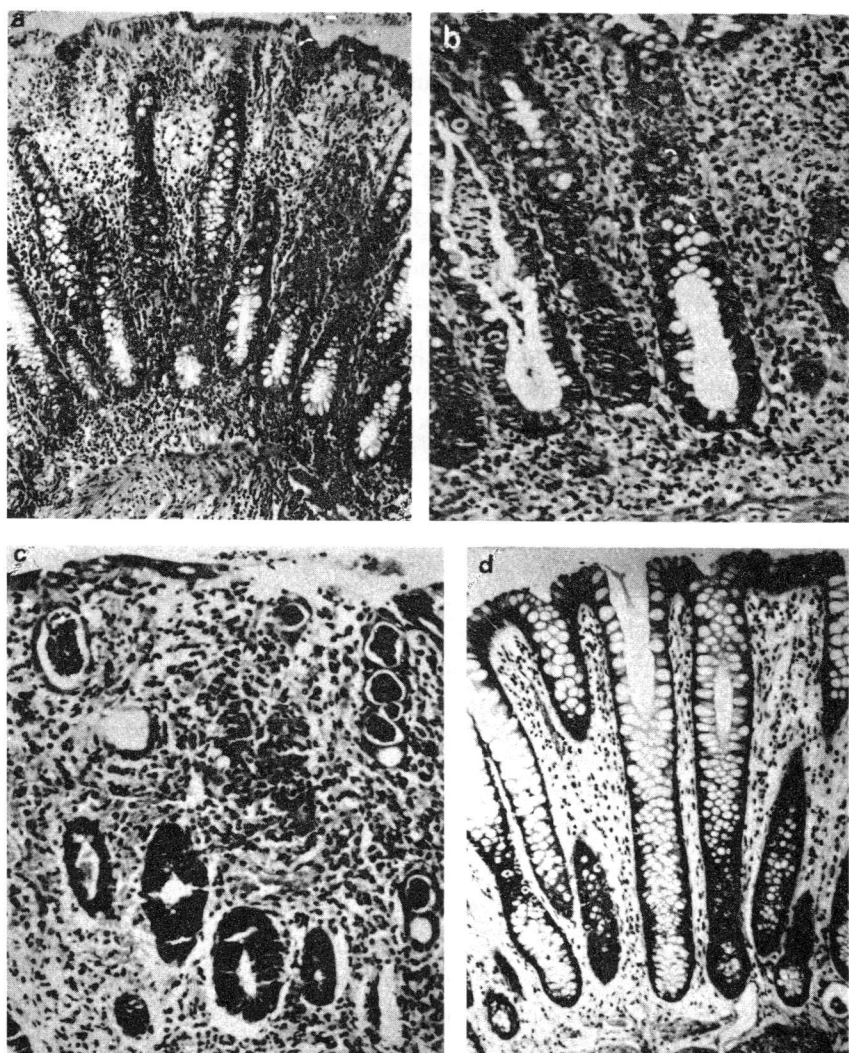

Figure 42.3 (a), (b) and (c) are from rectal biopsies from patients with Salmonella spp. infection. (a) Milder lesions: focal inflammation of mucosa with polymorphonuclear leucocytes in the lamina propria and mucosal capillaries, but no increase in chronic inflammatory cells. (H & E, 80×.) (b) More severe lesions: severe acute inflammation with polymorphs in the lamina propria infiltrating the crypt epithelium and present on the mucosal surface. There is an increase in chronic inflammatory cells but the goblet cell population is well preserved. (H & E, 135×.) (c) Severe focal abscesses tending to be localized in the crypt: there is marked depletion of mucus but crypt architecture is not distorted. The surface epithelium is flattened. (H & E, 150×.) (d) Normal mucosa. (H & E, 120×.) (a), (b) and (c) are reproduced from Day et al (74) with permission of the authors and the editor of *Histopathology*; (d) is reproduced by courtesy of B. C. Morson. (Reproduced with permission from P. C. B. Turnbull. Food poisoning with special reference to salmonella: its epidemiology, pathogenesis and control. *Clin Gastroenterol* 1979; 8(3).)

should be done in all severely ill patients. Coincidental inflammatory bowel disease should be suspected if bloody diarrhoea persists beyond 2 weeks despite the use of an appropriate antibiotic (e.g. ciprofloxacin). Sigmoidoscopic and barium contrast study findings are not discriminatory at this stage, but rectal biopsy is often helpful as crypt distortion and prominent goblet cell depletion are features of ulcerative colitis and are very rarely present in severe primary salmonella colitis.[74] When such a distinction is not possible, the patient should be treated with prednisolone and antibiotics continued. In those who respond promptly the diagnostic

dilemma can be resolved only by a repeat biopsy after 6 weeks. In primary salmonella colitis the rectal biopsy histology usually returns to normal by this time, but this is quite uncommon in ulcerative colitis.

TREATMENT

Most patients with salmonella enterocolitis have a short-lasting, self-limiting illness and require only increased fluid intake.

Antibiotics such as neomycin, colistin, ampicillin, chloramphenicol and co-trimoxazole do not influence the clinical illness and may prolong the duration of intestinal carriage. However, the 4-quinolone drugs (e.g. ciprofloxacin 500 mg b.d. for 5 days) have been shown to shorten the duration of the illness[90] and should be used in patients who are at high risk of developing severe enterocolitis and/or invasive illness, i.e. the elderly, patients who are immunocompromised or have gastric hypoacidity, aortic aneurysm, vascular graft(s), valve prosthesis or debilitating diseases. Antibiotics are definitely indicated in patients with suspected or confirmed septicaemia and/or metastatic infection(s). Severe colitis is another indication for therapy.

Chloramphenicol, co-trimoxazole and amoxycillin are also effective against invasive disease if the infective organism is sensitive. However, the incidence of infection due to salmonella organisms resistant to one or more of these drugs has increased in many parts of the world, including the UK and the USA. There is much geographical variation in the prevalence of the resistant strains and local knowledge of it is essential if these drugs are to be used (see Chapter 43).

Third generation cephalosporins (e.g. cefotaxime, ceftriaxone and cefoperazone) are highly effective and resistance to these drugs is rare. They are particularly suitable for use in children if 4-quinolone drugs are to be avoided.

The complication of colonic dilatation usually resolves without surgery.[85] Aortic salmonellosis generally requires surgical intervention.

Ciprofloxacin is also useful in eradicating persisting faecal carriage and should be given to food handlers.

PREVENTION

The main control measures are directed at maintaining high standards of hygiene in slaughterhouses and all areas of food preparation and distribution— both commercial and private. Raw meat and cooked food must be stored and handled separately. Thorough cooking of raw meat after adequate thawing is essential. Eggs should be boiled for 5 minutes and liquid egg for commercial use should be pasteurized. In the developing countries, adequate infection control procedures are essential in paediatric hospitals if the problem of endemic *Salmonella* spp. cross-infection is to be controlled.

Control of infection in the animal reservoir is a much more difficult problem. However, heat treatment of animal feeds, better standards of animal care and hygiene on the farm, and raising of infection-free flocks are some of the measures which will lower the contamination rates of flesh foods destined for human consumption.

Asymptomatic excretors who are handlers of unwrapped food meant for consumption without further cooking or reheating should be free of infection before returning to work. Others may do so or return to school once their diarrhoea has settled, provided their hygienic standards are adequate.

REFERENCES

1 Le Minor L & Popoff M Y. Request for an opinion. Designation of *Salmonella enterica* sp. nov, nom.rev, as the type and only species of the genus *Salmonella*. *Int J Syst Bacteriol* 1987; 37:465–468.

2 Parker MT. Salmonella. In Wilson G, Miles A & Parker M T (eds) *Topley and Wilson's Principles of Bacteriology, Virology and Immunity*, 7th edn. 1983: 332–355.

3 Christie AB. *Infectious Diseases: Epidemiology and Clinical Practice*, 3rd edn. Edinburgh: Churchill Livingstone, 1980.

4 Earampamoorthy S & Koff R S. Health hazards of bivalve-mollusk ingestion. *Ann Intern Med* 1975; 83:107–110.

5 Scottish Home and Health Department. *The Aberdeen Typhoid Outbreak, 1964*. Edinburgh: HMSO.

6 Hornick R B, Greiseman S E, Woodward T E,

Dupont H L, Dawkins A T & Snyder M J. Typhoid fever: pathogenesis and immunological control. *N Engl J Med* 1970; 283:686–691.

7 Gianella R A, Broitman S A & Zamcheck N. Influence of gastric acidity on bacterial and parasitic enteric infections. *Ann Intern Med* 1973; 78:271–276.

8 Gerichter C B. The dissemination of *Salmonella typhi*, *S. paratyphi A* and *S. paratyphi B* through the organs of the white mouse by oral infection. *J Hyg (Camb)* 1960; 58:307–319.

9 Sprinz H, Gangarosa E J, Williams M et al. Histopathology of the upper small intestines in typhoid fever. Biopsy study of experimental disease in man. *Am J Dig Dis* 1966; 11:615–624.

10 Huckstep R L. *Typhoid Fever and Other Salmonella Infections*. Edinburgh: Livingstone, 1962.

11 Butler T, Bell W R, Levin J, Linh N N & Arnold K. Typhoid fever: studies of blood coagulation,

bacteraemia and endotoxaemia. *Arch Intern Med* 1978; 138:407–410.

12 Hornick R B & Greiseman S. On the pathogenesis of typhoid fever. *Arch Intern Med* 1978; 138:357–358.

13 Edelman R & Levine MM. Summary of an international workshop on typhoid fever. *Rev Infect Dis* 1986; 8:329–349.

14 Kumar R, Malaviya A N, Murthy R G S, Venkataraman M & Mohapatra L N. Immunological study of typhoid: immunoglobulins, C_3, antibodies and leukocyte migration inhibition in patients with typhoid fever and TAB-vaccinated individuals. *Infect Immun* 1974; 10:1219–1225.

15 Sarasombath S, Banchuin N, Sukusol T, Rungpitarangsi B & Manasatif S. Systemic and intestinal immunities after natural typhoid infection. *J Clin Microbiol* 1987; 25:1088–1093.

16 Klugman K P, Gilberton I T, Koornhof H J et al. Vaccination advisory committee: protective activity of Vi capsular polysaccharide vaccine against typhoid fever. *Lancet* 1987; ii:1165–1169.

17 Mani V, Brennand J & Mandal B K. Invasive illness with *Salmonella virchow* infection. *BMJ* 1974; ii:143–144.

18 Rahaman M M & Alam A K M J. Rose spots in shigellosis caused by *Shigella dysenteriae* type I infection. *BMJ* 1977; ii:1123–1124.

19 Roy S K, Speelman P, Butler T, Nath S, Rahman H & Stoll B J. Diarrhoea associated with typhoid fever. *J Infect Dis* 1985; 151:1138–1143.

20 Teixeira R. Typhoid fever of protracted course. *Rev Inst Med Trop São Paulo* 1960; 2:65–70. Quoted by Prata A. Schistosomiasis. *Clin Gastroenterol* 1978; 7:49–75.

21 Farid Z, Bassily S, Kent D C et al. Chronic urinary Salmonella carriers with intermittent bacteraemia. *J Trop Med Hyd* 1970; 73:153–156.

22 Stanley P J, Flegg P, Mandal B K & Geddes A M. Open study of ciprofloxacin in enteric fever. *J Antimicrob Chemother* 1989; 23:789–792.

23 Archampong E Q. Operative treatment of typhoid perforation of the bowel. *BMJ* 1969; iii:273–276.

24 Angorn I B, Pillay S P, Hegarty M & Baker L W. Typhoid perforation of the ileum: a therapeutic dilemma. *S Afr Med J* 1975; 49:782–784.

25 Huckstep R L. Recent advances in the surgery of typhoid fever. *Ann R Coll Surg Engl* 1960; 26:207–230.

26 Gibney J. Typhoid perforation. *Br J Surg* 1989; 76:887–889.

27 Khosla S N. Typhoid hepatitis. *Postgrad Med J* 1990; 66: 923–925.

28 Calva J J & Ruiz-Palacois G M. Salmonella hepatitis: detection of salmonella antigens in the liver of patients with typhoid fever. *J Infect Dis* 1986; 154:373–374.

29 Hermans P, Gerard M, Laethem Y V, De Wit S & Clumeck N. Pancreatic disturbances and typhoid fever. *Scand J Infect Dis* 1991; 23:201–205.

30 Gupta F P, Gupta M S, Bhardwaj S & Chugh T D.

Current clinical patterns of typhoid fever: a prospective study. *J Trop Med Hyg* 1985; 88:377–381.

31 Osuntoken B O, Bademosi O, Ogunremi K & Wright S G. Neuropsychiatric manifestations of typhoid fever in 959 patients. *Arch Neurol* 1972; 27:7–13.

32 Breaky W R & Kala A K. Typhoid catatonia responsive to ECT. *BMJ* 1977; ii:357–359.

33 Ramachandran S, Wickremesinghe H R & Perera M V F. Acute disseminated encephalomyelitis in typhoid fever. *BMJ* 1975; i:494–495.

34 Baker N M, Mills A E & Rachman I. Haemolytic uraemic syndrome in typhoid fever. *BMJ* 1974; ii:84–87.

35 Sitprija V, Pipatanagul V, Boonpucknavig V & Boonpucknavig S. Glomerulitis in typhoid fever. *Ann Intern Med* 1974; 81:210–213.

36 Farid Z, Higashi G I, Bassily S & Milner W F. Immune-complex disease in typhoid and paratyphoid fevers. *Ann Intern Med* 1975; 83:432.

37 Naidoo P N & Yan C C. Typhoid polymyositis. *S Afr Med J* 1975; 49:1975–1976.

38 Cohen J I, Bartlett J A & Corey G R. Extra-intestinal manifestations of salmonella infections. *Medicine* 1987; 66:349–388.

39 Gadeholt H & Madsen S T. Clinical course complications and mortality in typhoid fever as compared with paratyphoid B. A survey of 2647 cases. *Acta Med Scand* 1963; 174:753.

40 Stuart B M & Pullen R L. Typhoid: clinical analysis of two hundred and sixty cases. *Arch Intern Med* 1946; 78:629–661.

41 Gilman R H, Terminel M, Levine M M, Hernandez-Mendoza P & Hornick R B. Relative efficacy of blood, urine, rectal swab, bone-marrow and rose-spot cultures for recovery of *Salmonella typhi* in typhoid fever. *Lancet* 1975; i:1211–1213.

42 Editorial. Typhoid and its serology. *BMJ* 1978; i:389–390.

43 Public Health Laboratory Service Report. The detection of the typhoid carrier state. *J Hyg (Camb)* 1961; 59: 231–247.

44 Brodie J. Antibodies and the Aberdeen typhoid outbreak of 1964. I. The Widal reaction. *J Hyg (Camb)* 1977; 79:161–180.

45 Doshi N & Taylor A G. Comparison of Vi indirect fluorescent antibody test with Widal agglutination method in the serodiagnosis of typhoid fever. *J Clin Pathol* 1984; 37:805–808.

46 Rai G P, Zacharia K & Shrivasta S. Comparative efficacy of indirect haemagglutination test, indirect fluorescent antibody test and enzyme linked immunosorbent assay in serodiagnosis of typhoid fever. *J Trop Med Hyg* 1989; 92:431–434.

47 Nardiello S, Pizzella T, Russo M & Galanti B. Serodiagnosis of typhoid fever by enzyme-linked immunosorbent assay determination of anti-*Salmonella typhi* lipopolysaccharide antibodies. *J Clin Microbiol* 1984; 20:718–721.

48 Sadallah F, Brighouse G, Guidice C D,

Drager-Dayal R, Hocine M & Lambert PH. Production of specific monoclonal antibodies to *Salmonella typhi* flagellin and possible application to immunodiagnosis of typhoid fever. *J Infect Dis* 1990; 161:59–64.

49 Rubin F A, McWhirter P D, Punjabi N H et al. Use of a DNA probe to detect *Salmonella typhi* in the blood of patients with typhoid fever. *J Clin Microbiol* 1989; 27:1112–1120.

50 Editorial. Typhoid carriers. *BMJ* 1964; i:1521–1522.

51 Scragg J N & Rubidge C J. Amoxycillin in the treatment of typhoid fever in children. *Am J Trop Med Hyg* 1975; 24:860–865.

52 Mandal B K. Modern treatment of typhoid fever. *J Infect* 1991; 22:1–4.

53 Herzog C. Chemotherapy of typhoid fever: a review of literature. *Infection* 1976; 4:166–173.

54 Rowland H A K. The complications of typhoid fever. *J Trop Med Hyg* 1961; 64:143–152.

55 Anand A C, Kataria V K, Singh W & Chatterjee S K. Epidemic multiresistant enteric fever in Eastern India. *Lancet* 1990; 335:352.

56 Adams D. Use of quinolones in paediatric patients. *Rev Infect Dis* 1989; 2 (supplement 5):S1113–1116.

57 Scully B E, Masao N, Ores C, Stanley D & Neu H C. Ciprofloxacin therapy in cystic fibrosis. *Am J Med* 1987; 82:196–201.

58 Soe G B & Overturf G D. Treatment of typhoid fever and other systemic salmonellosis with cefotaxime, ceftriaxone, cefoperazone and other newer cephalosporins. *Rev Infect Dis* 1987; 9:719–736.

59 Coovadia Y M, Gathiram V, Bhamjee A et al. An outbreak of multiresistant *Salmonella typhi* in South Africa. *Q J Med* 1992; 82:91–100.

60 Hoffman S L, Punjabi N H, Kumala S et al. Reduction of mortality in chloramphenicol treated severe typhoid fever by high dose dixamethasone. *N Engl Med J* 1984; 310:82–87.

61 Ferreccio C, Morris J G, Valdidieso C et al. Efficacy of ciprofloxacin in treatment of chronic typhoid carriers. *J Infect Dis* 1988; 157:1235–1239.

62 Gotuzzo E, Guerra J G, Benavente L et al. Use of norfloxacin to treat chronic typhoid carriers. *J Infect Dis* 1988; 157:1221–1225.

63 Bodhidatt L, Taylor D N, Thisyakorn U & Echeverria P. Control of typhoid fever in Bangkok, Thailand, by annual immunization of school children with parenteral typhoid vaccine. *Rev Infect Dis* 1987; 9:841–845.

64 Acharya I L, Lowe C U, Thapa R et al. Prevention of typhoid fever in Nepal with the Vi capsular polysaccharide of *Salmonella typhi*: a preliminary report. *N Engl J Med* 1987; 317:1101–1104.

65 Levine M M, Ferreccio C, Black R E, Germanier R and the Chilean Typhoid Committee. Large scale field trial of Ty21a live oral typhoid vaccine in enteric-coated capsules: a field trial in an endemic area. *Lancet* 1987; i:1049–1052.

66 Ferreccio C, Levine M M, Rodriguea H, Contreras R and the Chilean Typhoid Committee.

Comparative efficacy of two, three or four doses of Ty21a live oral typhoid vaccine in enteric-coated capsules: a field trial in an endemic area. *J Infect Dis* 1989; 159:766–769.

67 Simanjuntak C H, Paleologo F P, Punjabi N H et al. Oral immunisation against typhoid fever in Indonesia with Ty21a vaccine. *Lancet* 1991; 338:1055–1059.

68 Cowden J M. Salmonellosis and egg: public health, food poisoning and food hygiene. *Curr Opin Infect Dis* 1990; 3:246–249.

69 Rowe B & Threlfall E J. Antibiotic resistance in salmonella. *Microbiol Dig* 1986; 3:2–5 (Salmonella special March 1987 revision).

70 Baine W B, Gangarosa E J, Bennett J V et al. Institutional salmonellosis. *J Infect Dis* 1973; 128:357.

71 Mandal B K. Typhoid fever and other salmonellae. *Curr Opin Gastroenterol* 1986; 2:109–112.

72 Turnbull P C B & Richmond J E. A model of salmonella enteritis: the behaviour of *Salmonella eneritidis* in chick intestine studied by light and electron microscopy. *Br J Exp Pathol* 1978; 59:64–75.

73 Mandal B K & Mani V. Colonic involvement in salmonellosis. *Lancet* 1976; 1:887–888.

74 Day D W, Mandal B K & Morson B C. The rectal biopsy appearances in Salmonella colitis. *Histopathology* 1978; 2:117–131.

75 Rout W R, Formal S B, Dammin G J & Giannella R A. Pathophysiology of salmonella diarrhoea in the rhesus monkey: intestinal transport, morphological and bacteriological studies. *Gastroenterology* 1974; 67:59–70.

76 Gianella R A, Rout W R & Formal S B. Effect of indomethacin on intestinal water transport in salmonella-infected rhesus monkeys. *Infect Immun* 1977; 17:136–139.

77 Gianella R A. Importance of the intestinal inflammatory reaction in salmonella-mediated intestinal secretion. *Infect Immun* 1979; 23:140–145.

78 Acheson D W K. Enterotoxins in acute infective diarrhoea. *J Infect* 1992; 24:225–245.

79 McCullough N B & Eisele C W. Experimental human salmonellosis. 3. Pathogenecity of strains of *Salmonella newport*, *Salmonella derby* and *Salmonella bereilly* obtained from spray-dried whole egg. *J Infect Dis* 1951; 88:278–289.

80 Saphra I & Wasserman M. *Salmonella cholerae-suis*: a clinical and epidemiological evaluation of 329 infections identified between 1940 and 1954 in the New York Salmonella centre. *Am J Med Sci*; 228:525–533.

81 Mandal B K & Brennand J. Bacteraemia in salmonellosis: a 15 year retrospective study from a regional infectious diseases unit. *BMJ* 1988; 297:1242–1243.

82 Gulig P A. Virulence plasmids of *Salmonella typhimurium* and other salmonellae. Mini-review. *Microb Pathog* 1990; 8:3–11.

83 Fierer J, Krause M, Tauxe R & Guiney D. *Salmonella typhimurium* bacteraemia: association with the virulence plasmid. *J Infect Dis* 1992; 166:639–642.

84 Cowden J M, O'Mahoney M, Bartlett C L R et al. A national outbreak of *Salmonella typhimurium* DT 124 caused by contaminated salami sticks. *Epidemiol Infect* 1989; 103:219–225.

85 Schofield P F, Mandal B K & Ironside A G. Toxic dilatation of the colon in salmonella colitis and inflammatory bowel disease. *Br J Surg* 1979; 66:5–8.

86 Meadow W L, Schneider H & Beem M O. *Salmonella enteritidis* bacteraemia in childhood. *J Infect Dis* 1985; 152:185–189.

87 Young S W, Higashi G, Kamel R et al. Interactions of salmonellae and schistosomes in host–parasite relations. *Trans R Soc Trop Med Hyg* 1973; 67:797–802.

88 Granfors K, Jalkanen S, Lindberg A A et al. Salmonella lipopolysaccharide in synovial cells from patients with reactive arthritis. *Lancet* 1990; 335:685–688.

89 Buchwald D S & Blaser M J. A review of human salmonellosis II. Duration of excretion following infection with non-typhi salmonella. *Rev Infect Dis* 1984; 6:345–356.

90 Pichler H E T, Dirdle G, Stickler K & Wolf D. Clinical efficacy of ciprofloxacin compared with placebo in bacterial diarrhoea. *Am J Med* 1987; 82 (supplement 4A):329–332.

CHAPTER 43

RESISTANT GUT BACTERIA

E. J. Threlfall

Although in many countries reliable information is lacking, there is an ever increasing awareness of problems associated with drug resistance, and in particular multiple drug resistance, in enteric bacteria. The problem affects *Salmonella* spp., including not only *S. typhi* but also a range of other serovars, notably *S. typhimurium* and *S. wien* in developing countries and *S. typhimurium* and *S. virchow* in Britain, *Shigella* spp., especially *Sh. dysenteriae* 1, *Vibrio cholerae* O1 and to a lesser extent, *Escherichia coli* and *Campylobacter*.

SALMONELLAS (See also Chapters 3 and 42)

The occurrence of such resistance is of particular concern in *S. typhi* where treatment with an appropriate antibiotic is essential and should commence as soon as clinical diagnosis is made. However, the increasing occurrence of multiple resistance in serovars other than *S. typhi* has also had a profound effect in developing countries in the treatment of salmonella septicaemia in infants and young children, where since 1980 multiple resistant strains have been implicated in numerous outbreaks in hospital paediatric units.

SALMONELLA TYPHI

Typhoid fever is endemic in many developing countries, particularly in the Indian subcontinent, South and Central America and Africa. In contrast only 200–300 cases occur in the UK each year and the majority of infections are in patients who have returned from countries where *S. typhi* is endemic.[1] In 1948 chloramphenicol was introduced and in developed countries the use of this antibiotic for typhoid fever resulted in a reduction in the death rate from 10% to less than 2%. However, in the 1970s a series of outbreaks caused by chloramphenicol-resistant strains in countries in widely-separated geographical areas[2,3] gave rise to fears that the supremacy of this antibiotic might have become jeopardized.[4]

RESISTANCE TO CHLORAMPHENICOL

British isolates

Of 2356 strains of *S. typhi* isolated in the UK between 1978 and 1985, in only 6 (0.25%) was there clinically-significant resistance to chloramphenicol (minimum inhibitory concentration (MIC): >32 mg/l) (Table 43.1). As a result of these findings, in 1987 it was recommended that chloramphenicol should remain the first-line drug for typhoid fever in the UK and, in particular, that it should be used whilst the results of laboratory sensitivity tests were awaited.[5]

In the succeeding 4-year period 1986–1989 the occurrence of chloramphenicol-resistant *S. typhi* increased slightly and 12 of 790 (1.5%) isolates were resistant to this antibiotic[6] (Table 43.1). However, it was considered that the increase, from 0.25 to 1.5%, was not sufficient to warrant changing the recom-

Table 43.1 Isolations of chloramphenicol-resistant *Salmonella typhi* in the UK, 1978–1993.

Years	No. of isolates	Chloramphenicol resistant	
		No.	*%*
1978–1985	2356	6	0.25
1986–1989	790	12	1.5
1990–1993	872*	196	22.5

*Provisional figure.
Source: Laboratory of Enteric Pathogens.

mendation made in 1987 about the use of chloramphenicol.

The situation changed in 1990 when there was a dramatic increase in the number of chloramphenicol-resistant strains isolated in the UK. In that year 50 of 248 (20%) patients with *S. typhi* were found to be infected with chloramphenicol-resistant strains, the majority of which were also resistant to ampicillin and trimethoprim.[7] Most patients with chloramphenicol-resistant strains were infected with *S. typhi* of Vi-phage type M1 and had either acquired their infection(s) in Pakistan or had been in contact with patients who had recently returned from that country, although some strains of Vi-phage type E1 associated with patients who had recently returned from India were also identified.[7] The situation did not alter appreciably in the succeeding 3 years and from 1991 to 1993 between 21 and 25% of strains from patients with typhoid fever were resistant to chloramphenicol, ampicillin and trimethoprim. However, the proportion of strains belonging to Vi-phage type E1 increased and the majority of patients infected with strains of this phage type had recently returned from India.[8]

Isolates from other countries

Since 1989 chloramphenicol-resistant *S. typhi* have been isolated with increasing frequency in several countries. In India several outbreaks caused by chloramphenicol-resistant strains have been reported[9] and such strains have been isolated in Chandigarh in the north,[10] Calcutta in the east,[11] Kerala in the south-west,[12] Dindigul in the southeast[13] and also at Vellore[14] and Delhi[15] (Table 43.2). The most common Vi-phage type has been that of E1[8,9] but strains of phage types O, 28 and 51 have

Table 43.2 Outbreaks of chloramphenicol-resistant *Salmonella typhi*, 1989–1994.

Years	Country	Vi-phage type	Resistance
1989–1992	Pakistan	M1	C, A, Tm
1990–1994	India	E1, O, 51	C, A, Tm
1990	South Africa	A	C, A, K
1991	UK	M1	C
1991–1992	Egypt	C1, E2, D1-N	C, A, Tm
1991–1992	Kuala Lumpur	E1, B1, UVS	C, A, Tm
1993–1994	Philippines	*	C, Tm, K
1993–1994	Vietnam	*	C, A, Tm

C, chloramphenicol; A, ampicillin; Tm, trimethoprim; K, kanamycin; UVS, untypable Vi strain.
* Phage type not known.

been isolated.[9,11] In Pakistan the predominant multiresistant phage type is M1 and since 1989 there has been an extensive outbreak in Rawalpindi caused by strains of this phage type.[16] Chloramphenicol-resistant strains of Vi-phage types E1 and M1 linked to immigrant workers from the Indian subcontinent have also been isolated in several countries in the Arabian Gulf[17] and, in addition, multiresistant strains of different phage types have been isolated in Egypt (E2, C1 and D1-N),[18] Canada,[19] South Africa (Vi-phage type A),[20] Kuala Lumpur (E1, B1 and DVS/UVS), the Philippines[21] and Vietnam (Table 43.2).

PLASMIDS

In almost all chloramphenicol-resistant strains of *S. typhi* isolated in the UK since 1990, resistance to chloramphenicol, ampicillin and trimethoprim has been mediated by plasmids of the incompatibility (*inc*) H1 group with relative molecular mass (Mr) ranging from approximately 165 kilobases (kb) to 180 kb. A few strains have also been isolated which have been resistant to ampicillin and trimethoprim but sensitive to chloramphenicol, and in these strains resistance to these antimicrobials, previously presumably plasmid mediated, has become incorporated into the chromosome.[6] In strains isolated in other countries and examined in the Laboratory of Enteric Pathogens, in almost all instances the complete spectrum of resistance has been encoded by *inc* group H1 plasmids.

RECOMMENDATIONS FOR THERAPY

Resulting from the increased isolation of chloramphenicol-resistant strains since 1990, it has been stated that chloramphenicol should no longer be regarded as the automatic drug of choice for typhoid.[6,22,23] Since the great majority of chloramphenicol-resistant strains have also been resistant to trimethoprim and ampicillin, these drugs have also been compromised. However, with one exception, all chloramphenicol-resistant strains isolated in the UK since 1990 have been sensitive to ciprofloxacin with an MIC of <0.012 mg/l. With the possible exception of young children, it has therefore been recommended that, in the UK, physicians should consider 4-quinolone agents such as ciprofloxacin as the first-line drug(s) for the treatment of typhoid, particularly in travellers returning to the UK from areas where multiresistant strains are now common[7,22,23] and the efficacy of ciprofloxacin in the treatment of multiresistant typhoid fever has subsequently been confirmed in clinical trials.[24]

Although reservations about the promotion of ciprofloxacin as a first-line drug for the treatment of typhoid in developing countries have been expressed,[12] as yet the only documented report about the occurrence of resistance to ciprofloxacin in multiresistant *S. typhi* describes the appearance of resistance in a strain isolated in the UK following treatment of a patient with this antibiotic.[8] In view of the increasing occurrence and widespread distribution of strains of *S. typhi* with resistance to chloramphenicol, ampicillin and trimethoprim, the use of ciprofloxacin for multiresistant typhoid may therefore be justifiable, although monitoring for the appearance of resistance to ciprofloxacin and other new fluorquinolone drugs is essential.

OTHER *SALMONELLA* SEROVARS

In developed countries, including the UK, the majority of countries in Western Europe and the USA, salmonella infections, excluding those with *S. typhi* and *S. paratyphi*, are primarily zoonoses. When resistance is identified in strains isolated from humans, in the majority of instances it has been acquired in the primary animal reservoir as a result of the use of antimicrobials in animal husbandry. The most important serovars in the UK are *S. enteritidis*, *S. typhimurium* and *S. virchow* and the main method of spread is through the food chain. In general, person-to-person transmission is not of major importance in the spread of these serotypes. In most cases the clinical presentation is that of mild to moderate enteritis; the disease is usually self-limiting and antimicrobial therapy is seldom required. In contrast in developing countries, particularly in the Indian subcontinent, South-East Asia and South and Central America, and also in some countries in Africa, salmonella serovars such as *S. typhimurium*, *S. wien*, *S. johannesburg* and *S. oranienburg* have undergone changes both in their epidemiology and their clinical manifestations. An additional feature of these strains has been the possession of plasmid-mediated multiple drug resistance, often with resistance to seven or more antimicrobials.

Developing countries

Since 1970, multiresistant salmonellas have caused extensive outbreaks in many developing countries. The common pattern has been for several hospitals, often situated many miles apart, to be involved. The majority of outbreaks have occurred in neonatal and paediatric wards but community outbreaks in villages and small towns have also been reported. The clinical disease has been severe, with enteritis frequently accompanied by septicaemia, and in several outbreaks up to 30% mortality has been reported. Serovars involved include notably *S. typhimurium* in the Middle East[25] and the Indian subcontinent[26] and *S. wien* in Southern Europe, North Africa and India,[27,28] although infections caused by multiresistant strains belonging to several other serovars have also been reported (for review, see Rowe and Threlfall[29]). Strains have been resistant to up to ten antimicrobials and in recent years the incidence of strains of *S. typhimurium* with high-level resistance to nalidixic acid (MIC: >100 mg/l) and with reduced susceptibility to 4-quinolone antibiotics such as ciprofloxacin (MIC: 0.1 mg/l cp 0.0075 mg/l for nalidixic acid-sensitive strains) has increased dramatically in India.[30]

A particular feature of these infections has been the lack of involvement of an animal reservoir. Spread has been by person-to-person contact and antibiotic resistance has developed as a result of the use of antibiotics in human medicine, particularly in those countries where there is little control on the use of antibiotics. An example of the type of epidemic caused by multiresistant salmonellas is that which has occurred throughout India since 1977. The serovar involved has been *S. typhimurium* and strains have belonged to closely-related phage types. Outbreaks have occurred in both communities and in hospitals, particularly amongst neonates, although older children and adults have also been affected. The most common presentation has been severe enteritis; and cases of septicaemia have also been reported. Mortality was high in at least five outbreaks. The majority of strains have been resistant to at least seven antimicrobials including: ampicillin, chloramphenicol, gentamicin, kanamycin, streptomycin, sulphonamides, tetracyclines and trimethoprim (A, C, G, K, S, Su, T, Tm); resistance to furazolidone (Fu) and nalidixic acid (Nx) has also been common. With the exception of resistance to furazolidone and nalidixic acid, all resistances have been plasmid mediated and have been encoded by a plasmid of the *inc* FI*me* group. Such plasmids have also been identified in unrelated phage types of *S. typhimurium* which have caused similar outbreaks throughout the Middle East and in several countries in Africa, and in multiresistant strains of *S. wien* responsible for outbreaks in Europe, North Africa and India between 1978 and 1990.[27,28] In addition to coding for multiple drug resistance, such plasmids also carry genes coding for the production of the hydroxamate

Table 43.3 Resistance to specific antimicrobials in *Salmonella typhimurium*, *S. enteritidis* and *S. virchow* isolated from humans in England and Wales, 1993.

| Serotype | Total | *Per cent resistant to* | | | | | | | | | |
		A	C	G	K	S	Su	T	Tm	Fu	Cp
S. enteritidis	20668	4	0.1	0.1	<0.1	1	1	2	0.4	0.8	0.3
S. typhimurium	4843	39	33	2	3	41	53	57	16	4	1
S. virchow	1419	12	6	0.4	4	11	15	13	15	8	4

A, ampicillin; C, chloramphenicol; G, gentamicin; K, kanamycin; S, streptomycin; Su, sulphonamides; T, tetracyclines; Tm, trimethoprim; Fu, furazolidone; Cp, ciprofloxacin.
Source: Laboratory of Enteric Pathogens (figures are provisional).

siderophore aerobactin, which is a known virulence factor for some enteric and urinary tract pathogens.[31]

Antimicrobial therapy is often essential for the treatment of infections caused by these multiresistant strains, particularly when they cause extraintestinal infections. As yet, patients infected with these strains appear to be responding to treatment with some of the new 4-quinolone antibiotics, although decreased susceptibility in strains isolated in India has been reported (see above). There is also concern that the widespread use of nalidixic acid in the Indian subcontinent for the treatment of shigellosis (see below) is rapidly eroding the efficacy of such potentially life-saving drugs as ciprofloxacin.[30]

England and Wales

In contrast to the situation in developing countries, salmonella septicaemia is rare in England and Wales in other than a few serovars of limited epidemiological importance. Indeed, over the 10-year period 1981–1990 the occurrence of bloodstream invasion with the two most common serovars, *S. enteritidis* and *S. typhimurium*, was less than 2%.[32] However, salmonella septicaemia can be a life-threatening disease and resistance of strains to drugs of therapeutic importance can limit the choice of antimicrobials available for therapy.

In the 13-year period 1981–1993 *S. enteritidis*, *S. typhimurium* and *S. virchow* comprised over 70% of all human salmonella isolations identified in England and Wales. In these serovars the overall incidence of drug resistance has remained at between 22 and 24% but the incidence of multiple resistance (resistance to four or more antimicrobials) has increased from 3% in 1981[33] to 8% in 1993. Although drug resistance has declined in *S. enteriti-*

dis, it has increased in *S. typhimurium* and *S. virchow* and in particular, multiple resistance has increased from 6 to 39% in *S. typhimurium* and from 0.2 to 14% in *S. virchow* since 1981. These increases have been paralleled in isolates from food-producing animals.[34]

In *S. typhimurium*, multiple resistance has been particularly common in three definitive phage types (DTs), DTs 204c, 193 and 104. In DT 204c multiple resistance, including resistance to ampicillin, chloramphenicol and trimethoprim (A, C, Tm) is plasmid mediated and multiresistant strains possess at least three independent resistance plasmids;[35] in DT 193, multiple resistance (ASSuT) is also plasmid mediated but has become integrated into the *S. typhimurium* serovar-specific plasmid.[36] In contrast, in DT 104 multiple resistance (ACSSuT) is not plasmid mediated and appears to have become chromosomally integrated.[37] The three *S. typhimurium* phage types in which multiple resistance is most common in humans are those most prevalent in cattle. In contrast, for *S. virchow*, multiresistance is common in phage types associated with poultry, particularly in isolates from poultry-meat imported from France.[34]

Notable in strains isolated in 1993 was the high incidence of resistance to ampicillin, chloramphenicol, tetracyclines and trimethoprim in *S. typhimurium*, and to ampicillin, tetracyclines and trimethoprim in *S. virchow* (Table 43.3). Also of note was the increased incidence of resistance to quinolone drugs in *S. virchow*, and in particular to ciprofloxacin, now the therapeutic agent of choice for severe *Salmonella* spp. infections.

In contrast to the situation in developing countries, the use of antibiotics in food-producing animals has been an important factor in the development of multiple resistance in salmonellas isolated in Britain.

SHIGELLAS (See also Chapters 3 and 41)

In Britain

In a survey of the resistance to 13 antibiotics of strains of *Sh. dysenteriae, Sh. flexneri* and *Sh. boydii* isolated in England and Wales in the 4-year period 1979–1983, it was reported that 84% of 2753 strains were resistant to one or more drugs, with resistance to streptomycin, sulphonamides and tetracyclines occurring most frequently.[38] During the period of the survey, resistance to ampicillin, chloramphenicol and tetracyclines increased significantly, and particularly noteworthy was the increase in the incidence of resistance to trimethoprim, from 0.5% in 1978 to 17% in 1983. Resistance to trimethoprim has continued to increase, and of strains isolated between 1989 and 1991 almost 60% of isolates were resistant to this antimicrobial (T. Cheasty, personal communication).

It is important to note that *Sh. dysenteriae, Sh. flexneri* and *Sh. boydii* are not indigenous to England and Wales and the majority of infections have been identified either in patients with a history of recent foreign travel, particularly to the Indian subcontinent, or those who have had contact with recent travellers. Thus resistance in these serotypes does not reflect the use of antibiotics for the treatment of shigellosis in Britain. However, analysis of patients infected with trimethoprim-resistant strains in the 4-year period 1979–1983 revealed that fewer patients with strains resistant to trimethoprim had a history of foreign travel than did patients with strains sensitive to trimethoprim. On the basis of these observations it was concluded that the use of products containing trimethoprim in both Britain and developing countries had contributed to the increased incidence of trimethoprim-resistance in shigella strains isolated in Britain.[38]

In *Sh. sonnei*, which is indigenous to Britain, a different picture has emerged, with multiple resistance declining from 38% in 1972 to 8% in 1977.[39] It must, however, be realized that antibiotics are not recommended in the UK for the treatment of uncomplicated shigellosis and also that the occurrence of resistance in *Sh. sonnei* has not been monitored on a regular basis.

Other countries

Since 1969 multiresistant strains of *Shigella*, and in particular *Sh. dysenteriae* type 1 (Shiga's bacillus), have caused extensive outbreaks in many countries in Central America, Africa and the Indian subcontinent. The first major outbreak was that which occurred in Central America from 1969 to 1972 and the strain was resistant to chloramphenicol, streptomycin, sulphonamides and tetracyclines (R-type CSSuT). Over 10 000 deaths were reported. In the 1970s a series of outbreaks, although not on the same scale as the Central American outbreak but caused by strains of the same R-type, were reported in several countries in the Indian subcontinent (for review, see Rowe and Threlfall[29]). In all these outbreaks resistance to chloramphenicol, streptomycin, sulphonamides and tetracyclines was invariably plasmid mediated and was encoded by a plasmid of the *inc* B group.

The second major international outbreak occurred in Central Africa (Zaire, Rwanda, Burundi) from 1979 to 1982. Over 13 000 cases were reported in eastern Zaire between 1981 and 1982, with over 1700 deaths. The strain was of R-type ACSSuT and although resistances were plasmid encoded, the plasmids were of different incompatibility groups to that identified in the Central American and Indian strains.[40] Following the discontinuation of the use of tetracyclines and the introduction of co-trimoxazole early in 1981, plasmid-mediated resistance to the latter antimicrobial soon emerged.[41] Nalidixic acid was subsequently introduced in Zaire in November 1981 for the treatment of *Shigella* spp. dysentery, and the use of this antimicrobial resulted in a drop in case fatality rate from 4.6 to 2.0%.[41]

Since 1984 there have been reports of epidemics and outbreaks in several states in India of bacillary dysentery caused by multiresistant *Sh. dysenteriae* type 1. Of particular note was that which occurred in West Bengal in 1984,[42] in which the strains were resistant to ampicillin, chloramphenicol, tetracyclines and co-trimoxazole. Because of the appearance in such strains of resistance to ampicillin and co-trimoxazole, at that time the drugs of choice for first-line treatment of bacillary dysentery in India, nalidixic acid became the first line alternative treatment in the 1980s[43] and has subsequently been used extensively throughout India for this purpose. However, strains with resistance to nalidixic acid have now emerged on the Indian subcontinent,[44] thus undermining the use of this antimicrobial for the treatment of bacillary dysentery in that area. Although resistant to nalidixic acid, strains of *Sh. dysenteriae* type 1 isolated in India have been found to be highly susceptible to the fluoroquinolones and, for adults, a single (1 g) dose of ciprofloxacin coupled with standard rehydration therapy has been reported to be highly effective.[43]

In the USA, strains of *Sh. sonnei* have developed resistance to trimethoprim–sulphamethoxazole in response to antimicrobial therapy during the course of outbreaks,[45] and in 1987 a large outbreak of shigellosis, possibly affecting over 6000 people, was caused by a strain of *Sh. sonnei* resistant to ampicillin, tetracyclines, streptomycin and trimethoprim–sulphamethoxazole.[46] However, since antimicrobial susceptibility testing of *Shigella* spp. isolates is not routinely performed in the USA, the overall occurrence and persistence of such resistant strains is unknown.

RECOMMENDATIONS FOR THERAPY

Until 1984 ampicillin was widely regarded as the drug of choice for the treatment of severe bacillary dysentery, with trimethoprim the drug of choice for patients infected with ampicillin-resistant strains.[38] More recently, because of the increased prevalence of strains resistant to ampicillin and trimethoprim, nalidixic acid has been increasingly used in developing countries as a primary alternative.[47] However, if *Sh. dysenteriae* type 1 infection is suspected or nalidixic acid-resistant strains of *Shigella* have been identified, treatment with pivmecillinam has been recommended. For children, treatment with pivmecillinam or ceftriaxone has been suggested, although reservations have been expressed both about the cost of these antibiotics and about the non-availability of an oral formulation of ceftriaxone.[47] It has also been recommended that in developing countries, the newer quinolone drugs should be held in reserve for the treatment of strains resistant to nalidixic acid and pivmecillinam. For developed countries where resistance to ampicillin and co-trimoxazole is less common, it has been recommended that, should antibiotic therapy be indicated, children should continue to be treated with ampicillin or trimethoprim–sulphamethoxazole, and that adults should be treated with one of the quinolone drugs.[47] However, because of the rapidly increasing range of resistance in shigella strains, it has been strongly recommended that, whenever possible, antibiotic sensitivities should be determined before commencing treatment, as the choice of antibiotic for initial treatment is becoming increasingly limited.[38]

VIBRIO CHOLERAE (See also Chapters 3 and 41)

V. CHOLERAE O1 BIOTYPE EL TOR

The first protracted outbreak of *V. cholerae* O1 biotype El Tor with multiple drug resistance was that which occurred in Tanzania in 1977.[48] The strains were of R-type ACKSSuT and the appearance of resistance was attributed to the extensive use of tetracycline(s) for cholera prophylaxis in Tanzania. Outbreaks caused by drug-resistant strains of *V. cholerae* O1 biotype El Tor have subsequently been reported in Bangladesh in 1979–1980 and 1981, in Zaire in 1982–1983, and in Tanzania in 1983.[29] A variety of R-types have been identified and, in addition to the resistances given above, strains with additional resistance to gentamicin and trimethoprim have been identified in Bangladesh and Zaire. More recently, strains of *V. cholerae* O1 biotype El Tor with resistance to ampicillin, chloramphenicol, kanamycin, sulphonamides, tetracyclines and trimethoprim have been identified in epidemic cholera in Ecuador, South America,[49] and it has been subsequently reported that up to 36% of strains from this epidemic are now multiresistant.[50]

In all multiresistant strains of *V. cholerae* O1 biotype El Tor from outbreaks in Africa, Bangladesh and South America, the complete spectrum of resistance has been encoded by plasmids of the *inc* C group[49] and it appears that plasmids of this incompatibility group appear to have an affinity for *V. cholerae* similar to that shown by *inc* H1 plasmids for *S. typhi* (see above).

Although the therapy of choice for cholera is oral rehydration, when antimicrobial therapy is indicated doxycycline, a long-acting tetracycline, is recommended for adults and co-trimoxazole for children, with furazolidone, erythromycin and chloramphenicol considered to be effective alternatives.[51] The appearance of strains with resistance to three of the drugs of choice for the treatment of cholera in countries with low standards of hygiene is of some concern and reappraisal of the use of antimicrobials in some outbreak situations may now be necessary.

V. CHOLERAE O139

Since early 1993 there have been several reports of a large outbreak of cholera caused by *V. cholerae*

O139 in the Indian subcontinent. A limited study of strains isolated in the UK from travellers known to have recently returned from the Indian subcontinent demonstrated that these strains were resistant to streptomycin, sulphonamides and trimethoprim.[52] As with infections caused by *V. cholerae* O1, the therapy of choice for infections caused by non-O1 *V. cholerae* is oral rehydration, and the occurrence of resistance to streptomycin, sulphonamides and trimethoprim should have little effect on treatment regimens.

ESCHERICHIA COLI (See also Chapter 41)

The occurrence of antibiotic resistance in pathogenic *E. coli* has been documented elsewhere[29] and will not be discussed at length in this chapter. Plasmids have been identified which code for antibiotic resistance and the production of both heat-stable (ST) and heat-labile (LT) toxin,[53] and in a study of drug resistance among toxin-producing strains isolated in the Far East, 72% of strains were reported to be drug resistant and 44% multiresistant.[54]

The use of antibiotics for the treatment of *E. coli* infections is also a contentious issue (Chapter 3). There is little doubt that a number of antibiotics reduce the incidence and duration of diarrhoea in travellers,[55] and both ciprofloxacin[56] and norfloxacin[57] have been reported to be particularly effective. However, concern has been expressed that the widespread use of these antimicrobials for prophylaxis may reduce their efficacy in the long term.[58]

CAMPYLOBACTER (See also Chapter 41)

Because *Campylobacter jejuni* enteritis is usually a self-limiting disease, antibiotics are not usually administered except to septicaemic patients and those with other underlying complications. When antibiotic treatment is indicated, erythromycin has been the drug of choice.[59,60] Gentamicin, tetracyclines, chloramphenicol and furazolidone have also been used with some success, and gentamicin and chloramphenicol have been recommended for the treatment of patients with erythromycin-resistant strains.[61] In studies of the occurrence of resistance to different antimicrobials, only 0.5% of strains isolated in 1978 in a targeted study in the UK were resistant to erythromycin[62] but, in contrast, 10% of strains isolated in Sweden[63] and 9% of strains isolated in Belgium[64] in 1978 were erythromycin resistant.

The use of fluoroquinolone drugs for the treatment of a variety of acute diarrhoeal diseases, including campylobacter enteritis, has recently been advocated.[65,66] Of potential importance for human therapy is a reported increase of up to 11% in the incidence of fluoroquinolone resistance in campylobacters isolated from humans in the Netherlands following the extensive use of enrofloxacin in the poultry industry in that country.[67]

CONCLUSIONS

Multiple drug resistance is now common in pathogenic gut bacteria in both developing and developed countries throughout the world. The rapid emergence of resistance to the drugs of choice for diseases such as typhoid fever, bacillary dysentery and cholera is of particular concern. Although for the most part such resistance is plasmid mediated, a recent development is the emergence of strains with chromosomal resistance, not only to antibiotics such as chloramphenicol, ampicillin and trimethoprim, but also to some of the fluorquinolone drugs such as ciprofloxacin. In order to preserve the efficacy of such drugs for the treatment of life-threatening infections, it is essential that their usage should be strictly regulated and, whenever possible, reserved for treatment of severe infections which do not respond to more conventional antimicrobials.

REFERENCES

1 Anonymous. Typhoid and paratyphoid fevers. *OPCS Monitor* 1985; MB2 85/2:9–11.

2 Anonymous. Typhoid fever — Mexico. *MMWR* 1972; 21:177–178.

3 Paniker C K J & Vilma K N. Transferable chloramphenicol resistance in *Salmonella typhi*. *Nature* 1972; 239:109–110.

4 Anonymous. Chloramphenicol resistance in typhoid. *Lancet* 1973; ii:1008–1009.

5 Rowe B, Threlfall E J & Ward L R. Does chloramphenicol remain the drug of choice for typhoid? *Epidemiol Infect* 1987; 98:379–383.

6 Rowe B, Threlfall E J & Ward L R. Spread of multiresistant *Salmonella typhi*. *Lancet* 1990; 336:1065.

7 Rowe B, Ward L R & Threlfall E J. Treatment of multiresistant typhoid fever. *Lancet* 1991; 337:1422.

8 Rowe B, Ward L R & Threlfall E J. Ciprofloxacin and typhoid fever. *Lancet* 1992; 339:740.

9 Prakash K & Pillai P K. Multidrug-resistant *Salmonella typhi* in India. *APUA Newslett* 1992; 1:1–3.

10 Panigrahi D, Roy P & Sehgal R. Ciprofloxacin for typhoid fever. *Lancet* 1991; 338:1601.

11 Anand A C, Kataria V K, Singh W et al. Epidemic multiresistant enteric fever in Eastern India. *Lancet* 1990; 335:352.

12 Kumar P D. Ciprofloxacin for typhoid fever. *Lancet* 1991; 338:1143.

13 Threlfall E J, Ward L R, Rowe B et al. Widespread occurrence of multiple drug-resistant *Salmonella typhi* in India. *Eur J Clin Microbiol Infect Dis* 1992; 11:990–993.

14 Jesudasan M V & John R J. Multiresistant *Salmonella typhi* in India. *Lancet* 1990; 336:256.

15 Gupta B L, Bhujwala R A & Shrinwas. Multiresistant *Salmonella typhi* in India. *Lancet* 1990; 336:252.

16 Karamat K A. Multiple drug resistant *Salmonella typhi* and ciprofloxacin. In *Proceedings of the 2nd Western Pacific Congress on Infectious Diseases and Chemotherapy*. Thailand: Infectious Disease Association of Thailand, Western Pacific Society of Chemotherapy, 1990:480.

17 Wallace M & Yousif A A. Spread of multiresistant *Salmonella typhi*. *Lancet* 1990; 336:1065–1066.

18 Mourad A S, Metwally M, Nour El Deen A et al. Multiple-drug-resistant *Salmonella typhi*. *Clin Infect Dis* 1993; 17:135–136.

19 Hartnett N, McLeod S, AuYong Y et al. Emergence in Ontario, Canada, of multiresistant *Salmonella typhi* from South Asia. *Lancet* 1992; 340:177.

20 Coovadia Y M, Gathiram V, Bhamjee A et al. An outbreak of multiresistant *Salmonella typhi* in South Africa. *Q J Med* 1992; 82:91–100.

21 Superable J F T, Castillo M T G, Magboo F P et al. Multiresistant *Salmonella typhi* outbreak in Metro Manila, Philippines. In *Proceedings of the 2nd Asia Pacific Symposium on Typhoid Fever and other Salmonellosis*. Bangkok: Infectious Diseases Association of Thailand, 1994:76.

22 Threlfall E J, Rowe B & Ward L R. Occurrence and treatment of multi-resistant *Salmonella typhi* in the UK. *PHLS Microbiol Digest* 1992; 8:56–59.

23 Mandal B K. Modern treatment of typhoid fever. *J Infect* 1991; 22:1–4.

24 Wallace M R, Yousif A A, Mahroos G A et al. Ciprofloxacin versus ceftriaxone in the treatment of multiresistant typhoid fever. *Eur J Clin Microbiol Infect Dis* 1993; 12:907–910.

25 Anderson E S, Threlfall E J, Carr J M et al. Clonal distribution of resistance plasmid-carrying *Salmonella typhimurium*, mainly in the Middle East. *J Hyg* (Camb) 1977; 79:429–448.

26 Rowe B, Frost J A & Threlfall E J. Spread of a multiresistant clone of *Salmonella typhimurium* phage type 66/122 in South-east Asia and the Middle East. *Lancet* 1980; i:1070–1071.

27 Le Minor S. Apparition en France d'une épidémie à *Salmonella wien*. *Med Mal Infect* 1972; 2:441–448.

28 McConnell M M, Smith H R, Leonardopoulos J & Anderson E S. The value of plasmid studies in the epidemiology of infections due to drug-resistant *Salmonella wien*. *J Infect Dis* 1979; 139:178–180.

29 Rowe B & Threlfall E J. Drug resistance in gram-negative aerobic bacilli. *Br Med Bull* 1984; 40:68–76.

30 Lewin C S, Nandivadà L S & Amyes S G B. Multiresistant salmonella and fluoroquinolones. *J. Antimicrob Chemother* 1991; 27:147–149.

31 Carbonetti N H, Nicoletti, Visca P et al. Composite IS*1* elements encoding hydroxamate-mediated iron uptake in FI*me* plasmids from epidemic *Salmonella* spp. *J. Bacteriol* 1985; 162:307–316.

32 Threlfall E J, Hall M L M & Rowe B. Salmonella bacteraemia in England and Wales, 1981–1990. *J Clin Pathol* 1992; 45:34–36.

33 Ward L R, Threlfall E J & Rowe B. Multiple drug resistance in salmonellas isolated from humans in England and Wales: a comparison of 1981 with 1988. *J Clin Pathol* 1990; 43:563–566.

34 Threlfall E J, Rowe B & Ward L R. A comparison of multiple drug resistance in salmonellas from humans and food animals in England and Wales, 1981 and 1990. *Epidemiol Infect* 1993; 111:189–197.

35 Threlfall E J, Rowe B, Ferguson J L & Ward L R. Characterization of plasmids conferring resistance to gentamicin and apramycin in strains of *Salmonella typhimurium* phage type 204c isolated in Britain. *J Hyg (Camb)* 1986; 97:419–426.

36 Threlfall E J, Hampton M D, Chart H & Rowe B. Identification of a conjugative plasmid carrying antibiotic resistance and salmonella plasmid virulence (*spv*) genes in epidemic strains of *Salmonella typhimurium*. Lett Appl Microbiol 1994; 18:82–88.

37 Threlfall E J, Frost J A, Ward L R & Rowe B.

Epidemic in cattle of *S. typhimurium* DT 104 with chromosomally-integrated multiple drug resistance. *Vet Rec* 1994; 134:557.

38 Gross R J, Threlfall E J, Ward L R & Rowe B. Drug resistance in *Shigella dysenteriae, Sh. flexneri* and *Sh. boydii* in England and Wales: increasing incidence of resistance to trimethoprim. *BMJ* 1984; 288:784–786.

39 Gross R J, Rowe B, Cheasty T & Thomas L V. Increase in drug resistance in *Shigella dysenteriae, Sh. flexneri* and *Sh. boydii* isolated in England and Wales. *BMJ* 1981; 283:575.

40 Frost J A, Rowe B, Vandepitte J & Threlfall E J. Plasmid characterisation in the investigation of an epidemic caused by multiply-resistant *Shigella dysenteriae* type 1 in Central Africa. *Lancet* 1981; ii:1074–1076.

41 Frost J A, Rowe B & Vandepitte J. Acquisition of trimethoprim resistance in epidemic strains of *Shigella dysenteriae* type 1 from Zaire. *Lancet* 1982; i:963.

42 Pal S C. Epidemic bacillary dysentery in West Bengal, India, 1984. *Lancet* 1984; i:1462.

43 Bhattacharya S K, Battacharya M K, Dutta D et al. Single dose ciprofloxacin for shigellosis in adults. *J. Infect* 1992; 25:117–119.

44 Sen D, Dutta P, Deb B C & Pal S C. Nalidixic acid-resistant *Shigella dysenteriae* type 1 in Eastern India. *Lancet* 1988; ii:911.

45 CDC. Multistate outbreak of *Shigella sonnei* gastroenteritis — United States. *MMWR* 1987; 36:440–442, 448–449.

46 Wharton M, Spiegel R A, Horan J M et al. A large outbreak of antibiotic-resistant shigellosis at a mass gathering. *J Infect Dis* 1990; 162:1324–1328.

47 Bennish M L & Salam M A. Rethinking options for the treatment of shigellosis. *J Antimicrob Chemother* 1992; 30:243–247.

48 Mhalu M S, Mmari P W & Ijumba J. Rapid emergence of El Tor *Vibrio cholerae* resistant to antimicrobial agents during first month of fourth cholera epidemic in Tanzania. *Lancet* 1979; i:345–347.

49 Threlfall E J, Said B, Rowe B & Dàvalos-Pèrez A. Emergence of multiple drug resistance in *Vibrio cholerae* El Tor from Ecuador. *Lancet* 1993; 342:1173.

50 Weber J T, Mintz E D, Canizares R et al. Epidemic cholera in Ecuador: multidrug-resistance and transmission by water and seafood. *Epidemiol Infect* 1994; 112:1–11.

51 World Health Organization. *Guidelines for Cholera Control*. Geneva: WHO, 1993.

52 Cheasty T, Rowe B, Said B & Frost J A. *Vibrio cholerae* serogroup O139 in England and Wales. *Lancet* 1993; 307:1007.

53 McConnell M M, Willshaw G A, Smith H R et al.

Transposition of ampicillin resistance to an enterotoxin plasmid in an *Escherichia coli* strain of human origin. *J Bacteriol* 1979; 139:346–355.

54 Echeverria P, Verhaert L, Ulangco C V et al. Antimicrobial resistance and enterotoxin production among isolates of *Escherichia coli* in the Far East. *Lancet* 1978; ii:589–592.

55 Gross R J. *Escherichia coli* diarrhoea. In Smith G (ed.) *Topley and Wilson's Principles of Bacteriology, Virology and Immunity*, 8th edn, vol. 3. London: Edward Arnold, 1990: 470–487.

56 Ericsson C D, Johnson P C, DuPont H L et al. Ciprofloxacin or trimethoprim-sulfamethoxazole as initial therapy for travellers' diarrhoea. A placebo-controlled, randomized trial. *Ann Intern Med* 1987; 106:216–220.

57 Wistrom J, Jertborn M, Hedstrom S A et al. Short-term self-treatment of travellers' diarrhoea with norfloxacin: a placebo-controlled study. *J Antimicrob Chemother* 1989; 23:905–913.

58 Wood M J. The use of antibiotics in infections due to *Escherichia coli* O157:H7. *PHLS Microbiol Digest* 1991; 8:18–21.

59 McNulty C A M. The treatment of campylobacter infections in man. *J Antimicrob Chemother* 1987; 19:281–284.

60 Bibhat K, Mandal P, De Mol P & Butzler J-P. Clinical aspects of *Campylobacter* infection in humans. In Butzler J-P (ed.) Campylobacter *Infection in Man and Animals*. Boca Raton: CRC Press, 1984;22–30.

61 Rowe B & Gross R J. Salmonellosis, Campylobacter enteritis and Shigella dysentery. In Goodwin C S (ed.) *Microbes and Infections of the Gut*. Oxford: Blackwell, 1984:477–777.

62 Brunton W A T, Wilson A M M & MacRae R M. Erythromycin-resistant campylobacters. *Lancet* 1978; ii:1385.

63 Walder M & Fosgren A. Erythromycin-resistant campylobacters. *Lancet* 1978; ii:1201.

64 Vanhoof R, Vanderlinden N P, Dierickz R et al. Susceptibility of *Campylobacter fetus* subsp. *jejuni* to 29 antimicrobial agents. *Antimicrob Agents Chemother* 1978; 14:553–556.

65 Dupont H L, Corrado M & Sabbaj J. Use of norfloxacin in the treatment of acute diarrheal disease. *Am J Med* 1987; 82 (supplement 6B):79–83.

66 Pichler H E T, Stickler D G & Wolf D. Clinical efficacy of ciprofloxacin compared to placebo in bacterial diarrhea. *Am J Med* 1987; 82 (supplement 4A):329–332.

67 Endtz H P, Ruijs G J, van Klingeren B et al. Quinolone resistance in campylobacter isolated from man and poultry following the introduction of fluoroquinolones in veterinary medicine. *J Antimicrob Chemother* 1991; 27:199–208.

CHAPTER 44

BACTERIAL MENINGITIS

C. A. Hart

Bacterial meningitis is common in many areas of the tropics and has a significant mortality, especially in children (see also Chapter 8). The bacteria causing meningitis vary with geographic and climatic conditions, with age, and whether the illness is chronic

Table 44.1 Aetiology of acute meningitis.

Purulent	Lymphocytic
Neonatal	
Group B streptococcus	Herpes simplex virus
Listeria monocytogenes	Enteroviruses
Escherichia coli and other coliforms	
Salmonella spp.	
Pseudomonas aeruginosa	
Candida albicans	
Older individuals	
Neisseria meningitidis	*Mycobacterium tuberculosis*
Haemophilus influenzae	*Leptospira* spp.
Streptococcus pneumoniae	*Treponema pallidum*
Salmonella spp.	*Borrelia* spp.
L. monocytogenes	Enteroviruses
Naegleria fowleri	Mumps virus
Anaerobes	Arthropod-borne togaviruses
	Adenovirus
	Lymphocytic chroriomeningitis virus
	Human immunodeficiency virus

Table 44.2 Aetiology of chronic meningitis.

Bacteria	Fungi	Parasites
Mycobacterium tuberculosis	*Cryptococcus neoformans*	*Toxoplasma gondii*
Brucella spp.	*Histoplasma capsulatum*	Cysticercosis
Treponema pallidum	*Coccidiodes immitis*	
Borrelia burgdorferi	*Candida albicans*	
Neisseria meningitidis	*Actinomyces israelii*	

or acute (Tables 44.1 and 44.2). Outside the neonatal period the three major pathogens are: *Streptococcus pneumoniae*, *Haemophilus influenzae* and *Neisseria meningitidis*. Neonatal meningitis may also be caused by these organisms[1] but other bacteria such as *Escherichia coli*, *Str. agalactiae* (Group B streptococcus) and *Klebsiella pneumoniae* tend to predominate. The relative importance of *H. influenzae*, pneumococci and meningococci outside the neonatal period varies according to country; for example, in wet low lying regions *Str. pneumoniae* and *H. influenzae* predominate, whereas in dryer regions, for example the meningitis belt of sub-Saharan Africa, the meningococcus causes vast spreading epidemics.[2] *H. influenzae* meningitis is rare in individuals over 7 years of age. In addition to a high mortality rate, bacterial meningitis carries a high risk of neurological sequelae.

NEONATAL MENINGITIS

With improvements in and the more widespread availability of neonatal intensive care, neonates of increasing prematurity have a chance of survival. The premature neonate is not only immature in terms of pulmonary, alimentary and renal function but is also an immune-compromised host. This means that the neonate, and especially the premature neonate, is at increased risk of infection. Early bacterial meningitis is usually part of a syndrome of sepsis neonatorum with few specific signs in the premature neonate.[3] Once infection is established, convulsions, bulging fontanelle and neck stiffness may be detected.

GEOGRAPHICAL ASPECTS

Although some geographical variations in the incidence and microbiology of neonatal meningitis are reported, the variability relates more to the presence of neonatal intensive care units and thus whether the infection is hospital or community acquired. For example, in Nigeria, *Salmonella* spp. *Staphylococcus aureus* are the major pathogens[4,5] whereas in a neonatal intensive care unit in South Africa, *Klebsiella* spp. and *E. coli* were predominant.[6]

EPIDEMIOLOGY

The incidence of meningitis varies according to the prematurity of the neonate, and in some areas is apparently decreasing. In Durban the incidence was 1.27/1000 live births in 1981 and had fallen to 0.22/1000 live births in 1987.[6] A more recent survey in Oman revealed an incidence of 1/1000 live births.[7]

BACTERIOLOGY

The bacteria causing neonatal sepsis have altered considerably over the past 60 years.[8] This change in part reflects the changes in neonatal intensive care and in the availability of antibiotics of increasing potency and breadth of spectrum. In the first part of the twentieth century group A β-haemolytic streptococci, followed by *Staph. aureus*, were the major pathogens. After the introduction of penicillins Gram-negative bacteria such as *E. coli* and *Klebsiella* spp. emerged as significant pathogens. Then in the 1970s the importance of the group B streptococcus (*Str. agalactiae*) was realized and the existence of antibiotic-resistant coliforms became apparent. Latterly, low-virulence pathogens such as *Staph. epidermidis* have been shown to be capable of causing septicaemia and meningitis. In tropical countries this evolution has only been apparent in centres with neonatal intensive care units. Elsewhere primary pathogens such as *Salmonella* spp. *Str. agalactiae* and *Listeria monocytogenes* are more important.

PATHOGENESIS

In most cases the neonate first becomes colonized by the pathogen, which then translocates to produce bacteraemia. Bacteria can then lodge in the meninges to produce infection. In cases where infection presents within the first 48 hours of life the bacteria have been acquired from the birth canal or maternal perineum. Bacteria causing early overt infection include *Str. agalactiae*, *E. coli*, *L. monocytogenes* and *Salmonella* spp. These same bacteria may also cause meningitis occurring later in the neonatal period but more often bacteria such as *Pseudomonas* spp. and *Klebsiella* spp. are commonly encountered.

The premature neonate has defects in both humoral and cell-mediated immunity that predispose it to serious infection. For example, the neonate's phagocytes do not work efficiently and the activity of the complement cascade is only 50% of that of adults. At birth the neonate's own IgM production is 20% of adult levels, of IgG is 5% of adult levels and IgA production begins at birth. Thus the neonate also has defects in humoral immunity.

CLINICAL FEATURES

The early signs of meningitis in premature neonates are often indistinguishable from those of septicaemia. The signs of septicaemia in premature neonates are not specific to infection; for example, in one series of 139 episodes of septicaemia, pyrexia was present in only six episodes.[3] Signs that suggest neonatal meningitis, such as bulging fontanelle, stiff neck, convulsions or opisthotonos, are uncommon. For example, 17% of neonates with meningitis present with a bulging fontanelle, 33% with opisthotonos, 23% with neck stiffness and 12% with convulsions.[9–11] Thus to diagnose neonatal meningitis will require a high index of suspicion and part of the investigation of suspected neonatal septicaemia should include examination and culture of CSF.

The results of infection can be dire. The mortality rates associated with neonatal meningitis vary according to the gestational age. Thus meningitis in neonates of extremely low birth weight (<1000 g) is associated with mortality rates of up to 80%, and that in neonates of very low birth weight (<1500 g) is 20–30% in developed countries. In less well developed countries the mortality rates vary with gestational age from 46 to 90%.[6] Mortality rates are also greater if meningitis is due to Gram-negative bacilli.[6,12] Other acute complications include hydrocephalus, subdural effusions, deafness and blindness. Ventriculitis complicates Gram-negative bacillary meningitis in particular (70% of cases) and can make therapy very difficult. In long-term follow-up 5–10% of neonates with meningitis have severe neurological deficit.

DIAGNOSIS

The definitive diagnosis depends upon examination of cerebrospinal fluid taken either by lumbar or ventricular puncture. The interpretation of the findings depends upon a knowledge of what is normal in neonatal CSF. For example, in the first days of life 'normal' neonatal CSF may contain up to 30 white blood cells per cubic millimetre (60% polymorphs), up to 170 mg/dl protein and raised glucose. Unfortunately, for certain bacteria the early cellular and biochemical findings overlap with the 'normal'. For example, 30% of neonates with *Str. agalactiae* meningitis have a 'normal' cellular response.[13] In contrast, most (96%) of those with Gram-negative bacillary meningitis have an abnormal CSF. It follows that rapid detection of bacteria in CSF is of prime importance in diagnosing neonatal meningitis. Examination of Gram-stained smears will detect up to 80% of cases and provide information on the aetiology. Tests for detection of bacterial antigens are available for some bacteria. Both countercurrent immunoelectrophoresis and latex particle agglutination tests are available for detection of *Str. agalactiae*, *Str. pneumoniae*, *N. meningitidis*, *H. influenzae* and *E. coli* K1 antigens. In general the latter is more sensitive and convenient than the former but countercurrent immunoelectrophoresis can be less expensive.

Culture is the gold standard but will take 18–24 hours. It also has the advantage that it will provide information on the antimicrobial susceptibility.

MANAGEMENT

Neonates with meningitis may require elective ventilation and circulatory support but the mainstay of therapy is administration of antibiotics that achieve therapeutic levels in CSF. Because there is a large range of potential pathogens, blind initial therapy must cover as wide a spectrum as possible. Most neonatal intensive care units employ a combination of ampicillin and gentamicin. This, however, does have some drawbacks, especially in treating Gram-negative bacteria which may be resistant to ampicillin, and the CSF penetration of gentamicin even through inflamed meninges is not good.[14] Penicillin or ampicillin are sufficient for treating *Str. agalactiae* or *L. moncytogenes* meningitis and little resistance has developed. The susceptibility of Gram-negative bacilli to antibiotics is less predictable and varies from unit to unit and with time. A third generation cephalosporin such as ceftazidime or cefotaxime can prove useful.[6] Chloramphenicol, although effective against Gram-negative bacilli in vitro, is not uniformly effective in vivo since it is not bactericidal. Finally, instillation of gentamicin directly into the ventricles is not recommended for therapy of neonatal bacterial meningitis.[14]

PREVENTION

Prevention of neonatal meningitis can be difficult, firstly because so many different pathogens may be involved, and secondly the premature neonate is an immunoincompetent host. For prevention of *Str. agalactiae* sepsis two strategies are being investigated. Following the successful immunoprophylaxis of neonatal tetanus by actively immunizing the mother in the last trimester a similar study is being pursued using the group B streptococcal capsular polysaccharide. Vaginal irrigation with chlorhexidine prior to delivery has been shown to decrease the incidence of neonatal group B streptococcal sepsis.[15]

MENINGITIS IN OLDER INDIVIDUALS

Outside the neonatal period *N. meningitidis*, *Str. pneumoniae* and *H. influenzae* are responsible for over 90% of cases of acute bacterial meningitis. The remaining cases are due to a variety of bacteria, including both *Salmonella typhi* and non-typhi *Salmonella* spp. The latter can produce meningitis in the immunocompetent but may occur more commonly in the malnourished or in patients with sickle cell disease.[16]

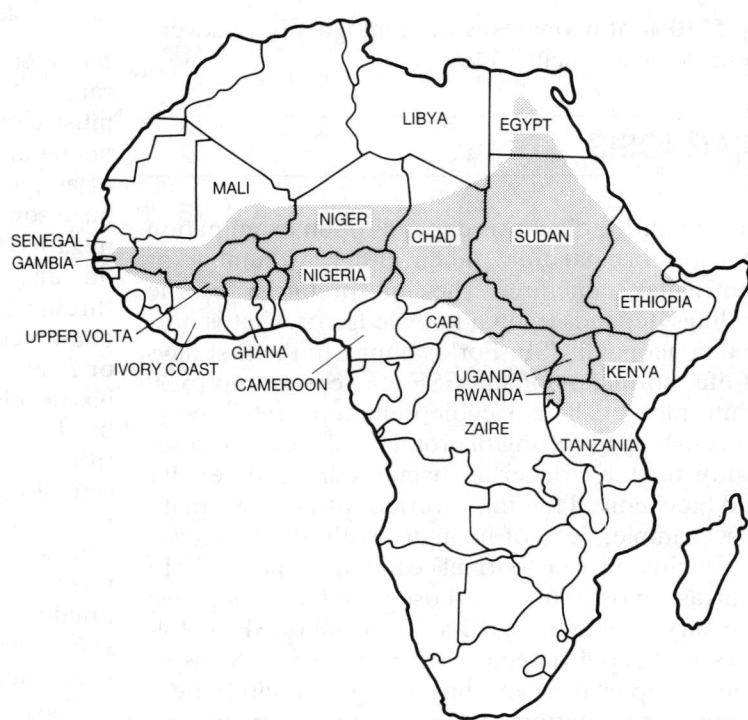

Figure 44.1 The 'meningitis belt' of sub-Saharan Africa where epidemics occur in 8–14-year cycles.

HISTORY

The history of meningitis covers only epidemics of 'cerebrospinal fever' with or without 'malignant purpuric fever', and this probably refers only to meningococcal disease. The meningococcus was first isolated in 1887 at autopsy and in 1896 in life. Thereafter, the individual pathogens were gradually isolated and the disease more clearly defined.

GEOGRAPHICAL ASPECTS

Acute bacterial meningitis is found throughout the world but the relative contribution of the three main pathogens varies considerably. The reasons for this variation are still unclear. In the meningitis belt of sub-Saharan Africa (Figure 44.1) epidemics of meningococcal meningitis occur with 8–14 year cycles. During epidemics the incidence rises to over 400 cases/100 000 population per year but even between epidemics the hyperendemic rate is over 40 cases/100 000 per year.[2] These cases are most often due to group A meningococci but occasionally group C meningococci can cause epidemics. In contrast, in certain parts of Africa such as Zaire (Table 44.3) and in temperate industrialized countries epidemics with group A meningococci are rarely reported. In low lying regions such as Zaire pneumococci are the major meningeal pathogens in all age groups.[21] *H. influenzae* is responsible for cases of meningitis in children under 5 years old in all regions of the world.

EPIDEMIOLOGY

For each of the three main pathogens spread is by droplet or exchange of saliva. Spread is facilitated by close contact. For example, household contacts of a case of meningococcal disease run a risk of developing infection which is 1245 times greater than that for the general population.[38] In most cases colonization of the nasopharynx precedes invasive disease. The incubation period can be as short as 2–3 days but secondary cases of meningococcal disease have been reported as long as 4 months after contact. However, in studies of secondary cases in households with an index case of meningococcal disease, 70% of secondary cases occur within the first week of contact, 13% in the second week, 6% in the third week and the remaining 11% from the fourth to tenth week.[38]

Although the incidence of pneumococcal and *H. influenzae* meningitis remains relatively constant, *N. meningitidis* is able to produce epidemics spreading through many parts of the world.[2] For example a clone of group A *N. meningitidis* (III-1) produced an

Table 44.3 Relative importance of meningeal pathogens.

| | Cases of meningitis (%)* | | | | | |
	N. meningitidis	S. pneumoniae	H. influenzae	Population	Years	Reference
Africa						
South Africa	31	22	16	M	1980–1982	17
Malawi	4	54	38	C	1983	18
Malawi	47	42	11	M	1983–1989	19
Zambia	23	38	6.3	M	1978–1981	20
Zaire	1.6	33	46	C	1958–1977	21
Nigeria	16	39	28	C	1976–1979	22
Ivory Coast	6.4	39	17	M	1971–1975	23
Libya	10	18	27	C	1981–1984	24
Senegal	11	29	20	M	1970–1979	25
Algeria	30	11	19	M	1969	26
Asia						
India	0	61	7	M	1972–1980	27
Malaysia	5.6	24	54	C	1985–1987	28
Thailand	5.6	47	39	C	1967–1968	29
Australasia						
Papua New Guinea	36	59	4	A	1974–1979	30
Vanuatu	35	33	23	C	1983–1988	31
Caribbean						
Jamaica	4.1	38	30	M	1965–1980	32
Puerto Rico	1.4	10	74	C	1976–1982	33
America						
Brazil	40	21	28	A	1973–1982	34
Chile	8.6	33	58	C	1972–1981	35
Panama	14	14	0	A	1975–1982	36
Europe						
UK (Merseyside)	57	14	30	C	1981–1990	UD
Denmark	41	19	8	A	1966–1976	37

A, adults; C, children; M, children and adults; UD, unpublished data.
*Percentage of bacteriologically proven cases.

epidemic of disease in China in the 1970s which spread to Nepal in 1982, causing an epidemic in 1983–1984. The same clone was responsible for epidemics in New Delhi (1985) and Pakistan (1985). It was then brought by hadjis to Mecca in (1987) (Figure 44.2). Clone III-1 was then disseminated throughout the world by hadjis returning home. In the African meningitis belt it initiated the 1988 epidemic but in other areas such as Europe and USA, despite up to 11% of returning pilgrims being carriers, it did not spread.

Although in Africa epidemic meningococcal disease occurs in the hot dry season this is not the sole determinant. Person-to-person spread of the meningococcus occurs as readily throughout the year and it is thought the seasonality of disease is related to increased invasiveness. This may reflect an effect

of the dust storms, extreme dryness and heat on the host's mucosal defences.

BACTERIOLOGY

NEISSERIA MENINGITIDIS

Meningococci are small ($0.8 \times 0.6\,\mu$m) non-motile Gram-negative cocci arranged in pairs with contiguous sides flattened.

Optimal growth of meningococci is achieved on enriched media (blood or chocolatized agar) in CO_2 (10%) in air at 37°C. Small convex greyish mucoid colonies are produced after 18–24 hours incubation. All pathogenic meningococci are piliated (protein

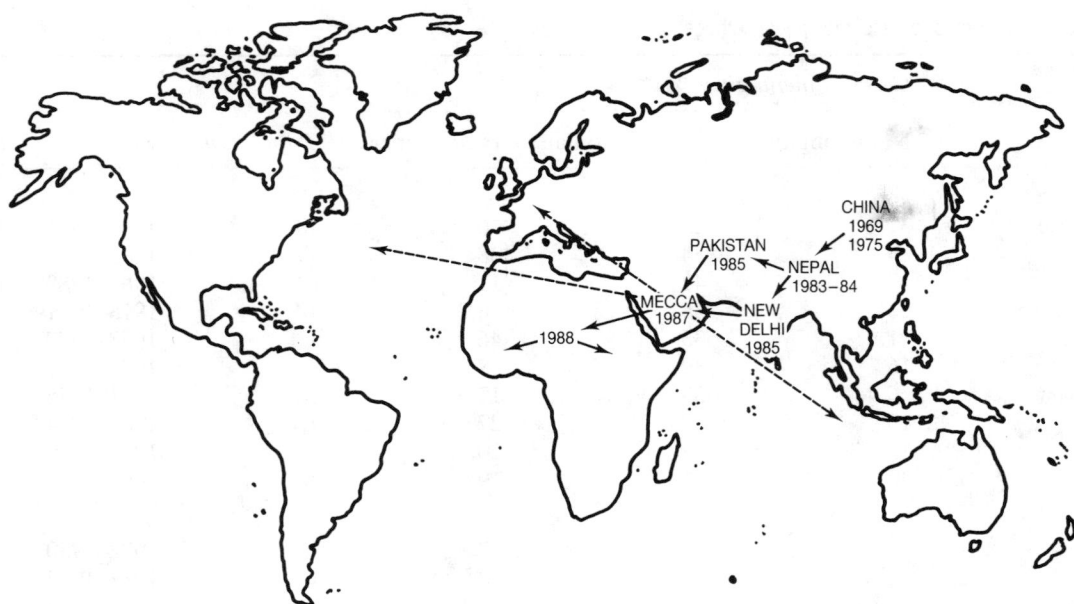

Figure 44.2   Intercontinental spread of clone III-1 of group A *N. meningitidis*.

spikes for attachment to mucous and endothelial surfaces) and capsulate. The capsules are acidic polysaccharides that allow the bacteria to evade phagocytic killing. There are nine different capsular serogroups (A, B, C, D, X, Y, Z, W-135 and 29E). Groups A, B and C are associated with most cases of meningitis. Groups A and C are associated with epidemics and group B with sporadic endemic disease. Groups B and C may be further typed on the basis of outer membrane proteins to provide further epidemiological information. Group A meningococci may be further subdivided by means of multilocus enzyme electrophoresis.[39]

HAEMOPHILUS INFLUENZAE

This is a small pleomorphic (1.5 × 0.4 µm) non-motile Gram-negative coccobacillus. It requires chocolatized blood agar and an atmosphere of CO_2 (10%) in air for growth and produces small convex greyish mucoid colonies after 18–24 hours. Only one of the capsulate strains of *H. influenzae* is able to produce invasive disease in the immunocompetent. This is *H. influenzae* (b) which possesses a polyribitol phosphate capsule. Although *H. influenzae* meningitis is rare in those over 5–7 years old it can still occur in adults.[30,34,37]

STREPTOCOCCUS PNEUMONIAE

These are lanceolate Gram-positive cocci (0.8 × 1.0 µm), usually arranged in pairs. They grow best on blood agar in CO_2 (10%) in air, where they produce either small draughtsman-like colonies or large transparent mucoid (like drops of water) α-haemolytic colonies. The latter are the more virulent strains. Pneumococci are sensitive to optochin which differentiates them from other α-haemolytic streptococci. There are over 80 different capsular types but the 23 included in the current capsular vaccine are responsible for 90–95% of cases of invasive disease. Pneumococci also produce an exotoxin, pneumolysin.

PATHOGENESIS

Each of the three main pathogens is able to colonize the nasopharynx. There is evidence to suggest that the risk of disease is greatest in the period immediately after colonization. Bacteria in the nasopharynx then translocate to enter the circulation. How this occurs is not clear, but for the meningococcus there is an association between respiratory tract infection with viruses or mycoplasma and meningitis.[40] The bacteria localize in the pia mater and set up an inflammatory response in the meninges and cerebrospinal fluid. The presence of capsule allows bacteria to survive longer in the circulation and meninges. Various components of the bacterial cell surface, such as teichoic acid in pneumococci, lipopolysaccharide (endotoxin) in meningococci and *H. influenzae* and peptidoglycan in all of them, induce secretion of a variety of factors such as tumour necrosis factor (TNF), interleukins 1 and 6 (IL-1, IL-6), eicosanoids, and platelet activating factor

(PAF). This results in potentiation of inflammation, further activation of neutrophils, further complement activation and increased permeability of the blood–brain barrier. This can then produce cerebral vessel thrombosis and vasculitis, cerebral oedema, intracranial hypertension and cerebral infarction. Finally the activated neutrophils consume large amounts of glucose and oxygen and deprive neuronal tissues of these essential components.

PATHOLOGY

The pathological features of acute bacterial meningitis are similar for each of the pathogens and have been well reviewed.[41] The principal feature is of a purulent exudate in the subarachnoid space which often damages the pia mater and the underlying superficial cortex. There is cerebral vessel vasculitis and thrombosis with neuronal damage and superficial encephalitis. There may also be damage to cranial and spinal nerves as they traverse the subarachnoid space.

CLINICAL FEATURES

The signs and symptoms of bacterial meningitis are those of infection and of inflammation of the meninges. The onset is sudden with fever in most cases but is often preceded by symptoms of upper respiratory tract infection. Meningeal irritation will become manifest by nausea, vomiting, headache, irritability, confusion, back pain and neck stiffness. In addition it may be possible to elicit Kernig's (pain on attempting to extend the knee with the hips flexed) or Brudzinski's (neck flexion producing flexion of the hips and knees) signs. It is unusual for all of these features to be present at once, especially in young patients or in the early stages of disease. For example in a review of over 1000 children with meningitis 1.5% showed no signs of meningeal irritation throughout their infection.[42]

Even early in infection there may be some evidence of mental dysfunction, ranging from drowsiness and lethargy to coma in fulminant infection. Convulsions may occur, especially in children. These are reported in up to 20% of children prior to admission and in 26–30% overall.

There may be signs of raised intracranial pressure reflected by headache, and in infants by bulging fontanelle or even diastasis of sutures. Papilloedema is not common in children.

Finally, inappropriate secretion of antidiuretic

Table 44.4 Complications of *H. influenzae* meningitis.

Complication	Cases (%)
Early	
Recurrent or persistent pyrexia	35–40
Subdural effusions	33
Inappropriate antidiuretic hormone secretion	50–80
Paralysis	16
Late	
Persistent paralysis	2–3
Relapse of meningitis	4
Visual impairment	2–3
Hearing deficit	10–15
Hypertension	2–3
Hydrocephalus	<1
Epileptic fits	7

hormone is a common occurrence (in up to 80% of cases) in childhood meningitis. This leads to water retention and may lead to a further rise in intracranial pressure.

Pneumococcal meningitis in particular is more likely to be associated with focal signs on admission.

DIFFERENTIAL DIAGNOSIS

Meningitis can be missed in its early stages, especially in children when there may be only subtle signs of meningism. It should be considered in any child with febrile convulsions or in patients suddenly becoming confused. Similar clinical features may be seen in cerebral malaria, typhus, relapsing fever and cerebral tumours. Viral, fungal or tuberculous meningitis may also present in a similar fashion. Examination of CSF will help to differentiate bacterial meningitis from the rest.

COMPLICATIONS

The mortality rates associated with bacterial meningitis vary according to the age of the patient and the infecting micro-organisms. For example, in one survey in Brazil the overall mortality in non-neonatal meningitis was 32% but rose to 48% in those aged 2–6 months and 40% in those aged from 6 months to 2 years.[34] The mortality rate from pneumococcal meningitis (57%) is highest, followed by *H. influenzae* meningitis (38%) with meningococcal meningitis (14%) having the lowest mortality. Overall mortality rates were much lower (19%) in a series reported from Malaysia.[28]

The acute and later sequelae of *H. influenzae* meningitis are shown in Table 44.4. Unfortunately, there are few long-term follow-up studies of bacterial meningitis in the tropics and most of the information is extrapolated from temperate zones. However, in one study in Malaysia, 47% of children attending follow-up at least once had neurological sequelae. The incidence of sequelae in *H. influenzae* and pneumococcal meningitis is similar and higher than that encountered in meningococcal meningitis. A proportion of children with *H. influenzae* meningitis redevelop pyrexia at day 5–6 of therapy. This can represent the formation of subdural effusion or abscesses but most often no reason is found.

MENINGOCOCCAL DISEASE

Although the mortality from meningococcal meningitis is relatively low, if infection is complicated by septicaemia it can prove rapidly fatal. The meningococcus continuously blebs off part of its outer membrane (Figure 44.3). Approximately 25% of the lipid in the outer membrane is lipo-oligosaccharide. This is a powerful endotoxin, and release of endotoxin produces activation of clotting and complement factors, activation of neutrophils and macrophages, with release of IL-1 (endogenous pyrogen), vasculitis and release of TNF. This can result in profound shock and bleeding from capillaries. On the skin this produces petechiae, purpura and ecchymoses which together with adrenal haemorrhage constitute the Waterhouse–Friedrichsen syndrome. The onset of disease is sudden with fever and progression through shock, purpura and coma, and death can be rapid (as fast as 2 hours). It is important to distinguish meningococcal meningitis from meningococcal meningitis with septicaemia or septicaemia alone,[43] since the management and pro-

gression of the two differ. Defects in the terminal components of the complement cascade (C6–9) and properdin predispose to the development of fulminant meningococcal septicaemia. The proportion of cases of meningococcal disease with a septicaemic component appears to be lower in tropical countries. For example only 4 of 112 (4%) of cases of meningococcal disease had septicaemia in one study in Sudan[44] and we have observed only four cases of septicaemia out of 700 cases of meningococcal disease in Malawi. A similarly low incidence of meningococcal septicaemia (5%) was observed in Nigeria.[45] In contrast only 24% of cases of meningococcal disease on Merseyside had no septicaemic component.[43] Whether this difference represents a true difference in susceptibility to meningococcal septicaemia, or is a reflection of the difficulties of recognizing a petechial rash on a dark skin, or patients in Africa with septicaemia are dying prior to reaching hospital is unclear.

Complications of meningococcal septicaemia include gangrene of the skin and extremities and arthritis, which can be purulent or immunologically mediated.

DIAGNOSIS

The definitive diagnosis of bacterial meningitis depends upon examination of CSF (Table 44.5). The CSF is usually turbid due to the presence of large numbers of neutrophils. However, in early infection low cell counts ($200/mm^3$) may cause the CSF to appear clear. A high CSF neutrophil count and protein concentration and low CSF glucose reflect the extent of inflammation and indicate a poorer prognosis. A specific aetiological diagnosis can be obtained rapidly by examining a Gram-stained smear of centrifuged CSF deposits. This will provide a specific diagnosis in 80–85% of cases. A useful, if expensive, adjunct to diagnosis is detection of bacterial capsular antigens (acidic polysaccharides). Countercurrent immunoelectrophoresis is less sensitive than latex particle agglutination, which has a sensitivity and specificity of 85–100% and 96–100% respectively, for detection of the appropriate micro-organism.[45,46]

CSF culture will take 18–24 hours but has the advantage of being relatively cheap and providing data on the antimicrobial susceptibility of the bacterium. Blood culture, if facilities are available, is a useful adjunct to diagnosis. Detection of antigen in urine or serum can also be of value for diagnosis of pneumococcal or *H. influenzae* meningitis but is less useful in meningococcal meningitis.[47]

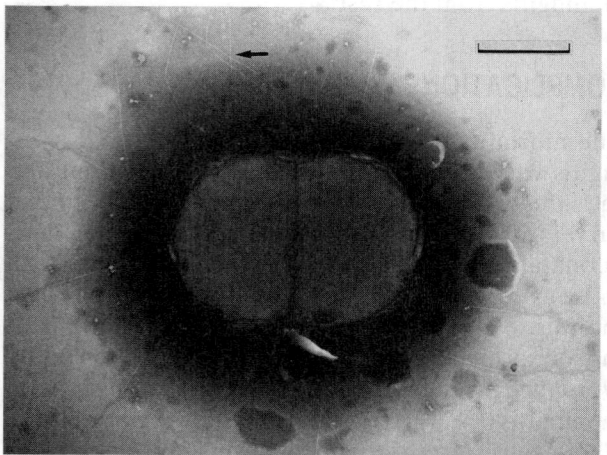

Figure 44.3 Transmission electronmicrograph of *N. meningitidis* showing pili (arrowed) and loss of the outer membrane by 'blebbing' (bar = 0.5 μm)

Table 44.5 Cerebrospinal fluid in meningitis.

	Normal	Bacterial Meningitis	Aseptic Meningitis
Volume (ml)	40–120	—	—
Appearance	Clear	Turbid	Clear to opalescent
Pressure (mmH$_2$O)	<180–200	<300	Normal
Protein (g/l)	0.15–0.4	0.5–6.0	0.5–1.0†
Mononuclear cells (× 10^6/l)	0–5	Can be raised	15–500
Neutrophils (× 10^6/l)	0	100–6000	<15
Glucose (mmol)*	2.2–3.3	0–2.2	2.2–3.3†

*Must be compared with blood glucose (should be 50–60% of blood glucose level).
†In tuberculous meningitis the CSF protein is often high and glucose low.

MANAGEMENT

Patients with meningitis should, where possible, be managed in hospital. Blood pressure and respiratory and pulse rates should be monitored regularly. The unconscious patient should be nursed so as to maintain an open airway. Fluid intake should be monitored to prevent dehydration (due to fever and poor fluid intake) or overhydration (due to inappropriate antidiuretic hormone secretion). If fits occur, appropriate anticonvulsants should be administered, bearing in mind that hepatic microsomal enzyme inducers such as phenobarbitone or phenytoin might increase the rate of conjugation of chloramphenicol and decrease blood levels. High dose intravenous dexamethasone (0.15 mg/kg 6-hourly for children or 12 mg/12 h for adults) has been shown to decrease mortality in pneumococcal meningitis[48] and decrease neurological sequelae and inflammation in H. influenzae meningitis.[49]

The efficacy of antimicrobial chemotherapy depends upon the penetration of the antibiotic into CSF (Table 44.6) and the susceptibility of the infecting micro-organism.

For blind initial therapy chloramphenicol has been shown to be as effective as a chloramphenicol–penicillin combination,[50] and a long-acting oily suspension of chloramphenicol as effective as ampicillin.[51] The oily suspension has the benefit of providing treatment even for those who abscond from hospital. Early antibiotic treatment even prior to hospital admission has been shown to improve outcome in bacterial meningitis.[52]

MENINGOCOCCAL MENINGITIS

Benzyl penicillin (300 000 units/kg per day) should be given intravenously or intramuscularly 6-hourly

Table 44.6 Penetration of antibiotics into cerebrospinal fluid.

Antibiotic	Serum level in CSF (%)	Therapeutic level
Penicillins		
Penicillin	2–6	+
Ampicillin	10	+
Cephalosporins		
Cephalothin	1–5	±
Cefuroxime	5–10	+
Cefotaxime	10–25	+
Ceftazidime	20	+
Ceftriaxone	5–10	+
Aminoglycosides		
Gentamicin	10–30	−
Netilmicin	20–25	−
Others		
Sulphadiazine	50–80	+
Sulphamethoxazole	25–30	±
Trimethoprim	30–50	+*
Tetracycline	25	+
Chloramphenicol	90	+
Ciprofloxacin	5–20	+†

*Not effective against N. meningitidis.
†Not effective against S. pneumoniae.

for up to 7 days. Chloramphenicol (75–100 mg/kg per day) is a useful alternative given 6-hourly orally or i.m. There are sporadic reports of penicillin insusceptible meningococci,[53] but most are still exquisitely sensitive.

PNEUMOCOCCAL MENINGITIS

Benzylpenicillin (400 000 units/kg per day) is given 6-hourly i.v. or i.m., usually for 10 days. Chloramphenicol can also be used in a regimen, as for meningococcal meningitis. The emergence of penicillin-resistant pneumococci is an increasing problem worldwide.[54,55] Meningitis due to such strains is unlikely to be treatable with penicillin. In some cases these penicillin-resistant pneumococci, although susceptible to chloramphenicol in vitro, are not eradicated by chloramphenicol in vivo.[55]

H. INFLUENZAE MENINGITIS

Chloramphenicol (75–100 mg/kg per day) should be given every 6 hours parenterally and subsequently may be given orally. Treatment is usually continued for 10 days. Ampicillin (200 mg/kg per day) is an alternative although this may be associated with higher morbidity. Strains of *H. influenzae* (b) resistant to ampicillin (5–10%) or chloramphenicol (5%) and even to both antibiotics[56] are emerging.

Although penicillin and chloramphenicol have the advantage of cheapness and ready availability in tropical countries, a recent randomized open study in Finland demonstrated that cephalosporins such as cefotaxime or ceftriaxone had a clear advantage over chloramphenicol.[57] However, these cephalosporins are expensive and none of the antibiotics was associated with a 100% cure rate.

MENINGOCOCCAL SEPTICAEMIA

The treatment of fulminant meningococcal septicaemia is difficult and requires intensive management. Clinical scoring systems such as the Glasgow Meningococcal Septicaemia Prognostic Score[58] are of value in assessing the severity of disease and identifying those at greatest risk of dying (Table 44.7). If possible, patients should be artificially ventilated electively and given plasma and inotropes such as dobutamine as well as penicillin. Dexamethasone does not alter the course of endotoxic shock.

PREVENTION

CHEMOPROPHYLAXIS

Chemoprophylaxis is used to prevent secondary cases of meningococcal and *H. influenzae* meningitis in household contacts of an index case. There is no evidence that it is beneficial in pneumococcal meningitis.

N. meningitidis

Reports from the USA prior to the availability of vaccination and chemoprophylaxis show that sec-

Table 44.7 Glasgow Meningococcal Septicaemia Prognostic Score (GMSPS).

	Points†
Blood pressure	3
<75 mmHg systolic <4 years	
<85 mmHg systolic >4 years	
Skin/rectal temperature difference >3°C	3
*Modified coma scale score** <8 or	3
deterioration of >3 points in 1 hour	
Deterioration in hour prior to scoring	2
Absence of meningism	2
Extending purpuric rash or widespread	
ecchymoses	1
Base deficit (capillary or arterial) >8.0	1

*Modified coma score. (1) *Eyes open*: spontaneously, 4; to speech, 3; to pain, 2; none, 1. (2) *Best verbal response*: orientated, 6; words, 4; vocal sounds, 3; cries, 2; none, 1. (3) *Best motor response*: obeys commands, 6; localized pain, 4; moves to pain, 1; none, 1. Add scores in (1) (2) and (3) to obtain coma score.
†A GMSPS of >8 predicts mortality with a sensitivity of 100% and specificity of 95%.

ondary attack rates of 4–10% within households were common.[59] More recently it has been shown that 10% of patients presenting with meningococcal meningitis in Nigeria were secondary cases.[60] Two strategies are employed. In the first phenoxymethylpenicillin or amoxycillin is given as pre-emptive therapy for 7 days. The rationale for this is that most secondary cases occur in the first week after contact.[38] This will not affect nasopharyngeal carriage nor will it prevent secondary cases after therapy has ceased.

The second strategy aims to eradicate nasopharyngeal carriage. Antibiotics that are effective in eradicating susceptible nasopharyngeal meningococci include sulphadiazine, minocycline, rifampicin, ciprofloxacin or ceftriaxone.[61] Resistance to sulphonamides limits the value of these agents and minocycline has a high incidence of side-effects and cannot be used in children, pregnancy or lactation.

Rifampicin has been used in Africa[62] and does eradicate carriage. It is given as a 2-day regimen orally (600 mg twice daily for adults, 10 mg/kg per day for children of 1–12 years and 5 mg/kg per day for children under 1 year). Disadvantages include emergence of resistant meningococci during treatment[62] and the possibility of compromising the use of rifampicin as a first-line drug in tuberculosis. Ciprofloxacin (500–700 mg orally) or ceftriaxone (125 mg i.m.) are given as single dose regimens and are as effective as rifampicin in eradicating carriage. Unless sulphonamides are used, chemoprophylaxis is expensive (ceftriaxone £4, ciprofloxacin £2, rifampicin £2.70, per regimen: UK 1992 prices). To use vaccines would be much more cost effective; however, vaccines are of no value in the immediate protection of household contacts since it will take 2 weeks or more to develop protective antibody levels.

H. influenzae

In the USA secondary attack rates in households by invasive *H. influenzae* in children under 5 years are 500–800 times greater than the endemic rate.[63] Chemoprophylaxis is by means of a 4-day regimen of rifampicin (20 mg/kg per day once daily). This is given to all household members where there is an index case and a child under 3 years, except for pregnant or lactating women and those with severe hepatic impairment.

VACCINE

The acidic capsular polysaccharides of each of the three bacteria are highly immunogenic and vaccines are available for all of them. The problems in using polysaccharide antigens is that they are T-cell-independent antigens, which means that the antibody response is IgM and IgG_2 and immunological memory is poor.

The immunogenicity of such vaccines is poor in young children. For example, in children under 4 years old the group A meningococcal polysaccharide vaccine had produced persistant protective antibody 1 year after immunization in 100%, in 52% after 2 years and 0% after 3 years, whereas in children of 4 years or older the corresponding figures were 85%, 75% and 67% respectively.[64]

H. influenzae (*b*)

The capsular polysaccharide of *H. influenzae* (b) (Hib) is polyribitol phosphate. The problem of poor immunogencity of the capsular antigen has been overcome by conjugating it to a protein (diphtheria or tetanus toxoid). This significantly improves the quantity and duration of antibody response, even in those under 2 years old.[65] The Hib vaccine can be given together with the triple (diphtheria, pertussis, tetanus) vaccine with no deleterious effects. Hib vaccine has been shown to have 74% efficacy in preventing invasive Hib infection and 76% efficacy in preventing Hib meningitis in children aged 18–59 months.[66] It also eliminates oropharyngeal carriage and thus provides hard immunity.

N. meningitidis

A meningococcal vaccine incorporating groups A and C capsular polysaccharides is available. Its use has proved effective in controlling epidemics of meningococcal disease in Asia, Africa and Latin America. Protective antibodies persist for up to 5 years in adults but only 1–2 years in children under 4 years old. The vaccine does not affect nasopharyngeal carriage[67] and thus does not provide herd immunity. It is likely that a conjugate vaccine which should give better and more prolonged protection to infants will be available in the future.

The group B meningococcal capsule is a homopolymer of *N*-acetylneuraminic acid (as is the *E. coli* K1 capsule) and is a self-antigen being found on human neuronal glycoproteins and glycolipids. Thus there is no group B capsular vaccine. Vaccines incorporating group B meningococcal outer membrane proteins have worked well in Cuba[68] but less so in Chile or Norway[69].

Str. pneumoniae

The pneumococcal vaccine incorporates 23 of the 84 pneumococcal capsular polysaccharides. These 23 serogroups are responsible for 90–95% of invasive penumococcal disease. The vaccine is not widely used and suffers from the same problems as other polysaccharide vaccines. Its use is confined to those who are about to have splenectomy or in patients with sickle cell disease. A protein conjugate vaccine is not available.

REFERENCES

1 de Louvois J, Blackbourn J, Hurley R & Harvey D. Infantile meningitis in England and Wales: a two year study. *Arch Dis Child* 1991; 66:603–607.
2 Moore PS. Meningococcal meningitis in Sub-Saharan Africa: a model for the epidemic process. *Clin Infect Dis* 1992; 14:515–525.
3 Hensey O J, Hart C A & Cooke R W I. Serious infection in a neonatal intensive care unit. *J Hyg* 1985; 95:289–297.

4 Barclay B. High frequency of *Salmonella* species as a cause of neonatal meningitis in Ibadan, Nigeria. *Acta Paediatr Scand* 1971; 60:540–544.

5 Longe A C, Omene J A & Okolo A A. Neonatal meningitis in Nigerian infants. *Acta Paediatr Scand* 1984; 74:477–481.

6 Coovadia Y M, Mayosi B, Adhikari M, Solwa Z & van den Ende J. Hospital acquired neonatal meningitis: the impacts of cefotaxime usage on mortality and of amikacin usage on incidence. *Ann Trop Paediatr* 1989; 9:233–239.

7 Rajab A & de Louvois J. Survey of infection in babies at the Khoula Hospital, Oman. *Ann Trop Paediatr* 1990; 10:39–43.

8 Freedman R M, Ingram D L, Gross I, Ehrenkranz R A, Warkshaw J B & Baltimore R S. A half century of neonatal sepsis at Yale: 1928 to 1978. *Am J Dis Child* 1981; 135:140–144.

9 Overall J C. Neonatal bacterial meningitis: analysis of predisposing factors and outcome compared with matched control subjects. *J Pediatr* 1970; 76:499–508.

10 Berman P H & Banker B Q. Neonatal meningitis: a clinical and pathological study of 29 cases. *Pediatrics* 1966; 38:6–18.

11 McCracken G H & Shinefield H R. Changes in the pattern of neonatal septicaemia and meningitis. *Am J Dis Child* 1966; 112:33–41.

12 McCracken G H & Mize S G. A controlled study of intrathecal antibiotic therapy in Gram negative enteric meningitis of infancy. *J Pediatr* 1976; 89:66–74.

13 Sarff L D, Platt L H & McCracken G H. Cerebrospinal fluid evaluation in neonates. Comparison of high risk infants with and without meningitis. *J Pediatr* 1976; 88:473–479.

14 McCracken G H, Mize S G & Threlkeld N. Intraventricular gentamicin therapy in Gram negative bacillary meningitis of infancy. *Lancet* 1980; i:787–791.

15 Burman L G, Christensen P, Christensen K et al. Prevention of excess neonatal morbidity associated with group B streptococci by vaginal chlorhexidine disinfection during labour. *Lancet* 1992; 340:65–69.

16 Webb D K H & Serjeant G R. Systemic Salmonella infections in sickle cell anaemia. *Ann Trop Paediatr* 1989; 3:169–172.

17 Liebowitz L D, Koornhof H J, Barrett M et al. Bacterial meningitis in Johannesburg—1980–1982. *S Afr Med J* 1984; 66: 677–679.

18 Borgstein A. Pyogenic meningitis in children at Queen Elizabeth Central Hospital Blantyre. *Malawi Med Quart J* 1984; 17:26–27.

19 Cuevas L E & Hart C A. Acute bacterial meningitis in Malawi. *Malawi Med J* 1991; 7:2–6.

20 Dube S D & Shenderov B A. Incidence and pattern of bacterial meningitis in Lusaka. *Cent Afr J Med* 1983; 29:100–103.

21 Omanga U, Nethihinyurwa M, Shako D et al. Aspectes étiologiques et évolutifs des méningites purulentes de l'enfant à Kinshasa: analyse de 471 cases. *Méd d'Afrique Noire* 1980; 27:25–34.

22 Babalola A A & Coker A O. Pyogenic meningitis among Lagos children: causative organisms, age, sex and seasonal incidence. *Cent Afr J Med* 1982; 28:14–18.

23 Couprie F & Chippaux-Hyppolite C. Les méningites purulentes à Abidjan. *Méd Armées* 1977; 5:823–828.

24 Elzouki A Y & Vesikari T. First international conference on infections in children in Arab countries. *Pediatr Infect Dis* 1985; 4:527–531.

25 Cadoz M, Denis F & Diop Mar I. Etude épidémiologiques des cas de méningites purulentes hospitalisés à Dakar pendant la décennie 1970–79. *Bull World Health Organ* 1981; 59:575–584.

26 Benhassine M & Mered B. Les méningites purulentes en Algérie: étude bactériologique de 133 cas. *Arch Inst Pasteur Algér* 1969; 47:13–26.

27 Bhat B V, Verma I C, Puri R K, Srinivasan S & Nalini P. Prognostic indicators in pyogenic meningitis. *Indian Pediatr* 1987; 24:977–983.

28 Choo K F, Ariffin W A, Ahmad T, Lim W L & Gururaj A K. Pyogenic meningitis in hospitalized children in Kelantan Malaysia. *Ann Trop Paediatr* 1990; 10:89–98.

28 Sunakorn P, Lexomboon U & Sindhurat S. Acute bacterial meningitis at the children's hospital Bangkok. *J Med Assoc Thai* 1969; 52:1001–1011.

30 Naraqi S. Aetiology of acute bacterial meningitis in the highlands and islands of Papua New Guinea. *Papua New Guinea Med J* 1980; 23:108–110.

31 McKay T. Experience of changing antibiotic protocol in childhood bacterial meningitis in Vanuatu. *Trop Doct* 1989; 19:158–159.

32 Sharma A, Sharma D & Prabhakar P. Infectious meningitis at the university hospital of the West Indies. Review of clinical and laboratory findings (1965–1980). *West Indian Med J* 1984; 33:14–30.

33 Munoz A I. Bacterial meningitis in pediatric patients: a five year experience. *Bol Asoc Med P R* 1982; 74:62–65.

34 Bryan J P, de Silva H R, Tavares A, Rocha H & Scheld W M. Etiology and mortality of bacterial meningitis in North Eastern Brazil. *Rev Infect Dis* 1990; 12:128–135.

35 Juliet C, Rodriguez G, Marti A & Burgos O V. Meningitis bacteriana en el nino: experiencia con 441 casos. *Rev Med Chil* 1983; 111:690–698.

36 Cherigo-Quiros E Z & Rodriguez-French A. Meningitis bacteriana en Hospital Santo Tomas (1975–1982). *Rev Med Panama* 1984; 9:35–44.

37 Bohr V, Hansen B, Jessen O et al. Eight hundred and seventy-five cases of bacterial meningitis. I: Clinical data, prognosis and the role of specialized hospital department. *J. Infect* 1983; 7:21–30.

38 De Wals P, Hertoghe L, Boree-Grimee I et al. Meningococcal disease in Belgium. Secondary attack rate among household, day-care nursery and pre-elementary school contacts. *J Infect* 1981; 3(supplement I):53–61.

39 Caugant D A, Froholm L O, Bovre K et al.

Intercontinental spread of a genetically distinctive complex of clones of *Neisseria meningitidis* causing epidemic disease. *Proc Natl Acad Sci USA* 1986; 83:4927–4931.

40 Moore P S, Hierholzer J, De Witt W et al. Respiratory viruses and mycoplasma as cofactors for epidemic group A meningococcal meningitis. *JAMA* 1990; 264:1271–1275.

41 Adams RD, Kubik CS & Bonner FJ. The clinical and pathological aspects of influenzal meningitis. *Arch Pediatr* 1948; 65:354–376.

42 Geisler P J & Nelson K E. Bacterial meningitis without clinical signs of meningeal irritation. *South Med J* 1982; 75:448–450.

43 Thomson A P J, Hart C A & Sills J A. Meningococcal disease in Liverpool children 1977–1987: mode of presentation. *Pediatr Rev Commun* 1990; 5:109–116.

44 Salih M A M, Ahmed H S, Karrar Z A et al. Features of a large epidemic of group A meningococcal meningitis in Khartoum, Sudan in 1988. *Scand J Infect Dis* 1990; 22:161–170.

45 Whittle H C & Greenwood B M. Meningococcal meningitis in the northern savanna of Africa. *Trop Doct* 1976; 6:99–104.

46 Cuevas L E, Hart C A & Mughogho G. Latex particle agglutination tests as an adjunct to the diagnosis of bacterial meningitis: a study from Malawi. *Ann Trop Med Parasitol* 1989; 83:375–379.

47 Holland S J, Marzouk O, Thomson A P J, Sills J A & Hart C A. Sensitivity and specificity of serum antigen detection for diagnosis of meningococcal disease in children. *Serodiagn Immunother Infect Dis* 1990; 4:345–349.

48 Girgis N I, Farid Z, Mikhail I A et al. Dexamethasone treatment for bacterial meningitis in children and adults. *Pediat Infect Dis J* 1989; 8:848–851.

49 Lebel M H, Freij B J, Syrogiannopoulos G A et al. Dexamethasone therapy for bacterial meningitis. *New Engl J Med* 1988; 319:964–971.

50 Shann F, Barker J & Poore P. Chloramphenicol alone versus chloramphenicol plus penicillin for bacterial meningitis in children. *Lancet* 1985; ii:681–701.

51 Pecoul B, Varine F, Keita M et al. Long acting chloramphenicol versus intravenous ampicillin for treatment of bacterial meningitis. *Lancet* 1991; 338:862–866.

52 Gedde-Dahl T W, Hoiby E A & Eskerud J. Unbiased evidence on early treatment of suspected meningococcal disease. *Rev Infect Dis* 1990; 12:973–992.

53 Esso D V, Fontanals D & Uriz S. *Neisseria meningitidis* strains with decreased susceptibility to penicillin. *Pediatr Infect Dis* 1987; 6:438–439.

54 Allen K D. Penicillin-resistant pneumococci. *J Hosp Infect* 1991; 17:3–13.

55 Friedland I R & Klugman K P. Failure of chloramphenicol therapy in penicillin-resistant pneumococcal meningitis. *Lancet* 1992; 339:405–408.

56 Coovadia Y M, Coovadia H M & van den Ende J. Meningitis due to beta-lactamase producing, chloramphenicol resistant *Haemophilus influenzae* type b in South Africa. *J Infect* 1986; 12:247–249.

57 Peltola H, Anttila M & Renkonen O K. Randomized comparison of chloramphenicol, ampicillin, cefotaxime and ceftriaxone for childhood bacterial meningitis. *Lancet* 1989; i:1281–1287.

58 Thomson A P J, Sills J A & Hart C A. Validation of the Glasgow Meningococcal Septicaemia Prognostic Score. A ten year retrospective survey. *Crit Care Med* 1991; 19:26–30.

59 French M R. Epidemiological study of 383 cases of meningococcal meningitis in the city of Milwaukee, 1927, 1928 and 1929. *Am J Public Health* 1931; 21:130–138.

60 Greenwood B M, Bradley A K & Cleland P G. An epidemic of meningococcal meningitis at Zaria, Northern Nigeria. *Trans R Soc Trop Med Hyg* 1979; 73:557–573.

61 Cuevas L E & Hart C A. Chemoprophylaxis of bacterial meningitis. *J Antimicrob Chemother* 1993; 31:79–91.

62 Blakebrough I S & Gilles H M. The effect of rifampicin on meningococcal carriage in family contacts in northern Nigeria. *J Infect* 1980; 2: 137–143.

63 Glode M P, Daum R S, Goldmann D A, Leclair J & Smith A. *Haemophilus influenzae* type b meningitis: a contagious disease in children. *BMJ* 1980; i:899–901.

64 Reingold A C, Broome C V, Hightower A W et al. Age specific differences in duration of clinical protection after vaccination with meningococcal polysaccharide A vaccine. *Lancet* 1985; ii:114–118.

65 Booy R & Moxon E R. Immunization of infants against *Haemophilus influenzae* type b in the UK. *Arch Dis Child* 1991; 66:1251–1254.

66 Wenger J D, Pierce R, Deaver K A et al. Efficacy of *Haemophilus influenzae* type (b) polysaccharide–diphtheria toxoid conjugate vaccine in US children aged 18–59 months. *Lancet* 1991; 338:395–398.

67 Blakebrough I S, Greenwood B M, Whittle H C, Bradley A K & Gilles H M. Failure of meningococcal vaccination to stop the transmission of meningococci in Nigerian schoolboys. *Ann Trop Med Parasitol* 1983; 77:175–178.

68 Sierra G V G, Campa H C, Varacel N M et al. Vaccination against group B *Neisseria meningitidis*: protection trial and mass vaccination results in Cuba. *NIPH Ann* 1991; 14:195–210.

69 Bjune G, Hoiby E A, Gronnesby J K et al. Effect of outer membrane vesicle vaccine against group B meningococcal disease in Norway. *Lancet* 1991; 338:1093–1096.

CHAPTER 45

BRUCELLOSIS

S. G. Wright

Brucellosis is a zoonotic infection due, most often, to one of three species of the genus *Brucella*: *B. melitensis*, *B. abortus* and *B. suis*.[1] *B. canis*, *B. ovis* and *B. neotomae* are also recognized. The first of these causes occasional infections in man. The infection has a worldwide distribution, predominantly in rural areas among pastoralist peoples. It occurs in urban settings when small numbers of animals are kept in compounds around houses. Eradication campaigns have been successful in a number of areas but these required much effort and often considerable expense.

BACTERIOLOGY

CHARACTERISTICS AND GROWTH

These organisms are aerobic, Gram-negative bacilli or coccobacilli. They are non-motile and non-spore forming. Brucellae grow slowly in vitro on enriched media, such as serum dextrose agar, optimally at 37°C. *B. abortus* and *B. ovis* grow better in the presence of added CO_2. Slow growth in vitro requires that cultures be maintained and subcultured blindly for up to 6 weeks before discarding clinical samples for culture. Isolates from clinical material have a smooth appearance to the colonies; this becomes rough after a time in culture. Catalase production is uniformly present and oxidase production is a common feature. For a detailed description of microbiological features see Corbel.[1]

LABORATORY INFECTIONS

Laboratory transmission of *Brucella* spp. is a well-recognized occurrence and in endemic areas staff are well aware of this. An organism identified as *Moraxella phenylpyruvica* with a probability of 90.5% using the API20NE microbiological test strip was subsequently found to be *B. melitensis* using agglutinating sera.[2] Laboratories in countries where *Brucella* spp. isolates are uncommon should be aware of this potential problem.

TAXONOMY

Several biovars are recognized for each of the three main pathogens; *melitensis* (3 biovars), *abortus* (9) and *suis* (5). These species and biovars represent the presently accepted taxonomy for the genus but DNA homology studies have shown such uniformity among the genus as to challenge the current concepts. This may lead to revision in time.

ANTIGENS AND CROSS-REACTIONS

In agglutination reactions two lipopolysaccharide surface antigens, designated A and M, have been defined. These are the most studied of a wide range of brucella antigens. A antigen predominates in *abortus* and *suis*, while M is the major antigen in *melitensis*.[1]

Antigenic cross-reactivity exists between brucellae and a number of other Gram-negative species including *Escherichia coli* O116, *Francisella tularensis*, *Pseudomonas maltophila*, *Vibrio cholerae*, *Yersinia enterocolitica* serogroup O9, and *Salmonella urbana*.

EPIDEMIOLOGY

ANIMAL INFECTIONS

The three main pathogenic species are fairly restricted in their host specificities, with bovines harbouring *abortus*, goats, camels and sheep infected with *melitensis* and pigs with *suis*. Cross-infection among these animals can occur but the resulting infections are short lived. Infection in utero or early in life usually results in lifelong infection.

Infection in animals often causes abortion soon after acquisition of the organism, and thereafter latent infection recrudesces with subsequent pregnancy, causing congenital infection or milk-borne infection in the offspring. This pattern is similar for cattle, goats and sheep. Among pigs the boar transmits infection to sows through semen. Brucellosis causes considerable economic losses through reduced fecundity, fetal losses and diminished milk production.

TRANSMISSION

Several routes of transmission are possible. Ingestion of infected, unpasteurized milk is most readily thought of and, as brucellae are very acid sensitive, it is convenient to think of milk neutralizing gastric acid, allowing organisms to survive transit through the stomach to the duodenum where they enter the mucosa. It has been suggested that persons taking antacid medications or H_2-receptor antagonists have an increased risk of infection. Soft cheeses and similar products made from unpasteurized milk also transmit infection because the shorter time for preparation does not allow the pH to fall sufficiently to kill the organisms. It is also likely that organisms can enter through the epithelium overlying lymphoid tissue in the nasopharynx.

Aerosols occurring in laboratories or through splashing of amniotic fluid or milk may be infective through inhalation or contact with conjunctiva or nasopharynx. Semen may also be a route of transmission between humans, as may blood transfusion and organ transplantation. Brucellae may be introduced through cuts and abrasions on the hands. Congenital infection is also reported, as is infection through human breast milk.

The vaccine strains used in animals are not attenuated for humans and may cause human disease from accidental inoculation. Brucellae are capable of surviving for prolonged periods in the environment and so inhalation of contaminated dusts in hot, dry countries may be a source of infection.

DISTRIBUTION AND INCIDENCE

The disease occurs in all areas of the world with few countries spared. As it is frequently present in rural communities the infection may well go unrecognized. The frequency of animal infections is a useful guide to the likely occurrence in man. Human brucellosis is present in the countries of southern Europe. For example in France the incidence varies between 1.07 and 18.4 per 100 000 of the populations of different regions. Brucellosis due to *B. melitensis* was particularly common in Saudi Arabia and Kuwait in the 1980s, with an incidence increasing from 1.15 to 42.8 per 100 000 over the decade—to 1984—in Kuwait.

Because of the animal origin of infection there is a strong occupational predisposition to infection among those having close contact with animals or their infected milk or tissues. Shepherds, cowherds, swineherds, veterinarians and their assistants, abattoir workers and those handling meat, etc. in kitchens are all at risk. Laboratory infections with brucella are a particular concern and must be borne in mind when assessing infections in veterinary or hospital laboratory workers.

Both sexes and all age groups are susceptible to infection. Infections among children represent the minority of cases. There is evidence of an increased occurrence among males compared with females, though a recent study from Saudi Arabia[3] showed a higher incidence among females than males at all age groups between 15 and 64 years. Over 65 years the incidence was higher in males.

PATHOGENESIS AND PATHOLOGY

Brucellae are facultatitive intracellular pathogens. Within the body they are phagocytosed by neutrophils which kill *B. abortus* and avirulent—but not virulent, *B. melitensis*.[4] Complement enhances

phagocytosis. Macrophages subsequently become parasitized by the organisms.

In mice, numbers of organisms in liver and spleen macrophages rise progressively during the first 14 days of infection and then decline dramatically with the development of T-cell reactivity. The T-cells concerned have a suppressor–cytotoxic phenotype. In mice that have apparently contained the infection small numbers of persisting organisms can be isolated and it seems possible that these persisting organisms may give rise to the relapses that occur in brucellosis.

Antibody responses to brucellae are capable of affecting the progression of infection in mice receiving antilipopolysaccharide or antipeptidoglycan antibodies prior to inoculation of organisms. Their contribution to controlling infection in man is uncertain.

The pathological feature in affected tissues is granuloma formation. As the organism is widely distributed through the bloodstream these are found in many tissues. There are no characteristic features of the granuloma and the differential diagnosis of febrile illnesses associated with granuloma formation is considerable. There may be progression to microabscess formation around these granulomas. Clinically apparent abscess formation is not uncommon and may occur in a range of tissues, including the vertebrae.

CLINICAL FEATURES

The incubation period is about 2–4 weeks. This has been gauged most accurately in instances of laboratory infection resulting from a broken culture flask. The initial illness is non-specific, with fevers, lethargy, anorexia and night sweats. This illness, while causing marked symptoms, is often not troublesome enough to bring the patient to seek medical advice. Often it is the appearance of localized disease that brings this about. In this early phase enlargement of liver and spleen, present in 27% of a large series of cases, with perhaps lymph node enlargement may be the only clinical evidence.[5]

One of the names given to this infection was 'undulant fever', so called because of the waxing and waning of fever in a cycle lasting 2–4 weeks. This is not usually seen currently because the diagnosis is made before a sufficient time has passed to see the undulations but it was apparent to physicians in the preantibiotic era. The *Lancet* for 9 September 1899 carried an article describing several cases, including that of Almroth Wright who had injected himself with a living culture of brucellae to test the efficacy of a killed vaccine he had previously received. He became ill 16 days later with a fever showing an undulant pattern with a cycle of 4 weeks between the first two peaks. Other cases described show a range of periodicity to the undulations. These and other reports show that, while spontaneous resolution after weeks or months of clinical illness occurs, there was a mortality associated with brucellosis, estimated at up to 7%.

SKELETAL DISEASE

Bone and joint involvement is a particularly common feature, certainly in *B. melitensis* infections which have been the subject of study in large series of cases reported in recent years.[5,6] Where peripheral joints are involved it is usually a large weight-bearing joint such as hip or knee. Pain is severe and the patient may not be able to walk. Sacroiliitis is also common. Often the organisms cannot be isolated from joint fluid, suggesting that this is a reactive arthritis. Arthritis in the knee may cause posterior rupture of the joint capsule, giving the appearances of a ruptured Baker's cyst. True infective arthritis occurs and this is more likely in joints with pre-existing degenerative or other disease. While these are the joints affected most often, any joint may be affected; examples are the sternoclavicular joint and costochondral junctions.

Involvement of the axial skeleton is common.[7] This may present with sciatica in young adults, most likely the result of inflammation and swelling of the affected intervertebral disc(s). Infection of adjacent vertebral bodies may lead to abscess formation. This may affect any part of the spine but the lumbar region is an area of predilection. The clinical presentation is very similar to that of tuberculosis, particularly when brucella causes paravertebral or psoas abscess, and careful distinction of the two conditions is necessary.

LOCALIZATION TO OTHER SITES

Epididymo-orchitis is frequent, occurring in about 7% of cases. Renal involvement occurs and brucellae can be cultured from the urine. Pulmonary disease is not common. Endocarditis is one of the most serious complications affecting either a normal valve, the aortic, or a previously diseased valve, usually the mitral.

Neurological disease is infrequent but can cause a wide range of manifestations, including papilloedema, cranial neuritis, focal or diffuse cerebritis, encephalopathy, meningoencephalitis, parkinsonian syndromes and transient ischaemic episodes and vasculitis. Spinal involvement may present with cord compression due to vertebral abscess, a cauda equina syndrome, myelitis and myelopathy; peripheral nerve involvement can cause sensory and/or motor abnormalities affecting either single or multiple nerve roots.

Rashes have been described, as has ocular infection. Brucellosis can cause abortion but this may be an effect of the febrile illness rather than a specific feature of this infection, as is seen for example in cattle with *B. abortus*.

BRUCELLA AND HUMAN IMMUNODEFICIENCY VIRUS

Brucellar spp. infections have occurred in a number of patients with human immunodeficiency virus (HIV) infection and the acquired immune deficiency syndrome (AIDS). This is perhaps not unexpected in view of the frequency of infections with intracellular organisms. Further experience will show how often this infection will complicate the course of AIDS.

CHRONIC BRUCELLOSIS

Chronic infection is a feature that has long been associated with brucellosis, causing both protracted fever and recrudescent infection over many years with symptom-free periods intervening. Ten per cent of a series of cases from Kuwait had symptoms for more than 1 year. In individual cases it can be difficult to assess, requiring careful clinical assessment and serological testing with the use of more invasive procedures such as bone marrow examination and liver biopsy, as indicated clinically. The association between brucellosis and depression is one that is widely held, though the evidence for it is far from clear.

LABORATORY INVESTIGATIONS

CULTURE

Isolation and identification of the organism proves the diagnosis.[1] Blood is most often taken for culture and in standard media with blind subculture every 5 days it commonly takes 12 days before isolation and may take up to 6 weeks. Positive results are obtained in 14–50% of cases. Prior administration of the commonly used antibiotics interferes with growth of *Brucella*. Culture of bone marrow aspirate may give higher yields, for example a positive culture on 90% of samples from a series of cases of acute infection in Chile.[8] Pus or tissue obtained at biopsy should also be cultured in the investigation of febrile patients.

SEROLOGY

Serological testing alone will often not be diagnostic and the result or a series of results obtained over a period must be considered in relation to the case under investigation.[9] Occasionally, entirely paradoxical results are obtained; for example, negative agglutination tests when the organism has been isolated in culture. While this apparently does occur, a more common explanation is the presence of blocking antibodies which bind but do not agglutinate. These account for the prozone phenomenon which causes negative agglutination reactions at low dilutions of the test sera. As the blocking antibodies are present at low titre their effects are readily diluted out and testing at high dilution will give a positive agglutination. Smooth strains of brucellae should be used as antigen.

AGGLUTINATION REACTIONS

These are carried out by incubating a standard suspension of brucellae with test sera and assessing the highest dilution at which agglutination can be seen. In general a titre of 1:160 or over is associated with infection, though it must be stated that a titre below this level does not exclude infection. The value of the method is extended by treating the test sera with 2-mercaptoethanol (2-me) before retesting as this destroys IgM.

If an initial high titre positive test is reduced to a low titre positive this suggests that IgM is the major antibody class producing the effect and that the infection is recent, while a titre that is not affected by 2-me is due to IgG antibody and the infection is more long standing. Predominantly 2-me-labile responses suggest a low chance of relapse after treatment. IgG agglutinins disappear over a period of up to 30 months after treatment.

For many countries this method of measuring brucella antibody responses will remain the standard for some time to come because of the relative ease with which the test can be performed and the absence of specialized laboratory equipment needed to do it.

ANTIGLOBULIN TEST

This is a Coombs' test in which non-agglutinating antibody is detected by adding an antihuman globulin after thorough washing of the non-agglutinated antigen. It gives higher yields of positivity in chronic infections.

ENZYME LINKED IMMUNOSORBENT ASSAYS

These tests are in the process of being developed and offer the chance to use more specifically defined subcellular antigens.[10] Antibody classes may be more readily identified. Internationally agreed standardization of these procedures is awaited.

POLYMERASE CHAIN REACTION

This technique, which produces the multiplication of predetermined specific nucleotide sequences, offers great potential for the microbiological diagnosis of brucellosis because brucellae tend to be difficult to isolate by standard culture methods and the laboratory risks of handling this organism are considerable. The method has been applied successfully, though there are still obstacles to doing this test in field conditions.

OTHER INVESTIGATIONS

Normochromic normocytic anaemia with a white count in the normal range showing more or less equal numbers of lymphocytes and granulocytes are usual findings in the peripheral blood. Liver function tests show elevation of the alkaline phosphatase associated with granulomatous inflammation in the liver. There may be some elevation of transaminases. Globulins increase and albumin levels decline—non-specific effects of inflammation.

Radiological changes accompany skeletal involvement. Abnormal technetium bone scans may indicate brucella-induced inflammation before there is radiographic evidence of damage to bones and joints. In the vertebrae there may be swelling of intervertebral discs, demonstrable on computerized tomography. Bone destruction is usually evident on plain radiographs, with destruction of anterior superior margins of vertebrae. With increasing duration of untreated infection osteophyte formation will appear in addition to destruction. Soft tissue swelling may be visible around the affected area. Madkour and Sharif[11] have reviewed these radiological changes.

TREATMENT

In recent years there have been several prospective randomized studies of the treatment of brucellosis. Overall these have shown that probably the best results are obtained by the use of streptomycin 1.0 g intramuscularly daily for 14–21 days, together with doxycycline 200 mg daily for 6–12 weeks. Longer duration of treatment is needed when there is evidence of joint, neurological or other severe organ involvement. Endocarditis is a particular problem and long-term antibiotic treatment is usually combined with valve replacement.

Children under the age of 8 years cannot be given

tetracyclines; co-trimoxazole together with an aminoglycoside or rifampicin should be in appropriate doses for the same periods. Co-trimoxazole should not be given alone as it is associated with an unacceptably high relapse rate. In pregnancy, rifampicin should be given.

Doxycycline is now as cheap as tetracycline and should be used because the single daily dose is so much more convenient. A single dose of streptomycin is usually acceptable. The use of netilmicin instead of streptomycin is recommended by some authors but this is much more expensive than the latter and has to be given twice daily. The fluorinated quinolones have not proved effective in brucellosis. The chemotherapy of brucellosis has been reviewed.[12]

Where there are abscesses the pus should be evacuated, particularly when there is evidence of cord compression.

PREVENTION

For individuals in endemic areas the boiling of milk before drinking it or using it to make other products is protective. However, this commonly requires a change in behaviour which is not easy to bring about. When commercial dairy enterprises are set up they should ideally be stocked with brucella-free cattle and kept free of infection with regular serological testing to ensure this. Brucella eradication schemes using the attenuated Rev-1 (*B. melitensis*) or S19 (*B. abortus*) vaccines to protect animals who show no seroreactivity to agglutination tests and, ideally, destruction of reactors, will ultimately lead to control and eradication of this zoonosis but continued surveillance is necessary to ensure that reinfection does not occur. Eradication has been successful in a number of European countries but the costs have been high due to compensation payments. However, these costs have to be set against the economic benefits among human and animal populations resulting from eradication. As yet there is no vaccine that can be used in man.

REFERENCES

1 Corbel M J. Microbiological aspects. In Madkour M M (ed.) *Brucellosis*. London: Butterworth, 1989:29–44.

2 Microbiological test strip (API20NE) identifies *Brucella melitensis* as *Moraxella phenylpyruvica*. *Commun Dis Rep* 1991; 1:165.

3 Cooper C W. The epidemiology of human brucellosis in a well defined urban population in Saudi Arabia. *J Trop Med Hyg* 1991; 94:416–422.

4 Young E J, Borchert M, Kretzer F L et al. Phagocytosis and killing of *Brucella* by human polymorphonuclear leukocytes. *J Infect Dis* 1985; 151:682–690.

5 Lulu A R, Araj G F, Khateeb M I et al. Human brucellosis in Kuwait: a prospective study of 400 cases. *Q J Med* 1986; 66:39–54.

6 Madkour M M, Rahman A, Talukder M A & Kudwah A. Brucellosis in Saudi Arabia. *Saudi Med J* 1985; 6:324–332.

7 Ariza J, Gudiol F, Valverde J et al. Brucella spondylitis: a detailed analysis based on current findings. *Rev Infect Dis* 1985; 7:656–664.

8 Gotuzzo E, Carrillo C, Guerra J & Llosa L. An evaluation of diagnostic methods for brucellosis: the value of bone marrow culture. *J Infect Dis* 1986; 153:122–125.

9 Young E J. Serologic diagnosis of human brucellosis: analysis of 214 cases by agglutination tests and review of the literature. *Rev Infect Dis* 1991; 13:359–372.

10 Araj G F & Kaufmann A F. Determination by enzyme linked immunosorbent assay of immunoglobulin G (IgG), IgM and IgA to *Brucella melitensis* with major outer membrane proteins and whole-cell heat-killed antigens. *J Clin Microbiol* 1989; 27:837–842.

11 Madkour M M & Sharif H. Bone and joint imaging. In Madkour M M (ed.) *Brucellosis*. London: Butterworth, 1989:90–104.

12 Hall W H. Modern chemotherapy for brucellosis in humans. *Rev Infect Dis* 1990; 12:1060–1099.

CHAPTER 46

BARTONELLOSIS

G. Scott

Alternative names: Oroya fever, Guaitara fever, Carrión's disease, Verruga peruana.

Carrión, a medical student, infected himself with tissue from Verruga peruana, a cutaneous eruption of haemangioma-like growths, and developed Oroya fever, an acute febrile haemolytic illness, and died, thus establishing the intimate link between these two disparate clinical conditions.[1]

GEOGRAPHICAL DISTRIBUTION

Proven bartonellosis has a remarkable focal distribution, only occurring between latitudes S 09 and 16 between altitudes 800 and 3000 m on the Western slopes of the Andes in Columbia, Peru and Ecuador.[2,3] Furthermore, the infection tends to cause outbreaks only in narrow valleys (quebradas) where the vector proliferates. *Bartonella*-like infections associated with febrile anaemia or dermal nodules have been reported from Thailand, Sudan, Niger, Pakistan and the eastern USA but their relationship to *Bartonella bacilliformis* is not clear. Many of these will have been due to *Rochalimaea* (now renamed *Bartonella*) infections.

AETIOLOGY

B. bacilliformis occurs in two forms: one is a rod-shaped, slightly curved, Gram-negative bacillary organism, $2 \times 0.5 \mu$m, staining well with Giemsa, often in branching rods and chains but never crossed, which occurs in a large proportion of the red cells (Figure 46.1) during Oroya fever. V- and Y-shaped forms probably represent dividing organisms. The other form is coccoid about 1 μm or less in diameter, oval or pear-shaped and containing chromatin granules. They occur singly or end-to-end in pairs or chains.

Though aggressively motile, they are difficult to detect in fresh blood. When dried films are 'shadowed' with palladium and examined by bright field microscopy it is found that the organisms lie in depressions in red cells; by electron microscopy lashing flagella are visible, each with a diameter of 20 nm, in bundles of up to ten flagellae for each organism.

Bartonella resemble *Rickettsia* since both are minute, pleomorphic, Gram-negative and, though found intracellularly in vivo, are able to grow on solid media.[4] Recent work has shown a tenuous link between *B. bacilliformis* and organisms variously thought to cause cat-scratch disease or bacillary angiomatosis. The organism is closely related to *Brucella abortus* and *Rochalimaea quintana* by 16S

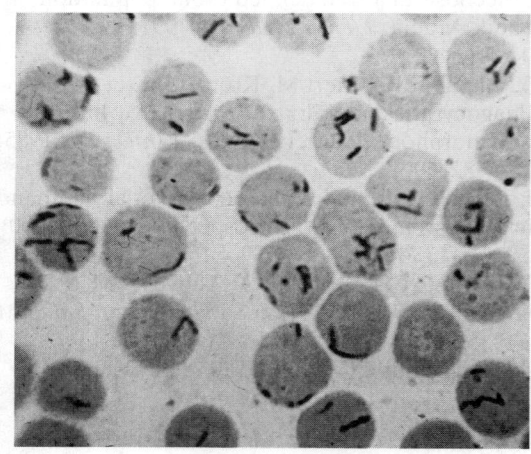

Figure 46.1 Bartonella bacilliformis in blood.

DNA hybridization[5] but a probe to detect a conserved region of *B. bacilliformis* by polymerase chain reaction from clinical specimens failed to recognize *Brucella abortus*.[6] More interestingly, *Rochalimaea* spp. have now been reclassified under the *Bartonellaceae*.[7] Thus when *Bartonella quintana* is transmitted by body louse (*Pediculus humanis corporis*) it is associated with trench fever, and *B. quintana* and *B. henselae* cause cat-scratch disease, bacillary angiomatosis, peliosis hepatis and disseminated infections in acquired immune deficiency syndrome (AIDS).[8] As yet the term bartonellosis is only applied to infections caused by *B. bacilliformis*.

Intravenous injection of *B. bacilliformis* into macaque monkeys causes irregular fever and anaemia, while the organisms can be demonstrated in the blood cells. Intradermal inoculation into the supraorbital tissues gives rise to verrugous nodules.

CULTURAL CHARACTERISTICS

Bartonella was first seen by Barton in 1909, then cultured on solid media from citrated blood of patients with Carrión's disease by Noguchi and Battistini in 1926. It is an obligate aerobe and grows best at 25–28°C on blood agar. Battistini's method of culture is simple: a small drop of blood from the finger of the patient is withdrawn into serum-agar or Noguchi's *Leptospira* medium, the vial sealed and incubated at 28°C. Colonies are visible in 5 or 6 days. *B. bacilliformis* is also readily cultivated in the allantoic fluid of the developing chick embryo at 25–28°C. The growth is rapid and abundant and the cultivated bodies are 0.6–1.6 μm in length. Zinsser's agar slant method for cultivation of rickettsiae may also be used.[9]

TRANSMISSION

Bartonella can be transmitted experimentally to monkeys and grey squirrels (*Citellus tridecemlineatus*). After inoculation of grey squirrels the organism could only be recovered for the first 24–48 hours and the animals were asymptomatic. Macaque rhesus monkeys were asymptomatic unless splenectomized and the blood from a patient with Oroya fever was then fatal.[9] *Bartonella*-like (*Haemobartonella muris*) bodies are found in the blood of healthy mice and certain rodents; they cannot be cultured and exist as a latent infection. They are transmitted by rat lice and after splenectomy cause an acute fatal anaemia resembling Oroya fever. A similar anaemia occurs in the dog after splenectomy when infected with *B. canis*. Verruga can be conveyed by inoculation to puppies and rabbits and *Bartonella* occurs as a natural infection in native American Indian dogs. However, human infection has not been clearly shown to be a zoonotic disease depending on a natural animal reservoir.

HUMAN RESERVOIR

It is probable that the main reservoir consists of asymptomatic human cases. *Bartonella* was cultured from seven of 81 students and three of these seven were asymptomatic. In the Verruga zone, 10–15% of people have been shown to be chronic carriers with positive blood cultures.[9,10] *B. bacilliformis* can be seen in the endothelial cells of cutaneous Verruga nodules, suggesting that they could act as a source of continuing infection to sandflies.

SANDFLY TRANSMISSION

The only proven vectors in man are New World sandflies, *Lutzomyia* spp.: *L. verrucarum* is the definitive vector.[11] Evidence incriminating *L. noguchii* (and *L. verrucarum*) was obtained when insects were collected in a Verruga district of Peru and sent to New York, where they were ground up in saline and injected intradermally into monkeys.[12] An outbreak of Oroya fever in the Mantaro valley of Peru occurred in the absence of *L. verrucarum* but *L. pescei* (rare below 2400 m) and *L. bicornutus* (rare above 2600 m) were identified as being prevalent in the area of the epidemic. The former species was thought to be more likely to be responsible for the outbreak because the cases occurred at higher altitudes.[13] In the Narino department of South-Western Colombia, the habits of *L. colombianus* are so like those of *L. verrucarum* that it may be a vector in this area. *L. noguchii* and *L. peruensis* are also suspected vectors.

The organisms adhere to the midgut of the sandfly in moderate numbers after feeding on infected patients and have been found occasionally on the proboscis of wild-caught sandflies, suggesting that transmission may be by mechanical inoculation during biting.

PATHOLOGY

RED BLOOD CELLS

The organisms invade erythrocytes, in which they multiply, causing destruction of the cells.[14] In severe cases, the blood count may drop in 3 or 4 weeks to 500 000/mm[3]. The anaemia is typically normocytic and hypochromic but may be macrocytic because of reticulocytosis or if there is associated dietary folate deficiency.[15] Destruction of the red cells is due to intravascular haemolysis; 50% of labelled erythrocytes have a half-life of 6 days (normal median survival 120 days). However, those red cells which survive this period have a normal survival rate. Normal erythrocytes injected into patients in the febrile anaemic phase behaved similarly, but red cells from a patient with Verruga peruana survived normally, suggesting that the patient had acquired resistance to the haemolytic process after cessation of the febrile stage.

There is an associated polymorphonuclear leucocytosis but without eosinophilia.

RETICULOENDOTHELIAL SYSTEM

The organism invade the cells of the reticuloendothelial system causing hyperplasia in the lymph glands, with proliferation of Kupffer cells of the liver and histiocytes in the spleen, bone marrow, kidneys, adrenals, pancreas, thyroid and testes. They also parasitize the endothelial lining cells of the blood and lymph vessels which may be so distended by closely packed masses of the parasites that infected cells can be detected on low-power microscopic examination of lymph glands, spleen, liver and intestines.[12] Marked changes are present in the liver, speen and bone marrow. In the liver, areas of degenerative and central necrosis are found around the hepatic veins. In the centre of the necrotic areas a yellow pigment resembling haemosiderin is present in abundance. The spleen is invariably enlarged and contains necrotic areas with pigment. The lymph glands contain large macrophage endothelial cells studded with bacteria. The bone marrow shows proliferation, necrosis and marked phagocytosis of the large endothelial cells. The malpighian bodies are not affected.

VERRUGA STAGE

The verrugous eruption is a sequela to the lesions in the reticuloendothelial system.[16] There is proliferation of the endothelium of the lymphatic channels which become obstructed by plasma cells and fibroblasts, but the structure is much more vascular than that of yaws which it otherwise resembles. The capillary blood vessels become dilated so that the granulomatous tumours are vascular, almost cavernous and apt to bleed profusely. Nodules of angioblasts around the blood vessels are characteristic of the disease. *B. bacilliformis* is seen in considerable numbers in the endothelial cells of cutaneous Verruga nodules, but distension of the cells is less than that seen in Oroya fever cases. Scanty bacteria may be found in blood corpuscles.

IMMUNITY

Recovery from the disease in any of its forms confers lasting immunity but this is not solely dependent on the presence of specific agglutinins in the blood.[17] Passage from the Oroya fever to the Verruga stage, which is a change in the host–parasite relationship resulting from the development of immunity, is accompanied by a diminution of symptoms. It was shown that graduated inoculation of verrugous material induces an artificial immunity.[12] In monkeys infected with Verruga tissue, splenectomy reverses the process and produces Oroya fever.

Serum antibodies which agglutinate the organism

in titres from 10 to 80 have been found in patients in both the Oroya fever and Verruga stages.[17,18] Cross-reactions occur with *Proteus* sp. OX19, OXK and OX2 (another tenuous link with rickettsiae). A strong agglutinating serum can be prepared for laboratory identification of *B. bacilliformis*.

Prophylactic inoculation with a formalinized suspension of *B. bacilliformis* resulted in partial immunity so that subsequent attacks of Oroya fever were modified.[17]

CLINICAL FEATURES[2]

NATURAL HISTORY

The spectrum of disease ranges from common asymptomatic carriage and to Verruga peruana, to the severe and often fatal Oroya fever.

SYMPTOMS AND SIGNS

OROYA FEVER

The incubation period of Oroya fever is about 3 weeks.[2,19] Its onset is insidious and is marked by malaise, soon followed by a rapidly developing anaemia and an irregular remittent pyrexia, associated with very severe pains in the head, joints and long bones. The bone pains are probably connected with the disturbances in the haemopoietic system. The initial fever is like that of malaria and the most severe illness resembles fulminating typhus and is known as the 'severe fever of Carrión'. The liver, spleen and lymph nodes are enlarged and tender.

A characteristic anaemia develops with a tendency to macrocytosis with nucleated red cells and a high reticulocytosis. In the febrile phase, most of the red cells contain numerous bacilliform organisms and there is a polymorphonuclear leucocytosis.

The death rate varies from 10 to 40%, death coming within 2 or 3 weeks of the onset of the disease. A terminal delirium is often noted. In those cases which proceed to the Verruga stage, the fever may last for 3 to 4 months. Superinfection with *Salmonella typhimurium* may prove fatal.[20]

VERRUGA PERUANA STAGE (LOCALIZED BARTONELLOSIS OR ERUPTIVE STAGE)

The latent interval subsequent to the development of Oroya fever is 30–40 days. Although Verruga is usually a sequel of Oroya fever, it may arise spon-

taneously as long as 2 months after exposure. The initial stages are characterized by rheumatic-like pains together with fever, the pains being like those of yaws only more severe. As in yaws, the constitutional symptoms subside on the appearance of the skin lesions. The eruption may be sparse or abundant, discrete or confluent. Some granulomas fail to erupt, others subside rapidly and others may continue to increase and then after remaining stationary for a time gradually wither, shrink and drop off without leaving a scar.

Two types of eruption are seen. The miliary eruption (Figure 46.2), not exceeding the size of a small pea, is found most abundantly on the face and extensor aspect of the extremities, less commonly on the trunk. A pink macule first appears, later darkening and becoming nodular. The Verruga artificially

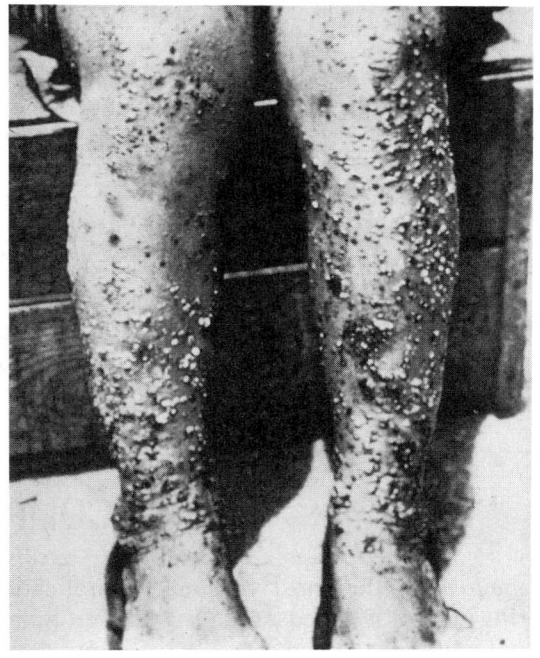

Figure 46.2 Verruga-like eruption in bartonellosis. (Courtesy of P. D. Marsden.)

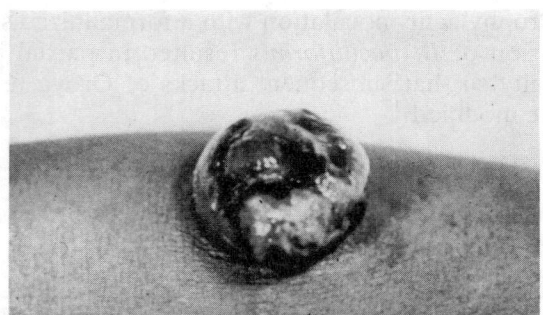

Figure 46.3   Giant nodule on the arm caused by bartonellosis. (Courtesy of P. D. Marsden.)

produced in monkeys by injection of *Bartonella* bodies is bright cherry-pink. The nodules, which are flat or somewhat pedunculated, are vascular and may develop on mucous surfaces in the mouth, oesophagus, stomach, intestine, bladder, uterus and vagina; hence the dysphagia which is a common symptom, and occasional haematemesis, melaena, haematuria and bleeding from the vagina.

The Oroya and Verruga stages frequently coexist and relapses of both the fever and the eruption may occur.

The nodular eruption (Figure 46.3) is rarer but more chronic than the miliary. Individual lesions can grow to the size of a pigeon's egg and may become strangulated and a source of danger from haemor-

rhage. This type does not invade the mucous membranes and is usually confined to the regions of the knees and elbows. It appears in crops and lasts 2–3 months. The mortality rate from Verruga is practically nil.

NEUROBARTONELLOSIS

Bartonella may invade the brain in large numbers in parasitized red cells.[21] The pathological changes are found in the ependyma and choroid plexus, the vessels of the meninges and in the neurones. Vascular changes include venous thrombosis, adventitious haemorrhage and characteristic glioepithelial verrucomas.

Clinically, nervous system involvement occurs during the haemolytic phase; the cerebral form presents as meningoencephalitis with or without convulsions and has a high mortality. The spinal form, which is less common, presents as spastic or flaccid paralysis which may leave permanent disability, and the neuronal forms appear during the Verruga stage arising from granulomas in the spinal or cranial nerves; these resolve with little or no disability. The cerebrospinal fluid shows raised protein with a pleocytosis and numerous intracellular *Bartonella*. Treatment is that of the systemic disease.

DIAGNOSIS

B. bacilliformis can be seen in the red cells on blood examination in the acute febrile stage(s) and in smears from Verruga. The organisms can be cultured from the blood on appropriate special media. Serology is of no practical use except perhaps in travellers who pass transiently through an endemic area.[18]

TREATMENT

Chloramphenicol (4.0 g daily in divided doses) is the antibiotic of choice. The fever subsides in 48 hours and there is a rapid return of the blood to normal.[22]

Other effective antibiotics include penicillin, tetracycline, streptomycin and co-trimoxazole.

COMPLICATIONS

Salmonellosis is the most frequent complication, occurring in 40–50% of cases of Oroya fever. Salmonella infection is shown by a worsening of the patient's condition and a recurrence of fever with gastrointestinal symptoms.

Other complications are thromboses, pleurisy, parotitis and meningoencephalitis; transitory arthralgia may precede the eruption.

DIFFERENTIAL DIAGNOSIS

The Oroya fever stage must be distinguished from other acute fevers like malaria, typhus, typhoid and acute haemolytic anaemia. The Verruga stage may resemble yaws or secondary syphilis. A single lesion may resemble a fibrosarcoma or angioma.

EPIDEMIOLOGY

HISTORY

It is probable that this disease existed in certain Andean valleys in north-west South America in pre-Columbian days. Many thousands died during the reign of the Inca Huayna Capac and it is possible that Pizarro's men also suffered from it.

The earliest account of this disease was that of Gago de Vadilla in 1630. In the 1870s when the central railway was being constructed from Lima to Oroya in Peru, a severe epidemic broke out among the construction workers, resulting in 7000 deaths. In 1906, out of 2000 men employed on tunnel work 200 perished. In 1885, the eponymous, Carrión, inoculated himself with blood from a Verruga nodule and died from Oroya fever, from which experiment Peruvian physicians deduced that Verruga and Oroya fever were different stages of the same disease.[1]

PRESENT STATUS

A considerable outbreak occurred in the Guaitara valley in southern Colombia near the Ecuador boundary in 1936, mainly in the valleys of the Mayo, Sambingo, Pacual and Juanambu tributaries in the Rio Patia. An outbreak with 200 deaths occurred in 1959 between January and April in the city of Anco which lies 2400 m above sea level in the valley of the Mantaro river in the Peruvian Andes.[13] Another outbreak with 28 symptomatic individuals (14 deaths) occurred between February and October 1987 in Shuapillar, also in Peru.[23] It is thought that Oroya fever has again become a serious problem in Peru following the cessation of spraying which was part of the malaria eradication programme.

The range of the infection is singularly limited and is confined to certain narrow valleys and ravines, the inhabitants of neighbouring places being exempt. The disease is acquired only at night and a single night's residence in an endemic area may be sufficient. During the outbreak in the 1870s on the central railway in Peru, infection could be avoided by leaving the endemic area before nightfall. The disease is most prevalent from January to April when streams are in flood, the air hot, still and moist, malaria epidemic and insect life abundant.

CONTROL

Control of the vector sandflies is easily obtained with DDT and sandflies have been eradicated from human habitations.[24]

REFERENCES

1 Schultz M G. Daniel Carrión's experiment. *N Engl J Med* 1968; 278:1323–1326.
2 Ricketts W E. Clinical manifestations of Carrión's disease. *Arch Intern Med* 1949; 84:751–781.
3 Dooley J R. Haemotropic bacteria in man. *Lancet* 1980; ii:1237–1239.
4 Peters D & Weigand R. Bartonellaceae. *Bacteriol Rev* 1955; 19:150–159.
5 Brenner D J, O'Connor S P, Hollis D G, Weaver R E & Steigerwalt A G. Molecular characterization and proposal of a neotype strain for *Bartonella bacilliformis*. *J Clin Microbiol* 1991; 29:1299–1302.
6 Maas M, Schreiber M & Knobloch J. Detection of *Bartonella bacilliformis* in cultures, blood and formalin preserved skin biopsies by use of the

polymerase chain reaction. *Trop Med Parasitol* 1992; 43:191–194.

7 Brenner D J, O'Connor S P, Winkler H H & Steigerwalt A G. Proposals to unify the genera *Bartonella* and *Rochalimaea*. *Int J Syst Bacteriol* 1993; 43:777–786.

8 Cockerell C J. *Rochalimaea* infections. *Curr Opinion Infect Dis* 1995; 130–136.

9 Weinman D J & Pinkerton H. Carrión's disease. Experimental production in animals. Natural sources of *Bartonella* in the endemic zone. Studies on *Phlebotomus* as the possible vector. *Proc Soc Exp Biol Med* 1938; 37:594–600.

10 Herrer A. Carrión's disease. Presence of *Bartonella bacilliformis* in the peripheral blood of patients with the benign form. *Am J Trop Med Hyg* 1953; 2:645–649.

11 Townsend C H T. The transmission of Verruga by *Phlebotomus*. *JAMA* 1913; 61:1717–1718.

12 Pinkerton H & Weinman D J. Carrión's disease. Behaviour of the etiological agent within cells growing or surviving in vitro. Comparative morphology of the etiological agent in Oroya fever and Verruga peruana. *Proc Soc Exp Biol Med* 1937; 37:587–593.

13 Herrer A & Blancas F. Estudios sobre la enfermedad de Carrión en el valle interandino del Matvjaro I. Observaciones entomologicas. *Rev Med Exp* 1959; 13:27–45.

14 Benson L A, Kar S, McLaughlin G & Ihler G M. Entry of *Bartonella bacilliformis* into erythrocytes. *Infect Immun* 1986; 54:347–353.

15 Reynafarje C & Ramos J. The haemolytic anaemia of human bartonellosis. *Blood* 1961; 17:562–578.

16 Arias-Stella J, Lieberman P H, Erlandson R A & Arias-Stella J Jr. Histology, immunohistochemistry and ultrastructure of the Verruga in Carrión's disease. *Am J Surg Pathol* 1986; 10:595–610.

17 Howe C. Carrión's disease. Immunologic studies. *Arch Intern Med* 1943; 72:147–167.

18 Knobloch J, Solano L, Alvarez O et al. Antibodies to *Bartonella bacilliformis* as determined by fluorescent antibody test, indirect haemagglutination and ELISA. *Trop Med Parasitol* 1985; 36:183–185.

19 Ricketts W E. Carrión's disease. A study of the incubation period in thirteen cases. *Am J Trop Med* 1947; 27:657–659.

20 Cuardra M. Salmonellosis complication in human bartonellosis. *Tex Rep Biol Med* 1956; 14:97–113.

21 Trelles J O. In Spillane JD (ed.) *Tropical Neurology*. Oxford: Oxford Medical Publications, 1973:387.

22 Urteaga B O & Payne E H. Treatment of the acute febrile phase of Carrión's disease with chloramphenicol. *Am J Trop Med Hyg* 1955; 4:507–511.

23 Gray G C, Johnson A A, Thornton S A et al. An epidemic of Oroya fever in the Peruvian Andes. *Am J Trop Med Hyg* 1990; 42:215–221.

24 Hertig M & Fairchild G B. Control of *Phlebotomus* in Peru with DDT. *Am J Trop Med* 1948; 28:207–230.

CHAPTER 47

TULARAEMIA

G. Scott

An acute febrile zoonotic infection. The causative organism is distinguished from other parvobacteria and has been named *Francisella tularensis* after Edward Francis, an American bacteriologist who studied the agent and pathogenesis.

Tularaemia is an infectious disease of rodents caused by *Francisella tularensis* which is transmitted from these animals to man by the bite of infected blood-sucking insects, by handling infected animals, by the ingestion of infected meat or water or by the inhalation of contaminated aerosols or dust. It is also known locally as deer fly fever, Pahvant Valley plague, rabbit fever, Ohara disease, yatobyo (Japan) or lemming fever.

GEOGRAPHICAL DISTRIBUTION

Human tularaemia has been recognized in relatively restricted geographical environments in North America, Europe and the former Soviet Republics and also to a lesser extent in Japan.[1]

AETIOLOGY

F. tularensis is a small, non-motile, aerobic Gram-negative, coccobacillus measuring $0.2 \times 0.2–0.7\,\mu$m. Some of the organisms pass through coarser bacterial filters. Possession of a capsule confers virulence and is seen consistently in isolates from human infections. The organisms stain in tissue preparation with Giemsa, but stain poorly with Gram; in smears from cultures they show up well with aniline gentian violet. Immunofluorescent techniques can be used to specifically identify the organisms in clinical material.[2]

The organism is not difficult to culture on chocolated blood agar rich in cystine, aerobically at 37°C, but it will not grow well on ordinary blood or nutrient agar. Most blood culture media will support growth but animal blood or spleen can be inoculated directly on to media enriched with cystine and thiamine with satisfactory results. Cystine agar consists of beef infusion agar (pH 7.6), to which 0.02% of cystine is added. Growth appears on about the third day and flourishes luxuriantly in subcultures without the addition of fresh animal tissue. The organism causes green staining of blood and brown staining of chocolated blood. To ensure the primary growth it is necessary that a piece of animal tissue be added to the medium. Tissue should be rubbed into agar and then left on the medium. Fermentation of glucose, laevulose, maltose and glycerine occurs with acid formation. Intraperitoneal injection of fresh capsulate isolates causes death in guinea-pigs in 5–10 days. Cultures of *F. tularensis* are very infectious to the microbiology staff and should be handled with great care.

There are two broad types of infection in man, one associated with a rabbit reservoir and a tick vector, with 5–7% mortality, and the other which is less virulent and is associated with rodents. Two biovars are recognized: *tularensis* (causing type A, the more serious infection) and *palaearctica* (causing type B or milder disease).[3] Type A predominates in North America, type B in Europe. It is not easy to separate the biovars in the laboratory.

TRANSMISSION

F. tularensis is transmitted in nature by a wide variety of routes but the three main ones appear to be: (1) between rodents in water and by close contact; (2) to carnivores by consumption of infected rodents; and (3) to birds and larger animals by ticks, biting flies and mosquitoes. Man acquires the infection by direct contact from skinning rabbits, by eating them as food and from tick, horse-fly and mosquito bites. Outbreaks may be associated with inhaled dust in rural areas, particularly where the rodent population increases and then becomes epizootically infected. It can also be easily acquired in the laboratory.

WATER-BORNE INFECTION

The infection is maintained among rodents mainly in water. The water is contaminated by dead animals and excreta and large numbers of rodents may be infected and die in this way.

INGESTION

Carnivora are infected chiefly from the consumption of sick, infected rodents which are easy to catch.

Domestic cats may become infected in this way and then transmit the organisms to man by biting.[4,5]

INSECT VECTORS

A wide variety of ticks can act as vectors. The nymph stages feed on small rodents and adults feed on larger mammals, including man. The infection persists during the development of the tick but infection is also transmitted transovarially. By this method infection can be maintained through the winter.

Dermacentor andersoni (wood tick), *D variabilis, D. occidentalis, Ixodes ricinus* and *Haemaphysalis leporispalustris* (rabbit tick) can all transmit the infection. *D. andersoni* is particularly important in the USA and *F. tularensis* is found in the intestinal lumen, in the cells of the gut wall, in the body fluids and in the faeces. The organism can also be transmitted by biting fleas, the deer fly (*Chrysops discalis*) as well as the stable fly (*Stomoxys calcitrans*), the squirrel flea (*Ceratophyllus acutus*), the rabbit louse (*Haemodipus ventricosus*) and the mouse louse (*Polyplax serratus*). The bacteria may be found in bed bugs or mites but it is not certain how important these are in transmission. *Aedes* and *Theobaldia* spp. mosquitoes have been shown to transmit *F. tularensis* under experimental conditions, and in Sweden *Aedes cinereus* does so in nature. Mosquitoes transmit the infection to and between birds.

PATHOLOGY

Since the disease is rarely fatal in man, the pathology is best seen in infected animals. The pathological appearances of infected guinea-pigs and rabbits at autopsy resemble those of plague. In an experimentally-infected guinea-pig, there is haemorrhagic oedema at the site of inoculation, blood-stained peritoneal exudate and a diffusely enlarged spleen with characteristic small necrotic foci. Similar lesions may be detected in the liver. On microscopic section of these organs, a dense infiltration with polymorphonuclear cells can be found but the organisms can be detected only with difficulty. In the spleen of the mouse, on the other hand, little or no leucocytic response occurs and *F. tularensis* can be demonstrated in large numbers. In the few recorded autopsies in man, nodules have been found in the lung and spleen.

IMMUNITY

There is a great deal of interest in the immunopathology of tularensis, a typical intracellular infection where cell-mediated immunity plays an important part in response to infection.[6-8] Infection induces long-lasting immunity in man and there is no record of a second generalized attack. However, local reinfection may occur and persistent infection in those treated with bacteriostatic antibiotics is not infrequent. Agglutinating antibodies appear in the serum in the second week and reach maximum between the fourth and eighth weeks, after which there is a gradual fall, but they may persist for as long as 11 years. Serum antibodies can be used in diagnosis but cross-reactions occur with *Brucella* *melitensis* and *B. abortus* (23% of tularaemia sera cross react with *B. melitensis* and *B. abortus* and 35% of *B. melitensis* and *B. abortus* with tularaemia). In 13% of cases of tularaemia, the serum agglutinates *Proteus* OX19 at a titre of 80 or over.

Type IV hypersensitivity can be demonstrated by an intradermal test employing a suspension of killed organisms, and peripheral lymphocytes proliferate in response to *F. tularensis* antigens.[9]

CLINICAL FEATURES

SUBCLINICAL INFECTIONS

Seroprevalence surveys during outbreaks and in areas of hyperendemicity reveal that the majority acquire *F. tularensis* asymptomatically or without a characteristic infection. In Sweden, up to 23% of a population studied had been infected, the infection being subclinical in a third of those with positive reactions. The disease presents in a number of ways depending on the route of infection. The incubation period is 1–10 days.

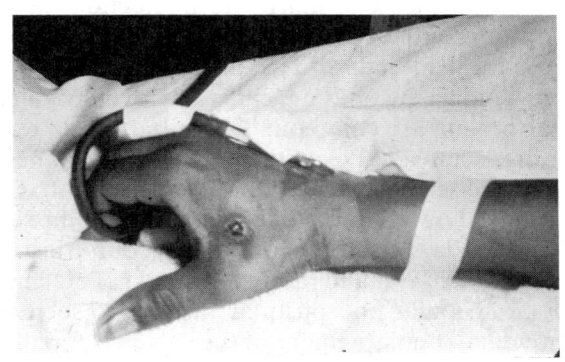

Figure 47.1   An ulcer on the hand in tularaemia. (Courtesy of WTIM.)

CUTANEOUS (ULCEROGLANDULAR) FORM (APPROXIMATELY 60% OF CASES)[10]

Local cutaneous disease results from infection from the bite of an infected tick or fly or direct contact of the broken skin with an infected source. An inflamed papule develops at the site of infection, which becomes pustular with a necrotic centre. This separates, leaving a punched-out ulcer (Figure 47.1) which is replaced by a scar on healing. Small sores on the hands are usually not diagnosed as tularaemia. Often, however, there is painful enlargement of the local lymph glands which may suppurate after 1–2 months and may remain enlarged for 2–3 months. A glandular form of the disease may be seen (in about 15% of cases) without any sore. Sometimes the local lesion is associated with general signs of infection such as fever and prostration.

OPHTHALMIC (OCULOGLANDULAR) FORM (1% OF CASES)

The site of entry of infection is the conjunctival sac, which is usually involved unilaterally. The patient may have rubbed the eyes while handling infected material or have been bitten on the eyelid by an infected insect. There is itching, lacrimation, photophobia and pain in the eye with swelling of the preauricular, parotid, submaxillary and cervical lymph glands. The eyelids become swollen and the conjunctiva red and covered with small discrete nodules and grey exudate. Punched-out ulcers develop and last for 2–3 weeks. Suppuration of the glands is common. Dacryocystitis and corneal ulcers occur, and permanent impairment of vision may follow.

ORAL AND ABDOMINAL FORM

This follows ingestion of infected meat or other food contaminated by rodent excreta. There is a necrotizing pharyngitis with abscesses on the roof of the mouth, fever, enlargement of local lymph glands and sometimes abdominal pain, vomiting and diarrhoea. Peritonitis may develop with persistent ascites, appendicitis or intestinal haemorrhage.

PNEUMONIC AND TYPHOIDAL (SEPTICAEMIC) FORMS (ABOUT 18% OF CASES)

This form may arise primarily from infection via the respiratory route or as a late result of dissemination from a local infection. The onset is sudden with severe headache, vomiting, chills and fever. Myalgia and arthralgia are common. The initial rise in temperature is above 40°C, with generalized weakness, aching, prostration, sweats and loss of weight. The fever may show an initial rise followed by remission and a secondary rise or a continuous course lasting usually 10–15 days, and rarely 3–4 weeks. Petechial, roseolar, papular and pustular rashes are seen. A slightly tender enlargement of the spleen is found in one-third of cases. There may be a moderate polymorphonuclear leucocytosis of $12–15 \times 10^9/1$, but more often in this infection the white count is normal.

In one-half of the cases, pulmonary symptoms develop. Pulmonary involvement results in dyspnoea and pleuritic pain. Milder forms resemble atypical pneumonia but may last for a month. There may be pleurisy, effusion, pneumonic consolidation or lobular bronchopneumonia with abscess and cavitation in severe cases and occasionally pericarditis. There is an associated enlargement of the bronchial and mediastinal glands.

Dissemination may lead to meningitis, which mimics tuberculous meningitis, or osteomyelitis.

COURSE

The infection is rarely fatal but in a series of severe untreated cases there was a mortality rate of 62% in pulmonary and 20% in typhoidal forms of the disease. The mean duration of fever in untreated cases is 26 days and adenopathy may last for 3–4 months. In one-third of cases, recovery is slow, the debilitating effect being very marked and lassitude persisting for months. *F. tularensis* may remain dormant intracellularly for years.

DIAGNOSIS

The diagnosis is suspected only by a keen clinical awareness of behavioural risk in the patient and a local geographical pathology. The differential diagnosis of the local form must be made from anthrax, plague, tick typhus and rat bite fever.[11] The organism is isolated from an ulcer or lymph node aspirate on enriched agar or broth or by inoculation into guinea-pigs, mice or rabbits, from whose tissues the organism may be isolated on special media as described. The organisms are rarely present in the blood.[12] A serological diagnosis may be attempted using agglutination tests with cultures of *F. tularensis* from the spleens of infected mice in a formalinized citrate suspension but cross-reactions with undulant and typhus fevers may occur.

The differential diagnosis of the pulmonary form of tularaemia[13] includes all the causes of atypical pneumonia, including legionellosis, psittacosis, Q fever, *Mycoplasma pneumoniae* and *Chlamydia pneumoniae*.

TREATMENT

Streptomycin is extremely effective: 1 g intramuscularly daily for 7 days will terminate the infection. Gentamicin is a suitable, less toxic alternative. The patient should be kept in bed for a time after subsidence of the fever and convalescence should be prolonged. More recently, tetracycline (250 mg four times daily for 2 weeks) has been preferred but there may be a relapse. Although erythromycin may be selected empirically to treat atypical pneumonia, and has been successful in tularaemia,[14] it is worth noting that some strains are constitutively resistant.

The fluoroquinolones are very active in vitro and have been successful in treating the few cases where they have been tried.[15,16]

EPIDEMIOLOGY

Tularaemia in man is essentially a rural infection and has a varying epidemiology according to the area in which it occurs and the method of transmission. Several important methods of acquisition have been identified.

1. Vector-borne: by ticks, tabanid flies and mosquitoes.
2. Trapping: from the skins of infected rodents, musk-rats and rabbits.
3. Hunting: from the consumption of rabbit meat.
4. Water-borne: from the water of streams infected by dead rats; well water infected by mice and field voles.
5. Agricultural: from working in haystacks contaminated by field voles and mice; processing of agricultural products; airborne transmission by contaminated dust.
6. Domestic: use of grain and other products contaminated by mice; from domestic cats.
7. Laboratory infections: presumably by the aerosol route or by accidental ingestion.
8. Wartime: trench and foxhole outbreaks.

Outbreaks in man invariably follow natural epizootics of different species of wild mammals.

NATURAL INFECTIONS

F. tularensis occurs as a natural infection of wild rodents, especially rats, field mice, hares and rabbits. It has an extremely wide host range and many other species of animals as well as birds can be infected.[17]

USA:	wandering shrew, grey fox, dog, cat, various ground squirrels (Pirote, Wyoming, Beechey's and Columbian), chipmunk, beaver, wood rat, white-footed mouse, meadow mouse and varieties (Sawatch and Tule) of musk-rat and brown rat (*Rattus norvegicus*), varying hare, jack rabbit, black-tailed jack rabbit, cottom-tail rabbit, sheep, calves, ruffed grouse, sharp-tailed grouse, bobwhite quail and horned owl.
Canada:	Richardson's ground squirrel, Osgood's white-footed mouse, Drummond meadow mouse, varying hare, white-tailed jack rabbit and Franklin's gull.
Sweden:	lemming and varying hare.
Central Europe:	rabbit and hare.
USSR (formerly):	introduced musk-rat, little ground squirrel, steppe lemming, water rat, continental vole, large water vole, house mouse, long-tailed field mouse and hamster.
Asia Minor:	continental vole, house and harvest mouse.
Japan:	local rabbit.

NORTH AMERICA

In North America the most important reservoirs of infection are the jack rabbit, hare and their relatives. The infection is found in Wyoming and Montana in streams contaminated by dead beavers, which have been found in large numbers. Man acquires the infection as a hunter from skinning rabbits, and preparing carcasses for cooking and also after tick and deer fly (*Chrysops discalis*) bites. Occasionally contact with sheep is the source of infection. The disease is most prevalent during the months of June, July and August.[18]

EUROPE

In Sweden the lemming and varying hare are the main reservoirs, and tularaemia is known as 'lemming fever'; it is caused by contact with infected water contaminated by the bodies and excreta of infected lemmings. Outbreaks have occurred in peasant women who go barefoot in summer and are bitten by numerous mosquitoes (*Aedes cinereus*). A very large outbreak involving 676 identified cases occurred in Sweden in the winter of 1966 in which the likely source was airborne dust from hay contaminated by vole faeces.[19] In Austria, the Czech and Slovak Republics and in Poland, the rabbit and hare are the main reservoirs. In France, the infection has become much more common since the introduction of hares from central Europe for sporting purposes. In northern Europe cases occur from July to October and in southern Europe from June to August.

THE FORMER USSR

In Russia, the water rat and introduced musk-rat, which spread widely in the Ukraine after the disturbance caused by the great tank battles of the Second World War (1939–45), are the main reservoirs. There was a great increase in the number of human infections after the war. In Central Asia *Microtus* and *Arvicola* are the predominant rat hosts.

PREVENTION

Prevention depends upon avoidance of the circumstances leading to infection in the various endemic areas. Rabbits should not be skinned without gloves and sick rabbits should not be eaten. However, proper cooking destroys the organism, as does prolonged freezing. Experimental work with *F. tularensis* in the laboratory must be undertaken with great caution. Killed and live attenuated vaccine strains have been used in the former Soviet Republics for years. Live attentuated vaccines are much more effective than killed ones and induce cell-mediated immunity.[9,20] They do not reduce the risk of ulceroglandular disease but simply the danger from bacteraemia.

REFERENCES

1 Ohara Y, Sato T, Fujita H, Ueno T & Homma M. Clinical manifestations of tularaemia in Japan: analysis of 1355 cases observed between 1924 and 1987. *Infection* 1991; 19:14–17.

2 Eigelsbach H T & McGann V G. Genus *Francisella*. In Krieg NR & Holt JG (eds) *Bergey's Manual of Systemic Bacteriology*, Vol. 1. Baltimore, MD: Williams & Wilkins, 1984: 394–399.

3 Uhari M, Syrjala H & Salminen A. Tularaemia in children caused by *Francisella tularensis* biovar *palaearctica*. *Pediatr Infect Dis J* 1990; 9:80–83.

4 Liles W C & Burger R J. Tularaemia from domestic cats. *West J Med* 1993; 158:619–622.

5 Cappelan J & Fong I W. Tularaemia from a cat bite: case report and a review of feline-associated tularaemia. *Clin Infect Dis* 1993; 16:472–475.

6 Tarnvik A. Nature of protective immunity to *Francisella tularensis*. *Rev Infect Dis* 1989; 11:440–451.

7 Surcel H M. Diversity of *Francisella tularensis* antigens recognised by human T lymphocytes. *Infect Immun* 1990; 58:2664–2668.

8 Karttunen R, Surcel H M, Andersson G, Eicre H P & Herve E. *Francisella tularensis*-induced in vitro gamma interferon, tumor necrosis factor alpha, and interleukin 2 responses appear within two weeks of tulareaemia vaccination in human beings. *J Clin Microbiol* 1991; 29:753–756.

9 Waag D, Galloway A, Sandstrom G et al. Cell mediated and humoral responses induced by scarification vaccination of human volunteers with a new lot of the live vaccine strain of *Francisella tularensis*. *J Clin Microbiol* 1992; 30:2256–2264.

10 Rohrbach B W, Westerman E & Istre G R. Epidemiology and clinical characteristics of tularaemia in Oklahoma, 1979–1985. *South Med J* 1991; 84:1091–1096.

11 Kostman J R & DiNubile M J. Nodular lymphangitis: a distinctive but often unrecognised syndrome. *Ann Intern Med* 1993; 118:883–888.

12 Hoel T, Scheel O, Nordahl S H & Sandvik T. Water- and airborne-*Francisella tularensis* biovar *palaearctica* isolated from human blood. *Infection* 1991; 19:348–350.

13 Scofield R H, Lopez E J & McNabb S J. Tularaemia pneumonia in Oklahoma 1982–1987. *J Okl State Med Assoc* 1992; 85:165–170.

14 Harrell R E Jr & Simmons H F. Pleuropulmonary tularaemia: successful treatment with erythromycin. *South Med J* 1990; 83:1363–1364.

15 Syrjala H, Schildt R & Raisaninen S. In vitro susceptibility of *Francisella tularensis* to fluoroquinolones and treatment of tularaemia with norfloxacin and ciprofloxacin. *Eur J Clin Microbiol Infect Dis* 1991; 10:68–70.

16 Scheel O, Hoel T, Sandvik T & Berdal B. Susceptibility pattern of Scandinavian *Francisella tularensis* isolates with regard to oral and parenteral antimicrobial agents. *Acta Pathol Microbiol Immunol Scand* 1993; 101:33–36.

17 Burrough A L, Holdenreid R, Longanecker D S & Meyer K F. A field study of latent tularaemia in rodents with a list of all known naturally infected vertebrates. *J Infect Dis* 1945; 76:115–119.

18 Cumming H S. La tularémie aux Etats-Unis. *Bull Off Int Hyg Publique* 1937; 29:2532–2535.

19 Dahlstrand S, Ringertz O & Zetterburg B. Airborne tularaemia in Sweden. *Scand J Infect Dis* 1971; 3:7–16.

20 Fortier A H, Slayter M V, Ziemba R, Meltzer M S & Nacy C A. Live vaccine strain of *Francisella tularensis*: infection and immunity in mice. *Infect Immun* 1991; 59:2922–2928.

CHAPTER 48

TETANUS

Michael D. Smith

Tetanus is a highly characteristic disease caused by a potent neurotropic toxin produced by *Clostridium tetani*, an ubiquitous organism found in soil throughout tropical and temperate regions of the world (see also Chapter 8). Despite being entirely preventable by immunization with a toxoid, it remains one of the leading causes of death in developing countries.

Although tetanus was described by Hippocrates, it was in the late nineteenth century that the nature of the disease was elucidated. Pirigov postulated that the cause was an infectious agent, and later a bacillus was described in smears from the wound of a patient with tetanus.[1] In 1884 Rattone demonstrated that the causative agent could be transmitted to rabbits by inoculation of pus from the man's infected wound. Nicolaier found that inoculation of animals with soil frequently produced the signs of tetanus, and Rosenbach (1886) described the classical 'drumstick' bacillus in pus from a human case. In 1889 Kitasato succeeded in isolating a pure culture of the organism, and subsequently Behring and Kitasato injected a culture filtrate into animals and produced an antibody that could neutralize the toxic agent.[2]

Tetanus is a generalized or localized hypertonia of skeletal muscles, frequently accompanied by paroxysmal muscular spasms. Tetanus is derived from the Greek *tetanos* (a muscular spasm), which in turn is derived from the Greek verb *teino* (to stretch).

EPIDEMIOLOGY

C. tetani is found worldwide, but the disease it causes is now primarily confined to developing countries where immunization is not available to the majority of the population at risk. In these countries tetanus remains one the most common infectious causes of death, particularly of neonates but also of children and young adults.

Tetanus occurs following the inoculation of spores of *C. tetani* into a wound or devitalized tissue. In neonatal tetanus the site of infection is invariably the umbilical stump which is contaminated by the local application of soil, cow dung and other substances, or from dirty instruments used to cut the umbilical cord. In children and adults the site of infection is commonly a laceration or puncture wound on the lower limb, which may be severe or trivial. Other portals of entry include, middle ear infections, postpartum or postabortion infections of the uterus, non-sterile intramuscular injections, animal bites, ear piercing and other ritual practices that puncture the skin. The site of entry is not evident in 10–20% of patients.[3]

It has been estimated that tetanus causes up to half a million deaths per year worldwide. In developing countries 70–80% of deaths occur in neonates although this age group accounts for only 20–30% of all cases of tetanus. In developed countries such as the USA a few cases of tetanus still occur each year but most occur in adults over 50 years of age in whom immunization is inadequate or who were never immunized.[4] A small but significant proportion of cases are intravenous drug addicts.

BACTERIOLOGY

C. tetani is a strictly anaerobic Gram-positive bacillus found in soil and animal faeces. When subjected to adverse conditions rounded terminal spores are formed; this gives the classical 'drumstick' appearance to the bacillus, although this is not always seen. *C. tetani* is described as Gram positive but from cultures more than 24 hours old it is readily decolorized and thus appears Gram negative. It is motile by means of numerous flagellae and when cultured on blood agar this results in swarming, giving a film with a feathery margin on the surface of the agar. Increasing the concentration of agar in the medium will inhibit swarming. Discrete colonies are flat, translucent and show a narrow zone of haemolysis.

The biochemical activity of *C. tetani* is limited. In general it does not ferment sugars, although some strains will ferment glucose. Gelatin is slowly hydrolysed but other proteins used in laboratory tests are not digested. Indole is produced slowly, but not hydrogen sulphide. Neither lecithinase nor lipase are produced. Gas–liquid chromatography of broth culture extracts reveals the major bacterial products to be acetic, butyric and proprionic acids.

Antibiotics to which the bacilli of *C. tetani* are susceptible include penicillin, erythromycin, clindamycin, tetracycline, chloramphenicol and metronidazole. The spores are very resistant to many physical and chemical agents. Spores may survive in boiling water for several minutes or longer (although they are destroyed by autoclaving at 121°C for 15–20 minutes), and they can survive desiccation, most household disinfectants and marked changes in pH. Spores are commonly found in soil from all areas of the world, and the organism may be found in animal and human faeces although isolation rates have varied widely.

Both toxigenic (toxin-producing) and nontoxogenic strains of *C. tetani* occur. Toxogenicity is associated with the presence of a single large plasmid[5] which contains the gene coding for toxin production.[6] The entire nucleotide sequence has been determined together with the amino acid sequence of the toxin,[7] which has some similarities with botulinum toxin.

PATHOGENESIS

When spores of *C. tetani* are introduced into healthy tissues they do not germinate and are removed by phagocytes. However, if spores are inoculated into damaged tissue, along with adjuvants such as soil, faeces, chemical substances or other bacteria, local oxygen tensions are lowered and favourable conditions are created for germination and vegetative growth.[2] Occasionally the organism may remain dormant, only to be activated months or years later, perhaps by minor trauma.

The typical features of tetanus result from a potent neurotoxin, tetanospasmin, which is produced during the growth phase of the organism and is released upon cell lysis. Tetanospasmin is a protein with a molecular weight of 150 000. Initially produced as a single chain, it is then cleaved by proteolytic enzymes to the 'extracellular' form which has a heavy chain and a light chain linked by a disulphide bond. If separated, neither the heavy chain nor the light chain alone are toxic.[8] The heavy chain is responsible for binding to cell receptors, and it is postulated that the light chain enters the cell producing the toxic effects.[9] Tetanus toxin binds selectively to gangliosides GD_{1b} and GT_{1b},[10] which are found only in neuronal cells, thus explaining the specific neurotoxicity.

Following uptake by neuronal cells the toxin travels by intra-axonal retrograde transport along α motor neurones. Upon reaching the spinal cord the toxin blocks inhibitory synapses, by preventing release of the mediators γ-aminobutyric acid (GABA) and glycine.[10] The removal of this inhibition allows uncontrolled motor neurone activity and stimulation of muscle contraction, resulting in the characteristic rigidity and spasms.

Whether a particular patient develops localized or generalized tetanus may depend upon the amount of toxin produced.[11] If large amounts of toxin are produced it is both transported by local neurones and spread by the lymphatic system into the general circulation. It is then accessible to motor neurones all over the body. Muscle groups with the shortest neurones, and thus quickest transport, will be affected first. This results in rigidity of the masseters followed by other muscles in a descending pattern. In local tetanus there may only be enough toxin for uptake by the local motor neurones. There is evidence that tetanospasmin can also cause flaccid paralysis by preventing acetylcholine release at the neuromuscular junction.[2,11] Although this possibly accounts for episodes of facial paralysis in cephalic tetanus, it is not important compared with central nervous system involvement.

CLINICAL PICTURE

Tetanus is characterized by muscular rigidity and spasms, which may remain localized but are most commonly generalized. There may be a variety of premonitory symptoms. The incubation period, i.e. the time from inoculation to the first symptom, is usually 1–2 weeks, but may vary between 1 day and several months. A short incubation period of 4 days or less generally indicates severe disease. The period between the first symptom and the development of muscular spasms is termed the onset period. Shorter onset periods, particularly less than 48 hours, are followed by more severe forms of tetanus.

The first symptom is usually trismus ('lockjaw'), an inability to open the mouth fully, which results from rigidity of the masseter muscles. Less common early symptoms include backache, neck stiffness, generalized or localized weakness, pains in the legs, abdominal cramps, dysphagia and facial paralysis. Headache, sweating and irritability may also occur.

As the disease progresses muscular rigidity develops elsewhere. This may begin with a few muscle groups (localized tetanus) but typically then spreads to other muscles, in a descending pattern from masseters to limbs, resulting in generalized tetanus. Rigidity of the facial muscles causes the characteristic sustained grinning expression known as 'risus sardonicus' (Figure 48.1). Neck stiffness may be prominent and resembles the board-like rigidity of meningitis. Rigidity in the vertebral muscles leads to exaggerated curvature of the spine, and rigidity in abdominal muscles may mimic that found in peritonitis. There is a progressive phasic increase in muscle tone with paroxysmal increases or spasms. These are intensely painful and vary in severity from a slight twitch to a generalized spasm with opisthotonos, adducted arms, clenched fists, extended legs and marked risus sardonicus. These spasms also involve the pharyngeal, laryngeal and respiratory muscles resulting in hypoxia and episodes of apnoea, during which the patient becomes cyanotic and may have a respiratory arrest. Pharyngeal and glottal spasms lead to aspiration of secretions. There is profuse sweating and salivation during the spasms. They usually last for a few seconds but sometimes for a minute or so, and in severe cases may be repeated every few minutes. Their onset may be triggered by physical stimuli such as pain, sudden noise and light, swallowing, and even light touch. Severity is assessed from the frequency, extent and duration of the spasms.

The patients are fully conscious except for brief periods during intense spasms, or may become delirious in the later stages, particularly if under heavy sedation. There is usually no high fever unless secondary infection occurs. In a minority of patients, particularly if partially immune, rigidity may remain localized to the area near the site of infection. One particular form of localized disease is 'cephalic tetanus', in which the manifestations are confined to the head and neck, including trismus, facial paralysis, nuchal rigidity and dysphagia.

Generalized tetanus is associated with the syndrome of sympathetic overactivity.[12] This results in tachycardia, arrhythmias, unstable hypertension, paroxysmal peripheral vasoconstriction, profuse sweating and fever. In the late stages there may be bowel ileus, and hypotension is often a preterminal event. There is increased urinary excretion of catecholamines.

Neonatal tetanus usually follows an infected umbilical stump, but rarely occurs after a non-sterile injection or surgical procedure. The incubation period can be very short (1–2 days) but usually averages 7–10 days. It commonly presents with difficulty in sucking, and progresses to a total inability to feed and then to the typical features of generalized tetanus[13] (Figure 48.2).

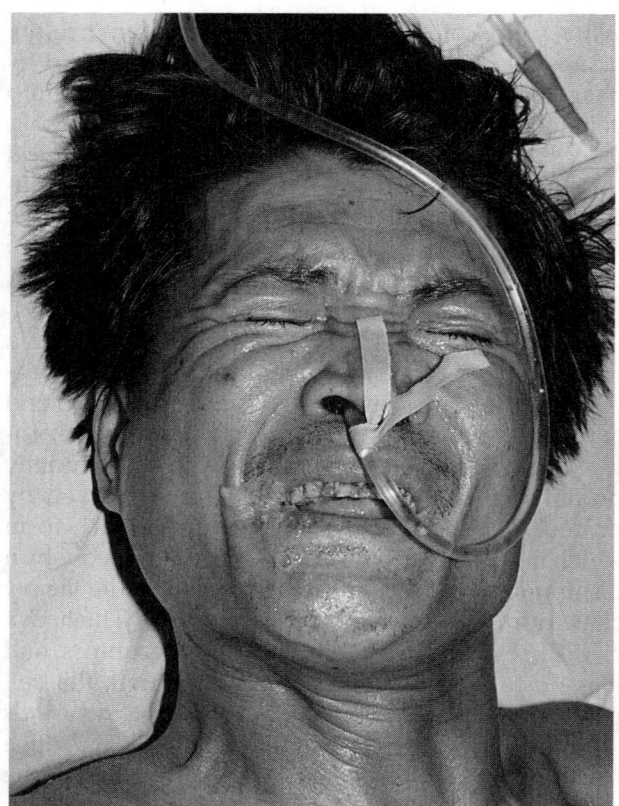

Figure 48.1   Tetanus: risus sardonicus with profuse salivation.

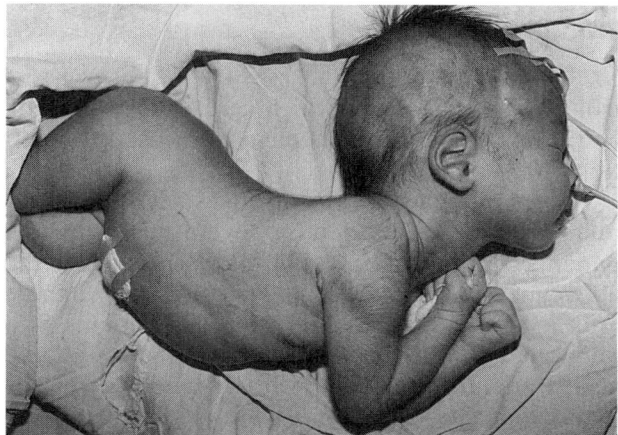

Figure 48.2 Neonatal tetanus: typical features of generalized tetanus resulting from an infected umbilical stump.

Secondary infections are a frequent complication of severe tetanus, most commonly related to the lower respiratory tract, urinary catheterization, intravascular cannulas or the original wound. Pneumonia occurs as a result of aspirated secretions, areas of atelectasis, heavy sedation, and intubation and mechanical ventilation. Haematemesis, due to acute gastric erosion or ulceration, is also common and usually occurs within the first few days. Other complications include pulmonary emboli, constipa-

tion, decubitus ulcers, compression fractures of vertebrae, rupture of muscles or tendons, and intramuscular haematoma formation.

The main causes of death are: pneumonia and respiratory failure, circulatory disturbances, haemorrhage and septicaemia.[14] In severe tetanus sudden death usually occurs during a generalized spasm. Mortality increases with the severity of the disease, extremes of age and the presence of secondary infections. Tetanus neonatorum has a mortality rate estimated at 65–90% depending on the available means of treatment.[13,15] The increasing use of modern intensive care facilities has significantly reduced the overall mortality of non-neonatal tetanus to 10% or less,[14,16] however mortality remains high (42%) for patients aged 50 years or older.[17] Various groups have devised schemes to judge a patient's chance of survival based on the rapidity of onset, clinical findings on admission and subsequent progress.[13,18]

For those who survive, the course of the disease may take 4 weeks or more in severe cases and some 2 weeks for milder cases. Residual effects include limb deformities due to residual contractures which improve with physiotherapy, and chest deformities due to vertebral fractures.[13] Temporary neurological sequelae following tetanus include irritability, sleep disturbance, fits and myoclonus.[19]

DIAGNOSIS

Diagnosis is based on the history and clinical findings which are characteristic. There are no confirmatory laboratory tests. Clinical suspicion is high if a wound has been sustained within the previous 2 weeks, but in many people this is not evident. A search for toxigenic *C. tetani* in the suspected focus of infection is usually unsuccessful. Even if isolated, the presence of *C. tetani* in a wound is not diagnostic for tetanus without the characteristic clinical picture. However, a definite history of immunization or adequate serum levels of antibody would argue against a diagnosis of tetanus.

Established generalized tetanus is not usually misdiagnosed. Strychnine blocks inhibitory reflexes in the spinal cord and strychnine poisoning closely mimics tetanus. There is usually a history of ingestion and symptoms may begin within 30 minutes;

toxicological tests can confirm the diagnosis. In the earlier stages of tetanus some of the clinical findings may be confused with other conditions.[13] Dental abscess, peritonsillar abscess or temporomandibular joint disease may simulate trismus. Nuchal rigidity may be confused with meningitis, but the cerebrospinal fluid in tetanus is normal. Facial paralysis may resemble Bell's palsy, and abdominal rigidity may suggest peritonitis. In tetany the characteristic spasms are confined to the hands and feet, and a low serum calcium will help the differentiation from tetanus. The early stages of rabies may be confused with the dysphagia of cephalic tetanus. Epilepsy is associated with clonic convulsions rather than the tonic spasms seen in tetanus. Dystonic reactions to phenothiazines may simulate trismus and may cause spasms of the back resembling opisthotonos.

MANAGEMENT

Once tetanus toxin has bound to its receptors in the central nervous system the effect cannot be reversed by any pharmacological manoeuvre. Therefore therapy is essentially supportive. The main aims of treatment are to relieve the patient's distress, to maintain the airway and adequate respiration, inhibit unbound toxin, and to prevent further toxin production. The extent to which these can be achieved will depend on the availability of resources. Where possible patients should be admitted to an intensive care unit equipped for assisted ventilation and intensive monitoring.

There are many sedative and muscle relaxing drugs which can alleviate the patient's symptoms, however the large doses that are often necessary may lead to depression of respiratory function and consciousness, which are undesirable and increase the risk of complications. If facilities for assisted ventilation are not available it is preferable to avoid heavy sedation, even if a few spasms occur, so that spontaneous respiration and consciousness are maintained. Patients need intensive nursing care with gentle attention but should be protected from loud noises, bright light, frequent examination or any other unnecessary manipulations which may provoke spasms.

Even in situations where mechanical ventilation is not available, a tracheostomy should be performed as soon as possible in generalized tetanus.[20] This will allow maintenance of the airway during laryngeal spasms, and provide access for removal of secretions from the respiratory tract. Profuse respiratory secretions are a problem in tetanus. The airway usually needs repeated suction, although this tends to provoke spasms. Also a nasogastric tube should be used for feeding, with a reduced risk of aspiration of gastric contents.

The benzodiazepines, and in particular diazepam, are used most frequently. They are both tranquillizer and muscle relaxant, and have a wide margin of safety. Diazepam may be given orally or intravenously. Bioavailability following oral administration is good, with almost complete absorption and peak plasma levels occurring within 30–90 minutes. Diazepam has a long terminal half-life of 72 hours. Doses of up to 20mg every 2–4 hours should be titrated to the patient's response and the desired level of sedation. Diazepam has also been given by intravenous infusion, but this can lead to prolonged coma if the dose is not properly titrated, therefore the newer short-acting benzodiazepine, midazolam, might be more suitable.[20] In severe cases diazepam alone may not be sufficient to con-trol muscle spasms, in which case chlorpromazine and other phenothiazines have been used in addition.

Neuromuscular blocking agents such as pancuronium bromide are used in the severest cases, where patients continue to have painful spasms despite the above measures. They can only be used where there are facilities for artificial ventilation. Patients who undergo paralysis and assisted ventilation should also be adequately sedated with a benzodiazepine or narcotic analgesic.[21] Dantrolene has been used to reduce spontaneous muscular spasms,[22] but it is potentially hepatotoxic if used for prolonged periods, and again requires additional sedatives. Intrathecal baclofen, a GABA agonist, has successfully suppressed spasticity in cases where diazepam failed.[23]

In patients with signs of autonomic instability, the manifestations of tachycardia, arrythmias and hypertension may be treated with propranolol or the combination of propranolol and bethanidine.[24] The combined α- and β-adrenergic blocker labetolol has also been used successfully,[25] but in other studies it has failed to stabIlize the blood pressure.[26] Other therapeutic measures, such as intravenous morphine[27] or continuous epidural blockade,[28] have succeeded in treating autonomic instability in a few patients.

Once the diagnosis of tetanus is made, human tetanus immune globulin (HTIG) should be given in order to neutralize any unbound toxin. Doses of 3000 units or more have been recommended,[3,9] however smaller doses (500 units) may be equally effective.[29] If HTIG is not available equine antiserum (10 000 units) should be given by the intramuscular or intravenous route. It does not appear to be any less effective than HTIG but subsequent adverse reactions are reported to occur in 5–50% of patients.[2]

Once tetanus toxin has entered the nervous system it is no longer accessible to neutralization by antitoxin administered systemically. However, any unbound toxin within the central nervous system may be accessible to antitoxin administered intrathecally. This approach was first used in 1914,[30] then abandoned because of dangerous side-effects. Interest resurfaced in the 1970s. One trial showed that the intrathecal administration of equine antiserum, in addition to the systemic route, reduced mortality from 14.5 to 4.5%.[31] Cisternal administration was no better than using the lumbar route. It was well tolerated, although high-dose steroids were also given. A later trial used intrathecal HTIG (250 units) in patients with early tetanus, resulting in a significant reduction in progression of the disease and subsequent mortality;[32] however, another trial by the same author failed to show any beneficial effect if given after the onset of spasms.[33] Although there were no side-effects with HTIG in either of these trials, it is not licensed for intrathecal administration, which remains experimental.

In order to prevent further growth and toxin production by *C. tetani*, an appropriate antibiotic should also be given. Either benzylpenicillin or procaine penicillin, for 5–10 days, are usually recommended. However, metronidazole was reported to be preferable in a single trial.[34] Additional antibiotics should be given according to the individual patient's clinical condition. A few hours after administering the antitoxin and antibiotic, any wound should be cleaned and debrided. Care should be taken to remove all foreign bodies, no matter how small.

Various general supportive measures are appro-priate. The maintenance of water, electrolyte and nutritional balance is important because patients are ill for prolonged periods, and the marked sweating leads to volume depletion. If the airway is protected by an endotracheal tube or tracheostomy, and there is no bowel ileus, a nasogastric tube can be inserted for enteral feeding. Intravenous fluids and electrolytes should also be given. Prophylactic heparinization is recommended to reduce the possibility of deep venous thrombosis and pulmonary emboli. Haematemesis, due to acute peptic ulceration, requires prophylactic use of histamine H_2-receptor antagonist, antacids or sucralfate. Dedicated nursing care is vital to monitor progress, maintain patient comfort and reduce the risks of complications. Frequent (2-hourly) turning of the patient may be necessary to avoid bedsores. Finally, the amount of toxin circulating in natural disease is insufficient to provoke an immunizing antibody response, so all patients should receive a course of tetanus toxoid to prevent recurrences.

PREVENTION

The prevention of tetanus depends on primary immunization and the thorough management of wounds in those people who have not been immunized or whose immune status is thought to be inadequate. In addition, health education and improved socioeconomic conditions are very important, for example the use of aseptic techniques in the management of the umbilical cord and the provision of adequate protective footwear.[9]

Tetanus toxoid is produced by formaldehyde treatment of the toxin (plain toxoid). Although it is a relatively good immunogen, the duration of antibody response is much improved by adsorption with aluminium hydroxide as an adjuvant. In many countries a course of three injections of adsorbed toxoid is given for active immunization. A protective antibody level is attained after the second dose but a third dose is recommended to ensure prolonged immunity. In the UK, the first dose is given at 2 months of age, followed by the second and third doses at 4 week intervals.[35] In the USA, a four-dose schedule is recommended, with intervals of 4–8 weeks between the first three doses, and the fourth dose 6–12 months later.[36] Adsorbed toxoid is available in combination with diphtheria toxoid and pertussis vaccine (DTP) for use in these immunization schedules of young children. A booster dose of tetanus and diphtheria toxoids (DT) is given at 4–6 years of age. Adults and older children who have not been immunized previously should also receive a primary course of three doses of adsorbed tetanus toxoid. Serum antitoxin levels of 0.01 unit/ml are usually considered protective, although tetanus has occurred in some patients with antitoxin levels of 0.01–1.0 unit/ml, but the disease is usually mild with a very low mortality.[37,38] In order to maintain levels above this minimum, additional booster doses of adsorbed tetanus toxoid should be given every 10 years. Reactions to tetanus toxoid are infrequent, and usually local and mild; however, they occur more often and may be more severe if booster doses are given more frequently than outlined.

Neonatal tetanus may be prevented by immunization of women during pregnancy. Two or preferably three doses of adsorbed toxoid should be given, with the last dose at least 2–4 weeks prior to delivery. Immunity is passively transferred to the fetus and the antibodies will remain long enough to protect the baby during the neonatal period. In subsequent pregnancies a single booster can be given at 6 months gestation, but if pregnancies are frequent boosters should only be given every 5 years.

One problem with these immunization schedules is their complexity. In the developing world, particularly in rural areas, people may not return for the second and subsequent doses, therefore a single dose regimen is desirable. This has been achieved by using much larger doses of toxoid or using a different adjuvant such as calcium phosphate.[37] However, the response is delayed and if used in pregnant women it should be given 6 months prior to delivery.

Prevention of tetanus also depends on the effective management of wounds. It is most important that wounds are thoroughly cleaned, all foreign material removed and non-viable tissue debrided. Particular attention should be given to tetanus-prone wounds. These include puncture wounds, burns, animal and human bites, wounds contaminated with soil or faeces, and any wound where treatment is delayed. These wounds should not be sutured: packing, frequent inspection and delayed primary closure is preferable.[2] Antibiotic chemoprophylaxis is of secondary importance to good surgical management and immunoprophylaxis. When indicated, a long-acting penicillin can be given. If the wound is infected with β-lactamase-producing staphylococci an appropriate alternative antibiotic such as erythromycin or flucloxacillin should be used.

A history of previous immunization should be sought as this will determine the exact type of immunoprophylaxis to be given. If the patient has received a full course or a booster of tetanus toxoid within the previous 5 years, a further dose should not be given unless the risk of tetanus developing is high. If the last dose was more than 10 years ago a further dose should be given, and if the last dose was 5–10 years ago a booster dose should probably be given for all but trivial wounds. Where there is doubt about any previous immunization or a full course was never completed, a full course of adsorbed tetanus toxoid should be commenced. In this case passive immunization with HTIG (250 units) should also be given for tetanus-prone wounds. If HTIG is not available, equine antiserum (1500 units) is an alternative. Very high-risk wounds are those with heavy soil or faecal contamination, extensive burns, or where foreign material or necrotic tissue cannot be removed; in these cases the dose of HTIG should be doubled to 500 units and a further dose may be given after 4 weeks if the wound is still not clean or healed. Both toxoid and immunoglobulin can be given at the same time providing that separate sites are used.

REFERENCES

1 Bytchenko B. Microbiology of tetanus. In Veronesi R (ed.) *Tetanus: Important New Concepts*. Amsterdam: Excerpta Medica, 1981: 28–39.

2 Smith J W G & Collee J G. Tetanus. In Smith R S and Easmon C S F (eds) *Topley and Wilson's Principles of Bacteriology, Virology and Immunity*, Vol. 3, 8th edn. London: Edward Arnold, 1990: 331–351.

3 Finegold S M, George W L & Mulligan M E. Tetanus. In Anaerobic infections, Part II. *Dis Mon* 1985; 31:82–88.

4 Centers for Disease Control. Tetanus: United States, 1987 and 1988. *MMWR* 1990; 39:37–41.

5 Laird W J, Aaronson W, Silver R P, Habig W H & Hardegree M C. Plasmid-associated toxogenicity in *Clostridium tetani*. *J Infect Dis* 1980; 142:623.

6 Finn C W, Silver R P, Habig W H, Hardegree M C, Zon G & Garon C F. The structural gene for tetanus neurotoxin is on a plasmid. *Science* 1984; 224:881–884.

7 Eisel U, Jarausch W, Goretski K et al. Tetanus toxin: primary structure, expression in *E. coli* and homology with botulinum toxins. *EMBO J* 1986; 5:2495–2502.

8 Hatheway C L. Toxogenic clostridia. *Clin Microbiol Rev* 1990; 3:66–98.

9 Collee J G & van Heyningen S. Systemic toxogenic diseases (tetanus, botulism). In Duerden BI &

Drasar BS (eds) *Anaerobes and Human Disease*. London: Edward Arnold, 1990: 372–394.

10 Mellanby J & Green J. How does tetanus toxin act? *Neuroscience* 1981; 11:281–300.

11 Kryzhanovsky G N. Pathophysiology. In Veronesi R (ed.) *Tetanus: Important New Concepts*. Amsterdam: Excerpta Medica, 1981: 109–182.

12 Kerr J H, Corbett J L, Prys-Roberts C, Crampton Smith A & Spalding J M K. Involvement of the sympathetic nervous system in tetanus: studies on 82 cases. Lancet 1968; ii:236–241.

13 Veronesi R & Focaccia R. The clinical picture. In Veronesi R (ed.) *Tetanus: Important New Concepts*. Amsterdam: Excerpta Medica, 1981: 183–206.

14 Edmonston R S & Flowers M W. Intensive care in tetanus: management, complications and mortality in 100 cases. *BMJ* 1979; i:1401–1404.

15 Salimpour R. Cause of death in tetanus neonatorum: study of 233 cases with 54 necropsies. *Arch Dis Child* 1977; 52:587–589.

16 Trujillo M H, Castillo A, Espana J, Manzo A & Zerpa R. Impact of intensive care management on the prognosis of tetanus: analysis of 641 cases. *Chest* 1987; 92:63–65.

17 Centers for Disease Control. Tetanus: United States, 1985–1986. *MMWR* 1987; 36:477–481.

18 Armitage P & Clifford R. Prognosis in tetanus: use

of data from therapeutic trials. *J Infect Dis* 1978; 138:1–8.

19 Illis L S & Taylor F M. Neurological and electroencephalographic sequelae of tetanus. *Lancet* 1971; i:826–830.

20 Rey M, Diop-Mar I & Robert D. Treatment of tetanus. In Veronesi R (ed.) *Tetanus: Important New Concepts*. Amsterdam: Excerpta Medica, 1981: 207–237.

21 Olsen K M & Hiller F C. Management of tetanus. *Clin Pharm* 1987; 6:570–574.

22 Tidyman M, Deamer R L & Mac N. Adjunctive use of dantrolene in severe tetanus. *Anesth Analg* 1985; 64:538–540.

23 Muller H, Borner U, Zierski J & Hemplemann G. Intrathecal baclofen for the treatment of tetanus-induced spasticity. *Anesthesiology* 1987; 66:76–79.

24 Prys-Roberts C, Kerr J H, Corbett J L et al. Treatment of sympathetic overactivity in tetanus. Lancet 1969; i:542–546.

25 Dundee J W & Morrow W F. Labetalol in severe tetanus. *BMJ* 1979; i:1121–1122.

26 Wesley A G, Hariparsad A G, Pather M et al. Labetalol in tetanus. The treatment of sympathetic nervous system overactivity. *Anaesthesia* 1983; 38:243–249.

27 Buchanan N, Cane R D, Wolfson G & De Andrade M. Autonomic dysfunction in tetanus: the effects of a variety of therapeutic agents, with special reference to morphine. *Intensive Care Med* 1979; 5:65–68.

28 Southorn P A & Blaise G A. Treatment of tetanus-induced autonomic nervous system dysfunction with continuous epidural blockade. *Crit Care Med* 1986; 14:251–252.

29 Blake P A, Feldman R A, Buchanon T M et al. Serologic therapy of tetanus in the United States, 1965–1971. *JAMA* 1976; 235:42–44.

30 Park W H & Nicoll M. Experiments on the curative value of the intraspinal administration of tetanus antitoxin. *JAMA* 1914; 63:235–241.

31 Sanders R K M, Joseph R, Martyn B & Peacock M L. Intrathecal antitetanus serum (horse) in the treatment of tetanus. *Lancet* 1977; i:974–977.

32 Gupta P S, Kapoor R, Goyal S, Batra V K & Jain B K. Intrathecal human tetanus immunoglobulin in early tetanus. *Lancet* 1980; ii:439–440.

33 Gupta P S & Kapoor R. Intrathecal use of human tetanus immunoglobulin. *Clinician* 1980; 44:127–133.

34 Ahmadsyah I & Salim A. Treatment of tetanus: an open study to compare the efficacy of procaine penicillin and metronidazole. *BMJ* 1985; 291:648–650.

35 Department of Health. *Immunisation against Infectious Disease*. London: HMSO, 1992.

36 Advisory Committee on Immunization Practices. Diphtheria, tetanus and pertussis: guidelines for vaccine prophylaxis and other preventive measures. *MMWR* 1985, 34:405–414, 419–426.

37 Veronesi R. Prophylaxis. In Veronesi R (ed.) *Tetanus: Important New Concepts*. Amsterdam: Excerpta Medica, 1981: 238–263.

38 Passen E L & Andersen B R. Clinical tetanus despite a 'protective' level of toxin-neutralizing antibody. *JAMA* 1986; 255:1171–1173.

CHAPTER 49

ANTHRAX

G. Scott

Anthrax (Greek: black) is a disease of domestic herbivores caused by the bacterium *Bacillus anthracis,* which lives in topsoil and which is ingested by the animals when grazing. Infection in man is rare considering the potential exposure to the organism and it presents as a local cutaneous lesion, gastro-intestinal infection or with overwhelming pneumonia and disseminated disease.

GEOGRAPHICAL DISTRIBUTION

Anthrax occurs worldwide but is 'endemic' in herbivorous livestock in certain regions. Domestic carnivores (dogs and cats) may be infected by eating contaminated carcasses. Human disease is most likely to occur in endemic regions (Iran,[1] Central Africa, South America, Russia) by direct contact with infected carcasses. Industrial cases may occur anywhere and reflect exposure to imported animal carcass products such as bone meal (which used to be used for making glues) or hides.

AETIOLOGY

B. anthracis is a large, non-motile, brick-shaped, aerobic, Gram-positive rod which has the capacity to make heat- and dry-resistant spores under adverse conditions. The spore is central and does not expand the bacterium. Spores may survive for decades in topsoil and resist high temperatures (e.g. 140°C in dry heat for 3 hours and 100°C in moist heat for 10 minutes). The organism may be provisionally identified by Gram stain of pus aspirated from a lesion and will grow in air within 24 hours to give large irregular colonies on simple media. The edge of the colony is sometimes likened to Medusa's head. The organism is then distinguished from other *Bacillus* spp. on chemical grounds and motility. Virulence is conferred by a capsule (which develops soon after germination in vivo and inhibits phagocytosis) and a complex exotoxin which is plasmid determined. The exotoxin is released by germinating spores and replicating organisms and consists of 'oedema' and 'lethal' factors together with a 'protective antigen' determinant.

EPIDEMIOLOGY AND TRANSMISSION

The sequence of events leading to the manifestation of anthrax in animals (and, usually subsequently, in man) is complex and not completely understood. In areas of endemicity, the soil may be heavily contaminated by spores. These spores originated from vast numbers of organisms shed from animals who died of the disease. The bacteria have to compete with other soil bacteria and rapid sporulation encouraged at high ambient temperature is critical to their survival. Vegetative forms die. Germination of spores occurs in conditions of high humidity, again encouraged by high temperature. In temperate conditions, although very humid, the temperature is rarely high enough to encourage either sporulation or germination so it is rare for the topsoil to become significantly contaminated. Most new veterinary infection is imported with animal food-stuffs. The organism may be transmitted by insects including house flies.[2,3]

If the summers are hot and dry, germination never occurs but the spores remain viable. If germination does occur after a period of rain followed by drought, animals will crop the grass down to the soil and be more likely to eat soil containing the organisms. Man will then tend to become infected during the dry season.[4] Infection of the animal is not well understood but it is thought that minor trauma from rough vegetation and soil itself in the mouth may cause a sufficient portal of entry. An infected animal which dies is loaded with vast numbers of bacteria.

Man acquires infection by direct inoculation of spores through breaks in the skin, by inhalation of spores or by ingestion of contaminated meat. There may be some person-to-person spread in peculiar circumstances: for example, an outbreak in the Gambia was in part traced to the use of communal loofahs when bathing,[4] and in the UK and Russia shaving brushes have been a source. In some areas, cutaneous disease is prevalent[3,4] but in others, the intestinal form is much more common[5] a difference which has not been fully explained.

CLINICAL PRESENTATION

CUTANEOUS

After an incubation period of 2–3 days there is a small papule in the skin, perhaps with a central vesicle at the site of inoculation. A bacteriological diagnosis can be made from this point onwards. The next day, there are vesicles around the central lesion which ulcerates and then dries leaving a black eschar. Atypically, there may be no vesicles. The eschar spreads to involve the vesicles as these dry up. There is no pain or even discomfort. The lesion does not discharge pus, but by the third day considerable local oedema has developed and the local lymph nodes are swollen. Anthrax lesions are common on the head and neck and exposed arms but rarely on the hands. If lesions of the neck are associated with massive oedema, they may cause respiratory obstruction (Figure 49.1). The lesion always resolves slowly, over a period of 2–6 weeks, despite appropriate antimicrobial treatment. The peripheral white cell count is usually normal.

PULMONARY

Classically the patient inhales spores from contaminated hides. Wool sorters must be generally very resistant to disease because in factory conditions, when opening bales, they would be expected to inhale about 1000 spores during an 8-hour shift, yet rarely contract the disease. It appears that workers who are continuously exposed become relatively resistant to infection. However, there have been occasional unexplained outbreaks, possibly associated with a very large inoculum.

After a short incubation period, pulmonary anthrax starts with fever and chills and the patient rapidly becomes cyanotic and short of breath. The lungs fill with interstitial fluid and the illness progresses inexorably to death over some days. The diagnosis is rarely made before death unless the history reveals occupational risk.

INTESTINAL

Common in Africa[5] but very rare elsewhere in the world, this is thought to arise by the consumption of contaminated meat. The presentation is non-

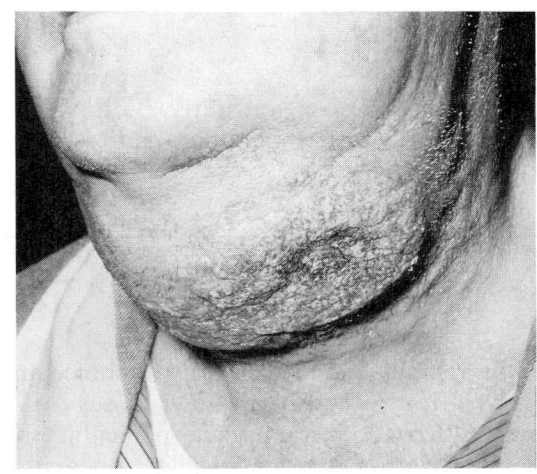

Figure 49.1 Anthrax pustule on the jaw.

specific with vomiting, diarrhoea and fever, occasionally with haematemesis and dysenteric stools. In autopsy cases an eschar may be found in the gut but most patients recover spontaneously.

OTHER SITES

Local lesions in the oropharynx may occur after eating contaminated meat—local severe oedema is again a prominent and life-threatening effect.[6] Bacteraemia may lead to infection at any site and will usually be fatal. Meningeal anthrax secondary to bacteraemia has been described.

PATHOLOGY

The organism is found in the capillaries. The malignant pustule is an area of local necrosis of the skin. In the lung, pulmonary oedema, haemorrhage, pleural effusion and mediastinitis are found but there is no single lesion. Generalized petechiae reflect vasculitis secondary to bloodstream spread.

Often the spleen is enlarged and infected in fatal cases. Patients make antibody to the organism after natural infection but the persistence of this antibody is very variable.

DIFFERENTIAL DIAGNOSIS

A typical cutaneous malignant pustule is easy to recognize. Other local lesions which may cause confusion include tick bites with local rickettsia infection, orf, tularaemia, cutaneous diphtheria and plague. A scraping must be done and examined microscopically, a common alternative cause for the lesion being *Streptococcus pyogenes* with *Staphylococcus aureus*. In the early stages the lesion is just a small spot with a vesicle and is unlikely to present to a doctor. Oropharyngeal anthrax may be confused with diphtheria. Anthrax must be a very rare cause of overwhelming pneumonitis, for which the differential diagnosis is huge. A diagnosis of anthrax would be entertained only in someone with occupational exposure.

DIAGNOSIS

The organism is seen on direct scraping and aspiration—little pus is obtained—and will grow rapidly on simple media. Blood cultures are also useful.

TREATMENT

Penicillin remains the proven drug of choice and is best given intravenously in high doses to sick patients. Otherwise intramuscular penicillin (short- and long-acting) or oral amoxycillin appears to be satisfactory—the vast majority of mild cases are going to recover anyway. Co-trimoxazole seems to be a useful alternative but the organism tends to be resistant to chloramphenicol. The clinical course of the severe illness is not materially modified by antibiotics.

PREVENTION

The population should be encouraged not to eat the meat of animals that become ill or die.[7,8] The spread of the disease from animals which have died of anthrax can be reduced by burying their carcasses in lime. Hides should be disinfected before export and occupational exposure reduced as far as possible by simple, sensible measures. There is no longer any place for the hyperimmune serum which used to be popular. However, a vaccine may be obtained for those at special risk of exposure[9] and live attenuated strains are under evaluation.[10] The protective antigen gene has recently been cloned into vaccinia and baculovirus vectors.[11]

REFERENCES

1 Amidi S, Dutz W, Kohout E & Ronaghy A. Human Anthrax in Iran. Report of 300 cases and review of the literature. *Z Tropenmed Parasitol* 1974; 25:96–104.

2 McKendrick D R A. Anthrax and its transmission in humans. *Cent Afr J Med* 1980; 26:126–129.

3 Turner M. Anthrax in humans in Zimbabwe. *Cent Afr J Med* 1980; 26:160–161.

4 Heyworth B, Ropp M E, Meinel H & Darlow H M. Anthrax in the Gambia: an epidemiological study. *BMJ* 1975; iv:79–82.

5 Fendall N R E & Grounds J G. The incidence and epidemiology of disease in Kenya. I. Some disease of social significance. *J Trop Med Hyg* 1965; 68:77–84.

6 Sirisanthana T, Navachareon N, Tharavichitkul P, Sirisanthana V & Brown A E. Outbreak of oral-oropharyngeal anthrax: an unusual manifestation of human infection with *Bacillus anthracis*. *Am J Trop Med Hyg* 1984; 33:144–150.

7 Kunanusont C, Limpakarnjanarat K & Foy H M. Outbreak of anthrax in Thailand. *Ann Trop Med Parasitol* 1990; 84:507–512.

8 Sekhar P C, Singh R S, Sridhar M S, Bhaskar C J & Rao Y S. Outbreak of human anthrax in Ramabhadrapuram village of Chittar district of Andhra Pradesh. *Indian J Med Res* 1990; 91:448–452.

9 Turnbull P C. Anthrax vaccines: past, present and future. *Vaccine* 1991; 9:533–539.

10 Ivins B E, Welkos S L, Knudson G B & Little S F. Immunization against anthrax with aromatic compound-dependent (Aro-) mutants of *Bacillus anthracis* and with recombinant strains of *Bacillus subtilis* that produce anthrax protective antigen. *Infect Immun* 1990; 58:303–308.

11 Iacono-Connors L C, Welkos S L, Ivins B E & Dalrymple J M. Protection against anthrax with recombinant virus-expressed protective antigen in experimental animals. *Infect Immun* 1991; 59:1961–1965.

CHAPTER 50

PLAGUE

Michael D. Smith and Nguyen Duy Thanh

Plague is an acute infectious disease caused by the organism *Yersinia pestis*. It is a zoonosis, transmitted mainly by the bite(s) of infected fleas. Wild rodents are the natural reservoir. In man the most common clinical presentation is bubonic plague (regional lymphadenitis) which accounts for over 90% of cases. Other forms include septicaemic plague without bubo, pneumonic plague (either primary or secondary to bacteraemia), meningitis and pharyngitis. Asymptomatic and minor self-limiting infections also occur.

Plague is best known as an ancient disease—pestilence, although it remains endemic in many parts of the world today. There have been three documented world pandemics. The first was in the sixth century. In the fourteen century, the Black Death swept across Europe killing between one-quarter and one-third of the entire population.[1] The third pandemic originated in China in 1860 and reached Hong Kong in 1894. It was here that the causative organism was successfully isolated by Alexandre Yersin (for a full account of this discovery, see Butler[2]). The pandemic spread—by rats on board ships, to South-East Asia, India, Africa and the Americas. The infection was then transmitted to sylvatic rodents, thus allowing it to become established in rural areas. In India there may have been up to ten million deaths by 1919. During the 1960s and early 70s there was a resurgence of plague in Vietnam, with a peak of over 4000 cases per year.[2]

EPIDEMIOLOGY

Plague is still reported consistently from several countries in Africa, Asia and South America, and the USA. During the years 1986–1990 the leading countries were: Tanzania (1758 cases), Vietnam (1186), Zaire (844) and Madagascar (553). Uganda reported an isolated outbreak of 340 cases in 1986. Brazil, Botswana, Bolivia and China each reported over 100 cases. In the USA a few cases occur every year.[3]

Foci of infection are maintained worldwide in natural animal reservoirs, and transmission by bites of infected fleas or ingestion of infected animals. In Asia and Africa the domestic black rat *Rattus rattus* and the brown sewer rat *R. norvegicus* remain the most important animal reservoir(s) for transmission of plague to man. Human plague may be presaged by a sudden 'die off' in these urban rodents. Dead rats dropping from the rafters of houses or warehouses is considered an ominous harbinger of disease in man. Other rodents maintain the infection in the field, for example *R. exulans* in Asia, and *Mastomys* spp. and gerbils in Africa. The most important flea vector involved in transmission is *Xenopsylla cheopis*, in which infection with *Y. pestis* causes a blocked proventriculus and regurgitation of organisms when taking a blood meal. In the USA, plague is maintained in sylvatic rodents such as ground squirrels, rock squirrels and prairie dogs. These animals may enter areas of human habitation directly, or the infected fleas may be carried by domestic cats and dogs.

A distinct seasonal pattern is seen. Most cases occur in warm dry periods when fleas are most abundant and humans are most likely to come into contact with the natural hosts. In Vietnam the peak months are March–April; in Tanzania, January–March; and in the USA, May–October.

BACTERIOLOGY

Y. pestis is a small Gram-negative coccobacillus, which commonly exhibits bipolar staining and pleomorphism, particularly in clinical specimens. The genus *Yersinia* belongs to the family Enterobacteriaceae. *Y. pestis* is non-motile and non-spore forming. Both in vivo and in culture on serum agar at 37°C a capsule-like envelope may be formed. It grows aerobically on many common culture media, including nutrient agar and blood agar, and forms tiny colourless, often granular, colonies after 24 hours at 37°C; there is no haemolysis. On MacConkey agar it appears as pinpoint non-lactose-fermenting colonies, which disappear after 2–3 days, presumably due to autolysis. Cultures in nutrient broth initially form a granular deposit, and if oil is floated on top of the broth stalactites form beneath the droplets. Growth is optimal at 28°C and is slightly enhanced by the addition of serum. Biochemically *Y. pestis* is catalase positive, oxidase positive and reduces nitrate, but does not hydrolyse urea. It does not utilize citrate, or produce indole. Glucose and mannitol are fermented, but not sucrose or lactose. On triple sugar–iron agar slants it produces an acid butt and an alkaline slope.

The organism is susceptible to adverse conditions but can survive for many months in the cool damp conditions of the soil in rodent burrows. Organisms are killed by heating at 56°C for 15 minutes, and by exposure to sunlight for 4 hours. They may survive drying for a few days, but survival is prolonged in dried blood and secretions.

PATHOGENESIS

Y. pestis produces a number of virulence factors encoded either chromosomally or on one of three plasmids.[4] A temperature-dependent coagulase is produced during infection of the flea, which causes clotting of blood in the proventriculus. As a consequence of this blockage of the flea's foregut, blood containing many organisms is regurgitated during subsequent attempts to feed. The coagulase is most active at temperatures below 30°C but is inactive at 35°C or above. Fleas are cold blooded and these observations may explain why transmission of plague ceases in the hot seasons in endemic areas.[5] Fraction 1 antigen is a capsular glycoprotein which enables the organism to evade phagocytosis; it is produced at 37°C but not below 27°C. Thus in the flea and when first inoculated into humans these organisms express capsular or fraction 1 antigen poorly and are easily phagocytosed, but not killed, by neutrophils and monocytes. However, subsequent generations express fraction 1 antigen fully, enabling them to avoid phagocytosis. The 'low calcium response', mediated by a 70 kb plasmid, occurs at 37°C but not 26°C, and is important for adaptation to an intracellular environment. This enables the bacterium to step down growth and initiate synthesis of various virulence factors under conditions of low calcium concentrations, such as found in the phagolysosome.[4] These include V and W antigens[6] which are present within the cyotoplasm or secreted from the cell, but not located on the cell surface. Their exact function is not known but they appear to maintain bacteriostasis and thus aid intracellular survival.[4] *Yersinia* outer membrane proteins (Yops) are also produced, of which types E and K appear to be important for virulence.[7]

Other virulence factors include: antigen 4 or 'pH 6' antigen,[8] pigment production and classical lipopolysaccharide endotoxin. The largest plasmid also encodes for a murine exotoxin which is essentially lethal for mice and rats only.

PATHOLOGY

The essential feature of plague in man is the bubo—an enlarged, congested and centrally necrotic lymph node. *Y. pestis* can be demonstrated in abundance in these lesions. Congestion and haemorrhage may be seen in most organs of the body, and extensive haemorrhages may be present in the mucosa of the gastrointestinal tract. In pneumonic plague the findings are of a haemorrhagic pneumonia and bloodstained fluid in the pleural cavities.

CLINICAL FEATURES

Historical accounts suggest that plague is one of the most virulent infections known to man, but subclinical cases are not uncommon and bubonic plague can be of mild or moderate severity. The incubation period is generally 2–5 but may be up to 15 days. With primary pneumonia the incubation period is often short, sometimes only 1 day, and the disease is rapidly fatal. In a small proportion of cases there is a prodromal stage of fever, weakness and anorexia. The initial manifestations are usually due to lymphadenitis in the nodes draining the site of a flea bite.

BUBONIC PLAGUE

This is the most common clinical form of plague. The clinical picture is characteristic. Typically, bubonic plague presents with a short prodrome of fever, malaise, anorexia and headache. Sometimes there is a dull ache at the site of future buboes, which will develop within 24 hours. The primary buboes will be found in different locations depending on the site of inoculation. The most common site is the groin (70–80%), with the femoral nodes more often involved compared to inguinal nodes.[9] Other primary sites are the axilla (14–20%), the cervical and submaxillary regions, and very rarely the clavicular, popliteal and epitrochlear nodes. Cervical and submaxillary node involvement is more often present in children. Buboes usually affect only one site but very occasionally two or more may be involved.

Development of the bubo is characterized by severe pain, swelling and marked tenderness of the affected lymph node. Individual nodes may attain the size of a hen's egg; sometimes clusters of nodes form a larger, more irregular swelling. There is surrounding oedema and the overlying skin is warm, reddened and adherent. The mass is immoveable and non-fluctuant, although, particularly if not treated with antibiotics, suppuration and abscess formation will occur during later stages. The buboes are generally so tender that the patient will hold the associated limb, or head, in such a position as to relieve the pressure.

The onset of fever in plague is often abrupt with the temperature rising rapidly to 39–40°C or even higher. Prostration and lethargy is marked. Sometimes there is agitation or even delirium. Vomiting and diarrhoea occur occasionally. Hepatomegaly is common but the spleen, although slightly enlarged, is not usually palpable.

In some patients small skin lesions such as vesicles and pustules may be seen in the region drained by the affected nodes. These may ulcerate or form an eschar, or rarely a carbuncle. *Y. pestis* can be isolated from these lesions. Although uncommon, perhaps the best-known skin manifestation is a patchy purpuric dermal necrosis which gave rise to the popular name 'Black Death'.

Laboratory findings include an elevated leucocyte count ($12000–22000/mm^3$) and toxic granulation of neutrophils. Eosinophilia is absent in the acute phase but is often noticed during convalescence. There is also laboratory evidence of disseminated intravascular coagulation.[10] Liver enzymes and bilirubin are frequently elevated, especially in more severe cases, although clinical jaundice is rare.

Although the picture of severe bubonic plague is distinctive, other infections can cause acute lymphadenitis. Staphylococcal and streptococcal infections will usually be associated with an obvious suppurative lesion or an area of lymphangitis in the region drained by the affected lymph nodes. In the USA tularaemia may cause confusion. Lymphogranuloma venereum and chancroid also cause inguinal lymphadenopathy; however the buboes are less painful and often fluctuant, and there are usually mild constitutional features.

Minor infections also occur and may go unnoticed. They may present with mild fever and less pronounced lymph node enlargement ('pestis minor'), which is self-limiting.

SEPTICAEMIC PLAGUE

Episodes of bacteraemia often occur in bubonic plague: in one study quantitative culture of small volumes of blood detected bacteraemia in 40% of cases.[11] Densities greater than $10^2/ml$ were associated with higher mortality.

The term 'septicaemic plague' denotes a severe acute illness characterized by a high density of organisms in the blood, without clinically apparent buboes. The bacteraemia may be so high (up to $10^7/ml$) that organisms are detectable in a peripheral blood smear. Septicaemic plague accounted for 11% of cases in the USA during the 1970s.[12] However, in New Mexico from 1980 to 1984, 25% of the 71 cases reported were septicaemic.[13] This was more likely to occur in people aged over 40 years. Symptoms include: fever, rigors, malaise and headache and are generally indistinguishable from those of other Gram-negative septicaemias. Gastrointestinal symptoms of nausea, vomiting, diarrhoea and abdominal pain are more frequent than in bubonic plague. The duration of illness is shorter than in bubonic plague and, if not treated appropriately, the patient rapidly becomes shocked and dies within a few days.

PNEUMONIC PLAGUE

Pneumonia in plague can occur in two forms, either as a primary pneumonia or secondary to bacteraemic spread in bubonic plague or septicaemic plague. The illness begins with intense headache and malaise, fever, vomiting and marked prostration and clouding of consciousness. In the initial stages there may be little to suggest pneumonia, but cough and dyspnoea develop with the production of watery, bloodstained sputum. Physical signs in the lungs are slight; there are reduced breath sounds and coarse crepitations at the bases. Respiratory failure ensues and the patient rapidly dies. Chest radiography shows evidence of multilobar consolidation or bronchopneumonia; there may be minimal pleural effusions. The discrepancy between gross radiographic abnormalities and minimal physical signs in the chest is characteristic. Pneumonia in plague has to be differentiated from the 'adult respiratory distress syndrome' that may occur in bubonic and septicaemic forms. Mortality in both types of plague pneumonia is extremely high and appropriate antibiotic treatment must be given within 24 hours of onset if the mortality rate is to be reduced.

Pneumonic plague is generally very uncommon, but it is the one form that may result in human-to-human transmission via infected droplets from patients with a productive cough. Where the climate is cool and humid, allowing infectious particles to persist, epidemics of pneumonic plague have occurred, such as that in Manchuria in 1910–1911. It is also a potential risk in laboratory workers handling cultures of *Y. pestis*. Primary pneumonia is so lethal that death can occur in as little as 1 day following exposure.

PLAGUE MENINGITIS

Primary plague meningitis is extremely rare. Most cases of meningeal involvement have occurred as a complication of inadequately treated bubonic plague, typically after 9–15 days. There is an associ-

ation between the presence of axillary buboes and the development of meningitis.[11] It is postulated that this may be due to spread by the lymphatic route, but bacteraemia is considered to be the means of spread from other sites.

Plague meningitis presents with symptoms and signs common to all types of pyogenic meningitis, including fever, headache, nausea, vomiting and neck stiffness. Examination of cerebrospinal fluid will show a predominately neutrophil leucocytosis, and *Y. pestis* is demonstrated by Gram stain and culture. Mortality is higher than in uncomplicated bubonic plague.

PHARYNGEAL OR TONSILLAR PLAGUE

This is a very rare variety of plague that possibly results from ingestion or inhalation of the organism. Usually the tonsils become swollen and inflamed. There is anterior cervical lymphadenopathy and swelling of the parotid area, with surrounding oedema. *Y. pestis* can be isolated from the throat. It should be distinguished from other common causes of acute tonsillitis and diphtheria.

ASYMPTOMATIC PLAGUE

Asymptomatic infections are probably not uncommon in endemic areas as demonstrated by serological surveys.[14] Asymptomatic carriage of the organism in the throat has also been documented.[15]

MORTALITY

The mortality rate from plague before the antibiotic era ranged from 50 to 95%. With the advent of effective antibiotic therapy the mortality rate fell dramatically. The overall fatality rate in cases reported to the World Health Organization during the last 15 years has been 9.6%.[3] In uncomplicated bubonic plague this may be as low as 5%, but in septicaemic plague documented in New Mexico the case fatality rate was 33%.[13] The prognosis is much worse in patients with pulmonary involvement and, in particular, primary pneumonia invariably remains fatal if treatment is delayed more than 24 hours.

DIAGNOSIS

The diagnosis of plague must be considered in anyone presenting with fever and localized lymphadenitis, without another obvious cause of infection, if they live in, or have returned from, an endemic area. Once plague is suspected, laboratory confirmation should be sought as quickly as possible so that appropriate therapy is given.

In most cases aspiration of a bubo will provide material for microscopic examination and culture. If no fluid or pus is obtained a small amount of saline can be injected and reaspirated. Smears may be stained with Wayson, Giemsa or Gram stains. A presumptive diagnosis of plague is made by demonstration of bipolar staining coccobacilli. This should be confirmed by culture, but rapid identification can be made by immunofluorescence using specific antibodies labelled with fluorescein.[16]

Blood cultures should always be taken, and in suspected pneumonic or meningeal plague specimens of sputum or cerebrospinal fluid should be processed in the same way as bubo aspirates. Speci-mens for culture should be inoculated on to blood agar and MacConkey agar, and also placed into an enrichment broth—with subculture after 24–48 hours. If required, material may also be inoculated into rats or mice, with culture of lymph nodes or spleen after death.

Serological diagnosis is also possible but antibodies may not be detectable when the patient first presents, however it is useful in culture-negative cases. Haemagglutinating antibodies appear after a week and may be detected by the passive haemagglutination test (PHA), which utilizes *Y. pestis* fraction 1 as the antigen. A single titre of $\geqslant 16$, or a fourfold rise, is very suggestive of plague.[2] Enzyme immunoassays have been developed for detection of both antibody and F1 antigen, which appear to be useful adjunctive diagnostic tests.[17] Other methods of serological testing such as latex particle agglutination and radioimmunoassay have also been described.[18,19]

TREATMENT

In clinically suspected cases appropriate antibiotic therapy should be started as soon as specimens have been taken for microbiological confirmation. Even bubonic plague can evolve quickly into a life-threatening disease. The response to treatment is dramatic provided the patient is not already moribund. Patients with pulmonary involvement are highly infectious and must therefore be kept in strict isolation, with precautions against air-borne spread, until at least 3 days of antibiotic(s) have been given and the patient is clinically improved.

Streptomycin, tetracycline and chloramphenicol are the antibiotics traditionally used in the treatment of plague, and they remain highly effective today. Streptomycin was established as the treatment of choice over 40 years ago; the regimen is 30 mg/kg per day in two divided doses, given intramuscularly, for 10 days. There is rapid defervescence of fever. This drug is potentially ototoxic and nephrotoxic; in elderly patients and those with renal impairment, the frequency of administration and total dosage should be reduced. Renal function should be monitored and blood taken for streptomycin levels, if available. There have not been any studies with the newer aminoglycosides.

Tetracycline is a satisfactory alternative, espe-cially in milder cases, when an oral drug is preferred. The dosage is 250–500 mg four times daily—for 10 days. Tetracycline is useful when prophylaxis is considered necessary. It should not be given to pregnant women or children up to 8 years of age, and should also be avoided in renal failure.

Chloramphenicol is the drug of choice for plague meningitis because it achieves good concentrations in the cerebrospinal fluid. An initial loading dose of 25 mg/kg is given intravenously, followed by 100 mg/kg per day in four divided doses. When the clinical condition permits, it can be administered orally for a course of 10 days.

Combinations of these antibiotics are often used in severe cases, although there may be no additional benefit because the individual antibiotics are highly effective and there is no evidence of resistance developing. The fluoroquinolone compounds appear to be highly active against *Y. pestis* in a murine model of infection,[20] although only one bacterial strain was studied. Although newer β-lactam antibiotics were also effective in this single experiment, they cannot be recommended for treatment until more data are available because they have not been successful in treating animal infections with the other yersinioses despite having good in vitro activity.[21]

PREVENTION

The control of plague depends upon public education, rodent and flea control measures and vaccination where appropriate. During an outbreak, active case finding and follow-up of contacts are essential.

The presence of food sources and shelter in areas of human habitation encourages rodents and may be associated with outbreaks of plague. There should be proper disposal of food and refuse; unused outbuildings, wood piles and other forms of shelter for rats should be removed.[22] People should be educated to avoid activities that will bring them into contact with rodents and their fleas. In areas of sylvatic plague, pet cats and dogs should be treated periodically with insecticides.

Surveillance should be undertaken to assess the potential for epizootic plague and the risk of transmission to man. This includes bacteriological monitoring of dead or sick rodents and the serological testing of 'sentinel animals' such as carnivores and dogs, which are more likely to have contact with plague-infected rodents. Enzyme linked immunosorbent assay (ELISA) techniques have advantages over PHA for serological surveillance,[23] and a specific DNA probe has also been developed.[24] A flea index (number of fleas per host animal) should be established. Specific rodent and flea control measures with the use of rodenticides and effective insecticides, although important, are most likely to be successful in the control of urban plague rather than sylvatic plague (which may cover a large area). Attempts at rodent control should be preceded by flea control measures because of the potential risk of increasing human exposure to plague-infected fleas. Houses and warehouses should be rat-proofed. Rat control on ships and in docks, by fumigation, poisoning and trapping, is very important in preventing the dissemination of plague.

An inactivated vaccine, consisting of formalin-killed *Y. pestis*, is available (from Greer Laboratories, Lenoir, NC, USA) for individuals working in high-risk areas. It should also be given to laboratory personnel who work with live cultures of *Y. pestis*. Two initial injections should be given 1–2 months apart, with booster doses every 6 months. Chemoprophylaxis with oral tetracycline is recommended for persons in close contact with plague *pneumonia*, and individuals contaminated in laboratory accidents.

REFERENCES

1 Slack P. The black death past and present. 2. Some historical problems. *Trans R Soc Trop Med Hyg* 1989; 83:461–463.

2 Butler T. *Plague and other Yersinia Infections*. New York: Plenum Press, 1983.

3 Anonymous. Human plague in 1990. *Weekly Epidemiol Rec* 1991; 66:321–324.

4 Brubaker R R. Factors promoting acute and chronic diseases caused by *Yersiniae*. *Clin Microbiol Rev* 1991; 4:309–324.

5 Cavanaugh D C. Specific effect of temperature upon transmission of the plague bacillus by the Oriental rat flea *Xenopsylla cheopis*. *Am J Trop Med Hyg* 1971; 20:264–273.

6 Une T & Brubaker R R. Roles of V antigen in promoting virulence in Yersiniae. *J Immunol* 1984; 133:2226–2230.

7 Straley S C. The plasmid-encoded outer-membrane proteins of *Yersinia pestis*. *Rev Infect Dis* 1988; 10:S323–S326.

8 Lindler L E, Klempner M S & Straley S C. *Yersinia pestis* pH6 antigen: genetic, biochemical and virulence characterization of a protein involved in the pathogenesis of bubonic plague. *Infect Immun* 1990; 58:2569–2577.

9 Butler T. A clinical study of bubonic plague: observations of the 1970 Vietnam epidemic with emphasis on coagulation studies, skin histology and electrocardiograms. *Am J Med* 1972; 53:268–276.

10 Butler T, Bell W R, Linh N N, Tiep N D & Arnold K. *Yersinia pestis* infection in Vietnam. I. Clinical and hematologic aspects. *J Infect Dis* 1974; 129:S78–S84.

11 Butler T, Levin J, Linh N N, Chau D M, Adickman M & Arnold K. *Yersinia pestis* infection in Vietnam. II. Quantitative blood cultures and detection of endotoxin in the cerebrospinal fluid of patients with meningitis. *J Infect Dis* 1976; 133:493–499.

12 Kaufmann A F, Boyce J M & Martone W J. Trends in human plague in the United States. *J Infect Dis* 1980; 141:522–524.

13 Hull H F, Montes J M, & Mann J M. Septicemic plague in New Mexico. *J Infect Dis* 1987; 155:113–118.

14 Legters L J, Cottingham A J Jr & Hunter D H. Clinical and epidemiologic notes on a defined

outbreak of plague in Vietnam. *Am J Trop Med Hyg* 1970; 19:639–652.

15 Marshall J D, Quy D V & Gibson F L. Asymptomatic pharyngeal plague infection in Vietnam. *Am J Trop Med Hyg* 1967; 16:175–177.

16 Winter C C & Moody M D. Rapid identification of *Pasteurella pestis* with fluorescent antibody. II. Specific identification of *Pasteurella pestis* in dried smears. *J Infect Dis* 1959; 104:281–287.

17 Williams J E, Arntzen L, Tyndal G L & Isaacson M. Application of enzyme immunoassays for the confirmation of clinically suspect plague in Namibia, 1982. *Bull World Health Organ* 1986; 64:745–752.

18 Suzuki S, Sakakibara H & Hotta S. Latex agglutination tests for measurement of antiplague antibodies. *J Clin Microbiol* 1977; 6:332–336.

19 Hudson B W, Wolff K & Butler T. The use of solid-phase radioimmunoassay techniques for serodiagnosis of human plague infection. *Bull Pan Am Health Organ* 1980; 14:244–250.

20 Bonacorsi S P, Scavizzi M R, Guiyoule A, Amouroux J H & Carniel E. Assessment of a fluoroquinolone, three β-lactams, two aminoglycosides, and a cycline in treatment of murine *Yersinia pestis* infection. *Antimicrob Agents Chemother* 1994; 38:481–486.

21 Lemaitre B C, Mazigh D A & Scavizzi M R. Failure of beta-lactam antibiotics and marked efficacy of fluoroquinolones in treatment of murine *Yersinia pseudotuberculosis* infection. *Antimicrob Agents Chemother* 1991; 35:1785–1790.

22 Mann J M, Martone W J, Boyce J M, Kaufmann A F, Barnes A M & Weber N S. Endemic human plague in New Mexico: risk factors associated with infection. *J Infect Dis* 1979; 140:397–401.

23 Shepherd A J, Leman P A, Hummitzsch D E & Swanepoel R. A comparison of serological techniques for plague surveillance. *Trans R Soc Trop Med Hyg* 1984; 78:771–773.

24 McDonough K A, Schwan T G, Thomas R E & Falkow S. Identification of a *Yersinia pestis* specific DNA probe with potential for use in plague surveillance. *J Clin Microbiol* 1988; 26:2515–2519.

CHAPTER 51

MELIOIDOSIS

D. A. B. Dance

Melioidosis is an infection caused by the bacterium *Burkholderia pseudomallei*. Although considered a rare disease, it has recently emerged as an important cause of illness and death in some tropical regions, particularly north-east Thailand.[1]

The causative organism was previously assigned to the genus, *Pseudomonas*.

HISTORY

Melioidosis was first described in Rangoon, Burma by Alfred Whitmore and C.S. Krishnaswami in 1912.[2] Whitmore's early studies elegantly fulfilled Koch's postulates for the motile bacillus that he isolated from the 'glanders-like' lesions of morphine addicts who had perished on the city's streets. The following year, William Fletcher isolated the organism during a distemper-like outbreak in the laboratory rodents at the Institute for Medical Research in Kuala Lumpur, although some years passed before he and Stanton recognized its identity with Whitmore's bacillus and revealed the infection to be widespread amongst man and animals in Malaya.[3] French workers in Indochina, recognizing that cases of melioidosis occasionally followed immersion in muddy water, later demonstrated that *B. pseudomallei* was a free-living environmental saprophyte.[4] Over 400 French and American soldiers subsequently contracted the disease whilst stationed in Vietnam.[5] Interest in the disease waned when American troops were withdrawn from South-East Asia, but has been rekindled by the recognition of increasing numbers of cases in north-east Thailand and northern Australia.[1,6]

EPIDEMIOLOGY

Melioidosis is endemic in South-East Asia and northern Australia, with seasonal peaks occurring during the annual rains. In north-east Thailand, *B. pseudomallei* accounts for almost 20% of community-acquired septicaemia, outnumbering cases caused by *Staphylococcus aureus* and *Escherichia coli* during the rainy season.[1] Sporadic cases have also arisen in the Indian subcontinent, Central Africa, Central and South America, the Caribbean and Pacific Islands, and Iran, and during the 1970s an epizootic occurred in France.[7] In endemic areas, *B. pseudomallei* is readily isolated from mud and surface water, particularly rice paddy.[8] Melioidosis is most common in people who have close contact with soil and water (e.g. rice farmers in Thailand, aboriginals in Australia), and is assumed to be acquired through inoculation, inhalation, aspiration or possibly ingestion of environmental organisms.[1,6] Iatrogenic and laboratory acquired infections have occurred occasionally,[9] but the disease is rarely transmitted to contacts of infected humans or animals.[10]

The seasonal nature of melioidosis has been interpreted as implying that most cases are recently acquired, with an incubation period of a few days or weeks. However, less than 10% of patients with septicaemic melioidosis in north-east Thailand could identify a specific episode of exposure.[1] One possible reason for this is the remarkable ability of *B. pseudomallei* to remain latent for periods of up to 26 years,[11] which has given rise to the nickname 'Vietnamese time-bomb'. The proportion of seropositive persons who are latently infected is unknown.

AETIOLOGY

B. pseudomallei is an ovoid, oxidase-positive, motile Gram-negative bacillus which often exhibits marked bipolarity microscopically. The organism was included in the genus *Pseudomonas* during the 1960s on the basis of its biochemical characteristics and nucleic acid composition.[12] It is closely related to *B. mallei*, the causative agent of glanders, with which it has antigenic cross-reactivity, and *B. cepacia*, with which it may occasionally be confused in culture. It grows readily on most routine culture media, giving off a sweet earthy smell. Other characteristics include arginine dihydrolase and gelatinase activity, growth at 42°C, the ability to use a wide range of carbon and energy sources, and intrinsic resistance to aminoglycosides, polymyxins and the early β-lactams. Only two serotypes have been described,[13] and no epidemiologically useful typing scheme is available.

PATHOGENESIS

Although severe melioidosis may occur in apparently normal individuals, the disease usually behaves as an opportunistic infection. Approximately 70% of cases in north-east Thailand have underlying diseases, most frequently diabetes mellitus or chronic renal failure.[1] Steroid therapy, liver disease and alcohol abuse, haematological malignancy and pregnancy may also predispose to melioidosis, and relapse of latent infection usually occurs at times of intercurrent stress.[11] It is thus possible that infection with the human immunodeficiency virus will unmask many more cases of latent melioidosis.

The result of exposure to *B. pseudomallei* varies markedly from case to case and depends on the balance between host immunity, the virulence of the bacterial strain, and the size and route of the inoculum. The possible outcomes are summarized in Figure 51.1. The relative contributions of individual virulence factors to the disease process have not been well characterized. Lipopolysaccharide and a heat-labile exotoxin[14] are likely to be important during the septicaemic phase, although their effects are probably mediated through host-derived cytokines such as tumour necrosis factor and the interleukins.[15,16] Haemolysins, proteases, lecithinase and lipase may cause local tissue damage,[17] and intracellular persistence may contribute to the long periods of latency and the refractory nature of the disease.[18]

PATHOLOGY

The initial lesion of melioidosis is a nodule which tends to undergo central necrosis as it enlarges: adjacent nodules often coalesce. The microscopic appearance of the lesions is not pathognomonic and forms a spectrum from abscess to granuloma depending on the duration of the illness and the response of the individual.[19] The nodules may occur in any tissue, but are most commonly found in the lungs, liver, spleen, lymph nodes, skin and soft tissues, and urinary tract. Pulmonary lesions are frequently surrounded by a zone of haemorrhage.[20] The bacteria can usually be demonstrated by Giemsa or Gram stain in acute lesions, but are scanty in the granulomas of chronic melioidosis.

CLINICAL FEATURES

The variable course and manifestations have made it difficult to develop a satisfactory clinical classification of melioidosis. Since up to 49% of the population in endemic areas has antibodies to *B. pseudomallei*,[21] the majority of infections are presumably mild or asymptomatic. Seroconversion has

Melioidosis – Natural History

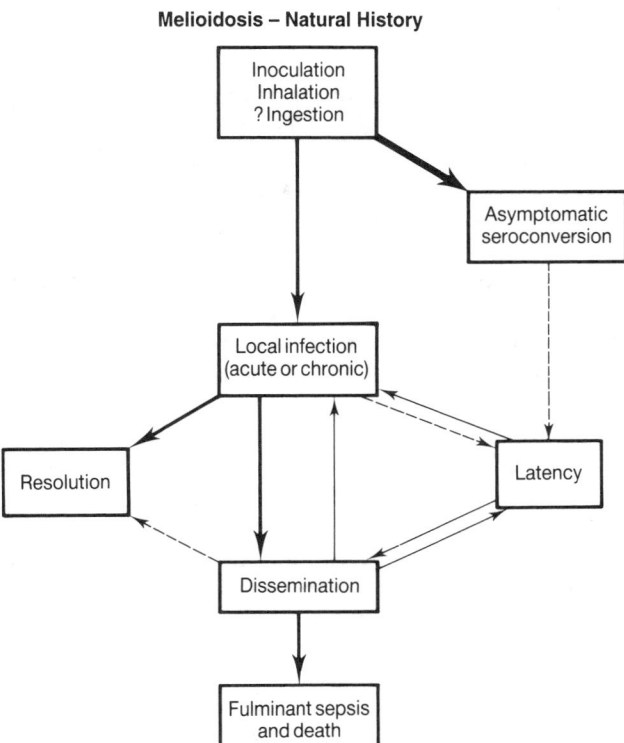

Figure 51.1   Natural history of melioidosis. The most common progression is represented by the broadest arrows. Dotted lines indicate rare or uncertain sequences of events.

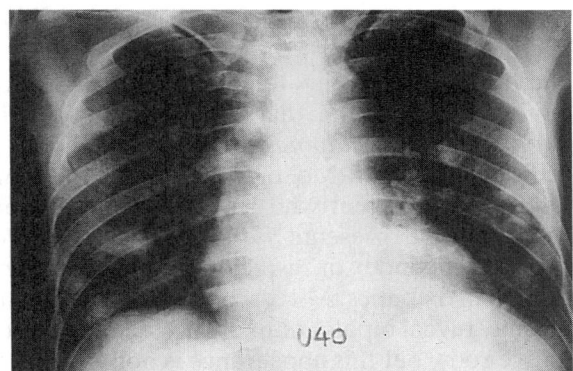

Figure 51.2   Septicaemic melioidosis. Widespread nodular shadowing representing blood-borne pneumonia.

most common pattern being widespread, nodular shadowing (Figure 51.2). Poor prognostic features include hypotension, absence of fever, leucopenia, azotaemia and abnormal liver function tests.[1]

LOCALIZED MELIOIDOSIS

The lung is the most common site for localized melioidosis. The most frequent form is a cavitating pneumonia accompanied by profound weight loss, which is often confused with tuberculosis or lung abscess, although mild bronchitis or bronchopneumonia may be the only manifestation(s). Any lung zone may be affected, although there is a predilection for upper lobe involvement.[23] Localized complications include: pneumothorax, empyema and purulent pericarditis, whilst progression to septicaemia is not uncommon.

Acute suppurative parotitis is a characteristic manifestation of melioidosis in children, accounting for approximately one-third of paediatric cases in north-east Thailand.[24] Parotid abscesses usually ensue and may rupture into the auditory canal. Facial nerve palsy and septicaemia are rare complications.

Localized *B. pseudomallei* infection may occur in any organ. Other presentations include: cutaneous and subcutaneous abscesses, lymphadenitis, osteomyelitis and septic arthritis, liver and/or splenic abscesses,[25] cystitis, pyelonephritis, prostatic abscesses, epididymo-orchitis, and, rarely, brain abscesses. Recently described forms include keratitis and neurological manifestations in the absence of a space occupying lesion.[26,27]

been associated with a flu-like illness.[22] Some of the more common forms of culture-positive melioidosis are described below.

SEPTICAEMIC MELIOIDOSIS

Sixty per cent of cases of culture-positive melioidosis are bacteraemic, and the majority of these are clinically septicaemic. Patients usually have a short history (median 6 days; range 1 day to 2 months) of fever and rigors.[1] Approximately half have evidence of a primary focus of infection, usually pulmonary or cutaneous. Diminished consciousness, jaundice and diarrhoea may also be prominent features. Initial investigations usually reveal anaemia, a neutrophil leucocytosis, coagulopathy and evidence of renal and hepatic impairment. Deterioration is often rapid, with the development of widespread metastatic abscesses, particularly in the lungs, liver and spleen, and metabolic acidosis with Kussmaul's breathing. Cutaneous or subcutaneous abscesses occur in approximately 10% of cases and an abnormal chest radiograph is found in 80% of patients, the

DIAGNOSIS

Melioidosis is difficult to diagnose on clinical grounds alone, so the diagnosis depends on the isolation of *B. pseudomallei* or the detection of specific antibodies. Melioidosis should be considered in any patient who has ever visited an endemic area and presents with septicaemia and/or abscesses. The index of suspicion should be particularly high in diabetics. Microscopy of pus, sputum or urine may reveal bipolar or unevenly staining Gram-negative rods, but this appearance is not specific for *B. pseudomallei*. Several methods for the detection of *B. pseudomallei* antigen(s) in clinical material are under development.

The organism should be sought in blood, pus, urine, sputum or any other specimen indicated by the patient's clinical presentation. The laboratory should be notified when melioidosis is suspected, since selective techniques may increase the isolation rate,[28] and the organism may be overlooked or discarded as a contaminant by the unwary. Furthermore, it is classified as a 'category 3' pathogen because of the risk of infection amongst laboratory staff.[9]

The indirect haemagglutination (IHA) test, which detects antibodies to heat-stable antigens (probably lipopolysaccharide), is the test most widely used for the detection of *B. pseudomallei* antibodies, although recently developed enzyme linked immunosorbent assays (ELISAs) for IgG appear to give similar results.[22] These tests are useful in patients from non-endemic areas in whom a single IHA titre of >1:40 at presentation is highly suggestive of melioidosis. In populations continually exposed to *B. pseudomallei*, the high background seropositivity reduces the predictive value of the test,[1] and in such patients only a rising or very high titre, or the presence of specific IgM can be taken as evidence of melioidosis.[22]

MANAGEMENT

GENERAL

Patients with septicaemic melioidosis require aggressive supportive treatment, with particular attention to correction of volume depletion and septic shock, respiratory and renal failure, and hyperglycaemia or ketoacidosis. Severe cases should ideally be managed in an intensive care unit. Corticosteroids are of doubtful benefit, but anti-endotoxin and anticytokine antibodies remain to be evaluated. Abscesses should be drained surgically whenever possible in both disseminated and localized disease.

SPECIFIC

B. pseudomallei is intrinsically resistant to the combination of penicillin and gentamicin which is often used empirically to treat patients with septicaemia in the tropics, and a complete failure to defervesce on this regimen may help to suggest the diagnosis in an endemic area. Conventional treatment has usually comprised antibiotics such as chloramphenicol, the tetracyclines and co-trimoxazole. Two recent studies have shown that ceftazidime, with or without co-trimoxazole, reduces the mortality of acute severe melioidosis compared with conventional combination regimens.[29,30] Other β-lactams with similar activity in vitro include imipenem, co-amoxiclav and the ureido-penicillins.[31] Treatment of severe cases should comprise ceftazidime (120 mg/kg per day in divided doses or an equivalent dose adjusted for renal function) for at least 2 weeks or until fever has subsided. In β-lactam allergic patients, conventional drugs [chloramphenicol 100 mg/kg per day and doxycycline 4 mg/kg per day, with or without co-trimoxazole (10 mg trimethoprim plus 50 mg sulphamethoxazole)] should be used. Thereafter, treatment with oral agents (co-amoxiclav or the conventional combination regimen as above) should be continued for between 6 weeks and 6 months in order to prevent relapse. Mild cases may be treated with these oral drugs alone.

PREVENTION

No *B. pseudomallei* vaccine has been developed for human use, although experimental vaccines have been used in animals.[32] Prevention is thus limited to the avoidance of contact with *B. pseudomallei* in the environment, particularly by 'at-risk' individuals such as diabetics. Whilst this is feasible in developed countries, it is impractical in the regions where melioidosis is most prevalent. The risk of cross-infection appears to be very low, but cases may be barrier nursed where facilities are available.

REFERENCES

1 Chaowagul W, White N J, Dance D A B et al. Melioidosis: a major cause of community-acquired septicemia in Northeastern Thailand. *J Infect Dis* 1989; 159:890–899.

2 Whitmore A & Krishnaswami C S. An account of the discovery of a hitherto undescribed infective disease occurring among the population of Rangoon. *Indian Med Gazette* 1912; 47:262–267.

3 Stanton A T & Fletcher W. *Melioidosis*, Studies from the Institute for Medical Research, Federated Malay States, 21. London: John Bale & Sons and Danielson, 1932.

4 Chambon L. Isolement du bacille de Whitmore à partir du milieu extérieur. *Ann Inst Pasteur* 1955; 89:229–235.

5 Sanford J P. *Pseudomonas* species (including melioidosis and glanders). In Mandell G I, Douglas R G & Bennett J E (eds) *Principles and Practice of Infectious Diseases*, 3rd edn. New York: Churchill Livingstone, 1990:1692–1696.

6 Ashdown L R. Epidemiological aspects of melioidosis in Australia. *Commun Dis Intell* 1991; 15:272–273.

7 Dance D A B. Melioidosis: the tip of the iceberg? *Clin Microbiol Rev* 1991; 4:52–60.

8 Strauss J M, Groves M G, Mariappan M & Ellison D W. Melioidosis in Malaysia. II. Distribution of *Pseudomonas pseudomallei* in soil and surface water. *Am J Trop Med Hyg* 1969; 18:698–702.

9 Schlech W F, Turchik J B, Westlake R E, Klein G C, Band J D & Weaver R E. Laboratory-acquired infection with *Pseudomonas pseudomallei* (melioidosis). *N Engl J Med* 1981; 305:1133–1135.

10 Kunakorn M, Jayanetra P & Tanphaichitra D. Man to man transmission of melioidosis. *Lancet* 1991; 337:1290–1291.

11 Mays E E & Ricketts E A. Melioidosis: recrudescence associated with bronchogenic carcinoma twenty-six years following initial geographic exposure. *Chest* 1975; 68:261–263.

12 Rogul M, Brendle J J, Haapala D K & Alexander A D. Nucleic acid similarities amongst *Pseudomonas pseudomallei*, *Pseudomonas multivorans*, and *Actinobacillus mallei*. *J Bacteriol* 1970: 101:827–835.

13 Dodin A & Fournier J. Antigènes précipitants et antigènes agglutinants de *Pseudomonas pseudomallei* (B. de Whitmore). 1. Complexe thermostable et complexe thermolabile. Typage sérologique. *Ann Inst Pasteur* 1970; 119:211–221.

14 Heckly R J. Differentiation of exotoxin and other biologically active substances in *Pseudomonas pseudomallei* filtrates. *J Bacteriol* 1964; 88:1730–1736.

15 Friedland J S, Suputtamongkol Y, Remick D G et al. Prolonged elevation of interleukin-8 and interleukin-6 concentrations in plasma and of leukocyte interleukin-8 mRNA levels during septicemic and localized *Pseudomonas pseudomallei* infection. *Infect Immun* 1992; 60:2402–2408.

16 Suputtamongkol Y, Kwiatkowski D, Dance D A B, Chaowagul W & White N J. Tumor necrosis factor in septicemic melioidosis. *J Infect Dis* 1992; 165:561–564.

17 Ashdown L R & Koehler J M. Production of hemolysins and other extracellular enzymes by clinical isolates of *Pseudomonas pseudomallei*. *J Clin Microbiol* 1990; 28:2331–2334.

18 Pruksachartvuthi S, Aswapokee N & Thankerngpol K. Survival of *Pseudomonas pseudomallei* in human phagocytes. *J Med Microbiol* 1990; 31:109–114.

19 Greenwald K A, Nash G & Foley F D. Acute systemic melioidosis. Autopsy findings in four patients. *Am J Clin Pathol* 1969; 52:188–198.

20 Piggott J A & Hochholzer L. Human melioidosis. A histopathologic study of acute and chronic melioidosis. *Arch Pathol* 1970; 90:101–111.

21 Khupulsup K & Petchclai, B. Application of indirect haemagglutination test and indirect fluorescent antibody test for IgM antibody for diagnosis of melioidosis in Thailand. *Am J Trop Med Hyg* 1986; 35:366–369.

22 Ashdown L R, Johnson R W, Koehler J M & Cooney C A. Enzyme-linked immunosorbent assay for the diagnosis of clinical and subclinical melioidosis. *J Infect Dis* 1989; 160:253–260.

23 Dhiensri T, Puapairoj S & Susaengrat W. Pulmonary melioidosis: clinical and radiologic correlation in 183 cases in northeastern Thailand. *Radiology* 1988; 166:711–715.

24 Dance D A B, Davis T M E, Wattanagoon Y et al. Acute suppurative parotitis in children caused by

Pseudomonas pseudomallei. J Infect Dis 1989; 159:654–660.

25 Vatcharapreechasagul T, Suputtamongkol Y, Dance D A B, Chaowagul W & White N J. *Pseudomonas pseudomallei* liver abscess: a clinical, laboratory and ultrasonographic study. *Clin Infect Dis* 1992; 14:412–417.

26 Siripanthong S, Teerapantuwat S, Prugsanusak W et al. Corneal ulcer caused by *Pseudomonas pseudomallei*; report of three cases. *Rev Infect Dis* 1991; 13:335–337.

27 Woods M L, Currie B J, Howard D M et al. Neurological melioidosis: seven cases from the Northern Territory of Australia. *Clin Infect Dis* 1992; 15:163–169.

28 Wuthiekanun V, Dance D A B, Wattanagoon Y, Suputtamongkol Y, Chaowagul W & White N J. The use of selective media for the isolation of *Pseudomonas pseudomallei* in clinical practice. *J Med Microbiol* 1990; 33:121–126.

29 White N J, Dance D A B, Chaowagul W, Wuthiekanun V & Pitakwatchara, N. Halving of mortality of severe melioidosis by ceftazidime. *Lancet* 1989; ii:697–700.

30 Sookpranee M, Boonma P, Susaengrat W, Bhuripanyo K & Punyagupta S. Multicenter prospective randomised trial comparing ceftazidime plus co-trimoxazole with chloramphenicol plus doxycycline and co-trimoxazole for treatment of severe melioidosis. *Antimicrob Agents Chemother* 1992; 36:158–162.

31 Dance D A B, Wuthiekanun V, Chaowagul W & White N J. The antimicrobial susceptibility of *Pseudomonas pseudomallei*. Emergence of resistance in vitro and during treatment. *J Antimicrob Chemother* 1989; 24:295–309.

32 Vedros N A, Chow D & Liong, E. Experimental vaccine against *Pseudomonas pseudomallei* infections in captive cetaceans. *Dis Aquatic Organisms* 1988; 5:157–161.

CHAPTER 52

DIPHTHERIA

N. J. White and T. T. Hien

DEFINITION

Diphtheria is an acute infectious disease of the tonsils, pharynx, larynx or nose, and occasionally of other mucous membranes or skin caused by *Corynebacterium diphtheriae*. The word diphtheria originates from the term 'diphtherite', which has a Greek root meaning skin or hide, and refers to the leathery appearance of the characteristic pharyngeal membrane.[1] The disease is caused by the local effects of destructive infection (usually in the naso-pharynx) and the distal effects of diphtheria toxin on the heart, peripheral nerves and kidneys. Death results from airways obstruction, myocarditis or polyneuritis. Diphtheria has declined dramatically in affluent countries over the past 70 years,[2,3] but it remains an important disease in many parts of the tropics and there has been a recent resurgence of the disease in what was western Russia.

BACTERIOLOGY

The diphtheria bacillus was first grown in pure culture by Loeffler in 1884. The causative organism, *C. diphtheriae* is a non-motile, non-capsulated, non-spore forming aerobic bacillus. Although it is described as Gram positive, it is easily decolorized and thus may appear Gram negative. On microscopy, *C. diphtheriae* exhibits considerable pleomorphism, ranging from the classical club shape to long slender bacilli, and the arrangement of organisms on a smear often resembles Chinese letters. The presence of metachromatic granules when stained by Loeffler's methylene blue or Albert's stains is characteristic, although this should not be relied upon for identification.

C. diphtheriae grows well on blood agar, but tellurite blood agar (Hoyle's medium) is recommended as this inhibits other respiratory flora and allows the characteristic colonial morphology of the three bioptypes (*gravis*, *intermedius* and *mitis*) to develop.[4] Although, as the name implies, toxigenic *gravis* strains are generally associated with more severe disease, in vitro *mitis* strains often produce more toxin than *gravis* or *intermedius* strains. Toxin production is very dependent on the composition of the growth medium. The iron content is particularly important. Young organisms produce more toxin than older organisms, and thus increased toxin production is associated with rapid growth. The association between biotype and severity is not constant. *C. diphtheriae* is further identified by biochemical reactions: acid is produced from glucose and maltose but only very rarely from sucrose; urea is not hydrolysed. The *gravis* biotype ferments starch.[5] Simple screening tests have been developed for identification of the pathogenic corynebacteria, which do not produce pyrazinamidase, but do produce cystinase (seen as a brown halo around colonies, when cystine is incorporated into modified Tinsdale's agar).[6]

PATHOGENESIS

The potential lethal effects of diphtheria in man are caused by an exotoxin. The toxigenicity of *C. diphtheriae* depends on the presence of a *tox*[+] phage (a lysogenic β-phage) which induces the organism to produce toxin. Harmless non-toxigenic strains of *C. diphtheriae*, lacking the *tox*$^+$ β-phage, can be converted to pathogenic toxigenic strains by infection with a lysogenic phage (in vitro). This process may also occur in vivo.[7]

Toxin production by corynebacteria is usually detected by the Elek's test[5] or guinea-pig inoculation, but recently enzyme immunoassays have been developed which are cheaper and easier.[8] It should be noted that diphtheria toxin can also be produced by *C. ulcerans* and this has also resulted in clinical diphtheria.[9]

Diphtheria exotoxin is a 62000 Da polypeptide which includes 2 segments: the active toxin moiety (A) and the binding (B) segment which binds to specific receptors on susceptible cells. The binding B portion attaches to the cell membrane allowing the active A portion to enter the cells where it catalyses a reaction which inactivates the transfer RNA (t-RNA) translocase 'elongation factor 2' (EF2), in eukaryotic cells. This factor is essential for reactions which transfer triplet codes from messenger RNA to amino acid sequences via t-RNA. Thus EF2 inactivation stops synthesis of the polypeptide chains. The diphtheria toxin affects all human cells but the most profound effects are on the myocardium (myocarditis), peripheral nerves (demyelination) and kidneys (acute tubular necrosis).

EPIDEMIOLOGY

The only known reservoir for *C. diphtheriae* is man. Diphtheria spreads from person to person, either from acute cases or from asymptomatic carriers. The principal modes of spread are by respiratory droplets or direct contact with secretions from the respiratory tract or exudate from infected skin. Fomites and dust are not important vehicles of transmission, but the organism can resist drying and can be isolated from floor dust in a ward or an infected room. Epidemics have been caused by milk contaminated by a human carrier. Some patients become carriers and continue to harbour *C. diphtheriae* for weeks or months or rarely for a lifetime.

The incidence of diphtheria in the Western world has decreased in the last 50–75 years (152 cases/100000 population in 1920 to 0.002/100000 in 1980 in the USA). As diphtheria began to decline before the immunization programme, and epidemics have occurred even in highly immunized populations, it seems that there are additional undefined factors contributing to the low incidence of diphtheria in affluent countries. Although the World Health Organization reports similar decreases in incidence worldwide, the disease is still a significant problem in many developing countries.

CLINICAL MANIFESTATIONS

Diphtheria is predominantly a disease of childhood.[10,11] After an incubation period of 2–5 days, diphtheria presents in a variety of different forms depending upon the location of the pseudomembrane. The grey-white membrane is the hallmark of the infection. It is caused by the destructive effects of the toxin on epithelial cells. The membrane is composed of a coagulum of leucocytes, bacteria, cellular debris and fibrin. It is adherent to underlying tissues and bleeds if pulled away. In clinical practice the disease can be divided into groups as follows: cutaneous, nasal, faucial, tracheolaryngeal and malignant diphtheria. Faucial diphtheria is the most common, whereas cutaneous diphtheria is relatively rare in endemic areas; but where the disease is rare, cutaneous diphtheria is relatively more common.

ANTERIOR NASAL DIPHTHERIA

The principal symptom is nasal discharge (100%). This is usually unilateral, thin at first, then purulent and bloody with excoriations of the nostril and skin above the upper lip. Nasal diphtheria is relatively common in infancy. It is often mild except when nasopharyngeal or faucial forms coexist.

FAUCIAL DIPHTHERIA

This is the most common form of diphtheria. The onset is usually slow, with moderate fever, malaise and sore throat (80%). Other symptoms may include nausea, vomiting and painful dysphagia. There is typically a patch or patches of greyish-yellow adherent membrane with a surrounding dull red inflammatory zone on one or both tonsils. At the beginning of the illness diphtheria can look like any type of tonsillitis, with only a small spot of membrane on one tonsil. The membrane may then extend to the uvula, soft palate, oropharynx, nasopharynx or larynx. The lymph nodes in the neck are slightly enlarged and painful and the neck may be slightly swollen. The foetor of diphtheria is characteristic and was once one of the four criteria for clinical diagnosis (membrane, foetor, lymphadenitis, oedema).[2]

TRACHEOLARYNGEAL DIPHTHERIA

Diphtheria of the larynx is usually secondary to faucial diphtheria (85%). Occasionally, there is no membrane on the pharynx at all. The initial symptoms include moderate fever (75%) with hoarseness (100%), unproductive cough and dyspnoea. Obstruction of breathing by the expanding membrane and associated oedema occurs gradually over approximately 24 hours. The severely affected child appears agitated, but is quiet, sweating and ominously cyanotic. The accessory muscles of respiration are used, with retraction of supraclavicular, substernal and intercostal tissues on inspiration. Without a tracheostomy the child will suffocate and die.

MALIGNANT DIPHTHERIA

This is the most severe form of diphtheria. The onset is more acute than in other forms. The patient becomes rapidly 'toxic', with high fever, rapid pulse, low blood pressure and cyanosis. Usually, extension of the membrane is more rapid, spreading from the tonsils to the uvula, then creeping forward across the hard palate, up the nasopharynx, or sometimes down the nostrils. Cervical adenitis and oedema produce the classical 'bull neck' appearance. The patient may bleed from the mouth, nose and skin. Cardiac involvement with heart block occurs earlier, within few days from the onset. More than one half of malignant diphtheria cases are fatal, and this high mortality has changed little with treatment.

CUTANEOUS DIPHTHERIA

Skin infections with *C. diphtheriae* are now more common than nasopharyngeal disease in the West. This particularly affects vagrants and alcoholics living in unhygienic conditions. The clinical features range from a simple pustule to a chronic non-healing ulcer with a grey, dirty, membrane. Toxic complications from these infections are infrequent, and when they do occur are more likely to manifest as neuritis than myocarditis.

OTHER SITES

Occasionally, clinical infections with *C. diphtheriae* may occur in other sites, such as ears, conjunctiva or vagina. Swabs of ear discharge from otitis media may occasionally grow *C. diphtheriae* but toxic manifestations are rare.

COMPLICATIONS

Severe diphtheria is a terrible disease. Even if patients survive the acute destructive phase of the infection, they are likely to die from the remote effects of the toxin. Patients recovering from diphtheria may die suddenly up to 8 weeks following the acute disease. The most prominent toxic complications of diphtheria are myocarditis and neuritis. The risk and the severity of toxin damage correlate with the extent of the pseudomembrane and the delay in administration of antitoxin. The frequency of cardiac involvement following laryngeal and malignant diphtheria is three- to eightfold higher compared with tonsillar diphtheria, and two- to threefold higher if antitoxin is given ≥48 hours from the onset of disease. Overall, approximately 10% of patients with diphtheria develop myocarditis, although two-thirds of patients with severe infection will have some evidence of cardiac involvement. The first evidence of cardiac toxicity usually occurs after the first week of illness.[12] Clinical signs include soft heart sounds, a gallop rhythm, and less commonly signs of congestive heart failure. Incompetent murmurs may develop as the ventricles dilate. The mortality of diphtheritic myocarditis is approximately 50%. ECG abnormalities are more common than clinical signs of myocarditis and include frequent supraventricular and ventricular ectopics, ST and T wave changes, varying degrees of heart block, and arrythmias. Patients with bundle branch block and complete heart block have a >80% increased mortality.

The exotoxin causes degeneration of the myelin sheath and axon cylinder of peripheral nerves. Polyneuritis is uncommon in mild diphtheria but occurs in approximately 7–10% of moderate and severe cases. Paralysis develops late, usually between 5 and 8 weeks after the onset of local symptoms. Paralysis of the soft palate is characteristic. This results in a nasal voice and regurgitation of ingested fluids through the nose. Later, blurred vision may occur because of paralysis of muscles of accommodation. Most neurological complications develop between the sixth and seventh weeks, when clinical progress seems to be otherwise satisfactory. Paralysis of the pharynx, larynx and respiratory muscles is the most common manifestation. Less common complications of diphtheria include acute tubular necrosis, endocarditis and secondary pneumonia. The overall mortality of diphtheria is approximately 5–10%, with a relatively higher rate in infancy and old age.

DIAGNOSIS

In many parts of the world, especially in developing countries, diphtheria is still a common disease. It should be considered in any patient with the following symptoms: tonsillitis and/or pharyngitis with pseudomembrane, hoarseness and stridor, cervical adenopathy or cervical swelling (bull neck), unilateral bloody nasal discharge or paralysis of the palate. Direct smears of infected areas of the throat are often made but these are unreliable. The diagnosis is confirmed by isolation and identification of *C. diphtheriae* from infected sites. The differential diagnosis includes streptococcal or viral pharyngitis and tonsillitis, and Vincent's angina. A common and sometimes tragic error is to diagnose tonsillar diphtheria as infectious mononucleosis, or a case of 'bull neck' (malignant diphtheria) as mumps.

TREATMENT

Emergency tracheostomy should be performed to relieve respiratory obstruction in laryngeal diphtheria. The procedure must not be delayed until the patient develops cyanosis. Agitation and the use of the accessory respiratory muscles are indications for immediate tracheostomy. Since the mortality of diphtheria increases with delay in antitoxin administration, treatment with diphtheria antitoxin should be started on clinical suspicion, without waiting for definitive laboratory confirmation. The dose of antitoxin depends on the site of primary infection, the extent of pseudomembrane and the delay between the onset and the antitoxin administration: 20000–40000 units for faucial diphtheria of <48 hours duration, or cutaneous infection; 40000–80000 units for faucial diphtheria of >48 hours duration, or laryngeal infection; 80000–100000 units for malignant diphtheria (bull neck, toxic state). Adrenaline should be available to cope with rare anaphylactic reactions to the antitoxin.

Antibiotics will stop toxin production and prevent further spread of organisms in the host. *C. diphtheriae* is susceptible to a variety of antibiotics including penicillin, cephalosporins, erythromycin and tetracycline. Erythromycin has been the most effective in eliminating the carrier state. The recommended antibiotic treatment regimens are penicillin G, 100000 units/kg twice a day, or erythromycin, parenterally or orally 5mg/kg four times daily.

Bed-rest is recommended during the acute phase, but there is no proof of its benefit. Close electrocardiographic monitoring is indicated, particularly after the first week, to detect cardiac involvement. If there is high-grade heart block then temporary pacing should be considered, although there have been no studies to determine whether this influences outcome. A recent study has suggested that carnitine may be beneficial by decreasing the incidence of myocarditis,[13] but additional evidence of its efficacy is required. The administration of corticosteroids is of no benefit.[14]

PREVENTION

Diphtheria is readily preventable by vaccine administration. This is included in the triple vaccine: diphtheria, tetanus and pertussus vaccine (DTP). The recommended primary course of immunization of children up to 7 years old consists of three doses: the first at 6–8 weeks old, the second at 3 months and the third at 4 months. A fourth dose is given 6–12 months after the third. A booster dose of diphtheria–tetanus (DT) vaccine is given at school entry. If primary immunization is delayed until 7 years of age, or is interrupted, a series of three doses of tetanus and diphtheria toxoid adsorbed (DT ads), which contains less diphtheria toxoid than DTP, should be completed: the second dose 4–8 weeks after the first; and the third 6–12 months later. Patients with diphtheria should receive active immunization after recovery. Close contacts should be screened for *C. diphtheriae* with throat swab culture. If the immunization status is unclear, they should be treated with an appropriate antibiotic if culture positive, and receive primary immunization according to their age. Immunity following immunization is assessed by the Schick test. A standardized sterile diluted filtrate from a culture of *C. diphtheriae* (the Schick test toxin) is injected intradermally (0.2 ml) into the flexor surface of the left forearm. An equal volume (0.2 ml) of heat-inactivated filtrate (Schick test control) is injected intradermally into the right forearm. The injection sites are inspected after 24–48 hours and again at 5–7 days. A lack of inflammation indicates adequate antitoxic immunity. Sometimes non-specific reactions (pseudoreactions) occur, but these are usually equal in both arms (i.e. toxin and control elicit an equal inflammatory reaction). Schick-negative patients are either resistant to disease, or with *gravis* and *intermedius* strains they may sometimes develop mild disease.

REFERENCES

1 English P C. Diphtheria and theories of infectious disease: centennial appreciation of the critical role of diphtheria in the history of medicine. *Pediatrics* 1985; 76:1–9.

2 Kwantes W. Diphtheria in Europe. *J Hyg (Camb)* 1984; 93:433–437.

3 Dixon J M S. Diphtheria in North America. *J Hyg (Camb)* 1984; 93:419–432.

4 Noble W C & Dixon J M S. *Corynebacterium* and other coryneform bacteria. In Parker T M & Duerden B I (Eds) *Topley and Wilson's Principles of Bacteriology, Virology and Immunity*, vol. 2, 8th edn. London: Edward Arnold, 1990: 103–118.

5 Brooks R & Joynson D H M. Bacterial diagnosis of diphtheria. *J Clin Pathol* 1990; 43:576–580.

6 Coleman G, Weaver E & Efstratiou A. Screening tests for pathogenic corynebacteria. *J Clin Pathol* 1992; 45:46–48.

7 Pappenheimer A M & Murphy J H. Studies on the molecular epidemiology of diphtheria. *Lancet* 1983; ii:923–926.

8 Hallas G, Harrison T G, Samuel D & Coleman G. Detection of diphtheria toxin in culture supernates of *Corynebacterium diphtheriae* and *C. ulcerans* by immunoassay with monoclonal antibody. *J Med Microbiol* 1990; 32:247–253.

9 Meers P D. A case of classical diphtheria due to *Corynebacterium ulcerans*. *J Infect* 1979; 1:139–142.

10 Hong N T, Phu V T & Hien T T. A study of 2597 cases of diphtheria treated at Cho Quan Hospital during 10 years (1976–85). *Ann Sci Rep Cho Quan Hosp Vietnam* 1985.

11 Naiditch M J & Bower A G. Diphtheria. A study of 1433 cases observed at the Los Angeles County Hospital. *Am J Med* 1954; 17:229–245.

12 Boyer N H & Weinstein L. Diphtheritic myocarditis. *N Engl J Med* 1948; 239:913–919.

13 Ramos A C M F, Elias P R D, Barrucand L & Silva J A F D. The protective effect of carnitine in human diphtheric myocarditis. *Pediatr Res* 1987; 18:815–819.

14 Thisyakorn U, Wongvanich J & Kumpeng V. Failure of corticosteroid therapy to prevent diphtheritic myocarditis or neuritis. *Pediatr Infect Dis* 1984; 3:126–128.

CHAPTER 53

ACTINOMYCOSIS

G. Scott

Actinomycosis is characterized by indolent abscesses that cross fascial planes, forming chronic sinuses which discharge pus containing (in 40% of cases) 'sulphur granules'.[1] The causative organisms are mouth flora, so the jaw is a characteristic site for infection; other sites include the appendix, lung and uterus but any organ may be infected.

GEOGRAPHICAL DISTRIBUTION

Because the organisms are part of the normal buccol flora, the infection may occur in any part of the world.

AETIOLOGY

The primary causative agents are Gram-positive anaerobic (or rarely facultatively aerobic), branching bacteria of the genera *Actinomyces* and *Arachnia*. These organisms used to be thought of as fungi because they branched and formed aerial mycelia. However, they are clearly bacteria, by being prokaryocytic, by the absence of typical fungal carbohydrates (e.g. chitin) in the cell wall and by their method of reproduction. The term is derived from *aktino* (Greek: ray), suggested by the spikes radiating from the edge of the sulphur granules. The first species described (*A. bovis*) from tumours of the jaws of cattle does not cause disease in man.

However, one or more of a number of species (*A. israelii* (the most important species named after the pioneering microbiologist Israel who first described sulphur granules from a lesion in man in 1878), *A. naeslundii*, *A. meyeri*, *A. viscosus*, *A. odontolyticus* and *Arachnia propionica*[2]) may cause human disease. These bacteria are rarely found alone in clinical specimens but are intimately associated with Gram-negative ones such as *Actinobacillus actinomycetemcomitans* and *Haemophilus aphrophilus* (both well known for causing endocarditis). Separating and identifying these bacteria is difficult even in the specialized laboratory.

CLINICAL PRESENTATION

Head and neck actinomycosis is unlikely to be recognized specifically when it presents early. If associated with local invasion from the mouth, there will be soft, relatively non-tender, swellings which grow insidiously and then break down and discharge to the outside. Some report that the abscesses look blue. Because the infection can spread unhindered by fascial planes, the abscesses may discharge anywhere in the region of the head and neck, including the tongue, palate or even scalp. Direct extension of the abscess may lead to invasion of the central nervous system. Infection in the thyroid has been recorded. Occasionally an actinomycetoma will develop more rapidly than usual but it will still be 'cold'.

When the patient presents, it may well be possible to get a history of predisposing dental work or it may be quite obvious that the patient has very poor dentition with extensive caries. Sometimes the infection is precipitated by trauma, such as dental extraction or even an external blow. Human bites or trauma to the fist from front teeth in a fight may cause local inoculation and infection.

Infection in the lungs spreads locally through to pleura, chest wall or mediastinum, and presumably follows the inhalation of a foreign body colonized with mouth flora. The presentation is one of constitutional upset associated with some symptoms referable to the chest (even haemoptysis) with an abnormal radiograph. Rare fatal disease is usually associated with invasion of myopericardium.

DISSEMINATION

Bloodstream spread of the organism most commonly occurs from established chronic infections at any site. This may lead to miliary multifocal infection and skin lesions. Extensive spread has been documented in association with malignant disease.

ABDOMINAL

One-quarter to one-half of all cases of actinomycosis involve an abdominal organ. There may be a precipitating event such as abdominal surgery, or internal (e.g. foreign body) or external trauma. The most usual antecedent surgery is for acute appendicitis and it is no surprise therefore that the most common site for infection is the ileocaecal region. The infection spreads gradually from the primary site, is very difficult to diagnose and may only become obvious when the infection points and discharges characteristic pus. Even then, a small discharging sinus may go unrecognized for years. Spread through the portal system leads to liver abscess which may spread insidiously through chest wall or diaphragm.

Pelvic or endometrial actinomycosis is rare but some cases were recognized in patients using intrauterine contraceptive devices. This is rather uncommon—beware the cytopathologist's report of the Papanicolaou stain of cervical smear suggesting that *Actinomyces* spp. are present.[3] This is not a sensitive or specific way of making the diagnosis. However, it is worth considering the diagnosis if patient with an intrauterine contraceptive device does develop indolent uterine or parauterine disease which is often initially considered to be a malignant tumour.

DIFFERENTIAL DIAGNOSIS

In extensive late disease, where sinuses are discharging pus with characteristic sulphur granules, the diagnosis should be obvious and can easily be confirmed in the laboratory. Sulphur granules may also be demonstrated in section by the histologist searching for presumed tumour: the organism will not be seen on haematoxylin and eosin stain but will require a silver or Gram stain (Figures 53.1 and 53.2). Several other organisms yield sulphur granules from pus but rarely are they as characteristically gritty, with the stellate radiations seen in *Actinomyces*. They include *Nocardia* spp. (which produce almost indistinguishable disease, more often in immunosuppressed patients, and demands rather different antimicrobial therapy): the sulphur granules in nocardiasis are grey and smooth. *Staphylococcus aureus* may cause chronic abscesses which discharge

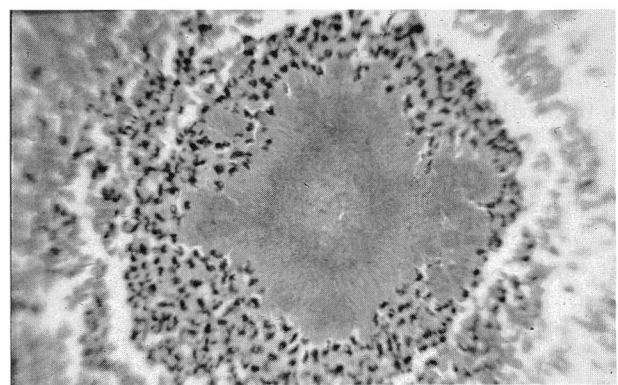

Figure 53.1 Sulphur granule stained with H & E.

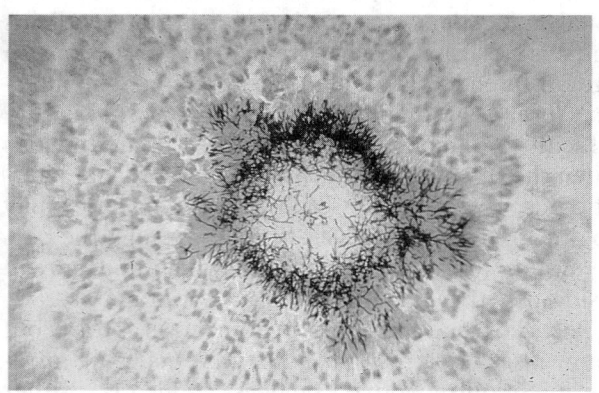

Figure 53.2   Sulphur granule stained with Gram stain, revealing typical central Gram-positive branching bacteria.

rather soft irregular yellow granules—a condition known as botriomycosis. Various fungi (e.g. *Streptomyces* spp.) may cause granules, and it is not unusual for these to be discharged from Madurella mycetoma, without any hint of *Actinomyces* spp. on culture.

Pulmonary disease will most often be diagnosed initially as tuberculosis or tumour. Nocardia and fungi are more important opportunistic pulmonary pathogens than *Actinomyces*, which most often affects otherwise healthy people. Abdominal disease may be misdiagnosed as appendix mass, Crohn's disease or ileocaecal tuberculosis.

Uterine disease, if not diagnosed early, may present with a massive tumour in a fixed pelvis, which will inevitably first be diagnosed as malignancy.

DIAGNOSIS

The diagnosis is by macroscopic and microscopic examination of pus and granules and culture—preferably prolonged, in anaerobic conditions at 37°C. Whereas most strains have classical branching bacillary morphology, some appear as pleomorphic coccobacilli. Pus should be cultured in thioglycollate broth with added rabbit serum or brain–heart infusion broth or trypticase soy agar. Complex semi-synthetic media may be more successful. Some species grow aerobically in carbon dioxide after a while but this is not reliable. Under optimal conditions, a fine aerial mycelium is seen at day 1, then the colony grows into a solid white block which collapses centrally over a period of 7–14 days, known (most appropriately) as a 'molar tooth'.

Most microbiologists will not bother to speciate the strain, although this can be done by chemical tests provided the bacterium can be separated from the concomitant Gram-negatives. Another method is to use species-specific conjugated antibody either on the original specimen or the cultured organism.[4,5] *Arachnia propionica* forms smaller, smoother colonies than *A. israelii*, and they are not molar-tooth shaped; the organism produces propionic acid which can be detected by gas–liquid chromatography.

TREATMENT

Actinomyces spp. are sensitive to a wide variety of antimicrobials, including penicillin which remains the drug of choice. Unfortunately, penicillin V is not well absorbed so is not suitable for initial therapy. High and prolonged dosage is indicated together with appropriate surgical drainage and debridement. Virtually every other simple antibiotic can be used as an alternative—sulphonamide, erythromycin, chloramphenicol and tetracycline being effective. There is little correlation between in vitro sensitivity tests and clinical results. Drugs relatively ineffective in vitro are often very effective in vivo. However, metronidazole is inactive. Clindamycin seems a logical choice, being active in vitro, well absorbed and penetrating into tissues and bone well, and might be the drug of choice when bone is involved.

PREVENTION

Actinomycosis is rare. Disease associated with poor dentition can naturally be prevented by improving dental hygiene. The association with intrauterine contraceptive devices is sufficiently rare that it should not be considered a contraindication to this method of contraception.

REFERENCES

1 Weese W C & Smith J M. A study of 57 cases of actinomycosis over a 36 year period. *Arch Intern Med* 1975; 135:1562–1568.

2 Brock D W, Georg L K, Brown J M et al. Actinomycosis caused by *Arachnia propionica*. Report of 11 cases. *Am J Clin Pathol* 1973; 59:66–77.

3 Spence M R, Gupta P K, Frost J K & King T M. Cytologic detection and chemical significance of *Actinomyces israelii* in women using intrauterine contraceptive devices. *Am J Obstet Gynecol* 1978; 131:295–298.

4 Slack J M & Gerencser M A. Two new serological groups of *Actinomyces*. *J Bacteriol* 1970;103:265–266.

5 Slack J M, Landfried S & Gerencser M A. Identification of Actinomyces and related bacteria in dental calculus by the fluorescent antibody technique. *J Dent Res* 1971; 50:78–82.

CHAPTER 54

ENDEMIC TREPONEMATOSES

O. P. Arya

The endemic or non-venereal treponematoses include: yaws, endemic syphilis and pinta. Their causative organisms, *Treponema pertenue* for yaws, *T. pallidum* for endemic syphilis and *T. carateum* for pinta, have remained up until the present time morphologically indistinguishable from *T. pallidum* which causes venereal syphilis (Chapter 13). Likewise, there are no differences in serology or response to penicillin. Nevertheless, there are significant clinical and epidemiological differences among these treponematoses. The discrepant manifestations of these biologically 'similar' organisms has generated considerable interest leading to academic disputes and much speculation and argument among medical historians. Hudson[1] recognized only *T. pallidum* and believed in an all-embracing concept (unitarian theory), i.e. all of the treponematoses were due to the same organism and that the differences were determined by the socioenvironmental conditions such as age, microclimate of skin, temperature and humidity. Others, including Hackett,[2] believe that these conditions are separate entities caused by different organisms. Whereas it is generally believed that the DNA profiles of the causative organisms of venereal syphilis, yaws and endemic syphilis are indistinguishable,[3] there may well be subtle morphological differences which remain to be characterized. In one study, *T. pertenue* and *T. pallidum* were reported to differ in at least one nucleotide.[4] The differences with regard to experimental infections in laboratory animals have also been described.

Infection with one organism may provide only partial protection against subsequent infection by another.

Endemic treponematoses were among the most predominant diseases in the preantibiotic era. Thus in the mid-twentieth century there were an estimated 50 million cases of yaws worldwide (half in Africa), over 1 million cases of endemic syphilis (mostly in North Africa and the eastern Mediterranean basin) and about a million cases of pinta confined to Central and South America. Discovery of long-acting penicillin preparations, which were cheap, safe and curative with a single intramuscular injection, made a cost-effective eradication programme possible. Consequently in 1948, the World Health Organization, in conjunction with UNICEF and many national governments, established a global control programme, first against yaws and later extended to include endemic syphilis and pinta. Mobile teams were formed, and over 50 million individuals were treated out of 160 million examined in 46 countries. As a result these diseases were brought under control or even eliminated from some areas. However, dismantling of the mobile teams and lack of active surveillance led to the persistence of endemic foci in some countries. From 1980, not surprisingly, reports began to appear of an alarming resurgence, notably of yaws and endemic syphilis, particularly in West Africa, Central Africa and to a lesser extent South-East Asia and the Western Pacific.[5–9] In some parts of the Central African Republic, the pygmy population has been suggested to harbour the main focus of yaws.[10] Sporadic cases were also being reported from some countries in the Americas.[11,12]

In some tropical areas, when yaws came under control, venereally-acquired syphilis had apparently become more prevalent, possibly because of immunological and sociocultural factors. Thus both yaws and venereally-acquired syphilis were being encountered in these areas, giving rise to diagnostic problems.

In addition to the similarities (morphologically, serologically, and in response to penicillin) mentioned above, the endemic treponematoses have some other common characteristics which include non-venereal transmission (mainly in childhood), a predominantly rural distribution associated with poverty, overcrowding, the absence of congenital transmission and the absence of involvement of cardiovascular and central nervous systems. (The occasional reports purporting to show evidence of involvement of cardiovascular and central nervous systems have attracted little support and positive serological tests in the newborn may be due to the passive transplacental transfer of IgG. Their differentiation, therefore, at the present time, is dependent on clinical and epidemiological aspects.

The *incubation period* of endemic treponematoses is similar to that of venereal syphilis.

YAWS (BUBA, FRAMBOESIA, PIAN)

The causative organism is *T. pertenue* which, at the present time, is morphologically indistinguishable from *T. pallidum* which causes veneral syphilis (Chapter 13).

EPIDEMIOLOGY AND MODE OF TRANSMISSION

Yaws is found in the warm, humid, tropical, predominantly rural areas of Africa, Central and South America, the Caribbean, and equatorial islands of South-East Asia, notably Indonesia, and Papua New Guinea, and has a limited distribution in some remote parts of India and Thailand. In endemic areas the prevalence of infectious yaws increases during the rainy season, when skin lesions tend to be more numerous.

Yaws occurs commonly among children aged 2–15 years, living in poor, overcrowded and insanitary conditions. The infection is transmitted from one person to another by direct skin-to-skin contact with material from infectious lesions. A lack of soap and water, clothes and footwear, and the presence of cuts and abrasions, and possibly flies settling on moist lesions, facilitate the spread of the disease. The treponemes cannot penetrate intact skin.

CLINICAL FEATURES

The course of yaws may be divided into early, latent (during which infectious relapses may occur) and late non-infectious stages.

EARLY STAGE (PRIMARY AND SECONDARY STAGE)

After an average incubation period of 21 days the *initial* or *primary* lesion ('mother yaw') appears at the site of entry of the organisms, usually on the exposed parts of the body such as legs, arms, face and neck. It begins as a papule and may develop into a large papilloma (Figure 54.1). It is usually round or

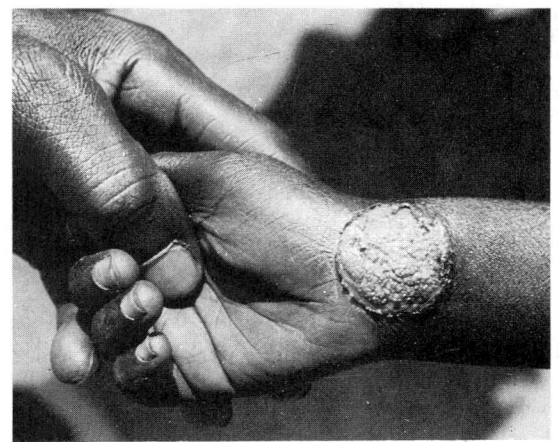

Figure 54.1   Yaws: initial lesion 'mother yaw'. (Courtesy of C. J. Hackett.)

oval and 2–5 cm in diameter. The lesion, which contains numerous treponemes, is painless but usually itchy, and may ulcerate or excoriate by scratching.

The primary lesion may last 3–6 months and heal with or without scar formation. Lymphatic spread may lead to lesions in the neighbouring areas, and haematogenous spread of the organisms may produce lesions elsewhere in the body.

Secondary lesions usually appear a few weeks to up to 2 years after the appearance of the primary lesion, and only rarely are there any constitutional disturbances such as fever, malaise, etc. The characteristic lesion is a papilloma, measuring 1–5 cm in diameter. The papule may ulcerate and the serum may dry to form a yellow-brown scab. The lesions are usually multiple and, after removal of the yellow crust, may appear as raspberry granulomas (framboesides) (Figures 54.2 and 54.3). They may be annular, discoid (Figure 54.4), crescentic or irregular in shape, and occur on any part of the body. Those occurring on the moist areas of the body, or at the mucocutaneous junctions, may resemble the condylomata lata of syphilis.

The secondary lesions, which tend to occur in crops, may last up to 6 months and heal without any

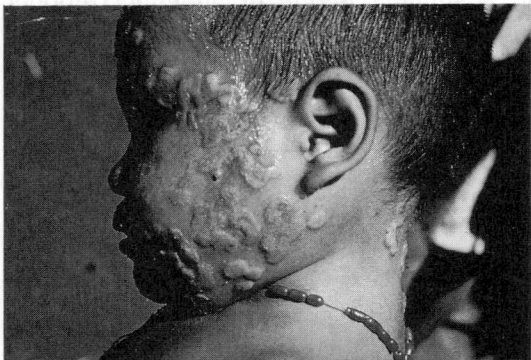

Figure 54.2 Cutaneous early yaws: papillomas. (Courtesy of C. J. Hackett.)

scars except when ulcerated and secondarily infected.

Other manifestations of early yaws include macular and minor papular lesions, especially in the dry season, mixed or polymorphous lesions, regional lymphadenopathy, and hyperkeratotic palmar and plantar lesions. The plantar and palmar skin may develop diffuse non-ulcerative dermatitis (Figure 54.5). Plantar papillomas usually take longer to erupt than those elsewhere on the skin and may make walking painful, resulting in a sideways crab-like gait (crab yaws). (Figure 54.6).

Infectious relapses may occur for up to 5, occasionally for up to 10 years or even longer. The serum exuding from the skin lesions described above contains many treponemes and these early lesions are therefore infectious.

Bone involvement is manifested by osteitis and periostitis; the affected bones are painful (worse at night) and tender. Dactylitis, i.e. osteoperiostitis of the proximal phalanges of the fingers (Figure 54.7), and swelling of the ulna as well as involvement of the long bones of the legs, are common in children. In very rare cases there is hypertrophic osteitis of the nasal process of the maxillae, giving rise to the

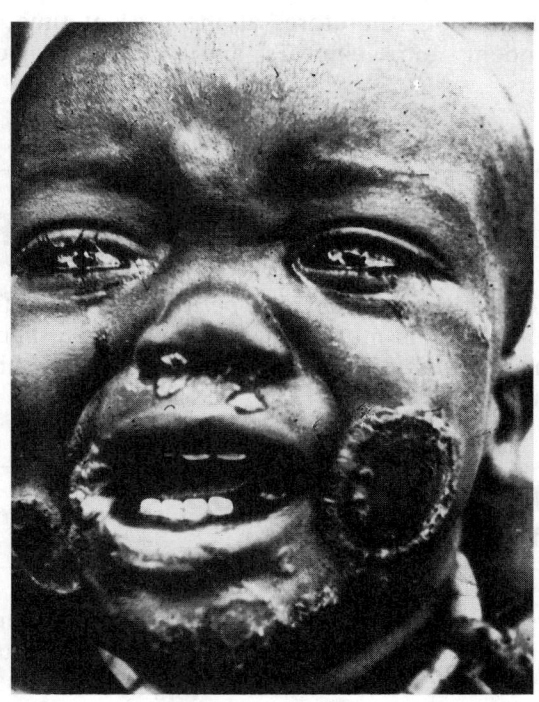

Figure 54.4 Cutaneous early yaws: papillomas. (Courtesy of C. J. Hackett.)

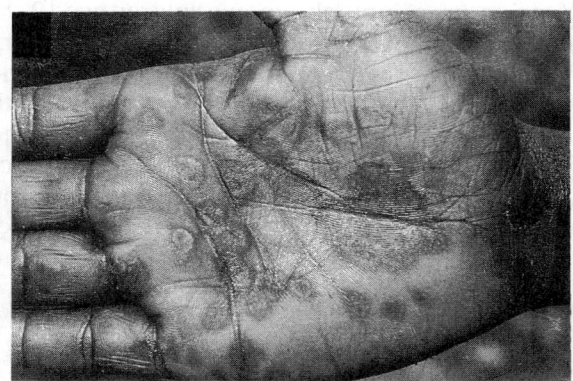

Figure 54.5 Indeterminate yaws: palmar hyperkeratosis.

swellings on both sides of the bridge of the nose, called *goundou* (Figure 54.8). In untreated cases the swellings may grow and obstruct the nostrils.

LATENT STAGE

The disease may then progress to latency, resulting eventually in spontaneous cure or persistent latency. Serological tests may remain positive, usually at low titres. Some patients develop late lesions after 5 or more years of untreated infection.

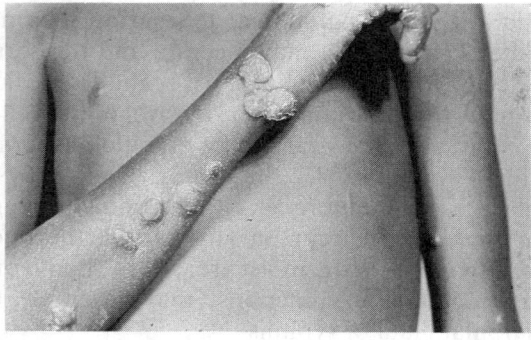

Figure 54.3 Cutaneous early yaws: papillomas. (Courtesy of C. J. Hackett.)

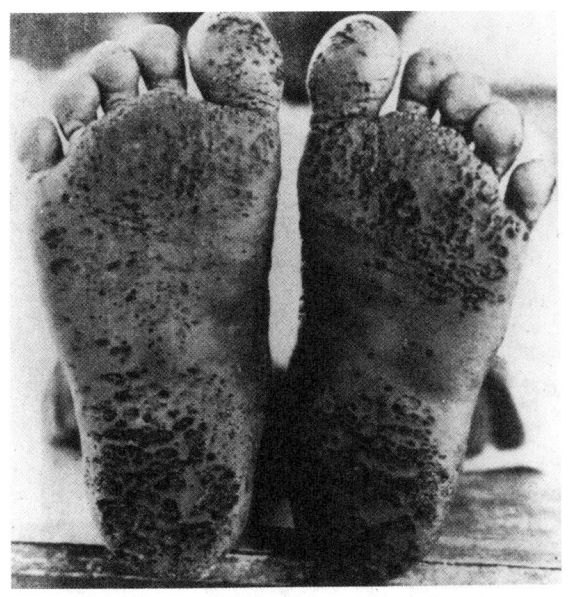

Figure 54.6   Indeterminate yaws: plantar hyperkeratosis (crab yaws).

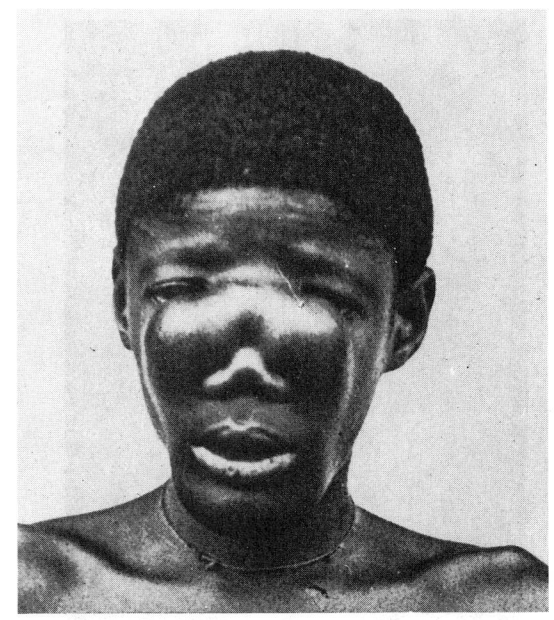

Figure 54.8   Early yaws: goundou. (Courtesy of C. J. Hackett.)

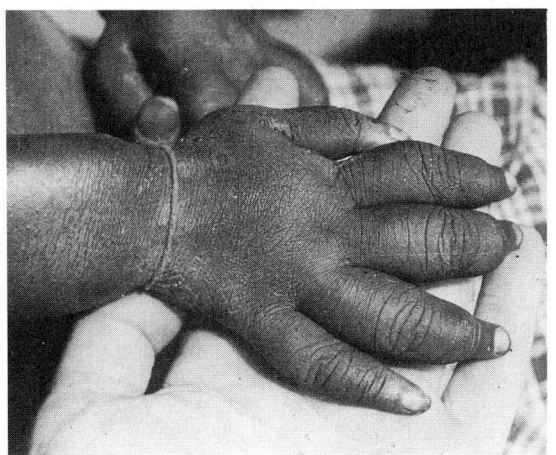

Figure 54.7   Early yaws: polydactylitis.

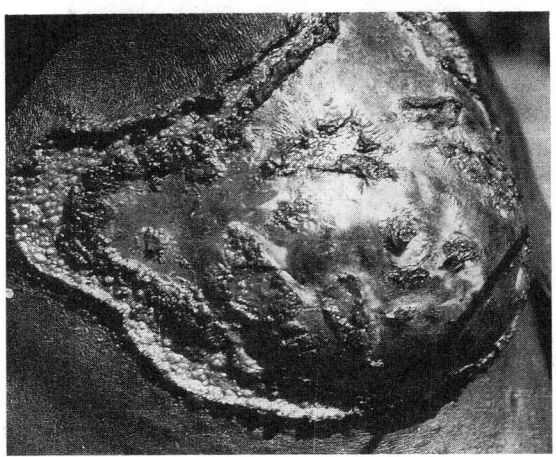

Figure 54.9   Late yaws: gumma of the right breast. (Courtesy of C. J. Hackett.)

LATE STAGE

The late stage is characterized by necrotic destructive lesions of the skin (Figure 54.9) and gummatous lesions of the bones (Figure 54.10) and overlying tissues, resulting in varying degrees of scarring and deformities. These lesions are similar to those of venereal syphilis (Chapter 13). The late manifestations include: hyperkeratosis of palms and soles with deep fissuring; juxta-articular subcutaneous fibrous nodules around the elbows and knees; bursitis (Figure 54.11); disfiguring lesions of the nasopharynx (rhinopharyngitis mutilans or gangosa) (Figure 54.12) as a result of ulceration of the palate or nasal septum progressing to perforation and destruction of the turbinates and pharynx, and secondary infection and offensive discharge; and sabre tibia (Figure 54.13) as a result of hypertrophic osteoperiostitis. Hyperkeratosis of palms and soles (Figure 54.6) and *goundou* (Figure 54.8) are much more pronounced in late yaws. The former may be accompanied by fissures and may be very painful. Eventually, there may be scarring and disfiguration of the hands and feet.

Congenital transmission does not occur, and the cardiovascular and nervous systems are considered

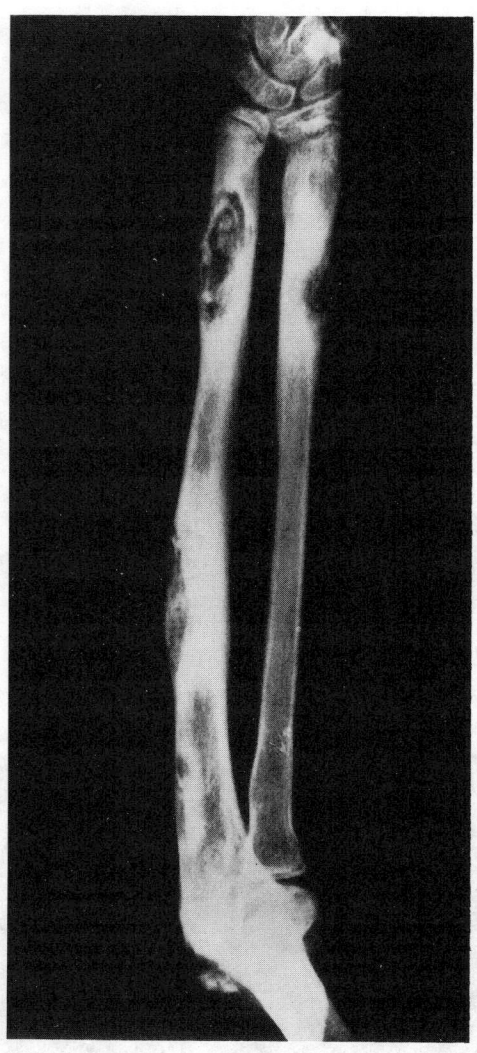

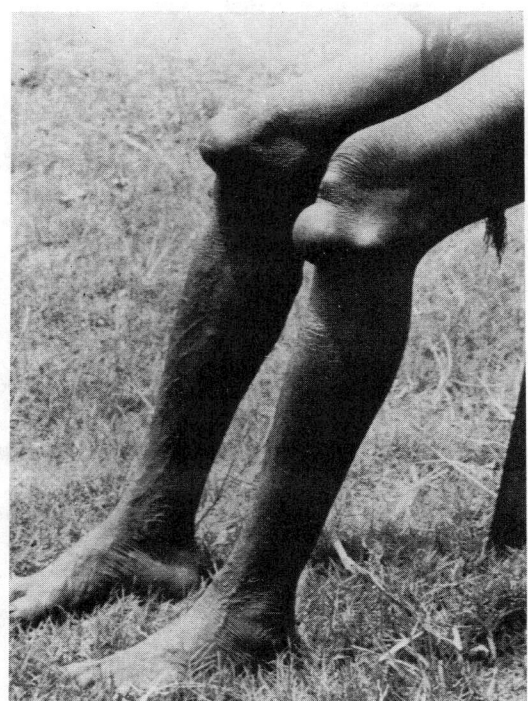

Figure 54.11   Late yaws: chronic bilateral prepatellar bursitis.

Figure 54.10   Late yaws: gummatous osteitis of radius and ulna. (Courtesy of C. J. Hackett.)

not to be affected. However, in one study, ocular and neurological abnormalities were noted in patients presumed to be suffering from late yaws.[13] Román and Román[14] renewed the controversy surrounding distinction(s) between syphilis and yaws. They further suggested that the resurgence of yaws provides an opportunity for further research in order to answer the various unresolved questions with regard to the natural history of endemic treponematoses. Moreover, rapid progress in this field should now be possible by the application of recent advances in recombinant DNA technology.

HISTOPATHOLOGY

Histological examination of biopsy specimens may show characteristic changes, and treponemes in

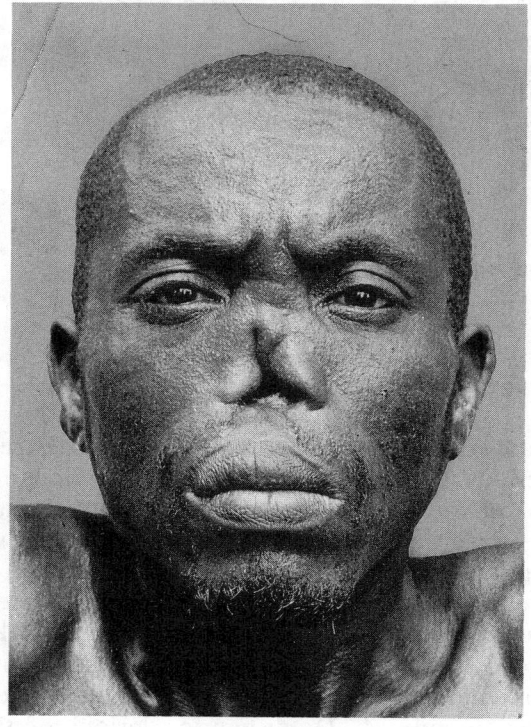

Figure 54.12   Late yaws: gangosa. (Courtesy of C. J. Hackett.)

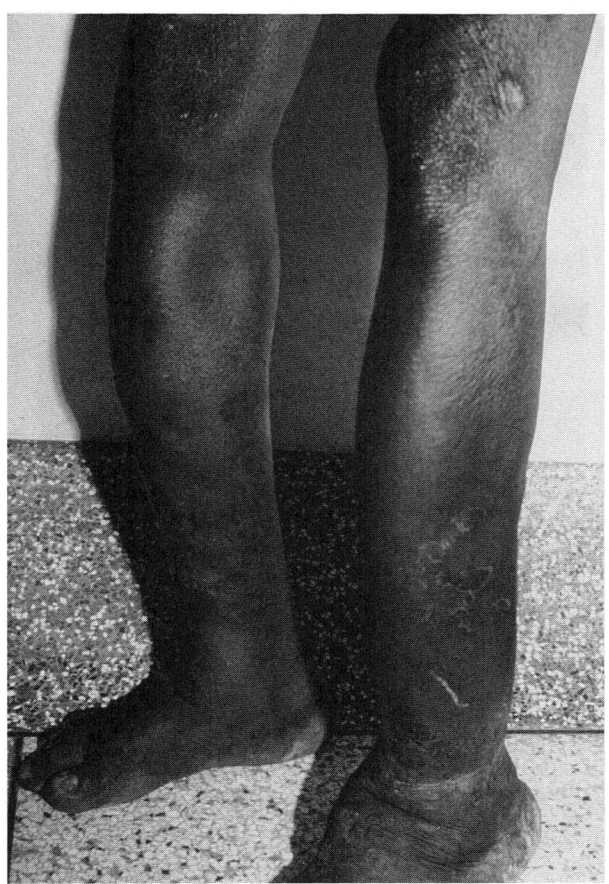

Figure 54.13 Late yaws: sabre tibia. (Reproduced with permission from Arya O. P., Osoba A. O. & Bennett F J. (eds) *Tropical Venereology*, 2nd edn. Edinburgh: Churchill Livingstone, 1988: 138.)

early stage lesions if the specimen is stained by a silver impregnation technique.[15] It is generally believed that the basic pathology in yaws is the same as in venereal syphilis. However, in yaws, endothelial proliferation seems to be much less marked; obliterative changes in the vessels are not encountered, and acanthosis is more prominent.[15]

Studies have been recently carried out to localize treponemes and characterize inflammatory infiltrate in skin biopsies from patients with early venereal syphilis and early infectious yaws.[16] Treponemes in yaws cases (from West Sumatra) were found to be mostly, but not exclusively, confined to the epidermis as opposed to early venereal syphilis lesions—in which the organisms were demonstrated largely in the dermal–epidermal junction as well as in the dermis. Using specific monoclonal antibodies, these same authors were also struck by the paucity of T and B lymphocytes in yaws specimens.

DIAGNOSIS AND DIFFERENTIAL DIAGNOSES

Dark-field examination of exudates from primary and secondary skin lesions will reveal motile treponemes which must be differentiated from saprophytic spirochaetes. Serological tests behave as in the case of venereal syphilis (Chapter 13). Radiography will demonstrate bony involvement in late lesions.

Clinical diagnosis of yaws in the presence of classical lesions is straightforward in endemic areas but differentiation from endemic syphilis may, occasionally, be difficult.

The common skin conditions to be differentiated include scabies, fungal infections, septic wounds, lichen planus, psoriasis, tungiasis, etc. Gummatous lesions should be differentiated from: tropical ulcer, fungating mycotic lesions, leishmaniasis, leprosy, neoplasm(s) and possibly other conditions. Juxta-articular nodules of onchocerciasis and dactylitis of tuberculosis and sickle cell disease should be distinguished by appropriate tests.

If differentiation from venereal syphilis is difficult—especially in latent cases, as may happen if an immigrant presents at a clinic in a temperate climate country and adequacy of any previous treatment is in doubt, then he/she should be treated as for syphilis. However, in view of the social implications, special care should be taken in communicating the diagnosis to the patient, who should be given a full explanation.

TREATMENT AND CONTROL

See pp. 948–949.

ENDEMIC SYPHILIS (BEJEL, FIRJAL)

EPIDEMIOLOGY AND MODE OF TRANSMISSION

The disease is endemic in the arid Sahelian areas of West Africa, with foci also in Zimbabwe, Botswana, and to a lesser extent among the nomadic people in the Arabian peninsula, and the aborigines of central Australia.

Endemic syphilis is primarily a disease of poor, rural communities living in unhygienic and over-crowded conditions. The majority of early cases are found in children aged 2–15 years who are the main reservoir of infection. The initial lesion is usually on the oral mucosa, and transmission is by direct contact through kissing and by indirect contact through eating and drinking utensils. The infection spreads easily among family groups and village communities from infected children to other children and pre-viously uninfected adults. The role of flies acting as vectors remains unproven.

There is no proof that congenital transmission occurs in endemic syphilis.

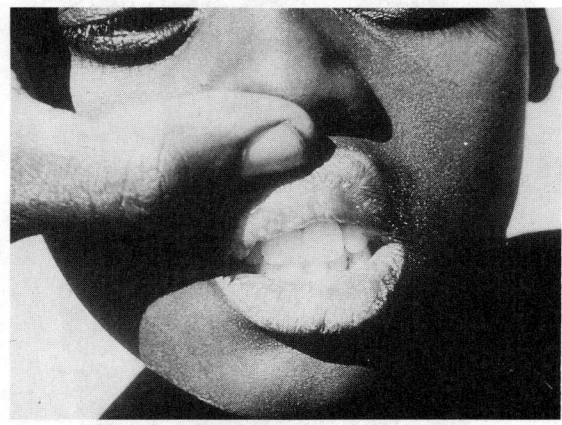

Figure 54.14 Early endemic syphilis: mucous papules on the buccal surface of the upper lip.

CLINICAL FEATURES

A primary lesion is rarely present in endemic syphilis. The earliest lesions encountered are the mucous

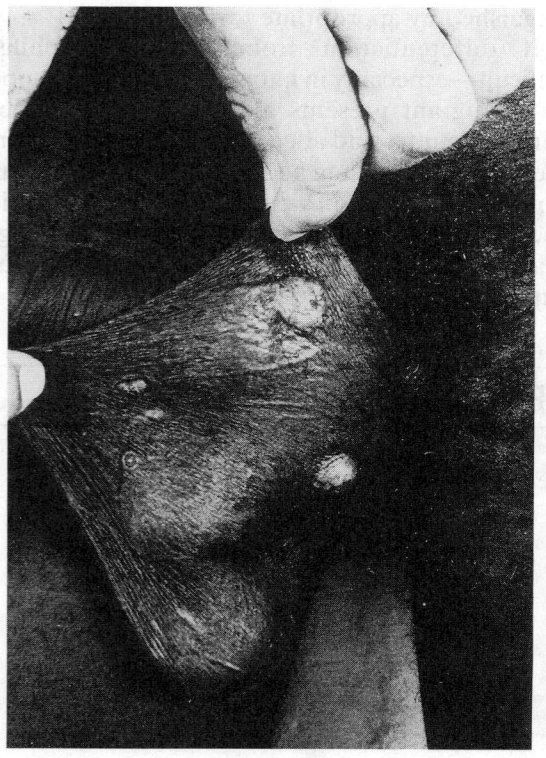

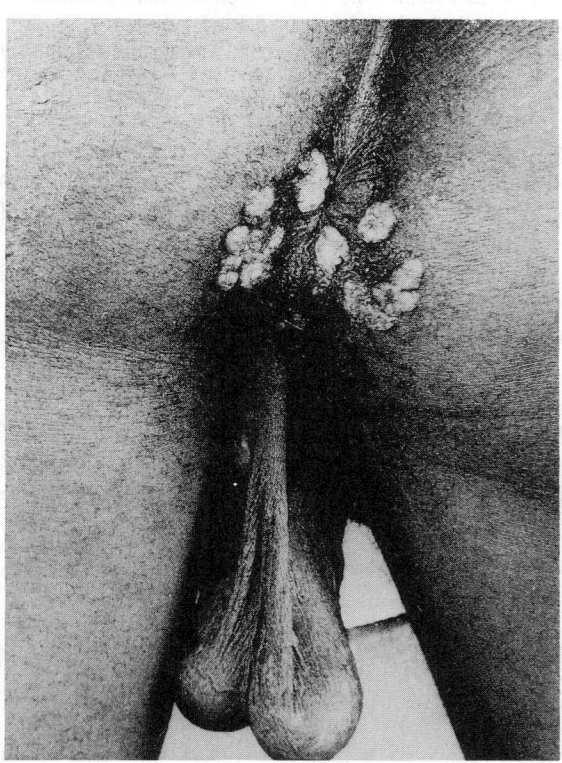

Figure 54.15 Early endemic syphilis: moist papules involving the anus and scrotum. (Courtesy of P. D. Marsden.)

patches—which are shallow painless ulcers on the lips (Figure 54.14) and in the oropharynx, when the patient may complain of sore throat and hoarseness of the voice—the latter due to laryngitis. Other early manifestations of the disease are osteoperiostitis of the long bones causing nocturnal bone pains—as in yaws, condylomata lata occurring in the moist areas of the body, e.g. anogenital area (Figure 54.15) and axillae, and angular stomatitis and split papules, and occasionally a generalized maculopapular and other forms of rash—as in venereal syphilis. Generalized lymph gland enlargement may also be encountered.

In untreated patients the early lesions tend to undergo healing with or without scarring, and the patient passes into the latent phase of the disease. Secondary relapses are uncommon. The period of latency is usually prolonged, after which some patients develop late lesions such as osteoperiostitis, and gummatous lesions. These result in ulceration and destruction of the skin and bones. As in yaws, destruction of the maxilla, palate and nasal bones results in 'gangosa'. Severe plantar and palmar kera-

tosis may be encountered, with ulceration and disability. Juxta-articular nodules also occur. There is, as yet, no convincing evidence of the involvement of cardiovascular and nervous systems in endemic syphilis. Recently, ocular manifestations were described in 17 patients (age range 37–73 years) with clinical findings consistent with bejel.[17]

DIAGNOSIS AND DIFFERENTIAL DIAGNOSIS

This is essentially the same as that for yaws.

TREATMENT AND CONTROL

See pp. 948–949.

PINTA (AZUL, CARATE, MAL DE PINTO)

EPIDEMIOLOGY AND MODE OF TRANSMISSION

Pinta, which affects skin principally, is confined to the underdeveloped rural areas of northern South America and Mexico. However, there is a paucity of data with regard to the current incidence.

The infection is acquired in childhood or early adolescence among people living in unhygienic conditions. Those aged 15–30 years, with long-standing skin lesions, comprise the main reservoir. Treponemes persist in these lesions for many years. The lesions tend to be dry but are itchy, and scratching may release serum with abundant treponemes. Transmission, as in the case of yaws, is believed to be by direct lesion-to-skin contact and facilitated by a breach in the recipient's skin. As in the case of other treponematoses, the role of flies in the transmission of pinta remains uncertain.

CLINICAL FEATURES

The primary lesion appears at the site of entry of the organisms, usually located on the exposed parts of the body such as arms, legs or face. It starts as an itchy erythematosquamous papule which enlarges slowly and is accompanied by satellite lesions. The regional lymph nodes are enlarged and painless.

The secondary stage develops several months after the initial lesion, with the appearance of erythematosquamous plaques either around the primary lesion or disseminated to other areas. These 'pintids' are painless but itchy. They undergo a variety of colour change(s) from red to copper colour, lead-grey and bluish-black. The lesions, of various sizes and colours, may be found anywhere on the body.

There is no latent stage.

The late lesions are characterized by varying degrees of hypochromia and atrophy around dys-

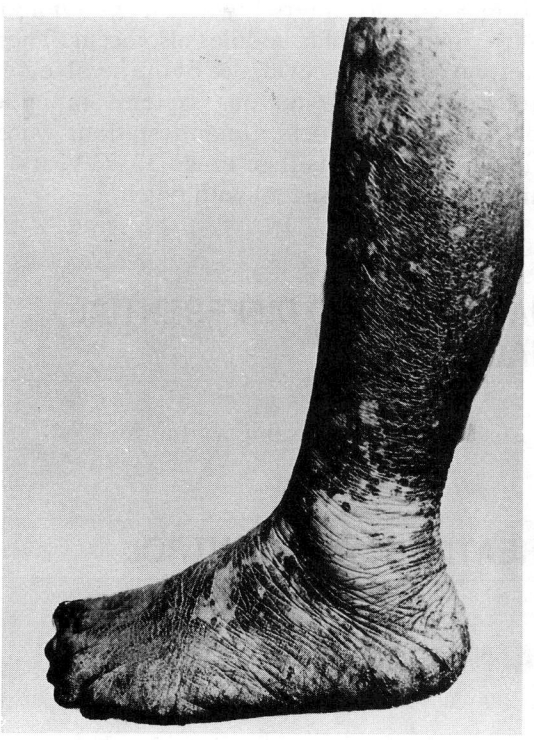

Figure 54.16   Late pinta: depigmentation of the fast and lower leg. (Courtesy of L. A. Leon.)

chromic and achromic lesions (Figure 54.16). Hyperkeratosis of the palms and soles, and juxta-articular nodes, are occasionally encountered but some experts dispute this, and consider that these patients may in fact be suffering from yaws. Leucoderma is the main complication, and this may result in social stigmas. There is no reliable evidence of systemic involvement.

DIAGNOSIS AND DIFFERENTIAL DIAGNOSIS

Diagnostic tests are the same as those for other endemic treponematoses, i.e. dark-field examination of the material from the early lesions, and serological tests. The histopathological picture is largely similar to that of yaws. In addition, the basal cells show loss of melanin and many melanophages may be present in the dermis.[18] The characteristic colour changes provide a clue to the diagnosis, but other conditions, such as vitiligo, pityriasis versicolor, leprosy, etc., should be excluded.

HUMAN IMMUNODEFICIENCY VIRUS INFECTION AND ENDEMIC TREPONEMATOSES

No information is at present available on the relationship between human immunodeficiency virus (HIV) infection and endemic treponematoses. However, immunological abnormalities associated with HIV infection have been reported to alter the course of syphilis, albeit in a minority of patients. These abnormalities may reactivate latent infection, decrease the latent period before onset of neurosyphilis, increase the severity of manifestations, alter serological responses and render conventional therapy inadequate.[19–21] It is highly likely that HIV infection will have similar influences on endemic treponematoses. The modified clinical manifestations and serological responses may cause difficulties in diagnosis.

Ulcerative lesions caused by syphilis are believed to facilitate HIV transmission. Likewise, yaws lesions might also enhance the risk of acquiring and transmitting HIV.

TREATMENT OF ENDEMIC TREPONEMATOSES

Penicillin is the agent of choice. Benzathine penicillin G is given as a single intramuscular injection in the upper outer quadrant of the buttock. The dose is 600 000 units for children under the age of 6 years, 1.2 million units for those aged 6–15, and 2.4 million units for adults.

Treatment in the early stage(s) will result in cure and complete resolution of manifestations, but treatment in the late stages will not reverse the damage that has already occurred. The lesions become non-infectious within 24 hours after administration of the antibiotic.

Erythromycin or tetracycline, 500 mg by mouth 4 times daily for 15 days, is recommended for those allergic to penicillin. Children between the ages of 8 and 15 years should receive half that dose. Tetracycline should not be given to pregnant women or to children below 12 years.

CONTACTS

See below.

FOLLOW-UP

After adequate treatment, in the large majority of patients, non-treponemal test (rapid plasma reagin (RPR) or Venereal Disease Research Laboratory (VDRL)) titres decline and the test becomes negative in due course. However, in a small proportion of patients, especially if treated in the late stages, the RPR or VDRL may remain positive at low titre (below 1:8). This is not an indication for further treatment. The specific tests (*T. pallidum* haemagglutination (TPHA) or fluorescent treponemal antibody absorption (FTA-ABS)), which remain reactive throughout life, play no part in assessment of the adequacy of treatment.

CONTROL OF ENDEMIC TREPONEMATOSES

There is no evidence of emergence of penicillin-resistant treponemes but this situation could change at any time; hence, the *control* of endemic treponematoses should be a priority.

The main method of control lies in identification of infectious cases and their treatment, as well as treatment of their immediate contacts. Clinical surveillance (requiring dark-field microscopy and RPR or VDRL tests) to detect the prevalence of active infection is the first step. The detection of latent disease will require serological tests.

The treatment policies recommended by the World Health Organization[22] are as follows:
1. If the prevalence of clinically active infection in the community is over 10%, give benzathine penicillin G to the entire population.
2. If the prevalence of clinically active cases is 5–10%, give benzathine penicillin G to the patients,

their contacts, and to all children below the age of 15 years.
3. If the prevalence of clinically active infection is under 5%, then treat all active cases as well as household and other obvious contacts with benzathine penicillin G.

Economic considerations may necessitate integration of treponematosis control activities into other public health programmes.

The standards of living and personal and environmental hygiene must be improved. Sustained surveillance, integrated into existing primary health care, must be maintained to detect and treat new or missed cases and their contacts, and treatment failures. This will necessitate surveys as well as strengthening of the primary health care infrastructure.

REFERENCES

1 Hudson E H. *Non-venereal Syphilis. A sociological and Medical Study of Bejel*. Edinburgh; Livingstone, 1958.
2 Hackett C J. On the origin of the human treponematoses. *Bull World Health Organ* 1963; 29:7–41.
3 Norris S J. Polypeptides of *Treponema pallidum*: progress toward understanding their structure, functional and immunologic roles. *Treponema Pallidum*—Polypeptide Research Group. *Microb Rev* 1993; 57:750–779.
4 Noordhoek G T, Hermans P W M, Paul A N et al. *Treponema pallidum* subspecies *pallidum* (Nichols) and *Treponema pallidum* subspecies *pertenue* (CDC 2575) differ in at least one nucleotide, comparison of two homologous antigens. *Microb Pathog* 1989; 6:29–42.
5 Editorial. Yaws again. *BMJ* 1980; 281:1090.

6 Editorial. Endemic treponematoses in the 1980s. *Lancet* 1983; ii:551–552.

7 Agadzi V K, Aboagye-Atta Y, Nelson J W, Perine P L & Hopkins D R. Resurgence of yaws in Ghana. *Lancet* 1983; ii:389–390.

8 Proceedings of Inter-Regional Meeting on Yaws and other Endemic Treponematoses. Cipanas, Indonesia, 22–24 July 1985. *Southeast Asian J Trop Med Public Health* 1986; 17(supplement 4):1–96.

9 Noordhoek G T, Engelkens H J, Judanarso J et al. Yaws in West Sumatra, Indonesia: clinical manifestations, serological findings and characterisation of new Treponema isolates by DNA probes. *Europ J Clin Microb and Infect Dis* 1991; 10:12–19.

10 Herve V, Kassa Kelembho E, Normand P, Georges A, Mathiot C & Martin P. Resurgence of yaws in Central African Republic. Role of the Pygmy population as a reservoir of the virus. *Bull Soc Pathol Exot* 1992; 85:342–346.

11 St John R K. Yaws in the Americas. *Rev Infect Dis* 1985; 7(supplement 2):266–272.

12 Guderian R H, Guzman J R, Calvopina M & Cooper P. Studies on a focus of yaws in the Santiago Basin, Province of Esmeraldas, Ecuador. *Trop Geogr Med* 1991; 43:142–147.

13 Lawton Smith J, David N J, Indgin S et al. Neuro-ophthalmological study of late yaws and pinta: II. the Caracas project. *Br J Vener Dis* 1971; 47:226–251.

14 Román G C & Román L N. Occurrence of cogenital cardiovascular, visceral, neurologic, and neuro-ophthalmologic complication in late yaws; a theme for future research. *Rev Infect Dis* 1986; 8:760–770.

15 Engelkens H J H, Vuzevski V D, Jubianto Judanaso et al. Early yaws; a light microscopic study. *Genitourin Med* 1990; 66:264–266.

16 Engelkens H J H, ten Kate F J W, Judanarso Jubianto et al. The localisation of treponemes and characterization of the inflammatory infiltrate in skin biopsies from patients with primary or secondary syphilis, or early infectious yaws. *Genitourin Med* 1993; 69:102–107.

17 Tabbara K F, Al Kaff A S & Fadel T. Ocular manifestations of endemic syphilis (bejel). *Ophthalmology* 1989; 96:1087–1091.

18 Marquez F & Pinta. In Canizares O (ed.) *Clinical Tropical Dermatology*. Oxford: Blackwell Scientific Publications. 1975: 86–92.

19 Johns D R, Tierney M & Felsenstein D. Alterations in the natural history of neurosyphilis by concurrent infection with the human immunodificiency virus. *N Engl J Med* 1987; 316:1569–1572.

20 Hicks C B, Benson P M, Lupton G P & Tramont E C. Seronegative secondary syphilis in a patient infected with the human immunodeficiency virus (HIV) with Kaposi sarcoma: a diagnostic dilemma. *Ann Intern Med* 1987; 107:492–495.

21 Musher D M, Hamill R J & Baughn R E. Effect of human immunodeficiency virus (HIV) infection on the course of syphilis and on the response to treatment (Review). *Ann Intern Med* 1990; 113:872–881.

22 World Health Organization. Treponemal infections. *World Health Organization* Technical Report Series 674, Geneva, 1982, 16–20.

FURTHER READING

Csonka G W. Clinical aspects of bejel. *Br J Vener Dis* 1953; 29:95–103.

Hackett C J & Loewenthal L J A. The Differential Diagnosis of Yaws, monograph no. 36. Geneva: World Health Organization, 1960.

Hudson E H H. Bejel: the endemic syphilis of the Euphrates Arab. *Trans R Soc Trop Med Hyg* 1937; 37:9–46.

Perine P L, Hopkins D R, Niemel P L A, St John R K, Causse G & Antal G M. *Handbook of Endemic Treponematoses: Yaws, Endemic Syphilis and Pinta*. Geneva: World Health Organization, 1984.

CHAPTER 55

OTHER SPIROCHAETAL DISEASES

G. C. Cook

RELAPSING FEVER

Relapsing fever is also known as recurrent fever, spirillum fever, tick fever and tick bite fever.

AETIOLOGY

The causative agents are two morphologically indistinct species of spirochaete: *Borrelia recurrentis* and *B. duttoni*; they are actively motile spiral organisms (6–10 × 0.4 μm) with 5–10 fairly regular, but loose waves (Figure 55.1). Multiplication is by transverse fission. They have tapering ends, but no flagella; electron microscopy reveals that each consists of a bundle of 12 filaments twisted round the spirochaete body, external to the cell wall, with a thin covering layer of viscid material. They have a rapid 'corkscrew' movement and can be visualized in blood films between the red cells, staining pink with Giemsa or Leishman reagents, and sometimes appearing beaded or granular. The organisms may assume irregular shapes, and appear tangled together towards the end of a pyrexial attack. They can be visualized by dark-ground illumination, grown with difficulty in enriched media[1,2] in the allantoic fluid of fertile hen's eggs, but are best demonstrated by animal inoculation. Susceptible animals include: newborn rabbits, monkeys, mice,[3] rats and ground squirrels; guinea-pigs are not normally susceptible.

Species differentiation

B. recurrentis infects lice, but not ticks; guinea-pigs are resistant except in East Africa. Sudanese strains are not infective to monkeys. *B. duttoni* involves soft ticks, which can infect lice and most rodents.

PATHOPHYSIOLOGY

Human cycle

During pyrexial attacks the spirochaetes appear in the blood, where they may be visualized in leucocytes; they disappear during a crisis, and can be detected only by animal inoculation. Resistant spirochaetes persist in the brain and other tissues until a fresh immunologically distinct strain proliferates and reaches the bloodstream.

Pathogenesis

Borrelia spp. enter the skin and subcutaneous tissues without causing a primary lesion; from there

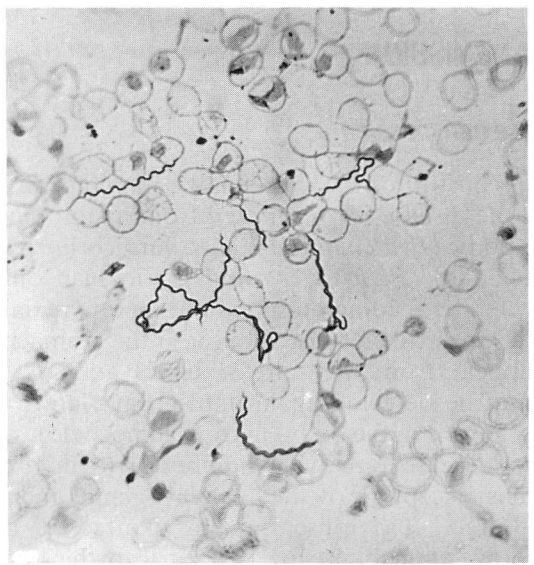

Figure 55.1 Borrelia recurrentis in a peripheral blood film.

they invade both systemic and lymphatic circulations. They multiply in blood, being phagocytosed by the reticuloendothelial system; there is no replication at extravascular sites. However, sequestration of platelets occurs in the bone marrow with thrombocytopenia; this is responsible for petechial rashes in the skin, and haemorrhages. In the liver there is intrahepatic biliary obstruction; hepatocellular involvement results in jaundice.

Fever is caused by large numbers of *Borrelia* spp. (they do not produce toxins), which are pyrogenic; the outer envelope is heat stable, and stimulates mononuclear cells to produce pyrogens. A Jarisch–Herxheimer reaction may occur spontaneously, or following treatment consequent on phagocytosis of a large number of *Borrelia* spp. Disseminated intravascular coagulation may also occur.

Morphology

General features at post mortem consist of: jaundice, congestion of organs—with petechial haemorrhages in the pleura, lungs, heart, brain, kidneys, stomach and intestine.

Borrelia spp. concentrate in the liver, where they multiply causing focal necrosis of parenchymal cells, which they invade. Fixed phagocytes do not respond to live *Borrelia* spp. but ingest dead ones. Shortly before a crisis the *Borrelia* spp. 'roll up' and are taken up by endothelial cells in the liver, spleen and bone marrow. Surviving *Borrelia* spp. remain in these organs, and also the brain, until the next relapse.

In the spleen *Borrelia* spp. accumulate and multiply in sinuses, causing cellular infiltration; they may enter endothelial cells, causing infarcts and necrosis; they can be demonstrated in infarcts. The spleen is large, soft and red; perisplenitis is common. *Borrelia* spp. may also be demonstrated in the kidneys.

In blood vessels, damage to the endothelium causes haemorrhage(s), which may present as petechiae.

A polymorphonuclear leucocytosis is present and *Borrelia* spp. may sometimes be visualized within polymorphs. The bone marrow is hyperaemic. Lymph glands may be involved.

Myocardium shows 'cloudy swelling'. Bronchopneumonia is common.

Borrelia spp. are neurotropic—involving the meninges and central nervous system. In infected animals they may be found in the brain (they are present in capillaries) and cerebellum as long as one year after infection. There are no changes in nerve cells, but there is intense microglial reaction in the cortex. Meningitis is sometimes present.

IMMUNITY

Immunologically, *Borrelia* spp. behave in a way comparable with the African trypanosome. Antigenic variation overcomes specific humoral antibodies to give rise to a series of relapses. When spirochaetes first enter in the bloodstream, IgM antibodies (agglutinins, immobilizing antibodies, spirochaeticidine, lysins and leucostatic antibodies which promote phagocytosis) specific to the antigenic *Borrelia* spp. type overwhelm the haematological forms but do not eradicate the organisms from the tissue(s). Remaining *Borrelia* spp., which are antigenically unstable, generate new antigens—only to be removed by fresh IgM antibodies specific to that type. This process leads to 'waves' of IgM antibodies succeeding one another; this is followed by the formation of IgG antibodies which lack specificity. Lytic activity is dependent on complement. There is no significant immunity to subsequent attacks of relapsing fever.

LOUSE-BORNE RELAPSING FEVER: EPIDEMIC (COSMOPOLITAN) TYPE

GEOGRAPHICAL DISTRIBUTION

The major endemic area lies in the highlands of Ethiopia[4–7] and Burundi; the infection can appear anywhere in areas of low endemicity in Peru and Bolivia, north-west and East Africa, India, Asia and China—wherever environmental conditions are suitable, and also in times of social unrest and war (Figure 55.2).

TRANSMISSION

Louse transmission

Man constitutes the only known mammalian host, and the disease is transmitted from man to man by the body (*Pediculus humanus* var. *corporis*) and head louse (*P. h.* var. *capitis*). Lice can only be infected by feeding on blood during a pyrexial episode. Spirochaetes are taken into the stomach and disappear from there in 24 hours at 28°C; they cannot be detected again until 6 days later, when they appear in the body cavity (haemocoele), where they increase rapidly in number(s) to involve all organs, except the ovaries, salivary glands and intestinal tract. The louse remains unaffected; spirochaetes can only escape by injury to the body or limbs. Lice are not infective until 6 days after a feed,

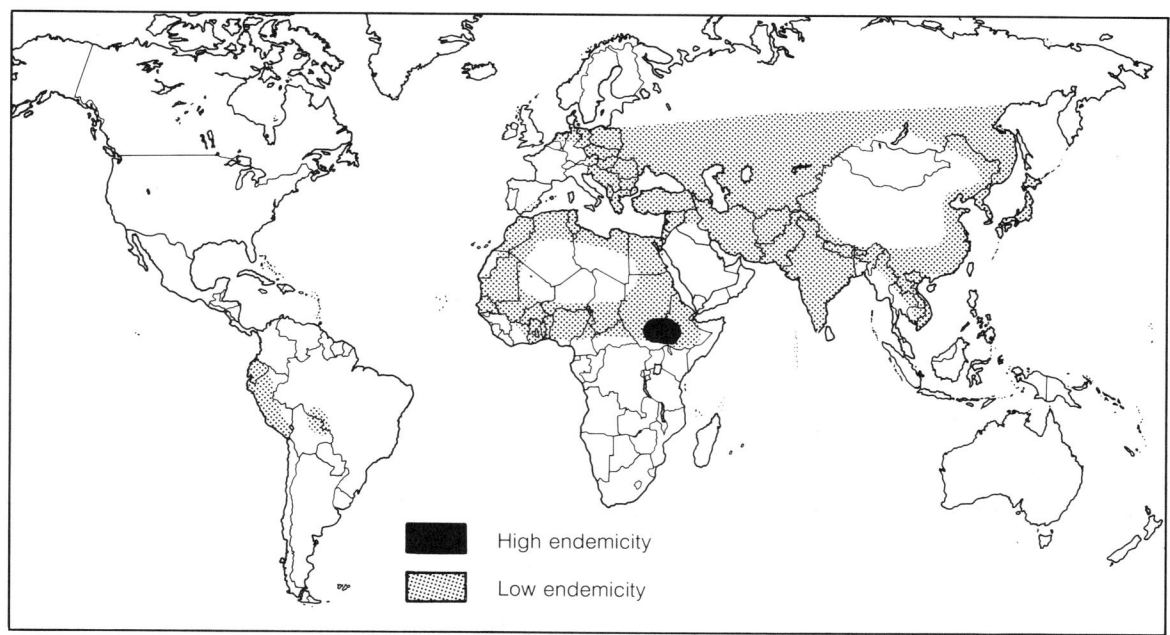

Figure 55.2 Geographical distribution of louse-borne relapsing fever (*Borrelia recurrentis*). (Courtesy of Department of Entomology, London School of Hygiene and Tropical Medicine.)

and man is infected by crushing lice on the skin—not by a bite. There is no transovarian transmission.

Congenital transmission

Transplacental transmission and abortion are by no means uncommon.

Transmission by blood transfusion

This has been recorded albeit rarely.

CLINICAL FEATURES

Natural history

Louse-borne relapsing fever can manifest as a severe disease, consisting of a febrile illness characterized by a primary attack of fever, followed by up to four relapses. There is a great variation in the degree of severity, varying from an asymptomatic parasitaemia to a severe febrile illness with death resulting from hepatic or cardiac failure. In some epidemics a mortality rate of up to 70% has been recorded.

Incubation period

This is 2–10 (usually 4–8) days.

Symptoms and signs

Onset is sudden, with chills and fever (temperature rises rapidly to 40.5°C or even higher), when the patient may become delirious.[5,6] He/she sits or lies on the bed or ground, silent, with a glazed expression and apathetic manner, and is mentally dull or confused. There is associated dizziness, severe headache[5,6] and pain in the back, chest, abdomen and legs (especially the calves) and joints. Nausea, vomiting and dysphagia are common. Dyspnoea is also common; it is loud and hissing and can be heard for some distance away from the patient; the diagnosis can be suspected from a distance. Cough is common; the sputum may contain *Borrelia* spp. The spleen becomes enlarged,[5] occasionally to such a degree that spontaneous rupture occurs. Hepatomegaly is present; jaundice is common. Bleeding often occurs into the skin (petechial rash),[5] over the flanks and shoulders, and into mucous membranes; epistaxis is common. During the first attack an erythematous rash may appear over the upper part of the body—resembling that of typhoid. Conjunctival vessels are congested and may bleed (clumps of adherent *Borrelia* spp. become impacted in capillaries, where they enmesh red cells, causing capillary rupture followed by haemorrhage). There may be widespread intravascular coagulation. Heavy albuminuria is usually present.

Liver function tests reflect extensive hepatocellular dysfunction.[5] Anaemia is present and a marked

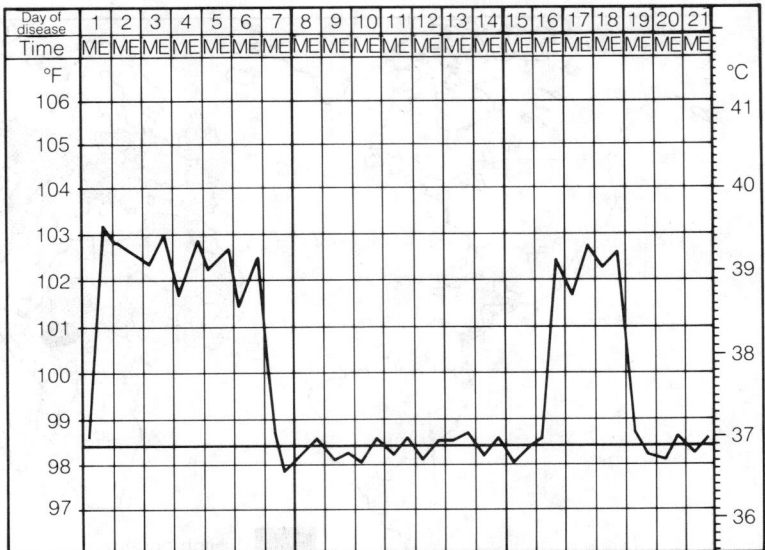

Figure 55.3 Temperature chart in a case of louse-borne relapsing fever. There is usually one relapse, and not more than four.

polymorphonuclear leucocytosis (15–30 × 10⁹/l) is apparent on a peripheral blood film.

CSF pressure is often elevated; a lymphocytic pleocytosis is common and *Borrelia* spp. may be present.

Fever lasts 5–7 days; temperature falls by crisis to 36°C or even lower (when there may be a state of collapse) and is accompanied by profuse sweating, diarrhoea, weakness and relief from associated symptoms.

Relapse occurs 5–9 days after the first attack in two-thirds of patients (Figure 55.3); it is less severe and there is no rash. A second relapse occurs in one-quarter of those infected, but more than four relapses are exceedingly unusual.

COMPLICATIONS

Complications include pneumonia (of lobar distribution),[5,6] which may be a major clinical feature, and nephritis, parotitis, diarrhoea, arthritis, neuropathy, acute ophthalmitis and iritis, meningoencephalitis, meningitis and meningism.

Cardiac involvement

Myocardial involvement[6] is not uncommon on the day of crisis; this is accompanied by a prolonged QTc, altered T waves, pulse >100/min, systolic blood pressure ≤90 mmHg, gallop rhythm, and reversed splitting of the second sound in the pulmonary area. A phase of critically low cardiac output (resulting from myocardial damage) may ensue; this usually resolves after treatment.

PROGNOSIS

Case mortality varies; it is usually around 2–9% but occasionally reaches 12%. Death usually occurs during the first febrile attack, as a result of prothrombin deficiency, hepatic coma, myocarditis or disseminated intravascular coagulation. During the initial crisis death may result from hyperpyrexia, with convulsions, heart failure, shock or cerebral oedema. Death is usually sudden and unexpected and may occur shortly after initiation of treatment.

DIFFERENTIAL DIAGNOSIS

In parts of East Africa, epidemics of febrile illness in which jaundice[5] is a feature often result from louse-borne relapsing fever. During the initial attack, other causes of febrile jaundice can present similarly: yellow fever (which does not usually present with jaundice as a major feature), viral hepatitis, leptospirosis, severe *Plasmodium falciparum* infection, typhoid fever, louse-borne typhus fever (with which it sometimes coexists in the same individual), trench fever and cerebrospinal meningitis (CSF has been known to reveal meningococci and *Borrelia* spp. in the same microscopical field). Following the initial attack, and during relapses,[5,6] other differential diagnoses are: relapsing typhoid fever, relapsing malaria (*P. vivax*), pyelonephritis, gallstones and kala-azar.

DIAGNOSIS

Borrelia spp. are usually detected in thick blood films obtained during a febrile attack. They may be isolated at any time by inoculation of blood or CSF into young rats or white mice, in which the blood yields a positive result within 2–3 days; guinea-pigs, adult rabbits and dogs are refractory.

Serological tests

These are unreliable; those for syphilis may give a false-positive result. A complement fixation test has been devised, and an immobilization test has proved sensitive; a fluorescent antibody test using *Borrelia* spp. antigen is less sensitive, and cross-reacts with *Treponema pallidum*.

TREATMENT

This consists of tetracycline, either alone or combined with penicillin.[5,6] Procaine penicillin (300 mg) plus tetracycline (500 mg) 6-hourly for 7 days is effective and safe. In Ethiopia a single oral dose of 500 mg tetracycline or erythromycin has proved effective. Intravenous tetracycline 250 mg is effective when oral therapy is contraindicated. A Jarisch-Herxheimer[5,6] reaction commonly occurs after administration of tetracycline and/or penicillin, especially after intravenous administration. The patient becomes restless, a rigor lasts 10–30 minutes with an abrupt temperature rise, and a rapid pulse rate, respiratory rate and raised blood pressure are accompanied by intense shivering; this is followed by a phase of flushing and profuse sweating when the blood pressure falls. The affected patient then becomes more comfortable and falls asleep; the temperature is normal the following day. *Borrelia* spp. disappear from peripheral blood about the time of the peak reaction. The mortality rate is low. Corticosteroids are ineffective, but meptazinol (an opioid antagonist with agonist properties) 300–500 mg intravenously reduces the severity of an attack. Intravenous fluid is often necessary to counteract dehydration.[6]

EPIDEMIOLOGY

Louse-borne relapsing fever behaves similarly to louse-borne typhus, with which it frequently coexists. It is a disease of great antiquity; epidemics have occurred in times of war. Refugees and major population migrations (with overcrowding and poor hygiene) favour epidemics. It has been estimated that there were 15 million cases in sub-Saharan Africa, Sudan, Ethiopia, eastern Europe and Russia between 1910 and 1945, with over five million deaths; the mortality rate reached up to 75%. It is a disease of overcrowding, cold and poor hygiene—

conditions which lead to heavy louse infection. It is also encountered in the tropics at high altitudes, where head lice may be important in transmission.

CONTROL

With modern delousing methods, using insecticides, epidemics should immediately be brought to a halt.[7] Insecticide powder is blown into the clothes of the population at risk to eliminate lice; heat sterilization of clothing kills the eggs. Personal prevention may be achieved by careful delousing, without crushing the lice, and avoidance of scratching. Lice cannot transmit infection by bite(s) or faeces (see Appendix IV).

TICK-BORNE RELAPSING FEVER

GEOGRAPHICAL DISTRIBUTION

Tick-borne relapsing fever has a wide distribution in both the Old[8] and New[9] Worlds, in five main areas (three in the Old World and two in the New); each has a specific *Borrelia* spp. tick vector complex (Figure 55.4).

AETIOLOGY

Seven species of *Borrelia* spp. are involved (Table 55.1).

TRANSMISSION

Ticks

The major mode of transmission is by soft ticks of the genus *Ornithodoros* (see Appendix IV).

Tick cycle
Both nymphs and adults transmit the infection via salivary glands (and bite), and by coxal fluid. *Borrelia* spp. penetrate the wall of the small intestine after being ingested during a blood meal; they subsequently invade the haemocoele and other organs, including salivary glands, coxal glands and ovary, where they multiply. Organisms are *not* found in tick faeces. Infection of a susceptible animal can take place via the bite of an infected tick—a relatively large puncture into which infective saliva is pumped, or which may be the portal of entry for coxal fluid

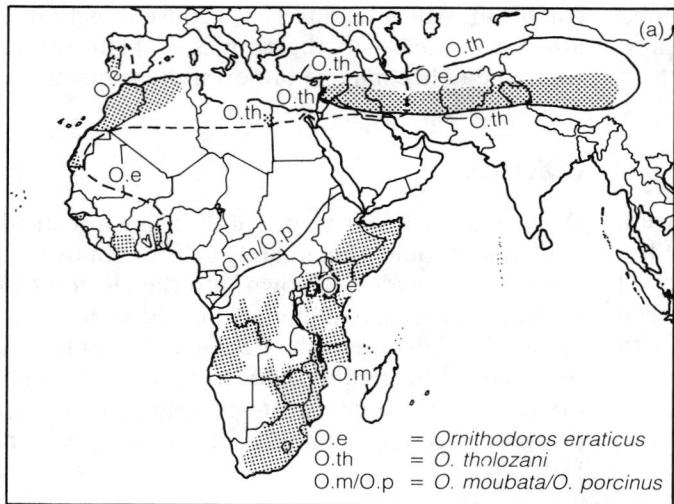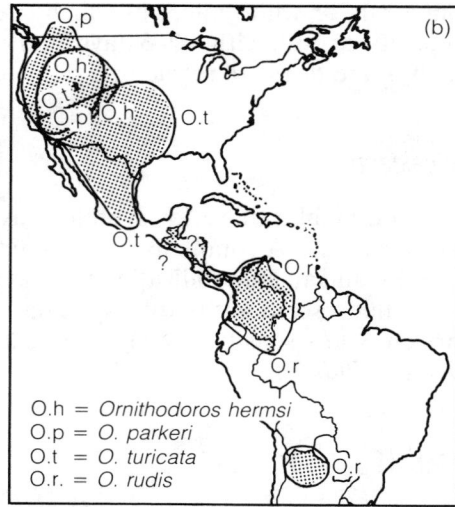

Figure 55.4 Geographical distribution of tick-borne (endemic) relapsing fever in (a) the Old and (b) New World. (Courtesy of Department of Entomology, London School of Hygiene and Tropical Medicine.)

Table 55.1 Species of *Borrelia* involved in tick-borne relapsing fevers.

Species	Vector	Geographical area
B. duttoni	O. moubata (O. m. porcinus and O. savignyi)	East, central and South Africa
B. hispanica	O. erraticus	Mediterranean region (part), North and West Africa, Portugal and Spain
B. persica	O. tholozani (= papillipes) including var. crossi	Mediterranean region (part), Tobruk, Cyprus, Israel, through Iran to Kashmir and Sinkiang province of western China
B. parkeri	O. parkeri	Central and western USA, Mexico
B. turicata	O. turicata	Central and western USA, Mexico
B. hermsi	O. hermsi	Central and western USA, Mexico
B. venezuelensis	O. rudis (= venezuelensis)	Northern, South and Central America southwards to northern Argentina

secreted during feeding. *O. moubata* nymphs transmit by both salivary and coxal fluid, while those of *O. turicata*, *O. parkeri*, *O. hermsi* and *O. tholozani* do not produce coxal fluid whilst feeding. Transmission can occur in less than one minute after tick attachment.

Transovarian transmission is usual; a tick remains infected for many years, transmitting the infection to its offspring. The organisms can perpetuate themselves enzootically in ticks (without the requirement of another host) for at least five generations.

Other methods of transmission

Borrelia spp. can enter through intact mucous membrane and skin. Accidental infection via the conjunctiva is also possible. Transfusion, transplacental transmission and infection via intravenous drug administration have all been recorded. *Borrelia* spp. can survive in lice and bed bugs; they do not develop further in these hosts.

Hosts

Man is the only source of infection for *O. moubata*; major sources of infection for other soft ticks are rodents, which live in open country, caves and burrows and do not infest human dwellings. Infection is transmitted to man only incidentally. Animal hosts include monkeys, squirrels, chipmunks, rats, hedgehogs and possibly bats and other cave-dwelling mammals.

IMMUNITY

Tick-borne relapsing fever is more serious in expatriates than indigenous people who have previously been exposed to the disease; neurological complications are far more common in visitors to an endemic area.

CLINICAL FEATURES

Natural history

Tick-borne relapsing fever is usually milder than the louse-borne form. The primary bout of fever is followed by several relapses (not exceeding 11) before the infection resolves. Mortality is low, but neurological complications (see below) are a significant feature. Recovery is usually complete; there are no long-term sequelae.

Incubation period

Although this may be short (1–2 days has been recorded in the Spanish form), it is more often longer—up to 14 days.

Symptoms and signs

Onset
The primary attack begins abruptly with severe headache and fever of up to 40°C. It may rarely be fulminating—leading to coma and death; it can also take the form of chronic low-grade fever. During this attack the spleen enlarges (45%) and infarcts; haemorrhage(s) may ensue. Hepatomegaly can also occur (11%) but jaundice is not as common as in the louse-borne form. There may also be diarrhoea, bronchitis and pneumonia. Massive haematuria, associated with nephritis, has been recorded in Israel.

Changes in peripheral blood
Borrelia spp. are less numerous in peripheral blood than in the louse-borne form. A polymorphonuclear leucocytosis is present. The initial attack may last 4–5 days (shorter in the African form), ending in a crisis; this can lead to 'collapse'.

Relapses

Relapses are characteristic of the tick-borne form. They may occur at intervals of a day or two, or may be separated by up to 3 weeks. Between three and six relapses are common, with up to 11 in the African form (Figure 55.5).

COMPLICATIONS

Neurological

Borrelia spp. causing tick-borne relapsing fever are neurotropic.[8] They may be present in CSF and can be detected by microscopic examination or animal inoculation. Various neurological syndromes may result—initially appearing at the end of the first bout of fever, or during relapses.

Cranial nerve involvement
This is the most common neurological complication. The seventh nerve is most frequently involved (22% in one series in North Africa); the third, fourth,

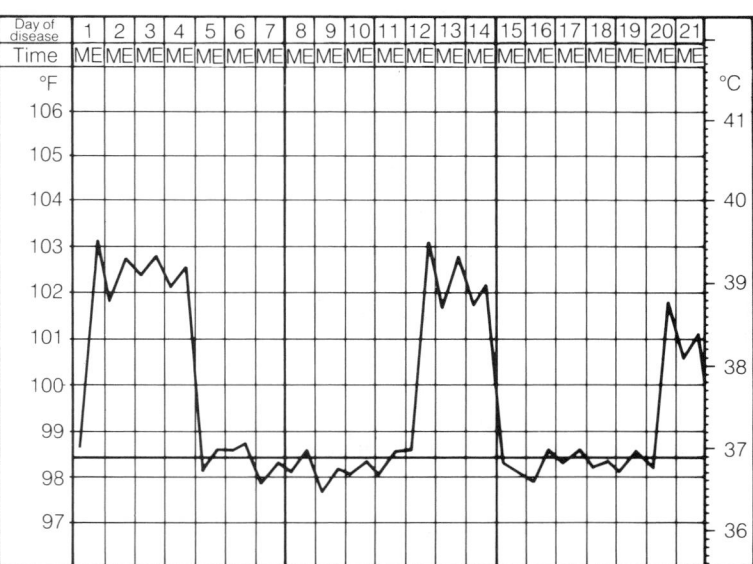

Figure 55.5 Temperature chart in tick-borne relapsing fever. There are usually 3–6 relapses; as many as 11 have been recorded.

fifth, sixth (with ophthalmoplegia) and the eighth (with deafness) nerves may also be affected.

Meningitic form

Lymphocytic meningitis and occasionally subarachnoid haemorrhage may occur. The CSF is under pressure; a pleocytosis is frequently present. This form is not uncommon in expatriates in the Dakar area.

Other cerebral syndromes

Hemiplegia, aphasia, encephalitis, optic atrophy, iritis and iridocyclitis are by no means uncommon. The spinal nerves may be involved, especially in *O. moubata* and *O. tholozani* infections. There may be seventh nerve involvement and sciatic neuralgia, with anaesthesia. Most cerebral complications resolve without residual deficit.

Other complications

Bronchitis, hepatic failure and arthritis may occur.

DIFFERENTIAL DIAGNOSIS

Other fevers should be distinguished, and between louse-borne relapsing fever and other relapsing fevers (rat-bite fevers); major differences between the tick-borne and louse-borne forms are summarized in Table 55.2.

DIAGNOSIS

In the febrile phase, *Borrelia* spp. can be visualized in a peripheral blood film; they are fewer than in the louse-borne form, and inoculation into mice and rats may be required for demonstration. Diagnosis is often difficult in the afebrile period; a history of travel and residence in a known infected camp or village is of value, and in a subsequent relapse *Borrelia* spp. can be demonstrated at the onset and peak of the febrile episode. Serological tests may be useful, as in louse-borne relapsing fever.

TREATMENT

Treatment is the same as that for louse-borne relapsing fever: tetracycline (a single 500 mg dose) or procaine penicillin (300 mg). Doxycycline has also been used.[8,9] The Jarisch-Herxheimer reaction is *not* a recognized complication, but can occur.[8,10]

EPIDEMIOLOGY

Tick-borne relapsing fever is an endemic disease found only in certain locations. In Central, East and South Africa—where man is the sole reservoir—it is present in human habitations and wherever man lives collectively, i.e. in certain types of house, staging camps for migrant workers, and in old camping sites. In East Africa, *O. moubata* consists of two types: one preferring to feed on chickens (which are not important in transmission) living in hot humid conditions, and the other preferring man and found in cooler, wetter locations (highlands)—where it is an important vector.

O. moubata porcinus—widely distributed in African dwellings at all altitudes in East Africa — feeds on man and favours a higher rainfall and a high relative humidity; it is a superior vector to *O. moubata*. *O. savignyi* prefers a hot, dry climate and infests market places and cattle byres around wells; here it comes into contact with man.

In North Africa, the eastern Mediterranean, central Asia and North and South America rodents constitute the major reservoir; infection is transmit-

Table 55.2 Major differences between tick-borne and louse-borne relapsing fevers*.

	Tick-borne	Louse-borne
Parasites in peripheral blood	Scanty	Numerous
Paroxysms (days)	Relatively short, not more than 5–7. Often chronic, irregular fever	Relatively long—up to 10
Relapses	Two or more	Two or less, often none
Vomiting	Only with meningitis	At any stage
Other symptoms	Lethargy, loss of weight, debility	Diarrhoea, jaundice, coma, severe haemorrhage
Neurological complications	Common. Cranial nerve palsies	Infrequent
Ocular complications	Papilloedema with meningitis	Infrequent
Illness	Less severe	More severe
Mortality (%)	Less than 10	May be high—up to 50

*After Cogill N F. *J R Army Med Corps* 1949; 93:2.

ted to man incidentally. Ticks live in animal burrows and caves, and in North America in holiday homes — where chipmunks live in roofs.

CONTROL

Control of infection where dwellings are the source of infection is effected by construction of concrete floors and improved walls so that ticks lack access. Ticks can be killed by insecticides;[11] they are relatively unaffected by DDT, but are susceptible to BHC (20 mg/900 cm^2) used to dust the floor. Old camping sites and mud houses should be avoided. Travellers must never sleep on the floor.[8]

Lyme disease, caused by the spirochaete *B. burgdorferi* in the eastern USA is described in Appendix IV.

RAT BITE FEVERS[12]

Two forms of fever have been described: (1) sodoku (sokosha),[13,14] named by Japanese workers and caused by *Spirillum minus (S. morsus-muris)*; and (2) Haverhill fever (infectious erythema), named by American workers and caused by *Actinobacillus muris* (formerly *Streptobacillus moniliformis*).

These are not strictly *tropical* diseases; their inclusion is because they are 'relapsing' diseases and can be confused with other infections.

SODOKU

GEOGRAPHICAL DISTRIBUTION

Most recorded cases have occurred in Japan; it is also present in Australia, Africa, the Americas and Europe.

AETIOLOGY

Spirillum minus is a short spiral organism (2–4 μm long), rather thick, and with regular rigid spirals and pointed ends continued into one or more flagella. It moves rapidly, resembling a vibrio, and is readily stained by methylene blue or Giemsa.

S. minus can be cultivated; subcultivation has been unsuccessful. It can be grown by intraperitoneal inoculation into guinea-pigs, mice and rats.

TRANSMISSION

S. minus parasitizes rats; they are healthy carriers. Transmission is from rat to man, although infection can be caused by the bite of cats, ferrets and bandicoots. Rat urine contaminating food constitutes a further vehicle of transmission.

PATHOLOGY

The organism enters at the site of the bite; local inflammation and even necrosis may be present. It is transmitted to regional lymph glands. In fatal cases neuronal degeneration has been recorded in brain, and degenerative changes in liver and kidneys.

CLINICAL FEATURES

Natural history

Sodoku consists of a relapsing fever which may subside spontaneously or continue for many months. It is a relatively mild disease; the mortality rate is about 10%.

Incubation period

The incubation period varies from 5 to 30 days—the average being 5–10 days.

Symptoms and signs

There is usually a history of a bite,[13] this heals, but may later break down to form an ulcer (Figure 55.6). Later, the scar and sometimes the surrounding tissues become inflamed, with formation of blebs and even necrosis. The lymphatics draining the area are involved and regional glands become swollen and tender. Onset of fever is characterized by rigors and malaise; the temperature gradually rises in 3 days to a maximum of 39.4–40°C; after a further 3-day period this ends in a crisis—accompanied by profuse sweating.

Following the primary attack a quiescent interval (5–10 days) ensues. One or more relapses—associated with similar symptoms and a characteristic purple papular exanthem, or urticaria, on the

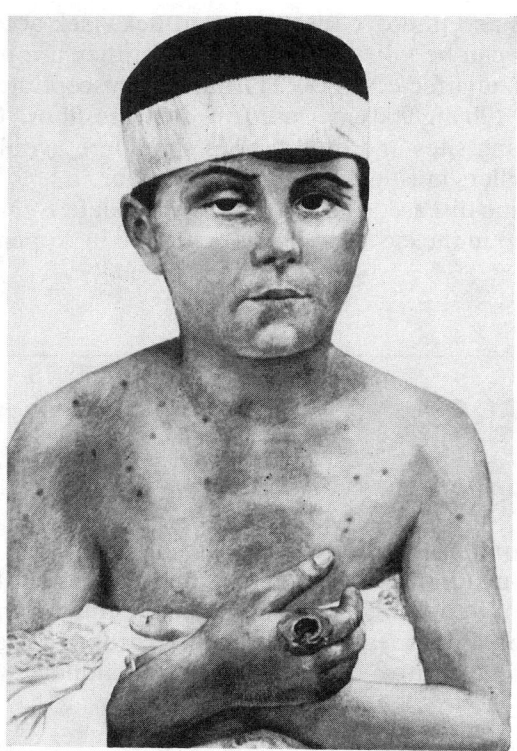

Figure 55.6   Rat bite fever produces an initial lesion at the site of the bite; this is followed by relapsing fever and rash. (Courtesy of WTIM.)

chest and arms—have been recorded. The eruption is sometimes nodular. With each bout of fever the cicatrix at the site of the original bite becomes inflamed.

In most cases the reflexes are increased; there may be pains in muscles and joints and hyperaesthesiae and oedema involving various parts of the body. Arthritis has been recorded. The mortality rate is about 10%. In fatal cases the terminal phase is ushered in by delirium, often followed by coma. Some cases subside spontaneously; others continue for months.

As in relapsing fever the organism can be demonstrated in peripheral blood during the febrile episode only, disappearing during apyrexial intervals. During the paroxysm there is an eosinophilia and moderate leucocytosis (e.g. 15×10^9/l). CSF pressure is increased.

DIFFERENTIAL DIAGNOSIS

Differential diagnosis is from the different forms of relapsing and trench fevers—with which the temperature chart (Figure 55.7) has much in common. In tropical countries the possibility of coexistent *Plasmodium* spp. infection should be taken into

account. Puffiness of the face accompanying the urticarial eruption may simulate acute nephritis.

The reaction occurring around the site of the scar can be confused with either erysipelas or cellulitis.

DIAGNOSIS

In many cases a diagnosis of rat bite fever can be fully established from the history, infiltration at the site of the bite, typical temperature chart, a characteristic rash and response to penicillin administration. Diagnosis can be confirmed either by darkground illumination (spirilla may be visualized in the exudate obtained from the site of the bite, or in serous fluid from the papule)[13] or a Giemsa-stained smear. It is seldom possible to demonstrate spirilla in a thick blood film. If a number of relapses have occurred, the most useful investigative procedure consists of demonstrating lytic antibodies. Absolute proof of clinical diagnosis may be obtained by inoculating the patient's blood, lymph gland or wound biopsy into a guinea-pig or mouse.

S. minus is not easily found in peripheral blood (although it does enter the bloodstream after a few days) but is found in exudate near the bite and in 'juice' from local lymph nodes. Inoculation of infected material into a mouse or rat produces a haematological infection, and in the guinea-pig a febrile disease. Dogs can be infected but remain asymptomatic. Monkeys and rabbits are susceptible. The spirilla are present in rat tongue muscle. Rats, mice and guinea-pigs may be healthy carriers.

Serology

Serum gives a weak positive treponemal serological reaction, and a positive Weil–Felix to proteus OXK strain.

TREATMENT

Infection responds rapidly to penicillin; a single injection (300 mg) of a repository penicillin[13,14] is adequate. Streptomycin and tetracycline are also effective.

EPIDEMIOLOGY

Single sporadic cases occur following a rat bite. Small epidemics can follow, when contaminated raw milk is the vehicle of infection.

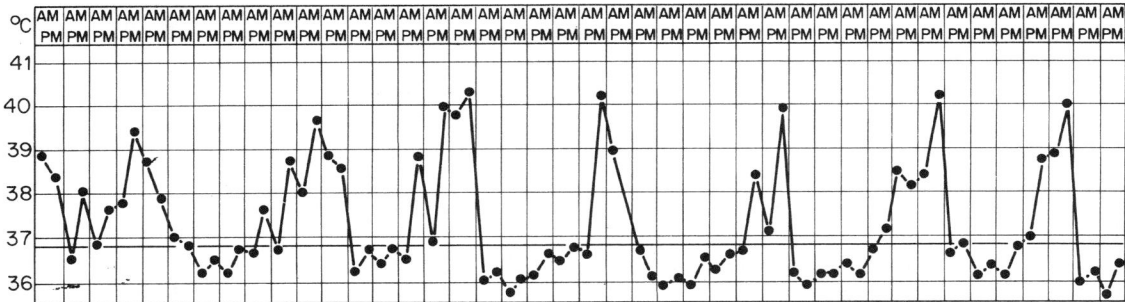

Figure 55.7 Temperature chart in rat bite fever, showing periodic relapses.

HAVERHILL FEVER

GEOGRAPHICAL DISTRIBUTION

Haverhill fever is present in the USA, Europe and elsewhere.[15-19]

AETIOLOGY

Actinobacillus muris (A. moniliformis, Streptobacillus moniliformis) is a natural 'parasite' of the nasopharynx of rats. It consists of a pleomorphic organism which forms slender, branching filaments $(1-3 \times 0.3-0.4\,\mu m)$; these break up to form chains of bacillus or coccoid bodies. It is a more common cause of rat bite fever than *S. minus*.

TRANSMISSION

Although infection can often be traced to a rat bite, transmission can occur via raw milk contaminated by rat urine; this has caused many epidemics.

PATHOLOGY

Little is known of the pathology; ulcerative endocarditis and subacute myocarditis have both been recorded. Hepatomegaly is usually present.

CLINICAL FEATURES

Natural history

Haverhill fever consists of a febrile illness, an erythematous rash (most prominent on hands and feet), arthralgia[15] and subsequent development of a sore throat. The fever may relapse and, untreated, continue for months.

Incubation period

The incubation period is 3–10 days; during this time gastrointestinal symptoms may be present.

Symptoms and signs

If bitten,[15,17] the wound has usually healed; this is followed by fever, extreme prostration, severe generalized muscular pain(s) and tenderness, headache and a generalized morbilliform rash[17]—most marked on the hands and feet. Generalized lymphadenopathy is present. Non-suppurative shifting arthritis[15] is characteristic. In untreated cases the disease may subside spontaneously after 9–10 days; it can continue with a prolonged relapsing fever accompanied by night sweats; this can recur for weeks or months at irregular intervals. Case mortality is about 10%, the cause usually being bacterial endocarditis and/or abscess formation.[19]

DIAGNOSIS (Table 55.3)

Differential diagnoses include: Coxsackie infection, meningococcal septicaemia and erythema multiforme. The organism can be isolated from blood by aerobic culture,[15] and subcultured on blood agar (in a carbon dioxide atmosphere) after 48 hours.

Serology

A. muris can be agglutinated by serum; a fluorescent antibody titre (IgM) at 1:400 has been obtained using an antigen consisting of *Actinobacillus* spp.

TREATMENT

Tetracycline (250 mg 6-hourly for 2 weeks) is the antibiotic of choice. Erythromycin is also effective.[16] Penicillin has also been used;[17,18] however, some coccobacillary variants are resistant to this agent.

Table 55.3   Differentiating features of sodoku and Haverhill fever.

	Sodoku	*Haverhill fever*
Transmission	Bite of rat	Bite of rat or other animal. Possibly contaminated food
Incubation period (days)	5–30	3–10 (average 5)
Wound from bite	Apparent healing, followed by chancre-like ulceration	Heals promptly
Lymph glands	Regional lymphadenitis	Not involved
Systemic manifestations	Regularly relapsing fever	Intermittent, but not regularly relapsing fever
	Generalized maculopapular rash	Macular, pustular and petechial eruption
	Varying degrees of prostration and debility	Varying degree(s) of prostration
	Arthritis very rare	Metastic arthritis fairly common
Laboratory findings	Polymorphonuclear leucocytosis	Same
	Secondary anaemia	Same
	Kahn test, usually +	Negative
	Isolation of *Spirillum* spp. by animal inoculation of blood or infected gland	Isolation of *A. muris* by blood culture and from pustules on veal infusion broth enriched with rabbit serum
	Agglutination test negative	Agglutination test with *A. muris* positive. Serum agglutinates a polyvalent antigen of the bacillus

REFERENCES

1 Morshed M G, Konishi H, Nishimura T & Nakazawa T. Evaluation of agents for use in medium for selective isolation of Lyme disease and relapsing fever *Borrelia* species. *Eur J Clin Microbiol Infect Dis* 1993; 12:512–518.

2 Cutler S J, Fekade D, Hussein K et al. Successful in-vitro cultivation of *Borrelia recurrentis. Lancet* 1994; 343:242.

3 Cadavid D, Bundoc V & Barbour A G. Experimental infection of the mouse brain by a relapsing fever *Borrelia* species: a molecular analysis. *J Infect Dis* 1993; 168:143–151.

4 Almaviva M, Hailu B, Borgnolo G, Chiabrera F, Tolesse G & Gebre B. Louse-borne relapsing fever epidemic in Arssi Region, Ethiopia: a six months survey. *Trans R Soc Trop Med Hyg* 1993; 87:153.

5 Borgnolo G, Denku B, Chiabrera F & Hailu B. Louse-borne relapsing fever in Ethiopian children: a clinical study. *Ann Trop Paediat* 1993; 13:165–171.

6 Borgnolo G, Hailu B, Ciancarelli A, Almaviva M & Woldemariam T. Louse-borne relapsing fever. A clinical and an epidemiological study of 389 patients in Asella Hospital, Ethiopia. *Trop Geogr Med* 1993; 45:66–69.

7 Sundnes K O & Haimanot A T. Epidemic of louse-borne relapsing fever in Ethiopia. *Lancet* 1993; 342:1213–1215.

8 Colebunders R, De-Serrano P, Van-Gompel A et al. Imported relapsing fever in European tourists. *Scand J Infect Dis* 1993; 25:533–536.

9 Spach D H, Liles W C, Campbell G L, Quick R E, Anderson D E Jr & Fritsche T R. Tick-borne diseases in the United States. *N Engl J Med* 1993; 329:936–947.

10 Liles W C & Spach D H. Late relapse of tick-borne relapsing fever following treatment with doxycycline. *West J Med* 1993; 158:200.

11 Vasil'eva I S & Gutova V P. A comparative evaluation of the sensitivity of the vector of tick-borne relapsing fever to pesticides by using the standard test paper. *Med Parazitol (Mosk)* 1993; Jan–Feb:31–32.

12 Dow G R, Rankin R J & Saunders B W. Rat-bite fever. *N Z Med J* 1992; 105:133.

13 Hinrichsen S L, Ferraz S, Romeiro M et al. Sodoku—a case report. *Rev Soc Bras Med Trop* 1992; 25:135–138.

14 Bhatt K M & Mirz N B. Rat bite fever: a case report from a Kenyan. *East Afr Med J* 1992; 69:542–543.

15 Fordham J N, McKay-Ferguson E, Davies A & Blyth T. Rat bite fever without the bite. *Ann Rheum Dis* 1992; 51:411–412.

16 Konstantopoulos K, Skarpas P, Hitjazis F et al. Rat bite fever in a Greek child. *Scand J Infect Dis* 1992; 24:531–533.

17 Rygg M & Bruun C F. Rat bite fever (*Streptobacillus moniliformis*) with septicemia in a child. *Scand J Infect Dis* 1992; 24:535–540.

18 Mathiasen T & Rix M. Rat bite—an infant bitten by a rat. *Ugeskr Laeger* 1993; 155:1475–1476.

19 Vasseur E, Joly P, Nouvellon M, Laplagne A & Lauret P. Cutaneous abscess: a rare complication of *Streptobacillus moniliformis* infection. *Br J Dermatol* 1993; 129:95–96.

CHAPTER 56

LEPTOSPIROSIS

G. Scott and T. J. Coleman

INTRODUCTION

Leptospirosis is an acute febrile illness common in many parts of the world. Most cases are mild or asymptomatic but the most severe illness, known as Weil's disease, may be associated with death through renal failure.[1-5] Leptospirosis is a world-wide zoonotic infection. It is known by many different local names (e.g. mud, swamp, sugar cane, Fort Bragg, Japanese autumnal fevers). The major reservoir is rodents and the organism is passed in their urine for months and can survive in fresh but not brackish water. Man is infected by contact with rodent urine or with the urine of other infected animals such as dogs and domestic farm animals, or with meat contaminated by urine.

AETIOLOGY

THE ORGANISM

The causative agents belong to the genus *Leptospira*, fine spiral bacteria of $0.1\,\mu$m diameter and 6–$20\,\mu$m in length.[6] The organism appears straight with one or both ends hooked (Figure 56.1). Spinning motility may disguise the spiral nature of the organisms on dark-ground examination.[7] *L. interrogans* comprises the parasitic and pathogenic strains which can cause disease in man and animals. This species can be divided into a large number of serovars and although var. *icterohaemorrhagiae* is thought classically more virulent and more likely to cause Weil's disease, severe forms of infection may occasionally occur in man, with any of >200 recognized serovars, each of which tends to a particular geographical distribution. The severity of infection is probably as much to do with dose and host susceptibility as to the strain involved. Common serovars causing sporadic infection in man include *canicola*, *hardjo*, *hebdomadis*, *grippotyphosa* and *pomona*.[5] Some serovars tend to show a particular geographical distribution and differences in the major maintenance host. For example, in the UK, *L. hardjo* is particularly associated with cattle explaining the observed increased risk of infection with this serovar in dairy farmers.

Free living saprophytic strains (*L. biflexa*) do not

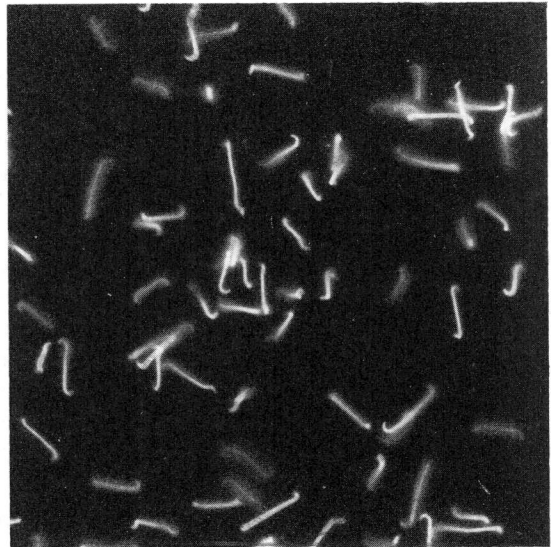

Figure 56.1 Leptospires under dark-ground illumination—characteristically hooked at both ends.

cause disease in man but their presence in the environment indicates that conditions exist under which strains pathogenic to man can survive. *L. biflexa* strains grow at 13°C and in the presence of β-azaguanine, both of which are inhibitory to *L. interrogans*, and are not pathogenic to hamsters.

CULTURE REQUIREMENTS

L. interrogans is an obligate aerobe which can be grown on various media which incorporate vitamins B_1 and B_{12}, long-chained fatty acids ($\geq C_{15}$) and ammonium salts. The optimal growth conditions are pH 7.2–7.6 with media enriched with fresh serum or albumin, with incubation at a temperature of 28–30°C. The organism survives in anticoagulated (but not citrated blood) for many days. However, it is unusual for laboratories to undertake the culture of leptospires routinely unless they are in a centre of endemic or epidemic infection.

CLASSIFICATION

Traditionally, the family of Leptospiraceae has been subdivided into two genera—the *Leptospira* and *Leptonema*. The genus *Leptospira* comprises three species, *L. interrogans* (pathogenic), *L. biflexa* (saprophytic) and *L. parva* (a single strain which is considered non-pathogenic but is serologically related to both other species).

The species *L. interrogans* is divided into many serovars and strains are identified by cross-agglutination–absorption with known strains using homologous antisera raised in rabbits. The test is labour intensive and therefore expensive. Major and unique antigens are currently being defined by raising monoclonal antibodies and these may be applied to the identification of certain specific serovars.

Chromatography of whole cell DNA digests may also be used to show dissimilarities between strains.[8,9] This welcome move away from (potentially variable) antigen characterization may well reveal even more strains contained in what are termed 'geno-' and 'subgeno-groups'. However, at present, classification based on serological differences rather than DNA-relatedness is most practical for clinical usage.

EPIDEMIOLOGY AND TRANSMISSION

The rat is the main host to leptospires. However, it is likely that every mammal has the potential to become a carrier of some serovar and is capable of spreading the disease among its own kind. There is a wide variety of interesting hosts described ranging from virtually every sort of small mammal with which man occasionally comes into contact (e.g. hedgehogs, rabbits, hares, house and field mice, voles, skunks, possums, coypus and mongooses) to reptiles (various frogs and snakes). Leptospirae have been found in migratory water birds and various insects. In maintenance hosts, the organisms continue to replicate in the renal tubules after primary infection and are excreted for months or years asymptomatically.

The greatest risk to man is from the carriage of leptospirosis in rats. Man acquires infection by direct or indirect contact with the urine of maintenance hosts, which include rodents and some domestic animals (e.g. dogs excreting *L. canicola*) and farm animals (e.g. cattle excreting *hardjo*), or by rat bites. Contact with urine-contaminated water is extremely important. In order for man to be infected, the organism has to gain entry and is reputed to be able to do so through intact waterlogged skin. This seems improbable in practice and it is much more likely that it actually enters through fresh cuts or grazes and possibly through mucous membranes. Eating food contaminated with rat urine is risky. Immersion in heavily contaminated fresh water carries a high risk; the number of organisms increases dramatically in the late summer in temperate climes, particularly in stagnant water. Bathing in canals carries a significant risk.[10] Working closely with infected animals also carries a risk, as does working physically in an environment heavily contaminated with rat urine (e.g. in mines or cutting down sugar cane) unless work practices are adopted to reduce the risk of skin contact.

The survival of leptospires in the environment is favoured by moist conditions and neutral or slightly alkaline pH. They survive in fresh water at neutral pH for up to 4 weeks but at pH 5, survival is reduced to 2 days. Comparison of workers in two rat-infested mines in Japan showed the seroprevalence of leptospirosis to be very high in the mine where the water was alkaline but low where the water was acid.

Common occupations associated with leptospirosis include mining, farming, veterinary medicine, fish farming and processing, sewage and canal work, cane harvesting, and trench warfare. Leptospirosis is known by many different local names (e.g. mud, swamp, sugar cane, Fort Bragg, Japanese autumnal fevers). Seroprevalence studies in high-risk populations in areas of hyperendemicity (e.g. many areas of sub-Saharan Africa) indicate that the infection is extremely unusual. More recently, the disease has been described in those taking part in recreational water sports such as canoeing or rafting in fast-flowing rivers or windsurfing. Recreational may now be more important than occupational exposure in developed countries.

Domestic animals such as dogs may be infected. Although human infection with *L. canicola* is most often contracted from dogs, the latter are more likely infected with and get overt disease from *L. icterohaemorrhagiae*. This observation demonstrates that an animal may be a maintenance host for one serovar and show no evidence of disease and yet is susceptible to other pathogenic serovars. Swine tend to be infected with *L. pomona* and become long-term maintenance hosts of this serovar. Other domestic farm livestock such as goats, horses, sheep and cattle are often chronically infected. The organism has been found in bull semen and is transmitted by natural and artificial insemination.[11]

PATHOLOGY AND IMMUNOLOGY

Leptospires disseminate widely after entering the body. In the most severe cases jaundice, bleeding and renal failure occur.[12] Virulence factors identified include hyaluronidase and a 'burrowing motility'. These could explain the ability of the organism to penetrate intact mucous membranes and perhaps the dissemination, but neither explains the pathological picture.

Whereas the first phase does not involve much inflammation, direct hepatocellular damage leads to jaundice, and tubular damage occurs by a yet undiscovered mechanism. The liver is not enlarged and microscopic damage ranges from no appreciable light microscopic changes, to unicellular damage with oedema, to multiple necrotic foci, seen only in those who die rapidly.[13] Regeneration of the liver begins rapidly and reorganization will have begun in a patient who dies late from renal failure. Renal changes include enlargement with oedema and subcapsular haemorrhage, and renal tubular necrosis.[14–16]

Haemorrhage may be present in any internal organ, and reflects endothelial damage and increased capillary fragility. The mechanism of damage in liver, kidneys and blood vessels is not known. Although much of the pathological change could be explained by cytotoxins, none has been demonstrated. The second phase of the illness is characterized by host immune response and includes immune complex glomerulonephritis and vasculitis with endothelial injury.

CLINICAL PRESENTATION

Most people who have been infected with leptospires do not remember an illness to account for seropositivity. It is likely that there are many mild influenza-like illnesses. Severe infection resulting in jaundice and renal failure is rare. In others infection may be asymptomatic. Although some serovars (e.g. *L. icterohaemorrhagiae*) tend to be associated with serious illness there is no 'serovar-specific presentation' in man. Some serovars such as *L. canicola* tend to cause transient lymphocytic meningitis rather than hepatorenal syndrome. Men are infected more often than women but this may simply reflect increased risk of occupational or recreational exposure rather than increased susceptibility. In many cases, leptospirosis follows a biphasic course.

EARLY NON-SPECIFIC BACTERAEMIC PHASE

The incubation period of natural infection is not known but in those few instances of laboratory accident or known single exposure risk the incubation period was 2–20 (median 11) days. There follows an acute febrile illness with chills, headache, myalgia, back pain, anorexia, nausea and vomiting. A sore throat is common and herpes simplex labialis may occur. Sometimes the acute phase is very severe, the patient is prostrate and has a persistently high fever (39–40°C) with exquisitely tender muscles, some cough and perhaps even haemoptysis, with dyspnoea and persistent vomiting. Abdominal pain is common and the patient tends to be constipated.

During this phase, leptospires may be cultured from blood and CSF but *not* the urine. Serological tests are negative. This so-called bacteraemic illness lasts around 4–7 days and, if mild, is followed by a remission lasting 2 days.

Wide dissemination of the organism in the acute phase leads to meningeal invasion. The organism can be seen in and cultured from the CSF and tissues. There may be a transient non-specific rash. A 'specific' rash has been described in Fort Bragg fever: this is transient pretibial raised erythematous patches (2–5 cm diameter) with some induration but much less tenderness than would be expected with erythema nodosum. It seems to be more common with *L. autumnalis* or *pomona* than with *canicola* or *icterohaemorrhagiae*. Myalgia and tender musculature, with raised serum creatine phosphokinase, and conjunctival suffusion are characteristic. There may be moderate hepatomegaly but splenomegaly is less common.

The platelet count may fall and thrombocytopenic purpurae and frank bleeding ensue. The urinalysis shows proteinuria but the creatinine clearance usually remains normal until tubular necrosis or glomerulonephritis occur.

SECOND PHASE

Following the initial illness, a second phase then begins, characteristically the patient having developed antibodies to the infecting organism, with meningeal or hepatorenal manifestations being prominent. In the severe form of the disease, the first and second phases merge imperceptibly with persistent high fever. The fever subsides in milder cases but then the patient deteriorates, becoming jaundiced and starting to bleed into the skin, mucous membranes and lungs. The liver enlargement is now more prominent. As the sclerae become icteric the suffused vessels glow orange. Purpurae and ecchymoses are seen. Oliguric renal failure, shock and myocarditis follow and are associated with a high

mortality.[14–16] The patient develops pulmonary oedema and subpleural pulmonary haemorrhages with haemoptysis. The ECG is abnormal, reflecting myopericarditis. The patient will deteriorate rapidly if significant gastrointestinal haemorrhage occurs.

Patients who develop oliguria then anuria with rising plasma creatinine require renal dialysis. The bilirubin is high but without marked enzyme abnormalities and the combination of high bilirubin and creatinine should immediately raise the question of leptospirosis. Renal failure is the usual cause of death but myocarditis, adrenal failure, haemorrhage and cerebral artery thrombosis may also be contributory. In those who are going to survive without renal support, the creatinine level begins to fall at the end of the second week of the illness, indicating rapid resolution of the tubular necrosis.

CENTRAL NERVOUS SYSTEM INVOLVEMENT

A patient may present predominantly with meningitis and the CSF contains moderate numbers of lymphocytes and mildly elevated protein without altered glucose. The presence of myalgia, conjunctival suffusion, slight jaundice and occasional petechiae can be clues to help move the diagnosis away from enterovirus infection. Cerebral arteritis is an unusual late complication—Moyamoya syndrome is caused by obstruction of the internal carotid arteries near the circle of Willis.

EYE INVOLVEMENT

The eyes are suffused and there may be subconjunctival haemorrhages during acute leptospirosis. Pathogenic *leptospires* may invade the eye during the acute febrile phase and this may be followed by uveitis weeks or months after recovery. More commonly a mild anterior iridocyclitis, blurring of the vitreous and haemorrhages in the retina can occur and result in disturbance to vision.

DIFFERENTIAL DIAGNOSIS

Jaundice and renal failure with an acute febrile illness should immediately suggest the diagnosis of leptospirosis and a full history of occupational, rec-

reational and animal exposure must be taken. In practice, most cases of jaundice will at first be thought to be due to viral hepatitis: a raised bilirubin with relatively unchanged enzymes and polymorphonuclear leucocytosis with negative viral serology should point away from viral infection. However, many other acute fevers are associated with jaundice (e.g. malaria, acute schistosomiasis, visceral leishmaniasis, melioidosis, plague, tularaemia and relapsing fever). The most important clinical clue is the link with renal failure. The haemolytic–uraemic syndrome may be caused by toxin produced by gut pathogens such as *Shigella* spp. and *Escherichia coli* (serotype O157) but dysentery is a prominent feature in such cases. If petechiae are present, then meningococcal disease must be excluded. Examination of the CSF is therefore very important if there is any hint of meningitis. Any patient with acute lymphocytic meningitis must have a good history for possible exposure taken.

DIAGNOSIS

It is unlikely that the early non-specific illness of leptospirosis will be diagnosed unless there is a clear suggestion of the diagnosis in some occupational or recreational exposure or if there is an outbreak. Clinical clues which may suggest the diagnosis over other causes of acute fever are disproportionate myalgia, jaundice, conjunctival suffusion, pretibial rash and lymphocytic meningitis. If the diagnosis is suspected at this early stage, liaise with the microbiologist to arrange blood and CSF to be examined under dark-field microscopy and for the special media to be prepared.[3] However, do not expect rapid results: cultures may take 2–3 weeks to prove positive. Many artefacts (e.g. RBC membranes) may resemble leptospires when blood cultures are viewed directly using dark-field microscopy. Culture into special media is more sensitive than direct microscopy. On days 1–4 of the illness, all blood cultures should be positive but on the fifth day only 50% will be positive, and thereafter none will be.[17]

The urine will be negative in the bacteraemic phase so is not worth testing until the illness has been underway for some 10 days. By then serological tests will be positive. Urine must be examined fresh and the leptospires will die if it is acid. A simple way of alkalinizing the urine is to give potassium citrate mixture, for example, as Cystopurin, one sachet (equivalent to 3 g) three times per day for 2 days, or sodium bicarbonate, 3 g every 2 hours, until the urine pH is >7. Some confusion will occur if there are protein fibrils in the urine associated with renal tubular damage—they look surprisingly like immobile leptospires. Viability and motility of the bacteria are therefore particularly important.

When the patient is jaundiced the bilirubin is markedly elevated but transaminases and alkaline phosphatase do not rise much beyond the upper limit of normal. The urine contains bilirubin and urobilinogen with some protein. The creatine phosphokinase is raised.[18] There is also a polymorphonuclear leucocytosis which is useful in distinguishing leptospirosis from acute viral hepatitis. The haemoglobin may fall, partly due to the infection and partly due to haemorrhage. As the illness develops, the albumin falls and globulin rises. The bleeding time is prolonged: the clotting is normal and bleeding is due to capillary fragility.[19] There is no consumption of clotting factors. Later a rise in prothrombin time reflects hepatocyte failure. The erythrocyte sedimentation rate rises in the second week.

Antibodies to leptospires do not rise until at least 6 days after the onset of symptoms.[2,20] After this, a single high titre (agglutination >100) may be of help but a rising titre is diagnostic. Reference laboratories may provide differentiation of the antibody into IgM and IgG.[21] Crude agglutination or complement fixation tests using a standardized polyvalent antigen are done in local laboratories. Reference laboratories perform more specific tests including one of a variety of enzyme linked immunosorbent assay (ELISA) techniques[22] or microagglutination against live or formalinized organisms (MAT) which aids differentiation between serovars.

SYNDROMES ASSOCIATED WITH OTHER SEROVARS

CANICOLA FEVER

Serovar *L. canicola* is more likely to cause lymphocytic meningitis than the hepatorenal syndrome and is rarely fatal.[23] If acquired in pregnancy, the fetus may abort. The disease is usually acquired from domestic dogs which can excrete the organism in the urine for years. Dogs may fall ill themselves on acquiring the infection and should be immunized against leptospirosis as puppies. A common symptom in the infected dog is polyuria, and the history of contact with dogs, other pets or farm animals must be sought from any patient with lymphocytic meningitis (or other symptom complex suggestive of leptospirosis). Pigs sometimes also acquire *L. canicola* but are usually asymptomatic.

OTHER SEROVARS

Outbreaks of infection with other serovars are geographically focal and become well recognized locally. Most cause symptoms which are nonspecific (headache, myalgia, fever, perhaps with mildly elevated bilirubin levels but rarely with overt jaundice). However, *L. autumnalis* is particularly associated with a Fort Bragg fever: curious pretibial, raised 2–4 cm erythematous patches which are much less tender than erythema nodosum and occur at the height of the illness.[24] However, pretibial fever may occur with other serovars (e.g. *pomona*) and there has been some confusion with legionellosis. *L. pomona*, a parasite predominantly of pigs, causes swineherds' disease, first described in Australia then in Switzerland, and behaves in man like canicola fever.

L. grippotyphosa causes swamp or mud fever and *bataviae* causes rice-field disease described in outbreaks first in Indonesia and later in Italy.

TREATMENT

Penicillin and other related β-lactam antibiotics (but not most cephalosporins or chloramphenicol) are active against experimental leptospirosis in animals.[25] Tetracyclines are also effective but there is some controversy as to whether penicillin is better than tetracycline in eliminating chronic renal infection. Penicillin (2 megaunits benzylpenicillin intravenously or intramuscularly every 6 hours) is probably the drug of choice in patients suspected of having leptospirosis but it used to be a widely held view that this would be ineffective if delayed beyond the first few days of the illness.[26] After all, after this time, the manifestations of the disease are probably immunologically mediated. However, recent placebo-controlled studies suggest that there is still an advantage in giving penicillin late (i.e. beyond the fourth day of the illness).[27] Tetracycline (e.g.

doxycycline, 100 mg q. 12 h p.o.)[28] or erythromycin (500 mg q. 12 h p.o.) are effective in patients allergic to penicillin.

For very ill patients, intensive care support may be necessary. Specific support therapy is required for anaemia due to bleeding and for renal failure. Haemodiafiltration is now favoured if resources permit but when resources are limited, peritoneal dialysis should be instituted to tide the patient over until the tubular necrosis has begun to resolve. A tendency to bleeding is not a contraindication to instituting haemodialysis. Parenteral feeding is important because of the hypercatabolic state of the febrile patient in renal failure.[15]

There are neglible risks to health care workers of acquiring the disease from an infected patient.

CONTROL AND PREVENTION

With over 200 pathogenic serovars and the fact that all animals may become infected, some chronically,

the eradication of leptospirosis is clearly impossible. However, there are three main ways in which the risk of leptospirosis in man can be reduced. First, domestic farm animals and pets can be immunized. This does not completely abolish the risk of an animal acquiring infection but significantly reduces the overall risk to man.[29] Secondly, risks in occupational exposure can be identified and addressed. Although classically described in sewer workers, leptospirosis is very rare in this group because protective clothing and simple hygienic precautions have been introduced. In general, farmers tend not to take similar precautions because of a misconception that the disease is not particularly associated

with this occupation. However, specific measures can be taken: for example, burning cane fields prior to harvest reduces the risk of the sharp young shoots cutting hands. Other simple measures such as removing rubbish from work and domestic environments will reduce the rodent population. Improved education of people at particular risk (e.g. farmers and those taking part in water sports) increases awareness and may enable earlier diagnosis and treatment. Thirdly, chemoprophylaxis (e.g. with doxycycline) can be used in groups at particularly high risk.[30]

REFERENCES

1 Turner L H. Leptospirosis I. *Trans R Soc Trop Med Hyg* 1967; 61:842–855.

2 Turner L H. Leptospirosis II. *Trans R Soc Trop Med Hyg* 1968; 62:880–899.

3 Turner L H. Leptospirosis III. *Trans R Soc Trop Med Hyg* 1970; 64:623–646.

4 Edwards G A & Domm B M. Human leptospirosis. *Medicine* 1960; 39:117–156.

5 Heath C W Jr, Alexander A D & Galton M M. Leptospirosis in the United States. Analysis of 483 cases in man 1949–1961. *N Engl J Med* 1965; 273:857–864.

6 Johnson R C & Faine S. *Leptospiraceae.* In Krieg N R & Holt J G (eds) *Bergey's Manual of Systemic Bacteriology*, vol. 1. Baltimore, MD: Williams & Wilkins, 1984: 62–67.

7 Cox P J & Twigg G I. Leptospiral motility. *Nature* 1974; 250:260–261.

8 Hookey J V, Waitkins S A & Jackman P J H. Numerical analysis of Leptospira DNA-restriction endonuclease patterns. *FEMS Microbiol Lett* 1985; 29:185–188.

9 Robinson A J, Ramadass P, Lee A & Marshall R B. Differentiation of subtypes within *Leptospira interrogans* serovars *hardjo*, *balcanica* and *tarassovi* by bacterial restriction-endonuclease DNA analysis (BRENDA). *J Med Microbiol* 1982; 15:331–338.

10 Hutchinson J H, Pippard J S, White M H G & Sheehan H L. Outbreak of Weil's disease in the British Army in Italy. *BMJ* 1946; 1:81–86.

11 Kiktenko V S, Balashov N G & Rodina V N. Leptospirosis infection through insemination of animals. *J Hyg Epidemiol Microbiol Immunol* 1976; 20:207–213.

12 Arean V M. The pathologic anatomy and pathogenesis of fatal human leptospirosis (Weil's disease). *Am J Pathol* 1962; 40:393–423.

13 Ramos-Morales F, Díaz-Rivera R S, Cintrón-Rivera A A, Rullán J A, Benenson A S & Acosta-Matienzo

J. The pathogenesis of leptospiral jaundice. *Ann Intern Med* 1959; 51:861–878.

14 Sitprija V. Renal involvement in human leptospirosis. *BMJ* 1968; ii:656–658.

15 Kennedy N D, Pusey C D, Rainford D J & Higginson A. Leptospirosis and acute renal failure: clinical experiences and a review of the literature. *Postgrad Med J* 1979; 55:176–179.

16 Lai K N, Aarons I, Woodroffe A J & Clarson A R. Renal lesions in leptospirosis. *Aust N Z J Med* 1982; 12:276–279.

17 Smith J. Weil's disease in the north-east of Scotland. *Br J Ind Med* 1949; 6:213–220.

18 Johnson W D, Silva I C & Rocha H. Serum creatine phosphokinase in leptospirosis. *JAMA* 1975; 233:981–982.

19 Edwards C N, Nicholson G D, Hassell T A, Everard C O R & Callender R J. Thromocytopenia in leptospirosis: the absence of evidence for disseminated intravascular coagulation. *Am J Trop Med Hyg* 1986; 35:352–354.

20 Cursons R T M, Pyke P A & Penniket J. The serological diagnosis of leptospirosis. *N Z J Med* 1982; 95:26–37.

21 Pappas M G, Ballou W R, Gray M R. Takafuji E T, Miller R N & Hockmeyer W T. Rapid serodiagnosis of leptospirosis using the IgM-specific dot-ELISA: comparison with the microscopic agglutination test. *Am J Trop Med Hyg* 1985; 34:346–354.

22 Watt G, Alquiza L M, Padre L P, Tuazon M L & Laughlin L W. The rapid diagnosis of leptospirosis: a prospective comparison of the dot enzyme linked immunosorbent assay and the genus-specific microscopic agglutination at different stages of illness. *J Infect Dis* 1988; 157:840–842.

23 McIntyre W I & Seiler H E. The epidemiology of canicola fever. *J Hyg (Camb)* 1953; 51:330–339.

24 Fraser D W, Glosser J W, Francis D P, Phillips C J,

Feeley J C & Sulzer C R. Leptospirosis caused by serotype *Fort-Bragg*. *Ann Intern Med* 1973; 79:786–794.

25 Alexander A D & Rule P L. Penicillins, cephalosporins and tetracyclines in treatment of hamsters with fatal leptospirosis. *Antimicrob Agents Chemother* 1986; 30:835–839.

26 Christie A B. Leptospiral infections. In *Infectious Diseases*, vol. 2, 4th edn. Edinburgh: Churchill Livingstone, 1982: 1173.

27 Watt G, Padre L P, Tuazon M L et al. Placebo-controlled trial of intravenous penicillin for severe and late leptospirosis. *Lancet* 1988; i:433–435.

28 McClain J B L, Ballou W R & Harrison S M. Doxycycline therapy for leptospirosis. *Ann Intern Med* 1984; 100:696–698.

29 Feigin R D, Lobes L A Jr, Anderson D & Pickering L. Human leptospirosis from immunized dogs. *Ann Intern Med* 1973; 79:777–785.

30 Takafuji E T, Kirkpatrick J W, Miller R N et al. An efficacy trial of doxycycline prophylaxis against leptospirosis. *N Engl J Med* 1984; 310:497–500.

CHAPTER 57

TUBERCULOSIS AND OTHER MYCOBACTERIAL DISEASES

Norman Horne

Tuberculosis is a disease of great antiquity. What were almost certainly tuberculous lesions have been found in the vertebrae of neolithic man in Europe, and of Egyptian mummies perhaps as early as 3700 BC.[1] The infectious agent, the tubercle bacillus, was discovered by Robert Koch in 1882.

Today tuberculosis has become the most important infectious disease in the world. The World Health Organization (WHO) estimates that about 1722 million people (one-third of the world population) are infected with tubercle bacilli. Furthermore, in 1990 eight million new cases of tuberculosis occurred, 95% of them in the developing world.[2] In early 1992 WHO estimated that approximately four million people had been infected with both *Mycobacterium tuberculosis* and the human immunodeficiency virus (HIV) since the beginning of the pandemic, 95% being in developing countries. The impact of the two epidemics on resource-poor countries has ominous social and medical implications and the already overstretched health services now have to face a tremendously increasing tuberculosis problem.[3] In 1982 Bignall[4] commented: 'The story of tuberculosis during the past 30 years has been one of triumph and tragedy—the triumph of the scientists who provided the means to control and ultimately eradicate the disease, and the tragedy of the widespread failure to exploit their discoveries.' These words were echoed almost a decade later:[5] 'The neglect of tuberculosis as a major public health priority over the last two decades is simply extraordinary. Perhaps the most important contribution to this state of ignorance was the greatly reduced clinical and epidemiological importance of tuberculosis in the wealthy nations.'

EPIDEMIOLOGY

Tuberculosis, like other new infections, when introduced into a susceptible population, takes the form of an epidemic wave. Unlike other infections the wave runs its course in about 300 years.

In England the present epidemic wave began in the sixteenth century and probably reached its peak about 1780 with the industrial revolution. The peak in Western Europe was probably reached in the early 1800s and in Eastern Europe some 80 years later. In North and South America the peak was reached about 1900 but it has not yet been reached in the developing countries of Asia and Africa except in a very few countries. The decline in tuberculosis in recent years led to its neglect as a major health priority, particularly by the wealthy nations. The problem had become so much smaller that there was discussion of possible elimination of the disease in some European countries by the middle of the twenty-first century. In an article[6] entitled 'Eradication of tuberculosis in Europe: so near and yet so far' in 1983 the following statement was made: 'forecasts that tuberculosis would disappear within a generation have been made for nearly a century, but it seems likely that several more generations will come and go before eradication is achieved.' This proved prophetic because 2 years later the USA observed for the first time a deviation from the expected logarithmic decline in tuberculosis. From then onwards America would see a progressive rise in new cases. In 1980 the increase over the previous year would be 4% and in 1990 a staggering 9.4%. Increases also took place in Western Europe (Table 57.1). In Scotland and Northern Ireland the previous decline has stopped. In America the acquired immune deficiency syndrome (AIDS) appears to be making a major impact on the upsurge. Deterior-

Table 57.1 Tuberculosis notification rates in industrialized countries.

Country	Lowest rate per 100 000	Most recent rate per 100 000	Increase (%)
Switzerland	13.8 (1986)	18.4 (1990)	33.3
Denmark	5.2 (1984)	6.8 (1990)	30.7
Italy	5.7 (1988)	7.3 (1990)	28.0
Norway	7.0 (1988)	8.5 (1991)	21.4
Ireland	15.1 (1988)	17.9 (1990)	18.5
Austria	17.8 (1989)	20.8 (1990)	16.8
Finland	15.5 (1990)	18.1 (1991)	16.7
USA	9.3 (1985)	10.4 (1991)	11.8
Netherlands	8.4 (1987)	9.2 (1990)	9.5
Sweden	6.4 (1988)	6.7 (1990)	4.6
UK	10.1 (1987)	10.5 (1991)	3.9

Source: Tuberculosis Programme, WHO/HQ, 1991.[7]

ation of public health services, socioeconomic decline and impoverishment are additional factors. However, in Denmark, the Netherlands, Norway, Sweden and Switzerland the increase is mainly in the foreign born. In England and Wales immigrants from the Indian subcontinent have a high incidence of tuberculosis.[8]

But the new situation is not confined only to numbers of new patients: it is also concerned with an increase in the number of patients harbouring resistant—often multiresistant—tubercle bacilli. On Wednesday 17 October 1990 the *New York Post* carried a startling four-inch high headline: 'Highly contagious tuberculosis close to epidemic level in the city.' An example of the problem comes from Kings County, Brooklyn. Of 246 patients (106 with an HIV risk) the overall resistance rate was 30.9%— primary 22.6%, secondary 49.2%. Multiple resistance was present in 43% and resistance to isoniazid

was reported in 90% and to rifampicin in 50%. There was no difference between HIV and non-HIV patients.[9] Further confirmation is contained in a survey from New York which found that isolates from a third of people with tuberculosis were resistant to one or more antituberculosis drugs, mainly rifampicin and isoniazid.[10] A serious drug-resistance problem is present in other parts of the world. If there is anxiety about the situation in certain parts of the developed countries, the mood is one of dismay so far as the developing countries are concerned. WHO estimates that about 1722 million people (one-third of the world population) are infected with tubercle bacilli. Furthermore in 1990 eight million new cases of tuberculosis occurred, 95% of them in the developing world and 5% in industrialized countries. Close to three million people die of this disease every year.[11] In early 1992 WHO estimated that approximately four million people had been infected with both tuberculosis and HIV since the beginning of the pandemic, 95% being in the developing countries. Whereas the largest number of cases is in Asia, the highest incidence rate is seen in sub-Saharan Africa. During a WHO meeting in 1990 Africa was described as 'lost'. No one questioned this description which was taken to mean there was no way of dealing with coinfection with HIV and the tubercle bacillus.[12]

Recent scientific and technical developments offer unprecedented opportunities for managing patients with tuberculosis. Only with a sustained effort and a serious social commitment to controlling the disease will we be able to reverse current trends and achieve a decline in tuberculosis again. A much larger contribution must be made by the developed countries.

A major contribution to the epidemiology of tuberculosis has been made by Styblo.[13]

BACTERIOLOGY AND PATHOLOGY

M. tuberculosis was first described by Robert Koch in 1892. Two main species are recognized, *M. tuberculosis* and *M. bovis*. A third species, *M. africanum* occurs in West and Central Africa. *M. tuberculosis* has an important feature in its ability to lie dormant for many years, the so-called 'persister'.[14]

Tubercle bacilli are long, curved, often beaded rods 4 μm or more in length and about 0.5 μm in diameter. Once stained with Ziehl–Neelsen fluorochromes they strongly resist decolorization with acid and alcohol. Culture is usually carried out on

Löwenstein–Jensen medium. Radiometric methods of culture are too expensive for developing countries. With the BACTEC system, a mean recovery time for *M. tuberculosis* was 8.7 days compared with 21 days for 90.7% and 42 days for 9.3% of the isolates on conventional methods.[15] The greatest potential of the BACTEC system would appear to be the early determination of susceptibility of tubercle bacilli, the early identification of non-tuberculous mycobacteria and the screening of experimental drugs.

A good culture service can increase the proportion of bacteriologically confirmed tuberculosis by 35–50% and such a service is desirable in all countries. It is, however, expensive and a degree of centralization may well be necessary in developing countries. Centralization also produces a higher standard of testing.

When tubercle bacilli are deposited in tissue there is a sequence of cellular events. First, there are inflammatory or exudative lesions consisting of vasodilatation and oedema and an influx of polymorphonuclear lymphocytes and macrophages to the area. The macrophages then undergo metamorphosis to form epithelioid cells. Langhans' multinucleated giant cells may then form. When the cells are arranged in a small sphere they are called tubercles. Thereafter caseation occurs and subsequently fibrosis takes place and some areas may undergo calcification.

RISK FACTORS

There are many risk factors, some more important than others.

Age and sex

Infants and young children of both sexes have weak defences and are prone to suffer from miliary tuberculosis and tuberculous meningitis. In developing countries the vast majority of cases occur between the ages of 15 and 59 years—the most economically productive individuals in society. In industrialized countries tuberculosis has shifted from being a disease of young women to a disease in old men.

Malnutrition

There is good evidence that malnutrition reduces resistance.

Toxic factors

Tobacco smoking, high alcohol consumption, corticosteroid and immunosuppressive drugs also reduce body defences.

Other diseases

Infection with HIV is a critical factor in the current situation. Diabetes, leukaemia, measles and whooping cough in children and chronic malaria and worm infestation are less important factors.

Poverty

Overcrowding increases significantly the risk of transmission of tubercle bacilli.[16]

TUBERCULOSIS IN CHILDREN (See also Chapter 15)

Children may be infected with tuberculosis in three different ways, the most common being infection via the lungs.

The main source of infection is through the *inhalation* of tubercle bacilli into the lungs from an infectious adult. Exceptionally the tubercle bacilli may lodge in the tonsil or adenoids and set up a primary lesion there. When young children are infected the source is usually from a family member or a neighbour. Other possible sources are schools, places of worship and of entertainment. The risk of infection is less in well-ventilated rooms but is larger in closed rooms, huts or small spaces.

Tubercle bacilli can be *ingested* in food or milk, causing a primary lesion in the intestine. *M. bovis* is commonly responsible, milk from infected animals being the source.

Cutaneous primary lesions may occur rarely, skin infections mainly occurring on exposed surfaces such as face or legs, less frequently on hands or feet (Figure 57.1).

THE PRIMARY COMPLEX

Tubercle bacilli enter the lung and multiply locally to form the *primary focus*. There is a local influx of

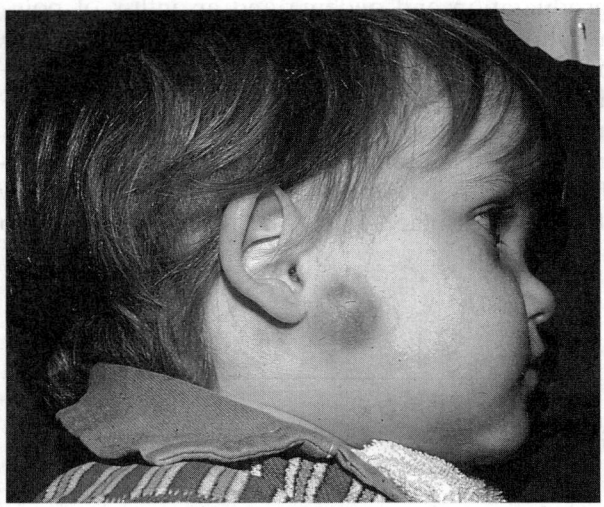

Figure 57.1   Cutaneous primary tuberculous lesion.

polymorphonuclear leucocytes and macrophages. After several weeks the macrophages predominate. These crowd together to form epithelioid cells to create the tubercle. Some macrophages fuse to form multinucleated or Langhans' giant cells. Lymphocytes surround the tubercle and caseous necrosis occurs in the centre. This may calcify subsequently. Haematogenous spread occurs, probably via the lymphatics, with seeding of bacilli to other parts of the lung and other organs. Studies with radioactive BCG suggest that within less than an hour of reaching the lung they are found in the regional lymph nodes.[17] The regional lymph nodes enlarge and there is spread to mediastinal, paratracheal and sometimes cervical nodes. These may rupture into bronchi, leading to pneumonitis-collapse, or trachea, causing suffocation. The lesions in the lung and nodes form the *primary complex*. Subsequent events are determined by a number of factors, of which age is the most important. Progression is most likely in the very young, children from 5 years old until puberty having greater resistance, though this is less true of acute miliary tuberculosis. Malnutrition is an important determining factor, as are other infections, especially measles and whooping cough. HIV infection has recently been added to factors lowering resistance. Some 3–6 weeks after primary infection the tuberculin test becomes positive.

Progression takes several forms which are illustrated in Figure 57.2. Rupture into the pleural space from a focus at the periphery of the lung with leakage of tubercle bacilli and caseous material results in *pleural effusion*. This can resolve without treatment but it is essential to treat pleural effusions with chemotherapy in order to prevent the occurrence of disseminated lesions in later life. If large

numbers of tubercle bacilli are present, an empyema may result. Enlarging nodes may perforate the pericardium to produce a *pericardial effusion*.

When resistance is poor the primary lesion may progress to form a *tuberculous pneumonia* which may cavitate. Less commonly, the primary lesion may enlarge to form a round (coin) lesion which subsequently calcifies. Concentric rings of *calcification* may be seen, or speckling: sometimes the whole lesion calcifies.

The enlarged *mediastinal nodes* are responsible for several clinical syndromes. They press upon and may erode the soft bronchi and cause *pneumonitis-collapse* of the relevant area of the lung. This is usually symptomless, though transient wheeze may be present. The segmental or lobar opacity present on chest radiography is due partly to collapse and partly to pneumonia, which is itself due to a hypersensitivity reaction to inhaled caseous material. In rare cases the enlarged nodes cause *obstructive emphysema* and, fortunately still rarer, nodes may erupt into the trachea causing suffocation. The majority of the lesions clear without permanent damage but in a few cases, especially when lower lobes are involved, *bronchiectasis* may result.

Occasionally enlarged cervical lymph nodes are due to a primary lesion in the tonsil or mouth.

The haematogenous phase which follows primary infection results, particularly in young malnourished children, in acute miliary tuberculosis, and in some children tuberculous meningitis. These are inevitably fatal diseases unless treated. Extrapulmonary disease may occur in later years in bones, lymph nodes, kidneys and other organs. These conditions are described in detail on pp. 983–992.

NATURAL HISTORY OF TUBERCULOUS INFECTION: THE TIMETABLE OF TUBERCULOSIS

With tuberculosis, as with any other disease, there are no absolute rules of behaviour but the pattern of disease development defined 45 years ago by Wallgren[18] describes in general terms the natural history of the disease before specific interventions were applied. Limited evidence from Africa and Asia suggests, surprisingly, that the latent period between primary infection and the development of pulmonary tuberculosis in adult life is much longer than is found in Europe.

Important confirmation of Wallgren's timetable is to be found in the account of the British Medical Research Council's tuberculosis vaccine trials.[19] Of the 12 867 participants left unvaccinated, 1335 were infected and 108 (8.1%) of those infected developed

A **Focus and complications**

Caseous nodes

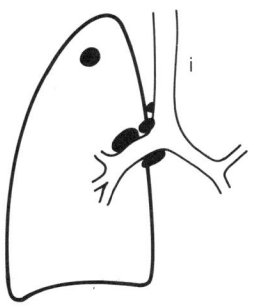
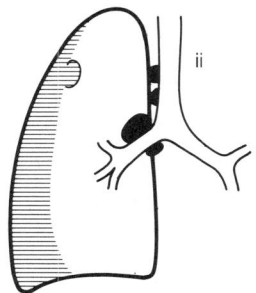
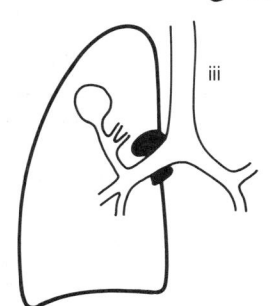
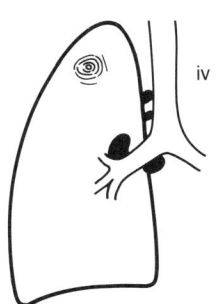

Primary complex.
Focus and regional glands

Rupture of focus into pleural
space with effusion; serous
occasionally purulent

Rupture of focus into
bronchus: cavitation

Enlarged focus sometimes
laminated 'round' or 'coin'
shadow

B **Mediastinal (regional) nodes and complications**

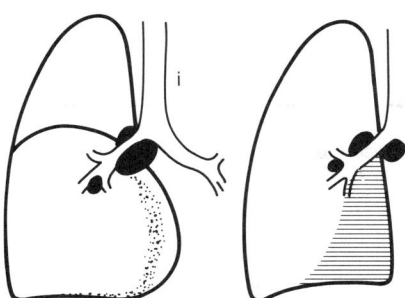
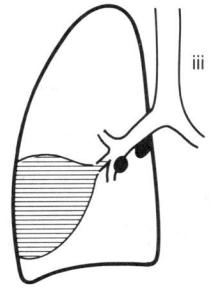
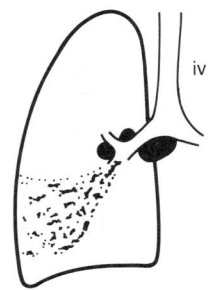
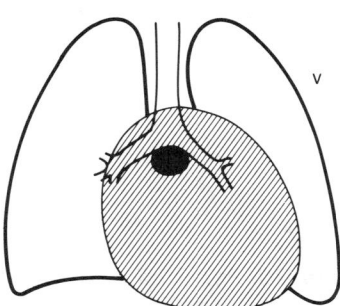

Incomplete
bronchial obstruction
(ball valve)
Inflation of middle
and lower lobes

Collapsed
lower lobe after
complete bronchial
obstruction without
consolidation

Collapse after
partial
consolidation
segmental
lesion

Erosion into
bronchus
inhalation and
areas of tuberculous
bronchopneumonia

Pericardial effusion post-rupture
of node through pericardium

C **Sequelae of bronchial complications**

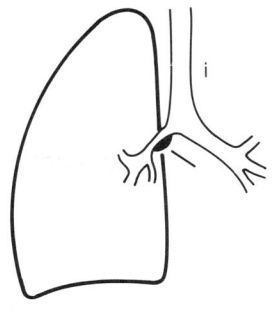
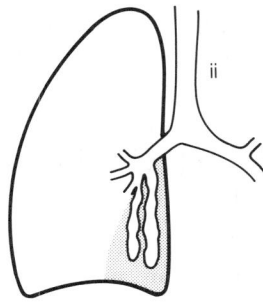
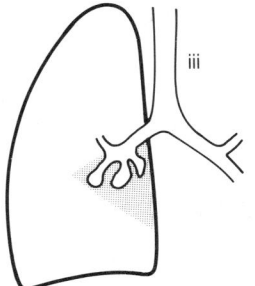
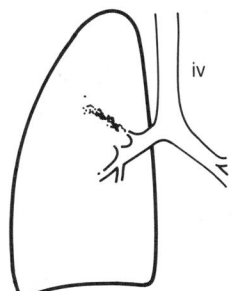

Structure of
bronchus

Cylindrical
bronchiectasis in
area of old collapse

Wedge shadow with
fibrosis and
bronchiectasis
following contracture
of segmental lesion

Linear scar of fibrosis
following segmental
lesion

Figure 57.2 The complications and sequelae of pulmonary primary lesions. (Reproduced with permission from Miller F.J.W. *Tuberculosis in Children*. Edinburgh: Churchill Livingstone, 1982.)

PATIENT'S DETAILS	HOSPITAL OR PHC LOCATION
Name	
Age yrs	Date
(d.o.b. / /)	Scored by:
Sex MF	
Weight kg	Nurse/Health Ass/Doctor
BCG scars 0/1/2/3	

SCORE CHART   (Circle box and write in score)

Children suspected of having tuberculosis

FEATURE	0	1	3	
LENGTH OF ILLNESS	LESS THAN 2 WEEKS	2–4 WEEKS	MORE THAN 4 WEEKS	
NUTRITION (WEIGHT)	ABOVE 80% FOR AGE	BETWEEN 60% AND 80%	LESS THAN 60%	
FAMILY TUBERCULOSIS PAST OR PRESENT	NONE	REPORTED BY FAMILY	PROVED SPUTUM POSITIVE	

SCORE FOR OTHER FEATURES IF PRESENT

Positive tuberculin test	3
Large painless lymph nodes; firm, soft, sinus in neck, axilla, groin	3
Unexplained fever, night sweats, no response to malaria treatment	2
Malnutrition, not improving after 4 weeks	3
Angle deformity of spine	4
Joint swelling, bone swelling or sinuses	3
Unexplained abdominal mass or ascites	3
CNS: change in temperament fits or coma (send to hospital if possible)	3

TOTAL SCORE

When score is 7 or more treat for tuberculosis – see notes.

Figure 57.3 Paediatric Tuberculosis Score Chart A. (Courtesy of Keith Edwards, University of Papua New Guinea. Reproduced with permission from Crofton et al.[20])

clinical tuberculosis in the 10 years following primary infection. Fifty-four per cent had developed disease within 1 year and 80% within 2 years of infection. Analysis of the data regarding time of onset of extrapulmonary disease related to primary infection confirmed Wallgren's timetable.

There are two other clinical features which are sometimes associated with primary infection: phlyctenular conjunctivitis and erythema nodosum.

PHLYCTENULAR CONJUNCTIVITIS

This occurs most commonly in the first year after primary infection. It begins with pain, conjunctival irritation, lacrimation and photophobia, usually unilaterally. One or more grey or yellow spots are found around the limbus of the cornea. A leash of small blood vessels extends to the edge of the conjunctival sac. The condition slowly recedes over the period of several days but often recurs. In severe attacks the cornea may become ulcerated. The pain is severe and there is marked intolerance to light. If secondary infection occurs, corneal scarring results. The condition is most likely to occur in young people between the ages of 5 and 15 years and is common in Africa, India and South-East Asia. It is also sometimes associated with haemolytic streptococcal infection.

ERYTHEMA NODOSUM (See also Chapters 2, 5 and 11)

This usually occurs in association with the primary infection and is rare below the age of 7 years. It appears to be much rarer in individuals with dark skin. It is a manifestation of hypersensitivity to tuberculoprotein. Other causes include streptococcal infections, certain drugs, sarcoidosis, leprosy, histoplasmosis and coccidiomycosis. It is more common in females. It may be accompanied by high fever and arthralgia affecting the larger joints, which

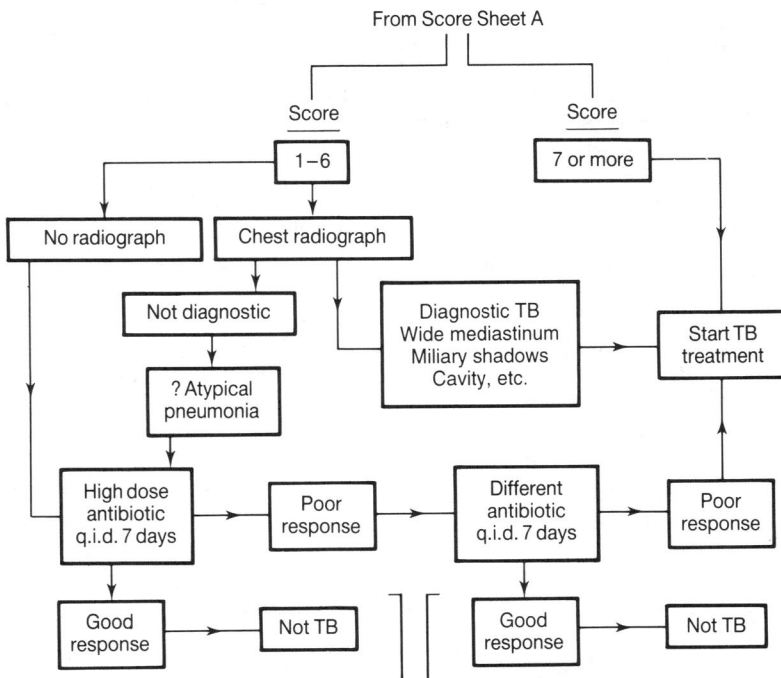

Figure 57.4 Paediatric Flow Chart B. (Courtesy of Keith Edwards, University of Papua New Guinea. Reproduced with permission from Crofton et al.[20]) For use when presentation suggests pneumonia and there are no other signs of tuberculosis (TB).

may be hot, swollen and tender. The erythrocyte sedimentation rate is high. Tender, dusky red, slightly nodular lesions 5–20 mm in diameter appear on the front of the legs below the knee. They feel deep to the skin and may become confluent. Recurrent crops may occur over a period of weeks. Lesions may also occur around the elbows and, rarely, on the breasts. The tuberculin test is usually strongly positive and if tuberculosis is suspected it may be wise to begin with only 1 TU of tuberculin. The condition responds well to treatment by chemotherapy: if arthralgia is severe, treatment with corticosteroids for a few days is very effective.

CLINICAL PRESENTATIONS OF TUBERCULOSIS IN CHILDREN

Many children have no recognizable symptoms or signs in association with the primary infection. Particularly in developing countries and in immigrants from Africa, Asia or certain areas of the Caribbean, it is very important to observe a high index of suspicion regarding the possibility of tuberculosis. Clinical features which should alert the physician are:

- Failure to gain weight or loss of weight.
- Loss of energy.
- Persistent cough and/or wheeze.
- Unexplained fever for more than a week.
- Swelling of the abdomen, especially if masses or fluid are present *or* chronic diarrhoea not responding to treatment for worms or giardiasis.
- A limp on walking; a stiff spine; a gibbus; swelling of bone or joint not due to trauma; a discharging sinus near a joint.
- A painless firm lymph node which may have smaller nodes adjacent to it; associated discharging sinus.
- One or more soft swellings under the skin which may ulcerate, usually with a clean base.
- Headache and irritability, occasional vomiting, desire to be left alone, gradually becoming less rousable.

Whereas in technically advanced countries the diagnosis can usually be made in the vast majority of patients, in many areas of the world diagnostic facilities are few and often unavailable. In such situations it is important to make the best possible assessment of the probability that the child is suffering from tuberculosis. This can usually be achieved by the use of a score chart. Several have been developed but one devised by Dr Keith Edwards in Papua New Guinea is particularly useful (Figure 57.3). If the score is 7 or more, treatment should be given. When the clinical presentation is pneumonia, the flow chart (Figure 57.4) is a guide to management.

EXTRAPULMONARY TUBERCULOSIS

These manifestations are described on pp. 981–992.

CONGENITAL TUBERCULOSIS

This is a very rare condition. Tuberculous disease in the mother is invariable though it may not be overt. The modes of infection are:

- Haematogenous infection via the umbilical vein.
- Aspiration or inhalation of infected amniotic fluid resulting in primary infection in the liver or lungs.

Recently phage typing has been used to establish the common identity of mycobacteria isolated from both mother and infant.[21]

Within 2 weeks the infant ceases to thrive. Respiratory distress and cyanosis due to bronchopneumonia or miliary disease occurs and fever, hepatosplenomegaly and lymphadenopathy are common. Obstructive jaundice due to nodes in the porta hepatis may occur. The tuberculin test is negative. Fine moist sounds are heard bilaterally and the radiograph of the chest shows signs of acute pneumonia or miliary shadows. Tubercle bacilli are very numerous. Diagnosis should be sought by examination of stomach washings or by biopsy of liver, lymph node or lung. Only half the infants affected survive. Immediate treatment by chemotherapy is imperative and corticosteroid treatment is indicated in seriously ill children.

HIV INFECTION AND AIDS AND TUBERCULOSIS IN CHILDREN

The most common route of infection is from mother to child during pregnancy or at birth. The risk of an infected mother passing on HIV to her child is between 24 and 40%, and may be higher if the mother has clinical AIDS. Other possible sources of infection are blood transfusions and contaminated syringes or needles. Streptomycin should therefore be avoided if possible. Breast feeding does not seem to be an important source of infection.

Tuberculous infection is more likely to spread in children with HIV infection. Tuberculous meningitis, miliary tuberculosis and diffuse lymphadenopathy are all more likely to occur. Counselling is an important aspect of management.

TREATMENT OF TUBERCULOSIS IN CHILDREN

Chemotherapy in children is the same as in adults, with appropriate adjustment in dosage, and is discussed in detail on pp. 997–1006.

Children who are known to have had a recent primary infection (by observation of tuberculin conversion) and children under the age of 5 years who have a strongly positive tuberculin reaction (grade III Heaf) because of the high risk of miliary and meningeal disease, should be given isoniazid 5 mg/kg once daily for a minimum of 6 months, so-called chemoprophylaxis.

Children with all forms of tuberculous disease should be given full treatment. Treatment may also be necessary for concurrent infections and anaemia. Many of the children in developing countries are malnourished and close attention to proper feeding and nutrition is required.[20]

POSTPRIMARY OR 'ADULT-TYPE' PULMONARY TUBERCULOSIS

In the developed countries most postprimary pulmonary tuberculosis occurs in middle-aged or elderly persons, the trend towards increasing age being significant in the last 20 years. In Edinburgh for example in 1985, 43% of patients with respiratory tuberculosis were aged 65 years or over, compared with 24% in 1975 and 16% in 1965. In developing countries it is most common in the 25–55 years age group.

The main presenting features of respiratory tuberculosis are as follows:

- None
- Cough
- Unresolved pneumonia
- Fever and sweating
- Sputum (mucoid or purulent)
- Haemoptysis
- Chest wall pain
- Breathlessness
- Localized wheeze
- Frequent 'colds'
- Loss of weight
- Lassitude
- Anorexia
- Dyspepsia
- Apical crackles
- Amenorrhoea.

Patients, even though they have quite extensive disease, may admit to no symptoms, and mild debility may be so gradual in onset that the patient may not notice it. These symptoms are not specific for tuberculosis. *Examination of the sputum for tubercle bacilli is therefore mandatory* and radiological examination should be carried out if facilities are available.

Physical signs are often absent, but careful examination may lead to a suspicion of tuberculosis. The most common finding is the presence of fine apical crackles. In advanced cases there may be dullness on percussion or bronchial breathing or localized wheeze. There may be signs of a pleural effusion. Clubbing of the fingers may be present, severe clubbing in advanced disease having been reported from Africa.[22] Pulmonary tuberculosis may be discovered in the course of investigation of other conditions, e.g. ischiorectal abscess, lymphadenopathy, cystitis.

INVESTIGATIONS

The most important and most reliable way of making the diagnosis is to find tubercle bacilli on *examination of a direct smear of sputum*. Three specimens should be examined if possible:

- The first spot specimen when the patient presents (lest he or she absconds thereafter).
- An early morning specimen consisting of all the sputum collected in the first 2 hours.
- A second spot specimen when the patient returns with the early morning specimen.

The physiotherapist may be able to help in obtaining a specimen and a specimen may sometimes be obtained following the inhalation from a nebulizer containing 3% (hypertonic) saline. Remember that a positive smear may be reported as a result of a laboratory or clerical error. An excellent account[23] of the detailed technique of sputum examination should be consulted.

Laryngeal swabs should be taken in pairs when no sputum is available. The operator should be gowned and masked. An alternative to laryngeal swabs is *gastric aspiration*: this method may be useful in children who rarely produce sputum.

Fibreoptic bronchoscopy specimen. Where the conventional methods of obtaining bacterial confirmation of suspected tuberculosis have failed, flexible fibreoptic bronchoscopy[24] can be used to provide direct smear- or culture-positive specimens from bronchial washings, bronchial brushings or transbronchial biopsies.[25,26]

Mediastinoscopy can prove valuable, especially in Asians and Africans. Tubercle bacilli can sometimes be obtained from *pleural fluid* or *pleural biopsy*.

Sometimes *thoracotomy* is required especially if there is a single nodular (coin) lesion present.

Culture of tubercle bacilli. Facilities for culture are non-existent in many parts of the world but it may be possible to send specimens to central laboratories. Drug resistance testing is used less for adjusting treatment in the individual than for establishing the pattern of drug resistance in the community. Culture on Löwenstein–Jensen medium takes 3–6 weeks to give a result but a new method gives quicker results. Rapid diagnosis is now possible within 2–6 days by using a radiometric culture (BACTEC) system.[15]

Haematological and biochemical examination. The white blood cell count is not usually elevated unless secondary infection is present. Normochromic normocytic anaemia may be present. Mild abnormalities of liver function are not uncommon in moderate or advanced disease.

Tuberculin test. This is usually positive but it may be negative in as high as 8% of individuals.[27] The tuberculin test is less valuable as a diagnostic tool in many poorer countries, due to malnutrition. Furthermore the existence of mycobacteria other than *M. tuberculosis* may cause confusion. A positive tuberculin test is more valuable in diagnosis in a young child.

Radiological examination. Exceptionally pulmonary tuberculosis may be present with a normal radiograph. This occurs when a positive sputum is associated with localized postprimary endobronchial tuberculosis.[28] Opacities strongly suggestive of adult-type tuberculosis are as follows, though all may be mimicked by other diseases, especially carcinoma.[29] The abnormalities in primary tuberculosis are described on pp. 973–974.

- Upper zone patchy shadows, unilateral or bilateral, with or without:
- Cavitation, especially if multiple (Figure 57.5).
- Calcification. Remember that pneumonia and lung tumours may occur at the site of a previous healed tuberculous lesion.
- Diffuse small nodular opacities (miliary tuberculosis).

Other types of opacity which may be due to tuberculosis are:

- Oval or round shadows (coin lesions). These sometimes show small areas of calcification: this does not exclude bronchial carcinoma.
- Hilar or paratracheal lymph nodes: rare in Europeans (except when AIDS coexists) but may be present in Asians and Africans.

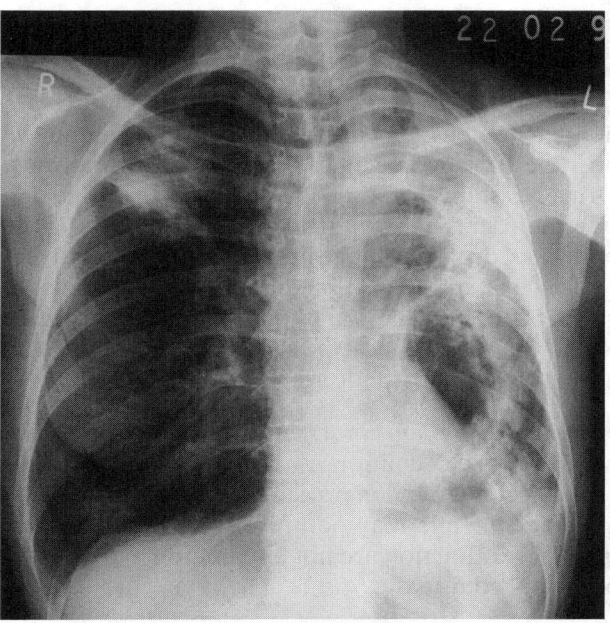

Figure 57.5   Extensive pulmonary tuberculosis with cavitation.

- Mycetoma or 'fungus ball'—the mass falls away from the cavity wall to leave a halo shadow.

Tomography is sometimes of value in determining the presence of cavities, enlarged mediastinal lymph nodes or calcification in a coin lesion.

The radiological features in patients with AIDS may be different (see pp. 992–994).

COMPLICATIONS

The following are the main complications of pulmonary tuberculosis:

- Pleural effusion and empyema.
- Pneumothorax due to a ruptured focus.
- Chronic obstructive airways disease and cor pulmonale secondary to extensive fibrotic disease. Early treatment prevents this complication.
- Tuberculous laryngitis and tuberculous enteritis due to inhalation and ingestion of sputum containing large numbers of tubercle bacilli.
- Amyloidosis, which is now extremely rare.

- Aspergilloma. Healed thin-walled cavities may become infected with *Aspergillus fumigatus*. A ball of fungus is seen within the cavity. Recurrent haemoptysis occurs, sometimes fatal. If pulmonary function permits, surgical resection may occasionally be successful.
- Spread to other organs. Always examine the testes, urine and lymph nodes.

DIFFERENTIAL DIAGNOSIS

Tuberculosis enters into the differential diagnosis of many pulmonary diseases. The main conditions are pneumonia, carcinoma of bronchus, lung abscess and pulmonary infarct.

In pneumonia, the symptoms are usually of recent onset and fever is common. If sputum smears are negative for tubercle bacilli, a non-tuberculous antibiotic should be prescribed and a radiograph taken after 2–3 weeks. If no significant improvement has taken place, tuberculosis (or tumour) is the likely diagnosis.

Carcinoma of the bronchus may present with a consolidated area distal to a proximal tumour, and it may be cavitated. If sputum smears are negative, examination of sputum for malignant cells and bronchoscopy, if available, should be carried out. An isolated, solid, rounded opacity often presents a problem in diagnosis and if there is any doubt about the diagnosis thoracotomy is mandatory. Tumours may cavitate and thus present diagnostic difficulty. Tomography may help by demonstrating an irregular or polypoid wall. Patients with lung abscess are usually feverish and ill and have a large quantity of sputum. Organisms such as *Staphylococcus aureus* or *Klebsiella pneumoniae* may be isolated from sputum and blood. If smears are negative for tubercle bacilli, lung abscess is likely to be the cause.

MANAGEMENT

The management of pulmonary tuberculosis including chemotherapy is described on pp. 997–1006.

TUBERCULOUS PLEURAL EFFUSION AND EMPYEMA

Tuberculous pleural effusion occurs as a result of spread from a peripheral tuberculous focus or more rarely from an intercostal node into the pleural space. It may occur: (1) contemporaneously with the primary lesion, in which case the effusion is usually quite small and relatively transient; (2) as a postprimary phenomenon 1–2 years after primary infection; (3) in the older age group when it may develop into an empyema. If a large focus ruptures, a bronchopleural fistula forms and a pyopneumothorax develops.

CLINICAL FEATURES

The main clinical features are: chest pain, which is accentuated by breathing becoming, in the later stages, a dull ache over the lower chest; fever, which is often mild and transient; breathlessness on exertion; slight irritating cough. There is dullness on percussion over the lower chest and diminished air entry. If there is a large effusion, the mediastinum may be shifted to the side opposite to the effusion.

Radiologically, a small effusion (about 100 ml) shows as a blunting of the costophrenic angle. Large effusions are denser at the base, tailing up into the axilla. Subpleural effusions mimic a high diaphragm: on the left side the stomach bubble will resolve the problem, on the right a lateral decubitus radiograph may be necessary. An interlobar effusion may simulate a tumour. In hydropneumothorax a characteristic fluid level will be seen.

Occasionally an *empyema* ruptures into the chest wall to form a cold abscess. Such an abscess may also result from rupture of an intercostal node. The tuberculin test is usually positive in young people.

INVESTIGATION AND DIAGNOSIS

The diagnosis is usually made by aspiration of fluid from the pleural space. Obtaining a large amount of fluid for bacteriological examination enhances the diagnostic rate. Bedside inoculation of pleural fluid is claimed to increase culture yield substantially.[30] If facilities exist, pleural biopsy by means of an Abrams punch[31] should be carried out, the material being sent for histological examination. The taking of four or five bites enhances the chances of a positive finding.[32] If the fluid is removed at a rapid rate the patient may become breathless; rarely pulmonary oedema may ensue. Alternatively the dyspnoea may be due to a pneumothorax.

DIFFERENTIAL DIAGNOSIS

The main conditions to be considered are:

- Tumour (malignant cells in sputum or pleural effusion; diagnostic bronchoscopy).
- Pneumonia complicated by effusion (effect of antibiotics).
- Cardiac failure (usually bilateral: diuretics).
- Amoebic abscess if right sided.
- Pulmonary embolism and infarction.

MANAGEMENT

Most tuberculous pleural effusions resolve satisfactorily. However, pleural effusion is a marker of dissemination of tubercle bacilli: consequently chemotherapy must always be administered. Corticosteroid treatment is valuable by reducing the number of aspirations required; aspiration is usually necessary only once. Rarely a fibrothorax occurs with shrinkage of the chest wall and traction of the mediastinum to the affected side.

Needle aspiration may be effective in empyema but surgical drainage is often required and may need to be followed by decortication.

DISSEMINATED TUBERCULOSIS

There are four varieties of disseminated tuberculosis, each with its own distinctive features:

- Acute (classical) miliary tuberculosis.
- Cryptic miliary tuberculosis.
- Non-reactive tuberculosis.
- Chronic disseminated tuberculosis.

The main features of acute and cryptic miliary tuberculosis are shown in Table 57.2.

ACUTE MILIARY TUBERCULOSIS

This is an acute, progressively fatal illness unless treated with chemotherapy. In past years it affected young children[34]—and still does in many developing countries—but the epidemiology has changed dramatically elsewhere, more than one-third of patients being over 65 years of age.[35]

In addition to the symptoms shown in Table 57.2,

Table 57.2 Main features of acute and cryptic miliary tuberculosis.

Features	Acute miliary	Cryptic miliary
Constitutional symptoms (fever, malaise, loss of weight)	Marked and rapidly progressive	Slight initially and slowly progressive
Chest radiograph (miliary shadows)	Present except in first 2–3 weeks	Absent until very late
Choroidal tubercles (see Figure 57.7)	Present in 15%	Absent
Hepatosplenomegaly	Present in 20–30%	Absent
Tuberculin test	Positive becoming negative (see text)	Often negative
Meningitis	Present in 10%	Rarely: terminal stages
Diagnostic biopsy	Seldom required	Bone marrow,[33] liver, bronchial
Haematological disorder	Anaemia, rarely	Anaemia common; bizarre haematology sometimes presenting feature
Hypokalaemia, hyponatraemia	Present	Common
Adult respiratory distress syndrome	Rare	Absent
Sources of isolation of tubercle bacilli	Laryngeal swabs, gastric lavage, bronchial lavage, urine. Blood culture in AIDS	Bone marrow, liver
Identifiable contact	40%	None
Age	Any age	Usually elderly

headache, haemoptysis and abdominal pain are occasional complaints.

The radiograph of the chest shows diffuse miliary nodular shadows which appear more numerous in the central and basal areas. These may be absent in the first 2–3 weeks of illness. Enlarged mediastinal nodes may be present if the miliary disease occurs soon after primary infection (Figure 57.6) and larger pulmonary shadows typical of adult-type tuberculosis may be present in other cases. Rarely small bilateral pleural effusions may be present.

Choroidal tubercles[36] should always be looked for when examining a patient, particularly a child, suspected of having miliary tuberculosis or anyone with an unexplained fever. The presence of choroidal tubercles (Figure 57.7) is a very valuable diagnostic sign. The tubercles may be single or multiple. They are usually greyish-white or yellowish in colour and 0.5–3 mm in diameter and are generally located in the posterior pole. The centre of the tubercle becomes white and pigmentation occurs as the lesions regress. Multiple and frequent examination by direct ophthalmoscopy is essential. The pupils should be dilated and up to 30 minutes should be

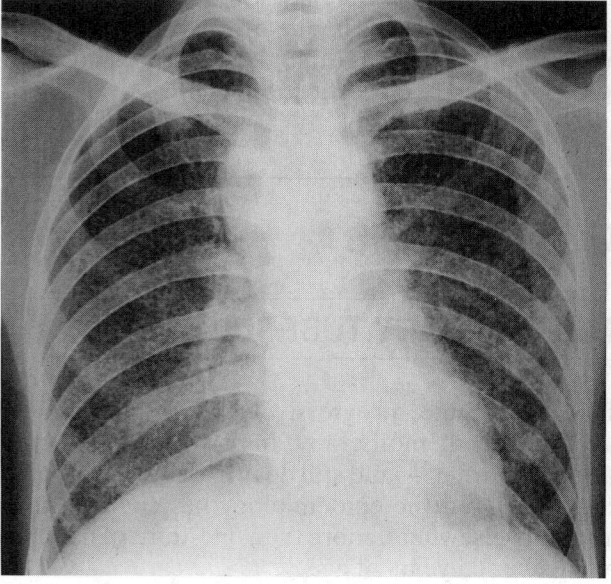

Figure 57.6 Miliary tuberculosis. Note persistent paratracheal node.

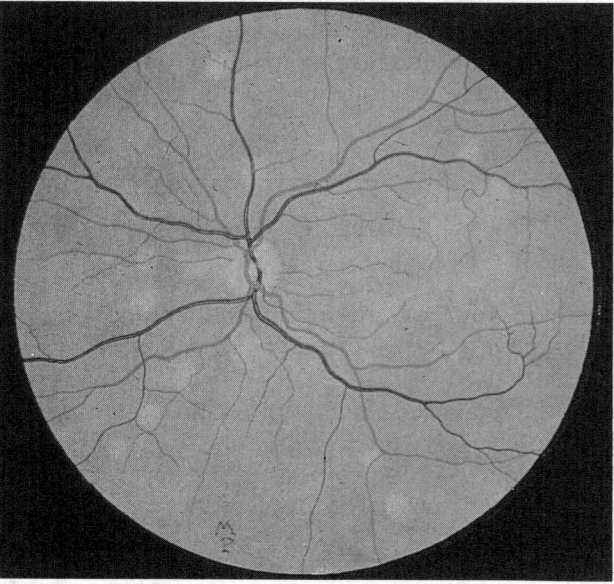

Figure 57.7 Choroidal tubercles.

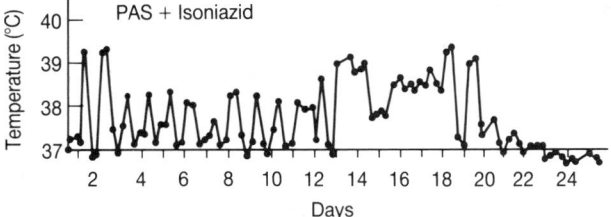

Figure 57.8 Cryptic miliary tuberculosis diagnosed because the patient improved with specific antituberculosis treatment. Man, aged 70 years, with continued fever, anaemia, a negative tuberculin test and no direct evidence of miliary tuberculosis: no abnormal clinical signs and an apparently normal chest radiograph. Usual investigations for fever of unknown origin negative. Using treatment with PAS and isoniazid (which would not affect other infections) his temperature fell and his blood count returned to normal.

spent in examination of the choroid. Children may need to be sedated. The tuberculin test may be positive early in the illness but becomes negative as the disease advances, only to become positive again if treatment is successful.

It is valuable to culture material for tubercle bacilli from several sites (Table 57.2) in order to identify the type of mycobacteria and the susceptibility to individual drugs. Smears are rarely positive. Miliary lesions of the skin are seen rarely and take the form of papules, macules or purpuric lesions.

Differential diagnosis includes pneumonia due to viruses or *Mycoplasma pneumoniae* in acute miliary disease, and sarcoidosis, histoplasmosis and coccidiomycosis in cryptic miliary disease. Where there is diagnostic difficulty, a 'test of cure' with *para*-aminosalicylic acid (PAS) or ethambutol plus isoniazid should be applied (Figure 57.8).

Treatment. Acute miliary tuberculosis responds well to chemotherapy. Corticosteroids should be added in seriously ill patients. A satisfactory response is observed in 2–3 weeks.

CRYPTOGENIC MILIARY TUBERCULOSIS

Cryptogenic disseminated tuberculosis is characterized by an insidious onset and progression which unobtrusively undermines general health but may not arouse the patient's concern until an advanced stage has been reached. The clinical features are shown in Table 57.2. Pyrexia is not invariable but when present is commonly intermittent and unspectacular; anaemia is common; the tuberculin test is frequently negative and diagnosis frequently depends upon biopsy techniques. The diagnosis is sometimes arrived at following investigation of haematological disorders—pancytopenia, leukaemoid reactions, myelofibrosis, polycythaemia.

NON-REACTIVE TUBERCULOSIS

This is rare but many of the reported cases have come from Africa or Asia. It is an acute malignant form of tuberculous septicaemia. Histologically the lesions are necrotic, with very large numbers of tubercle bacilli present. The patient is extremely ill. The chest radiograph sometimes shows no miliary lesions. The tuberculin test is negative. Unusual blood disorders may be present. The diagnosis is often missed, and the patient dies rapidly.

CHRONIC DISSEMINATED TUBERCULOSIS

This is a distinct form of tuberculosis in which involvement of individual organs, e.g. wrist followed by lymph nodes, testis and kidney, occurs at intervals over a period of months or years. With the advent of chemotherapy this form has become increasingly rare.

TUBERCULOUS MENINGITIS (See also Chapter 8)

With the decline in the incidence of tuberculosis, tuberculous meningitis has become relatively rare in developed countries. Its very rarity presents a problem as the diagnosis may be forgotten. Those most at risk are individuals from high prevalence areas; it is more common in infants and children. Pulmonary (especially miliary) tuberculosis and other manifestations of extrapulmonary disease may coexist. Infections with atypical mycobacteria, especially *M. avium-intracellulare*, in patients with AIDS has become an increasingly serious problem.

Table 57.3 Investigations in tuberculous meningitis.

- Chest radiograph
- Tuberculin test
- Examination of the CSF
  —Appearance—under pressure; clear or slightly opalescent: 'spider-web' clot
  —Cell count—rising to 400/mm^3, mainly lymphocytes (in the first 48 hours polymorphs may predominate)
  —Protein concentration, rising to 80–400 mg/100 ml
  —Glucose falling, sometimes to zero
  —Careful smear examination (Ziehl–Neelsen) for tubercle bacilli and culture (50–80% positive)

  Remember that:

  —The first CSF examination may reveal no abnormality and the examination should be repeated
  —There are often fluctuations in the level of cells and protein from day to day
  —These levels may be reduced if the patients are taking corticosteroid drugs
- Radiographic examination of the skull, scanning or an encephalogram may reveal calcification in a tuberculoma or a degree of ventricular enlargement
- Retinoscopy—choroidal tubercles
- Computerized tomography
- Examination of lymph nodes, liver and spleen

CLINICAL FEATURES

Tuberculous meningitis usually has an insidious onset. The initial symptoms are general malaise, low-grade fever, intermittent headache and vomiting. Subsequently fever becomes more marked, headache becomes persistent and the patient becomes drowsy. There is neck stiffness and oculomotor palsies may occur. At a later stage involuntary movements, hemiplegia, increased drowsiness and evidence of hydrocephalus ensue, proceeding to decerebration and death. Untreated, death usually occurs in 3–6 weeks. The important investigations are shown in Table 57.3. The usual clinical manifestations of tuberculous meningitis may be muted, absent or obscured in AIDS, though it has been reported that infection with HIV does not influence the clinical presentation or outcome.[37]

The tuberculin test is often negative, especially in advanced disease. The retina should be very carefully examined for choroidal tubercles, and the presence of an enlarged liver and spleen should be sought. The CSF glucose may be normal, especially in the early stages. A rare manifestation is tuberculous spinal arachnoiditis, secondary to spinal caries, characterized by radiculomyelopathy.

DIFFERENTIAL DIAGNOSIS

Diagnosis is often difficult but early diagnosis is essential if a good prognosis is to be expected. Miliary shadows in the radiograph or the presence of typical lymph nodes or enlarged liver and spleen enhance the likelihood of tuberculosis being the correct diagnosis. Pyogenic (untreated or partially treated) or fungal meningitis or involvement of the meninges by carcinoma or reticulosis will also have to be considered.

PROGNOSIS

Tuberculous meningitis is a very serious disease, four out of ten patients with advanced (grade III) disease failing to survive. Even in well-equipped centres there is a mortality of 5%. There is an important morbidity from cranial nerve involvement, monoplegia or hemiplegia, behaviour disturbances and impairment of mental faculties.

TREATMENT

Chemotherapy should be commenced with isoniazid 10 mg/kg (5 mg/kg in Indian patients), rifampicin 10 mg/kg, pyrazinamide 35 mg/kg and ethambutol 25 mg/kg *or* streptomycin 10 mg/kg. Prothionamide 15 mg/kg may be valuable in areas where there is a high incidence of isoniazid-resistant strains as it penetrates into the CSF. Intrathecal treatment has virtually been abandoned. If progress is satisfactory ethambutol (or streptomycin) and pyrazinamide can be stopped after 2–3 months, rifampicin and isoniazid being continued for 9 months at least. If rifampicin is not available substitute thiacetazone 4 mg/kg and continue treatment for 12 or preferably 18 months. Corticosteroids should be given to all patients other than those in stage 1 of the disease. Preoccupation with chemotherapy and corticosteroid therapy should not blind the physician to the possible need for neurosurgical intervention.[38]

TUBERCULOMA OF THE BRAIN

A tuberculoma usually presents with symptoms compatible with a space-occupying lesion. Laboratory findings are often normal but elevation of CSF protein is common. Radiological studies including computerized studies (CT) are essential. Surgical removal is commonly carried out, covered by anti-tuberculosis drugs.

TUBERCULOSIS OF SUPERFICIAL LYMPH NODES

Mycobacterial infection and inflammation of the cervical, axillary, intercostal and inguinal lymph nodes is most commonly due to *M. tuberculosis*. In developed countries in children the infecting organisms are usually atypical mycobacteria (opportunist mycobacteria) most frequently *M. avium-intracellulare*.[39] In Africans and Asians, the disease is most common in younger age groups, whereas in countries such as Britain it is more common in the elderly. The cervical nodes are most frequently affected—more than 90%. A primary lesion is rarely identified and the condition may be blood borne. If supraclavicular nodes are involved they usually arise as a result of spread from mediastinal nodes.

CLINICAL FEATURES

The enlargement of the nodes is usually slow and painless. There is often a larger node surrounded by a number of smaller ones. The nodes may become matted together and the skin becomes fixed over them. A cold abscess may then form and discharge with the production of a sinus. Diffuse lymph node involvement may be encountered in children with a reduced immunity due to AIDS and in acute miliary tuberculosis in children. Fever may be present if there is extensive involvement of mediastinal nodes as well. Constitutional symptoms occur in less than 20% of patients. Search should be made for evidence of tuberculosis elsewhere: a chest radiograph is an essential part of diagnosis. The tuberculin test is usually positive, except in infection by opportunistic mycobacteria. Differential tuberculin testing with different antigens may be helpful in some cases.

TREATMENT

Chemotherapy is very effective. Until recently 9 months of rifampicin and isoniazid supplemented by ethambutol for the first 2 months was the current treatment of choice,[40] but 6 months has now been shown to be equally effective.[41] Uneventful resolution of the condition can be expected in 70% of patients. Nodes may appear and enlarge during treatment. Fluctuation, discharge, sinus formation and scar breakdown occur in the minority. At the end of treatment 10% may be left with residual nodes. After chemotherapy fresh nodes may appear, usually transiently. Such events do not imply relapse and are thought to be due to variation in tuberculin sensitivity or secondary bacterial infection from the upper respiratory tract.[42] Surgical treatment should be reserved for relief of discomfort and to avoid sinus formation: a small incision is to be preferred to aspiration, as healing is more satisfactory. Resection of a node may be required if the diagnosis is in doubt and is usually curative in solitary nodes caused by atypical mycobacteria.[43]

DIFFERENTIAL DIAGNOSIS

This is extensive, and includes other infections, neoplasms, sarcoidosis, lymphoma and branchial cysts. Because lymph nodes contain few bacilli bacteriological diagnosis is obtained in less than 60% of patients. Biopsy may eventually be required to establish the diagnosis. It is essential that a portion of the node be sent for bacteriological examination—before fixation! If diagnostic facilities are poor, treatment should be commenced and progress observed.

ABDOMINAL TUBERCULOSIS (See also Chapter 3)

Abdominal tuberculosis is common in developing countries, especially in females, but it is rare in industrialized countries, except in immigrants. It may arise from a primary infection in the gastro-intestinal tract with spread to mesenteric nodes, from haematogenous dissemination from other sites or from swelling sputum containing large numbers of tubercle bacilli, causing tuberculous enteritis. Oesophageal and gastric tuberculosis are extremely rare, as is colitis in the absence of ileocaecal involvement. It may present as a stricture making differentiation from a carcinoma difficult. Treatment with chemotherapy may help to resolve the problem if surgical facilities are not available. Ischiorectal abscess is also rare but is often missed unless biopsy specimens are taken for histological examination. The most common presentation is an abdominal mass (or masses) with ascites. The fallopian tubes may become involved leading to infertility.

CLINICAL FEATURES

Loss of weight and appetite are very common. There may be fever, night sweats, diarrhoea and amenorrhoea. Pain and swelling of the abdomen occur and abdominal masses may be felt, especially in hyperplastic ileocaecal tuberculosis. Ascites is common and attacks of intestinal obstruction may occur. The Mantoux test is commonly positive. The diagnosis has often to be made on clinical grounds and the response to chemotherapy. Where facilities permit, radiographic examination (straight radiograph and barium meal and follow-through examination), culture of aspirated fluid and peritoneal biopsy may prove positive in up to 75% of cases.[44] Laparotomy is probably the most reliable method of diagnosis, a success rate of 94% having been recorded.[45]

The outcome is usually very satisfactory though infertility may be a complication. Corticosteroids should be given where there is a large effusion or intestinal obstruction present.

BONE AND JOINT TUBERCULOSIS (See also Chapter 14)

Skeletal tuberculosis is now comparatively rare in developed countries and occurs mainly in immigrants. In developing countries it is more frequently to be found in children, whereas elsewhere it is more common in adults. The most commonest locations are the spine (50%); the hip (15%) and the knee (15%). Multiple skeletal lesions may be present in people of African or Asian origin.

THE SPINE

The lesions develop following haematogenous spread. In about 70% of patients two adjacent vertebral bodies are involved; in 20% three or more. The disease commences in the anterior superior or inferior angle of the body and spreads to an adjacent body. The disc becomes involved and the disc space becomes narrowed (Figure 57.9). The spinal cord may be compressed and cause associated neurologi-

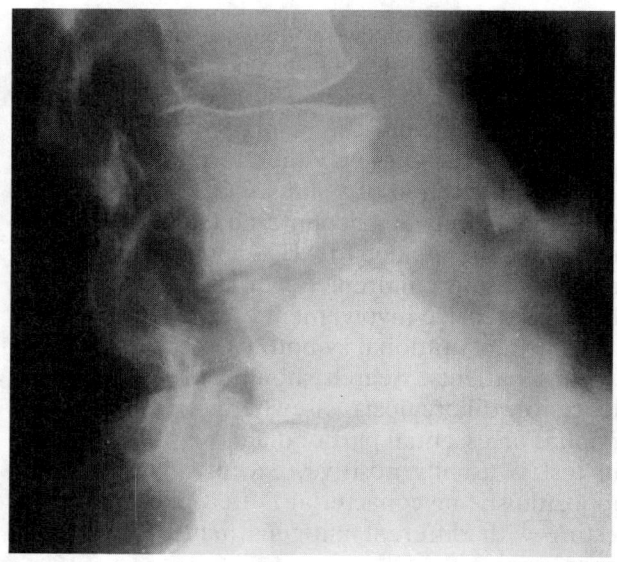

Figure 57.9 Spinal tuberculosis. Note involvement of two adjacent vertebrae and loss of joint space.

cal signs. The most common site is T10 and the frequency decreases the further the lesion is above or below T10. The first symptom is pain. To reduce this the child or adult holds the back stiffly and refuses to pick up anything from the floor unless he or she bends the knees, keeping the back straight. In the early stages the pain is relieved or ameliorated by rest. In cervical lesions the patient avoids turning the head and may sit with the head cupped in the hands. An abscess may appear behind the sternomastoid muscle or bulge into the pharynx. When the thoracic region is involved, the back is stiff and there is spasm of the muscle mass. Unwillingness to pick something off the floor is characertistic. Later there may be a visible lump and angling of the spine—the so-called gibbus—due to the collapse of the vertebrae. If abscess formation occurs it usually tracks intercostally or posteriorly and may cause paraplegia. If the lumbar region is involved the abscess may appear as a swelling above or below the inguinal ligament or in the upper thigh (psoas abscess). Paraplegia may ensue. In malnourished children, there may be fever and lymphadenopathy. There is often a long delay in making the diagnosis.[46]

INVESTIGATIONS AND DIFFERENTIAL DIAGNOSIS

In the absence of radiological facilities, treatment should be started if tuberculosis seems to be a likely diagnosis. Radiographic examination should be made by anteroposterior and lateral views of the spine. Coned views and tomography may be required in the diagnosis of early lesions. The anterosuperior and inferior angles are most frequently involved and the pedicle and articular facets may be affected. There is much less sclerosis present than in other infectious diseases of bone. Loss of disc space occurs early (Figure 57.9). A paravertebral abscess may be demonstrated: in mid-thoracic disease this may be misdiagnosed as a mediastinal tumour. Radiography of the chest should be carried out as it may reveal active or inactive pulmonary disease or a tumour. It is important not to jump to the conclusion that a segmental or lobar collapse is due to tumour: bronchoscopy may be necessary to establish the diagnosis. In experienced hands, needle biopsy may be useful. Blood tests for staphylococcal, streptococcal, typhoid and paratyphoid and brucellosis should be carried out when the diagnosis is in doubt.

The tuberculin test is usually positive but may be negative, particularly in malnourished children.

TREATMENT

Chemotherapy is very effective in the treatment of spinal tuberculosis and ambulant treatment has been shown to have a very high (90%) success rate in countries with few sophisticated facilities.[47] There is no evidence that frames, plaster beds, prolonged recumbency, followed by plaster jackets and spinal supports are of value in patients who are receiving adequate chemotherapy. Hodgson and Stock[48] developed the concept of radical operation supplemented by chemotherapy in 1956, often referred to as the Hong Kong operation. This requires highly specialized surgical and anaesthetic skills. In developing countries, most patients are treated—and most of them successfully—by ambulant chemotherapy. When special facilities do not exist immobilization is required only in cervical disease, provided careful monitoring to detect any deformity is carried out. In more advanced disease many surgeons prefer to remove diseased bone and disc material followed by anterior inlay grafting. Radical surgery limits the degree to which kyphosis develops. Three to six weeks rest in bed thereafter is often recommended. Progressive paraplegia is an urgent indication for operative treatment.

TUBERCULOSIS OF OTHER JOINTS

Presenting symptoms are pain, swelling of the joint and muscle wasting. Radiological examination may be unhelpful, the diagnosis being made by examination of synovial fluid or biopsy. Karlen[49] described well-bordered cystic lesions with a sclerotic zone in long bones in young children and it is frequently reported from Africa. The lesions show large numbers of tubercle bacilli. Hard painless swellings, which do not affect the overlying skin, develop over the site of the bony lesions, particularly in long bones. Chemotherapy may be used diagnostically. Immobilization is required very occasionally.

GENITOURINARY TUBERCULOSIS (See also Chapter 7)

Tuberculosis of the kidney, unlike most other extrapulmonary manifestations of the disease, does not become clinically manifest until a long time after primary infection in a large number of cases—more than 5 years in two-thirds of patients and more than 15 years in a quarter of cases.[50] For reasons that are ill understood it is relatively rare in developing countries.[51]

CLINICAL PRESENTATION

Most commonly patients present with symptoms of bladder inflammation: frequency, dysuria, haematuria or renal colic. Constitutional symptoms are the exception rather than the rule.

In an investigation of 150 patients with renal tuberculosis between 1965 and 1970, hypertension was found in 12 of the patients. Once patients were placed on antituberculosis chemotherapy there was steady regression of hypertension in 11 of the 12 patients. There was a lack of responsiveness to hypotensive drug regimens.[52] Patients with carcinoma and renal tuberculosis occurring in the same kidney have been reported but the association of these two diseases is extremely uncommon. Symptomatic chronic renal failure occurs very rarely and only where there is extensive disease. However, it has been observed that in 131 patients with urogenital tuberculosis 43% had a subclinical impairment of creatinine clearance.[53]

INVESTIGATION AND DIFFERENTIAL DIAGNOSIS

EXAMINATION OF THE URINE

In the early stages of the disease there may be pyuria. As the disease progresses, proteinuria may be observed and varying amounts of pus and blood are found.

The diagnosis of renal tuberculosis depends on the isolation of *M. tuberculosis* from the urine. At least three (and preferably six) consecutive morning specimens should be cultured. Smear examination can be misleading as harmless non-pathogenic acid-fast bacilli are frequently found in urine. Positive smear examination should not be accepted as diagnostic unless there is clear evidence pointing to tuberculosis. If smear-negative, culture for non-tuberculous bacteria should be carried out, if pos-

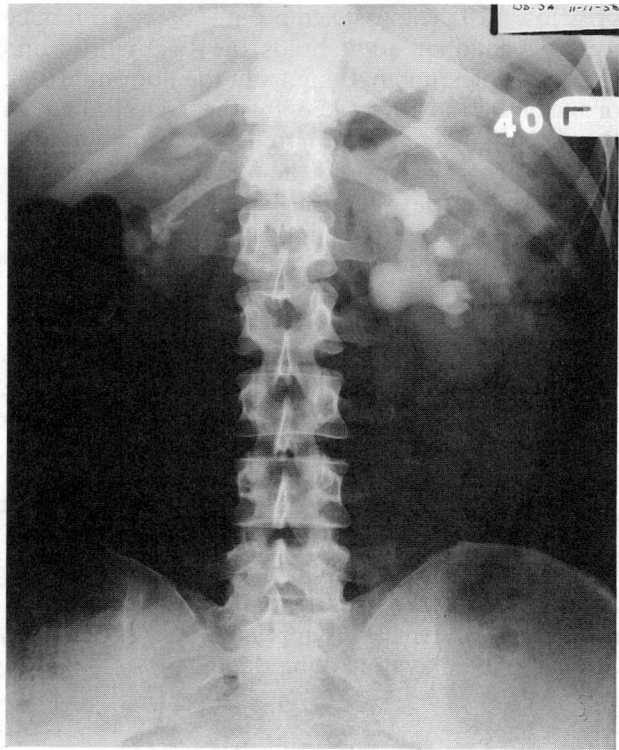

Figure 57.10   Renal tuberculosis. Note loss of calyceal architecture and ureteric obstruction.

sible, and treatment for simple cystitis given. If there is no clinical improvement antituberculosis treatment should be considered.

RADIOLOGICAL EXAMINATION

Typical pyelographic appearances are shown in Figure 57.10. Retrograde pyeloureterography, tomography, isotope venography and cystoscopy should be employed selectively. A detailed account of these investigations is given by Weinstein.[54]

Concurrent pulmonary tuberculosis is present in 5% of patients and a radiograph of the chest should be taken. The tuberculin test is rarely helpful. Careful examination of the genital tract is essential. Patients may give a history of previous tuberculous disease, e.g. pleural effusion. Rarely other sites, e.g. spine or lung, may be affected.

MANAGEMENT

Genitourinary tuberculosis can almost always be managed on an outpatient basis. A scheme of man-

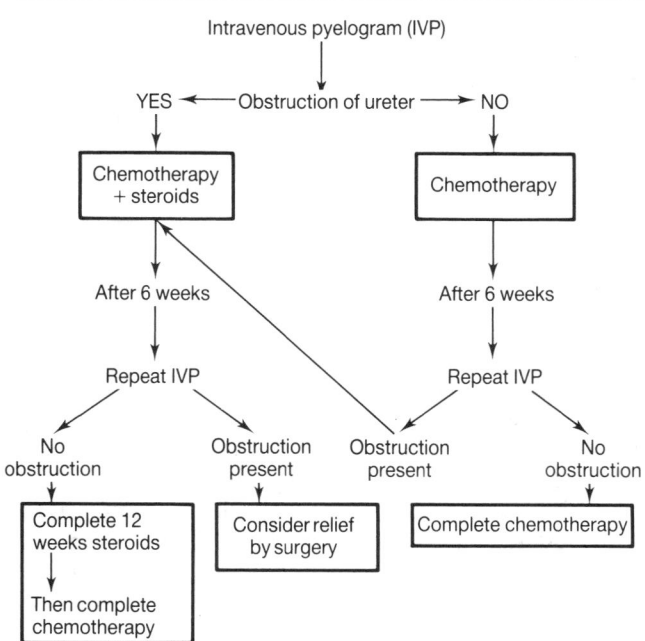

Figure 57.11 Management of renal tuberculosis.

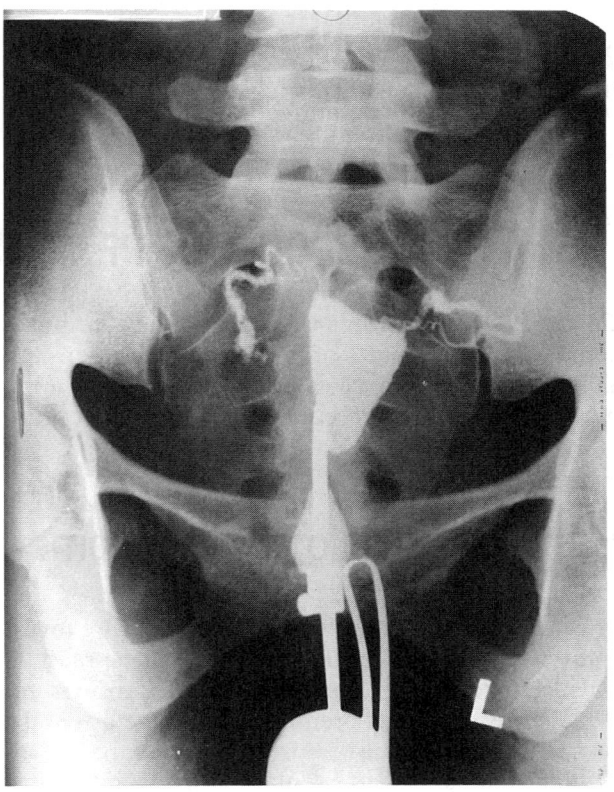

Figure 57.12 Genital tuberculosis. Hysterosalpingogram showing distortion of fallopian tubes.

agement is shown in Figure 57.11; management of ureteric obstruction is vital.[55]

Standard chemotherapy should be given for 6 months. If corticosteroid treatment is indicated prednisolone should be administered in a dose of 40 mg daily for 2 weeks, 30 mg for 2 weeks and 20 mg until it is shown at 6 weeks whether the obstruction has been relieved or not. If it has, the dose may be reduced gradually over the next 6 weeks. If pain and frequency are severe, prednisolone (20 mg daily) for 1–2 weeks usually gives effective relief.

If the ureter remains obstructed surgical relief may be obtained by bouginage, Davis intubation or surgical reconstruction of the ureter. Nephrectomy is very rarely required.[55]

PROGNOSIS

Provided that patients take chemotherapy as recommended the prognosis is excellent, the exception being in instances where there is extensive destruction of both kidneys.

GENITAL TUBERCULOSIS IN THE MALE

Epididymitis is the most common presentation of male genital tuberculosis but the testes, prostate and seminal vesicles may also be involved. The diagnosis may become apparent in the investigation of infer-

tility.[56] A palpable mass lesion is present in most patients and rectal examination is essential. Primary sterility is present in 10% of patients. In the presence of prostatitis, tuberculosis may be spread by semen.[57]

GENITAL TUBERCULOSIS IN THE FEMALE

This manifestation of tuberculosis usually arises from blood-borne dissemination of tubercle bacilli after primary infection, but rarely it arises as a result of infection by a male with genitourinary tuberculosis.

About 90% of cases arise during the period of active ovarian function, the fallopian tubes being involved in about 85% of patients. The tubes become distorted, thickened and retort-shaped (Figure 57.12), and the endometrium of the uterus becomes involved. The ovary, cervix and, rarely, the vulva may also be affected.

Primary sterility is the most common presentation. It is usually asymptomatic but there may be pain if there is a tubal abscess. There may be amenorrhoea or irregular menstruation.

The main investigation is by hysterosalpingography. Culture of urine, cervical discharge and menstrual blood should be carried out; endometrial biopsy is frequently definitive.

Chemotherapy results in healing of the disease, but alone rarely allows conception. Microsurgical procedures have recently improved the prognosis in infertile couples.

TUBERCULOUS PERICARDITIS (See also Chapter 5)

Tuberculous pericarditis is on the whole rare but is common in some parts of the world, e.g. Transkei. Tubercle bacilli may reach the pericardium via the bloodstream but more commonly through rupture of a mediastinal node.

ACUTE TUBERCULOUS PERICARDITIS

The most prominent early clinical features are fever, chest pain and pericardial friction. Widespread T-wave changes are present in the electrocardiogram. When effusion occurs breathlessness develops and a rapid paradoxical pulse, low blood pressure, raised jugular venous pressure, enlarged liver and ascites are present. Radiological examination shows a large pericardial effusion and often a small pleural effusion. Echocardiography, which is safe, rapid and non-invasive, is the most sensitive method of diagnosis.[58] Other helpful procedures are ECG, pericardial aspirate, culture and biopsy. The tuberculin test is usually positive.

There is a significant mortality from tuberculous pericarditis. Pericardiocentesis should be performed without delay if tamponade develops, and chemotherapy commenced immediately with a standard form of treatment. Corticosteroids should also be given when a noticeable decrease in heart size often occurs in 2–3 days. Prednisolone 80 mg daily should be maintained for 5–7 days and be progressively reduced to discontinuation in 6–8 weeks.

The patient may proceed to develop constrictive pericarditis, the thickened and often calcified pericardium forming a rigid casing around the heart (Figure 57.13). The heart is small and there are signs of congestive cardiac failure. In a controlled trial in Transkei of 143 patients with active tuberculous constrictive pericarditis, the group given steroids as well as chemotherapy fared significantly better than those treated with chemotherapy alone. Clinical improvement was significantly more rapid. Death occurred in 2% of steroid-treated patients and in 11% in the placebo group. Pericardectomy was required in 21 and 30% respectively for persisting or deteriorating severe constriction.[59]

Cardiovascular tuberculosis is well reviewed by Crocco.[60]

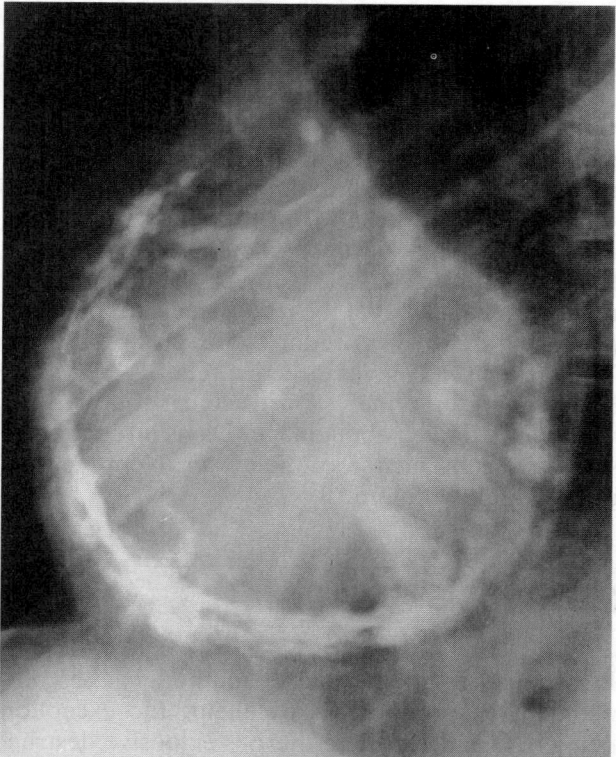

Figure 57.13   Constrictive tuberculous pericarditis.

CUTANEOUS MYCOBACTERIOSIS (See also Chapter 11)

Skin lesions caused by mycobacteria are comparatively rare and few clinicians, other than dermatologists, have sufficient experience to make a confident diagnosis. A high index of suspicion is necessary.

The nomenclature—tuberculosis colliquativa cutis and tuberculosis cutis miliaris acuta are good examples—must deter all but the most ardent classicists. Beyt and his colleagues[61] have proposed a relatively simple working classification.

The first group includes all the lesions caused by inoculation from an exogenous source. In patients not previously exposed to tubercle bacilli, usually children, a primary cutaneous lesion (see Figure 57.1) is associated with enlarged regional lymph nodes and the nodes may ulcerate. In patients who have been infected before, the lesion results in a hyperkeratotic papule without adenopathy—'the prosector's wart'.[62]

The second group includes all lesions from an endogenous source:

- Scrofuloderma—the fistulous openings of sinuses originating in nodes, bones, epididymis.
- Orificial cutaneous tuberculosis—where the source of tuberculous material is passed through body orifices: the mouth, rectum and vagina.

Ischiorectal abscesses are sometimes haematogenous in origin.

The third group are those which occur as a result of haematogenous spread: lupus vulgaris, multiple abscesses or nodules (in AIDS) and miliary skin lesions.

There is another group—the tuberculides—which was specifically omitted by Beyt and his colleagues as they are considered to be hypersensitivity phenomena. Erythema nodosum and papulonecrotic tuberculide come into this category.

Skin lesions are sometimes caused by mycobacteria other than tubercle bacilli. Examples are necrotic indolent ulcers on the legs of children in Africa[63] and Australia,[64] and the so-called 'swimming bath' ulcer caused by *M. marinum* (*balnei*).

Cutaneous lesions respond well to chemotherapy, appropriate adjustments being made if lesions are due to mycobacteria other than tubercle bacilli.

Leprosy is discussed in Chapter 58.

OCULAR TUBERCULOSIS (See also Chapter 10)

Primary exogenous infections are rare but may occur in the lids or conjunctiva. By far the most common form of ocular involvement results from haematogenous dissemination from a distant site to involve the uveal tract (iris, ciliary body and choroid). *Choroidal tubercles* are described on p. 982, and *phlyctenular conjunctivitis* on p. 976.

Primary infection of the eye. If tubercle bacilli develop under the upper or lower eyelid of a child who has not been previously infected they multiply and form a tuberculous primary infection. Caseation occurs and small yellow lesions will be seen on everting the eyelid. The eye becomes irritable and the lid becomes swollen. Spread occurs by the lymphatics and the preauricular node enlarges. It may soften and form an abscess. Treatment is the same as for any other primary site. *Acute tuberculous panophthalmitis* is very rare. It usually occurs in people with chronic illness or in malnourished children. The common presentation is painless progressive visual loss. The cornea becomes cloudy.

The diagnosis is frequently missed, the condition being thought to be due to metastatic carcinoma. Enucleation of the eye may be necessary eventually.

In *tuberculous uveitis* mutton-fat keratotic precipitates on the posterior aspect of the cornea and iris nodules are present. Similar appearances are seen in brucellosis, sarcoidosis and toxoplasmosis. An isoniazid therapeutic test has been described.[65]

In *tuberculous retinitis* a vitreous opacification and a grey-white retinal lesion may be observed. Retinal perivasculitis (Eales disease) has also been linked with tuberculosis.

TREATMENT

All forms of ocular disease respond well to chemotherapy. The addition of corticosteroids at an early stage may prevent destruction of tissue with loss of vision and possible loss of the eye.

TUBERCULOSIS OF UPPER RESPIRATORY TRACT

Although lesions in the upper respiratory tract, especially the larynx, are commonly associated with advanced pulmonary tuberculosis, primary lesions do occur and painless enlargement of a lymph node may be the presenting feature. The lesions may also occur as a result of haematogenous dissemination. Primary lesions of the gum have been reported and they may also be found in the nose[66], tonsil, epiglottis and ear. Bacilli may be swept into the eustachian tube when an infant or young child is feeding. A focus develops in the ear and the ear discharges. Spread to the mastoid may occur. The possibility of tuberculosis should be borne in mind in any chronic upper respiratory condition, especially if there is lymphadenopathy.

The larynx is the most common organ involved, usually resulting from sputum heavily infected with tubercle bacilli. Pain is prominent and may be severe and may stop the patient from eating. Hoarseness occurs and the voice becomes a moist whisper. Laryngeal tuberculosis may occur in older patients in the absence of active lung disease, often being misdiagnosed as tumour, the correct diagnosis being by biopsy.[67] Treatment by chemotherapy is very effective and the addition of corticosteroids causes rapid alleviation of pain.

RARER FORMS OF EXTRAPULMONARY DISEASE

Tuberculosis may affect any organ in the body. Organs rarely affected are the adrenals, breast, thyroid and liver. Tuberculosis may also be associated with hypercalcaemia and the syndrome of inappropriate antidiuretic hormone secretion.[68]

Tuberculosis of the *adrenals* causes possibly only 20% of adrenal destruction, 75% being due to idiopathic or autoimmune disease. The main clinical features are weakness, weight loss, hyperpigmentation, hypotension, amenorrhoea and gastrointestinal symptoms. Hyperpigmentation occurs, especially over pressure areas, e.g. elbows and lower thoracic spine, and also in patches in the mouth—a particularly valuable sign in races with naturally pigmented skin. The diagnosis is made by the appropriate tests of adrenocortical function. A radiograph of the abdomen frequently demonstrates calcified opacities in the adrenals. If facilities exist, ultrasonography and computed tomography are the best ways of diagnosing adrenal enlargement. Treatment with chemotherapy is effective but hormonal replacement is also necessary.

Tuberculosis of the *breast* presents as a painless craggy mass, the diagnosis usually being made on biopsy.[69] A breast abscess may stem from caseation of intercostal nodes.

Tuberculosis of the *thyroid* usually presents as a nodule or abscess.[70]

The *liver* is frequently involved in tuberculosis but involvement is rarely manifested as a clinical entity. Diffuse granulomas are present in acute miliary tuberculosis: 75–100% in autopsy series and 25–100% in needle biopsy specimens. Tuberculomas are rare and may cause fever, malaise and weight loss; hepatomegaly is frequently present. Disease of the bile ducts is rare, as is tuberculosis involving the gallbladder. Hepatic lesions are to be found in the majority of patients with AIDS and the liver is commonly involved in congenital tuberculosis. An extensive account of tuberculosis of the liver and biliary tract is given by Lewis and Zimmerman.[71]

HUMAN IMMUNODEFICIENCY VIRUS-ASSOCIATED TUBERCULOSIS

The association between tuberculosis and HIV presents an immediate and grave public health and socioeconomic threat, particularly in the developing world.[72] In early 1992 WHO estimated that approximately 4 million people had been infected with both *M. tuberculosis* and HIV since the beginning of the pandemic, 95% being in developing countries. The association between tuberculosis and HIV is evident from the high incidence of tuberculosis, estimated at 5–8% per year among HIV-infected persons, the high seroprevalence among patients with tuberculo-sis, the high recurrence of tuberculosis among AIDS patients and the coincidence of increased tuberculosis notifications with the spread of the epidemic in several African countries.

In many developing countries tuberculosis has now emerged as the most common opportunistic disease associated with AIDS. Between 20 and 40% of AIDS patients in Africa, 18% of patients in Haiti and up to 25% in some Latin American countries have clinical tuberculosis during the course of HIV infection.[3] In the USA the figure is about 4% of

AIDS cases reported nationally, though the figure in selected areas such as Florida and New York was much higher. However, HIV does not yet appear to be directly implicated in England and Wales.[73] A dramatic increase in the number of cases of tuberculosis due to HIV infection is predicted for sub-Saharan Africa in the 1990s.[74]

The overlap between tuberculosis and HIV has ominous social and medical implications, particularly for the resource-poor countries. The development of tuberculosis is often a marker for the presence of AIDS.[75]

CLINICAL FEATURES

It is important to recognize that the clinical features in patients infected by HIV show certain variations from the normal patterns of disease.

In Africa, surveys in Kenya[76] and Tanzania[77] between 1964 and 1984 provide reliable information on the pattern of tuberculosis before the AIDS epidemic. In 1964 almost 90% had pulmonary disease; of those with extrapulmonary disease 85% had lymphadenopathy (mainly cervical), bone and joint disease or pleural effusion. Miliary tuberculosis was uncommon. Now extrapulmonary disease appears to be more common, especially in forms which were previously rare, such as pericarditis, peritonitis and miliary disease. For instance in Bangui, Central African Republic, extrapulmonary tuberculosis and mediastinal lymphadenopathy were significantly more common in HIV-positive (60–65%) compared with HIV-negative (25%) patients with tuberculosis.[78]

Patients with both HIV infection and pulmonary tuberculosis may present with typical radiographic features. However, many show predominantly lower lobe disease, large mediastinal nodes and air–fluid levels. Pleural effusion is common. The radiographic abnormalities may change rapidly. Miliary tuberculosis is not uncommon. Sputum is often smear negative and aggressive diagnostic methods, which are more dangerous to health workers, may be required to try to prove the diagnosis.

Tubercle bacilli may be obtained from blood cultures (almost unknown in seronegative individuals) or from faeces, especially in opportunistic mycobacterial infections.

Generalized lymphadenopathy is more frequent. For example in Uganda tuberculous lymphadenopathy used to be relatively uncommon. In 1983, only 6 of 120 new patients with tuberculosis seen in Mulago Hospital, Kampala, over 6 months had lymphadenopathy, whereas in 1986 16 patients were

seen with this form of disease in 6 weeks, all of whom were HIV positive.[79] The clinical features of tuberculous meningitis and the mortality rate (20%) are similar, the disease being more common in seropositive (10%) compared with seronegative (2%) patients. Abscesses in unusual sites (brain, testis and chest wall) may be encountered.[80]

The tuberculin test is often negative and is reflected in the non-reactive histological features which are often encountered.

TREATMENT

The response to treatment is as good in seropositive individuals provided that the tubercle bacilli are initially sensitive to the drugs being used. However, in a segment of the population (intravenous drug users, the homeless) drug-resistant infections are now prevalent. It is important where possible to identify the drug susceptibility pattern. This is also important in relation to the identification of opportunistic mycobacteria (especially the MAIS (*M. avium–intracellulare–scrofulaceum*) complex) which is frequently the cause of death in AIDS patients. Treatment should be commenced with four drugs, rifampicin, isoniazid, pyrazinamide and ethambutol, for 2 months and at least until the drug sensitivity pattern is known, after which pyrazinamide and ethambutol may, if appropriate, be withdrawn. It is generally recommended that treatment be continued for 6 months after the last positive sputum culture and some authorities recommend treatment with isoniazid alone indefinitely thereafter. If the organism belongs to the MAIS complex, treatment should be continued for 2 years. In drug abusers and those whose compliance is poor a fully supervised regimen is recommended. If the standards of sterilization are suspect the safety of streptomycin must be taken into consideration. A guide to sterilization and high level disinfection methods is available.[81] Streptomycin is no longer available in some areas. Drug hypersensitivity, particularly to thiacetazone, is more common in AIDS.

CHEMOPROPHYLAXIS

Preventive tuberculosis chemotherapy has not been recommended for developing countries in the past, primarily because the limited resources as regards both health staff and drugs had to be reserved for treatment of acute tuberculosis. In addition it was difficult to identify high-risk groups, aside from contacts, among the vast numbers of tuberculosis-infected persons. The risk of a dually infected person developing tuberculosis is not known precisely but is probably six times higher in HIV seropositive individuals in the early stages of the disease and is likely to be very much higher in the later stages. The significance of a 'positive' tuberculin test is affected by previous BCG vaccination and many HIV seropositive individuals are anergic, increasingly so as the disease progresses. Another salient factor is the local prevalence of drug-resistant infections, particularly to isoniazid, which may render prophylaxis ineffective. In countries where the national tuberculosis programme strategies include chemoprophylaxis, dual infection with HIV and *M. tuberculosis* should be considered as an indication for chemoprophylaxis. An additional consideration for recommending preventive therapy is that by doing so the risk of infection to health care workers is diminished. Practical details regarding isoniazid chemoprophylaxis are described on p. 1004.

Preventive therapy is likely to be more cost effective than treatment of tuberculosis cases that will recur in the future in the HIV–tuberculosis coinfected pool. For instance of the estimated 3.1 million dually infected persons in sub-Saharan Africa, one million will develop tuberculosis in the next 10 years. In terms of drug costs only this would require approximately $34 million calculated at the rate of $34 per patient in Africa. By contrast the cost of isoniazid for all HIV–tuberculosis coinfected persons would be about $6 million, as a 6-month supply of isoniazid costs less than $2 per person.

It may now be possible to provide preventive therapy by establishing voluntary HIV and tuberculin testing centres. These centres should not only identify dually infected individuals but provide them with preventive therapy. In this area, collaboration between national tuberculosis and AIDS programmes is essential.

BCG VACCINATION

BCG is widely used in the developing world for the prevention of disseminated tuberculosis. Isolated case reports describing adverse reactions associated with BCG among children and adults with HIV infection have raised concern about its safety. The potential benefits from BCG would appear to outweigh theoretical risks. The current recommendation by WHO is that for asymptomatic HIV-infected individuals where the risk of tuberculosis is high, BCG is recommended at birth or as soon as possible thereafter, in accordance with standard policies for non-HIV-infected children, but for symptomatic HIV-infected individuals BCG should be withheld.[82] However, the Immunisation Practices Advising Committee in the USA shows greater caution, discouraging BCG vaccination in all seropositive children, whether symptomatic or not. A similar view is held in Britain.[83]

Tuberculosis and human immunodeficiency virus infection in developing countries is well reviewed by Harries.[84]

NON-TUBERCULOUS MYCOBACTERIAL DISEASE

Disease due to *M. leprae* is not considered in this context. Disease caused by mycobacteria other than *M. tuberculosis*, *M. bovis* or *M. africanum* are becoming increasingly important, especially in the context of AIDS. Little progress was made in the identification and classification of these mycobacteria until Runyon[85] divided the strains he encountered in clinical practice into four groups on the basis of growth rate and pigmentation. This classification is rarely used nowadays, the International Working Group of Mycobacterial Taxonomy having classified over 40 species of mycobacteria. Only 16 species of mycobacteria are clearly pathogenic to man but several others may be. These are listed in Tables 57.4 and 57.5. These infectious organisms are often

Table 57.4 Opportunistic mycobacteria which commonly cause disease and their common sites.

Species		Usual site
M. kansasii		Lung
M. avium		
M. intracellulare	MAIS	Lung, nodes, disseminated
M. scrofulaceum	complex	disease (AIDS)
M. xenopi		Lung
M. malmoense		Lung
M. szulgai		Lung, nodes
M. simiae		Lung
M. fortuitum		Soft tissue, skin
M. marinum		Skin
M. ulcerans		Skin

Table 57.5 Opportunistic mycobacteria which are likely to be contaminants but may very rarely cause disease.

Species	Usual site
M. gordonae	Lung
M. terrae	Lung
M. chelonei	Injection abscess, post-cardiac surgery, post-renal transplantation osteoarticular
M. flavescens	Lung
M. gastri	Lung

referred to as atypical mycobacteria but perhaps a more appropriate name is opportunistic mycobacteria as they often require some form of tissue damage or immunosuppression before they can cause disease. They are also referred to as anonymous, non-tuberculous or MOTT (mycobacteria other than tuberculous). It is essential that, where facilities exist, acid-fast bacilli isolated from clinical specimens are identified rapidly and accurately to ensure that correct chemotherapy is prescribed, to ensure that unnecessary chemotherapy with relatively toxic drugs is not given, to avoid unnecessary contact tracing, and to avoid labelling a patient as tuberculous who does not have the disease. Even now a certain stigma still attaches to tuberculosis.

Opportunistic mycobacteria are ubiquitous in the environment, occurring in water, soil and dust and in association with birds, swine and cattle. Identification is made on the basis of their rate of growth, colonial appearance (including light sensitivity), optimal temperature for growth and a series of sophisticated tests, including drug sensitivity tests, which allow characterization to be made.[86] Many of the species show multiple drug resistance. At the present time, these infections are more common in the industrialized world than in the developing world but they are likely to become more so in developing countries with the tragic spread of the AIDS epidemic. They cause non-specific sensitization to tuberculin which can obscure the use of the tuberculin test in diagnosis. Identification of the group or complex is usually sufficient for clinical purposes.

The main clinical presentations are pulmonary, cervical adenopathy, skin infections, local abscesses and disseminated disease.

PULMONARY DISEASE

The clinical features are similar to those of classical tuberculosis. Patients are most often middle-aged to elderly males (the exception being young adults with HIV infection) and present with cough, sputum, malaise and loss of weight, occasionally with haemoptysis. Many are asymptomatic. Fever and a poor clinical condition are present in AIDS patients. The typical radiological features are fibrosis with cavitation in 80% of non-AIDS patients, with slow progress. In AIDS patients the radiograph may be normal in 35%, and the opacities are often diffuse and rapidly changing.[87] Two isolates at 7 days interval are usually required to establish the diagnosis and to indicate a requirement for treatment. The natural history of pulmonary disease is variable. *M. kansasii* infections are commonly progressive though there may be a tendency to intermittent healing.

CERVICAL LYMPHADENOPATHY

Non-tuberculous mycobacteria involve the lymphatic system most commonly in the cervical nodes in children between the ages of 1 and 5 years.[88] The large majority of cases are due to the MAIS complex but *M. kansasii* may be responsible. The nodes are almost always unilateral and there are rarely any systemic symptoms. The site is usually the submandibular or submaxillary nodes; very rarely the preauricular, axillary or inguinal nodes may be affected. Progress to disseminated disease may occur and may be fatal. Differential tuberculin testing with material prepared from appropriate antigens may be helpful in children.[89] Lymph node involvement is now commonly seen in AIDS patients, abdominal nodes being affected from time to time. Localized cervical nodes are best treated by total excision: they should not be aspirated as sinus formation commonly follows this procedure. It has been suggested that excision of localized nodes need not be followed by chemotherapy.

SKIN AND SOFT TISSUE INFECTIONS

Four of the non-tuberculous mycobacteria are responsible for skin and soft tissue infections: *M. ulcerans* and *marinum* especially, *M. fortuitum* and *chelonei* less commonly.

M. ulcerans is the cause of a superficial ulcer called the Buruli ulcer. It is seen only in tropical areas of the world (Central Africa and tropical parts of Australia, New Guinea and Mexico). The lesion is self-limiting but can lead to considerable disability because of the contraction that occurs on healing. The only effective treatment is excision of the ulcer followed by skin grafting but this facility is rarely available in the endemic area. It has been known for 40 years that infection by *M. marinum* can cause slowly evolving, usually solitary, nodules which sometimes ulcerate. They occur in swimmers at sites of trauma. They occur especially on the elbows, knees and dorsum of the feet and hands. Occasionally the lesions spread to resemble sporotrichosis. The source, in addition to swimming pools,[90] may be aquaria.[91] Chemotherapy is usually very effective. *M. fortuitum* and *M. chelonei* have also been implicated as a cause of abscesses.

BURSAE, JOINT, TENDON SHEATHS, BONES

Chronic granulomatous lesions of these tissues may rarely be caused by non-tuberculous mycobacteria.[92] Osteoarticular involvement due to *M. chelone8* has been described.[93]

DISSEMINATED DISEASE

Patients with AIDS are shown to be increasingly vulnerable to widespread disseminated disease due to non-tuberculous mycobacteria. The predominant species is the MAIS complex but *M. kansasii* is responsible occasionally. Sometimes there are few symptoms but patients may complain of fever, abdominal pain and diarrhoea. Pulmonary symptoms are often minimal. All systems may be involved, especially miliary involvement of the lungs, bone marrow, liver and bowel. The meninges are rarely affected. Blood and bone marrow cultures are important ways of diagnosing MAIS infection in AIDS patients, and faecal acid-fast smears and cultures may also be useful.

TREATMENT

The treatment of patients with opportunistic mycobacterial infections presents considerable problems both because the organism is frequently resistant to many antituberculosis drugs and also because of the lack of controlled trials of therapy. General guidelines only can be given; patients must be treated on an individual basis and experimental combinations of drugs may have to be used.

Patients with *M. kansasii* seem to respond well to treatment with rifampicin, isoniazid and ethambutol. However, treatment for 9–15 months with rifampicin and ethambutol only has been shown to be effective[94] and in a prospective study in 158 patients treated with rifampicin and ethambutol for only 9 months one had a positive culture in the last 3 months of therapy. Relapse occurred in 9% of patients, half of whom were poorly compliant in treatment.[95] Patients may well have had treatment for several weeks with rifampicin, isoniazid, pyrazinamide and possibly ethambutol before the true nature of the isolate is recognized. Prothionamide, capreomycin, kanamycin and cycloserine have been used in treatment failures. Surgical treatment, even when possible, is rarely indicated.

Treatment of patients with infection with the *M. avium* complex is even more problematical. The exception is infection of cervical nodes in young children, when surgical excision is usually curative. General guidelines for management may be expressed as follows. In those patients with mild localized forms of the disease, a proven indolent course and few or no symptoms, observation alone is usually sufficient. Surgical treatment may be considered. In patients who have moderate disease, especially if cavitated, or who are worsening, treatment with rifampicin, isoniazid and ethambutol should be started and continued for 18–24 months. In patients who are deteriorating and in those with disseminated disease, as in AIDS, kanamycin, prothionamide and cycloserine may be added and consideration given to the use of rifabutin, clofazimine and the quinolones. The success rate varies from 25 to 90% and relapse is frequent. A fatal outcome is very frequent in patients with AIDS. If relapse occurs the same drug regimen should be used again and continued indefinitely. Drug toxicity is a major problem in multidrug regimens containing the more toxic drugs, particularly in patients with AIDS. Infections due to *M. szulgai* respond similarly to those from *M. kansasii* and usually respond to treatment with rifampicin and ethambutol with or without isoniazid. *M. fortuitum* and *M. cholonei* are very resistant to standard antituberculosis drugs. Promising results have been obtained by the use of doxycycline, amikacin, sulphadiazine, gentamicin and cefoxitine. The best results are obtained by using four drugs if possible.[96] *M. xenopi* is often susceptible to isoniazid, rifampicin, ethambutol and streptomycin. Chemotherapy may be necessary in *M. marinum* infections if spontaneous recovery does not take place. Rifampicin and ethambutol should be given until the lesions are completely cleared.

Treatment of opportunist mycobacterial infections is often very difficult but it does offer success in many cases. Treatment demands diligence and persistence by both patient and physician. An excellent account of the diagnosis and treatment of disease caused by non-tuberculous mycobacteria has been published by the American Thoracic Society.[97]

TREATMENT

CHEMOTHERAPY

The main aim of treatment is cure. Prior to the introduction of chemotherapy, 75% of patients with sputum smear-positive disease would die within 5 years. Modern chemotherapy is so effective that if proper drug regimens are prescribed and the patient is wholly co-operative in treatment then cure takes place in 100% of patients with initially drug-sensitive tubercle bacilli and in the majority of patients who have drug-resistant organisms. A subsidiary but nevertheless important aim is to render the patient non-infectious and thus prevent spread of disease.

RATIONALE OF CHEMOTHERAPY OF TUBERCULOSIS

In earlier 'standard' chemotherapy using streptomycin, *para*-aminosalicylic acid (PAS) and isoniazid, drug combinations were selected with a view to preventing drug resistance. The organisms were eventually killed or died out after many months of treatment. The new concept of short-term chemotherapy is different, the object being to select combinations of drugs that are rapidly sterilizing.

It is of crucial importance, especially for patients harbouring large bacterial populations, to prevent further bacterial multiplication so that the disease is brought under control as soon as possible. This not only saves the lives of patients and prevents disastrous gross lung destruction, but it also limits the dissemination of infection in the community. Treatment with three or four drugs in the initial phase will almost always prevent the emergence of drug-resistant mutants and will, with few exceptions, secure a successful outcome in patients with initially drug-resistant infection, preventing the emergence of 'persisters'.[14] A good regimen is one that largely overcomes the influence of initial drug resistance.[98] The use of drugs with a high sterilizing effect in the continuation phase is designed to eliminate relapse.[99] The practical implication of these principles is discussed below.

DRUGS AND REGIMENS

The chemotherapy of pulmonary tuberculosis demands not only a detailed knowledge of the individual drugs which are effective but also of the regimens which are essential to a successful outcome of treatment.

It is almost 35 years since it was established that with appropriate combinations of drugs administered for a sufficiently long period of treatment, and given strict compliance by the patient, treatment would be 100% effective in patients with initially sensitive organisms,[100] and relapse would be rare.[101] Earlier effective regimens have, however, been superseded by short-term chemotherapy. The short-term regimens now recommended have the advantages of reducing chronic toxicity, of making compliance by the patient easier, of being highly effective even in the presence of initial infection with drug-resistant organisms, and making relapse highly unlikely even in patients complying with treatment for periods as brief as 4 months.[102] Monotherapy must never be used except in chemoprophylaxis.

Short-course chemotherapy is applicable to all forms of the disease. Certain minor modifications (e.g. meningitis) or additions (e.g. corticosteroids) apply to some sites of disease. It is important therefore to consult the section relating to particular sites before embarking on treatment.

For more detailed information on drugs and regimens, the reader is referred to other texts.[103–105]

DRUGS USED IN CHEMOTHERAPY

The drugs available for the treatment of tuberculosis fall conveniently into two groups:

1. Those commonly used in previously untreated patients:

    Isoniazid (H)   Pyrazinamide (Z)
    Rifampicin (Rifampin,   Streptomycin (S)
      USA) (R)   Thiacetazone (T)
    Ethambutol (E)

2. Those used if primary treatment has failed:

    Cycloserine (CYC)   Capreomycin (CAP)
    Prothionamide (PRO)   Viomycin (VIO)

Table 57.6 Chemotherapy for newly-diagnosed patients: drugs—preparation and dosage.

Drug*	Preparation	Daily		Intermittent	
		Adults	Children	Adults	Children
Isoniazid	Tablet 50 mg; 100 mg Syrup 50 mg/5 ml Ampoule 50 mg in 2 ml	300 mg 10 mg/kg in miliary/ meningitis† 5 mg/kg: chemoprophylaxis	10 mg/kg	15 mg/kg (max. 750 mg) plus pyridoxine 10 mg	15 mg/kg (max. 750 mg) plus pyridoxine 10 mg
Rifampicin	Capsule 150 mg, 300 mg Syrup 150 mg/5 ml Ampoule 300 mg i.v.	<50 kg: 450 mg >50 kg: 600 mg	10 mg/kg (max. 600 mg)	600–900 mg	10 mg/kg (max. 600 mg)
Pyrazinamide	Tablet 500 mg	<50kg: 1.5 g 50–74 kg: 2.0 g >75 kg: 2.5 g	35 mg/kg	Thrice weekly <50 kg: 2.0 g >50 kg: 2.5 g Twice weekly <50 kg: 3.0 g >50 kg: 3.5 g	Thrice weekly 50 mg/kg Twice weekly 75 mg/kg
Ethambutol	Tablet 100 mg; 400 mg	15 mg/kg	If over 12 years of age, as for adults	Thrice weekly 30 mg/ kg Twice weekly 45 mg/ kg	If over 12 years of age as for adults
Streptomycin	Vial 1 g	<50 kg: 0.75 g >50 kg: 1.0 g (0.75 g if over 40 years of age)	20 mg/kg	<50 kg: 0.75 g >50 kg: 1.0 g	20 mg/kg (max. 0.75 g)
Thiacetazone	Tablet 50 mg	150 mg	4 mg/kg	Unsuitable	Unsuitable

*All drugs should be given in a single dose.
†Reduce to 5 mg/kg in Indian patients.
Combined preparations of isoniazid and rifampicin are available. For fixed dose preparations of isoniazid, rifampicin and pyrazinamide see p. 1002.

Ethionamide (ETH)   Kanamycin (KAN)
Para-aminosalicylic acid   Newer drugs
   (PAS)   (p. 1000)

The dosage, adverse effects and drug interactions are summarized in Tables 57.6–57.8. The adverse effects are amplified in the following notes.

Isoniazid

The advantages of isoniazid are that it is a very powerful bactericidal drug, it has very few adverse effects, and it is very cheap.

Highly effective concentrations of the drug are obtained in all tissues, including the CSF. There is no cross-resistance with other drugs. The rate of conversion to an inactive form—acetylation—varies in different races but is extremely rarely of practical importance in standard treatment. However, slow inactivators are more likely to suffer from the complication of peripheral neuropathy. *Adverse effects* of isoniazid are uncommon. Generalized skin rashes rarely occur. *Peripheral neuropathy* (tingling and numbness of hands and feet) is the main adverse effect. It is more common in malnourished patients and with high doses. It can be treated by giving 100–200 mg pyridoxine daily and can be prevented by giving 10 mg pyridoxine daily. It is worth while giving routine pyridoxine with high dosage isoniazid (for instance in twice-weekly treatment), if there is much malnutrition and if toxic effects are frequent locally. The national programme may make recommendations about this.

Rifampicin (Rifampin, USA)

There is no cross-resistance to other antituberculosis drugs. Highly effective concentrations are obtained in all tissues, with moderate levels in the CSF. Although the cost is higher than most other initial drugs, the results are so good that chemotherapy may be cheaper per cured case.

It should, if possible, be taken half an hour before breakfast. If nausea is a problem, it should be taken last thing at night. All patients should be warned

Table 57.7 Chemotherapy for newly-diagnosed patients: drugs—adverse effects*.

Drug	Common adverse effects	Drug interactions
Isoniazid	Peripheral neuropathy Cutaneous hypersensitivity Hepatitis Elevation of hepatic enzymes	Phenytoin
Rifampicin (Rifampin, USA)	Nausea and vomiting Hepatitis Toxic reactions in intermittent therapy Turns body secretions and urine orange	Oral contraceptives, coumarin drugs, corticosteroids (dose should be doubled), digoxin, oral hypoglycaemics, methadone
Pyrazinamide	Hepatitis Arthralgia (hyperuricaemia) Photosensitivity Nausea, anorexia, vomiting	
Ethambutol	Retrobulbar neuritis (dose related)	
Streptomycin	Giddiness, ataxia, tinnitus, deafness (eighth cranial nerve damage) Nephrotoxicity Pregnancy—avoid	Potentiation of neuromuscular blocking agents
Thiacetazone	Nausea and vomiting Cutaneous reactions (often severe) Conjunctivitis	

*These are amplified in the text.

Table 57.8 Second-line drugs.

Drug	Dosage	Common adverse effects
Ethionamide Prothionamide	Less than 50 kg: 750 mg (250 mg in the morning and 500 mg immediately before going to sleep at night: this helps to avoid nausea) 50 kg or more: 1.0 g (500 mg 2 × daily: but many patients can only tolerate 250 + 500 mg as above)	Gastrointestinal; metallic taste in mouth
Sodium *para-* aminosalicylate (PAS)	10–12 g divided into two equal doses daily	Gastrointestinal; fever and rash
Cycloserine	250 mg 2 × daily increasing to 250 mg 3 × daily	Confusion, convulsions, suicide
Capreomycin Kanamycin Viomycin	As streptomycin (Table 57.6); monitor serum urea and electrolyte concentrations	As streptomycin; hypolcalcaemia, hypomagnesaemia. Ototoxicity less common

that *rifampicin colours the urine, sweat and tears orange*.

Cutaneous reactions in the form of mild flushing and itchiness of the skin, and occasionally a rash, occur very infrequently. These reactions are often so mild that the patient desensitizes himself or herself without the drug having to be stopped.

Hepatitis is extremely uncommon unless the patient has a history of liver disease or alcoholism. It is wise if possible to estimate liver function from time to time in such patients. A significant rise in bilirubin may occur in patients with congestive cardiac failure.

The following syndromes occur mostly in patients

having *intermittent treatment*. They may also rarely occur in patients who have been *prescribed* daily treatment but *take* the drugs intermittently.

- 'Influenza' syndrome: shiveriness, malaise, headache and bone pain.
- Thrombocytopenia and purpura: platelets fall to a very low level and haemorrhages occur. It is essential to stop treatment immediately.
- Respiratory and shock syndrome: shortness of breath, wheeziness, fall in blood pressure, collapse. Corticosteroids may be required.
- Acute haemolytic anaemia and renal failure.

Rifampicin should never be given again if the shock syndrome, acute haemolytic anaemia or acute renal failure has occurred.

Rifampicin and *pregnancy* is discussed on p. 1003.

Streptomycin

Streptomycin is not absorbed from the intestine so it has to be given by intramuscular injection. It diffuses readily into most body tissues. The concentrations are very low in normal CSF but the levels are higher in the presence of meningitis. It does, however, cross the placenta. Providing syringes and staff to inject the drug add to the cost. The *nurse* who gives the injections must wear gloves, otherwise there is a risk of the development of *skin reactions*.

HIV can be spread by infected needles. If a new needle cannot be used for every patient, or if you cannot be sure that sterilization is absolutely reliable, ethambutol should be substituted for streptomycin. This is particularly important if you are working in an area which has a high prevalence of AIDS. Do not, however, use ethambutol in young children: they may not tell you that their sight is failing.

Damage to the vestibular apparatus is manifested by giddiness. It may start suddenly and, if acute, there may also be vomiting. Unsteadiness is more marked in darkness and there may be nystagmus. It is more likely to occur in older patients: attention to dosage is thus very important. *Treatment must be stopped immediately*. The damage to the nerve may be permanent if the drug is not withdrawn when the symptoms start. If the drug is stopped immediately, symptoms usually clear over weeks. *Deafness* occurs extremely rarely.

Anaphylaxis: injection may be followed by tingling around the mouth, nausea and occasionally by sudden collapse. Streptomycin *should be avoided*, if at all possible, in *pregnancy* because it may cause *impaired hearing* in the child.

Ethambutol

Ethambutol is a bacteriostatic drug. It is mainly used to prevent the emergence of drug resistance to the main bactericidal drugs (isoniazid, rifampicin and streptomycin). *It is essential not to give more than the recommended dose*. Never give ethambutol to young children who are unlikely to tell you they are losing their sight. Avoid also in renal failure.

The main and possibly very serious adverse reaction is *progressive loss of vision* caused by retrobulbar neuritis. When the patient begins treatment *warn him or her about possible decrease in vision*. Failing eyesight will be noticed even before any abnormality is seen when the eye is examined with the ophthalmoscope. The drug must be stopped immediately. If this is done there is every chance sight will be recovered. If treatment is continued the patient may become completely blind.

Pyrazinamide

Pyrazinamide is very valuable in short course treatment and in meningitis. The most common side-effects are hepatotoxicity and arthralgia. *Hepatotoxicity* may be discovered only on carrying out routine biochemical tests. Anorexia, mild fever, tender enlargement of liver and spleen may be followed by jaundice. If severe hepatitis occurs do not give the drug again.

For arthralgia simple treatment with aspirin is often sufficient: allopurinol is required for the treatment of gout.

Thiacetazone (Tb1)

Thiacetazone is a weak drug but is very valuable as a companion drug in preventing the development of isoniazid resistance. It is relatively cheap, remains stable in high temperatures and is easier to dispense and store than PAS. It is poorly tolerated by the Chinese population of Hong Kong and Singapore, poorly tolerated by Europeans and surprisingly well tolerated in East African countries and in South America. Severe reactions may occur in patients with HIV infection. Natural resistance to thiacetazone occurs in certain countries. It should be used only in communities where it has been shown to be effective and to be of low toxicity.

'Second-line drugs'

These drugs may have to be used in retreatment when there is resistance, or probable resistance, to the drugs used in standard treatment. Most of the drugs are unpleasant for the patient. They are difficult to use effectively. The drugs are ethionamide/prothionamide, PAS, cycloserine, kanamycin and capreomycin. Dosage and main side-effects are shown in Table 57.8. PAS is now unobtainable in a number of countries.

Newer experimental drugs

New drugs active against *M. tuberculosis* are urgently required to treat the increasing numbers of patients with drug-resistant organisms but also to try to reduce the period of treatment necessary for cure. Only those drugs belonging to the fluoroquinolone and macrolide classes have demonstrated unequivocal activity against isoniazid- and rifampicin-resistant mycobacteria. Rifamycin derivatives and phenazines are of potential interest.

Of the fluoroquinolones, *ofloxacin* (300–600 mg daily) has a definite but limited activity, though sparfloxacin may prove to be more effective. Of the phenazines, clofazimine has a bacteriostatic effect against *M. tuberculosis* and *M. avium*. The initial dose is 200 mg daily, increased according to tolerance to 400 mg daily. Doses larger than 100 mg should not be continued for more than 3 months. The skin and urine become reddish. *Rifapentin* is very effective but shows cross-resistance to rifampicin. *Rifabutin* may be beneficial for the treatment of *M. avium* infections and for this reason is often used in the compassionate care of *M. avium* disseminated infection in AIDS patients.[106]

Amikacin, an aminoglycoside, is a potent inhibitor of growth of *M. tuberculosis* in vitro. The dose is 15 mg/kg per day in two divided doses. It has the same toxicity as streptomycin.

The administration of the newer drugs is best guided by a specialist.

MANAGEMENT OF REACTIONS TO ANTITUBERCULOSIS DRUGS

These are important because they cause discomfort to patients and interrupt treatment.

Hypersensitivity (Allergic) Reactions

These rarely occur in the first week of treatment. They are most common in the second to fourth weeks. They are much less frequent with isoniazid, rifampicin and ethambutol than with streptomycin and thiacetazone. Very rarely patients become allergic to all three drugs in a regimen. Treatment should be stopped immediately unless the reaction is very mild.

There are various degrees of reaction:

- *Mild*: itching of the skin only; this is often the only sign of rifampicin allergy.
- *Moderate*: fever and rash. The rash is often mistaken for measles or scarlet fever. If severe the skin looks blistered and resembles urticaria.
- *Severe*: in addition to fever and rash there may be generalized swelling of lymph nodes, enlargement of liver and spleen, swelling round the eyes and swelling of the mucous membranes of the mouth and lips. High fever, a generalized blistering rash and ulceration of the mucous membranes of the mouth, genitals and eyes (Stevens–Johnson syndrome) may occur. This is a rare but dangerous reaction seen particularly to thiacetazone, and in patients with HIV infection. Very rarely there may be chronic eczema involving the limbs and occurring after the eighth week. This is almost always due to allergy to streptomycin.

Management

Immediate. If the only complaint is mild itching, treatment can usually be continued as the patient desensitizes him- or herself; give antihistamine drugs if available.

If there is *fever* and *rash*, stop all drugs and give an antihistamine drug if available.

If there is a *very severe reaction*, stop all drugs. Immediate treatment should be given with:

- hydrocortisone 200 mg i.v. or i.m. followed by:
- dexamethasone 4 mg i.v. or i.m. followed by:
- prednisolone 15 mg three times a day, reducing the dose gradually every 2 days according to the patient's response;
- i.v. fluids as required.

Desensitization is rarely required because another effective drug can be substituted. Desensitization is a tedious and complicated procedure.[107]

CHEMOTHERAPY FOR NEWLY DIAGNOSED PATIENTS

In the following paragraphs, the figures preceding the symbols of the drugs refer to the duration in months, e.g. 2EHR. The subscript indicates the degree of intermittency, e.g. H_2R_2 indicates that the drugs are given twice weekly.

National tuberculosis programme

If the country in which you are working has a national tuberculosis programme[108] the regimen or regimens it recommends should be used. In some programmes the regimens may be different for sputum-negative patients or for children.

If there is no national tuberculosis programme the regimen now recommended by the International Union Against Tuberculosis and Lung Disease (IUATLD) and approved by WHO should be used. It is a 6-month regimen, suitable for *countries with a low rate of initial drug resistance*:

- Isoniazid (H) plus rifampicin (R) plus pyrazinamide (Z) for the first 2 months followed by isoniazid and rifampicin for 4 months (see Table 57.6 for dosage). The shorthand form for this regimen is 2HRZ/4HR.

Give all three drugs together in a single dose daily, if possible on an empty stomach. In many countries combined preparations of rifampicin and isoniazid are available. There is now good evidence to suggest that 4 months of treatment is adequate in patients who are smear negative, whether their initial sputum cultures are positive or negative.[109]

A recent development is the *fixed dose combination* of isoniazid, rifampicin and pyrazinamide. Use of this modality simplifies the regimen. These drugs are effective and have been shown to have no greater degree of toxicity than single drug administration. They avoid the risk inherent in lapsing into monotherapy, which may result in the emergence of drug resistance, and minimize risks associated with prescription errors. A minor disadvantage is that having accustomed patients to one form of medication in the initial phase it is necessary to make an adjustment to a different formulation in the second phase.

Unfortunately fixed dose combination preparations have been marketed for which the biological availability of the drugs has been shown to be inadequate. *It is essential to use only those preparations for which biological studies have been carried out and have shown that serum drug concentrations are not altered by the combination.*[110]

The situation is further compounded by the fact that, worldwide, there are five different formulations of Rifater. For this reason consultation of the manufacturer's literature is advised. The same contraindications and warnings apply to fixed dose combinations as do to their individual constituents.

Four-drug regimen

In populations with a higher rate of initial drug resistance add a fourth drug for the first 2 months: either *streptomycin* (S) or *ethambutol* (E).

- Never give ethambutol 25 mg/kg for more than 2 months. If continued after that, lower the dose to 15 mg/kg.
- Avoid ethambutol in young children who may not tell you about losing their vision.

These regimens can then be written briefly as 2SHRZ/4HR or 2EHRZ/4HR. Each would give four drugs for the first 2 months. This would usually be effective even if the patient's tubercle bacilli were resistant to rifampicin as well as isoniazid. In some national tuberculosis control programmes in Africa one of the above is used as a *retreatment regimen*. The regimen is used for any patient who has missed more than a month of routine treatment.

Recommendations

The above regimens are recommended for both pulmonary and non-pulmonary tuberculosis in both adults and children. There are some minor modifications in tuberculosis meningitis (p. 984) and pericarditis (p. 990).

Supervision

If at all possible try to make sure that each dose is fully supervised, at least for the first 2 months. This may be done by a health worker at a clinic or even, if necessary, by a volunteer or member of the patient's family. In some countries it is felt that it can only be done effectively in a hospital, hostel[111] or hutted village for nomadic populations.[112] This aspect, which is so important to success, is discussed further on p. 1004.

Eight-month regimen

In several African countries with tuberculosis control programmes assisted by the IUATLD the routine treatment is an 8-month regimen as follows.

First 2 months:

1. Isoniazid, rifampicin and pyrazinamide as above, often given in hospital.
2. If you work in a country with a high rate of initial drug resistance, add a fourth drug, preferably ethambutol in Africa, in order to avoid the AIDS risk from streptomycin injections.

After the first 2 months follow this by *6 months* of:

1. Isoniazid plus thiacetazone (Tb1).
2. If the patient develops side-effects to Tb1, give isoniazid and ethambutol (15 mg/kg) or isoniazid alone to complete 8 months treatment.

This regimen is also recommended by WHO. It can be summarized as 2HRZ/6HT or 2EHRZ/6HT.

In the national control programmes in Africa where there was close supervision of the first 2 months of intensive treatment, 85% of patients treated with these regimens became sputum negative by 2 months and the rest in a further 2–3 weeks. In previous 1-year regimens without rifampicin or pyrazinamide only 50% were negative by 2 months.[111]

Intermittent or partly intermittent short-course regimens

It is essential to note that the dose of drugs used in an intermittent regimen is different from that used in daily treatment (see Table 57.6).

Alternatives to daily short course chemotherapy are as follows: $2HRZ/4H_3R_3$, $2HRZ/4H_2R_2$, $2E_3H_3R_3Z_3$ or $2S_3H_3R_3Z_3/4H_3R_3$. Ethambutol should be added to the first two of these regimens where there is a high incidence of initial drug resistance. These regimens should not be used unless there is a reasonable prospect of patient compliance. The danger of transmission of HIV infection by injections of streptomycin must also be considered.

Twelve-month regimens without rifampicin

These are summarized in Table 57.9 as some countries are still using them. WHO and the IUATLD now recommend that they cease to be used as soon as possible.

Table 57.9 Standard long-term regimens given for 8–12 months.

Initial phase*	Continuation phase†
2SHRZ	6HT
2SHRZ	$6S_2H_2Z_2$
2SHP	10HP
2SHT	10HT
2SHE	10HE
2SHR	7HR
2EHR	7HR
9HR	—
2SHP	$10H_2S_2$
2SHT	$10H_2S_2$
2HR	$10H_2S_2$

*1–3 months, usually in hospital.
†check Table 57.6 for intermittent dosage.
For definition of abbreviations see note on p. 1001.

Special situations

Renal failure

Treatment of patients with renal failure requires special care. Rifampicin and isoniazid are reasonably safe but special dosage is required for treatment with streptomycin and ethambutol.[113]

Liver impairment and liver failure

Many of the drugs are hepatotoxic. Rifampicin requires special attention. It has been shown that in patients with cirrhosis bilirubin concentrations exceeding $50\,\mu mol/l$ should be an indication for reduction in rifampicin dosage. Alcoholics, the elderly, malnourished children and children under 2 years of age handle rifampicin less efficiently and liver function tests should be monitored regularly in these patients as reduction in dosage may be required. There is no need to perform liver function tests in other patients.

Pregnancy

Streptomycin is potentially ototoxic to the fetus and may cause impairment of hearing. It should be avoided, as should capreomycin, kanamycin and viomycin. Ethionamide and prothionamide have been shown to be teratogenic and must not be used.

Some controversy surrounds the effect of rifampicin on the fetus. However, in a review[114] of the adverse effects in pregnancy it is stated: 'There is no evidence that the dosage of rifampicin used in clinical practice has a teratogenic effect.' The author agrees with the statement made by the Committee on Chemotherapy of Tuberculosis[115] that: 'the administration of these drugs (isoniazid, ethambutol and rifampicin) are not indications for therapeutic abortion.'

MANAGEMENT OF PATIENTS WITH DRUG-RESISTANT ORGANISMS

Patients may have infections with drug-resistant tubercle bacilli, either from initial infection or as a result of failure of chemotherapy, which is usually due to failure of compliance. As treatment of such patients is expensive and very difficult to treat even by specialized physicians, some national programmes have to regard these patients as untreatable.

It is only possible to set out general principles here.

In determining appropriate treatment of patients whose primary treatment has failed, the following principles are important in coming to a decision.

1. It is important to obtain as accurate a chemotherapy history as possible and try to assess the degree of compliance. This can be very difficult.
2. Where facilities exist, information regarding the resistance pattern is obviously important.
3. The 'reserve' drugs are costly, may not be obtainable locally and have unpleasant side-effects.
4. Treatment failure is often due to non-compliance and supervised regimens are to be preferred.
5. There is good evidence that three drugs—or even four—give better results than two.
6. The newer drugs, rifabutin and the oxyquinolones are very expensive and have only a limited place in treatment.
7. The duration of treatment should be 12 months after sputum has become smear negative.
8. If sensitivity tests are available, appropriate adjustment of treatment should be made.
9. Such problems are best handled by specialists, who often find them difficult themselves!

Detailed practical advice on the management of drug-resistant tuberculosis has been published.[116]

GENERAL MANAGEMENT

Rest

The vast majority of patients do not require rest and can continue at work.

Segregation

Patients become non-infectious within 2 weeks of treatment containing rifampicin and isoniazid[117] and sputum smear-positive patients require only 2 weeks segregation, with the possible exception of those dealing with children. Segregation is required in drug-resistant patients.

Hospitalization

The majority of patients can be managed as outpatients, the exceptions being severely ill patients, those with mechanical or investigative problems and those with severe drug reactions. A chest radiograph should be taken at the end of treatment, and sputum examination 2 months previously. However, in some developing countries the cure rate has been increased from approximately 45 to 80% by the provision of cheap inpatient facilities in hostel beds or in hutted camps, as in the Manyata project amongst the nomads in Kenya.[112]

Compliance

This can be considerably enhanced by a friendly, encouraging attitude of all staff in clinics, by careful and repeated explanation of what is required of the patient, by pill counts at each clinic visit, occasional urine testing for the presence of drugs and the enlistment of the help of relatives and friends. Other factors which influence compliance include anxiety about jobs, poverty, alcoholism, stigma of the disease and ignorance. Failure of treatment is not always the fault of the patient. The prescription of bad treatment is sometimes responsible. Doctors, nurses and health workers have crucial roles in obtaining maximum compliance.

An excellent account of the problems of compliance has been given by Fox.[102]

CHEMOPROPHYLAXIS

The administration of drugs to prevent the development of tuberculosis evolved following the discovery of a cheap very effective drug of relatively low toxicity, isoniazid. Chemoprophylaxis is generally subdivided into primary or infection prophylaxis, e.g. breast-fed infant of infectious mother, in which drugs are administered to persons believed to be uninfected with tubercle bacilli, and secondary or disease prophylaxis where drugs are given to individuals who are already infected in order to prevent the development of disease. Mass community prophylaxis is no longer thought to be appropriate. The effectiveness of isoniazid has been demonstrated in a number of controlled trials.[118] Recommendations regarding the groups of individuals who would benefit from prophylaxis would be straightforward were it not for the fact that isoniazid therapy is sometimes associated with hepatitis and that prolonged treatment is difficult to sustain, particularly in patients who believe themselves to be healthy.

At one time chemoprophylaxis was considered inadvisable for developing countries but the view has changed recently. For current practice the national treatment programme (if available) should be consulted. Guidelines for chemoprophylaxis in children are given by the British Thoracic Association.[119]

In developed countries individuals who should be considered for prophylaxis include:

- Tuberculin-positive children under 5 years of age because of their vulnerability to miliary disease and tuberculous meningitis.
- Individuals who have undergone recent tuberculin conversion.
- Breast-fed infants of sputum-positive mothers.
- Patients with certain clinical conditions in which tuberculosis is more likely to develop, e.g. HIV infection, Hodgkin's disease, asthma (prolonged treatment with prednisolone at a dose of 10 mg or more per day), leukaemia and those being treated with anticancer drugs.
- Household and other close contacts under 35 years of age of newly diagnosed sputum-positive patients, though some authorities prefer annual radiographic examination for 1–2 years.
- Immigrant children from countries where tuberculosis is common—grade 3 and 4 Heaf test reactors, whether or not previously vaccinated with BCG, and grade 2 reactors who have no evidence of previous vaccination.
- All tuberculin-positive reactors under 35 years old.

The latter is the most controversial indication and is applied with various degrees of fervour. It is not applied in the UK or Europe but published guidelines for preventive isoniazid therapy in the USA recommend its unrestricted use in tuberculin reactors below the age of 35 years.[120] This upper limit is chosen because the incidence of isoniazid-induced hepatitis rises appreciably above this age. Snider and Tabas[121] have reported a compilation of 177 deaths in the USA from isoniazid-associated hepatitis, a significant proportion of the mortality (46 of the deaths) occurring among persons less than 35 years of age. This has led Israel[122] from Philadelphia, USA to comment: 'other advanced countries should think twice before adopting the American practice of widespread preventive therapy lest they encounter more fatalities from the "friendly fire" of INH.'

In general, chemoprophylaxis is administered as isoniazid 5 mg/kg to a maximum of 300 mg in a single dose daily for a minimum of 6 months, though some authorities recommend a duration of 12 months. Isoniazid may not be effective in areas where there is a high incidence of primary drug resistance. Supplies of the drug should be issued monthly, enquiry being made at each visit regarding possible symptoms of hepatotoxicity. Methods of trying to ensure compliance are discussed on p. 1004. Some AIDS programmes advise administration of isoniazid alone to patients infected with HIV but without obvious tuberculosis. Further research is needed to evaluate this. Further research is also required regarding the efficacy of only three months chemoprophylaxis with rifampicin and isoniazid and rifampicin and pyrazinamide.[106] The shorter period would improve compliance. The debate as to how and when chemoprophylaxis is to be applied is likely to continue.

Patients with radiographic evidence of doubtfully active disease should be given standard treatment; chemoprophylaxis is inappropriate in such circumstances.

CORTICOSTEROIDS AND TUBERCULOSIS

Corticosteroids should never be used in the treatment of tuberculous patients unless effective chemotherapy is being given concurrently. The evolution of corticosteroid treatment in tuberculosis has been described by Horne,[123] and its current application has been reviewed by Alzeer and FitzGerald.[124]

The indications for steroid treatment are as follows:

- *Hypersensitivity reactions* to drugs, particularly if they are life threatening.
- *Life-threatening tuberculosis*. Few physicians would withhold steroid treatment from patients who seem to be in imminent danger of dying from the disease.
- Treatment of *pleural*, *pericardial* and *peritoneal* tuberculosis. *Pleural* effusions resolve more quickly and a single aspiration usually suffices.[125] Fibrothorax and chest deformity can be avoided. No advantage is to be gained by intrapleural injections. In *pericardial* effusions the fluid is more rapidly absorbed and the haemodynamic effects of the fluid controlled more quickly. Mortality is lower.[59] *Peritoneal* effusions absorb more rapidly and the serious complications of intestinal obstruction may be minimized.[126]
- *Pulmonary tuberculosis*. All investigators are agreed that the rate of clinical improvement and of radiographic clearing are hastened by steroid treatment but the advantages conferred are insufficient to warrant steroids in routine treatment.[127] The exception is the seriously ill patient.
- Several studies using both short-term and long-term end-points have shown that corticosteroids increase survival and reduce long-term sequelae in patients with *tuberculous meningitis*, although mortality and morbidity remain high.[128]
- *Renal tuberculosis*. Steroid treatment has a defi-

nite place in the management of acute cystitis and in ureteric obstruction.[55]

- *Lymph node tuberculosis*. The main indication is in the management of life-threatening enlargement of mediastinal nodes associated with tracheal obstruction, especially in children. Where there is a large abscess in the neck threatening skin necrosis, steroids may be of value in avoiding scarring and ugly sinuses.
- *HIV infection*. The use of steroids in patients who are already immunocompromised would seem illogical. However, a recent report described a dramatic response in an HIV-positive patient with continued hectic fever and weight loss despite being treated with drugs to which the tubercle bacilli were sensitive.[129] Attention has recently been drawn to the importance of considering the possibility of mineralocorticoid deficiency in patients with AIDS-related infections.[130]
- *Other conditions*:
  —destructive ocular lesions to preserve sight;
  —laryngeal lesions to ameliorate pain;
  —replacement therapy in Addison's disease;
  —life-threatening reaction to tuberculin.

DOSAGE

The recommended dose in the literature varies widely but the following seems to be a reasonable level:

- Moribund patients: hydrocortisone 100–200 mg i.v., repeated if necessary, plus steroids as below. Severely ill and meningitis: 60–80 mg orally daily (children 1–3 mg/kg).
  Other forms: 40 mg daily (children 1–3 mg/kg).
- Subsequent dosage: this should be tapered by 5 mg daily at weekly intervals, depending upon clinical progress, to a total of 12 weeks.

REACTIVATION OF TUBERCULOSIS DUE TO CORTICOSTEROID THERAPY

Long-term treatment with steroids may allow 'persistent' mycobacteria to multiply and cause pulmon-
ary or disseminated disease. The classical features of progressive tuberculosis may mimic the disease for which steroids have been prescribed. Death from unsuspected tuberculosis in immunosuppressed patients is not uncommon.[131] Patients at risk may suffer from conditions such as polymyalgia rheumatica, temporal arteritis, systemic lupus erythematosus, chronic active hepatitis, rheumatoid arthritis, haemodialysis, renal transplantation, lymphoma, various cancers and, rarely, asthma in dosage in excess of 10 mg daily. A high degree of suspicion of the development of tuberculosis in such patients is essential. Chemoprophylaxis should be considered.

SURGICAL TREATMENT

At the present time there are few indications for surgical treatment.

In pulmonary disease surgical resection requires consideration and may be desirable if there is no contraindication, such as impaired ventilatory function, in the following circumstances:

- Uncooperative patients.
- When drug resistance exists and there is intolerance to all drugs.
- When there are recurrent infections and life-threatening haemoptysis even though sputum negativity has been obtained.
- Mycetoma associated with *Aspergillus fumigatus*.
- In primary tuberculosis, as an emergency when mediastinal nodes obstruct the trachea.
- Empyema.
- When difficulty is encountered in differentiating tumour from tuberculosis.
- Rarely in infections due to mycobacteria other than tubercle bacilli.

Surgical treatment for extrapulmonary disease is discussed under the appropriate heading.

TUBERCULOSIS CONTROL PROGRAMMES

By far the most important control measure is *good case finding*, especially of smear-positive individuals combined with *good chemotherapy*, preferably with short-course regimens. This has a substantial impact on the chain of transmission. By comparison the
effect of BCG in preventing smear-positive cases in developing countries is between 0.3 and 2.0% per year.[132] Bad or inadequate chemotherapy will greatly increase the prevalence of acquired and primary drug resistance and may result in a tubercu-

Table 57.10 Major control measures in tuberculosis.

Control measure	Method	Comment
Bovine	Tuberculosis-free herds	Infection from other animals rare
	Pasteurization of milk	
Human		
Case-finding	Bacteriological examination	Especially sputum smears; other excreta of little epidemiological importance
	Radiographic examination	Mass radiography; selective radiography (see Table 57.11)
	Examination of contacts	Especially those of smear-positive patients
	Treatment and isolation	—
	Tuberculin testing of children	—
	Examination of immigrants	—
	General medical services	Identify half or more of notified cases
Increasing host defences	BCG vaccination	—
	Improvement in socioeconomic conditions	
Interruption of progression of infection to disease	Chemoprophylaxis	Treatment or surveillance of 'inactive' or untreated pulmonary lesions

losis problem uncontrollable by current methods of treatment. The quality of treatment programmes is thus of the utmost importance. In a study of treatment programmes in Taiwan, Korea, South India and Kenya, quiescence of the disease at 1 or 2 years was achieved in only about 60–65% of all patients under treatment. Deaths numbered 10–16% and chronic bacillary excretors remained high at approximately 25%.[133] In some programmes the success rate achieved by routine treatment services with regimens which are theoretically 100% effective have fallen to levels of the order of 50%. In Tanzania this proportion was increased to about 80% in patients who were 'hospitalized' for the initial 2 months.[111] The situation in sub-Saharan Africa is extremely grave, where for instance 40% of AIDS patients suffer from tuberculosis.[134] Augmentation of case finding in developing countries may be achieved by promoting greater awareness about the problem amongst health professionals, house-to-house surveys by health workers on a single occasion of suspects with recurrent symptoms, interrogation of village elders regarding suspects, and questioning of mothers in maternity hospitals regarding household members who have relevant symptoms.

Sophisticated measures for tuberculosis control are often difficult to undertake in developing countries. Excellent detailed accounts of control measures applicable to developed countries have been published for Britain[135] and the USA.[136] The major control measures are shown in Tables 57.10 and 57.11. The possibility of the recurrence of microepidemics must be borne in mind.[137]

CONTACT EXAMINATION

Contact examination can be summarized as follows. Maximum notification is essential[138] and information from bacteriologists and pathologists as well as physicians and surgeons should be sought. In one

Table 57.11 Selective radiography.

- Selective radiography
  High yield groups:
      General practitioner referrals
      Detainees in prisons and borstals
      Patients in hospitals for the mentally ill
      Contacts of infectious cases
      Inhabitants of lodging houses
      Immigrants
      Men over 45 years
  Danger groups:
      Persons working with children
      Doctors, dentists, nurses, medical auxiliaries
      Persons in service industries, e.g. barmen, waitresses
- Surveys of special groups, e.g. in miniepidemics[137] in schools and nursing homes

series 14% of sputum smear-positive and 27% of all cases were not notified.[139] In most reports 10–14% of all notifications have been detected by contact screening, contacts being 10–60 times more likely to have the disease than the general population.

Close contacts (defined as those who share a household with the infectious patient and others judged to have had an important degree of contact) are investigated by inquiry into BCG vaccination status, tuberculin testing and chest radiography. Those who are tuberculin negative should be retested in 8 weeks and, if still negative, given BCG if under 35 years of age or at special risk. Chemoprophylaxis should be given to tuberculin-positive children under 16 years and Asians and others from high prevalence areas under 35 years. Follow-up examination should be carried out at 1 year except in persons originating from high prevalence areas, when surveillance should be continued for 2 years. Special attention should be given to immigrants from high prevalence areas: BCG should be given at birth to immigrant children. Casual contacts do not normally require follow-up examination. Contact examination of contacts of extrapulmonary disease is unproductive.[140] Departure from standard contact procedures are not recommended but much unnecessary screening can be avoided if a rational approach is adopted.[141] A comparison of diagnostic tools and their case-finding applicability is shown in Table 57.12.

The impact of HIV-associated tuberculosis on resource-poor countries has ominous social and medical implications. In order to respond to this urgent problem the highest priority must be given to strengthening national control programmes in high-prevalence countries. The cure rate must be significantly improved by early diagnosis and treatment of the largest possible number of patients. Two other major strategies which need consideration include BCG vaccination, which has been proved safe,[142] and preventive chemotherapy for HIV-infected individuals. However, a number of issues have to be addressed before the latter intervention can be implemented in developing countries.

BCG (BACILLE CALMETTE–GUÉRIN) VACCINE

Vaccination against tuberculosis currently consists of the intracutaneous injection of BCG vaccine. This organism is named after two French investigators responsible for its development from an attenuated strain of *M. bovis* early this century. It was first used in an oral form in Paris in 1921.[143] It is an important component of tuberculous control programmes. Its purpose is to replace virulent natural infection with avirulent BCG organisms and thus to prepare the body defences. It does not prevent infection but limits multiplication and dissemination of mycobacteria following infection.[144]

THE VACCINE

BCG vaccine (intradermal) is supplied in the form of multidose ampoules containing a white freeze-dried plug which on reconstitution disperses to form an opalescent liquid. It is reconstituted with 1 ml of distilled water. The reconstituted vaccine should be allowed to stand for 1 minute, must not be shaken and not allowed to stand in sunlight. It should be used within 4 hours.

BCG (percutaneous) contains many more viable bacilli and must not be used for intradermal injection. *Isoniazid-resistant BCG* is available for infants where separation from the mother is inadvisable. Isoniazid should be given for 6 weeks.

METHODS OF VACCINATION

The intradermal method is most widely used. Strict attention to sterile technique is essential, and antiseptics and detergents should not be used to clean the skin. In adults 0.1 ml and in neonates 0.05 ml of vaccine is injected intradermally into the upper arm at the junction of the upper and middle thirds. A satisfactory vaccination raises a weal of 5 mm or more. No dressing is required. A small papule develops in 14–21 days. A shallow ulcer may form. Healing usually occurs in 6–12 weeks. A simple dry gauze dressing may be required if a persistent ulcer forms; the ulcer heals following the local application of isoniazid or erythromycin.[145] Multiple-puncture vaccination with percutaneous vaccine gives a very high tuberculosis conversion rate. No untoward reaction occurs if tuberculin-positive individuals are vaccinated.

PRECAUTIONS AND CONTRAINDICATIONS

Vaccination must be avoided in any conditions where immunological deficiency exists or if corticosteroid treatment is being given. It is thus contraindicated in well-developed AIDS. The situation in respect of HIV infection is discussed on p. 994. Diffuse eczema and infected dermatoses are contraindications. BCG should be temporarily withheld in tuberculin-negative contacts as they may be in the preallergic state.

BCG is a live vaccine and should not be adminis-

Table 57.12 Comparison of diagnostic tools and their case-finding applicability.

Diagnostic tool	Advantages	Disadvantages	Sensitivity*	Specificity*	Cost	General
Tuberculin test	1. Is simple to organize. 2. Can be administered to large numbers at a single session	1. Needs expertise to administer and read the test properly 2. Applicable only to non-BCG vaccinated persons 3. Results not available until after 72 hours	High	Low	Low	Only useful for epidemiological work†
Radiology	1. Comparatively simple to take and not messy 2. Result available same day or next day 3. Gives a visual impression and a record for future comparison	1. Very expensive to install equipment and difficult to maintain 2. Needs well-trained technicians and very experienced interpreters 3. Radiographic reading shows much inter- and intraindividual variation 4. Needs large numbers to examine to justify cost: therefore is only suitable for urban areas	High	Low	High	Can be used for diagnosis and as a screening tool for selecting persons to be examined bacteriologically
Sputum microscopy	1. Can be installed easily and inexpensively 2. Procedure is simple, practical and highly applicable 3. Can be installed even in rural areas 4. Result is specific 5. Result is available while the patient waits and treatment can be started there and then	1. Sputum collection and smear preparation may be regarded as 'messy' 2. Patient may have no sputum or may not produce a good specimen	Moderate	Moderate	Low	Is an ideal diagnostic tool in 'passive' case finding and for use after radiological examination of patients with abnormal chest radiograph shadows
Sputum culture	1. Can pick out early infectious cases 2. Drug sensitivity of the bacilli can be determined 3. Result highly specific	1. Is very expensive to install and maintain 2. Is so complicated that only a few centres can do it 3. Needs high degree of training 4. Result not available until after 4 weeks‡	High	Very high	High	Is useful mainly for specialized needs, case finding in countries with a low prevalence of the disease and community drug-resistance studies

*The comparison is based on studies on 'symptomatics' attending health institutions in a high-prevalence country.
†It can also be valuable in diagnostic work.
‡Results can be obtained earlier nowadays.
Reproduced with permission from *Tuberculosis Control*. Pan American Health Organisation, 1986.

tered at the same time as yellow fever, measles, rubella, mumps and smallpox vaccines. At least 3 weeks should elapse between BCG vaccine and these vaccines, and no vaccination or inoculation should be given in the same arm for 4 months.

COMPLICATIONS

Reference has already been made to local abscess formation. Suppurative lymphadenitis is usually due to faulty technique, is more common in infants and in individuals with HIV infection. Surgical excision is rarely required. Keloid formation is more common in Israelis, Asians and Africans. Lupus vulgaris at the site of vaccination is rare, as is erythema nodosum. Osteitis has been reported in Scandinavian children almost exclusively and usually manifests itself about a year after vaccination.[146] Death from disseminated BCG, which may be fatal, is exceedingly rare and is usually seen in those with immunological disorders.

EFFICACY OF VACCINE

The initial reaction to the use of BCG was scepticism, but in recent years scepticism has given way to controversy.

The protection afforded by BCG in various populations has shown enormous variation. In England and Wales the protection afforded to 14-year-old children was high (77%)[147] whereas in Puerto Rico[148] and Georgia and Alabama[149] it was low (29 and 6% respectively). In Chingleput, South India[150] no protection was demonstrated, but this trial failed to obtain evidence of the possible benefit of BCG given to children. Several recently conducted case–control studies have confirmed the protection given to children, especially in the prevention of meningitis. BCG is protective against meningitis in developed countries.[151] Discussion continues as to whether the differences in level of protection are due to differences in the strains of vaccine used, the high prevalence of possible protection by opportunistic mycobacterial sensitization in some areas, faulty study design or severe malnutrition.

POLICY AND PRACTICE

The policy which is adopted is different in developing and industrially advanced communities.

In developing countries, despite conflicting evidence of its efficacy, BCG is recommended by WHO to be given to all newly born children as early in life as possible, including when the mother is known to be or suspected of being HIV infected.[152] BCG should be withheld from individuals with symptomatic HIV infection. In some areas serious consideration is given to revaccination on entering school or leaving school, without prior tuberculin testing. The relevant national tuberculosis programme should be consulted in this context.

The coverage of BCG in developed countries varies from considerable to minimal and selective. In Britain the evidence that BCG protects against tuberculosis is conclusive. A large randomized controlled trial of BCG in 14-year-olds, started in 1950, showed protective efficacy averaging 77% over 20 years of follow-up. Since 1953 schoolchildren have routinely received BCG at the age of about 13 years and retrospective cohort analyses in 1973, 1978 and 1983 showed an efficacy of about 75% throughout the period.[153] A decision to abandon this policy has been shelved pending further assessment of the epidemiological situation, with special reference to HIV infection. Compulsory vaccination of neonates has been abandoned in Sweden and Czechoslovakia.

There are some specific indications for BCG vaccination which are independent of the local epidemiological situations:

- Newborn and young children in immigrant communities originating from countries with a high incidence of tuberculosis, e.g. Asians in Britain and Haitians in USA.
- Health workers, including students and nurses.
- Close contacts of infectious patients.
- Persons, especially children, proceeding to areas of the world where prevalence remains high.

It has been suggested that immunotherapy with *Myobacterium vaccae* may improve the results of treatment.[154] Properly controlled trials will be required to establish whether it is effective or not.

TUBERCULIN TESTING

When tuberculin is injected into the skin of an infected person a delayed local reaction develops in 24–48 hours. The response may be suppressed by a number of conditions, e.g. malnutrition, viral infections, HIV, measles, chickenpox, glandular fever, cancer, severe infections (including tuberculosis), sarcoidosis, chronic renal failure and the presence of corticosteroids and anticancer drugs. False results may be due to faulty storage of the material or faulty technique.

Two types of tuberculin are available: PPD-S and PPD-RT23, which is commonly used in survey work. The strength of PPD is expressed in international units (iu). *Undiluted tuberculin is for use only in the Heaf test.*

MANTOUX TEST

In diagnostic work, if tuberculosis is suspected it is best to begin with 5 iu. The same dose can be used for survey work. A strictly intracutaneous injection of 0.1 ml of the appropriate tuberculin solution is made in the skin of the volar or dorsal aspect of the forearm using a no. 25 or 26 needle. Do not clean the arm with acetone or ether. A weal about 7 mm in diameter is raised. The test should be read after 72 hours. If the individual is a positive reactor an area of induration surrounded by erythema will develop. The transverse diameter of the palpable induration should be measured and recorded, e.g. Mantoux 12 mm, the area of erythema being disregarded. A reaction of 10 mm or more to 5 iu PPD-S or 1 iu PPD-RT23 is usually regarded as positive. A negative test does not exclude tuberculosis as a number of conditions suppress the response.

HEAF TEST

The Heaf gun which is used in this test consists of six spring-loaded needles which, when fired, pierce the skin through a drop of undiluted PPD. The 'magnetic' type of gun is the best to use.

Using a dropper place a drop of undiluted PPD on the volar aspect of the forearm. The length of the needles should be adjusted (2 mm for adults, 1 mm for children) and the end-plate and needles dipped into a shallow dish containing spirit, which should then be ignited. Cool for not less than 10 seconds as burns have been misinterpreted as positive tests.

Then place the end-plate firmly over the drop of tuberculin and depress the handle of the gun.

The test should be read at 48–72 hours, though a strong reaction will still be visible at 7 days. Record the result according to the following criteria:

Grade 0   No reaction
Grade I   Palpable induration around at least four points
Grade II   Papules have formed a ring
Grade III A solid area of induration has been formed
Grade IV   There are shiny vesicles over the solid area

Grades III and IV are regarded as definitely positive, grade II probably so.

In survey work using the Mantoux test the criteria for a positive reaction will be determined by the national tuberculosis programme. In diagnostic work a diameter of less than 10 mm is usually regarded as negative, though this does not exclude tuberculosis because of the several conditions which may suppress the response. A diameter of over 15 mm in a child who has had BCG is regarded as positive and probably indicates that the child has been infected with tubercle bacilli. A 'positive' test does not necessarily indicate that disease is present.

REFERENCES

1 Morse D, Brothwell D R & Ucko P J. Tuberculosis in ancient Egypt. *Am Rev Resp Dis* 1964; 93:524–530.

2 Kochi A. The global situation and the new control strategy of the World Health Organization. *Tubercle* 1991; 72:1–6.

3 Narain J P, Raviglione M C & Kochi A. HIV-associated tuberculosis in developing countries: epidemiology and strategies for prevention. *Tuberc Lung Dis* 1992; 73:311–321.

4 Bignall J R. Failure to control tuberculosis: a personal view. *Bull Int Union Tuberc* 1982; 57:122–125.

5 Murray C J L. Social, economic and operational research on tuberculosis: recent studies and some priority questions. *Bull Int Union Tuberc Lung Dis* 1991; 66:149–156.

6 Horne N W. Eradication of tuberculosis in Europe: so near and yet so far. *Eur J Resp Dis* 1983; supplement 126:169–173.

7 World Health Organization Office of Information. *Tuberculosis Notification Rates in Industrialized Countries*. Press Release WHO/40, 17 June 1992.

8 Medical Research Council Cardiothoracic Epidemiology Group. National survey of notifications of tuberculosis in England and Wales. *Thorax* 1992; 47:770–775.

9 Chawla P K, Clapper P J, Kamholz S L et al. Drug-resistant tuberculosis in an urban population including patients at risk from human immunodeficiency virus. *Am Rev Resp Dis* 1992; 146:260–284.

10 Freiden T R, Sterling T, Pablos-Mendez A et al. The emergence of drug-resistant tuberculosis in New York City. *N Engl J Med* 1993; 328:521–526.

11 Grzybowski S. Tuberculosis in the third world. *Thorax* 1991; 46:689–691.

12 Stanford J, Grange J M & Pozniak A. Is Africa lost? *Lancet* 1991; 338:557–558.

13 Styblo K. *Epidemiology of Tuberculosis*. Selected Papers, 24. Royal Netherlands Tuberculosis Association, The Hague, The Netherlands, 1991, pp 1–117.

14 Grange J M. The mystery of the mycobacterial 'persister'. *Tuberc Lung Dis* 1992; 73:249–251.

15 Heifets L, Iseman M & Lindholm-Levy P. Application of rapid methods (BACTEC system) in

clinical mycobacteriology and in the search for new drugs. *Bull Int Union Tuberc Lung Dis* 1988; 63:19.

16 Spence D P S, Williams C S D, Hotchkiss J A & Davies P D O. Tuberculosis and poverty. *Thorax* 1992; 47:849P (abstract).

17 Strom L. A study of the cutaneous absorption of BCG vaccine labelled with phosphate in subjects with or without immunity. *Acta Tuberc Scand* 1955; 31:141–145.

18 Wallgren A. The timetable of tuberculosis. *Tubercle* 1948; 29:245–251.

19 Medical Research Council. BCG and vole bacillus in the prevention of tuberculosis in adolescence and early adult life. *Bull World Health Organ* 1972; 46:371–381.

20 Crofton J, Horne N & Miller F. *Clinical Tuberculosis*. London: Macmillan, 1992: 80–82.

21 Snider D E, Jones W D & Good R C. The epidemiological usefulness of phage-typing *Myco. tuberculosis*. *Am Rev Resp Dis* 1984; 130:1095–1099.

22 Macfarlane J T, Ibrahim M & Tor-Agbidye S. The importance of finger-clubbing in pulmonary tuberculosis. *Tubercle* 1979; 60:45–48.

23 International Union Against Tuberculosis and Lung Disease. *Technical Guide for Sputum Examination for Tuberculosis by Direct Microscopy*. Paris: IUATLD, 1978.

24 Neff T A. Bronchoscopy and Bactec for the diagnosis of tuberculosis. *Am Rev Resp Dis* 1984; 133:962–966.

25 Stenson W, Aranda C & Bevelaqua F A. Transbronchial biopsy culture in pulmonary tuberculosis. *Chest* 1983; 83:883–885.

26 Sarkar, S K, Sharma T N, Purohit S D et al. The diagnostic value of routine culture of bronchial washings in tuberculosis. *Br J Dis Chest* 1982; 76:358–361.

27 Maher J, Kelly P, Hughes P & Clancy L. Skin anergy and tuberculosis. *Resp Med* 1992; 86:481–484.

28 Ip M S M, Yo S Y, Lam W K et al. Endobronchial tuberculosis revisited. *Chest* 1986; 89:727–730.

29 Van den Brande P, Lambrechts M, Tack J et al. Endobronchial tuberculosis mimicking lung cancer in elderly patients. *Resp Med* 1991; 85:107–109.

30 Maartens G & Bateman E D. Tuberculous pleural effusions: increased culture yield with bedside inoculation of pleural fluid and poor diagnostic value of adenosine deaminase. *Thorax* 1991; 46:96–99.

31 Mungal I P F, Cowan P N, Cooke N T et al. Multiple pleural biopsy with the Abrams needle. *Thorax* 1980; 35:600–603.

32 Abrams L D. A pleural biopsy punch. *Lancet* 1958; i:30–32.

33 Prout S & Benatar R. Disseminated tuberculosis: a study of 62 cases. *S Afr Med J* 1980; 58:835–842.

34 Debré R. Miliary tuberculosis in children. *Lancet* 1952; ii:545–549.

35 Proudfoot A T, Akhtar A J, Douglas A C et al. Miliary tuberculosis in adults. *BMJ* 1969; ii:273–276.

36 Illingworth R S & Lorber J. Tubercles of the choroid. *Arch Dis Child* 1956; 31:467–470.

37 Berenguer J, Moreno S, Laguna F et al. Tuberculous meningitis in patients infected with the human immunodeficiency virus. *N Engl J Med* 1992; 326:668–672.

38 Humphries M. The management of tuberculous meningitis. *Thorax* 1992; 47:577–581.

39 Editorial. Scrofula today. *Lancet* 1983; i:335–336.

40 British Thoracic Research Committee. Short course chemotherapy for tuberculosis of lymph nodes: final report at 5 years. *Br J Dis Chest* 1988; 82:282–284.

41 Ormerod L P on behalf of British Thoracic Society Research Committee. Six months versus nine months chemotherapy for tuberculosis of the lymph nodes: final results. *Thorax* 1993; 48:423 (abstract).

42 Editorial. The treatment of superficial tuberculous lymphadenitis. *Tubercle* 1990; 71:1–3.

43 White M P, Bangash H, Goel K M & Jenkins P A. Non-tuberculous mycobacterial lymphadenitis. *Arch Dis Child* 1986; 61:368–371.

44 Lambrianides A L, Ackroyd N & Shorey B A. Abdominal tuberculosis. *Br J Surg* 1980; 67:39–57.

45 Wells A D, Northover J M A & Howard E R. Abdominal tuberculosis: still a problem today. *J R Soc Med* 1986; 79:151–153.

46 Walker C F. Failure of early recognition of skeletal tuberculosis. *BMJ* 1968; i:682–684.

47 Medical Research Council. Five year assessment of controlled trials of ambulatory treatment, debridement and anterior spinal fusion in the management of tuberculosis of the spine. *J Bone Joint Surg [Br]* 1978; 60:163–170.

48 Hodgson A R & Stock F E. Anterior spinal fusion. *Br J Surg* 1956; 44:266–271.

49 Karlen A. On cystic tuberculosis of bone. *Acta Scand Orthop* 1960; 31:163–167.

50 Ustvedt H J. Tuberculosis of the kidney. *Nord Med* 1946; 31:1755–1758.

51 Ormerod L P. Why does genitourinary tuberculosis occur proportionately less than expected in the Indian subcontinent ethnic population in the United Kingdom. *Thorax* 1992; 48:876P (abstract).

52 Chowdhury B K. Hypertension as a presenting feature of renal tuberculosis. *J Urol* 1974; 111:282–283.

53 Wisnia L G, Kukolj S, Lopez de Santa Mario J et al. Renal function damage in 131 cases of urogenital tuberculosis. *Urology* 1978; 11:457–461.

54 Weinstein A J. Genito-urinary tuberculosis. In Schlossberg D (ed.) *Tuberculosis*, 2nd edn. New York: Springer, 1988:110–112.

55 Horne N W & Tulloch W S. Conservative management of renal tuberculosis. *Br J Urol* 1975; 47:481–487.

56 Sole-Balcells E, Jimenez-Cruz F, Saenz de Cabezon J et al. Tuberculosis and infertility in men. *Eur Urol* 1977; 3:129–131.

57 Lattimer J K. Renal tuberculosis. *N Engl J Med* 1965; 273:208–311.

58 Berger M, Bobak L, Jelvah M et al. Pericardial effusion diagnosed by echocardiography. *Chest* 1978; 72:1744–1749.

59 Strang J I G, Kakaza H H S, Gibson D G et al. Controlled trial of prednisolone as adjuvant treatment of tuberculous constrictive pericarditis in Transkei. *Lancet* 1987; ii:1418–1422.

60 Crocco J A. Cardiovascular tuberculosis. In Schlossberg D (ed.) *Tuberculosis*, 2nd edn. New York: Springer, 1988: 133–137.

61 Beyt B E Jr, Ortbals D W, Santa Cruz D J et al. Cutaneous mycobacteriosis: analysis of 34 cases with a new classification of the disease. *Medicine* 1981; 60:95–99.

62 Hoyt E M. Primary inoculation tuberculosis. *JAMA* 1981; 245:1556–1561.

63 Uganda Buruli Group. Clinical features and treatment of pre-ulcerative Buruli lesions (*Mycobacterium ulcerans* infection). *BMJ* 1970; ii:390–393.

64 Radford A J. *Mycobacterium ulcerans* in Australia. *Aust N Z J Med* 1975; 5:162–169.

65 Abrams A B & Schlaetal T F. The role of the isoniazid therapeutic test in tuberculous uveitis. *Am J Ophthalmol* 1982; 94:511–515.

66 Rao S, Rau P V P, Sahoo R C et al. Primary nasal tuberculosis. *Tuberc Lung Dis* 1992; 73:305.

67 Hunter A M, Millar J W, Wightman A J A et al. The changing pattern of laryngeal tuberculosis. *J Laryngol Otol* 1981; 95:393–398.

68 Arnstein A R. Endocrine and metabolic aspects of tuberculosis. In Schlossberg D (ed.) *Tuberculosis* 2nd edn. New York: Springer, 1988:193–194.

69 Vaishnar P & Mathuswary P. Tuberculosis of the breast. *Am Rev Resp Dis* 1982; 125(S):181.

70 Emery P. Tuberculous abscess of the thyroid with recurrent nerve palsy. Case report and review of the literature. *J Laryngol Otol* 1980; 94:553–558.

71 Lewis J H & Zimmerman H J. Tuberculosis of the liver and biliary tract. In Schlossberg D (ed.) *Tuberculosis*, 2nd edn. New York: Springer, 1988:149–169.

72 Styblo K. The global aspects of tuberculosis and HIV infection. *Bull Int Union Tuberc Lung Dis* 1990; 65:28–32.

73 Nisar M, Narula M, Beeching N et al. HIV-related tuberculosis in England and Wales. *Tuberc Lung Dis* 1992; 73:200–202.

74 Schulzer M, FitzGerald J M, Enarson D A et al. An estimate of the future size of the tuberculosis problem in sub-Saharan Africa resulting from HIV infection. *Tuberc Lung Dis* 1992; 73:52–58.

75 Perronne A, Ghoubontni A, Leport C et al. Should pulmonary tuberculosis be an AIDS-defining diagnosis in patients infected with HIV? *Tuberc Lung Dis* 1992; 73:39–44.

76 Kenya/British Medical Research Council Co-operative Investigation. Tuberculosis in Kenya 1984; a third national survey and a comparison with earlier surveys in 1964 and 1974. *Tubercle* 1989; 56:269–294.

77 Tanzanian/British Medical Research Council Collaborative Study. Tuberculosis in Tanzania: a national survey of newly notified cases. *Tubercle* 1985; 66:161–178.

78 Cathebras P, Vohito J A, Yeta M L et al. HIV infection among patients in Bangui (Central African Republic): a prospective study. XIIth International Congress for Tropical Medicine and Malaria. *Int Congress Ser* 1988; 810:66

79 Nambuya A, Sewankambo N, Mugerwa J et al. Tuberculous lymphadenitis associated with human immunodeficiency virus (HIV) in Uganda. *J Clin Pathol* 1988; 41:93–96.

80 Reichman L B. HIV infection: a new face of tuberculosis. *Bull Int Union Tuberc Lung Dis* 1988; 63:19–24.

81 *WHO AIDS Series No. 2*. Geneva: WHO, 1988.

82 World Health Organization. Special programme on AIDS and expanded programme on immunization. Joint statement: consultation on human immunodeficiency virus (HIV) and routine childhood immunization. *Weekly Epidemiol Rec* 1987; 62:297–309.

83 Department of Health, Welsh Office, Scottish Home and Health Department. *Immunisation Against Infectious Disease*. London: HMSO, 1990:72–89.

84 Harries A D. Tuberculosis and human immunodeficiency virus infection in developing countries. *Lancet* 1990; i:387–390.

85 Runyon E F. Anonymous mycobacteria in pulmonary disease. *Med Clin N Am* 1959; 43:273–290.

86 Yeager H Jr. Clinical syndromes and diagnosis of tuberculous ('atypical') mycobacterial infection. In Schlossberg D (ed.) *Tuberculosis*, 2nd edn. New York: Springer, 1988:202–211.

87 Papillon F, Huchon G, Labrune G et al. Non-tuberculous mycobacterial diseases of the lung in a pulmonology department. *Bull Int Union Tuberc Lung Dis* 1988; 63:17–19.

88 Lincoln E M & Gilbert L A. Disease in children due to mycobacteria other than *M. tuberculosis*. *Am Rev Respir Dis* 1972; 105:683–714.

89 Hsu K H K. Atypical mycobacterial infections in children. *Rev Infect Dis* 1981; 3:1075–1080.

90 Philpott J A Jr, Woodborne A R, Philpott O S et al. Swimming pool granuloma. A study of 290 cases. *Arch Dermatol* 1963; 88:158–162.

91 Adams R M, Remington J S, Steinberg J *et al*. Tropical fish aquariums: a source of *Mycobacterium marinum* infections resembling sporotrichosis. *JAMA* 1970; 211:457–461.

92 Kelly D H, Weed L A & Lipscomb R P. Infections of tendon sheaths, bursae, joints and soft tissues by acid fast bacilli other than tubercle bacilli. *J Bone Joint Surg* 1963; 45:1521–1530.

93 de Haler R, Fritsch D & Kobel T. Infections due to

Mycobacteria chelonei. Bull Int Union Tuberc Lung Dis 1988; 63:23.

94   Banks J, Hunter A M, Campbell I A et al. Pulmonary infection with *Mycobacteria kansasii* in Wales 1970–79; review of treatment and response. *Thorax* 1983; 38:271–274.

95   Campbell I A for BTS Research Committee. BTS Study of the treatment of *M. kansasii* pulmonary disease. *Thorax* 1993; 48:423 (abstract).

96   Wallace R J Jr, Swenson J M, Silcox V A et al. Treatment of non-pulmonary infections due to *Mycobacterium fortuitum* and *Mycobacterium chelonei* on basis of in vitro susceptibilities. *J Infect Dis* 1985; 152:500–514.

97   American Thoracic Society. Diagnosis and treatment of disease caused by non-tuberculous mycobacteria. *Am Rev Resp Dis* 1990; 142:940–952.

98   Fox W. Short course chemotherapy for tuberculosis. In Flenley D C (ed.) *Recent Advances in Respiratory Medicine 2*. Edinburgh: Churchill Livingstone, 1980:197–199.

99   Fox W. Short course chemotherapy for tuberculosis. In Flenley D C (ed.) *Recent Advances in Respiratory Medicine 2*. Edinburgh: Churchill Livingstone, 1980:183–203.

100   Crofton J. 'Sputum conversion' and the metabolism of isoniazid. *Am Rev Tuberc Resp Dis* 1958; 77:869–870.

101   Ross J D, Horne N W, Grant I W B et al. Hospital treatment of pulmonary tuberculosis. A follow up study of patients admitted to Edinburgh hospitals in 1953. *BMJ* 1953; 1:237–240.

102   Fox W. Compliance of patients and physicians: experience and lessons from tuberculosis. *BMJ* 1983; 287:33–36, 101–103.

103   Horne N W. *Modern Drug Treatment of Tuberculosis*, 7th edn. London: Chest, Heart and Stroke Association, 1990.

104   Crofton J, Horne N W & Miller F. *Clinical Tuberculosis*. London: Macmillan, 1992.

105   Committee on Treatment of the International Union Against Tuberculosis and Lung Disease. Anti-tuberculosis regimens of chemotherapy. *Bull Int Union Tuberc Lung Dis* 1988; 63:60–64.

106   Grosset J. Present and new drug regimens in chemotherapy and chemoprophylaxis of tuberculosis. *Bull Int Union Tuberc Lung Dis* 1990; 65:86–91.

107   Horne N W. *Modern Drug Treatment of Tuberculosis*, 7th edn. London: Chest, Heart and Stroke Association, 1990:32–35.

108   International Union Against Tuberculosis and Lung Disease. *Tuberculosis Guide for High Prevalence Countries*, 2nd edn. Paris: IUATLD, 43–47.

109   Hong Kong Chest Service/Tuberculosis Research Council Madras/British Medical Research Council. A controlled trial of 3-month, 4-month and 6-month regimens of chemotherapy for sputum smear negative pulmonary tuberculosis. *Am Rev Resp Dis* 1989; 139:871–876.

110   Acocella G. The use of fixed dose combinations in anti-tuberculosis chemotherapy. Rationale for their application in daily, intermittent and paediatric regimens. *Bull Int Union Tuberc Lung Dis* 1990; 65:77–83.

111   Chum H J. The Tanzania National Tuberculosis/Leprosy Programme in the face of HIV infection. *Bull Int Union Tuberc Lung Dis* 1990/1991; 66 (supplement): 53–55.

112   Idukitta G O & Bosman M C J. The tuberculosis manyatta project for Kenya nomads. *Bull Int Union Tuberc Lung Dis* 1989; 64:44–47.

113   Horne N W. *Modern Drug Treatment in Tuberculosis*, 7th edn. London: Chest, Heart and Stroke Association, 1990:46–47.

114   Girling D K & Hitze K. Adverse effects of rifampicin. *Bull World Health Organ* 1979; 57:45–49.

115   Committee on Chemotherapy of Tuberculosis. Standard therapy for tuberculosis 1985. *Chest* 1985; 87 (supplement 2):117S.

116   Crofton J. The prevention and management of drug resistant tuberculosis. *Bull Int Union Tuberc* 1987; 62:6–10.

117   Jindani A, Aber V R, Edwards E A & Mitchison D A. The early bactericidal activity of drugs in patients with pulmonary tuberculosis. *Am Rev Resp Dis* 1980; 121:139–148.

118   Ferebee S H. Controlled chemoprophylaxis trials in tuberculosis. A general review. *Adv Tuberc Res* 1970; 17:28–106.

119   Ormerod L P for a Sub-committee of the Joint Tuberculosis Committee. Chemotherapy and management of tuberculosis in the United Kingdom: recommendations of the Joint Tuberculosis Committee of the British Thoracic Society. *Thorax* 1990; 45:403–408.

120   Centers for Disease Control. The use of preventive therapy for tuberculosis infection in the United States. *MMWR* 1990; 39 (no. RR-8):9–12.

121   Snider D E & Tabas G J. Isoniazid associated hepatitis deaths; a review of available information. *Am Rev Resp Dis* 1992; 145:494–497.

122   Israel H L. Chemoprophylaxis for tuberculosis. *Resp Med* 1993; 87:81–83.

123   Horne N W. A critical evaluation of corticosteroids in tuberculosis. *Adv Tuberc Res* 1966; 15:1–54.

124   Alzeer A H & FitzGerald J M. Corticosteroids and tuberculosis: risks and use as adjunct therapy. *Tuberc Lung Dis* 1993; 74:6–11.

125   Aspin J & O'Hara H. Steroid treated tuberculous pleural effusions. *Br J Tuberc Dis Chest* 1958; 52:81–83.

126   Singh M, Bhargave A N & Jain K P. Tuberculous peritonitis. *N Engl J Med* 1969; 281:1091–1094.

127   Tuberculosis Research Committee. Study of chemotherapy regimens of 5 and 7 months duration and the role of corticosteroids in the treatment of sputum positive patients with pulmonary tuberculosis in South India. *Tubercle* 1983; 64:73–91.

128   Girling D J, Derbyshire J H, Humphries M J &

O'Maloney G. Extrapulmonary tuberculosis. *Br Med Bull* 1988; 44:738–756.

129 Masud T & Kemp E. Corticosteroids in treatment of disseminated tuberculosis in patient with HIV infection. *BMJ* 1988; 296:464–465.

130 Guy R J C, Turberg Y, Davidson R N et al. Mineralocorticoid deficiency in HIV infection. *BMJ* 1989; 298:496–497.

131 Millar J W & Horne N W. Tuberculosis in immunocompromised patients. *Lancet* 1979; ii:1176–1178.

132 Styblo K & Meijer J. Impact of BCG vaccination programmes in children and young adults on the tuberculosis problem. *Tubercle* 1976; 57:17–43.

133 Grzybowski S & Enarson D A. The fate of cases of tuberculosis under various treatment programmes. *Bull Int Union Tuberc* 1978; 53:70–75.

134 De Cock K M, Soro B, Coulibaly I M et al. Tuberculosis and human immunodeficiency virus infection in sub-Saharan Africa. *JAMA* 1992; 268:1581–1587.

135 Sub-Committee of the Joint Tuberculosis Committee of the British Thoracic Society. Control and prevention of tuberculosis in Britain: an updated code of practice. *BMJ* 1990; 300:995–999.

136 American Thoracic Society. Control of tuberculosis in the United States of America. *Am Rev Resp Dis* 1992; 146:1623–1633.

137 Veen J. Microepidemics of tuberculosis: the stone in the pond principle. *Tuberc Lung Dis* 1992; 73:73–76.

138 Reider H L. Misbehaviour of a dying epidemic: a call for less speculation and better surveillance. *Tuberc Lung Dis* 1992; 73:181–183.

139 Sheldon C D, King K, Cock H et al. Notification of tuberculosis: how many cases are never reported? *Thorax* 1992; 47:1015–1018.

140 Capewell S & Leitch A G. The value of contact procedures for tuberculosis in Edinburgh. *Br J Dis Chest* 1984; 78:317–329.

141 Leitch A G. Rationalising tuberculosis contact tracing in low prevalence areas. *Resp Med* 1992; 86:371–374.

142 Lallemant-Le Couer S, Lallemant M, Cheynier D et al. Bacillus Calmette Guérin immunization in infants born to HIV-I-seropositive mothers. *AIDS* 1991; 5:195–199.

143 Lugosi L. Theoretical and methodological aspects of BCG vaccine from the discovery of Calmette and Guérin to molecular biology: a review. *Tuberc Lung Dis* 1992; 73:252–261.

144 Sutherland I & Lindgren I. The protective effect of BCG vaccination as indicated by autopsy studies. *Tubercle* 1979; 60:225–230.

145 Hanley S P, Gumb J & Macfarlane J T. Comparison of erythromycin and isoniazid in treatment of adverse reactions to BCG vaccination. *BMJ* 1985; 290:970–971.

146 Bottinger M, Romanus V, De Verdier J et al. Osteitis and other complications caused by generalised BCG-itis. *Acta Paediatr Scand* 1982; 71:471–479.

147 Hart P D'A & Sutherland I. BCG and vole bacillus vaccines in the prevention of tuberculosis in adolescence and early adult life. Final report to the Medical Research Council. *BMJ* 1977; ii:293–295.

148 Comstock G W, Livesay V T & Woolpert S F. Evaluation of BCG vaccination among Puerto Rican children. *Am J Public Health* 1974; 64:283–291.

149 Comstock G W, Woolpert S F & Livesay V T. Tuberculosis studies in Muscogee County, Georgia. Twenty year evaluation of a community trial of BCG vaccination. *Public Health Rep* 1976; 91:276–280.

150 Tuberculosis Preventive Trial. Trial of BCG vaccines in South India for tuberculosis prevention. *Bull World Health Organ* 1979; 57:819–827.

151 Wasz-Hockert O, Genz H, Landmann H et al. The effects of systematic BCG vaccination of newborns in the incidence of post primary tuberculous meningitis in childhood. *Bull Int Union Lung Dis* 1988; 63:49–51.

152 World Health Organization. *Statement on AIDS and tuberculosis*, WHO/GPA/INF/89.4. Geneva: WHO, 1989.

153 Springett V H & Sutherland I. BCG vaccination of schoolchildren in England and Wales. *Thorax* 1990; 45:83–88.

154 Onyebujah P C, Abdulmumini T, Robinson S et al. Immunotherapy with *Mycobacterium vaccae* as an addition to chemotherapy for the treatment of pulmonary tuberculosis under difficult conditions in Africa. *Resp Med* 1995; 89: 199–207.

CHAPTER 58

LEPROSY

S. K. Noordeen and V. K. Pannikar

GEOGRAPHICAL DISTRIBUTION

ESTIMATED NUMBER OF LEPROSY CASES

It is not easy to estimate the number of cases of leprosy in the world. Case diagnosis and definition are not always clear or consistent and the enumeration of cases in many regions of the world is incomplete or irregular. Despite these difficulties, estimates are extrapolated from data on registrations from time to time. The World Health Organization (WHO) estimates for 1966 and 1976 were 10.8 and 10.6 million cases respectively; prevalence in the 1980s was estimated at 10–12 million cases. The current estimate (1994) is 2.4 million cases, a reduction of over three-quarters since the 1980s, mainly due to the widespread application of multidrug therapy in leprosy control.[1]

POPULATION AT RISK

Approximately 2.2 billion people live in areas where leprosy is an important problem, i.e. where the estimated prevalence is over 1 case per 10 000 persons, and thus may be considered at significant risk of contracting the disease.

REGISTERED CASES

Information on leprosy cases registered for treatment is much more reliable than that on estimated cases, as it is based on actual records. There had been a very steady increase in the number of registered cases between 1966 and 1985; 2.8 million for 1966, 3.6 million for 1976, and 5.4 million for 1985.

The last figure represented an increase of 49.1% over 1976, and 89.6% over 1966. The prevalence of registered cases had correspondingly increased from 0.84 cases per 1000 population in 1966 to 0.88 in 1976, and 1.2 in 1985.[2] However, since 1985 there has been a steady decline so that by 1994 the total number of registered cases was 1.67 million, representing a reduction of about 69%.[1]

Although information on registered cases appears to be more reliable as it is based on actual records, there are several problems in evaluating this information for the purpose of leprosy control. Firstly, all registered cases are not necessarily under regular treatment, and even among patients who collect their drugs from the clinics there is a proportion who do not consume the drugs as expected. The next problem in evaluating information on registered cases is that often it is not updated. Inactive cases continue to remain in the registers, either because of patients lost to follow-up or the inability to assess periodically a patient's clinical and bacteriological condition. In addition, there are also the problems of duplicate registration of patients in more than one clinic. However, the situation appears to have improved in recent years, partly as a result of the introduction of multidrug therapy. This has made it necessary for workers responsible for leprosy control to review their records and to classify patients according to their bacteriological state. In this connection, the definition of a case of leprosy as one requiring or under treatment, made by the WHO Expert Committee on Leprosy in 1988, has improved the situation further.[3]

The distribution of registered cases, prevalence rates, the proportion of cases and new cases detected in the WHO regions as of 1994 are shown in Table 58.1. Although only a proportion of the estimated cases ever get registered for treatment, the information on registered cases reflects, to a large extent, the leprosy situation in any given region and its relative importance *vis-à-vis* other regions.

Table 58.1   Distribution of registered leprosy cases, by WHO Region, 1994.

WHO region	Registered cases	Prevalence per 10 000	Percentage of total	New cases detected	Case detection per 10 000
Africa	149 212	2.78	8.93	39 654	0.74
Americas	267 196	3.55	15.99	38 364	0.51
South-East Asia	1 170 763	8.47	70.10	495 344	3.58
Europe	4 927	0.06	0.28	74	0.001
Eastern Mediterranean	22 575	0.53	1.35	5 168	0.12
Western Pacific	56 824	0.35	3.40	12 329	0.08
World	1 671 497	3.01	100.00	590 933	1.06

AETIOLOGY

The aetiological agent in leprosy is *Mycobacterium leprae*. It is a strongly acid-fast, rod-shaped organism with parallel sides and rounded ends. In size and shape it closely resembles the tubercle bacillus. It occurs in large numbers in the lesions of lepromatous leprosy, chiefly in masses within the lepra cells, often grouped together like bundles of cigars or arranged in a palisade. Chains are never seen. Most striking are the intracellular and extracellular masses, known as globi, which consist of clumps of bacilli in capsular material.

Under the electron microscope the bacillus appears to have a great variety of forms. The most common is a slightly curved filament, 3–10 μm in length, containing irregular arrangements of dense material, sometimes in the shape of rods. Short rod-shaped structures can also be seen (identical with the rod-shaped inclusions within the filaments) and also dense spherical forms. Some of the groups of bacilli can be seen to have a limiting membrane.

It is believed that only leprosy bacilli which stain with carbol-fuchsin as solid acid-fast rods are viable and that bacilli which stain irregularly are probably dead and degenerating. The differences are valuable pointers in biopsy specimens to the effects of treatment. In patients receiving standard multidrug therapy, a very high proportion of bacilli are killed within days, which suggests that many of the manifestations of leprosy, including reactions of the erythema nodosum type—which follow initial treatment, must be due in part to antigens from dead organisms rather than living bacilli. We therefore need drugs which will help the body to dispose of dead leprosy bacilli.

Two indices[4] which depend on observation of *M. leprae* in smears from skin or nasal smears are useful in assessing the amount of infection, and the viability of the organisms and also the progress of the patient under treatment. They are the morphological index and the bacteriological index.

THE BACTERIOLOGICAL INDEX (BI)

This is an expression of the extent of bacterial load. It is calculated by counting 6–8 stained smears under the 100× oil immersion lens in a smear made by slitting the skin with a sharp scalpel and scraping it; the fluid and tissue obtained are spread fairly thickly on a slide and stained by the Ziehl–Neelsen method and decolorized (but not completely) with 1% acid alcohol. The results are expressed on a logarithmic scale.

1+ At least 1 bacillus in every 100 fields.
2+ At least 1 bacillus in every 10 fields.
3+ At least 1 bacillus in every field.
4+ At least 10 bacilli in every field.
5+ At least 100 bacilli in every field.
6+ At least 1000 bacilli in every field.

The bacteriological index is valuable because it is simple and is representative of many lesions, but it is affected by the depth of the skin incision, the thoroughness of the scrape and the thickness of the film.

A more accurate and reliable index of the bacillary content of a lesion is given by the logarithmic index of biopsies (LIB). This is mainly used in research and details should be sought in the original paper.[4] These indices help to assess the state of patients at the beginning of treatment and to assess progress.

THE MORPHOLOGICAL INDEX (MI)

This is calculated by counting the numbers of solid-staining acid-fast rods. Only the solid-staining bacilli are viable. It is not unusual for solid-staining *M. leprae* to reappear for short periods in patients being successfully treated with drugs. It is important to recognize that measurement of MI is liable to observer variation and therefore not always reliable.

CULTURE IN VITRO

Claims of successful culture have been made in the past but none have been substantiated and *M. leprae* has not yet been successfully cultured in vitro. There have been many reports of cultivation in artificial media of acid-fast bacilli from the skin or other tissues of leprosy patients and many authors have claimed such bacilli to be true leprosy bacilli, but no satisfactory evidence of this has been produced. Most of the organisms isolated in culture from lepromatous tissues appear to be mycobacteria related to the *M. avium* complex.

CULTURE IN VIVO

NORMAL MICE

The mouse footpad inoculation method developed by Shepherd is still the chief method of culture in vivo. Inoculation of 10^4 bacilli into the hind-footpads yields 10^6 bacilli after 5–6 months, although no clinical disease develops. During the logarithmic phase the mean generation time is 10–20 days, which is consistent with the natural history of disease in man and is responsible for the long time of several months taken to measure multiplication in the footpad test.[5] No subsequent local increase in bacterial numbers takes place and the bacilli slowly degenerate.

The mouse footpad has been used to test the minimum concentration of drugs necessary and the sensitivity of the bacilli to new drugs. It is a valuable tool for measuring drug resistance in patients.

IMMUNOLOGICALLY DEFICIENT MICE

Rees et al[6] have developed an experimental lepromatous leprosy model in animals by inoculating thymectomized irradiated (TR) mice. The generation time remained unchanged but the bacilli continued to multiply until 10^8–10^9 bacilli per footpad were obtained after 9–12 months. The histological picture is that of lepromatous leprosy, and numerous bacilli can be found in the liver and spleen, although the main spread is to the nose, tail, front paws and ears. The TR mouse has been used to detect small numbers of viable organisms (3–10 viable out of an inoculum of 10^5) and is used to detect 'persisters' after 12 months.

THE NINE-BANDED ARMADILLO (*DASYPUS NOVEMCINCTUS*)

An important development has been the discovery that the nine-banded armadillo can be infected with *M. leprae*[7] and this animal has become the main source of *M. leprae* for biochemical and immunological research, including development of a vaccine. The armadillo has a primitive immunological system and a low body temperature. Intravenous inoculation produces widespread disseminated disease, with yields from the liver and spleen reaching 10^{12} organisms per gram of tissue.

TRANSMISSION

Leprosy is known to occur at all ages from early infancy to very old age. The youngest age reported for the occurrence of leprosy is 3 weeks in Martinique.[8] The youngest case seen by the authors was in an infant of 2.5 months, where the diagnosis of leprosy was confirmed by histopathology. Occurrence of leprosy, presumably for the first time, is not uncommon even after the age of 70 years.

SEX DISTRIBUTION

Although leprosy affects both sexes, in most parts of the world males are affected more frequently than females, often in the ratio of 2:1. This preponderance of males is observed in as diverse geographic situations as India, the Philippines, Hawaii, Venezuela and Cameroon. Doull et al,[9] from their studies in the Philippines, have also pointed out that the difference is a true difference due to higher incidence among males, and not due to differing duration of disease for the two sexes. If it were the latter case, the sex-specific prevalence could be different even with the same sex-specific incidence. It should be pointed out that the male preponderance in leprosy is not universal and there are several areas, particularly in Africa, where there is either equal occurrence of leprosy in the two sexes or occasionally even a higher prevalence among females. Such situations have been observed in Uganda, Nigeria, Malawi, Gambia, Burkina Faso, Zambia, Thailand and Japan.

THE PREVALENCE POOL

The prevalence pool of leprosy in a population in general is in a constant flux resulting from inflow and outflow. The inflow is contributed by the occurrence of new cases, relapse of cured cases and immigration of cases. The outflow is mainly through cure or inactivation of cases, death of cases and emigration of cases. Of the various factors that influence the prevalence pool, the importance of inactivation of disease and mortality are less well recognized.

INACTIVATION OF DISEASE

Where leprosy treatment facilities exist, inactivation or cure due to specific treatment is an important mode of elimination of cases from the prevalence pool. Even in the absence of specific treatment, a majority of patients, particularly of the tuberculoid and indeterminate types, tend to be cured spontaneously. An early study in India had shown that, over a period of 20 years, the extent of spontaneous regression among children with tuberculoid leprosy was about 90%. A study in Culion Island in the Philippines showed that, among children, self-healing occurred in 77.7% of cases.[10] A later study in South India involving long-term follow-up of a high endemic population showed that, among newly detected tuberculoid cases of all ages and both sexes, the rate of inactivation was 10.9% per year, the bulk of inactivation in the study being spontaneous.[11]

MORTALITY IN LEPROSY

Mortality in leprosy is often not considered important because the disease is rarely an immediate cause of death. However, leprosy patients are exposed to increased mortality risks due to its indirect effects. In a study in Cebu, Philippines,[12] it was found that the mortality rate for lepromatous patients was four times that of the general population, and that the situation for non-lepromatous patients was very similar to that of the general population. A comparative study of lepromatous patients, non-lepromatous patients and the general population from the same rural area in South India[13] showed that the standardized death rate for lepromatous patients was three-and-a-half times that of the general population, the non-lepromatous patients themselves having a mortality risk which was twice that of the general population. In that population, leprosy was found to contribute to about 1% of all deaths.

RESERVOIR OF INFECTION

The human being is the only known reservoir of infection in leprosy, except for the fact that naturally occurring disease with organisms indistinguishable from *M. leprae* has also been detected among wild armadillos in parts of the southern USA.[14] Up to 5% of armadillos in Louisiana have been found to have clinical disease, with about 20% having serological evidence of *M. leprae* infection.[15] The epidemiological significance of the armadillo is generally considered to be negligible in spite of occasional cases reported among individuals giving a history of handling armadillos.[16] Among human beings it is the lepromatous cases that carry the largest load of organisms, the maximum load reaching over 7 billion organisms per gram of tissue. Patients with non-lepromatous cases carry a very much smaller bacillary load, probably not exceeding 1 million organisms in total. In addition to clinically identified cases, the occurrence of acid-fast bacilli in the skin[17,18] and nasal mucosa of healthy subjects[19] have also been reported. The evidence that the acid-fast bacilli found on such 'carriers' is *M. leprae* is not conclusive, although there is some evidence that persons who carry such acid-fast bacilli have a higher chance of developing the disease, as found during their follow-up.[18]

PORTAL OF EXIT OF *M. LEPRAE*

The two portals of exit of *M. leprae* often described are the skin and the nasal mucosa. However, the relative importance of these two portals is not clear. It is true that the lepromatous cases show large numbers of organisms deep down in the dermis. However, whether they reach the skin surface in sufficient numbers is doubtful. Although there are reports of acid-fast bacilli being found in the desquamating epithelium of the skin, Weddell et al[20] have reported that they could not find any acid-fast bacilli in the epidermis, even after examining a very large number of specimens from patients and contacts.

Regarding the nasal mucosa, its importance was recognized as early as 1898 by Schäffer,[21] particularly that of the ulcerated mucosa. The quantity of bacilli from nasal mucosal lesions in lepromatous leprosy was demonstrated by Shepard[22] as large, with counts ranging from 10 000 to 10 000 000. Pedley[23] reported that the majority of lepromatous patients showed leprosy bacilli in their nasal secretions as collected through blowing the nose. Davey and Rees[24] indicated that nasal secretions from lepromatous patients can yield as much as 10 million viable organisms per day.

VIABILITY OF *M. LEPRAE* OUTSIDE THE HUMAN HOST

The possibility of discharge of *M. leprae* from the nasal mucosa raises the question of survival of the discharged organisms outside the human host. Davey and Rees[24] reported that *M. leprae* from the nasal secretions can survive up to 36 hours or more. Desikan[25] reported on the survival of *M. leprae* in nasal secretions under tropical conditions for up to 9 days. Such survival of the organisms suggests the possibility of contaminated clothing and other fomites acting as sources of infection.

PORTAL OF ENTRY OF *M. LEPRAE*

The portal of entry of *M. leprae* into the human body is not definitely known. However, the two portals of entry seriously considered are the skin and the upper respiratory tract.

With regard to the respiratory route of entry of *M. leprae*, the evidence in its favour is on the increase in spite of the long-held belief that the skin was the exclusive portal of entry. Rees and McDougall[26] succeeded in the experimental transmission of leprosy through aerosols containing *M. leprae* in immune-suppressed mice, suggesting a similar possibility in humans. Successful results have also been reported on experiments with nude mice when

M. leprae were introduced into the nasal cavity by topical application.[27]

In summary, although no firm conclusions can be reached with regard to the portal of entry, entry through the respiratory route appears most probable, although other routes, particularly broken skin, cannot be ruled out.

SUBCLINICAL INFECTION IN LEPROSY

In spite of the fact that as yet there is no simple immunological test to identify subclinical infection with sufficient specificity and sensitivity, evidence accumulated in the past few years clearly indicates that subclinical infection does occur in leprosy, as in many other communicable diseases. This evidence has mainly come from limited studies with in vitro tests for cell-mediated immunity such as the lymphocyte transformation test (LTT) and serological tests for detecting humoral antibodies such as phenolic glycolipid I-based enzyme linked immunosorbent assay (ELISA).

In addition to the above, skin tests with various preparations of lepromin, and more recently with soluble antigens from *M. leprae*, have also provided useful information on the occurrence of subclinical infection, although the specificity of these tests, particularly of integral lepromin, has been rather questionable. Zuniga et al,[28] using a soluble skin test antigen prepared by the Convit method, have found that skin test positivity in a part of Venezuela was 19% among the general population (non-contacts), 36% among contacts outside the household and 48% among household contacts. The gradation of reactivity clearly suggests the correlation between exposure and possible subclinical infection. However, in India[29] no difference was seen in the distribution of skin test reactions to soluble antigens among cases, contacts and the general population.

INCUBATION PERIOD

In leprosy both the reference points for measuring the incubation period and the times of infection and onset of disease are difficult to define; the former because of the lack of adequate immunological tools and the latter because of the insidious nature of the onset of leprosy. Even so, several investigators have attempted to measure the incubation period for leprosy. The minimum incubation period reported is as short as a few weeks and this is based on the very occasional occurrence of leprosy among young infants.[8] The maximum incubation period reported is as long as 30 years, or over, as observed among war veterans known to have been exposed for short periods in endemic areas but otherwise living in non-endemic areas.

METHOD OF TRANSMISSION OF LEPROSY

The exact mechanism of transmission of leprosy is not known. At least until recently, the most widely held belief was that the disease was transmitted by contact between persons with leprosy and healthy persons. More recently the possibility of transmission by the respiratory route is gaining ground. There are also other possibilities, such as transmission by insects, which cannot be completely ruled out.

The term 'contact' in leprosy is generally not clearly defined. All that we know at present is that individuals who are in close association or proximity with leprosy patients have a greater chance of acquiring the disease. It is with reference to this observation that the early workers appear to have used the term 'contact' as the method of transmission. However, it is the definition of contact by later workers, with qualifications such as 'skin to skin', 'intimate', 'repeated', etc., that has made it appear as if the disease could be acquired only under such conditions, and that the transmission involved some kind of 'inunction' or rubbing in of the organisms from the skin of affected persons into the skin of healthy subjects. Certainly, there is no proof that transmission takes place only through such inunction.

In general, closeness of contact is related to the dose of infection, which in turn is related to the occurrence of disease. Of the various situations that promote close contact, contact within the household is the only one that is easily identified. The actual incidence among contacts and the relative risk for them appear to vary considerably in different studies. Attack rates for contacts of lepromatous leprosy have varied from 6.2 per 1000 per year in Cebu[9] to 55.8 per 1000 per year in a part of South India.[30]

The possibility of transmission of leprosy through the respiratory route has gained increasing attention in recent years. It is based on (1) the inability to find organisms on the surface of the skin; (2) the demonstration of a large number of organisms in the nasal discharge; (3) the high proportion of morphologically intact bacilli in the nasal secretions; (4) the evidence that *M. leprae* could survive outside the human host for several hours or days; and (5) the ability to infect experimental animals through the nasal route.

FACTORS DETERMINING CLINICAL EXPRESSION AFTER INFECTION

There is evidence that not all people who are infected with *M. leprae* develop leprosy. The factors that determine clinical expression after infection appear to be as important as the factors that determine infection after exposure. Of the many possible factors that determine clinical expression of disease, a few are discussed below.

is the role of genetics *vis-à-vis* other factors in determining this clinical expression.

GENETIC FACTORS

Genetic factors have been considered for a long time in leprosy. This is largely due to the observation of clustering of leprosy around certain families, and the failure to understand why certain individuals develop lepromatous leprosy while other develop non-lepromatous leprosy. Admittedly, it is the host factors that play a key role. However, what is not clear

ROUTE OF INFECTION

Studies by Shepard et al[31] in the mouse footpad model suggest that the route of entry of the organism may, to some extent, determine the occurrence of leprosy. This is based on the observation that, while intradermal administration of killed *M. leprae* sensitizes the animal, intravenous administration of killed *M. leprae* tends to tolerize the animal, as studied through skin test reactivity. This also raises the possibility of tuberculoid and lepromatous leprosy being the result of different routes of entry of the organisms.

REINFECTION

The occurrence of leprosy, presumably for the first time, in older individuals in endemic areas has raised the possibility of reinfection in these individuals, since it is difficult to believe that they remained uninfected for such a long time in an endemic area. However, this occurrence in the older age groups can also be explained by the possibility that the disease in these persons represents reactivation of old undetected primary disease following waning of previously acquired immunity. Since there is no evidence of a distinct primary disease occurring in leprosy as in tuberculosis, the hypothesis of reinfection gains some importance. Further, the occurrence of relapse in lepromatous leprosy also suggests, at least in a proportion of relapsed individuals, the possibility of reinfection. There is nothing to prevent these immune-deficient inactive patients living in endemic areas from succumbing to fresh infection. In the absence of a method for the identification of strain variations of *M. leprae*, the hypothesis on reinfection will remain untested.

PRIOR INFECTION WITH OTHER MYCOBACTERIA

There is some evidence that, as in tuberculosis, the atypical environmental mycobacteria and possibly *M. tuberculosis* play a role in the occurrence of leprosy. This is possibly due to antigenic overlap between *M. leprae* and other mycobacteria. The varying degrees of protection given by BCG against leprosy in different geographic areas, and the limited protection seen among natural tuberculin-positive reactors in the BCG study in Uganda,[32] support this possibility. Rook et al[33] have gone further and have suggested that the protective efficacy of BCG in different areas may be enhanced or diminished depending upon the local environmental mycobacteria, some acting synergistically with BCG and some antagonistically.

HUMAN IMMUNODEFICIENCY VIRUS INFECTION AND LEPROSY

It is now well recognized that human immunodeficiency virus (HIV) infection has created a serious situation with regard to the incidence of tuberculosis. Case–control studies carried out in several parts of Africa have clearly shown that the substantial increase in pulmonary tuberculosis is attributable to HIV infection. This is also true for atypical mycobacteriosis. Although a similar situation is possible with regard to leprosy there is only limited information on this so far. There have been many anecdotal reports of leprosy and HIV infection occurring together. However, good case–control studies are able to provide an answer to the question of HIV infection as a risk factor for clinical leprosy. In a detailed review of the situation, Lucas[34] concluded that clinical leprosy does not appear to be more frequent in HIV-positive than in HIV-negative individuals in areas where both infections are endemic. There have also been other reports[35,36] reaching the same conclusion. One of the problems identified recently in interpreting HIV serodiagnosis information based on ELISA and/or Western Blot is the possibility of a significantly higher rate of false-positive results[37,38] occurring in sera from lepromatous leprosy patients.

CLASSIFICATION OF LEPROSY

Leprosy is mainly classified on the basis of clinical manifestations but it may also be classified by the pathological reaction of the tissues and the number of bacilli contained in them. When leprosy bacilli gain access to the tissues they may quickly be destroyed by the protective phagocytes of the host.

If the bacilli do obtain a foothold the defence mechanisms of the host (varying from effective to poor) may create an early reaction, which is named 'indeterminate' because the lesion is too immature to be classifiable. This may persist for months or years or go on to complete healing, or to one of the fairly clear-cut forms of clinical leprosy.

The more definitive forms of leprosy show a continuous spectrum of severity according to the immune status of the host, from the tuberculoid form, in which resistance is high, to the lepromatous form at the other pole, in which resistance is low. Between these extremes there is a borderline (sometimes known as dimorphous) form which may show some characters of tuberculoid and some of lepromatous leprosy.

Table 58.2 Histological classification of leprosy.

Histological feature	TT	BT	BB	BL	LL
Granuloma	Epitheloid cells with or without giant cells, in foci	Like TT	Epitheloid cells but no giant cells	(a) Histiocytes evolving to epitheloid cells; scanty foamy change. Lymphocytes scanty (b) Histiocytes sometimes foamy; no large globi. Many lymphocytes	*Active*: Macrophages round or spindle-shaped, with very many bacilli *Regressive*: Histiocytes with fatty change; foam cells or globi often large; multinucleate
Lymphocytes	Dense zone of infiltration round foci of granuloma	Like TT	Usually scanty. If present they are diffusely spread through granuloma	(a) Scanty (b) Numerous occupying whole segments of granuloma, or forming perineural cuffs	Scanty, diffuse
Nerves	Those in granuloma usually destroyed beyond recognition. Occasional caseation	Greatly swollen by Schwann cell proliferation. Perineural sheath intact	Moderate Schwann cell proliferation. Sheath intact	No cell proliferation in nerve bundle, which is often structureless. May be infiltration of histiocytes in perineurium	May show structural damage but not infiltration or cuffing
Subepidermal zone	Granuloma extends to basal layer of epidermis. No clear zone	Clear subepidermal zone, usually narrow	Clear subepidermal zone, broad or narrow	Like BB	Like BB
Bacilli in granuloma	None seen	0–3+	3–5+	5 or 6+	5 or 6+

TT, tuberculoid; BT, borderline tuberculoid; BB, borderline; BL, borderline lepromatous; LL, lepromatous.
After Ridley and Jopling.[39]

This differentiation into three forms, which can be made clinically, has been widely accepted and is adequate for many purposes but the general spectrum of the disease may be further divided, histologically and to some extent clinically, into five grades.[39] This classification is shown in Tables 58.2 and 58.3. Leprosy may also be classified according to the bacillary presence and this is extensively used in deciding treatment and in prognosis.

Multibacillary (MB) leprosy contains all lepromatous (LL), borderline lepromatous (BL) and borderline (BB) patients and also those borderline tuberculoid (BT) patients positive for *M. leprae* in the skin smears.

Paucibacillary (PB) leprosy contains indeterminate (I), tuberculoid (TT) and also those BT patients who are smear negative.

The polar forms, TT and LL, are relatively stable but the borderline form is unstable. Without treatment it tends to deteriorate to lepromatous. After treatment it sometimes reverts.

A subdivision of the LL group into LLp (polar lepromatous) and LLs (subpolar lepromatous) is now accepted. Clinically a patient with LLs will have

Table 58.3 Clinical classification of leprosy.

TT	BT	BB	BL	LL
Lesions consist of a few macules and/or plaques. Plaques tend to be large, have a rough dry hairless surface and well-defined edges from which there is a gradual slope to a flattened centre Distribution of lesions asymmetrical	May be confused clinically with TT but differentiated by: (a) lesions more numerous, surface less dry and rough, edges less well defined, and hair growth may be sight; and (b) annular lesions common, the peripheral band of tissue being raised and having well-defined outer and inner edges	Macules and plaques are intermediate in number and size between TT and LL. 'Punched-out' lesions are characteristic. Annular lesions occur as in BT Distribution of lesions asymmetrical	May be confused clinically with LL but differentiated by: (a) macules and plaques not consistently small, edges less vague, and less tendency to bilateral symmetry; some may have 'punched-out' appearance; (b) papules and nodules unusual and few; nodules may be dimpled; and (c) rare and less marked are iritis and keratitis, nasal ulceration, madarosis, thickened ear lobes, testicular damage and bone changes	Macules, papules, nodules and plaques may all be present. Lesions small, multiple, distributed bilaterally and symmetrically with smooth shiny surface. Macules and plaques have vague edges and no hair loss. May be nasal ulceration, iritis and keratitis, madarosis, leonine facies, thickened ear lobes, testicular damage, oedema of legs, and bone changes in limbs and skull
Lesions markedly anaesthetic	Lesions moderately anaesthetic	Lesions show mild anaesthesia	Some lesions may show slight patchy anaesthesia	Lesions not anaesthetic
Nerve thickening early, often single. First manifestations may be neural	Nerve thickening early, more numerous than in TT. First manifestations may be neural	Nerve thickening early, more numerous than in BT. First manifestations may be neural	Nerve thickening early, more numerous than in BB. First manifestations may be neural	Nerve thickening (and damage) late and tends to be bilateral and symmetrical (e.g. glove and stocking anaesthesia). First manifestations never neural
Lepromin test strongly positive	Lepromin test moderately or weakly positive	Lepromin test negative	Lepromin test negative	Lepromin test negative

TT, tuberculoid; BT, borderline tuberculoid; BB, borderline; BL, borderline lepromatous; LL, lepromatous.
After Ridley and Jopling.[39]

typical early lepromatous lesions and also some typical lesions of borderline type, with one or more thickened nerve trunks with or without evidence of nerve dysfunction.[40] Whereas LLp is immunologically stable, LLs is not. During chemotherapy LLs may become bacteriologically negative sooner than LLp. The two types can be differentiated histologically.[41]

PATHOLOGY

PATHOLOGICAL CHANGES

In very early infection the acid-fast bacilli proliferate in the fixed cells of the dermis and thereafter monocytes from the blood migrate towards the bacilli, engulfing and disintegrating them. Leprosy bacilli may also enter nerves, causing focal damage related to the blood vessels near their site of entry into the nerves. They spread along the fine fibres of cutaneous nerve twigs and are carried centripetally, multiplying and bursting into the endoneural spaces where they are phagocytosed by histiocytes. In this way an incipient infection may be eradicated, although this is less likely once the bacilli have gained a foothold in nerves. If a skin lesion develops, a biopsy specimen at this stage shows foci of inflammatory cellular exudate, mainly around the finest nerve fibres in plexuses in the dermis. The exudate is determined by the ability of the host to react immunologically and it consists of lymphocytes, histiocytes and other cells; clinically it is marked on the skin by wheal-like papules or pink or pale macules. This is the *indeterminate* stage of infection, which usually occurs in children in whom resistance has not been determined and which may last for months, or resolve, or progress to *tuberculoid*, *dimorphous (borderline)* or *lepromatous* leprosy, depending on the immunological response of the body.

In lepromin-negative persons (whose resistance is poor) the histiocytes gradually change into lepra cells which in more severe cases become foamy; the ingested bacilli are not destroyed. In lepromin-positive persons (whose resistance is good) the histiocytes change into epithelioid cells after ingesting the bacilli, which they destroy.

Although the manner of evolution of these cells containing *M. leprae* is important, the mediators of immunity are the lymphocytes, and although the lymphocytes in skin lesions are not all immunologically active, the numbers present in tuberculoid and borderline lesions are significant indications of the degree of resistance to the infection.

TUBERCULOID LEPROSY

The change from indeterminate to tuberculoid leprosy involves the appearance of groups of epi-

thelioid cells (derived from histiocytes) inside fine nerve twigs and the formation of sharply circumscribed foci of these cells in the dermis, often surrounded by a zone of lymphocytes, which are fairly numerous. The epithelioid cells often coalesce to form giant cells. The epidermis is thinner than normal and there are foci of inflammatory cells reaching the epidermis without a clear space. In the dermis the granulomatous cords follow the lines of neurovascular bundles (see Figure 58.7). The nerve bundles in the skin are swollen by proliferation of Schwann cells, which develop into epithelioid cells. The nerves become difficult to recognize; they occasionally undergo caseation, which does not occur in leprosy except in nerves.

Acid-fast bacilli are very rare in the cells of the inflammatory exudate in tuberculoid leprosy, except in reaction phases, but bacilli may be found in the active extending margin of a tuberculoid macule.

The most consistent feature of tuberculoid leprosy is the early involvement of peripheral nerves. In the upper extremity this often goes on to weakness and paralysis of the intrinsic muscles of the hand (main-en-griffe) and in the leg to drop foot. Damage to the sympathetic nerves leads to slow atrophy and absorption (osteoporosis) of the small bones of the hands and feet through interference with vasodilatation.

BORDERLINE LEPROSY

Indeterminate leprosy often goes on to the borderline form in which large hypopigmented patches appear, often on the limbs, usually with loss of sensations of touch and temperature. Satellite macules with varying degrees of sharpness in the edges also appear; they are usually small. Acid-fast bacilli can always be found in these lesions. The lepromin reaction is variable but is usually weakly positive.

The histological picture shows features intermediate between those of lepromatous and tuberculoid lesions. There is an inflammatory reaction with cellular exudate in the superficial layers of the dermis; it consists of small round cells, histiocytes and clumps of epithelioid cells but no giant cells. Nerves may show large numbers of bacilli and round cells or epithelioid cells with few bacilli, i.e. they may re-

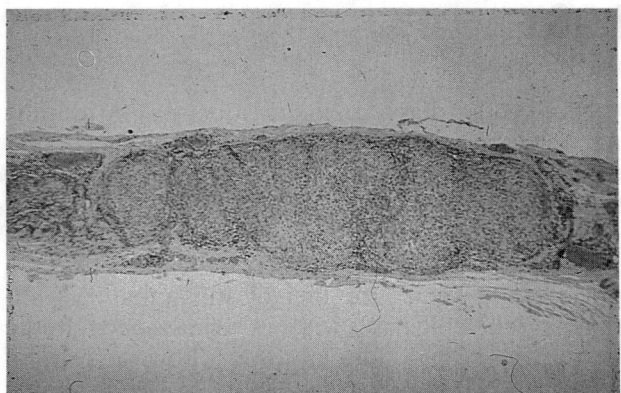

Figure 58.1   Nerve lesions (low power) of tuberculoid leprosy. (Courtesy of the late S.G. Browne.)

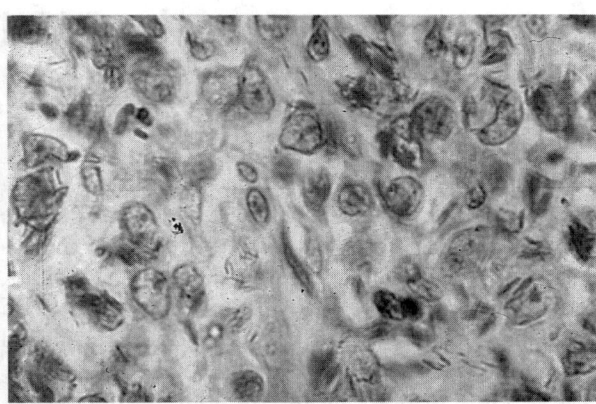

Figure 58.3   Skin lesions of lepromatous leprosy (high power) showing the lepra cellular tissue. (Courtesy of the late S.G. Browne.)

LEPROMATOUS LEPROSY

In fully developed lepromatous disease large areas of the dermis are converted into continuous sheets of chronic inflammatory tissue containing enormous numbers of bacilli in slabs of lepra (Virchow) cells (derived from histiocytes) (Figure 58.3), interspersed with groups of mononuclear and plasma cells. Lymphocytes are scanty. The subepidermal zone of the dermis is clear of infiltrate. The disease is now systemic, the bacilli being transported by blood or lymph nodes, liver, spleen and bone marrow, where miliary lepromas and even large lepromas may be found and subcutaneous veins may be involved.

The mucous membrane of the upper respiratory tract from the nose to the larynx, including the root of the tongue and the peritonsillar tissues, is heavily infiltrated in advanced lepromatous leprosy. It is oedematous, thickened and ulcerated and the nasal cartilages may be perforated. If the disease regresses as a result of treatment, the skin lesions heal in a remarkable manner.

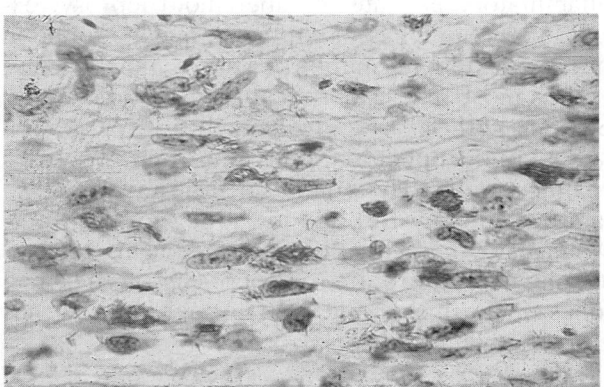

Figure 58.2   Nerve lesions (high power) of lepromatous leprosy. (Courtesy of the late S.G. Browne.)

semble nerves in lepromatous or tuberculoid disease (Figures 58.1 and 58.2). This dimorphous leprosy is unstable and tends to progress to the lepromatous form if not treated.

IMMUNITY

Protective immune response in leprosy is based upon cellular immune mechanisms and leprosy bacilli are killed or eliminated only by this mechanism. Although not killed by humoral antibodies, leprosy bacilli stimulate the production of humoral antibodies against various constituent antigens. The type of leprosy produced depends on the ability to produce and develop cell-mediated immunity (CMI). CMI (mediated by lymphocytes) is strong in tuberculoid leprosy but weak or absent in lepromatous leprosy.[42] However, antibodies are produced plentifully in lepromatous leprosy but their immunological role is unclear. Tuberculoid leprosy patients give a positive lepromin test showing the immune response to *M. leprae*. The histological picture shows numerous lymphocytes and epithelioid cells, whereas lepromatous patients show little cellular reaction (Figure 58.3). The inability of a small proportion of individuals to mount an effective CMI response to *M. leprae* may be due to genetic factors, as shown by some that HLA types do play a part in the process.[43,44] Leprosy patients can resist other infections so that the anergy is specific, as demonstrated in lymphocyte transformation tests using *M. leprae* as antigen.[45]

Studies on T lymphocyte subpopulations have shown that the distribution of T-helper and T-suppressor cells varies in the different types of leprosy and that the distribution of helper and suppressor cells in tuberculoid leprosy resembles that found in sarcoidosis.[46] Whereas macrophage function in lepromatous leprosy is satisfactory, there is a deficiency in lymphokines.[47] *M. leprae* possesses a number of antigens which are specific[48] but they have a wide variation in sensitivity in immunological tests. In tuberculoid leprosy CMI is intact but aberrant, resulting from delayed recognition of *M. leprae* antigens.

LEPROMIN

The lepromin test is used frequently in leprosy. Lepromin is a reagent derived from human nodular lepromatous or infected armadillo tissue and it represents a suspension of the bacilli together with cellular matter from the host tissues. Lepromin is injected intradermally in a dose of 0.1 ml. Standard Mitsuda lepromin contains 160 million leprosy bacilli per millilitre.

Reactions to lepromin are of two kinds.
1 The early (Fernandez) reaction, which becomes positive in 48 hours and shows erythema and infiltration 10–15 mm in diameter (+ reaction), 15–20 mm (++) or over 20 mm (+++).
2 The late (Mitsuda) reaction, read at 4–5 weeks, positive results giving + reaction (3–5 mm), ++ (6–10 mm) or +++ (over 10 mm or a reaction of any size which ulcerates).

It is generally understood that the early (Fernandez) reaction is an allergic reaction similar to the tuberculin reaction. It is positive in all forms of leprosy (unlike the Mitsuda reaction), but most strongly positive in the tuberculoid form. It is a reflection of the sensitivity of the tissues to the protein of the leprosy bacilli. The late (Mitsuda) reaction, however, is an index of resistance. Dharmendra lepromin, much used in India, is a purified suspension of *M. leprae* extracted with chloroform–ether. The early (Fernandez) reaction is best seen when this lepromin is used.

The Mitsuda reaction is strongly positive in tuberculoid leprosy, usually negative or weakly positive in borderline leprosy and almost invariably negative in lepromatous leprosy. It is sometimes positive in persons who have never been in contact with the leprosy bacillus and the test is therefore of no diagnostic value. A positive result indicates resistance to leprosy bacilli; a negative result in a patient with the disease is a sign of poor resistance. Reversal of a negative to a positive Mitsuda test in a leprosy patient is taken as a sign of increased resistance and therefore of improved prognosis.

BACILLAEMIA

Bacillaemia occurs in leprosy. Of 240 biopsy specimens from leprosy patients in India, 21% of those with lepromatous disease had shown leprous granulomas in the liver;[49] BT, BB and BL patients gave intermediate results. This indicates that bacillaemia occurs even in the 'immune' group. Acid-fast bacilli have also been seen in the liver in BT, BB, BL and LL groups, even when treatment had produced negative bacterial indices in the skin.

CLINICAL FEATURES

NATURAL HISTORY

The natural history of leprosy is very variable. The majority of people who come into contact with infectious lepromatous patients develop no symptoms or signs of infection, although the lymphocyte transformation test shows that a majority will have experienced infection, which they overcome. The majority of those who experience clinical effects mount a strong CMI response and develop tuberculoid leprosy. A minority who mount a weak CMI response or none at all develop lepromatous leprosy, a chronic progressive disseminated infection. A proportion of cases mount varying degrees of CMI response and develop borderline or indeterminate leprosy, and may then swing one way or the other on the pendulum, downgrading or upgrading, depending upon changes in the immunological response.

SYMPTOMS AND SIGNS

The mode of onset is very variable. An early lesion may occur as a vague ill-defined hypopigmented patch with some anaesthesia. The disease can also occur with multiple infiltrated patches or just diffuse skin infiltration. In certain instances leprosy can manifest itself as areas of anaesthesia in the skin with no skin patches.

Spontaneous healing may take place in a very high proportion of early lesions of childhood and this is quite common in some communities; however, a definite diagnosis is an indication for treatment.

As compared with tuberculosis, one of the chief characteristics of leprosy is the absence of toxicity; enormous numbers of bacilli may be present in the body with few signs. The local inflammatory reactions to lepra bacilli vary within wide limits. Thus, in one patient the disease may be so localized that it affects one small skin area or its main nerve supply. There may be acute inflammatory swelling, local pain and trophic, sensory and other disturbances. Bacilli can be demonstrated with great difficulty. In contrast, some cases show involvement of almost the whole body, so that a preparation taken from any part of the skin may reveal numerous bacilli, although the patient is not acutely ill and is able to go about and work normally. The nerves are not noticeably thickened and superficially the skin appears normal. At any stage during invasion sudden exanthematous reactions may appear, accompanied by fever and general symptoms.

The *chronic onset* is so gradual and insidious that the disease has advanced to a considerable extent before any abnormality is evident. There may be tenderness, tingling or thickening of a nerve, an area of anaesthesia, perhaps with some change in the appearance of the skin, insensitiveness to burning, formication, tingling or numbness of extremities. Discoloured skin patches may be mistaken for eczema or ringworm; these may at first be small, gradually increasing in size.

In *acute onset*, which is much less common, there are occasionally multiple lesions with less diffused margins, which tend to spread rapidly and which contain very numerous bacilli. The first noticeable sign may be an evanescent rash. The onset may be determined by occurrence of some other acute disease or physiological change or stress, e.g. extra

strain imposed on the body during puberty, parturition and the menopause.

LEPROMATOUS LEPROSY

This is the type of leprosy seen in persons with a negligible resistance; leprosy bacilli are widely disseminated throughout the skin, nerves and reticuloendothelial system. In addition, there may be bacillary invasion of eyes, testes, bones and mucous membranes of mouth, nose, pharynx, larynx and trachea.

SKIN LESIONS

These are multiple, small and symmetrically distributed; they take the form of macules, infiltrations (plaques), papules and nodules (Figure 58.4), all of which may be present in the same patient at the same time once the disease has become well established. The pure diffuse type is an exception and will be described later.

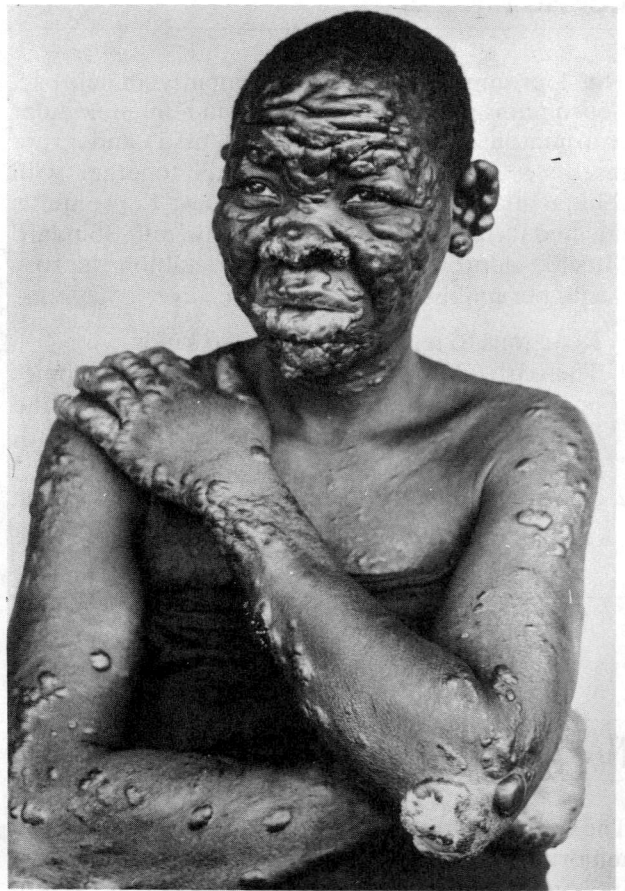

Figure 58.4 Nodular skin lesions of lepromatous leprosy. (Courtesy of the late S.G. Browne.)

The earliest skin lesions are macules; they are level with the skin and therefore cannot be palpated. They are small, circular or elliptical; they are erythematous in light skins, sometimes with a coppery or purple hue, and coppery in dark skins, sometimes with a faintly hypopigmented background. They have a smooth and shiny surface, their edges are indistinct and they are not anaesthetic or anhidrotic. Owing to the fact that these macules are often difficult to see and are not associated with itching or anaesthesia, they may be ignored by the patient. They may be situated on any part of the body, but are unusual in the axillae, groins, perineum, on the external genitalia or on the scalp. They are most commonly found on the face, buttocks and extremities; on the limbs the flexor surfaces may be involved as well as the extensor, and the palms and soles as well as the backs of hands and feet.

Infiltrated lesions are raised above the level of the skin and give a sensation of thickening when gripped between finger and thumb. Their distribution and colouring are the same as those of lepromatous macules, except that they do not appear on palms and soles because of the thickness and tightness of the skin. They are raised in the centre and slope away peripherally to merge imperceptibly with the surrounding skin, have a smooth and shiny surface, and do not exhibit sensory loss, unless situated in a region of skin which is already anaesthetic as a result of peripheral nerve damage. Papules and nodules make their appearance as the disease advances and particularly favour the face, ears and buttocks. Ears should always be carefully examined, for the lobes are more constantly affected than any other part and appear thickened quite early in the course of the disease, such thickening being readily confirmed by palpation with finger and thumb. Advanced infiltration and nodulation of the face give rise to leontiasis or 'leonine facies', in which the normal wrinkles on the forehead and cheeks have become deep furrows. Nodules and infiltrations may undergo superficial necrosis and ulceration and large ulcers may form on the lower legs when leprous infiltration of the skin is associated with chronic bilateral lymphoedema, secondary to massive bacillary invasion of the lymphatics. Thinning of the eyebrows is common, commencing in the lateral half and sometimes progressing to complete loss of eyebrows and eyelashes (supercilliary and ciliary madarosis).

One particular variety of skin infiltration requires separate mention, namely the pure diffuse type described by Lucio and Alvarado in Mexico in 1852 and later by Latapi in 1938. The skin of the whole body becomes diffusely infiltrated (no macular stage being observed), rendering it stiff and smooth, as in scleroderma. There is no obvious disfigurement, apart from loss of eyebrows and eyelashes which always occurs, but there may be widespread small telangiectases; nasal destruction may develop and sometimes there is alopecia and loss of body hair. Laryngeal ulceration has been recorded but cutaneous nodules and ocular involvement are absent. Mexican physicians have described, in these patients, a unique form of lepra reaction known as 'Lucio's phenomenon', in which painful, purpuric, ulcerating patches appear on the skin, becoming crusted and leaving scars.[40] This may be differentiated from the erythema nodosum leprosum (ENL) reaction by the absence of fever and leucocytosis, absence of tender lesions, and a good response to antileprosy drugs, but not to thalidomide. It may also be distinguished histologically.[50,51]

NERVE INVOLVEMENT

Nerve involvement, in the absence of skin involvement, has not been described in lepromatous leprosy, but combined dermal and neural changes are a usual finding. Nerves do not show signs of damage as early as in the other types of leprosy, but nerve thickening and associated sensory or motor dysfunction can usually be demonstrated as the disease advances. As sensory loss is often more pronounced than muscular wasting, patients continue to use the affected limbs and the skin suffers much damage from repeated trauma owing to insensitivity to pain. Thus the hands become scarred from injuries and burns and trophic ulcers develop on the soles of the feet. Nerve thickening, like skin involvement, tends to be bilateral and symmetrical but there may be a difference in degree on the two sides. It is found in those peripheral nerves which are superficial in some part of this course, the thickening being localized to the superficial portion, e.g. the great auricular nerves in the neck (Figure 58.5), the

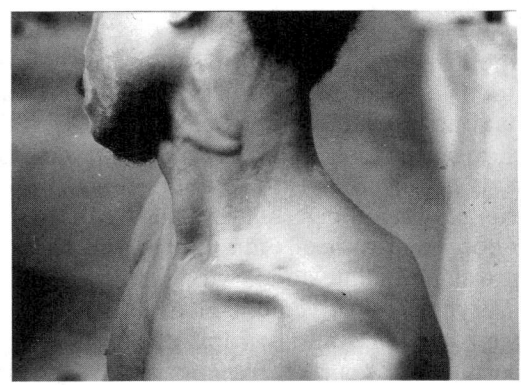

Figure 58.5 Gross enlargement of the auricular nerve in tuberculoid leprosy. (Courtesy of the late S.G. Browne.)

supraclavicular nerves as they cross the clavicles, the ulnar nerves just above the elbows, the antebrachial cutaneous nerves in the forearms, the radial and median nerves at the wrists, the femoral cutaneous nerves, the common peroneals as they wind round the necks of the fibulae, the superficial peroneals in front of the ankles and the posterior tibial nerves immediately below the internal malleoli.

The earliest sensory disturbances may take the form of paraesthesia, hyperaesthesiae and hyperalgesia, to be followed later by impairment of light touch, temperature or pain sensation. All three modalities should be tested when examining a patient, as sometimes only one is affected (dissociated anaesthesia); in such a case it is usually the ability to differentiate between hot and cold which is lost first. Loss of position sense, vibration sense and tendon reflexes may occur, but not commonly. Muscle wasting may produce deformities such as claw hand (ulnar nerve), main-en-griffe (combined ulnar and median nerves), drop foot (common peroneal nerve) and facial palsy (facial nerve), but careful examination of muscles will show evidence of weakness long before paralysis occurs.

Involvment of autonomic nerves manifests itself in the early stages by slight oedema of the hands or feet; more marked vasomotor disturbance develops later, causing the skin of hands and feet to be puffy and cyanosed.

OTHER TISSUES INVOLVED IN LEPROMATOUS LEPROSY

Nails of fingers and toes

These are affected when trophic changes take place in digits, and appear dry, lustreless, narrowed and longitudinally ridged.

Mucous membranes

The patient may complain of nasal discharge, possibly bloodstained, and of blocking of the airway; examination reveals hyperaemia and swelling of the mucosa, together with nodules or ulcers on the nasal septum. Ulceration leads to septal perforation and later to cartilage destruction and consequent 'saddle-nose' deformity. Nodules may also form on the lips, tongue, palate and larynx, leading to ulceration. Laryngeal involvement gives rise to hoarse cough, husky voice and stridor. Oedema of the glottis, occurring as part of a reactional state, used to be a dreaded complication in the presulphone era, calling for immediate tracheotomy. Perforation of

the palate may occur in the absence of syphilis or yaws. Jopling[40] stresses the importance of nasal symptoms (stuffiness, crust formation, bloodstained discharge) and of bilateral oedema of the legs as early signs which may point to a diagnosis of lepromatous leprosy long before the appearance of the classical skin lesions.

Eye

Visual impairment and blindness occur frequently in leprosy patients, particularly in those with advanced lepromatous leprosy. Leprosy is the third leading cause of blindness worldwide. The major complications leading to blindness from leprosy are the following.

- *Corneal changes* are exposure keratitis due to lagophthalmos, and reduced or absent corneal sensation, both predisposing to corneal ulceration and scarring. The early stages can be recognized by fine punctate superficial spots on the cornea. Secondary bacterial infection or a foreign body may subsequently cause a corneal ulcer.
- *Iris involvement* may be either in the acute form of iridocyclitis, which occurs as part of the ENL reaction, or a chronic process. The acute form causes pain, photophobia and pericorneal redness. If acute iritis is untreated it may smoulder on as a chronic iritis, with posterior synechiae formation and small irregular pupil. A chronic insidious form of iridocyclitis frequently occurs in lepromatous leprosy. Early in the disease process, 'flare' (cloudiness of aqueous fluid) and cells can be detected in the anterior chamber, if examined with a slit lamp. This form of chronic iridocyclitis will tend to lead to iris atrophy and a regular pinpoint pupil without posterior synechiae formation.
- *Cataract* may be caused by or made worse by iridocyclitis or the use of systemic steroids in reaction, and intraocular invasion with bacilli.

Bones

Changes in bones in lepromatous leprosy are confined to the skull and limbs. In the limbs the changes are almost solely concentrated in the hands and feet and are due to a combination of factors which include: (1) deposition of bacilli; (2) neurotrophic atrophy; (3) repeated trauma resulting from analgesia; (4) disuse owing to paralysis and contractures; (5) secondary infection from trophic ulceration; and (6) generalized osteoporosis of hormonal origin. Deposition of bacilli in the medullary cavities, the periosteum and the nutrient vessels gives rise to bone cysts, enlarged nutrient foramina, aseptic necrosis and spindle-shaped leprous dactylitis closely simulating that of tuberculosis or syphilis. Leprous periostitis of the tibia, fibula and ulna has been described. Neurotrophic atrophy affecting the hands is localized to the phalanges. Metacarpals and carpal bones are spared. In the feet the atrophic changes are localized to the metatarsals and phalanges, commencing in the proximal phalanges or in the heads of the metatarsals. In the proximal phalanges the diaphyses become gradually thinned by rarefying osteitis, known as 'concentric bone atrophy', so that eventually there is but a fine needle of bone left. This may be followed by disappearance of the affected bones and the shortened toes are connected to the foot by soft tissue only. In the metatarsals absorption begins at the distal ends, which become thinned and pointed—the 'sucked candystick' appearance. The tarsal bones are spared.

Sensory loss results in repeated trauma, both major and minor, and this is an important contributory factor to the production of bone atrophy and absorption. Brand[52] states: 'By far the greatest proportion of finger absorption is secondary to burns and trauma which follow anaesthesia.' In addition, sensory loss can lead to the development of Charcot joints in the fingers, toes, wrists or ankles.

Muscle paralysis can lead to disuse and, in neglected cases, to fibrous or bony ankylosis of the interphalangeal, metacarpophalangeal and metatarsophalangeal joints. Disuse also results in osteoporosis due to decreased osteoblastic activity.

Secondary infection commonly follows neglected trophic ulceration of feet or hands and can result in pyogenic osteomyelitis.

Generalized osteoporosis may follow defective production of testosterone as a result of testicular damage.

Changes in the skull in lepromatous leprosy consist of atrophy of the anterior nasal spine and the maxillary alveolar process, probably caused by a combination of aseptic necrosis, due to leprous endarteritis, and pyogenic osteomyelitis, due to gross ulceration in the nose.

Reticuloendothelial system

Lymph glands may be enlarged and painless with the consistency of soft rubber, particularly the femoral, inguinal and epitrochlear glands, but occasionally one or more glands become very swollen and tender as part of a reactional state. The reticuloendothelial elements of the abdominal viscera are invaded by bacilli, especially in the spleen and liver, and the red marrow is similarly invaded. Lymphoedema of the lower legs may occur, giving rise to elephantiasis in neglected cases.

Testes

Testicular atrophy may occur, resulting in sterility and gynaecomastia.

Kidneys

Glomerulonephritis, interstitial nephritis and pyelonephritis may occur. Renal amyloidosis is a prevalent complication in some geographical areas but is uncommon in others; it appears to be related to the severity and frequency of type 2 lepra reactions (ENL).

Serological tests for syphilis are usually positive in lepromatous leprosy but the *Treponema pallidum* immobilization (TPI) test remains negative in the absence of syphilis.

TUBERCULOID LEPROSY

This is the type of leprosy seen in persons with a good resistance and may be purely neural or combined neural and dermal. The infection is never widespread but is localized to one area or to a few areas asymmetrically. Affected nerves are thickened, sometimes irregularly, and there are associated sensory or motor changes depending on the type of nerve involved. Sensory disturbance occurs as described under lepromatous leprosy, except for the fact that it occurs earlier in the course of the disease. If the patient complains of sensory disturbance, such as paraesthesiae or anaesthesia, a search must be made for palpable thickening of the nerve responsible for the sensation of that area, e.g. face (trigeminal nerve), neck (great auricular nerve), forearm (antebrachial cutaneous nerve), fifth finger (ulnar cutaneous nerve), hand (median nerve at the wrist), thigh (femoral cutaneous nerve), lower leg (common peroneal nerve at the neck of the fibula), dorsum of foot (superficial peroneal nerve) and sole of foot (posterior tibial nerve just below the internal malleolus).

Loss of position sense, vibration sense and tendon reflexes occur rarely. Motor changes are shown by muscle weakness or wasting and must be sought in the face, the intrinsic muscles of the hand and the dorsiflexors of the foot. It is extremely rare for the dorsiflexors of the wrist to be affected, owing to the

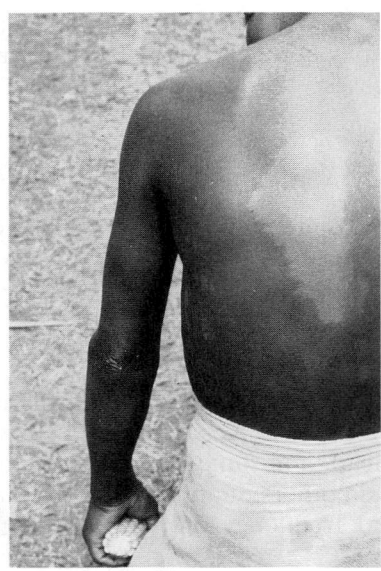
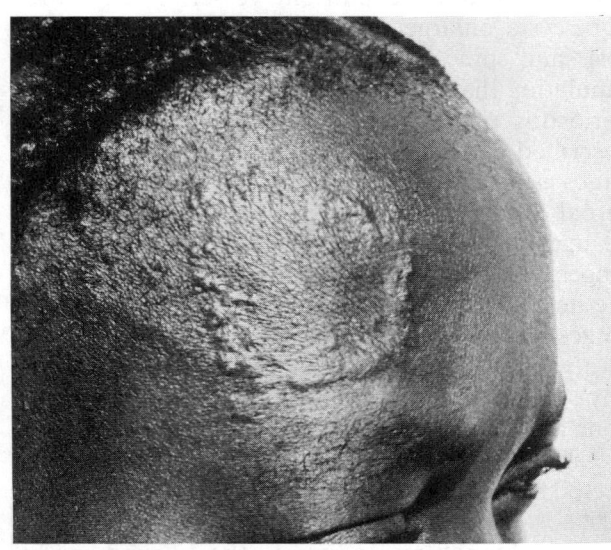

(a)   (b)

Figure 58.6   Skin lesions of tuberculoid leprosy: (a) macular; (b) infiltrated. (Courtesy of the late S.G. Browne.)

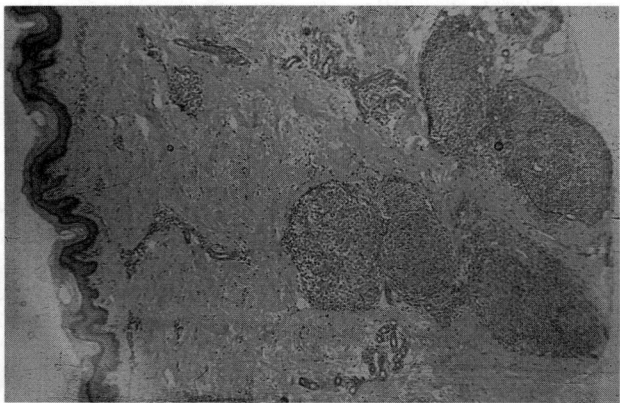

Figure 58.7   Skin lesions of tuberculoid leprosy (high power). (Courtesy of the late S.G. Browne.)

fact that the radial nerve in the arm and forearm follows a deep course among the muscles and is therefore rarely involved. It is interesting to note that the same nerve, when it becomes superficial at the end of its course, often becomes thickened and can be palpated as a firm mobile cord as it lies against the lower end of the radius. Abscesses in the course of affected nerves are not uncommon in tuberculoid leprosy.

Skin lesions take the form of macules or infiltrations (plaques) (Figures 58.6 and 58.7). A tuberculoid macule is erythematous on fair skins and hypopigmented (not depigmented) on dark ones, has a dry and rather rough surface, its edges are well defined, and it is anaesthetic (except on the face) and anhidrotic. Infiltrated lesions are erythematous, whether on fair or dark skins, sometimes with a coppery, brownish or purple hue, have a dry and

rather rough surface, which may be irregular or pebbled, are sometimes scaly, have well-marked sensory loss and have edges which are raised and clear-cut while the centres show variable flattening. In dark skins the colouring of the lesions obscures the underlying hypopigmentation. Central healing and peripheral extension give rise to annular lesions in which the *outer* edges are raised and well defined and the *inner* ones are flattened and indistinct.

Lesions of tuberculoid leprosy are usually few, large and asymmetrically situated; they favour the face, extensor surfaces of limbs, back and buttocks, while tending to avoid the chest, abdomen, scalp and flexor aspects of limbs. If palms or soles are involved the lesions are not raised owing to the thickness and tightness of the skin. Sometimes one or two small 'satellite' lesions are seen in the vicinity of a large plaque and may look like nodules, but the fact that they are less elevated in the centre than at the edges can be confirmed by palpation. Thickened cutaneous nerves may be palpated in the vicinity of the lesions, but tissues other than skin and nerves are not involved directly. The eye may suffer indirectly from corneal ulceration when there is damage to the facial nerve (exposure keratitis) and also when there is damage to the trigeminal nerve (neuropathic keratitis). Loss of eyebrows does not occur unless there is an infiltrated lesion traversing the eyebrow, and then the loss of hair is confined to that portion of the eyebrow, which is actually covered by the lesion.

Bone changes in hands or feet are less common than in the lepromatous type as leprosy bacilli are not deposited in the bones or their nutrient arteries; also, the early development of muscle wasting and

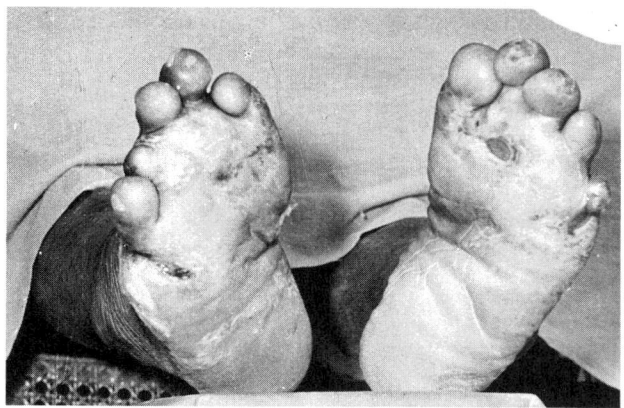

Figure 58.8 Trophic ulceration and deformity of the feet. (Courtesy of the late S.G. Browne.)

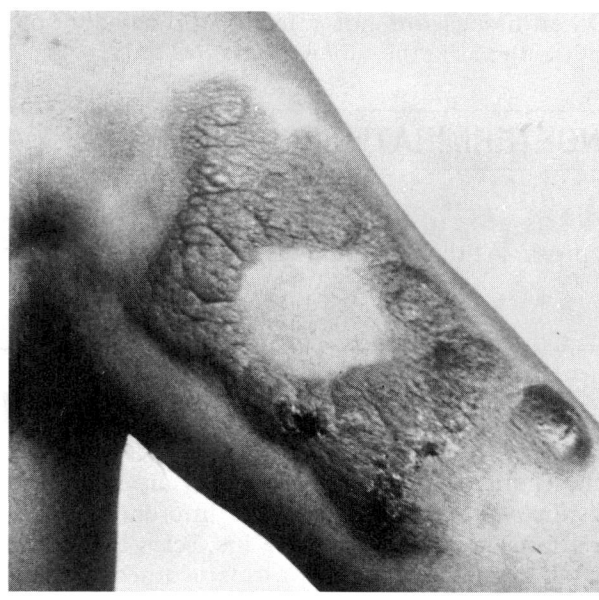

Figure 58.9 Borderline leprosy. (Courtesy of the late S.G. Browne.)

paralysis results in disuse and therefore reduced risk of repeated trauma. However, neuropathic atrophy may occur in the phalanges of fingers or in the metatarsals and phalanges of feet but, unlike the changes in lepromatous leprosy, they are never bilateral and symmetrical. Bone changes secondary to disuse, to loss of sensation and to trophic ulceration may occur as described under lepromatous leprosy. Trophic ulcers of the feet are common (Figure 58.8).

BORDERLINE (DIMORPHOUS) LEPROSY

This is the type of leprosy seen in persons with a limited or variable resistance and usually presents with skin and nerve involvement. At the Sixth International Congress of Leprosy in Madrid (1953)[53] the existence of a pure neural form was not accepted, but careful observation since then has proved that a polyneuritic form does exist.

The infection is neither as strictly localized as in tuberculoid leprosy nor as widespread as in the lepromatous type but is somewhere between the two. Some patients remain dimorphous throughout but others progress to one or other of the two polar types, depending on immunological factors not yet understood.

Skin lesions are macular, infiltrated or both, the earliest lesions being macules which are erythematous in fair skins or hypopigmented (sometimes with an erythematous periphery) in dark skins. They may appear on trunk or limbs but have a predilection for the back; in number and character they are intermediate between the two polar types. Careful testing will reveal impairment of sensation in some if not all of the macules.

Infiltrated lesions have their own distinctive features in which the characteristics of the two polar types are merged. They are moderate in number, asymmetrical in distribution, their erythema has an admixture of purple or brown, their surface is smooth and often shiny and they slope away peripherally from raised centres. The edges are well defined in places and indefinite in others.

Some of these infiltrations may take the form of bands, annular lesions and small nodules. Annular lesions have a characteristic form in which an oval area of normal looking but anaesthetic skin is surrounded by a band of infiltrated tissue of varying width, the *inner* edge being raised and clear-cut (giving the oval area a punched out appearance), the *outer* merging imperceptibly with the surrounding skin. These should not be mistaken for annular tuberculoid lesions for in the latter the outside edges are raised and clear-cut while the inner edges are indistinct. Sometimes there is an oval band of infiltrated tissue, even in width, and more raised in the central part of the band, which has well-defined outer and inner edges. Infiltrated lesions are invariably anaesthetic and may be found on any part of the body, with the exception of axillae, groins, perineum and scalp, but favour the limbs and buttocks (Figure 58.9).

Nerve involvement can always be demonstrated in borderline leprosy, and neurological symptoms such as paraesthesiae and hyperalgesia often precede the onset of skin manifestations. Nerves are involved asymmetrically and show palpable thickening and impaired function (sensory, motor or both).

Other tissues are not affected directly but only indirectly, as in the tuberculoid type.

INDETERMINATE LEPROSY

This is an early phase in the natural history of leprosy. At this stage the disease has not yet determined into which type it is going to evolve. Lesions are macular, macules being nondescript with uncharacteristic histology and absence of bacilli.

DIFFERENTIAL DIAGNOSIS

The characteristic marks of leprosy are sufficiently distinctive, but they have to be differentiated from psoriasis, seborrhoeic dermatitis, scars from burns or other injuries, various forms of tinea, eczema, lichen planus, pellagra and filarial disease. Blastomycosis produces skin lesions reminiscent of leprosy. Differentiation from syphilis and yaws may not always be so easy. Syphilitic and yaws skin lesions may often closely resemble the maculae of leprosy but the absence of sensory changes and reaction to treatment are sufficiently distinctive. The VDRL reaction alone cannot always be depended upon in differential diagnosis as syphilis and leprosy may coexist; also a false-positive reaction is not uncommon in lepromatous leprosy. Leprophilia is the name given to a hysterical condition with false anaesthesia developed by a peculiar kind of psychoneurotic who craves for sympathy.

The early lesions of mycosis fungoides might possibly be mistaken for early nodular leprosy, and leucoderma is not infrequently associated with leprosy in the popular mind. It is extremely common, especially in India and in Africa, and unfortunate sufferers are sometimes to be found in leprosy institutions. Depigmentation in leucoderma, however, is more complete and sensory changes are absent. Lupus vulgaris and other tuberculides are very likely to be mistaken for leprosy lesions and in both diseases acid-fast bacilli are difficult to demonstrate. Lupus evinces a greater tendency to scar formation and there are no sensory changes.

Cutaneous leishmaniasis and, in South America, espundia may be mistaken for leprosy. The lesions on the skin of the face tend to concentrate round the mouth and nose and form a more raised margin than those in leprosy. Demonstration of the Leishman–Donovan body will always settle the matter but leishmanial lupus-like lesions on the ears may cause difficulty. Burns and other injuries may leave behind anaesthetic scars.

Polyneuritic leprosy affecting the hands has to be differentiated from syringomyelia, in which analgesia and loss of heat sense are accompanied by retention of sense of touch and normal sweat function. The absence of nerve swelling and tenderness is important. The nerve injuries caused by trauma of the ulnar nerve or by cervical rib may possibly be called into question, but can be settled by X-ray examination. Meralgia paraesthetica (Bernhardt's syndrome) may cause anaesthesia of the antero-lateral region of the thigh and Raynaud's disease can cause trophic changes in the extremities. Familial hypertrophic interstitial neuritis (Déjérine–Scottas disease) may cause confusion because of the characteristic thickening of peripheral nerves, together with sensory and motor changes in the limbs. Anaesthesia of the feet, leading to trophic ulceration and mutilation, can occur in diabetes, tabes, familial sensory radicular neuropathy and primary amyloidosis involving peripheral nerves. Von Recklinghausen's disease (neurofibromas) may sometimes resemble leprosy. Scarring and anaesthesia caused by extensive herpes zoster on the chest may give rise to difficulty. Scleroderma, localized or diffuse, may be confused with lepromatous leprosy but madarosis is not present, nerves are not thickened, acid-fast bacilli are absent from smear and skin biopsy is diagnostic. The absence of fever and the presence of neural signs should differentiate tuberculoid leprosy in reaction from erysipelas. Erythema nodosum leprosum may be mistaken for other forms of erythema nodosum or for the Weber–Christian syndrome (a relapsing, febrile, non-suppurative, nodular panniculitis). Sarcoidosis can resemble tuberculoid leprosy but there is no sensory loss and no nerve thickening. Although a peripheral neuropathy has been reported complicating sarcoidosis, there is no nerve thickening. Granuloma annulare may simulate tuberculoid leprosy but there is no sensory loss or nerve thickening and the histological appearances are different. Granuloma multiforme may resemble tuberculoid leprosy; it appears to be localized to Nigeria. There is no sensory loss or nerve thickening and the histological appearances are different.

DIAGNOSIS

The diagnosis of leprosy rests upon three cardinal signs and an awareness of the disease:

1 Palpable thickened nerves
2 Demonstration of anaesthesia
3 Demonstration of *M. leprae* in skin, nasal mucous membrane or biopsy.

Leprosy should be considered in any untypical or unfamiliar skin disorder in a patient from an endemic area and in any obscure neurological disorder.

Thickened nerves may be felt on palpation and tenderness elicited by pressing sharply with the finger. The ulnar nerve is commonly affected above the elbow; the common peroneal at the head of the fibula behind the knee; the superficial peroneal in front of the ankle; the terminal branch of the radial as it passes over the lower end of the radius; the posterior tibial below the inner malleolus; the great auricular as it runs parallel to the external jugular vein; and the branches of any particular nerve supplying a tuberculoid lesion.

To test sensation the patient should be blindfolded. For testing anaesthesia to light touch a feather or a nylon filament should be used; analgesia is tested by pinprick, using an area of normal skin as control. The two-pin test is often positive when the test is negative. Loss of thermal sensation is important and can be elicited by using a test tube containing hot water and another containing iced water. Hyperaesthesia and paraesthesia may precede anaesthesia to light touch. *The possibility of leprosy should be considered in any patient presenting with a painless burn, injury or ulcer of one limb.*

BACTERIOLOGICAL EXAMINATION

This is essential in order to establish proof of the disease and to assist in correct classification; it consists in carrying out a series of smears from the lesions. The slit-scrape method is recommended and is carried out as follows. The lesion is cleaned with ether and a fold is firmly held between thumb and forefinger of the left hand (to render it avascular); with a small-bladed scalpel an incision is made about 5 mm long and 3 mm deep, pressure of the fingers being maintained; the blade is then turned at right angles to the cut and the wound is scraped several times so that tissue fluid and pulp collect on one side of the blade; this is *gently* smeared on a glass slide. Smears are fixed by heat and are then stained by the Ziehl–Neelsen technique. By this method acid-fast bacilli will always be found in lepromatous leprosy and frequently in the borderline form, but will usually be absent in the tuberculoid type and in the indeterminate group. Nasal scrapings have been advocated in the past but experience has shown that skin smears are far more valuable in diagnosis. In untreated lepromatous leprosy they are always positive but bacilli disappear from the nose more quickly after chemotherapy than they do from the skin. Nasal scrapings are always negative in BB, BT and TT leprosy and negative in most BL cases.

For routine purposes no more than three smears are necessary, one from each ear lobe and one from the edge of one of the active lesions.

SKIN BIOPSY

Biopsy of the skin is essential for correct classification as it enables the histological changes in the skin to be studied. In addition several biopsies carried out at regular intervals provide a valuable method of assessing prognosis and treatment. In carrying out a biopsy the most active part of the lesion must be chosen; this will be at the edge of the lesion in tuberculoid leprosy and in the centre in the lepromatous type. After ensuring local anaesthesia with 2% procaine a portion of skin is removed with a scalpel or by a skin biopsy punch possessing a circular cutting edge, 5–7 mm in diameter. It is essential that the incision should reach the subcutaneous fat, otherwise the deeper layers of the dermis may not be included in the biopsy material. Paraffin sections are stained with haematoxylin and eosin to show the histological changes and, with the Ziehl–Neelsen method, to demonstrate acid-fast bacilli. A nerve biopsy will be necessary in a purely neural case or where a skin biopsy has not given sufficient information; a thickened sensory nerve is chosen, such as the great auricular in the neck, the antebrachial cutaneous in the forearm, the radial at the lateral aspect of the wrist, the femoral cutaneous in the thigh, the sural in the leg or the superficial peroneal on the dorsum of the foot.

SUBSIDIARY SIGNS

Anhidrosis is characteristic of chronic cases and is usually present in tuberculoid macules. In doubtful cases pilocarpine 0.2 ml of 1 in 1000 solution is injected intradermally in a suspected patch and a similar amount in adjacent healthy skin. Both areas are then painted with tincture of iodine and, when dry, powdered with starch. The control area sweats, turning the starch blue. Absence of sweat at the point of injection indicates leprosy.

The histamine test of Rodriguez is somewhat similar in slight or early cases. A drop of 1 in 1000 solution of histamine is placed within the margin of the suspected area and a second outside. A prick is made with a needle through the drops. A red flare appears in normal skin. This test can be of great value in a purely neural case with sensory loss in one or more limbs, for it will exclude hysteria and organic disease of the central nervous system, such as syringomyelia. In all those conditions a red flare develops in the anaesthetic skin, but no flare appears if the anaesthesia is due to leprosy or other forms of peripheral neuritis.

LEPRA REACTIONS

The sudden exacerbation of the disease referred to as reactional state has been described and interpreted in different ways, although it essentially relates to the immune status of the patient. It is important to remember that simple extension or regression of lesions does not constitute the true leprosy reaction. The two essential types of reaction are erythema nodosum leprosum (ENL) or type 2 reaction in lepromatous leprosy (LL, BL), and reversal or type 1 reaction in borderline leprosy (BT, BB, BL).

The reactions in leprosy are all acute episodes associated with alterations in the immunological balance between the bacilli and the host. The reactions that take place in borderline and lepromatous leprosy are described by Ridley[54] as follows:

● *Borderline*: downgrading and reversal (both associated with changes in cell-mediated immunity).
● *Lepromatous*: erythema nodosum leprosum (associated with humoral mechanisms).

DOWNGRADING

This is a relatively uncommon type of reaction and is immunologically unfavourable, associated with movement towards lepromatous leprosy and occurs only in untreated patients.

Histological features include: increase in bacilli; loss of the usual compact focalization of the granuloma; and intracellular and extracellular oedema.

REVERSAL

This is immunologically favourable and occurs in near-lepromatous and borderline patients when the bacterial load is diminished by treatment.

Clinical features are similar in both downgrading and reversal reactions. They may appear rapidly and violently. There may be fever (in severe reaction) possibly lasting several months. Erythema and swelling of skin lesions occurs and possibly ulceration. Hands and feet may be swollen and acutely tender. Nerve involvement is common; lesions are very tender. Gross paralysis may develop in a few days. New lesions (towards the tuberculoid type in reversal reactions) may occur. The nasal passages may be blocked by swollen mucosa. The patient may be in a miserable state.

Histological features may be seen in marked reversal cases (in mild cases there is little histological sign). These include: decrease in bacilli; change of host cells towards the epithelioid form; necrosis in severe reactions; oedema in and around the granuloma, which enlarges; and dermal reaction.

ERYTHEMA NODOSUM LEPROSUM

This may be precipitated by intercurrent infection or other stress factors. It is not an indication of shift in immunological status. It occurs usually when patients have been under treatment and the bacterial load has fallen, the bacilli are disintegrating and releasing antigenic material and are relatively numerous in the circulating blood. It is probably associated with humoral mechanisms and represents a manifestation of the Arthus phenomenon.

Clinical features include: fever; transient crops of small painful red nodules lasting a few days; painful red plaques if severe, with necrosis and ulceration; enlargement of lymph nodes, liver and spleen; iridocyclitis, orchitis and painful enlargement of nerves (neuralgia); swollen joints; and nephritis occasionally.

These manifestations are found mostly where bacilli are common, except the lesions in joints, kidneys and possibly the eyes. Changes in the kidneys, apparently due to deposition of antigen–antibody complexes within the nephrons, tend to occur in patients subject to severe reactional states. The nephrons may be destroyed.

Histological features: reaction is not in the major skin lesions but in small, clinically unapparent lesions with few bacilli. Polymorphs are present and predominant. Oedema is marked. Cellular disintegration is marked. Lymphocytes appear later. Nerve involvement with polymorphs occurs and there is infiltration of bacilli into walls of large vessels and necrosis of small vessels. Dermal reaction can be intense.

TREATMENT

Treatment should be started as soon as a definite diagnosis has been made and the case classified as multibacillary (LL, BL or BB) or paucibacillary (BT, TT or indeterminate). Multidrug therapy (MDT) is now the standard treatment of leprosy.

It is probably unwise to begin treatment in very anaemic patients, in whom it should be delayed until the haemoglobin has been increased to 5 g/dl. Once the diagnosis is established most patients can be treated on an outpatient basis. Lepromatous patients need not be kept isolated as they are not discharging any viable bacilli with rifampicin treatment. Tuberculoid patients are not infectious. Modern drug therapy has led to the establishment of country-wide treatment programmes as part of leprosy control.

DRUGS FOR TREATMENT OF LEPROSY

Several drugs are available for treatment and two or more are given concurrently as standard treatment.

DAPSONE (DDS; 4,4'-diaminodiphenylsulphone)

Dapsone is slowly bactericidal. The dose is 6–10 mg/kg weekly, i.e. a dose of 100 mg daily for adults and suitably reduced for children. The drug may be given to all patients in full dosage from the start of treatment.

Side-effects

These are uncommon but include haemolytic anaemia, methaemoglobinaemia, hepatitis, skin conditions including fixed eruptions, exfoliative dermatitis, together with systemic symptoms, slight or severe. Subjects with a deficiency of glucose-6-phosphate dehydrogenase (G6PD) are more susceptible to haemolysis than are normal subjects. Agranulocytosis has been reported in patients taking dapsone for other conditions in much larger doses than are usually given in leprosy.

Dapsone by itself is no longer used as it once was and this is due to two factors: slow and limited effectiveness with treatment and the development of dapsone resistance.

Prevalence of dapsone resistance

Secondary dapsone resistance has been detected wherever it has been employed in monotherapy—the highest incidence so far being 40% in central Burma.[55] For this reason treatment with only one drug is no longer possible.

Persistence of M. leprae

It has been found that a small number of dapsone-sensitive bacilli may persist in the body for many years, leading to relapse up to 20 years later.[56]

RIFAMPICIN

This antibiotic, an addition to leprosy therapy in 1970, has proved its value. It is a strongly bactericidal drug. An early report[57] showed that it rapidly reduced the morphological index (MI) of bacilli in skin to zero in 5 weeks, compared with 5 months in control patients with lepromatous leprosy receiving dapsone. Rifampicin is rapidly effective in relieving nasal symptoms in lepromatous leprosy and in healing ulceration resulting from the breaking down of nodules.[40] Rifampicin is effective given monthly[40] in a dose of 600 mg every 4 weeks on an empty stomach.

Side-effects

Rifampicin may produce a reddish-brown colour in urine, sputum and sweat. Other side-effects include nausea, abdominal discomfort, 'flu' syndrome and, rarely, toxic effects on the liver.

It should be noted that the effects of steroids are reduced by rifampicin and the drug also impairs the effectiveness of oral contraceptives.[58]

The first two cases of rifampicin resistance were reported in 1976[59] and subsequently other cases have been reported in patients given rifampicin monotherapy.

CLOFAZIMINE (Lamprene; B 663 (Geigy); G 30320)

This is a rimino compound derived from phenazine dye. It appears to have a remarkable action on ENL and on the course of lepromatous leprosy itself.

Clofazimine has been given by mouth in doses of 100–300 mg daily for long periods to patients in reaction, formerly dependent on corticosteroids, and the steroids have been reduced gradually and eventually abandoned completely, with good clinical and bacteriological results. Once reaction is controlled the dose can be reduced.[60] If reaction does break through the dose should not be reduced but should be increased. Clofazimine has now been found effective in previously untreated lepromatous leprosy in doses of 100 mg two or three times each week. In the standard MDT it is given in a daily dose of 50 mg supplemented by a monthly loading dose of 300 mg.

Clofazimine is slowly eliminated from the body. The main adverse reaction is deep and persistent redness followed by pigmentation of the skin, which is resented by patients with light skins but not by others who appreciate its therapeutic value. It not only controls ENL but also improves the clinical condition, the bacillary index and the morphological index. It may rarely cause abdominal pain and diarrhoea. Because of occasional reports of serious adverse effects in patients who have received this drug in high dosage of more than 100 mg daily, larger doses should be given for as short a period as possible and only under supervision. A few cases of fatal diarrhoea have been reported[61] when dosage has been continued for many months or years. No confirmed cases of clofazimine resistance have been reported.

THIOAMIDES (ethionamide and prothionamide)

Ethionamide and prothionamide are given in a dosage of 250–500 mg daily; larger doses cause gastrointestinal upsets and jaundice. The usual dose is 375 mg daily after the main meal. They kill M. leprae faster than dapsone but more slowly than rifampicin. Resistance can develop after years of single drug treatment.[62] The most important toxic effect is hepatotoxicity, particularly when given together with rifampicin; the drug is therefore recommended for use only in exceptional situations.

FLUOROQUINOLONES

Although a large number of fluoroquinolones have been developed, most interest has focused on ofloxacin. Like all fluoroquinolones, ofloxacin interferes with bacterial DNA replication by inhibiting the A subunit of the enzyme DNA gyrase. It was used in a clinical trial by Ji and Grosset[63] at a dose of 400 mg daily. A single dose had moderate bactericidal activity; 22 doses killed 99.99% of the viable M. leprae. Ofloxacin is well absorbed, reaching peak serum concentration after 2 hours, and has a half-life of 7 hours. Most of the dose is excreted unchanged in the urine. Side-effects include nausea, diarrhoea and other gastrointestinal complaints, and a variety of central nervous system complaints including insomnia, headaches, dizziness, nervousness and hallucinations. Serious problems are infrequent and do not usually require discontinuation of the drug.

MINOCYCLINE

Minocycline is the only member of the tetracycline group of antibiotics that has significant bactericidal activity against M. leprae. This may be because of its lipophilic properties, which allow it to penetrate cell walls.[64] The standard dose is 100 mg daily, which gives a peak serum level that exceeds the minimum inhibitory concentration of minocycline against M. leprae by a factor of 10–20. Its bactericidal activity against M. leprae is greater than that of clarithromycin, but much less than that of rifampicin.[65] It was shown to be very effective clinically when administered as monotherapy in patients with lepromatous leprosy, although 2 months of therapy were required before all patients became negative for M. leprae, as determined in the mouse footpad model.[66]

Like other tetracyclines, minocycline inhibits protein synthesis via a reversible binding at the 30S ribosomal subunit, thereby blocking the binding of aminoacyl transfer RNA to the messenger RNA ribosomal complex. It is well absorbed, with a half-life of 11–23 hours. Side-effects include discoloration of teeth in infants and children, occasional pigmentation of the skin and mucous membranes, various gastrointestinal symptoms and central nervous system complaints, including dizziness and unsteadiness.

MACROLIDES

Several members of this group, including erythromycin, have been evaluated as antileprosy drugs, but only clarithromycin shows significant promise at this time. Studies in the mouse footpad model have demonstrated the potent bactericidal activity of clarithromycin, but it is clearly less bactericidal than rifampicin.[64] When clarithromycin was administered at a dose of 500 mg daily to lepromatous patients, 99% of bacilli were killed within 28 days and 99.9% by 56 days.[67]

Clarithromycin is readily absorbed from the gastrointestinal tract and converted to its active metabolite, 14-hydroxyclarithromycin. A single dose of 500 mg produces a peak serum concentration in 1–4 hours, with a half-life of 6–7 hours. About 38% of the dose is excreted in the urine and 40% in the faeces. Tissue concentrations are higher than those in serum.

Clarithromycin inhibits bacterial protein synthesis by linking to the 50S ribosomal subunit, thereby preventing elongation of the protein chain. It is relatively non-toxic. Gastrointestinal irritation, nausea, vomiting and diarrhoea are the most common problems, but they usually do not necessitate discontinuation of the drug.

OTHER DRUGS

With the possible exception of fusidic acid,[68] other drugs available or currently under study with known activity against *M. leprae* are much less potent than those mentioned above. They include amoxicillin plus clavulanic acid, brodimoprim, thioacetazone and deoxyfructoserotonin.

TREATMENT REGIMENS

Antileprosy drugs are no longer given alone and multidrug regimens are necessary to overcome dapsone resistance, prevent resistance to other drugs, particularly rifampicin in cases with a significant bacterial load and to encourage compliance. Two standard regimens are recommended.[69]

MULTIBACILLARY LEPROSY

For adults:
Rifampicin 600 mg once a month supervised.
Dapsone 100 mg daily self-administered.
Clofazimine 50 mg daily self-administered, plus 300 mg once a month supervised.

For others:
Dapsone 1–2 mg/kg daily
Rifampicin 450 mg < 35 kg, 300 mg < 20 kg, 150 mg < 12 kg.

As an alternative to 50 mg daily of clofazimine, 100 mg may be given every other day.

This triple drug regimen must be given for a fixed period of 2 years. Relapsed smear-positive patients should also be treated for 2 years.

PAUCIBACCILLARY LEPROSY

Rifampicin 600 mg supervised once a month for 6 doses.
Dapsone 100 mg daily self-administered for 6 months.

TREATMENT OF COMPLICATIONS INCLUDING REACTIONAL STATES

The main therapeutic weapons in the treatment of reactional states are steroids, clofazimine and, where not contraindicated, thalidomide.

ENL (type 2 reaction)

Antileprosy drugs must be continued in full dosage throughout treatment. Mild ENL cases can be treated as outpatients. If there is any nerve tenderness the affected limb should be rested. Analgesics should be given as required, and the patient should be seen regularly at least once every 2 weeks. In particular, eyes should be checked at each visit to ensure that the patient is not developing iridocyclitis.

The following drugs may be of value in the management of mild ENL:

- Chloroquine
- Stibophen injection

- Acetylsalicylic acid or other similar mild analgesics, as required.

Patients suffering from severe ENL reaction, should be referred to hospital. Drugs that are effective against such reaction are steroids, thalidomide and clofazimine.

Steroids may be used in repeated short courses[55] but in chronic ENL steroids may be given together with clofazimine or thalidomide. The usual course of steroids in the form of prednisolone is 30–40 mg daily for 1–2 weeks, followed by reducing the daily dose by 5–10 mg every 2 weeks.

One point about treatment with corticosteroids is that when such patients complain of abdominal pain or diarrhoea, trophozoites of *Entamoeba histolytica* can often be found in their stools. These exacerbations of amoebic colitis respond to standard antimoebic treatment and do not indicate cessation of steroid treatment.[70] The development of the hyperinfection syndrome of strongyloidiasis does demand immediate withdrawal of corticosteroids.

Thalidomide is also an effective drug in the treatment of ENL reaction. The initial dose is usually 200–400 mg daily, given as a single bedtime dose to exploit its sedative action. The dosage can be reduced to 50–100 mg daily after 1–2 weeks. Thalidomide has few toxic effects; the contraindication for its unsupervised use derives from its teratogenicity, and it should therefore not be given to women of child-bearing age. All patients must be fully informed of its side-effects and this drug must be given only under close supervision. Where strict supervision and appropriate use of thalidomide cannot be assured, it should not be utilized.

In addition to its antileprosy effect, clofazimine has an anti-inflammatory action which is useful in controlling type 2 lepra reaction.[40] It is slower in its effect than steroids and takes 4–6 weeks to exert its full effect. The initial dose is usually 100 mg three times daily. An average course of clofazimine is:

100 mg three times daily for 1 month;
100 mg twice daily for 1 month;
100 mg daily thereafter.

The continuous administration of a high dosage of clofazimine can produce, apart from skin discoloration, gastrointestinal disorders, the most serious being ileitis and intestinal obstruction.

REVERSAL (type 1 reaction)

Treatment in type 1 reactions may be urgent because of the possibility of permanent nerve damage and should be instituted without delay with corticosteroids. In tuberculoid and dimorphous leprosy the reactionary state is less severe but the lesions may become painful or ulcerate and a peripheral nerve may be involved with pain and weakness. Antileprosy treatment should be continued in full dosage. Analgesics will be required for the pain associated with the neuritis characteristic of the type 1 lepra reaction. The most effective drugs against severe type 1 reactions are steroids, prednisolone being the most commonly used. A suggested average course is:

weeks 1 and 2, prednisolone 40 mg daily;
weeks 3 and 4, prednisolone 30 mg daily;
weeks 5 and 6, prednisolone 20 mg daily;
weeks 7 and 8, prednisolone 15 mg daily;
weeks 9 and 10, prednisolone 10 mg daily;
weeks 11 and 12, prednisolone 5 mg daily.

In very severe reactions, and particularly in prolonged neuritis, prompt and adequate treatment with steroids is essential; a higher dosage may be used for a longer period, and must be adjusted to the clinical response. The affected limb may need splinting to rest painful nerves. If a nerve abscess develops it should be aspirated or incised. Lesions which ulcerate require appropriate dressings.

TREATMENT OF EYE COMPLICATIONS

Protection must be afforded to those patients with lagophthalmos by use of goggles or sunglasses. Frequent use of artificial tear drops during the day and ointments or oily drops at night is advocated. In early stages, active exercises to help the patient close the eyelids frequently and fully may be very useful. In the late or established cases, with lid gap of more than 5 mm, surgery is indicated. The standard procedure is lateral tarsorrhaphy.

The treatment of the acute form of iridocyclitis is with topical application of atropine and steroids. Acute leading to chronic iridocyclitis needs to be treated, often for extended periods of time. The treatment should include topical atropine and steroids, to which 5% phenylephrine should be added to stimulate pupillary dilatation. In cases of severe complications optical iridectomy may be necessary to restore some vision.

PREVENTION AND MANAGEMENT OF DEFORMITIES

Primary deformity is due to the activity of the disease, for instance to erosion of the phalanges due to lepromatous granulomas. Secondary deformity is due to damage which the patient inadvertently self-inflicts as a consequence of anaesthesia or paralysis.

The results of nerve involvement in leprosy lead to ulceration, paralysis and deformity of the limbs so often that the prevention of correction or the deformities involve a multitude of special techniques up to full orthopaedic surgery. A discussion of these complicated treatments is outside the scope of this book and surgeons who wish to study the subject are referred to books on surgery in leprosy by Carayon et al,[71] Fritschi[72] and McDowell and Enna,[73] and to the book on foot problems by Brand.[52]

It is important to keep the hands under constant examination for swelling, sensation and function and to ensure as far as possible that they are protected from trauma during the period when decalcification of the bones may be taking place.

Examination by X-ray is essential for complete assessment. The same is true of the feet, but in the feet deep plantar damage may occur before anaesthesia is complete and nerve damage must therefore be recognized when loss of localization of light touch occurs on the sole. Plantar damage and ulceration can be prevented, partly by provision of footwear with rigid wooden soles and soft insoles and by the use of Plastazote insoles placed inside orthopaedic shoes.[74] It is important regularly to scrape away the callus which forms over a healed ulcer. Dry, cracked skin can be treated by soaking in water for several hours each day and then covering with soft paraffin. Ulcers can be treated by rest, dressings and antibiotics; a plaster cast may obviate the need for more than a few days bed-rest. Foot drop needs special surgical measures such as tendon transplantation for correction.

PROGNOSIS

Leprosy in its milder forms is a self-healing disease; it is also curable. Of those who become infected, only a small proportion develop overt signs. Its old terrible reputation is justifiable only in extreme cases.

In *macular tuberculoid leprosy* the prognosis after treatment is excellent, though with severe hypopigmentation the pigment may not return to completely healed lesions, and if anaesthesia is extensive, sensation may not be restored completely, even after complete cure.

In *infiltrated tuberculoid leprosy* the prognosis is also excellent after treatment but if nerves have been grossly enlarged there may be some permanent anaesthesia and the patient should be trained to protect the hands and feet because of the risk of permanent ulceration or deformity.

In *lepromatous leprosy* the prognosis is now much better than ever before. The earlier the treatment is instituted, the better the prognosis. If the patient suffers from acute ENL, especially if this goes on to progressive reaction, the prognosis is not good. In advanced lepromatous leprosy permanent sequelae—deformity, paralysis or paresis from nerve injury, damage to the eyes—may occur, although modern treatment can do much to prevent these.

In *infiltrated borderline leprosy* the prognosis should be guarded at first; there is a tendency to severe deformity after reactional borderline lesions. Moreover, this form may go on to lepromatous leprosy. This borderline group is particularly prone to lead to serious deformities; the patients need careful attention.

With modern treatment, including drug treatment, surgery and physiotherapy, much deformity can be avoided or relieved.

Relapse may occur, especially when full courses of treatment are not observed. Clinically, a relapse shows itself by the appearance of new skin lesions, erythematous papulonodules, and these are accompanied by the presence of morphologically normal leprosy bacilli in skin smears and sections from the lesions and in nasal mucus. These lesions should not be mistaken for those of ENL, which are often tender and disappear in a few days. Only small numbers of granular bacilli are found in an ENL lesion.

CONTROL

OBJECTIVES AND STRATEGY

The objectives of leprosy control are threefold:

1 To interrupt transmission of the infection, thereby reducing the incidence of disease so that it no longer constitutes a public health problem.
2 To treat patients in order to achieve their cure and, where possible, complete rehabilitation.
3 To prevent the development of associated deformities.

The strategy of leprosy control involves essentially secondary prevention through early detection of cases and treatment of patients with effective drugs so that the reservoirs of infection can be eliminated and transmission of infection interrupted. So far, there is no primary preventive strategy available for leprosy, although BCG itself is known to have some protective effect against the disease, particularly in certain parts of the world. The widespread application of WHO-recommended MDT since the early 1980s has had a significant impact in reducing the disease burden in the world, raising hopes of eliminating the disease as a public health problem by the year 2000.

MULTIDRUG THERAPY

Prompt treatment of all existing and newly detected cases with multidrug therapy (MTD) is the principal method currently used for control of leprosy. Until the 1980s, leprosy control was based on treating patients with dapsone, with limited results. Many leprosy control programmes were faced with the problem of increasing secondary and primary resistance of *M. leprae* to the drug dapsone. In order to cope with this problem a WHO Study Group on Chemotherapy of Leprosy for Control Programmes that met in 1981[69] recommended MDT for both multibacillary and paucibacillary patients. This essential change in the strategy of leprosy control has now been generally endorsed by the governments of countries where leprosy is endemic and by international and other non-governmental voluntary organizations that support leprosy control activities.

The coverage of leprosy patients with MDT has rapidly increased over the past few years and by 1994 had reached 54.6% of total registered cases.[1] The increasing acceptability of MDT among national health services and leprosy patients is due to: (1) the fixed, and relatively short duration of treatment; (2) the low level of treatment-related side-effects; (3) the very low relapse rates following completion of treatment;[75,76] (4) the high level of acceptance of clofazimine in spite of the discoloration produced by the drug; and (5) significant reduction in frequency and severity of lepra reactions. One more positive consequence of MDT is the considerable increase in the proportion of self-reporting cases at an early stage of the disease. This in turn has led to a reduction in the number and degree of deformities among new cases.

CASE FINDING

The most cost-effective approach for case finding is the promotion of self-reporting of suspect lesions through increased community awareness about the disease and its curability. This should be supported by efficient and easily accessible treatment services for the community. Special efforts may be needed to identify cases in high endemic areas. These may include organization of active case finding activities, such as population survey and school survey. Peripheral health service staff should be adequately trained to recognize signs of leprosy and to initiate treatment with an appropriate MDT regimen.

PATIENT AND COMMUNITY EDUCATION

For MDT regimens to be implemented successfully, however, a good health education programme must be developed and maintained, using all available resources, including the mass media. Before starting MDT, patients should be informed of the treatment they will receive, the possibility of side-effects, lepra reactions or disabilities occurring, and what to do if such problems arise. Patients should also be advised about the consequences of interrupting or stopping MDT. This information is essential to ensure that patients co-operate with health workers. Throughout their treatment patients should be advised about how to take care of insensitive hands, feet and eyes.

Because the risk of relapse after completion of the MDT regimens has been shown to be negligible,[77] it is not necessary to carry out routine surveillance of patients. Instead, patients should be taught, at the time of release from treatment, to recognize the early signs of possible relapse or reactions and to report promptly for treatment.

IMMUNOPROPHYLAXIS

The value of any antileprosy vaccine in reducing the incidence of the disease will depend very much upon its effectiveness in preventing infection, and thus the disease, in uninfected individuals (immunoprophylactic effect), and in preventing disease in infected individuals (immunotherapeutic effect), as well as the proportion of these two populations in any community.

With regard to the role of BCG in leprosy, information based on the results of five large field studies conducted in Myanmar, India, Malawi, Papua New Guinea and Uganda, showed that the protective effect varied from 80% (Uganda) to 20–30% (Myanmar and India). In all these studies the observed protective effect of BCG was primarily against paucibacillary leprosy.

Attempts to develop a vaccine against leprosy are primarily based on the assumption that induction of a cell-mediated immune response to *M. leprae* will lead to protection against the bacillus. A double-blind trial on the protective effect of *M. leprae* plus BCG, compared with BCG alone, in a high-risk population comprising about 30 000 contacts did not provide conclusive results.[78] A similar large-scale, long-term immunoprophylactic trial is currently in progress in Malawi.

Vaccines based on other mycobacteria studied in India have shown that killed vaccine preparations based on cultivable mycobacteria belonging to the *M. avium* complex (the 'ICRC' bacilla and mycobacterium 'W') are capable of producing skin test conversion responses to lepromin in human subjects.[79,80]

HOUSEHOLD CONTACTS OF PATIENTS

Household contacts of leprosy patients are at significant risk for the development of the disease. Thus, contacts of newly diagnosed cases should be examined for evidence of leprosy at that time. They should then be advised of the early signs of the disease and told to return if any suspect skin, motor, sensory or other lesions occur. Chemoprophylaxis with antileprosy drugs is not recommended for contacts of leprosy patients in leprosy control programmes.

FUTURE PROSPECTS

Because of the opportunities available, as well as the need, the 44th World Health Assembly, which met in May 1991, adopted a resolution to eliminate leprosy as a public health problem by the year 2000, and defined elimination as attaining a level of prevalence below one case per 10 000 population. This is considered to be an achievable goal provided leprosy control efforts are sufficiently intensified.

REFERENCES

1 World Health Organization. *Weekly Epidemiol Rec* 1994; 20–21.
2 Noordeen S K & Lopez Bravo L. *World Health Stat Q* 1986; 39:122–128.
3 World Health Organization. WHO Expert Committee on Leprosy. Sixth Report. *WHO Tech Rep Ser* 1988; 768.
4 Ridley D S. *Trans R Soc Trop Med Hyg* 1967; 61:596.
5 Rees R J W. *Trans R Soc Trop Med Hyg* 1967; 61:581.
6 Rees R J W, Waters M F R, Weddell A G M et al. *Nature* 1967; 215:599–602.
7 Kirchheimer W F, Storrs E E & Binford C H. *Int J Lepr* 1972; 40:229.
8 Montestruc E & Berdonneau R. *Bull Soc Pathol Exot Filiales* 1954; 47:781–783.
9 Doull J A, Guinto R S, Rodriguez J N et al. Int J Lepr 1942; 10:107–131.
10 Lara C B & Nolasco J O. *Int J Lepr* 1956; 24:245–263.
11 Noordeen S K. *Lepr India* 1975; 47:85–93.
12 Guinto R S, Doull J A, de Guia L et al. Int J Lepr 1954; 22:273–284.
13 Noordeen S K. *Indian J Med Res* 1972; 60:439–445.
14 Walsh G P, Meyers W M, Binford C H et al. Lep Rev 1981; 52(supplement 1):77–83.
15 Truman R W, Shannon E J, Hagstad H V et al. Am J Trop Med Hyg 1986; 35:588–593.
16 Lumpkin L R III, Cox G F & Wolf J E Jr. *J Am Acad Dermatol* 1983; 9:899–903.

17 Figueredo N & Desai S D. *Indian J Med Sci* 1949; 3:253–265.

18 Chatterjee B R. *Lepr India* 1976; 48:643–644.

19 Chacko C J G, Mohan M, Jesudasan K et al. Abstract presented at the XIth Biennial Conference of the Indian Association of Leprologists, 1979, Madras, India.

20 Weddell A G M, Palmer E & Rees R J W. *Lepr Rev* 1963; 34:156–158.

21 Schaffer I. *Arch Dermato Syphilis* 1898; 44:159–174.

22 Shepard C C. *Am J Hyg* 1960; 71:147–157.

23 Pedley J C. *Lepr Rev* 1973; 44:33–35.

24 Davey T F & Rees R J W. *Lepr Rev* 1974; 45:121–134.

25 Desikan K V. *Lepr Rev* 1977; 48:231–235.

26 Rees R J W & McDougall A C. *J Med Microbiol* 1977; 10:63–68.

27 Chehl S, Job C K & Hastings R C. *Am J Trop Med Hyg* 1985; 34:1161–1166.

28 Zuniga M, Castellazzi Z, Lambert P et al. Paper presented at the conference and workshop on Pathogenesis and Immunotherapy of Leprosy, 1982, Caracas, Venezuela.

29 Gupte M D, Anantharaman D S, Nagaraju B et al. Lepr Rev 1990; 61:132–144.

30 Noordeen S K & Neelan P N. *Indian J Med Res* 1978; 67:515–527.

31 Shepard C C, Walker L L, Van Landingham R M et al. Infect Immun 1982; 38:673–680.

32 Stanley S J, Howland C, Stone M M et al. J Hyg (Camb) 1981; 87:233–248.

33 Rook G A W, Bahr G M & Stanford J L. *Tubercle* 1981; 62:63–68.

34 Lucas S. *Lepr Rev* 1993; 64:97–103.

35 Leonard G, Sangare A, Verdier M et al. J Acquir Immune Defic Syndr 1990; 3:1109–1113.

36 Ponnighaus J M, Mwanjasi L J, Fine P E M et al. Int J Lepr 1991; 59:221–228.

37 Shiv Raj L, Patil S A, Girdhar A et al. Int J Lepr 1988; 56:546–551.

38 Andrade V L, Avelleira J C, Marques A et al. Int J Lepr 1991; 59:125–126.

39 Ridley D S & Jopling W H. *Int J Lepr* 1966; 34:255.

40 Jopling W H. *Handbook of Leprosy*, 2nd edn. London: Heinemann, 1978.

41 Ridley D S. *Bull World Health Organ* 1974; 51:451.

42 Turk J L. *Immunology in Clinical Practice*. London: Heinemann, 1969.

43 Eden W, Van Vries R R P, Mehra N K et al. J Infect Dis 1980; 141:693–701.

44 Eden W, Van Vries R R P, de Marao J D et al. Hum Immun 1982; 4:343–350.

45 Godal T, Lofgren M & Negassi K. *Int J Lepr* 1972; 40:243–250.

46 Narayanan R B, Bhutani L K, Sharma A K et al. Clin Exp Immunol 1983; 51:421–430.

47 Haregewoin A, Godal R, Mustafa A S et al. Nature 1983; 303:542–544.

48 Harboe M. *Int J Lepr* 1982; 50:342–350.

49 Karat A B A, Job C K & Rao P S S. *BMJ* 1971; 1:307.

50 Rea T H & Levan N E. *Arch Dermatol* 1978; 114:1023.

51 Rea T H & Ridley D S. *Int J Lepr* 1979; 47:161.

52 Brand P. *Insensitive Feet: A Practical Handbook on Foot Problems in Leprosy*. London: Leprosy Mission, 1966.

53 International Congress of Leprosy. *Int J Lepr* 1953; 21:484.

54 Ridley D S. *Lepr Rev* 1969; 40:77.

55 Pearson J M H. *Int J Lepr* 1981; 49:417–420.

56 Waters M F R. In Gilles H M (ed.) *Recent Advances in Tropical Medicine*. Edinburgh: Churchill Livingstone, 1984.

57 Rees R J W, Pearson J M H & Waters M F R. *BMJ* 1970; 1:89.

58 Jopling W H & Pettit J H S. *Int J Lepr* 1979; 40:229.

59 Jacobson R R & Hastings R C. *Lancet* 1976; ii:1304.

60 Browne R G. *Lepr Rev* 1966; 37:141.

61 Jopling W H. *Lepr Rev* 1976; 47:1–3.

62 Browne S G. *Int J Lepr* 1965; 33:267–273.

63 Ji B & Grosset J H. *Acta Lepr* 1991; 7:321–326.

64 Ji B, Perani E G & Grosset J H. *Antimicrob Agents Chemother* 1991; 35:579–581.

65 Gelber R H. *J Infect Dis* 1987; 156:236–239.

66 Gelber R H et al. BMJ 1992; 304:91–92.

67 Ji B et al. J Infect Dis 1993; 168:188–190.

68 Franzblau S G, Biswas A N & Harris E B. *Antimicrob Agents Chemother* 1992; 36:92–94.

69 World Health Organization. *WHO Tech Rep Ser* 1982; 675.

70 Goodwin C S. *BMJ* 1969; iii:174.

71 Carayon A, Bourrel P & Languillon J. *Surgery in Leprosy*. Paris: Masson, 1964.

72 Fritschi E P. *Reconstructive Surgery in Leprosy*. Bristol: Wright, 1971.

73 McDowell F & Enna C. *Surgical Rehabilitation in Leprosy and Other Peripheral Nerve Disorders*. Baltimore, MD: Williams & Wilkins, 1974.

74 Jopling W H. *Lepr Rev* 1969; 40:175.

75 Ekambaram V & Rao M K. *Indian J Lepr* 1991; 63:34–42.

76 Becx-Bleumink M. *Int J Lepr* 1992; 60:421–435.

77 World Health Organization. *Risk of relapse in leprosy*. WHO/CTD/LEP/94.1. Geneva: WHO.

78 Convit J, Sampson C & Zuniga M et al. Lancet 1992; 339:446–450.

79 Deo M G et al. Int J Lepr 1983; 51:540–549.

80 Talwar G P & Fotedar A. *Int J Lepr* 1983; 51:550–552.

SECTION 5D
MYCOTIC INFECTIONS

CHAPTER 59

FUNGAL INFECTIONS

R. J. Hay

The fungi are well recognized causes of disease in most parts of the world. The best known of the infections caused by these eukaryotic organisms are superficial, and include common diseases such as dermatophytosis or ringworm and candidosis. However extensive, deforming and potentially fatal deep or systemic infections can also occur.[1]

Fungi are eukaryotic organisms which possess a nucleus and full complement of intracellular organelles such as Golgi apparatus and mitochondria. They are characterized by the presence of a polysaccharide-based cell wall. There are two principal types of fungi, the yeasts and moulds. Yeasts are single cells which reproduce by a process of bud formation to give rise to single daughter cells. With fungi that form hyphae, the mycelial or mould fungi, chains of cells are formed and cells remain in contiguity. Some fungi, known as the dimorphic fungi, exist as either a yeast or mycelium at different stages of their life cycles. Examples of these organisms include most of the major respiratory pathogens such as *Histoplasma capsulatum* and *Coccidioides immitis*. The formation of specialized vegetative or reproductive structures or spores is very typical of fungi, but while these are formed by pathogenic fungi in laboratory cultivation media and are of major importance in the recognition of organisms they are not produced in vivo. The principal exception is the formation of thick-walled vegetative cells within the hyphae of certain pathogenic fungi such as the dermatophytes, the development of which appears to aid survival.

Fungi can cause human disease in a number of different ways, such as the production of toxins, the possession of sensitizing antigens (allergens) or by the invasion of tissue. Fungal toxins have been recognized for many years in large thallic fungi such as the rye ergot (ergotamine). More pharmacologically potent toxins may also be produced by fungi such as *Aspergillus flavus* contaminating stored foodstuffs. These mycotoxins—*A. flavus* produces amongst others a series of aflatoxins—are particularly potent. Aflatoxin-associated hepatitis and hepatic necrosis has been reported from many parts of the developed and developing worlds, including a large outbreak in Kenya where stored grain was implicated as a source. The outer cell wall of most fungi is potentially allergenic as it contains a number of polysaccharide antigens. These occur in some of the organisms that produce air-borne spores, such as *Aspergillus*, *Alternaria* and *Penicillium* species, and hay fever or asthma due to such organisms is estimated to account for up to 15% of respiratory allergies. The third mechanism of disease production is the invasion of tissue. These different modes of pathogenesis cannot always be neatly separated and in some instances two, or even three, are all present. For instance in primary infections of histoplasmosis symptoms due to immune complex deposition, such as arthritis or erythema multiforme, may be involved.

Invasive diseases caused by fungi are known collectively as the mycoses and they affect predominantly superficial, subcutaneous or deep tissues. These are known as the superficial, subcutaneous or systemic mycoses, respectively.

The distribution of mycoses is affected by a number of factors: the presence of the organisms in the environment, host immunity, frequency of exposure and the availability of invasive or immunosuppressive medical technology. These influence the spread of fungal disease in the tropics as well as in temperate climates. The main superficial mycoses are common in the tropics. The subcutaneous infections, which occur through implantation of pathogenic organisms via injury, are largely confined to the tropics and subtropics. The main systemic mycoses due to respiratory pathogens such as *H. capsulatum* occur in the tropics, while systemic opportunistic infections caused by organisms such as *Aspergillus* are probably more common in temperate areas where there is a greater use of medical techniques involving severe immunosuppression.

SUPERFICIAL MYCOSES

Superficial infections caused by fungi are common in all environments. They are a particular problem in the tropics as their prevalence is higher. While on occasions this is due to the existence of endemic foci of specific diseases such as tinea imbricata or tinea capitis, there is also a real increase in prevalence of certain infections. Factors such as climate, humidity of the skin surface and the $P\text{CO}_2$ concentration may all affect the expression of these diseases.

The main superficial infections are dermatophytosis or ringworm, superficial candidosis and pityriasis (tinea) versicolor (Table 59.1). However, other conditions such as foot infection caused by *Scytalidium dimidiatum* (*Hendersonula toruloidea*) as well as the hair shaft infections, white and black piedra, and tinea nigra are also seen. The former in particular is common although frequently it passes unrecognized in the tropics. Otomycosis, a superficial infection of the external auditory meatus, is also common. Oculomycosis, in particular mycotic keratitis, occurs in both temperate as well as tropical environments but poses a frequent and difficult management problem in the tropics (see Chapter 10).

DERMATOPHYTOSIS

The dermatophyte or ringworm fungi are common causes of superficial infections.[2] They are mould fungi which have become adapted to parasitize the skin by attacking the keratin by elaborating proteases with keratin specificity. They can invade epidermis but remain confined to the stratum corneum as well as the hair shaft or nail plate. There are three pathogenic genera of dermatophyte in humans: *Trichophyton*, *Microsporum* and *Epidermo-*

Table 59.1 Superficial mycoses.

Dermatophytosis (ringworm, tinea)
Superficial candidosis (thrush)
Malassezia infections: pityriasis versicolor,
    Malassezia folliculitis, (seborrhoeic dermatitis)
Scytalidium infections
Less common
    Tinea nigra
    White piedra
    Black piedra
    Alternariosis
    Onychomycosis due to mould fungi
Otomycosis
Keratomycosis

phyton. These organisms normally cause exogenous infections originating from outside the human host. There are three main sources: other humans, animals or soil, known respectively as anthropophilic, zoophilic or geophilic. Examples of possible animal hosts are cats and dogs (*M. canis*), cattle (*T. verrucosum*), monkeys (*T. simii*) and rodents (*T. mentagrophytes*).

PATHOGENESIS

The pathogenesis of dermatophytosis is fairly well understood. The fungi invade after adhering to stratum corneum cells. Factors which encourage fungal invasion include increased environmental humidity and CO_2 content, both of which may occur in a tropical environment. Less is known about those factors which determine human susceptibility; generally it is thought that most individuals are susceptible to infection.[3] The presence of medium chain length fatty acids in sebaceous material may, however, prevent hair shaft invasion by dermatophytes in postpubertal children. There is evidence that susceptibility to tinea imbricata may be mediated via an autosomal recessive gene.[4] In addition, patients with persistent treatment unresponsive dermatophytosis affecting the palms and soles are significantly more likely to be atopic than others.[5] Resistance is largely mediated via non-specific factors such as an increase in epidermal turnover, unsaturated transferrin or by activation of T-cell-mediated immunity. Patients with the acquired immune deficiency syndrome (AIDS), for instance, although not apparently showing an increased incidence of infection, may have clinically atypical and extensive lesions.[6]

The clinical features of dermatophytosis are well known. The normal term for this infection is tinea, followed by the Latin for the appropriate part of the body affected (tinea capitis, head; tinea cruris, groin, etc.). The archetypal lesion is a round scaly plaque with a more pronounced edge containing scales and papules, sometimes known as tinea circinata.

EPIDEMIOLOGY

In most tropical countries dermatophytosis is common.[7-11] The main types of infection seen are tinea corporis, tinea cruris and tinea capitis. Tinea pedis is considered to be less common in many parts of the tropics. However, there are several features of the epidemiology of foot infections which may be relevant.[12] Occlusion of the feet with shoes or socks predisposes to infection, although a higher proportion of the populace may have asymptomatic infections of their soles. In areas of the tropics where there is industrial activity, such as in the mining or petroleum industries, the incidence of foot infections may be much higher. There are a number of different organisms which can cause this type of infection, ranging from dermatophytoses to *Candida* spp., Gram-negative bacteria and erythrasma, a Gram-positive bacterial infection.[13] For instance in eastern Saudi Arabia there is a high rate of *Candida* infection in the toe-web spaces rather than dermatophytosis.[14] Populations of organisms on the feet, particularly those affecting the interdigital spaces, may vary from time to time and one may replace another to cause infection; the term 'dermatophytosis complex' has been coined to describe this phenomenon.[13]

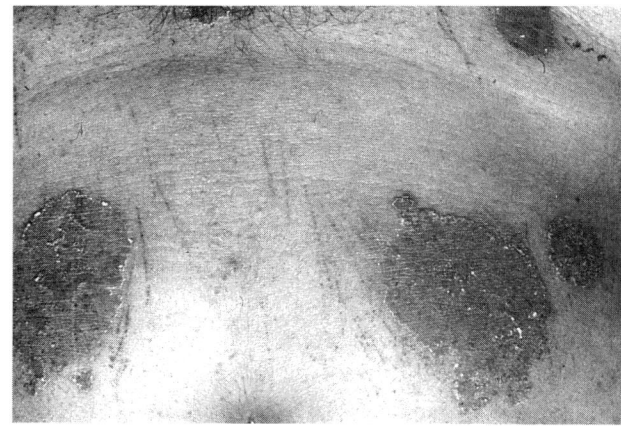

Figure 59.1   Tinea corporis due to *Trichophyton rubrum*.

LABORATORY DIAGNOSIS

The diagnosis of dermatophytosis can be confirmed by demonstrating the organisms in skin scrapings or hair or nail samples taken from lesions.[2,15] Scrapings are generally best removed with a blunt scalpel from the edge of lesions. They are mounted in 5–10% potassium hydroxide and are then scanned with a microscope. The organisms are seen in scrapings as chains of cells forming hyphae. In addition, they grow on simple mycological media such as Sabouraud's agar and their gross and microscopic morphology is used to distinguish the different species.

CLINICAL FEATURES

Tinea corporis

This presents with a scaly and itchy rash affecting the trunk or proximal limbs. The typical lesion is a circular scaling patch with some central clearance (Figure 59.1). However, in many lesions the main abnormalities, scaling or papule/pustule formation, are seen at the edge where an intact or broken rim can just be made out. Tinea corporis lesions may be very large and affect a wide area on the back and chest. In patients with AIDS the symptoms and signs may be reduced considerably.[16]

Tinea imbricata is a specific type of tinea corporis caused by the fungus *T. concentricum*.[17] It is endemic in remote and humid tropical areas in the West Pacific and parts of Malaysia, India and South America. Lesions are characterized by the develop-

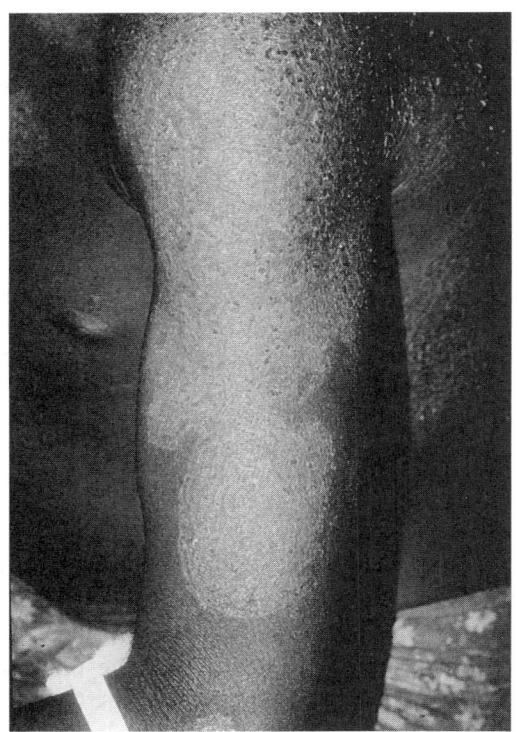

Figure 59.2   Tinea imbricata.

ment of multiple concentric rings of scales which may cover a large area of the body from an early age (Figure 59.2). Other patterns include diffuse desquamation with large scales and lichenification. This infection is notoriously difficult to eradicate from patients who are living in endemic areas.

Localized lesions respond to one of the azole antifungals such as clotrimazole or econazole. Whitfield's ointment is also effective in many patients. Oral therapy is generally needed for extensive disease or tinea imbricata; the main choices are griseofulvin, itraconazole or terbinafine.

Tinea capitis

Tinea capitis or scalp ringworm is endemic in many developing countries. It can be caused by either anthropophilic or zoophilic fungi.[18] Generally in rural areas anthropophilic organisms are more common and this is true for large areas of India, Latin America and Africa.[19] By contrast, in the Middle East and in some South American countries, particularly in cities, zoophilic infections are being seen more frequently, usually caused by *M. canis*. The difference between the two types is in their transmission, with those originating from human sources being more easily transmitted from child to child, causing small or large epidemics of disease. In many communities in Africa, for instance, scalp ringworm is endemic.[20–22]

Tinea capitis is an infection generally confined to prepubertal children. With most anthropophilic fungi the infections present insidiously with diffuse or circumscribed areas of hair loss. Scaling may be minimal and hairs are broken at scalp level, leaving a swollen black dot in the hair follicle (Figure 59.3). More scaly types which resemble seborrhoeic dermatitis, but highly inflammatory lesions (kerion) are occasionally seen. The course of disease is indolent but lesions normally clear at puberty. The zoophilic organisms are generally more inflammatory and scaling with hair loss is obvious. Lesions are often quite itchy and inflammatory crusts cover the lesions. Children (and adults) may carry the organisms without appearing to produce clinical lesions.[23,24]

Favus is a specific form of scalp ringworm caused by *T. schoenleinii*. It is found mainly in isolated pockets in parts of North and South Africa, the Middle East and South America. The infection is characterized by the formation of large crusts, scutula, over the scalp. Hairs are often retained until late in the course of the disease but their loss may be permanent. The crust is often white or yellowish in colour and confluent; the hair appears to be covered by a large area of matted material.

The diagnosis of this infection can be confirmed by examining scrapings from the patient's scalp and by culture.[25] Some causes of dermatophytosis affecting hairs, notably those due to *Microsporum* spp., lead to the appearance of greenish fluorescence in scalp hairs when they are illuminated with a filtered ultraviolet (Wood's) light.

The best treatment for dermatophytosis affecting the scalp is oral; topically applied drugs are seldom

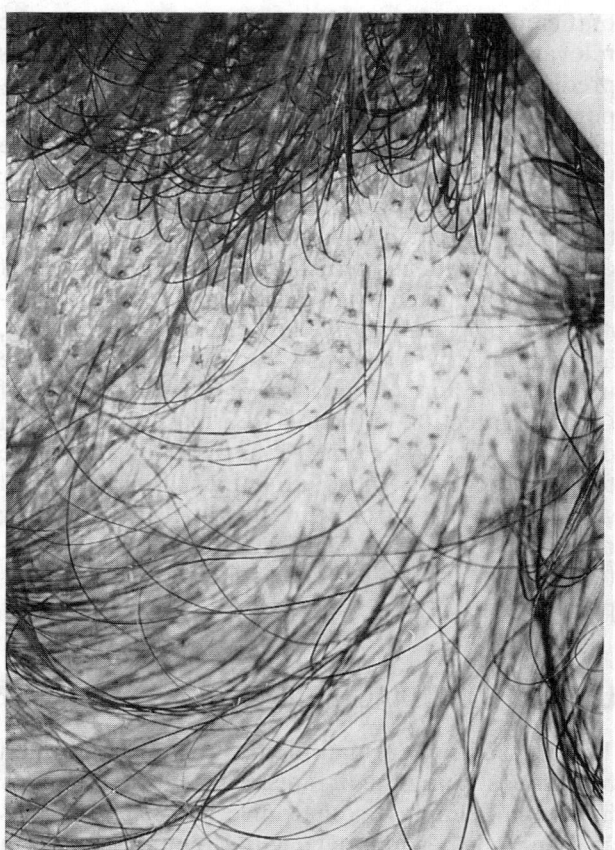

Figure 59.3 Scalp ringworm (tinea capitis) due to *Trichophyton violaceum* showing the 'black dot' appearance.

effective.[22] Griseofulvin in a dose of 10–15 mg/kg daily is the usual agent.[26,27] The normal duration of therapy is 6–8 weeks. However, in some cases it is possible to use a single dose of 1 g daily, which can be given under supervision to large numbers of children in a school.[18] There has been less experience to date with the newer oral agents such as itraconazole and terbinafine.

Tinea cruris

Dermatophytosis affecting the groin, tinea cruris or jock itch, is common in most tropical countries. It is almost always caused by anthropophilic species of dermatophytes, mainly *T. rubrum* and *E. floccosum*. Sometimes these infections may appear to reach epidemic proportions in certain groups such as soldiers or prisoners. The usual lesion is an itchy rash with a raised border extending from the groin down the upper thigh, and on occasions into the natal cleft. In women it may extend around the waist area. Treatment with topically applied antifungal creams such as clotrimazole or micronazole or half strength Whitfield's ointment work well in most cases.[28]

Tinea pedis

Dermatophytosis affecting the feet is very common in most temperate climates; however it is less important in developing countries. There is some evidence that carriage of certain dematophyte fungi on the feet may be higher, although symptoms are often minimal. The most common sites of infection are the interdigital spaces, usually those of the lateral toes. The main symptoms are itching and occasionally pain. There may be erosions affecting this area. If there are severe erosive changes, particularly if there is greenish discoloration of the area, Gram-negative bacteria such as *Pseudomonas* spp. may be implicated. Other possibilities include *Candida* and *Scytalidium* species or erythrasma, a bacterial infection caused by *Corynebacterium minutissimum*.

The usual treatment for toe-web dermatophytosis is a topically applied antifungal. Good results can be obtained with a range of compounds including Whitfield's ointment, azoles such as clotrimazole or micronazole, or terbinafine. For infections of the sole requiring treatment oral therapy with griseofulvin, terbinafine or itraconazole are preferable.

Onychomycosis

Nail plate invasion caused by dermatophytes is common in temperate countries, where it may affect 3–4% of the population. The prevalence of this infection in the tropics is unknown. It normally occurs together with sole or web-space infections and is most common on the toe-nails. The usual causes are anthropophilic fungi such as *T. rubrum*. The affected nails become thickened and opaque; distal erosion of the nail plate occurs in long-standing cases[29] (Figure 59.4). Superficial invasion of the nail plate

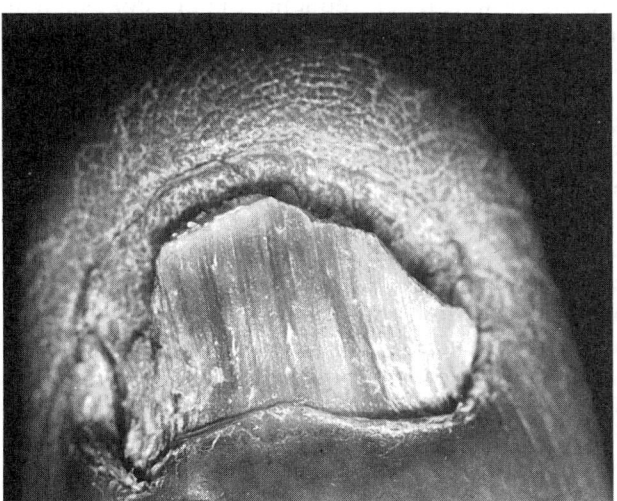

Figure 59.4 Onychomycosis due to a dermatophyte.

caused by dermatophytes, such as *T. interdigitale*, or moulds such as *Acremonium* or *Fusarium* spp., are seen more frequently in the tropics.[30] This is called superficial white onychomycosis. Therapy is difficult with few nail infections responding to topical antifungals, although in the early stages some will clear with tioconazole or amorolfine nail solutions. The most common oral treatment, griseofulvin, is associated with a high relapse rate when toe-nails are involved. It may have to be used for 12–18 months. The newer oral drugs terbinafine (250 mg)[31] or itraconazole (200 mg)[32] produce higher recovery rates in shorter periods (3 months). They are also more expensive than griseofulvin.

SUPERFICIAL CANDIDOSIS

Superficial infections due to *Candida* spp. are common in a tropical environment and include oral and vaginal as well as skin infections.[33] The principal pathogen is *C. albicans*, although other species such as *C. tropicalis*, *C. parapsilosis*, *C. krusei* and *C. glabrata* may also cause human infections. *C. albicans* forms filaments or hyphae during the process of tissue invasion. The disease is seen worldwide, although some clinical varieties are more common in warm climates than others. For instance interdigital candidosis is more common in the tropics,[14] whereas onychomycosis without paronychia due to *Candida* is mainly seen in colder climates.

PATHOGENESIS AND EPIDEMIOLOGY

C. albicans is a normal commensal of the mouth, gastrointestinal tract and vagina. Carriage rates vary but 15–60% of normal individuals, depending on the group surveyed, have commensal carriage in the mouth. Somewhat lower percentages have colonization of the gastrointestinal tract or vagina.[34] Survival of the organisms in these sites depends on a variety of factors, including their ability to adhere to mucosal cells and compete with commensal bacteria. Factors which disturb this balance favour either elimination or growth and subsequent invasion by the organism. They can usually be explained logically. For instance, use of antibiotics eliminates other members of the commensal flora of the mouth and bowel and allows *Candida* to invade. Depression of either T-lymphocyte or neutrophil-mediated immunity allows the organisms to grow and invade following inhibition of normal control mechanisms. The main exception is vaginal candidosis where most women with the infection have no detectable predisposition.

CLINICAL FEATURES

The main clinical forms of superficial disease are oropharyngeal, vaginal and cutaneous candidosis. In addition, chronic mucocutaneous candidosis is a condition which may appear as a rare chronic infection in predisposed patients. Systemic candidosis is a serious infection generally confined to compromised patients. It will be discussed elsewhere (see page 1069).

Oropharyngeal candidosis

Oral infection is seen in all countries, particularly in infants, the elderly and immunocompromised patients, including those with AIDS.[35] It occurs in breast-fed and bottle-fed infants and may be a complication of malnutrition, in which it can affect the reintroduction of feeding because of soreness of the mouth. As a complication of human immunodeficiency virus (HIV) infection, the appearance of oropharyngeal candidosis is a common manifestation of the development of AIDS. In some African countries the emergence of oral candidosis is one of the most important early signs of AIDS.

There are a number of different clinical types of oropharyngeal candidosis.[36,37] These are largely distinguished by their chronicity and clinical appearances. Acute pseudomembranous candidosis presents with white plaques on the epithelium that are inflamed and easily detached. The scattered nature of these appearances is suggestive of the speckling on a thrush's breast, hence its common name 'thrush'. This may present as an acute infection in infants, the elderly or in patients who are immunocompromised, such as those with AIDS. In the last group and in patients with chronic mucocutaneous candidosis the condition is often persistent and refractory to therapy—chronic pseudomembranous candidosis.

In some individuals plaques are not formed but the mucosal surface appears red and glazed, acute erythematous candidosis also known as acute atrophic oral candidosis. This may occur in patients with AIDS.[37,38] In patients presenting with inflammatory changes and oral discomfort associated with dentures (denture sore mouth), persistent erythema associated with Candida is a common feature—chronic erythematous candidosis. In smokers, chronic candidosis may have additional features such as the appearance of irregular white plaques, which cannot be detached, on the tongue and other areas of the mouth—chronic plaque-like candidosis. Histologically this contains epithelial atypia and, in some patients, oral carcinomas have developed. A few patients with chronic oral Candida infection may develop a pebbly appearance on the mucosa—chronic nodular candidosis.

Any of the above changes can be accompanied by splitting at the corners of the mouth (angular cheilitis), which in these cases may be due to Candida infection. This is an important and common sign of candidosis and can be spotted easily.

In most patients the main focus of infection is the buccal mucosa, but in severely infected individuals there is involvement of the tongue or pharynx, as well as the oesophagus. Oesophageal candidosis is mainly seen in patients with AIDS, leukaemia or chronic mucocutaneous candidosis. While it may present with retrosternal pain on swallowing it is often silent. Secondary oral infection due to Candida may occur in patients with epithelial abnormalities such as hyperkeratosis or ulceration due to lichen planus, pemphigus and other conditions such as oral submucous fibrosis, mainly seen in Indian patients.

Vaginal candidosis

Vaginal Candida infection is normally caused by C. albicans although other Candida spp. such as C. glabrata or C. tropicalis have also been cultured.[33] While it can occur in pregnant women or diabetics, one of the features of this condition is that there is usually no underlying abnormality to be found. Severely immunocompromised women do not usually show a higher frequency of persistent vaginal infections than appropriate control groups, although persistent vaginal infection has been reported in some women with AIDS.

The main clinical forms of vaginal candidosis are similar to those seen in the oral mucosa, most commonly an acute (pseudomembranous or erythematous) form.[34] However, chronic relapsing or persistent vaginal candidosis and secondary vaginal candidosis can all occur.[39] The symptoms of the acute types vary from a creamy discharge to itching and dyspareunia. Recurrent infections are unfortunately common and occasionally they are persistent. The clinical appearances are varied but the main variations are the presence or absence of soft white plaques (thrush). Secondary candidosis may occur in those with underlying mucosal disease such as pemphigoid, lichen planus or Behçet's syndrome.

Candida intertrigo

The skin is only indirectly involved in vaginal infection when there is spread of infection to the vulva and the perineum. In this case a prominent red rash in the groin and on the upper surface of the thighs may appear together with satellite pustules and papules. The same can occur in other sites such as beneath the breasts and around the umbilicus. In some cases there is no underlying skin abnormality, although groin candidosis in males and females is more common in diabetics. Eczema or psoriaris affecting the skin flexures may be accompanied by secondary candidosis.

Interdigital candidosis

Infection of the finger or toe-web spaces by *Candida* is more common in hot climates. It may be the most common type of foot infection in army groups in the tropics. Lesions are white with soggy-looking skin which is superficially eroded. Between the toes *Candida* may be a secondary invader in a lesion primarily caused by a dermatophyte (see p. 1054). Lesions on the fingers are mainly seen in women and a relationship between repeated washing and cooking has been suggested; it is also more common in the overweight individual.

Candida *infection and nappy dermatitis*

Nappy rash in infants is a form of irritant eczema which is often secondarily infected with, amongst other organisms, *C. albicans*. The presence of yeasts may be suspected by the appearance of satellite pustules and this is confirmed by culturing the organisms from swabs of the area.

Candidosis of the nails

Paronychia are acute or chronic infections of the nail folds caused by *Candida* spp. such as *C. albicans* or *C. parapsilosis*.[40] These are common in the tropics. They occur in patients who are likely to immerse their hands frequently in water or whose occupations involve cooking. In addition to swelling of the nail fold, pain and intermittent discharge of pus, the lateral border of the nail may be undermined with onycholysis (Figure 59.5). Other causes of paronychia are staphylococcal and Gram-negative bacterial infections. The latter often coexist with *Candida* spp.

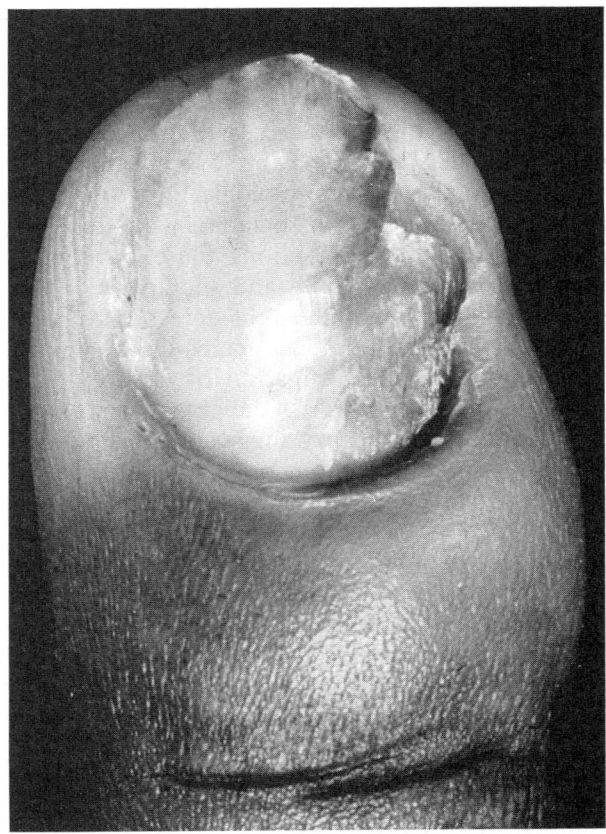

Figure 59.5   Chronic *Candida* paronychia.

Table 59.2   Classification of chronic mucocutaneous candidosis (CMC).

Childhood onset
Inherited CMC: autosomal recessive type, autosomal dominant type
CMC associated with polyendocrinopathy (usually hypoparathyroidism, hypoadrenalism or hypothyroidism)
Idiopathic CMC

Adult onset
CMC associated with thymoma, systemic lupus erythematosus

Chronic mucocutaneous candidosis

The rare syndrome of chronic mucocutaneous candidosis (CMC) (Table 59.2) usually presents in childhood or infancy with oral, nail and cutaneous candidosis which recurs despite treatment.[41] Other chronic skin infections such as warts (papilloma viruses) and dermatophytosis may also appear. An adult form also exists.

The oral lesions are usually of the chronic pseudomembranous or plaque types. The skin may be covered with crusted plaques—the so-called *Candida* granulomas—particularly where the infection has spread to the face or scalp. The finger-nail changes involve the nail plates, nail folds and periungual skin, all of which may be severely damaged.

A large number of immunological abnormalities have been described in association with this condition but with few exceptions these have been found to change with time and therapy. For this reason it is likely that the real defect(s) in most patients with this condition remains unknown and the immunological investigation of children with CMC is not necessary unless they have very extensive infections or a history suggestive of abnormal responses to other infections, such as chickenpox or severe staphylococcal boils. Here it is worth excluding functional leucocyte abnormalities, such as chronic granulomatous disease, although such patients usually have a history of internal infection. With the exception of bronchiectasis most patients with CMC do not have internal disease, although the most severely affected patients may later develop systemic infections such as tuberculosis.

LABORATORY DIAGNOSIS

The diagnosis of superficial candidosis can be confirmed by direct microscopy (see Dermatophytosis) of skin scrapings or swabs. Both yeasts and hyphae can be seen. *Candida* spp. can be distinguished on culture by assimilation and fermentation reactions.[15]

TREATMENT

Candida infections respond well to a range of antifungals available in cream, vaginal tablet or oral pastille forms.[27] These include the polyene antifungals such as amphotericin B or nystatin and azole drugs (econazole, clotrimazole, ketoconazole, miconazole). Gentian violet is still used in some areas but the response to treatment is much slower than with the specific antifungals. Patients with AIDS may respond poorly to topical therapy and orally absorbed antifungals, such as fluconazole (50–100 mg daily),[42] ketoconazole (200–400 mg daily)[43] or itraconazole (100–200 mg daily),[44] given intermittently are used. There is a risk that if some of these oral drugs are used continuously in such patients in the face of continuing disease microbial resistance will develop. Oral antifungal therapy is also needed for patients with CMC.

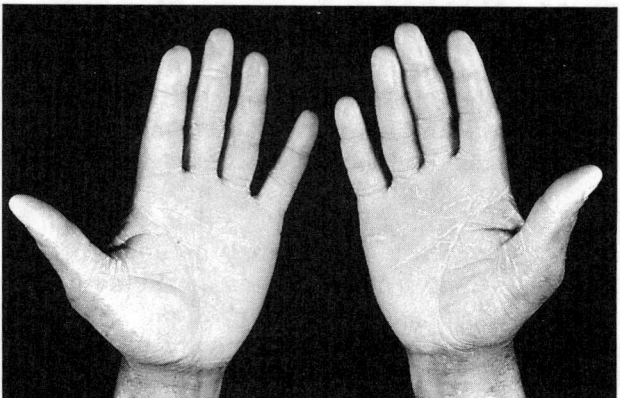

Figure 59.6   Palm infection caused by *Scytalidum*. This mimics dermatophytosis.

SCYTALIDIUM INFECTIONS

Scytalidium dimidiatum (*Hendersonula toruloidea*), a plant pathogen found in the tropics and subtropics, and *Scytalidium hyalinum*, which has only been isolated from humans, cause infections of the skin which mimic the dry-type infections caused by *T. rubrum*.[45] Both fungi are inhibited by cycloheximide which is commonly incorporated into mycological media and this may explain why their existence has only been established in recent years. These infections have mainly been reported in immigrants from tropical areas to temperate countries, although infection in the tropics may be more common than previously believed.[46] Recent studies from Nigeria, for instance, have suggested that this is a common infection in both dermatological outpatients and industrial groups such as mine workers. Infections have been reported from West and East Africa, India and Pakistan, Thailand, Hong Kong and several countries in Latin America.

The infection presents with scaling of soles and palms and cracking between the toe webs (Figure 59.6). Nail dystrophy is common and onycholysis without significant thickening is often seen; some patients have nail-fold swelling. The clinical features of *S. dimidiatum* and *S. hyalinum* infections are indistinguishable. Lesions are often asymptomatic.

It is important to recognize these infections because they are common in some areas and do not respond to most antifungal drugs. The laboratory diagnosis follows similar lines to that used in dermatophytosis—skin scrapings and culture.[47] The appearances of these fungi in skin scrapings is characteristic as they are sinuous and irregular. They do not grow on media containing cycloheximide, which is often used to suppress growth of contaminant fungi.

Treatment of these infections is difficult. Nail disease does not respond to any of the antifungal agents. Responses of skin infection have been recorded with a number of compounds such as Whitfield's ointment, econazole or terbinafine, although relapse is common.

MALASSEZIA YEAST INFECTIONS

The *Malassezia* or *Pityrosporum* (lipophilic) yeasts are skin-surface commensals which have also been associated with certain human diseases, the most common of which are pityriasis versicolor, *Malassezia* folliculitis and seborrhoeic dermatitis and dandruff.[48] In addition these organisms rarely cause systemic infections, usually in neonatal infants receiving intravenous lipid infusions.

There are a number of Malassezia species. On culture media they are oval or round yeasts and their distribution on the skin surface differs. An oval type is the dominant form on the scalp, a round form on the trunk. At present it is not clear whether these are variants of the same or separate species. In addition, the formation of short stubby hyphae by round yeasts on the skin surface is a feature of the development of pityriasis versicolor and this form is named *Malassezia furfur*. Occasionally oval yeasts without hyphae have been found to cause pityriasis versicolor. The taxonomy of these fungi, therefore, remains in doubt.

Pityriasis versicolor

The pathogenesis of pityriasis versicolor is still ill understood. The disease occurs in young adults and older individuals but is less common in childhood.[49] Pityriasis versicolor is a common disease in the tropics and elsewhere in otherwise healthy patients and there is no evidence of immunosuppression in these groups. However, it has also been associated with Cushing's syndrome and immunosuppression associated with organ transplantation, but not with AIDS. The pigmentary changes which characterize this infection are thought to follow the inhibition of melanin formation by substances, such as azeleic acid, produced when the yeast is present within epidermis. The infection is very common in the tropics and incidence rates of over 70% have been reported in some studies. Generally this disease is associated with warm climates and sun exposure.

The rash consists of multiple hypo- or hyperpigmented, occasionally red, macules which are distributed across the upper trunk and back; with time these coalesce. The lesions are asymptomatic and scaly. Patients usually notice this infection because of its unsightly appearance. The hypopigmented lesions may be confused with vitiligo but here there is complete loss of pigmentation. The presence of scaling and partial loss of pigment is, however, typical of pityriasis versicolor.

Lesions can also be highlighted by shining a Wood's light on the area. They fluoresce with a yellowish light, although this is generally a weak response and complete darkness as well as a powerful light source are necessary. Alternatively, scrapings from the lesions will show the characteristic organisms which consist of clusters of round yeasts closely associated with short stubby hyphae. These are normally viewed in 10% potassium hydroxide treated mounts, although the addition of Parker Quinck ink to the potassium hydroxide is an easy stain to apply and it highlights the fungi well.

Malassezia folliculitis

A second condition associated with *Malassezia* yeasts is an itchy folliculitis on the back and upper trunk which often appears after sun exposure. *Malassezia* folliculitis is a clinically distinct condition most often seen in teenagers or young adult males. Lesions are itchy papules and pustules which are often widely scattered on the shoulders and back. The condition has to be distinguished from acne as it does not respond to the same range of treatments.

Seborrhoeic dermatitis

Lipophilic yeasts of the genus *Malassezia* are part of the normal skin flora and therefore any evidence that they are either directly or indirectly implicated in the pathogenesis of common skin diseases such as dandruff (scalp scaling) or seborrhoeic dermatitis is difficult to assess. However, these yeasts are found in large quantities in the scales of seborrhoeic dermatitis and dandruff. Most patients with seborrhoeic dermatitis or dandruff respond to treatment with azole antifungal agents and this coincides with the disappearance of the yeasts. Some patients with seborrhoeic dermatitis have been reported to have significantly raised levels of antibody to these organisms. Seborrhoeic dermatitis is one of the earliest and most consistent abnormalities seen in patients with AIDS[50] but it is also common in perfectly healthy individuals. This association has also been seen in some tropical areas such as Latin America.

The main clinical feature of seborrhoeic dermatitis is the appearance of erythema, together with greasy scales in the scalp, eyebrows and eye lashes, in the nasolabial folds, behind the ears and over the sternum.

TREATMENT

Treatment of *Malassezia* infection can usually be accomplished using topical azole antifungals such as clotrimazole (cream) or ketoconazole (cream or shampoo). Oral therapy with ketoconazole or itraconazole is also a possibility. Cheaper alternatives include selenium sulphide (1–2%) or 20% sodium hyposulphite solution. In the case of seborrhoeic dermatitis, topically applied azole antifungals will produce significant improvements; other possibilities include: topical tar-based preparations and corticosteroids.

RARER SUPERFICIAL INFECTIONS

White piedra is a chronic infection of the hair shafts caused by a yeast, *Trichosporon beigelii*.[51] It is generally sporadic and rare and the infection is mainly seen in genital hair. It may also affect the axilla and scalp. The lesions are soft yellowish nodules around the hair shafts.[52] This disease can be seen in temperate and tropical areas. It is usually asymptomatic and is noticed on routine inspection. Trichomycosis axillaris, in which hairs in the axillae are covered with a soft yellowish coating, is caused by a bacterial infection associated with excessive sweating. It is generally easily controlled with an antiperspirant.

Black piedra caused by *Piedraia hortae* is a rare infection confined to the tropics. Here, scalp hairs are surrounded by a dense black concretion containing spores, thus forming a small nodule.[53] The disease has been reported in both humans and apes. Once again the infection is generally asymptomatic.

Tinea nigra is an infection of palmar or plantar skin caused by a black yeast, *Phaeoannelomyces werneckii*. It is mainly seen in the tropics but can present in Europe and the USA. The main differential diagnosis is an acral melanoma as it presents as a flat pigmented mark on the hands or feet. If the lesion is scraped with a glass slide or scalpel it can be shown to be scaly. Lesions are usually solitary. The presence of pigmented hyphae in skin scrapings is typical. Tinea nigra responds to a variety of treatments including Whitfield's ointment and azole creams.

Alternaria spp. cause a rare form of skin granuloma, often presenting with ulceration in normal or immunocompromised patients. The lesions are most often located over exposed sites such as the dorsum of the hands. It has been seen in patients with AIDS.

Scopulariopsis brevicaulis causes a form of onychomycosis and may occasionally be isolated from toe-web spaces. The onychomycosis is generally confined to the great toe-nail which develops a light tan discoloration. Other fungi may also be isolated from dystrophic nails. These include species of *Fusarium*, *Aspergillus* and *Pyrenochaeta*. Generally they are secondary invaders of already dystrophic nails; however, if they are isolated from this source repeatedly, treatment or nail removal is appropriate. *Acremonium* and *Fusarium* spp., in particular, are sometimes associated with superficial nail-plate invasion (superficial white onychomycosis) in the tropics.

OTOMYCOSIS

Otomycosis or otitis externa caused by fungi is seen in most tropical areas. The most common cause is *A. niger*,[54] which forms an inflammatory mat in the external auditory meatus, with loss of hearing and serous secretion. This can be removed carefully with a wax hook through an otoscope. Occasionally other fungi may secondarily infect this site, particularly if multiple antibiotics have previously been used.

SUBCUTANEOUS MYCOSES

Subcutaneous fungal infections are diseases which are mainly confined to the tropics and subtropics (Table 59.3). While they are seldom common, their diagnosis and management is difficult and they therefore attract a disproportionate share of attention. These infections are generally caused by direct introduction of organisms through the skin into the dermis or subcutaneous tissues and for this reason they are often called 'mycoses of implantation'. They generally remain confined to their site of introduction, only spreading by contiguity; however, there are rare examples where the infection disseminates beyond this area to affect distal sites. In addition, the disease, sporotrichosis, has both a

Table 59.3 Subcutaneous mycoses.

Mycetoma
Chromoblastomycosis (chromomycosis)
Sporotrichosis
Lobomycosis
Subcutaneous zygomycosis
due to *Basidiobolus*
due to *Conidiobolus*

subcutaneous and a systemic form, in the latter instance the infection spreading from a primary pulmonary focus.

MYCETOMA

Mycetoma (madura foot) is a chronic subcutaneous infection caused by actinomycetes or fungi in which the organisms form into aggregates (called grains), attracting an inflammatory response in the deep dermis and subcutaneous tissue and leading to the development of draining sinuses communicating with the overlying skin and causing osteomyelitis.[55] Those mycetomas caused by actinomycetes are called actinomycetomas; those caused by fungi, eumycetomas (mycotic mycetomas) (Table 59.4). The disease was first described by the German physician and explorer Kaempfer in 1663 during a visit to southern India where he recorded a condition known as paracal or foot anthill. However, the most thorough early description was by Godfrey in Madras in 1864. Following his description of the disease, the infective nature of the process and the presence of fungi in lesions were discovered shortly afterwards.

EPIDEMIOLOGY

Mycetoma is generally a disease seen in the tropics or subtropics, although cases are described from other zones.[55,56] It is more often seen in areas where there is a low annual rainfall. The main sites for this infection are Mexico, Central and northern South America, Africa, the Middle East and India. Cases are reported less frequently in the Far East, the USA and in Europe, where most patients are immigrants from elsewhere. The main causes of mycetoma are shown in Table 59.4. Organisms prevalent in certain areas are shown; however, cases may rarely be seen outside these endemic zones. As a general principle the main causes of mycetoma in Central America are *Nocardia* spp.,[57] whereas in most African countries and the Indian subcontinent

Madurella mycetomatis is the most common cause. The causes of mycetoma are generally classified according to organism, namely fungi (eumycetoma) or actinomycetes (actinomycetoma), and by grain colour—black, red or pale, e.g. red grain actinomycetoma is an infection caused by *Actinomadura pelletieri*. The proportion of pale grain eumycetomas is higher in temperate areas and in addition many of the fungi isolated are sterile moulds which cannot be identified because of a lack of distinguishing characteristics.

Mycetoma is more common in males than females and generally affects adults. It is also mainly seen in agricultural workers, although this is not invariable. There is no evidence to suggest that patients with mycetoma are in any way predisposed and the majority appear to have no underlying reason for developing this chronic infection. There is evidence that the organisms are spread from the environment via a penetrating injury such as a thorn prick. The fungal causes of mycetoma have been isolated from plants and plant debris; *Nocardia* species have been isolated from soil. It appears that the organisms possess mechanisms for survival in the human host which allow them to evade defences. Some of the mechanisms of adapation include the deposition of intra- or extracellular melanin, cell wall thickening and immunomodulation.[58]

CLINICAL FEATURES

The earliest sign of a mycetoma is the appearance of a small symptom-free dermal or subcutaneous swelling.[55,56] It is difficult to give an accurate estimate of incubation periods as few patients give a history of a penetrating injury. However, it may take several years before the first sign of disease, a painless subcutaneous nodule, is seen. With time this slowly enlarges and sinuses appear on its upper surface (Figure 59.7). Pain may occur prior to rupture of sinuses on to the skin surface and in the early stages these dry up. Chronically discharging sinuses may be formed in well-established lesions. At this stage there is considerable woody swelling affecting the site, accompanied by deformity.

The main areas affected are those subject to trauma such as the feet, lower legs and hands. *Nocardia* spp. are prominent amongst causes of lesions on the chest and back; *Streptomyces somaliensis* is the most common cause of head and neck lesions. Dissemination is rare, although some infections may become very extensive and spread widely over a limb. The only threat to life is where they involve the skull.

Radiological changes include cortical thinning or

Table 59.4 Causes of mycetoma.

Organism	Colour of grain	Common distribution
Fungi		
Madurella mycetomatis	Black	Africa, Middle East, India
M. grisea	Black	Central and South America, Caribbean
Pseudallescheria boydii	White/yellow	Anywhere, USA and Europe
Fusarium or *Acremonium* spp.	White/yellow	Anywhere
Aspergillus nidulans	White/yellow	Sudan, elsewhere
Dermatophytes	White/yellow	Anywhere
Neotestudina rosati	White/yellow	Africa
Actinomycetes		
Actinomadura madurae	White/yellow	Africa, Middle East, elsewhere
A. pelletieri	Red	Africa, India, elsewhere
Streptomyces somaliensis	White/yellow	Africa, Middle East, elsewhere
Nocardia spp.	Small white/yellow	Americas, elsewhere

hypertrophy, periosteal proliferation and lytic lesions.[59]

DIFFERENTIAL DIAGNOSIS

Mycetomas may be mistaken for osteomyelitis caused by bacteria or actinomycosis. Actinomycosis is an infection caused by *Actinomyces israelii*, *A. bovis* or other actinomycetes such as *Arachnia propionica*. The infections are usually located close to the sites where these organisms can be carried, such

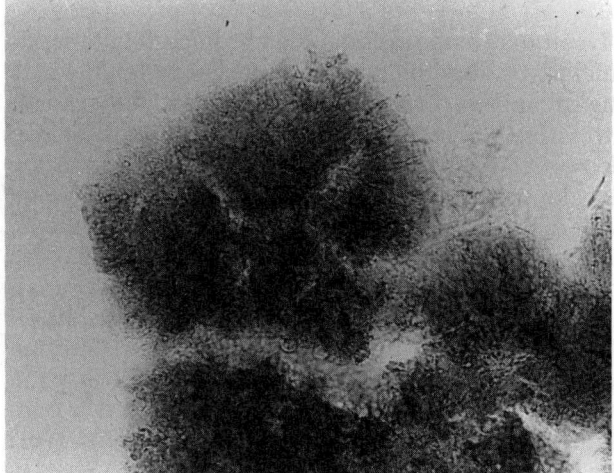

Figure 59.8 Direct microscopy in potassium hydroxide (10%) of a black grain eumycetoma. (40×).

as the oral cavity, chest, and, within the abdominal cavity, around the caecum. Pelvic actinomycosis occasionally follows use of intrauterine contraceptive devices. Rarely actinomycosis arises in other sites where it may mimic mycetoma and the grains or sulphur granules discharged by lesions are typical.

LABORATORY DIAGNOSIS

The laboratory diagnosis of mycetoma depends on the demonstration of grains of the organisms.[60] These are generally obtained by opening a sinus where there is a small amount of pus beneath the skin surface, using a sterile needle. The grains can usually be seen with the naked eye in the pus and blood from the sinus tract. They can be processed as follows:

- *Direct microscopy*. Grains are mounted in 5–10% potassium hydroxide (Figure 59.8). They can

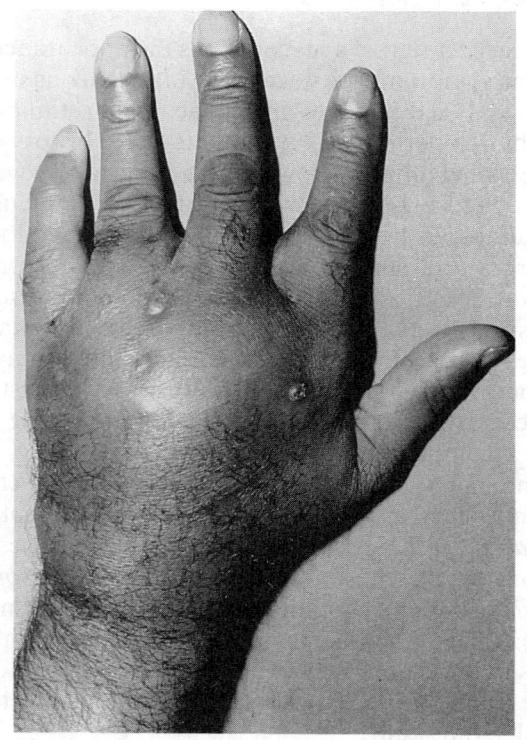

Figure 59.7 Mycetoma affecting the hand due to *Madurella grisea*.

gently be squashed. As a general rule if the filament can be seen with the 40× objective the cause is a fungus. However, if they are not visible the cause is likely to be an actinomycete.

- Grains can be taken for *histology* and embedded after formalin fixation. The pathology laboratory should be shown were the grains are, otherwise they may be discarded prior to fixation.[61] The appearance of many grains is typical in haematoxylin and eosin stained sections and the use of special fungal stains such as periodic acid–Schiff or methenamine silver is not strictly necessary.
- Grains can be *cultured* on a variety of media and the appearances of the fungi or actinomycetes is typical, although a specialist laboratory will be needed for their identification.
- *Serology*. Patients may form specific antibodies to the causative fungi. Overall serology is mainly useful in following the course of treatment in actinomycete infections because there is some cross-reactivity which may confuse the results if they are used as the sole means of diagnosis.

The main aim of laboratory diagnosis is to separate fungal and actinomycete causes because the treatment of each is different.

TREATMENT

The treatment of mycetoma depends on knowing whether the cause is an actinomycete or a fungus.[62] The actinomycetes respond to a variety of antibiotics such as sulphonamides and sulphones or co-trimoxazole. For many infections it is advisable to use a second-line drug such as rifampicin or streptomycin. Alternatives include amikacin, ciprofloxacin and imipenem for difficult cases. Most of these infections will respond to therapy although *Str. somaliensis* is notoriously resistant to therapy in some cases. Here, alternative regimens include combined sodium fusidate and sulphonamide.

Treatment of eumycetomas is more difficult. About 40–50% of infections due to *Madurella mycetomatis* respond to ketoconazole 200–400 mg daily. Other possibilities include griseofulvin (500–1000 mg daily) and itraconazole 200–400 mg daily. Although surgery remains an option the most effective approach is amputation and if the patient is not incapacitated by the infection, which is usually the case, removal of a limb, for instance, may do more harm than good. This is especially true where facilities for artificial limbs and rehabilitation are poor. Generally mycetomas are only slowly progressive and are seldom life threatening. It may be better for the patient to receive no treatment in these circumstances.

CHROMOBLASTOMYCOSIS

There are a number of fungal infections which are caused by pigmented fungi, known as dematiaceous fungi.[63] Generally these organisms contain melanin or secrete extracellular melanin into the environment. The production of melanin is of evolutionary importance as it allows these fungi to withstand environmental changes such as drought, heat or cold. There are a number of different infections caused by dematiaceous fungi but the most common is chromoblastomycosis (chromomycosis).

EPIDEMIOLOGY AND PATHOGENESIS

Chromoblastomycosis is a chronic infection caused by pigmented fungi which form specialized cells, muriform or sclerotic cells, in tissue (Table 59.5).[64] It involves the dermis and epidermis where a variety of pathological changes occurs, ranging from pseudoepitheliomatous hyperplasia to granuloma formation. The organisms which cause this infection are found in the natural environment in plant debris or forest detritus. The main range of chromoblastomycosis involves the tropics and subtropics and the incidence of infection is highest in countries with ahigh rainfall. The disease is mainly seen in countries of Central and northern South America, parts of Africa, particularly the east coast of southern Africa, the Far East, Japan and the West Pacific.[63] Cases have been recorded outside these areas, and in northern Europe they have even been seen in Finland. The infection is most common in males and in agricultural workers.

Like mycetoma there is no evidence of underlying predisposition in those with chromoblastomycosis. The infection is believed to gain entry via an abrasion, although there are no animal models of the infection to establish this as the chief mode of entry.

CLINICAL FEATURES

The hallmark of chromoblastomycosis is warty proliferation of the skin. The early lesions are small nodules or papules which slowly enlarge.[65,66] They become raised and verrucose and adjacent nodules

Table 59.5 Causes of chromoblastomycosis.

Fonsecaea pedrosoi
F. verrucosa
Cladosporium carrionii
Rhinocladiella aquaspersa

amalgamate to form a complex of warty growth (Figure 59.9). Other lesions are flatter and plaque-like and extend slowly, sometimes healing with central scarring. Cyst-like changes and mycetoma-like lesions are also seen. The lesion are asymptomatic, although with necrosis of keratin there is often an unpleasant smell associated with them. Long-standing lesions can cause considerable deformity at the site infected and rarely squamous carcinomas can develop.

The main sites affected are those on peripheral locations such as hands, feet and lower legs. The infection spreads locally and bloodstream dissemination is very rare. Occasionally, deep infections with the same organism have been reported.

DIFFERENTIAL DIAGNOSIS

The changes of chromoblastomycosis are typical, although there are some features which may be confused with other processes. For instance, early lesions may resemble other warty conditions such as papilloma virus infections or tuberculosis verrucosa. In extensive chromoblastomycosis the chronic changes may superficially resemble mossy foot secondary to lymphoedema. However, in the latter condition the changes are diffusely distributed over the skin surface.

LABORATORY DIAGNOSIS

The process of identification of chromoblastomycosis follows standard mycological lines:

- *Direct microscopy* of skin scrapings. These should be taken from the surface of lesions. The pigmented muriform cells with transverse septa can be seen in potassium hydroxide-treated specimens (Figure 59.10).
- *Biopsy*. The histopathology of chromoblastomycosis is characteristic. The epidermis shows pseudepitheliomatous hyperplasia with some attempt at transepidermal elimination of fungi. The latter can also be seen in granulomas or neutrophil abscesses in the dermis.
- *Culture*. Although the organisms grow readily on conventional mycological media they are black moulds which are difficult to identify because of the close resemblance of many of their specific features, such as sporulation. Often it is necessary to send cultures to specialist laboratories.[67] However, the diagnosis can be made on histopathological grounds alone.

TREATMENT

The treatment of chromoblastomycosis has changed over recent years. Generally it is inadvisable to use surgical excision unless the lesion is very small and chemotherapy is also used. The reason is that the infection may spread within the scar.

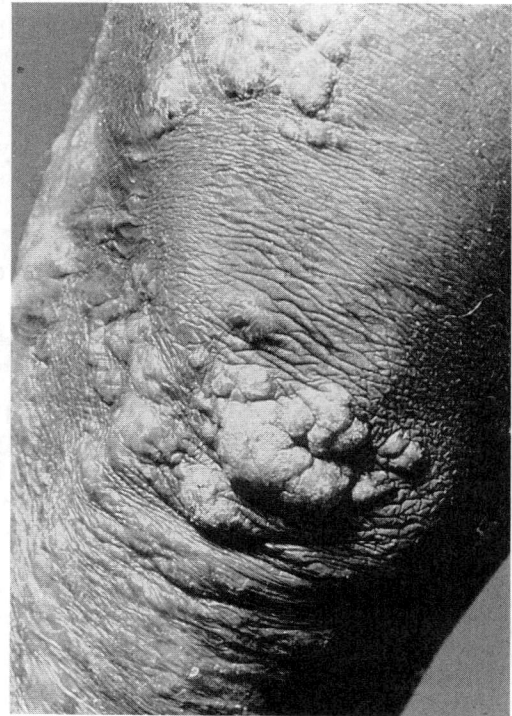

Figure 59.9 Chromoblastomycosis.

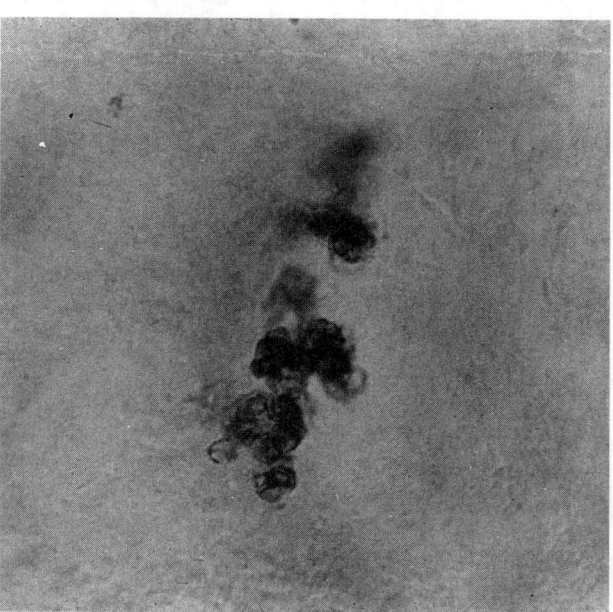

Figure 59.10 Direct microscopy in potassium hydroxide (10%) of a skin scraping from a case of chromoblastomycosis showing the muriform cells. (40×).

The commonly used drugs are itraconazole (100–400 mg daily) or flucytosine 150 mg/kg in a patient with normal renal function). Thiabendazole is an alternative. A combination of flucytosine and itraconazole is probably most successful in late and extensive cases, although itraconazole has been reported to be effective in some patients with early disease, particularly if the organisms are *Cladosporium carrionii*. A further approach to therapy is the use of local heat applied from heat-retaining gels or pocket hand-warmers. The heat must not be sufficient to burn the patient but high enough to be just comfortable.

PHAEOHYPHOMYCOSIS

Phaeohyphomycosis is another infection due to pigmented fungi in the skin. Cases are diffusely distributed through most tropical countries but are not common. Generally the infection presents with large cysts around the lower or upper limbs and these can mimic ganglia or Baker's cysts.[67]

The organisms are implanted from the environment and in some of these cysts there are fragments of plant material. Each cyst is surrounded by a fibrous capsule but contains palisading granulomas and a necrotic centre. The fungi are present as irregular mycelial fragments whose pigmentation may be very variable and occasionally it is necessary to use specific fungal stains. Occasionally this form of infection is seen in immunocompromised patients, particularly those receiving systemic corticosteroids.

The treatment is excision.

SPOROTRICHOSIS

Sporotrichosis, the infection caused by the dimorphic fungal pathogen *Sporothrix schenckii*, is widely distributed through the tropical world.[68] It may present either as a cutaneous infection or on occasion as a deep mycosis (see below). Extensive disseminated cutaneous infections are seen in patients with AIDS.[69]

EPIDEMIOLOGY

Sporotrichosis was first described in the USA and subsequently in Europe but although it is seen in the central and southern USA the main foci of infection are in Mexico, Central and South America, Africa and Japan. Scattered cases are seen in the Far East and Australia. The organism is part of an extensive group of soil and plant pathogens, the *Sporothrix* and *Sporotrichum* species. The ability of *Sporothrix schenckii* to invade animals is unique, as is its dimorphism whereby it exists as a mould at room temperature and in the environment but as a yeast in animal tissue.[68]

Exposure to infection is usually sporadic, although small outbreaks of infection have been described in certain occupational groups, such as florists, packers, plant workers, fishermen and armadillo hunters. There are also focal areas where the disease appears to be hyperendemic in Guatemala,[70] Peru and South Africa. The reason for this is not clear, although in South Africa contamination of pit props has been reported to cause disease in mine workers.

Sporotrichosis affects both males and females and can also infect children and infants.

CLINICAL FEATURES

There are a variety of different clinical forms of sporotrichosis.[71,72] Some infections appear to resolve spontaneously, although the frequency of this occurrence is unknown. Certain patients develop fixed lesions which are usually solitary ulcerated granulomas on exposed sites, including the face. Small satellite lesions frequently develop around the edge of these larger granulomas. Ulcers enlarge slowly. A second form of cutaneous sporotrichosis is called lymphangitic because the infection spreads from a primary granuloma or ulcer along the course of local lymphatics. Secondary lesions formed along the lymphatic path may discharge or ulcerate. Other forms of infection may mimic chronic leg ulcers and lupus vulgaris. Disseminated deep lesions of sporotrichosis may affect other body sites such as the joints, lungs and meninges.[73] While most of these patients do not have major underlying conditions, alcoholism or diabetes is seen in some.

In patients with AIDS these infections may spread to involve multiple skin sites with large numbers of ulcers or nodules.[71]

DIFFERENTIAL DIAGNOSIS

Leishmaniasis may resemble either of the two principal forms of sporotrichosis and where this condition is endemic some physicians advise using a sporotricin intradermal skin test to orientate the direction of investigation. This is read after 48 hours, like a tuberculin reaction. Atypical mycobacterial infection may cause similar changes, particularly *Mycobacterium marinum* which spreads along lymphatics.

LABORATORY DIAGNOSIS

Sporotrichosis differs from the other subcutaneous mycoses in that culture is the most reliable mode of diagnosis because there are few organisms present in lesions and these may be difficult to find.[68]

- *Direct microscopy* seldom has a role to play although it may be used to screen for amastigotes of *Leishmania* spp.
- *Culture. Sporothrix schenckii* grows well on Sabouraud's agar and will form characteristic spores. Samples from swabs, curettings and biopsies are all suitable. They should be taken from the edge of lesions.
- *Biopsy*. The histopathology shows a mixed granulomatous and polymorphonuclear response. Organisms are scattered in this infiltrate, although some are surrounded by a refractile eosinophilic halo called an asteroid body. In some centres an immunofluorescence test is available using specific antibody conjugates for application to fixed biopsy tissue.
- *Sporotricin* skin test. This is used to orientate the investigation. It is an intradermal reaction. The agent is prepared from polysaccharide antigens of the organism. Uninfected patients from endemic areas may also have positive responses.

TREATMENT

The main treatment for sporotrichosis is potassium iodide made up in a saturated solution. The starting dose is 1–2 ml given three times daily and increased drop by drop to a maximum of 4–6 ml three times a day. The slow increase is necessary because of the unpleasant taste and the possibility of symptoms of iodism: nausea, dry mouth, altered taste, swollen salivary glands. The normal duration of therapy is at least 2 months and often up to 4 months. Alternatives are itraconazole in doses of 100–200 mg daily or terbinafine 250 mg daily.

SUBCUTANEOUS ZYGOMYCOSIS

Subcutaneous zygomycosis (phycomycosis) comprises two separate diseases, those caused by *Basidiobolus* and *Conidiobolus*.[74] Generally the clinical features of these infections are distinct, as are their epidemiology and age prevalence.

Subcutaneous zygomycosis due to *Conidiobolus* (conidiobolomycosis, rhinoentomophthoromycosis) is uncommon but is found in different tropical areas of the West Indies, South America, Africa and Southern India.[75,76] The causative organism is usually *C. coronatus*, a fungus which is an insect pathogen. The usual focus of infection is within the nasal cavity and the infection spreads from the turbinates to involve the subcutaneous tissues of the face and neck with a hard painless swelling. The deformity may be grotesque. This is infection seen mainly in adults.

Subcutaneous zygomycosis is also caused by *Basidiobolus* (subcutaneous phycomycosis, basidiobolomycosis). The usual cause of this infection is *B. ranarum*, a pathogen of amphibians and reptiles. The site of infection is usually confined to the limb girdles or proximal limbs.[77,78] It is mainly seen in Central, East and West Africa and chiefly infects children. Once again the swelling is deforming and has a woody consistency.

In both diseases the histology is similar, with a dense infiltrate of eosinophils in the subcutis and large strap-like hyphae contained in granulomas.

The treatment is either ketoconazole or itraconazole, although an alternative includes the use of saturated potassium iodide.

LOBOMYCOSIS

Lobomycosis is a rare infection, seen in Central and South America, caused by *Loboa*, a fungus which has not been cultured to date.[79] The infection is seen in subcutaneous tissues and presents with plaques and keloid-like scars. The only treatment is excision. The epidemiology of the infection is unusual as it is seen mainly in remote areas[80] and the same infection has also been seen in sea or freshwater dolphins. Rarely squamous carcinomas may develop in long-standing lesions.

SYSTEMIC MYCOSES

The systemic mycoses are fungal infections which involve deep organs. While some, often referred to as the endemic mycoses, affect healthy individuals, others are opportunistic infections which occur in patients with some underlying predisposition. In recent years systemic mycoses, such as cryptococcosis and histoplasmosis, have become prominent as secondary complications in patients with AIDS, although it is of interest that other systemic mycoses have not increased in this population. Generally in most developed countries the opportunistic infections are more common but in many tropical areas the endemic systemic fungal infections are seen more frequently.

ENDEMIC SYSTEMIC MYCOSES

The main endemic mycoses are shown in Table 59.6. The most common of these are histoplasmosis, blastomycosis, coccidioidomycosis and paracoccidioidomycosis. Infections due to *Penicillium marneffei* are rarer, but have probably been confused in the past with histoplasmosis because of their remarkable histological resemblance. The usual route of entry of all organisms in this group is the lung, although direct implantation into the skin after an accident is also possible. Each disease has a defined endemic area and their pathogenesis is similar. The majority of people exposed to infection are merely sensitized to the organism and develop delayed-type hypersensitivity to the fungus, seen on intradermal testing with an appropriate antigen (the *asymptomatic form*). In some patients there is a primary illness which appears to follow massive exposure to the organisms (the *acute pulmonary form*). *Chronic pulmonary forms* of these diseases may also occur and they closely resemble pulmonary tuberculosis. Dissemination from the primary lung focus may also take place. It may be a rapid event followed by widespread infiltration of organs (*acute disseminated form*). The infection in such cases progresses rapidly and the disease may be fatal unless treatment is instituted. Acute disseminated forms are most likely to occur in patients who are immunosuppressed (AIDS, lymphoma) but may also be seen in infants and others. More slowly progressive forms also occur and have to be monitored carefully (*chronic disseminated forms*). While generally they only spread slowly, in some situations they may begin to disseminate. In some infections, histoplasmosis and coccidioidomycosis for example, disseminated and pulmonary forms do not generally coexist. *Primary cutaneous infections* are rare and generally follow laboratory or postmortem room accidents.

HISTOPLASMOSES

The classification of histoplasmosis in man is somewhat complicated. There are two main types.[81] The first, sometimes called classical or small form histoplasmosis, is caused by *H. capsulatum* var. *capsula-*

Table 59.6   Systemic mycoses.

Mycosis	Organism
Endemic respiratory infections	
Histoplasmosis	*Histoplasma capsulatum* var. *capsulatum*
African histoplasmosis	*H. capsulatum* var. *duboisii*
Blastomycosis	*Blastomyces dermatitidis*
Coccidioidomycosis	*Coccidioides immitis*
Paracoccidioidomycosis	*Paracoccidioides brasiliensis*
Infection due to *Penicillium marneffei*	
Opportunistic infections	
Systemic candidosis	*Candida albicans, C. tropicalis, C. glabrata*, etc.
Aspergillosis	*Aspergillus fumigatus, A. flavus, A. niger*
Cryptococcosis	*Cryptococcus neoformans*
Zygomycosis	Species of *Absidia, Rhizopus* and *Rhizomucor*
Others: infections due to *Fusarium, Trichosporon*	

tum. This is a dimorphic fungus whose yeast phase forms are those present in tissue. The disease is endemic throughout much of the world, with the exception of Europe, and presents with pulmonary and disseminated infection affecting the lungs, reticuloendothelial system and mucosal surfaces. The yeast forms seen in tissue are small (2–4 μm in diameter). It will be referred to hereafter as histoplasmosis. The second form, African or large-form histoplasmosis caused by *H. capsulatum* var. *duboisii*, only occurs in Africa.[82] The yeasts found in tissue are large (12–20 μm) and the main signs of infection follow dissemination to lymph nodes, skin and bones. The organisms isolated from both are identical in culture and so are regarded as variants of a single species, *H. capsulatum*.

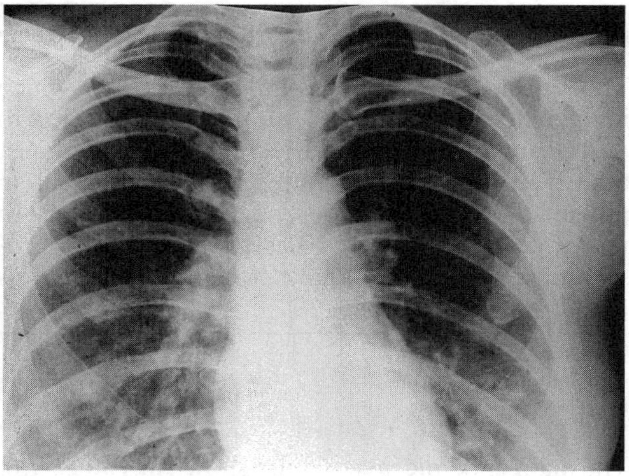

HISTOPLASMOSIS

Histoplasmosis is an infection caused by the dimorphic fungus, *H. capsulatum* var. *capsulatum*. The organism can be found in soil or areas where large numbers of birds or bats have roosted, including barns, caves and under the eaves of houses. There is no association with any one particular bat species in the tropics. The endemic areas include parts of the USA, West Indies, Central and South America, Africa, India and the Far East.[81] Apart from the USA the endemic areas with the highest incidence of new infections occur in Central and South America. The role played by birds and bats in the propagation of the organism is complicated. It is thought that their excreta provides the necessary milieu for growth of organisms present in the environment, although bats can also be infected. Exposure in man is usually sporadic, although occasionally the disease is seen in groups of exposed patients such as cave explorers or farm workers.

Defence against *H. capsulatum* is largely by cell-mediated responses. The organism is about 2–4 μm in diameter and can be taken up by macrophages. The infection may therefore be prolonged in individuals with defective T-lymphocyte-mediated responses, including those with AIDS.

Clinical features

The majority of patients who acquire histoplasmosis remain asymptomatic, the only sign of past exposure being a positive intradermal histoplasmin test which is read after 48 hours. This test is used for studying the epidemiology of infection but has little value as a diagnostic procedure because it only indicates exposure and many patients with active infection appear to be anergic.

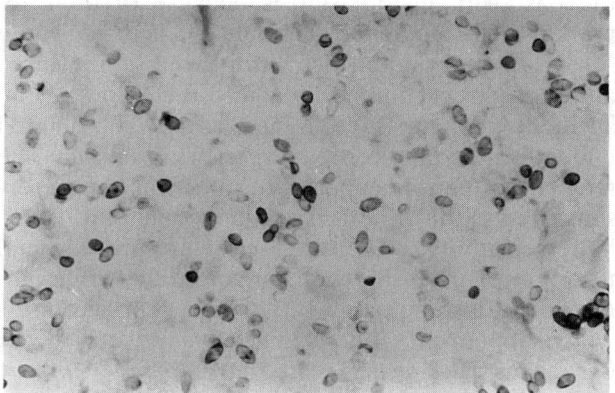

Figure 59.11   Acute pulmonary histoplasmosis.

Figure 59.12   *Histoplasma capsulatum* in a lung lesion. Gomori (methenamine silver) (GMS 100×.)

The acute pulmonary form of histoplasmosis often follows exposure to a site containing numerous *Histoplasma* spores such as a cave. Patients develop an acute febrile illness 10–14 days after exposure. There is cough, chest pain, joint pains and, in some cases, erythema multiforme. Radiologically there is often diffuse mottling and in some cases hilar enlargement (Figure 59.11). Normally, spontaneous recovery occurs and no treatment is given except supportive measures. However, very rarely in some patients the disease progresses and disseminates.

Some patients may be found on routine radiography to have solitary or multiple asymptomatic pulmonary nodules which are surgically removed in order to distinguish them from a carcinoma. These are then found to contain *Histoplasma* yeasts (Figure 59.12). Once again therapy is not necessary. A second type of chronic pulmonary disease produces focal consolidation and cavitation, usually in one or

4

Table 59.7 Use of laboratory tests in histoplasmosis.

Type	Tests
Acute pulmonary	Serology (after 14–18 days), culture, chest radiography
Chronic pulmonary	Culture (sputum), serology, chest radiography
Acute disseminated	Culture (bone marrow, blood, sputum, skin)
	Serology* (including antigen detection)
	Histopathology†
Chronic disseminated	Culture (ulcers)
	Serology (often negative)
	Histopathology

*In acute forms of histoplasmosis titres of complement fixation test antibodies greater than 1:64 indicate a risk of dissemination.
†Some laboratories can carry out immunofluorescence on fixed tissue using conjugated anti-*Histoplasma* antibodies to identify the organisms.

both apices and seen on radiography. This closely resembles pulmonary tuberculosis. The main symptoms, such as cough, chest pain and haemoptysis, are also similar. In the early stages some recovery can occur but later in established cases there is slow progression of the inflammatory lesion which can encroach on other lung areas. This form of histoplasmosis is not often seen in the tropics.

Acute disseminated histoplasmosis affects the bone marrow and lymph glands as well as the liver and spleen.[83] Patients present with fever, weight loss, malaise and hepatosplenomegaly. There may be evidence of bruising and purpura. Diffuse pulmonary infiltrates and small skin papules and ulcers can also occur. This type of histoplasmosis will progress to death if unchecked. Acute forms of disseminated histoplasmosis are seen in patients with AIDS.[84,85] In the latter groups the symptoms may be non-specific (weight loss and fever), although some clues such as hepatosplenomegaly or multiple skin lesions (nodules, papules, ulcers) may be seen. A more indolent type of disseminated histoplasmosis is seen in otherwise healthy individuals. They usually present with either oral ulceration or hypoadrenalism. The latter should be sought in such patients. Chronic disseminated histoplasmosis may present years after the patient has left an endemic area. The oral ulcers are persistent and painful. Laryngeal involvement, meningitis and endocarditis can also occur.

Laboratory diagnosis

The organisms of *H. capsulatum* are very small and difficult to visualize direct microscopy but they can sometimes be seen in bone marrow or blood smears stained with Giemsa. They can be grown readily from sputum or other sources such as bone marrow in appropriate cases. Blood cultures are sometimes positive in patients with AIDS. The organisms grow as moulds at room temperature and have to be converted into yeast phase at 37°C. As this process is slow a more rapid test involving the detection of antigen leached from culture, the exoantigen test, is available. Serology has a useful role in diagnosis. There are complement fixation tests for histoplasmosis as well as an immunodiffusion test, both of which use standardized reagents. These tests can be used in diagnosis and as a guide to prognosis. A new test of particular value in patients with AIDS has been developed for the detection of circulating *Histoplasma* antigen, but it is not widely available. Histopathology is also useful. *Histoplasma* are small oval yeasts up to 5 μm in diameter. They are usually found intracellularly. In patients with AIDS they tend to be more pleomorphic in size and shape.

A guide to the use of diagnostic tests in the different forms of histoplasmosis is seen in Table 59.7.

Treatment

The asymptomatic forms of histoplasmosis do not require therapy. Therapy is also usually withheld in acute pulmonary forms, although supportive treatment such as bed-rest and fluids may be given where necessary. The value of antifungals in these types is not known, although itraconazole would be a possible choice. Chronic pulmonary histoplasmosis and chronic disseminated histoplasmosis are usually treated with either ketoconazole or itraconazole. The role of fluconazole in this infection is not as yet clear. Itraconazole (200–400 mg daily) can also be given in more rapidly disseminating types of infection. An alternative is amphotericin B (0.6–1.0 mg/kg daily) in the disseminated types. In patients with AIDS it is necessary to use long-term suppressive therapy with itraconazole or intermittent amphotericin B after induction of remission, otherwise relapse will normally occur.

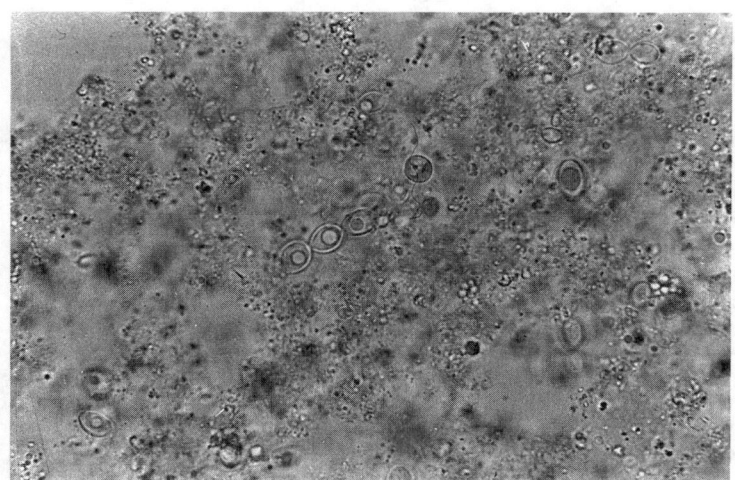

Figure 59.13   African histoplasmosis. Direct microscopy in potassium hydroxide (10%) of pus from a skin ulcer. (40×.)

AFRICAN HISTOPLASMOSIS

African histoplasmosis, as the name suggests, is confined to Africa. It is caused by *H. capsulatum* var. *duboisii*, which resembles the other variant but forms larger yeasts in tissue.[82] The infection is not common but occurs in Central and West Africa south of the Sahara and north of the Zambezi river. The ecological source of this fungus is unknown. It is thought that, as with the other type of histoplasmosis, it gains entry through the lungs.

The patient usually presents with focal disease affecting the skin, bone or a lymph gland. Alternatively multiple sites may be affected, including the gastrointestinal tract, lungs and other mucosal surfaces. This form is more rapidly progressive.

The disease is diagnosed by the presence of large oval yeasts (8–14 μm) seen in direct microscopy (Figure 59.13) or histopathological examination of biopsied lesions. The organism can be isolated in culture. Serology is generally negative.

The main agents are itraconazole, ketoconazole or even amphotericin B. Sulphonamides have also been used in some cases where there has been limited spread.

BLASTOMYCOSIS

Blastomycosis is a systemic fungal infection caused by *Blastomyces dermatitidis*, a dimorphic pathogen.[86] The disease is mainly found in the USA and Canada but cases have also been seen in Africa, India and the Middle East. As with histoplasmosis the main portal of entry is via the respiratory tract. Yeast phase organisms cause disease.

EPIDEMIOLOGY

B. dermatitidis has only occasionally been isolated from the natural environment, usually in North America and in sites where there is a risk of flooding, such as river banks.[87] The organism has not been isolated from such sources in Africa and its ecological niche here is unknown. The infection was first described in the USA and subsequently it became known as North American blastomycosis, until the first case was described from North Africa. Since then cases have been described from a variety of African countries from the north coast (e.g. Algeria) to Namibia.[88] The largest number of cases have been seen in Zimbabwe. It is not clear whether the disease differs in different geographic areas, but in African cases the principal signs of the disease are those of disseminated infection affecting the bone or skin. There is also evidence that the organisms from African and US sources are antigenically different although morphologically identical. Other cases have been detected in the Middle East,[89] India[90] and Europe.

CLINICAL FEATURES

The main clinical features of infection follow a somewhat similar pattern to those seen with histoplasmosis.

There is no commercially available skin test for blastomycosis but the use of experimental antigens has suggested that subclinical exposure is present in endemic areas. There is an uncommon acute pulmonary form of the infection which presents with acute respiratory symptoms—cough, pleuritic pain and fever. This is most often seen in children and has not been described in the tropics.[86]

The chronic pulmonary type of blastomycosis

presents with focal consolidation and cavitation in the chest with symptoms of cough, fever and weight loss. This may be confused radiologically with pulmonary tuberculosis. Unlike histoplasmosis this may coexist with disseminated lesions of blastomycosis. Disseminated blastomycosis is most often seen in the tropics. The main sites of dissemination are the skin and bones. Skin lesions may be ulcers, abscesses, granulomas or crusted plaques which heal with scar formation. The bones involve are principally axial skeletal bones, such as vertebrae, and spinal cord compression may occur as a result of this infection. Dissemination also occurs in the immunocompromised patient.[91]

LABORATORY DIAGNOSIS

The diagnosis of this infection is based on direct microscopy at suitable sites as well as sputum and culture. *B. dermatitidis* is a dimorphic fungus which grows as a mould at room temperature but as a yeast at 37°C. Histological changes of blastomycosis are typical as the yeasts produce a characteristic broad-based bud.

TREATMENT

Therapy of blastomycosis involves the use of either itraconazole (200–400 mg daily) or ketoconazole (200–400 mg daily). Intravenous amphotericin B is an alternative (0.6–1.0 mg/kg daily).

COCCIDIOIDOMYCOSIS

Coccidioides immitis is a soil organism, geographically confined to semidesert areas of the New World.[92] The infection consists of a respiratory disease which may spread to other sites. Coccidioidomycosis may affect both healthy and immunocompromised patients.

EPIDEMIOLOGY

This infection is seen mainly in a geological zone known as the lower Sonoran life zone where there is a low annual rainfall and a characteristic vegetation including cacti and creosote bushes. The disease is confined to the semidesert areas of the New World in the USA, Central America (Honduras, Guatemala), Colombia, Venezuela, Argentina and Paraguay. The first case was described in Argentina but subsequent work centred around a Californian focus

in the San Joaquin valley. The infecting form is an arthrospore which is inhaled but is transformed in the host into a spore-like structure, the spherule. This is a large 50–80 μm diameter spore containing small endospores which are released by rupture of the spherule; they can develop into further spores.

CLINICAL FEATURES

Infection follows inhalation. Once again in the endemic area a significant proportion of the populace appear to be subclinically sensitized, e.g. up to 70% in California.[93] The primary infection, when it is symptomatic, may present with fever, weight loss, cough and chest pains. Arthralgia, conjunctivitis and erythema nodosum or erythema multiforme may all develop. The radiological changes vary from minimal focal consolidation to pleural effusion to massive hilar adenopathy. This clinical type is usually self-resolving, although progression is much more likely in American Indians, Blacks or mestizos. Pregnant women are also at risk from dissemination. An extensive pneumonia may follow infection in patients with depressed T-lymphocyte function, such as those who have received organ transplants. Chronic pulmonary nodules or cavitation may also occur.[92] The latter is characteristically thin-walled on radiography. Dissemination is also seen. Dissemination of coccidioidomycosis often affects the joints or meninges, but skin and other organs may also be affected. Skin changes include ulcers and granulomas as well as warty papules and nodules. Meningitis is a chronic process which clinically mimics tuberculous infection. It is notoriously difficult to treat. In patients with AIDS prolonged pneumonia and disseminated infections can both occur.[94]

LABORATORY DIAGNOSIS

The diagnosis depends on the identification of spherules in smears, biopsies or sputum as well as on the growth of the organism. *C. immitis* is a white mould fungus which is easily spread by aerosol. It is therefore a potential laboratory hazard and laboratory staff should be forewarned if this is being considered diagnostically. There are also a number of useful serological tests (complement fixation, immunodiffusion and immunoelectrophoresis).

TREATMENT

The treatment of coccidioidomycosis has been changing in recent years, with an increasing reliance on the use of ketoconazole, itraconazole and fluconazole. Intravenous amphotericin B is an alternative. The responses of widely disseminated infection and meningitis to these treatments are generally poor.

PARACOCCIDIOIDOMYCOSIS

Paracoccidioidomycosis or South American blastomycosis is a sytemic fungal infection which is confined to Central and South America.[95] It causes a range of pulmonary and systemic symptoms but is a sporadically occurring infection caused by the dimorphic fungus *Faracoccidioidomycosis brasiliensis*. Yeast phase organisms are visualized in tissue.

EPIDEMIOLOGY

The main areas where this disease is present are Colombia, Venezuela, Ecuador, Brazil and Argentina, but other South and Central American countries may be involved. Skin testing reveals that the distribution of sensitization in the community is patchy, and seldom more than 25% have positive skin tests. Both sexes may be sensitized but this infection is very much more common in men than women. The process of transformation from hyphal (environmental) phase to yeast phase *P. brasiliensis* is partly regulated by an intracytoplasmic oestrogen receptor. The natural source of the organism is unknown.

CLINICAL FEATURES

The presence of a small group of healthy individuals in an endemic area with positive skin test reactions suggests that there is a subclinical form of this disease.[96] The main clinical types are named after those parts of the body predominantly affected, such as pulmonary, lymphonodular, mucocutaneous or mixed. In chronic pulmonary infection there is often widespread and extensive infiltration followed by severe fibrosis. There is also dissemination to other sites such as the oral or nasal mucosa or lymph nodes.[97] These are the mucosal (mucocutaneous) or lymphatic forms, respectively, but the most common variety is a mixed type where there are multiple foci of infection. Usually all are only slowly pro-

gressive. On mucosal surfaces this infection produces large erosions and ulcers, less commonly warty papules. All these forms of infection are virtually confined to males. While in most patients paracoccidioidomycosis is an indolent infection, an agressive widespread form of disease occurs occasionally in younger patients. Paracoccidioidomycosis is rare in patients with AIDS.

LABORATORY DIAGNOSIS

The infection is diagnosed by demonstrating presence of the characteristic yeast forms in sputum, smears or biopsies. These yeasts form multiple buds, often appearing around the periphery of a parent cell. The organism is a dimorphic fungus which can be isolated in culture. At room temperature it grows as a mycelial form and has to be converted on enriched agar into the yeast phase at 37°C. Immunodiffusion and complement fixation tests are also available.

TREATMENT

The main treatments are ketoconazole (200 mg daily) and itraconazole (100–200 mg daily), but intravenous amphotericin B is an alternative. The latter may be necessary in the widespread aggressive forms of infection. In some cases sulphonamides can be tried.

INFECTION DUE TO *PENICILLIUM MARNEFFEI*

P. marneffei is a fungus which is a pathogen of a species of rodent found in China and South-East Asia. It causes a disease which grossly resembles histoplasmosis in both otherwise healthy and immunocompromised patients.[98] The main sites affected are the lungs, skin, liver, spleen and bone marrow. The organisms resemble *Histoplasma* spp. but do not form buds, individual cells being divided by septa. The organism has a characteristic appearance in culture. The main therapeutic agents are itraconazole or amphotericin B. Penicillinosis may be seen in patients with AIDS.

SYSTEMIC OPPORTUNISTIC PATHOGENS

The main opportunistic fungi are listed in Table 59.8. In industrialized countries they are a major problem in severely ill patients, particularly those with neutropenia and those receiving solid organ or bone marrow transplants. They are also seen in intensive care units. In addition to these, some infections such as cryptococcosis are presemt in patients with AIDS. In the tropics less attention has been paid to some of these opportunists, such as candidosis and aspergillosis, with some important exceptions;[99] by contrast, cryptococcosis is recognized to be a common and increasingly important problem everywhere. For more detailed information on these infections the reader is referred to other texts.[100]

SYSTEMIC CANDIDOSIS

Systemic *Candida* infections occur in a variety of patients, particularly those who are neutropenic, such as leukaemia patients, those who have received major surgery and patients receiving long-term intravenous feeding. The importance of these infections in the tropics is largely unknown. Their management is discussed elsewhere.[100]

ASPERGILLOSIS

Aspergillosis is a disease caused by species of the genus *Aspergillus*, principally *A. fumigatus*, *A. flavus* and *A. niger*. There are a number of different clinical syndromes caused by these fungi which occur in temperate and tropical climates alike. Aspergilli are well-recognized causes of allergic pulmonary disease, either when inhaled as spores (extrinsic asthma) or when growing within airways where, in susceptible individuals, they may cause a form of intrinsic asthma known as allergic bronchopulmonary aspergillosis.[101] The latter causes reversible bronchoconstriction in the early stages but thereafter irreversible pulmonary damage may occur. This type of disease has been recorded in India amongst other tropical areas. A form of aspergillosis seen regularly in tropical areas is the development of a fungus ball in patients with pulmonary cavitation, usually secondary to tuberculosis. This colonizing ball may elicit an inflammatory response and in a minority of patients (15%) will cause haemoptysis, often of great severity.[102] The other mode of pathogenesis by *Aspergillus* is through invasion of tissue. This is mainly a problem in the severely neutropenic patient. However, there is one invasive *Aspergillus* syndrome which is mainly seen in the tropics—invasive paranasal *Aspergillus* granuloma.

Invasive *Aspergillus* granuloma of the paranasal sinuses is a slowly progressive infection affecting the sinuses, orbit and brain.[103,104] It is seen mainly in Africa and the Middle East and in most patients is caused by *A. flavus*. The patient presents with headache, nasal obstruction and orbital swelling with, in some cases, proptosis. In later stages invasion of the brain may ensue. On radiography a mass can be seen in the maxillary or ethmoid sinuses with erosion of the bones of the base of the skull and orbit. These changes can be confirmed with computerized tomography. If nuclear magnetic resonance imaging is available the infiltrated area contains a typically dense mass. If the lesions are biopsied the main change is a hard progressive granulomatous mass with fibrosis. Scattered fungal fragments can be seen in giant cells, using a methenamine silver stain, and the organism can be isolated in culture. Serology (immunodiffusion) is often positive. The main differential diagnosis is consists of other *Aspergillus*-related illnesses. The presence of an intrasinus mass without bone erosion may be due to an aspergilloma or dense colonization with aspergilli. In this instance presence of the organism may not be of pathological significance. The decision is difficult as unless numerous fragments of tissue are examined the more sinister changes of fibrosis will not be seen. Aggressive paranasal sinus invasion may also occur in neutropenic patients.

The main treatment for paranasal *Aspergillus* granuloma is surgical removal of as much of the tumour as is possible, followed by long-term therapy with itraconazole (200–400 mg daily). This may have to be extended for 6–24 months and, if available, serology is a helpful way of monitoring. An alternative therapeutic option is amphotericin B but long-term therapy is not possible with this drug.

Table 59.8 Opportunistic systemic mycoses.

Systemic candidosis
Aspergillosis
Mucormycosis
Cryptococcosis
Less common
    Systemic infections due to *Trichosporon, Hansenula, Fusarium, Bipolaris*

MUCORMYCOSIS

Fungi belonging to the genera *Absidia*, *Rhizopus* and *Rhizomucor*, and less commonly other groups, may cause an aggressive paranasal, pulmonary or disseminated infection in predisposed groups such as diabetic or neutropenic patients.[105] This infection, known as mucormycosis, is seen in temperate as well as tropical countries and may cause the rapid demise of a patient unless there is prompt surgical intervention and treatment with intravenous amphotericin B. It may also present with orbital cellulitis or as a necrotizing wound infection. In malnourished children it may cause a necrotizing gastrointestinal infection.

Treatment with amphotericin B combined, where possible, with surgical debridement offers the best chance of recovery.

CRYPTOCOCCOSIS

Cryptococcosis is a systemic infection caused by an encapsulated yeast fungus, *Cryptococcus neoformans*. Its distribution is worldwide and it generally presents with meningitis or some other manifestation of extrapulmonary dissemination. While it may cause disease in otherwise healthy individuals, it is also a pathogen of patients with defective T-lymphocyte function, such as patients with AIDS, lymphoma or those eceiving corticosteroid therapy.

EPIDEMIOLOGY AND PATHOGENESIS

There are two variants of *C. neoformans*: *C. neoformans* var. *neoformans* and *C. neoformans* var. *gattii*.[106,107] The *neoformans* variety causes disease in immunocompromised patients including those with AIDS, and is found in most countries. Its ecological niche appears to be soil or areas where there are large amounts of pigeon excreta, from which this fungus can be isolated. The presumed route of entry is via inhalation. The *gattii* form is seen mainly in tropical areas in otherwise healthy individuals. It has been reported from Africa, the Far East, Papua New Guinea and Australia. This organism has only recently been isolated from the environment from debris from certain species of *Eucalyptus*. In addition to the differences in distribution there are no clear differences in their clinical behaviour apart from the predilection of the *neoformans* variety for patients with AIDS.[108]

It is difficult to ascertain infection rates, although there is evidence from the use of experimental skin

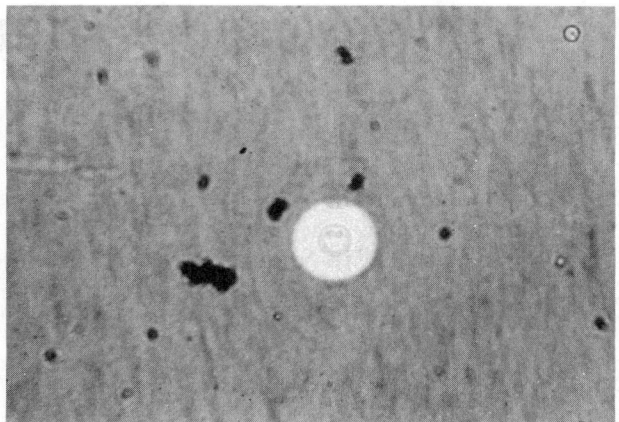

Figure 59.14   Cryptococcal cell in CSF. (India ink, 100×.)

test reagents that subclinical sensitization may be seen in the general population, as with other systemic mycoses such as histoplasmosis. Infection rates in the tropics are not known and appear to be variable, even in patients with AIDS. There is evidence that in Zaire that about 12% of those with AIDS have circulating cryptococcal antigen, indicating active infection. However, in AIDS patients in Kenya the incidence is lower; in Zambia the infection is again more common. The scientific basis for these fluctuations is unknown. However, clustering of cases may occur and has been seen for instance in Papua New Guinea where the disease is mainly caused by *C. neoformans* var. *gattii*.

CLINICAL FEATURES

Cryptococcal infection may present with pulmonary infection—cough, chest pain and fever.[107] However, pulmonary lesions are more often present as an incidental, and symptomless, finding in a patient with other manifestations of cryptococcosis. The main presentation of this infection in the non-AIDS patient is with meningitis, although headache and neck stiffness may not be severe; but other signs such as confusion, drowsiness, photophobia and cranial nerve palsies may be seen. Other signs of dissemination such as papular or ulcerative skin lesions, lytic bone deposits and prostatitis may be found. In patients with AIDS the symptoms of meningitis are often minimal and fever may be the main clinical sign, together with malaise and tiredness.[109]

LABORATORY DIAGNOSIS

The laboratory diagnosis of cryptococcosis is straightforward. It depends on the demonstration of the organism(s) by staining smears, CSF or sputum with Indian ink (Figure 59.14) or nigrosin. The capsule surrounding the organism displaces the dense strain and the surrounding clear halo seen with the microscope is typical of *Cryptococcus*. The organism can be cultured readily on conventional mycological media such as Sabouraud's agar, although it may take 3–12 days for the yeasts to be recognizable. Sources of culture material include: CSF, sputum and biopsies. In patients with AIDS blood cultures may also be positive. There is no clinical advantage in identifying the different varieties.

The quickest method of diagnosis is the use of the antigen detection test using antibody sensitized latex particles. It is used to detect capsular antigen in serum or CSF. The test is specific and will produce a positive response in 30 minutes. It can also be used to follow the course of therapy. Biopsy material will also show the large yeast cells using periodic acid–Schiff or Grocott stains; the mucicarmine stain is specific for cryptococcal cells, which it stains pink.

TREATMENT

The main therapy in the non-AIDS patient is a combination of intravenous amphotericin B (0.4–0.8 mg/kg daily) and flucytosine (120–150 mg/kg daily divided in four doses). The response in most patients is good but therapy may have to be continued for 4–6 weeks, and sometimes longer. The treatment of the AIDS case is more complex. Few treatments can produce permanent recovery and the usual strategy is to start with a period of induction therapy followed by long-term suppression to prevent relapse. At present the best choice of drugs is still unclear. Many units will use an initial period of amphotericin (0.4–0.8 mg/kg daily), with or without flucytosine, for 2 weeks, followed by long-term daily suppressive therapy with fluconazole(200–400 mg) or itraconazole (200–300 mg). Fluconazole may also be used to produce remission on its own, although the correct dose is not clearly established.

OTHER MYCOSES

Other opportunistic infections with fungi are seen in different countries and are not specifically associated with the tropics. Again they usually occur in the neutropenic patient. They include infection with *Trichosporon*, *Fusarium* and *Bipolaris* spp. These diseases are generally uncommon, but carry a high mortality.

OCULOMYCOSIS (See also Chapter 10)

Infections of the eye caused by fungi are regularly seen in the tropics. Generally they involve the cornea and follow contamination of a traumatic external injury (keratomycosis[110]). The chief causes in the tropics are filamentous fungi of the genera *Fusarium*, *Aspergillus*, *Curvularia*, *Acremonium* and *Penicillium*. Less commonly yeasts such as *Candida* spp. are implicated. Patients usually present with pain in the eye and photophobia. There is often an obvious ulcer, although it may be necessary to demonstrate this with slit-lamp microscopy. The ulcer may be covered with slough and there are small satellite ulcers around the edge. Surrounding chemosis and a hypopyon may also be present. If the condition is not treated, severe intraocular infection followed by glaucoma, blindness and perforation of the globe will occur. Scrapings from the ulcer will readily show the presence of fungal hyphae and these can then be isolated on Sabouraud's medium. It is very important to establish the presence of fungi in such cases of keratitis because their management is very different to that used for bacteria.

Intensive application of antifungal drops such as econazole (1%) in arachis oil, clotrimazole or natamycin every few hours is advised. Oral itraconazole may help in some infections although it is seldom useful where *Fusarium* is involved. Mechanical debridement may also be useful in some cases. Keratomycosis is a preventable cause of blindness if recognized and treated as soon as possible.

REFERENCES

1 Rippon J W. *Medical Mycology*, 2nd edn. Philadelphia: W B Saunders, 1985.
2 Rebell G & Taplin D. *Dermatophytes: Their Recognition and Identification*, 2nd edn. Miami: University of Miami Press, 1976.
3 de Vroey C. Epidemiology of ringworm (dermatophytosis) *Semin Dermatol* 1985; 4:185–200.
4 Serjeantson S & Lawrence G. Autosomal recessive

inheritance of susceptibility to tinea imbricata. *Lancet* 1977; i:13–15.

5 Hay R J. Chronic dermatophyte infections. I. Clinical and mycological features. *Br J Dermatol* 1982; 106:1–6.

6 Torssander J, Karlsson A, Morfeldt-Mason L et al. Dermatophytosis and HIV infection — study in homosexual men. *Acta Derm Venereol* 1988; 68:53–59.

7 Amer M, Taha M, Tossan Z & El-Garf A. The frequency of causative dermatophytes in Egypt. *Int J Dermatol* 1981; 20:431–434.

8 Bhardway G, Hajini G H, Khan I A et al. Dermatophytosis in Kashmir, India. *Mykosen* 1987; 30:135–138.

9 Blank H, Taplin D & Zaias N. Cutaneous *Trichophyton mentagrophtyes* infections in Vietnam. *Arch Dermatol* 1969; 99:135–144.

10 Gugnani H C & Njoku-Obi A N U. Tinea capitis in school children in East Nigeria. *Mykosen* 1986; 29:132–144.

11 Karaoui R, Selim M & Mousa A. Incidence of dermatophytosis in Kuwait. *Sabouraudia* 1979; 17:131–137.

12 Howell S A, Clayton Y M, Phan Q G & Noble W C. Tinea pedis: the relationship between symptoms and host characteristics. *Microbiol Ecol Health & Dis* 1988; 1:131–138.

13 Leyden J J & Kligman A M. Interdigital athletes foot: the interaction of dermatophytes and residual bacteria. *Arch Dermatol* 1978; 114:1466–1472.

14 Al-Sogair S M, Moawad M K & Al-Humaidan Y M. Fungal infection as a cause of skin disease in the Eastern Province of Saudi Arabia: tinea pedis and tinea manuum. *Mycoses* 1991; 34:339–344.

15 Evans E G V & Richardson M D (eds). *Medical Mycology. A Practical Approach*. Oxford: IRL Press, 1989.

16 Pernicario C & Peters M S. Tinea faciale mimicking seborrheic dermatitis in a patient with AIDS. *N Engl J Med* 1986: 314:315–316.

17 Hay R J, Reid S, Talwat E & MacNamara K. Endemic tinea imbricata—a study on Goodenough Island, PNG. *Trans R Soc Trop Med* 1984; 78:246–251.

18 Clayton Y M. Scalp ringworm (tinea capitis). In Verbov J L (ed.) *Superficial Fungal Infections*. Manchester: MTP Press, 1986:1–8.

19 Rippon J W. Epidemiology and emerging patterns of dermatophyte species. *Curr Top Med Mycol* 1985; 1:208–234.

20 Vanbreusegehem R. *Trichophyton soudanense* infection in and outside Africa. *Br J Dermatol* 1968; 80:140–148.

21 Verhagen A R. Distribution of dermatophytes causing tinea capitis in Africa. *Trop Geogr Med* 1973; 26:101–120.

22 Wright S & Robertson V J. An institutional survey of tinea capitis in Harare, Zimbabwe and a trial of miconazole cream versus Whitfield's ointment in its treatment. *Clin Exp Dermatol* 1986; 11:371–377.

23 Ive F A. The carrier state of tinea capitis in Nigeria. *Br J Dermatol* 1966; 78:219–221.

24 Babel D & Baughman S A. Evaluation of the adult carrier state in juvenile tinea capitis caused by *Trichophyton tonsurans*. *J Am Acad Dermatol* 1989; 21:1209–1212.

25 Krowchuk D P, Lucky A W & Primmer S I. Current status of the identification and management of tinea capitis. *Pediatrics* 1983; 72:625–631.

26 Davies R R, Griseofulvin. In Speller D C E (ed.) *Antifungal Chemotherapy*. Chichester: Wiley, 1980:149–182.

27 Roberts S O B. Treatment of superficial and subcutaneous mycoses. In Speller D C E (ed.) *Antifungal Chemotherapy*. Chichester: Wiley, 1980:255–283.

28 Clayton Y M & Connor B L. Comparison of clotrimazole cream, Whitfield's ointment and nystatin ointment for the topical treatment of ringworm infections, pityriasis versicolor, erythrasma and candidiasis. *Br J Dermatol* 1973; 89:297–303.

29 Zaias N. Onychomycosis. *Arch Dermatol* 1972; 105:262–274.

30 Zaias N. Superficial white onychomycosis. *Sabouraudia* 1966; 5:99–103.

31 Goodfield M J D, Rowell N R, Forster R A et al. Treatment of dermatophyte infection of the finger- and toe-nails with terbinafine (SF 86-327, Lamisil), an orally active fungicidal agent. *Br J Dermatol* 1989; 121:753–758.

32 Willemsen M, de Donker P, Willems J et al. Post treatment itraconazole levels in the nail. *J Am Acad Dermatol* 1992; 26:731–735.

33 Odds F C. *Candida and Candidosis*. London: Baillière Tindall, 1988.

34 Gough P M, Warnock D W, Turner A et al. Candidosis of the genital tract in non-pregnant women. *Eur J Obstet Gynecol Reprod Biol* 1985; 19:237–246.

35 Torssander J, Morfeldt-Mauson L, Biberfeld G et al. Oral *Candida albicans* in HIV infection. *Scand J Infect* 1987; 189:291–295.

36 Samaranayake L P & MacFarlane T W (eds). Oral *Candidosis*. London: Wright, 1990.

37 Pindborg J J. Classification of oral lesions associated with HIV infection. *Oral Surg Oral Med Oral Pathol* 1989; 67:292–295.

38 Greenspan D & Greenspan J S. Oral mucosal manifestations of AIDS. *Dermatol Clin* 1987; 5:733–737.

39 Sobel J D. Recurrent vulvovaginal candidiasis. *N Engl J Med* 1986; 315:1455–1458.

40 Frain-Bell W. Chronic paronychia. Short review of 590 cases. *Trans St John Hosp Derm Soc* 1957; 38:29–30.

41 Dwyer J M. Chronic mucocutaneous candidiasis. *Ann Rev Med* 1981; 32:491–497.

42 Grant S M & Clissold S P. Fluconazole: a review of its pharmacodynamic and pharmacokinetic

properties, and therapeutic potential in superficial and systemic mycoses. *Drugs* 1990; 39:877–916.

43 Jones H E (ed.) *Ketoconazole Today. A Review of Clinical Experience*. Manchester: ADIS Press, 1987.

44 Grant S M & Clissold S P. Itraconazole: a review of its pharmacodynamic and pharmacokinetic properties and therapeutic use in superficial and systemic mycoses. *Drugs* 1989; 37:310–344.

45 Hay R J & Moore M K. Clinical features of superficial fungal infections caused by *Hendersonula toruloidea* and *Scytalidium hyalinum*. *Br J Dermatol* 1984; 110:677–683.

46 Gugnani H C, Nzelibe F K & Osunkwo I C. Onychomycosis due to *Hendersonula toruloidea* in Nigeria. *J Med Vet Mycol* 1986; 24:239–241.

47 Moore M K. Morphological and physiological studies of isolates of *Hendersonula toruloidea Nattrass* cultured from human skin and nail samples. *J Med Vet Mycol* 1988; 26:25–39.

48 Faergemann J. Lipophilic yeasts in skin disease. *Semin Dermatol* 1985; 4:173–184.

49 Roberts S O B. Pityriasis versicolor; a clinical and mycological investigation. *Br J Dermatol* 1969; 81:315–326.

50 Mathes B M & Douglas M C. Seborrheic dermatitis in patients with acquired immunodeficiency syndrome. *J Am Acad Dermatol* 1985; 13:947–951.

51 Kaiter D C A, Tschen J A, Cernoch P L et al. Genital white piedra; epidemiology, microbiology and therapy. *J Am Acad Dermatol* 1986; 14: 982–993.

52 Lassus A, Kanerva L, Stubbs S et al. White piedra. *Arch Dermatol* 1982; 118:208–211.

53 Adam B A T, Soo-Hoo T S & Chong K C. Black piedra in West Malaysia. *Australas J Dermatol* 1977; 18:45–47.

54 Pahwa V K, Chamiyal P C & Suri P N. Mycological study of otomycosis. *Indian J Med Res* 1983; 77:334–338.

55 Mahgoub E S & Murray I G. *Mycetoma*. London: Heinemann, 1973.

56 Mariat F, Destombes P & Segretain G. The mycetomas: clinical features, pathology, etiology and epidemiology. *Contrib Microbiol Immunol* 1977; 4:1–39.

57 Lavalle P. Micetomas; la experiencia mexicana. Problemas actuales. In *Proceedings of the Second International Symposium on Mycetomas*, Taxco, 1987:66–73.

58 Wethered D B, Markey M A, Hay R J et al. Ultrastructural and immunogenic changes in the formation of mycetoma grains. *J Med Vet Mycol* 1986; 25:39–46.

59 Davies A G M. The bone changes of Madura foot. Observations on Uganda Africans. *Radiology* 1958; 70:309–315.

60 Palestine R F & Rogers R S. Diagnosis and treatment of mycetoma. *J Am Acad Dermatol* 1982; 6:107–111.

61 Destombes P. Histological diagnosis of mycetoma

granules. *Proceedings of the First International Symposium on Mycetoma*, Venezuela, 1978:80–94.

62 Mahgoub E S. Medical management of mycetoma. *Bull World Health Organ* 1976; 54:303–310.

63 Bayles M A H. Chromomycosis. *Baillière's Clin Trop Med Commun Dis* 1989; 4:45–70.

64 Banks I S, Palmieri J R, Lanoie L, Connor D H & Meyers W M. Chromomycosis in Zaire. *Int J Dermatol* 1985; 24:302–307.

65 Carrion A L. Chromoblastomycosis and related infections. *Int J Dermatol* 1975; 14: 27–32.

66 Romero A & Trejos A. La cromoblastomicosis en Costa Rica. *Rev Biol Trop* 1953; 1:95–115.

67 McGinnis M R. Chromoblastomycosis and phaeohyphomycosis; new concepts, diagnosis and mycology. *J Am Acad Dermatol* 1983; 8:1–16.

68 de Albornoz M C B. Sporotrichosis. *Baillière's Clin Trop Med Commun Dis* 1989; 4:71–96.

69 Bibler M R, Luber H J, Clueck H I et al. Disseminated sporotrichosis in a patient with HIV infection after treatment for acquired factor VIII inhibitor. *JAMA* 1986; 256:3125–3126.

70 Mayorga R, Caceres A, Toriello G et al. Etude d'une endémie sporotrichosique au Guatemala. *Sabouraudia* 1978; 16:185–198.

71 Auld J C & Beardmore G L. Sporotrichosis in Queensland: a review of 137 cases at the Royal Brisbane Hospital. *Aust J Dermatol* 1979; 20:14–22.

72 Itoh M, Okamoto S & Kanya H. Survey of 260 cases of sporotrichosis. *Dermatologica* 1986; 172:203–213.

73 Brian M & Strom R. Multiarticular sporotrichosis. *JAMA* 1978; 240:556–557.

74 Baker R D, Seabury J H & Schneidau J D. Subcutaneous and cutaneous mucormycosis and subcutaneous phycomycosis. *Lab Invest* 1962; 11:1091–1102.

75 Martinson F D. Clinical, epidemiological and therapeutic aspects of entomophthoromycosis. *Ann Soc Belg Méd Trop* 1972; 52:329–342.

76 Segura J J, Gionzale K, Berrocal J et al. Rhinoentomophthoromycosis; report of the first two cases observed in Costa Rica (Central America) and review of the literature. *Am J Trop Med Hyg* 1981; 30:1078–1084.

77 Joe L K & Eng N I T. Subcutaneous phycomycosis: a new disease found in Indonesia. *Ann N Y Acad Sci* 1969; 89:4–16.

78 Kamalam A & Thambiah A S. Muscle invasion by *Basidiobolus haptosporus. Sabouraudia*. 1984; 22:273–277.

79 Baruzzi R G & Marcopito L F. Lobomycosis. *Baillière's Clin Trop Med Commun Dis* 1989; 4:97–112.

80 Baruzzi R G, Lacaz C S & Souza F A A. Historia natural da doenca de Jorge Lobo. Ocorrencia entre os indios Caiabi (Brasil Central). *Rev Inst Med Trop São Paulo* 1979; 21:302–338.

81 Goodwin R A, Loyd J E & DesPrez R M. Histoplasmosis in normal hosts. *Medicine* 1981; 60:231–266.

82 Drouhet E. African histoplasmosis. *Baillière's Clin Trop Med Commun Dis* 1989; 4:221–247.

83 Goodwin R A, Shapiro J L, Thurman G H et al. Disseminated histoplasmosis. *Medicine* 1980; 59:1–33.

84 Wheat L J, Slama T G, Norton J A & Zeckel M L. Histoplasmosis in the acquired immune deficient syndrome. *Am J Med* 1985; 78:203–210.

85 Barton E N, Roberts L, Ince W E et al. Cutaneous histoplasmosis in the acquired immunodeficiency syndrome: a report of three cases from Trinidad. *Trop Geogr Med* 1988; 40:153–157.

86 Sarosi G A & Davies S F. Blastomycosis. *Am Rev Respir Dis* 1979; 120: 911–938.

87 Klein B S, Vergeront J M, Weeks R J et al. Isolation of *Blastomyces dermatitidis* in soil associated with a large outbreak of blastomycosis in Wisconsin. *N Engl J Med* 1986; 314:529–534.

88 Emerson P A, Higgins E & Branfoot A. North American blastomycosis in Africans. *Br J Dis Chest* 1984; 78:286–291.

89 Kingston M, El-Mishad M M & Ashraf A M. Blastomycosis in Saudia Arabia. *Am J Trop Med Hyg* 1980; 29:464–466.

90 Randhawa H S, Khan Z V & Gaur S N. *Blastomyces dermatitidis* in India. First report of its isolation from clinical material. *Sabouraudia* 1983; 21:215–221.

91 Recht L D, Davies S F, Eckman M R et al. Blastomycosis in immunosuppressed patients. *Am Rev Respir Dis* 1982; 125:359–362.

92 Drutz D J & Catanzaro A. Coccidioidomycosis. Parts I and II. *Am Rev Respir Dis* 1978; 117:559–585, 727–771.

93 Gifford J & Catanzaro A. A comparison of coccidioidin and spherulin skin testing in the diagnosis of coccidioidomycosis. *Am Rev Respir Dis* 1981; 124:440–444.

94 Bronniman D A, Adam R D, Galgiani J N et al. Coccidioidomycosis in the acquired immunodeficiency syndrome. *Ann Intern Med* 1987; 106:373–379.

95 Del Negro G, Lacaz C S, Fiorillo A M (eds). *Paracoccidioidomicose*. São Paulo: Sarvier, 1982.

96 Franco M F, Host–parasite relationship in paracoccidioidomycosis. *J Med Vet Mycol* 1978; 25:5–18.

97 Restrepo A, Robledo M, Giraldo R et al. The gamut of paracoccidioidomycosis. *Am J Med* 1976; 61:33–42.

98 Jayanetra P, Nitiyanant P, Ajello L et al. Penicillinosis marneffei in Thailand; report of five human cases. *Am J Trop Med Hyg* 1984; 33:637–644.

99 Hay R J. Opportunistic fungal infection in the tropics. *Ballière's Clin Trop Med Commun Dis* 1989; 4:249–267.

100 Warnock D & Richardson M D (eds). *Fungal Infections in the Compromised Patient*. Chichester: Wiley, 1989.

101 Attapattu M C. Allergic bronchopulmonary aspergillosis in a chronic asthmatic. *Ceylon Med J* 1983; 28:251–270.

102 Bovornkitti S, Pacharee P, Chatvanich K et al. Aspergilloma in a bronchogenic cyst. A case report. *J Med Assoc Thai* 1984; 53:211–215.

103 Martinson F D, Ali A F & Clarke B M. Aspergilloma of the ethmoid. *J Laryngol Otol* 1970; 84:857–861.

104 Veress B, Malik O A, El Tayeb A A et al. Further observations on the primary paranasal aspergillus granuloma in the Sudan. *Am J Trop Med Hyg* 1973; 22:765–772.

105 Bahadur S, Ghosh P, Chopra P et al. Rhinocerebral phycomycosis. *J Laryngol Otol* 1983; 97:267–270.

106 Bennett J E, Kwon-Chung K J & Howard D H. Epidemiologic differences among serotypes of *Cryptococcus neoformans*. *Am J Epidermiol* 1977; 10:582–586.

107 Dupont B. Cryptococcosis. *Baillière's Clin Trop Med Commun Dis* 1989; 4:113–124.

108 Swinne D & de Vroey C. Epidémiologie de la cryptococcose. *Rev Iberica Micol* 1987; 4:77–83.

109 Kovacs J A, Kovacs A A, Polis M et al. Cryptococcosis in the acquired immunodeficiency syndrome. *Ann Intern Med* 1985; 103:533–538.

110 Thomas P A. Keratomycosis. *Baillière's Clin Trop Med Commun Dis* 1989; 4:269–286.

CHAPTER 60

PNEUMOCYSTIS CARINII INFECTION

R. Miller

HISTORY

When it was first described over 50 years ago in premature babies and malnourished infants *Pneumocystis carinii* pneumonia was known as plasma cell interstitial pneumonitis, a descriptive term based on the appearances of the lung at autopsy. Patients typically presented with a non-productive cough and relentlessly progressive dyspnoea, but they rarely had fever. Examination of the chest was usually normal and the chest radiograph frequently showed diffuse bilateral infiltrates. Death due to respiratory failure occurred in the majority of cases. It was not until the mid-1950s that *P. carinii* was identified as the causative agent. The organism had originally been identified in 1911 by Chagas in guinea-pigs and man. In the mid-1990s *P. carinii* pneumonia is now a major cause of opportunistic infection in patients with human immunodeficiency virus (HIV) infection (see also Chapter 12).

RISK FACTORS FOR THE DEVELOPMENT OF *P. CARINII* PNEUMONIA

P. carinii pneumonia (PCP) develops most frequently in individuals with T-lymphocyte immunodeficiency. *P. carinii* causes sporadic disease in patients immunosuppressed by the effects of malignancy such as leukaemia and lymphoma, or the treatment thereof, or because of immunosuppressive therapy given either to prevent rejection following organ transplantation or to treat vasculitis; sporadic disease also occurs in those with hypogammaglobulinaemia. Epidemic PCP occurs in patients infected with HIV. Rarely, individuals with no evidence of immunosuppression develop PCP (Table 60.1).

Table 60.1 Risk groups for pneumocystis pneumonia.

1 Sporadic disease
  Patients receiving chemotherapy (for leukaemia, lymphoma)
  Immunosuppressed organ transplant recipients (kidney, heart–lung, heart)
  Immunosuppression for inflammatory disorders (vasculitis)
  Hypogammaglobulinaemia
2 Epidemic disease
  Associated with HIV infection
3 No apparent risk factors

HISTOPATHOLOGY

Pulmonary infection with *P. carinii* is characterized by a foamy intra-alveolar exudate which is associated with a plasma cell interstitial infiltrate. Two forms of *P. carinii* may be identified. By using Grocott's methaminine silver, toluidine blue O or cresyl violet stains, thick-walled cysts (6–7 μm in diameter), each containing 4–8 sporozoites, are seen to lie freely within the alveolar exudate (Figure 60.1). The exudate itself consists largely of thin-walled irregularly shaped single nucleated trophozoites (2–5 μm in size) which are best shown with Giemsa stain or electron microscopy. Both forms of *P. carinii* may also be demonstrated by use of indirect immunofluorescence with monoclonal antibodies raised against *P. carinii*. Unusually interstitial fibrosis, granulomatous inflammation, diffuse alveolar damage, intrapulmonary cyst formation and extrapulmonary pneumocystosis may occur.

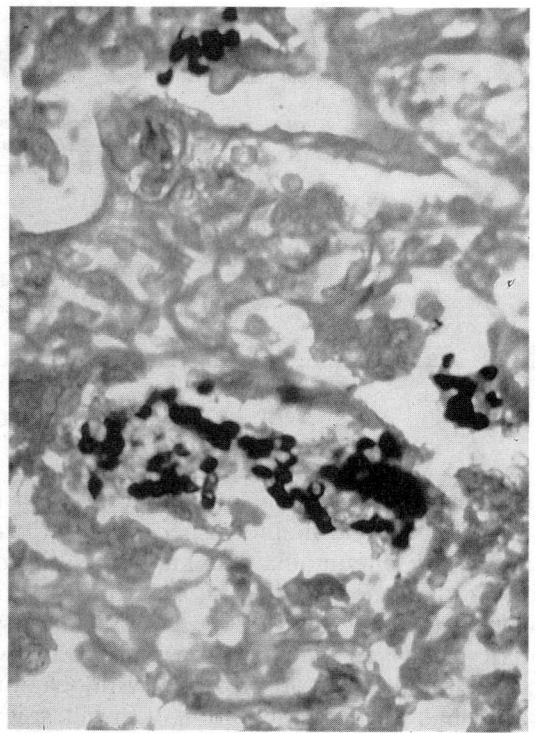

Figure 60.1 Transbronchial biopsy showing cysts of *P. carinii*. (Grocott's methenamine silver, 200 ×.)

IS *P. CARINII* A FUNGUS OR A PROTOZOON?

Based on its morphology, the inability to culture the organism in vitro and its response to antiprotozoal but not antifungal drugs, *P. carinii* has been taxonomically regarded as a protozoon. Use of the molecular biological techniques of cloning and sequencing to compare several chromosomal and mitochondrial genes from *P. carinii* and from many different fungi representing all seven phyla now suggest that *P. carinii* is a member of the fungal kingdom and that

different 'types' of *P. carinii* infect man and other host species. Infection in some hosts, for example in humans, appears to be clonal, whereas rats and ferrets may be simultaneously coinfected with two types of *P. carinii*. In experiments which have attempted to grow *P. carinii* from one host species in the lungs of another host, cross-infection has been unsuccessful, suggesting that there is host specificity for different types of *P. carinii*.

IS *P. CARINII* PNEUMONIA DUE TO REINFECTION OR REACTIVATION?

The majority of healthy children and adults have antibodies to *P. carinii*, suggesting that asymptomatic infection occurs in childhood and that PCP in an immunosuppressed individual arises by reactivation of latent infection. However, studies using mono-

clonal antibodies and DNA detection with *P. carinii*-specific primers have failed to identify *P. carinii* in autopsy lung tissue or bronchoalveolar lavage fluid of healthy individuals; *P. carinii* in low levels has been detected in the lungs of only 20% of patients immunosuppressed by HIV and other causes with respiratory symptoms and diagnoses other than PCP. *P. carinii* DNA has been identified in the air of rural and hospital locations. These data, together with others showing host specificity, support the hypothesis that clinical infection in the immunosuppressed human host is not a zoonosis, and arises by reinfection, rather than by reactivation of latent infection.

CLINICAL PRESENTATION

Patients typically present with progressive exertional dyspnoea, a non-productive cough and fever of several days or weeks duration which is often associated with a sensation of inability to take in a deep breath. In patients immunosuppressed by HIV infection symptoms are usually of longer duration than in patients immunosuppressed by other causes. Auscultation of the chest is usually normal; rarely fine inspiratory crackles may be heard. Table 60.2 shows typical and atypical features for patients presenting with PCP.

Table 60.2 Presentation of *P. carinii* pneumonia.

Typical features	Atypical features
Progressive exertional dyspnoea over days or weeks	Sudden onset of dyspnoea over hours
Dry cough ± mucoid sputum	Cough productive of purulent sputum Haemoptysis Pleuritic chest pain
Inability to take in a deep breath not due to pleuritic pain Fever ± sweats Tachypnoea	
Examination of the chest Normal breath sounds or fine end inspiratory basal crackles	Signs of focal consolidation, pleural effusion, or wheeze
Chest radiograph Normal or perihilar haze } early presentation or bilateral interstitial shadowing or alveolar-interstitial changes or 'white out' (marked alveolar consolidation with sparing of apices and costophrenic angles) } late presentation	

Arterial blood gases

	Pao_2	$Paco_2$
Early	Normal	Normal or hypocarbia
Late	Hypoxaemia	Normal or hypercarbia

Reproduced with permission from Malin A S & Miller R F. *Pneumocystis carinii* pneumonia: presentation and diagnosis. *Rev Med Microbiol* 1992; 3:80–87.

INVESTIGATIONS

NON-INVASIVE INVESTIGATIONS

These investigations have moderate to high sensitivity but lack specificity.

CHEST RADIOLOGY

In early pneumonia the chest radiograph may be normal; with later presentations and with more severe disease diffuse perihilar interstitial infiltrates are seen (Figure 60.2). These appearances may progress to diffuse bilateral air space (alveolar) consolidation resembling pulmonary oedema (Figure 60.3). With delayed presentation or untreated severe disease the lungs may show confluent alveolar shadowing ('white out') throughout both lungs, with sparing of the costophrenic angles and apices. The chest radiographic appearances in PCP may change rapidly from being normal at presentation to markedly abnormal over a period of only 2–3 days. Atypical radiographic features are seen in up to 20% of patients with PCP; these include cystic air space and pneumatocoele formation, unilateral consolidation, lobar infiltrates, nodules, mediastinal lymphadenopathy, pleural effusions and upper zone infiltrates resembling tuberculosis (Figure 60.4). Although the chest radiograph is a very sensitive

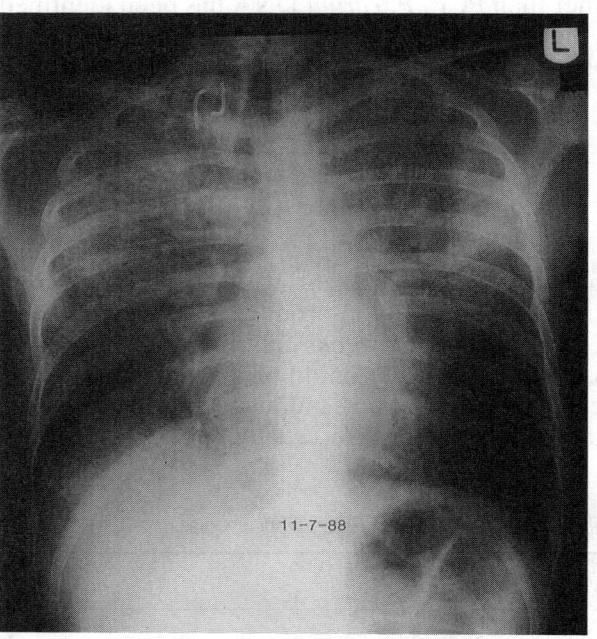

Figure 60.3 Extensive bilateral shadowing in a patient with severe pneumocystis pneumonia.

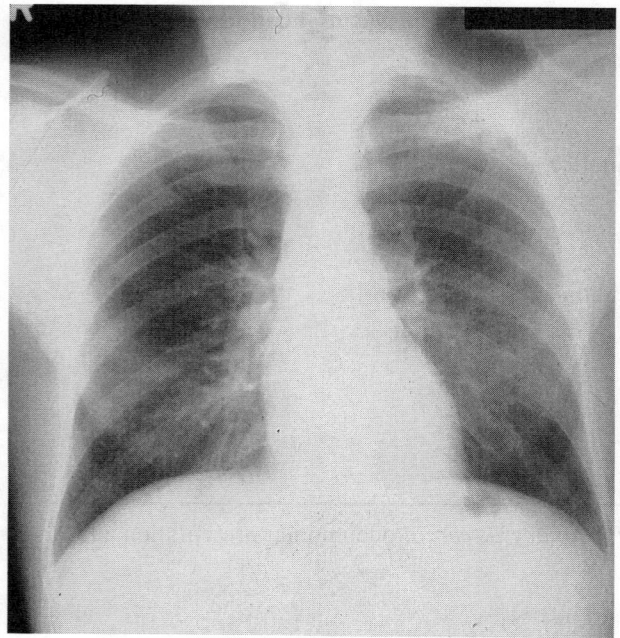

Figure 60.2 Perihilar shadowing in a patient with early pneumocystis pneumonia.

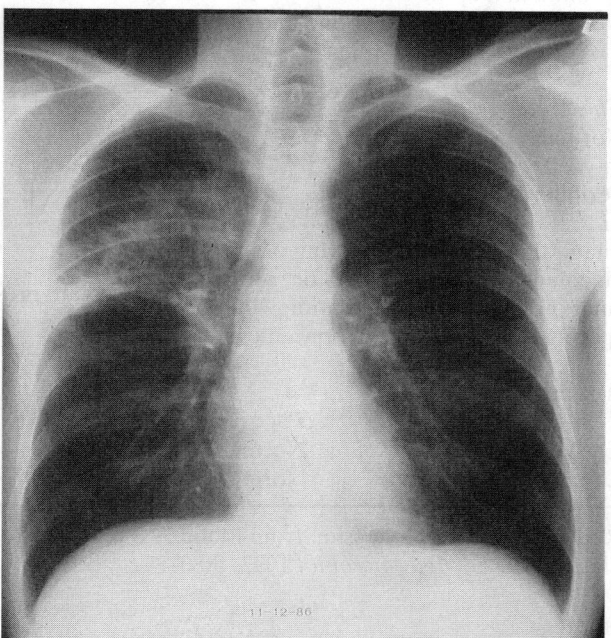

Figure 60.4 Atypical appearances of upper lobe consolidation—mimicking tuberculosis, in a patient with pneumocystis pneumonia.

way of detecting PCP, these typical and atypical radiographic appearances may also occur in other fungal, mycobacterial and bacterial infections and in non-infectious conditions such as pulmonary Kaposi's sarcoma (KS) and non-specific interstitial pneumonitis (NIP). With treatment of PCP, improvements in the chest radiographic appearances are not usually apparent for 7–10 days. After treatment some radiographs remain abnormal for many months in the absences of symptoms; others show residual fibrosis or postinfectious bronchiectasis.

ARTERIAL BLOOD GASES

In early PCP, even though the arterial oxygen tension (Pao_2) may be normal or near normal, hypocarbia (indicating hyperventilation) may be present. With progression of the pneumonia hypoxia may occur (Table 60.2). The occurrence of hypercarbia in the hypoxaemic patient with PCP is an ominous sign and implies that there is severe respiratory compromise. By performing arterial blood gas analysis the alveolar–arterial oxygen gradient $D(A–a)o_2$ may be calculated. The $D(A–a)o_2$ gradient is widened in over 90% of patients with PCP. Both hypoxaemia and a widened $D(A–a)o_2$ gradient may occur in bacterial and mycobacterial infections, NIP and KS as well as in PCP.

EXERCISE OXIMETRY

The need for repeated arterial puncture is avoided if the arterial oxygen saturation is measured using a transcutaneous oximeter. In immunosuppressed patients with respiratory symptoms, normal or near normal chest radiographs and normal resting Pao_2, values exercise-induced arterial desaturation is a sensitive and specific method of detecting PCP. A normal exercise test (with no desaturation) virtually excludes a diagnosis of PCP.

PULMONARY FUNCTION TESTS

The carbon monoxide transfer factor (TLCO) is frequently reduced to ≤70% in patients with PCP but similar values are also found in other opportunistic infections and in some HIV-infected individuals without respiratory disease.

LACTATE DEHYDROGENASE

Serum lactate dehydrogenase (LDH) enzyme levels are raised in the majority of patients with PCP and a normal value makes the diagnosis unlikely. Raised LDH levels may occur in bacterial pneumonia and pulmonary KS.

NUCLEAR MEDICINE TESTS

Technetium diethylenetriamine pentaacetic acid (DPTA) clearance. The rate of alveolar to capillary clearance of technetium DTPA aerosol is significantly increased in HIV-positive patients with PCP, in contrast to those with bacterial and mycobacterial infections and pulmonary KS. This test has a high sensitivity and specificity for the diagnosis of PCP. Its clinical usefulness is limited as it is not routinely available in most centres.

Gallium-67 citrate scanning. Diffuse or focal accumulation of gallium-67 citrate occurs in patients with PCP and other inflammatory conditions, including bacterial and mycobacterial infection and lymphoid interstitial pneumonitis; gallium does not accumulate in KS lesions so imaging the lungs may help to distinguish PCP or other infections from pulmonary KS in the immunosuppressed patient who has an abnormal chest radiograph. The main limitation of the test is that imaging takes up to 72 hours.

INVASIVE INVESTIGATIONS

SPUTUM INDUCTION

Immunosuppressed patients with suspected PCP rarely expectorate sputum spontaneously, but sputum may be obtained by inhalation of an aerosol of hypertonic (2.7%, 3 Normal) saline generated by an ultrasonic nebulizer. The success rate for this technique varies considerably between centres. A high diagnostic yield depends on a number of factors, including patient selection (if only those with a high index of suspicion for PCP are studied then the yield is high). Careful patient preparation (in particular rigorous cleansing of the mouth before the procedure) and deployment of an experienced nurse or physiotherapist to supervise the procedure increases the success rate. In prospective studies that have compared sputum induction with bronchoscopy and bronchoalveolar lavage the yield for PCP and other pathogens from sputum induction is approximately half of that obtained by bronchoscopy. Some patients find sputum induction is an unpleasant procedure and experience cough, nausea and retching, or dyspnoea. Unpredictable arterial blood desaturation may occur during inhalation of saline and persists for up to 20 minutes after the procedure. The patient's arterial oxygen saturation should be measured with an oximeter during sputum induction.

FIBREOPTIC BRONCHOSCOPY

Fibreoptic bronchoscopy with bronchoalveolar lavage (BAL) and transbronchial biopsy (TBB) have a high diagnostic yield when used in the investigation of immunocompetent and immunosuppressed patients with radiographically diffuse pneumonia. Early in the acquired immune deficiency syndrome (AIDS) epidemic both BAL and TBB were routinely used in order to diagnose PCP in other pathogens. With the realization that BAL alone had a very high yield for *P. carinii*, and that performing TBB added very little additional diagnostic information yet was associated with pneumothorax (in up to 20% of cases, which occurred whether or not fluoroscopic screening was used), haemorrhage (which was sometimes fatal) and sudden falls in Pao_2 which occasionally required ventilatory support, the technique was used less frequently. At bronchoscopy the majority of AIDS centres now routinely only perform BAL. Treatment should never be deferred pending results of bronchoscopy in a patient with suspected PCP as significant clinical deterioration may occur. Cysts of *P. carinii* persist in the lung for many days after the start of antimicrobial therapy so the diagnostic yield from BAL remains high.

OPEN LUNG BIOPSY

Before the onset of AIDS and in the early years of the AIDS epidemic this technique, which has a high diagnostic yield in immunosuppressed patients with diffuse pulmonary disease, was routinely used to diagnose PCP. The observed high yield from bronchoscopy and BAL means that the technique is now rarely necessary. Open lung biopsy is still occasionally performed in HIV-positive patients with diffuse pneumonia and negative results from two or more bronchoscopies and in patients who deteriorate despite treatment for a bronchoscopically confirmed pathogen.

EMPIRICAL THERAPY

Some physicians have suggested that it is not necessary to perform invasive tests, including bronchoscopy, in HIV-infected patients presenting with symptoms, chest radiographic and arterial blood gas abnormalities typical of PCP, and that such patients may be treated empirically, with bronchoscopy reserved for those who fail to respond or deteriorate on therapy and those who have presentations atypical for PCP. Others have argued strongly that bronchoscopic confirmation of the diagnosis is mandatory is every case. Both strategies appear equally effective in clinical practice.

DNA AMPLIFICATION

Applied to clinical samples of BAL and induced sputum, DNA amplification using *P. carinii*-specific oligonucleotides has been shown in prospective studies to be more sensitive than conventional methenamine silver staining for the diagnosis of PCP in patients immunosuppressed by HIV and other causes. Another study has shown that PCP may be diagnosed from saliva by DNA amplification in almost 80% of patients with bronchoscopically confirmed PCP. DNA amplification tests for detection are not currently available commercially.

PROGNOSIS

Several clinical and laboratory features are predictive of a poor outcome in an HIV-infected patient with PCP. These include at admission no prior knowledge of HIV status, presentation with a second or subsequent episode of PCP, a history of respiratory symptoms of more than 4 weeks duration, tachypnoea (>30 breaths/min), evidence of poor oxygenation ($Pao_2 < 7.0$ kPa or $D(A-a)o_2 \geq 4.0$ kPa), marked chest radiographic abnormalities, peripheral blood leucocytosis (WBC $> 10.8 \times 10^9$/l), a low serum albumin (<35 g/l) and raised serum LDH enzyme levels (>300 iu/l). After admission and investigation the identification of a copathogen in induced sputum or BAL fluid, the presence of >5% neutrophilia in BAL fluid, marked interstitial oedema in TBB specimens and raised serum LDH enzyme levels (that remain elevated despite treatment) are also predictive of a poor outcome.

TREATMENT

An assessment of the severity of the pneumonia, using the history, examination findings and results of arterial blood gas estimations and the chest radiograph (Table 60.3), will enable decisions to be made about choice of therapy; this also identifies those patients who will benefit from adjunctive glucocorticoids (see below). In patients with Glucose 6-phosphate dehydrogenase deficiency co-trimoxazole, dapsone and primaquine should not be used as they increase the risk of haemolysis.

trimoxazole is associated with a reduced toxicity profile but no reduction in efficacy. It is not clear why there is such a high frequency of adverse reactions to co-trimoxazole in patients immunosuppressed by HIV infection compared with patients immunosuppressed by other causes but it may be due to HIV-induced changes in acetylator status, accumulation of toxic metabolites such as hydroxylamines, or glutathione deficiency.

CO-TRIMOXAZOLE

High dose co-trimoxazole ($100 \, \text{mg} \, \text{kg}^{-1} \, \text{day}^{-1}$ sulphamethoxazole and $20 \, \text{mg} \, \text{kg}^{-1} \, \text{day}^{-1}$ trimethoprim) given in 2–4 divided doses orally or intravenously for 21 days is the first choice therapy for PCP of all grades of severity. Because of the potential for severe marrow toxicity zidovudine and ganciclovir should be stopped while patients are receiving high dose co-trimoxazole. Adverse reactions to co-trimoxazole, which are usually first evident at 6–14 days of treatment, are common and include neutropenia and anaemia in up to 40% of patients, rash in 25%, fever in over 20% and abnormal liver function is approximately 10%. Co-administration of folic or folinic acid does not reduce or prevent haematological toxicity and may be associated with increased therapeutic failure. Dose reduction, to 75% of the dose given above, of co-

PENTAMIDINE

Intravenous pentamidine ($4 \, \text{mg} \, \text{kg}^{-1} \, \text{day}^{-1}$) by single infusion for 21 days is second-line therapy in PCP of whatever severity. Pentamidine is not routinely given by intramuscular injection because of the risk of sterile abscesses. Compared with high-dose co-trimoxazole, intravenous pentamidine is of almost equivalent efficacy but has a greater toxicity profile. Up to 60% of patients receiving pentamidine develop nephrotoxicity (usually an isolated elevation of serum creatinine), approximately half develop leucopenia, and hypotension and nausea/vomiting both occur in up to 25%. Hypoglycaemia occurs in approximately 20% of patients. Reduction of the dose to $3 \, \text{mg} \, \text{kg}^{-1} \, \text{day}^{-1}$ does not compromise efficacy and reduces toxicity. There are no therapeutic advantages in combining high dose co-trimoxazole and intravenous pentamidine therapy;

Table 60.3 Grading of severity of *P. carinii* pneumonia.

	Mild	*Moderate*	*Severe*
Symptoms and signs	Increasing exertional dyspnoea with or without cough and sweats	Dyspnoea on minimal exertion, occasional dyspnoea at rest, fever with or without sweats	Dyspnoea at rest, tachypnoea at rest, persistent fever, cough
Blood gas tensions (room air)	Pao_2 normal, Sao_2 falling on exercise	Pao_2 8.1–11 kPa	$Pao_2 < 8.0$ kPa
Chest radiograph	Normal or minor perihilar infiltrates	Diffuse interstitial shadowing	Extensive interstitial shadowing with or without diffuse alveolar shadowing ('white out') sparing costophrenic angles and apices

Sao_2, arterial oxygen saturation—measured with a transcutaneous oximeter.
Reproduced with permission from Miller and Mitchell *Pneumocystis carinii pneumonia. Thorax* 1992; 47:305–314.

indeed the combination has a much higher toxicity profile than either drug used alone.

OTHER THERAPY

Several other treatments are available if co-trimoxazole or pentamidine are not tolerated by the patient or if treatment fails (Table 60.4).

DAPSONE WITH TRIMETHOPRIM

The combination of dapsone (100 mg/day) and trimethoprim (20 mg kg^{-1} day^{-1}) is as effective as oral co-trimoxazole (dose as above) and is better tolerated. Rash, nausea and vomiting, and asymptomatic methaemoglobinaemia (due to dapsone) are the major side-effects with this combination. Approximately 50% of patients develop mild hyperkalaemia (<6.1 mmol/l). The drug has not been shown to be of benefit in severe disease.

CLINDAMYCIN WITH PRIMAQUINE

This combination was originally used to 'salvage' patients with mild and moderate severity disease who failed to respond to co-trimoxazole or pentamidine. It is now used in doses of clindamycin 300–450 mg four times daily and primaquine 15mg once daily, both given orally; it is as effective as oral dapsone/trimethoprim and co-trimoxazole for initial treatment of mild and moderate severity PCP. In severe disease clindamycin is usually given intravenously in doses of 450–600 mg four times daily. Almost two-thirds of patients develop a rash and approximately 25% develop diarrhoea. If diarrhoea occurs the stool should be analysed for the presence of *Clostridium difficile* toxin.

Table 60.4 Treatment of *P. carinii* pneumonia.

First choice	Co-trimoxazole
Second choice	Intravenous pentamidine
Alternative therapy	Dapsone and trimethoprim Clindamycin and primaquine Atovaquone
Less often used alternative therapy	Trimetrexate Eflornithine Nebulized pentamidine
Moderate and severe disease	Adjunctive steroids

ATOVAQUONE

Oral atovaquone at a dose of 750 mg three times daily is less effective than either oral high-dose co-trimoxazole or intravenous pentamidine for mild and moderate severity PCP but is better tolerated than either drug. There are no data to support its use in patients with severe disease. Common adverse reactions include: rash, nausea/vomiting and constipation. Absorption of atovaquone from the gastrointestinal tract is poor; taking the tablets with food increases their absorption.

TRIMETREXATE

Trimetrexate, a methotrexate analogue at a dose of 45 mg m^2 per day i.v. (given with folinic acid 20 mg/m^2 four times daily by mouth — to protect human cells from trimetrexate-induced toxicity) is less effective than co-trimoxazole for treatment of moderate and severe PCP; the two regimens have similar rates of toxicity. Trimetrexate is also used to 'salvage' patients who have failed to respond to co-trimoxazole and intravenous pentamidine; in this situation approximately two-thirds of patients respond to therapy.

EFLORNITHINE

Intravenous eflornithine (400 mg kg^{-1} day^{-1} in divided doses) is used as 'salvage' therapy in patients deteriorating despite treatment with intravenous co-trimoxazole or pentamidine. In this situation it is >60% effective; major side-effects include neutropenia and phlebitis.

NEBULIZED PENTAMIDINE

This form of therapy is now only rarely used to treat mild and moderate severity PCP; it should not be used to treat severe disease. Patients given nebulized pentamidine (600 mg/day) for 21 days respond to therapy very slowly; reductions in fever and dyspnoea and improvements in radiographic appearances and blood gases may take more than 14 days. There is a greater relapse rate of PCP in patients treated with nebulized pentamidine than there is in those given parenteral therapy. Development of extrapulmonary pneumocystosis may not be suppressed by this form of treatment as very little drug is absorbed systemically. If nebulized pentamidine is used to treat PCP some groups have advocated combining it with intravenous pentamidine (doses as above) for the first 3–5 days of therapy to ensure rapid accumulation of the drug within the lungs.

CORTICOSTEROIDS

Adjunctive therapy with glucocorticoids for patients with moderate and severe PCP has been shown to reduce the likelihood of respiratory failure (by half) and death (by one-third). Corticosteroids probably act by reducing the body's intrapulmonary inflammatory response to *P. carinii*. It is recommended (National Institutes of Health Consensus Statement, 1990) that glucocorticoids are given to HIV-infected patients with proven or suspected PCP who have a Pao_2 of ≤ 9.3 kPa or $D(A-a)o_2 \geq 4.7$ kPa (both measured while the patient is breathing room air). Corticosteroid treatment should begin at the start of specific antipneumocystis therapy. In some patients treatment will begin on a presumptive basis and it is necessary to confirm the diagnosis as soon as possible. Several regimens have been used, the most common being oral prednisolone 40 mg twice daily for 5 days, thereafter 40 mg once daily for days 6–10 and then 10 further days of 20 mg daily. Intravenous methylprednisolone may be given at 75% of these doses; alternatively, higher doses may be given for a shorter period of time, i.e. methylprednisolone 1 g once daily for 3 days and 0.5 g on days 4–6, followed by oral prednisolone 40 mg once daily reducing to zero over 10 days. There is no evidence that adjunctive corticosteroids are of benefit in patients with mild PCP.

GENERAL MANAGEMENT

Patients with mild PCP may be treated with oral co-trimoxazole as outpatients under close supervision of a physician. If oral co-trimoxazole is not tolerated, despite clinical recovery, treatment may be changed to oral clindamycin/primaquine, dapsone/trimethoprim or atovaquone, or the co-trimoxazole may be given intravenously. All patients with moderate and severe PCP should be treated in hospital with intravenous co-trimoxazole or pentamidine and adjunctive corticosteroids. If by 7–10 days the patient does not respond to either regimen, or deteriorates before this time, he or she should be switched to the other drug. If there is still no evidence of response intravenous clindamycin with oral primaquine, intravenous trimetrexate with oral folinic acid or intravenous eflornithine should be used. All hypoxaemic patients with PCP should receive supplemental oxygen therapy via a tight-fitting face mask in order to maintain the $Pao_2 > 8.0$ kPa. If an inspired oxygen concentration of 60% fails to maintain the $Pao_2 \geq 8.0$ kPa, non-invasive ventilatory support with continuous positive airways pressure (CPAP) ventilation, either by nasal or face mask, may be used. If CPAP ventilation fails to maintain oxygenation, or the $Paco_2$ rises, or the patient tires, mechanical ventilation should be considered. The decision to carry out mechanical ventilation is not an easy one to make as the prognosis of patients with severe PCP and respiratory failure who fail to respond to specific therapy and adjunctive steroids and who are ventilated remains extremely poor. Most centres would mechanically ventilate patients with a first episode PCP and those rapidly deteriorating following bronchoscopy.

CHEMOPROPHYLAXIS

With progressive immunosuppression and falls in CD4 (T-helper lymphocyte) counts, HIV-infected individuals are at increased risk of developing PCP. *Primary* prophylaxis is given to prevent a first episode of PCP, to patients who have CD^4 counts $<0.20 \times 10^9$/l or a CD^4:total lymphocyte count <1.5, or HIV-related constitutional symptoms (such as fever or oral candida) regardless of CD^4 count, and to those with other AIDS-defining diseases such as KS. *Secondary* prophylaxis is given in order to prevent a recurrence.

CO-TRIMOXAZOLE

Co-trimoxazole 960 mg once daily, or three times a week is the first choice regimen for both primary and secondary prophylaxis. This combination may also protect against bacterial infections and reactivation of cerebral toxoplasmosis, and does not interact adversely with zidovudine. Rash, which occurs in about 20% of individuals, is the most common adverse reaction. Before considering a change to an alternative agent for prophylaxis in a patient who has developed an adverse reaction to co-trimoxazole, it is worth attempting desensitization to the drug.

NEBULIZED PENTAMIDINE

Nebulized pentamidine at a dose of 300 mg per month using a jet nebulizer is the second choice for primary and secondary prophylaxis. It is less effective than co-trimoxazole (doses as above) for both indications. It is important to use a nebulizer (such as the Respirgard II) that produces an aerosol of pentamidine droplets that are small enough to deposit in the alveoli rather than in the upper airways and oropharynx (where pentamidine may cause adverse reactions—including cough, hypersalivation and bronchoconstriction). A bronchodilator, for example 200 μg of salbutamol given via a metered dose inhaler, should be given before nebulized pentamidine to reduce these adverse effects. Because nebulization induces coughing, there are concerns that the procedure may increase the risk of nosocomial transmission of respiratory diseases, such as tuberculosis, to staff of other immunosuppressed patients; nebulization of pentamidine in hospitals and outpatient clinics should therefore take place away from other patients, ideally in a separate room with an extractor fan. Medical and nursing staff may experience adverse reactions (as above) if they remain in the room with the patient during nebulization. There is minimal systemic absorption of pentamidine when it is given by a nebulizer, so it may not prevent extrapulmonary pneumocystosis.

DAPSONE

Dapsone, at a dose of 50–100 mg daily, has been shown to have an equivalent efficacy to nebulized pentamidine (dose as above) but is less well tolerated. The addition of pyrimethamine, 25–50 mg per week, does not confer any additional protection against PCP but it may protect against reactivation of cerebral toxoplasmosis.

OTHER DRUGS

Sulfadoxine 1 g and pyrimethamine 500 mg given once a week is less effective than the regimens listed above. Pentamidine given intravenously or intramuscularly may cause severe side-effects—including muscle abscess, hypotension and hypoglycaemia. It has been used at a dose of 300 mg given every 2–4 weeks in patients who are intolerant of other prophylactic regimens.

FURTHER READING

Anonymous. Prevention and treatment of *Pneumocystis carinii* pneumonia in patients infected with HIV. *Drug Ther Bull* 1994; 32:12–15.

Hopkin J M. *Pneumocystis carinii*. Oxford: Oxford University Press, 1991.

Jeffrey A A, Bullen C & Miller R F. Intensive care management of *Pneumocystis carinii* pneumonia. *Care Crit Ill* 1993; 9:258–260.

Malin A & Miller R F. Diagnosis and investigation of *Pneumocystis carinii* pneumonia. *Rev Med Microbiol* 1992; 3:80–87.

Miller R F & Mitchel D M. *Pneumocystis carinii* pneumonia: AIDS and the lung update 92. *Thorax* 1992; 47:305–314.

Stringer J R. The identity of *Pneumocystis carinii*: not a single protozoan, but a diverse group of exotic fungi. *Infect Agents Dis* 1993; 2:109–117.

Waltzer P D (ed.). *Pneumocystis carinii* pneumonia. *Lung Biology in Health and Disease*, Series No. 69, 2nd edn. New York: Marcel Dekker, 1993.

SECTION 5E
PROTOZOAN INFECTIONS

Sir Ronald Ross published his autobiography in 1923; he subtitled the work: . . . *the great malaria problem and its solution*. Few, if any, would then have believed that *Plasmodium* spp. infection would remain a potentially greater health problem in the tropics the better part of a century later! This disease is very far from 'solved', and with growing expanses of tropical and subtropical terrain becoming endemic to this protozoan parasitosis, together with the continuing emergence of parasite-resistance to most of the available chemoprophylactic and chemotherapeutic agents, the health problems presented by this infection worldwide are probably greater today than was the case in Ross' time. In fact we have been forced back to the most fundamental form of prophylaxis—avoidance of mosquito bites between dusk and dawn! This section opens with a detailed account of *Plasmodium* spp. infection—dominated by *P. falciparum*—and steers the reader through the chemoprophylactic maze: efficacy *versus* safety. Chemotherapy also leaves much to be desired and the brunt of the attack is back to quinine—first listed in the London Pharmacopoeia in 1677—following its introduction into Europe from Peru. And, as with all parasitic infections—both protozoan and helminthic—a satisfactory vaccine (applicable both to the developing country scenario and the traveller) seems far away.

The trypanosomiases—both African and South American—also present major problems as they did in Manson's day. Basic research continues on *Trypanosoma brucei*, but in chemotherapy the only gleam of hope lies in eflornithine—effective in west Africa, but not east or central. *T. cruzi* infection continues to be a major problem in South America; although chemotherapy in the early stage(s) of the infection yields moderately satisfactory results, the 'end-stage' disease remains unamenable to chemotherapy (or any other effective measure). *Leishmania* spp., which also figured prominently in the first edition of this text, remains a problem in both its visceral and cutaneous forms; fortunately, chemotherapy has progressed (albeit slowly), and modern methods of management are proving promising.

A major problem worldwide involves the gastrointestinal protozoan infections (well covered in this section). Small-intestinal disease is dominated by *Giardia lamblia* (the mechanism[s] of pathogenicity remains unclear—despite an enormous amount of research), whilst colorectal disease in tropical locations is largely dominated by *Entamoeba histolytica* infection. Significant progress has been made in this latter infection; the suggestion by Emile Brumpt in 1925 of two strains of the parasite—one pathogenic and the other not—has been (largely) confirmed by recent molecular biological observations. The 5-nitroimidazole compounds have revolutionized management in both of these gastrointestinal infections.

This section also highlights several other important protozoan infections; however, very little progress has been made in *prevention*! Following his seminal work which demonstrated the complete life-cycle of avian *Plasmodium* spp. infection, Ross devoted most of energies to *prevention* of the disease; sadly, advances in this area have been exceedingly slow—not only with this protozoan infection, but with most others also.

CHAPTER 61

MALARIA

Nicholas J. White

Malaria is the most important parasitic disease of man. The human disease is a protozoan infection of red blood cells transmitted by the bite of a blood-feeding female anopheline mosquito. Malaria, or ague as it was commonly known, has been described since antiquity. Hippocrates is usually credited with the first clear description amongst occidental writers: In *Epidemics* he distinguished different patterns of fever, and in his *Aphorisms* he describes the regular paroxysms of intermittent fever. In Europe seasonal periodic fevers were particularly common in marshy areas, and were frequently referred to as 'paludial' (L. *palus* marshy ground; Fr. *paludisme*). In the early nineteenth century miasmatic influences were believed to cause a variety of diseases. Malaria was thought by Italian writers to be caused by the offensive vapours emanating from the Tiberian marshes.[1] The word 'malaria' comes from the Italian, and means literally 'bad air'. Indeed the cause of the seasonal periodic fevers was a continuous source of debate until the late nineteenth century.[2] The work of Meckel, Virchow and Frerichs had established that the pigment (mistakenly thought to be melanin) observed in the blood of some patients with periodic fever resulted from the destruction of red blood corpuscles. This same pigment caused the characteristic grey discoloration of the internal organs in patients dying from this disease. In the 1870s, medicine slowly moved towards the germ theory of disease, following the pioneering work of Koch. In 1879, Edwin Klebs and Corrado Tommasi-Crudelli reported the identification of a bacterial cause of malaria. Recovery of the 'organism', *Bacillus malariae*, from patients with malaria was confirmed by several influential Italian physicians and pathologists—and similar reports began to appear in the USA. It was not surprising, therefore, that the report of a French Army surgeon working in Algeria, claiming that malaria was caused by a parasite, was treated initially with some scepticism.[3] On the 20 October 1880 (or in a later publication he gives the date as 6 November) Charles Louis Alphonse Laveran was examining the fresh blood of a patient with ague, and observed moving bodies (he was probably watching gametocyte exflagellation) which he surmised correctly were parasites of the red blood cells. The transmissability of the infection in blood was proved 4 years later by Gerhardt, but the route of natural infection was not discovered until the next decade. Following the suggestion of Manson, a young Scottish physician in the Indian Medical Service, Ronald Ross, began to investigate the possibility that malaria could be transmitted by mosquitoes. In 1897 he reported the presence of pigmented bodies in the gut of a certain species of mosquito fed on patients with malaria.[4] He speculated that these might represent the parasite stage in the mosquito (he was in fact describing the oocysts) but, because of difficulties in obtaining these 'unusual' mosquitoes and his transfer to Calcutta, he was unable to characterize the complete life cycle, i.e. transmission from human to mosquito to human. After many years of study, Ross finally proved the existence of the complete life cycle involving a mosquito in the malaria of canaries. He identified the dapple-winged or anopheles mosquito as the vector of human malaria, although by the time Ross finally had the opportunity to demonstrate *Plasmodium falciparum* sporogony in anopheline mosquitoes in Sierra Leone, Bignami[6] and his colleagues had succeeded in infecting a healthy volunteer with *P. falciparum* from mosquito bites in Rome. Both Laveran and Ross received Nobel Prizes for their respective discoveries.

Until the nineteenth century malaria was found in northern Europe, North America and Russia—and transmission in Southern Europe was intense. Since then it has been eradicated from these areas, and the number of cases in the Middle East, China and the Indian subcontinent has fallen, but elsewhere in the tropics there has been a resurgence of the disease[1] and the number of cases worldwide continues to increase. This has been accompanied by increasing resistance of the anopheline vector to insecticides, and of the parasite to the antimalarial drugs. Approximately 270 million people suffer from malaria, and there are between 1 and 2.5 million deaths each year. Most of these deaths are in African children.

Four species of the genus *Plasmodium* infect

Table 61.1 Human malaria parasites.

	P. falciparum	*P. vivax*	*P. ovale*	*P. malariae*
Exoerythrocytic hepatic phase of development (days)	5.5	8	9	15
Erythrocytic cycle (days)	2	2	2	3
Hypnozoites (relapses)	No	Yes	Yes	No
Number of merozoites per hepatic schizont	30 000	10 000	15 000	2000
Erythrocyte preference	Young RBCs but can invade all ages	Reticulo-cytes	Reticulo-cytes	Old RBCs
Maximum duration of untreated infection (years)	2	4	4	40

RBC, red blood cell.

humans, although occasional infections with errant primate malarias may occur also.[4] The individual characteristics of the four species of human malaria parasites are shown in Table 61.1. Almost all deaths and severe disease are caused by *P. falciparum*. This parasite appears to be a relatively recent evolutionary acquisition of man (perhaps within the past 10 000 years). In phylogenetic terms, it is closest to the avian malarias (*P. lophurae*, *P. gallinaceum*).[8]

Its propensity to kill has been cited as an example of evolutionary immaturity, although for such a widespread infection this is debatable. The three 'benign' malarias, *P. vivax*, *P. ovale* and *P. malariae*, all lie close together on the evolutionary tree near the other primate malarias.[8] Severe disease with these species is very unusual, although occasionally patients will die from rupture of an enlarged spleen.[9]

GEOGRAPHICAL ASPECTS

DISTRIBUTION

Malaria is found throughout the tropics. In Africa, *P. falciparum* predominates, as it does in Papua New Guinea and Haiti, whereas *P. vivax* is more common in Central and parts of South America, North Africa, the Middle East and the Indian subcontinent. The prevalence of both species is approximately equal in other parts of South America, East Asia and Oceania. *P. vivax* is rare in sub-Saharan Africa, whereas *P. ovale* is rare outside West Africa. *P. malariae* is found in most areas, but is relatively uncommon outside Africa. Malaria was once endemic in Europe and northern Asia, and was introduced to North America, but it has been eradicated from these areas. In northern China and adjacent countries *P. vivax* strains (*P. vivax* hibernans) with long incubation periods and long intervals (10–12 months) between relapses may still be found.

EPIDEMIOLOGY

THE VECTOR

Malaria is transmitted by some species of anopheline mosquitoes. Malaria transmission does not occur at temperatures below 16°C, or above 33°C, and at altitudes greater than 2000 m because development in the mosquito (sporogony) cannot take place. The optimum conditions for transmission are high humidity and an ambient temperature between 20 and 30°C. Although rainfall provides breeding sites for mosquitoes, excessive rainfall may wash away mosquito larvae and pupae.[10]

The epidemiology of malaria is complex and may vary considerably even within relatively small geographic areas. Malaria transmission to man depends on several interrelated factors.[10,11] The most important pertain to the anopheline mosquito vector, and in particular its longevity. As sporogony (development of the sporozoite parasites in the vector) takes over a week (depending on ambient temperatures), the mosquito must survive for longer than this after feeding on a gametocyte-carrying human, if malaria is to be transmitted. Macdonald gave the following formula for the likelihood of infection based on the sporozoite rates,[11,12] i.e. the proportion of anopheline mosquitoes with sporozoites in their salivary glands.

$$S = \frac{P^n ax}{ax - \log_e P}$$

where P = the probability of mosquito survival through 1 day; n = the duration, in days, of the extrinsic cycle of the parasite in the mosquito; a = average number of blood meals on man per day, and x = the proportion of bites infective to man. The probability of a mosquito surviving n days is given by

$$\frac{P^n}{-\log_e P}.$$

The inoculation rate, or the mean daily number of bites (h) received by sporozoite-bearing mosquitoes is given by

$$h = mabs$$

where m = anopheline density in relation to man, and b = proportion of bites that are infectious. The reproduction rate of the infection (r) or the number of secondary cases resulting from a primary case is then given by

$$r = \frac{ma^2 b P^n}{-z \log_e P}\left(1 - \frac{ax}{ax - \log_e P}\right)$$

where z is the recovery rate, or the reciprocal of the duration of human infectivity. This is usually estimated at 80 days for $P.\ falciparum$ in a non-immune subject, i.e. $z = 0.0125$. The term

$$1 - \frac{ax}{ax - \log_e P}$$

refers to the proportion of anopheline mosquitoes 'not yet infected'. When transmission is very low (i.e. $x \to 0$) then the basic reproduction rate (r_0) reduces to

$$r_0 = \frac{ma^2 b P^n}{-z \log_e P}.$$

Thus, as a general approximation, malaria transmission is directly proportional to the density of the vector, the square of the number of times each day that the mosquito bites man, and the tenth power of the probability of the mosquito surviving for 1 day. The model described by MacDonald has certain theoretical limitations (it has been refined in recent years to accommodate these), but it does illustrate certain fundamental points of practical relevance to control or eradication programmes. The importance of vector longevity in determining transmission is clearly important and focuses control measures on the adult mosquito. At very high levels of transmission (i.e. $r \to 100$) there is considerable reserve in the system and large reductions in r reduce malaria by a negligible amount—but as r approaches the critical value of 1 (below which the disease dies out), small reductions in r have large effects on the amount of malaria. Control programmes can be very effective in these circumstances—as indeed they were in Europe where r was certainly low in many areas, and the vector rested inside houses and could be attacked with residual insecticides.

Vectors differ considerably in their natural abundance, feeding and resting behaviours, breeding sites, flight ranges, choice of blood source (many anopheline vectors also bite animals), and vulnerability to environmental conditions and insecticides. Thus there is also considerable variation in their ability to transmit malaria (the vectorial capacity). Of the nearly 400 species of anopheline mosquitoes (many of which are species complexes), approximately 80 can transmit malaria, 66 are considered natural vectors, and about 45 are considered important vectors.[10] Each vector has its own behaviour patterns, for example in South-East Asia mosquitoes of the *Anopheles dirus* complex are an important cause of 'forest fringe' malaria. They breed in the tree collections of water, and are consequently vulnerable to deforestation, or too little or too much rainfall, but they are difficult to attack with insecticides. *A. stephensi*, the principal vector in the Indian subcontinent, breeds in wells or stagnant water and can be controlled by treating breeding sites with insecticides or polystyrene balls. The most effective malaria vectors (such as the *A. gambiae* complex) are hardy, long lived, naturally occur in high densities, and bite humans frequently. Malaria is often seasonal, coinciding with the rainy season which provides water for mosquito breeding and increased humidity favouring mosquito survival. Other factors, which are not well understood, also influence mosquito populations and lead to fluctuations in the prevalence of malaria.

THE HUMAN HOST

The behaviour of man also plays an important role in the epidemiology of malaria.[11] There must be a human reservoir of gametocytes to transmit the infection. In areas of high transmission infants and young children are more susceptible to malaria than the more immune older children and adults. Parasite densities are higher and gametocytaemia is detected more frequently in children. This younger age group probably represents the main reservoir and also the main recipient of infection. Those in the older age group also have asymptomatic infections but parasite densities are much lower. The endemicity of malaria is defined traditionally in terms of the spleen or parasite rates in children aged between 2 and 9 years.[7]

- Hypoendemic: spleen rate or parasite rate 0–10%.
- Mesoendemic: spleen or parasite rate 10–50%.
- Hyperendemic: spleen or parasite rate 50–75% and adult spleen rate is also high.
- Holoendemic: spleen or parasite rate over 75%, and adult spleen rate low. Parasite rates in the first year of life are high.

In areas which are holoendemic or hyperendemic for *P. falciparum*, such as much of tropical Africa or coastal New Guinea, people are infected repeatedly throughout their lives.[12,13] There is considerable morbidity and mortality during childhood. In The Gambia, where people are infected once each year on average (a relatively low figure for the African continent), malaria has been estimated to cause 25% of deaths between 1 and 4 years of age,[14] but eventually, if the child survives, a state of 'premunition' is achieved where infections cause little or no problems to the host. Thus a form of immunity develops which is sufficient to control, but not prevent the infection. The slow rate at which premunition is acquired may be a function of age.[15] Non-immune adults entering an area of intense transmission acquire premunition more rapidly than children. Falciparum malaria infections are more severe in pregnancy, particularly in primigravidae,[16,17] and may be augmented by iron supplementation.[18]

CLINICAL EPIDEMIOLOGY

Babies develop severe malaria relatively infrequently (although, if they do, the mortality is high). The factors responsible for this include passive transfer of maternal immunity,[19] and the high haemoglobin F content of the infants' erythrocytes which retards parasite development.[20] In holoendemic areas the baby is inoculated repeatedly with sporozoites during the first year of life, but the blood stage infection is seldom severe.[12] People may receive up to two infectious bites per day. In this epidemiological context the main clinical impact of falciparum malaria is to cause severe anaemia in the

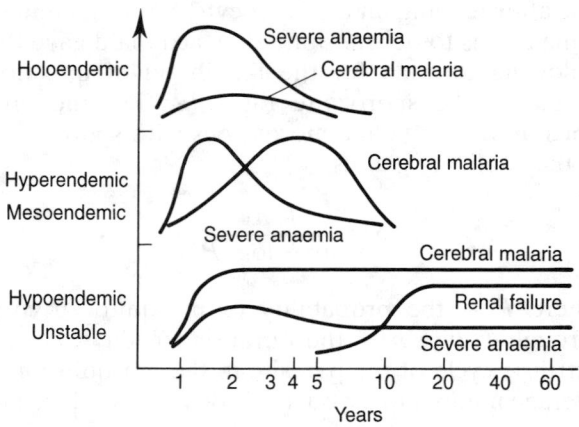

Figure 61.1 Relationship between age and the clinical presentations of severe falciparum malaria at different levels of malaria transmission.

1–3-year age group (Figure 61.1). With less intense or more variable or unstable transmission the age range affected by severe malaria extends to older children, and cerebral malaria becomes a more prominent manifestation of severe disease.[21,22] In hyperendemic and holoendemic areas indigenous adults never develop severe malaria, unless they leave the transmission area and return years later (and even then malaria is seldom life threatening). Immunity is constantly boosted and effective premunition prevents parasite burdens reaching dangerous levels. Nearly all infections in adults are asymptomatic. In terms of the mathematical models presented earlier, an index of malaria transmission stability is given by $a/-\log_e P$; values of >2.5 indicate stable transmission.

Where transmission of malaria is low, erratic, markedly seasonal, or focal, symptomatic infections are more common. A state of premunition is often not attained. Symptomatic disease occurs at any age and cerebral malaria is a prominent manifestation of severe disease at all ages. This is termed 'unstable' malaria.[11] In many areas the transmission of malaria varies considerably over short distances, and severe disease is common when non-immune individuals enter these areas (e.g. woodcutters in South America and South-East Asia where malaria is of the 'forest fringe' type).

Malaria is usually a 'rainy season disease' coinciding with increased mosquito abundance. However, in some areas parasite rates (i.e. the proportion of people with positive blood smears) are relatively constant throughout the year, but the majority of cases occur during the wet season.[25] In Europe, before eradication, falciparum malaria was common in spring and in late summer and autumn, and was termed 'aestivo–autumnal malaria'.[24] The intensity of transmission or 'endemicity' can change. For example in Africa, the sub-Sahelian drought has reduced rainfall and mosquito transmission in countries such as Senegal and The Gambia. In the 1960s transmission was intense, and severe disease was rare in children over 3 years of age.[19,25] Today, transmission has fallen to levels found in areas of unstable endemicity, such as some areas of South-East Asia[14] and cases of cerebral malaria occur occasionally in indigenous adults. Deforestation, population migration and changes in agricultural practice have profound effects on malaria transmission. Urban malaria is becoming an increasing problem in many countries.

Malaria can also behave as an epidemic disease carrying a high mortality.[11] Epidemics are caused by migrations (i.e. introduction of suceptible hosts), the introduction of new vectors, or changes in the habits of the mosquito vector or the human host. Epidemics have occurred in North India, Sri Lanka, South-East Asia, Madagascar and Brazil (when the formidable African vector *A. gambiae* was inadvertently imported from Africa in the 1930s).

With increasing international air travel and worsening antimalarial drug resistance, imported cases of malaria in tourists, travellers and immigrants are now common. Fortunately this has not led to the reintroduction of malaria to areas from where it had earlier been eradicated (although the vector, and thus the potential, remains). Imported malaria is often misdiagnosed, and severe presentations of falciparum malaria are not uncommon. Malaria may also be transmitted by blood transfusion, transplantation, or through needle-sharing among intravenous drug addicts.

AETIOLOGY

PRE-ERYTHROCYTIC DEVELOPMENT

Infection with human malaria begins when the feeding female anopheline mosquito inoculates plasmodial sporozoites at the time of feeding.[7,26] The small motile sporozoites are injected during the phase of probing as the mosquito searches for a vascular space before aspirating blood. In most cases, relatively few sporozoites are injected (approximately 8–15) but up to 100 may be introduced in some instances.[27,28] Most sporozoites come from the larger salivary ducts and represent only a small fraction of the total number in the salivary gland. After injection they enter the circulation, either directly or via lymph channels, and rapidly target the hepatic parenchymal cells. Within 45 minutes of the bite all sporozoites have either entered the hepatocytes or have been cleared. Each sporozoite bores into the hepatocyte and there begins a phase of asexual reproduction. This stage lasts on average between 5.5 (*P. falciparum*) and 15 days (*P. malariae*) before the hepatic schizont ruptures to release merozoites into the bloodstream.[7] In some instances the primary incubation period can be much longer. In *P. vivax* and *P. ovale* infections a proportion of the intrahepatic parasites do not develop, but instead rest inert as sleeping forms or 'hypnozoites', to awaken weeks or months later, and cause the relapses which characterize infections with these two species. During the pre-erythrocytic or hepatic phase of development considerable asexual multiplication takes place and many thousands of merozoites are released from each ruptured infected hepatocyte. However, as only a few liver cells are infected, this phase is asymptomatic for the human host.

ASEXUAL BLOOD-STAGE DEVELOPMENT

The merozoites liberated into the bloodstream closely resemble sporozoites. They are motile ovoid forms which rapidly invade red cells. The process of invasion involves attachment to the erythrocyte surface, orientation so that the apical organelle, the rhoptry, abuts the red cell, and then interiorization takes place by a wriggling or boring motion inside a vacuole composed of the invaginated erythrocyte membrane. Once inside the erythrocyte the parasite lies within the erythrocyte cytosol surrounded by its own plasma membrane, and a surrounding parasitophorous vacuolar membrane. It has recently been suggested that the parasite may be connected directly to the surrounding plasma by a parasitophorous duct, but this is disputed. The attachment of the merozoite to the red cell is mediated by a specific erythrocyte surface receptor. In *P. vivax* this is related to the Duffy blood group antigen Fy[a] or Fy[b].[29,30] The absence of these phenotypes in West Africans, or people who originate from that region, explains their resistance to infection with *P. vivax*, and the absence of vivax malaria in West Africa. The receptors for *P. falciparum* have not been identified with certainty. The glycophorins, a family of membrane sialoglycoproteins, are probably involved as red cells from subjects with some abnormal glycophorins resist infection.[30,31] The red cell surface receptors for *P. malariae* and *P. ovale* are not known.

During the early stage of development (<12 hours) the small 'ring forms' of the four parasite species often appear similar under light microscopy. The young developing parasite looks like a signet ring or, in the case of *P. falciparum*, like a pair of stereo-headphones, with darkly staining chromatin in the nucleus, a circular rim of cytoplasm, and a pale central food vacuole. Parasites are freely motile within the erythrocyte. As they grow they consume the erythrocyte's contents (most of which is haemoglobin). Proteolysis of haemoglobin within the digestive vacuole releases amino acids which are taken up and utilized by the growing parasite for protein synthesis, but the liberated haem poses a problem. When haem is freed from its protein scaffold it oxidizes to the toxic ferric form. Toxicity is avoided by spontaneous polymerization to an inert crystalline substance, haemozoin.[32] The digested products, mainly the brown or black insoluble pigment haemozoin, can be seen within the digestive vacuole of the growing parasite. To obtain amino acids and other nutrients and to control the electrolytic milieu in the infected erythrocyte the parasite inserts specific transporters and chemicals in the red cell membrane. These and other disruptions make the red cell more permeable. The infected erythrocyte becomes progressively less elastic and deformable and more spherical as the parasite grows.[33]

At approximately 24–26 hours of development *P. falciparum* parasites begin to exhibit a high molecular weight strain-specific variant antigen on the surface of the infected red cell which mediates attachment to vascular endothelium.[34] This is associated with knob-like projections from the erythrocyte membrane. These red cells then disappear from the circulation by attachment or 'cytoadherence' to the walls of venules and capillaries in the vital organs. This process is called 'sequestration'. The other three 'benign' human malarias do not cytoadhere and all stages of development are seen in peripheral blood.

As *P. vivax* grows it enlarges the infected red cell, and red granules appear throughout the erythrocyte. These are known as Schüffner's dots. Similar dots are also prominent in *P. ovale*, which also distorts the shape of the infected erythrocyte (hence its name). *P. malariae* produces characteristic 'band forms' as the parasite grows. It is usually present at low parasitaemias. High parasitaemias (over 2%) are usually caused by *P. falciparum*.[7] Approximately 36 hours after merozoite invasion (or 54 hours in *P. malariae*) repeated nuclear division takes place to form a 'segmenter' or schizont (the term 'meront' is etymologically more correct). Eventually the growing parasite occupies the entire red cell, which has become circular, rigid, depleted in haemoglobin and full of merozoites. This then ruptures; between 6 and 36 merozoites are released, destroying the remnants of the red cell (Table 61.1). These rapidly reinvade other red cells and start a new asexual cycle. Thus the infection expands logarithmically. The asexual life cycle is 48 hours for *P. falciparum*, *P. vivax* and *P. ovale*, and 72 hours for *P. malariae*.

SEXUAL STAGES AND DEVELOPMENT IN THE MOSQUITO

After a series of asexual cycles, a subpopulation of parasites develops into sexual forms (gametocytes) which are long lived and motile. This process (gametocytogony) takes about 4 days in *P. vivax* infections, and more than 10 days in *P. falciparum*. The male-to-female gametocyte sex ratio for *P. falciparum* is approximately 1:4.[35] Following ingestion in the blood meal of a biting female anopheline mosquito, the male and female gametocytes become activated.[2] The male gametocytes undergo rapid nuclear division and each of the eight nuclei formed associates with a flagellum (20–25 μm long). The motile male microgametes then separate and seek the female macrogametes. Fusion and meiosis then takes place to form a zygote. Within 24 hours the enlarging zygote becomes motile and this form (the ookinete) penetrates the wall of the mosquito midgut (stomach) where it encysts (as an oocyst). This spherical bag of parasites expands by asexual division to reach a diameter of approximately 500 μm, i.e. it is visible to the naked eye. During the early stage of oocyst development there is a characteristic pigment pattern and colour that allows speciation (and caught the eye of its discoverer, Ronald Ross, in 1897), but these patterns become obscured by the time the oocyst has matured to contain thousands of fusiform motile sporozoites. The oocyst finally bursts to liberate myriads of sporozoites into the coelomic cavity of the mosquito. The sporozoites then migrate to the salivary glands to await inoculation into the next human host during feeding. The development of the parasite in the mosquito is termed sporogony, and takes between 8 and 35 days depending on the ambient temperature and species of parasite and mosquito. Obviously the longevity of the mosquito is a critical factor in determining its vectorial capacity (see above).

MOLECULAR GENETICS

Inheritance in plasmodium is similar to that in other eukaryotes. Haploid and diploid generations alternate. The haploid genome of *P. falciparum* is divided among 14 chromosomes. A large number of genes have now been cloned and sequenced on the long and winding road towards the development of a malaria vaccine. Many of the sequenced genes have encoded antigenic polypeptides, and, to the chagrin of the vaccine developers, as in other protozoan parasites, many of these antigens have been found to be polymorphic.[35] As sexual reproduction is an obligatory part of the parasite life cycle, the opportunity for genetic diversity arises from the recombination that occurs during meiosis in the mosquito.[36] Self-fertilization is common in *P. falciparum* (i.e. the fusion of male and female gametocytes originating mitotically from the same haploid cell), but the extent to which self-fertilization or heterozygous recombination occur in natural populations is unresolved.[37] Antigenic diversity is necessary for the parasite to elude the host immune system.[36] The mechanisms maintaining genetic diversity within the parasite genome are many and complex. Some of the polymorphic antigens identified are encoded by single gene copies in the haploid genome. These polypeptide antigens are characterized by tandem repeat sequences. Unequal crossing over during recombination can generate completely different sequences of these repeats. As these repeat sequences are primary antibody targets, their variation provides antigenic diversity. Another mechanism for generating antigenic diversity is intragenic recombination between two parental alleles. Recent evidence suggests that the variant surface protein which mediates cytoadherence (PFEMP1) is the main antigen, determining the parasite population structure during chronic falciparum malaria infections. It has been suggested that the diversity of these immunodominant variant repeat sequences interferes with the selection of high affinity antibody responses, and perpetuates low-affinity responses in malaria, and this delays the development of effective immunity.[38] Immune selection also provides the selective pressure to maintain diversity in T- and B-cell epitopes through a high frequency of non-synonymous base mutations during the asexual development of malaria parasites.

THE INFECTION

GENETIC FACTORS PROTECTING AGAINST MALARIA

In 1949, J.B.S. Haldane suggested that people who were heterozygous for red cell abnormalities such as thalassaemia or sickle cell disease might be protected against malaria.[39] This would explain the high gene frequencies for the haemoglobinopathies in tropical areas. A state of 'balanced polymorphism' would exist, whereby the loss of the disadvantaged homozygotes would be offset by the survival advantage in heterozygotes. There is now good evidence from detailed epidemiological studies that this hypothesis is correct. The greatest protection is conferred by sickle cell trait, and melanesian ovalocytosis.[40] These patients' cells resist parasite invasion (in the case of sickle cell trait under low oxygen tensions), and once invaded the AS cells sickle readily, facilitating clearance by the reticuloendothelial system. The protective effect conferred by the thalassaemias or glucose-6-phosphate dehydrogenase (G6PD) deficiency (which share a geographical distribution with malaria) is weaker, and in some epidemiological studies has not been apparent. The mechanism of protection is also less well understood. Red cells from patients with α thalassaemia are invaded normally by *P. falciparum*, but they bind greater numbers of antibody molecules to the erythrocyte surface than infected normal cells and may therefore be cleared from the circulation more readily.[40] In addition the rate of decline of haemoglobin F in the first year of life is slower in α- and β-thalassaemia heterozygotes.

Erythrocytes containing high haemoglobin F concentrations do not support parasite growth well. Melanesian ovalocytic erythrocytes both resist invasion by malaria parasites and provide a hostile intraerythrocytic ionic milieu for development. The mechanisms whereby the other haemoglobinopathies or red cell abnormalities protect against malaria remain controversial.

Certain human leucocyte antigens (HLAs) are rare in Northern Europeans, but common in West Africans. Two of these, the class I antigen HLA-BW53 and the class II antigen HLA-DR B1* 1302, may also confer protection against severe malaria.[42] HLA molecules present processed antigenic peptides to cytotoxic T lymphocytes. HLA-B53-restricted cytotoxic T cells recognize a conserved nonamer peptide from a pre-erythrocytic (liver) stage-specific malaria antigen (LSA-1).[43] This suggests that cytotoxic T-lymphocyte responses to the pre-erythrocytic stages of malaria may be important in immunity, and would explain how possession of HLA-B53 might confer a survival advantage.

EXPANSION OF THE INFECTION

When the hepatic meronts rupture, they liberate approximately 10^5–10^6 merozoites into the circulation (i.e. the product of 5–100 successful sporozoites). These invade passing red cells immediately. In non-immune subjects the multiplication rate in *P. falciparum* usually exceeds 10 per cycle (i.e. >50% efficiency) and often reaches twentyfold per cycle during the subsequent expanding phase of the infection (Figure 61.2). For the first few cycles the host is unaware of the brewing infection. On average parasites are detectable in the blood by microscopy on the 11th day after sporozoite inoculation (the diligent microscopist can detect 20–50 parasites/μl reliably on Giemsa-stained thick films). At this stage the host may still feel well, or may complain of vague non-specific symptoms of malaise, headache, myalgia, weakness or anorexia.[44,45] On average the fever begins 2 days later, but in some cases fever precedes detectable parasitaemia. The rise in parasite count is logarithmic initially, with a rising sine wave pattern of parasitaemia,[46] but in most cases the parasite expansion terminates abruptly to limit the infection at a parasitaemia of 10^4–10^5/μl (Figure 61.2). Only *P. falciparum* has the capacity for untrammelled multiplication, and parasitaemias may exceed 50% in some cases. Several factors converge to limit parasite multiplication. The host mobilizes specific and non-specific immune defences. The parasite

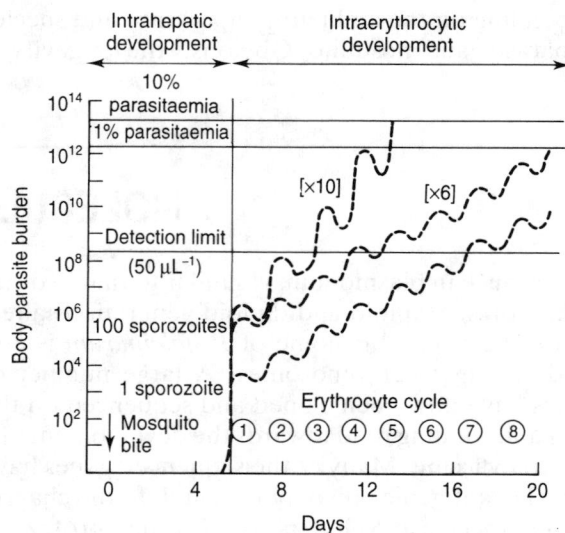

Figure 61.2 Logarithmic expansion of malaria infection in vivo. The body burden represents the total number of parasites in the body following infection of an adult of 50 kg. The infection rapidly reaches a lethal burden at high multiplicaton rates unless restrained. Maximum recorded multiplication rates are approximately × 20 in vivo (from White & Krishna: *Transactions of the Royal Society of Tropical Medicine & Hygiene* 1989, with permission).

meronts are also damaged by high fevers and this alone could explain the brake on parasite expansion.[47] The availability of suitable red cells is exhausted: *P. vivax* and *P. falciparum* prefer younger red cells and *P. malariae* prefers older cells. Thus the untreated infection increases exponentially, then the rate of expansion decelerates rapidly, parasitaemia fluctuates, settles around a plateau, then declines and continues for several weeks or months at low levels before finally being eliminated. Although natural infections often contain two or more, genetically different parasite strains, development tends to be relatively synchronous from the outset.[48] Further synchronization takes place in untreated infections in non-immune subjects, such that merogony ('sporulation') takes place within 1–2 hours. This is associated with fever and rigors (the 'paroxysm'). Although one 'brood' predominates, in *P. falciparum* there is usually at least one minor 'brood' or subpopulation cycling 24 hours our of phase with the major brood.

The periodicity of malaria is enshrined in the terminology of the fever pattern. *P. malariae* has a 72-hour life cycle, and in untreated infections the paroxysm occurred on the fourth day (using the Greek system the previous paroxysm is considered to occur on day 1). This is termed 'quartan malaria'. The other malarias are termed tertian (fever on the third day; 48-hour asexual cycle). *P. falciparum* often synchronized to a daily fever spike (quotidian fever), presumably caused by two broods of approximately equal size oscillating 24 hours out of phase, or failed to synchronize at all.[44–46] The classic descriptions of malaria symptomatology derive largely from detailed clinical observations made in the late nineteenth and early twentieth centuries, the experience with artificial infections in early chemotherapy studies, and the use of malaria therapy in the treatment of neurosyphilis.[49,50] In malaria therapy non-immune adults were artificially infected, by mosquito bite or transfusion, and the infection with *P. falciparum* or *P. vivax* was left untreated, or if symptoms were severe, was judiciously titrated with quinine. Nowadays these characteristic fever charts are seen rarely because malaria is treated promptly. It was apparent from these studies and later animal experiments[51] that some strains of *P. falciparum* were more virulent than others. For example, the now extinct European strains were notorious. The virulence factors of malaria parasites have not been characterized, but probably include multiplication capacity, cytoadherence and rosetting ability, the potential to induce cytokine release, antigenicity, and antimalarial drug resistance.

PARASITE BIOMASS

Malaria is readily diagnosed from the blood film stained with a Romanowsky dye. In the benign malarias (where sequestration is considered not to occur) the number of parasites in the body may be estimated simply by multiplying the parasitaemia by the estimated blood volume. In *P. falciparum* the microscopist can see only the first half of the asexual life cycle. In the second half the parasitized cells are sequestered. As a consequence there may be large discrepancies between the number of parasites in the peripheral (circulating) blood and the number of parasites in the body (the parasite burden) (Figure 61.3).[48,52] This has often puzzled and misled clinicians; some patients appear to tolerate high parasitaemia with little adverse effects, whereas others die with low parasite counts. The clue to the discrepancy lies both in the immune status of the host and in the stage of development of parasites on the peripheral blood smear.[53] A predominance of more mature parasites indicates that a greater proportion are sequestered, and carries a worse prognosis for any parasitaemia than a predominance of younger forms. In synchronous *P. falciparum* infections the peripheral blood parasite numbers fall at the time of sequestration, and rise abruptly at the time of merogony (when a predominance of tiny rings are

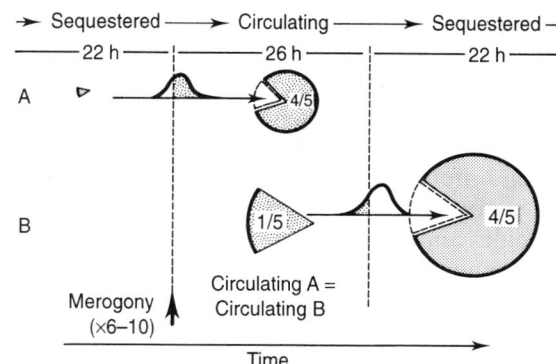

Figure 61.3 The problem of assessing the parasite burden from the peripheral parasitaemia in *P. falciparum* malaria. Sequestration hides the parasites causing harm. Two patients A and B have the same parasitaemia. In patient A, most of the parasites are circulating, and only a few from the previous cycle have yet to undergo merogony. In patient B, most of the parasites have already sequestered and only 20% of the biomass still circulates. There are over 60 times more parasites in patient B than in patient A. The clue lies in the stage distribution (shown crossing the hatched lines) of the circulating parasites which will be more mature in patient B (from Silamut & White: *Transactions of the Royal Society of Tropical Medicine & Hygiene* 1993: 87:436–443).

seen).[53] The other explanation for the ability to tolerate high parasitaemias without apparent adverse effects relates to the development of 'antitoxic' immunity.[54] The host adapts to repeated infection by producing less cytokines for a given quantum of parasites (see below).[55] Eventually a state is reached where infections are asymptomatic. This is called premunition.

IMMUNITY

The precise mechanisms controlling malaria infections are still incompletely understood. It was apparent from the era of malaria therapy, when malaria infections were used to treat neurosyphilis, that a strain-specific immunity developed which protected against rechallenge with the same strain, but did not protect from challenge with a different strain.[50,56] Immunity, as distinct from premunition, may be reached when there has been exposure to all local strains of malaria parasites. This is difficult to quantify as there is no in vitro correlate of either antitoxic or strain-specific immunity to malaria. In controlling the acute infection non-specific host defence mechanisms and the development of more specific cell-mediated and humoral responses are both important. Protective antibodies inhibit parasite expansion through co-operation with the monocyte–macrophage series by binding to parasitized erythrocytes and then activating these cells' Fc receptors.[58] Non-specific effector mechanisms include the activation of phagocytic cells (including neutrophils) to release toxic oxygen species[59] and nitric oxide,[60] both of which are parasiticidal. The reaction of these oxygen intermediates with lipoproteins produces lipid peroxides.[61] These are more stable cytotoxic molecules and are unaffected by antioxidants. There is also augmentation of splenic clearance function: both filtration[62] and Fc receptor-mediated phagocytosis are increased.[63,64] Infected erythrocytes are more rigid[33,65] and more opsonized than uninfected red cells as they express both host- and parasite-derived neoantigens on the erythrocyte surface. However, the parasite proteins expressed on the red cell surface undergo antigenic variation,[36,38,66,67] and this is probably instrumental in avoiding complete immune clearance and sustaining the infection. The monocyte–macrophage series appear to be the most important immune effector cells in the direct attack on parasitized erythrocytes and merozoites, although neutrophils may also play a role.

THE IMMUNE RESPONSE

Following natural infection there is a transient humoral response to sporozoite antigens; sporozoite antibodies decline, with a half-life of 3–4 weeks.[68] In areas of high transmission sporozoite antibody levels tend to plateau between 20 and 30 years of age, and do not correlate with premunition. The role of a cytotoxic T-cell immune response to the pre-erythrocytic liver stages in humans is not known,

although several lines of evidence including the recent discovery that HLA-B53 is associated with protection from severe malaria, and that HLA-B53-restricted T lymphocytes recognize a liver stage antigen LFA-1, suggests that it may be important.[42,43] Strain-specific immunity to the asexual stage parasites develops slowly during natural untreated infections, but does provide good protection against rechallenge.[50,56] However, parasite populations are diverse, and cross-strain protection is initially weak or negligible. The development of immunity in endemic areas may represent the gradual acquisition of a repertoire of immunological memory for the range of local parasites. This involves strain transcending immunity sufficient to ameliorate disease (antitoxic immunity) and a more strain-specific immunity which protects from or ameliorates the infection. The relative importance of humoral and cellular immunity in man in this complex process has not been defined clearly.[57] Infusion of hyperimmune serum to patients with acute malaria can reduce or eliminate parasitaemia,[69–71] mainly through opsonization, phagocytic cell activation and cytotoxicity, and augmentation of ring-form infected erythrocyte clearance.[72] Immune serum also reduces parasite multiplication by agglutinating merozoites. Cell-mediated immunity is undoubtedly important as well, both in controlling the infection and in retaining immunological memory, but the complex interaction of specific and non-specific cellular immune responses has yet to be unravelled in human infections. It is of interest that malaria does not seem to be worsened by the acquired immune deficiency syndrome (AIDS).[73]

PATHOPHYSIOLOGY

The pathophysiology of malaria results from destruction of erythrocytes, the liberation of parasite and erythrocyte material into the circulation, and the host reaction to these events. *P. falciparum* malaria-infected erythrocytes also sequester in the microcirculation of vital organs, interfering with microcirculatory flow and host tissue metabolism.

TOXICITY CYTOKINES

For many years malariologists hypothesized that parasites contained a toxin which was liberated at

meront rupture, and caused the symptoms of the paroxysm. No toxin in the strict sense of the word has been identified, but malaria parasites do induce release of cytokines in much the same way as bacterial endotoxin.[74,75] A glycolipid material with many of the properties of bacterial endotoxin is released on meront rupture.[76–78] This material appears to be associated with the glycosylphosphatidylinositol anchor which covalently links proteins including the malaria parasite surface antigens to the cell membrane lipid bilayer.[79] The limulus lysate assay, a test of endotoxin-like activity, is often positive in acute malaria. These parasite products, like endotoxin, induce activation of the cytokine cascade. Cells of the macrophage–monocyte series, and possibly endothelium, are stimulated to release cytokines. Initially tumour necrosis factor (TNF), which plays a pivotal role, and interleukin (IL)-1 are produced and these in turn induce release of other pro-inflammatory cytokines including IL-6 then IL-8.[76] Cytokines are responsible for many of the symptoms and signs of the infection, particularly fever and malaise. Plasma concentrations of the cytokines are elevated in both acute vivax and falciparum malaria.[80–82] In established vivax malaria, which tends to synchronize earlier than *P. falciparum*, a pulse release of TNF occurs at the time of meront rupture and this is followed by the characteristic symptoms and signs of the 'paroxysm', i.e. shivering, cool extremities, headache, chills, a spike of fever, and sometimes rigors followed by sweating, vasodilatation and defervescence.[83]

Cytokines are currently a subject of considerable interest, but the interpretation of blood concentration data is difficult. In the case of TNF, the assays (other than bioassays) available until recently measured both bioactive and inactive forms of TNF and also TNF bound to soluble receptors. They did not assess the effects of circulating inhibitors. Cytokine levels measured by enzyme linked immunosorbent assay (ELISA) or indirect fluorescent antibody test (IRMA) fluctuate widely over a short period of time, and are high in both *P. vivax* and *P. falciparum*; indeed some of the highest TNF concentrations recorded in malaria occur during the paroxysms of synchronous *P. vivax* infections.[83] Nearly all the TNF measured in these assays is bound to soluble receptors; there is usually little or no bioactivity. Nevertheless there is a positive correlation between cytokine levels and prognosis in severe falciparum malaria.[80–82] Whether this is a cause or an effect of severe disease remains to be seen.

Cytokines appear to play an important role in the pathogenesis of cerebral symptoms in murine models of severe malaria,[84] but these models are clinically and pathologically unlike human cerebral malaria. There is no direct nitric oxide evidence that cytokines cause coma in humans (although mechanisms involving release within the central nervous system and consequent inhibition of neurotransmission can be hypothesized). Cytokines may also be involved in placental dysfunction, suppression of erythropoiesis and inhibition of gluconeogenesis, and almost certainly cause fever in malaria.[85,86] Tolerance to malaria, or premunition, reflects both immune regulation of the infection and also reduced production of cytokines in response to malaria ('antitoxic immunity'). Cytokines may up-regulate the endothelial expression of vascular ligands for *P. falciparum*-infected erythrocytes and thus promote cytoadherence. They may also be important mediators of parasite killing by activating leucocytes, and possibly other cells, to release toxic oxygen species,[87] nitric oxide, by generating parasiticidal lipid peroxides, and by causing fever. Thus, whereas high concentrations of cytokines appear to be harmful, lower levels probably benefit the host. The availability of monoclonal anti-TNF and other cytokine antibodies should help to dissect their role in malaria pathogenesis.

SEQUESTRATION

The process whereby erythrocytes containing mature forms of *P. falciparum* adhere to microvascular endothelium ('cytoadherence') and thus disappear from the circulation is known as sequestration (Figure 61.4). This phenomenon is also seen in the simian malarias *P. coatneyi* and *P. fragile* infecting rhesus monkeys. Sequestration is thought to be central to the pathophysiology of falciparum malaria.[18,88,89] Cytoadherence begins at the middle of the parasites' 48-hour asexual life cycle. As a consequence, whereas in the other malarias of man mature parasites are commonly seen on blood smears, these forms are rare in falciparum malaria, and often indicate serious infection.[53] Sequestration occurs predominantly in the venules of vital organs. It is not distributed uniformly throughout the body, being greatest in the brain, particularly the white

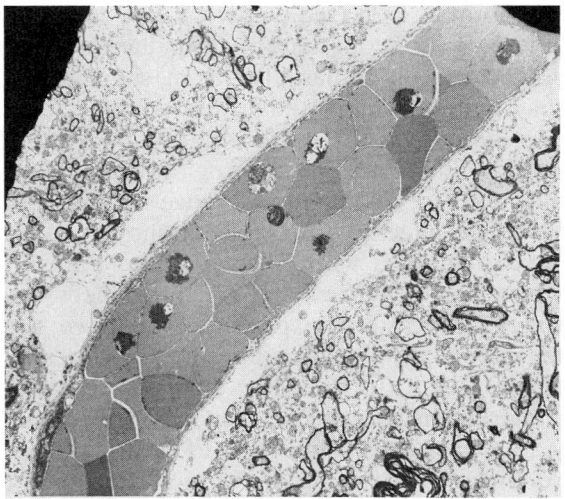

Figure 61.4 Electron micrograph (× 4320) showing densely packed sequestered parasitized erythrocytes in a cerebral venule, from a fatal case of cerebral malaria. Note that electron dense deposits are evident on the cell membranes of most of the erythrocytes. This indicates that all these red cells contain *P. falciparum* parasites, but the bodies of the parasites have been missed on the section (courtesy of D. Ferguson).

matter, prominent in the heart, liver, kidneys, intestines and adipose tissue, and least in the skin.[90] Cytoadherence and the related phenomenon of rosetting lead to microcirculatory obstruction in falciparum malaria. The consequences of microcirculatory obstruction are reduced oxygen and substrate supply, leading to anaerobic glycolysis and lactic acidosis.[89]

CYTOADHERENCE

Cytoadherence is mediated by a family of strain-specific, high molecular weight parasite-derived proteins termed *P. falciparum* erythrocyte membrane protein 1 or Pf EMP₁.[91–93] This protein (molecular mass 240–260 kDa) is exported to the surface of the infecting erythrocyte where it is anchored through the membrane to a submembraneous accretion of parasite-derived histidine-rich protein.[34] These accretions cause humps or knobs on the surface of the red cell, and these are the points of attachment to vascular endothelium. The protuberances are not essential for cytoadherence. A small subpopulation of naturally occurring parasites do not induce surface knobs, and parasites can be selected in culture which are knob negative (K−) but still cytoadhere.[94,95] However, most natural parasite isolates are knob positive (K+). A protein similar to Pf EMP₁ named sequestrin (molecular mass 270 kDa) has recently been identified on the surface of infected red cells using anti-idiotypic antibodies raised against one of the putative vascular receptors CD36 (see below).[96] The central role of Pf EMP₁ or sequestrin in cytoadherence is not accepted by all; it has also been suggested that cytoadherence is mediated by altered red cell membrane components.[93] In culture, most parasites lose the ability to cytoadhere after several cycles of replication. In vivo, cytoadherence may be modulated by the spleen.[97] This has been shown in *Saimiri* monkeys infected with *P. falciparum*. Parasitized erythrocytes do not cytoadhere in splenectomized monkeys. Occasionally patients who have had a splenectomy develop falciparum malaria, and in some of these cytoadherence does not occur[98] and all stages of the parasite are seen in peripheral blood smears. The adhesive protein, Pf EMP₁, is present in relatively low amounts on the red cell surface. It is the only parasite protein unequivocally present on the outside of the erythrocyte. It is a trypsin-sensitive antigen, and has been shown to undergo antigenic variation within cloned parasite lines.[99] Approximately 2% of the parasites switch to a different antigenic phenotype each asexual cycle.

There are two other candidates for the 'glue' which binds parasitized red cells to endothelium. The protein MESA may also be partially expressed on the surface of the red cell. The other possibility is that a modified form of the red cell cytoskeleton protein band 3 (the major erythrocyte anion transporter) is the adhesin.[93]

VASCULAR ENDOTHELIAL LIGANDS

Several different sticky proteins present on the surface of vascular endothelium have been shown to bind parasitized red cells (Figure 61.5). This property of cytoadherence can be studied in vitro with cells expressing the potential ligands on their surface (e.g. melanoma cells, human umbilical vein endothelial cells or COS cells) or with the immobilized purified candidate ligand proteins. Probably the most important of these proteins is the leucocyte differentiation antigen CD36;[95,100–102] nearly all freshly obtained parasites bind to CD36.[103] Binding is increased at low pH (<7.0) and in the presence of high calcium concentrations.[104,105] CD36 is present on vascular endothelium and monocytes/macrophages. The intercellular adhesion molecule (ICAM1), which is also the receptor for rhinovirus attachment, will also bind parasitized erythrocytes.[106] This is an attractive alternative as expression of ICAM1, but not CD36, can be

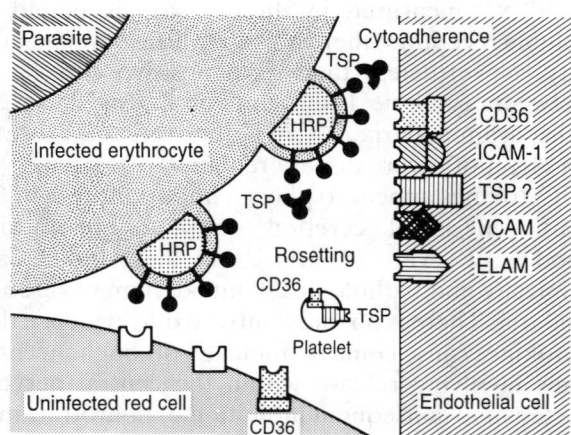

Figure 61.5 Schematic illustration of cellular adhesion in falciparum malaria. For cytoadherence (red cell to vascular endothelium) more than five potential vascular receptors for the adhesive variant surface protein Pf.EMP 1 have been identified (see text). The molecules on the red cell surface involved in rosetting (infected red cell to infected red cell) appear to be different to those causing cytoadherence. CD36: cellular differentiation antigen 36, ICAM 1: intercellular adhesion molecule 1, TSP: Thrombospondin, VCAM 1; vascular cell adhesion molecule 1, ELAM 1 (E-selectin) Endothelial leukocyte adhesion molecule 1, HRP: histidine rich protein.

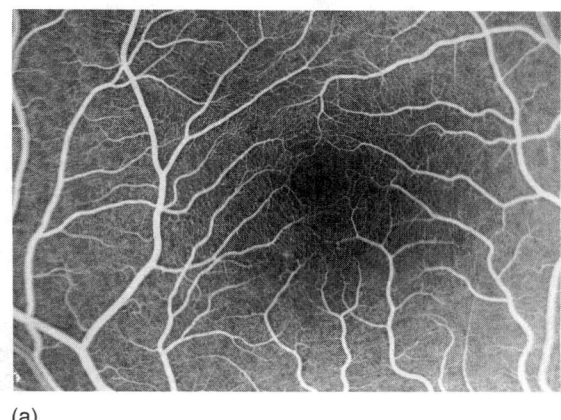
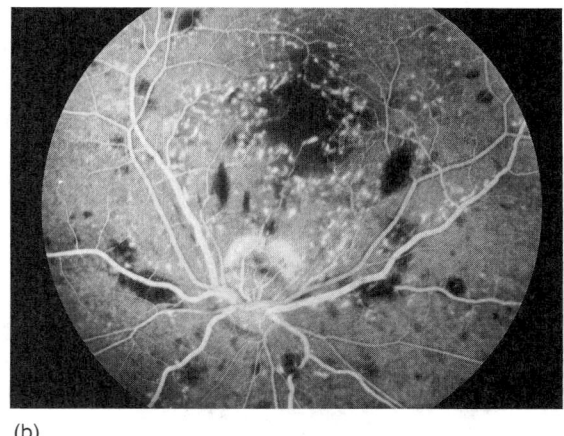

(a)   (b)

Figure 61.6 (a) Retinal angiogram in cerebral malaria showing disruption of the usually symmetrical 'Spider's web' array of vessels around the macula, presumably because of microvascular obstruction. (b) Late phase angiogram showing haemorrhages (dark) and fluoroscein leakage (white) from the retinal microvasculature in cerebral malaria. (From White N. J. and Ho M.; *Advances in Parasitology* 1992; 31:83–173 with permission.)

upregulated by cytokines (notably TNF), and would provide a plausible pathological scenario whereby cytokine release enhances cytoadherence. At physiological shear rates (i.e. those likely to be encountered in the human microcirculation) the binding forces ($c. 10^{-10}$ N) are similar for CD36 and ICAM1.[107,108] For both, the forces of attachment are lower than those required for detachment, which suggests postattachment alterations to increase adhesion. Thrombospondin (a natural ligand to CD36) will also bind to some parasitized red cells,[109,110] and recently the ubiquitous proteins VCAM and ELAM have also been shown to bind in some circumstances.[111] Although CD36 fulfils many of the criteria for the major vascular ligand in falciparum malaria, the usual conformation and antigenic form of CD36 is not present on the surface of cerebral vascular endothelium, whereas it is present elsewhere. Recent pathology studies have shown colocalization of CD36 expression and sequestration of parasitized erythrocytes in vessels outside the brain; but in cerebral vessels there was colocalization of ICAM1 with sequestration. Other as yet unidentified vascular receptors are also present, as sequestration also occurred in vessels expressing none of the five potential ligands indentified so far. Thus ICAM1 appears to be the major vascular ligand in the brain involved in cerebral sequestration and CD36 is probably the major ligand in other organs. This is supported by observations that CD36 binding of parasites from patients with acute falciparum malaria does not correlate with the development of cerebral malaria,[104,112] but does correlate with severe disease involving other vital organs. The relative importance of the various potential vascular ligands in the pathophysiology of severe falciparum malaria and the precise role of the spleen[113] remain to be determined. As there is such considerable variability in the cytoadherence determinants in both the parasite and the host, severe malaria and the pattern of organ involvement may reflect the result of a particular host–parasite combination.

ROSETTING

Erythrocytes containing mature parasites also adhere to uninfected erythrocytes.[114,115] This process leads to the formation of 'rosettes' when suspensions of parasitized erythrocytes are viewed under the microscope (Figure 61.7). Rosetting shares some characteristics of cytoadherence.[114–118] It occurs mainly at the middle of the asexual life cycle and it is trypsin-sensitive. But parasite species which do not sequester do rosette and unlike cytoadherence, rosetting is inhibited by certain heparin subfractions and calcium chelators. Furthermore, whereas all fresh isolates of *P. falciparum* cytoadhere, not all rosette. The forces required to separate a rosette are approximately five times greater than those required to separate cytoadherent cells.[108] When known rosetting parasite lines (K+ R+) are perfused through the rat mesocaecum, an ex vivo model for the study of vascular perfusion,[88] they cause significantly more microvascular obstruction than isolates which cytoadhere but do not rosette (K+ R−).[119] Rosetting in *P. falciparum* infections is associated with cerebral malaria.[120,121] If blood is taken from patients with acute falciparum malaria and incu-

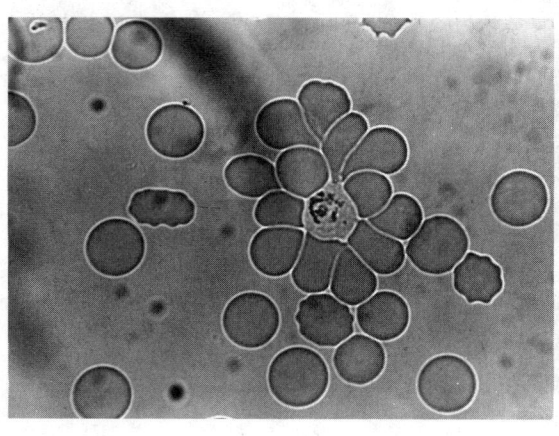
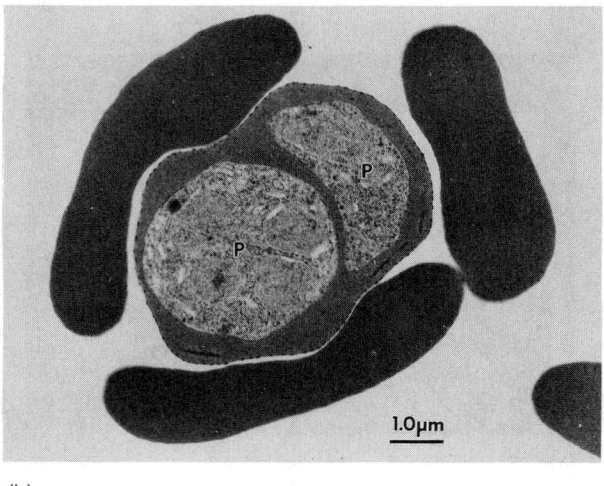

(a)   (b)

Figure 61.7 Rosetting. (a) Uninfected red cells bind to a *P. vivax* infected erythrocyte (courtesy of R. Udomsangpetch). (b) Transmission electron micrograph of a rosette formed around a *P. falciparum* infected erythrocyte (courtesy of D. Ferguson).

bated, such that the parasites mature, then isolates from patients with cerebral malaria rosette more, and the corresponding serum is less likely to have antirosetting antibodies, than blood from patients with uncomplicated falciparum malaria.[120] Thus rosetting appears to be associated with parasites causing cerebral malaria, and increased cytoadherence with other vital organ dysfunction. It has been suggested that rosetting might encourage cytoadherence by reducing flow (shear rate), which would enhance anaerobic glycolysis, reduce pH and facilitate adherence of infected erythrocytes to venular endothelium. Rosetting tends to start in venules, and this could certainly reduce flow. The adhesive forces involved in rosetting could also impede forward flow of uninfected erythrocytes as they squeeze past sticky cytoadherent parasitized red cells in capillaries and venules.[89] The mechanical obstruction or 'static hindrance' would be compounded by the lack of deformability of the adherent, and circulating parasitized red cells.

DEFORMABILITY

As the parasite matures inside the erythrocyte, the normally flexible biconcave disc becomes progressively more spherical and rigid.[33] The reduction in deformability results from reduced membrane fluidity, increasing sphericity, and the enlarging and relatively rigid intraerythrocytic parasite.[122] Infected red cells are less filterable than uninfected cells. However, reduced deformability alone cannot account for microvascular obstruction as it would lead to obstruction at the mid-capillary (i.e. the

smallest internal diameter in the vasculature) and could not explain sequestration in venules.[89]

IMMUNOLOGICAL PROCESSES

It has been suggested that severe malaria, and in particular cerebral malaria, results from specific immune-mediated damage. This is unlikely. There is no pathological evidence in man for vasculitis with a cellular infiltrate in or around the cerebral vessels. Indeed, fatal falciparum malaria is remarkable for the lack of extravascular pathology. Although some glomerular abnormalities have been noted in fatal malaria,[120] the clinical and pathological findings suggest that acute tubular necrosis, and not acute glomerulonephritis, is the cause of renal dysfunction. The pathogenesis of pulmonary oedema is uncertain—as it is for the adult respiratory distress syndrome in other conditions—but it is unlikely to involve a specific immune-mediated process. Despite the enormous intravascular antigenic load in malaria, with the formation of immune complexes and variable complement depletion,[121–124] there is little evidence of a specific immunopathological process in severe malaria.

Acute malaria infections are associated with malaria antigen-specific unresponsiveness.[55,128,129,130]. This selective paresis is one of the factors contributing to the slow development of an effective and specific immune response in malaria. Acute malaria is characterized by non-specific polyclonal B-cell activation. There is a reduction in circulating T cells with an increase in the γ/δ T-cell subset,[131] but other T-cell proportions are usually normal.[132] Although

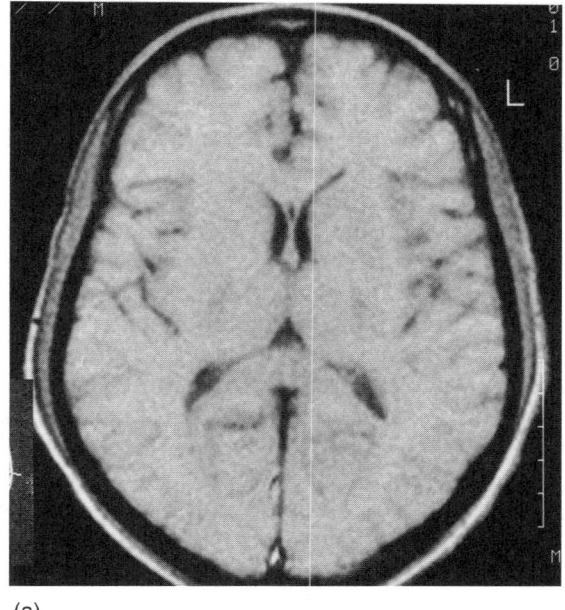

(a)

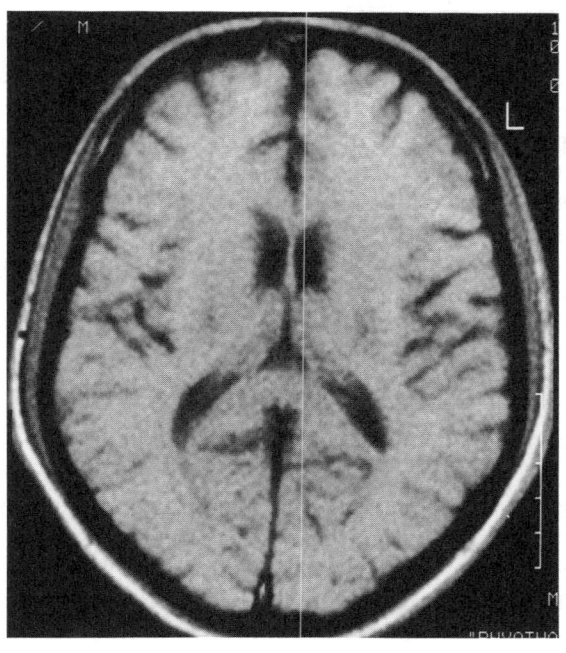

(c)

(b)

Figure 61.8 T_1 weighed magnetic resonance imaging (550/25 TR/TE) of the brain in a 28-year-old man with cerebral malaria. (a) During coma showing slight swelling. (b) Following recovery of consciousness showing shrinkage. (c) 135 days later the brain is normal. There was no evidence of cerebral oedema on T_2 weighted images. The acute swelling was interpreted as representing increased intracerebral blood volume (from Looareesuwan et al. *Clinical Infectious Diseases* 1995; 21, with permission).

residents of hyperendemic or holoendemic malarious areas have hypergammaglobulinaemia, most of this antibody is not directed against malaria antigens. In non-immune individuals, the acute antibody response to infection often comprises mostly IgM or IgG_2, isotypes which are unable to arm cytotoxic cells and thus kill asexual malaria parasites.[133] These observations have led to the suggestion that malaria induces an immunological 'smokescreen' with broad-spectrum and non-specific acti-

vation that interferes with the orderly development of a specific cellular immune response.[132] In severe malaria there is evidence of a broader immune suppression, with defects in monocyte and neutrophil chemotaxis, reduced monocytic phagocytic function and a tendency to bacterial super-infection.[133–136]

In the nephrotic syndrome associated with chronic *P. malariae* infections, malarial antigen and immune complexes can be eluted from the kidney, indicating a role for quartan malaria in this condition.[137] Why some children are affected but the majority are not remains unresolved.

PERMEABILITY

There is evidence of a mild generalized increase in systemic vascular permeability in severe malaria.[138] In the past it was suggested that cerebral malaria resulted from an increase in cerebral capillary permeability which led to brain swelling, coma and death.[139,140] It is now clear from imaging studies that the majority of adults and children with cerebral malaria have no evidence of cerebral oedema.[141] However, the role of raised intracranial pressure in cerebral malaria remains unclear. Whereas 80% of adults have opening pressures at lumbar puncture which are in the normal range (<200 mm CSF), 80% of children have elevated opening pressures (>100 mm CSF: the normal range is lower in children)[142,144] and intracranial pressure may rise transiently to very high levels. Some patients with cerebral malaria die from acute respiratory arrest with neurological signs that are compatible with brain stem compression. The clinical findings are not conclusive as these signs are also common, and may persist for many hours, in survivors. The elevation in opening pressure is usually not great (in general it is much lower than in pyogenic meningitis), and there is no difference between these lumbar puncture opening pressures in surviving children and fatal cases.[144,145] Studies of computerized tomography or magnetic resonance imaging have generally shown slight brain swelling in crebral malaria (compatible with an increased intracerebral blood volume), but no evidence of cerebral oedema[436,437] (Figure 61.8). Other studies have also failed to detect major alterations in blood–brain barrier permeability.[142,146] Thus, raised intracranial pressure probably arises from an increase in cerebral blood volume, independent of permeability. This results from circulating blood required to maintain cerebral perfusion and the considerable sequestered biomass of intracerebral parasites. Children may be particularly vulnerable as after the skull sutures have fused, there is less space for cranial expansion than in adults. The relationship between intracerebral pressure and volume is non-linear (i.e. once the brain has expanded to fill the skull, only small further increases in volume cause large increases in intracranial pressure). The possibility that a sudden rise in intracranial pressure accounts for some deaths cannot be excluded.

PATHOGENESIS OF COMA

The cause of coma in cerebral malaria is not known. There is undoubtedly an increase in cerebral anaerobic glycolysis with cerebral blood flows that are inappropriately low for the arterial oxygen content, increased cerebral metabolic rates for lactate, and increased CSF concentrations of lactate,[147,148] but these changes do not provide sufficient explanation for coma.[89] Presumably the metabolic milieu created adjacent to the sequestered and highly metabolically active parasites interferes with neurotransmission but how this occurs is not known. Cytokines increase production of nitric oxide, a potent inhibitor of neurotransmission, by leucocytes, smooth muscle cells, microglia and vascular endothelium through induction of the enzyme nitric oxide synthase. Local synthesis of nitric oxide could well be relevant to the impairment of consciousness. Coma in malaria is not caused by raised intracranial pressure.

RENAL FAILURE

There is renal cortical vasoconstriction and consequent hypoperfusion in severe malaria with renal impairment.[149] Acute tubular necrosis presumably results from renal microvascular obstruction consequent upon sequestration in the kidney. Significant glomerulonephritis is very rare.[150–152] The role of local cytokine release and altered regulation of renal microvascular flow is uncertain. Massive haemolysis compounds the insult in blackwater fever complicating severe malaria.[153–155]

PULMONARY OEDEMA

Despite intense sequestration in the myocardial vessels, pump function is remarkably well preserved in severe malaria. Pulmonary oedema in malaria results from a sudden increase in pulmonary capillary permeability that is not reflected in other vascular beds.[138,156,157] The pulmonary capillary wedge pressure is usually normal and the threshold for the development of pulmonary oedema is relatively low. The cause of this increase in permeability is not known.

FLUID SPACE AND ELECTROLYTE CHANGES

Following rehydration the plasma volume is increased in moderate and severe malaria.[158,160]

Total body water and extracellular volume are normal. Plasma renin activity, aldosterone and antidiuretic hormone concentrations are elevated, reflecting an appropriate activation of homeostatic mechanisms to maintain adequate circulating volume in the presence of general vasodilatation and a falling haematocrit. Although some reports have suggested that the secretion of antidiuretic hormone may be inappropriate,[161] direct measurements have refuted this. Mild hyponatraemia and hypochloraemia are common, but serum potassium concentrations are usually normal.

ANAEMIA

The pathogenesis of anaemia is multifactorial.[162,163] There is obligatory destruction of red cells containing parasites at merogony. There is also accelerated destruction of non-parasitized red cells that parallels disease severity.[164,165] In severe malaria anaemia develops rapidly; the rapid haemolysis of unparasitized red cells is a major contributor to the decline in haematocrit.[164–166] The haemolytic anaemia is compounded by bone marrow dysfunction;[167–169] dyserythropoeisis persists for days or weeks following acute malaria and reticulocyte counts are usually low in the acute phase of the disease.[168,169] Although there is evidence of a lowered threshold for splenic clearance of abnormal erythrocytes,[62–64] the factors that trigger removal of uninfected erythrocytes have not been identified. In simian malarias there is evidence of an inversion of the erythrocyte membrane lipid bilayer in uninfected erythrocytes,[170] but this has not been studied in man. The role of antibody (i.e. Coombs'-positive haemolysis) in anaemia is unresolved.[167,171–173] The majority of studies to date do not show increased red cell immunoglobulin binding in malaria, but in the presence of a lowered recognition threshold for splenic clearance, this might be difficult to detect (see below). Red cell survival is shortened in malaria[164–166] and this is unaffected by corticosteroids.[174]

COAGULOPATHY AND THROMBOCYTOPENIA

There is accelerated coagulation cascade activity with accelerated fibrinogen turnover, consumption of antithrombin III, and increased concentrations of fibrin degradation products.[174–178] In severe infections the prothrombin and partial thromboplastin times may be prolonged, and in 5% of patients bleeding may be significant.[89] Thrombocytopenia is caused by increased splenic clearance.[179] The role of platelet-bound antibody in this process is controversial.[180–182] Platelet turnover is increased. There has been evidence of platelet activation in some studies,[181] but not others.[183] Erythrocytes containing mature parasites may activate the coagulation cascade directly,[184] and cytokine release is also procoagulant. It has also been suggested that disseminated intravascular coagulation (DIC) is important in the pathogenesis of severe malaria,[175,185–187] but detailed prospective clinical and pathogenesis studies have refuted this. Coagulation cascade activity is directly proportional to disease severity,[178] but hypofibrinogenaemia resulting from DIC is significant in approximately 5% of patients with severe malaria, and lethal haemorrhage is unusual. Intravascular thrombus formation is observed rarely at autopsy in fatal cases.

BLACKWATER FEVER (Figure 61.9)

This is a poorly understood condition in which there is massive intravascular haemolysis and the passage of 'Coca-Cola'-coloured urine. Blackwater (urine) occurs in three circumstances: (1) when patients with G6PD deficiency take oxidant drugs irrespective of whether they have malaria or not; (2) occasionally when patients with G6PD deficiency have malaria and receive quinine treatment; and (3)

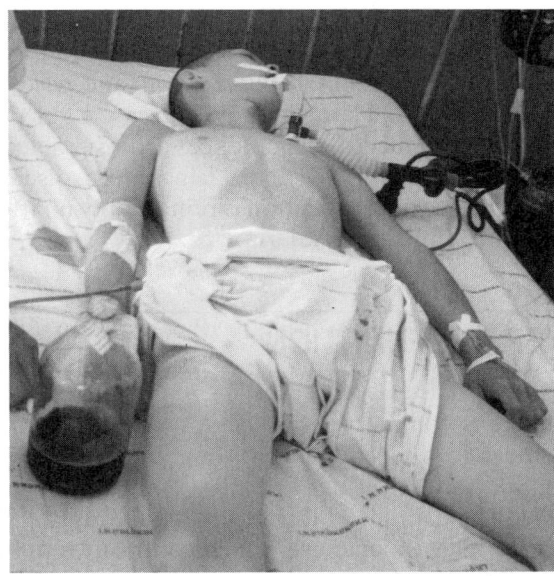

Figure 61.9 'Blackwater fever'. A 25-year-old man with severe malaria, pulmonary oedema, renal impairment and massive haemolysis.

in some patients with severe quinine-treated falciparum malaria who have normal erythrocyte G6PD levels. How quinine causes blackwater in these last two situations is not known as it is not an oxidant drug. G6PD-deficient red cells are particularly susceptible to oxidant stress as they are unable to synthesize adequate quantities of NADPH through the pentose shunt. This leads to low intraerythrocytic levels of reduced glutathione, and both alterations in the erythrocyte membrane and increased susceptibility to organic peroxides.

THE SPLEEN

There is considerable splenic enlargement in malaria, and an increased capacity to clear red cells from the circulation both by Fc receptor-mediated (immune) mechanisms[6e,64] and by recognition of reduced deformability (filtration).[65] The spleen may also modulate cytoadherence.[97] It plays a central role in limiting the acute expansion of the malaria infection by removing parasitized erythrocytes, and this has led to the suggestion that a failure to augment splenic clearance sufficiently rapidly may be a factor in the development of severe malaria.[48,52]

GASTROINTESTINAL DYSFUNCTION

Minor stress ulceration of the stomach and duodenum is common in severe malaria. The pattern of malabsorption of sugars, fats, and amino acids suggests reduced splanchnic perfusion.[188–191] This results from both gut sequestration and visceral vasoconstriction. There may be increased gut permeability or reduced local defences against bacterial toxins, or even whole bacteria in severe disease. Antimalarial drug absorption is remarkably unaffected in uncomplicated malaria.[192]

LIVER DYSFUNCTION

Jaundice is common in adults with severe malaria, and there is other evidence of hepatic dysfunction, with reduced clotting factor synthesis, reduced metabolic clearance of the antimalarial drugs, and a failure of gluconeogenesis which contributes to lactic acidosis and hypoglycaemia. Nevertheless, true liver failure (as in fulminant viral hepatitis) is very unusual. There is sequestration in the hepatic microvasculature, and in very severe infections liver blood flow is reduced.[191] Liver blood flow values less than 15 ml/kg per minute are associated with elevated venous lactate concentrations,[193] which suggests a flow limitation to lactate clearance and thus a contribution of liver dysfunction to lactic acidosis. However, many patients with acute falciparum malaria have elevated liver blood flow values. There is no relationship between liver blood flow and impairment of antimalarial drug clearance. Jaundice in malaria appears to have haemolytic, hepatitic and cholestatic components. Cholestatic jaundice may persist well into the recovery period.

METABOLIC DYSFUNCTION

In severe malaria arterial, capillary, venous and CSF concentrations of lactate rise in direct proportion to disease severity. Indeed the venous lactate concentration 4 hours after admission to hospital is the best prognostic indicator in severe malaria. Lactic acidosis is an important cause of death. It results from several discrete processes: the tissue anaerobic glycolysis consequent upon microvascular obstruction; a failure of hepatic and renal lactate clearance; and the production of lactate by the parasite.[89,194,195] Mature malaria parasites consume up to 70 times as much glucose as uninfected cells, and over 90% of this is converted to L+ lactic acid (plasmodia do not have the complete set of enzymes necessary for the citric acid cycle). Interestingly, up to 6% of the lactic acid appears as D− lactate, but this does not contribute materially to the acidosis.[196] Calculations based on glucose and lactate turnover in man indicate that the majority of the lactic acid produced in malaria derives from host rather than parasite sources. Lactate levels also rise after generalized convulsions. Hyperlactataemia is accompanied by hyperalaninaemia, reflecting the impairment of gluconeogenesis through the Cori cycle.[197–199] Lactate and alanine are the major gluconeogenic precursors. Triglyceride and free fatty acid levels are also elevated in acute malaria,[200] and plasma concentrations of ketone bodies are raised in patients who have been unable to eat.[198,199] In severe malaria there is dysfunction of all organ systems, particularly those with obligatory high metabolic rates. The endocrine glands are no exception. Pituitary–thyroid axis abnormalities result in the 'sick euthyroid' syndrome and also parathyroid dysfunction.[201] Mild hypocalcaemia is common[202,203] and hypophosphataemia may be profound in the very seriously ill.[202] By contrast, the pituitary–adrenal axis appears normal in acute malaria.[204]

HYPOGLYCAEMIA

Hypoglycaemia is associated with hyperlactataemia and shares the same pathophysiological aetiology: an increased peripheral requirement for glucose consequent upon anaerobic glycolysis (the Pasteur effect) and the increased metabolic demands of the febrile illness;[205] the obligatory demands of the parasites which use glucose as their major fuel (increased demand); and a failure of hepatic gluconeogenesis and glycogenolysis (reduced supply).[89,197–199] Hepatic glycogen is exhausted rapidly: stores in fasting adults last approximately 2 days, but children only have enough for 12 hours. In patients treated with quinine, this is compounded by quinine-stimulated pancreatic β-cell insulin secretion.[197,199,206,207] Hyperinsulinaemia is balanced by a reduced tissue sensitivity to insulin,[208] which returns to normal as the patient improves. This probably explains why quinine-induced (hyperinsulinaemic) hypoglycaemia tends to occur after the first 24 hours of treatment, whereas malaria-related hypoglycaemia (with appropriate suppression of insulin secretion) is often present when the patient with severe malaria is first admitted. Hypoglycaemia contributes to nervous system dysfunction, and in cerebral malaria is associated with residual neurological deficit in survivors.[21]

PLACENTAL DYSFUNCTION

Pregnancy increases susceptibility to malaria. This is probably caused by a suppression of systemic and placental cell-mediated immune responses.[209] There is intense sequestration of *P. falciparum* infected erythrocytes in the placenta[210] and maternal anaemia. This leads to placental insufficiency.[211–217] Fetal growth is retarded. In areas of intense transmission low birth weight and a possible increase in the risk of stillbirth are confined to primigravidae. With lower levels of transmission (i.e. less immunity) the risk extends to other pregnancies[218] and there is a propensity to develop severe malaria with a high incidence of fetal death.[220] The effects of the benign malarias on placental pathology or fetal development have not been defined.

BACTERIAL INFECTION

Patients with severe malaria are vulnerable to bacterial infections, particularly of the lungs and urinary tract (following catheterization). Postpartum sepsis is also common. Spontaneous Gram-negative septicaemia may occur but is rare;[219–220] however, salmonella septicaemias are an important complication of otherwise uncomplicated falciparum malaria in African children.[221]

PATHOLOGY

As the benign human malarias are rarely fatal there is very little information available on the pathology of these infections. Unfortunately this is not the case for *P. falciparum* malaria.

In fatal malaria the microvasculature of the vital organs is packed with erythrocytes containing mature forms of the parasite. There is abundant intra- and extraerythrocytic pigment[222–228] and organs such as the liver, spleen and placenta may be grey-black in colour. Sequestration is not uniformly distributed; it tends to be greatest in the brain and heart,[90,229] followed by the gut, kidney, adipose tissue, liver, lungs and least of all in bone marrow and skin. There is remarkably little extravascular pathology in malaria.

BRAIN

If the patient dies from the acute infection the brain is commonly slightly swollen with multiple small petechial haemorrhages throughout the white matter.[222–228,230] Haemorrhages are unusual in the grey matter. Large haemorrhages or infarcts are rare. There is usually no evidence of tentorial or foramen magnum herniation. Nearly every capillary and venule is packed with erythrocytes containing mature forms of the parasite (whereas these are seen rarely in peripheral blood smears).[89] This sequestration is particularly prominent in the white matter, although the tissue is much less vascular than the grey matter. The degree of cerebral sequestration and the intensity of erythrocyte packing is greater in cerebral malaria than in fatal malaria in which the patient was not comatose.[90,229] A large quantity of intra- and extraerythrocytic pigment is evident. In the white matter, accumulations of glial cells are seen surrounding haemorrhagic foci (Dürck's granuloma) where vessels appear to have been occluded by a mass of parasitized cells, and then ruptured. At the ultrastructural level the erythrocytes are seen to be packed closely together and the infected red cells are adherent to the vascular endothelium by attachment of knob-like surface projections to the endothelial surface.[90,229,231] Occasional fibrin strands are seen but there is a striking absence of platelets[90] and no evidence for leucocyte aggregation, i.e. there is no evidence of thrombus formation or vasculitis. On immunofluorescent staining malarial antigens may be seen on the endothelial basement membrane,[231,232] but the significance of this observation is uncertain (i.e. does it reflect pathology in vivo or postmortem artefact?). In some cases there are only a few, or no parasites in the cerebral vessels. This occurs when death was several days after parasite clearance.

HEART AND LUNGS

Despite intense sequestration in the myocardial microvasculature the heart is remarkably normal, although in anaemic patients it is commonly pale and dilated. As in all other organs, extravascular pathological changes are rare. In adults there is often evidence of pulmonary oedema. Hyaline membrane formation suggests leakage of proteinaceous fluid.[157] There is moderate sequestration[233,234] and sometimes leucocyte aggregates are seen. There may be secondary bacterial pneumonia.

LIVER AND SPLEEN

The liver is generally enlarged and may be black from malaria pigment. There is congestion of the centrilobular capillaries with sinusoidal dilatation and Kupffer cell hyperplasia.[235] Sequestration of parasitized erythrocytes is associated with variable cloudy swelling of the hepatocytes and perivenous ischaemic changes, and sometimes centrizonal necrosis. Hepatic glycogen is often present despite hypoglycaemia. In uncomplicated malaria the liver histology is often normal.[236,237] The spleen is often

dark or black from malaria pigment, enlarged, soft and friable. It is full of erythrocytes containing mature and immature parasites.[238] There is evidence of reticular hyperplasia and architectural reorganization.[239] The soft and acutely enlarged spleen of acute lethal infections contrasts with the hard fibrous enlargement associated with repeated malaria.

KIDNEYS

The kidneys are often slightly swollen. In adults there are commonly tubular abnormalities consistent with ischaemia. There is sequestration, particularly in the glomerular capillaries,[189] and sometimes mesangial and endothelial cell proliferative changes are seen. Immunofluorescent studies show immunoglobulin deposition on the glomerular capillary basement membranes.

ALIMENTARY TRACT

Upper gastrointestinal bleeding from erosions may occur in severe malaria. There is intense sequestration in the gut,[189] and visceral ischaemia may explain the acute abdominal pain that sometimes occurs in severe malaria. Despite this, drug absorption is often remarkably normal.

BONE MARROW

Dyserythropoeitic change is prominent in all the acute malarias.[167–169,240] Bone marrow macrophages contain pigment, and erythrophagocytosis may be seen. Iron is usually plentiful. The platelet and white cell series are usually normal.

PLACENTA

The placenta may be black from malaria pigment even if the mother is asymptomatic throughout pregnancy. Large numbers of mature parasites are seen on crush smears,[241] although the peripheral blood smear may be negative. There is often trophoblastic thickening, macrophage infiltration and perivillous fibrin deposition.[242,244]

CLINICAL FEATURES

The clinical manifestations of malaria are dependent on the previous immune status of the host. In areas of intense *P. falciparum* malaria transmission, asymptomatic parasitaemia is usual in adults (premunition). Severe malaria never occurs in this age group: it is confined to the first years of life, and becomes progressively less frequent with increasing age. The rate at which age-specific acquisition of premunition occurs is proportional to the intensity of malaria transmission. In areas with a constant high-level *P. falciparum* transmission (e.g. average infected anopheline biting frequencies of daily up to monthly), severe malaria occurs predominantly between 6 months and 3 years of age; mild symptoms are seen in older children, and adults are asymptomatic and have low parasitaemias. Malaria is common in pregnancy, but is asymptomatic (although anaemia may be severe), but the birth weight of babies born to primagravidae is reduced significantly. Spleen rates will be high (>50%) in children between 2 and 9, corresponding with the epidemiological terms hyperendemic and holoendemic malaria. Severe anaemia in infancy is the most common presentation of severe falciparum malaria in these circumstances. With lower or more seasonal or unstable transmission patterns the age distribution of severe malaria shifts upwards, severe malaria is seen in older children as well, and cerebral malaria becomes the most prominent manifestation. Spleen rates in children are lower than 50%. With even lower or more sporadic patterns of transmission, and when non-immunes travel to endemic areas, symptomatic disease is seen at all ages.

INCUBATION PERIOD

Precise data on the incubation period of malaria comes from the detailed studies of malaria therapy for neurosyphilis, and also the many hundreds of volunteer experiments conducted between the turn of the century and 1965 (Table 61.2).[44–46,49,50] In the majority of mosquito-transmitted infections several heavily infected anophelines were allowed to bite. The sporozoite inocula were therefore probably larger than those received in most naturally acquired (autochthonous) infections. The shortest incubation period documented was reported by Shute[245] in a sailor who docked briefly in West Africa and developed malaria 3 days later. Primary incubation periods can be long, particularly if the infection is suppressed by partially effective chemoprophylaxis.

Table 61.2 Malaria incubation periods in malaria therapy and volunteer studies.

	Prepatent period (days)	Incubation period (days)
P. falciparum	11.0 (2.4)	13.1 (2.8)
P. vivax	12.2 (2.3)	13.4 (2.7)
P. malariae	32.7*	34.7*
P. ovale	12.0	14.1

Values are mean (SD).
*These data are taken from artificially induced malaria data in Boyd (1948); naturally acquired infections are considered to have an incubation period of between 13–28 days.

Most tropical strains of *P. vivax* had similar incubation periods to *P. falciparum* but some strains from cooler countries had extremely long incubation periods. The primary infection began 9–12 months after sporozoite inoculation. This coincided with the short summer-time mosquito breeding season in these cold countries. These strains of *P. vivax* (e.g. *P. vivax* hibernans) acquired in northern and eastern Europe, Russia, central and northern China, and North Korea are now nearly extinct.

In the artificial infection experiments the differences in recorded incubation periods between strains of the same plasmodia species were small, although a negative correlation was apparent between the probable dose of sporozoites and the duration of the prepatent period (the time from sporozoite inoculation until the first positive blood film). The incubation period (time from sporozoite inoculation to fever) was prolonged by ineffective antimalarial treatment or prophylaxis—which reduced the effective multiplication rate. In simultaneous infection with *P. falciparum* and *P. vivax*, the former suppresses the latter, and the primary vivax malaria infection may not appear until several weeks later.[44] Sometimes the reverse occurs and *P. vivax* suppresses *P. falciparum*. In many areas outside Africa *P. falciparum* and *P. vivax* are both common and coexistent infections are frequent. For example in Thailand approximately 30% of patients with *P. falciparum* malaria will have a subsequent symptomatic infection with *P. vivax* within 2 months of their primary falciparum malaria, but without further exposure to malaria infection.[252]

The durations of the prepatent and incubation periods are also strongly influenced by previous exposure, i.e. 'immunity'. Effective immunity both reduces effective multiplication, which prolongs the prepatent period, and raises the threshold at which symptoms occur (premunition), which prolongs the incubation period. In vivax malaria the symptom threshold is raised disproportionately in immune individuals, i.e. the gap between the prepatent and incubation period widens.

PYROGENIC DENSITY

The parasitaemia at which fever (>37.3°C) occurs is termed the 'pyrogenic density'. This varies widely: some non-immune patients will become febrile before parasites are visible on blood smears (i.e. the incubation period is shorter than the prepatent period), whereas immune adults can on occasions tolerate up to 100 000 *P. falciparum* parasites/µl without fever. The pyrogenic density for *P. vivax* is generally lower than that of *P. falciparum*; in 76% of cases reported by Kitchen[44] the pyrogenic density was <100 parasites/µl. In *P. falciparum* infection average pyrogenic densitites in non-immunes can be as high as 10 000/µl, but it must be remembered that only half the life cycle circulates in falciparum malaria. The parasites in the blood smear are the circulating parasites in the generation subsequent to that which underwent pyrogenic merogony, and they are therefore an underestimate of the total parasite burden. The pyrogenic density is a marker of immunity. High pyrogenic densities indicate premunition, and a lower risk of severe disease. There are less data on pyrogenic densities in *P. malariae* infections, but it appears that they are higher than for *P. vivax*; values over 500/µl were found in 38% of Boyd's cases. There are limited data on *P. ovale*, but the available evidence suggests a pyrogenic density similar to *P. vivax*.

UNCOMPLICATED MALARIA

The clinical features of uncomplicated malaria are common to all four species, although there is a suggestion that *P. vivax*, which tends to synchronize rapidly, may cause more severe symptoms early in the course of the infection. *P. ovale* and *P. malariae* both have a more gradual onset than *P. vivax*. *P. falciparum* is unpredictable: the onset ranges from gradual to fulminant. The first symptoms of malaria are non-specific and resemble influenza. They are similar for all four species of *Plasmodium*. Headache, muscular ache, vague abdominal discomfort, lethargy, lassitude and dysphoria often precede fever by up to 2 days. The temperature rises erratically at first, with shivering, mild chills, worsening headache and malaise, and loss of appetite. Chil-

dren are irritable, lethargic and anorexic. If the infection is left untreated the fever in *P. vivax* and *P. ovale* regularizes to a 2-day cycle (tertian), and *P. malariae* fever spikes occur every 3 days (quartan pattern). *P. falciparum* remains erratic for longer, and may never regularize to a tertian pattern. These terms derive from the Greek practice of inclusive reckoning, in which the beginning of the fever is considered day 1. Thus, a tertian fever recurs every *third* day and a quartan fever every *fourth* day, with intervals of 2 and 3 days respectively. Some infections consist of two broods cycling 24 hours out of phase and in these there is a daily fever spike (quotidian fever). Even more complex fever patterns are described in detail in the early literature.

The classical malaria fever charts (which graced earlier editions of this textbook), and the teeth-chattering rigors and profuse sweats that characterized the 'paroxysm', are relatively unusual today as malaria therapy of neurosyphilis is no longer practised (penicillin is more effective and more pleasant), and symptomatic infections are treated as soon as they are diagnosed. In a true paroxysm the temperature usually rises steeply from a normal or slightly elevated level to exceed 39°C. As the temperature begins to rise there is intense headache and muscular discomfort. The patient feels cold, clutches at blankets, and curls up shivering and uncommunicative (the chill). There is peripheral vasoconstriction, and often 'goose-pimples'. Within minutes the limbs begin to shake and the teeth chatter, and the temperature climbs rapidly to a peak (usually between 39 and 41.5°C). The rigor usually last 10–30 minutes, but can last up to 90 minutes. By the end of the rigor there is peripheral vasodilatation and the skin feels hot. A profuse sweat then breaks out. The blood pressure is relatively low and there may be symptomatic orthostatic hypotension.[257–259] The patient feels exhausted and may sleep. Defervescence usually takes 4–8 hours. Paroxysms with rigors are more common in *P. vivax* (Figure 61.10) and *P. ovale* than in *P. falciparum* or *P. malariae* malaria. True rigors are unusual in naturally acquired faciparum malaria. As the infection continues the spleen and liver enlarge and anaemia develops. The patient loses weight. If no treatment is given the natural infection stabilizes for several weeks or months and then gradually resolves. The duration of illness is proportional to the level of immunity and differs between the parasite species. Mild abdominal discomfort is common in malaria, and rarely patients may appear to have an 'acute abdomen'. Constipation or diarrhoea may occur. In some areas watery diarrhoea is a prominent manifestation. However, there is usually no difficulty distinguishing malaria from gastroenteri-

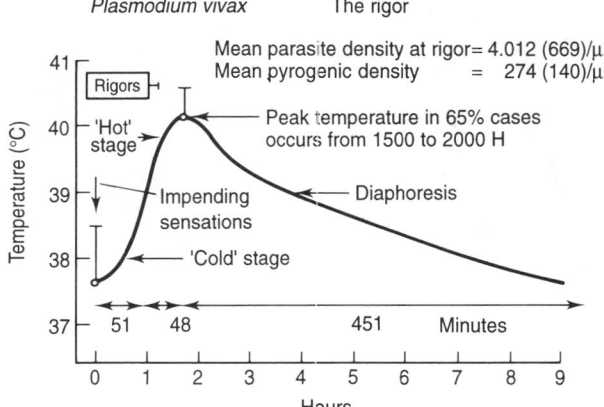

Figure 61.10   The rigor of *P. vivax* malaria. The time course of signs and symptoms is taken from Kitchen & Puttnam *Journal of the National Malaria Society* 1946; 5:57–78. True rigors are rare in *P. falciparum* malaria and occur only after the infections with the other three parasites have synchronized sufficiently.

tis. A dry cough has been reported in some series, but this is not as prominent as in typhoid, and on chest examination there is no other clinical evidence of respiratory tract involvement. However, the respiratory rate may be raised, particularly in children, and this can give rise to diagnostic confusion in primary health care facilities where respiratory rate is used as the only criterion for the diagnosis of acute respiratory infection. In routine clinical practice in malarious areas of the tropics, malaria is the most common cause of fever in children and is the most likely diagnosis in a febrile patient with no obvious respiratory or abdominal abnormalities. In travellers returning from such areas any fever must be considered to be malaria unless proved otherwise. In semi-immune patients low-grade fever may be the only complaint in malaria. In tropical practice malaria is so common that it must be excluded in any febrile patient.

RELAPSE

Both *P. vivax* and *P. ovale* have a tendency to relapse after resolution of the primary infection. Relapse, which results from maturation of persistent hypnozoites in the liver, must be distinguished from recrudescence of the primary infection because of incomplete treatment. *P. falciparum* is the usual cause of recrudescent infections and these tend to arise 2–4 weeks following treatment (but this can be as long as 10 weeks following mefloquine treatment). Relapses occur weeks or months (or even years) after the primary infection. The pattern of relapse is determined largely by the geographic

origin of the infection. Subtropical *P. vivax* tends to have long gaps between relapses (as in Patrick Manson's famous experiment where he infected his son with *P. vivax*, and relapsed 9 months later) whereas tropical strains have short intervals (3–6 weeks). The symptoms of a relapse start more abruptly than in the primary infection as the infection is more synchronous. They may begin with an abrupt chill or rigor. Primaquine will eradicate hypnozoites in over 80% of patients but, if it is not given, relapse occurs in approximately half of those infected. The proportion of cases relapsing and the intervals between relapses vary between strains.

MALARIA IN PREGNANCY

In areas of intense transmission the principal impact of falciparum malaria in pregnancy is an increased incidence of anaemia and a reduction in birth weight (approximately 170 g on average) of babies born to primigravidae.[19,212] Thus a greater proportion of babies have low birth weights (<2.5 kg). Despite intense sequestration of parasites in the placenta,[210] the mothers are usually asymptomatic. In areas with less transmission (mesoendemic or hypoendemic) symptomatic disease occurs and pregnant women are at an increased risk of severe falciparum malaria,[89] particularly in the second and third trimesters. The adverse effects of malaria on birth weight now extend to the first three pregnancies (and in non-immunes, probably to all pregnancies).[218] If pregnant women develop severe malaria, fetal loss is common, and the maternal mortality is also high. Acute pulmonary oedema and hypoglycaemia are particular complications. The mortality of cerebral malaria in pregnancy is approximately 50%, compared with approximately 20% in non-pregnant adults. The adverse effects of *P. vivax* on pregnancy have not been defined adequately.

MALARIA IN CHILDREN (Figure 61.11)

The majority of childhood malaria infections present with fever and malaise, and respond rapidly to antimalarial treatment. Severe falciparum malaria is rare in infancy, although when it does occur the mortality is high. In young children the progression of falciparum malaria can be rapid. Generalized seizures are more common in *P. falciparum* than *P. vivax* malaria, even in the absence of other signs

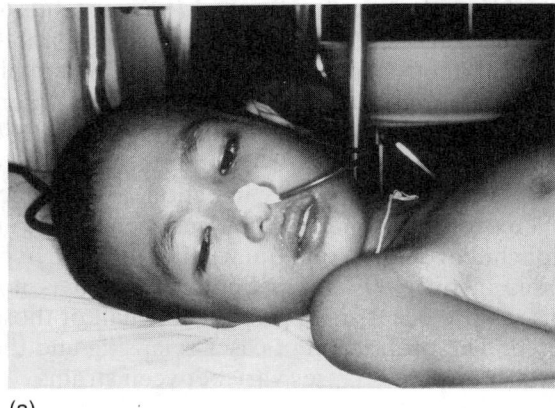
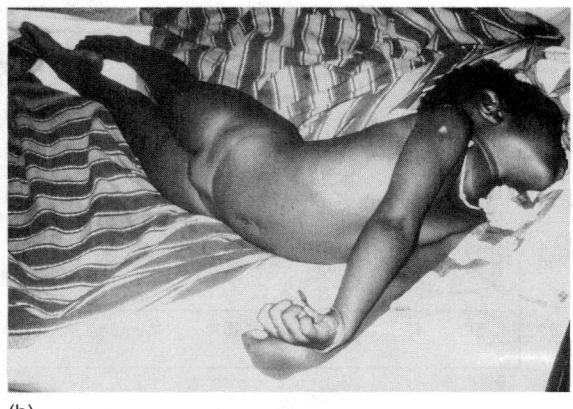

(a)   (b)

Figure 61.11 (a) A 6-year-old Thai boy with cerebral malaria. His father was admitted at the same time with cerebral malaria—both survived. (b) A 3-year-old Gambian girl with cerebral malaria and opisthotonos (courtesy Jane Crawley).

of cerebral involvement. Coma, convulsions, lactic acidosis, hypoglycaemia and severe anaemia are common presenting features of severe malaria in childhood. At the bedside, the presence of respiratory distress or deep coma defines children at high risk of dying. In areas of intense transmission profound anaemia is the usual manifestation of severe malaria, and this occurs in the 1–3-year age group. Severe malaria is rare in older children. In areas of less stable transmission cerebral malaria becomes the predominant manifestation of severe disease, and the age range shifts upwards. Jaundice and pulmonary oedema are unusual in young children, and renal failure is very rare (a dramatic difference compared with adults). As a consequence fluid balance is less of a problem than in adults, although intravenous fluid administration must be carefully supervised in small children and hypovolsemia treated promptly. Convulsions are common, particularly in the <3-year age group, and should be treated promptly. Aspiration pneumonia is a potentially lethal sequel. Phenobarbitone prevents convulsions in adults but the dose and effectiveness in children have yet to be determined. We give all comatose children a single intramuscular injection of phenobarbitone (7 mg/kg) but this dose may be insufficient. Hypoglycaemia is common, and is often accompanied by lactic acidosis. The blood glucose should be checked frequently and, where possible, continuous intravenous infusions of 5% or 10% dextrose given as a preventative measure.

In general children tolerate the antimalarial drugs better than adults, and their symptoms resolve more quickly. The temptation to estimate body weight by 'eye' should be resisted, and all children should be weighed so that the doses of antimalarial drugs can be given on a mg/kg basis. (Although administration of drugs adjusted to surface area is theoretically preferable, antimalarial doses have been devised on the basis of body weight.) Children with acute malaria vomit readily, particularly if the temperature is high. Oral antimalarial treatment is more likely to be retained if the child is cool and calm before drug administration. In busy tropical clinics only a minority of patients can be admitted to hospital, and many children with moderately severe malaria have to be treated on an outpatient basis. It is common practice to administer a single dose of parenteral chloroquine or quinine and to send the patient home with the remainder of the oral regimen, and to give the parents advice to return if the child deteriorates further. In this situation there is a danger of significant iatrogenic hypotension if the child is kept upright (e.g. on the mother's back). If possible the child should be observed for at least 2 hours following parenteral drug administration and reassessed before discharge.

SEVERE MALARIA

Death from acute *P. vivax*, *P. ovale* or *P. malariae* infections is very rare. Occasionally already debilitated patients may succumb, and fatal haemorrhage may follow a ruptured spleen[9] (either traumatic or spontaneous), but these events are very uncommon. There have been many case reports of 'cerebral vivax malaria' but none of these is entirely convincing, i.e. clinical details were sketchy, or coexistent falciparum malaria could not be excluded. If it does occur it must be rare. On the contrary falciparum malaria is a potentially lethal infection. The progression to severe disease can be rapid. In young children presenting with cerebral malaria a history of less than 1 day's illness is common. Severe malaria is rare in malnourished children and often seems to strike down the healthiest people. The great malariologist Ettore Marchiafava noted over 100 years ago how common severe malaria was in the 'hale and hearty' Italian shepherds who descended from the malaria-free mountains to the malarious valleys every autumn.[247] In adults, patients with severe malaria usually have a history of being ill for several days before admission to hospital.

The following definition of severe falciparum malaria has been proposed by a working group convened by the World Health Organization (WHO).[248]

1. Cerebral malaria—unrousable coma not attributable to any other cause in a patient with falciparum malaria. The coma should persist for at least 30 minutes after a generalized convulsion to make the distinction from transient postictal coma.
2. Severe anaemia—normocytic anaemia with haematocrit <15% or haemoglobin <5 g/dl in the presence of parasitaemia more than 10 000/μl. If anaemia is hypochromic and/or microcytic, iron deficiency and thalassaemia/haemoglobinopathy must be excluded. (These criteria are rather generous; a parasitaemia of >100 000/μl might be a more appropriate threshold.)
3. Renal failure—defined as a urine output of less than 400 ml in 24 hours in adults, or 12 ml/kg in 24 hours in children, failing to improve after rehydration, and a serum creatinine of more than 265 μmol/l (>3.0 mg/dl). (In practice, for initial assessment, the serum creatinine alone is used.)
4. Pulmonary oedema or adult respiratory distress syndrome.
5. Hypoglycaemia—defined as a whole blood glucose concentration of less than 2.2 mmol/l (40 mg/dl).
6. Circulatory collapse or shock—hypotension (systolic blood pressure <50 mmHg in children aged 1–5 years or <70 mmHg in adults), with cold clammy skin or core–skin temperature difference >10°C.
7. Spontaneous bleeding from gums, nose, gastrointestinal tract, etc., and/or substantial laboratory evidence of DIC.
8. Repeated generalized convulsions—more than two observed within 24 hours despite cooling. (In young children, these may be febrile convulsions, and the other clinical and parasitological features need to be taken into account.)
9. Acidaemia—defined as an arterial pH <7.25, or acidosis defined as a plasma bicarbonate concentration <15 mmol/l.
10. Macroscopic haemoglobinuria—if definitely associated with acute malaria infection and not merely the result of oxidant antimalarial drugs in patients with erythrocyte enzyme defects such as G6PD deficiency. (This is difficult to ascertain in practice: if the G6PD status is checked following massive haemolysis, the value in the remaining red cells may be normal even in mild G6PD deficiency. This definition is not very useful.)
11. Postmortem confirmation of diagnosis. In fatal cases a diagnosis of severe falciparum malaria can be confirmed by histological examination of a postmortem needle necropsy of the brain. The characteristic features, found especially in cerebral grey matter, are venules/capillaries packed with erythrocytes containing mature trophozoites and schizonts of *P. falciparum*. (These features may not be present in patients who die several days after the start of treatment, although there is usually some residual pigment.)

One or more of the above features in the presence of asexual parasitaemia defines severe falciparum malaria. Other manifestations of severe malaria which (according to the WHO document) do not in themselves define the condition in all geographical areas and age groups include the following.

1. Impairment of consciousness less marked than unrousable coma. (However, any impairment of consciousness must be treated seriously.)
2. Prostration or weakness, so that the patient cannot sit or walk, with no obvious neurological explanation. ('Cannot' should be distinguished from 'does not want to'!)
3. Hyperparasitaemia—the relation of parasitaemia to severity of illness is different in different populations and age groups, but in general very high parasite densities are associated with increased risk of severe disease, e.g. >5% parasitaemia is dangerous in non-immunes, but may be well tolerated in semi-immune children. (In practice, any parasitaemia over 2% carries an increased risk of a fatal outcome, and most authorities would regard a parasitaemia over 10% as indicating a potentially dangerous infection irrespective of the other features.)
4. Jaundice—detected clinically or defined by a serum bilirubin concentration >50 μmol/l (3.0 mg/dl).
5. Hyperpyrexia—rectal temperature above 40°C in adults and children. (Sustained hyperpyrexia in severe malaria indicates a poor prognosis.)

In severe malaria there is often evidence of multiple vital organ dysfunction, and more than one of the above criteria are fulfilled. Physicians should not worry unduly about definitions or semantics. They should treat any patient about whom they are worried as having severe malaria, even if they do not fall clearly into one of the above categories.

CEREBRAL MALARIA

This may be defined strictly as unrousable coma (i.e. there is a non-purposeful response or no response to a painful stimulus) in falciparum malaria. In practice any patient with altered consciousness should be treated for severe malaria. Although cerebral malaria is the most prominent feature of severe falciparum malaria, some patients with ultimately lethal infections never lose consciousness until they die. In cerebral malaria the onset of coma may be sudden, often following a generalized seizure, or gradual, with initial drowsiness, confusion, disorientation, delirium or agitation, followed by unconsciousness. Extreme agitation is a poor prognostic sign in falciparum malaria. The length of the prodromal history is usually several days in adults, but in children can be as short as 6–12 hours. A history of convulsions is common.[249]

On examination the patient is febrile and unrousable. There may be some passive resistance to hand flexion, but the board-like rigidity of meningitis is not found, and there are no other signs of meningeal irritation. There may be anaemia, which in some cases, particularly children, may be profound. Conversely jaundice is relatively unusual in children but common in adults. Signs of bleeding are unusual (<5%) and indicate a poor prognosis. The patient is usually warm, dry and well perfused peripherally, with a low–normal blood pressure and a sinus tachycardia. Skin perfusion is variable, intermittent 'goose-pimples' are common in association with cutaneous vasoconstriction. Sustained hyperventilation is a poor prognostic sign as it indicates metabolic acidosis if the chest is clear, or pneumonia or pulmonary oedema if it is not. The liver and spleen are commonly enlarged, but soft. Massive splenomegaly is not found. There is no lymphadenopathy and no rash. The clinical features are usually of a symmetrical encephalopathy. Focal signs are unusual. On examination of the nervous system the gaze is usually normal or divergent (but there is no evidence of extraocular muscle paresis) (Figure 61.12). The pupils are usually mid-size and equally reactive and the fundus is unremarkable. Papilloedema is rare (<1% cases) but retinal haemorrhages may be seen in 15% of cases[250] (more if indirect

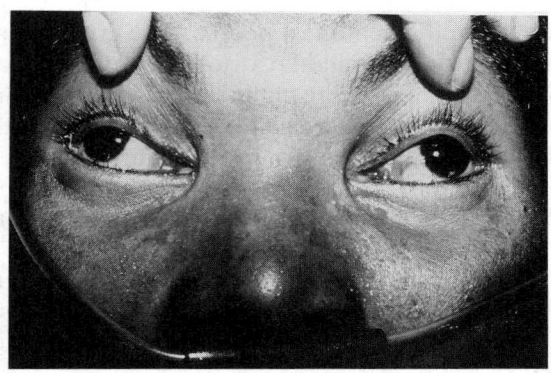

Figure 61.12   Divergent gaze in a 42-year-old Burmese woman with cerebral malaria.

ophthalmoscopy is used). The haemorrhages are often flame shaped, and may have a pale centre resembling Roth spots. They rarely affect the macula. In adult patients the corneal reflexes are usually preserved but in children with deep coma they may be lost (a poor prognostic sign). There may be forced jaw closure with repetitive spontaneous teeth grinding (bruxism). The jaw jerk is sometimes brisk and there is often a pout reflex. Other frontal release signs are very unusual. Cranial nerve abnormalities are rare. Tone may be increased, decreased or normal. Likewise the reflexes can be brisk or depressed. The abdominal reflexes are invariably absent, the cremasteric reflexes often preserved, and the plantar responses extensor in approximately half the patients. Patients may exhibit phasic increases in tone with extensor posturing of the decorticate (arm flexed, legs extended), or more usually decerebrate (arms and legs extended) types. The back may arch as in opisthotonus, with sustained, usually upward and lateral, ocular deviation. The posturing is commonly associated with noisy hyperventilation. Generalized or sometimes focal seizures may occur. The duration of coma varies considerably but overall is shorter in children (average 1 day) than in adults (average 2–3 days).

Untreated cerebral malaria is probably uniformly fatal. The overall mortality of treated cerebral malaria obviously depends on the referral practices and medical facilities available, but in reported studies averages 15% in children and 20% in adults (but up to 50% in pregnancy).[89] Some series have reported lower mortalities, but in these the definition of cerebral malaria has been more 'generous', i.e. they have included patients who were obtunded or delirious but not unrousable. Hospitals acting as secondary or tertiary referral centres often experience higher mortalities as they see a residue of more severe patients. The later the patient is referred, the higher the mortality. In the Vietnam war, the mortality of acute falciparum malaria was higher in soldiers who had returned to the USA than it was in Vietnam.[251] Obviously the diagnosis was made much more rapidly in Vietnam where physicians were well aware of malaria, than in the USA where they were not.

CASE HISTORY

A 2-year-old girl is brought to a provincial African hospital by her mother in the afternoon. She has had two generalized convulsions in the morning, and she was unrousable after the first of these. Her mother noticed she did not eat the previous evening and that she had a fever, but before that she appeared to be well (although the mother had been working in the fields the previous day, and so could not be exact as to the time when symptoms began). After the first convulsion the child has been taken to a health centre where a presumptive diagnosis of malaria was made, and a single intramuscular injection of chloroquine given before the child was referred on to hospital. In the past the child had received her immunizations, and had received treatment for malaria in the previous rainy season. She had also had several febrile episodes which the mother had treated at home with chloroquine and traditional medicines, and these had resolved without complications.

On examination the child was unrousably comatose with only a non-localized motor response to a painful stimulus (Blantyre coma score 1).[249] She was not anaemic or jaundiced, and she weighed 8 kg. The blood pressure was 85/65 mmHg, the pulse 138/min, and the rectal temperature 40.1°C. The child was not clinically dehydrated. The respiratory rate was 52/min with use of accessory muscles of respiration and flaring of the alar nasae. There were coarse breath sounds, particularly over the left lung field. The spleen tip was palpable and the liver 3 cm enlarged. There was some passive resistance to head flexion, but no other evidence of meningeal irritation. On fundoscopy a flame-shaped haemorrhage with a pale centre was visible adjacent to the superior nasal artery in the left eye. The optic discs were flat. The eyes were divergent. Positive findings on examination of the central and peripheral nervous systems were a pout reflex, a symmetrical increase in tone, and extensor plantar responses. Intermittent extensor posturing of the 'decerebrate' type, with extended arms and legs, sustained upward gaze, and hyperventilation lasting 10–15 seconds, occurred every 5 minutes. Blood was taken and an intravenous infusion of 5% dextrose water

was started. A glucose oxidase stick test indicated the blood glucose was only 1.1 mmol/l; 8 ml (0.5 g/kg) of 50% dextrose was given by slow intravenous injection and the infusion was changed to 10% dextrose. There was no improvement in her clinical condition. The haematocrit was read as 36% and the parasitaemia on brief microscopic examination of the thin film was heavy; a subsequent count gave a value of 136/1000 red cells. Over 20% of the parasites were mature trophozoites, i.e. parasite-associated pigment was visible, and over 5% of the neutrophils contained phagocytosed pigment. Chloroquine-resistant falciparum malaria is prevalent in the area, and so an infusion of quinine dihydrochloride was started. A loading dose of 160 mg (20 mg salt/kg) was drawn up (as close as possible to 0.53 ml of a 300 mg/ml solution in a 1 ml syringe) and injected into a 120 ml burette (infusion chamber) with 10% dextrose and set to run at 30 ml/hour. (The hospital was fortunate to have a stock of paediatric infusion sets but if these had not been available, the quinine could have been given by intramuscular injection.) A single intramuscular injection of phenobarbital 7 mg/kg was then given. A lumbar puncture was performed; the CSF was clear, there was free rise and fall with respiration, and the opening pressure was recorded as 140 mm CSF. Tepid sponging brought the rectal temperature down to 38.3°C. The posturing lessened in intensity and frequency. The vital signs remained stable over the next 4 hours and the chest remained clear, but the respiratory rate increased to 60/min. The bed was wet, indicating that urine had been passed. A repeat blood glucose at 4 hours was 3.2 mmol/l. At 5 hours the blood pressure was 80/50, pulse 150/min, temperature 37.7°C and respiratory rate 62/min. The coma score was still 1, and the neurological signs were unchanged. Twenty minutes later the respiration became ataxic, and then stopped. She could not be resuscitated.

Comment

This child with cerebral malaria had several poor prognostic features on admission to hospital: deep coma, convulsions, extensor posturing, hyperventilation, hyperparasitaemia, a predominance of mature parasites on the peripheral blood smear, pigment in peripheral blood leucocytes and hypoglycaemia. The admitting physician was aware immediately that the outlook was bleak from the combination of coma and respiratory distress. The short history and absence of anaemia together with the high parasite count suggest a fulminant infection. The predominance of mature parasites suggests the possibility of a much greater sequestered parasite biomass than that evident from the peripheral parasitaemia. She was hypoglycaemic and almost certainly had lactic acidosis. Although the best available parenteral antimalarial treatment was started as soon as the diagnosis was made, irreversible pathological processes may already have taken place. As in many fatal cases in children, the exact cause of the final respiratory arrest was not known.

CONVULSIONS

Seizures are common, particularly in young children. They are particularly associated with falciparum malaria even in uncomplicated infections. In the majority of cases the child recovers uneventfully following one or two generalized convulsions, but some patients do not recover consciousness rapidly (<30 minutes) and remain unrousable (cerebral malaria). Focal seizures may also occur, but they are less common. Aspiration pneumonia is a common and preventable sequel to grand mal seizures. (Repeated grand mal seizures in cerebral malaria are associated with residual neurological sequelae.)

POSTMALARIA NEUROLOGICAL SYNDROMES

In approximately 3% of adults and 10% of children there is a persistent neurological deficit following cerebral malaria (Figure 61.13).[21,249] In children this is associated with profound and protracted coma, anaemia, hypoglycaemia and prolonged convulsions. In approximately 60% of cases there is a hemiparesis with variable hemisensory deficit and sometimes hemianopia. Cortical blindness, diffuse cortical damage, tremor and occasionally cranial

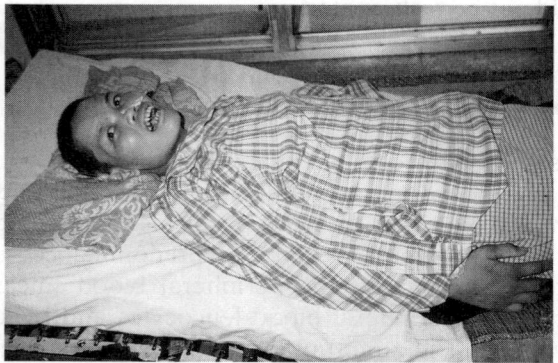

Figure 61.13 Permanent global residual neurological deficit following prolonged hypoglycaemia in a 33-year-old Vietnamese woman who had cerebral malaria in pregnancy. She had received intravenous quinine but despite parenteral glucose administration became repeatedly hypoglycaemic.

nerve palsies may occur.[21,249,252,253] Six months later complete recovery from postcerebral malaria neurological deficit has occurred in 50% of cases, partial recovery has occurred in 25% of cases, and the remainder of patients have not recovered.[21] The possibility that cerebral malaria causes persistent subclinical intellectual deficits in survivors has not been explored.

Rarely patients who recover from cerebral malaria may lapse into coma again, usually after a period of 1–2 days when they are rousable. In this condition the CSF protein may be elevated (200–300 mg/dl) and there is sometimes an increase in CSF lymphocytes. There may be residual neurological deficit on recovery. A variety of other late neurological complications may occur. These include psychosis, encephalopathy, tremor and cerebellar dysfunction. These postmalaria neurological syndromes may also follow uncomplicated malaria and could account for some of the cases previously attributed to mefloquine or chloroquine neurotoxicity. The conditions are self-limiting and usually resolve over several days, or sometimes 1–2 weeks. The syndrome of cerebellar ataxia occurring 2–3 weeks after acute uncomplicated malaria appears to be relatively common in Sri Lanka.[253,254] It too is usually self-limiting with recovery over a few weeks.

ACUTE RENAL FAILURE

In some adult patients with severe malaria acute oliguric renal failure and other vital organ dysfunction is present on admission, whereas in others renal dysfunction becomes evident as the patient recovers from the acute phase of severe disease.[152,256–258] In the former fulminant presentation there is a high incidence of associated hepatic dysfunction and metabolic acidosis, and pulmonary oedema is the usual terminal event. The blood pressure is normal. Jaundice is common and there may be a bleeding tendency. There may be slight proteinuria, but the urine sediment is unremarkable. The subacute presentation carries a better prognosis. The patient may be oliguric or sometimes polyuric. The serum creatinine rises over a period of days until either dialysis is required because of hyperkalaemia or uraemic complications such as bleeding, pleural or pericardial effusions, encephalopathy or intractable vomiting, or there is gradual resolution with an increase in urine output. In the subacute presentation of acute renal failure parasitaemia may have cleared following antimalarial treatment before the patient is referred to hospital.[152] Although acute renal failure is a common complication of malaria in adults living in areas of low or unstable transmission, it is rare in children. Indeed in high-transmission areas it is almost unheard of. Renal failure is also associated with haemoglobinuria in patients with massive haemolysis[258] (see below, Blackwater Fever).

METABOLIC ACIDOSIS

Hyperventilation with increased inspiratory effort and a clear chest on auscultation (Kussmaul's breathing) suggests metabolic acidosis. This may result from renal failure in adults, but more usually there is a primary ('type B') lactic acidosis. The outlook is poor. Although blood pressure and tissue perfusion is usually adequate initially, hypotension commonly ensues.

BLACKWATER FEVER

The sinister reputation of blackwater fever derives from the high mortality (20–30%) documented in Europeans and Asians working in colonial Africa in the first half of the twentieth century.[154,155,258,259] Approximately half of these deaths were caused by renal failure. G. R. Ross,[259] writing from Southern Rhodesia (Zimbabwe), described blackwater fever as 'a disease to blanch the cheek of the bravest', and such was its reputation that magistrates considered it as an excuse for a felony! Today the mortality is much lower. Indeed the passage of black or dark-brown–red urine (blackwater) is often not associated with significant renal impairment. Blackwater is usually transient and resolves without complications, but in severe cases renal failure may develop.[260] This behaves as acute tubular necrosis. Blackwater results from massive haemolysis. Transfused blood is also rapidly haemolysed. The mortality is highest when blackwater fever is associated with severe malaria and other evidence of vital organ dysfunction. Patients with blackwater fever and severe anaemia often have a slate-grey appearance, and their plasma may be red (haemoglobinaemia).

ACUTE PULMONARY OEDEMA

Hyperventilation or Kussmaul's breathing (sometimes termed respiratory distress) is a poor prognostic sign in malaria. In the tachypnoea associated with high fever, breathing is shallow compared with the ominous laboured hyperventilation associated with metabolic acidosis, pulmonary oedema or pneumonia. Acute pulmonary oedema may develop at any time in severe falciparum malaria. It is particularly common in pregnant women, but rare in children. This is one form of the adult respiratory distress syndrome,[156,157,261–263] and in some cases may be difficult to distinguish clinically from aspiration pneumonia. The central venous pressure and pulmonary artery occlusion pressures are usually normal (unless the patient has been overhydrated) and the heart sounds are normal. The chest radiograph shows increased interstitial shadowing and a normal heart size.

HYPOTENSION

The majority of patients with severe malaria are febrile, with a high cardiac output, a low systemic vascular resistance and a low–normal blood pressure. They are usually warm and well perfused. Patients with severe disease may develop sudden hypotension and become shocked. This is called 'algid malaria'.[264,265] In a proportion of cases there is bacterial septicaemia, but in the majority blood cultures are negative. Shock usually responds temporarily to saline infusion and inotropes, but pulmonary oedema may be provoked if too much salt is given and left sided filling pressures (pulmonary artery wedge pressures) rise above 15 mmHg. The overall mortality is high. Orthostatic hypotension is common in acute uncomplicated malaria.[266,267] It is associated with impaired reflex cardioacceleration and is worsened by the quinoline antimalarial drugs.[268]

HYPOGLYCAEMIA

Hypoglycaemia is either asymptomatic in severely ill patients, or presents as a further deterioration in the level of coma.[197–199,269] In severe malaria the usual signs of sweating and increased sympathetic nervous system activity are commonly absent or indistinguishable from the signs of malaria. Hypoglycaemia occurs in approximately 8% of adults and 30% of children with cerebral malaria. The clinical response to glucose is usually unimpressive. In pregnant women with quinine-stimulated hyperinsulinaemic hypoglycaemia, the clinical features of hypoglycaemia are usually evident, and the patient responds dramatically to glucose. Hypoglycaemia can be prevented by intravenous dextrose infusions.

ANAEMIA

The degree of anaemia and the rate at which it develops vary enormously. The haemoglobin concentration may fall by up to 2 g/dl each day. Anaemia is a particular problem in children, where it may lead to high-output cardiac failure and sudden death. These complications are particularly likely with haemoglobin concentrations below 4 g/dl (12% haematocrit). Some patients appear to tolerate severe malarial anaemia relatively well. These patients usually have an underlying chronic anae-mia, and have adapted to increased oxygen carriage (right-shifted oxygen dissociation curve). Thus it is both the absolute haemoglobin concentration and the magnitude of the fall that determine the clinical consequences.

LATER PROBLEMS

Patients with severe malaria may have persistent fever after parasite clearance. Although a proportion of cases have an identifiable chest or urinary tract infection, or in children blood cultures may grow *Salmonella* spp.,[221] the majority of cases have no clear explanation and the fever eventually resolves in a few days without further treatment.

LABORATORY FINDINGS

HAEMATOLOGY

There is a progressive normochromic normocytic anaemia. The white count is usually normal, but may be raised in very severe malaria, and very occasionally there is a leucoerythroblastic picture. There is slight monocytosis and eosinopenia, with reactive eosinophilia in the weeks following the acute infection.[271] The platelet count is reduced in all acute malarias, usually to around 100 000/μl, but thrombocytopenia is profound in some cases.[179–183] Fibrinogen levels are usually elevated—a reduction indicates significant DIC. The fibrin degradation products are elevated.[175–177] There is evidence of increased coagulation cascade activity through intrinsic pathway activation with antithrombin III depletion that is proportional to disease severity and there may be prolongation of the prothrombin and partial thromboplastin times.[178,438] Polymorphonuclear leucocyte elastase levels are elevated in severe infection, suggesting[272] neutrophil activation.

ACUTE PHASE PROTEINS

The C-reative protein, orosomucoid (α_1-acid glycoprotein) and fibrinogen levels are raised, and immunoglobulin levels rise while albumin falls. Cytokine levels are raised in acute malaria; there are increased concentrations of circulating cytokine receptors, and there is an increase in urinary neopterin.[273]

BIOCHEMISTRY

There may be mild hyponatraemia[274] but the potassium is normal. The serum bicarbonate is often reduced and the anion gap widens in proportion to the acidosis. In adults the serum creatinine and blood urea may be raised, with an increased urea to creatinine ratio. Total and conjugated bilirubin may be elevated, the transaminase concentrations are often raised, and there may also be slight elevation of the hepatic alkaline phosphatase concentration. In children the 5-nucleotidase is raised in proportion to disease severity. Creatine phosphokinase, myoglobin and plasma urate levels are elevated in adults and children with severe malaria.[275] The serum calcium may be low and hypophosphataemia may be profound in severe infections.[202] Hypoglycaemia may occur, and in the absence of quinine treatment this is accompanied by elevated ketones, raised lactate and alanine, and low insulin levels.[197–199] Lactate levels in arterial or venous blood, or CSF, are elevated in proportion to disease severity.[148]

CEREBROSPINAL FLUID

The CSF is usually normal in cerebral malaria, but moderately raised concentrations of protein are common (sometimes up to 200 mg/dl). There may be up to 10 cells/μl, and on occasions up to 50 are seen (all lymphocytes). The lactate concentration is raised in proportion to disease severity, and the glucose is often slightly low relative to blood.[148,277,278] If the patient is deeply jaundiced the CSF may appear yellow.

PROGNOSTIC FACTORS

The prognostic factors listed in Table 61.3 reflect vital organ dysfunction and the magnitude of the parasite burden. They are not absolute, and in fatal cases several factors usually coexist. Some of the apparently poor prognostic factors can have a benign explanation. Hyperventilation (respiratory distress) is usually a bad sign (indicating pulmonary oedema, pneumonia or metabolic acidosis), but tachypnoea can result from high fever alone (the tidal volume is lower). Upper gastrointestinal bleeding in cerebral malaria may also occur spontaneously. The prognostic implications of severe anaemia depend on the rate at which the haematocrit falls, the coexisting parasitaemia and the stage of the infection. If anaemia develops gradually then even haemoglobin values less than 5 g/dl (packed cell volume <15%) can be surprisingly well tolerated as there is time for homeostatic adaptations such as the right shift in the oxygen dissociation curve, the increase in cardiac index and the fall in

Table 61.3 Features indicating a poor prognosis in severe *P. falciparum* malaria.

Clinical

Agitation	Deep coma
Hyperventilation	Convulsions
Hypothermia (<36.5°C)	Anuria
Sustained hyperthermia (>39°C)	Jaundice
Bleeding	Shock
Severe anaemia (PCV <15%)	

Laboratory
Biochemistry

Hypoglycaemia	<2.2 mmol/l
Hyperlactataemia	>5 mmol/l
Acidosis	Arterial pH <7.3, serum HCO_3 <15 mmol/l
Serum creatinine	>265 μmol/l
Total bilirubin	>50 μmol/l
Liver enzymes	sGOT (AST) ×3 upper limit of normal
	sGPT (ALT) ×3 upper limit of normal
	5-Nucleotidase ↑
Muscle enzymes	CPK ↑
	Myoglobin ↑
Urate	>600 μmol/l

Haematology

Leucocytosis	>12 000/μl
	Severe anaemia (PCV <15%)
Coagulopathy	Platelets <50 000/μl
	Prothrombin time prolonged >3 s
	Prolonged partial thromboplastin time
	Fibrinogen: <200 mg/dl

Parasitology
Hyperparasitaemia >100 000/μl—increased mortality
                          >500 000/μl—high mortality
>20% of parasites are pigment-containing trophozoites and schizonts
>5% of neutrophils contain visible pigment

PCV, packed cell volume; sGOT (AST), serum glutamic oxaloacetic transferase (aspartate aminotransferase); sGPT (ALT), serum glutamic pyruvic transaminase (alanine aminotransferase); CPK, creatine phosphokinase.

systemic vascular resistance. Hypotension is a poor prognostic sign only when associated with poor tissue perfusion. Patients, particularly children, with acute malaria often have very low blood pressures but they are warm and well perfused. The biochemical measures are in general proportional to severity, but individual abnormalities can have other explanations. For example, hypoglycaemia carries a fivefold higher mortality in severe malaria, but in pregnant women treated with quinine hypoglycaemia may occur in uncomplicated infections because of quinine-stimulated hyperinsulinaemia. The concentration of lactate in venous or arterial blood or CSF in linearly proportional to the severity of disease. In terms of predictive prognostic value the venous lactate concentration has the best sensitivity and specificity. Although deep jaundice is usually a bad sign, some adult patients develop a profound cholestatic jaundice without other evidence of vital organ dysfunction.

Parasitaemia has traditionally been used as a measure of severity since the classic studies of Field and colleagues in Kuala Lumpur, Malaysia.[278–279]

They established that *P. falciparum* parasite counts over 100 000/μl were associated with an increased risk of dying, and that the mortality of a count over 500 000/μl was 50%. The distribution of parasite counts in severe malaria is shifted to higher parasitaemias in children living in areas of intense transmission, compared with non-immune adults. For example, parasite counts over 200 000/μl are not uncommon in ambulant semi-immune children who are mildly ill, whereas parasitaemias in this range are usually associated with severe disease in non-immune adults. The sensitivity and specificity of parasitaemia alone as a prognostic indicator is limited, but can be improved by staging parasite development (more mature parasites—worse prognosis), and noting the number of polymorpho-nuclear neutraphil leucocytes which contain pigment (>5%—poorer prognosis).[53] For any parasitaemia the prognosis is worse if >20% of parasites contain visible pigment, and better if >50% of parasites are at the tiny ring stage. In severe malaria if >5% of neutrophils contain visible pigment the prognosis is worse.

DIAGNOSIS

BLOOD SMEARS

Malaria is diagnosed by microscopic examination of the blood. It is not a clinical diagnosis. Thick and thin blood films are made on clean, grease-free glass slides (Figure 61.14). Having written the patient's name, time and date, the glass slide can be cleaned by breathing on the surface and wiping with a clean cloth. The patient's finger should be cleaned with alcohol, allowed to dry, and then the side of the finger tip should be pricked with a sharp sterile lancet or needle. Two drops of blood are placed at one end of the slide. The thin film is made immediately by placing the *smooth* leading edge of a second (spreader) slide in the central drop of blood, adjusting the angle (less blood—more acute) and, whilst holding the edges of the slide, smearing the blood with a swift and steady sweep along the surface. If the blood drop is too large, the spreader slide should be dunked in the drop, then 'jumped' to the slide surface carrying a smaller amount of blood—and then smeared. Making good thin films requires some practice. Anaemic blood smears poorly. The thick film should be stirred in a circular motion with the

corner of the second slide until clotting takes place. The thick film must be of uneven thickness, but it should be possible to read the hands, but not the figures, of a watch face through the film.

INTRADERMAL SMEARS

Chinese researchers have shown that smears from intradermal blood may contain more mature forms of *P. falciparum* than the peripheral blood.[280] This is considered to allow a more complete assessment of severe malaria. The intradermal smears may also be positive or may show pigment containing leucocytes after the blood smear is negative. In terms of diagnostic sensitivity the intradermal smear is similar to the bone marrow (i.e. slightly more sensitive than peripheral blood). The smears are taken (Figure 61.15) from multiple intradermal punctures with a 25 G needle on the volar surface of the upper forearm. The punctures should not ooze blood spontaneously, but sero-sanguinous fluid can be expressed on to the slide by squeezing.

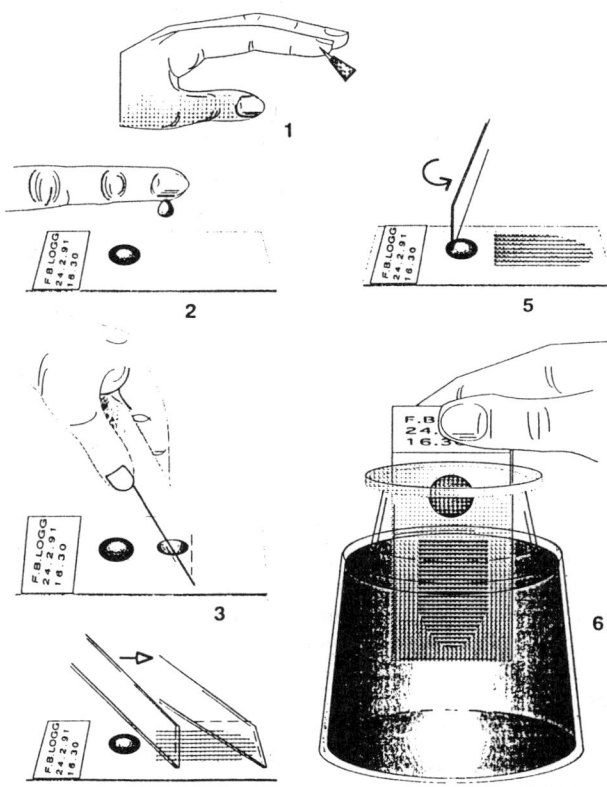

Figure 61.14   Making a peripheral blood smear.

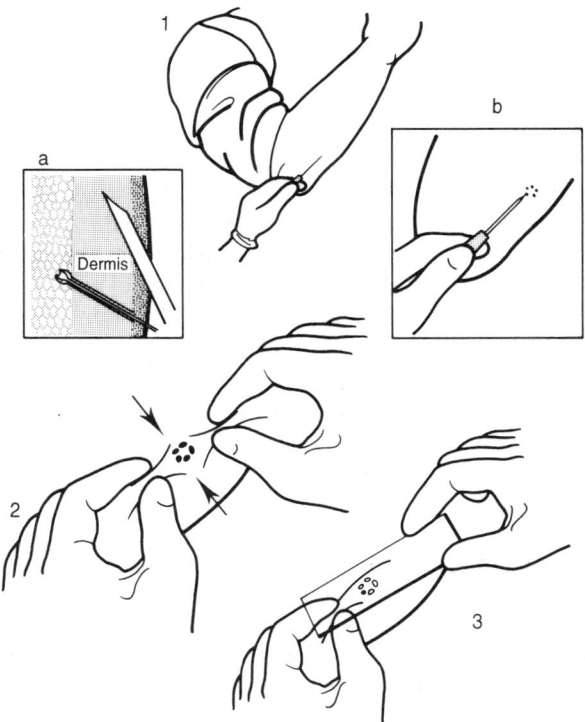

Figure 61.15   Making an intradermal smear.

STAINING AND READING

The thick film should be dried thoroughly otherwise it may wash away during staining. The thin film is then fixed in anhydrous methanol (taking care *not* to fix the thick film). Giemsa's stain buffered to a pH of 7.2 makes the best malaria slides, but for optimum results the stain should be left on the slide for 30 minutes. Field's stain is quicker, but the thin and thick films are treated differently.[281] The thin film is immersed in the red stain (Field's B) for 6 seconds, then gently washed off for 5 seconds, then immersed in the blue stain (Field's A) for 3–4 seconds and then gently washed off (5 seconds). The reverse order applies to the thick film: the slide is first immersed in the blue stain (Field's A) for 5 seconds, then gently washed off (5 seconds) then the red stain (Field's B) for 5 seconds, then gently washed off (5 seconds). Slides should be dried in a slide rack before examining under oil immersion at a magnification of ×1000.

Before going to oil immersion on the microscope, the slide should be scanned briefly under low magnification to identify the best area for detailed examination. For the thin film, the tail of the film should be examined; for the thick film the area of optimum thickness and staining and least artefact is chosen. The thick film is approximately 30 times more sensitive than the thin film, although sensitivity and specificity depend to a great extent on the experience of the microscopist, the quality of the slides, stains and microscope, and the time spent examining the slide. Artefacts are common and often confusing. Speciation of malaria at the trophozoite stage is easier on the thin film, although gametocytes and schizonts are more likely to be seen on the thick film. The thin film is more accurate for parasite counting. The number of parasitized red cells per 1000 red cells should be counted. If there are two parasites in one red cell, this is counted as one. At low parasitaemias (<5/1000 on the thin film) the thick film should be counted; the number of parasites per 200, or preferably 500 white cells is noted. These figures can then be corrected by the total red cell and white cell counts to give the number of parasites per unit blood volume (μl). If the white count is not available then the count is assumed to be 8000/μl.. An alternative is to count all parasites in a fixed volume of blood.[282] In severe malaria parasitaemias are usually high, and the stage of parasite development should be assessed on the thin film. The proportion of asexual parasites containing visible pigment (i.e. mature trophozoitas and schizonts) should be counted. The presence of pigment in neutrophils and monocytes should also be noted. In patients who have already

Table 61.4 Morphological characteristics of human malaria parasites.

	P. falciparum	P. vivax	P. ovale	P. malariae
Asexual parasites	Usually only ring forms seen. Fine blue cytoplasm oval, circular, comma-shaped or occasionally squeezed to the edge of the cell (appliqué form). One or two chromatin dots Parasitaemia may exceed 2%	Irregular large fairly thick rings becoming very pleomorphic as the parasite matures. One chromatin dot	Regular dense ring enlarges to compact blue mature trophozoite. One chromatin dot	Dense thick rings, maturing to dense round trophozoites or rectangular or band-form trophozoites. Pigment associated with rings and trophozoites. Large red chromatin dot or band. Low parasitaemia usual
Meronts	Rare in peripheral blood. 8–32 merozoites, dark brown-black pigment	Common. 12–18 merozoites, orange brown pigment	8–14 merozoites, brown pigment	8–10 merozoites, black pigment
Gametocytes	Banana-shaped. Male: light blue. Female: darker blue. Red-black nucleus with few scattered blue-black pigment granules in cytoplasm	Round or oval. Male: round, pale blue. Female: oval, dark blue. Triangular nucleus, few orange pigment granules	Large round dense blue like *P malariae*, but prominent James' dots. Brown pigment	Large oval-shaped. Male: pale blue. Female: dense blue. Large black pigment granules
Red cell changes	Normal size. As parasite matures cytoplasm becomes pale, the cells become crenated, and a few small red dots appear over the cytoplasm (Maurer's clefts)	Enlarged. Pale red Schüffner's dots increase in number as parasite matures	Cells become oval with tufted ends. Prominent James' dots	Normal size and shape. No red dots

received antimalarial treatment, pigment may still be present in leucocytes after clearance of parasitaemia, and this is an important clue to the diagnosis. Monocytes containing pigment are cleared more slowly than pigment containing neutrophils.

The morphological characteristics of human malaria parasites are given in Table 61.4.

OTHER TECHNIQUES

Unlike mature red cells, malaria parasites contain DNA and RNA. This can be stained with fluorescent dyes and visualized under ultraviolet light microscopy, or, with appropriate filters, seen under ordinary light. In the QBC® technique blood samples are taken into a specialized capillary tube containing acridine orange stain and a float. Under high centrifugal forces (14000 *g*) the infected eryth-

rocytes, which have a higher buoyant density than uninfected cells, become concentrated around the float. Using a modified lens adaptor (Paralens®) with its own light source, the acridine orange fluorescence from malaria parasites can be visualized through an ordinary microscope.[283] In some series this system has proved more sensitive than conventional light microscopy, although it does not give parasite counts or speciation with accuracy, and it is relatively expensive. DNA probes have also been developed for malaria diagnosis, but their utility outside epidemiological surveys is uncertain. Detection of malaria antibody can be useful in some circumstances, such as confirmation of earlier infection, but has no place in acute diagnosis.

Recently a rapid and simple stick test based on a monoclonal antibody against *P. falciparum* histidine rich protein 2 has performed as well as microscopy in field studies.

POSTMORTEM DIAGNOSIS

The diagnosis of cerebral malaria post mortem can be confirmed from a brain smear.[248] A needle aspirate or biopsy is obtained through the superior orbital foramen or the foramen magnum. A smear of grey matter is examined after staining the slide in the same way as for a thin blood film. Capillaries and venules are identified microscopically under low power, and examined under high power. If the patient died in the acute stage of cerebral malaria the vessels are packed with erythrocytes containing mature parasites and a large amount of pigment.

THE ANTIMALARIAL DRUGS

HISTORY

Extracts of the plant qinghao (*Artemesia annua*), known as qinghaosu, have been used in traditional medical practice in China for over two millenia. In AD 340 Ge Hong described use of qinghao infusions for the treatment of fever in the famous *Handbook of Emergency Treatments*. Thereafter qinghao is mentioned frequently in the Chinese materia medica as a treatment for agues. The antimalarial properties of qinghaosu were rediscovered in 1971 when low temperature ethylether extracts of the plant were shown to have activity against experimental rodent malaria.[286] On the other side of the world another medicinal plant came to medical attention during the reign of the Count of Cinchon as Viceroy of Peru between 1628 and 1629 (Figure 61.16). Legend has it that the Viceroy's wife, the Countess, was afflicted by ague in Lima. She was a well known and popular figure and news of her illness spread inland. It eventually reached Lloxa where a Spaniard was in governorship. He knew of a local remedy obtained from the bark of a tree and sent it to the ailing Countess. The therapeutic result was excellent; she improved rapidly, and was so impressed that she ordered the bark in quantity and dispensed it to the poor of Lima who commonly suffered from the dangerous tertian fevers. The pulverized bark became known as 'los polvos de la Condeca' or the Countess' powder, and Linnaeus subsequently named the tree from which the bark was obtained 'Cinchona' in honour of the Countess. Sadly the detective work of one A.W. Haggis, reported in 1941,[287] has shown that 'the fabulous story of the Countess of Cinchon' is almost certainly

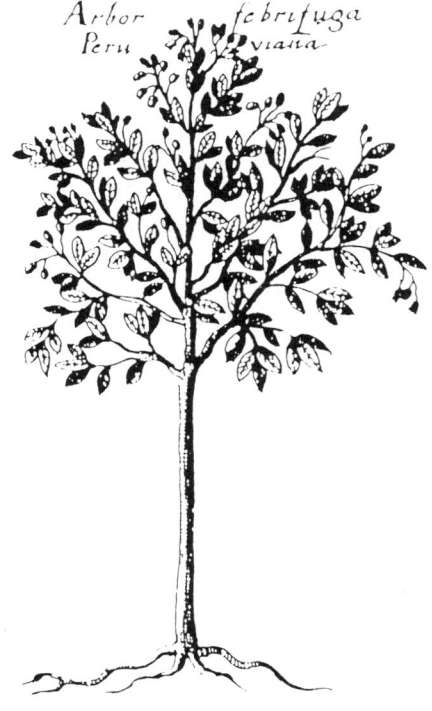

(a)

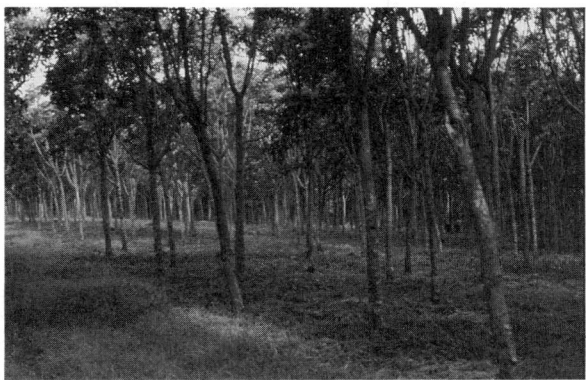

(b)

Figure 61.16 (a) The 'Arbor febrifuga Peruviana'. 'In the district of the city of Loja, diocese of Quito, grows a certain kind of large tree, which has a bark like cinnamon, a little more coarse and very bitter: which ground to powder is given to those who have fever, and with only this remedy, it leaves them' (Bernabé Cobo S. J. *Historia del Nuevo Mundo*; 1582–1657. (b) A Cinchona plantation in Zaire today.

a romantic fable. Nevertheless, it is likely that the bark was introduced to Europe by the Fathers of the Society of Jesus around the time of the story, or even earlier (*c.* 1630) and was widely promoted in Europe by the Jesuit Cardinal Juan de hugo. For these reasons it became known as Jesuit's bark. Not everyone was convinced by the new remedy, and when in 1653 Archduke Leopold of Austria relapsed 1 month after being cured of double quartan fever, his personal physician Jean-Jacques Chifflet began a bitter polemic on the merits of the bark which was to last for 200 years. Much of the dispute stemmed from the fact that many considered all fevers had the same cause, and clearly not all responded to Jesuit's bark. It was probably Torti in 1712 who first stated that the bark was 'specific solely for the ague'.

Another source of debate, and one that is still active today, was dosage. Sir Robert Talbor (Talbot) was one of the few physicians who was not afraid to give the bark in large and repeated doses, and when he cured the Dauphin (the son of Louis XIV) with his 'remède anglais' his fame spread far and wide. He subsequently treated Charles II of England successfully with the same medicament. Others were less enthusiastic. Many protestants believed the bark to be a poison disseminated by the Jesuits. The dose–response question was clarified in 1768 by Lind, who demonstrated clearly that in order to get best results the bark should be given in full doses as soon as the disease was diagnosed. (Advice that has stood the test of time.)

In 1820 the French chemists Pierre Pelletier and Joseph Caventou isolated the alkaloid quinine from cinchona bark. Purification of the various cinchona alkaloids allowed standardization of dosage. Adequate doses could now be given in relatively small amounts of pure drug, but by the middle of the nineteenth century enormous doses (up to 100–150 grains over 2 days) were being prescribed. Toxicity was common and the popularity of the medicine fell. Gradually, however, the diagnosis of agues and the prescription of cinchona alkaloids became more rational and logical. The new colonial powers recognized the importance of cinchona, and improved methods of horticulture resulted in better yields of the alkaloids from the cultivated trees. The Dutch took the lead and vast plantations of high yielding *Cinchona ledgeriana* were started in the East Indies (principally in Java).[288]

Laveran, having identified haematozoa as the cause of paludism, later concluded that quinine cured the disease by killing the newly discovered parasites. This theory encountered considerable resistance in the years immediately following its publication. In 1880 Bacelli described the intravenous method of administering quinine (although there is evidence that this route had been used for 50 years before that). Laveran considered intravenous injection to be dangerous, giving rise to both local and general complications, and was only justified in 'the most grave and pernicious disease'. He also confirmed the earlier observations of Thomas Willis (1659) that cinchona cured the acute attacks of ague, but did not prevent relapses, and also appeared to have no effect on crescents (gametocytes of *P. falciparum*).[289] The eminent Italian malariologists subsequently showed that quinine prevented asexual blood-stage development but could not stop sporulation of formed segmenters (meronts).

In England in 1856 William Henry Perkin discovered analine purple (mauve) whilst attempting to synthesize quinine from coal tar products. Later in Germany, the antimicrobial properties of those newly discovered aniline dyes were investigated. In 1890 Ehrlich showed that methylene blue had antimalarial activity against *P. cathemerium* in canaries, but the dye proved disappointing in clinical practice, and structural modifications did not lead to compounds with improved activity. During the Great War (1914–1918) whole armies were immobilized in the Balkans because of malaria, and there were heavy losses in Mesopotamia, East Africa and the Jordan Valley. The British and French armies used quinine extensively, and despite frequent objections to the bitter medicament many lives were saved. The military and strategic importance of antimalarial drugs stimulated much research immediately after the war.[290] In the early 1920s the resurgent German chemical industry again focused its attention on new antimicrobial compounds. The first synthetic antimalarial was discovered in 1926. This was an aminoquinoline compound, pamaquine, also known as plasmoquine or plasmochin, a precursor of the 8-aminoquinoline primaquine. Pamaquine was followed by the acridine compound mepacrine (quinacrine) in 1932, and the structurally related 4-aminoquinoline, chloroquine, in 1934. Initially chloroquine was rejected as being too toxic for human use, and the research team at Bayer were asked to produce a safer compound. They then produced 3-methylchloroquine (Sontoquine) but, despite clinical studies, these compounds were generally unavailable at the outbreak of the Second World War.

Malaria research has often been tied to warfare. Armies fighting in tropical theatres of war usually lose more men to malaria than bullets.[290] At the outset of the Second World War, the Allies knew their position was precarious in the tropics as most of the world's cinchona was grown in Java,[291] and this was vulnerable to Japanese invasion. They embarked upon a tremendous combined research effort into the development and evaluation of new antimalarials. In the event Java did fall to the Japanese, but widespread use of mepacrine (quinacrine) prophylaxis by the Allied soldiers proved highly effective (albeit somewhat toxic) and probably saved the day. Information on chloroquine was, in fact, available to the Allied Powers through prewar reciprocal arrangements between the pharmaceutical companies, Bayer and Winthrop, but lay buried in documents until the defection of two French soldiers in North Africa in 1943. They brought with them a German antimalarial, later identified as Sontoquine. However, chloroquine was not fully evaluated until the end of the war.[292]

An entirely separate line of research in the UK led to the discovery in 1945 of the antimalarial biguanides, proguanil and subsequently chlorproguanil. These compounds were later shown to inhibit the plasmodial enzyme dihydrofolate reductase (DHFR). Researchers at the Wellcome Research Laboratories synthesizing purine analogues developed the antimitotic compound 6-mercaptopurine (and later azathioprine) and in 1952 discovered the antiprotozoal DHFR inhibitor pyrimethamine. This same line of research later developed trimethoprim, which has considerably greater affinity for bacterial DHFR (but also inhibits the plasmodial enzyme), and also allopurinol, acyclovir and zidovudine (AZT).

By the early 1950s the 4-aminoquinolines chloroquine, and to a much lesser extent amodiaquine, had become the treatment of choice for all malaria throughout the world. Pyrimethamine was used in treatment, and chloroquine, pyrimethamine and proguanil were used for prophylaxis. Primaquine was given to prevent relapses of P. vivax and P. ovale.[293] The cinchona alkaloids were little used outside francophone Africa, and with the discontinuation of quinine, blackwater fever became a rarity. This was the heyday of the malaria eradication era,[294] and with the tremendous successes in Europe and many urban areas of the tropics, interest in the development of new antimalarial drugs waned rapidly.

However, within years of the introduction of pyrimethamine, resistance was noted in both P. falciparum and P. vivax (vivax malaria is intrinsically pyrimethamine resistant). Quinine resistance had been first reported from Brazil in 1910[295] but antimalarial resistance was not treated seriously until chloroquine resistance in P. falciparum developed almost simultaneously in South-East Asia and South America in the early 1960s. At first this was low grade and sporadic, but inexorably resistance increased and spread. The expanding tide of antimalarial drug resistance, together with the looming conflict in Vietnam and the manifest failure of the eradication programme prompted a massive US army-led research effort to screen and test new antimalarial compounds. Most of the compounds developed were structurally related to the known quinoline antimalarials. Mefloquine and halofantrine are the result of this effort. Since then there has been very little research on new antimalarial drugs. An 8-aminoquinoline compound which is less toxic and more active than primaquine has been developed by the American army research programme.[297] A naphthaquinone compound (atovaquone, a modification of a compound discovered over 40 years ago) appears to be a safe and effective antimalarial (although resistance develops rapidly),[298] and the Chinese have produced several interesting synthetic antimalarial compounds structurally related to existing drugs. The most promising of these is pyronaridine, which has structural similarities to amodiaquine, but is active against multidrug-resistant malaria, and also benflumetol. These have not been used outside China.[229]

The most important development in recent years has been the rediscovery and development of the drugs related to artemisinin (qinghaosu) in China.[286,300,301] These drugs are structurally unrelated to existing antimalarials. They are rapidly effective and appear to be safe, and may be the best drugs available for the treatment of severe malaria.[302–304] Artemisinin and the derivatives artemether and artesunate have been used widely in China for over a decade. In the West, the derivatives arteether[305] and artelinic acid[366] have been developed, and have proved effective in animal studies.

During the 1970s chloroquine resistance in P. falciparum increased in South-East Asia and South America, and also became more widespread. By the early 1980s chloroquine was no longer effective in many countries, and the first ominous reports of resistance on the east coast of Africa appeared.[307,308] Since then chloroquine resistance has spread across Africa, and now few countries in the tropics are unaffected. Pyrimethamine resistance has consolidated, and the synergistic combination with sulphonamides is also no longer effective in many countries. In 1984 mefloquine replaced quinine as the treatment of choice for falciparum malaria in Thailand. This was the first country in which mefloquine was used widely. It was introduced in combination with sulfadoxine and pyrimethamine in order to delay the onset of resistance. However, since 1988 mefloquine resistance has developed rapidly in Thailand[309] and adjacent Cambodia and western Burma, while sensitivity to quinine has declined gradually (Figure 61.17). Some strains of P. falciparum isolated in West Africa appear to be primarily resistant to mefloquine[310] (i.e. before the drug has been used). Indeed, *P. falciparum* has been able to develop resistance to all available antimalarial drugs with alarming speed. There is a real possibility that untreatable strains of *P. falciparum* could appear before the beginning of the next millenium.[308] To compound the situation, significant chloroquine resistance in *P. vivax* has also been reported recently in Oceania.[309]

ANTIMALARIAL TREATMENT (Figure 61.17)

In general the antimalarial drugs are more toxic than antibacterials, i.e. the therapeutic ratio is narrower, but serious adverse effects are rare.[312] The available antimalarials fall into three broad groups: the quinoline-related compounds (quinine, quinidine, chloroquine, amodiaquine, mefloquine, halofantrine, primaquine); the antifols (pyrimethamine, proguanil, chlorproguanil, trimethoprim); and the artemisinin compounds (artemisinin, artemether, artesunate). Of these, the artemisinin drugs have the broadest time window of action on the asexual malarial parasites, from medium-sized rings to early schizonts, and produce the most rapid therapeutic responses.[313,314] Several antibacterial drugs also have antiplasmodial activity, although in general their action is slow, and they are used in combination with the antimalarial drugs. These are the sulphonamides and sulphones, the tetracyclines and the macrolides. The tetracyclines are particularly useful as they retain activity against multidrug-resistant parasites. Patients with acute malaria may have up to 10^{12} parasites in the circulation. Even with killing rates per cycle of 99.99% it will take at least three life cycles (6 days) to eradicate all the parasites. Thus antimalarial treatment must usually provide therapeutic drug concentrations for 7 days to effect a cure in non-immune subjects.[52] However, in semi-immune subjects, the host defences collaborate with antimalarial treatment to eradicate residual parasites, and shorter courses of treatment or lower doses of long-acting drugs may be effective.[315]

MODE OF ACTION AND MECHANISMS OF RESISTANCE

Pyrimethamine and the antimalarial biguanides interfere with folic acid synthesis in the parasite by inhibiting the bifunctional enzyme dihydrofolate reductase–thymidilate synthase (DHFR). Sulphonamides act at the previous step in the synthetic pathway by inhibiting dihydropteroate synthetase. Resistance to pyrimethamine in *P. falciparum* was reported within a few years of its introduction.[316] *P. vivax* is intrinsically relatively insensitive to these drugs. DHFR resistance is associated with point mutations in the DHFR gene which lead to reduced affinity (100–1000 times less) of the enzyme complex for the drug.[317] Interestingly mutations conferring pyrimethamine resistance do not necessarily confer cycloguanil resistance, and vice versa.[318,319] As only a single- or double-step mutation is required to move from 'sensitivity' to 'resistance', DHFR resistance occurs readily.

The mode of action of the quinoline antimalarials has been a source of controversy for years. These drugs are weak bases, and they concentrate in the acid food vacuole of the parasite,[320] but this in itself does not explain their antimalarial activity.[321] Chloroquine intercalates DNA, but only at concentrations (1–2 mmol/l) much higher than required to kill parasites (10–20 nmol/l). Chloroquine also binds to ferriprotoporphyrin IX, a product of haemoglobin degradation, and it has been suggested that this complex could be toxic to the parasite.[322] However, there seems to be no difference between the ferriprotoporphyrin IX produced by resistant and sensitive parasites. Recently it has been shown that the quinoline antimalarials selectively inhibit haem

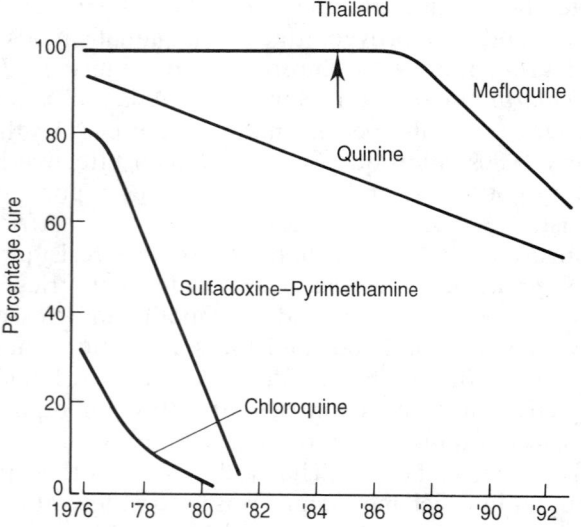

Figure 61.17 Antimalarial resistance at its worst. The decline in antimalarial drug efficacy on the borders of Thailand. The arrow marks the introduction of mefloquine in November 1984. Treatment efficacy depends not only on the sensitivity of the infecting parasites, but also the duration therapeutic antimalarial concentrations are present in blood (pharmacokinetics, compliance), and the background immunity of the patient.

polymerization.[323] This is an essential defence mechanism for the parasite to detoxify haem, and inhibition of this process is therefore a plausible explanation for the selective antimalarial action of these drugs.[324]

Chloroquine resistance is associated with reduced concentrations of drug in the acid food vacuole. The resistant parasites pump chloroquine out 40–50 times faster than drug-sensitive parasites. This efflux mechanism is similar to that found in multi-drug resistant (MDR) mammalian tumour cells, and is mediated by an ATP-requiring transmembrane pump, *P. glycoprotein*. Genes encoding these proteins in neoplastic cells have been sequenced, and similar genes have been identified in *P. falciparum*. But although these MDR genes are amplified in most quinine and mefloquine resistant parasites, the relationship between MDR and chloroquine resistance is inconsistent.[325–327] Furthermore, in other experiments involving careful cloning and genetic crossover of parasites, chloroquine resistance did not cosegregate with the MDR genes.[327–329] Kinetic modelling of chloroquine uptake and efflux rates also does not support the role of an MDR pump in chloroquine resistance.[330] From an epidemiological standpoint multiple unlinked mutations are probably required for the development of chloroquine resistance.

The chloroquine efflux mechanism in resistant parasites can be inhibited by a number of structurally unrelated drugs: calcium channel blockers, tricyclic antidepressants, phenothiazines, cyproheptadine, etc. whereas mefloquine resistance is reversed by perfluridol which does not reduce chloroquine efflux.[331,332] This has given hope that chloroquine resistance might be reversed, but so far clinical evaluations have been disappointing and this hope has not been translated into clinical practice. In in vitro studies of antimalarial drug sensitivity resistance to mefloquine, quinine and halofantrine is linked, but as suggested by their different susceptibility to reversing agents, chloroquine resistance and mefloquine resistance are not linked. Indeed there is some evidence that increasing mefloquine resistance is associated with increased susceptibility to chloroquine.[333,334] The mechanism of action of the artemisinin drugs appears to involve oxidative damage. Parasiticidal activity is dependent on the integrity of the peroxide bridge. How these drugs induce ring form-infected erythrocyte clearance is not known. Low level resistance can be induced experimentally, but the mechanisms have not been characterized.

How does resistance arise naturally? Wild populations of *P. falciparum* are genetically diverse with heterogenous sensitivity to the antimalarial drugs.[335] Human infections are usually polyclonal. Resistance is thought to arise from spontaneous chromosomal point mutations which are independent of drug pressure but, once formed, these more resistant mutants have a survival advantage in the presence of antimalarial drugs.[336] Models of the development of drug resistance predict that, if maximally effective treatment is given to more than 25% of the population in areas of intense transmission, resistance will arise rapidly.[337,338] In theory the use of drug combinations delays the onset of resistance, but only if the resistance genes are rare, free recombination can occur between them, and less than 25% of the population receive treatment.[337] Resistant parasites will be selected when parasites are exposed to subtherapeutic drug concentrations. This occurs if there is widespread use of the drug, and if doses are inadequate. It is also inevitable if the drug is eliminated slowly from the body.[308] Inadequate dosing occurs if there is poor compliance, or unregulated distribution and prescribing. Slowly eliminated drugs such as mefloquine ($T_{\frac{1}{2}}\beta$ 3 weeks) or chloroquine ($T_{\frac{1}{2}}\beta$ 2 months) persist in blood and act as a selective pressure for months after drug administration. In Africa approximately 250 000 kg or 170×10^6 adult treatment doses of chloroquine are consumed annually.[339] Thus in many parts of the continent the majority of the population has chloroquine in the blood at any time. Drug pressure is intense. At low levels of resistance it is reinfections that encounter these subtherapeutic levels, but as resistance increases the chances that a resistant mutant will escape the primary therapeutic assault increases. Cross-resistance is another important potential source of drug pressure. At present there are a number of important, but unanswered, practical questions concerning resistance. We do not know if mefloquine resistance drives quinine resistance, how important the cross-resistance between mefloquine and halofantrine is, whether chloroquine sensitivity might return if the drug pressure was removed, or whether widespread trimethoprim–sulphamethoxazole use for bacterial infections encourages antimalarial antifol resistance.

The drugs used for the treatment of severe malaria all act predominantly in the middle third of the life cycle when there is the greatest increase in parasite synthetic and metabolic activity.[313,314,340] The antifols act a little later, but none of the drugs will prevent rupture and reinvasion once the meront (schizont) has formed (the widely used term schizontocidal is therefore incorrect). Young rings are also relatively drug resistant (particularly to quinine and pyrimethamine). The artemisinin compounds have the broadest time window of antimalarial action, and the most rapid in vivo activity.[314] These

Table 61.5 Antimalarial drugs: salt–base equivalents.

	Salt (mg)	Base (mg)
Chloroquine sulphate	204	150
Chloroquine diphosphate	242	150
Chloroquine hydrochloride	184	150
Amodiaquine dihydrochloride	261	200
Mefloquine hydrochloride	274	250
Quinine sulphate	363	300
Quinine bisulphate	508	300
Quinine hydrochloride	405	300
Quinine dihydrochloride	366	300
Quinine hydrobromide	366	300
Quinine ethylcarbonate	366	300
Quinidine sulphate	217	200
Quninidine bisulphate	234	200
Quinidine gluconate	289	200
Primaquine phosphate	26	15

compounds, and chloroquine, induce accelerated clearance of ring form-infected erythrocytes, and reduce subsequent cytoadherence, whereas quinine does not.[48,52]

QUININE

Quinine is a bitter powder obtained from the bark of the cinchona tree. It is widely used as a flavouring (tonic water, bitter lemon) and as a treatment for night cramps, as well as for malaria. Contrary to widespread belief quinine is not antipyretic. Quinine is usually formulated as the dihydrochloride salt for parenteral administration, and as the sulphate, bisulphate, dihydrochloride, ethylcarbonate, hydrochloride or hydrobromide salts for oral administration. Unlike the other antimalarials, and somewhat confusingly, quinine doses are usually prescribed as weights of salt rather than base (the different salts have different base contents) (Table 61.5). Quinine acts principally on the mature trophozoite stage of parasite development. It does not prevent sequestration or further development of formed meronts and does not kill the pre-erythrocytic or sexual stages of *P. falciparum*.

PHARMACOKINETICS (Table 61.6)

Quinine is well absorbed after oral or intramuscular administration.[192,341–343] Peak levels are usually reached within 4 hours (more rapidly if the intramuscular injections are diluted) (Figure 61.18). In acute malaria the total apparent volume of distribution (V_d) is contracted and systemic clearance reduced in proportion to disease severity.[192,344,345] As a result blood concentrations are higher in uncomplicated malaria than in healthy subjects, and highest in severe malaria. The elimination half-life is approximately 18 hours in cerebral malaria, 16 hours in uncomplicated malaria and 11 hours in health.[345,346] In children and pregnant women the apparent volume of distribution is relatively smaller and elimination is more rapid.[192,344] Quinine is a base and is bound principally to the acute phase plasma pro-tein α_1-acid glycoprotein. Plasma protein binding is increased in malaria from approximately 75–80% in healthy subjects to over 90% in severe malaria.[347–349] Red cell concentrations vary between one-third and one-half of corresponding plasma concentrations,[350] and concentrations in breast milk and cord blood are approximately one-third of those in plasma.[351] The therapeutic range has not been well defined but total plasma concentrations of between 8 and 15 mg/l are certainly safe and effective. Toxicity is increasingly likely with plasma concentrations over 20 mg/l (free quinine >2 mg/l). Approximately 80% of the administered drug is eliminated by hepatic biotransformation, and the remaining 20% is excreted unchanged by the kidney.[345] Although systemic clearance is reduced in severe malaria, this 80:20 proportion is preserved. The principal metabolite 3-hydroxyquinine is biologically active, but the more polar metabolites are either less active, or inactive as antimalarials.

TOXICITY

Minor adverse effects are common with quinine but serious toxicity is remarkably rare in the treatment of malaria. Quinine is extremely bitter and therefore unpleasant to take, and regularly produces a symptom complex known as 'cinchonism'. This comprises tinnitus, high-tone hearing impairment, nausea, dysphoria and often vomiting. As a consequence compliance with the 5–7-day regimens required for cure is poor. Quinine predictably prolongs repolarization in skeletal and cardiac muscle and this is reflected in the electrocardiograph as prolongation of the QT_c interval.[352] This can be used as a pharmacodynamic measure of toxicity. However, significant conduction or repolarization abnormalities are rare and iatrogenic dysrhythmias are extremely uncommon. Quinine, like the other quinoline antimalarials, exacerbates malaria-induced orthostatic hypotension, but iatrogenic supine hypotension is rare. Blindness, resulting from retinal ganglion cell toxicity, and deafness are common following self-

Table 61.6 Pharmacokinetic properties of the antimalarial drugs.

Drug	Absorption: time to peak p.o.	i.m.	Peak plasma protein Oral dose (mg/kg)	Level (mg/l)	Binding (%)	V_d/f (l/kg)	Clearance/f (ml kg^{-1} min^{-1})	$T_{\frac{1}{2}}\beta$ (hours)	Notes
Uncomplicated malaria									
Quinine	6	1	10	8	90	0.8	1.5	16	Protein binding increased. V_d and clearance further reduced in severe malaria. Rate of i.m. absorption proportional to concentration
Quinidine	1	—	10	5	85	1.3	1.7	10	—
Chloroquine	5	0.5	10	0.12	55	100–1000	2.0	30–60 days	Concentrated in red cells, white cells and platelets. Kinetics unaffected by disease severity
Mefloquine	17	—	15	0.2	>98	19	0.4	20 days	Whole blood and plasma concentrations similar
Halofantrine	15	—	8	0.9	>98	—	7.5	113	Metabolized to active desbutyl metabolite which is eliminated more slowly
Pyrimethamine	12	41	1.25	0.5	—	—	0.33	81	—
Healthy subjects									
Primaquine	3	—	0.6	0.15	—	3	6	6	Unidentified active metabolite.
Proguanil (Chloroguanide)	3	—	3.5	0.17	—	24	19	16	Prodrug for active triazine metabolite cycloguanil which is eliminated more rapidly
Pyrimethamine	4	—	0.3	0.35	—	2.9	0.4	85	—

poisoning,[352,353] but rare in malaria treatment. Perhaps the most important toxic effect of quinine is its stimulatory action on the pancreatic β-cell.[198,206,207,355] This causes hyperinsulinaemic hypoglycaemia. It is particularly common in pregnant women but may occur in any severely ill patient, particularly if intravenous glucose solutions are not given. Contrary to popular opinion, quinine does not induce premature labour at therapeutic doses.[219] Quinine is rarely associated with a variety of allergic reactions, notably immune thrombocytopenia. Blackwater fever is undoubtedly associated with quinine use, but the underlying pathophysiological mechanism is not understood.[356]

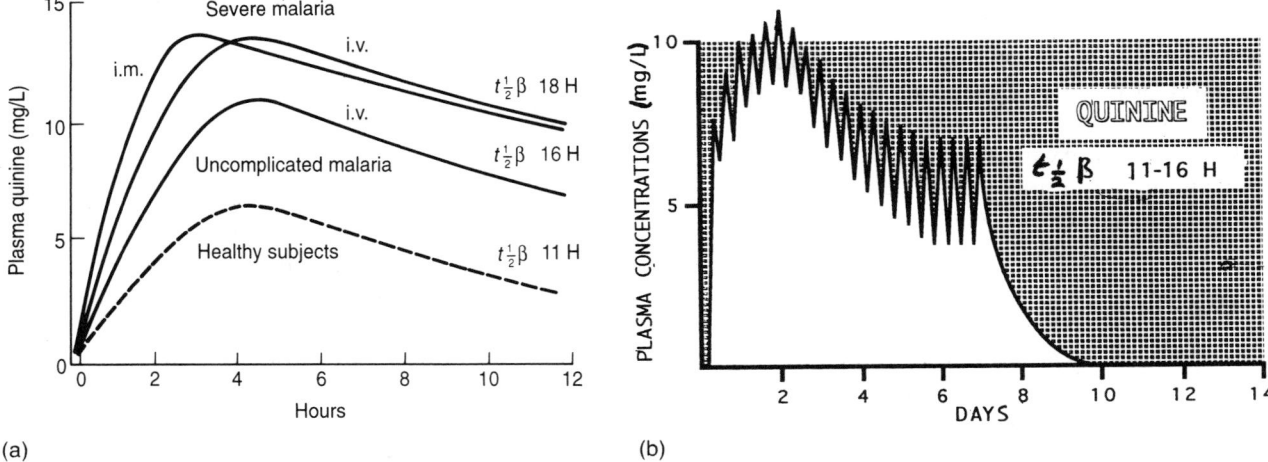

(a)

(b)

Figure 61.18 Quinine plasma concentrations. (a) Time profiles in malaria and in healthy subjects following a single dose of 20 mg salt/kg (from White N. J. *British Journal of Clinical Pharmacology* 1992; 34:1–10 with permission). (b) During the treatment of malaria.

USE

Parenteral quinine should be given by rate-controlled intravenous infusion in either · 0.9% saline, 5% or 10% dextrose, or by deep intramuscular injection. It should never be given by intravenous injection (as it causes hypotension.) The initial doses (mg/kg) in children and pregnant women are the same as in non-pregnant adults, although in areas with resistant parasites it has been recommended that the dose be increased in children to 15 mg salt/kg from day 4 to day 8 to prevent recrudescent infection.[357] In severe malaria treatment should begin with a loading dose so that therapeutic levels are reached as quickly as possible.[358] If adequate treatment has been given before referral to hospital (i.e. >15 mg/kg in the preceding 24 hours) the loading dose is unnecessary. If lower doses have been given the full loading dose should be administered. In severe malaria quinine doses should be reduced by one-third to one-half after 48 hours if there is no clinical improvement, or if there is acute renal failure. This prevents blood concentrations accumulating to toxic levels. Intramuscular quinine is painful and sclerosant if given undiluted (300 mg/ml). It should be diluted in sterile water 1:3 to 1:5 and given to the anterior thigh, not the buttock (to avoid the risk of sciatic nerve damage), using strict aseptic technique.

QUINIDINE

Quinidine is the dextrorotatory diastereoisomer of quinine. It is intrinsically more active as an antimalarial, but is also more cardiotoxic.

PHARMACOKINETICS (Table 61.6)

Oral quinidine is well absorbed in malaria.[359] The V_d and systemic clearance are significantly greater than for quinine,[360,361] and the free fraction in plasma is approximately twice that of quinine. As for quinine, systemic clearance and V_d are reduced in malaria in proportion to disease severity.

TOXICITY

Quinidine has a greater effect on the cardiovascular system, approximately equal stimulatory effect on the pancreatic β cell, and causes less deafness than quinine. Systemic hypotension and myocardial conduction and repolarization abnormalities (widening of the QRS complex and greater than 25% pro-

longation of the ECC QT_c interval) are more common in patients receiving parenteral quinidine compared with those receiving quinine treatment.[360] Electrocardiographic monitoring is advisable (this is unnecessary for quinine).[362] The spectrum of adverse effects is otherwise similar to quinine.

USE

Quinidine should be given for the treatment of severe chloroquine-resistant falciparum malaria if quinine or qinghaosu derivatives are not available. The usual salt is quinidine gluconate. It should be given by careful rate-controlled intravenous infusion with continuous electrocardiographic monitoring.[362] The infusion should be stopped or the rate reduced if the ECG shows >25% prolongation of the QTc interval or >50% widening of the QRS complex. There are no data on intramuscular quinidine in malaria. Oral quinidine is given in the same doses of base equivalent as for quinine (Table 61.6).

CHLOROQUINE

Chloroquine is a 4-aminoquinoline. It is formulated as sulphate, phosphate and hydrochloride salts, and is prescribed in weights of base content. Various liquid formulations are available for paediatric use. Chloroquine can be given by intravenous infusion, intramuscular or subcutaneous injection, orally, or by suppository. Chloroquine acts mainly on the large ring-form and mature trophozoite stages of the parasite. It is more rapidly acting than quinine. Chloroquine is also used in the treatment of hepatic amoebiasis, and for some collagen-vascular and granulomatous diseases, notably rheumatoid arthritis (where hydroxychloroquine is preferred).

PHARMACOKINETICS (Table 61.6)

Chloroquine has complex pharmacokinetic properties with an enormous V_d (resulting from extensive tissue binding) and a very long elimination phase.[363,364] The terminal elimination half-life is 1–2 months. As a consequence the blood concentration profile during malaria is determined mainly by distribution rather than elimination processes.[365,366] Chloroquine is well absorbed by mouth[367] and is very rapidly absorbed following subcutaneous or intramuscular injection, such that absorption may outpace distribution, and transiently toxic concentrations may occur.[365,366] To circumvent this, intravenous chloroquine is administered by constant-rate infusion, and subcutaneous or intramuscular chloroquine given in small (2.5–3.5 mg base/kg) frequent injections. A suppository formulation has been developed which also has good bioavailability.[368] Chloroquine is approximately 55% bound to plasma protein. The principal metabolite of chloroquine, desethylchloroquine, has approximately equivalent antimalarial activity. This is of relevance to prophylactic, but not therapeutic efficacy.

TOXICITY

Chloroquine is generally well tolerated. Oral chloroquine may induce nausea or dysphoria and visual disturbances. Orthostatic hypotension may be accentuated. Pruritus is particularly troublesome in dark-skinned patients and may be dose limiting.[369] Very rarely chloroquine may cause an acute and self-limiting neuropsychiatric reaction. In prophylaxis cumulative doses over 100 g (>5 years prophylaxis) are associated with an increased risk of retinopathy.[370,371] Residents on long-term chloroquine prophylaxis should probably have regular ophthalmological checks after taking the drug for 5 years, of if they experience any visual loss. Myopathy is rare at the doses used in antimalarial prophylaxis. Parenteral chloroquine may cause hypotension if administered too rapidly or a large dose (>3.5 mg base/kg) is given by intramuscular or subcutaneous injection. In self-poisoning, chloroquine produces hypotension, arrhythmias and coma. Diazepam is a specific antidote.[372]

USE

Chloroquine is still the drug of choice for sensitive malaria parasites. It is therefore used widely for *P. vivax*, *P. malariae* and *P. ovale*, but is being progressively replaced for *P. falciparum* treatment. The time-honoured oral chloroquine regimen of 25 mg base/kg spread over three days (10, 10, 5 or 10, 5, 5, 5 mg/kg at 24-hour intervals)[339] can be condensed into 36 hours of drug administration.[373] Intravenous chloroquine should only be used if the infusion rate can be monitored carefully, otherwise intramuscular or subcutaneous administration is safer.

AMODIAQUINE

Amodiaquine is also a 4-aminoquinoline with a similar mode of action to chloroquine. It is more active against resistant isolates of *P. falciparum*, but it is also more toxic.

PHARMACOKINETICS

Oral amodiaquine undergoes extensive first-pass metabolism to the biologically active metabolite desethylamodiaquine.[374] This exerts the principal antimalarial activity. Like chloroquine, desethylamodiaquine is extensively distributed and slowly eliminated. There are no parenteral formulations commercially available, although a structurally similar compound, amopyraquine, is available for intramuscular administration in some countries.

TOXICITY

Prophylactic use of amodiaquine is associated with an unacceptably high incidence of serious toxicity. Approximately 1 in 2000 patients develop agranulocytosis.[375] Serious hepatotoxicity has also been reported. Minor adverse effects are similar to those of chloroquine, although pruritus is less of a problem.

MEPACRINE (QUINACRINE)

Mepacrine is structurally similar to chloroquine. It has the same side chain, but is an acridine instead of a quinoline. It is more toxic and less effective than chloroquine. It should not be used as an antimalarial.

CINCHONINE AND CINCHONIDINE

These methylated natural cinchona alkaloids have no advantages over quinine and quinidine.

MEFLOQUINE

Mefloquine is a fluorinated 4-quinoline methanol compound. It has two asymmetric carbon atoms and is used clinically as a 50:50 racemic mixture of the erythroisomers. These have equal antimalarial activity. The parasiticidal action is similar to that of quinine. Mefloquine is very insoluble in water. It is available as tablets, which should be kept dry. There are no parenteral or paediatric liquid formulations. Mefloquine has been combined with pyrimethamine and sulfadoxine, but this combination preparation offers no advantage over mefloquine alone, and carries the potential for severe sulphonamide toxicity.[376]

PHARMACOKINETICS (Table 61.6)

Mefloquine is moderately well absorbed, extensively distributed, and slowly eliminated.[377,378] It is highly (>98%) bound to plasma proteins.[379] Mefloquine is cleared principally by hepatic biotransformation to inactive metabolites. The terminal elimination half-life is approximately 3 weeks. Blood concentrations are higher in malaria than in healthy subjects and are reduced in diarrhoea (probably by interruption of enterohepatic recycling). Mefloquine clearance is increased in pregnancy.[380] The pharmacokinetics in adults and children are similar.[381]

TOXICITY

Nausea, vomiting, dizziness, weakness and dysphoria are relatively common.[382,383] Although children are more likely to vomit immediately after receiving mefloquine, they otherwise tolerate the drug better than adults. Women, in particular, commonly complain of dizziness and dysphoria for up to 4 days after receiving mefloquine treatment.[383] Mefloquine exacerbates malarial orthostatic hypotension. When used as a prophylactic, mefloquine is associated with an approximate 1:15 000 incidence of acute and self-limiting neuropsychiatric reactions[384,386] (convulsions, psychosis, encephalopathy). The incidence following antimalarial treatment is approximately ten times higher.

USE

Mefloquine is used for the single-dose oral treatment of uncomplicated multidrug-resistant falciparum malaria. The dose ranges from 15 mg base/kg in semi-immunes and 25 mg/kg in non-immune patients and should be repeated if the patient vomits within 1 hour. The higher dose should be split (15 mg/kg stat. followed by 10 mg/kg 8–12 hours later). Mefloquine is used for antimalarial prophylaxis at a dose of approximately 4 mg base/kg once weekly for both adults and children.

HALOFANTRINE

Halofantrine is a 9-phenanthrene methanol. It has one asymmetric carbon atom and is used as a race-

mate. The enantiomers have equal antimalarial activity. Halofantrine is intrinsically more potent than quinine or mefloquine. It is available as tablets and a suspension for paediatric use.

PHARMACOKINETICS (Table 61.6)

Halofantrine is poorly and erratically absorbed. Furthermore, absorption appears to be 'saturable', i.e. with individual doses over 8 mg/kg no increment in blood concentrations occurs. Absorption is increased by fats.[387] Halofantrine is extensively distributed and cleared largely by hepatic biotransformation. The terminal elimination half-life is about 1–3 days in healthy subjects and approximately 4 days in patients with malaria.[388] There is extensive first-pass metabolism to a biologically active desbutyl metabolite. This is eliminated more slowly ($T_{\frac{1}{2}}$ 3–7 days) than the parent compound and undoubtedly contributes to antimalarial activity.

TOXICITY

Halofantrine is very well tolerated. Diarrhoea may be provoked by high doses. Halofantrine slows atrioventricular conduction and produces the 'quinidine effect' on myocardial repolarization: a significant dose-related prolongation of the ECG QT interval. This is increased by previous treatment with mefloquine. Halofantrine has been associated with sudden death, presumably resulting from ventricular tachyarrhythmias. There are no data for pregnancy, so halofantrine should not be used.

USE

When used at standard doses (8 mg/kg given three times at 6–8 hour intervals, and repeated one week later in non-immune patients), to patients with a normal resting electrocardiogram, halofantrine is safe and effective in areas with fully sensitive malaria parasites. In multi-drug resistant areas, higher total doses are required but these are associated with an unacceptable risk of cardiotoxicity. Halofantrine should not be used to treat recrudescent infections following mefloquine treatment.

PYRIMETHAMINE

Pyrimethamine is a DHFR inhibitor. It is used most widely in combination with long-acting sulphonamides such as sulfadoxine and sulfalene. The DHFR

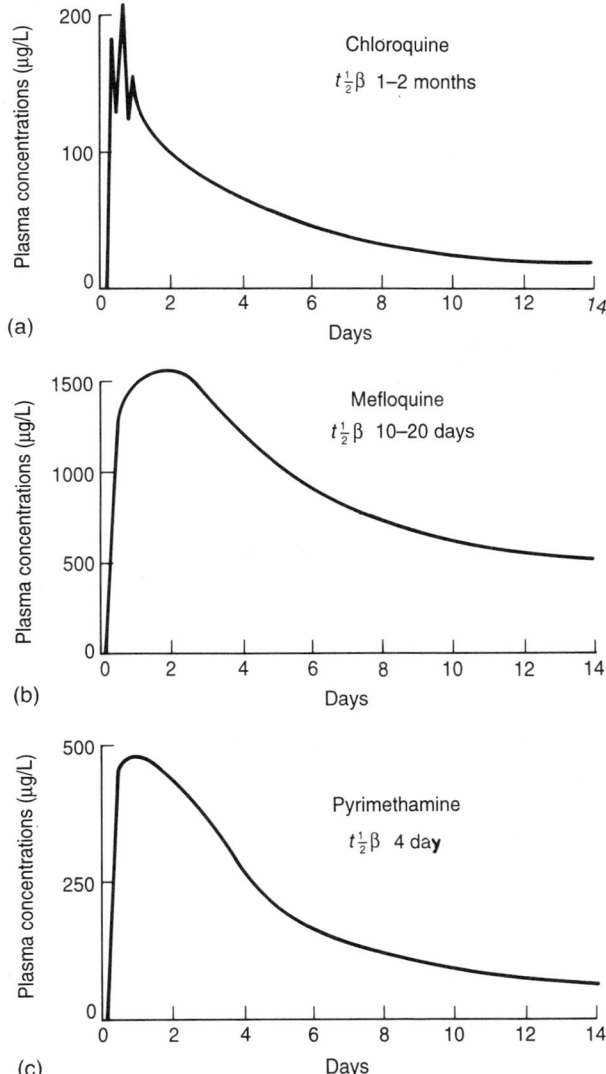

Figure 61.19 Plasma concentration time profiles following treatment doses of (a) chloroquine (b) mefloquine (c) pyrimethamine.

inhibitors inhibit development of the mature trophozoite stage of the asexual parasite, in addition to having pre-erythrocytic and sporontocidal activities. Pyrimethamine is also used for the treatment of toxoplasmosis.

PHARMACOKINETICS (Table 61.6)

Pyrimethamine is well absorbed, and is eliminated over several days ($T_{\frac{1}{2}}$ 3 days), allowing single-dose treatment.[192,392] Following intramuscular injection absorption is as rapid as after oral administration but blood concentrations are lower, which suggests incomplete intramuscular bioavailability.[392]

TOXICITY

Pyrimethamine is very safe and well tolerated. Occasionally megaloblastic anaemia, neutropenia or thrombocytopenia may develop in patients with pre-existing folate deficiency. The toxicity of the widely used combinations with long-acting sulphonamides (sulfadoxine, sulfalene) or sulphones (dapsone) is almost entirely related to the sulpha components.[393,394] The sulphonamides may cause severe skin reactions, hepatitis, blood dyscrasias and other allergic reactions. The sulphones commonly cause methaemoglobinaemia, and also rarely cause blood dyscrasias.[394]

USE

Combinations of pyrimethamine with long-acting sulphonamides should not be used for prophylaxis, whereas the sulphone combination, which appears to be safer (at a once weekly dose), is used for prophylaxis but not treatment. Pyrimethamine alone is no longer used as a prophylactic as resistance is widespread. The combinations are also used for the single-dose treatment of chloroquine-resistant falciparum malaria known to be sensitive to pyrimethamine–sulphonamide. This is well tolerated, cheap and efficient. The risks of serious sulpha toxicity are relatively low for treatment. The role of the intramuscular preparation of pyrimethamine–sulfadoxine is uncertain.

PRIMAQUINE

Primaquine is an 8-aminoquinoline used for its actions against the hypnozoites of *P. vivax* (to prevent relapse) and the gametocytes of *P. falciparum* (to prevent transmission). Primaquine also has activity against asexual stage parasites.

PHARMACOKINETICS (Table 61.6)

Primaquine is well absorbed. It is cleared by hepatic biotransformation[395] to the more polar metabolite carboxyprimaquine with an elimination half-life of 7 hours. It is not known whether primaquine itself or its metabolites are responsible for the action against *P. vivax* hypnozoites.

TOXICITY

Nausea, headache, vomiting and abdominal discomfort are relatively common particularly if higher doses ($\geqslant$30 mg) are taken on an empty stomach. Chest pain, weakness, visual disturbances and pruritus occur occasionally. Methaemoglobinaemia is rare. The principal toxicity of primaquine is oxidant haemolysis in patients with G6PD deficiency[396,397] (indeed, this is how the enzyme deficiency was originally discovered). Primaquine is contraindicated in pregnancy.

PROGUANIL/CHLORPROGUANIL

Proguanil (chloroguanide) and the dichlorobiguanide chlorproguanil are considered the safest of all antimalarials. They are DHFR inhibitors, and are only available as tablets.

PHARMACOKINETICS (Table 61.6)

Proguanil and chlorproguanil are well absorbed. Both compounds are prodrugs for the active triazine metabolites cycloguanil and chlorcycloguanil. These in turn are metabolized to the inactive metabolites chloro- and dichlorophenylbiguanide respectively.[398,399] As the parent compounds are eliminated more slowly than the metabolites the profile of antimalarial activity resulting from the cyclic metabolites is determined by the parent drug distribution and elimination. Approximately 3% of Caucasian and African populations, but up to 20% of Orientals, fail to convert the parent compounds to their active metabolites. This is related to a genetic polymorphism in the IIC subfamily of the cytochrome P450 mixed-function oxidase system.[400] The same enzyme hydroxylates the anticonvulsant mephenytoin. The conversion of proguanil to the active metabolite is reduced in pregnancy.[401]

TOXICITY

The antimalarial biguanides are very well tolerated. They occasionally cause mouth ulcers, and hair loss has been reported.[402] Two patients with renal failure, in whom the drugs may have accumulated, developed pancytopenia following prophylactic administration of proguanil.[403]

USE

Proguanil is used as a prophylactic taken once daily, often in combination with chloroquine. Chlorproguanil was once recommended as a once-weekly prophylactic, but pharmacokinetic studies suggest it should be given once daily. It is also used in combination with dapsone as a treatment of falciparum malaria.[404]

QINGHAOSU (Figure 61.20)

Qinghaosu is also known as artemisinin.[301] It is a sesquiterpene lactone peroxide extracted from the leaves of the shrub *Artemesia annua*. Two derivatives are widely used: the oil-soluble methyl ether artemether, and the water-soluble hemisuccinate derivative artesunate. These drugs are the most rapidly acting of known antimalarials; they also have a broad time window of antimalarial effect from ring forms to the mature trophozoites. They produce rapid parasite clearance and appear to be very safe in clinical practice.[300,304,405,406] In animal studies they are much less toxic than the quinoline antimalarials, but there are insufficient data from clinical studies to provide precise estimates of their toxic potential. Artemisinin is available as capsules of powder or as suppositories. Artemether is formulated in peanut oil for intramuscular injection. Artesunate is formulated either as tablets or as dry powder of artesunic acid for injection, supplied with an ampoule of 5% sodium bicarbonate. The powder is dissolved in the sodium bicarbonate, to form

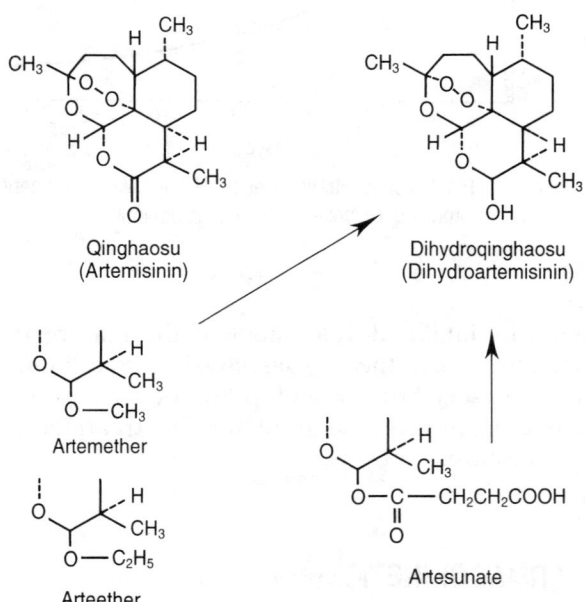

Figure 61.20 Qinghaosu: the parent compound artemisinin and the three derivatives. The oil soluble ethers, artemether and arteether, and the water soluble artesunate are all converted in vivo to a common biologically active metabolite dihydroartemisinin. The peroxide bridge in the sesquiterpene structure is essential for antimalarial activity (from Hien & White *Lancet* 1993; 341:603–608).

sodium artesunate, and then diluted in 5% dextrose or normal saline for intravenous or intramuscular injection. Arteether is a very similar compound to artemether. It is the oil-soluble ethyl ether and will be given by intramuscular injection. Artelinic acid is a water-soluble second-generation compound under development. Both these compounds have been developed in the West. Neither have yet undergone clinical trials.

PHARMACOKINETICS

There are no generally available, reliable and reproducible assays for these drugs. Recently there has been considerable progress with HPLC methods that use reductive mode electrochemical detection and bioassay. Current evidence suggests good absorption and rapid elimination, with half-lives in minutes for the water soluble artesunate and hours for artemether and arteether.[407,408] All the drugs except artemisinin are hydrolysed to the active metabolite dihydroartemisinin,[303] which has an estimated elimination half-life of approximately 45 minutes.

TOXICITY

The artemisinin-related compounds have been remarkably well tolerated in clinical evaluations. There has been no documented toxicity. In volunteer studies a depression of reticulocyte counts has been noted,[409] and this has also been a consistent feature of animal studies. The principal toxicity in animals has been a dose-related selective pattern of neurotoxicity affecting brain stem nuclei. Cardiac and gut toxicity has also occurred in animals, usually with higher doses. However, the therapeutic ratio is much greater than for the quinoline antimalarials, and there has been no hint of these effects in clinical practice.

USE

Parenteral artesunate and artemether have consistently produced rapid therapeutic results in severe malaria. Comparative studies have shown that they predictably give faster parasite and fever clearance times than other antimalarial drugs. Artemether and artesunate are given by intramuscular injection.[405,410] Artesunate is also given by intravenous bolus injection. Rectal artemisinin suppositories have also proved rapidly effective in severe malaria. The optimum use of oral artemisinin and oral artesunate is less clear. These drugs are also rapidly effective and can be combined with longer-acting drugs (e.g. mefloquine) to accelerate the initial therapeutic response and increase overall cure rates.[411] There is some concern that if the oral artemisinin derivatives are used alone, then resistance to these valuable compounds may develop rapidly.

ANTIBACTERIALS WITH ANTIMALARIAL ACTIVITY

The sulphonamides and sulphones inhibit plasmodial folate synthesis by competing for the enzyme dihydropteroate synthetase. They are usually used in combination with pyrimethamine or the antimalarial biguanides. The tetracyclines are consistently active against all species of malaria. The macrolides are active in vitro. Azithromycin has been evaluated as prophylaxis and clindamycin has proved effective in the treatment of falciparum malaria in Africa and South America,[412] although erythromycin and spiramycin have not potentiated the activity of quinine in Thailand. Rifampicin also has a weak antimalarial effect in vivo. These drugs all act relatively slowly, and they are therefore used in combination with more rapidly acting agents. The fluoroquinolones have some antimalarial activity, but despite one promising sentinel report, subsequent clinical experience has proved uniformly disappointing.

CHOICE OF DRUGS (Tables 61.7 and 61.8)

In severe malaria, rapidly acting parenteral treatment should be given. Quinine is the mainstay of treatment, although the presence of low-grade chloroquine resistance does not contraindicate use of chloroquine in severe malaria. It is likely that the artemisinin drugs will become first-line antimalarials

Table 61.7 Treatment of uncomplicated malaria.

Malaria	Drug treatment
P. vivax[1], *P. malariae*, *P. ovale*[1], known chloroquine-sensitive *P. falciparum*	Chloroquine 10 mg base/kg stat. followed by: (a) 5 mg/kg at 12, 24 and 36 h; or (b) 10 mg/kg at 24 h, 5 mg/kg at 48 h
Chloroquine-resistant *P. falciparum* known to be sensitive to sulfadoxine–pyrimethamine (SP)	Pyrimethamine 1 mg/kg + sulfadoxine 20 mg/kg (single dose) 3 tablets in an adult
Chloroquine-resistant *P. vivax*[1*] and chloroquine- and SP-resistant *P. falciparum*	(a) Quinine 10 mg salt/kg three times daily plus tetracycline 4 mg/kg four times daily or doxycycline 2.5 mg/kg once daily for 7 days[2]; or (b) Mefloquine 15 mg base/kg (single dose) in semi-immunes. For non-immune patients a second 10 mg/kg dose should be given 8–24 hours later
Mefloquine-resistant *P. falciparum*	(a) Quinine + tetracycline or doxycycline (b) Oral artesunate 4 mg/kg daily for 3 days + mefloquine 25 mg base/kg (15 mg/kg stat., 10 mg/kg 8–24 hours later).

*This refers to truly resistant infections, thus far reported only in Oceania, and should not be confused with relapse. Primaquine 22.5 mg (base) adult dose should be given once daily for 14 days for radical cure.

General points
A. Mefloquine and artesunate should not be given in the first trimester and halofantrine and tetracycline should not be used at any time in pregnancy, and sulfadoxine should not be used near term.
B. Vomiting is less likely if the patient's temperature is lowered before oral drug administration.
C. In semi-immune subjects shorter courses of quinine (3–5 days) combined with tetracycline (7 days) may be effective.
D. In renal failure the dose of quinine should be reduced by one-third to one-half after 48 hours, and doxycycline but *not* tetracycline should be prescribed.
E. The doses of all drugs are unchanged in children and pregnant women.

Specific points
1. Patients with *P. vivax* and *P. ovale* infections should also be given primaquine 0.25 mg base/kg daily (0.375 mg base/kg in Oceania) for 14 days. In mild G6PD deficiency 0.75 mg base/kg should be given once weekly for 6 weeks.
2. None of the tetracyclines should be given to pregnant women or children under 8 years of age.

for severe malaria over the next few years. In uncomplicated malaria the choice of drugs depends on local patterns of sensitivity, background immunity, availability, rate of action, toxicity and cost. The decision of when to change drug recommendations in the face of increasing resistance is a difficult one. In areas of intense transmission, reinfection is inevitable and the initial therapeutic response is often satisfactory, but infections recur with increasing frequency and anaemia does not recover. In these areas malaria-related morbidity rather than parasitological measures should determine treatment policies.

Table 61.8   Treatment of severe malaria.

	Hospital intensive care unit (ICU)	Health clinic: no intravenous infusion	Rural health clinic: no injection facilities
Known chloroquine-sensitive *P. falciparum*	Chloroquine 10 mg base/kg infused intravenously at constant rate over 8 hours followed by 15 mg base/kg over 24 hours	Chloroquine 3.5 mg base/kg 6-hourly or 2.5 mg base/kg 4-hourly by i.m. or s.c. injection. Total dose 25 mg base/kg	Artemisinin suppositories 10 mg/kg at 0 and 4 hours followed by 7 mg/kg at 24, 36, 48 and 60 hours; or nasogastric chloroquine as for oral regimen
Chloroquine-resistant *P. falciparum*	*Quinine* Quinine dihydrochloride 7 mg salt/kg infused over 30 minutes followed by 10 mg/kg over 4 hours; or 20 mg salt/kg infused over 4 hours. Maintenance dose: 10 mg salt/kg infused over 2–8 hours at 8-hour intervals*	Quinine dihydrochloride 20 mg salt/kg diluted 1:2 with sterile water given by split injection into both anterior thighs. Maintenance dose: 10 mg/kg 8-hourly*	
	Quinidine 10 mg base/kg infused over 1 hour followed by 0.02 mg base/kg per hour. Electrocardiographic monitoring advisable	—	—
	Artemisinin derivatives Artemether 3.2 mg/kg stat. by i.m. injection followed by 1.6mg/kg at 24-hour intervals; or artesunate 2 mg/kg stat. by i.v. injection followed by 1 mg/kg at 12-hours then 1 mg/kg daily	As for hospital ICU: artesunate can also be given by i.m. injection	Artemisinin suppositories 10 mg/kg at 0 and 4 hours followed by 7 mg/kg at 24, 36, 48 and 60 hours

*The dosage interval for quinine in Africa where *P. falciparum* is highly quinine sensitive is 12 hours.
General points
A. If in doubt, consider the infection as chloroquine-resistant although halofantrine should not be given within 6 weeks of mefloquine treatment.
B. Infusions can be given in 0.9% saline, 5% or 10% dextrose/water.
C. Infusion rates for the quinoline antimalarials should be carefully controlled.
D. Oral treatment should start as soon as the patient can swallow reliably enough to complete a full course of treatment.

ANTIMALARIAL DRUG INTERACTIONS

Antimalarial drug interactions have not been defined adequately. Mefloquine, halofantrine, quinidine and quinine are structurally similar and may compete for blood and tissue binding sites. Cardiotoxicity is assumed to be additive. It is also recommended that mefloquine should not be given to people also receiving quinine to avoid adverse cardiovascular effects, but in practice this toxicity has not been observed. Parenteral quinine is commonly given to patients who have received mefloquine previously without apparent complications, but this important potential interaction needs further study. It has been reported that quinine and chloroquine antagonize each other's antimalarial activities, but there is no evidence for this, or indeed a cardiotoxic interaction, in practice.[413] There is no evidence that the structurally disimilar antimalarials interact.

CASE HISTORY

A 31-year-old married female aid worker returned from a project in rural western Cambodia. One week later she developed headache, malaise and low-grade fever. She was found to have a *P. falciparum* infection; the peripheral blood parasite count was 35 000/μl, and she was referred to hospital. She had no relevant past medical history. She had been taking chloroquine and proguanil antimalarial prophylaxis regularly since the beginning of her project 2 months previously. On examination she was listless and febrile (oral temperature 38.9°C) but there were no other abnormal clinical findings. As she was able to take fluids and there were no signs of severe malaria, she was given oral mefloquine (25 mg base/kg) in a single dose on arrival at hospital, but 15 minutes later she vomited. The dose was therefore repeated and this time the drug was retained. The next morning her fever was higher (up to 40.4°C) and the parasite count had risen to 78 500/μl, but she remained lucid and able to sit and drink. Thereafter, the fever gradually subsided, the parasite count fell, and she felt steadily better. The fever clearance time was 84 hours and the parasite clearance time 108 hours. Eighteen days after discharge (24 days after treatment), she was readmitted with fever. A blood smear was again positive for *P. falciparum*; the count was 1800/μl. She said that her period was late, and a pregnancy test proved positive. She was readmitted and treated with oral quinine sulphate 10 mg salt/kg three times daily. Her fever and parasitaemia resolved within 4 days and she was discharged with instructions to finish a 7-day course of treatment. Three weeks later she returned to hospital with a recurrence of symptoms. On examination she was apyrexial but gave a history of fever, and she was clinically anaemic. The spleen tip was palpable. The blood smear was again positive (count 560/μl). She admitted having taken quinine for only 5 days in total because she was continually nauseated, felt the drug gave her a constant buzzing in the ears and made her dizzy. She was readmitted to hospital and given a supervised 7-day course of quinine. Her haematocrit was 27% and the blood film was normochromic and normocytic. Iron and folic acid treatment was started. Thereafter she made an uncomplicated recovery, had no further recrudescences of malaria, and 7 months later delivered a healthy baby girl weighing 3.0 kg.

Comment

This case illustrates several points.

- Chloroquine and proguanil prophylaxis are in-completely effective in this area of multidrug-resistant *P. falciparum*. Chloroquine should have prevented *P. vivax* (up to 50% of the malaria in this area was *P. vivax*), and proguanil may have had some effect against *P. falciparum*, but protection would have been partial at best.

- Vomiting after administration of oral antimalarials to patients with high fever is common. If possible the fever should have been brought down with antipyretics and tepid sponging and the patient made comfortable before being given the mefloquine. Although the 25 mg/kg dose should have been divided (15 mg/kg stat., 10 mg/kg 12 hours later), this does not reduce the incidence of vomiting. If vomiting occurs within 1 hour the dose should be repeated, as was done in this case.

- Parasitaemia may rise over the 24 hours following treatment with quinoline antimalarials or pyrimethamine–sulfadoxine. This does not mean the infection is resistant. It is a reflection of the timing of drug administration and synchroncity of the infection. Merogony is not prevented if most of the parasites are mature meronts when the drugs are started. A change to parenteral treatment is indicated only if the patient deteriorates clinically and fulfils the criteria for severe malaria, or cannot take oral medication. R_3 resistance (see below) is assessed at 48 hours.

- This patient's infection was mefloquine resistant. Blood concentrations of mefloquine would have been higher if the dose had been divided, and might have cured the infection. However, highly mefloquine-resistant strains of *P. falciparum* are now prevalent in western Cambodia and eastern Thailand. These infections respond poorly to treatment with mefloquine alone, but usually respond either to a combination of oral artesunate (10–12 mg/kg over 3–5 days) and mefloquine (25 mg/kg), or a 7-day course of quinine and tetracycline. However, this patient was pregnant: quinine is the only drug recommended in this situation. The suggested treatments for recrudescent infections are shown in Figure 61.20a.

- Treatment failure rates with quinine alone are over 50% in non-immune pregnant women with falciparum malaria acquired in this area. Poor compliance is a major contributor to this poor therapeutic response, as in this case. A further recrudescence after the second course of quinine would not have been unexpected.

- Anaemia is a common consequence of treatment failure in malaria, and a particular complication of malaria in later pregnancy.

- Although malaria consistently reduces birth weight, the effects in this case are difficult to assess as her infection occurred early in pregnancy.

ASSESSMENT OF THE THERAPEUTIC RESPONSE

UNCOMPLICATED MALARIA

In defining criteria for resistance to the aminoquinoline antimalarial drugs, the WHO has described three grades of resistance following treatment.[414]

(low grade) R_1: Recrudescence of the infection between 7 and 28 days of completing treatment following initial resolution of symptoms and parasite clearance.
(high grade) R_2: Reduction of parasitaemia by >75% at 48 hours, but failure to clear parasites within 7 days.
R_3: Parasitaemia does not fall by >75% within 48 hours.

These criteria are useful for all the antimalarial drugs but have several limitations. It is often difficult to follow patients for 28 days. Furthermore, in endemic areas it may be impossible to distinguish recrudescence from reinfection. A simple and practical alternative in high-transmission areas is to assess after 2 weeks. This '14-day test' may be used to compare different drug regimens, but will always underestimate resistance.

The other limitations of the classification are:

- R_1 resistance. Recrudescent infections may recur up to 2 months or more following treatment (i.e. after the 28-day 'limit').
- Therapeutic failure may result from inadequate dosing, failure to absorb the antimalarial, vomiting or host pharmacokinetic factors.[415] Unless the blood concentration of antimalarial drug is measured at the time of recrudescent infection, these factors cannot be excluded.
- R_2 resistance. This category is very broad. Parasitaemia may clear very slowly in some patients (often a harbinger of resistance). The patient improves clinically but a few parasites may still be present at day 7. These may clear by day 9 without further treatment. Alternatively, in highly resistant infections parasitaemia may fall for 1–2 days, then rise alarmingly, with deterioration in the patient's condition.
- R_3 resistance. In occasional cases treatment is started at a time when synchronous merogony is either taking place or about to occur. The parasite count rises considerably and by 48 hours has not fallen by >75% of the initial value (even though the parasites are drug sensitive) but will do so over the next few hours.[45]

In uncomplicated malaria the immediate therapeutic response is usually assessed by the parasite and fever clearance times.

PARASITE CLEARANCE TIME (PCT)

This is the time between beginning antimalarial treatment and the first negative blood slide. The accuracy of the measurement depends on the frequency with which blood slides are taken and the quality of microscopy. The PCT is directly proportional to the admission parasitaemia.[52] The time taken for parasitaemia to fall to half of the admission value (PCT_{50}) and to fall to 10% of the admission value (PCT_{90}) are also useful comparative measures.

FEVER CLEARANCE TIME (FCT)

This is the time from beginning antimalarial treatment until the patient is apyrexial. This is easier said than read! Fever does not come down linearly—it often fluctuates erratically. The method and site of measurements should be standardized and the use of antipyretics documented. One approach is to record when temperature first falls below 37.5°C (FCT_A), and then when the temperature falls and remains below 37.5°C for 24 hours (FCT_B).

SEVERE MALARIA

In addition to parasite and fever clearance the rate of clinical recovery should be assessed. In unconscious patients the Glasgow Coma Score should be assessed 4–6-hourly and the times to reach scores of 8, 11 and 15 recorded. Modified scales have been devised for children. The time to drink, sit, walk and leave hospital should also be documented. The changes in venous lactate and in adults' serum creatinine can also be followed and used as measures of the therapeutic response.

IN VITRO SENSITIVITY TESTING

P. falciparum can be cultured in vitro, whereas the other malaria parasites cannot. Short-term culture over one cycle is relatively easy, requiring simple culture media, a candle jar and an incubator. Antimalarial drug susceptibility can be tested by measuring the inhibition of development to the schizont stage, or the degree of inhibition of radio-labelled ³hypoxanthine uptake.[416] This is a useful epidemiological tool, but it does not predict the clinical response to treatment because it does not take into account individual differences in antimalarial pharmacokinetics, immunity or stage of disease.

RETREATMENT OF RECRUDESCENT INFECTIONS

A suggested algorithm is shown in Figure 61.21. It is important to try and differentiate true resistance from a failure of drug compliance or absorption or inadequate dosing. Subsequent treatment policy depends on local drug availability and health policies. Chloroquine failures will respond to sulfadoxine–pyrimethamine in some areas. In others, quinine or mefloquine should be given. In multidrug-resistant areas recrudescent infections are common, but quinine and tetracycline taken properly for 7 days will still cure over 80% of recrudescent infections. Some infections are very difficult to cure, and cumulative drug toxicity becomes more likely. The combination of artesunate (10–20 mg/kg over 3–5 days) and mefloquine (25 mg/kg) is also effective, in primary treatment of mefloquine resistant infections but for recrudescences, artesunate should be used alone as there is an increased incidence of serious central nervous system reactions if mefloquine is used again in treatment.

Recrudescence following:	Treat with
Chloroquine	→ Sulphadoxine-pyrimethamine ↘
Sulphadoxine-pyrimethamine	→ Mefloquine
Mefloquine ± Artesunate	→ Quinine ± tetracycline ↘ Artesunate (12 mg/kg over 7 days)

Figure 61.21

MANAGEMENT

Where possible, a definite species diagnosis should be obtained by microscopic examination of the blood smear. If there is any doubt, *Plasmodium falciparum* infection should be assumed. The management of malaria depends very much on the health facilities available and the endemicity of disease, i.e. the likely immune status of the patient. For example, in areas of intense transmission asymptomatic parasitaemia is common in older children and adults, and fever is more likely to be the result of some other infection. On the other hand fever may precede detectable parasitaemia in non-immune adults or young children. The blood film should be rechecked in suspected cases. 'Blood smear-negative malaria' is a common diagnosis in the tropics—but one to be avoided. Other infections are more likely. In uncomplicated malaria it is safe to wait, seek other causes for the symptoms, and repeat the blood smears. In severely ill patients antimalarial treatment should be started, but other diagnoses sought. Patients may remain unconscious or develop renal failure after parasite clearance, but there is usually a clear history of previous treatment, and malaria pigment may still be found in peripheral blood leucocytes or intradermal smears. If the temperature is high on admission (>38.5°C) then symptomatic treatment with antipyretics and tepid sponging brings symptomatic relief, and also reduces the likelihood that the patient will vomit the oral antimalarials. This is particularly important for young children who are less likely to have a seizure and much more likely to tolerate oral antimalarials when their temperature has been lowered and they are quiet and calm.

BENIGN MALARIAS

Although *P. vivax*, *P. ovale* or *P. malariae* rarely kill, the disease can be moderately severe, requiring initial parenteral treatment. More usually oral treatment with chloroquine (Table 61.8) leads to resolution of the fever within 2–3 days. The total dose is usually 25 mg base/kg, although 15 mg base/kg is sufficient. The initial dose is 10 mg base/kg and this is followed at 12-hour intervals with subsequent doses of 5 mg/kg. Chloroquine-resistant *P. vivax* is now a significant problem on the island of New Guinea. These infections respond to quinine or mefloquine. Primaquine is also given to patients with *P. vivax* or *P. ovale* to prevent relapse. The usual adult dose is 15 mg base/day (0.25 mg/kg) for 14 days but 22.5 mg base/day is needed for the relatively resistant Chesson strain (found in Oceania).[417] Primaquine is unnecessary if the patient is going to return immediately to an endemic area, and should not be given to pregnant or lactating women or patients with known severe variants of G6PD deficiency. If mild variants of G6PD deficiency are known or likely then primaquine should be given in a dose of 0.75 mg/kg (45 mg) once weekly for 6 weeks.

P. FALCIPARUM MALARIA

Uncomplicated falciparum malaria can be treated on an outpatient basis in the same way as the other malarias. The choice of drugs will depend on the local pattern of resistance where the infection was acquired. Because of the propensity for *P. falciparum* infections to kill, careful assessment of severity is most important. There is obviously a distribution of severity from asymptomatic parasitaemia to fulminant lethal malaria. In practice any patient who is unable to take oral medication will require parenteral treatment and careful observation, and any impairment of consciousness should be treated seriously. The progression to cerebral malaria can be rapid, particularly in children.

MANAGEMENT OF SEVERE *P. FALCIPARUM* MALARIA

Severe malaria is a medical emergency. The airway should be secured in unconscious patients, an intravenous infusion should be started, and other resuscitation measures taken. The patient should be weighed so that the antimalarials can be given on a body weight basis (for adults, a simple method is for the stretcher-bearers to stand on bathroom scales with, and without, the patient.) Immediate measurements of blood glucose (stick test), haematocrit, parasite count and, in adults, renal function (blood urea or creatinine) should be taken. Blood should be taken for cross-match, and later (if available) full blood count, platelet count, clotting studies and full biochemistry. The venous lactate is a very useful prognostic index. Arterial blood pH and gases should be measured in patients who are hyperventilating. Parenteral antimalarial treatment should be given as soon as possible. Where there are adequate nursing facilities the antimalarial drugs should be given by intravenous infusion. The quinoline antimalarials (chloroquine, quinine, quinidine) are compatible with saline or dextrose solutions. They should never be given by bolus intravenous injection. Artesunate should be given by intravenous or intramuscular injection, and artemether by intramuscular injection only. The assessment of fluid balance is critical in severe malaria. Overhydration may produce pulmonary oedema, whereas underhydration may contribute to shock or precipitate or worsen renal impairment. In adults there is often a very thin dividing line between the two, and careful and frequent evaluations of the jugular venous pressure, peripheral perfusion, venous filling, skin turgor and urine output should be made. Where there is uncertainty over the jugular venous pressure, and if nursing facilities permit, a central venous catheter should be inserted and the pressure (CVP) measured directly. The CVP should be maintained between 0 and 5 cm. If the venous pressure is elevated (usually because of overenthusiastic fluid administration), the patient should be nursed with the head at 45° and intravenous frusemide given. Convulsions should be treated promptly with intravenous or rectal diazepam or intramuscular paraldehyde. All unconscious patients should receive a single intramuscular injection of phenobarbitone 5–7 mg/kg (larger doses up to 20 mg/kg may be needed in children).[418]

When these immediate measures have been completed a more detailed clinical examination should be conducted, with particular note of the level of consciousness and record of the coma score. Several coma scores have been advocated. The Glasgow coma score is suitable for adults, and the simple Blantyre modification[249] is readily performed in children. Unconscious patients must have a diagnostic lumbar puncture to exclude bacterial meningitis. The opening pressure should be recorded and the rise and fall with respiration noted (or the Quickenstedt test performed). The CSF should be sent for microscopic analysis, culture, and measurement of glucose, lactate and protein. Subsequent observations should be as frequent as possible and should include vital signs, with an accurate respiratory rate, and assessment of the coma score. The blood glucose should be checked, using rapid stick tests every 4 hours if possible, until recovery of consciousness.

CEREBRAL MALARIA

There is no specific treatment for cerebral malaria. Many adjuvant therapies have been suggested, including heparin, low molecular weight dextran, mannitol, urea, prostacyclin, pentoxifylline (oxpentifylline), des Ferrioxamine, anti-TNF antibody, cyclosporine and hyperimmune serum, but none has been proved to be beneficial. High-dose corticosteroids have been shown to be of no benefit in two studies, and harmful in one.[419,420] Specific management includes care of the unconscious patient, prevention and rapid treatment of convulsions, treatment of hyperpyrexia, and early detection and treatment of other manifestations or complications of severe malaria. Hypoglycaemia should be suspected in any patient who deteriorates suddenly, and this should be treated empirically if glucose stick tests are unavailable. Supervening bacterial infections are common, particularly chest infections and catheter-related urinary tract infections, and spontaneous Gram-negative septicaemia may occur occasionally. Aspiration pneumonia commonly follows generalized seizures. Patients should be nursed on their sides, and turned frequently. Most children will recover consciousness within 2 days, and most adults within 3 days. Rarely adults may remain unconscious for as long as 10 days. Obviously with longer periods of coma complications such as pressure sores and secondary infections become increasingly likely. The role of raised intracranial pressure in cerebral malaria has been re-examined recently. Although approximately 80% of children with cerebral malaria have moderately elevated pressures at lumbar puncture (whereas in adults 80% of pressures are in the normal range), the role of osmotic agents remains uncertain. Most authorities consider

that these should be used only if there is clear clinical evidence of raised intracranial pressure.

FLUID BALANCE

There is evidence of renal impairment in approximately 50% of adults admitted with severe malaria. In the majority of these there will be a transient period of oliguria, followed by uncomplicated recovery, but a minority will progress to established acute tubular necrosis.[421] Rarely polyuric renal failure develops. Patients with severe malaria are very vulnerable to fluid overload and the physician treads a narrow path between underhydration, and thus worsening renal impairment, and overhydration, with the risk of precipitating pulmonary oedema. Following admission patients should be rehydrated carefully to a CVP of between 0 and 5 cm with 0.9% (normal) saline or other isotonic electrolyte solutions. Thereafter the daily fluid requirements will depend on urine output (± diarrhoea) and insensible losses, which can be considerable in febrile patients nursed in hot environments. Water and glucose are provided by 5% or 10% dextrose solutions. It is not possible to generalize on initial fluid requirements as these can vary from deficits of several litres, to patients who are admitted oliguric and unconscious but well hydrated with a slightly elevated jugular venous pressure. Each patient's requirements should be assessed individually. If there is no CVP line it is well worth spending some time establishing clearly the level of the jugular venous pressure. If blood glucose is less than 4 mmol/l then 10% glucose should be started following saline replacement; if it is less than 2.2 mmol/l then hypoglycaemia should be treated immediately (0.3–0.5 g/kg of glucose). The fluid regimen must also be tailored around infusion of the antimalarial drugs. Some physicians prefer to put the 24-hour quinine maintenance dose in one 500 ml bottle of 0.9% saline or 5% dextrose water and infuse this at constant rate, whilst adjusting fluid balance as necessary through a separate piggy-backed line. It is rarely necessary to give potassium or other electrolyte supplements. Many patients will require blood transfusion. The exact criteria for transfusion will depend on blood availability, but in general if the haematocrit falls below 20% then blood should be given. In severe malaria where there is a danger of overhydration, packed cells only should be transfused. In practice if blood is allowed to sediment in a bag or bottle, only the cells are given. Frusemide (0.3 mg/kg) can be given with each unit.

ACUTE RENAL FAILURE

If the patient remains oliguric (<0.4 ml of urine/kg per hour) despite adequate rehydration, and the blood urea or creatinine are rising or already high, then fluids should be restricted to replace insensible losses only. Dialysis should be started early when there is evidence of multiple organ dysfunction. The role of dopamine and loop diuretics in preventing the progression of renal failure is controversial. Renal failure is hypercatabolic in the acute phase of the disease, and once conventional indications for dialysis have been reached (i.e. hyperkalaemia, volume overload, metabolic acidosis, uraemic complications) the patient may deteriorate quickly. An ECG should be performed if acute renal failure is suspected and an immediate blood potassium measurement is unavailable. If there are signs of hyperkalaemia (peaked T waves, widening of the QRS complex) then calcium, and glucose plus insulin, should be given immediately. The exact indications for beginning dialysis require careful clinical appraisal and some experience—but in general, if there is doubt, dialysis should be started. The tempo of disease is faster in patients with acute disease and multiple organ dysfunction, and dialysis should be started earlier than in those whose renal failure develops after other acute manifestations have resolved. Haemodialysis or haemofiltration are preferable to peritoneal dialysis, but the latter is adequate in most cases.[421] The addition of hypertonic dextrose to the peritoneal dialysate can be used to remove excess fluid, and also to provide glucose in hypoglycaemic cases. The efficiency of peritoneal dialysis often improves after the first 24 hours. Reduced peritoneal clearance is thought to be related to sequestration in the peritoneal microvasculature during the acute phase. Peritonitis (cloudy dialysis effluent) is relatively common if dialysis is continued for more than 72 hours. The dose of quinine should be reduced by between one-third and one-half on the third day of treatment. Tetracycline is contraindicated, but doxycycline can be given. The median time to recovery of urine flows (>20ml/kg per 24 hours) is 4 days.[152] The overall prognosis and rate of recovery is better in oliguric than in anuric cases (Figure 61.22).

Patients with blackwater fever should be managed in the same way as other patients. Parenteral quinine should not be stopped unless an artemisinin derivative is available for substitution. Urinary alkalinization is not recommended. Blood transfusion is often needed but the increase in haematocrit is often less than predicted because of brisk haemolysis of the transfused cells. If the patient is volume over-

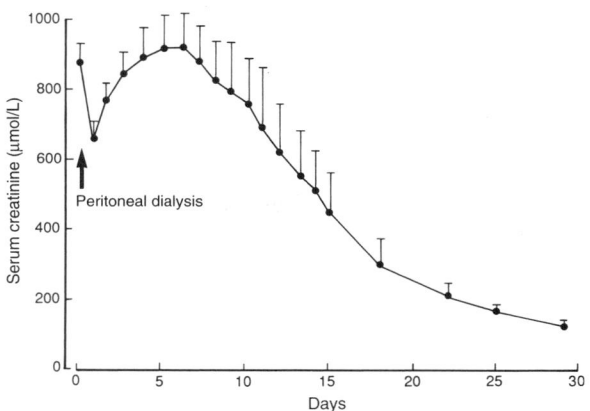

Figure 61.22 Recovery from malarial acute renal failure. This results from acute tubular necrosis. Many patients will not become oliguric, despite a rising serum creatinine in the first few days of hospitalization, and can be managed conservatively.

loaded, but needs blood, then dialysis or haemofiltration must be given first to create enough vascular 'space' for the blood. Packed cells should be given and the transfusion administered as slowly as possible.

ACUTE PULMONARY OEDEMA

This grave manifestation of severe malaria commonly coexists with acute renal failure. The differential diagnosis includes pneumonia, if there are abnormal chest signs, and metabolic acidosis, if the chest is clear. Tachypnoea is a serious sign in malaria; occasionally it results from high fever alone, in which case breathing is shallow, but more usually there is hyperventilation (Kussmaul's breathing) and the implications are serious. Patients with acute pulmonary oedema should be nursed upright and given oxygen, and the right-sided filling pressures should be reduced with whichever treatments are available (loop diuretics, opiates, venodilators, venesection, haemofiltration, dialysis). The right-sided pressure should be reduced to the lowest level compatible with an adequate cardiac output. Positive pressure ventilation should be started if the patient becomes hypoxic.

HYPOGLYCAEMIA

Ideally, blood glucose should be checked 4-hourly while patients are unconscious. Hypoglycaemia should be treated by slow intravenous injection of

0.5–1 ml/kg of 50% dextrose water, and prevented by administering a 10% dextrose infusion at 1–2 mg/kg per hour. Quinine-stimulated hyperinsulinaemia may be blocked by somatostatin or its synthetic analogue, if available. If possible, serum potassium should be checked frequently in hypoglycaemic patients receiving quinine and hypertonic dextrose solutions.

LACTIC ACIDOSIS

Hypovolaemia should be corrected, but in many cases there is a type B lactic acidosis with adequate blood pressure and warm peripheries. Venous, arterial and CSF concentrations of lactate rise in proportion to disease severity. Lactic acid accumulation is buffered initially, but decompensation often occurs in severe malaria. The role of sodium bicarbonate in the treatment of metabolic acidosis has declined from established practice to the controversial. Now most authorities either do not give sodium bicarbonate at all, or give it once only in very severe acidosis (e.g. pH <7.15). The pyruvate dehydrogenase activator dichloroacetate has proved promising in preliminary clinical trials, but its role in treatment remains to be defined. Ideally, dialysis should be started as soon as possible.

BLEEDING

Patients with cerebral malaria may have haematemesis or a bloody nasogastric aspirate because of acute gastric erosions. The incidence of upper gastrointestinal bleeding has declined since the discontinuation of high-dose corticosteroids in cerebral malaria. The role of prophylactic antacids, H_2 blockers, sulfacrate or omeprazole has not been studied. Approximately 5% of patients with cerebral malaria develop clinically significant DIC. These patients should be given fresh blood transfusions and vitamin K.

BACTERIAL SUPERINFECTION/ CONTINUED FEVER

Patients with secondary pneumonia should be given empirical treatment with a third-generation cephalosporin, unless admitted with clear evidence of aspiration, in which case penicillin or clindamycin is adequate. Children with persistent fever despite parasite clearance may have a systematic salmonella infection. Urinary tract infections are common in catheterized patients. Antibiotic treatments should depend on likely local antibiotic sensitivity patterns. Sustained high fever in severe malaria is a poor prognostic sign. Continued fever after parasite clearance is common; antibiotic treatment is only indicated if the patient becomes severely ill or there is a definite focus of infection.

CASE HISTORY

A 46-year-old Brazilian forestry official was admitted to a large provincial hospital with a 5-day history of fever and malaise. Four days previously he had attended a health clinic and was told he had malaria. An intramuscular injection was given, and he was given three large white tablets to take immediately. A further six tablets were prescribed: two to be taken every 4–6 hours. On direct questioning he said that the injection was not painful (and looked like water), that the tablets were not particularly bitter, and that he did not have subsequent ringing in the ears or deafness. His symptoms did not improve, and so he left for the city. When he arrived (the previous morning), he was still febrile and felt ill so he consulted his private practitioner who gave him more white tablets (two to be taken three times daily) and red/yellow capsules (one to be taken four times daily). He found this medicine extremely bitter. By the time of admission he had taken four white tablets and two capsules, but had vomited twice the previous evening.

On examination he was lucid, but slightly agitated, jaundiced and anaemic. His oral temperature was 38.7°C. He was slightly dehydrated; the blood pressure was 100/70 and the pulse 120/min. The cardiovascular and respiratory systems were normal, but the liver and spleen were both enlarged. The haematocrit was 24%, the thick blood film showed a heavy *P. falciparum* parasitaemia with gametocytes, and the thin film count was 58/1000 red cells (no mature parasites with pigment were seen). An urgent serum creatinine was 4.1 mg/dl (360 μmol/l) and blood glucose 72 mg/dl (4.0 mmol/l). The admitting physician put up an intravenous infusion and, after considering the history of previous treatment, gave a loading dose of quinine dihydrochloride (20 mg salt/kg) over 4 hours. This was followed by further infusions of 10 mg/kg 8-hourly. The next day the serum creatinine had risen to 5.5 mg/dl (485 μmol/l), with a blood urea nitrogen of 120 mg/dl, but the serum potassium was 4.6 mmol/l and the urine output 1500 ml (positive balance 1200 ml). The parasite count was 22/1000 red cells. The following day the serum creatinine was 6.3 mg/dl (554 μmol/l), the potassium 4.8 mmol/l and the urine output 1800 ml, but the fever had improved and the patient felt better. The quinine dose was reduced to 10 mg/kg 12-hourly. Thereafter the patient improved steadily, and the serum creatinine fell. The fever clearance time was 74 hours and parasite clearance time 82 hours. The patient was discharged after 10 days with a serum creatinine of 260 μmol/l. He was given doxycycline 100 mg daily for 7 days to take as an outpatient. One week later he was well, with a serum creatinine of 180 μmol/l.

Comment

This patient had severe malaria. The admitting physician was confronted with the common question of whether to give a loading dose of quinine or not. She decided that at the patient's first consultation the injection given was probably an antipyretic (and even if it had been quinine—which is painful if undiluted, and yellow in colour—it would not have altered her decision). 'Four days ago' would correspond to approximately five half-lives (5 × 18 hours) in severe malaria, i.e. if peak concentrations after the injection were 15 mg/l, then 4 days later they

would be less than 1 mg/l). She thought on balance that the antimalarial treatment had probably been sulfadoxine–pyrimethamine (three tablets), and the other tablets antipyretics. On the previous day, however, he had probably been given quinine and tetracycline, and, despite having vomited, he could have absorbed up to 1200 mg (four tablets) of quinine. Her decision then was difficult: the patient might have a plasma quinine concentration as high as 6 mg/l, but it was probably lower, and it could be that she was wrong about the drugs he had been prescribed. On the other hand, he was clearly sick and in need of urgent treatment. In practice, quinine toxicity is unusual in the treatment of severe malaria. If plasma quinine levels are over 3 mg/l on admission a loading dose is unnecessary and should not be given, but precise information is rarely available. As in this case, the admitting physician has to make an educated guess.

Although this patient's malaria infection responded well to treatment, and his urine output remained good, his renal function deteriorated initially. When renal function deteriorates steadily but there is no other evidence of vital organ failure, and urine output is adequate, then a careful 'watch and wait policy' is reasonable until an indication for dialysis arises. In the acute phase of severe malaria with multiple organ failure there should be a lower threshold for starting dialysis. In this case the patient fortunately turned the corner and made a good recovery with conservative management.

MALARIA IN PREGNANCY

SEVERE MALARIA

Pregnant women in the second and third trimesters are more likely to develop severe malaria, often complicated by pulmonary oedema and hypoglycaemia. Fetal death and premature labour are common. The role of early caesarean section for the viable live fetus is unproven, but recommended by many authorities. Obstetric advice should be sought at an early stage, the paediatricians alerted, and the blood glucose checked frequently. Hypoglycaemia is often recurrent if the patient is receiving quinine. The antimalarial drugs should be given in full doses. Severe malaria may also present immediately following delivery. Postpartum bacterial infection is a common complication in these cases. Falciparum malaria has also been associated with severe mid-

trimester haemolytic anaemia in Nigeria. This often requires transfusion, in addition to antimalarial treatment and folate supplementation.

UNCOMPLICATED MALARIA

Symptomatic malaria in pregnancy requires hospitalization where possible. Premature labour may occur and pregnant women receiving quinine are liable to develop hypoglycaemia. Chloroquine, pyrimethamine, proguanil and quinine are considered safe in pregnancy, and sulphonamides are safe until term (where there is the theoretical risk of causing kernicterus in the newborn). Mefloquine is still under evaluation, but preliminary experience is encouraging. Halofantrine and the tetracyclines should not be used. Where necessary (i.e. in areas with mefloquine resistant *P. falciparum*) the artemisin derivatives can be used after the first trimester. In areas with resistant *P. falciparum*, treatment failure rates are higher in pregnant women than in non-pregnant adults. Close follow-up is essential. Women in malarious areas should be encouraged to attend weekly antenatal clinics where blood smears and haematocrit can be checked, in addition to routine obstetric assessment. If effective in the area, antimalarial prophylaxis should be given.

BREAST FEEDING

Nearly all the antimalarial drugs appear in breast milk, but the actual amounts excreted are small. Primaquine should be avoided, but otherwise there seems no reason to discourage breast feeding in women receiving antimalarial drugs.

MALARIA IN CHILDREN

Although maternal malaria is very common, congenital malaria is surprisingly rare given the high frequency with which placental smears are positive in endemic areas, and the not infrequent finding of parasites in cord blood smears. Nevertheless, it may occur with any of the four human malarias. Congenital falciparum malaria is seldom severe. Congenital *P. vivax* or *P. ovale* infections do not require radical treatment as there are no pre-erythrocytic stages in the baby, primaquine should not be given to neonates.

Severe malaria is relatively uncommon in the first 6 months of life, although when it does occur the mortality is high. In young children malaria presents as a febrile illness without focal signs. In *P. falciparum* infections, convulsions are an important complication in the first 3 years. They are twice as common as in *P. vivax* malaria, despite similar fever profiles. The progression to cerebral malaria in young children can be very rapid. Recovery is also rapid compared with adults. In areas of intense transmission, severe anaemia in the 1–3-year age group is the principal manifestation of severe falciparum malaria. A comparison of the relative frequencies of complications in adults and children is shown in Table 61.9.

Children receive the brunt of malaria's assault on humans. Most of the deaths from malaria are in children and most of those are in Africa. Malaria is also an important cause of morbidity, failure to thrive, and probably increased susceptibility to other infections. Whether cerebral malaria, malaria-associated convulsions, or the debilitating effects of repeated weakening febrile illnesses and anaemia cause intellectual retardation needs to be determined. In general children tolerate the antimalarial drugs better than adults. In severe malaria fluid balance is also easier as renal failure is very unusual. However, the small volumes of intravenous fluid required and the difficulties of providing adequate nursing in the tropics often mean that intramuscular, subcutaneous or suppository administration of antimalarial drugs is preferable. Children may deteriorate very rapidly in severe malaria and sudden death is common in cerebral malaria, but, if they survive, recovery is also more rapid than in adults.

Table 61.9 Relative incidence of severe falciparum malaria complications.

	Non-pregnant adults	Pregnant women	Children
Anaemia	+	++	+++
Convulsions	+	+	+++
Hypoglycaemia	+	+++	+++
Jaundice	+++	+++	+
Renal failure	+++	+++	−
Pulmonary oedema	++	+++	+

MALARIA WITH LIMITED RESOURCES

Most patients with severe malaria are not admitted to hospital; they are treated at home or at rural health clinics. Where intravenous infusions cannot be given, intramuscular administration is acceptable for all the antimalarials. It is essential that sterile technique is adhered to fully. Where injections are not possible then oral or, if a tube is available, nasogastric instillation should be attempted, pending transfer of the patient. Artemisinin and chloroquine are available as suppositories in some countries and these are simple and effective alternatives to parenteral administration.

Most malaria in the world is either untreated or treated inadequately by self-medication. Education of the public sector and the private commercial sector is vitally important, and coherent and efficient schemes for drug purchase and distribution are essential. The problem is simple: most tropical countries cannot afford to buy sufficient antimalarial drugs for their needs.[422] The annual per capita expenditure on antimalarial drugs in most of sub-

Table 61.10   Cost of antimalarial treatment for a 60 kg adult (1991).

Drug	$US
Halofantrine	5.31
Mefloquine	1.92
Quinine	1.47
Sulfadoxine–pyrimethamine	0.13
Chloroquine	0.08

Saharan Africa is less than $US5. An adult (60 kg) course of chloroquine costs $US0.08, but a 1-day course of halofantrine is $US5.31 (Table 61.10). The economic implications of deteriorating chloroquine resistance in poor countries are horrendous.

In order to slow the pace of resistance it is essential that whoever gives antimalarial treatment (parent, relative, village health worker, shop assistant) ensures a full course of treatment is administered. This is obviously much easier for single dose antimalarial treatment.

PREVENTION

PERSONAL PREVENTION

The chances of being bitten by a malaria-infected female anopheline mosquito can be reduced considerably by simple measures. Covering exposed skin surfaces and remaining indoors or under a net at peak biting times will obviously reduce exposure. For example most mosquitoes feed at night; sleeping indoors under insecticide (permethrin, deltamethrin)-treated bed-nets reduces morbidity and mortality in malarious areas. A single impregnation of a cotton or nylon mosquito net will provide protection for 1 year.[423] Nylon tends to retain permethrin and deltamethrin better than cotton. The nets can be washed and can tolerate small tears or holes without markedly reducing the protective effects. The benefits conferred by bed-nets depend greatly on the biting habits of the mosquito, the size and constitution of the nets, whether they are impregnated with insecticide, and a variety of sociological factors that determine actual use of the nets in practice. The protective efficacy of unimpregnated bed-nets is variable and depends very much on the way in which they are used (Do they have holes? Are they tucked under the mattress? etc.). The use of mosquito nets impregnated with pyrethroid insecticides such as permethrin or deltamethrin has proved remarkably effective in some areas. In a recent study from The Gambia, use of insecticide-treated bed-nets reduced overall childhood mortality by 60%,[424] whereas earlier studies had shown malaria to account for approximately one-quarter of deaths in this age group, i.e. the reduction in mortality was over twice that expected.[425] This suggests that the debilitating effects of malaria may predispose to other infections, and consequent mortality. As a consequence many countries have taken up impregnated bed-net programmes as an important component of their antimalaria strategy. However, impregnated nets do not work in some areas, presumably because of different human and mosquito behaviour. Other simple preventive measures, including the application of permethrin or deltamethrin to clothing or the use of insect repellants such as diethyltoluamide (DEET) on exposed skin surfaces, are also effective and need not be prohibitively expensive. DEET is generally very safe. Coconut oil and DEET 'soap bar' preparations are available which are cheap, stable and readily applied. Houses can be mosquito proofed by using wire-mesh grilles over windows, and designed in such a way as to discourage mosquito ingress. All these measures reduce the chances of an infection, but they do not eliminate it.

CHEMOPROPHYLAXIS

Although the early colonists devised many ingenious methods of taking quinine regularly (including 'Indian tonic water'), they were generally neither pleasant nor fully effective. Quinine (a poor prophylactic) was relied upon by armies and colonists until after the Great War. The subsequent discovery of mepacrine in 1934 gave the Allied Powers an efficacious, albeit rather toxic, prophylactic which prevented malaria effectively during the Second World War. However, it was the introduction of chloroquine, the antimalarial biguanides, and subsequently pyrimethamine after the war, that finally brought safe and effective antimalarial prophylaxis. The DHFR inhibitors (pyrimethamine, proguanil, chlorproguanil) inhibit parasite development in the liver (pre-erythrocytic activity) and in the erythrocyte. They are sometimes called causal prophylactics. These drugs also inhibit development in the mosquito (sporontocidal activity). Chloroquine, later amodiaquine, and more recently mefloquine inhibit asexual blood-stage development but do not prevent development of the liver stages. They are called suppressive prophylactics. These drugs also have gametocytocidal activity against *P. vivax*, *P. malariae* and *P. ovale*, but not *P. falciparum*.

Antimalarial prophylaxis must be taken regularly to ensure therapeutic antimalarial concentrations are maintained (see world map in Chapter 18, Figure 18.7, for current World Health Organization recommendations for antimalarial prophylaxis by region). Increasing drug resistance in recent years has meant that prophylactic drugs can no longer be relied upon, particularly in areas of multiple drug resistance such as South-East Asia and South America.[426] The recommended prophylactic drug regimens are shown in Table 61.11. When prescribing antimalarial prophylaxis to travellers, it is important to emphasize that no antimalarial is completely effective, and that a febrile illness could still be malaria. It is essential that prophylaxis is taken regularly, and for most drugs continued for 4 weeks after leaving the transmission area. It is prudent to begin prophylaxis 1 week before departing for a malarious area so that tolerance to the drug regimen can be assessed, and therapeutic concentrations are

Table 61.11 Antimalarial chemoprophylaxis.*

Chloroquine-sensitive malaria†	
Chloroquine	5 mg base/kg weekly, or 1.5 mg base/kg daily
and/or	
Proguanil	3 mg/kg daily
Chloroquine-resistant malaria	
Mefloquine	3.5 base/kg/weekly
or	
Doxycycline	1.5 mg/kg daily

*Detailed local knowledge of *P. falciparum* antimalarial susceptibility and malaria risk should always be obtained.
†Some European authorities advise the combination of weekly chloroquine and daily proguanil for many areas, including those with moderately resistant strains of *P. falciparum*.
The WHO currently recommend chloroquine alone for Central America, north of the Panama Canal, some parts of the Middle East, and northern China, and chloroquine plus proguanil for the remainder of the Middle East, the Indian Subcontinent, Malaysia, Indonesia and the Philippines. Elsewhere mefloquine is recommended except for the border areas where doxycycline is preferred.

present on arrival. In anglophone countries, chloroquine is prescribed weekly, but in francophone countries it is given once daily (this is theoretically preferable). Mefloquine and pyrimethamine are taken once a week and proguanil and doxycycline daily. Amodiaquine, quinine, sulfadoxine–pyrimethamine and the artemisinin drugs should not be used for prophylaxis.

In situations where the risk of infection is low, or there are no effective antimalarial available or there is brief repeated exposure to intermediate or high transmission (e.g. aircrews), travellers can be advised to carry a treatment course of antimalarial drugs with them. If they become ill, and there are no medical facilities for malaria diagnosis and treatment, the treatment course is self-administered.

The use of antimalarial prophylaxis by the inhabitants of malarious areas remains controversial. It is generally agreed that pregnant women should take antimalarial prophylaxis if there is a significant risk of malaria, but that other adults should not. Chloroquine, pyrimethamine and proguanil are all considered safe in pregnancy. Mefloquine is still undergoing evaluation; it is not yet approved. Tetracyclines are contraindicated in pregnancy. The use of antimalarial prophylaxis by children living in an endemic area has been shown to reduce mortality; in The Gambia administration of pyrimethamine and dapsone (Maloprim) in the 1–4-year age group reduced mortality by 25%.[425] Despite this encouraging result, this practice has not been generally adopted.

About 20% of patients taking prophylactic anti-malarial drugs report some adverse effects.[427] These are usually minor and do not require a change in prophylaxis. Nausea is the most common side-effect. Dizziness is particularly associated with mefloquine, visual disturbances with chloroquine, and photosensitivity with doxycycline. The risks of neuropsychiatric reactions or seizures are approximately 1:10 000, and appear similar for mefloquine and chloroquine.[427]

PROGRESS TOWARDS A MALARIA VACCINE

Despite considerable effort and expense, a generally available and highly effective malaria vaccine is unlikely in the near future.[428] Indeed the original goals of a vaccine producing sterile immunity (like the polio or yellow fever vaccines) without natural boosting may be unrealistic (and in some cases unwanted). The path of vaccine development has proved long and strewn with pitfalls, but there has been progress. Research has concentrated on all stages of the parasite life cycle: the sporozoite, the liver stage, the asexual blood stage, and the gametocyte. The genes coding for the circumsporozoite protein of *P. falciparum*, the major surface antigen of the sporozoite, were cloned and sequenced in 1984. The central region of the protein consists of a series of tetrapeptide repeats, nearly all of which are NANP. Two vaccines based on this repeat sequence have already been tried in man, but with only limited success, and others are being constructed. The early vaccines lacked T-cell epitopes and produced only transient antibody responses. Current strategies to improve the immune response to these constructs include coupling the NANP repeats with known T-cell epitopes from the circumsporozoite protein, or from non-malarial proteins such as pseudomonas toxin A, or fusion with other 'boosters' such as the non-structural protein of influenza A virus or monophosphoryl lipid A. The vehicle for vaccines also plays an important role in immunogenicity and presentation in alum or in liposomes augments the antibody response. For the development of a blood-stage vaccine, work has concentrated on two merozoite surface antigens (MSP_1 and MSP_2), the ring-infected erythrocyte surface antigen, and to a lesser extent proteins associated with the rhoptries, and the parasitophorous vacuole. A vaccine consisting of a combination of synthetic peptides containing a number of defined blood-stage antigenic epitopes has already been tested extensively in South America. Large-scale clinical trials are now in progress with this and candidate sporozoite vaccines. Transmission blocking vaccines directed against the gametocytes and *P. vivax* sporozoite vaccines are also under development. At present it seems unlikely that these various vaccines will give complete or long-lasting protection. In endemic areas they will be part of the overall antimalaria strategy. Indeed, rather than preventing infection in areas of intense transmission (and thus interrupting the natural acquisition of immunity), their principal benefit may be to attenuate infection and prevent death rather than disease.

CHRONIC COMPLICATIONS OF MALARIA

Malaria is a major cause of chronic ill health in the tropics, particularly in childhood. Repeated attacks of malaria cause anaemia, failure to thrive, and probably also contribute to vulnerability to other infections and retard educational development. Chronic malaria is associated with certain specific syndromes.

QUARTAN NEPHROPATHY (See also Chapter 7)

The nephrotic syndrome, with albuminuria, hypoalbuminaemia, oedema and variable renal impairment, is common in the tropics.[429] Repeated or continuous *P. malariae* infection is associated with childhood nephrotic syndrome in West Africa and Papua New Guinea. In the past, quartan nephropathy was also described in eastern Asia. It has disappeared from countries where *P. malariae* has been eradicated, such as Guyana, where Giglioli first described the relationship between malaria and nephrosis. This strong epidemiological association has been supported by pathological studies,[429,430] although it is not known why certain individuals develop quartan nephropathy whereas the majority of those infected with *P. malariae* do not. The other species of malaria are also suspected of causing occasional glomerulonephritis, but the evidence is less convincing than for *P. malariae*.

PATHOLOGY

Quartan nephropathy is a chronic soluble immune complex nephropathy. Renal biopsy reveals a variety of abnormalities. There is commonly thickening of the subendothelial aspect of the basement membrane, giving rise to a double contour of argyrophilic fibrils. The changes are segmental initially. The capillary lumens narrow and become obliterated. On electron microscopy the basement membrane is irregularly thickened with lacunae of electron-dense material. Immunofluorescent study[429] shows IgG and IgM along the capillary walls. In two-thirds of cases this is accompanied by C3 and other complement components. Coarse granular deposits with IgG3 are more common than fine granular or linear staining, which is more associated with IgG2, and a poor response to cytotoxic therapy. In acute disease *P. malariae* antigens are demonstrable in approximately one-third of cases, but these are not evident in long-standing nephrosis. The severity of the glomerulonephritis is usually graded: <30% glomeruli involved, grade I; 30–75% glomeruli involved + tubular atrophy, grade II; and >75% of glomeruli involved, with extensive tubular pathology grade III. Very occasionally adults develop a proliferative glomerulonephritis. This is not seen in children.

CLINICAL FEATURES

The pattern of renal involvement varies from asymptomatic proteinuria to full-blown nephrotic syndrome. Oedema, ascites or pleural effusions are usual presenting features. Anaemia and hepatosplenomegaly are common, and many patients have fever on admission. The blood pressure is usually normal; the urinary sediment may show granular or hyaline casts in addition to proteinuria, but haematuria or red cell casts are rare. The disease usually progresses inexorably to renal failure over 3–5 years. Spontaneous remission is rare. Antimalarial treatment does not prevent progression,[470] and cor-

ticosteroids are usually ineffective. Some cases respond to cytotoxic therapy.

HYPERREACTIVE MALARIAL SPLENOMEGALY (See also Chapters 3 and 6)

This is also widely known as the tropical splenomegaly syndrome. It occurs where transmission of malaria is intense and has been reported throughout the tropics.[431] The highest incidence of hyperreactive malarial splenomegaly (HMS) yet reported is in the Upper Watut Valley of Papua New Guinea, where 80% of adults and older children have large spleens. Genetic factors undoubtedly also play a role because within a malarious area the geographical distribution of HMS does not follow closely that of malaria transmission.

PATHOLOGY

There is gross splenomegaly with normal architecture, and lymphocytic infiltration of the hepatic sinusoids with Kupffer cell hyperplasia. The massively enlarged spleen leads to hypersplenism with anaemia, leucopenia and thrombocytopenia. There is a polyclonal hypergammaglobulinaemia with high serum concentrations of IgM. High titres of malaria antibodies, and a variety of autoantibodies (antinuclear factor, rheumatoid factor) are usually present. The hypergammaglobulinaemia is believed to result from polyclonal B-cell activation in the absence of adequate numbers of CD8+ suppressor T cells,[432,433] which have been removed by an antibody-dependent cytotoxic mechanism. Cell-mediated immune responses are otherwise normal. Immunoglobulin gene rearrangements have been demonstrated in a subgroup of patients with HMS.[434] This indicates clonal lymphoproliferation and the potential for progression to malignant lymphoma or leukaemia.

CLINICAL FEATURES

Most patients present with abdominal swelling and a dragging sensation in the abdomen. The malaria blood slide is usually negative. The large, hard spleen is vulnerable to trauma. Acute left-sided abdominal pain suggests splenic infarction. The liver is also enlarged. Anaemia is often symptomatic and associated with pancytopenia (hypersplenism), and there is an increased susceptibility to bacterial infections. The long-term prognosis of HMS is not good, with an increased mortality from infection.

TREATMENT

The enlarged spleen usually regresses over a period of months with effective antimalarial prophylaxis. The liver also returns to normal, and the IgM levels fall. Treatment is required for the duration of malaria exposure. Splenectomy is only recommended if there is an unequivocal failure of prophylaxis given for at least 6 months and there is severe hypersplenism.

BURKITT'S LYMPHOMA (See also Chapter 32)

In some countries, Burkitt's lymphoma is the most common malignancy of childhood. It is an uncon-

trolled proliferation of B lymphocytes, and is associated with Epstein–Barr (EB) virus infections and malaria. The epidemiological association between malaria and Burkitt's tumour is very strong. EB virus infections are widespread in the tropics, and in most countries over 80% of children have serological evidence of infection by the age of 3 years. Normally, progression of EB virus infection in B lymphocytes is controlled by virus-specific cytotoxic T cells (the atypical mononuclear cells of infectious mononucleosis). This EB virus cytotoxic T-cell response is decreased significantly during acute malaria, and there is increased proliferation of EB virus-infected lymphocytes.[435] This may predispose to malignant transformation.

MALARIA CONTROL

In his classic work on the prevention of malaria, Ronald Ross (1910) noted that in approximately 550 BC Empedocles rid the Sicilian town of Selinus from a pestilence by draining the nearby marshes. Hippocrates (400 BC) knew that stagnant water and marshlands were unhealthy, and that people living nearby would have enlarged spleens. The principles of drainage and land-fill to control disease have continued since Roman times. The early attempts at joining the Atlantic and Pacific oceans were thwarted by disease, of which malaria was a major contributor, but during the final building of the Panama Canal, malaria was almost eradicated from the Canal Zone by a vigorous combination of felling, drainage, house screening, pesticide use and antimalarial drugs. In recent years the practices of vector control have evolved, and environmental management and modification have come to the fore, both for disease control and for agricultural and other economic purposes. This is a complex and multidisciplinary field. Only a brief outline of the various approaches to malaria control will be described here.

WATER LEVEL MANAGEMENT

The oldest method of vector control drainage remains the most cost effective, particularly in relatively dry areas where there is a high ratio of population to standing water. The practical aspects of drainage are beyond the scope of this book. Water level management to flush out mosquito breeding areas, and to provide a hostile aquatic environment for mosquito egg and larval development, is an alternative to drainage. Changing water salinity or allowing organic matter pollution may also reduce vector populations. As always, major alterations to the environment should not be undertaken lightly: short-term benefits may be offset by long-term problems.

HUMAN BEHAVIOUR

Mosquitoes cannot fly far; most anophelines cannot fly more than 4 km, and in general they remain within 2 km of their breeding sites. If humans do not live near breeding sites, the chances of infection are reduced. Many vectors bite inside houses, and the design and protection offered by the dwelling are important determinants of malaria risk. Wire-mesh screens and other mosquito proofing measures are effective, but expensive, and may also reduce ventilation. The use of mosquito-proof bed-nets prevents human–vector contact, but they are considerably more effective in preventing malaria when impregnated with insect repellents or insecticides. Pyrethroid insecticide (permethrin, deltamethrin)-impregnated nylon nets are best. The use of insect repellents applied to exposed skin is also effective, and can be relatively cheap (e.g. diethyltoluamide)), where domestic species of anophelines exist (e.g. *A. stephensi* in India). Water jars, tanks or containers should be closed to prevent mosquito access.

IMAGOCIDES

Although chemical agents, such as the larvicide Paris green, and pyrethrum insecticides had been widely used for vector control before the Second World War, the discovery of 2,2-bis-(*p*-chlorophenyl)-1,1,1-trichloroethane (DDT), with excellent activity against the adult mosquito (imagocidal activity), was a major advance in malaria control. DDT has residual imagocidal activity, which pyrethrum did not. It could be sprayed on the interior of houses, and would kill or deter mosquitoes for many months afterwards. DDT, along with two other chlorinated hydrocarbon residual insecticides, gamma benzene hexachloride (gamma HCH) and dieldrin, were the principal weapons in the campaign to eradicate malaria and they had a tremendous impact on health and development in the tropics. Imagocides can be classified into three general categories.

1. *Pyrethrins and pyrethroids*. The naturally occurring compounds are light sensitive and unstable, but the new synthetic pyrethroids (permethrin, deltamethrin) are both highly toxic to mosquitoes and stable, giving good residual activity.
2. *Chlorinated hydrocarbons*. (DDT, gamma HCH, dieldrin) are widely used as water-dispersible powders which form an aqueous suspension suitable for spraying. Resistance, human toxicity and ecological concerns have restricted the use of DDT in recent years. Dieldrin is now considered too toxic to humans and it is no longer used.
3. *Anticholinesterases*. These comprise the organophosphorous compounds (malathion, fenitrothion) and the carbamates (propoxur, trimethacarb, bendiocarb). Although resistance to

the organophosphates has limited use in some areas, these compounds are still distributed widely. Malathion is the cheapest and most widely used. The anticholinesterases pose a potential health hazard to spraying teams, despite their wide therapeutic ratios.

Imagocides are also classified either by their portal of entry to the body of the mosquito, or to the method of application. Residual insecticides are applied as a deposit on to surfaces where the mosquitoes will rest (e.g. walls, ceilings). Space sprays fill the air with a mist or fog of insecticide. The choice of insecticide and application method will be determined by the sensitivity and behaviour of the local vectors and the nature of the environment. The anopheline mosquito vectors have countered these chemical assaults by changing their behaviour (resting and feeding preferences) and evolving resistance to the insecticides. This has had drastic consequences: reduced effectiveness; the necessity for more expensive replacements (to which resistance has also developed in some species); a disinclination of the chemical industry to invest further in a difficult and often unprofitable field; and as a consequence an inability of impecunious governments to pay for the new insecticides. Over 50 vector species are resistant to one or more of the organochlorine insecticides, and over ten are resistant to the organophosphates. Most important, *A. gambiae s.l.*, the dominant vector in Africa, has developed resistance to organochlorine insecticides in many areas. In Central America *A. albimanus* has developed multiple insecticide resistance. In India the major vectors, *A. culicifacies* and *A. stephensi*, have become resistant to the organochlorines and malathion.

LARVICIDING

With the problems besetting use of residual imagocidal insecticides, there has been renewed interest in methods of larval control in recent years. These include environmental and water manipulation to prevent creation of mosquito breeding sites, the use of larvivorous fish and bacterial toxins, and the application of chemical agents. Mineral oils were the first larvicides to be employed, and diesel oil is still widely used today. Many of the imagocidal compounds described above are also used for larvicides. However, the organochlorines were highly effective but are no longer recommended because of their adverse environmental impact, and the development of resistance. The organophosphorous compounds are used widely and are relatively safe; for example, compounds such as temephos are safe to warm-blooded animals and fish and can be used to treat potable water.

OVERALL APPROACH

The objectives of a malaria control programme will depend on the prevailing epidemiological situation, the availability of resources and feasibility. The first priority is the reduction of mortality by making available facilities and personnel for diagnosis and treatment. The second priority is to reduce malaria morbidity (such programmes should focus on malaria in childhood and malaria in pregnancy). The third priority is to try and reduce transmission in the most appropriate and cost-effective way. The fourth is to anticipate and prevent the development of epidemics. Having 'secured' the situation, it is also necessary to secure those areas free from malaria to prevent re-establishment of the infection. Finally, and in a carefully planned and multifaceted programme, work to eliminate the disease should begin.

REFERENCES

1 Bruce-Chwatt L J. History of malaria from prehistory to eradication. In Wernsdorfer W H & McGregor I (eds) *Malaria: Principles and Practice of Malariology*. Edinburgh: Churchill Livingstone, 1988:1–59.

2 Smith D C & Sanford L B. Laveran's germ: the reception and use of a medical discovery. *Am J Trop Med Hyg* 1988; 34:2–20.

3 Laveran C L A. Note sur un nouveau parasite trouvé dans le sang de plusieurs malades atteints de fièvre palustre. *Bull Acad Méd* 1880; 9:1235.

4 Ross R. On some peculiar pigmented cells found in two mosquitos fed on malarial blood. *BMJ* 1897; 2:1786–1788.

5 Ross R. *The Prevention of Malaria*, 2nd Edn. London: Murray.

6 Bignami A. Come si prendono le febbri malariche. *Boll R Acad Med Roma* 1899; 25:17–46.

7 Garnham P C C. *Malaria Parasites and Other Haemosporidia*. Oxford: Blackwell, 1966.

8 Waters A P, Higgins D G & McCutchan T F. *Plasmodium falciparum* appears to have arisen as a result of lateral transfer between avian and human hosts. *Proc Natl Acad Sci USA* 1991; 88:3140–3144.

9 Covell G. Spontaneous rupture of the spleen. *Trop Dis Bull* 1955; 52:705–723.

10 Gillies M T. Anopheline mosquitos: vector behaviour and bionomics. In Wernsdorfer W H & McGregor I (eds) *Malaria: Principles and Practice of Malariology*. Edinburgh: Churchill Livingstone, 1988:453–485.

11 Molineaux L, Muir D A, Spencer H C & Werndorfer W H. The epidemiology of malaria and its measurement. In Wernsdorfer W H & McGregor I (eds) *Malaria: Principles and Practice of Malariology*. Edinburgh: Churchill Livingstone, 1988:999–1090.

12 MacDonald G. *The Epidemiology and Control of Malaria*. London: Oxford University Press.

13 Cattani J A, Tulloch J L, Vrbova H et al. The epidemiology of malaria in a population surrounding Madang. Papua New Guinea. *Am J Trop Med Hyg* 1986; 35:3–15.

14 Greenwood B M, Bradley A K, Greenwood A M et al. Mortality and morbidity from malaria among children in rural areas of The Gambia, West Africa. *Trans R Soc Trop Med Hyg* 1987; 81:478–486.

15 Baird J K, Jones T R, Danudirgo E W et al. Age dependent acquired protection against *Plasmodium falciparum* in people having two years exposure to hyperendemic malaria. *Am J Trop Med Hyg* 1991; 45:65–76.

16 Brabin B J. Analysis of malaria in pregnancy in Africa. *Bull World Health Organ* 1983; 61:1005–1016.

17 Nosten F, ter Kuile F, Malankirri L et al. Malaria in pregnancy in an area of unstable endemicity. *Trans R Soc Trop Med Hyg* 1991; 85:424–429.

18 Oppenheimer S J, Gibson F D, Macfarland S B et al. Iron supplementation increases prevalence and effects of malaria: report on clinical studies in Papua New Guinea. *Trans R Soc Trop Med Hyg* 1986; 80:603–612.

19 McGregor I A. Epidemiology, malaria and pregnancy. *Am J Trop Med Hyg* 1984; 33:517–525.

20 Pasvol G, Weatherall D J & Wilson R J M. Effects of fetal hemoglobin on susceptibility of red cells to *Plasmodium falciparum*. *Nature* 1977; 270:171–173.

21 Brewster D, Kwiatkowski D & White N J. Neurological sequelae of cerebral malaria in childhood. *Lancet* 1990; 336:1039–1043.

22 Hendrickse R G, Hasan A H, Olumide L O & Akinkunmi A. Malaria in early childhood. An investigation of five hundred seriously ill children in whom a 'clinical' diagnosis of malaria was made on admission to the Children's Emergency Room at University College Hospital, Ibadan. *Ann Trop Med Parasitol* 1971; 65:1–20.

23 Lindsay S W, Wilkins H A, Zieler H A et al. Ability of *Anopheles gambiae* mosquitos to transmit

malaria during the dry and wet seasons in an area of irrigated rice cultivation in The Gambia. *J Trop Med Hyg* 1991; 94:313–324.

24 Marchiafava E. *Am J Trop Med Hyg* 1932;

25 McGregor I A. Consideration of some aspects of human malaria. *Trans R Soc Trop Med Hyg* 1965; 59:145–152.

26 Garnham P C C. Malaria parasites of man: life cycles and morphology. In Wernsdorfer W H & McGregor I (eds) *Malaria: Principles and Practice of Malariology*. Edinburgh: Churchill Livingstone, 1988:61–69.

27 Ponnudurai T, Lensen A H W, van-Gemart G J A et al. Feeding behaviour and sporozoite ejection by infected *Anopheles stephensi*. *Trans R Soc Trop Med Hyg* 1991; 85:175–180.

28 Rosenburg R & Wirtz R A. An estimation of the number of sporozoites ejected by a feeding mosquito. *Trans R Soc Trop Med Hyg* 1990; 84:209–212.

29 Miller L H, Mason S J, Clyde D F & McGinniss M H. The resistance factor to *P. vivax* in Blacks: the duffy blood group genotype. *N Engl J Med* 1976; 295:302–304.

30 Miller L H. Genetically determined human resistance factors. In Wernsdorfer W H & McGregor I (eds) *Malaria: Principles and Practice of Malariology*. Edinburgh: Churchill Livingstone, 1988: 487–500.

31 Hadley T J, Klotz F W & Miller L H. Invasion of erythrocytes by malaria parasites: cellular and molecular overview. *Ann Rev Microbiol* 1986; 40:451–477.

32 Slater A F G. Malaria pigment. *Exp Parasitol* 1992; 74:362–365.

33 Cranston H A, Boylan C W, Carroll G L et al. *Plasmodium falciparum* maturation abolishes physiologic red cell deformability. *Science* 1984; 223:400–402.

34 Leech J H, Barnwell J W, Miller L H & Howard R J. Identification of a strain-specific malarial antigen exposed on the surface of *Plasmodium falciparum* infected erythrocytes. *J Exp Med* 1984; 159:1567–1575.

35 Read A F, Nanara A, Nee S et al. Gametocyte sex ratios as indirect measures of outcrossing rates in malaria. *Parasitology* 1992; 104:387–395.

36 Kemp D J, Cowman A F & Walliker D. Genetic diversity in *Plasmodium falciparum*. *Adv Parasitol* 1990; 29:75–149.

37 Day K P, Koella J C, Nee S et al. Population genetics and dynamics of *Plasmodium falciparum*: an ecological view. *Parasitology* 1992; 104:535–552.

38 Anders R F. Multiple cross reactivities amongst antigens of *Plasmodium falciparum* impair the development of protective immunity against malaria. *Parasite Immunol* 1986; 8:529–539.

39 Haldane J B S. Disease and evolution. *Ric Sci* 1949; 19 (Supplement):68–75.

40 Hill A V S. Malaria resistance genes: a natural selection. *Trans R Soc Trop Med Hyg* 1992; 86:225–226.

41 Luzzi G A, Merry A H, Newbold C I et al. Surface antigen expression on *Plasmodium falciparum* infected erythrocytes is modified in α- and β-thalassaemia. *J Exp Med* 1991; 173:785–791.

42 Hill A V S, Bennett S, Allsopp C E M et al. Common West African HLA antigens are associated with protection from severe malaria. *Nature* 1991; 352:595–600.

43 Hill A V S, Elvin J, Willis A C et al. Molecular analysis of an HLA–disease association: HLA-B53 and resistance to severe malaria. *Nature* 1992; 360:434–439.

44 Kitchen S F. Symptomatology: general considerations and falciparum malaria. In Boyd M F (ed.) *Malariology*, vol. 2. Philadelphia: W B Saunders, 1949:996–1017.

45 James S P, Nichol W D & Shute P G. A study of induced malignant tertian malaria. *Proc R Soc Med* 1932; 25:1153–1186.

46 Fairley N H. Sidelights on malaria in man obtained by subinoculation experiments. *Trans R Soc Trop Med Hyg* 1947; 40:521–676.

47 Kwiatkowski D & Nowak M. Periodic and chaotic host parasite interaction in human malaria. *Proc Natl Acad Sci USA* 1990; 88: 5111–5113.

48 White N J, Chapman D & Watt G. The effects of multiplication and synchronicity on the vascular distribution of parasites in falciparum malaria. *Trans R Soc Trop Med Hyg* 1992; 86:590–597.

49 Wagner-Jauregg D. The treatment of general paresis by inoculation of malaria. *J Nerv Ment Dis* 1922; 55:369–375.

50 Jeffery G M. Epidemiological significance of repeated infections with homologous and heterologous strains and species of Plasmodium. *Bull World Health Organ* 1966; 35:873–882.

51 Schmidt L H. *Plasmodium falciparum* and *Plasmodium vivax* infections in the owl monkey (*Aotus trivirgatus*). 1. The course of untreated infections. *Am J Trop Med Hyg* 1978; 27:671–702.

52 White N J & Krishna S. Treatment of malaria: some considerations and limitations of the current methods of assessment. *Trans R Soc Trop Med Hyg* 1989; 83:767–777.

53 Silamut K & White N J. The relationship of stage of parasite development to prognosis in falciparum malaria. *Trans R Soc Trop Med Hyg* (1993; 87:436–443).

54 Playfair J H L, Taverne J, Bate C A W & de Souza J B. The malaria vaccine: anti-parasite or anti-disease immunity. *Immunol Today* 1990; 11:25–27.

55 Riley E M, Andersson L, Otoo N et al. Cellular immune responses to *Plasmodium falciparum* antigens in Gambian children during and after an acute attack of falciparum malaria. *Clin Exp Immunol* 1988; 73:17–22.

56 Ciuca M, Baluf L & Chelarescu-Vierum. Immunity in malaria. *Trans R Soc Trop Med Hyg* 1934; 27:619–622.

57 Brown K N, Berzins K, Jarra W & Schetters T. Immune responses to erythrocytic malaria. *Clin Immunol Allergy* 1986; 6:227–249.

58 Bouharoun-Tayoun H, Attanath P, Sabcharoen A et al. Antibodies that protect humans against *P. falciparum* blood stages do not on their own inhibit parasite growth *in vitro* but act in cooperation with monocytes. *J Exp Med* 1990; 172:1633–1641.

59 Nnalue, N A & Friedman M J. Evidence for a neutrophil-mediated protective response in malaria. *Parasite Immunol* 1988; 10:47–58.

60 Rockett K A, Awburn M A & Aggarwal B B. In vivo induction of nitrite and nitrate by tumor necrosis factor, lymphotoxin and interleukin-1: possible role in malaria. *Infect Immun* 1992; 60:3725–3730.

61 Rockett K A, Targett G A T & Playfair J H L. Killing of blood-stage *Plasmodium falciparum* by lipid peroxides from tumor necrosis serum. *Infect Immun* 1988; 56:3180–3183.

62 Looareesuwan S, Ho M, Wattanagoon Y et al. Dynamic alterations in splenic function in falciparum malaria. *N Engl J Med* 1987; 317:675–679.

63 Lee S H, Looareesuwan S, Wattanagoon Y et al. Antibody dependent red cell removal during *P. falciparum* malaria: the clearance of red cells sensitised with IgG anti-D. *Br J Haematol* 1989; 73:396–402.

64 Ho M, White N J, Looareesuwan S et al. Splenic Fc receptor function in host defence and anaemia in acute falciparum malaria. *J Infect Dis* 1990; 161:555–561.

65 Lee M V, Ambrus J L, De Souza J M & Lee R V. Diminished red blood cell deformability in uncomplicated human malaria. A preliminary report. *J Med* 1982; 13:479–485.

66 Hommel M & Semoff S. Expression and function of erythrocyte-associated surface antigens in malaria. *Biol Cell* 1988; 64:183–203.

67 Marsh K & Howard R. Antigens induced on erythrocytes by *P. falciparum*. Expression of diverse and conserved determinants. *Science* 1986; 231:150–153.

68 Webster H K, Brown A E, Chuenchitra C et al. Characterisation of antibodies to sporozoites in *Plasmodium falciparum* malaria and correlation with protection. *J Clin Microbiol* 1988; 26:923–927.

69 Cohen S, McGregor I A & Carrington S. Gamma globulin and acquired immunity to human malaria. *Nature* 1961; 192:735–737.

70 McGregor I A, Carrington S & Cohen S. Treatment of East African *P. falciparum* malaria with West African human gamma-globulin. *Trans R Soc Trop Med Hyg* 1963; 50:170–175.

71 Sabcharoen A, Burnouf T, Ouattara D et al. Parasitologic and clinical response to immunoglobulin administration in falciparum malaria. *Am J Trop Med Hyg* 1991; 45:297–308.

72 Taliaferro W H & Mulligan M W. The histopathology of malaria with special reference to the function and origin of the macrophages in defence. *Indian Med Res Mem* 1937; 29:1–138.

73 Butcher G A. HIV and malaria: a lesson in immunology. *Parasitol Today* 1992; 8:307–311.

74 Kwiatkowski D, Cannon J, Manogue K et al. Tumour necrosis factor production in falciparum malaria and in association with schizont rupture. *Clin Exp Immunol* 1989; 77:361–366.

75 Clark I A, Virelizier J-L, Carswell E A & Wood P R. Possible importance of macrophage-derived mediators in acute malaria. *Infect Immun* 1981; 32:1058–1066.

76 Bate CAW, Taverne J & Playfair J H L. Malaria parasites induce TNF production by macrophages. *Immunology* 1988; 64:227–231.

77 Bate C A W, Taverne J & Playfair J H L. Soluble malarial antigens are toxic and induce the production of tumour necrosis factor in vivo. *Immunology* 1989; 66:600–605.

78 Bate C A W, Taverne J, Dave A & Playfair J H. Malaria exoantigens induce T-independent antibody that blocks their ability to induce TNF. *Immunology* 1990; 70:315–320.

79 Schofield L & Hackett F. Signal transduction in host cells by a glycosylphosphatidylinositol toxin of malaria parasites. *J Exp Med* 1993; 177:145–153.

80 Kern P, Hemmer C J, Van Damme J et al. Elevated tumor necrosis factor alpha and interleukin 6 serum levels as markers for complicated *Plasmodium falciparum* malaria. *Am J Med* 1989; 87:139–143.

81 Grau G E, Taylor T E, Molyneux M E et al. Tumor necrosis factor and disease severity in children with falciparum malaria. *N Engl J Med* 1989; 320:1586–1591.

82 Kwiatkowski D, Hill A V S, Sambou I et al. TNF concentrations in fatal cerebral, non-fatal cerebral, and uncomplicated *Plasmodium falciparum* malaria. *Lancet* 1990; 336:1201–1204.

83 Karunaweera N D, Grau G E, Gamage P et al. Dynamics of fever and serum levels of tumour necrosis factor are closely associated during clinical paroxysms in *Plasmodium vivax* malaria. *Proc Natl Acad Sci USA* 1992; 89:3200–3203.

84 Grau G E, Piguet P F, Vassalli P & Lambert P H. Tumour necrosis factor and other cytokines in cerebral malaria: experimental and clinical data. *Immunol Rev* 1989; 112:49–70.

85 Clark I A & Chaudhri G. Tumour necrosis factor may contribute to the anaemia of malaria by causing dyserythropoiesis and erythrophagocytosis. *Br J Haematol* 1988; 70:99–103.

86 Clark I A & Chaudhri G. Tumor necrosis factor in malaria-induced abortion. *Am J Trop Med Hyg* 1988; 39:246–249.

87 Malhotra K, Salmon D, Le Bras J & Vilde J L. Susceptibility of *Plasmodium falciparum* to a peroxidase-mediated oxygen-dependent microbicidal system. *Infect Immun* 1988; 56:3305–3309.

88 Raventos-Suarez C, Kaul D K, Macaluso F &

Nagel R L. Membrane knobs are required for the microcirculatory obstruction induced by *Plasmodium falciparum*-infected erythrocytes. *Proc Natl Acad Sci USA* 1985; 82:3829–3833.

89 White N J & Ho M. The pathophysiology of malaria. *Adv Parasitol* 1992; 31:34–173.

90 MacPherson G G, Warrell M J, White N J et al. Human cerebral malaria: a quantitative ultrastructural analysis of parasitized erythrocyte sequestration. *Am J Pathol* 1985; 119:385–401.

91 Magowan C, Wollish W, Anderson L & Leech J. Cytoadherence by *Plasmodium falciparum*-infected erythrocytes is correlated with the expression of a family of variable proteins on infected erythrocytes. *J Exp Med* 1988; 168:1307–1320.

92 Howard R J & Gilladoga A D. Molecular studies related to the pathogenesis of cerebral malaria. *Blood* 1989; 74:2603–2618.

93 Sherman I W, Crandall I & Smith H. Membrane proteins involved in the adherence of *Plasmodium falciparum* infected erythrocytes to the endothelium. *Biol Cell* 1992; 74:161–178.

94 Biggs B A, Culvenor J G, Ng J S et al. *Plasmodium falciparum*: cytoadherence of a knobless clone. *Exp Parasitol* 1989; 69:189–197.

95 Biggs B A, Gooze L, Wycherley K et al. Knob-independent cytoadherence of *Plasmodium falciparum* to the leucocyte differentiation antigen CD36. *J Exp Med* 1990; 171:1983–1992.

96 Ockenhouse C F, Klotz F W, Tandon N N & Jamieson G A. Sequestrin, a CD36 recognition protein on *Plasmodium falciparum* malaria-infected erythrocytes identified by anti-idiotype antibodies. *Proc Natl Acad Sci USA* 1991; 88: 3175–3179.

97 David P H, Hommel M, Miller L H et al. Parasite sequestration in *Plasmodium falciparum* malaria: spleen and antibody modulation of cytoadherence of infected erythrocytes. *Proc Natl Acad Sci USA* 1983; 80:5075–5079.

98 Israeli A, Shapiro M & Ephros M A. *Plasmodium falciparum* malaria in an asplenic man. *Trans R Soc Trop Med Hyg* 1987; 81:233–234.

99 Biggs B A, Gooze L, Wycherley K et al. Antigenic variation in *Plasmodium falciparum*. *Proc Natl Acad Sci USA* 1991; 88:9171–9174.

100 Barnwell J W, Asch A S, Nachman R L et al. A human 88-kD membrane glycoprotein (CD36) functions in vitro as a receptor for a cytoadherence ligand on *Plasmodium falciparum* infected erythrocytes. *J Clin Invest* 1989; 84:765–772.

101 Oquendo P, Hundt E, Lawler J & Seed B. CD36 directly mediates cytoadherence of *Plasmodium falciparum* parasitized erythrocytes. *Cell* 1989; 58:95–101.

102 Panton L J, Leech J H, Miller L H & Howard R J. Cytoadherence of *Plasmodium falciparum*-infected erythrocytes to human melanoma cell lines correlates with surface OKM5 antigen. *Infect Immun* 1987; 55:2754–2758.

103 Ockenhouse CF, Ho M, Tandon N N et al. Molecular basis of sequestration in severe and uncomplicated *Plasmodium falciparum* malaria. Differential adhesion of infected erythrocytes to CD36 and CD54 (ICAM-1). *J Infect Dis* 1991; 164:163–169.

104 Marsh K, Marsh V M, Brown J et al. *Plasmodium falciparum*: the behavior of clinical isolates in an in vitro model of infected red blood cell sequestration. *Exp Parasitol* 1988; 65:202–208.

105 Crandall I, Smith H & Sherman I W. *Plasmodium falciparum*: the effect of pH and Ca^{2+} concentration on the in-vitro cytoadherence of infected erythrocytes to amelanotic melanoma cells. *Exp Parasitol* 1991; 73:362–368.

106 Berendt A R, Simmons D L, Tansey J et al. Intercellular adhesion molecule-1 is an endothelial cell adhesion receptor for *Plasmodium falciparum*. *Nature* 1989; 341:57–59.

107 Wick T M & Louis V. Cytoadherence of *Plasmodium falciparum* infected erythrocytes to human umbilical vein and human dermal microvascular endothelial cells under shear conditions. *Am J Trop Med Hyg* 1991; 42: 578–586.

108 Nash G B, Cooke B M, Marsh K et al. Rheological analysis of the adhesive interactions of red blood cells parasitised by *Plasmodium falciparum*. *Blood* 1992; 79:798–807.

109 Roberts D D, Sherwood J A, Spitalnik S L et al. Thrombospondin binds falciparum malaria parasitised erythrocytes and may mediate cytoadherence. *Nature* 1985; 318:64–66.

110 Rock E P, Roth E F, Rojas-Corona R R et al. Thrombospondin mediates the cytoadherence of *Plasmodium falciparum*-infected red cells to vascular endothelium in shear flow conditions. *Blood* 1988; 71:71–75.

111 Ockenhouse C F, Tegoshi T, Maeno et al. Human vascular endothelial cell adhesion receptors for *Plasmodium falciparum*-infected erythrocytes: roles for endothelial leukocyte adhesion molecule 1 and vascular cell adhesion molecule 1. *J Exp Med* 1992; 176:1183–1189.

112 Ho M, Singh B, Looareesuwan S et al. Clinical correlates of in vitro *Plasmodium falciparum* cytoadherence. *Infect Immun* 1991; 59:873–878.

113 Hommel M, David P & Oligino L. Surface alterations of erythrocytes in *Plasmodium falciparum* malaria. Antigenic variation, antigenic diversity and the role of the spleen. *J Exp Med* 1983; 157:1137–1148.

114 David P H, Handunnetti S M, Leech J H et al. Rosetting: a new cytoadherence property of malaria-infected erythrocytes. *Am J Trop Med Hyg* 1988; 38:289–297.

115 Handunnetti S M, David P H, Perera K L R L & Mendis K N. Uninfected erythrocytes form 'rosettes' around *Plasmodium falciparum* infected erythrocytes. *Am J Trop Med Hyg* 1989; 40:115–118.

116 Udomsangpetch R, Wahlin B, Carlson J et al. *Plasmodium falciparum*-infected erythrocytes form

spontaneous erythrocyte rosettes. *J Exp Med* 1989; 169:1835–1840.

117 Hasler T, Handunnetti S M, Aguiar J C et al. In vitro rosetting, cytoadherence and microagglutination properties of *Plasmodium falciparum* infected erythrocytes from Gambian and Tanzanian patients. *Blood* 1990; 76:1845–1852.

118 Wahlgren M, Carlson J, Ruangjirachuporn W et al. Geographical distribution of *Plasmodium falciparum* erythrocyte rosetting and frequency of rosetting antibodies in human sera. *Am J Trop Med Hyg* 1990; 43:333–338.

119 Kaul D K, Roth E F, Nagel R L et al. Rosetting of *Plasmodium falciparum* infected red blood cells with uninfected red blood cells enhances microvascular obstruction under flow conditions. *Blood* 1991; 78:812–819.

120 Carlson J, Helmby H, Hill A V S et al. Human cerebral malaria: association with erythrocyte rosetting and lack of anti-rosetting antibodies. *Lancet* 1990; 336:1457–1460.

121 Ho M, Davis T M E, Silamut K et al. Rosette formation of *P. falciparum* infected erythrocytes from patients with acute malaria. *Infect Immun* 1991; 59:2135–2139.

122 Nash G B, O'Brien E, Gordon-Smith E C & Dormandy J A. Abnormalities in the mechanical properties of red blood cells caused by *Plasmodium falciparum*. *Blood* 1989; 74:855–861.

123 Bhamarapravati N, Boonpucknavig S, Boonpucknavig V & Yaemboonruang C. Glomerular changes in acute *Plasmodium falciparum* infection. *Arch Pathol* 1973; 96:298–293.

124 Adam C, Geniteau M, Gougerot-Pocidalo M et al. Cryoglobulins, circulating immune complexes and complement activation in cerebral malaria. *Infect Immun* 1981; 31:530–535.

125 Neva F A, Howard W A, Glew R H et al. Relationship of serum complement levels to events of the malarial paroxysm. *J Clin Invest* 1974; 54:451–460.

126 Petchclai B, Chutanondh R, Hiranras S & Benjapongs W. Activation of classical and alternate complement pathways in acute falciparum malaria. *J Med Assoc Thai* 1977; 60:174–176.

127 Phanuphak P, Hanvanich M, Sakultamrung R et al. Complement changes in falciparum malaria infection. *Clin Exp Immunol* 1985; 59:571–576.

128 Ho M, Webster H K, Looareesuwan S et al. Antigen-specific immuno-suppression in human malaria due to *Plasmodium falciparum*. *J Infect Dis* 1986; 153:763–771.

129 Ho M, Webster H K, Green B et al. Defective production of and response to interleukin 2 in acute falciparum malaria. *J Immunol* 1988; 141:2755–2759.

130 Riley E M, MacLennan C, Kwiatkowski D K & Greenwood B M. Suppression of in-vitro lymphoproliferative responses in acute malaria patients can be partially reversed by indomethacin. *Parasite Immunol* 1989; 11:509–517.

131 Ho M, Webster H K, Tongtawe P et al. Increased gamma/delta T cells in acute falciparum malaria. *Immunol Lett* 1990; 25:139–142.

132 Ho M & Webster H K. T cell responses in acute falciparum malaria. *Immunol Lett* 1990; 25:135–138.

133 Bouharoun-Tayoun H & Druilhe P. *Plasmodium falciparum* malaria: evidence for an isotype imbalance which may be responsible for delayed acquisition of protective immunity. *J Clin Microbiol* 1992; 60:1473–1481.

134 Brasseur P, Agrapart M, Ballett J J et al. Impaired cell mediated immunity in *Plasmodium falciparum* infected patients with high parasitaemia and cerebral malaria. *Clin Immunol Immunopathol* 1983; 27:38–50.

135 Druilhe P, Brasseur P, Agrapart M et al. T-cell responsiveness in severe *Plasmodium falciparum* malaria. *Trans R Soc Trop Med Hyg* 1983; 77:671–672.

136 Ward K N, Warrell M J, Rhodes J et al. Altered expression of human monocyte Fc receptor in *Plasmodium falciparum* malaria. *Infect Immun* 1984; 44:623–626.

137 Allison A C, Houba V, Hendrickse R G et al. Immune complexes in the nephrotic syndrome of African children. *Lancet* 1969; ii:1232–1237.

138 Davis T M E, Suputtamongkol Y, Spencer J L et al. Measures of capillary permeability in acute falciparum malaria: relation to severity of infection and treatment. *Clin Infect Dis* 1992; 256–266.

139 Maegraith B G & Fletcher A. The pathogenesis of mammalian malaria. *Adv Parasitol* 1972; 10:49–75.

140 Migasena P & Areekul S. Capillary permeability function in malaria. *Ann Trop Med Parasitol* 1987; 81:549–560.

141 Looareesuwan S, Warrell D A, White N J et al. Do patients with cerebral malaria have cerebral oedema? A computed tomography study. *Lancet* 1983; i:434–437.

142 Warrell D A, Looareesuwan S, Phillips R E et al. Function of the blood–cerebrospinal fluid barrier in human cerebral malaria: rejection of the permeability hypothesis. *Am J Trop Med Hyg* 1986; 35:882–889.

143 Newton C R J C, Kirkham F J, Winstanley P A et al. Intracranial pressure in African children with cerebral malaria. *Lancet* 1991; 337:573–576.

144 Waller D, Crawley J, Nosten F et al. Intracranial pressure in childhood cerebral malaria. *Trans R Soc Trop Med Hyg* 1991; 85:362–264.

145 White N J. Lumbar puncture in cerebral malaria. *Lancet* 1991; 338:640–641.

146 Badibanga B, Dayal R, Depierreux M et al. Etude des principaux facteurs immunologiques et de la barrière hémato-méningée au cours de la malaria cérébrale chez l'enfant en pays d'endémie (Zaire). *Ann Soc Belg Med Trop* 1986; 66:23–27.

147 Warrell D A, White N J, Veall N et al. Cerebral anaerobic glycolysis and reduced cerebral oxygen

transport in human cerebral malaria. *Lancet* 1988; ii: 534–538.

148 White N J, Warrell D A, Looareesuwan S et al. Pathophysiological and prognostic significance of cerebrospinal-fluid lactate in cerebral malaria. *Lancet* 1985; i:776–778.

149 Arthachinta S, Sitprija V & Kashemsant U. Selective renal angiography in renal failure due to infection. *Aust J Radiol* 1974; 18:446–452.

150 Boonpucknavig V & Sitprija V. Renal disease in acute *Plasmodium falciparum* infection in man. *Kidney Int* 1979; 16:44–52.

151 Hartenblower D L, Kantor G L & Rosen V J. Renal failure due to acute glomerulonephritis during falciparum malaria. Case report. *Milit Med* 1972; 137:74–76.

152 Trang T T M, Phu N H, Vinh H et al. Acute renal failure in severe falciparum malaria. *Clin Infect Dis* 1992; 15:874–880.

153 Barratt J O W & Yorke W. An investigation into the mechanism of production of blackwater. *Ann Trop Med Parasitol* 1909–1910; 3:1–256.

154 Maegraith B G. *Pathological Processes in Malaria and Blackwater Fever*. Oxford: Blackwell, 1948:348–349.

155 Maegraith B G. Recent advances in tropical medicine: blackwater fever. *West Afr Med J* 1952; 1:4–10.

156 James M F M. Pulmonary damage associated with falciparum malaria: a report of ten cases. *Ann Trop Med Parasitol* 1985; 79:123–138.

157 Charoenpan P, Indraprasit S, Kiatboonsri S et al. Pulmonary edema in severe falciparum malaria. Hemodynamic study and clinicophysiologic correlation. *Chest* 1990; 9:1190–1197.

158 Brooks M H, Malloy J P, Bartelloni P J et al. Pathophysiology of acute falciparum malaria. Correlation of clinical and biochemical abnormalities. *Am J Med* 1967; 43:735–744.

159 Chongsuphajaisiddhi T, Kasemuth R, Tajavanija S & Harinasuta T. Changes in blood volume in falciparum malaria. *Southeast Asian J Trop Med Public Health* 1971; 2:344–350.

160 Malloy J P, Brooks M H, Barry K G et al. Pathophysiology of acute falciparum malaria. II. Fluid compartmentalization. *Am J Med* 1967; 43:745–750.

161 Ogunye O & Ghadebo A O. Syndrome of inappropriate antidiuretic hormone (SIADH) in measles and malaria infections. *Trop Geogr Med* 1981; 33:165–168.

162 Zuckerman A. Recent studies on factors involved in malarial anaemia. *Milit Med* 1966; 131 (supplement):1201–1216.

163 Perrin L H, Mackey L J & Miecher P A. The hematology of malaria in man. *Semin Hematol* 1982; 19:70–82.

164 Looareesuwan S, Davis T M E, Pukrittayakamee S et al. Erythrocyte survival in severe falciparum malaria. *Acta Trop* 1991; 48:263–270.

165 Davis T M E, Krishna S, Looareesuwan S et al. Erythrocyte sequestration and anaemia in severe falciparum malaria. Analysis of acute changes in venous haematocrit using a simple mathematical model. *J Clin Invest* 1990; 86:793–800.

166 Looareesuwan S, Merry A H, Phillips R E et al. Reduced erythrocyte survival following clearance of malarial parasitaemia in Thai patients. *Br J Haematol* 1987; 67:473–478.

167 Abdallah S, Weatherall D J, Wickramasinghe S N & Hughes M. The anaemia of *P. falciparum* malaria. *Br J Haematol* 1980; 46:171–183.

168 Phillips R E, Looareesuwan S, Warrell D A et al. The importance of anaemia in cerebral and uncomplicated falciparum malaria: role of complications, dyserythropoiesis and iron sequestration. *J Med* 1986; 58:305–323.

169 Knuttgen H J. The bone marrow of non-immune Europeans in acute malaria infection: a topical review. *Ann Trop Med Parasitol* 1987; 81:567–576.

170 Joshi P, Alam A, Chandra R et al. Possible basis for membrane changes in non parasitised erythrocytes of malaria infected animals. *Biochim Biophys Acta* 1986; 862:220–222.

171 Facer C A, Bray R S & Brown J. Direct Coombs' antiglobulin reactions in Gambian children with *Plasmodium falciparum* malaria. I. Incidence and class specificity. *Clin Exp Immunol* 1979; 35:119–127.

172 Facer C A. Direct Combs' antiglobulin reactions in Gambian children with *Plasmodium falciparum* malaria. II. Specificity of erythrocyte bound IgG. *Clin Exp Immunol* 1980; 39:279–288.

173 Merry A H, Looareesuwan S, Phillips R E et al. Evidence against immune haemolysis in falciparum malaria in Thailand. *Br J Haematol* 1986; 64:187–194.

174 Charoenlarp P, Vanijanonta S & Chat-Panyaporn P. The effect of prednisolone on red cell survival in patients with falciparum malaria. *Southeast Asian J Trop Med Public Health* 1979; 10:127–131.

175 Jaroonvesama N. Intravascular coagulation in falciparum malaria. *Lancet* 1972; i:221–223.

176 Horstmann R D & Dietrich M. Haemostatic alterations in malaria correlate with parasitaemia. *Blut* 1975; 51:329–333.

177 Sucharit P, Chongsuphajaisiddhi T, Harinasuta T et al. Studies on coagulation and fibrinolysis in cases of falciparum malaria. *Southeast Asian J Trop Med Public Health* 1975; 6:33–39.

178 Pukrittayakamee S, White N J, Clemens R et al. Activation of the coagulation cascade in falciparum malaria. *Trans R Soc Trop Med Hyg* 1989; 83:762–766.

179 Skudowitz R B, Katz J, Lurie A et al. Mechanisms of thrombocytopenia in malignant tertian malaria. *BMJ* 1973; ii:515–518.

180 Kelton J G, Keystone J, Moore J et al. Immune-mediated thrombocytopenia of malaria. *J Clin Invest* 1983; 71:832–836.

181 Essien E. The circulating platelet in acute malaria infection. *Br J Haematol* 1989; 72:589–590.

182 Looareesuwan S, Davis J G, Allen D L et al. Thromboeytopenia in malaria. *Southeast Asian J Trop Med Public Health* 1992; 23:44–50.

183 Supanaranond W, Davis T M E, Dawes J et al. In-vivo platelet activation and anomalous thrombospondin levels in severe falciparum malaria. *Platelets* 1992; 3:195–200.

184 Udeinya I J & Miller L H. *Plasmodium falciparum*: effect of infected erythrocytes on clotting time of plasma. *Am J Trop Med Hyg* 1987; 37:246–249.

185 Punyagupta S, Srichaikul T, Nitiyanant P & Petchclai B. Acute pulmonary insufficiency in falciparum malaria: summary of 12 cases with evidence of disseminated intravascular coagulation. *Am J Trop Med Hyg* 1974; 23:551–559.

186 Reid H A & Nkrumah F K. Fibrin-degradation products in cerebral malaria. *Lancet* 1972; i:218–221.

187 Borochovitz D, Crosley A & Metz J. Intravascular coagulation with fatal haemorrhage in cerebral malaria. *BMJ* 1970; ii:710.

188 Karney W W & Tong M J. Malabsorption in *Plasmodium falciparum* malaria. *Am J Trop Med Hyg* 1972; 21:1–5.

189 Olsson R A & Johnston E H. Histopathologic changes and small bowel absorption in falciparum malaria. *Am J Trop Med Hyg* 1969; 18:355–359.

190 Segal H E, Hall A P, Jewell J S et al. Gastrointestinal function, quinine absorption and parasite response in falciparum malaria. *Southeast Asian J Trop Med Public Health* 1974; 5:499–503.

191 Molyneux M E, Looareesuwan S, Menzies I S et al. Reduced hepatic blood flow and intestinal malabsorption in severe falciparum malaria. *Am J Trop Med Hyg* 1989; 40:470–476.

192 White N J. Clinical pharmacokinetics of the antimalarial drugs. *Clin Pharmacokinet* 1985; 10:187–215.

193 Pukrittayakamee S, White N J, Davis T M E et al. Hepatic blood flow and metabolism in severe malaria: the clearance of intravenously administered galactose. *Clin Sci* 1992; 82:63–70.

194 Jensen M D, Conley M & Helstowski L D. Culture of *Plasmodium falciparum*: the role of pH glucose and lactate. *J Parasitol* 1983; 69:1060–1067.

195 Pfaller M A, Parquette A R, Krogstad D J & Nguyen-Dinh P. *Plasmodium falciparum*: stage-specific lactate production in synchronized cultures. *Exp Parasitol* 1982; 54:391–396.

196 Vander Jagt D, Hunsaker L A, Campos N M & Baack B R. D-lactate production in erythrocytes infected with *Plasmodium falciparum*. *Mol Biochem Parasitol* 1990; 42:277–284.

197 White N J, Warrell D A, Chanthavanich P et al. Severe hypoglycaemia and hyperinsulinaemia in falciparum malaria. *N Engl J Med* 1983; 309:61–66.

198 White N J, Miller K D, Marsh K et al. Hypoglycaemia in African children with severe malaria. *Lancet* 1987; i:708–711.

199 Taylor T E, Molyneaux M E, Wirima J J et al. Blood glucose levels in Malawian children before

and during the administration of intravenous quinine in severe falciparum malaria. *N Engl J Med* 1988; 319:1040–1047.

200 Onongbu I C & Onyeneke E C. Plasma lipid changes in human malaria. *Tropenmed Parasitol* 1983; 34:193–196.

201 Davis T M E, Supanaranond W, Pukrittayakamee S et al. The pituitary–thyroid axis in severe falciparum malaria. *Trans R Soc Trop Med Hyg* 1990; 84:330–335.

202 Davis T M E, Pukrittayakamee S, Woodhead J S et al. Calcium and phosphate metabolism in acute falciparum malaria. *Clin Sci* 1991; 81:297–304.

203 Petithory J C, Lebeau G, Galeazzi G & Chauty A. L'hypocalcémie palustre. Etudes des corrélations avec d'autres parametres. *Bull Soc Pathol Exot Filiales* 1983; 76:455–462.

204 Brooks M H, Barry K G, Cirksen W J et al. Pituitary–adrenal function in acute falciparum malaria. *Am J Trop Med Hyg* 1969; 18:872–877.

205 Davis T M E, Looareesuwan S, Pukrittayakamee S et al. Glucose turnover in severe falciparum malaria. *Metabolism* 1993; 42:334–340.

206 Okitolonda W, Delacollette C, Malengreau M & Henquin J C. High incidence of hypoglycaemia in African patients treated with intravenous quinine for severe malaria. *BMJ* 1987; 295:716–718.

207 Davis T M E, Karbwang J, Looareesuwan S et al. Comparative effects of quinine and quinidine on glucose metabolism in normal man. *Br J Clin Pharmacol* 1990; 30: 397–403.

208 Davis T M E, Pukrittayakamee S, Supanaranond W et al. Glucose metabolism in quinine-treated patients with uncomplicated falciparum malaria. *Clin Endocrinol (Oxf)* 1990; 33:739–749.

209 Riley E M, Schneider G, Sambou I & Greenwood B M. Suppression of cell-mediated immune responses to malaria antigens in pregnant Gambian women. *Am J Trop Med Hyg* 1989; 40:131–144.

210 Bray R S & Sinden R E. The sequestration of *Plasmodium falciparum* infected erythrocytes in the placenta. *Trans R Soc Trop Med Hyg* 1979; 73:716–719.

211 Jelliffe E F P. Low birth weight and malarial infection of the placenta. *Bull World Health Organ* 1968; 38:69–78.

212 Brabin B J. Analysis of malaria in pregnancy in Africa. *Bull World Health Organ* 1983; 61:1005–1016.

213 Menon R. Pregnancy and malaria. *Med J Malaysia* 1972; 27:11–119.

214 McGregor I A, Wilson M E & Billewicz W Z. Malaria infection of the placenta in The Gambia, West Africa: its incidence and relationship to stillbirth, birthweight and placental weight. *Trans R Soc Trop Med Hyg* 1983; 77:232–244.

215 Bray R S & Anderson M J. Falciparum malaria and pregnancy. *Trans R Soc Trop Med Hyg* 1979; 73:427–431.

216 Archibald H M. The influence of malaria infection

of the placenta on the incidence of prematurity. *Bull World Health Organ* 1956; 15:842–845.

217 Anagnos D, Lanoie L O, Palmieri J R et al. Effects of placental malaria on mothers and neonates from Zaire. *Parasitol* 1986; 72:57–64.

218 Nosten F, ter Kuile F, Malankirri L et al. Malaria in pregnancy in an area of unstable endemicity. *Trans R Soc Trop Med Hyg* 1991; 85:424–429.

219 Looareesuwan S, Phillips R E, White N J et al. Quinine and severe falciparum malaria in late pregnancy. *Lancet* 1985; ii:4–8.

220 Bygbjerg I C & Lanng C. Septicaemia as a complication of falciparum malaria. *Trans R Soc Trop Med Hyg* 1982; 76:705.

221 Mabey D C W, Brown A & Greenwood B M. *Plasmodium falciparum* malaria and *Salmonella* infections in Gambian children. *J Infect Dis* 1987; 155:1319–1321.

222 Marchiafava E & Bignami A. *On Summer–Autumnal Fever*. London: New Sydenham Society, 1894.

223 Dudgeon L S & Clarke C. A contribution to the microscopical histology of malaria. *Lancet* 1917; ii:153–156.

224 Dudgeon L S & Clarke C. An investigation on fatal cases of pernicious malaria caused by *Plasmodium falciparum* in Macedonia. *Q J Med* 1918; 12:372–390.

225 Gaskell J F & Millar W L. Studies on malignant malaria in Macedonia. *Q J Med* 1920; 13:381–426.

226 Kean B H & Smith J A. Death due to aestivo-autumnal malaria. A resumé of one hundred autopsy cases 1925–1942. *Am J Trop Med Hyg* 1944; 24:317–322.

227 Edington G M. Pathology of malaria in West Africa. *BMJ* 1967; i:715–718.

228 Spitz S. Pathology of acute falciparum malaria. *Milit Med* 1946; 99:555–572.

229 Pongponratn E, Riganti M, Punpoowong B & Aikawa M. Microvascular sequestration of parasitised erythrocytes in human falciparum malaria — a pathological study. *Am J Trop Med Hyg* 1991; 44:168–175.

230 Oo M M, Aikawa M & Than T. Human cerebral malaria: a pathological study. *J Neuropathol Exp Neurol* 1988; 46:223–231.

231 Igarashi I, Oo M M, Stanley H et al. Knob antigen deposition in cerebral malaria. *Am J Trop Med Hyg* 1987; 37:511–515.

232 Boonpucknavig V, Boonpucknavig S, Udomsangpetch R & Nitiyanant P. An immunofluorescent study of cerebral malaria. *Arch Pathol Lab Med* 1990; 114: 1028–1034.

233 Duarte M I S, Corbett C E P, Boulos M & Amata Neto V. Ultrastructure of the lung in falciparum malaria. *Am J Trop Med Hyg* 1985; 34:31–35.

234 Feldman R M & Singer C. Non-cardiogenic pulmonary edema and pulmonary fibrosis in falciparum malaria. *Rev Infect Dis* 1987; 9:134–139.

235 Deller J J, Cifarelli P S, Berque S & Buchanan R. Malaria hepatitis. *Milit Med* 1967; 132:614–620.

236 De Brito T, Barone A A & Earia R M. Human liver biopsy in *P. falciparum* and *P. vivax* malaria. A light and electron microscopy study. *Virchows Arch* 1969; 348:220–229.

237 Corcoran T E, Hegstrom G J, Zoeckler S J & Keil P G. Liver structure in non fatal malaria. *Gastroenterology* 1953; 24:53–62.

238 Pongponratn E, Riganti M, Harinasuta T & Bunnag D. Electron microscopic study of phagocytosis in human spleen in falciparum malaria. *Southeast Asian J Trop Med Public Health* 1989; 20:31–39.

239 Weiss L. The spleen in malaria; the role of barrier cells. *Immunol Lett* 1990; 25:165–172.

240 Wickramasinghe S N, Looareesuwan S, Nagachinta B & White N J. Dyserythropoiesis and ineffective erythropoiesis in *Plasmodium vivax* malaria. *Br J Haematol* 1989; 72:91–99.

241 Clark H C. The diagnostic value of the placental blood film in aestivo-autumnal malaria. *J Exp Med* 1915; 22:427–444.

242 Walter P, Gavin J F & Blot P. Placental pathologic changes in malaria. *Am J Pathol* 1982; 109:330–342.

243 Philippe E & Walter P. Les lésions placentaires du paludisme. *Arch Fr Pediatr* 1985; 42 (supplement): 921–923.

244 Galbraith R M, Fox, Hsi B et al. The human materno-fetal relationship in malaria. II. Histological, ultrastructural and immunopathological studies of the placenta. *Trans R Soc Trop Med Hyg* 1980; 74:61–72.

245 Shute P G. Malaria. *B M J* 1951; 11: 1280.

246 Looareesuwan S, White N J, Chittamas S et al. High rate of *Plasmodium vivax* relapse following treatment of falciparum malaria in Thailand. *Lancet* 1987; ii: 1052–1055.

247 Marchiafava E & Bignami A. *On Summer–Autumnal Fever*. London: New Sydenham Society, 1894.

248 World Health Organization. Division of Control of Tropical Diseases: Severe and Complicated Malaria. *Trans R Soc Trop Med Hyg* 1990; 84 (supplement 2):1–65.

249 Molyneux M E, Taylor T E, Wirima J J & Borgstein J. Clinical features and prognostic indicators in paediatric cerebral malaria: a study of 131 comatose Malawian children. *Q J Med* 1989; 71:441–459.

250 Looareesuwan S, Warrell D A, White N J et al. Retinal haemorrhage, a common physical sign of prognostic significance in cerebral malaria. *Am J Trop Med Hyg* 1983; 32:911–915.

251 Dover A S & Western K A. Fatalities due to malaria in the United States, 1966–1969. *J Infect Dis* 1970; 121:573–575.

252 Omanga U, Ntihinyurwa M, Shako D & Mashako M. Les hémiplégies au cours de l'accès pernicieux a *Plasmodium falciparum* de l'enfant. *Ann Pediatr* 1983; 30:294–296.

253 Collomb H, Rey M, Dumas M et al. Les

hémiplégies au cours du paludisme aigue. *Bull Soc Med Afr Noire* 1967; 12:791–795.

254 De Silva H J, Gamage R, Herath H K N et al. A delayed onset cerebellar syndrome complicating falciparum malaria. *Ceylon Med J* 1986; 31:147–150.

255 Senanayake N. Delayed cerebellar ataxia: a new complication of falciparum malaria. *BMJ* 1987; 294:1253–1254.

256 Dukes D C, Sealey B J & Forbes J L. Oliguric renal failure in blackwater fever. *Am J Med* 1948; 45:899–903.

257 Canfield C J. Renal and hematologic complications of acute falciparum malaria in Vietnam. *Bull N Y Acad Med 1969*; 45:1043–1057.

258 Blackie W K. Blackwater fever. *Clin Proc* 1944; 3:272–312.

259 Ross G R. Blackwater fever in Southern Rhodesia in retrospect. *Cent Afr Med J* 1962; 8:294–297.

260 Stone W J, Hanchett J E & Knepshield J R. Acute renal insufficiency due to falciparum malaria. *Arch Intern Med* 1972; 129:620–628.

261 Brooks M H, Kiel F W, Sheehy T W & Barry K G. Acute pulmonary edema in falciparum malaria. *N Engl J Med* 1968; 279:732–737.

262 Gurman G, Schlaeffer F, Alkan M & Heilig I. Adult respiratory distress syndrome and pancreatitis as complications of falciparum malaria. *Crit Care Med* 1988; 16:205–206.

263 Fein L A, Rackow E C & Shapiro L. Acute pulmonary edema in *Plasmodium falciparum* malaria. *Am Rev Respir Dis* 1978; 118:425–429.

264 Sullivan J. Pernicious fever: febris algida and febris comatosa. *Med Times Gaz* 1876; 1:277–279.

265 Gage A. Algid malaria. *Ther Gaz* 1926; 50:77–81.

266 Butler T & Weber D M. On the nature of orthostatic hypotension in acute malaria. *Trans R Soc Trop Med Hyg* 1973; 22:439–442.

267 Kofi-Ekue J M, Phiri D E D, Mukunyandela M et al. Severe orthostatic hypotension during treatment of malaria. *BMJ* 1988; 296:396.

268 Supanaranond W, Davis T M E, Pukrittayakamee S et al. Abnormal circulatory control in falciparum malaria: the effects of antimalarial drugs. *Eur J Clin Pharmacol* 1993; 44:325–329.

269 Migasena S. Hypoglycaemia in falciparum malaria. *Ann Trop Med Parasitol* 1983; 77:323–324.

270 Das B A, Satpathy S K, Mohanty D et al. Hypoglycaemia in severe falciparum malaria. *Trans R Soc Trop Med Hyg* 1988; 82:197–201.

271 Davis T M E, Ho M, Supanaranond W et al. Changes in the peripheral blood eosinophil count in falciparum malaria. *Acta Trop* 1991; 48: 243–245.

272 Pukrittayakamee S, Clemens R, Pramoolsinsap C et al. Polymorphonuclear leukocyte elastase in *Plasmodium falciparum* malaria. *Trans R Soc Trop Med Hyg* 1992; 86:598–601.

273 Kern P, Hemmer C J, Gallati M et al. Soluble tumour necrosis factor receptors correlate with parasitemia and disease severity in human malaria. *J Infect Dis* 1992; 166:930–934.

274 Miller L H, Makaranond P. Sitprija V et al. Hyponatraemia in malaria. *Ann Trop Med Parasitol* 1967; 61:265–279.

275 Miller K D, White N J, Lott L A et al. Biochemical evidence of muscle injury in African children with severe malaria. *J Infect Dis* 1989; 159:139–142.

276 White N J, Miller K D, Brown J et al. Prognostic value of CSF lactate in cerebral malaria. *Lancet* 1987; i:1261.

277 White N J & Looareesuwan S. Cerebral malaria. In Kennedy P G E & Johnson R T (eds) *Infections of the Nervous System*. London: Butterworth, 1987:118–143.

278 Field J W & Niven J C. A note on prognosis in relation to parasite counts in acute subtertian malaria. *Trans R Soc Trop Med Hyg* 1937; 30:569–574.

279 Field J W. Blood examination and prognosis in acute falciparum malaria. *Trans R Soc Trop Med Hyg* 1949; 43:33–68.

280 Li Q Q, Guo X, Jian N et al. Development state of *Plasmodium falciparum* in the intradermal, peripheral and medullary blood of patients with cerebral malaria. *Natl Med J Chin* 1983; 63:692–693.

281 White N J & Silamut K. Rapid diagnosis of malaria. *Lancet* 1989; i:435.

282 Earle W C & Perez M. Enumeration of parasites in the blood of malaria patients. *J Lab Clin Med* 1983; 17:1123–1130.

283 Rickman L S, Long G W, Oberst R et al. Rapid diagnosis of malaria by acridine orange staining of centrifuged parasites. *Lancet* 1989; i:68–71.

284 Wongsrichanali C, Pornsilapatip J, Namsiripongpun V et al. Acridine orange fluorescent microscopy and the detection of malaria in populations with low density parasitemia. *Am J Trop Med Hyg* 1991; 44:17–20.

285 Barker R H, Suebsang L & Rooney W. Specific DNA probe for the diagnosis of *P. falciparum* malaria. *Science* 1986; 230:1434–1436.

286 Editorial. Rediscovering wormwood, qinghaosu, for malaria. *Lancet* 1992; 339:649–651.

287 Haggis A W. Fundamental errors in the early history of cinchona. *Bull Hist Med* 1941; 10:568–592.

288 Duran-Reynolds M G. *The Fever Bark Tree*. New York: Doubleday, 1946.

289 Dawson W T. Cinchona alkaloids and bark in malaria. *Int Clin* 1930; 2:121–149.

290 Melville C H. The prevention of malaria in war. In Ross R (ed.) *The Prevention of Malaria*, 2nd edn. London: Murray, 1911:577–599.

291 Taylor N. *Cinchona in Java*. New York: Greenberg, 1945.

292 Coatney G R. Pitfalls in a discovery: the chronicle of chloroquine. *Am J Trop Med Hyg* 1963; 12:121–128.

293 Covell G. Chemotherapy of malaria. *WHO Monogr Ser* 1967; 27.

294 Pampana E J. *A Textbook of Malaria Eradication*, 2nd edn. London: Oxford University Press, 1969.

295 Nocht B & Werner H. Beobachtungen uber relative Chininresistenz bei Malaria aus Brasilien. *Dtsch Med Wochenschr* 1910; 36:1557–1560.

296 Rozman R S & Canfield C J. New experimental antimalarial drugs. *Adv Pharmacol Chemother* 1979; 16:1–43.

297 World Health Organization. Practical chemotherapy of malaria. *WHO Tech Rep Ser* 1990; 805.

298 Hammond D J, Burchell J R & Pudney M. Inhibition of pyrimidine biosynthesis de novo in *Plasmodium falciparum* by 2-(4-*t*-butylcyclohexyl)-3-hydroxy-1, 4-naphthaquinone in vitro. *Mol Biochem Parasitol* 1985; 14:97–109.

299 Ding G S. Recent studies on antimalarials in China: a review of literature since 1980. *Int J Exp Clin Chemother* 1988; 1:9–22.

300 Qinghaosu Antimalarial Coordinating Research Group. Antimalarial studies on qinghaosu. *Chin Med J* 1979; 92:811–816.

301 Klayman D L. Qinghaosu (artemisinin). An antimalarial drug from China. *Science* 1985; 228:1049–1055.

302 Jiang J B, Li G Q, Gao X B et al. Antimalarial activity of mefloquine and qinghaosu. *Lancet* 1982; ii:285–288.

303 Lee I S & Hufford C D. Metabolism of antimalarial sequiterpene lactones. *Pharmacol Ther* 1990; 48:345–355.

304 Li G Q, Guo X B & Jiang R. Clinical studies on treatment of cerebral malaria with qinghaosu and its derivatives. *J Tradit Chin Med* 1982; 2:124–130.

305 Shwe T, Myint P T, Htut Y et al. The effect of mefloquine-artemether compared with quinine on patients with complicated falciparum malaria. *Trans R Soc Trop Med Hyg* 1988; 82:665–667.

306 Hien T T & White N J. Qinghaosu, *Lancet* 1993; 341:603–608.

307 Watkins W M, Percy M, Crampton J M et al. The changing response of *Plasmodium falciparum* to antimalarial drugs in East Africa. *Trans R Soc Trop Med Hyg* 1988; 82:21–26.

308 White N J. Antimalarial drug resistance: the pace quickens. *J Antimicrob Chemother* 1992; 30:571–585.

309 Nosten F, ter Kuile F, Chongsuphajaisiddhi T et al. Mefloquine-resistant falciparum malaria on the Thai–Burmese border. *Lancet* 1991; 337:1140–1143.

310 Simon F, Le-Bras J, Gaudebout C & Girard P M. Reduced sensitivity of *Plasmodium falciparum* to mefloquine in West Africa. *Lancet* 1988; i:467–468.

311 Rieckmann K H, Davis D R & Hutton D C. *Plasmodium vivax* resistance to chloroquine? *Lancet* 1989; ii:1183–1184.

312 White N J. Drug treatment and prevention of malaria. *Eur J Clin Pharmacol* 1988; 34:1–14.

313 Yayon A, Vande Waa J A, Yayon M et al. Stage dependent effects of chloroquine on *Plasmodium falciparum* in vitro. *J Protozool* 1983; 30:642–647.

314 ter Kuile F, White N J, Holloway P et al. *Plasmodium falciparum*: in vitro studies of the pharmacodynamic properties of drugs used for the treatment of severe malaria. *Exp Parasitol* 1993; 76:85–95.

315 York W & Macfie J W S. Observations on malaria made during treatment of general paralysis. *Trans R Soc Trop Med Hyg* 1924:12–44.

316 Clyde D F & Shute G T. Resistance of East African varieties of *Plasmodium falciparum* to pyrimethamine. *Trans R Soc Trop Med Hyg* 1954; 48:495–500.

317 Peterson D S, Walliker D & Wellems T. Evidence that a point mutation in dihydrofolate reductase-thymidylate synthase confers resistance to pyrimethamine in falciparum malaria. *Proc Natl Acad Sci USA* 1988; 85:9114–9118.

318 Peterson D A, Milhous W K & Wellems T E. Molecular basis of differential resistance to cycloguanil and pyrimethamine in *Plasmodium falciparum* malaria. *Proc Natl Acad Sci USA* 1990; 87:3018–3022.

319 Foote S J, Galatis D & Cowman A F. Aminoacids in the dihydrofolate reductase–thymidylate synthase gene of *Plasmodium falciparum* involved in cycloguanil resistance differ from those involved in pyrimethamine resistance. *Proc Natl Acad Sci USA* 1990; 87:3014–3017.

320 Krogstad D & Schlesinger P H. Acid vesicle function, intracellular pathogens and the action of chloroquine against *Plasmodium falciparum*. *N Engl J Med* 1987; 317:542–549.

321 Krugliak M & Ginsburg H. Studies on the antimalarial mode of action of quinoline-containing drugs: time dependence and irreversibility of drug action, and interactions with compounds that alter the function of the parasite's food vacuole. *Life Sci* 1991; 49:1213–1219.

322 Chou A C, Chevli R & Fitch C D. Ferriprotoporphyrin IX fulfills the criteria for identification as the chloroquine receptor of malaria parasites. *Biochemistry* 1980; 19:1543–1549.

323 Slater A F C & Cerami F. Inhibition by chloroquine of a novel haem polymerase enzyme activity in malaria trophozoites. *Nature* 1992; 355:167–169.

324 Wellems T. Malaria. How chloroquine works. *Nature* 1992; 355:108–109.

325 Foote S J, Thompson J K, Courman A F & Kemp D J. Amplification of the multidrug resistance gene in some chloroquine-resistant isolates of *Plasmodium falciparum*. *Cell* 1989; 57:921–930.

326 Wilson C M, Serrano A E, Walsey A et al. Amplification of a gene related to mammalian mdr genes in drug resistant *Plasmodium falciparum*. *Science* 1989; 244:1184–1186.

327 Newbold C. The path of drug resistance. *Nature* 1990; 345:202–203.

328 Wellems T E, Walker-Jonah A & Panton L J.

Genetic mapping of the chloroquine-resistant locus on *Plasmodium falciparum* chromosome 7. *Proc Natl Acad Sci USA* 1991; 88: 3382–3386.

329 Wellems T E. Molecular genetics of drug resistance in *Plasmodium falciparum* malaria. *Parasitol Today* 1991; 7:110–112.

330 Ginsburg H & Stein W D. Kinetic modelling of chloroquine uptake by malaria infected erythrocytes. Assessment of the factors that may determine drug resistance. *Biochem Pharmacol* 1991; 41:1463–1470.

331 Martin S K, Oduola A M J & Milhous W K. Reversal of chloroquine resistance in *Plasmodium falciparum* by verapamil. *Science* 1987; 235:899–901.

332 Salama A & Facer C A. Desipramine reversal of chloroquine resistance in wild isolates of *Plasmodium falciparum*. *Lancet* 1990; 335:164–165.

333 Brasseur P, Kouamouo J, Brandicourt O Patterns of in-vitro resistance to chloroquine, quinine, and mefloquine of *Plasmodium falciparum* in Cameroon 1985–1986. *Am J Trop Med Hyg* 1988; 39:166–172.

334 Warsame M, Wernsdorfer W H, Payne D & Bjorkman A. Susceptibility of *Plasmodium falciparum* in vitro to chloroquine, mefloquine, quinine and sulfadoxine/pyrimethamine in Somalia: relationship between the responses to different drugs. *Trans R Soc Trop Med Hyg* 1991; 85:565–569.

335 Thaithong S. Clones of different sensitivities in drug resistant isolates of *Plasmodium falciparum*. *Bull World Health Organ* 1983; 61:709–712.

336 Wernsforfer W H. The development and spread of drug resistant malaria. *Parasitol Today* 1991; 7:296–303.

337 Curtis C F & Otoo L N. A simple model of the build up of resistance to mixtures of antimalarial drugs. *Trans R Soc Trop Med Hyg* 1986; 80:889–892.

338 Cross A P & Singer B. Modelling the development of resistance of *Plasmodium falciparum* to antimalarial drugs. *Trans R Soc Trop Med Hyg* 1991; 85:349–355.

339 World Health Organization. Practical chemotherapy of malaria. *WHO Tech Rep Ser* 1990; 805.

340 Zhang Y, Asante K S & Jung A. Stage dependent inhibition of chloroquine on *Plasmodium falciparum* in vitro. *J Parasitol* 1986; 72:830–836.

341 Supanaranond W, Davis T M E, Pukrittayakamee S et al. Disposition of oral quinine in acute falciparum malaria. *Eur J Clin Pharmacol* 1991; 40:49–52.

342 Waller D, Krishna S, Craddock C et al. The pharmacokinetic properties of intramuscular quinine in Gambian children with severe falciparum malaria. *Trans R Soc Trop Med Hyg* 1990; 84:488–491.

343 Mansor S M, Taylor T E, McGrath C S et al. The safety and kinetics of intramuscular quinine in

Malawian children with moderately severe falciparum malaria. *Trans R Soc Trop Med Hyg* 1990; 84:482–488.

344 Sabcharoen A, Chongsuphajaisiddhi T & Attanath P. Serum quinine concentrations following the initial dose in children with falciparum malaria. *Southeast Asian J Trop Med Public Health* 1989; 13:689–692.

345 White N J, Looareesuwan S, Warrell D A et al. Quinine pharmacokinetics and toxicity in cerebral and uncomplicated falciparum malaria. *Am J Med* 1982; 73:564–572.

346 White N J, Chanthavanich P, Krishna S et al. Quinine disposition kinetics. *Br J Clin Pharmacol* 1983; 16: 399–404.

347 Silamut K, White N J, Warrell D A & Looareesuwan S. Binding of quinine to plasma proteins in falciparum malaria. *Am J Trop Med Hyg* 1985; 34:681–686.

348 Silamut K, Molunto P, Ho M et al. Alpha-one acid glycoprotein (orosomucoid) and plasma protein binding of quinine in falciparum malaria. *Br J Clin Pharmacol* 1991; 32:311–315.

349 Mansor S M, Molyneux M E, Taylor T E et al. Effect of *Plasmodium falciparum* malaria infection as the plasma concentration of alpha acid glycoprotein and the binding of quinine in Malawian children. *Br J Clin Pharmacol* 1991; 32:317–325.

350 White N J, Looareesuwan S & Lavansiri K. Red cell quinine concentrations in falciparum malaria. *Am J Trop Med Hyg* 1983; 32:456–460.

351 Phillips R E, Looareesuwan S, White N J et al. Quinine pharmacokinetics and toxicity in pregnant and lactating women with falciparum malaria. *Br J Clin Pharmacol* 1986; 21:677–683.

352 White N J, Looareesuwan S & Warrell D A. Quinine and quinidine: a comparison of EKG effects during the treatment of malaria. *J Cardiovasc Pharmacol* 1983; 5:173–177.

353 Dyson E H, Proudfoot A T, Prescott L F & Heyworth R. Death and blindness due to overdose of quinine. *BMJ* 1985; 291:31–33.

354 Boland M E, Brennand-Roper S M & Henry J A. Complications of quinine poisoning. *Lancet* 1985; i:384–385.

355 Henquin J C, Horeman B, Henquin M et al. Quinine-induced modifications of insulin release and glucose metabolism by isolated pancreatic islets. *FEBS Lett* 1975; 57:280–284.

356 Bruce-Chwatt L J. Quinine and the mystery of blackwater fever. *Acta Leiden* 1987; 55:181–196.

357 Chongsuphajaisiddhi T, Sabcharoen A & Attanath P. In-vivo and in-vitro sensitivity to quinine in Thai children. *Ann Trop Paediatr* 1981; 1:21–26.

358 White N J, Warrell D A, Looareesuwan S et al. Quinine loading dose in cerebral malaria. *Am J Trop Med Hyg* 1983; 32:1–5.

359 White N J, Looareesuwan S, Warrell D A et al. Quinidine in falciparum malaria. *Lancet* 1981; ii:1069–1072.

360 Phillips R E, Warrell D A, White N J et al. Intravenous quinidine for the treatment of severe falciparum malaria. Clinical and pharmacokinetic studies. *N Engl J Med* 1985; 312:1273–1278.

361 Karbwang J, Davis T M E, Looareesuwan S et al. A comparison of the pharmacokinetic and pharmacodynamic properties of quinine and quinidine in healthy Thai males. *Br J Clin Pharmacol* 1993; 35:265–271.

362 Miller K D, Greenberg A E & Campbell C C. Treatment of severe malaria in the United States with a continuous infusion of quinidine gluconate and exchange transfusion. *N Engl J Med* 1989; 321:65–70.

363 Gustafsson L L, Walker O, Alvan G et al. Disposition of chloroquine in man after single intravenous and oral doses. *Br J Clin Pharmacol* 1983; 15:471–479.

364 Frisk-Holmberg M, Bergqvist Y, Termond E & Domeij-Nyberg B. The single dose kinetics of chloroquine and its major metabolite desethyl-chloroquine in healthy subjects. *Eur J Clin Pharmacol* 1984; 26:521–530.

365 White N J, Watt G, Bergqvist Y & Njelesani E. Parenteral chloroquine in the treatment of falciparum malaria. *J Infect Dis* 1987; 155:192–201.

366 White N J, Miller K D, Churchill F C et al. Chloroquine treatment of severe malaria in children: pharmacokinetics, toxicity, and revised dosage recommendations. *N Engl J Med* 1988; 319:1493–1500.

367 Walker O, Daurodu A H, Adeyokunnu A A et al. et al. Plasma chloroquine and desethylchloroquine concentrations in children during and after chloroquine treatment for malaria. *Br J Clin Pharmacol* 1983; 16:701–705.

368 Minker F & Iran J. Experimental and clinicopharmacological study of rectal absorption of chloroquine. *Acta Physiol Hung* 1991; 77:237–248.

369 Ward S A, Helsby N A, Skjelbo E et al. The activation of the biguanide antimalarial proguanil cosegregates with the mephenytoin oxidation polymorphism. A panel study. *Br J Clin Pharmacol* 1991; 31:689–692.

370 Easterbrook M. Ocular effects and safety of antimalarials. *Am J Med* 1988; 85 (supplement 4a): 23–29.

371 Peruval S P B & Meancock I. Chloroquine: ophthalmological safety and clinical assessment in rheumatoid arthritis. *BMJ* 1968; 3:579–584.

372 Riou B, Barriot P, Rimailho A & Band F J. Treatment of severe chloroquine poisoning. *N Engl J Med* 1988; 316:1–6.

373 Pussard E, Lepers J P, Clavier F et al. Efficacy of a loading dose of oral chloroquine in a 36-hour treatment schedule for uncomplicated *Plasmodium falciparum* malaria. *Antimicrob Agents Chemother* 1991; 35:406–409.

374 Winstanley P, Edwards G, Orme ML'E & Breckenridge A M. The disposition of amodiaquine

in man after oral administration. *Br J Clin Pharmacol* 1987; 23:1–7.

375 Hatton C S, Peto T E A, Bunch C et al. Frequency of severe neutropenia associated with amodiaquine prophylaxis against malaria. *Lancet* 1986; i:411–414.

376 White N J. Combination treatment for *P. falciparum* prophylaxis. *Lancet* 1987; i:680–681.

377 Desjardins R E, Pamplin C L, Von Bredow J et al. Kinetics of a new antimalarial. Mefloquine. *Clin Pharmacol Ther* 1979; 26:372–379.

378 Karbwang J & White N J. Clinical pharmacokinetics of mefloquine. *Clin Pharmacokinet* 1990; 19:264–279.

379 Looareesuwan S, White N J, Warrell D A et al. Studies of mefloquine bioavailability and kinetics using a stable isotope technique: a comparison of Thai patients with falciparum malaria and healthy Caucasian volunteers. *Br J Clin Pharmacol* 1987; 24:37–42.

380 Nosten F, Karbwang J, White N J et al. Mefloquine antimalarial prophylaxis in pregnancy: dose finding and pharmacokinetic study. *Br J Clin Pharmacol* 1990; 30:79–85.

381 Nosten F, ter Kuile F, Chongsuphajaisiddhi T et al. Mefloquine pharmacokinetics and resistance in children with acute falciparum malaria. *Br J Clin Pharmacol* 1991; 31:556–559.

382 Slutsker L M, Khoromana C D, Payne D et al. Mefloquine therapy for *Plasmodium falciparum* malaria in children under 5 years of age in Malawi: in vivo/in vitro efficacy and correlation of drug concentration with parasitological outcome. *Bull World Health Organ* 1990; 68:53–59.

383 ter Kuile F, Nosten F, Thieren M et al. High-dose mefloquine in the treatment of multidrug-resistant falciparum malaria. *J Infect Dis* 1992; 166:1393–1400.

384 Bjorkman A, Steffen R, Armengaud M et al. Malaria chemoprophylaxis with mefloquine. *Lancet* 1991; 337:1479–1480.

385 Luxemburger C, Nosten F, ter Kuile F et al. Mefloquine for drug-resistant malaria. *Lancet* 1991; 338:1268.

386 Weinke T, Trautman M, Held T et al. Neuropsychiatric side effects after the use of mefloquine. *Am J Trop Med Hyg* 1991; 45:86–91.

387 Milton K A, Edwards G, Ward S A et al. Pharmacokinetics of halofantrine in man: effects of food and dose size. *Br J Clin Pharmacol* 1989; 28:71–77.

388 Veenendaal J R, Parkinson A D, Kere N et al. Pharmacokinetics of halofantrine and *n*-desbutylhalofantrine in patients with falciparum malaria following a multiple dose regimen of halofantrine. *Eur J Clin Pharmacol* 1991; 41:161–164.

389 Watkins W M, Oloo J A, Lury J D et al. Efficacy of multiple dose halofantrine in treatment of chloroquine resistant falciparum malaria in children in Kenya. *Lancet* 1988; ii:247–250.

390 Wirima J, Khoromana C, Molyneux M E & Gilles H M. Clinical trials with halofantrine hydrochloride in Malawi. *Lancet* 1988; ii:250–252.

391 Shanks C D, Watt C, Edstein M D et al. Halofantrine given with food for falciparum malaria. *Trans R Soc Trop Med Hyg* 1992; 86:233–234.

392 Winstanley P, Watkins W M, Newton C R J C et al. The disposition of oral and intramuscular pyrimethamine/sulphadoxine in Kenyan children with high parasitaemia but clinically non-severe falciparum malaria. *Br J Clin Pharmacol* 1992; 33:143–148.

393 Miller K D, Lobel H O, Satriale R F et al. Severe cutaneous reactions among American travellers using pyrimethamine-sulfadoxine (Fansidar®) for malaria prophylaxis. *Am J Trop Med Hyg* 1986; 35:451–458.

394 Bjorkman A & Phillips-Howard P A. Adverse reaction to sulfa drugs: implications for malaria chemotherapy. *Bull World Health Organ* 1991; 69:297–304.

395 Mihaly G W, Ward S A, Edwards C et al. Pharmacokinetics of primaquine in man: identification of the carboxylic acid derivative as a major plasma metabolite. *Br J Clin Pharmacol* 1984; 17:441–446.

396 Carson P E, Flangan C L, Ickes C E & Alving A S. Enzymatic deficiency in primaquine sensitive erythrocytes. *Science* 1956; 124:484–485.

397 Chan T K, Todd D & Tsao S C. Drug-induced haemolysis in glucose-6-phosphate dehydrogenase deficiency. *BMJ* 1976; ii:1227–1229.

398 Watkins W M, Chulay J D, Sixmith D G et al. A preliminary pharmacokinetic study of the antimalarial drugs proguanil and chlorproguanil. *J Pharm Pharmacol* 1987; 39:261–265.

399 Wattanagoon Y, Taylor R B, Moody R R et al. Single dose pharmacokinetics of proguanil and its metabolites in healthy adult volunteers. *Br J Clin Pharmacol* 1987; 24:775–780.

400 Helsby N A, Ward S A, Edwards C et al. The pharmacokinetics and activation of proguanil in man: consequences of variability in drug metabolism. *Br J Clin Pharmacol* 1990; 30:593–598.

401 Wangboonskul J, White N J, Nosten F et al. Single dose pharmacokinetics of proguanil and its metabolites in pregnancy. *Eur J Clin Pharmacol* 1993; 44:247–251.

402 Watkins W M, Brandling-Bennett Nevill C G, Carter J Y et al. Chlorproguanil/dapsone for the treatment of non-severe *Plasmodium falciparum* infection in Kenya. *Trans R Soc Trop Med Hyg* 1988; 82:398–403.

403 Harries A D, Forshaw A I & Friend H M. Malaria prophylaxis among British residents of Lilongwe and Kasungu districts, Malawi. *Trans R Soc Trop Med Hyg* 1988; 82:690–692.

404 Boots M, Phillips M & Curtis J R. Megaloblastic anaemia and pancytopenia due to proguanil in

patients with chronic renal failure. *Clin Nephrol* 1982; 18:106–108.

405 Li G Q. Clinical studies on artemisinin suppository and on artesunate and artemether. In Shen J X (ed.) *Antimalarial Drug Development in China.* Beijing: National Institute of Pharmaceutical Research and Development, 1989:69–73.

406 Li G Q, Guo X B, Fu L C & Jian H X. A summary of clinical studies on the treatment of malaria with qinghaosu suppositories. In Li G Q, Guo X B & Yang F (eds) *Clinical Trials on Qinghaosu and its Derivatives*, Vol 1. Guangzhou: College of Traditional Chinese Medicine, Sanya Tropical Medicine Institute, 1990:17–22.

407 Yang S D, Ma J M, Sun J H et al. Clinical pharmacokinetics of a new effective antimalarial artesunate, a qinghaosu derivative. *Chin J Clin Pharmacol* 1986; 1:106–109.

408 Song Z Y & Zhao K C. Determination of artemisinin (qinghaosu) and its active derivatives in biological materials and studies on the pharmacokinetics of these compounds. In Shen J X (ed.) *Antimalarial Drug Development in China.* Beijing: National Institute of Pharmaceutical Research and Development, 1989:37–44.

409 Canfield C J. The development of artemether by the scientific working group on the chemotherapy of malaria in antimalarial drug development in China. In Shen J X (ed.) *Antimalarial Drug Development in China*. Beijing: National Institute of Pharmaceutical Research and Development, 1989:75–84.

410 Hien T T, Phu N H, Mai N T H et al. An open randomised comparison of intravenous and intramuscular artesunate in severe falciparum malaria. *Trans R Soc Trop Med Hyg* 1992; 86:584–585.

411 Looareesuwan S, Viravan C, Vanijanonta S et al. Randomised trial of artesunate and mefloquine alone and in sequence for acute uncomplicated falciparum malaria. *Lancet* 1992; 339:821–824.

412 Kremsner P G, Zotter G M, Feldmeier H et al. A comparative trial of three regimens for treating uncomplicated falciparum malaria in Acre, Brazil. *J Infect Dis* 1988; 158:1368–1371.

413 Molyneux M E, Taylor T E, Thomas C G et al. Efficacy of quinine for falciparum malaria according to previous chloroquine exposure. *Lancet* 1991; 337:1379–1380.

414 World Health Organization. Chemotherapy of malaria and resistance to antimalarials. Report of a WHO Scientific Group. *WHO Tech Rep Ser* 1973; 529:30–35.

415 Looareesuwan S, Charoenpan P, Ho M et al. Fatal *Plasmodium falciparum* malaria after an inadequate response to quinine treatment. *J Infect Dis* 1990; 161:577–580.

416 Webster H K, Boudreau E F, Pavanand K et al. Antimalarial drug susceptibility testing of *Plasmodium falciparum* in Thailand using a

microdilution radioisotope method. *Am J Trop Med Hyg* 1985; 34:228–235.

417 Arnold J, Alving A S, Hockwald R S et al. The effect of continuous and intermittent primaquine therapy on the relapse rate of Chesson strain vivax malaria. *J Lab Clin Med* 1954; 43:429–438.

418 White N J, Looareesuwan S, Phillips R E et al. Single dose phenobarbitone prevents convulsions in cerebral malaria. *Lancet* 1988; ii:64–66.

419 Warrell D A, Looareesuwan S, Warrell M J et al. Dexamethasone proves deleterious in cerebral malaria. A double blind trial in 100 comatose patients. *N Engl J Med* 1982; 306:313–319.

420 Hoffman S L, Rustama D, Punjabi N H et al. High-dose dexamethasone in quinine-treated patients with cerebral malaria: a double-blind, placebo-controlled trial. *J Infect Dis* 1988; 158:325–331.

421 Canfield C J, Miller L H, Bartellino P J et al. Acute renal failure in *Plasmodium falciparum* malaria. Treatment by peritoneal dialysis. *Arch Intern Med* 1968; 122:199–203.

422 Foster S D. Pricing, distribution and use of antimalarial drugs. *Bull World Health Organ* 1991; 69:349–363.

423 Lindsay S W & Gibson M E. Bednets revisited — old idea, new angle. *Parasitol Today* 1988; 4:270–272.

424 Alonso P L, Lindsay S W, Armstrong J R M et al. The effect of insecticide-treated bed nets on mortality of Gambian children. *Lancet* 1991; 337:1499–1502.

425 Greenwood B M, Greenwood A M, Bradley A K et al. Comparison of two strategies for control of malaria within a primary health care programme in the Gambia. *Lancet* 1988; i: 1121–1128.

426 Bjorkman A & Phillips-Howard P A. The epidemiology of drug resistant malaria. *Trans R Soc Trop Med Hyg* 1990; 84:177–180.

427 World Health Organization. Review of central nervous system adverse effects related to the antimalarial drug mefloquine (1985–1990). WHO/MAL/o1.1063. Geneva: *WHO*, 1991.

428 Chulay J D. Development of sporozoite vaccines for malaria. *Trans R Soc Trop Med Hyg* 1989; 83 (supplement):61–66.

429 Hendrickse R G, Adeniyi A, Edington G M et al. Quartan malarial nephrotic syndrome. Collaborative clinicopathological study in Nigerian children. *Lancet* 1977; i:1143–1149.

430 Gilles H M & Hendrickse R G. Nephrosis in Nigerian children: role of *Plasmodium malariae* and effect of antimalarial treatment. *B M J* 1963; ii:27–31.

431 Crane G. Tropical splenomegaly. Part II Oceania. *Clin Haematol* 1981; 10:976–982.

432 Piessens W F, Hoffman S L, Wadee A A et al. Antibody mediated killing of T suppressor lymphocytes as a possible cause of macroglobulinemia in the tropical splenomegaly syndrome. *J Clin Invest* 1985; 75:1821–1827.

433 Hoffman S L, Piessens W F, Ratiwayanto S et al. Reduction of suppressor T-lymphocytes in the tropical splenomegaly syndrome. *N Engl J Med.* 1984; 310:337–341.

434 Bate I, Bedu-Addo G, Bevan D H & Rutherford T R. Use of immunoglobulin gene rearrangements to show clonal lymphoproliferation in hyper-reactive malarial splenomegaly. *Lancet* 1991; 337:505–507.

435 Lam K M C, Syed N, Whittle H & Crawford D H. Circulating Epstein–Barr virus-carrying B cells in acute malaria. *Lancet* 1991; 337:876–879.

436 Newton C R, Peshu N, Kendall B. Brain swelling and ischaemia in Kenyans with cerebral malaria. *Arch Dis Child* 1994; 70:281–287.

437 Looareesuwan S, Wilairatana P, Krishna S et al. Magnetic resonance imaging of the brain in cerebral malaria. *Clin Infect Dis* 1995, in press.

438 Clemens R, Pramoolsinsap C, Lorenz R. Activation of the coagulation cascade in severe malaria through the intrinsic pathway. *Br J Haematol* 1994; 87:100–105.

439 Alonso P L, Smith T, Schellenberg J A et al. Randomised trial of SPF66 vaccine against *Plasmodium falciparum* malaria in children in southern Tanzania. *Lancet* 1994; 344:1175–1181.

CHAPTER 62

BABESIOSIS

Peter L. Chiodini

Babesia spp. are protozoan parasites of domestic and wild animals. They are members of the phylum Apicomplexa, order Piroplasmida, family Babesiidae.

Most human cases of babesiosis are due to *Babesia bovis*, *B. divergens* or *B. microti*. *B. caucasica* has also been reported to infect humans, but Hoare[1] considered it to be synonymous with *B. bovis*. He also regarded *B. divergens* as a synonym of *B. bovis* but this has not been adopted, thus Kakoma and Mehlhorn[2] recognize *B. divergens* and *B. bovis* as separate species. There is one case reportedly due to *B. canis*,[3] and a new *Babesia*, known for the moment as WA1, has been isolated from a patient in Washington State, USA.[4]

LIFE CYCLE

Human babesiosis is a zoonosis acquired by tick bite when individuals accidentally interact with the natural life cycle of the parasite. Humans represent dead-end hosts for *Babesia* spp.

BOVINE BABESIAS

Sporozoites are injected into the bloodstream by tick bite and penetrate erythrocytes. In contrast to the malaria life cycle, no tissue stage has ever been demonstrated for *B. bovis* or *B. divergens*. Within the erythrocyte the parasites vary in appearance, being oval, round or pear shaped.

Ring forms especially may be confused with malaria parasites, especially *Plasmodium falciparum*. However, *Babesia* does not form pigment and does not cause alterations in red cell morphology or staining, such as the Maurer's clefts of *P. falciparum*, the Schüffner's dots of *P. vivax* or the James's dots of *P. ovale*. *Babesia* multiplies in the red cell by budding (*Plasmodium* by schizogony). Release of daughter parasites is followed by reinvasion of fresh erythrocytes and further asexual multiplication.

Some of the sporozoites injected by the tick vector follow a different path of intraerythrocytic development, growing slowly and 'folding' to form accordion-like structures, thought to be gametocytes[2] which are destined to undergo further development in the tick vector.

Within the gut of the tick the accordion-like stage is able to resist digestion and eventually fuses with another, to form a zygote. Further development outside the intestine occurs in a variety of tissues, the salivary glands and ovaries being especially important for transmission.

Sporozoites in tick salivary glands are injected into the mammalian host at the next blood meal. Transovarial transmission of *B. bovis* also takes place so that newly hatched larvae are already infected. Trans-stadial transmission to nymph and then to adult stages can then take place.

BABESIA MICROTI

In the small mammal host of *B. microti*, sporozoites from the tick vector first enter lymphocytes and undergo merogony, the daughter parasites of which then enter erythrocytes.[2] There is no published report of this intralymphocytic stage in human *B. microti* infections.

B. microti does not undergo transovarial transmission,[2] but once a larva has become infected from a mammalian host it is able to pass on the infection trans-stadially to the nymph.

EPIDEMIOLOGY

Human infection follows tick bite or, rarely, blood transfusion[5] or transplacental/perinatal infection.[6] Each *Babesia*–vector–mammalian host system has its own characteristics and the ecology and bionomics of the vector tick define the pattern of risk for the human population.[7]

EUROPEAN CASES

Infection with *B. divergens* (14) or *B. bovis* (2) accounts for 16 of the 19 cases reported. One case was reportedly due to *B. microti*.[3] The vector of *B. divergens* is *Ixodes ricinus*[7] and of *B. microti* in England is *I. trianguliceps*, in contrast to the situation in the USA, where *B. microti* is transmitted by *I. dammini*. All 14 of the *B. divergens* and one of the two *B. bovis* infected patients had been splenectomized previously.[3] One patient with *B. microti* infection had an intact spleen.

There is an association of human *B. bovis* infection with exposure to land grazed by infected cattle[8] for occupational or recreational purposes.

NORTH AMERICAN CASES

Almost all the cases have been due to *B. microti*. Most reports have come from the north-eastern coastal region of the USA,[9] with some from Wisconsin[10] and sporadic reports from California and Georgia.[11]

B. microti infects the mouse *Peromyscus leucopus*, the preferred host for the larva of *I. dammini*. Nymphs of this tick feed either on *Peromyscus* or on the deer *Odocoileus virginianus*, which does not appear to be susceptible to *B. microti*. Adult *I. dammini* prefer to feed on *Odocoileus*. Humans appear to become infected via nymphs and the peak month for transmission is June, which coincides with their active feeding period.

The vector for *B. microti* in North America is *I. dammini*,[12] which is also the vector for *Borrelia burgdorferi*, the causative agent of Lyme disease. Infection of the same patient with *B. microti* and Lyme disease can occur.[13]

B. microti in North America can infect previously healthy individuals with intact spleens. The infection is more severe in splenectomized individuals.[14] Benach and Habicht[13] studied common risk factors for babesiosis in 17 patients. They found no association with a particular blood group. Age was an important risk factor. The presence of a significant medical history (including splenectomy, cancer, cancer therapy, autoimmune disease, endocrinopathies and previous parasitic disease) was noted in 10 of the 17 cases. The mean age of patients with significant medical histories (47.7 years) was significantly less than of those who were previously healthy (63.4 years).

Two cases of *B. microti* infection have been reported from human immunodeficiency virus (HIV)-positive patients, one of whom had also been splenectomized. Persistent parasitaemia and severe disease were noted.[15,16]

PATHOLOGY

Haemolytic anaemia, jaundice due to unconjugated hyperbilirubinaemia, frank haemoglobinuria and acute renal failure due to acute tubular necrosis are all features of *B. bovis* infection in splenectomized individuals.[8,17,18] Thrombocytopenia has been recorded.[19]

B. microti infection also results in haemolytic anaemia. Its presence in splenectomized as well as intact patients indicates that hypersplenism alone

cannot explain the occurrence of haemolytic anaemia. Scanning electron microscopy of human blood infected with *B. microti* has revealed substantial damage to the erythrocyte membrane, with protrusions, inclusions and perforations evident, suggesting that red cell destruction is parasite mediated.[20] C3 and C4 levels were suppressed in acute *B. microti* infections.[21]

CLINICAL FEATURES

BABESIA BOVIS/DIVERGENS

The incubation period varies from 1 to 4 weeks. The patient may feel vaguely unwell at first,[17] but by the time the diagnosis has been made is usually very ill, with fever, prostration, jaundice, anaemia and haemoglobinuria.[8] Nausea, vomiting and diarrhoea are also recorded.[17,18] Finding an operation scar gives a clue to previous splenectomy. Infection is sometimes unsuspected and, given the fulminant nature of this condition, may not be confirmed until after the patient has died[8] or the diagnosis is felt to be *P. falciparum* malaria when intraerythrocytic parasites are seen in the blood film. Other misdiagnoses include leptospirosis and viral hepatitis.[17] Thus, for the diagnosis to be made early, babesiosis should be considered in the differential diagnosis of any splenectomized patient in whom exposure to tick bites is a possibility.

BABESIA MICROTI

Most human infections are subclinical.[22] Where clinical illness develops, the incubation period is 1–3 weeks, occasionally up to 6 weeks, for tick-transmitted infections[23] and 6–9 weeks for post-transfusion cases.[24] The illness usually begins gradually, with anorexia and fatigue, plus fever (without periodicity), sweating, rigors and generalized myalgia. Physical examination may reveal only fever but may also show mild splenomegaly and sometimes mild hepatomegaly.[11]

Given the non-specific nature of the clinical findings, human infection with *B. microti* cannot be diagnosed with certainty on clinical grounds alone. A history of tick bite is helpful but is not elicited in most cases.[13] However, public knowledge of Lyme disease, which shares the same vector with *B. microti* in the USA, can raise awareness of tick-transmitted disease(s). The relatively localized geographical distribution of human *B. microti* infections in the USA means that local physicians may become very aware of the infection but it may be missed by those practising in non-endemic areas in other countries.

LABORATORY DIAGNOSIS

Definitive diagnosis depends upon finding parasites on blood film examination. Hamster inoculation and serodiagnosis have also been deployed.

BLOOD FILM EXAMINATION

BABESIA BOVIS/DIVERGENS (Figure 62.1)

B. divergens was separated from *B. bovis* as a result of the predominance of paired forms, diverging at a wide angle of up to 180°, situated on the periphery of the red cell.[1] In addition, *B. divergens* is smaller ($0.4 \times 1.5 \mu m$) than *B. bovis* ($2.4 \times 1.5 \mu m$). However, the parasites are pleomorphic and their size can vary depending upon the host they infect.[1]

B. bovis/divergens are pear shaped, oval or round and may exist in pyriform pairs. In fulminant human cases *B. divergens* takes the form of rings, loops, clubs, rods, pyriform and amoeboid shapes. Occasional divergent forms are seen. There may be 1–8 parasites per red cell.[17] Parasitaemia as high as 70% has been reported from a fatal case.[18] The 'Maltese cross' form is unique to *Babesia* among members of the Apicomplexa, but in its absence it may be very difficult to distinguish young ring forms of *Plasmodium* spp., especially *P. falciparum*. The absence of pigment cannot be relied upon as *young*

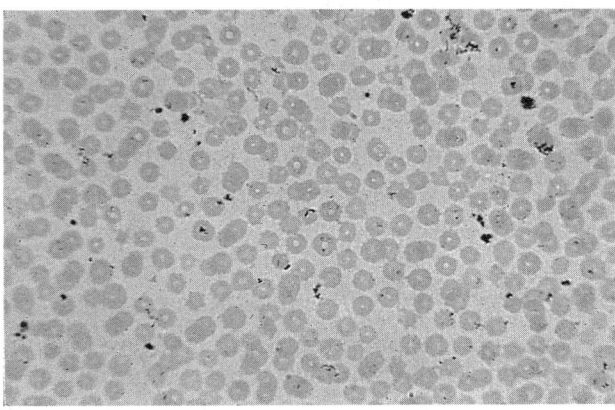

Figure 62.1   *Babesia divergens* in calf blood.

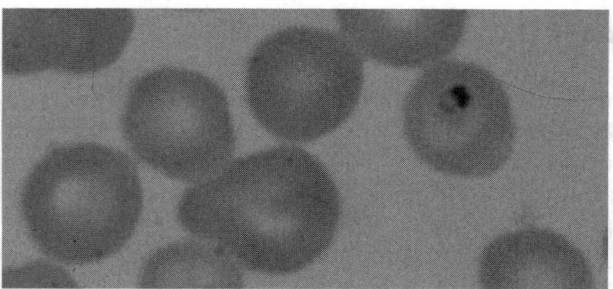

Figure 62.2   Babesia microti in human blood.

rings of *Plasmodium* spp. do not exhibit pigment. If cultured in vitro, *P. falciparum* will develop pigment but *Babesia* will not. *Babesia* are smaller than malaria parasites, and in some of the larger rings there is a white vacuole, instead of the pink vacuole containing erythrocyte stroma seen in malaria.[8] *Babesia* does not form schizonts.

BABESIA MICROTI (Figure 62.2)

Ring, rod-shaped, pyriform, amoeboid and 'Maltese cross' forms are seen.[1] In heavy infections different stages may be noted in the same red cell. Intraerythrocytic stages measure approximately $2 \times 1.5 \mu m$. In very high parasitaemias extracellular merozoites with plentiful cytoplasm were found singly or as a syncytial structure.[20]

Peak parasitaemia varies between less than 1% to approximately 10%[11] but a splenectomized patient who was also taking systemic steroids developed a *B. microti* parasitaemia of 85%.[20]

OTHER LABORATORY FINDINGS

BABESIA BOVIS/DIVERGENS

Anaemia, leucocytosis, haemolysis, unconjugated hyperbilirubinaemia and raised blood urea are found. Reticulocytosis occurs in response to the haemolytic anaemia. Frank haemoglobinuria is evident.[17,18]

BABESIA MICROTI

Anaemia may be mild to moderately severe, ranging from 5.8 to 11.6 g/dl in one series.[11] Serum haptoglobin may be reduced and the reticulocyte count increased, supporting the view that most of the anaemia is due to haemolysis. Total white blood cell counts are low or normal and there may be thrombocytopenia.[11]

Mean and differential lymphocyte counts and percentages of B lymphocytes and levels of T lymphocytes with the IgG Fc receptor were elevated in acute infection. Polyclonal hypergammaglobulinaemia was found. Levels of serum IgG, IgM and C1q binding were significantly increased; C3 and C4 levels and haemolytic activity were reduced in acute-phase sera.[21]

There may be mild elevation of serum glutamic oxaloacetic transaminase (aspartate aminotransferase), alkaline phosphatase and bilirubin.[11]

ELECTRON MICROSCOPY

This technique is not helpful for routine diagnosis of human babesiosis but can provide useful confirmation of the nature of the infection. Transmission electron microscopy of *B. microti* from a splenectomized patient also receiving systemic steroids showed considerable pleomorphism. All developmental stages were seen in both reticulocytes and mature erythrocytes. The same study identified convoluted cells with many free ribosomes, thought to represent an early gametocyte stage.[20]

SERODIAGNOSIS

The indirect fluorescent antibody test (IFAT) is available for bovine babesia and for *B. microti*. However, serology should not be seen as an alternative to blood film examination, especially in view of the fulminant nature of bovine babesia infection in splenectomized patients. Demonstration of parasites in a blood film provides unequivocal proof of current infection. Some *B. microti* infections may have low level or transient parasitaemia[22] and serology has a useful part to play in establishing the diagnosis. Ruebush et al[22] defined individuals with IFAT titres to *B. microti* of greater than or equal to 64 as seropositive. In patients with acute *B. microti* infection, IFAT titres were greater than or equal to 1 in 1024, and fell to 1 in 256 or 1 in 64 over 8–12 months. The possibility of cross-reaction with antimalarial antibody must be borne in mind when serological results are interpreted.[25] The *B. microti* IFAT has a reported 88–96% sensitivity and 90–100% specificity.[26]

POLYMERASE CHAIN REACTION

This technique has been applied to the diagnosis of *B. microti*, with a reported test sensitivity of approximately three merozoites.[27]

ANIMAL INOCULATION

This is not routinely used for diagnosis of individual cases but *B. microti* from human cases can be isolated in hamsters,[11] and *B. divergens* from a fatal human case was successfully passaged to gerbils and to a splenectomized calf.[18]

CLINICAL COURSE AND TREATMENT

BABESIA BOVIS/DIVERGENS

Untreated, infection of splenectomized humans with bovine babesias leads to fulminant illness and death. Specific treatment remains difficult and is based upon anecdotal case reports. Diminazene (Berenil) is active against *Babesia* in animals and was used in a case of human *B. divergens* infection, but the patient died.[28] Successful treatment of *B. divergens* (5% parasitaemia) in a splenectomized patient with pentamidine plus co-trimoxazole has been recorded.[28] Quinine and chloroquine plus pyrimethamine have proven ineffective.[18]

Brasseur and Gorenflot[29] reported successful treatment of three cases with massive exchange blood transfusion (2–3 blood volumes) followed by intravenous clindamycin and oral quinine.

BABESIA MICROTI

In most instances patients suffer a mild illness from which they recover spontaneously. Recovery can be prolonged, with several months of fatigue and malaise.[11] Where illness is severe enough to merit treatment, oral quinine 650 mg every 8 hours plus clindamycin 300–600 mg i.v or i.m every 6 hours (adult doses), for 7–10 days, is regarded as the treatment of choice,[3,30] although it is not universally effective.[31] Paediatric dosage: is oral quinine 25 mg/kg per day and intravenous or intramuscular clindamycin 20 mg/kg per day.[32]

Chloroquine is unhelpful. Diminazene was used in one case and the patient recovered but developed neurological complications resembling the Guillain–Barré syndrome.[33]

Whole blood or red cell exchange transfusion has produced a rapid and substantial fall in parasitaemia[34] and its use as an adjunct to chemotherapy should be considered in severely ill patients with high parasitaemias, especially splenectomized patients infected with bovine babesias.

PREVENTION

There is no vaccine licensed for human use. Prevention of human babesiosis depends upon avoidance of tick bite: avoidance of tick habitats; wearing appropriate clothing to cover the lower part of the body; use of insect repellent, e.g. diethyltoluamide and permethrin impregnated clothing; and prompt removal of ticks found on the person. In endemic areas, awareness of the possibility of transfusion-transmitted *Babesia* infection should be maintained so that those thought to be potentially infected with *Babesia* can be excluded from donation, but routine screening of donor blood is not yet established.

REFERENCES

1 Hoare C A. Comparative aspects of human babesiosis. *Trans R Soc Trop Med Hyg* 1980; 74:143–148.

2 Kakoma I & Mehlhorn H. *Babesia* of domestic animals. In Kreier J P (ed.) *Parasitic Protozoa* 7, 2nd edn. San Diego: Academic Press, 1994: 141–216.

3 Telford S R III, Gorenflot A, Brasseur P & Spielman A. Babesial infections in man and wildlife. In Kreier J P & Baker J R (eds) *Parasitic Protozoa 5*, 2nd edn. San Diego: Academic Press, 1993: 1–47.

4 Thomford J W, Conrad P A, Telford S R et al. Cultivation and phylogenetic characterisation of a newly recognised human pathogenic protozoan. *J Infect Dis* 1994; 169:1050–1056.

5 Popovsky M A. Transfusion-transmitted babesiosis. *Transfusion* 1991; 31:296–298.

6 Esernio Jenssen D, Scimeca P G, Benach J L & Tenenbaum M J. Transplacental/perinatal babesiosis. *J Pediatr* 1987; 110:570–572.

7 Donnelly J. Human babesiosis. *Trans R Soc Trop Med Hyg* 1980; 74:158.

8 Garnham P C C. Human babesiosis: European aspects. *Trans R Soc Trop Med Hyg* 1980; 74:153–155.

9 Meldrum S C, Birkhead G S, White D J, Benach J L & Morse D L. Human babesiosis in New York State: an epidemiological description of 136 cases. *Clin Infect Dis* 1992; 15:1019–1023.

10 Steketee R W, Eckman M R, Burgess E C et al. Babesiosis in Wisconsin: a new focus of disease transmission. *JAMA* 1985; 253:2675–2678.

11 Ruebush T K II. Human babesiosis in North America. *Trans R Soc Trop Med Hyg* 1980; 74:149–152.

12 Spielman A, Clifford C M, Piesman J & Corwin M D. Human babesiosis on Nantucket Island, USA: description of the vector *Ixodes (Ixodes) dammini* n.sp (Acarina: Ixodidae). *J Med Entomol* 1979; 15:218–234.

13 Benach J L & Habicht G S. Clinical characteristics of human babesiosis. *J Infect Dis* 1981; 144:481.

14 Rosner F, Zarrabi M H, Benach J L & Habicht G S. Babesiosis in splenectomised adults. Review of 22 reported cases. *Am J Med* 1984; 76:696–701.

15 Ong K R, Stavropoulos C & Inada Y. Babesiosis, asplenia and AIDS. *Lancet* 1990; 336:112.

16 Benezra D, Brown A E, Polsky B, Gold J W M & Armstrong D. Babesiosis and infection with human immunodeficiency virus (HIV). *Ann Intern Med* 1987; 107:944.

17 Cotton Kennedy C. Human babesiosis: summary of a case in Ireland. *Trans R Soc Trop Med Hyg* 1980; 74:156.

18 Williams H. Human babesiosis. *Trans R Soc Trop Med Hyg* 1980; 74:157.

19 Uhnoo I, Cars O, Christensson D & Nystrom Rosander C. First documented case of human babesiosis in Sweden. *Scand J Infect Dis* 1992; 24:541–547.

20 Sun T, Tenenbaum M J, Greenspan J et al. Morphologic and clinical observations in human infection with *Babesia microti*. *J Infect Dis* 1983; 148:239–248.

21 Benach J L, Habicht G S & Hamburger M I. Immunoresponsiveness in acute babesiosis in humans. *J Infect Dis* 1982; 146:369–380.

22 Ruebush T K II, Juranek D D, Chisholm E S, Snow P C, Healy G R & Sulzer A J. Human babesiosis on Nantucket Island. Evidence for self-limited and subclinical infections. *N Engl J Med* 1977; 297:825–827.

23 Ruebush T K II, Juranek D D, Spielman A, Piesman J & Healy G R. Epidemiology of human babesiosis on Nantucket Island. *Am J Trop Med Hyg* 1981; 30:937–941.

24 Popovsky M A, Lindberg L E, Syrek A L & Page P L. Prevalence of *Babesia* antibody in a selected blood donor population. *Transfusion* 1988; 28:59–61.

25 Ruebush T K II, Chisholm E S, Sulzer A J & Healy G R. Development and persistence of antibody in persons infected with *Babesia microti*. *Am J Trop Med Hyg* 1981; 30:291–292.

26 Krause P J, Telford S R, Ryan R et al. Diagnosis of babesiosis: evaluation of a serologic test for the detection of *Babesia microti* antibody. *J Infect Dis* 1994; 169:923–926.

27 Persing D H, Mathiesen D, Marshall W F, Telford S R & Spielman A. Detection of *Babesia microti* by polymerase chain reaction. *J Clin Microbiol* 1992; 30:2097–2013.

28 Raoult D, Soulayrol L, Toga B, Dumon H & Casanovna P. Babesiosis, pentamidine and cotrimaxozole. *Ann Intern Med* 1987; 107:944.

29 Brasseur P & Gorenflot A. Human babesiosis in Europe. *Mem Inst Oswaldo Cruz* 1992; 87:131–132.

30 Gelfand J A. Babesia. In Mandell G L, Bennett J E & Dolin R (eds) *Principles and Practice of Infectious Diseases*, 4th edn. New York: Churchill Livingstone, 1995: 2497–2500.

31 Anonymous. Clindamycin and quinine treatment for *Babesia microti* infections. *MMWR* 1983; 32:65–71.

32 Wittner M, Rowin K S, Tanowitz H B et al. Successful chemotherapy of transfusion babesiosis. *Ann Intern Med* 1982; 96:601–604.

33 Ruebush T K II, Rubin R H, Wolpow E R, Cassady P B & Schultz M G. Neurologic complications following the treatment of human *Babesia microti* infection with diminazene aceturate. *Am J Trop Med Hyg* 1979; 28:184–189.

34 Jackoby G A, Hunt J V, Kosinski K S et al. Treatment of transfusion-transmitted babesiosis by exchange transfusion. *N Engl J Med* 1980; 303:1098–1100.

CHAPTER 63

AFRICAN TRYPANOSOMIASIS IN MAN

D. H. Molyneux, V. Pentreath and F. Doua

African human trypanosomiases are caused by parasites of the genus *Trypanosoma* (subgenus *Trypanozoon*). The organisms are flagellate protozoa and in the new classification of the subkingdom Protozoa are in the phylum Sarcomastigophora, order Kinetoplastida. This order contains those parasites which are characterized by the possession of a kinetoplast and also includes the *Leishmania* parasites. The organisms responsible for human trypanosomiasis in Africa belong to the species *Trypanosoma brucei*, a complex of organisms transmitted to man by the bite of tsetse flies, *Glossina*. Trypanosomiasis of man is usually referred to as 'sleeping sickness' and is characterized by a range of symptoms which initially only affect the haemolymphatic system, but after varying periods of time following infection, also involve the central nervous system (CNS). The meningoencephalitic or late stage produces a wide range of signs and symptoms associated with the CNS pathology. The name sleeping sickness derives from the comatose, somnolent state characteristic of patients in the terminal stage of the disease.

GEOGRAPHICAL DISTRIBUTION

Sleeping sickness is endemic only in areas where *Glossina* species are found. The ecological limit of *Glossina* distribution is approximately a line from 14°N from Senegal in the West to 10°N in southern Somalia in the East and 20°S corresponding to the northern fringes of the Kalahari and Namibian Deserts. The distribution of *Glossina* is determined by climate through its effect(s) on vegetation, and recently it has been possible to define the limits of distribution more precisely by reference to temperature and humidity means. It is anticipated that satellite technology will be of increasing use in defining fly distribution in relation to habitats. Comparison of such images over time will, in association with geographical information system (GIS) techniques, be of value in predicting tsetse distribution in relation to changes in ecology.[1] Rogers and Randolph[1] and Rogers and Williams[2] correlated data from meteorological satellites which produce normalized vegetation-type indices (NDVI) related to photosynthetically active vegetation on a continent-wide scale, with *Glossina* abundance in both savanna (*G. morsitans*) and riverine (*G. palpalis/G. tachinoides*) habitats. NDVI values correlated with *Glossina* size; decrease in *Glossina* size is associated with increased mortality.

There are 23 species of *Glossina* and a number of subspecies. While all are capable of acting as vectors of trypanosomes which cause human sleeping sickness (as well as animal pathogenic trypansomes), the disease is transmitted by two groups of flies: the *G. palpalis* group (subgenus *Nemorhina*), which transmit *T. b. gambiense* and are associated with the chronic form of the disease; and the *G. morsitans* group, which are associated with the transmission of *T. b. rhodesiense* in endemic situations. In Uganda, epidemic *T. b. rhodesiense* was transmitted by the riverine tsetse fly, *G. fuscipes*. The major vectors and their geographical distribution are listed in Table 63.1. The current distribution of sleeping sickness in Africa is shown in the map (Figure 63.1). Jordan[3] provides an up-to-date summary of *Glossina* biology and control.

Glossina spp. infest approximately $10 \times 10^6 \text{ km}^2$ or about one-third of the African continent; sleeping sickness is endemic in 36 countries and, while 20 000–50 000 cases are recorded annually, it is believed this is an underestimate, particularly because

Table 63.1 Major vectors of *T. b. gambiense* and *T. b. rhodesiense* and geographical distribution.

T. b. gambiense

G. palpalis subspecies: *palpalis, gambiensis*
Angola, Benin, Burkina Faso, Cameroon, Central African Republic, Congo, Gabon, Gambia, Ghana, Guinea, Guinea-Bissau, Ivory Coast, Liberia, Mali, Niger, Nigeria, Senegal, Sierra Leone, Togo, Zaire

G. tachinoides
Benin, Burkina Faso, Cameroon, Central African Republic, Chad, Ethiopia, Ghana, Guinea, Ivory Coast, Mali, Niger, Nigeria, Sudan, Togo

G. fuscipes subspecies: *quanzensis, martinii*
Angola, Cameroon, Central African Republic, Chad, Congo, Ethiopia, Uganda, Zaire

T. b. rhodesiense

G. morsitans: subspecies *morsitans, centralis*
Angola, Botswana, Burundi, Malawi, Mozambique, Rwanda, Tanzania, Zambia, Zimbabwe

G. pallidipes
Burundi, Ethiopia, Kenya, Malawi, Mozambique, Rwanda, Sudan, Tanzania, Uganda, Zambia, Zimbabwe

G. swynnertoni
Kenya, Tanzania

G. fuscipes subspecies: *fuscipes*
Ethiopia, Kenya, Uganda

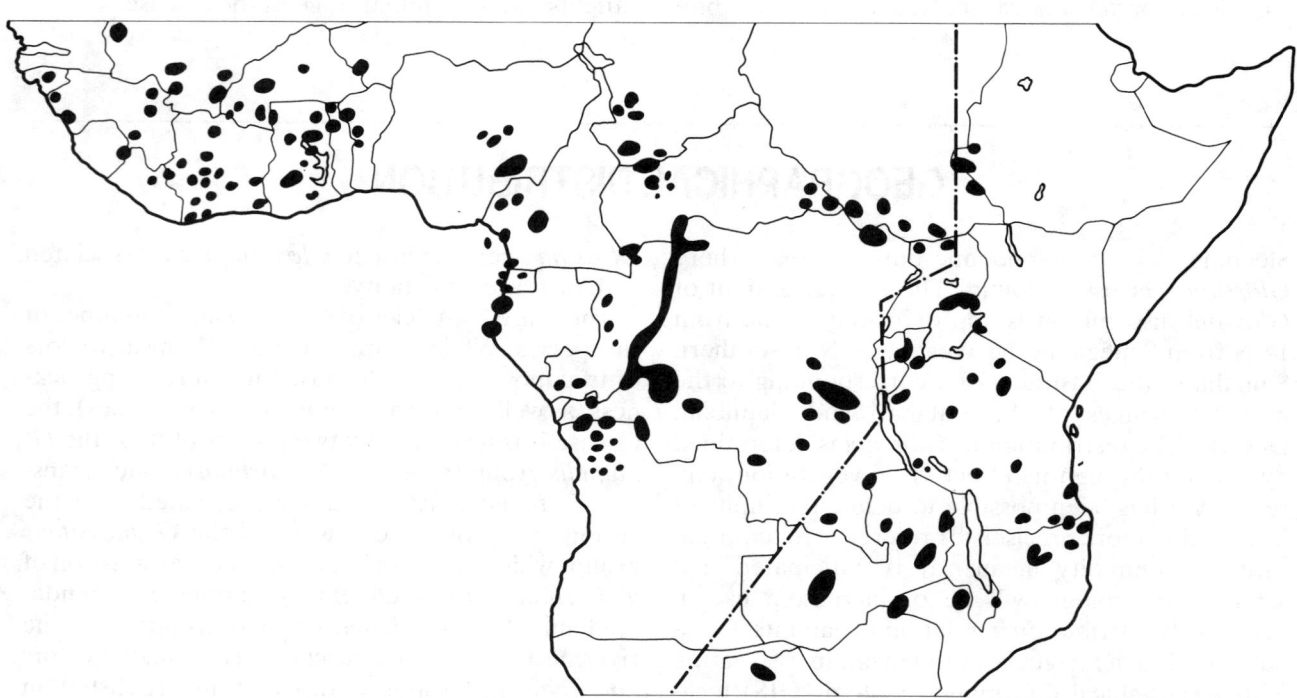

Figure 63.1 Distribution of trypanosomiasis foci in Africa. *T. b. gambiense* areas of distribution to left of dotted line in West and Central Africa; *T. b. rhodesiense* to right of line in East and South Africa.

surveillance has been reduced as public health services have been under economic constraints and because priority has been given to other problems such as malaria and the human immunodeficiency virus (HIV). This situation was highlighted by the last World Health Organization (WHO) Expert Committee report.[4] The report details up-to-date country information in active foci of the disease and provides numbers of reported cases and recent documented trends. It is emphasized that current figures suffer from reduced surveillance in over 200 known foci, inadequate reporting when passive detection systems are used, shortage of trained personnel and the logistic and financial constraints which prevent endemic foci being regularly surveyed. Since the WHO[4] report the continued pressure on, and in some areas further deterioration of health services suggests the likelihood that sleeping sickness will be an increasing public health problem, compounded by political and social upheavals in endemic countries. The public health importance of sleeping sickness is frequently underestimated; while the quoted figure emanating from WHO[4] referred to 15 000–20 000 new cases annually, the actual number of cases may be in excess of ten times that figure. This estimate is based on information available from highly endemic countries where control services have been reduced or broken down completely. The number of deaths has been estimated in the World Development Report as 55 000/year[5]. Death from sleeping sickness is inevitable if the disease is untreated; for this reason epidemics will cause serious social disruption and economic loss to communities who are deprived of treatment because hospitalization is neither feasible nor available. Indeed the problem of drug supply is a major consideration in view of the costs of treatment. The economic and social impact of sleeping sickness has been little studied but the World Development Report has calculated that the disability of adjusted life years lost (DALYS) is 17.8×10^5. DALYS combine healthy life years lost through premature mortality with those of disability. Comparative figures for DALYS in sub-Saharan Africa regarding vector-borne diseases place African sleeping sickness as the third most important contributor to the global burden of parasitic disease after malaria (315.1) and schistosomiasis (34.9). It can be predicted that over the coming years (mid-1990s), in countries where health services are so depleted, sleeping sickness will cause severe social disruption in many rural areas of sub-Saharan Africa. The surveillance and information systems used in the past to detect and contain epidemics will no longer be sustained and even passive systems of surveillance, regarded as minimal, will suffer through lack of skilled human resources and motivation. The cost and difficulty of obtaining drugs will add to the problem; even simple methods of vector control (impregnated traps and targets) are not sustainable without outside funds.

AETIOLOGY

T. brucei subspecies trypanosomes of the subgenus Trypanozoon are morphologically indistinguishable. However, since the 1970s much research has been undertaken to define more precisely, using a range of biochemical and molecular methods, markers which might define clinical disease and epidemiology. The problems which these extensive studies have addressed are the identity and potential infectivity to humans of trypanosomes circulating in domestic and game animals and those isolated from Glossina, and the different organisms circulating in epidemic and endemic situations.

T. brucei morphology is described by Hoare[6,7] (Figure 63.2). Parasites are pleomorphic, extracellular in the blood and tissues and vary in length from 12 to 42 μm; they have a small subterminal kinetoplast and a free flagellum. Parasite multiplication is impaired by specific antibodies produced by the host, resulting in a decrease in the parasitaemia. However, some parasites escape the immune response by the mechanism of antigenic variation, a mutation which enables the trypanosomes to produce an antigenically different surface coat.[8] The result is a fluctuating parasitaemia with progressive and multiple pathological changes which vary in pattern and intensity with

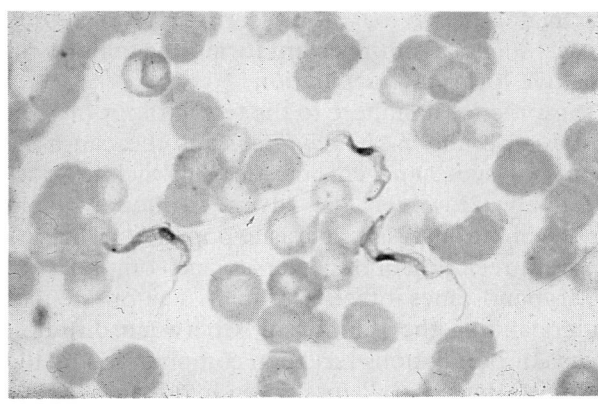

Figure 63.2   T. brucei in blood.

the different parasite strains, host, population and individual characteristics.

T. brucei organisms are infective to laboratory animals: inoculation of infective material from human and animal reservoir hosts and Glossina produce infections in a range of laboratory animals—mice, rats, rabbits, guinea-pigs and the multimammate rat (Mastomys natalensis). However, chronic T. b. gambiense infections are less infective, and frequently parasites in man from some locations (in particular Cameroon) have not proved infective to a range of hosts. This has resulted in the development of an in vitro culture technique[9] for isolation of parasites which multiply in a culture medium. This technique, known as KIVI (kit for in vitro isolation), together with the use of *Glossina* membrane feeding to produce procyclic (tsetse mid-gut) forms, has enabled studies on the characterization of such isolates to be undertaken. The parasites are produced in sufficient numbers by this method to enable isoenzyme characterization to be carried out.

It is generally recognized that *T. b. brucei* is the animal infective form of the subgenus *Trypanozoon* not infective to man. *T. b. brucei* is lysed by human serum; this is associated with high-density lipoprotein molecules which are trypanocidal.[10] The lytic effect of human serum was the basis for the development of the blood incubation infectivity test (BIIT).[11] This test involved incubation of trypanosomes in human serum prior to inoculation into rats; potentially human-infective trypanosomes developed infection in rats, whereas *T. b. brucei*, which is non-infective to man, was lysed by human serum and did not develop infection in recipient rats. The BIIT was modified for studies in *T. b. gambiense* by the use of *M. natalensis* as a recipient animal because it is more easily infected with avirulent parasite stocks.[12–14] The most recent development of BIIT was by Jenni and Brun,[15] who introduced an in vitro test in which the viability of the test organism is compared in parallel cultures containing 20% heat-inactivated horse or rabbit serum. The method detects single serum-resistant forms in a majority of sensitive forms in a population.

It is practice to adhere to the terminology of *T. b. rhodesiense* and *T. b. gambiense* as the causative agents of acute and chronic sleeping sickness, respectively. However, the advent of modern technology in the analysis of parasite populations has led to an appreciation of the diversity and complexity of the trypanosomes infective to man. The problem of understanding the relationships between different demes or populations has been compounded by the demonstration that *T. brucei* can hybridize in *Glossina* in the laboratory;[16] hybridization has also been achieved in vitro,[17] while the location of hybridization in a natural cycle appears to be in the mid-gut of *Glossina*.[18] Markers for identification of parasite stocks in hybridization studies are isoenzymes and restriction fragment length polymorphisms of endonuclease-digested DNA. Neither the frequency of hybridization in the wild nor its significance in terms of epidemiology and patterns of drug resistance are yet known. What is clear is that the precise mechanisms and location of the event will be difficult to resolve.

These studies have provoked extensive discussion

on the genetics of wild populations of parasites and the relative importance of clonality[19] and sexuality in such populations. The most extensively used technique for characterization of trypanosomes is isoenzyme electrophoresis. Extensive studies of nearly 1000 parasite stocks have been undertaken. Several reviews summarize the results[20,21] and attempts to reduce the number of enzymes used to identify subspecies and strain groups have been introduced.[22,23] The application and use of modern techniques in the epidemiology of trypanosomiasis are described by Gibson and Miles.[24] Principal zymodemes recognized in *Trypanozoon* were originally proposed by Gibson et al. (1980) and, although there is a tendency to remain committed to the use of *T. b. rhodesiense* and *T. b. gambiense* as nomenclature, it may be appropriate to consider recognizing strain groups if an association between geographical distribution, clinical features and particular zymodemes becomes apparent. Strain groups are made up of zymodemes characteristic of specific localities which, when subjected to numerical taxonomic analysis, cluster in dendrograms which provide an indication of the degree of genetic identity. The groupings proposed by Stevens and Godfrey[22] are corroborated by DNA methods,[24,25] while similar results were obtained using two different methods (the Jaccardi coefficient and the Nei method) to construct a dendrogram of relationships. The groupings of the subgenus *Trypanozoon*, after over a decade of molecular and biomedical studies, suggest that *T. b. gambiense* and *T. evansi* (the equine and camel parasite) can be regarded as distinct subspecies and species respectively. *T. b. brucei* is subdivided into strain groups 'bouaflé', 'sindo', 'kiboko' and 'kakumbi'; bouaflé is the most diverse of these groups and is also found in West African animals. Some of the stocks of bouaflé are infective to man, some potentially so; some isolates of bouaflé are also found in East Africa. The relationship between *T. b. rhodesiense* and *T. b. brucei* is complex. *T. b. rhodesiense* in the classical sense is divided into Zambezi and Busoga strain groups with characteristic isoenzyme profiles and DNA banding.[26] The Zambezi group of isolates from man in Zambia is of relatively low virulence; Busoga stocks are from man in northern and central areas of *T. b. rhodesiense* distribution; the Busoga zymodeme may also be found in West Africa, being more enzymically variable than Zambezi, with an affinity to the non-human infective group bouaflé.

It can be expected that, with enhanced identification and diagnostic methods such as the polymerase chain reaction (PCR), analysis of small numbers of organisms could be undertaken to further enhance the numbers of samples analysed without recourse to growing large numbers of parasites for later analysis. In such circumstances a more precise definition of the organisms infecting man may be important for treatment.

TRANSMISSION

T. brucei subspecies are transmitted to mammalian hosts by the bite of tsetse flies (*Glossina*). A complex developmental cycle in the fly (see Ref. 27) terminates in the presence of infective metacyclic trypanosomes in the lumen of the salivary glands. Metacyclic trypanosomes reach the skin of the mammalian host during the probing and feeding process. Development in the tsetse fly involves a complex series of changes to the morphology, physiology and biochemistry of the parasite. The factors influencing the development of the trypanosome in *Glossina* are complex: Maudlin[27] describes in detail the mechanisms involved. These mechanisms involve lectins present in *Glossina* mid-gut and haemolymph, the presence of *Rickettsia*-like organisms, and molecular signals influencing parasite transformation, establishment and maturation. Different species of *Glossina* have lectins with different carbohydrate-binding specificities: *G. morsitans* flies have *N*-acetylglucosamine-specific lectins as, when glucosamine is fed to *G. morsitans*, elevated mid-gut infection rates with *T. brucei* are found;[28] *G. palpalis* subspecies have galactose-specific lectins, while different subspecies of *G. palpalis* have different molecules that have both trypanolytic and agglutinogenic properties.[29] The ecological and behavioural factors influencing infection of *Glossina* with trypanosomes are listed by Molyneux.[30]

Infected *Glossina* have been demonstrated to have altered probing behaviour as a result of infection with trypanosomes; the presence of trypanosomes prevents rapid engorgement and probing continues, hence *Glossina* extrudes infective forms during the probing process.[31] Changes in probing behaviour by other pathogen-infected vectors have been reviewed by Molyneux and Jefferies.[32]

The possibility of non-cyclical or mechanical transmission by biting insects as well as *Glossina* has been suggested, although there is only circumstantial evidence to support the idea. Mechanical transmission has been suggested as the reason for the clustering of cases in a household or where cases are found outside the normal habitat or range of *Glossina*.

Congenital infection of *T. b. gambiense* from the mother to the newborn rarely occurs but plays no significant epidemiological role. Acquisition of infection by transfusion is theoretically possible, although it has not been recorded in Africa.

EPIDEMIOLOGY

T. B. GAMBIENSE

The epidemiology of *T. b. gambiense* has been reviewed by Molyneux;[33] more detailed studies since this review have involved the extensive biochemical analysis of trypanosome stocks from different areas of West and Central Africa,[21] while Mehlitz[14] reviewed the studies of animal reservoirs of *T. b. gambiense*. *T. b. gambiense* is endemic throughout West and Central Africa and is frequently associated with foci (foyers) of infection which historically were recognized as areas where prevalence was often tenfold higher. Transmission of *T. b. gambiense* is associated with particular sites, usually near riverine vegetation, river crossings, water collection points, washing sites, sacred forests, and villages adjacent to rivers or lakes (Figure 63.3). *T. b. gambiense* transmission is 'site associated', and intense transmission was considered to occur particularly at the end of the dry season when contact between humans and *G. palpalis* was most frequent; flies required regular blood meals and humans were always available at these particular sites. In more humid forest regions, however, *G. palpalis* distribution is more widespread and hence transmission sites are less well localized. Human fly contact is less intense and *Glossina* can live for several weeks; once infected a fly can infect each time it bites, hence a single infected *Glossina* could infect many individuals at a particular site (Figure 63.4).

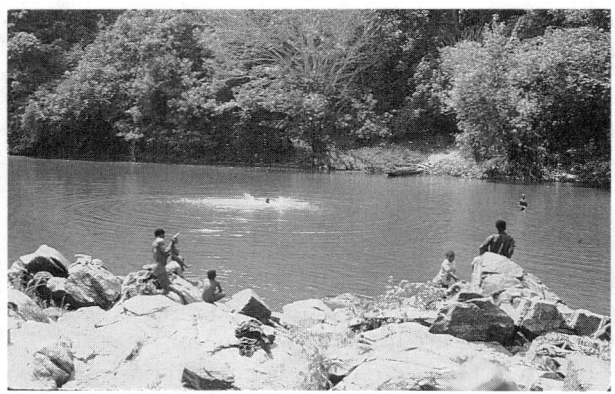

Figure 63.3 Typical site of transmission of *T. b. gambiense* where human fly contact is high; people gather to wash and cross the river. Habitat of *G. palpalis*.

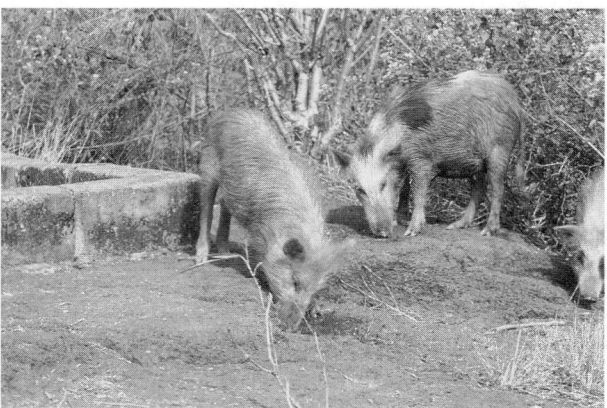

Figure 63.5 Domestic pigs: potential reservoir hosts of *T. b. gambiense* in West Africa.

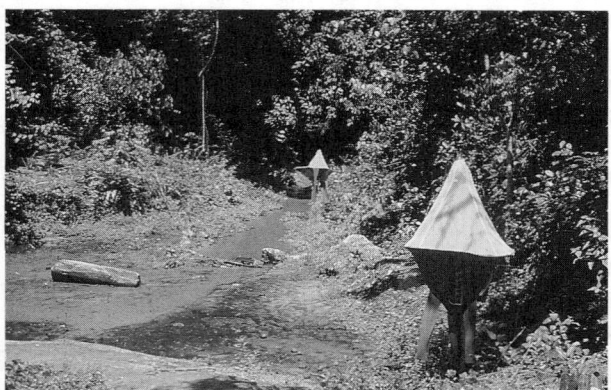

Figure 63.4 Traps in Congo placed adjacent to riverine transmission site habitat of *G. palpalis* group flies. Tsetse traps and targets such as this have been impregnated with insecticides to control transmission in several countries in West and Central Africa.

The most recent categorization of *T. b. gambiense* places this organism in a particular strain group; all isolates from humans in West and Central Africa in this group are comprised of six zymodemes (stocks with characteristic isoenzyme profiles). There are, however, chronic infections of man from the Ivory Coast, the most sampled area, which are now placed in the bouaflé strain group and which belong to the same zymodeme as stocks isolated from a range of wild and domestic animals.[13,23] This suggests that classical *T. b. gambiense* of man is not normally associated with animals; however a pig isolate from Liberia and a sheep isolate from Congo are biochemically similar to *T. b. gambiense*, but a second 'non-gambiense'[34] organism causing chronic infections of man with an animal reservoir also occurs in West Africa. Animal reservoirs of the bouaflé strain group, consisting of some 16 zymodemes, are pigs, dogs and cattle (Figure 63.5). Most isolations have

been made from pigs. Game animal species which are hosts of bouaflé parasites are kob (*Kobus kob*) and hartebeeste (*Alcelaphus buselaphus*); isolates of bouaflé have also been obtained from *G. palpalis*. Early experimental studies (reviewed by Molyneux[33,35]) demonstrated that a range of domestic and wild animals were capable of being infected with isolates of *T. b. gambiense* from man, although the strain group to which these isolates belonged are not known. Recent decades have seen a considerable increase in our understanding of the complex interrelationships of the subgenus *Trypanozoon*. Earlier studies were handicapped by a lack of methods for parasite identification and isolation. Isoenzymes and DNA methods have provided a strong base for future detailed epidemiological studies, particularly using PCR, to identify precisely the strain group from small amounts of parasite material from humans, mammals or *Glossina*; more representative sampling will be assisted by the development of the KIVI[9] which will enable stocks of parasite previously difficult to isolate (particularly those from Cameroon) to be identified to strain groups. Table 63.2 lists the animals which have been found infected with *T. b. gambiense* and the bouaflé strain group which are known to be infective to man and cause chronic disease in West and Central Africa. It is important to emphasize that the frequency with which man is infected from animal hosts cannot be determined.

T. b. rhodesiense

THE ENDEMIC SITUATION

T. b. rhodesiense is the cause of acute sleeping sickness. It is distributed from Uganda and Kenya in

Table 63.2 Known or suspected reservoir hosts of *T. b. gambiense*.

Host	*Country*	*Identification method(s)*
Dog	Fernando Po	Volunteer
	Liberia	BIIT*
		Isoenzyme
Pig	Liberia	BIIT
	Ivory Coast	Isoenzyme
	Zaire	DNA probe
Sheep	Congo	BIIT
		Isoenzyme
		DNA probe
Cattle	Burkina Faso	BIIT
		Isoenzyme
		DNA probe
	Nigeria	BIIT
Kob (*Kobus kob*)	Burkina Faso	BIIT
		Isoenzyme
		DNA probe
Hartebeeste (*Alcelaphus buselaphus*)	Burkina Faso	BIIT
		Isoenzyme
		DNA probe
Chicken	Ivory Coast	BIIT

*BIIT, blood incubation infectivity test.

the northern part of East Africa to Botswana in the south. Recent biochemical and molecular studies have identified two main strain groups associated with acute sleeping sickness, Zambezi and Busoga, the strain groups representing the southern and northern area of distribution respectively. Zambezi strains from Zambia and Malawi are often less virulent than Busoga because in Zambia and Malawi trypanosomes are found in the blood of humans who are not necessarily symptomatic.[36]

Sleeping sickness is endemic throughout eastern and south-eastern Africa and humans are infected by the bite of *Glossina* spp. associated with woodland savanna habitats (Figure 63.6). The *G. morsitans* group, particularly *G. pallidipes* and *G. swynnertoni*, as well as *G. morsitans* itself, are the vectors; these species are preferentially bovid feeders and are not attracted to humans. Savanna *Glossina* spp. therefore only feed on humans when other hosts are not available and when they are 'hungry'. The classical view of the epidemiology of *T. b. rhodesiense* trypanosomiasis is that specific groups of people are associated with infection, usually those whose activities or occupations bring them into more frequent contact with savanna *Glossina* in savanna woodland or thicket habitat in which game animals are abundant; examples of such groups are honey gatherers (Figure 63.6), fisher-

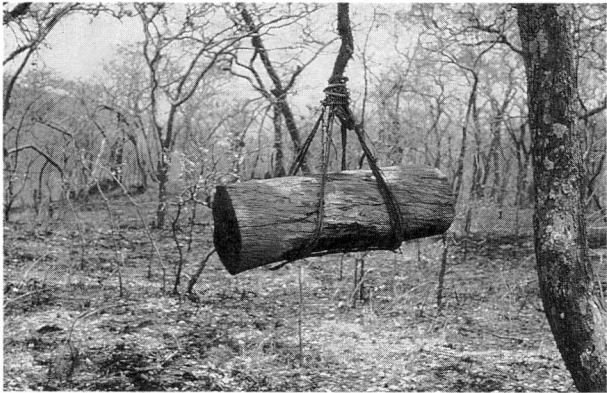

Figure 63.6 Savanna woodland in Malawi, showing beehive used by honey gatherers who are regarded as a high-risk group due to frequent contact with *G. morsitans* which feed predominantly on game animals in this habitat.

men, game wardens, poachers and firewood collectors. *T. b. rhodesiense* is a zoonosis; the known reservoir hosts are listed in Table 63.3 (Figure 63.7). The relationship between *T. b. brucei* and *T. b. rhodesiense* is difficult to define precisely as markers of human infectivity have been elusive, although Hide et al,[26] using repetitive DNA sequences, have demonstrated that not only are Zambian strains different from those in Kenya and Uganda, but that in a cluster analysis stocks from non-human sources

Table 63.3 Known or suspected reservoir hosts of *T. b. rhodesiense*.

Host	Location	Identification method(s)
Bushbuck (*Tragelaphus scriptus*)	Nyanza, Kenya	Volunteer
Hartebeeste (*Alcelaphus buselaphus*)	Serengeti, Tanzania	BIIT* Volunteer
Lion	Serengeti, Tanzania	BIIT Volunteer
Hyaena (*Crocuta crocuta*)	Serengeti, Tanzania	
Cattle	Alego, Kenya Busoga, Uganda Lambwe Valley, Kenya	Volunteer Isoenzyme Isoenzyme
Dog	Busoga, Uganda	Isoenzyme
Reedbuck (*Redunca redunca*)	Lambwe Valley, Kenya	BIIT
Waterbuck (*Kobus ellipsiprymnus*)	Tanzania Zambia	BIIT BIIT
Sheep	Lambwe Valley, Kenya	BIIT
Goat	Lambwe Valley, Kenya	BIIT

*BIIT, blood incubation infectivity test.

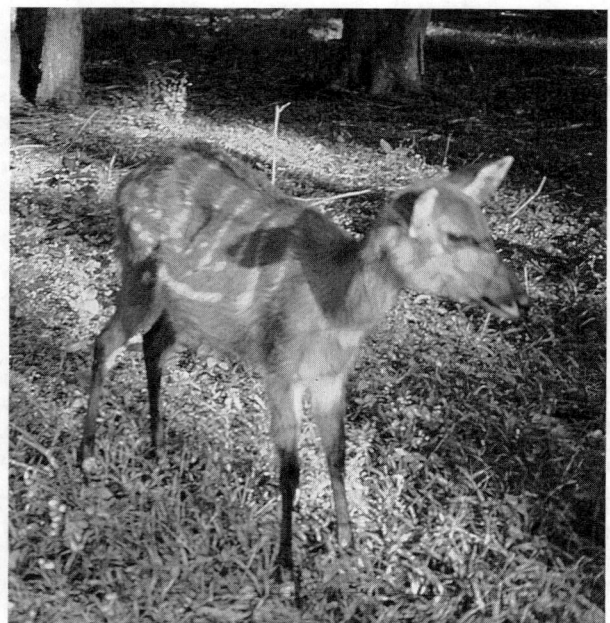

Figure 63.7 Bushbuck (*Tragelaphus sciriptus*), an important wild reservoir host of *T. b. rhodesiense*.

in the same area were separable from stocks from humans, and although no isoenzyme markers for human infectivity have been found, human stocks present consistent profiles within a locality. Cibulskis (1992) recommends the use of the zymodeme concept in relation to human infectivity in East Africa.

Analysis of the zymodemes of *T. brucei* from the Lambwe Valley, Kenya by Cibulskis,[37] using a contingency table approach, has suggested that particular zymodemes are associated with particular mammalian hosts and that such relationships are stable, at least over a 32-month period. Earlier studies in this locality showed that the *T. brucei* population changed during the sleeping sickness outbreak in 1980[38,39] showing that outbreaks arose from within the locality rather than through the introduction of strains from outside. In the context of the experimental finding of sexual recombination in *T. brucei*, Cibulskis[37] suggests that genetic exchange has an important role in the macroevolution of *T. brucei* populations, a view that differs from that of Tibayrenc et al[19] who consider sexual reproduction predominant in establishing clones stable in space and time; Cibulskis[37] considers *T. brucei* populations evolve clonally over short time periods, and clones or zymodemes possess characteristics which remain stable. In *T. brucei*, zymodemes tend to have a limited capacity to disperse, as indicated by an analysis of distribution of nearly 900 stocks.[21]

EPIDEMIC *T. b. rhodesiense*

Epidemics of acute disease have been observed over many decades but most recently in Busoga, Uganda.

This epidemic involved around 8000 cases per year in the mid-1980s but now appears to have been controlled through a combination of interventions: intense surveillance, diagnosis and treatment, and vector control (aerial spraying and trapping). The epidemic in Busoga was believed to be caused by a change in the agriculture of the area when cotton and coffee production ceased and the land was not cultivated, allowing the weed *Lantana camara* to become abundant. This shrub provided a suitable habitat for *G. f. fuscipes* to invade Busoga from the lakeside habitat where it was characteristically found. A similar invasion of *G. f. fuscipes* occurred in Alego, Kenya[40,41] and was associated with an earlier epidemic. In both these epidemics cattle have been implicated as reservoir hosts,[38,39,41] while detailed analysis of zymodemes has allowed the characterization of these parasites into the strain group Busoga, with a smaller number of isolates belonging to the Zambezi strain group which is more characteristic of Zambia. The movement of *G. f. fuscipes* flies into peridomestic situations in East Africa, associated with cattle or possibly also pigs as a reservoir, parallels peridomestic populations of West African riverine flies where, in humid areas,

peridomestic *G. palpalis* group flies are associated with domestic pig populations living close to or within villages.[42]

In Zambia epidemics of *T. b. rhodesiense* are characterized by the change in male:female:child ratio of infection which will be closer to unity, contrasting with the endemic situation when sporadic cases are associated with males who are traditionally likely to penetrate tsetse habitats. Epidemics arise when *G. morsitans* becomes more closely associated with humans by dispersing towards villages in the rainy season, as a result of humans settling close to abundant tsetse populations or through a close association of game animals with human settlements.

The importance of microepidemiological studies is emphasized by the existence of hot-spots of transmission. In the Lambwe Valley, Kenya, the major reservoir host, the bushbuck (*Tragelaphus scriptus*), and the vector, *G. pallidipes*, are closely associated as a result of the strong feeding preference of *G. pallidipes* for bushbuck, and the high infection rate of *Trypanozoon* in bushbuck and the abundance of *G. pallidipes* result in pockets of transmission of human infective parasites.[43]

DIAGNOSIS

Many of the symptoms of sleeping sickness, particularly in the early stages, are similar to those caused by other infectious organisms and toxaemic conditions. Because chemotherapy causes a significant risk, particularly in the late stage of treatment when the parasite has invaded the CNS, diagnosis of the stage of the disease is critical. Mortality is frequently recorded at between 5 and 10% during treatment; hence, if sleeping sickness is suspected, positive identification of the parasite is essential before commencing chemotherapy.

Several immunodiagnostic procedures have been developed as potential preliminary and alternative screens. These methods offer the possibility of examining large numbers of the at-risk population, from which positive suspects can then be examined by the more rigorous methods of parasite detection.

PARASITES IN BLOOD, TISSUES AND CSF

Freshly prepared blood films are used for the rapid detection of parasites in circulating blood. Wet

blood films require examination of blood under a coverslip for the detection of parasite movement. Stained thick films are, however, the most sensitive of the blood film methods. Because parasites may only be present in the blood in low numbers, concentration techniques based on centrifugation or filtration using cellulose columns have been developed. The most widely used techniques are the microhaematocrit centrifugation method, followed by examination of the buffy coat, either directly or using a long working-distance objective, and the minianion exchange centrifugation technique. The latter method requires passage of blood through a DEAE-52 anion exchange column. The red blood cells are retained on the column, while the trypanosomes pass through the column in an appropriate buffer and are then centrifuged. The haematocrit method has been modified and its sensitivity enhanced in the quantitative buffy coat (QBC) technique, which is now considered to be of great value for parasitological diagnosis,[44] being at least as sensitive as other concentration methods.

A major problem with both *T. b. gambiense* and *T. b. rhodesiense* is that trypanosomes may only be present in small numbers in the blood, both acute and chronic infections having fluctuating aparasitaemic periods. It is important to recognize that the parasites' preferred environment is within the lymphoid and connective tissue spaces, where numbers do not necessarily correlate with parasitaemia. In some suspected cases it may be necessary to continue examination of blood samples for several days, especially in patients without fever. In a group of 12 patients with *T. b. gambiense* who were seropositive, parasitological examinations were made daily for some 14 days before all positive parasitological identifications were achieved. As an indirect aid to this problem blood or other tissue materials may be inoculated into animals—mice, rats, rabbits, *M. natalensis* and guinea-pigs. If parasitaemia develops in the recipient animal, parasites may be isolated in greater numbers for further studies. However, this procedure is time consuming. Alternatively a KIVI may be used.[9]

In *T. b. gambiense* suspects with enlarged cervical lymph glands, aspirates of glands may be examined directly under the microscope. Occasionally parasites can be detected in bone marrow aspirate if they are not found in blood, lymph tissue or CSF. Smears of bone marrow are stained before microscopy.

Because the prognosis is significantly worse once the parasite has entered the CNS, accurate assessment of the stage of the disease is essential. Unfortunately diagnosis is dependent upon direct analysis of CSF, which again may be negative even though the blood–CSF and blood–brain barriers have been breached. Multiple centrifugation procedures considerably increase the likelihood of detection. Centrifugation of the fresh CSF must be undertaken rapidly (within 10 minutes) because the parasites appear to be more fragile than those in blood. The analysis of CSF normally includes the additional criteria of raised leucocyte count and elevated protein levels, which in health are low (i.e. leucocytes <3 cells/mm^3; protein <40 mg%) but which become markedly increased in inflammatory CNS disorders, including late-stage sleeping sickness. Different authorities have presented varying values as their standard for diagnosis of CNS involvement, but widely accepted criteria are: (1) the presence of trypanosomes; and/or (2) leucocytes $\geqslant 5$ cells/mm^3; and/or (3) protein $\geqslant 40$ mg%. Only rarely are large numbers of trypanosomes present in the CSF; this may be associated with haemorrhage because CSF is not a favourable environment for parasite survival. If sleeping sickness has already been diagnosed, an elevated leucocyte count and/or protein level in the CSF in the absence of parasites is an indicator(s) of CNS involvement.

The sequential approach to serological and parasitological diagnosis of *T. b. gambiense* would be: card agglutination test for trypanosomiasis (CATT), gland puncture, thick blood film, microhaematocrit miniamine exchange column and QBC. In *T. b. rhodesiense* it would be wet film, thick film, microhaematocrit and QBC.

IMMUNODIAGNOSTIC METHODS

A number of serological methods have been developed for the screening of populations for sleeping sickness suspects, from which further parasitological examination can be made. It is also desirable to develop alternatives to the laborious and sometimes difficult detection of trypanosomes in the blood or CSF. Several techniques have been developed for the measurement of antibodies to trypanosomes and for antigen detection.[45] Patients with sleeping sickness produce a range of antibodies directed against variant surface glycoproteins (VSGs) as well as other antigens. The diversity of VSG is relatively limited for *T. b. gambiense*, where most of the parasite population expresses a limited number of predominant variant antigen types (VATs) early in infection, regardless of the geographic location. Serological tests have been developed which are based on direct agglutination, haemagglutination, gel precipitation, immunofluorescence and enzyme linked immunosorbent assays (ELISA). The most widely used tests to date have been indirect immunofluorescence and the CATT, using a VAT found in the majority of *T. b. gambiense* isolates. The presence of a VAT and/or elevated IgM in the CSF correlates directly with the trypanosome infection of CSF. Unfortunately such a prevalent VAT does not occur with *T. b. rhodesiense* and serodiagnosis relies on the detection of relatively small amounts of antibody against the invariant surface antigens, for which tests lack both specificity and sensitivity. Alternatively, diagnosis of sleeping sickness may be based on the detection of antibodies against more precise parasite markers, such as enzymes. This approach, termed anti-parasite enzyme-specific antibody assay, has recently been used for parasite acid phosphatase.[46] The test also cross-reacts with phosphatase from *Leishmania*, although this should not interfere with diagnosis of sleeping sickness in most endemic regions of Africa, apart from southern Sudan where visceral leishmaniasis as well as trypanosomiasis is endemic. Emphasis on detection of antigens as a means of diagnosis has been pursued recently with an antigen detection system using monoclonal antibodies against a procyclic invariant antigen.[45] The reagent has been tested in a multicentre study[47] for diagnosis of *T. b. rhodesiense* in serum and CSF. The test sites in Tanzania, Uganda and Zambia involved material from parasitically confirmed cases; the overall detection rate exceeded 91% and there was no cross-reactivity with other common disease agents. The antigen detection system is linked to a sandwich ELISA methodology using monoclonal antibody-coated polystyrene tubes, followed by incubation in the test serum, treatment with peroxidase-labelled monoclonal antibodies, and subsequent exposure to H_2O_2 substrate and chromogen. The positive reactions were those which developed a visible colour change. CSF antigens were also detected in a similar way.

The availability of immunodiagnostic tests developed with high quality reagents, such as CATT and the antigen-capture ELISA, have demonstrated that it is possible to produce tests which are sufficiently sensitive and simple to use under field conditions. The challenge is to ensure availability, cost-effectiveness and competent use in active surveillance or at fixed health centres as a primary filter for the reliable identification of patients for whom parasitological diagnosis and chemotherapy should be continued.

CLINICAL SYMPTOMS AND SIGNS

There is considerable variation in the clinical picture of African trypanosomiasis, with many symptoms being non-specific. The acute and chronic forms of the disease vary more in terms of the degree and rate of onset of signs and symptoms than in the symptoms themselves. Infection is characterized by initial intermittent fevers, gradual involvement of the reticuloendothelial system and the endocrine system, and later the development of neurological symptoms. Several reviews of the clinical picture have been published.[48–50] The initial stage in virulent *T. b. rhodesiense* disease is the chancre which develops at the site of the bite of *Glossina* (Figure 63.8). This is a local swelling, appearing several days after the bite, and is characterized by local heat, oedema, erythema and tenderness. There is desquamation at the periphery; the chancre lasts several weeks and trypanosomes can be detected in the chancre fluid. As the chancre progresses the skin becomes hyperpigmented and can remain so for several years. Chancres are not seen in chronic *T. b. gambiense* and seem characteristic of the virulent Busoga strain group of *T. b. rhodesiense*.

Within a few days of the tsetse bite, fever develops as a consequence of the invasion of the blood by parasites. The incubation period between the bite and the onset of fever varies, with recorded times as short as a few hours following the chancre or up to several weeks. The early stages of the disease are subsequently characterized by relatively non-specific symptoms in what is known as the haemolymphatic stage. Irregular febrile episodes are accompanied by headaches, malaise, weight loss, muscle and joint pains, pruritus, anaemia, rash and deep hyperaesthesia (Kerandel's sign). Facial oedema, endocrine disorders (for example, sterility,

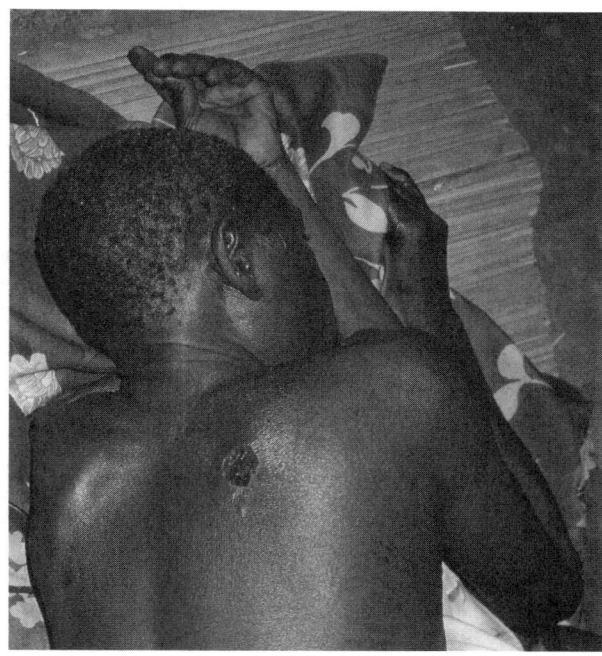

Figure 63.8 Comatose patient with sleeping sickness showing two chancres on shoulder blades.

impotence, or amenorrhoea and abortion in women), cardiac abnormalities, enlarged lymph glands, moderate splenomegaly and hepatomegaly, and involvement of the digestive system are among the variety of other features which are associated with the disease. Some of these are described in more detail below. However, as pointed out earlier, the manifestations of sleeping sickness are extremely variable: in some cases many symptoms are barely noticeable or absent, in others a particular symptom or cluster of symptoms may be markedly aggravated. There is also a general and significant difference in the time course of the disease: most cases óf *T. b. rhodesiense* run an acute or subacute course which is fatal in a few months from damage to the heart or viscera; those due to *T. b. gambiense* frequently extend to a chronic course of several years, leading to the extensive nervous system involvement of classic sleeping sickness.

Although sleeping sickness is associated with a large and varied range of symptoms none appears to be truly pathognomonic. The lymph gland enlargement occurs near the site of the infective bite, but becomes general. The adenopathy in chronic disease characteristically involves the supraclavicular and posterior groups. The enlarged neck glands are sometimes easily visible (Winterbottom's sign). In acute disease the axillary and epitrochlear ·glands but not the cervical glands are involved. The peculiar deep hyperaesthesia (Kerandel's sign), with pain shortly following soft-tissue compression, associated for example with daily knocks and bumps but out of all proportion to the pressure, is almost pathognomonic but does not occur in all patients. Local oedema of the face, in the lower eyelids and extending to give a puffy, swollen and somewhat dumb expression, is alsó characteristic and progressive, but again many patients with both forms of the disease may be unaffected. The lesions may extend into the eyes, producing interstitial keratitis and conjunctivitis, especially with *T. b. rhodesiense* infection(s). The cardiac abnormalities are obvious suggestive symptoms; an early tachycardia may progress to extensive damage, with pericardial effusions and pancarditis involving all layers, valves and conducting systems, as described by Poltera et al.[51] Not surprisingly the ECG tracings may have marked abnormalities. Many other signs also contribute to the clinical picture of sleeping sickness. These include: enlargement of the liver and spleen, endocrine dysfunctions, anaemia and rashes (erythematous circinate patches, about 7–10 cm diameter, occurring mainly on the trunk and shoulder and difficult to detect on dark skin) but they are inconstant and relatively common in other tropical diseases and are not in themselves of much diagnostic value. Sleeping sickness is also frequently associated with intercurrent infections, for example of the respiratory system causing bronchopneumonia. Such infections significantly complicate the clinical presentation.

The nervous system involvement is progressive and manifests several peculiar features of the chronic and late stages of the disease. Trypanosomes cannot usually be detected in the CSF for some time after initial infection: 3–4 weeks for *T. b. rhodesiense* and several months for *T. b. gambiense*. Neurological symptoms such as headache, irritability, mood changes and altered EEG, may, however, occur within a few days of infection during the initial febrile period, thus preceding parasite entry into the CSF. The early changes correlate with the widespread meningeal inflammation which occurs in both forms of the disease. As the disease progresses the signs of nervous system involvement become more marked, with progressive mental deterioration, mood changes and, particularly in *T. b. gambiense* infection, the classical reversal of sleep patterns with daytime somnolence leading to permanent sleep, coma and eventually death. Motor functions become seriously impaired, with abnormal movements (dyskinesia, choreoathetosis and convulsions) and altered gait. The picture may resemble that of parkinsonism, with the subject being able to walk only with sticks and with help. Speech is impaired.

The profound neurological changes correlate with progression from meningitis to encephalitis. As described above, this is most extensive in *T. b. gambiense* infection, with its natural duration of 2 years or more, for which there is a large and fascinating literature describing a variety of mental changes. The pattern is one of a basic lethargy from which bouts of mania, delirium, paranoia and schizoid and aggressive behaviour (likened to the general paralysis of the insane) may occur. Patients with sleeping sickness have been found in psychiatric institutions—with their trypanosomiasis undiagnosed. Presumably the different patterns correlate with the extent, location and intensity of the meningoencephalitis. In *T. b. rhodesiense* infection, with a normal duration of only 6–9 months, the late-stage encephalitis and marked neurological symptoms are not seen, although there may be some drowsiness, tremors and unsteadiness preceding the terminal coma. Again, in both diseases concurrent infections due to a range of other organisms have been recorded and these may significantly contribute to, or modify the clinical picture. Some of the characteristic symptoms of sleeping sickness are summarized in Table 63.4.

Table 63.4 Clinical symptoms of sleeping sickness (After Molyneux et al,[93]).

Chancre related
Localized erythema, tenderness, heat

Parasitaemia related
Periodic fever
Headache
Joint pains and muscle ache
Lymphadenopathy
Weight loss
Pruritus
Erythema
Anaemia

Organ related
Oedema: peripheral, ascites, lung oedema, pericardial effusion
Cardiac changes: non-specific ECG changes, congestive heart failure and distension
Endocrinological: amenorrhoea, abortion, impotence, anorexia
Digestive tract: diarrhoea
Nervous system: altered reflexes, hyperaesthesiae, paraesthesiae, epileptiform fits, mental disorders, insomnia/
somnolence, ataxia/dyskinesia, slurred speech, pareses/paralysis, cheiroral reflexes

DIFFERENTIAL DIAGNOSIS

Owing to the many clinical variations of sleeping sickness it is difficult to describe a 'typical' case of the disease; differential diagnosis might therefore seem of unusual importance. The chancre, rashes, febrile responses, swollen glands, anaemia, wasting and neurological changes are similar to those of many familiar conditions, ranging from trivial insect bites to tuberculous lymphadenopathy, Hodgkin's disease, brucellosis, relapsing fever, malaria, infectious mononucleosis, typhoid, viral encephalitis, tuberculous meningitis, neurosyphilis, etc. In practice, however, the positive identification of parasites in blood or CSF, following their examination once there is suspicion of sleeping sickness, renders the differential diagnosis less of a problem.

PREGNANCY AND CHILDREN

Fetal transmission, although uncommon, is well documented for *T. b. gambiense* but no reported cases are known for *T. b. rhodesiense*. The disease in children is similar to that in adults.

MORTALITY

There have been reports of 'healthy carriers' and spontaneous termination of a *T. b. gambiense* infection but these are probably due to anomalous or atypical parasite strains. Generally in such cases the follow-up has not been adequate to justify the claim(s). Although in some relatively resilient patients without other intercurrent infections mild cases may progress very slowly over many years; in the absence of precise diagnostic criteria and suitable follow-up it would be inappropriate to term these subclinical. The possibility for spontaneous recovery cannot be excluded, but it is, however, clear that such a phenomenon could only occur in the early stages. Once the disease has progressed to involvement of the CNS, death is inevitable without treatment.

IMMUNITY

Although humans are immune to infection by some common trypanosome parasites of animals, for example *T. congolense* and *T. vivax*, there is no direct evidence for innate or acquired immunity to *T. b. rhodesiense* or *T. b. gambiense*. The degree of resistance which develops in some districts after prolonged exposure may be due to several factors, including non-specific parasite antigen(s) and altered parasite virulence.

PATHOLOGY AND PATHOGENESIS

Sleeping sickness produces multiple pathological changes that involve most organs and systems. The changes are progressive and their gross anatomy, histology, physiology, biochemistry and immunology have been extensively described. The damage results from a complex interplay of factors between the different systems. The parasite escapes the immune response by varying the surface glycoprotein coat, thus exposing the host to altered antigenic variants, and by inducing generalized suppression of immunological functions. Many human studies have been made from postmortem material, which provides information chiefly on the end-stage of the disease (for reviews of the gross pathology, see refs. 52 and 53). Studies have also been made on a variety of animal models in order to elucidate the initiating lesions and pathogenesis; they are of considerable value in advancing understanding of the human condition.

The disease affects principally the haemolymphatic system. An obvious major feature is the general increase in perivascular cellularity characteristic of the inflammatory process due to an infiltration of monocytes, lymphocytes and plasma cells. This is associated with widespread haemorrhage(s) and tissue oedema. Particularly rapid changes occur in the heart with *T. b. rhodesiense* disease; myocarditis extends to a generalized involvement of all cardiac layers, including the conducting and valvular systems.[53a] There is marked infiltration of plasma cells, amongst which are morular cells. These are large plasma cells with vacuolated cytoplasm and pycnotic nuclei, first described in sleeping sickness by Mott,[54] and which have subsequently become known as Mott morular cells. Their presence in the blood, bone marrow or CSF has been considered pathognomonic. The cardiac damage extends to fibrosis and myocytolysis, and secondary infections may contribute to the cardiac lesions. In the chronic forms of the disease perivascular infiltrations also become a marked feature of the CNS involvement with meningoencephalitis. The major features of the pathological alterations are listed in Table 63.4 and summarized in the following sections.

HAEMATOLOGICAL MANIFESTATIONS

The haematological manifestations are of great complexity. A number of central and fundamental changes are associated with the varying effects of changing parasitaemia, the parasite virulence and its metabolic and breakdown products, the extent of other organ failure(s), and the presence of other concurrent infections and the immune state of the host. Patients have markedly altered plasma albumin:globulin ratios; the macroglobulinaemia is characteristic of both the Gambian and Rhodesian forms and has been extensively documented. The increases are highest for IgM with the first parasitaemia; IgG responses are not so marked. Thereafter there is a progressive suppression which is selective for the IgG production, but with the IgM levels remaining high. Another obvious change in plasma is the increase in total lipid content, which in rabbits may be up to four times that of non-infected animals. Large amounts of cholesterol and β-lipoprotein(s) are present. The alterations in serum lipoprotein may result from the decreased thyroid output. There are also increases in free fatty acids (e.g. linoleic, oleic, palmitic and stearic) which may be generated from lysed trypanosomes. Disturbances of other plasma constituents (e.g. decrease of calcium and bicarbonate, increase of phosphate, urea and creatinine) indicate renal damage. Glomerulonephritis has been observed in experimental animals, although gross pathological changes to the kidney are not a usual feature of patients with sleeping sickness. The presence of increased enzymes in plasma, such as aspartate transaminase and creatinine phosphokinase—again in animal models, may correlate with generalized cell destruction.

The aetiology of the anaemia in sleeping sickness is multifactorial, with haemolysis, haemodilution and disordered and/or non-compensatory erythropoiesis having continued with variable contributions during the infection.[55] Haemolysis is largely responsible, with the phagocytosis of red cells that have become coated with immune complexes in the spleen sinusoids and by the Kupffer cells of the liver. The liver is enlarged in approximately 25% of patients, but how much this is due to secondary infection is again difficult to assess. The haemolysis may also result in part from haemolytic factors liberated by the trypanosomes. As infection progresses the blood and plasma volumes become progressively enlarged, thus causing a haemodilution effect. This appears to be an almost constant sequel to splenic enlargement. Red cell production by the bone marrow is significantly reduced. The defect here is associated with a failure of iron incorporation into the red cell precursors, with a large excess of storage iron not employed for haemoglobin synthesis.

Patients may also have a moderate leucocytosis; differential counts regularly show monocytosis, lymphocytosis and plasmacytosis. The large Mott morular cells may also be present.

Blood homeostasis becomes seriously disturbed. The disease is commonly associated with minor haemorrhages and multiple petechiae, although these are rarely sufficiently severe to be life threatening. The pathogenesis is associated with vascular injury, coagulopathy with increased fibrinolysis, and thrombocytopenia (see ref. 55). The vascular injury may be brought about by the release of pharmacologically active mediators, which are summarized below. The coagulopathy is most common in acute *T. b. rhodesiense* disease and consists of thrombosis, haemorrhage, tissue necrosis and microangiopathic anaemia, which have been attributed to the condition termed disseminated intravascular coagulation. Fibrinogen and fibrin degradation products are present at increased levels, and may be detected in the urine if there is renal damage. In both types of the disease there are decreased platelet numbers, platelet clumping and altered aggregatory responses. The thrombocytopenia may result from increased destruction of platelets, failure of platelet production, or their abnormal distribution or dilution loss. In addition the blood becomes hyperviscous. Unfortunately the mechanisms underlying these complex changes are in the main not understood. This would seem inevitable in view of the complexities imposed by the multiple and overlapping cascade systems involved, the variations in parasite virulence, the differences in individual responses to the parasite and the high frequency of several intercurrent infections.

IMMUNOLOGICAL MANIFESTATIONS

The cellularity and architecture of the lymphoid organs are severely altered, especially in the later stages of infection. At the gross level there is splenomegaly, lymphadenopathy and thymic atrophy. For the spleen and lymph nodes this is largely due to the hyperplasia of lymphoid and mononuclear cells; increases in spleen size have also been noted to correlate with the degree of anaemia. In animal models the B-cell spleen areas become massed, with large lymphoid cells and immature and mature plasma cells. T-cell areas also become infiltrated with macrophages and plasma cells. T cells, B cells and null cells increase around peaks of parasitaemia. As discussed above, the removal of erythrocytes which have become coated with immune complexes, or in some manner sensitized in the infected circulation, by the macrophages (in the extended splenic vascular network) may largely account for the anaemia. The bone marrow is also disrupted, with marked depletion of the stem cells. Similar changes occur in the lymph nodes, but generally later in infection than the spleen, with a marked filling with plasma cells and lymphoblasts. The alterations in lymphoid architecture have been summarized by Bancroft and Askonas.[56] Another important feature is the marked infiltration of various tissues, including lymphoid organs and brain areas, with CD8+ T cells, which is discussed in more detail below.

Because the pathogenesis is ultimately linked to the inability of the untreated patient to remove the parasite, considerable efforts have been made to elucidate the ways in which the parasite interacts with the immune system, upsetting the balance of cytokines and other mediator substances and thus allowing pathology to develop. Trypanosome VSG determinants stimulate B cells through T-cell independent and T-cell dependent pathways. The resulting antibodies to the surface coat cause immune lysis of the trypanosomes, with their destruction being completed mainly by the liver Kupffer cells. The parasitaemia decreases to a low, generally undetectable level. However, the heterologous antigenic variants (less than 0.1% of each peak population) survive to repopulate the blood and other tissues. As each VAT population is eliminated, the VAT-specific immunoglobulins (IgG and IgM) decline to low levels, but the invariant trypanosome antibodies

Table 63.5   Alterations in cytokine/prostaglandin network in trypanosomiasis.

Activated macrophages	↑ IL-1 release (PG-dependent) ↑ PGE_2 (transient) ↑ TNF-α
T cells	↑ IFN (CD8+ cells) ↑ IL-2 production (macrophage PG mediated) ↑ IL-2 receptor expression (macrophage mediated)
Serum	↑ GM-CSF (transient) ↑ $PGF_{2\alpha}$
Brain	↑ TNF (expression) ↑ IL-1, IL-4, IL-6 (expression) ↑ MIP-1 (expression) ↑ PGD_2 (CSF) ↑ PGD_2 and PGE_2 production (astrocytes)

GM-CSF, granulocyte-macrophage colony stimulating factor;
MIP-1, macrophage inflammatory protein 1.
Sources: Fierer et al;[64] Hunter et al;[65] Mutayoba et al;[66] Oka et al;[67] Pentreath et al;[68] Sileghem et al.[59,60]

(especially the IgM) remain high due to their maintained stimulation. The regulation of the immunoglobulin responses is complex,[57] but the antigen non-specific changes appear most closely linked to the immunopathology. During developing parasitaemia several lymphocyte populations (including B cells and suppressor and helper T cells) and macrophages are non-specifically stimulated. The cells proliferate and the B and T cells' responsiveness to a range of non-parasite-related antigens become increased, but strangely the ability to induce T-cell dependent B cell responses declines, with progressive impairment of T cell helper, suppressor and cytotoxic functions until the disease continues with only the T-independent B cell functions operating, which are usually enhanced. The parasite thus induces the paradoxical changes of polyclonal stimulation coupled with immunosuppression. The T-cell dependent immune responses to the persistent trypanosome antigens are depressed, but the active T-independent B cell responses to the VSG surface epitopes still control successive parasitaemias.

It has, however, become clear, largely from work in rodent models, that macrophages have a key involvement in this progressive immunosuppression. These cells become unable to present antigens normally to T cells and are generally suppressive to T-cell activities. The immunosuppression can be transferred to uninfected animals via a relatively small number of macrophages from infected animals.[58] The possible mechanisms behind the suppressive activity include faulty processing of trypanosome antigens and their inadequate presentation with major histocompatibility (MHC) class II products (Ia antigen presentation). In accord with this, antigen processing may be reduced at early stages of the disease and Ia expression has been reported to be increased or decreased during the infection.

Attention has been turned to the altered secretion by macrophages and other cell types of immunoregulatory cytokines and other mediators which, by analogy with other tropical diseases, may be in part responsible for the faulty immune response and other aspects of the pathogenesis. Some of the altered patterns of cytokine formation in different tissues and cells are summarized in Table 63.5. Interleukin (IL)-1 secretion by macrophages from infected mice is markedly increased rather than decreased, which is due to enhanced IL-1 release rather than synthesis.[59] In lymph nodes, T-cell proliferation is suppressed by at least two separate effector mechanisms which block T-cell regulatory effects;[60] the proliferation of IL-2 production is severely depressed by prostaglandin (PG)-producing macrophages (i.e. IL-2 production is restored by PG synthesis inhibitors), and IL-2-receptor expression on both CD4+ and CD8+ cells is blocked by a PG-independent suppressive mechanism, with no influence on IL-2 secretion. IL-1 activates PG synthesis, thus limiting its own production, and thus the inhibition of IL-2 production may be in part caused by the increased IL-1. *T. b. brucei* also activate macrophages to produce TNF α, which has trypanostatic activity.[61] Other studies implicate interferon (IFN)-γ. In experimental rodent models the disease is associated with a prominent infiltration of many tissues by CD8+ T cells. Selective depletion of these cells suppresses parasite growth and increases survival of the infected ani-

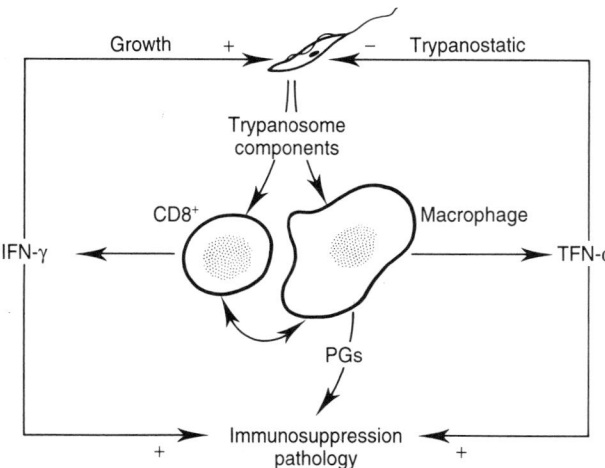

Figure 63.9 Interactions between *T. b. brucei*, CD8+ T cells and macrophages in experimental rodent trypanosomiasis. Substances from *T. b. brucei* activate CD8+ cells to produce INFγ, and macrophages to produce TNFα. The responses of the two cell types may be facilitated by these cytokines and by local contact signals. IFNγ promotes parasite growth, activates macrophages, suppresses T cell proliferation and inhibits CD4 cell activation by blockage of 1L-2 receptors. Activated macrophages produce TNFγ, which is trypanostatic, and prostaglandins which may block 1L-2 secretion from the CD4 cells, thus enhancing the immunosuppression. Although other types of cytokines are involved, this type of model provides valuable insights into the immunopathology of sleeping sickness. The model summarizes information from Bakhiet et al,[91] Lucas et al[61] and Sileghem et al.[60]

mals[62]. The CD8+ cells are responsible for production of IFN-γ which is a potent activator of macrophages and can suppress T-cell proliferation. In addition the observation has been made that IFN-γ has a growth promoting effect on *T. b. brucei*. The interesting possibility is therefore raised that IFN-γ released by CD8+ T cells may provide both an immunosuppressive signal and a stimulus for parasite growth in the infiltrated tissues, for example in the lymphoid tissues where the parasite is known to reside preferentially.[62] Some of these features are summarized in Figure 63.9.

Another important question is the nature of the substance(s) which triggers the suppressive behaviour of macrophages and altered cytokine production. Trypanosome-specific antibody does not seem to be directly involved.[58] Both parasite contact and soluble factor(s) derived from *T. b. rhodesiense* suppress IL-2 receptor expression on lectin-stimulated human peripheral blood mononuclear cells.[63] A diffusible molecule which may directly activate CD8+ T cells to produce IFN-γ also appears to be released from *T. b. brucei*. The substance has an apparent molecular weight of 41–46 kDa, and could act directly on the CD8+ molecule itself[62] (Figure 63.10).

The modifications to the cytokine/mediator network and the associated changes in immune performance offer another valuable approach to understanding the immunopathology. However, because the different mediators in the network are regulated in mutual and complex ways, it is difficult to pin-point a primary and crucial role for any individual substance, if indeed such a situation should exist. Unfortunately, to date only a few of the known mediator substances have been investigated—mainly in the animal models, with very little information available for the human sleeping sickness patient, and it is also likely that many more immune mediator substances await discovery.

NEUROLOGICAL MANIFESTATIONS

In sleeping sickness complex neuropathology usually develops, manifesting a wide and varied range of symptoms. Some general distinctions can be made between the chronic *T. b. gambiense* form and the acute *T. b. rhodesiense* form; in the former the disease may progress to an extensive meningoencephalitis and comatose state of somnolence, from which the disease is named, but in the acute disease encephalitis may not occur as the patient may succumb to cardiac failure or another cause before it is reached. The neuropathological changes summarized in Table 63.6 are therefore most applicable to the chronic *T. b. gambiense* disease. Another feature of great clinical importance concerns post-treatment encephalopathy which occurs in an estimated 10% of cases, often causing death. This reaction may follow treatment with the organic arsenic melarsoprol, which crosses the blood–brain barrier and which is still the drug of choice for patients with CNS involvement. The post-treatment reaction may be due to the release of antigens released from parasites killed inside the brain, or more likely results from subcurative therapy leaving surviving parasites in the CNS, which in turn provoke a violent inflammatory response.[69]

The choroid is damaged early in the disease, with parasites occupying the stromal spaces and spilling into the CSF. The CSF does not provide a particularly favourable medium for parasite survival, especially in the late disease stages when its composition may be altered by large amounts of immunoglobulin and many lymphocytes. The parasites may then have access, via the CSF circulating through the subarachnoidal spaces over the brain surface, to the perivascular extensions (Virchow–Robin spaces) which pass into the brain. It seems likely that this

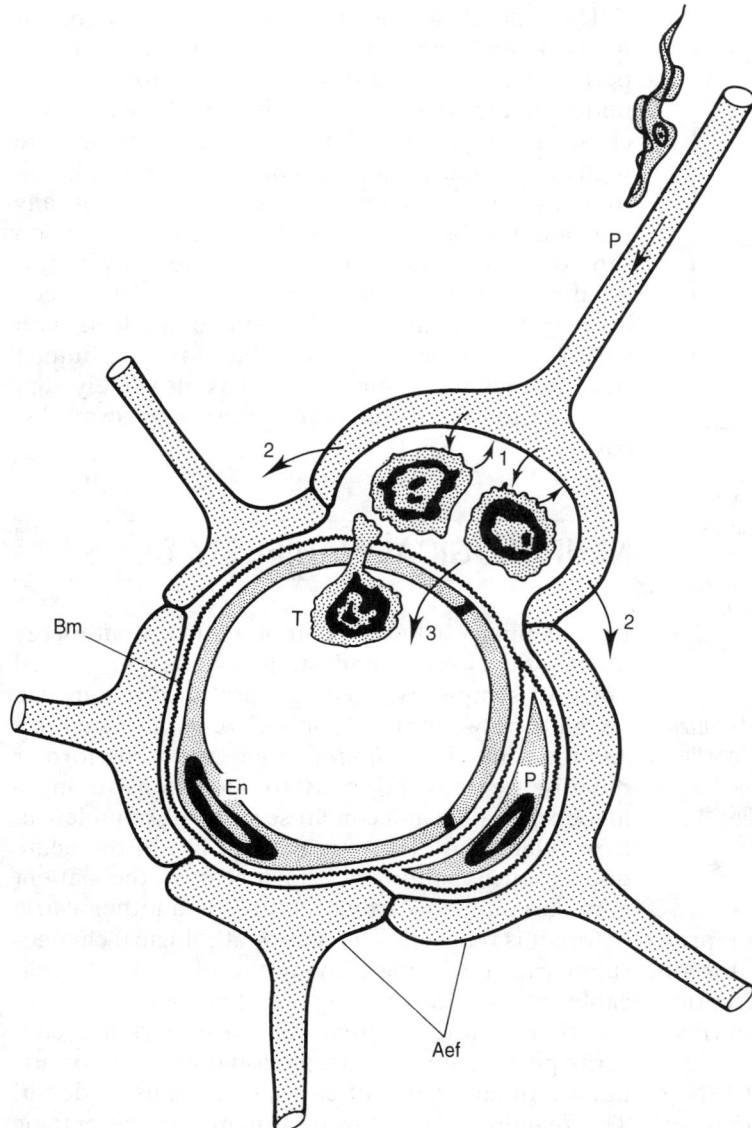

Figure 63.10 The blood–brain interface in the CNS and the possible roles of astrocytes in trypanosomiasis; capillary endothelial cells (En) form a monolayer with adjacent cells joined by tight junctions. Pericytes (P) are located along, and frequently enclosed by the basement membrane (Bm). Pericytes may be microglial cell precursors or have immune roles such as antigen presentation. The astrocyte end-feet (Aef) are joined by gap junctions to form a continuous layer around the capillary. Activated T cells (T) are able to migrate across the endothelium and basement membrane, where they make contact with the astrocyte end-feet. The astrocytes are well positioned to transport and present antigens from parasites (P) which enter the parenchyma. The secretion of cytokines and other mediators by the activated astrocytes may (1) (arrows) sustain the local inflammatory response with lymphocyte proliferation or suppression in the perivascular cuffs; may (2) (arrows) promote local astrocyte and microglial proliferation, pericyte development into microglia or affect other structures locally in the parenchyma to produce disease symptoms (e.g. somnolence); or (3) (arrow) modify the blood–brain barrier and signal further lymphocyte entry. (Reproduced with permission from Pentreath).[78]

Table 63.6 Neuropathological changes in African trypanosomiasis.

Meningitis
Choroid plexus breakdown
Parasite entry into circumventricular areas (regions with reduced blood–brain barrier)
CD8+ T-cell infiltration and MHC class I induction in circumventricular areas, and supraoptic and paraventricular hypothalamic nuclei
Astrocyte activation
Perivascular cuffing (astroglial and microglial hyperplasia, macrophages, plasma cells, T-helper/inducer cells)
Immune complex deposition and complement activation
Blood–brain barrier breakdown
Autoantibody production (e.g. against myelin basic protein, cerebrosides and gangliosides)
Altered EEG to permanent delta wave form
Regional changes in monoamine transmitters
Altered cytokine/prostaglandin/mediator expression and production

This list is not exhaustive but includes the major changes observed in human and the animal models. Meningitis and choroid plexus breakdown are early events, but the remainder of the changes are not necessarily in chronological order. For references see text.

Table 63.7 Alterations in monoamines in brains of mice with chronic trypanosomiasis.

	DA	NA	HVA	5-HT	5H1AA
Cerebellum	—	↑	—	—	—
Brain stem	↑	↑	—	↓	↑
Hypothalamus	—	—	—	↑	↑
Striatum	—	↑	↑	—	—
Hippocampus	—	↑	↑	—	—
Cortex	—	—	—	↓	↑

No significant alterations in the cholinergic system have been recorded.
DA, dopamine; NA, noradrenaline; HVA, homovanillic acid;
5-HT, 5-hydroxytryptamine; 5-HIAA, 5-hydroxy indole acetic acid.
Sources: Amole et al[92] and Stibbs and Curtis.[76]

represents the point of departure from meningitis to encephalitis. Perivascular cuffing becomes a prominent feature in the brain. This may be very obvious in the brain stem and cerebellum, although human encephalitis does not appear to become preferentially localized in specific regions.[79] The cuffs are comprised of complexes of macrophages, plasma cells, morular cells, T helper/inducer cells and hyperplasic astrocytes and microglia. The numbers, ratios and intensities of the encephalic cuffs show no consistent pattern in any brain region in different patients, but there is a general increase in severity during the chronic infection. The extent to which trypanosomes may actually penetrate the parenchyma is unclear, but this may be a relatively rare occurrence for most areas of the CNS except in the terminal disease stages. In the rodent model parasites appear selectively to invade areas with a reduced blood–brain barrier (e.g. pineal, median eminence, area postrema and other circumventricular areas), and it has been suggested that this distribution may correlate with some of the neurological manifestations, for example sensory disturbances, neuroendocrine dysfunctions and altered sleep patterns.[71] Studies on the rodent model, using dye tracers, also show that there is progressive damage to the blood–brain barrier. Not surprisingly, the EEG tracings show profound alterations. In late-stage patients the recordings are dominated by large, slow-wave oscillations resembling the delta-wave sleep state.[72]

Considerable effort has been spent searching for mechanisms which may produce and control pathogenesis and account for the neurological changes. Unfortunately the studies have been hampered by a general lack of knowledge regarding the immunology of the CNS. The presence of brain-specific antibodies in the sera of patients and rodent models may indicate an autoimmune process.[73,74] For example, autoantibodies against myelin proteins could cause the demyelination observed in some chronic cases. Alternatively the autoantibodies may represent specific antiparasite antibodies which cross-react with brain-specific antigens, or the release of autoantigens from the CNS caused by parasite damage or inflammatory responses. Immune complex deposition in the brain, perhaps associated with intracranial immunoglobulin synthesis[75] and subsequent complement activation, is another potential cause of damage, although there is disagreement over some of the findings. In the rodent model the circumventricular regions, supraoptic and paraventricular hypothalamic nuclei become infiltrated with CD8+ T cells and show marked MHC class I induction.[71] Such areas may relate to some of the clinical symptoms. The levels of several monoamine transmitters and their metabolites become significantly altered in localized brain regions of infected animals[76] (Table 63.7) and these may again be associated with some of the neurological manifestations.

More recently attention has focused on cytokines and other mediator substances, and the involvement of astrocytes in the control of inflammatory responses in nervous tissue. These cells are capable of secreting a range of cytokines, PGs and mediator substances. Astrocyte activation and subsequent alterations in the secreted substances have been implicated in several disease and pathological states of the CNS. Astrocyte activation is an obvious feature of late-stage sleeping sickness. In the rodent model the astrocyte activation appears to be associated with increased expression of tumour necrosis factor (TNF)-α, IL-1 and IL-4, amongst others[65] (see Table 63.5). During measurements of cytokines and immune mediators in the CSF of late-stage patients infected with *T. b. gambiense* some large increases in PGD_2 were found.[68] PGD_2 is one of the ultimate sleep-regulating substances,[77] and astrocytes are known to be potent producers of PGD_2 when stimulated by different active substances—including parasite products.

The advancing field of neuroimmunology offers exciting prospects for understanding the nervous system changes in sleeping sickness. Although it seems likely that astrocytes have key roles in co-ordinating the inflammatory responses, particularly in the perivascular cuffs,[78] other resident cell types (including endothelial cells, pericytes and microglia) are almost certainly involved. The CNS pathogenesis will probably be found to result from complex cytokine-mediated interactions between these cells, the immune cells from the blood, the blood–brain barrier and the trypanosomes.

PATHOGENIC SUBSTANCES FROM TRYPANOSOMES

The success of African trypanosomes is largely due to their ability to parasitize the blood and tissue spaces of the host in a relatively innocuous manner without (at least in the short term) producing serious lesions. The parasites certainly do not produce potent toxins of any sort, as has been established from a large number of investigations. However, they do release a range of active products, especially in their dead or dying state(s), which could account for the progressive pathological changes (see ref. 79) (Table 63.8). More specifically it is possible that particular parasite components may have properties which activate characteristic or precise biochemical and immune changes in the host, for example the production of a particular cytokine. Such a specific, primary modification could thus initiate a large range of secondary or downstream changes which manifest the chronic disease state, in a similar way for example, to that in which the lipopolysacharide (LPS) components of bacterial cell walls are primary substances in the pathogenesis of septicaemia.

Living trypanosomes metabolize tryptophan to

Table 63.8 Trypanosome products.

Variable antigenic coat, exoantigens
Phospholipase A_1
Proteases (especially cysteine)
Saturated fatty acids (B-cell mitogens)
Aromatic amino acid derivatives (e.g. tryptophol)
Endotoxins with LPS-like activity
Undefined proteins and phospholipids implicated in host responses

Sources: Alafiatayo et al,[82] Tizard et al.[79]

tryptopol and other indole derivatives which are secreted into the blood and which have some sleep-inducing properties. They also release surface antigens (exoantigens) which stimulate antibody production, combining with them to form immune complexes. These may in turn lead to activation of complement and the kallikrein–kinin system, causing release of bradykinins, histamine and other potentially damaging substances.[80] Some of the antigens may bind to erythrocytes, provoking sensitization to lysis by antitrypanosome antibodies. However, most attention has been given to substances in dead or dying trypanosomes because the clinical observations suggest that the symptoms are exacerbated when parasitaemia falls rapidly as a result of immune or chemotherapeutic trypanolysis. Proteases and phospholipases are two damaging groups of enzymes whose release may cause widespread non-specific damage, especially to the endothelium. As yet undefined LPSs, some of which may activate complement, and free fatty acids, which could have a range of damaging effects including immunosuppression, have also been implicated. In addition, there are reports of various mitogenic, haemolytic, hepatotoxic and inflammatory substances which could correlate with certain aspects of the pathology in different animals.[79] For example studies with *T. b. brucei* in the rodent model indicate the presence of a 41–46 kDa molecule, termed *T. brucei*-derived lymphocyte-triggering factor, which may selectively activate CD8+ T cells to produce IFN-γ.[62] Unfortunately the significance and possible causal connections of the various substances are not understood. It must also be kept in mind that most of the studies have been based on 'test-tube' extractions and purifications, which may bear little resemblance to the breakdown products or internalized products which are manifest in the infected host.

Another important area concerns the possible role(s) of non-specific substances, such as endotoxins, in the pathogenesis of sleeping sickness. In relation to this the great similarities of many features of sleeping sickness to other protozoan and bacterial infections have frequently been noted.[81] Studies with the rodent model, and more recently patients from the Ivory Coast, suggest that serum and CSF endotoxin may be markedly elevated during the disease.[82] Because the endotoxins were evaluated by the *Limulus* amoebocyte lysate (LAL) test, they share properties with classical bacterial and some other protozoal endotoxins. The source(s) of the raised endotoxins is not yet clear, though parasite fragments, intercurrent infections, or release into blood from the damaged intestinal walls are potential possibilities.

TREATMENT AND MANAGEMENT

For several decades the treatment of African human trypanosomiasis has always evoked concern, particularly regarding the best and appropriate use of available trypanocides. Most drugs in regular use have an origin dating back at least 50 years and concern is continually expressed about the lack of availability of a drug which is not only safe and effective but also usable in the context of current health service resources in Africa. Kuzoe[83] has provided a useful summary of the current problems regarding the chemotherapy of sleeping sickness; Table 63.9 is reproduced from his paper. A recent supplement covering all aspects of chemotherapy of African trypanosomiasis has recently been published.[84] This series of review papers should be consulted for detailed information on topics related to chemotherapy of human sleeping sickness, such as developments in rational drug design, mode of action of candidate trypanocides, and the use of in vitro assays for evaluation of drug sensitivity.

Two drugs, suramin and pentamidine, are currently used for the treatment of early-stage disease; both of these compounds are used for treatment of *T. b. gambiense*, but only suramin is effective in *T. b. rhodesiense*. The dose regimens used are summarized in Table 63.9. These two compounds are only of use in early-stage disease as they do not penetrate the blood–brain barrier and should only be used as the sole treatment in patients whose CSF parameters are normal (cells less than $5/mm^3$; protein level less than 40mg%; trypanosome negative).

Pentamidine, an aromatic diamidine (lomidine in French-speaking countries), is used for patients with *T. b. gambiense* and is administered by the intramuscular or intravenous route. There have been records of lack of susceptibility to pentamidine in some areas and in these circumstances suramin is used. The dosages used are 4 mg/kg; 7–10 injections are given daily or on alternate days. Side-effects of pentamidine, recently recorded by Doua and Boa[85] in a study of 150 cases of *T. b. gambiense* in the Ivory Coast, were minor and consisted largely of digestive problems (nausea, loss of appetite, diarrhoea, colic, hypersalivation) in 24% (36/150); seven (4.6%) patients were febrile during treatment, four had headaches, two dizziness and two acute asthenia. One patient in the group had pruritus and one convulsions. One case of diabetes mellitus was recorded, while one succumbed during treatment in a state of hyperthermia. Relapse or reinfection was observed in three cases.

Pentamidine has been used in chemoprophylaxis when control of sleeping sickness in at-risk populations was achieved by 6-monthly intramuscular inoculations. This method of control has been abandoned but the use of pentamidine in this way may have provoked resistance and masked infections, making diagnosis difficult. Pentamidine has not been used in *T. b. rhodesiense* endemic areas as this organism appears to be resistant to the drug, although the mode of action of the compound on trypanosomes is not fully understood.

Suramin is a polyanionic compound used in the early stages of *T. b. rhodesiense* disease but also in *T. b. gambiense* when there is a possibility of pentamidine-resistant strains of trypanosome circulating in the area. Caution in administration of suramin is necessary in areas of endemic onchocerciasis; skin snipping and test dosing (4 mg/kg) may be appropriate to avoid reactions to suramin in patients with this infection.

Suramin is administered intravenously at a dose of 20 mg/kg; five injections usually are given at intervals of 5–7 days. Side-effects are: hypersensitivity reactions, fever, cutaneous eruption, desquamation and arthritis.

MELARSOPROL (ARSOBAL; MEL B)

Melarsoprol has remained the drug of choice for the treatment of late-stage sleeping sickness due to both *T. b. gambiense* and *T. b. rhodesiense*. This trivalent arsenical compound is effective, however, in both early and late stages and is administered at a dose of 3.6 mg/kg per day. A variety of different regimens of treatment are listed by WHO.[4] However, in a recent study of 350 patients in the Ivory Coast, Doua and Boa[85] used the following regimen: day 1, $\frac{1}{3}$ of the dose; day 2 $\frac{2}{3}$ dose; day 3 full dose; day 4 full dose. The patients received three series of four intravenous injections in each series. Prior to the melarsoprol regimen patients received an intramuscular dose of pentamidine, corticosteroid treatment, anthelmintic treatment, nutrititive supplementation for those in poor nutritional state and anticonvulsive prevention. Minor side-effects were febrile episodes, pruritus and subcutaneous cellulitis, sometimes with necrosis at the site of the injection due to leakage. Arsenical encephalopathy arises between the first and 15th day of treatment and was observed in 14/350 patients.

Arsenical encephalopathy is manifested by sudden loss of consciousness, with or without convulsions and fever. Of the series under study by Doua

Table 63.9 Chemotherapy of African trypanosomiasis.

Drug	Pentamidine	Suramin	Melarsoprol	Eflornithine	Nifurtimox‡
Introduced	1937	1922	1949	1990	—
Chemical status	Diamidine	Sulphated naphthylamine	Arsenical	Difluoromethyl-ornithine	Nitrofuran
Route of administration	Intramuscular	Intravenous	Intravenous	Intravenous	Oral
Effective in relation to disease stage	Early-stage *T. b. gambiense*	Early-stage *T. b. gambiense* and *T. b. rhodesiense*	Early or late *T. b. gambiense* and *T. b. rhodesiense*	Early or late *T. b. gambiense*	Arsenical-resistant *T. b. gambiense*
Dosage regimen	4 mg/kg body weight >10 daily injections	20 mg/kg body weight 5–7 injections every 5–7 days	3.6 mg/kg body weight 3–4 series of 4 injections separated by 1 week	400 mg/kg body weight 100 mg every 6 hours for 14 days	10 mg/kg body weight daily 60–90 days
Resistant strains	+	+	+	*T. b. rhodesiense* refractory	Unknown
Side-effects	Vomiting, hypotension, hypoglycaemia	*Pyrexia, joint pains, rash, desquamation	Encephalopathy, diarrhoea	Diarrhoea, anaemia, thrombo-cytopenia	Convulsions, psychosis, vomiting, neuralgia, polyarthritis, paraesthesia
Cost of drug/treatment ($US)	100†	15	47	266	60–100
Costs of complementary drugs ($US)	—	—	130 if encephalopathy occurs	200, i.v. fluid, perfusion kits, etc.	—
Hospitalization costs ($US)	60 (12 days)	120 (30 days)	150 (30 days)	70 (14 days)	Not available
Total costs $US	160	175	197 (or 327)	536	—

*Test dose in onchocerciasis areas.
†Pentamidine is presently being supplied by WHO at a nominal cost through the courtesy of Rhône Poulenc—the manufacturer.
‡Nifurtimox has not been widely used in African trypanosomiasis. Figures are based on best estimates from use in Chagas' disease.
+Resistance to drugs exists.

and Boa,[85] 20 (5.7%) died during treatment, seven of reactive encephalopathy, three of Lyell syndrome and ten of trypanosomiasis itself. The last patients were in a coma on arrival at the hospital in the terminal stage of the disease. The figures usually quoted for death during treatment range from 5 to 10%. Follow-up of arsenical-treated cases is necessary and in this series 326 were followed up; there was a relapse rate of 3.7% (12 cases).

There is considerable variation in the regimens for treatment.[4] In addition the use of corticosteroids has also been a controversial topic in sleeping sickness treatment; the most recent evidence available suggests that in *T. b. gambiense* the use of cortico-

steroid reduces the incidence of encephalopathy—the cause of which remains unknown.[86–88]

TREATMENT OF ARSENICAL-INDUCED SIDE-EFFECTS[4]

1. *On the first manifestation of signs of encephalopathy*
Transfer the patient to a quiet, well-ventilated room, provided with oxygen facilities if possible. Connect an intravenous drip with a 50 g/l isotonic

glucose solution. Administer a 200–250 g/l mannitol solution or any hypertonic solution as a 10-minute 'flash' injection of 150 ml via the infusion tube (for children 10 ml/kg). This treatment may be repeated every 6 hours should the coma persist or recur. Give 25iu intravenously or intramuscularly, of a synthetic adrenocorticotrophin (ACTH) substitute, e.g. tetracosactide (fast-acting); if none of these is available, give 50 mg of prednisolon intravenously. Should the ACTH injection provoke an allergic reaction, 0.1–0.5 mg of adrenaline—by slow intravenous injection, or intravenous corticosteroids should be used. Administer by the parenteral route (e.g. frusemide, 20 mg intravenously). Give only in the case of fever and administer initially by the intravenous route (e.g. lysine acetylsalicylate, 10–40 mg/kg per day).

2. *In the case of convulsions*
Give 0.4 mg/kg diazepam intravenously, immediately followed by further slow administration (0.2 mg/kg per hour), adding the drug to the infusion fluid. Phenobarbitol may be given intramuscularly at a dose of 4 mg/kg per day, but it is active only after several hours and is therefore indicated for long-term rather than immediate treatment. When convulsions persist in spite of treatment, increase the dose of the anticonvulsant and administer extra doses by 'flash' injections each time a new attack of convulsions threatens.

3. *In the case of external or internal haemorrhage(s)*
If mucosal or conjunctival bleeding occurs: (1) interrupt any corticosteroid treatment; and (2) administer a haemostatic drug, such as etamsylate, 5 mg/kg intramuscularly per day, or carbazochrome, 1 mg/kg per day added to the infusion fluid (e.g. adrenaline, 0.02 mg/kg subcutaneously; see below).

4. *Adrenaline injections as a routine procedure*
The routine use of adrenaline for the treatment of encephalopathy may be envisaged, providing the patient does not have coronary insufficiency, a cardiac rhythm disturbance or heart failure. It should be administered subcutaneously at a dose of 0.04 mg/kg at 2-hourly intervals until the condition has improved.

5. *General guidelines*
Permanent surveillance of the patient will provide the best hope of successful treatment and should include observation and recording of the patient's reactions every 30 minutes, as follows:
   (a) consciousness level (response to verbal communications, or, more specifically, to his or her name; response to contact and environmental stimuli);
   (b) pupil response (normal, mydriasis or myosis);
   (c) vegetative functions (temperature, pulse/respiration rates);
   (d) renal function (urine volume in relation to liquid intake).

6. *In the case of prolonged loss of consciousness (3 hours)*
   (a) Implement long-term reanimation procedures.
   (b) Ensure energy intake by administering infusion solutions, e.g. infuse Ringer's lactate, glucose solution or plasma substitute.
   (c) Provide for electrolytic equilibration: potassium, sodium, calcium and vitamins.
   (d) Prevent acidosis by daily infusion of 250 ml of 14 g/l sodium bicarbonate solution.
   (e) Prevent secondary infection(s) by administration of broad-spectrum antibiotics.
   (f) Apply general nursing procedures for the prevention of secondary pneumonia and bedsores, such as regular rotation of the patient's position, frequent washing and changes of bed linen.

Treatment using melarsoprol requires the patient to be under medical care in view of the problems associated with treatment; this also requires additional facilities and skills as well as drug availability, good diagnostic facilities and methods for follow-up. The problems of provision of such facilities within the existing constraints on health services in Africa are clearly evident. Many cases, if not the majority, do not have access even to a diagnostic facility, while adequate treatment must be out of reach of the vast majority. The costs of treatment, which include trypanocidal drugs, supportive therapies, hospitalization costs and medical care, are a severe drain on African health care services. Such provision is only likely to be provided in future by external support or by private providers such as non-governmental organizations.

ALTERNATIVE TREATMENTS

Melarsoprol-resistant cases, or relapsed cases who do not respond to further arsenical therapy in *T. b. gambiense* infection can now be treated with eflornithine (dimethyl difluorornithine), a potent inhibitor of polyamine synthesis. This compound, developed as an antitumour agent, is now registered as 'Ornidyl' for use in sleeping sickness due to *T. b. gambiense*. Extensive studies in melarsoprol-refractory cases in Sudan and the Ivory Coast have demonstrated the efficacy of the compound in patients previously regarded as untreatable.[85,89,90]

Eflornithine is administered at a dose of 100 mg/kg i.v. every 6 hours in an isotonic saline infusion for 14 days, followed at 21–30 days by an oral dose of 75 mg/kg every 6 hours. In a recent trial of 126 patients in the Ivory Coast, all in late-stage disease, different regimens were used.[85] Forty-five were treated by the above regimen, while 81 patients only received the intravenous regimen—57 at a dose of 100 mg/kg every 6 hours and 24 at 200 mg/kg every 12 hours. Side-effects, similar to those found by earlier workers,[89] in the i.v./oral regimen were diarrhoea (64.4%), anaemia (35.5%) and intercurrent infection(s) (28.9%); in addition, patients reported abdominal pain, vomiting, dizziness, convulsions and thrombocytopenia. There was a reduced number of side-effects in the patients who only received the intravenous regimen.

Intercurrent infections occurred mainly in melarsoprol-resistant patients and were cured with antibiotics; side-effects are reversible after treatment ends, and the only case of mortality registered by Doua and Boa[85] was a patient with anaemia 24 months after treatment.

While eflornithine is clearly a safer compound than melarsoprol, its cost and the intensity of medical care and support facilities required mean that the cost of treatment (drug $US210; intravenous fluid, perfusion kit, etc. $US200; hospitalization costs $US70 per 14-day treatment period) is outside the capacity of national health services. Eflornithine is not effective alone in *T. b. rhodesiense* infections, although the first report of successful treatment using a combination therapy with suramin has been reported (see ref. 83). The continued availability of eflornithine is in doubt in view of its cost and the limited market for its use. The search for a drug which is safe, efficacious, cheap and deliverable without recourse to intense medical supervision or long hospitalization remains the hope.

NIFURTIMOX

This compound, which is used for treatment of acute *T. cruzi* infections (Chagas' disease) (Chapter 64), has been used for treatment of melarsoprol-resistant *T. b. gambiense* with some success; Pepin et al[86] have extended earlier studies with variable results. Nifurtimox is also toxic at therapeutic doses.

PROGNOSIS, COMPLICATIONS AND SEQUELAE

Clear distinction must be made, as far as is possible, between cases with early or secondary stage infection. For both *T. b. rhodesiense* and *T. b. gambiense* the prognosis following treatment with suramin or pentamidine is excellent, provided there is no CNS involvement. Achievement of cure is lessened with even marginal CNS signs. An additional risk is then imposed by the likely use of a more toxic drug (e.g. melarsoprol). Nevertheless cure rates of at least 90% are achievable in severely advanced infection(s).

Relapse may be signalled by deterioration with headache, fever and other neurological symptoms, and this may be confirmed by immunodiagnosis of CSF and assessment of its leucocyte and protein content. However, it should be noted that both cell and protein content of CSF may remain elevated for several months after chemotherapy in cured patients. Relapses after treatment with suramin or pentamidine should be treated with melarsoprol or eflornithine. Patients who relapse after melarsoprol should receive a second course of the same drug, or eflornithine. All relapsed patients should be treated with antibiotics to minimize secondary infection(s).

Patients treated in both the early or late stage disease should, if possible, be maintained under surveillance for two to three years. Sequelae occur only rarely even if there is marked mental impairment before chemotherapy. The patient may suffer from irritability or insomnia. In rare instances more serious disturbances such as attacks of violent behaviour have been reported.

REFERENCES

1   Rogers D J & Randolph S F. *Nature* 1991; 351:739–741.

2   Rogers D J & Williams B G. *Parasitology* 1993; 106:S77–S92.

3   Jordan A M. *Trypanosomiasis Control and African Rural Development*. London: Longman, 1986: 357.

4   World Health Organization. Epidemiology and control of African trypanosomiasis. *WHO Tech Rep Ser* 1986; 739.

5   World Development Report. Investing in Health World Development Indication. The World Bank, 1993: 329.

6   Hoare C A. The mammalian trypanosomes of Africa (Chapter 1); Systematic description of mammalian trypanosomes of Africa (Chapter 2). In Mulligan H W (ed.) *The African Trypanosomiases*. London: Allen & Unwin, 1970: 3–23; 24–59.

7   Hoare C A. *The Trypanosomes of Mammals: A Zoological Monograph*. Oxford: Blackwell, 1972: 749.

8   Vickerman K. *Nature* 1978; 273:613–617.

9   Aerts D, Truc P, Penchennier L, Claes Y & Le Ray B. *Trans R Soc Trop Med Hyg* 1992; 86:394–395.

10 Rifkin M R. *Proc Natl Acad Sci USA* 1978; 75:3450–3454.

11 Rickman L R & Robson J. *Bull World Health Organ* 1970; 42:911.

12 Gibson W C, Mehlitz D, Lanham S M & Godfrey D G. *Tropenmed Parasitol* 1978; 29:335–345.

13 Mehlitz D, Zillman U, Scott C M & Godfrey D G. *Tropenmed Parasitol* 1982; 33:113–118.

14 Mehlitz D. *Etudes et Syntheses de L'Iemvt No. 18: Le Reservoir Animal de la Maladie du Sommeil à Trypanosome brucei gambiense*. Paris: IEMVT, 1986: 156.

15 Jenni L & Brun R. *Acta Trop* 1982; 39:281–284.

16 Jenni L, Marti S, Schweizer J et al. *Nature* 1986; 322:173–175.

17 Schweitzer J, Tait A & Jenni L. *Parasitol Res* 1988; 75:98–101.

18 Schweitzer J & Jenni L. *Acta Tropica* 1991; 48:319–321.

19 Tibayrenc M, Kjellberg F & Ayala F J. *Proc Natl Acad Sci USA* 1990; 87:2413–2418.

20 Gibson W C, de Marshall T F & Godfrey D G. *Adv Parasitol* 1980; 18:175–246.

21 Godfrey D G, Baker R D, Rickman L R & Mehlitz D. *Adv Parasitol* 1990; 29:1–74.

22 Stevens J R & Godfrey D G. *Parasitology* 1992; 104:75–86.

23 Stevens J R, Lanham S M, Allingham R & Gashumba J K. *Ann Trop Med Parasitol* 1992; 86:9–28.

24 Gibson W C & Miles M A. *Br Med Bull* 1985; 41:115–121.

25 Paindavoine P, Pays E, Laurent M et al. *Parasitology* 1986; 92:31–50.

26 Hide G, Buchanan N, Welburn S, Maudlin I, Barry J D & Tait A. *Exp Parasitol* 1991; 72:430–439.

27 Maudlin I. *Adv Dis Vector Res* 1991; 7:117–148.

28 Maudlin I & Welburn S. *Tropenmed Parasitol* 1987; 38:167–170.

29 Stiles J K, Ingram G A, Wallbanks K, Molyneux D H, Maudlin I & Welburn S. *Parasitology* 1990; 101:369–376.

30 Molyneux D H. *Adv Parasitol* 1977; 15:1–82.

31 Jenni L, Molyneux D H, Livesey J L & Galun R. *Nature* 1980; 283:383–385.

32 Molyneux D H & Jefferies D. *Parasitology* 1986; 92:721–736.

33 Molyneux D H. African trypanosomiasis. *Clin Trop Med Commun Dis* 1986; :535–555.

34 Gibson W C. *Parasitol Today* 1986; 2:255–257.

35 Molyneux D H. *Ann Soc Belg Med Trop* 1973; 53:605–618.

36 Buyst H. *Ann Soc Belg Méd Trop* 1977; 57:349–359.

37 Cibulskis R. *Parasitology* 1992; 104:99–109.

38 Gibson W C & Gashumba J K. *Trans R Soc Trop Med Hyg* 1983; 77:114–118.

39 Gibson W C & Wellde B T. *Trans R Soc Trop Med Hyg* 1985; 79:671–676.

40 Willett K. *Trans R Soc Trop Med Hyg* 1965; 59:374–386.

41 Onyango R J, van Hoeve K & de Raadt P. *Trans R Soc Trop Med Hyg* 1966; 60:175–182.

42 Baldry D A T. *Insect Science and its Application* 1980; 1:85–93.

43 Allsop R. *Bull World Health Organ* 1972; 47:735–746.

44 Bailey J W & Smith D H. *Trans R Soc Trop Med Hyg* 1992; 86:630.

45 Nantulya V. *Parasite Immunol* 1989; 11:69–75.

46 Borowy N K, Schnell D, Schäfer C & Overath P. *J Infect Dis* 1991; 164:422–425.

47 Komba E, Odiit M, Mbulamberi D B, Chimfurembe E C & Nantulya V M. *Bull World Health Organ* 1992; 70:57–61.

48 Duggan A J & Hutchinson M P. *J Trop Med Hyg* 1966; 69:124–131.

49 Collomb H. *Gaz Méd Fr Sci Med Pratpgen* 1957; 64:1069–1078.

50 Poltera A A. *Br Med Bull* 1985; 41:169–174.

51 Poltera A A, Cox J N & Owor R. *Br Heart J* 1976; 38:827–837.

52 Apted F I C. Clinical manifestations and diagnosis of sleeping sickness. In Mulligan H W (ed.) *The African Trypanosomiases*. London: Allen & Unwin, 1970: 587–601.

53 Ormerod W E. Pathogenesis and pathology of Trypanosomiasis in man. In Mulligan H W (ed.) *African Trypanosomiases*. London: Allen & Unwin, 1970: 587–601.

53a Poltera A A & Cox J N. *Virchows Archiv [A]* 1977; 375:53–70.

54 Mott F W. Report of the Sleeping Sickness Commission of the Royal Society, 1906; 7:3–45.

55 Jenkins G C & Facer C A. Hematology of African trypanosomiasis. In Tizard I (ed.) *Immunology and Pathogenesis of Trypanosomiasis*. Boca Raton: CRC Press, 1985: 13–44.

56 Bancroft G J & Askonas B A. Immunobiology of African trypanosomiasis in laboratory rodents. In Tizard I (ed.) *Immunology and Pathogenesis of Trypanosomiasis*. Boca Raton: CRC Press, 1985: 75–102.

57 Mansfield M. Immunology of African trypanosomiasis. In Wyler D G (ed.) *Modern Parasite Biology*. New York: W H Freeman, 1990: 222–246.

58 Borowy N K, Sternberg J M, Schrieber D, Nonnengasser C & Overath P. *Parasite Immunol* 1990; 12:233–246.

59 Sileghem M, Darji A, Hamers R & De Baetselier P. *Immunology* 1989a; 68:137–139.

60 Sileghem M, Darji A, Hamers R, Van de Winkel, M & De Baetselier P. *Eur J Immunol* 1989b; 19:829–835.

61 Lucas R, Mayez S, Songa B et al. *Res Immunol* 1993; 144:370–376.

62 Olsson T, Bakhiet M & Kristensson K. *Parasitol Today* 1992; 8:237–239.

63 Sztein M B & Kierszenbaum F. *Immunology* 1991; 73:180–185.

64 Fierer J, Salmon J A & Askonas B A. *Clin Exp Immunol* 1984; 58:548–556.

65 Hunter C A, Jennings F W, Kennedy P G E & Murray M. *Lab Invest* 1992; 67:635–642.

66 Mutayoba B M, Meyer H H D, Osaso J & Gombe S. *Theriogenology* 1989; 32:545–555.

67 Oka M, Nagasawa H, Ito Y & Himeno K. *Clin Exp Immunol* 1989; 78:285–291.

68 Pentreath V W, Rees K, Owalabi O A, Philip K A & Doua F. *Trans R Soc Trop Med Hyg* 1990; 84:795–799.

69 Jennings F W, Hunter C A, Kennedy P G E & Murray M. *Trans R Soc Trop Med Hyg* 1993; 87:224–226.

70 Adams J H, Haller L, Boa F Y, Doua F, Dago A & Konia K. *Neuropathol Appl Neurobiol* 1986; 12:81–94.

71 Schultzberg M, Olsson T, Samuelson F B, Machlen J & Kristensson K. *J Neuroimmunol* 1989; 24:105–112.

72 Hamon J F, Seri B, Doua F, Camara P & Aba L. *Pharmacol Biochem Behav* 1990; 36:831–835.

73 Asonganyi T, Lando G & Ngu J L. *Ann Soc Belg Méd Trop* 1989; 69:213–221.

74 Poltera A A. *Trans R Soc Trop Med Hyg* 1980; 74:706–715.

75 Lambert P H, Berney M & Kazyumba G. *J Clin Invest* 1981; 67:77–85.

76 Stibbs H H & Curtis D A. *Ann Trop Med Parasitol* 1987; 81:673–679.

77 Hayaishi O. *Ann N Y Acad Sci* 1989; 559:374–381.

78 Pentreath V W. *Parasitol Today* 1989; 5:215–218.

79 Tizard I, Nielsen K H, Seed J R & Hall J E. *Microbiol Rev* 1978; 42:661–681.

80 Boreham P F L. Autocoids: their release and possible roles in the pathogenesis of African trypanosomiasis. In Tizard I (ed.) *Immunology and Pathogenesis of Trypanosomiasis*. Boca Raton: CRC Press, 1985: 45–66.

81 Goodwin B M. *Lancet* 1974; i:435–436.

82 Alafiatayo R A, Crawley B, Oppenheim B A & Pentreath V W. *Parasitology* 1993; 107:49–53.

83 Kuzoe F A S. *Acta Trop* 1993; 54:13–162.

84 Brun R. Editorial. Advances in chemotherapy of African trypanosomiasis. *Acta Trop* 1993; 54:3–4.

85 Doua F & Boa F. Yapo. *Acta Trop* 1993; 54:163–168.

86 Pepin J, Milord F, Meurice F, Ethier L, Loko L & Mpia B. *Trans R Soc Trop Med Hyg* 1992; 86:254–256.

87 Pepin J, Milord F, Khonde A, Niyonsenga T, Loko L & Mpia B. *Trans R Soc Trop Med Hyg* 1994; 88:447–452.

88 Pepin J, Milord F, Khonde A N et al. *Trans R Soc Trop Med Hyg* 1995; 89:92–97.

89 Van Nieuwenhoeve S, Schechter P J, Declerq J, Bone G, Burke J & Sjoerdsma A. *Trans R Soc Trop Med Hyg* 1985; 79:692–698.

90 Doua F, Boa Y F, Schechter P J et al. *Am J Trop Hyg* 1987; 37:525–533.

91 Bakhiet A.-M. O. *Immunopathogenesis of experimental African trypanosomiasis. Interactions between* Trypanosoma brucei brucei, *CD*+ T cells and interferon gamma*. Stockholm: Karolinska Institute, 1993.

92 Amole B, Sharpless N, Wittner W & Tanowitz H B. *Ann Trop Med Parasitol* 1989; 83:225–232.

93 Molyneux D H, de Raadt P & Seed J R. African human trypanosomiasis. *Adv Trop Med VSI* 1984; 1:39–62.

CHAPTER 64

AMERICAN TRYPANOSOMIASIS

Philip D. Marsden

Human trypanosomiasis is the most geographically restricted of the great endemic protozoan diseases. African trypanosomiasis occurs in Africa because the 22 surviving tsetse flies (*Glossina*) are restricted to that continent. There is evidence in Californian shales of a fossil New World *Glossina* which may have fed on primitive ungulates.

Conversely American trypanosomiasis only occurs in the New World because virtually all triatomine bugs, the natural vectors, are localized in the American continent. One exception is *Triatoma rubrofasciata* which appears to have been spread around the world by sailing ships. This bug has been reported even from Japan.

How *Trypanosoma cruzi* infection became a major health problem in Latin America is a matter for speculation. Possibly the triatomine bug–trypanosome association is the more long-standing since close analogies can be found between flagellates and reduviid bugs both in plant-sucking and insect-predatory analogous hemipterous families. From these ancestors arose bugs feeding on mammalian blood, a distinct advantage in reproductive terms compared with plant juices or insect haemolymph. Possibly the earliest examples of such Hemiptera are those associated with bats, among which exist several *T. cruzi*-like organisms.[1] The subfamily Triatominae evolved in its turn, furnishing all important vectors.[2] Of such vectors the most important is *Triatoma infestans* and a brief consideration of its vector success will have to serve to illustrate the historical progress of *T. cruzi* transmission. In the Valley of Cochabamba in Bolivia it can still be found associated with the nests of sylvatic animals (e.g. rodents, opossums). The latter are probably ancient hosts, just as they were early in the mammalian evolutionary scale. They show a high tolerance with prolonged parasitaemias with *T. cruzi* and little pathology. In addition, infected marsupials have been caught within 200 miles of New York, and the geographical distribution of such infected animals extends south throughout the Americas, limited only by the cold of the Arctics. Thus *T. cruzi* exists in all Latin American countries.

Human activities in the Cochabamba Valley created a scarcity of animal reservoirs, resulting in *Triatoma infestans* occupying man's own dwellings and feeding on human blood. Triatominae rarely show a marked host preference in captivity. In the wild, conquest of a suitable epidemiological niche is important and *Triatoma infestans* is most successful as an infester of cracks in the walls of poor housing. It dislocates other triatomine occupants for reasons that are unclear. *Triatoma infestans* is also an opportunist traveller in human clothing, baggage and transport and it is probably thus that it migrated to become the dominant domestic vector by the 1970s, reigning over an area encompassing Bolivia, southern Peru, Paraguay, Uruguay, northern Chile and Argentina. The most striking recent migration, however, was its sweep through central Brazil, including the states of São Paulo, Minas Gerais and Goiás, to reach the southern limits of Maranhão.

This history is repeated with other important vector species under slightly different circumstances in different parts of Latin America. Man's rapacious environmental exploitation, with destruction of animal reservoirs, and the construction of poor quality housing due to the poverty of rural workers, are monotonous facts in most countries. Chagas' disease is the inevitable result of senseless exploitation of the environment to little benefit of the mass of the local population. The sugar, coffee and beef booms of Brazil are examples of the results of the process of clearing natural vegetation to plant a monoculture crop, resulting in domiciliary invasion by triatomine bugs. Many rural areas of South America have now become so unproductive of crops that only goats can find enough to eat. Amazonian Indians have been lucky—only sporadic accidental *T. cruzi* infections being registered in their region. This is not only because they usually build houses without walls, for ventilation, but they also have an alert sense of how to handle their environment without destroying the ecological balance. Current events in Amazonia could change this picture in terms of Chagas' disease.[3]

HISTORY

Few doubt today that the contribution of Carlos J. Chagas, in unravelling a complex life cycle and realizing its implications in rural populations of the state of Minas Gerais, Brazil, was medical science of a high order. Sent to investigate a malaria epidemic in the interior of the state, he listened to the complaints of householders regarding a nocturnal bloodsucking bug living in the house fabric. Capturing some of these red and black bugs, identified today as *Panstrongylus megistus*, he found flagellates in their intestinal dejecta. He inoculated these into marmosets at the Manguinhos Institute in Rio de Janeiro, and named the trypanosome which appeared in the peripheral blood of these animals *T. cruzi* after his mentor, Oswaldo Cruz.

Further work with colleagues at Manguinhos revealed a true tissue form of the parasite, an amastigote dividing by binary fission forming nests or pseudocysts of the parasite, particularly in heart muscle fibres. Chagas then arranged a small field laboratory in a railway carriage in Lassance, an endemic area of the state of Minas Gerais. It was here that he recognized the first patients with the acute form of the disease. One of these children, for usually children acquire the acute phase, survived to live into old age (Berenice) showing the unpredictable nature of the infection.[4] Chagas[5] announced his great discovery to the world in a classic paper in the *Memórias do Instituto Oswaldo Cruz*. Then followed a whole series of seminal publications in which he described the cardiovascular and digestive symptoms in man, identified further insect vectors and established that the infection existed in both domestic and wild animal reservoirs. Prata[6] has edited a valuable *collectanea* of these rare papers. In 1913 Guerreiro and Machado[7] described a serological test for detecting the frequent occult infections.

Chagas succeeded Cruz as director of the famous Instituto Oswaldo Cruz in Rio de Janeiro, and administrative matters limited the amount of time he could devote to research. Also, in certain quarters, his discoveries were doubted. For example Krause in Argentina went to a non-endemic area and was unable to confirm Chagas' findings. Certainly in the early decades of the twentieth century the impact of Chagas' discovery of a new form of myocarditis did not receive the attention it deserved, but he was championed by Salvador Mazza and colleagues[8] of Argentina, who found transmission by breast milk and confirmed many of Chagas' findings. Chagas himself never lost interest in *T. cruzi* infection(s) and felt not only that it was an important endemic South American disease but that the probable solution lay in a better understanding of the vector, which proved correct. Brumpt[9] pointed out that the unusual susceptibility of triatomine bugs enable laboratory-reared uninfected specimens to be used in xenodiagnosis.

The key advance in the control of Chagas' disease came with Müller's discovery of the residual action of chlorinated hydrocarbon insecticides. Confirmed by Busvine at the London School of Hygiene and Tropical Medicine, great interest was aroused in residual spraying of houses to combat a variety of insect vectors, among which triatomine bugs seemed particularly vulnerable by nature of their domiciliation. This proved to be the case with the pioneering field studies of Emmanuel Dias.[10] Today this remains the major weapon for control.

Brazilian workers played an important role from the beginning, but major contributions have also come from Argentina, Venezuela and Chile. The difficulty for the reader of this textbook in the past was finding an author who dominated languages sufficiently to get a clear picture of the current situation; also, the English were preoccupied with African trypanosomiasis. Chagas is only known to have submitted one presentation in English—to the Chicago Medical Society.[11] His scientific contributions have acted as a worldwide stimulus to young workers to take up an interest in this fascinating protozoan infection.[12] His memory is commemorated every year by a sophisticated scientific meeting in Caxambu, Minas Gerais, where new work on all aspects of *T. cruzi* infections are presented and summarized in a special supplement of the *Memórias do Instituto Oswaldo Cruz*.[13] The last of the many bibliographies of relevant publications is referenced here.[14]

GEOGRAPHICAL DISTRIBUTION

Table 64.1 and Figure 64.1 detail the distribution of serologically positive individuals in Brazil and the geographical distribution of the five most important vector bugs, respectively.[15,16] Calculation of the number of serologically positive individuals is based on relatively small population surveys in other countries and extrapolation to the general population and is bound to be inaccurate. Only in Brazil was a large nationwide survey done. This showed heavy foci in central and southern Brazil.

However, positive serology does not indicate disease but only infection with *T. cruzi*. The pathogenicity of different isolates of *T. cruzi* varies very much geographically in terms of their disease manifestations. Cardiopathy and megasyndromes are relatively common on the high central plateau of Brazil. Many such patients are seen in Brasília and Goiânia. In Venezuela and Central America megasyndromes are virtually unknown. Cardiomyopathy has a variable geographical distribution but in central Brazil as many as 50% of positive seroreactors may show ECG abnormalities.

According to the literature there are also geographical differences in the therapeutic response to specific chemotherapy with nifurtimox or benznidazole, patients from countries of the Cone Sul responding better than Brazilian equivalents.

Figure 64.1 shows that Amazonia is spared important vector domiciliation; therefore Chagas' disease is not a problem in the Amazonas forest, although many sylvatic cycles of transmission exist.[17] The reason why *Triatoma infestans* has never managed to establish itself in Belém, despite frequent arrival by passive transport, could be related to temperature determinants.

Table 64.1. The distribution of serologically positive individuals in Brazil.

Distribution by region	Total number of boroughs	Total number of neighbourhoods	Number of boroughs with estimates of prevalences over 0%	Estimate of prevalence per 100
North				
Rendônia	2	172	3	0.41
Acre	7	132	7	2.39
Amazonas	11	767	36	1.88
Roraima	2	151	2	0.31
Pará	83	2110	46	0.56
Amapá	5	177	—	—
North-East				
Maranháo	130	2136	51	0.12
Piaui	114	1191	103	4.04
Ceara	141	2224	93	0.84
Rio Grande do Norte	140	1009	110	1.78
Paraiba	171	1466	150	3.48
Pernambuco	163	2003	144	2.79
Alagoas	94	915	70	2.48
Sergipe	74	600	60	5.97
Bahia	331	4778	301	5.44
*South-East**				
Minas Gerais	717	5344	574	8.83
Espirito Santo	52	629	27	0.32
Rio de Janeiro	61	587	35	1.75
South				
Parana	290	3175	245	4.00
Santa Catarina	197	1130	130	1.39
Rio Grande do Sud	234	1895	189	8.84
*Centre/West***				
Mato Grosso	34	1355	31	2.82
Mato Grosso do Sud	50	473	43	2.46
Goiás	219	2110	210	7.40

*Excluding Sâo Paulo.
**Excluding Federal District.
Reproduced from Camargo et al.[15]

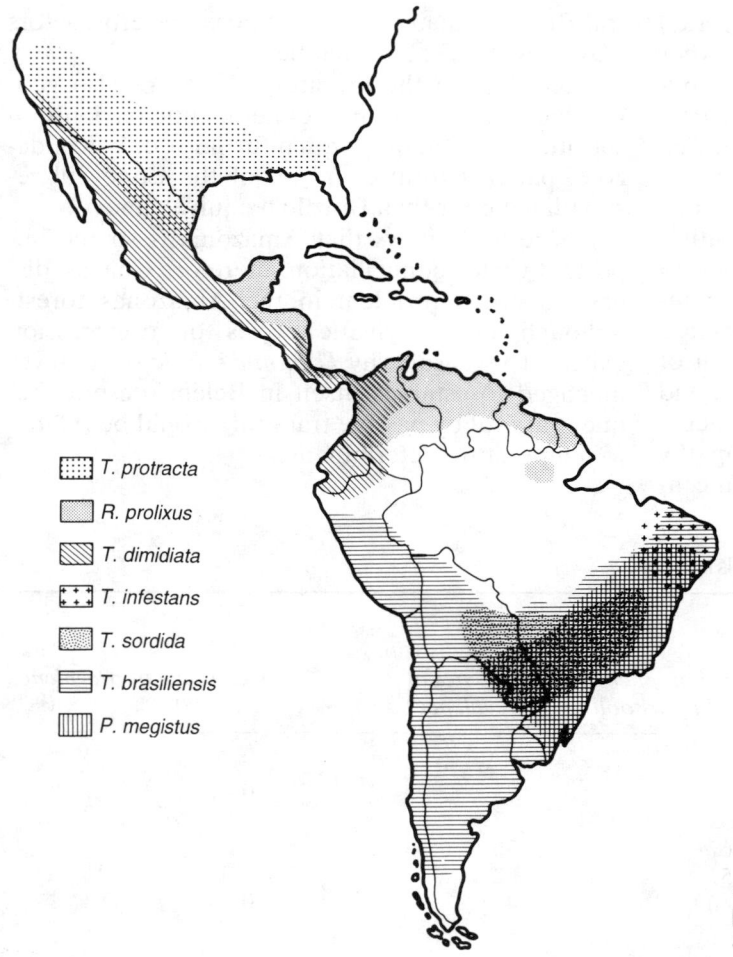

T. protracta

R. prolixus

T. dimidiata

T. infestans

T. sordida

T. brasiliensis

P. megistus

Figure 64.1 Distribution of the five major triatomine vectors, plus *R. prolixus* and *R. megistus*, in Latin America. (After Sherlock.[16])

The two dominant vectors of the north of South America, namely *Triatoma dimidiata* in the east and *Rhodnius prolixus* in the west, extend up into Central America. As one travels north into Central America documentation of the classical human pathology becomes rarer, although human infection certainly exists. There has recently been evidence of a small epidemic of human *T. cruzi* infection on the west coast of Mexico.

The situation in the USA is modified by three factors:

1. A high standard of living and good housing.
2. Sylvatic cycles are normally divorced from human contact.

3. Laboratory evidence of low pathogenicity of North American isolates of *T. cruzi* in experimental animals.

Occasionally transmission to man of *T. cruzi* is documented by North American triatominae, particularly in the south-west. Immigration from most Central American countries and Mexico has resulted in the introduction of a human infected reservoir to the USA, and some of these patients eventually develop cardiac pathology.[18] With the current migration of the Brazilian population from rural areas to the periphery of large towns, suburban transmission, even with bug-infested houses, is a threat.[19]

AETIOLOGY

T. cruzi is a polymorphic trypanosome with both broad, intermediate and narrow forms. It appears that all are infective to bugs, unlike the *brucei* group.

The posteriorly placed kinetoplast is so large as to distort the membrane of the cell. Only one wave of detectable parasitaemia occurs in the acute phase, after which the primed immune response reduces circulating trypanosome numbers to below microscopically detectable levels. Antigenic variation of the trypanosome coat does not occur as in *T.brucei*.

T. cruzi is usually introduced by skin contamination with infected triatomine bug faeces containing metacyclic trypanosomes. Many factors influence whether such stercorarian transmission will occur, such as number and type of infective organisms, skin microclimate, host factors, etc.[20] Children often live for years in bug-infested houses before acquiring infection, showing that there is much chance in this occurrence.

Once trypanosomes have penetrated skin macrophages they round up to form amastigotes which multiply every 10 hours by binary fission. The duration of this phase will depend on the host cell invaded. In muscle cells (a known tropism) it lasts about 5 days, with the formation of a pseudocyst containing up to several hundred parasites. Rupture results in death of many but others assume the circulating trypanomastigote form which infects other cells. This process proceeds indefinitely during the life of the host. Only these two forms occur at body temperature. Dvorak[21] advanced the understanding of this basic protozoology when he showed that clones of one isolate of *T. cruzi* had very different parasitological qualities in terms of infectivity to the insect vector, pathology in the vertebrate host, etc. It appears then that this ancient protozoan has developed many biological subtypes even within single isolates. Isolates have been isoenzymatically characterized into five zymodemes, some of which are more associated with sylvatic cycles and others with human, but this has not been of much help to the clinician because such zymodemes cannot be linked to a specific clinical picture.[17]

The life cycle of *T. cruzi* in the invertebrate host is more complex than in the mammalian host and can only be mentioned here. Some triatomine bugs are extremely susceptible to infection, even with small numbers of flagellates. These, being ingested by the bug during a meal, round up in the stomach to form spheromastigotes. Epimastigote forms make their appearance in the mid-gut, while the rectum contains metacyclic trypanosomes as well. The flagellates in the rectum congregate at the entrance of the malpighian tubules. The process of differentiation is variable, depending on the size of the blood meal, the stock and the number of flagellates ingested, but takes at least 10 days. At a further feed the size of the blood meal stimulates abdominal stretch receptors, resulting in rectal contraction and defecation. Early-defecating bug species are especially dangerous in terms of transmission.

T. cruzi can be cultivated in artificial media held at the arthropod body temperature (26°C) and, after exponential growth, differentiation into epimastigotes and trypanomastigotes occurs, as in the insect gut.

Trypanomastigotes pass through mucous membranes with relative ease, not only on invasion, but may be excreted in the acute phase (e.g. opposum urine, human tears, etc.). Laboratory workers should wear protective clothing, masks and glasses.[22]

EPIDEMIOLOGY

This textbook will be used mainly by doctors outside endemic areas who are interested only in the diagnosis and treatment of the occasional individual case, so, within the space allowed, comments must necessarily be brief. Triatominae are true bugs or hemipterans (worth defining because Americans are inclined to use the term 'bug' indiscriminately). It is a mistake to think that transmission will be uniform in a known endemic area. This is not the case, due to a multitude of environmental, vector, parasite and host factors.[20] Bug infestation of a house without *T. cruzi* transmission is not uncommon. In terms of triatomine efficiency of transmission to man of *T. cruzi* in Brazil, the risk could be summarized thus:

Triatoma infestans > *Panstrongylus megistus* > *Triatoma brasiliensis* > *Triatoma pseudomaculata*.

Triatoma infestans is most effective because of the high bug densities attained and the ability to dislocate other species. *P. megistus* achieves high density trypanosome infections but is mainly sylvatic in southern Brazil and almost entirely domiciliated in the north-east. *Triatoma brasiliensis* and *Triatoma pseudomaculata* exist in the peridomicile as well as the domicile and are therefore more difficult to control. North of the Amazonian forest *R. prolixus* appears a greater threat as a vector than *Triatoma dimidiata*, due to its prolix multiplication in houses and its existence in many sylvatic niches such as the palm fronds that are frequently thrown on roofs. *Triatoma dimidiata* like domiciliated *P. megistus*, prefers the lower 1.5 metres of wall (bed level).

Domestic animals may be important in maintaining cycles of *T. cruzi*; dogs are especially so because they often breed in the house and follow man's sleep rhythm. Bugs are found in the house fabric near such blood-meal sources but humans dominate because of their bulk and somnolent nocturnal habit. Domiciliated triatomines have two primary objectives: to hide from their enemies, especially during daylight, and to take a maximal nocturnal blood meal as rapidly as possible in order to pass, with successive meals, through each of the five larval stages. With an extra large meal they then achieve adulthood with wings that enable them to migrate for mating and to start fresh colonies. They are efficient syringe-type feeders, engorging in minutes. Triatominae have many enemies in the wall fabric: ants, spiders, scorpions, lizards, a minute wasp (*Telenomus* sp.) which parasitizes eggs, etc.[23] Cats are frequently infected because they eat infected rodents that eat infected bugs, but they have little importance in maintaining *T. cruzi* cycles in the house because they hunt at night. Goats are said to be important peridomiciliary reservoirs in the Argentinian chaco. Pigs, horses and cows are not important reservoirs. Chickens resist *T. cruzi* infections and are excellent bug predators. The multitude of wild animal reservoirs has been reviewed elsewhere;[24] the opossum is the most important of these because it is frequently infected and builds its nest in the peridomicile (Figure 64.2).

There is a relationship between the quality of housing and the presence of bugs (Figure 64.3). Cracked mud walls are ideal hiding places, as are thick palm roofs for certain bug species. Large families (more blood sources) and poor domestic hygiene also facilitate the maintenance of domestic colonies of triatominae. Houses which receive many visitors also have a high risk of bug infestation. The author has often seen triatominae leaving the clothing, baggage, umbrellas, etc. of casual visitors to hide in the wall.

Community attitudes are of great importance, especially in ensuring control and protecting the family future. In the past, houseowners were too often casual in assessing the importance of the familiar bug to hand: 'My grandfather had this and he lived to ninety', used to be a common reply as we drank an evening glass.

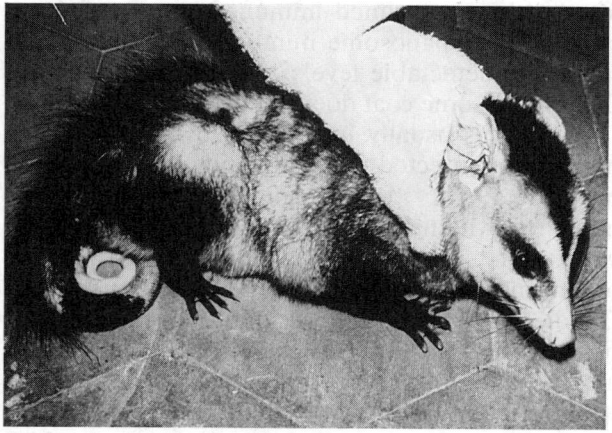

Figure 64.2   Oppossum (*Didelphis* sp.): an important peridomiciliary reservoir of *T. cruzi*.

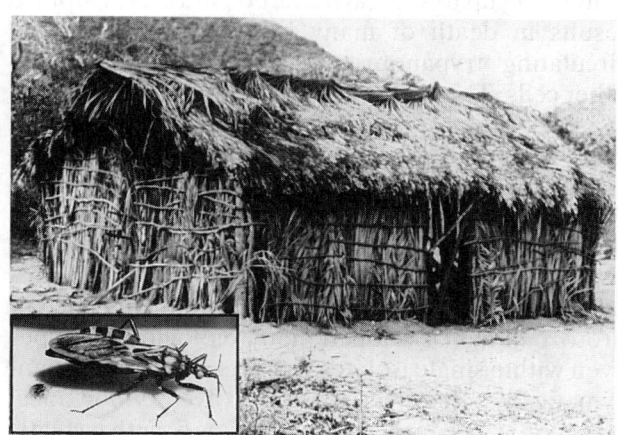

Figure 64.3   A house which on demolition had more than 1000 *Triatoma infestans*. The insert shows an adult bug.

Finally, in epidemiology one must emphasize that *T. cruzi* is a highly infectious protozoan and sometimes infects without the route being clear, as in the case of an infected animal handler in New York. Oral transmission occurs, as in the example of a cluster of acute cases at a farm party in northern Brazil at which contaminated sugar-cane juice was drunk.[25] There have been over 50 infections among research workers but these have never been fully reported because of delicate political considerations.

PATHOGENESIS AND PATHOLOGY

There are analogies between African and American trypanosomiasis. In both, the phases of infection can be divided into three:

1. Phase of local multiplication.
2. Phase of tissue dissemination.
3. Phase of organ localization.

LOCAL MULTIPLICATION

Some metacyclic trypanosomes in infected bug faeces engulfed by skin macrophages resist the intracellular environment and, dividing by binary fission, form the first generation of the multiplying forms of *T. cruzi*. For obvious ethical reasons the minimum dose of trypanosomes necessary to infect man is not known as it is for African trypanosomes. Possibly a single one directly inoculated into the bloodstream during transfusion is sufficient. The early phase of infection has been extensively studied in animals. The trypanosomal chancre or chagoma of *T. cruzi* inoculation is clinically detectable in fewer than half infected patients. Romaña's sign, where the conjunctiva is the portal of entry, is explained by the habit of covering the child at night leaving only the face exposed, where the bug feeds and defecates. On waking the child often rubs faeces into the eye. Step sections of the orbit in experimental studies of Romaña's sign show rapid dissemination via the orbital muscle to the bloodstream, and in some cases even to the optic nerve.[26] The lacrimal gland and preauricular lymph gland are parasitized and enlarged. Romaña's sign, presenting as unilateral bipalpebral brawny oedema is slow to resolve, in a matter of 10 days, differentiating it from allergic conditions. By the time this sign is present there are amastigote nests in the myocardium because the second phase is rapid. Chagomas on other parts of the body are indurated erythematous swellings and should always be needled because trypanosomes may be demonstrated.

Unusual forms of the acute phase include those transmitted via the intestinal tract (mother's milk, contaminated food) where, of course, no inoculation chagoma is present. This is also the case in congenital Chagas' disease. Since the first phase merges into the second, acute Chagas' disease will be discussed in the next section.

TISSUE DISSEMINATION

Again animal studies show that, given a sufficient inoculum of a pathogenic strain, all tissues, even the

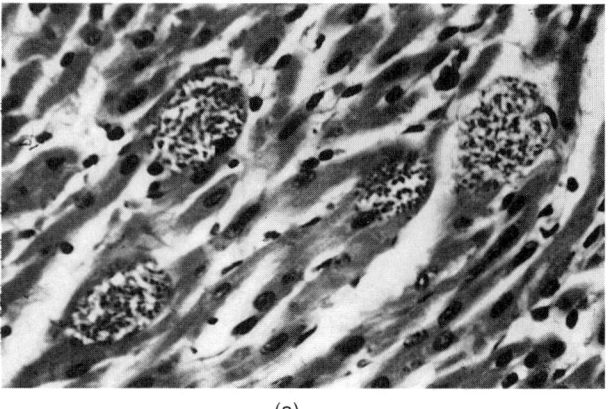

(a)

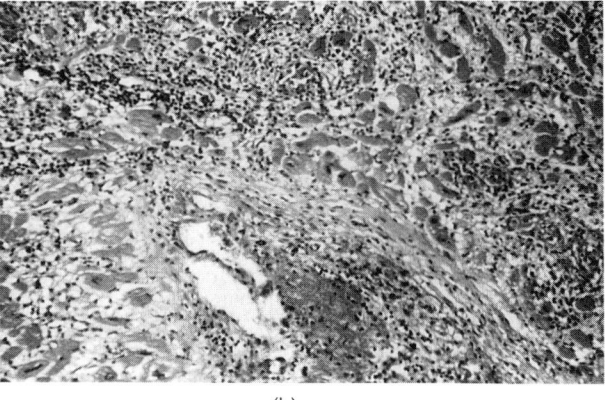

(b)

Figure 64.4 Myocardium at two phases of *T. cruzi* infection. (a) Acute phase: many pseudocysts with amastigotes; no inflammatory reaction. (b) Chronic phase: no visible parasites; massive myocardial fibre destruction with intense lymphocytic infiltration and some areas of haemorrhage.

pituitary gland, may be the site of amastigote nests.[26] Normally in humans, because the dose is small, the predilection for muscle, especially the walls of the cardiac auricles, is an early manifestation. Early generation of pseudocysts shows no lymphocyte or plasma cell infiltration, just amastigotes in a swollen cardiac fibre. However, there is rapidly (within a few cycles) tissue evidence of a profound cellular immune alert with mononuclear cell infiltration (Figure 64.4). The mystery is that this brisk immune response suppresses but does not eradicate the infection.

These early months of infection, when parasite multiplication is at its maximum, are believed to be the period during which the degree of tissue damage determines the subsequent evolution of the disease in future decades. Destruction of autonomic ganglia in the smooth muscle of the gut will govern subsequent aperistalsis. Destruction of the Purkinje fibres and ganglia of the conducting system of the heart results in arrhythmias; however, cardiac fibre destruction is a chronic process continuing over years and leading to the major manifestation of the next phase.[27]

ORGAN LOCALIZATION

THE HEART

This is the major site of pathology because the muscle of all four cavities constitutes the site of amastigote multiplication since the initial phase. With the passage of time amastigotes become so scarce that autoimmune mechanisms have been evoked to explain continued muscle fibre destruction with haemorrhage and necrosis. *T. cruzi* is said to share common antigens with cardiac muscle.[28] What is not in doubt is that in a proportion of chronically infected patients (10–50%) progressive chronic cardiomyopathy leads eventually to dilatation and pump failure. Conduction defects are common, and a valuable early sign of a poor prognosis. Macroscopically the chronic chagasic heart is flabby and thin walled and may contain an apical aneurysm or mural thrombosis[29].

THE GUT

A similar process of involvement of the smooth muscle of the gut and its parasympathetic ganglia leads to disorganized muscular contraction and aperistalsis. Köberle[30] was a key researcher in clarifying this aspect in the rich pathological material in Ribeirão Preto. The parts of the gut with solid food residues are particularly affected, namely the oesophagus and sigmoid colon. Aperistalsis also affects the cardiac sphincter.

Megasyndromes are described rarely from other parts of the bowel, and even other hollow viscera such as the gallbladder and urinary bladder.

OTHER SYSTEMS

A recent advance, again a Brazilian contribution, has been to localize the sites where residual amastigote nests are multiplying to give an intermittently positive subpatent parasitaemia. The wall of the suprarenal vein, which carries a high dose of corticoids, has usually been found to be parasitized in patients with chronic infection.[31] Although pseudocysts and resultant inflammation have been found in many other organs in animals, actual clinical sequelae of such involvement are rare in humans.

CLINICAL FEATURES

ACUTE PHASE

Figure 64.5 illustrates both Romaña's sign and a chagoma, examples of sites of initial infection. Unilateral orbital oedema should always suggest acute Chagas' disease in an endemic area.

More difficult are the acute cases without a detectable portal of entry. This phase must be considered in the differential diagnosis of any unknown fever in children from an area where transmission occurs. Tachycardia is disproportionate to the fever and peripheral oedema is common. The younger the child the more frequent are the systemic signs of lymphadenopathy, hepatosplenomegaly, anaemia and rarely a morbilliform rash. There is usually no difficulty in detecting circulating motile trypanosomes in thick fresh blood smears but a simple Strout concentration, centrifuging the serum from clotted blood, is more sensitive than direct micro-

scopy. Serology will not be helpful in the early phases of infection.

A useful routine clinical investigation is the white cell count, which often shows a lymphocytosis. Liver and muscle enzymes may be elevated and muscle biopsy may show parasites. Apart from tachycardia the ECG may show alterations in ventricular repolarization, subepicardiac ischaemia and first-degree atrioventricular block. Acute phase infection is not usually fatal and often passes unperceived. After a few weeks the patient settles into the more chronic phase. However, subacute progression is described, with the rapid onset of heart muscle failure and/or arrhythmia, leading eventually to a rapid demise.

With the advent of fast international travel dissemination of carriers of trypanosomes is occurring, as witnessed by the number of transfusion cases in non-endemic areas. Rarely (less than 5%) acute disease is associated with meningoencephalitis or

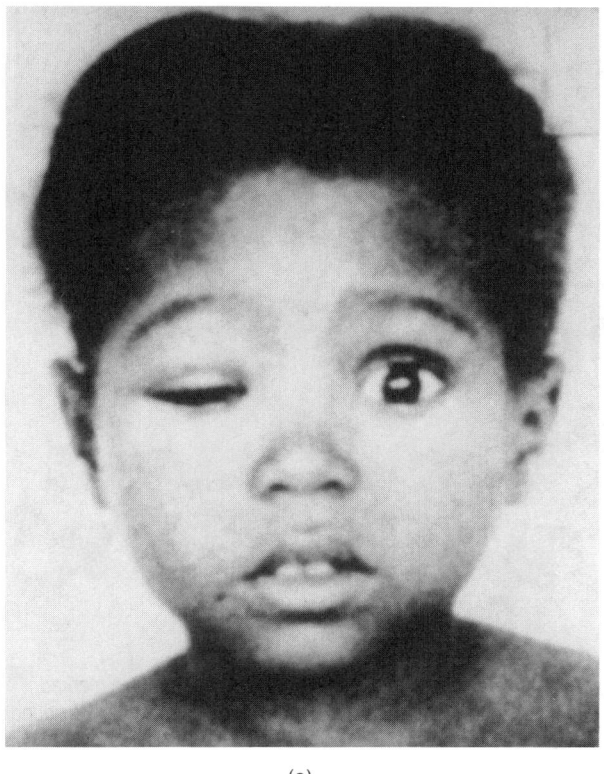

(a)

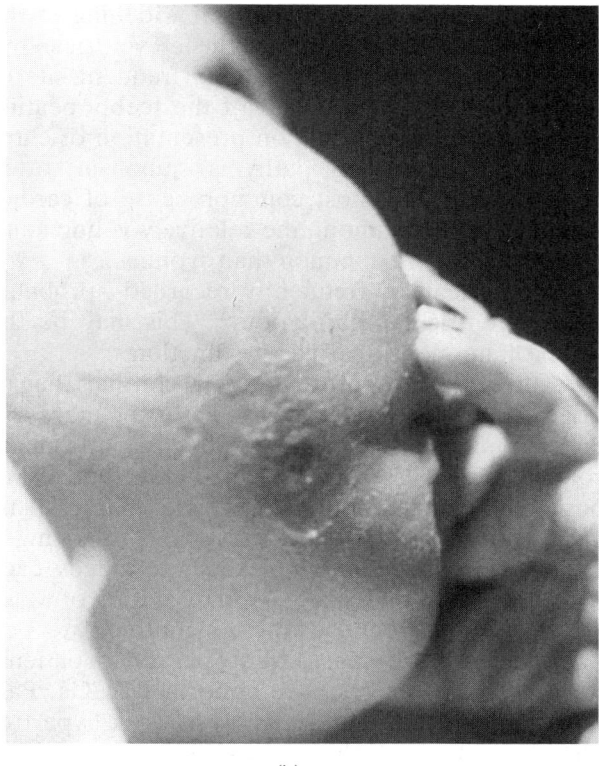

(b)

Figure 64.5   (a) Romaña's sign, and (b) an inoculation chagoma on a baby's chin, from which trypanosomes were isolated.

heart failure; both are bad prognostic signs. By the time clinical manifestations of acute Chagas' disease occur, amastigotes are multiplying in the heart muscle and the ECG may already show abnormalities.

CHRONIC PHASE

In an endemic area many patients cannot remember the acute phase of the disease, which occurs in childhood and is dismissed as a common febrile illness. Chronic chagasic cardiomyopathy is established decades before the pump is prejudiced. It is usually adult males at the age of maximal physical activity (30–40 years) when they are having to support young families, who commence with their first cardiac decompensation. This is one of the tragedies of Chagas' disease. In the area of Mambaí, Goiás, where I have worked since 1973, 34% of the population have positive serology but only a third of these have abnormal ECGs, with extrasystoles and various degrees of atrioventricular block as common findings. Some defects of conduction are more specific than others for Chagas' disease; for example right complete bundle branch block with left anterior hemiblock (Figure 64.6). About 20% of posi-

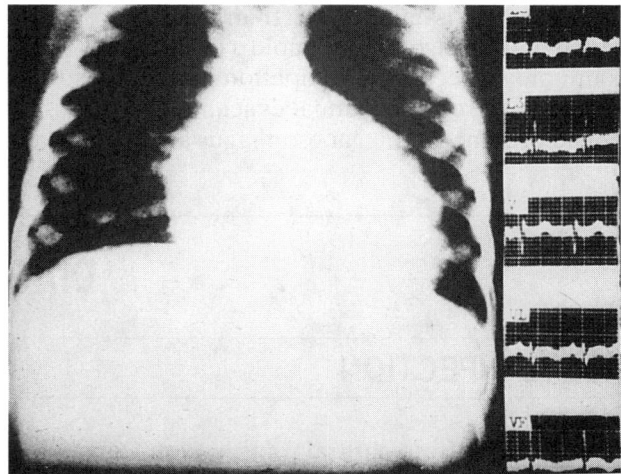

Figure 64.6   Chagas' disease: left, radiograph showing generalized cardiomegaly; right, ECG, which is so important in predicting prognosis.

tive seroreactors will enter into the phase of ventricular decompensation before the age of 50 years. Pump failure is biventricular for it is a pancardiomyopathy, so pulmonary congestion is not common. Functional valvular incompetence is common due to the widening of the mitral and tricuspid valve rings caused by the cardiac dilatation. A small apical aneurysm develops, as a result of widening of the great spiral muscular bundle of the left ventricle, but rarely ruptures. It is, however, a frequent site of thrombosis, as are the walls of the feebly beating ventricles. Another common presentation of chronic chagasic cardiomyopathy is embolism, often cerebral. It is the most common cause of cardiovascular accident among the relatively young adult patients, far more common than syphilis.

Sudden death is frequently recorded—probably due to ventricular fibrillation.[32] This may be the result of autonomic cardiac dysfunction.[33]

Another frequent presentation of chronic Chagas' disease in our area of central Goiás is the megasyndromes, especially megaoesophagus and megacolon.[34] Megaoesophagus occurs in less than 5% of positive seroreactors and there is a characteristic history of progressive difficulty in swallowing—especially of dry foods. In the late stages each mouthful has to be accompanied by a drink of water to effect stomach entry. These symptoms are well known in endemic areas. Twenty per cent of patients with megaoesophagus have abnormal ECGs. Parotid gland enlargement, possibly a 'work hypertrophy' to facilitate deglutition or else similar to that seen in malnutrition, gives rise to the 'cat face' (Figure 64.7). Megaoesophagus is classified by Rezende into four grades. Severe grades are often associated with malnutrition.

Megacolon is even rarer than megaoesophagus and it is the distal or sigmoid colon that is most commonly affected. Constipation may be of such a degree as to require manual evacuation.

The presence of megaoesophagus and megacolon

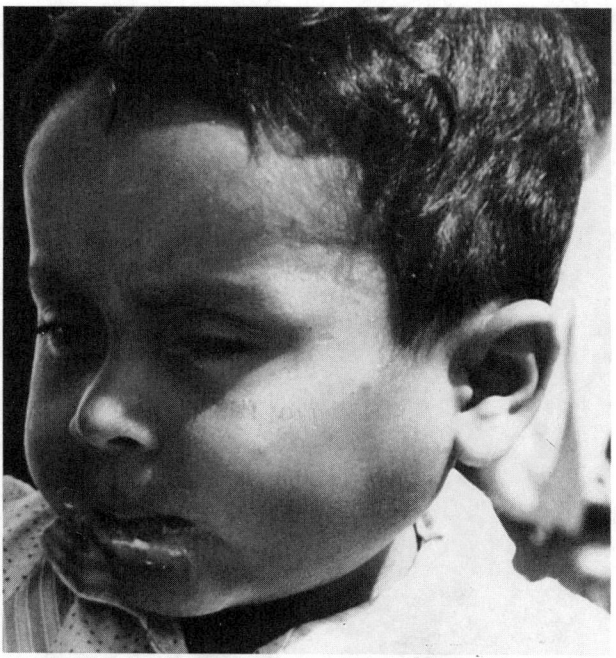

Figure 64.7   'Cat face' due to parotid gland enlargement in marked megaoesophagus. Note that such megasyndromes can occur in young patients.

is confirmed by radiological studies using barium contrast media.

Many other syndromes have been attributed to *T. cruzi* infection, including endocrine and exocrine gland functional abnormalities and central nervous system damage—in the chronic phase. For details the reader is referred to a more detailed text.[35]

DIAGNOSIS

ACUTE INFECTION

This can arise from natural transmission, congenital infection, blood transfusion, oral transmission or laboratory accident. Diagnosis in this phase is not usually difficult. More than 90% of cases will have *T. cruzi* visible on direct fresh smears. Strout concentration can be done if this fails, followed by xenodiagnosis if available. If not, cultures in NNN medium (Difco blood agar with 10% defibrillated rabbit blood) held at 26°C should be examined weekly. Subinoculation of young mice may also reveal circulating trypanosomes after 7–14 days. Serology only converts after 1 month in the sequence haemagglutination, fluorescence, complement fixation. The sensitivity and specificity of these tests has been reviewed.[36]

CHRONIC INFECTION

After the initial wave of parasitaemia, circulating trypanosomes become subpatent. Xenodiagnosis is the best method of recovering them. I use 40 1st instar clean *Dipetalogaster maximus*, dissected 30 days after feeding, and believe this species to be the most sensitive agent.[37] Xenodiagnosis literature is poor because standard criteria are not adopted. It is possible that the local bug species could be a more effective agent in certain areas. Some species, e.g.

R. prolixus, are prone to cause nasty skin reactions but there is no place for artificial xenodiagnosis. Xenodiagnosis is more likely to be positive soon after the acute phase, and the patients can be divided (like experimental animals) into high and low yielders in terms of xenodiagnosis.[38,39]. Whether this has any reflection on prognosis is unknown.

If xenodiagnosis is not available, culture in NNN medium and mouse subinoculation can be tried but the yields are less. Xenodiagnosis has three main uses:
1. To check serology.
2. To isolate strains.
3. To evaluate chemotherapy.

Even the author's unit, which has a large xeno facility, does not use it routinely because of the expense.

Serology is the usual way of confirming the presence of a chronic infection. It is as important as in the treponematoses. The fact that this remains positive for life, suggests that antigenic stimulation of specifically activated lymphocytes continues. This serology is an important laboratory investigation in our hospital in central Brazil but it is still far from perfect, as evidenced by the fact that more than one of the three tests is recommended (indirect haemogglutination, immunofluorescence, complement fixation). False positives occur with malaria, leprosy and leishmaniasis. The polymerase chain reaction promises well for the future but in spite of intensive research it is still not available as a routine test. Serological tests depending on the presence of cardiac autoantibodies and live trypanosome immobilization have not fulfilled their promise as indicators of progressive cardiomyopathy. If we had an indicator to measure this, perhaps a more rational approach to treatment could be devised for the chronic phase. Reference serology centres exist in Rio de Janeiro and at the Centers for Disease Control and Prevention (CDC), Atlanta, GA, USA.

TREATMENT

Specific treatment of *T. cruzi* infection employs one of two drugs: nifurtimox ('Lampit') or benznidazole ('Rochagan'). The manufacturers, Bayer and Roche respectively, have made little profit from these compounds despite huge development costs. This is because affected patients do not have the money! Thus these drugs are at present very difficult to obtain. Nifurtimox is available by arrangement with CDC. There should now be a similar service in each continent because many parasitic diseases, including this one, travel well.

Nifurtimox is given in an oral dose of 10 mg/kg body weight daily in three divided doses, after meals, for at least 30 days. Its effect can be rapidly demonstrated in acute cases, with disappearance of parasitaemia and, in some, negativation of serology. Some recommend treatment for up to 3 months and at a higher dose of 15 mg/kg body weight per day. Children tolerate the drug better than adults. Side-effects are anorexia and weight loss and, at a high dose, haemolytic anaemia associated with glucose-6-phosphate dehydrogenase deficiency, peripheral neuritis and psychosis.

Benznidazole is now preferred in central Brazil because the local isolates of *T. cruzi* seem to be more susceptible to it. At an oral dose of 5–10 mg/kg body weight per day for 30–60 days photosensitive skin rashes occur in 50% of patients, and peripheral neuritis is seen towards the end of treatment. It is available in many local pharmacies.

Since the beginning of the nifurtimox trials in Chile and Argentina it has been noted that there are differences in treatment response in different parts of South America. Also, carefully controlled studies with repeated xenodiagnosis in chronic cases show that parasitological cure is achieved in only about half the patients in central Brazil.[40,41] For this reason, and the fact that there is little evidence as yet that chronic phase patients benefit from specific treatment, most experienced physicians refuse to treat these patients with such toxic drugs, neither of which is licensed in either Europe or the USA because of mutagenicity.

All are agreed, however, that such treatment in the acute phase is valuable in reducing the degree of parasitic involvement of the tissue, especially in such target tissues as the heart and the smooth muscle of the gut. For this reason steps should be taken internationally to make one of these drugs available for clinicians with responsibility for acute cases of Chagas' disease. In the centre of what is one of the greatest foci of pathogenic Chagas' disease today, in Brasília, I only see acute disease associated with blood transfusion, congenital transmission, etc. People with chronic Chagas' disease are travelling and such cases can occur anywhere today. Drugs should also be available in any laboratory working with *T. cruzi*.

SYMPTOMATIC TREATMENT

CHRONIC CHAGASIC CARDIOMYOPATHY

As it is a panmyocarditis it does not on the whole respond well to conventional therapy. Bed-rest, digitalis and diuretics usually produce a marked initial improvement under ward conditions. Beta blockers are not advised in trying to control arrhythmias but emergency treatment of ventricular fibrillation requires procainamide, adenosine, etc. In patients with marked arrhythmia, such as complete atrioventricular block associated with Stokes–Adams attacks, a cardiac pacemaker may be inserted with benefit, especially in those with a normal cardiac size radiologically. Transplantation is contraindicated because immunosuppression will reactivate the chronic trypanosome infection. Embolism or evidence of thrombosis may necessitate anticoagulant therapy. Most importantly, the physician must take time with the patient to explain the nature of the tissue injury and how life must be modified accordingly, with the avoidance of hard physical exercise, emotional upheaval, etc. This is difficult with the average patient who is an illiterate tiller of the soil. A serological screen of the family is indicated if the patient has been living in a bug-infested house.

MEGASYNDROMES

Although mechanical dilatation with weighted bougies may help megaoesophagus, and manual clearance of faeces megacolon, patients with progressive disease usually come to surgery. For megaoesophagus a Thal operation with excision of the spastic cardiac sphincter, cardioplasty and anastomosis of the oesophagus and stomach gives good results. For megasigmoid an excision procedure produces relief. Cardiac function must be assessed before undertaking such procedures.

EVOLUTION AND PROGNOSIS

Evolution in both the acute and chronic phases depends on a variety of variables implicit in the initial inoculum and the host response to it.[20] There is evidence that superinfection with different *T. cruzi* stocks can occur and this could also influence outcome.[42]

Cardiac failure is a bad sign and 50% of patients will die within 2 years of their first attack, despite adequate treatment. Failure is mainly right-sided and acute left ventricular failure is uncommon because the basic lesion is a panmyocarditis. Marked degrees of atrioventricular block also carry a poor prognosis. Continuous Holter recordings have shown that such patients pass through a series of cardiac arrhythmias, including fibrillation and flutter, in a 24-hour period.

Megaoesophagus, if of marked degree, may cause overspill of food remnants into the bronchial tree with repeated bronchopneumonia, especially in the young. Intestinal delay can precipitate hyperinfection with *Strongyloides stercoralis* if this infection is present. Megacolon can present with spurious diarrhoea due to fluid faecal loss around a large impacted bolus; abdominal examination will detect the bolus. Volvulus of the sigmoid is a recognized complication.

PREVENTION AND CONTROL

Although, as is usually the case, this topic is the last to be considered, it is of primary concern in arresting the sinister implications of Chagas' disease for Latin America.[43] The history of control is very sad for although the answer was found in the 1940s domiciliated vector control is still wanting in many countries. This relates in part to the history of the region, for it has produced a sharply stratified society based on material values where the rich pay little attention to the predicament of the poor.[44]

The control of Chagas' disease has to be a central government decision. This decision was taken in Brazil in 1983 and was based on a national serological survey and detailed records of vector invasion of rural Brazilian houses.[45] Money was provided from the national insurance scheme and the result is an outstanding example of organized vector control which is now in its consolidation phase.[46] There were three phases to the programme:

1. Epidemiological research to determine important foci in terms of human infection and domiciliated bugs.
2. An attack phase of spraying with residual insecticides. Today a whole series of efficient pyrethroid insecticides is available.
3. A vigilance phase to prevent bug return to the house or invasion by another species, with a further insecticide spray if necessary.

It is the third phase that is the most difficult to implement and maintain as interest tends to wane.[47] To avoid this, community participation is essential and our group in Brasília has been active in devising and sustaining better vigilance methods.[48] How well these will work at a national level remains to be seen. House improvement is a final measure. Constructing new houses is too expensive but replastering (using a non-cracking formulation devised for the area) is effective for problem houses. The houseowner must participate in this reform.

The Brazilian success in Chagas' disease control has stimulated other affected countries such as Bolivia to initiate a national programme, especially against the major vector T. infestans, which is especially vulnerable because it is rarely recorded outside the peridomicile.

Meanwhile people infected in childhood have begun to travel. Therefore any pregnant Latin American mother should be asked about blood-sucking bugs in the house in childhood. They are usually well known and a photograph or specimens should be kept in the outpatient department for demonstration purposes. An affirmative reply warrants serology, even though less than 2% of serologically positive mothers will produce a congenitally infected child. Blood screening with similar serology will avoid such acute cases as occurred in a 4-year-old child with leukaemia who was infected in New York by a bottle of Bolivian blood. A serious laboratory accident with T. cruzi is an indication for immediate specific therapy which can be discontinued if serology is negative at 30 days.

Where blood has to be sterilized for T. cruzi because it cannot be discarded, 0.25 g of gentian violet per litre added to it for 24 hours in the bank is sufficient to kill any trypanosomes present.[49]

CONCLUSION

We live in stirring times and it is possible that by the year 2000 domiciliated triatomine control will have reached most of rural Latin America. Table 64.2 shows an estimate of the dimension of the problem.[50] Surely this must be a high priority for health ministries of afflicted countries, and a case for real investment for the future.

TRYPANOSOMA RANGELI

In a practical textbook of tropical medicine T. rangeli is more of nuisance value—in terms of confusion with T. cruzi. Reports of T. rangeli emanate mainly from Venezuela (where it was initially described), Columbia, Peru and Central America.[51] However, the literature shows it to be much more widely distributed, with a number of reports from Brazil, even in the south.

The slender trypanosome with a small kinetoplast can occasionally be found in human blood. It divides by binary fission. Characteristic elongated epimastigotes are produced in the bug. It appears to have no amastigote phase and is not pathogenic in man. Its importance rests in the confusion it can cause if it is not recognized at isolation. On xenodiagnosis T. rangeli invades the haemolymph of the bug and infects the salivary gland, so anterior dissection will settle the point. It is also pathogenic to triatomine bugs, frequently killing them. A second point of confusion is to what extent an occult human infection with T. rangeli will produce positive seroreactors for T. cruzi. This point has never been satisfactorily settled with conventional serology, although specific monoclonal antibodies have been developed.[52] As we wait for the polymerase chain reaction to be routinely employed in doubtful T. cruzi serology we hope for clarification.

Table 64.2. Chagas' disease in Latin America.

Country	Total population (millions)	Rural (%)	Estimated cases (millions)	Main vector
Argentina	26.393	21	2.640	*T. infestans*
Belize	0.145	ND	0.003	*T. dimidiata*
Bolivia	4.647	77	1.858	*T. infestans*
Brazil	119.024	36	6.300	*T. infestans*
Chile	10.857	20	0.367	*T. infestans*
Colombia	0.026	29	0.217	*R. prolixus*
Costa Rica	2.110	59	0.130	*T. dimidiata*
Ecuador	6.521	58	0.180	*T. dimidiata*
El Salvador	4.300	60	0.322	*T. dimidiata*
French Guiana	0.080	ND	0.021	*R. pictipes?*
Guatemala	7.110	64	0.730	*T. dimidiata*
Guyana	0.835	73	0.208	*R. prolixus?*
Honduras	3.400	68	0.213	*R. prolixus*
Mexico	69.900	34	3.798	*T. barberi*
Nicaragua	2.400	52	0.114	*T. dimidiata*
Panama	1.630	49	0.226	*R. pallescens*
Paraguay	2.880	56	0.397	*T. infestans*
Peru	16.800	42	0.643	*T. infestans*
Suriname	0.352	ND	0.147	*R. pictipes?*
Uruguay	2.886	17	0.278	*T. infestans*
Venezuela	13.913	30	4.865	*R. prolixus*
Total	322.233	36	24.697	

T., *Triatoma*; R., *Rhodnius*; ND, no data available.
Reproduced from Schofield.[50]

REFERENCES

1 Hoare C A *The Trypanosomes of Mammals*. Oxford: Blackwell, 1972: 749.

2 Lent H & Wygodzinsky P. Revision of the Triatominae (Hemiptera Reduviidae) and their significance as vectors of Chagas' disease. *Bull Am Mus Nat Hist* 1974; 163:123–520.

3 Coura J R. Chagas' disease as endemic to the Amazon basin: risk or hypothesis. *Rev Soc Bras Med Trop* 1990; 23:67–70.

4 Salgado J A, Garces P N, Oliveira C F & Galizzi J. Revisão clínica atual do primeiro caso humano descrito da doença de Chagas. *Rev Inst Med Trop São Paulo* 1962; 4:330–337.

5 Chagas C. Tripanozomiaze humana. Estudos sobre a morfologia e o ciclo evolutivo do *Schizotrypanum cruzi* N. Gen N. Sp. agente etiológico de nova entidade morbida do homem. *Mem Inst Oswaldo Cruz* 1909; 1:159–218.

6 Prata A. Carlos Chagas. Coletânea de trabalhos científicos. *Coleção Temas Bras* 1981; 6:883.

7 Guerreiro C & Machado A. Da reação de Bordet e Gengou na moléstia de Carlos Chagas como elemento diagnóstico. *Bras Med* 1913; 27:225–226.

8 Mazza J, Montana A, Benitez C & Janzi E Z. Transmission del *Schizotrypanum cruzi* al nino por leche de la madre con enfermedad de Chagas. *MEPRA* 1936; 28:41–46.

9 Brumpt E. Le xenodiagnostic application au diagnostic de quelques infections parasitaires et en particulier à la trypanosomose de Chagas. *Bull Soc Pathol Exot* 1912; 7:706–710.

10 Dias E. *Um Ensaio de Profilaxia da Moléstia de Chagas* Rio de Janeiro: Imprensa Nacional 1945:116.

11 Chagas C. American trypanosomiasis. Study of the parasite and the transmitting insect. *Proc Inst Med Chicago* 1921; 3:220–242.

12 Pan American Health Organization. *American trypanosomiasis research*, Scientific Publication No. 318. Washington, DC: PAHO, 1976.

13 Caxambu – XVIIIth Meeting for basic research in Chagas' disease. *Mem Inst Oswaldo Cruz* 1991; 86(supplement 1):312.

14 Dvorak J A, Gibson C C & Mackelt A. *A Bibliography on Chagas' Disease 1968–1984*. Washington, DC: National Institute of Health, 1985:397.

15 Camargo M E, Da Silva G R, Castilho E A & Silveira A C. Inquérito sorológico da prevalência de

infecção chagásica no Brasil 1975–1980. *Rev Inst Med Trop São Paulo* 1984; 26:192–204.

16 Sherlock I A. In Brener A & Andrade Z (eds) *Trypanosoma cruzi e Doença de Chagas*. Rio de Janeiro: Guanabara Koogan, 1979:83.

17 Miles M A Transmission cycles and the heterogenicity of *Trypanosoma cruzi*. In Lumsden W H R & Evans D A (eds) *Biology of the Kinetoplastidae*, vol. 2. London: Academic Press, 1979:117–196.

18 Hagar J M & Rahimtoola S H. Chagas heart disease in the United States. *New Engl J Med* 1991; 325:763–767.

19 Coura J R. Doença de Chagas como endemia urbana. In Cançado J R & Chuster R (eds) *Cardiopatia Chagásica*. Belo Horizonte: Fundação Carlos Chagas, 1985; 356–361.

20 Marsden P D. The transmission of *Trypanosoma cruzi* infection to man and its control. In Croll N A & Cross J H (eds) *Human Ecology and Infectious Diseases*. London: Academic Press, 1983, 253–289.

21 Dvorak J. Single cell isolates of *Trypanosoma cruzi*. How and why? *Rev Soc Bras Med Trop* 1985; 18(supplement 1):15–24.

22 Marsden P D. *Compendium of Symposium on American Trypanosomiasis Research*, Scientific Publication No. 318. Washington, DC: Pan American Health Organization, 1976:397–402.

23 Barrett T V. Parasites and predators of Triatominae. In *American Trypanosomiasis Research*, Scientific Publication No. 318. Washington, DC: Pan American Health Organization, 1976:24–300.

24 Barretto M P. Epidemiologia. In Brener Z & Andrade Z (eds) *Trypanosoma cruzi e Doença de Chagas*. Rio de Janeiro: Guanabara Koogan, 1979:89–151.

25 Yasuda M A S, Marcondes C B, Guedes L A et al. Possible oral transmission of acute Chagas' disease in Brazil. *Rev Inst Med Trop São Paulo* 1991; 33:351–358.

26 Marsden P D & Hagstrom J W C. Experimental *Trypanosoma cruzi* infection in Beagle puppies: the effect of variations in the dose and source of infecting trypanosomes and the route of inoculation on the course of infection. *Trans Soc Trop Med Hyg* 1968; 61:816–824.

27 Andrade A A & Andrade S G. Patologia. In Brener Z & Andrade Z (eds) *Trypanosoma cruzi e Doença de Chagas*. Rio de Janeiro: Guanabara Koogan, 1979:199–248.

28 Teixeira A R L. Imunopatologia da doença de Chagas. In *Anais do Simpósio sobre Moléstia de Chagas*. Pub. ACIESP 16. Academia de Ciências do Estado de São Paulo, 1979:56–71.

29 Raso P, Chapadeiro E, Tafuri W L, Lopes E R & Rocha A. Anatomia patológica da cardiopatia crônica. In *Cardiopatia Chagásica*. Cançado J R & Chuster R (eds) Belo Horizonte: Fundação Carlos Chagas, 1985:41–53.

30 Köberle F. Chagas' disease and Chagas' syndromes: the pathology of American trypanosomiasis. *Adv Parasitol* 1968; 6:63–116.

31 Teixeira V P A. Comparison of the occurrence of *Trypanosoma cruzi* nests in the adrenal gland vein and other tissues and its relationship with myocarditis in human chronic infection. *Rev Soc Bras Med Trop* 1989; 22:229–230.

32 Prata A, Lopes E R & Chapadeiro E. Características da morte súbita tida como não esperada na doença de Chagas. *Rev Soc Bras Med Trop* 1986; 19:9–12.

33 Junqueira L F. Sobre o possível papel da disfunção autonômica cardíaca na morte súbita associada a doença de Chagas. *Arg Bras Cardiol* 1991; 56:420–434.

34 Rezende J. Clínica. Manifestações Digestivas. In Brener Z & Andrade Z (eds) *Trypanosoma cruzi e Doença de Chagas*. Rio de Janeiro: Guanabara Koogan, 1979:312–361.

35 Marsden P D. Chagas' disease: clinical aspects. In Gilles H M (ed.) *Recent Advances in Tropical Medicine*. Edinburgh: Churchill Livingstone, 1984:63–77.

36 Camargo M E & Takeda G K F. Diagnóstico de laboratório. In Brener Z & Andrade Z (eds) Rio de Janeiro: Guanabara Koogan, 1979:175–198.

37 Marsden P D. *Dipetalogaster maxima* or *D.maximus* as a xenodiagnostic agent. *Rev Soc Bras Med Trop* 1986; 19:205–207.

38 Miles M A, Marsden P D & Pettit L E et al. Experimental *Trypanosoma cruzi* infection in rhesus monkeys. III. Electrocardiagraphic and histological findings. *Trans Soc Trop Med* 1979; 73:528–532.

39 Castro C N. Influência da parasitemia no quadro clínico da doença de Chagas. *Rev Pat Trop* 1980; 9:73–136.

40 Canaçado J R. Tratamento específico. In Cançado J R & Chuster R (eds) *Cardiopatia Chagásica*. Belo Horizonte: Fundação Carlos Chagas, 1985:327–355.

41 Ferreira H O. Treatment of the indeterminate form of Chagas' disease with Nifurtimox and Benznidazole. *Rev Soc Bras Med Trop* 1990; 23:209–211.

42 Macêdo V. Influência da exposição à reinfecção na evolução da doença de Chagas (estudo longitudinal de cinco anos). *Rev Pat Trop* 1976; 5:33–115.

43 Marsden P D. Selective primary health care: strategies for control of disease in the developing world. XVI. Chagas' disease. *Rev Infect Dis* 1984; 6:855–865.

44 Marsden P D. South American trypanosomiasis and leishmaniasis: endemic disease of continental dimensions affecting poor, neglected and underfunded people. In England P T & Sher A (eds) *The Biology of Parasitism*, Vol. 9, MBL Lectures in Biology. New York: Alan R Liss, 1988; 77–92.

45 Fiúsa Lima J T. Incremento do programa de controle da doença de Chagas no Brasil. *Rev Soc Bras Med Trop* 1983; 16:128–129.

46 Dias J C P. Control of Chagas' disease in Brasil. *Parasitol Today* 1987; 3:336.

47 Garcia-Zapata M T A & Marsden P D. Chagas' Disease. In Gilles H M (ed.) *Clin Trop Med Comm Dis*. 1, 3. Saunders, London.

48 Garcia-Zapata M T, Marsden P D, Virgens D & Soares V A. Epidemiological vigilance with community participation in the control of the vectors of Chagas' disease in Goiás, Central Brazil. *Rev Argent Microbiol* 1988; 20(supplement): 106–117.

49 Souza H M. The present state of chemoprophylaxis in transfusional Chagas' disease. *Rev Soc Bras Med Trop* 1989; 22:1–3.

50 Schofield C J. Control of Chagas' disease vectors. *Br Med Bull* 1985; 41:187–194.

51 D'Alessandra-Bacigalupo A, Saravia N G. *Trypanosoma rangeli*. In Kreier J P & Baker J R (eds) *Parasitic Protozoa*. San Diego: Academic Press, 1992.

52 Anthony R L, Lody T S & Constantine N T. Antigenic differentiation of *Trypanosoma cruzi* and *Trypanosoma rangeli* by means of monoclonal-hybridoma antibodies. *Am J Trop Med Hyg* 1981; 30:1192–1197.

CHAPTER 65

LEISHMANIASIS

A. D. M. Bryceson

Leishmaniasis is caused by infection with parasites of the genus *Leishmania*. Leishmaniasis is not a single disease but a 'variety of syndromes' that are 'complex and cosmopolitan'.[1] These syndromes are widespread geographically and often represent zoonotic infections with variable penetration to man. They occur in numerous zoogeographical zones, each of which is characterized by its own biological complex of parasite, reservoir and vector, and their intimate relationship in that particular ecological setting (Table 65.1). So successful has *Leishmania* been in adapting to circumstances that its species have established themselves in forest and desert, mountain and plain, town and country. The several patterns of human disease reflect this diversity to some extent, but are limited by the capabilities of the host's immune response to the intracellular infection, and modified by the subtleties of the parasite's means of subverting it.

Table 65.1 Epidemiology of leishmaniasis: distribution, reservoirs and vectors.

Organisms	Geography	Reservoir	Vector
Old World			
L. donovani	North-east India, Bangladesh, Burma	Humans	*Phlebotomus argentipes*
L infantum	Mediterranean basin, Middle East, China, central Asia	Dogs, foxes, jackals	*P. perniciosus, P. ariasi*
L. donovani (Africa)	Sudan, Kenya, Horn of Africa, ? Senegambia	? Rodents in Sudan, ? canines, ? humans	*P. orientalis, P. martini*
L. major	Semideserts in Middle East, north India, Pakistan, North Africa, central Asia	Gerbils (*Rhombomys, Meriones* et al.)	*P. papatassi*
L. major	Sub-Saharan savanna, Sudan	Rodents (especially *Arvicanthus, Tatera*)	*P. duboscqi*
L. tropica	Towns in Middle East, Mediterranean basin, central Asia	Humans	*P. sergenti*
L. aethiopica	Highlands of Kenya, Ethiopia	Hyraxes (*Procavia, Heterohyrax*)	*P. longipes, P. pedifer*
New World			
L. chagasi	Central America, northern South America, esp. Brazil, Venezuela	Foxes, dogs, opossums (*Didelphys*)	*Lutzomyia longipalpis*
L. mexicana	Yucatan, Belize, Guatemala	Forest rodents (esp. *Ototylomys*)	*Lu. olmeca*
L. amazonensis	Tropical forests of South America	Forest rodents (esp. *Proechimys, Oryzomys*)	*Lu. flaviscutellata*
L. braziliensis	Tropical forests of South and Central America	? Forest rodents, peridomestic animals	*Psychodopygus wellcomei,* et al., *Lutzomyia* spp., *Lu. umbratilis*
L. guyanensis	Guyana, Surinam, into Brazil	Sloths (*Choleopus*) arboreal anteaters, (*Tamandua*)	*Lu. umbratilis*
L. panamensis	Panama, Costa Rica, Colombia	Sloths (*Choleopus*)	*Lu. trapidoi* et al.
L. peruviana	West Andes of Peru, Argentine highlands	Dogs	*Lu. verrucarum, Lu. peruenis*

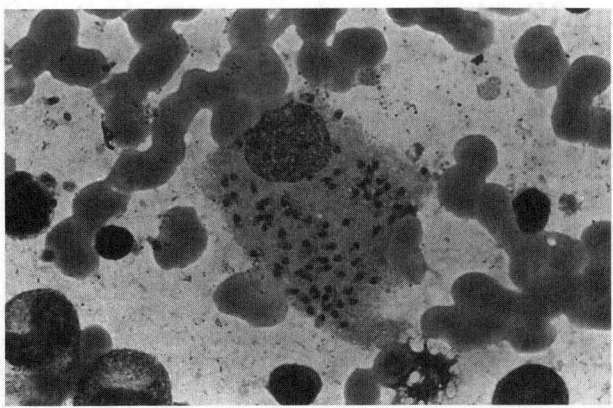

Figure 65.1 Intracellular amastigotes of *Leishmania* in the smear of a bone marrow aspirate from a patient with visceral leishmaniasis.

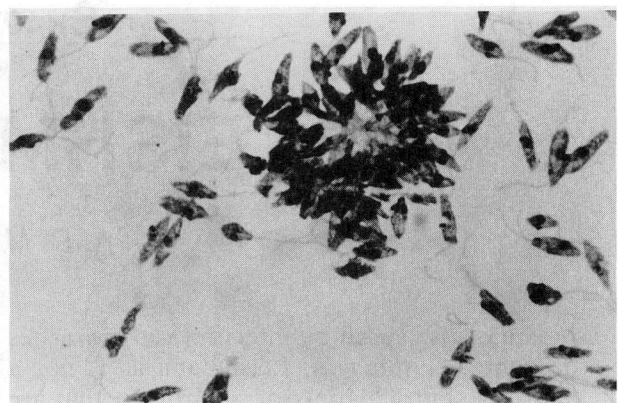

Figure 65.2 Promastigotes of *Leishmania* in culture medium showing nucleus kinetoplast and flagellum.

AETIOLOGY

THE PARASITE

Leishmania are transmitted between long-lived vertebrate hosts by short-lived phlebotomine sandflies, and have a cycle of development in each. In the vertebrate, *Leishmania* are in their amastigote form (Figure 65.1), round or oval bodies with a maximum diameter of 2.5–6.8 μm, without a flagellum. In the sandfly, and in artificial culture medium, they are in the promastigote form, long slender motile bodies, 10–20 × 1.5–3 μm, with an anterior flagellum of equal or greater length.

A trilaminar membrane encloses the cytoplasm, which contains the nucleus, kinetoplast and basal body from which arises the flagellum (Figure 65.2). These structures are visible by light microscopy. Multiplication of each form is by binary fission.

SPECIATION AND IDENTIFICATION

There are at least 30 species of *Leishmania*, of which 12 named and several unnamed species infect man.[2] Speciation was originally on geographical and clinical grounds, later modified by morphology, by behaviour in sandflies, hosts and culture, by biotypes and life cycles, by antibody responses to antigens (in particular monoclonal antibodies), and by genetic methods. Genomic identification is through DNA analysis, especially hybridization techniques. Phenotypic identification is through analysis of electrophoretic mobility of isoenzymes secreted in culture, a given pattern identifying a zymodeme. Zymodeme analysis extends identification beyond

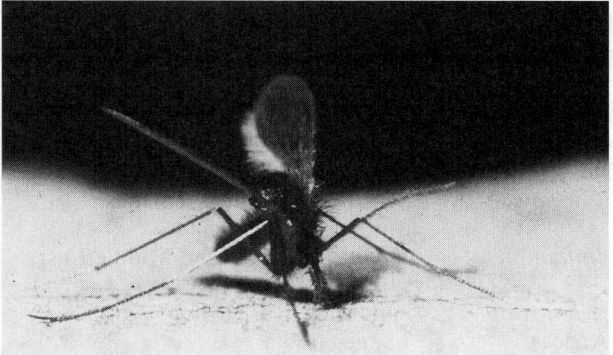

Figure 65.3 *Phlebotomus ariasi*, the vector of *Leishmania infantum* in southern France. (Courtesy R. Killick-Kendrick.)

the species level, and shows differences within a species that may reflect geographical identity,[3] tropism[4] and adaptability to altered host resistance.[5] DNA techniques have been refined for use on small numbers of parasites that may be obtained directly from reservoir hosts or sandflies.[6,7]

LIFE CYCLE[8,9]

In the sandfly

Ingested amastigotes transform into promastigotes and pass to the hindgut in New World sandflies, or midgut in Old World sandflies. Over the next 4–7 days they migrate to the foregut, developing into infective metacyclic forms. During this process, three molecules in particular are heavily expressed on the surface membrane and are thought to be important for infectivity. Lipophosphoglycan forms a matrix or glycocalyx and protects the promastigote from lysis by host complement, which is deposited as C3b on the glycocalyx, and helps establish the parasite in the host macrophage.[10] Lipophosphoglycan shows some variability between leishmanial species, and is secreted in quantity into culture medium, and has been used to type *Leishmania*.[11] The other two molecules are the major glycoprotein gp63[12] and an acid phosphatase.[13] Metacyclic promastigotes are inoculated with sandfly saliva, which increases infectivity.[14]

In the host

Mouthparts of sandflies tear tissue, thus creating a tiny pool of blood from which they feed and into which promastigotes are deposited; it is not known precisely how promastigotes enter macrophages in this situation. However, in vitro experiments suggest that lipophosphoglycan and gp63 bind to specific lectin receptors on the macrophage surface membrane through their carbohydrate moieties. Promastigotes activate complement through the classical pathway. C3b is deposited on its surface and is recognized by a macrophage receptor. The macrophage extrudes its membrane to engulf the promastigote, forming a parasitophorous vacuole. This vacuole contains lysosomal hydrolases, cathepsins and β-glucuronidase secreted by the macrophage, and is therefore a classical phagolysosome. The amastigote survives, however. This is thought to be due largely to its secretions of acid phosphatase and phospholipase, which maintain an acid environment (pH 5.0), while a proton pump in its membrane pushes out hydrogen ions, maintaining the intracellular pH at 6.2. The pump also pulls in glucose and amino acids. Various enzymes secreted by the amastigote salvage host purines, catabolize fatty acids, peptides and amino acids, and protect it against oxidants.

Parasitization of the macrophage 'down-regulates' the host's cell-mediated response, by reducing the expression of class II molecules on the macrophage surface and increasing the requirement of interferon-γ for microbial killing. The amastigote resists killing by oxygen radicals, which are the classical end-mechanism of cell-mediated immunity, but is killed by nitrous oxide produced from L-arginine.[15] Several leishmanial antigens are expressed on the macrophage surface. Gp63 seems to be important for the induction of a successful immune response, while the carbohydrate moiety of lipophosphoglycan may be immunosuppressive.[16]

RESERVOIR HOSTS[17,18]

With notable exceptions, the leishmaniases are normally zoonoses of wild animals, usually rodents, edentates or canines, which include the domestic dog. In a given cycle of transmission there is usually a restricted number of primary reservoir hosts that are capable of maintaining the cycle, but secondary hosts may extend the range of that cycle, for example dogs for *L. chagasi*. Accidental hosts may be found infected but are unimportant from the point of view of maintaining the cycle, e.g. man for *L. major*. The condition of post-kala-azar dermal leishmaniasis (PKDL) makes man a genuine reservoir of infection for *L. donovani* in India, capable of maintaining the parasite throughout interepidemic periods. Acute cases of visceral leishmaniasis (VL) in India and Africa, but not in Europe, may also serve as reservoirs. Most natural reservoir hosts are well adapted to leishmanial infection and develop mild lesions, most commonly on the skin, that persist for many years and do no harm. Dogs are an exception, developing visceral disease with *L. infantum*, which eventually kills them. Where reservoir and vector share the same habitat precisely, for example *P. papatassi* and the gerbil, transmission (of *L. major*) is intense, and the risk of accidental human infection is high. Where the habitats are separate but overlapping, as with *Lutzomyia umbratilis* (which breeds on the ground) and the arboreal sloths and anteaters, transmission may be less intense and the risk of accidental human infection (with *L. guyanensis* in this example) correspondingly less.

SANDFLY VECTORS[19]

In the Old World sandfly vectors belong to the genus *Phlebotomus* (Figure 65.3), and in the New World to the genera *Lutzomyia* and *Psychodopygus*. Sandflies breed in organic detritus in a variety of sites, which include rodent burrows, forest leaf litter, and human and animal manure. The breeding sites of many species is unknown. Breeding, and thus sandfly populations, depend on temperature in cool climates and rainfall in hot climates. Thus transmission of leishmaniasis is often seasonal. Sandflies rest in a variety of sites, which may bring them into close contact with man. For example, *P. argentipes* rests in cattle sheds that may abut on to houses in Indian villages, while *P. martini* rests in eroded termite hills in Kenya which may be distant from houses. Sandflies may fly up to 2 km or be carried further on wind, thus extending the area of transmission. Vector species vary in their degree of anthropophilia or zoophilia and in their efficiency as transmitters to man.

Sandflies feed mostly on plant juices containing sugars. Parous female sandflies need at least two blood meals to permit maturation of eggs. Infected sandflies live for up to 30 days, not as long as do uninfected flies but long enough for three or four gonadotrophic cycles and six or eight blood meals. The gut of infected flies may be partially blocked by the infection, which induces them to probe repeatedly, thereby increasing the risk of transmission. Sandflies are fastidious in their requirements for temperature, humidity and still air. The majority of species bite at night, perhaps only during a few hours; some bite at dawn and dusk; a few will bite in daylight. Thus type and timing of human activity are important determinants of infection.

TRANSMISSION

Man is normally infected by the bite of an infected sandfly. Factors that affect the risk of transmission are discussed in the preceding section and in the individual sections under Epidemiology below. Rarely, VL has been transmitted by blood transfusion, sexual intercourse,[20] accidental or deliberate inoculation in the laboratory[21] or congenitally.[22] In addition, cutaneous leishmaniasis (CL) has been transmitted by deliberate scarification as a form of immunization,[23] and through suckling.[24] Secondary cases within a family are otherwise almost unknown.

EPIDEMIOLOGY

The behaviour of leishmaniasis in a given area reflects the behaviour of the human population in relation to the cycle of transmission, be that zoonotic or anthroponotic (Figure 65.5). The population at risk will differ in each situation, and may depend upon one or more factors, which include:

- Proximity of residence to sandfly breeding and resting sites.
- Type of housing.
- Occupation.
- Extent of exposure to sandfly bites.
- Age, as an expression of endemicity, risk of exposure or independently.
- Natural resistance, which may be genetic or acquired from previous infection individually or as a part of the herd. Immunity may be reduced by extrinsic factors such as nutrition,[25] natural disasters, intercurrent epidemics of influenza[26] or human immunodeficiency virus (HIV).[27]

There are no data on variation of parasite virulence within a given species, but some species would seem to be more infectious than others. The availability of the parasite to sandflies varies greatly. Zoonotic reservoirs usually provide a stable chronic source of infection, although rodent populations may vary considerably. Human reservoirs are less reliable and decline as epidemics decline, due to death, treatment and the acquisition of herd immunity, unless there is a chronic interepidemic reservoir, as in PKDL or leishmaniasis recidivans. In zoonotic infections humans make a negligible contribution to force of transmission.

The efficiency of transmission by sandflies, or vectorial capacity, defined as the number of infective bites delivered per human per annum, also varies greatly.[28] It depends upon density and seasonality of sandfly populations and their longevity and flight range. Populations of sandflies that live alongside an efficient reservoir, such as *P. papatassi* with gerbils, are likely to be highly infectious. Vectors in cycles of transmission remote from man, for example in the forest canopy, are less likely to infect man. Vectors vary in their degree of anthrophilia and zoophilia.[29] Quantitative data on transmission are scanty, and mathematical models of transmission are rudimentary, but have been applied to zoonotic CL in Russia[30] and to epidemic VL in India.[26]

The impact of these factors is considered below.

L. infantum[18] is responsible for VL in the Mediterranean basin, western Asia, and eastern China, in a broad belt between 30°N and 45°N. Affected areas are separated by large unaffected areas. The infection is enzootic in dogs, especially domestic dogs but feral dogs may be important in the Middle East, and foxes in southern Europe,[31] and North Africa. Man is ineffective as a reservoir, but the skin of infected dogs is rich in parasites that are readily available to sandflies. Rates of infection in dogs, currently range between 1% in parts of France and Spain and 24% in part of Tuscany.[32] Canine infection does not necess-

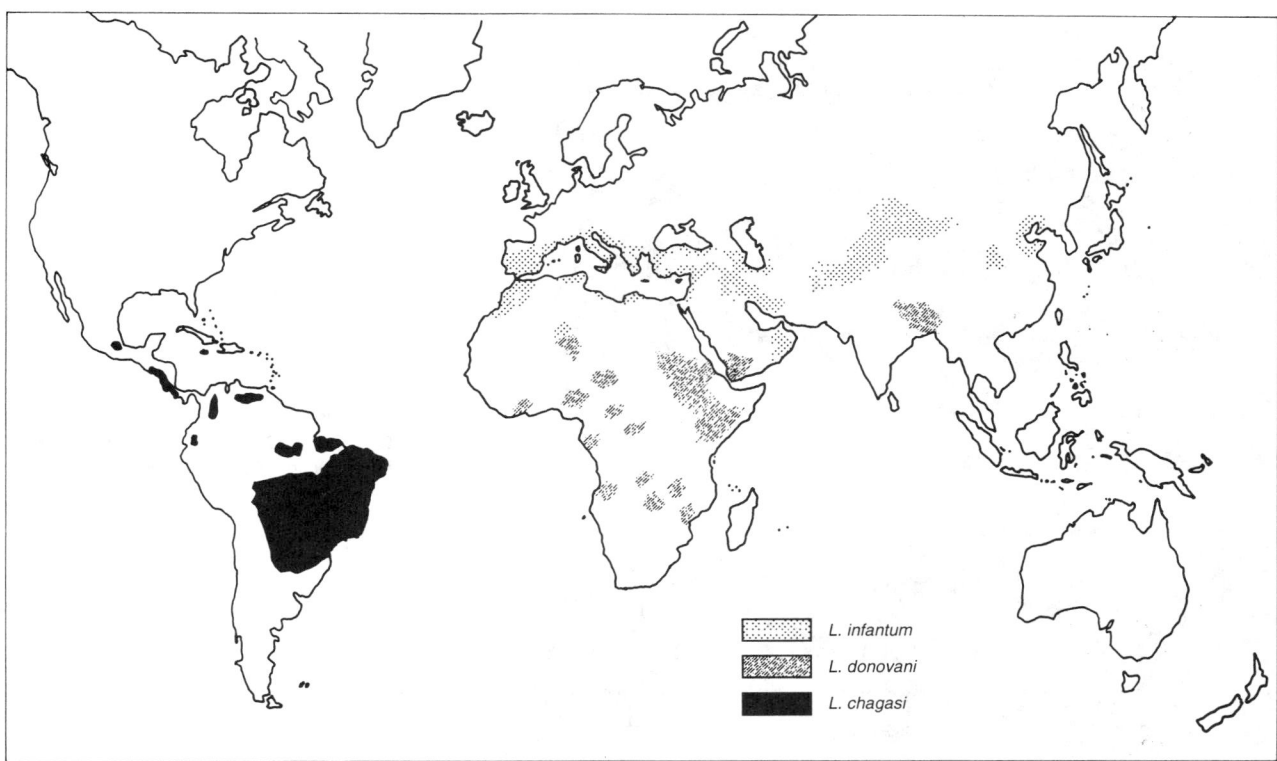

Figure 65.4 Distribution of visceral leishmaniasis.

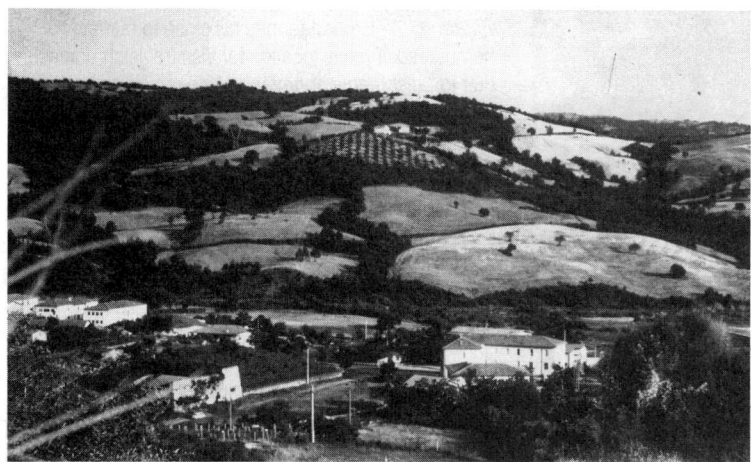

Figure 65.5 Bacinello in Tuscany, Italy. Typical location for sporadic visceral leishmaniasis due to *Leishmania infantum* in southern Europe.

arily lead to human infections[33] and is often patchy, small outbreaks of disease appearing and disappearing. This pattern may possibly reflect the spread of infection by foxes and the availability of breeding sites for the vectors. Little is known of the precise breeding and resting sites of the main vectors *P. perniciosus* and *P. ariasi*, but they have adapted a wide range of habitats, and bite man readily.

In China,[34] VL due to *L. infantum* used to be extremely common in the Huange (Yellow) and Changjiang (Yangtze) River valleys, affecting man and dogs, but was controlled by vigorous public health measures aimed at both sources of infection, and the disease has been virtually eradicated here. There is still an extensive area of infection in the hills of east and central China. The vector is *P. chinensis*, and the racoon dog is an additional reservoir.[35] Anthroponotic VL, probably due to *L. donovani*, occurs sporadically in the deserts of Xinjiang, and over the huge North China Plain.

Throughout its area of distribution, VL due to *L. infantum* is most commonly found in young children under the age of 5 years. This may reflect endemicity and domestic transmission, as is suggested by posi-

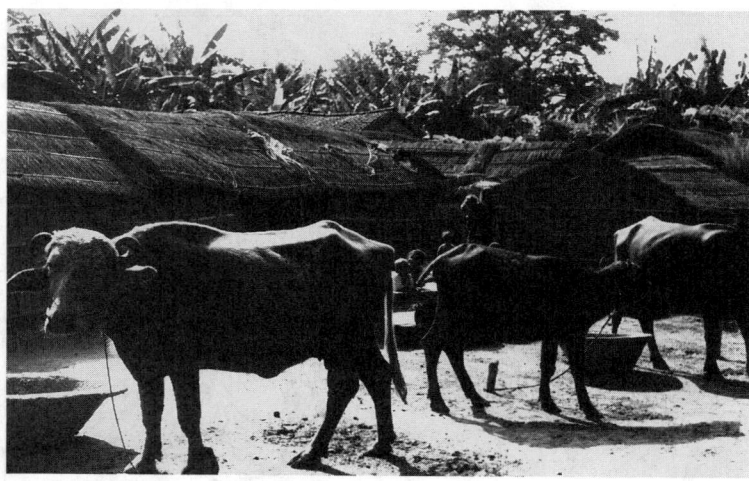

Figure 65.6 Village in Bihar showing close association between people and cattle. Typical location for epidemic visceral leishmanis in the Ganges Valley.

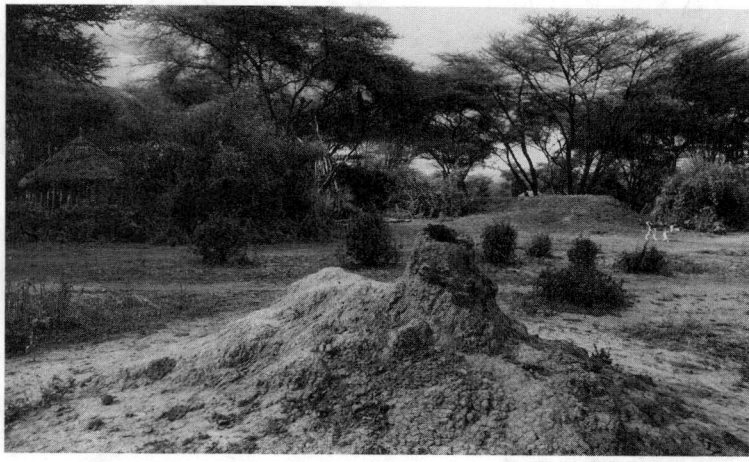

Figure 65.7 Eroded termite hill close to human homestead. Typical location for visceral leishmaniasis due to *Leishmania donovani* in Kenyan Northern Rift Valley.

tive leishmanin skin test rates of up to 30% in adults in some foci,[36] but infantile cases are relatively common among tourists, suggesting an infantile predisposition. Non-immune adults are susceptible, and postprimary disease occurs in immuno-suppressed adults in endemic areas.[27]

L. donovani causes anthroponotic VL, or kala-azar, in the Indian subcontinent and in some parts of China.[18] Man is the only known reservoir. There are two distinct areas of the disease: the most important is the epidemic area of the north-east, but there are more stable foci of sporadic cases in valleys of the Himalayan foothills, Rajasthan, and northern Gujerat.[37] Little is known of the epidemiology in these small foci. Epidemic VL occurs in the Ganges–Brahamaputra valleys (Figure 65.6), affecting especially Bihar, west Bengal, Bangladesh and Assam, and at times spreading as far south as Madras and Burma. In western Assam the cycles have had a periodicity of about 15 years, possibly reflecting waning of herd immunity, but in most of Assam, Bihar and Bengal epidemic peaks have been separated by 30–45 and 20 years. This suggests that the

disease may be becoming more stable, perhaps associated with endemicity due to the presence of cases of PKDL, but is then destabilized by extrinsic factors such as famine and epidemics of malaria and influenza.[26] Cases of PKDL are thought to represent the interepidemic reservoir. Cases of VL are infectious to sandflies before treatment.

Mass spraying of DDT to control malaria may have been responsible for the virtual elimination of VL from the epidemic areas in the 1950s, but the incidence began to increase in 1971, reaching epidemic proportions in 1977, when 70 000 cases were reported from Bihar alone. The disease affects especially the 10–29-year-old age group, males more commonly than females in the ratio 6:1.[38] In epidemics, cases are often clustered in households. The vector *P. argentipes* rests in cattle sheds which are often closely attached to houses; a subpopulation of the fly is anthropophilic. It breeds in organic detritus on the ground.

In sub-Saharan Africa *L. donovani* causes enzootic VL, especially in southern Sudan, the borders of Ethiopia, Somalia and northern Kenya (Figure

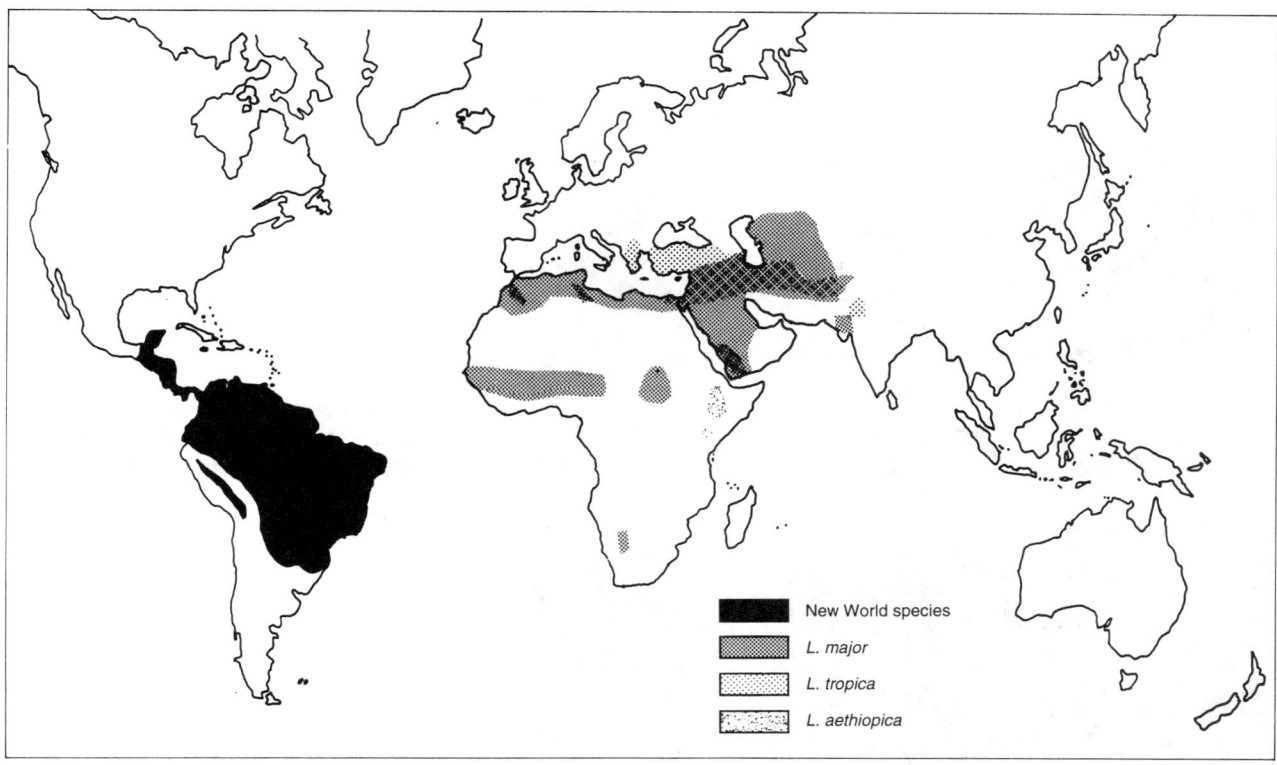

Figure 65.8   The distribution of cutaneous leishmaniasis.

65.7). The main enzootic foci would seem to be in *Acacia–Balanites* woodland. In Sudan *P. orientalis* transmits the infection among certain rodents, while in Kenya *P. martini*[39] has been found infected and capable of transmitting the infection;[21] it rests in eroded termite hills, and cases cluster around these.[40] It bites on hot humid evenings without wind. Sporadic cases of human VL occur in these areas. Epidemics of human VL have been recorded in Sudan within and beyond these natural foci. *P. orientalis* is a ferocious human biter, at rates up to 600 bites per man per hour. An epidemic began in 1982 in western Upper Nile region of Sudan, associated with famine and displacement through civil war. Seroprevalence of 23% was recorded.[41] Thousands of patients have been treated in centres in Khartoum and Leer, and over 40 000 people have died.[42] In Kenya the random appearance of VL in 8–12-year-old boys reflects the enzootic state, while in epidemics there is a wider age range with domestic focalization, suggesting anthroponotic transmission in huts. The finding of infected dogs[43] may be incidental as they are not thought to be an efficient reservoir of the African parasite.[44] Rare cases of VL have also been recorded from Gambia and Senegal, where dogs may be the reservoir,[45] and from Niger, Chad, Central African Republic, Zambia, Malawi,

Zaire and Angola, where nothing is known of their epidemiology.

L. chagasi is responsible for VL in the New World.[17,46] The main endemic area is north-east Brazil, where transmission is rural and peridomestic. The vector *Lutzomyia longipalpis* rests and feeds in chicken houses, but readily bites dogs and man, thus setting up a cycle of transmission. Foxes (*Cerdocyonthous*) introduce the parasite from the forest. Little is known of the natural cycle in the wild, but the opposum *Didelphis marsupialis* has been found infected with *L. chagasi* in Colombia.[47] Male children are most commonly affected.[48]

In other parts of South and Central America VL is scanty and sporadic. Cases have been reported from Mexico, Honduras, El Salvador, Colombia, Venezuela and Bolivia. The disease is commonly in young adults, presumably infected from a zoonotic cycle.

L. major is responsible for most zoonotic CL of the Old World (Figure 65.8). It is endemic throughout the flat hot semideserts and dry silt valleys of North Africa, the Middle East and the Arabian peninsula through to Rajasthan in India and north to Turkmenia, Uzbekistan, Tadjikistan and Kazakhstan. A second belt runs across the west of sub-Saharan Africa, and reappears in central Sudan and northern Kenya.[49] Genetically a stable species,

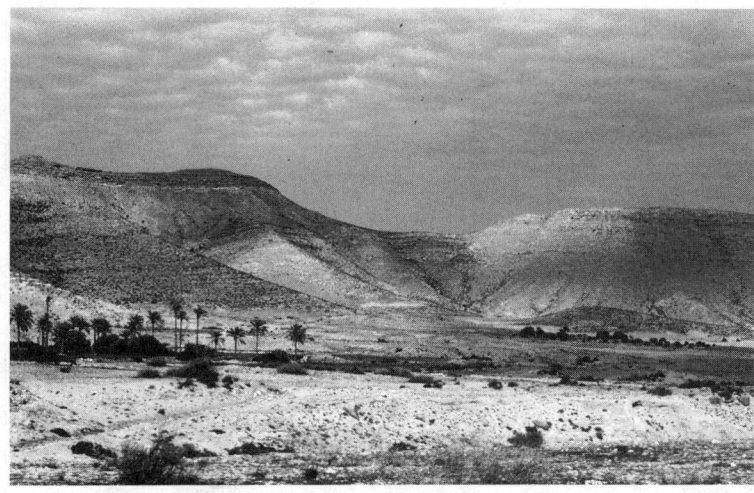

Figure 65.9 The oasis of Rabta in Libya. Typical location for cutaneous leishmaniasis due to *Leishmania major* in north Africa. (Courtesy R. Ashford.)

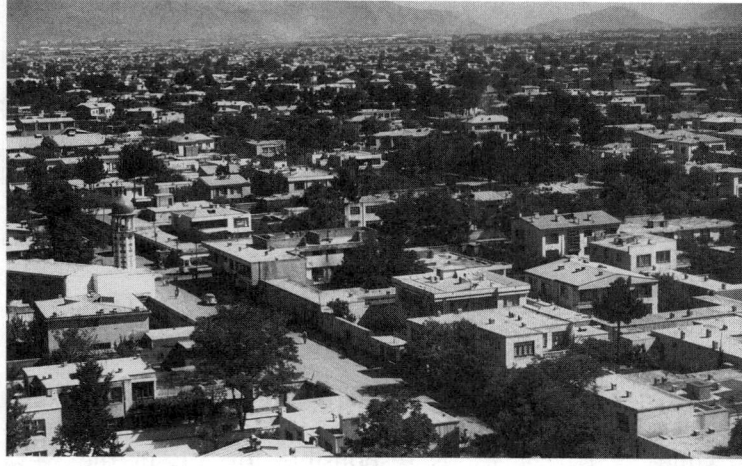

Figure 65.10 Kabul City. Typical location of cutaneous leishmaniasis due to *Leishmania tropica* in the Middle East. (Courtesy R. Ashford.)

some zymodeme variation has been found in Israel, Saudi Arabia and India.[50] North of the Sahara, the reservoirs are the gerbils, especially *Rhombomys opimus*, throughout the range, supported by jirds (*Meriones* spp.) and fat rats (*Psammomus* spp.). Gerbils live in complex burrows up to 3 m deep in the soft soil, in colonies of 10–15 animals, with a mean life span of 12 months. Gerbil populations may vary by a factor of 50, but colonies are stable over decades, even centuries. Infection rates with *L. major* are commonly about 2%, sometimes 20%. Infections are on non-hairy skin, especially ears, and tend to persist throughout the animal's life (Figure 65.9). *P. papatassi* is the most important vector. It is widespread, abundant, aggressive and lives in gerbil burrows and human habitations, biting at dawn and dusk. *P. sergenti*, although widespread, probably plays a secondary role.[51] Transmission is greatest between April and June. The incidence of infection in susceptible humans varies from nil to 100%. All ages are affected. People are at risk in expanding towns and new settlements, or on entering the desert as hunters, soldiers or tourists. Epidemics of CL

may occur, for example at an oasis, for no apparent reason after years of quiescence.[52]

South of the Sahara the infection is less prevalent. Several rodents serve as reservoirs, notably *Arvicanthus* and *Tatera*, but rates of infection are low and the infection is visceral. Human infection is not common, but epidemics have occurred in Sudan. The vector throughout the area is *P. duboscqi*,[53] which lives in rodent burrows.

L. tropica is responsible for anthroponotic cutaneous leishmaniasis of the Old World. It extends round the Mediterranean basin from Greece eastwards, as far north as Serbia and Romania, through Turkey,[54] the Middle East (Figure 65.10), and west Asia to Afghanistan, Pakistan and India as far as Delhi, and on the whole of the northern African littoral. The climatic range is wide. Zymodeme analysis shows marked genetic variation.[55] Transmission is urban, in towns and villages. Man is the principal, possibly only, reservoir. *L. tropica* has been isolated from viscera of *Rattus rattus* in Iraq, and from skin of dogs in India, Russia and Morocco,[56] but the role of these animals as reservoirs is

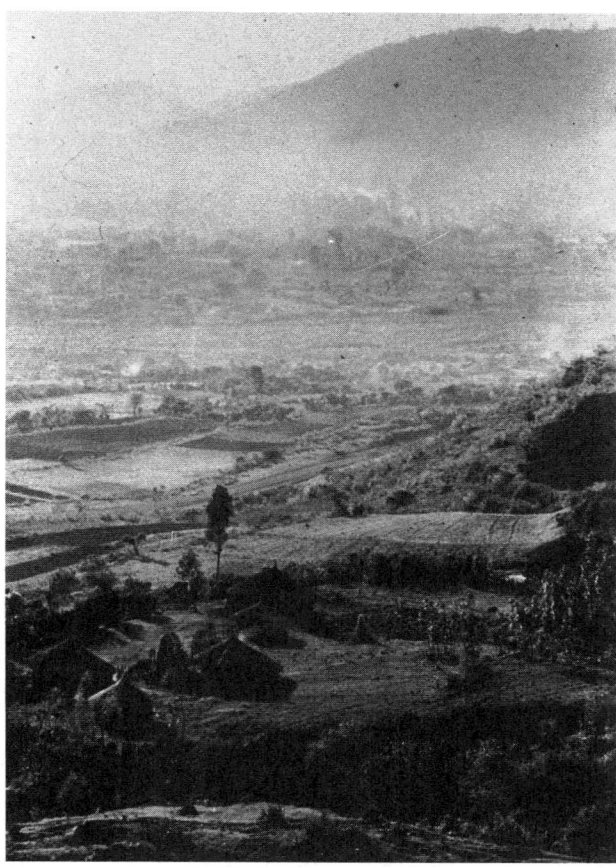

Figure 65.11   Village of Wurgesa in the Ethiopian highlands. Typical location for cutaneous leishmaniasis due to *Leishmania aethiopica*.

uncertain. The most important vector is *P. sergenti*, which is found in greater density in urban than in rural areas. It bites within and without houses, especially in the early evening and at dawn. Transmission peaks in late summer. *P. papatassi* also transmits the infection in the Middle East and North Africa. In affected towns the whole population is at risk, and in the past every adult bore the scar of a sore contracted in childhood. There are innumerable local names for the disease. Rarely, *L. tropica* has been isolated from cases of VL in India, Kenya and Saudi Arabia,[57] and from cases of mucosal leishmaniasis (ML).[58]

L. aethiopica is responsible for cutaneous leishmaniasis in the highlands of Ethiopia (Figure 65.11), western Kenya and eastern Uganda, between 1500 and 2700 metres above sea level, on the rocky escarpments and gorges, and the fertile rolling hill country. The parasite seems to be the least immunogenic of the Old World cutaneous species, and may be capable of suppressing the human immune response, with the production of rare cases of diffuse cutaneous leishmaniasis (DCL). The zoonotic reservoirs are the hyraxes *Procavia habessinica* and *Heterohyrax brucei*, which inhabit rocky outcrops and holes in ancient wild fig trees.[59] Up to 27% have been found infected, bearing mild skin lesions. The vectors, *P. longpipes* and *P. pedifer* live in hyrax burrows, crevices and caves and bite hyrax, cattle and man readily. Up to 15% of parous female flies have been found infected in hyrax burrows. People are most commonly bitten while sitting outside their houses, especially on warm, moist evenings when the flight range is greatest, but they may also be bitten near the rock outcrops or in their houses at night. Thus all ages and sexes are at risk. Up to 40% of the population bear scars of healed lesions, usually on the face, and over 70% are positive to leishmanin by adulthood.[60]

Cutaneous leishmaniasis in Namibia.[61] Two unnamed species of *Leishmania* have been found, one in man and *P. rossi*, and the other in the rock hyrax *Procavia capeses*, but the cycles and epidemiology are not understood. Isolated cases of CL have been reported from Angola, Zaire and Tanzania.

In the New World, at least six species of *Leishmania* cause CL, and three ML. With the exception of *L. peruviana* their geographical distributions overlap, which has made it difficult to sort out their life cycles and epidemiological patterns, and the picture is still incomplete.[17,29,46] The disease is common and grossly underreported. It is zoonotic, and human infections are usually associated with opening up the forest. This leads to destruction of biotypes and a fall in incidence of infection. However, some cycles of transmission are adapting to the new situations so that in some places human disease is increasing.

L. braziliensis is the most common and most serious cause of CL in Central and South America. It is endemic throughout the hot humid natural forest and, as a result of changes in reservoirs and vectors, is becoming adapted to secondary forest and to the suburbs of towns.[62] It is found in Belize, Guatemala, Honduras, Costa Rica, Panama, Peru, Argentina, Bolivia, Paraguay, Colombia and Venezuela, throughout the Amazonian forest below a height of 2000 metres, and in hot forests of the pacific coast of Colombia, and Central America. *L. braziliensis* is heterogeneous, showing marked zymodeme variation. The natural forest reservoirs have not been identified, despite intensive search, but incidental infections have been found in many genera. In its suburban setting, dogs and equines are probably the reservoirs.[63] There are many species of sandfly vectors, most importantly *Psychodopygus welcomei* and *Lu. whitmani*, which bite in the forests, and *Lu. intermedia* which will bite in houses. They are all anthropophilic. Young adult males are most at risk as they develop the forest. In Brazil 63 000 cases were reported over a ten-year period,

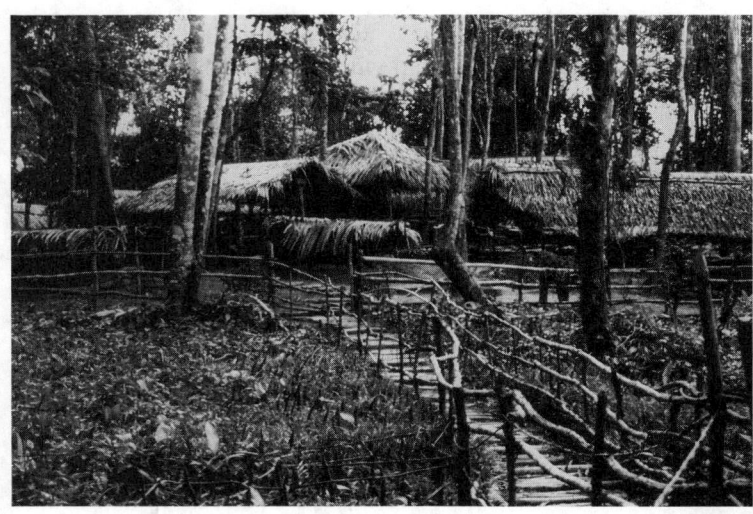

Figure 65.12 Encampment in forest clearing in Belize. Typical location for cutaneous leishmaniasis due to *Leishmania braziliensis*. (Courtesy D. A. Evans.)

and in Ecuador 4000 cases over 4 years, but there are no good incidence data. The majority of cases are of CL, but in Colombia 25% of new cases presenting for treatment are ML, and in Ecuador 7%. Rates for ML subsequent to CL have in the past been put as high as 80% but are more usually under 10%.

L. panamensis is the dominant parasite of Central America, being found in Costa Rica, Honduras, Nicaragua, Panama, Colombia and the Pacific coast of Ecuador. Its natural host is the two-toed sloth *Choleopus hoffmanni*, which lives in the forest canopy, descending at night to defecate and urinate.[64] Numerous other wild species and dogs have been found infected incidentally. Infection rates as high as 48% have been found in sloths close to houses of infected people in Panama.

The principal vectors, *Lu. ylephiletor*, *Lu. trapidoi* and *Lu. shannoni* rest between the tree buttresses, where man becomes an accidental host.[65] In endemic areas, incidence rates between 20 and 200/100 000 are reported. In an epidemic at one microfocus in Costa Rica, 22% of non-immune soldiers were infected within three nights,[66] while in eastern Colombia 60% of the population became infected within 6 years of the introduction of the infection.

L. guyanensis is restricted to the Amazonian forests of Brazil, Colombia, French Guiana, Guyana and Surinam. Its natural hosts are the arboreal sloth *Choleopus didactylus* and anteater *Tamandra tetradactyla*, with *Choleopus marsupialis* amplifying the infection peridomestically. The main vectors, *Lu. umbratilis* and *Lu. anduzei*, rest between the tree buttresses. In French Guiana young male adults are most at risk, entering the forest for soldiering, hunting, road work and settlement. Infections are most common after the rains, in April–May and November–December.[67] In Panama about 2–5% of cases will later develop ML.[68]

L. mexicana is most prevalent in the Yucatan peninsula of Mexico, but extends through Guatemala, Honduras, and Panama to Colombia. A closely related parasite is found in Texas, and the Dominican Republic.[69] Numerous rodents that inhabit the forest floor serve as reservoirs, including *Ototylomus* spp., *Heteromys* spp., *Nyctomys* spp. and *Sigodon* spp. The rate of infection is high. The vector *Lu. olmeca olmeca* rests in the forest litter and will bite man if disturbed. The incidence among adult males who work in the Yucatan forests is 500/100 000, and 90% become leishmanin positive.[70] The pinna of the ear is the most common site of infection. Rare cases of DCL occur,[71] especially in the Dominican Republic, where no self-healing forms have yet been reported.

L. amazonensis occurs throughout the Amazon forests of Brazil, Bolivia, Colombia, Ecuador, Peru, French Guiana and Venezuela. It exhibits some zymodeme variation and its cycle of transmission has become adapted to secondary forest and to plantations. Rodents of the forest floor, especially *Proechimys* spp. and *Oryzomis* spp., commonly carry inapparent skin infections, and the intensity of infection is high. The vector, *Lu. flavisculleta*, is widespread but not anthropophilic. Human infections occur throughout the area, but are relatively rare, and there is a disproportionately high rate of cases of DCL, suggesting that the parasite is not well adapted to man. Cases of VL have also been attributed to *L. amazonensis*.[72]

L. peruviana is responsible for cutaneous leishmaniasis in the high valleys of the Andes of Peru and the Argentinian highlands, at an altitude of 1200–3000 metres. It is generally recognized as a separate species but isoenzyme analysis cannot distinguish it from *L. braziliensis* (Figure 65.12). It affects villagers and rural workers. The dog is thought to be the urban reservoir, but there is probably a wild reservoir in the forest galleries that accompany the steep mountain streams. About 2000 cases are reported annually in Peru. There are no reported cases of ML. *Lu. peruviana* and *Lu. verrucarum* are the vectors.

CUTANEOUS AND MUCOSAL LEISHMANIASIS

PATHOGENESIS[73]

Leishmania multiply in cells of the mononuclear phagocyte system, which includes blood monocytes, macrophages, histiocytes, epithelioid cells, Kupffer cells and reticuloendothelial cells in spleen and lymphoid tissue. Inoculated promastigotes are phagocytosed in the skin and transform into amastigotes and start to divide. One of three events follows:

(1) Parasites are killed by a successful immune response and the person becomes immune to reinfection by that species.
(2) A local infection is established which persists until the host's immune response eradicates it or is overwhelmed, permitting dissemination.
(3) The infection metastasizes through the bloodstream to the viscera (viscerotropic species), oronasal mucosa (*L. braziliensis* commonly, others rarely)[74] or skin (especially *L. aethiopica* and *L. mexicana* if cell-mediated immunity fails). Distant metastasis via the lymphatics is rare as parasites are destroyed in lymph nodes.

CUTANEOUS LEISHMANIASIS

In any early lesion of CL, infected macrophages are infiltrated or surrounded by lymphocytes and plasma cells, following which one or more patterns may develop.[75,76] Ridley has identified five types, but they are not necessarily sequential, and more than one pattern may be seen in an individual case.[77] The patterns reflect the nature of the immune response, rather than the species of *Leishmania*. The non-specific early pattern (type III) may linger, especially with *L. aethiopica* infections, which tend to persist with little ulceration or crusting. Lysis of individual infected macrophages may contain the infection.[78] When *L. braziliensis* lesions show this pattern, there is a high rate of secondary mucosal disease.[78] The most common pattern in self-healing CL is of microfoci of epithelioid cells and necrosis, whereby infected macrophages are destroyed (type

II). This occurs when a particular ratio of plasma cells to lymphocytes has accumulated, and involves deposition of immune complexes on the macrophage surface.[79]

Chronicity is associated with the development of a classical tuberculoid pattern, with epithelioid cell granulomas and scanty parasites (type IV). It is especially associated with recidivans leishmaniasis[80] and ML in Ethiopia.[81] In this situation parasites are digested by macrophages as a result of classical cell-mediated immune mechanisms, involving the production by lymphocytes of interleukin 2 and interferon-γ,[82–84] and the generation of intracellular nitric oxide from L-arginine.[85] Usually, the epidermis breaks down and the resulting ulcer is filled with a crust or exudate of cell debris, dead and live parasites and serum. Rejection of parasitized macrophages may be a fourth way for the elimination of the infection. When cell-mediated immunity fails, the infiltrate consists entirely of heavily parasitized macrophages, many of which are vacuolated, and a variable number of plasma cells (type 1). This pattern characterizes DCL,[81] a condition in which specific cell-mediated immunity is not expressed,[86] and in which adherent suppressor cells have been found.[87] Thus there is a histological spectrum in leishmaniasis, based on immunity, but it differs from that seen in leprosy and is not expressed across its whole range by any one species.[88]

Epidermal changes also reflect the development and type of immune response. The epidermis thickens and pseudoepitheliomatous hyperplasia may be striking. In the dermis, collagen is swollen and disrupted; later there is an influx of fibroblasts and healing is accompanied by fibrosis. Some lesions due to *L. braziliensis* are accompanied by vasculitis and fibrinous exudate.

Animal experiments indicate that resistance and susceptibility,[89] type of disease[90] and immunopathology[91] are genetically controlled and vary according to the strain of mouse infected with a given species of *Leishmania*. Genetic susceptibility in man is poorly understood. In Venezuela HLA class I haplotypes HLA-Bw22 and HLA-DQw3 are associated with 12- and 4-fold increases, respectively, in risk of acquiring CL.[92]

POST-KALA-AZAR DERMAL LEISHMANIASIS

Indian PKDL is characterized by dermal infiltration with histiocytes, plasma cells and lymphocytes that is variable in distribution, extent and intensity. It is more intense and parasites are more numerous in the nodular variety. Epidermal changes are not marked and there is no ulceration.[93] As a rule, viscera are spared. Immunoglobulin and antibody responses are less marked than in VL, and tend towards normal in the more chronic cases.[94] Specific cell-mediated responses to leishmanial antigens are less consistently and less severely suppressed than in VL, and non-specific responses are normal.[95] These abnormalities take longer to normalize after treatment than in VL. The basis of the change from viscerotropism to dermotropism and of the delicate prolonged balance between infection and immunity that characterize Indian PKDL have not been explained.

In Africa PKDL is characterized by a tuberculoid histology, scanty parasites and a positive leishmanin test. It represents recognition and destruction of residual cutaneous parasites by the emergent cellular immune response.

MUCOSAL LEISHMANIASIS

The early lesion is in the deep mucosa of the nose or mouth. An infiltrate of lymphocytes and plasma cells develops around small arterioles whose endothelial cells contain amastigotes.[96] The inflammation extends towards the mucosal surface and may assume any of the various histological patterns that are seen in CL, especially the necrotic.[97] Necrosis and endarteritis may cause severe mutilating destruction of tissue. More granulomatous lesions cause enlargement and protuberance of nose and lips, and occlusion of the pharynx, and even larynx. Cell-mediated hypersensitivity is strong and the leishmanin test positive.

CLINICAL FEATURES

The incubation period ranges from a few days to several months, sometimes over a year; experimentally, this is determined by the size of the inoculum.[98] One or more lesions appear on uncovered parts of the body. The face, neck, arms and legs are the most common sites. At the site of inoculation a nodule appears, erythematous in pale skins. As it grows, a golden, brown or blood-stained crust forms centrally, which may persist or fall away, leaving an

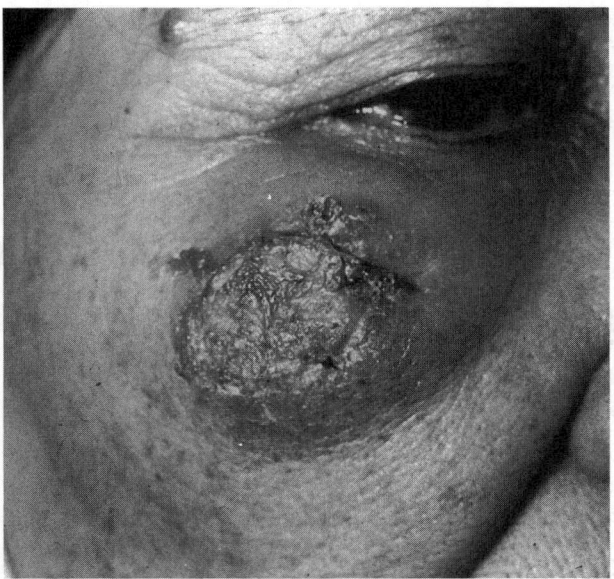

Figure 65.13 Cutaneous leishmaniasis due to *Leishmania major*, Iran. Typical sore with golden crust and surrounding erythema.

ulcer, which usually has a raised edge. The sore remains in this stage for a variable time, often without further growth, before healing, leaving a depressed, mottled scar. Secondary bacterial infection is unimportant. Satellite lesions are common. The lesions are not normally painful but may irritate at first. They may disfigure or disable if scarring is severe, especially over a joint or on the face. Healing is normally accompanied by lifelong immunity to the same species of parasite. Recurrence may represent relapse associated with old age or depressed immunity, or reinfection with a different zymodeme.[99,100] This pattern is basic to all self-healing sores but the natural history differs between species of *Leishmania*, and there tend to be characteristic, but inconstant, clinical differences.[101]

CUTANEOUS LEISHMANIASIS

CL due to *L. major* has an incubation period of 1 week to 2 months. Lesions necrose rapidly and tend to be inflamed and exudative 'wet sores', (Figures 65.13 and 65.14). They reach their maximum size, usually 3–6 cm over 2–3 months, and heal within 3–5 months. Lesions are most common on the limbs.[102,103] Lesions on lips or nose do not spread to the mucosae. During epidemics the disease tends to be more severe, with multiple lesions, often deeply ulcerated, affecting people of all ages and both sexes equally,[52,104] and lesions along the draining lymphatics are common.

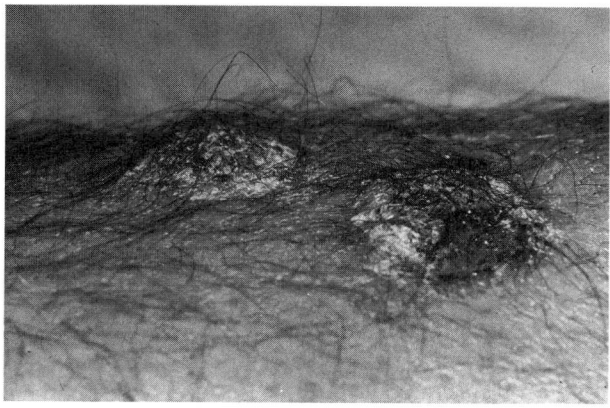

Figure 65.14   Cutaneous leishmaniasis due to *Leishmania major*, Saudi Arabia. Dense crusts conceal the underlying ulcer.

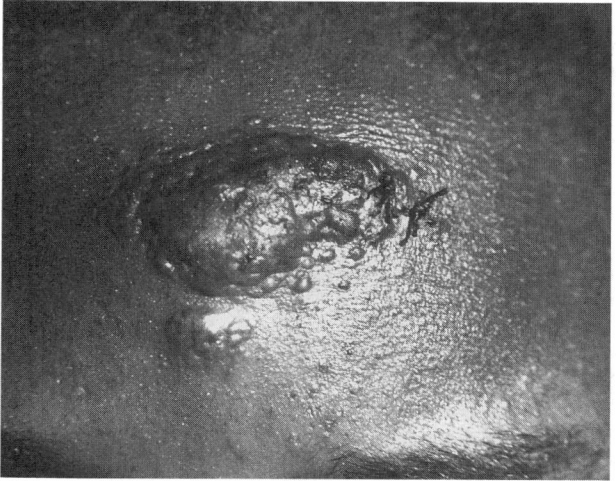

Figure 65.16   Cutaneous leishmaniasis due to *Leishmania aethiopica*, Kenya. Typical large nodule with numerous small satellite papules.

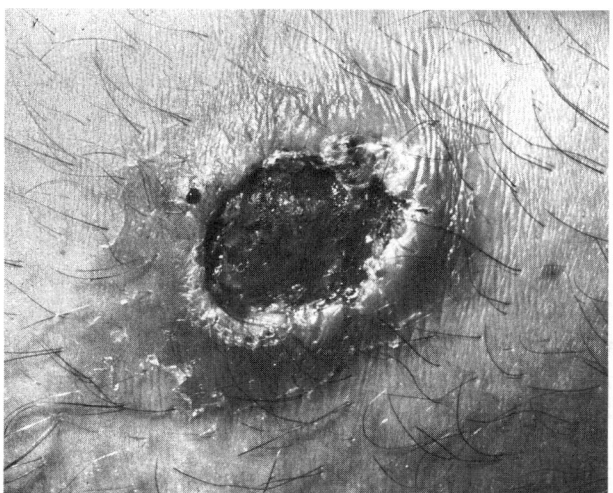

Figure 65.15   Cutaneous leishmaniasis due to *Leishmania major*, Israel. Typical ulcer with raised edge.

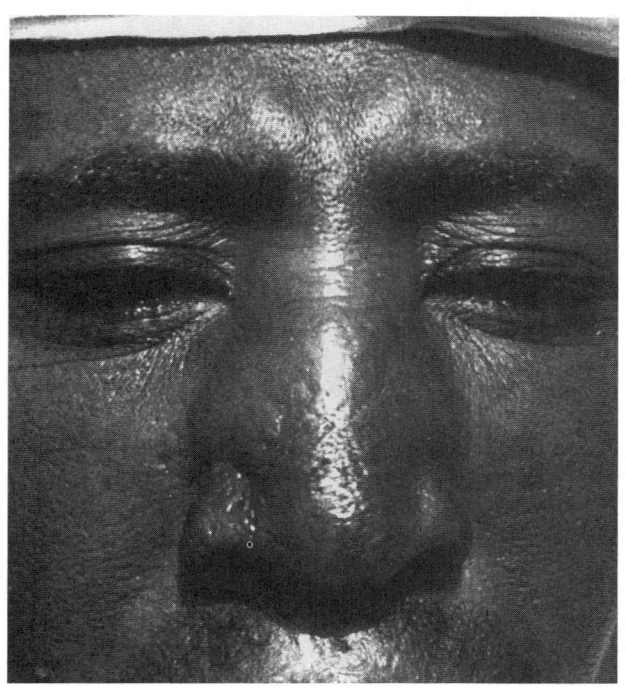

Figure 65.17   Mucocutaneous leishmaniasis due to *Leishmania aethiopica*, Ethiopia. Showing characteristic expansion of nose and upper lip.

CL due to *L. tropica* is slower in evolution and less severe. The incubation period is normally 2–4 months but may be as long as 2 years. The initial nodule may develop little satellite papules. It reaches its maximum diameter of 1–2 cm over 8–12 months, crusting slowly, and heals within 10–14 months, occasionally longer, and a few become very persistent. Lesions are commonly on the face; children are commonly affected.[102,105]

CL due to *L. infantum*[106] and *L. chagasi*[107] is even less aggressive. The incubation period may exceed 1 year. The lesions are nodular, may never ulcerate and last from 1–3 years. They are most common on the face. Mucosal lesions of the nose, mouth and larynx occur rarely.[108]

CL due to *L. aethiopica* causes solitary lesions centrally on the face. Satellite papules accumulate to produce a spreading nodule (Figure 65.18), tumour or plaque that may not crust or ulcerate but heals slowly over 2–5 years.[60] If the lesion is at the mucocutaneous border of the nose or mouth, the infection may spread along the mucocutaneous margins, producing expansion of the lips or nose (Figure 65.17), and persist for many years, though without the severe destruction that characterizes mucocutaneous disease in South America; nor does the disease spread further into the oronasal cavities.[81]

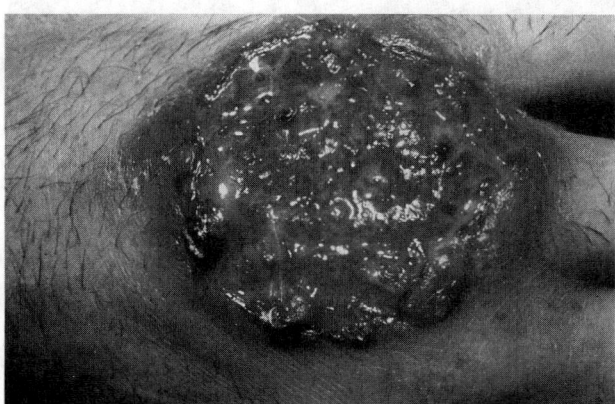

Figure 65.18 Large ulcer on dorsum of hand due to *Leishmania braziliensis* from Belize.

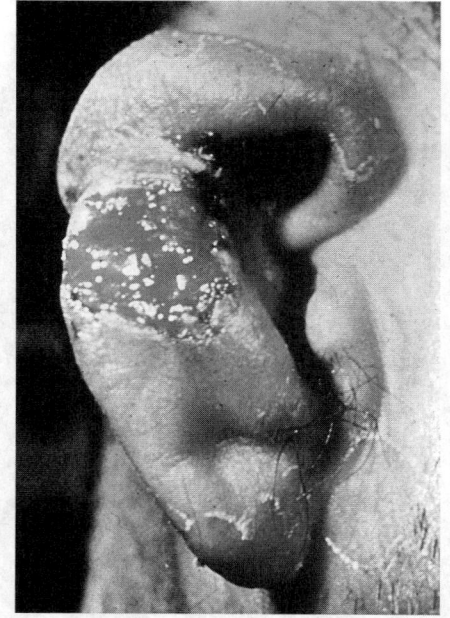

Figure 65.19 'Chiclero ulcer'. Cutaneous leishmaniasis eroding the cartilage of the pinna, due to *Leishmania mexicana*, Mexico. (Courtesy L. Ash.)

CL due to *L. braziliensis* causes deep, usually single, rapidly developing ulcers with raised red edges, especially on the limbs (Figure 65.18).[109,110] Eighty per cent of sores heal within 1 year,[111] but the infection is common and many people have sores that last up to 10 years. Up to 15% of patients present with recrudesences or second infections.[100] Sores may appear unexpectedly at the site of an injury.

CL due to *L. guyanensis* is commonly known as 'pian bois' or bush yaws. Lesions are often multiple, on the trunk or limbs, and associated in up to half the cases with lymphatic spread. Lymph vessels are palpably thickened and contain nodules that may ulcerate, so producing chains of ulcers.[112] Facial lesions may be associated with alarming brawny oedema.[113]

CL due to *L. panamensis*[114] is also associated with lymphatic and lymph node involvement, and sores may persist for many years.

CL due to *L. peruviana* is known as 'uta'. Lesions are usually on the face, single, in children, and heal in 3–6 months. Most adults in endemic areas bear scars. The infection does not metastasize to the mucosae but a primary sore on the nostril or lip may run along the mucocutaneous margin.

CL due to *L. mexicana*[114,115] commonly causes sores on the side of the face or behind the ears (Figure 65.19), that heal in 6–8 months (chiclero ulcer). When they occur on the pinna of the ear, however, the infection becomes chronic, cartilage is invaded, and the pinna is slowly destroyed over many years.

CL due to *L. amazonensis*[116] lesions are usually solitary, without lymphatic involvement, but little is known of their natural history.

Four forms of CL do not heal spontaneously.

DIFFUSE CUTANEOUS LEISHMANIASIS[81,117]

This occurs in about 1 per 10 000 infections with *L. aethiopica* (Figure 65.20),[118] a much greater proportion of cases with *L. amazonensis*, and is the rule with the parasite of the Dominican Republic.[119] The primary lesion does not ulcerate but, after a period of months or years, spreads slowly locally and through the bloodstream to other parts of the skin, especially the cooler extensor surfaces of the limbs, and face, producing nodules, plaques and hypopigmented macules that may resemble lepromatous leprosy and cause grotesque deformity. External genitalia may be affected but mucosae, eyes and internal organs are spared. The disease progresses for many years and spontaneous healing is rare.

LEISHMANIASIS RECIDIVANS[80]

Relapsing, recidivans or lupoid leishmaniasis represents persistence of the infection in the face of a vigorous immune response and is a rare complication of infection with *L. tropica*. Red-brown or yellow-brown papules appear in or around the scar of a healed sore and continue to ulcerate, heal and reappear over many years. They may form a plaque, resembling lupus vulgaris, that covers relatively large areas of skin (Figure 65.21). Keloidal, verru-

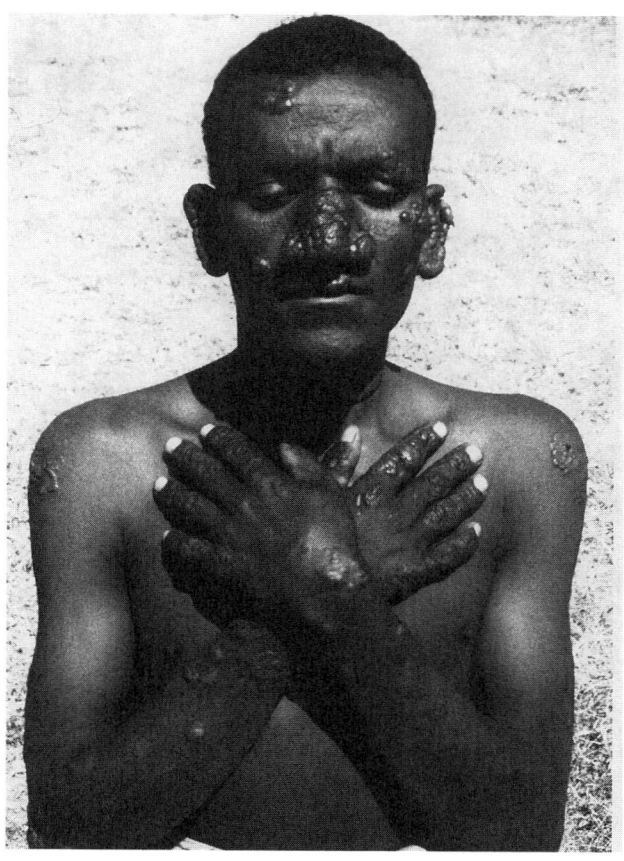

Figure 65.20   Diffuse cutaneous leishmaniasis due to *Leishmania aethiopia*, Ethiopia. Showing widespread semi-symmetrical dissemination of nodules.

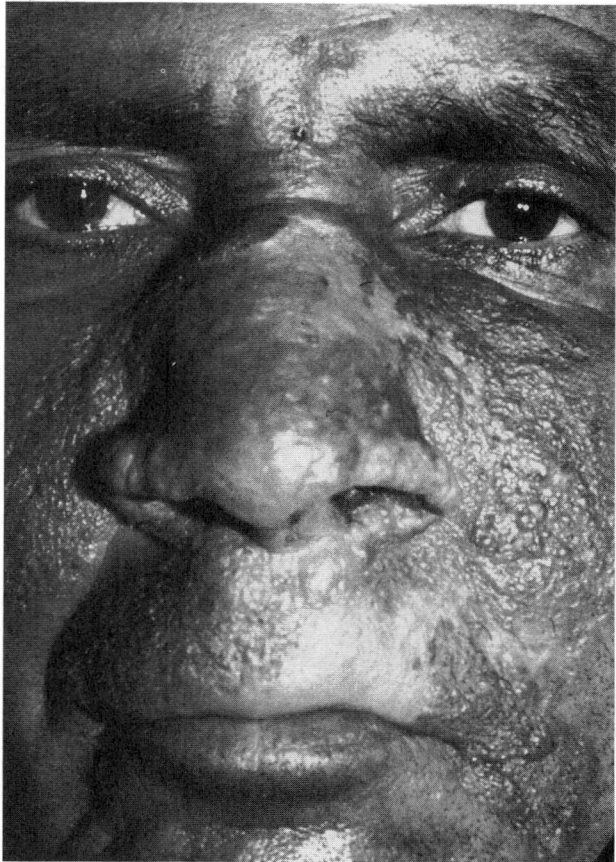

Figure 65.21   Leishmaniasis recidivans due to *Leishmania tropica*, Baghdad, Iraq, showing central scarring with persistent peripheral papules. (Courtesy Dr Ahmed.)

cous and psoriaform lesions are described. The lesions are often worse in the summer months.

POST-KALA-AZAR DERMAL LEISHMANIASIS[120]

This is a sequel to infection with *L. donovani*. Most patients give a history of previous treatment for VL, some of a clinical self-healing febrile illness compatible with VL, and others no such history. Attack rates of PKDL following VL are quoted at 6–20% in India and 2–5% in East Africa. Cases are occasionally seen in China. Increasing incidence may be associated with progression from epidemicity to endemicity.[26]

In India the onset is insidious. Lesions commonly start to appear after an interval of 1–2 years, sometimes longer,[121] and diagnosis may be delayed for 20 years.[122] Hypopigmented macules appear over chin, lips, neck, extensor surfaces of arms, inner sides of thighs, and eventually all over the body, sparing the scalp, palms, soles, axillae and perineum. Consequently, or independently, nodules develop in a similar distribution. External genitalia and the mu-

cosa of nose, mouth and occasionally pharynx may be affected. Verrucous, papillomatous, xanthomatous and gigantic nodular forms are described.[123] PKDL progresses over many years and seldom heals spontaneously. Clinically, PKDL may be confused with lepromatous leprosy, but peripheral nerves are not involved and slit-skin smears fail to show acid-fast bacilli (Figures 65.22 and 65.23).

In East Africa PKDL commonly occurs at the end of the course of treatment for VL, presenting as a transient papular rash over face and forearms or as a crop of well-defined rounded papules, less than 5 mm in diameter, that heal spontaneously within a few months. Rarely, late onset and clinical features resemble Indian PKDL.[124] The differential diagnosis is against sarcoidosis and tuberculosis.

AMERICAN MUCOSAL LEISHMANIASIS[109,114,125]

Between 2 and 40% of patients with cutaneous ulcers due to *L. braziliensis* (Figure 65.24), and a much smaller proportion of those due to *L. guyan-*

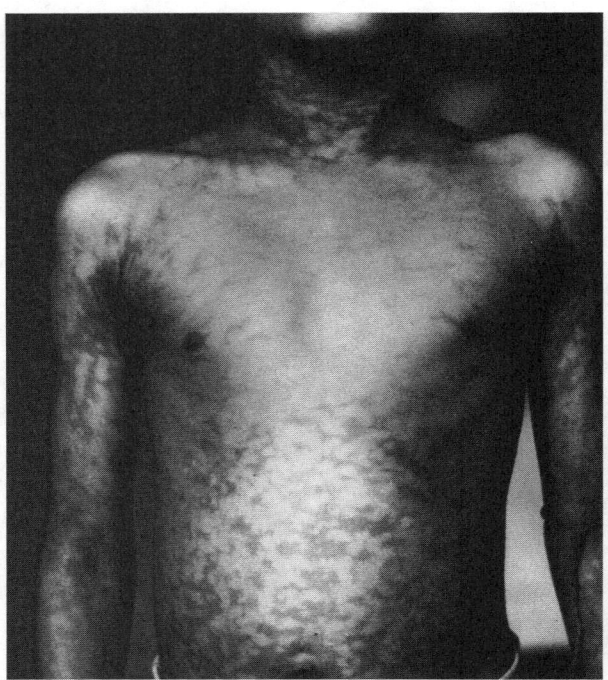

Figure 65.22   Post kala-azar dermal leishmaniasis. Widespread macules typical of early PKDL in India.

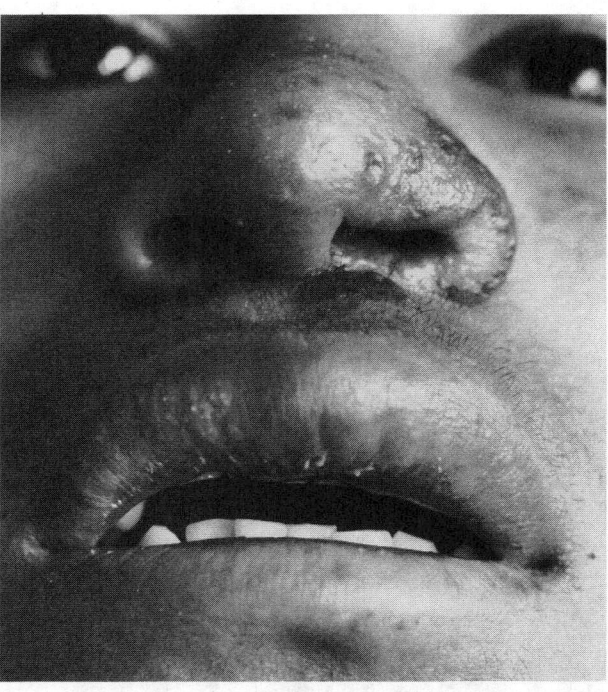

Figure 65.24   Mucosal leishmaniasis due to *Leishmania braziliensis*, Peru. Showing expansion of the upper lip and spread of the disease from the nasal mucosa onto the skin.

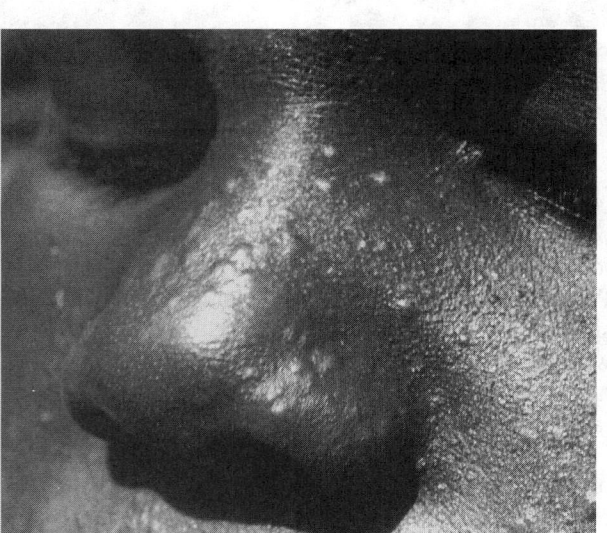

Figure 65.23   Post kala-azar dermal leishmaniasis, Kenya. Showing typical small papules on the face.

ensis and *L. panamensis*,[46] will develop metastatic mucosal lesions, often about the time that the ulcer heals. Young adult males who have had multiple or chronic primary lesions, particularly above the waist, are at greatest risk. The condition may be worse in those of Negro origin.[126] Fifty per cent of

mucosal lesions arise within 2 years of the appearance of the ulcer, and 90% within 10 years. Delays of up to 35 years are recorded.[127] About 15% of cases of ML give no previous history of a skin lesion. Most commonly the nasal mucosa is affected anteriorly, and in a third of cases another site is also involved: the pharynx, larynx and upper lip, in order of frequency.

The initial lesion is a nodule, usually on the anterior septum or inferior turbinate, and the initial symptom is of nasal obstruction or epistaxis. The septum perforates early, the nasal cartilage may collapse and the destructive lesion spreads at a variable speed to involve oronasopharyngeal mucosa down to and sometimes beyond the larynx, causing dysphonia and predisposing to pneumonia. The infection spreads from the mucosa to the mucocutaneous junctions of the lips and nose, and sometimes on to the surrounding facial skin or conjunctiva. If hypertrophy predominates, a grossly protuberant nose and mouth develop, a condition known as espundia (Portuguese: a sponge); if ulceration predominates, there is severe mutilation. Nasal, pharyngeal and laryngeal obstruction from exuberant growth or fibrotic stenosis are serious, even fatal complications. Death may also ensue from secondary sepsis, pneumonia or starvation. Spontaneous healing is unusual.[128]

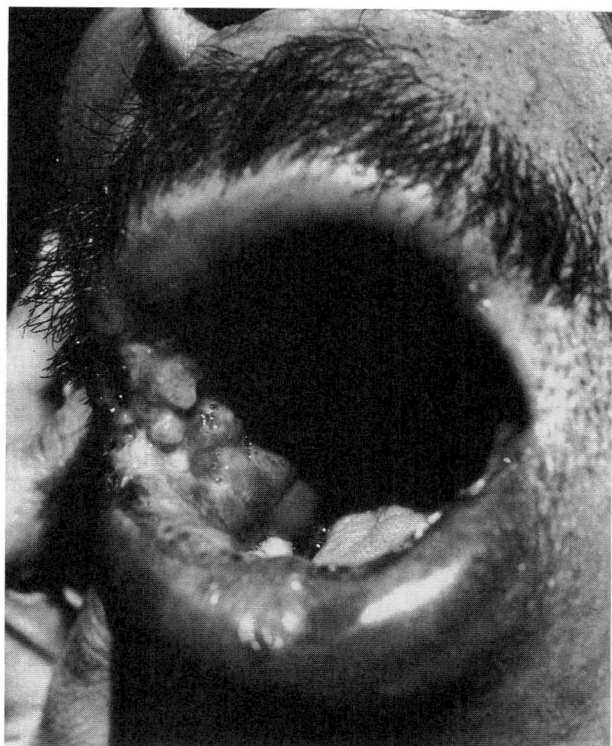

Figure 65.25 Mucosal leishmaniasis due to *Leishmania braziliensis*, Peru—showing extensive nodular infiltration on the buccal mucosa.

LABORATORY FINDINGS

PARASITOLOGICAL DIAGNOSIS

Leishmania may normally be isolated from up to 80% of sores during the first half of their natural course.[60,129] After that, parasitological diagnosis becomes more difficult. From a nodular lesion, or the nodular edge of the lesion, tissue is best obtained by the slit-skin smear, as in leprosy. The nodule is grasped firmly between finger and thumb to exclude blood, and an incision a few millimetres long is made into the dermis. The scalpel blade is used to scrape tissue juice, not blood. The material obtained is used to inoculate culture media and to make smears on slides, which are fixed and stained with Giemsa, Wright's or Leishman's stain. The culture media most commonly employed are diphasic rabbit-blood agar media or supplemented insect tissue culture media, but different species may have particular requirements and cultures may need to be established on several media to maximize the chance of growth.[130,131] Exudate or scrapings from the base of an ulcer may also be treated similarly, but secondary bacterial or fungal infection may contaminate the cultures.

Biopsy specimens may be used to make im-pression smears, cultured or inoculated into hamsters, or, least efficient, sent for histological examination. Immunoperoxidase staining helps to identify scanty parasites in tissue sections.[132]

For cutaneous lesions smears and culture are usually adequate, but for mucosal lesions biopsy and hamster inoculation are best, with a yield approaching 50%.[129,133] Species identification is important in areas where there is a risk of *L. braziliensis* infection (Figure 65.25). Isoenzyme methods are best developed but too slow for immediate clinical value. Monoclonal antibodies[134] and DNA probes[135] are simpler, quicker and available in some reference laboratories.

IMMUNODIAGNOSIS

Leishmanin is a suspension of washed promastigotes in a solution of 0.5% phenol in saline. To be valid the antigen must be standardized against cases and controls in the endemic area.[136] The leishmanin test is performed by inoculating 0.1 ml leishmanin into the volar surface of the forearm and measuring the area of induration 48–72 hours later. The test is positive in well over 90% of cases of CL and ML, but less frequently in *L. aethiopica* infections or in cases of ML with multiple sites of disease.[129]

Antibodies may be detected in low titre in a proportion of cases of CL but serology is not of practical value for diagnosis.[137] In ML, however, antibodies are more consistently and readily detected, and are useful for diagnosis. Enzyme linked immunosorbent assay (ELISA) is highly specific and sensitive.[138] The indirect immunofluorescence test (IFAT) is less sensitive but particularly useful in assessing progress and detecting relapse after treatment.[139]

TREATMENT[140]

SIMPLE SORES

General considerations

Most simple sores, especially from the Old World, will heal spontaneously without complications and may not need treatment; but treatment may accelerate healing and reduce the severity of scarring. Indications for treatment include sores on disfiguring or disabling sites, such as the face or over a joint, multiple sores, or sores at a site where healing is likely to be slow, for example, on the lower leg or pinna. Sores that might be due to *L. braziliensis* require systemic treatment to prevent espundia. CL associated with an immune defect, as in leishmaniasis recidivans or DCL, or possibly HIV-infected individuals, may not heal untreated. No single method of treatment is suitable for all forms of the disease.

Local treatment

Physical methods

These include surgical excision,[141] curettage,[142] heat[143] and freezing.[144] Surgery is suitable only for small facial lesions, and in competent hands produces a more acceptable scar. Curettage under local anaesthetic permits healing in 3–6 weeks, according to the size of the sore. Heating to 39–41°C kills dermatotropic species of *Leishmania* and maximizes the efficiency of lymphocytes and macrophages, thus accelerating natural healing. It is necessary to maintain this temperature for many hours over several days. Methods of delivering heat are cumbersome and unsuitable for routine use; they include plastic sacks containing water circulating from a thermostatically controlled water bath, thermostatically controlled pads and infrared. Heat is a useful supplement to systemic treatment when healing is slow, for example on a cool extremity. Cryotherapy, using liquid nitrogen or carbon dioxide snow, is suitable for small well-defined lesions with little surrounding inflammation.

Chemical methods

Aminosidine ointment (15% with 15% urea in white soft paraffin) cures up to 80% of Old World sores if applied for up to 12 weeks.[145] A preparation of aminosidine 15% and methylbenzethonium chloride 12% cures 77% of sores due to *L. major* within 10 days, but may cause unacceptable inflammation.[146] Careful infiltration of sodium stibogluconate or meglumine antimoniate into the edge and base of the lesion is effective against small sores or larger chronic sores without significant inflammation. Using a 1 ml syringe and very fine needle, less than 1 ml suffices for a 2 × 3 cm lesion.[147,148] A second or third injection at intervals of 2–3 days may be needed.

Systemic treatment

Antimonials remain the most generally useful and available treatment (see p. 1073 for details). Dermatotrophic species of *Leishmania* are normally sensitive at conventional dosage, with the exception of *L. aethiopica*, although there is a wide range of sensitivity in vitro among New World isolates,[149] including instances of primary resistance. Isolates from relapsed patients are 10–17 times less susceptible than primary isolates, and are therefore often unresponsive to treatment. The regimen given on Table 65.5 is suitable for most previously untreated cases, although some recommend a full 20 mg Sb/kg body weight for *L. braziliensis* and *L. panamensis*.[150] Three weeks is usually adequate but if response is slow treatment should be continued longer. It is important not to undertreat lesions due to *L. braziliensis*; serology is useful in follow-up. Persistent or rising titres of antibodies detected by immunofluorescence are strongly indicative of relapse.[139] The upper limit of 850 mg Sb per dose, as recommended by the World Health Organization (WHO),[151] should be disregarded.

Other drugs are less well established, and no generalizations may be made. Success has been claimed for allopurinol against sores due to *L. panamensis* in Colombia,[152] and for ketoconazole in a dose of 600 mg daily for 30 days against *L. panamensis* in Panama,[153] and *L. mexicana* and against *L. major* in Sinai.[154] Itraconazole has a better pharmacokinetic profile than ketoconazole but data on efficacy are scanty. Dapsone in a dose of 200 mg daily for 4 weeks cured 82% of CL sores in India.[155]

There are no indications for *immunotherapy* in simple CL, although local injections of interferon-γ increase histological markers of cellular immunity.[148]

LEISHMANIASIS RECIDIVANS

Local or systemic injections of antimonials, as for simple CL, are usually curative.[156]

DIFFUSE CUTANEOUS LEISHMANIASIS

Treatment needs to be prolonged until the last parasite has been eliminated. In practice this means until slit-skin smears from several sites have become negative, and for a further 2–4 months.[157] *L. aethiopica* responds to aminosidine, but the relapsed parasite is less sensitive by a factor of four. Treatment should be with aminosidine in a dose of 15 mg/kg body weight and sodium stibogluconate (see Table 65.5) daily.[158] Alternatively, pentamidine should be given in a dose of 4 mg salt per kg body weight by intramuscular injection once weekly.[157] Similar principles should be applied to DCL in Latin America, where antimonials are by contrast of value in previously untreated cases. In both situations concurrent heat treatment has been found helpful.[143] It would seem logical to follow chemotherapy with immunotherapy.

MUCOSAL LEISHMANIASIS

ML due to *L. braziliensis* is difficult to treat. It responds slowly and relapse rates are high after treatment with antimonials given in the WHO recommended dose of 20 mg Sb/kg body weight daily for 28 days: 30% overall or 90% in advanced cases with laryngeal involvement.[159,160] The prognosis is worse in patients who have previously received antimony, in many of whom the disease has become unresponsive to antimonials, and in patients with intercurrent disease. For previously untreated cases without laryngeal involvement, antimonials should be given at 20 mg Sb/kg body weight daily for 6–8 weeks. When there is laryngeal involvement, or in previously treated cases, amphotericin should be used in a dose of 1 mg/kg body weight by intra-venous infusion on alternate days for 6–8 weeks.[140] Ideally treatment should be monitored by laryngoscopy, biopsy and serology. Liposomal amphotericin and aminosidine are under trial. The first few doses of an effective drug may induce laryngeal oedema, which should be treated with corticosteroids for a few days. Later, plastic surgery may be necessary to correct residual defects.

TREATMENT OF POST-KALA-AZAR DERMAL LEISHMANIASIS

In well-nourished Kenyan children the condition is self-healing and no further treatment is necessary. In the epidemic situation in malnourished patients in Sudan, and in India, the condition persists. There are no clear published guidelines for treatment. In principle, treatment with an antimonial should be given in a dose of 20 mg Sb/kg daily for 3–4 months.[140]

VISCERAL LEISHMANIASIS

PATHOGENESIS

SUSCEPTIBILITY AND RESISTANCE

In the endemic situation there are about 30–100 subclinical infection for every case of VL,[161,162] but fewer in the epidemic situation of Sudan.[163] Healing is associated with the development of tuberculoid granulomas in the liver, the transient appearance of antibodies and the acquisition of leishmanin posi-tivity.[161] Risk factors for the development of VL include malnutrition[25] and immune depression due to organ transplantation, haematological neoplasia, corticosteroid treatment and HIV infection.[27]

IMMUNOLOGY

Established VL represents the failure of specific cell-mediated immunity to control the infection. The leishmanin test is negative, as are in vitro tests of lymphocyte responses to leishmanial antigens, as judged by transformation,[164] and of the production of interferon-γ.[165–168]

There is a general depression of cell-mediated immune responses, shown by reduced responses to intradermal antigens.[164] This depression, together with malnutrition and leucopenia, probably under-lies the high rate of secondary infections that are the common causes of death in VL, notably measles, tuberculosis, pneumococcal disease, bronchopneu-monia and cancrum oris.[168]

HISTOPATHOLOGY

Parasites multiply more or less freely in mono-nuclear phagocytic cells throughout the visceral reti-culoendothelial system, notably the spleen, liver, bone marrow and lymphoid tissue.[169,170] In the

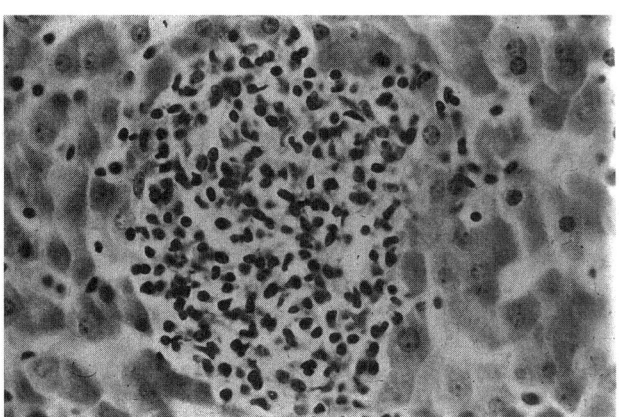

Figure 65.26 Liver biopsy showing granuloma composed of lymphocytes and epithelioid cells in a patient with self-healing visceral leishmaniasis. (Courtesy S. Pampiglione.)

spleen, the red pulp is heavily infiltrated, and the germinal centres atrophic. Infarcts are common. In the liver, Kupffer cells are hypertrophied, hyperplastic and heavily parasitized and push out into the sinusoids. In a heavy infection this may reach as far as centrilobular veins. If venous congestion is severe there may be patchy necrosis of groups of hepatocytes, but severe hepatocellular damage is rare.[170] In other cases discrete granulomas are found in the lobules and portal tracts, comprising macrophages, plasma cells and lymphocytes, but without epithelioid cell differentiation (Figure 65.26). Parasites are scanty and hepatocytes normal.[171] A fibrogenic response may develop, with intralobular proliferation of reticulin fibres and deposition of collagen bands, which may lead to multifocal perisinusoidal fibrosis. Cirrhosis is a rare complication of long-standing VL. Lymph nodes show sinusoidal cell proliferation and parasitization and depletion of germinal centres.[169] Duodenal and jejunal mucosa is thickened and the villi blunted; the submucosa is infiltrated with parasitized macrophages, plasma cells and lymphocytes.[172] The bone marrow is usually hyperplastic, but with some dyserythropoiesis and maturation arrest.[173] Parasites may be found in apparently normal skin and circulate in the blood.[174] Three-quarters of patients coming to autopsy show interstitial pneumonitis with mononuclear cells, which may contain amastigotes or leishmanial antigen.[175]

CLINICAL PATHOLOGY

This cellular infiltration and parasitization of the reticuloendothelial system is accompanied by typical cellular and biochemical changes in the blood, and sometimes secondary tissue pathology, that may or may not lead to significant physiological disturbance. Globulins are overproduced, especially immunoglobulin IgG and IgM, whose mean values may be five times and twice those of the local norms, respectively.[176] Some of this immunoglobulin is antileishmanial antibody.[177] Some represents B-cell polyclonal activation with the production of many autoantibodies to various proteins and haptens[178] and cytoplasmic and nuclear antigens.[179] Complement is activated, complement levels are reduced[176] and immune complexes present in high titre, notably cryoglobulins and rheumatoid factor.[180] Immune complex-mediated disease is, however, rare, but includes uveitis[181] and nephritis.[182,183] In patients without proteinuria renal biopsies show mesangial thickening and deposition of complexes containing IgG and complement, but no cellular infiltration. A proportion of cases have proteinuria. About 5% of Indian cases

show reversible impairment of renal function.[183] Fatal cases show interstitial nephritis.[184]

Biochemical tests of liver function show normal levels of hepatocellular enzymes.[172] Plasma albumin is greatly reduced, often to below 2.0 g/l, but it is not known if this is due to reduced synthesis, increased catabolism or intestinal loss. Prothrombin levels are usually normal. Differences in findings between different reports may reflect differing expressions of underlying liver disease from other causes. Epistaxis is common early in the disease; its pathogenesis is not understood. Haemorrhage late in the disease is probably due to a combination of deficient clotting factors, and thrombocytopenia. Disseminated intravascular coagulation is rare.[185] Diarrhoea is a common complaint in some reports.[186] Leishmanial enteritis may cause malabsorption and diarrhoea[172] and the diarrhoea may be severe in advanced cases. Secondary intestinal infections are probably common. Wasting of muscle and fat[187] and avitaminosis[188] follow. There have been no measurements of cardiac or pulmonary function in VL.

Pancytopenia is the rule. Erythrocytes are sequestered in the spleen and have a shortened half-life, due to haemolysis.[189] Immune lysis and ineffective erythropoiesis may contribute to the anaemia.[173] Reticulocytosis is suppressed. Haemoglobin levels are commonly around 7 g/dl, and often below 4 g/dl. Anaemia may come on rapidly. Neutrophils are similarly sequestered and destroyed prematurely and the marginal granulocyte pool is enlarged.[190] Leucocyte counts of $2-3 \times 10^3$/dl are common. Eosinophils are suppressed. Platelets are also sequestered and destroyed, and counts typically fall to $100-150 \times 10^9$/dl.

CLINICAL FEATURES[186,191]

The established disease presents a fairly uniform pattern but the onset tends to differ between indigenous and expatriate individuals. The features found on presentation reflect the severity and chronicity of the infection, its complications and the intercurrent infections endemic to that geographical area (Table 65.2).

The clinical incubation period ranges from 3 weeks to over 2 years,[192] but 2–4 months is average. Postprimary cases can occur in the immunosuppressed many years after infection.[193]

In expatriates, and early in epidemics, the onset is usually acute[194] with the sudden appearance of acute fever and rigors in 96%. Malaise, headache, dizziness, anorexia, cough or diarrhoea may occur early in a few patients but there are no specific symptoms

Table 65.2 Clinical features of established visceral leishmaniasis.

Feature	%*
Fever	100
Abdominal pain	80
Diarrhoea	45
Cough	76
Epistaxis	51
Weight loss	100
Oedema	27
Splenomegaly	100
Hepatomegaly	75
Lymphadenopathy	
India	5
Africa	84
Jaundice	5
Hyperpigmentation	
Europeans	0
Indians	70

*Maximum prevalence in literature cited.

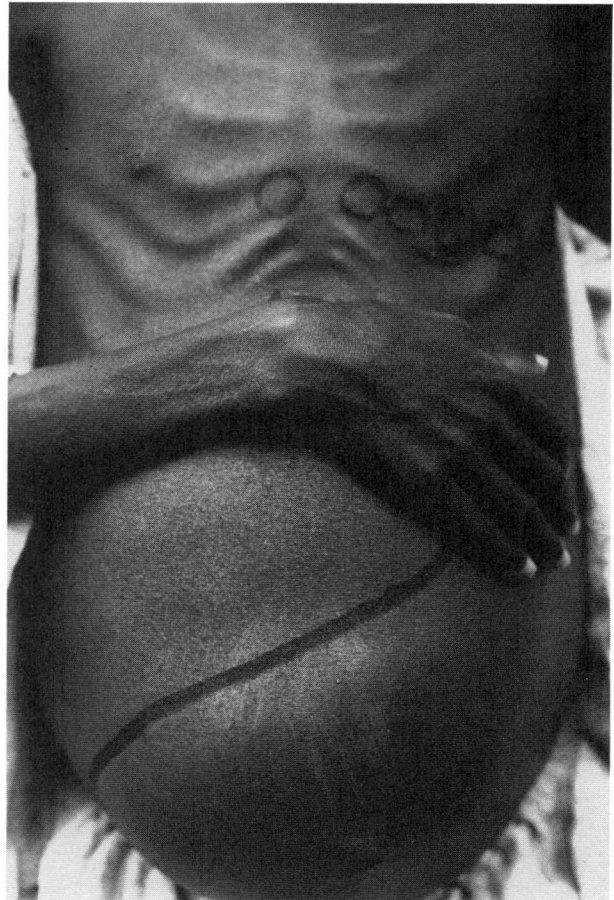

Figure 65.27 Visceral leishmaniasis in a Kenyan child showing wasting, hyperpigmentation of the hand and splenomegaly. The line marks the upper border of the grossly enlarged spleen which extended into the right iliac fossa.

and the differential diagnosis rests among malaria, brucellosis, bacterial endocarditis, typhoid, miliary tuberculosis and haemopoietic malignancy.[194,195] In indigenous people in an endemic area the onset is equally commonly insidious,[196,197] such that the patient may not seek attention for up to a year.

Physical examination early on shows splenomegaly in over 90% of patients and hepatomegaly in 75%, the spleen being disproportionately enlarged and sometimes extending into the pelvis. In a few patients in Africa peripheral lymph nodes will be palpably enlarged.

As the disease progresses physical features accumulate. In Sudan and in the Mediterranean littoral the disease may present as afebrile lymphadenopathy. Abdominal pain is usually due to the enlarged spleen. Cough and diarrhoea may indicate intercurrent infection. Epistaxis is common and occasionally severe but other forms of haemorrhage are rare. Jaundice may be due to chronic leishmanial inflammation or to intercurrent hepatitis. Oedema may be part of a syndrome comprising hair and skin changes, resembling kwashiorkor. Skin lesions are uncommon in Mediterranean VL.[198] Occasionally in Africa there may be a primary skin lesion before or during the febrile disease. In India the majority of patients develop darkening, even blackening of the skin, affecting especially the face, hands and upper torso (kala-azar = black sickness). This is seen, although with greater difficulty, in a proportion of Africans, but not in Europeans. Retinal haemorrhage and uveitis are seen occasionally.

In an endemic area[161,199] the infection may cause only mild non-specific symptoms such as malaise, tiredness and intermittent hepatosplenomegaly. Some will recover spontaneously within 3 years, and others, especially if malnourished,[25] develop classical VL.

COURSE AND PROGNOSIS

Gradually the patient becomes exhausted and emaciated and the abdomen more distended by liver and spleen. Intercurrent infections supervene, notably pneumococcal otitis, pneumonia and septicaemia, tuberculosis, measles, and locally endemic infections such as brucellosis, bacillary and amoebic dysentery, and cancrum oris (Table 65.3). Untreated, 80–90% of patients die. Treated, only the desperately sick die. Usually there are no seque-

Table 65.3 Intercurrent infections and complications of visceral leishmaniasis.

Measles
Pneumonia—especially pneumococcal
Bacillary dysentery
Brucellosis
Tuberculosis
Severe epistaxis
Malabsorption
Severe malnutrition
Nephritis
Uveitis
Retinal haemorrhage
Post-kala-azar dermal leishmaniasis
Death
    0–50% treated
    85–90% untreated

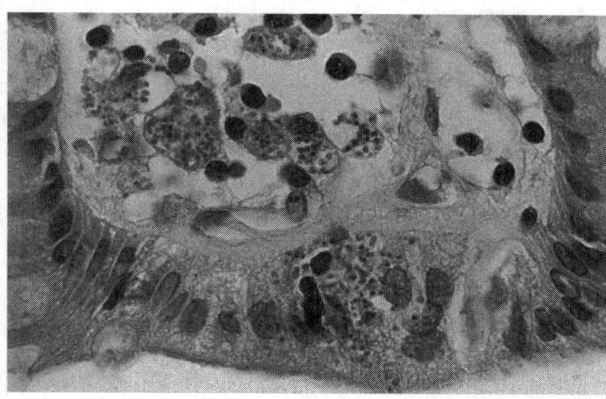

Figure 65.28 Rectal biopsy showing heavy parasitisation with amastigotes in a patient with visceral leishmaniasis and the acquired immune deficiency syndrome. (Courtesy S. Lucas.)

lae, although cirrhosis has been reported.[171] Most patients become sensitive to leishmanin and are presumed to be immune.[166] PKDL develops in up to 5% of cases in Africa and up to 20% in India.

VL has also been associated with other forms of immune suppression, notably in renal transplant patients.[27]

VISCERAL LEISHMANIASIS IN THE IMMUNOSUPPRESSED

Since 1986 VL has been recognized as a complication of infection with HIV.[200,201] VL is thought to represent reactivation of latent infection in a proportion of cases, and in others the failure to express cellular immunity to a new infection. The problem is greatest in southern Europe, where HIV and *L. infantum* are both endemic, and has been reported in Brazil.

In Spain 50% of adults with VL are HIV positive, and it is estimated that 3% of HIV-infected individuals will acquire VL.[202] The cardinal signs of VL in this situation are unexplained fever, splenomegaly and leucopenia, but the presentation may not be typical. Often the parasite is found by chance, for example in a rectal or skin biopsy taken for other purposes, or in bronchiolar lavage (Figure 65.28).[203] The bone marrow is teeming with parasites but two-thirds of cases have no detectable antileishmanial antibodies. In 90% of cases the CD4 count is under $0.3 \times 10^6/l$, and the CD4:CD8 ratio is under 1.[204] The disease responds slowly to treatment. Relapse is common.

DIAGNOSIS[205]

PARASITOLOGICAL DIAGNOSIS

Leishmania may be isolated by the techniques described in Appendix V from samples of tissue or blood. Approximate diagnostic yields are given on Table 65.4. Splenic aspiration is the most sensitive method. It is simple, safe and virtually painless if proper procedures are observed: the prothrombin

Table 65.4 Diagnostic yield of *Leishmania* isolated by aspiration from different sites in patients with visceral leishmaniasis.

Site	Positive (%)
Spleen	over 95
Liver	75–85
Bone marrow	64–85
Enlarged lymph node	64
Buffy coat—India	67–99
Buffy coat—Africa	50

time should be normal and platelets above $40 \times 10^9/l$. Palpate the spleen and mark its outline. Using a 1.25 inch (3 cm) 21 gauge needle attached to a 5 ml disposable syringe, penetrate the skin over the spleen, pull the plunger back 1 ml, plunge the needle into the spleen upwards at an angle of 45° and withdraw *instantly*, maintaining the suction throughout. The tiny amount of material obtained is adequate to inoculate two culture tubes and make 2–4 smears. The pulse and blood pressure are monitored for 8 hours, while the patient remains in bed. In stained smears parasites are usually extracelluar and, if scanty, demand a long careful search. For research or for the management of difficult cases, for example with the acquired immune deficiency syndrome (AIDS) or drug resistance, it is useful to quantitate parasites on a logarithmic scale to assist in subsequent monitoring.[206] Culture is 1 log more sensitive than smears.

Bone marrow aspiration is most commonly used but requires special needles and is painful and not suitable for quantitation or parasitological monitoring after treatment. Lymph node aspiration has been found useful for routine field diagnosis in Sudan.

Occasionally *Leishmania* are identified by chance in biopsies of liver, bone marrow, lymph node or jejunal mucosa.

IMMUNOLOGICAL DIAGNOSIS

Antibodies are readily detectable by several techniques. Indirect immunofluorescence, countercurrent immunoelectrophoresis, ELISA, and direct agglutination tests (DAT) are positive in 97–100% cases.[207–209] Specificity varies from about 70% with DAT, 90% with countercurrent, and approaches 100% with ELISA. ELISA is especially useful for field work as samples may be collected on filter papers and eluted directly into microtitre wells. The assay is performed at a predetermined dilution of serum and there is no need for incubators or refrigeration.[210,211] Complement fixation and the older aldehyde tests are much less sensitive and specific. The leishmanin test is negative.

TREATMENT[140,212]

GENERAL CONSIDERATIONS

VL is an intracellular infection in a patient who has failed to express cellular immunity. The patient requires treatment with an effective drug for an adequate duration. *Leishmania* show different sensitivities to drugs between and among species, and individual patients respond to treatment at different rates. Optimum regimens may be different in different endemic areas, and can only be defined by locally established relapse rates, which should be under 2%.

Pentavalent antimonials generally remain the drug of choice for reasons of cost, availability, efficacy and familiarity. However, antimony resistance has become a serious problem in the epidemics in India and Sudan.[213,214] HIV coinfected individuals commonly relapse after antimonial treatment. Aminosidine, amphotericin B, and liposomal amphotericin are useful alternatives. Pentamidine should be kept in reserve.

CHEMOTHERAPY OF PREVIOUSLY UNTREATED IMMUNOCOMPETENT PATIENTS

Pentavalent antimonials

Two preparations are available, sodium stibogluconate, containing 100 mg Sb/ml and meglumine antimoniate containing 85 mg Sb/ml. They are equal in efficacy and toxicity when used in equivalent Sb doses. They may be given by intramuscular or intravenous injection. The main elimination half-life is about 2 hours and 90% of the drug is excreted in the urine within 8 hours, but there is a slow accumulation of, presumably, trivalent antimony which may contribute to cumulative toxicity.[215] Toxicity normally relates to total dose and includes anorexia, musculoskeletal pain, minor T wave and ST segment changes on the electrocardiogram, slow rise in hepatic enzymes and slow fall in circulating leucocytes. None is serious and they do not require monitoring at conventional dosage. Doses in excess of 20 mg Sb/kg body weight daily require monitoring, especially for prolongation of the Q–T interval, which may precede a dangerous arrythmia.[216] Idiosyncratic toxicity includes pancreatitis and exfoliative dermatitis. For previously untreated patients, the regimen recommended by WHO is suitable: 20 mg Sb/kg body weight for 3–4 weeks.[151] The upper limit of 850 mg should, however, be ignored, as should package inserts that recommend 10 mg Sb/kg Pentostam, or 28 mg Sb/kg Glucantime. Adults tolerate antimonials poorly compared with children. At this dosage, 80% suffer arthralgia and 30% anorexia,[159] and the schedule on Table 65.5 may be more appropriate.[218] In areas of antimony resistance, notably Bihar, the full 20 mg Sb/kg should be given for up to 40 days. In other areas about 1% of previously

Table 65.5 Simplified dose regimens for pentavalent antimonials based on body surface area (BSA) according to the formula BSA m^2 = 0.1 $\sqrt[3]{kg^2}$ whereby a 20 kg child receives 20 mg Sb/kg @ 542 mg Sb/m^2 (adapted from ref. 218.)

Nearest weight of patient (kg)	Calculated dose (mg Sb)	Recommended dose (ml (mg Sb))	
		Pentostam*	Glucantime†
90	1088	11.0 (1100)	13.0 (1105)
80	1006	10.0 (1000)	12.0 (1020)
70	925	9.5 (950)	11.0 (935)
60	832	8.5 (850)	10.0 (850)
50	737	7.5 (750)	9.0 (765)
40	635	6.5 (650)	7.5 (637)
30	524	5.0 (500)	6.0 (510)
20	400	4.0 (400)	5.0 (425)
10	252	2.5 (250)	3.0 (255)
5	159	2.0 (200)	2.5 (212)

*Pentostam (Burroughs Wellcome) = sodium stibogluconate solution, containing 100 mg Sb/ml.
†Glucantime (Special) = meglumine antimoniate solution containing 85 mg Sb/ml.

untreated patients will be unresponsive, due to antimony-resistant parasites.[150]

Aminosidine (paromomycin)

This is a conventional aminoglycoside antibiotic (Gabbromycina, Carlo-Erba Farmitalia, Milan, Italy) that has a unique action against *Leishmania*. It is not toxic in conventional dosage in patients with normal renal function but has the potential for renal and ototoxicity common to all aminoglycosides. It is an acceptable first-line alternative for VL due to *L. infantum* or *L. donovani* in India and Kenya, given in a dose of 14 mg/kg body weight daily by intramuscular injection or intravenous infusion over 90 minutes, once daily for 3–4 weeks.[219] Aminosidine given with antimonials may be more effective than either drug alone.[214,220] In vitro it is synergistic with antimonials.

Amphotericin B desoxycholate

This (the conventional preparation) is 400 times more potent than antimonials against *Leishmania*. It damages ergosterol, the major cell membrane sterol of amastigotes. In its conventional dose of 1 mg/kg body weight by intravenous infusion on alternate days it commonly causes anaemia and renal glomerular and tubular damage, as well as rigors and venous thrombosis, which has limited its value as a second line drug for leishmaniasis, especially when prolonged courses are necessary. It has, however, proved effective and non-toxic in cases of Indian VL in a dose of 0.5 mg/kg on alternate days for 14 doses.[221]

Liposomal amphotericin B

One formulation, Ambisome (Vestar, San Dimas, CA, USA) is being licensed for use in leishmaniasis. Experimentally, it achieved concentrations in the liver and spleen ten times those achieved by conventional amphotericin, and is one-tenth as toxic.[222] It is effective and non-toxic in cases of VL due to *L. infantum* in a dose of 3 mg/kg by intravenous infusion for ten daily doses.[223] Lower doses may also prove to be effective. The speed of response and lack of toxicity would make this drug the choice for VL if it were shown to be effective in other endemic zones, and if it were less expensive.

CHEMOTHERAPY OF PREVIOUSLY TREATED, RELAPSED PATIENTS

If antimonials are to be used, the dose should be 20 mg Sb/kg once daily for 60 days. Any further relapse should be treated as for antimony resistance.

CHEMOTHERAPY OF PATIENTS UNRESPONSIVE TO ANTIMONY OR MULTIPLY RELAPSED

The choice lies between aminosidine, amphotericin B, liposomal amphotericin, or pentamidine in a dose of 4 mg salt/kg two or three times a week.[224] Pentamidine is associated with hypotension, hypo-glycaemia, injection abscesses, renal damage and diabetes. There may be an adjunctive role for interferon-γ.[225]

CHEMOTHERAPY OF PATIENTS WHO ARE IMMUNOINCOMPETENT DUE TO HIV INFECTION OR IMMUNOSUPPRESSIVE DRUGS

Conventional courses of treatment, even of liposo-mal amphotericin, are seldom curative; relapse is the rule, often with drug resistance. There are no data on long-term maintenance treatment.

SUPPORTIVE MEASURES

Owing to the chronicity of the infection, patients are usually well adapted to anaemia and increased plasma volume. Blood transfusion is not required except in the case of heart failure, when packed cells may be administered slowly under diuretic cover. Known or suspected haematinic deficiencies should be corrected. In malarious areas a suitable antima-larial may be given. Intercurrent infection must be sought and treated.

MONITORING THE RESPONSE TO TREATMENT

The patient usually feels better and becomes afe-brile within a few days. Haematological indices start to improve during the second week. Haemoglobin, serum albumin and body weight are the most useful indicators of progress. The spleen may take up to 1 year to regress completely. Persistent or recurrent splenomegaly indicates relapse or a second con-dition, such as malaria, schistosomiasis or cirrhosis. In previously untreated patients parasitological assessment is not normally necessary.

In relapsed, and especially unresponsive and immunoincompetent patients, treatment should be continued until parasitological cure, and for several weeks longer. Parasitological cure is best assessed by quantitation of parasites in splenic aspirates, taken every 1–2 weeks, according to the rate of response.[206] The patient must be monitored for toxic effects of the chosen drug.

PREVENTION AND CONTROL OF THE LEISHMANIASES[151,226]

PROTECTION OF THE INDIVIDUAL

Travellers and tourists should avoid endemic areas during the season of transmission. Within endemic areas measures should be taken to avoid sandfly bites. These include: not camping or sleeping out near gerbil burrows, using fine mesh bed nets impregnated with permethrin, applying insect repel-lent creams to exposed skin, wearing long sleeves and trousers against day-biting sandflies.

'Vaccination' with live virulent *L. major* has been practised traditionally in the Middle East for centur-ies, and recently by armed forces, in order to pro-duce controlled immunizing infections at innocuous sites.[23] Such vaccines, however, have not been stan-dardized and are not generally available. Vacci-nation with attenuated or dead organisms, or with defined antigens, is in its infancy.[227]

CONTROL IN THE COMMUNITY

Three methods of control are available: treatment or destruction of animal reservoirs of infection (in-cluding man), sandfly control and vaccination.[228] Their application in a given situation will depend upon the local epidemiology of the infection and the biology of reservoir and vector. Guidelines have been established.[229]

Domestic canine reservoirs of VL may be identi-fied by serological tests[230] and treated or eliminated. On the island of Elba diagnosis and treatment of infected dogs led to a fall in incidence of canine VL from 12 to 5%,[231] but the effect on human incidence is unknown and there is a theoretical risk of encour-aging antimony-resistant organisms because dogs invariably relapse.

Rodent reservoirs have been controlled in the Middle East and former USSR by the destruction of gerbils and their burrows.[226] This method also elim-inates resident sandflies and reduces the incidence of human CL by a factor of 10. Rodent control is not practicable in the forests of Latin America.

Human reservoirs of CL due to *L. tropica*, and of VL due to *L. donovani* in India, may be controlled by mass active case finding and treatment. These methods eradicated CL in Azerbaijan,[226] and may be supplemented by residual spraying of microfoci of sandfly vectors. Case finding and treatment has not proved successful on its own in India, unless supported by spraying, because of the infectivity of early cases and the difficulty in diagnosing and treating cases of PKDL.[232]

Sandflies are extremely susceptible to standard residual insecticides and have, so far, not become resistant to them.[233] Spraying of sandfly resting sites has proved a successful method of control where such sites are peridomestic, as with *P. argentipes* in India, and partially successful where they are focal, as with *P. papatasi* in the former USSR and *P. martini* in Kenya.

Successful control, in a given focus, is likely to depend on the application of more than one suitable method, coupled with education of the population at risk.

REFERENCES

1 Garnham P C C. Introduction. In Peters W & Killick-Kendrick R (eds) *The Leishmaniases in Biology and Medicine*, vol. 1. Orlando: Academic Press, 1987: xiii–xxv.

2 Lainson R & Shaw J J. Evolution, classification and geographical distribution. In Peters W & Killick-Kendrick R (eds) *The Leishmaniases in Biology and Medicine*, vol. 1. Orlando: Academic Press, 1987: 1–120.

3 Gramiccia M, Gradoni L, di Martino L, Romano R & Ercolini D. Two synoptic zymodemes of *Leishmania infantum* cause human and canine visceral leishmaniases in the Naples area, Italy. *Acta Trop* 1992; 50:357–359.

4 Gramiccia M, Ben-Ismail R, Gradoni L, Ben Rachid M S & Ben Said M. A *Leishmania infantum* enzymatic variant, causative agent of cutaneous leishmaniasis in north Tunisia. *Trans R Soc Trop Med Hyg* 1991; 85:370–371.

5 Gramiccia M, Gradoni L & Troiani M. HIV-Leishmania co-infection in Italy. Isoenzyme characterization of *Leishmania* causing visceral leishmaniasis in HIV patients. *Trans R Soc Trop Med Hyg* 1992; 86:161–163.

6 Rodgers M R, Popper S J & Wirth D F. Amplification of kinetoplast DNA as a tool in the detection and diagnosis of leishmaniasis. *Exp Parasitol* 1990; 71:267–275.

7 Laskay T, Gemetchu T, Teferedegn H & Frommel D. The use of DNA hybridization for the detection of *Leishmania aethiopica* in naturally infected sandfly vectors. *Trans R Soc Trop Med Hyg* 1991; 85:599–602.

8 Alexander J & Russell D G. The interaction of *Leishmania* species with macrophages. *Adv Parasitol* 1992; 31:179–231.

9 Molyneux D H & Killick-Kendrick R. Morphology, ultrastructure and life cycles. In Peters W & Killick-Kendrick R (eds) *The Leishmaniases in Biology and Medicine*, vol. 1. Orlando: Academic Press, 1987; 121–176.

10 Sacks D L. The structure and function of the surface lipophosphoglycan on different developmental stages of *Leishmania* promastigotes. *Infect Agents Dis* 1992; 1:200–206.

11 Schnur L F, Chance ML, Ebert F, Thomas S C & Peters W. Biochemical and serological taxonomy of visceral leishmaniasis. *Ann Trop Med Parasitol* 1981; 75:131–144.

12 Bordier C. The promastigote surface protease of *Leishmania. Parasitol Today* 1987; 3:151–153.

13 Gottlieb M & Dwyer D M. *Leishmania donovani*: surface membrane acid phosphatase activity of promastigotes. *Exp Parasitol* 1981; 52:117–128.

14 Titus R G & Ribeiro J M C. Salivary gland lysates from the sandfly *Lutzomyia longipalpis* enhance leishmanial infectivity. *Science* 1988; 239:1306–1308.

15 Liew F Y. Regulation of cell-mediated immunity in leishmaniasis. *Curr Top Microbiol Immunol* 1990; 55:53–64.

16 Gorczynski R M. Do sugar residues contribute to the antigenic determinant responsible for protection and/or abolition of protection in leishmania-infected BALB/c mice? *J Immunol* 1986; 137:1010–1016.

17 Shaw J J & Lainson R. Ecology and epidemiology: New World. In Peters W & Killick-Kendrick R (eds) *The Leishmaniases in Biology and Medicine*, vol. 1. Orlando: Academic Press, 1987: 291–363.

18 Ashford R W & Bettini S. Ecology and epidemiology: Old World. In Peters W & Killick-Kendrick R (eds) *The Leishmaniases in Biology and Medicine*, vol. 1. Orlando: Academic Press, 1987: 366–424.

19 Lewis D J & Ward R D. Transmission and vectors. In Peters W & Killick-Kendrick R (eds) *The Leishmaniases in Biology and Medicine*, vol. 1. Orlando: Academic Press, 1987: 235–262.

20 Symmers WStC. Leishmaniasis acquired by contagion. A case of marital infection in Britain. *Lancet* 1960; i:127–132.

21 Manson-Bahr P E C, Southgate B A & Harvey A E C. Development of kala-azar in man after inoculation with a leishmania from a Kenya sandfly. *BMJ* 1963; i:1208–1210.

22 Nyakundi P M, Muigai R, Were J B O, Oster C N, Gachihi G S & Kirigi G. Congenital visceral leishmaniasis: case report. *Trans R Soc Trop Med Hyg* 1988; 82:564.

23 Gunders A E. Vaccination: past and future role in control. In Peters W & Killick-Kendrick R (eds) *The Leishmaniases in Biology and Medicine*, vol. 2. Orlando: Academic Press, 1987: 929–941.

24 Marsden P D, Almeida E A, Llanos-Cuentas E A et al. Leishmania braziliensis braziliensis infection of the nipple. *BMJ* 1985; 290:433–434.

25 Cerf B J, Jones T C, Badaro R, Sampaio D, Teixeira R & Johnson Jr. W D. Malnutrition as a risk factor for severe visceral leishmaniasis. *J Infect Dis* 1987; 156:1030–1033.

26 Dye C & Wolpert D M. Earthquakes, influenza and cycles of Indian kala-azar. *Trans Soc Trop Med Hyg* 1988; 82:843–850.

27 Fernandez-Guerrero M L, Aguado J M, Buzon L et al. Visceral leishmaniasis in immunocompromised hosts. *Am J Med* 1987; 83:1098–1102.

28 Dye C. Leishmaniasis epidemiology: the theory catches up. *Parasitol Today* 1992; 104:S7–S18.

29 Lainson R. The American leishmaniases: some observations on their ecology and epidemiology. *Trans R Soc Trop Med Hyg* 1983; 77:569–596.

30 Lysenko A J & Beljaev A E. Quantitative approaches to epidemiology. In Peters W & Killick-Kendrick R (eds) *The Leishmaniases in Biology and Medicine*, vol. 1. Orlando: Academic Press, 1987: 263–288.

31 Rioux J A, Albaret J L, Houin R, Dedet J P & Lanotte G. Ecologie des leishmanioses dans le sud de la France. 2. Les réservoirs selvatiques. Infestation spontanée du renard (*Vulpes vulpes L.*). *Ann Parasitol Hum Comp* 1968; 43:421–428.

32 Gradoni L, Pozio E, Bettini S & Gramiccia M. Leishmaniasis in Tuscany (Italy). III. The prevalence of canine leishmaniasis in two foci of Grosseto Province. *Trans R Soc Trop Med Hyg* 1980; 74:421–422.

33 Pozio E, Gradoni L, Bettini S & Gramiccia M. Leishmaniasis in Tuscany (Italy) VI. Canine leishmaniasis in the focus of Monte Argentario (Grosseto). *Acta Trop* 1981; 38:383–393.

34 Minter D M. Visceral Leishmaniasis. In Manson-Bahr P E C & Bell D R, (eds) *Manson's Tropical Diseases*, 19th edn. London: Baillière Tindall, 1987: 1305–1308.

35 Zhi-biao X, Zhi-chang D, Wen-kai C et al. Discovery of naturally infected racoon dog, wild animal reservoir host of leishmaniasis in China. *Chin Med J* 1982; 95:329–330.

36 Pampiglione S, Manson-Bahr P E C, La Placa M, Borgatti M A & Musumeci S. Studies in Mediterranean leishmaniasis. 3. The leishmanin skin test in kala-azar. *Trans R Soc Trop Med Hyg* 1975; 69:60–68.

37 Aggarwal P & Wali J P. Kala-azar in North India—nine years' experience. *Trans R Soc Trop Med Hyg* 1988; 82:415.

38 Thakur C P, Kumar M & Pathak P K. Kala-azar hits again. *J Trop Med* 1981; 84:271–276.

39 Perkins P V, Githure J I, Mebrahtu Y et al. Isolation of *Leishmania donovani* from *Phlebotmus martini* in Baringo District, Kenya. *Trans R Soc Trop Med Hyg* 1988; 82:695–700.

40 Wijers D J B & Kiilu G. Studies on the vector of kala-azar in Kenya, VIII. The outbreak in Machakos District; epidemiological features and a possible way of control. *Ann Trop Med Parasitol* 1984; 78:597–604.

41 Penman H G. Epidemic visceral leishmaniasis in Southern Sudan. *Lancet* 1989; 344:1222–1223.

42 Lockwood N J. Sudan: Kala-azar should be in the news. *Lancet* 1994; 338:624–625.

43 Mutinga M J & Ngoka J M. The isolation and identification of leishmanial parasites from domestic dogs in the Machakos District of Kenya, and the possible role of dogs as reservoirs of kala-azar in East Africa. *Ann Trop Med Parasitol* 1980; 74:140–143.

44 Mansour N S, Stauber L A & McCoy J R. Leishmaniasis in the Sudan Republic. 29. Comparison and epidemiological implications of experimental canine infections with Sudanese, Mediterranean, and Kenyan strains of *Leishmania donovani*. *J Parasitol* 1970; 56:468–472.

45 Desjeux P, Bryan J H & Martin-Saxton P. Leishmaniasis in The Gambia. 2. A study of possible vectors and animal reservoirs, with the first report of a case of canine leishmaniasis in The Gambia. *Trans R Soc Trop Med Hyg* 1983; 77:143–148.

46 Grimaldi G, Tesh R B & McMahon-Pratt D. A review of the geographical distribution and epidemiology of leishmaniasis in the new world. *Am J Trop Med Hyg* 1989; 41:687–725.

47 Corredor A, Gallego J F, Tesh R B et al. Didelphis marsupialis, an apparent wild reservoir of *leishmania donovani chagasi* in Colombia, South America. *Trans R Soc Trop Med Hyg* 1989; 83:195.

48 Magalhaes P A, Mayrink W, Costa C A et al. Calazar na zona do Rio Doce-Minas Gerais. Resultados de mediadas profilaticas. *Rev Med Trop Sao Paulo* 1980; 22:197–202.

49 Muigai R, Githure J I, Gachihi G S, Were J B O, Leeuwenburg J & Perkins P V. Cutaneous leishmaniasis caused by *Leishmania major* in Baringo District, Kenya. *Trans R Soc Trop Med Hyg* 1987; 81:600–602.

50 Le Blancq S M, Schnur L F & Peters W. Leishmania in the Old World: 1. The geographical and hostal distribution of *L. major* zymodemes. *Trans R Soc Trop Med Hyg* 1986; 80:99–112.

51 Dedet J P. Les leishmanioses en Afrique du nord. *Bull Inst Pasteur* 1979; 77:49–82.

52 Belazzoug S. Une épidémie de leishmaniose cutanée dans la region de M'sila (Algérie). *Bull Soc Pathol Exot* 1982; 75:497–504.

53 Beach R, Kiilu G, Hendricks L, Oster C & Leeuwemburg J. Cutaneous leishmaniasis in Kenya: transmission of *Leishmania major* to man by the bite of a naturally infected *Phlebotomus duboscqi*. *Trans R Soc Trop Med Hyg* 1984; 78:747–751.

54 Gramiccia M, Bettini S & Yarasol S. Isoenzyme characterization of *Leishmania* isolates from human cases of cutaneous leishmaniasis in Urfa, south-east Turkey. *Trans R Soc Trop Med Hyg* 1994; 78:568.

55 Lanotte G, Rioux J A, Maazoun R, Pasteur N, Pratlog F & Lepart J. Application de la méthode numerique à la taxonomie du genre. *Ann Parasitol Hum Comp* 1981; 55:635–643.

56 Dereure J A, Rioux J A, Gallego J F et al. Leishmania tropica in Morocco: infection in dogs. *Trans R Soc Trop Med Hyg* 1991; 85:595.

57 Mebrahtu Y, Lawyer P A, Githure J I et al. Visceral leishmaniasis unresponsive to Pentostam caused by *Leishmania tropica* in Kenya. *Am J Trop Med Hyg* 1989; 41:289–294.

58 Lanotte G, Rioux J A & Pratlong F. Ecologie des leishmanioses dans le sud de la France 14. Les leishmanioses humaines en Cevennes. Analyse clinique et biologique des forms viscerales et musqueuses. *Ann Parasitol Hum Comp* 1981; 55:575–592.

59 Ashford R W, Bray M A, Hutchinson M P & Bray R S. The epidemiology of cutaneous leishmaniasis in Ethiopia. *Trans R Soc Trop Med Hyg* 1973; 67:568–601.

60 Lemma A, Foster W A, Gemetchu T, Preston P M, Bryceson A & Minter D M. Studies on leishmaniasis in Ethiopia I. Preliminary investigations into the epidemiology of cutaneous leishmaniasis in the highlands. *Ann Trop Med Parasitol* 1969; 63:455–472.

61 Grove S S. Leishmaniasis in South West Africa/ Namibia to date. *S Afr Med J* 1989; 75:290–292.

62 Oliveira-Neto M P, Pirmez C, Rangel E, Schubach A & Grimaldi G. An outbreak of American cutaneous leishmaniasis (*Leishmania braziliensis braziliensis*) in a periurban area of Rio de Janeiro City, Brazil: clinical and epidemiological studies. *Mem Inst Oswaldo Cruz* 1988; 83:427–435.

63 Aguilar C M, Rangel E F, Grimaldi G & Momen H. Human, canine and equine leishmaniasis caused by *Leishmania braziliensis* in an endemic area in the state of Rio de Janeiro. *Mem Inst Oswaldo Cruz* 1987; 82:143.

64 Herrer A & Christensen H A. *Leishmania braziliensis* in Panamanian two-toed sloths, *Choloepus hoffmani*. *Am J Trop Med* 1980; 29:1196–1200.

65 Christensen H A & De Vasquez A M. The tree-buttress biotope: a pathobiocenose of *Leishmania braziliensis*. *Am J Trop Med Hyg* 1982; 31:243–251.

66 Sanchez J L, Diniega B M, Small J W et al. Epidemiologic investigation of an outbreak of cutaneous leishmaniasis in a defined geographic focus of transmission. *Am J Trop Med Hyg* 1992; 47:47–54.

67 Dedet J P, Pradinaud R & Gay F. Epidemiological aspects of human cutaneous leishmaniasis in French Guiana. *Trans R Soc Trop Med Hyg* 1989; 83:616–620.

68 Christensen H A, Fairchild G B, Herrer A, Johnson C M, Young D G & De Vasquez A M. The ecology of cutaneous leishmaniasis in the Republic of Panama. *J Med Entomol* 1983; 20:463–484.

69 Schnur L F, Walton B C & Bogaert-Diaz H. On the identity of the parasite causing diffuse cutaneous leishmaniasis in the Dominican Republic. *Trans R Soc Med Hyg* 1983; 77:756–762.

70 Andrade-Narvaez F J, Simmonds-Diaz E, Rico-Aguilar S et al. Incidence of localized cutaneous leishmaniasis (chiclero's ulcer) in Mexico. *Trans R Soc Trop Med Hyg* 1990; 84:219–220.

71 Velasco O, Savarino S, Walton B C, Gam A A & Neva F A. Diffuse cutaneous leishmaniasis in Mexico. *Am J Trop Med Hyg* 1989; 41:280–288.

72 Barral A B, Pedral-Sampaio D, Grimaldi G et al. Leishmaniasis in Bahia, Brazil: evidence that *Leishmania amazonensis* produces a wide spectrum of clinical disease. *Am J Trop Med Hyg* 1991; 44:536–546.

73 Ridley D S. Pathology. In Peters W & Killick-Kendrick R (eds) *The Leishmaniases in Biology and Medicine*, vol. 2. Orlando: Academic Press, 1987: 666–695.

74 Kanan M W & Ryan T J. Endonasal localization of blood borne viable and non viable particulate matter. *Br J Dermatol* 1975; 92:475–477.

75 Ridley D S. The pathogenesis of cutaneous leishmaniasis. *Trans R Soc Trop Med Hyg* 1979; 73:150–159.

76 Ridley D S. A histological classification of cutaneous leishmaniasis and its geographical expression. *Trans R Soc Trop Med Hyg* 1980; 74:515–521.

77 Bittencourt A L & Barral A. Evaluation of the histopathological classifications of American cutaneous and mucocutaneous leishmaniasis. *Mem Inst Oswaldo Cruz* 1991; 86:51–56.

78 Ridley M J & Wells C W. Macrophage–parasite interaction in the lesions of cutaneous leishmaniasis. *Am J Pathol* 1986; 123:79–85.

79 Ridley M J & Ridley D S. Cutaneous leishmaniasis: immune complex formation and necrosis in the acute phase. *Br J Exp Pathol* 1984; 65:327–336.

80 Pettit J H S. Chronic (lupoid) leishmaniasis. *Br J Dermatol* 1962; 74:127–131.

81 Bryceson A D M. Diffuse cutaneous leishmaniasis, the clinical and histological features of the disease in Ethiopia, I. *Trans R Soc Trop Med Hyg* 1969; 63:708–737.

82 Modlin R L, Taplia F J, Bloom B R et al. In situ characterization of the cellular immune response in American cutaneous leishmaniasis. *Clin Exp Immunol* 1985; 60:241–248.

83 Sadick M D, Locksley R M & Raff H V. Development of cellular immunity in cutaneous leishmaniasis due to *Leishmania tropica*. *J Infect Dis* 1984; 150:135–138.

84 Rada E, Trujillo D, Castellanos P L & Convit J. Gamma interferon production induced by antigens in patients with leprosy and American cutaneous

leishmaniasis. *Am J Trop Med Hyg* 1987; 37:520–524.

85 Green S J, Meltzer M S, Hibbs J B & Nacy C A. Activated macrophages destroy intracellular *Leishmania major* amastigotes by an L-arginine-dependent killing mechanism. *J Immunol* 1990; 144:278–283.

86 Bryceson A D M. Diffuse cutaneous leishmaniasis in Ethiopia III. Immunological studies. *Trans R Soc Trop Med Hyg* 1970; 64:380–393.

87 Petersen E A, Neva F A, Oster C N & Diaz H B. Specific inhibition of lymphocyte-proliferation responses by adherent suppressor cells in diffuse cutaneous leishmaniasis. *N Engl J Med* 1982; 306:387–390.

88 Kerdel-Vegas F & Essenfeld-Yahr E. Histopatologia de la leishmaniasis americana. *Med Cutan* 1966; 1:267–275.

89 Blackwell J M. A murine model of genetically controlled host responses to leishmaniasis. In *Ecol Genet of Host–Parasite Interact* London: The Linnean Society, 1985: 147–153.

90 Barral A, Petersen E A, Sacks D L & Neva F A. Late metastatic leishmaniasis in the mouse. *Am J Trop Med Hyg* 1983; 32:277–285.

91 Andrade Z A, Reed S G, Roters S B & Sadigursky M. Immunopathology of experimental cutaneous leishmaniasis. *Am J Pathol* 1984; 114:137–148.

92 Lara M L, Layrisse Z, Scorza J V et al. Immunogenetics of human American cutaneous leishmaniasis. *Hum Immunol* 1991; 30:129–135.

93 Majumdar T D. Post kala-azar dermal leishmaniasis. *Dermatol Int* 1967; 6:174–177.

94 Haldar J P, Saha K C & Ghose A C. Serological profiles in Indian post kala-azar dermal leishmaniasis. *Trans R Soc Trop Med Hyg* 1981; 75:514–517.

95 Neogy A B, Nandy A, Ghosh Dastidar B & Chowdhury A B. Modulation of the cell-mediated immune response in kala-azar and post kala-azar dermal leishmaniasis in relation to chemotherapy. *Ann Trop Med Parasitol* 1988; 82:27–34.

96 Klotz O & Lindenberg H. The pathology of leishmaniasis of the nose. *Am J Trop Med* 1923; 3:117–141.

97 Ridley D S, De Magalhaes A V & Marsden P D. Histological analysis and the pathogenisis of mucocutaneous leishmaniasis. *J Pathol* 1989; 159:293–299.

98 Griffiths W A D. Old World Cutaneous leishmaniasis. In Peters W & Killick-Kendrick R (eds) *The Leishmaniases in Biology and Medicine*, vol. 2. Orlando: Academic Press, 1987; 617–633.

99 Killick-Kendrick R, Bryceson A D M, Peters W, Evans D A, Leaney A J & Rioux J A. Zoonotic cutaneous leishmaniasis in Saudi Arabia: lesions healing naturally in man followed by a second infection with the same zymodeme of *Leishmania major*. *Trans R Soc Trop Med Hyg* 1985; 79:363–365.

100 Saravia N, Weigle K, Segura I et al. Recurrent

lesions in human *Leishmania braziliensis* infection: reactivation or reinfection? *Lancet* 1990; 336:398.

101 Bryceson A D M. Clinical variations associated with various taxa of Leishmania. In Rioux J (ed.) *Leishmania*. Proceedings of the International Colloquium on Taxonomy and Phylogeny. Montpellier: *IMEEE*, 1986:221–228.

102 Kozevnikov P V. Two nosological forms of cutaneous leishmaniasis. *Am J Trop Med Hyg* 1963; 12:719–724.

103 Nadim A & Faghih M. The epidemiology of cutaneous leishmaniasis in the Isfahan province of Iran. *Trans R Soc Trop Med Hyg* 1968; 61:534–549.

104 El-Safi S H, Peters W, El-Toam B, El-Kadarow A & Evans D A. Studies on the leishmaniases in the Sudan. 2. Clinical and parasitological studies on cutaneous leishmaniasis. *Trans R Soc Trop Med Hyg* 1991; 85:457–464.

105 Schewach-Millet M, Fisher B K & Semah D. Leishmaniasis recidivans treated with sodium stibogluconate. *Cutis* 1981; 28:67–89, 94.

106 Belazzoug S, Ammar-Khodja A, Belkaid M & Tabet-Derraz O. La leishmaniose cutanée du nord de L'Algérie. *Bull Soc Pathol Exot* 1985; 78:615–622.

107 Ponce C, Ponce E, Morrison A et al. Leishmania donovani chagasi: new clinical variant of cutaneous leishmaniasis in Honduras. *Lancet* 1991; 337:67–69.

108 Borzoni F, Gradoni L, Gramiccia M, Maccioni A, Valdes E & Loddo S. A case of lingual and palatine localization of a viscerotropic *Leishmania infantum* zymodeme in Sardinia, Italy. *Trop Med Parasitol* 1991; 42:193–194.

109 Llanos-Cuentas E A, Marsden P D, Lago E L, Barreto A C, Cuba C C & Johnson W D. Human mucocutaneous leishmaniasis in Tres Bracos, Bahia, Brazil. An area of *Leishmania braziliensis* transmission. II. Cutaneous disease. Presentation and evolution. *Rev Soc Bras Med Trop* 1984; 17:169–177.

110 Desjeux P, Mollinedo S, Le Pont F, Paredes A & Ugarte G. Cutaneous leishmaniasis in Bolivia. A study of 185 human cases from Alton Beni (La Paz Department). Isolation and isoenzyme characterization of 26 strains of *Leishmania brasiliensis brasiliensis*. *Trans R Soc Trop Med Hyg* 1987; 81:742–746.

111 Marsden P D, Llanos-Cuentas E A, Lago E L et al. Human mucocutaneous leishmaniasis in Tres Bracos, Bahia, Brazil. An area of *Leishmania braziliensis braziliensis* transmission. III. Mucosal disease presentation and initial evolution. *Rev Soc Bras Med Trop* 1984; 17:179–186.

112 Dedet J P. Cutaneous leishmaniasis in French Guiana: a review. *Am J Trop Med Hyg* 1990; 43:25–28.

113 Low-A-Chee R M, Rose P & Ridley D S. An outbreak of cutaneous leishmaniasis in Guyana: epidemiology, clinical and laboratory aspects. *Ann Trop Med Parasitol* 1983; 77:255–260.

114 Walton B C. American cutaneous and

mucocutaneous leishmaniasis. In Peters W & Killick-Kendrick R (eds) *The Leishmaniases in Biology and Medicine*, vol. 2. Orlando: Academic Press, 1987: 638–661.

115 Biagi F F. The treatment of Mexican cutaneous leishmaniasis (chicele ulcer). *Med Mex* 1954; 33:436–438.

116 Silveira F T, Lainson R, Shaw J J, De Souza A A, Ishikawa E A & Braga R R. Cutaneous leishmaniasis due to *Leishmania (Leishmania) amazonensis* in Amazonian Brazil, and the significance of a negative Montenegro skin-test in human infections. *Trans R Soc Trop Med Hyg* 1991; 85:735–738.

117 Convit J & Kerdel-Vegas F. Disseminated cutaneous leishmaniasis. *Arch Dermatol* 1965; 91:439–447.

118 Bryceson A D M. Diffuse cutaneous leishmaniasis in Ethiopia III. Immunological studies. *Trans R Soc Trop Med Hyg* 1970; 64:380–393.

119 Diaz H B, Martinez D, Quinones M & de Esteves F N. Anergic leishmaniasis in the Dominican Republic. Study of 20 cases. *Ann Bras Dermatol* 1985; 60:229–236.

120 Acton H W & Napier L E. Post-kala-azar dermal leishmaniasis. *Ind J Med Res* 1927; 15:97–106.

121 Takahashi S & Sato T. Disseminierte kutane Leishmaniose. *Hautarzt* 1981; 32:459–462.

122 Munro D D, Vivier A & Jopling W H. Post kala-azar dermal leishmaniasis. *Br J Dermatol* 1972; 87:374–378.

123 Morgan F M, Watten R H & Kuntz R E. Post-Kala-Azar dermal leishmaniasis. A case report from Taiwan (Formosa). *J Formosan Med Assoc* 1962; 61:282–291.

124 Rashid J R, Chunge C N, Oster C N, Wasunna K M, Muigai R & Gachihi G S. Post-kala-azar dermal leishmaniasis occurring long after cure of visceral leishmaniasis in Kenya. *East Afr Med J* 1986; 365–371.

125 Marsden P D. Mucosal leishmaniasis (espundia Escomel, 1911). *Trans R Soc Trop Med Hyg* 1986; 60:859–876.

126 Walton B C & Valverde L. Racial differences in espundia. *Ann Trop Med Parasitol* 1974; 73:23–29.

127 Walton B C, Chinel L V, Eguia Y & Eguia O. Onset of espundia after many years of occult infection with *Leishmania braziliensis*. *Am J Trop Med Hyg* 1973; 22:696–698.

128 Marsden P D, Badaro R, Netto E M & Casler D. Spontaneous clinical resolution without specific treatment in mucosal leishmaniasis. *Trans R Soc Trop Med Hyg* 1991; 85:221.

129 Cuba C C, Llanos-Cuentas E A, Barreto A C et al. Human mucocutaneous leishmaniasis in Tres Bracos Bahia, Brazil. An area of *Leishmania braziliensis braziliensis* transmission. I. Laboratory diagnosis. *Rev Soc Bras Med Trop* 1984; 17:161–167.

130 Schnur L F & Jacobson R L. Parasitological techniques. In Peters W & Killick-Kendrick R (eds) *The Leishmaniases in Biology and Medicine*, vol. 1. Orlando: Academic Press, 1987: 499–541.

131 Miles E A. Leishmania-culture and biochemical comparisons—some difficulties. In Chance M L & Walton B C (eds) *Biochemical Characterization of Leishmania*. Geneva: UNDP/World Bank/WHO Special Programme for Research and Training in Tropical Diseases: 1982: 123–137.

132 Sells P G & Burton M. Identification of *Leishmania* amastigotes and their antigens in formalin fixed tissue by immunoperoxidase staining. *Trans R Soc Trop Med Hyg* 1981; 75:461–468.

133 Weigle K A, De Davalos M, Heredia P, Molineros R, Saravia N G & D'Alessandro A. Diagnosis of cutaneous and mucocutaneous leishmaniasis in Colombia: a comparison of seven methods. *Am J Trop Med Hyg* 1987; 36:489–496.

134 Hanham C A, Zhao F, Shaw J J & Lainson R. Monoclonal antibodies for the identification of New World Leishmania. *Trans R Soc Trop Med Hyg* 1991; 85:220.

135 Gramiccia M, Smith D F, Angelici M C, Ready P D & Gradoni L. A kinetoplast DNA probe diagnostic for *Leishmania infantum*. *Parasitol Today* 1992; 105:29–34.

136 Leeuwenburg J, Bryceson A D M, Mbugua G G & Siongok T K Arap. The use of the leishmanin skin test to define transmission of leishmaniasis in Baringo District, Kenya. *East Afr Med J* 1983; 60:81–84.

137 El Safi S H & Evans D A. A comparison of the direct agglutination test and enzyme-linked immunosorbent assay in the sero-diagnosis of leishmaniasis in the Sudan. *Trans R Soc Trop Med Hyg* 1989; 83:334–337.

138 Guimaraes M C S, Celeste B J, Franco E L, Cuce L C & Belda W Jr. Evaluation of serological diagnostic indices for mucocutaneous leishmaniasis: immunofluorescence tests and enzyme-linked immunoassays for IgG, IgM and IgA antibodies. *Bull World Health Organ* 1989; 67:643–648.

139 Walton B C. Evaluation of chemotherapy of American leishmaniasis by the indirect fluorescent antibody test. *Am J Trop Med Hyg* 1980; 29:747–752.

140 Bryceson A D M. Therapy in man. In Peters W & Killick-Kendrick R (eds) *The Leishmaniases in Biology and Medicine*, vol. 2. Orland: Academic Press, 1987: 847–895.

141 Kurban A K, Farah F S & Chaglassian H T. The treatment of cutaneous leishmaniasis. *Dermatol Int* 1967; 6:168–171.

142 Currie M A. Treatment of cutaneous leishmaniasis by curettage. *BMJ* 1983; 287:1083–1156.

143 Neva F A, Petersen E A, Corsey R, Bogaert H D & Martinez D. Observations on local heat treatment for cutaneous leishmaniasis. *Am J Trop Med Hyg* 1984; 33:800–804.

144 Bassiouny A, El Meshad M, Talaat M, Kutty K & Metawaa B. Cryosurgery in cutaneous leishmaniasis. *Br J Dermatol* 1982; 107:467–474.

145 Bryceson A D M, Murphy A & Moody A H. Treatment of cutaneous leishmaniasis of the Old World with aminosidine ointment: results of an open study in patients in London. *Trans R Soc Trop Med Hyg* 1994; 88:226–228.

146 El-On J, Halevy S, Grunwald M H & Weinrauch L. Topical treatment of Old World cutaneous leishmaniasis caused by *Leishmania major*: a double-blind control study. *J Am Acad Dermatol* 1992; 27:227–231.

147 Duperrat B, Puissant A, Fischer R, Badillet G & Mascaro J M. Leishmaniose cutanée plurifocale traite par Glucantime interlesionelle. *Bull Soc Fr Dermatol Syphiligr* 1966; 73:219–220.

148 Harms G, Chehade A K, Douba M et al. A randomized trial comparing a pentavalent antimonial drug and recombinant interferon-gamma in the local treatment of cutaneous leishmaniasis. *Trans R Soc Trop Med Hyg* 1991; 85:214–216.

149 Grogl M, Thomason T N & Franke E D. Drug resistance in leishmaniasis: its implication in systemic chemotherapy of cutaneous and mucocutaneous disease. *Am J Trop Med Hyg* 1992; 47:117–126.

150 Herwaldt B L & Berman J D. Recommendations for treating leishmaniasis with sodium stibogluconate (pentostam) and review of pertinent clinical studies. *Am J Trop Med Hyg* 1992; 46:91–255.

151 WHO Expert Committee. *Control of the Leishmaniases*. Geneva: WHO, 1990.

152 Martinez S & Marr J. Alopurinol in the treatment of American cutaneous leishmaniasis. *N Engl J Med* 1992; 326:741–744.

153 Saenz R E, Paz H & Berman J D. Efficacy of ketoconazole against *Leishmania braziliensis panamensis* cutaneous leishmaniasis. *Am J Med* 1990; 89:147–155.

154 Norton S, Frankenburg S & Klaus S N. Cutaneous leishmaniasis acquired during military service in the Middle East. *Arch Dermatol* 1992; 128:83–87.

155 Dogra J. A double-blind study on the efficacy of oral dapsone on cutaneous leishmaniasis. *Trans R Soc Trop Med Hyg* 1991; 85:212–213.

156 Schewach-Millet M, Fisher B K & Semah D. Leishmaniasis recidivans treated with sodium stibogluconate. *Cutis* 1981; 28:67–89, 94.

157 Bryceson A D M. Diffuse cutaneous leishmaniasis: II. Treatment. *Trans R Soc Trop Med Hyg* 1970; 64:369–379.

158 Teklemariam S, Hiwot A G, Frommel D, Miko T L, Ganlov G & Bryceson A. Aminosidine and its combination with sodium stibogluconate in the treatment of diffuse cutaneous leishmaniasis caused by *Leishmania aethiopica*. *Trans R Soc Trop Med Hyg* 1994; 88:334–339.

159 Franke E D, Wignall F S, Cruz M E et al. Efficacy and toxicity of sodium stibogluconate for mucosal leishmaniasis. *Ann Int Med* 1990; 113:934–940.

160 Netto E M, Marsden P D, Llanos-Cuentas E A et al. Long-term follow-up of patients with *Leishmania (Viannia) braziliensis* infection and treated with Glucantime. *Trans R Soc Trop Med Hyg* 1990; 84:367–370.

161 Pampiglione S, Manson-Bahr P E C, Giungi F, Giunti G, Parenti A & Canestri Trotti G. Studies on Mediterranean Leishmaniasis 2. Asymptomatic cases of visceral leishmaniasis. *Trans R Soc Trop Med Hyg* 1974; 68:447–453.

162 Ho M, Siongok T K, Lyerly W H & Smith D H. Prevalence and disease spectrum in a new focus of visceral leishmaniasis in Kenya. *Trans R Soc Trop Med Hyg* 1982; 76:741–746.

163 Seaman J, Ashford R W, Schorscher J & Dereure J. Visceral leishmaniasis in southern Sudan: status of healthy villagers in epidemic conditions. *Ann Trop Med Parasitol* 1992; 86:481–486.

164 Ho M, Koech D K, Iha D W & Bryceson A D M. Immunosuppression in Kenyan visceral leishmaniasis. *Clin Exp Immunol* 1983; 51:207–214.

165 Meller-Melloul C, Farnarier C, Dunan S et al. Evidence of subjects sensitized to *Leishmania infantum* on the French Mediterranean coast: differences in gamma interferon production between this population and visceral leishmaniasis patients. *Parasite Immunol* 1991; 13:531–536.

166 Ho J L, Badaro R, Schwartz A et al. Diminished in vitro production of interleukin-1 and tumor necrosis factor-alpha during acute visceral leishmaniasis and recovery after therapy. *J Infect Dis* 1992; 165:1094–1102.

167 Karp C L, El-Safi S H, Wynn T A et al. In vivo cytokine profiles in patients with kala-azar. *J Clin Invest* 1993; 91:1644–1648.

168 Meleney H E. The histopathology of kala-azar in the hamster, monkey, and man. *Am J Pathol* 1925; 1:147–168.

169 Veress B, Malik O A, Satir A A & Hassan A M. Morphological observations on visceral leishmaniasis in the Sudan. *Trop Geogr Med* 1974; 26:198–203.

170 Khaldi F, Bennaceur B, Ben Othman H, Achouri E, Ayachi R & Regaieg R. Les formes sévères d'atteinte hépatique au cours de la leishmaniose viscérale. *Arch Fr Pediatr* 1990; 47:257–260.

171 Duarte M I S & Corbett C E P. Histopathological patterns of the liver involvement in visceral leishmaniasis. *Rev Inst Med Trop São Paulo* 1987; 29:131–136.

172 Muigai R, Gatei D G, Shaunak S, Wozniak A & Bryceson A D M. Jejunal function and pathology in visceral leishmaniasis. *Lancet* 1983; ii:476–479.

173 Wickramasinghe S N, Abdalla S H & Kasili E G. Ultrastructure of bone marrow in patients with visceral leishmaniasis. *J Clin Pathol* 1987; 40:267–275.

174 Saran R, Gupta A K & Prasad L S N. A search for leishmania in normal skin and blood of kala-azar patients from Bihar, India. *J Commun Dis* 1988; 20:89–90.

175 Duarte M I S, da Matta V L R, Corbett C E P,

Laurenti M D, Chebabo R & Goto H. Interstitial pneumonitis in human visceral leishmaniasis. *Trans R Soc Trop Med Hyg* 1989; 83:73–76.

176 Ghose A C, Haldar J P, Pal S C, Mishra B P & Mishra K K. Serological investigations on Indian kala-azar. *Clin Exp Immunol* 1980; 40:318–326.

177 Mauel J & Behin R. Immunity: clinical and experimental. In Peters W & Killick-Kendrick R (eds) *The Leishmaniases in Biology and Medicine*, vol. 2. Orlando: Academic Press, 1987: 732–775.

178 Galvao-Castro B, Sa Ferreira J A, Marzochi K F, Marzochi M C, Coutinho S G & Lambert P H. Polyconal B cell activation, circulating immune complexes and autoimmunity in human American visceral leishmaniasis. *Clin Exp Immunol* 1984; 56:58–66.

179 Argov S, Jaffe C L, Krupp M, Slor H & Shoenfeld Y. Autoantibody production by patients infected with *Leishmania. Clin Exp Immunol* 1989; 76:190–197.

180 Pearson R D, De Alencar J E, Romito R, Naidu T G, Young A C & Davis J S I V. Circulating immune complexes and rheumatoid factors in visceral leishmaniasis. *J Infect Dis* 1983; 147:1102.

181 El-Hassan A M, El-Sheikh E A, Eltoum E A et al. Post kala-azar anterior uveitis: demonstration of *Leishmania* parasites in the lesion. *Trans R Soc Trop Med Hyg* 1991; 85:471–473.

182 De Brito T, Hoshino-Shimizu S, Amato Neto V, Duarte I S & Penna D O. Glomerular involvement in human kala-azar. *Am J Trop Med Hyg* 1975; 24:9–18.

183 Prasad L S N, Sen S & Ganguly S K. Renal involvement in kala-azar. *Indian J Med Res* 1992; [A]95:43–46.

184 Duarte M I S, Silva M R R, Goto H, Nicodemo E L & Amato Neto V. Interstitial nephritis in human kala-azar. *Trans R Soc Trop Med Hyg* 1983; 77:531–537.

185 Blount E R, Hartmann R & Nernoff J. Kala-azar as a cause of disseminated intravascular coagulation. *Clin Pediatr* 1980; 19:139–140.

186 Rees P H & Kager P A. Visceral leishmaniasis and post-kala-azar dermal leishmaniasis. In Peters W & Killick-Kendrick R (eds) *The Leishmaniases in Biology and Medicine*, vol. 2. Orlando: Academic Press, 1987: 584–596.

187 Harrison L H, Naidu T G, Drew J S, Eduardo de Alencar J & Pearson R D. Reciprocal relationships between undernutrition and the parasitic disease visceral leishmaniasis. *Rev Infect Dis* 1986; 8:447–453.

188 Sen Gupta P C, Sanyal N N, Bhattacharyya B & Mathen K K. Avitaminosis in kala-azar. *Indian Med Gaz* 1952; 87:444–448.

189 Woodruff A W, Topley E, Knight R & Downie C G B. The anaemia of kala-azar. *Br J Haematol* 1972; 22:319–329.

190 Musumeci S, D'Agata A, Schiliro G & Fischer A. Studies of the neutropenia in kala-azar: results in two patients. *Trans R Soc Trop Med Hyg* 1976; 70:500–503.

191 Zijlstra E, Siddig Ali M, El-Hassan A M et al. Kala-azar in displaced people from southern Sudan: epidemiological, clinical and therapeutic findings. *Trans R Soc Trop Med Hyg* 1991; 85:365–369.

192 Jopling W H. Long incubation period in kala-azar. *BMJ* 1955; ii:1013.

193 Broeckaert-van Orshoven A, Michielsen P & Vandepitte J. Fatal leishmaniasis in renal-transplant patient. *Lancet* 1979; ii:740–741.

194 Most H M & Lavietes P H. Kala-azar in american military personnel. *Medicine* 1947; 26:221–285.

195 Lee C U & Chung H L. A clinical study of the early manifestations of Chinese kala-azar. *Chin Med J* 1935; 49:1281–1300.

196 Cole A C E. Kala-azar in East Africa. *Trans R Soc Trop Med Hyg* 1944; 37:409–435.

197 Maru M. Clinical and laboratory features and treatment of visceral leishmaniasis in hospitalized patients in northwestern Ethiopia. *Am J Trop Med Hyg* 1979; 28:15–18.

198 Schiliro G, Russo A, Musumeci S & Sciotto A. Visceral leishmaniasis following a skin lesion in a six-year-old Sicilian girl. *Trans R Soc Trop Med Hyg* 1978; 72:656–657.

199 Badaro R, Jones T C, Carvalho E M et al. New perspectives on a subclinical form of visceral leishmaniasis. *J Infect Dis* 1986; 154:1003–1011.

200 Montalban C, Martinez-Fernandez R, Calleja J L et al. Visceral leishmaniasis (kala-azar) as an opportunistic infection in patients infected with the human immunodeficiency virus in Spain. *Rev Infect Dis* 1989; 11:655–660.

201 Altes J, Salas A, Riera M et al. Visceral leishmaniasis: another HIV-associated opportunistic infection? Report of eight cases and review of the literature. *AIDS* 1991; 5:201–207.

202 Alvar J, Gutierrez-Solar B, Molina R et al. Prevalence of *Leishmania* infection among AIDS patients. *Lancet* 1992; 339:1427.

203 Romeu J, Sirera G, Ferrandiz C, Carreres A, Condom M J & Clotet B. Visceral leishmaniasis involving lung and a cutaneous Kaposi's sarcoma lesion. *AIDS* 1991; 5:1272.

204 del Mar Sanz M, Rubio R, Casillas A et al. Visceral leishmaniasis in HIV-infected patients. *AIDS* 1991; 5:1272–1273.

205 Manson-Bahr P E C. Diagnosis. In Peters W & Killick-Kendrick R (eds) *The Leishmaniases in Biology and Medicine*, vol. 2. Orlando: Florida, Academic Press, 1997:704–728.

206 Chulay J D & Bryceson A D M. Quantitation of amastigotes of *Leishmania donovani* in smears of splenic aspirates from patients with visceral leishmaniasis. *Am J Trop Med Hyg* 1983; 32:475–479.

207 Aikat B K, Sehgal S, Mahajan R C et al. The role of counter immunoelectrophoresis as a diagnostic tool in kala-azar. *Indian J Med Res* 1979; 70:592–597.

208 Mittal V, Bhatia R & Sehgal S. Serodiagnosis of Indian kala-azar: evaluation of IFA, ELISA and CIEP tests. *J Commun Dis* 1991; 23:131–134.

209 Zijlstra E E, Siddig Ali M, El-Hassan A M et al. Direct agglutination test for diagnosis and sero-epidemiological survey of kala-azar in the Sudan. *Trans R Soc Trop Med Hyg* 1991; 474:476.

210 Jahn A & Diesfeld H J. Evaluation of a visually read ELISA for serodiagnosis and sero-epidemiological studies of kala-azar in the Baringo District, Kenya. *Trans R Soc Trop Med Hyg* 1983; 77:451–454.

211 Ho M, Leeuwenburg J, Mbugua G, Wamachi A & Voller A. An enzyme-linked immunosorbent assay (ELISA) for field diagnosis of visceral leishmaniasis. *Am J Trop Med Hyg* 1983; 32:943–946.

212 Olliaro P L & Bryceson A D M. Practical progress and new drugs for changing patterns of leishmaniasis. *Parasitol Today* 1993; 9:323–328.

213 Thakur C P, Kumar M, Kumar P, Mishra B N & Pandey A K. Rationalisation of regimens of treatment of kala-azar with sodium stibogluconate in India: a randomised study. *BMJ* 1988; 296:1557–1561.

214 Seaman J, Pryce D, Sondorp H E, Moody A, Bryceson A D M & Davidson R N. Epidemic visceral leishmaniasis in Sudan: a randomized trial of aminosidine plus sodium stibogluconate versus sodium stibogluconate alone. *J Infect Dis* 1993; 168:715–720.

215 Chulay J D, Fleckenstein L & Smith D H. Pharmacokinetics of antimony during treatment of visceral leishmaniasis with sodium stibogluconate or meglumine antimoniate. *Trans R Soc Trop Med Hyg* 1988; 82:69–72.

216 Chulay J D, Spencer H G & Mugambi M. Electrocardiographic changes during treatment of leishmaniasis with pentavalent antimony (sodium stibogluconate). *Am J Trop Med Hyg* 1985; 34:702–709.

218 Anabwani G & Bryceson A D M. Visceral leishmaniasis in Kenyan children. *Indian Paediatr* 1982; 197:819–822.

219 Scott J A G, Davidson R N, Moody A H et al. Aminosidine (paromomycin) in the treatment of leishmaniasis imported into the United Kingdom. *Trans R Soc Trop Med Hyg* 1992; 86:617–619.

220 Chunge C N, Owate J, Pamba H O & Donno L. Treatment of visceral leishmaniasis in Kenya by aminosidine alone or combined with sodium stibogluconate. *Trans R Soc Trop Med Hyg* 1990; 84:221–225.

221 Mishra M, Biswas U K, Jha D N & Khan A B. Amphotericin versus pentamidine in antimony-unresponsive kala-azar. *Lancet* 1992; 340:1256–1257.

222 Croft S L, Davidson R N & Thornton E A. Liposomal amphotericin B in the treatment of visceral leishmaniasis. *J Antimicrob Chemother* 1991; 28:111–118.

223 Davidson R N, di Martino L, Gradoni L et al. Liposomal amphotericin B (AmBisome) in Mediterranean visceral leishmaniasis: a multi-centre trial. *Q J Med* 1994; 87:75–81.

224 Thakur C P, Sinha G P, Sharma V, Pandey A K, Kumar M & Verma B B. Evaluation of amphotericin B as a first line drug in comparison to sodium stibogluconate in the treatment of fresh cases of kala-azar. *Indian J Med Res* 1993; 97:170–175.

225 Badaro R, Falcoff E, Badaro F S et al. Treatment of visceral leishmaniasis with pentavalent antimony and interferon gamma. *N Engl J Med* 1990; 322:16–21.

226 Vioukov V N. Control of transmission. In Peters W & Killick-Kendrick R (eds) *The Leishmaniases in Biology and Medicine*, vol. 2. Orlando: Academic Press, 1987: 909–926.

227 Modabber F. Development of vaccines against leishmaniasis. *Scand J Infect Dis Suppl* 1990; 76:72–78.

228 Marsden P D. Selective primary health care: strategies for control of disease in the developing world. XIV. Leishmaniasis. *Rev Infect Dis* 1984; 6:736–745.

229 Desjeux P. *Information on the Epidemiology and Control of the Leishmaniases by Country or Territory*. Geneva: WHO, 1992.

230 Ashford D A, Badaro R, Eulalio C et al. Studies on the control of visceral leishmaniasis: validation of the falcon assay screening test-enzyme-linked immunosorbent assay (fast-ELISA) for field diagnosis of canine visceral leishmaniasis. *Am J Trop Med Hyg* 1993; 48:1–8.

231 Gradoni L, Gramiccia M, Mancianti F & Pieri S. Studies on canine leishmaniasis control. 2. Effectiveness of control measures against canine leishmaniasis in the Isle of Elba, Italy. *Trans R Soc Trop Med Hyg* 1988; 82:568–571.

232 Thakur C P & Kumar K. Post kala-azar dermal leishmaniasis: a neglected aspect of kala-azar control programmes. *Ann Trop Med Parasitol* 1992; 86:355–359.

233 Lane R P. Contribution of sandfly control to leishmaniasis control. *Ann Soc Belg Med Trop* 1991; 71:65–74.

CHAPTER 66

TOXOPLASMOSIS

Richard E. Holliman

Toxoplasma gondii is an obligate intracellular parasite that causes infection in most mammals worldwide. Human infection is usually mild or asymptomatic but toxoplasmosis represents a life-threatening disease in the immunocompromised patient.

HISTORY

The organism was first described when Nicolle and Manceaux[1] found the parasite in the liver and spleen of a North African rodent, the gondii (*Ctenodactylus gundi*) in 1908. An association was made with human disease when Jankû[2] observed parasitic cysts in the retina of a child with hydrocephalus and microphthalmia. Wolf and Cowen[3] demonstrated the significance of congenital toxoplasmosis, while the discovery by Pinkerton and Weinman[4] of postnatal infection followed in 1940. Sabin and Feldman[5] developed the first reliable serological assay, the dye test, in 1948. This test allowed studies to establish the prevalence and clinical spectrum of the infection.

EPIDEMIOLOGY

The prevalence of antibodies specific to *T. gondii* is directly proportional to the age of the population, indicating that infection is acquired throughout life. The incidence of infection shows marked geographical variation: a quarter of pregnant women in England will have serological evidence of exposure to the parasite, whereas three-quarters of pregnant French women will have been infected.[6] These differences are associated with diet, climate and cat contact so that toxoplasmosis is most common in warm, wet areas with a large cat population where meat is eaten lightly cooked or raw. Many developed countries have noted a decline in the prevalence of the disease in recent years which may be associated with the practice of freezing meat and the introduction of intensive farming techniques which separate cats from livestock.

AETIOLOGY

T. gondii is a coccidian parasite which has a sexual cycle in the intestinal epithelium of the definitive host, members of the cat family, and an asexual cycle in secondary hosts, such as birds, rodents and other mammals (including man).

PARASITOLOGY

The characteristic form of toxoplasma is the crescent-shaped trophozoite, 6 μm in length and

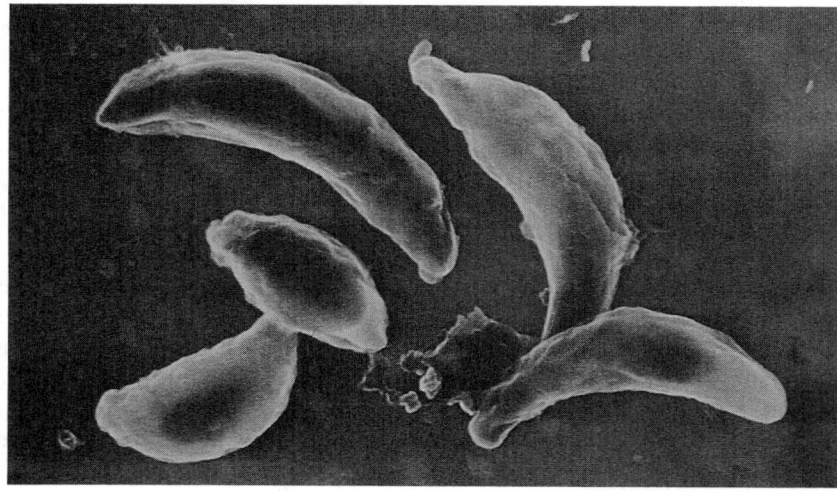

Figure 66.1 Trophozoites of *T. gondii* (scanning electron micrograph).

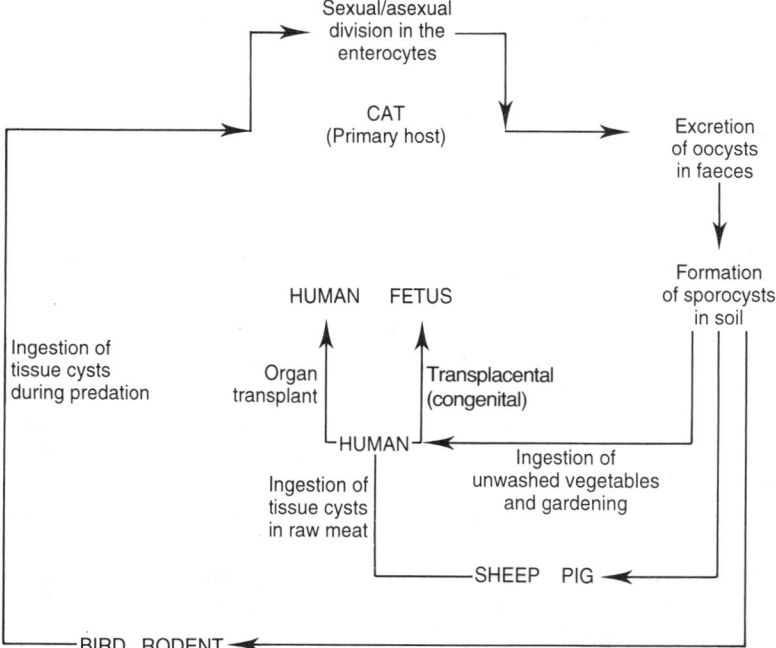

Figure 66.2 Transmission of toxoplasmosis.

3 μm wide, containing a single nucleus (Figure 66.1). *Toxon*, the Greek word for an arc or bow, the incidence of parasitaemia and the original animal source provide the derivation of the proper name *Toxoplasma gondii*.

Sexual and asexual multiplication of toxoplasma occurs in the enterocytes of felids and leads to the excretion of oocysts in their faeces. The oocysts sporulate within 3–4 days to form the infectious sporocyst. The sporocyst can retain viability for over 1 year in moist soil. Ingestion of the sporocyst by a secondary host is followed by release of tachyzoites which disseminate via the blood and lymphatic system, and by active cell invasion. Asexual multiplication of tachyzoites occurs in all nucleated cells, leading to disruption and invasion of adjoining cells.

Eventually a tissue cyst forms, consisting of a cyst wall (partly parasite, partly host in origin), and up to several thousand bradyzoites. The bradyzoite is morphologically similar to the tachyzoite but shows greatly reduced metabolic activity. Predation of the secondary host completes the life cycle. Tissue cysts release their contents in the gut lumen of the cat and the active tachyzoites invade the intestinal epithelium.[6,7]

TRANSMISSION (Figure 66.2)

Human infection is acquired by ingestion of tissue cysts in raw or poorly cooked meat, notably lamb and pork, or ingestion of sporocysts derived from cat faeces contaminating soil or inadequately washed vegetables. Rarely, infection can be acquired via an organ transplant.

PATHOGENESIS

The tachyzoite actively invades the cell and generates the formation of a parasitophorous vacuole which does not fuse with intracellular organelles, thereby avoiding destruction.[8] The tachyzoites divide by binary fission, forming an intracellular pseudocyst which distorts the host cell and ultimately leads to cellular disruption. The tachyzoites released in this process invade adjacent cells. Eventually tissue cysts form, containing quiescent bradyzoites. Periodic excystation occurs, controlled by mechanisms which are not established. Release of toxoplasma results in cellular destruction due to invasion and disruption by tachyzoites as well as damage associated with the host immune response.

Immunity is predominantly cell mediated. Activated macrophages and T cells play a central role while interferon-γ and other cytokines induce an effective immune response.[9] Specific antibody in the presence of complement eliminates extracellular parasites.

PATHOLOGY

Lesions observed at histopathological examination result from the dissemination of the parasite in the circulation, cytolytic action of the organism and the immune response of the host. Tissue necrosis is associated with thrombosis of small vessels.

Lymphadenopathy in the immunocompetent individual shows follicular hyperplasia and collections of mononuclear cells, usually at the periphery of the node. The normal tissue architecture is preserved and the parasites are rarely identified unless immunohistochemical stains are used.[10] The immunosuppressed patient, by contrast, may have abundant toxoplasma in the tissues. In cases of toxoplasmic encephalitis with the acquired immune deficiency syndrome (AIDS), cerebral tissues show central necrosis with surrounding astrocytosis. Pseudocysts are seen at the necrotic margins.[11] Necrosis, thrombosis and pseudocysts are present in the heart, liver, lung and brain of immunosuppressed patients with disseminated toxoplasmosis.

Congenital toxoplasmosis can be generalized or predominantly localized in the CNS. Brain tissue shows encephalitis with multiple infarcts and necrosis, particularly in the cortex, basal ganglia and periventricular areas. Characteristic glial nodules are formed. Focal calcification with zones of necrosis are present in severe disease of prolonged duration.[12] The infected placenta has chronic inflammation in the decidua and focal reaction within the villi.[13] Infected ocular tissue shows destruction of areas of the retina, with proliferation of pigment at the borders of lesions during healing. Occasionally parasites may be seen at the margins.[14]

CLINICAL FEATURES

THE IMMUNOCOMPETENT PATIENT

In most cases of toxoplasmosis the source of infection cannot be identified but the usual incubation period is between 1 and 3 weeks. The majority of individuals suffer no discernible illness and the acute infection passes unnoticed. The most common presentation of symptomatic toxoplasmosis is painless cervical lymphadenopathy, which may be accompanied by fever. Fewer persons experience generalized lymphadenopathy with malaise and myalgia which follows a course of relapse and remission over several weeks or months. The differential diagnosis includes lymphoma and infectious mononucleosis. Rarely, cutaneous rash, arthralgia, pericarditis or acute chorioretinitis may be associated with post-natal toxoplasma infection.[15] Some studies have suggested a link between hepatitis and toxoplasmosis but this remains contentious.[16]

CONGENITAL INFECTION

The incidence and presentation of acute toxoplasmosis in the pregnant woman does not differ from that of the population as a whole. Consequently, most infections pass unrecognized unless systematic screening is undertaken. The primary risk of congenital toxoplasmosis is associated with maternal parasitaemia and subsequent placentitis. As parasitaemia is normally limited to less than 20 days' duration, the greatest risk of fetal infection is associated with maternal infection acquired during pregnancy. A number of cases of congenital toxoplasmosis have been reported where the mother acquired the infection well before conception, but this is likely to be a rare event. The rate of maternal–fetal transmission of infection rises as the gestational age at the time of maternal infection progresses. The risk of fetal infection is 25% when the mother acquires her infection during the first trimester, and 65% if maternal infection is acquired in the third trimester. Conversely, the risk of severe fetal damage is highest if the infection crosses the placenta in early pregnancy.[17]

The features of congenital toxoplasmosis range from a severely damaged infant, with death in the perinatal period, to an infected but clinically unaffected child. Severe congenital toxoplasmosis presents with hydrocephalus, mental retardation, cerebral calcification and retinochoroiditis. Skin rash, hepatitis, pneumonia, myocarditis and myositis may be present.[18] Only 10% of all congenitally infected infants suffer such severe disease. Limited studies suggest most children born with congenital infection will develop ocular disease in later life, regardless of the clinical status at birth.[19]

OCULAR TOXOPLASMOSIS

Most cases of ocular toxoplasmosis result from periodic reactivation of infection established in the prenatal period. Excystation of the parasite is associated with acute inflammatory episodes and progressive retinal damage occurs. Retinal lesions may be apparent at birth but most often present as late sequelae in the second and third decades of life. Severe congenital disease is associated with microphthalmia, cataract, strabismus and nystagmus. The characteristic lesion is that of necrotizing retinitis, which appears as yellow-white 'cotton-wool' patches in the fundus during acute episodes. The lesions appear 'punched out' and pigmented when quiescent. The degree of visual disturbance depends on the location of the lesions within the retina. The differential diagnosis of ocular toxoplasmosis includes: colobomatous defect, intraocular haemorrhage, defects of retinal blood vessels, retinoblastoma and glioma.[20]

TOXOPLASMOSIS AND AIDS

Toxoplasmosis is the most common cause of focal brain lesions and one of the most frequent opportunistic infections in patients with AIDS. Most cases result from secondary reactivation of a chronic, previously quiescent infection associated with impairment of the individual's immune function. Features of cerebral infection predominate and the characteristic presentation is that of fever, persistent headache, deterioration of mental status and focal neurological signs. Retinochoroiditis, following extension of CNS infection, and pulmonary disease (presenting with cough and dyspnoea) are also described. Disseminated infection involving the heart, liver, CNS and lungs may be found at post mortem.[21] The differential diagnosis of cerebral toxoplasmosis with AIDS includes: lymphoma, cryptococcal infection and bacterial brain abscess. Human immunodeficiency virus (HIV)-infected patients with residual cell-mediated immune function (pre-AIDS) may present with an indolent illness comprising malaise, chronic headache and lymphadenopathy, usually associated with primary toxoplasma infection.

TOXOPLASMOSIS AND ORGAN TRANSPLANTATION

Toxoplasmosis represents a life-threatening complication to organ graft recipients. Severe toxoplasma infection in association with solid organ transplantation (heart, heart–lung, liver and kidney) is restricted to the recipient without pre-existing immunity to toxoplasma (seronegative) who is given an organ containing viable cysts of the parasite (seropositive donor). The frequency of infection in such 'mismatches' reflects the likelihood of the organ transplant containing cysts. Consequently, infection is most frequent after cardiac transplant and least common in association with renal transplantation. The infected recipient develops fever, deterioration of consciousness and signs of respiratory failure—reflecting disseminated disease, usually 3–6 weeks after the operation.[22]

As the duration of parasitaemia following acute infection is limited, blood transfusion will rarely transmit toxoplasmosis. The risk is greater after granulocyte transfusion. Toxoplasmosis associated with bone marrow transplant is a rare event and is usually due to reactivation of the recipient's previously quiescent, chronic infection. Fever, CNS signs and pulmonary dysfunction are characteristic findings 15–150 days after transplantation.[23]

DIAGNOSIS

In most instances the non-specific nature of the signs and symptoms of toxoplasmosis does not permit reliable diagnosis based solely on the clinical findings. However, due to the diversity of toxoplasma infection, investigations must be selected which are appropriate to that patient group.[24] Suitable test selections are given in Table 66.1.

ISOLATION

T. gondii can be isolated from infected tissues by animal inoculation or tissue culture. Intraperitoneal injection into mice is a highly sensitive diagnostic method but results are only available 3–6 weeks after inoculation. Tissue culture is less sensitive but produces a result within 10 days.[25]

PARASITE DETECTION

Histological examination can be helpful, particularly following excision of enlarged lymph nodes or biopsy of a cerebral lesion in AIDS. The sensitivity of these investigations is improved if immunohistochemical studies are employed.[26] A number of antigen detection methods has been developed utilizing

Table 66.1 Investigation of toxoplasmosis.

	Parasite isolation	Histology	Parasite detection	Serology	Other
Immunocompetent patient					
Lymphadenopathy	—	Excision biopsy	—	IgG, IgM	—
Pregnancy	—	—	—	IgG, IgM, IgA, avidity tests	—
Ocular disease	—	—	Ocular fluid	IgG, local antibody production	—
Immunosuppressed patient					
Fetus	Amniotic fluid, blood cells	—	Blood cells	IgM, IgA	Total IgM, liver function tests
Neonate	Placenta, blood cells	—	Blood cells	Sequential IgG assessment, IgM, IgA	Radiology of brain, ocular examination
AIDS	Brain biopsy	Brain biopsy	Brain biopsy	IgG	Radiology of brain, therapeutic trial
Organ transplant					
Heart/lung/liver/ kidney	Tissue biopsy, bone marrow	Tissue biopsy	—	IgG, IgM	—
Bone marrow	Bone marrow, blood cells	—	Bone marrow	—	Therapeutic trial

enzyme linked immunosorbent assay (ELISA) and agglutination systems.[27] Antigen detection is most valuable when investigating the immunocompromised when the serological response is altered. The limitation of antigen detection has been the relative lack of sensitivity of the assay. Methods based on the detection of toxoplasma DNA by hybridization with specific probes or amplification using the polymerase chain reaction may represent a considerable advance.[28]

SEROLOGY

A wide range of antibody detection methods are available and serology is often the investigation of choice. *T. gondii* contains a large number of membranous and cytoplasmic antigens which are incorporated into the different serological assays in variable proportions. It is not possible to compare antibody levels recorded by different tests. Whole organisms are used as the antigen source in the dye test, direct agglutination test and fluorescent antibody assay. Disrupted organisms are fixed to carrier particles in the indirect haemagglutination test and latex agglutination test and provide the antigen source for ELISA-based systems.[24]

The presence of specific IgG indicates prior exposure to the parasite and the potential for reactivation in the immunocompromised. Specific IgM, IgA or low avidity IgG is associated with more recent infection of the immune competent individual. The dye test remains the 'gold standard' test but the availability of this bioassay is restricted.

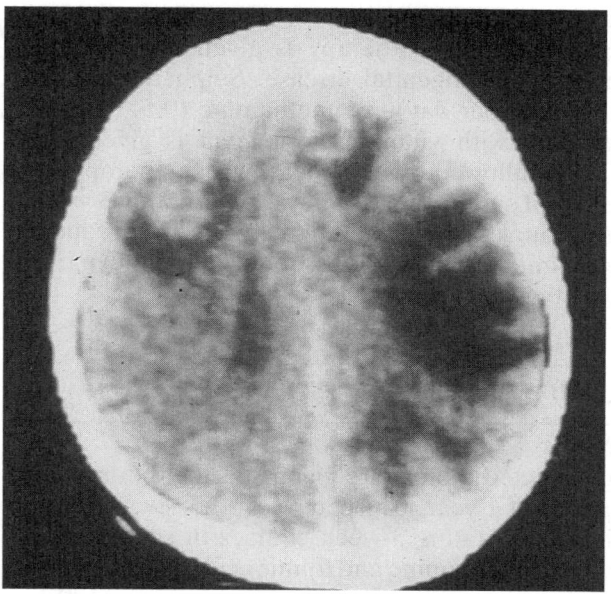

Figure 66.3 Computerized tomography of the brain in cerebral toxoplasmosis associated with AIDS.

OTHER METHODS

Cell-mediated immunity can be measured by a skin test or in vitro assays but has limited clinical applications. Computerized tomography of the brain is useful in the investigation of patients with congenital toxoplasmosis and AIDS (Figure 66.3). Therapeutic trials of antiparasite drugs may be required to confirm the diagnosis of toxoplasmosis in the profoundly immunosuppressed.[21]

MANAGEMENT

None of the agents currently available for clinical use shows activity against the encysted form of the parasite. Consequently, treatment is directed against the active tachyzoite form and complete eradication of the parasite is not attempted.[29]

IMMUNOCOMPETENT PATIENTS

Specific therapy has *not* been shown to be effective in otherwise healthy individuals and is rarely indicated in view of the potential toxicity of antitoxoplasma agents. Therapy may be considered when the illness is protracted or unusually severe. Sulpha-

diazine (2 g/day) with pyrimethamine (25 mg/day) is given by the oral route. Sulphadimidine may be substituted for sulphadiazine. Vitamin supplementation consisting of folinic acid (15 mg twice weekly) or yeast tablets BPC (8 tablets twice weekly) is given to prevent bone marrow toxicity.[30]

THE PREGNANT WOMAN

The macrolide antibiotic spiramycin should be given at a dose of 3 g/day throughout the confinement to reduce the risk of transplacental passage of the parasite. If fetal infection is confirmed by cordocentesis, antiparasite therapy is given to reduce the severity of congenital disease. Sulphadiazine (50–100 mg/kg per day)–pyrimethamine (0.5–1.0 mg/kg per day) with vitamin supplement is given for 3 weeks, followed by a further 3 weeks' therapy consisting of spiramycin (3 g/day). Alternating 3 weeks' drug courses are given until delivery. The frequency of pyrimethamine dosing is reduced if bone marrow toxicity is demonstrated.[31]

CONGENITAL INFECTION

All infected infants are given specific therapy until the age of 1 year, irrespective of the severity of the disease. Rotating 3-week courses of sulphadiazine with pyrimethamine and folinic acid (doses as for the pregnant woman) followed by spiramycin (100 mg/kg per day) are given.[32] The role of corticosteroids is not established.

OCULAR DISEASE

Quiescent lesions noted beyond the age of 1 year require observation only. When active inflammation is noted sulphadiazine (2 g/day) or clindamycin (1.2 g/day) given with pyrimethamine (25 mg/day) and vitamin supplementation is advised. Treatment is continued for 10 days after inflammation subsides. Systemic corticosteroids are usually administered during the antiparasite therapy.[33] Laser or cryotherapy may be used in an attempt to limit the spread of a lesion across the retina.

TOXOPLASMOSIS WITH AIDS

Acute therapy comprises sulphadiazine (4–8 g/day)–pyrimethamine 50–75 g/day) with vitamin supplements continued for 6 weeks. Clindamycin (2.4–4.8 g/day) can be substituted if severe sulphonamide toxicity is experienced. Reduced dose maintenance therapy is given after an acute episode to prevent relapse.[34] Dapsone (200 mg/day) is also suitable for this purpose.

ORGAN TRANSPLANT RECIPIENTS

Seronegative recipients of a seropositive heart, heart–lung or liver donor should be given pyrimethamine (25 mg/day) prophylaxis for 6 weeks after the operation to prevent primary infection.[35] When significant disease is established in any organ graft recipient high-dose therapy, similar to that given in AIDS, is indicated. Maintenance therapy is not required unless the period of immunosuppression is likely to be prolonged.

PREVENTION AND CONTROL

HEALTH EDUCATION

Women contemplating pregnancy or shown to be seronegative after conception should be given guidance to reduce the risk of acquiring toxoplasmosis during pregnancy. Foods eaten without further preparation, such as vegetables and fruit, should be washed to remove contaminating soil and sporocysts. Gloves should be worn when gardening or emptying cat litter trays. Meats that might contain tissue cysts should be cooked until well done and hand-washing after preparing raw meat should be emphasized.[36] Similar advice can be given to HIV-infected individuals.

Previously, deliberate exposure to the parasite prior to puberty was encouraged in some areas by the habit of eating raw meat. This practice is no longer considered ethical due to the risk of reactivated infection should the individual later become immunosuppressed.

VACCINATION

Short-lived immunity can be induced when using non-viable toxoplasma, while viable organisms of reduced pathogenicity are associated with chronic infection and potential reactivation.[37] Field trials of non-cyst-forming strains of T. gondii in sheep are in progress but there is presently no vaccine suitable for humans.

ANTENATAL SCREENING

Any screening programme should be evaluated in four main areas: frequency and severity of the disease; sensitivity, specificity, performance and cost of diagnosis; effectiveness of management; adminis-trative structure. In France, a programme based on IgG seroconversion is in operation and similar schemes have been promoted in other countries.[38] Further research is required to establish the harm:benefit ratio of screening for toxoplasmosis in pregnancy before the diversion of scarce funds from other health projects can be justified.

REFERENCES

1 Nicolle C & Manceaux L. Sur une infection à corps de leishman (où organisme voisins) du gondii. *C R Acad Sci* 1908; 147:763–766.

2 Jankû J. Pathogensa a pathologiká anatomie tak nazvaného vrozeného kolobomu zluté skurny v oku normálne velikém a mikrophthalmickém s nálezem parazitu v sítnici. *Cas Lék Ces* 1923; 62:1021–1027.

3 Wolf A & Cowen D. Granulomatous encephalomyelitis due to an encephalitozoan (encephalitozoic encepholomyelitis). A new protozoan disease of man. *Bull Neurol Inst N Y* 1937; 6:306–371.

4 Pinkerton H & Weinman D. Toxoplasma infection in man. *Arch Pathol* 1940; 30:374–392.

5 Sabin A B & Feldman H A. Dyes as microchemical indicators of a new immunity phenomenon affecting a protozoan parasite. *Science* 1948; 108:660–663.

6 Remington J S & Desmonts G. In Remington J S & Klein J O (eds) *Infectious Diseases of the Fetus and Newborn Infant*. London: W B Saunders, 1990: 89–195.

7 Dubey J P & Beatie G P. *Toxoplasmosis of animals and man* (Homo sapiens). Boca Raton: CRC Press, 1988: 41–60.

8 Joiner K. Cell attachment and entry by *Toxoplasma gondii*. *Behring Inst Mitt* 1991; 88:20–26.

9 Suzuki Y, Orellana M A, Schreiber R D & Remington J S. Interferon gamma, the major mediator of resistance against *Toxoplasma gondii*. *Science* 1988; 240:516–518.

10 Fleck D G & Kwantes W. *The Laboratory Diagnosis of Toxoplasmosis*. Public Health Laboratory Service Monograph 13. London: HMSO, 1980.

11 Luft B J, Brooks R G, Conley F K, McCabe R E & Remington J S. Toxoplasmic encephalitis in patients with acquired immune deficiency syndrome. *JAMA* 1984; 257:913–917.

12 Frenkel J K. Toxoplasma: mechanisms of infection, laboratory diagnosis and management. *Curr Top Pathol* 1971; 54:27–75.

13 Elliot W G. Placental toxoplasmosis: report of a case. *Am J Clin Pathol* 1970; 53:413–417.

14 Hogan M J. *Ocular Toxoplasmosis*. New York: Columbia University Press, 1951: 86.

15 Kean B H. Clinical toxoplasmosis—50 years. *Trans R Soc Trop Med Hyg* 1972; 66:549–571.

16 Weitberg A B, Alper J C, Diamond I & Flegiel Z. Acute granulomatous hepatitis in the course of acquired toxoplasmosis. *N Engl J Med* 1979; 300:1093–1096.

17 Carter A O & Frank J W. Congenital toxoplasmosis: epidemiological features and control. *Can Med Assoc J* 1986; 135:618–623.

18 Eichwald H. *A Study of Congenital Toxoplasmosis*. Munksgaard: Copenhagen, 1960: 41–49.

19 Koppe J G, Loewer-Sieger D H & de Roever-Bonnet H. Results of 20 year follow-up of congenital toxoplasmosis. *Lancet* 1986; 1:254–255.

20 de Jong P T. Ocular toxoplasmosis: common and rare symptoms and signs. *Int Ophthalmol* 1989; 13:391–397.

21 Holliman R E. Toxoplasmosis and the acquired immune deficiency syndrome. *J Infect* 1988; 16:121–128.

22 Wreghitt T G, Hakim M, Gray J J et al. Toxoplasmosis in heart and heart and lung transplant recipients. *J Clin Pathol* 1987; 42:194–199.

23 O'Driscoll J C & Holliman R E. Toxoplasmosis and bone marrow transplantation. *Rev Med Microbiol* 1991; 2:215–222.

24 Holliman R E. The diagnosis of toxoplasmosis. *Serodiagn Immunother Infect Dis* 1990; 4:83–93.

25 Hughes H P, Hudson L & Fleck D G. In vitro culture of *Toxoplasma gondii* in primary and established cell lines. *Int J Parasitol* 1986; 16:317–322.

26 Conley F K & Junkins K A. Immunohistological study of the anatomic relationship of toxoplasma antigens to the inflammatory response in the brains of mice chronically infected with *Toxoplasma gondii*. *Infect Immun* 1981; 31:1184–1192.

27 van Knapen F & Panggabean S O. Detection of circulating antigens during acute infections with *Toxoplasma gondii* by enzyme-linked immunosorbent assay. *J Clin Microbiol* 1977; 6:545–547.

28 Savva D, Morris J C, Johnson J D & Holliman R E. Polymerase chain reaction for detection of *Toxoplasma gondii*. *J Med Microbiol* 1990; 32:25–31.

29 McCabe R E & Oster S. Current recommendations and future prospects in the treatment of toxoplasmosis. *Drugs* 1989; 38:973–987.

30 Krick J A & Remington J S. Toxoplasmosis in the adult—an overview. *N Engl J Med* 1978; 298:550–553.

31 Couvreur J & Desmonts G. Toxoplasmosis. In MacCleod C L (ed.) *Parasitic Infections in Pregnancy and the Newborn*. Oxford: Oxford University Press, 1988; 112–142.

32 Wilson C B. Treatment of congenital toxoplasmosis. *Pediatr Infect Dis J* 1990; 9:682–683.

33 Dutton G N. Recent developments in the prevention and treatment of congenital toxoplasmosis. *Int Ophthalmol* 1989; 13:407–413.

34 Navia B A, Petito C K, Gold J W, Cho E S, Jordan B D & Price R W. Cerebral toxoplasmosis complicating the acquired immune deficiency syndrome: clinical and neuropathological findings in 27 patients. *Ann Neurol* 1986; 19:224–238.

35 Holliman R E, Johnson J D, Adams S & Pepper J R. Toxoplasmosis and heart transplantation. *J Heart Lung Transplant* 1991; 10:608–610.

36 Carter A O, Gelmon S B, Wells G A & Toepell A P. The effectiveness of a prenatal education programme for the prevention of congenital toxoplasmosis. *Epidemiol Infect* 1989; 103:539–545.

37 Overnes G, Nesse L L, Waldeland H, Lougren K & Gudding R. Immune response after immunisation with an experimental *Toxoplasma gondii* ISCOM vaccine. *Vaccine* 1991; 9:25–28.

38 McCabe R E & Remington J S. Toxoplasmosis: the time has come. *N Engl J Med* 1988; 318:313–315.

CHAPTER 67

INTESTINAL PROTOZOA

Michael J. G. Farthing, Ana-María Cevallos and Paul Kelly

Human intestinal protozoan infections are found worldwide both in developing countries and the industrialized world. Pathogenic intestinal protozoa produce disease by infecting the small or large intestine, or both. Intestinal protozoa are found in highest prevalence in developing countries, where they are responsible for a substantial burden of disease. The small intestinal protozoa, *Giardia lamblia* and *Cryptosporidium parvum* have their major impact in children, while the large bowel pathogen, *Entamoeba histolytica* infects all age groups but has its most profound effects in adults. The epidemiology of intestinal protozoan infection has developed rapidly with the increase in acquired immunodeficiency states, particularly that relating to cytotoxic chemotherapy for cancer and human immunodeficiency virus (HIV) infection and the acquired immune deficiency syndrome (AIDS). Interestingly, some of the protozoa, particularly *Cryptosporidium* and *Isospora belli*, have a profoundly increased morbidity in immunodeficiency states, whereas the severity of disease due to giardiasis and amoebiasis is little affected.

The world of human intestinal pathogenic protozoa continues to expand. Human infection with *Cryptosporidium parvum* was first recognized in 1976, since when several new pathogenic protozoa have been discovered in man, namely the microsporidia (*Enterocytozoon bieneusi, Septata intestinalis*) and *Cyclospora cayatenensis*. As methods of detection improve it seems likely that other human protozoan pathogens will emerge.

Despite the prevalence of human protozoan enteropathogens, their history has evolved gradually during the nineteenth and twentieth centuries, with major advances occurring since the 1970s when it has been possible to culture some in the laboratory. The coccidia, however, have largely resisted attempts at in vitro culture, presumably because of their more complex life cycle. The pathogenic potential of these protozoa has been vigorously debated; during the first half of the twentieth century for example, the clinical importance of *Giardia lamblia* was still seriously questioned, even by eminent parasitologists such as Dobell. The fact that these infections are responsible for significant intestinal disease in humans, with profound morbidity, and in some cases mortality, is now well established, although as yet parasite biology and mechanisms of pathogenesis are still not clearly established. For many of the protozoa the host immune response remains poorly defined, as are the mechanisms involved in eradication and the development of protective immunity. As yet there is no candidate vaccine for any of the intestinal protozoa. It is likely that the next decade will produce great advances in our understanding of many of these questions, with commensurate progress in treatment and prevention.

THE SARCODINA (AMOEBAE)

The subphylum Sarcodina is characterized by organisms that move by pseudopodia or by locomotive protoplasmic flow without discrete pseudopodia; flagella, when present, are usually restricted to developmental or other temporary stages. Most species are free living, such as *Acanthamoeba* and *Naegleria*. However, many species such as *Entamoeba histolytica, E. coli, E. hartmanni, E. gingivalis, Dientamoeba fragilis, Endolimax nana* and *Iodamoeba bütschlii* have been definitely established as parasites of man. All live in the large intestine, except *E. gingivalis*, which is found in the mouth.

ENTAMOEBA HISTOLYTICA

Amoebiasis, the infection caused by the parasitic protozoan, *E. histolytica*, is reported to affect around 480 million people around the world.[1] The majority of these individuals are asymptomatic, with the organism existing as a harmless commensal in the intestine. However, about 10% develop disease, usually in the colon and less frequently in the liver. In 1875, Löch[2] in St Petersburg described the clinical and autopsy findings of a case of fatal dysentery and identified the amoebae. Although he was able to infect a dog with this organism, he was not able to mimic the disease produced in his patient and failed to recognize the relationship. In 1890, William Osler[3] reported the case of a young man who contracted dysentery and developed an hepatic abscess that led to his death. One year later, Councilman and Lafleur[4] conducted a detailed study of patients with amoebic dysentery and hepatic abscess. They confirmed the pathogenic role of amoebae and created the terms 'amoebic dysentery' and 'amoebic liver abscess'. Schaudinn[5] differentiated E. histolytica from E. coli in 1903. In 1913, Walker and Sellards[6] definitively established the pathogenicity of E. histolytica by feeding cysts to volunteers. Brumpt[7] in 1925 was the first to suggest that the differences in symptomatology and in the global distribution of invasive amoebiasis were due to the presence of two species of amoeba, morphologically indistinguishable one from another, but with different pathogenic potential. He distinguished the two species based on their pathogenicity in humans and in experimentally infected kittens. He suggested the term E. dysenteriae for the pathogenic amoeba and E. dispar for the non-pathogenic. Because Brumpt was unable to distinguish morphologically between the two proposed species and because there was growing evidence that cysts obtained from asymptomatic carriers could produce experimental infection, his explanation gained little support. It regained favour only after Sargeaunt and associates[8,9] were able to distinguish pathogenic strains of E. histolytica from non-pathogenic strains on the basis of isoenzyme typing. Using this typing method, other virulence markers have been described. In 1993, Diamond and Clark,[10] using all of the biochemical, immunological and genetic evidence for distinguishing pathogenic from non-pathogenic strains of E. histolytica, redescribed E. histolytica Schaudinn, 1903, formally separating it from E. dispar Brumpt, 1925. If the presence of two species within E. histolytica is widely accepted, the epidemiological data available and the natural history of both infections would need to be re-evaluated.

THE ORGANISM

Taxonomy

The Committee on Systematics and Evolution of the Society of Protozoology has placed E. histolytica in the phylum Sarcomastigophora, subphylum Sarcodina, superclass Rhizopoda, class Lobosea, subclass Gymnamoebia, order Amoebida and suborder Tubulina.[11] More recently its phylogenetic status has been questioned and it has been suggested that E. histolytica should be reclassified within a new (sub)kingdom, the Archezoa, which would incorporate all existent organisms whose ancestors branched off the main eukaryotic line before protomitochondria were incorporated, such as Giardia and Vairimorpha.[12]

Structure

The trophozoite is distinguished from other intestinal amoebae by morphological characteristics of diagnostic importance. It ranges in size from 10 to 60 μm. Two zones can be recognized within the cytoplasm: an outer zone or ectoplasm and an inner zone or endoplasm. The ectoplasm is clear, refractive and sharply separated from the endoplasm. The endoplasm contains abundant vesicles embedded in a cytoplasmic matrix, which gives them the appearance of ground glass. The cytoplasmic vesicles sometimes contain ingested red blood cells in various stages of disintegration. Trophozoites have no rough endoplasmic reticulum or Golgi system, present in other eukaryotic cells. Ribosomes appear to be ordered in helical arrays. The cytoskeleton is characterized by microfilaments, generally found immediately below the plasma membrane at the sites of attachment of the amoeba to the substrate and where phagocytic channels are formed. The nucleus is not usually visible, although it may be faintly discerned as a finely granular ring in the unstained amoeba. When stained with haematoxylin, trichrome or Lawless stain, details of nuclear structure may be observed. The nucleus is spherical and 4–7 μm in diameter. The nuclear membrane is clearly defined; its inner surface is lined with uniform and closely packed fine granules of chromatin. In the centre of the nucleus is a small mass of chromatin, the karyosome. A clear halo surrounding the karyosome and a 'linin' network giving a 'cartwheel' appearance has been described but they probably represent fixation artefacts.

In fresh isolates, E. histolytica can move as fast as 5 μm per second. Trophozoites move by means of pseudopodia, cytoplasmic protrusions which may be formed at any point on the surface of the organism. Actively moving trophozoites have a well-defined morphological polarity. The clear glass-like ecto-plasm flows out to form the pseudopodium, slowly followed by the more granular endoplasm as the amoeba moves in the direction in which it was extruded. The pseudopodial extension is accompanied by recycling of the cytoplasm and formation of a posterior appendix, commonly referred to as the uroid. The uroid accumulates capped ligands as bacteria, lectins or antibodies and, by an unknown mechanism, is detached from the amoeba without damaging the parasite.

The precyst amoebae are colourless, round or oval cells that are smaller than the trophozoite but larger than the cyst. They may be distinguished by a rounded single nucleus, absence of ingested material and lack of a cyst wall. The cytoplasm usually contains deposits of diffuse glycogen and, occasionally, chromatoid bodies are seen. The nuclear morphology is often confusing at this stage and it is best to rely upon either trophozoites or cysts for specific identification.

The cysts are round or oval, slightly asymmetrical hyaline bodies, $10-16\,\mu m$, with a smooth, refractive, non-staining wall about $0.5\,\mu m$ thick. The immature cyst has a single nucleus, about one-third of its diameter, while the mature infective cyst contains four smaller nuclei, rarely more. The nuclei may at times appear as small refractive spheres within the cytoplasm of the unstained cyst, but more often they are not visible. The cytoplasm of the young cysts contains vacuoles with glycogen and chromatoid bodies. These chromatoid bodies, so named because they stain with haematoxylin like the chromatin of the nucleus, are reported to contain ribonucleic and deoxyribonucleic acids and phosphates, and tend to disappear as the cyst matures, so that they may be absent in about half of the cysts. When stained with iodine, the cytoplasm of the cyst will be yellow-green to yellow-brown in colour; the nuclear membrane and karyosome are distinct and light brown. Chromatoidal bars do not stain and appear as clear spaces in the cytoplasm. If glycogen is present in the cytoplasm it will stain a dark yellow-brown.

Microbiology

The main reservoir of *E. histolytica* is man, although morphologically similar amoebae may be found in primates, dogs and cats. The complete life cycle of *E. histolytica* consists of four consecutive stages: the trophozoite, precyst, cyst and metacyst. The cyst is resistant to gastric acid, and on ingestion it passes into the small intestine. The amoeba within the cyst becomes active in the neutral or alkaline environment of the small intestine. The cyst wall is digested, probably by the digestive enzymes within the lumen of the gut. The encysted amoeba becomes very active, separates from the cyst wall and rapidly divides into the number of organisms corresponding to the number of nuclei present, usually four. They rapidly undergo division to form eight uninucleate trophozoites which are smaller than the trophozoites seen in the colon. They are carried into the caecum where they complete their maturation. They multiply by binary fission, the nucleus dividing by modified mitosis. As the amoebae pass down the colon they become dehydrated and assume a spherical shape known as a precyst. A thin cyst wall is secreted, forming an unripe cyst. Two mitotic divisions occur, resulting in a cyst that contains four nuclei. They are evacuated in the stool and discharged into the environment. Cysts remain viable and infective for several days in faeces and water, but are easily killed by desiccation.

Robinson's[13] medium for the cultivation of amoebae in association with bacteria has been widely used for the isolation and characterization of amoebae. Diamond's[14] medium allows the cultivation of pathogenic *E. histolytica* without bacteria or other living organisms, that is axenically. So far, all efforts to grow non-pathogenic strains axenically have been fruitless. Optimum growth occurs at 35–37°C at pH 7.0, and under reduced oxygen tension. Culture of amoebae directly from faecal specimens for diagnostic purposes is possible, but bacterial flora must be added to the culture and therefore is not in routine use.

All strains of *E. histolytica* are able to adhere to host cells and induce proteolysis of the host's cellular matrix in vitro. However only some strains are able to invade in vivo. This crucial difference in clinical behaviour has led to the classification of *E. histolytica* trophozoites in two groups: pathogenic (P) and non-pathogenic (NP). P *E. histolytica* can be discriminated from NP *E. histolytica* on the basis of the migration of six isoenzymes (hexokinase, phospho-glucomutase, aldolase, acetylglucosaminidase, peptidase and NAD-diaphorase)[15] (Figure 67.1). They can also be identified by monoclonal antibodies against several proteins: the 96kDa antigen,[16] the 29–30kDa antigen,[17,18] the Gal/GalNAc adherence lectin,[19] the EDG (electron-dense granules)[20] antigen, the 81–84 kDa antigen[21] and an uncharacterized antigen.[22] They can also be separated by the use of genetic markers such as: (1) dot hybridization with probe P145;[23] (2) fragment pattern length polymorphism of genomic DNA probed with the 125 kDa antigen,[24] actin,[24] cysteine-proteinase,[25] super-

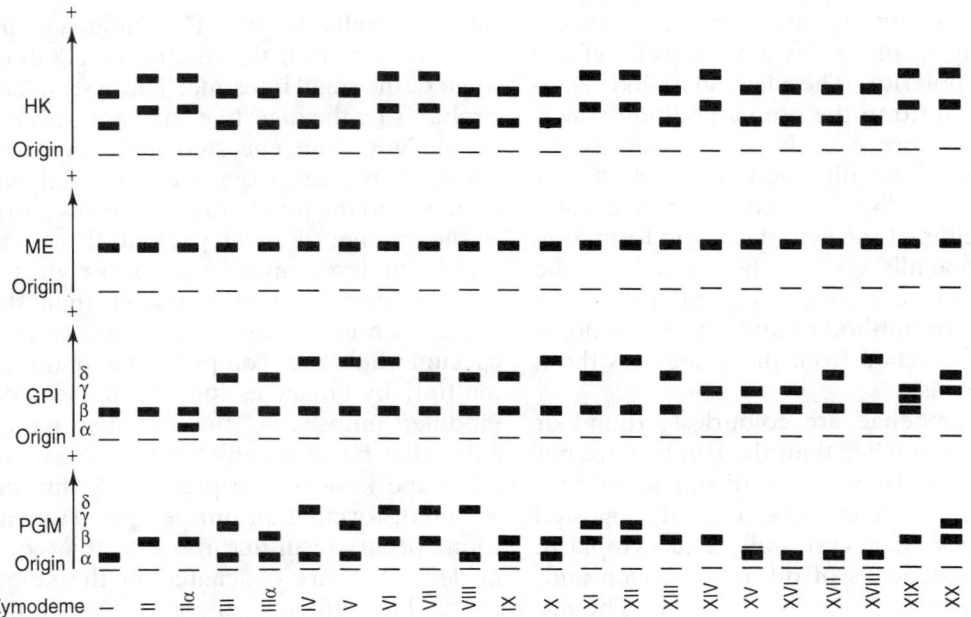

Figure 67.1   Zymodemes of *E. histolytica* identified by using GPI (EC 5.3.1.9), L-malate:NADP$^+$ oxidoreductase (ME; oxaloacetate decarboxylating) (EC 1.1.1.4.0), PGM (EC 2.7.5.1) and HK (EC 2.7.1.1). Pathogenic zymodemes include II, IIα, VI, VII, XI, XII, XIII, XIV, XIX and XX. Non-pathogenic zymodemes include I, III, IIIα, IV, V, VIII, IX, X, XV, XVI, XVII, XVIII and (not shown) XXI. (Reproduced from Bruckner.[56])

oxide dismutase[26] or ribosomal genes;[27,28] (3) restriction enzyme digestion of polymerase chain reaction (PCR) amplification products of the small subunit rRNA,[29] the 29–30 kDa antigen[30] or 125 kDa antigen genes;[31] and (4) PCR amplification of gene fragments with oligonucleotides specific for the small subunit rRNA[29] or 29–30 kDa antigen[32] genes.

There are two hypotheses to explain the biological difference between P and NP isolates. The first sustains that P and NP isolates are in fact two different species of *Entamoeba*. The second suggests that a commensal *E. histolytica* is capable, under special conditions, of conversion into an invasive pathogen. Currently the most accepted hypothesis is that non-pathogenic strains represent a different species of *Entamoeba*. Diamond and Clark[10] in 1993 published a redescription of *E. histolytica* Shaudinn, 1903, excluding NP isolates which they proposed should be reclassified as *E. dispar* Brumpt, 1925.

Metabolism

E. histolytica is one of the most primitive eukaryotes, lacking mitochondria, cytochromes, peroxisomes, Golgi apparatus, rough endoplasmic reticulum, typical lysosomes and organized cytoskeleton. It is not an obligate anaerobe because it does consume oxygen and will grow in an environ- ment containing up to 5% oxygen. Carbohydrates are the main source of energy for the parasite. The uptake of glucose involves a specific transport system that provides approximately 100 times the amount incorporated by endocytosis.[33] Glucose is degraded to pyruvate via the Embden–Meyerhof pathway. The principal end-products of the anaerobic carbohydrate metabolism are ethanol and carbon dioxide; lactate is not produced and lactate dehydrogenase has not been reported. In many of the glycolytic reactions inorganic pyrophosphate, rather than ATP, is used as an energy source. Amoebic trophozoites also have an aerobic metabolism and display high affinity for oxygen.[34] Despite the lack of mitochondria and tricarboxylic acid cycle, electrons are transferred from reduced substrates to molecular oxygen through a succession of carriers, including flavins and non-haem iron.

Synthesis of nucleic acids depends on the salvage of preformed purines as *E. histolytica* lacks a *de novo* purine pathway. It is also able to salvage pyrimidine bases although it is able to synthesize them *de novo*.[35] It is estimated that there is 0.5 pg of DNA per nucleus with a genomic size of 4.0×10^8 bp.[36] Several copies of rDNA are present as extrachromosomal circular elements. The number of copies in the different strains varies. These circular rDNA contain two large repetitive regions. The polymorphism of these regions have been useful as probes for strain identification.[23]

Genetics

There is increasing evidence to suggest that there are two distinct species of *E. histolytica*. Many biological, immunological and genetic differences between P and NP isolates have been described.

Biological differences include: differences in susceptibility to complement-mediated lysis and phagocytic capacity. Non-pathogenic *E. histolytica* is always resistant to complement. However pathogenic *E. histolytica* in axenic culture are susceptible to complement lysis, whereas when grown in the presence of human sera or after passage through animals they become resistant. In general, pathogenic amoebae engage in active erythrophagocytosis, whereas non-pathogenic amoebae ingest few red blood cells. Only P isolates can be grown axenically.

Immunological differences

Monoclonal antibodies against the Gal/GalNAc adherence lectin revealed that four of six epitopes on P isolates were not present on NP forms.[19] Monoclonal antibodies against the 81/84 kDa antigen,[21] against the 29/30 kDa antigen[17] and against electron-dense granules[20] have been found to react only with P isolates.

Genetic differences

Analysis of the taxonomic relationship between P and NP strains based on the isoenzyme profiles of 14 loci clearly demonstrated that P and NP isolates fall into two genetically distinct groups, and that several enzymes unambiguously distinguished between the two.[37] Significant genetic divergence has also been found for the inferred amino acid sequences for the cysteine proteinases,[25] superoxide dismutase[26] and 29/30 kDa antigens. Partial sequencing of the small subunit ribosomal RNA genes demonstrated a genetic distance of 2.2%, a difference greater than that occurring between human and mice.[29] Southern blots of restriction enzyme digested total DNA from several P and NP isolates using recombinant ribosomal DNA probes revealed consistent pattern differences between the two forms. P isolates encode for a cysteine proteinase gene (ACP1) absent in NP isolates.[38] The presence of the ACP1 gene correlated with increased proteinase expression, activity and an in vitro cytopathic effect.

Despite the compelling evidence discussed above for two species, there are factors which do not support this hypothesis. The conversion of the isoenzyme patterns of certain cloned and uncloned NP isolates to those of the P form during attempts to axenize NP amoebae has been reported.[39,40] Reversion back to the NP pattern was accomplished by reassociating the amoebae with their original flora. The conversion of the isoenzyme patterns was accompanied by a parallel alteration in virulence from avirulent to virulent. These converted NP strains resemble typical P amoeba at the immunological and DNA levels.[23,28,29] It was speculated that: 'all *E. histolytica* strains contain copies of the same sequences in their genomes, but changes in certain conditions of growth may cause the amoeba to amplify different elements and express modified amoebic components and behaviours which would remain undetected under other culture conditions of growth.' Using PCR techniques, evidence was presented for the existence of one or a few tandemly repetitive P145 elements characteristic of P isolates in an NP isolate.[41] However, copies of the NP-specific B133 repetitive elements could not be demonstrated in P amoebae. In another study, the presence of a P rRNA gene by PCR was sought in an NP isolate without success.[29] Other attempts to alter isoenzyme patterns and to convert NP isolates into P isolates have failed, including studies using the two isolates reported in the conversion papers.

More research is clearly needed to explain why, if NP isolates are able to adhere to host cells and induce proteolysis in vivo, they do not invade in vivo. It is also necessary to investigate if NP isolates can convert to P isolates in vivo. Genetic exchange between isolates with different zymodemes has been demonstrated in vitro.[42] The possibility that this may also occur in vivo, particularly between P and NP isolates because they frequently coexist, should be explored.

EPIDEMIOLOGY

E. histolytica has a worldwide distribution and is endemic in most countries with low socioeconomic conditions. It is the third leading parasitic cause of death after malaria and schistosomiasis. It has been estimated that approximately 480 million people, or 12% of the world's population, are infected and that the annual mortality is 40 000–110 000 persons.[1] However, there is a wide variation in prevalence, depending on the population studied, from around 1% in industrialized countries to 50–80% in the tropics. There are very few data looking, specifically, at the prevalence of pathogenic strains; in one study the prevalence of asymptomatic carriage of *E. histolytica* was 10% and of pathogenic strains only 1%.[43] Recognized high-risk groups include travellers, immigrants, migrant workers, immunocompromised individuals, sexually active male homosexuals, individuals in mental institutions, prisons and, possibly, children in day-care centres. In

Western countries the high prevalence of infection in homosexual men is determined by an increase in infection with non-pathogenic strains; however, in Japan infection with pathogenic strains is not uncommon. Severe infections occur in very young children, pregnant women, the malnourished and individuals taking corticosteroids. Patients with AIDS do not have an increased risk of severe infection.

Infection occurs via the faecal–oral route, food and drink becoming contaminated through exposure to human faeces. Food-borne outbreaks of disease are due to insanitary handling of food and its preparation by infected individuals. Therefore it is not surprising that prevalence is high in places where human faeces are used for fertilizer. Cyst carriers are the main reservoir of infection. Epidemics occur when raw sewage contaminates water supplies. Sexual transmission also occurs.

PATHOGENESIS

E. histolytica has the capacity to destroy almost all tissues of the human body. The intestinal mucosa, the liver, and, to a lesser extent, the brain and skin are the most commonly affected. Even cartilage and bone can be eroded by *E. histolytica* trophozoites. Several virulence factors have been identified, such as adhesion molecules, toxins, contact-dependent cytolysis, proteases and phagocytic activity.

To produce damage, trophozoites must first colonize the colon. The presence of bacteria is essential for colonization as they provide an environment with low oxygen tension and probably supply other metabolic needs. Trophozoites must then penetrate through the mucous layer and adhere to the host cells. *E. histolytica* enhances mucus secretion, alters its composition and depletes goblet cells of mucin, thereby making epithelial surfaces more vulnerable to invasion. Trophozoites adhere to colonic mucins and host cells through the *N*-acetyl-D-galactosamine-inhibitable lectin a 260 kD protein, also known as the Gal/GalNAc adherence lectin, composed of a 170 kDa and a 35 kDa subunits.[44] The 170 kDa subunit is immunologically similar to the integrins.[45] They also possess several receptors that recognize proteins in the extracellular matrix; two of these receptors recognize fibronectin and another three recognize collagen.[46] Contact of trophozoites with the extracellular matrix induces the release of cysteine proteases[47] and electron-dense granules[48] that contain collagenase. Cysteine proteinases can degrade cellular attachment and matrix proteins such as collagen, laminin and fibronectin.[49] There is a direct correlation between the amount of protein-

ase activity and the pathogenicity of the amoeba. *E. histolytica* has a potent cytolytic activity on target cells which is contact dependent. Putative *E. histolytica* contact-dependent cytotoxins include the *N*-acetyl-D-galactosamine-inhibitable adherence lectin, a pore-forming peptide and lysodiacylphospholipids resulting from phospholipase A activity.[46] Cytolysis of adherent target cells by *E. histolytica* is dependent on parasite microfilament function, phospholipase A enzyme activity and maintenance of an acid pH in amoebic intracellular vesicles. The ability of pathogenic *E. histolytica* to phagocytose is undoubtedly related to their virulence. Pathogenic amoebae ingest lysed and living cells. In general, pathogenic amoebae engage in active erythrophagocytosis; in contrast, non-pathogenic amoebae and those of low virulence ingest few red blood cells. Amoebae rendered defective in phagocytic capacity lose their virulence.

Invasion of the colonic and caecal mucosa by *E. histolytica* begins in the interglandular epithelium. This is a site of low resistance where intestinal cells are normally shed as the final stage in the renewal of the epithelium. Cell infiltration around invading amoebae leads to rapid lysis of inflammatory cells and tissue necrosis; thus, acute inflammatory cells are seldom found in biopsy samples or in scrapings of rectal mucosal lesions. Ulceration may deepen and progress under the mucosa. Further progression of the lesion may produce loss of the mucosa and submucosa and eventually perforation of the colon.

Amoebae probably spread from the intestine to the liver through the portal circulation. The presence and extent of liver involvement bears no relationship to the degree of intestinal amoebiasis, and these conditions do not necessarily coincide. The early stages of hepatic amoebic invasion have not been studied in humans. In experimental animals, inoculation of *E. histolytica* trophozoites into the portal vein produces multiple foci of neutrophil accumulation around parasites, followed by focal necrosis and granulomatous infiltration. As the lesions extend in size the granulomas are gradually substituted by necrosis, until the lesions coalesce and necrotic tissue occupies progressively larger portions of the liver. Hepatocytes close to the early lesions show degenerative changes which lead to necrosis, but direct contact of liver cells with amoebae is very rarely observed. It is thought that liver damage is not caused directly by the amoebae but rather by the lysosomal enzymes of lysed polymorphonuclear cells (PMNs) and monocytes that accumulate around the parasite. During experimental infection, hypocomplementaemic and leucopenic animals demonstrate reduced amoebic-induced liver damage when compared with normal animals.

In severe cases, especially in patients treated with corticosteroids, amoebic trophozoites can be found in virtually every organ of the body, including the brain, lungs and eyes.

IMMUNITY

Infection with pathogenic *E. histolytica* produces a marked immune response which results in the development of protective immunity. Recurrence of invasive colitis or amoebic abscess is unusual. De Leon[50] monitored more than 1000 patients with amoebic liver abscess for 5 years and found a recurrence rate of 0.29%. The risk of recurrence is increased if treatment fails to eradicate the pathogenic amoeba from the colon.[51] Patients with AIDS surprisingly do not appear more susceptible to amoebic disease than patients without AIDS; amoebic lesions in AIDS patients do not differ from those in non-AIDS patients. Intestinal invasion by *E. histolytica* results in a prompt local secretory antibody response followed by a systemic antibody response. Circulating antibodies can be demonstrated as early as 1 week after the onset of invasive amoebiasis in humans and experimental animals. All immunoglobulin classes are involved but there seems to be a predominance of IgG_2 antibodies. Various studies have revealed both elevated and decreased complement levels in humans and experimental animals with invasive amoebiasis. Such inconsistency contrasts with the consistent observation that virulent and non-virulent strains of *E. histolytica* are equally capable of activating the complement system by both pathways; the classical is more vigorous than the alternative pathway, even in the presence of antibody. In vitro the activated complement is lethal to the virulent amoebae, while non-virulent amoebae do not succumb to complement-mediated lysis. During infection *E. histolytica* trophozoites are continuously exposed to the complement system. Complement resistance is mediated in part by the Gal/GalNAc adherence lectin. The adhesin binds to C8 and C9 and inhibits their assembly and therefore C5b–9-mediated lysis. The immune complex disappears from the amoebic surface, probably by capping, as the biochemical analysis of the uroid reveals the presence of complement components. Also, resistance of pathogenic *E. histolytica* to complement lysis decreases after incubation with either cytochalasin B or trypsin, and after glutaraldehyde fixation. This suggests that intact membrane mobility and a trypsin-sensitive surface component are necessary to inhibit the activation of the alternative complement pathway.

There is a two-wave inflammatory cellular reaction elicited by axenic amoebae, namely an immediate infiltration by PMNs followed several hours later by mononuclear cells.

CLINICAL FEATURES (See also Chapter 3)

The clinical spectrum of intestinal *E. histolytica* infection ranges from asymptomatic carrier state or acute colitis, to fulminant colitis with perforation. Infection with non-pathogenic strains of *E. histolytica* is always asymptomatic. Infection with pathogenic strains is usually symptomatic. Cysts of pathogenic and non-pathogenic *E. histolytica* have been found in the stool of asymptomatic cyst passers.

Asymptomatic infection

Asymptomatic cyst carriage of both pathogenic and non-pathogenic strains has been well documented. The majority will clear the infection spontaneously. An epidemiological study in a semirural area in South Africa showed that 90% of asymptomatic carriers of pathogenic strains cleared the infection within a year, the remaining 10% developed amoebic colitis.[52]

Intestinal amoebiasis (Table 67.1)

The onset is insidious, except in fulminating cases, with abdominal discomfort, loose motions or frank diarrhoea, not necessarily with blood or excessive mucus. In more severe cases the stools rapidly become bloodstained with mucus. Tenesmus occurs

Table 67.1 Symptoms and findings in acute colitis.

	%
Symptoms	
Duration of symptoms (weeks)	
0–1	48
2–4	37
>4	15
Diarrhoea	100
Dysentery	99
Abdominal pain	85
Low back pain	66
Physical findings	
Fever	38
Abdominal tenderness	83

Source: Adams E B & MacLeod I N. Invasive amebiasis. I. Amebic dysentery and its complications. *Medicine* 1977; 56:315–323.

in half of the patients and is always associated with rectosigmoid involvement. Constitutional symptoms are not prominent. On physical examination tenderness may be localized anywhere in the lower abdomen but is usually over the caecum, transverse colon or sigmoid. The liver may be slightly enlarged and tender. Rectosigmoidoscopy and colonoscopy of mild or moderate cases usually reveals the presence of small ulcers (3–5 mm in diameter) that most frequently involve the caecum and rectum but may be scattered throughout the colon and are especially numerous in the region of the flexures. Rarely the disease may involve the terminal ileum. The ulcers are initially superficial with hyperaemic borders and a necrotic base covered with a yellowish exudate. There is normal mucosa between sites of invasion. However, diffuse inflammation has also been described, making firm diagnosis on gross appearance difficult. On rare occasions involvement of the blood vessels at the base of the ulcer may produce brisk bleeding. More rarely an ulcer may perforate and the patient may die of peritonitis. Extensive inflammatory polyposis has been demonstrated as a complication of amoebic colitis and this may be a source of confusion with idiopathic inflammatory bowel disease.[53] Acute amoebic dysentery must be differentiated from bacterial colitis caused by *Shigella* sp., *Salmonella* sp., *Campylobacter jejuni*, enteroinvasive and enterohaemorrhagic *Escherichia coli* and *Yersinia enterocolitica*.

In surgical specimens ulcers look flat and oval in shape, without induration of the underlying bowel wall. Histologically, there is non-specific diffuse inflammation around the superficial ulcerations. As the disease advances, the classically described flask-shaped ulcers with undermined edges are formed. The lamina propria is infiltrated by plasma cells, lymphocytes, neutrophils and eosinophils. There is oedema and focal haemorrhage. The infiltrate also involves the surface epithelium, and frequently there is an overlying exudate within which trophozoites may be found (Figure 67.2).

Fulminant colitis is the result of confluent ulceration and necrosis of the colon. The clinical picture is virtually indistinguishable from fulminant ulcerative colitis. The bowel is dilated, particularly in its transverse portion. The patient is extremely febrile and toxic and shows signs of hypovolaemia and electrolyte imbalance. Despite the severity of the illness, amoebae may not be readily recovered from the stools in these patients. Surgical specimens reveal extensive areas of necrosis within which some patches of intact, hyperaemic mucosa are found.

An amoeboma, or amoebic granuloma, may result from repeated invasion of the colon by *E. histolytica*, complicated with pyogenic infection.

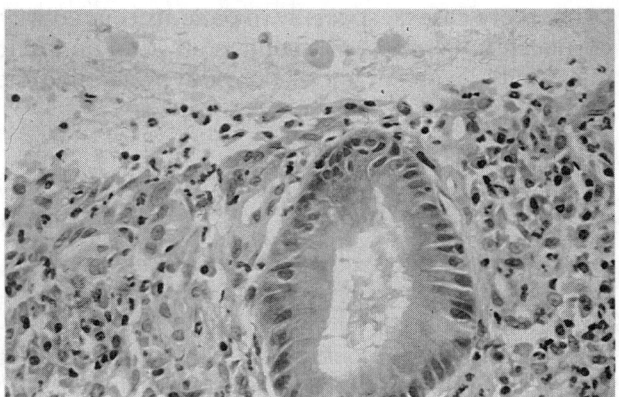

Figure 67.2 Colonic mucosa showing superficial ulceration with amoebic invasion. (H & E, 400×.) (Courtesy of Paola Domizio, Department of Morbid Anatomy, St Bartholomew's Hospital.)

Amoebomas may be found anywhere in the colon but are more frequent at the caecum (40%) and rectosigmoid junction (20%). Lesions are usually single and involve a short segment of the colon. These mass lesions are often mistaken for malignancies and may occasionally be palpable. Histologically the amoeboma is non-fibrotic and contains granulation tissue with lymphocytes, plasma cells, eosinophils and giant cells. There is remarkably little inflammation and most of the swelling is due to oedema. Amoebae are scanty and difficult to demonstrate. Fibrous tissue is formed later.

Amoebic liver abscess (Table 67.2)

This is the most common extraintestinal form of invasive amoebiasis. Amoebic abscesses may be found in all age groups, but are ten times more frequent in adults than in children, and are more frequent in males than in females. They are more common in the poorest sectors or urban populations. Approximately 20% of patients have past histories of dysentery. About 10% of patients have diarrhoea or dysentery at the time of diagnosis of amoebic liver abscess. The parasite can be detected in faeces in less than 50% of the cases if standard microscopy is used; the prevalence rises to 75% if culture is used.[51] The onset of symptoms is usually abrupt, with pain in the upper abdomen and high fever. The pain is intense and constant, radiating to the scapular region and right shoulder; it increases with deep breathing, coughing, or when the patient rests on the right side. When the abscess is localized on the left lobe, pain occurs on the left side of the abdomen and may radiate to the left shoulder. Localized tenderness in the region of the abscess, most commonly at the lower right intercostal spaces,

Table 67.2 Symptoms and findings in amoebic liver abscess.

	%
Symptoms:	
Duration of symptoms (weeks)	
<2	37–66
2–4	20–40
4–12	16–42
>12	5–11
Pain	90
Diarrhoea and/or dysentery	14–66
Weight loss	33–53
Cough	10–32
Dyspnoea	4
Physical findings	
Localized tenderness	80–95
Enlarged liver	43–93
Fever	75–98
Rales, rhonchi	8–47
Localized intercostal tenderness	40
Epigastric tenderness	22
Swelling over the liver	10
Jaundice	10–25
Laboratory findings	
Increased bilirubin	10–25
White blood cells $>10 \times 10^9$/l	63–94
Elevated transaminases	26–50
Elevated alkaline phosphatase	38–84
Increased ESR	81

Source: Martinez-Palomo A. *The Biology of Entamoeba histolytica*. Chichester: University Research Press/Wiley, 1982.

is frequent even in the absence of diffuse liver pain. Fever is present in most cases; it varies between 38° and 40°C, frequently in spikes but sometimes constant over several days, with rigors and profuse sweating. Anorexia, weight loss, nausea, vomiting and fatigue may all be present. Mild jaundice is quite common but severe obstructive jaundice is rare. Hepatomegaly may not be detected in patients with amoebic abscess of the dome of the liver because the enlargement is upward. Amoebic abscess and cirrhosis may coexist so a hard liver does not exclude the diagnosis. Movement of the right side of the chest and diaphragm is restricted and there is hypoventilation of the right lower lobe of the lung. This is frequently associated with atelectasis or effusion in the right chest. The presentation may be so abrupt that it can be confused with an acute surgical abdomen. The usual clinical diagnosis in such a case is acute cholecystitis or appendicitis. Differential diagnosis with pyogenic liver abscess should be established, particularly in non-endemic areas.

Lesions are usually single and most are found in the right lobe of the liver in the posterior, external and superior portions. The incidence of amoebic abscesses of the left lobe ranges from 5 to 21%. The liver abscess has a thin capsular wall with a necrotic centre composed of a thick fluid, an intermediate zone of coarse stroma and an outer zone of nearly normal tissue. Typically, abscess fluid is odorless, resembling 'chocolate syrup' or 'anchovy paste', and bacteriologically sterile, although secondary bacterial invasion may occur. Microscopic examination of the abscess fluid reveals granular eosinophilic debris with no or few cells; amoebae tend to be located at the periphery of the abscess. Liver abscesses may heal, rupture or disseminate. Mortality has been estimated to be around 0.2–2.0% in adults and 26% in children.[54]

Invasive amoebic lesions in humans, whether localized in the large intestine, liver or skin, almost invariably heal without the formation of scar tissue, if properly treated. The absence of fibrotic tissue following necrosis is particularly striking in the liver. The complete anatomical and functional restitution of liver integrity after treatment of liver abscess has been assessed by scintillography.

Peritoneal amoebiasis

This is caused by the rupture of a hepatic liver abscess or, less frequently, by perforation of the caecum. It is characterized by a sudden increase in abdominal pain, frequently generalized, which resembles that of septic peritonitis. A plain abdominal radiograph will reveal the presence of free air in the peritoneal cavity. In some instances the perforation may be smaller and the abdominal signs are more localized.

Pericardial amoebiasis

Pericardial involvement is the most serious complication of an amoebic liver abscess. It occurs in less than 1% of all amoebic liver abscesses, especially of the left lobe. Although there may be a presuppurative stage that is associated with a sterile effusion, perforation of the abscess into the pericardium is usually followed by progressive tamponade or the sudden development of shock. Although the mortality from pericardial involvement has decreased from more than 90% to less than 40%, it is still frequently necessary to perform open drainage because of the development of loculations and thickened pericardium.

Pleuropulmonary amoebiasis

Invasion of the pleural cavity or the lung parenchyma is most commonly due to extension from a liver abscess and occurs in less than 1% of those with amoebic dysentery, in 3% of all autopsies on people dying of amoebiasis and in 15% of patients with liver abscess. Haematogenous spread is rare. The first clinical symptoms are those of the liver abscess, followed by severe pain in the lower chest, often radiating to the right shoulder. There may be dyspnoea and non-productive cough. Bronchohepatic fistulas are characterized by expectoration of large amounts of dark-brown material. Superimposed bacterial infections are common.

Cerebral amoebiasis

Cerebral involvement has been documented in 1.2–2.5% of patients who have amoebiasis at autopsy but in less than 0.1% of patients whose cases are reported in studies of large clinical series. Although the symptoms of cerebral amoebiasis depend on the site and size of the lesion, as many as 50% of patients may have abrupt onset of symptoms and die of cerebellar involvement or rupture within 12–72 hours. The availability of metronidazole, which penetrates the blood–brain barrier, should greatly improve the prognosis of this unusual complication.

Genitourinary amoebiasis

Renal amoebiasis, a rare complication of amoebic liver abscess, is thought to occur by rupture of a hepatic abscess, haematogenous spread from lesions in the liver or lungs, or extension through the lymphatics. Patients who have renal amoebiasis usually respond well to aspiration and medical therapy. Genital lesions also occur infrequently and are usually caused by fistulas from a liver abscess or rectocolitis. Typically, lesions are painful, punched out ulcers with profuse discharge. Medical treatment is usually sufficient for resolution of the lesions.

Cutaneous amoebiasis

This results from perforation of an abscess or intestine into the skin. It may also develop from surgical wounds infected secondarily with an internal amoebic lesion or in the perineal–genital area. Histologically there is ulceration with extensive necrosis in the base, pseudoepitheliomatous hyperplasia at the margins, and a non-specific inflammatory infiltrate extending into the deep dermis and subcutaneous tissues beneath the ulcer base. Sometimes there is extensive pseudoepitheliomatous hyperplasia involving much of the lesion with only small punctate areas of ulceration. This may resemble verrucous carcinoma. *E. histolytica* may be found in the overlying exudate.

DIAGNOSIS AND DIFFERENTIAL DIAGNOSIS

Detection of the parasite (See also Appendix II)

Amoebiasis, although often suspected clinically, requires confirmation in the laboratory by finding cysts and trophozoites in the stools or trophozoites in the various tissues. The detection of the organism depends on appropriate specimen collection, processing and examination by trained personnel (Table 67.3).

Table 67.3 Laboratory diagnosis of *E. histolytica* (after ref. 56).

Sample	Fixative	Examination	Stain
Stool	PVA, 10% formalin, Schaudinn's fixative, sodium acetate–acetic acid formalin	Concentrate, permanently stained slide	Gomori trichrome, iron haematoxylin
Sigmoid colon	PVA, Schaudinn's fixative	Permanently stained slide	Gomori trichrome, iron haematoxylin
Aspirate			
Direct	None	Wet mount with or without enzyme digest	
Fixed	PVA, Schaudinn's fixative	Permanently stained slide	Gomori trichrome, iron haematoxylin, periodic acid–Schiff, haematoxylin and eosin
Biopsy	Formalin	Routine histology	

PVA, polyvinyl alcohol with either $HgCl_2$ or $CuSO_4$; with periodic acid–Schiff organism stains intensely pink and has a distinct outline, but cytoplasmic and nuclear details are obscured. Haematoxylin and eosin stain cytoplasm pink and nucleus blue; in sections the nucleolus may not always be present.

Stools

Examination for ova and parasites in a minimum of three stool specimens, using concentration and permanent stain techniques, is the standard method of detection and identification of the organism. If possible, the stools should be examined before the administration of antimicrobial, antidiarrhoeal and antacid preparations or barium because all these agents may interfere with the recovery of amoebae. Fresh samples may be examined for detection of trophozoites containing erythrocytes. However, this is only useful if the sample is examined within 30 minutes of the passage of the specimen. When using fresh samples, three types of wet mount preparations should be made from each specimen: mounts in saline solution (to observe amoebic motility in a warm specimen); mounts in saline plus iodine (to differentiate *E. histolytica* cysts from other amoebic species and helminth ova); and mounts in saline plus methylene blue (to distinguish cysts from leucocytes, which stain blue). It is advisable always to confirm the diagnosis by using a permanent-stained slide (iron haematoxylin or trichrome). The presence of trophozoites of *E. histolytica* containing ingested red blood cells is diagnostic of amoebiasis. However, the presence of cysts in a patient with gastrointestinal symptoms does not necessarily indicate a causative effect. Non-pathogenic strains cannot be distinguished microscopically from pathogenic amoebae. *E. hartmanni* is morphologically identical to *E. histolytica* and can only be positively identified by measuring its size.

Examination of material scraped or aspirated from mucosal surfaces during sigmoidoscopy may reveal the presence of trophozoites. Microscopic examination of wet preparations may be difficult because of the need for low light intensity and difficulties in differentiating the unstained *E. histolytica* from other amoebae and from inflammatory cells (Table 67.4). The mucosal material may also be smeared, fixed and stained with trichrome stain. Fixation of stool smears can be achieved by immersion of the slide in Schaudinn's solution or by adding 2–3 drops of polyvinyl alcohol to the mucosal material directly on the slide, mixing it, and allowing the slide to air dry.

Culture of amoebae is a more sensitive technique than microscopic examination of faeces and allows for determination of zymodeme patterns to distinguish pathogenic from non-pathogenic strains. At present this technique is not practical for routine clinical laboratories. Results are not available for 4 days or more. Monoclonal antibodies and DNA probes that distinguish between pathogenic and non-pathogenic *E. histolytica* have been described but are only available in research centres.

A promising enzyme linked immunosorbent assay (ELISA) for the identification of pathogenic *E. histolytica* in stools is being developed. The assay is based on detection of epitopes of the 170 kDa adhesin present only in pathogenic strains of *E. histolytica*. Specificity and sensitivity of the assay for pathogenic *E. histolytica* are calculated around 97 and 100%, respectively. More studies are needed to confirm its value in the diagnosis of infection with pathogenic amoebae. If commercially developed, it would be particularly useful in the management of asymptomatic carriers, as would allow to discriminate between P and NP strains.

Sigmoidoscopy

This is of value in symptomatic cases. The mucosal lesions should be aspirated and the material examined for trophozoites. Biopsies may be taken from the edge of the ulcers and stained with periodic acid–Schiff solution.

Liver aspirate

This should be collected in a number of different containers as it is obtained from the abscess. The amoebae are sparse in necrotic material from the centre of the abscess, but they are more abundant on the marginal walls and are therefore more commonly found in the last portions of aspirated material. Demonstration of the organism is often extremely difficult because trophozoites may be trapped in viscous pus or debris and will not exhibit typical motility.

Laboratory investigations (See also Appendix V)

In mild cases of colitis laboratory tests are normal. With severe disease leucocytosis is present. About 75% of patients with amoebic liver abscesses have white blood cells counts $>10000/mm^3$. The occasional patient with leucopenia will usually have long-standing disease and may have underlying alcoholism or folate deficiency. Eosinophilia is not associated with extraintestinal amoebiasis. Anaemia is common, particularly in patients who have chronic amoebic liver abscesses. The level of alkaline phosphatase is elevated in more than 75% of patients, particularly in those with long-standing disease. Levels of transaminases may be elevated in 50%, especially those with acute disease or complications. The levels of transaminases usually return to normal soon after therapy is initiated, although alkaline phosphatase may remain elevated for several months. In extraintestinal amoebiasis, organisms may or may not be found in the stool; therefore,

Table 67.4 Differential characteristics of host cells, *E. coli* and *E. hartmanni*, commonly mistaken for *E. histolytica*, in wet preparations (after ref. 56).

Cell	Diameter or length (µm)	Motility	Nucleus		Cytoplasm appearance (stained)	Inclusions
			No.	Visibility / Nucleus: cytoplasm ratio		
E. histolytica Trophozoites	10–60	Progressive with hyaline fingerlike pseudopodia; may be rapid	1	Hard to see in unstained preparations (1:10–1:12)	Ground glass appearance. Clear differentiation of ectoplasm and endoplasm; vacuoles usually small.	Presence of erythrocytes diagnostic
Cysts	10–20	None	1–4	1:2–1:3	Clear	Chromidial bodies (stained) may be present; usually elongate with blunt, smooth rounded edges; round or oval
E. coli Trophozoites	15–50	Sluggish, non-directional; blunt, granular pseudopodia	1	Often visible in unstained preparation	Granular, little differentiation into ectoplasm and endoplasm; usually vacuolated	Bacteria, yeast cells other debris
Cysts	10–35	None	1–8	≥16 nuclei seen occasionally	Clear	Chromidial bodies (stained) may be present, less frequently than in *E. histolytica*; splinter shape with rough pointed ends
E. hartmanni Trophozoites	6–10	Progressive, with hyaline finger-like pseudopodia; may be rapid	1	Hard to see in unstained preparations; 1:10–1:12	Ground glass appearance. Clear differentiation of ectoplasm and endoplasm; vacuoles usually small	Can only be differentiated from *E. histolytica* by direct measurement of either trophozoite or cyst
Cysts	5–8	None	1–4	1:2–1:3	Clear	—
Host cells PMNs	Average 16	None	1	2–4 segments; if lobed, nucleus fragments may mimic the four nuclei found in *E. histolytica* cyst (1:1).	Granular	None
Macrophages	20–60; may be 5–10	Sluggish	1	Large, may be irregular in shape (like monocyte); may mimic *E. histolytica* trophozoite; can also ingest erythrocytes	Coarse; may be highly vacuolated	Usually contain ingested debris, PMNs and erythrocytes

the presence of antibodies against *E. histolytica* may be useful. Antibody response is present in 85–95% of patients with invasive disease. There is a good correlation between infection with pathogenic zymodemes and positive serological results. Virtually all known serological tests have been employed to detect antiamoebic antibody, including immunofluorescent antibody tests, indirect haemagglutination tests, radioimmunoassay, countercurrent immunoelectrophoresis and ELISAs. ELISAs are the most sensitive and do not give false-negative results in patients with amoebic liver abscesses. ELISA is also specific, giving only 3.6% false-positive results in controls living in endemic areas. The results of serological tests may be negative in patients who present acutely and should be repeated in 5–7 days. Serological responses measured by agar gel diffusion, countercurrent immunoelectrophoresis and ELISA usually become negative within 6–12 months, although they may persist for over 3 years. However, results of IHAs may remain positive for more than 10 years after clinical and parasitological cure, even in the absence of reinfection. Therefore these tests should be interpreted with caution as antibody may be present for prolonged periods, and in areas of high endemicity a high prevalence of seropositivity already exists. Clinical laboratories should check with their local health authorities for guidelines for use and interpretation of serological tests.

Radiology

Radiological changes in the colon consist of mucosal oedema, haustral blunting and ulceration, usually localized to one part of the colon. Ulcers are initially shallow but may deepen and assume a 'collar-button' or flasked-shaped appearance. There may be toxic dilatation of the colon. Amoebomas manifest as an intraluminal mass, an annular lesion or irregularity of the bowel wall with lack of normal distensibility. Differential diagnosis with carcinoma may be difficult; rapid disappearance of the lesion after treatment favours the diagnosis.

In patients with hepatic involvement, a plain radiograph of the thorax may reveal elevation of the right hemidiaphragm, pleural reaction obscuring the right costophrenic angle. Radiologically, unruptured abscesses do not show a fluid level, and calcification of the liver parenchyma is very rare. Non-invasive radiographic studies have dramatically increased early diagnosis of amoebic liver abscesses and their potential complications. The isotope liver scan is very useful as it becomes positive within the first days of illness, often prior to other imaging techniques. Presumably these early changes reflect either a focal decrease in blood supply or injury to the Kupffer cells rather than liquefaction necrosis. Ultrasonography of an amoebic liver abscess typically reveals a round or oval hypoechoic area that is contiguous to the liver capsule and without signifi-

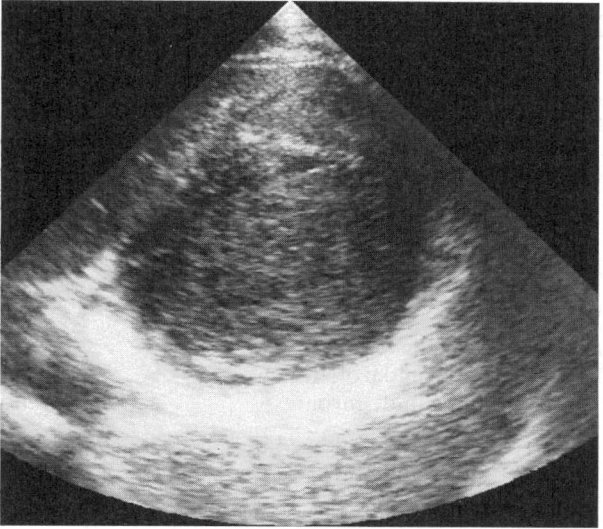

Figure 67.3   Liver ultrasonograph demonstrating an amoebic hepatic abscess. (Courtesy of Alison McLean.)

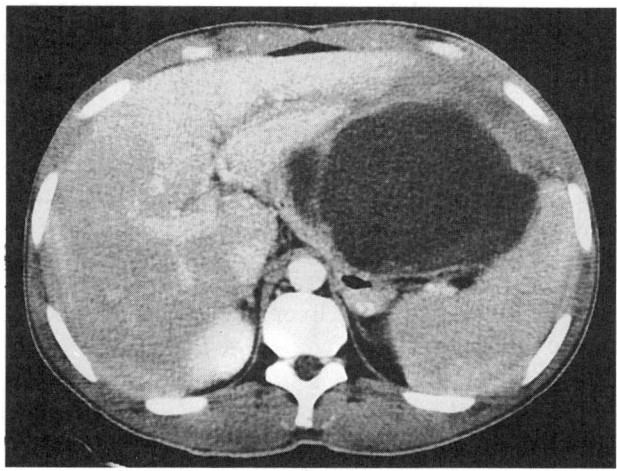

Figure 67.4   Computerized tomograph of the liver demonstrating a left lobe amoebic abscess. (Courtesy of Alison McLean.)

cant wall echoes (Figure 67.3). Computerized tomography and magnetic resonance imaging are also sensitive studies for demonstrating amoebic liver abscesses (Figure 67.4). More than 80% of patients who have symptoms of an abscess for more than 10 days have a single lesion of the right lobe of the liver, while 50% of patients who present acutely may have multiple lesions. Abscesses resolve slowly and may increase in size during the first few weeks after therapy, even with successful treatment. The ultrasonographic abnormalities resolve within 6 months in two-thirds of the patients with amoebic liver abscess, however 10% remain abnormal for more than one year after treatment. The differential diag-

Table 67.5 Treatment of amoebiasis.

		Adult dosage	Paediatric dosage ($mg\ kg^{-1}\ day^{-1}$)
Asymptomatic intestinal carrier			
1st choice	diloxanide furoate	500 mg t.i.d. × 10 days	20 (divided in 3 doses × 10 days)
2nd choice	paromomycin	25–30 mg kg^{-1} day^{-1} in 3 doses × 7–10 days	25–30 (divided in 3 doses × 7–10 days)
or	iodoquinol	650 mg t.i.d. × 20 days	20–40 (divided in 3 doses × 20 days)
Intestinal infection			
1st choice	metronidazole followed by	750–800 mg t.i.d. × 10 days	35–50 (divided in 3 doses × 10 days)
	diloxanide furoate*	500 mg t.i.d. × 10 days	20 (divided in 3 doses × 10 days)
	tinidazole followed by	2 g/day × 2–3 days	50–60 (× 3 days)
	diloxanide furoate*	500 mg t.i.d. × 10 days	20 (divided in 3 doses × 10 days)
2nd choice	paromomycin	25–30 mg kg^{-1} day^{-1} in 3 doses × 7–10 days	25–30 (divided in 3 doses × 7–10 days)
Amoebic liver abscess			
1st choice	metronidazole followed by	750–800 mg t.i.d. × 10 days	35–50 (divided in 3 doses × 7–10 days)
	diloxanide furoate*	500 mg t.i.d. × 10 days	20 (divided in 3 doses × 10 days)
or	tinidazole followed by	2 g/day × 3–5 days	50–60 (×5 days)
	diloxanide furoate*	500 mg t.i.d. × 10 days	20 (divided in 3 doses × 10 days)
2nd choice	dehydroemetine followed by	1–1.5 mg kg^{-1} day^{-1} (max. 90 mg/day) i.v. × 5 days	1 (×10 days maximum)
	diloxanide furoate*	500 mg t.i.d. × 10 days	20 (divided in 3 doses × 10 days)

*Paromomycin or iodoquinol may be used as an alternative to diloxanide furoate.

nosis includes pyogenic liver abscess, gallbladder disease and sepsis.

TREATMENT

Two classes of drugs are used in the treatment of amoebic infections. Luminal amoebicides, such as diloxanide furoate and iodoquinol, act on organisms in the intestinal lumen and are not effective against organisms in tissue. Tissue amoebicides, such as metronidazole, dehydroemetine and chloroquine, are effective in the treatment of invasive amoebiasis but less effective in the treatment of organisms in the bowel lumen (Table 67.5).

Asymptomatic patients

In non-endemic areas, asymptomatic patients may be treated with diloxanide furoate, paromomycin or iodoquinol. Iodoquinol and its analogue iodochlor-hydroxyquin are effective against intraluminal amoebae but have been reported to cause myelo-

optic neuropathy after long-term use. The value of treatment of asymptomatic carriers in endemic areas is questionable because of the high rate of reinfection.

Intestinal infection

Metronidazole is the drug of choice for amoebic colitis as it is very effective against the trophozoite; however, it has little effect on cyst and therefore treatment should be followed by a luminal agent such as diloxanide furoate. Tinidazole may be used instead of metronidazole.

Liver abscess

Metronidazole or tinidazole followed by diloxanide furoate is the treatment of choice. The potential cardiovascular and gastrointestinal adverse effects of dehydroemetine and emetine limit their use and they are only used as second-line treatment. Higher relapse rates are associated with chloroquine than with other therapeutic agents.

Table 67.6 Indications for aspiration of amoebic liver abscess.

Formal indications
To rule out a pyogenic abscess, particularly with multiple lesions
As adjunct to medical therapy (no response after 72 hours)
If rupture is believed to be imminent
Abscess in the left lobe where the risk of rupture is increased

Possible indications
To reduce the period of disability[55] (further trials are necessary to confirm this indication)

Aspiration of the abscess may be necessary in some cases (Table 67.6). However, the need of open surgical drainage has decreased since the success of percutaneous drainage. Surgery should be reserved for patients with rupture of their abscess, with bacterial superinfection, or when an abscess which needs drainage cannot be approached.

PREVENTION

The control of invasive amoebiasis could be achieved through improvement of living standards and the establishment of adequate sanitary conditions in countries where the disease is prevalent. Methods of attack should aim at: (1) the community, through the improvement of environmental sanitation including water supply, adequate disposal of faeces, food safety and health education to prevent faecal–oral transmission; and (2) the individual, through early detection and treatment in cases of infection and disease.

Cysts remain viable and infective for several days in faeces and may survive in soil for at least 8 days at 34–38°C, and for 1 month at 10°C. They also remain infective in fresh water, sea water, sewage and wet soil. Cysts survive up to 45 minutes in faecal material lodged under the fingernails but are killed within 1 minute by desiccation on the surface of the hands. Amoebic cysts are destroyed by exposure to 200 parts/10^6 of iodine, 5–10% acetic acid, and heating at temperatures above 68°C. They can be removed from water by sand filtration but are not killed by the quantity of chlorine ordinarily used to purify water; therefore chlorination alone cannot prevent epidemics originating from faecal contamination of water. In places where purification of water supplies is inadequate, boiling for 10 minutes will kill all cysts.

In the past, mass chemotherapy of high-risk populations has been attempted but with only partial success. Mass treatment of carriers is impractical because treatment with luminal antiamoebic drugs is prolonged, which reduces compliance, and the probability of reinfection in endemic areas is high. In non-endemic areas, asymptomatic carriers should be treated. Individual chemoprophylaxis for travellers is not indicated because the possibility of acquiring the infection has been shown to be very low (4%) and the risk of acquiring a pathogenic strain is only 0.3%.[57]

There is no vaccine available against amoebiasis. Several antigenic fractions of *E. histolytica* have been developed as possible immunogens. These have different degrees of purity and are used in conjunction with a variety of adjuvants. As yet these have been tried only in animal models.

ENTAMOEBA DISPAR (as redescribed by Diamond and Clark[10])

If the existence of *E. dispar* is widely accepted, it should be considered as morphologically identical to *E. histolytica*. The terms *E. dispar* and 'non-pathogenic *E. histolytica*' would become synonymous (see *E. histolytica*; strain differences). However, the authors suggest that applying the term non-pathogenic to *E. dispar* may be inaccurate. They claim that this amoeba may be capable of inducing focal intestinal lesions in experimental animals such as kittens, gerbils and guinea-pigs. Infection with *E. dispar* may coexist with infection with *E. histolytica*. Up to 20% of *E. dispar* infections may lead to seropositivity for standard immunodiagnosis of *E. histolytica*. Unfortunately, diagnosis requires use of specific laboratory tests not yet available for routine use. Prospective epidemiological studies are needed to establish the natural history of infection and its potential pathogenicity.

ENTAMOEBA MOSHKOVSKII ('*E. HISTOLYTICA*-LIKE' AMOEBAS)

E. moshkovskii was originally isolated from sewage in Moscow by Tshalaia[58] and subsequently reported in many parts of the world. *E. moshkovskii* is described as morphologically indistinguishable from *E. histolytica* but is isolated from free-living sources, usually in the sediment of sewage polluted waters. Similar amoebae have been isolated from humans and were grouped under the name of 'E. histolytica-like amoebae'. The best known of these is the 'Laredo' strain. Initially, they were thought to represent atypical E. histolytica. Numerous studies revealed differences between these strains and true E. histolytica, including a lack of serological cross-reactivity, dissimilar DNA base composition, and distinctive isoenzyme profiles. Recently analysis of the small subunit ribosomal RNA gene suggested that these amoebae are strains of E. moshkovskii and are not closely related to E. histolytica.[59] This amoeba has a wide temperature tolerance, multiplying at 10–37°C. It produces contractile vacuoles in hypotonic media and is highly resistant to amoebicidal drugs.

ENTAMOEBA CHATTONI

This amoeba frequently infects apes and monkeys, in which it causes no clinical symptoms. Asymptomatic infection in individuals who are in close contact with monkeys has been reported.[60]

ENDOLIMAX NANA

Endolimax nana is a cosmopolitan and common intestinal amoeba of man, primates and pigs that can be confused with E. histolytica. Endolimax nana is non-pathogenic. The trophozoites are small (6–15 μm in diameter). Movement is by pseudopodia but this fails to produce directional locomotion. The cysts are from 8 to 10 μm in diameter and have a refractile cyst wall. The details of nuclear structure and the appearance of the cytoplasm closely resemble those of Iodamoeba bütschlii. Usually there is only one nucleus in trophozoites but there are four nuclei in immature cysts. Endolimax nana has no chromidial body in stained samples, and the nuclear membrane appears devoid of peripheral chromatin.

IODAMOEBA BÜTSCHLII

Iodamoeba bütschlii is the most common amoeba of swine, and the pig was probably its original host. It is also frequently found in humans and monkeys. Trophozoites vary greatly in size, ranging from 6 to 20 μm in diameter. The cytoplasm contains one or more glycogen mass(es) that may be seen after iodine staining, as well as bacteria, yeasts and debris; red blood cells are never ingested. The nucleus is usually not visible but permanent stains will reveal a characteristic appearance with a large central karyosome surrounded by a ring of small chromatin granules. Cysts of I. bütschlii are 8–15 μm in diameter, commonly ovoidal or irregularly pyriform in shape. The cysts are distinctive in preparations stained with iodine because of the constant presence of the large, sharply outlined and dense glycogen-containing vacuole. Only one nucleus is found in most cysts.

I. bütschlii is non-pathogenic; only exceptionally has the presence of this parasite been linked to symptomatic infection in man. As is the case with other amoebae commonly found in the human colon, I. bütschlii has a distinct isoenzyme profile.

DIENTAMOEBA FRAGILIS

Infection with Dientamoeba fragilis may be associated with gastrointestinal symptoms, such as diarrhoea and abdominal pain, but most cases are asymptomatic. D. fragilis is a small (6–12 μm) cosmopolitan parasite. Only trophozoites are known; they can be differentiated from other intestinal amoebae by the presence of two nuclei in the majority of them. However, around 30–40% of organisms are mononucleate and may be confused with Blastocystis hominis, which is more common.[61] Trichrome stains should always be performed. Culture is possible and the parasite can be differentiated by its distinct isoenzyme profile. This organism is now considered to be an aberrant trichomonad flagellate, not an amoeba.[62]

THE MASTIGOPHORA (FLAGELLATES)

GIARDIA INTESTINALIS

Giardia intestinalis (syn. *lamblia*, *duodenalis*) is the most common human protozoan enteropathogen throughout the world. The question as to whether this organism was a true pathogen or merely a commensal was debated for many decades but there is now compelling evidence to indicate that infection with this parasite can cause both acute and chronic diarrhoea.[63–65] Intestinal malabsorption can be severe, and in children chronic infection may be associated with retardation of growth and development. Molecular and genetic analysis of the parasite has shown that *Giardia* has a unique place in evolution as it is probably the first organism to emerge from the prokaryotic to the eukaryotic state.[66] Our knowledge of this parasite has expanded rapidly since it was first cultured in the 1970s but many aspects of its biology and interactions with its mammalian hosts remain unanswered. There is no satisfactory explanation for the diverse clinical spectrum seen in giardiasis, which ranges from asymptomatic carriage to persistent diarrhoea with malabsorption. As yet no virulence factors have been identified and thus a clear explanation of pathogenesis is lacking. In addition, despite extensive investigation in animal models and to some extent during human infection, the key immunological determinants for clearance of acute infection and the development of protective immunity remain poorly defined. The increasing evidence that this infection may be a zoonosis and can be transmitted, not only by person-to-person contact but through water supplies, means control within the environment is an important public health issue which needs to be tackled not only in the developing world but also in industrialized nations.

THE ORGANISM

Taxonomy

Giardia is in the subphylum Sarcomastigophora, the superclass Mastigophora and in the order Diplomonadida.[67] *Giardia* belongs to the family Hexamitidae which contains six genera, three of which, including *Gardia*, are exclusively parasitic. Members of the genus *Giardia* have an adhesive disc on the ventral surface, unlike other members of the family Hexamitidae. There are three major morphological

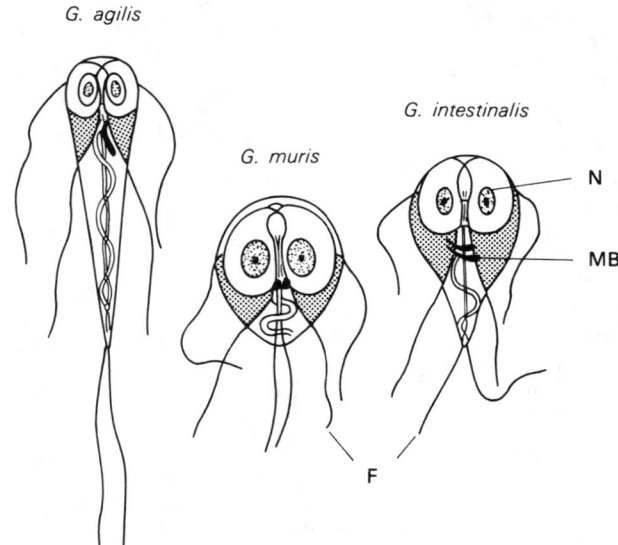

Figure 67.5   *G. agilis*, *G. muris* and *G. intestinalis*. N, nucleus; MB, median body; F, flagellum.

subtypes of *Giardia*: *G. agilis* from amphibians, *G. muris* from mice and *G. intestinalis* from humans and some other vertebrates (Figure 67.5). These different types can be distinguished by the overall shape and dimensions of the trophozoite body and also by the distinctive shapes of the median bodies. Two other *Giardia* isolates have been described: *G. psittaci* isolated from a budgerigar and *G. ardeae* from the great blue heron. Again these can be distinguished from the other subtypes by an absence of the ventrolateral flange in the former and a single (rather than a double) caudal flagellum in the latter.

The chemotaxonomy of *Giardia* has been explored using a variety of techniques, including antigen, isoenzyme and DNA analysis. These approaches have clearly shown that *Giardia* isolates differ from one to another, although the sensitivity of the techniques varies. DNA fingerprinting using the bacteriophage M13 genome as a probe may be one of the more sensitive approaches and has been used to demonstrate changes in genotype during chronic infection.[68] These techniques have also shown similarities between human and animal isolates, supporting the view that giardiasis may be a zoonosis.

Structure

Giardia exists as a trophozoite which colonizes the proximal small intestine and is responsible for the

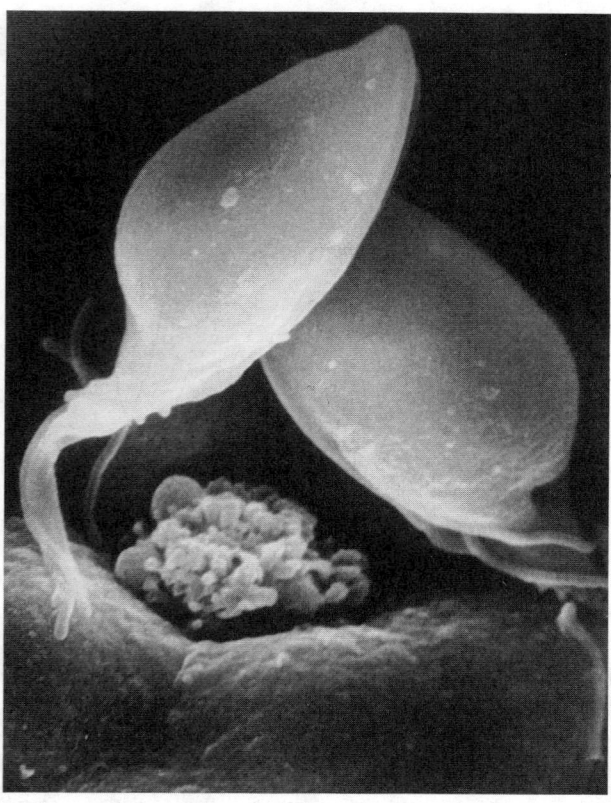

Figure 67.6 Scanning electron micrograph showing two *G. intestinalis* trophozoites.

Giardia trophozoites are largely devoid of cytoplasmic organelles, the major structure being multiple ovoid vacuoles which appear to resemble lysosomes, containing a variety of hydrolases, including acid phosphatase, proteinases and DNAases and RNAases. Other structures include what may be a primitive Golgi apparatus which is involved in protein sorting, bacterial endosymbionts and a 35 nm double-stranded RNA virus. The role of these organisms in *Giardia*'s life cycle has not been established.

Cysts are ovoid or elliptical, approximately 7–10 μm in length. The cyst wall is composed of a layer of fibrils arranged as a felt-like web. There is controversy as to whether *N*-acetylglucosamine or galactosamine is the major cyst wall sugar.[70] The cyst contains two or four nuclei; a median body and cytoskeletal components can usually be identified. The cyst is able to survive in a cool, moist environment for weeks or even months.

Microbiology

The life cycle of *Giardia* is simple, involving the ingestion of cysts in contaminated water or food or through direct person-to-person contact, infection being initiated with as few as 10–100 cysts. Excystation occurs in the proximal small intestine where the trophozoite multiplies. The cycle is completed when encystation occurs in the distal small intestine and colon, and cysts are excreted again into the environment in faeces at a concentration of approximately 150 000–20 000 cysts per gram of faeces.

Colonization involves three processes, namely excystation, attachment to the intestinal epithelium and multiplication. Excystation is thought to be triggered by low pH and duodenal and pancreatic secretions. The intracellular vacuoles have been observed to discharge their contents during excystation, suggesting that hydrolases are required to complete the process.

Giardia attaches to the intestinal epithelium, probably by a variety of mechanisms, although it seems likely that the ventral disc plays a major part, either by flagella-generated hydrodynamic forces beneath the disc or by direct disc movement mediated by its contractile proteins, particularly those in the peripheral regions of the disc.[71] Pharmacological disruption of microfilament function inhibits attachment, supporting a central role for the ventral disc. However, like many micro-organisms, *Giardia* possesses a mannose-binding surface lectin which appears to exist as a prolectin in the cytoplasm which is activated by trypsin.[72,73] This lectin has been purified and shown to have a molecular weight of

production of diarrhoea and malabsorption, and the cyst which is able to exist outside the host in a suitable environment and is the form of the parasite by which giardiasis is usually transmitted.

The trophozoite, when fixed for light microscopy, is 12–15 μm long and 5–9 μm wide (Figure 67.6). It has two nuclei and four symmetrically placed flagella originating from basal bodies at the anterior pole of the nuclei. The median body is found posteriorly and varies in shape according to subtype (see Figure 67.5). A median body contains cytoskeletal proteins, including the giardins, actin and α-actinin. The trophozoite has a convex dorsal surface and a concave ventral surface containing the ventral disk. This organelle is unique to *Giardia* and is a rigid structure consisting of microtubules, cross-bridges attached to microtubules and microribbons which run perpendicularly to both the microtubules and the cross-bridges. The disc contains a variety of cytoskeletal proteins, including the family of giardins, actin, α-actinin, myosin and tropomyosin.[69] These proteins give the disc flexibility and allow it to change shape, a process which is thought to be important for attachment. The flagella have the usual eukaryotic structure consisting of nine pairs of microtubules with two central single microtubules.

28–30 kDa. Experiments in attachment models using mammalian intestinal epithelial cells or culture cell lines suggest that both disc and lectin-mediated mechanisms are important, at least in vitro.

Giardia trophozoites divide by binary fission but the mechanisms by which growth is controlled and the factors which are essential for growth remain poorly defined. Bile has been shown to promote growth of *Giardia* both in vivo and in vitro.[74] This probably relates to *Giardia*'s absolute requirement for preformed phospholipid, uptake being facilitated by the presence of conjugated bile salts. Bile salt uptake has been shown to occur by an active transport process, suggesting that a specific carrier may be present in the surface membrane. Other factors which are known to be essential for growth include a carbohydrate source, usually glucose, and a low partial pressure of oxygen.

The final stage of the life cycle, encystation, can also be completed in vitro following exposure of trophozoites to high concentrations of conjugated bile salts and myristic acid at neutral pH. Thus, bile and bile salts may have a dual role in the parasite life cycle, on one hand promoting growth and multiplication, while at the same time ensuring that the parasite completes its life cycle by encystation.

None of these in vitro studies of the parasite life cycle would have been possible without the ability to culture the parasite in vitro. This was first achieved axenically in 1970 by Meyer[75] using a complex, undefined medium containing serum. This medium has been modified slightly since then; the most widely used medium is TYI-S-33 which includes casesin digest (typticase), yeast extract, iron as ferric ammonium citrate, dextrose, bovine serum, ascorbic acid, bile salts and cysteine. *Giardia* may be cultured in screw-capped glass tubes or flasks, ensuring only a small air space to maintain a low oxygen concentration.

Metabolism

Following the development of methods for axenic cultivation of *Giardia*, knowledge of the parasite's biochemistry and metabolism expanded rapidly. *Giardia* lacks mitochondria and mitochondrial enzymes and respires in the presence of oxygen by a flavin, iron–sulphur protein-mediated electron transport system. Glucose is the major energy source which is converted to pyruvate by Embden–Meyerhof and hexose monophosphate shunt pathways.[76] Glucose is metabolized incompletely to carbon dioxide, ethanol and acetate. In strictly anaerobic environments, alanine is produced from pyruvate and ketoglutarate, whereas in the presence of low oxygen concentrations ethanol production increases and alanine production is reduced.

Giardia predominantly acquires membrane and other lipids from the culture medium and has little or no capacity for in vivo synthesis. Trophozoites can use exogenous arachidonic acid for phosphatidyl-inositol synthesis.

Giardia is unable to synthesize purines and pyrimidines, which distinguishes it from most other eukaryotes. *Giardia* relies therefore on salvage pathways for both of the nucleic acids which must be synthesized exogenously. Pyrimidines are taken up by active transport processes, one for uridine and cytosine and another for thymidine.[77]

The calcium-binding protein, calmodulin, has been detected in *Giardia* trophozoites and probably has a similar function in maintaining intracellular calcium homeostasis as it does in other eukaryotes.

Genetics

Restriction fragment length polymorphism analysis and DNA fingerprinting have demonstrated marked genetic heterogeneity in *Giardia* isolates from animals and humans.[64] Detailed genetic analysis of the organism has, however, been hindered by a lack of a defined growth medium with nutritional auxotrophs or drug-resistant mutants. A stable transformation with foreign DNA is also not easy to achieve in protozoa. Information on the genetics of *Giardia* derives predominantly from analysis of the few genes that have been cloned.

Light microscopy has indicated the presence of four chromosomes, while pulsed-field gel electrophoresis indicates that there are at least five sets of chromosomes, often with additional minor bands.[78] Chromosome size varies between 1 and 4×10^6 bp, giving a total of 1.2×10^7 bp for the five chromosomes. Densitometric scanning of restriction endonuclease digests of *Giardia* DNA produce a similar genome size. *Giardia* nuclei appear to be haploid, and thus genetic diversity is explained on the basis of clonal divergence.

The G + C content of the *G. intestinalis* genome has been estimated to be 42–48%, of the protein-coding gene sequences to be 49 to >60% and of the rDNA gene to be 75%.[64] The non-coding regions are relatively A + T rich. *Giardia* rRNAs are smaller than other eukaryotes and eubacteria. The rDNA gene is only 5566 bp in *G. intestinalis* and slightly larger in *G. muris* and *G. ardeae*. Sequence analysis of the 16S-like RNA has demonstrated *Giardia*'s intermediate position between prokaryotes and eukaryotes.

EPIDEMIOLOGY

Giardiasis is found worldwide but in high prevalence in the developing world, where prevalence rates can reach 20–30%. Prevalence rates can often underestimate the overall impact of a pathogen. In rural Guatemala 45 children were followed from birth through the first 3 years of life; all were found to have giardiasis during this period and many had recurrent and prolonged infections with the parasite.[79] Prevalence in Peruvian children reached 40% by the age of 6 months, and stool examination confirmed prevalence rates of about 20% in children in Zimbabwe and Bangladesh. Age-specific prevalence rises throughout infancy and childhood, only declining in adolescence.[80] In the industrialized world prevalence varies between 2 and 5%, although within these low prevalence areas there may be localized regions of higher prevalence.

Age appears to be a risk factor for susceptibility to giardiasis, infection being more common in infants and young children, although giardiasis is rare during the first 6 months of life, particularly where breast feeding is practised. Undernutrition may increase the susceptibility to infection, as indicated by a study in Gambian children with chronic diarrhoea and malnutrition in which 45% had giardiasis compared with only 12% of healthy age- and sex-matched controls.[81]

Giardiasis is well recognized to occur in travellers, although overall it accounts for no more than 5% of cases of traveller's diarrhoea. However, 30% of travellers to the former Soviet Union were positive for *Giardia* in one study and more than 40% of Scandinavian visitors to St Petersburg acquired the infection.[82] Travelling within the USA may be hazardous, particularly for skiers in Colorado and visitors to National Parks, especially if they drink the apparently clean surface water.

Individuals with hypo- or agammaglobulinaemia are at risk of chronic giardiasis but individuals with HIV and AIDS do not seem to be at particularly increased risk of developing symptomatic disease, although carriage rates are generally higher than in the general population. These observations are consistent with the view that secretory immunity in the intestinal lumen is more important for clearance than cell-mediated responses within the intestinal mucosa.

A key factor in transmission of giardiasis is the ability of the cyst to survive for long periods in a suitable environment outside the host. Surface water in many parts of the world, including North America and Europe, are contaminated with *Giardia* cysts, which are not inactivated by chlorination alone. Interruption of the ancillary water purification procedures can lead to contamination of municipal water supplies and has been shown to account for many of the reported epidemics of water-borne giardiasis.[83,84] Water-borne transmission has also been shown to occur in swimming pools. Despite these epidemics, water-borne transmission probably represents a relatively small proportion of the total infections worldwide. Food has also been shown to be a vehicle for transmission of giardiasis, although again this is probably a relatively uncommon route of transmission.

Direct person-to-person spread by faecal–oral transmission certainly accounts for the high prevalence of giardiasis in day-care centres, schools and residential institutions, where prevalence may be as high as 35%. Person-to-person spread is also known to occur as a result of sexual contact.[85]

The major reservoirs of *Giardia* cysts are the human host and contaminated surface water. There is increasing evidence that a variety of domestic and wild animals carry *Giardia* spp. which are genotypically indistinguishable from human isolates. Although there is as yet no direct evidence that transmission has occurred from animals to humans, the higher prevalence of *Giardia* in companion animals which are in close contact with humans, particularly children in the home, makes this a strong possibility.[86]

PATHOGENESIS

As yet no specific virulence factors have been identified in *Giardia* and thus no unifying hypothesis for pathogenesis has yet emerged. Current evidence suggests that *Giardia* is able to perturb mucosal structure and function; at the same time there may be additional factors operating in the intestinal lumen which may also contribute to diarrhoea and malabsorption[87,88] (Table 67.7).

Mucosal factors

Disruption of intestinal structure

In human giardiasis the full spectrum of abnormalities of villous architecture have been described, ranging from normal to subtotal villous atrophy (Figure 67.7). A majority of infected individuals have relatively mild abnormalities of villous architecture, with associated crypt hyperplasia. Infections in experimental models produce similar changes but, as in human infection, the abnormalities are generally mild. The gerbil provides a good model for studying small intestinal structure and function as weanling gerbils develop diarrhoea and by the sixth day of infection have villous shortening

Table 67.7 Pathogenesis of giardiasis: possible mechanism.

Mucosal factors
Direct damage by trophozoites
  Microvilli
  Disaccharidases
  Transport proteins
Parasite products
  Proteases
  Lectin
Immune mediated
  T-cell activation

Luminal factors
Bacterial overgrowth
Inhibition of digestive enzymes
Bile salt deconjugation
Bile salt uptake by trophozoites

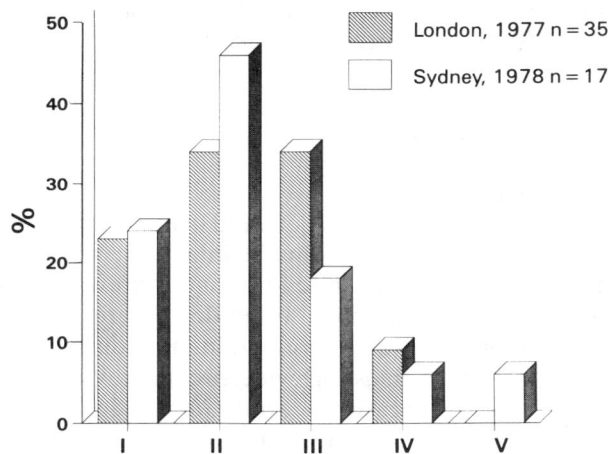

Figure 67.7 Percentage of patients with giardiasis with normal (I), mild (II), moderate (III) and severe (IV) partial villous atrophy, and subtotal villous atrophy (V).

in the duodenum and crypt hyperplasia throughout the small intestine.[89] However, as with murine giardiasis there is no associated mucosal inflammation.

Even in the absence of gross changes in villous architecture, ultrastructural abnormalities such as shortening and disruption of microvilli have been described in both humans and the gerbil model. Recent work in a neonatal rat model of giardiasis confirmed the reduction in villous height and an increase in crypt depth.

These morphological abnormalities are associated with reduction in disaccharidase activities. In animal models diarrhoea is at its peak when disaccharide activities are most profoundly reduced.[90]

Intestinal dysfunction

Intestinal solute and electrolyte absorption is impaired in gerbil and neonatal rat models of infection. Perfusion of a lactose-containing solution in neonatal rats exaggerated the abnormalities of water and electrolyte absorption and also showed impaired glucose absorption compared with non-infected controls. In vitro studies in Ussing chambers and in brush-border membrane vesicles from infected mice provide further support for an impairment of glucose and amino acid transport.

Mechanisms of mucosal injury

A variety of mechanisms have been proposed to explain these structural and functional abnormalities of the intestinal mucosa.[87,88] Attachment of *Giardia* trophozoites to the epithelium can disrupt and distort microvilli, particularly in murine giardiasis. It seems unlikely that this degree of disruption can account for the widespread changes of microvillous membrane surface area and other abnormalities of villous architecture observed in the small intestine.[87,88]

There is some evidence to suggest that *Giardia* trophozoites produce cytopathic substances that might be responsible for this disruption of epithelial structure and function. *Giardia* is known to produce a variety of proteinases which could find cleavage sites in proteins of the microvillous membrane. *Giardia* also has a mannose-binding surface lectin which could interact with mannose residues on relatively immature enterocytes and again contribute to epithelial damage. Other dietary plant lectins are known to be able to produce substantial abnormalities of villous architecture.

There is increasing evidence to suggest that T-cell activation within the intestinal mucosa can produce villous atrophy.[91,92] This mechanism is thought to operate in graft-versus-host disease and in coeliac disease. T-cell activation in normal human fetal small intestinal explants with pokeweed mitogen or with an anti-CD3 antibody results in villous atrophy, crypt hyperplasia and increased interleukin (IL)-2 production, confirming T-cell activation. Further support for this hypothesis has been obtained from studies of experimental *G. muris* infection in athymic nu/nu mice. Despite prolonged infection the alteration of villous:crypt cell ratio is less severe in T-cell deficient mice compared with immunocompetent controls.[92] When lymphocytes from the spleen of immunologically intact mice are injected into athymic infected mice, histological abnormalities in the small intestine become more apparent. Reduction in the villous:crypt cell ratio does occur to some extent in immunocompromised mice before reconstitution, and thus it seems likely that T-cell-independent mechanisms are also involved.

Luminal factors

Bacterial overgrowth

Giardiasis has been associated with increased numbers of aerobic and/or anaerobic bacteria in the upper small intestine of the indigenous Indian population or in travellers to the Indian subcontinent.[93,94] Bacterial overgrowth can produce architectural abnormalities in the small intestine similar to those seen in giardiasis and thus may have a role in the pathogenesis of mucosal damage.

Bile salt deconjugation

Conjugated bile salts have an important role in dietary fat absorption but if deconjugated by luminal bacteria they lose their detergent properties and can damage cell membranes. One study in Indian patients with giardiasis showed evidence of bile salt deconjugation, although this was not confirmed by a further study of patients in the UK. *Giardia* itself does not have the ability to deconjugate bile salts.

Bile salt uptake

As discussed previously, bile salts have an important role in *Gardia*'s life cycle. There is evidence to suggest that the organism takes up bile salts during growth by an energy-requiring active transport process, possibly involving a membrane carrier.[95] Although the precise metabolic advantages to the parasite have not been defined, a secondary effect of this process could be the depletion of intraluminal bile salt, thus impairing micellar solubilization of dietary fats and at the same time inhibition of pancreatic lipase, which is dependent on bile salts for full expression of hydrolytic activity.

Pancreatic enzyme inhibition

Several studies have suggested that concentrations of pancreatic enzymes in the duodenum are reduced in patients with giardiasis. Although there is no evidence of primary pancreatic failure in giardiasis, *Giardia* trophozoites are able to inhibit trypsin and lipase activity in vitro.[96,97] The precise mechanisms by which the organism achieves this have not been established, although it seems likely that this may relate to a direct effect of *Giardia* proteinases on the secreted pancreatic proteins.

Until specific virulence factors have been identified it is unlikely that the relative importance of these mucosal and luminal mechanisms in pathogenesis will be established. At present it seems reasonable to assume that the process is multifactorial, involving a combination of varying degrees of mucosal injury combined with disruption of the luminal phases of digestion and absorption.

IMMUNITY

Studies in experimental models and limited studies in human giardiasis have made it possible to attribute essential roles to the immune system in the eradication of acute infection and to determine, at least in part, the determinants of persistent infection in an otherwise immunocompetent host. There is increasing evidence to suggest that immunological factors are important in protecting mammalian hosts from reinfection, and thus the development of protective immunity. It seems unlikely that a single infection provides long-lasting protective immunity because age-specific prevalence increases throughout childhood and into early adolescence, suggesting that multiple exposures to the parasite are required before protection is achieved.

Giardia antibodies

Serum antibody

Anti-*Giardia* IgG can be detected in more than 80% of patients with symptomatic infection; antibody titres may remain elevated for months or even years after primary infection. In endemic areas anti-*Giardia* IgG titres are increased in individuals without infection, suggesting widespread previous exposure to the parasite.[98] Anti-*Giardia* IgM titres increase early in infection and then decline rapidly.[99] Studies in India and The Gambia indicate that only 30% of patients with infection have detectable anti-*Giardia* IgA.[100] Giardiasis has also been associated with raised total serum IgE, although in one case where this was investigated in depth this was not directed towards *Giardia* but possibly to food antigens as a result in increased intestinal permeability following acute giardiasis.[101] Similar patterns in antibody responses have been demonstrated in murine and neonatal rat models of giardiasis.

Secretory antibody

The secretory (s) IgA response in giardiasis is likely to be the most important aspect of immune response for parasite clearance. This is probably the reason why individuals with immunoglobulin deficiency have persistent giardiasis which is often refractory to treatment.[102] Specific sIgA has been detected on the surface of *G. lamblia* trophozoites in human jejunal biopsies and in human jejunal fluid. Anti-*Giardia* sIgA has also been detected in human milk and saliva, and epidemiological evidence suggests that the presence of these antibodies may contribute to protection from giardiasis in breast-fed infants.

Experimental infections in mice and neonatal rats support a role for sIgA and IgG antibodies in parasite clearance.[103] Administration of anti-IgM to mice produces a profound reduction in sIgA and results in chronic giardiasis. Protective effects of immune milk have also been demonstrated experimentally in mice. However, anti-*Giardia* sIgA is clearly not the only determinant of chronic infection since C3H/He mice develop persistent infection despite normal concentrations of anti-*Giardia* sIgA.

Giardia *antigens*

The surface antigen profile varies between *Giardia* isolates and this may be one contributory factor to the delay in achieving protective immunity to this parasite.[104,105] Thus, ideally all studies seeking to identify immunodominant antigens should relate to the serum or secretory antibody responses to the particular isolate in each given infection. This is extremely difficult and probably impossible to achieve on a wide scale. A variety of antigens (24–225 kDa) have been detected by immunoprecipitation and immunoblotting techniques using polyclonal antisera, monospecific antisera and monoclonal antibodies. Some antigens have been studied in more depth, particularly a 170 kDa surface antigen which has been partly cloned and sequenced. This is one of a series of cysteine-rich proteins which appear to be immunogenic, although their role in the parasite clearance of protective immunity has not been established.

An 82–88 kDa surface antigen has also been studied by several groups and is known to be a target for the immune response in human giardiasis. Recently a *Giardia* heat shock antigen has also been shown to be important in human giardiasis[106] and failure to produce an antibody response to this antigen may be an important factor leading to persistent infection.[106] Expression of this antigen is now known to occur not only following a temperature shift but also on exposure to the physical and chemical environment found in duodenal fluid.[106] This antigen has been recently identified to be homologous with hsp70, a highly conserved family of heat shock proteins found throughout the animal kingdom and shown to be important determinants of the host immune response in other bacterial and parasitic infections.

Giardia has also been shown to be able to vary expression of certain of its surface antigens in both experimental and human infection and this may be a way in which the parasite evades immune clearance. Further evidence is required before it can be established whether this mechanism is relevant in humans in vivo.

Cell-mediated immunity

Cellular immune responses are thought to be important in the immune response to this parasite, although evidence largely stems from work in animal models. Increased numbers of lamina propria and intraepithelial lymphocytes have been reported in both experimental giardiasis and in human infection, although an increase in absolute lymphocyte numbers does not appear to be a prerequisite for parasite clearance. There have, however, been no detailed studies on lymphocyte phenotype in human giardiasis.

T lymphocytes

The most compelling evidence of a role for T lymphocytes in parasite clearance has been obtained from the natural history of murine giardiasis in the athymic nu/nu T-cell-deficient mouse.[92] Infection is prolonged in this strain but can be eradicated by reconstitution with lymphocytes from syngeneic mice with normal immune function. These experiments have suggested that CD4 cells are critically important for the ability of mice to clear *G. muris* infection and may be involved in switching B-cell IgM to IgA production during infection. Genetic factors are also important because immunocompetent mice with different genetic backgrounds vary in their susceptibility to infection with *G. muris* and in their ability to eradicate infection.

B lymphocytes

Total B-cell numbers increase in human small intestinal mucosa infected with *G. intestinalis*, IgM-bearing cells being the predominant subtype. IgM cells are prominent early in infection and in nodular lymphoid hyperplasia of the small intestine, which occurs in some patients with giardiasis. A further study found only IgA and IgG cells, although this may reflect differences in sampling time because it would be expected that, during the later stages of infection, IgM-producing cells would switch to IgA production.

Mast cells, macrophages and polymorphonuclear leucocytes

Mast cell deficiency prolongs experimental infection in mice but the role of mast cells in human infection has not been established. Macrophages may also act as effector cells, their phagocytic activity for *Giardia* trophozoites being increased in the presence of specific antibodies. Neutrophils from patients with giardiasis also exhibit antibody-dependent cell-mediated cytotoxicity (ADCC) against *Giardia* trophozoites in vitro.

Integrated immune response in giardiasis

The immune system would appear to have a role in parasite clearance during acute infection, the control of mucosal invasion and ultimately the development of protective immunity. Current evidence suggests that anti-*Giardia* sIgA has a major role in clearing *Giardia* from the gut lumen, possibly by trophozoite agglutination and/or inhibition of flagella motility.[107] Monoclonal antibodies have been shown to be directly cytotoxic to *Giardia* trophozoites and it is likely that ADCC may occur within the intestinal lumen.[108]

Invasion of the intestinal epithelium by *Giardia* trophozoites is a rare event but a variety of mechanisms will be available within the mucosa to inhibit this process; these include cytotoxic intraepithelial lymphocytes, ADCC and the complement system.[109]

The immunological determinants of long-term protective immunity remain to be discovered. Clinical and experimental evidence suggests that secretory antibody in the intestinal lumen is likely to be important, although the antigenic determinants are as yet not defined. Preliminary evidence suggests that *Giardia* heat shock antigen, one of the family of hsp70 proteins, may be involved.

CLINICAL FEATURES (See also Chapter 3)

The most common form of giardiasis is asymptomatic carriage. This is particularly prevalent in highly endemic areas in the developing world, although is well recognized as occurring in parts of Europe and North America where the infection is common. Such individuals appear to suffer no ill effects from the parasite, although there have been no systematic studies of the subclinical impact of such an infection. It is unclear whether asymptomatic infections relate to carriage of 'non-pathogenic' strains or whether the host is able to maintain parasite numbers at a level below expression of clinical disease without complete clearance of the infection.

Table 67.8 Symptoms of acute giardiasis in travellers.

Clinical features	Patients (%)
Diarrhoea	95
Weakness	76
Weight loss	68
Abdominal pain	69
Nausea	60
Steatorrhoea	56
Flatulence	35
Vomiting	29
Fever	17

Acute giardiasis has been well characterized in individuals travelling from areas of low to high endemicity.[65] Symptoms usually begin within 3–20 days (mean 7 days) of arrival within a high-risk area and in the vast majority recovery occurs within 2–4 weeks. In up to 25% of travellers with giardiasis, symptoms may persist for 7 weeks or more. Diarrhoea is the major symptom and is usually watery initially but subsequently develops the features of steatorrhoea, often associated with nausea, abdominal discomfort, bloating and weight loss (Table 67.8).

Although giardiasis is self-limiting in the majority of healthy, immunocompetent individuals, a proportion, possibly 30–50%, go on to have persistent diarrhoea, usually with features of steatorrhoea.[65] Weight loss can be profound, with losses of 10–20% of the usual or ideal body weight. In symptomatic patients with persistent diarrhoea, 50% will have biochemical evidence of fat malabsorption and possibly of other nutrients, including vitamin A and vitamin B_{12} (Table 67.9). Secondary lactase deficiency is well recognized as occurring in human giardiasis and in experimental models and may take many weeks to recover even after clearance of the parasite.

Clinical complications of giardiasis

Retardation of growth and development

A series of hospital-based studies have clearly shown the potential of giardiasis to impair growth and development in infants and young children.[79,110] This is a highly selected population, biased towards more severely affected children, and thus does not give any indication as to the impact of giardiasis in the community. Several studies from Central America and West Africa suggest that giardiasis does have an independent inhibitory effect on child growth but it is difficult to arrive at firm

Table 67.9 Intestinal malabsorption in giardiasis.

Study	Location	No. of subjects	Subjects with normal results (%)				
			D-*xylose*	*Lactose*	*Fat*	*Vitamin B_{12}*	*Vitamin A*
Veghelyi, 1939	Hungary	14	—	—	71	—	—
Katsampes, 1944	USA	15	—	—	—	—	100
Cantor, 1967	Argentina	20	—	—	25	—	—
Hoskins, 1967	USA	6	50	100	40	100	—
Alp, 1969	Australia	5	20	20	100	—	—
Barbieri, 1970	Brazil	11*	27	—	82	—	—
Ament, 1972	USA	77	—	—	66	100	—
Cowen, 1973	USA	3	100	—	60	100	—
Tewari, 1974	India	30	23	—	50	6	—
Rabassa, 1975	Cuba	50	62	27	34	—	—
Wright, 1977	UK	40	45	—	35	—	—
Tandon, 1977	India	63	4	—	27	0	—
Hartong, 1979	USA	12	55	—	64	60	—
Mahalanabis, 1979	India	4	79	—	50	—	100
Mean (%)			47	49	55	61	100

*Asymptomatic children.

conclusions because within these populations many other factors are contributing to undernutrition and impaired development.

Allergic and inflammatory conditions

Lymphoid nodular hyperplasia has been associated with chronic giardiasis and immune deficiency. There is no clear indication as to the precise pathogenetic relationship between these phenomena, although there is some evidence to suggest that a common feature may be a predominance of IgM-producing B cells possibly as a result of the failure to switch from IgM to IgA production within the intestine. IgE-mediated allergic phenomena are uncommon in giardiasis, unlike many helminth infections, although occasional cases have been described.

Protein-losing enteropathy

This is a rare occurrence in giardiasis but has been described in children in West Africa and may contribute to undernutrition.[111]

DIAGNOSIS

Clinically, giardiasis is often suggested by a typical history which often includes a period of recent foreign travel. The main differential diagnoses include other causes of intestinal malabsorption such as tropical sprue and coeliac disease. Other infective causes of persistent diarrhoea include strongyloidia-

sis, cryptosporidiosis, microsporidiosis and that due to the new coccidian parasite, *Cyclospora cayatenensis*. Many clinicians will treat giardiasis empirically with a nitroimidazole derivative, even without achieving a firm microscopic diagnosis.

Microscopy

Giardia cysts and occasionally *Giardia* trophozoites are detected in faecal specimens by light microscopy, which continues to be the gold standard for the diagnosis of giardiasis. Faecal specimens are examined, either fresh or fixed with polyvinyl alcohol formalin, and then stained with trichrome or iron haematoxylin. Cyst detection can be improved by concentration techniques using formalin–ethyl acetate or zinc sulphate. Immunofluorescent anti-cyst antibodies have been used to assist the detection of cysts in faecal specimens. Examination of multiple faecal specimens increases the chances of making a positive diagnosis, with up to 70% of positive stools detected following examination of a single faecal specimen, rising to 85% when at least three separate stool specimens are examined. Trophozoites are usually found only in freshly passed watery diarrhoea. Trophozoites can also be detected microscopically in duodenal fluid and, although overall this technique has a lower sensitivity than faecal microscopy, it does complement the latter, in that some patients with negative stool microscopy will have a positive duodenal aspirate.[112] Tropho-

Table 67.10 Drug treatment of giardiasis.

Drug	Adults	Children	Efficacy (%)
Metronidazole	2 g (single dose) daily, 3 days or 400 mg three times daily, 5 days	15 mg/kg per day (max. 750 mg), 10 days	>90
Tinidazole	2 g single dose	50–75 mg/kg single dose	>90
Mepacrine (quinacrine)	100 mg three times daily, 5–7 days	2 mg/kg three times daily, 5–7 days	>90
Furazolidone	100 mg four times daily, 7–10 days	2 mg/kg three times daily, 7–10 days	>80

zoites may also be detected by endoscopic brush cytology or in mucosal impression smears of small intestinal biopsies.

Faecal antigen ELISA

Sensitive and specific ELISAs for *Giardia* antigens have been developed and some of these assays are now marketed commercially.[113,114] Sensitivity and specificity are reported to be 87–100%. However, further studies are awaited to determine whether their use can be widely recommended in routine diagnostic laboratories. False positives, however, are almost always reported in these assays and the interpretation of these findings is difficult. Enthusiasts for the test will regard this as 'microscopy-negative' giardiasis, but the pessimist will merely regard this as a true false positive, possibly due to the presence of cross-reacting faecal antigens. It seems likely, however, that microscopy-negative cases of giardiasis do exist and the more sensitive methods of detection such as ELISA or DNA-based diagnostic techniques will eventually prove the case.[115,116]

Serology

Anti-*Giardia* IgG titres are not helpful in diagnosis since they are commonly found to be increased in non-infected individuals in endemic areas.[98] Anti-*Giardia* IgM titres are usually only elevated in infected individuals and have been shown to be useful in a research setting for detecting individuals with acute giardiasis in endemic areas such as India and The Gambia. Sensitivity and specificity decrease, however, in children with persistent diarrhoea, in some of whom anti-*Giardia* IgM titres persist for several months.

DNA-based techniques

Specific DNA probes for *Giardia* are now available, although preliminary studies suggest that there may be difficulties in liberating DNA from *Giardia* cysts.[116] Amplification techniques such as PCR may be able to overcome these difficulties.

TREATMENT

In many healthy, immunocompetent individuals giardiasis is a self-limiting illness, with the parasite being eradicated by host defence mechanisms without specific treatment. Administration of an antigiardial drug will generally reduce the severity of symptoms and the duration of the illness.[64,117] Although symptomatic patients with giardiasis are generally offered antimicrobial chemotherapy, the question as to whether asymptomatic patients, particularly those in an endemic area, should be treated continues to be discussed. Since the development of in vitro culture techniques for *Giardia* isolates, methods have been developed to assess drug sensitivity in vitro.[118] However, the precise relationship between indices of drug susceptibility in vitro and the subsequent behaviour of the drug in vivo has not been clearly established. Treatment failures do occur and it is thought that at least some of these episodes are related to drug resistance.

Three classes of drugs are commonly used to treat giardiasis, namely the nitroimidazole derivatives, the acridine dyes, such as mepacrine, and the nitrofurans such as furazolidone.[64] Some commonly used treatment regimens for adults and children are shown in Table 67.10. Nitroimidazole derivatives are probably the drugs of choice, particularly when used as short-course regimens. Mepacrine has a similar efficacy but is generally less well tolerated. Furazolidone has a lower efficacy but is popular for the treatment of giardiasis in childhood as it has relatively few adverse effects and is available as a

Table 67.11 Adverse effects of antigiardial drugs.

Drugs	Adverse effects
Metronidazole and tinidazole	Nausea, vomiting, metallic taste, gastrointestinal disturbances, rashes, urticaria and angioedema *Rarely* drowsiness, headache, dizziness, ataxia *Prolonged* use, peripheral neuropathy Disulfiram-like reaction with alcohol *Avoid* in pregnancy and breast feeding
Mepacrine (quinacrine)	Gastrointestinal disturbances, dizziness, headache, nausea and vomiting Occasionally toxic psychosis *Prolonged* use, yellow discoloration of skin, sclerae and urine, chronic dermatoses, hepatitis and aplastic aneamia *Avoid* in pregnancy, hepatic impairment, psoriasis, the elderly and history of psychosis
Furazolidone	Nausea, vomiting Haemolysis in glucose-6-phosphate dehydrogenase deficiency

suspension. The adverse effects of these agents are summarized in Table 67.11.

The variety of other chemotherapeutic agents have been assessed in vitro and some have also been used in the clinical setting. The benzimidazole drugs appear to have some antigiardial activity which almost certainly relates to their ability to inhibit cytoskeletal function. Albendazole has been shown to have antigiardial activity in vitro[119] and recent clinical trial data would support its value in human infection. Other drugs such as sodium fusidate,[120] D and DL-propranolol,[121] mefloquine, doxycycline and rifampicin have all been shown to have antigiardial activity,[122] although the majority have not been subjected to rigorous evaluation in clinical practice.

PREVENTION

It seems highly unlikely that *Giardia* spp. will ever be eliminated from the environment, since they can survive for weeks or months outside the host in water or a moist environment and it is now well established that surface water in many parts of the world is contaminated with *Giardia* cysts. This reservoir could potentially maintain the animal reservoir of *Giardia*, which is increasingly thought to be another potential source of human infection. Despite vigilance about water quality, it is vital to ensure that contaminated surface water collecting grounds are appropriately treated before water enters the public water supply. Attention to personal hygiene in order to break the faecal–oral cycle is also important, particularly in residential institutions and day-care centres.

There is compelling evidence that breast feeding protects against giardiasis; this can be partly attributed to passive immunization. Whether active immunization in the form of a vaccine is feasible, or even appropriate, continues to be evaluated. Parenteral immunization with adjuvants can protect experimental animals from challenge with *G. intestinalis*, and the epidemiological evidence in humans that protective immunity does eventually develop, probably over a number of years, suggests that immunological approaches to prevention are feasible. However, it is unclear as to why the development of protective immunity following natural infection appears to require repeated exposure to the organism. It is possible that this is related, at least in part, to the variable antigenic profiles of different *Giardia* isolates. In addition, it is known that the expression of certain *Giardia* antigens can vary during both experimental and human infection, thus providing a way in which the organism may evade the host immune response. Failure to mount an antibody response to *Giardia* heat shock antigen in children with chronic diarrhoea in The Gambia suggests that impaired response may also be a factor. Clearly all of these issues need to be taken into account in planning a vaccine development strategy.

NON-PATHOGENIC FLAGELLATES

There are a number of other flagellates that are found in humans that do not appear to cause disease. *Trichomonas hominis* is commonly found in faeces of individuals living in the developing world. Only the trophozoite form is recognized; it varies from 5 to 14 μm in length. There is a single nucleus, anterior to which are basal bodies from which arise 3–4 flagella.

Chilomastix mesnili occurs as both cysts and trophozoite and is larger than *Trichomonas hominis*, being usually 10–15 μm in length, although it may occasionally be as large as 20 μm. The trophozoite has a large spiral longitudinal cleft anteriorly and an anterior single nucleus. Basal bodies at the anterior pole of the nucleus give rise to three anterior flagella, two fibrils which support the margins of the longitudinal cleft (the mouth), and to a fourth flagellum which moves within the longitudinal cleft. There are no cytoskeletal elements, the parasite maintaining its shape by a pellicle. The cyst is pear-shaped and approximately 18 μm in length. Internal structures are apparent in the stained cyst in which one or two nuclei may be observed.

Rare, non-pathogenic flagellates include *Embadomonas intestinalis* and *Enteromonas hominis*.

THE CILIOPHORA

Members of this class are all relatively large in size, are covered by short, hair-like organelles called cilia, which give the organism its motility. They have two nuclei, one somatic and one germinal. Reproduction is by binary fission, although conjugation does occur when nuclear material is exchanged between parasites. The only ciliate that is pathogenic to humans is *Balantidium coli*.

BALANTIDIUM COLI

Balantidium coli is the largest and probably least common protozoan pathogen of humans.[123] It can cause a severe, life-threatening colitis which is potentially avoidable by appropriate antibiotic therapy. Fatalities are almost invariably due to diagnostic imprecision.[124]

THE ORGANISM

B. coli exists as a trophozoite (usually found in stools of acute infection) and cysts, which become more apparent in chronic infection or asymptomatic carriers. The trophozoite is oval in shape, about 17 μm long and 15 μm wide. In its favoured host, the pig, trophozoites may reach 200 μm in length, when they can be seen with the aid of a hand lens or in some cases with the naked eye. The trophozoite is covered with cilia which propel the organism through the fluid contents of the intestinal lumen. At the anterior end of the trophozoite there is a cytostome (a mouth) leading into the cytopharynx which extends approximately one-third of the body length. Posteriorly there is a cytopyge (anus).

There are two nuclei, a larger macronucleus and a smaller micronucleus which lies in the concavity of the macronucleus. There are two contractile vacuoles connected by a canal. Intracellular organelles are limited, the major features being food vacuoles which circulate through the endoplasm. The trophozoite multiplies by lateral transverse fission, which may be preceded by conjugation, in which nuclear material is exchanged between trophozoites.

B. coli forms a large spherical cyst which may reach 60 μm in diameter. Cysts can survive outside the mammalian host for several weeks in moist conditions but are rapidly destroyed in hot, dry conditions. Infection is usually transmitted by the cyst.

EPIDEMIOLOGY

The parasite is found in northern and southern hemispheres, although it is most commonly reported in tropical and subtropical regions, particularly Central and South America, Iran, Papua New Guinea and the Philippines. Prevalence is usually less than 1%, although higher rates are reported in hyperendemic areas and some residential institutions. *B. coli* is found in many mammals other than man, particularly pigs and monkeys. Swine appear to be the most important animal reservoir for human disease, although enteric disease does not seem to occur in this host. The largest reported endemic of balantidiasis, involving 110 persons, resulted from gross contamination of ground and surface water supplies by pig faeces after a severe typhoon.[125] Communities which live in close association with swine tend to have increased prevalence of the disease because carriage by pigs has been estimated to be 40–90%.

PATHOGENESIS

The trophozoite is able to invade the distal ileal and colonic mucosa to produce intense mucosal inflammation and ulceration. The mechanisms involved are not clearly understood, although it is considered that the motile trophozoite is able to penetrate the mucosa and submucosa and even in some instances the muscle layers of the colon. Invasion is thought to be facilitated by the enzyme, hyaluronidase, produced by the parasite. The resulting inflammation may be partly mediated by other products liberated by the parasite and possibly by recruitment of mucosal inflammatory cells, particularly neutrophils.

CLINICAL FEATURES

In many respects the illness produced by infection with *B. coli* closely resembles amoebic colitis. Clinical presentation occurs in three forms: (1) the asymptomatic carrier state, most commonly seen in persons in institutional care and possibly accounting for up to 80% of all infections; (2) acute and acute fulminant colitis; and (3) chronic infection. In the acute form, diarrhoea with blood and mucus begins abruptly and may be associated with nausea, abdominal discomfort and marked weight loss.[126] Proctosigmoidoscopy reveals inflammatory changes, including discrete ulceration, although the rectum is not invariably involved. The illness can progress rapidly, accompanied by fever and prostration, and lead to death, usually due to peritonitis from colonic perforation. A protracted course with intermittent diarrhoea but only occasional blood in the stools is typical of the chronic form of the disease. A few cases of balantidial appendicitis have been reported.

DIAGNOSIS AND DIFFERENTIAL DIAGNOSIS

The large motile trophozoites are the predominant form of the parasite excreted in faeces and these can often be seen with the aid of a hand lens. Trophozoites may also be obtained from material from the margins of ulcers seen in the rectum at proctosigmoidoscopy. The macroscopic appearances at sigmoidoscopy do not, however, distinguish balantidiasis from other forms of infective or non-specific inflammatory bowel disease. Specific antibody responses to the parasite can be detected in serum but the value of serological tests in clinical diagnosis has not been clearly determined.

TREATMENT

The most commonly used treatment is tetracycline 500 mg four times daily for 10 days. The parasite is also sensitive to bacitracin, ampicillin, metronidazole and paramomycin.[127] Surgery may be required in fulminant disease, as in amoebiasis, although a conservative approach should be taken wherever possible.

THE COCCIDIA

CRYPTOSPORIDIUM PARVUM

Tyzzer[128] in 1907 was the first to describe an organism of this genus with a short account of *Cryptosporidium muris* in the gastric mucosa of laboratory mice. He identified the mode of transmission as faecal–oral, and provisionally classified the organism with the coccidia. A further report in 1912 by the same author demonstrated a similar parasite in the small intestine; as he was unable to cross-infect from one site to the other with the two organisms, he recognized that they were different species. This latter organism is *C. parvum*.

Following this early description, the organism was regarded as non-pathogenic until 1955, when a syndrome of fatal diarrhoea in turkeys was described, and then in 1971 a similar disorder in calves was recognized. The first report in man was in 1976,[129] and its identification in patients with AIDS in the 1980s cast it firmly in the role of an 'opportunist'. It is now recognized to represent a substantial threat to HIV-infected individuals, with a lifetime risk of infection of around 10%, but it is also responsible for substantial outbreaks of water-borne diarrhoea in the immunocompetent, and for diarrhoea in travellers and in children.

THE ORGANISM

Taxonomy

C. parvum is a protozoan, of the phylum Apicomplexa, class Sporozoasida, subclass Coccidiasina, order Eucoccidiorida. There are four other species in the genus: *C. muris*, which parasitizes rodents, some cattle and a gazelle; *C. nasorum*, which affects

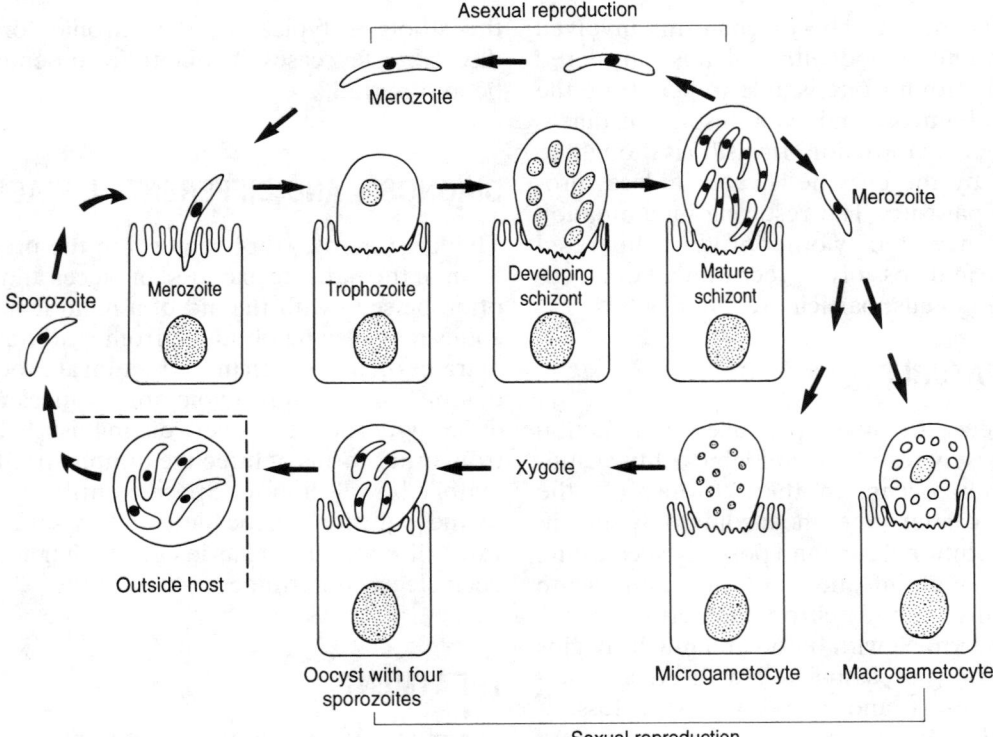

Figure 67.8 Life cycle of *C. parvum*.

fish; and two avian species, *C. meleagridis* and *C. baileyi*. *C. parvum* infects man, cattle, sheep, goats, deer, horses, buffaloes, cats and other non-mammalian vertebrates.[130]

Structure and ultrastructure

It is characteristic of these coccidia that the life cycle (Figure 67.8) includes merogony, gametogony and sporogony, and takes place within a vertebrate host. The ingested form is the oocyst, which has probably already sporulated before shedding. Excystation takes place in the small intestine, with four sporozoites being released from each oocyst. These are actively motile and penetrate the enterocyte. Electron micrographs show that the trophozoite takes up an intracellular but extracytoplasmic position (Figure 67.9).[131] Merogony or schizogony leads to the liberation of eight merozoites from the cell in the first cycle and four in the second, and direct invasion of neighbouring enterocytes takes place, magnifying the infection. Sexual multiplication takes place, leading to the formation of the zygote, and subsequently to the development of thin-walled oocysts (20%) and thick-walled oocysts (80%). Thick-walled oocysts are excreted in the faeces, but it is thought that thin-walled oocysts may lead to auto-infection.[132]

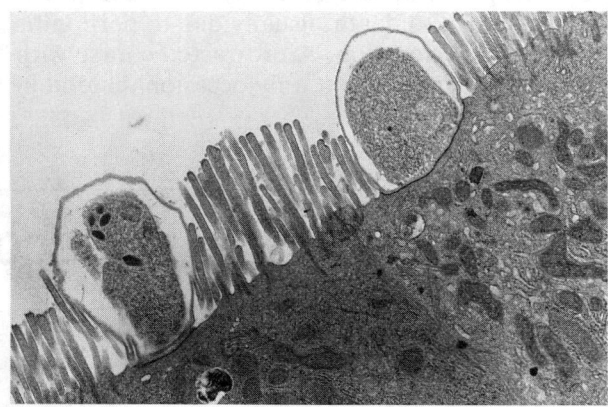

Figure 67.9 Transmission electron micrograph of *C. parvum* trophozoites in distal duodenal mucosa. The trophozoites occupy an intracellular but extracytoplasmic position. (20 000×.) (Courtesy of Graham McPhail.)

Genetics

Scanty information is available on the genetic make-up of *C. parvum* as there is no way of amplifying parasite material in vitro for analysis. However, some progress has been made, largely through the use of genomic libraries.[133] The genes which encode actin, tubulin, thymidylate synthase, topoisomerase, 18S rRNA and a few surface proteins (of unknown function) have been isolated. As yet there are no data on genes responsible for pathogenicity or virulence. However, there is genetic evidence for variation between isolates, based on restriction fragment length polymorphism analysis of genomic DNA and of isoenzymes.

EPIDEMIOLOGY

Immunocompetent individuals

Substantial evidence has accumulated implicating *C. parvum* in outbreaks of water-borne diarrhoea[134] and in stable endemic childhood diarrhoea among the poor of the developing world. Traveller's diarrhoea may result from infection with this parasite.[135] The evidence for the water-borne nature of the infection comes from epidemics that have occurred along water distribution patterns and the finding that oocysts can be detected in the water supply by filtration of large volumes through $1\,\mu m$ pores. As cryptosporidiosis is a common pathogen in calf and lamb diarrhoea, it is probably a zoonosis, transmitted in surface run-off water contaminated by calf faeces. Chlorination of water at usual levels fails to inactivate oocyst. It is probably this resistance to chlorination which allowed transmission of 70 cases following contamination of a swimming pool in the UK, and in a similar outbreak reported from California.

Data from the Public Health Laboratory Service in North Wales,[136] based on diagnostic laboratory returns, shows an age distribution of infection, with a peak between 1–5 years and a marked reduction over the age of 35 years. The incidence is seasonal and varies with rainfall. Cryptosporidial infection is a common cause of diarrhoea outbreaks in children, and these may cluster in nurseries. The spring peak in incidence in the UK closely parallels that observed for lambs, according to reports from the Central Veterinary Laboratories. Cases have been identified in which the only apparent transmission opportunity has been exposure to horse manure used as garden fertilizer. Veterinary students have an increased risk of infection, as do dairy farmers compared with other farming groups. Indirect transmission has occurred to young urban children from the clothing of mechanical digger operators returning home with boots and clothes soiled by farm manure.[136]

Cryptosporidiosis is an important contributor to childhood diarrhoea, with prevalences among children with diarrhoea of 1–3% in the industrialized world and 4–17% in developing countries. Figures of 1–13% have been reported in several studies from China.[137] In the developed world cryptosporidiosis

is found in outbreaks clustered around day-care nurseries. In a careful prospective study in Guinea-Bissau, cryptosporidia were found in 6.1% of acute (less than 2 weeks) diarrhoea and 15% of chronic diarrhoea, with a relative mortality in children with cryptosporidial diarrhoea in the first year of life of 2.9.[138]

Serological studies show that exposure to cryptosporidial infection is common. In a study of IgM and IgG antibody responses to the parasite, Ungar et al[139] found IgG-specific antibodies in 13/15 immunocompetents with cryptosporidiosis, and 26/26 patients with cryptosporidiosis and AIDS. Presumed uninfected individuals were negative in 57/60. Sera from 9/44 (21%) of Ecuadorian children with diarrhoea were positive, as were almost 50% of sera from adults with other parasitic diseases.

Insight into the transmission and pathobiology of the infection arises from the report of an outbreak of cryptosporidiosis in Denmark in 1990.[140] The setting was an infectious disease ward with a mixed population of HIV-seropositive and -seronegative patients; the index case was a demented seropositive man with cryptosporidial diarrhoea who contaminated an ice machine with faeces. None of the 73 HIV-seronegative inpatients became infected, but in 57 HIV-positive patients the attack rate was 18 (32%); 17 of these had AIDS. The mean incubation time was at least 13 days.

Immunodeficient individuals

Infection is acquired by the faecal–oral route. The course of the illness is variable, and depends largely, but not entirely, on the degree of immune deficiency, as measured by the CD4 cell count in the peripheral blood.[141]

Cryptosporidiosis first came to prominence as a problem in the context of AIDS, to the extent that chronic cryptosporidial diarrhoea is a case-defining diagnosis for AIDS. Table 67.12 shows a summary of the studies that have examined relative contributions of protozoal infections to the AIDS-related diarrhoea. Infections other than protozoa have been described, particularly salmonellae, shigellae, and in Africa, *Strongyloides stercoralis*. The contribution of viruses to the diarrhoea is uncertain at present. Differences in the proportions of specific infections found in patients in Africa and in patients in developed countries may reflect the more advanced stage of immune deficiency which the latter group reach before death, as well as the overall prevalence of the infection in the environment. Given the number of cases in which no infection is found, the significance of any coprodiagnostic

Table 67.12   Summary of studies of prevalence of protozoa in HIV-related diarrhoea in different geographical areas.

	Percentage of cases in which protozoan identified	
	Africa + Caribbean*	Industrial countries†
C. parvum	27	12
I. belli	13	0.5
Microsporidia	5‡	27§
G. intestinalis	2	5
E. histolytica	2	5

*Means of 11 studies from Haiti, Zaire, Uganda, Burundi, Zambia and Mali.
†Means of 15 studies from UK, USA, France, Germany, Holland and Australia.
‡Only two studies included a search for microsporidia.
§Some of these studies were of selected patients and the prevalence is raised artefactually.

finding is uncertain, and there are those who believe that many intestinal infections are incidental, and that the real culprit is 'HIV enteropathy'.[142]

PATHOGENESIS

Human studies on the distribution of infection are limited. Blanshard et al[141] showed that C. parvum is detected less frequently in duodenal and rectal biopsies than in faeces. In children with normal immune function, Phillips et al[143] found trophozoites in jejunal biopsies by light or scanning electron microscopy in seven out of nine patients with chronic diarrhoea (defined as >14 days) and malnutrition due to cryptosporidiosis. Goodgame et al[144] studied 12 patients with AIDS-related intestinal cryptosporidiosis and found no parasites on duodenal biopsy in four; in two patients the entire biopsy surface was covered; in the remainder, a partial covering was observed. They found that the total daily count of shed oocysts varied by only one order of magnitude, and correlated significantly with the proportion of duodenal biopsy surface covered. There was no relationship between oocyst shedding rate and stool volume. In their study, most duodenal biopsy specimens showed normal villous architecture.

Studies in piglets suggest that the infection moves along the gut in a caudal direction.[145] The heaviest infections were seen in the distal jejunum and ileum, moving to the colon with time, and were associated with partial villous atrophy, crypt hyperplasia and an inflammatory infiltrate in the lamina propria.

Electron microscopy of the infection shows that the presence of the trophozoites leads to destruction of the microvilli (Figure 66.9), which is associated with a reduction in disaccharidase activity.[143] Detailed ultrastructural work in a guinea-pig model of infection[131] shows the initial event to be attachment of the sporozoite to the microvillus, followed by invagination of the protozoan into an envelope of host cell origin. Subsequently the parasite induces conformational changes in the host membrane, which eventually breaks down with the formation of a 'feeder organelle' by which the parasite communicates directly with host cytoplasm.

Experiments in germ-free lambs showed that the villous architecture was normal in jejunum and ileum during colonization, until the appearance of sexual stages of the life cycle. At this point the villi were reduced in height and became fused, an inflammatory infiltrate appeared in the lamina propria and diarrhoea commenced.[133]

Cryptosporidial infection has been associated with increased numbers of mitotic figures in the crypts and villous atrophy. In the normal human intestine, cell maturation takes place during migration up the crypt and along the length of the villous. This process is accompanied by the change from a crypt cell generating net water and salt secretion to a villous cell with net salt and water absorption. Maturation is also accompanied by the synthesis of a normal complement of brush-border enzymes, including disaccharidases, lipases and alkaline phosphatase. According to the 'enterocyte immaturity hypothesis',[146] the repopulation of the villous with immature enterocytes leads to the failure of digestion and absorption seen in many protozoal small bowel parasitoses.

It has been assumed that, because some conspicuous individuals have high sodium and water losses in stool, often quoted at up to 20 litres/day, the principal mechanism of diarrhoea must be a cholera-like jejunal secretory state: 'diarrhoea in the human appears to be mostly due to hypersecretion of fluid and electrolytes from the proximal small intestine into the gut lumen.'[147] Animal perfusion studies in a neonatal piglet model of cryptosporidiosis do not support this hypothesis, nor do studies in humans using a jejunal perfusion technique.[148] It has been suggested that ileal malabsorption of bile salts may have a role in the pathogenesis of the diarrhoea.

IMMUNITY

Studies on the gastrointestinal specific immune responses to cryptosporidial infection in man are limited. Immunoblotting using postinfection serum, hyperimmune bovine colostrum and monoclonal antibodies has identified a range of antigens on the surface of the oocyst and the sporozoite. Various techniques reveal around 17 proteins on the surface of the oocyst, and between 20 and 40 antigens on the surface of the sporozoite. Most of these potential antigens are glycoproteins, with a molecular weight range between 15 and >900 kDa, and a dense cluster in the range 20–25 kDa. One of these glycoproteins, GP900, appears to be the target of protective antibodies in hyperimmune bovine colostrum.[133]

The majority of cases of chronic cryptosporidiosis occur in patients with HIV-induced immunosuppression. Chronic diarrhoea has been reported in congenital hypogammaglobulinaemia and in IgG_2 deficiency,[149] and severe combined immune deficiency.[147] Chronic diarrhoea may also follow administration of immunosuppressive drugs and usually resolves on withdrawal.

CLINICAL FEATURES

Early reports considered the infection in the context of AIDS as 'unremitting, profuse diarrhoea lasting for months', but this is an oversimplification. The clinical picture of infection is variable, and there is variation in disease severity even after accounting for the degree of immune deficiency by blood CD4 cell count. It is now established that patients with AIDS may carry heavy parasite burdens asymptomatically, and transient infection is not uncommon. However, a substantial proportion of patients present with diarrhoea, abdominal cramps and vomiting. About 8% of patients in London had fulminant diarrhoea, with collapse and severe dehydration due to the passage of high volumes of diarrhoea. The majority of patients in this study had stool volumes of 500–1500 ml/24 h, with stool frequency of 2–10 per day.[150] There is no way of clinically distinguishing patients with cryptosporidiosis from those with any other chronic diarrhoeal illness. The natural history of the infection in the West is that of a remitting and relapsing diarrhoea. In one study, 11/38 patients with HIV-related cryptosporidiosis underwent spontaneous remission lasting more than 2 months. These patients had higher peripheral blood CD4 cell counts than those who did not.[151] In a series of patients in Lusaka, Zambia, the median duration of diarrhoea at presentation with cryptosporidiosis was 5 months, with 60% admitting to intermittent diarrhoea (P. Kelly, personal observations). Among the patients studied by Colebunders et al,[152] in a series of Zairean patients, 89% had intermittent diarrhoea and the mean duration was 9 months; no difference was demonstrated between patients with cryptosporidiosis and those with other forms of HIV-related diarrhoea.

Patients in all areas of the globe show considerable wasting as AIDS progresses, but it is difficult to discern how much can be attributed to any particular infection. There is certainly anorexia in AIDS, and oral and oesophageal candidiasis exacerbate the problem. There is no evidence that cryptosporidiosis is associated with a greater degree of nutritional impairment than any other enteric manifestation of AIDS. Phillips et al,[143] however, showed an association between cryptosporidial infection and nutritional impairment in immunocompetent children. Children in Guinea-Bissau who were undernourished were not more likely to develop the infection.[138]

Some patients develop small bowel disease alone, while others may also have involvement of the biliary tract. The first large study of biliary disease in AIDS[153] described a syndrome of sclerosing cholangitis, sometimes associated with cholecystitis. This may be associated with cryptosporidial infection of the biliary tract, with microsporidiosis (see below), with cytomegalovirus, or it may be impossible to identify a cause. The disorder usually occurs in patients with chronic diarrhoea and is associated with progressive right upper quadrant abdominal pain. The patients tend to have had other opportunistic infections by this stage of the HIV infection. Biochemical tests of hepatic damage usually show elevated serum alkaline phosphatase and γ-glutamyltransferase concentrations in the absence of jaundice. Transaminases may or may not be elevated. Ultrasonographic examination of the liver may show irregularly dilated intrahepatic bile ducts. The definitive test is endoscopic retrograde cholangiopancreatography, which shows this distortion of the biliary anatomy, with or without papillary stenosis. Forbes et al[154] found cryptosporidia in 13/20 cases, and estimated that up to one in six of all cases of AIDS-related cryptosporidiosis may also have sclerosing cholangitis. This sort of study is unlikely to be carried out in the tropics, but there may be undiagnosed cases amongst patients with AIDS, usually presenting with chronic right upper quadrant pain.

DIAGNOSIS

Current diagnostic methods rely heavily on the identification of the oocysts in faeces. Three staining methods are in common use: auramine staining, modified Ziehl–Neelsen staining and immunofluorescence using monoclonal antibodies to oocysts. These techniques are relatively insensitive. The threshold of reliable (100%) detection was found to be 10 000 cysts/g in watery stool, but in formed stool thresholds were 50 000/g by immunofluorescence and 500 000/g by acid-fast staining.[155]

ELISAs which incorporate antioocyst antibodies to detect cryptosporidial antigen in faeces have been developed. There is a problem in knowing what to use as a reference standard, but two analyses suggest sensitivities of 82.3%[156] and 93%.[157] The specificity of such assays (which would be expected to be more sensitive than the reference standard, i.e. microscopy) is difficult to interpret. Two different assays using PCR have been published for detection of DNA in stool or biopsies,[158] but this is still a research tool.

Serological tests have been described, but have not reached the stage of routine use. The ELISA technique has been mentioned above, and an indirect fluorescent antibody test (IFAT) has been developed which will detect serum antibodies to oocyst antigens.[159] The IFAT was positive in 50% of AIDS patients with gastrointestinal complaints and 24.6% of non-AIDS patients.

TREATMENT

There is no effective treatment which will eradicate cryptosporidial infection. Approximately 80 drugs have been tested without success. The most promising agent to date is paromomycin, and trials are under way to assess its efficacy. The most important aspect of treatment is fluid and electrolyte replacement with oral rehydration solutions, although intravenous therapy may be necessary. Symptomatic treatment with codeine phosphate or powerful opiates should be given readily, according to resources. Octreotide, a long-acting somatostatin analogue, has been used with some success in patients refractory to opiates. Response rates vary but average 40–50%. Hyperimmune bovine colostrum has been found to have some effect when administered enterally, and studies are under way to determine its efficacy.

PREVENTION

When dealing with a disease affecting mainly the immunocompromised it is difficult to evaluate measures directed at reduction of incidence. On the basis of what little we know about transmission, it would seem prudent to advise those at risk, including HIV-infected individuals to boil all drinking water, and to avoid swimming in public water. There is no immediate prospect of effective immunization against the infection.

Prevention of nosocomial or laboratory-acquired infection requires strict attention to containment and generous washing of any contaminated areas. Disposables should be used where possible. The oocysts are resistant to many disinfectants, but are reliably inactivated by boiling, freezing, drying and 3% hydrogen peroxide.[160]

ISOSPORA BELLI

This coccidian was first described in 1915 but has received much less attention in the world literature than cryptosporidia, probably because of its comparative rarity in the developed world. It has recently attracted interest because of its identification in patients with AIDS. The infective form of the parasite is the oocyst, which releases sporozoites, leading to a small bowel infection. The parasite there takes up an intracellular location and undergoes merogony and sporogony.

EPIDEMIOLOGY

The route of transmission of the parasite is not established but faecal–oral spread seems likely. Infection is uncommon in the developed world, as reflected in the prevalences in European and North American AIDS patients (compared with Africans) shown in Table 67.12. In Paris, in a series of 3500 patients from the tropics studied before the HIV pandemic, only five (0.1%) cases of isosporiasis were found. A survey of 55 421 stool specimens in Chile over a 10-year period revealed only 452 (0.8%) positives.[161]

PATHOGENESIS

Isosporiasis is associated with mild to a subtotal villous atrophy. This is seen in patients with AIDS, but was also reported before the HIV pandemic.[162] Inflammatory cells and eosinophils are seen in the lamina propria.

CLINICAL FEATURES

As with cryptosporidiosis, isosporiasis leads to a self-limiting diarrhoea in the immunocompetent, and chronic diarrhoea in the immunocompromised. The illness in the apparently immunocompetent may be prolonged, extending to 20 years in one report.[163] There is little evidence regarding the frequency with which isosporiasis spontaneously remits in AIDS. In AIDS, isosporiasis is associated with wasting and dehydration. The most thorough analysis is that of De Hovitz et al,[164] in which 15 patients with *Isospora belli* were identified among 131 Haitian AIDS patients whose main complaints were watery diarrhoea, cramping abdominal pain and nausea.

DIAGNOSIS

Diagnosis rests on stool examination using wet preparations and modified Ziehl–Neelsen acid-fast stained smears. The oocysts appear oval, larger than cryptosporidial oocysts (20–30 × 11–19 μm), and have two easily identified sporoblasts. The oocysts also fluoresce with the phenol auramine stain under ultraviolet light. The parasites may also be recognized in small bowel biopsies, visible within enterocyte cytoplasmic vacuoles under electron microscopy and light microscopy.[162]

TREATMENT

Treatment with oral co-trimoxazole (sulphamethoxazole 800 mg and trimethoprim 160 mg) four times daily for 1 week eliminated the parasite from stool in most cases, with an interruption in diarrhoea.[164] Unfortunately this was followed by relapse in 50%, usually within 12 weeks on the whole. Retreatment was usually effective. Prophylactic co-trimoxazole may be necessary. Pyrimethamine–sulphonamide combinations (such as fansidar) are also effective.[163,165] There is little information on the regimen of choice for those who are intolerant of the sulphonamide.

SARCOCYSTIS SPECIES

Infection with this coccidian, formerly known as *Isospora hominis*, is uncommonly recognized. The parasite is similar to *Isospora belli* in its biology,[161] but the life cycle requires alternating infection of intermediate hosts, such as cattle and pigs, and definitive hosts, such as humans. In Strasbourg the infection was present in 286 patients over a 5-year period, representing 0.4–1.5% of all stool specimens. The infection has not so far been recognized in AIDS. In the Strasbourg series, 30% of cases had peripheral eosinophilia. Biopsy specimens may show in eosinophilic infiltrate. Sporocysts are recognized in stool with the same stains as are used for isosporiasis, but the cysts are smaller (15 × 10 μm).

CYCLOSPORA CAYETANENSIS

During the mid 1980s a new intestinal pathogen was identified in the stools of individuals with persistent diarrhoea; these were initially known as cyanobacterium-like bodies.[166] It has subsequently become evident that this organism is a member of the coccidia, of the genus *Cyclospora*. The organism has been tentatively named, *Cyclospora cayetanensis*.[167]

THE ORGANISM

Until the recent reports in humans, organisms of the genus *Cyclospora* have only been identified in reptiles, myriapods, insectivores and rodents. Oocysts of the human parasite differ morphologically from these animal species and it thus appears that the human isolate is a new species. Each oocyst has two sporocysts. Sporulation has been effected in vitro after 7–13 days in culture. Excystation results in the liberation of two sporozoites which are crescent-shaped, approximately 9 μm in length and 1.2 μm in width.[167] The ultrastructural characteristics of the oocysts are entirely consistent with other members of the coccidia. The complete life cycle of the parasite remains to be described.

EPIDEMIOLOGY

Cyclospora spp. were first identified in individuals with a history of foreign travel and those infected with HIV. Seasonal outbreaks were described in Nepal among foreign residents and travellers and a small outbreak has been reported in medical staff in a Chicago hospital. Since these initial observations a more detailed study in Nepal has revealed new information about the infection. As yet the global prevalence of the infection is unknown, although a prevalence of 4–7% has been reported in foreign residents in Nepal, with peak prevalence rates occurring during the warmer months with higher rainfall.[168] The incubation period is quite short, ranging from 1 to 7 days. Transmission appears to be by the faecal–oral route, water being the most important vehicle identified to date.

PATHOGENESIS

The mechanism by which this organism produces diarrhoea has not been clearly established. However, the organism takes up an intracellular location within enterocytes, and histological examination of small intestinal biopsies has demonstrated mild reduction in villous height, with associated mucosal inflammation and increased numbers of intraepithelial lymphocytes.[169] No specific virulence factors have yet been identified.

CLINICAL FEATURES

There is increasing epidemiological evidence that *Cyclospora cayetanensis* is responsible for persistent diarrhoea in both immunocompetent and immunocompromised individuals. Diarrhoea can last for 1–8 weeks and may be associated with abdominal pain, nausea, vomiting and anorexia. Abdominal gas and bloating are also commonly associated features.[167,168] In prolonged infection weight loss can be profound. Other than the persistence of symptoms there are no specific features that can distinguish cyclospora diarrhoea from other causes of persistent diarrhoea.

DIAGNOSIS

Oocysts can be detected in stool by light microscopy and can be induced to sporulate in the presence of 5% potassium dichromate solution.[167] Cyst concentration techniques can be used to increase the chances of cyst identification and typical features of the *Cyclospora* spp. can be detected by transmission electron microscopy. Parasites can also be detected in small intestinal biopsies by transmission electron microscopy.

Differential diagnosis includes other parasitic infections such as giardiasis, cryptosporidiosis, microsporidiosis and tropical sprue. A careful search for these parasites in faeces and in small intestinal biopsies is required to identify these infective agents.

TREATMENT

No specific therapy has been identified for the treatment of *Cyclospora cayetanensis* infection in humans.

PREVENTION

Epidemiological studies suggest that the major vehicle for the transmission of *Cyclospora* spp. oocysts is in water. Travellers should be advised to heed the usual advice regarding the drinking of tap water in tropical and subtropical climates. As yet there are no data on the susceptibility of sporocysts to chlorination, although it is likely that, like other members of the protozoa, this is an unreliable way of inactivating cysts. However, boiling water for 10 minutes should lead to their destruction.

THE MICROSPORA

ENTEROCYTOZOON BIENEUSI

Infection with this organism was first reported in 1985 by Modigliani et al,[170] who found the parasite in electron micrographs of small intestinal biopsies. Infection in humans had not been reported before the syndrome of AIDS-related diarrhoea was recognized, but various microsporidia infect other species of vertebrates and invertebrates. Since the first report, many cases have been identified, and microsporidial infection is prominent among those infections to which the HIV-infected individual is susceptible.

THE ORGANISM

Microsporidia constitute their own phylum within the protozoa, distinct from the coccidia which are part of the phylum Apicomplexa. They are obligate intracellular spore-forming organisms with a wide range of hosts.

Infection is acquired via the spore. Following ingestion, the spore extrudes a polar tube (possibly through increased intracellular pressure), through which sporoplasm is passed, infecting any enterocytes penetrated by the tube.[171] This infection of the enterocyte is followed by proliferation by binary fission (merogony), with the meront in an intracytoplasmic position, surrounded by a simple membrane. Microsporidia have a few elements of endoplasmic reticulum but no mitochondria.[172] Ribosomal molecular analysis indicates that the ribosomes are of prokaryotic size (70S), and RNA sequence analysis demonstrates considerable divergence from the ribosomal structure of most eukaryotes, suggesting that, like *G. intestinalis*, microsporidia evolved early along a divergent path from other protozoa. Merogony overlaps with sporogony, which leads to the development of spores.

These are about $1.5 \times 0.9\,\mu$m in size, and are shed in the faeces.

EPIDEMIOLOGY

The prevalence of infection with microsporidia in studies of patients with AIDS diarrhoea is shown in Table 67.12. It is important to note that different diagnostic tools were used and that some of the patient series were subject to selection. There are no reports of the infection outside the setting of AIDS, and there is no evidence for infection of animals other than humans.

PATHOGENESIS

Morphological studies of biopsies of infected small bowel reveal multiple meronts and sporonts in the host cell, often around the nucleus. Cells thus infected are apparently healthy at first, but the development of the later stages of sporogony is associated with enterocyte degeneration, vacuolation and loss of the brush border. These cells are subsequently sloughed off into the lumen, where the spores are liberated after cytolysis. Adjacent, uninfected cells are not apparently damaged.[173] Infection of enterocytes with microsporidia is seen only on the villi, not in the crypts. Villous atrophy occurs, possibly through increased enterocyte loss.[172] It is not known whether adjacent spread of infection occurs from cell to cell. There is no synchrony of life cycles amongst different organisms parasitizing the same cell.

Infection is confined to the small bowel, principally from the distal duodenum to the ileum.[174] One study has demonstrated an equal prevalence of microsporidial infection in biopsies from HIV-infected homosexual men without diarrhoea as in a group with diarrhoea, casting doubt on the causal association of the parasite and diarrhoea.[175] Another study showed microsporidia only in patients with diarrhoea.[176] Studies in patients have demonstrated diminished D-xylose absorption[177] compared with patients with AIDS-related diarrhoea without microsporidiosis, but serum vitamin B_{12} concentrations were not reduced.

IMMUNITY

Immune responses to this parasite have not as yet been formally studied. Intestinal infection with *Enterocytozoon bieneusi* appears, however, to be confined to patients with AIDS, indicating the likely importance of the immune system in controlling human infection.

CLINICAL FEATURES

Enterocytozoon bieneusi infection occurs rarely outside the context of AIDS diarrhoea. Among 38 HIV-seropositive patients with the infection, only one did not have diarrhoea,[178] and most series do not report any asymptomatic infections. Patients in this Australian study had a mean duration of diarrhoea of 7 months and a mean peripheral blood CD4 cell count of 40×10^6/l. The volume of the diarrhoea is variable, and is associated with anorexia, nausea and crampy abdominal pain.[176,177] This is probably true of all forms of AIDS-related diarrhoea.

There are several reports in the literature of a sclerosing cholangitis-like syndrome,[177,179] indistinguishable from that associated with cryptosporidiosis (q.v.).

DIAGNOSIS

The original and 'gold standard' technique for diagnosis is electron microscopy of small bowel biopsies. Early meronts are recognized by the paler appearance of the cytoplasm relative to that of the host cell (Figure 67.10). The hallmark of the late meront or sporont is the development of the characteristic electron-dense polar tube, which has about 5–7.5 coils. Other characteristics include the presence of electron-lucent inclusions (ELIs) and electron-dense discs (EDDs). Spores are identifiable by their intensely osmophilic walls.

Light microscopic diagnosis of histological sections of small bowel biopsy material is possible using careful scanning of sections stained with Giemsa,[173] Brown–Brenn or Unna blue. Biopsies obtained

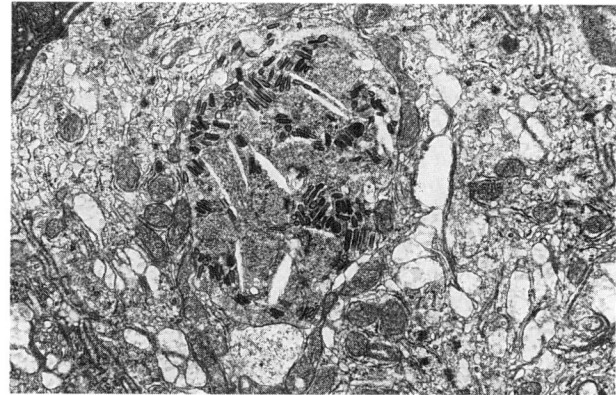

Figure 67.10 Meront of *Enterocytozoon bieneusi*, showing EDDs. (20 000×.) (Courtesy of Graham McPhail.)

from the distal duodenum are perfectly adequate, and either light or electron microscopy provides a more sensitive diagnostic tool than stool examination.[180]

Detection of spores in stool has become possible by the use of a chromotrope.[181,182]

TREATMENT

Treatment with metronidazole is largely ineffective, and other therapies have also failed. However, uncontrolled reports suggest that albendazole is the treatment of choice.[183] Albendazole inhibits microtubule formation, and thus reduces cell division and possibly polar tube action. Treatment is in high dose (400 mg twice daily for 4 weeks). Most patients seem to respond, although it is important to be aware of natural fluctuations in diarrhoea severity, with relapse after about 1 month after discontinuation of treatment. Placebo-controlled studies are awaited.

ENCEPHALITOZOON SPP.

Unlike *Enterocytozoon bieneusi*, *Encephalitozoon* spp. are widespread amongst other vertebrates. *Encephalitozoon cuniculi* is the best known, and differs from *Enterocytozoon bieneusi* in that all stages lie within a parasitophorous vacuole, and it does not cause enteropathy. Five human cases have been recorded, three with neurological disorders, one with hepatitis, and one with peritonitis in a patient with AIDS.[171] However, serological testing for *Encephalitozoon cuniculi* indicates that exposure to this microsporidian may in fact be quite common.[184]

Recently, infection with *Enterocytozoon hellem* has been described in patients with AIDS, with corneal infection and disseminated disease involving lungs and kidneys but not the gastrointestinal tract.

Another microsporidian has been reported in patients with AIDS in developed countries and in Africa. The first case was of chronic diarrhoea due to an organism resembling, but distinct from, *Encephalitozoon cuniculi*. Subsequently it has become apparent that this microsporidian is capable of dissemination, leading to an interstitial nephritis. The microsporidia may be found in lamina propria macrophages, and free spores can be found in the renal vasculature and the portal vein. The spores are then shed in the urine. One of the characteristics of this organism is its development within a parasitophorous vacuole which is septated. For this reason, some authors have referred to it by the name *Septata intestinalis*.[185] The parasite seems to be more sensitive to albendazole than are the other microsporidia.

REFERENCES

1 Walsh J A. Problems in recognition and diagnosis of amebiasis: estimation of the global magnitude of morbidity and mortality. *Rev Infect Dis* 1986; 8:228–238.

2 Löch F D. Massive development of amebas in the large intestine. Translated and reprinted in *Am J Trop Med Hyg* 1875; 24:383–392.

3 Osler, W. On the *Amoeba coli* in dysentery and in dysenteric liver abscess. *Johns Hopkins Hosp Bull* 1890; 1:53–54.

4 Councilman W T & Lafleur H A. Amoebic dysentery. *Johns Hopkins Hosp Rep* 1891; 2:395–548.

5 Schaudinn F. Untersuchungen über die Fortpflanzung einiger Rhizopoden. (Vorläufige Mittheilung.) *Arb Kaiserlichen Gesundheitsamte* 1903; 19:547–576.

6 Walker E L & Sellards A W. Experimental entamoebic dysentery. *Philippine J Sci B Trop Med* 1913; 8:253–330.

7 Brumpt E. Etude sommaire de l' 'Entamoeba dispar' n. sp. Amibe à kystes quandrinuclées, parasite de l'homme. *Bull Acad Med (Paris)* 1925; 94:943–952.

8 Sargeunt P G, Williams J E & Grene J D. The differentiation of invasive and non-invasive *Entamoeba histolytica* by isoenzyme electrophoresis. *Trans R Soc Trop Med Hyg* 1978; 72:519–521.

9 Sargeunt P G & Williams J E. Electrophoretic isoenzyme patterns of the pathogenic and nonpathogenic intestinal amoeba of man. *Trans R Soc Trop Med Hyg* 1979; 73:225–227.

10 Diamond L S & Clark C G. A rediscription of *Entamoeba histolytica* Schaudinn, 1903 (Emended Walker, 1911) separating it from *Entamoeba dispar* Brumpt, 1925. *J. Eukaryot Microbiol* 1993; 40:340–344.

11 Levine N D, Corliss J O, Cox F E G et al. A newly revised classification of the protozoa. *J Protozool* 1980; 27:37–58.

12 Cavalier-Smith T. In Schenk H E A & Schwemmler W (eds) *Endocytobiology II*. Tubingen: de Gruyter, 1983: 1027–1034.

13 Robinson G L. The laboratory diagnosis of human parasitic amoebae. *Trans R Soc Trop Med Hyg* 1968; 62:285–294.

14 Diamond L S. Techniques of axenic cultivation of *Entamoeba histolytica* Schaudinn, 1903 and *E. histolytica*-like amoeba. *J Parasitol* 1968; 54:1047–1056.

15 Sargeunt P G. The reliability of *Entamoeba histolytica* zymodemes in clinical diagnosis. *Parasitol Today* 1987; 3:40–43.

16 Torian B F, Reed S L, Flores B M et al. The 96-kilodalton antigen as an integral membrane protein in pathogenic *Entamoeba histolytica*: potential differences in pathogenic and nonpathogenic isolates. *Infect Immun* 1990; 58:753–760.

17 Tachibana H, Kobayashi S, Kato Y, Nagakura K, Kaneda Y & Takeuchi T. Identification of a pathogenic isolate-specific 30000-M_r antigen of *Entamoeba histolytica* by using a monoclonal antibody. *Infect Immun* 1990; 58:955–960.

18 Reed S L, Flores B M, Batzer M A et al. Molecular and cellular characterization of the 29-kilodalton peripheral membrane protein of *Entamoeba histolytica*: differentiation between pathogenic and nonpathogenic isolates. *Infect Immun* 1992; 60:542–549.

19 Petri W A, Jackson T F H G, Gathiram V et al. Pathogenic and nonpathogenic strains of *Entamoeba histolytica* can be differentiated by monoclonal antibodies to the galactose-specific adherence lectin. *Infect Immun* 1990; 58:1802–1806.

20 Muñoz M de L, Lamoyi E, León G et al. Antigens in electron-dense granules from *Entamoeba histolytica* as possible markers for pathogenicity. *J Clin Microbiol* 1990; 28:2418–2424.

21 Gonzalez-Ruiz A, Haque R, Rehman T et al. A monoclonal antibody for distinction of invasive and noninvasive clinical isolates of *Entamoeba histolytica*. *J Clin Microbiol* 1992; 30:2807–2813.

22 Strachan W D, Spice W M, Chiodini P L, Moody A H & Ackers J P. Immunological differentiation of pathogenic and non-pathogenic isolates of *Entamoeba histolytica*. *Lancet* 1988; i:561–563.

23 Garfinkel L I, Giladi M, Huber M et al. DNA probes specific for *Entamoeba histolytica* possessing pathogenic and nonpathogenic zymodemes. *Infect Immun* 1989; 57:926–931.

24 Tannich E, Horstmann R D, Knobloch J & Arnold H H. Genomic DNA differences between pathogenic and nonpathogenic *E. histolytica*. *Proc Natl Acad Sci USA* 1989; 86:5118–5122.

25 Tannich E, Scholze H, Nickel R & Horstmann R D. Homologous cysteine proteinases of pathogenic and nonpathogenic *Entamoeba histolytica*. *J Biol Chem* 1991; 266:4798–4803.

26 Tannich E, Bruchaus I, Walter R D & Horstmann R D. Pathogenic and nonpathogenic *Entamoeba histolytica*: identification and molecular cloning of an iron-containing superoxide dismutase. *Mol Biochem Parasitol* 1991; 49:61–72.

27 Que X & Reed S L. Nucleotide sequence of a small subunit ribosomal RNA (16S-like rRNA) gene from *Entamoeba histolytica*: differentiation of pathogenic from nonpathogenic isolates. *Nucleic Acids Res* 1991; 19:5438.

28 Cruz-Reyes J A, Spice W M, Rehman T, Gisborne E & Ackers J P. Ribosomal DNA sequences in the differentiation of pathogenic and non-pathogenic isolates of *Entamoeba histolytica*. *Parasitology* 1992; 104:239–246.

29 Clark C G & Diamond L S. Ribosomal RNA genes of 'pathogenic' and 'nonpathogenic' *Entamoeba histolytica* are distinct. *Mol Biochem Parasitol* 1991; 49:297–302.

30 Tachibana H, Ihara S, Kobayashi S, Kaneda Y, Takeuchi T & Watanabe Y. Differences in genomic DNA sequences between pathogenic and non-pathogenic isolates of *Entamoeba histolytica* identified by the polymerase chain reaction. *J Clin Microbiol* 1991; 29:2234–2239.

31 Tannich E & Burchard G D. Differentiation of pathogenic from non pathogenic *Entamoeba histolytica* by restriction fragment analysis of a single gene amplified *in vitro*. *J Clin Microbiol* 1991; 29:250–255.

32 Tachibana H, Kobayashi S, Takekoshi M & Ihara S. Distinguishing pathogenic isolates of *Entamoeba histolytica* by polymerase chain reaction. *J Infect Dis* 1991; 164:825–826.

33 Serrano R & Reeves R E. Glucose transport in *Entamoeba histolytica*. *Biochem J* 1974; 144:43–48.

34 Weinbach E C & Diamond L S. *Entamoeba histolytica*: I. Aerobic metabolism. *Exp Parasitol* 1974; 35:232–243.

35 Albach R A. Nucleic acids of *Entamoeba histolytica*. *J Protozool* 1989; 36:197–205.

36 Byers T J. Molecular biology of DNA in *Acanthamoeba*, *Amoeba*, *Entamoeba*, and *Naegleria*. *Int Rev Cytol* 1986; 99:311–314.

37 Blanc D S. Determination of taxonomic status of pathogenic and nonpathogenic *Entamoeba histolytica* zymodemes using isoenzyme analysis. *J Protozool* 1992; 39:471–479.

38 Reed S, Bouvier J, Pollak A S et al. Cloning of a virulence factor of *Entamoeba histolytica*. Pathogenic strains possess a unique cysteine proteinase gene. *J Clin Invest* 1993; 91:1532–1540.

39 Mirelman D, Bracha R, Chayen A, Aust-Kettis A & Diamond L S. *Entamoeba histolytica*: effect of growth conditions and bacterial associates on isoenzyme patterns and virulence. *Exp Parasitol* 1986; 62:142–148.

40 Andrews B J, Mentzoni L & Bjorvatn B. Zymodeme conversion of isolates of *Entamoeba histolytica*. *Trans R Soc Trop Med Hyg* 1990; 84:63–65.

41 Mirelman D, Bracha R, Wexler A & Chayen A. Changes in isoenzyme patterns of a cloned culture of nonpathogenic *Entamoeba histolytica* during axenization. *Infect Immun* 1986; 54:827–832.

42 Blanc D, Nicholls R & Sargeunt P G. Experimental production of new zymodemes of *Entamoeba*

histolytica supports the hypothesis of genetic exchange. *Trans R Soc Trop Med Hyg* 1989; 83:787–790.

43 Gathiram V & Jackson T F G H. Frequency distribution of *Entamoeba histolytica* zymodemes in a rural South African population. *Lancet* 1985; i:719–721.

44 Ravdin J I. *Entamoeba histolytica*: from adherence to enteropathy. *J Infect Dis* 1989; 159:420–429.

45 Adams S A, Robson S C, Gathiram V et al. Immunological similarity between the 170kD amoebic adherence glycoprotein and human β2 integrins. *Lancet* 1993; 341:17–19.

46 Guillén N. Cell signalling and motility in *Entamoeba histolytica*. *Parasitol Today* 1993; 9:364–369.

47 Reed S L, Keene W E & McKerrow J H. Thiol proteinase expression and pathogenicity of *Entamoeba histolytica*. *J Clin Microbiol* 1989; 27:2772–2777.

48 Muñoz M de L, Lamoyi E, León G et al. Antigens in electron-dense granules from *Entamoeba histolytica* as possible markers for pathogenicity. *J Clin Microbiol* 1990; 28:2418–2424.

49 Schulte W & Scholze H. Action of the major protease from *Entamoeba histolytica* on proteins of the extracellular matrix. *J Protozool* 1989; 36:538–543.

50 De Leon A. Pronóstico tardío en el absceso hepático amibiano. *Arch Invest Med* 1970; 1:205–206.

51 Irusen E M, Jackson T F H G & Simjee A E. Asymptomatic intestinal colonization by pathogenic *Entamoeba histolytica* in amebic liver abscess: prevalence, response to therapy and pathogenic potential. *Clin Infect Dis* 1992; 14:889–893.

52 Gathiram V & Jackson T F H G. A longitudinal study of asymptomatic carriers of pathogenic zymodemes of *Entamoeba histolytica*. *S Afr Med J* 1987; 72:669–672.

53 Berkowitz D & Bernstein L H. Colonic pseudopolyps in association with amoebic colitis. *Gastroenterology* 1975; 68:786–789.

54 Carrada Bravo T. Invasive amebiasis as a public health problem. *Bol Med Hosp Infant Mex* 1989; 46:139–148.

55 Freeman O, Akamaguna A & Jarikre L N. Amoebic liver abscess: the effect of aspiration on the resolution or healing time. *Ann Trop Med Parasitol* 1990; 84:281–287.

56 Bruckner D A. Amebiasis. *Clin Microbiol Rev* 1992; 5:356–369.

57 Weinke T, Friedrich-Jänicke B, Hopp P & Janitschke K. Prevalence and clinical importance of *Entamoeba histolytica* in two high-risk groups: travelers returning from the tropics and male homosexuals. *J Infect Dis* 1989; 161:1029–1031.

58 Tshalaia L E. Contributions to the study of *Entamoeba moshkovskii*. *Med Parazitol (Mosk)* 1947; 16:60–69.

59 Clark C G & Diamond L S. The Laredo strain and other *Entamoeba histolytica*-like amoeba are *Entamoeba moshkovskii*. *Mol Biochem Parasitol* 1991; 46:11–18.

60 Sargeaunt P G, Patrick S & O'Keeffe D. Human infections of *Entamoeba chattoni* masquerade as *Entamoeba histolytica*. *Trans R Soc Trop Med Hyg* 1992; 86:633–634.

61 Ash L R & Orihel T C. *Atlas of Human Parasitology*, 3rd edn. Chicago: ASCP Press, 1990.

62 Camp R R, Mattern C F T & Honigberg B M. Study of *Dientamoeba fragilis* Jepps & Dobell. I. Electron microscopic observations of the binucleate stages. II. Taxonomic position and revision of the genus. *J Protozool* 1974; 21:69–82.

63 Farthing M J G. Host–parasite interactions in human giardiasis. *Q J Med* 1989; 70:191–204.

64 Adam R D. The biology of *Giardia* spp. *Microbiol Rev* 1991; 55:706–732.

65 Farthing M J G. Giardiasis as a disease. In Reynoldson J A, Thompson R C A & Lymbery A J (eds) *Giardia: From Molecules to Disease and Beyond*. London: CAB International, 1993: 15–37.

66 Kabnick K S & Peattie D A. *Giardia*: a missing link between prokaryotes and eukaryotes. *Am Sci* 1991; 79:34–43.

67 Meyer E A. Taxonomy and nomenclature. In Meyer E A (ed.) *Giardiasis*. Amsterdam: Elsevier, 1990: 51–60.

68 Carnaby S, Katelaris P H, Naemm A & Farthing M J G. Genotypic heterogeneity within *Giardia lamblia* isolates demonstrated by M13 DNA fingerprinting. *Infect Immun* 1994; 62:1875–1880.

69 Peattie D A, Alonso R A, Hein A & Caulfield J P. Ultrastructural localization of giardins to the edges of disk microribbons of *Giardia lamblia* and the nucleotide and deduced protein sequence of alpha-giardin. *J Cell Biol* 1989; 109:2323–2335.

70 Jarroll E L, Manning P, Lindmark D G, Coggins J R & Erlandsen S L. *Giardia* cyst wall-specific carbohydrate: evidence for the presence of galactosamine. *Mol Biochem Parasitol* 1989; 32:121–132.

71 Erlandsen S L & Feely D E. Trophozoite motility and the mechanism of attachment. In Erlandsen S L & Meyer E A (eds) *Giardia and Giardiasis*. New York: Plenum Press, 1984: 33–60.

72 Farthing M J G, Pereira M E A & Keusch G T. Description and characterization of a surface lectin from *Giardia lamblia*. *Infect Immun* 1986; 51:661–667.

73 Lev B, Ward H, Keusch G T & Pereira M E A. Lectin activation of *Giardia lamblia* by host protease: a novel host–parasite interaction. *Science* 1986; 232:71–73.

74 Farthing M J G, Keusch G T & Carey M C. Effects of bile and bile salts on growth and membrane lipid uptake by *Giardia lamblia*: possible implication for pathogenesis of intestinal disease. *J Clin Invest* 1985; 76:1727–1732.

75 Meyer E A. *Giardia lamblia*: isolation and axenic cultivation. *Exp Parasitol* 1976; 39:101–105.

76 Jarroll E L, Muller P J, Meyer M R & Kranz P. Glucose metabolism in *Giardia lamblia*. *Mol Biochem Parasitol* 1981; 2:187–196.

77 Wang C C & Aldritt S. Purine salvage networks in *Giardia lamblia*. *J Exp Med* 1983; 158:1703–1712.

78 Adam R D, Nash T E & Wellems T E. The *Giardia lamblia* trophozoite contains sets of closely related chromosomes. *Nucleic Acids Res* 1988; 16:4555–4567.

79 Farthing M J G, Mata L, Urrutia J J & Kronmal R A. Natural history of *Giardia* infection of infants and children in rural Guatemala and its impact on physical growth. *Am J Clin Nutr* 1986; 43:393–403.

80 Oyerinde J P O, Ogunbi O & Alonge A A. Age and sex distribution of infections with *Entamoeba histolytica* and *Giardia intestinalis* in the Lagos population. *Int J Epidemiol* 1977; 6:231–234.

81 Sullivan P B, Marsh M N, Phillips M B et al. Prevalence and treatment of giardiasis in chronic diarrhoea and malnutrition. *Arch Dis Child* 1991; 66:304–306.

82 Jokipii L & Jokipii A M. Giardiasis in travelers: a prospective study. *J Infect Dis* 1974; 30:295–299.

83 Craun G F. Waterborne outbreaks of giardiasis. Current status. In Erlandsen S L & Meyer E R (eds) *Giardia and Giardiasis*. New York: Plenum Press, 1984: 243–261.

84 Jephcott A E, Begg N T & Baker I A. Outbreak of giardiasis associated with mains water in the United Kingdom. *Lancet* 1986; i:730–732.

85 Owen R L. Direct fecal–oral transmission of giardiasis. In Erlandsen S L & Meyer E A (eds) *Giardia and Giardiasis*. New York: Plenum Press, 1984: 329–339.

86 Winsland J K D, Nimmo S, Butcher P D & Farthing M J G. Prevalence of *Giardia* in dogs and cats in the United Kingdom: survey of an Essex veterinary clinic. *Trans R Soc Trop Med Hyg* 1989; 83:791–792.

87 Katelaris P H & Farthing M J G. Diarrhoea and malabsorption in giardiasis: a multifactorial process. *Gut* 1992; 33:295–297.

88 Farthing M J. Diarrhoeal disease: current concepts and future challenges. Pathogenesis of giardiasis. *Trans R Soc Trop Med Hyg* 1993; 87(Suppl 3):17–21.

89 Buret A, Hardin J A, Olson M E & Gall D G. Pathophysiology of small intestinal malabsorption in gerbils infected with *Giardia lamblia*. *Gastroenterology* 1992; 103:506–513.

90 Gillon J, Al Thamery D & Ferguson A. Features of small intestinal pathology (epithelial cell kinetics, intraepithelial lymphocytes, disaccharidases) in a primary *Giardia muris* infection. *Gut* 1982; 23:498–506.

91 MacDonald T T & Spencer J. Evidence that activate mucosal T cells play a role in the pathogenesis of enteropathy in human small intestine. *J Exp Med* 1988; 167:1341–1349.

92 Roberts-Thomson I C & Mitchell F G. Giardiasis in mice. I. Prolonged infections in certain mouse strains and hypothymic (nude) mice. *Gastroenterology* 1978; 75:42–46.

93 Tandon B N, Tandon R K, Satpathy B K & Shriniwas. Mechanism of malabsorption in giardiasis: a study of bacterial flora and bile salt deconjugation in upper jejunum. *Gut* 1977; 18:176–181.

94 Tomkins A M, Drasar B S, Bradley A K & Williamson W A. Bacterial colonization of jejunal mucosa in giardiasis. *Trans R Soc Trop Med Hyg* 1978; 72:33–36.

95 Halliday C E, Clark C & Farthing M J. Giardia-bile salt interactions *in vitro* and *in vivo*. *Trans R Soc Trop Med Hyg* 1988; 82(3):428–432.

96 Katelaris P H, Seow F & Ngu M C. The effect of *Giardia lamblia* trophozoites on lipolysis *in vitro*. *Parasitology* 1991; 103:35–39.

97 Seow F, Katelaris P H & Ngu M. The effect of *Giardia lamblia* trophozoites on trypsin, chymotrypsin and amylase *in vitro*. *Parasitology* 1993; 106:233–238.

98 Farthing M J G, Goka A K J, Butcher P D & Arvind A S. Serodiagnosis of giardiasis. *Serodiagn Immunother* 1987; 1:233–238.

99 Goka A K J, Rolston D D K, Mathan V I & Farthing M J G. Diagnosis of giardiasis by specific IgM antibody enzyme-linked immunosorbent assay. *Lancet* 1986; ii:184–186.

100 Goka A K J, Rolston D D K, Mathan V I & Farthing M J G. Serum IgA response in human *Giardia lamblia* infection. *Serodiagn Immunother* 1989; 3:273–277.

101 Farthing M J G, Chong S & Walker-Smith J A. Acute allergic phenomena in giardiasis. *Lancet* 1984; ii:1428.

102 Snider D P & Underdown B J. Quantitative and temporal analyses of murine antibody response in serum and gut secretions to infection with *Giardia muris*. *Infect Immun* 1986; 52:271–278.

103 Heyworth M F. Intestinal IgA responses to *Giardia muris* in mice depleted of helper T lymphocytes and in immunocompetent mice. *J Parasitol* 1989; 75:246–251.

104 Adam R D, Aggarwal A, Lal A A, de la Cruz V F, McCutchan T L & Nash T E. Antigenic variation of a cysteine-rich protein in *Giardia lamblia*. *J Exp Med* 1988; 167:109–118.

105 Nash T E & Keister D B. Differences in excretory–secretory products and surface antigens among 19 isolates of *Giardia*. *J Infect Dis* 1985; 152:1166–1171.

106 Char S, Cevallos A M & Farthing M J G. An immunodominant antigen of *Giardia lamblia* is a heat shock protein. *Biotechnol Ther* 1992; 3:151–157.

107 Char S, Cevallos A M, Yamson P, Sullivan P B, Neale G & Farthing M J G. Impaired IgA response to *Giardia* heat shock antigen in children with persistent diarrhoea and giardiasis. *Gut* 1992; 34:38–40.

108 Smith P D, Keister D B & Elson C O. Human host

response to *Giardia lamblia*. II. Antibody-dependent killing *in vitro*. *Cell Immunol* 1983; 82:308–315.

109 Deguchi M, Gillin F D & Gigli I. Mechanism of killing of *Giardia lamblia* trophozoites by complement. *J Clin Invest* 1987; 79:1296–1302.

110 Farthing M J G, Mata L J, Urrutia J J & Kronmal R A. Giardiasis: impact on child growth. In Walker-Smith J A & McNeish A S (eds) *Diarrhea and Malnutrition in Childhood*. London: Butterworth, 1986: 68–78.

111 Sullivan P B, Lunn P G, Northrop-Clewes C A & Farthing M J G. Parasitic infection of the gut and protein-losing enteropathy. *J. Pediatr Gastroenterol Nutr* 1992; 15:404–407.

112 Goka A K J, Rolston D D K, Mathan V I & Farthing M J G. The relative merits of faecal and duodenal juice microscopy in the diagnosis of giardiasis. *Trans R Soc Trop Med Hyg* 1990; 84:66–67.

113 Green E L, Miles M A & Warhurst D C. Immunodiagnostic detection of *Giardia* antigen in faeces by a rapid visual enzyme-linked immunosorbent assay. *Lancet* 1985; ii:691–693.

114 Addiss D G, Sanders C A, Sonnad S S et al. Stool diagnosis of giardiasis using a commercially available enzyme immunoassay to detect *Giardia*-specific antigen 65 (GSA 65). *J Clin Microbiol* 1989; 27:1137–1142.

115 Char S & Farthing M J G. DNA probes for diagnosis of enteric infection. *Gut* 1991; 32:1–3.

116 Butcher P D & Farthing M J G. DNA probes for the faecal diagnosis of *Giardia lamblia* infections in man. *Biochem Soc Trans* 1988; 17:363–364.

117 Davidson R A. Issues in clinical parasitology: the treatment of giardiasis. *Am J Gastroenterol* 1984; 79:256–261.

118 Crouch A A, Seow W K & Thong Y H. Effect of twenty-three chemotherapeutic agents on the adherence and growth of *Giardia lamblia* in vitro. Trans R Soc Trop Med Hyg 1986; 80:893–896.

119 Meloni B P, Thompson R C A, Reynoldson J A & Seville P. Albendazole: a more effective anti-gardial agent *in vitro* than metronidazole or tinidazole. *Trans R Soc Trop Med Hyg* 1990; 84:375–379.

120 Farthing M J G & Inge P M G. Anti-giardial activity of the bile salt-like antibiotic sodium fusidate. *J Antimicrob Chemother* 1986; 17:165–171.

121 Farthing M J G, Inge P M G & Pearson R M. Effect of D-propranolol on growth and motility of flagellate protozoa. *J Antimicrob Chemother* 1987; 20:519–522.

122 Crouch A A, Seow W K, Whitman L M & Thong Y H. Sensitivity *in vitro* of *Giardia intestinalis* to dyadic combinations of azithromycin, deoxycline, mefloquine, tinidazole and furazolidone. *Trans R Soc Trop Med Hyg* 1990; 84:246–248.

123 Arean V M & Koppisch E. Balantidiasis: a review and report of cases. *Am J Pathol* 1956; 32:1089–1115.

124 Samranwetaya P, Dechakaisaya S & Tangchai P. Fatal balantidal colitis. Report of a case. *J Med Assoc Thai* 1972; 55:259–262.

125 Walzer P D, Judson F N, Murphy K B, Healy G R, English D K & Schultz M G. Balantidiasis outbreak in Truk. *Am J Trop Med Hyg* 1973; 22:33–41.

126 Baskerville L. Balantidium colitis. Report of a case. *Am J Dig Dis* 1970; 15:727–731.

127 Garcia-Laverde A & De Bonilla L. Clinical trials with metronidazole in human balantidiasis. *Am J Trop Med Hyg* 1975; 24:781–783.

128 Tyzzer E E. A sporozoan found in the peptic glands of the common mouse. *Proc Soc Exp Biol Med* 1907; 5:12–13.

129 Nime F A, Burek J D, Page D L & Hoescher M A. Acute enterocolitis in a human being infected with the protozoan *Cryptosporidium*. *Gastroenterology* 1976; 70:592–598.

130 Current W L & Bick P H. Immunobiology of *Cryptosporidium* spp. *Pathol Immunopathol Res* 1989; 8:141–160.

131 Marcial M A & Madara J L. Cryptosporidium: cellular localization, structural analysis of absorptive cell–parasite interactions in guinea pigs, and suggestion of protozoan transport by M Cells. *Gastroenterology* 1986; 90:583–594.

132 Angus K W. Cryptosporidiosis and AIDS. *Baillière's Clin Gastroenterol* 1990; 4:425–440.

133 Petersen C. Cellular biology of *Cryptosporidium parvum*. *Parasitol Today* 1993; 9:87–91.

134 Smith H V & Rose J B. Waterborne cryptosporidiosis. *Parasitol Today* 1990; 6:8–12.

135 Katelaris P & Farthing M J G. Cryptosporidiosis—an emerging risk to travellers. *Trav Med Int* 1992; 1:10–14.

136 Casemore D P. Epidemiological aspects of human cryptosporidiosis. *Epidemiol Infect* 1990; 104:1–28.

137 Zu S X, Zhu S Y & Li J F. Human cryptosporidiosis in China. *Trans Roy Soc Trop Med Hyg* 1992; 86:639–640.

138 Molbak K, Hojlyng N, Gottschau A et al. Cryptosporidiosis in infancy and childhood mortality in Guinea Bissau, West Africa. *BMJ* 1993; 307:417–420.

139 Ungar B L P, Soave R, Fayer R & Nash T E. Enzyme immunoassay detection of IgM and IgG antibodies to Cryptosporidium in immunocompetent and immunocompromised persons. *J Infect Dis* 1986; 153:570–577.

140 Ravn P, Lungren J D, Kjaeldgaard P et al. Nosocomial outbreak of cryptosporidiosis in AIDS patients. *BMJ* 1991; 302:277–280.

141 Blanshard C, Jackson A M, Shanson D C, Francis N & Gazzard B. Cryptosporidiosis in HIV seropositive patients. *Q J Med* 1992; 85:813–823.

142 Gazzard B G & Blanshard C. Diarrhoea in AIDS and other immunodeficiency states. *Baillière's Clin Gastroenterol* 1993; 7:387–419.

143 Phillips A D, Thomas A G & Walker-Smith J A.

Cryptosporidium, chronic diarrhoea and the proximal small intestinal mucosa. *Gut* 1992; 33:1057–1061.

144 Goodgame R W, Genta R M, White A C & Chappell C L. Intensity of infection in AIDS associated cryptosporidiosis. *J Infect Dis* 1993; 167:704–709.

145 Vitovec J & Koudela B. Pathogenesis of intestinal cryptosporidiosis in conventional and gnotobiotic piglets. *Vet Parasitol* 1992; 43:25–36.

146 Buret A, Gall D G, Nation P N & Olson M E. Intestinal protozoa and epithelial cell kinetics, structure and function. *Parasitol Today* 1990; 6:375–380.

147 Tzipori S. Cryptosporidiosis in perspective. *Adv Parasitol* 1988; 27:63–129.

148 Kelly P, Thillainayagam A V, Keating J et al. Jejunal water and electrolyte transport in AIDS-related cryptosporidiosis. *Gut* 1993; 34:S69.

149 Jacyna M R, Parkin J, Goldin R & Baron J H. Protracted enteric cryptosporidial infection in selective immunoglobulin A and saccharomyces opsonin deficiencies. *Gut* 1990; 31:714–716.

150 Connolly G M, Dryden M S, Shanson D C & Gazzard B G. Cryptosporidial diarrhoea in AIDS and its treatment. *Gut* 1988; 29:593–597.

151 McGowan I, Hawkins A & Weller I. The natural history of cryptosporidial diarrhoea in HIV infected patients. *AIDS* 1993; 7:349–354.

152 Colebunders R, Francis H, Mann J M et al. Persistent diarrhea, strongly associated with HIV infection in Kinshasa, Zaire. *Am J Gastroenterol* 1987; 82:859–864.

153 Teixidor H S, Godwin T A & Ramirez E A. Cryptosporidiosis of the biliary tract in AIDS. *Radiology* 1991; 180:51–56.

154 Forbes A, Blanshard C & Gazzard B. Natural history of AIDS related sclerosing cholangitis: a study of 20 cases. *Gut* 1993; 34:116–121.

155 Weber R, Bryan R T, Bishop H S, Wahlquist S P, Sullivan J J & Juranek D D. Threshold of detection of Cryptosporidium oocysts in human stool specimens: evidence for low sensitivity of current diagnostic methods. *J Clin Microbiol* 1991; 29:1323–1327.

156 Ungar BLP. ELISA for detection of cryptosporidial antigens in faecal specimens. *J Clin Microbiol* 1990; 28:2491–2495.

157 Chapman P A, Rush B & McLauchlin J. An EIA for detecting cryptosporidia in faecal and environmental samples. *J Med Microbiol* 1990; 32:233–237.

158 Webster K. Molecular methods for detection and classification of *Cryptosporidium. Parasitol Today* 1993; 9:263–266.

159 Tsaihong J C & Ma P. Comparison of an indirect fluorescent antibody test and stool examination of diagnosis of cryptosporidiosis. *Eur J Clin Microbiol Infect Dis* 1990; 9:770–773.

160 Casemore D P, Blewett D A & Wright S E. Cleaning and disinfection of equipment for gastrointestinal flexible endoscopy: interim recommendations of a working party of the British Society of Gastroenterology. *Gut* 1990; 31:1156–1157 (letter).

161 Stürchler D. Parasitic diseases of the small intestinal tract. *Baillière's Clin Gastroenterol* 1987; 1:397–424.

162 Brandborg L L, Goldberg S B & Breidenbach W C. Human coccidiosis—a possible cause of malabsorption. *N Engl J Med* 1970; 283:1306–1313.

163 Trier J S, Moxey P C, Schimmel E M & Robles E. Chronic intestinal coccidiosis in man: intestinal pathology and response to treatment. *Gastroenterology* 1974; 66:923–935.

164 De Hovitz J A, Pape J W, Boncy M & Johnson W D. Clinical manifestations and therapy of *Isospora belli* infection in patients with AIDS. *N Engl J Med* 1986; 315:87–90.

165 Pape J W, Verdier R I & Johnson W D. Treatment and prophylaxis of *Isospora belli* infections in patients with AIDS. *N Engl J Med* 1989; 320:1044–1047.

166 Shlim D R, Cohen M T, Taton M, Rajah R, Long E G & Ungar B L. An algae-like organism associated with an outbreak of prolonged diarrhea among foreigners in Nepal. *Am J Trop Med Hyg* 1991; 45:383–389.

167 Ortega Y R, Sterling C R, Gilman R H, Cama V A & Diaz F. Cyclospora species—a new protozoan pathogen of humans. *N Engl J Med* 1993; 328:1308–1312.

168 Hoge C W, Shlim D R, Rajah R et al. Epidemiology of diarrhoeal illness associated with coccidian-like organism among travellers and foreign residents in Nepal. *Lancet* 1993; 341:1175–1179.

169 Bendall R P, Lucas S, Moody A, Tovey G & Chiodini P L. Diarrhoea associated with cyanobacterium-like bodies: a new coccidian enteritis of man. *Lancet* 1993; 341:590–592.

170 Modigliani R, Bories C, le Charpentier Y et al. Diarrhoea and malabsorption in AIDS: a study of four cases with special emphasis on opportunistic protozoan infections. *Gut* 1985; 26:179–187.

171 Canning E U & Hollister W S. *Enterocytozoon bieneusi* (Microspora): prevalence and pathogenicity in AIDS patients. *Trans Roy Soc Trop Med Hyg* 1990; 84:181–186.

172 Cali A & Owen R L. Intracellular development of *Enterocytozoon*, a unique microsporidian found in the intestine of AIDS patients. *J Protozool* 1990; 37:145–155.

173 Peacock C S, Blanshard C, Tovey D G, Ellis D S & Gazzard B G. Histological diagnosis of intestinal microsporidiosis in patients with AIDS. *J Clin Pathol* 1991; 44:558–563.

174 Orenstein J M, Tenner M & Kotler D P. Localization of infection by the microsporidian *Enterocytozoon bieneusi* in the gastrointestinal tract of AIDS patients with diarrhoea. *AIDS* 1992; 6:195–197.

175 Rabeneck L, Gyorkey F, Genta R M, Gyorkey P, Foote L W & Risser J. The role of microsporidia in the pathogenesis of HIV-related chronic diarrhea. *Ann Intern Med* 1993; 119:895–899.

176 Eeftinck-Shattenkerk J K M, Van Gool T, Van Ketel R J et al. Clinical significance of small intestinal microsporidiosis in HIV-1 infected individuals. *Lancet* 1991; 337:895–898.

177 Molina J M, Sarfati C, Beauvais B et al. Intestinal microsporidiosis in HIV infected patients with chronic unexplained diarrhea: prevalence and clinical and biologic features. *J Infect Dis* 1993; 167:217–221.

178 Field A S, Hing M C, Millikan S T & Marriott D J. Microsporidia in the small intestine of HIV-infected patients. A new diagnostic technique and a new species. *Med J Aust* 1993; 158:390–394.

179 Pol S, Romana C A, Richard S et al. Microsporidia infection in patients with HIV and unexplained cholangitis. *N Engl J Med* 1993; 328:95–99.

180 Beauvais B, Sarfati C, Molina J M, Lesourd A, Lariviere M & Derouin F. Comparative evaluation of five diagnostic methods for demonstrating microsporidia in stool and intestinal biopsy specimens. *Ann Trop Med Parasitol* 1993; 87:99–102.

181 Weber R, Bryan R T, Owen R L, Wilcox C M, Gorelkin L & Visvesara G S. Improved light microscopical detection of Microsporidia spores in stool and duodenal aspirates. *N Engl J Med* 1992; 326:161–166.

182 Van Gool T, Hollister W S, Eeftinck-Schattenkerk J K M et al. Diagnosis of microsporidiosis by recovery of spores from faeces. *Lancet* 1990; 336:697–698.

183 Blanshard C, Ellis D S, Tovey D G, Dowell S & Gazzard B. Treatment of intestinal microsporidiosis with albendazole in patients with AIDS. *AIDS* 1992; 6:311.

184 Hollister W S & Canning E U. An ELISA for detection of antibodies to *Encephalitozoon cuniculi* and its use in determination of infections in man. *Parasitology* 1987; 94:209–219.

185 Cali A, Kotter D P & Orenstein J. *Septata intestinalis* n.g., n.s.p., an intestinal microsporidian associated with chronic diarrhoea and dissemination in AIDS patients. *J Eukaryot Microbiol* 1993; 40:101–112.

CHAPTER 68

POTENTIALLY PATHOGENIC FREE-LIVING AMOEBAE

D. C. Warhurst

For many years the only amoeba thought to be of significance in human disease was the obligate parasite *Entamoeba histolytica*. It is now recognized that facultatively parasitic free-living amoebae, normally found in soil and water, cause three important diseases in man: primary amoebic meningoencephalitis (PAM), granulomatous amoebic encephalitis (GAE) with invasion of other tissues, and chronic amoebic keratitis (CAK). Both PAM and CAK occur in healthy individuals while GAE and related diseases are associated with immunodeficient states.[1]

The free-living amoebae concerned belong to three groups: amoeboflagellates, Acanthamoebidae and Leptomyxida.

AMOEBOFLAGELLATES

Naegleria fowleri which causes PAM, is found worldwide in warm fresh water, normally feeding on bacteria. Its life cycle has three stages; the feeding, growing, multiplying form or trophozoite found on surfaces of vegetation and mud; the rapidly motile biflagellate form found in the surface layers of water; and the dormant cyst form found in the same locations as the trophozoite. Experimental and epidemiological evidence supports the infectivity to man of the trophozoite and flagellate. Infection takes place through the olfactory epithelium of the nose when the organisms are inhaled in contaminated water, usually during swimming, penetrate the epithelium and pass along the olfactory nerve branches in the cribriform plate to enter the meninges where they multiply in the perivascular Virchow–Robin spaces. Trophozoites penetrate the substance of the brain, ingesting cerebral tissue. The symptoms and features of the CSF are characteristic of a purulent bacterial meningitis, but there is no response to antibacterials. Coma culminates in death. The application of specific therapy after early

diagnosis of the condition has led to recovery in only four of more than 144[2] recorded cases. Although relatively few cases of PAM are recorded, the disease is significant among those associated with recreational water use, particularly because of its almost invariably fatal outcome. In the 2-year period 1989–1990, three cases of PAM were reported among 1062 cases of illness associated with recreational water use in the USA.[3]

ACANTHAMOEBIDAE

Acanthamoeba spp. which cause GAE and CAK are found worldwide and also feed on bacteria, but they are not necessarily associated with warm water, and can also multiply in brackish conditions. The life cycle consists only of the trophozoite and cyst forms, and either of these can be a source of infection for man. Several species of the genus have been isolated from human tissue, and the ubiquitous distribution of these organisms means that human exposure is widespread. For example, it is estimated that humans inhale one of the resistant cysts every day.[4] As a corollary of this wide exposure, the organism finds it difficult to colonize man, and infections are generally restricted to the immunodeficient or to immunoprivileged sites, the most common of which is the cornea. Infections are generally of a chronic type and there is a marked granulomatous tissue reaction. Successful treatment by medical or surgical means is so far restricted to ocular infection. It is estimated that more than 200 cases of CAK have been recorded since 1974.

ACANTHAMOEBA AND UPPER RESPIRATORY INFECTION

Association of *Acanthamoeba* with upper respiratory infections was suspected in the 1960s[5] and the organism has been regularly isolated from oronasal swabs. Several strains isolated from room and outside air using a slit sampler were found to be cytopathic to mammalian cell cultures.[4] Although there is a suggestive link between the isolation of *Acanthamoeba* from the upper respiratory tract and nose bleeding, rhinitis and upper respiratory infections, the connection has not yet been convincingly drawn. It may be argued that, in some cases at least, isolations from the nose represent trapped air-borne cysts, and not active infections.

LEPTOMYXIDA

Among more than 56 case reports of GAE, mainly due to infection with *Acanthamoeba* spp., are a few cases of infection with leptomyxid free-living amoebae (now designated *Balamuthia mandrillaris*). The predisposing factors are apparently similar to those for systemic *Acanthamoeba* infection, and the life cycle of the leptomyxids also resembles that of these amoebae. Nothing is yet known about treatment, and diagnosis may prove difficult. These amoebae are not known to cause CAK.[6]

ASSOCIATION OF FREE-LIVING AMOEBAE WITH *LEGIONELLA* AND OTHER BACTERIA

Acanthamoeba spp. and *Naegleria* spp. can harbour pathogenic micro-organisms such as *Legionella*[7,8] and the cholera vibrio[9] and are thought capable of serving as chlorine-resistant infection reservoirs for these organisms in water supplies. The short incubation period, non-pneumonic form of legionellosis, 'Pontiac fever', and 'humidifier fever' are both thought to be linked to hypersensitivity reactions to free-living amoebae in air-conditioning systems.[10,11]

PRIMARY AMOEBIC MENINGOENCEPHALITIS

CLINICAL FEATURES[12]

In the first documented case of infection, *Naegleria* was found disseminated in many tissues,[13,14] but this is the only such report and the patient was severely malnourished. *N. fowleri* is normally restricted to the central nervous system.

The illness begins 3–7 days after exposure to contaminated water, in patients previously of good health, with headache and slight pyrexia, in some cases associated with sore throat and rhinitis. Over the next 3 days the disease progresses, with rising fever and increasing headache, vomiting and stiff neck. The severely disorientated or comatose patient is admitted to hospital with a diagnosis of acute pyogenic meningitis. Lumbar puncture reveals a purulent CSF but no bacteria are demonstrated. The CSF pressure is generally raised. No response is noted to antibacterials. Deep coma is followed by cardiorespiratory failure and death ensues.[15] Haemorrhagic pulmonary oedema may develop during the course of the disease and this is thought to be neurogenic.[16] In addition, myocarditis may be detected at post mortem.[17]

Although involvement with water sports antecedes most cases, some fatal infections reported from Australia have been acquired from the mains water supply. In one US case,[14,18] the patient, a narcotic addict who had recently had teeth extracted, had no history of water contact other than with public water supplies; and a Nigerian farmer is thought to have become infected after ritual nose rinsing with water from a local pond.[19]

DIAGNOSIS

The major problem in diagnosis of PAM is to distinguish between it and other encephalitides of rapid onset such as meningococcal, acute tubercular and viral meningitis. Distinction from all but non-tubercular bacterial meningitis is relatively straightforward because on CSF examination there is a markedly raised cell count, mainly polymorphonuclear cells. In tubercular or viral meningitis the cellular increase, when present, is composed mainly of mononuclear cells. The presence of erythrocytes in CSF has been suggested as characteristic of PAM, but evidence so far does not confirm its specificity and, in addition, erythrocytes may accidentally contaminate CSF during the lumbar puncture procedure. CSF protein is generally above 1 g/l and may be up to 10 g/l, and this contrasts with viral meningitis where low values are usually found. Glucose may be lower than normal, as in bacterial meningitis, but this is not a useful diagnostic feature.

It is recommended that in investigation of CSF from meningitis cases a fraction of the CSF should be put on one side while the film is being stained for bacteria, so that if bacteria are not seen the CSF can be examined in wet film in more detail. Observation of the CSF under a coverslip is a procedure which may give much information. First, in the case of bacterial meningitis, the presence of bacteria may be observed directly, before cultures have grown. If no bacteria are seen, amoebic trophozoites may be discovered. Here there is scope for error. Highly active mononuclear or other white cells may be found in the CSF, and unless careful observation is made to detect the large granular nucleus and the non-progressive movement of the mammalian cells, the cells may be mistaken for amoebae. In CSF, *Naegleria* moves actively at a rate of 1–3 body lengths per minute. The movement is progressive and the body is elongated like a slug during movement, with characteristic explosive protrusion of a clear pseudopodium on alternate sides of the anterior. Warming the wet preparation may be a useful method of stimulating movement.

As well as wet microscopy, examination of cytospin films stained by a Romanovsky stain should be carried out. An acridine orange stain with examination under the fluorescent microscope[16] may also be useful to differentiate the amoebae from leucocytes, the small nucleus and large area of reddish foamy cytoplasm of the amoebae being particularly noteworthy.[20]

To confirm the diagnosis after treatment has been instituted, cultures of the CSF sample upon 1.5% non-nutrient agar coated with washed *Escherichia coli* bacteria and maintained in a moist box at 37°C overnight should be examined. The agar may be made up in distilled water or ideally in the dilute amoeba saline solution of Page:[21]

NaCl	0.12 g
$MgSO_4.7H_2O$	0.004 g
$CaCl_2.2H_2O$	0.004 g
Na_2HPO_4	0.14 g
KH_2PO_4	0.136 g

in 1 litre distilled water, autoclaved in 100 ml aliquots and stored at room temperature.

N. fowleri will grow in cell cultures used in the usual virus isolation techniques, and these may be used as an isolation method. It is important to ensure that antifungals such as amphotericin (Fungizone) are not included in the cultures.

N. fowleri-specific monoclonal antibodies have been developed which are likely to prove valuable in diagnosis,[22] and isoenzyme,[23] restriction digestion[24]

and polymerase chain reaction (PCR) techniques for identification of *N. fowleri* from environmental and pathological material have been described.[25]

TREATMENT

There is a shortage of successful treatments on which to base recommendations. However, in all except one of four successfully treated cases, success followed the institution of a high-dose regimen of amphotericin B after early diagnosis of the infection. Three patients with 'primary amoebic meningoencephalitis' treated at Bristol, UK, in 1970,[26] of whom two survived, did not have a characteristic disease course, and in any case the infections were not proved to have been caused by *N. fowleri*;[27] therefore they will not be considered here.

It is informative to compare two case histories in female children of 9 (case 2, Table 68.1) and 11[33] years of age. A mild headache was the first indication of the disease, with no upper respiratory symptoms noted.

Treatment in the former case was successful. The patient had been swimming in a hot spring where a fatal case of PAM had been acquired in 1971.[34] Before admission the patient had a 3-day history of symptoms, initially headache, followed by nausea, vomiting and increasing lethargy. On the morning of admission she was unresponsive. A diagnosis of bacterial meningitis was made on the cell count and chemical features of the CSF. Cells with amoeboid movement were observed in the CSF and in stained preparations[35] in the County Hospital to which she was transferred, and a diagnosis of PAM was made. The treatment was begun while the patient was responsive to pain and to tactile stimulation. Although nuchal rigidity and diffuse papilloedema were present, muscle tone and deep tendon reflexes were normal. Serum electrolytes, blood urea nitrogen and glucose were within normal limits, and significantly, computerized tomography showed cerebral oedema was mild. Combination drug treatment was successful in achieving removal of detectable amoebae from the CSF and stabilization of the patient's condition after 3 days. During the remainder of her stay in hospital the patient's condition continued to improve, although after discharge some decrease in pain sensation in the left leg was noted, which resolved within 2 months, while the CSF remained abnormal for several months. Subsequent cases in the USA treated with a similar though not identical regimen have not survived.[36]

The second patient, at Bath Spa, UK, was also admitted to hospital with a 3-day history of head-

Table 68.1. Details of four successfully-treated cases of primary amoebic meningoencephalitis.

Location	Culture proof	Delay (cerebral oedema, coma, etc.)	Antiamoebic drug treatment
Case 1 S. Australia[28]	Yes	>3 days (coma, responding to painful stimuli)	Amphotericin B: $1.0\,mg/kg^{-1}\,day^{-1}$ i.v. × 5, then 0.5 mg intrathecally and a ventricular reservoir fitted to allow 10 doses of 0.1 mg on alternate days, with Stemetil premedication. The intraventricular amphotericin dose was mixed with CSF prior to administration (K. Anderson, personal communication)
Case 2 California[30]	Yes	3 days (mild: coma, responding to painful stimuli)	Amphotericin B: $1.5\,mg/kg^{-1}\,day^{-1}$ i.v. in 2 divided doses for 3 days then $1\,mg/kg^{-1}\,day^{-1}$ for 6 days. For the first 2 days 0.15 mg amphotericin was given per day intrathecally and then 0.1 mg every other day for 8 days; miconazole intravenously $350\,mg/m^2$ of body surface per day in 3 divided doses for 9 days; miconazole intrathecally, 10 mg/day and then 10 mg every other day for 8 days, and rifampicin orally at $10\,mg/kg^{-1}\,day^{-1}$ in 3 divided doses for 9 days. Dexamethasone and phenytoin were given respectively for increased intracranial pressure and for seizures
Case 3 Pennsylvania[31]	No	<13 hours (mild)	Amphotericin B: 75 mg/day i.v. (weight not given, but adult male). Oral rifampicin by nasogastric tube, 600 mg twice a day. In addition on the next day, an Ommaya reservoir was fitted to give intrathecal amphotericin B: 0.1 mg with 0.25 mg dexamethasone in 0.4 ml dextrose and water, on every other day. Therapy continued for 10 days
Case 4 Northern Thailand[32]	No, on six, occasions	1–2 days (purposefully responsive to painful stimuli. No evidence of cerebral oedema)	Amphotericin B: $0.5\,mg/kg^{-1}\,day^{-1}$ i.v. for 14 days, rising from $10–50\,mg/kg^{-1}\,day^{-1}$; oral rifampicin (600 mg/day) and oral ketoconazole (800 mg/day) for 1 month cured the patient, with no recurrence

ache and a 1-day history of pyrexia, vomiting and blurred vision. She had swum in a warm mineral water pool 6 days previously. The patient was drowsy, with slight neck stiffness. Eye movements and fundi were normal. Thus the clinical condition on admission to hospital was apparently no worse than in the first case. On the basis of purulent CSF and other characteristic features a diagnosis of pyogenic meningitis was made, and treatment with antibacterial antibiotics was instituted. The condition of the patient deteriorated during the next few hours, and convulsions began to occur which were controlled with phenytoin, diazepam and intramuscular paraldehyde. The optic fundi remained normal, but cerebral oedema was assumed to be present, and mannitol was given intravenously. Respiratory arrest occurred 20 hours after admission, and at 36 hours identification of amoebae was made in the CSF, followed by culture, and antiamoebic therapy (amphotericin B 0.5 mg/kg per day by single 6-hourly i.v. infusion, concurrently with sulphadimidine and rectal metronidazole) was begun. Amphotericin B (0.15 mg) was administered through a ventricular catheter. Although it had been planned to increase the intravenous amphotericin dose to 1 mg/kg per day, poor urinary output and rising blood urea led to only 0.6 mg/kg being achieved. On day 3, 0.05 mg amphotericin was given, and on day 4, 0.1 mg intraventricularly. Although amoebae were then absent from the CSF (and not detected by culture), the patient did not wake from her coma and died on day 5 after cardiac arrest.

A significant difference between the two cases is that the clinicians and laboratory staff in the first were aware of the possibility of PAM, having seen an earlier fatal case acquired from the same stream, and identification of amoebae in the CSF was made soon after the patient was admitted to hospital. Differences in the treatment may also have been significant, in particular the initial lower intravenous dose of amphotericin in the fatal case, but early diagnosis is clearly to be aimed at. It is, however, important to note that studies on DNA from the isolate from the Californian case indicate that the *N. fowleri* involved was an unusual variety which had a restriction pattern that diverges most from all other strains tested.[24]

Recommendations for treatment were made by Duma.[37] The administration of amphotericin B should not be delayed once diagnosis of the condition has been made. In addition, the approach that is normally made to intravenous amphotericin treatment for other conditions, that is, to start at a lower dose (0.25–0.5 mg/kg per day) and increase it cautiously to detect idiosyncrasy and delay kidney damage, is inappropriate. After a low trial dose the maximum dose possible should be given immediately, by slow intravenous infusion. Judging by the intrathecal dose of amphotericin B used in case 1, it appears that there is some scope for increase. It is recognized that children can tolerate higher doses of amphotericin B than adults (see also references 38 and 39). The Thai report, however, maintains that a gradual increase in amphotericin dose is best. An argument maintained by Ferrante[40] is that too high a dose of the drug leads to lysis of amoebae and an adverse immunological reaction to the released foreign protein. However, it may be relevant to point out that the Thai case is abnormal in several respects. No history of swimming or exposure to water could be elucidated, although as the patient was a gardener hose-pipe spray exposure might have been responsible. Also the patient was older than usual (61 years) and may have acquired some immunity. Another significant point is that six unsuccessful attempts were made to culture the amoebae. However, the prompt institution of rifamycin and ketoconazole oral therapy may be significant. Ferrante's point is probably best addressed by the judicious use of corticosteroids to moderate the inflammatory reaction, as in cases 2 and 3.

It is important to monitor the blood urea nitrogen value daily during amphotericin treatment, and the manufacturers recommend that if this rises above 17.8 mmol/l (50 mg/dl), or the creatinine above 310 μmol/l (3.5 mg/dl), one day of therapy should be omitted and the next dose lowered. Amphotericin B methyl ester, a less toxic modification of the drug, though active in vitro, has not been found effective in protecting experimental mice.[41]

THE USE OF DRUG COMBINATIONS

In in vitro and animal studies a potentiative synergism of amphotericin with tetracycline,[42,43] miconazole[44] and rifampicin[45] has been reported. The rationale for using combination drug treatment with miconazole is supported by in vitro studies carried out on the strain of *N. fowleri* isolated from the CSF in the Californian case, since synergism was seen with amphotericin. Synergism was not demonstrated between rifampicin and amphotericin, but there was clearly an additive effect, while the effects of rifampicin and miconazole were apparently mildly antagonistic. In the view of the present author there is still some doubt as to whether combination drug treatments are really necessary, but providing there is no evidence of antagonism with amphotericin B there seems no reason not to try them. It is worth noting that for *Candida albicans*, miconazole is antagonistic to amphotericin B,[46] but this was not seen for *N. fowleri*. Ketoconazole appears to be an alternative to miconazole and potentially less toxic.

PATHOLOGY AND PATHOGENESIS

N. fowleri injures nerve cells by two alternate mechanisms: trogocytosis (ingestion of the cytoplasm through a feeding cup); and contact-dependent lysis due to alteration of the permeability of the target cell by lytic proteins. Cell death is due to the release of ions, followed later by the loss of large macromolecules.[47]

The pathogenic process in the brain is probably similar to that in bacterial meningitis. An inflammatory reaction develops in the meninges and the cellular influx leads to damage of the cellular functions of the blood–brain barrier. In addition there is damage to the integrity of the barrier due to direct invasion of amoebae into the brain tissue, which occurs without obvious cellular reaction.

Although it probably has no relevance to the pathogenesis of PAM, it is interesting to note that even non-pathogenic species of *Naegleria* harbour an agent capable of causing cytopathic changes in cultured vertebrate cells. The agent is termed NACM (*Naegleria* amoeba cytopathic agent) and is a protein of 35 kDa. NACM shows the features of an infectious agent, with some similarity to a prion.[48]

IMMUNOLOGY

Reciprocal titres in the indirect fluorescent antibody test of 5 to 20 were found in a survey of normal human sera in New Zealand.[49] It will probably be concluded that for such low titres to be found in such a sensitive test indicates little exposure and probable cross-reactivity with antigens from related or unrelated species. The disease course is too rapid in the majority of clinical cases for humoral antibody to be stimulated, but it has been demonstrated in a recovered case. Although a low total serum IgA level has been postulated to be a predisposing factor in infection,[50] this has not been confirmed.[51] Evidence has been obtained experimentally in BALB/c mice that immunity can be transferred by immune spleen cells but not by immune serum.[52] However, an earlier study did show transfer by immune serum.[53] There is experimental evidence that immunity is manifested at the nasal mucosa by polymorphonuclear leucocytes, which kill the amoebae, and also by the shedding of necrotic epithelium.[54]

Although the amoebae are unaffected by recombinant human interleukin 1 or tumour necrosis factor,[55] the latter stimulates the adherence of neutrophils to *N. fowleri*, with destruction of the amoeba. This is independent of complement or specific immunoglobulin. Ingestion of neutrophils by trophozoites was observed following more prolonged incubation, particularly in the absence of tumour necrosis factor. Ability of trophozoites to ingest host neutrophils may represent a virulence factor.[56]

The trophozoites are killed by complement[57] in the bloodstream, and this probably explains the usual restriction to the CNS.

EPIDEMIOLOGY

N. fowleri has been isolated from thermally elevated aquatic environments worldwide, but temperature factors associated with occurrence of the amoeba remain relatively undefined. It is interesting that, although *N. fowleri* will grow well at temperatures up to 45°C, cysts are not readily produced at high temperatures, in contrast to the non-pathogenic species *N. lovaniensis*,[58] which also grows at 45°C. This may perhaps explain the persistence of *N. fowleri* in areas of fluctuating temperature or exposure to a temperature gradient. At Bath Spa[59] *N. fowleri* was isolated from water in an area where warm water mixed with cool, and only *N. lovaniensis* in a site where the water was uniformly at a high

temperature. In a recent study of a newly created cooling reservoir (Clinton Lake, Illinois) before and after thermal additions from a nuclear power plant, *N. fowleri* was isolated from the thermally elevated arm but not from the ambient-temperature arm of the reservoir. The probability of isolating thermophilic *Naegleria* and pathogenic *N. fowleri* increased significantly with temperature. Repetitive DNA restriction fragment profiles of the *N. fowleri* Clinton Lake isolates and a known *N. fowleri* strain of human origin were homologous.[60] This suggests that even in temperate areas we can expect *N. fowleri* colonization of any newly introduced heated freshwater habitats, such as warm pools.

PREVENTION

In the North Island of New Zealand the bathing places fed by hot springs are generally lined with earth, and the only preventive measures which are applicable are warnings not to immerse the head. These are presented to the public in graphic notices around the pools. In the UK, the contaminated pools associated with the Bath Spa mineral spring have been closed for bathing, and a borehole has been drilled into the aquifer, allowing hot water to reach the surface uncontaminated.

WATER TREATMENT

Filtration

Treatment of raw water to be used for drinking purposes by coagulation and filtration is generally effective for removal of organisms which do not multiply in the environment, such as bacterial pathogens, *E. histolytica* and *Giardia*. In the case of the potentially pathogenic free-living amoebae, even one organism which passes through the filter is significant, since unlimited multiplication is possible in the 'purified' water. Chemical or physical disinfection is therefore the only suitable approach.

Physical treatment

N. fowleri is not usually isolated from waters at temperatures below 25°C. The cysts and trophozoites are killed by temperatures above 60°C. Attractive recreational waters generally exceed 25°C and are at well below amoebicidal temperatures. The amoebae will grow at a wide range of pH in culture, although growth halts below pH 4.6 and above pH 9.5. Ultraviolet radiation appears ineffective in preventing *Naegleria* or bacterial contamination of swimming pools.[61]

Chemical treatment

It has been noted that *N. fowleri* will not grow in brackish water. Concentrations of sodium chloride of more than 0.75% will inhibit growth. It has also been shown experimentally that high concentrations of calcium (40–60 mmol/l) are inhibitory.[62]

The cysts of *N. fowleri*, like those of *E. histolytica* and *Giardia*, need a free chlorine residual concentration (mg/l) × time (minutes) factor (CT factor) in the region of 40 for 99.9% inactivation,[63] i.e. 4 mg/l for 10 minutes or 2 mg/l for 20 minutes. (Depending on the amount of organic material capable of reacting with chlorine present in the water, an initial quantity of chlorine added will produce different residual concentrations of chlorine available for microbial inactivation. In any experimental study it is therefore important to determine the residual concentration of chlorine which remains after the experiment. This level only is relevant in determination of microbial sensitivity. The pH of the water is also relevant, since the active chemical species HOCl, hypochlorous acid, decreases in concentration as pH is raised.) However, the trophozoites are killed by lower chlorine residuals in the antibacterial region of 0.5–1 mg/l. Disinfection efficiency of chlorine is inversely related to pH, and these values are valid up to pH 7.5, but not higher. It is also important to note that chlorination is less efficient at lower temperatures. If bacterial growth is prevented, and this can be confirmed in water masses by a low or nil total plate count, growth of the amoebae should not be possible. It is still possible, however, that bacteria and amoebae may be growing on and in surfaces not adequately in contact with the disinfectant. For example, in the Czechoslovakian series of infections associated with a chlorinated swimming pool, the amoebae were being harboured in unchlorinated water behind a false wall at one end of the pool.[64] In the Bath Spa episode there was a channel of communication between contaminated unchlorinated warm spring water flowing under the swimming pool and the chlorinated contents. The South Australian series of PAM cases were apparently infected from the public water supply, which was piped over desert after chlorination and thus lost its chlorine content and allowed amoebae to grow. The problem was solved by introducing supplementary chlorination points along the desert pipeline.[65] In addition, the disinfectant monochloramine has been used because it is more persistent than chlorine itself.[66] Ozonation has been tested with some success.[67]

Although the problem of eliminating *Naegleria* from swimming pools seems immense, this is a much more serious problem for natural waters than for artificial pools, where careful design and proper maintenance should be able to achieve effective control.[68]

GRANULOMATOUS AMOEBIC ENCEPHALITIS

The first hard evidence for involvement of *Acanthamoeba* in human cerebral granulomatous disease was reported in the early 1970s.[69,70] Several species of the genus have now been identified in human pathological material. The organism produces infections in various tissues in the immunocompromised or debilitated, including those with the acquired immune deficiency syndrome (AIDS).

CLINICAL FEATURES

The incubation period is generally prolonged. The signs and symptoms are typical of a variety of conditions resulting from space-occupying lesions in the brain and include hemiparesis, seizures and, in about 70%, altered mental ability (stupor or lethargy, and later disorientation, irritability and combativeness). The predisposing factors include use of corticosteroids (42%), antibiotics, chemotherapy, alcoholism, AIDS, diabetes and pregnancy.[12] Although the disease is generally found in immunocompromised states and is prolonged and chronic, acute *Acanthamoeba* meningoencephalitis has been seen associated with *Acanthamoeba* keratitis and uveitis in a child.[71]

Martinez[72] reviewed 15 cases of GAE known or assumed to be due to *Acanthamoeba*. The patients, six female and nine male, were aged 5 to 58 years, 11 were white and four black, and their illnesses lasted from 7 to 120 days. In six cases there was a history of chronic skin ulceration or other visceral or superficial lesion. The symptoms were those of a focal or diffuse encephalopathy, with meningeal irritation.

Fever, mental abnormalities, seizures, headache and hemiparesis were predominant. On admission to hospital none of these patients was in coma, in contrast to the situation often found with PAM. Cirrhosis or other liver disease was also present in 3/15 patients; pneumonitis, diabetes, Hodgkin's disease and glucose-6-phosphate dehydrogenase deficiency were also seen. Apart from antibiotic treatment, eight (53%) had been given corticosteroids. Six had been given cancer chemotherapy, three radiation therapy, three were alcoholic and two of the four females of child-bearing age were pregnant. Fifty-six cases have now been reported as due either to *Acanthamoeba* or some other free-living amoeba causing GAE.[6]

No patient in this series had any recent history of swimming or water sports.

LEPTOMYXID AMOEBAE

The involvement of this soil amoeba group in disease was not discovered until 1989, when Visvesvara was able to detect and culture an unusual amoeba[73] in the brain of a baboon showing symptoms similar to those of meningoencephalitis and GAE, and it soon became clear that several human GAE cases which had been thought to be caused by *Acanthamoeba*, but where the amoebae in sections did not stain with *Acanthamoeba*- or *Naegleria*-specific serum, were in fact of leptomyxid origin. Subsequently, an infection was seen in an AIDS case.[74]

DIAGNOSIS

The characteristics of the disease can mimic a deep mycosis with systemic dissemination. In the five cases reviewed by Jager and Stamm there was frontal headache, fluctuating coma, with or without significant history of a predisposing disease. The route of infection of the brain in the Hodgkin's lymphoma case they reviewed is thought to have been intranasal, since there were basal cortical changes in the brain, with the olfactory lobes affected. Presence of amoebae in the vessel walls gives rise to a vasculitis of an allergic type. Dead and dying organisms are found, and there is evidence of a foreign body giant cell reaction. It is noteworthy that amoebic cysts are seen in the tissues in GAE and CAK, unlike the situation in *Naegleria* PAM.

The CSF cell count was raised in all patients, lymphocytes being markedly elevated, composing 19–100% of the cells present. Glucose concentrations, where measured, were not appreciably lowered, as would be found in bacterial meningitis or PAM.

Although amoebic trophozoites have been reported in CSF in a few cases of GAE, there is no doubt that this is an extremely unusual finding.

In view of the chronic nature of the infection and the invasive character of attempts to obtain biopsy specimens, the ideal initial investigation would seem to be serological. Kenney[69] examined 1000 sera collected on a routine basis from patients in a New York hospital and found two which reacted at a high titre with *A. culbertsoni* antigen in a complement fixation test. One of the patients had suffered from gastrointestinal problems, and there was little other evidence to incriminate amoebae. (It is interesting to note that we have recently seen a case of *A. culbertsoni* infection in the small intestinal wall of a Malaysian patient.) The other died of a cerebrovascular accident, and amoebae similar to *Acanthamoeba* were demonstrated at postmortem histological examination of the brain. This case illustrates the probable usefulness of antibody tests in the diagnosis of systemic *Acanthamoeba* infections.

Cerebral biopsy is not an uncommon procedure, and specific polyclonal antibody has been used on wax-embedded sections in immunofluorescence[75] or immunoperoxidase techniques. *Acanthamoeba*-specific monoclonal antibodies which are likely to prove valuable in diagnosis have been developed.[22]

Cultures (as above for *Naegleria*) may be made from (ideally unfrozen) biopsy material and incubated at 37°C for up to a week under humid conditions. Leptomyxid amoebae apparently do not grow well under these conditions, but they, *Naegleria* and *Acanthamoeba* can be isolated in cell cultures. Attempts at culture from CSF can also be made.

The detection of restriction fragment length polymorphisms in *Acanthamoeba* mitochondrial DNA is valuable for the study of relationships between cultured isolates. This can be carried out on whole-cell DNA extracts (see below, Chronic *Acanthamoeba* Keratitis).

PCR techniques for the identification of *Acanthamoeba* isolates at the generic and specific level have been described[76] but these are not currently available for detection of the organism in clinical material.

TREATMENT

As yet there has been no successful treatment of systemic *Acanthamoeba* infection in man. There are reports of the successful use of rifampicin and of paromomycin in treatment of infections in mice.[77] Since both these agents may be used parenterally in treatment of other diseases, the time appears to be right for a trial in man.

Sulphadiazine will protect but not cure mice. It should also be remembered that the diamidine drugs are very highly active in vitro, and since some experience of the use of such agents as pentamidine and hydroxystilbamidine in pneumocystosis and leishmaniasis exists, it would seem sensible to try these out.

PATHOLOGY AND PATHOGENESIS

Acanthamoeba probably injures cells by two mechanisms: trogocytosis (ingestion of the cytoplasm

through a feeding cup); and contact-mediated lysis of cellular components due to secreted enzymes. Much of the pathology is probably related to attraction of a granulomatous cellular response. It has been shown that collagenase, for example, is effective in attracting cells into the cornea (see below, Chronic *Acanthamoeba* Keratitis).

IMMUNOLOGY

Reciprocal titres of up to 80 in the indirect fluorescent antibody test were found in a survey of normal human sera in New Zealand.[49]

CHRONIC *ACANTHAMOEBA* KERATITIS

Acanthamoeba is present in all types of environments throughout the world. Since its cysts are resistant to drying, the chance of cyst inoculation into a mucous surface is high. The cornea is an immunoprivileged site, because there is no direct contact with the blood, and it is possible for cysts or trophozoites of this organism to infect corneal stroma.

Acanthamoeba keratitis or keratouveitis presents a serious diagnostic and treatment problem to ophthalmologists. Since the first reports from the UK and the USA in the early 1970s, many further cases have been seen in Europe, the USA and other countries. The major part of the increase in developed countries is probably related to contact-lens use and is related to direct inoculation of amoebic trophozoites or cysts into the cornea during insertion of the contaminated lens.

CLINICAL FEATURES

The first ocular infections[78,79] were thought to be associated with trauma to the cornea, leading to invasion of the amoebae, and were not linked to contact-lens use. However, 85% of *Acanthamoeba* eye infections in a recent US survey were in hard or soft contact-lens wearers.[80]

Symptoms characteristically mimic those of her-

pes keratitis, although the condition is generally more painful than the viral disease.

Retrospective studies of keratitis material in London prior to 1973 failed to reveal any earlier cases.[81]

Lang and von Heimburg-Elliger[82] in 1991 reviewed 108 literature case reports: eight (7%) patients were wearing hard contact lenses; 19 (17%) remembered trauma; four (4%) had visited a hot tub; 61 (56%) needed penetrating keratoplasty, 11 (10%) rekeratoplasty; five (5%) eyes were enucleated; in 21 (19%) of the patients the diagnosis was made on histological grounds.

Acanthamoeba keratitis has occurred in both male and female patients aged from 23 to 67 years. Inflammation of the cornea (keratitis) is seen, generally with a larger or smaller epithelial defect. Accumulation of pus in the anterior chamber (hypopyon) is a common feature, together with a ring infiltrate. Following erosion of the cornea the posterior membrane (Descemet's membrane) may bulge forwards (descemetocele) and may perforate, releasing the aqueous humour. There may also be secondary infection with bacteria, graft rejection, swelling of the conjunctiva (chemosis) or accumulation of blood in the anterior chamber (hyphema). Secondary glaucoma (increased intraocular tension related to inflammation of the ciliary body) may complicate the disease.[83]

The disease runs a slow relapsing course; often a

ring abscess is persistent, epithelial breakdown is recurrent, and the hypopyon waxes and wanes.

DIAGNOSIS[84]

Clinical signs have been confused not only with those of other infective entities but also with those due to topical anaesthetic abuse.[85]

Diagnosis may be made by observation of characteristic cysts in wet mounts (10% KOH wet mount is reported to be satisfactory[86]) of corneal ulcer scrapings, and subsequent culture. Cultures made from superficial scrapings of the cornea, or from punch biopsies,[87] are valuable. Suggestive but not conclusive evidence for the infection is obtained when the amoeba is isolated from the contact lenses themselves, the cases or washing fluid. The fluorescent dye Calcofluor has been used to stain the cysts in smears.

The temperature of the eye is lower than that of the rest of the human body, therefore *Acanthamoeba* strains that grow at lower temperatures may also contribute to infection. Recent evidence indicates that perhaps only a limited number of species cause ocular disease. Delineation of the exact species of *Acanthamoeba* which cause keratitis is a prerequisite for the study of the ecology of the keratitis-producing amoebas.[88]

Restriction endonuclease digestion of *Acanthamoeba* whole-cell DNA was used to study the relationship between 33 morphologically identical strains from keratitis cases (30 strains), contact-lens storage containers (two strains), and soil (one strain). Samples digested with *Bgl*II, *Eco*RI or *Hind*III and separated by agarose gel electrophoresis contained detectable mitochondrial DNA restriction fragment length polymorphisms. By comparing these, the strains could be assigned to seven multiple-strain and three single-strain groups. The largest of these contained nine strains, eight of which were isolated in keratitis cases in various locations worldwide and may indicate a group particularly associated with keratitis.[89]

EPIDEMIOLOGY

Acanthamoeba is ubiquitous in air,[4] soil and water. In a study of the moist areas in physiotherapeutic departments of ten hospitals, 61% of the swabs taken in those areas were positive for one or several species of amoebae cultivated on NN agar according to Page. Forty-seven strains of *Acanthamoeba* and only two non-pathogenic strains of *Naegleria* were isolated. Six of the 47 strains of *Acanthamoeba* isolated revealed pathogenic characters in mice.[90]

TREATMENT

The most effective therapeutic drugs so far examined have been the diamidines—propamidine and dibromopropamidine.[91] It is important to remember that *Acanthamoeba*, unlike *Naegleria*, encysts in infected tissues. Clinical cure generally utilizes medication in combination with surgical procedures, such as keratoplasty or, sometimes, debridement.[92] Anti-inflammatory corticosteroids are thought to increase the susceptibility of the eye to *Acanthamoeba* infection, but the judicious use of them in conjunction with drug treatment has been valuable in many cases. This problem is discussed with respect to several eye infections by Stern and Buttross.[93]

The first patient treated successfully at Moorfields Eye Hospital had a 4-month history of suppurative keratitis, associated with an epithelial defect, hypopyon and secondary glaucoma. *Acanthamoeba* was isolated from the eye on three occasions. Intensive therapy with propamidine isethionate (0.1%) drops hourly by day and night, with dibromopropamidine ointment (0.15%) 4-hourly, was instituted. After 9 days, although corneal improvement was noted, signs of toxicity, including reddening of the eye and swelling of the lids, were seen. The intensive propamidine treatment was discontinued, neomycin drops were instilled 4-hourly day and night, and the 4-hourly dibromopropamidine treatment was continued. After a month the epithelium had healed and 4-hourly prednisolone drops were added, with steady improvement in the corneal inflammation. The treatment was tapered off over a further month, leaving only the neomycin drops, which were continued for 1 year, when some toxic signs developed (limbal follicles, with some increased palpebral conjunctival hyperaemia and cellularity, but no signs of skin irritation). Following cessation of all topical therapy, 4 months elapsed, with disappearance of limbal and conjunctival signs and no recurrence of the disease. Twenty-two months after initial presentation a penetrating keratoplasty (corneal graft) was carried out. The excised corneal disc showed no special changes and no morphologically identifiable *Acanthamoeba* on light and electron microscopical examination. Using the indirect fluorescent antibody technique and rabbit anti-*Acanthamoeba* serum it was possible to see small curved arcs, which probably represented fragments of cyst wall.

Propamidine isethionate drops were instilled four times a day for 2 months, in addition to the usual postoperative topical steroids and antibiotics. There was no evidence of adverse effect(s) on the graft or the remainder of the eye. The graft remained clear for a further 9 months, when a rejection episode developed which was readily controlled with topical corticosteroids. Because of persisting secondary glaucoma, the intraocular pressure needed to be controlled using timolol maleate (0.25%) drops twice daily.

The initial intensive treatment probably need not be continued for more than 1 week because intensive therapy with propamidine may give rise to corneal toxicity.[94] More recent observations confirm the effectiveness of propamidine (or dibromopropamidine) and neomycin.[95] However, a recent case was successfully treated with propamidine isethionate and 'Neosporin' (neomycin/polymyxin/gramicidin) at 30-minute intervals for 11 and 9 days,[96] whereas in seven other cases 1% miconazole topically was used successfully in triple therapy with a less intensive course of the other two agents.[97] Earlier studies at Moorfields and in my laboratory showed that the gramicidin component of 'Neosporin' was irritating and relatively non-toxic to amoebae. A recent successful regimen used neomycin, polymyxin and dibromopropamidine together with gentamicin.[98]

An early report of the efficacy of oral ketoconazole (200 mg twice a day) and topical miconazole[99] encouraged the use of these antifungals, which have shown some success. Miconazole or ketoconazole drops have been used, with or without 'Neosporin' drops.[100] In a more recent study the new antifungal itraconazole was used orally with topical 0.1% miconazole hourly during the day. The therapy was successful after 5, 8 and 9 weeks in three patients.[101]

Resistance to topical dibromopropamidine was observed in a case of bilateral keratitis. Eradication of amoebae was finally achieved following prolonged topical therapy and two corneal grafts in each eye. Paromomycin, benzethonium chloride, clotrimazole and R11/29 (a phenanthridinium compound) were continued topically for 3 months postoperatively. There were no further recurrences during a 14 month follow-up. Drug sensitivities were performed for three isolates of *Acanthamoeba* spp. (group II), which demonstrated the development of resistance to dibromopropamidine. In addition the resistant isolates were temperature-sensitive mutants which would not grow at temperatures above 30°C.[102]

A novel treatment with a polyhexamethylene biguanide biocide, first shown to be active on free-living amoebae in the early 1970s,[103] 'Baquacil' or 'ReNu', has recently shown promise in the elimination of *Acanthamoeba* from the human eye. It is active at low concentrations against the cysts,[104] unlike most other agents, and this means that it attacks one of the main sources of treatment failure because drug treatment may stimulate encystment.[105,106]

Animal models of *Acanthamoeba* keratitis have recently been developed and will be important in understanding the pathogenic mechanisms involved in the disease and in testing new drug treatments. It may be that improvements will be possible when the host response is better understood.[107]

PATHOLOGY AND PATHOGENESIS

Parasite-conditioned medium contains both collagenase and lower concentrations of other proteolytic enzymes. However, most of the collagenolytic and pathogenic activity is directly attributable to specific collagenase. Intrastromal injection of sterile, *Acanthamoeba*-conditioned culture medium into naive Lewis rats produces corneal lesions clinically similar to and closely resembling those found in biopsy specimens of human patients diagnosed with acanthamoebic keratitis. There is moderate-to-severe neutrophil infiltration, disruption of stromal lamellae and oedema. *Identical pathological sequelae have been produced by intrastromal injection of purified collagenase (25 units/ml).*[108]

In acanthamoebic keratitis the organisms apparently depend on the cellular components of the cornea as substrates for growth.[109]

Commensal bacteria on the eyelids, conjunctiva and tear film may have a role in pathogenesis.[110] This may also be the case for viruses. Many cases of human keratitis due to *Acanthamoeba* spp. have a pseudoherpetic appearance and the infection is known to have followed herpes infection in some cases. After herpetic and amoebic coinfection rabbits show severe corneal lesions, and when the viral infection is treated the amoebic coinfection progresses unchecked with severe lesions until day 37 postinfection, with numerous trophozoites and cysts.[111] This may have significant implications in human disease. However, experimental infections have also been established in the rabbit without coinfection with herpes,[112] and several rat models have now been described.[113] In the Wistar rat model the inflammatory cell profile was observed to change at intervals. In tissue sections the cellular response consisted of neutrophils on the first day but predominantly macrophages on the following days.

Some T lymphocytes but no B lymphocytes were observed.[114]

IMMUNOLOGY

Immunity against these amoebae involves a combination of complement, antibody and cell-mediated immunity. Evidence suggests that the major mechanism is activation of phagocytic cells, especially neutrophils, by lymphokines and opsonization of the amoebae by antibody which promotes an antibody-dependent cellular destruction of the organism.[115]

PREVENTION OF CONTACT-LENS-RELATED *ACANTHAMOEBA* EYE INFECTION

There can be little doubt that the reason for the increase in case numbers of *Acanthamoeba* keratitis in the developed world since the 1970s has been the introduction of contact lenses, and of soft contact lenses in particular.[116] It is becoming clear that the type of lens and the way the lenses are handled by the patient may be crucial in raising the risk of infection. Adequate means for lens cleaning, disinfection, rinsing and storage need to be available. In addition, for patients who are careless or persist in using non-sterile rinsing solutions, it has been suggested that an adequate method of disinfection will be of great help in preventing *Acanthamoeba* infection.[117]

When storage cases for contact lenses of 102 asymptomatic lens wearers were tested for contamination by bacteria and free-living amoebae, 43 had significant counts of viable bacteria. Seven had contamination by acanthamoebae.[118] In a recent study, infection of the eye by *Acanthamoeba* has been conclusively linked to the contact-lens storage container, the home-made saline solution and the kitchen cold water tap. The authors recommend that the use of home-made saline solutions and the rinsing of contact lenses in tap water be strongly discouraged.[119]

Unfortunately, many contact lens users receive poor lens care instructions or cannot be relied on to follow appropriate routines. Finding a foolproof means of lens disinfection for them is critical. Recently, several disinfection systems were tested against *A. castellanii* and *A. polyphaga* cysts and trophozoites to see which might prove most effective. Effective systems included heat disinfection at 70–80°C for 10 minutes, 3% hydrogen peroxide for 2–3 hours, 0.001% thimerosal with edetate for 4 hours, 0.005% benzalkonium chloride with edetate for 4 hours, and either 0.001% chlorhexidine for 4 hours or 0.004% chlorhexidine for 1 hour.

Problems associated with chemical disinfection (with, for example 3% hydrogen peroxide) of plastic contact lenses include lens fit alterations, which may lead to epithelial trauma. In addition antimicrobial chemicals need to be rinsed, neutralized or degraded after use, as they can injure the corneal and conjunctival epithelium.[120]

Adherence of cysts and trophozoites to the contact lens is probably important in mediation of infection. Trophozoites of *A. polyphaga* adhered in vitro to low and high water content non-ionic soft contact lenses. Adherence was greater to high water content soft lenses. Cyst attachment occurred only to the soft lenses, and was higher for the high water content lenses. Attachment of cysts to each lens tested was significantly lower than that of trophozoites. Recommended cleaning procedures using two commercial solutions (10% sodium tridecyl ether sulphate for rigid gas permeable lenses; EDTA and sorbic acid for soft contact lenses) removed all adherent trophozoites and cysts from lenses. Correctly applied lens cleaning agents may reduce the risk of infection.[121]

The use of disposable hydrogel contact lenses, which are worn continuously and then discarded, is thought to protect against lens-related infection. But if lenses are removed during the period of use, or rinsed or stored in tapwater or well water, this protective effect may be lost.[122]

Chlorhexidine may also have a role in treatment of *Acanthamoeba* keratitis.[123]

REFERENCES

1 Warhurst D C. Pathogenic free-living amoebae. *Parasitol Today* 1985; 1:24–28.
2 Ma P, Visvesvara G S, Martinez A J, Theodore F H, Daggett P M & Sawyer T K. *Naegleria* and *Acanthamoeba* infections: review. *Rev Infect Dis* 1990; 490–513.

3 Herwaldt B L, Craun G F, Stokes S L & Juranek D D. Waterborne-disease outbreaks, 1989–1990. *MMWR* 1991; 40:1–21.

4 Kingston D & Warhurst D C. Isolation of amoebae from the air. *J Med Microbiol* 1969; 2:27–36.

5 Warhurst D C. Ryan virus and the lipovirus: examples of *Acanthamoeba (Hartmannella)* contamination of cell cultures. *Parasitol Today* 1989; 5:161–162.

6 Visvesvara G S & Stehr-Green J K. Epidemiology of free-living ameba infections. *J. Protozool* 1990; 37:25S–33S.

7 Rowbotham T J. Preliminary report of the pathogenicity of *Legionella pneumophila* for freshwater and soil amoebae. *J Clin Pathol* 1980; 33:1179–1183.

8 Kilvington S & Price J. Survival of *Legionella pneumophila* within cysts of *Acanthamoeba polyphaga* following chlorine exposure. *J Appl Bacteriol* 1990; 68:519–525.

9 Thom S, Warhurst D C & Drasar B S. Association of *Vibrio cholerae* with fresh water amoebae. *J Med Microbiol* 1992; 36:303–306.

10 Rowbotham T J. Pontiac fever explained. *Lancet* 1980; ii:969.

11 Humidifier fever: report of MRC Symposium 1976. *Thorax* 1977; 32:635–663.

12 Martinez A J. Clinical manifestations of free-living amoeba infections. In: Rondanelli E G (ed.) *Amphizoic Amoebae: Human Pathology*. Padua: Piccin Press, 161–177.

13 Derrick E H. A fatal case of generalized amoebiasis due to a protozoon closely resembling if not identical to *Iodamoeba buetschlii. Trans R Soc Trop Med Hyg* 1948; 42:191–198.

14 Stamm W P. The staining of free-living amoebae by indirect immunofluorescence. *Ann Soc Belg Med Trop* 1974; 54:321–325.

15 Carter R F. Primary amoebic meningoencephalitis. An appraisal of present knowledge. *Trans R Soc Trop Med Hyg* 1972; 66:193–213.

16 Miller G, Cullity G, Walpole I, O'Connor J & Masters P. Primary amoebic meningoencephalitis in Western Australia. *Med J Aust* 1982; 1:352–357.

17 Markowitz S M, Martinez A J, Duma R J & Shiel F O M. Myocarditis associated with primary amebic meningoencephalitis. *Am J Clin Pathol* 1974; 62:619–628.

18 Patras D & Andujar J. Meningoencephalitis due to *Hartmannella (Acanthamoeba). Am J Clin Pathol* 1966; 46:226–233.

19 Lawande R V, MacFarlane J T, Weir W C & Awunor-Renner C. A case of primary amebic meningoencephalitis in a Nigerian farmer. *Am J Trop Med Hyg* 1980; 29:21–25.

20 Medley S. Acridine orange: method for diagnosis of amoebic meningitis? *Med J Aust* 1980; 2:635.

21 Page F C. Taxonomic criteria for limax amoebae, with descriptions of 3 new species of *Hartmannella* and 3 of *Vahlkampfia. J. Protozool* 1967; 14:499–521.

22 Flores B M, Garcia C A, Stamm W E & Torian B E. Differentiation of *Naegleria fowleri* from *Acanthamoeba* species by using monoclonal antibodies and flow cytometry. *J Clin Microbiol* 1990; 28:1999–2005.

23 Kilvington S, Mann P G & Warhurst D C. Differentiation between *Naegleria fowleri* and *N. lovaniensis* using isoenzyme electrophoresis of aspartate aminotransferase. *Trans R Soc Trop Med Hyg* 1984; 78:562–563.

24 De Jonckheere J F. Characterization of *Naegleria* species by restriction endonuclease digestion of whole-cell DNA. *Mol Biochem Parasitol* 1987; 24:55–66.

25 McLaughlin G L, Vodkin M H & Huizinga H W. Amplification of repetitive DNA for the specific detection of *Naegleria fowleri. J Clin Microbiol* 1991; 29:227–230.

26 Apley J, Clarke S K R, Roome A P C H et al. Primary amoebic meningoencephalitis in Britain. *BMJ* 1970; i:596–599.

27 Saygi G, Warhurst D C & Roome A P C H. A study of amoebae isolated from the Bristol case of primary amoebic encephalitis. *Proc R Soc Med* 1973; 66:277–282.

28 Anderson K. & Jamieson A. Primary amoebic meningoencephalitis. *Lancet* 1972; ii:379.

30 Seidel J S, Harmatz P, Visvesvara G S, Cohen A, Edwards J & Turner J. Successful treatment of primary amebic meningoencephalitis. *New Engl J Med* 1982; 306:346–348.

31 Brown R L. Successful treatment of primary amebic meningoencephalitis. *Arch Intern Med* 1991; 151:1201–1202.

32 Poungvarin N & Jariya P. The fifth nonlethal case of primary amoebic meningoencephalitis. *J Med Assoc Thai* 1991; 74:112–115.

33 Cain A R R, Wiley P E, Brownell B & Warhurst D C. Primary amoebic meningoencephalitis. *Arch Dis Child* 1981; 56:140–143.

34 Hecht R H, Cohen A H, Stoner J & Irwin C. Primary amebic meningoencephalitis in California. *Calif Med* 1972; 117:69–73.

35 Boyle A L, Friedman T A, Braustein H. & Tomasulo M. Rapid diagnosis of primary amoebic meningoencephalitis due to *Naegleria*: detection of organisms with bacterial stains. *J Clin Pathol* 1979; 32:306–307.

36 Stevens A R, Shulman S T, Lansen T A, Cichon M J & Willaert E. Primary amebic meningo-encephalitis: a report of two cases and antibiotic and immunologic studies. *J Infect Dis* 1981; 143:193–199.

37 Duma R J. Disease caused by free-living amoebae. *Infect Dis Newslett* 1989; 8:25–32.

38 Drutz D J. Rapid infusion of amphotericin B: is it safe, effective and wise? *Am J Med* 1992; 93:119–121.

39 Cruz J M, Peacock J E, Loomer L et al. Rapid intravenous infusion of amphotericin B: a pilot study. *Am J Med* 1992; 93:123–130.

40 Ferrante A. Free living amoebae: pathogenicity and immunity. *Parasite Immunol* 1991; 13:31–47.

41 Ferrante A. Comparative sensitivity of *Naegleria fowleri* to amphotericin B and amphotericin B methyl ester. *Trans R Soc Trop Med Hyg* 1982; 76:476–478.

42 Thong Y H, Rowan-Kelly B, Ferrante A & Shepherd C. Synergism between tetracycline and amphotericin B in experimental amoebic meningoencephalitis. *Med J Aust* 1978; 1:663–664.

43 Thong Y H. Delayed treatment of primary amoebic meningoencephalitis with amphotericin B and tetracycline. *Trans R Soc Trop Med Hyg* 1979; 73:806–808.

44 Thong Y H. Chemotherapy for primary amebic meningoencephalitis. *N Engl J Med* 1982; 306:1295–1296.

45 Thong Y H, Rowan-Kelly B & Ferrante A. Treatment of experimental *Naegleria* meningoencephalitis with a combination of amphotericin B and rifamycin. *Scand J Infect Dis* 1979; 11:151–153.

46 Schachter L P, Owellen R J, Rathbun H K & Buchanan B. Antagonism between miconazole and amphotericin-B. *Lancet* 1976; ii:318.

47 Marciano-Cabral R, Zoghby K L & Bradley S G. Cytopathic action of *Naegleria fowleri* amoebae on rat neuroblastoma target cells. *J Protozool* 1990; 37:138–144.

48 Dunnebacke T H & Dixon J S. NACM, a cytopathogenic protein from *Naegleria gruberi*, EGs; purification, production of monoclonal antibody, and the immunoidentification of a product that develops in NACM-treated vertebrate cell cultures. *J Protozool* 1990; 37:11S–16S.

49 Cursons R T M, Brown T J, Keys E A, Moriarty K M & Till D. Immunity to pathogenic free living amoebae: role of humoral antibody. *Infect Immun* 1980; 29:401–407.

50 Cursons R M, Keys E A, Brown T M, Learmonth J, Campbell C & Metcalf P. IgA and primary amoebic meningoencephalitis. *Lancet* 1979; i:223–224.

51 Cain A R R, Mann P G & Warhurst D C. IgA and primary amoebic meningoencephalitis. *Lancet* 1979; i:441.

52 Ahn M H & Min D Y. [Resistance to *Naegleria fowleri* infection passively acquired from immunized splenocyte, serum or milk.] *Kisaengchunghak Chapchi* 1989; 27:79–86.

53 Thong Y H, Ferrante A, Shepherd C & Rowan-Kelly B. Resistance of mice to *Naegleria* meningoencephalitis transferred by immune serum. *Trans R Soc Trop Med Hyg* 1978; 72:650–652.

54 Thong Y H, Carter R F, Ferrante A & Rowan-Kelly B. Site of expression of immunity to *Naegleria fowleri* in immunized mice. *Parasite Immunol* 1983; 5:67–76.

55 Fischer-Stenger K, Cabral G A & Marciano-Cabral F. The interaction of *Naegleria fowleri* amoebae with murine macrophage cell lines. *J Protozool* 1990; 37:168–173.

56 Michelson M K, Henderson W R Jr, Chi E Y, Fritsche T R & Klebanoff S J. Ultrastructural studies on the effect of tumor necrosis factor on the interaction of neutrophils and *Naegleria fowleri*. *Am J Trop Med Hyg* 1990; 42:225–233.

57 Rowan-Kelly B, Ferrante A & Thong Y H. Activation of complement by *Naegleria*. *Trans R Soc Trop Med Hyg* 1980; 74:333–336.

58 Aufy S, Kilvington S, Mann P G & Warhurst D C. Improved selective isolation of *Naegleria fowleri* from the environment. *Trans R Soc Trop Med Hyg* 1986; 80:350–351.

59 Kilvington S, Mann P G & Warhurst D C. *Pathogenic Naegleria Amoebae in the Waters of Bath: A Fatality and its Consequences*. Bath: Bath City Council, 1991, 89–96.

60 Huizinga H W & McLaughlin G L. Thermal ecology of *Naegleria fowleri* from a power plant cooling reservoir. *Appl Environ Microbiol* 1990; 56:2200–2205.

61 De Jonckheere J F. Hospital hydrotherapy pools treated with ultraviolet light: bad bacterial quality and presence of thermophilic Naegleria. *J Hyg (Camb)* 1982; 88:205–214.

62 Brown T M & Cursons R T M. Prophylaxis. In E G Rondanelli (ed.) *Amphizoic Amoebae: Human Pathology*, Chapter 10. Padua: Piccin Press, 1987: 217–236.

63 Chang S L. Resistance of pathogenic *Naegleria* to some common physical and chemical agents. *Appl Environ Microbiol* 1978; 35:368–375.

64 Kadlec V, Cerva L & Skvarova J. Virulent *Naegleria fowleri* in an indoor swimming pool. *Science* 1978; 201:1025.

65 Dorsch M M, Cameron A S & Robinson B S. The epidemiology and control of primary amoebic meningoencephalitis with particular reference to South Australia. *Trans R Soc Trop Med Hyg* 1983; 77:372–377.

66 Esterman A, Roder D M, Cameron A S, Robinson B S, Walters R P, Lake J A & Christy P E. Determinants of the microbiological quality of South Australian Swimming Pools. *Appl Env Microbiol* 1984; 47: 325–328.

67 Cursons R T M, Brown T J & Keys E A. Effect of disinfectants on pathogenic free-living amoebae: in axenic conditions. *Appl Environ Microbiol* 1980; 40:401–407.

68 Lyons T B & Kapur R. Limax amoebae in public swimming pools of Albany, Schenechtady and Rensselaen counties, New York: their concentration, correlations and significance. *Appl Environ Microbiol* 1977; 33:551–555.

69 Kenney M. The Micro-Kolmer complement fixation test in routine screening for soil ameba infection. *Health Lab Sci* 1971; 8:5–10.

70 Jager B V & Stamm W P. Brain abscesses caused by free living amoeba probably of the genus

Hartmannella in a patient with Hodgkin's disease. *Lancet* 1972; ii:1343–1345.

71 Jones D B, Visvesvara G S & Robinson N M. *Acanthamoeba polyphaga* keratitis and Acanthamoeba uveitis associated with fatal meningoencephalitis. *Trans Ophthalmol Soc UK* 1975; 95:221–232.

72 Martinez A J. Is Acanthamoeba encephalitis an opportunistic infection? *Neurology* 1980; 30:567–574.

73 Visvesvara G S, Martinez A J, Schuster F L et al. Leptomyxid ameba, a new agent of amebic meningoencephalitis in humans and animals. *J Clin Microbiol* 1990; 28:2750–2756.

74 Anzil A P, Rao C, Wrzolek M A, Visvesvara G S, Sher J H & Kozlowski P B. Amebic meningoencephalitis in a patient with AIDS caused by a newly recognized opportunistic pathogen, leptomyxid ameba. *Arch Pathol Lab Med* 1991; 115:21–22.

75 Warhurst D C. *Naegleria* and *Acanthamoeba* in tissue sections. In J M B Edwards, C E D Taylor & A H Tomlinson (eds) *Immunofluorescence techniques in Diagnostic Microbiology*. London: HMSO, 1982: 46–48.

76 Vodkin M , Howe D K, Visvesvara G S & McLaughlin G L. Identification of *Acanthamoeba* at the generic and specific levels using the polymerase chain reaction. *J Protozool* 1992; 39:378–385.

77 Mazur T, Kasprzak W & Zagarska-Nowak G. Sensitivity of limax amoebae to some antiparasitic drugs II Activity in vivo. *Wiadomosci Parazitologiczne* 1983; 29: 271–272.

78 Nagington J, Watson P G, Playfair T J, McGill J, Jones B R & Steele A D McG. Amoebic infection of the eye. *Lancet* 1974; ii:1537–1540.

79 Visvesvara G S, Jones D B & Robinson N M. Isolation, identification, and biological characterization of *Acanthamoeba polyphaga* from a human eye. *Am J Trop Med Hyg* 1975; 24:784–790.

80 Stehr-Green J K, Bailey T M & Visvesvara G S. The epidemiology of *Acanthamoeba* keratitis in the United States. *Am J Ophthalmol* 1989; 107:331–336.

81 Ashton N & Stamm W P. Amoebic infection of the eye: a pathological report. *Trans Ophthalmol Soc UK* 1975; 95:214–220.

82 Lang G E & von Heimburg-Elliger A. [Acanthamoeba keratitis in hard contact lens wearers. Case report and review of the literature of 108 cases.] *Klin Monatsbl Augenheilkd* 1991; 198:290–294.

83 Hirst L W, Green W R, Merz W et al. Management of *Acanthamoeba* keratitis: a case report and review of the literature. *Ophthalmology* 1984; 91:1105–1111.

84 Visvesvara G S. Acanthamoebiasis and Naegleriosis. In Balows A, Hausler W J, Ohashi M & Turano A (eds) *Laboratory Diagnosis of Infectious Disease*. New York: Springer, 1988: 723–730.

85 Rosenwasser G O, Holland S, Pflugfelder S C et al. Topical anesthetic abuse. *Ophthalmology* 1990; 97:967–972.

86 Sharma S, Srinivasan M & George C. Diagnosis of acanthamoeba keratitis—a report of four cases and review of literature. *Indian J Ophthalmol* 1990; 38:50–56.

87 Lee P & Green W R. Corneal biopsy. Indications, techniques, and a report of a series of 87 cases. *Ophthalmology* 1990; 97:718–721.

88 De-Jonckheere J F. Ecology of *Acanthamoeba*. *Rev Infect Dis* 1991; 13 (supplement):S385–S387.

89 Kilvington S, Beeching J R & White D G. Differentiation of *Acanthamoeba* strains from infected corneas and the environment by using restriction endonuclease digestion of whole-cell DNA. *J Clin Microbiol* 1991; 29:310–314.

90 Michel R & Menn T. [*Acanthamoeba, Naegleria* and invertebrates in wet areas of physiotherapy equipment in hospitals.] *Zentralbl Hyg Umweltmed* 1991; 191:423–437.

91 Wright P, Warhurst D C & Jones B R. *Acanthamoeba* keratitis successfully treated medically. *Brit J Ophthalmol* 1985; 69:778–782.

92 Osato M S, Robinson N M, Wilhelmus K R & Jones D B. In vitro evaluation of antimicrobial compounds for cysticidal activity against *Acanthamoeba*. *Rev Infect Dis* 1991; 13 (supplement):S431–S435.

93 Stern G A & Buttross M. Use of corticosteroids in combination with antimicrobial drugs in the treatment of infectious corneal disease. *Ophthalmology* 1991; 98:847–853.

94 Johns K J, Head W S & O'Day D M. Corneal toxicity of propamidine. *Arch Ophthalmol* 1988; 106:68–69.

95 Maudgal P C. Acanthamoeba keratitis: report of three cases. *Bull Soc Belg Ophthalmol* 1989; 231:135–148.

96 John T, Lin J & Sahm D F. Acanthamoeba keratitis successfully treated with prolonged propamidine isethionate and neomycin–polymyxin–gramicidin. *Ann Ophthalmol* 1990; 22:20–23.

97 Berger S T, Mondino B J, Hoft R H et al. Successful medical management of *Acanthamoeba* keratitis. *Am J Ophthalmol* 1990; 110:395–403.

98 Beattie A M, Slomovic A R, Rootman D S & Hunter W S. Acanthamoeba keratitis with two species of *Acanthamoeba*. *Can J Ophthalmol* 1990; 25:260–262.

99 Hirst L W, Green W R, Merz W et al. Management of *Acanthamoeba* keratitis: a case report and review of the literature. *Ophthalmology* 1984; 91:1105–1111.

100 Sharma S, Srinivasan M & George C. Acanthamoeba keratitis in non-contact lens wearers. *Arch Ophthalmol* 1990; 108:676–678.

101 Ishibashi Y, Matsumoto Y, Kabata T et al. Oral

itraconazole and topical miconazole with debridement for *Acanthamoeba* keratitis. *Am J Ophthalmol* 1990; 109:121–126.

102 Ficker L, Seal D, Warhurst D & Wright P. Acanthamoeba keratitis—resistance to medical therapy. *Eye* 1990; 4:835–838.

103 Warhurst D C & Singer M. Inhibition of growth of Naegleria by a swimming pool additive. *Trans R Soc Trop Med Hyg* 1975; 69:7.

104 Kilvington S. Activity of water biocide chemicals and contact lens disinfectants on pathogenic free-living amoebae. *Int Biodeterioration* 1990; 26:127–138.

105 Kim B G, McCann P P & Byers T J. Inhibition of multiplication of *Acanthamoeba castellanii* by specific inhibitors of ornithine decarboxylase. *J Protozool* 1987; 34:264–266.

106 Byers T J, Kim B G, King L E & Hugo E R. Molecular aspects of the cell cycle and encystment in Acanthamoeba. *Rev Inf Dis* 1991; 13:S378–S384.

107 Badenoch P R. The pathogenesis of *Acanthamoeba* keratitis. *Aust N Z J Ophthalmol* 1991; 19:9–20.

108 He Y G, Niederkorn J Y, McCulley J P et al. In vivo and in vitro collagenolytic activity of *Acanthamoeba castellanii*. *Invest Ophthalmol Vis Sci* 1990; 31:2235–2240.

109 Stopak S S, Roat M I, Nauheim R C et al. Growth of acanthamoeba on human corneal epithelial cells and keratocytes in vitro. *Invest Ophthalmol Vis Sci* 1991; 32:354–359.

110 Larkin D F & Easty D L. External eye flora as a nutrient source for *Acanthamoeba*. *Graefes Arch Clin Exp Ophthalmol* 1990; 228:458–460.

111 Paniagua-Crespo E, Tsouria-Belaid A, Bellon C, Jacquemin J L & Simitzis-Le-Flohic A M. [Amoebic keratitis caused by *Acanthamoeba* sp. May HSV1 infection play a role?] *J Fr Ophthalmol* 1991; 14:25–31.

112 Cote M A, Irvine J A, Rao N A & Trousdale M D. Evaluation of the rabbit as a model of *Acanthamoeba* keratitis. *Rev Infect Dis* 1991; 13 (supplement):S443–S444.

113 Larkin D F & Easty D L. Experimental *Acanthamoeba* keratitis: I. Preliminary findings. *Br J Ophthalmol* 1990; 74:551–555.

114 Larkin D F & Easty D L. Experimental *Acanthamoeba* keratitis: II. Immunohistochemical evaluation. *Br J Ophthalmol* 1991; 75:421–424.

115 Ferrante A. Free living amoebae: pathogenicity and immunity. *Parasite Immunol* 1991; 13:31–47.

116 Meisler D M & Rutherford I. Acanthamoeba and disinfection of soft contact lenses. *Rev Infect Dis* 1991; 13 (supplement):S410–S412.

117 Moore M B. Acanthamoeba keratitis and contact lens wear: the patient is at fault. *Cornea* 1990; 9 (supplement):S33–S35.

118 Larkin D F, Kilvington S & Easty D L. Contamination of contact lens storage cases by *Acanthamoeba* and bacteria. *Br J Ophthalmol* 1990; 74:133–135.

119 Kilvington S, Larkin D F, White D G & Beeching J R. Laboratory investigation of *Acanthamoeba* keratitis. *J Clin Microbiol* 1990; 28:2722–2725.

120 Chandler J W. Biocompatibility of hydrogen peroxide in soft contact lens disinfection: antimicrobial activity vs. biocompatibility—the balance. *CLAO J* 1990; 16 (supplement):S43–S45.

121 Kilvington S & Larkin D F. Acanthamoeba adherence to contact lenses and removal by cleaning agents. *Eye* 1990; 4:589–593.

122 Heidemann D G, Verdier D D, Dunn S P & Stamler J F. *Acanthamoeba* keratitis associated with disposable contact lenses. *Am J Ophthalmol* 1990; 110:630–634.

123 Hay J, Kirkness C M, Seal D V and Wright P. Drug resistance and Acanthamoeba keratitis: the quest for alternative antiprotozoal chemotherapy. *Eye* 1994; 8:555–563.

CHAPTER 69

TRICHOMONAL INFECTION

G. C. Cook

Trichomonas vaginalis is a pathogenic protozoan with a very high degree of site specificity[1]—the lower female genitourinary tract. Infection may or may not be symptomatic; it is sexually transmitted. In women $<10^4$, and in men 4×10^6 organisms can produce an infection. Related organisms are: *T. tenax* and *Pentatrichomonas hominis*—they colonize the gums and colon, respectively—however, neither is of proven pathogenicity.

First visualized by Donné in 1836, *T. vaginalis* was first shown, using inoculation studies, to be patho-genic in the early twentieth century.[1] It is an ovoid organism, $10–20\,\mu m$ wide; 'twitching' motility is brought about by four anterior flagella and a recurrent flagellum (embedded in an undulating membrane, which runs along two-thirds of the cell). It is actively phagocytic; optimal growth occurs under moderately anaerobic conditions. Reproduction is by binary fission; unlike many pathogenic protozoa, cysts are *not* formed. When subjected to either in vitro or in vivo study, a strain variation in virulence becomes apparent.

DISTRIBUTION AND EPIDEMIOLOGY

Infection occurs worldwide, in both urban and rural settings. In the 1970's, the World Health Organization estimated an annual world incidence of 180 million cases; however, this infection is not notifiable, and any data on prevalence are therefore highly unreliable. In sexually transmitted disease (STD) clinics, overall figures varying from 7 to 32% have been recorded.[1] In some prostitutes figures of up to 80% have been noted. Highest prevalence figures are in groups with a high level of sexual activity. In tropical populations recorded prevalence has varied from 3.1% in Manila university students to 15–20% in clinic populations studied in Asia and Africa.[1] Three studies from Nigeria give an insight into the prevalence of infection in West Africa.[2–4] Infection was detected in 505 (24.7%) out of 2048 urine specimens submitted by students at a 'higher institution'; 374 (74%) occurred in women and 131 (26%) in men.[2] At Jos, infection rates of 37.6% and 24.8% were recorded in groups of urban and rural women;[3] 250 were examined in each group. Specimens from 2224 adult women examined at the cytology clinic, University College Hospital, Ibadan, revealed an infection rate of 9.8%. At Dar-Es-Salaam, Tanzania, an investigation of 359 gynaecological inpatients revealed that those infected with *T. vaginalis* had an almost threefold higher risk of being infected with the human immunodeficiency virus (HIV).[5] In men, in whom the disease is usually asymptomatic and self-limiting (see below), meaningful prevalence figures are virtually non-existent. The organism is frequently coexistent with another infection, e.g. candidiasis, gonorrhoea, syphilis or HIV infection;[5] it is therefore important to screen an infected woman for another STD(s), which not infrequently has a greater medical significance. Although non-venereal transmission of *T. vaginalis* is rare, the organism can survive for several hours in a moist environment. Perinatal infection in about 5% of female babies born (vaginally) to infected mothers is recorded.

PATHOGENESIS AND PATHOLOGY

The organism involves squamous (not columnar) epithelium; only rarely can it be isolated from the endocervix, but the urethra is involved in 90% of infected cases.[1] It has been demonstrated in the epididymis and prostate rarely, and occasionally causes non-gonococcal (tetracycline-resistant) urethritis (NGU). *T. vaginalis* is associated with large numbers of polymorphonuclear neutrophils (PMNs) (which together with macrophages are able to kill the organism) and consequent vaginal discharge. The organism is not invasive, existing either free in the vaginal cavity or adherent to epithelium; in about 50% of cases microscopic haemorrhage can be visualized using an appropriate technique. Local IgA is usually detectable (see below); however, serum antibody concentration remains low, and is of no use diagnostically (see below).

CLINICAL ASPECTS

The classical presentation consists of vulvo-vaginitis.[6–9] In experimentally-induced infection the incubation period ranges from 3 to 28 days. Although 50–90% of infected women are sympto-matic, it is frequently difficult to attribute symptoms directly to *T. vaginalis* because another organism(s) is coexistent. In 50–75% of those infected a vaginal discharge (often frothy and greenish-yellow,[3] and sometimes odorous) is present; 25–50% of women suffer from vulval irritation,[2,3] and 50% experience dyspareunia; mild dysuria is sometimes present. Lower abdominal discomfort is described by 10% of infected women; it may be accompanied by salpingi-tis, but this may have a different aetiology, possibly another STD. A yellowish vaginal discharge is pres-ent in 50–75% of those infected, but vulval erythema is present in less than one-third.

In men, although NGU may be present,[10–13] the majority of cases are asymptomatic.[2] When sympto-matic, infection may resemble NGU of another aetiology;[12,13] it is recognized because there is fail-ure of response to standard chemotherapeutic regi-mens. *T. vaginalis* can be detected in 70% of men who have experienced sexual intercourse with an infected woman within the previous 48 hours. It is one of several STDs to affect male homosexuals.[14] Involvement of the epididymis and prostate are rare events.

While a small percentage of female infants born to infected mothers may be infected (see above), *T. vaginalis* infection in older children may indicate sexual abuse.

In the long term *T. vaginalis* infection is benign. There is no good evidence that it directly predis-poses to cervical carcinoma; an associated organ-ism(s), e.g. a papillomavirus,[8] may, however, be implicated.

DIAGNOSIS

A definitive diagnosis depends on demonstration of the parasite in a specimen from a symptomatic woman (see above)—who in many cases has had sexual intercourse with a 'new' partner. (Recent use of an antibiotic(s) suggests the possibility of a *Candida* spp. infection.) Presence of another STD should be sought by careful examination of the vulva using a speculum; further examination after tricho-moniasis has been treated may also reveal an associ-ated (coexistent) infection. Vaginal inflammation is present with both *T. vaginalis* and *Candida* spp. infection, but not in bacterial vaginosis.[6,8,15,16] The cervix should be examined for evidence of cervicitis and a purulent or mucopurulent discharge.

T. vaginalis can be demonstrated using a vaginal swab. The specimen can either be transferred directly to a microscope slide, or the swab agitated in a tube containing about 1 ml saline.[17] The organism can be cultured using a variety of media.

Normal vaginal pH is ≤4.5; this is maintained in most women suffering from vulvovaginal candidia-sis. However, more than 75% of women with a *T. vaginalis* infection,[2,3] and also bacterial vagino-sis,[1,15] have a pH >4.5. Cervical discharge has an elevated pH, therefore that in vaginal material may be artificially elevated; recent coitus also significantly elevates pH (semen is significantly more alkaline than vaginal secretion). Following determination of pH, several drops of 10–20% potassium hydroxide can be added to the discharge obtained in the speculum; a pungent, fishy, amine-like odour will be produced in 75% of women with a *T. vaginalis* infection, and most with bacterial vaginosis;[15] this test is, however, negative in vulvovaginal candidiasis.

For a definitive diagnosis microscopic examination of vaginal discharge is mandatory; a drop of wet-mount preparation should be examined under a coverslip.[17,18] In a *T. vaginalis* infection the flora consists of rods or coccobacilli, while epithelial cells are clean and PMNs plentiful; motile (decreasing in older, cooled preparations) *T. vaginalis* can be visualized in 40–80% of those infected. Gram-staining is virtually useless for recognition of *T. vaginalis*; Giemsa is 50% sensitive, and an acridine orange technique about 60% sensitive. Use of a routine Papanicolaou technique[18] on a cervical specimen detects *T. vaginalis* in 60–70% of cases. Newer fluorescent antibody techniques[17] possess a sensitivity of 80–90%, when compared with culture. In bacterial vaginosis the normal flora consisting of rods is replaced by coccobacilli (which encrust the epithelial cells); few PMNs are present.

In men, diagnosis is usually difficult;[19] occasionally a wet-mount preparation of urethral discharge reveals motile organisms. The most effective method of diagnosis is by culture (see below) of a urethral specimen or urine sediment following prostatic massage.[11]

Culture techniques (which have a sensitivity >95%) are not widely used, but these increase the detection rate.[20,21] *T. vaginalis* grows best on a suitable medium in an anaerobic environment at 37°C; selective growth can be achieved by addition of an appropriate antibiotic(s). Recently, an enzyme linked immunosorbent assay has been compared with wet-mount and culture techniques for detecting *T. vaginalis*;[21–24] culture proved to be the most sensitive. Other recently developed techniques include: employment of monoclonal antibodies;[17] a molecular probe for identification of *T. vaginalis* DNA;[22] a polymerase chain reaction;[23] and detection of anti-*T. vaginalis* antibodies in cervical secretions and serum samples.[24,25]

Local IgA is detectable in most infected women (see above)[21,24,25] but this does not give rise to significant elevation of serum concentration.

TREATMENT

T. vaginalis is usually highly sensitive (minimal inhibitory concentration $\leq 1\,\mu g/ml$) to the 5-nitroimidazole compounds,[26] but not to most other antimicrobial agents. Recently, however, relative resistance in some strains of these compounds has been demonstrated.[9,17]

In women, the agent most usually prescribed is metronidazole,[6,9,14,15,27–29] with a recommended dose regimen of 2.0 g as a single dose; this cures 85%, and when the sexual partner is treated simultaneously this rises to 95%. Another regimen utilizes a single-day split dose of 1.6 g. A regimen of 250 mg three times a day for 7 days seems to give a comparable result. In men, the 7-day course is of proven efficacy, and the single-dose regimen has not been adequately assessed. Metronidazole possesses significant side-effects (see Chapter 67), including the subsequent development of a *Candida* spp. infection. Although there is no evidence of teratogenicity in *Homo sapiens*, metronidazole should generally be avoided during the first trimester of pregnancy.[17] A 100% cure rate has been recorded using nimorazole (4 g in two equally divided doses 24 hours apart).[26] Experience with tinidazole is limited[17,26,30,31] but results using a single-dose regimen are encouraging; it has the advantage of being significantly less expensive, and possesses minimal side-effects. Clotrimazole 100 mg intravaginally at night usually relieves symptoms; a 7-day course only cures about 20%. Clindamycin is another alternative.[15] Mebendazole, furazolidone and anisomycin may all be effective in 5-nitroimidazole-resistant *T. vaginalis*;[32] however, 'prospective, randomized, double-blind, active-control comparative studies' are required.[33]

Use of condoms is very effective in prevention of infection.[2] A spermatocide, nonoxynol 9—present in many vaginal preparations—possesses significant trichomonacidal properties.[32]

REFERENCES

1 Rein M F. Trichomoniasis. In Strickland G T (ed.) *Hunter's Tropical Medicine*, 7th edn. Philadelphia: W B Saunders, 1991: 582–586.

2 Anosike J C, Onwuliri C D, Inyang R E et al. Trichomoniasis amongst students of a higher institution in Nigeria. *Appl Parasitol* 1993; 34:19–25.

3 Ogbonna C I, Ogbonna I B, Ogbonna A A & Anosike J C. Studies on the incidence of *Trichonomas vaginalis* amongst pregnant women in Jos area of Plateau State, Nigeria. *Angew Parasitol* 1991; 32:198–204.

4 Konje J C, Otolorin E D, Ogunniyi J D, Obisesan K A & Ladipo G A. The prevalence of *Sardnerella vaginalis*, *Trichomonas vaginalis* and *Candida albicans* in the cytology clinic at Ibadan, Nigeria. *Afr J Med Sci* 1991; 20:29–34.

5 Meulen J ter, Mgava H N, Chang-Claude J et al. Risk factors for HIV infection in gynaecological inpatients in Dar es Salaam, Tanzania, 1988–1990. *East Afr Med J* 1992; 69:688–692.

6 Kent H L. Epidemiology of vaginitis. *Am J Obstet Gynecol* 1991; 165:1168–1176.

7 Sobel J D. Vulvovaginitis. *Dermatol Clin* 1992; 10:339–359.

8 Hatch K D. Vulvar and vaginal disorders. *Curr Opin Obstet Gynecol* 1992; 4:904–906.

9 Heine P & McGregor J A. *Trichomonas vaginalis*: a reemerging pathogen. *Clin Obstet Gynecol* 1993; 36:137–144.

10 Fowler J E Jr. Urethritis in men. *Semin Urol* 1991; 9:15–27.

11 Saxena S B & Jenkins R R. Prevalence of *Trichomonas vaginalis* in men at high risk for sexually transmitted diseases. *Sex Transm Dis* 1991; 18:138–142.

12 Krieger J N, Jenny C, Verdon M et al. Clinical manifestations of trichomoniasis in men. *Ann Intern Med* 1993; 118:844–849.

13 Krieger J N, Verdon M, Siegel N & Holmes K K. Natural history of urogenital trichomoniasis in men. *J Urol* 1993; 149:1455–1458.

14 Levine G I. Sexually transmitted parasitic diseases. *Prim Care* 1991; 18:101–128.

15 Majeroni B A. New concepts in bacterial vaginosis. *Am Fam Physician* 1991; 44:1215–1218.

16 Hart G. Factors associated with trichomoniasis, candidiasis and bacterial vaginosis. *Int J STD AIDS* 1993; 4:21–25.

17 Lossick J G & Kent H L. Trichomoniasis: trends in diagnosis and management. *Am J Obstet Gynecol* 1991; 165:1217–1222.

18 Weinberger M W & Harger J H. Accuracy of the Papanicolaou smear in the diagnosis of asymptomatic infection with *Trichomonas vaginalis*. *Obstet Gynecol* 1993; 82:425–429.

19 Krieger J N, Verdon M, Siegel N, Critchlow C & Holmes K K. Risk assessment and laboratory diagnosis of trichomoniasis in men. *J Infect Dis* 1992; 166:1362–1366.

20 Boeke A J, Dekker J H & Peerbooms P G. A comparison of yield from cervix versus vagina for culturing *Candida albicans* and *Trichomonas vaginalis*. *Genitourin Med* 1993; 69:41–43.

21 Sharma P, Malla N, Gupta I, Ganguly N K & Mahajan R C. A comparison of wet mount, culture and enzyme linked immunosorbent assay for the diagnosis of trichomoniasis in women. *Trop Geogr Med* 1991; 43:257–260.

22 Rubino S, Muresu R, Rappelli P et al. Molecular probe for identification of *Trichomonas vaginalis* DNA. *J Clin Microbiol* 1991; 29:702–706.

23 Riley D E, Roberts M C, Takayama T & Krieger J N. Development of polymerase chain reaction-based diagnosis of *Trichomonas vaginalis*. *J Clin Microbiol* 1992; 30:465–472.

24 Romia S A & Othman T A. Detection of antitrichomonal antibodies in sera and cervical secretions in trichomoniasis. *J Egypt Soc Parasitol* 1991; 21:373–381.

25 Bhatt R, Pandit D & Deadhar L. Detection of serum antitrichomonal antibodies in urogenital trichomoniasis by immunofluorescence. *J Postgrad Med* 1992; 38:72–74.

26 Chunge C N, Kangethe S, Pamba H D & Dwate J. Treatment of symptomatic trichomoniasis among adult women using oral nitroimidazoles. *East Afr Med J* 1992; 69:398–401.

27 Hager W D & Rapp R P. Metronidazole. *Obstet Gynecol Clin North Am* 1992; 19:497–510.

28 Drug-resistant *Trichomonas vaginalis*. *Commun Dis Rep CDR Weekly* 1993; 3:141.

29 Ikeh E I, Bello C S & Ajayi J A. In vitro susceptibility of *Trichomonas vaginalis* strains to metronidazole—a Nigerian experience. *Genitourin Med* 1993; 69:241–242.

30 Hamed K A & Studemeister A E. Successful response of metronidazole-resistant trichomonal vaginitis to tinidazole. A case report. *Sex Transm Dis* 1992; 19:339–340.

31 D-Prasertsawat P & Jetsawangsri T. Split-dose metronidazole or single-dose tinidazole for the treatment of vaginal trichomoniasis. *Sex Transm Dis* 1992; 19:295–297.

32 Livengod C H & Lossick J G. Resolution of resistant vaginal trichomoniasis associated with the use of intravaginal nonoxynol-9. *Obstet Gynecol* 1991; 78:954–956.

33 McCutchan J A, Ronald A R, Corey L & Handsfield H H. Evaluation of new anti-infective drugs for the treatment of vaginal infections. Infectious Diseases Society of American and the Food and Drug Administration. *Clin Infect Dis* 1992; 15 (supplement 1): S115–S122.

SECTION 5F
HELMINTHIC INFECTIONS

Helminthic infections traditionally dominated the discipline of tropical medicine; this followed Manson's great interest in and seminal work on lymphatic filariasis. It is not therefore inappropriate that the first contribution to this section should address the filariases. Soil-transmitted helminthiases (also nematode infections) are extremely common in a tropical context and their true importance is undoubtedly underrated as far as clinical manifestations, morbidity and socioeconomic sequelae are concerned.

Schistosomiasis is a disease of colossal relevance worldwide; one estimate is that 200 million individuals suffer from hepatosplenic disease caused by this group of trematodes (flukes)—involving the gastrointestinal (and liver) and urinary tracts. Numerically, other trematodes are of lesser importance; the majority of these are localized to South-East Asia.

Intestinal cestode (tapeworm) infections are by and large benign but when they assume the role of systemic infections—caused by the larval stages (most importantly hydatidosis and neurocysticercosis)—significant pathology frequently ensues.

This section illustrates very clearly how writing and teaching of the traditional discipline followed upon parasitological and hence taxonomic classification(s). The filariases and schistosomiases, for example, both consist of several divergent *clinical* entities. To a physician it makes little or no sense to group gastrointestinal and urinary forms of schistosomiasis together. Similarly, do lymphatic filariasis, onchocerciasis, loiasis, dracontiasis and *Mansonella perstans* infections have anything in common to the clinician? Surely the time has come for a reorientation!

Diagnosis and management of helminthic infections has advanced almost beyond recognition since the early 1970s. Improved serological techniques have simplified the diagnosis of several of these—including filariasis, schistosomiasis, hydatidosis and neurocysticercosis; regrettably such techniques are not yet available for most of the intestinal infections (with the exception of strongyloidiasis), and a search for adult worms and/or their eggs remains the sole method for diagnosis. In chemotherapy, the newer benzimidazoles (for most nematode infections) were introduced in the 1960s, praziquantel (for schistosomiasis and other trematode and cestode infections) in the 1970s, and ivermectin (for onchocerciasis and to a lesser extent, other filariases) in the 1980s. Much remains to be accomplished, however, in *preventive* strategies for this extremely important group of human infections.

CHAPTER 70

FILARIASES

J. E. McMahon and P. E. Simonsen

The filariases result from infection with vector-borne tissue-dwelling nematodes called filariae. Depending on the species, adult filariae may live in the lymphatics, blood vessels, skin, connective tissues or serous membranes. The females produce larvae (microfilariae) which live in the bloodstream or skin. All true filariae infecting man (superfamily Filarioidea; family Onchocercidae) are transmitted by dipteran vectors. The guinea worm (superfamily Dracunculoidea) is not a true filaria, but is included in this section as a related nematode transmitted by arthropod vectors. A summary of the common filarial worms infecting man and the common disease symptoms is shown in Table 70.1. A few species of animal filariae may accidentally infect man. The transmission of human filariae is confined to warm climates, a high temperature being necessary for the parasites to develop in the vectors.

The pattern of the life cycle of all species of filariae is shown in Figure 70.1. Detailed life cycles of the species infecting man are given in Appendix III. The infective form is the third-stage larva which is transmitted by the vector. The rate of growth and differentiation of worms and longevity of both microfilariae and adult worms differ markedly between different species. Some adult worms may live as long as 20 years. A high specificity of the filaria–vector and the filaria–host relationships has evolved over a long period of time.

From the public health point of view onchocerciasis and lymphatic filariasis are the most important filarial infections. Dracunculiasis (guinea worm infection) results in severe ulceration, and Calabar swellings and other clinical manifestations of loiasis may have severe consequences for the patient.

Table 70.1 Characteristics of filarial parasites and guinea worm and common clinical manifestations in humans.

Species	Distribution	Vectors	Main location of adults	Main location of microfilariae	Common disease symptoms
Wuchereria bancrofti	Tropics	Mosquito spp.	Lymphatics	Blood	Hydrocoele Lymphadenitis Elephantiasis
Brugia malayi	East and South-East Asia South India	Mosquito spp.	Lymphatics	Blood	Lymphadenitis Elephantiasis
Brugia timori	Indonesia	Mosquito spp.	Lymphatics	Blood	
Loa loa	West and Central Africa	Chrysops spp.	Connective tissue	Blood	Calabar swellings
Mansonella perstans	Africa Central and South America	Culicoides spp.	Body cavities Serous membranes	Blood	Usually symptomless
Mansonella streptocerca	Central and West Africa	Culicoides spp.	Skin	Skin	Usually symptomless
Mansonella ozzardi	Central and South America	Culicoides spp. Simulium spp.	Peritoneal cavity Serous membranes	Blood and skin	Usually symptomless
Onchocerca volvulus	Africa Central and South America	Simulium spp.	Skin	Skin	Dermatitis, Nodules Eye lesions
Dracunculus medinensis	Africa India	Copepods	Connective tissues including skin	—	Ulceration

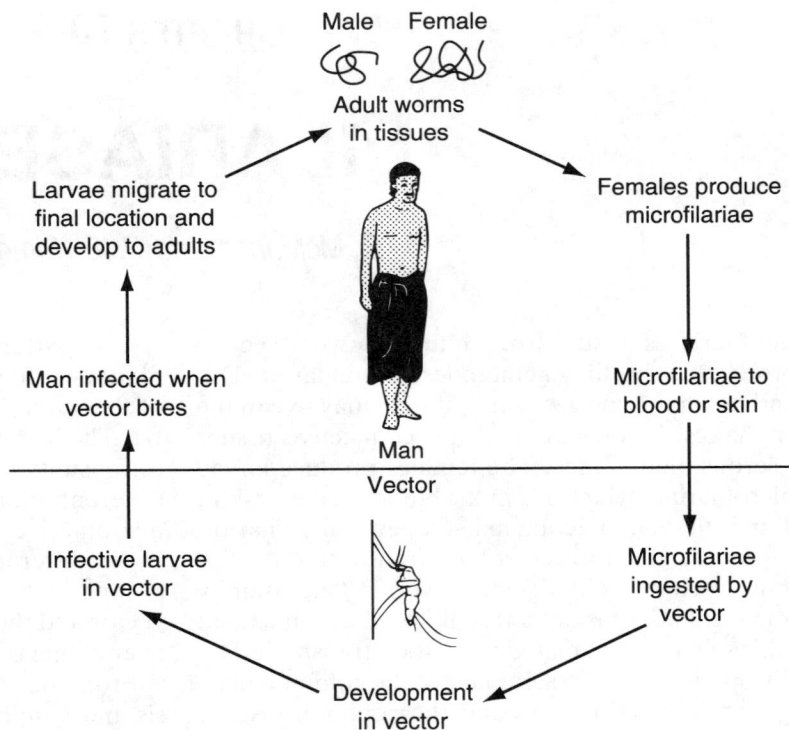

Figure 70.1 General life cycle of filariae.

LYMPHATIC FILARIASIS

Lymphatic filariasis results from infection with filarial worms. Three species, *Wuchereria bancrofti*, *Brugia malayi* and *B. timori*, cause this infection in humans. Infection with *W. bancrofti* is sometimes called bancroftian filariasis while brugian filariasis refers to infection by the other two species. *W. bancrofti* is much more widespread than the *Brugia* spp. (Figure 70.2).

HISTORICAL BACKGROUND

Our present knowledge of filariasis owes much to the investigations carried out towards the end of the nineteenth and the beginning of the twentieth centuries. Two distinguished pioneers of this period were Sir Patrick Manson and Dr Friedrich Fülleborn. In contrast to the present era, information available during the working lives of these men was very limited. They compensated for this lack of information by acute observation and the critical thinking ability that is exemplified in their writings. As early as 1878 Patrick Manson speculated that filariasis was transmitted by mosquitoes.

Microfilariae were first described by Demarquay in 1863.[2] In 1868 Wucherer found microfilariae in the urine of a patient with haematochyluria.[3] Adult worms were found by Bancroft in 1876 and named *Filaria bancrofti*.[4] In 1921 this species was included in the genus *Wuchereria*.

Examination of specimens of adult worms thought to be *Wuchereria* revealed a new species subsequently called *Brugia malayi* (1960).[5] Adult worms of the parasite formerly known as Timor microfilaria have been described. The species has been named *B. timori*.[6]

A detailed history of lymphatic filariasis has been produced.[7]

LIFE CYCLE AND TRANSMISSION

For details of the life cycles of the three causal parasites of lymphatic filariasis and of the mosquito vectors transmitting this infection in different geographical zones, see Appendices III and IV.

The adult worms reside in the lymphatics of the human host. Female *W. bancrofti* measure 80–100 × 0.25 mm and the male 40 × 0.1 mm. The adult *Brugia* spp. have only half of this dimension. Micro-

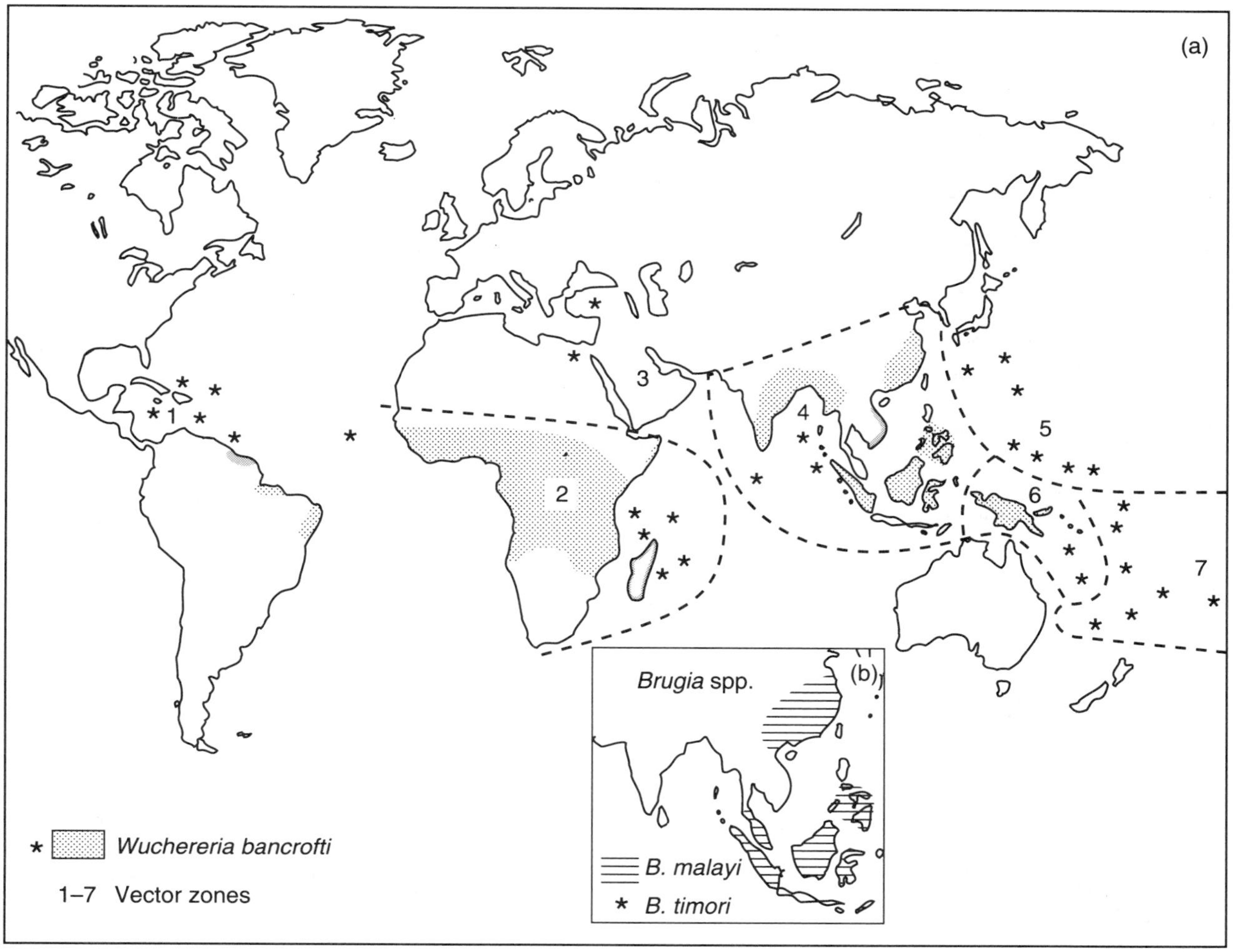

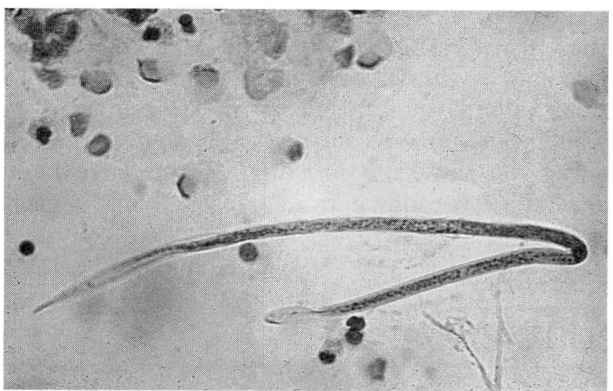

Figure 70.2 Geographical distribution of human lymphatic filariasis. (a) Bancroftian filariasis. (b) Brugian filariasis. For vector species in the different zones, see Appendix IV. (After WHO.[1])

filariae are produced from ova in the uterus of the female worm. They are sheathed and measure on average $260 \times 8\,\mu$m (Figures 70.3 and 70.4). Microfilariae appear in the blood after a minimum of 8 months in *W. bancrofti* and 3 months in *B. malayi*.

Microfilariae are ingested by the vector female mosquito during a blood meal. They exsheath in the mosquito stomach, becoming first-stage larvae which penetrate the stomach wall of the mosquito and migrate to the thorax muscles. There they develop through two moults to the infective third-stage larvae ($1500 \times 20\,\mu$m). The development in the mosquito takes a minimum of 10–12 days. Mature infective larvae then migrate to the mouthparts of the mosquito and they enter the skin of the human host, probably through the puncture site made by the proboscis of the vector when it takes its blood meal. The larvae migrate to the lymphatics and develop to adult worms which may live and produce microfilariae for more than 20 years, but on average the life span is shorter.

PERIODICITY

Like many filarial species, *W. bancrofti*, *B. malayi* and *B. timori* exhibit a daily periodicity in the

Figure 70.3 Microfilaria of *W. bancrofti*, in thick blood film stained with Giemsa.

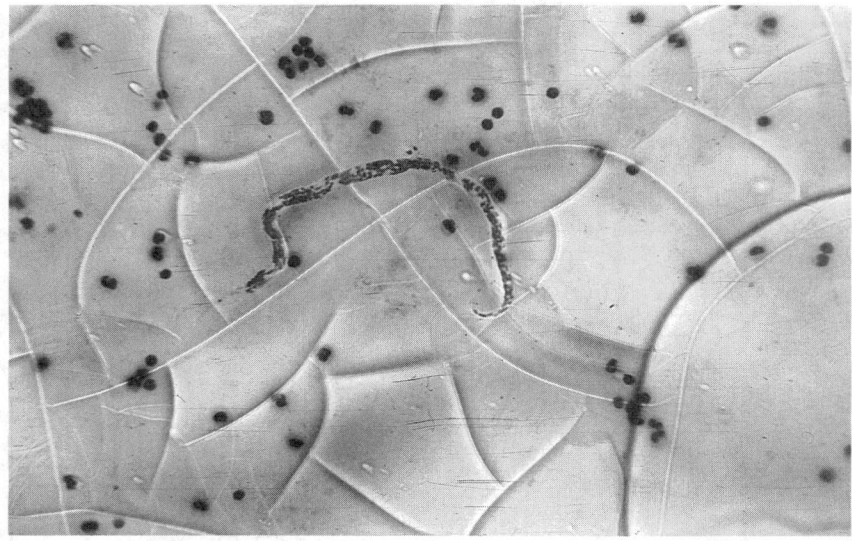

Figure 70.4 Microfilaria of *B. malayi*, in thick blood film stained with Giemsa.

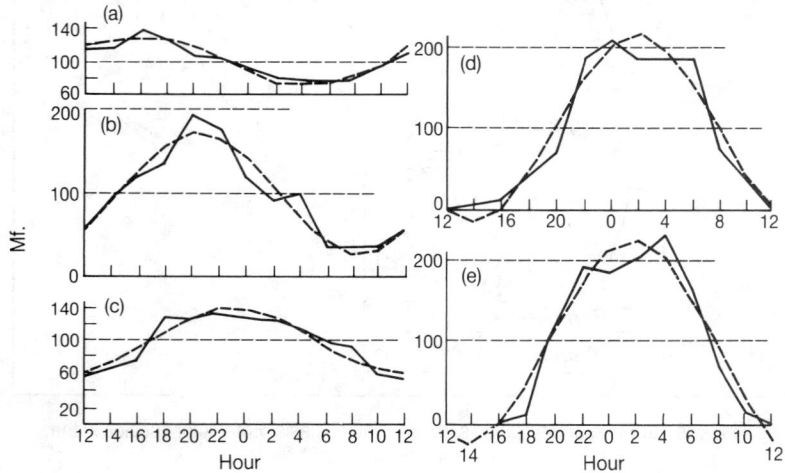

Figure 70.5 Observed (—) and theoretical (---) periodicity of microfilariae in peripheral blood. (a) Diurnally subperiodic *W. bancrofti* in the South Pacific. (b) Nocturnally subperiodic *W. bancrofti* from West Thailand. (c) Nocturnally subperiodic *B. malayi* in the Philippines. (d) Nocturnally periodic *B. malayi* in Malaysia. (e) Nocturnally periodic *W. bancrofti* in Malaysia. (Reproduced from WHO.[9])

concentration of microfilariae in the peripheral blood of the host. The different periodicities of microfilariae correspond with the biting habits of their principal vector. This adaptation enhances their chances of onward transmission. The details of microfilarial periodicity are discussed in Appendix III.

Microfilarial periodicity was studied in detail by Hawking. Depending on whether the highest microfilarial density over a 24-hour period occurs during the night or the day, periodicity is termed nocturnal or diurnal. Hawking and Denham[8] emphasized the need for care in the use of terms such as subperiodic, non-periodic and semiperiodic, which have been used to qualify these two major forms of periodicity.

In most areas the periodicity of both *W. bancrofti* and *B. malayi* is nocturnal, with peak concentrations in the blood around midnight and none or very few at midday (Figure 70.5). In these areas, the parasites are transmitted by night-biting mosquitoes. There also exist diurnally subperiodic and nocturnally sub-

periodic forms of *W. bancrofti*, where microfilariae are present continuously in the peripheral blood but where the concentrations are higher than average during day and night respectively. A strain of *B. malayi* also exhibits nocturnal subperiodicity (Figure 70.5).

The periodicity is due to a biological rhythm inherent in the microfilariae but influenced by the circadian rhythm of the host. Microfilaraemia of nocturnally periodic *W. bancrofti* ceases to be periodic in persons who start work at night and sleep during the day, and in patients who have been hospitalized for long periods.

CLINICAL FEATURES

Lymphatic filariasis manifests in both acute and chronic forms and may be with or without fever. The onset is usually sudden but may be slow and insidious.

BANCROFTIAN FILARIASIS

Common clinical manifestations of bancroftian filariasis are adenolymphangitis, involvement of the spermatic cord (funiculitis, lymphocoel, epididymoorchitis), hydrocoele, elephantiasis, chyluria and tropical pulmonary eosinophilia (TPE).

Lymphangitis and adenitis

Episodes of acute lymphangitis and adenolymphangitis, accompanied by fever and chills, become recurrent, occurring several times within a year. In most endemic areas groin glands and lymphatics of the male genitalia are frequently affected. Although the lymphangitis is often retrograde there are important exceptions, e.g. in East Africa.[10]

A painless lymphadenovarix of the inguinal or femoral glands is not uncommon. Glands are often matted together and have a soft rubbery texture.

Funiculitis and hydrocoele

Recurring attacks of funiculitis or epididymoorchitis may lead to hydrocoele formation. Following the early episodes the swelling around the testis disappears completely but over the years the tunica vaginalis becomes thickened and there is progressive enlargement of the hydrocoele (Figure 70.6). Other lesions of the spermatic cord include lymphocoele, lymphangiectasis and lymphadenovarix. Whether homologous lesions involving the ovary or fallopian tubes occur in female subjects is unknown. Filarial lymphangitis of the broad ligament was described in Queensland,[11] and in Guyana live adult worms were reported in lymphatics accompanying the ovarian vessels.[12] As bacterial salpingitis is common in women in the tropics, clinical differentiation of the cause(s) of deep pelvic pain is difficult.

Abscess formation

Sterile abscesses (more common in subperiodic *W. bancrofti* infections) may occur deep to the rectus fascia in the lower abdomen. Infected lymph nodes may suppurate. Painful lumps may occur due to

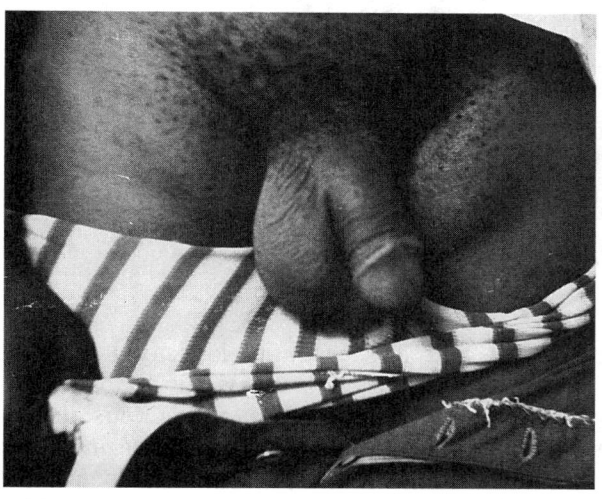

(a)

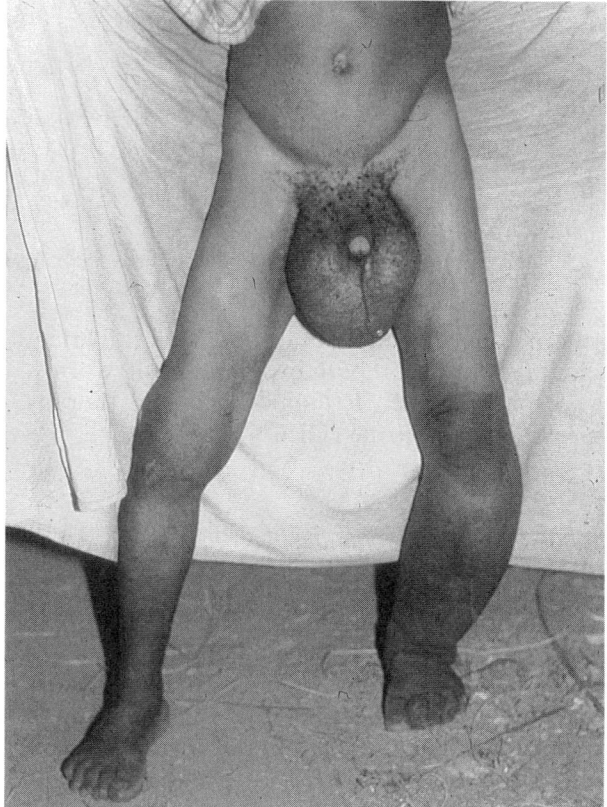

(b)

Figure 70.6 Lymphatic filariasis: hydrocoele. (a) Early; (b) advanced.

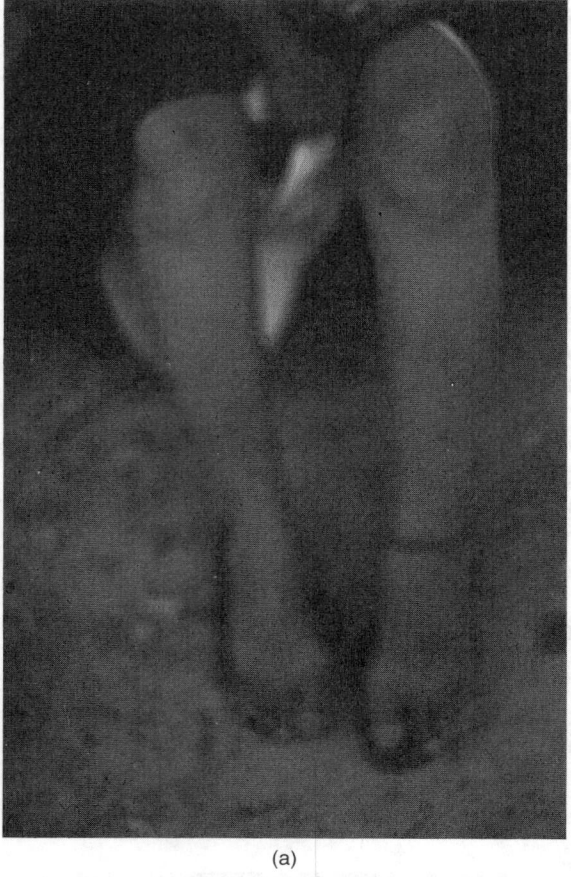

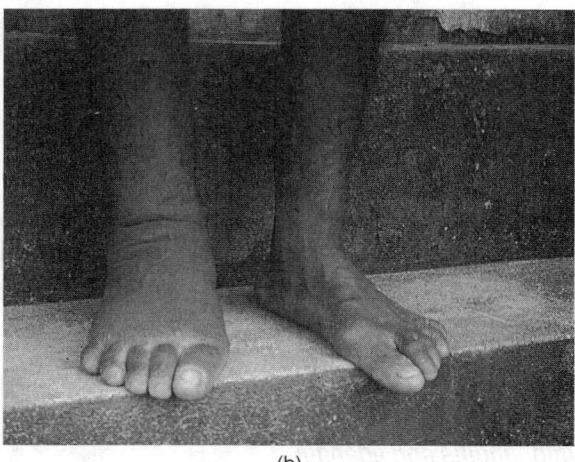

(b)

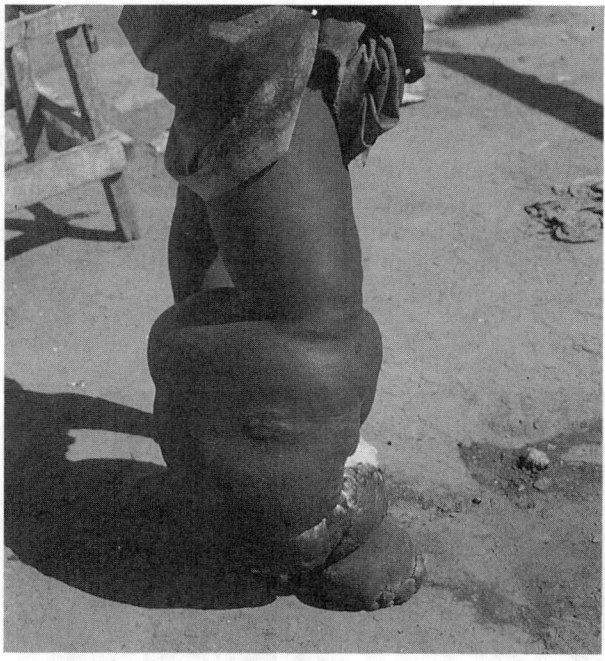

(c)

Figure 70.7 Lymphatic filariasis: elephantiasis of the leg. (a) Stage 1; (b) stage 2 (Courtesy of N. Kolstrup); (c) stage 3.

granulomatous reactions around microfilariae, developing worms or perhaps even adult worms. This is especially likely to happen following therapy with diethylcarbamazine (DEC).

Lymphoedema and elephantiasis

Lymphoedema progressing to elephantiasis most commonly affects the lower limbs (Figure 70.7). The upper limbs (Figure 70.8), scrotum, penis, vulva and breasts (Figure 70.9) may also be affected. Early attacks are usually characterized by adenitis and pitting oedema. In the legs loss of contour is first observed around the ankles (stage 1). Following initial attacks the limb returns to normal. Over several years the oedema becomes non-pitting with

thickening and loss of skin elasticity (stage 2). Further progression leads to evident elephantiasis with dermatosclerosis and papillomatous lesions (stage 3). These three stages are shown in Figure 70.7. The development of elephantiasis may be arrested at any stage. It commences in one leg but often becomes bilateral.

Scrotal elephantiasis can be graded as follows (Figure 70.10): stage 1, lymphoedema; stage 2, muddy scrotum; stage 3, thickened skin with loss of elasticity; and stage 4, evident elephantiasis with gross deformation.

Chyluria

Chyluria, the presence of chyle in the urine, follows the rupture of dilated lymphatics into the urinary

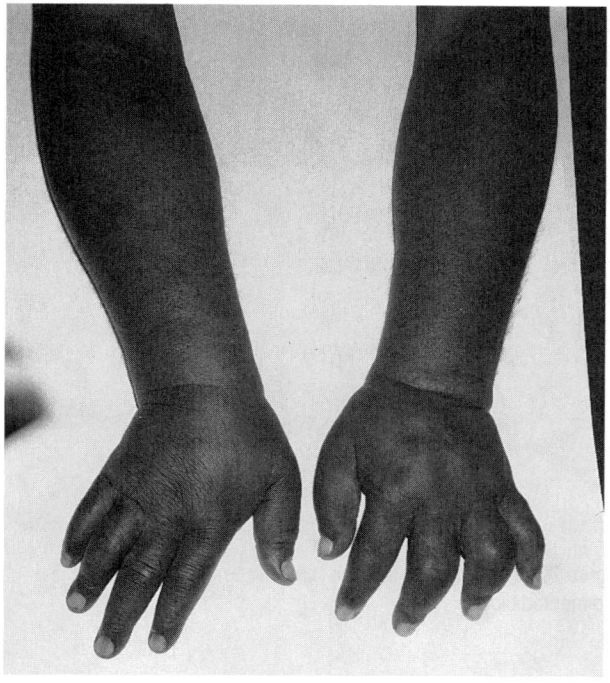

Figure 70.8 Lymphatic filariasis: elephantiasis of the arm.

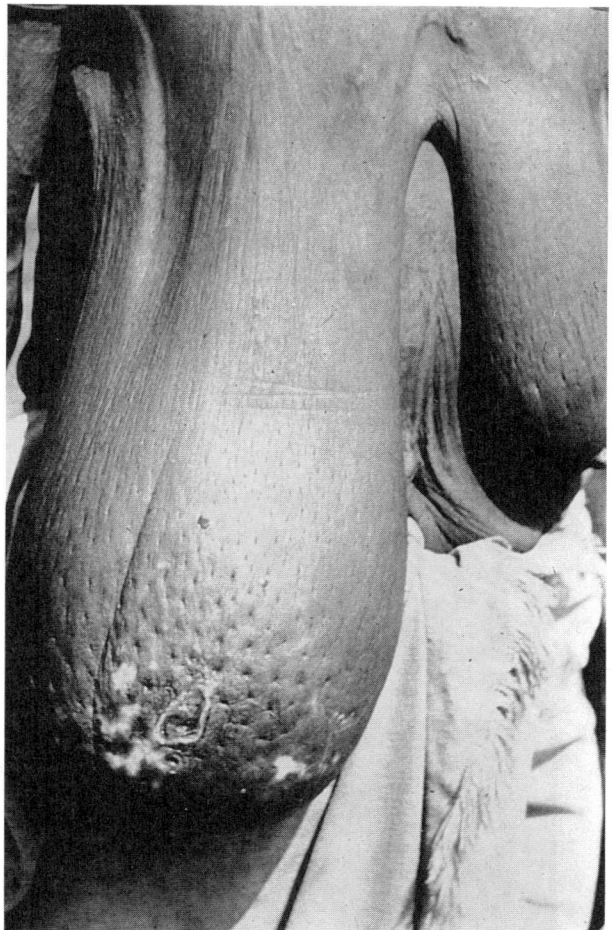

Figure 70.9 Lymphatic filariasis: elephantiasis of the breast.

tract. The most common sites for this rupture are the urinary pelvis and bladder. Chylous urine is milky in appearance (Figure 70.11). The obstruction to lymph flow is due to blockage of the retroperitoneal lymph nodes below the cysterna chyla. The onset may be insidious or sudden. Retention of urine from the presence of chylous or blood clots may be the first symptom. Chyluria is more pronounced after a heavy meal containing fat. The urine is often white in the morning and red later in the day.

Prolonged chyluria results in loss of weight and subcutaneous fat, hypoproteinaemia, lymphopenia and anaemia. In most areas endemic for filariasis the prevalence of chyluria is low.

Apart from chyluria, chylous reflux following obstruction to abdominal lymphatics may produce chylocoele (chyle in the tunica vaginalis), lymphadenovarix of the spermatic cord, scrotal dermal chylorrhoea, chylous ascites, chylous diarrhoea and other chylous complications.

Monoarticular arthritis

Monoarthritis is common in filarial endemic areas. The knee joint is most frequently affected, followed by the ankle. The joint becomes painful, warm and tender and the condition is indistinguishable from other forms of arthritis. A rapid cure follows treatment with DEC. Other evidence for a filarial aetiology comes from the Pacific: in a drug trial in Irian

Jaya, pain and swelling in the knees followed DEC therapy. Before bancroftian filariasis disappeared from Australia it was reported that adenitis of the popliteal space was frequent in infected persons. The resulting obstruction could cause a lymphatic fistula into the synovial sac.

Occult filariasis

The term occult filariasis refers to those conditions occurring in areas endemic for filariasis, in which the classical condition of lymphatic pathology is not present and where microfilariae are not found in the blood, but in which adult worms, microfilariae or other larval stages may be seen in the tissues. TPE is a classical example of occult filariasis.

Tropical pulmonary eosinophilia

TPE is characterized by clinical and immunological hyperresponsiveness. It occurs in both adults and children, is more common in males than females and

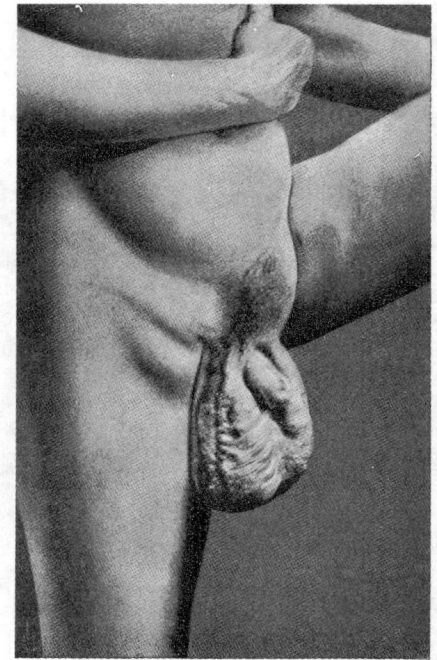

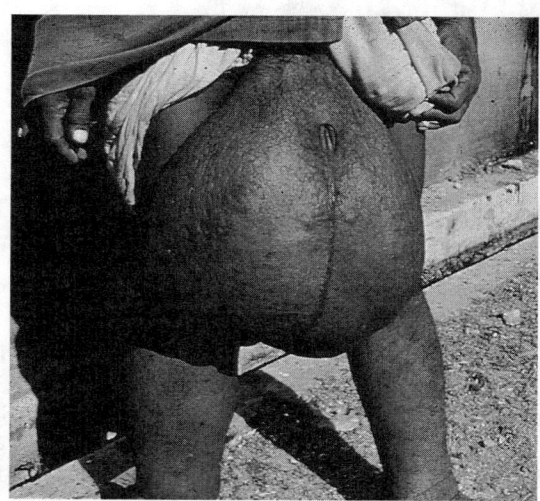

Figure 70.10   Lymphatic filariasis: elephantiasis of the scrotum. (a) Stage 1; (b) Stage 4 (see text).

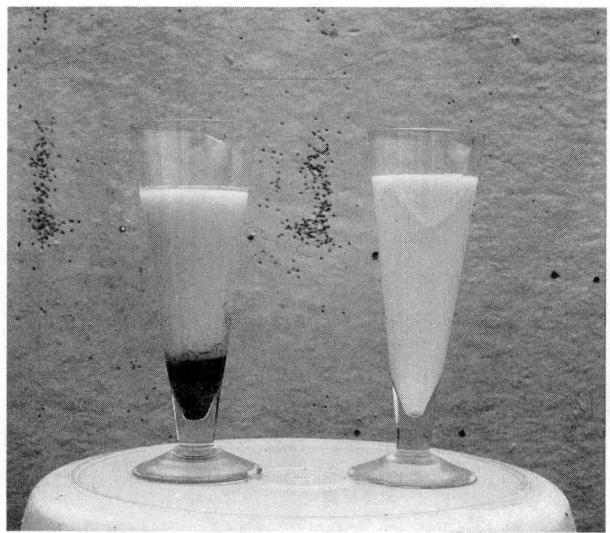

Figure 70.11   Lymphatic filariasis: chyluria—milky urine with sedimented blood.

in persons of Indian and Indonesian descent. Patients present with paroxysmal cough and wheezing that is worse at night, low-grade fever, scanty sputum production but occasional haemoptysis, adenopathy and extreme blood eosinophilia. This hypereosinophilia is the most constant feature of the syndrome. Absolute eosinophil counts range from 3000 to 60 000 cells/mm^3 of blood. The level of eosinophilia is not related to the severity of symptoms. There is radiological evidence of diffuse miliary lesions. Extrapulmonary manifestations occur in some patients and include splenomegaly, lymphadenopathy and hepatomegaly.

In many cases of TPE lung function is impaired, with a reduction in the vital capacity, total lung capacity and residual volume.

Others

Scattered reports associate endomyocardial fibrosis, tenosynovitis, thrombophlebitis, nerve palsies, dermatoses and glomerulonephritis with filariasis. These conditions sometimes coexist with filariasis and may be atypical manifestations of other diseases conditioned by pre-existing filarial infection. Recently it has been shown that haematuria (usually microscopic) occurs in many microfilaraemic persons.[13] The pathogenesis probably relates to immune complexes deposited on the basement membrane of the renal glomeruli.

BRUGIAN FILARIASIS

The main difference in the clinical manifestations between brugian and bancroftian filariasis is the rarity of hydrocoeles and other genital lesions in areas endemic for *B. malayi*. Chyluria is another sign not associated with *B. malayi*.

Elephantiasis of the legs in *B. malayi* infections is often confined to below the knee, whereas in infections with *W. bancrofti* the thigh as well as the lower leg is frequently involved. In Brugian filariasis in Indonesia, Malaysia and Thailand infected lymph nodes may suppurate. In India or other countries where *B. malayi* is endemic abscess formation is rarely encountered.

B. timori produce similar clinical manifestations to those seen in infections due to *B. malayi*, i.e. scrotal lesions are almost absent and elephantiasis tends to be below the knee. However, foci of *B. timori* infections have been reported in which prevalence of abscesses in lymph glands and lymph vessels is high and elephantiasis rates are 15%.[14]

DIFFERING CLINICAL MANIFESTATIONS

The clinical manifestations of lymphatic filariasis differ markedly, not only between species of parasite and between geographical zones but also in infections with the same species in the same endemic area.

Asia and the Pacific

Most cases of TPE have been reported from India and some other South and South-East Asian countries.

In Indonesia elephantiasis of the arms due to bancroftian filariasis is rare, whereas in islands of the Western Pacific rates of this lesion may be high. In Fiji the epitrochlear gland was affected in 22% of the population.[15]

In areas of Papua New Guinea endemic for bancroftian filariasis a high microfilaraemia (>30%) tends to be associated with a low clinical sign rate. Hydrocoele rates of 7% contrast markedly with prevalences of above 50% associated with *W. bancrofti* infection in East Africa.

In a village in Irian Jaya, 36% of persons with elephantiasis had microfilaraemia.[16] Similar foci have been reported in Samoa. This contrasts with results from other areas of the Pacific as well as those from other geographical areas where microfilaria rates are low in persons with elephantiasis.

In Tahiti acute attacks of adenolymphangitis in bancroftian filariasis commence around the age of 6 years. This is in contrast to the much later onset of this clinical manifestation in most other endemic areas.

Africa

In Africa, genital lesions and elephantiasis are the most common signs. In most countries accurate information on the distribution of bancroftian filariasis is lacking. There is a focus in the Nile delta of Egypt where there is a much greater frequency of chyluria and haemochyluria than in the rest of Africa. The prevalence of chyluria in the Egyptian focus is higher in urban than in rural areas.[17]

In East Africa, funiculitis, hydrocoele and elephantiasis, in that order, are the most common signs (J. E. McMahon, personal communication). The prevalence of both chyluria and the TPE is low. At a weekly filariasis clinic conducted over a 5-year period on the East African coast only five cases of chyluria and two of TPE were seen.

In West Africa sign rates tend to be lower than in East Africa. The overall hydrocoele rate in the coastal region of Liberia was 14.7%;[18] in villages in the Gambia it was 9%.[19] In Sierre Leone, where onchocerciasis is endemic over most of the mainland, lymphatic filariasis tends to be absent. On the island of Bonthe, where there is no onchocercal transmission, lymphatic filariasis is endemic. A small study revealed a microfilariae rate of 7% and hydrocoele and elephantiasis rates to be 9 and 2% respectively (J. E. McMahon, personal communication).

The Americas

In the Americas in general the prevalence of microfilaria and sign rates are low. Hyperendemic foci exist in Haiti.

DIAGNOSIS

A sudden onset of fever, acute groin pain with swollen tender lymph glands and oedematous swelling of the legs distinguishes an acute attack of filarial elephantiasis from the many other causes of fever and adenitis which occur in tropical countries. In many areas endemic for lymphatic filariasis retrograde lymphangitis accompanies these episodes.

Blood samples taken from patients with elephantiasis, whether acute or chronic, are often negative for microfilariae.

CLINICAL AND DIFFERENTIAL DIAGNOSIS

Scrotal swellings

Funiculitis
This presents as acute pain and swelling of the spermatic cord. It may be unilateral or bilateral. Funiculitis in areas endemic for lymphatic filariasis is usually filarial in origin.

The condition needs to be differentiated from funiculitis due to bacterial infections. The pain of filarial funiculitis usually radiates up and backwards or it may pass downwards to the testis. In East

Africa the tender swelling usually lacks signs of acute inflammation, i.e. local heat, redness and general fever. Funiculitis may be accompanied by epididymitis and/or hydrocoele formation. A hydrocoele may commence in the absence of funiculitis and presents as a tense tender swelling surrounding the testis. Funiculitis often becomes chronic, presenting as a tender thickened spermatic cord.

Chronic hydrocoele

Inguinal hernias are the most common scrotal swelling needing to be distinguished from hydrocoele. If the hernia is irreducible then the translucency test and the inability of the examiner to get above the swelling distinguish it from hydrocoele. Both irreducible hernias and hydrocoeles often exist in the same patient.

Obstructed hernias, tumours of the testis, tuberculosis and other bacterial infections of the epididymis, *Schistosoma haematobium* of the cord and acute lymphadenitis of the groin glands need to be distinguished from genital lesions of filarial origin.

Scrotal elephantiasis

Although the grade 4 stage of scrotal elephantiasis mentioned above is evident, grades 1 to 3 need to be distinguished from other conditions which affect the scrotal skin. Grades 1 and 2 are stages of lymph scrotum and must be distinguished from fungal infections and scrotal oedema due to onchocerciasis, and grade 3 must be distinguished from the thickened skin that results from the intense itching and scratching in scabies infections.

Leg elephantiasis

Among peasant communities the most common conditions needing to be distinguished from grades 1 and 2 are old ankle fractures with deformities and chronic osteomyelitis (particularly if no discharging sinus is present). Other conditions to be differentiated are onchocerciasis, swollen limbs due to congestive cardiac failure, subacute nephritis or blockage of venous (thrombosis) or lymphatic (tuberculosis, leprosy) systems and Kaposi's sarcoma. In all these conditions the patient's history greatly assists in differentiating them from filarial elephantiasis. The oedema of cardiac failure and subacute nephritis has a painless onset and is bilateral. Secondary carcinoma of lymph glands and surgical ablation may result in elephantiasis of the limbs.

An endemic form of leg elephantiasis occurs in Africa at altitudes which preclude a filarial aetiology. Silica, absorbed through the plantar skin of bare-footed peoples, affects the lymphatic vessels (see Chapter 28). Non-filarial tropical elephantiasis has also been reported from South and Central America.

Tropical pulmonary eosinophilia

Differentiation has to be made from bronchial asthma, pulmonary tuberculosis, miliary tuberculosis, allergic disease from inhaled dust (farmer's lung), pulmonary aspergillosis, eosinophilic lung reaction to drugs and eosinophilic leukaemia. TPE must also be distinguished from helminth infections that have a stage of the life cycle that involves lung tissue—*Ascaris*, *Strongyloides*, *Schistosoma* spp. and trichinosis. Confusion may also arise with visceral larva migrans caused by *Toxocara*. A rapid beneficial response to DEC therapy distinguishes TPE from the above-mentioned conditions.

PARASITOLOGICAL DIAGNOSIS

Adult worms are only rarely recovered from the tissues, and parasitological diagnosis is usually based on recovery of microfilariae from the patient's blood. Amicrofilaraemia does not exclude filarial disease, nor does microfilaraemia denote it. In individuals there is no relationship between microfilarial density and severity of disease. Microfilariae frequently occur in hydrocoele fluid and may occasionally be seen in urine or other body fluids.

For parasitological diagnosis of lymphatic filariasis, a blood specimen should be obtained at the time of the day when the peak concentration of microfilariae is expected (e.g. between 21.00 and 03.00 for nocturnally periodic forms). Many techniques have been described for demonstrating microfilariae in blood samples (see also Appendix V). The counting chamber technique is fast, quantitative and cheap.[20] In Tanzania 0.1 ml of finger-prick blood is added to a tube containing 3% acetic acid. Microfilariae are counted in a counting chamber under the low power of a compound microscope. If only one species of filaria is present in the area, this technique is the most suitable for routine hospital diagnosis as well as for field surveys. The counting chamber technique is relatively more sensitive than examining 1 or more millilitre of venous blood by the membrane filtration technique.[20] This greater relative sensitivity could result from the slower flow of blood in the peripheral cutaneous system compared with that in the veins.[20,21] Species identification of the microfilariae may be difficult with the counting chamber technique.

In areas where more than one species of blood microfilariae exist, staining techniques are recommended. These are simple to perform but sensitivity is rather low due to the small amount of blood examined and loss of microfilariae during the staining procedure. Microfilariae of *W. bancrofti*, *B. malayi* and *B. timori* have sheaths (see Figures 70.3 and 70.4). Microfilariae of *W. bancrofti* measure on average $260 \times 8 \mu m$, whilst those of *B. malayi* are slightly shorter and can be distinguished from microfilariae of *W. bancrofti* by the two isolated nuclei at the tip of the tail and the absence of nuclei in the cephalic space (see Appendix III). Microfilariae of *B. timori* are longer than those of *B. malayi*. *B. timori* have a length-to-width cephalic space ratio of 3:1. Apart from microfilariae of *W. bancrofti*, two other species of microfilariae found in the blood in parts of Africa are those of *Loa loa* and *Mansonella perstans*. Staining with Giemsa or haematoxylin enables microfilariae of these species to be differentiated morphologically. *M. perstans* and *M. ozzardi* microfilariae also occur in the blood in South America and the West Indies.

The membrane (Nuclepore) filtration techniques are sensitive and excellent if the high cost of filters can be afforded. Staining of filters enables identification of the microfilariae. The techniques are impractical for field surveys since venous blood is needed. If filters are not available for examination of large quantities of blood, the Knott concentration technique may be used as an alternative, highly sensitive test (see Appendix V).

Recent developments in parasitological techniques include: (1) a technique for preserving blood specimens for membrane filtration;[22] (2) a technique for staining of microfilarial sheaths in thick blood smears with fluorescein-conjugated lectins to enable rapid detection of microfilariae;[23] and (3) the commercial development of a microhaematocrit tube technique, incorporating acridine orange in the tube, for fast and easy diagnosis of malaria parasites in blood samples. This technique may also be used for finding microfilariae in the blood.[24]

The diethylcarbamazine provocative test

Nocturnally periodic microfilariae of *W. bancrofti* and *B. malayi* may be provoked, by the administration of DEC, to enter the peripheral blood in the daytime. This test was adapted in East Africa for diagnostic purposes, epidemiological surveys and the preliminary screening of potential antifilarial drugs. In Tanzania, 45–60 minutes is the optimum time for examination after the administration of a dose of 2 mg/kg of DEC, whereas 6 mg/kg induces a peak of microfilariae in the peripheral circulation 15 minutes after drug administration.[25,26]

In contrast to its daytime action on nocturnally periodic *W. bancrofti*, the administration of DEC at night reduces the microfilaraemia. A similar reduction occurs following the daytime administration of the drug to diurnally subperiodic *W. bancrofti*. In persons on normal daily activities the daytime DEC provocative method is as sensitive a method for detecting microfilariae of the nocturnally periodic *W. brancrofti* as examination of night blood. In hospitalized patients and others whose sleep rhythms have been altered the test is of little use.

The test has an important practical use in obtaining a clear reflection of the prevalence and density of the microfilariae in a community in areas where it is difficult to obtain the co-operation of peoples for night blood surveys. When the daytime provocative test was compared with the non-provocative night examination, although densities of microfilariae in individuals were considerably lower in the day test, day and night densities were highly correlated ($r = 0.83$).[26] The dose of 2 mg/kg of DEC is readily acceptable to the people in coastal East Africa. Because of the risk of a severe Mazzotti reaction the test is contraindicated in onchocerciasis endemic regions.

IMMUNOLOGICAL DIAGNOSIS

Filarial worms induce a wide range of immune reactions in the host. Several immunodiagnostic techniques, including the indirect fluorescent antibody test (IFAT) and enzyme linked immunosorbent assay (ELISA), have been developed for lymphatic filariasis.[27] Homologous *W. bancrofti* antigen is not available, and *B. malayi* and various animal filariae are used for antigen preparation. At present, however, immunodiagnosis is of little practical use in lymphatic filariasis, due to low sensitivity and specificity of the tests. Cross-reactions to other nematode infections are common, and the tests cannot distinguish past and present infection. Most people living in endemic areas are positive for antibodies to crude filarial antigens due to the constant exposure to infection. Immunodiagnosis may be of value in diagnosing visitors to endemic areas who develop symptoms of lymphatic filariasis but have no microfilaraemia.

Development of new, specific and sensitive immunodiagnostic tests is a priority in filariasis research: these include tests which can diagnose prepatent infections, amicrofilaraemic adult worm infections and infections with low microfilaraemias. Cross-reactions in serodiagnostic tests have been reduced through detection for specific IgE and IgG4 antibodies.[28–30] Monoclonal antibody-based tests for circulating antigens show promise in the diagnosis of filarial infection,[31–33] and a kit for highly specific detection of circulating *W. bancrofti* antigens is now commercially available (JCU Tropical Biotechnology, Australia). A number of recombinant filarial antigens have also been produced. They are currently being tested for their diagnostic value, and new methods are being developed using DNA probes to identify microfilariae in body fluids and filarial larvae in the mosquito vectors.

PATHOLOGY AND IMMUNOLOGY

Most of the pathology associated with lymphatic filariasis is limited to the lymphatics. A spectrum of manifestations is seen in endemic regions (Figure 70.12). On one hand are people with no signs of infection or disease and asymptomatic microfilaria carriers, and, on the other, those who develop signs of lymphatic responsiveness to adult worms, with fever, and who later develop chronic lymphatic pathology.[34] In the case of TPE there is a vigorous immune response directed against the microfilariae, with consequent pathology.

The majority of individuals in endemic areas mount an immunological response to filarial antigens, due to the constant exposure. However, infected persons and/or persons with clinical manifestations of lymphatic filariasis (except those with TPE) are in general less immunologically responsive to filarial antigens when compared with uninfected persons from the same endemic environment.[35,36] This hyporesponsiveness is manifested in both the humoral and cellular immune response, and it appears to be limited to filarial antigens. It is most prominent in patients with microfilaraemia, and its existence is presumably important for the successful persistence of the parasites within the host.

There is now increasing evidence, mainly from experimental filariasis in the nude mouse,[37] that the damage to the lymphatic vessels is mediated both by an inflammatory response to the adult worms as well as by a direct action of the parasites or their released products on the lymphatic tissues. Experiments have shown that immunodeficient nude mice infected with brugian parasites, develop, *in the absence of inflammation*, marked lymphatic dilatation with subsequent lymphoedema. Reconstitution of these immunodeficient mice by immunocompetent cells from filaria-sensitized normal mice results in an *inflammatory* granuloma reaction around the parasites, with subsequent obstruction of the lymphatics and lymphoedema.[37] Apparently, the parasites themselves may induce endothelial cell proliferation and lymphatic dilatation, whereas the host inflammatory reactions around the parasites result in local granuloma formation and obstruction of the lymphatics.

Few histological studies have been made on human lymphatic tissues from filaria-infected persons from endemic areas. Extensive studies were conducted on tissues from expatriates (American servicemen), from a non-endemic zone, who acquired infection when they entered endemic areas in the Pacific during the Second World War.[38] The obstructive, obliterative inflammatory reactions around dead parasites in the reconstituted nude mice parallel the findings found in tissues from these expatriates. On the other hand, parasite-induced reactions in the nude mice parallel some of the clinical findings from East Africa, where the non-inflammatory nature of many of the acute clinical manifestations have been noted.[10]

The intermittent development of lymphoedema may be related to bursts of metabolic activity of the worms, or to the release of provocative substances by worms which have sustained mechanical trauma. Blockage of the lymph vessels and successive lymphatic hypertension lead to oedema and subsequent formation of lymphatic collaterals. Protein-rich fluid accumulates in the subcutaneous tissues and eventually sets up fibrotic reactions.

The formation of tortuous collateral lymphatics and the apparent development of new vessels has been demonstrated by lymphangiographs in persons with clinical symptoms from endemic areas.[39] Recent studies, using lymphoscintigraphy, have shown that even asymptomatic individuals whose only manifestation of infection is microfilaraemia have dilated lymphatics and compromised lymphatic function.[40] This may reflect the direct effect of the parasites on lymphatics, causing dilatations and proliferation. A recent study examining lymphatic tissue of infected asymptomatic patients from an endemic region showed a minimal or no inflammatory activity around adult worms and microfilariae.[41]

Prenatal sensitization of the fetus by infected mothers has been demonstrated to occur in human lymphatic filariasis.[42] Evidence from studies on animal models, as well as from human populations

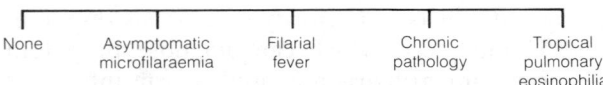

Figure 70.12 Spectrum of clinical manifestations of lymphatic filariasis in endemic areas. (After Ottesen.[34])

migrating from non-endemic to endemic areas, suggests that prenatal sensitization may affect the later course of infection and disease in the offspring.[43,44] It is possible that this may partly account for the difference in clinical response between people native to an endemic area and migrants to that area. Prenatal exposure may also explain why children born of microfilaraemic mothers appear to have a higher chance of developing microfilaraemia later, than do those born of amicrofilaraemic mothers.[45]

In contrast to most other people in filariasis endemic areas, patients with TPE are immunologically hyperresponsive to filarial antigens.[46,47] Laboratory studies demonstrate high serum levels of filaria-specific IgG and IgE, and marked peripheral blood eosinophilia. The manifestations of TPE are most marked in the lungs, and lung biopsies have shown inflammatory foci around degenerating microfilariae. These findings, together with the absence of circulating microfilariae, suggest that an antibody-mediated mechanism of microfilaria destruction occurs in the lungs of these patients. If left untreated, TPE may progress to a chronic stage with interstitial fibrosis and permanent loss of lung function.

Protective immunity has not been proved in lymphatic filariasis. However, there is evidence that some individuals in endemic areas develop resistance to the microfilarial or the infective larval stages of the parasite. In filaria endemic areas, a proportion of the amicrofilaraemic persons (with or without symptoms) produce antibodies to the microfilarial sheath, whereas such antibodies are not seen in patients harbouring microfilariae.[48–50] This close correlation between antisheath antibodies and amicrofilaraemia, together with evidence from animal models,[51–54] suggest that these persons may have developed a resistance mechanism against the microfilarial stage of the parasite. Furthermore,

recent observations indicate that a proportion of adults in endemic areas develop resistance to infective larvae.[55,56] In Papua New Guinea, protection was seen to correlate with the presence of an antibody binding to the surface of the infective-stage larvae.

TREATMENT

The treatment of filariasis mainly consists of chemotherapy and/or symptomatic treatment. A new surgical technique utilizing lymphovenous drainage procedures shows promise for the treatment of elephantiasis (see below).

CHEMOTHERAPY

The drug most commonly used is diethylcarbamazine citrate (DEC, Hetrazan, Banocide, Notezine). It is a microfilaricidal agent also capable of killing adult *W. bancrofti*, *B. malayi* and *B. timori* (Table 70.2). Ivermectin for the treatment of lymphatic filariasis is currently being evaluated.

DEC exerts no direct lethal action on the microfilariae but apparently modifies them so that they are removed by the host's immune system. It is administered orally. The recommended dose is 6 mg/kg body weight daily, in three divided doses after food, for 12 days. The microfilariae usually rapidly decrease in the blood after the start of treatment and then increase, usually at reduced intensity, after some months. Drug reactions, due to dying parasites, may commence a few hours after the start of treatment. They are less severe in bancroftian filariasis than in brugian filariasis. There are two groups of reactions, systemic and local, both with and without fever. Systemic reactions include headache,

Table 70.2 The effect of diethylcarbamazine and ivermectin on microfilariae and adults of human filarial parasites.

Drug	Stage	Wuchereria bancrofti *and* Brugia spp.	Loa loa	Mansonella perstans	Mansonella streptocerca	Mansonella ozzardi	Onchocerca volvulus
Diethyl-carbamazine	Microfilaria	++	++ *	−	++	−	++ *
	Adult	+	+	−	++	−	−
Ivermectin	Microfilaria	++	++	−	?	++	++
	Adult	?	?	?	?	?	?

−, No effect;
+, few are eliminated;
++, most are eliminated;
?, unknown.
*, Severe side effects may occur.

joint and body pain, dizziness, anorexia, malaise and vomiting. Fever and systemic reactions tend to be related to the intensity of infection. Giving the drug in repeated small doses or spacing the doses reduces the severity of the reactions. Localized drug reactions include lymphadenitis, abscess formation and transient lymphoedema. In bancroftian filariasis funiculitis, epididymitis and hydrocoele formation also occur. These local reactions tend to occur later and last longer than the systemic effects. Interruption of treatment is not usually necessary. The passing of *Ascaris* worms is often a beneficial side-effect of DEC therapy.

Side-effects of DEC therapy are reduced when treatment is spaced: for example, when single doses (6 mg/kg) are given once weekly, twice monthly or monthly. Recently follow-up examinations following a single dose of DEC (100 mg to adults and 50 mg to children) revealed reductions in microfilaraemias of 52, 65 and 82% at 1, 3 and 6 months respectively (P. E. Simonsen and D. W. Meyrowitsch, personal communication).

DEC treatment of microfilaraemic patients and those with acute symptoms may prevent development of chronic obstructive disease. Treatment may be repeated about every 6 months for as long as the person remains microfilaraemic or has symptoms. There may be severe reactions to DEC in persons infected with *Onchocerca volvulus* or *Loa loa*. Therefore special care must be taken in areas where these two parasites occur.

The recommended treatment for TPE is a 3-week course of DEC. Following DEC therapy most patients show improvement but not complete resolution of TPE.[57]

Due to its efficiency in killing microfilariae of *O. volvulus*, studies have been initiated to test the efficiency of ivermectin against *W. bancrofti* and *B. malayi* (Table 70.2). Preliminary results have shown that a single oral dose of ivermectin (150 µg/kg body weight) effectively removes microfilariae of *W. bancrofti*, but there is no evidence of a macrofilaricidal effect and microfilariae reappear in the blood faster than after treatment with a full dose of DEC. In brugian filariasis the fall in microfilaraemia was much more gradual than is the case in bancroftian filariasis.[40] Side-effects of ivermectin therapy are similar to those mentioned above for DEC. Should further investigations confirm low drug toxicity, in particular low neurotoxicity, ivermectin may soon be commonly used for the treatment of lymphatic filariasis.

A compound called 'coumarin' has been investigated in India and China. In clinical trials this product appears to have caused reductions in oedema and other clinical signs of elephantiasis.[40,58]

SYMPTOMATIC TREATMENT

In conjunction with DEC therapy symptomatic treatment—analgesics/antipyretics and bed-rest—are useful measures for treating acute attacks of filarial fever and lymphadenitis. Elevation of the affected limb, special massage, the application of an elastic bandage or stocking and prevention of superficial bacterial and fungal infections all assist in the management of lymphoedematous limbs.

SURGICAL TREATMENT

Prior to any surgical procedure a course of DEC is recommended. Chronic hydrocoeles require excision and eversion of the sac. In scrotal elephantiasis the surgical removal of the grossly elephantoid skin and scrotal tissues with preservation of the penis and testicles has proved very worthwhile. Surgical treatment of limb elephantiasis has generally proved unsuccessful. Earlier techniques involving the excision of redundant tissue from severely affected limbs generally led to long-term results that were unsatisfactory. More beneficial responses have been obtained recently with lymphovenous procedures, followed by removal of excess subcutaneous and fatty tissue from the affected extremities and adequate postural drainage and physiotherapy.[59] In chyluria, if conservative approaches using DEC therapy and restriction of dietary fats are not helpful, then surgery is indicated. This may include disconnection of the renal hilar lymphatics by nephropexy.

EPIDEMIOLOGY

The distribution of the three causal parasites of lymphatic filariasis, *W. bancrofti* (bancroftian filariasis), *B. malayi* and *B. timori* (brugian filariasis), is shown in Figure 70.2. *W. bancrofti* is distributed throughout the tropical regions of Asia, Africa, the Americas and the Pacific and is particularly prevalent in areas with hot and humid climates. *B. malayi* is found in South-East Asia, and in areas of south-west India and South and Central China, whereas *B. timori* only occurs on some small islands in Indonesia. It is difficult to estimate the total world prevalence of lymphatic filariasis because, in many countries, accurate information is not available. It is thought that about 750 million people are living in endemic areas and that at least 79 million are infected.[40] Lymphatic filariasis has disappeared from North America, Japan and Australia, and in some countries, especially China, recent control programmes have greatly decreased the prevalence. It continues to be a major public health problem in most of southern and South-East Asia, in Africa, and in a number of Caribbean and Pacific Islands. In recent years the prevalence in many urban areas has increased due to increase in both human and vector populations in these areas.

The epidemiology of *W. bancrofti* and *B. malayi* infections varies in different geographical areas, especially with respect to the prevalence and intensity of infection, the transmission pattern and the clinical manifestations. Differences in vectorial capacity is an important factor influencing these epidemiological parameters in different endemic areas. There are also differences in the response of the host (see p. 111), as well as inherent differences in the parasite, e.g. three strains of *W. bancrofti* and two strains of *B. malayi* have been recognized on the basis of differences in periodicity of the microfilariae. It is also possible that variation in worm habitat preferences within the host's lymphatic system may contribute to differences in clinical manifestations.

In most areas the microfilariae of *W. bancrofti* are nocturnally periodic, being adapted to transmission by night-biting *Culex* and *Anopheles* mosquitoes. A diurnal subperiodic form is found in the South Pacific[60] and in the Andaman and Nicobar Islands (India),[61] whereas a nocturnally subperiodic form is found in Thailand.[62] *B. malayi* occurs both in a nocturnal periodic and a nocturnal subperiodic form, whereas *B. timori* is nocturnally periodic.[63] The subperiodic forms are transmitted by vectors biting mainly during the daytime.

The vector distribution for all geographical zones is shown in Appendix IV. *Culex quinquefasciatus* is the principal vector of *W. bancrofti* in urban and semiurban areas of southern and South-East Asia, East Africa and America. Increased pollution of fresh water bodies and the introduction of pit latrines, which favour breeding of this mosquito, has led to increased transmission in many areas. *C. quinquefasciatus* is an endophilic night biter. There is no evidence that it is transmitting filariasis in West Africa. In rural areas of Asia and Africa *Anopheles* spp. are the main vectors, with the *A. gambiae* complex and *A. funestus* being the most important vectors in Africa. The main vectors of the *Anopheles* spp. bite indoors at night and breed in open rather clean water.

In the South Pacific islands the predominant vectors of *W. bancrofti* belong to day-biting *Aedes* spp., especially *Ae. polynesiensis*. The majority of these mosquitoes bite outdoors and breed in small temporary water collections: tree holes, empty cans and bottles, coconut shells, plant axils and crab holes. In Papua New Guinea night-biting *Anopheles* spp. are the principal vectors. Because of the heterogeneous nature of filariasis within this region (microfilaraemias and clinical manifestations of bancroftian filariasis differ markedly from area to area) the South Pacific has been divided into four epidemiological zones: Micronesian, Papuan, Polynesian and New Caledonian.[64]

The nocturnally subperiodic form of *B. malayi* is transmitted by *Mansonia* mosquitoes in dense swamp forest areas. This form is commonly found also in wild monkeys. Nocturnally periodic *B. malayi* has been reported only from man. It is transmitted in open plains and agricultural areas, mainly by *Mansonia* spp. mosquitoes, although in some areas species of *Anopheles* and *Aedes* also play a role. The larvae and pupae of *Mansonia* mosquitoes obtain their oxygen directly from the cells of certain species of aquatic plants present in clean water bodies. Survival of the *Mansonia* spp. is dependent on the association with the plants. Increased pollution has in some places led to a decrease in breeding of *Mansonia*, with a subsequent drop in transmission of *B. malayi*. *Mansonia* spp. prefer to feed outside and biting usually commences shortly after dusk. *A. barbirostris* is the only mosquito to date to have been identified as a vector of *B. timori*.

Characteristic broad patterns of microfilaraemia and disease are seen in affected populations in endemic areas.[65–69] An example of this pattern in a highly *W. bancrofti* endemic East African village is seen in Figure 70.13. Usually microfilaraemia starts to appear in children about 5 years of age. The prevalence then rises with increasing age and commences to level out above the age of 30 years. The prevalence rarely goes above 40–50% in any age group. It may decrease slightly in older persons. Signs of disease begin to develop around the onset of puberty or in early adult life, with recurrent attacks of fever, lymphadenitis, lymphangitis (sometimes retrograde), and in males funiculitis. Hydrocoeles also begin to appear around this age. The prevalence of signs rises steadily and in highly endemic areas the majority of elderly males may have hydrocoeles. In stable endemic communities elephantiasis is mainly seen in older people, but younger persons may also be affected.

Cross-sectional surveys, although providing important information on the distribution of infection and disease in the affected population, only give a static view of the situation. In reality there is a dynamic sequel in development of infection and disease. Many of the people who are amicrofilaraemic during the survey have been positive for microfilariae previously, or will become so later. Also,

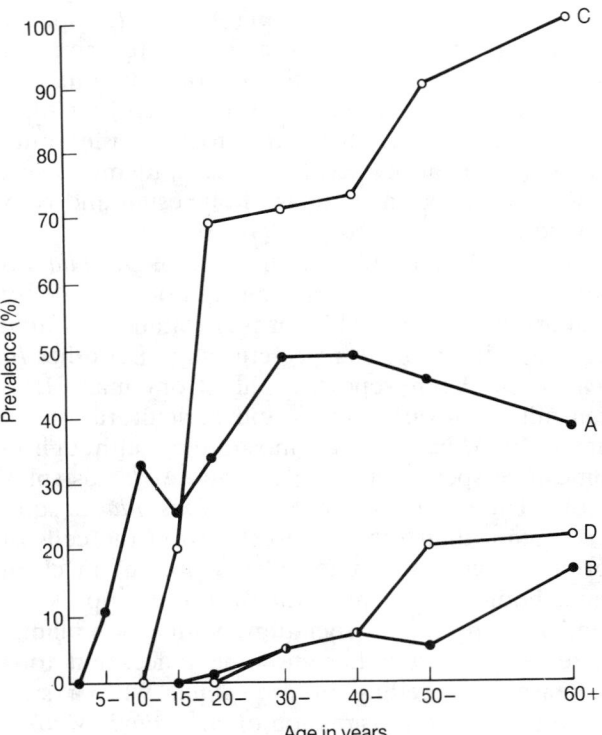

Figure 70.13 Microfilaraemia and clinical manifestations of *W. bancrofti* in an endemic village on the coast of north-east Tanzania. Prevalence of microfilaraemia (A) and elephantiasis (B) in the whole population and the prevalence of hydrocoele (C) and scrotal elephantiasis (D) among the males. Rates of arm and breast elephantiasis were 1 and 0.5% respectively. (Based on McMahon et al.[65])

clinical manifestations often develop late in the course of infection, when some people have already reached the amicrofilaraemic stage. In many surveys the prevalence and intensity of microfilaraemia has been slightly higher in males than in females. In a recent analysis this was shown to be especially significant for the 20–39-year age group.[70] It was suggested that hormonal factors in females of reproductive age makes them more resistant to infection than males of the same age group.

Exposure to intense transmission over long periods is necessary before a patent infection with microfilariae is acquired. Visitors to endemic from non-endemic areas only rarely develop microfilaraemia, but they may acquire adult worms. Expatriates, exposed to intense transmission, may develop symptoms faster than is the case with resident natives of that endemic area.[38] During the Second World War 40 000 American service personnel were exposed to infection with *W. bancrofti*. More than 10 000 cases of disease were diagnosed, but microfilaraemia developed in less than ten of these.[71]

Humans are only infected by mosquitoes carrying infective larvae. Microfilariae can be transmitted in blood transfusions and will circulate in the recipient's blood for weeks, during which time they maintain their periodicity. Congenital transmission of microfilariae has been reported but seems to be of little significance. Congenital transmission of other stages of the parasite does not occur. There is no evidence for zoonotic infections of *W. bancrofti* under natural conditions. Recently leaf monkeys (*Presbytis* spp.) have been infected with *W. bancrofti* in the laboratory.[72] A closely related species, *W. kalimantani*, has been recovered from leaf monkeys in Indonesia[73] but as far as is known this species does not infect man. On the other hand, many species of *Brugia* infect animals, and some of these may occasionally also infect man. The nocturnally periodic form of *B. malayi* has only been reported from man, but the subperiodic form is found also in a wide variety of domestic and wild animals (monkeys, cats), at least in Malaysia.[63] There appears to be no animal reservoir of *B. timori*.

CONTROL

The objective of filariasis control is to reduce morbidity, thereby eliminating filariasis as a public health problem. Successful programmes for the control of lymphatic filariasis must be based on a thorough understanding of the distribution and dynamics of the disease in the targeted population. The diverse characteristics of communities in endemic foci, as well as differences in vector, parasite and disease parameters, do not permit a simple, uniform approach to control that is applicable in all, or even most, situations.

The main methods used in the control of filariasis are chemotherapy and mosquito control. To achieve success in a control programme it is necessary for the community to be actively involved. To ensure community participation a preparatory phase is necessary, during which community leaders and motivated persons are identified and approached for the purpose of obtaining their co-operation in the programme. Adequate health education is given on the nature of the disease and on the methods used for its control.

CHEMOTHERAPEUTIC CONTROL

Chemotherapeutic regimens of DEC have been used for several decades for the control of bancroftian and brugian filariasis. The efficacy and side-effects of DEC are discussed on pp. 115–116. DEC is relatively cheap, it rapidly reduces the prevalence of microfilaraemia, and it also has some effect on the adult worms.

Therapy to a community may consist of selective or mass treatment. In mass treatment DEC is administered to the total population (except infants, pregnant women or persons with debilitating conditions) in that community. In mass treatment campaigns there is no need to conduct parasitological diagnoses prior to treatment. Thus cost is reduced. The amicrofilaraemic infections and persons with low microfilarial densities who may have been falsely negative in a diagnostic test are included for treatment. In selective treatment microfilarial carriers and/or people with clinical manifestations of filariasis are identified by large-scale screening. Subsequently, DEC is given only to those who are positive. Selective treatment is mainly suitable for areas with low endemicity.

In control programmes DEC may be administered in the normal intensive regimens of therapy. The total dosage may be lowered, or single doses given. The drug may be administered in widely spaced doses or it may be added to salt. Spaced doses effectively reduce microfilaraemias and have fewer and less severe side-effects than the more intensive regimens. In Kenya and Tanzania, once weekly, once monthly and bi-monthly doses were administered for periods up to one year. Total doses ranged from 36 to 72 mg/kg body weight.[74-76] Single doses of 3 or 6 mg/kg body weight, given once a year against subperiodic *W. bancrofti* in Tahiti, have been shown to reduce microfilarial loads by 80–90%.[77] Control programmes with DEC-medicated salt have successfully controlled lymphatic filariasis in parts of China and Taiwan.[40,78] Recent comparative trials in Tanzania have shown that a monthly low dose of DEC (100 mg to adults and 50 mg to children) or administration of medicated cooking salt (0.3% DEC) were more effective in reducing microfilaraemias over a 1-year follow-up period than the recommended standard intensive regimen (see pp. 115–116) (P. E. Simonsen and D. W. Meyrowitsch, personal communication).

MOSQUITO CONTROL

The feasibility and value of vector control as one of the components of filariasis control depends upon the local epidemiological conditions, including the species of vectors, their biting, resting and breeding habits and the type of environment, e.g. rural or urban. Effective vector control rapidly reduces transmission, but because it is slow to reduce the prevalence of filariasis in a population, vector con-

trol measures in integrated programmes should be preceded by, or combined with chemotherapy. DEC therapy rapidly reduces the prevalence of microfilariae.

The main antivector measures that have been used in the control of filariasis are environmental control of breeding sites, larviciding and the use of insecticides against adult mosquitoes. Environmental management varies from the filling in of temporary pools and clearing of refuse which collects water, to the construction of drainage systems in urban areas. *C. quinquefasciatus* breeds in highly polluted water and plays a major role in the transmission of *W. bancrofti* in urban and semiurban areas. As well as its importance in urban transmission, in some villages on the East African coast *C. quinquefasciatus* has become the principal vector of filariasis.[65] This problem is often caused by the construction of pit latrines which become potential breeding sites for *C. quinquefasciatus*. It has been controlled by a combination of larviciding and simple to more complex environmental measures. A new method, aimed at controlling *C. quinquefasciatus* in stagnant water, especially cesspits and latrines, utilizes a layer of expanded polystyrene beads which float on the water surface and prevent the mosquito larvae from breathing (Figure 70.14). This method has proved to be long lasting and has been successful in filariasis control in Zanzibar.[79] Environmental management involving a strong element of community participation has been successful in a recent control programme for lymphatic filariasis in Pondicherry, India.[80]

Anopheles vectors are responsible for transmission of much rural filariasis. In areas where malaria and filariasis transmission depend on the

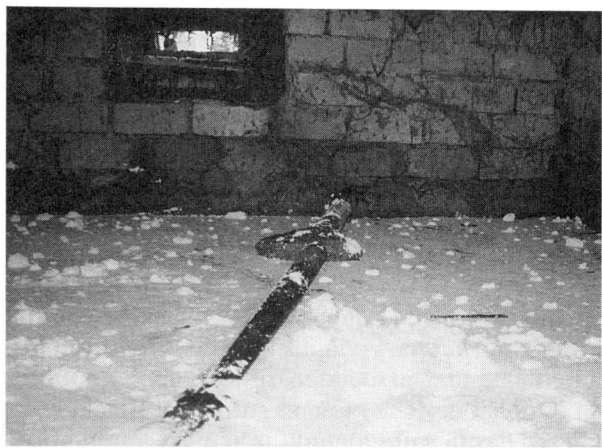

Figure 70.14 Flooded cellar (heavily infested with *C. quinquefasciatus*) in Zanzibar after treatment with polystyrene beads. (Courtesy of C. Curtis.)

same *Anopheles* species or vectors with similar bionomics, filariasis control may benefit from malaria vector control programmes. In the Solomon Islands, bancroftian filariasis was eliminated as a result of a malaria control programme utilizing residual insecticides against *Anopheles* mosquitoes.[81]

Residual insecticides have also been used against *Mansonia* vectors in India.[1] However, due to variability in feeding behaviour and resting places of *Mansonia* mosquitoes, control using insecticides is not very effective. Because *Aedes* vectors bite mainly by day and have scattered and inaccessible breeding sites, vector control in the absence of chemotherapy is not recommended.

Disadvantages of using chemical insecticides in control schemes may include their high cost, development of resistance by the target organisms and environmental damage. Despite these problems insecticides remain the major weapon in the control of vectors. The use of pyrethroid-impregnated bed-nets can significantly reduce morbidity due to malaria and impregnated bed-nets are being evaluated for the control of lymphatic filariasis.[40] Several biological control methods are also being assessed. *Bacillus sphaericus*, a spore-forming bacteria, shows promise for vector control.

PROPHYLAXIS

In India a prophylactic effect of DEC in *W. bancrofti* has been shown.[40] Progress towards the prevention of filariasis by immunization is slow. Even in animal models little information is available about the mechanism of protective immunity in lymphatic filariasis.

ONCHOCERCIASIS

Onchocerciasis (river blindness) results from infection with *Onchocerca volvulus*. Man is the natural host and the vectors are species of blackflies (*Simulium* spp.).

Since the early 1970s, an enormous amount of information has been generated by the activities of the Onchocerciasis Control Programme (OCP) in West Africa. Despite the information that is now available, our knowledge of the aetiology of the blinding eye lesions, and the factors that govern their progression, remains meagre.

HISTORICAL BACKGROUND

In 1875, in the Gold Coast (now Ghana), microfilariae were described by O'Neill.[82] These microfilariae were in the skin of Africans suffering from 'craw-craw'. Later (1893) Leuckart named the parasite *Filaria volvulus*. Robles,[83] working in Guatemala, first associated subcutaneous nodules with eye lesions. The pioneer studies of Blacklock[84] in Sierra Leone culminated in the next landmark— the discovery of the life cycle of *O. volvulus*. A detailed history of onchocerciasis has been written.[85]

GEOGRAPHICAL DISTRIBUTION

It is estimated that about 17.5 million persons worldwide are infected with *O. volvulus* (C. P. R. Ramachandran, personal communication, 1994) (Figures 70.15 and 70.16). More than 95% of all cases are in Africa in a zone that spreads from west to east. This band extends between 15° N and 15° S in the west, widening towards the east to reach the lower southern latitude in Malawi. Nigeria accounts for over one-third of the global prevalence of onchocerciasis.

Foci in Guatemala and Mexico of about 55 000 infected persons exist mainly on the Pacific slope of the Sierra Madra between altitudes of 500 and 1500 m. Smaller foci have been found in Venezuela, Columbia, Brazil, Ecuador, Yemen and Saudi Arabia.

LIFE CYCLE, TRANSMISSION AND DISTRIBUTION IN HUMANS

The general filarial life cycle is shown in Figure 70.1. For details of the life cycle of *O. volvulus*, see Appendix III.

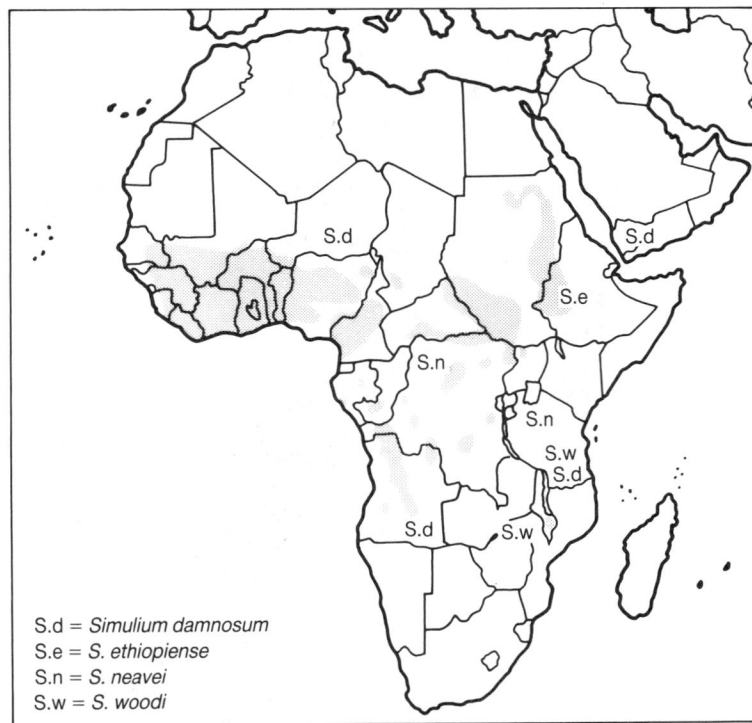

S.d = *Simulium damnosum*
S.e = *S. ethiopiense*
S.n = *S. neavei*
S.w = *S. woodi*

Figure 70.15 Geographical distribution of onchocerciasis in Africa and the Arabian Peninsula.

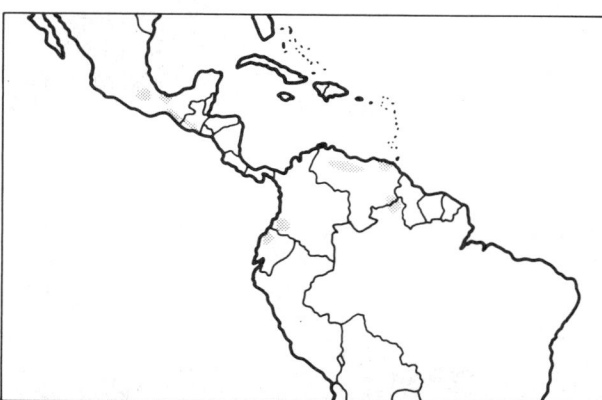

Figure 70.16 Geographical distribution of onchocerciasis in Central and South America.

Adult worms live in subcutaneous nodules or are free in the skin. The ratio of adult females ...es in nodules is about 3:1. The adults are slender white worms, the male 2.5 cm × 0.2 mm and the females 35–70 cm × 0.4 mm. The female produces sheathless microfilariae measuring 300 × 0.8 μm with a sharply pointed precurved tail (Figure 70.17a).

Microfilariae are mainly found in the upper dermis and in nodules but may also appear in blood, urine or any body fluid, particularly after treatment with DEC.

Microfilarial loads may be as high as 2000/mg of skin. They are common in the eye, with direct spread from adjacent skin appearing to be their main mode of entry. Other routes into the eye may be by the bloodstream, along the sheath of the posterior ciliary vessels and perhaps the cerebrospinal fluid along the optic sheath.[86]

Microfilariae present in the skin are ingested by the *Simulium* vector when feeding. Some of the ingested microfilariae migrate from the gut of the blackfly into the thoracic muscles and develop into infective larvae over a period of 6–8 days (for a description of the development in the fly, see Appendix III and for the life history of *Simulium* see Appendix IV). Transmission of infective larvae occur when the fly takes its next blood meal. Infection in humans begins with this penetration of the skin by infective larvae. They develop over several months to adult worms. The gravid female then releases microfilariae, which are found in the skin after a prepatent period of 7–34 months following the introduction of infective larvae.[87]

Simulium flies can only breed in well-oxygenated water. The gravid female oviposits into free-flowing rivers and streams, particularly in rapids, and transmission mainly takes place near these locations. Hence the name 'river blindness'.

Transmission in utero of microfilariae of *O. volvulus* has been reported.[88]

CLINICAL FEATURES

The main clinical manifestations of onchocerciasis are dermatitis, eye lesions and nodule (onchocer-

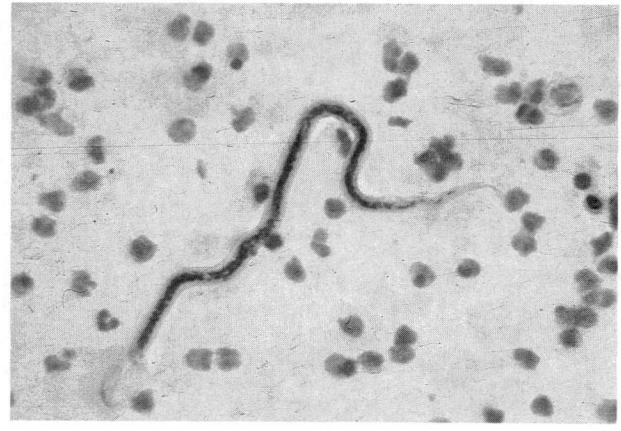

(a)

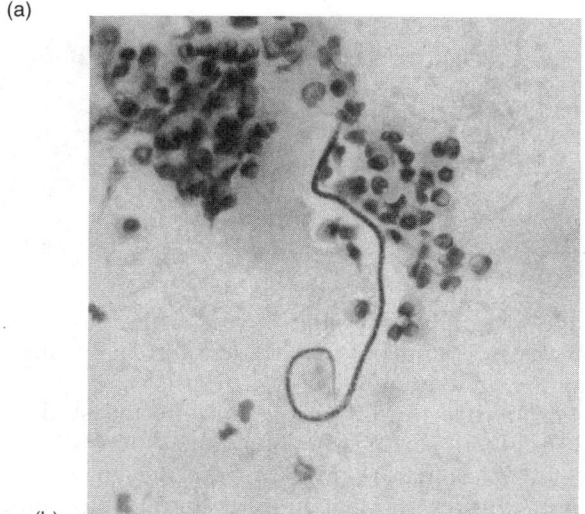

(b)

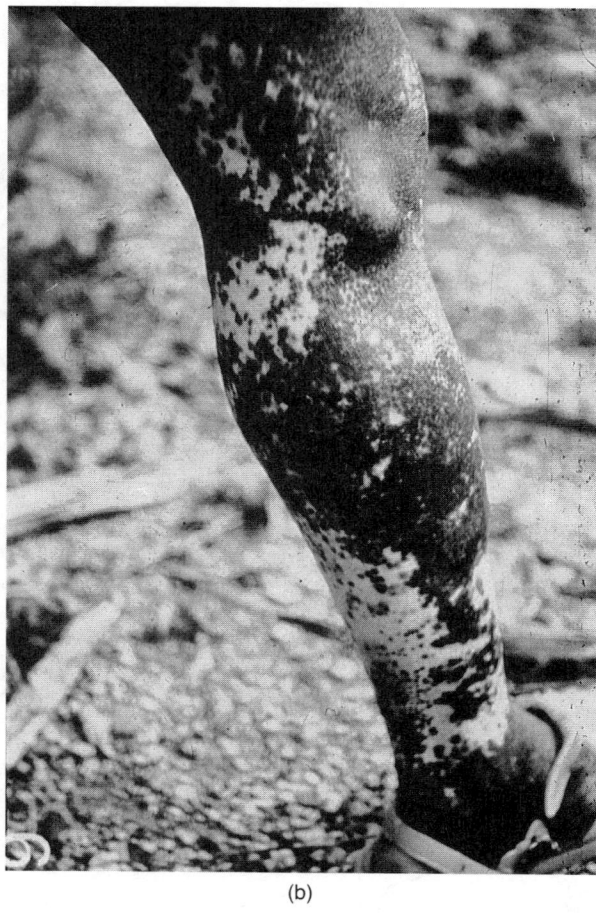

(b)

Figure 70.17   Skin microfilariae: (a) *O. volvulus*; (b) *M. streptocerca*; (c) See Figure 70.38 for *M. ozzardi*.

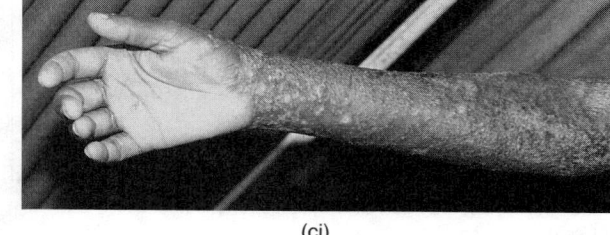

(ci)

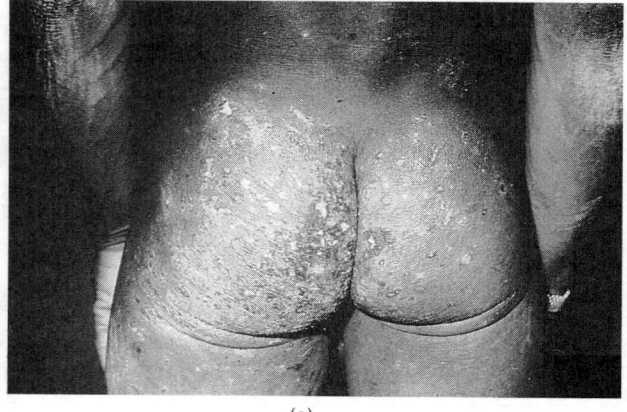

(a)

Figure 70.18   Onchocerciasis: skin lesions. (a) Papule formation and scratching (Courtesy of WHO); (b) depigmentation and leopard skin (Courtesy of WHO); (c) eczematoid dermatitis: (i) arm, (ii) leg. (Courtesy of D. Morgan.)

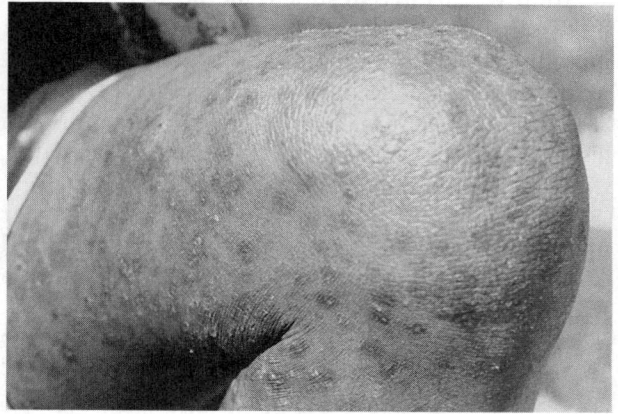

(cii)

coma) formation. There is a broad spectrum of both skin and ocular lesions. Many persons who have microfilariae in the skin, especially those with light infections, have no symptoms or signs.

SKIN LESIONS

Dermal changes occur when the microfilariae are undergoing destruction and vary from a few papules to the extensive pigmentary and chronic atrophic changes of presbyderma (premature aged appearance).

Frequently a combination of skin atrophy, hypo- and hyperpigmentation exist in the same person. Papules are due to microabscess formation and may disappear within a few days or spread. Usually the rash is confined to one anatomical quarter of the body or to a 'butterfly' distribution on the buttocks. The resulting pruritus can be very intense ('gale filarienne', filarial itch). A range of skin lesions is shown in Figure 70.18.

The more chronic changes are probably related to the repeated occurrence of local pathology around dying parasites. A condition called leopard skin (Figure 70.18b) may occur. This results from loss of pigment, degeneration of the dermal collagen and thinning of the epidermis. Leopard skin particularly affects the pretibial regions, where trauma or scratching following the bites of *Simulium* flies may exacerbate, or even cause, the depigmentation of this condition.

In Africa, the skin lesions are most common over the lower limbs but may cover the whole body. A localized eczematoid dermatitis with hyperkeratosis and pigmentary changes may occur. In the later stages there is a heavy lichenification and thickening of the skin (xeroderma or lizard skin).

Sowda

Sowda (Figure 70.19), from the Arabic for black or dark, is a localized form of onchocerciasis. It is common in the Yemen but is also found in the northern Sudan and in West Africa. It has been described in Guatemala.

Sowda is the result of a strong immune response on the part of the host. The condition is usually localized to one limb but both legs and/or arms or the trunk may be involved. It is characterized by intense itching. The involved skin becomes swollen and darkened and covered with scaly papules. Local lymph glands are enlarged. Microfilariae are extremely difficult to find in skin snips.

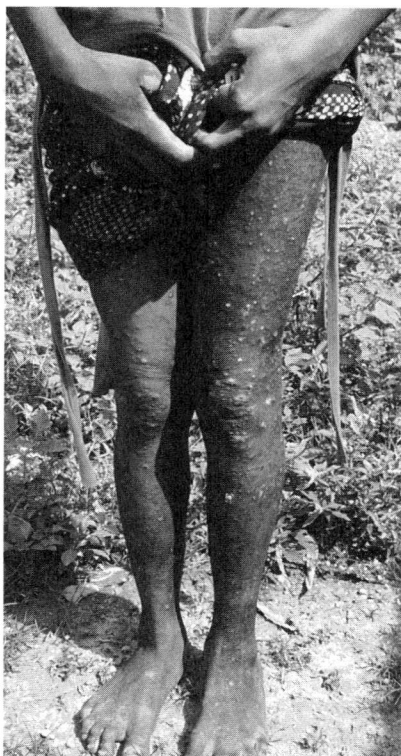

Figure 70.19 Onchocerciasis: Sowda. (Courtesy of D. Morgan.)

NODULES

Nodules are subcutaneous granulomas resulting from the tissue reaction around adult worms. They are painless, round to oval, firm, smooth, vary in size from a few millimetres to several centimetres and are often matted together in clumps (Figure 70.20).

In Africa 80% of nodules occur on the body prominences of the pelvic girdle (iliac crest, coccyx, sacrum and greater trochanter). Others occur on the abdomen, chest wall, head or limbs (Figure 70.21).

In Central America nodules are commonly found on the head. It is believed that the location of the nodules reflects the biting habits of the vector flies. Nodules do not cause medical problems unless they press on vital areas. Large clumps are often aesthetically displeasing to the patient. Some, perhaps one-quarter of nodules, are not detectable.

EYE LESIONS

Many changes in both anterior and posterior segments can occur in the eyes of infected individuals. The more serious lesions may progress to blindness (see p. 127 and Chapter 10).

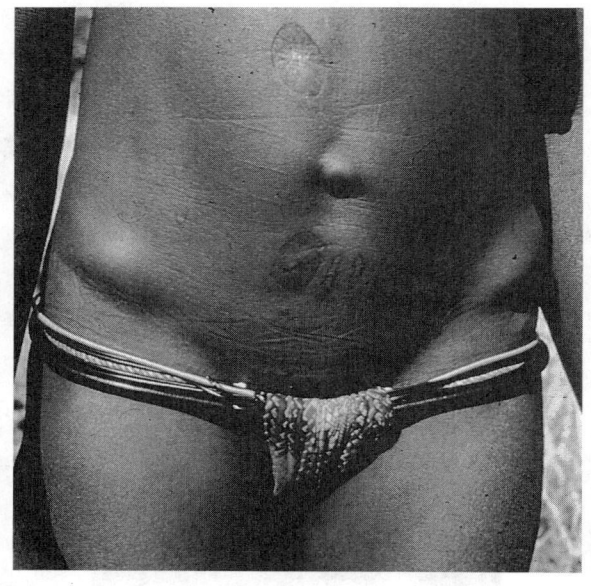

(a)

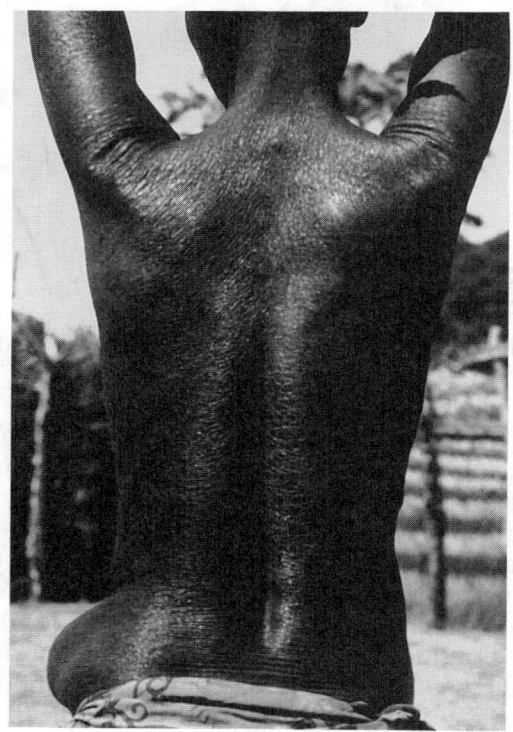

(b)

Figure 70.20 (a) and (b) Onchocerciasis: clumps of nodules over iliac crests. (Courtesy of the Institute of Child Health, London.)

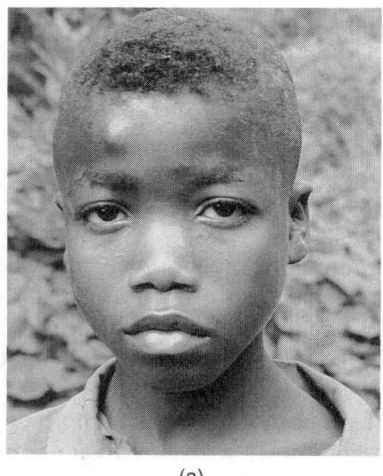

(a)

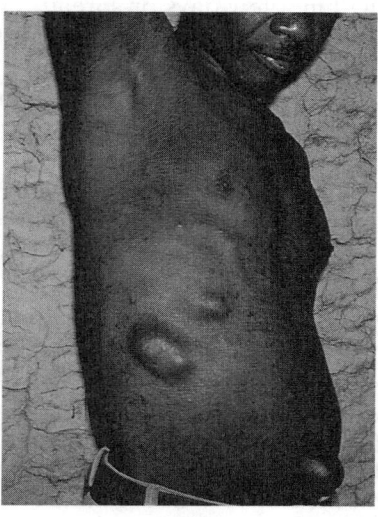

(b)

Figure 70.21 Onchocerciasis: nodule on (a) head; (b) lower chest. (Courtesy of D. Morgan.)

Anterior segment lesions

Punctate keratitis (snowflake opacities) occurs as an acute inflammatory reaction around microfilariae (Figure 70.22). It appears to be the corneal equivalent of the discrete papule reactions seen in the skin. Punctate keratitis is more common in the younger

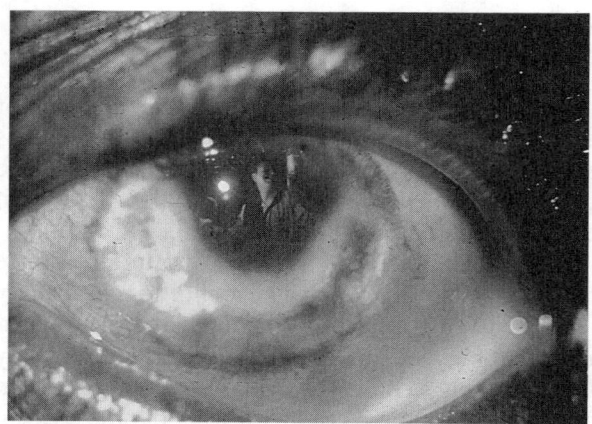

Figure 70.22 Onchocerciasis: punctate keratitis. (Courtesy of the Institute of Child Health, London.)

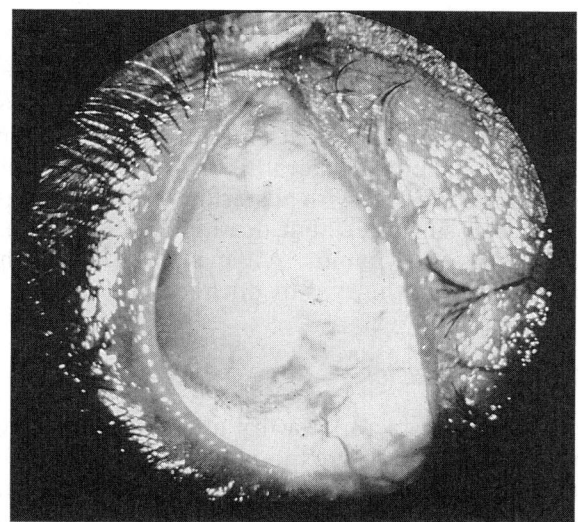

Figure 70.23 Onchocerciasis: sclerosing keratitis. (Courtesy of the Institute of Child Health, London.)

age groups. These lesions are reversible. In sclerosing keratitis, vascular infiltrates begin at the limbus and pass inwards, resulting in a cellular organization and excessive scarring of the cornea which causes blindness (Figure 70.23).

Microfilariae dying in the ciliary body give rise to iridocyclitis and the formation of synechiae. Inflammation of the uveal tract also contributes to iridial pathology.

Posterior segment lesions

Both optic nerve atrophy and choroidoretinitis of the posterior segment may result in blindness. Lesions of choroidoretinitis range from unequivocal inflammatory process to exclusively atrophic lesions with atrophy of the retinal pigment epithelium and of the choriocapillaris and hyperpigmentation of the pigment epithelial layer.[89]

Advanced optic nerve atrophy is usually signified by a large glaucoma cup. Optic nerve atrophy rather than choroidoretinal degeneration is considered to be an important cause of both decreased visual acuity and visual field constriction. Acceleration of optic nerve damage may follow treatment with DEC. In fact, with any of the eye lesions, exacerbation associated with the death of microfilariae may be a complication of drug therapy.

CLINICAL PICTURE IN FOREST AND SAVANNA ZONES OF WEST AFRICA

Clinical manifestations (skin and eye lesions) are known to differ widely in varied endemic geographi-

cal areas. Surveys in the United Cameroun Republic showed the prevalence of sclerosing keratitis and blindness to be much higher in savanna than in forest areas.[90] The OCP considered that there was a gradation from very severe ocular lesions in the dry (Sudan)-type savanna, to moderately severe in wet savanna areas, to a much lower prevalence of eye lesions in forest zones. However, surveys conducted in Sierra Leone by the Medical Research Council Laboratory revealed the prevalence of blindness and sclerosing keratitis to be higher in the forest than in the savanna areas of that country.[91–93] (Figure 70.24).

Similar results in Sierra Leone have since been reported by OCP.[94] These studies emphasize the need for epidemiological studies to be conducted prior to instituting control measures. Reasons for the higher prevalence of blinding lesions in forest than in savanna regions of Sierra Leone include the siting of villages away from *Simulium damnosum* s.l. breeding sites and a less dense and more scattered population in the northern savanna.

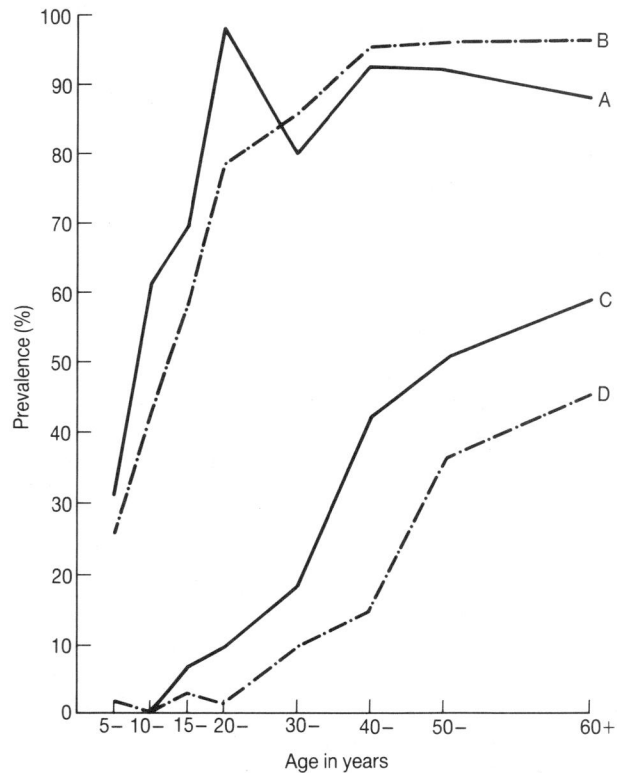

Figure 70.24 Onchocerciasis: the prevalence of onchocerciasis based on the presence of microfilariae in iliac crest and/or canthus skin snips in males (A) and females (B), and the prevalence of blindness and/or severe eye lesions in males (C) and females (D) as seen in rain forest villages of Sierra Leone. (After McMahon et al.[91–93])

PATHOGENESIS OF BLINDING EYE LESIONS

Following years of controversy among ophthalmologists concerning the ocular manifestations of onchocerciasis, it is now accepted that the main blinding lesions are the anterior segment changes (sclerosing keratitis and iritis) and the posterior segment lesions (choroidoretinitis and optic atrophy). Possible parasite, host and environmental factors of relevance to the pathogenesis and the difference in prevalence of the different lesions in various ecological zones are given below.

Parasite factors

A more virulent strain of parasite may be transmitted in dry savanna than in wet forest areas. A marked differentiation of DNA of the forest and savanna strains has been demonstrated.[95]

A study conducted in West Africa revealed a close association between microfilariae at three sites (outer canthus, cornea and anterior chamber) and sclerosing keratitis and iritis.[91] The association with the posterior segment lesion optic atrophy was also significant but in both the savanna and forest areas of the study the association with choroidoretinitis was either absent or very weak. This lack of association between choroidoretinitis and microfilariae could reflect a different pathogenesis for this compared with the other three lesions. In anterior segment lesions there is direct contact between the microfilariae and tissues.[91] The inflammatory pathological reaction associated with sclerosing keratitis is considered to be associated with the death of microfilariae. In contrast to their presence in the cornea, microfilariae have rarely been seen in the retina in vivo. Microfilariae were seen in the vitreous humour in 6% of persons examined[90] and experimental evidence has been produced to show that choroidoretinal degenerative changes occur in rabbits following intravitreal injection of microfilariae of *O. volvulus*.[96] An excellent ophthalmological study in humans noted that atrophic changes may be the predominant changes in choroidoretinitis.[89] It seems feasible that the slow death of microfilariae in the vitreous humour over months or years may produce a slower reaction in the choroidoretinal tissue than that produced when microfilariae are in direct contact with the tissue. It is possible that microfilariae secrete a substance toxic to retinal tissue. Studies in areas where transmission of onchocerciasis has been interrupted by vector control have shown that an important factor in predisposing to blindness was the presence of a heavy load of microfilariae in the eye at the initial examination.[97]

Host factors

The role of the immune response of the host in the pathogenesis of eye lesions is not understood. At present more evidence exists for the inflammatory reaction of sclerosing keratitis having an immune basis than is the case with posterior segment lesions. It has been suggested that nutritional deficiencies, particularly of vitamin A, may aggravate the damage done to the eyes by onchocerciasis.

Environmental factors

Environmental factors—a dry atmosphere, photophobic effect, dust or exposure to higher levels of ultraviolet radiation—may in combination or separately result in damage to the cornea.[91] All of these factors are likely to be higher in dry savanna than in rain forest zones.

PATHOLOGY AND IMMUNOLOGY

Large numbers of live microfilariae may be present in the skin without inducing any tissue reaction (Figure 70.25). Pathology in the skin and in the anterior segment of the eye is caused mainly by dying and dead microfilariae.

The initial lesions comprise foci of inflammatory reactions around degenerating microfilariae, composed mainly of eosinophils, neutrophils and macrophages.[98,99] IgG antibodies, immune complex formation and complement activation on the surface of the microfilariae may be involved in attracting the immunocompetent cells.[100] The dermal tissue between the early focal lesions shows no changes. Later, dermal fibroblasts increase in numbers, leading to fibrosis, and the normal collagen and elastic fibres of the dermis are gradually replaced by hyalinized scar tissue. There may also be loss of pigment in the skin. The histological appearance of the skin in advanced cases closely resembles the skin of very

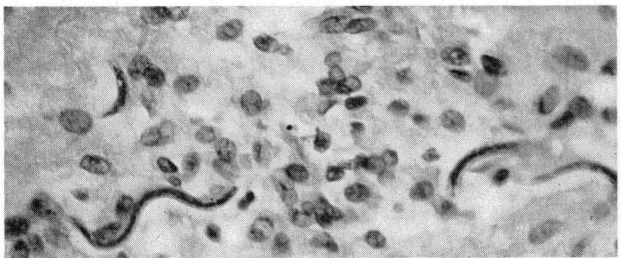

Figure 70.25   Onchocerciasis: microfilariae of *O. volvulus* in subcutaneous tissue.

old subjects, i.e. presbyderma. Some of the skin damage observed in onchocerciasis patients may also be caused by the mechanical effects of scratching, by toxins inoculated when blackflies take a blood meal or by secondary infections.

In the skin condition Sowda there is a very marked immunological response, the most striking histopathological feature being the presence of an extensive inflammatory cell infiltrate of the upper dermis.[101] Sclerosis and oedema of the dermis may be prominent features. Microfilariae are extremely difficult to find in tissue sections.[35,102,103]

Using a slit lamp, live microfilariae can be seen in the cornea of the eye. There is no visible tissue response to their presence. Dead microfilariae give rise to foci of inflammation which cause the characteristic punctate ('snowflake') keratitis, with opacities around each microfilaria. The major pathology of the anterior segment is due to sclerosing keratitis. Chronic inflammation and vascularization leading to scarring eventually results in complete opacification of the cornea. This process normally starts from each side and from below (see Chapter 10) and resembles an inflammatory immune response. The aetiology of the posterior segment lesions is less clear. Autoantibodies against retinal proteins, cross-reacting with antibodies against *Onchocerca* antigens, were thought to be involved, but a recent study showed no relationship between the antiretinal antibody levels and the occurrence of choroidoretinitis in ocular onchocerciasis.[104] There is no evidence that DEC treatment worsens already existing posterior segment lesions. This is in contrast to its effect in sclerosing keratitis, where dying microfilariae accelerate pathogenesis.

Some adult worms are found free in the subcutaneous tissues but most are contained in nodules. Nodules are essentially granulomatous reactions around adult worms. They often have separate chambers containing several worms. Nodules have thick fibrous walls with a variable degree of cellular infiltration (Figure 70.26). Calcification may occur in older nodules and in dead worms. Lipid-filled macrophages occupy zones adjacent to the centre of nodules.[105] Lipid accumulation was not found to be related to the clinical status of the patient. The origin and functional significance of this lipid is unknown.

Due to constant exposure the humoral responses of people living in areas endemic for onchocerciasis are usually marked.[35,106] Patients with different clinical forms of onchocerciasis show a different recognition of antigens.[107] Patients with Sowda often have stronger IgG3 responses to *Onchocerca* antigens than persons with other clinical manifestations of onchocerciasis.[103] *Onchocerca* antigens

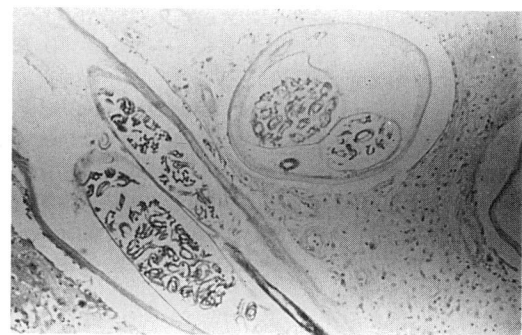

Figure 70.26 Onchocerciasis: adult *O. volvulus* in nodule. (Courtesy of H. Zaiman.)

have been demonstrated in the breast milk of *O. volvulus*-infected women.[108] Antibodies mediating cellular killing of microfilariae and infective larvae in vitro have been observed in sera from some persons living in endemic areas.[100,109] The presence of such antibodies may indicate that immune elimination of larval stages occurs in some infected individuals, although protective immunity has not been proved in onchocerciasis.

There is evidence that most patients with onchocerciasis have a diminished cellular responsiveness to *O. volvulus* antigens in comparison to apparently uninfected persons from the same endemic areas and to patients with the more localized Sowda.[102,110,111] This relative hyporesponsiveness seems to be broader and less specific than that found in patients with lymphatic filariasis. Diminished cellular immune responses to tetanus and BCG vaccinations and an increased prevalence of lepromatous leprosy have been reported from areas endemic for *O. volvulus* infection.[112]

DIAGNOSIS

CLINICAL DIAGNOSIS

For the diagnosis and differential diagnosis of onchocercal eye lesions see Chapter 10.

The pruritic onchodermatitis (filarial itch) must be distinguished from: infection with *Mansonella streptocerca*, in which the lower limbs are rarely affected; scabies, where the typical burrows and mites can be found between the fingers; insect bites which come on early after residence in the tropics; prickly heat; contact dermatitis; and sycosis cruris, a chronic low-grade bacterial infection of the legs. In heavy infections of long standing the skin changes must be differentiated from tertiary yaws, superficial mycoses, leprosy and chronic eczema.

Scrotal oedema of onchocerciasis may be confused with lymph scrotum (see Figure 70.10) of lymphatic filariasis.

Painlessness, firmness and extreme mobility are characteristic of onchocercomas. However, some nodules, particularly those on the head, become fixed due to adherence to underlying tissues. Nodules must be distinguished from enlarged lymph glands, lipomas, dermal cysts, ganglia and neurofibromas.

Ultrasonography

Ultrasound scanning has proved capable of distinguishing onchocercal nodules in the tissues of patients.[113,114] This technique may be especially useful for detecting deep non-palpable nodules.

Mazzotti test

This test involves the administration of a small dose (usually 50 mg for an adult) of DEC by mouth. The death of microfilariae in the skin results in a reaction between 20 minutes and 24 hours later of intense pruritus, with the appearance of a skin rash or the exacerbation of an existing one. This test may precipitate serious complications and is not recommended as a routine diagnostic procedure. Either false-negative or false-positive results may also occur. The Mazzotti test can assist diagnosis when onchocerciasis is suspected in persons with a negative skin snip.

A Mazzotti patch test using a topical application of DEC has been devised. The administration of DEC in lotion form may produce more severe reactions than administration by the oral route. The patch method is dangerous and should not be used.

PARASITOLOGICAL DIAGNOSIS

The diagnosis is made by demonstrating microfilariae that have emerged from bloodless skin snips. Although most persons with clinical signs have positive skin snips this is not always the case. The optimal site for the biopsy depends on the geographical area. In Africa, the preferred bodily site is from the iliac crest or below, whereas in Mexico the skin over the scapula or deltoid region is favoured. Two to four skin snips are taken. When epidemiological and clinical studies of onchocercal eye lesions are being conducted, it is important to take a skin snip from the outer canthus.

After cleaning the skin with spirit and allowing to dry, a razor blade can be used to shave off the tip of a dome of skin that has been elevated with a needle. Alternatively a Walser corneoscleral punch is used to produce skin snips with an average weight of

1.0 mg. Punches must be very carefully sterilized before reuse. Snips should be immersed in isotonic saline, not water.[115] Microfilariae that have emerged after 10–20 minutes are counted under the low power of a compound microscope. Teasing the skin is unnecessary. Subsequent digestion of the snip by collagenase revealed that more than 80% of microfilariae had emerged prior to digestion.[115] Microfilariae of *O. volvulus* are 270–320 μm long, unsheathed, and have a characteristic head and a pointed tail (see Figure 70.17). They must be differentiated from the smaller skin-dwelling microfilariae of *M. streptocerca* in Africa and *M. ozzardi* in South America. Blood microfilariae—*Wuchereria bancrofti*, *Loa loa* and *M. perstans*—occasionally appear in skin snips contaminated by blood.

IMMUNODIAGNOSIS

Several immunodiagnostic tests have been devised for onchocerciasis, including those based on IFAT and ELISA techniques.[116] The source of antigen used is mainly adult *O. volvulus* isolated from nodules, or adult worms or microfilariae of *O. gibsoni* or *O. gutturosa* from cattle. Generally, immunodiagnosis based on detection of antibodies to crude antigens is of limited practical use due to the low specificity and sensitivity of the tests. Cross-reactions to other nematode infections are common and the tests cannot distinguish between past and present infections. In endemic areas, where the population is continuously exposed to infection, most people are positive to the tests. Such tests may be of value in assisting in the diagnosis of onchocerciasis in persons from non-endemic areas who have visited an endemic area.

The development of specific and sensitive immunodiagnostic tests is a priority in onchocerciasis research. The specificity of tests has been improved by detection for specific IgE and IgG4 antibodies[28,117] and for circulating antigens.[118,119] Tests utilizing specific recombinant antigens are being developed,[120] and an ELISA based on a cocktail made from three of these antigens has shown a high sensitivity and 100% specificity.[121] Tests utilizing another cloned *O. volvulus* antigen are able to detect human infections long before the appearance of microfilariae.[122]

A polymerase chain reaction technique with high specificity for *O. volvulus* DNA has recently been developed.[123] In addition to identifying worm DNA from infected humans, this technique is capable of detecting *O. volvulus* larvae in extracts of blackfly vectors. DNA probes to distinguish blinding and non-blinding forms of onchocerciasis are also being field tested.

TREATMENT

DRUG TREATMENT

For more than 40 years, DEC has been the drug of choice for the treatment of onchocerciasis. It has recently been replaced by ivermectin (Mectizan). Both these drugs have a strong microfilaricidal effect (see Table 70.2). A potential macrofilaricidal activity of higher dosage regimens of ivermectin needs further investigation.

Metrifonate, mebendazole and other benzimidazole derivatives that are antifilarial are less effective than DEC or ivermectin and are largely being replaced by ivermectin. Suramin, although largely used as a macrofilaricide, also has some microfilaricidal effects. Fatalities due to drug toxicity may occur and its use is not recommended. Toxic reactions include exfoliative dermatitis, ulceration of the mouth and tongue, prolonged high fever, severe prostration and heavy albuminuria. A new macrofilaricidal drug Amocarzine (CGP 6140) is presently undergoing clinical trials.

Diethylcarbamazine

In 1947, DEC was found to be an effective microfilaricide in onchocerciasis.[124] Adverse reactions subsequently known as 'Mazzotti reactions' have been used diagnostically to detect the presence of *O. volvulus* infection. DEC has little demonstrable effect on parasite metabolism but is intricately associated with the host's immune response. There is no evidence that it has any effect on adult worms.

Adverse reactions associated with DEC therapy may be local (pruritus, skin rash, exacerbation of eye lesions) or systemic effects. These include fever, headache, joint and muscle pains, postural hypotension, collapse, respiratory distress or vertigo. The reactions induced by DEC are considered to be due to an accelerated destruction of microfilariae. Because of the severity of some of the reactions, DEC is being replaced by ivermectin as the microfilaricide of choice in onchocerciasis.

If DEC is administered, the clinical severity of reactions can be reduced by starting treatment with very low doses, which are then gradually increased, and by the use of antiinflammatory drugs. The initial dose of DEC recommended for the first 1–2 days is 25 mg or 50 mg for an adult (0.5–1.0 mg/kg). This is increased to 100 mg (2.0 mg/kg) twice daily for 5–7 days so that the total drug dose given is approximately 1.3 g (30 mg/kg). Betamethazone is the drug of choice for damping down inflammatory reactions.

Aspirin can be very useful for the treatment of severe side-effects of DEC.

Ivermectin

Ivermectin in a single oral dose of 150 μg/kg body weight causes a rapid elimination of microfilariae from the skin.[125] More than 80% of skin microfilariae are eliminated in the first 48 hours and this then slowly increases to 97%. The disappearance of microfilariae from the eye is much more gradual than microfilarial reduction in the skin. Retreatment may be necessary and follow-up skin snips should be examined 6–12 months after the initial treatment.

Adverse reactions resemble, but appear to be much less severe than, those associated with DEC therapy. The frequency of side-effects reported by various investigators varies between less than 10 and 60%. In a forest zone in Sierra Leone[126] the most common side-effect of ivermectin was the passing of ascaris worms! Other effects in descending order of frequency were: itching and/or rash, muscle and/or joint pains, fever, headache, swelling of the limbs, joint or face, dizziness, tender lymphadenopathy, conjunctivitis and tender nodules. Other investigators have noted severe postural hypotension and bronchoconstriction to be side-effects of ivermectin therapy. These conditions are reported to be transient and to respond to symptomatic management.

The single dose ivermectin regimens used by investigators has no known long-lasting effect on mature worms, but the drug causes intrauterine degeneration and temporary sequestration of unborn microfilariae.[127] Multiple monthly or twice yearly doses kill a small proportion of male and female adult worms.[128]

Ivermectin shows promise as an effective microfilaricidal drug for the treatment of onchocerciasis. It has fewer side-effects, especially ocular complications, than DEC. More information is needed on possible drug toxicity and total dosage of ivermectin required to kill adult worms and the frequency and spacing of doses for preventing further ocular and dermal lesions in infected persons. Because neurotoxic reactions in dogs appear to be related to the concentration of ivermectin within the central nervous system, information is needed as to whether, in humans, the blood–brain barrier for ivermectin could be dangerously lowered.

NODULECTOMY

Nodulectomy has only limited use because many worms are present outside the nodules and some nodules are not palpable. Head nodules should be excised because their presence increases the risk of blindness.

EPIDEMIOLOGY

ENDEMICITY

Many different criteria have been used for defining the level of endemicity of onchocerciasis in a population. The OCP classify levels as sporadic, hypo-, meso- or hyperendemic on the basis of the age-standardized microfilarial prevalence being <10, 10–29, 30–59 and 60+%, respectively.

In a hyperendemic zone of Sierra Leone the following criteria were used to evaluate the true prevalence of onchocerciasis: (1) microfilariadermia in skin snips; (2) the presence of at least one nodule (Table 70.3) or any other clinical sign of onchocerciasis; and (3) microfilariae in the anterior chamber or cornea of the eye. Combining these criteria, based on the presence of at least one of them, the overall prevalence of onchocerciasis increased by 10% compared with when the prevalence was based on the microfilarial rate alone.[93]

Some investigators consider that the risk of ocular complications relates more closely to the annual transmission potential (ATP) than to the level of endemicity. The ATP is the total number of infective larvae of *O. volvulus* which could be inoculated into one person in a year should all the flies biting him or her transmit their total load of infective larvae.[129] Although a useful quantitative measure of the transmission of onchocerciasis, the ATP is a gross overestimate of the number of larvae actually inoculated.

Some factors involving parasite, host and vector that are important for understanding the epidemiology of onchocerciasis are mentioned below.

Parasite

The microfilariae of *O. volvulus* are morphologically indistinguishable throughout the range of the parasite. In West Africa there are at least four different patterns of acid phosphatase distribution on isoenzyme analysis, and significant differences between forest and savanna strains.[131,132] There is such a degree of *Onchocerca–Simulium* adaptation that there is incompatibility between parasite strains and vectors from different geographical areas.[133] Blinding lesions are more severe in the dry savanna than in forest areas and there is evidence that a forest strain has lower ocular pathogenicity than a savanna strain. However, when considering the pathogenicity of eye lesions, as well as possible strain difference of the parasite it is also important to consider environmental factors that may be involved (see p. 126). The relation between onchocercal eye lesions and the presence of microfilariae in the skin and orbital tissues is discussed on p. 124.

Host

Human host factors to be considered are occupation, seasonal migration, changes in habits or in economic or social standing of the population, concurrent infections and differences of prevalence in different age, sex and racial groups. For example, in the Yemen a severe form of Sowda occurs. Also in Ecuador, in the same endemic area American Indians were more likely than Blacks to have generalized atrophic changes of the skin.[134]

Vector

Crucial factors in the transmission of onchocerciasis are the density, biting and infectivity rates and flight range of the vectors.

AFRICAN ONCHOCERCIASIS

Members of the *Simulium damnosum* complex are the predominant vectors in most of the endemic areas of Africa (see Appendix IV). In parts of East and Central Africa species of *S. neavei* also transmit the infection.

Flies of the *S. damnosum* complex breed in large rivers or small streams where there is an adequate velocity of water, adequate food supplies and suitable attachment sites (rocks, sticks, trailing vegetation). A primary larval habitat is rivers in which exposed rocks create 'white water' rapids. Female blackflies generally restrict their flight to within a

Table 70.3 The prevalence of pruritus and nodules by age and sex as seen in a rain forest village of Sierre Leone endemic for onchocerciasis. (After McMahon et al.[130])

Age (years)	No. examined	% with pruritus	% with nodules
1–4	70	1.4	0.0
5–9	82	2.4	8.5
10–14	67	6.0	20.9
15–19	29	20.7	31.0
20–29	68	30.9	44.1
30–39	73	30.1	54.8
40–49	79	46.8	79.7
50–59	59	50.8	89.8
60+	71	50.7	85.9
Total	598	26.6	46.3

few kilometres of breeding sites and bite most intensely in the immediate vicinity. However, with the assistance of prevailing winds they may migrate several hundred kilometres from one river basin to another.

The female flies feed mainly on man but in some areas blood meals are also taken from animals, particularly bovines, horses and small ruminants. *S. damnosum* s.l. is a complex of numerous sibling species which differ in bionomics and vectorial capacity. They are very similar morphologically but can be distinguished by the banding patterns of their larval chromosomes.

West Africa

The six main West African members of the *S. damnosum* complex can be separated in three pairs. The pairs are: *S. damnosum* s.s./*S. sirbanum*; *S. sanctipauli*/*S. soubrense*; and *S. yahense*/*S. squamosum*. The geographical distribution of these species is considerably influenced by local climatic and ecological characteristics. The first two are termed 'savanna' species, and the other four 'forest' species. The *S. damnosum* s.s./*S. sirbanum* pair occupy the savanna zone as far as 14° N, which is also the northern limit of the endemic area for onchocerciasis. These species may find their way into forest areas along the major water courses. The *S. sanctipauli*/*S. soubrense* pair is forest dwelling but spreads into the savanna up to 10° N. *S. yahense* is limited to small forest water courses and *S. squamosum* has a focal distribution in forest and savanna with a preference for small or medium-sized rivers in hilly and mountainous areas.

In the dry savanna, transmission of onchocerciasis is seasonal. This contrasts to a much longer transmission period in wet savanna and in forest areas.

Entomological surveys in the southern (forest) area of Sierra Leone between 1983 and 1987 revealed only a very limited distribution of savanna flies.[135-137] However, a more recent survey of blackfly breeding sites by the OCP showed that *S. damnosum* s.s. and *S. sirbanum* were widespread in both the northern and southern parts of Sierra Leone.[138] This invasion of savanna flies into forest areas of Sierra Leone appears to be a completely new phenomenon which may have major epidemiological consequences. Rainfall in Sierra Leone has shown a fluctuating decrease since 1949. The reasons postulated for this decline include sunspot activity, removal of the tropical rain forest and a reduction in atmospheric moisture related to changes in wind speed and wind patterns.[137] In West Africa ecological changes subsequent to this decrease in rainfall have probably encouraged the extension of the geographic range of savanna species of *S. damnosum* s.l. into areas previously only inhabited by forest species.

East and Central Africa

The most important vectors in East and Central Africa belong to the *S. damnosum* complex, but vectors of the *S. neavei* group also transmit onchocerciasis in Ethiopia, Tanzania, Uganda and parts of Zaire. This group includes all *Simulium* species with larvae and pupae that become attached to riverine crabs of the genus *Potamonautes*. In Tanzania, *S. woodi* is the most important vector within the *S. neavei* group. In the Tukuyu valley and Mahenge mountains transmission is by *S. damnosum* s.l.[139,140] In East Africa onchocerciasis rarely causes blindness.

Recently, a marked increase in the prevalence of onchocerciasis in Uganda has been reported (C. P. Ramachandran, personal communication, 1994).

CENTRAL AND SOUTH AMERICAN ONCHOCERCIASIS

In Latin America (see Figure 70.16) there are seven medically important species of the *Simulium amazonicum* group. A detailed study of their distribution, biology and role as vectors of human onchocerciasis (and mansonelliasis) has recently been published.[141] Similar studies have been made on the *S. exiguum* complex.[142]

Mexico and Guatemala

The principal vector is *S. ochraceum* s.l. It breeds in small streams at altitudes between 500 and 1500 m. Transmission is mainly confined to the dry season. In some foci there are many head nodules, and eye involvement is common.

Brazil, Venezuela, Columbia and Ecuador

The relative importance of onchocerciasis in some South American countries is difficult to assess because of conflicting data and the lack of recent epidemiological surveys. *S. exiguum* s.l. is the most widespread vector, occurring in all the known onchocerciasis foci of South America.

In Brazil, onchocerciasis occurs in the north, in the Amazonia, in a focus bordering Venezuela. The prevalence of onchocerciasis in this focus is not known.

In Venezuela, clinical manifestations in northern and eastern foci are mild and *S. metallicum* s.l. is the principal vector. In the south, onchocerciasis occurs in both highland and lowland areas, being hyperendemic in some groups of Yanomana Indians. *S. guianense* s.l. is the main vector in the highlands and *S. oyapockense* s.l. in the lowlands.

In the Western Andes, in Columbia, where *S. exiguum* s.l. is the vector, lesions are mild.

In Ecuador, onchocerciasis occurs in the northwestern coastal province of Esmeraldas and in particular it affects both Chachi Indians and the Black population of the Santiago river basin. Due to the presence of an efficient vector—*S. exiguum* s.l.—and migration of infected individuals, onchocerciasis is increasing in prevalence and becoming more widespread.[143] Severe skin and eye lesions exist in both races. Surveys show 60% of nodules occur on the pelvic girdle and 21.6% on the head[144] and blindness attributable to onchocerciasis to be 0.4%; iridocyclitis, optic atrophy and chorioretinopathy are 1.5, 5.1 and 28.0%, respectively.[145]

CONTROL

Antivector control, particularly larviciding of breeding sites, has been the main control measure used in onchocerciasis. To date all macrofilaricidal drugs have been too toxic for mass drug treatment against the parasite. As side-effects of the microfilaricide, DEC, may also be severe, it has not been widely used in control schemes. Ivermectin shows promise of being of value both in mass chemotherapeutic regimens and as a clinical prophylactic.

VECTOR CONTROL

Since 1974, the OCP has been engaged in a large scale attempt to control the savanna species of the vectors of onchocerciasis in seven West African countries (Burkino Faso, Benin, Côte d'Ivoire, Ghana, Mali, Niger and Togo) in the Volta River Basin area.[146] Successful vector control by aerial larviciding of *Simulium* breeding sites has reduced the parasite to such a level that it is close to being eliminated from the hyperendemic foci of the core area of the programme. The campaign has markedly reduced the incidence of skin and eye lesions, and the deterioration of existing eye lesions has also decreased.

The emergence of resistance to larvicides being applied and the reinvasion of treated areas from non-controlled areas are major problems that have been encountered. Attempts to counter the resistance problem have involved alternating the larvacides being used, whilst extension of the programme into countries to the west and south has reduced the reinvasion problem.

It is very important to know the environmental impact of larvicidal control. The continued use of larvicides over 20 years may have serious ecological problems. At least in the medium term temephos seems to have had no detrimental effects on fish. The cost of such a large control scheme is high. During wet seasons, a fleet of up to 11 helicopters and two fixed-wing aircraft operate over 23 000 km of rivers. The programme is now turning its emphasis to mass treatment with ivermectin.

Vector control programmes that have been on a much smaller scale than the OCP have been conducted in several African countries. *S. neavei* has been entirely eradicated from Kenya by larvicidal treatments, except for a small focus on the Ugandan border. Transmission has been completely interrupted and no new cases of onchocerciasis have been reported in any of the districts since the elimination of the vector.

CHEMOTHERAPEUTIC CONTROL

Community trials in several endemic areas have shown that ivermectin is acceptable for mass treatment.[147–150] It reduces the microfilarial burden and thus transmission in the community. Research is underway to assess the epidemiological impact of various dosage schemes of ivermectin. Currently a dose of 150 μg/kg body weight every 6 months or once yearly is being encouraged. [The manufacturer of ivermectin (Merck) has made the drug available free of charge through the Mectizan Donation Committee to governmental and non-governmental health care organizations involved in onchocerciasis control programmes.] Treatment is contraindicated in pregnant women, breast-feeding women with infants under 3 months old, children under 5 years old, or persons with serious acute or chronic illnesses.

Treatment with ivermectin resulted in regression of both early and advanced lesions of the anterior segment of the eye. Lesions of the posterior segment remained stable.[151] A single dose of the drug results in significant improvement of severe onchocercal skin disease.[152] As an additional benefit it reduces the prevalence and intensity of *Ascaris* infections.[153] There is evidence that repeated doses of ivermectin kill adult worms.[128]

Following the initial field testing of ivermectin, the OCP has now started large-scale distribution for morbidity control in the programme area.[146] Nigeria has initiated a nationwide onchocerciasis control programme with large-scale ivermectin treatment.[154] Numerous smaller control programmes utilizing mass treatment have been started in endemic areas. [The River Blindness Foundation, a voluntary organization established in the USA in 1990, distribute ivermectin to persons with onchocerciasis in the Third World, and is now involved in onchocerciasis control programmes in several African, and Central and South American countries.]

NODULECTOMY

Nodulectomy campaigns have been encouraged in some countries, especially in those where head nodules are common. The impact of such campaigns on ocular disease can be difficult to assess; for example, in Guatemala, where systematic campaigns have been associated with decreased blindness, other factors, particularly changes in socioeconomic conditions, may have decreased man–vector contact.

OTHER FILARIAL INFECTIONS

In addition to the filarial worms resulting in human lymphatic filariasis and onchocerciasis, four other species of filariae commonly infect man. These are *Loa loa*, *Mansonella perstans*, *M. streptocerca* and *M. ozzardi* (see Table 70.1). A few species of animal filariae cause rare zoonotic infections in man.

LOA LOA

Loa loa is a filarial parasite of man in parts of West and Central Africa.[155] It is commonly known as the 'eye-worm', since adult worms are occasionally seen to move across the eye of the patient.

LIFE CYCLE AND TRANSMISSION

Adult *L. loa* live and move around in the connective tissues of man. They frequently wander through the subcutaneous tissues and may sometimes pass beneath the conjunctiva of the eye. The females measure $50–70 \times 0.5$ mm and the males $30–35 \times 0.4$ mm. More detailed morphology is given in Appendix IV. The sheathed microfilariae circulate in the blood and measure $230–300 \times 6–8 \mu m$ (Figure 70.27).

Human *L. loa* is transmitted by tabanid flies of the genus *Chrysops*. The microfilarial periodicity is adapted to the day-biting habits of the vectors. It is diurnal, with peak concentration in the peripheral blood around noon (Figure 70.28). Microfilariae ingested by the vectors during feeding penetrate the stomach wall of the flies and migrate to the fat body where they develop in 8–10 days. Infective larvae (2 mm $\times 25 \mu m$) then move via the thorax to the proboscis. The larvae burrow into the skin of the human host when the vector feeds. The minimum prepatent period (until appearance of microfilariae)

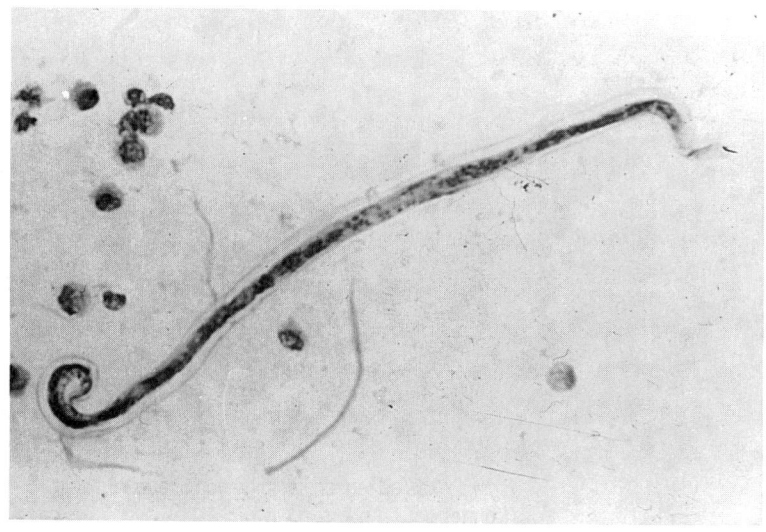

Figure 70.27　Microfilaria of *L. loa* stained with haematoxylin.

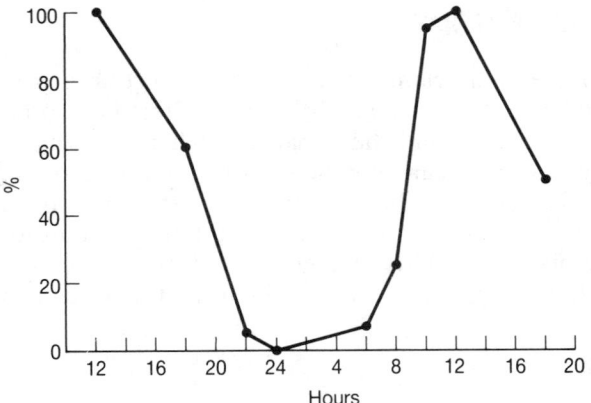

Figure 70. 28   Periodicity of *L. loa* microfilariae in the peripheral blood.

is 5 months, but it can be much longer, and adult worms may live for 17 years or more.

CLINICAL FEATURES

The most common clinical manifestations of loiasis are Calabar swellings. Adult worms may be noticed when they pass under the conjunctiva of the eye (Figure 70.29) or under the skin (Figure 70.30).[156–158] They usually appear and then disappear within 10–15 minutes, leaving no trace behind. Hypereosinophilia, especially in expatriates, is common. Calabar swellings (Figure 70.31) are most commonly observed on the wrists and ankles, but they may appear anywhere on the body. The swellings are usually 5–20 cm in diameter, painless, and do not pit on pressure. They may last from a few hours to several days. Usually one swelling occurs at a time, and may recur at irregular intervals for years after the patient has left the endemic area. Calabar swellings probably reflect the host's response to parasite antigens at the site of the swellings. Other common symptoms include fatigue, generalized pruritus and arthralgia. The death of an adult worm may occasionally cause a localized abscess. Dead worms sometimes calcify and are then easily seen on X-ray.

More serious complications can occur when *L. loa* invade the central nervous system and other vital organs. An epidemiological correlation has been observed between loiasis and the occurrence of endomyocardial fibrosis, and it is possible that hypereosinophilia induced by the infection may lead to the cardiac damage.[159] Nephropathy and encephalopathy are less common pathological changes. Nodules in the conjunctiva, swelling of the eyelids and proptosis were previously reported from Uganda as complications of loiasis. However, histological evidence has shown that these lesions are due to *M. perstans*.[160] For ocular loiasis, see Chapter 10.

As in other filarial infections, expatriates entering an endemic area are more troubled by clinical manifestations than are the indigenous inhabitants. However, the prevalence of microfilaraemia is apparently lower in expatriates than in the local inhabitants.[158]

DIAGNOSIS

The appearance of characteristic Calabar swellings in persons who live in an endemic area or who have visited such an area, or a history by the patient of a worm having crossed the eye, is strongly suggestive of *L. loa* infection.

Other helminths may migrate under the skin and cause cutaneous reactions. Swellings produced by *M. perstans* are similar to Calabar swellings. Cutaneous larva migrans (caused by *Strongyloides* or hookworm larvae) moves slowly, causes intense

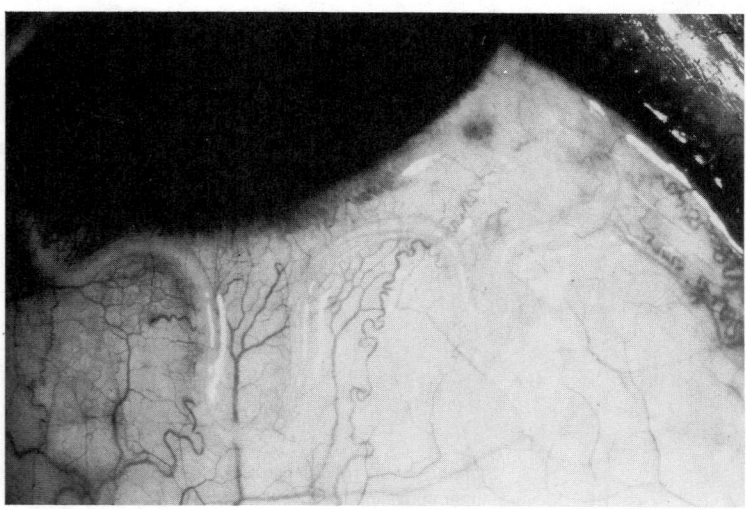

Figure 70.29   Transocular migration of adult *L. loa*. (Courtesy of J. Anderson.)

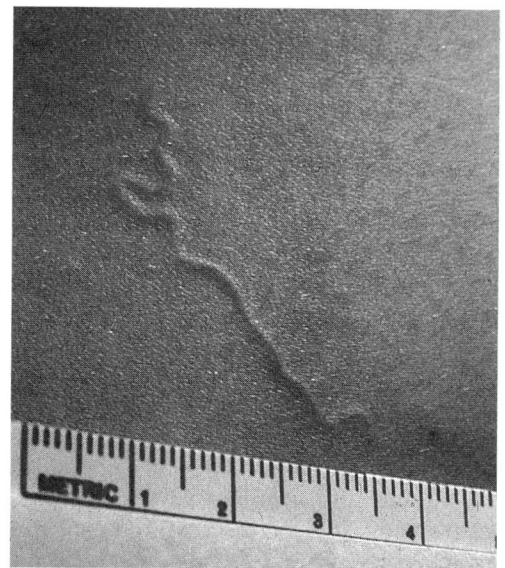

Figure 70.30 L. loa migrating under the skin. (Courtesy of P. G. P. Manson-Bahr.)

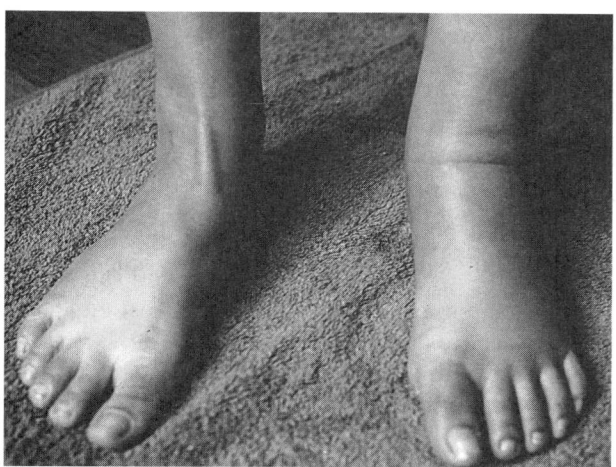

Figure 70.31 Calabar swelling.

irritation and leaves multiple tracks which may last for hours or even weeks. Subcutaneous *L. loa* causes little or no reaction, is usually single and only appears transiently for a few minutes. Guinea worm is a very large worm which can be palpated under the skin. In the eye, *L. loa* is subconjunctival and much larger than *Toxocara*, which may appear in the anterior chamber.

L. loa infections can be parasitologically diagnosed by removal of adult worms from the skin or conjunctiva, but it is usually done by identification of the characteristic microfilariae in the blood (see Figure 70.27). Microfilariae are, however, absent in many persons with clinical loiasis.[161] The optimal time for taking a blood sample is around noon, when the concentration of microfilariae in the peripheral blood is highest (see Figure 70.28). The various techniques for concentration and examination of the blood for microfilariae mentioned under lymphatic filariasis can also be used for *L. loa*. The sheath of *L. loa* microfilariae stains with haematoxylin but not with Giemsa. Other characteristic features used in the identification of the microfilariae are indicated in Appendix III.

As in other filarial infections, there is no reliable immunodiagnostic test for *L. loa* because of low sensitivity and cross-reactions with other filarial species.

IMMUNOLOGY

Most infected individuals show a high antibody titre to filarial antigens in IFAT and ELISA,[158,162] and maternal antibodies can be demonstrated in babies born in endemic areas.[163] The proteinuria and haematuria observed in some loiasis patients may be caused by an immune complex-induced glomerulonephritis.[157]

Antibodies recognizing a surface antigen on *L. loa* microfilariae have been demonstrated in persons with amicrofilaraemic adult infections, whereas these antibodies were not present in microfilaraemic persons from the same endemic area.[164] Amicrofilaraemic adult infections may thus result from the development of an immune response specifically eliminating the microfilarial stage of the parasite. Some cases may also be due to single sex infections.

TREATMENT

DEC rapidly eliminates microfilariae of *L. loa* from the blood (see Table 70.2) in dosages varying from 5 to 10 mg/kg body weight divided daily into three doses for 2–4 weeks. DEC has some effect on adult worms, but complete cure may require repeated treatment with this drug regimen. Side-effects may include fever, malaise, angio-oedema and pruritus. In patients with high microfilaraemia, the side-effects can be severe, and there is a risk of severe central nervous system complications. When treating heavy infections it is recommended to start with very small doses of DEC combined with administration of steroids. Because of the danger of inducing Mazzotti reactions, care must be taken when

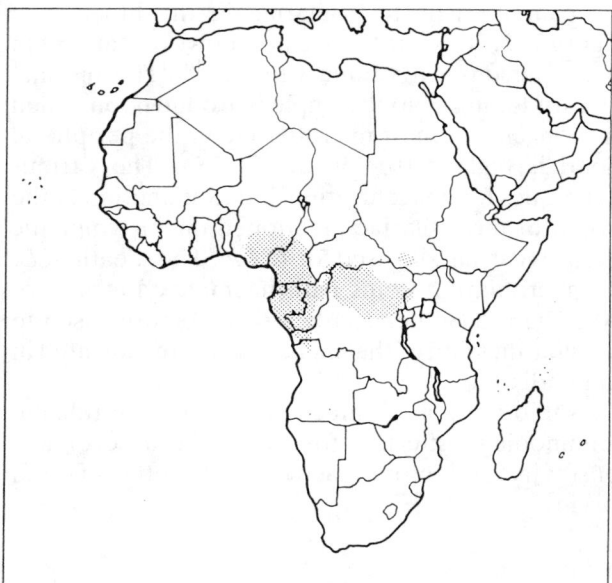

Figure 70.32   Geographical distribution of *L. loa*.

patients with loiasis are also infected with *O. volvulus*.

Mebendazole in low doses has been shown to reduce significantly microfilaraemia in persons with heavy *L. loa* infections.[165] Side-effects were low.

Recently, ivermectin given in dosages of 200–400 μg/kg body weight has been reported to be a safe and efficient microfilaricide.[166,167]

EPIDEMIOLOGY

Human loiasis occurs only in Africa, where transmission is confined to the rain forest and swamp forest areas of West and Central Africa (Figure 70.32). The vectors breed in these areas. It is estimated that 20–30 million people reside in endemic areas. The parasite was previously also observed in the more western rain forests of Sierre Leone, Liberia, Ivory Coast and Ghana, but it has not been reported from these countries for many years and it may have disappeared spontaneously.[155]

Human *L. loa* is transmitted by day-biting female tabanid flies of the genus *Chrysops*, mainly *C. silacea* and *C. dimidiata*. Other species of *Chrysops* are of local importance, especially in the periphery of the transmission zone. *Chrysops* flies rest in the forest canopy and are attracted mainly by movement, dark colours and wood smoke. They lay their eggs in swamps and river edges below the forest trees, and the larvae move about in the mud. Larval development is slow, taking up to a year or more to reach the adult stage. Transmission takes place mainly during the wet season. More information on the vectors and their bionomics is given in Appendix IV.

The possible existence of an animal reservoir for *L. loa* has been extensively studied. Species of forest-dwelling primates, including the mandril and several species of *Cercopithecus*, harbour filariae which closely resemble *L. loa*. The periodicity of these parasites is nocturnal. Monkeys can be infected with the human parasite, which retains its diurnal periodicity in the new host. The non-human primate *Loa* are transmitted by species of *Chrysops* which are only feeding at night on monkeys living in the canopy, whereas blood meal analyses have shown that *C. silacea* and *C. dimidiata* do not feed on non-human primates. Thus it appears that, in nature, human and monkey *L. loa* comprise two distinct transmission complexes, and that the parasite is not a zoonosis.

The microfilaria rate in children tends to be low. In adults, it gradually rises with age, but even in old age rarely exceeds 40%.[168,169] Despite the lack of microfilaraemia, many children harbour the adult parasites, which occasionally cross the eye. Within an endemic community, the microfilarial prevalence is commonly higher in males than in females.

CONTROL

Methods to control loiasis include environmental modifications, personal protection and vector control. No large-scale control programmes have been conducted.

The siting of houses and plantations should be established some distance from the forest edge and swamps where the vectors breed. The larvae of *Chrysops* live in the mud and can be destroyed there with insecticides. However, this method is impractical.

The wearing of light-coloured clothing and frequent application of insect repellent will reduce the risk of bites by the flies. Personal prophylaxis with a 300 mg dose of DEC once a week has recently proven efficient in expatriates working in endemic areas.[170]

MANSONELLA PERSTANS

M. perstans is a human filarial parasite, widely distributed in Africa as well as in parts of Central and South America and in the Caribbean (Figure

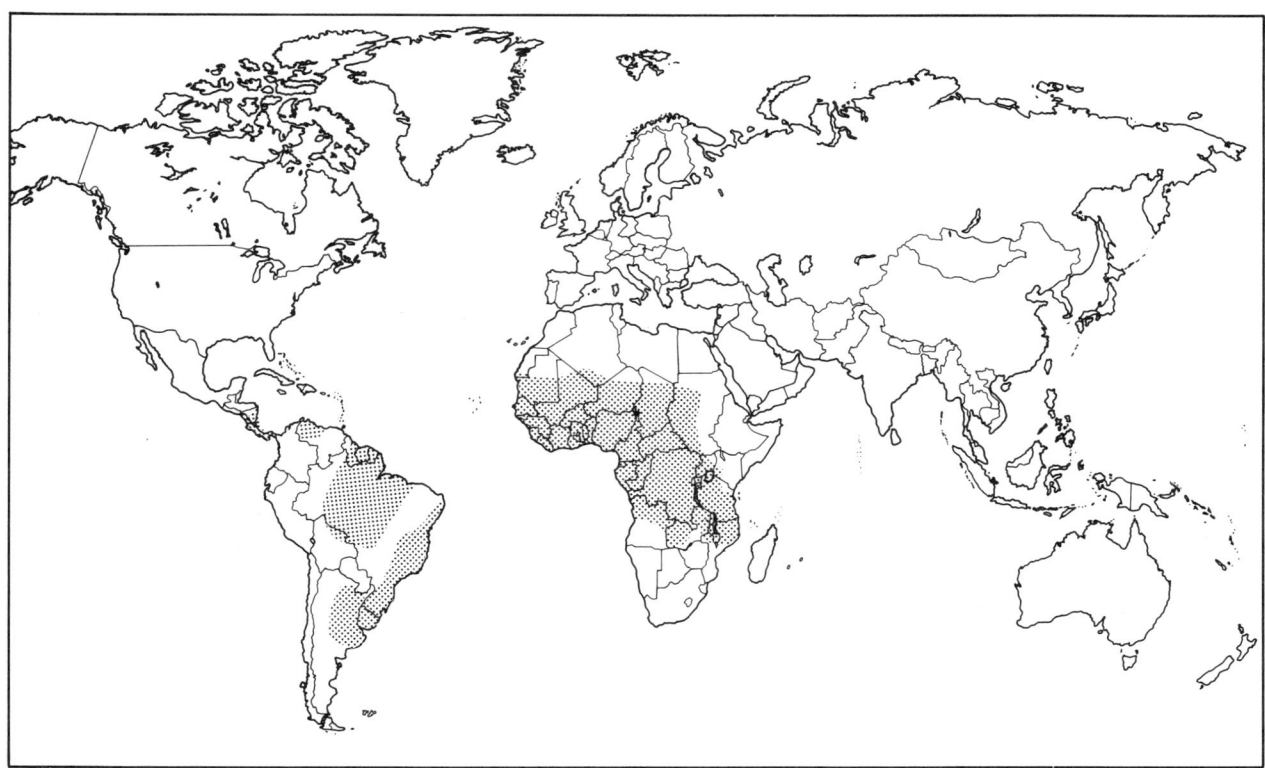

Figure 70.33 Geographical distribution of *M. perstans*. (Courtesy of the Department of Entomology, London School of Hygiene and Tropical Medicine.)

70.33). It is transmitted by tiny biting midges of the genus *Culicoides*. Rarely have adult worms been recovered from humans. They live in the serous cavities, mainly the peritoneal cavity, and usually cause no symptoms. Occasionally they have been found subcutaneously. The adult female measures 70–80 × 0.1 mm and the male 35–45 × 0.06 mm. Microfilariae (200 × 4.5 μm) are unsheathed, non-periodic, and circulate in the blood (Figure 70.34). For more detailed morphology, see Appendix III.

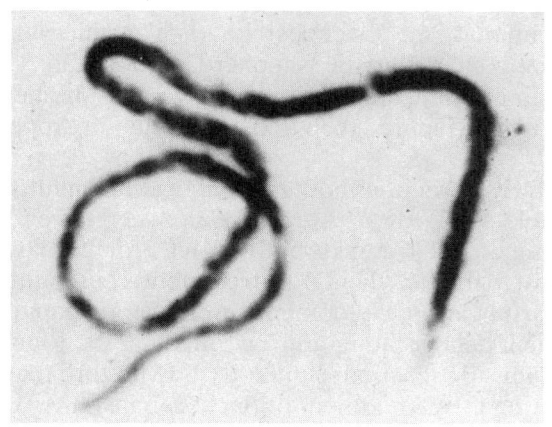

Figure 70.34 Microfilaria of *M. perstans*.

In the vector, following a blood meal, the ingested microfilariae develop to the infective stage. Infective larvae penetrate the skin of humans when the vector feeds again. The time from infection until appearance of microfilariae in the blood of humans is unknown.

M. perstans infections are largely non-pathogenic, but a variety of clinical manifestations can occur in some infected individuals. Symptoms are more common in expatriates coming to endemic areas from non-endemic ones. Transient swellings resembling the Calabar swellings of loiasis occur. Other manifestations are pruritus, fever, and pain or ache in bursae and/or joint synovia. Severe abdominal pain, especially in the liver region, may occur. Nodules in the conjunctiva, swelling of the eyelids and proptosis have also been attributed to *M. perstans* infections.[160] Eosinophilia is present in many cases of infection. It is likely that some of the pathological changes observed are induced by immune responses to the infection.

Diagnosis is by recovering the microfilariae (Figure 70.34) from the blood. Blood samples may be obtained at any time of the day, and techniques similar to those used for concentration and examination of blood samples for the diagnosis of lymphatic filariasis are utilized. For morphological features of the microfilariae, see Appendix III.

DEC or ivermectin have little or no effect on *M. perstans* infections (see Table 70.2). Mebendazole has proved effective in eliminating the microfilariae in a dose of 100 mg two to three times daily for 28–45 days.[165]

Very few studies have been carried out on the epidemiology of *M. perstans* infections. In some localities high prevalences and intensities of microfilaraemia are found. The microfilarial prevalence is generally lower in children than in adults, and males are usually more frequently infected than females.[168,169] Microfilarial prevalences can reach more than 80% in adults in highly endemic areas.

The main vector in Africa is *C. grahami*, but other species of *Culicoides* also play a role. The species of *Culicoides* transmitting *M. perstans* in the New World have not been identified.[170] *M. perstans* is found commonly in chimpanzees and gorillas, but it is also widespread in areas where there are no large apes.

MANSONELLA STREPTOCERCA

M. streptocerca is a filarial parasite of man, having a limited distribution in Central and West Africa (Figure 70.35). The adult worms inhabit the dermis of the upper thorax and shoulders, but they have rarely been recovered and very few have been examined in detail. The adult female measures 27 × 0.075 mm and the male 17 × 0.05 mm. The microfilariae

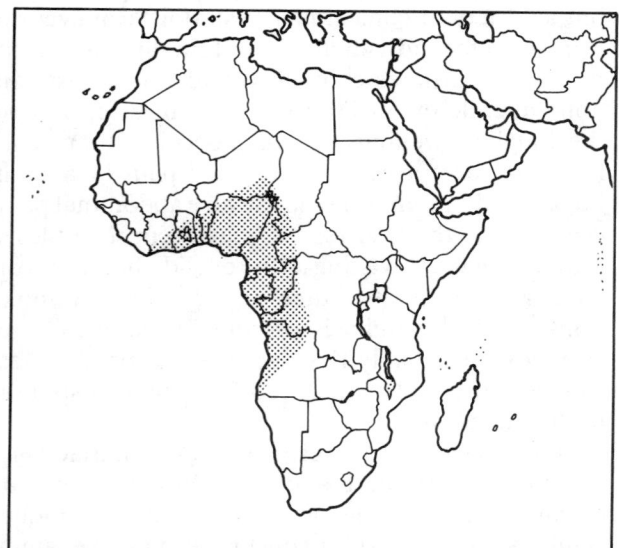

Figure 70.35 Geographical distribution of *M. streptocerca*. (Courtesy of the Department of Entomology, London School of Hygiene and Tropical Medicine.)

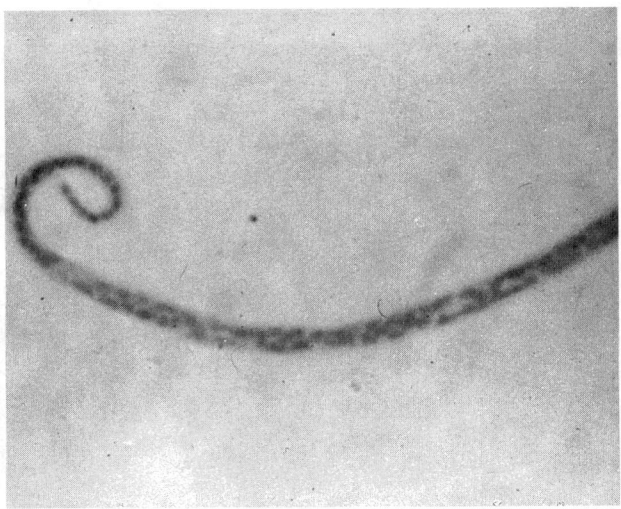

Figure 70.36 Microfilaria of *M. streptocerca*.

(Figure 70.36) also inhabit the dermis. They are unsheathed, measure 180–240 × 3–5 μm and exhibit no periodicity.

M. streptocerca is transmitted by tiny biting midges of the genus *Culicoides*, the most common vector probably being *C. grahami*.[171] Complete development in the vector has been observed experimentally to take 9 days. Information on the development of *M. streptocerca* in the human host is lacking, and the prepatent period is unknown.

The infection generally causes few clinical manifestations. Dermatitis is the most common sign and is most marked over the thorax and shoulders.[172] It is characterized by pruritus, hypopigmented macules and papules. Microscopically, infected skin shows dilated dermal lymphatics, and it has been suggested that *M. streptocerca* might be a cause of lymphoedema and elephantiasis. Clinically the infection must be distinguished from onchocerciasis and leprosy.

Diagnosis is made by finding the unsheathed microfilariae of *M. streptocerca* in skin snips (for the technique, see Onchocerciasis). The microfilariae have a characteristic 'shepherd's crook' tail. Other distinguishing features of the microfilariae are shown in Figure 70.36 and mentioned in Appendix III.

DEC eliminates both microfilariae and adults (see Table 70.2) of *M. streptocerca* when given in a dosage of 2–6 mg/kg body weight for 21 days. In most patients, the DEC treatment causes intense pruritus and development of cutaneous papules in which degenerating adult worms may be found.[172] Other side reactions similar to the Mazzotti reaction during DEC treatment of onchocerciasis may occur but are not common.

Adults and microfilariae of *M. streptocerca* are

found in the skin of chimpanzees, but whether the infection is a zoonosis is not known.

MANSONELLA OZZARDI

M. ozzardi is a human filarial parasite found only in the New World. Foci exist in Central America, in northern South America and in some Caribbean islands (Figure 70.37). Few adult female worms (65–80 × 0.25 mm) have been recovered from the peritoneal cavity of man. The microfilariae (Figure 70.38) measure 200 × 4.5 μm. They are unsheathed, nonperiodic, and are found in both blood and skin.

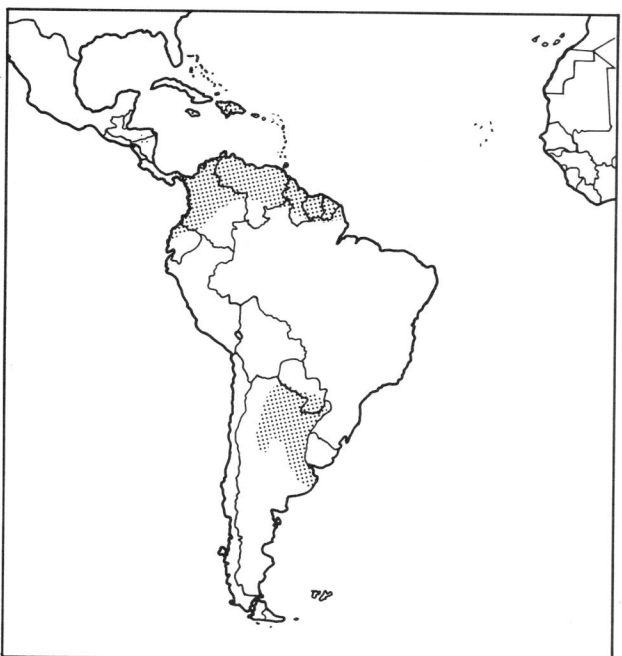

Figure 70.37 Geographical distribution of *M. ozzardi*. (Courtesy of the Department of Entomology, London School of Hygiene and Tropical Medicine.)

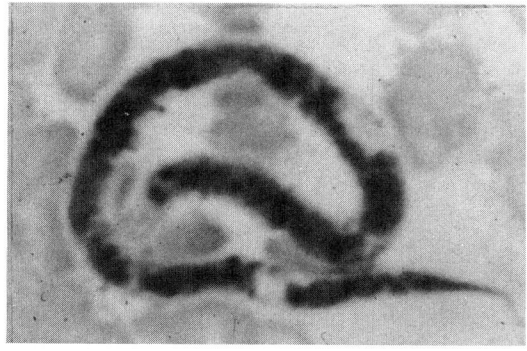

Figure 70.38 Microfilaria of *M. ozzardi*.

Two groups of vectors have been shown to transmit *M. ozzardi* infections. In the Caribbean islands the vectors are biting midges of the genera *Culicoides*, whereas in the Amazon basin *Simulium* blackflies have been incriminated.[171] The development of the parasite has been studied in the vectors and in experimental infections in patas monkeys. In the monkeys the prepatent period was 5–6 months. Natural *M. ozzardi* infections have not been reported from animals. In endemic foci, human infections tend to be highly prevalent, with the microfilarial infection rates increasing with age.[173,174]

Most people infected with *M. ozzardi* are symptomless. However, symptoms of severe articular pain, headache, fever and pruritus have been reported.[175] Eosinophilia is common. Individuals in endemic areas have high titres of antibodies against filarial antigens.[176]

The infection is diagnosed by finding the microfilariae in blood or in skin biopsies.[177] The techniques described under lymphatic filariasis and onchocerciasis can be used. For characteristics of the microfilariae, see Figure 70.38 and Appendix III. DEC has little or no effect on *M. ozzardi* infections (see Table 70.2), but a single dose of ivermectin (140 μg/kg body weight) has recently been reported to be effective in eliminating microfilariae in a patient.[178]

RARE FILARIAL INFECTIONS

Man occasionally becomes infected with species of filariae normally found in animals. Among these zoonotic infections, those due to *Dirofilaria* spp. are the most frequently reported and the most widespread.

DIROFILARIASIS

Dirofilaria spp. are natural parasites of various species of carnivores. In these hosts, the microfilariae circulate in the blood. Transmission is by mosquitoes. In human infections, parasite development is impaired and no microfilariae are produced.[179]

Pulmonary dirofilariasis

D. immitis is a filarial parasite of dogs. It is transmitted worldwide, except in cold climates. In the dog, adult *D. immitis* inhabit the right ventricle of the heart, where they may occur in large coiled masses. Pulmonary dirofilariasis in man results from infection with *D. immitis*. In man, the parasite may develop partially in the right ventricle of the heart before being swept into the pulmonary artery. Typically a spherical nodule 1–3 cm in diameter is discovered in the lungs on routine radiography (a 'coin lesion') or at autopsy. A single worm, usually necrotic and sometimes calcified, is present in the lumen of the artery. Most patients are asymptomatic. When present, symptoms include cough, chest pains, eosinophilia, haemoptysis and fever. Diagnosis is usually based on biopsy. Serological diagnosis has not been very successful. The only treatment is surgical excision.

Subcutaneous dirofilariasis

D. repens is a natural parasite of dogs and cats in warmer climates of the Old World. It has not been reported from America. In the normal hosts, adult worms are located in the subcutaneous tissues. In man, occasional infections may result in formation of subcutaneous nodules consisting of a degenerating immature worm surrounded by granulomatous tissue. Nodules occur in many parts of the body, especially the breasts, arms, legs, scrotum, eyelid and conjunctiva. The nodules may occasionally be slowly migrating. Immunodiagnosis has not proved useful, and diagnosis is by biopsy. Treatment is by surgical removal of the nodule.

In North America, two other species of *Dirofilaria*, *D. tenuis* and *D. ursi*, which are natural parasites of racoons and bears respectively, have been reported to cause subcutaneous dirofilariasis in man.

OTHER RARE FILARIAL INFECTIONS

Human infections with *Brugia* parasites have occasionally been reported from countries where transmission of human *Brugia* spp. does not occur. This includes infections acquired in Africa and America. These *Brugia* parasites are believed to be of animal origin.[40]

Microfilariae with no resemblance to those of human filarial species have been reported from humans. Cases of encephalopathy with microfilariae found in the cerebrospinal fluid were described from Zimbabwe. The microfilariae were shown to be *Meningonema peruzzi*, a filarial parasite of cercopithecus monkeys.[180] Microfilariae similar to *Microfilaria rodhaini* from chimpanzees were recovered in skin biopsy specimens from humans during a survey in Gabon.[181] Microfilariae of unknown species found in the blood of American Indians in a remote jungle area in Venezuela were named *Microfilaria bolivarensis*.[182] In a survey in north-western Zaire, many villagers had microfilariae of unknown species in the blood. These were named *Microfilaria semiclarum*.[183] A comprehensive list of helminth parasites recovered from man, including filariae, has been produced.[184]

DRACUNCULIASIS (GUINEA WORM)

Dracunculiasis or guinea worm disease in man results from infection with *Dracunculus medinensis*.

LIFE CYCLE AND TRANSMISSION

D. medinensis is a nematode parasite related to filarial worms. The vectors are cyclopoid copepods (water fleas), which are tiny free-swimming crustaceans usually found in abundance in natural fresh water bodies. Humans acquire the infection by drinking water containing the vectors infected with guinea worm larvae.[185] The presence of guinea worm in an area is therefore essentially due to the poor quality of drinking water.

Adult female *D. medinensis* (up to 60–80 cm long and 1.5–2.0 mm in thickness) inhabit the subcutaneous connective tissues of man. They may be located anywhere on the body but in the late stage of infection they are usually attracted to the legs and feet. At this stage most of the interior of the worm is occupied by the uterus, which contains thousands of first-stage larvae. A blister is formed on the skin of the host around the anterior end of the worm, and, when exposed to water, the blister ruptures. The female guinea worm will protrude its anterior end from the ulcer and discharge first-stage larvae (640 × 23 μm) into the water. It remains protruding for the following 2–6 weeks (Figure 70.39), releasing larvae each time it is immersed in water. After this period it dies.

The larvae are infective in fresh water for 5–6 days, and for further development must, within this period, be swallowed by a copepod of the right species. The larva penetrates the gut wall, and in the haemocoel it moults twice. It can reach the infective third stage (450 × 14 μm) in about 2 weeks. Vectors

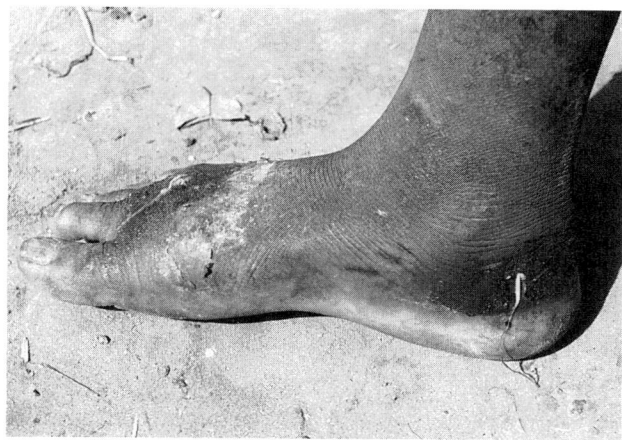

Figure 70.39 Mature adult female guinea worm protruding from a foot. (Courtesy of P. Bloch.)

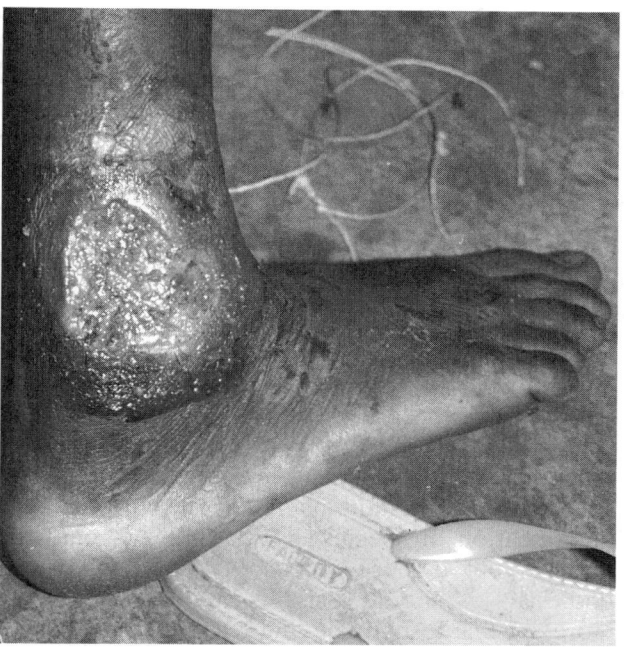

Figure 70.40 Secondarily infected guinea worm ulcer. (Courtesy of P. Bloch.)

that contain third-stage larvae become sluggish and sink to the bottom of a pond. Many species of cyclopoid copepods have been found naturally infected in various parts of the world, mainly being of the genera *Mesocyclops* and *Thermocyclops*.[186,187]

In man, vectors ingested in drinking water are dissolved by the gastric juice. The guinea worm infective larvae are released and penetrate the stomach or intestine of the new host. After a period in the abdominal cavity, the larvae enter the connective tissues, where they develop to mature worms. Mating occurs about 3 months after the initial infection, and the males, which are much smaller than the females (1–4 cm × 0.4 mm), die shortly thereafter. The females move about in the connective tissues and usually reach the lower extremities between 8 and 10 months after infection.

CLINICAL FEATURES

There are usually no symptoms in the prepatent period. The first sign appears a few days before the worm pierces the skin. The dermis becomes elevated and a blister develops. The patient feels a burning sensation and itching, which he or she tries to relieve by placing the affected part in water. On exposure to water the blister ruptures, the anterior part of the worm protrudes and *Dracunculus* larvae are discharged into the water.

The worm is most frequently located in the foot or lower leg, but may appear on arms, breasts, head, back, scrotum or anywhere on the body surface. When it is close to joints it may cause arthritis. Further inflammation, or the calcification of worms,

may cause joints of legs and feet to become stiff, thereby crippling the patient. In many cases, sometimes 50% or more, the ulcer caused by the parasite becomes secondarily infected with bacteria (Figure 70.40), and a spreading cellulitis may develop. Tetanus infection is a serious complication of guinea worm infection.

Inflammation around it makes the whole worm difficult to extricate before the uterus is empty of larvae. Provided there is no secondary infection, the ulcer heals spontaneously after extrication of the empty worm. If broken, the remainder of the worm withdraws into the host tissue, causing a severe inflammatory reaction followed by an ulcer and later scar tissue. Usually only a single worm appears in the patient annually, but up to 20 or more can appear at the same time in one individual.

Some female worms fail to emerge and die in the body. Usually they become encysted and calcify, and are then only apparent on X-ray. Dead or ruptured worms may lead to formation of a sterile subcutaneous abscess. Migration of worms to vital organs can cause serious consequences. Such migrations are rare.

DIAGNOSIS

Guinea worm infections cannot be diagnosed in the prepatent period, i.e. for the first 8–10 months of infection. Shortly before appearance the adult female worm can sometimes be seen or palpated under the skin. A clinical diagnosis is made by examining the guinea worm ulcer and observing the female protruding from the blister (see Figure 70.39). The appearance of the blister, with local itching and burning pain, makes diagnosis simple, even for the sufferer. Active larvae can be obtained by immersing the protruding adult female in a small tube or container with water. The first-stage larvae, with their characteristic pointed tails (see Appendix III), can then be observed under the microscope.

Serology is of no practical use in diagnosis. Due to constant exposure, all persons in endemic areas usually have high antibody titres, and cross-reactions to other nematode antigens reduce the specificity of immunodiagnostic tests.[188] Recent identification of species-specific antigens, and the finding of higher specificity of IgG4 antibodies,[188–190] should assist in the development of more specific tests, including tests for diagnosis of prepatent infections. High eosinophilia is commonly observed in guinea worm infections. Dead calcified worms are easily seen on radiological examination.

IMMUNOLOGY

There is no evidence of acquired immunity—people in endemic areas suffer from infections year after year. Whether the vigorous antibody response mentioned above has any effect on the course of the infection is unknown.[188–190]

TREATMENT

The traditional method of slow extraction of the emergent guinea worm is usually the most effective. The protruding part of the female worm is attached to a small stick which is twisted a small amount each day until the worm has been removed (Figure 70.41). Care should be taken not to break the worm. Administration of antibiotics and cleaning and dressing of the ulcers are important in reducing secondary infections, and tetanus vaccination is recommended.

A technique for surgical extraction of guinea worm prior to eruption through the skin has recently been described.[191] In the field, surgical removal of unerupted worms resulted in a significant decrease in guinea worm associated disability.

No anthelminthic treatment is available. Some drugs, especially niridazole (given orally at 12.5 mg/

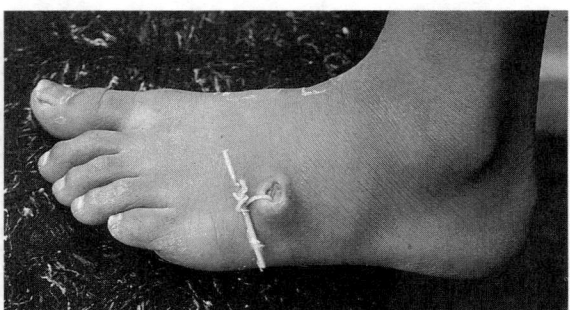

Figure 70.41   Traditional method of removal of guinea worm.

kg body weight daily) have been reported to reduce inflammation around the worm, thereby allowing easier extraction. Chemotherapeutic drug trials have recently been carried out in an animal model, including trials with DEC and ivermectin, but no significant effects of any of the drugs were observed.[192]

EPIDEMIOLOGY

Human guinea worm infections were previously much more widespread, but the distribution is now limited to the Sahelian and sub-Sahelian areas of Africa, to the Indian subcontinent and the Arabian peninsula (Figure 70.42), with most cases being seen in West Africa. About 140 million people are living in areas where transmission occurs, and about 10 million people are thought to be infected annually.[193]

The occurrence of guinea worm infection is associated with the use of small sources of water in semiarid countries. Humans contract the infection by drinking the water containing infected cyclopoid copepods, and again contribute to transmission by immersing the guinea worm ulcer in water, thereby allowing the release of first-stage larvae. In the Sahelian region of Africa, transmission mainly occurs in small surface water pools used for collecting drinking water and for washing. In many places of India, guinea worm infection is associated with step wells, which the inhabitants enter via a series of steps, immersing their feet regularly in the water, so that transmission and infection are occurring from the same source.

The transmission of guinea worm is frequently seasonal,[187,194] with the majority of patent infections and infected copepods occurring within a few months of the year (Figure 70.43). The seasonality is closely related to the rainfall. In the arid areas the transmission usually coincides with the rainy season, when surface water is available, whereas in wet

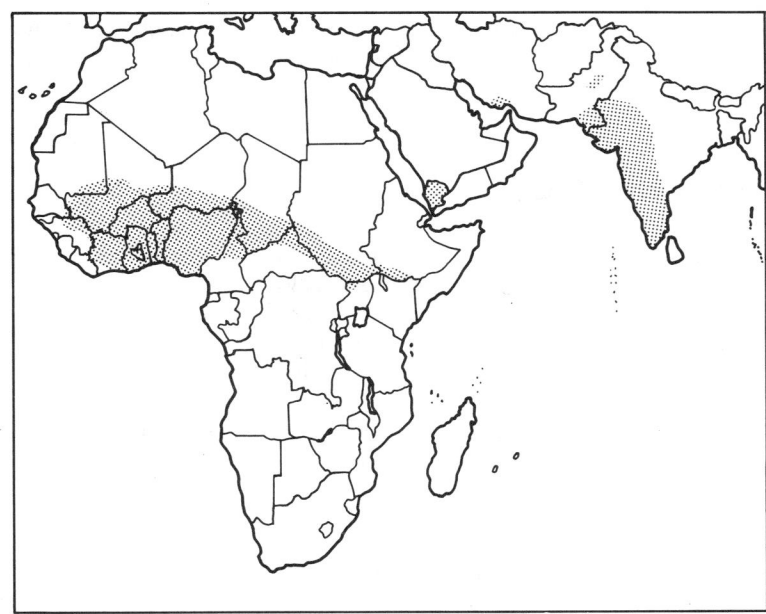

Figure 70.42 Geographical distribution of guinea worm. (Courtesy of the Department of Entomology, London School of Hygiene and Tropical Medicine.)

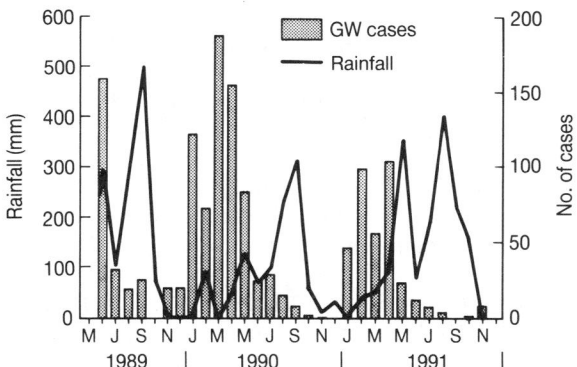

Figure 70.43 Seasonal variation in rainfall and number of guinea worm ulcers in a village in the northern region of Ghana. (Courtesy of P. Magnussen.)

areas transmission is most intense in the dry season, when drinking water sources are few. The incidence of infection varies from area to area, but where endemicity is high, 50% or more of the population may be affected by the infection every year. However, even in highly endemic areas, some people never experience guinea worm infections, although they use the same drinking water source as the rest of the population. There is considerable variation in sex prevalence between different endemic areas. Persons aged between 15–40 years are mostly affected. The transmission season often coincides with the peak period of agricultural work.[190] Since a large proportion of the farmers may be incapacitated, guinea worm infection can severely reduce agricultural output.

Parasites resembling *D. medinensis* are seen in animals, especially in dogs, but there is no evidence that they are a reservoir of infection for man.

CONTROL

Due to its simple life cycle, and the apparent lack of an animal reservoir, the control of guinea worm seems feasible. The United Nations-supported International Drinking Water and Sanitation decade (1981–1990) raised global attention to the possibility of eradicating the infection by improving the quality of human drinking water, and in 1986 the World Health Organization declared guinea worm the next human infection to be eradicated after smallpox. Many organizations are presently involved in programmes to eliminate the infection.[196]

Provision of safe drinking water in the form of boreholes is the most expensive, but also the most effective measure, and has been shown to give dramatic reductions in the incidence of guinea worm infection.[197] As well as efforts being made to improve drinking water sources, other measures to control guinea worm transmission are health education and chemical vector control. Health education focuses on drinking water as the source of infection and on the importance of boiling or filtering the water before use. Special monofilament nylon material has been produced for filtering water.[198] A much cheaper filtering method relies on a layer of tightly woven cotton cloth. To prevent infestation of the water with guinea worm larvae, health education also emphasizes the reasons why people with guinea worm ulcers should avoid entering water sources. Vector control can be achieved in ponds and wells by applying the insecticide temephos (Abate).[199]

REFERENCES

1 World Health Organization. WHO expert committee on filariasis. *WHO Tech Rep Ser* 1984; 702.

2 Demarquay J N. Note sur une tumeur des bourses contenant un liquide laiteux (galactocèle de Vidal) et referment des petits êtres vermiformes que l'on peut considérer comme des helminthes hematoides à l'état d'embryon. *Gaz Méd Paris* 1863; 18:665–667.

3 Wucherer O E. Noticia preliminar sobre vermes de una especie ainda não descripta, encontrados na urina de doentes de hematuria intertropical bo Brazil. *Gaz Med Bahia* 1868; 3:97–99.

4 Cobbold T S. Discovery of the adult representative of microscopic filariae. *Lancet* 1877; ii:70–71.

5 Buckley J J. On *Brugia* gen. nov. for *Wuchereria* spp. of the 'malayi' group, i.e. *W. malayi* Brug, 1927, *W. pahangi* Buckley and Edeson, 1956, and *W. patei* Buckley, Nelson and Heisch, 1958. *Ann Trop Med Parasitol* 1960; 54:75–77.

6 Partono F, Purmono A, Dennis D T, Atmosoedjono S, Oemijati S & Cross J H. *Brugia timori* sp.n. (Nematoda: Filarioidea) from Flores Island, Indonesia. *J Parasitol* 1977; 63:540–546.

7 Grove D I. *A History of Human Helminthology.* London: CAB International, 1990: 597–640.

8 Hawking F & Denham D A. The distribution of human filariasis throughout the world. Part I. The Pacific Region including New Guinea. *Trop Dis Bull* 1976; 73:347–373.

9 World Health Organization. *Control of Lymphatic Filariasis. A Manual for Health Personnel.* Geneva: WHO, 1987.

10 Wijers D J B & McMahon J E. Early signs and symptoms of Bancroftian filariasis in males at the East African Coast. *East Afr Med J* 1976; 53:57–63.

11 Cilento R W. *Tropical Diseases in Australia*, 2nd edn. Brisbane: Smith & Patterson, 1942.

12 Romiti C. The primary aspect of the disease syndrome of bancroftian filariasis in British Guiana. *West Indian Med J* 1956; 5:113–119.

13 Dreyer G, Ottesen E A, Galdino E et al. Renal abnormalities in microfilaraemic patients with Bancroftian filariasis. *Am J Trop Med Hyg* 1992; 46:745–751.

14 Dennis D T, Partono F, Purmono, Atmosoedjono S & Saroso J S. Timor filariasis: epidemiologic and clinical features in a defined community. *Am J Trop Med Hyg* 1976; 25:797–802.

15 Manson-Bahr P H (ed.) Parasites of the lymphatic system and connective tissue: Filariasis. In *Manson's Tropical Diseases*, 14th edn. London: Cassell & Co, 1957: 755.

16 Rook H D E. Filariasis in the village of Inanwatan (South coast of the Vogel Kop. Nederlands, New Guinea). *Trop Geogr Med* 1959; 11:313–331.

17 Southgate B A. Bancroftian filariasis in Egypt. *Trop Dis Bull* 1979; 76:1045–1068.

18 Brinkmann U K. Infektionen mit *Wuchereria bancrofti* in Marschall Territory, einem Küstengebiet Liberias. *Z Tropenmed Parasitol* 1972; 23:369–386.

19 Knight R. Current status of filarial infections in The Gambia. *Ann Trop Med Parasitol* 1980; 74:63–68.

20 McMahon J E, Marshall T F C, Vaughan J P & Abaru D E. Bancroftian filariasis: a comparison of microfilariae counting techniques using counting chamber, standard slide and membrane (nuclepore) filtration. *Ann Trop Med Parasitol* 1979; 73:457–464.

21 Eberhard M L, Roberts I M, Lammie P J & Lowrie R C. Comparative densities of *Wuchereria bancrofti* microfilaria in paired samples of capillary and venous blood. *Trop Med Parasitol* 1988; 39:295–298.

22 Dickerson J W, Eberhard M L & Lammie P J. A technique for microfilarial detection in preserved blood using nuclepore filters. *J Parasitol* 1990; 76:829–833.

23 Rao U R, Lowrie R C, Vickery A C, Kwa B H & Nayar J K. A direct fluorescence technique for the rapid detection of sheathed microfilariae in blood smears. *Int J Parasitol* 1990; 20:1099–1103.

24 Long G W, Rickman L S & Cross J H. Rapid diagnosis of *Brugia malayi* and *Wuchereria bancrofti* filariasis by an acridine orange/microhematocrit tube technique. *J Parasitol* 1990; 76:278–281.

25 McMahon J E. The examination-time/dose interval in the provocation of nocturnally periodic microfilariae of *Wuchereria bancrofti* with diethylcarbamazine and the practical uses of the test. *Tropenmed Parasitol* 1982; 33:28–30.

26 McMahon J E, Marshall T F C, Vaughan J P & Kolstrup N. Tanzania filariasis project: a provocative day test with diethylcarbamazine for the detection of microfilariae of nocturnally periodic *Wuchereria bancrofti* in the blood. *Bull World Health Organ* 1979; 57:759–765.

27 Ambroise-Thomas P & Peyron F. Filariasis. In Walls K W & Schantz P M (eds) *Immunodiagnosis of Parasitic Diseases*, vol. I: Helminthic Diseases. London: Academic Press, 1986: 233–253.

28 Weiss N, Hussain R & Ottesen E A. IgE antibodies are more species specific than IgG antibodies in

human onchocerciasis and lymphatic filariasis. *Immunology* 1982; 45:129–137.

29 Lal R B & Ottesen E A. Enhanced diagnostic specificity in human filariasis by IgG4 antibody assessment. *J Infect Dis* 1988; 158:1034–1037.

30 Kwan-Lim G, Forsyth K P & Maizels R M. Filarial specific IgG4 response corellates with active *Wuchereria bancrofti* infection. *J Immunol* 1990; 4298–4305.

31 Weil G J, Jain D C, Santhanam S et al. A monoclonal antibody-based enzyme immunoassay for detecting parasite antigenemia in bancroftian filariasis. *J Infect Dis* 1987; 156:350–355.

32 More S J & Copeman D B. A highly specific and sensitive monoclonal antibody-based ELISA for the detection of circulating antigen in bancroftian filariasis. *Trop Med Parasitol* 1990; 41:403–406.

33 Forsyth K P, Spark R, Kazura J et al. A monoclonal antibody-based immunoradiometric assay for detection of circulating antigen in bancroftian filariasis. *J Immunol* 1985; 134:1172–1177.

34 Ottesen E A. Immunopathology of lymphatic filariasis in man. *Springer Semin Immunopathol* 1980; 2:373–385.

35 Ottesen E A. Immunological aspects of lymphatic filariasis and onchocerciasis in man. *Trans R Soc Trop Med Hyg* 1984; 78(supplement):9–18.

36 Ottesen E A. Filariasis now. *Am J Trop Med Hyg* 1989; 41:9–17.

37 Vickery A C, Albertine K H, Nayar J K & Kwa B H. Histopathology of *Brugia malayi*-infected nude mice after immune reconstitution. *Acta Trop* 1991; 49:45–55.

38 Michael P. Filariasis among navy and marine personnel: report on laboratory investigations. *US Navel Med Bull* 1944; 42:1059–1074.

39 Cohen L B, Nelson G, Wood A M, Manson-Bahr P E C & Bowen R. Lymphangiography in filarial lymphoedema and elephantiasis. *Am J Trop Med Hyg* 1961; 10:843–848.

40 World Health Organization. Lymphatic filariasis: the disease and its control. Fifth report of the WHO Expert Committee on Filariasis. *WHO Tech Rep Ser* 1992: 821.

41 Jungmann P, Figueredo-Silva J & Dreyer G. Bancroftian lymphadenopathy: a histopathologic study of fifty-eight cases from Northeastern Brazil. *Am J Trop Med Hyg* 1991; 45:325–331.

42 Weil G J, Hussain R, Kumaraswami V, Tripathy S P, Phillips K S & Ottesen E A. Prenatal allergic sensitization to helminth antigens in offspring of parasite-infected mothers. *J Clin Invest* 1983; 71:1124–1129.

43 Klei T R, Blamchard D P & Coleman S U. Development of *Brugia pahangi* infections and lymphatic lesions in male offspring of female jirds with homologous infections. *Trans R Soc Trop Med Hyg* 1986; 80:214–216.

44 Partono F, Purmono, Pribadi W & Soewarta A. Epidemiological and clinical features of *Brugia timori* in a newly established village, Karakuak, West Flores, Indonesia. *Am J Trop Med Hyg* 1978; 27:910–915.

45 Lammie P J, Hitch W L, Allen E M W, Hightower W & Eberhard M L. Maternal filarial infection as risk factor for infection in children. *Lancet* 1991; 337:1005–1006.

46 Rohatgi P K & Smirniotopoulos T T. Tropical eosinophilia. *Semin Respir Med* 1991; 12:98–106.

47 Nutman T B, Vijayan V K, Pinkston P et al. Tropical pulmonary eosinophilia: analysis of antifilarial antibody localized to the lung. *J Infect Dis* 1989; 160:1042–1050.

48 Subrahmanyam D, Mehta K, Nelson D S, Rao Y V B G & Rao C K. Immune reactions in human filariasis. *J Clin Microbiol* 1978; 8:228–232.

49 Simonsen P E. *Wuchereria bancrofti* in Tanzania: immune reactions to the microfilarial surface, and the effect of diethylcarbamazine upon these reactions. *Trans R Soc Trop Med Hyg* 1985; 79:852–858.

50 McGreevy P B, Ratiwayanto S, Tuti S, McGreevy M M & Dennis D T. *Brugia malayi:* relationship between anti-sheath antibodies and amicrofilaraemia in natives living in an endemic area of South Kalimantan, Borneo. *Am J Trop Med Hyg* 1980; 29:553–562.

51 Johnson P, Mackenzie C D, Suswillo R R & Denham D A. Serum-mediated adherence of feline granulocytes to microfilariae of *Brugia pahangi* in vitro: variations with parasite maturation. *Parasitol Immunol* 1981; 3:69–80.

52 Mehta K, Sindhu R K, Subrahmanyam D & Nelson D S. IgE-dependent adherence and cytotoxicity of rat spleen and peritoneal cells to *Litomosoides carinii* microfilariae. *Clin Exp Immunol* 1980; 41:107–114.

53 Weiss N. Studies on *Dipetalonema viteae* (Filaroidea). I. Microfilaraemia in hamsters in relation to worm burden and humoral immune response. *Acta Trop* 1978; 35:477–485.

54 Weil G J, Powers K G, Parbuoni E L, Line B R, Furrow R D & Ottesen E A. *Dirofilaria immitis.* VI. Antimicrofilarial immunity in experimental filariasis. *Am J Trop Med Hyg* 1982; 31:477–485.

55 Day K P, Gregory W F & Maizels R M. Age-specific acquisition of immunity to infective larvae in a bancroftian filariasis endemic area of Papua New Guinea. *Parasitol Immunol* 1991; 13:277–290.

56 Vanamail P, Subramanian S, Das P K et al. Estimation of age-specific rates of acquisition and loss of *Wuchereria bancrofti* infection. *Trans R Soc Trop Med Hyg* 1989; 83:689–693.

57 Rom W N, Vijayan V K, Cornelius M J et al. Persistent lower respiratory tract inflammation associated with interstitial lung disease in patients with pulmonary eosinophilia following conventional treatment with diethylcarbamazine. *Am Rev Respir Dis* 1991; 142:1088–1092.

58 Jamal S, Casley-Smith J R & Casley-Smith J R. The effects of 5,6 benzo-[a]-pyrone (coumarin) and

DEC on filaritic lymphoedema and elephantiasis in India. Preliminary results. *Ann Trop Med Parasitol* 1989; 83:287–290.

59 UNDP/World Bank/WHO Special Programme for Research and Training in Tropical Diseases. *Lymphatic pathology and immunopathology in filariasis: Report on the twelfth meeting of the scientific working group on filariasis*, TDR/FIL-SWG (12)/85.3. Geneva: WHO, 1985.

60 Ramalingam S. The epidemiology of filarial transmission in Samoa and Tonga. *Ann Trop Med Parasitol* 1968; 62:305–323.

61 Russal S, Das M & Rao C K. Filariasis in Andaman and Nicobar Islands. Part I. Survey findings: Non cowry, Terressa, Chawra, Carmicobar and Port Blair. *J Commun Dis* 1975; 7:15–30.

62 Khamboonruang C, Pan-In S, Somboon P et al. Bancroftian filariasis in Tambol Na-Sai, Amphoe Li, Lamphun Province: a preliminary survey for microfilaraemia. *J Med Assoc Thai* 1989; 72:321–324.

63 Ramachandran C P. The epidemiology and control of Brugian filariasis in South East Asia: an update. *Ann Soc Belg Med Trop* 1981; 61:257–268.

64 Iyengar M O T. *Epidemiology of filariasis in the South Pacific*, Technical Paper No. 148. Noumea: South Pacific Commission, 1965.

65 McMahon J E, Magayuka S A, Kolstrup N et al. Studies on the transmission and prevalence of Bancroftian filariasis in four coastal villages of Tanzania. *Ann Trop Med Parasitol* 1981; 75:415–431.

66 Wijers D J B. Bancroftian filariasis in Kenya. I. Prevalence survey among adult males in the Coast Province. *Ann Trop Med Parasitol* 1977; 71:313–331.

67 Rao C K, Datta K K, Sundaram R M et al. Epidemiological studies on bancroftian filariasis in East Godavari district (Andhra Pradesh): baseline filariometric indices. *Indian J Med Res* 1980; 71:712–720.

68 Raccurt C P, Mojon M & Hodges W H. Parasitological, serological, and clinical studies of *Wuchereria bancrofti* in Limbe, Haiti. *Am J Trop Med Hyg* 1984; 33:1124–1129.

69 Grove D I, Valeza F S & Cabrera D B. Bancroftian filariasis in a Philippine village: clinical, parasitological, immunological, and social aspects. *Bull World Health Organ* 1978; 56:975–984.

70 Brabin L. Sex differentials in susceptibility to lymphatic filariasis and implications for maternal child immunity. *Epidemiol Infect* 1990; 105:335–353.

71 Wartman W B. Filariasis in American Armed Forces in World War II. *Medicine* 1947; 26:333–394.

72 Palmieri J R, Connor D H, Purmono A, Dennis D T & Marwoto H. Experimental infection of *Wuchereria bancrofti* in the silvered leaf monkey *Presbytis cristatus* Eschscholtz 1821. *J Helminthol* 1982; 56:243–245.

73 Palmieri J R, Purmono A, Dennis D T & Marwoto H A. Filarid parasites of South Kalimantan (Borneo), Indonesia. *Wuchereria kalimantani* sp.n. (Nematoda: Filarioidea) from the silvered leaf monkey, *Presbytis cristatus* Eschscholtz 1921. *J Parasitol* 1980; 66:645–651.

74 Kolstrup N, McMahon J E, Magayuka S A, Mosha F W, Bushrod F M & Bryan J H. Control measures against Bancroftian filariasis in coastal villages in Tanzania. *Ann Trop Med Parasitol* 1981; 75:433–451.

75 Wijers D J B & Kaleli N. Bancroftian filariasis in Kenya. V. Mass treatment given by members of the local community. *Ann Trop Med Parasitol* 1981; 78:383–394.

76 McMahon J E. Chemotherapy with diethylcarbamazine and levamisole in Bancroftian filariasis. *Tropenmed Parasitol* 1981; 32:250–252.

77 Cartel J L, Celerier P, Spiegel A, Burucoa C & Roux J F. A single diethylcarbamazine dose for treatment of *Wuchereria bancrofti* carriers in French Polynesia: efficacy and side effects. *Southeast Asian J Trop Med Public Health* 1990; 21:465–470.

78 Fan P. Eradication of Bancroftian filariasis by diethylcarbamazine-medicated common salt on Little Kinmen (Liehyu District), Kinmen (Quemoy) Islands, Republic of China. *Ann Trop Med Parasitol* 1990; 84:25–33.

79 Maxwell C A, Curtis C F, Haji H, Kisumku S, Thalib A I & Yahya S A. Control of bancroftian filariasis by integrating therapy with vector control using polystyrene beads in wet pit latrines. *Trans R Soc Trop Med Hyg* 1990; 84:709–714.

80 Rajagopalan P K, Panicker K N & Das P K. Control of malaria and filariasis vectors in South India. *Parasitol Today* 1987; 3:233–241.

81 Webber R H. Eradication of *Wuchereria bancrofti* infection through vector control. *Trans R Soc Trop Med Hyg* 1979; 73:722–724.

82 O'Neil J. On the presence of filaria in 'craw-craw'. *Lancet* 1875; i:265–266.

83 Robles R. Enfermedad nueva en Guatemala. *Juventud Med* 1917; 17:97–115.

84 Blacklock D B. The development of *Onchocerca volvulus* in *Simulium damnosum*. *Ann Trop Med Parasitol* 1926; 20:1–48.

85 Grove D I. *A History of Human Helminthology*. London: CAB International, 1990: 661–691.

86 Duke B O, Vincellette J & Moore P J. Microfilariae in the cerebrospinal fluid and neurological complications during treatment for onchocerciasis with diethylcarbamazine. *Trop Med Parasitol* 1976; 27:125–132.

87 Prost S. Latence parasitaire dans l'onchocercose. *Bull World Health Organ* 1980; 58:923–925.

88 Brinkmann U K, Kramer P, Presthus G T & Sawadogo B. Transmission in utero of microfilariae of *Onchocerca volvulus*. *Bull World Health Organ* 1976; 54:708–709.

89 Bird A C, Anderson J, Fuglsang H, Hamilton P J S

& Marshall T F de C. Morphology of posterior segment lesions of the eye in patients with onchocerciasis. *Br J Ophthalmol* 1976; 60:2–20.

90 Anderson J, Fuglsang H, Hamilton P J S & Marshall T F de C. Studies on onchocerciasis in The United Cameroon Republic. II. Comparison of onchocerciasis in rain-forest and Sudan-savanna. *Trans R Soc Trop Med Hyg* 1974; 68:209–222.

91 McMahon J E, Sowa S I, Maude G H & Kirkwood B R. Onchocerciasis in Sierra Leone. 3. Relationships between eye lesions and microfilarial prevalence and intensity. *Trans R Soc Trop Med Hyg* 1988; 82:601–605.

92 McMahon J E, Sowa S I, Maude G H, Hudson C M & Kirkwood B R. Epidemiological studies of onchocerciasis in savanna villages of Sierra Leone. *Trop Med Parasitol* 1988; 39:260–268.

93 McMahon J E, Sowa S I, Maude G H, Hudson C M & Kirkwood B R. Epidemiological studies of onchocerciasis in forest villages of Sierra Leone. *Trop Med Parasitol* 1988; 39:251–259.

94 World Health Organization. *Onchocerciasis Control Programme in West Africa: progress report*, JPC 11.2 OCP/PR/90. Geneva: WHO, 1990.

95 Ertmann K D, Unnasch T R, Greene B M et al. A DNA sequence specific for forest-form *Onchocerca volvulus*. Nature 1987; 327:415–417.

96 Garner A. Pathology of ocular onchocerciasis: human and experimental. *Trans R Soc Trop Med Hyg* 1976; 70:374–377.

97 Dadzie K Y, Remme J, Rolland A & Thylefors B. The effect of 7–8 years of vector control on the evolution of ocular onchocerciasis in West African savanna. *Trop Med Parasitol* 1986; 37:263–270.

98 Mackenzie C D, Williams J F, Sisley B M, Steward M W & O'Day J. Variations in host responses and the pathogenesis of human onchocerciasis. *Rev Infect Dis* 1985; 7:802–808.

99 Gibson D W, Connor D H, Brown H L et al. Onchocercal dermatitis: ultrastructural studies of microfilariae and host tissues, before and after treatment with diethylcarbamazine (Hetrazan). *Am J Trop Med Hyg* 1976; 25:74–87.

100 Greene B M, Taylor H R & Aikawa M. Cellular killing of microfilariae of *Onchocerca volvulus*: eosinophil and neutrophil-mediated immune serum-dependent destruction. *J Immunol* 1981; 127:1611–1618.

101 World Health Organization. WHO expert committee on onchocerciasis. *WHO Tech Rep Ser* 1987: 752.

102 Bartlett A, Turk J, Ngu J, Mackenzie C D, Fuglsang H & Anderson J. Variation in delayed hypersensitivity in onchocerciasis. *Trans R Soc Trop Med Hyg* 1978; 72:372–377.

103 Cabrera Z, Buttner D W & Parkhouse R M E. Unique recognition of a low molecular weight *Onchocerca volvulus* antigen by IgG3 antibodies in chronic hyper-reactive oncho-dermatitis (Sowda). *Clin Exp Immunol* 1988; 74:223–229.

104 Van der Lelij A, Rothova A, Stilma J S, Vetter J C M, Hoekzema R & Kijlstra A. Humoral and cell-mediated immune response against retinal antigens in relation to onchocerciasis. *Acta Leiden* 1990; 59:271–283.

105 Gatrill A J, Mackenzie C D, McMahon J E, Williams J F & Guderian R H. A histocytochemical study of the macrophages present in tissue responses to adult *Onchocerca volvulus*. *Histochem J* 1987; 19:509–519.

106 Greene B M, Gbakima A A, Albiez E J & Taylor H R. Humoral and cellular immune responses to *Onchocerca volvulus* infections in humans. *Rev Infect Dis*, 1985; 7:789–795.

107 Lucius R, Buttner D W, Kirsten C & Diesfield H J. A study of antigen recognition by onchocerciasis patients with different clinical forms of disease. *Parasitology* 1986; 92:569–580.

108 Petralanda I, Yarzabal L & Piessens W F. Parasite antigens are present in breast milk of women infected with *Onchocerca volvulus*. *Am J Trop Med Hyg* 1988; 38:372–379.

109 Leke R G, Boto, Labdo & Ngu J L. Immunity to *Onchocerca volvulus*. Serum mediated leucocyte adherence to infective larvae in vitro. *Trop Med Parasitol* 1989; 40:39–41.

110 Gallin M, Edmonds K, Ellner J J et al. Cell mediated immune responses in human infection with *Onchocerca volvulus*. *J Immunol* 1988; 140:1999–2007.

111 Ward D J, Nutman T B, Zea-Flores G, Portocarrero C, Lujan A & Ottesen E A. Onchocerciasis and immunity in humans: enhanced T cell responsiveness to parasite antigen in putatively immune individuals. *J Infect Dis* 1988; 157:536–543.

112 Kilian H D & Nielsen G. Cell-mediated and humoral immune response to tetanus vaccinations in onchocerciasis patients. *Trop Med Parasitol* 1989; 40:285–291.

113 Homeida M A, Mackenzie C D, Williams J F & Ghalib H W. The detection of onchocercal nodules by ultrasound technique. *Trans R Soc Trop Med Hyg* 1986; 80:570–571.

114 Leichsenring M, Troger J, Nelle M, Buttner D W, Darge K & Doehring-Schwerdtfeger E. Ultrasonographical investigations of onchocerciasis in Liberia. *Am J Trop Med Hyg* 1990; 43:380–385.

115 Goddard J. *Studies in diagnostic field techniques in Sierra Leone for the identification of microfilariae of* Onchocerca volvulus. Thesis, Fellowship of Institute of Medical Laboratory Sciences, 1986: 74.

116 Mackenzie C D, Burgess P J & Sisley B M. Onchocerciasis. In Walls K V & Schantz P M (eds) *Immunodiagnosis of Parasitic Diseases*, vol. I: Helminthic Diseases. London: Academic Press, 1986: 255–289.

117 Weil G J, Ogunrinade A F, Chandrashekar R & Kale O O. IgG4 subclass antibody serology for onchocerciasis. *J Infect Dis* 1989; 161:549–554.

118 Chandrashekar R, Ogunrinade A F, Alvarez R M, Kale O O & Weil G J. Circulating immune

complex-associated parasitic antigens in human onchocerciasis. *J Infect Dis* 1990; 162:1159–1164.

119 Schlie-Guzman M A & Rivas-Alcala A R. Antigen detection in onchocerciasis: correlation with worm burden. *Trop Med Parasitol* 1989; 40:47–50.

120 Ramachandran C P. Improved immunodiagnostic tests to monitor onchocerciasis control programmes: a multicenter effort. *Parasitol Today* 1993; 9:76–79.

121 Bradley J E, Trenholme K R, Gillespie A J et al. A sensitive serodiagnostic test for onchocerciasis using a cocktail of recombinant antigens. *Am J Trop Med Hyg* 1993; 48:198–204.

122 Lobos E, Weiss N, Karam M, Taylor H R, Ottesen E A & Nutman T B. An immunogenic *Onchocerca volvulus* antigen: a specific and early marker of infection. *Science* 1991; 251:1603–1605.

123 Meredith S E O, Lando G, Gbakima A A, Zimmerman P A & Unnasch T R. *Onchocerca volvulus*: application of the polymerase chain reaction to identification and strain differentiation of the parasite. *Exp Parasitol* 1991; 73:335–344.

124 Mazzotti L & Hewitt R. Tratamiento de la onchocercosis por el cloruro del 1-dietilcarbamil-4-metilpiperazine (Hetrazan). *Med Mex* 1947; 28:3–6.

125 Awadzi K, Dadzie K Y, Klager S & Gilles H M. The chemotherapy of onchocerciasis. XIII. Studies with onchocerciasis patients in northern Ghana, a region with long lasting vector controls. *Trop Med Parasitol* 1989; 40:361–366.

126 Whitworth J A, Morgan D, Maude G H & Taylor D W. Community-based treatment with ivermectin. *Lancet* 1988; ii:97–98.

127 Jenkins D C. Ivermectin in the treatment of filarial and other nematode infections of man. *Trop Dis Bull* 1990; 87:R1–R9.

128 Duke B O L, Zea-Flores G, Castro J, Cupp E W & Nuños B. Comparison of the effects of a single dose and four six-monthly doses of ivermectin on adult *Onchocerca volvulus*. *Am J Trop Med Hyg* 1991; 45:132–137.

129 Duke B O L. Studies on factors influencing the transmission of onchocerciasis in the biting cycles, infective biting density and transmission potential of 'forest' *Simulium damnosum*. *Ann Trop Med Parasitol* 1968; 62:95–106.

130 McMahon J E, Davies J B, White M D, Goddard J M, Beech-Garwood P A & Kirkwood B R. Onchocerciasis in Sierra Leone 1: studies on the prevalence and transmission in Gbaiima village. *Trans R Soc Trop Med Hyg* 1986; 80:802–809.

131 Braun-Munziger R A & Southgate B A. Preliminary studies on the histochemical differentiation of strains of *Onchocerca volvulus* microfilariae in Togo. *Bull World Health Organ* 1977; 55:569–575.

132 Omar M S & Garms R. Histochemical differentiation of filarial larvae found in *Simulium damnosum* s.l. in West Africa. *Tropenmed Parasitol* 1981; 32:259–264.

133 Duke B O L, Lewis D J & Moore P J. Transmission of forest and Sudan-savanna strains of *Onchocerca volvulus* from Cameroon by *Simulium damnosum* from various West African bioclimatic zones. *Ann Trop Med Parasitol* 1966; 60:318–336.

134 Hay R J, Mackenzie C D, Guderian R, Noble W C, Proana J R & Williams J F. Onchodermatitis: correlation between skin disease and parasitic load in an endemic focus in Ecuador. *Br J Dermatol* 1989; 121:187–198.

135 Post R J & Crosskey R W. The distribution of the *Simulium damnosum* complex in Sierra Leone and its relation to onchocerciasis. *Ann Trop Med Parasitol* 1985; 79:169–194.

136 Davies J B, Beech-Garwood P A, Thomson M C & McMahon J E. Onchocerciasis transmission levels and *Simulium damnosum* complex biting activity at riverside and rice field sites in Sierra Leone. *Med Vet Entomol* 1988; 2:357–369.

137 Thomson M C, Davies J B, Bockarie M J, Beech-Garwood P A, Kandehe J & Post R. Invasion of savanna *Simulium damnosum* s.l. into southern Sierra Leone in 1988. *Bull Entymol* in press.

138 Baker R H, Guillet P, Seketeli A et al. Progress in controlling the reinvasion of windborne vectors into the western area of the Onchocerciasis Control Programme in West Africa. *Philos Trans R Soc London [Biol]* 1990; 328:731–747.

139 Pedersen E M & Maegga B T. Quantitative studies on the transmission of *Onchocerca volvulus* by *Simulium damnosum* s.l. in the Tukuyu Valley, South West Tanzania. *Tropenmed Parasitol* 1985; 36:249–254.

140 Pedersen E M & Kolstrup N. The epidemiology of onchocerciasis in the Tukuyu Valley, South West Tanzania. *Tropenmed Parasitol* 1986; 37:35–38.

141 Shelley A J. Biosystematics and medical importance of the *Simulium amazonicum* group and the *S. exiguum* complex in Latin America. In Service M W (ed.) *Biosystematics of Haematophagous Insects*. Systematics Association Special Volume No. 37, Oxford: Clarendon Press, 1988: 203–220.

142 Shelley A J. Vector aspects of the epidemiology of onchocerciasis in Latin America. *Ann Rev Entomol* 1988; 33:337–366.

143 Guderian R H & Shelley A J. Onchocerciasis in Ecuador: The situation in 1989. *Mem Inst Oswaldo Cruz, Rio de Janero* 1992; 87:405–415.

144 Guderian R H, Beck J, Guevara A E, Chico M H & Lazo R S. Oncocercosis en El Ecuador: Los Oncocercomas II. Prevalencia en los Focos de Emeraldas, Universidad de Guayaquil, 1989; 77:17–36.

145 Cooper P J, Proano R, Beltran C, Anselmi M & Guderian R H. Onchocerciasis in Ecuador: ocular findings in *Onchocerca volvulus* infected individuals. *Br J Ophthalmol* in press

146 Webbe G. The Onchocerciasis Control Programme. *Trans R Soc Trop Med Hyg* 1992; 86:113–114.

147 Remme J, Baker R H A, De Sole G, Dadzie K Y

et al. A community trial of ivermectin in the onchocerciasis focus of Asubende, Ghana. I. Effect on the microfilarial reservoir and the transmission of *Onchocerca volvulus*. *Trop Med Parasitol* 1989; 40:367–374.

148 Taylor H R, Pacqué M, Muños B & Greene B M. Impact of mass treatment of onchocerciasis with ivermectin on the transmission of infection. *Science* 1990; 250:116–118.

149 Whitworth J A G, Morgan D, Maude G H, Luty A J F & Taylor D W. A community trial of ivermectin for onchocerciasis in Sierra Leone: clinical and parasitological responses to four doses given at six-monthly intervals. *Trans R Soc Trop Med Hyg* 1992; 86:277–280.

150 Collins R C, Gonzales-Peralta C, Castro J et al. Ivermectin: reduction in prevalence and infection intensity of *Onchocerca volvulus* following biannual treatments in five Guatemalan communities. *Am J Trop Med Hyg* 1992; 47:156–169.

151 Dadzie K Y, Remme J & De Sole G. Changes in ocular onchocerciasis after two rounds of community-based ivermectin treatment in a holo-endemic onchocerciasis focus. *Trans R Soc Trop Med Hyg* 1991; 85:267–271.

152 Pacqué M, Elmets C, Dukuly Z D et al. Improvement in severe onchocercal skin disease after single dose ivermectin. *Am J Med* 1991; 90:590–594.

153 Whitworth J A G, Morgan D, Maude G H, McNicholas A M & Taylor D W. A field study of the effect of ivermectin on intestinal helminths in man. *Trans R Soc Trop Med Hyg* 1991; 85:232–234.

154 Edungbola L D. Onchocerciasis control in Nigeria. *Parasitol Today* 1991; 7:97–99.

155 Pinder M. *Loa loa*: a neglected filaria. *Parasitol Today* 1988; 4:279–284.

156 Noireau F, Apembet J D, Nzoulani A & Carme B. Clinical manifestations of loiasis in an endemic area in the Congo. *Trop Med Parasitol* 1990; 41:37–39.

157 Carme B, Mamboueni J P, Copin N & Noireau F. Clinical and biological study of *Loa loa* filariasis in Congolese. *Am J Trop Med Hyg* 1989; 41:331–337.

158 Nutman T B, Miller K D, Mulligan M & Ottesen E A. *Loa loa* infection in temporary residents of endemic regions: recognition of a hyper-responsive syndrome with characteristic clinical manifestations. *J Infect Dis* 1986; 154:10–18.

159 Ive F A, Willis A J P, Ikeme A C & Brockington I F. Endomyocardial fibrosis and filariasis. *Q J Med* 1967; 36:495–516.

160 Baird J K, Neafie R C & Connor D H. Nodules in the conjunctiva, bung-eye, and bulge-eye in Africa caused by *Mansonella perstans*. *Am J Trop Med Hyg* 1988; 38:553–557.

161 Dupont A, Zue-N'dong J & Pinder M. Common occurrence of amicrofilaraemic *Loa loa* filariasis within the endemic region. *Trans R Soc Trop Med Hyg* 1988; 82:730.

162 Egwang T G, Dupont A, Leclerc A, Akue J P & Pinder M. Differential recognition of *Loa loa* antigens by sera of human subjects from a loiasis endemic area. *Am J Trop Med Hyg* 1989; 41:664–673.

163 Goussard B, Ivanoff B, Frost E, Garin Y & Bourderiou C. Age of appearance of IgG, IgM, and IgE antibodies specific for *Loa loa* in Gabonese children. *Microbiol Immunol* 1984; 28:787–792.

164 Pinder M, Dupont A & Egwang T G. Identification of a surface antigen on *Loa loa* microfilariae the recognition of which correlates with the amicrofilaraemic state in man. *J Immunol* 1988; 141:2480–2486.

165 Hoegaerden M V, Ivanoff B, Flocard F, Salle A & Chabaud B. The use of mebendazole in the treatment of filariases due to *Loa loa* and *Mansonella perstans*. *Ann Trop Med Parasitol* 1987; 81:275–282.

166 Chippaux J P, Ernould J C, Gardon J, Gardon-Wendel N, Chandre F & Barberi N. Ivermectin treatment of loiasis. *Trans R Soc Trop Med Hyg* 1992; 86:289.

167 Martin-Prevel Y, Cosnefroy J Y, Tshipamba P, Ngari P, Chodakewitz J A & Pinder M. Tolerance and efficacy of single high-dose ivermectin for the treatment of loiasis. *Am J Trop Med Hyg* 1993; 48:186–192.

168 Noireau F, Carme B, Apembet J D & Gouteux J P. *Loa loa* and *Mansonella perstans* filariasis in the Chaillu mountains, Congo: parasitological prevalence. *Trans R Soc Trop Med Hyg* 1989; 83:529–534.

169 Hoegaerden M V, Chabaud B, Akue J P & Ivanoff B. Filariasis due to *Loa loa* and *Mansonella perstans*: distribution in the region of Okondja, Haut-Ogoou Province, Gabon, with parasitological and serological follow-up over one year. *Trans R Soc Trop Med Hyg* 1987; 81:441–446.

170 Nutman T B, Miller K D, Mulligan M et al. Diethylcarbamazine provides effective prophylaxis for human loiasis. *N Engl J Med* 1988; 319:752–756.

171 Linley J R, Hoch A L & Pinheiro F P. Biting midges (Diptera: Ceratopogonidae) and human health. *J Med Entomol* 1985; 20:347–364.

172 Meyers W M, Connor D H, Harman L F, Fleshman K, Moris R & Neafie R C. Human streptocerciasis. A clinico-pathologic study of 40 Africans (Zairans) including identification of the adult filaria. *Am J Trop Med Hyg* 1972; 22:528–545.

173 Nathan M B, Tikasingh E S, Nelson G S, Santiago A & Davies J B. The prevalence and distribution of *Mansonella ozzardi* in coastal north Trinidad, WI. *Trans R Soc Trop Med Hyg* 1979; 73:299–302.

174 Raccurt C, Lowrie R C & McNeeley D F. *Mansonella ozzardi* in Haiti. I. Epidemiological survey. *Am J Trop Med Hyg* 1980; 29:803–808.

175 McNeeley D F, Raccurt C P, Boncy J & Lowrie R C. Clinical evaluation of *Mansonella ozzardi* in Haiti. *Trop Med Parasitol* 1989; 40:107–110.

176 Katz S P, Raccurt C P, Lowrie R C, Boncy J & Leiva L M. *Mansonella ozzardi* in Haiti. IV.

Evaluation of antibody reactivity to heterologous antigens. *Am J Trop Med Hyg* 1986; 35:303–307.

177 Raccurt C, Lowrie R C, Boncy J & Katz S P. *Mansonella ozzardi* in Haiti. III. A comparison of the sensitivity of four sampling methods in detecting infections. *Am J Trop Med Hyg* 1982; 31:275–279.

178 Nutman T B, Nash T E & Ottesen E A. Ivermectin in the successful treatment of a patient with *Mansonella ozzardi* infection. *J Infect Dis* 1987; 156:662–665.

179 Boreham P F L. Dirofilariasis in man. In Boreham P F L & Atwell R B (eds) *Dirofilariasis*. Boca Raton: CRC Press, 1988: 218–226.

180 Orihel T C. Cerebral filariasis in Rhodesia: a zoonotic infection? *Am J Trop Med Hyg* 1973; 22:596–599.

181 Richard-Lenoble D, Kombila M, Bain O, Chandenier J & Mariotte O. Filariasis in Gabon: human infections with *Microfilaria rodhaini*. *Am J Trop Med Hyg* 1988; 39:91–92.

182 Godoy G A, Orihel T C & Volcan G S. *Microfilaria bolivarensis*: A new species of filaria from man in Venezuela. *Am J Trop Med Hyg* 1980; 29:545–547.

183 Fain A. *Dipetalonema semiclarum* sp. nov. from the blood of man in the republic of Zaire (Nematoda: Filarioidea). *Ann Soc Belg Med Trop* 1974; 54:195–207.

184 Coombs I & Crompton D W T. *A Guide to Human Helminths*. London: Taylor & Francis, 1991.

185 Muller R. *Dracunculus* in Africa. In Macpherson C N L & Craig P S (eds) *Parasitic Helminths and Zoonoses in Africa*. London: Unwin Hyman, 1991: 204–223.

186 Muller R. Life cycle of *Dracunculus medinensis*. In *Opportunities for Control of Dracunculiasis*. Washington: National Academy Press, 1985: 13–18.

187 Steib K & Mayer P. Epidemiology and vectors of *Dracunculus medinensis* on northwest Burkina Faso, West Africa. *Ann Trop Med Parasitol* 1988; 82:189–199.

188 Bloch P, Simonsen P E & Vennervald B J. The antibody response to *Dracunculus medinensis* in an endemic human population of northern Ghana. *J Helminthol* 1993; 67:37–48.

189 Fagbemi B O & Hillyer G V. Immunodiagnosis of dracunculiasis by Falcon assay screening test-enzyme-linked immunosorbent assay (FAST-ELISA) and by enzyme-linked immunoelectrotransfer blot (EITB) technique. *Am J Trop Med Hyg* 1990; 43:665–668.

190 Garate T, Kliks M M, Cabrera Z & Parkhouse R M E. Specific and cross-reacting antibodies in human responses to *Onchocerca volvulus* and *Dracunculus medinensis* infections. *Am J Trop Med Hyg* 1990; 42:140–147.

191 Rohde J E, Sharma B L, Patton H, Deegan C & Sherry J M. Surgical extraction of guinea worm: Disability reduction and contribution to disease control. *Am J Trop Med Hyg* 1993; 48:71–76.

192 Eberhard M L, Brandt F H, Ruitz-Tiben E & Hightower A. Chemoprophylactic drug trials for treatment of dracunculiasis using the *Dracunculus insignis*–ferret model. *J Helminthol* 1990; 64:79–86.

193 Hopkins D R. Dracunculiasis. In Warren K S & Mahmoud A A F (eds) *Tropical and Geographical Medicine*. New York: McGraw-Hill, 1990: 439–442.

194 Smith G S, Blum D, Huttly S R A, Okeke N, Kirkwood B R & Feachem R G. Disability from dracunculiasis: effect on mobility. *Ann Trop Med Parasitol* 1989; 83:151–158.

195 Belcher D W, Wurapa F K, Ward W B & Lourie I M. Guinea worm in southern Ghana: its epidemiology and impact on agricultural productivity. *Am J Trop Med Hyg* 1975; 24:243–249.

196 Hopkins D R, Ruiz-Tiben E, Kaiser R L, Agle A N & Withers P C. Dracunculiasis eradication: beginning of the end. *Am J Trop Med Hyg* 1993; 49:281–289.

197 Edungbola L D, Watts S J, Alabi T O & Bello A B. The impact on a Unicef-assisted rural water project on the prevalence of Guinea worm disease in Asa, Kwara State, Nigeria. *Am J Trop Med Hyg* 1988; 39:79–85.

198 Sullivan J J & Long E G. Synthetic-fibre filters for preventing dracunculiasis: 100 versus 200 micrometres pore size. *Trans R Soc Trop Med Hyg* 1988; 82:465–466.

199 McCullough F S. Cyclopoid copepods: their role in the transmission and control of dracunculiasis. In *Opportunities for Control of Dracunculiasis*. Washington: National Academy Press, 1985: 65–76.

CHAPTER 71

SOIL-TRANSMITTED HELMINTHS (GEOHELMINTHS)

H. M. Gilles

These are intestinal nematodes, part of the development of which takes place outside the body—in the soil.

Soil-transmitted nematodes are of great importance in the health of many populations in developing countries where the frequency of infection is a general indication of the local level of development of hygiene and sanitation. These nematodes are usually found as multiple infections and measures against and treatment of one closely affect the others. They may be divided into three types according to their life cycle.

TYPE 1 DIRECT

Embryonated eggs are passed; they hatch and reinfect within 2–3 hours by being carried from the anal margin to the mouth and either do not reach the soil or, if they do, do not require a period of development there. This group includes *Enterobius vermicularis* (threadworm) and *Trichuris trichiura* (whipworm).

TYPE 2 MODIFIED DIRECT

Eggs are passed out in the stool and undergo a period of development in the soil before being ingested, where they hatch, releasing larvae which penetrate the mucous membrane(s) of the stomach and enter the circulation to reach the lungs, passing up the respiratory tract to enter the oesophagus reaching the intestine where they become adult. These include *Ascaris lumbricoides* (roundworm) and *Toxocara canis*.

TYPE 3 PENETRATION OF THE SKIN

In this group eggs are passed in the stools to the soil, where they hatch into larvae which undergo further development before they are ready to penetrate the skin and reach the circulation and lungs which they penetrate to enter the respiratory tract; they move up to enter the oesophagus and reach the small intestine, where they become adult. *Ancylostoma* (hookworm) and *Strongyloides stercoralis* belong to this group, but differ in that *Strongyloides* larvae are passed in the stool and autoinfection can occur at the anal margin, or independent development take place in the soil where they can exist in the absence of any further cycle through man.

TYPE 1 DIRECT (*ENTEROBIUS, TRICHURIS*)

ENTEROBIASIS (THREADWORM, PINWORM, OXYURIASIS)

GEOGRAPHICAL DISTRIBUTION

Enterobius vermicularis has a worldwide distribution.

AETIOLOGY

The adult *Enterobius vermicularis* (Figure 71.1, Chapter 3 and Appendix III) are small and white with a double bulb oesophagus and a mouth surrounded by a cuticular expansion; the skin is transversely striated. The female (9–12 mm) has a long, pointed tail and a slit-like vulva in the anterior quarter of the body. The male, which is much smaller (2.5 mm), has a posteriorly curved third and a blunt caudal extremity. The egg (Figure 71.2) measures 50–54 × 20–27 mm and has a characteristic shape, flattened on one side. It is almost colourless with a bean-shaped double contour shell containing a fully formed embryo.

LIFE CYCLE (see Appendix III)

There is no multiplication inside the body. The mature female has a life duration of 37–93 days and when the ovary is full of eggs she migrates down to the anus, from which she emerges to lay the eggs on the perianal skin and on the perineum. The eggs which are ingested in faecal material lodged under the fingernails hatch in the stomach and larvae emerge which rapidly grow to 140–150 μm in length. They pass through the intestine to the caecum and appendix where they invade the glandular crypts and mature. The whole cycle takes 2–4 weeks.

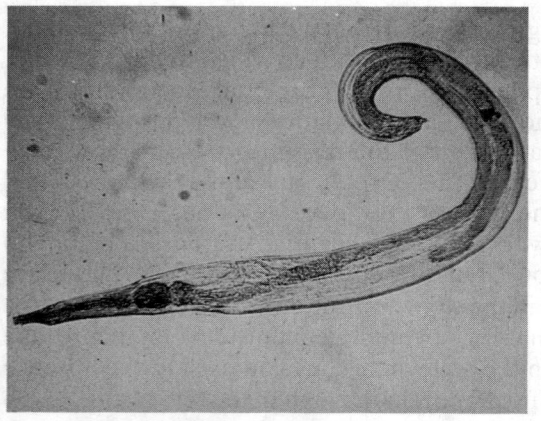

Figure 71.1 Adult *Enterobius vermicularis* (threadworm, pinworm).

TRANSMISSION

There are four possible ways of transmission; the most common is by direct transmission from the anal and perianal region to the mouth by fingernail contamination and by soiled nightclothes. A second way is by exposure to viable eggs on soiled bed linen and other contaminated objects in the environment. A third way is via the mouth or nose from contaminated dust in which embryonated eggs have been detected. The fourth way is by retroinfection[1] in which eggs hatch on the anal mucosa and larvae migrate up the bowel.

PATHOLOGY

The adult worm lives in the upper part of the colon, especially the caecum and lower ileum, where minute ulcerations may develop at the site of attachment of the adult worms to the caecal and appendiceal mucosa. At times haemorrhages occur and secondary infection causes ulcers and submucosal abscesses. Symptoms are caused when gravid females migrate out of the anus on to perianal skin to deposit eggs, where they cause pruritus.

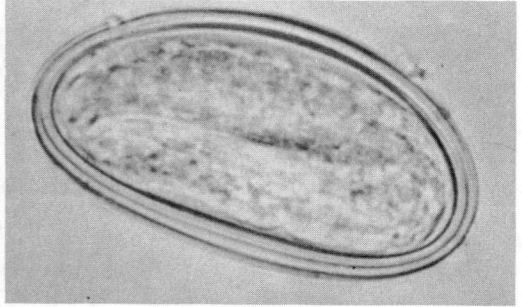

Figure 71.2 Egg of *Enterobius vermicularis*, as laid partially embryonated.

ECTOPIC LESIONS

Occasionally *Enterobius* is found in the female genital organs and more rarely in the ear and nose. Rarely worms can invade the abdominal cavity and cause threadworm granulomas of the liver,[2] ovary, kidney, spleen and lung. Chronic pelvic peritonitis has been described.[3] The route by which *Enterobius* gains access to these organs is not clear but may be via the fallopian tubes or haematogenous spread. Direct infection following abdominal operations may also occur. The granuloma which forms around the female and eggs consists chiefly of lymphocytes with a few eosinophils but no giant cells. Four cases of eosinophilic granuloma of the large bowel and omentum have been ascribed to *Enterobius*.

CLINICAL FEATURES

NATURAL HISTORY

In the majority of infections *Enterobius* lives out its normal life span in the caecum and appendix, migrates down to the anus and deposits its eggs, and the larvae re-establish themselves in the host, causing few or no symptoms.

SYMPTOMS AND SIGNS

Pruritus ani is the main symptom and varies from mild itching to acute pain which occurs mainly at night. The pruritus provides scratching of the perianal region resulting in excoriation and secondary infection.

Vulvitis may be caused by pinworms entering the vulva causing a mucoid discharge and *pruritus vulvi*.

General symptoms are insomnia and restlessness, and a considerable proportion of children show loss of appetite, loss of weight, irritability, emotional instability and enuresis. There is usually no eosinophilia or anaemia.

DIAGNOSIS

The diagnosis is made by finding the characteristic eggs (see Figure 71.2) in the faeces (5% only), perianal scrapings or swabs from under the fingernails, or by finding adult worms round the anus, usually at night.

FAECAL EXAMINATION (See also Appendix V)

Eggs are present in the faeces of no more than 5% of infected individuals.

A Sellotape swab has been devised with which it is possible to obtain eggs by scraping the perianal area. Enclosed in a container, it may be sent through the post and examined at leisure. The Sellotape is mounted in water or 0.1 mol sodium hydroxide on a slide, covered with a coverslip and examined.

The Scotch tape method, in which eggs adhere to a sticky surface, is very popular (see Appendix V).

TREATMENT

The whole family must be treated to avoid reinfection. Chemotherapy must be combined with education, and personal hygiene aimed at preventing autoinfection. Although it is simple to effect a temporary cure, eradication may prove difficult because of reinfection from the contaminated environment or from asymptomatic members of the same household. Eradication may necessitate repeated courses of treatment for up to a year or more.

CHEMOTHERAPY

Albendazole is the treatment of choice, as a single oral dose of 400 mg or 10–14 mg/kg for children.

Mebendazole is as effective in a single oral dose of 100 mg. It is available 'over the counter'.

Pyrantel pamoate (Combantrin) 10 mg/kg may be given as a single oral dose and repeated every 6 weeks until the environment is clear.

During treatment it is important to prevent reinfection. The child must sleep in cotton clothes and gloves and the fingernails must be kept short and scrubbed. Other members of the family or school should also be treated.

EPIDEMIOLOGY

Enterobiasis is worldwide in distribution and is a group infection, more common in children than adults. It occurs in family groups or institutions, such as asylums and schools, especially under crowded conditions. When one infection is found it is likely that there are others also. Although it is a human infection, chimpanzees, gibbons and marmosets can all be infected.

TRICHURIASIS (*TRICHURIS TRICHIURA*) (WHIPWORM)

GEOGRAPHICAL DISTRIBUTION

Trichuris trichiura occurs worldwide. It is estimated that 755 million people in the world are infected.[4]

AETIOLOGY

Trichuris trichiura is a greyish-white worm, often slightly pink, which lives in the caecum and appendix. The male (30–45 mm long) has an attenuated anterior portion containing a cellular oesophagus which is half as long again as the thicker posterior portion, and a caudal extremity curved through 360° with a single spicule in the sheath which is studded with spines (Figure 71.3). The female (30–35 mm long) has the posterior half occupied by a stout uterus packed with eggs. The egg (50 × 22 μm) is brown with a characteristic band shape and a single shell with a plug at each end; it contains a single embryo (Figure 71.4).

LIFE CYCLE (See Appendix III)

The worms live in the caecum where they maintain their position by transfixing a superficial fold of mucosa and lie embedded in mucus between the intestinal villi. The egg is laid unsegmented, and embryonation takes at least 21 days. It can withstand low temperatures but not desiccation. Infection is direct from stale faeces. The egg hatches after being swallowed in the intestine, where the shell is digested by intestinal juices and the larva emerges in the small intestine; it penetrates the villi and develops for a week until it re-emerges and passes to the caecum and colorectum, where it attaches itself to the mucosa and becomes adult.

TRANSMISSION

Transmission is direct from mature eggs to the mouth via fingers contaminated from infected soil.

PATHOLOGY

When there are only a few worms there is little damage but with heavy infections they spread throughout the colon to the rectum. They cause haemorrhages, mucopurulent stools and symptoms of dysentery with rectal prolapse.[5]

Trichuris is frequently associated with *Ascaris* and hookworm and a secondary infection with *Entamoeba histolytica* causes further ulceration.

CLINICAL FEATURES

NATURAL HISTORY

In the vast majority of infections, which are light, the worms live harmlessly in the caecum and appendix but when the infection is heavy (more than 10 000/g of faeces) there can be marked symptoms and signs.

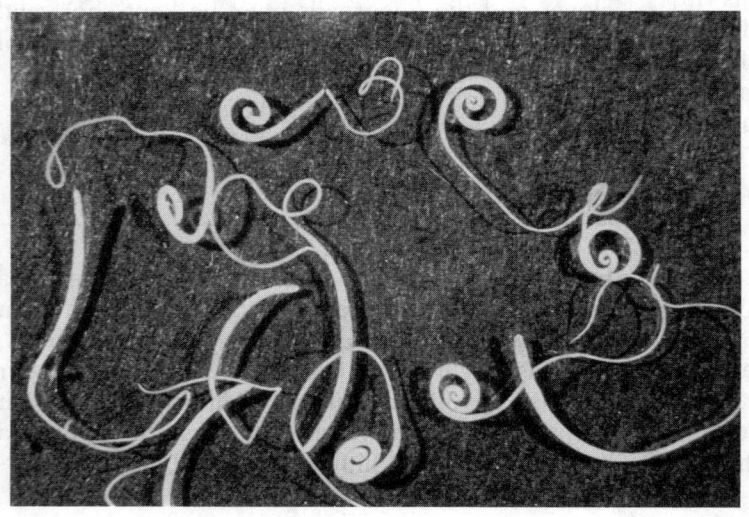

Figure 71.3 Adult *Trichuris* worms (whipworms), male and female. (Courtesy H. Zaiman.)

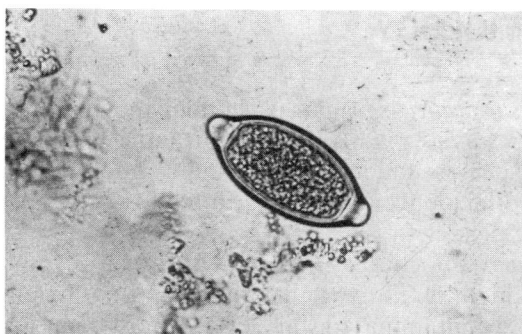

Figure 71.4   Egg of *Trichuris*. (Courtesy WTIM.)

INCUBATION PERIOD

The prepatent period from ingestion of eggs to the appearance of eggs in the stool is 60 days.

SYMPTOMS AND SIGNS

In light infections there are no symptoms, but when associated with *Ascaris* or hookworm mild symptoms occur. Epigastric pain, vomiting, distension, flatulence, anorexia and weight loss may occur.[6] Pain in the epigastrium and right iliac fossa is common.[7] When associated with *Entamoeba histolytica*, *Balantidium coli* or shigellosis, symptoms are highly aggravated and dysenteric symptoms occur. Anaemia and low serum albumin is more pronounced in double infections with *Trichuris* than in amoebic infections alone.[8] There is usually no eosinophilia which, if pronounced, usually denotes a concurrent *Toxocara* infection, with which it is often associated.

Trichuris *dysentery*

In heavy infections, as seen in the southern USA, the West Indies and South-East Asia, infection may extend from the caecum to the rectum and there may be quite a severe dysentery with blood and mucus in the stools (Figure 71.5) and prolapse of the rectum (Figure 71.6). These infections, which are often associated with amoebiasis, respond well to anthelmintic treatment. In severe massive infantile trichuriasis digital clubbing, hypoproteinaemia, severe anaemia and growth retardation are common.[9]

DIFFERENTIAL DIAGNOSIS

In severe infection the clinical picture may resemble hookworm disease, acute appendicitis or amoebic dysentery.

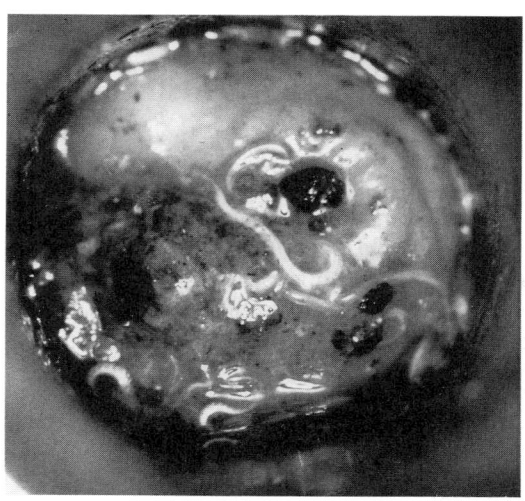

Figure 71.5   Proctoscopic view of *Trichuris* worms causing dysentery.

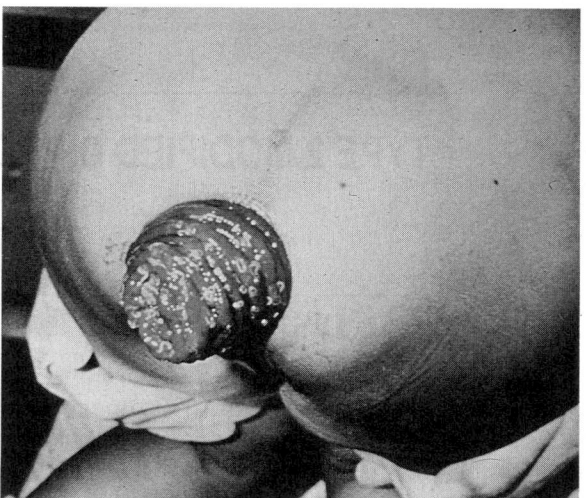

Figure 71.6   Prolapse of the rectum in *Trichuris* dysentery.

DIAGNOSIS

The diagnosis is made by finding the characteristic eggs in the stool (see Figure 71.4) by direct smear or by concentration methods (see Appendix V). An egg count (see Appendix V) will reveal the degree of infection and 30 000 eggs/g of faeces or more is a heavy infection[5] which would indicate the presence of several hundred worms and the production of symptoms.

Proctoscopy in cases of dysentery will show numerous worms attached to the mucosa—which is reddened and ulcerated where they are responsible for the dysentery.

Radiological appearances

In some cases a 'honeycomb' appearance of the small intestine has been seen with the appearances of Crohn's disease; deformity of the intestine is most marked in the proximal colon but also present in the ileum and appendix.

TREATMENT

Mebendazole is the drug of choice. A single oral dose of 600 mg will reduce the egg count by over 85% and is as efficient as the standard dose of 100 mg twice daily for 3 days.[10]

Albendazole is equally effective at a single dose of 400 mg

EPIDEMIOLOGY

Trichuris trichiura is primarily a human infection but *Trichuris suis* of pigs is indistinguishable from the human species and can infect man. There is an increased incidence of *Trichuris* infection in people handling pigs.

Trichuris infection is common in areas of high rainfall, high humidity, dense shade and poor sanitation and contaminated soil. It is the most common soil-transmitted helminthic infection in Malaysia. The greatest prevalence is in children of primary school age who pollute the soil around the house and who develop heavy worm burdens. *Trichuris* infection is often associated with *Ascaris* and *Toxocara*, the epidemiology of which is similar.

Control is the same as that for *Ascaris*: avoidance of soil pollution and periodic mass chemotherapy (see pp. 182–184). Regional differences in susceptibility of *Trichuris trichiura* to albendazole seem to occur and it would be therefore prudent to evaluate local sensitivity when planning mass chemotherapy.[11]

TYPE 2 MODIFIED DIRECT (*ASCARIS, TOXOCARA*)

ASCARIS

GEOGRAPHICAL DISTRIBUTION

Ascaris lumbricoides (roundworm) is one of the most common and most widespread human infections. Possibly one in four of the world's population is infected. It occurs in Asia, Central and South America, Europe, Africa and North America.

The prevalence of *Ascaris* varies in different parts of the world. In China and South-East Asia it is highly prevalent. In the central Asian republics of the former USSR it is common in humid areas. In Central and South America the average rate of infection is 45%, and in parts of Africa 95%. In Europe and the southern USA it is low.

AETIOLOGY AND LIFECYCLE (Figure 71.7)

Ascaris lumbricoides (Figure 71.8) is a comparatively large worm (female 20–25 cm × 3–6 mm; male

15–31 cm × 2–4 mm) which inhabits the small intestine (the morphology is described in Appendix III). Eggs (Figure 71.9) are laid in the small intestine and are passed out as immature ova containing no segmented or differentiated embryo. In damp soil an embryo develops at 36–40°C in 2–4 months (at the optimum of 25°C in 3 weeks); it lies coiled up in the egg, undergoing one moult before being hatched as an infective second stage rhabditiform larva in the small intestine when the egg is swallowed (see Appendix III). Here the rhabditiform larva penetrates the mucous membrane, enters the bloodstream—reaching the lungs via the right heart where it cannot pass through the lung capillaries, so that it burrows through the alveolar wall to enter the respiratory tract. From here it is carried up the trachea to the larynx, where it moves over the epiglottis and enters the oesophagus, and is swallowed a second time to reach the small intestine. The whole process takes 10–14 days, during which time the larva moults twice, the fourth moult taking place between the 25th and 29th days. Larvae may reach the intestine as early as the fifth day. In man the

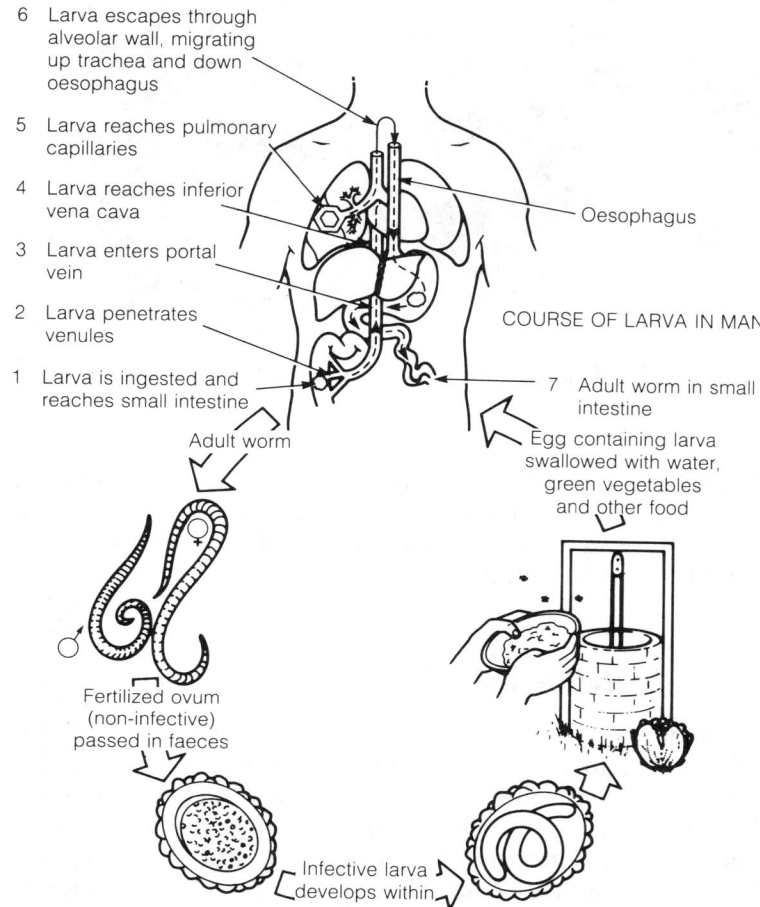

6 Larva escapes through alveolar wall, migrating up trachea and down oesophagus

5 Larva reaches pulmonary capillaries

4 Larva reaches inferior vena cava

3 Larva enters portal vein

2 Larva penetrates venules

1 Larva is ingested and reaches small intestine

Oesophagus

COURSE OF LARVA IN MAN

7 Adult worm in small intestine

Egg containing larva swallowed with water, green vegetables and other food

Adult worm

Fertilized ovum (non-infective) passed in faeces

Infective larva develops within ovum

Figure 71.7 Life cycle of *Ascaris lumbricoides* (roundworm). (Courtesy WTIM.)

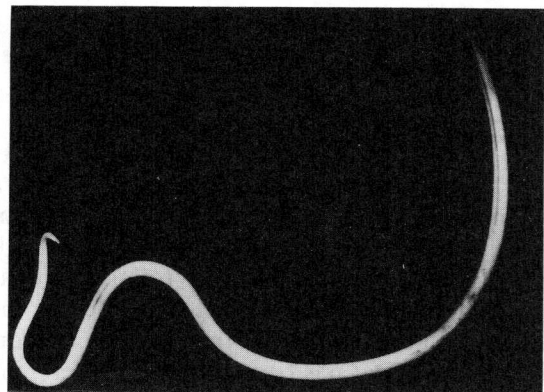

Figure 71.8 Adult *Ascaris* worm (roundworm). (Courtesy WTIM.)

period from infection to the first passage of ova in the stool is 60 to 70 days.

ASCARIS SUUM

Ascaris suum is almost indistinguishable from human *Ascaris* and man is not a normal host but

Ascaris pneumonia is common in pigs and a proportion of similar respiratory troubles in people associated with pigs may be due to *Ascaris suum*. Although *Ascaris suum* can infect humans, man is not its normal host; double infections may occur and eosinophilic granuloma of the bowel may be caused by *Ascaris suum*.

TRANSMISSION

Infection is acquired from ingestion of eggs in contaminated soil, usually by children when playing around the house situated in suitable soil.

PATHOLOGY

Pathology may be caused by migrating larvae or adults.

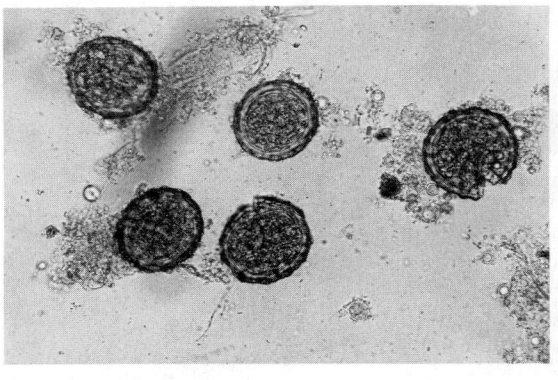
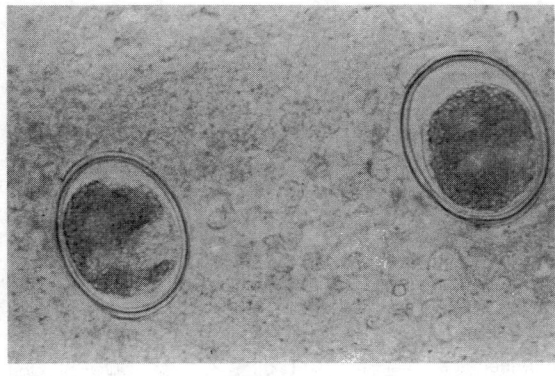

(a) **(b)**

Figure 71.9 Eggs of *Ascaris lumbricoides* (roundworm). (a) Fully formed, fertile, in stool (courtesy WTIM). (b) Decorticated from liver abscess (courtesy M. L. Chu).

MIGRATING LARVAE (LARVAL ASCARIASIS)

Migrating larvae cause symptoms from their actual physical presence and the immune reactions they elicit.

Ascaris *pneumonia*

Damage to the lungs occurs during the migration of larvae on their way to the intestine. 'Löffler's syndrome' may be produced with fever, cough, sputum, asthma, eosinophilia and radiological pulmonary infiltration. In 1956 it was concluded that the majority of cases of Löffler's syndrome were due to larval ascariasis.[12] Segments of fourth stage larvae can be seen in the bronchioles associated with infiltration with polymorphonuclear and eosinophilic leucocytes with scattered Charcot–Leyden crystals usually associated with lysed eosinophils.

Other organs

Small areas of necrosis with eosinophils may be found in the liver.[13] Migrating larvae have been recovered from aspirated gastric juice and sputum. If the larvae reach the general circulation they may cause localized symptoms resembling those of visceral larva migrans caused by *Toxocara canis*. Larvae may wander into the brain, eye or retina,[14] causing granulomas simulating *Toxocara canis*. In small children ascariasis is frequently associated with *Toxocara*. Hundreds of larvae have been removed from a swelling in the neck (but see lagochilascariasis, p. 167).

ADULT WORMS

Adult worms by themselves cause little pathology in their normal habitat (small intestine). Heavy infec-

tions can cause intestinal colic which is the most important complaint. Aggregate masses of worms may cause volvulus, intestinal obstruction (Figure 71.10) or intussusception.

WANDERING ASCARIDS

Wandering ascarids may reach abnormal situations and cause acute symptoms: ileus from mechanical obstruction, perforation of the bowel in the ileocaecal region, acute appendicitis from a worm blocking the lumen, diverticulitis, gastric or duodenal trauma, blocking of the ampulla of Vater with pancreatic necrosis, blocking of the common bile duct with obstructive jaundice, entry into the liver parenchyma and liver abscess, invasion of the genital tract and oesophageal perforation.

Ascaris *liver abscess*

Ascaris liver abscess is caused by female *Ascaris* worms migrating up the common bile duct into the liver where they die, releasing eggs. Histologically there is a granulomatous reaction round the dead worm with release of the eggs which can be demonstrated in the abscess as smooth, oval bodies from which the outer coat has been digested (see Figure 71.9b). In some parts of the world *Ascaris* liver abscess is more common in young children than amoebic abscess.

Peritoneal lesions

Granulomatous masses may form around the eggs released from the female worms which have escaped into the peritoneum and mimic tuberculous perito-

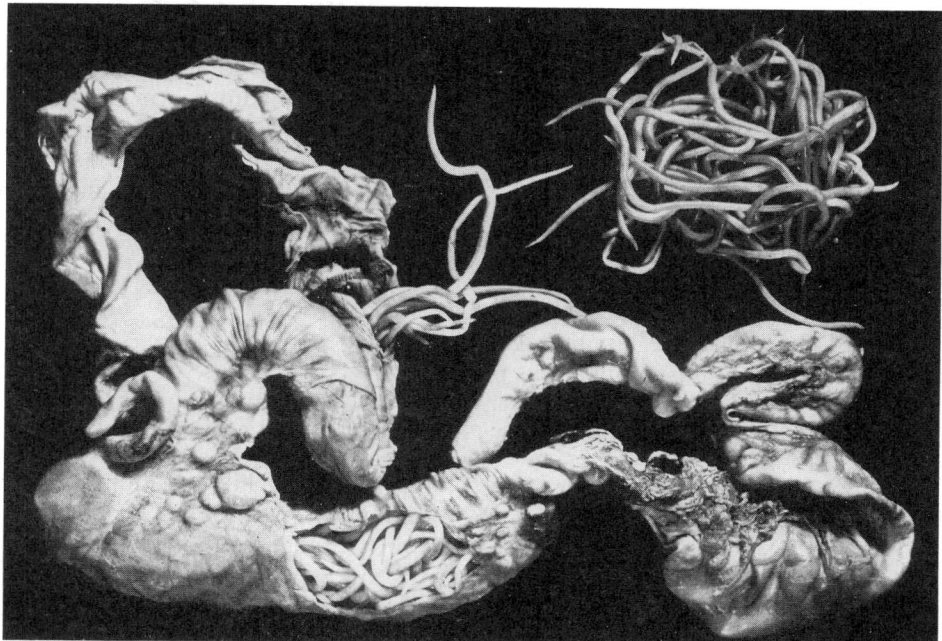

Figure 71.10 Impacted mass of adult *Ascaris* worms in the small intestine causing fatal intestinal obstruction.

nitis.[15] An eosinophilic granuloma of the bowel may be caused by *Ascaris suum*.

Biliary ascariasis

Biliary ascariasis is not uncommon in the Philippines where 20% of patients treated surgically for biliary disease are found to have live or dead *Ascaris* worms in the biliary tract and in South Africa where it is common in children.[16] The symptoms are acute onset of right upper abdominal pain, sometimes with fever and jaundice from recurrent cholangitis. Adult worms may be demonstrated on plain radiographs, by barium meal or by intravenous cholangiography. At post mortem cholangitis or liver abscess may be found. Good results follow anthelmintic treatment after the acute symptoms have subsided with supportive treatment. Adult worms, larvae and ova may all initiate stone formation and can be found in the core of many bile duct stones.[17]

IMMUNOPATHOLOGICAL EFFECTS

Many infected individuals manifest a sensitivity to the antigens of *Ascaris* and entry to a laboratory where worms are being dissected is enough to cause conjunctivitis, urticaria and asthma. The skin of these people is extremely sensitive to minimal doses of *Ascaris* antigen and gives an immediate hypersensitivity reaction, often with urticaria and erythematous lesions.

The passage of adult worms in sensitive persons may give rise to intense anal pruritus, vomiting of worms, and oedema of the glottis.

It has been postulated that the high serum IgE levels found in *Ascaris* might inhibit the development of bronchial asthma but this has been shown not to be the case.[18]

INDIRECT EFFECTS

Micro-organisms may be carried by adult worms on their migration from the bowel and a relationship between *Ascaris* infection and the incidence of poliomyelitis has been suggested.

NUTRITIONAL RELATIONSHIPS

Ascariasis may contribute to protein–energy malnutrition. From calculations in an experimental study in man[19] it has been estimated that in children infected with 13–40 worms approximately 4 g of protein are lost per day from a daily diet containing 35–50 g of protein. Kwashiorkor has been associated with *Ascaris* infection from the time when it was first recognized as a nutritional syndrome. *Ascaris* infection may contribute to vitamin A deficiency and children suffering from night blindness have shown rapid improvement in their eye symptoms within a few days of therapeutic elimination of the worms. Infected children have also been shown to excrete a significantly lower amount of vitamin C after a test dose of ascorbic acid. *Ascaris* can also adversely affect normal growth.[20,21]

IMMUNITY

Man acquires only partial immunity to reinfection, and animals can be protected using extracts of adults and larvae.[22] The main immune reaction is humoral and is directed against the migrating larval stage. The reaction to adult worms in unusual locations is cellular.

LARVAL MIGRATORY STAGES

The antigens which elicit antibodies are released at the moulting period between the second and third larval stages when there is a great increase in IgE. A further response is elicited in the bowel between the fourth and fifth stages, at which time there may be a marked loss of worm burden; this may be a regulatory mechanism in natural infections.

ADULT STAGE

Adult worms in the bowel elicit no response but when they wander into the tissues the reaction is cellular and results in a granuloma. Immediate hypersensitivity to adult *Ascaris* antigens develops in some people.

CLINICAL FEATURES

NATURAL HISTORY

Most *Ascaris* infections are symptomless but heavy infections in childhood give rise to symptoms. These heavy infections are controlled by immunity, or by diminished exposure, so that adults have much lighter infections, although reinfection can occur throughout life.

INCUBATION PERIOD

The incubation period from infection after swallowed eggs to the first appearance of eggs in the stools is 60–70 days. In larval ascariasis pulmonary symptoms occur 4–16 days after infection.

SYMPTOMS AND SIGNS

Light infections do not usually cause symptoms, though a single adult worm can cause a liver abscess or block the common bile duct. Acute manifestations are roughly proportional to the number of worms harboured and serious disease may be caused when the burden amounts to 100 worms or more.

Larval ascariasis

Ascaris pneumonia
During the migratory stages the larvae cause a pneumonitis 4–16 days after infection—with fever, cough, sputum and radiological infiltration of the lungs. There is a high eosinophilia and larvae can be found in the sputum or gastric juice—especially if a quantity is collected, digested with trypsin and centrifuged. Seasonal attacks of *Ascaris* pneumonia have occurred in Saudi Arabia following the onset of spring rains and the restarting of transmission.[23] The pneumonitis is of short duration, about 3 weeks (in contrast to tropical pulmonary eosinophilia (TPE) which lasts for many months). There may be asthma, which can be so intense as to cause status asthmaticus,[13] and the liver may be affected, becoming enlarged and tender.

General symptoms
On reaching the general circulation larvae may cause symptoms similar to those of *Toxocara canis*. Neurological disorders including convulsions, meningism and epilepsy, palpebral oedema, insomnia and tooth grinding during the night may occur. When the larvae wander into the brain they cause granulomas—presenting as small tumours in the eyes, retina or brain.

Adult ascariasis

The major manifestation of adult ascariasis is small bowel obstruction (Figure 71.10), which usually occurs in children, and as many as 1000 worms have been removed from one patient. Gastrointestinal discomfort, colic and vomiting are quite common. Ascariasis is the most common cause of abdominal surgical emergency in children in South Africa and Rangoon.[24,25]

Migratory adult worms
Adult worms tend to migrate when their environment is disturbed. In the presence of tetrachlorethylene, anaesthetics or fever they migrate and wander into the bile ducts, ampulla of

Vater, appendix, perineal sinuses and eustachian tubes. They can cause volvulus and gangrene of the bowel, intestinal perforation and peritonitis, acute pancreatitis, suppurative cholangitis, liver abscess, acute cholecystitis and obstructive jaundice.

For these reasons it is important not to give tetrachlorethylene when there is a possibility of *Ascaris* infection and to deworm children when they are ill and febrile or before giving an anaesthetic.

DIAGNOSIS

A diagnosis can be made from passage of worms in the stool or by finding eggs in faeces.

Fertile eggs are oval and measure about 60 × 45 μm. The shell is transparent, is surrounded by an outer mamillated shell stained by bile pigments and contains an unsegmented embryo (see Figure 71.9a).

Unfertile eggs are longer and narrower (90 × 40 μm), have a thinner shell, more irregular outer covering and are found in about two-thirds of infections, due either to a shortage or absence of males. In male infections no eggs are passed in the stool.

Decorticated eggs are usually found in ectopic sites where they have had the outer shell removed and present as smooth oval objects (see Figure 71.9b).

EOSINOPHILIA

In larval ascariasis there is a high eosinophilia but in adult infections there is little or none. If a marked eosinophilia occurs in adult infections then an associated *Toxocara* or *Strongyloides* infection must be suspected.

ADULT WORMS

Sometimes the passage of an adult worm from the nose, mouth or anus will be reported and causes distress. The size and shape will distinguish it from other worms, especially tapeworms which may be noticed by patients.

RADIOGRAPHY

Radiographic examination 4–6 hours after an opaque meal displays the worms as cylindrical filling defects or as string-like shadows produced by the opaque substance which the worms have ingested.

SEROLOGICAL DIAGNOSIS

Specific antibodies have been detected in persons infected with *Ascaris lumbricoides* and the following tests have been used for the detection of infection: complement fixation, precipitin, agar-gel diffusion, immunoelectrophoresis and the radioallergosorbent test. Hypersensitivity to *Ascaris* is well recognized, and cutaneous tests have been used in man as diagnostic aids. There is a lack of correlation between the immunological reaction(s) and the presence of eggs in faeces, but in pigs the incidence of positive reactions increases with the severity of the pathology produced by the migrating parasites.[26] Since there is much cross-reactivity with other helminthic antigens, immunodiagnosis is of little help in *Ascaris* infection, either adult or larval.

DIFFERENTIAL DIAGNOSIS

The syndrome of pulmonary symptoms, radiological lung infiltration and hypereosinophilia are common to a number of helminthic and other infections.

Larval ascariasis must be distinguished from *Toxocara*, hookworm, *Strongyloides*, schistosomiasis and TPE. Essentially, larval ascariasis is a short-term illness lasting 2–3 weeks with a rapidly falling eosinophilia.

Toxocara (see pp. 163–166)
Often associated with *Ascaris*, *Toxocara* causes the visceral larva migrans (VLM) syndrome which persists for many months with a persistently high eosinophilia, and lung symptoms are not prominent. Wandering *Toxocara* larvae cause almost identical lesions of the brain and eye as *Ascaris* and can be diagnosed by specific serological tests.

Hookworm (see pp. 167–174)
The invasive stage of hookworm lasts 2–3 months, subsiding gradually, ova being found in the stool from 42 days onwards. It may be preceded by a localized eruption on the legs (ground itch).

Schistosomiasis (see Chapter 72)
The invasive stage of schistosomiasis (Katayama syndrome) can last 2–3 months. There is usually splenomegaly and specific serology is available for diagnosis.

Tropical pulmonary eosinophilia (see Chapter 70)
TPE may closely resemble *Ascaris* pneumonia. It occurs mainly in adults, has a much longer duration and specific filarial serological tests will be positive (older tests using less specific antigens cross-reacted with *Ascaris*). It responds rapidly to diethylcarbamazine.

Other eosinophilic lung syndromes

Pulmonary aspergillosis, drug reactions and eosinophilic leukaemia are all more chronic.

TREATMENT

Treatment is effective only against the adult worms. Although the vast majority of *Ascaris* infections cause few, if any, symptoms it is easy to treat and it is wise to treat any established infection. The drugs of choice are as follows:
Albendazole: for children 2–5 years a single dose of 200 mg; for older children and adults, one dose of 400 mg is given.
Mebendazole: 100 mg twice daily for *one* day only.
Levamisole: a single dose of 5 mg/kg body weight.
Pyrantel pamoate (Combantrin): a single dose of 10 mg/kg body weight.

They are best given between meals, without any special diet, fast, or use of purgatives before or after therapy.

TREATMENT OF COMPLICATIONS

Ascaris *pneumonitis*[27]

This responds dramatically to prednisolone therapy. Anthelmintics should be given 2 weeks after lung involvement.

Biliary ascariasis[27]

Conservative treatment—antispasmodics, analgesics, gastric decompression via a nasogastric tube, administration of intravenous fluids—is usually successful. An anthelmintic, preferably in soluble form and quick-acting (levamisole, pyrantel) is given when the acute phase of the illness is over and intestinal function restored. If this fails, surgical removal is needed.

Intestinal obstruction[27]

Here again, conservative treatment is the first choice—antispasmodics, gastric decompression, intravenous fluids, liquid paraffin and anthelmintics—and is usually successful. If surgical intervention is decreed necessary because of fever, tachycardia, visible peristalsis, severe pain or lack of remission within 48 hours of conservative treatment, this should be as conservative as possible, e.g. careful unknotting of the worm bolus and milking of the worms into the colon. Rarely is enterotomy required.

EPIDEMIOLOGY

Ascaris eggs develop best in shady damp soil. They are resistant to cold and to disinfectants in the strengths normally used. They are killed by direct sunlight and by temperatures above 45°C. Infection is spread by faecal pollution of the soil.

In endemic areas three distinct trends in the prevalence and intensity of endemic ascariasis in man have been observed:[28]

1. High prevalence (over 60%) in the whole population over 2 years, with the intensity of infection lower in adults; a common and constant exposure to invasive *Ascaris* eggs by dirty hands and contaminated food.
2. Moderate prevalence (below 50%) with its peak at preschool or early school ages and low values in adults; a household or family type of transmission probably prevails.
3. Overall prevalence low (below 10%) and infections tend to have a focal distribution related to particular housing and sanitary conditions or agricultural and behavioural practices.

Ascariasis is spread countrywide in a few regions where climatic and social conditions are almost uniform; in many other countries, its distribution is stratified. Thus, in the 'shanty' overcrowded towns of non-industrialized societies with poor hygiene prevalence may be higher in urban than in rural areas. In drier areas of the tropics, transmission is limited to the short rainy season. Coprophagous arthropods, e.g. dung beetles, cockroaches and animals can spread the infection widely by ingesting and excreting viable eggs.

Apart from the spatial differences in *Ascaris* prevalence at the level of country, village and family, there is considerable difference in intensity of infection among individuals, giving a negative binomial distribution.[29] The reasons for such individual predisposition—spatial, behavioural, genetic—are still unknown.

Epidemic ascariasis caused by the use of raw sewage for agricultural purposes, waste-water irrigated vegetables[30] and contaminated imported vegetables has been reported.

Sporadic ascariasis as a result of holiday travel to endemic areas—association with infected immigrants and infection from imported fresh vegetables and fruits has been described.[31]

Although the basic epidemiology of the geohelminths is relatively straightforward, their *quantitative epidemiology* is more complex. Some of the important features can be summarized as follows:

- The distribution of worm numbers per person tends to be highly aggregated in form. Thus, most individuals harbour a few parasites, while only a few harbour heavy burdens.[32]
- Worm fecundity appears to decline as the burden within an individual increases.[33]
- For *Ascaris* and *Trichuris*, changes in the average intensity of infection with age tend to be convex, with infection rising in childhood and declining in

adulthood, while in *hookworm* there is a steady rise in intensity with age.[34]

- Predisposition of heavily infected individuals within a community due to a variety of possible factors, e.g. behavioural, social, nutritional or genetic.[35,36,37]

The complex interplay of these aspects has been addressed mathematically in order to predict the results of intervention by chemotherapy.[38,39] Several studies have now confirmed the association between a broad range of nematodal species and growth in children, in various parts of the world.[40–45] The immunoepidemiology of intestinal helminthic infections has recently attracted the attention of several scientists.[46–50]

CONTROL

Control is based on a combination of personal hygiene, proper disposal of faeces, health education and chemotherapy (see pp. 182–184).

TOXOCARIASIS

Toxocariasis in man is the result of infection with the dog *Ascaris—Toxocara canis*—which does not undergo normal development in man but is arrested at the larval stage, causing toxocariasis, VLM or ocular toxocariasis.

AETIOLOGY

Toxocara canis is a roundworm infection in dogs. The morphology resembles that of *Ascaris lumbricoides* (see pp. 156–157), the males being 4–6 cm long and the female 6.5–10 cm long. The eggs, which are pitted superficially, measure $85 \times 75\,\mu m$, being larger than those of *Ascaris*. They are not found in man, only in dog faeces and contaminated soil.

GEOGRAPHICAL DISTRIBUTION

Toxocara canis infection in dogs has a worldwide distribution and infection rates vary from 2 to 90%.

Visceral larva migrans, which was first described in the southern USA,[51] has been recognized mainly in the southern and eastern USA but also in Europe, the Caribbean, Mexico, Hawaii, the Philippines, Australia, South Africa and eastern Europe.

Ocular toxocariasis (granulomatous ophthalmitis), first described in the USA,[52] has been recognized in many parts of the world and serological surveys have shown many cases of ocular toxocariasis in Britain.[53]

LIFE CYCLE

In the dog the life cycle is similar to that of *Ascaris* in man except that transplacental infection of puppies takes place in pregnant bitches and the puppies born with a patent infection shed numerous eggs from birth. In contrast, adult dogs excrete few eggs. Dogs are infected by ingesting the eggs from soil or as puppies at birth so that the whole cycle may be maintained in a small flat without any access to the outside.

In man, who is not the normal host, the eggs hatch in the stomach and second stage larvae penetrate the mucosa to enter the circulation via the mesenteric vessels, reaching the intestinal viscera and liver where they are held up in the capillaries, but may pass into the general circulation through the lungs and end up in the brain, eye and other organs. In these organs as well as the liver the larvae are eventually held up and destroyed by a granulomatous reaction which blocks their further migration and causes pathology. In the human host the larvae do not grow or moult but can remain alive for as long as 11 years—as has been shown experimentally.

TRANSMISSION

The main source of infection is puppies, which excrete large numbers of eggs. Infection is acquired by children playing in contaminated soil or in playgrounds—as in *Ascaris* infection, and is encouraged by the habit of earth eating (pica). Direct infection from handling puppies is also important.

PATHOLOGY

The pathology depends upon the density of infection. In heavy infections in childhood the syndrome of VLM is produced, whereas lighter infections cause ocular toxocariasis, found in later life.

VISCERAL LARVA MIGRANS

In heavy infections in children the second stage larvae, which are 450 μm × 16–20 μm in diameter, are arrested mostly in the liver where they cause few or many miliary lesions.[54] These lesions are composed of granulomas which can be seen as white subcapsular nodules the size of millet seeds. Other sites are the lungs, kidneys, heart, striated muscle, brain and eye. Microscopically the granulomas contain a centre of closely packed eosinophils and histiocytes surrounded by larger histiocytes with pale vesicular nuclei, sometimes arranged in a palisade-like manner. Occasionally there is an atypical multinucleate giant cell. Living second stage larvae may sometimes be demonstrated in recent granulomas but more usually only the remains can be seen. Less commonly they reach the lungs or brain where similar lesions can be seen.

OCULAR TOXOCARIASIS

In the eye the granulomatous reaction forms a large subretinal mass with a superimposed patch of chor-

oiditis which can closely resemble a retinoblastoma (for further details see Chapter 10).

IMMUNITY

In the abnormal host (man) the larvae elicit both a humoral and cellular response. Antibodies are formed which cause a quantitative rise in immunoglobulins, mostly IgG but also IgM (the globulin may be so elevated that a positive formol gel test can be shown) and IgE, and there is a peripheral eosinophilia. The larvae themselves elicit a cell-mediated granulomatous response causing the granulomas so typical of the infection. In the dog immunity to reinfection develops so that adult dogs pass few or no eggs.

CLINICAL FEATURES

NATURAL HISTORY

Following infection from ingested eggs which hatch in the stomach the larvae migrate to the liver where they may be arrested, or continue and reach other organs. In most cases the larva is destroyed without causing any trouble but in some cases it can survive for many years, and on its wanderings may eventually cause a lesion. Unless the infection is heavy and the VLM syndrome is produced, most cases of infection never cause any trouble. Heavy infections cause VLM, which can be self-limiting or cause death in a few cases. Lesions in the eye can produce severe loss of vision and even complete loss of sight in the affected eye.

INCUBATION PERIOD

An incubation period cannot be determined but in heavy infections (VLM) it is similar to that of *Ascaris*. In light infections many years may pass before the ocular granuloma presents itself.

SYMPTOMS AND SIGNS

There are two main clinical presentations: VLM and ocular toxocariasis (granulomatous ophthalmitis).

Visceral larva migrans[55]

This is seen most commonly in younger children. The child becomes unwell with an enlarged liver, fever and asthma. There is a marked hypereosinophilia and there can be pulmonary signs (radiological mottling), cardiac dysfunction, nephrosis and neurological lesions (fits, epilepsy, pareses and transverse myelitis). There is a great increase in the serum globulin and the eosinophil count is raised to $10-20 \times 10^9$/litre. In many urban areas where lead paint is used this is ingested with soil with the habit of pica and signs of lead poisoning may accompany VLM (blue lines on the gums and anaemia).

Progress

Most cases of VLM recover naturally after two years but some die, and postmortem examination will reveal extensive lesions in the liver and sometimes the brain.

Ocular toxocariasis[56]

The retinal lesion presents as a solid retinal tumour often at or near the macula. In the early stages it is raised above the level of the retina and closely mimics a retinal neoplasm. Later when the acute phase has subsided the lesion remains a clear-cut circumscribed area of retinal degeneration. Formerly these lesions were designated tuberculous, exanthematous or neoplastic. If the lesion is central the visual acuity is reduced or central vision may be lost (see Chapter 10).

Strabismus due to macular damage is often the presenting symptom. Low-grade iridocyclitis with posterior synechiae may develop and progress to general endophthalmitis and detachment of the retina. The second stage larva may rarely be seen with a slit-lamp microscope in the anterior chamber of the eye. Secondary glaucoma may result.

DIFFERENTIAL DIAGNOSIS

VLM must be distinguished from other migrating helminths, larval ascariasis (much shorter duration), strongyloidiasis (much longer duration), TPE (pulmonary symptoms are more marked and found in adults).

Ocular toxocariasis must be distinguished from a retinal tumour (retinoblastoma) and other causes of choroiditis (toxoplasmosis). All cases of retinoblastoma in children should have a serological test to exclude toxocariasis. The enzyme linked immunosorbent assay (ELISA) has a sensitivity of 90% and a specificity of 91% at a diagnostic titre of 1:8 in ocular toxocariasis. Vitreous toxocara antibody can also be measured.[57]

DIAGNOSIS

A history of exposure with puppies is important. The most consistent laboratory findings in VLM are: eosinophilia, leucocytosis, a decreased albumin:globulin ratio and an increase in IgG, IgH, anti-A or anti-B isohaemagglutinin titres.

DEMONSTRATION OF LARVAE

This is very difficult and seldom achieved. Larvae of portions of degenerate larvae may be seen at the centre of the granuloma in liver biopsy or postmortem material. A larva has been demonstrated in the cerebrospinal fluid[58] in a case of meningitis.

Liver biopsy may show a granuloma containing many eosinophils which can be suggestive but which must be distinguished from a *Schistosoma mansoni* granuloma. In biopsy and postmortem material *Ancylostoma braziliense* and *Ancylostoma caninum*, which usually invade the skin, can occasionally enter man via the intestinal tract and form granulomas in the viscera. Autoinfection with *Strongyloides* may cause a similar picture. Immunofluorescent staining of histological sections may be necessary to differentiate them.

SEROLOGY

The difficulty with serological diagnosis has always been to obtain an antigen specific to *Toxocara* second stage larvae which does not cross-react with other tissue helminths. A specific antigen has been obtained from the secretory/excretory products of second stage *Toxocara canis* larvae which is both sensitive and specific.[59] It has been used in ELISA,[60] which is now the test of choice, but human A and B blood group substances share similarities with parasite-derived antigen which has raised some doubts as to the specificity of the test.

ELISA[53]

Using larval antigens the sensitivity of the ELISA is 78% and specificity is 93% in VLM, providing the serum is first absorbed with *Ascaris suum* to remove cross-reacting antibodies.[61] A strong positive result is greater than 1.5 times screening level.

Other tests which have been used are passive haemagglutination and immunofluorescence. A radioallergosorbent test has been used to detect larva specific IgE.[62] The skin sensitivity test has been abandoned.

OCULAR TOXOCARIASIS

In addition to serum and vitreous toxocara antibody determinations, fluorescein angiography, ultrasonography or computerized tomography should be carried out to differentiate retinoblastoma from ocular larva migrans.

TREATMENT

Two drugs are used in treatment: diethylcarbamazine and thiabendazole.

DIETHYLCARBAMAZINE

This is the drug of choice. Diethylcarbamazine is given orally 3 mg/kg body weight three times daily for 21 days.

THIABENDAZOLE

Thiabendazole is given orally 50 mg/kg body weight daily in three divided doses for 7–28 days depending upon the tolerance shown to the drug.

In VLM the high eosinophilia may persist for months after clinical cure, which is shown by subsidence of the fever and hepatomegaly. Once overcome, relapses do not occur and second infections are unlikely. In ocular toxocariasis the addition of corticosteroids may be needed (see Chapter 10). Loss of vision can be arrested but lost vision not restored.

EPIDEMIOLOGY

Toxocara canis is a common inhabitant of adult dogs and puppies. Puppies are infected by second stage larvae in utero and are born with established intestinal infection. The puppies excrete eggs on to the ground which are ingested by small children along with *Ascaris* and *Trichuris* ova and, in urban areas in the USA, lead products found in old paint. Toxocariasis is often associated with *Ascaris* and *Trichuris* infection, and in urban areas with signs of lead poisoning. The most common age of infection is around 2½ years and the infection is patent from about 3 to 5 years of age. It is uncommon at a later age unless an unusual habit of dirt eating is present, as in mental defectives. Ocular toxocariasis is found at a later age. A statistical association between the incidence of *Toxocara* infection, as shown by skin sensitivity tests, and poliomyelitis and epilepsy has been demonstrated.[63] This is probably due to the introduction of the viral agents from the intestine by the migrating second stage larvae.

CONTROL

Control rests upon control of infection in dogs, especially puppies, which are the main agent(s) of infection, and regular treatment of dogs and bitches as well as newborn puppies with anthelmintics is essential when there are children in the house. Dogs should be denied access to sandpits in the back yard and playgrounds.

LAGOCHILASCARIASIS

GEOGRAPHICAL DISTRIBUTION

Lagochilascariasis is a rare infection of man, who is an accidental host. Cases have been described from South and Central America and the Caribbean.[64]

AETIOLOGY

Lagochilascaris minor is a parasite of the opossum (see below). The adult worms live in cavities in the submucosa of the small intestine and eggs containing infective larvae pass out in the stool where they are ingested by mice and other small mammals. The larvae hatch in the intestine and migrate to skeletal muscle where they mature and wait to be ingested by the definitive host, the opossum.

TRANSMISSION

Man becomes infected either by ingesting eggs from the soil or eating the intermediate host. A case reported from Tobago was thought to have acquired the infection through eating the raw meat of the manakou opossum.

PATHOLOGY

In man, *Lagochilascaris* causes subcutaneous abscesses on the head and neck, and lesions in the nasopharynx. The tonsils and lymphoid tissue are replaced by granulomatous tissue containing epithelioid granulomas with larvae and eggs. Abscesses form in the neck which discharge pus.

CLINICAL FEATURES

Early symptoms are recurrent tonsillitis, a feeling of worms crawling at the back of the throat and even discharge of small white worms from the mouth.

Tender tumours which swell and eventually burst discharging pus and worms form in the cervical region.

DIAGNOSIS

Adult worms can be recognized by a longitudinal furrow along the lateral line (see Appendix III).

TREATMENT

Most anthelmintics are ineffective but levamisole was curative in one case.[64]

TYPE 3 PENETRATION OF THE SKIN (*ANCYLOSTOMA, STRONGYLOIDES, TRICHOSTRONGYLUS*)

ANCYLOSTOMIASIS (HOOKWORM)

Hookworm disease (ancylostomiasis) is caused by two hookworms *Ancylostoma duodenale* and *Necator americanus* and is an extremely common infection; in many cases the nematodes, which are often present in huge numbers attached to the small intestine, from which they suck blood and protein, causing disease (hookworm anaemia, hookworm disease).

GEOGRAPHICAL DISTRIBUTION

The hookworm occurs in all tropical and subtropical countries.[65]

A. duodenale is essentially a parasite of southern Europe, the north coast of Africa, northern India, north China and Japan. It was introduced by migration into Paraguay around 3000 BC by Japanese fishermen[66] and is the predominant hookworm in coastal Peru and Chile. It has been introduced into Western Australia and into areas where *N. americanus* is the predominant human hookworm, southern India, Myanmar, Malaya, the Philippines, Indonesia, Polynesia, Micronesia and Portuguese West Africa.

N. americanus is the predominant hookworm of western, central and southern Africa, southern Asia, Melanesia and Polynesia. It is widely distributed in the southern USA, the islands of the Caribbean, Central America and northern South America where it was introduced by slaves from Africa.

AETIOLOGY

Two species of hookworm, *A. duodenale* and *N. americanus*, infect man.

ANCYLOSTOMA DUODENALE

A. duodenale is a small cylindrical white, grey or reddish-brown (from ingested blood) thread-like worm (Appendix III). Both male and female worms have a buccal capsule containing two pairs of teeth (cf. *N. americanus*) for attaching to the small intestinal mucosa. The male (0.8–1.1 × 0.4–0.5 cm) has a copulatory bursa at the rear end consisting of an umbrella-like expansion of the cuticle (Appendix III). The female (1–1.3 × 0.6 cm) is slightly larger and has the body cavity occupied by the ovary and coiled uterine tubes packed with eggs. The vulva is in the posterior third of the body. The maximum egg output occurs 15–18 months after infection; the interval between infection and final disappearance

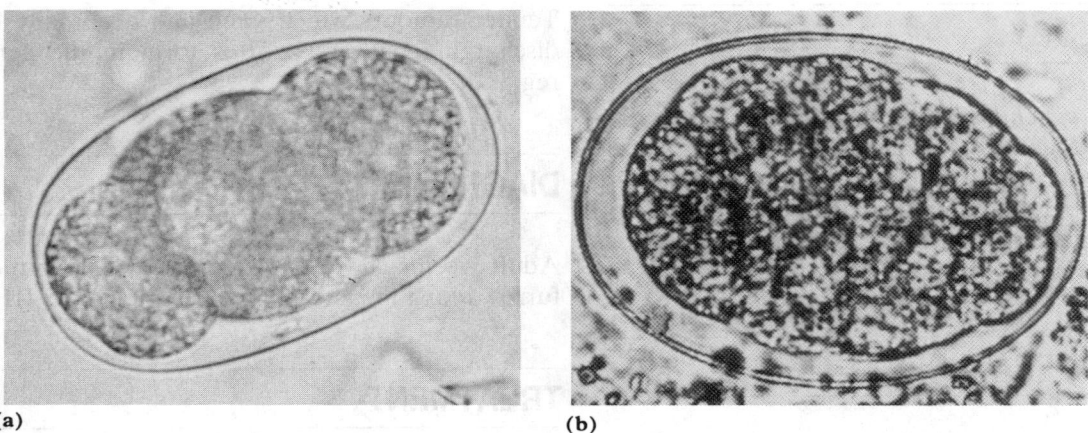

(a) **(b)**

Figure 71.11 Hookworm eggs. (a) Immature egg showing developing larva (courtesy J. S. Tatz). (b) Mature egg (courtesy WTIM).

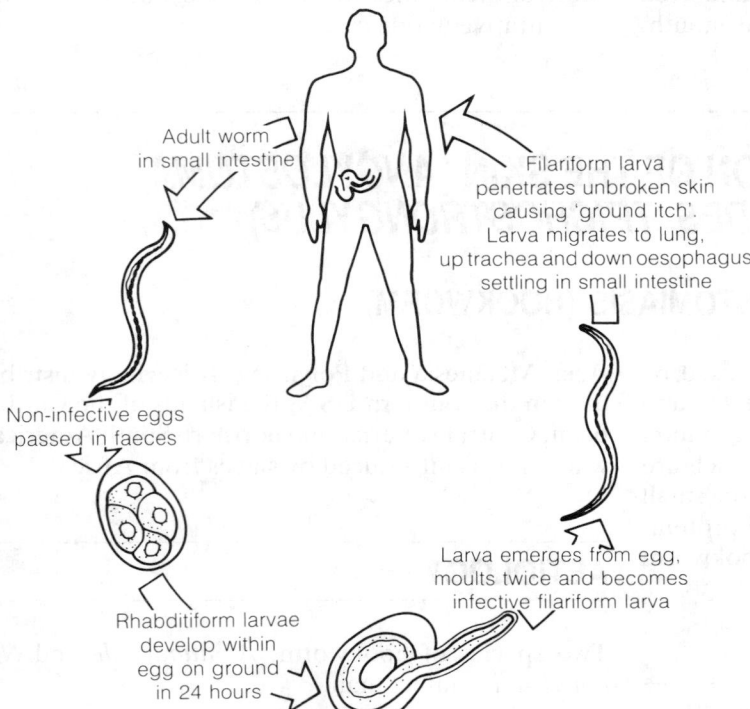

Adult worm
in small intestine

Filariform larva
penetrates unbroken skin
causing 'ground itch'.
Larva migrates to lung,
up trachea and down oesophagus
settling in small intestine

Non-infective eggs
passed in faeces

Rhabditiform larvae
develop within
egg on ground
in 24 hours

Larva emerges from egg,
moults twice and becomes
infective filariform larva

Figure 71.12 Life cycle of hookworm (Courtesy WTIM).

of eggs from the stool with death of the worm averages 6 years. The female produces 25–35 000 eggs each day and some 18–54 million during its lifetime. (For full morphological description, see Appendix III.) The eggs (50–60 μm × 35–40 μm) are elliptical with a transparent shell and when freshly laid contain two to four segments (blastomeres) (Figure 71.11).

NECATOR AMERICANUS

N. americanus closely resembles *A. duodenale* but it is shorter and more slender (0.9–1.1 × 0.4 cm) and can be distinguished from *A. duodenale* by the

position of the vulva in the female which is in the anterior third of the body (Appendix III) and the buccal capsule which is smaller than that of *A. duodenale*, has cutting plates instead of teeth. The egg is slightly larger than that of *A. duodenale* (64–75 × 36–40 μm). The female necator lays 6000–20 000 eggs daily and has a life duration on average of 5 years.

LIFE CYCLE (Figure 71.12)

The eggs are deposited into the lumen of the intestine containing two, four or eight blastomeres and are passed out in the faeces where, if deposited in damp shaded soil, they hatch into *rhabditiform* (first stage) larvae (Figure 71.12) which are free living and have a bulbed oesophagus. They feed avidly on bacteria. The larva moults on the third day and the oesophagus disappears on the fifth day, the larva becoming elongated and fully developed at 20–30°C. It then moves away from the faeces into the soil and moults to form a *filariform* (infective) larva (Figure 71.12) which has a simple muscular oesophagus and a protective sheath. The larva moves towards oxygen and cannot survive in water. The larvae are most numerous in the upper 2.5 cm of soil but can ascend from deeper layers. Protected from desiccation they can live in warm damp soil for 2 years. Direct sunlight, drying, or salt water are fatal. When the filariform larva comes into contact with the skin of the host it penetrates it and enters the bloodstream, reaching the lungs on the third day. Breaking through the alveoli it enters the bronchioles, moves up the trachea, down the oesophagus to the stomach and small intestine. During this migration the third moult takes place and the buccal capsule is formed. It arrives in the intestine on the seventh day and a fourth moult takes place, the buccal capsule assumes the adult form and the worm attaches to the mucosa of the small intestine, where it can be seen at post mortem as a small thread-like structure containing a small red lining of ingested blood. In 3–5 weeks it becomes sexually mature and the female produces fertile eggs. Adult worms live from 1–9 years and produce 30 000 eggs per day (necator 9000 eggs daily).

The life cycles of *Ancylostoma* and *Necator* are similar except that:

- *A. duodenale* can infect by ingestion as well as via the skin.
- *N. americanus* infects only through the skin.
- Migrating larvae of *N. americanus* grow and develop in the lungs, whereas those of *Ancylostoma* do not.

TRANSMISSION

Infection is normally acquired via the skin (percutaneous route) from *filariform* (infective) larvae in the soil contaminated by human faeces; or orally via the ingestion of contaminated food. However, other methods of transmission which are comparatively unimportant have been suggested:

- Through eating uncooked meat containing the larvae of *A. duodenale* which have migrated into the muscles of the animal, where they can survive for 26–34 days.[67]

- Via human milk (hypobiosis as in *A. caninum* in puppies).

The migrating infective filariform larvae of *A. duodenale* are arrested in their development and migrate to the mammary gland where they are excreted in the milk and infect the child.[68] Third stage infective filariform larvae of *N. americanus* have been found in the milk but none of the infected mothers were found to have infected babies.[69]

A. duodenale further differs from *N. americanus* in possessing the ability to remain within the host as a larval stage for many months before finally developing to an adult, thus bridging seasons which are inappropriate for transmission.[68]

PATHOLOGY

Ancylostoma causes pathology at three stages of infection (the first two caused by larval hookworm usually seen only in expatriates who receive a primary infection):

1. Vesiculation and pustulation at the site of entry (ground itch). This is usually mild or absent in the tropics except in expatriates.
2. Asthma and bronchitis during migration through the lungs with small haemorrhages into the alveoli and eosinophilic and leucocytic infiltration.
3. *Established infection*—seen in the inhabitants of endemic areas leading to hookworm anaemia and hookworm disease.

HOOKWORM ANAEMIA

The classical anaemia of hookworm infection is a hypochromic microcytic anaemia, the relationship of which to hookworm infection has long been debated. The main theories which have been put forward as to the causation of anaemia are chronic blood loss and depletion of iron stores with deficiency of iron intake and toxic factors.

Hookworms have been shown to produce active suction impulses 120–200 times per minute and evidence indicates that the hookworm is indeed an habitual blood-sucker and needs serum.[70] The blood loss has been estimated as 0.03 ml/day per worm in *N. americanus* and 0.15 ml/day per worm in *A. duodenale* infections.[70] There is a significant relationship between the level of haemoglobin and the worm burden, which depends upon the level of iron stores in the body. A significant negative correlation between plasma ferritin levels and hookworm burden, using the worm expulsion method, has been reported.[71] Hookworm anaemia is of the iron deficiency type and responds dramatically to iron salts by mouth and also to removal of the hookworm burden, but after a much longer period. Light infections may cause anaemia where the iron intake is deficient and anaemia may also be caused in spite of the presence of an adequate iron intake, provided that the worm burden is heavy enough. A folate deficiency may be present, masked by the severe iron deficiency anaemia, and become overt only when this has been corrected.

Little is known about the anaemia which develops in light primary infections. It may be related to that which develops in pups infected with *A. caninum* and be of immunological origin.

HYPOPROTEINAEMIA

Loss of protein is an important feature of hookworm anaemia, which is a cause of protein-losing enteropathy and the oedema of hookworm disease which does not respond to diuretics.[72] The protein loss, which is in excess of the red cell loss and is closely related to the hookworm load, is caused by a limited capacity for albumin synthesis as well as loss caused by anaemia and other factors such as liver disease.

HOOKWORM ENTEROPATHY

There have been conflicting reports on the role of hookworm in tropical malabsorption states. Structural abnormalities of the villi reverting to normal after deworming have been shown in Puerto Rico[73] and India,[74] but no changes were reported from Africa.[75] It has been suggested that it is the associated hypoalbuminaemia which is the cause of the enteropathy.

PATHOLOGICAL ANATOMY

In fatal cases the pathological changes are those of severe anaemia. There is plenty of fat in the usual situations. The appearance of plumpness is further increased by a greater or lesser amount of generalized oedema. There may be an effusion in one or more of the serous cavities. The heart is dilated and flabby. The liver is fatty and the kidneys and all other organs pale.

If the postmortem examination has been made within an hour or two after death the hookworms, in numbers ranging from a few dozen up to many hundreds, will be found attached by their mouths to the mucous surfaces of the lower part of the duodenum, jejunum and perhaps the upper part of the ileum. If the examination has been delayed for some time the parasites will have loosened their hold and are then found in the mucus coating the bowel. Many small extravasations of blood, some fresh, others of long standing, are seen in the mucous membrane and a minute wound in the centre of each extravasation represents the point at which a hookworm had been attached. Old extravasations are indicated by punctiform pigmentation. Occasionally streaks or large clots of blood are found in the lumen of the bowel and severe melaena may occur in children. The hookworms secrete some anticoagulant substance and may move from spot to spot, thereby increasing the damage and blood loss. The worms themselves may be seen in situ to show thin red streaks from fresh red blood in the intestinal canal; at other times they will be iron grey owing to the deposition of haemosiderin granules in the intestine.

IMMUNITY

Dogs develop partial protective immunity towards *A. caninum* which in endemic areas can cause a 50% mortality from anaemia in early life. Pups that survive to adult life retain only minimal intestinal infection. After a single infection with 1000 irradiated *A. caninum* larvae significant immunity can be demonstrated by worm counts following challenge with unirradiated larvae, but there was not evidence of protective immunity in a volunteer repeatedly exposed to infection with *A. duodenale*[76] and no evidence of protective immunity in a field study. Primary infections in man may cause fever, eosinophilia and a moderate anaemia, even when the infection is light. Such light infections do not cause symptoms of anaemia in the indigenous inhabitants of endemic areas, suggesting that a partial immunity has developed. Immediate hypersensitivity develops in hookworm infections and a skin test using an antigen prepared from *N. americanus* larvae has been used in Venezuela to indicate both prevalence and load of hookworm infection.[77] Fluorescent antibody titres rise with primary infections and then decline but there is no correlation between titres and worm loads and cross-reactions occur with *Strongyloides*.

Whereas there is good evidence that immunity plays a role in controlling infections with *A. caninum* and *A. ceylanicum*[78] in dogs, observations in communities living in endemic areas are not compatible with the existence of a vigorous, long-lasting protective immunity to hookworm infections.[75,79] There is, in fact, little to indicate that infections in man are curtailed by immune phenomena.[75] A comprehensive review of this subject has recently been published.[80]

CLINICAL FEATURES

NATURAL HISTORY

After the establishment of adult worms in the intestine the females start to lay eggs. The number of eggs passed bears a direct relation to the number of female worms. The higher the worm load the greater the blood loss so that where iron intake is satisfactory then up to 100 worms may cause no symptoms. With worm loads of 500–1000 then significant blood loss and anaemia will result, even in the presence of an adequate iron intake. It has been suggested that the relative freedom from hookworm anaemia shown by the African population of West, South and Central Africa is due to the use of iron cooking pots, which is also responsible for haemosiderosis, whereas in East Africa, where aluminium pots are mostly used, haemosiderosis is not found but hookworm anaemia is common. Light infections cause little trouble, but in a minority symptoms result from heavy infections.

INCUBATION PERIOD

In larval ancylostomiasis symptoms appear 1–2 weeks after the primary infection, and in established infection eggs appear from the 42nd day onwards after infection.

SYMPTOMS AND SIGNS

Larval hookworm

This is seen in a primary infection, most usually in non-immune expatriates. It is not so common or so marked as *larval ascariasis*.

At the site of entry of the infective larvae there is a 'ground itch', which consists of an irritating vesicular rash limited to the exposed portion(s) of the body, usually the soles of the feet or the hands. After 1–2 weeks pulmonary symptoms develop with a dry cough and asthmatic wheezing. Fever and a high degree of eosinophilia are found. These symptoms gradually disappear and ova of hookworm can be seen on or about day 42 after infection. The whole episode is self-limiting, lasting not more than 2–3 months.

Light infection (100 worms or under)

The main effects of light infections may be seen in Europeans and other expatriates who have arrived recently in an endemic area. The practitioner in the tropics should always be on the look-out for these cases, especially in children. Minor degrees of anaemia induce a tendency to fatigue and lassitude and digestive disturbances are common. Any of these symptoms in the presence of an eosinophilia should lead to the suspicion of infection. In indigenous people most light infections are asymptomatic.

Established infection in indigenous people

The essential symptoms of hookworm infection are connected with progressive iron deficiency anaemia associated with gastric and intestinal dyspepsia but not wasting. An early symptom is epigastric pain or discomfort which may be relieved by food and may be mistaken for duodenal ulcer. Although many people who suffer from irregular abdominal pain may possess hookworm ova in their stools it does not necessarily follow that hookworm infection is the cause of the abdominal pain.

The taste may be perverted, some patients exhibiting and persistently gratifying an unnatural craving for such things as earth, mud or lime (pica or geophagy). The stools may contain blood, and frank melaena may occur in children. The occult blood test is always positive in the stools in cases where symptoms are caused by hookworm.

When the iron deficiency anaemia develops then symptoms of anaemia occur. The mucous surfaces and the skin become pale. The face is puffy and the feet and ankles swollen and there may be generalized oedema caused by the hypoalbuminaemia. There is lassitude, breathlessness, palpitations, tinnitus and vertigo, mental apathy, depression and liability to syncope. There is often koilonychia. There is a high output failure and haemic murmurs can be heard over the heart, which is seen to be enlarged on radiographic examination. A minority of patients have a slow pulse, collapsed veins, severe oedema that often affects the face and arms, and ascites. They look ill, continuously feel cold and are hypothermic (body temperature less than 36°C).[75] Hookworm anaemia is a common cause of heart failure in the tropics and may easily be confused with rheumatic carditis. Ophthalmoscopic examination may reveal retinal haemorrhages. An irregular fever may be found in any severe anaemia.

The anaemia is typical of iron deficiency (see Chapter 6). The haemoglobin is reduced to a greater degree than the red cell count. The mean corpuscular volume is decreased and the mean corpuscular haemoglobin concentration may fall to as low as 22. The red cells show microcytosis and severe hypochromia. The serum iron is greatly reduced and the total iron-binding capacity of the serum greatly raised, indicating that iron stores are very low. There is no marked poikilocytosis or leucocytosis, although there may be an eosinophilia of 7–14%. The serum albumin is reduced in heavy infections. Because of the persistent anaemia, growth and development become stunted in children.

The rate of progress varies in different cases. In some a high degree of anaemia and even death may result within a few weeks or months of the appearance of the first symptoms. More frequently the disease is chronic, ebbing and flowing or slowly progressing through a long series of years.

INFANTILE HOOKWORM DISEASE

Most cases of hookworm in infants have been reported from China and the majority have been caused by *A. duodenale*.[81] The clinical features include diarrhoea with bloody stools, melaena, anorexia, vomiting, pallor and massive haemorrhage. The mortality is up to 12%.

Transmission occurs in a variety of ways: transmammary, laying infants on contaminated soil, infected diapers consisting of a cloth bag stuffed with soil containing hookworm larvae, and rarely transplacental infection.

DIFFERENTIAL DIAGNOSIS

In countries where hookworm infection is endemic, eggs may be found in faeces in any number of conditions which are not causally related. In these conditions an egg count is essential to determine the worm load (see below). Light infections in expatriates associated with moderate eosinophilia and mild anaemia must be differentiated from other helminth infections: *Schistosoma mansoni*, *Fasciola hepatica* and other liver flukes and *Strongyloides* The epigastric pain associated with hookworm infection may suggest duodenal ulcer or pancreatitis and any patient from an endemic area with epigastric symptoms who has hookworm ova in the stool should be treated, since in many cases the symptoms will disappear without the need for any further investigation.

Severe hookworm anaemia must be distinguished from other iron deficiency anaemias, and generalized anasarca from kwashiorkor and the nephrotic syndrome.

DIAGNOSIS

The diagnosis is made by finding eggs in the stool (see Figure 71.11). Rhabditiform larvae may be found in stale stools and be mistaken for *Strongyloides* in which larvae only and not eggs are found in the stool (see pp. 176–180). The eggs may be confused with those of *Trichostrongylus* which are more translucent and smaller. In light infections concentration methods are necessary, such as zinc sulphate concentration, formol ether or the Kato smear (see Appendix V). The worm load can be estimated by an egg count (Stoll egg count method, see Appendix V). Since *A. duodenale* lay an average 25 000 eggs per day, the number of eggs in a gram of stool multiplied by the daily stool weight in grams divided by 25 000 will give the estimated worm load. An egg count of 2500/g is significant and will be associated with symptoms. Less than 25 worms is insignificant while 500–1000 worms invariably cause disease.

OTHER DIAGNOSTIC TESTS

Barium meal studies will not reveal the worms but radiological abnormality of the duodenum is closely related to haemoglobin levels in hookworm patients.[82] Serological diagnosis is not practical since there are so many cross-reactions with other helminths.

TREATMENT

Treatment consists of elimination of the parasites and treatment of the anaemia, if present. Treatment of the anaemia is the first priority but there is no reason why both objectives should not be proceeded with concurrently if non-toxic anthelmintics are used. Suggestions in the past that one drug might be best for one species and another for the other do not apply to modern drugs. Light asymptomatic infections in children should be treated if possible. In adults they are often left untreated, especially if reinfection is probable.

Treatment is usually directed against the adult stages but there is evidence that albendazole in a single dose of 400 mg is active against the preintestinal larval stages of *N. americanus*.[83]

ELIMINATION OF ADULT PARASITES

In the past it was necessary to examine post-treatment stools for 48 hours and examine any worms passed to determine whether the infection in the area was *A. duodenale* or *N. americanus,* since the latter was much more resistant to treatment. With the more modern drugs this is no longer necessary. It is not usually necessary to remove all worms but to reduce the worm load significantly. The drug of choice is albendazole.

Albendazole. This is effective against both *A. duodenale* and *N. americanus*. A single dose of 400 mg will produce an 80% reduction in egg count and 200 mg daily for 3 days will give 100% cure. It is also highly effective against *Ascaris* and is therefore especially suitable for mass treatment.

Mebendazole. A regimen of 100 mg twice daily for 3 days is highly effective against both *A. duodenale* and *N. americanus*.

Levamisole. A single dose of 150 mg orally or 2.5 mg/kg body weight is less effective against *N. americanus*.

Pyrantel pamoate (Combantrin). A single dose of 10 mg/kg body weight is given.

Bephenium hydroxynaphthoate (Alcopar). This has now largely been superseded but a single dose of 5 g will eradicate *A. duodenale* but three or more consecutive doses are necessary for *N. americanus*.

Tetrachlorethylene. The sole advantage of tetrachlorethylene is that it is cheap. It has to be given in a high dosage, 6 ml, which is relatively toxic and is now little used because of the danger with concurrent *Ascaris* infection and the relative low cost of the broad-spectrum anthelmintics.

TREATMENT OF ANAEMIA

The anaemia is treated by the administration of iron by mouth, either in the form of ferrous sulphate of gluconate, 200 mg three times daily, which should be continued for 3 months after a normal haemoglobin level has been achieved. This will restore the iron reserves to normal.

After starting iron therapy, a reticulocyte response may be seen in about 1 week. In most cases the haemoglobin will rise by 1.0 g per week. Folic acid, 5 mg daily, should be given for at least 1 month to cover the erythopoeitic response. Many patients in the tropics fail to correct the haemoglobin fully and develop macrocytosis if this is not done.

Parenteral iron—iron–dextran complex or iron–poly (sorbitol gluconic acid) complex—may be used in patients who cannot tolerate oral iron, in patients where compliance is in doubt or in patients in whom regular follow-up is difficult or unlikely.

EPIDEMIOLOGY AND CONTROL

The only reservoir of infection is man and the propagation of hookworm infection depends upon an adequate source of infection in the human population, the deposition of eggs in a favourable environment for extrinsic development of the parasite, appropriate conditions of the soil (moisture and warmth) to allow larvae to develop and suitable conditions for the infective larvae to penetrate the skin. In many tropical and subtropical countries transmission is perennial but in cooler and drier climates transmission may take place in the warmer or wet seasons. In some temperate climates local environmental conditions may allow transmission, as in the Cornish tin mines in the past and in the Rand in South Africa today. Cultural and agricultural practices such as the use of human faeces for fertilizer provide good opportunities for infection.

The methods which are employed to determine the amount of hookworm in a community are determination of the *prevalence* and *intensity* of infection by stool surveys and egg counts from which the worm burden can be calculated. These surveys will show whether the infection in the community is low grade, moderate or severe. Soil pollution in the area must also be studied and filariform larvae of hookworm can be demonstrated in soil by the Baermann method or they can be cultured (see Appendix V). Studies of the nutritional level of the community, especially the haemoglobin level, must also be undertaken.

Because of logistic and social difficulties, estimates of worm numbers by chemotherapeutic expulsion in an age-stratified host population have been very few, most studies having relied on an indirect measure of parasite abundance, the density of eggs in the stools. A recent study in Zimbabwe,[32] in which the intensity of infection was measured directly by parasite expulsion, showed a steady rise in intensity with age, resembling those previously reported with a similar technique from India and Papua New Guinea. I believe that a similar pattern will also be found in areas where worm loads are appreciably higher.[75]

The basis of prophylaxis and control is described on pp. 182–184.

CUTANEOUS LARVA MIGRANS (CREEPING ERUPTION, SANDWORM, PLUMBER'S ITCH, DUCKHUNTER'S ITCH)

Cutaneous larva migrans is a cutaneous eruption resulting from exposure of the skin to the infective filariform larvae of non-human hookworms (*A. braziliense, A. caninum*) and *Strongyloides* of the nutria and racoon. The infective larvae cannot complete their normal life cycle in the human host but persist under the skin, without developing further, where they cause cutaneous larva migrans.

GEOGRAPHICAL DISTRIBUTION

Creeping eruption occurs in most warm humid tropical and subtropical areas, being especially common in the southern USA, along the coast of the Gulf of Mexico and Florida. It is also common on the coasts of West, South and East Africa, South-East Asia, India, Malaysia, Sri Lanka and Thailand.

AETIOLOGY

ANCYCLOSTOMA

A. braziliense is the hookworm of dogs and cats. It is smaller than *A. duodenale* (female 1 cm and male 8.5 mm long), the internal pair of ventral teeth are smaller and the dorsal rays in the copulatory bursa are distinctive (Figure III.62). The eggs are indistinguishable from those of human hookworms. The life cycle is similar to that of *A. duodenale* but man is an unsuitable host and the third stage larva does not enter the bloodstream but wanders under the skin, causing cutaneous larva migrans.

A. caninum is the dog hookworm. Its life history is similar to that of *A. braziliense*.

STRONGYLOIDES

Filariform larvae of *S. stercoralis* can re-enter the skin as part of autoinfection around the anus and buttock where they cause larva currens, a rash rather like that of cutaneous larva migrans.

S. myopotami (nutria) and *S. procyornis* (racoon) all produce similar lesions in the human host[84] in which they cannot complete their normal lifecycle. The lesions are more persistent.

TRANSMISSION

Infection is acquired from damp contaminated soil through the skin of that part of the body in contact with the soil (foot, abdomen).

PATHOLOGY

The filariform larvae are unable to penetrate below the stratum germinativum of human skin where they form a tunnel with the corium as a floor and the stratum granulosum as a roof. Local eosinophilia and round cell infiltration occurs round the tunnel and may persist for months. Rarely the larvae reach the lungs where they cause transitory pulmonary symptoms and eosinophilia and may be recovered from bronchial washings. They do not mature in the intestine.

IMMUNITY

Little is known about immunity. There is no protective immunity and people can be infected more than once.

CLINICAL FEATURES

NATURAL HISTORY

The larvae wander under the skin and can persist for months before they eventually die.

INCUBATION PERIOD

Symptoms start immediately after penetration of the skin, a matter of a few hours only.

SYMPTOMS AND SIGNS

There is a red itchy papule at the site of entry which becomes elevated and vesicular. The larvae move several millimetres to a few centimetres each day and leave tunnels which become dry and crusted. The track is linear and twists and turns (Figure

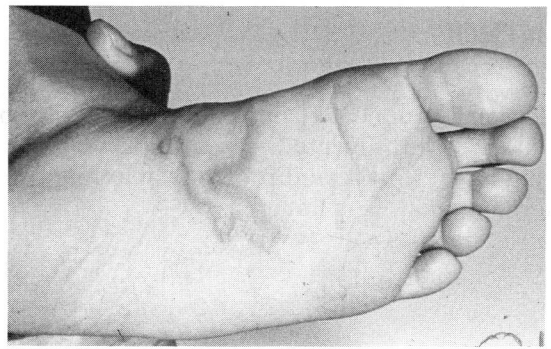

Figure 71.13 Cutaneous larva migrans (*A. braziliense*).

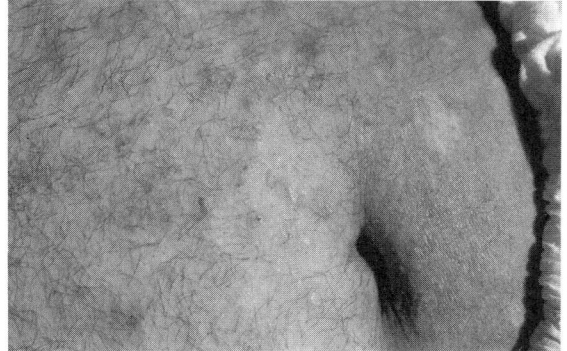

Figure 71.14 Multiple burrows of cutaneous larva migrans (creeping eruption).

71.13). It causes an intense pruritus and the skin is scratched and becomes secondarily infected. The lesions may be single or multiple. The most common sites are the hands and feet with *A. braziliense* but the abdomen is often infested in plumber's itch and the lesions may be very numerous indeed (Figure 71.14).

The lesions produced by non-human hookworms (cutaneous larva migrans) are well defined, move very slowly and persist for months. There is little surrounding flare and the track is indurated. In contrast the lesions produced by *Strongyloides* (larva currens) are less well defined, have a red flare on the outside, move much more rapidly and persist for a few hours only.

DIAGNOSIS

Creeping eruptions can be caused by *Strongyloides stercoralis* (larva currens, see p. 179), *Gnathostoma spinigerum* (see Chapter 8), cutaneous myiasis (*Hypoderma bovis* and *Hypoderma lineatum*, see Chapter 79), warble fly maggots (*Gasterophilus*, see Chapter 79), and cutaneous *Fasciola hepatica* (see Chapter 73).

The diagnosis is clinical. *Ancylostoma* larva migrans is usually situated on the foot or toe (see Figure 71.13) and lasts for months, moving very slowly. *Strongyloides* (larva currens) is situated on the buttocks and trunk and lasts for hours only, moving comparatively quickly. Non-human *Strongyloides* is usually situated on the trunk and abdomen and can persist for many months. *Loa loa* causes no cutaneous reaction and appears and disappears in a matter of minutes. There is usually no eosinophilia but if there is then internal migration of the larvae can be suspected. It is not possible to retrieve the larva since it is invariably in advance of its track and impossible to isolate. There are no serological tests.

TREATMENT

Thiabendazole is the drug of choice. It is given in a dose of 25 mg/kg twice daily for 5 days. A further 5 days treatment may be necessary after 2 days rest.[85] Itching should cease in 24 hours and the rash disappears in 10 days. *Strongyloides* responds better than hookworms to treatment. Other dosage schedules are 50 mg/kg as a single dose weekly until the lesions disappear.[86,87]

Topical thiabendazole[88] is given by grinding up a 0.5 g tablet with 5 g of petroleum jelly and applying liberally over the track of the worm daily for 5 days.

Mebendazole is sometimes effective given in a dosage of 100 mg three times daily for 7 days. Albendazole is also effective.

Metriphonate can be given topically: 10% in petroleum jelly and covered with plastic over the worm tracks, left on overnight.

In a recent randomized trial a simple 12 mg dose of ivermectin was found to be more effective than a single dose of 400 mg of albendazole.[89]

EPIDEMIOLOGY

The source of infection is soil contaminated with dog and cat faeces underneath beach houses on stilts, exposure taking place when people crawl underneath to repair facilities (plumber's itch) or bathe with bare feet and walk along the sand above the high water mark (sandworm) or expose themselves to mounds contaminated by nutria and racoons in the marshes (duckhunter's itch). In subtropical countries exposure is most common during the summer months and early autumn.

CONTROL

Little can be done to control dogs and cats but infection can be prevented by wearing sandals above the high water mark and protective clothing when underneath houses in hot areas.

STRONGYLOIDIASIS

GEOGRAPHICAL DISTRIBUTION

S. stercoralis has a worldwide distribution in the tropics and subtropics. It is highly prevalent in parts of tropical Brazil, Colombia and South-East Asia. In temperate climates it is not uncommon in inmates of institutions, such as mental hospitals, prisons and the mentally retarded children's homes. It has become a serious problem in individuals receiving suppressive treatment.

AETIOLOGY

Strongyloidiasis is caused by *S. stercoralis* (see Appendix III), a nematode worm which has two forms, one parasitic and the other free living. There are three developmental forms: adult, rhabditiform larva and filariform (infective) larva.

LIFE CYCLE (Figure 71.15)

There are two lifecycles in which reproduction takes place: an internal sexual cycle involving parasitic worms and the external sexual cycle involving free-living worms.

Internal sexual cycle

The adult female parasitic worm (2.5 × 0.034 mm) tapers anteriorly and ends in a conical tail. There is an oesophagus occupying a quarter of the body which has two bulbs divided by a constriction. The vulva lies in the posterior third of the body and there is a prominent uterus containing 50 eggs (50–58 × 30–34 μm) (Appendix III). The male exists but disappears from the bowel soon after oviposition and eggs can be produced parthenogenetically (as happens with *S. ratti*). The eggs hatch immediately in the

bowel into male and female rhabditiform larvae which pass out in the faeces to continue the external sexual cycle.

External sexual cycle

The free-living rhabditiform larvae (p. 177) develop into free-living adults which copulate in the soil and produce eggs. The free-living forms have a double bulbed muscular oesophagus. The free-living female is smaller (1 × 0.05 mm) than the parasitic female, the vulva lies posteriorly and the uterus contains eggs measuring 70 × 40 μm (Appendix III). The male form measures 0.7 × 0.035 mm. The rhabditiform larvae produced by both parasitic and free-living forms are indistinguishable and develop into filariform (infective) larvae (Figure 71.16) which can remain alive in the soil for many weeks.

INFECTION AND AUTOINFECTION

Under unsuitable conditions the external sexual cycle may be omitted and the filariform larvae infect the definitive host via the skin or buccal mucosa, as in *Ancylostoma* or *Necator*. The larvae travel up to the lungs, enter the bronchi, cross over the glottis and pass to the small intestine where they mature into parasitic adults.

Autoinfection

Autoinfection, which results in multiplication in the host indefinitely, arises in one of two ways. The filariform larvae do not pass out in the stools but reinvade the bowel or skin. The other way is when the filariform larvae lodge in the bronchial epithelium and produce further progeny. Autoinfection leads to a build-up in the body of the population so that the worms can maintain themselves in the absence of any further infection from an external

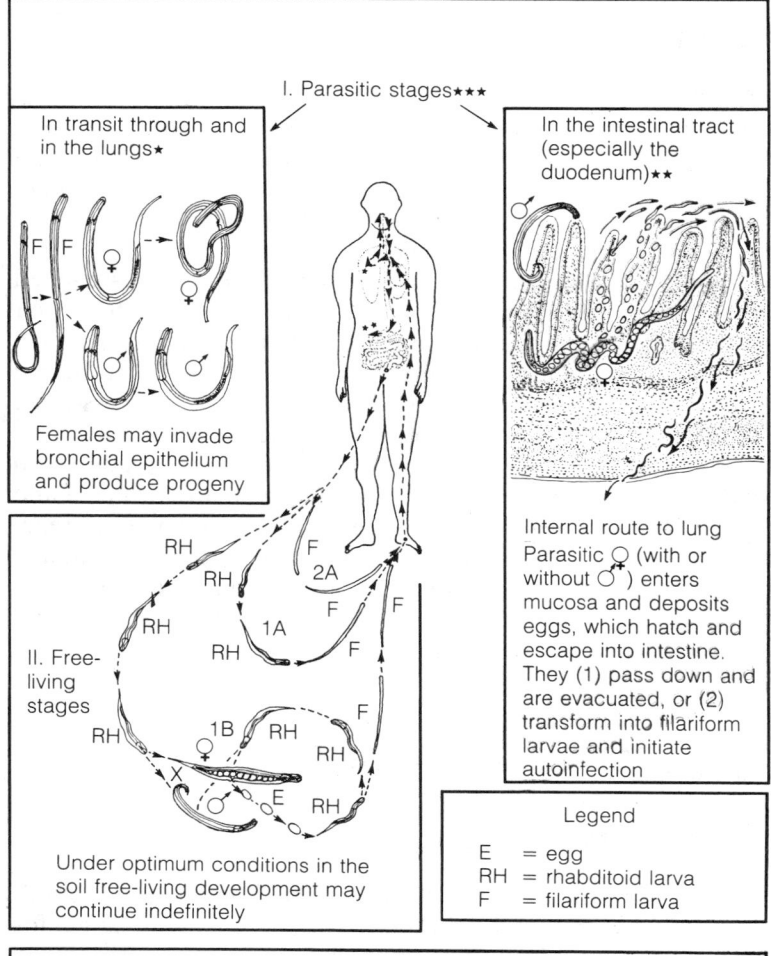

I. Parasitic stages★★★

In transit through and in the lungs★

F F ♀ ♀ ♂ ♂

Females may invade bronchial epithelium and produce progeny

In the intestinal tract (especially the duodenum)★★

Internal route to lung

Parasitic ♀ (with or without ♂) enters mucosa and deposits eggs, which hatch and escape into intestine. They (1) pass down and are evacuated, or (2) transform into filariform larvae and initiate autoinfection

II. Free-living stages

RH
RH
RH
RH
F
2A
F
1A
F
F
RH
1B
RH
♀ ♂
X
RH
RH
♂ ♀
E

Under optimum conditions in the soil free-living development may continue indefinitely

Legend

E = egg
RH = rhabditoid larva
F = filariform larva

Methods of infection

1. Filariform larvae enter skin in contact with soil
   A. Following direct RH→ F larval development
   B. Following free-living cycle in the soil
2. Filariform larvae develop before leaving patient
   A. Following deposition on the soil, enter exposed skin
   B. Enter perianal skin and initiate autoinfection
   C. Enter intestinal mucosa, migrate to lung and initiate autoinfection

Figure 71.15 Life cycle of *Strongyloides stercoralis*.

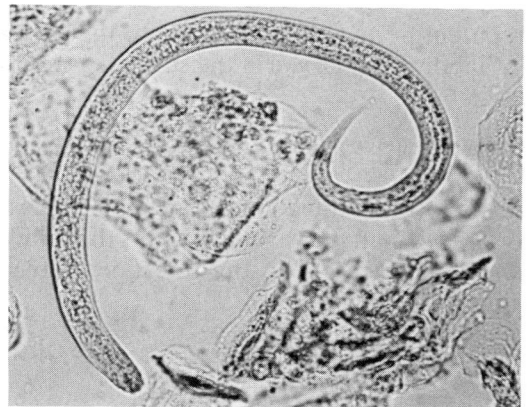

Figure 71.16 *S. stercoralis*. Rhabditiform larva in stool. (Courtesy J. S. Tatz).

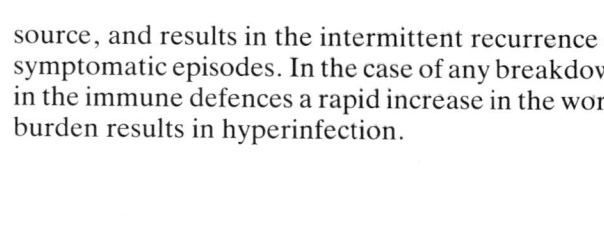

source, and results in the intermittent recurrence of symptomatic episodes. In the case of any breakdown in the immune defences a rapid increase in the worm burden results in hyperinfection.

PATHOLOGY

The pathogenic effects begin with the entry of the infective larvae into the skin. The filariform larvae cause petechial haemorrhages at the site of invasion accompanied by intense pruritus, congestion and oedema. The larvae migrate into cutaneous blood vessels and are carried to the lungs. In the lungs they enter the alveoli and pass up the respiratory tree where they may be delayed by the host response, become adults and invade the bronchial epithelium. Passing through the lungs the young worms may cause symptoms resembling those of bronchopneumonia with some lobular consolidation.

When they have become lodged in crypts in the intestine the females mature and invade the tissues of the bowel wall but rarely penetrate the muscularis mucosae, and move in tissue channels beneath the villi, where the eggs are deposited. The eggs hatch out and first stage larvae work towards the lumen of the bowel and are passed out in faeces.

In heavy infections the first stage larvae, instead of passing out in the faeces, develop in the intestine, bore into the wall of the duodenum and jejunum and develop to the adult stage, producing ova, while encysted in the bowel. From here they spread throughout the lymphatic system to the mesenteric lymph glands and can enter the general circulation and be found in the liver, lungs, kidneys and gallbladder wall. The ileum, appendix and colon are sites of reinvasion and here the worms cause granulomas with a central necrotic area often containing a degenerate larva. The mesenteric glands may be similarly affected. The lungs may show abscesses and the liver may be enlarged with small pinpoint larval granulomas. The larvae may carry microorganisms and an overwhelming septicaemia caused by *Escherichia coli* has been caused in this way. In light infections jejunal biopsy has shown oedema, cellular infiltration and eosinophilic infiltration of the mucosa with partial villous atrophy.[61] At post mortem, ulceration and atrophy of the mucosa are seen with numerous adult worms in the wall of the duodenum and jejunum. At times filariform larvae fail to break out of the alveoli, gain access to the general circulation and can invade the brain, intestine, lymph glands, liver, lungs and, rarely, myocardium.

TRANSMISSION

Infection is acquired originally from contaminated soil via free-living filariform infective larvae. Once established further infection may be acquired from the colon or anal skin from parasitic infective larvae. The transmission of *Strongyloides* through the milk has been demonstrated in several animal species and it is possible that this occurs in man.

IMMUNITY

Immunity to reinfection develops in most individuals after a primary infection and the *Strongyloides* adults and larvae are confined to the small intestine and the worm load is controlled. Immunity is both antibody and cell mediated.

Humoral antibody-mediated immunity is elicited by the secretions of the infective larvae with a type I response, an eosinophilic tissue response, and a peripheral eosinophilia—often with urticarial rashes. Antibodies are produced which cross-react with many other helminths, including filariae.

Cell-mediated immunity is elicited by adult and larval worms in the tissues, which are localized and destroyed by a cell-mediated granulomatous reaction. If cell-mediated immunity is depressed for any reason, such as immunodepressive states of drugs, then a generalized hyperinfection results causing massive strongyloidiasis.

CLINICAL FEATURES

NATURAL HISTORY

In the majority of cases a small population of adult worms maintains itself in the small intestine for many years (30 or more) in the absence of any further infection from the outside causing recurrent symptoms when filariform larvae enter the perianal skin, and cause a recurrent rash (larva currens)—sometimes associated with urticaria. In a small minority of cases the defences of the body break down and a generalized severe infection ensues.

INCUBATION PERIOD

The prepatent period from infection to the appearance of rhabditiform larvae in the stools is 1 month.

SYMPTOMS AND SIGNS

The vast majority of infections in endemic areas are symptomless. When for various reasons the number of *Strongyloides* present in the intestine increases then symptoms develop.

Diarrhoea

Watery mucous diarrhoea may develop, the degree of which depends on the intensity of the infection, its duration and the ability of the host tissue(s) to encapsulate the worms. Frequently, diarrhoea alternates with constipation.

Strongyloides *enteropathy*

Malabsorption of fat and vitamin B_{12} with chronic diarrhoea[90] and protein-losing enteropathy with malabsorption,[91] which were all rapidly reversed by anthelmintic treatment, have been described and the mechanism suggested is a hypersensitivity reagin-like reaction with the liberation of histamine and increased capillary permeability and oedema of the lamina propria.[90] In massive strongyloidiasis the lacteals of the small bowel may be so involved that their obstruction causes malabsorption.

Hypereosinophilia

When autoinfection takes place, hypereosinophilia and pulmonary symptoms resembling TPE may occur.

Skin rashes

These are of two types. One, occurring around the anus and anywhere on the trunk, is a linear eruption (larva currens) in which the larvae migrate under the skin causing an itching rash with a larval track which is not indurated and has a red flare at the edge which moves quite rapidly, disappearing in a few hours (Figure 71.17), in contrast to the more indurated and persistent track of non-human hookworm (cutaneous larva migrans). The second form is urticaria caused by allergy to the larvae penetrating the skin in an individual who has already been sensitized. The creeping type of eruption, which is seen mainly in infections from Indo-China and was common in prisoners of war in the Far East in the 1939–45 war, can last for 30 years or more.

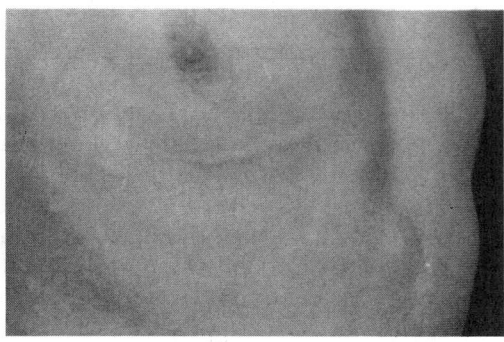

Figure 71.17 Skin rash (larva currens) of *Strongyloides stercoralis*.

Massive *strongyloidiasis*

In persons debilitated by disease, malnutrition or serious illness, especially in institutions, serious illness and sometimes death may result from massive invasion of the tissues by strongyloides.[92] Treatment with immunosuppressive drugs for lymphoma and other conditions may produce the same result.[93] First stage larvae develop in the duodenum and jejunum, bore into the bowel wall, become adult and produce ova. In this way the number of strongyloides is immensely increased and infective larvae invade the tissues and circulate, causing massive strongyloidiasis. There is a severe diarrhoea, often with malabsorption, oedema, liver enlargement and paralytic ileus. In these cases encephalopathy is common and pyogenic meningitis with strongyloides larvae in the meninges has been described.[94,95] Fatal bowel infarction has occurred.[96] Prompt treatment with albendazole or thiabendazole will save some of these patients. Two comprehensive reviews on disseminated strongyloidiasis have recently appeared.[97,98]

LABORATORY FINDINGS

Towards the end of the early stage of infection there is a high leucocytosis up to 25×10^9/litre; an eosinophilia of $10–12 \times 10^9$/litre is characteristic. Later when the infection is chronic there is a moderate eosinophilia which may persist for years. In generalized massive strongyloidiasis the eosinophilia disappears and is an indication of poor prognosis.

DIFFERENTIAL DIAGNOSIS

Strongyloidiasis must be differentiated from other tissue-invading helminths: *Ascaris*, ancylostomiasis and liver flukes. Disseminated strongyloidiasis may closely resemble tropical pulmonary eosinophilia, especially since serology cross-reacts (see Chapter 70). Larva currens resembles cutaneous larva migrans but in distinction from it in larva currens the rash is situated mainly round the buttocks and on the trunk, lasts only a few hours and may occur intermittently for many years.

DIAGNOSIS

Only adults or rhabditiform larvae (Figure 71.16) appear in the stools or duodenal drainage. They can be demonstrated by the formol ether method or cultured in charcoal at 26°C for a week (see Appendix III).

A modified agar plate method has recently been described which is considered to be superior to the filter paper method in detecting *Strongyloides*.[99]

The differentiation of the rhabditiform larvae from hookworm and *Trichostrongylus* is shown in Appendix III. Radiological diagnosis is not much used but the appearances have been described by Louisey and Barton.[100] Other methods of diagnosis are a modified Beesmann technique; the agar plate culture method; ELISA and serum IgG reactivity to larval proteins of *Strongyloides stercoralis*.[101,102]

SEROLOGY

There is considerable cross-reaction with other helminths and filariae. The filarial complement fixation test is positive in 45% of larva currens[103] and in 65% of acute cases but may be negative in massive strongyloidiasis. A sensitive ELISA test is also in use.

A gelatin particle indirect agglutination test is considered to be more convenient than the micro-ELISA for mass screening for strongyloidiasis.[105]

Immunofluorescence

The filarial fluorescent antibody test cross-reacts and is sometimes useful in diagnosis.

TREATMENT

Strongyloides should usually be treated whether or not the infection is giving rise to symptoms. It should be looked for and treated especially in immunosup-pressed patients, for example those on corticosteroid therapy or persons from endemic areas in whom transplantation is being contemplated. Albendazole, 400 mg once or twice daily for 3 days, is the drug of choice. Both thiabendazole and mebendazole are effective. Massive strongyloidiasis responds very effectively.[106] Thiabendazole is effective in a dose of 25 mg/kg twice daily for 3 days. Mebendazole 100 mg three times a day for 7 days has proved moderately effective, but 2–4 weeks treatment is needed to achieve high cure rates. Ivermectin in a single dose of 200 mg/kg has proved even more effective in a recent study.[107]

EPIDEMIOLOGY

Man is the most important host of *Strongyloides* but dogs and chimpanzees have been found infected with strains indistinguishable from those of man. Larvae are unable to survive temperatures below 8°C, or above 40°C or desiccation. Strongyloidiasis thrives in conditions of overcrowding on damp soil in tropical conditions such as in rural villages in South-East Asia. It was very common amongst prisoners of war in Burma and Indo-China in the Second World War (1939–45), but it may also become established in deep mines in cold climates.

CONTROL

Control methods are the same as for other soil-transmitted helminths (see pp. 182–184).

STRONGYLOIDES FÜLLEBORNI

GEOGRAPHICAL DISTRIBUTION

Strongyloides fülleborni is widely distributed in monkeys and in Pygmies in Zaire and Zambia in forested areas. In Papua New Guinea human infection is widely distributed in western Papua New Guinea, along the Fly river and in the eastern highlands in forested areas.

AETIOLOGY

S. fülleborni can be distinguished from *S. stercoralis* by the prominent vulvar lips, narrowing behind the vulva and a prominent oesophagus. Eggs are passed in the stool in contrast to *S. stercoralis* and resemble those of hookworm, for which they are commonly mistaken. There are probably two strains of the parasite, one in Africa and the other in Papua New Guinea. The life cycle is similar to that of *S. stercoralis*.

TRANSMISSION

Transmission is similar to that of *S. stercoralis*—from contaminated soil; although in infants the route has not been determined, transmission via the placenta or milk has been suggested.

PATHOLOGY

Pathology as far as is known, is similar to that of *S. stercoralis*; although heavy populations may build up without ill effect in infants abdominal symptoms with oedema may result, causing 'swollen belly' sickness, probably from protein loss.

SYMPTOMS AND SIGNS

In most cases there are no symptoms; 24% of pygmies in Zaire were found to be passing ova[108] and very heavy infections were found without any evidence of disease. In infants in Papua New Guinea 'swollen belly' sickness is characterized by respiratory distress, abdominal distension, generalized oedema and variable disturbance of gastrointestinal function.

DIAGNOSIS

Ova resembling hookworm can be demonstrated in faeces, and distinction from hookworm ova made by culturing stool to obtain adults and then identify them.

TREATMENT

Thiabendazole and mebendazole are effective—as used in *S. stercoralis* infection. Plasma infusions to correct hypoproteinaemia may be necessary.

EPIDEMIOLOGY

S. fülleborni is a zoonosis infecting monkeys and apes in tropical Africa where it is common in human populations in the rain forest. Although it is a zoonosis, interhuman transmission may occur, and 24% of pygmies have been found infected.[108] In Papua New Guinea infection, which is abundant in children from 3 to 5 years old, is rare in adults; there it is confined to mainly forested areas in western New Guinea, along the Fly river and in the eastern highlands which suggest a zoonosis, although no animal host has been identified. The distribution, incidence, transmission and chemical signs of a new subspecies *Strongyloides fülleborni kellyi* has recently been described from Papua New Guinea.[109]

TRICHOSTRONGYLIASIS

GEOGRAPHICAL DISTRIBUTION

Normally a parasite of sheep and goats, human infection with *Trichostrongylus* is widespread in Central Africa, Egypt and in Asia and India, Assam, Indonesia and Japan.

AETIOLOGY

Three species can infect man: *Trichostrongylus colubriformis*, *Trichostrongylus orientalis* and, more rarely *Trichostrongylus probolurus*. The female worm ($5–8 \times 0.07$ mm) is slender and pink with a posterior vulva (Appendix III); the male ($4–5 \times 0.07$ mm) has bilobed copulatory bursa and two spicules. The mouth is unarmed. The parasites are situated in the duodenum and jejunum where they are not attached to the bowel but are a half to a third buried in mucus. The eggs, which have a transparent hyaline shell and resemble those of hookworm but are larger ($85 \times 115\ \mu$m), are passed in the stool in the morula stage and are remarkably resistant to desiccation and cold. The life cycle is similar to that of hookworm but they do not migrate through the lungs. Adults mature in the intestine within 25–30 days.

TRANSMISSION

Infection is acquired through the skin or mouth from contaminated food or drink.

PATHOLOGY

Little is known about pathology and none has been observed, even in individuals with heavy egg counts.

SYMPTOMS AND SIGNS

These are few but mild anaemia and general ill health may result.

DIAGNOSIS

Diagnosis is made by finding eggs in faeces and adults after treatment.

TREATMENT

Levamisole is the drug of choice and is given as a single oral dose of 2.5 mg/kg. Thiabendazole is less effective. Albendiazole has not been tested.

EPIDEMIOLOGY

Trichostrongylus colubriformis is a parasite of sheep and goats and is common in some areas where sheep and goats are kept: up to 70% of the inhabitants may be infected.

Trichostrongylus orientalis is common among people who look after donkeys and goats and the use of human excreta as fertilizer in Asia is responsible for the high level of infection.

COMMUNITY CONTROL OF GEOHELMINTHS

The five basic essentials needed for controlling geohelminth infections at the community level are: (1) chemotherapy; (2) sanitation; (3) health education; (4) community participation; and (5) monitoring and evaluation.

CHEMOTHERAPY

There are now several anthelmintics active against the geohelminths. They have a broad spectrum of activity, which makes them particularly useful for community control, since polyparasitism is more common than monoparasitism in most of the countries where geohelminths are endemic. They are relatively non-toxic, they can be given orally, and are effective in a single dose if reduction in intensity of infection rather than absolute cure is the main objective.

For countries that adopt a national 'essential drugs' policy and take advantage of the joint UNICEF–WHO initiative for the procurement of 'essential drugs', the cost is now low. The clinical pharmacology of the most commonly used broad-spectrum anthelmintics is given on pp. 184–185.

In general, pregnant women and children under 2 years of age or weighing under 10 kg should not be included in community control chemotherapeutic campaigns. These are high-risk groups in the tropics, and a fatality occurring within days of drug administration, even if unrelated, is frequently attributed to the event and can adversely affect community participation.

In countries where transmission of soil-transmitted helminths is seasonal, the time of the campaign is important. In these circumstances, two treatments, the first after the start of the wet season, e.g. 8 weeks, and the second after the end of the rains, e.g. 8 weeks, will reduce the risk of reinfection during the subsequent dry season. In countries where transmission is perennial, more frequent treatments may be required, e.g. 3–4 times yearly, which would naturally increase the cost of the campaign.

The strategy of chemotherapeutic interventions should be integrated with the other activities of the local health services: for example primary health care programmes; immunization programmes; child health programmes; family planning programmes; school health programmes; and in *appropriate circumstances* e.g. when age-infection of intensity distribution overlap, in a multiple infection delivery approach.

Since reduction in morbidity is the primary objective of chemotherapy the limitations of the multiple infection delivery approach are obvious when it is appreciated that the age distribution of infection intensity varies substantially between the parasite species:[110] the peak intensities of *Ascaris* and *Trichuris* occur in children under 10 years of age; of schistosomes in the age group 10–20 years; of hookworms in adults over 20 years of age.

Three chemotherapeutic strategies can be used: *mass chemotherapy*, i.e. treatment of all persons if the prevalence of infection is 50% or over; *selective population chemotherapy*, i.e. treatment of *all* infected persons at the time of a survey; *targeted chemotherapy*, i.e. treatment of specific groups likely to suffer the greatest morbidity.

SANITATION

Marked improvements in environmental hygiene are the ultimate answer to the control and elimination of geohelminth infections, but for many countries in the tropics these are relatively expensive and long-term objectives.

In the medium term, however, many varieties of affordable latrines are available, e.g. ventilated improved pit latrines, double-vault latrines. These have proved to be culturally acceptable in many countries; they are easy to install, operate and maintain.[111,112] Further, they allow adequate composting of human excretion as fertilizer.

The impact of the water-sanitation decade in several countries should play an important role in the control of geohelminths. It must be appreciated that the effect of sanitation is slow to develop, and that therefore periodic anthelmintic treatment should be maintained until sanitation has had an impact on transmission.[113]

HEALTH EDUCATION

Human behaviour is of great importance in the transmission of geohelminths and the success or failure of control programmes often hinges on the modification of behavioural patterns. Health education must target its activities on this crucial criterion, aiming to determine which local culture and practices are conducive to the transmission of infection and need to be modified to reduce the risk. If beneficial cultural practices are identified, these should be reinforced to enhance compliance. As many people as possible should be involved in the planning process, particularly women, who in the past have often been ignored. Improvements in personal hygiene should be actively encouraged. Modern audiovisual technology may be used when appropriate.

COMMUNITY PARTICIPATION

This is crucial for the success of any control programme. Active participation of the community in the planning and execution of any intervention is mandatory. The schedule should suit the convenience of the community and be discussed and agreed by them.

MONITORING AND EVALUATION

Monitoring and evaluation are mandatory and should be used to review or revise any control programme. In view of the severe financial constraints for health care in most developing countries, the cost-effectiveness of any strategy used should be determined wherever possible.

Targeted chemotherapy implemented within an existing health infrastructure has been shown to achieve an overall reduction in the prevalence and intensity of *Ascaris* and *Trichuris* infection in children aged 2–15 years at one-fifth of the drug purchase cost of mass chemotherapy, and with few of the attendant costs of drug delivery.[114]

CLINICAL PHARMACOLOGY OF ANTHELMINTIC DRUGS[115,116,117]

The drugs most commonly used for the community control of the soil-transmitted helminths are albendazole, mebendazole, pyrantel and levamisole. They are all broad-spectrum anthelmintics, although their efficacy against the individual geohelminths varies.[118] Their spectrum of activity against the various nematodes is shown in Table 71.1.

These safe and orally administered, single-dose broad-spectrum anthelmintics have revolutionized our concepts for the community control of the geohelminths.

ALBENDAZOLE

This is now the most widely used anthelmintic for the community control of multiple geohelminth infections and is the newest of the benzimidazole derivatives.

It is poorly absorbed from the gastrointestinal tract and is rapidly and extensively metabolized by the liver to sulphoxide and sulphone metabolites.

The sulphoxide metabolite is an active anthelmintic and may be responsible for most of the drug effects in vivo.

Albendazole is not detectable in plasma after oral administration. It is known to be teratogenic and embryotoxic in some animals. It should not be administered during confirmed or suspected pregnancy. In women of child-bearing age albendazole should be administered no more than 7 days after the start of the last menstrual period.

Adverse effects are mild and transient. They include epigastric pain, diarrhoea, headache, nausea, vomiting, dizziness, constipation, pruritus and dry mouth.

MEBENDAZOLE

Mebendazole is effective against adult worms and larval stages. It selectively inhibits glucose uptake in nematodes; this results in increased utilization of helminth glycogen and deprivation for the worms of their main source of energy.

Oral absorption is limited by its poor solubility.

The small amount absorbed is metabolized extensively by the liver to inactive compounds.

Teratogenic and embryotoxic effects in animals have been recorded; it is therefore not recommended in pregnancy.

Adverse effects include transient gastrointestinal discomfort and headache.

Mebendazole sometimes stimulates *Ascaris* worms to emerge from the mouth and nostrils, which alarms the patients unless they are forewarned.

PYRANTEL

Pyrantel owes its activity to its action on the neuromuscular system of the worms. It paralyses the worms, which are then expelled in the faeces.

It is poorly absorbed from the gastrointestinal tract, with less than 15% excreted in the urine as unchanged drug and metabolites and 70% excreted unchanged in the faeces.

It should be stored in tight, light-resistant containers.

Adverse effects include mild gastrointestinal discomfort, headache, dizziness, drowsiness, insomnia and skin rash.

Pyrantel and piperazine are antagonistic and should not be administered concurrently.

LEVAMISOLE

Levamisole causes a spastic paralysis of susceptible nematodes, resulting in their elimination from the intestine.

It is rapidly absorbed from the gastrointestinal tract, achieving peak plasma levels within 2 hours, and is eliminated within 3 days. Much of the absorbed drug is metabolized in the liver.

Adverse effects include abdominal pain, nausea, vomiting, dizziness and headache.

Table 71.1 Spectrum of activity of antinematode drugs.

	Albendazole	Pyrantel	Mebendazole	Levamisole
Ascaris lumbricoides	+++	+++	+++	+++
Trichuris trichiura	++	++	++	+
Necator americanus	+++	++	++	++
Ancyclostoma duodenale	+++	+++	+++	+++
Strongyloides stercoralis	++	+	+	+

+++, High; ++, moderate; + low.

OTHER NEMATODES FOR WHOM MAN IS NOT THE NORMAL HOST

TRICHINOSIS (*TRICHINELLA SPIRALIS*)

GEOGRAPHICAL DISTRIBUTION (Figure 71.18)

Trichinosis has a worldwide distribution and is important as an infection of man in Europe and the USA. It is less important in the tropics but occurs in both east and west sub-Saharan Africa. It is an important cause of disease and death in the Arctic where polar explorers have died as a result of trichinosis. *It is not a soil-transmitted helminth infection.*

AETIOLOGY

Trichinella spiralis occurs in two forms: adult and cystic.

The adult *T. spiralis* (Appendix III) is a white worm just visible to the naked eye which inhabits the small intestine. The male (1.6 × 0.04 mm) has a cloaca situated posteriorly between two caudal papillae. The female (3–4 × 0.06 mm) has a vulva in the anterior fifth, an ovary in the posterior half of the body and a coiled uterine tube in the anterior portion.

LIFE CYCLE (See Appendix III)

The female lives for 30 days and is viviparous. The eggs (20 μm) live in the upper uterus and the larvae (100 × 6 μm) break out, living free in the uterine cavity. One female produces more than 1500 larvae. The larvae, which emerge as early as 4–7 days after infection, continue to be produced for 4–16 weeks. They make their way via the lymphatics and blood circulation to the right heart and lungs where they enter the arterial circulation and reach striated muscle, where they encyst.

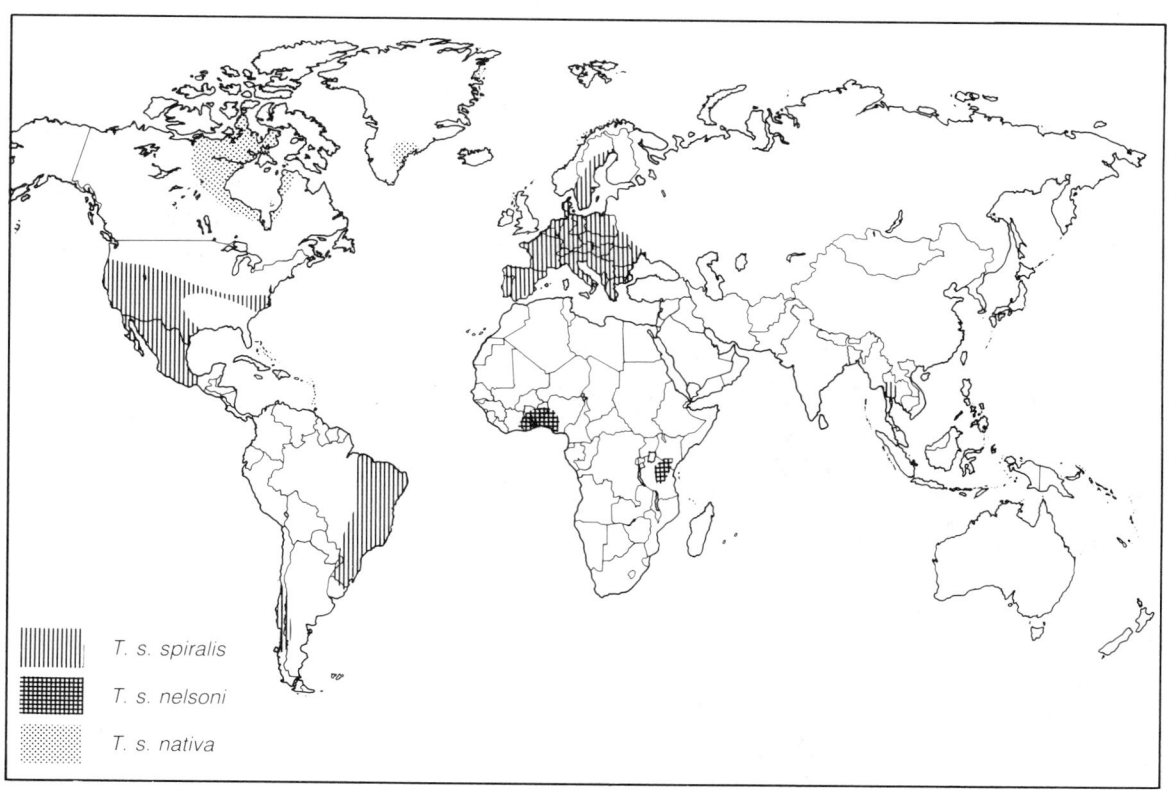

T. s. spiralis

T. s. nelsoni

T. s. nativa

Figure 71.18 Geographical distribution of trichinosis.

Cystic stage

The cyst is formed by the larva encapsulated by the host tissue. The capsule is an adventitious ellipsoidal sheath with blunt ends resulting from cellular reaction around the tightly coiled larva (Figure 71.19). The long axis parallels that of the muscle fibres and host amino acids nourish it so that it can remain alive for many years. In man calcification may take place after 6 months and lead to death of the larva. When consumed by a carnivorous host the cysts are digested in the stomach and after encysting the larvae, which are resistant to gastric juice, invade the duodenal and jejunal mucosa where they penetrate the columnar epithelium and develop into adults after 36 hours. The period between infection and the encysting stage in the muscles is 17–21 days.

SPECIES AND STRAINS OF *TRICHINELLA*

T. spiralis contains three subspecies which can infect man. They are indistinguishable morphologically but vary in their host specificity and can be distinguished enzymatically.[119]

- *T. spiralis spiralis* of temperate regions with domestic pigs the source of human infection.
- *T. spiralis nativa* of the Arctic regions; a parasite of carrion feeding carnivores; polar bears and walruses are the main sources of human infection.
- *T. spiralis nelsoni* in Africa and southern Europe in wild carnivores with wild pigs the source of human infection.

T. s. nativa is very resistant to freezing and *T. s. nelsoni* and *T. s. nativa* have a low infectivity for domestic pigs and rats.

TRANSMISSION

Transmission is by mouth from eating undercooked meat.

T. S. SPIRALIS

Human infection is acquired from eating undercooked pork from infected pigs. The pigs are infected from eating raw garbage or perhaps from eating rats which themselves become infected from garbage.

T. S. NATIVA

Human infection is acquired from eating bear meat (the top predator), polar bear in the Arctic and brown bears in sub-Arctic regions of the former USSR and North America. Walrus meat can also be infective. Polar explorers have died as a result of eating polar bear meat.

T. S. NELSONI

Human infection results from eating bush-pig or wart-hog meat which are themselves infected from carrion.

PATHOLOGY

The capsule of the infective larva is digested in the intestine since it is resistant to the gastric juice and penetrates the duodenal and jejunal mucosa where

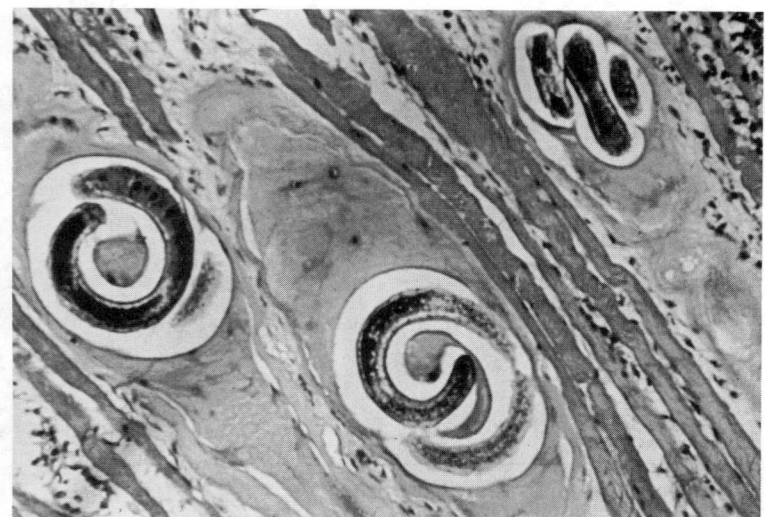

Figure 71.19   Larvae of *T. spiralis* in muscle.

the amount of trauma and irritation depends upon the number of larvae. This will cause the symptoms of the *enteric phase*.

After 5–7 days the worms mature and the females discharge larvae to the tissues, causing symptoms of the *migratory* or *invasive* stage. Later the larvae encyst causing symptoms of the *encystment* stage. Larvae only encyst in striated muscle but travel through the brain and heart muscle where they are unable to encyst.

STRIATED MUSCLE

Larvae, after travelling through the circulation, encyst in muscles of the diaphragm, masseters, intercostals, laryngeal, tongue and ocular muscles. At first there is a basophilic degeneration of the muscle fibres followed by formation of a hyaline capsule around the larva with an inflammatory infiltrate of lymphocytes and a few enosinophils (Figure 71.19). Foreign body giant cells may be present. The infiltrate subsides and fat is deposited at the poles and after 6 months calcification takes place, eventually leading to death of the larva.

BRAIN

Larvae migrate through the brain and meninges causing leptomeningitis, granulomatous nodules in the basal ganglia, medulla, cerebellum and perivascular cuffing in the cortex. They can be found in the cerebrospinal fluid with a raised cell count and increased protein.

HEART

The larvae cause considerable damage on passage through the myocardium, cellular infiltration and necrosis with subsequent fibrosis of the myocardial bundles.

IMMUNITY

NATURAL IMMUNITY

Natural immunity is confined to cold-blooded animals with a temperature below 37°C.

ACQUIRED IMMUNITY

A well-marked immunity to reinfection develops after the first infection but it is necessary for the infective larvae to develop through to the adult stage before immunity is produced, which is both anti-adult and antilarval. Cell-mediated immunity is largely responsible but humoral antibodies develop.[120] Immunized mice respond rapidly to challenge infections with an inflammatory reaction in the bowel and the elimination of adult worms. Cellular immunity can be transferred by cellular elements and diminished by corticosteroids, adrenalectomy and whole body irradiation.

A type I hypersensitivity reaction is responsible for most of the pathology of the migratory or invasive phase, fever, oedema, rash, hypereosinophilia and tissue damage. Immune complexes are not apparently important. Humoral antibodies develop and are used in diagnosis. Cellular immunity is responsible for sealing off the cysts during the stage of encystment. Both immediate and delayed hypersensitivity can be demonstrated by skin tests.

CLINICAL FEATURES

NATURAL HISTORY

Trichinosis is a self-limiting infection lasting in light infections 2–3 weeks and in heavy ones at the most 2–3 months. Except in heavy infections mortality is low. Light infections are often asymptomatic and routine examination of diaphragms at autopsy have shown a significant number containing calcified cysts in endemic areas.

INCUBATION PERIOD

From eating infected meat the development of symptoms during the enteric phase is up to 7 days after infection and for the migratory phase from 7 to 21 days.

SYMPTOMS AND SIGNS

The symptomatology depends upon the level of infection and can be related to the number of larvae per gram of muscle. Light infections (subclinical) up to ten larvae, moderate 50 to 500 larvae and severe and possibly fatal infections more than 1000. In symptomatic cases symptoms develop in three stages: enteric (invasion of the intestine) phase, migration of the larvae (invasive phase) and a period of encystation in the muscles.

Enteric phase

Irritation and inflammation of the duodenum and jejunum where the larvae penetrate causes nausea, vomiting, colic and sweating, resembling an attack of acute food poisoning. There may be a maculopapular skin rash, and in a third of cases symptoms of a pneumonitis occur between the second and sixth day, lasting about 5 days.

Migratory (invasion) phase

The cardinal symptoms and signs of this phase are severe myalgia, periorbital oedema and eosinophilia. There is difficulty in mastication, breathing and swallowing due to the involvement of the muscles and there may be some muscular paralysis of the extremities. There is a high remittent fever with typhoidal symptoms, splinter haemorrhages under the nails and in the conjunctivae and blood and albumin in the urine. Characteristically there is a hypereosinophilia from the 14th day which decreases after a week and persists at a lower level. An absence of eosinophilia denotes a poor prognosis. The lymph glands may be enlarged as well as the parotid and submental glands. Occasionally there is splenomegaly. In severe cases there may be subpleural, gastric and intestinal haemorrhages.

Myocardial complications

Myocardial complications are frequent and may lead to congestive heart failure 4–8 weeks after infection; between the second and fifth week sudden death from dysrhythmia or congestive heart failure with peripheral oedema may occur. Pericardial effusion is common. Most cases recover completely but a few continue with chronic cardiac disability.

Neurological complications

During the passage of larvae through the central nervous system symptoms of meningitis, meningoencephalitis and focal cerebral lesions may develop. Ocular disturbances, diplegia, deafness and a syndrome resembling motor neurone disease, epileptiform attacks and coma may occur in very heavy infections.

Encystment phase

This is the third stage and may be severe. There may be cachexia, oedema and extreme dehydration. During the second month after infection there is a decrease in muscle tenderness, fever and itching subside and congestive heart failure may appear.

Damage to the brain may persist with protean neurological signs which may clear up later or persist. Gram-negative septicaemia from organisms introduced by the larvae, permanent hemiplegia[121] and Jacksonian epilepsy 10 years after an attack of trichinosis have been described.

PROGNOSIS

Death is unusual except in cases of heart failure when it occurs during the sixth and seventh week from exhaustion, heart failure, pneumonitis, peritonitis or nephritis. Persistent leakage of larval antigen leads to a continued low eosinophilia and circulating antibody with positive serology and immediate and delayed hypersensitivity.

DIFFERENTIAL DIAGNOSIS

Trichinosis resembles many conditions: typhoid, encephalitis, myositis and tetanus; due to the association with a high eosinophilia it closely resembles the tissue stages of schistosomiasis (Katayama syndrome), hookworm, *Strongyloides* and other helminthic infections. Trichinosis may also resemble collagen disorders such as periarteritis nodosa and acute rheumatoid arthritis.

DIAGNOSIS

Diagnosis is made by demonstrating larvae and by serology.

DEMONSTRATION OF LARVAE

Larvae have been isolated from peripheral blood in the early stages of the migration phase by mixing blood with dilute acetic acid and centrifuging. Larvae may be demonstrated in muscle by trichinoscopy.

Trichinoscopy

This can only be used when the encystment phase has started from 7 days after infection onwards. Samples (1 cm^2) of deltoid, biceps, gastrocnemius or pectoralis major are digested with 1% pepsin and 1% hydrochloric acid for several hours at 37°C, filtered or centrifuged and the number of larvae per gram of muscle estimated. Larvae can also be seen on muscle pressed between two slides, which is more useful in the first 3 weeks of the disease.

Xenodiagnosis can be performed by feeding diaphragmatic tissue to uninfected albino white rats and examining them 1 month later.

BIOCHEMICAL TESTS

In the acute phase there are serum enzyme changes with a rise in the creatine phosphokinase, lactate dehydrogenase and myokinase levels.[122]

SEROLOGY

Circulating antibody can be detected as early as 2 weeks in heavy infections and 3–4 weeks in lighter infections. Titres fall markedly after 1–2 years but decrease before this. The bentonite and latex (BFT and LFT) tests, indirect fluorescent antibody test (IFAT) and ELISA are now used. The antigens used are larval antigens originally extracted in Coca's fluid or an acid-soluble protein fraction—Melcher antigen[123]—but more refined antigens are becoming available.

BFT and LFT

The BFT and LFT are tests of choice. Bentonite and latex particles are added to trichinella extract and glycerine solution. The reagents are stable and the tests are easily and quickly performed. They detect antibody during the acute stage of the disease[124,125] becoming positive about day 15. A titre of 1:5 is diagnostic.

Immunofluorescence

The IFAT becomes positive at high titre from 2 to 3 weeks after infection, falling to a lower level after 3 months.

ELISA

The ELISA has proved most useful, being highly sensitive.

A 'sandwich' ELISA technique based on detection of circulating antigen(s) was shown to be highly sensitive and specific in the serodiagnosis of human trichonellosis.[126]

TREATMENT

Treatment is directed against the larvae and the immune reaction they invoke.

LARVICIDAL

Mebendazole. Prolonged oral high dosage mebendazole has proved effective. A dose of 20 mg/kg body weight 6-hourly for 2 weeks has proved larvicidal and may have to be repeated.[127]

IMMUNOSUPPRESSION

In severe life-threatening infections the immune response must be controlled, and prednisone 20 mg three times daily is given, initially reducing and finally discontinuing over a period of 2–3 weeks. Some cases are resistant to prednisone. Old calcified larvae do not need treatment.

EPIDEMIOLOGY (Figure 71.20)

Man is not the normal host of *T. spiralis* and becomes infected only after eating raw or undercooked flesh. The usual type, *T. s. spiralis*, found in Europe and North America is an infection of the black and brown rats by which it is propagated. These rats are cannibalistic and may be eaten by domestic pigs which infect man when raw or undercooked pork is eaten. This type is common wherever uncooked sausage is eaten, especially in Germany and other areas of the world to which Germans have travelled, for example, North America and Chile.

Clinical illness is most likely to occur when sausage prepared from a single heavily infected pig is eaten by a family or community. Where the meat has been diluted by uninfected meat then the disease is mild or subclinical. In the USA two outbreaks occurred in 1956 and one in 1957[128] and a severe epidemic occurred in England in Liverpool in 1953. Under the conditions developed by man for raising and fattening pigs, garbage which contains unsterilized pig scraps and other trimmings is the most common source of infection in pigs in the USA at the present time. Another possible source is the ingestion of faeces of other infected animals, mice, rats, foxes and other pigs at a time when mature larvae are becoming established in the intestinal wall. The majority of infections are symptomless and Link[129] has estimated 350 000 new infections in the USA annually, of which only 16 000 produced symptoms.

Temperate zone: *T.s. spiralis*

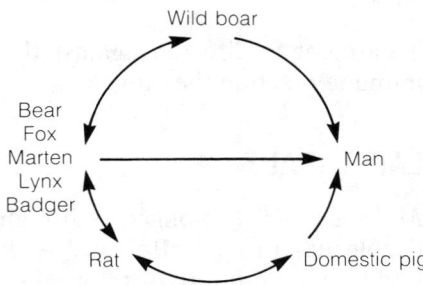

Africa: *T.s. nelsoni*

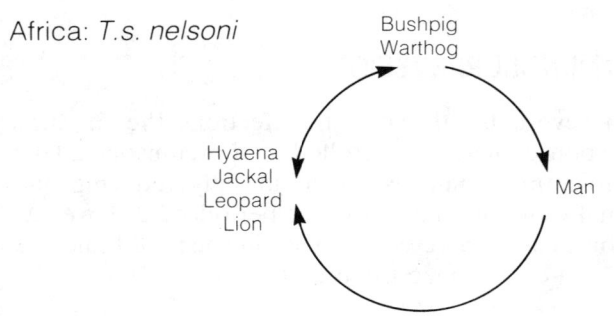

Arctic: *T.s. nativa*

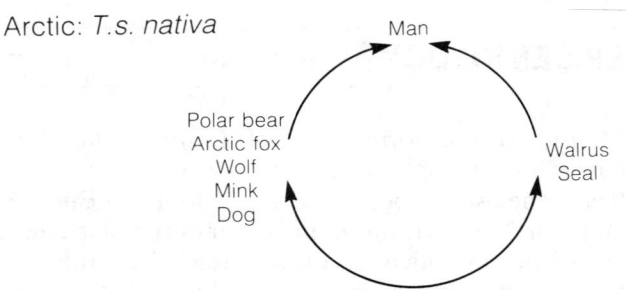

Figure 71.20 Epidemiology of *T. spiralis*.

It is estimated that subclinical trichinosis can be demonstrated in 20% of the population in the USA and 1% in England by digestion of material obtained at autopsy.

T. s. nativa is found mainly in Alaska and the northern regions of the world.[130] Here trichinosis is found in the white whale, walrus, hair seal, tree squirrel, black and white polar bear, dog, wolf, fox and wolverine. The polar bear, which is at the top of the Arctic food pyramid, is usually heavily infected and is the usual source, along with the black and brown bear, of human infections. Bear meat is eaten as a luxury and as an essential food in polar regions and whole expeditions have died of trichinosis after eating polar bear meat. Two epidemics have been reported from Alaska as a result of the consumption of black bear meat.[131] In 1947 an epidemic occurred in Greenland with 300 cases and 33 deaths caused by eating walrus meat.

T. s. nelsoni is found in Africa south of the Sahara where it has been described from East Africa[132] and Senegal. The infection is found in bush pigs (*Potamochoerus porcus*) and in the lion, leopard, cheetah and hyena. Man is infected by eating bush pig; domestic pigs are not infected.

PREVENTION

The main method of prevention is thorough cooking of all meat and regular meat inspection by means of trichinoscopy of all pork. Effective treatment of pork may be instituted by means of refrigeration. Storage of pork in deep freeze units at −18°C to −15°C is effective. The cysts are destroyed by storage at −15°C for 20 days, −20°C for 10 days, −25°C for 6 days and immediately by quick freezing at −37°C.[133]

Cooking of all garbage will prevent the infection in pigs and dressed pork may be irradiated by cobalt-60 or caesium-137, which kills the cysts. In the Arctic and sub-Arctic regions bear meat should be avoided.

REFERENCES

1 Schüffner W. Die Bedeutung der Staubinfektion für die Oxyuriasis. Richtlinien der Therapie und Prophylaxe. *Munch Med Wochenschr* 1944; 31:411–414.

2 Daly J J & Baker G F. Pinworm granuloma of the liver. *Am J Trop Med Hyg* 1984; 33:62–64.

3 Pearson R D, Irons R P & Irons R P Jr. Chronic pelvic peritonitis due to the pinworm *Enterobius vermicularis*. *JAMA* 1981; 245:1340–1341.

4 Muller R. *Worms and Disease. A Manual of Medical Helminthology*. London: Heinemann, 1975.

5 Jung R & Beaver P C. Clinical observations on *Trichocephalus trichuris* (whipworm) infestation in children. *Pediatrics* 1952; 8:548–557.

6 Wolfe M S. Oxyuris, trichostrongylus and trichuris. *Clin Gastroenterol* 1978; 7:201–217.

7 Swartzwelder J C. Clinical *Trichocephalus trichuris* infection; analysis of 81 cases. *Am J Trop Med* 1939; 19:473–481.

8 Gilman R H, Davis C & Fitzgerald F. Trichuris infection and amoebic dysentery in Orang Alsi children. A comparison of the two diseases. *Trans R Soc Trop Med Hyg* 1976; 70:313–316.

9 Kan S P. Efficacy of single doses of mebendazole in the treatment of *Trichuris trichiura* infection. *Am J Trop Med Hyg* 1983; 32:118–122.

10 Callender J et al. Development levels and nutritional status of children with the *Trichuris trichiura* dysentery syndrome. *Trans R Soc Trop Med Hyg* 1993; 87:528–9.

11 Hall A & Nahar Q. Albendazole and infections with *Ascaris lumbricordes* and *Trichuris trichiura* in children in Bangladesh. *Trans R Soc Trop Med Hyg* 1994; 88:110–112.

12 Loeffler P. Transient lung infiltrations with blood eosinophilia. *Arch Int Allergy* 1956; 8:54–59.

13 Beaver P C & Danaraj T J. Pulmonary ascariasis resembling eosinophilic lung. Autopsy report with description of larvae in the bronchioles. *Am J Trop Med Hyg* 1958; 7:100–111.

14 Parsons H E. Nematode chorioretinitis: report of a case. *Arch Ophthalmol* 1952; 6:799–800.

15 Reddy C R M, Venkateswar Rao D V, Sarma E N B & Swamy G M N. Granulomatous peritonitis due to *Ascaris lumbricoides* and its ova. *J Trop Med Hyg* 1975; 78:146–149.

16 Louw J H. Biliary ascariasis in childhood. *S Afr J Surg* 1974; 4:219–225.

17 Batu A T, Myint S, Myint A et al. Ascaris larvae and ova in the core of bile-duct stones in Rangoon. *Trans R Soc Trop Med Hyg* 1975; 69:167 (letter).

18 Carswell F, Meakins R H & Harland P S E G. Parasites and asthma in Tanzanian children. *Lancet* 1976; ii:706–707.

19 Venkatachalam P S & Patwardhan V N. The role of *Ascaris lumbricoides* in the nutrition of the host: effect of ascariasis on digestion of protein. *Trans R Soc Trop Med Hyg* 1976; 47:169–176.

20 Stephenson L S, Crompton D W T, Latham M C et al. Relationship between *Ascaris* infection and growth of malnourished pre-school children in Kenya. *Am J Clin Nutr* 1980; 33:1165–1172.

21 Thein-Hlaing, Thane-Toe, Than-Shaw, Myint-Luin. A controlled chemotherapeutic intervention trial on the relationship between *Ascaris lumbricoides* infection and malnutrition in children. *Trans R Soc Med Hyg* 1991; 85:523–528.

22 Williams J F & Soulsby E J L. Antigenic analysis of the developmental stages of *Ascaris suum*. *Exp Parasitol* 1970; 27:150–162, 362–367.

23 Gelpi A P & Mustafa A. Seasonal pneumonitis with eosinophilia. A study of larval ascariasis in Saudi Arabia. *Am J Trop Med Hyg* 1967; 16:646–657.

24 Loue J H. Abdominal complications of *Ascaris lumbricoides* infection in children. *Br J Surg* 1966; 53:510–521.

25 Thein-Hlaing. *Ascaris lumbricoides* infection in Burma. In Crompton D W T, Neisheim M C & Pawlowski Z S (eds) *Ascariasis and its Public Health Significance*. London: Taylor & Francis, 1985:83–112.

26 Soulsby E J L. Intradermal tests on pigs with antigens prepared from *Trichinella spiralis* and *Ascaris lumbricoides*. *Br Vet J* 1957; 113:447–449.

27 Pawlowski Z S. Ascaris. In Pawlowski Z S (ed.) *Intestinal Helminthic Infections*, vol. 12, no. 3. London: Baillière Tindall, 1987; 595–615.

28 Crompton D W T & Pawlowski Z S. Life history and development of *Ascaris lumbricoides* and the persistence of human ascariasis. In Crompton D W T, Neisheim M C & Pawlowski Z S (eds) *Ascariasis and its Public Health Significance*. London: Taylor Francis, 1985:9–23.

29 Croll N A & Ghadiriam E. Wormy persons: contributions to the nature and patterns of overdispersion with *Ascaris lumbricoides*, *Ancyclostoma duodenale*, *Necator americanus* and *Trichuris trichiura*. *Trop Geogr Med* 1981; 33:241–248.

30 Shuval H T, Yekutial P & Fattal B. Epidemiological evidence for helminth and cholera transmission by vegetables irrigated with waste water: Jerusalem — a case study. *Water Sci Technol* 1984; 17:433–442.

31 Denham D A. *Ascaris lumbricoides* in English school children. *Trans R Soc Trop Med Hyg* 1984; 78:566–567 (letter).

32 Anderson R M & Schad G A. Hookworm burdens and faecal egg counts: an analysis of the biological basis of variation. *Trans R Soc Trop Med Hyg* 1985; 79:812–825.

33 Schad G A & Anderson R M. Predisposition of hookworm infection in humans. *Science* 1985; 228:1537–1540.

34 Bradley M, Chandiwana S K, Bundy D A P & Medley G F. The epidemiology and population biology of *Necator americanus* infection in a rural community in Zimbabwe. *Trans R Soc Trop Med Hyg* 1992; 86:73–76.

35 Wakelin D. Genetics, immunity and parasitic survival. In Rollinson D & Anderson A M (eds) *Ecology and Genetics of Host–Parasite Interactions*. London: Academic Press, 1985:39–54.

36 Chan L, Bundy D A P & Kan S P. Aggregation and predisposition to *Ascaris lumbricoides* and *Trichuris trichiura* at the familiar level. *Trans R Soc Trop Med Hyg* 1994; 88:46–48.

37 Chan L, Kan S P & Bundy D A P. The effect of repeated chemotherapy on age-related predisposition to *Ascaris lumbricoides* and *Tichuris trichiura*. *Parasitology* 1992; 38:323–326.

38 Anderson R M & May R M. Helminth infections in humans: mathematical models, population dynamics and control. *Adv parasitol* 1985; 24:1–101.

39 Thein-Hlaing, Than-Saw & Myat-Lay-Kyin. The impact of three monthly age-targeted chemotherapy on *Ascaris lumbricoides* infection. *Trans R Soc Trop Med Hyg* 1991; 85:519–522.

40 Linillater J M et al. Absorption of carbohydrate

from rice in *Ascaris lumbricoides* infected Burmese village children. *J Trop Paced* 1992; 38:323–326.

41 Theine – H Laing et al. A controlled chemotherapeutic intervention trial on the relationship between *Ascaris lumbricoides* infection and malnutrition in children. *Trans R Soc Trop Hyg* 1991; 85:523–528.

42 Medley G, Gayeth A L & Bundy D A P. A quantitative framework for evaluating the effect of community treatment on the morbidity due to ascariasis. *Parasitology* 1993; 106:211–221.

43 Crompton D W T. Ascariasis and childhood malnutrition. *Trans R Soc Trop Med Hyg* 1992; 86:577–579.

44 Hall A. Intestinal parasitic worms and the growth of children. *Trans R Soc Trop Med Hyg* 1993; 87:241–242.

45 Thein H Laing. The effect of targeted chemotherapy against ascariasis on the height of children in rural Myamar. *Trans R Soc Trop Med Hyg* 1994; 88:433.

46 Brophy P M & Pritchard D I. Immunity to helminths: ready to tip the biochemical balance? *Parasite Immunology* 1992; 8:419–422.

47 Woodhouse M E J. A theoretical framework for the immunoepidemiology of helminth infection. *Parasite Immunology* 1992; 14:563–578.

48 Bundy D A P. Immunoepidemiology of intestinal helminthic injections; 1. The global burden of intestinal nematode disease. *Trans R Soc Trop Med Hyg* 1994; 88:259–261.

49 Needham C S & Lillywhite J E. Immunoepidemiology of intestinal helminthic injections; 2. Immunological correlates with patterns of *Trichuris* infection. *Trans R Soc Trop Med Hyg* 1994; 88:262–264.

50 MacDonald T T et al. Immunoepidemiology of intestinal helminthic injections; 3. Mucosal monophases and cybolline production in the colon of children with *Trichuris trichiura* dysentery. *Trans R Soc Trop Med Hyg* 1994; 88:265.

51 Beaver P C, Synder C H, Carrera G M et al. Chronic eosinophilia due to visceral larva migrans: report of 3 cases. *Pediatrics* 1952; 9:7–19.

52 Wilder H C. Nematode endophthalmitis. *Trans Am Acad Ophthalmol* 1950; 55:99–109.

53 Ree G H, Voller A & Rowland H A K. Toxocariasis in the British Isles 1982–3. *BMJ* 1984; 288: 628–629.

54 Dent J H, Nichols R L, Beaver P C et al. Visceral larva migrans with case report. *Am J Pathol* 1956; 32:777–803.

55 Beaver P C. The nature of visceral larva migrans. *J Parasitol* 1969; 55:3–12.

56 Woodruff A W. Toxocariasis. *BMJ* 1970; 3:663–669.

57 Biglan A W, Glickman L T & Lobes L A Jr. Serum and vitreous *Toxocara* antibody in nematode ophthalmitis. *Am J Ophthalmol* 1979; 88:898–901.

58 Wang C, Huang C Y, Chang P H et al. Transverse myelitis associated with larva migrans: finding of larva in cerebrospinal fluid. *Lancet* 1983; i: 423 (letter).

59 Bisseru B & Woodruff A W. The detection of circulating antibody in human toxocara infection using the indirect fluorescent antibody test. *J Clin Pathol* 1968; 21:449–455.

60 Savigny D H, Voller A & Woodruff A W. Toxocariasis: serological diagnosis by enzyme immunoassay. *J Clin Pathol* 1979; 32:284–288.

61 Glickman L T, Schanz P M, Dombroske R et al. Evaluation of serodiagnostic tests for visceral larva migrans. *Am J Trop Med Hyg* 1978; 27:492–498.

62 Brunello F, Genchi C & Falangiani P. Detection of larva-specific IgE in human toxocariasis. *Trans R Soc Trop Med Hyg* 1983; 77:279–280.

63 Woodruff A W, Bisseru B & Bowe J C. Infection with animal helminths as a factor in causing poliomyelitis and epilepsy. *BMJ* 1966; 1:1576–1579.

64 Botero D & Little M D. Two cases of Lagochilascaris infection in Colombia. *Am J Trop Med Hyg* 1984; 33:381–386.

65 Faust E C & Russell P F. *Craig & Faust Clinical Parasitology*, 7th edn. Philadelphia: Lea & Febiger, 1964.

66 Manter H W. Some aspects of the geographical distribution of parasites. *J. Parasitol* 1967; 53:3–9.

67 Schad G A, Murrell K D, Fayer R et al. Paratenesis in *Ancylostoma duodenale* suggests possible meat-bone human infection. *Trans R Trop Med Hyg* 1984; 78:203–204.

68 Schad G A, Chowdhury A B, Dean C G et al. Arrested development in human hookworm infections: an adaptation to a seasonally unfavourable external environment. *Science* 1973; 180:52–54.

69 Setasuban P, Punsri P & Muennoo C. Transmammary transmission of *Necator americanus* lava in the human host. *Southeast Asian J Trop Med Public Health* 1980; 11:535–538.

70 Roche H & Layrisse M. The nature and causes of 'hookworm anaemia'. *Am J Trop Med Hyg* 1966; 15:1031–1102.

71 Pritchard D I, Quinnell R J, Moustafa M et al. Hookworm (*Necator americanus*) infection and storage iron depletion. *Trans R Soc Trop Med Hyg* 1991; 85:235–238.

72 Brumpt L C & Ho-Thi-Sang. Pathogénie des oedémes de l'anémie ankylostomique et leur guérison par le traitement vermifuge. *Bull Soc Pathol Exot* 1955; 48:46–50.

73 Sheehy T W, Meroney W H, Cox R S et al. Hookworm disease and malabsorption. *Gastroenterology* 1962; 42:148–156.

74 Burman N N, Sehgal A K, Chakravarti R N et al. Morphological and absorption studies of small intestine in hookworm infestation (ankylostomiasis). *Indian J Med Res* 1970; 58:317–325.

75 Gilles H M, Watson-Williams E J & Ball P A J. Hookworm infection and anaemia. An

epidemiological, clinical and laboratory study. *Q J Med* 1964; 33:1–24.

76 Ball P A J & Bartlett A. Serological reactions to infections with *Necator americanus*. *Trans R Soc Trop Med Hyg* 1969; 63:362–369.

77 De Hurtado I & Layrisse M. Epidemiologic role of skin hypersensitivity in hookworm disease. *Am J Trop Med Hyg* 1968; 17:72–78.

78 Carroll S M & Grove D I. Resistance of dogs to re-infection with *Ancylostoma ceylanicum* following anthelmintic therapy. *Trans R Soc Trop Med Hyg* 1985; 79:519–523.

79 Pritchard D I, McKean P G & Schad G A. An immunological and biochemical comparison of hookworm species. *Parasitol Today* 1990; 6:154–156.

80 Behnke J M. Immunology. In Gilles H M & Ball P A J (eds) *Hookworm Infections*. Amsterdam: Elsevier, 1991:93–155.

81 Wang Chang-i. Parasitic diarrhoeas in China. *Parasitol Today* 1988; 10:284–287.

82 Rowland H A K. Dyspepsia, duodenitis and hookworm infection. *Trans R Soc Trop Med Hyg* 1966; 60:481–485.

83 Cline B L, Little M D, Bartholomew R K et al. Larvicidal activity of albendazole against *Necator americanus* in human volunteers. *Am J Trop Med Hyg* 1984; 33:387–394.

84 Little M D. Dermatitis in a human volunteer infected with *Strongyloides* of nutria and racoon. *Am J Trop Med Hyg* 1965; 14:1007–1009.

85 Miller M J & Maynard G R. 'Creeping eruption' treated by thiabendazole. *J Can Med Assoc* 1967; 97:860–861.

86 Katz R, Ziegler J & Blank H. The natural course of creeping eruption and treatment with thiabendazole. *Arch Dermatol* 1965; 91:420–424.

87 London I D. The treatment of creeping eruption with thiabendazole: report of 23 cases . *South Med J* 1965; 58:1026–1028.

88 Harland P S E G, Meakins R H & Harland R H. Treatment of cutaneous larva migrans with local thiabendazole. *BMJ* 1977; ii:772 (letter).

89 Caumes E et al. A randomised trial of ivermectin versus albendazole for the treatment of cutaneous larva migrans. *Am J Trop Med Hyg* 1993; 49:641–644.

90 O'Brien W. Intestinal malabsorption in acute infection with *Strongyloides stercoralis*. *Trans R Soc Trop Med Hyg* 1975; 60:69–77.

91 Laudanna A A, Polack M, Betarello A et al. Evidence of protein-losing enteropathy in strongyloidiasis. *Rev Inst Med Trop Sâo Paulo* 1973; 15:222–226.

92 Bras G, Richards R C, Irvine R A et al. Infection with *Strongyloides stercoralis* in Jamaica. *Lancet* 1964; ii:1257–1260.

93 Rogers W A Jr & Nelson B. Strongyloidiasis and malignant lymphoma. 'Opportunistic infection' by a nematode. *JAMA* 1966; 195:685–687.

94 Wilson S & Thompson A E. A fatal case of strongyloidiasis. *J Pathol Bacteriol* 1964; 87: 169–176.

95 Wilson S & Thompson A E. A fatal case of strongyloidiasis with *Strongyloides* larvae in the meninges. *Trans R Soc Trop Med Hyg* 1975; 70:497–499.

96 Ali-Khan Z & Seemayer T A. Fatal bowel infarction and sepsis: an unusual complication of systemic strongyloidiasis. *Trans R Soc Trop Med Hyg* 1975; 69:473.

97 Cook G C. *Strongyloides stercoralis* hyperinfection syndrome: how often is it missed? *Q J Med* 1987; 64:625–629.

98 Genta R M. Global prevalence of strongyloidiasis: critical review with epidemiologic insights into the prevention of disseminated disease. *Rev Infect Dis* 1989; 11:755–767.

99 Koga K, Kasura S, Khamboomuang C et al. A modified agar plate method for detection of *Strongyloides stercoralis*. *Am J Trop Med Hyg* 1991; 45:518–521.

100 Louisey C L & Barton C J. The radiological diagnosis of *Strongyloides stercoralis* enteritis. *Radiology* 1971; 98:535–541.

101 Convey et al. Serum IgG reactivity with 41-, 31- and 28-KDa larval proteins of *Strongyloides stercoralis* in individuals with strongyloides. *J Inf Diseases* 1993; 168:784–787.

102 Girud de Kaminsky R. Evaluation of three methods for laboratory diagnosis of *Strongyloides stercoralis* infection. *J Parasitology* 1993; 79:277–280.

103 Gill G V & Bell D R. *Strongyloides stercoralis* infection in former Far East prisoners of war. *BMJ* 1979; ii:572–574.

104 Gam A A, Neva F A & Krotoski W A. Comparative sensitivity and specificity of ELISA and IHA for serodiagnosis of strongyloidiasis with larval antigens. *Am J Trop Med Hyg* 1987; 37:157–161.

105 Sato Y, Toma H, Kiyuna S & Shiroma Y. Gelatin particle indirect agglutination test for mass examination for strongyloidiasis. *Trans R Soc Trop Med Hyg* 1991; 85:515–518.

106 Cahill K M. Thiabendazole in massive strongyloidiasis. *Am J Trop Med Hyg* 1967; 16:451–453.

107 Datry A et al. Treatment of *Strongyloides stercoralis* infection with invermeotin compared with albendazole: results of an open study of 60 cases. *Trans R Soc Trop Med Hyg* 1994; 88:344–345.

108 Pampiglione S & Riccardi M. The presence of *Strongyloides fülleborni* von Linstow, 1905 in man in Central and East Africa. *Parassitologia* 1971; 13:257–269.

109 Ashfad R W, Basnish G & Viney M E. *Strongyloides fuellebovni kelli*: Infection and disease in Papua New Guinea. *Parasitology Today* 1992; 8:314–318.

110 Bundy D A P, Chandiwana S K, Homeida M M A

et al. The epidemiology implications of a multiple-infection approach to the control of human helminth infections. *Trans R Soc Trop Med Hyg* 1991; 85:274–276.

111 Wimblad V & Kilama W. *Sanitation Without Water*. London: Macmillan for the Swedish International Development Agency, 1985.

112 Cairncross S. Small scale sanitation. *Ross Inst Trop Hyg Bull* 1989; 8:60.

113 Bradley M, Chandivana S K & Bundy D A P. The epidemiology and control of hookworm infection in the Burma Valley area of Zimbabwe. *Trans R Soc Trop Med Hyg* 1993; 87:145–147.

114 Bundy D A P, Wong M S, Louis L L & Horton J. Control of geohelminths by delivery of targeted chemotherapy through schools. *Trans R Soc Trop Med Hyg* 1990; 84:115–120.

115 Cook G C. Anthelmintic agents: some recent developments and their clinical application. *Postgrad Med J* 1991; 67:16–22.

116 Karbwang J & Harinasuta T. *Handbook of Antiparasitic Drugs*. Bangkok: SEAMED-TROP MED, 1992.

117 James D B & Gilles H M. *Human Antiparasitic Drugs. Pharmacology and Usage*. Chichester: Wiley, 1985.

118 Albonico M et al. A randomised control trial comparing mebendazole and albendazole against ascariasis, trichuris and hookworm infections. *Trans R Soc Trop Med Hyg* 1994; 88:585–589.

119 Flockhart H A, Harrison S E, Robinson A R et al. Enzyme polymorphism in *Trichinella*. *Trans R Soc Trop Med Hyg* 1982; 76:541–554.

120 Larsh J E Jr. The present understanding of the mechanism of immunity of *Trichinella spiralis*. *Am J Trop Med Hyg* 1967; 16:123–132.

121 Spink W W. Cardiovascular complications of trichinosis. *Arch Intern Med* 1935; 56:238–249.

122 Hennekeuser H H, Pabst K, Poeplau W et al. Zur klinik und Therapie der Trichinose. Boebachtung an 47 Patienten während einer Epidemie. *Dtsch Med Wochenschr* 1968; 93:867–873.

123 Melcher L R. Antigenic analysis of *Trichinella spiralis*. *J Infect Dis* 1943; 71:31–39.

124 Anderson R I, Sadun E H & Schoenbeckler M J. Cholesterol–lecithin slide (TsSF) and charcoal card (TsCC) flocculation tests using an acid soluble fraction of *Trichinella spiralis* larvae. *J Parasitol* 1963; 49:642–647.

125 Kagan I G. Trichinosis: a review of biologic, serologic and immunologic aspects. *J Infect Dis* 1960; 197:65–93.

126 Nishiyama T, Araki T, Mizieno N et al. Detection of circulating antigens in human trichinellosis. *Trans R Soc Trop Med Hyg* 1992; 86:292–293.

127 Levin M L. Treatment of trichinosis with mebendazole. *Am J Trop Med Hyg* 1983; 32:980–983.

128 Dauer C C & Davids D G. 1958 summary of disease outbreaks. *Public Health Rep Wash* 1959; 74:715–720.

129 Link V B. Trichinosis: a health and economic problem. *Public Health Rep Wash* 1953; 68:417–418.

130 Rausch R. Animal-borne diseases. *Public Health Rep Wash* 1953; 68:533–534.

131 Maynard J E & Pauls E P. Trichinosis in Alaska. A review and report of two outbreaks due to bear meat with observations on serodiagnosis and skin testing. *Am J Hyg* 1962; 76: 252–261.

132 Forrester A T T, Nelson G S & Sander G. The first record of an outbreak of trichinosis in Africa and south of the Sahara. *Trans R Soc Trop Med Hyg* 1961; 33:503–513.

133 Kagan I G. Trichinosis in the United States. *US Public Health Rep* 1959; 74:159–162.

CHAPTER 72

SCHISTOSOMIASIS

Andrew Davis

The term human schistosomiasis indicates a complex of acute and chronic parasitic infections caused by mammalian blood flukes (*Schistosoma*). These infections are transmitted by specific aquatic or amphibious snails in a wide variety of freshwater habitats.

The various species of the genus *Schistosoma* are members of the family Schistosomatidae, dioecious digenean parasites whose habitat is the blood–vascular system of vertebrates. The family is divided into three subfamilies, the Schistosomatinae, Bilharziellinae and Gigantobilhaziinae and contains 12 genera, of which several are confined to birds and five to mammals; only *Schistosoma* is associated with man.

A general feature of the family is that the female is longer and more slender than the male and is normally carried in a ventral groove, the gynaecophoric canal, formed by ventrally flexed lateral outgrowths of the male body. Of all the mammalian blood flukes, the genus *Schistosoma* has achieved the greatest geographical distribution and diversification.[1]

Of the 16 species of schistosomes known to infect man or animals, only five are responsible for the overwhelming proportion of human infections: *Schistosoma haematobium, S. intercalatum, S. mansoni, S. japonicum* and *S. mekongi*. Rarely other zoophilic species or hybrids may be found in man.[2]

The five principal species infecting man are subdivided into three groups characterized by the size and appearance of the eggs produced by the female schistosome:

- Eggs with a terminal spine, *S. haematobium, S. intercalatum.*
- Eggs with a lateral spine, *S. mansoni.*
- Rounded or ovoid minutely spined eggs, *S. japonicum* and *S. mekongi.*[2]

HISTORY

S. HAEMATOBIUM

Chronic haematuria and various bladder disorders occurred in Egypt and Mesopotamia from the earliest times in association with the agricultural civilizations of the great river valleys. Haematuria was described in the Gynaecological Papyrus of Kahun, written in the mid-XIIth dynasty period, about 1900 BC. Many remedies for haematuria were recorded from the time of the Ebers Papyrus and it can be assumed that the condition was widespread.[3] Calcified ova of the parasite were demonstrated in the kidneys of two Egyptian mummies of the XXth dynasty (1250–1000 BC).[4] During the Napoleonic invasion of Egypt, 1799–1801, symptoms of the disease in troops were rife.[5] Yet it was not until 1851 that the causal agent (*Distoma haematobium*, now *Schistosoma haematobium*), a blood fluke, was found in a mesenteric vein during a postmortem examination at the Kasr el Aini hospital in Cairo by Theodor Bilharz.[6]

S. MANSONI

In 1902 Manson[7] found lateral-spined eggs in the faeces of a West Indian patient in London and postulated the existence of a second species of blood fluke. Subsequent controversy between A. Looss and L. W. Sambon, eminent scientists of the day, was resolved by the work of Leiper[8] at El Marg, a village in the present Qualyubia Governorate, just north of Cairo, in 1915, who established beyond doubt the existence of two distinct species of schistosome and the presence of snail intermediate hosts belonging not only to two different genera but to two different subfamilies. In the New World eggs with a lateral spine were found in Bahia (Brazil) in 1904 and described in 1908[9] and in Venezuela in 1906.[10]

S. JAPONICUM

In 1847, the clinical entities 'Kabure itch' and 'Katayama syndrome' were described in a village in Hiroshima Prefecture in Japan,[11] whilst in 1904 Katsurada[12] recovered worms from the portal system of a cat and named the species *Schistosomum japonicum*. From 1909 to 1915 the biology of this parasite, its life cycle and the pathology it caused were elucidated and described by Japanese and other investigators.[13–16]

The infection was recognized clinically in both China[17] and the Philippines in the early years of the twentieth century[18] and in Sulawesi, Celebes in the 1930s.[19]

In China the *Oncomelania* intermediate hosts were discovered in 1924[20] and in the Philippines in 1932.[21]

S. INTERCALATUM

Suspicion arose in 1923 that, since some cases of human 'intestinal' schistosomiasis in the Yakusu area near Kisangani in present-day Zaire showed an atypical clinical picture and possessed an unusual egg morphology, a species distinct from *S. haematobium* was involved.[22] Follow-up of this work led to a description in 1934 of a new species, *S. intercalatum*, of which the snail intermediate host was a member of the *Bulinus africanus* group.[23]

S. MEKONGI

Described initially in 1978,[24] the parasite causes human schistosomiasis in an, as yet, restricted area in Laos and Kampuchea (Cambodia).

The intermediate host, *Tricula aperta*, is aquatic and is not susceptible to strains of *S. japonicum*.[25] A monograph provides the most authoritative account of the species to date.[26]

GEOGRAPHICAL ASPECTS (Figures 72.1 and 72.2)

S. haematobium is endemic in 52 countries of the Old World; on the African continent, in the Eastern Mediterranean including the Arabian peninsula; on many of the Indian Ocean islands and in Western Asia.[27] In India, a focus of urinary schistosomiasis was described at Gimvi, in the Ratnagiri district, Maharashtra State.[28] A re-examination in 1981 was confirmatory[29] but a combined Indian Government/World Health Organization (WHO)/World Bank mission in 1985 found only two persons infected in 352 examined using Nuclepore filtration of urine. The presumed intermediate host, a freshwater limpet, *Ferrissia tenuis* was found in all water bodies of major human water contact.[30]

S. mansoni infection occurs in 53 countries ranging from the Arabian peninsula, numerous countries in the African continent, particularly the Nile valley neighbours, Sudan and Egypt, to the New World: Brazil, Surinam, Venezuela and seven islands in the Caribbean.[27]

In 40 countries, double infections with *S. mansoni* and *S. haematobium* are endemic.[27]

S. japonicum infection in man is found only in mainland China, Indonesia (Lindu lake valley and the Napu valley in Central Sulawesi) and the Philippines. There is no evidence of recent transmission in Japan and Thailand. A parasite resembling *S. japonicum* (*S. malayensis*), transmitted by *Robertsiella kaporensis*, has been found in man[31] in Pahang State, Malaysia. Wild rats are the only known natural host and it is thought that man is not an important host for this parasite.

S. intercalatum has been reported from seven countries of Central and West Africa.[27]

S. mekongi is endemic on Khong Island, Lao People's Democratic Republic and in some areas of Democratic Kampuchea.[27]

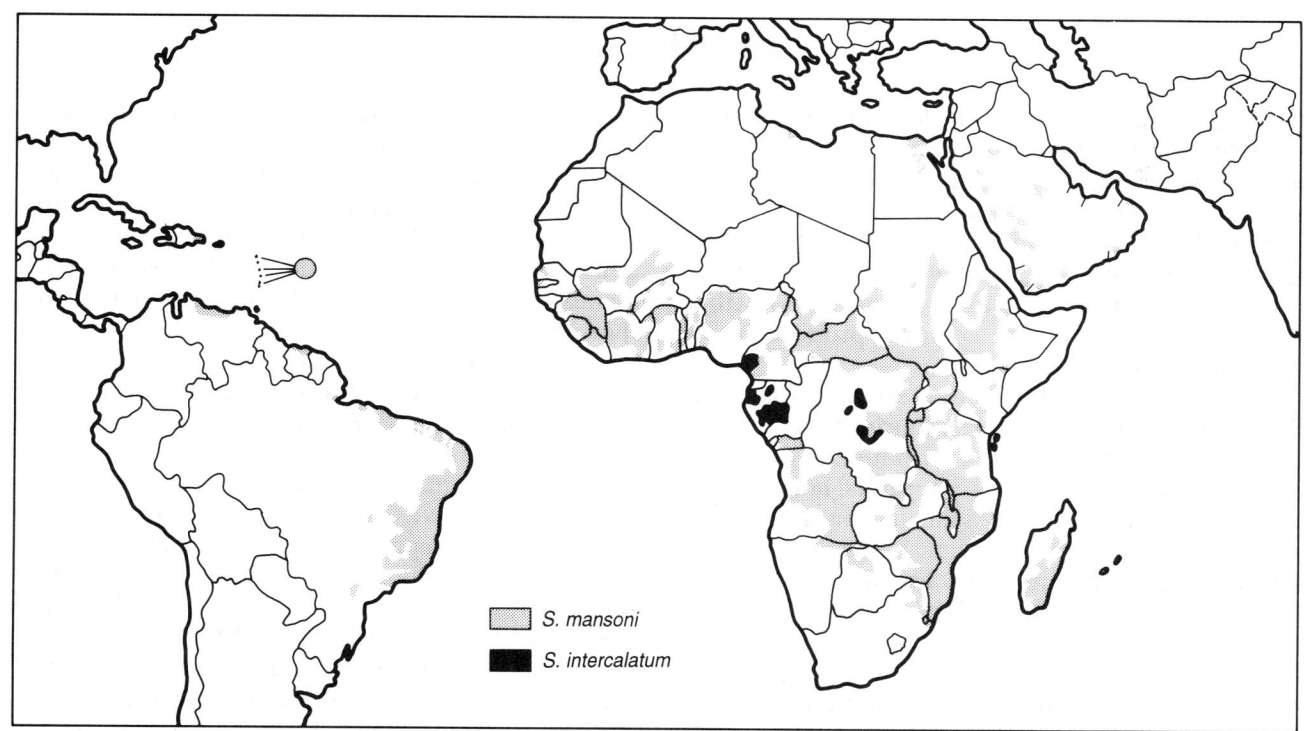

Figure 72.1   Global distribution of schistosomiasis due to *Schistosoma mansoni* and *S. intercalatum*, 1985.

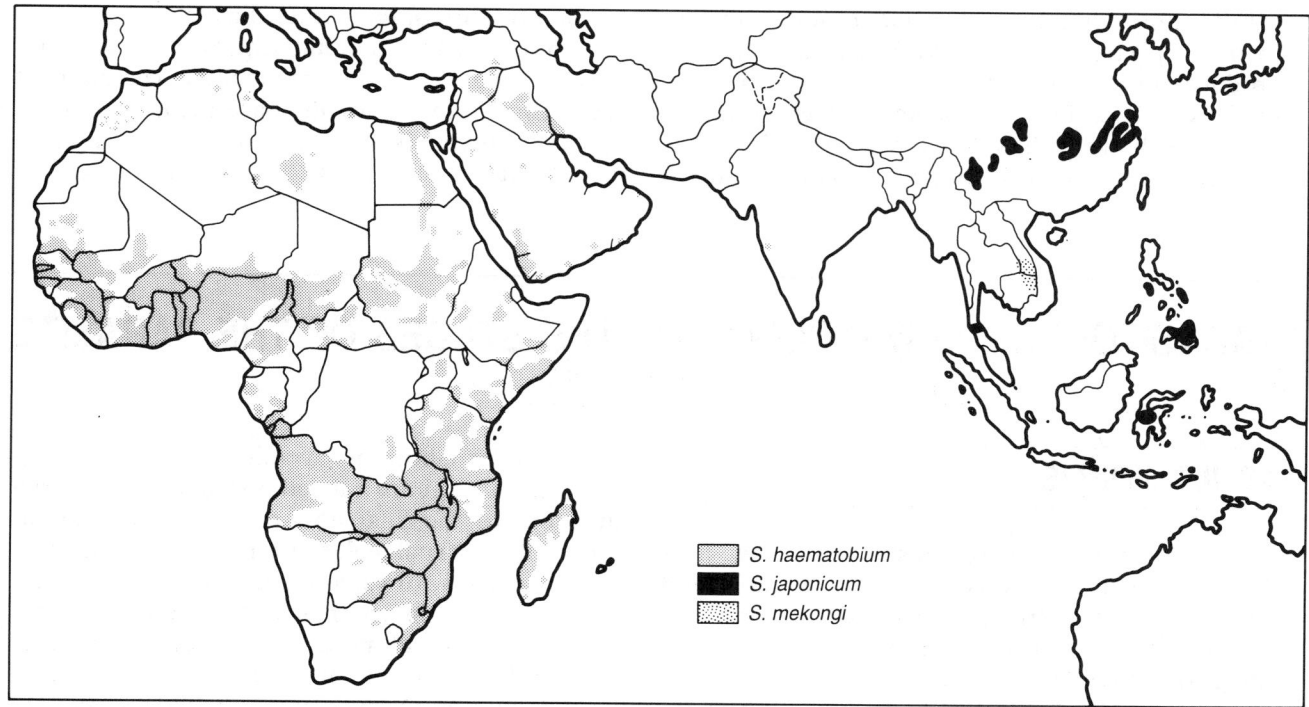

Figure 72.2   Global distribution of schistosomiasis due to *Schistosomiasis haematobium* and *S. japonicum*, 1985.

AETIOLOGY

Of the five species of the genus *Schistosoma* responsible for most human infections, *S. mansoni*, *S. japonicum* and *S. mekongi* inhabit the pericolonic venules within the distribution of the portal venous system. The eggs of *S. mansoni* are characterized by a laterally placed spine; those of *S. japonicum* and *S. mekongi* are smaller and are round or ovoid with a rudimentary spine. All these species produce 'intestinal' or 'rectal' schistosomiasis.

S. haematobium inhabits the terminal venules in the wall of the bladder, the genitourinary system and the pelvic plexus within the distribution of the inferior vena cava; its eggs have a terminal spine and it causes 'urinary' or 'vesical' schistosomiasis.[32]

Neither *S. haematobium* nor *S. mansoni* are restricted exclusively in their anatomical vascular habitats within the distributions respectively of the inferior vena caval or the portal venous systems. *S. haematobium* can exist in the perirectal venules and its eggs are found in the stools, although almost invariably they are dead. *S. mansoni* may live in the pelvic plexus and its eggs can be detected in urine ('Mansonuria'), although this is an uncommon finding during epidemiological surveys.

Much less is known on human infection with *S. intercalatum* than is the case with the other species. Two geographical strains ('Cameroon' and 'Zaire') have been described,[33,34] each with distinct and different intermediate snail hosts and patterns of egg distribution within the host. *S. intercalatum* appears to be a species distinct from *S. haematobium*; it produces terminal-spined eggs of characteristic morphology and the clinical syndrome of infection is that of a lower bowel colitis, i.e. lower abdominal pain with either dysentery or diarrhoea. This should be qualified with the reminder that many cases are asymptomatic. Its geographical distribution is restricted to Central and West Africa. Natural hybridization between *S. intercalatum* and *S. haematobium* has been described.[35–37] Experimentally, hybridization between *S. mansoni* and *S. intercalatum* in a monkey (*Erythrocebus patas*) from Nigeria has been reported.[38]

S. mekongi is, as yet, confined to Laos and Kampuchea (Cambodia), is transmitted by an aquatic intermediate host, *Tricula aperta*, and is also found in dogs.

Infrequently, man is infected by schistosomes which normally live in other mammalian hosts,[32] e.g. *S. bovis*, a member of the *S. haematobium* complex and a common parasite in cattle and sheep; *S. mattheei*, which has multiple hosts in both domestic and wild animals in Southern Africa; *S. margrebowiei*, a parasite frequent in antelopes in Central Africa. Such infections in humans are seldom of pathological significance but suggestions have been advanced that they may confer a relative type of immunity (heterologous immunity) against *S. mansoni* and *S. haematobium* infections in areas where all species coexist.[39,40]

The cercariae of certain avian blood flukes, *Trichobilharzia*, *Gigantobilharzia* and *Ornithobilharzia*, may penetrate human skin producing cercarial dermatitis of 'swimmer's itch'. Outbreaks may occur in either tropical or temperate climates but development of cercariae into adult schistosomes does not occur in man. Even less frequently, cercariae of adult schistosomes normally parasitic in mammals, e.g. *S. douthitti* from rodents and *S. spindale* from water buffaloes, may cause a similar syndrome.

PARASITOLOGY AND BIOLOGY OF THE STAGES OF THE PARASITE
(Table 72.1)

ADULT WORMS

In nature, a population of schistosomes in the final definitive host usually comprises both male and female worms (Figure 72.3). Since the genus *Schistosoma* differs from most digenetic trematodes in being dioecious, a consequence of heteromorphic chromosomes in the ovum,[41] a population could conceivably be unisexual (male or female worms only). Under laboratory conditions, single miracidial snail infections carried through to cercarial infections of the final host result in either populations of unisexual males or unisexual females.[42]

Adult worms, of separate sex, are small, with a species variation in length of 6–28mm and in breadth of 0.25–1 mm. In all species the outer integument of the female is smooth, while that of the male *S. haematobium* and *S. mansoni* is covered with minute spines or tubercles. The outer surface of the male *S.*

Table 72.1 Comparison of principal features of *Schistosoma* spp. infecting man.

Item	S. japonicum	S. mekongi*	S. mansoni	S. haematobium	S. intercalatum
Adult worms					
Location of adult in host	Mesenteric veins	Mesenteric veins	Mesenteric veins	Vesical plexus	Mesenteric veins
Length of posterior gut caecum	Medium	Medium	Very long	Short	Short
Male					
Length (mm)	10–20	~15	6–13	10–15	11–14
Width (mm)	0.55	0.41	1.10	0.90	0.3–0.4
No. of testes	6–7	6–7	4–13 (6–9)†	4–5	2–7 (4–5)†
Tubercles	Absent	Absent?	Coarse	Fine	Fine
Female					
Length (mm)	20–30	~12	10–20	16–26	10–14
Width (mm)	0.30	0.23	0.16	0.25	0.15–0.18
Ovary: Position in body	Middle	Rear half	Front third	Rear third	Rear half
Uterus: Position in body	Front half	Front half	Front half	Front two-thirds	Front two-thirds
Length	Short	Short	Very short	Long	Long
Number of eggs	50–200	10+	1–2	10–50	5–60
Mature egg					
Shape	Round	Round	Ovoid	Ovoid	Ovoid
Size (μm)	60 × 100	57 × 66	61 × 140	62 × 150	61 × 176
Spine	Lateral (reduced)	Lateral (reduced)	Lateral (prominent)	Terminal (prominent)	Terminal (prominent)
Normally passed in	Faeces	Faeces	Faeces	Urine	Faeces (and urine)
Eggs per female per day	3500	?	100–300	20–300	150–400
Reaction of egg shell to Ziehl–Neelson stain‡	+ve	?	+ve	−ve	+ve
Intermediate host snail	*Oncomelania*	*Tricula*	*Biomphalaria*	*Bulinus*	*Bulinus*

*From experimental animal infections.   †Usual range.   ‡In histological sections.
Courtesy of R. F. Sturrock, Department of Medical Parasitology, London School of Hygiene and Tropical Medicine.
Reproduced with permission from Jordan P, Webbe G & Sturrock R F (eds) *Human Schistosomiasis*. Wallingford: CAB International, 1993.

japonicum is non-tuberculated.[32] The tegument of the adult parasite, derived from that of the penetrating infective cercarial stage, has unusual structural features, of great significance in the ability of the fluke to withstand immunological attacks by the host.[42]

Adult worms possess an oral sucker opening into the alimentary tract, and a more posteriorly situated ventral sucker used for attachment to the endothelium of blood vessels. In the male, a distinctive large ventral groove, the gynaecophoric canal, encloses the female during pairing.

The digestive system consists of a short oesophagus opening into an intestine that divides anterior to the ventral sucker and reunites behind the gonads as a blind posterior gut caecum.[43] The black gut contents contain haematin derived from ingested blood.

The excretory system consists of flame cells, collecting tubules and an excretory bladder with a terminal pore.

The male reproductive system comprises four or five pairs of dorsally situated testes opening to the exterior through a vas deferens and seminal vesicle through an infolded cirrus.[42]

In females the reproductive system consists of a pear-shaped ovary in the mid-body line from which the oviduct runs anteriorly to join the common reproductive duct formed after fusion with a vitelline duct. The common duct enters the ootype which in turn opens into the uterus which eventually opens to the exterior just below the ventral sucker.[42]

The life span of the adult worm in humans is not known accurately. In the past, stress was laid on evidence of longevity with periods quoted ranging from 18 to 28 years[44] to more than 30 years.[45] Since the 1970s, epidemiological studies of the egg outputs of groups of infected people, in the absence of

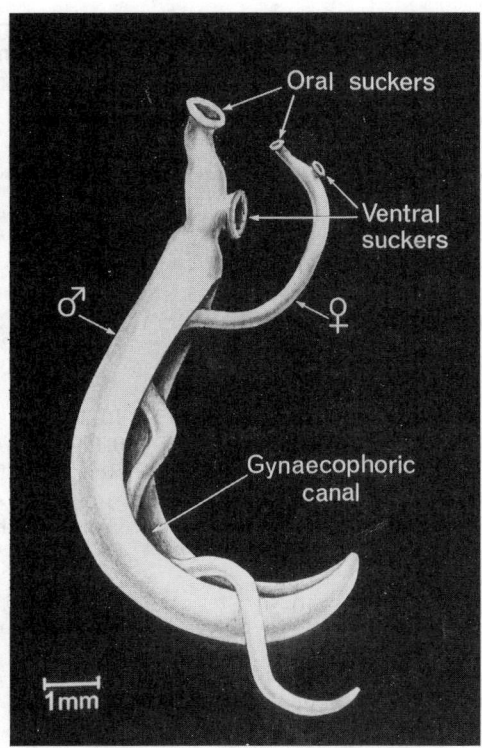

Figure 72.3   Male and female schistosomes. (Courtesy of WTIM.)

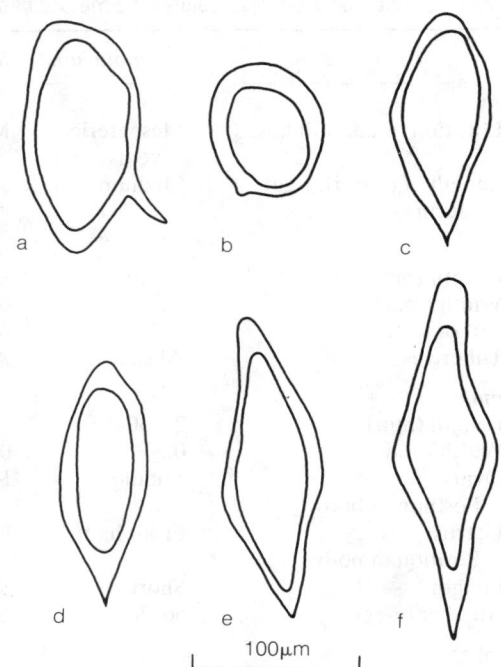

Figure 72.4   Eggs of *Schistosoma* spp. (a) *S. mansoni*; (b) *S. japonicum*; (c) *S. haematobium*; (d) *S. intercalatum*; (e) *S. mattheei*; (f) *S. bovis*.

treatment or in the absence of reinfection after successful treatment, have suggested that a proportion of children, in particular, cease to pass eggs in the excreta within a relatively short time. This has been interpreted as indicative of the mortality of established worm burdens and has led to the popular (but not necessarily correct) current concept of the mean length of life of the female schistosome being of the order of 3–8 years.[46]

Detailed reviews of the somewhat fragmentary knowledge of the physiology, biochemistry, genetic constitution and molecular biology are given in specialist publications.[47,48]

EGGS

A general description of egg morphology is given in the section on Aetiology; their microscopic appearance is diagnostic of the parent schistosome species (Figure 72.4) and they are laid by fertilized female schistosomes intravascularly towards the periphery of the capillary venules. Eggs are non-operculate, possess a spine, and contain an embryo, the miracidium, which develops within the egg within a period of some 16 days. As a rough generalization it is supposed that approximately 50% of eggs pass

through the walls of the bladder, the genitourinary apparatus or the colon to be excreted in urine or faeces and the remainder are retained within the tissues. The latter die about 21 days after oviposition. Excreted eggs usually contain embryos seen to be viable by observation of flame cell, ciliary or whole body movement on microscopy. In a suitable environment of fresh water and warmth (10–30°C), the embryos (miracidia) hatch and leave the egg through slits induced partly by their own activity and partly by osmotic effects.

An adult *S. haematobium* female produces 20–200 terminal spined eggs per day, *S. mansoni* produces 100–300 or more lateral spined eggs per female per day and *S. japonicum* produces 500–3500 ovoid eggs with a rudimentary lateral 'knob' per female per day.[2] The fecundity of *S. intercalatum* (another terminal spined species) and *S. mekongi* (ovoid eggs with a rudimentary lateral spine) is unknown.[2]

MIRACIDIA

Although miracidia of different species differ in size, they have similar morphological features and behavioural patterns. Details are given in specialist texts.[49]

On hatching from an egg in appropriate conditions, miracidia swim actively (at 2 mm/s), have behavioural patterns similar to those of the molluscan intermediate hosts and are infective to snails for 8–12 hours.

INTRAMOLLUSCAN DEVELOPMENT

There appear to be two main mechanisms by which miracidia locate the intermediate snail host: miracidial responses to the main physical responses present in the environment and their response to chemical stimuli originating from snail hosts. The considerable amount of published experimental work on these topics is reviewed in specialist texts.[43,49]

After contact, miracidia penetrate the body surface of the snail through a secretion from the apical gland cells; penetration is initiated by the papilla, the miracidial boring movement probably being assisted by lytic enzymes secreted from the gut.[43] Penetration occurs via the foot of the snail in 70%, other points of entry being either the tentacle or the edge of the mantle.[49] In *S. japonicum* penetration points are found over the whole of the cephalopedal area.[49]

After penetration, the ciliated surface of the miracidium disappears and, in an appropriate species of snail, a mother sporocyst develops near the entry site. If the snail is not a potential host, miracidia are destroyed by phagocytic action. Only a small proportion of entering miracidia develop to mature mother sporocysts.

At 96 hours the mother sporocyst is an elongated sac filled with germinal cells and small centrally located vacuoles; at 8 days it has undergone further considerable growth. Germ cells are budded off from the epithelial lining; these develop into daughter sporocysts that migrate to other parts of the body of the snail, mainly through the loose connective tissue, to the digestive gland. Further germ ball production occurs, resulting in the final form of the larvae, the cercariae.

Due to this asexual multiplication process within mother and daughter sporocysts, thousands of cercariae are formed, all of the same sex, and all originating from a single miracidium.

A proportion of infected snails have a shortened life span or become sterile. Some exhibit self-cure and their egg laying returns to normal; some die.

From the time of miracidial penetration, production of mature cercariae occurs after 4–5 weeks in *S. mansoni* infection, 5–6 weeks in *S. haematobium* and 7 weeks or longer in *S. japonicum*. Numerous physical, environmental and biological factors account for these variations in time.[43]

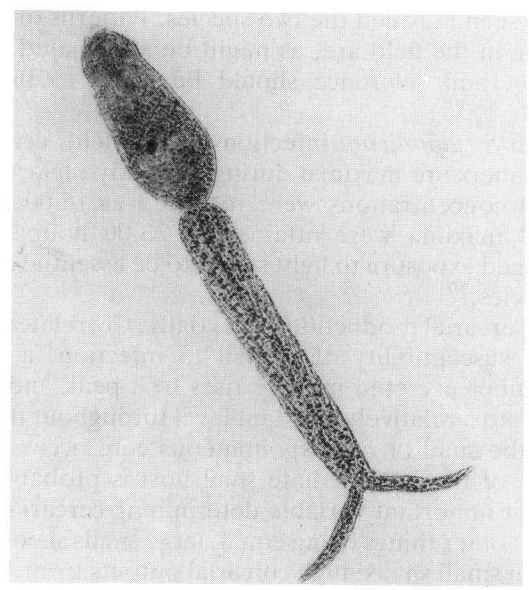

Figure 72.5   Schistosome cercaria. (Courtesy of O. D. Standen.)

CERCARIAE

All cercariae originating from one miracidium are of the same sex; when mature they emerge from the snail as a free-swimming stage adaptable to invasion of the definitive host (Figure 72.5).

Cercariae are furcocercous (brevifurcate), have no eye spots or pharynx, are less than 1 cm in length, have a muscular oral sucker occupying about one-third of the body and a small ventral sucker or acetabulum. Their trilaminar tegument is covered with minute spines and hairs; the digestive system has a mouth in the centre of the oral sucker, an oesophagus and a pair of dorsally-placed caeca; behind the oral sucker is a mass of nerve fibres from which three pairs of nerves emerge: the excretory system consists of flame cells, collecting tubules, an excretory bladder and one pair of protonephridia in the tail. Six pairs of cephalic glands subserve the emergence from the snail and penetration of the host skin, aided by enzymatic secretions which have an adhesive function as the cercariae move over the skin in host location.

CERCARIAL PRODUCTION

In *S. haematobium* and *S. mansoni* the main stimulus for the release of cercariae is light, usually at temperatures between 10 and 30°C. Cercariae can however be shed in small numbers in the dark. In the laboratory, marked differences in shedding patterns are seen between the two species. Patterns of shedding in the field are, as might be anticipated, variable, and reference should be made to biology texts.[43,49]

In *S. japonicum* infections in the field, cercarial numbers are maximal during the early night; minimal concentrations were recorded at 15.00 hours and maxima were attained at 23.00 hours. Prolonged exposure to light seems to be essential in this species.[50]

Cercarial production varies daily. Correlated with the susceptibility of a snail to infection, a small number excreted initially rises to a peak and then falls to a relatively constant level throughout the life of the snail or until spontaneous cure occurs. The size of the intermediate snail host is probably the most important variable determining cercarial output; other things being equal, large snails shed more than small snails; high cercarial outputs from *Biomphalaria glabrata* are common: 1000–3000 cercaria per day; African *Biomphalaria* spp. shed some 500 cercariae daily and rarely exceed 1500; among the larger *Bulinids*, similar numerical shedding occurs but rarely is 2000 cercariae per day exceeded.

In *S. japonicum* infections, the snail hosts are much smaller and estimates of natural shedding in *Oncomelania hupensis quadrasi* were as low as 15 per day although, under particular conditions, 160 per day were obtained.[50] In Japan, *O. h. nosophora* is thought to produce many more cercariae than *O. h. quadrasi*.

Cercarial life span is short: 36–48 hours. Since they are non-feeding organisms dependent on their large glycogen reserves, adverse environmental variables stimulating glycogen usage reduce cercarial viability.

Water velocity studies relating cercarial penetration and infection rates have produced anomalous results; patently most cercariae are infective to vertebrate hosts encountered under field conditions.

SCHISTOSOMULA

After cercariae penetrate human skin (or pharyngeal mucosa), a rapid process aided by lytic substances from the penetration glands, they lose their tails and become schistosomula. A remarkable additional transition is that from a 'fresh water environment' to a 'salt water environment' within the body.

Schistosomula are thus tailless and worm-like in appearance, shed the glycocalyx, and the skin becomes the seven-layered membrane of the adult worm, consisting of two closely opposed lipid bilayers.[49,51] They then traverse the subcutaneous tissues within 48 hours, penetrate the peripheral lymphatics or venous channels, are transported to the right side of the heart and lungs, where the peak concentration is attained in 5–7 days. Further development in length and surface area occur. Whilst controversy on the route of migration of schistosomula from the lungs to the hepatic portal system has existed for 60 years,[51] more recent evidence suggests that lung development adapts schistosomula for intravascular migration and subsequently the parasites exit the lungs in the direction of blood flow, pass to the left side of the heart, are then distributed to systemic organs in proportion to cardiac output, i.e. a totally intravascular route. Those parasites entering splanchnic organs penetrate capillary networks rapidly, enter the hepatic portal venous system and most are trapped in the liver. The parasites distributed to organs supplied by the systemic circulation eventually return to the lungs in venous blood.[51] This implies that individual organisms may make repeated circuits of the pulmonary–systemic circulation before entering a blood vessel leading to the hepatic portal system. On arrival in the hepatic portal system the majority of schistosomula begin to feed on blood, increase in mass and, from a primary location in the smallest hepatic portal distributaries, grow and move upstream into larger vessels.[51] The parasites shorten in dimension, experience a marked loss in motility and undergo various metabolic changes and, once schistosomula have transformed to adult worms in the liver, lose their ability to undertake intravascular migration.[52]

In experiments with *S. mansoni*, pairing occurred 28–35 days after infection. This was succeeded by migration of paired adults to egg-laying sites in the distribution of the mesenteric superior and inferior veins, or the veins of the vesical and pelvic plexus.

LIFE CYCLE

The life cycle of all species of schistosome infecting man has a common pathway from a sexual generation of adult schistosomes within the vascular system of the definitive host, an asexual phase in the freshwater intermediate snail host and a return to man via cercarial invasion of the skin or mucosa on a

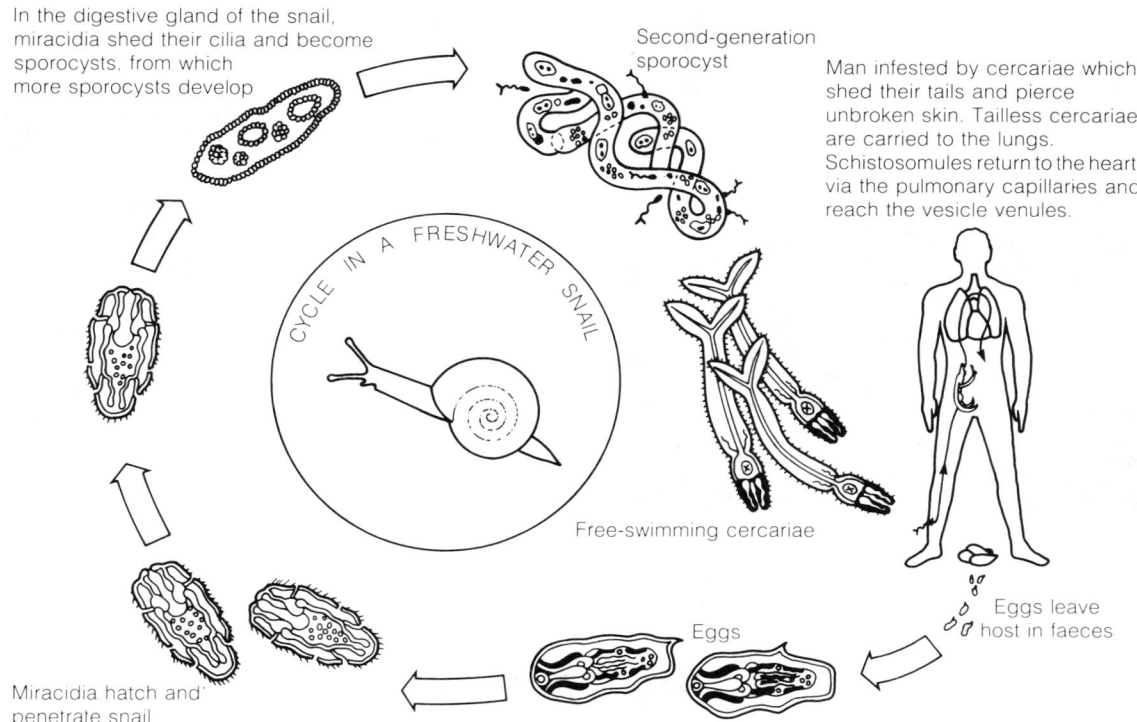

In the digestive gland of the snail, miracidia shed their cilia and become sporocysts, from which more sporocysts develop

Second-generation sporocyst

Man infested by cercariae which shed their tails and pierce unbroken skin. Tailless cercariae are carried to the lungs. Schistosomules return to the heart via the pulmonary capillaries and reach the vesicle venules.

CYCLE IN A FRESHWATER SNAIL

Free-swimming cercariae

Eggs leave host in faeces

Eggs

Miracidia hatch and penetrate snail

Figure 72.6   Life cycle of *S. mansoni*. (Courtesy of WTIM.)

host's exposure to cercarial infested fresh water (Figure 72.6).

Adult schistosomes, living as pairs within capillary blood vessels, the slender filiform females held in the gynaecophoric canal of the males, copulate and the females produce eggs daily throughout their life, the numbers varying with the species (see Aetiology).

Eggs, the microscopic appearance of which is diagnostic of the parent schistosome species, are laid intravascularly toward the peripheral branches of the capillary venules. Partly mature at oviposition, some eggs pass through the vessel wall, aided by their spine and cytolytic secretions, into the lumen of the genitourinary tract (*S. haematobium*) or the bowel (*S. mansoni*, *S. japonicum*, *S. mekongi*, *S. intercalatum*) and reach the external world in the excreta (urine and/or faeces). Other eggs, which are the immune-stimulating and pathogenic agents in the tissues, embolize from their intravascular origin to liver, lung and many other sites.

When viable schistosome eggs are excreted and reach fresh water, either by direct deposition or by being washed in from a neighbouring site, in a suitable environment of warmth and light, then the larvum within each egg becomes active and, aided by osmosis, the egg ruptures or 'hatches'; the larvum, now termed a miracidium, emerges. Miracidia are mobile organisms swimming actively by means of ciliary movements. Miracidial behaviour is related in

a general way to the ecology of the snail intermediate host and adaptive behavioural patterns have been described. During a short life span, miracidia are infective to snail intermediate hosts for some 8–12 hours, and must find a suitable freshwater snail for continuance of the life cycle; such snails (intermediate hosts) are specific for each species of schistosome.

Miracidia then penetrate the soft tissues of the snail, influenced by numerous variables, including chemotaxis, relative numbers of larvae and snails within a water body, length of contact time and physical characteristics of the surrounding medium, i.e. water temperature, velocity of flow, turbulence and the presence of ultraviolet light.

Usually, only one or two miracidia undergo further intramolluscan development, producing a sacculate mother sporocyst which in turn produces daughter sporocysts. This is followed by migration to the digestive gland of the snail and subsequent cercarial development.

After an incubation period within the snail, the time of which varies with the species and the surrounding physical environment, cercariae escape from the daughter sporocysts and emerge from the snail under suitable conditions of temperature, light and pH.

Free-swimming fork-tailed cercariae, about 1 mm in length, penetrate human skin or mucosa (Figure 72.7) when man is exposed to infested water and,

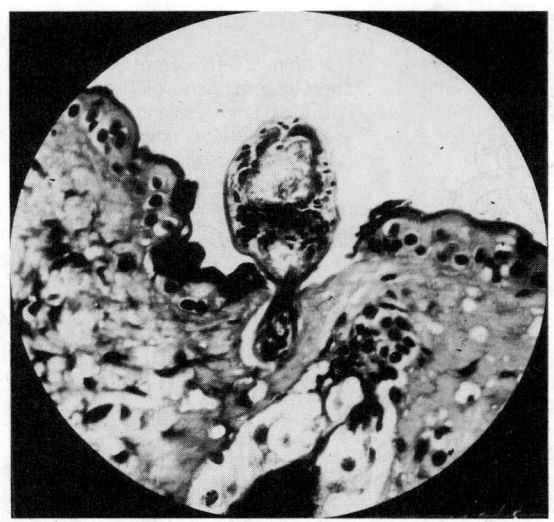

Figure 72.7   Cercarial penetration in schistosomiasis. (Courtesy of O. D. Standen).

after passage through the tissues as schistosomula, will develop into a male or female schistosome.

Throughout their long life snails continue to produce a reasonably constant output of cercariae; many thousands can originate from a single miracidium.

After migration of schistosomula to the portal vascular system, further growth occurs in the intrahepatic vessels. Pairing of male and female schistosome takes place on sexual maturity, with subsequent migration to the preferred sites of egg deposition: *S. mansoni* and *S. intercalatum* in the distribution of the inferior mesenteric veins; *S. japonicum* and *S. mekongi* in the distribution of the superior and inferior mesenteric veins; and *S. haematobium* in the distribution of the vesical veins and the pelvic plexus. Egg deposition begins and the cycle is complete.

INTERMEDIATE HOSTS

The biology of the snail intermediate hosts (Figures 72.8–72.10) of the schistosomes is a complex subject covered in numerous specialist texts to which reference should be made for specific details.[2,53–60]

The snail host range of schistosomes is comparatively limited. Successful parasitism of the approxi-

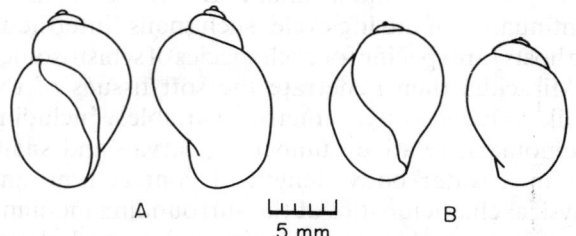

Figure 72.8   Snails of the *Bulinus* genus hosts of *S. haematobium*. A, *Bulinus truncatus* group. B, *B. africanus* group.

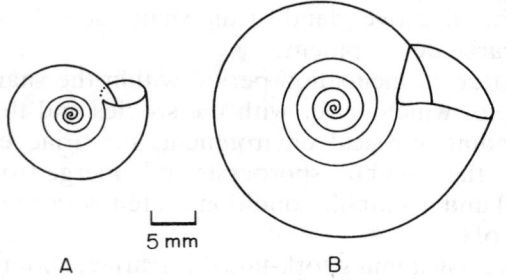

Figure 72.9   Snails of the *Biomphalaria* genus hosts of *S. mansoni*. A, *Biomphalaria alexandrina*. B, *B. glabrata*.

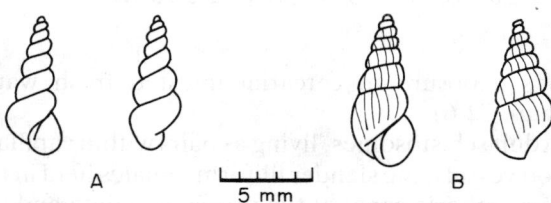

Figure 72.10   Snails of the *Oncomelania* genus host of *S. japonicum*. A, *Oncomelania hupensis nosophora*. B, *O. h. hupensis*.

mately 18 recognized species of schistosome depends on the ability of the parasite to develop in a small number of species of intermediate host within only ten genera.[58]

Although the schistosomes and their intermediate hosts can be divided roughly into groups reflecting their zoogeographical distribution and host specificity, the situation is complicated since the distribution of schistosomes does not exactly match that of the potential intermediate hosts.[58]

INTERMEDIATE HOSTS OF *S. HAEMATOBIUM*

S. haematobium is transmitted by some 30 nominal species of the genus *Bulinus*, classified into four species-groups: *Bulinus africanus*, an important group medically as species within the group are intermediate hosts of *S. haematobium* in Africa south of the Sahara and, additionally, some cattle schistosomes; the *B. forskalii* group is distributed in a pan-African fashion with representatives found in Arabia and in some Indian Ocean islands; the *B. truncatus/tropicus* complex, again of pan-African distribution, extends from Malawi to East, West and North Africa and the Middle East as far as Iran; a small group, *B. reticulatus*, is found patchily in Africa, e.g. in Ethiopia, and in isolated habitats in the Arabian peninsula.

INTERMEDIATE HOSTS OF *S. INTERCALATUM*

Of the two biologically distinct strains of *S. intercalatum* known to exist, one is transmitted by snails of the *Bulinus africanus* group and occurs in a restricted area in north-east Zaire; the other is transmitted by *B. forskalii* and occurs in Cameroon and Gabon. Each strain is unable to develop in a snail with which the other is compatible and, additionally, there are differences in prepatent periods and in certain enzyme patterns of the parasite.[2]

INTERMEDIATE HOSTS OF *S. MANSONI*

S. mansoni is transmitted by species of the genus *Biomphalaria*, widely distributed in the Old World throughout Africa, the Nile valley, the Arabian peninsula but not in Iraq or Iran. In the New World the genus is found in the southern USA, several Caribbean islands (notably Puerto Rico, St Lucia, Guadeloupe and the Dominican Republic) and on the South American continent in Brazil, Surinam and Venezuela.

The framework for the taxonomic status was described in 1978[60] and four species-groups are still recognized. In the Old World the *Biomphalaria pfeifferi* group has several forms and is found in all parts of Africa south of the Sahara, the Malagasy Republic, in Aden, Yemen and Saudi Arabia; the *choanomphala* group has only a few forms restricted to certain of the great natural African lakes; the *alexandrina* group has a scattered distribution in Africa and is common in the Sudan and Egypt. *B. sudanica* has both East and West African species components.

In the New World, the genus *Biomphalaria* is represented by some 20 species but of these, only *B. glabrata* (Say), *B. straminea* (Dunker) and *B. tena-*

gophila (Orbigny) have been found to be naturally infected with *S. mansoni*.

PARASITE–INTERMEDIATE HOST RELATIONSHIPS

There are many complex and complicated variations in the relationships between schistosomes and their intermediate hosts; parasite infectivity is as important as intermediate host susceptibility and differences in relationships occur even within limited geographical areas. Both environmental and genetic factors play parts in influencing the transmission of a schistosome through a particular species of snail.

The genera *Bulinus* and *Biomphalaria* are aquatic snails and are identified on the basis of various conchological, anatomical and biological characters. This is a highly specialized field and requires biological expertise. The snails are found in many different habitats including permanent or semipermanent small ponds, marshes, swamps, rivers and streams and large permanent water bodies such as lakes, dams, irrigation channels and rice fields. Their biology varies with their environment and requires lengthy study to elucidate the details.

Cross-fertilization is usual in aquatic snail intermediate hosts but they are in fact hermaphrodites and are capable of self-fertilization. Ova are laid in water as egg masses some 5–10 mm in diameter. Hatching of free-living snails occurs in 1–2 weeks; a steady growth ensues and maximal size and maturity is seen in 3–6 months. Snail intermediate hosts have an enormous reproductive potential since egg laying continues throughout life and lifespans have wide variations in the different species, e.g. *Bulinus globosus* infected with *S. haematobium* lived for 400 days,[61] *Biomphalaria pfeifferi* infected with *S. mansoni* survived for 213 days.[62]

INTERMEDIATE HOSTS OF *S. JAPONICUM*

S. japonicum is transmitted by amphibious snails, populations of polytypic *Oncomelania hupensis*, of which there are six subspecies: *O. h. hupensis* in mainland China; *O. h. quadrasi* in the Philippines; *O. h. nosophora* in Japan; *O. h. lindoensis* in Sulawesi, Indonesia; and in Taiwan where schistosomiasis is confined to animals and does not exist in man, *O. h. formosana* and *O. h. chiui*.[56] A genus *Tricula aperta* from the subfamily Triculinae transmits *S. mekongi*.

The oncomelanid shell differs markedly in size and shape from those of the aquatic snails (Figure 72.10) and oncomelanid snails have very different biological characteristics. They are dioecious, lay their eggs mainly at night and above the water on a solid-phase location. The separate sexes copulate repeatedly and the female is able to lay eggs more than 3 months after isolation from the male.[50] In the Philippines the average longevity is 66 days but in other endemic areas snails may survive for 12 months or longer. Egg laying and hatching are continuous throughout the year.

AESTIVATION

Both aquatic and amphibious snails have the capacity to survive out of water for weeks, or in some cases, for months; this phenomenon, termed 'aestivation', has important consequences on the epidemiology of the infection and its control; immature infections of both *S. mansoni* and *S. haematobium* can be carried through from one wet season to another, thus perpetuating the transmission cycle.

EPIDEMIOLOGY OF HUMAN SCHISTOSOMIASIS

Involving a definitive host in man, an intermediate host in various species of aquatic or amphibious snails, a freshwater environment which man contaminates with excreta through insanitary habits, and from which infection is also acquired through repeated water contact by means of many occupational and recreational activities, the epidemiology and epidemiological dynamics of schistosomiasis is heterogeneous and complicated.[32]

The parasites need the internal environments of the two hosts, definitive and intermediate, to complete the sexual and asexual phases of the life cycle respectively, and the free-living larval stages present in the common aquatic environment are the linking infective factors.[63]

Transmission is influenced by numerous variables, the major ones being:

1. The distribution, biology and population dynamics of the intermediate snail host(s).
2. The patterns and extent of environmental contamination with human excreta which in turn depend on the prevalence and intensity of human infection and the socioeconomic and hygienic background.
3. Human water contact activities, pattern and duration.
4. The host–parasite relationship in man and the role of protective immune mechanisms.[64]

Of all the parasitic infections of man, schistosomiasis is one of the most widespread, as illustrated by data advanced by WHO.[2,27] The disease ranks second only to malaria in terms of socioeconomic and public health importance in many tropical and subtropical areas. It is second to none in prevalence among water-borne diseases and is most common in rural areas of developing countries, with an estimated 200 million infected globally in 76 countries and 600 million exposed to infection due to a low socioeconomic status on a background of poverty and ignorance, with resultant poor housing, lack of potable water, inadequate hygienic conditions, few if any sanitary facilities and a multitude of activities bringing a population into contact with water into which eggs are passed and in which are found intermediate snail hosts, e.g. domestic, hygienic, occupational, recreational or religious. Thus transmission begins. Children are particularly important as reservoirs of infection because of their indiscriminate excretory habits, particularly urination while swimming, and their unrivalled opportunities for water contact in hot climates.

Schistosomiasis is not invariably a rural disease; expanding populations in periurban fringes of cities overwhelm the available sanitation and are thus at risk of transmission; examples are not infrequent within the boundaries of the modern cities of Africa. The infection may also occur from movements of infected people into refugee camps where endemic foci may be initiated.

Major factors associated with the spread and intensification of schistosomiasis are its links with water development projects, particularly man-made lakes and irrigation schemes since these are often sites of population immigrations for farming and fishing, so much a feature of the present tropical scene.

In many countries, schistosomiasis is not a notifiable disease and prevalence figures (i.e. the proportion of subjects infected at a given point in time) are frequently gross underestimates. The advanced clinical symptoms, signs and associated complications known to occur do not represent the full picture of infection in a community. Moreover, intensities of infection (i.e. measures of worm burdens in a group or in a community usually inferred by the surrogate technique of quantitative egg counting in stools or urine) are extremely variable. Whilst in general there is a good correlation between intensity of infection and the pathology produced, expressed as morbidity, exceptions occur and many cases of schistosomiasis are uncovered only during a purposive survey or incidentally in the investigation of another complaint.

This generalized correlation between prevalence and intensity of infection means that, for all practical purposes, the higher the prevalence, the greater the mean intensity of infection in a sample.

The epidemiology of schistosomiasis shows wide variations within any endemic country. Focality is a major feature of the epidemiology and surprising differences of prevalence and intensity of infection occur between neighbouring geographic environments. This makes broad generalized descriptions of the status of the infection within a country difficult and also renders many comparisons between countries invalid. The epidemiology can change rapidly in any endemic area as a result of water resource development projects of any type.

Community-based studies of schistosomiasis usually demonstrate that age-specific prevalences and intensities of infection are highly positively skewed, this phenomenon being more marked in *S. haematobium* than in *S. mansoni* and even less so in *S. japonicum*, while data for *S. intercalatum* and *S. mekongi* are as yet too fragmentary to allow definitive statements.

In urinary schistosomiasis (*S. haematobium*) prevalence rises rapidly from the age when youngsters begin to wander afield.[32] The peak prevalence and intensity of infection occur in children aged from 10 to 14 years of age and thereafter successive decades see a progressive lowering of prevalence to much lower levels. Some 60–70% of all infected persons lie within the age range 5–14 years and the heaviest infections occur similarly in this age range.

In endemic areas of *S. mansoni* prevalences and intensities of infection are maximal in the 10–24-year age group. Although reductions occur with increasing age, prevalence levels remain at higher levels than those seen in *S. haematobium* infections. Some 5–25% of the infected population excretes at least 50% of the total number of eggs contaminating the environment and the majority of heavily infected children lie in the 10–14-year age group. In a high proportion of those with over 800 eggs per gram of faeces, an enlarged liver and spleen are present.[2]

The explanation of the reduction in prevalence and intensity of infection in older age groups in endemic areas of *S. haematobium* and *S. mansoni* depends on multiple factors: immune mechanisms

certainly contribute; tissue fibrosis prevents eggs from reaching the exterior; a proportion of the body population of infecting worms will have died. Apart from occupational water contact, exposure to cercarial infested water is likely to be less with increasing age.[32] The exact roles played by immune, pathological, parasitological and environmental, ecological and human behavioural mechanisms and their possible interactions are uncertain and remain a topic for constant debate among various 'lobby protagonists'.

In *S. japonicum* infection 'typical' age-distribution and intensity patterns do not seem to occur. This doubtless reflects epidemiological variations between areas within a country and also between countries and perhaps the many animals which can act as reservoir hosts.

Bimodal prevalence peaks in the 10–14-year and 35–44-year age groups have been documented.[2]

ANIMAL RESERVOIRS

Some 31 wild mammals and 13 domestic animals have been shown to be infected with *S. japonicum* in China[65] but only rarely has their role in transmission been evaluated. Yet they cannot be considered negligible for, based on the total animal population, prevalence, mean daily egg output and hatchability, the dog, cow, pig, rat, carabao (water buffalo) and goat were, in decreasing order of magnitude, estimated to be responsible for some 25% of the total potential environmental contamination, while man was thought to provide 75% in the Philippines.[50]

In striking contrast, man is the only definitive host of *S. haematobium*. The few infections with this parasite reported in Primates, Arteridactyla or Rodentia can be considered as incidental and of no epidemiological importance.

Many reports exist of infection with *S. mansoni* in a wide range of mammals (Primates, Insectivora, Arteriodactyla, Marsupilia, Rodentia, Carnivora, Edentata). Evidence implicating their role in maintenance of transmission of the parasite is, with two exceptions, lacking. In Tanzania, it was considered that baboons were maintaining the parasite among themselves[66] and there is good reason to believe that *S. mansoni* is maintained by both rats (*Rattus rattus*, a known reservoir host) and man in a natural habitat in Guadeloupe[67,68] and in some areas in Brazil.[1]

In *S. mekongi* infections, dogs are known to be a reservoir host.[26]

IMMUNITY

Neither sex nor age confers immunity and all races are susceptible to infection. The female adult schistosomes lay eggs after pairing and deposit them in the capillary habitat for many years. Thus schistosomiasis is a chronic disease with morbidity produced by granulomatous reactions to eggs deposited in the tissues. Primary infections occur early in life. Although the host is presented with new and heavy antigenic burdens when cercariae invade and schistosomula are maturing, few infected persons are diagnosed as having the clinical picture of the acute febrile illness known as 'acute toxaemic' schistosomiasis or 'Katayama syndrome'.

The development of acquired immunity in schistosomal infections is slow and inefficient and differs from the immediate and complete immunity of the type occurring after common childhood viral or bacterial infections.[69] The reasons for this are unclear but IgG and IgM antibodies antagonize the protective effects of the immune system in young children and may be related to the slow development of immunity faced with a number of potentially protective responses.[70–74]

After the primary infection in childhood, numerous reinfections occur in subsequent years and are largely unopposed. Since schistosomes do not replicate within the human host, this results in a rapid acquisition of high worm loads, high egg outputs and resultant morbidity and pathology. Yet it is well known from community-based surveys that prevalences and intensities of infection progressively decrease in the teenage years and successive decades see a decline of prevalence to much lower levels. One theory advanced to explain the age distributions of prevalence and intensity in whole populations was that the decrease in older age groups might be due to changing social habits resulting in reduced human water contact.[75] Other factors involved may be tissue fibrosis, preventing eggs from reaching the exterior, and the death of various proportions of the body population of infecting worms, which, additionally, would account for the phenomenon of 'loss of infection' encountered during epidemiological surveys, i.e. the failure to detect eggs in excreta on successive surveys in persons who were previously egg positive.[63]

Despite enormous amounts of recent experimental, immunological and clinicoepidemiological research inputs into the explanation of acquired immunity or antischistosome resistance in schistosomiasis, a wide variety of basic questions remain.[76]

A high proportion of adults in endemic areas who have acquired their primary infection in childhood possess immunity to superinfections and usually show few clinical signs. Although this immunity is protective against schistosomula and adult worms, it causes characteristic lesions of the infection when directed against eggs.

Protective immunity directed against cercariae and schistosomula reduces the numbers surviving to adulthood. Two mechanisms are involved: an antibody-dependent cell-mediated cytotoxicity process, itself dependent on eosinophils and IgG; and a process involving IgE and macrophages.

Concomitant immunity in experimental terms describes the resistance, partial or total, of an actively infected host to a subsequent challenge infection by the same type of organism. Adult worms evade the immune responses by adding a layer of host-specific antigens to their tegmental membranes. Adult worms of a primary infection are unharmed by cercarial challenge but the invading parasite forms of the challenge infection tend to be destroyed.[69] Concomitant immunity occurs in schistosome infections and challenges in many experimental hosts and in man.[76]

Further explanatory progress was made through longitudinal field studies involving detailed quantitation of egg outputs and water contact in children and the technique of reinfection studies. Chemotherapy is given to remove existing infections; the levels of newly acquired infections (reinfections) are observed, quantitated and related to water contact and degree of exposure. These techniques produced strong evidence that age-dependent resistance to reinfection is distinct from age-dependent exposural change, in two areas, the Gambia and Kenya, for both *S. haematobium* and *S. mansoni* infection. For example, in the Gambia, changes in intensity of infection with time were compared in two communities, in one of which transmission had been interrupted by mollusciciding. In this area the mean life span of the worms was 3–4 years, allowing the comparison in the untreated (control) area of the numbers of eggs deposited by worms over the same 3-year period. The acquisition of new infections by adults over 25 years of age was 1000-fold less than that of 5–8-year-old children. This difference could not be attributed to a 1000-fold reduction of water contact in the adults, thus suggesting age-dependent acquisition of immunity to superinfection.[77–80]

Thus the role of acquired immunity in limiting schistosome infections in communities in areas endemic for *S. haematobium* and *S. mansoni* has been placed on a firmer footing. However, the immunity is probably not absolute, is evident only after years of exposure to infection and some data suggest that it occurs earlier in areas of high prevalence and intensity.

The balance of the immune response in the early years of exposure to infection is directed towards production of blocking antibodies, which may be IgM, IgG_2, or IgG_4. Protective antibodies, IgE or other IgG isotypes, are detected in both older children and adults who appear to be resistant to infection.[81]

PATHOGENESIS

The lesions occurring during this long-lived infection are caused largely by schistosome eggs. Adult worms are impervious to the immune system of the host and by themselves cause little or no pathology. Yet they excrete antigens, e.g. the gut-associated soluble antigen which is found in the sera of patients with schistosomiasis and which is now used both as a marker for infection and as an indicator of therapeutic success through estimation of the cathode-associated antigen.[82]

Schistosome eggs cannot traverse capillary beds unaided because they measure up to $70\,\mu$m in width. Slightly less than half of the eggs are laid into the lumen of the gut or urinary tract. The remainder are laid in the walls of the organ or embolize into the portal radicles or lung arterioles. Collateral vascular bypasses enable eggs to reach many other organs in the body.

At oviposition, eggs are immature but miracidial maturation takes place in a few days. Soluble egg antigens (SEA) originating from the secretory glands of miracidia enclosed within eggs diffuse out through submicroscopic pores in the eggshell and induce an acute host hypersensitivity response. The immunopathology of schistosomiasis is considered to be due to granuloma formation around tissue-deposited eggs and is a manifestation of delayed hypersensitivity through a T-cell mediated immune response.

During an active infection, a range of early, mature and involuting granulomas is present.[83] Granulomas vary with the immune status of the host: in primary infections with marked reactions to soluble egg antigens, large florid granulomas occur with some central necrosis. The florid granuloma is composed of the schistosome egg surrounded by cellular aggregates of eosinophils, mononuclear phagocytes, lymphocytes, neutrophils, plasma cells and fibroblasts. Activated macrophages cluster close to the eggshell whilst lymphocytes and plasma cells are peripherally placed. Fibroblasts appear early, and throughout the lengthy involution process, replace other cell types.[83] Many granulomas are of sizes much greater than those of schistosome eggs.

After the acute phase of some 3 months, modulation of host immune responses to soluble egg antigens results in relatively small granulomas which have fewer surrounding eggs.

There are consistent and strong correlations of high organ and tissue egg loads and severe pathology in quantitative autopsy studies in *S. haematobium* and *S. mansoni*,[84,85] and clinicoepidemiological findings are in agreement. Other factors may operate, e.g. direct and indirect fibroblastic proliferation and induced abnormalities of types I and III collagen.

Thus the pathology of schistosomiasis results from collections of granulomas, from fibroblastic lesions obstructing vessels and fibroinflammatory swellings containing millions of eggs.[83] Unlike early granulomas, these late obstructive and fibrous lesions respond poorly to chemotherapy.

There is a plethora of systemic host responses to schistosome infection since cercariae, schistosomula, adult worms and eggs all generate multiple antigens to which the host immune system responds through immunocompetent cells. Antibodies specific to each stage are long lived and persist after successful chemotherapy. Several defined schistosome antigens have been detected; the most useful in clinical work is the cathode-associated antigen. Other antigens are complexed to immunoglobulins and can be found at various sites, e.g. schistosomal nephropathy.[86]

Von Lichtenberg[83] has strikingly contrasted the pathogenetic variables and prognosis in the hepatosplenomegaly of the early infection resulting from cell proliferation with florid granulomas, reticuloendothelial hyperplasia and diffuse inflammatory infiltrates, all reversible by specific chemotherapy, with the hepatosplenomegaly of the advanced disease induced by fibrovascular pathology with periportal fibrosis, portal hypertension and its associated effects on the spleen in which the prognosis is far less dependent on chemotherapy but more on surgical alleviation of a mechanical obstructive condition.

The influence of genetic factors on immunopathology and on protective immunity remains unclear.

While two studies in Egypt[87] and the Philippines[88] suggested a relationship between severe disease and specific HLA haplotypes, the association was not found in Brazil.[89] Yet a more recent Brazilian study demonstrated that host genetic factors were implicated in human resistance to *S. mansoni* in one specific focus.[90] No firm generalizations can yet be made.

PATHOLOGY

It is useful to consider the pathology and pathophysiology of the various schistosome infections within the stages of the life cycle and their time frames:

1. Cercarial invasion and schistosomular migration.
2. Maturation of schistosomes, pairing and commencement of egg laying.
3. Established infection with continuous egg laying.
4. Late stages and complications.

Attempts to link discrete clinical entities with these stages should be made only with the realization that the apparently endless series of epidemiological, immunological and physiological interactions encountered, particularly in endemic areas, make resultant associations and correlations less than clear-cut. Frequently much clearer relationships between clinical expressions and pathophysiological derangements are seen in non-immune visitors, transients or immigrants who become infected in endemic areas. In parallel, infected travellers or holidaymakers returning to temperate locations may present clear pictures of infection acquired in endemic zones.

Cercarial invasion of the skin or mucosal penetration on exposure to infested water, particularly when the quantum of infection is high, can occur in less than 15 minutes; the clinical complement of cercarial dermal invasion is a schistosome (cercarial or allergic) dermatitis which last for 24–48 hours. The pathophysiological response is the initiation of the first mechanisms of the immune response with marked eosinophilia and an antibody-dependent cell-mediated cytotoxic process involving IgG.

At widely different times, ranging from 2 to 16 weeks after cercarial invasion, during the migration of schistosomula, their maturation, pairing and initiation of egg laying, the clinical manifestation of acute toxaemic schistosomiasis or Katayama syndrome may arise. Worm and/or egg antigens produce a marked antigenic stimulus with rapidly rising antibody levels and an increase in serum IgG, IgA and IgM. Circulating immune antigen–antibody complexes are found and may be deposited in glomeruli, producing immune complex glomerulopathy. The whole clinical picture is one resembling the acute serum sickness syndrome.

At variable times after infection, from some 2 months onward, the stage of established infection occurs, with continuous egg laying associated with the 'classical' symptoms and signs of established schistosomiasis. Soluble egg antigens from miracidia in the eggs provoke a T-lymphocyte-mediated host response which, in time, results in the characteristic granuloma with eosinophils prominent in the destruction of the eggs.

After some years, changes in clinical symptoms and physical signs appear and there is superimposition of late stage complications, e.g. obstructive uropathy, hydronephrosis and pyelonephritic renal failure in *S. haematobium* or portal hypertension which may be 'compensated' or 'decompensated' with ascites, and hepatosplenomegaly with or without gastrointestinal variceal bleeding in *S. mansoni*, *S. japonicum* and *S. mekongi* infections. Modulation by T suppressor lymphocytes and antibody blockade diminish host immune response over time; fibroblasts stimulate collagen production and fibrotic complications involving a variety of anatomical sites, e.g. periportal hepatic fibrosis and obstructive uropathy, ensue.

PATHOLOGY OF ESTABLISHED INFECTION

S. HAEMATOBIUM

Urinary bladder

The urinary bladder is the most frequently affected organ. Cystoscopy, surgery or autopsy reveal the gross lesions, which are often multiple. A hyperaemic mucosa on cystoscopy is universal. 'Sandy patches' occur in one-third; these are raised greyish-yellow mucosal irregularities associated with heavy egg deposition and surrounded by dense fibrous tissue. Calcification may occur. They are sited most commonly at the trigone and near the ureteric orifices.[91]

Other raised lesions are granulomas, nodules and

polyps which may be sessile or pedunculated and are related to local heavy tissue egg loads. Focal granulomas are of pin-head size with the customary histological appearances.

Vesical ulcers are less common and can vary in size from a small irregular defect to an irregular deep transverse fissure. They occur mainly on the posterior wall of the bladder.

Many degrees of bladder muscle hypertrophy are found at autopsy but specific associations with tissue egg loads or local lesions are lacking; muscle hypertrophy appears to be more frequent in cases with obstructive uropathy. Obstructive lesions from fibrosis of the neck of the bladder in periurethral granulomatous reactions are a common complication, as are bladder calculi.

Bladder calcification is common and is often encountered both in clinical practice and in radiological surveys. Calcification is linear, occurring along lines of deposited eggs. Calcified bladders usually retain normal elasticity.

Ureters

Although the ureters are less frequently affected than the bladder, their involvement is important for it leads to morbidity and is the forerunner of obstructive uropathy. Tissue egg loads in the ureters are greater in cases with obstructive uropathy than in those without.[91,92] Arguments on whether unilateral disease predominates more on the left than the right have continued for at least a decade. In a quantitative analysis, tissue egg burdens were much higher in the right lower ureter than in the left, but unilateral obstructive uropathy occurred equally on both sides.[91,92] Bilateral ureteric involvement is the rule.

The histopathology of ureteric lesions resembles that of bladder lesions. Granulomatous lesions resolve and lead to ureteral fibrotic stenosis. Rising back pressure proceeds to hydroureter, with or without hydronephrosis, the collective title of which is obstructive uropathy. This condition predisposes to *Escherichia coli* or *Salmonella* urinary tract infection which can lead to chronic pyelonephritis and Gram-negative septicaemia.[93,94]

Genital organs

Since *S. haematobium* parasitizes the vesical plexus, eggs are not uncommonly found in both male and female genital organs, but the long-running debate of their functional significance has not yet been concluded. In males the mean *S. haematobium* egg count per gram of seminal vesicle tissue was 20 000 in one investigation.[91] The resultant enlargement,

muscular hypertrophy and fibrosis produced an increase in weight of the seminal vesicles which correlated with the presence of obstructive uropathy.[91] Much less commonly affected were the prostate, testes, epididymis and penis. A causal role for these lesions in the production of male infertility has not been substantiated.

In females, the finding of eggs in the female genital organs is similarly frequent; eggs are found in the vulva, vagina and cervix, where ulcerating, polypoid or nodular lesions may be seen. Nodules in the perineal skin are not rare. The internal female genital organs, ovaries, fallopian tubes and uterus are much less commonly affected. In Malawi, gynaecological complications of schistosomiasis were considered a significant cause of female morbidity, particularly when the lower genital tract was involved; ovarian, uterine and tubal pathology were not major causes of morbidity but diagnosis was difficult.[95] There is a dearth of recent reports associating ectopic pregnancy or infertility and *S. haematobium* infection.[96]

Schistosomiasis has little impact on female infertility and rarely renders a woman anovulatory despite the proximity of eggs to the gonads, tubes and uterus.[83]

Gastrointestinal tract

S. haematobium eggs are frequent in the gastrointestinal tract, their density being highest in the appendix with a gradual decrease in density down to the distal tract. Polyps have been recorded in the rectosigmoid colon in an autopsy study of *S. haematobium* cases; the polyps were inflammatory and often ulcerated.[97]

S. haematobium eggs are often seen in rectal biopsy material but are usually dead.

Kidney

Although schistosomal granulomas are rare in the parenchyma, renal lesions occur as a sequel of obstructive uropathy and are manifest as pyelonephritis.

Schistosomal antigens in mesangial areas of the glomeruli in uncomplicated cases of *S. haematobium* infection have been observed by immunofluorescent microscopy as well as granular deposits of IgG, IgM and C3, yet there was a lack of basement membrane changes, an absence of clinical renal disease and normal renal function tests.[98] There remains doubt about whether *S. haematobium* causes a specific nephropathy in the face of other mechanisms of renal failure.[99] A reversible nephrotic syndrome in

S. haematobium complicated by *Salmonella* infection has been described.[100]

Lung

Pulmonary arteritis and cor pulmonale are rare in pure *S. haematobium* infection, yet egg granulomas are frequently encountered at autopsy.[96]

Ectopic lesions

Migration of *S. haematobium* within the vascular system and subsequent egg laying may produce a variety of ectopic lesions.

It was formerly considered that *S. haematobium* in Egypt was not a cause of Symmers' periportal hepatic fibrosis (despite the common finding of *S. haematobium* granulomas in the liver). More recent studies, and in particular those using ultrasonography, have shown that *S. haematobium* in Egypt does indeed cause schistosomal hepatic fibrosis, characterized by periportal fibrosis, hepatic granulomas, cellular infiltration of the portal tracts and obstruction and substitution of portal radicles by granulomas.[101,102]

Cutaneous deposition of *S. haematobium* eggs is not uncommon and has been recognized for decades.[103] Papular or nodular lesions occur in many sites, most frequently in the genital and perineal areas but also in the neck, chest and abdominal wall.[104-108]

Other sites of ectopic lesions are the central nervous system (CNS), an occurrence less frequent than in infections due to *S. japonicum* or *S. mansoni*. The finding of eggs of *S. haematobium* in the CNS without clinical sequelae is not rare; eggs appear to produce minimal or no histological reaction, in contrast to the production of inflammatory responses when laid elsewhere.[109] The spinal cord is affected more often than the brain.[96,109]

Rare and curious lesions have been described, e.g. multiple *S. haematobium* egg deposition in the pericardium, causing a fibrous pericarditis,[110] and the demonstration of an adult *S. haematobium* worm in the choroid plexus.[111]

Bladder cancer and S. haematobium infection

Despite at least 14 reviews of the relationship between bladder cancer and *S. haematobium* infection published since the early 1980s, the aetiological significance of the parasite in the causation of this cancer remains a topic for argument.[96]

In Egypt, where *S. haematobium* has been hyperendemic for centuries and despite the fact that the prevalence and intensity of infection has decreased rapidly and substantially since the 1960s, cancer in a bladder infected with schistosomiasis occupies the primary rank among all recorded cancers.[112] In certain other countries, e.g. Iraq, coastal Kenya, Ghana, Malawi, Mozambique, Zambia and Zimbabwe, a consistent association between the presence of *S. haematobium* and bladder carcinoma seems to exist. Yet in Nigeria, South Africa and Saudi Arabia, all countries with moderate or high prevalences of *S. haematobium*, the association is not present; bladder cancer is no more frequent than in non-endemic countries.

When cancer is associated with urinary schistosomiasis the tumour may occur at any site in the bladder, yet it rarely originates in the trigone, a frequent site of origin in non-schistosomal cancers and the most common site of 'sandy patches' and heavy egg deposition.

Schistosomal bladder cancer occurs in an age group significantly younger than that in which cancer occurs in non-schistosomal areas.

The histopathology of cancer in association with schistosomiasis is dominated by squamous cell tumours, in contrast to the more common transitional cell carcinoma encountered in non-schistosomal areas.[84,96,113] Most squamous cell cancers in schistosomal bladders are fairly well differentiated, largely indolent and localized, spreading directly through the bladder wall with late and infrequent lymphatic spread. Bloodstream metastasis is rare. This picture contrasts sharply with that of transitional cell carcinoma.

Bladder cancer has been produced experimentally in monkeys and baboons infected with *S. haematobium*,[114,115] species not known for the common occurrence of bladder tumours. Yet two large consecutive autopsy series conducted in Cairo showed no differences of significance in the frequency or type of urothelial malignancies in patients with and without urinary schistosomiasis.[91,97]

Several mechanisms have been suggested to explain the suspected role of *S. haematobium* in bladder cancer, none of which is proven; for example, fibrosis induced by schistosome eggs may induce proliferation, abnormal hyperplasia and metaplasia, all possible precancerous changes, in epithelial cells;[116] chronic urinary bacterial infection and production of nitrosamines, well-known bladder carcinogens, from their precursors in urine;[117] urinary stasis allowing concentration of endogenous carcinogens leading to their absorption from urine and exposure of the bladder epithelium;[118,119] raised urinary β-glucuronidase levels originating from miracidia and adult schistosomes liberating carcinogenic amines in urine.[113]

In summary, carcinogenic change associated with *S. haematobium* occurs only after many years of infection. The schistosomal infection is considered as a tumour promoter, potentiating carcinogenesis, rather than as a direct inducer. The various cofactors necessary for neoplasia are not known with any certainty.

However, arguments against an association between urinary schistosomiasis and bladder cancer still remain.[120] Possibly the next few decades will provide clarification of any relationship. Large scale population-based chemotherapy directed at control of morbidity would be expected to lower cancer incidence rates in the worst affected of the endemic countries and studies to this end are in place. The critical problem will be the acquisition of accurate and acceptable population-based incidence figures of bladder cancer.

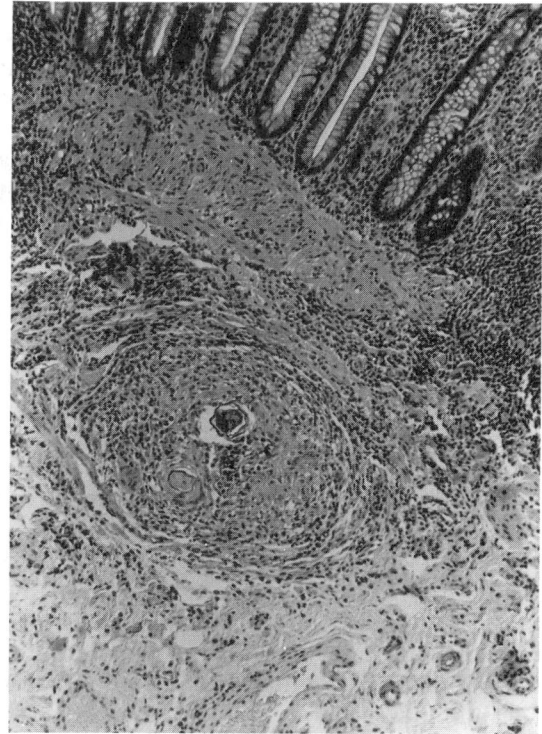

Figure 72.11 Schistosomal granuloma (*S. mansoni*) of bowel. The structureless mass at the centre is an egg.

S. MANSONI

A range of chronic lesions is found, from scattered granulomas of the intestinal tract to gross periportal hepatic fibrosis (Symmers' pipe-stem fibrosis; bilharzial clay pipe-stem fibrosis).

Focal granulomas and fibrosis may occur in any part of the intestinal tract, most frequently in the rectosigmoid colon since the preferred habitat of adult *S. mansoni* is in the tributaries of the inferior mesenteric vein. These lesions rarely lead to gross clinical symptoms. Pathology in the small bowel is not as severe as in the large gut, even though in late stage infections, particularly in Egypt and Brazil, there was a shift in egg deposition from the colon to the small intestine at autopsy.[85]

Colonic polyposis, a syndrome peculiar but not exclusive to Egypt, occurs in young patients and is directly related to intensity of infection. The colon and rectum are the sites of multiple pedunculated polyps with associated mucosal swelling, hyperaemia and oedema. The concentration of eggs within the polyps is much higher than in other sites in the intestine. The clinical accompaniments are significant blood and protein losses producing anaemia, chronic diarrhoea, tenesmus and a protein-losing enteropathy.

Occasionally, pseudotumours of schistosomal eggs surrounded by extensive fibrous tissue occur in *S. mansoni* and are termed 'bilharziomas'. Sites of predilection are the omentum, mesenteric lymph

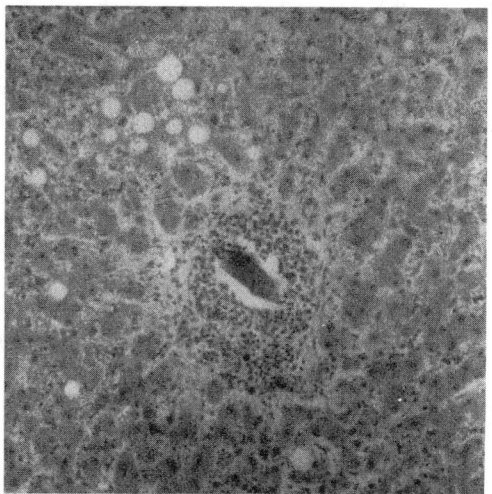

Figure 72.12 Schistosomal granuloma (*S. mansoni*) in liver. The structureless mass at the centre is an egg. (Courtesy of B. H. Kean.)

nodes, paracaecal region and infrequently the wall of the gut.

Schistosomal granulomas in bowel and liver are illustrated in Figures 72.11 and 72.12.

Hepatosplenic schistosomiasis

The major, and undoubtedly the most important complication of chronic *S. mansoni* infection is periportal hepatic fibrosis; since the basic pathology is sited in and around the portal tracts and the hepatic parenchyma is normal in uncomplicated cases, the term cirrhosis is inappropriate. A cut section of the liver, which may or may not be enlarged, shows macroscopic wide bands of fibrosis around portal tracts, resembling the stems of a number of clay pipes; the surface of the liver may be smooth, granular or nodular. Between portal fields, the hepatic parenchyma does not exhibit the nodularity of Laënnec's cirrhosis.

Deposited eggs produce granulomas with surrounding inflammatory infiltrates in connective tissue surrounding the hepatic veins, proximal to presinusoidal vessels. Affected portal tracts become blocked with granulomas and disorganized by inflammation, fibrosis and pyelophlebitis.[83] Eggs, an eosinophilic infiltrate, schistosomal pigment and/or organizing thrombi are found. The accumulation of egg granulomas around sites of blockage lead to further portal enlargement and simultaneously the hepatic arteries enlarge and push out new branching capillaries. Thus the presinusoidal portal hypertension produces a compensatory arterial flow. Total intrahepatic blood flow remains within normal limits, with maintenance of hepatocellular integrity. The diminished portal blood flow from portal hypertension is compensated for by the increase in hepatic arterial supply and the rich capillary arterial network around the portal branches which communicates with the portal vein.[121] There remain unexplained discrepancies between clinical and pathological interpretations of the arterial origin of the hepatic capillary network.[121]

Hepatic fibrosis results from accumulation of collagen in the liver[122] and may originate in proliferation of collagen-synthesizing cells, increase in synthesis by existing cells or deficiency in collagen degradation.[123] In experimental animals the amount of collagen in the liver increases in parallel with egg granuloma formation;[124] in human hepatic schistosomiasis there is increased collagen content and marked collagen synthesis in wedge liver biopsy material when compared with control tissue.[125]

The natural course of periportal fibrosis is slow and is termed 'compensated' since liver cell function tests show only slight abnormalities, if any. Over time, the consequences of portal hypertension with splenomegaly and variceal haemorrhage, with or without ascites, appear, although hepatic decompensation does not develop until an advanced stage of the process.

Spleen

Splenomegaly is the usual accompaniment of hepatic schistosomiasis and is due to portal venous hypertension, chronic passive congestion and reticuloendothelial hyperplasia. Focal infarcts and trabecular haemorrhages may occur and the spleen is tough and fibrotic. Hypersplenism may produce a pancytopenia or a leucoerythroblastic anaemia. The spleen may become enormously enlarged (Egyptian splenomegaly in the older literature) as in kala-azar (visceral leishmaniasis) or the myeloproliferative syndromes.[83] Lymphomas have been reported occasionally.[126]

Lungs and heart

Pulmonary hypertension caused by granulomatous pulmonary arteritis originating from large-scale embolization of eggs is commonly the result of pipe-stem fibrosis with extensive portocaval shunts occurring in *S. mansoni* or *S. japonicum* infections. This may produce schistosomal cor pulmonale. Strangely, and despite a direct access to the lungs via the inferior vena cava, cor pulmonale occurs less frequently in pure or mixed *S. haematobium* infection than would be anticipated.[96] There are fewer reports of cor pulmonale in *S. japonicum* than in *S. mansoni* despite the similar pathogenetic mechanisms.[121]

Granulomatous inflammation occludes distal pulmonary arterial branches and eventually produces a rise in pulmonary arterial pressure with right ventricular hypertrophy and strain; the smaller arterioles show fibrointimal sclerosis; fibrinoid necrosis and angiomatoid formation is widespread in alveolar tissue. This complication arises in long-standing cases of heavy infection and presents clinically as congestive heart failure arising in chronic cor pulmonale.

Kidney

Renal lesions (schistosomal nephropathy; glomerulonephritis), consisting of deposition of immune complexes of host immunoglobulins with adult worm or egg antigens in the glomerular mesangium and basement membrane, occur in *S. mansoni* infection. A variety of glomerular lesions have been found at autopsy in hepatosplenic patients.[127] Mild proteinuria is common in chronic *S. mansoni* infection, and, in hepatosplenic cases, progressive nephropathy leading to renal failure occurs in a small proportion but the clinical course is slow and the greater risks are from the hepatic complications.[83]

Amyloidosis has been demonstrated in renal biopsy material from patients with the nephrotic syndrome and schistosomiasis in Egypt.[128]

Egg deposition in the kidney is rare and is not thought to be responsible for any renal pathology.

Central nervous system

Various forms of 'neurological schistosomiasis' occur in infections due to *S. mansoni*, *S. japonicum* and *S. haematobium*. Yet in view of the global total of infected people, CNS localization is rare. Eggs of all three species have been found in the brain and spinal cord and adult worms have been demonstrated at various sites.

'Cerebral' schistosomiasis has traditionally been associated with *S. japonicum* infection but eggs of *S. mansoni* and *S. haematobium* have also been found in the brain, rather more frequently with *S. mansoni*. The route of infection is thought to be via Batsons's valveless intervertebral plexus or by arterial egg embolism.[129] Eggs may be present in the CNS with little or no histological reaction and in a randomly selected series of hepatosplenic schistosomiasis coming to autopsy, one-quarter had *S. mansoni* eggs in the brain;[129] these cases may be symptom free.

Myelopathy with various motor and/or sensory presentations occurs, more commonly in *S. mansoni* than in *S. haematobium*, and cord transection with paraparesis is well known. Not infrequently, spinal cord schistosomiasis is recognized in the acute toxaemic stages which occur in tourists and transient visitors to endemic areas on their return to temperate climates after a short tropical stay.

Other ectopic lesions

Cutaneous lesions due to *S. mansoni* are rare but papular or nodular lesions at different sites are known.

In Egypt, genital lesions are not uncommonly found at autopsy.[89] Placental schistosomiasis has been reported from Brazil.[130]

S. JAPONICUM

The intestinal and hepatic lesions of *S. japonicum* are in general similar to those occurring in *S. mansoni* but with several specific differences. The primary lesion is a T-cell-mediated granuloma formation around the eggs but modulation of the granuloma size is largely antibody mediated, whereas in *S. mansoni* cell mediation is the dominant mechanism.

The adult worms are located in the branches of the inferior mesenteric vein and in the superior haemorrhoidal vein[131] and an adult female deposits 1000–3500 eggs per day in highest density in the large intestine and, in descending order, in the rectum, sigmoid and descending colon. The small intestine is relatively lightly affected.[132]

Knowledge of pathological anatomy, gross and microscopic, in *S. japonicum* lags behind that of *S. mansoni* since autopsy studies are fewer, currently are seldom performed in the endemic countries of *S. japonicum* and, in the broad public health sense, schistosomiasis has been progressively declining as a cause of death for some decades.[227]

Gastrointestinal lesions in experimental animals are focal and isolated and are interspersed with normal bowel. Segmental lesions occur in man and multiple findings are common, including mucosal hyperplasia, pseudopolyposis, ulceration and thickening of the intestinal wall.

Gastric schistosomiasis is seen frequently in surgical or biopsy specimens. Subclinical cases are probably common but unrecognized owing to non-diagnostic symptoms and insensitive diagnostic techniques.

Macroscopic hepatic changes in the chronic phase parallel those in *S. mansoni* infection. The liver is frequently enlarged with an irregular surface. On cross-section the characteristic wide bands of fibrous tissue surrounding the larger portal tracts are seen and Symmers' periportal (clay pipe-stem) fibrosis is found at autopsy. Microscopically the picture is one of chronic pseudotubercles with chronic inflammation, cellular infiltrates around eggs, extensive fibrosis and neovascularization in the portal tracts. The accompanying manifestations of portal hypertension, i.e. splenomegaly, with or without gastro-oesophageal varices, with or without bleeding, are to be anticipated.

Although *S. japonicum* eggs are often found in the lung and obliterative pulmonary arteritis is similar to that seen in *S. mansoni*, clinical cor pulmonale has not been reported as frequently as in *S. mansoni* infection.[133]

In contrast to *S. mansoni* and *S. haematobium*, the brain is more commonly affected in *S. japonicum* infection, yet spinal cord involvement appears to be less frequent. The cerebral lesions are held to be caused by intracrarial egg deposition or embolism via a vascular route.

In the first half of this century, schistosomal dwarfism with retardation of growth and sexual development was recognized as a not uncommon occurrence in China. This syndrome is rare in modern times.

Cancer and S. japonicum infection

Epidemiological studies have not demonstrated any direct relationships between gastric cancer and *S. japonicum* infection.[227]

The situation regarding a relationship between colonic or rectal cancer and *S. japonicum* is much more complex. Case–control studies in China and in the Philippines and epidemiological cross-sectional surveys in China have suggested both positive and negative associations. One case–control study in China showed a strong association between *S. japonicum* infection and rectal cancer but no association between colonic cancer and a history of *S. japonicum* infection.[227]

No definitive conclusions can be reached from the studies to date. Improved designs of further studies are essential for clarification.

A similar position exists on the presence or absence of a relationship between primary liver cell cancer and schistosomiasis. The ubiquity of hepatitis B infection, a known precancerous condition, in endemic areas of *S. japonicum* has complicated study designs. Again, the correlation is speculative.

S. MEKONGI

Although the clinical manifestations of *S. mekongi* are similar to those of *S. japonicum*, the morbidity and pathology resulting from the former is compounded by the presence of *Opisthorcis viverrini* in endemic areas of *S. mekongi*. Objective descriptions of detailed pathology in man are lacking.

S. INTERCALATUM

Confined in its endemic distribution to six countries (Cameroon, Guinea, Gabon, Congo, Zaire and Angola) along the gulf of Guinea, with sporadic cases occurring in Burkina Faso and Nigeria, more information on experimental animal infections exists than does pathological description.[134]

The disease is mild, and in proctoscopy on hospital inpatients the rectal and colonic mucosa was considered abnormal in 47 of 85 patients. Nonspecific lesions predominated: mucosal congestion, oedema, bleeding and/or ulceration. In liver biopsies, granulomatous lesions, of a size smaller than those in *S. mansoni* infection, were seen in the portal tracts. Tissue reaction to eggs was slight or absent in some patients. No portal hypertension was seen.[135]

CLINICAL FEATURES

GENERAL

To the clinician, particularly in the tropics, schistosomiasis can be a frustrating infection. With the exception of haematuria in urinary schistosomiasis there is no one diagnostic symptom or sign; even the commonly described various symptoms and signs are rarely pathognomonic. Schistosomiasis is a collection of infections of protean manifestations.

Whereas clinical medicine is taught in the context of classical descriptions of symptoms and signs, these were, in the past, culled from classical and advanced cases. This is rarely the rule in practice, for classical and advanced cases represent only a small proportion of an extensive frequency distribution of clinical syndromes. 'Classical' cases of schistosomiasis are in a minority; many patients have non-specific symptoms and many more are symptom free or ignore their symptoms and are only discovered on purposive surveys or during investigations for some unrelated complaint. This is due to the biological phenomenon of the overdispersed distribution of parasites within hosts; this aggregated distribution means that, in any population of hosts, there exists only a small proportion of 'heavy' infections with 'typical' symptoms and that the majority of cases are moderate or light infections with a corresponding freedom from symptoms or even a complete lack of symptoms.

While it is useful to consider schistosomiasis within the 'classical' stages of the life history, i.e. cercarial invasion, transformation of schistosomula and maturation of adults, established infections, late stages and complications, to attempt to link clinical pointers to these stages, it should be realized that the stages merge into each other and are rarely clear-cut, particularly in endemic areas in semi-immunes. Non-immune visitors to endemic areas or transients who become infected often provide a clearer clinical description than residents of endemic zones.

SYNDROMES COMMON TO ALL SCHISTOSOME INFECTIONS

CERCARIAL DERMATITIS

Seldom if ever described in indigenous inhabitants of endemic areas, especially in Africa, and only rarely in non-immune visitors, cercarial dermatitis more commonly occurs on exposure to avian cercariae where symptoms are more intense than in cases exposed to human schistosomal cercarial-infested waters.

Arising within a few minutes of exposure and receding within 24–72 hours, itching (pruritus) of the skin is the prime symptom, accompanied in some cases by erythema and/or a papular eruption. The condition can occur after exposure to any of the five common schistosomes infecting man.

ACUTE SCHISTOSOMIASIS

Also termed acute toxaemic schistosomiasis, Katayama syndrome or Katayama fever, after the Katayama region in Hiroshima prefecture, Japan, where it was originally described, this acute illness can be found after exposure to any of the schistosomes infecting man but is most marked in primary infections in non-immune individuals.

Recent reports from China indicate that this acute syndrome due to *S. japonicum* is not limited to uninfected individuals living in an endemic area at the time of first exposure but may occur even in those with an active chronic infection or persons with a recent history of infection and documented treatment and cure.[227]

In the acute syndrome due to *S. mansoni*, a diminution in transmission produced by control measures has led to a relative increase in reports of acute cases and this phenomenon has been observed in Puerto Rico and Venezuela.

Acute schistosomiasis is much less commonly reported in *S. haematobium* infection and there are no data on its occurrence in *S. intercalatum* or *S. mekongi*.

Since the incubation periods of the different schistosome infections are not known accurately and have been the subject of numerous estimates, only broad descriptions of the time phases of the occurrence of the syndrome after initial cercarial exposure can be given.

In *S. japonicum*, the mean period between exposure to infection and the onset of fever in 105 people with no previous history of infection and with only a single day's exposure to infested water was 41.5 days, with a range of 14–84 days.[227]

In *S. mansoni*, the incubation period of the Katayama syndrome ranges from 4 to 87 days but is generally between 3 and 7 weeks.[121]

Surprisingly short incubation periods may be encountered in non-immunes who become infected in endemic areas, e.g. within 35 days of returning from Botswana, symptoms occurred in 12 of 13 US travellers with a history of water contact; symptoms lasted 1–30 days (mean 8 days) and 9 of 11 had eggs of *S. mansoni* in the stools during the symptomatic period,[136] three Dutch non-immunes infected in Mali developed illness within 1–4 weeks after exposure and all had both *S. mansoni* and *S. haematobium* eggs in the stools at 12 weeks.[137]

The clinical picture is one of an acute pyrexial illness; continuing fever is a prime characteristic; the patient feels ill and may have rigors, sweating, general myalgia and headache. An urticarial skin rash may appear and lymphadenopathy or other non-specific signs can occur. Anorexia, nausea, abdominal discomfort and loose stools or diarrhoea, sometimes with mucus or blood, are not rare. The liver is frequently slightly enlarged and tender and a slightly enlarged spleen occurs in about one-third of patients.

A cough with, on physical examination, dry or moist rales, is frequent and an intense eosinophilia is almost invariably present.

Cerebral symptoms may appear and the occurrence of spinal cord syndromes or suggestive initial symptoms is an indication for urgent investigative measures.

ESTABLISHED INFECTIONS

S. HAEMATOBIUM (URINARY SCHISTOSOMIASIS)

With the proviso that many patients will have minimal symptoms, the cardinal complaint is recurrent painless haematuria. Other urinary tract symptoms may precede or be associated, e.g. burning on micturition, frequency, suprapubic discomfort or pain. Bladder involvement may lead to precipitancy, dribbling or incontinence. In fact, in an endemic area, any urinary tract symptom is an indication to explore for the presence of *S. haematobium*. Yet in many countries in Africa, in the young age groups and early teenagers, macroscopic haematuria may be virtually universal; in boys it provokes little comment and is regarded as a natural sign of puberty and an approach to manhood.

In the phase of established infection it is common practice to recognize two stages: (1) an active stage in children, adolescents and young patients, with egg deposition in many organs and egg excretion in the urine with proteinuria and haematuria, macroscopic or microscopic; and (2) in older patients, urinary egg excretion is sparse or absent but extensive pathology has developed. Even in the later stages of obstructive uropathy, symptoms may be absent or minimal. Chronic bladder lesions may produce persistent urinary dribbling and occasionally multiple fistulas in the perineum, with the picture of the 'watering can scrotum', although this phenomenon is much rarer nowadays than in the past, coincidental with the widespread use of chemotherapy at the peripheral level of health care.

Surveys have shown wide regional variation in coexistent bacteriuria; when present the predominant organisms are *E. coli*, *Klebsiella* spp., *Pseudomonas* spp. and *Salmonella* spp.

In Egypt, recurrent *Salmonella* bacteraemia is a well-recognized complication of *S. haematobium*. Patients with urinary schistosomiasis presenting with a recurrence of salmonellosis should first be treated for their *S. haematobium* infection.[138]

In the later stages of obstructive uropathy, hydronephrosis may develop and cause renal parenchymal dysfunction which, added to urinary tract infection, leads to impaired kidney function.[139] The ominous relationship between bilateral schistosomal uropathy, bacteriuria with impairment of hydrogen ion excretion, non-functioning kidneys and mortality has been well described.[139]

S. INTERCALATUM (INTESTINAL OR URINARY SCHISTOSOMIASIS)

In comparison with *S. haematobium* or *S. mansoni* infection, clinical symptoms of disease are commonly mild or absent and it is not regarded as a serious public health problem.[140,141] Active infection is seen in children and adolescents and only in those with egg excretion in excess of 400 eggs per gram of faeces is pathology detected.

The usual clinical presentation is one of diarrhoea, often with blood in the faeces and lower abdominal pain or discomfort. Yet some cases may present with haematuria and, in a report from Nigeria, *S. intercalatum* eggs were found in the urine, but not in faeces, in 6% of 1709 people surveyed.[142] The known existence of natural hybridization between *S. intercalatum* and *S. haematobium* can produce atypical clinical pictures with ectopic localization of worms.[143]

S. MANSONI/S. JAPONICUM/S. MEKONGI (INTESTINAL SCHISTOSOMIASIS)

The wide spectrum of clinical presentations has been emphasized in recent decades by the increasing use of community-based surveys as tools of investigation, in contrast with the customary descriptions of infection and disease rooted in hospital patients. Many, if not the majority of persons infected with *S. mansoni* are symptom free or have minimal and nonspecific symptoms, findings again in agreement with the known epidemiological/biological distribution of the parasite in the human host.

Clinical features are encountered in only a small proportion of persistent or heavy infections. Intestinal disease is shown by a chronic or intermittent diarrhoea with blood in the stools, abdominal discomfort or pain and colicky cramps. Severe dysentery is rare but certainly does occur. Secondary symptoms of fever, weakness, fatigue, anorexia and weight loss are frequent.

In epidemiological surveys there are significant correlations between visible or occult blood in the stools, abdominal pain and diarrhoea.

Hepatomegaly, often of the left lobe, and splenomegaly are frequent accompaniments. In the later stages of infection, there occurs a chronic catarrhal state of the intestine with a swollen, granular mucosa and loose stools with blood and/or mucus or an intermittent dysenteric syndrome.

The primary complications of polyposis and hepatosplenic schistosomiasis have their own symptomatology: polyposis produces what is in effect a severe chronic dysentery with blood and protein loss. Intussusception and/or rectal prolapse may occur.

Hepatosplenic schistosomiasis, often remarkably symptom free, presents as upper abdominal discomfort, left upper abdominal pain or a swelling of the abdomen. Physical signs include a firm enlargement of the liver, often with splenomegaly. The spleen may become greatly enlarged, sometimes extending downwards past the umbilicus into the left iliac fossa, and may even at times fill most of the abdomen. Ascites may be present but the classical signs of hepatocellular disease, spider-web angiomas, gynaecomastia, palmar erythema, jaundice and alterations in hair distribution are not present in 'pure' schistosomal disease. They may, however, be found where hepatitis B or C coexist with schistosomal periportal fibrosis and lead to posthepatitic hepatocellular damage. In advanced cases, endocrine changes may be found: growth retardation, infantilism, retarded bone age, all probably due to hypopituitarism. Amenorrhoea, early menopause, infertility and loss of libido have been attributed to a similar cause.[121]

A not uncommon primary presenting sign of hepatosplenic disease in schistosomiasis is haematemesis from gastro-oesophageal varices. It may occur without warning or may be preceded by a feeling of weakness or upper abdominal discomfort; patients have classical signs of acute blood loss with sweating, pallor, thirst, somnolence and a lowered blood and pulse pressure. In many cases melaena follows and this acute episode may precipitate ascites and/or peripheral oedema. Fatalities may occur with the primary haemorrhage if treatment is not available; multiple recurrent haemorrhagic episodes are usual. Unless complicated by hepatitis B, liver function remains good and hepatic encephalopathy does not develop. Where mixed infections of *S. mansoni* and hepatitis B coexist then the downhill clinical course is correspondingly rapid and the typical signs of hepatocellular failure appear with, in parallel, a poor prognosis.

S. JAPONICUM/S. MEKONGI

While infections with the oriental schistosomes follow a broadly similar clinical course to *S. mansoni*, several distinct differences emerge. In general, infection with *S. mekongi* is milder than that with *S. japonicum*. Hepatosplenomegaly is common but cerebral and cardiopulmonary complications are not reported.

In the past there have been more hospital-based clinical studies of *S. japonicum* than community-based investigations. Hence the clinical descriptions have been slanted towards advanced cases.

In fact, at least half of patients infected by *S. japonicum* are asymptomatic. General symptoms, fatigue, weakness, non-specific abdominal discomfort, irregular bowel movements or intermittent diarrhoea are frequent. Chronic diarrhoea is said to be a common symptom and lower abdominal pain a frequent complaint.[132]

The later signs of hepatosplenic schistosomiasis evolve as do those in *S. mansoni*. Although schistosomal dwarfism was not uncommon in China in the first half of the twentieth century, it has become a rarity nowadays. Cardiopulmonary and renal complications are well known.

The main difference clinically is the occurrence of cerebral schistosomiasis in *S. japonicum*. Spinal cord involvement appears less frequently than in *S. mansoni* but such generalizations are difficult if not impossible to confirm scientifically.

In the acute phase of cerebral schistosomiasis the presenting symptoms and signs are those of a meningoencephalitis with pyrexia, headache, vomiting, blurred vision and disturbed consciousness. In the established or chronic phase of the infection, several distinct neurological presentations are recognized: most common is epilepsy which may be generalized but is more frequently jacksonian in type; signs suggestive of a space occupying lesion or a stroke are also described. Computerized tomography and electroencephalography, with or without operational biopsy, are diagnostic.

DIFFERENTIAL DIAGNOSIS

In an infection of such diverse clinical manifestations it is scarcely surprising that schistosomiasis in any of its forms can be confused with many other disease processes. Acute schistosomiasis (Katayama syndrome) must be differentiated from typhoid (leucopenia, no eosinophilia), brucellosis, malaria, leptospirosis and numerous other causes of pyrexia of uncertain origin. Pyrexia and eosinophilia occur in trichinosis, tropical eosinophilia, visceral larva migrans and infections with *Opisthorcis, Paragonimus* and *Clonorchis* spp.

In the established stage, *S. haematobium* must be distinguished from renal tuberculosis with haematuria, haemoglobinurias, cancer of the urogenital tract and other infections such as acute nephritides.

S. mansoni, with its common presentation of non-specific abdominal symptoms, may suggest peptic ulcer, biliary disease or pancreatitis; in such cases symptoms disappear after antischistosomal treatment.

Lower abdominal conditions to be excluded are the various forms of dysentery, particularly amoebic dysentery, ulcerative colitis and non-schistosomal polyposis.

The differential diagnosis of hepatosplenic schistosomiasis is wide and embraces all causes of hepatomegaly and splenomegaly, separately and combined. The marked splenic enlargement of portal hypertension due to periportal fibrosis must be distinguished from kala-azar (visceral leishmaniasis), certain of the chronic leukaemias or myeloproliferative syndromes, some of the haemoglobinopathies, e.g. thalassaemias, and the tropical splenomegaly syndrome.

In endemic areas schistosomiasis must always be considered as one of the causes of cor pulmonale and virtually any neurological presentation but particu-larly the various forms of epilepsy and the different types of myelopathy or spinal cord compression.

A sound knowledge of local or regional epidemio-logical patterns of parasitic and other infectious diseases and a high index of suspicion contribute greatly to the avoidance of diagnostic error.

DIAGNOSIS

A definitive diagnosis is made by the direct visual demonstration of the eggs of the parasite in body excretions or secretions, overwhelmingly stool (Figures 72.13–72.16) and urine; or alternatively in material from rectal biopsy or biopsies from liver or surgically removed tissue. A sensitive direct diagnosis can also be made by hatching tests in which swimming miracidia originating from excreted eggs can be seen with the naked eye. This is an indication beyond doubt that the eggs are viable and have originated from living fertilized female schistosomes.

A recent addition to direct diagnostic techniques is the detection of schistosome antigens in serum or urine, i.e. circulating anodic antigen (CAA) and circulating cathodic antigen (CCA). These two glycoprotein circulating antigens associated with the gut of the adult worm are well characterized, are genus specific and their presence indicates active infection in cases of *S. mansoni, S. haematobium* or *S. intercalatum* infection. They are detected by enzyme immunoassay and have virtually 100% speci-

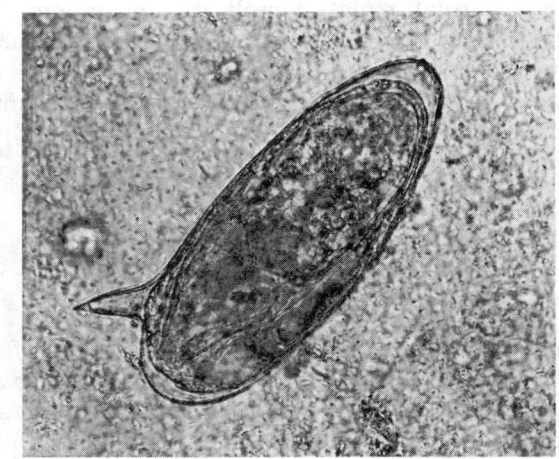
Figure 72.14   Egg of *S. mansoni.* (Courtesy of O. D. Standen.)

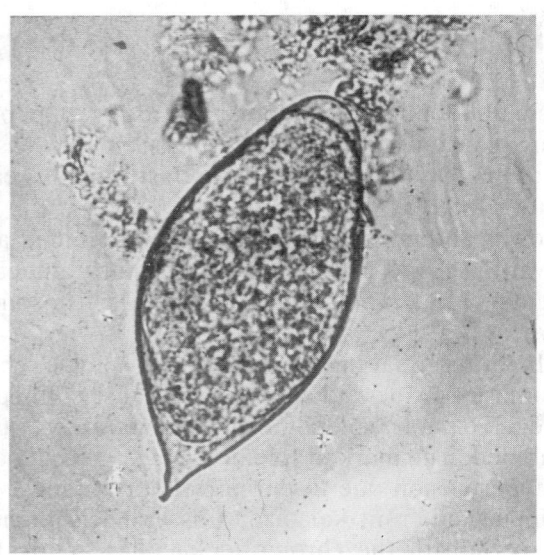
Figure 72.13   Egg of *S. haematobium.* (Courtesy of WTIM.)

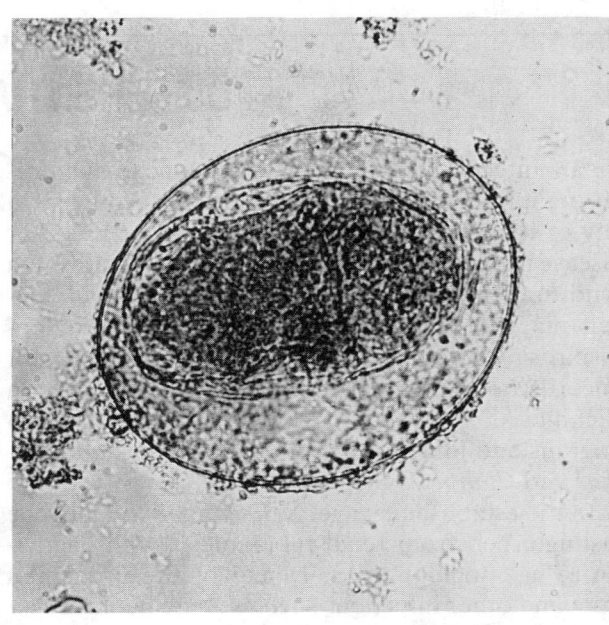
Figure 72.15   Egg of *S. japonicum.* (Courtesy of WTIM.)

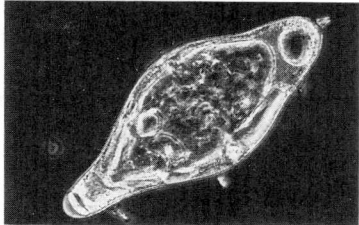

Figure 72.16   Egg of *S. intercalatum*. (Courtesy of V. R. Southgate.)

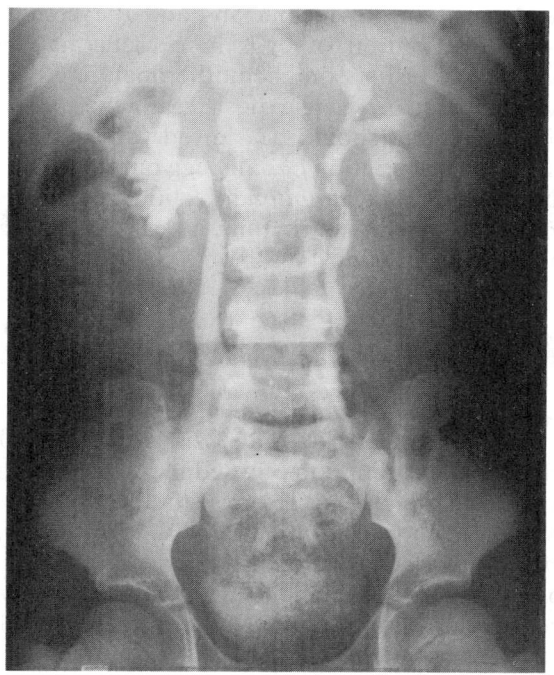

Figure 72.18   Dilated ureters, calcified bladder and hydronephrosis caused by *Schistosoma* infection. (Courtesy of D. M. Forsyth.)

DIRECT DIAGNOSTIC TECHNIQUES

PARASITOLOGICAL DIAGNOSIS

No single optimal technique applicable to all situations exists. Most of the current techniques can be interpreted qualitatively or quantitatively depending on the diagnostic setting. Quantitative techniques are virtually always used in research, in experimental chemotherapy and clinical trials, in epidemiological surveys and in evaluation of intervention measures.

In an individual clinical setting it is customary to examine repeated specimens of excreta parasitologically (in practice, three) before declaring a patient 'negative'. Confirmation of a diagnosis by hatching tests demonstrates that the eggs are viable and an active infection exists; dead eggs only in the excreta are not an indication for chemotherapy.

EGG COUNTING

The direct demonstration of eggs provides an enormous advantage over all other diagnostic techniques since specificity is obviously maximal, yet a slavish belief in the absolute virtues of quantitative diagnosis is scarcely justified. Egg counts are merely indirect estimates of worm load; they vary in time

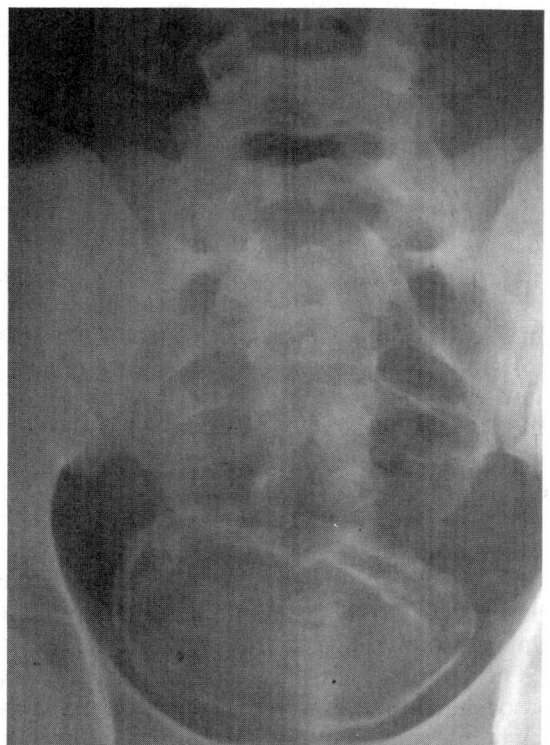

Figure 72.17   Calcification of the bladder in late *S. haematobium* infection.

ficity and very high sensitivity. Patently they offer new possibilities for epidemiological and postchemotherapeutic monitoring but are expensive, are 'high technology', need complex reagents and require standardization and controlled trials before operational use in control programmes. At present they are used at the research level in individual patients or in small groups.[144–148]

All other methods of diagnosis, be they clinical, immunological, radiological (Figures 72.17 and 72.18) or endoscopic without biopsy, are essentially indirect.

and place and with technicians and the assumed Poisson distribution of eggs in excreta may not hold.[149] Conclusions on chemotherapeutic efficacy of drugs based on single post-treatment examinations of excreta should be viewed with cynicism; coefficients of variation of daily egg output are very high and, in *S. haematobium* infections, egg output is subject to a circadian rhythm; it peaks and is least variable from 10.00 to 14.00 hours.

DIAGNOSIS OF *S. HAEMATOBIUM* INFECTION

Ova of *S. haematobium* are usually detected easily in the urine. A qualitative diagnosis is made by the microscopic examination of a sedimented or centrifuged urine specimen. Exercise before specimen collection is unnecessary. Eggs of *S. mansoni* or *S. intercalatum* are found not infrequently in the urine. In one series, 15% of patients with a sole *S. mansoni* infection had 'mansonuria', but this is unusually high.[150]

Nowadays, filtration techniques, giving a quantitative estimation of egg excretion, have tended to replace simple sedimentation and/or centrifugation and are certainly the 'norm' in epidemiological studies. Currently urine samples are passed through filter paper,[151,152] polycarbonate[153,154] or a polyamide material[155,156] by a variety of syringes or pumps. The principle common to all is that eggs are retained on the filter and can be counted with or without staining. Many different stains are in use; preferences are largely personal; eggs may be 'stored' in preservative or a preservative–stain mixture.[152] As with all techniques, problems arise during field usage. False epidemiological results may occur from loss of eggs during bulk transport of dried filter papers,[157] and, in a small but significant proportion, eggs are retained on polyamide filters (Nytrel) even after careful washing in attempts to reuse them. As a general rule, any filter should be used once only and then discarded.

DIAGNOSIS OF INTESTINAL DWELLING SCHISTOSOMES

In infections with *S. mansoni*, *S. japonicum*, *S. mekongi* and *S. intercalatum*, where eggs are excreted in the faeces, simple comminution of the stool and sedimentation before microscopy is a reliable diagnostic technique. Direct saline microscopy of stool has a very low diagnostic sensitivity due to the small size of the faecal sample examined.

Many concentration techniques have been described.[158–162] All involve removal of fat, faecal debris and mucus and, of necessity, require more sophisticated laboratory facilities. They find their optimal use in the detection of 'light' infections where egg excretion is at a low intensity or is intermittent. In South Africa a popular and efficient technique for egg recovery from stools in both medical and veterinary practice is based on twin nylon gauze filters and the use of water pressure to break up faecal material. Claims of high sensitivity have been advanced.[163]

Nowadays, the cellophane thick faecal smear, the Kato technique or one of its numerous modifications,[164,165] has become a standard diagnostic tool in both clinical and epidemiological studies. Essentially a semiconcentration–clearing–staining process, it is a simple microscopic method examining 20–50 mg of stool, depending on the template used, and is quantitative, thus permitting international comparisons of data. It can be performed in the field and can be used at a primary health care level. The prepared slide takes some time to clear; this varies with ambient temperature and humidity. Slides can be stored for at least 1 week, often longer, the time again being variable so that assessments of technicians' counts can be incorporated into a quality control system. A further advantage lies in its use in the diagnosis and counting of eggs of many intestinal nematodes or cestodes, e.g. *Ascaris lumbricoides*, *Trichuris trichuria*, *Taenia* spp. and hookworms, although to assess hookworm loads counts must be made 15–30 minutes after slide preparation because eggs of hookworm disappear due to solution from the Kato slides after this period and assessment is useless after an hour. The exact details of the procedure must be calibrated for each working location, taking into account environmental variables, resources and local skills. Disadvantages of the Kato technique are that watery or diarrhoeal stools cannot be processed and dietary habits may result in hard fibrous stools that are difficult to process. Additionally, there is a definite limit of sensibility of 50–100 eggs per gram of stool detectable by a single smear.

A variant of a thick smear technique for *S. mansoni* infections is the glass sandwich technique[166,167] which has been used widely in the Sudan and Malawi. The technique requires no reagents and it has been suggested it is more cost-effective than other similar quantitative methods. A small-scale experiment showed no significant differences in egg recoveries or in methods, readers or slides prepared from the same stool specimens and processed by either the Kato or the glass sandwich technique.[168] Further comparisons on a larger scale are needed and one disadvantage of this technique is limited to use in restricted endemic areas; hence comparison of findings with other endemic areas is, at present, invalid.

MIRACIDIAL HATCHING

Described originally by Fulleborn in 1921,[169] and in routine use in biological and experimental chemotherapeutic studies for decades, it is surprising that more attention has not been given to this technique in clinical medicine since hatching is generally accepted as the most sensitive of all parasitological diagnostic methods in all forms of schistosomiasis. It remains essential for adequate post-treatment evaluation in clinical trials. However, adaptation to field studies has been uncommon because standardization and quantification are more difficult than in those techniques where eggs can be simply counted. Yet is it salutary to recall that diagnosis and follow-up of treated cases in the huge Chinese control programmes of the 1960s and 1970s were based on the use of a 'nylon network running water sedimentation technique'—essentially a field-adapted hatching process.[170,171]

The relative ease of isolation of eggs from urine led to many more attempts to quantify hatching procedures in *S. haematobium* than in *S. mansoni* infections. As a rough estimate of the numbers of hatchable eggs, the miracidiascope was used as a macroscopic technique routinely for surveys in Southern Africa.[172,173,174] More sensitive and accurate hatching techniques have followed[175,176] and further refinements are appearing;[177,178,179] undoubtedly the use of 'wet' preparations has complicated field standardization but hatching retains its primacy as the most sensitive tool in *S. haematobium* infections.

In *S. mansoni* infection, many variants of hatching techniques exist, some semiquantitative, all possessing high sensitivity.[180,181,182] In *S. japonicum* endemic areas in China, miracidial hatching is widely used for both epidemiological surveys and as indictors of parasitological cure after chemotherapy.[227]

RECTAL BIOPSY

Used for decades as a simple direct diagnostic technique at the individual clinical level, rectal biopsy may be employed in addition to faecal examination and provides an effective way of visualizing eggs. Small biopsy specimens of mucosa are soaked in water and examined microscopically as a crush preparation. In the intestinal dwelling species, egg viability can often be determined by observation of flame cell or miracidial movement within the eggshell. Biopsies may be taken from rectal valves via a crocodile forceps or, a much simpler procedure, with a curette and rectoscope: the mucosa is pulled over the end of the rectoscope and cut off with the curette.[180]

Ova of *S. haematobium* in rectal snips are usually non-viable and black.

In Brazil, the oogram technique (a quantitative rectal biopsy with division of eggs into developmental stages) is commonly used. If an oogram is used in addition to faecal examination in an assessment of the effects of antischistosomal drugs, it can be confidently predicted that estimates of 'cure rates' based solely on excretal examination will be considerably reduced.[183]

OTHER BIOPSY SITES

As expected, schistosome ova are frequently found in other biopsy locations, e.g. liver, bladder, cervix, vagina, perineum and skin, and indications for a biopsy of such sites lie at the individual clinical level.

INDIRECT DIAGNOSTIC TECHNIQUES

A high index of epidemiological suspicion with appropriate physical or radiological signs, seroimmunological assessment of antibody levels by a variety of assays or, in *S. haematobium* infections, the detection of red blood cells and protein in the urine in subjects in endemic areas, all remain indirect diagnostic techniques.

CHEMICAL REAGENT STRIPS

Indirect diagnostic techniques are used most frequently in *S. haematobium* infections in which the application of chemical reagent strips (CRS) in a semiquantitative fashion is highly useful as a direct diagnostic surrogate in endemic areas of the disease where a positive result is interpreted as indicating an active infection.

Reagent strips in current use have ranges of sensitivity of 5–15 red blood cells per microlitre and 0.015–0.03 mg of haemoglobin per 100 ml urine. They use a peroxide compound and orthotolidine as a chromogen. The colour distinction between negative and the first level of reactivity on the strips is well defined, and in the presence of blood the colour indicators show distinct changes from yellow or pale orange to green or blue.[184] False-positive reactions occur in myoglobinuria and in the presence of bacterial peroxidases resulting from heavy bacteriuria, and inhibition of the reactions may occur if urinary ascorbic acid levels exceed 10 mg/100 ml urine.

CRS measuring levels of proteinuria semiquantitatively use tetrabromophthalein ethylester with a buffer. The colour discrimination between negative and the first level of proteinura is, however, not well defined. Precise assessment of colour change from yellow–green to green–blue is difficult. False positives occur in alkaline urines or when quinine or a quinine derivative is present. False negatives have occurred in strongly acid urines with Bence Jones proteinuria or urines containing predominantly γ-globulin.

Many experiences of the use of CRS in endemic areas of S. haematobium[185–188] have confirmed the consistent and significant correlation between reagent strip reactions indicating haematuria and/or proteinuria and increasing intensity of egg output.

Good predictive values resulting from high sensitivity and specificity emphasize the limitations of conventional single microscopic examinations at very low egg output levels and confirm the validity of CRS in detecting those with a 'high' egg output, i.e. over 50 eggs/10 ml urine in this case.[189] CRS can be used in areas of both high and low transmission patterns and find an optimal use in the detection of those with 'heavy' infections, a priority for chemotherapy. The use of CRS can be expected to increase at primary health care level in programmes of morbidity control in S. haematobium.

IMMUNODIAGNOSIS

Serodiagnostic techniques are used for the detection of either specific antibodies or genus-specific antigens.

Antibodies to adult worm, schistosomular, cercarial or egg antigens are detected by a multiplicity of procedures including various forms of enzyme linked immunosorbent assay (ELISA), radioimmunoassay (RIA), indirect immunofluorescence test (IFAT), gel precipitation techniques (GPT), indirect haemagglutination (IHA), latex agglutination (LAT) and circumoval precipitin tests (COPT), which have superseded the older Cercarienhüllen reactions (CHR) and complement fixation tests (CFT).

In general, antibody detection techniques have been less useful to the practising physician and epidemiologist than the techniques of direct parasitological diagnosis. Their basic disadvantage is that they all point to past exposure to mammalian, or in rare instances, avian schistosomes without indicating the duration, activity or quantum of infection. Further disadvantages are an absence of globally agreed criteria of performance and standards, the necessity for expensive equipment, costly or labile reagents, the need for skilled technical personnel and the slow diminution of specific antibody level after treatment, thus reducing their value as a

marker of chemotherapeutic success. Each laboratory in endemic or non-endemic areas has tended to use its own particular antigen and assay procedure. WHO has conducted several collaborative studies[190,191] in attempts to improve the technology and to standardize both antigens and procedures. Agreement is not yet in sight. A most useful summary of the current position has been given.[192]

In striking contrast very real advances have been made in antigen detection. Improvements in the production of monoclonal antibodies led to the new diagnostic tests of CAA and CCA detection in serum and urine. These are discussed above.

RADIOLOGY

As a form of indirect diagnosis, various radiological procedures for detecting morbidity from a schistosome infection have long been in use in hospital practice and have included plain abdominal radiographs to detect bladder calcification, intravenous pyelography to detect bladder and ureteral changes or obstructive uropathy, isotope renography, computerized tomography for cerebral schistosomiasis, myelography for suspected cord damage and portal venography for hepatosplenic schistosomiasis with portal venous hypertensive changes. Complications such as upper gastrointestinal bleeding may require the use of specialized techniques, including upper abdominal ultrasonography, splenoportography and nuclear isotopic studies of hepatic blood flow. The indications for a particular investigation lie at the individual patient level and are the responsibility of the physician in charge.

ULTRASONOGRAPHY

Major changes in the diagnostic approach in individual patients and in the epidemiological assessment of schistosomal morbidity in communities have occurred in parallel with the introduction and expanded use of ultrasonography.

The technique is non-invasive, simple, portable, has no biological hazard to the patient or the operator and either complements or is an alternative diagnostic measure to many invasive techniques. With the exception of hydroureter, ureteral calculi and bladder calcification, it has, in comparison with other diagnostic procedures, high specificity and sensitivity, is superior to physical examination in measuring liver and spleen size and is the best technique for grading schistosomal periportal fibrosis, portal hypertension, hydronephrosis, urinary bladder wall lesions and renal and bladder stones.[193] A recent extensive review of technical and clinical experience is available.[194]

Following field use of portable ultrasonography, particularly in Egypt where it is widely used, an agreed protocol for standardized investigations and methods of reporting was produced by WHO.[195]

It has been demonstrated in community studies that sonographic lesions of periportal fibrosis in *S. mansoni*, with thickening of portal tracts and portal vein walls, correlated with the number of eggs in the stool.[196] Fine measurements of hepatic pathology are possible and are superior to clinical examination.[197] Where available, ultrasonography should replace clinical grading and physical examination as a preferred method of assessing liver and spleen size.[197]

The sonographic patterns of schistosomal hepatic fibrosis are characteristic and are distinct from those of other hepatic diseases. Schistosomiasis can now be distinguished from cirrhosis with confidence.[198]

Additionally, an ultrasonographic scoring system is of clinical use in the prediction both of oesophageal varices and the likelihood of bleeding from them.[199]

An interesting outcome of ultrasonographic studies has been the demonstration that *S. haematobium* can cause mild degrees of schistosomal periportal fibrosis in an area where *S. mansoni* does not exist;[101] this confirms an observation, first made in 1974 in upper Egypt, that hepatosplenic disease caused by *S. haematobium* is a distinct entity.[100]

The use of abdominal ultrasonography in the measurement of the decrease in morbidity produced by population-based chemotherapy programmes can be expected to grow dramatically.

TREATMENT

In no other parasitic diseases have there been such major advances in chemotherapy as have occurred since the 1960s in the treatment of schistosomiasis. The introduction and widespread use, at both the individual patient level and in large-scale community-based operations, of the current highly effective, orally administered, well-tolerated antischistosomal drugs have provided physicians, epidemiologists and public health practitioners with therapeutic opportunities not in existence at the end of the 1960s.

The primary objective of chemotherapy is the cure of the individual patient by eradication of the infection (or the infection with two species) from which he or she suffers. Cure leads to cessation of egg deposition, the pathogenic agent in the tissues, and this prevents additional organ damage; existing lesions will, in the vast majority of cases, regress. In large scale community-based chemotherapy, where compromises on dosage may have to be made to ensure a viable delivery system and optimal population coverage, the main aim is to reduce the community egg load by the greatest amount possible; individual cure may or may not occur; the community benefits as a whole by the block of the egg–miracidium–snail stage of the biological cycle, which reduces transmission by minimizing excretal pollution of water supplies and thus diminishes cercarial contamination of human water contact sites; of even greater importance is the reduction of community morbidity caused by schistosomiasis; nowa-

days this can be measured and the success of interventions can be evaluated accurately.

Antischistosomal drugs can be divided into two categories:

1. The one drug effective against all species of schistosome infecting man, praziquantel.
2. The monospecific drugs effective against only one species of schistosome, i.e. oxamniquine, effective only against *S. mansoni*, and metriphonate, used solely in *S. haematobium* infections. (Although metriphonate does in fact have some activity against *S. japonicum* and *S. mansoni*, it is not used in their treatment and conventionally is termed a monospecific antischistosomal drug).

These three antischistosomal compounds are all on the WHO List of Essential Drugs and much experience has been accumulated in their large-scale use in recent years. The older drugs, e.g. antimonials, niridazole, hycanthone, can be regarded as defunct.

PRAZIQUANTEL

The drug of choice, it is effective against all schistosome species occurring in man. It is also effective in the other snail-borne trematode infections, clonorchiasis, paragonimiasis and opisthorciasis, and in infections due to the adult cestodes, *Taenia solium*, *T. saginata*, *Hymenolepis nana* and *Diphylloboth-*

rium spp. It is active against the secondary larval stages of *T. solium* in man, dermal cysticercosis and neurocysticercosis, but has little or no effect in ocular cysticercosis. It is not active in the human secondary larval infections of *Echinococcus* spp. and it is generally ineffective in *Fasciola hepatica* infections. There is no therapeutic activity in protozoan or nematode infections, including the filariae.

Praziquantel is available as 600 mg tablets Biltricide (Bayer AG), Distocide (Shin Poong Pharmaceutical Co. Ltd); as Cysticide (E. Merck, 500 mg); as Cesol or Cestox (E. Merck, 150 mg); and as Cestocide (Shin Poong Pharmaceutical Co. Ltd., 150 mg). In the People's Republic of China, the drug is produced as a 200 mg tablet named Pyquiton for use within the country. Since the expiry of the patent, other suppliers have become available.

Although dosage is standardized in large-scale epidemiologically-based morbidity control programmes, there is frequently a variation in dose in the treatment of an individual patient.

In field programmes, a single oral dose of 40 mg/kg is effective in *S. haematobium*, *S. mansoni* and *S. intercalatum* infections.

For *S. japonicum* and *S. mekongi* infections either three doses each of 20 mg/kg given at 4-hourly intervals or two doses each of 30 mg/kg given at 4- or 6-hourly intervals is used, i.e. a total dose of 60 mg/kg. Although the usual total dose of *S. mekongi* is 60 mg/kg there is evidence that repeated treatment at this dose level may be necessary for cure of this species.[200–203]

For treatment of individual patients with heavy infections by *S. mansoni* (over 800 eggs per gram of stool) a total dose of 50 or 60 mg/kg, given in two equal doses 4–6 hours apart, may be needed. Single doses are best given after food and, if possible, in the evening.

Patient tolerance is extremely good and virtually all trials have confirmed the absence of toxicity in the liver, kidney, haemopoetic or other body organs and functions. Yet minor side-effects do occur: those related to the gastrointestinal tract are epigastric or generalized abdominal pain or discomfort, nausea, rarely vomiting, anorexia and loose stools. These side-effects are mild, transient, and even if their incidence is high, rarely if ever require medication. A rare event in patients heavily infected with *S. mansoni* or *S. japonicum* is the passage of blood in the stools after praziquantel treatment. The explanation is unknown; it occurs a few hours after dosage but recovery is rapid without clinical sequelae.

Headache and dizziness may be encountered as may fever, fatigue, pruritus or a transient skin eruption, none of which is serious nor lasting. Side-effects in field treatments tend to be more frequent in foci of intense transmission but should not be used as an argument for reduction of dose.

'Cure' rates are high; it can be expected that with the appropriate dose they will be around 80% in small groups. However, in large-scale field operations where supervision is of necessity less stringent and where compliance may be difficult to ensure, then rates of about 50% will be found when a single oral dose of 40 mg/kg is used; egg reduction in the excreta of those not cured should exceed 90% of pretreatment output.

METRIPHONATE

Metriphonate is an organophosphorus compound used in the treatment of *S. haematobium* infection. It has some activity against *S. mansoni*, *S. japonicum*, various intestinal nematodes, onchocerciasis and both dermal and cerebral cysticercosis but is never normally given in the treatment of these parasitic infections in man. The sole indication is in the treatment of *S. haematobium* infection.

Both metriphonate and trichlorfon, an insecticidal formulation of the same substance, act as prodrugs to form the direct acetylcholinesterase inhibitor dichlorvos, which is the active ingredient.

Despite early concerns on toxicity, a large toxicological literature has been built up since the 1950s when the compound was first used as an agricultural insecticide, and safety in man is firmly established. The mechanism of action is complex and somewhat obscure. It is available as a white scored tablet containing 100 mg of active substance (Bilarcil; Bayer AG).

The standard dose is 7.5 or 10.0 mg/kg body weight, given in three oral doses at an interval of 14 days, i.e. a total dose of 22.5 or 30.0 mg/kg. Which dose is preferred depends on the cure rates obtained in local experience of its use. When egg output is measured quantitatively the cure rates on these regimens are inversely proportional to the pretreatment intensity of infection and vary from 50 to 90% in different population samples with *S. haematobium* infection. Some low intensity infections are cured after one or two doses and relapses are uncommon.[204,205]

In the late 1970s and early 1980s, after the first major use of metriphonate in the control of epidemic urinary schistosomiasis on Lake Volta, Ghana, where repetitive population-based chemotherapy was given to infected patients annually for 5 years,[206] numerous large-scale chemotherapeutic programmes for control of *S. haematobium* were implemented on the African continent. These programmes of very large-scale drug administration constituted a unique phenomenon in schistosomiasis morbidity control at that time and provided evidence of the safety of metriphonate (dichlorvos) in human medicine. Modest therapeutic effects on hookworm infections, when these coexist with schistosomiasis, offer a useful peripheral gain.

Patient tolerance to metriphonate is extremely good; like other organophosphorus compounds it inactivates the enzyme destroying acetylcholine, thus allowing the chemical neurotransmitter to persist. Cholinergic symptoms (fatigue, muscle weakness, tremor, sweating, abdominal colic, nausea and vomiting, diarrhoea and bronchospasm) are extremely rare during treatment. If they do occur their severity is mild and spontaneous disappearance in a few hours is the general rule. No treatment is necessary. A constant effect of metriphonate treatment is depression of acetylcholinesterases in erythrocytes and plasma. This is not correlated with the incidence or severity of side-effects and appears to be an inescapable pharmacological adjuvant effect. There is no need in normal clinical practice to undertake pretreatment acetylcholinesterase measurements but when patients are exposed to other anticholinergic agents, e.g. organophosphorus sprays in malaria campaigns, which may produce a cumulative lowering effect on the enzyme, then it would be a wise precaution to check the pretreatment enzyme level.

Metriphonate is a cheap and useful treatment for *S. haematobium* infection. It can be used in outpatients and in small field programmes where a good delivery system exists. Although limited by a dosage system extending over 1 month, which inevitably leads to many uncompleted treatments, and also tending to be replaced by praziquantel for ease of delivery, it remains a safe, well-tolerated drug of moderate therapeutic efficacy.

OXAMNIQUINE

A tetrahydroquinoline compound distantly related to hycanthone, oxamniquine is effective against *S. mansoni*. In animal models it proved inactive against *S. japonicum* and early trials in man showed virtually no activity against *S. haematobium* or *S. mattheei*.

In the animal studies one peculiarity was that male worms proved more susceptible than female worms. Egg laying by surviving females ceased in the absence of males after successful treatment, thus removing the basic pathogenetic mechanism in *S. mansoni*.[207,208]

Oxamniquine is available as capsules of 250 mg or as a syrup containing 50 mg/ml and is marketed as Mansil in South America or Vansil in Africa. In the USA, capsules have a yellow body marked PFIZER 641 with a dark green cap marked VANSIL. Shelf-lives are 5 years for capsules and 3 years for the syrup.

Oxamniquine is used in all stages, from acute toxaemic to chronic and complicated *S. mansoni* infections, with good results.

Advanced *S. mansoni* with hepatosplenomegaly, portal hypertension and/or ascites responds well and in schistosomal polyposis there are great improvements in both the associated anaemia and protein-losing enteropathy.[209,210,211]

High cure rates (60–90% in different samples) are seen after oxamniquine treatment of uncomplicated *S. mansoni* infections.

From 1975 to 1979 oxamniquine was used in a major campaign in Brazil when some five million doses were given in the field programmes with high cure and very good tolerance.[212]

The dose of oxamniquine varies with geographic origin of the *S. mansoni* infection, the age and hence the surface area of the patient. In South America, adults are given 15 mg/kg body weight as a single oral dose; in children 20 mg/kg is preferred, given in two divided portions each of 10 mg/kg with an interval of 4–6 hours between doses. If practicable, the drug should be given after food or just before sleep.

With *S. mansoni* occurring on the African continent only those strains of West African origin are given the same doses as in South America. In Egypt, Sudan and southern Africa, a total dose of 60 mg/kg body weight is used, either as 15 mg/kg twice daily for 2 days, or as 20 mg/kg once daily for 3 days. In East Africa, total doses of 30 or 40 mg/kg are given in split regimens over 1 or 2 days.

In general oxamniquine is well tolerated. There are virtually no contraindications but classes of patients exist who require close monitoring. Patients with a history of any form of epilepsy must be supervised for 48 hours after treatment since a small number of epileptiform convulsions have been reported, as have generalized seizures after the drug, fortunately without sequelae and with clinical and electroencephalographic recovery.

As with many other drugs, treatment during the first 4 months of pregnancy should not be given.

Any patient whose occupation involves care of heavy machinery or is employed in the transport industry, e.g. pilots, truckers, etc., should be placed off work for 48 hours after treatment.

Side-effects are uncommon; dizziness, drowsiness and headache are most frequent but last for some 4–6 hours only. Hallucinations and a state of excitement are very rare events. Although abdominal discomfort, vomiting and diarrhoea do occur, there is no constant statistical correlation and, in practice, adverse effects have had no influence on compliance in field programmes.

A harmless orange-red discoloration of the urine may occur but is transitory, and a syndrome of peripheral blood eosinophilia, scattered pulmonary infiltrates and increased immune complexes in serum with urinary excretion of schistosomal antigens is known in Egypt but has not been described in other locations.[213]

An eosinophilia after treatment occurs commonly and is maximal in 7–10 days; it represents a reaction to dead or dying schistosomes. Changes in hepatic enzyme levels may be seen but no constant pattern exists.

In summary, oxamniquine is a highly useful drug for treatment of all forms of *S. mansoni*, including many advanced and complicated syndromes. Resistance to oxamniquine is known in South America but is not yet a public health problem since such patients are treated successfully with praziquantel.[214]

ASSESSMENT OF CHEMOTHERAPY

Assessment of patients treated for schistosomiasis is conducted by repeated clinical observation, evaluation of symptomatic improvement and diminution or disappearance of physical, radiological, particularly ultrasonographic, and endoscopic signs.

Direct parasitological examinations of urine, stool or rectal biopsy are essential and should be performed on repeated specimens of excreta (three) at about 6–8 weeks and 4–6 months after treatment, by a selection of appropriate techniques detailed above.

Follow-up is simple if no reinfection risk is present; the explanation of the presence of viable eggs in the excreta at 4–6 months is less clear in endemic areas where transmission persists and may be due to a maturing prepatent infection unaffected by chemotherapy, a true reinfection or a therapeutic failure. It is not always easy to decide which event, or even combination of events, is responsible. Increased use of antigen detection techniques, e.g. CAA, CCA, offer real possibilities for clarification of these problems.

SPECIAL CLINICAL SYNDROMES AND TREATMENT

NEUROLOGICAL SCHISTOSOMIASIS

The efficacy and safety of modern antischistosomal drugs has led to early treatment of encephalopathies or myelopathies or other spinal cord syndromes reasonably suspected, even if not proven, to be due to schistosomiasis. This improves prognosis since cord damage in myelopathy is closely related to time of diagnosis.

An ELISA using keyhole limpet haemocyanin distinguishes between antibody responses in acute and chronic schistosomal infection[215] and CAA detection can be diagnostic where eggs are not yet excreted. These two diagnostic techniques should be used when available; unfortunately they are, as yet, restricted to certain high technology centres.

The use of corticosteroids in schistosomal myelopathy remains controversial. Laminectomy is an important intervention in acute paraplegia with spinal compression or block, or in deteriorating clinical circumstances during conservative treatment.

In *S. japonicum*, cerebral schistosomiasis should be localized with modern imaging techniques and treated with praziquantel which is safe and effective. Computerized tomography demonstrates resolution of intracerebral masses, regression of cerebral oedema and subsequent disappearance of epilepsy.[216] Appropriate neurosurgical supervision should be on hand.

ACUTE TOXAEMIC SCHISTOSOMIASIS (KATAYAMA SYNDROME)

Early diagnosis of a suspicious clinical presentation can now be made with the keyhole limpet haemocyanin antibody and CAA antigen techniques. Disputes remain whether steroids should be added to specific drug treatment with praziquantel or oxamniquine and the position has not yet been resolved. As a general principle, patients should be treated with praziquantel, which is effective in all species.

ASSOCIATED SALMONELLOSIS

The chronic bacteraemia due to *Salmonella typhi* or *S. paratyphi* is due to attachment of the bacteria to the integument or in the gut of the adult schistosome. Although clinical response to antibiotics is good, bacteraemia will recur unless the underlying schistosomiasis is treated. The therapeutic response to antischistosomal drugs is good.

ASSOCIATED HEPATITIS

Even if, in hepatosplenic schistosomiasis, there is serological or other evidence of an associated hepatitis B infection (or C, D or E), and activity of the schistosomiasis is still present, it is worthwhile treating the latter with praziquantel.

PORTAL HYPERTENSION

Chemotherapy is but one part of patient care since complications are mainly due to the mechanical obstructive pathology resulting from periportal fibrosis. Where eggs are still found in the excreta, treatment with praziquantel is indicated and gives the usual response.

GASTROINTESTINAL BLEEDING

Admission to a specialized centre is essential since that is where skills in assessment, immediate resuscitation, fibreoptic endoscopy, balloon tamponade and/or endoscopic sclerotherapy are present. The treatment of this complication is beyond the scope of the general physician and is preferably a matter for specialists in this area of intensive care. Emergency portocaval shunts have fallen into disrepute as a high proportion of operative deaths may occur and, in the survivors, there is frequently a loss of shunt patency and/or encephalopathy. A selective distal splenorenal shunt has been claimed to offer a lower haemorrhage recurrence rate and an improved survival rate.[217]

The clinical application of β-adrenergic blockade using non-selective beta blockers (e.g. propranolol) for the prevention of an initial gastrointestinal haemorrhage in either cirrhosis or portal hypertension from schistosomal periportal fibrosis is ambiguous. It is not yet clear which clinical variables are the best predictors of response to beta blockers.

In endemic rural areas the major difficulty is diagnosing the presence of oesophageal varices in the absence of a history or an actual bleed, for the necessary diagnostic facilities are not there. Thus referral to a specialized centre possessing the essential facilities is the optimal, if Elysian, form of management.

SCHISTOSOMIASIS WITHOUT EGGS

This title describes cases where no ova can be found but there exists a high index of clinical suspicion of a schistosomal infection, usually based on an epidemiological history of exposure, existing cases in fellow members of a group, an unexplained eosinophilia in a presenting suspect and a suggestive or suspicious seroimmunodiagnostic test.

In endemic areas of *S. haematobium* the presence of a positive test for microhaematuria on CRS testing is taken as indicative of infection.

Again the simplicity of use of modern drugs has clarified many difficult diagnostic situations and frequently one treats 'on suspicion alone', a practice justifiable only when exhaustive efforts to reach a parasitological or serological diagnosis have failed.

Detailed monographs on the properties of antischistosomal drugs and their use in clinical and field practice have been produced.[218–221]

PREVENTION AND CONTROL

Both prevention and control depend on an area-specific, species-specific and epidemiologically-specific mixture of intervention methods. The characteristics of endemic areas, the transmission patterns, the infecting parasite species and strains, the intermediate snail host(s) and the behavioural customs of the human communities and their socio-economic backgrounds all contribute a multiplicity of interactions to produce a vast mosaic of transmission and epidemiological pictures. An accurate diagnosis of all of these variables, quantitative when possible, is necessary before entering into prevention and control programmes. The aims of both prevention and control are:

1. The reduction in the number of eggs excreted from infected people reaching waters which harbour the intermediate snail hosts; this is dependent on health education, the provision and use of adequate sanitary facilities and specific antischistosomal chemotherapy for infected individuals and communities.
2. The reduction in the probability of miracidial/snail contact; this relies on all factors in (1),

appropriate modifications of the aquatic environment and reduction of intermediate snail host numbers by application of chemical molluscicides or use of suitable biological control means.

3. The reduction of cercarial densities, which will occur as a result of all the preceding actions but overwhelmingly from the employment of molluscicides.

4. The reduction of the probability of cercariae locating a definitive host, again due to the cumulative effects of all of the preceding factors plus the reduction of human water contact with infected water bodies by the provision of adequate domestic or peridomestic water supplies and the substitution of safe recreational water sites.

5. The reduction of the longevity of the adult worms in the host, a function of chemotherapy.

Multiple overlaps are obvious in these processes and conventionally stress in 'prevention' is directed towards health education and the provision of adequate sanitation and water supplies supplemented by environmental improvements. 'Control' is dominated by chemotherapy and molluscicides. Yet integration of these interventions is essential for success and each endemic focus or region requires an individual clinicoepidemiological, zoogeographic, sociological and environmental approach based on the common principles listed above.

In the past, emphasis was given to 'transmission control', largely through repetitive mollusciciding. This was expensive; molluscicides did not achieve total kills of snails and their eggs in operationally difficult terrains and the techniques require skilled biologists and technical personnel. Epidemiological extrapolation of the successes of modern chemotherapy and the employment of simple low-cost diagnostic techniques led inevitably to a reappraisal of the strategy and tactics of control. Many control operations implemented through a single disease control mechanism are simply beyond the financial and human resources of the great majority of endemic countries, as was the case with malaria eradication. A strategy of schistosomiasis control has now evolved which stresses repetitive population-based chemotherapy, aimed at 'morbidity control' rather than 'transmission control'. It is implemented through delivery systems by the peripheral health care workers in the primary health care system adopted by all countries and many successes have been documented which have been evaluated by epidemiological, parasitological and ultrasonographic tools. However, the naive supposition that chemotherapy alone will provide the definitive answer to schistosomiasis control is not substantiated. In such a multifaceted socioeconomic, biological and clinical syndrome, 'control' needs population-based chemotherapy as a spearhead but also needs to be reinforced by such snail control measures as required by epidemiological criteria. Reinfection is a risk that is ever present against a backcloth of unchanging socioeconomic conditions since the constraints of achieving total population coverage with drugs and the less than absolute cure rates mean that egg deposition continues, albeit at a much lower level, and therefore transmission persists.

Add to this the difficulties in environmental improvement, the provision of sanitation and water supplies and the deployment of continuing health education, and the 'control' of schistosomiasis implying a permanent cessation of transmission is clearly a Herculean task. Patently the constraining factors are political and economic and not technical.

A summary of the current rationale for control and data on its employment are provided in the last two reports of the WHO Expert Committee.[2,222]

MOLLUSCICIDING

The use of molluscicides in the control of schistosomiasis is a highly specialized field. Synthetic molluscicides are virtually restricted nowadays to one compound, niclosamide (Bayluscide, Bayer AG), and although other chemicals lethal to snails exist, their practical use is minimal. Although many molluscicides of plant origin are known,[223] the eventual outlook for the isolation, characterization, toxicological screening, large-scale production and distribution of their active ingredients for use in endemic countries is blurred.

A useful specialist text on indications, technical use, application in different habitats and evaluation of molluscicides has been produced by WHO.[224]

Molluscicides will continue in use as one of the integral specific control tools but techniques have changed markedly from the 'blanket application' to a much more focused approach guided by the epidemiological criteria of high prevalence, high intensity and rapidity of reinfection rates in any particular focus or area of infection.

VACCINES AND VACCINATION

The limitations of current control measures have changed the old aims of 'transmission control', with implied eradication after cessation of transmission, to the current strategy of 'morbidity control', with an uncertain diminution of transmission but recognition that some residual will continue.

These factors, added to the virtually unchanging

socioeconomic circumstances in many endemic countries and added to the recent explosion of new techniques in biotechnology, led to the huge rise in research aimed at the production of vaccines against schistosomiasis or the pathology produced. While advances in molecular biology have led to the identification and characterization of an impressive number of schistosome antigens, progress in human vaccination studies has lagged behind those in animal models. One view emerging is that a vaccine, even with a long-term protective effect, would probably be insufficient as a sole control mechanism but would need to be given in conjunction with chemotherapy and other control methods.[69]

The antigenic identities of the biologically active molecules currently selected as candidates for schistosomal vaccine development are: a variant of the isoenzyme glutathione *S*-transferase (Sm28 GST);

paramyosin (Sm97); an irradiation-associated vaccine antigen (IrV-5) (both muscle proteins); the glycolytic enzyme triose-phosphate isomerase (TPI); and the membrane antigen Sm23 and a fatty acid binding protein (FABP)-14 (Sm14).[225,226]

A vaccine programme of sequential steps of preclinical development, independent testing of antigens, human correlate studies, scale-up and subsequent field trials has been initiated by WHO/TDR.[226] There remain, however, many unanswered questions on the immunology of schistosomiasis and on the mechanisms of protection when it exists, and there lie ahead formidable challenges on large-scale antigen production and the improvement of the current modest levels of protection achieved to date.

It will be some years before vaccines in man evolve from the present enthusiastic hope to realistic practical usage in the field.

REFERENCES

1 Rollinson D & Southgate V R. The genus *Schistosoma:* a taxonomic appraisal. In Rollinson D & Simpson A J G (eds) *The Biology of Schistosomes. From Genes to Latrines.* London: Academic Press, 1987:1–4.

2 World Health Organization. The control of schistosomiasis. *WHO Tech Rep Ser* 1985; 728:1–49.

3 Farooq M. Historical development. In *Epidemiology and Control of Schistosomiasis (Bilharziasis).* Basel: Karger, 1973:2.

4 Ruffer M A. Note on the presence of *Bilharzia haematobia* in Egyptian mummies of the 20th dynasty 1220–1000 BC. *BMJ* 1910; 2557,i:16.

5 Larrey D J. (Haematurie) *Mémoires de Chirurgie Militaire et Campagnes.* Paris: Smith, 1812–1817.

6 Ein Beitrag zur Helminothographia Lumana, aus brieflichen Mitteldungen des Dr Bilharz in Cairo. *Z Wiss Zool* 1853; 4:59–62. English translation in Kean B H, Mott K E and Russel A J (eds) *Tropical Medicine and Parasitology*, vol. 2. Ithaca: Cornell University Press, 1978:475.

7 Manson P. Report of a case of bilharzia from the west Indies. *BMJ* 1902; ii:1894–1895.

8 Leiper R T. *Researches on Egyptian Bilharziosis.* (A report to the War Office on the Results of the Bilharzia Mission in Egypt, 1915). 1918. London: John Bale Sons and Danielson, 1918: 1–140. Reprinted from *J R Army Med Corps* 1915; XXV:1,147, 253; 1916; XXVII:171; 1918; XXX:235.

9 Silva M. Piraja da. La schistosomose à Bahia. *Arch Parasitol* 1908; 13:231–302. Contribution to the study of schistosomiasis in Bahia, Brazil (English

translation of original paper). *J Trop Med Hyg* 1909; 12:159–164.

10 Soto V R. *Naturateza de la disenteria en Caracas.* Doctoral thesis, no. 63, 1906.

11 Fujii Y. *Chugai Iji Shimpo* 1847; 691:55 (in Japanese).

12 Katsurada, F. *Schistosomum japonicum*, a new parasite of man by which an endemic disease in various areas of Japan is caused. *Annot Zool Japan* 1904; 5:146–160.

13 Miyagaawa Y. *Mitte Med Fak Univ Tokyo* 1913; 1383;1–3 (in Japanese).

14 Miyairi K & Suzuki M. *Tokyo Iji Shinshi* 1913; 1386:1 (in Japanese).

15 Miyairi K & Suzuki M. *Mitte Med Fak Kais Univ Kyushu (Fukuoka)* 1914; 1:187.

16 Leiper R T & Atkinson E L. Observations on the spread of Asiatic Schistosomiasis. *Chin Med J* 1915; 29:143–149.

17 Logan O T. Three cases of infection with *Schistosoma japonicum* in Chinese subjects. *J Trop Med Hyg* 1906; 9:294–296.

18 Woolley P G. The occurrence of schistosomiasis japonicum vel cattoi in the Phillipine islands. *Philippine J Sci* 1906; 1:83–90.

19 Brug S L & Tesch J W. Parasitic worm infestations in inhabitants around Lake Lindoe, Celebes. *Geneeskd T Ned Ind* 1937; 77:2151–2158.

20 Faust E C & Meleney H E. Studies on schistosomiasis japonica. With a supplement on the molluscan hosts of the human blood fluke in China and Japan, and species liable to be confused with them, by Nelson Anandale. *Am J Hyg* (Monogr Ser) 1924; 3:1–339.

21 Tubangui M A. The molluscan intermediate host in the Philippines of the oriental blood fluke *Schistosoma japonicum. Phillipine J Sci* 1932; 49:295–304.

22 Chesterman C C. Note sur la bilharziose dans la region de Stanleyville (Congo belge). *Ann Soc Belg Méd Trop* 1923; 3:73.

23 Fisher A C. A study of the schistosomiasis of the Stanleyville district of the Belgian Congo. *Trans R Soc Trop Med Hyg* 1934; 28:277–306.

24 Voge M, Bruckner D & Bruce J I. *Schistosoma mekongi* sp. n. from man and animals compared with four geographic strains of *Schistosoma japonicum. J. Parasitol* 1978; 64:577–584.

25 Liang Y S & Kitikoon V. Susceptibility of *Lithoglyphopsis aperta* to *Schistosoma mekongi* and *Schistosoma japonicum.* In Bruce J I, Sornmani S, Asch H L & Crawford K A (eds) The Mekong Schistosome. *Malacol Rev* 1980; supplement 2:53–60.

26 Bruce J I, Sornmani S, Asch H L & Crawford K A (eds) The Mekong Schistosome. *Malacol Rev* 1980; supplement 2:282.

27 Doumenge J P, Mott K E, Cheung C et al. *Atlas de la Répartition Mondiale des Schistosomiases* (Atlas of the global distribution of schistosomiasis). Talence, CEGET-CRNS, Geneva, WHO; Talence, PUB 1987; 400.

28 Gadgie R K & Shah S N. Human schistosomiasis in India. Discovery of an endemic focus in the Bombay State. *Indian J Med Sci* 1952; 6:760–763.

29 Sathe B D, Mukerji S, Gaitonde B B & Renapurkar D M. Reinvestigation of an old focus of schistosomiasis in Gimvi village, District Ratnagiri, in Maharashtra State, India. *Bull Haffkine Inst* 1981; 9:34–37.

30 World Health Organization. Assessment of the risk of introduction of schistosomiasis in water resources development projects and a survey of schistosomiasis in Gimvi, Ratnagiri District, Maharashtra State, India. A report of a joint mission. British Museum (Natural History), Haffkine Institute, Maharashtra State Directorate of Health, National Institute of Communicable Diseases, World Bank, World Health Organization; 13–22 November 1985. *Weekly Epidemiol Rec* 1985; 60:43.

31 Davis G M & Greer G J. A new genus and two new species of Triculinae (Gastropoda Prosobranchia) and the transmission of a Malaysian mammalian *Schistosoma* sp. *Proc Acad Nat Sci Philadelphia* 1980; 132:245–276.

32 Davis A. Schistosomiasis. In Robinson D (ed.) *Epidemiology and The Community Control of Disease in Warm Climate Countries*, 2nd edn. Edinburgh: Churchill Livingstone, 1985:389–412.

33 Brown D S, Sarfati C, Southgate V R, Ross G C & Knowles R J. Observations on *Schistosoma intercalatum* in southeast Gabon. *Z Parasitenkd* 1984; 70:243–253.

34 Wolfe M S. *Schistosoma intercalatum* infection in an American family. *Am J Trop Med Hyg* 1974; 23:45–50.

35 Wright C A, Southgate V R, van Wijk H B & Moore P J. Hybrids between *Schistosoma intercalatum* and *S. haematobium* in Cameroon. *Trans R Soc Trop Med Hyg* 1974; 68:413–414.

36 Burchard G D & Kern P. Probable hybridization between *S. intercalatum* and *S. haematobium* in Western Gabon. *Trop Geogr Med* 1985; 37:119–123.

37 Southgate V R, van Wijk H B & Wright C A. Schistosomiasis at Loum, Cameroon: *Schistosoma haematobium, S. intercalatum* and their natural hybrid. *Z Parasitenk* 1976; 49:145–159.

38 Kuntz R E, McCullough B, Huang T C & Moore J A. *Schistosoma intercalatum*, Fisher 1934 (Cameroon) infection in the patas monkey. (*Erythrocebus patas*, Schreber, 1775). *Int J Parasitol* 1978; 8:65–68.

39 Nelson G S, Amin M A, Saoud M F A & Teesdale C. Studies on heterologous immunity in schistosomiasis. 1. Heterologous schistosome immunity in mice. *Bull World Health Organ* 1968; 38:9–17.

40 Amin M A, Nelson G S & Saoud M F A. Studies on heterologous immunity in schistosomiasis. 2. Heterologous schistosome immunity in rhesus monkeys. *Bull World Health Organ* 1968; 38:19–27.

41 Short R B. Sex and the single chromosome. *J Parasitol* 1983; 69:3–22.

42 Erasmus D A. The adult schistosome: structure and reproductive biology. In Rollinson D & Simpson A J G (eds) *The Biology of Schistosomes. From Genes to Latrines.* London: Academic Press, 1987:51–82.

43 Webbe G. The Life Cycle of the Parasites. In Jordan P & Webbe G (eds) *Schistosomiasis, Epidemiology, Treatment and Control.* London: Heinemann, 1982:50–78.

44 Christopherson J B. Longevity of parasitic worms. The term of living existence of *Schistosoma haematobium* in the human body. *Lancet* 1924; i:742–743.

45 Chabasse D, Bertrand G, Leroux J P, Gouthery N & Hocquet P. Bilharziose à *Schistosoma mansoni* evolutive découverte 37 ans après l'infection. *Bull Soc Pathol Exot Filiales* 1985; 78:643–647.

46 World Health Organization. Immunology of schistosomiasis. *Bull World Health Organ* 1974; 51:553–595.

47 Simpson A J G. Schistosome molecular biology. In Rollinson D & Simpson A J G (eds) *The Biology of Schistosomes. From Genes to Latrines.* London: Academic Press, 1987:147–161.

48 Rumjanek F D. Biochemistry and physiology. In Rollinson D & Simpson A J G (eds) *The Biology of Schistosomes. From Genes to Latrines.* London: Academic Press, 1987:163–183.

49 Jourdane J & Théron A. Larval development: eggs to cercariae. In Rollinson D & Simpson A J G

(eds) *The Biology of Schistosomes. From Genes to Latrines*. London: Academic Press, 1987:83–113.

50 Pesigan T P, Farooq M, Hairston N G et al. Studies on *Schistosoma japonicum* infection in the Philippines. 1. General considerations and epidemiology. *Bull World Health Organ* 1958; 18:345–455.

51 Wilson R A. Cercariae to liver worms: development and migration in the mammalian host. In Rollinson D & Simpson A J G (eds) *The Biology of Schistosomes. From Genes to Latrines*. London: Academic Press, 1987:115–146.

52 Miller P & Wilson R A. Migration of the schistosomula of *Schistosoma mansoni* from the lungs to the hepatic portal system. *Parasitology* 1980; 80:267–288.

53 Wright W H. Geographical distribution of Schistosomes and their intermediate hosts. In Ansari N (ed.) *Epidemiology and Control of Schistosomiasis (Bilharziasis)*. Basel: Karger, 1973:32–249.

54 Hairston N G. The dynamics of transmission. In Ansari N (ed.) *Epidemiology and Control of Schistosomiasis (Bilharziasis)*. Basel: Karger, 1973:250–336.

55 Brown D S. *Freshwater Snails of Africa and their Medical Importance*. London: Taylor & Francis, 1980:1–488.

56 Webbe G. The intermediate hosts and host–parasite relationships. In Jordan P & Webbe G (eds) *Schistosomiasis, Epidemiology, Treatment and Control*. London: Heinemann, 1982:16–49.

57 Malek E A. *Snail Hosts of Schistosomiasis and Other Snail-Transmitted Diseases in Tropical America: A Manual*, Scientific Publication No. 478, Pan American Health Organization, World Health Organization. Geneva: WHO, 1988:1–316.

58 Southgate V R & Rollinson D. Natural history of transmission and interactions. In Rollinson D & Simpson A J G (eds) *The Biology of Schistosomes. From Genes to Latrines*. London: Academic Press, 1987:347–378.

59 Sobhon P & Upatham E Suchart. *Snail Hosts, Life-Cycle and Tegmental Structure of Oriental Schistosomes*, UNDP/World Bank/WHO Special Programme for Research and Training in Tropical Diseases. Geneva: WHO, 1990:1–321.

60 Mandahl-Barth G. *An appraisal of the present taxonomic status of* Biomphalaria *and* Bulinus *in Africa and the Near East*. SCHISTO/WP 78:5. Geneva: WHO (Unpublished document).

61 Fryer S E. *Studies on the epidemiology of a Nigerian strain of* Schistosoma haematobium *with particular reference to the molluscan hosts*. PhD thesis, University of Wales, 1986: pp 253.

62 Meulemann E A. Host–parasite interrelationships between the freshwater pulmonate *Biomphalaria pfeifferi* and the trematode *Schistosoma mansoni*. *Neth J Zool* 1972; 22:355–427.

63 Jordan P & Webbe G. Epidemiology. In Jordan P & Webbe G (eds) *Schistosomiasis: Epidemiology,*

Treatment and Control. London: Heinemann, 1982: 227–292.

64 Wilkins H A. Epidemiology of schistosome infections in man. In Rollinson D & Simpson A J G (eds) *The Biology of Schistosomes. From Genes to Latrines*. London: Academic Press, 1987:379–397.

65 Cheng T H. Schistosomiasis in mainland China. A review of research and control programs since 1949. *Am J Trop Med Hyg* 1971; 20:26–53.

66 Fenwick, A. Baboons as reservoir hosts of *Schistosoma mansoni*. *Trans R Soc Trop Med Hyg* 1969; 63:557–567.

67 Combes C & Delattre P. Principaux paramètrés de l'infestation des rats (*Rattus rattus* et *Rattus norvegicus*) par *Schistosoma mansoni* dans un foyer de schistosomiase intestinale de la region caraibe. *Oecol Appl* 1981; 2:63–79.

68 Rollinson D, Imbert-Establet D & Ross G C. *Schistosoma mansoni* from naturally infected *Rattus rattus* in Guadeloupe: identification, prevalence and enzyme polymorphism. *Parasitology* 1986; 93:39–53.

69 Bergquist R. Prospects of vaccination against schistosomiasis. *Scand J Infect Dis Suppl* 1990; 76:60–71.

70 Butterworth A E. Immunity in human schistosomiasis. In Prospects for immunological intervention in human schistosomiasis. *Proceedings of a Meeting of the Scientific Working Group on Schistosomiasis*, 26–28 May 1986, Geneva. *Acta Trop* 1987; (supplement 12):31–40.

71 Khalife J, Capron M, Grzych J-M, Butterworth A E, Dunne D W & Ouma J H. Immunity in human schistosomiasis mansoni. Regulation of protective immune mechanisms by IgM blocking antibodies. *J Exp Med* 1986; 164:1626–1640.

72 Butterworth A E, Bensted-Smith R, Capron A et al. Immunity in human schistosomiasis mansoni: prevention by blocking antibodies of the expression of immunity in young children. *Parasitology* 1987; 94:281–300.

73 Butterworth A E, Fulford A J C, Dunne D W, Ouma J H & Sturrock R F. Longitudinal studies on human schistosomiasis. *Philos Trans R Soc Lond [Biol]* 1988; 321:495–511.

74 Capron A, Dessaint J P, Capron M, Ouma J H & Butterworth A E. Immunity to schistosomes: progress toward vaccine. *Science* 1987; 238:1065–1072.

75 Dalton P R. A socioecological approach to the control of *Schistosoma mansoni* in St Lucia. *Bull World Health Organ* 1976; 54:587–595.

76 Colley D G & Colley M D Protective immunity and vaccines to Schistosomiasis. *Parasitol Today* 1989; 5:350–354.

77 Wilkins H A, Goll P H, Marshall T F de C & Moore P J. Dynamics of *Schistosoma haematobium* infection in a Gambian community. 1. The patterns of human infection in the study area. *Trans R Soc Trop Med Hyg* 1984; 78:216–221.

78 Goll P H, Wilkins H A & Marshall T F de C.

Dynamics of *Schistosoma haematobium* infection in a Gambian community. 2. The effect on transmission of control of *Bulinus senegalensis* by the use of niclosamide. *Trans R Soc Trop Med Hyg* 1984; 78:222–226.

79 Wilkins H A, Goll P H, Marshall T F de C & Moore P J. Dynamics of *Schistosoma haematobium* in a Gambian community. 3. Acquisition and loss of infection. *Trans R Soc Trop Med Hyg* 1984; 78:227–232.

80 Butterworth A E & Hagan P. Immunity in human schistosomiasis. *Parasitol Today* 1987; 3:11–16.

81 Hagan P. Reinfection, exposure and immunity in human schistosomiasis. *Parasitol Today* 1992; 8:12–16.

82 De Jonge N, Gryseels B, Hilberath G W, Krijger F W, Polderman A M & Deelder A M. Detection of circulating anodic antigen by ELISA for seroepidemiology of schistosomiasis mansoni. *Trans R Soc Trop Med Hyg* 1988; 82:591–594.

83 von Lichtenberg F. Consequences of infections with schistosomes. In Rollinson D & Simpson A J G (eds) *The Biology of Schistosomes: From Genes to Latrines.* London: Academic Press, 1987:185–232.

84 Smith J H & Christie J D. The pathobiology of *Schistosoma haematobium* in humans. *Hum Pathol* 1986; 17:333–345.

85 Cheever A W, Kamel I A, Elwi A M, Mosimann J E & Danner R. *Schistosoma mansoni* and *S. haematobium* infections in Egypt. II. Quantitative parasitologic findings at necropsy. *Am J Trop Med Hyg* 1977; 26:702–716.

86 Hoshino-Shimizu S, Brito T & Kanamura H Y. Human schistosomiasis: *Schistosoma mansoni* antigen detection in renal glomeruli. *Trans R Soc Trop Med Hyg* 1976; 70:492–496.

87 Abdel-Salam E, Ishaak S & Mahmoud A A F. Histocompatibility linked susceptibility for hepatosplenomegaly in human schistosomiasis mansoni. *J Immunol* 1979; 123:1829–1851.

88 Sazazuki T, Ohuta N, Kanoeoka R & Kojima S. Association between an HLA haplotype and low responsiveness to schistosomal worm antigen in man. *J Exp Med* 1979; 152:314–318.

89 Pereira D M da S M. *Sistemas HLA, ABO e Rhe caracteristicas racais em patientes com hepatosplenomegalia equistossomotica.* Thesis, University of Brazilia, 1979: pp 152.

90 Abel L, Demenais F, Prata A, Souza A E & Dessein A. Evidence for the segregation of a major gene on human susceptibility/resistance to infection by *Schistosoma mansoni. Am J Hum Genet* 1991; 48:959–970.

91 Smith J H, Kamel I A, Elwi A & von Lichtenberg F. A quantitative post mortem analysis of urinary schistosomiasis in Egypt. I. Pathology and pathogenesis. *Am J Trop Med Hyg* 1974; 23:1054–1071.

92 Smith J H, Elwi A, Kamel I A & von Lichtenberg F. A quantitative post mortem analysis of urinary schistosomiasis in Egypt. II. Evolution and

epidemiology. *Am J Trop Med Hyg* 1975; 24:806–822.

93 Farid Z. Chronic urinary Salmonella carriers with intermittent bacteraemia. *J Egypt Public Health Assoc* 1970; 45:157–160.

94 Farid Z, Trabolsi B & Hafez A. *Escherichia coli* bacteraemia in chronic schistosomiasis. *Ann Trop Med Parasitol* 1984; 78:661–662.

95 Wright E D, Chiphangi J & Hutt M S R. Schistosomiasis of the female genital tract. A histopathological study of 176 cases from Malawi. *Trans R Soc Trop Med Hyg* 1982; 76:822–829.

96 Chen, M G & Mott K E. Progress in the assessment of morbidity due to *Schistosoma haematobium*. A review of recent literature. In *Progress in Assessment of Morbidity Due to Schistosomiasis. Trop Dis Bull* 1989; 86:R1–R36.

97 Cheever A W, Kamel I A, Elwi A M, Mosimann J E, Danner R & Sippel J E. *Schistosoma mansoni* and *S. haematobium* infections in Egypt. III. Extrahepatic pathology. *Am J Trop Med Hyg* 1978; 27:55–75.

98 Higashi G I, Abdel-Salam E, Soliman M, Abdel-Meguid A E & El-Ghadban H. Immunofluorescent analysis of renal biopsies in uncomplicated *Schistosoma haematobium* infections in children. *J Trop Med Hyg* 1984; 87:123–129.

99 Sadigursky M, Andrade Z A, Danner R, Cheever A W, Kamel I A & Elwi A M. Absence of schistosomal glomerulopathy in *Schistosoma haematobium* infection in man. *Trans R Soc Trop Med Hyg* 1976; 70:322–323.

100 Farid Z, Higashi G I, Bassily S, Young S W & Sparks H A. Chronic salmonellosis, urinary schistosomiasis and massive proteinuria. *Am J Trop Med Hyg* 1972; 21:578–581.

101 Nafeh M A, Medhat A, Swifae Y et al. Ultrasonographic changes of the liver in *Schistosoma haematobium* infection. *Am J Trop Med Hyg* 1992; 47:225–230.

102 Nooman Z M, Nafeh M A, El-Kateb H, Atta S M & Ezzat E S. Hepatosplenic disease caused by *Bilharzia haematobium* in Upper Egypt. *J Trop Med Hyg* 1974; 77:42–48.

103 Girges R. *Schistosomiasis (Bilharziasis).* London: John Bale Sons and Danielson, 1934:161–162.

104 Adeyemi-Doro F A B, Osoba A O & Junaid T A. Perigenital cutaneous schistosomiasis. *Br J Vener Dis* 1979; 55:446–449.

105 Develoux M, Blanc L, Veller J M & Cenac A. Bilharziose cutanée thoracique. *Ann Dermatol Vener* 1987; 114:695–697.

106 Hull P R & Hay I T. Peri-umbilical cutaneous schistosomiasis: a case report. *S Afr Med J* 1979; 53:654.

107 Macdonald D M & Morrison J G L. Cutaneous ectopic schistosomiasis. *BMJ* 1976; ii:619–620.

108 Obasi O E. Cutaneous schistosomiasis in Nigeria. An update. *Br J Dermatol* 1986; 114:597–602.

109 Scrimgeour E M & Gajdusek D C. Involvement of the central nervous system in *Schistosoma mansoni*

and *S. haematobium* infection, a review. *Brain* 1985; 108:1023–1038.

110 van der Horst R. Schistosomiasis of the pericardium. *Trans R Soc Trop Med Hyg* 1979; 73:243–244.

111 Chitiyo M E. Schistosomal involvement of the choroid plexus. *Cent Afr J Med* 1972; 18:45–47.

112 Elsebai I. Parasites in the aetiology of cancer: bilharziasis and bladder cancer. *CA* 1977; 27:100–106.

113 Lucas S B. Squamous cell carcinoma of the bladder and schistosomiasis. *East Afr Med J* 1982; 59:345–351.

114 Kuntz R E, Cheever A W & Myers B J. Proliferative epithelial lesions of the urinary bladder of nonhuman primates infected with *Schistosoma haematobium*. *J Natl Cancer Inst* 1972; 48:223–235.

115 Hicks R M, James C & Webbe G. Effect of *S. haematobium* and *N*-butyl-*N*-(4-hydroxy butyl) nitrosamine on the development of urothelial neoplasia in the baboon. *Br J Cancer* 1980; 42:730–755.

116 Brand K G. Schistosomiasis-cancer: etiological considerations. *Acta Trop* 1979; 36:203–214.

117 Hicks R M, Ismael M M, Walters C L, Beecham P T, Rabie M F & El Alamy M A. Association of bacteriuria and urinary nitrosamine formation with *Schistosoma haematobium* infection in the Qualyub area of Egypt. *Trans R Soc Trop Med Hyg* 1982; 76:519–528.

118 Bhagwandeen S B. Schistosomiasis and carcinoma of the bladder in Zambia. *S Afr Med J* 1976; 50:1616–1620.

119 Cheever A W. Schistosomiasis and neoplasia. *J Natl Cancer Inst* 1978; 61:13–18.

120 Attah E B & Nkposong E O. Schistosomiasis and carcinoma of the bladder: a critical appraisal of causal relationship. *Trop Geogr Med* 1976; 28:268–272.

121 Chen M G & Mott K E. Progress in assessment of morbidity due to *Schistosoma mansoni* infection. *Progress in Assessment of Morbidity Due to Schistosomiasis*. Reviews of recent literature. *Trop Dis Bull* 1988; 85:R1–R56.

122 Warren K S. The kinetics of hepatosplenic schistosomiasis. *Semin Liver Dis* 1984; 4:293–300.

123 Dunn M A & Kamel R. Hepatic schistosomiasis. *Hepatology* 1981; 1:653–661.

124 Warren K S. The relevance of schistosomiasis. *N Engl J Med* 1980; 303:203–206.

125 Dunn M A, Kamel R, Kamel I A et al. Liver collagen synthesis in schistosomiasis mansoni. *Gastroenterology* 1979; 76:978–982.

126 Andrade Z A & Abreu W N. Follicular lymphoma of the spleen in patients with hepatosplenic schistosomiasis mansoni. *Am J Trop Med Hyg* 1971; 20:237–243.

127 Andrade Z A, Andrade S G & Sadigursky M. Renal changes in patients with hepatosplenic

schistosomiasis. *Am J Trop Med Hyg* 1971; 20:77–83.

128 Barsoum R S, Bassily S, Solimann M M, Ramzy M F, Milad A M & Hassaballa A. Renal amyloidosis and schistosomiasis. *Trans R Soc Trop Med Hyg* 1979; 73:367–374.

129 Pitella J E H & Lana-Peixoto M. Brain involvement in hepatosplenic schistosomiasis mansoni. *Brain* 1981; 104:621–632.

130 Bittencourt A L, Almeida M A C, Inues M A F & Motta C D C. Placental involvement in schistosomiasis mansoni; report of four cases. *Am J Trop Med Hyg* 1980; 29:571–575.

131 Chen M G. Relative distribution of *Schistosoma japonicum* eggs in the intestine of man: a subject of inconsistency. *Acta Trop* 1990; 48:163–171.

132 Mao S P, He Y X, Yang Y Q et al. *Schistosoma japonicum* and schistosomiasis japonica. In Wu Z J, Mao S P & Wang J W (eds) *Chinese Medical Encyclopaedia, Parasitology and Parasitic Diseases*. Shanghai: Shanghai Publishing House for Sciences and Technology, 1984:44–55 (in Chinese).

133 Santos A T. The present status of schistosomiasis in the Philippines. *Southeast Asian J Trop Med Public Health* 1984; 15:439–445.

134 Garin D, Chapalain J C, Thierry J, Perrier Gros Claude J D, Peyron F & Courtois D. Le point sur *Schistosoma intercalatum*. *Méd Trop* 1990; 50:433–440.

135 van Wijk H B & Elias E A. Hepatic and rectal pathology in *Schistosoma intercalatum* infection. *Trop Geogr Medicine* 1975; 27:237–248.

136 Centers for Disease Control. Acute schistosomiasis in US travelers returning from Africa. *MMWR* 1990; 39:141–148.

137 Stuiver P C. Acute schistosomiasis (Katayama fever). *BMJ* 1984; 288:221–222.

138 Farid Z, Bassily S, Kent D C, Sanborn W R, Hassan A & Abdel-Wahab M F. Chronic urinary salmonella carriers with intermittent bacteraemia. *Am J Trop Med Hyg* 1970; 73:153–156.

139 Farid Z, Kilpatrick M E & Ishak E A. *S. haematobium* and *S. intercalatum*. Clinical and pathological aspects. In Webbe G, Jordan P & Sturrock R F (eds) *Human Schistosomiasis*, 3rd edn. Oxford: Commonwealth Agricultural Bureau 1993; 159–193.

140 Simarro P P, Sima F O & Mir M. African trypanosomiasis and *Schistosoma intercalatum* infection in Equatorial Guinea: comparative epidemiology and feasibility of integrated control. *Trop Med Parasitol* 1989; 40:159–162.

141 Simarro P P, Sima F O & Mir M. Urban epidemiology of *Schistosoma intercalatum* in the city of Bata, Equatorial Guinea. *Trop Med Parasitol* 1990; 41:254–256.

142 Arene F O, Ukpeibo E T & Nwanze E A. Studies on schistosomiasis in the Niger Delta; *Schistosoma intercalatum* in the urban city of Port Harcourt, Nigeria. *Public Health* 1989; 103:295–301.

143 Corachan M, Escosa R, Mass J, Ruiz L & Campo

E. Clinical presentations of *Schistosoma intercalatum* infestation. *Lancet* 1987; i:1139.

144 Deelder A M, De Jonge N, Boerman O C et al. Sensitive determination of circulating anodic antigen in *Schistosoma mansoni* infected individuals by an enzyme-linked immunosorbent assay using monoclonal antibodies. *Am J Trop Med Hyg* 1989; 40:268–272.

145 De Jonge J, Fillié Y E, Hilberath G W et al. Presence of the schistosome circulating anodic antigen (CAA) in urine of patients with *Schistosoma mansoni* or *S. haematobium* infections. *Am J Trop Med Hyg* 1989; 41:563–569.

146 De Jonge N, Schommer G, Krijger F W et al. Presence of circulating anodic antigen in serum of *Schistosoma intercalatum*-infected patients from Gabon. *Acta Trop* 1989; 46:115–120.

147 De Jonge N, Rabello A L T, Krijger F W et al. Levels of the schistosome circulating anodic and cathodic antigens in serum of schistosomiasis patients from Brazil. *Trans R Soc Trop Med Hyg* 1991; 85:756–759.

148 Kremsner P G, De Jonge N, Simarro P P et al. Quantitative determination of circulating anodic and cathodic antigens in serum and urine of individuals infected with *Schistosoma intercalatum*. *Trans R Soc Trop Med Hyg* 1993; 87:167–169.

149 Braun-Munzinger R A & Southgate B A. Repeatability and reproducibility of egg counts of *Schistosoma haematobium* in urine. *Trop Med Parasitol* 1992; 43:149–154.

150 Cook J A & Jordan P. Excretion of *Schistosoma mansoni* eggs in the urine. *Trans R Soc Trop Med Hyg* 1970; 64:793–794.

151 Bell D R. In *East African Institute for Medical Research: Annual Report 1961–62*. Kenya: Government Printer, 1962:24.

152 Dazo B C & Biles J E. Two new field techniques for detection and counting of *Schistosoma haematobium* eggs in urine samples. *Bull World Health Organ* 1974; 51:399–408.

153 Peters P A, Warren K S & Mahmoud A A F. Rapid accurate quantification of schistosome eggs via nuclepore filters. *J Parasitol* 1976; 62:154–155.

154 Peters P A, Mahmoud A A F, Warren K S, Ouma J H & Arap Siongkok T K. Field studies of rapid accurate means of quantifying *Schistosoma haematobium* eggs in urine samples. *Bull World Health Organ* 1976; 54:159–162.

155 Mott K E, Baltes R, Bambahga J & Baldassini B. Field studies of a reusable polyamide filter for detection of *Schistosoma haematobium* eggs by urine filtration. *Trop Med Parasitol* 1982; 33:227–228.

156 Mott K E. A reusable polyamide filter for diagnosis of *S. haematobium* infection by urine filtration. *Bull Soc Pathol Exot* 1983; 76:101–104.

157 Braun-Munzinger R A & Rohde R. False epidemiological results from the bulk transport of dried filter paper in urinary schistosomiasis. *Trop Med Parasitol* 1986; 37:286–289.

158 Ritchie L S. An ether sedimentation technique for routine stool examinations. *Bull US Army Med Dept* 1948; 8:326.

159 Hunter G W III, Hodges E P, Jahnes W G, Diamond L S & Ingalls J W. Studies on schistosomiasis. II. Summary of further studies on methods of recovering eggs of *S. japonicum*. *Bull US Army Med Dept* 1948; 8:128–131.

160 Blagg W, Schaegel, E L, Mansour N S & Khalaf G I. A new concentration technique for the demonstration of protozoa and helminthic eggs in the faeces. *Am J Trop Med Hyg* 1955; 4:23–28.

161 Knight W B, Hiatt R A, Cline B L & Ritchie L S. A modification of the formol–ether concentration technique for increased sensitivity in detecting *Schistosoma mansoni* eggs. *Am J Trop Med Hyg* 1970; 25:818–823.

162 Allen A V H & Ridley D S. Further observations on the formol–ether concentration technique for faecal parasites. *J Clin Pathol* 1970; 23:545–546.

163 Visser P S & Pitchford R J. A simple apparatus for rapid recovery of helminth eggs from excreta with special reference to *Schistosoma mansoni*. *S Afr Med J* 1972; 46:1344–1346.

164 Komiya Y & Kobayashi A. Evaluation of Kato's thick smear technique with a cellophane cover for helminth eggs in faeces. *Jpn J Med Sci Biol* 1966; 19:59–64.

165 Katz N, Chaves A & Pellegrino J. A simple device for quantitative thick smear technique in schistosomiasis mansoni. *Rev Inst Med Trop São Paulo* 1972; 14:397–400.

166 Teesdale C H & Amin M A. Comparison of the Bell technique, a modified Kato thick smear technique and a digestion method for the field diagnosis of schistosomiasis mansoni. *J Helminthol* 1976; 59:17–20.

167 Teesdale C H & Amin M A. A simple thick smear technique for the diagnosis of *Schistosoma mansoni* infection. *Bull World Health Organ* 1976; 54:703–705.

168 Chitsulo L, Teesdale C H & Dixon H. Comparison of the Teesdale glass sandwich and Kato–Katz techniques for the diagnosis of *Schistosoma mansoni*: a double-blind study. *Trop Med Parasitol* 1990; 41:447–449.

169 Fulleborn F. Über den Nachweis der *Schistosomum mansoni*: Eir in Stuhle. *Arch Schiffs Tropenkr Hamburg* 1921; 25:334–340.

170 Fun-Zhi. *Schistosomiasis Shou Chai*, 2 edn. (Prevention and control of schistosomiasis handbook compiled by the Revolutionary Committee of Shanghai Schistosomiasis Research Institute.) Shanghai: Peoples Press, 1971: Edition 2, 140 (in Chinese).

171 Shanghai Municipal Institute for Prevention and Treatment of Schistosomiasis. *Handbook on the Prevention and Treatment of Schistosomiasis*. (Translated by the US Department of Health, Education and Welfare, Public Health Service,

National Institutes of Health.) DHEW Publication No. (NIH) 77-1290, 1977:61–69.

172 Gorman S, Meeser S V, Ross W F & Blair D M. The macroscopic diagnosis of urinary schistosomiasis. *S Afr Med J* 1947; 21:853–854.

172 Meeser S V, Ross W F & Blair D M. Further observations on the macroscopic diagnosis of urinary schistosomiasis. *J Tropical Med Hyg* 1948; 51:54–59.

174 Weber M C. Miracidial hatching. *Cent Afr J Med* 1973; 19 (supplement 9):11–14.

175 Davis A. Field trials of 'Ambilhar' in the treatment of urinary bilharziasis in schoolchildren. *Bull World Health Organ* 1966; 35:827–835.

176 Davis A. Comparative trials of antimonial drugs in urinary schistosomiasis. *Bull World Health Organ* 1968; 38:197–227.

177 Braun Munzinger R A & Southgate B A. Egg viability in urinary schistosomiasis. I. New methods compared with available methods. *J Trop Med Hyg* 1993; 96:22–27.

178 Braun-Munzinger R A & Southgate B A. Egg viability in urinary schistosomiasis. II. Simplifying modifications and standardization of new methods. *J Trop Med Hyg* 1993; 96:71–75.

179 Braun-Munzinger R A & Southgate B A. Egg viability in urinary schistosomiasis. III. Repeatability and reproducibility of new methods. *J Trop Med Hyg* 1993; 96:179–185.

180 Newsome J. Recent investigations into the treatment of schistosomiasis by Miracil D in Egypt. *Trans R Soc Trop Med Hyg* 1951; 44:611–634.

181 Upatham E S, Sturrock R F & Cook J A. Studies on the hatchability of *Schistosoma mansoni* from a naturally infected human community on St Lucia, West Indies. *Parasitology* 1976; 73:253–264.

182 Zicker F, Katz N & Wolf J. Availiaçao do teste de ecloso de miracidios na equistossoma mansonica. *Rev Bras Malariol Doencas Trop* 1977; 30:65–75.

183 Da Cunha A S. A availiaçao terapéutica da oxamniquine na equistossomose mansoni humana pelo metodo do oograma por biopsia de mucosa rectal. *Rev Inst Med Trop* Sâo Paulo 1982; 24:88–94.

184 World Health Organization. *Diagnostic techniques in schistosomiasis control*. WHO/SCHISTO/83.69 Parasitic Diseases Programme. Geneva: WHO 1983:1–36 (unpublished document).

185 Briggs M, Chatfield M, Mummery D & Briggs M. Screening with reagent strips. *BMJ* 1971; iii:433–434.

186 Wilkins H A, Goll P, Marshall T F de C & Moore P J. The significance of proteinuria and haematuria in *Schistosoma haematobium* infection. *Trans R Soc Trop Med Hyg* 1979; 73:74–80.

187 Pugh R N H, Bell D R & Gilles H M. Malumfashi endemic diseases research project. XV. The potential medical importance of bilharzia in Northern Nigeria: a suggested rapid, cheap and effective solution for control of *Schistosoma*

haematobium infection. *Ann Trop Med Parasitol* 1980; 74:597–613.

188 Feldmeir H, Doehring E & Dafallah A A. Simultaneous use of a sensitive filtration technique and reagent strips in urinary schistosomiasis. *Trans R Soc Trop Med Hyg* 1982; 76:416–421.

189 Savioli L, Hatz C, Dixon H, Kisumbu U M & Mott K E. Control of morbidity due to *Schistosoma haematobium* on Pemba Island: egg excretion and haematuria as indicators of infection. *Am J Trop Med Hyg* 1990; 43:289–295.

190 Mott K E & Dixon H. Collaborative study on antigens for immunodiagnosis of schistosomiasis. *Bull World Health Organ* 1982; 60:729–753.

191 Mott K E, Dixon H, Carter C E et al. Collaborative study on antigens for immunodiagnosis of *Schistosoma japonicum* infections. *Bull World Health Organ* 1987; 65:233–244.

192 Bergquist R. In Bergquist R (ed.) *Immunodiagnostic Approaches in Schistosomiasis*. Chichester: Wiley, 1992:1–8.

193 Abdel-Wahab M F & Strickland G T. Abdominal ultrasonography for assessing morbidity from schistosomiasis. 2. Hospital studies. *Trans R Soc Trop Med Hyg* 1993; 87:135–137.

194 Hatz C, Jenkins J M & Tanner M. Ultrasound in schistosomiasis. *Acta Trop* 1992; 51:1–97.

195 World Health Organization. *Meeting on ultrasonography in schistosomiasis. 1991*. UNDP/ World Bank/WHO Special Programme for Research and Training in Tropical Diseases. TDR/ SCH/ULTRASON/91.3, CTD/91.3. Geneva: WHO, 1–32 (unpublished document).

196 Abdel-Wahab M F, Esmat G, Narooz S I, Yoseri A, Struewing J P & Strickland G T. Sonographic studies of schoolchildren in a village endemic for *Schistosoma haematobium*. *Trans R Soc Trop Med Hyg* 1990; 84:69–73.

197 Abdel-Wahab M F, Esmat G, Farrag A, El-Boraey Y A & Strickland G T. Grading of hepatic schistosomiasis by the use of ultrasonography. *Am J Trop Med Hyg* 1992; 46:403–408.

198 Abdel-Wahab M F, Esmat G, Milad M, Abdel-Razek S & Strickland G T. Characteristic sonographic patterns of schistosomal hepatic fibrosis. *Am J Trop Med Hyg* 1989; 40:72–76.

199 Abdel-Wahab M F, Esmat G, Farrag A, El-Boraey Y A & Strickland G T. Ultrasonographic prediction of esophageal varices in schistosomiasis mansoni. *Am J Gastroenterol* 1993; 88:560–563.

200 Ajana F, Dei-Cas E, Colin J J et al. La bilharziose humaine à *Schistosoma mekongi*; problèmes diagnostiques et theŕapeutiques. *Méd Mal Infect* 1986; 3:141–146.

201 Chidiac C, Beaucaire G, Mouton Y, Caillaux M & Fournier A. Echecs au praziquantel dans le traitement des bilharzioses; intér
t de la biopsie de muqueuse rectale et du suivi prolonge. *Méd Mal Infect* 1986; 5:380–384.

202 Duong T H, Furet Y, Lorett G, Barrakes A,

Arbeille B & Combescot C. Traitement de la bilharziose à *Schistosoma mekongi* par le praziquantel. *Méd Trop* 1988; 48:39–43.

203 Manoury V, Guillemot F, Mathieu-Chandelier C et al. Bilharzioses à *Schistosoma mekongi* diagnostiquées par biopsie rectale et traitées par praziquantel; à propos de 5 cases. *Gastroenterol Clin Biol* 1990; 14:1032–1033.

204 Davis A & Bailey D R. Metrifonate in urinary schistosomiasis. *Bull World Health Organ* 1969; 41:209–224.

205 Plestina R, Davis A & Bailey D R. Effect of metrifonate on blood cholinesterases in children during the treatment of schistosomiasis. *Bull World Health Organ* 1972; 46:747–759.

206 World Health Organization. Research on the epidemiology and methodology of schistosomiasis control in man-made lakes (RAF/71/217). *Project Findings and Recommendations*. Report prepared for the United Nations Development Programme and the Governments of Ghana and Egypt. Geneva: WHO, 1979:PDP/79.2.

207 Foster R & Cheetham B L. Studies with the schistosomicide oxamniquine (UK-4271). I. Activities in rodents and in vitro. *Trans R Soc Trop Med Hyg* 1973; 67:674–684.

208 Foster R, Cheetham B L & King D F. Studies with the schistosomicide oxamniquine. (UK-4271.) II. Activity in primates. *Trans R Soc Trop Med Hyg* 1973; 67:685–693.

209 Bassily S, Farid Z, Higashi G I & Watten R H. Treatment of complicated schistosomiasis mansoni with oxamniquine. *Am J Trop Med Hyg* 1978; 27:1284–1286.

210 Farid Z, Higashi G I, Bassily S, Trabolsi B & Watten R H. Treatment of advanced hepatosplenic schistosomiasis with oxamniquine. *Trans R Soc Trop Med Hyg* 1980; 74:400–401.

211 Abaza H H, Hammouda N, Abd Rabbo H & Shafei A Z. Chemotherapy of schistosomal polyposis with oxamniquine. *Trans R Soc Trop Med Hyg* 1978; 72:602–604.

212 Machado P A. The Brazilian control programme for schistosomiasis control. 1975–1979. *am J Trop Med Hyg* 1982; 31:76–86.

213 Higashi G I & Farid Z. Oxamniquine fever: drug induced or immune complex reaction? *BMJ* 1979; 2:830.

214 Katz N, Rocha R S, De Souza C P et al. Efficacy of alternating therapy with oxamniquine and praziquantel to treat *Schistosoma mansoni* in children following failure of first treatment. *Am J Trop Med Hyg* 1991; 44:509–512.

215 Mansour N M, Omer Ali P, Farid Z, Simpson A J G & Woody J W. Serological differentiation of acute and chronic schistosomiasis mansoni by antibody responses to keyhole limpet haemocyanin. *Am J Trop Med Hyg* 1989; 41:338–344.

216 Watt G, Adapon B, Long G W, Fernando M C, Ranoa C P & Cross J H. Praziquantel in treatment of cerebral schistosomiasis. *Lancet* 1986; ii:529–532.

217 Ezzatt F A, Abu-Elmagd K M, Aly M A et al. Selective shunt versus nonshunt surgery for management of both schistosomal and nonschistosomal variceal bleeders. *Ann Surg* 1990; 212:97–108.

218 Davis A. Metriphonate. In Dollery C (ed.) *Therapeutic Drugs*, vol 2. Edinburgh: Churchill Livingstone, 1991: M164–M170.

219 Davis A. Oxamniquine. In Dollery C (ed.) *Therapeutic Drugs*, vol. 2. Edinburgh: Churchill Livingstone, 1991: O42–O45.

220 Wegner D H G. Praziquantel. In Dollery C (ed.) *Therapeutic Drugs*, vol. 2. Edinburgh: Churchill Livingstone, 1991: P189–P195.

221 Davis A. Antischistosomal drugs and clinical practice. In Jordan P, Webbe G & Sturrock R F (eds) *Human Schistosomiasis*, 3rd edn. Oxford: CAB International, 1993:367–404.

222 World Health Organization. The control of schistosomiasis. Second report of the WHO Expert Committee. *WHO Tech Rep Ser* 1993; 830: pp 1–86.

223 Mott K E (ed.) *Plant Molluscicides*. Published on behalf of the UNDP/World Bank/WHO Special Programme for Research and Training in Tropical Diseases. Chichester: Wiley, 1987:1–326.

224 McCullough F S. *The use of mollusciciding in schistosomiasis control*. WHO/SCHISTO/92.107. Geneva: WHO, 1992:1–34 (unpublished document).

2225 World Health Organization. *Meeting on strategies for the development of a schistosomiasis vaccine*. UNDP/World Bank/WHO Special Programme for Research and Training in Tropical Diseases. TDR/SCH/VAC-DEV/91.3. Geneva: WHO, 1991:1–11 (unpublished document).

226 Bergquist N R. Controlling schistosomiasis by vaccination: a realistic option? *Parasitology Today* 1995; 11:191–194.

227 Cheng M G & Mott K E. Progress in assessment of morbidity due to *Schistosoma japonicum*. A review of recent literature. In *Progress in assessment of morbidity due to schistosomiasis*. From *Trop Dis Bull* 1988; 85:R1–R45.

CHAPTER 73

FOOD-BORNE TREMATODES

Melissa R. Haswell-Elkins and David B. Elkins

The liver flukes (*Fasciola, Opisthorchis, Clonorchis*), lung flukes (*Paragonimus*) and intestinal flukes (*Fasciolopsis, Echinostoma, Heterophyes*) are important causes of human disease.[1] Although these are commonly thought of as 'tropical' parasites, some species are not limited to hot climates. An extreme example is *Opisthorchis felineus* which is commonly acquired through the consumption of raw frozen fish in Siberia. The availability of freshwater flora and fauna and a preference for eating them raw or incompletely cooked are the most important factors determining their distribution in man.

All food-borne trematodes are hermaphroditic and have oral and ventral suckers for attachment. Their life cycles are complex and involve one or more intermediate hosts (the first always being a snail) and several morphological stages (Figure 73.1). Although differing in anatomical location in the final host and therefore causing different diseases, transmission to man occurs almost exclusively through the consumption of raw foods harbouring the infective stage. In contrast, schistosomes have two sexes and enter their final hosts by active penetration.

Among the thousands of food-borne trematodes, hundreds may infect man, and new species are still being discovered.[1–3] Because most species also parasitize other animals and are of veterinary importance, the term 'accidental' is sometimes used to describe human infections. The term is appropriate for some representatives, such as *Fasciola*—which usually occur in outbreaks, or flukes rarely reported in humans, e.g. *Watsoni, Dicrocoelium, Eurytrema*. However, estimates that 70–100 million people harbour food-borne trematodes[4] argue against a major role of chance in most infections.

The endemic areas of these parasites often overlap, since people often enjoy many kinds of raw food. For example, adult worms of 13 food-borne trematode species (plus *Taenia saginata*) were found by expulsion chemotherapy in 224 residents of a single village in north-east Thailand.[3] Up to seven species have been reported in a single individual.[2] Some authors have reported an association between 'tastiness' of fish and the season or species with the

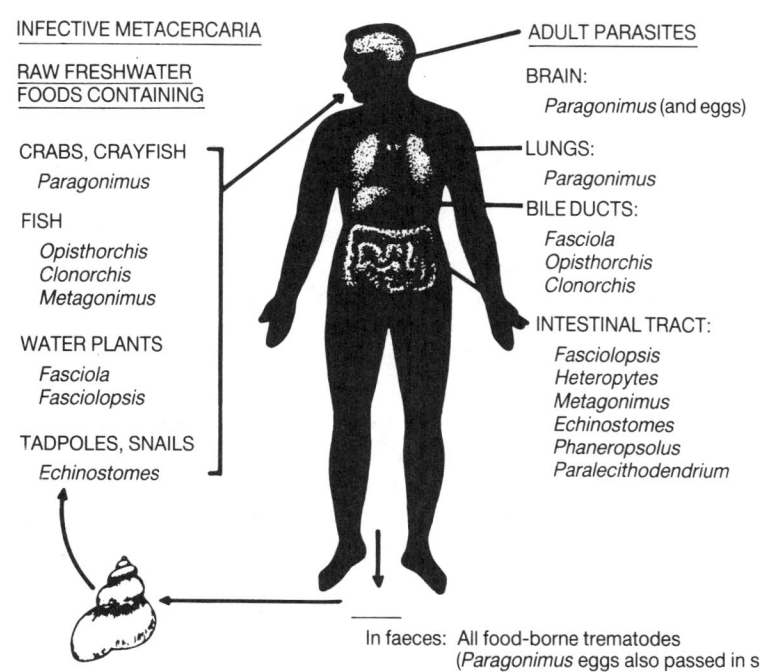

INFECTIVE METACERCARIA

RAW FRESHWATER
FOODS CONTAINING

CRABS, CRAYFISH
  Paragonimus

FISH
  Opisthorchis
  Clonorchis
  Metagonimus

WATER PLANTS
  Fasciola
  Fasciolopsis

TADPOLES, SNAILS
  Echinostomes

ADULT PARASITES

BRAIN:
  Paragonimus (and eggs)

LUNGS:
  Paragonimus

BILE DUCTS:
  Fasciola
  Opisthorchis
  Clonorchis

INTESTINAL TRACT:
  Fasciolopsis
  Heteropytes
  Metagonimus
  Echinostomes
  Phaneropsolus
  Paralecithodendrium

In faeces: All food-borne trematodes
(*Paragonimus* eggs also passed in sputum)

Figure 73.1 Diagrammatic representation of the life cycle of the major food-borne trematode infections of man. Drawn by Banchob Sripa.

highest intensity of infective stages.[5] This may reflect an influence of human taste preference on parasite life cycles.

Food-borne trematodes have received less attention than other helminth infections, perhaps because of their focal distribution and lack of acute symptoms. However, some authors have mistakenly reported them as comparatively benign, which is certainly not the case for the liver flukes and *Paragonimus*, as reviewed here. Severity of disease is associated with worm burden, except perhaps in the case of ectopic infections.

Due to increasing tourism and migration, infections previously confined to endemic areas are increasingly being reported in non-endemic countries.[6,7] Fortunately life cycles are not becoming established in new countries. There are, however, numerous reports of endemic areas growing larger due to domestic migration, and increasing availability/preference for raw foods.[8–10] On the other hand, as newly industrialized countries alter their natural environment and pollute their river systems, native snail, crustacean and fish fauna are becoming adversely affected.[11,12] Night-soil and manure, potentially containing fluke eggs, are being replaced by chemical fertilizer. Thus risk of infection by eating 'wild' foods might be gradually replaced by risk of exposure to potentially hazardous chemicals.

Efforts to control food-borne parasites were revolutionized by the drug praziquantel, which is now inexpensive and widely available. However, in addition to anthelmintic treatment to cure current infection, improvements in sanitation and health promotion to encourage the cooking of foods involved in transmission are important components of control to hinder reinfection. Although the latter sounds simple, eating habits of all people often have cultural and social significance and are difficult to change.[11]

LIVER FLUKES

OPISTHORCHIASIS AND CLONORCHIASIS

AETIOLOGY

The human liver flukes, *Clonorchis sinensis, Opisthorchis viverrini* and *O. felineus*, remain important public health problems in many endemic areas where they infect at least 20 million people.[8,10,13,14] *O. guayaquilensis* has been reported in a small human focus in Ecuador.[1] In addition to their association with hepatobiliary disease, *O. viverrini* and *C. sinensis* are major aetiological agents of bile duct cancer.[15–21] This is a leading cause of death in northeast Thailand.[17]

The three major flukes have similar adult and egg morphologies, life cycles and pathogenesis (Figures 73.1 and 73.2). Distinction between them is generally based on the flame cell pattern of the adult worms.[22]

HISTORY AND SEMINAL DISCOVERIES

Human infection with these flukes was first discovered in 1875 (*C. sinensis*), 1892 (*O. felineus*) and the early 1900s (*O. viverrini*).[1] The close association between bile duct carcinoma and *O. viverrini* and *C. sinensis* was first researched by Hoeppli,[18] Viranuvatti and Mettiyawongse[19] and Hou.[20] Thamavit et al established a laboratory model of cholangiocarcinoma in hamsters exposed to *O. viverrini* infection and low doses of *N*-dimethylnitrosamine.[21] The very high incidence of this cancer in an endemic area of Thailand has now been documented by Vatanasapt et al.[17]

LIFE CYCLE

The adult parasites live in the smaller intrahepatic bile ducts of their final hosts—which include humans, cats, dogs and other wild and domestic fish-eating mammals. Eggs pass down the bile duct and into the faeces and can also be found in the gallbladder. Eggs are fully embryonated upon excretion, and hatch into miracidia after being ingested by snails. Generally fewer than 1–2% of snails are infected.[14,23] The miracidia transform into sporocysts and rediae which multiply, then become free-swimming cercaria which exit the snail and attach, penetrate and encyst in susceptible species of fish. Most belong to the family Cyprinidae. Wide variation in the prevalence (up to 100%) and intensity of metacercaria is found between seasons, types of water bodies and species of fish.[14,22] Metacercaria are infective to humans and other mammals if consumed uncooked. The metacercaria excyst, migrate up the duodenum through the ampulla of Vater and

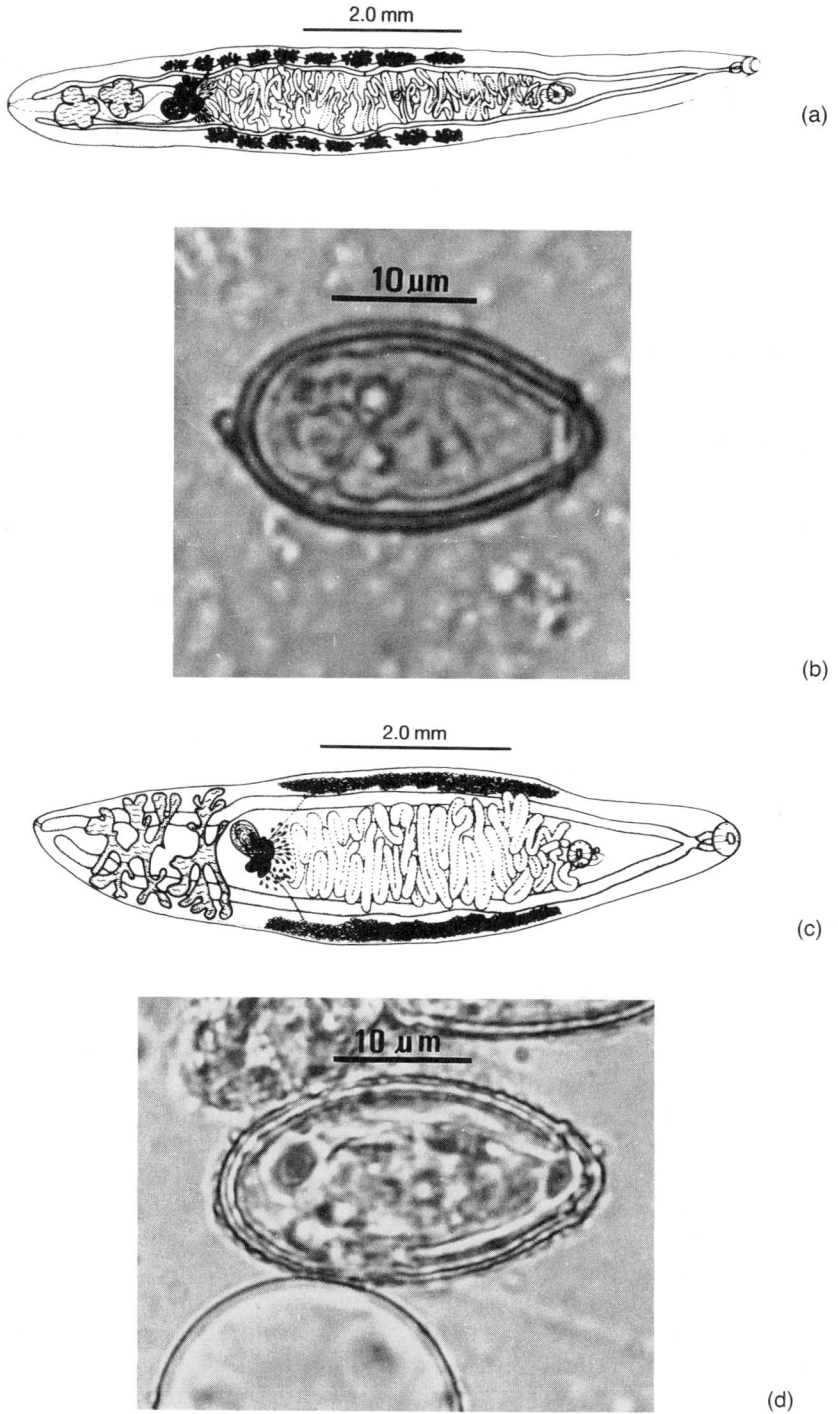

Figure 73.2 (a) Adult stage worm of *Opisthorchis viverrini*. Drawn by Sasithorn Kaewkes. (b) Egg of *O. viverrini*. Photograph by Sasithorn Kaewkes. (c) Adult stage worm of *Clonorchis sinensis*. Drawn by Sasithorn Kaewkes. (d) Egg of *C. sinensis*. Photograph by Sasithorn Kaewkes.

the extrahepatic biliary system to the intrahepatic bile ducts where they mature. The prepatent period is about 1 month and the adults may live many years.[1,7,14]

EPIDEMIOLOGY

Humans become infected with *Opisthorchis* and *Clonorchis* through the consumption of raw or undercooked cyprinoid fish. Geographical and age-related patterns of human infection therefore overlap with this dietary habit.

O. felineus is prevalent in animals throughout Europe, and has been reported in humans from eastern Germany, Poland and mainly in the former Soviet Union.[1,24] Most recent information comes from Siberia, notably the Tyumen and Khanty regions, where high prevalences and intensities are reported.[25,26] Residents and immigrants to the endemic focus in Siberia enjoy eating thinly sliced frozen or lightly salted cyprinoid fish.

O. viverrini infects an estimated seven million people, or approximately 35%, of the 20 million people in north-east Thailand and is also common in Laos.[8,27,28] Recent reports show an increase in the average prevalence of infection in northern Thailand—up to 26% in 1992.[8]

Raw fish dishes are a well-established dietary tradition of Laos people and the ethnic Laos in north-east Thailand. Fresh fish dishes may contain large numbers of metacercaria and are eaten occasionally. Uncooked fermented fish, which is eaten daily, also contain metacercaria, but its importance as a source of infection is unclear.

C. sinensis, although largely eliminated from Japan and drastically reduced in Korea, remains prevalent and may be increasingly common in parts of Taiwan, Hong Kong, Vietnam and China.[9,10,14,15] Human infection occurs in 24 Chinese provinces, with one major focus in the south (especially Guangdong and Guangsxi provinces) and another in the north-east (Henjian).[10] Generally the Chinese enjoy eating raw fish dipped in hot rice porridge, or children catch and eat them during play. This latter practice results in an unusual age-related pattern of infection, whereby most infection occurs in children. Generally, however, prevalence and intensity of infection rises with age, with most initial infections occurring in the early teens, and may be higher in males than females.[14,16,24]

Thus despite widespread availability of praziquantel and massive control efforts, these liver flukes remain common and may be spreading to new areas with increased consumption of raw fish.

CLINICAL FEATURES

Most chronically infected individuals have few specific signs or symptoms, except an increased frequency of palpable liver, as shown in community-based studies using physical examination.[14,26,29–31] Haematological and biochemical features are unremarkable, even in heavy infections. Ultrasonography, however, reveals a high frequency of gallbladder enlargement, sludge, gallstones and poor function in asymptomatic individuals.[30,31]

Symptomatic cases of *Opisthorchis* and *Clonorchis* infection generally experience pain in the right upper quadrant, diarrhoea, loss of appetite, indigestion and fullness. Severe cases may present with weakness, lassitude, weight loss, ascites and oedema. Complications may include cholangitis, obstructive jaundice, intra-abdominal mass, cholecystitis and gallbladder or intrahepatic stones.[13,14,24,31,32] Such stones are particularly frequent in clonorchiasis.

The most important clinical manifestation of liver fluke infection is an enhanced susceptibility to cholangiocarcinoma. Case–control studies in Thailand suggest a fivefold increased risk during infection of any intensity, while heavily infected people may face a 15-fold risk.[33] This is reflected in a sixfold and tenfold higher incidence of cholangiocarcinoma (in females and males, respectively) in an endemic province of Thailand above that of a non-endemic area.[17] While such a dramatic increase is not reported for *Clonorchis* infection, there is ample evidence that this fluke is also strongly associated with cholangiocarcinoma.[14,15,31]

A special feature of *O. felineus* infection, not often reported for the other species, is acute opisthorchiasis.[24] This is characterized by hepatosplenomegaly and tenderness, eosinophilia up to 40%, and chills and fever. It occurs early in infection and may be associated with primary exposure to a large dose of metacercaria.

PATHOLOGY AND PATHOGENESIS

Liver enlargement and dilated subcapsular bile ducts with thick fibrotic walls can be seen grossly in heavily infected cases.[1,13,14–16,18,20,34] Microscopically, bile duct pathology is characterized by desquamation of epithelial cells of secondary and tertiary ducts and chronic inflammation with infiltration of lymphocytes, monocytes, eosinophils and plasma cells. Epithelial hyperplasia may lead to the formation of glands lined with columnar epithelial cells beneath the epithelial lining. In severe cases, adenomatous hyperplasia, periductal fibrosis and goblet cell metaplasia may be seen. Inflammation, necrosis and atrophy of hepatic cells has also been reported.

The pathology of fluke-associated cholecystitis consists of fibrosis of the gallbladder wall, mast cell infiltration and mucosal hyperplasia. Parasites and eggs have been observed in the nidus of gallbladder and intrahepatic stones.[13]

It remains unclear whether liver flukes mediate tissue damage directly via mechanical or chemical irritation, or whether the pathogenesis is immune mediated.[16,35] Elevated levels of parasite-specific IgG occur frequently in gallbladder disease and cholangiocarcinoma.[30,35,36] Increased endogenous production of *N*-nitroso compounds or hepatic activation of dietary carcinogens, plus chronic hyperplasia of the bile duct epithelium, may enhance susceptibility to cancer.[15,16,21,36,37]

DIAGNOSIS AND INVESTIGATIONS

Egg counts have traditionally been used to diagnose liver fluke infection, most often using the Kato thick smear, Stoll's dilution or quantitative formalin ethyl acetate concentration technique. All three techniques effectively detect moderate and heavy infections. However, comparative studies in low intensity areas have shown that a single reading of the concentration and dilution techniques detect about 70% of infections, while the sensitivity of Kato is considerably lower (45%).[38] Worm burden and egg count correlate closely, with an estimated egg output of 53 per gram of faeces per worm (using Stoll's dilution technique).[39] Stoll's egg counts are roughly eightfold higher than those of the concentration technique.

Although egg detection is almost always used in surveys and treatment programmes, several immunodiagnostic tests have been described.[13,14,40] Antigen detection enzyme linked immunosorbent assays (ELISAs) using specific monoclonal antibodies against secretory antigens have shown promise,[40] while those based on parasite-specific antibody levels are neither sensitive nor specific. DNA probes have also been developed but these require radioactive labelling.[40]

MANAGEMENT

Treatment with praziquantel at 40 mg/kg body weight in a single dose is effective against opisthorchiasis and clonorchiasis.[14,24,41,42] This regimen has been used most commonly in large-scale treatment programmes. Reports from China, however, indicate that higher doses (120 mg/kg over 2 days) are needed to cure heavy *Clonorchis* infections.[42] Side-effects, such as dizziness, vomiting and abdominal pain, occur frequently but are transient and rarely severe. Most abnormalities of the gallbladder are also eliminated by elimination of the parasite.[43] Praziquantel may be dangerous for people with early cholangiocarcinoma, since the sudden expulsion of many worms may aggravate obstruction. No such cases have been reported, but caution should be exercised. The drug hexachloroparaxylol (Chlox-

yle) has also been used extensively for the treatment of *O. felineus*,[24] but it may be less effective than praziquantel.[42]

PREVENTION AND CONTROL

Prevention of *Opisthorchis* infection can be facilitated by treatment (to reduce the excretion of eggs), sanitation (to prevent eggs from reaching water sources) and health education (to discourage the eating of raw fish).[11] Control of snail vectors by molluscicides is not considered feasible because of their widespread distribution and resistance to adverse conditions.[23] To be most effective, health education should be designed and delivered in a culturally sensitive manner with the aim of affecting behaviour change as well as simply providing information. Large-scale efforts in each of these areas by the Ministries of Public Health in many of the endemic countries have probably had a major impact on the intensity of all three infections.

FASCIOLIASIS

Fasciola infections are common in domestic ruminants and wildlife throughout the world and cause massive economic loss in the livestock industry.[44,45] Humans usually become infected by eating aquatic plants grown in water contaminated with faeces from animals harbouring *Fasciola*. The morbidity and epidemiology have recently been reviewed by Chen and Mott.[46]

HISTORY AND SEMINAL DISCOVERIES

Fasciola hepatica was the first trematode to be described—500 years before most others (de Brie, 1379; cited in reference 1). Its complete life cycle was identified by Leuckart (1882) and Thomas (1883); this greatly facilitated the elucidation of other trematode life cycles. Elegant studies by Isseroff and colleagues examined the role of proline in the pathogenesis of bile duct fibrosis and dilatation, and anaemia of *F. hepatica* in mice.[47]

AETIOLOGY AND LIFE CYCLE

F. hepatica (the sheep liver fluke) and *F. gigantica* (mainly of cattle) cause fascioliasis in humans. The parasites vary in adult and egg size and shape

(Figure 73.3) and species of the snail host of the family Lymnaeidae. *F. hepatica* is common in temperate and subtropical areas, especially in sheep-raising areas, and human infections are relatively common in Europe (especially France, Spain and Portugal), the Middle East (particularly Egypt), Central and South America (Cuba, Peru) and Africa.[44,46] *F. gigantica* occurs in South and South-East Asia and Africa. The two coexist in some countries, and differentiation often is difficult.

The adult worm lives in the bile duct of the final host and eggs are excreted in the faeces of the host. The eggs undergo further development upon reaching a water body; miracidium then hatch and penetrate a suitable snail host. After multiplication as sporocysts and rediae, free-swimming mature cercariae exit the snail, attach to aquatic vegetation and become metacercarial cysts. These cysts establish infection upon ingestion by man and other mammals. They excyst in the duodenum, then migrate through the intestinal wall, into the body cavity, through Glisson's capsule across the liver parenchyma and into the bile ducts, where they may live for many years. Eggs are excreted 3–4 months after ingestion. Generally the life cycle is maintained by domestic animals, particularly by sheep for *F. hepatica* and cattle/buffalo for *F. gigantica*; it is completed in 4–6 months.

EPIDEMIOLOGY

Fortunately infection in humans is a relatively rare event, even where prevalence among domestic animals is high. However, during outbreaks a high proportion of exposed people become infected.[48,49] Human infection with *Fasciola* is apparently dependent on temperature (10–30°C for *F. hepatica*) and the frequency of humans eating plants (mainly watercress) from water bodies contaminated with animal faeces. High humidity and rainfall favour transmission.[44–46,48–50]

Since fascioliasis has been reported mainly in case reports rather than in community-based studies, it is difficult to assess the extent of infection within areas where cases are reported. The frequency of infection is undoubtedly underreported since eggs are often not detected by faecal examination; investigations following outbreaks have identified asymptomatic infections amongst those with severe symptoms and misdiagnoses are common.[46,48–50] Outbreaks of *F. hepatica* are most often associated with consumption of wild watercress, while cultivated watercress may be free from infection. Infection might also be acquired from contaminated drinking water or cooking utensils.[50]

PATHOGENESIS

These parasites cause considerable mortality in sheep and cattle, and human morbidity—which is dependent on the number of worms and stage of infection.[44,46,47,51] The acute phase occurs during migration of the immature flukes through the liver. Severe pathology results from parasite ingestion and destruction of parenchymal tissue, haemorrhage, parasite death and inflammatory responses largely mediated by eosinophils. Repair mechanisms can lead to extensive fibrosis, increased pressure atrophy of the liver and periportal fibrosis.

The chronic phase, during which parasites are

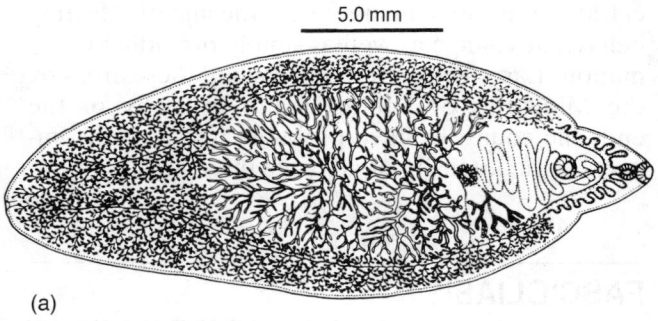

5.0 mm

(a)

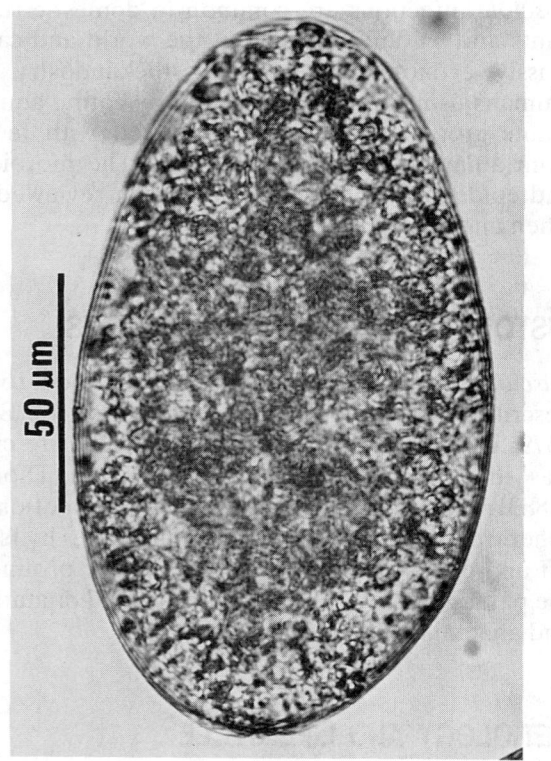

50 μm

(b)

Figure 73.3 (a) Adult stage worm of *Fasciola hepatica*. Drawn by Sasithorn Kaewkes. (b) Egg of *F. hepatica*. Photograph by Sasithorn Kaewkes.

present in the bile ducts, tends to be less severe. Tissue change, including bile duct proliferation, dilatation and fibrosis, is largely caused by mechanical obstruction of the ducts, inflammatory responses and the activity of proline, which the fluke excretes in large quantity.[47] Proline may facilitate movement of the parasite through the narrow ducts. Anaemia may result from blood loss through bile duct lesions. Death is uncommon, but is usually caused by haemorrhaging in the bile duct and case reports suggest it occurs more frequently in children.[46]

Flukes that migrate out of the intestine but do not locate in the liver can form ectopic lesions in many tissues.[46,51] These nodules, granulomas or migration tracts are often misdiagnosed as malignant tumours or gastric ulcers.

PATHOLOGY

Multiple yellow nodules of necrotic tissue (1–4 mm in diameter) and linear lesions through the parenchyma infiltrated with eosinophils and Charcot–Leyden crystals can be observed, probably as a result of inflammatory reaction(s) to dead parasites and migration, respectively.[46,51] Proliferation, dilatation, fibrosis and calcification of the bile ducts, plus sequelae of partial obstruction, may occur during the chronic phase of infection. Dead flukes are sometimes observed inside calcified areas of tissue, and granulomas and abscesses can form around eggs trapped in the parenchymal tissue. Eosinophils may infiltrate the gallbladder wall, which may be thickened and oedematous with perimuscular fibrosis. Stones are often present in the gallbladder during infection. Self-cure appears to occur frequently and may result from inflammation and calcification.

CLINICAL FEATURES

Where cases are symptomatic, diarrhoea, upper abdominal pain or pain in the right costal margin, urticaria, malaise, weight loss, coughing, fever and night sweats may begin approximately 2 months following ingestion of metacercaria and 1–2 months prior to the onset of egg excretion.[44,46,48–52] The signs of this acute phase of infection are hepatomegaly, splenomegaly, anaemia, weakness and marked peripheral eosinophilia, up to 80%.

Adult flukes in the bile ducts may be associated with cholangitis and calculous or acalculous cholecystitis. Through their large size and the inflammatory and fibrotic response, the infection may cause obstruction leading to cholestatic jaundice, nausea, pruritus, abdominal pain, hepatomegaly and fatty

food intolerance. In severe cases, ascites with blood and severe anaemia may ensue. Since these moderate signs and symptoms do not differ from cholangitis and cholecystitis of other causes, the infection often goes unnoticed until worms are observed at surgery or histopathology. Eosinophilia and a history of eating water plants should be considered in the differential diagnosis.

DIAGNOSIS AND INVESTIGATIONS

Fascioliasis has been diagnosed by observation of eggs during faecal examination, by parasite-specific antibody detection in a variety of immunodiagnostic assays, by radiological methods and by laparotomy. Dietary history is also helpful, particularly in investigating outbreaks.

Examination of faeces for eggs is of limited use[44,46,48–52] since eggs are not excreted during the invasive stage of infection, when many patients present with severe symptoms. Often eggs are undetectable during the chronic phase, but whether the techniques used are insensitive for very low egg outputs in light infections (<100 eggs per gram) or eggs are not being produced is unclear. Clearly if eggs are being excreted, sensitivity of the stool examination can be increased by using an optimum technique (Weller–Dammin's modification and the AMS III technique) and by examining several fields for eggs and several faecal samples.[46] Differentiation of eggs from *F. hepatica*, *F. gigantica*, echinostomes and *Fasciolopsis* can be difficult (see Figures 73.3b, 73.4b and 73.5b,d). In addition to the faeces, eggs can also be found in duodenal contents and bile and in histological sections.

A further problem with faecal examination is that eggs may be detected after ingestion of liver from infected animals. This does not indicate infection; thus positive cases should be reconfirmed if liver has been eaten recently.[1]

Immunodiagnostic tests using every available technique have been reported in the literature, from skin tests to antibody and antigen detection assays.[46,53,54] Most claim excellent sensitivity (90%), but cross-reactivity with other trematode infections is a problem in areas where they coexist. *Fasciola*-specific ELISAs using partially purified fluke antigens are available.[53,54]

The advantage of immunodiagnosis over parasitological techniques is that they can detect early, prepatent infections as well as chronic ones with little or no egg output. In contrast to other infections, levels of antibody in ELISAs appear to drop rapidly after successful treatment, so the assays tend to detect only active infection. Immunofluorescence and counterimmunoelectrophoresis assays are recommended for early detection because of their high sensitivity in the invasive phase.

Clinical diagnosis is often difficult because presentations are not markedly different from hepatobiliary disease of other origin(s).[46,48,52] Clinicians may not think about fascioliasis where human infections are uncommon. In temperate climates, outbreaks are almost invariably associated with eating wild watercress. The finding of multiple, related cases with similar diet histories and high-risk occupation (e.g. sheep farmers) may provide supporting evidence. In tropical areas where consumption of gathered water plants is frequent, this may be of limited use. Laparotomy and radiological imaging by ultrasonography, endoscopic retrograde cholangiopancreatography and percutaneous cholangiography may be useful.[52,55–57] These allow visualization of the lesions of acute and chronic fascioliasis and sometimes eggs (by laparotomy) or worms in the hepatobiliary system.

MANAGEMENT

The treatment of fascioliasis remains highly problematic, in contrast to other trematode infections, requiring high or multiple doses of drugs with significant side-effects.[46,58–61] Efficacy is often variable and difficult to assess. These problems result from differing sensitivities of the adult and migrating worms, the size and thick tegument of *Fasciola*, impaired hepatic function, and varying clinical presentations.

Treatment with the drug bithionol, is effective against fascioliasis at a dose of 30–50 mg/kg body weight per day in three divided doses on alternate days for a duration of 10–15 days.[55,58,59] Success against acute infection has been reported for dehydroementine at a dose of 1 mg/kg daily for 10 days given intramuscularly or subcutaneously.[46,48] Moderate to severe side-effects have been observed;

both drugs and multiple courses are often required.[59]

While some reports claim success with praziquantel and mebendazole treatment, it is generally considered that these drugs are not effective against fascioliasis even at high doses.[52] The discrepancy may be due to difficulty in assessing parasite death and to coincidental self-cure during follow-up.

Triclabendazole is often effective at a dose of 10 mg/kg taken after meals, but may require multiple doses in persistent cases. This compound may become the drug of choice.[52,60]

Depending on the presentation of the patient, other drugs given before the fasciolicide appear to facilitate recovery. Prednisone (5–10 mg/day) may alleviate toxaemia, while antibiotics are often required to treat acute cholangitis due to secondary bacterial infection.[59,61] Chloroquine was previously used because it rapidly relieves symptoms of acute disease[46,48] but does not kill the flukes.

PREVENTION AND CONTROL

Ultimate control of *Fasciola* must focus on strategic treatment of livestock and other herbivorous animals that maintain the life cycle.[44–46] This is being considered by some countries and would also reduce the economic loss to the parasite.[45] Control of the snail vectors using molluscicides is not considered practical in most situations. Health education to discourage human consumption of raw wild watercress and other edible water plants may be effective in areas where the disease is prevalent. Strict controls on commercial production of water plants—as has been instituted in some Western countries, would help to prevent the expansion of endemic areas. Increased awareness by clinicians of the problem and its diagnostic difficulties, plus data from community-based studies assessing seroprevalence, may help quantify the extent to which fascioliasis affects human health.

INTESTINAL FLUKES

FASCIOLOPSIASIS

Fasciolopsiasis is caused by the giant intestinal fluke, *Fasciolopsis buski*.[1] It is in the same family as *Fasciola*, and its life cycle and morphology are similar (Figure 73.4). However, *Fasciolopsis* infection is largely confined to Asian countries, namely southern China, India, Bangladesh, Thailand, Malaysia, Borneo, Sumatra and Myanmar, and may reach high prevalences within endemic areas. The parasite attaches to the intestinal wall of man and pig. Light infections are less pathogenic than those of *Fasciola* and more easily diagnosed and treated. Heavy infections can be severe.

HISTORY AND SEMINAL DISCOVERIES

The life cycle was first described by Nakagawa (1921) and Barlow (1925).[1] Detailed studies in Thailand were by Sadun and Maiphoom[62] and Manning et al.[63] Jaroonvesama et al.[64] identified many important factors which determine fasciolopsiasis endemicity.

LIFE CYCLE

In contrast to *Fasciola*, the final host range of *F. buski* is limited and many mammals are refractory.[1,65] Humans and pigs become infected through the consumption of viable metacercaria attached to the seed pods of water plants. These include: the water caltrops, water hyacinth, water chestnut, water bamboo, lotus roots, wild rice shoots, etc. Although metacercaria are not present on the edible seed of these plants, ingestion occurs during removal of the pods with the teeth and lips. Metacercaria are also found free on the surface of ponds, and infection may occur from drinking water.[66]

F. buski excysts in the duodenum and the escaping larvae attach to the duodenal and jejunal wall. The larvae become mature adults in 3 months and produce large numbers (an estimated 10 000–25 000 per day per worm) of large, yellow, operculated eggs (Figure 73.4). If these eggs reach water sources, further development and embryonation occurs over 3–7 weeks, then miracidia hatch and enter snail intermediate hosts (family Planorbidae). After multiplication as sporocysts and redia, free-swimming cercaria attach and encyst on seed pods.

EPIDEMIOLOGY

In Thailand, infection is largely confined to low-lying areas in the central region(s) with heavy rainfall and extensive flooding, which leads to faecal contamination of the water.[62–65] Elsewhere the use of pig or human faeces for fertilization is associated with endemicity.[66] Prevalences are highest in areas with cultivation or year-round availability of water caltrops and other aquatic vegetation and where people enjoy eating the nuts raw. Chinese investi-

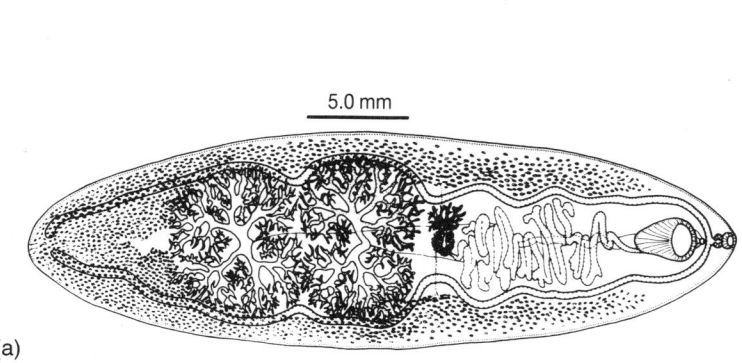

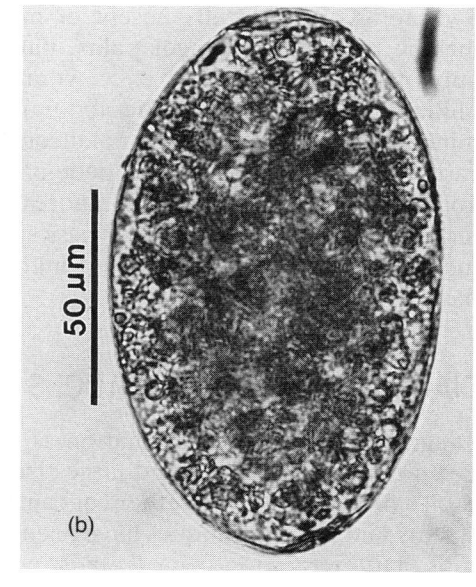

Figure 73.4   (a) Adult stage worm of *Fasciolopsis buski*. Drawn by Sasithorn Kaewkes. (b) Egg of *F. buski*. Photograph by Sasithorn Kaewkes.

gators have emphasized the importance of contaminated drinking water as a source of infection.[66]

Community-based prevalences generally reach 20%, with a typical peak in children over 5 years of age and little difference between sexes.[62–64,67,68] Children are often more frequently and heavily infected than adults since they enjoy gathering and eating water plants during play.[67–69]

PATHOGENESIS AND PATHOLOGY

Eosinophils accumulate at the site of parasite attachment on the jejunal or duodenal wall where mechanical injury and inflammation lead to ulcer formation.[1,51,65] These ulcers sometimes bleed due to capillary damage or become abscesses. Mild infection in healthy people is associated with lower haematocrit and serum levels of vitamin B_{12}, but no apparent change in other nutrients.[64,70] This may result from parasite sequestering of vitamin B_{12} or its impaired absorption from the damaged intestinal mucosa.

Although a few parasites cause little damage, the presence of many (hundreds to thousands) is associated with severe pathology and sometimes acute intestinal obstruction. Extensive intestinal ulceration may interfere with digestion, and cause malabsorption, leading to severe malnutrition and wasting. Oedema also occurs in severe cases; it may result from toxic parasite metabolites, allergic reactions or from hypoalbuminaemia secondary to electrolyte and protein imbalance from chronic malabsorption.

CLINICAL FEATURES

Symptoms are generally absent or mild, and may include: diarrhoea, hunger pains, flatulence, poor appetite, mild abdominal colic, vomiting, eosinophilia and fever.[1,51,62–65] The abdominal pain may mimic that of peptic or duodenal ulcer. Late, severe cases present with ascites or oedema of the face, abdomen and legs, anaemia, anorexia, weakness and vomiting and patients may pass stools containing large amounts of undigested material. Deaths have been reported.

DIAGNOSIS AND INVESTIGATIONS

Diagnosis by faecal examination is not difficult, given the large quantity and large size of the eggs. Stoll's dilution, formalin ether concentration, direct smears and Kato techniques have been used successfully. Differentiation from *Fasciola* eggs is difficult

(Figures 73.3b and 73.4b), so that a dietary and clinical history should also be considered.

MANAGEMENT

In the past, hexylresorcinol crystoids, tetrachloroethylene and dichlorophen were used for treatment of fasciolopsis with varying effectiveness.[65,69] Praziquantel is now the treatment of choice, with high efficacy at a dose of 15 mg/kg body weight.[42,65–69] In heavily infected cases there may be some danger of exacerbating obstruction or acute toxaemia with treatment, such that conservative treatment is advised.

PREVENTION AND CONTROL

In Indonesia, community-based praziquantel treatment has been used to control infection.[67,68] However, migration and fairly rapid reinfection following treatment (prevalences approached pretreatment levels within 12 months) confounded efforts to control infection by chemotherapy alone.

Weng et al[66] advocate the use of fermented, instead of fresh, silage for feeding pigs in endemic areas since metacercaria are sensitive to both heat and salt. Drying the plants may also be effective. Sterilizing or prohibiting the use of human and pig faeces for fertilizer and improved sanitation would help interrupt the life cycle. Refraining from using the mouth to peel the vegetables, then boiling for a few seconds, or careful washing after peeling them with hands or knife would reduce human infection. Filtering drinking water may prevent some infection. Health education should help people recognize the problem as well as indicate acceptable ways to avoid infection, since most infections are mild.

Successful control efforts in one country in China reduced the prevalence from 76% in 1951, to 24% in 1976.[13]

ECHINOSTOMIASIS

Fifteen species of echinostomes have been recorded in man, and the most common appear to be *E. ilocanum, E. revolutum, E. malayanum, E. echinatum* and *E. hortense* (Figure 73.5).[1,71–74] Although they are considered of minor medical importance, infections with these parasites reach high prevalences in endemic areas. The literature on human infections is limited and has been reviewed.[73]

LIFE CYCLE

These parasites have a highly variable and wide host range. Humans become infected with echinostomes through the consumption of raw or incompletely cooked freshwater snails, clams, fish and tadpoles harbouring metacercaria. The parasite lives in the intestine of the definitive host, and eggs are excreted in faeces. Snails are the first intermediate host, then after a brief free-swimming stage, cercaria encyst within a second intermediate host which may be another mollusc, fish or amphibian larvae. Aquatic birds are the most important final host of most species.

EPIDEMIOLOGY

Most human infections occur in Asia in areas where raw or incompletely cooked molluscs and fish are eaten. Infection is common in Korea, Indonesia, the Philippines, Malaysia, Taiwan and Thailand.[1,71–77] Reported prevalences in endemic communities generally range from 1 to 30%.[11,74,76] Infection may be clustered in families who prefer raw foods, and there is a tendency for those infected with *Opisthorchis* also to harbour echinostomes in north-east Thailand.[75]

DIAGNOSIS

The large, unembryonated, operculated eggs of echinostomes can be observed in faeces and are difficult to differentiate from those of *Fasciola* and *Fasciolopsis* (Figures 73.3b, 73.4b and 73.5b,d). Adult worms can be recovered from faeces following treatment.[72,77] This allows for positive differentiation based on morphology, of which the predominant feature is the collar of spines around

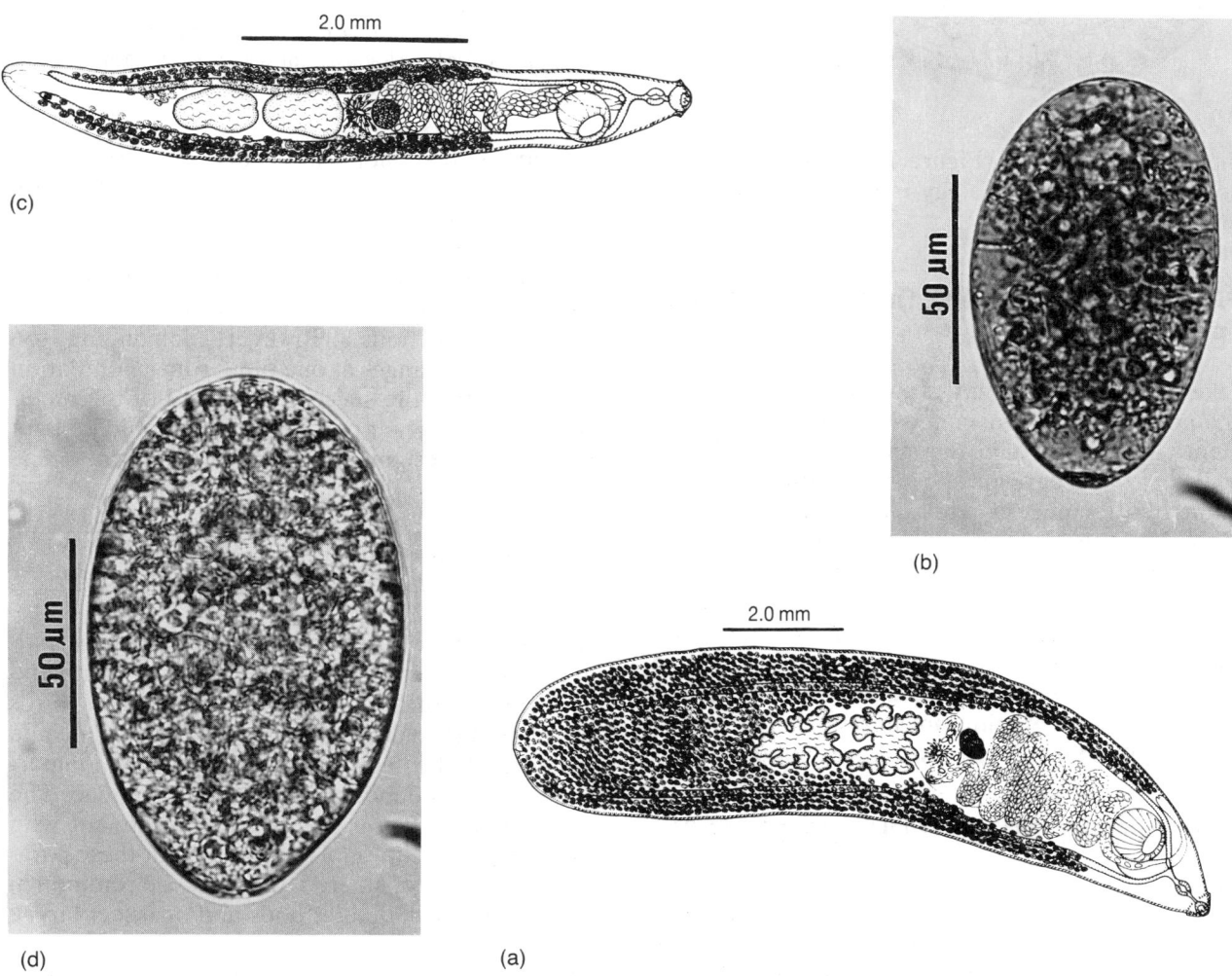

Figure 73.5 (a) Adult stage worm of *Echinostoma ilocanum*. Drawn by Sasithorn Kaewkes. (b) Egg of *E. ilocanum*. Photograph by Sasithorn Kaewkes. (c) Adult stage worm of *E. malayanum*. Drawn by Sasithorn Kaewkes. (d) Egg of *E. malayanum*. Photograph by Sasithorn Kaewkes.

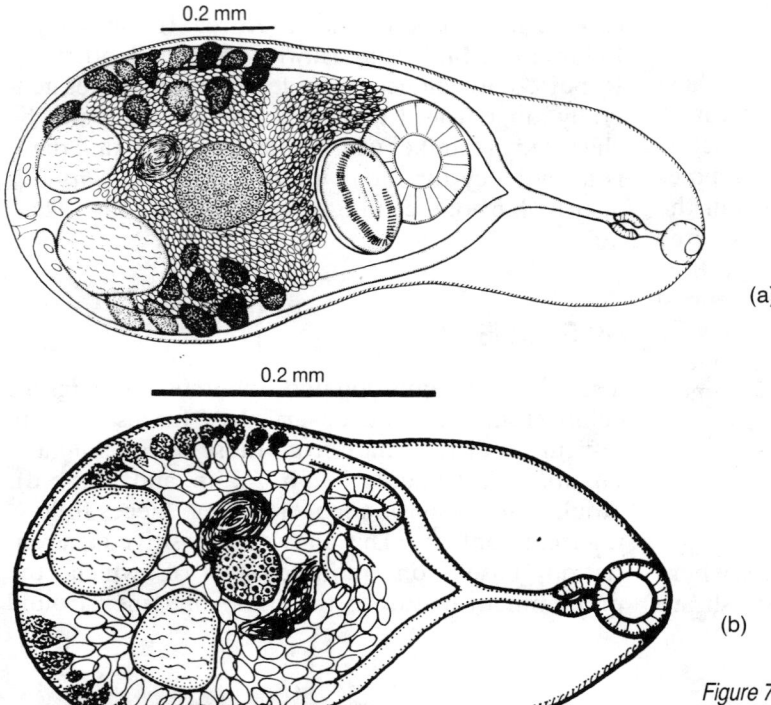

0.2 mm

(a)

0.2 mm

(b)

Figure 73.6   (a) Adult stage worm of *Heterophyes heterophyes*. Drawn by Sasithorn Kaewkes. (b) Adult stage worm of *Metagonimus yokogawai*. Drawn by Sasithorn Kaewkes.

the oral sucker[1,71,72] (Figure 73.5a,c). It should be noted that the morphology may be altered by the drug.[72,75]

PATHOGENESIS, PATHOLOGY AND CLINICAL FEATURES

Like *F. buski*, the major pathological lesions of echinostomes are associated with parasite attachment deep between the villae of the jejunal wall.[51,71,73,74] There may be inflammation and ulceration of the mucosa where the parasites locate. However, echinostomes are not highly pathogenic to humans and there are only a few reports of clinical aspects of this infection. While light burdens are asymptomatic, heavy infections may cause diarrhoea, eosinophilia, abdominal discomfort and anorexia. These symptoms apparently do not develop into the life-threatening presentations that are described (albeit rarely) in fasciolopsis infection.

MANAGEMENT, PREVENTION AND CONTROL

Infections are relatively easily cured with mebendazole, albendazole, praziquantel, bithionol, hexylresorcinol crystoids and niclosamide.[73,74] Treatment with praziquantel at 15 mg/kg is recommended in areas where other trematodes are present, due to its broad efficacy, safety and ease of use.[71–73,76,77] In

these areas, drug application may be provided to facilitate control of echinostomiasis together with other trematode infections.

Prevention can be supplemented by health education to discourage the consumption of raw or incompletely cooked fish and molluscs, as for other fish-borne infections. However, demanding too many dietary changes at one time from a population may jeopardize the successful control of the medically most important parasites. This should be kept in mind when designing health promotion strategies.

HETEROPHYIASIS

There are a large number of small or minute intestinal flukes, measuring less than 2.5 mm in length and just visible to the eye, which parasitize man, birds and other mammals[1,72] (Figure 73.6). These include members of the families Heterophyidae, Plagiorchiidae, Lecithodendridae and Microphallidae. The examination of faeces passed after treatment with praziquantel or bithionol has shown that these parasites previously considered 'rare' may be common in areas where raw aquatic foods and/or insect larvae are eaten.[2,3,78] Species of *Heterophyes, Haplorchis, Metagonimus, Carneophallus* may cause disease in man.[1,51,78] Due to their similarity these parasites are covered here under the term 'heterophyids'.

AETIOLOGY AND LIFE CYCLE

Heterophyes heterophyes, *Metagonimus yokogawai*, *Haplorchis taichui*, *Haplorchis pumilio* and *Stellantchasmus falcatus* are a few of the many heterophyids known to infect man.[1,72,78] The first two species are thought to be the most important medically.

Adult heterophyids live deeply embedded in the intestinal mucosa of mammals and birds where they produce fully embryonated eggs which are excreted in faeces. Upon ingestion by a freshwater snail (*Melania*, *Semisulcospira* and others), the larvae escape, undergo multiplication, then exit as cercaria. The cercaria penetrate and encyst within many species of fresh and brackish water fish or shrimps.[78,79] Humans become infected while eating fish or shrimps harbouring viable metacercaria, which become mature adults within 5–10 days. An average of 10 000 metacercaria of *Metagonimus yokogawai* are found in the sweetfish (*Plecoglossus altivelis*) during the 'eating season' in Korea.[5,79]

EPIDEMIOLOGY

Heterophyids are mainly found in Asia (Japan, Korea, Laos, Thailand, Taiwan, Philippines, China), Hawaii, Siberia, Turkey and the Balkans.[1,2,3,28,72,78,79] Little has been reported about their epidemiology in humans beyond geographic distribution and life cycle.[2,3] Food habits and access to rich aquatic fauna are the important determinants of human infection.

Metagonimus yokogawai infects 1.2% of the Korean population, and is common (5–20% prevalence) in riverside communities where raw sweetfish is enjoyed.[5,79] Another species, *Heterophyes nocens*, which utilizes brackish water intermediate hosts, was found in 42% of residents from a Korean island.

PATHOGENESIS, PATHOLOGY AND CLINICAL SYMPTOMS

These are similar for different species. Most infections are asymptomatic or accompanied by mild intestinal discomfort, which may include mucous diarrhoea, colicky pains, intermittent neurasthenia and lethargy.[1,51,78] These probably result from mild inflammation with mainly eosinophils, superficial necrosis, excessive mucus secretion and bleeding at the site of attachment. Movement of the parasite's spiny surface may contribute to ulceration, and hyperplasia in the mesenteric lymph nodes may also cause abdominal pain.

Symptoms are most frequent in heavy infections, but they subside spontaneously after approximately 1 month, although the flukes remain.[5] Upon further infection, symptoms may recur, giving rise to occasional episodes of diarrhoea in endemic areas.

One special aspect of heterophyid pathogenesis is the involvement of eggs. These embed deeply in the intestinal wall, eliciting eosinophil and neutrophil infiltration. The eggs (and sometimes adult worms) may then enter nearby lymphatics or blood vessels and be transported to other sites—notably the heart, spinal cord or brain, lungs, liver and spleen.[51,78,80] Eggs become trapped and elicit granulomatous lesions and fibrosis. Signs of heterophyid myocarditis may include cardiac enlargement, cough, dyspnoea, cyanosis, fatigue, oedema and ascites, palpitation, loss of reflexes and abnormal heart sounds. Eggs or worms in the spinal cord or brain may cause neurological disease, transverse myelitis and loss of sensory and motor function.

DIAGNOSIS

Diagnosis is usually based on the recovery of eggs in faeces, but there are many problems. The daily egg output is low (35–45) and light infections (<100 worms) are easily missed. Extraintestinal cases of heterophyiasis may be discovered at surgery or autopsy, and then only after careful searching. Distinction between species of heterophyids and *Clonorchis* and *Opisthorchis* by egg is exceedingly difficult. However, recent publications have helped establish criteria for differentiation.[3,81,82] The recovery of adult worms from post-treatment stools allows a definitive diagnosis, but this procedure is extremely tedious due to their minute size.[2,3]

Antibodies against heterophyids cross-react with those against *O. viverrini* in ELISA.[83] However, antibody recognition patterns visualized by immunoblotting may differ and help to distinguish liver fluke from heterophyid infections.[83]

MANAGEMENT

Niclosamide, bithionol and tetrachloroethylene were previously used, but praziquantel is now the drug of choice. A single dose of 10–20 mg/kg is highly effective.[78,79]

PREVENTION AND CONTROL

Like other fish-borne trematodes, treatment with praziquantel, combined with health education to encourage cooking of fish and other aquatic foods, is important. More studies are required on the frequency and spectrum of clinical consequences in order to assess the amount of resources that should be allocated for control. Although the ability of the parasites to cause fatal disease is clear, the actual frequency of this has recently received very little attention.

LUNG FLUKES

PARAGONIMIASIS

These flukes are distributed widely, and infect an estimated ten million people in China alone.[84-91] Infection can cause severe respiratory or cerebral disease, depending on intensity, duration and site where the parasites become lodged.

AETIOLOGY

Although there are many lung flukes of mammals, only *Paragonimus* spp. infect man. Their taxonomy is unclear, but it is generally agreed that seven or eight species are of major medical importance in fairly distinct geographic areas[84] (Figure 73.7). These include *P. westermani, P. miyazakii, P. skrjabini* and *P. heterotremus* in Asia, *P. africanus* and *P. uterobilateralis* in Africa and *P. mexicanus* (and *P. ecuadoriensis*) in Latin and South America. Countries with significant numbers of cases include China, Taiwan, Thailand, Japan, Nigeria, Cameroon, Peru and Ecuador.[84-91]

LIFE CYCLE

Paragonimus lives in the lungs of some mammals—mainly wild and domestic cats, but also dogs, mon-

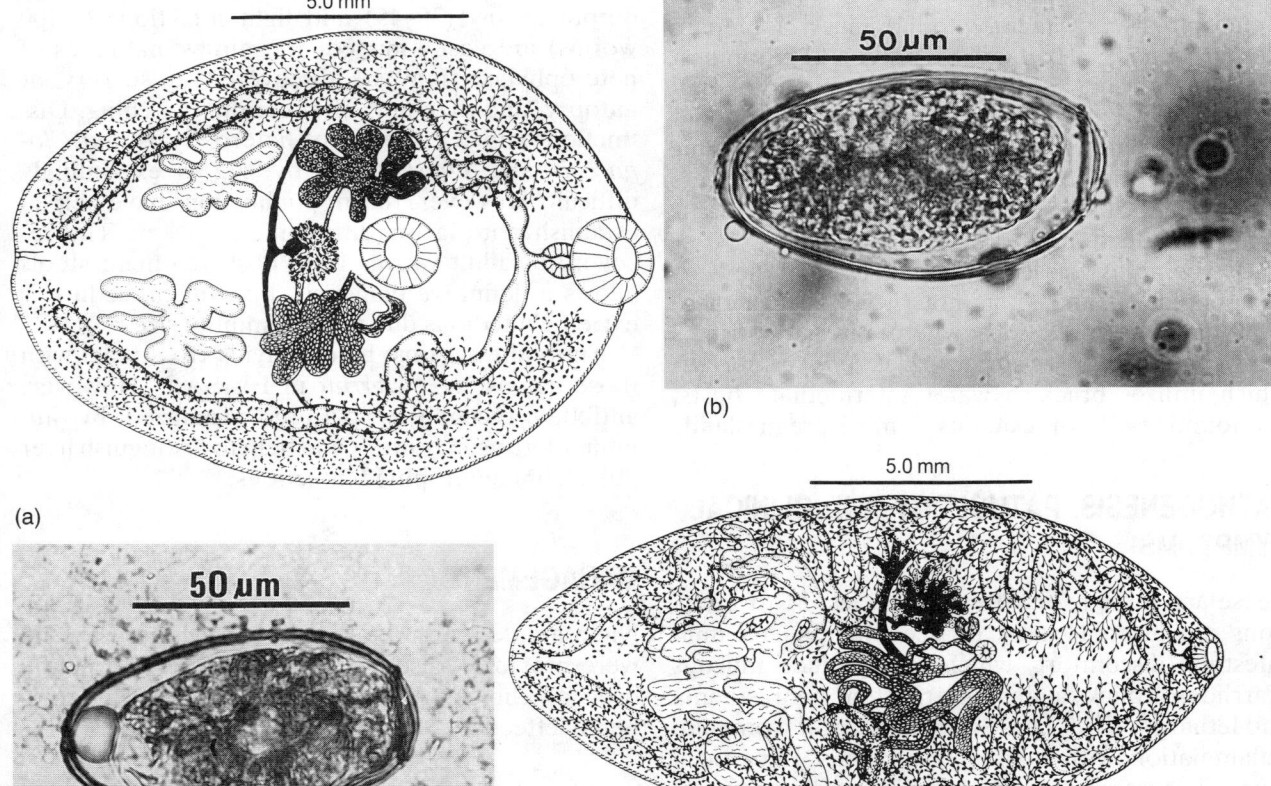

Figure 73.7 (a) Adult stage worm of *Paragonimus westermani*. Drawn by Sasithorn Kaewkes. (b) Egg of *P. westermani*. Photograph by Sasithorn Kaewkes. (c) Adult stage worm of *P. heterotremus*. Drawn by Sasithorn Kaewkes. (d) Egg of *P. heterotremus*. Photograph by Sasithorn Kaewkes.

keys and humans. Parasite eggs are coughed up from the lungs and either expectorated in the sputum, or swallowed and excreted in the faeces. When these eggs reach water, further development occurs until miracidia hatch; they then penetrate a snail host (mainly species of Thiaridae and Pleuroceridae). Multiplication and development occur in the snail until cercaria are produced. These may enter the second intermediate host, namely potamid or other crabs, crayfish and one species of shrimp, while free-swimming or during consumption of the snail by the crustacean. The cercaria encyst in the gills, liver and muscle tissue of the crab and require about 2 months to become infective metacercaria. When the crabs are eaten by a final mammalian host, the cysts excyst in the small intestine, penetrate the intestinal wall, travel from the peritoneum to the subperitoneal tissue, passing through the diaphragm to the lungs—where they mature in 2 months. Adult worms may live for 20 years. Due to aberrant migration, larvae sometimes become lodged in ectopic sites, e.g. brain, abdomen, groin, skin or heart.

In some mammals which serve as paratenic hosts, the larvae exit the small intestine and lodge without further development in muscle tissue.[84–88] When a final mammalian host consumes the paratenic host, the larvae survive passage through the stomach and escape through the intestinal wall. Migration to the lungs then results in maturation and egg excretion.

EPIDEMIOLOGY

Human infection most often results from consumption of raw or incompletely cooked pickled, wine- or brine-soaked crabs, crayfish and shrimps harbouring metacercaria.[84–88] Alternatively, transmission may occur via eating wild boar, pigs, or small animals harbouring preadult worms. Metacercaria may also be ingested during preparation of these foods via contamination of hands or utensils. In addition to dietary preferences, raw crab meat and juice are thought to have medicinal properties for enhancing fertility, reducing fever and treating measles.[87] This last practice once caused high levels of infection in Korean children, while Philippine children enjoy eating incompletely roasted crabs.[86]

Although endemic pockets are still being discovered in Korea, the number infected has dropped dramatically in recent years.[87] High prevalences of infection (up to 45%) were observed during a skin test survey in endemic communities in Korea in 1959. The infection is endemic throughout China, although again, vigorous control efforts have successfully reduced prevalences in some areas.[88,89] Surveys in the Philippines found prevalences of 0.5–

12% in human communities, while 50–100% of crabs in endemic areas harbour *Paragonimus*.[86] Significant prevalences have been reported recently from parts of Nigeria (16.8%) and Cameroon (2.1–28.6%).[90] Although eating raw food is not a widespread habit in India, 39 cases of *Paragonimus* were recently reported from Manipur State.[91]

PATHOGENESIS AND PATHOLOGY

The site of pathology of paragonimiasis depends upon the migratory route of the larvae and the tissue in which they lodge.[1,51,84,85,92,93] Inflammatory responses to the adult worms, immature worms and eggs are similar, regardless of location. Resulting lesions are granulomatous, beginning with leucocyte (mainly eosinophil) infiltration and finally resulting in thick cysts or abscesses and ultimately calcification. The parasites live within these fibrotic, greyish-white capsules (1.5–5 cm in diameter) in pairs or triplets, surrounded by thick, blood-streaked fluid and numerous eggs. Later, the capsules may be empty or fluid filled. Eggs trapped in the tissue may also provoke granulomas at the periphery of the necrotic area. The capsules occur most frequently in the upper right quadrant of the lungs and, in the fewer cases of cerebral involvement, the posterior portion of the brain is usually affected.

In both human and experimental infections there appears to be a subsidence of inflammation in later periods.[92] This may be due to modulation of the immune response.

CLINICAL FEATURES

Pulmonary infection is accompanied by a chronic productive cough, with brownish purulent sputum containing streaks of blood and parasite eggs in *P. westermani*, *P. heterotremus* and African and American paragonimiasis. Chest pain and night sweats may also occur. The signs mimic bronchiectasis, bronchopneumonia, or tuberculosis not responding to antibiotics. Eosinophilia of 20–25% is common.

Pleural effusion and pneumothorax with marked eosinophilia in the exudate and peripheral blood occur particularly frequently in *P. miyazakii* infections in Japan. Although there may be a persistent cough, neither brownish sputum nor eggs are expelled in *P. skrjabini* and *P. miyazakii* infections.

Cerebral paragonimus may cause eosinophilic meningitis, which is characterized by headache, convulsions of the focal Jacksonian type, hemiplegia and visual impairment with insidious onset.[51,85,94] Most cases involve males under 10 years of age.

Flukes in the spinal cord may cause spastic paraplegia. Pulmonary symptoms (cough with brownish sputum) usually accompany cerebral disease. Cutaneous paragonimiasis occurs when the parasites lodge in subcutaneous tissue, forming painless, mobile swellings which may contain immature worms. The patient may also exhibit mild pulmonary abnormalities. This manifestation occurs frequently in *P. skrjabini* infection, which does not localize to the lungs.

Sometimes the flukes migrate through the peritoneal cavity eliciting the formation of multiple nodules (abdominal paragonimiasis) which often appear similar to malignant tumours.

Mortality has been reported, either due to parasites and resulting abscesses in the heart or to fulminating infection in the abdominal cavity.

DIAGNOSIS AND INVESTIGATIONS

The clinical signs are fairly pathognomonic, particularly when diet history and residence in an endemic area are known, but misdiagnosis is commonly due to unfamiliarity with the disease.[6,91] Tests to rule out tuberculosis, skin tests and sputum smear and culture are helpful in differentiation.[6,91] Eggs of *Paragonimus* may be found in the faeces, sputum, gastric washings or tissue. Blood in the sputum contains sufficient eggs to be visualized by direct smear. Sputum without blood should be collected over 24 hours, centrifuged and the sediment dissolved in 3% sodium hydroxide for examination for eggs.[86] Eggs may not be present in the sputum of infected children or elderly people, but faecal examination using a concentration technique may reveal eggs. Adult worms might be expectorated after treatment or found in skin lesions.

Skin and immunodiagnostic tests using parasite antigens are highly sensitive and useful for surveys and in diagnosing the infection(s).[85,91,95] Complement fixation tests and ELISA detect early as well as chronic infection and titres decline rapidly (becoming negative in 1-2 months) after cure. These tests therefore assist in assessing cure following treatment.[95]

Radiological investigations—particularly plain radiography and computerized tomography, are useful in diagnosing pulmonary disease. Lesions typically show a nodular or ring shadow, patchy infiltration and cavities.[91,93] In eosinophilic meningitis, computerized tomography reveals a 'soap bubble appearance' of dilated ventricles and multiple dense calcification and calcified cystic lesions.[94]

MANAGEMENT

Long regimens of bithionol, totalling 10-15 doses of 30 mg/kg body weight on alternate days and niclofan (2 mg/kg, single dose) are effective and have been used widely. Praziquantel is now the drug of choice, with a course of 3×25 mg/kg body weight for 3 days being nearly 100% effective against all species.[88-90,95-97] Side-effects are usually mild and pulmonary abnormalities decrease within 4 months. Caution is required in the treatment of cerebral disease; one such patient became comatose for 48 hours, while others showed no severe effects.[42,97] Preliminary studies have also shown triclabendazole to be effective.[98]

PREVENTION AND CONTROL

In addition to drug treatment, health education to discourage the consumption of raw crustaceans is recommended—particularly addressing the special danger of infection to children. Increased recognition of the problem by health workers and the population may facilitate earlier treatment and dietary change. Folk beliefs regarding medicinal properties of raw crabs, plus the inability of rapid dry cooking or soaking in brine, soy sauce or alcohol to kill the parasites may require special attention in health promotion messages.

REFERENCES

1 Beaver P C, Jung R C & Cupp E W. *Clinical Parasitology*, 9th edn. Philadelphia: Lea & Febiger, 1984:406-414.
2 Radomyos P, Bunnag D & Harinasuta T. Worms recovered in stools following praziquantel treatment. *Drug Res* 1984; 34:1215-1217.
3 Kaewkes S. The epidemiology and taxonomy of minute intestinal flukes in Northeast Thailand. *PhD Thesis, University of Queensland*, 1993.
4 Anon. Introduction "The wormy world". In Hillyer G V & Hopla C E (section eds) *Section C: Parasitic Zoonoses Volume III. CRC Handbook Series in Zoonoses*, CRC Press: 1982.

5 Cho S Y, Kang S Y & Lee J B. Metagonimiasis in Korea. *Drug Res* 1984; 34:1211–1213.

6 Johnson J R, Boeck R, Paulson D & Godes J. Paragonimiasis in Hmong refuges—Minnesota. In Hillyer G V and Hopla C E (section eds) *Section C: Parasitic Zoonoses Volume III*. CRC Press: 1982: 165–166.

7 Papillo J L, Leslie K O & Dean R A. Cytologic diagnosis of liver fluke infestation in a patient with subsequently documented cholangiocarcinoma. *Acta Cytolog* 1989; 33:865–869.

8 Jongsukuntigul P, Chaychumsri W, Techamontrikul P, Cheeradit P & Suratawanich P. [Studies on prevalence and intensity of intestinal helminth and liver fluke in Thailand in 1991.] *Report of a national survey by the Helminth Division, Ministry of Public Health,* Thailand (in Thai).

9 Chen E R. Clonorchiasis in Taiwan. In Cross J H (ed.) *Emerging Problems in Food-borne Parasitic Zoonosis: Impact on Agriculture and Public Health.* Thai Watana Panich Press Co Ltd, 1991: 184–185.

10 Xiaopeng L. Food-borne parasitic zoonoses in the People's Republic of China. In Cross J H (ed.) *Emerging Problems in Food-borne Parasitic Zoonosis: Impact on Agriculture and Public Health.* Thai Watana Panich Press Co, 1991: 31–35.

11 Seo B S. Socio-economic and cultural aspects of human trematode infections in Korea. *Drug Res* 1984; 34:1116–1118.

12 Cross J H. Changing patterns of some trematode infections in Asia. *Drug Res* 1984; 34:1224–1126.

13 Rim H J. Clonorchiasis. In Hillyer G V and Hopla C E (section eds.) *Section C: Parasitic Zoonoses Volume III*. CRC Press: 1982: 17–32.

14 Rim H J. The current pathobiology and chemotherapy of clonorchiasis. *Korean J Parasitol Suppl.* 1986; 24:1–141.

15 Kim Y I. Liver carcinoma and liver fluke infection. *Drug Res* 1984; 34:1121–1126.

16 Haswell-Elkins M R, Satarug S & Elkins D B. Liver fluke infection and cholangiocarcinoma in Northeast Thailand. *J Gastroenterol Hepatol* 1992; 7:538–548.

17 Vatanasapt V, Uttaravichien T, Mairiang E, Pairojkul C. Chartbanchachai V, Haswell-Elkins M R. Northeast Thailand: A region with a high incidence of cholangiocarcinoma. *Lancet* 1990; 1:116–117.

18 Hoeppli R. Histological changes in the liver of sixty-six Chinese infected with *Clonorchis sinensis. Chin Med J* 1933; 47:1125–1141.

19 Viranuvatti V & Mettiyawongse S. Observation of two cases of opisthorchiasis in Thailand. *Ann Trop Med Parisitol* 1953; 47:291–293.

20 Hou P C. The relationship between primary carcinoma of the liver and infestation with *Clonorchis sinensis. J Path Bact* 1956; 72:239–246.

21 Thamavit W, Bhamarapravati N, Sahaphong S, Vajrasthira S & Angsubhakorn S. Effects of dimethylnitrosamine on induction of cholangiocarcinoma in *Opisthorchis viverrini* infected Syrian golden hamsters. *Cancer Res* 1978; 38:4634–4639.

22 Wykoff D E, Harinasuta C, Juttijudata P & Winn M M. *Opisthorchis viverrini* in Thailand—the life cycle and comparison with *O. felinius. J Parasitol* 1965; 51:207–214.

23 Brockelman W Y, Upatham E S, Viyanant V, Ardsungnoen S & Chantanawat R. Field studies on the transmission of the human liver fluke, *Opisthorchis viverrini,* in Northeast Thailand: population changes of the snail intermediate host. *Int J Parasitol* 1986; 16:545–552.

24 Rim H J. Opisthorchiasis. In Hillyer G V and Hopla C E. (section eds.) *Section C: Parasitic Zoonoses Volume III.* CRC Press: 1982:109–121.

25 Klimshin A A, Krivenko V V & Potseluev A N. [Data on the ecology and epidemiology of opisthorchiasis in various geographic zones of the Tyumen region.] In Sovremennoe sostoyanie problemy opistorkhoza. *Leningrad: Leningradskii NII Epidemiologii i Mikrobiologii im. Pastera:* 1981; pp 9–12. (In Russian, as cited in Heminthol Abstr.)

26 Bronshtein A M. [Communication 2. Morbidity of opisthorchiasis and diphyllobothriasis in the indigenous population of the Kyshik village in the Khanty-Mansiisk Autonomic region.] *Med Parazit (Mosk).* 1986; 3:44–48 (In Russian, as cited in Helminthol Abstr.)

27 Elkins D B, Haswell-Elkins M R, Zoulek G et al. The prevalence and intensity of infection with the liver fluke, *Opisthorchis viverrini* in Northeast Thailand. *Acta Tropica,* submitted.

28 Giboda M, Ditrich O, Scholz T, Viengsay T & Bouaphanh S. *Opisthorchis* and *Haplorchis* infections in Laos. *Trans R Soc Trop Med Hyg* 1991; 85:538–540.

29 Upatham E S, Viyanant V, Kurathong S et al. Relationship between prevalence and intensity of *Opisthorchis viverrini* infection, and clinical symptoms and signs in a rural community in northeast Thailand. *Bull WHO* 1984; 62:451–461.

30 Mairiang E, Elkins D B, Mairiang P et al. Relationship between intensity of *Opisthorchis viverrini* infection and hepatobiliary disease detected by ultrasonography. *J Gastroenterol Hepatol* 1992; 7:17–21.

31 Working Group. IARC Monographs on the evaluation of carcinogenic risks to humans. Volume 61: Some bacterial and parasitic infections. *International Agency for Research on Cancer,* 1995, in press.

32 Pungpak S, Riganti M, Bunnag D & Harinasuta T. Clinical features in severe opisthorchiasis viverrini. *Southeast Asian J Trop Med Pub Hlth* 1985; 16:405–409.

33 Haswell-Elkins M R, Mairiang E, Mairiang P et al. Cross-sectional study of *Opisthorchis viverrini* infection and cholangiocarcinoma in communities within a high risk area in Northeast Thailand. *Int J Cancer* 1994; 58:1–5.

34 Pairojkul C, Sithithaworn P, Sripa B et al. Risk

groups for opisthorchiasis—associated cholangiocarcinoma indicated by a study of worm burden-related biliary pathology. *Kan-Tan-Sui* 1991; 22:111–120.

35 Haswell-Elkins M R, Sithithaworn P, Mairiang E et al. Immune responsiveness and parasite-specific antibody levels in people with hepatobiliary disease associated with *Opisthorchis viverrini* infection. *Clin Exp Immunol* 1991; 84:213–218.

36 Srivatanakul P, Parkin M, Sukarayodhin S & Masathien C. Cholangiocarcinoma: association with *Opisthorchis viverrini* and CA 19-9 antigen. *Thai Cancer J* 1990; 16:35–38.

37 Srianujata S, Tonbuth S, Bunyaratvej S, Valyasevi A, Promvanit N & Chaivatsagul W. High urinary excretion of nitrate and N-nitrosoproline in opisthorchiasis subjects. In Bartsch H, O'Neill I K & Schulte-Hermann R (eds) *The Relevance of Nnitroso compounds in human cancer: exposure and mechanisms* (IARC Scientific Publ No 84), IARC, Lyon, 1987: 544–546.

38 Zavoikin V D, Plyushcheva G L, Nikiforova T F, Shurandin A S, Filinyuk A A & Sbagaida T P. [Evaluation of the efficacy of faecal examination techniques in the diagnosis of opisthorchiasis. Communication 1.] *Med Parazit* (Mosk). 1984; 3:13–16. (In Russian, as cited in Helminth Abstr.)

39 Sithithaworn P, Tesana S, Pipitgool V et al. Relationship between faecal egg count and worm burden of *Opisthorchis viverrini* in humans. *Parasitology* 1991; 102:277–281.

40 Sirisinha S, Chawengkirttikul R, Sermswan R, Amornpant S, Mongkolsuk S & Panyim S. Detection of *Opisthorchis viverrini* by monoclonal antibody-based ELISA and DNA hybridization. *Am J Trop Med Hyg* 1991; 44:140–145.

41 Bunnag D & Harinasuta T. Studies on the chemotherapy of human opisthorchiasis: III. Minimum effective dose of praziquantel. *Southeast Asian J Trop Med Pub Hlth* 1981; 12:413–417.

42 Sui F, Shu-hua X & Catto B A. Clinical use of praziquantel in China. *Parasitol Today* 1988; 4:312–315.

43 Mairiang E, Haswell-Elkins M R, Mairiang P, Sithithaworn P & Elkins D B. Reversal of biliary tract abnormalities associated with *Opisthorchis viverrini* infection following praziquantel treatment. *Trans R Soc Trop Med Hyg* 1993; 87:194–197.

44 Boray J C. Fascioliasis. In Hillyer G V and Hopla C E (section eds.) *Section C: Parasitic Zoonoses Volume III*. CRC Press: 1982: pp 71–88.

45 Srihakim S & Pholpark M. Problem of fascioliasis in animal husbandry in Thailand. In Cross J H (ed.) *Emerging Problems in Food-borne Parasitic Zoonosis: Impact on Agriculture and Public Health*. Thai Watana Panich Press Co, 1991: 352–355.

46 Chen M G & Mott K E. Progress in assessment of morbidity due to *Fasciola hepatica* infection: A review of recent literature. *Trop Dis Bull* 1990; 87:R1–R38.

47 Wolf-Spengler M L & Isseroff H. Fascioliasis: bile duct collagen induced by proline from the worm. *J Parasitol* 1983; 69:290–294.

48 Hardman E W, Jones R L H & Davies A H. Fascioliasis—a large outbreak. *BMJ* 1970; 3:502–505.

49 Ripert C, Tribouley J, Luong Dinh Giap G, Combe A & Laborde M. [Epidemiology of human fascioliasis in south west France.] *Bull Soc Franc Parasitol* 1987; 5:227–230 (in French).

50 Chen M G. *Fasciola hepatica* infection in China. In Cross J H (ed.) *Emerging Problems in Food-borne Parasitic Zoonosis: Impact on Agriculture and Public Health*. Thai Watana Panich Press Co. Ltd, 1991: 356–360.

51 Gutierrez Y. *Diagnostic Parasitology of Parasitic Infections with Clinical Correlations*. Philadelphia: Lea & Febiger, 1990: 359–392.

52 Patrick K M & Isaac-Renton J. Praziquantel failure in treatment of Fasciola hepatica. *Can J Infect Dis* 1992; 3:33–36.

53 Shaheen H I, Kamal K A, Farid Z, Mansour N, Boctor F N & Woody J N. Dot-enzyme-linked immunosorbent assay (Dot-ELISA) for the rapid diagnosis of human fascioliasis. *J Parasitol* 1989; 75:549–552.

54 Hillyer G V & Serrano A. Fractionation of *Fasciola hepatica* tegument antigens and their application to the serodiagnosis of experimental fascioliasis by the enzyme-linked immunosorbent assay. *J Helminthol* 1986; 60:173–178.

55 Takeyama N, Okumura N, Sakai Y et al. Computed tomography findings of hepatic lesions in human fascioliasis: report of two cases. *Am J Gastroenterol* 1986; 81:1078–1081.

56 Beers B van, Pringot J, Geubel A, Trigaux J P, Bigaignon G & Dooms G. Hepatobiliary fascioliasis: noninvasive imaging findings. *Radiology* 1990; 174:809–810.

57 Uribarren R, Borda F, Munoz M & Riveropuente A. Laparoscopic findings in eight cases of liver fascioliasis. *Endoscopy* 1985; 17:137–138.

58 Farag H F, Salem A, Al-Hifni S A & Kandil M. Bithionol (Bitin) treatment in established fascioliasis in Egyptians. *J Trop Med Hyg* 1988; 91:240–245.

59 Farid Z, Mansour N, Kamal M, Kamal K, Safwat Y & Woody J N. The treatment of acute fascioliasis infection in children. *Trop Geo Med* 1990; 42:95–96.

60 Wessely L, Reischig H L, Heinerman M & Stempka A. Human fascioliasis treated with triclabendazole (Fasinex) for the first time. *Trans R Soc Trop Med Hyg* 1988; 82:743–745.

61 Rakhmanov E R. [Combined treatment of patients with chronic fascioliasis complicated by bacterial infection of the bile ducts.] *Meditsinskaya Parazit.* (Mosk.) 1987; 2:32–33 (in Russian, as cited in Helminthol Abstr).

62 Sadun E H & Maiphoom C. Studies on the epidemiology of the human intestinal fluke, *Fasciolopsis buski* (Lankester) in central Thailand. *Am J Trop Med Hyg* 1953; 2:1070–1084.

63 Manning G S, Sukhawat K, Viyanant V, Subhakul

M & Lertprasert P. *Fasciolopsis buski* in Thailand, with comments on other intestinal parasites. *J Med Ass Thailand* 1969; 52:905–913.

64 Jaroonvesama N, Charoenlarp K, Areekul S, Aswapokee N & Leelarasmee A. Prevalence of *Fasciolopsis buski* and other parasitic infection in residents of three villages in Sena District, Ayudhaya Province, Thailand. *J Med Ass Thailand* 1980; 63:493–499.

65 Rim H J. Fasciolopsiasis. In Hillyer G V & Hopla C E (section eds.) *Section C: Parasite Zoonoses Volume III*. CRC Press, 1982; 89–97.

66 Weng Y L, Zhuang Z L, Jiang H P, Lin G R & Lin J J. [Studies on ecology of *Fasciolopsis buski* and control strategy of fasciolopsiasis.] *Chinese J Parasitol Parasit Dis* 1989; 7:108–111 (In Chinese, cited in Helminthol Abstr).

67 Handoyo I, Ismuljowono B, Darwis F & Rudiansyah. Evaluation of post-treatment control of fasciolopsiasis in Sei Papuyu village of Babirik Subdistrict, Hulu Sungai Utara Regency, South Kalimantan Province, Indonesia. *Trop Biomed* 1987; 4:125–127.

68 Handoyo I, Ismuljowono B, Darwis F & Rudiansyah. Further survey of fasciolopsiasis in Babirik Subdistrict, Hulu Sungei Utara Regency, South Kalimantan Province. *Trop Biomed* 1986; 3:119–123.

69 Bunnag D, Radomyos P & Harinasuta T. Field trial on the treatment of fasciolopsiasis with praziquantel. *Southeast Asian J Trop Med Pub Hlth* 1983; 14:216–219.

70 Jaroonvesama N, Charoenlarp K & Areekul S. Intestinal absorption studies in *Fasciolopsis buski* infection. *Southeast Asian J Trop Med Pub Hlth* 1986; 17:582–586.

71 Rim H J. Echinostomiasis In Hillyer G V & Hopla C E (section eds.) *Section C: Parasitic Zoonoses Volume III*. CRC Press: 1982: 53–69.

72 Waikagul J. Intestinal fluke infections in Southeast Asia. In Cross J H (ed.) *Emerging Problems in Food-borne Parasitic Zoonosis: Impact on Agriculture and Public Health*. Thai Watana Panich Press Co. Ltd, 1991:158–162.

73 Huffman J E & Fried B. Echinostoma and Echinostomiasis. *Adv Parasitol* 1990; 29:215–269.

74 Carney W P. Echinostomiasis—a snail-borne intestinal trematode zoonosis. In Cross J H (ed.) *Emerging Problems in Food-borne Parasitic Zoonosis: Impact on Agriculture and Public Health*. Thai Watana Panich Press Co. Ltd, 1991:206–211.

75 Tangtrongchitr A & Monzon R B. Eating habits associated with *Echinostoma malayanum* infections in the Philippines. In Cross J H (ed.) *Emerging Problems in Food-borne Parasitic Zoonosis: Impact on Agriculture and Public Health*. Thai Watana Panich Press Co. Ltd, 1991:212–216.

76 Phathihutthagon W, Sornmani S, Imphan P & Srithabut P. [Studies on the prevalence and reinfection rate of *Echinostoma* spp in an irrigated area.] *J Parasit Trop Med Ass Thailand* 1984; 7:12–16 (in Thai).

77 Radomyos P, Bunnag D & Harinasuta T. *Echinostoma ilocanum* (Garrison, 1908) Odhner, 1911, infection in man in Thailand. *Southeast Asian J Trop Med Pub Hlth* 1982; 13:265–269.

78 Velasquez C C. Heterophyidiasis. In Hillyer G V and Hopla C E (section eds.) *Section C: Parasitic Zoonoses Volume III*. CRC Press, 1982:99–107.

79 Chai J Y & Lee S H. Intestinal trematodes infecting humans in Korea. In Cross J H (ed.) *Emerging Problems in Food-borne Parasitic Zoonosis: Impact on Agriculture and Public Health*. Thai Watana Panich Press Co. Ltd, 1991:163–170.

80 Africa C, Leon W D E & Garcia E Y. Intestinal heterophyidiasis with cardiac involvement: a contribution to etiology of heart failure. *J Philipp Islands Med Assoc* 1935; 15:358–361.

81 Lee S H, Hwang S W, Chai J Y & Seo B S. Comparative morphology of eggs of heterophyids and *Clonorchis sinensis* causing human infections in Korea. *Korean J Parasitol* 1984; 22:171–180.

82 Ditrich O, Giboda M, Scholz T & Beer S A. Comparative morphology of eggs of the Haplorchiinae (Trematoda: Heterophyidae) and some other medically important heterophyid and opisthorchiid flukes. *Folia Parasitol* 1992; 39:123–132.

83 Ditrich O, Kopacek P, Giboda M, Gutvirth J & Scholz T. Serological differentiation of human small intestinal fluke infections using *Opisthorchis viverrini* and *Haplorchis taichui* antigens. In Cross J H (ed.) *Emerging Problems in Food-borne Parasitic Zoonosis: Impact on Agriculture and Public Health*. Thai Watana Panich Press Co. Ltd, 1991:174–178.

84 Miyazaki I. Paragonimiasis. In Hillyer G V & Hopla C E (section eds.) *Section C: Parasitic Zoonoses Volume III*. CRC Press: 1982; pp 143–164.

85 Yokogawa M. Paragonimiasis. In Hillyer G V & Hopla C E (section eds.) *Section C: Parasitic Zoonoses Volume III*. CRC Press: 1982; pp 123–142.

86 Cabrera B D. Paragonimiasis in the Philippines: current status. *Drug Res* 1984; 34:1188–1192.

87 Choi D W. Paragonimus and paragonimiasis in Korea. *Korean J Parasitol* 1990; 28:79–102.

88 Zhi-Biao X. Studies on clinical manifestations, diagnosis and control of paragonimiasis in China. In Cross J H (ed.) *Emerging Problems in Food-borne Parasitic Zoonosis: Impact on Agriculture and Public Health*. Thai Watana Panich Press Co. Ltd, 1991:345–348.

89 Lien-Yin H E. Advance in studies of *Paragonimus* and paragonimiasis in China. *Abstracts Vol 1 of the XIIIth International Congress for Tropical Medicine and Malaria*. 1992: Pattaya, pp 58–59.

90 Pozio E. Current status of food-borne parasitic zoonoses in Mediterranean and African regions. In Cross J H (ed.) *Emerging Problems in Food-borne Parasitic Zoonosis: Impact on Agriculture and Public Health*. Thai Watana Panich Press Co. Ltd, 1991:85–87.

91 Singh T S, Mutum S S & Razaque M A. Pulmonary paragonimiasis: clinical features, diagnosis and treatment of 39 cases in Manipur. *Trans R Soc Trop Med Hyg* 1986; 80:967–971.

92 Weina P J & England D M. The American lung fluke, *Paragonimus kellicotti*, in a cat model. *J Parasitol* 1990; 76:568–572.

93 Vanijanonta S, Bunnag D & Harinasuta T. Radiological findings in pulmonary paragonimiasis heterotremus. *Southeast Asian J Trop Med Pub Hlth* 1984; 15:122–128.

94 Jaroonvesama N. Differential diagnosis of eosinophilic meningitis. *Parasitol Today.* 1988; 88:262–266.

95 Tsuji M, Fujino T & Yokogawa M. Immunodiagnosis and chemotherapy of paragonimiasis. *Abstracts Vol 1 of the XIIIth International Congress for Tropical Medicine and Malaria* 1992: Pattaya, p. 60.

96 Udonsi J K. Clinical trials of praziquantel in pulmonary paragonimiasis due to *Paragonimus uterolateralis* in endemic populations of the Igwun Basin, Nigeria. *Trop Med Parasitol* 1989; 40;65–68.

97 Vanijanonta S, Bunnag D & Harinasuta T. *Paragonimus* spp. in Thailand: Pathogenesis, Clinic and Treatment. *Drug Res* 1984; 34:1186–1188.

98 Guderian R H, Calvopina M & Poltera A A. Triclabendazole chemotherapy for pulmonary paragonimiasis in Ecuadorian patients. Preliminary results. *Abstracts Vol 2 of the XIIIth International Congress for Tropical Medicine and Malaria* 1992: Pattaya, p. 37.

CHAPTER 74

INTESTINAL CESTODES

G. G. Baily

Tapeworms or cestodes are an ancient class of highly specialized flatworm parasites. Their ancestors diverged from free-living flatworms to parasitize the earliest vertebrates in Cambrian times, and subsequently followed all the complexities of vertebrate evolution so that there are now innumerable species subtly adapted to the behaviour, diet and immunology of their hosts. Most cestodes require at least two host species to support the different stages of their life cycles. Adult tapeworms inhabit the gut of a vertebrate animal (the definitive host), with four species adapted specifically to humans. The tapeworm consists of a scolex equipped with suckers, grooves (bothria) or hooks which are the means of attachment to the intestinal wall. This is connected by an actively growing neck region (the strobila) to a chain of a variable number of segments or proglottids which are progressively more mature towards the distal end of the worm. The mature proglottids, which form the bulk of the worm, are largely composed of hermaphrodite sexual organs and generate large numbers of eggs. A single *Taenia saginata* adult, for example, may produce 50 000 eggs daily for 10 years or more.

Cyclophyllidean cestodes typically have an exclusively terrestrial life cycle with a single intermediate host, which may be vertebrate or invertebrate. The intermediate host is infected by ingesting eggs which hatch into invasive larvae (oncospheres) in the gut, migrate into the host tissues and develop into one of the many distinctive, often cyst-like, morphologies of cestode larvae. The life cycle is completed if the intermediate host is eaten by a suitable definitive host in which the protoscolex of the larva can develop in the gut into a new adult tapeworm.

The Pseudophyllidean cestodes have a more complex life cycle. The first intermediate host is typically an aquatic invertebrate which is infected by the procercoid larval stage of the parasite. When the invertebrate is ingested by a suitable second intermediate host, likely to be a fish or reptile, the parasite develops into an invasive, worm-like, plerocercoid larva. This may then ascend the food chain through a series of further second intermediate hosts until finally reaching a suitable carnivorous vertebrate definitive host in which it can develop into an adult tapeworm. Tapeworms and larvae from both these cestode families can infect humans.

Because the relationship between the parasite and its host is central to the survival and propagation of the worm, but likely to be of more marginal significance to the host population, phenomena related to this ancient and highly adapted parasitism tend to have evolved predominantly according to the needs of the worm. Thus it is in the interests of the propagation of the worm that its definitive host should be long lived and active, disseminating eggs as widely as possible. Tapeworm infections tend therefore to be of trivial importance to the health of the host. In contrast, the worm's life cycle is only completed when the infected intermediate host is eaten, which may well occur more readily if the function of the intermediate host is disrupted. Larval cestode infections are consequently amongst the most serious helminthic diseases.

TAPEWORMS OF HUMANS

TAENIA SAGINATA

T. saginata is the beef tapeworm (Figure 74.1). Man is the only definitive host, and cattle are the significant intermediate hosts (Figure 74.2), though a variety of ungulates have been reported as being infected. The larval stage is a translucent fluid-filled bladder or cysticercus between 5 and 10 mm in diameter but, unlike the *T. solium* cysticercus, it has never been reliably described in a human. The adult is a large, white tapeworm that can reach 10 m in

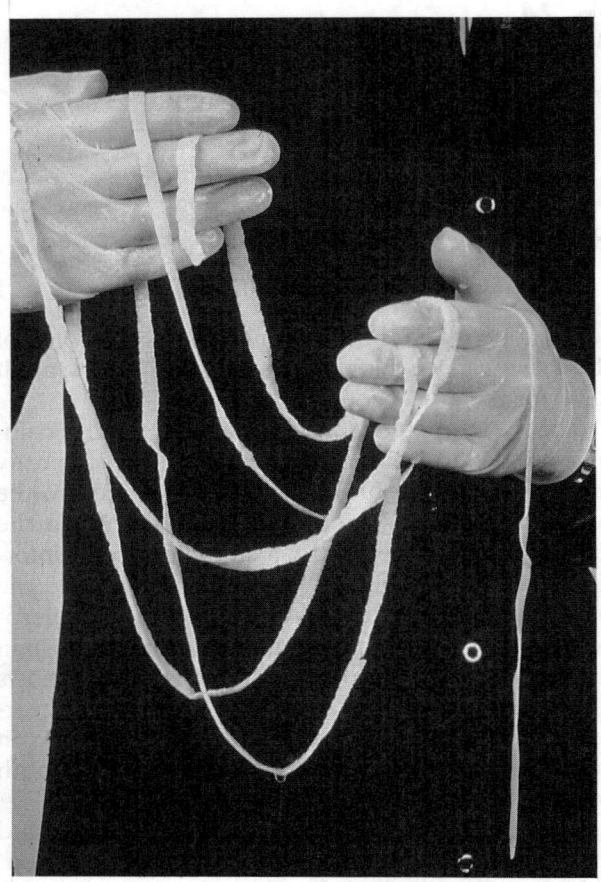

Figure 74.1   Adult beef tapeworm (*T. saginata*). (Courtesy of G. S. Nelson.)

length, though more typically 2–5 m, weighing around 20–30 g. The scolex is equipped with suckers but not hooks (Figures 74.3 and 74.4D). Mature proglottids detached from the distal end of the worm are highly motile and their independent emergence from the anus is the principal cause of symptomatology. An infected individual commonly harbours more than one worm. Human infection is acquired by eating undercooked beef. Cattle are infected when their feed or grazing is contaminated by human faeces.

PREVALENCE AND DISTRIBUTION

Originally a ubiquitous parasite, transmission has been prevented in developed countries by the sanitary disposal of human faeces and the detection of infected meat at abattoirs. It remains common elsewhere, especially in poorer communities where raw or undercooked beef is traditionally eaten. Highland Ethiopia is an area of intense transmission.

CLINICAL FEATURES

T. saginata carriers are often aware of motile proglottids which can be felt emerging from the anus unbidden and may cause some distress. They are also conspicuous in the faeces because of their motility. Otherwise infection is largely asymptomatic. A number of 'irritable bowel-type' symptoms, particularly abdominal pain but also nausea, distension and anorexia, have been attributed to the parasite but these are so common in the general population that causality is difficult to prove. Occasionally segments of worm may be vomited. Eosinophilia is not a feature of established infection.

DIAGNOSIS AND TREATMENT

Taenia eggs have a characteristic appearance (Figure 74.5) and can be detected by faecal microscopy. Since all *Taenia* ova are very similar they are not easily speciated, although they can be distinguished on Ziehl–Neelson staining. Soluble *Taenia* antigens can be detected in faeces but present methods tend to be cross-reactive between species.[1] Intact proglottids in reasonable condition can be speciated by the number of uterine branches. A single dose of praziquantel at 10 mg/kg is effective therapy. Niclosamide has also been used extensively.

TAIWAN *TAENIA*

An adult *Taenia* morphologically identical to *T. saginata* infects indigenous highland people in Taiwan in areas where there are no cattle. Cysticerci a little smaller than those of *T. solium* or *T. saginata* have been found in a number of mammalian species, including pigs, in which they have a strong tropism for the liver.[2] Molecular genetic studies confirm the parasite to be distinct from the other human taeniids.[3] It is probably distributed widely in East Asia.

TAENIA SOLIUM

Man is the only known definitive host for the pork tapeworm, *T. solium*—with pigs serving as intermediate host. The adult tapeworm is somewhat smaller than *T. saginata* and the scolex is markedly different being armed with two encircling rows of curved hooklets (Figures 74.4C and 74.6) which can also be identified on the protoscolex of the cysticercus. Detached proglottids are much less motile and

Taenia saginata

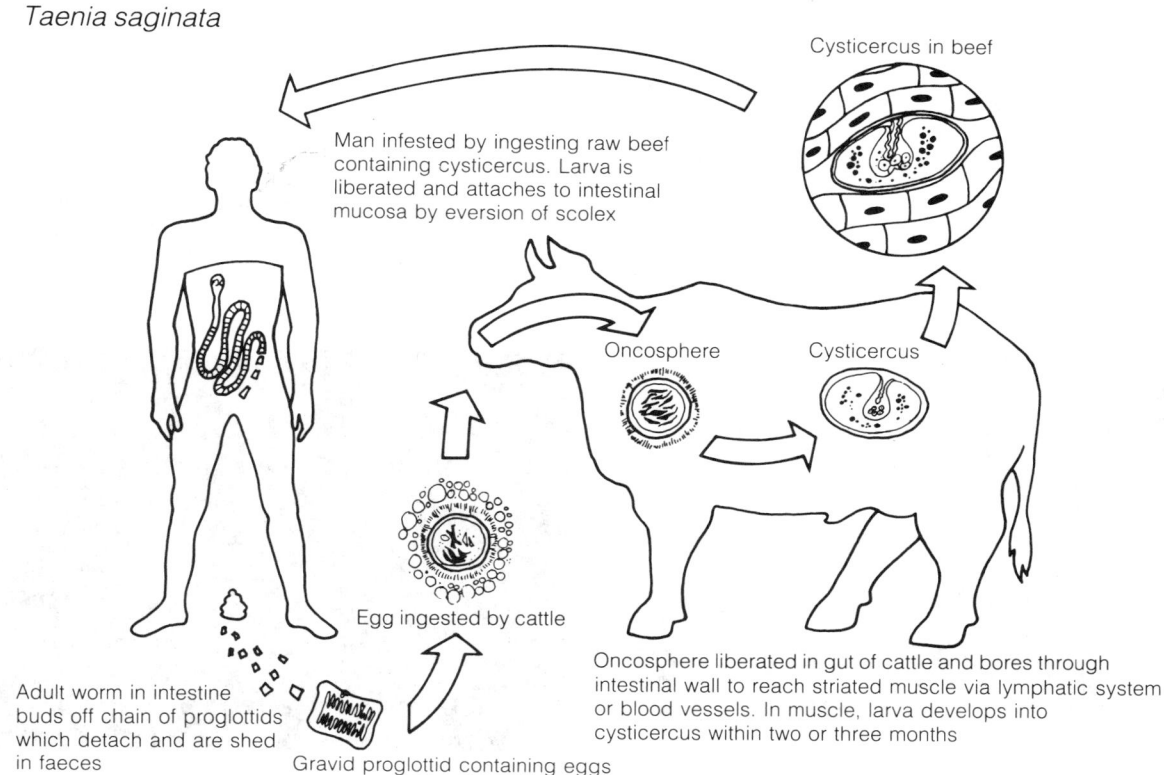

Cysticercus in beef

Man infested by ingesting raw beef containing cysticercus. Larva is liberated and attaches to intestinal mucosa by eversion of scolex

Oncosphere   Cysticercus

Egg ingested by cattle

Adult worm in intestine buds off chain of proglottids which detach and are shed in faeces

Gravid proglottid containing eggs

Oncosphere liberated in gut of cattle and bores through intestinal wall to reach striated muscle via lymphatic system or blood vessels. In muscle, larva develops into cysticercus within two or three months

Figure 74.2   Life cycle of *T. saginata*. (Courtesy of WTIM.)

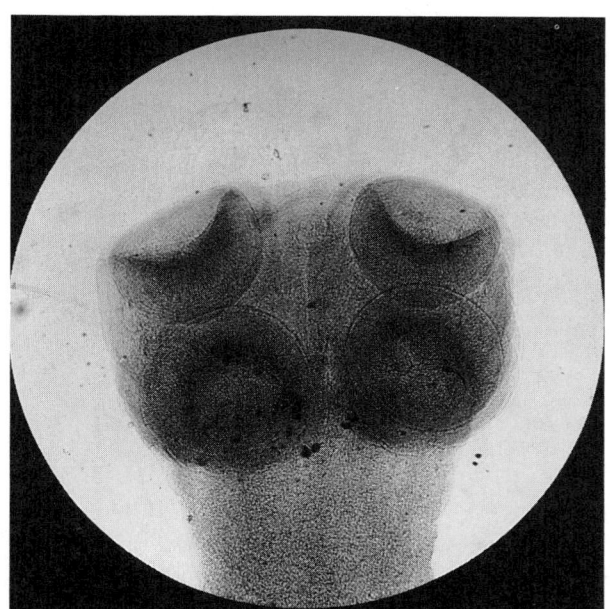

Figure 74.3   *T. saginata* (unarmed tapeworm) scolex. Suckers without hooklets. (Courtesy WTIM.)

consequently less likely to be noticed than are those of *T. saginata*. The chief significance of the parasite is that humans are readily infected by the larval cysticerci as well as the adult worm, giving rise to human cysticercosis. This is discussed, together with the transmission, prevalence and control of the parasite, in Chapter 76.

CLINICAL FEATURES

The great majority of *T. solium* carriers are unaware of their infection and it is detected only by screening. Minor abdominal symptoms may occur, as with *T. saginata*. However, carriers carry a substantial risk of acquiring cysticercosis by faeco-oral autoinfection and members of their household are also at increased risk.[4]

DIAGNOSIS AND TREATMENT

The detection and speciation of *Taenia* infections has been discussed above—under *T. saginata*. Treatment is also similar for the two infections, with praziquantel 10 mg/kg being the drug of choice. It has previously been common practice to combine antihelmintic therapy for *T. solium* with a purgative since eggs of the dying worm were believed to constitute a risk of cysticercosis through internal autoinfection. No evidence has ever emerged to support this hypothesis and purgation is no longer regarded as necessary.

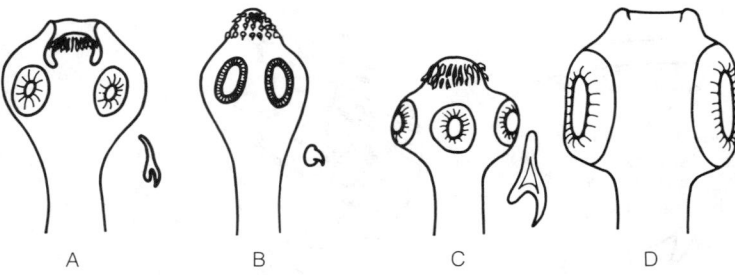

Figure 74.4 Heads of human cestodes, showing suckers and, when present, the arrangement of the hooklets. A, *Hymenolepis nana*. B, *Dipylidium caninum*. C, *Taenia solium*. D, *Taenia saginata*.

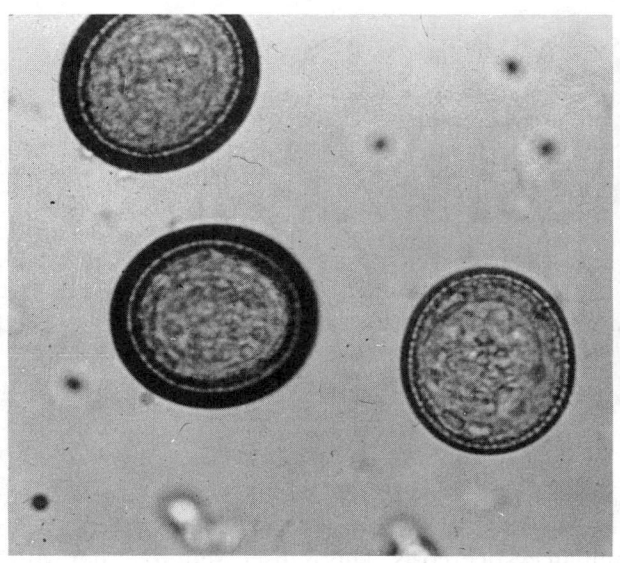

Figure 74.5 *Taenia* ova. (Courtesy of WTIM.)

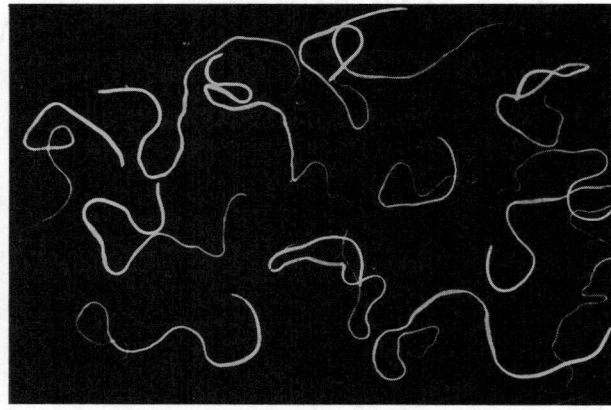

Figure 74.7 *H. nana* (dwarf tapeworm). (Courtesy of WTIM.)

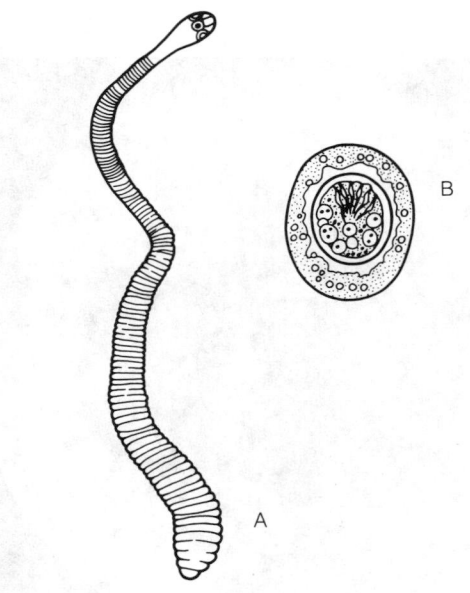

Figure 74.8 *H. nana* (dwarf tapeworm). Magnified. A, adult. B, egg.

HYMENOLEPIS NANA

The dwarf tapeworm *H. nana* (Figures 74.7 and 74.8) is unique amongst cestodes in that the life cycle is maintained between humans without the necessity for any other host species; indeed, the same indi-

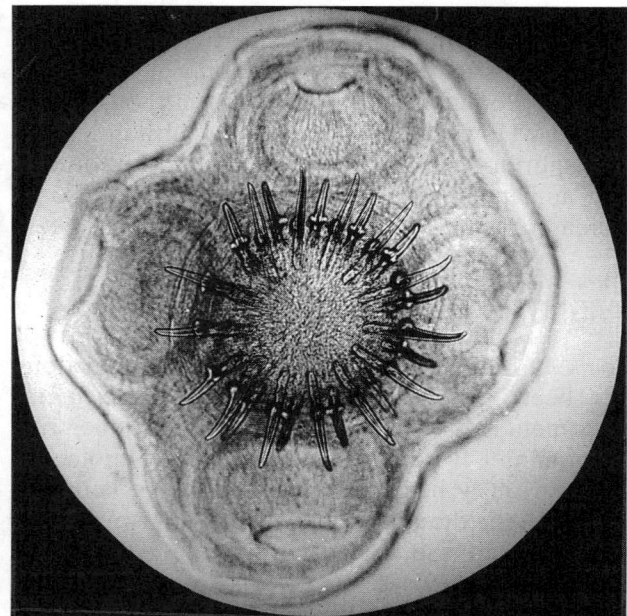

Figure 74.6 *T. solium* (pig tapeworm) (armed tapeworm). Scolex showing hooklets. (Courtesy of WTIM.)

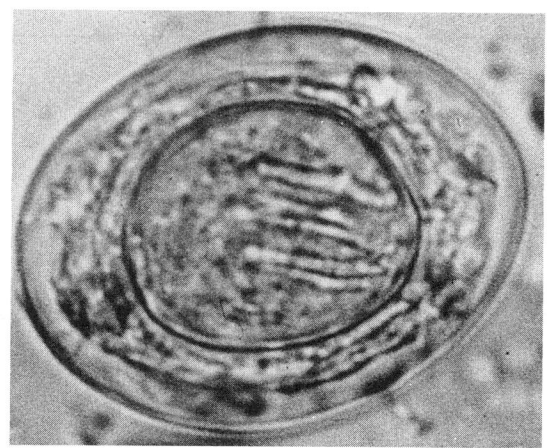

Figure 74.9   *H. nana* (dwarf tapeworm). Ovum. (Courtesy of WTIM.)

vidual acts as intermediate and definitive host. Ingested ova (Figure 74.9) are activated by the gut and invade the small intestinal mucosa where they encyst within a villus. Within 3–4 days the protoscolex of this cercocyst evaginates to become the scolex of an adult worm (Figure 74.4A). This attaches to the intestinal wall, the remainder of the worm developing to a mature length of 3–4 cm over about a month, after which egg production begins. Detached proglottids degenerate during passage through the intestine, releasing their cargo of ova, and are not seen in the faeces. Infections involving several hundred worms are common. Spread is by faecal-oral transmission with autoinfection, particularly amongst children, amplifying the intensity of infection. Rodents may act as an alternative definitive host and insects are capable of infection with the larval stage but neither of these appear to be important in parasite transmission.

PREVALENCE AND DISTRIBUTION

H. nana is a very common parasite in warm climates where sanitation is poor, particularly in children, amongst whom prevalences often exceed 10%.

CLINICAL FEATURES

A variety of symptoms have been attributed to *H. nana* infection, including abdominal pain and anorexia as well as systemic complaints such as irritability and headache. Eosinophilia is common. Several reports have associated infection with growth retardation.[5] It is difficult to be certain whether these features are truly a direct result of the parasite or whether it is acting as a marker of faecal-oral infec-

tion, insanitation and poverty, but heavy infections probably do have significant clinical consequences.

DIAGNOSIS AND TREATMENT

Diagnosis is by detecting the characteristic ova on faecal microscopy. The cercocyst stage is in contact with the host immune system and consequently, unlike other tapeworm infections, there is a sufficiently predictable humoral response for serology to be of some diagnostic value. An enzyme linked immunosorbent assay (ELISA) has been developed with sensitivity of about 80%.[6] There is extensive cross-reaction with other cestode infections. A single dose of praziquantel is effective therapy. At least 20 mg/kg is recommended. Niclosamide has also been widely used. Mebendazole only gives cure rate around 50%.

CONTROL

As with other faecal-oral infections, control depends on sanitation and education.

DIPHYLLOBOTHRIUM LATUM

Man can act as definitive host for a variety of pseudophyllidean tapeworms of the genus *Diphyllobothrium* (Table 74.1). Various tiny aquatic invertebrates, especially *Cyclops* water fleas, are the first intermediate host for these parasites (Figure 74.10). The plerocercoid larvae ascend to the apex of the aquatic food chain, with species specificity in their adaptation to particular larger carnivorous fish. Definitive hosts include birds and marine and terrestrial mammals. *D. latum*, the fish tapeworm, is the species adapted to humans; bears and other terrestrial carnivores may act as paratenic hosts but man is generally the host that is significant in transmission. It is a large (up to 10 m), slightly translucent tapeworm (Figure 74.11) inhabiting the small intestine where it attaches by means of two longitudinal slit-like suckers or bothria (Figure 74.12). Infections are commonly multiple and occasionally there may be more than a hundred individual worms. The largest recorded total length of *D. latum* tapeworm(s) expelled from one patient is 330 m.[7] The preferred second intermediate hosts are temperate freshwater fish, especially pike, perch and burbot.[8] Human infection is acquired by eating undercooked fish. Both freezing and cooking effectively destroy the parasite.

Table 74.1 Species of *Diphyllobothrium* infecting humans.

Species	Second intermediate host	Principle definitive host	Known range
D. latum	Pike, perch, etc.	Man	Widespread, but especially Russia
D. dendriticum	Char, salmon, trout	Gulls	Throughout subarctic region
D. klebanovskii	Pacific salmon	Marine mammals	Eastern Siberia
D. cordatum	?	Bearded seal	Greenland, Alaska
D. dalliae	Blackfish	Canines?	Alaska, eastern Siberia
D. ursi	Pacific salmon	Bears	Alaska, Canada
D. nihonkaiense	Pacific salmon	Marine mammals?	Japan

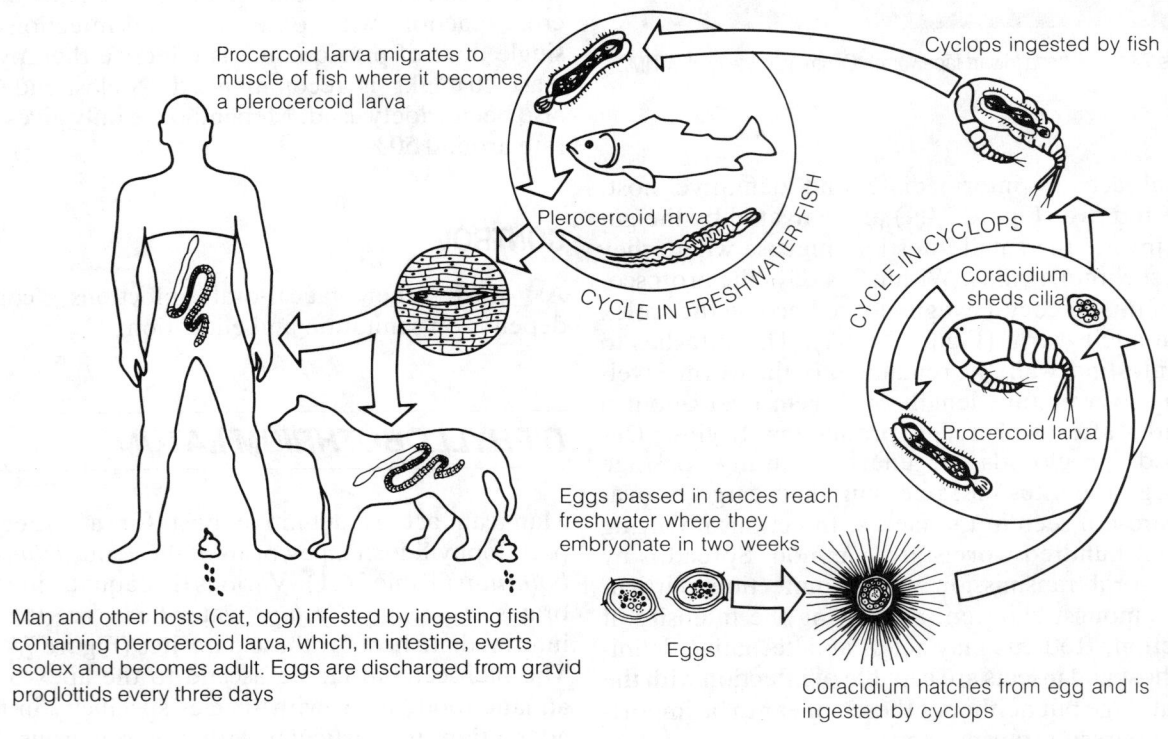

Diphyllobothrium latum

Procercoid larva migrates to muscle of fish where it becomes a plerocercoid larva

Cyclops ingested by fish

Plerocercoid larva

CYCLE IN FRESHWATER FISH

CYCLE IN CYCLOPS

Coracidium sheds cilia

Procercoid larva

Eggs passed in faeces reach freshwater where they embryonate in two weeks

Eggs

Man and other hosts (cat, dog) infested by ingesting fish containing plerocercoid larva, which, in intestine, everts scolex and becomes adult. Eggs are discharged from gravid proglottids every three days

Coracidium hatches from egg and is ingested by cyclops

Figure 74.10 Life cycle of *D. latum*. (Courtesy of WTIM.)

PREVALENCE AND DISTRIBUTION

Although the disease is reported from many parts of the world, most transmission occurs in Russia. The original heartland of *D. latum* infection extended from eastern Scandinavia across northern Russia and into western Siberia. Historically there have also been intense foci of transmission in the Danube delta in Romania and in the lakes of northern Italy and western Switzerland. Transmission no longer occurs in Western Europe and has been successfully controlled in Finland, where more than 20% of the entire nation was infected as recently as 1950.[9] In Russia there have been control programmes but also setbacks so that transmission continues to be common, with some extension of the range of the para-

site resulting from changes to the river systems by engineering projects. The parasite has also been spread very widely by human migration so that low-intensity transmission has been recorded from many parts of the world, including the smaller lakes of central North America and several parts of South America, especially Chile.

CLINICAL FEATURES

As with other tapeworm infections, carriers experience few if any symptoms. A controlled study in Finland showed that some of the minor symptoms traditionally attributed to infection—including abdominal pain, were not significantly associated with

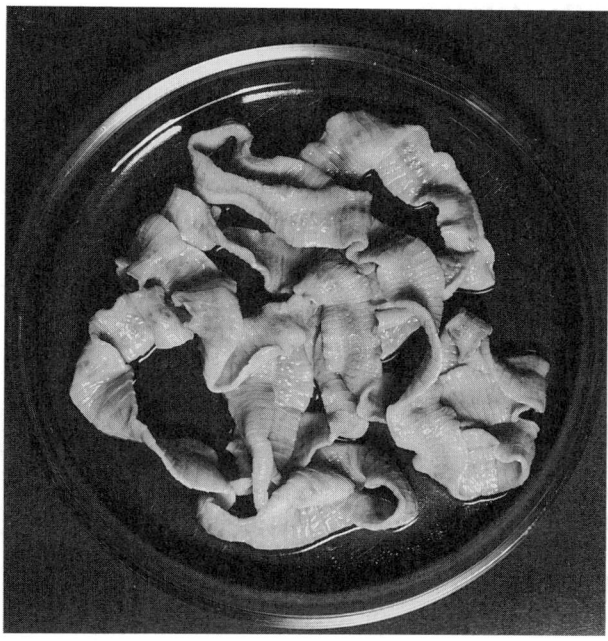

Figure 74.11   *D. latum* (fish tapeworm). Adult. (Courtesy of WTIM.)

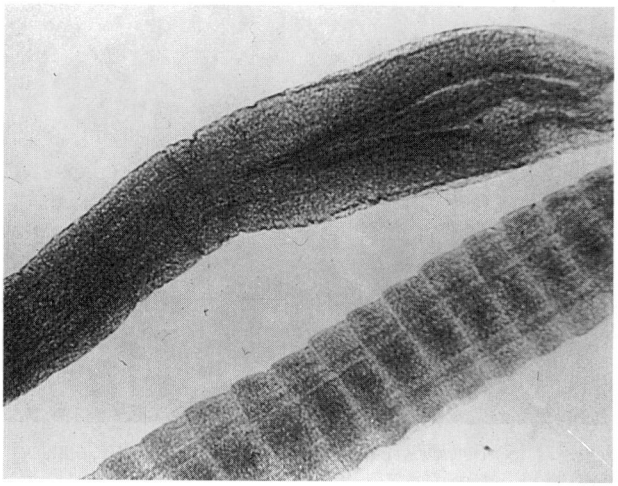

Figure 74.12   *D. latum* (fish tapeworm). Scolex without suckers or hooks but two grooves (bothria) which attach to the mucosa. (Courtesy of WTIM.)

carriage, although diarrhoea, headache and non-specific malaise all appeared to be somewhat more common.[9] Proglottids are seldom noticed in the faeces but occasionally carriers may become aware of their infection through the spontaneous expulsion of a whole worm.

Tapeworm anaemia

In the nineteenth century a condition was first described in which pernicious anaemia, at that time a

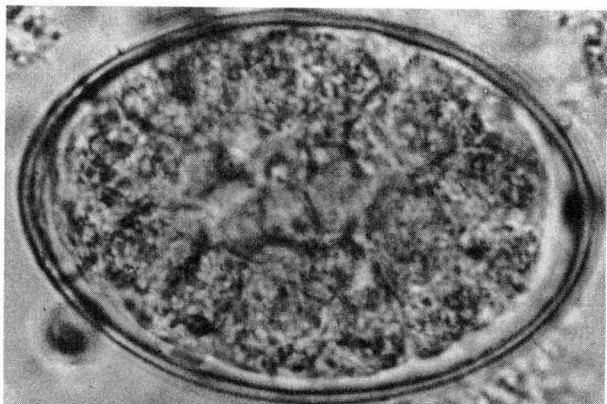

Figure 74.13   *D. latum* (fish tapeworm). Ovum. (Courtesy of D. S. Ridley.)

fatal disease, was associated with *D. latum* infection and in some instances improved dramatically after eradication of the worm. In the twentieth century the condition has been described exclusively from Finland and by the time that the modern understanding of the pathogenesis of megaloblastic anaemias had become established, tapeworm anaemia was already rapidly disappearing there. Our understanding of this disease is therefore tentative and, since there has been no recognized case for more than 20 years, will probably remain so. It seems clear that tapeworm anaemia was caused by vitamin B_{12} deficiency. It was strongly associated with gastritis and achlorhydria but neither of these were necessary conditions for its development, and intrinsic factor, as demonstrated by the earliest physiological methods, does not seem to have been deficient.[9] It is most probable that worms were simply competing with the host for vitamin B_{12}, with clinical consequences most likely to follow when absorption was already marginal. There is also some evidence of a familial predisposition.

DIAGNOSIS AND TREATMENT

Ova (Figure 74.13) are detected by faecal microscopy with an estimated sensitivity of 95% for a single examination. *Diphyllobothrium* ova are morphologically similar and cannot be speciated by microscopy. Praziquantel is the preferred therapy, a single dose of 10 mg/kg being effective. Niclosamide has been extensively used in the past.

CONTROL

Control has been effectively achieved in many areas by the mass detection and treatment of human cases, improved sanitation and education with regard to dietary habits.

ZOONOTIC TAPEWORMS

HYMENOLEPIS DIMINUTA

Rats are the definitive host for this parasite, with insects, principally fleas, acting as intermediate hosts. Man, usually a child, is infected by accidentally ingesting infected fleas. Adult worms can then develop to egg-producing maturity in the human gut, reaching a length of up to 6 cm. Human infection is uncommon but probably worldwide. Known clinical consequences are limited to eosinophilia and minor abdominal pain. Diagnosis is by stool microscopy, the ova (Figure 74.14) differing slightly from those of *H. nana*. Praziquantel is said to be effective.

DIPYLIDIUM CANINUM

A ubiquitous tapeworm of dogs, with their fleas acting as intermediate host(s), this parasite is very similar to *H. diminuta*, as an uncommon zoonotic infection of children who have accidently ingested dog fleas. A medium-sized tapeworm, up to 40 cm, can develop to maturity in the human gut (Figure 74.15). Motile proglottids the size of rice grains are passed intact in the stool; free ova (Figure 74.16) are difficult to detect. Infection is most often asymptomatic and there are no known serious consequences. Treatment is with praziquantel.

DIPHYLLOBOTHRIUM SPECIES

A number of species of *Diphyllobothrium* other than *D. latum* have been reported as infecting man (Table 74.1). *D. dendriticum* is the cause of human diphyllobothriasis amongst the indigenous people of the subarctic region where it infects salmonid fish, especially arctic char.[8] Gulls are the most significant definitive hosts. Prevalences of 30% and more have commonly been recorded in Canadian Inuit commu-

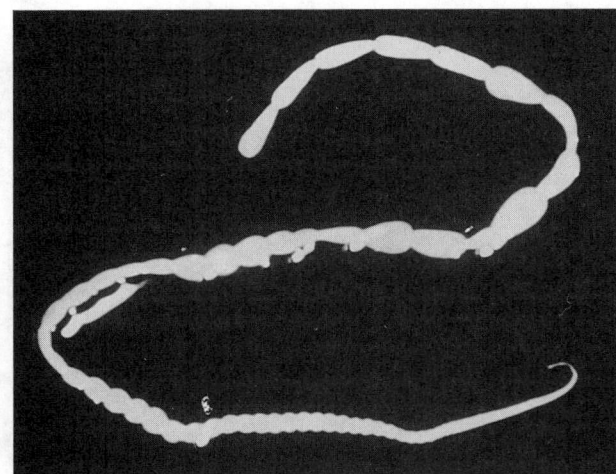

Figure 74.15   Dipylidium caninum (dog tapeworm). Adult. (Courtesy of WTIM.)

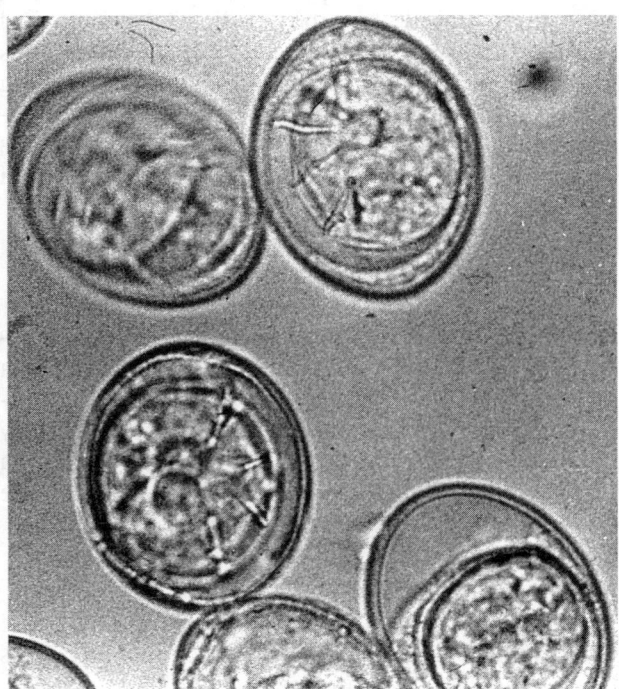

Figure 74.14   H. diminuta (rat tapeworm). Ova. (Courtesy of H. Zaiman.)

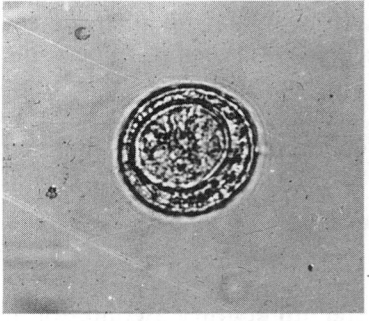

Figure 74.16   Egg of *Dipylidium caninum.*

nities. Several other parasites infect humans around the northern Pacific, through Pacific salmon,[10] including *D. klebanovskii* which is the principal parasite in the Russian Far East. The clinical consequences of these infections have not been well studied but are considered to be minor.

REFERENCES

1 Allan J C, Avila G, Garcia-Noval J, Flisser A & Craig P S. Immunodiagnosis of taeniasis by coproantigen detection. *Parasitology* 1990; 101:473–477.

2 Fan P C, Chung W C, Lin C Y & Wu C C. The pig as intermediate host for Taiwan *Taenia* infection. *J Helminthol* 1990; 64:223–231.

3 Zarlenga D S, McManus D P, Fan P C & Cross J H. Characterization and detection of a newly described Asian taeniid using cloned ribosomal DNA fragments and sequence amplification by the polymerase chain reaction. *Exp Parasitol* 1991; 72:174–183.

4 Diaz-Camacho S, Candil-Ruiz A, Uribe-Beltran A & Willms K. Serology as an indicator of *Taenia solium* tapeworm infections in a rural community in Mexico. *Trans R Soc Trop Med Hyg* 1990; 84:563–566.

5 Khalil H M, el Shimi S, Sarwat M A, Fawzy A F & el Sorougy A O. Recent study of *Hymenolepis nana* infection in Egyptian children. *J Egypt Soc Parasitol* 1991; 21:293–300.

6 Castillo R M, Grados P, Carcamo C et al. Effect of treatment on serum antibody to *Hymenolepis nana* detected by enzyme-linked immunosorbent assay. *J Clin Microbiol* 1991; 29:413–414.

7 Ostling G. Treatment of tapeworm infection with desaspidin, a new phloroglucinol derivative isolated from Finnish fern. *Am J Trop Med Hyg* 1961; 10:855–858.

8 Curtis M A & Bylund G. Diphyllobothriasis: fish tapeworm disease in the circumpolar north. *Arctic Med Res* 1991; 50:18–25.

9 von Bonsdorff B. *Diphyllobothriasis in Man*. London: Academic Press, 1977.

10 Rausch R L, Scott E M & Rausch V R. Helminths in eskimos in western Alaska, with particular reference to *Diphyllobothrium* infection and anaemia. *Trans R Soc Trop Med Hyg* 1967; 61:351–357.

CHAPTER 75

ECHINOCOCCOSIS/ HYDATIDOSIS

Bruno Gottstein and Jürg Reichen

The larval stages of two small tapeworms, *Echinococcus granulosus* and *E. multilocularis*, cause the main forms of hydatid disease in man. The two diseases, called cystic hydatid disease and alveolar hydatid disease, respectively, differ pathologically and clinically so much that they will be considered separately in this chapter. A third section will be devoted to some rarer species, in particular *E. vogeli*.

ECHINOCOCCUS GRANULOSUS

BIOLOGY

E. granulosus is a small cestode tapeworm approximately 3–6 mm in length when fully mature. The life cycle of *E. granulosus* is shown in Figure 75.1. The tapeworm lives as an intestinal parasite firmly attached to the mucosa of the small intestine of dogs or occasionally, other carnivores. Following infection by peroral ingestion of protoscolices originating from fertile hydatid cysts, sexual maturity of adult-stage tapeworms is reached within 4–5 weeks. This period, also known as prepatency, is followed by shedding of gravid proglottids—each containing several hundred eggs—or of eggs into the faeces of definitive hosts. Such eggs are infective for intermediate hosts immediately after their release into the surroundings. Following ingestion of *Echinococcus* eggs by susceptible intermediate animal hosts (those of importance for human medicine are predominantly domestic ungulates) and humans, an early stage larva, the oncosphere, is released from the egg envelope. The oncosphere penetrates through the intestinal epithelium into the lamina propria and corresponding blood vessels; it is subsequently transported passively through blood or lymph vessels to primary target organs such as liver and lung(s). At this location the oncosphere matures into a vesicle, which grows expansively by concentric enlargement. The final result is a fully mature metacestode or hydatid cyst; this is usually a fluid-filled, unilocular cyst, but multiple, communicating chambers also occur. The cyst consists of an inner germinal and nucleated layer supported externally by a tough, elastic, acellular laminated layer of variable thickness, surrounded by a host-produced fibrous adventitial layer (Figure 75.2). Occasionally, cysts may abut and coalesce, forming groups or clusters of cysts of variable size. In humans especially, where unusually large cysts may develop, daughter cysts can form within the primary cyst. The endogenous formation of brood capsules and protoscolices is a prerequisite for termination of the life cycle. Protoscolices will grow to the adult stage once ingested by a definitive host.

DISTRIBUTION AND EPIDEMIOLOGY

Infections with *E. granulosus* in definitive and intermediate hosts occur worldwide. A so-called 'European' form,[2] primarily involving synanthropic hosts in its cycle, has an almost universal distribution. This form is related to major public health or economic problems in many rural areas of the world. Another 'northern' form[2] is prevalent in northern parts of the North American continent and Eurasia. Endemic areas are mainly related to tundra and taiga and delineated by the southern limits of the boreal forest. Epidemiologically relevant is the fact that *E. granulosus* is distributed within only a few animals,

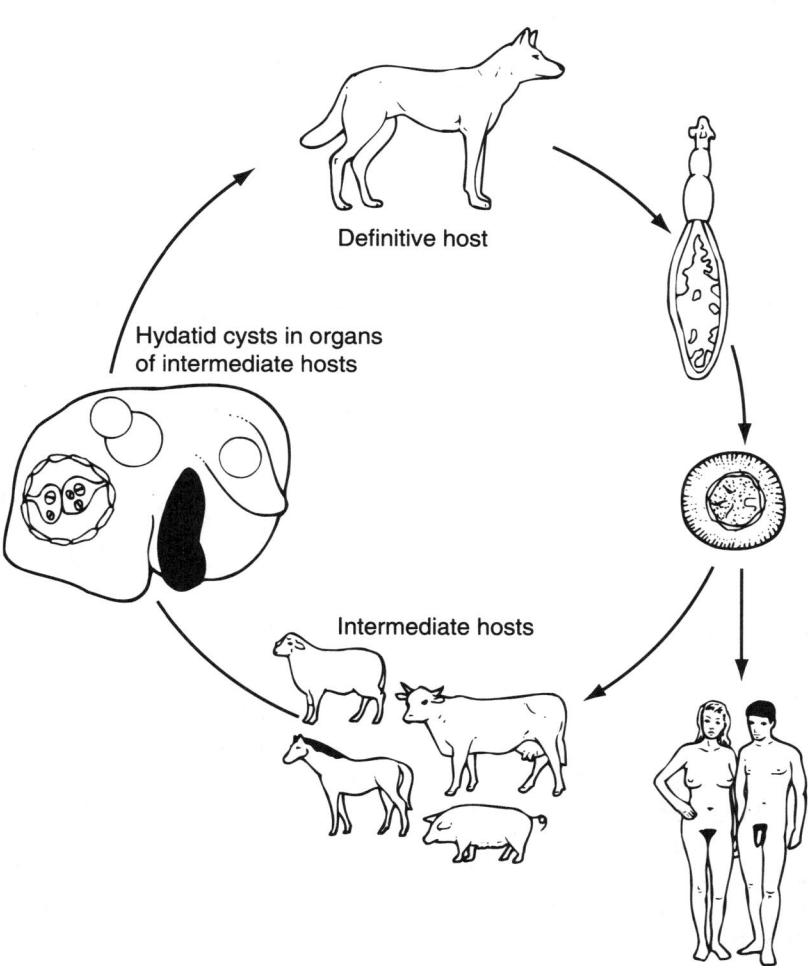

Figure 75.1 Life cycle of *E. granulosus*. Adult tapeworms living in the small intestine of dogs produce proglottids containing tapeworm eggs. These are infective for intermediate hosts, with mainly liver and lungs being affected. Man can become accidentally infected as an intermediate host. The hydatid cysts contain brood capsules with protoscolices which will develop into adult tapeworms in the definitive host.

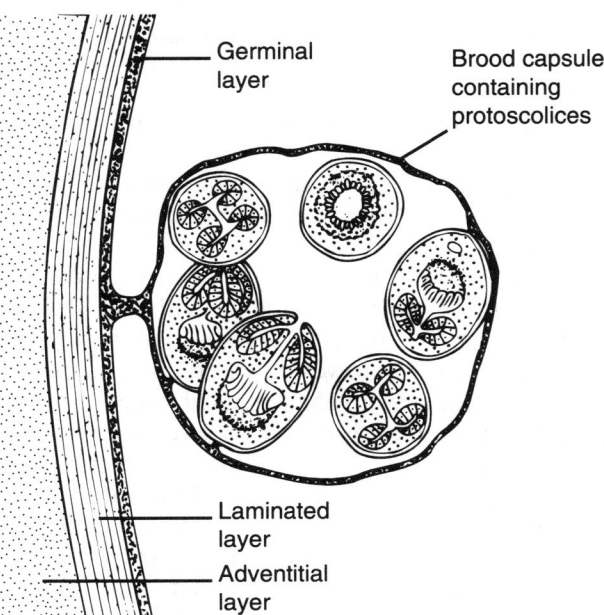

Figure 75.2 Metacestode of *E. granulosus*. Cross-section (schematic) through a hydatid cyst with a brood capsule and protoscolices produced by asexual multiplication. (Adapted from Morseth.[1])

which, however, harbour large numbers of protoscolices—so-called superspreaders. There is no crowding effect or parasite-induced host mortality and the respective numerical distribution does not contribute to the regulation of either adult or larval parasite populations. The following factors are considered to be relevant for determining the prevalence of parasite occurrence and the diseases induced by it: the parasite's biotic potential and the host's acquired immunity, are mechanisms responsible for egg dispersal, the climate determining their survival.

Measurement of the socioeconomic impact of echinococcosis/hydatidosis represents an important challenge, which frequently becomes highly relevant for calculating the cost:benefit ratio of possible activities for the control or eradication of *Echinococcus* spp. In humans, the quantifiable items are those connected with preoperative diagnosis, surgical treatment, hospitalization, postsurgical examination and drugs.[3] In some countries the cost of hospitalization alone involves 45 patient-days at an estimated cost of US$ 2000.[4,5] This is bound to increase in cases complicated by infection, rupture

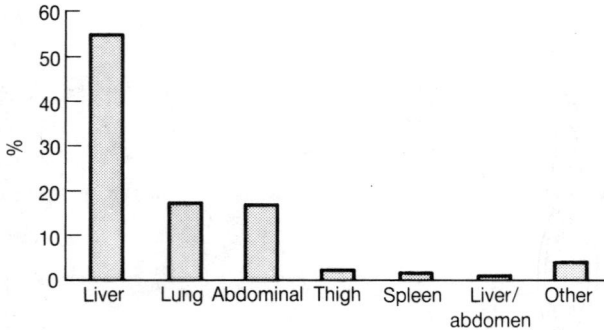

Figure 75.3 Localization of cysts of *E. granulosus* in 159 patients reported by McPherson et al.[7] For further details see text.

or unusual localizations or in patients with relapse.[4] In such complicated cases—given that the site and treatment involved could mean the loss of an organ, cause irreversible sequelae, or even threaten the life of the patient—the cost can be comparable with that of surgical treatment of cancer.[3] The convalescent period should also be considered as an economic loss in view of the well-documented fact that a high proportion of cases occur in actively working persons, which means that the contribution of their labour to the economy of their countries is lost.

Globally, incomplete data exist on the overall prevalence of human cystic echinococcosis. Regions with good documentation of the prevalence in defined geographical areas include: the whole Mediterranean area, the Kenyan Turkana district, large foci in South America but also many other zones over all continents. An updated review and summary of cases in countries of all five continents has been presented.[6]

CLINICAL DIAGNOSIS AND NATURAL HISTORY

Over 50% of *E. granulosus* cysts are located in the liver; other common localizations include the lungs and peritoneal cavity. The localization of cysts in a large series reported by MacPherson et al[7] is depicted in Figure 75.3. Less usual localizations include the kidneys,[8] bones,[7,9] breasts,[10] heart,[11] spleen,[7] pancreas,[7] and organs of the head and neck[12–14] including the brain.[15]

Symptoms are most often related to the expansive growth of the cysts. In agreement with their preferred localization the most frequent initial symptom is abdominal pain[16–19] (Table 75.1). Allergic phenomena are also quite frequent and may lead, following cyst rupture, to anaphylactic shock.[20] Fever and jaundice indicate cholangitis related to rupture of a cyst into the biliary tree; this is the presenting symptom in 5–25% of patients.[16–19, 21–24] Even in the absence of obstruction, hydatid cysts are frequently in communciation with the biliary tree.[23]

In most cases, imaging procedures together with serology will yield the diagnosis.[7] Sonography is the diagnostic procedure of choice; however, false positives can occur in up to 10%, the main confusion arising in the differentiation between hydatid and benign congenital cysts.[25] Diagnostic features of hydatid disease include separation of the membrane from the wall, daughter cysts and collapsed cysts.[25–28] In contrast, hydatid 'sand', often described as pathognomonic, can also be found in simple hepatic cysts.[25] Computerized tomography (CT), where available, is superior for the detection of extrahepatic disease,[29] while nuclear magnetic resonance imaging (NMR) does not appear to add any diagnostic benefit.[30] Ultrasonography is also very helpful in following treated patients, successfully treated cysts becoming hyperechogenic.[31]

Aspiration cytology using trichrome staining of the filtrated aspirate reveals the acid-fast hooklets.[32] Cytology appears particularly helpful in detecting pulmonary[33] and renal[8] involvement. Viability of aspirated protoscolices can be determined by microscopic demonstration of flame cell activity.

Serological diagnosis will be considered in the next section; a human basophil degranulation test has been reported to be helpful in difficult cases[34] but data about its specificity and sensitivity are lacking. Otherwise, laboratory examinations are not particularly helpful in establishing the diagnosis, with the exception of determination of IgE and eosinophilia in cases of ruptured cysts presenting with allergic symptoms.

Life expectancy in successfully operated patients appears to be normal; patients with extrahepatic disease seem to fare no worse than those with hepatic disease.[35] However, when patients present with complications, in particular cholangitis, there is an appreciable mortality.[19] Most hydatid cysts grow slowly; the best data on their natural evolution have been generated by Romig et al;[36] these authors have followed 36 patients sonographically over a year. The results of their study are depicted in Figure 75.4. Of particular interest is the fact that 13.6% of cysts either disappeared or collapsed spontaneously. This has to be taken into account when evaluating results of chemotherapy, although special attention should be given to the biological particularities of the parasite strain present in the Turkana district.[37]

Table 75.1 Signs and symptoms of *E. granulosus* infection.

Authors	n	Pain (%)	Hepatomegaly (%)	Fever/allergy (%)	Cholangitis (%)
AURC[16]	306	70	9	4	16
Elhamel[17]	23	90	—	—	16
Magistrelli et al.[18]	135	79	68	30	14
Schaefer and Khan[19]	42	—	7	7	

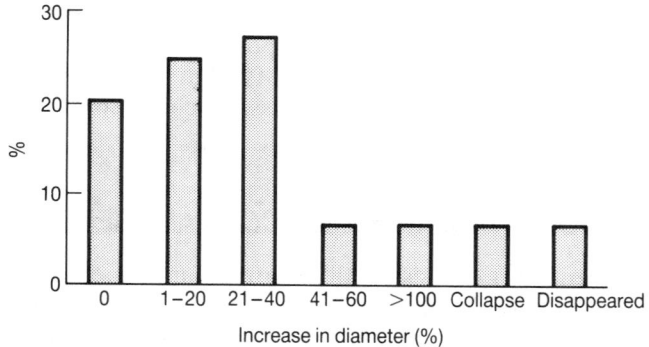

Figure 75.4 Evolution of untreated hydatid cysts followed by sonography for 12 months. Forty-four cysts in 36 patients were evaluated; 29 cysts grew, nine were static and six collapsed or disappeared. (Adapted from Romig et al.[36])

SEROLOGICAL AND MOLECULAR DIAGNOSIS

Immune responses in the host have been widely used to diagnose infection or disease. The selection of a particular immunodiagnostic test for that purpose primarily involves consideration of the diagnostic operating characteristics of the technique. The diagnostic sensitivity and specificity of the tests mostly used vary according to the:

1. Nature, purity and quality of the antigen.
2. Nature of patients' immunoglobulins (isotypes, etc.) or cell subpopulations specified in the test.
3. Sensitivity of the selected technology.

ANTIBODY TESTS

Most serological tests for immunodiagnosis of cystic echinococcosis employ *E. granulosus* antigen(s) for serum antibody detection. In particular, the use of widely available *E. granulosus* hydatid fluid antigen was reported to be diagnostically relatively sensitive (75–94%) for the indirect hemagglutination test (IHA)[38,39] and enzyme linked immunosorbent assay (ELISA).[40] One of the most specific immunodiagnostic approaches for cystic echinoccosis (*E. granulosus*) relies upon the demonstration of serum antibodies precipitating an antigen called 'antigen 5' by immunoelectrophoresis or a similar technique.[41]

Experimental studies indicate that antibodies to 'antigen 5' are among the first detectable antibodies after infection.[41–43] Diagnostic sensitivities with respect to hepatic cystic echinococcosis have been reported to vary between 50 and 80%.[44] Antibodies to antigen 5 also occur in serum of human patients with neurocysticercosis[45] and alveolar echinococcosis.[46] Comparative studies in Swiss patients have shown 58% of patients with alveolar echinococcosis to be 'arc 5'-positive, compared with 74% of patients with cystic echinococcosis.[47] Despite further investigation by various approaches using monoclonal antibodies and/or immunoblotting[58–50] or molecular biological techniques[51–52] there is evidence for a lack of species specificity and of diagnostic sensitivity due to the absence of anti-antigen 5 antibodies in a proportion of patients.

Other attempts to further characterize *E. granulosus* antigenic components and to identify corresponding antigens with optimal diagnostic characteristics included the finding of a low molecular subunit of an antigen B,[53] which, however, was found not to be species specific.[49] Resolution of *E. granulosus* hydatid cyst fluid by SDS-PAGE resulted in the immunoblot finding of relatively specific diagnostic components with various molecular masses.[54–56] Another approach to improving the characteristics of serological assays for *E. granulosus* consisted of chromatographic fractionation of hydatid cyst fluid; this resulted in a partially purified 20 kDa antigen, resembling that of antigen B. This antigen was postulated be be species specific for *E. granulosus*;[57] however, further evaluation of these agents will need to be undertaken to demonstrate their immunodiagnostic suitability.

In summary, the strategy for immunodiagnosis of cystic echinococcosis presently recommended is to rely upon a diagnostically sensitive test such as ELISA employing hydatid fluid antigen. Positive test results, dependent upon the geographical origin of the patient and the implied problems of cross-reactivity due to potential infection with other parasite species, have subsequently to be confirmed by tests demonstrating antibody activity against antigen 5 or other specific antigenic components, as discussed above, e.g. immunoblotting.

The demonstration of parasite-specific IgE has attracted particular attention due to its well known relevance in helminthic diseases[58–60] but has exhibited no significant immunodiagnostic advantage. Beside problems of diagnostic sensitivity and specificity due to cross-reactions, there is accumulating evidence for false-positive antibody reactions not related to infections with heterologous helminth species, but to malignancies,[61] the presence of anti-P1 antibodies,[62] and liver cirrhosis.[63]

Early diagnosis of persons with asymptomatic echinococcosis is a prerequisite for efficient management of the disease. Consequently, serological screening has been offered to populations in many areas. The tests most widely used were based upon the arc-5 detection due to its relative good specificity for areas non-endemic for *E. multilocularis* (see reference 44 for review). However, many studies have clearly demonstrated the limits of using serology alone in epidemiological studies; this is particularly true in areas where seropositivity is low among patients with cystic echinococcosis, such as the Turkana district in Kenya.[64] Recent studies therefore employed what can currently be considered to be the optimal epidemiological tool: ultrasound examination for abdominal cystic echinococcosis, if possible combined with immunodiagnosis.[26,65]

Serological studies to follow patients with cystic echinococcosis postoperatively have given much emphasis to the specific determination of parasite-specific antibody isotypes.[60,66] However, the contribution of serology for monitoring the course of the disease is limited and requires use of imaging techniques to provide an accurate prognostic and diagnostic judgement.

ANTIGEN TESTS

These are based mainly on the determination of circulating immune complexes by, for example, enzyme immunoassays; their diagnostic sensitivity ranges between 33 and 85%.[55,67,68] It has been suggested that these tests are more useful than antibody-based tests to monitor the course of disease, to determine viability of the parasite, and to assess the radicality of surgical removal of parasite lesions.[69]

CELL-MEDIATED IMMUNITY

Early work to assess cell-mediated immunity in cystic echinococcosis has relied mainly on skin tests and basophil degranulation tests (see reference 44

for review). They have largely been supplanted by newer tests due to the remarkable developments in basic cellular immunology making possible the elucidation of parasite-specific host cellular immune responses. Siracuso et al[70] studied the in vitro lymphoproliferative response to *E. granulosus* antigen stimulation in 40 patients with cystic echinococcosis and found no correlation between serological and lymphoproliferative results. Diagnostic sensitivity of positive test reactions was 75% for both serology and lymphocyte proliferation. The fact that some seronegative patients had a positive proliferation assay and vice versa suggests that addition of lymphocyte-specific immunoassays could improve the diagnostic yield.

RECOMBINANT *ECHINOCOCCUS* ANTIGENS

Recent approaches in the search for defined and specific protein antigens concentrated on the cloning and expression of *Echinococcus* genes in suitable vectors.[71] A cDNA expression library was screened with parasite-specific antibodies in order to identify bacterial clones producing recombinant antigens bearing relevant B-cell epitopes. Thus, an *E. granulosus* cDNA library derived from protoscolex mRNA was established using the *Escherichia coli* expression vector λ-gt11 and successfully screened with sera from patients with cystic echinococcosis. Several clones producing diagnostically highly sensitive fusion proteins could thereby be identified.[72] The cloning of an *E. granulosus* gene encoding for an antigen 5 component has already been mentioned (see above).[51]

MOLECULAR DIAGNOSIS

Molecular biological techniques have rapidly evolved and permit the identification of parasite species-specific or even stage-specific nucleic acid sequences. This technology is limited in its application due to its technical complexity and thus focuses mainly on the characterization of *Echinococcus* isolates or strains, providing epidemiological rather than clinical information. A variety of such DNA probes has been developed and used by several groups to characterize, identify or group different strains of *E. granulosus*[72–74] or *E. multilocularis*.[75] Apart from the restricted availability of these probes, a major problem remains the limited sensitivity of the hybridization and labelling techniques used. These technical limitations have been virtually eliminated by an extraordinary new tool, the polymerase chain reaction (PCR). Its sensitivity can be further enhanced by additional techniques such as reamplification with internal primers or Southern dot hybridization with sensitively labelled nucleotide probes. As an example, the nucleic acid sequence of an *Echinococcus* DNA probe pAL1[75] served to derive oligonucleotide primers suitable for use in PCR amplification of specific target sequences from diagnostic *Echinococcus* genomic DNA,[76] allowing the differentiation of *E. granulosus* from *E. multilocularis* parasite material of any parasite stage and origin.

IMMUNOLOGY AND PATHOLOGY

Cystic echinococcosis or hydatidosis of humans refers to infection with larval *E. granulosus*. Well delineated primary cysts are formed in different organs. Tissue damage results from gradual replacement of host tissue by the growing cysts and in some instances by vascular compromise. The histology of a typical, viable hydatid cyst due to *E. granulosus* is depicted in Figure 75.2. The germinal layer contains live parasites; it is surrounded by a parasite-derived laminated layer. The latter is periodic acid–Schiff-positive due to its rich amino sugar content.[77] The germinal layer differentiate into protoscolices; sometimes, only acid-fast-positive hooklets are demonstrable. The parasite evokes an immune response leading to formation of a host-derived collagenous capsule which often calcifies. Growth is expansive by an increase in cyst size. Bursting of the cysts, which can develop pressures of up to 80 cmH$_2$O,[78] can lead to haematogenous metastasis or implantation in the peritoneal cavity. The initial inflammatory response of the liver to live parasites is infiltration by eosinophils and mononuclear cells. In older cysts, there is usually virtually no inflammatory reaction. There is often pressure atrophy of the surrounding parenchyma. Cholestasis may be present in the liver. The cyst fluid often contains protoscolices (hydatid sand), granulae and occasionally free daughter cysts.

The primary site of the host–parasite interaction is the host's gastrointestinal mucosa. Little information is available on the immune response in man against migrating and subsequently established oncospheres and their development to the metacestode of *E. granulosus*. Diagnosis of hydatid disease is usually made at a stage where a fully developed and still proliferating metacestode has already induced an immune response of the host (see reference 79 for review). Cellular and humoral immune responses in man can vary enormously, as evidenced for example by the different patterns of parasite antigens recognized by different patients and during the course of disease.[49,80] These disparities are probably related to human and/or parasite genetic diversity, unlike the uniform genetic background of most experimental animals.[79]

Investigations of the cell-mediated immune response in murine cystic echinococcosis have demonstrated polyclonal B-cell activation[81] and a marked drop in the percentage of T cells[82] but an increase in suppressor cell activity.[83] Cytotoxicity of splenic T lymphocytes directed against the metacestode has been demonstrated.[84] There is impairment of the host defence potential, presumably by formation of anti-HLA reactive host antibodies.[85] The host's potential to develop a parasite-specific cellular response appears to be modulated by parasite-derived effector substances.[49,86] Local immune modulation by the parasite has been shown to enhance susceptibility to mycobacterial infections close to the site of parasite lesions.[87]

TREATMENT

SURGERY

Surgery remains the mainstay in the treatment of hydatid disease. Cystectomy and pericystectomy offer the best chance for cure and should be undertaken wherever possible.[88] Occasionally, formal hepatic resection will be required.[89] Radical surgery—either pericystectomy or resection—is possible in 50–85% of cases.[16,17,88–90] In the absence of complications this can be achieved with little mortality and an acceptable morbidity.

Whatever procedure is chosen, care has to be taken to avoid spillage of cyst content, which is the main predictor of recurrent disease. To achieve this, the peritoneal cavity should be carefully protected,[88] and the cyst evacuated and sterilized with scolicidal agents. The use of formalin and hypertonic saline should be abandoned since they can induce caustic injury to the biliary tree;[91–93] formalin and hypertonic saline have also been associated with severe acidosis and hypernatraemia, respectively.[19] Currently-used scolicidal agents include chlorhexidine, hydrogen peroxide, ethanol and cetrizamide.[19,88] Pretreatment with benzimidazole compounds has been proposed to avoid the use of dangerous scolicidal agents[94] and to decrease the rate of recurrence;[95] however, both of these contentions remain to be proven in larger series (see below).

Radical surgery—hepatectomy or pericystectomy—has relatively low relapse rates, ranging from 8.5 to 22%,[18,35,88,96,97] whereas relapse occurs in up

Table 75.2 Recurrence rates (as a percentage of the total series) after surgery for *E. granulosus.*

Authors	n	Radical* (%)	Non-radical† (%)
Behrns and van Heerden[90]	23	0	50
Magistrelli et al[18]	119	16.9	4.2
Morel et al[89]	42	2.4	27.3

*Includes formal hepatic resections and total pericystectomy.
†Includes different procedures such as capitonnage or partial pericystectomy.

to 75% after non-radical surgery[90] (Table 75.2). Local recurrence has been ascribed to the formation of exogeneous daughter cysts which are left behind in the case of non-radical surgery.[18]

Rupture into the biliary tree has been successfully treated with choledochojejunostomy or T-tube drainage;[22,98,99] in a comparative series, choledochojejunostomy was found to result in fewer instances of recurrent jaundice than T-tube drainage.[99] Recently, endoscopic sphincterotomy with or without nasobiliary drainage has been successfully used in the treatment of obstructive jaundice due to biliary rupture.[100–104] Sphincterotomy is also useful in case of postoperative biliary leaks.[104] Pulmonary cysts are often the result of infected or ruptured hepatic cysts; its surgical treatment consists of wedge resection or lobectomy.[105] Recurrence of pulmonary disease appears to be rare.[97,105]

INTERVENTIONAL RADIOLOGY

Several recent reports have advocated the use of cyst puncture under sonographic or CT guidance with instillation of hypertonic saline[106–108] or ethanol.[109,110] The follow-up in all these series was relatively short, however, and although none of the series recorded spillage of cyst content this remains a distinct possibility. For this reason, some authors used concomitant benzimidazole therapy.[106,110] Development of a biliary fistula has been observed after alcohol injection in 1 of 16 patients.[110] Even more worrisome is the potential for inducing anaphylactic shock. Again, this complication has not yet occurred but Gargouri et al[107] observed allergic phenomena in 7 of 37 patients treated with cyst puncture and lavage.

PHARMACOTHERAPY

Two benzimidazole compounds—mebendazole and albendazole—and praziquantel, have activity against *E. granulosus* in vitro and in animal models.[111,112] No controlled studies have ever been performed in man but large series with the benzimidazoles have been published (see Table 75.3). Albendazole appears preferable to mebendazole because of its better bioavailability.[113,114] Both drugs penetrate into the cysts[115,116] but sometimes heroic doses are needed to achieve a therapeutic plasma concentration of mebendazole.[117] Mebendazole should be given after a fat-rich meal and levels monitored 4 hours after the morning dose.[115] Plasma levels of mebendazole are unrelated to dose;[117,118] the generally accepted therapeutic levels are around 250 nmol/l.[119] The therapeutic level of albendazole sulphoxide, the major active metabolite in serum[114,120] has not been defined; better absorption of albendazole when given with a fatty meal has also been reported.[121] Cholestasis increases the blood levels of both drugs.[122,123] Most investigators use albendazole in cycles of 4 weeks, followed by a drug-free interval of 2 weeks; initially, this was proposed to diminish toxicity. Another rationale for giving albendazole in cycles rather than as a continuous course is autoinduction of its metabolism.[120]

Side-effects of the two drugs appear to be similar and include mainly leucopenia, hair loss and hepatotoxicity.[120,123–125] For both benzimidazoles it appears likely that they are not truly parasiticidal but rather parasitostatic agents. Thus, in those treated with mebendazole for 1 year, viable scolices could be found in at least 50% of patients in spite of therapeutic drug levels.[115] The figures appear somewhat better for albendazole because prior to surgical excision only 1 of 14 patients had viable protoscolices when treated for longer than 1 month, as opposed to two patients treated only for a few weeks.[94] In a large multi-centre report viable cysts were found at surgery in 10.6% of patients treated with albendazole for an average of 2.5 cycles.[126]

In a comparative, multicentre trial albendazole appeared to be slightly superior to mebendazole, in particular for extrahepatic sites.[124] In this trial, 68 of 112 patients were followed for at least 1 year; 39 and 14% of patients treated with albendazole (10 mg/kg per day) or mebendazole (increasing dose up to 4.5 g/day), respectively, were deemed to be treatment successes, as judged by disappearance or a major decrease in cyst size. The corresponding figures for favourable effects (meaning a decrease in cyst size or disappearance of some but not all cysts) was 39 and 64%, while treatment failures were 22 and 23%, respectively. Tolerance of the drugs was similar, side-effects occurring in 18 and 20% of patients treated with mebendazole and albendazole, respectively. This trial suffers from the fact that mebendazole levels were not measured and there-

Table 75.3 Effect of benzimidazole treatment on *E. granulosus*.

Authors	n (patients)	Dose per day	Treatment (months)	Follow-up	Success (%)*
Mebendazole					
Bartoloni et al[127]	52	50 mg/kg	—	> 5 years	100
Davis et al[124]	22	4.5 g	6	1 year	78
Kammerer and Schantz[128]	15	200 mg/kg	—	3–7 years	66
Messaritakis et al[129]	39	200 mg/kg	3	5 years	51
Schantz et al[130]	127	Variable	Variable	—	74
Teggi et al[131]	70	—	—	6 months	64
Todorov et al[9]	44	50 mg/kg	6–24	30 months	48
Albendazole					
Choudhuri et al[132]	7	10 mg/kg	4	—	14
Cossetto et al[133]	4	400 mg	6	—	100
Davis et al[124]	46	10 mg/kg	4	1 year	78
De Rosa and Teggi[134]	46	12 mg/kg	3	6–42 months	76
Horton[126]	253	800 mg	3	—	79
Morris et al[135]	22	10 mg/kg	—	—	68
Okelo[136]	12	10 mg/kg	2	—	100
Saimot et al[137]	10	14 mg/kg	Variable	—	50
Todorov et al[9]	35	10 mg/kg	4	33 months	74

*Success is defined as either disappearance or clear-cut regression of cysts, assessed by sonography. The remainder were failures, defined as unchanged or progressive radiological appearance.

fore the dose was not adjusted in the individual patients.

The World Health Organization (WHO) trial and other series evaluating mebendazole[9,124,127–131] and/or albendazole[9,132–137] are summarized in Table 75.3; this table should be read with some caution since it is possible that collaborators of the WHO trial published part or all of their patients independently. The same holds true for the report by Horton;[126] this report from the manufacturer of albendazole compiles records of a large number of patients treated on a compassionate basis; again, it stands to reason that some of these patients had been reported individually by the different investigators but it is not possible to confirm this. The early experience with different benzimidazoles has been compiled in a workshop reported by Schantz et al;[130] some of the series reported therein were later published as full papers and are given in Table 75.3. Therapeutic failures have clearly been described with both drugs; combining all the studies in Table 75.3, a slight advantage seems to emerge in favour of albendazole.

The data about mebendazole are quite mixed, success being defined as radiological disappearance or decrease in cyst size, ranging from 48 to 100%.[9,124,127–129] Most investigators used fixed dosing and did not adjust for blood levels. Given the slow growth of *Echinococcus* cysts,[36] a follow-up of at least 1 year is required to assess the value of any

pharmacological treatment of this disease. As already suggested by the data on cyst viability at surgery in treated patients, long-term follow-up indicates that mebendazole is only parasitostatic since Kammerer and Schantz[128] reported a 20% relapse rate after completion of therapy. The drug has also been used in children[129] and the response rate of 51% is comparable with that seen in adult series.

Disregarding the report by Choudhuri et al,[132] success, as defined above, after albendazole ranges from 66 to 100%.[9,126,132–137] Complete cyst disappearance was observed in 22% of patients with hepatic cysts.[135] Serum levels were not monitored and from the compilation in Table 75.3 it remains unclear whether higher doses of albendazole could increase the response rate.

Cyst size is a main determinant for response to either benzimidazole, small cysts responding better than large cysts, while cyst location, with the exception of bone, appears not to be major determinant.[9] Bone cysts appear to be a problematic indication for pharmacological therapy in the experience of different investigators.[9,137]

Recently, a few case reports demonstrating beneficial effects of praziquantel have appeared.[138,139] This is of particular interest in combination since it is more potent than either agent alone in an animal model of peritoneal spillage in vivo.[111] However, Piens et al[139] treated nine patients prior to surgery with two 10-day courses of praziquantel. The drug could not be detected in the cyst fluid and as many cysts remained vital as in an untreated control group, shedding doubt on the efficacy of praziquan- tel alone as a scolicidal agent. This may be due to the fact that praziquantel acts on protoscolices but not on the germinal layer.

ECHINOCOCCUS MULTILOCULARIS

BIOLOGY

The natural cycle of *E. multilocularis* (Figure 75.5) typically involves red and artic foxes as definitive hosts. Other carnivores such as the domestic dog or cat can occasionally be involved in the cycle as definitive hosts. As for *E. granulosus*, the adult-stage tapeworms attach to the mucosa of the small intestine. The fully developed parasite ranges between 1.2 and 4.5 mm in length and usually consists of between two and six (mean five) proglottids. The hermaphroditic adults reach sexual maturity in about 4 weeks. Egg production starts as early as 28 days after infection of definitive hosts.[140] Gravid proglottid uteri contain round-to-ovoid eggs 30–36 μm in diameter, with a single fully differentiated oncosphere embedded in an oncospheral membrane and surrounded by a thick embryophore. Such proglottids, and the free eggs released on their rupture, are shed in the faeces of infected definitive hosts. Eggs released into the environment show a high degree of longevity and resistance to degradation. When ingested by a suitable intermediate host (small mammals such as microtine and arvicolid rodents, occasionally muskrats and others), digestive processes and other factors in the host gut result in hatching and release of the oncosphere, which subsequently becomes activated—probably by the surface active properties of bile. The activated oncosphere penetrates the epithelial border of the intestinal villi and enters venous and lymphatic vessels, followed by distribution to other anatomical sites. Most of the oncospheres develop in the liver; some may reach lungs or other organs. Maturation to the asexually proliferating metacestode includes degeneration of the oncospheral tissue, cellular proliferation, vesicularization and creation of a germinative membrane with formation of a central cavity and a peripheral laminated layer, followed later by

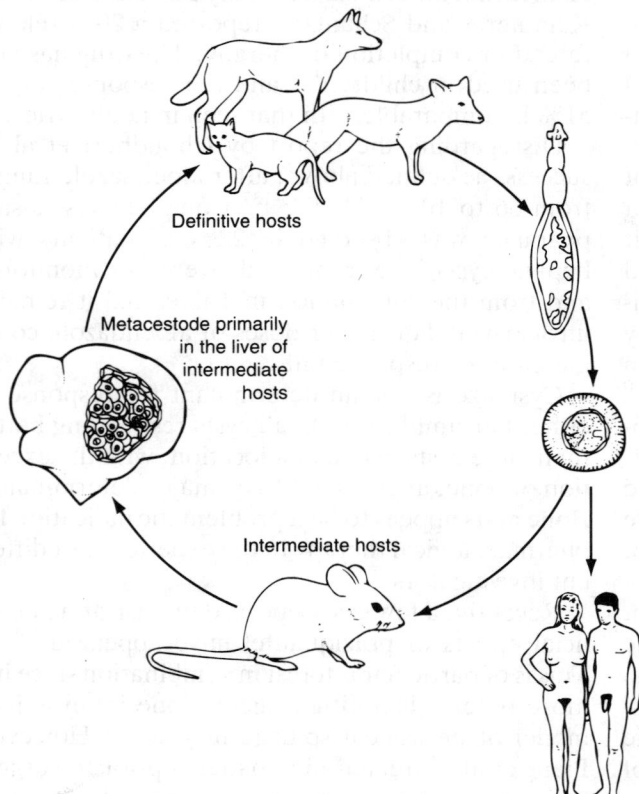

Definitive hosts

Metacestode primarily in the liver of intermediate hosts

Intermediate hosts

Figure 75.5 Life cycle of *E. multilocularis.* Foxes are the most important definitive hosts, occasionally replaced by dogs and cats. Tapeworm proglottids, containing tapeworm eggs, are passed into faeces. Rodents are the main intermediate hosts, man becoming infected accidentally. The main target organ is the liver, harbouring the parasitic metacestode lesion which consists of vesicles containing protoscolices. Single vesicles are surrounded by an outer laminated layer and have an inner germinal layer budding into protoscolices containing brood capsules.

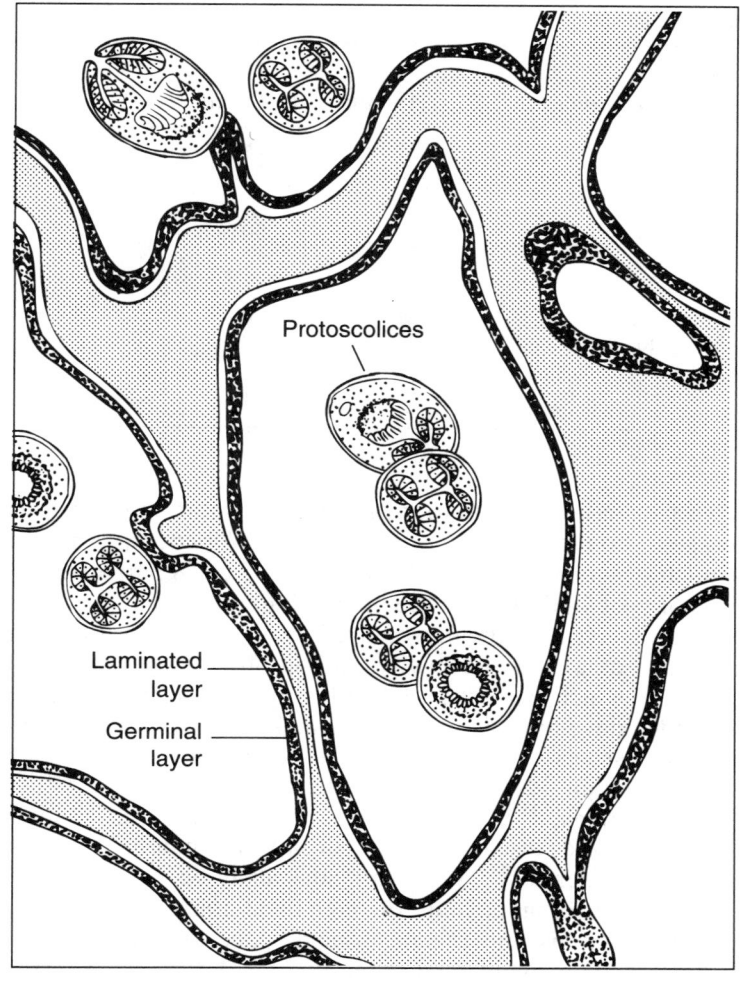

Figure 75.6   Cross-section of the metacestode of *E. multilocularis*. (Adapted from Brumpt.[141])

Protoscolices

Laminated layer

Germinal layer

endogenous and exogenous proliferation of metacestode tissue. A typical *E. multilocularis* lesion is illustrated in Figure 75.6.

Production of protoscolices may take place within 2–4 months, but may also be lacking, depending on the intermediate host species or strains. For completion of the life cycle, definitive hosts must ingest the mature infective metacestode containing protoscolices. Digestion of the infected tissue is followed by liberation of protoscolices with invaginated scolex. Pepsin and bile salts stimulate rapid evagination of the scolex, which is then able to attach firmly to the intestinal mucosa.

DISTRIBUTION AND EPIDEMIOLOGY

E. multilocularis occurs only in the Northern hemisphere; in North America the cestode is present in subarctic regions of Alaska and Canada, including St Lawrence Island and some others.[2] There is apparently an expansion of this original focus since the parasite has been discovered recently in the states of Illinois, Nebraska,[142] Alberta, Saskatchewan, Iowa, South Dakota, Montana, Wyoming, and even as far south as South Carolina.[143]

In Europe areas with relatively frequent reports of alveolar echinococcosis in humans encompasses central and eastern France, Switzerland, Austria and Germany. These main European endemic areas have previously been regarded as isolated foci, but recent data suggest that they might be linked to each other and to other Eurasian or Asian areas where *E. multilocularis* has been reported.

The Asian areas with *E. multilocularis* prevalence include the tundra zone ranging from the White Sea eastwards to the Bering Strait, covering large parts of the former Soviet Union. The southern borders are documented by cases reported in the latitudinal zone starting from Turkey, eastwards through Afghanistan, Iran, India, China and Mongolia to northern parts of Japan. One of the best updated overviews on the global distribution of *E. multilocularis* has been provided by WHO guidelines.[144]

At the global level scant data exist on the overall prevalence of human alveolar echinococcosis. The

Table 75.4 Signs and symptoms of *E. multilocularis* infection.

Authors	n (patients)	Pain (%)	Hepatomegaly (%)	Abscess (%)	Cholangitis (%)
Akinoglu et al[151]	39	'most'	'most'	10	18
Ammann et al[150]	60	37	30	—	30
Bresson-Hadni et al[147]					
Before 1983	50	80	50	—	50
After 1983	30	60	30	—	30
Kasai et al[160]	60	—			
Stage I*	6	0	0	0	0
Stage II	37	35	89	—	19
Stage III	17	47	94	—	71
Wilson and Rausch[145]	33	60	79		21

*Stages I, II and III refer to the asymptomatic, progressive and terminal periods, respectively.

annual incidence of the populations at risk in western Alaska, including St Lawrence Island, averages 28 new cases per 100 000 inhabitants;[145] this is much lower in Switzerland, with an annual incidence of 0.18/100 000.[146] Similar data were reported from France, Germany and Austria.[144] The prevalence in France is 4.4/100 000.[147]

In contrast to the relatively stable prevalence and incidence in Europe and Alaska, Japan reported spread of both parasite and disease in its northern areas: between 1937 and 1982, 129 cases of alveolar echinococcosis had been reported on Rebun Island; since then, the disease has spread to Hokkaido and Honshu Islands with a total of 264 and 60 new cases, respectively, registered up to 1988.[144,148] One of the highest incidences has been reported from China with an 8.8% seroprevalence.[149]

CLINICAL DIAGNOSIS AND NATURAL HISTORY

The primary manifestations of *E. multilocularis* are related to the liver, which is affected in 92–100% of all cases.[145,150–152] The most frequent presenting symptoms are listed in Table 75.4. Expansive and infiltrative growth of the parasite leads to non-specific abdominal pain, hepatomegaly and jaundice. In about 15% the parasite is discovered in asymptomatic patients, or there are only unspecific symptoms such as fatigue and weight loss.[150] As a result of screening programmes since 1983, more asymptomatic patients are being discovered in France[147] (Table 75.4). Occasionally, manifestations of portal hypertension, either variceal bleeding and/or ascites, is the first manifestation.[151] Invasion of the hepatic veins can lead to a Budd–Chiari syndrome.[153,154] Rarely, neurological mani-

festations due to invasion of the spine or metastasis to the brain are present. Thus, Weber et al[155] found neurological manifestations in 5 of 78 patients; in 3 of 78 they were the presenting symptoms.

One of the most feared complications is infection of a necrotic cavity and/or obstructed bile ducts which are associated with very high mortality due to development of septic shock.[147,151] Distant metastases can occur late in the disease; these have been described in brain,[145,150,151] spine,[151,155] lungs,[145,150,151,156] bone,[150,151] and eyes.[13] Metastatic disease occurs in approximately 10% of patients.[147] Growth can also be expansive—invading the lungs through the diaphragm, the porta hepatis and the peritoneal space and retroperitoneum, which can extend as far down as the testes encasing the ureters in the process.[157]

Mortality of untreated *E. multilocularis* has been reported to be 63–93% at 10 years.[139,145] Biologically, *E. multilocularis* behaves as a slowly growing, malignant tumour. The median growth rate was 15 ml/year with a range of 3.8–221 ml/year.[158] These figures were obtained from morphometric analysis of serial CT scans in seven patients, who had presumably undergone radical surgery; individual values are shown in Figure 75.7.

Laboratory investigations are not very helpful in diagnosis, with the exception of immunological tools (see below). IgE levels are elevated in 61%,[159] while eosinophilia is quite rare, occurring in only 10% of patients.[147] Evidence of cholestasis is frequently present, while transaminases are only rarely and moderately elevated, in particular when there is central necrosis.[147]

Among the imaging procedures, ultrasonography and CT are of greatest diagnostic value. Calcifications on plain abdominal radiographs may give the first clue as to the aetiology of the disease; the percentage of calcified lesions increases from 33 to 100% as the disease progresses.[160] On sonography, hyperechogenic and hypoechogenic zones are found in the lesion(s).[161] Since the cysts are quite small, no cystic appearance can be expected. Similar findings can be found on CT: the lesions are typically not enhanced with contrast medium;[161] the characteristic lesion has been called a 'geographic map' with irregular contours and alternating hypodense and hyperdense areas, reflecting necrosis and calcification, respectively.[161] CT is felt by some authors to be superior to ultrasonography in delineating the anatomy of parasite localization.[162] Hilar involvement can lead to liver atrophy which is easily visualized by CT.[163] Ultrasonography is 84% sensitive and specific in areas of high prevalence[149] and is the preferred imaging procedure for mass screening programmes.[149,162] As with *E. granulosus*, MRI adds little to diagnosis, in particular because microcalcifications are not visualized by this technique.[164,165]

SEROLOGICAL AND MOLECULAR DIAGNOSIS

ANTIBODY TESTS

Until recently most serological tests for immunodiagnosis of human alveolar echinococcosis employed heterologous *E. granulosus* antigen(s). This was partly because *E. granulosus* antigen could be obtained easily from many sources worldwide and because many diagnostic laboratories primarily investigated the more frequent cystic echinococcosis. Alternatively, *E. multilocularis* metacestode tissue was used as a source for *Echinococcus* antigen. Thus, specific antigen fractions from *E. multilocularis* were isolated by affinity chromatography,[166]

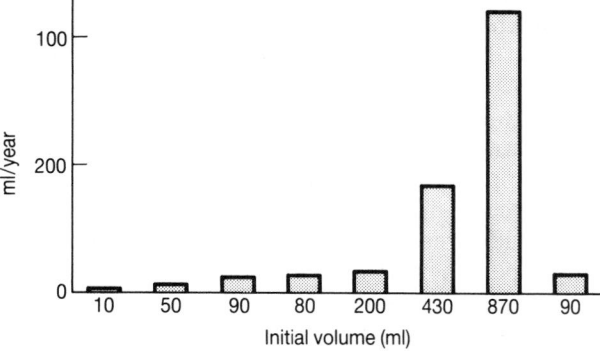

Figure 75.7 Growth rate of *E. multilocularis* in eight patients with recurrence after supposedly radical surgery. The initial volume of parasite was that observed when patients entered the trial. The volume and growth rate were obtained from serial morphometric analysis of CT scans. (Adapted from Luder et al[158] as published in Reichen et al[125] with permission from the author and the publishers.)

which proved to be more specific than heterologous *E. granulosus* antigen. The resulting fractions (Em1- and Em2-antigen) were successfully used to differentiate human cystic from alveolar echinococcosis.[167] Later on, the antigenic component of the Em2-antigen fraction was purified and used for the development of a monoclonal antibody against Em2-antigen.[168] Attempts to differentiate both forms of echinococcosis serologically have also been undertaken by others using various techniques.[169–171]

The improvements achieved in the sensitivity and specificity of these tests enabled reliable large-scale serosurveys in different endemic areas, such as Switzerland[146] and Alaska,[172] to be undertaken. Seroepidemiological studies in Alaska have shown that Em2-ELISA detected not only asymptomatic cases of human alveolar echinococcosis seronegative by other techniques,[173] but also unique cases in which the metacestode lesion had died at an apparently early stage of infection.[174]

Serological diagnosis is of particular interest in the surveillance of operated or pharmacologically-treated patients. Early tests, although exhibiting a decrease after surgery, were of limited clinical use.[175] In contrast, antibody measured by the Em2-ELISA declined dramatically within months after successful radical operation.[38,172] An exceptional immunological situation was found in patients receiving orthotopic liver transplantation:[153] serum antibodies were immediately eliminated by abundant blood transfusions coupled to immunosuppressive therapy. Patients with remaining residual foci of extrahepatic parasite tissue had extremely high recurrence rates due to immunosuppression and interruption of chemotherapy with antiparasitic benzimidazoles; this was accompanied by reappearance of anti-*Echinococcus* serum antibodies.[176]

Serological diagnosis is not very helpful in monitoring chemotherapy of alveolar echinococcosis.[150,172,175,177] A trend towards a decrease in specific antibody concentration(s) could be observed in regressive forms of disease, whereas specific serum antibody concentrations of patients with non-resectable lesions and/or palliative surgery and a progressive course remained elevated or increased. Parasite-specific antibody isotypes may better correlate with clinical findings than results of classical serological tests, especially with regard to IgA and IgE.[147,160]

CELL-MEDIATED IMMUNITY

The in vitro determination of lymphocyte proliferation in response to stimulation with *E. multilocu-*

laris antigens has been proposed as a diagnostic alternative to antibody detection in alveolar echinococcosis.[178] A progressive decrease in the capacity for responding to parasite-specific lymphocyte stimulation was observed in most of the patients with regressive course of disease. On the other hand, an increase of stimulation indices was usually shown to be associated with a progression of the liver lesion(s).[178] Another study showed that the in vitro lymphoproliferative response to *E. multilocularis* antigen stimulation was very high in cured patients who had radical surgery or patients with dead lesions; it was significantly lower in patients with either palliative or no surgery.[178]

RECOMBINANT *ECHINOCOCCUS* ANTIGEN

Various recombinant *E. multilocularis* antigens have been constructed, including the antigens II/3-10,[179,180] EM10,[181] EM4 and pEM10.[182] A preliminary large-scale evaluation of the recombinant antigen II/3-10 in ELISA resulted in diagnostic operating characteristics suggesting suitability for immunodiagnosis of alveolar echinococcosis in humans. Significant improvement was obtained by developing a hybrid test (designated Em2plus-ELISA) using simultaneously recombinant II/3-10 and Em2-antigen.[183]

MOLECULAR DIAGNOSIS

A PCR-based test to discriminate between *E. granulosus* and *E. multilocularis* at the level of parasite nucleic acids has been discussed (see above). Using the two *E. multilocularis* oligonucleotides BG1 and BG2 (corresponding to a 2.6 kbp fragment), a study of 14 individual isolates of *E. multilocularis* and other cestodes revealed the test to be specific for all *E. multilocularis* isolates.[76] Another *E. multilocularis* primer set—BG1 and BG3 defining a 0.3 kbp fragment—was found to be genus specific, i.e. indicative of *E. multilocularis*, *E. granulosus* and *E. vogeli*; this test was sensitive enough to detect approximately 2.5 pg template DNA and is currently already used in field studies.[184] A similar approach focused on the U1 snRNA gene repeat of *E. multilocularis*,[185] applying it to a PCR test for the identification of single *E. multilocularis* eggs.[186]

PATHOLOGY AND IMMUNOLOGY

The typical lesion (see Figure 75.6) is a mass of fibrous tissue with a multitude of cavities ranging from a few millimetres to centimetres in size.[147] Histologically, the characteristic lesion in man consists of a thin but marked laminated layer with or without a germinal layer; this is accompanied by a granulomatous reaction.[147] In contrast to infections in rodent hosts, lesions from infected humans rarely exhibit protoscolices, brood capsules or calcareous bodies. Immunocytochemical demonstration of *E. multilocularis* antigen(s) on biopsy or autopsy specimens is helpful and highly sensitive but it remains positive in patients having undergone successful chemotherapy and is thus not a measure of parasite viability.[187] In complicated cases, evidence of secondary biliary cirrhosis and/or cholangitis will be found. Recently, amyloid has been described in 2 out of 2 kidneys and 2 of 6 livers.[188]

As for *E. granulosus*, the primary site of interaction between *E. multilocularis* and its host is the mucosa of the gastrointestinal tract. Scarce information is available on the immune response against migrating and subsequently established oncospheres and their development into larvae of *E. multilocularis* in humans. Therefore, the following considerations will focus on the immune response to fully developed and often rapidly proliferating metacestodes.

Many patients with *E. multilocularis* infection respond with a marked synthesis of parasite-specific antibodies, including all isotypes of immunoglobulins. There is no evidence that specific antibodies have a direct restricting role on the growth of the metacestode. However, protoscolices and oncospheres of *E. multilocularis* can be lysed by antibody-mediated complement inactivation. Increased levels of total and parasite-specific serum IgE have been demonstrated;[189] some of this specific IgE is bound to circulating basophils and forms the basis of a degranulation test.[165] In spite of these phenomena, immediate-type hypersensitivity reactions have never been observed, not even during surgical manipulations or needle biopsies of the liver.[147] Antibodies appear to be involved in the rare chronic granulomatous course of the disease.

In contrast to antibodies, T-lymphocyte interactions appear to be of immunopathophysiological significance. Thus, a specific cellular immune response had already been shown by proliferation in vitro of peripheral blood mononuclear cells of *E. multilocularis* patients.[178,190] More direct information addressing the potential site of host-parasite interplay was obtained by Vuitton et al,[191] who showed that the periparasitic granuloma—mainly composed of macrophages, myofibroblasts and T cells, contains a large number of CD^4-positive lymphocytes in patients with so-called 'abortive' or 'died out' lesions, whereas in patients with active metacestodes the number of CD[8+] cells was increased. An association between lymphoproliferative responsiveness and mechanisms of resistance or susceptibility to *E. multilocularis* infections has also been suggested by comparative in vitro lymphocyte stimulation assays in patients with different courses of disease.[189]

The concept that T lymphocytes are the main determinant of host response is supported by different findings in animal models of alveolar echinococcosis. Thus, depletion of T cells enhances metastasis formation in mice.[192] In congenitally athymic nude mice, *E. multilocularis* develops very rapidly, and the host tissue reaction is much less than in heterozygote mice.[193] Activated macrophages appear to be key participants in immune response as they could be seen to adhere to the metacestode.[194] Alkarmi and Behbehani[195] suggested that the parasite survives by actively impairing cellular mechanisms of recognition and neutrophil chemotaxis in experimentally infected mice. This effect was attributed to phlogistic and chemotactic properties of *E. multilocularis* antigens, which may also modulate the intense inflammatory response and amyloidogenesis in alveolar echinococcosis.[196]

Susceptibility and resistance to infection with *E. multilocularis* metacestodes may depend upon genetically based immunological factors, as evidenced by marked differences in susceptibility to infection in different mouse strains; strains with particular susceptibility include AKR,[197] Balb/c and C57BL/6.[198] Relatively resistant inbred mouse strains include A/J[198] and C57BL/10.[197,198] However, reports are quite contradictory concerning the degree of susceptibility or resistance of several mouse strains; this could reflect a more complex situation concerning potential strain or isolate variation of the parasite.

Immunosuppression may also play some role in murine alveolar echinococcosis. Thus, a decline of peritoneal lymphocytes, monocytes and eosinophils, replaced subsequently by neutrophils, was observed during the phase of *E. multilocularis* proliferation,[199] although mechanisms responsible for these effects could not be elucidated. Analysis of the phenotypic patterns of cells within the periparasitic granulomas in susceptible and resistant mice showed that susceptibility was associated with the persistence of numerous LY4 (CD[4+]) lymphocytes and a low number of macrophages, whereas the periparasitic granulomas of resistant animals showed elevated numbers of LY2 (CD[8+]) T cells.[200] More recent data demonstrated the potential of the parasite to induce suppression of T-cell proliferation by LY2 T cells.[201]

TREATMENT

The mainstay of treatment remains surgical; in contrast to *E. granulosus*, interventional radiology and endoscopic procedures are rarely used.

SURGERY

Hepatic resection is the treatment of choice but this is possible only in 15–58% of cases.[147,151,160,175,201] Due to earlier diagnosis, the incidence of radically resectable cases has increased from 10 to 40% in a recent series.[147] Even in presumed radical surgery, recurrences can occur in 10–20%.[151,202] This is due to microlesions and root-like parasite protrusions extending far into apparently healthy tissue.[203] In patients where eradication is impossible, a good quality of life can be achieved when adequate biliary drainage is provided.[147,204]

Among palliative procedures, marsupialization[151,160] and biliary–digestive anastomoses or T-tube drainage for intrabiliary rupture[151] and cholangitis[202,204] have been used with success. Portal hypertension occasionally requires treatment with portosystemic shunt.[147,153,204] Metastatic disease, in particular in the brain, is sometimes amenable to surgical resection.[205]

Recently, hepatic transplantation has been proposed for patients with inoperable disease;[153] in this series of 17 patients, actuarial survival was 75% at 15 months; the operation was felt to be radical in nine patients[153] but serological and radiological recurrence was later reported in three of these patients, one succumbing to recurrent disease.[176] An ELISA directed against Em2 has been reported to reliably predict radical surgery.[39] However, anti-Em2 antibodies correlate with the presence of parasite only, not with its viability[174] (see above).

PHARMACOTHERAPY

In animal models the same three drugs discussed in the preceding section, namely mebendazole, albendazole and praziquantel, have some activity against *E. multilocularis*.[206] Praziquantel was the most effective scolicidal agent but did not inhibit cyst growth; albendazole was the most active agent in inhibiting cyst growth.[206]

The results of some clinical studies with mebendazole[130,150,151,207–209] and albendazole[125,126,210,211] are reported in Table 75.5; for the earlier trials, the reader is referred to the reports of a workshop.[130] Assessing efficacy in treatment of *E.*

Table 75.5 Effect of benzimidazole treatment on *E. multilocularis*.

Author	n	Dose	Follow-up (years)	Failure (%)*
Mebendazole				
Akinoglu et al[151]	19	50 mg/kg	1–6	63
Ammann et al[150]	57	Variable[†]	1–9	33
Davis et al[207]	54	40 mg/kg	1–12	22
Kern[208]	8	50 mg/kg	—	13
Rausch et al[209]	8	40 mg/kg	10	50
Albendazole				
Horton[126]	35	800 mg	1	11
Liu et al[211]	15	20 mg/kg	1–5	13
Reichen et al[125]	12	600 mg	1–5‡	17
Wilson et al[210]	*2*	*800 mg*	*<1*	*0*

*Failure is defined as either radiological progression, development of metastatic disease or death.
†Mebendazole dose adjusted to reach therapeutic levels.
‡Updated from the preliminary report.[125.]

multilocularis is even more difficult than in *E. granulosus* since viability of the parasite cannot easily be judged in vivo, spontaneous death of parasite has been described,[174] and radiological regression is rare.[158] Therefore, radiological progression and/or death are the only hard end-points as treatment failures;[150] these are recorded in Table 75.5. Quite convincing evidence that mebendazole affects the growth rate has been provided by Luder et al:[158] these authors found a negative growth rate in 4 of 6 treated patients, which is significantly different from the growth rate in untreated patients.[158] Similarly, Rausch et al[209] in a long-term follow-up on ten patients found a reduction in cyst size in 4 out of 8, as opposed to progression and/or development of distant metastases in 15 of 16 historical controls. The same reservations invoked earlier should apply when interpreting the data in Table 75.5, i.e. one cannot be assured that some of the patients described have not been reported elsewhere. No report comparing mebendazole with the better bioavailable albendazole has yet appeared; such a trial is, however, underway.[207] The data in Table 75.5 appear to give a slight edge to albendazole but, again, longer observation is needed to arrive at a definitive verdict.

It remains unclear whether any of the benzimidazoles are truly parasitostatic. Recurrence after discontinuation of mebendazole treatment was observed in 7 of 19 patients.[152] Inoculation of autopsy material from two patients treated with mebendazole failed to demonstrate growth, while growth was observed in 8 of 11 untreated patients; however, duration of treatment of at least 2 years is needed to observe such favourable effects, and viable material was found in patients treated for up to 48 months.[212] In contrast, in two patients treated for a short time with albendazole no growth could be observed,[210] which is in contrast to our own experience.[125] Finally, benzimidazole treatment has been found to render some patients—initially judged to be unresectable—fit for radical surgery.[213]

OTHER *ECHINOCOCCUS* SPECIES

ECHINOCOCCUS VOGELI

E. vogeli is maintained primarily in a silvatic predator–prey cycle which includes the bush dog and occasionally domestic dogs as definitive host and pacas as intermediate hosts. Humans are rarely infected. The metacestode of *E. vogeli* is polycystic and fluid-filled with a tendency to form multichambered conglomerates; the predilection site in the intermediate host is the liver. Endogenous proliferation and convolution of both germinal and laminated layers leads to the formation of secondary subdivisions of the primary vesicle, including production of brood capsules and protoscolices. The geographical distribution of *E. vogeli* includes the northern half of South America.

Polycystic hydatid disease due to *E. vogeli* in

humans has been reported from Argentina, Brazil, Colombia, Ecuador, Panama and Venezuela. While the most frequent primary site is the liver, primary polycystic infections have also occurred elsewhere in the abdominal cavity, in the lungs and in other thoracic organs.[214,215] Patients with polycystic echinococcosis usually present with a painful right hypochondrial mass, jaundice or an hepatic abscess, rarely with signs and symptoms of pulmonary disease—in particular cough and haemoptysis.[215] Commonly, the evolution of the disease is rather benign; recovery was reported following surgical resection, and sometimes spontaneously.[214] Laboratory tests rarely reveal eosinophilia; antibodies against homologous and heterologous (*E. granulosus*) antigens may help in diagnosis. In inoperable cases, albendazole yields much the same result(s) as in *E. granulosus* with cure or improvement observed in 4 of 6 patients in a recent small series.[216]

ECHINOCOCCUS OLIGARTHRUS

E. oligarthrus infects only felids (mainly the cougar, the jaguar, the ocelot, the jaguarundi and Geoffroyi's cat) as definitive hosts, with the larval stage occurring in subcutaneous muscles of large South American rodents such as agoutis and pacas. The metacestode is, like *E. vogeli*, polycystic and fluid filled. There is less subdivision into secondary chambers and the laminated layer is significantly thinner than that of *E. vogeli*. So far one single infection with larval *E. oligarthrus* has been reported in a human patient in Venezuela.[217]

ACKNOWLEDGEMENTS

Supported by grants from the Swiss National Science Foundation to J.R. (32.30168.90) and to B.G. (31–29651.90).

REFERENCES

1 Morseth D J. Fine structure of the hydatid cyst and protoscolex of *Echinococcus granulosus*. *J Parasitol* 1967; 53:312–325.

2 Rausch R L. Life-cycle patterns and geographic distribution of Echinococcus species. In Thompson RCA (ed.) *The Biology of Echinococcus and Hydatid Disease*. London: Allen & Unwin, 1986: 44–80.

3 Attanasio E, Ferretti G & Palmas C. Hydatidosis in Sardinia: review and recommendations. *Trans R Soc Trop Med Hyg* 1985; 79:154–158.

4 Commission of the European Community A. *Disease in Farm Livestock: Economics and Policy*. Report EUR 11285. Luxembourg: 1987.

5 Food and Agriculture Organization of the United Nations. *Cost/Benefit Analysis for Animal Health Programmes in Developing Countries*. Report of FAO Expert Consultation: 1990.

6 World Health Organization. *WHO Guidelines for Diagnosis, Surveillance and Control of Echinococcosis*. WHO/CDS/VPH/88/78. Geneva: WHO, 1988.

7 Macpherson C N L, Romig T, Zeyhle E, Craig P S & Watschinger H. Observations on human echinococcosis (hydatidosis) and evaluation of transmission factors in the Maasai of northern Tanzania. *Ann Trop Med Parasitol* 1989; 83:489–497.

8 Gogucs O, Beduk Y & Topukccu Z. Renal hydatid disease. *Br J Urol* 1991; 68:466–469.

9 Todorov T, Mechkov G, Vutova K et al. Factors influencing the response to chemotherapy in human cystic echinococcosis. *Bull World Health Organ* 1992; 70:347–358.

10 Ouedraogo E G. Hydatid cyst of the breast. 20 cases. *J Gynecol Obstet Biol Reprod (Paris)* 1986; 15:187–194.

11 Shields D A. Multiple emboli in hydatid disease. *BMJ* 1990; 301:213–214.

12 Kalovidouris A, Gouliamos A, Andreou et al. Primary hydatid disease of the infratemporal fossa and the parotid gland. *Radiologe* 1985; 25:235–236.

13 Williams D F, Williams G A, Caya J G, Werner R P & Harrison T J. Intraocular *Echinococcus multilocularis*. *Arch Ophthalmol* 1987; 105:1106–1109.

14 Touhami M, Benkirane M & Ouazzani H. Hydatidose cervico-faciale. A propos de neuf cas. *Rev Laryngol* 1985; 106:187–190.

15 Sierra J, Oviedo J, Berthier M & Leiguarda R. Growth rate of secondary hydatid cysts of the brain. *J Neurosurg* 1985; 62:781–782.

16 AURC, ARC, ACAPEM, Chipponi J & Huguier M. Hydatid disease of the liver in France: epidemiology, diagnosis and surgical treatment. *Gastroenterol Clin Biol* 1986; 10:419–423.

17 Elhamel A. Pericystectomy for the treatment of hepatic hydatid cysts. *Surgery* 1990; 107:316–320.

18 Magistrelli P, Masetti R, Coppola R, Messia A, Nuzzo G & Picciocchi A. Surgical treatment of

hydatid disease of the liver. *Arch Surg* 1991; 126:518–523.

19 Schaefer J W & Khan M Y. Echinococcosis (hydatid disease): lessons from experience with 59 patients. *Rev Infect Dis* 1991; 13:243–247.

20 Werczberger A, Colhman J, Wertheim G, Gunders A E & Chowers I. Disseminated echinococcosis with repeated anaphylactic shock. *Chest* 1979; 74:482–484.

21 Kattan Y B. Intrabiliary rupture of hydatid cysts of the liver. *Br J Surg* 1975; 62:885–890.

22 Alper A, Ariogul O, Emre A, Uras A & Oekten A. Choledocho-duodenostomy for intrabiliary rupture of hydatid cysts of liver. *Br J Surg* 1987; 74:243–245.

23 Van Steenbergen W, Fevery J, Broeckaert L et al. Hepatic echinococcosis ruptured into the biliary tract. *J Hepatol* 1987; 4:133–139.

24 Yilmaz E & Gokok N. Hydatid disease of the liver: current surgical management. *Br J Clin Pract* 1990; 44:612–615.

25 Harris K M, Morrisl D L, Tudor R, Toghill P & Hardcastle J D. Clinical and radiographic features of simple and hydatid cysts of the liver. *Br J Surg* 1986; 73:835–838.

26 MacPherson C N L, Romig T, Zehyle E, Rees P H & Were J B O. Portable ultrasound scanner versus serology in screening for hydatid cysts in a Nomadic population. *Lancet* 1987; ii:259–261.

27 Pant C S & Gupta R K. Diagnostic value of ultrasonography in hydatid disease in abdomen and chest. *Acta Radiol* 1987; 28:743–745.

28 Lewall D B & McCorkell S J. Hepatic echinococcal cysts: sonographic appearance and classification. *Radiology* 1985; 155:773–775.

29 el Tahir M I, Omojola M F, Malatani T, al Saigh A H & Ogunbiyi O A. Hydatid disease of the liver: evaluation of ultrasound and computed tomography. *Br J Radiol* 1992; 65:390–392.

30 Marani S A, Canossi G C, Nicoli F A, Alberti G P, Monni S G & Casolo P M. Hydatid disease: MR imaging study. *Radiology* 1990; 175:701–706.

31 Bezzi M, Teggi A, De Rosa F et al. Abdominal hydatid disease: US findings during medical treatment. *Radiology* 1987; 162:91–95.

32 Hira P R, Lindberg L G, Francis I, Shweiki H, Shaheen Y & Leven B K. Diagnosis of cystic hydatid disease: Role of aspiration cytology. *Lancet* 1988; ii:655–657.

33 Frydman C P, Raissi S & Watson C W. An unusual pulmonary and renal presentation of echinococcosis. Report of a case. *Acta Cytol* 1989; 33:655–658.

34 Huguier M, Leynadier F, Houry S, Lacaine F & Dry J. Human basophil degranulation test in liver hydatidosis. *Dig Dis Sci* 1987; 32:1354–1357.

35 Sullivan M, Delbridge L, Reeve T S & Crummer P. Hydatid disease at Royal North Shore Hospital: results of surgical treatment. *Aust N Z J Surg* 1987; 57:177–180.

36 Romig T, Zeyhle E, Macpherson C N L, Rees P H & Were J B O. Cyst growth and spontaneous cure in hydatid disease. *Lancet* 1986; i:861.

37 Thompson R C A & Lymbery A J. The nature, extent and significance of variation within the genus Echinococcus. *Adv Parasitol* 1988; 27:209–258.

38 Hess U, Eckert J & Froehlich A. Vergleich serologischer Methoden für die Diagnose der zystischen and alvelaeren Echinokokkose des Menschen. *Schweiz Med Wochenschr* 1974; 104:853–859.

39 Gottstein B, Tschudi K, Eckert J & Ammann R. Em2-ELISA for the follow-up of alveolar echinococcosis after complete surgical resection of liver lesions. *Trans R Soc Trop Med Hyg* 1989; 83:389–393.

40 Gottstein B, Schantz P M, Todorov T, Saimot A G & Jacquier P. An international study on the serological differential diagnosis of human cystic and alveolar echinococcosis. *Bull World Health Organ* 1986; 64:101–105.

41 Capron A, Yarzabal L, Vernes A. & Fruit J: Le diagnostique immunologique de l'echinoccose humaine. *Path Biol* 1970; 18:357–365.

42 Yong W K & Heath D D. Arc 5 antibodies in sera of sheep infected with *Echinococcus granulosus*, *Taenia hydatigena* and *Taenia ovis*. *Parasite Immunol* 1979; 1:27–38.

43 Conder G A, Anderson F L & Schantz P M. Immunodiagnostic tests for hydatidosis in sheep: evaluation of double diffusion, immunoelectrophoresis, indirect hemagglutination, and intradermal tests. *J Parasitol* 1980; 66:577–584.

44 Schantz P M & Gottstein B. Echinococcosis. In Walls K W & Schantz P M (eds) *Immunodiagnosis of Parasitic Diseases*. Orlando: Academic Press, 1986: 69–107.

45 Varela-Diaz V M, Coltorti E A & D'Alessandro A. Immunoelectrophoretic tests showing *Echinococcus granulosus* arc 5 in human cases of *E. vogeli* and cysticercosis multiple myeloma. *Am J Trop Med Hyg* 1978; 27:554–557.

46 Varela-Diaz V M, Eckert J, Rausch R L, Coltorti E A & Hess U. Detection of the *Echinococcus granulosus* diagnostic arc 5 in sera from patients with surgically confirmed *E. multilocularis* infection. *Parasitol Res* 1977; 53:183–188.

47 Gottstein B, Witassek F & Eckert J. Neues zur Echinokokkose. *Schweiz Med Wochenschr* 1986; 116:810–817.

48 Di Felice G, Pini C, Afferni C & Vicari G. Purification and partial characterization of the major antigen of *Echinococcus granulosus* (antigen 5) with monoclonal antibodies. *Mol Biochem Parasitol* 1986; 20:133–142.

49 Lightowlers M W, Liu D, Haralambous A & Rickard M D. Subunit composition and specificity of the major cyst fluid antigens of *Echinococcus granulosus*. *Mol Biochem Parasitol* 1989; 37:171–182.

50 Chamekh M, Facon B, Dissous C, Haque A & Capron A. Use of a monoclonal antibody specific

for a protein epitope of *Echinococcus granulosus* antigen 5 in a competitive antibody radioimmunoassay for diagnosis of hydatid disease. *J Immunol Methods* 1990; 134:129–137.

51 Facon B, Chamekh M, Dissous C & Capron A. Molecular cloning of an *Echinococcus granulosus* protein expressing an immunogenic epitope of antigen 5. *Mol Biochem Parasitol* 1991; 45:233–240.

52 Chamekh M, Gras-Masse H, Bossus M et al. Diagnostic value of synthetic peptide derived from echinococcus granulosus recombinant protein. *J Clin Invest* 1992; 89:458–464.

53 Leggatt G R, Yang W & McManus D P. Serological evaluation of the 12 kDa subunit of antigen B in *Echinococcus granulosus* cyst fluid by immunoblot analysis. *Trans R Soc Trop Med Hyg* 1992; 86:189–192.

54 Maddison S E, Slemenda S B, Schantz P M, Fried J A, Wilson M & Tsang V C W. A specific diagnostic antigen of Echinococcus granulosus with an apparent molecular weight of 8 kDa. *Am J Trop Med Hyg* 1989; 40:377–383.

55 Kanwar J R, Kaushik S P, Sawhney I, Kamboj M, Mehta S & Vinayak V K. Specific antibodies in serum of patients with hydatidosis recognized by immunoblotting. *J Med Microbiol* 1992; 36:46–51.

56 Verastegui M, Moro P, Guevara A, Rodriguez T, Miranda E & Gilman R H. Enzyme-linked immunoelectrotransfer blot test for diagnosis of human hydatid disease. *J Clin Microbiol* 1992; 30:1557–1561.

57 Al Yaman F & Knobloch J. Isolation and partial characterization of species-specific and cross-reactive antigens of *Echinococcus granulosus* cyst fluid. *Mol Biochem Parasitol* 1989; 37:101–108.

58 Matossian R M, Kane G J, Chantler S N, Batty I & Sarhadian H J. The specific immunoglobulin in hydatid disease. *Immunology* 1972; 22:423–430.

59 Wattal C, Mohan C & Agarwal S C. Evaluation of specific immunoglogulin E by enzyme-linked immunosorbent assay in hydatid disease. *Int Arch Allergy Appl Immunol* 1987; 87:98–100.

60 Pinon J M, Poirriez J, Lepan J, Geers R, Penna R & Fernandez D. Value of isotypic characterization of antibodies to *Echinococcus granulosus* by enzyme-linked immuno-filtration assay. *Eur J Clin Microbiol* 1987; 6:291–295.

61 Dar F K, Buhidma M A & Kidwai S A. Hydatid false positive serological test results in malignancy. *BMJ* 1984; 288:1197.

62 Ben-Ismail R, Rouger P, Carme B, Gentilini M & Salmon C. Comparative automated assay of anti-P1 antibodies in acute hepatic distomiasis (fasciolasis) and in hydatidosis. *Vox Sang* 1980; 38:156–168.

63 Iacona A, Pini C & Vicari G. Enzyme-linked immunosorbent assay (ELISA) in the serodiagnosis of hydatid disease. *Am J Trop Med Hyg* 1980; 29:95–99.

64 Craig P S, Zeyhle E & Romig T. Hydatid disease: research and control in Turkana. II. The role of immunological techniques for the diagnosis of hydatid disease. *Trans R Soc Trop Med Hyg* 1986; 80:183–192.

65 Coltorti E A, Guarnera E, Larrieu C, Santillan G & Aquino A. Seroepidemiology of human hydatidosis: use of dried blood samples on filter paper. *Trans R Soc Trop Med Hyg* 1988; 82:607–610.

66 Baldelli F, Papili R, Francisci D, Tassi C, Stagni G & Pauluzzi S. Postoperative surveillance of human hydatidosis: evaluation of immundiagnostic tests. *Pathology* 1992; 24:75–79.

67 Craig P S & Nelson G S. The detection of circulating antigen in human hydatid disease. *Ann Trop Med Parasitol* 1984; 78:219–227.

68 Gottstein B. An immunoassay for the detection of circulating antigens in human echinococcosis. *Am J Trop Med Hyg* 1984; 33:1185–1191.

69 Eckert J & Gottstein B. Advances in diagnostic and investigational procedures for parasitic zoonoses. In Dunsmore J D (ed.) *Tropical Parasitoses and Parasitic Zoonoses*. Perth: WAAVP, 1983: 73–90.

70 Siracuso A, Teggi A, Quinteri F, Notargiacomo S, De Rosa F & Vicari G. Cellular immune response of hydatid patients to *Echinococcus granulosus* antigen. *Clin Exp Immunol* 1988; 72:400–405.

71 Lightowlers M W. Immunology and molecular biology of Echinococcus infections. *Int J Parasitol* 1990; 20:471–478.

72 Yap K W, Thompson R C A & Pawlowski I D. The development of nonradioactive total genomic probes for strain and egg differentiation in taenid cestodes. *Am J Trop Med Hyg* 1988; 39:472–477.

73 Rishi A K & McManus D P. Genomic cloning of human *Echinococcus granulosus* DNA: isolation of recombinant plasmids and their use as genetic markers in strain characterization. *Parasitology* 1987; 94:369–383.

74 Lymbery A J & Thompson R C A. Genetic differences between cysts of *Echinococcus granulosus* from the same host. *Int J Parasitol* 1989; 19:961–964.

75 Vogel M, Mueller N, Gottstein B, Flury K, Eckert J & Seebeck T. *Echinococcus multilocularis*: characterization of a DNA probe. *Acta Trop* 1991; 48:109–116.

76 Gottstein B & Mowatt M R. Sequencing and characterization of an *Echinococcus multilocularis* DNA probe and its use in the polymerase chain reaction. *Mol Biochem Parasitol* 1991; 44: 183–194.

77 Korc K, Hierro J, Lasalvia E, Falco M & Calcagno M. Chemical characterization of the polysaccharide of the hydatid membrane of *Echinococcus granulosus*. *Exp Parasitol* 1967; 20:219–224.

78 Yalin R, Aktan A O, Yegen C & Doeslueoglu H H. Significance of intracystic pressure in abdominal hydatid disease. *Br J Surg* 1992; 79:1182–1183.

79 Heath D D. Immunobiology of Echinococcus infections. In Thompson R C A (ed.) *The Biology of Echinococcus and Hydatid Disease*. London: Allen & Unwin, 1986: 164–188.

80 Furuya K, Nishizuka M, Honma J et al. Prevalence

of human alveolar echinococcosis in Hokkaido as evaluated by Western blotting. *Jpn J Med Sci Biol* 1990; 43:43–49.

81 Cox D A, Marshall-Clarke S & Dixon J B. Activation of murine B cells by *Echinococcus granulosus*. *Immunology* 1989; 67:16–20.

82 Wangoo A, Ganguly N K & Mahajan R C. Lymphocyte subpopulations and blast transformation studies in experimental hydatidosis. *Indian J Med Res* 1987; 85:149–153.

83 Riley E M & Dixon J B. Experimental *E. granulosus* infection in mice: immunocytochemical analysis of lymphocyte populations in local lymphoid infections during early infection. *Parasitology* 1987; 94:523–532.

84 Wangoo A, Ganguly N L & Mahajan R C. Specific T-cell cytotoxicity in experimental *E. granulosus* infected mice. *Indian J Med Res* 1987; 86: 588–590.

85 Ameglio F, Saba F, Bitti A et al. Antibody reactivity to HLA classes I and II in sera from patients with hydatidosis. *J Infect Dis* 1987; 156:673–676.

86 Annen J, Koehler P & Eckert J. Cytotoxicity of *Echinococcus granulosus* cyst fluid in vitro. *Parasitol Res* 1981; 65:79–88.

87 Ellis M E, Sinner W, Asraf Ali M & Hussain Qadri S M. Echinococcal disease and mycobacterial infection. *Ann Trop Med Parasitol* 1991; 85:243–251.

88 Langer J C, Rose D B, Keystone J S, Taylor B R & Langer B. Diagnosis and management of hydatid disease of the liver. A 15-year North American experience. *Ann Surg* 1984; 119:412–417.

89 Morel P, Robert J & Rohner A. Surgical treatment of hydatid disease of the liver: a survey of 69 patients. *Surgery* 1988; 104:859–862.

90 Behrns K E & van Heerden J A. Surgical management of hepatic hydatid disease. *Mayo Clin Proc* 1991; 66:1193–1197.

91 Kehila M, Korbi S, Tlili K et al. Les cholangites sclérosantes secondaires et les séquelles biliaires fibrosantes du kyste hydatique du foie. *Med Chir Dig* 1989; 18: 467–476.

92 Teres J, Gomez-Moli J, Bruguera M, Visa J, Bordas J M & Pera C. Sclerosing cholangitis after surgical treatment of hepatic echinococcal cysts. A report of three cases. *Am J Surg* 1984; 148:694–697.

93 Belghiti J, Benhamou J P, Houry S, Grenier P, Huguier M & Fekete F. Caustic sclerosing cholangitis. A complication of the surgical treatment of hydatid disease of the liver. *Arch Surg* 1986; 121:1162–1165.

94 Morris D L. Pre-operative albendazole therapy for hydatid cyst. *Br J Surg* 1987; 74:805–806.

95 French C M. Mebendazole and surgery for human hydatid disease in Turkana. *East Afr Med J* 1984; 61:113–119.

96 Little J M, Hollands M J & Ekberg H. Recurrence of hydatid disease. *World J Surg* 1988; 12:700–704.

97 Cangiotti L, Giulini S M, Muiesan P, Begni A & Tiberio G. Hydatid disease of the liver: long-term results of surgical treatment. *J Chir* 1991; 12:501–504.

98 Dadoukis J, Gamvros O & Aletras H. Intrabiliary rupture of the hydatid cyst of the liver. *World J Surg* 1984; 8:786–790.

99 Xynos E, Zoras O-J L, Pechlivanidis G, Neonakis E & Vassilakis J S. Intrabiliary rupture of hydatid cyst of the liver. *Dig Surg* 1990; 7:148–152.

100 Leong S, Kim Y I, Gray R, Kortan P & Haber G. Endoscopic and surgical management of intrabiliary rupture of hydatid liver cyst. *Can J Gastroenterol* 1992; 6:135–139.

101 Shemesh E & Friedman E. Radiologic and endoscopic appearance of intrabiliary rupture of hydatid liver disease. *Digestion* 1987; 36:96–100.

102 Vignote M L, Mino G, DelaMata M, DeDios J F & Gomez F. Endoscopic sphincterotomy in hepatic hydatid disease open to the biliary tree. *Br J Surg* 1990; 77:30–31.

103 al Karawi M A, Yasawy M I & el Shiekh Mohamed A R. Endoscopic management of biliary hydatid disease: report on six cases. *Endoscopy* 1991; 23:278–281.

104 Iscan M & Duren M. Endoscopic sphincterotomy in the management of postoperative complications of hepatic hydatid disease. *Endoscopy* 1991; 23:282–283.

105 Novick R J, Tchervenkov C I, Wilson J A, Munro D D & Mulder D S. Surgery for thoracic hydatid disease: a North American experience. *Ann Thorac Surg* 1987; 43:681–686.

106 Acunas B, Rozanes I, Celik L et al. Purely cystic hydatid disease of the liver: treatment with percutaneous aspiration and injection of hypertonic saline. *Radiology* 1992; 182:541–543.

107 Gargouri M, Ben Amor N, Ben Chehida F et al. Percutaneous treatment of hydatid cysts (*Echinococcus granulosus*). *Cardiovasc Intervent Radiol* 1990: 13:169–173.

108 Khuroo M S, Zargar S A & Mahajan R. *Echinococcus granulosus* cysts in the liver: management with percutaneous drainage. *Radiology* 1991; 180:141–145.

109 Filice C, Pirola F, Brunetti E, Dughetti S, Strosselli M & Foglieni C S. A new therapeutic approach for hydatid liver cysts. *Gastroenterology* 1990; 98:1366–1368.

110 Giorgio A, Tarantino L, Franica G et al. Unilocular hydatid liver cysts: treatment with US-guided, double percutaneous aspiration and alcohol injection. *Radiology* 1992; 184:705–710.

111 Chinnery J B & Morris D L. Effect of albendazole sulphoxide on viability of hydatid protoscolices in vitro. *Trans R Soc Trop Med Hyg* 1986; 80:815–817.

112 Taylor D H & Morris D L. Combination chemotherapy is more effective in postspillage prophylaxis for hydatid disease than either albendazole or praziquantel alone. *Br J Surg* 1989; 76:954.

113 Braithwaite P A, Roberts M S, Allan R J &

Watson T R. Clinical pharmacokinetics of high dose mebendazole in patients treated for cystic hydatid disease. *Eur J Clin Pharmacol* 1982; 22:161–169.

114 Marriner S E, Morris D L, Dickson B & Bogan J A. Pharmacokinetics of albendazole in man. *Eur J Clin Pharmacol* 1986; 30:705–708.

115 Luder P J, Witassek F, Weigand K, Eckert J & Bircher J. Treatment of cystic echinococcosis (*Echinococcus granulosus*) with mebendazole: assessment of bound and free drug levels in cyst fluid and of parasite vitality in operative specimens. *Eur J Clin Pharmacol* 1985; 28:279–285.

116 Morris D L, Chinnery J B, Geogiou G, Stamatakis G & Golematis B. Penetration of albendazole suphoxide into hydatid cysts. *Gut* 1987; 28:75–80.

117 Luder P J, Siffert B, Witassek F, Meister F & Bircher J. Treatment of hydatid disease with high oral doses of mebendazole. Long-term follow-up of plasma mebendazole levels and drug interactions. *Eur J Clin Pharmacol* 1986; 31:443–448.

118 Bekhti A. Serum concentrations of mebendazole in patients with hydatid disease. *Int J Clin Pharmacol Ther Toxicol* 1985; 23:635–641.

119 Witassek F, Burkhardt B, Eckert J & Bircher J. Chemotherapy of alveolar echinococcosis: comparison of plasma mebendazole concentrations in animals and man. *Eur J Clin Pharmacol* 1981; 20:427–433.

120 Steiger U, Cotting J & Reichen J. Albendazole treatment of echinococcosis in humans: effects on microsomal metabolism and drug tolerance. *Clin Pharmacol Ther* 1990; 47:347–353.

121 Lange H, Eggers R & Bircher J. Increased systemic availability of albendazole when taken with a fatty meal. *Eur J Clin Pharmacol* 1988; 34:315–317.

122 Witassek F & Bircher J. Chemotherapy of larval echinococcosis with mebendazole: microsomal liver function and cholestasis as determinants of plasma drug levels. *Eur J Clin Pharmacol* 1983; 25:85–90.

123 Cotting J, Zeugin T, Steiger U & Reichen J. Albendazole kinetics in patients with echinococcosis: delayed absorption and impaired elimination in cholestasis. *Eur J Clin Pharmacol* 1990; 38:605–608.

124 Davis A, Dixon H & Pawlowski Z S. Multicentre clinical trials of benzimidazole carbamates in human cystic echinococcosis (phase 2). *Bull World Health Organ* 67:503–508.

125 Reichen J, Cotting J & Steiger U. Pharmaco-therapy of hepatic hydatid disease. In Bianchi L, Gerok W, Maier K P & Deinhardt F (eds) *Infectious Diseases of the Liver*. Dordrecht: Kluwer, 1990: 235–245.

126 Horton R J. Chemotherapy of *Echinococcus* infection in man with albendazole. *Trans R Soc Trop Med Hyg* 1989; 83:97–102.

127 Bartoloni C, Tricerri A, Guidi L & Gambassi G. The efficacy of chemotherapy with mebendazole in human cystic echinococcosis: long-term follow-up of 52 patients. *Ann Trop Med Parasitol* 1992; 86:249–256.

128 Kammerer W S & Schantz P M. Long term follow-up of human hydatid disease (*Echinococcus granulosus*) treated with a high-dose mebendazole regimen. *Am J Trop Med Hyg* 1984; 33:132–137.

129 Messaritakis J, Psychou P, Nicolaidou P, Karpathios T, Syriopoulou B & Fretzayas A. High mebendazole doses in pulmonary and hepatic hydatid disease. *Arch Dis Child* 66:532–533.

130 Schantz P M, Van den Bossche H & Eckert J. Chemotherapy for larval echinococcosis in animals and humans: report of a workshop. *Z Parasitenkd* 1982; 67:5–26.

131 Teggi A, Capozzi A, & De Rosa F. Treatment of *Echinococcus granulosus* hydatid disease with mebendazole. *J Chemother* 1989; 1:310–317.

132 Choudhuri G, Prasad R, Tantry B V, Sharma M P & Tandon R K. Poor response to long-term albendazole therapy of hydatid liver cysts. *Scand J Infect Dis* 1989; 21:323–325.

133 Cossetto D, Gruenewald S, Antico V & Little J M. Albendazole treatment of recurrent hydatid disease: serial evaluation with ultrasound. *Aust N Z J Surg* 1989; 59:933–936.

134 De Rosa F & Teggi A. Treatment of *Echinococcus granulosus* hydatid disease with albendazole. *Ann Trop Med Parasitol* 1990; 84:467–472.

135 Morris D L, Dykes P W, Marriner S et al. Albendazole: objective evidence of response in human hydatid disease. *JAMA* 1985; 253:2053–2057.

136 Okelo G B A. Hydatid disease: research and control in Turkana. III. Albendazole in the treatment of inoperable hydatid disease in Kenya: a report on 12 cases. *Trans R Soc Trop Med Hyg* 1986; 80:193–195.

137 Saimot A G, Cremieux A C, Hay J M et al. Albendazole as a potential treatment for human hydatidosis. *Lancet* 1983; ii:652–656.

138 Henrikson T H, Klungsoyr P & Zerihun D. Treatment of disseminated peritoneal hydatid disease with praziquantel. *Lancet* 1989; i:272.

139 Piens M A, Persat F, May F & Mojon M. Praziquantel in human hydatidosis. Evaluation by preoperative treatment. *Bull Soc Pathol Exot Filiales* 1989; 82:503–512.

140 Thompson R C A & Eckert J. Observations on *Echinococcus multilocularis* in the definitive host. *Parasitol Res* 1987; 69:335–345.

141 Brumpt E. *Précis de Parasitologie*, Chartres (France): Imprimerie Durand, Vol. 1. 1936.

142 Ballard N B & Van de Vusse J. *Echinococcus multilocularis* in Illinois and Nebraska. *J Parasitol* 1983; 69:790–791.

143 Kazakos K R & Schantz P M. *Proceedings of the International Workshop on Alveolar Hydatid Disease*. Atlanta: Department of Health and Human Services, 1990: 13–14.

144 World Health Organization. *Report of the WHO informal consultation on* Echinococcus

multilocularis *research*. WHO/CDS/VPH/88.78. Geneva, WHO: 1988.

145 Wilson J F & Rausch R L. Alveolar hydatid disease: a review of clinical features of 33 indigenous cases of *E. multilocularis* infection in Alaskan eskimoes. *Am J Trop Med Hyg* 1980; 29:1340–1355.

146 Gottstein B, Lengeler C, Bachmann P et al. Sero-epidemiologic survey for alveolar echinococcosis (by Em2 ELISA) of blood donors in an endemic area of Switzerland. *Trans R Soc Trop Med Hyg* 1987; 81:960–964.

147 Bresson-Hadni S, Miguet J P, Vuitton D et al. L'échinococcose alvéolaire hépatique humaine. *Sem Hôp Paris* 1988; 64:2692–2701.

148 Kamiya M. Infectious diseases transmitted by dogs to humans. *Asian Med J* 1988; 31:87–93.

149 Craig P S, Deshan L, Macpherson C N L et al. A large focus of alveolar echinococcosis in central China. *Lancet* 1992; 340:826–831.

150 Ammann R, Tschudi K, von Ziegler M et al. Langzeitverlauf bei 60 Patienten mit alveolaerer Echinokokkose unter Dauertherapie mit Mebendazol (1976–1985). *Klin Wochenschr* 1988; 66:1060–1073.

151 Akinoglu A, Demiryurek H & Guzel C. Alveolar hydatid disease of the liver: a report on thirty-nine surgical cases in eastern Anatolia, Turkey. *Am J Trop Med Hyg* 1991; 45:182–189.

152 Ammann R W, Hirsbrunner R, Cotting J, Steiger U, Jacquier P & Eckert J. Recurrence rate after discontinuation of long-term mebendazole therapy in alveolar echinococcosis (preliminary results). *Am J Trop Med Hyg* 1990; 43:506–515.

153 Bresson-Hadni S, Franza A, Miguet J P et al. Orthotopic liver transplantation for incurable alveolar echinococcosis of the liver: report of 17 cases. *Hepatology* 1991; 13:1061–1070.

154 Robotti G C, Meister F & Schroeder R. Budd–Chiari Syndrom bei Leberechinockokkose. *Fortschr Geb Roentgenstr Nuklearmed Erganzungsband* 1985; 142:511–513.

155 Weber M, Vespignani H, Jacquier P et al. Neurological manifestations of alveolar echinococcosis. *Rev Neurol (Paris)* 1988; 144:104–112.

156 Etievent J P, Vuitton D, Allemand H, Weill F, Gandjbackhch I & Miguet J P. Pulmonary embolism from a parasitic cardiac clot secondary to hepatic alveolar echinococcosis. *J Cardiovasc Surg* 1986; 27:671–674.

157 Strohmaier W L, Bichler K H, Wilbert D M & Seitz H M. Alveolar echinococcosis with involvement of the ureter and testis. *J Urol* 1990; 144:733–734.

158 Luder P J, Robotti G, Meister F P & Bircher J. High oral doses of mebendazole interfere with growth of larval echinococcus multilocularis lesions. *J Hepatol* 1985; 1:369–377.

159 Vuitton D, Bresson-Hadni S & Lenys D. IgE dependent humoral immune response in *Echinococcus multilocularis* infection: circulating and basophil-bound specific IgE against Echinococcus antigens in patients with alveolar echinococcosis. *Clin Exp Immunol* 1988; 71:247–252.

160 Kasai Y, Koshino I, Kawanishi N, Sakamoto H, Sasaki E & Kumagai M. Alveolar echinococcosis of the liver. Studies on 60 operated cases. *Ann Surg* 1980; 192:145–152.

161 Didier D, Weiler S, Rohmer P et al. Hepatic alveolar echinococcosis: correlative US and CT study. *Radiology* 1985; 154:179–186.

162 Choji K, Fujita N, Chen M et al. Alveolar hydatid disease of the liver: computed tomography and transabdominal ultrasound with histopathological correlation. *Clin Radiol* 1992; 46:97–103.

163 Rozanes I, Acunacs B, Celik L, Minareci O & Gokmen E. CT in lobar atrophy of the liver caused by alveolar echinococcosis. *J Comput Assist Tomogr* 1992; 16:216–218.

164 Claudon M, Bessieres M, Regent D et al. Alveolar echinococcosis of the liver: MR findings. *J Comput Assist Tomogr* 1990; 14:608–614.

165 Duewell S, Marincek B, von Schulthess G K & Ammann R. MRT and CT in alveolar echinococcosis of the liver. *ROFO* 1990; 152:441–445.

166 Gottstein B, Eckert J & Fey H. Serological differentiation between *Echinococcus granulosus* and *Echinococcus multilocularis* infections in man. *Z Parasitenkd* 347–356; 69:69.

167 Gottstein B. Purification and characterization of a specific antigen from *Echinococcus multilocularis*. *Parasite Immunol* 1985; 7:201–212.

168 Deplazes P & Gottstein B. A monoclonal antibody against *Echinococcus multilocularis* Em2 antigen. *Parasitology* 1991; 103:41–49.

169 Knobloch J, Lederer I & Mannweiler E. Species-specific immunodiagnosis of human echinococcosis with crude antigens. *Eur J Clin Microbiol* 1984; 3:554–555.

170 Auer H, Picher O & Aspoeck H. Combined application of enzyme-linked immunosorbent assay (ELISA) and indirect hemagglutination test (IHA) as a useful tool for the diagnosis and postoperative surveillance of human alveolar and cystic echinococcosis. *Zentralbl Bakteriol Hyg* 1988; A270:313–325.

171 Furuya K, Nishizuka M, Honma H et al. Prevalence of human alveolar echinococcosis in Hokkaido as evaluated by Western blotting. *Jpn J Med Sci Biol* 1990; 43:43–49.

172 Lanier A P, Trujillo D E, Schantz P M, Wilson J F, Gottstein B & McMahon B. Comparison of serologic tests for the diagnosis and follow-up of alveolar hydatid disease. *Am J Trop Med Hyg* 1987; 37:609–615.

173 Gottstein B, Schantz P M & Wilson J F. Serologic screening for *Echinococcus multilocularis* infections with ELISA. *Lancet* 1985; i:1097–1098.

174 Rausch R L, Wilson J F, Schantz P M & McMahon

B J. Spontaneous death of *Echinococcus multilocularis*: cases diagnosed serologically (by Em2 ELISA) and clinical significance. *Am J Trop Med Hyg* 1987; 36:576–585.

175 Schantz P M, Wilson J F, Wahlquist S P, Boss L P & Rausch R L. Serologic test for diagnosis and post-treatment evaluation of patients with alveolar hydatidosis (*Echinococcus multilocularis*). *Am J Trop Med Hyg* 1983; 32:1381–1386.

176 Bresson-Hagni S, Miguet J-P, Lenys D et al. Recurrence of alveolar echinococcosis in the liver graft after liver transplantation. *Hepatology* 1992; 16:279–280.

177 Knobloch J, Biedermann H & Mannweiler E. Serum antibodies in patients with alveolar echinococcosis before and after therapy. *Trop Med Parasitol* 1985; 36:155–156.

178 Gottstein B, Mesarina B, Tanner I et al. Specific cellular and humoral immune responses in patients with different long-term courses of alveolar echinococcosis (infection with *Echinococcus multilocularis*. *Am J Trop Med Hyg* 1991; 45:734–742.

179 Vogel M, Gottstein B, Mueller N & Seebeck T. Production of a recombinant antigen of *Echinococcus multilocularis* with high immunodiagnostic sensitivity and specificity. *Mol Biochem Parasitol* 1988; 31:117–126.

180 Mueller N, Gottstein B, Vogel M, Flury K & Seebeck T. Application of a recombinant *Echinococcus multilocularis* antigen in an enzyme-linked immunosorbent assay for immunodiagnosis of human alveolar echinococcosis. *Mol Biochem Parasitol* 1989; 36:151–160.

181 Frosch P M, Frosch M, Pfister T, Schaad V & Bitter-Suermann D. Cloning and characterization of an immunodominant major surface antigen of *Echinococcus multilocularis*. *Mol Biochem Parasitol* 1991; 48:121–130.

182 Leggatt G R & McManus D P. Sequence homology between two immunodiagnostic fusion proteins from *Echinococcus multilocularis*. *Int J Parasitol* 1992; 22:831–833.

183 Gottstein B, Jacquier P, Bresson-Hadni S & Eckert J. Improved primary immunodiagnosis of alveolar echinococcosis in humans by an enzyme-linked immunosorbent assay using using the Em2plus-antigen. *J Clin Microbiol* 1993; 31:373–376.

184 Blunt D S & Hildreth M B. Use of the polymerase chain reaction for the identification of *Echinococcus multilocularis* fecal eggs. *Annual Meeting of the American Society of Parasitology* 1992; 67.

185 Bretagne S, Robert B, Vidaud D, Goossens M & Houin R. Structure of the *Echinococcus multilocularis* U1 snRNA gene repeat. *Mol Biochem Parasitol* 1991; 46:285–292.

186 Bretagne S, Guillou J P, Morand M & Houin R. Detection of *Echinococcus multilocularis* DNA in fox faeces using DNA amplification. *Parasitology* 1993; 106:193–199.

187 Condon J, Rausch R L & Wilson J F. Application of the avidin–biotin immunohistochemical method for the diagnosis of alveolar hydatid disease from tissue sections. *Trans R Soc Trop Med Hyg* 1988; 82:731–735.

188 Ali Khan Z & Rausch R L. Demonstration of amyloid and immune complex deposits in renal and hepatic parenchyma of Alaskan alveolar hydatid disease patients. *Ann Trop Med Parasitol* 1987; 81:381–392.

189 Gottstein B, Eckert J & Woodtli W. Determination of parasite-specific immunoglobulins using the ELISA in patients with echinococcosis treated with mebendazole. *Parasitol Res* 1984; 70:385–389.

190 Bresson-Hadni S, Vuitton D A, Lenys D, Liance M, Racadot E & Miguet J P. Cellular immune response in *Echinococcus multilocularis* infections in humans. I. Lymphocyte reactivity of Echinococcus antigens in patients with alveolar echinococcosis. *Clin Exp Immunol* 1989; 78:61–66.

191 Vuitton DA, Bresson-Hadni S, Laroche L et al. Cellular immune response in *Echinococcus multilocularis* infection in humans. II. Natural killer cell activity and cell subpopulations in the blood and in the periparasitic granuloma of patients with alveolar echinococcosis. *Clin Exp Immunol* 1989; 78:67–74.

192 Baron R W & Tanner C E. The effect of immunosuppression on secondary *Echinococcus multilocularis* infections in mice. *Int J Parasitol* 1976; 6:37–42.

193 Kamiya H, Kamiya M, Ohbayashi M & Nomura T. Studies on the host resistance to infection with *E. multilocularis*. 1. Difference of susceptibility of various rodents, especially of congenitally athymic nude mice. *Jpn J Parasitol* 1980; 29:87–100.

194 Baron R W & Tanner C E. *Echinococcus multilocularis* in the mouse: the in vitro protoscolicidal activity of peritoneal macrophages. *Int J Parasitol* 1977; 7:489–495.

195 Alkarmi T & Behbehani K. *Echinococcus multilocularis*: inhibition of murine neutrophil and macrophage chemotaxis. *Exp Parasitol* 1989; 89:16–22.

196 Alkarmi T O & Ali Khan Z. Chronic alveolar hydatidosis and secondary amyloidosis: pathological aspects of the disease in four strains of mice. *Br J Exp Pathol* 1984; 65:405–417.

197 Liance M, Vuitton D A, Guerret-Stocker S, Carbillet J P, Grimaud J A & Houin R. Experimental alveolar echinococcosis. Suitability of a murine model of intrahepatic infection by *Echinococcus multilocularis* for immunological studies. *Experientia* 1984; 40:1436–1439.

198 Lubinski G & Desser S S. Growth of the vegetatively propagated strain of larval *Echinococcus multilocularis* in C57L/J, B6AF1 and A/J mice. *Can J Zool* 1963; 42:1213–1216.

199 Devouge M & Ali Khan Z. Intraperitoneal murine alveolar hydatidosis: relationship between size of

the larval cyst mass, immigrant inflammatory cells, splenomegaly and thymus involution. *Tropenmed Parasitol* 1983; 34:15–20.

200 Bresson-Hadni S, Liance M, Meyer J P, Houin R, Bresson J L & Vuitton D A. Cellular immunity in experimental *Echinococcus multilocularis* infection. II. Sequential and comparative phenotypic study of the periparasitic mononuclear cells in resistant and sensitive mice. *Clin Exp Immunol* 1990; 82:378–383.

201 Kizaki T, Ishige M, Kobayashi S et al. Suppression of T-cell proliferation by CD8+ T cells induced in the presence of protoscolices of *Echinococcus multilocularis* in vitro. *Infect Immun* 1993; 61: 525–533.

202 Partensky C, Landraud R, Valette P-J, Bret P & Paliard P. Radical and nonradical hepatic resection for alveolar echinococcosis: report of 18 cases. *World J Surg* 1990; 14:654–659.

203 Eckert J, Thompson R C A & Mehlhorn H. Proliferation and metastases formation of larval *Echinococcus multilocularis*. I. Animal model, macroscopical and histological findings. *Parasitol Res* 1983; 69:737–748.

204 Mosimann F. Is alveolar hydatid disease of the liver incurable? *Ann Surg* 1980; 192:118–123.

205 Aydin Y, Barlas O, Yolacs C et al. Alveolar hydatid disease of the brain. Report of four cases. *J Neurosurg* 1986; 65:115–119.

206 Taylor D H, Morris D L, Reffin D & Richards K S. Comparison of albendazole, mebendazole and praziquantel chemotherapy of *Echinococcus multilocularis* in a gerbil model. *Gut* 1989; 30:1401–1405.

207 Davis A, Pawlowski Z S & Dixon H. Multicentre clinical trials of benzimidazolecarbamates in human echinococcosis. *Bull World Health Organ* 1986; 64:383–388.

208 Kern P. Human echinococcosis: follow-up of 23 patients treated with mebendazole. *Infection* 1983; 11:17–24.

209 Rausch R L, Wilson J F, McMahon B J & O'Gorman M A. Consequences of continuous mebendazole therapy in alveolar hydatid disease—with a summary of a ten-year clinical trial. *Ann Trop Med Parasitol* 1986; 80:403–419.

210 Wilson J F, Rausch R L, McMahon B J, Schantz P M, Trujillo D E & O'Gorman M. Albendazole therapy in alveolar hydatid disease: a report of favorable results in two patients after short-term therapy. *Am J Trop Med Hyg* 1987; 37:162–168.

211 Liu Y H, Wang X G & Chen Y T. Preliminary observation of continuous albendazole therapy in alveolar echinococcosis. *Chin Med J [Engl]* 1991; 104:930–933.

212 Wilson J F, Rausch R L, McMahon B J & Schantz P M. Parasiticidal effect of chemotherapy in alveolar hydatid disease: review of experience with mebendazole and albendazole in Alaskan Eskimos. *Clin Infect Dis* 1992; 15:234–249.

213 Ammann R W. Improvement of liver resectional therapy by adjuvant chemotherapy in alveolar hydatid disease. Swiss Echinococcosis Study Group (SESG). *Parasitol Res* 1991; 77:290–293.

214 D'Alessandro A, Rausch R L, Cuello C & Aristizabal N. *Echinococcus vogeli* in man, with a review of polycystic hydatid disease in Colombia and neighbouring countries. *Am J Trop Med Hyg* 1979; 28:303–317.

215 Meneghelli U G, Martinelli A L C, Llorach V M A, Bellucci A D, Magro J E & Barbo M L P. Polycystic hydatid disease (*Echinococcus vogeli*). Clinical, laboratory and morphological findings in nine Brazilian patients. *J Hepatol* 1992; 14:203–210.

216 Meneghelli U G, Martinelli A L C, Bellucci A D et al. Polycystic hydatid disease (*Echinococcus vogeli*): treatment with albendazole. *Ann Trop Med Parasitol* 1992; 86:151–156.

217 Lopera R D, Melendez R D, Fernandez I, Sirit J & Perera M P. Orbital hydatid cyst of *Echinococcus oligarthrus* in a human in Venezuela. *J Parasitol* 1989; 75:467–470.

CHAPTER 76

CYSTICERCOSIS

G. G. Baily

TRANSMISSION

Cysticercosis consists of infection with the small, bladder-like larvae of the pork tapeworm, *Taenia solium*. The life cycle of this parasite is maintained between man, the only definitive host able to harbour the adult tapeworm, and pigs infected with cysticerci (Figure 76.1). Unfortunately humans can also readily be infected with cysticerci and this is the cause of all the significant morbidity associated with the parasite. The tapeworms are acquired through eating undercooked pork containing cysticerci. Human cysticercosis, however, is a faecal-oral infection acquired by ingesting eggs excreted in the faeces of a human tapeworm carrier. Individuals harbouring an adult *T. solium* are at high risk of acquiring cysticercosis, probably through faecal-oral autoinfection. It has long been hypothesized that internal autoinfection might also occur as a result of reverse peristalsis, allowing taenia eggs to travel from the small bowel to the stomach and thus become activated and invasive. Little evidence has emerged to support this.

Cysticercosis was originally a ubiquitous disease occurring wherever pigs and humans existed in association and is probably of great antiquity: Aristotle gives a clear description of the condition in pigs.[1] It was once common in central Europe, with

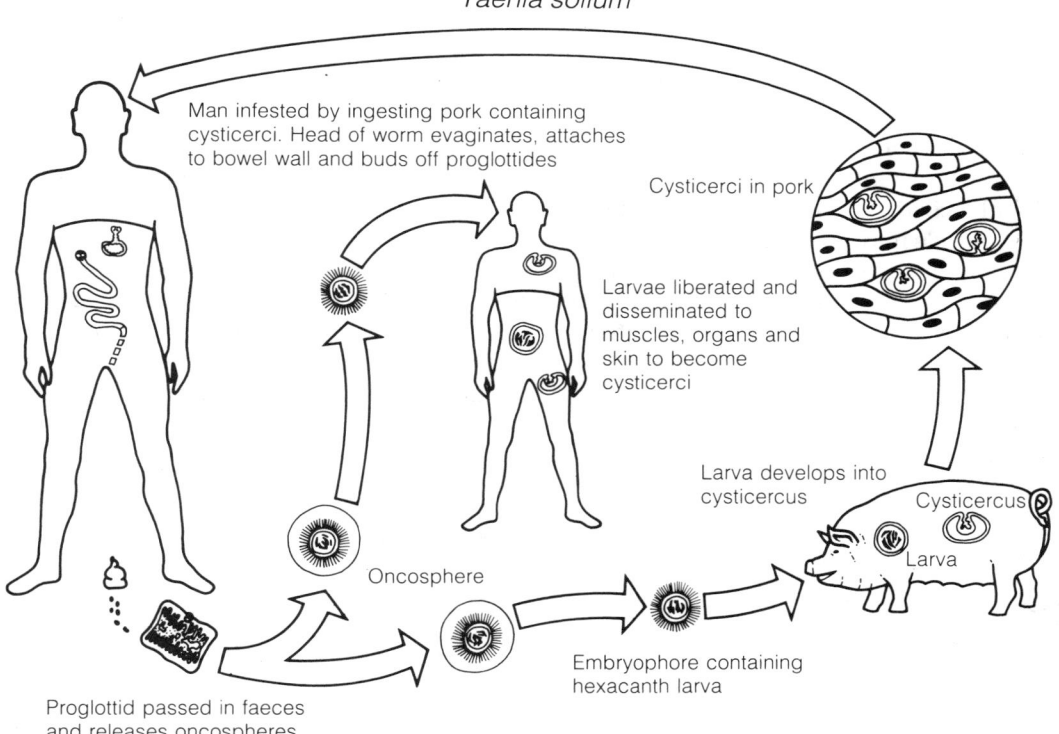

Taenia solium

Man infested by ingesting pork containing cysticerci. Head of worm evaginates, attaches to bowel wall and buds off proglottides

Cysticerci in pork

Larvae liberated and disseminated to muscles, organs and skin to become cysticerci

Larva develops into cysticercus

Cysticercus

Larva

Oncosphere

Embryophore containing hexacanth larva

Proglottid passed in faeces and releases oncospheres

Figure 76.1 The life cycle of *T. solium*. (Courtesy of WTIM.)

autopsy rates of 2% in Berlin[2] in the first half of the nineteenth century, coinciding closely with the 1.9% now described in Mexico City, an area of current high prevalence.[3] The parasite has long since been all but eradicated from the most developed countries but it remains common in Central and South America, South Asia and China. It appears to have a patchy distribution in Africa, with some areas of very high prevalence, but it is rare in the Islamic countries of North Africa and South-West Asia. In the 1970s an epidemic of cysticercosis occurred amongst the highland people of Irian Jaya[4] after the introduction of the parasite into a culture where pigs are of central importance and hygiene is primitive. The problem was first identified because of a dramatic increase in the incidence of severe burns related to individuals falling into domestic fires whilst fitting.

PATHOLOGY

Ingested taenia eggs, activated by gastric and duodenal environments, develop into invasive larvae, termed oncospheres, in the small intestine. These migrate across the intestinal wall and are probably carried by the bloodstream to the sites at which they eventually settle and mature into cysticerci, a process which takes approximately 2 months. Although cysticerci may occur anywhere in the body the distribution is not random. There is a preference for subcutaneous tissues, muscle and the central nervous system. The basis of this tropism as with other migratory larval helminths, is not understood. Cystercerci vary from a few millimetres to 2 cm or more across but are typically a little less than 1 cm, the largest cysts tending to be intracranial, particularly in the ventricles and the larger subarachnoid spaces. Established cysticerci that are neither actively growing nor degenerating elicit very little host immune response. The typical appearances in the brain is of the cyst surrounded by compressed, laminated host tissue with only a slight inflammatory infiltrate (Figure 76.2).[5] Dead, calcified or hyalinized cysts may be surrounded by a similar host-derived capsule. However, new (and therefore growing), and very large or degenerating cysts may all be associated with a much more extensive inflammatory response.

· CLINICAL FEATURES

The morbidity of cysticercosis is almost entirely due to central nervous system disease. Subcutaneous cysts are of only cosmetic significance. A heavy parasite load in muscle may give rise to some aching[6] but this is not common. Serious problems are confined to those anatomical sites where a small space occupying lesion, with or without some inflammation, can give rise to a major disturbance in function. Such sites include the eye and, very rarely, the conducting system of the heart, but overwhelmingly neurocysticercosis is the principal clinical problem.

NEUROCYSTICERCOSIS

Although autopsy rates for neurocysticercosis in areas of high prevalence may approach 2%, the majority of these cases have had no symptoms in life attributable to the infection.[3] When symptoms do occur, much the most common manifestation is epilepsy. Studies from endemic areas suggest that cysticercosis is a major cause of epilepsy, accounting for up to a half of late-onset cases,[7–9] and it is particularly prominent as a cause of focal epilepsy in children. However, any neurological syndrome attributable to one or more small space occupying lesions can occur, including focal weakness, extrapyramidal disorders and global changes in mental state.

MENINGITIS

Careful dissection in postmortem series has shown that 80% of intracranial cysticerci are in contact with the meninges.[5] Since they are often sited deep in the cerebral sulci, this may not be apparent from in vivo imaging. It is not therefore surprising that some abnormality of the CSF is found in approximately

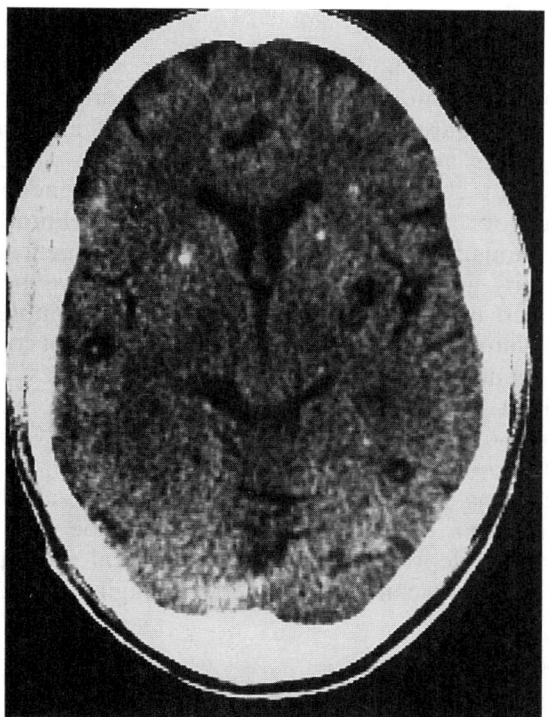

Figure 76.2 Calcified and visible cerebral cysticerci, some with the protoscolex visible as a central opacity.

50% of cases of neurocysticercosis—usually a mild pleocytosis or raised protein. However, in a minority of cases the clinical presentation may fall within the territory of chronic meningitis, with headache and global changes in cerebral function associated with markedly abnormal CSF. Fever, neck stiffness and cranial nerve palsies are not features. Thus more than 5% of cases of chronic or subacute meningitis in childhood were attributed to cysticercosis in a series from south India.[10] A persistently high CSF protein is associated with a poor prognosis, often with progression to hydrocephalus and without surgical intervention, consequent dementia and blindness.

ENCEPHALITIS

When there are many lesions in the brain, and particularly if the inflammatory response is brisk, the presentation may resemble subacute encephalitis.[11] In children in particular the inflammatory response may dominate the clinical picture, with a rapidly progressive illness over a few weeks charac-terized by fitting, a variety of focal neurological abnormalities, global mental deterioration and raised intracranial pressure.

VENTRICULAR DISEASE

Intraventricular cysts occur in about 15% of cases[5] and can cause diagnostic difficulties. They give rise to episodes of obstructive hydrocephalus which may spontaneously remit and recur due to the ball-valve effect of cysticerci intermittently occluding the ventricular outlet foramina. Untreated, however, most cases will progress to sustained hydrocephalus.

SPINAL DISEASE

A variety of spinal cord syndromes has been reported in association with cysts in and around the cord and the cauda equina. The most common presentation is of progressive paraplegia developing over a period of weeks.

DISAPPEARING LESIONS

There have been reports, mainly from India, of single small enhancing lesions on computerized tomography (CT), seen commonly in patients presenting for the first time with epilepsy but disappearing within a few months of follow-up. Many causes have been suggested for these lesions, including tuberculosis, but it seems from both serological evidence and a limited series of excision biopsies[12] that cysticerci are most often responsible.

OCULAR CYSTICERCOSIS

The parasite appears to have a tropism for the eye although estimates of the incidence of ocular disease vary widely. In 1964 Shanchez Fontan was able to describe 70 cases of ocular disease from Mexico.[5] The great majority of cysts were subretinal or in the vitreous humour but they could occur at any site. The initial presentation is most often as a scotoma but if the inflammatory reaction is marked, vision may be lost.

DIAGNOSIS

The clinical diagnosis of neurocysticercosis is often difficult as there is nothing specific about the neurological presentation. The presence of extracranial cysticerci may provide an important clue to the diagnosis. Subcutaneous cysts (Figure 76.3) can be palpated and, if in doubt, excised for histological examination. Cysts in striated muscle are in a more stressful environment than those in the central nervous system and die and calcify more rapidly. Spindle-shaped calcifications, particularly in the large proximal muscles (Figure 76.4), may be visible on radiography. However, such clues are often absent. Spinal cysticerci may be demonstrated on myelography (Figure 76.5). Otherwise support for the diagnosis must be obtained from serology or by imaging the parasites within the brain.

SEROLOGICAL DIAGNOSIS

Many serological methods have been described for cysticercosis using most of the conventional serodiagnostic techniques and a wide variety of antigens. Enzyme linked immunosorbent assays (ELISAs) are now widely used, with either whole T. solium cysts[13] (obtained from pigs) or cyst fluid[14] as antigen. Sensitivity and specificity vary according to the population studied, the performance being less impressive in areas of high endemicity or where other helminths are prevalent. Sensitivity with present ELISA techniques exceeds 80% even in endemic areas but cross-reactivity with other helminthic infections,[15] particularly hydatidosis and taeniasis, remains a problem. Improved results have been claimed using more purified and therefore potentially more specific antigens but these have not come into general use. The detection of antibodies[16] or antigen[17] in the CSF in combination with conventional serology marginally improves overall sensitivity.

Existing tests, however, are already a valuable clinical tool. In endemic areas they can be used to screen epileptic and other neurological patients. Positive cases can be confirmed by imaging and may

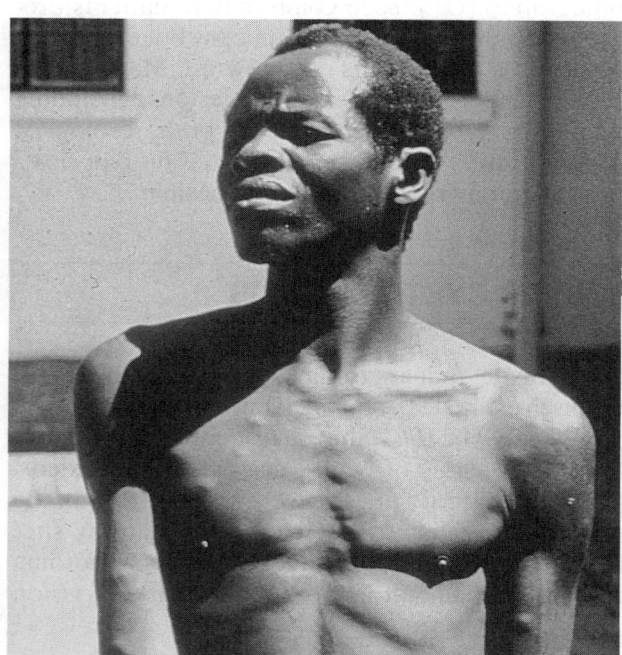

Figure 76.3 Readily visible sub-cutaneous cysticerci. (Courtesy of WTIM.)

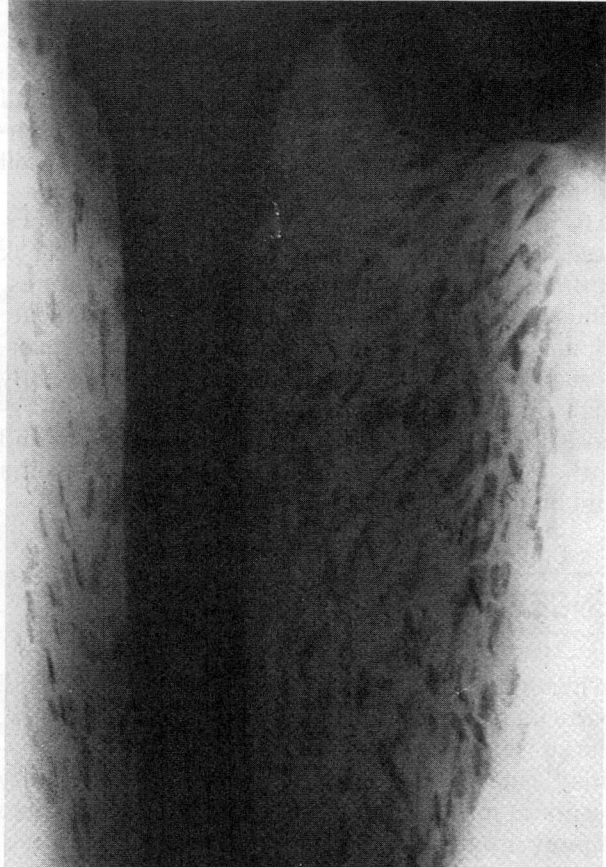

Figure 76.4 Very large numbers of calcified cysticerci in the thigh muscle.

then benefit from specific treatment. In a series of 630 patients seen at neurology clinics in Zimbabwe, 12% had antibodies detected by ELISA. The test had a positive predictive value of 87% and a negative predictive value of 85% for active neurocysticercosis potentially amenable to treatment.[18]

IMAGING

Modern imaging techniques have proved very powerful in demonstrating the presence of cysticerci in the brain and have also taught us a good deal about the natural history of the disease. A number of appearances have been described on CT.

- Calcified lesions.
- Small (<2 cm) hypodense lesions.
- Similar hypodense lesions with a bright central spot representing the protoscolex within the cyst. This is visible in a little under half of such lesions.
- Similar-sized lesions showing ring or disc enhancement. The natural history of these enhancing lesions is that they are likely to disappear from the CT image within 12 months.
- Occasionally there may be much larger cysts, up to 6 cm across, in which case other cestode larvae such as hydatid and coenurosis as well as racemose cysticercosis (see below) should be considered.

Magnetic resonance imaging has also proved valuable,[18] particularly, as with other pathologies, in demonstrating posterior fossa and spinal lesions. It is also superior for imaging ventricular cysts which, having a similar radiodensity to CSF, are not easily visualized on CT.

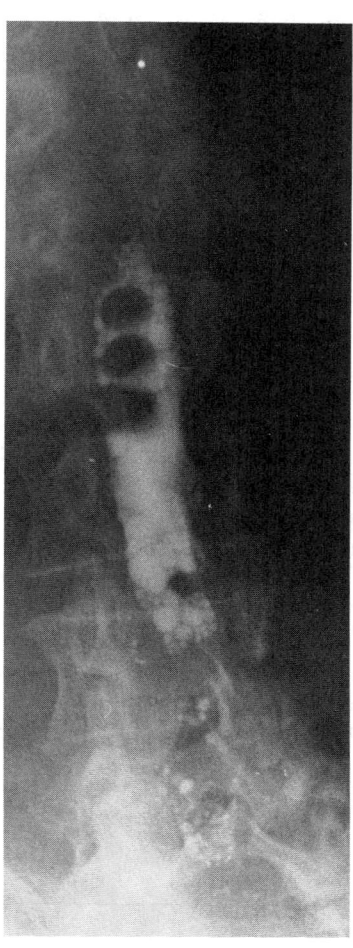

Figure 76.5 Cysticerci around the cauda equina on myelography.

MANAGEMENT

Until the 1980s there was no drug therapy that was known to be effective against cysticercosis. Treatment was therefore mostly symptomatic, although surgical intervention to remove cysts or to deal with their consequences, such as hydrocephalus, was sometimes appropriate. Since that time it has been shown that praziquantel is effective both in reducing the number of cysts present on CT[19] and in eliminating subcutaneous cysts.[20] The extent to which this leads to clinical benefit is more problematical and the exact role of praziquantel remains the subject of debate. In adults with parenchymal cysts demon-

strated by CT which do not show significant enhancement, there is clear evidence of both radiographical and clinical improvement after praziquantel 50 mg/kg daily for 15 days.[19] In almost all other groups of patients, however, information is either contradictory or lacking. Patients with calcified cysts on CT, even though they may persist in having epilepsy, are unlikely to gain any benefit from anthelmintic treatment. Markedly enhancing parenchymal lesions, which constitute the most common appearance in children, have been shown to disappear spontaneously from the CT image within a year.[21] From this observation it has been suggested that children can generally be managed with symptomatic treatment and corticosteroids to reduce the local inflammatory response and that praziquantel is unnecessary.[22] This very benign view of childhood cysticercosis reflects experience with imported disease in North America. In contrast, numerous reports from tropical countries have shown that a proportion of children have chronic disease and frequently relapsing symptoms; some of these develop severe neurological consequences such as hydrocephalus.[23] Whether enhancing lesions that disappear from the CT image have truly gone or have simply ceased to be visible because of a decrease in the inflammatory response is also a matter for debate.[23] Each case must be judged on its merits but on the available evidence it would seem reasonable that enhancing parenchymal lesions present in a child can be managed without praziquantel but with close follow-up.

Surgical excision is still conventionally recommended for intraventricular cysts,[24] although isolated reports exist of successful medical treatment.[25] Information on the use of praziquantel in meningeal and spinal disease remains very limited.

The significant adverse effects of praziquantel therapy appear to be directly related to the damage inflicted on cysticerci, which precipitates an acute inflammatory response. This may result in cerebral oedema and raised intracranial pressure, particularly if there are many cysts. Typically, a severe headache arises—sometimes within a few hours of commencing therapy but more often after 2–4 days. If treated symptomatically most of these will resolve without sequelae but a minority will develop a severe acute illness with cerebral infarction, and deaths[20] having been reported. Concomitant use of corticosteroids in substantial doses is effective in suppressing this in most (though not all) cases but steroids also have the unwanted effect of decreasing the uptake of praziquantel into the cysts. Although it has not been universally adopted, on balance the use of high-dose corticosteroids with praziquantel appears the safest option.

More recently albendazole has been assessed as an alternative to praziquantel. In substantial doses (15 mg/kg daily for a month) albendazole appears to have an equivalent or perhaps slightly more potent effect on reducing cysts present on CT.[26,27] Adverse effects are also similar and presumably occur through a comparable mechanism. The ideal dose of both drugs remains uncertain. Much shorter courses of praziquantel, e.g. 50 mg/kg daily for 8 days, have been shown to be effective in small numbers of cases. Similarly, 8 days of albendazole appears to be of equivalent efficacy to the original 1 month.[27] These shorter courses of anthelmintics, repeated after a period of months if necessary, offer the promise of a less expensive regimen for developing countries but they require much more extensive evaluation before they can be generally recommended.

CONTROL

Control of the parasite has been achieved in developed countries by the interruption of its life cycle at two points. The systematic inspection of pork meat and the removal of infected carcasses from the food chain effectively prevent human tapeworm infection. In addition, improvements in public health have ensured the sanitary disposal of human faeces, and eliminated the source of infection for both human and porcine cysticercosis. In contrast, in developing countries pigs often live in close association with man, rooting around for food within village compounds, and in some areas are deliberately fed human faeces (Figure 76.6). Animals are likely to be slaughtered within the village and there may be no understanding of the health significance of 'measely' pig meat. The difficulties of introducing good sanitation and modern abattoir practices into poor communities are considerable. In Africa, how-

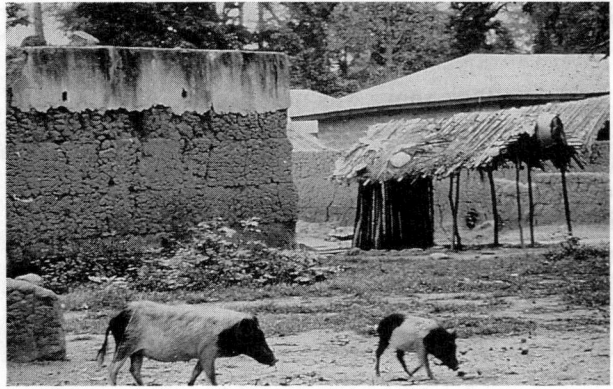

Figure 76.6 Pigs scavenging for food in an African village. (Courtesy of WTIM.)

ever, there is hope that transmission may be reduced as a by-product of mass treatment campaigns directed against schistosomiasis—using praziquan- tel. This should have a substantial impact on the incidence of adult tapeworm infection(s).

RACEMOSE CYSTICERCOSIS

Occasionally cestode larvae that are not easily ascribed to any particular parasite are found in the human brain. One characteristic appearance is of a cluster of interconnected grape-like cysts which have no identifiable protoscolex; they are usually situated in the cisterna magna or the ventricles and are often of considerable bulk. This is known as racemose cysticercus. Since it is the protoscolex which provides much of the basis for the identifi- cation of larval cestodes it has been difficult to be certain from which parasite racemose cysticerci are derived. Some appear to resemble cases of proven human coenurosis due to *T. multiceps*,[28] except for the absence of scolices. A similar sterile budding coenurus has been observed in an immunosup- pressed mouse deliberately infected with *T. seria- lis*.[29] However, circumstantial evidence suggests that most cases of racemose cysticercosis are due to the aberrant development of *T. solium* cysticerci. Pathological series show that typical *T. solium* cysti- cerci and racemose cysticerci are often found in the same individual, and occasionally intermediate forms with a single bud and a degenerating scolex can be found.[5]

Racemose cysticercosis is a serious condition fre- quently leading to hydrocephalus, as well as produc- ing local inflammatory and mass effects. Limited experience with praziquantel suggests that medical therapy is difficult and that surgery may retain a place in management.[30]

REFERENCES

1 Cook G C. Neurocysticercosis: parasitology, clinical presentation, diagnosis and recent advances in management. *Q J Med* 1988; 68:575–583.

2 Henneberg R. Die tierischen Parasiten des Zentralnervensystem. In Lewandowsky M (ed.) *Handbuch der Neurologie*. Berlin: Springer, 1912.

3 Mahajan R C. Geographical distribution of human cysticercosis. In Flisser A, Willms K, Laclette J P, Larralde C, Ridaura C & Beltran F (eds) *Cysticercosis. Present State of Knowledge and Perspectives*. New York: Academic Press, 1982: 39– 46.

4 Gajdusek D C. Introduction of *Taenia solium* into West New Guinea with a note on an epidemic of burns from cysticercus epilepsy in the Ekari people of the Wissel Lakes area. *Papua New Guinea Med J* 1978; 21:329–342.

5 Rabiela-Cervantes M T, Rivas-Hernandez A, Rodriguez-Ibarra J, Castillo-Medina S & Cancino Fde M. Anatomopathological aspects of human brain cysticercosis. In Flisser A, Willms K, Laclette J P, Larralde C, Ridaura C & Beltran F (eds) *Cysti- cercosis. Present State of Knowledge and Perspectives*. New York: Academic Press, 1982: 179–200.

6 McGill R J. Cysticercosis resembling myopathy. *Lancet* 1948; ii:728–730.

7 Medina M T, Rosas E, Rubio-Donnadieu F & Sotelo J. Neurocysticercosis as the main cause of late-onset epilepsy in Mexico. *Arch Intern Med* 1990; 150:325–327.

8 Powell S J, Proctor E M, Wilmot A J & Macleod I N. Cysticercosis and epilepsy in Africans: a clinical and serological study. *Ann Trop Med Parasitol* 1966; 60:152–158.

9 Chopra J S, Kaur U & Mahajan R C. Cysticercosis and epilepsy: a clinical and serological study. *Trans R Soc Trop Med Hyg* 1981; 75:518–520.

10 Chandramuki A & Nayak P. Sub acute and chronic meningitis in children: an immunological study of cerebrospinal fluid. *Indian J Pediatr* 1990; 57:685– 691.

11 Rangel R, Torres B, del Bruto O & Sotelo J. Cysticercotic encephalitis: a severe form in young females. *Am J Trop Med Hyg* 1987; 36:387–392.

12 Chandy M J, Rajshekhar V, Ghosh S et al. Single small enhancing CT lesions in Indian patients with epilepsy: clinical, radiological and pathological considerations. *J Neurol Neurosurg Psychiatry* 1991; 54:702–705.

13 Mohammed I N, Heiner D C, Miller B L, Goldberg M A & Kagan I G. Enzyme-linked immunosorbent assay for the diagnosis of cerebral cysticercosis. *J Clin Microbiol* 1984; 20:775–779.

14 Baily G G, Mason P R, Trijssenar F E J & Lyons N F. Serological diagnosis of neurocysticercosis: evaluation of ELISA tests using cyst fluid and other

components of *Taenia solium* cysticerci as antigens. *Trans R Soc Trop Med Hyg* 1988; 82:295–299.

15 Pammenter M D, Epstein S R & Rees R T. Cross reactions in the immunodiagnosis of schistosomiasis and cysticercosis by a cerebrospinal fluid enzyme-linked immunosorbent assay. *Trans R Soc Trop Med Hyg* 1992; 86:51–52.

16 Corona T, Pascoe D, Gonzalez-Barranco D, Abad P, Landa L & Estanol B. Anticysticercus antibodies in serum and cerebrospinal fluid in patients with cerebral cysticercosis. *J Neurol Neurosurg Psychiatry* 1986; 49:1044–1049.

17 Estrada J J, Almon Estrada J & Kuhn R E. Identification of *Taenia solium* antigens in cerebrospinal fluid and larval antigens from patients with neurocysticercosis. *Am J Trop Med Hyg* 1989; 41:50–55.

18 Manson P, Houston S, Gwanzura L. Neurocysticercosis: Experience with diagnosis by ELISA serology and computerised with tomography in Zimbabwe. *Cent Afr J Med* 1992; 38:149–154.

19 Sotelo J, Escobedo F, Rodriguez-Carbajal J, Torres B & Rubio-Donnadieu F. Therapy of parenchymal brain cysticercosis with praziquantel. *N Engl J Med* 1984; 310:1001–1007.

20 Pham Huang The & van Knapen F. Preliminary report of praziquantel treatment of cysticercosis patients in Vietnam. *Acta Leiden* 1989; 57:229–233.

21 Mitchell W G & Crawford T O. Intraparenchymal cerebral cysticercosis in children: diagnosis and treatment. *Pediatrics* 1988; 82:76–82.

22 Moodley M & Moosa A. The treatment of neurocysticercosis: is praziquantel the new hope? *Lancet* 1989; i:262–263.

23 Lopez-Hernandez A & Garaizar C. Analysis of 89 cases of infantile cerebral cysticercosis. In Flisser A, Willms K, Laclette J P, Larralde C, Ridaura C & Beltran F (eds) *Cysticercosis. Present State of Knowledge and Perspectives*. New York: Academic Press, 1982: 127–137.

24 Hanlon K A, Vern B A, Tan W S, Passen E & Jafar J J. MRI in intraventricular neurocysticercosis. *Infection* 1988; 16:242–244.

25 Allcut D A & Coulthard A. Neurocysticercosis: regression of a fourth ventricular cyst with praziquantel. *J Neurol Neurosurg Psychiatry* 1991; 54:461–462.

26 Cruz M, Cruz I & Horton J. Albendazole versus praziquantel in the treatment of cerebral cysticercosis. *Trans R Soc Trop Med Hyg* 1991; 85:244–247.

27 Sotelo J, del Brutto O H, Penagos P et al. Comparison of therapeutic regimen of anticysticercal drugs for parenchymal brain cysticercosis. *J Neurol* 1990; 237:69–72.

28 Jung R C, Rodriguez M A, Beaver P C, Schental J E & Levy R W. Racemose cysticercus in human brain. *Am J Trop Med Hyg* 1981; 30:620–624.

29 Lachberg S, Thompson R C A & Lymbery A J. A contribution to the etiology of racemose cysticercosis. *J Parasitol* 1990; 76:592–594.

30 Baily G G & Levy L F. Racemose cysticercosis treated with praziquantel. *Trans R Soc Trop Med Hyg* 1989; 83:95–96.

CHAPTER 77

OTHER LARVAL CESTODE INFECTIONS

G. G. Baily

COENUROSIS

Taenia multiceps is a parasite of dogs, with sheep being the principal intermediate host. The larval metacestode takes the form of a coenurus, a single cyst with multiple invaginated protoscolices which may grow to be several centimetres in diameter. In sheep these often develop in the hindbrain, giving rise to the condition known as 'staggers'. Other closely related *Taenia* species also give rise to a coenurus which may be morphologically indistinguishable. Human coenurosis is a rare but often serious condition. The parasite has a tropism for the brain and eye,[1] though many extracranial sites have also been described.

PREVALENCE AND DISTRIBUTION

Cases have been reported from a wide geographical area but are nowhere other than rare. Most reports have been from Africa and South America but there have also been cases in Europe (notably Sardinia) and North America. Extracranial localization has been most frequent in reports from tropical Africa, whilst reports from South Africa and elsewhere have been almost entirely of central nervous system involvement, giving rise to the suspicion that there is some heterogeneity amongst the causative parasites.[2]

CLINICAL FEATURES

Neurological features are those of a substantial intracranial mass lesion accompanied by varying degrees of inflammation. The cisterna magna is a particularly common site, and is associated with basal arachnoiditis and hydrocephalus. Untreated, there is usually progressive neurological disease and a poor outcome. Eye involvement may result in loss of vision.

DIAGNOSIS AND TREATMENT

Intracranial lesions appear on computerized tomography as clear cysts 2 cm or more in diameter without a discernable internal structure. Definitive diagnosis can only be made by histology; it is distinguished from cysticercosis and hydatidosis by the presence of both multiple protoscolices and a ridged cuticle. Occasionally the protoscolices may have degenerated, in which case the condition is difficult to distinguish from racemose cysticercosis. Surgical excision has been curative in some cases. The possible role of praziquantel remains undetermined but it has been used with some success in sheep.[3]

SPARGANOSIS

Plerocercoid larvae of the *Spirometra* genus of pseudophyllidean cestodes are capable of infecting man. These organisms resemble *Diphyllobothrium* spp. in their life cycles, with canines or other terrestrial carnivores as definitive hosts, a procercoid larval stage in the water flea *Cyclops* and plerocercoids

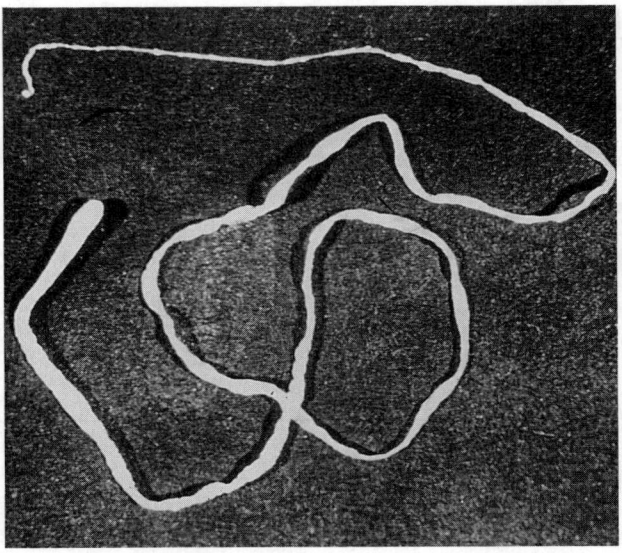

Figure 77.1 Spirometra mansonoides. Plerocercoid larva. (Courtesy of H. Zaiman.)

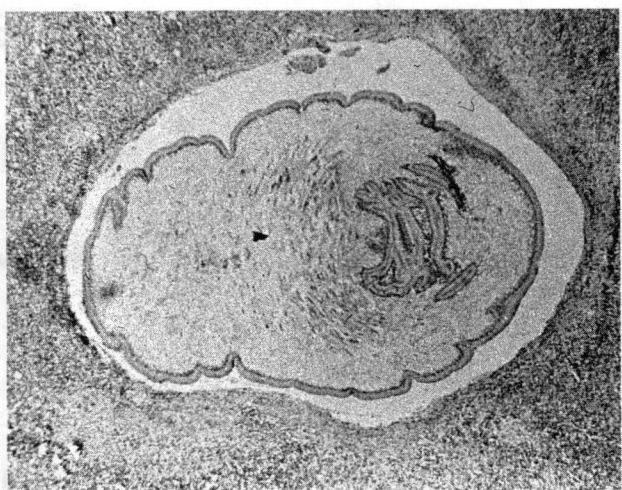

Figure 77.2 Sparganosis. Cross-section showing typical tapeworm morphology. A dense eosinophilic infiltration is present in the adjacent muscle. (Courtesy H. Zaiman.)

naturally infecting reptiles, amphibians and small mammals. Human sparganosis has been attributed to several species, including *S. mansoni*, *S. mansonoides* and, in Africa, *S. theileri*. Human infection occurs either by the ingestion of procercoid-infected invertebrates in drinking water, by ingestion of plerocercoids through eating uncooked frogs or snakes or possibly by direct transfer of a plerocercoid from fresh frog or snake tissue applied to wounds or inflamed eyes, as is the custom in some parts of East Asia. The plerocercoid, or sparganum, is a motile worm of very variable size (between 1 and 50 cm) but is more typically a few centimetres in length and 1–2 mm in width (Figure 77.1). It excites a brisk inflammatory response as it migrates through host tissues; in some instances it is found to be contained within a cyst or abscess cavity.[4] Multiple infections occur.

PREVALENCE AND DISTRIBUTION

This is an uncommon condition but has been recorded very widely in the tropics and subtropics. South-East Asia and East Africa are the areas of highest prevalence. Autochthonous cases are reported from North and South America.

CLINICAL FEATURES

The typical history is of inflammatory, sometimes migratory, subcutaneous swellings. These may break down to discharge the worm. Eosinophilia is common but not invariable (Figure 77.2). The most frequently described sites are the chest and legs. Involvement of the periorbital tissues may cause damage to the eye. Penetration of larvae into the brain—where they cause an intense local inflammatory lesion with invariably major neurological consequences, is uncommon but well described.[4]

DIAGNOSIS AND TREATMENT

The condition must be distinguished from that caused by other migratory helminths producing swellings, such as in gnathostomiasis and loiasis. Serological methods have been developed but they are not specific. Excision and identification of the worm remains necessary for a clear diagnosis. Excision is also the only effective treatment of the parasite, wherever situated, including the brain. No drug therapy has been shown to be beneficial and the killing of the worm within the tissues may not in any case be a desirable goal as it is likely to lead to much more intense inflammation in the short term.

PROLIFERATIVE SPARGANOSIS

A very rare variant of sparganosis has been described, from both Asia and the Americas, in which the parasite buds and proliferates, either as an expanding mass or as multiple small disseminated lesions. Clinically there may be numerous small cutaneous nodules or larger painful tumours. The lesions contain worm-derived structures, some clearly resembling a typical sparganum but of very variable morphology. The condition is slowly progressive, with death resulting from deep organ involvement. There is no known treatment; praziquantel and mebendazole have failed in one case.[5]

REFERENCES

1 Raper A B & Dockeray G C. Coenurus cysts in man: five cases from East Africa. *Ann Trop Med Parasitol* 1956; 50:121–128.
2 Templeton A C. Anatomical and geographical location of human coenurus infection. *Trop Geogr Med* 1971; 23:105.
3 Verster A & Tustin R C. Treatment of cerebral coenurosis in sheep with praziquantel. *J S Afr Vet Assoc* 1990; 61:24–26.
4 Holodniy M, Almenoff J, Loutit J & Steinberg G K. Cerebral sparganosis: case report and review. *Rev Infect Dis* 1991; 13:155–159.
5 Torres J R, Noya O O, Noya B A, Mouliniere R & Martinez E. Treatment of proliferative sparganosis with mebendazole and praziquantel. *Trans R Soc Trop Med Hyg* 1981; 75:846–847.

SECTION 5G
ECTOPARASITES

SECTION 5G
ECTOPARASITES

CHAPTER 78

LEECHES AND LEECH INFESTATION

G. B. White

GEOGRAPHICAL DISTRIBUTION

Land leeches are common in South-East Asia, the Pacific Islands, the Indian subcontinent and South America. Aquatic leeches have a worldwide distribution.

AETIOLOGY

Leeches which attack man have the following position in the animal kingdom:

Phylum	Annelida
Class	Hirudinea
Order	Gnathobdellida
Family	Hirudinidae

Gnathobdellid leeches are invertebrates, having a smooth cuticle, a mouth lacking a proboscis but with three jaws, two suckers (one surrounding the mouth, the other at the posterior end) and powerful muscles, circular and longitudinal. They attach themselves by the posterior sucker, the anterior end moving about freely. When unfed they are usually about 2.5 cm long and 5 mm thick; some are bigger. When full of blood they are dark, bloated objects.

The muscular jaws are covered with chitin and produce a characteristic triradiate wound in the skin of the victim. The mouth leads to a pharynx, with salivary glands which secrete the anticoagulant hirudin, a crop in which ingested blood can be stored, a stomach, intestine, rectum and anal pore near the posterior sucker. The excretory system consists of 17 paris of nephridia. There is a vascular system and a nervous system.

Leeches are hermaphrodites, each one possessing testes and ovaries, the spermatozoa of one individual being deposited during copulation on the cuticle (to migrate through the tissues to reach the ovary) or into the vagina of the other member of the copulating pair. Some leeches deposit egg masses on objects submerged in water, others form a cocoon to be deposited in water or mud, from which the young hatch and attach themselves to water plants. Others carry their young until they are able to suck.

Leeches which attack man may be divided into two classes: *land leeches*, which have powerful jaws which can penetrate the skin so that they can attach anywhere on the external surface of the body, and *aquatic leeches*, which have weak jaws and require soft tissues to feed on. They gain entrance to orifices such as the pharynx and vagina.

LAND LEECHES

Land leeches live in the vegetation of tropical rain forests and tend to breed near springs, streams and wells frequented by cattle, horses and other vertebrates. The species noted for attacks on man include *Haemadipsa zelanica, H. sylvestris* and *H. picta*. Land leeches attach themselves to the skin and feed; when fed they fall off on to the ground, having remained attached for a comparatively short time.

CLINICAL FEATURES

The punctures made in the skin by land leeches are painless and remain open and bleeding after the leech has gone; healing is slow. Leeches take much more blood than they need and if they remain attached, or are numerous, they can take so much that the patient becomes seriously anaemic and may die from loss of blood.

TREATMENT

Leeches which attach themselves to the skin must be induced to detach, but they must not be simply pulled off because they may then leave behind their jaws, which could become the starting point of destructive ulceration. Drops of strong salt solution, alcohol or strong vinegar applied around the mouth,

or heat from a lighted match or cigarette applied to the body will cause the leach to release its hold. The wound can then be treated with a styptic and an antiseptic.

PREVENTION

People in countries where land leeches are common should, when travelling in infested country, wear boots and trousers thick enough to prevent access by the leeches to the skin. Additional protection is afforded if the garments or the skin are treated with repellents such as diethyl toluamide (DEET), dimethyl or dibutyl phthalate (DMP, DBP) or inda-lone. DEET and DBP last longer on clothing and, if applied about once every 2 weeks at the rate of 28 ml per set of garments, or about $4\,\text{ml}/30\,\text{cm}^2$, are good repellents. On the skin, repellents are effective for only 3–5 hours, less if sweating is excessive. These repellents should not be used on synthetic fabrics which they can dissolve.

AQUATIC LEECHES

Aquatic leeches live exclusively in fresh water. Species feeding on man include *Limnatis nilotica*, which is large and haunts quiet water and ponds, and *L. maculosa. Phytobdella catenifera, Dinobdella ferox* and *Myxobdella africana* occur in sub-Saharan Africa.[1] Aquatic leeches deposit their eggs on water plants and the young may be seen in the water. They do not all require a mammalian host, and can exist on amphibians. Young leeches enter orifices such as the nose and pharynx where they attach themselves for prolonged periods until they become adult, when they drop off into the water. They are more danger-ous than land leeches because they are more likely to cause severe anaemia.

CLINICAL FEATURES

Aquatic leech infestation is less common than land leech infestation, but may be much more harmful. Aquatic leeches can enter the mouth or nostrils during drinking or washing and can also attack the conjunctiva, the vulva, vagina and urethra in per-sons bathing in infested water.

Having entered the mouth or nostrils the leech can quickly pass to the nasopharynx, epiglottis or oesophagus, and even to the trachea and bronchi. When attached to the mucous membrane the leech secretes anticoagulant and engorges. The result is bleeding, according to the site of attachment—epistaxis, haemoptysis or haematemesis—which may lead to severe anaemia. A leech in the nares may also give prolonged headache; if in the larynx there is a cough with bloody discharge, hoarseness, dyspnoea, pain and even suffocation. Leeches in the pharynx or oesophagus may cause difficulty in swallowing.

TREATMENT

In treating leech infestation of the upper respiratory passages an attempt should be made to see the leech. If it is in the posterior pharynx, larynx, trachea or bronchi, the patient should be positioned so that the leech cannot fall back and block the lower passages. If it is in the nares or upper pharynx it can be paralysed with cocaine and extracted directly. If lower down, a pair of long hooked forceps can be introduced through a laryngoscope and the leech pulled out gently, but tracheostomy may be necessary. If in the oesophagus the leech should be visualized through an eosophagoscope and treated with cocaine; it will then fall into the stomach where the gastric juice will kill it. For a leech in the genitourinary tract, irrigation with strong salt solution may make it release its hold.

PREVENTION

To avoid attack by aquatic leeches it is necessary to wear appropriate clothing and apply repellents, and to drink only water which has been filtered, strained through fine gauze or boiled.

Although they suck blood, leeches have not been incriminated in transmitting infection.

REFERENCE

1 Cundall D B, Whitehead S M & Hechtel F O P. *Trans R Soc Trop Med Hyg* 1986; 80:940–944.

CHAPTER 79

MYIASIS

G. B. White

Myiasis is caused when fly maggots (larvae of Diptera) invade living tissue or when they are harboured in the intestine or bladder.

Clinically, maggots causing myiasis may attack three parts of the body:

1 *Cutaneous tissue*. Some species of maggots cause furuncles (subcutaneous myiasis), invade sores and wounds (wound myiasis), burrow under the skin (dermal myiasis, a cause of creeping eruption) or suck blood.
2 *Body cavities*. Other species invade the nasal passages (nasal myiasis), mouth, ears and accessory passages, enter the orbit of the eye (ocular myiasis) or penetrate the anus or vagina.
3 *Gut lumen*. If accidentally ingested, fly eggs or larvae may survive passage through the stomach and bowel to emerge in the stool (intestinal myiasis).

Parasitologically, myiasis-producing flies can be divided into three categories (see also Appendix IV):

1 *Obligatory myiasis producers*. For some fly species, it is essential for the larvae to develop in living tissue because they are unable to develop elsewhere. These obligate parasites are highly specialized insects, the larvae of which have developed highly sophisticated mechanisms to avoid the host's immune system.
2 *Facultative myiasis producers*. These larvae usually develop on carrion but may invade wounds. They may be primary invaders which initiate myiasis; secondary invaders, entering tissue only when the animal has become infested; or tertiary, which only become involved later when decomposition is advanced.
3 *Accidental myiasis producers*. These eggs or larvae are accidentally ingested and are not killed in the intestine.

CUTANEOUS TISSUE MYIASIS

BLOOD SUCKERS (CONGO FLOOR MAGGOT) (See also Appendix IV)

GEOGRAPHICAL DISTRIBUTION

The adult fly *Auchmeromyia luteola* (see Appendix IV) is widely distributed throughout tropical Africa from 18°N to 26°S, from northern Nigeria and southern Sudan to Natal, from sea level to 2250 m in both dry and wet climates.

AETIOLOGY

The Congo floor maggot is the larval stage of *Auchmeromyia luteola* (see Appendix IV), an orange-buff coloured 'blowfly' covered with numerous small hairs which give it a smoky look. It has a stoutly built body 10–12 mm long.

Life cycle

The adult fly sits motionless among the thatch, beams and cobwebs of the roof of huts where it is protected by its colour and is difficult to see. Human faeces is its most important source of food. It lays eggs in the crevices of mud floors, favouring those contaminated by urine, 3 weeks after its emergence from the pupa. The larva which emerges from the egg is dirty white, semitransparent, 15 mm long and composed of 11 segments. This stage is known as the Congo floor maggot (see Appendix IV). The larva is mobile and merges from its hiding place to take blood meals from the host, which must be hairless and immobile, such as a sleeping human, aardvark or nestling birds. It feeds by scraping with its mouth hooks until it reaches a blood vessel. The first segment then retracts and its sucker is then applied. After feeding it becomes conspicuously red as it is filled with blood and retreats into a crack in the floor, under the mats on which people sleep, or burrows in the earth to a depth of up to 8 cm. Congo floor maggots feed mainly at night and drop off at once if disturbed. They can be recognized by the characteristic shape of the spiracles (see Figure IV. 17A). When ready to pupate the larva selects a suitable place and lies dormant. The pupa is dark reddish-brown with an oblong body 9–10 × 4.5 mm and this stage lasts 2–3 weeks.

CLINICAL FEATURES

The bite is painless. Blood loss has never been found sufficient to cause anaemia. No infections are known to be transmitted by its bite.

PREVENTION

Sleeping on a bed raised above the floor is sufficient to prevent attack. House-spraying with residual insecticide should be applied to eliminate infestations.

SUBCUTANEOUS MYIASIS

The maggot penetrates the skin; no previous lesion is necessary. Two species of fly are the cause; both are obligatory myiasis producers: *Cordylobia anthropophaga* (family Calliphoridae) in Africa and *Dermatobia hominis* (family Cuterebridae) in South America.

1. *CORDYLOBIA ANTHROPOPHAGA* (TUMBU FLY, PUTSI FLY, VER DU CAYOR) (See also Appendix IV)

GEOGRAPHICAL DISTRIBUTION

The tumbu fly occurs throughout sub-saharan Africa and has been recorded from southern Spain.

AETIOLOGY

Cordylobia anthropophaga (see Appendix IV) is a large robust yellow-brown fly, 7–12 mm long resembling the adult of the Congo floor maggot (*Auchmeromyia luteola*), difficult to distinguish from numerous other species of flies. *C. anthropophaga* is an obligate parasite. Adults are active in the early morning and late afternoon, laying eggs on sandy ground or contaminated clothing. The eggs hatch and the larvae which emerge invade the subcutaneous tissue and undergo three moults or instars (see Appendix IV); complete development in the subcutaneous tissues takes 8–12 days. The larvae emerge and fall to the ground where they pupate in 24 hours and the adult hatches after 10–20 days, according to temperature. The pupa has a characteristic shape with a truncated end. Rodents and dogs are the usual larval hosts and man is infected only accidentally.

TRANSMISSION

The female fly lays its eggs in two batches on sandy ground contaminated with urine or faeces, also on clothing (although such clothing may appear clean). Clothing laid on the ground to dry is affected but not clothing hanging in bright sunlight, because the eggs are only laid in shaded areas. The eggs are not laid directly on the skin.

On hatching, the small first-stage larvae hold themselves erect and can remain alive without food for about 9 days. The larvae, which are sensitive to both heat and vibration, become attached to a host and immediately begin to penetrate the unbroken skin, taking about 1 minute. Penetration, which is painless, may involve any part of the body but most commonly occurs on the back, head and neck in man. Larvae are acquired from lying on the ground or from clothing, and infection is more common in children. Dogs are an important domestic reservoir.

IMMUNITY

There is a localized degree of immunity which has been experimentally produced in guinea-pigs. There are no antibodies and no general immunity. Larvae penetrating the immune area die in 40 hours and grafted skin retains its immunity

CLINICAL FEATURES

Initially the lesion starts as a small papule containing the larva which may be itchy or pricking at intervals. As the papule increases in size the symptoms recur and may keep the patient awake at night. Serous fluid may be exuded and local lymphadenopathy may occur. There may be fever and general malaise. The lesion, which resembles a boil, grows over a period of 6 days, the larva being noticed by the time the third stage has been reached. While in the host (8–12 days) the larva has its posterior segment

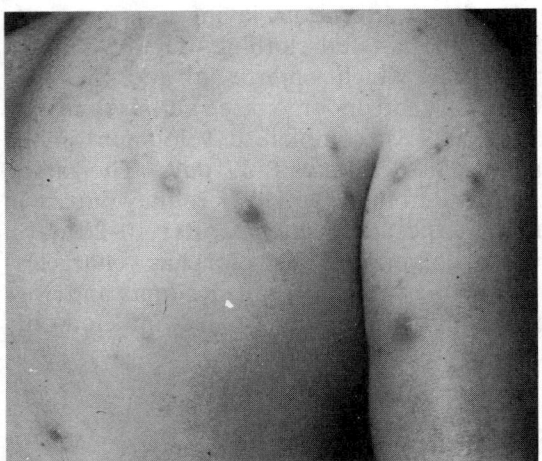

Figure 79.1   Lesions of tumbu fly (*Cordylobia anthropophaga*).

(bearing the respiratory spiracles) protruding from the aperture, but this can be withdrawn when touched. There may be numerous lesions resembling boils situated on the arms, scrotum and other parts of the body coinciding with areas of contact with contaminated clothing. Close inspection of the lesions will reveal that instead of a pustular head the lesions terminate in a 1–3 mm dark line, the site of the respiratory spiracles of the larva (Figure 79.1).

DIAGNOSIS

C. anthropophaga causes less pain than that of an ordinary boil, and the appearance of the spiracles is diagnostic. In case of doubt, the surface of the lesion should be covered with Vaseline, glycerine or oil. The appearance of bubbles clinches the diagnosis.

TREATMENT

The larvae can be removed by squeezing the boil, assisted by first covering the spiracles with a layer of paraffin oil to stop the oxygen supply. Mature larvae will then wriggle partly out, and can be finally removed by exerting firm digital pressure on each side. Early lesions are best left to develop for a few days, as immature larvae are reluctant to emerge. Rupture of the larvae by injudicious attempts at extraction may cause a severe inflammatory response.

PREVENTION

All clothing and towels should be ironed on *both* sides, and drip-dry clothes should be hung indoors with the windows closed[1] to prevent contact with the flies.

2. *DERMATOBIA HOMINIS* (VER MACAQUE, BERNE, EL TÓRSALO, BEEFWORM, HUMAN BOT FLY)

(See Appendix IV)

GEOGRAPHICAL DISTRIBUTION

Dermatobia hominis is widely distributed throughout Central and South America from Mexico to Argentina and Chile. It is especially common on the forested eastern slopes of the Andes in Colombia. It attacks a wide range of hosts and is a devastating pest of livestock in some areas.

AETIOLOGY

The adult fly is a large bluish-grey fly 1.5 cm long (see Appendix IV) with a strong flight, found primarily on the edge of tropical forests, particularly hilly areas of secondary forest between 160 and 3000 m. The adult *D. hominis*, on attaining maturity, lays its eggs directly on other insects or foliage, but especially on day-flying mosquitoes such as *Psorophora*, flies (*Sarcophaga*, *Musca* and *Stomoxys*) and ticks (*Amblyoma*). The packets of eggs adhere to the insect's thorax and are thus conveyed to the new host (usually cattle, dogs or humans). This characteristic is called phoresis or 'hitch-hiking'.

The larva remains in the egg until it senses warmth, whereupon it rapidly 'hatches' and penetrates the host's skin in 5–10 minutes, remaining at the site of penetration. Each larva penetrates individually and a small nodule develops around it with a central pore through which the larva breathes. The second stage larva has a characteristic shape which makes it difficult to remove. The duration of larval development is uncertain but probably lasts from 6 to 12 weeks in man, during which it grows slowly feeding on tissue exudate. It then emerges and drops to the ground and pupates.

CLINICAL FEATURES

Cutaneous swellings, each harbouring one larva, usually occur on exposed areas (although the flies can penetrate clothing) and are found most commonly on the head but also elsewhere on the body. In the orbit the larva can cause serious pathology and is a cause of ophthalmomyiasis (Chapter 10). Lesions can be multiple and 12 have been reported on one individual. The lesion is an inflamed swelling 2–3 cm in diameter, at the apex of which can be seen the small black spiracles from which exudes a seropurulent fluid containing the dark faeces of the larva. The lesions are very painful and itchy but do not suppurate, because the bacteriostatic activity of the gut of the larva prevents undesirable overgrowth of pyogenic bacteria.

DIAGNOSIS

Diagnosis is made by examining the lesion for the characteristic spiracles and the faecal-stained serous exudate.

COMPLICATIONS

Loss of the eye can occur in opthalmomyiasis. A fatal cerebral myiasis can occur in children but is rare.

TREATMENT

Occasionally the first-stage larva can be removed (as in *Cordylobia*) but more often surgical removal is necessary with second- and third-stage larvae. The larvae are best removed by a cruciate incision and care must be taken not to go through the central hole and damage the larva, portions of which must not be left in the wound.

CONTROL

In Brazil *D. hominis* has been controlled with insecticides including DDT, pyrethroids and Toxaphene. In Curaçao males sterilized by radiation were released to render the females sterile after mating (since females mate only once). After 2 years of the sterile male release programme the fly was exterminated in a similar manner to the cattle screw-worm, *Callitroga hominivorax*, which has been eradicated from North America by this method.

DERMAL MYIASIS OR CREEPING ERUPTION

Dermal myiasis is caused by the maggots of horse and cattle bot flies which are obligatory myiasis producers (whereas in man the maggots cannot develop further) producing tunnels in the epidermis in which they may wander for some time.

AETIOLOGY

Gasterophilus spp. (horse bots, warble flies)
(See also Appendix IV)

Gasterophilidae are common parasites of horses, and sometimes man, especially people who look after horses. The eggs are laid on the hair of the host or on grasses. On contact with skin, the larvae promptly penetrate, but do not develop beyond the first instar causing a swelling and a wandering tunnel in the lower epidermis in which they may wander for a long time.

Hypoderma spp. (cattle bots) (See also Appendix IV)

Hypoderma ovis and *H. lineatum* (Oestridae) are parasites of cattle and cause creeping eruption in persons connected with cattle. The eggs are deposited on the hair of cattle and hatch within a week. The larvae penetrate more deeply into the subcutaneous tissues than those of *Gasterophilus* sp. and have been reported to have invaded the nervous system.

CLINICAL FEATURES

The tunnels caused by *Gasterophilus* sp. maggots resemble the lesions caused by *Ancylostoma braziliense* (cutaneous larva migrans). They itch but do not discharge unless infected. Lesions caused by *Hypoderma* are deeper, producing a swelling resembling a boil. The maggots migrate slowly for considerable distances. *H. ovis* has been reported to invade the central nervous system.

DIFFERENTIAL DIAGNOSIS

Other causes of a creeping eruption are cutaneous larva migrans caused by *Ancylostoma*, *Strongyloides* (Chapter 71), *Gnathostoma* (Chapter 8) and *Fasciola hepatica* (Chapter 73). But *Strongyloides* is transient and very fast moving (hence 'larva currens'), whereas *Gnathostoma* and *Fasciola* larvae do not usually tarry in the skin for long before moving deeper.

For veterinary diagnosis, an increasing number of specific enzyme linked immunosorbent assay (ELISA) tests are becoming available for identifying the presence and identity of bot and warble flies causing myiasis.

Gasterophilus larvae can be identified if a small amount of clear mineral oil is smeared over the lesion. The larva can then be seen and identified by the black transverse bands of spines on its body.

TREATMENT

Gasterophilus larvae, when identified, can be removed with a needle. *Hypoderma* larvae can be removed through a cruciform incision.

BODY CAVITY MYIASIS

NASAL MYIASIS

GEOGRAPHICAL DISTRIBUTION

Nasal myiasis occurs most commonly in Asia, less commonly in Africa.

AETIOLOGY

Chrysomyia bezziana (Old World screw fly) is the most common cause, but *Oestrus ovis* (sheep nasal bot fly), *Rhinoestrus purpureus* (Russian gadfly), *Callitroga hominivorax*, *C. americana* (New World screw fly) are other causes (see Appendix IV).

PATHOLOGY

The flies are obligatory myiasis producers. The female flies lay eggs in the nasal cavity, especially where there is a chronic nasal discharge. The larvae require living tissue in which to develop. After the eggs hatch the larvae burrow into the tissue, even to the nasal bone, within a few hours.

CLINICAL FEATURES

The initial symptoms are tickling, sneezing, pain and nasal obstruction. Epistaxis is common, but the discharge soon becomes purulent and fetid. Destruction and erosion of the nose or mouth may facilitate larval migration to the brain with meningitis and death. A mortality of 8% has been recorded in cases of *Callitroga hominivorax* nasal infection.

DIAGNOSIS

The maggots can be seen with a nasal speculum and extracted for examination. They should be preserved in 70% alcohol and sent to a laboratory to be identified by their spiracles (see Appendix IV), or kept alive and hatched to permit identification.

Precise identification is academic unless control measures are intended and is of no practical importance to the patients.

TREATMENT

A few drops of 15% chloroform in light vegetable oil applied to the nasal passages will cause the larvae to appear, when they can be removed with forceps. In advanced cases the nasal sinuses may have to be opened surgically.

CONTROL

Callitroga hominivorax has been eradicated from some areas by the large-scale release of male flies sterilized by gamma radiation.

MYIASIS OF THE EAR

The same species may invade the ear, causing pain and discomfort accompanied by deafness and tinnitus and the drum can be perforated.

OCULAR MYIASIS (OPHTHALMOMYIASIS)
(See also Chapter 10)

External ophthalmomyiasis, where conjunctivitis only results, is caused by *Oestrus* spp. (sheep bots) or *Wohlfahrtia* spp.

Internal ophthalmomyiasis can be caused by *Dermatobia hominis*, *Oestrus ovis* (sheet bot), *Gasterophilus* spp., *Rhinoestrus* spp. (horse bots) and *Hypoderma* spp. (cattle bots). However, *Oestrus ovis* mainly attacks the conjunctivae (external ophthalmomyisais). The female fly strikes the eye, depositing eggs almost instantaneously while on the wing. Larvae are deposited on the conjunctiva at the inner canthus of the eye, the nasal openings or the lips. The larvae, which do not survive for more than 10 days, developing no further, are actively motile, possessing characteristic hooks which cause conjunctival irritation. They can be removed under direct vision after applying topical anaesthetic.

Internal ophthalmomyiasis involving the orbit and eye can be very destructive, leading to the loss of the eye (Chapter 10).

MYIASIS OF THE ANUS AND VAGINA

Wohlfahrtia spp. (flesh fly) (see Appendix IV) can lay their eggs in large numbers round the anus and vagina of adults and children in poor hygienic circumstances where there are soiling and sores in the anogenital region. Large numbers of maggots can develop within a few hours.

WOUND MYIASIS

AETIOLOGY

This includes myiasis produced by both obligatory and facultative myiasis producers. Larvae of several groups of flies usually associated with carrion have been found in wounds and gangrenous tissues, where they act as facultative parasites feeding on necrotic tissue, although occasionally they may attack living tissues.

Larvae of the facultative parasites *Calliphora, Lucilia, Phormia, Musca* and *Fannia* spp. are found living in moist folds of skin and enter sores and wounds. At one time it was practice to use the larvae of carefully cultivated *Lucilia* to cleanse wounds by removal of infected tissue, and this practice can still be appropriate for cases where antibiotics are ineffective and surgery impractical.[2]

In southern Europe, Russia, the Middle East and Africa *Wohlfahrtia magnifica* (Old World flesh fly or sheep maggot) is the common species and *W. vigil* (New World flesh fly) in the New World. In India, the Far East and sub-Saharan Africa *Chrysomyia bezziana* and in the New World *Callitroga hominivorax* (see above) are the most frequent agents of wound myiasis. These flies are obligatory myiasis producers, relying on living tissue for their survival.

UROGENITAL MYIASIS

Mistaken diagnosis of urinary myiasis is not uncommon, due to a larva from a contaminated vessel in which urine has been collected, or which has been introduced into the urine after it was passed; but there have been genuine cases in which larvae have been passed via the urethra from the bladder. If the vulva or vaginal area in women is infested, there are obvious opportunities for larvae to enter the bladder. The flies concerned are usually of the genera *Psychoda, Musca, Calliphora* and *Sarcophaga*.[3]

INTESTINAL MYIASIS

Eggs, and sometimes larvae, of many species of flies are deposited on foodstuffs, and sometimes survive the journey down the intestinal tract. They may then develop in the folds of mucous membrane, even causing some irritation (pain, vomiting, diarrhoea) or even ulceration before being evacuated. If deposited around the anus, such larvae may crawl into the rectum to complete their feeding inside the body. This kind of infestation may persist for months, producing severe anxiety as well as internal irritation. The larvae can be recognized in the faeces, sometimes in vomit.

The flies usually implicated include species of *Musca, Fannia, Chrysomyia, Calliphora* and *Lucilia*. Prevention entails the careful covering of food. Treatment with purgatives will aid elimination, and ivermectin would be worth a trial.

REFERENCES

1 Radcliffe W. *BMJ* 1972; ii:164.
2 Sherman R A & Pechter E A. *Med Vet Entomol* 1988; 2:225–230.
3 Lane R P & Crosskey R W (eds). *Medical Insects and Arachnids*. London: Chapman & Hall, 1993.

CHAPTER 80

JIGGER FLEAS

G. B. White

GEOGRAPHICAL DISTRIBUTION

Originally found in Central and South America the jigger has now spread to West and East Africa and parts of the Indian subcontinent.

AETIOLOGY (Appendix IV)

Tunga penetrans (the sand flea, jigger flea, chigoe, chique) is the cause, the female being adapted for an intracutaneous permanent attachment to the host (man, pig, poultry and other animals). As with other fleas, the larvae are free-living, dusty or sandy soil being best for *T. penetrans*. Adults are also free-living at first, when copulation occurs. The fertilized female then finds a suitable host and tries to penetrate crevices in the skin, such as cracks in the soles of the feet (Figure 80.1), between the toes and especially around the toenails. Any part of the human anatomy can be affected. By means of the mouth-parts, the female *Tunga* becomes firmly attached and soon swells to the size and shape of a small white pea. Somehow the host skin envelops the jigger, which lies below the stratum corneum but above the stratum granulosum, leaving only the posterior spiracles exposed to the air. Only when the jigger is almost mature and distended, after 8–12 days, does the infection begin to irritate. Severe inflammation and ulceration ensues, so that scratching helps to expel large numbers of white eggs from the jigger (see also Appendix IV).

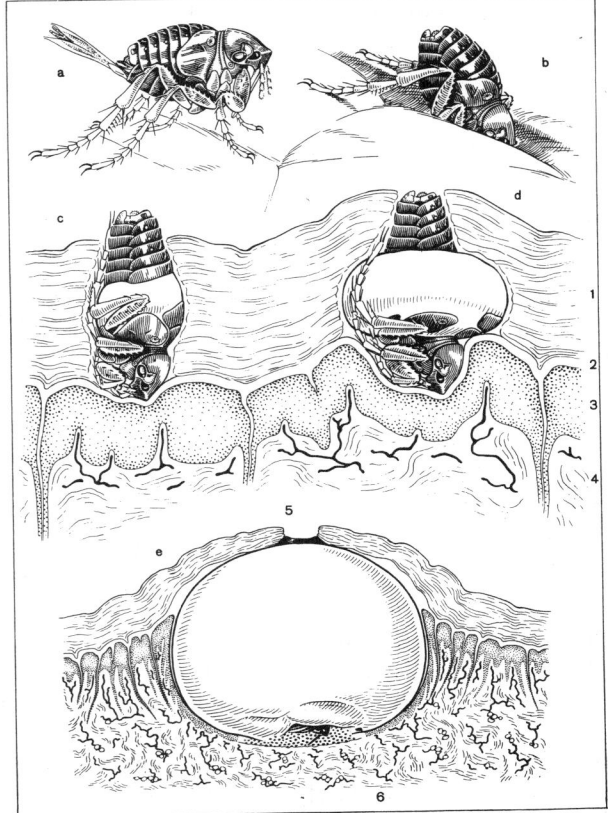

Figure 80.1 The sand flea or jigger.

CLINICAL FEATURES

The jigger seldom attacks the leg above the dorsum of the foot, but no part of the body escapes. The soles (Figure 80.2), the skin between the toes and that of the roots of the nails are favourite situations. Usually only one or two jiggers are found at a time, but occasionally they are present in hundreds, the little pits left after extraction or expulsion being sometimes so closely set that parts of the surface may look like a honeycomb. During her gestation the jigger causes a considerable amount of irritation. Pus may form around her distended abdomen, which now raises the integument into a pea-like elevation. After the eggs are laid the skin ulcerates and the jigger is expelled, leaving a small sore which may become seriously infected or lead to tetanus. Ulceration is common and may follow removal of the jigger or natural extrusion of the egg sac. The ulcer commences as a tiny pit and, as it extends, the sloping edge may develop into a septic ulcer. It remains more or less circular in outline, except under the nail or nail margin, where the outline is more irregular and a pocket of pus forms beneath it.

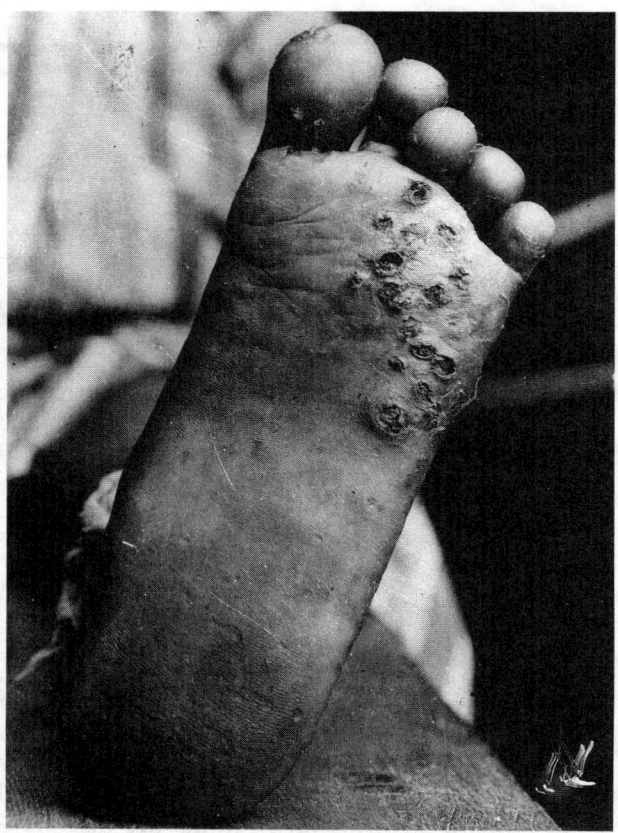

Figure 80.2   Jiggers in the sole of the foot.

TREATMENT

The mature female jigger should be removed carefully using a sterile needle, so as to pick out the jigger without bursting it. Inexpert attempts at removal may lead to severe secondary infection.

PREVENTION (Appendix IV)

Affected areas of soil may be burnt off in an effort to kill the fleas, or residual insecticide applied to infested areas. Since female jiggers are not good jumpers, human infestation is normally confined to the feet. Daily inspection of the interdigital clefts, roots of nails and soles of feet should cause freshly burrowing female jiggers to be detected and removed before they have grown much. To prevent attack, foot-enveloping shoes (not 'flip-flops' or sandals) are effective, and a more sensible solution than repellents.

CHAPTER 81

SCABIES

G. B. White

GEOGRAPHICAL DISTRIBUTION

Scabies is a worldwide infection generally associated with unhygienic life style, due to shortage of washing water, irrespective of climate.

AETIOLOGY

Sarcoptes scabiei, the itch or scabies mite (Acari: Sarcoptidae), causes human scabies. The same species is the aetiological agent of sarcoptic mange in dogs, horses and other animals.[1]

The female *S. scabiei* (0.3–0.4 mm) is twice the size of the male (0.2 mm) (see Appendix IV). The gravid female lays her oval eggs ($15 \times 100 \mu$m) in a burrow in the skin. The eggs give rise to adults 10–14 days later after passing through the larval and one or two nymphal stages. The nymphs moult, become sexually mature and pair off on the surface of the skin. The adults live for 4–5 weeks.

TRANSMISSION

Transmission is from person to person by direct skin contact and through bedding and clothing. Scabies is often transmitted sexually. The newly fertilized female is the infective agent.

PATHOLOGY

Both males and females of *S. scabiei* make short burrows, but it is only the fertilized female which makes a permanent burrow in the horny layers of the skin with the female at the end (see Appendix IV). Pathology is the result of sensitization of the host to the mites and their excretions.

A vesicle is present at the entry point of the tunnel in which eggs and faeces are deposited. The larvae hatch out after 3–4 days, when they leave the burrow for the skin surface for food and shelter in the hair follicles. After 4–5 days the adults mate and the female burrows into the cuticle of the skin to complete the cycle.

The population of mites builds up over 2–4 months and a fully developed case of scabies may have no more than 20 adult mites, often less. When sensitization of the host occurs, a generalized rash develops. Infiltration with eosinophils is found round the burrows, and foci of lymphocytes and histiocytes can be found deep in the corium after cure.

CLINICAL FEATURES (Chapter 11)

INCUBATION PERIOD

There is an incubation period of 6–8 weeks before symptoms appear.

SYMPTOMS AND SIGNS

The first stage is a small (1–3 mm), slightly raised, itchy papule which develops at the site of each mite. Scratching may destroy the mote and convert the papule into a pustule. Local sensitization is followed by the appearance of a rash.

The generalized rash of scabies is an itchy erythematous rash, the distribution of which does not correspond to the site of the mites. It is a phenomenon of hypersensitivity in which it may be impossible to demonstrate mites. The eruption occurs most commonly in the axiallae, around the waist, inner aspect of the thighs and back of the legs, from which it may spread all over the body. It commonly occurs in reinfection and the number of mites present may be small.

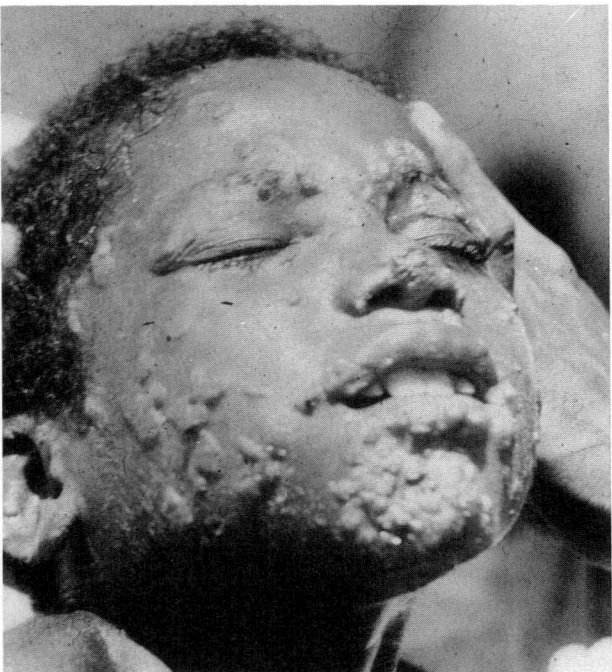

Figure 81.1   Crusted scabies. (Courtesy of P. Rotmil.)

IMMUNOSUPPRESSION AND CRUSTED SCABIES

Evidence for acquired immunity to scabies comes from the way that, in immunosuppressed persons, the mites escape control and multiply considerably, leading to encrustation of the skin, a condition known as crusted or Norwegian scabies. Steroid therapy to control undiagnosed itching may change ordinary into crusted scabies.

This is a severe type of scabies accompanied by profuse crusting and hyperkeratotic plaques (Figure 81.1). It is common in the tropics and used to be common in leprosy. Burrows are not formed and a large number of scabies mites may be present on the surface of the skin.

SCABIES IN CHILDREN

Scabies in children is atypical. During the first year of life the lesions are general and resemble pemphigus, the buttocks and perineum being most often severely affected. Burrows are often impossible to find and secondarily infected excoriations and scattered pustules are the most characteristic lesion (Figures 81.1 and Plate 11.11).

SARCOPTIC MANGE (ANIMAL SCABIES)

This is sometimes contracted by man by contact with dogs, cats and cattle infested with zoonotic races of *Sarcoptes*. They may be distinguished from human scabies by the distribution of papules and vesicles on the arms, shoulders, trunks and thighs and by the absence of burrows on the hands. Sarcoptic mange responds rapidly to treatment with ivermectin or sulphur.

IMPORTANT COMPLICATION: NEPHRITIS

Secondary infection of scabies lesions is very common, especially in children. Scabies infected with nephritogenic strains of β-haemolytic streptococci is an important cause of glomerulonephritis, and in some parts of the world may be a more frequent cause of nephritis than streptococcal throat infection. Secondarily infected scabies should always be treated with a course of antibiotic at the same time as antiscabetic treatment.

DIFFERENTIAL DIAGNOSIS

Scabies in the tropics is atypical in appearance, especially in children, in whom crusted scabies may be very difficult to distinguish from eczema and pyoderma. Itching is severe in scabies, in which it may be possible to identify burrows. In adults onchocerciasis (also intensely pruritic) and lepromatous leprosy (with which scabies may coexist) must be thought of.

DIAGNOSIS

Scabies burrows between the fingers may be seen with a magnifying glass. After opening a burrow, the mite at the end can be extracted with a needle and examined under mineral oil. Scrapings from ulcers may reveal mites or eggs.

TREATMENT (See also Chapter 11)

All members of the family in contact with the patient should be treated at the same time. In addition to affected areas of the head, it is important to treat the whole body from the neck down. Mites are found only above the neck in infants.

Benzyl benzoate 20% emulsion should be applied from the neck down after a bath and allowed to dry, when the clothes may be put on again. After 24 hours a second bath should be taken and the clothes and bedclothes washed in the meantime. A second treatment should be given 1 week later. Crusted lesions should first be removed with a mixture of sulphur and salicylic acid. Secondary infection is treated with a 5-day course of penicillin.

NBIN emulsion concentrate consists of 68% benzyl benzoate, 6% DDT, 12% benzocaine and 14% polysorbate 80. This requires a dilution of 1:15 in water before use.

Tetmosol (tetraethylthiuram monosulphide) in a 5% solution can be sued as benzyl benzoate. In soap form it is of little value.

Crotamiton (Eurax) is applied daily for 5 days and is suitable for infants. It is more expensive but has powerful antipruritic properties.

Lotions of 0.5% malathion or 1% BHC are also effective, and sting less than benzyl benzoate.

EPIDEMIOLOGY AND CONTROL

Human scabies waxes and wanes in incidence over 15–20 year cycles, probably due to changing immunity patterns. Scabies is widespread in the tropics, especially among children. Infection is associated with poor hygiene, the result of inadequate water supply.

Good personal hygiene, plus the search for and treatment of infected families is the best form of control in the community.

Prevention can be obtained by avoidance of skin contact with infected persons and clothing. People able to wash themselves frequently do not suffer much from scabies.

REFERENCE

1 Arlian L G. Biology, host relations, and epidemiology of *Sarcoptes scabei. Ann Rev Entomol* 1989; 34:139–161.

CHAPTER 82

LOUSE INFESTATION

G. B. White

Three species of louse are parasitic to man:
Pediculus humanus (body louse)
Pediculus capitis (head louse)
Phthirus pubis (crab louse).
Pediculus humanus and *P. capitis* are morphologically similar but have different habits. Although experimental interbreeding is possible this does not happen in nature. The majority of lice are host specific, and although lice from domestic animals may be found on man they do not persist. Most lice do not survive for long when removed from the host.

PEDICULUS HUMANUS (BODY LOUSE)

AETIOLOGY

P. humanus is larger (0.4 mm) than *P. capitis* (0.3 mm) and there are minor morphological differences (Figures 82.1 and 82.2). The female *P. humanus* sometimes attaches her eggs (nits) to body hair, but more often cements them to cloth fibres, usually along seams and folds in garments. The female lice produce an average of four to five eggs per day during their life of up to 1 month. The nymphs hatch in 8 days, becoming adult after three moults in 18 days. Nymphs and adults take blood meals two to five times a day throughout life.

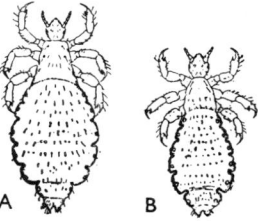

Figure 82.2   A, Female *Pediculus humanus*. B, Female *Pediculus capitis*.

TRANSMISSION

Pediculus infestation is usually acquired through close contact with lousy persons, shared clothes and bedding. Lice tend to leave patients with fever and sweating, thus promoting the spread of disease. They avoid light and leave a corpse as it becomes cold.

CLINICAL FEATURES

Body lice cause itching and a generalized red maculopapular rash. Scratching may cause secondary infection and impetigo may result. *P. humanus* is the sole transmitter of louse-borne typhus (*Rickettsia prowazeki*), trench fever (*Rickettsia quintana*) (Chapter 39) and louse-borne relapsing fever (*Borrelia recurrentis*) (Chapter 54).

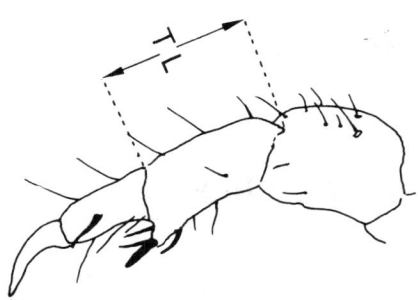

Figure 82.1   The second leg of *Pediculus*, showing the length of the tibia (TL). In *P. capitis*, TL = approximately 0.3 mm and in *P. humanus* TL = approximately 0.4 mm.

DIAGNOSIS

Eggs (nits) should be searched for on body hair. Adults, nymphs and eggs should be looked for in the seams and folds of clothing.

PEDICULUS CAPITIS (HEAD LOUSE)

P. capitis females cement their eggs (nits) to the base of head hairs, and growth of the hair eventually brings the empty egg cases into view after the eggs have hatched. They are confined to the scalp.

TRANSMISSION

This is by close contact, usually head-to-head transfer.

CLINICAL FEATURES

Head lice seldom cause noticeable signs or symptoms, and infestation is principally a hygienic and aesthetic nuisance. In heavy infections some dermatitis of the scalp can result from scratching. *P. capitis* is not known to be a vector for any disease.

DIAGNOSIS

Diagnosis is by searching for the presence of 'nits' in the hair or observing the lice themselves.

PHTHIRUS PUBIS (CRAB LOUSE)

Crab lice occur worldwide, and are found exclusively on man.

AETIOLOGY

Phthirus is shorter and broader then *Pediculus* and has massive claws on the second and third legs by which it clings to hair (Figure 82.3). It is most commonly found in the genital and inguinal regions, but may be found on any of the body hair except the scalp, including the beard, chest hair and eyelashes. It cannot survive off the host for more than 24 hours.

TRANSMISSION

This is by sexual and close personal contact.

CLINICAL FEATURES

Infection is normally noticed following irritation caused by the bite. Sometimes a characteristic small 'blue spot' (2–3 mm across) may result from the bite, different from the red spot caused by pediculid lice. *P. pubis* is not known to be the vector of any disease.

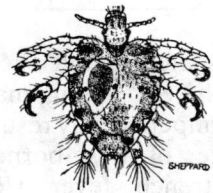

Figure 82.3 Female *Phthirus pubis*, showing the contained ovum. (12×.)

CONTROL OF LICE AND THE TREATMENT OF LOUSY PATIENTS

PEDICULUS

Destruction of the lice and eggs on clothes is most efficiently achieved by heating to 60°C for 30–40 minutes. For practical purposes, 70°C for 30 minutes is recommended. Particular attention should be paid to folds and pleats and the application of a hot iron to these is useful. Head lice may be removed by combing with a fine louse-comb, used with soft soap to remove nits. The most efficient comb of this type (Sacker patent) is now in short supply, but others are available, though for best effect they should be used in conjunction with chemical treatments. Chemical methods of control (both species) include application of DDT or permethrin dusts, or malathion, carbaryl and other insecticides prepared as suitable lotions or shampoos that are commercially available. As insecticide resistance is becoming a problem in many areas, WHO susceptibility tests should be made before widespread application of an insecticide. Such tests should be made on the target population. Resistance in one of the pediculids in a given area does not imply similar resistance in the other.

PHTHIRUS

Chemical methods, as outlined above, are normally used for this species. Resistance to insecticides is rare.

CHAPTER 83

ARTHROPOD DERMATOSES, STINGS, BITES, ALLERGIES AND NEUROSES

G. B. White

ACARINE DERMATOSIS

Intense irritation and dermatitis, somewhat resembling that produced by scabies, can result from various mites (Acari) living as temporary ectoparasites on the skin of man. The most common occurrence of such infestation is among workers associated with stored food products in which the mites occur as pests. The more familiar of these are grocer's itch caused by *Glycyphagus domesticus*, baker's itch (*Acarus siro*) and copra itch (*Tyrophagus putrescentiae*). *Pyemotes tritici (= ventricosus)*, the grain or straw itch mite (Figure 83.1), causes an urticarial and papular eruption of exposed parts of the body in those who handle grain, cottonseeds, beans and especially straw. These mites give rise to a severe pruritus, especially on the trunk. A lotion of warm water and vinegar or a saturated solution of picric acid in 90% alcohol will relieve the irritation.

An application of 5% betanaphthol ointment is a preventative treatment and a dilute phenol solution will kill the mites. *Dermatophagoides* mites have been recorded as causing an unusually severe dermatitis in man. In one case infestation of the scalp persisted for 7 years. Among the constituents of house dust it has been found that *Dermatophagoides* produced the most potent allergen. Bites of thrombiculid mites, or chiggers, cause a parasitic dermatitis known as trombidiosis or scrub-itch. This condition is an allergic reaction to the saliva of the mite and can be caused by about 15 species, mostly belonging to the genera *Eutrombicula, Schoengastia* and *Neoschoengastia*. Trombiculid bites can be prevented by mite repellents such as diethyltoluamide (see also Chapter 11).

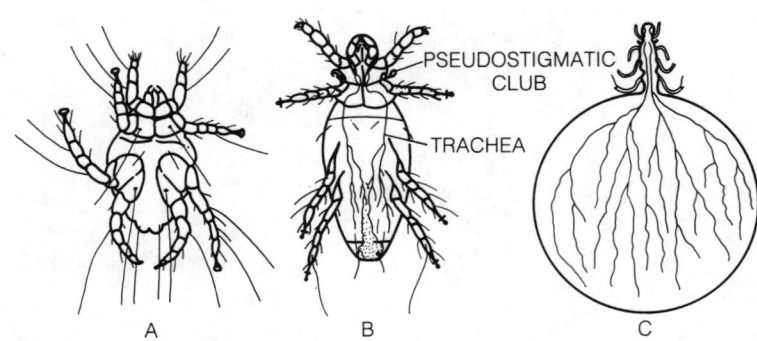

Figure 83.1 Pyemotes tritici. A, Male. B, Female. C, Pregnant female with brood sac. (80×)

TICKS

Extensive subcutaneous haemorrhages can be caused by the anticoagulant inoculated with the saliva of ticks.

BUTTERFLY AND MOTH DERMATOSES

Various moth and butterfly caterpillars, usually of the families Arctiidae, Lymantriidae, Saturniidae, Megalopygidae, Notodontidae and Nymphalidae, possess urticating hairs which can cause dermatitis. These hairs penetrate the skin and poison may be injected through them from attached glands. The poisons include histamine and cause irritation which can be severe if mucous membranes are affected, for example when detached hairs enter the eye and give rise to nodular conjunctivitis.[1] Both larvae and adults can be involved.

In Papua New Guinea and northern Australia the moth *Ochrogaster lunifer* has caused epidemics of urticaria among troops. In Brazil flannel moths (Megalopygidae) are well known urticators. In the Panama Canal Zone the urticating caterpillars of *Megalopyge lanata* produce rapidly developing eosinophilia (8–22%), numbness and vesication. The 'puss caterpillar', *Megalopyge opercularis*, causes thousands of cases of dermatitis in children in Texas, necessitating the closure of schools. In Japan, some 300 000 people were affected by the moth *Euproctis flava*. In Israel *Thaumetopoea pinivora* causes trouble every year in February and May and caterpillar dermatitis is also common in northern Kenya (Figure 83.2).

Urticating hairs may become detached from the caterpillar and the cocoon spun by the caterpillar before pupation. Such detached hairs may retain their urticating properties for a long time. If inhaled these hairs may cause dyspnoea and if ingested may give rise to stomatitis. In Africa *Anaphe renata* (Notodontidae) and related moths have both imago and larva clothed with detachable irritating hairs.

Caterpillars of the Venezuelan saturniid moth *Lonomia achelous* inject, through their hairs, a

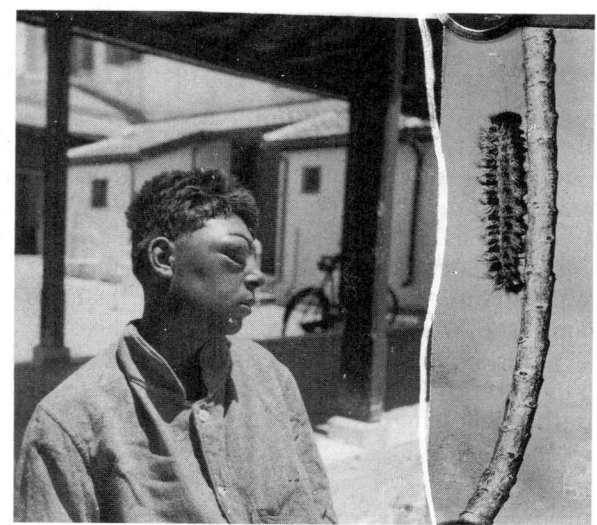

Figure 83.2   Urticating dermatitis caused by contact with a processionary caterpillar of the moth *Thaumetopoea wilkinsoni*.

powerful anticoagulant if handled or even brushed against and long-lasting fibrinolytic bleeding results.[2]

In Africa and Asia some adult moths of the families Pyralidae, Geometridae and Noctuidae feed upon the eye discharges of various mammals, including man. Although their probosces cannot penetrate live tissue, they may well be vectors of mammalian epidemic keratoconjunctivitis and other eye diseases. In Malaya one noctuid fruit-piercing moth *Calyptra eustrigata* can penetrate mammalian skin and suck blood and must therefore be considered a potential vector of disease or producer of allergic reaction.[3]

BEETLE DERMATITIS

Beetle larvae of the family Dermestidae have urticating hairs which produce a dermatitis. Since these beetles are pests of stored products, dockers unloading ships' cargoes have developed dyspnoea and erucic stomatitis from the inhalation and ingestion of detached hairs.

The family Meloidae contains some species known as blister beetles because their body fluids contain cantharidin, a cytotoxic principle which causes vesicular dermatitis when applied to the skin. The best known species is the so-called Spanish fly, *Lytta vesicatoria*, and in India *Mylabris cichorii* and *Epicauta hirticornis* are troublesome. In the Gilbert Islands severe blistering is caused by the coconut beetles *Sessinia collaris* and *Ananca decolor* of the family Oedemeridae. The bushmen of South Africa use body fluids from the larvae of the chrysomelid beetle *Diamphidia nigroornata* as a lethal arrow poison which causes death from a general paralysis. Staphylinid beetles of the genus *Paederus* cause urticaria and blistering and minute species of the genera *Atheta* and *Oxytelus* fly in numbers and may enter the eye, causing a burning sensation.

OTHER INSECTS

Other insects causing dermatitis are ceratopogonid flies (biting midges) of the genus *Culicoides*. In Brazil *C. paraensis* is a public health problem in this way and in El Salvador an increase in biting *Culicoides* was correlated with decreasing standards of sanitation and the cessation of a control campaign against the breeding sites of the mosquito *Aedes aegypti*. In Japan there are records of eczema following the bites of *C. erairai* and long-lasting sores (3–4 months) following bites by *C. obsoletus*. Mosquito bites in persons sensitized to their saliva can cause troublesome chronic ulcers which will respond dramatically to topical steroids. Sandflies and black flies can similarly cause quite severe reactions in sensitized persons which will respond quite readily to steroid ointment such as betamethasone valerate. An irritant vesicular rash, superficially resembling scabies, can be caused by Thysanoptera (see also Appendix IV).

BEE AND WASP STINGS

The stings of bees, wasps and hornets may produce a mild reaction easily soothed with an ice-pack, diluted vinegar or antihistamine ointment. They may be very serious in the case of multiple stinging or of stings in the mouth. Some people react violently to bee stings and may become increasingly hypersensitive with each successive sting. In such cases anaphylaxis may result which can be fatal. Massive anaphylaxis causes muscular paralysis and suggests a curare-like action on synapses of muscle end-plates. The antidote is an injection of adrenaline.

People extremely sensitive to bee stings should always have access to a pressurized bronchodilator spray and use two puffs when breathing in and this procedure can be repeated in 15 minutes. Such patients, however, may quickly become faint and lose consciousness and should be immediately taken into medical care.[4,5]

Bee and wasp venoms contain histamine, acetylcholine and enzymes (phospholipase A and hyaluronidase); the more superficial aspects of a sting are due to the histamine. The African honey-bee *Apis mellifica adansonii* is abundant in equatorial and warm temperate southern Africa and is a fairly aggressive species. In 1956 this species was introduced into South America and hybridization with local bees has produced an extremely aggressive race of Brazilian honey-bees. The spread of these bees has been very rapid from South America to the USA. A number of fatalities have resulted from the abundance and special behavioural characteristics of the bee. The slightest disturbance near the hive can cause hundreds of bees to become airborne; they may then sting any animal or human within 100 m of the apiary and may pursue fleeing victims for over a kilometre.[6]

In the honey-bee the sting is torn out by the act of stinging but the poison gland, which is attached to the sting, continues to inject venom into the wound. For this reason the sting should be carefully removed as soon as possible and the remaining venom expressed from the gland with forceps.

Sometimes stingless social bees (*Melipona*, etc.) are prone to aggressive mass biting and some neotropical species squirt caustic fluid, but these insects are rarely more than a nuisance. Some tiny stingless sweat-bees (*Trigona*) can be annoying in the African savanna regions, because of their numbers and persistence, are sometimes mistaken for *Simulium* (black flies).

Wasps (*Vespula*) and hornets (*Vespa*) can sting repeatedly because, unlike the honey-bee, the sting is not torn out by the action of stinging. Wasp venom contains a higher proportion of histamine and 5-hydroxytryptamine (serotonin) which is distinctly more active than that of the honey-bee. *Scleroderma nipponensis* (Bethylidae), in one incident in Japan, attacked 340 people, who were left with reddish swellings and injuries leading to suppuration and

lymphangitis. Some parasitic wasps of the family Ichneumonidae such as *Ophion, Netelia* and *Ichneumon* can inflict painful stings. Sensitive patients may be ill for some weeks following these stings.

Paper-wasps of the genus *Polistes* also cause many fatalities in the New World. These wasps build their nests under the eaves of houses or in ornamental shrubs and trees where people are likely to be exposed to their stings.

Arthropod venoms are dealt with in Chapter 22 by Beard[8] and Bucherl and Buckley.[9]

POISONOUS HONEY

Occasionally the honey produced by hive-bees, wild honey bees, bumble-bees and stingless bees may be toxic if particular plants are foraged or if polluted liquid resources are used in the absence of clean drinking water (which should be provided in the case of honey-bees).

ANTS

Ants can bite, sting and squirt formic acid. Mostly the attacks of ants produce only mild effects, but, as in wasps, the stinging apparatus is a modified ovipositor which can be extracted after each sting and used repeatedly; multiple stinging may induce an anaphylactic response. Some ants may also be mechanical transmitters of disease; for example, Pharaoh's ants (*Monomorium pharaonis*) have been found to carry *Salmonella, Pseudomonas, Staphylococcus, Streptococcus* and *Clostridium* spp. in hospitals.[10]

The venom of ants is largely proteinaceous but in the south-eastern USA *Solenopsis richteri* is a dangerous fire-ant in which the venom is non-proteinaceous and exhibits necrotic activity resembling the bites of *Loxosceles* spiders. When a colony is disturbed the ants erupt in thousands and 3000–5000 stings may be administered in a matter of seconds. Allergic reactions to such stings, and anaphylactic shock, may sometimes result in death of sensitive individuals. The subject is reviewed by Gurney.[11]

OTHER BITES AND ALLERGIES

Skin reactions of both immediate and delayed hypersensitivity type were common following the bite of *Triatoma infestans* and *T. maxima* in Brazil where the former was the major man-biting triatomid (Hemiptera). The reactions were severe enough to prevent the use of these bugs for xenodiagnosis.[12]

Other orders containing insects capable of inflicting bites or stings include other Hemiptera (plant bugs) and some Orthoptera. Chicken bugs in Mexico (*Haematosiphon inodorus*) and Brazil (*Ornithocoris toledo*) attack poultry but may incidentally bite

man and may produce a polymorphous dermatitis with pustules, scabs and linear scars. The bite of the giant water-bugs (Belostomatidae) may be nearly as severe as a bee sting. Many other bugs will bite if incautiously handled. The larger coreid and pentatomid bugs can squirt a jet of irritant fluid from the metathoracic glands into the eye of the beholder which can cause a very painful reaction for a day or two.

The bites of several insects not mentioned above may also produce allergic reactions. Recorded cases involve adult flies of the rhagionid genus *Symphoromyia* and larvae of Therevidae[13] and Tabanidae[14] (Diptera) and the possibility of such reactions following the bite of almost any insect must be considered; if possible suspected specimens should be collected and identified by a specialist.

In addition to bites, other allergic reactions are not uncommon. Inhalant allergens may be acquired from acarine sources in house dust (especially from *Dermatophagoides pteronyssinus*) or among stored products from the grain weevil *Sitophilus granarius* or the Mexican bean weevil *Zabrotes subfasciatus*.

Some aquatic insects such as Ephemeroptera and Trichoptera emerge in vast numbers and their cast exuviae are fragmented and windborne and become inhalant allergens. Chironomidae ('green nimitti') have also been associated with asthma and other allergic symptoms along the Nile.[15] Terrestrial counterparts causing similar allergies are the prolific aphids.

Allergic reactions to the bites and stings of insects and other arthropods are treated by Frazier[16] and Frazier and Brown.[17] Tu[18] surveys the whole field of arthropod poisons, allergens and venoms.

For the identification of arthropods of medical importance Lane and Crosskey[19] should be consulted.

NEUROSES

Many people have a morbid fear of insects and the extreme manifestation of this is in delusory parasitosis (Ekbom's syndrome), also loosely referred to as parasitophobia, acarophobia or entomophobia. In these cases patients suffering from dermatitis artefacta, usually of emotional origin, believe that they are infested with insects or other parasites which cause the itching. They then scratch the affected parts until the skin breaks down. Further skin damage may be caused by the overuse of disinfectants or insecticides. Such cases are difficult, and best treated by a psychiatrist, but every effort should be made to establish that there are in fact no minute biting insects such as *Culicoides* or allergen-producing mites or insects, particularly of the type bearing or shedding urticating hairs. The possibility of inanimate allergens such as paint should also be carefully investigated. Cases of delusory parasitosis may follow an actual infestation by fleas or other arthropods, by seeing or reading about ectoparasites in the popular media,[20,21] or by emotional disturbances.[22] Some success in treating this difficult condition has recently been claimed from use of the drug pimozide. A common feature of these cases is that the persistence of the sufferer often results in a second member of the household presenting similar symptoms, which adds credence to their claims.

Sometimes there are group outbreaks of imagined biting insects, a phenomenon which has only received attention in the 1980s.[22] In these cases 'phantom biters' may persist for 2 or 3 years in offices or small factories where several people work together. The causative agent may be carpet fibres, fragments of glass fibre lampshades or the coverings of wires on telephone switchboards. Spraying *during working hours* (even with water) has sometimes proved effective in these cases. Here again extreme care should be taken that an actual infestation of mites or minute insects in not the cause.

REFERENCES

1 Watson P G & Sevel D. *Br J. Ophthalmol* 1966; 50:209–217.

2 Arocha-Pinango C L & Layrisse M. *Lancet* 1969; i:810–812.

3 Bänziger H. *Mitt Schweiz Ent Ges* 1980; 53:127–142.

4 Frankland A W. Bee sting allergy. *Bee World* 1976; 57:145–150.

5 Hoffman D R. *Cutis* 1977; 19:763–767.

6 Michener C D. The Brazilian bee problem. *Ann Rev Entamol* 1975; 20:399–416.

7 Taylor O R. *Bee World* 1977; 58:19–30.

8 Beard R L. *Ann Rev Entamol* 1963; 8:1–18.

9 Bucherl W & Buckley E E. *Venomous Animals and Their Venoms, III. Venomous Invertebrates.* London: Chapman & Hall, 1971.

10 Beatson S H. *Lancet* 1972; i:425–427.

11 Gurney A B. Some stinging ants. *Insect World Digest* 1975; Sept./Oct.:19–25.

12 Costa C H N, Costa M T, Weber J N et al. *Trans R Soc Trop Med Hyg* 1981; 75:405–408.

13 Smith K G V. *Lancet* 1979; i:391–392.

14 Otsuru M & Ogawa S. *Acta Med Biol* 1959; 7:37–50.

15 Cranston P S, Gad-El-Rab M & Kay A B. *Trans R Soc Trop Med Hyg* 1981; 75:1–4.

16 Frazier C A. *Insect Allergy. Allergic and Toxic Reactions to Insects and other Arthropods*. St Louis: W H Green, 1969.

17 Frazier C A & Brown F K. *Insects and Allergy*. Norman: University of Oklahoma Press, 1980.

18 Tu A T (ed.). *Handbook of Natural Toxins*, vol. 2. *Insect Poisons, Allergens and Other Invertebrate Venoms*. New York: Marcel Dekker, 1984.

19 Lane R P & Crosskey R W. *Medical Insects and Arachnids*. London: Chapman & Hall, 1993.

20 Busvine J R. *Insects and Hygiene*, 3rd edn. London: Chapman and Hall, 1980.

21 Mester H. Das Syndrom des wahnhaften Ungezieferbefalls. *Agnew Parasitol* 1977; 18:70–84.

22 Lyell A. *Br J Dermatol* 1983; 108:485–499.

APPENDICES

APPENDICES

IMMUNOLOGICAL ASPECTS OF TROPICAL DISEASES

J. H. L. Playfair

The words 'tropical disease' are enough to strike fear into many hearts, conjuring up mysterious chronic infections that seem to pursue their debilitating and often disfiguring course regardless of prophylactic or therapeutic intervention. One only has to contrast poliomyelitis and malaria—the one now essentially preventable by a vaccine and (perhaps optimistically) targeted for global eradication by the year 2000, the other on the increase among one-third of the world's population and escaping from all forms of control in many areas. More than any other aspect, it is the immunology of these two diseases that underlies the opposite trends in their incidence. This chapter aims to describe the principal interactions between tropical infectious diseases and the immune system, illustrating each with examples; to cover all possible combinations would require a large textbook, of which there are several available (see References). Emphasis will be on infections either restricted to, or more serious in, the tropics; the term 'parasite' will be used in the broader sense to include viruses, bacteria and fungi.

Immunology impinges on the practice of tropical medicine in four main ways. First, as already mentioned, protective immunity to particular tropical infections is frequently inadequate and sometimes non-existent; this affects both the normal course of the disease and the prospects for vaccination. Second, the prolonged ineffective immune responses can give rise to serious immunopathological consequences. Third, people afflicted with these infections often suffer a general immunodeficiency that weakens their response to normally mild infections. Fourth, the monitoring of immune responses, even when they are not protective, can often be of great help in diagnosis and management.

PROTECTIVE AND NON-PROTECTIVE IMMUNITY

The mechanisms that normally protect against infection are conveniently classified as (1) external barriers, (2) natural immune defences, and (3) adaptive immune responses. Transmission by blood-sucking insects is a good example of how a resourceful parasite overcomes the external skin barrier and simultaneously solves the problem of spreading in a thinly-populated country, but of course it also restricts the parasite to areas where the vector flourishes. The faecal–oral route, used by many parasitic organisms, is all the more effective in tropical countries where water supplies are not yet highly organized. Both vector-borne and water-borne transmission offer alternative ways of controlling an infection, though this is usually much easier said than done.

Natural immune mechanisms are those ever present and unaffected by prior contact; they include the phagocytes and natural killer (NK) cells, complement and other acute phase proteins, and the interferons (which will be considered later, together with the other cytokines). It is important to appreciate that these are generally very successful in limiting infection, though there are some interesting examples of evasion, particularly by protozoa, such as the ability of *Entamoeba histolytica* to expel the complement membrane attack complex and so avoid lysis, the escape of *Leishmania* spp. from the macrophage phagosome to reside in the more hospitable environment of the cytoplasm, and the inhibition of phagosome–lysosome fusion by *Toxoplasma gondii*. Nevertheless, only a tiny minority of potential parasites actually succeed in gaining a foothold in man. When they do, the responsibility for dislodging them passes to the adaptive immune system.

Adaptive immunity operates rather differently in that it uses the highly specific T and B lymphocytes to recognize the invading parasite, respond and retain memory. These make use of two quite separate recognition systems. The B-cell receptor (antibody) detects the three-dimensional shape of protein or carbohydrate molecules, whereas the T-cell receptor detects small linear peptides (about nine amino acids long) held in the groove of the major histocompatibility complex (MHC) molecules on the surface of certain cells. The way in which these two systems function and interact has far-reaching implications for the whole adaptive immune response. For extracellular parasites, antibody is usually the most effective type of response, whereas intracellular parasite infections call for one or other of the cell-mediated responses. These will now be considered separately.

ANTIBODY RESPONSES

It is very rare for a parasite not to induce an antibody response. Even the higher eukaryotic organisms such as protozoa and helminths display large numbers of antigens foreign to man, who as a general rule makes antibody to most of them. Indeed, serum antibody is a most useful guide to infection, the general principle being that a predominance of IgM is a sign of recent infection. It has often been proposed that parasites adapt to their hosts by mimicking their antigens, and in support of this is the remarkable number of parasite–host cross-reactions, nowadays increasingly analysed at the amino acid sequence level. However, there is little firm evidence that such mimicry actually serves to reduce the host response; on the contrary it often stimulates the host to respond by making autoantibody, and some immunologists feel that most autoimmune diseases are in fact initiated in this way, though the offending organism has been identified only in a few cases—the group β-haemolytic *Streptococcus* in rheumatic carditis and *Trypanosoma cruzi* in the carditis and neuritis of Chagas' disease, for example.[1]

As mentioned earlier, antibody is only likely to be effective when the parasite (or a parasite product such as a toxin) is in the extracellular compartment—blood, tissue spaces, secretions, etc. Even then, however, the existence of an antibody response does not ensure parasite disposal. The antibody may be of the wrong class or subclass (isotype) or of inadequate amount or affinity. Many of the effects of antibody rely on attachment of the antibody molecule not only to the antigen but also to phagocytes and/or complement, and here IgG is the most desirable isotype. Isotype switching and affinity maturation are both dependent on help from T cells, as is the development of memory. The involvement of T as well as B cells in antibody responses is therefore crucial, and protein antigen sequences from parasites are increasingly being analysed for antigenic portions, or 'epitopes', with the characteristic B-cell or T-cell recognition patterns; this is felt to be particularly important when identifying antigens for incorporation into vaccines (see below). However, one interesting class of antigens induce antibody without help from T cells; these are the 'T-independent' antigens, which are mainly repetitive carbohydrates and give rise to exclusively IgM responses without memory or affinity changes. This type of antibody is particularly characteristic of responses to the carbohydrate capsules of bacteria and was probably the first to evolve. Its importance in eukaryotic infections is hard to judge except when T cells are deficient, but the surprising lack of effect of the acquired immune deficiency syndrome (AIDS) on the severity of malaria might be a case in point, though there are other possible explanations for this (see below).

It is also, of course, essential for the antibody to have access to the antigens of the parasite, and here the 'tropical' protozoa and helminths have evolved some of the most sophisticated evasion mechanisms, ranging from the almost continuous antigenic variation of the African trypanosomes to the cloistered existence of *Echinococcus granulosus* in its hydatid cyst, into which neither lymphocytes nor antibody penetrate. Some more examples are illustrated in Table I.1.

There is great current interest in the T cells that help B cells, and a concept increasingly gaining ground is that they constitute a distinct subpopulation of CD4 T cells, referred to as TH2 in contrast to the TH1 cells whose main function is to activate macrophages (see below). These differences in biological activity are related to the secretion of different cytokines (interleukins, interferons, etc.) and, for example, the enormous levels of IgE antibody in patients with helminth infections is thought to reflect an imbalance resulting in too much TH2 and not enough TH1, though it is arguable that IgE is useful in worm infections by virtue of its ability to generate local inflammation and perhaps also bind to macrophages.

One rather undesirable effect of antibody is, via binding to Fc receptors, the enhanced uptake into macrophages of organisms that thrive there; the most striking example of this is dengue virus. Another interesting point in relation to Fc receptors is that, despite many years of careful experiment, the role of the IgG–eosinophil combination in killing helminths in vivo is still controversial.

CELL-MEDIATED RESPONSES

This term includes two very different types of response, linked by the fact that they involve T cells but not antibody, and that they depend on the recognition of antigens from intracellular parasites which are otherwise hidden from view. The cytotoxic T cell, usually of the CD8 phenotype, is well known for its antiviral potential, while the activation of macrophages and other myeloid cells, mainly by CD4 T cells, operates against intracellular parasites of all kinds.

The best-studied example of protective CD8 T-cell-mediated cytotoxicity is probably Epstein–Barr (EB) virus infection, where the cytotoxic T cell is responsible for killing the EB virus-infected B cells and terminating the disease infectious mononucleosis. If this does not happen, according to one theory, malignant transformation may occur in the B cells, and this may explain the link between EB virus, malaria and Burkitt's lymphoma—the role of the malaria being to inhibit T cell function.[2] However, cytotoxic T cells have recently been implicated in a number of non-viral infections, including *Theileria* (East Coast fever) in cattle, where they kill lymphocytes harbouring the protozoa, and *Mycobacterium leprae*, where they kill Schwann cells and liberate the bacteria, which may then be taken up by macrophages and killed or, alternatively, simply render the infection more widespread. There is no established example of a CD8 T cell directly killing an infectious organism, and it seems unlikely since the CD8 T-cell receptor is specifically tuned to recognize foreign peptides in the groove of the MHC class I molecule (in man, HLA-A, -B or -C). One of the problems with T-cell-mediated cytotoxicity has been proving that it operates in vivo, and associated with this is the fact that even in vitro it is quite cumbersome to demonstrate.

Macrophage activation by T cells is better established and is of the greatest possible value in those infections where the parasite has the ability to survive inside the normally destructive phagocytic cell, as is the case in several important chronic infections (Table I.2). Classically a macrophage unable to limit the growth within it of, for example, *Leishmania* spp. parasites, becomes able to do so when stimulated by interferon (IFN)-γ secreted by CD4 T cells; the presence of large numbers of these T cells can be demonstrated by a positive delayed-type hypersensitivity skin test, using antigens from

Table I.1 Some parasite evasion mechanisms.

Immune mechanism	Evasion strategy	Examples
Complement	Cell wall protected	*Salmonella* spp.
	Lytic complex expelled	*Leishmania* spp.
Phagocytosis	Capsule formation	*Haemophilus* spp.
	Phagolysosome blocked	Toxoplasmosis
	Oxygen radicals neutralized	Malaria
	Escape into cytoplasm	*Leishmania* spp.
	Difficult to kill	Mycobacteria
	Phagocytes destroyed	*Staphylococcus* spp. (toxins)
Antibody	Intracellular habitat	Mycobacteria
		Viruses
	Cyst formation	*Echinococcus granulosus*
	Antigen mimicry	?
	Antigenic variation	
	by mutation	Influenza, poliovirus, HIV
	by recombination	Influenza
	by gene switching	Trypanosomes
		Borrelia spp.
		Brucella spp.
	Antibody binding factors	Staphylococcus protein A
	Antibody destroyed	Bacterial proteases
T cells	Inhibition of MHC expression	Herpesvirus
		Adenovirus
	TH2 stimulation	Leprosy
	Polyclonal activation	*Staphylococcus* spp. (enterotoxins)
T and B cells	Host antigen uptake	Schistosomiasis
	Tolerance	Congenital cytomegalovirus?
	Immunosuppression	Measles, HIV
		EB virus
		Trypanosomes
		Malaria
		Toxoplasmosis

Table I.2 Some important persistent intracellular infections.

Parasite	Site of persistence	Clinical result
Herpesvirus, varicella zoster virus	Dorsal root ganglia	Recurrence
Hepatitis B	Liver	Chronic hepatitis carrier state hepatoma
EB virus	B cells	Burkitt's lymphoma
	Nasal epithelium	Nasopharyngeal cancer
HIV	T cells	AIDS
	Macrophages	
M. tuberculosis	Macrophages	Recurrence
Salmonella typhi	Macrophages	Systemic spread Carrier state
Brucella	Macrophages	Chronic infection
Toxoplasma	Macrophages	Chronic infection
Trypanosoma cruzi	Macrophages	Chronic infection
Leishmania	Macrophages	Chronic infection
Plasmodium vivax	Hepatocytes	Recurrence

Table I.3 Some activities of T lymphocytes that are mediated by cytokines.

Cytokine	Target cell	Result
IFN-γ, IL-4	Macrophage	Activation Parasite killing MHC class II increased
IFN-γ, IL-2	NK cell	Activation Virus killing
IL-1 to -6	B cell	Antibody formation
IL-5	Eosinophil	Activation Worm killing?
IL-2	CD^4 T cell CD^8 T cell	Clonal T cell growth Clonal T cell activation

the parasite in question. This somewhat oversimplifies the situation, since cytokines other than IFN-γ can activate macrophages, cells other than macrophages can be activated by cytokines, and cells other than CD^4 T cells can make these. Table I.3 illustrates some of the combinations that have been shown to be effective.

Here again the distinction between TH1 and TH2 CD^4 T cells has profound significance. For optimum control of intracellular infections the TH1 subset is required, but in certain situations it is the TH2 subset which seems to be preferentially stimulated, with the result that copious antibody is made (which is of no benefit), while macrophage activation and parasite killing are reduced or absent. Leprosy is a perfect example of this, the lepromatous form representing the TH2 and the tuberculous form the TH1 pattern of response—though the latter can also be responsible for serious tissue damage and there is still much to learn about the response in healthy contacts, who appear to have achieved the right solution without going to either extreme. Leishmaniasis is another disease where the same reasoning can be applied.

The concept of T-cell subsets distinguished by the pattern of cytokines they release has also begun to make sense of the always rather mysterious phenomenon of T-cell-mediated suppression. In general, cytokines made by TH1 cells (e.g. IFN-γ) inhibit those made by TH2 cells (e.g. interleukin (IL)-4, IL-6) with the result that antibody formation is suppressed. Contrariwise, IL-4 and IL-10 made by TH2 cells will inhibit TH1 cells—which is probably what happens in lepromatous leprosy. Thus it is no longer necessary to postulate a special lineage of 'suppressor T cells' but the phenomenon of suppression is a real one, with very real practical value; for instance it may be possible to 'switch' an inappropriate response to an appropriate one by administration of the right cytokine or cytokine inhibitor, which is why the pharmaceutical industry is busy producing monoclonal anti-cytokine antibodies, soluble receptors, etc.

IS IMMUNITY EVER PROTECTIVE?

The combination of inappropriate immune responses with sophisticated parasite evasion ensures that virtually all protozoa and helminths can avoid elimination; the only case of 'proper' self-cure with resulting immunity, in the sense that we expect it with, for example, the childhood viruses, is seen with Old World cutaneous leishmaniasis (oriental sore). However, it is nowadays accepted that the reduced parasite load with age in malaria and schistosomiasis is genuinely due to the development of a partial state of immunity, though the exact mechanisms in both cases are controversial. It should be remembered that there are also bacterial infections where immunity is precarious (e.g. tuberculosis) or non-existent (e.g. syphilis), and viral infections where it is ineffective in practice because of extensive antigenic variation (e.g. influenza, human immunodeficiency virus (HIV)).

VACCINATION

It is a safe generalization that when protective immunity develops following infection a vaccine is likely to succeed. The question is whether vaccines will ever succeed against infections that do not induce good immunity. Opinion fluctuates on this point, but is at present guardedly optimistic. Great efforts are going into the production and testing of vaccines against malaria, schistosomiasis, leishmaniasis[3] and leprosy[4] and at the research level filariasis and trypanosomiasis are targeted, though with less certain prospects. A summary of some current malaria trials and plans is given in Table I.4. In view of the extent to which industry is backing off even well-established vaccines, mainly on grounds of cost

Table I.4. Some candidate malaria vaccines.

Source of antigen	Desired response	Problems	Status
Sporozoite	Blocking antibody	Need for 100% efficiency	Two trials
Liver stage	Cytotoxic T cells?	Need for 100% efficiency	Experimental
Merozoite	Blocking antibody	Antigenic diversity	Two trials
Infected red cell	Antibody	Antigenic diversity	Experimental
	Non-specific toxicity Cytokines?	Effectiveness?	Experimental
Gametocyte	Antibody	Transmission blocking only	Experimental
Gametes	Cytokines?		
Toxic molecules	Neutralizing antibody	Not antiparasite	Experimental
Attenuated parasite	Full immunity	Reversion Transmissibility?	Experimental

and risk, this activity on behalf of tropical vaccines is a subject for admiration, for which the World Health Organization deserves much of the credit, having resolutely supplied both financial and moral support since the 1970s.

Another controversial issue is what type of vaccine to use. The three published malaria vaccine trials used simple peptides, either synthetic or recombinant, in one case coupled to tetanus toxoid to supply T-cell epitopes, and usually injected with alum as adjuvant. Protection was moderate but significant. The next generation of vaccines will probably incorporate T-cell epitopes from the parasite itself. Malaria is unusual among protozoa for its complex life cycle, all stages of which are being considered as potential targets, as well as vaccines that would block transmission or operate against the toxic effects only (Table I.4). At the opposite extreme is a *Leishmania* spp. vaccine simply composed of killed promastigotes mixed with BCG, which is claimed to be as protective as 60 days of chemotherapy. The traditional practice of 'leishmanization' (exposure to mild lesions on the lines reputedly used by the ancient Chinese for smallpox) has encouraged some workers to think in terms of attenuated vaccines that might ultimately replace the wild population, as attenuated (Sabin) polio virus vaccine is doing, but the logistic problems are immense.

IMMUNOPATHOLOGY

Immune responses that do not achieve their purpose within a few weeks very often cause tissue damage to the host, and nowhere is this more true than with chronic tropical infections. All four of the classical types of hypersensitivity are seen (Table I.5), and sometimes they are responsible for almost all the symptoms of infection. Schistosomiasis is an example where, judging by single-sex experiments in animals, the worms themselves are perfectly well tolerated but their eggs, deposited in the liver or bladder wall, induce T-cell-mediated granulomas that can ultimately kill the patient. Hydatid disease is an infection in which the symptoms are due mainly to the large space-occupying cysts (largely a host fibrotic response to the worms), with the added possibility, upon cyst rupture, of life-threatening anaphylaxis due to the encounter of massive amounts of worm antigen and IgE-loaded mast cells. In *Plasmodium falciparum* malaria there has always been debate as to the cause of the very diverse symptoms, and interest is currently being focused on the possibility that many of them may be secondary to the overproduction of cytokines, notably tumour necrosis factor (TNF). TNF has been found in the blood of severely ill malaria patients, and the levels correlate with the incidence of cerebral malaria and of hypoglycaemia. In animal models, evidence has also been obtained for a role of TNF in pulmonary oedema and anaemia. However, a clinical trial of monoclonal antibody to TNF furnished statistically significant evidence for a role of TNF only in fever, and larger numbers will be needed to establish further correlations.[5] The roles of other cytokines such as IL-1, which resembles TNF in many of its actions, and of IFN-γ, also deserve investigation.

Table I.5 Some immunopathological consequences of infection.

Hypersensitivity type*	Mechanism involved	Examples
I (allergic) (anaphylactic)	IgE Mast cells, basophils	Ascaris (lung) Schistosomiasis (swimmers' itch) Hydatid cyst rupture
II (antibody-mediated)	IgG Complement Autoantibody	Malaria anaemia? *Trypanosoma cruzi* Streptococci
III (complex mediated)	Immune complexes Complement Neutrophils	Malaria (kidney) Trypanosomiasis Schistosomiasis Streptococci
IV (cell-mediated)	T cells Macrophages Eosinophils Cytokines	Schistosomiasis (egg granuloma) Tuberculosis Tuberculoid leprosy (granuloma) Lymphatic filariasis

*Gell and Coombs' classification.

IMMUNODEFICIENCY

The much more serious course run by certain worldwide diseases in tropical countries, for example measles, meningococcal infection and gastroenteritis, is mainly due to the lowered immune status of the patients. Often it is not possible to pinpoint the reason for this, since inhabitants of the tropics are exposed to such a large number of different causes of immunodeficiency. Tables I.6 and I.7 list the most important of these, and it can be seen that the two major categories are malnutrition and infection—which of course frequently occur together.

The links between nutrition and immunity are much more complex than might be supposed. Many diseases are undoubtedly more severe in patients who are malnourished or underweight, measles being among the most striking examples. Occasionally the opposite is true, as in the case of malaria, where iron deficiency inhibits the growth of the parasite and restoration of nutrition may induce a flare-up of the infection. A distinction is usually made between calorie deprivation and protein deprivation, the latter being generally more serious because both cell-mediated and antibody responses are impaired. There are also specific effects of deficiencies of iron, zinc, copper and vitamins on immune performance (see Table I.6). For a fuller discussion of this topic the reader is referred to specialist textbooks.[6,7]

Immunosuppression as a result of infection is extremely common, though it has usually proved very difficult to analyse the precise mechanisms involved, some of which have only been properly demonstrated in vitro (Table I.7). Thanks to the existence of animal models, malaria and African trypanosomiasis have been studied in particular detail, and the reality of the problem is well illustrated by the finding that treatment of even quite mild malaria improves the ability of patients to respond to unrelated vaccines (pneumococcal and meningococcal). Measles has long been known to suppress T-cell responses and predispose to secondary infection, but all previous examples have been put in the shade by HIV, the most immunosuppressive and the most intensively studied parasite ever.

AIDS AND TROPICAL INFECTIONS

The impact of AIDS in the tropics has, of course, been catastrophic. The original assumption that all the complications were due to a simple infection and destruction of CD^4 T cells has turned out to be greatly oversimplified, and current research is also focused on the effects of HIV on macrophages, antigen-presenting cells, B cells and the cytokine network. It was a protozoan (or perhaps, according to recent data, fungal) infection, *Pneumocystis carinii*, that first drew attention, at the beginning of the 1980s, to the impending AIDS epidemic, and this strange parasite remains a major cause of death in AIDS patients in the developed world, along with *Toxoplasma*, *Cryptococcus*, *Cryptosporidium* and other previously rare organisms. However, in tropical countries it is mycobacterial infections which have been most dramatically enhanced by AIDS, not only *Mycobacterium tuberculosis* but also the normally well-controlled *M. avium*, while some other parasites have been surprisingly unaffected. Malaria, for instance, shows virtually no change in either the density or the severity of infection, and nor, so far, do intestinal parasites such as *Entamoeba* or *Giardia*, or the major helminths.[8] Parasite immunologists are still digesting the implications of these unexpected findings, which seem to point to a particularly suppressive effect of HIV on those T cells that are concerned with parasites inhabiting macrophages, though *Pneumocystis* remains a puzzle because the parasite lives extracellularly in the lung alveoli. A sinister aspect of the relationship between HIV and *M. avium* is that each infection appears to enhance both the growth of the

Table I.6   Some immunodeficiency syndromes secondary to malnutrition.

Deficiency	Immune components affected	Effect on disease
Calorie (marasmus)	Neutrophils Complement T cells	Bacterial infections Virus infections Tuberculosis
Protein–calorie (kwashiorkor)	T cells Antibody Macrophages	All infections Vaccines
Iron	Neutrophils	Bacterial infections Malaria reduced?
Zinc, copper	T cells	Most infections Tuberculosis Fungal infections
Vitamin A	T cells	Most infections Tuberculosis

Table I.7 Some infections that cause immunodeficiency.

Infection	Immune components affected	Effect on disease
HIV	CD^4 T cells, macrophages	Opportunistic infection *Pneumocystis corinii* *Toxoplasma gondii* Tuberculosis
Measles	T cells, neutrophils	Pneumonia, otitis
Leprosy	T cells (TH1 only?)	Dissemination
Malaria	Antibody T cells	Vaccines impaired Burkitt's lymphoma?
Trypanosomiasis (African)	Antibody	Bacterial infection

Table I.8 Viruses, cancer and immunity.

Virus implicated	Tumour	Immune or other component
EB virus	Burkitt's lymphoma Nasopharyngeal carcinoma	Immunosuppression by malaria? High EB virus antibody Dietary carcinogens?
Hepatitis B	Hepatic carcinoma	Neonatal tolerance to virus? Aflatoxins
Papilloma	Cervical carcinoma	
Cytomegalovirus?	Kaposi's sarcoma	Immunosuppression by HIV

other within macrophages and the clinical progress of the disease, and it has been proposed that these effects are mediated by cytokines such as IL-1 and TNF.

IMMUNODEFICIENCY AND CANCER

Some of the best evidence for a role of the immune system in preventing malignancy comes from tropical conditions. In four tropical tumours a virus has been implicated, and in two, Burkitt's lymphoma and Kaposi's sarcoma, immuno-deficiency appears to be a contributory factor (Table I.8). Burkitt's lymphoma was recognized by Burkitt himself to have a very similar distribution to malaria in Africa and Papua New Guinea, and although the full aetiology is still not established, one plausible theory is that malaria suppresses the normal cytotoxic T-cell response against the EB virus-infected B cells. The precise stage at which the well-known translocation of the c-*myc* proto-oncogene to one or other of the immunoglobulin gene loci occurs is not clear.[2] Kaposi's sarcoma is found mainly in patients with T-cell deficiencies, including AIDS. However Kaposi's sarcoma is not particularly associated with malaria, nor is Burkitt's lymphoma with AIDS, which again emphasizes the range of different defects to which T cells are susceptible.

IMMUNODIAGNOSIS

Most tropical infections are diagnosed by a combination of clinical and microbiological/parasitological skills, and though numerous immunodiagnostic methods exist, they nearly all suffer from imprecision due to non-specificity.[9] This applies equally to skin tests and laboratory assays for serum antibody. The detection of parasite antigen by mono-clonal antibodies represents a definite step forward, since these reagents can usually be made specific for antigens unique to one parasite species. They have also proved invalu-able for charting the distribution of, for example, variant populations of trypanosomes or malaria parasites, and in studies in which correlations have been looked for between clinical protection and particular serum antibodies, as a prelude to the choice of antigens for vaccines. The poly-merase chain reaction enables the detection of DNA or RNA from numbers of organisms far too small to be picked up in any other way, but must be regarded as still experi-mental.[10]

REFERENCES

1 Rose N R, Beisel K W, Herskowitz A et al. Cardiac myosin and autoimmune myocarditis. *Ciba Found Symp* 1987; 129:3–18.

2 Facer C A & Playfair J H L. Malaria. Epstein–Barr virus, and the genesis of lymphomas. *Adv Cancer Res* 1989; 53:33–72.

3 Playfair J H L, Blackwell J M & Miller H R P. Parasitic diseases. In Moxon R (ed.) *Modern Vaccines*. London: Edward Arnold, 1990: 129–136.

4 Fine P E M & Rodrigues L C. In Moxon R (ed.) *Modern Vaccines*. London: Edward Arnold, 1990: 67–74.

5 Kwiatkowski D, Molyneux M E, Stephens S. et al. Anti-TNF therapy inhibits fever in cerebral malaria. *Quart J Med* 1993; 86:91–98.

6 Greenwood B M & Whittle H C. *Immunology of Medicine in the Tropics*. London: Edward Arnold, 1981.

7 Chandra R K & Newberne P M. *Nutrition, Immunity and Infection*. London: Plenum Press, 1977.

8 Lockwood D N J & Weber J N. Parasite infections in AIDS. *Parasitol Today* 1989; 5:310–316.

9 Houba V (ed.) Immunological investigation of tropical parasitic diseases. *Practical Methods in Clinical Immunology*, vol 2. Edinburgh: Churchill Livingstone.

10 Hayden J D, Ho S A, Hawkey P M, Taylor G R & Quirke P. The promises and pitfalls of P C R. *Rev Med Microbiol* 1991; 2:129–137.

APPENDIX II

PARASITIC PROTOZOA

J. R. Baker

Protozoa can be broadly defined as single-celled organisms which have animal-like nutrition (i.e. they do not contain photosynthetic pigment). Structurally, protozoa are equivalent to a single animal cell; functionally, they are equivalent to a whole animal. Each protozoan cell has all the normal metazoan cellular organelles: nucleus, mitochondria, ribosomes, Golgi apparatus, etc., although some may have been lost in certain specialized organisms. Many protozoa also possess unique organelles not found in metazoa.

Parasites can, equally broadly, be defined as organisms which live within organs or tissues of other organisms during some or all stages of their life cycle, and obtain nutrients either from the host organism's food supply or from its tissues. The processes by which these nutrients are digested, and the processes of respiration by which protozoa obtain their energy, do not differ fundamentally from those operating in other animal cells.

All protozoa reproduce asexually, by various forms of division—binary or multiple—or by budding; some also reproduce sexually, usually by division after some form of genetic exchange. Some parasitic protozoa utilize only one species of host in their life cycle, others require two. If only asexual reproduction occurs in one host, and sexual reproduction in the other, the former is termed the intermediate host and the latter is called the definitive host. Irrespective of this terminology, if one host is much smaller than the other it is often referred to as the vector. This is especially true, anthropocentrically, in human medicine, when the mosquito (for example) which infects a human being with malaria is referred to as the vector even though, on the preceding definition, it is also the definitive host. Non-human (usually mammalian) hosts which may be infected with the same stages of a parasite as the human, and from which the latter may acquire infection either directly or via a vector, are termed reservoir hosts.

There is, unfortunately, no agreement among experts about taxonomic schemes for protozoa. An attractively simple scheme, which none the less takes account of modern developments in tracing relationships between groups, is that devised by Cox[1] shown in abbreviated form in Table II.1. The four major groups are based on the type (or absence) of their locomotory organelles. The groups contain one or more phyla, each of which is (hopefully) a reasonably homogenous assemblage.

Most parasites are rarely, if ever, significantly harmful to their hosts. These are of marginal importance in human medicine, except in so far as they may be mistaken for other, potentially more harmful, forms. Even those which are capable of causing severe illness or death of the host do not necessarily always do so. The host–parasite relationship can be thought of as a delicate balance which may easily be tipped in favour of one partner or the other.

Table II.1 Classification of the major protozoan parasites of humans (based on that of Cox[1]).

Flagellates (locomotion by flagella)
  Phylum Metamonada: *Giardia, Trichomonas*
  Phylum Kinetoplasta: *Leishmania, Trypanosoma*
  Incertae sedis*: *Naegleria*

Amoebae (locomotion by pseudopodia)
  Phylum Rhizopoda: *Entamoeba, Acanthamoeba*

Sporozoa (locomotion by 'gliding'—no obvious locomotory organelle)
  Phylum Apicomplexa (or Sporozoa)
    Class Coccidea: *Toxoplasma, Sarcosystis, Isospora*
    Class Haemosporidea: *Plasmodium*
    Class Piroplasmea: *Babesia*

Microsporidia (with unicellular resistant spores)
  Phylum Microsporea: *Encephalitozoon, Nosema, Pleistophora, Enterocytozoon, Septata*

Ciliates (locomotion by cilia)
  Phylum Ciliophora: *Balantidium*

---

*Of uncertain taxonomic position.

MALARIA PARASITES (See also Chapter 61)

Four species of the genus *Plasmodium* infect humans: *P. falciparum*, *P. malariae*, *P. ovale* and *P. vivax*; the diseases they cause are known, respectively, as malignant tertian malaria, quartan malaria, ovale tertian malaria and benign tertian malaria.

LIFE CYCLE AND MORPHOLOGY

The life cycle of *P. vivax* is shown in Figures II.1 and II.2. When an infected mosquito bites a human, malaria sporozoites are injected with the insect's saliva. Within 30 minutes they have entered liver parenchyma cells (possibly via the Kupffer cells). *P. vivax* and *P. ovale* produce two kinds of sporozoites, those which continue their development inside the hepatic cells immediately, and others (hypnozoites) which remain dormant for some time before doing so (see below). Sooner or later the sporozoites commence nuclear division, and are then known as meronts (or schizonts). After producing several thousand nuclei, the meront undergoes cytoplasmic division to form a large number of small, uninucleate merozoites. Mature liver (exoerythrocytic) meronts may be as large as 50–60 μm in diameter (Figure II.3). The merozoites are freed by the rupture of the meront and enter the circulation, where they penetrate erythrocytes. They are

now known as trophozoites. Very young trophozoites consist of a small hollow sphere of cytoplasm with a central vacuole and one small nucleus; when viewed through a microscope in optical section they resemble a tiny signet ring, and hence are often referred to as 'ring forms'. Electron microscopy has shown that the trophozoites are contained within a parasitophorous vacuole, the limiting membrane of which is formed, at least in part, by the erythrocyte's surface membrane, which is invaginated by the entering merozoite and then becomes separated from the cell surface. As the trophozoite grows, the central vacuole disappears and the characteristic black or brown malarial pigment begins to appear. This pigment is formed by the insoluble iron-containing part of the haemoglobin molecule, ingested by the parasite as it feeds on its host cell's cytoplasm.

As the trophozoite continues to grow, its nucleus begins to divide: it, too, becomes a meront but this time the division process (merogony or schizogony) produces only 24 (or fewer) merozoites. The number depends on the species (Table II.2, which also lists other characteristics of the exo- and intraerythrocytic forms of the four species). When these intraerythrocytic merozoites are released by the rupture of the containing erythrocyte, they rapidly enter other erythrocytes and the cycle of erythrocytic merogony is repeated, unless terminated by the host's immune response or its death,

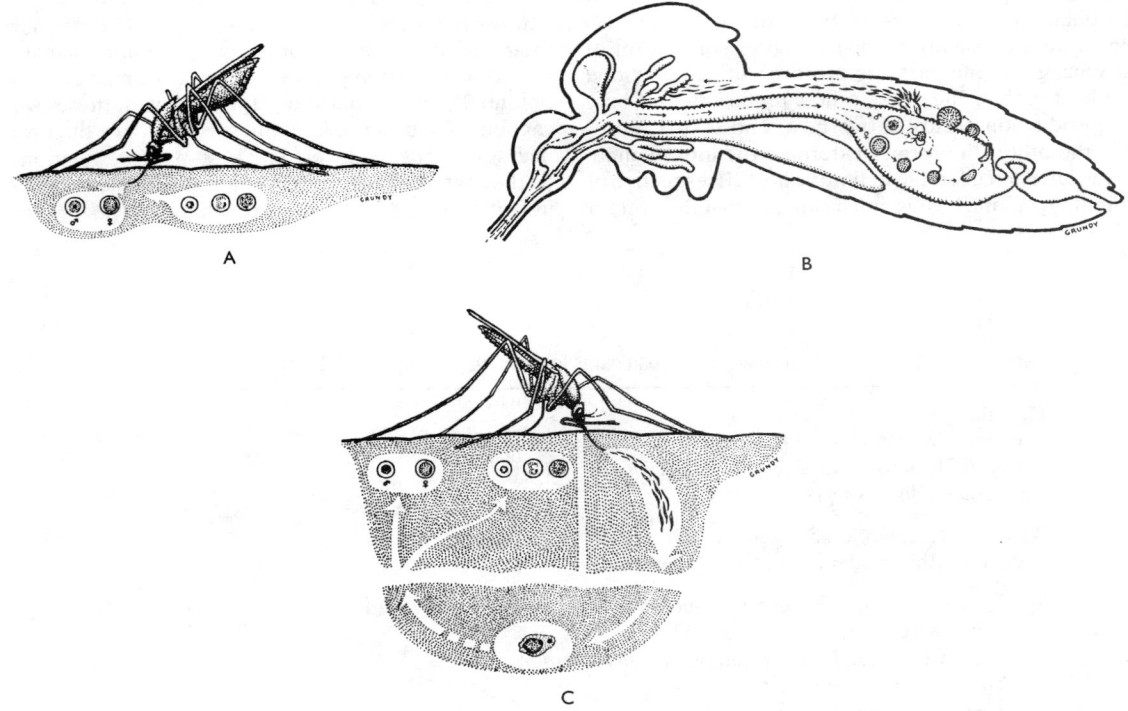

Figure II.1 Life cycle of the malaria parasite. A, Female *Anopheles* ingests gametocytes while feeding on the blood of an infected person; B, gametogony and sporogony occur within and on the stomach of the mosquito, culminating in the appearance of sporozoites in the salivary glands one week or more later (see Figure II.2); C, the infective mosquito injects sporozoites into the blood of the next person on whom it feeds. The sporozoites then enter the liver cells, within 30 minutes or so, to commence exoerythrocytic merogony (schizogony), unless they are dormant hypnozoites of *P. vivax* or *P. ovale* (see text). Depending on the species, exoerythrocytic merogony is completed in 5½ to 15 days (see Table II.2), and the emerging merozoites enter erythrocytes to initiate the erythrocytic phase of the life cycle; in non-immune subjects, a clinical attack of malaria usually develops within 2 to 5 days. (The diagrams of mosquitoes and parasites are not to scale.) (Drawing by J. Hull Grundy).

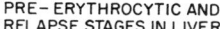

PRE – ERYTHROCYTIC AND
RELAPSE STAGES IN LIVER

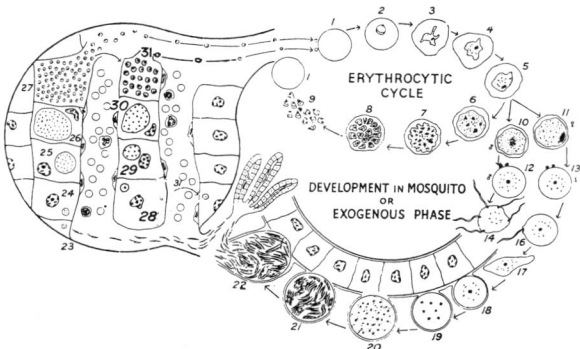

Figure II.2 Diagrammatic representation of the life cycle of malaria parasites. 1, Normal erythrocytes; 2–5, erythrocytes containing young parasites (trophozoites); 6–8, erythrocytic merogony (schizogony); 9, rupture of cell containing mature meront (schizont) with release of merozoites into the plasma and subsequent reinvasion of other erythrocytes. 10, 11, Microgametocyte (male) and macrogametocyte (female) within erythrocytes; 12, 13, extracellular gametocytes in the stomach of a female *Anopheles*; 14, production of eight male microgametes by the microgametocyte ('exflagellation'); 15, the macrogametocyte matures into a macrogamete; 16, one microgamete fertilizes the macrogamete; 17, the resulting motile zygote (ookinete) penetrates the wall of the mosquito's stomach; 18–21, the ookinete encysts on the outer surface of the stomach to form an oocyst, which undergoes sporogony to produce hundreds of sporozoites. 22, The mature oocyst ruptures, releasing the sporozoites into the mosquito's haemocoel, where they enter the cells and ducts of the salivary glands (22a). When the mosquito next feeds, sporozoites are injected with the saliva into the host's bloodstream. 23–27, The sporozoites enter hepatocytes and commence exoerythrocytic merogony, culminating in the release of merozoites back into the bloodstream, where they enter erythrocytes (1, 2) to start the erythrocytic merogony cycle. With *P. vivax* and *P. ovale*, some sporozoites are of a special type (hypnozoites); these remain dormant as unicellular bodies within hepatocytes for up to many months. 28, Liver cell containing a hypnozoite; 29–31, subsequent exoerythrocytic merogony of the hypnozoite, with release of merozoites into the blood to initiate a relapse.

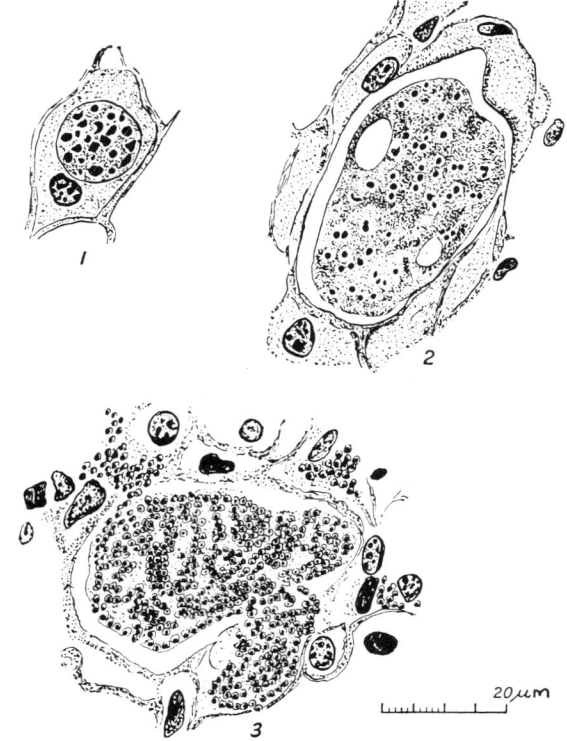

Figure II.3 Exoerythrocytic meronts of malaria parasites in liver parenchyma cells (hepatocytes). 1. *P. cynomolgi* (a species which infects monkeys but not humans) on the fifth day of its development. 2. *P. vivax* on the seventh day. 3. *P. vivax* on the eighth day; the meront is mature and merozoites can be seen escaping into the blood sinuses.

or by chemotherapy. *P. vivax* and, to a lesser extent, *P. ovale* cause the host red blood cell to enlarge and, in the case of *P. ovale*, it seems to become easily deformed; during the making of a thin blood film, the host cell may be drawn out into an irregular oval, hence the parasite's specific name. Other changes may become apparent in the host cell: marks (visible when stained) appear on the surface membrane. These may be very fine and faint (Ziemann's stippling), fine but more distinct (Schüffner's dots), or relatively large and coarse and fewer in number (Maurer's clefts) (Table II.2).

Not all the merozoites develop into another generation of meronts. Some grow into the sexual cells or gametocytes. The male or microgametocyte has paler cytoplasm and a larger, less intensely staining nucleus than the female macrogametocyte. The latter has cytoplasm which stains more intensely blue with Romanovsky stains because it contains a much larger number of ribosomes than does the male. The gametocytes do not develop any further in the human host; under natural conditions their continued development

depends on their being ingested by a feeding female mosquito of the genus *Anopheles* (male mosquitoes do not feed on blood).

In the mosquito's stomach the mature gametocytes leave their host red cells and become gametes. This process is imperceptible in the female, but the male gametocyte produces eight long motile male gametes (microgametes) by a process known as 'exflagellation'. The process is rapid; within a few minutes at most, the male nucleus has divided into eight, and eight lashing flagella erupt from the gametocyte's surface. One nucleus enters each flagellum, which possibly also possesses a mitochondrion, and the 'flagella' (now uninucleate microgametes) break free and swim through the blood meal in search of a female. All stages of *Plasmodium* within the vertebrate host are haploid, as are the gametes. After fertilization of a macrogamete by one microgamete, within the mosquito's midgut, a diploid zygote is formed. This zygote elongates and glides (in a fashion not fully understood) through the blood meal and into one of the cells of the midgut wall, in which it rounds up and secretes a thin cyst wall around itself. The motile zygote is called an ookinete, but once it has encysted it becomes an oocyst. The oocyst enlarges considerably, bulging outwards into the mosquito's haemocoel but still remaining within the basement membrane of the midgut wall. At the same time it undergoes a series of nuclear divisions, the first of which is a reduction (meiotic) division, followed by cytoplasmic cleavage in a

Table II.2 Species of *Plasmodium* which infect humans.

Species	Geographical distribution	Duration of merogony		No. of merozoites per meront		Main morphological characteristics of erythrocytic forms				
		Exoerythrocytic (days)	Erythrocytic (hours)	Exoerythrocytic	Erythrocytic	'Ring' form	Trophozoite	Meront	Gametocyte	Host erythrocyte*
P. vivax	Worldwide, in tropical, subtropical and warmer temperate regions	8	48	~10 000	12–24	At least one-third diameter of erythrocyte	Amoeboid	10 μm diameter	Round or ovoid, male: 9 μm, female: 10–11 μm	Enlarged, stippled ('Schüffner's dots')
P. malariae	Worldwide but scattered, mainly tropical and subtropical	14–15	72	~15 000	6–12	At least one-third diameter of erythrocyte	Compact, often bandlike	7 μm diameter	Round or ovoid, 7 μm	Not enlarged; very faint ('Ziemann's') stippling after prolonged staining only
P. ovale	Tropical Africa; also occasionally in other parts of tropics and subtropics (possibly of exogenous origin)	9	48	~15 000	6–12 (12–24 in relapses)	At least one-third diameter of erythrocyte	Compact	7 μm (larger in relapses)	Round or ovoid, 9 μm	Slightly enlarged, stippled ('Schüffner's dots'); may be distorted and elongated
P. falciparum	Worldwide, in tropics, subtropics and warmer temperate regions	5½	48	~30 000	8–24	Very small at first; two nuclei commonly; some apparently on edge of cell (accolé forms)	Compact; rarely seen in peripheral blood	5 μm; rarely seen in peripheral blood	Crescentic, male: 9–11 μm long, female: 12–14 μm	Not enlarged; often with fewer larger dots ('Maurer's clefts')

*These alterations do not develop until some growth of the parasite has occurred.

fashion similar to that undergone by the exoerythrocytic meront. The process within the oocyst, however, is termed sporogony and the resulting small, elongate, uninucleate cells are the sporozoites; several thousand are produced within each oocyst.

The sporozoites are then liberated from the rupturing oocyst into the mosquito's haemocoel, from where some, at least, find their way to the salivary glands in the insect's thorax. They penetrate the salivary gland lumen, and are injected into the bloodstream of the next vertebrate on which the mosquito feeds. The developmental cycle in the mosquito takes between about 1 and 4 weeks, depending on the ambient temperature (the higher the temperature, the shorter the cycle).

GEOGRAPHICAL DISTRIBUTION

P. falciparum is the most common species in tropical and subtropical areas, and may sometimes be found in warmer temperate regions. *P. malariae* is also distributed in the tropics and subtropics, but is less common than *P. falciparum* and its distribution tends to be patchy. *P. ovale*, the least common malaria parasite of humans, is probably restricted to Africa; the few cases reported from the western Pacific region may have been introduced or the result of a chance transmission from an imported case.

P. malariae is the only human malaria parasite to have another natural vertebrate host, the chimpanzee (*Pan troglodytes*), but this is of little, if any, epidemiological significance. The other species can experimentally infect splenectomized chimpanzees and monkeys (e.g. *Aotus* and *Macaca*).

PATHOGENESIS

The characteristic fever peaks of malaria result from synchronization of the intraerythrocytic merogony cycle. Simultaneous rupture of many erythrocytes, with the concomitant release of parasite debris and malarial pigment, causes a rise in fever. Destruction of the erythrocytes also leads to anaemia. Hepatic meronts do not seem to be pathogenic.

Erythrocytes infected with *P. falciparum* also adhere to the walls of capillaries, possibly due to their developing knoblike protrusions (visible by electron microscopy only); this can lead to capillary blockage and rupture, with haemorrhage into the surrounding tissue. Another consequence of this adhesion of infected cells is that it is rare for stages of *P. falciparum* other than ring-form trophozoites and gameto-

cytes to be seen in films of peripheral blood, as the older trophozoites and meronts are sequestered in the small blood vessels.

The enlargement of the spleen, which is a characteristic of malaria, results from proliferation of the host's mononuclear phagocytic system in response to the presence of the parasite.

Untreated malaria (if not fatal) is notoriously persistent, with recurring bouts of fever sometimes lasting for many years. In infections with *P. vivax* or *P. ovale* these recurrences may result from the reactivation of dormant hypnozoites lying within the hepatocytes, even when parasites have been eliminated from the blood by chemotherapy or the host's immune response. In a subspecies of *P. vivax*, *P. v. hibernans*, all the sporozoites are hypnozoites. The first clinical attack of malaria therefore does not occur until several months after the infective mosquito bite. This was an adaptation for survival of the parasite in a cooler climate, in which adult mosquitoes did not survive through the winter and so the parasite could not be transmitted to another host. *P. v. hibernans* is now restricted to temperate zones around the Mediterranean sea, in the Middle East and parts of China, but its range used to extend as far north as the Netherlands and southern England (the malaria parasite which existed in England was certainly *P. vivax*, but it is only assumed that it was *P. v. hibernans*).

Hypnozoites do not exist in *P. falciparum* or *P. malariae*. Recurrences of clinical malaria in patients infected with these species are due to the survival of small numbers of erythrocytic parasites, which persist at a low level until the host's immune response wanes sufficiently to permit their multiplication to a level sufficient to cause clinical illness once more. There is evidence that at least some species of *Plasmodium* can undergo antigenic variation—a structural change in their surface antigen—rather like the process in trypanosomes (see below), but it is less well understood in malaria parasites.

DIAGNOSIS

A clinical diagnosis, based on recurrent fever and splenomegaly, needs confirmation by the finding of parasites in stained thin or (usually) thick blood films. Serodiagnosis is also used, especially in surveys, but again needs confirmation by blood film examination as a positive serological test does not necessarily indicate active infection. The tests used include indirect immunofluorescence (IFAT), enzyme linked immunosorbent assay (ELISA) and indirect haemagglutination (IHA). IFAT is probably the best, but needs expensive equipment for fluorescence microscopy.

TRYPANOSOMES (See also Chapters 63 and 64)

Trypanosomes (genus *Trypanosoma*) are elongated protozoa with a single flagellum. They share with the leishmanial parasites (see below) the possession of an unusually large amount of mitochondrial DNA, which forms a structure

called the kinetoplast lying within the mitochondrion and, measuring from one to several micrometres in diameter, easily visible by light microscopy. The ordinal name, Kinetoplastida, is derived from the name of this organelle.

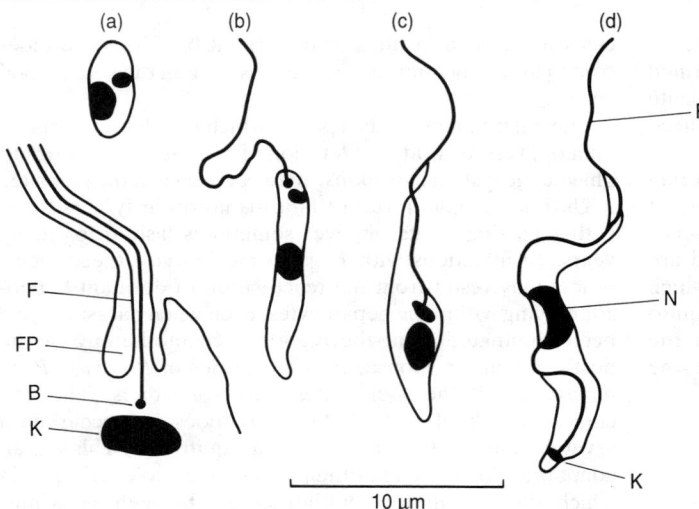

Figure II.4   The various forms which may develop in the life cycle of species of *Leishmania* and *Trypanosoma*. (a) Amastigote (= micromastigote), (b) promastigote, (c) epimastigote, and (d) trypomastigote (only the first two occur in *Leishmania*). B, basal body; F, flagellum; FP, flagellar pocket; K, kinetoplast; N, nucleus. (Slightly modified from Baker J R. *Companion to Microbiology* (Bull A T & Meadow P M editors) London 1987: Longman, pp. 431–457.)

LIFE CYCLE AND MORPHOLOGY

Like malaria parasites, trypanosomes have two hosts in the course of their life cycle: a vertebrate and an invertebrate vector. In the vertebrate host trypanosomes can exist in two forms (Figure II.4). The first is elongate, motile and extra-cellular; the origin of the flagellum is near the posterior end of the cell and the flagellum emerges through the flagellar pocket to run forwards along the margin of the cell, to which it is attached by a series of hemidesmosomes. As the flagellum undulates, it pulls out the surface membrane of the cell into a thin membrane-like structure called the undulating membrane. At the anterior end of the cell the flagellum may terminate or it may extend further forward. This form is called a trypomastigote. The second form is a non-motile, intracellular, more or less spherical cell called an amastigote (or micromastigote), which has at the most a very short, rudimentary flagellum.

Other stages may develop in the invertebrate host (Figure II.4). These include epimastigotes, in which the flagellar origin is close to the nucleus near the centre of the elongate cell, from whence it extends forward to form, as in the trypomastigote, an undulating membrane, and promasti-gotes, in which the flagellar origin is anterior and there is consequently no undulating membrane. In some species sphaeromastigotes also develop; these are small and spheri-cal, but differ from amastigotes in having a flagellum coiled around the outside of the cell.

As far as is known, trypanosomes reproduce only by binary fission; they are uninucleate except when in the process of division. There is good evidence that some form of genetic exchange occurs, at least in the species *T. brucei*, during the course of development in the vector, but this appears to be an occasional process and details are completely unknown.

Three species of *Trypanosoma* can infect humans: *T. brucei*, *T. cruzi* and *T. rangeli*; they are classified in three distinct subgenera—*Trypanozoon*, *Schizotrypanum* and *Tejeraia*, respectively.

TRYPANOSOMA BRUCEI

LIFE CYCLE AND MORPHOLOGY

In the vertebrate host (humans and other mammals), only trypomastigotes occur. These are variable in form (pleomor-phic) (Figures II.5 and II.6); long, slender cells with a considerable length of free anterior flagellum appear to be those which undergo longitudinal binary fission in the blood and tissue fluids of the host, while shorter, broader ('stumpy') forms, with little or no free anterior flagellum, seem not to divide while in the vertebrate but serve to continue the life cycle in the vector, a large blood-sucking dipteran fly of the genus *Glossina*. There are intermediate forms between these two extremes, although it is probable that, while slender forms transform into the broader forms, the reverse does not occur. (This interpretation of the signifi-cance of the forms, while probably generally accepted, is not universally agreed and is, to some extent, still speculative.)

Once ingested with its blood meal by a *Glossina* (tsetse fly), both sexes of which feed exclusively on blood, the trypomastigotes elongate still more to form the so-called procyclic trypomastigotes. These forms undergo binary fission, and have a fully active, large single mitochondrion and a functional Krebs' cycle, as do the subsequent stages which develop in the vector, apart from the final, metacyclic forms. The stages occurring in the mammal, however, pos-sess only an inactive mitochondrion and their respiration, though aerobic, is glycolytic and proceeds only as far as the production of pyruvate.

The procyclic trypomastigotes are at first confined within the peritrophic membrane, a chitinous tube which lines the tsetse's midgut and surrounds its blood meal, but they later appear outside this membrane but still within the midgut, presumably to prevent their being expelled with the fly's faeces. They also appear in the anterior portion of the midgut (the proventriculus), and eventually they reach the lumen of the salivary glands. The details of the route by which they reach the glands are still controversial. In the salivary glands,

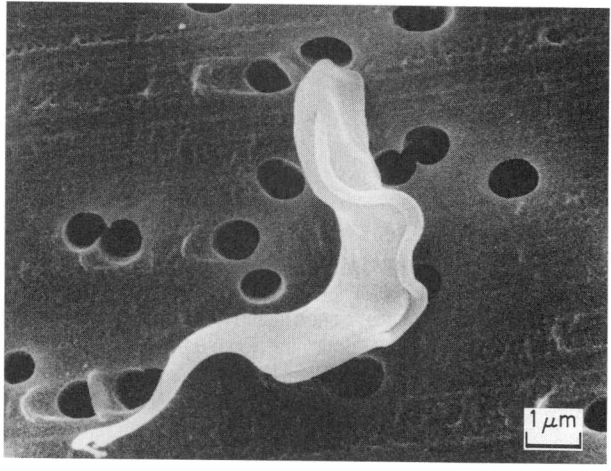

(a)

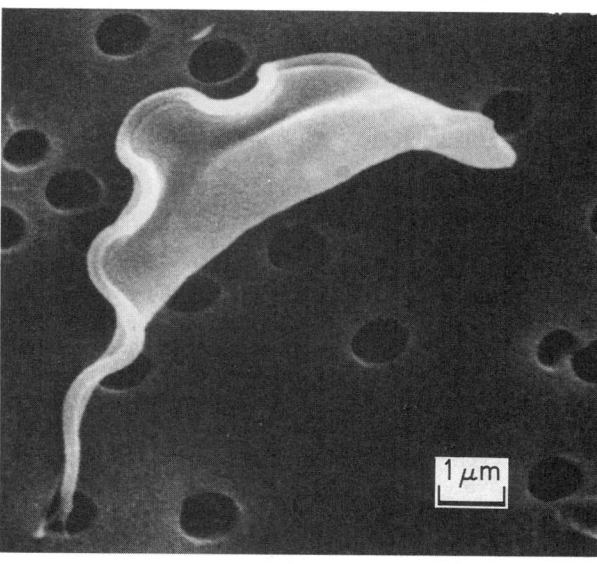

(b)

Figure II.5 Scanning electron micrographs of (a) long slender form and (b) short stumpy form of *Trypanosoma brucei*. (Micrographs by L. Tetley from Vickerman K & Tetley L. *Ann Soc Belge Méd Trop* 1977; 57: 441.)

epimastigotes appear, attached by their flagella to the wall of the glands. The epimastigotes eventually change again into short trypomastigotes, with at most a very short, free flagellum; these are the infective metacyclic trypomastigotes, which are injected with the fly's saliva into the next mammal on which it feeds (Figure II.7). The metacyclic trypomastigotes appear to respire in a similar fashion to the forms which live in the mammal, without participation of the single mitochondrion. Another way in which the metacyclic forms resemble those in the vertebrate is in their possession of a glycoprotein coat on the outer surface of the cell membrane (which is not present on procyclic trypomastigotes or epimastigotes). The life cycle in the tsetse fly takes about 2–3 weeks from ingestion of trypomastigotes to the appearance of metacyclic forms in the salivary glands.

Under natural conditions, for reasons not fully understood, in only a very small percentage of flies which ingest trypanosomes is the life cycle completed (fewer than 1%); in most flies the trypanosomes either fail to become established in, or fail to develop beyond, the midgut. However, once a fly does become infective (with trypomastigotes in its salivary glands), it appears to remain so for the rest of its life.

After injection into a susceptible mammal by the feeding fly, the metacyclic trypomastigotes transform into slender forms and commence division. At first they are more or less restricted to the tissue fluid around the site of the bite, where they cause the development of an inflamed trypanosomal chancre, but after a few days they spread throughout the body via the bloodstream and ultimately penetrate the central nervous system (CNS) and appear in the cerebrospinal fluid (CSF).

In the vertebrate host's bloodstream, antibodies are produced against the protein of the trypanosomes' surface glycoprotein coat and these antibodies, in the presence of complement, lyse the parasites. However, the molecular architecture of the coat is genetically controlled, and by complex processes of gene rearrangement and deregulation it is repeatedly changed. The 'new' coat is not recognized by the host's antibodies, and parasites bearing it can continue to multiply until fresh antibody specific for the restructured coat appears. Parasitaemia thus forms a series of waves, each wave consisting of a different variant antigenic type (VAT) of trypanosome. The process of changing the surface glycoprotein (also known as the variant surface glycoprotein or VSG) can occur at least 100 times or more, and may be limitless. This antigenic variation does not occur in a rigidly fixed sequence, but neither is it entirely random; much still remains to be learned about the details of the process. Its occurrence, needless to say, bedevils attempts to develop an effective antitrypanosome vaccine.

GEOGRAPHICAL DISTRIBUTION

T. brucei is restricted to tropical Africa because its vectors, *Glossina* spp., are similarly restricted. Within these limits, however, it is by no means evenly distributed. *Glossina* and, therefore, *T. brucei*, do not occur at altitudes above about 1800 metres at the most, almost certainly due to the temperature.

The infraspecific taxonomy of *T. brucei* is at present (1995) in a state of flux and somewhat confused. The 'classical' view that there were three species of tsetse-transmitted trypanosomes in Africa, *T. brucei*, *T. rhodesiense* and *T. gambiense* (with only the latter two infecting humans), has long been discarded in favour of a closer relationship, the three categories being reduced to subspecies of *T. brucei*. Even this view is now seen to be too simplistic, and current thinking is that *T. brucei* is composed of a number of 'strain groups', which are not neatly correlated with infectivity or non-infectivity to humans. It is, however, possible to recognize strain groups which more or less correspond to the three subspecies. Perhaps the most homogeneous is *T. b. gambiense*, an essentially West African group of strains which have in common the ability to infect humans as well as other mammals. There is a more diffuse assemblage of strain groups of East African origin which may conveniently be referred to as *T. b. rhodesiense*, but not all of these groups infect humans. Finally, a third rather diffuse assemblage of

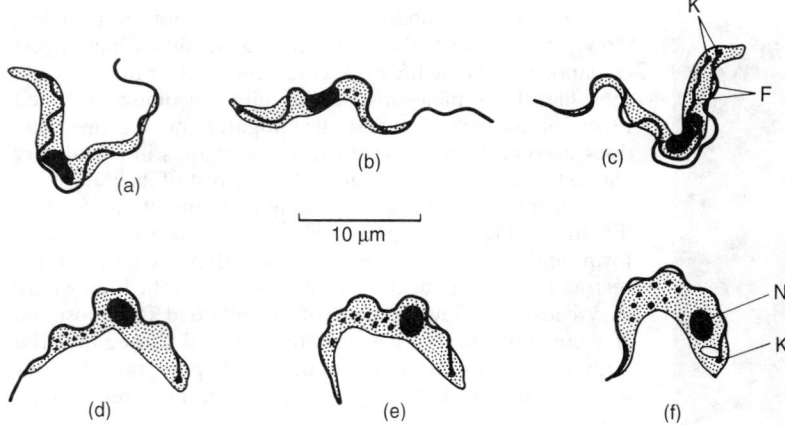

Figure II.6 *Trypanosoma brucei* in peripheral blood of an experimentally infected rat. A, B: long slender forms; C: dividing form; D, E: short stumpy forms; F: posteronuclear short stumpy form. F, flagellum; K, kinetoplast; N, nucleus. (From Baker J R. *Parasitic Protozoa,* 2nd edition. London: Hutchinson, 1973.)

strain groups, which can perhaps be regarded as *T. b. brucei*, is again largely West African in distribution; human infectivity is uncommon in this assemblage, but cannot entirely be ruled out. It is possible that the character of human infectivity is labile and inconstant within both *T. b. rhodesiense* and *T. b. brucei*, with the strain groups of the former being predominantly human-infective while those of the latter are not. Strains of the *T. b. gambiense* type seem to have spread eastwards across Africa, and there is an area of overlap between them and those of the *T. b. rhodesiense* type around the northern and eastern shores of Lake Victoria.

In general terms, *T. b. gambiense* is predominantly an infection of humans, transmitted by tsetse flies of the *G. palpalis* group from human to human, though reservoirs of infection undoubtedly exist among domestic animals (e.g. pigs) and wild ungulates. Since *G. palpalis* usually inhabits vegetation fringing rivers, transmission of the trypanosomes to humans commonly occurs at places where they come into frequent contact with the tsetse—at village watering places, fords, etc. Because of this, infection tends to be equally common in men, women and children.

By contrast, the strain groups forming *T. b. rhodesiense* are predominantly parasites of wild ungulates and domestic cattle, with humans being 'accidental' hosts. The parasite is therefore much less focally distributed than *T. b. gambiense*, and may be found across wide areas of the East African savanna; it is predominantly associated with tsetse of the *G. morsitans* group, which can survive under much drier conditions than can *G. palpalis*. Transmission of *T. b. rhodesiense* to humans is much less 'domestic' than that of *T. b. gambiense*, and usually cases of infection are more common in men than in women and children.

PATHOGENESIS

The types of disease produced in humans by *T. b. gambiense* and *T. b. rhodesiense* are essentially very similar, although the latter produces a much more acute disease, and can be described together.

After initial restriction to the chancre, the trypanosomes spread throughout the blood and lymph systems and give rise to a more or less acute febrile illness. Lymphadenopathy is common, and swollen cervical lymph glands constitute 'Winterbottom's sign', a classic indication of *T. b. gambiense* infection. After a period of weeks (*T. b. rhodesiense*), months or even years (*T. b. gambiense*), the parasites penetrate the CNS and multiply there in the capillaries, tissue fluid and CSF. At no stage of the infection do they enter cells of the host (except when ingested by phagocytes, in which they do not survive). Presumably in response to the repeated antigenic challenge resulting from the parasites' antigenic variation, large amounts of IgM are secreted into the blood plasma in the early stage of infection and, after invasion of the CNS, IgM also appears in the CSF. In the brain tissue there is massive lymphocytic infiltration in the arachnoid membrane and the pia mater which, in section, appears as a characteristic perivascular cuff around the brain capillaries. In addition to small round cells, the cuff often contains large plasma cells in the final stage of immunoglobulin secretion, the so-called morula (= mulberry) or Mott cells.

It is this meningoencephalitis which is responsible for the somnolence and coma which gave the disease its name 'sleeping sickness', and which is ultimately responsible for the death of the untreated patient.

DIAGNOSIS

Clinical diagnosis may be supported by a range of immunological tests, including IFATs, complement fixation tests, ELISAs and agglutination procedures. A commercial card agglutination test (CATT) is available.

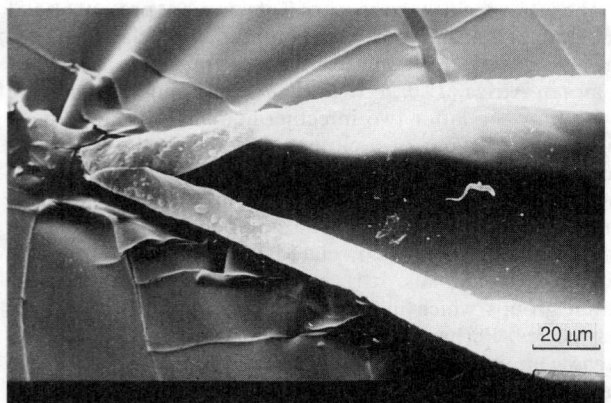

Figure II.7 Scanning electron micrograph showing *Trypanosoma brucei* in the tip of the proboscis (labrum) of *Glossina morsitans*. (From Molyneux D H. *Insect Sci Application* 1980; 1: 39.)

Final confirmation of active infection, however, depends on demonstration of the parasites, either microscopically or by isolation in laboratory rats or mice; cultivation in vitro is difficult and rarely used diagnostically. In the early infection, blood or lymph gland exudate is examined; the latter is likely to be more helpful in the chronic disease caused by *T. b. gambiense*. In the later stage, CSF obtained by lumbar puncture should be examined; if the CNS has been invaded, the CSF will contain scanty trypanosomes (which can sometimes be visualized by centrifugation), an increased number of lymphocytes (>5 cells/mm^3), morula cells and IgM.

Motile trypanosomes can be seen at magnifications of 400 or more in fresh preparations of blood, lymph or CSF, or stained preparations (thick blood films are better than thin films) may be examined at a magnification of 1000. Isolation by inoculation of blood, lymph or CSF into laboratory rats or mice is reliable for *T. b. rhodesiense*, but less so for *T. b. gambiense* which does not readily infect rodents; unweaned rats should be used, if possible, if isolation of *T. b. gambiense* is attempted.

TRYPANOSOMA CRUZI

LIFE CYCLE AND MORPHOLOGY

With this species both trypomastigotes and intracellular amastigotes develop in infected mammals, the former in the bloodstream and the latter mainly in macrophages and muscle cells. The trypomastigotes do not multiply but disseminate the infection around the body of the mammalian host and also serve to infect the vectors (large blood-sucking bugs of the subfamily Triatominae, family Reduviidae (Hemiptera); both sexes feed exclusively on blood). Trypomastigotes ingested by a feeding bug change into epimastigotes in the midgut, undergo division, and are moved back along the bug's gut as the blood meal is digested. In the hindgut they transform into small metacyclic trypomastigotes (which do not divide); these forms are expelled when the bug defecates while, or just after, feeding, and enter through the wound made by the bug's proboscis. The insects often feed on sleeping persons, and faecal matter may be transferred by the scratching or rubbing fingers of a sleepy child (or adult) to the eye; the trypomastigotes may then penetrate the conjunctiva.

T. cruzi can infect many mammals in addition to humans; dogs and cats, and wild animals living in or near houses such as rodents, armadillos, racoons, opossums and vampire bats may serve as reservoirs of human infection.

Once within a mammal the metacyclic trypomastigotes enter the host's cells, either actively or by being phagocytosed. If they are phagocytosed, the phagosome membrane seems to disintegrate, freeing the trypanosome, which thus evades digestion within a phagolysosome. The trypomastigotes then become rounded amastigotes (sometimes, perhaps more correctly, called micromastigotes, as they do possess a rudimentary intracellular flagellum) and divide by repeated binary fission until they fill, and then rupture, the host cell. Before its rupture, however, the contained parasites have retransformed into small trypomastigotes, which elongate after their liberation into trypomastigotes which are about 20 μm long and have a sharply pointed posterior end and an anterior extension of the flagellum beyond the end of

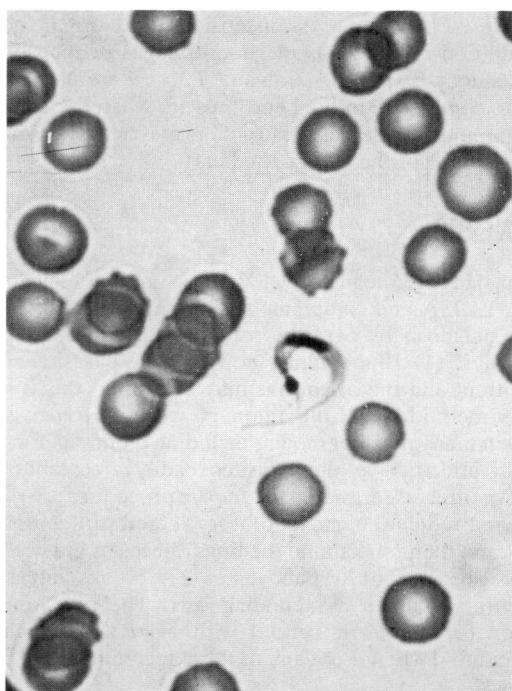

Figure II.8 Giemsa-stained bloodstream form of *Trypanosoma cruzi*. (Courtesy of the Department of Medical Parasitology, London School of Hygiene and Tropical Medicine.)

the cell (Figure II.8). On stained blood films these trypomastigotes often adopt a curved **C** shape. Marked pleomorphism, as in *T. brucei*, is not seen, though some workers believe that two forms can be distinguished—slender forms destined to reinvade host cells and broader forms which infect the vectors. There is no evidence of genetic exchange in *T. cruzi*.

GEOGRAPHICAL DISTRIBUTION

T. cruzi is widely distributed throughout continental South America and in Central America and the southern USA, between about latitudes 25°N and 38°S. The parasite has been isolated from wild mammals in the southern USA but few, if any, indigenous human cases have been reported. The disease is essentially one of poverty, poor quality housing being associated with bug infestation and, therefore, the risk of infection.

PATHOGENESIS

The initial sign of infection is often a swelling (chagoma) at the portal of entry of the trypanosomes. When this is the conjunctiva, and the swelling involves the eye, it is known as Romaña's sign. A more or less acute, rarely fatal, febrile illness is followed by the chronic phase, during which repeated intracellular multiplication cycles continually destroy the host's cells. Not only the cells containing amastigotes are destroyed, but also neighbouring cells, probably as part of an autoimmune phenomenon; neurones are particularly vulnerable. If the intracellular groups of amastigotes (pseudocysts) are concentrated in the oesophagus or colon, peristalsis may be interfered with and gross distension of the organ ensues; the condition is known as megaoesophagus or megacolon. The pseudocysts of some strains of *T. cruzi* are particularly prone to congregate in the heart muscle, when the resulting neuronal and muscle cell destruction may lead to thinning and weakening of the wall of the heart.

DIAGNOSIS

Clinical signs are inconclusive. Various immunological tests (IFAT, ELISA and complement fixation) are used. Confirmatory diagnosis by parasite isolation can be attempted in three ways. (1) Blood films: however, as parasitaemia is intermittent and the organisms may be scanty, this is not a reliable method. (2) Cultivation in vitro: *T. cruzi* grows readily in many nutrient media, including blood-agar media. (3) Cultivation in vivo: the parasites readily infect laboratory mice. An often used, simple diagnostic procedure is to allow uninfected reduviid bugs, laboratory reared, to feed on the patient and then to examine the bugs' faeces or gut contents for the presence of trypanosomes 3–4 weeks later; this procedure is known as xenodiagnosis. The possibility of infection (or double infection) with *T. rangeli* should be borne in mind when using any of these techniques.

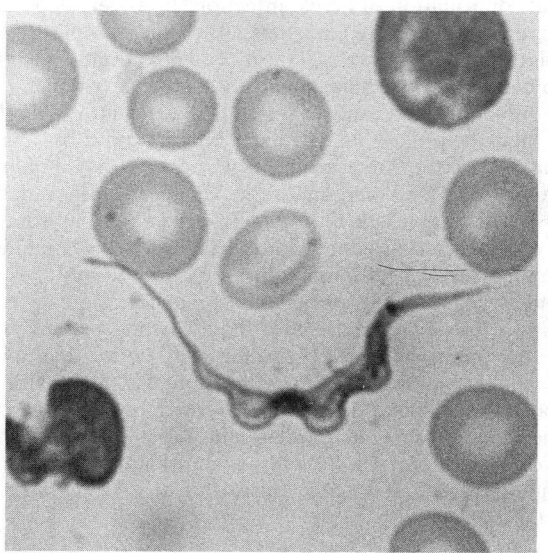

Figure II.9 Giemsa-stained blood stream form of *Trypanosoma rangeli*. (Photograph by Nester Añez, Imperial College of Science, Technology and Medicine, University of London.)

TRYPANOSOMA RANGELI

T. rangeli occurs in South America but its distribution is more patchy than that of *T. cruzi*. Although it infects humans, it is apparently entirely non-pathogenic and its only medical importance lies in the possibility of it being mistakenly diagnosed as *T. cruzi*, either in human or insect hosts, as it also shares reduviid bugs as vectors. The forms seen in humans are trypomastigotes only; they are longer than those of *T. cruzi*, measuring about 30 μm (Figure II.9). In bugs the parasite differs from *T. cruzi* by completing its development in the haemolymph and salivary glands, from whence it is transmitted to mammals by direct inoculation in the insect's saliva—like *T. brucei*. The metacyclic trypomastigotes which

develop in the bug's salivary glands (and in cultures in vitro) are also longer than those of *T. cruzi*. Unusually amongst trypanosomes, *T. rangeli* is pathogenic to its invertebrate host.

Apart from morphological differentiation *T. rangeli* can be distinguished from *T. cruzi* with the aid of monoclonal antibodies (although the two species have some common antigens), differential complement-mediated lysis, and isoenzyme electrophoresis. A relatively simple method of distinguishing the two trypanosomes involves the electrophoresis of whole cell DNA which has been digested with the restriction endonuclease *Bsp*RI; *T. rangeli* yields two fragments of about 1800 and 1900 base pairs which *T. cruzi* does not, while the latter provides a fragment of about 350 base pairs which *T. rangeli* lacks.[2]

LEISHMANIAL PARASITES (See also Chapter 65)

These parasites, species of the genus *Leishmania*, are classified in the same family (Trypanosomatidae) as the trypanosomes. Like them, they alternate between two hosts—a vertebrate and an invertebrate; however, the only forms which develop in the former are intracellular amastigotes, and those which develop in the invertebrate (insect) vector are promastigotes (Figure II.10). Promastigotes are elongate, motile flagellates with the flagellar origin and kinetoplast at the anterior end of the cell and the nucleus more or less in the middle. Both forms divide by binary fission and there is no evidence of sexual reproduction.

The vectors of all the species of *Leishmania* which infect humans are small insects (sandflies) of the genera *Phlebotomus* (in Africa, Asia and Europe) and *Lutzomyia* and *Psychodopygus* (in South and Central America); as with

mosquitoes, only female sandflies feed on blood. The species of *Leishmania* which infect humans can be divided into two major groups on the basis of their pathological behaviour—those which infect internal organs (liver, spleen, bone marrow) and cause visceral leishmaniasis (the *L. donovani* complex) and those which are restricted to the skin (dermis), causing cutaneous leishmaniasis (the *L. mexicana* and *L. braziliensis* complexes and three ungrouped species, *L. tropica*, *L. major* and *L. aethiopica*).[3]

LIFE CYCLE AND MORPHOLOGY

All the species infecting man are very similar morphologically. The rounded or oval amastigotes are smaller than those

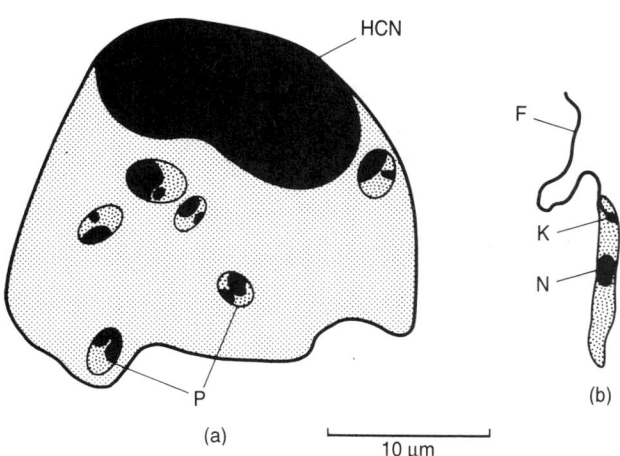

(a)

(b)

10 μm

Figure II.10 Leishmania sp. A, amastigotes (P) in a macrophage. HCN, host cell nucleus; B, promastigote in culture. F, flagellum; K, kinetoplast, N, nucleus. (From Baker J R. *Parasitic Protozoa*, 2nd edition. London 1973: Hutchinson.)

of *T. cruzi*, about 2–4 μm in diameter, and the promastigotes vary considerably in length from about 15 μm to 30 μm. After a feeding sandfly ingests amastigotes (presumably within monocytes or macrophages), the parasites escape from the cell and transform into promastigotes, which colonize the insect's midgut (Figure II.11). In one subgenus of *Leishmania* (*Viannia*), there is also a phase of promastigote development in the sandfly's hindgut. Finally, the promastigotes spread forwards into the foregut of the vector, and its proboscis, where the so-called metacyclic promastigotes are formed. These are injected with the fly's saliva when it next feeds on a mammal.

In the mammalian host the promastigotes enter phagocytes, either actively or passively, and transform into amastigotes. Unlike those of *T. cruzi*, the amastigotes remain enclosed within a phagosome which fuses with a lysosome but they somehow resist digestion by the lysosomal enzymes (or inhibit their production) and survive and multiply within the phagolysosome. When the host cell is full, it ruptures and the released amastigotes re-enter other phagocytes to continue the process. In the *L. donovani* complex the fixed liver phagocytes known as Kupffer cells also become infected.

VISCERAL LEISHMANIASIS

GEOGRAPHICAL DISTRIBUTION

Visceral leishmaniasis (sometimes known as kala-azar) occurs in South America in the southern tropical zone, in tropical East Africa, the North African littoral and the Mediterranean coastal region of southern Europe, and in parts of India and central Asia. In South America, it is caused by *L. chagasi*, which also infects dogs and wild Canidae, which may act as reservoir hosts; the vectors are sandflies of the genus *Lutzomyia*. In Asia and sub-Saharan Africa the causative species is *L. donovani* and the vectors are species of *Phlebotomus*; in parts of Africa the parasite also infects dogs

and certain rodents, while in India it seems that humans are the only vertebrate hosts. In countries bordering the Mediterranean sea, visceral leishmaniasis is caused by another, closely related species—*L. infantum*; this species is also transmitted by *Phlebotomus* spp., and dogs are important reservoirs of infection. All these species of *Leishmania* belong to the subgenus *Leishmania*.

PATHOGENESIS

Infection of cells of the monocyte/phagocyte system leads to extensive hyperplasia of the system, with gross enlargement of the liver and spleen and progressive interference with their function and with the haematopoietic functions of the bone marrow.

DIAGNOSIS

Confirmatory diagnosis depends on parasite isolation by microscopical examination of Giemsa-stained smears, or by in vitro inoculation into cultures of biopsy material obtained by puncture of the spleen or, more safely, the bone marrow (usually of the sternum). Most of the common blood-agar diphasic culture media are satisfactory, and the parasites grow as promastigotes.

CUTANEOUS LEISHMANIASIS

GEOGRAPHICAL DISTRIBUTION

L. major causes cutaneous leishmaniasis in Asia and tropical Africa, and possibly also in parts of North Africa; its vectors are *Phlebotomus* spp. and its reservoir hosts are rodents of various species (usually the gerbil *Rhombomys opimus* in Asia). *L. aethiopica* occurs only in East and north-east Africa, with hyraxes (*Procavia* and *Heterohyrax* spp.) as the main reservoir hosts and *Phlebotomus* spp. as vectors. *L. tropica* infects humans (and possibly dogs) in parts of Asia (the Middle East and north-eastern India), and probably also in parts of North Africa and southern Europe (including Greece) around the Mediterranean sea; it is transmitted by *Phlebotomus*.

In Central and South America cutaneous leishmaniasis is caused by a range of species, some as yet ill defined and unnamed; the more important species are listed in Table II.3.

The African and Asian species, and all those in South America, which cause cutaneous leishmaniasis are members of the subgenus *Leishmania* except for the *L. braziliensis* complex of species (Table II.3), which are classified in the subgenus *Viannia*. All the South American species except *L. braziliensis* are transmitted by species of *Lutzomyia*; *L. braziliensis* is transmitted by *Psychodopygus*.

PATHOGENESIS

In the cutaneous leishmaniases, parasitized macrophages are normally restricted to the dermis and mucous membranes. Lesions may range from a single, self-healing ulcer to wide-

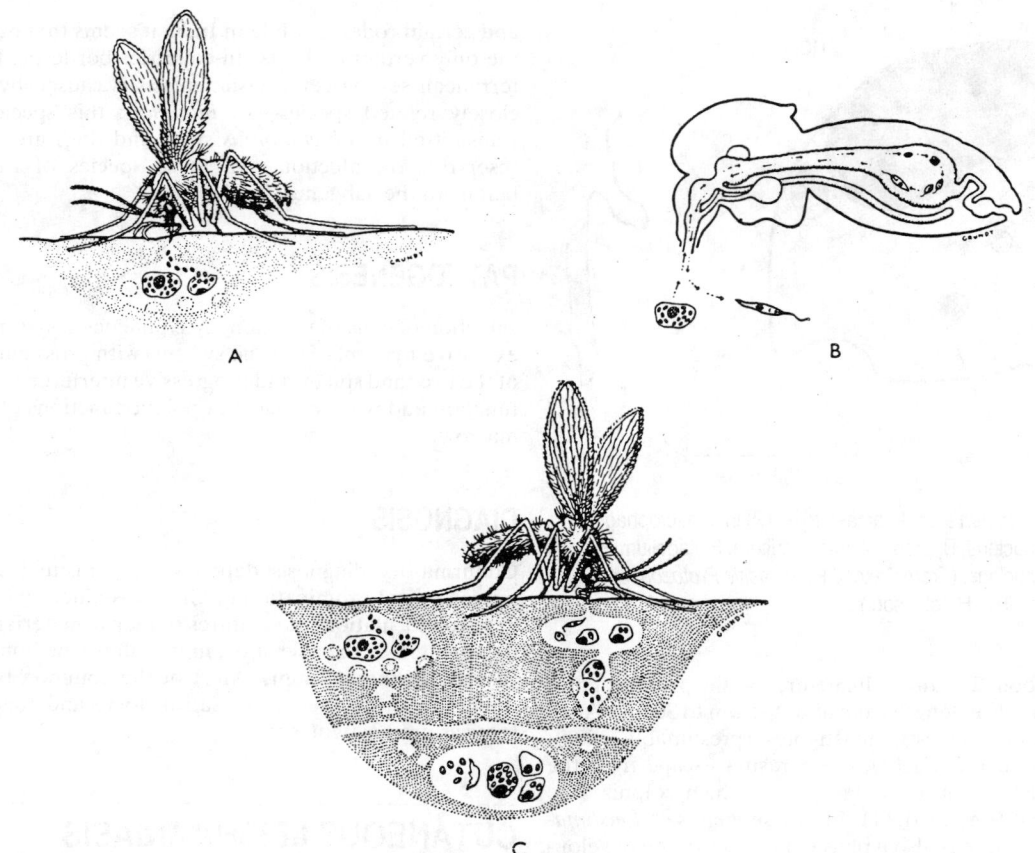

Figure II.11 Life cycle of *Leishmania* spp. A, feeding female sandfly ingests amastigotes from an infected vertebrate. B, the amastigotes develop into promastigotes, undergo division, and migrate forwards to the pharynx of the sandfly. C, when the sandfly next feeds on blood it injects promastigotes into the wound. The developmental cycle in the sandfly takes about ten days. (The diagrams of sandflies and parasites are not to scale.) (Drawing by J. Hull Grundy.)

Table II.3 Main species of *Leishmania* causing human cutaneous leishmaniasis in Central and South America (based on Lainson and Shaw[4]).

Parasite	Locality	Reservoir hosts
Subgenus *Leishmania*		
L. mexicana complex		
L. mexicana	Central America	Rodents
L. amazonensis	Northern Brazil	Rodents
L. venezuelensis	Venezuela	—
L. pifanoi*	Venezuela	—
Subgenus *Viannia*		
L. braziliensis complex		
L. braziliensis†	Brazil, Venezuela	?Rodents, opossum,‡ sloth§
L. guyanensis	South America, north of the Amazon river	Sloth,§ anteater¶
L. panamensis	Panama, Costa Rica, Colombia	Sloth‖
L. peruviana	Peru, Argentina	Dog

*So far known only from cases of diffuse cutaneous leishmaniasis; identity uncertain.
†Causes cutaneous and mucocutaneous leishmaniasis.
‡*Didelphis marsupialis.*
§*Choloepus didactylus.*
¶*Tamandua tetradactylus.*
‖*C. hoffmanni.*

spread ulceration over much of the body surface (diffuse cutaneous leishmaniasis or DCL), which sometimes results from infection with *L. aethiopica* or *L. pifanoi* (the latter having been isolated only from cases of DCL, although it presumably causes ordinary cutaneous leishmaniasis as well). *L. braziliensis* has a tendency to invade mucocutaneous junctions, particularly those of the nasopharynx and palate, where it causes the disfiguring lesions of mucocutaneous leishmaniasis or espundia. *L. peruviana* occurs at high altitudes in the Peruvian Andes; it causes cutaneous leishmaniasis with a characteristic dry sore on the skin, called uta.

Infection with human immunodeficiency virus (HIV) and the ensuing development of the acquired immune deficiency syndrome (AIDS) markedly reduces or destroys the immunological response to infection with *Leishmania*, leading to widespread dissemination of skin lesions and even invasion of the viscera by *Leishmania* spp. which have hitherto caused inapparent or localized infections.

DIAGNOSIS

As with visceral leishmaniasis, confirmatory diagnosis depends on detection of the parasites either by microscopical examination of Giemsa-stained slides or by cultivation in vitro. Suitable material can be obtained by puncture of the margin of a suspect lesion with a hypodermic needle attached to a syringe containing a small amount of physiological saline. The aspirate contained in the needle is then expelled on to a microscope slide or into a tube of culture medium (usually blood-agar).

ENTAMOEBA HISTOLYTICA (See also Chapter 67)

LIFE CYCLE AND MORPHOLOGY (Figure II.12)

E. histolytica inhabits the lumen of the large intestine of humans (and other primates, dogs, cats, pigs and rodents), where it may cause amoebic dysentery. The parasite also sometimes invades the mucosa and other viscera. The trophozoite is motile, irregular in shape, measures about 10–40 μm in diameter, and reproduces by binary fission. Sexual reproduction is unknown, but there is some evidence of genetic exchange. The trophozoites may contain red blood

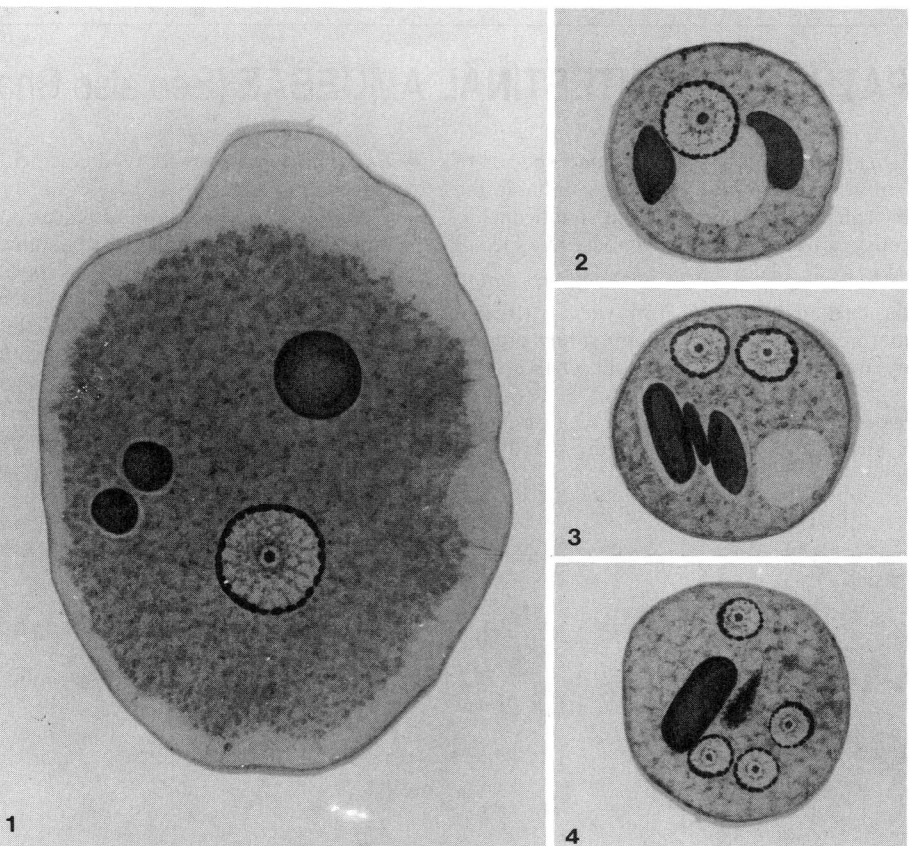

Figure II.12 *Entamoeba histolytica*. 1, Active amoeboid trophozoite with ingested erythrocytes; the nucleus is also visible. 2–4, Cysts with one, two and four nuclei respectively, and chromatoid bodies (semicrystalline ribosomal masses).

cells in food vacuoles. Transmission is by ingestion of the resistant cyst, which is excreted in the host's faeces, with contaminated food or water. The mature cyst is 9.5–15.5 μm in diameter, spherical, and contains four nuclei; often, but not always, it also contains paracrystalline aggregations of ribosomes, the 'chromatoid bodies', which appear as rods with blunt, rounded ends. They stain with iodine or haematoxylin stains, but appear glass-like in fresh specimens. Cysts develop only in the intestinal lumen, not within the tissues.

It has long been known that many persons who harbour intestinal amoebae which are morphologically indistinguishable from *E. histolytica* may show no sign or symptom of amoebiasis. Such persons may be found in all countries, tropical and temperate, while clinical amoebiasis is more or less restricted to the tropics.

In 1925 Brumpt[4] suggested that two morphologically identical parasites existed: *E. histolytica*, which could invade tissues and hence become pathogenic; and *E. dispar*, which could not. The topic has been debated ever since, with some workers believing that the pathogenic and non-pathogenic forms were interconvertible. The careful work of Sargeaunt and his collaborators,[5] who pioneered the classification of *E. histolytica* isolates into zymodemes by means of enzyme electrophoresis, provided the basis for a scientific appraisal of the situation. It is now clear that two distinct populations exist, one potentially pathogenic and the other not, corresponding to the 'classical' *E. histolytica* and Brumpt's *E. dispar*.

PATHOGENESIS

Amoebae in the gut lumen are not significantly harmful, but if, for reasons unknown, they penetrate the intestinal mucosa they multiply within flask-shaped ulcers and lead to haemorrhage and mucosal damage. When this occurs, the amoebae feed on red blood cells, which may be seen within the organisms. A bloody dysentery (amoebic dysentery) ensues, which can be differentiated from the bloody dysentery resulting from bacterial infection by the absence of the large numbers of pus cells characteristic of the latter.

The amoebic ulcers erode blood vessels (hence the haemorrhage), and thus amoebae may enter the circulation and be carried to other organs. Here they may become established, and form so-called amoebic 'abscesses', which are not true abscesses since they are bacteriologically sterile. The liver is the organ most commonly affected in this way, but the lungs and (rarely) brain may also be invaded.

DIAGNOSIS

Confirmatory diagnosis by identification of amoebae may be made either by direct microscopical examination of faecal specimens (fresh or concentrated) or by cultivation of the organisms in suitable media. Serological techniques can be used to detect tissue invasion, but rarely if ever detect infection with parasites living in the gut lumen only.

NON-PATHOGENIC INTESTINAL AMOEBAE (See also Chapter 67)

In addition to *E. dispar*, five other well-defined species of amoebae, none of which is pathogenic, may inhabit the human alimentary canal. Their only medical significance is that they may be mistaken for *E. histolytica*; these five species are listed below (Figure II.13).

- *E. coli*: cysts larger than those of *E. histolytica*, with eight nuclei when mature; chromatoid bars are rarely present but, when they are, they are thin and splinter-like, with pointed ends.
- *E. hartmanni*: cysts smaller than those of *E. histolytica*, but with four nuclei and chromatoid bodies of the *E. histolytica* type.

- *Endolimax nana*: small, oval cysts with four nuclei but no chromatoid bars.
- *Iodamoeba buetschlii*: uninucleate cyst, often containing a large glycogen vacuole which stains dark brown with iodine but appears clear in fresh specimens.
- *E. gingivalis*: unlike all the above-mentioned species, this amoeba inhabits the mouth (and so should not be confused with *E. histolytica*); it forms no cyst, transmission presumably being by direct contact or by the sharing of drinking vessels, etc.

The aberrant flagellate *Dientamoeba fragilis* (see p. 1574) resembles an amoeba as it lacks a flagellum, but it is binucleate and does not produce a cyst.

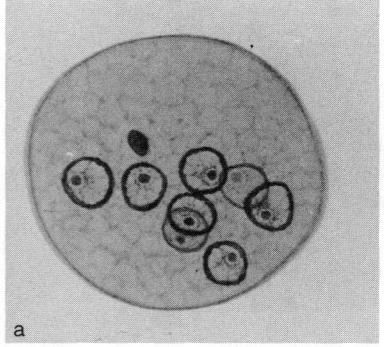 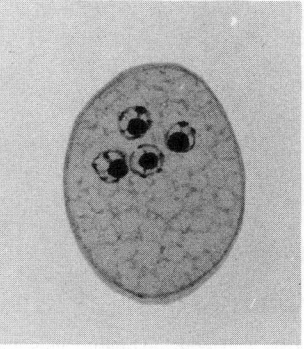 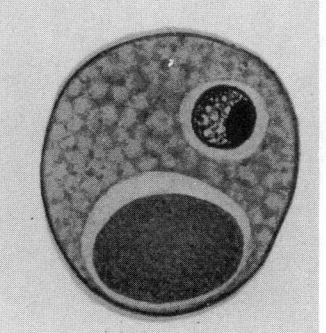

Figure II.13   Cysts of non-pathogenic intestinal amoebae. a: *Entamoeba coli*; b: *Endolimax nana*; c: *Iodamoeba buetschlii*.

GIARDIA DUODENALIS (See also Chapter 67)

LIFE CYCLE AND MORPHOLOGY

The motile trophozoite has two nuclei, four pairs of flagella, and one or two curved median bodies of unknown function (sometimes incorrectly called parabasal bodies) (Figures II.14 and II.15); it is 10–20 μm long, 5–10 μm broad and 2–4 μm thick. Reproduction is by binary fission; no sexual process is known.

The infective stage is an oval cyst, 6–10 × 8–14 μm (Figure II.14), which is excreted in the faeces and ingested with contaminated food or water. The cyst contains four small nuclei, grouped at one end, and a confused jumble of flagella, median bodies and etc. in the centre.

Giardia has a worldwide distribution; the species infecting humans is also known as *G. intestinalis* or *G. lamblia*, though *G. duodenalis* appears to be zoologically correct.

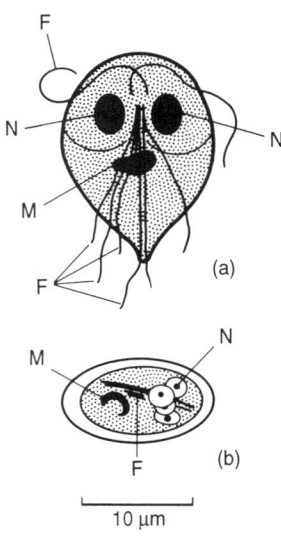

Figure II.14 Giardia sp. Trophozoite (a) and cyst (b), stained with Giemsa's stain. F, flagellum; M, median body; N, nuclei. (From Baker J R. *Parasitic Protozoa*, 2nd edition. London: Hutchinson, 1973.)

PATHOGENESIS

Trophozoites are attached to the mucosal surface of the duodenum or upper ileum by an oval, ventral anterior disc or 'sucker'; they do not penetrate the mucosa but may damage it if they are numerous, leading to villous atrophy and acute watery (not bloody) diarrhoea.

DIAGNOSIS

Giardiasis can be confirmed by demonstrating cysts in faecal specimens; they are often numerous, and usually easily recognizable even in unstained saline preparations, but iodine staining makes the internal structure more easily visible.

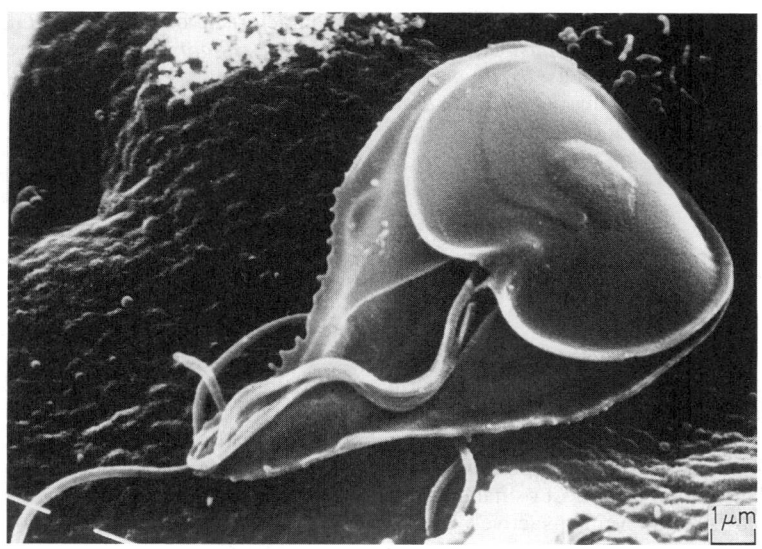

Figure II.15 Scanning electron micrograph of a trophozoite of *Giardia duodenalis* from a jejunal biopsy. (By kind permission of K. Vickerman, University of Glasgow.)

TRICHOMONAS VAGINALIS (See also Chapter 69)

LIFE CYCLE AND MORPHOLOGY

The trophozoites are oval, 14–17 × 5–15 μm, and have a single nucleus, four anterior flagella and a single lateral flagellum which runs back along the surface of the cell, to which it is attached to form a conspicuous undulating membrane supported by a marginal filament (Figure II.16). The lateral flagellum ends about half way along the cell, which also contains a prominent central rod or axostyle. Multiplication is by binary fission, with no sexual process.

No cyst is formed, the trophozoite being transmitted directly during sexual intercourse.

PATHOGENESIS

T. vaginalis inhabits the vagina and urethra. It is more commonly pathogenic in women than in men, though it may cause a mild urethritis or prostatitis.

DIAGNOSIS

Clinical diagnosis may be confirmed by demonstration of the trophozoites in Giemsa-stained smears made from swabs of

vaginal (or urethral) discharge. If they are not readily found, the swab can be placed in a tube of medium for cultivation of the parasites in vitro.

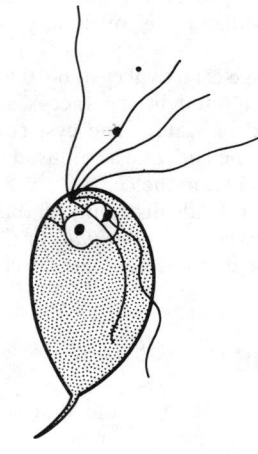

Figure II.16 Trophozoite of *Trichomonas* sp.

NON-PATHOGENIC INTESTINAL FLAGELLATES (See also Chapter 67)

As with the amoebae, there are other, non-pathogenic flagellates which may inhabit the human alimentary tract and which may be confused with *Giardia duodenalis*.

One of these species, *Trichomonas tenax*, inhabits the buccal cavity, but the others all live in the intestine. *Dientamoeba fragilis* is an aberrant flagellate which looks like an amoeba; it is binucleate but lacks a flagellum and median bodies. The other non-pathogenic flagellates (*Chilomastix mesnili*, *Enteromonas hominis*, *Retortamonas intestinalis* and *Pentatrichomonas hominis*) all have between one and six flagella and a single nucleus; *P. hominis* looks rather like *T.*

vaginalis but can be distinguished from it by the difference in habitat.

All these species except *T. tenax*, *P. hominis* and *D. fragilis* form cysts, which can be distinguished from those of *G. intestinalis* by their round shape and lack of the remains of flagella, etc., which are so characteristic of the cyst of *G. intestinalis*. The cysts of all except *E. hominis* have only one nucleus; *E. hominis*, like *G. intestinalis*, has four, but—unlike *G. intestinalis*—these are not usually grouped at one end of the cyst.

TOXOPLASMA GONDII (See also Chapter 66)

T. gondii has two distinct life cycles which usually take place in vertebrate hosts belonging to different genera. The 'normal' apicomplexan life cycle of merogony, gametogony and sporogony occurs only in domestic cats and a few closely related species, within epithelial cells of the small intestine; the cat is therefore referred to as the 'definitive' host. Oocysts, measuring about 11 × 13 μm, are voided in the cat's faeces and, when mature, contain two spherical sporocysts, each containing four elongate sporozoites.

If a mature oocyst is swallowed by another susceptible animal (the 'intermediate' host), which can be any warm-

blooded vertebrate (mammal or bird), the sporozoites are liberated by the action of the host's digestive juices and the secondary life cycle commences. (This also can occur in cats.)

The sporozoites emerge from the oocyst in the intermediate host's small intestine, pass through the mucosa and enter (either actively or passively) macrophages. The macrophage's lysosomes are inhibited from fusing with the phagosomes containing the parasites, which thus survive and begin to divide rapidly until the host cell is filled with small, crescentic, uninucleate parasites known as tachyzoites or endozoites, each measuring about 5 × 1–2 μm (Figure II.17).

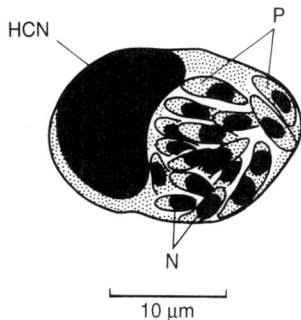

Figure II.17 *Toxoplasma gondii:* pseudocyst in a macrophage; a Giemsa-stained smear of mouse peritoneal fluid. (Reproduced from Baker J R. *Parasitic Protozoa*, 2nd edition. London: Hutchinson, 1973.)

The infected macrophage, referred to as a pseudocyst, eventually disintegrates and the liberated tachyzoites enter other macrophages and repeat the process. This constitutes the acute phase of the infection. Unless the host dies or is treated, the acute phase is immunologically controlled and the infection moves into the chronic phase. The parasites invade cells other than macrophages (including muscle cells and neurones) and secrete a thin but tough cyst wall, within which they continue to divide, though more slowly; the organisms within this cyst are called bradyzoites or cystozoites; the cyst may attain a diameter of 60 μm.

If a non-feline host eats uncooked meat or prey containing these tissue cysts, the bradyzoites are liberated in the duodenum and repeat the extraintestinal cycle after passing through the mucosal wall. However, if a cat ingests tissue cysts in its prey, or if infected raw meat or offal is fed to it, the cystozoites enter duodenal cells and begin the 'normal' apicomplexan life cycle. This intestinal cycle consists of a limited number of merogony cycles, with each batch of merozoites entering other duodenal cells to repeat the process, until the final generation of merozoites commences the sexual cycle of gametogony and fertilization within the duodenal cells, culminating with sporogony within the developing oocyst (which is secreted around the fertilized zygote). Sporogony is completed, with the production of two sporocysts each containing four sporozoites, as the oocyst passes down the cat's gut and in the expelled faeces. Oocysts can survive in the external environment for at least 1 year.

PATHOGENESIS

Infected cats show no obvious sign of illness. In humans the acute phase of infection (tachyzoites multiplying in macrophages) usually results in mild to moderate febrile illness with lymphadenopathy, except in immunocompromised persons (e.g. those with AIDS), in whom the infection may become generalized and fatal. The chronic phase is symptomless and, unless the patient becomes subsequently immunocompromised, appears to remain active but quiescent for the rest of the individual's life.

T. gondii is one of the few parasites that can cross the placenta, though only if the pregnant woman has an acute infection. Infection in utero is uncommon (probably fewer than 1 case per 1000 livebirths), but its effects on the fetus may be severe, with gross brain damage resulting from uncontrolled proliferation of the tachyzoites, leading to hydrocephaly and, often, death. If infection occurs later in pregnancy its effect may be mild, with retinopathy the only sign in the baby (often discovered by accident when the adult has an ophthalmological examination for some other reason).

DIAGNOSIS

Parasites may be isolated by inoculation of biopsy material (e.g. tonsil or an enlarged lymph gland) into mice, with microscopical examination of the murine peritoneal fluid as a Giemsa-stained smear after 3–4 weeks (unless the mice sicken and die earlier). Pseudocysts and artificially liberated tachyzoites will be seen. There are several serological tests for anti-*Toxoplasma* antibodies, but these remain positive throughout the chronic phase of infection and so do not necessarily indicate acute infection unless two similar tests, performed a few weeks apart, reveal a sharply rising titre. The tests used include complement fixation, agglutination (of killed tachyzoites), IFAT, and the so-called Sabin–Feldman dye test, which depends on the fact that living tachyzoites which have been exposed to specific antibody and complement are rendered unreceptive to methylene blue, which readily stains normal live organisms. This test is little used now because its dependence on living tachyzoites makes it potentially hazardous for the technician.

Serological evidence indicates that between 25 and 35% of the population of so-called 'developed' countries have anti-*Toxoplasma* antibodies, indicative of past infection. Reactivated acute toxoplasmosis is one of the more common, often fatal, complications of AIDS.

SARCOCYSTIS (See also Chapter 67)

Sarcocystis spp., though common parasites of herbivores and rodents, are not significant as parasites of humans. *Sarcocystis* is related to *Toxoplasma* and has a similar life cycle, though it differs in that each species has only a very limited range of intermediate hosts and extraintestinal development does not occur in the definitive host. The zooites are larger than those of *T. gondii*, being 10–15 μm long, and the tissue cysts, which occur only in muscle cells, may be very long—even visible macroscopically.

Humans are definitive hosts of *S. bovihominis* and *S. suihominis*, the intermediate hosts of which are oxen and pigs, respectively (as the specific names indicate). A few early records of human infection with tissue cysts (sarcocysts) suggest that humans can rarely, perhaps accidentally, act as intermediate hosts for one or more other species of *Sarcocystis*.

Isospora belli, a coccidian parasite of the human intestine which rarely causes mild diarrhoea, may be a stage in the life cycle of another, as yet unidentified, species of *Sarcocystis*.

PATHOGENESIS

Infection of the human intestine with *S. bovihominis* or *S. suihominis* may cause moderately severe diarrhoea, which is, however, self-limiting. Infection of the muscle with sarcocysts is usually symptomless but may, if intense, lead to some muscular weakness.

BABESIA (See also Chapter 62)

Species of *Babesia*, commonly known as piroplasms, are small intraerythrocytic apicomplexan parasites which occur commonly in cattle, sheep, horses, insectivores and rodents in many parts of the world but do not normally infect humans; they are transmitted by ticks (Arthropoda, Acarina), usually members of the family Ixodidae ('hard' ticks).

The small parasites ($1-2 \mu m$) multiply within red blood cells by binary fission, and some species (e.g. *B. microti* of voles) may also invade lymphocytes for one merogonic cycle before entering red cells.

A very few (perhaps 50–100) cases of *Babesia* infection have been reported in humans in North America and Europe. North American infections have all been due to *B. microti* of voles (insectivores of the genus *Microtus*), and the patients have recovered. In Europe, all the (few) infected persons had previously undergone splenectomy at some time, and most of them died; some (perhaps all) of the infections acquired in Europe were due to the cattle parasite *B. divergens*. No successful treatment is known for human babesiosis.

Diagnosis depends on recognizing the parasites in stained blood films, where they may be difficult to distinguish from young trophozoites of *Plasmodium*, though *Babesia* never contains pigment.

PNEUMOCYSTIS CARINII (See also Chapter 60)

The taxonomic position of *Pneumocystis* is uncertain. Study of its ribosomal RNA suggests close affinity with the fungi, rather than its being an 'odd' protozoan. It has been recorded in humans, dogs and rodents in all continents (except Antarctica); in Africa it appears to be uncommon.

The parasites are about $5-6 \mu m$ in diameter, uninucleate and spherical; they live extracellularly in lung alveolae. Binary fission has been described, though details of the life cycle are sparse and somewhat conflicting. Cyst-like, spherical bodies about $10 \mu m$ in diameter are formed in the lung alveolae, and are thought to be the infective phase. Transmission presumably occurs by droplet infection.

Infection is probably common but symptomless, unless the parasites become sufficiently numerous to block the alveolae with a foamy mass composed of plasma cells, parasites and mucus. This may occur in immunologically incompetent or immunocompromised persons, such as sickly or premature babies, persons receiving immunosuppressive therapy, or those afflicted with AIDS; *Pneumocystis carinii* pneumonia is perhaps the most common cause of death of patients, with AIDS.

FACULTATIVELY PARASITIC AMOEBAE (See also Chapter 68)

Two species of amoebae which are normally free living (i.e. non-parasitic) in water or mud are known to have occasionally infected human patients, and a third species is suspected of doing so.

Naegleria fowleri inhabits warm, fresh water, and has three stages in its life cycle: amoeboid form, flagellate form, and cyst. A few human infections due to *N. fowleri* are known, apparently resulting from amoebae being forced up the patient's nose while he or she was swimming or jumping in infected water, and then penetrating the nasal mucosa and migrating up the olfactory nerve to the brain. In the brain they multiply extensively (as amoeboid trophozoites only) and cause considerable damage, which is usually fatal. The condition is known as primary amoebic encephalitis (PAM). PAM is more common in tropical and subtropical areas, but infection can occur in artificially (or naturally) heated waters in colder countries; overall, however, it is rare (fewer than 200 cases are known). A related species, *N. australiensis*, can cause experimental PAM in mice and is therefore also suspected of being a potential, if not actual, facultative parasite of humans.

Acanthamoeba culbertsoni has also been reported as causing infection of the brain, in fewer than 50 humans. The parasite has no flagellated stage, and normally lives in damp soil or, as the cyst, in dry and dusty soil. Infection probably occurs when trophozoites in mud, or perhaps cysts in dry, dusty soil, are ingested or inhaled through the mouth. The most common manifestation of *Acanthamoeba* infection is a relatively mild pharyngitis, which has been reported in a limited number of young children and even fewer adults in the USA. It is thought the children may have acquired the infection while crawling or playing with soil. In a very few individuals (fewer than 50), *Acanthamoeba* infection of the brain has been reported post mortem; most of these persons were immunocompromised in some way, and probably amoebae from an initial pharyngeal infection were able to penetrate the mucosa and find their way to the brain; the resulting condition is known as granulomatous amoebic encephalitis.

Recent work has shown that *Acanthamoeba* spp. can infect the cornea of persons using soft contact lenses, presumably as a result of contamination of the wash solutions. There have also been a few cases of keratitis due to *Acanthamoeba* infection apparently unassociated with the use of contact lenses.

BALANTIDIUM COLI (See also Chapter 67)

LIFE CYCLE AND MORPHOLOGY

B. coli is the only known ciliate parasite of humans. Its natural habitat is the large intestine of domestic pigs and its distribution is worldwide. The large, oval, flattened trophozoites (60–70 × 40–60 μm; Figure II.18) are covered with short, hair-like cilia, by means of which they swim; they reproduce both asexually by transverse binary fission and sexually by the complicated process known as conjugation (unique to ciliates). Like almost all ciliates, *B. coli* has two nuclei: a large, polyploid macronucleus and a small, haploid micronucleus which is involved in sexual reproduction (dur-

ing which process the macronucleus degenerates, to be reformed by one of the progeny of the micronuclear fusion and subsequent fission which occurs during conjugation). Large, spherical cysts (50–60 μm in diameter) are formed and excreted in the faeces. Human infection presumably usually results from ingestion of cysts with contaminated food or water; person-to-person transmission has never been conclusively demonstrated.

PATHOGENESIS

Normally the ciliate lives harmlessly in the lumen of the pig's large intestine. Sometimes, however, perhaps as a result of concomitant infection with some other pathogen such as *Salmonella*, the trophozoites penetrate into the submucosa and form large, flask-shaped ulcers like those caused by *E. histolytica*. Bloody dysentery then ensues. A similar sequence of events probably occurs in humans, although symptomless infections of the gut lumen only have not yet been reported from humans (perhaps because no one has looked for them).

DIAGNOSIS

The large cysts, with their correspondingly large macronucleus, are easily recognized in fresh or stained faecal preparations. *B. coli* grows in most of the common culture media used for *Entamoeba*, but recourse to this technique is seldom necessary.

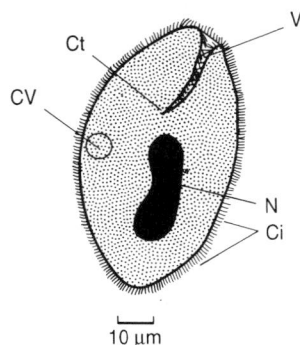

Figure II.18   Balantidium coli: trophozoite from a culture in vitro (the micronucleus is not visible in this specimen). (Reproduced from Baker J R. *Parasitic protozoa*, 2nd edition. London: Hutchinson, 1973.)

CRYPTOSPORIDIUM PARVUM (See also Chapter 67)

LIFE CYCLE AND MORPHOLOGY

C. muris is an apicomplexan parasite which was thought to be restricted to non-human mammals, including domestic cattle and rodents. Since 1976, however, the parasite has been reported in increasing numbers of patients throughout the world, more commonly in children and immunocompromised adults.

C. muris is transmitted by a resistant oocyst in the faeces of infected persons or animals, ingested with contaminated food or water. Four sporozoites emerge from the oocyst in the small intestine, enter cells of the microvillous border, and undergo merogony and, finally, gametogony. The parasites remain intracellular, though they lie very superficially just below the host cell's plasmalemma. The gametes fuse to form a diploid zygote, which then encysts to become an oocyst, only 4–6 μm in diameter.

Some oocysts, with thin walls, apparently mature and 'hatch' while still within the first host's intestine, which the emergent sporozoites then reinfect, enabling the infection to build up to a very high level unless it is controlled immunologically. Other oocysts, with thicker walls, are excreted and serve to transmit the infection orally to a fresh host. Human infections usually result from person-to-person transmission, but domestic animals and rodents may sometimes act as reservoir hosts.

PATHOGENESIS

Damage to the small intestinal mucosa, resulting from the successive cycles of merogony, leads to diarrhoea which, in immunologically competent persons, is usually self-limiting; neither blood nor pus cells are present in the stool. In immunodeficient persons (including patients with AIDS), the infection may progress unchecked, and severe, intractable and even life-threatening diarrhoea may result, with stool volumes up to 25 litres per day. Pulmonary cryptosporidiosis has been occasionally recorded, possibly as a result of inhalation of oocysts in vomit.

DIAGNOSIS

Confirmation of diagnosis depends on recognition of oocysts in faeces. The small size of the oocysts makes this difficult; they may be more readily found after concentration of faeces by flotation techniques followed by staining with acid-fast stains such as Ziehl–Neelsen.

MICROSPORIDA (See also Chapter 67)

Species which are known to infect humans are *Septata intestinalis*, *Enterocytozoon bieneusi*, *Encephalitozoon cuniculi*, *Nosema connori* and perhaps a species of *Pleistophora*. Microsporida in general are predominantly parasites of fish and insects, to which they may be very pathogenic; a few species are known to infect mammals.

LIFE CYCLE AND MORPHOLOGY

The infective stages of Microsporida are small spores, about 5 × 2 μm in size, which are usually ingested orally. The ingested spore ejects a hollow, tubular polar filament which introduces (rather in the manner of a hypodermic syringe) the infective contents of the spore, the sporoplasm (which is believed to be uninucleate, although this has not been conclusively demonstrated), into the cytoplasm of a host cell. Within the host cells (which may be of many different types), successive cycles of merogony, followed by sporogony, occur, resulting in the production of many more spores.

PATHOGENESIS

Encephalitozoon cuniculi is a common parasite of rodents, rabbits (*Oryctolagus*) and carnivores and it has been rarely reported from monkeys. Two cases of human infection are known—one from Japan and one from Sweden. Serological surveys have revealed a high prevalence (up to about 40%) of positive reactions to *E. cuniculi* antigen among persons with tropical experience, and particularly those with malaria or tuberculosis. The significance of this is not clear.

N. connori was described as a new species from an immunodeficient human infant in 1974; other species of *Nosema* are common parasites of arthropods (*N. apis* is a serious pathogen of honey-bees).

There have been two reports of Microsporida infecting human corneas. One case, in an immunodeficient man in the USA, was identified as a species of *Pleistophora*, a genus which normally infects fish and amphibians. In these cases it is likely that the spores were introduced directly into the eye, rather than being ingested orally.

All these cases of human infection were presumably 'accidental', the species involved normally being parasites of other animals. One of the other species involved in human infection, *Enterocytozoon bieneusi*, was first described in 1985 and is being found in an increasing (though still small) number of patients with AIDS; it has not yet been reported from any other species, and may be a genuine parasite of humans rather than an accidental infection with a parasite from some other host. Another species of *Enterocytozoon* has, however, been described from salmonid fish. *E. bieneusi* inhabits the mucosal cells of the small intestine. It seems likely that, with the increasing spread of infection with the human immunodeficiency viruses, the prevalence of infection with *E. bieneusi* will also increase; it is associated with severe, intractable diarrhoea.

Another species infecting humans has been described recently (1993) in five patients with AIDS in the USA; it was placed into a new genus, *Septata*, as *S. intestinalis*. Like *E. bieneusi*, this species inhabits human enterocytes but is also found in the kidney and gallbladder, and it differs morphologically from *E. bieneusi*. It is, however, rather similar to *Encephalitozoon*, and its distinction from this genus awaits confirmation.

DIAGNOSIS

Diagnosis of infection with *E. bieneusi* and *S. intestinalis* has, so far, been based on detection of the parasites in biopsy material.

REFERENCES

1 Cox F E G. Systematics of parasitic protozoa. In Kreier J P & Baker J R (eds) *Parasitic Protozoa,* 2nd edn, vol. 1. San Diego: Academic Press, 1991: 55–80.

2 Vallejo G A, Chiari E, Macedo A M & Pena S D J. A simple laboratory method for distinguishing between *Trypanosoma cruzi* and *Trypanosoma rangeli. Trans R Soc Trop Med Hyg* 1993; 87: 165–166.

3 Lainson R & Shaw J J. Evolution, classification and geographical distribution. In Peters W & Killick-Kendrick R (eds) *The Leishmaniases in Biology and Medicine.* London: Academic Press, 1987: 1–120.

4 Brumpt E. Etude sommaire de l'*Entamoeba dispar* n. sp. amibe à kystes quadrinuclées, parasite de l'homme. *Bull Acad Méd* 1925; 94: 942–952.

5 Sargeaunt P G. '*Entamoeba histolytica*' is a complex of two species. *Trans R Soc Trop Med Hyg* 1992; 86: 348.

FURTHER READING

Gilles H M & Warrell D A. *Bruce-Chwatt's Essential Malariology*, 3rd edn. Sevenoaks: Edward Arnold, 1993.

Kreier J P & (for vols 1–3) Baker J R. *Parasitic Protozoa*, 2nd edn, vols. 1–9 (vol. 10 in preparation). San Diego: Academic Press, 1991–1994.

Molyneux D H & Ashford R W. *The Biology of* Trypanosoma *and* Leishmania, *Parasites of Man and Domestic Animals.* London: Taylor & Francis, 1983.

Muller R & Baker J R. *Medical Parasitology.* Philadelphia/London: Lippincott/Gower, 1990.

Orihel T C & Ash C R. *Parasites in Human Tissues.* Chicago: ASCP Press, 1995.

Peters W & Gilles H M. *A Colour Atlas of Tropical Medicine and Parasitology,* 3rd edn. London: Wolfe, 1989.

Peters W & Killick-Kendrick R. *The Leishmaniases in Biology and Medicine*, vols 1 & 2. London: Academic Press, 1987.

Ravdin J I (editor). *Amebiasis. Human Infection by* Entamoeba histolytica. New York: John Wiley, 1988.

Rondinelli E G & Scaglia M. *Atlas of Human Protozoa.* Milan: Masson, 1993.

Taylor E R & Baker J R (eds). In vitro *Methods for Parasite Cultivation.* London: Academic Press, 1987.

Wernsdorfer W H & McGregor I (eds). *Malaria: Principles and Practice of Malariology.* Edinburgh: Churchill Livingstone, 1989.

APPENDIX III

MEDICAL HELMINTHOLOGY

V. R. Southgate

TREMATODES (See also Chapters 72 and 73)
Subclass Digenea (Carus, 1863)

FASCIOLA HEPATICA

Fasciola hepatica (Linnaeus, 1758) is a parasite of sheep and cattle causing 'liver rot'. It is also found in various species of domesticated and wild herbivores.

DISTRIBUTION

Worldwide.

PARASITOLOGY (Figure III.1)

Pale grey with dark borders, it measures 2.3 cm × 8–13 mm. The anterior extremity is narrow, containing the oral sucker; the ventral sucker is larger than the oral and situated 3 mm from the anterior extremity. Branched intestinal caeca with diverticula are present. The ovary is racemose, placed anterior to the testes in the posterior end of the body. The uterus is short and anterior to the ovary. An exsertile cirrus is present and the genital pore is median.

The *egg* (Figure III.2) is operculated, 130–140 × 63–90 μm, ovoid, brown and tanned and contains the ovum and yolk cells. A ciliated eye-spotted miracidium develops in about 3 weeks and enters freshwater amphibious lymnaeid snails (see below).

LIFE CYCLE (Figure III.3)

Snail hosts

Lymnaea truncatula (Europe, western Asia and highland southern Africa), *L. viator*, *L. diaphana* (South America),

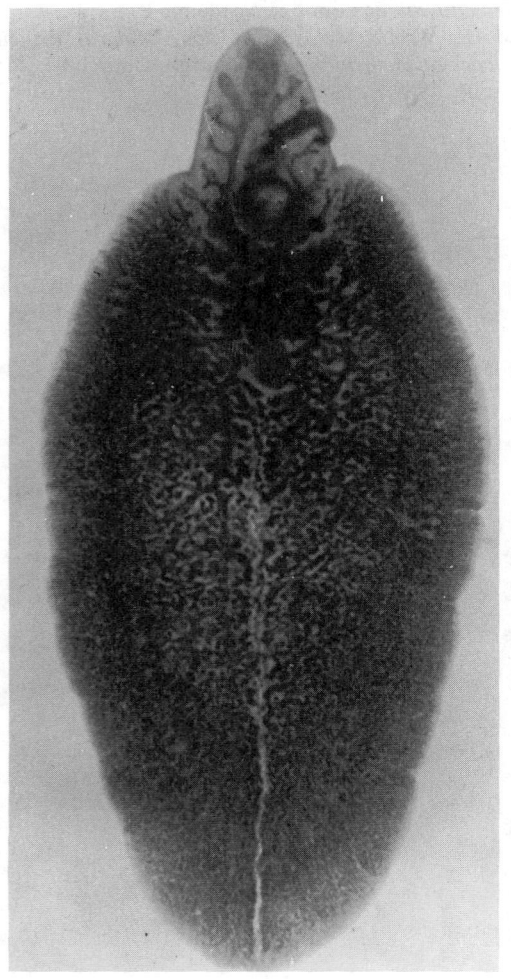

Figure III.1   Adult *Fasciola hepatica*. (Courtesy of H. Zaiman.)

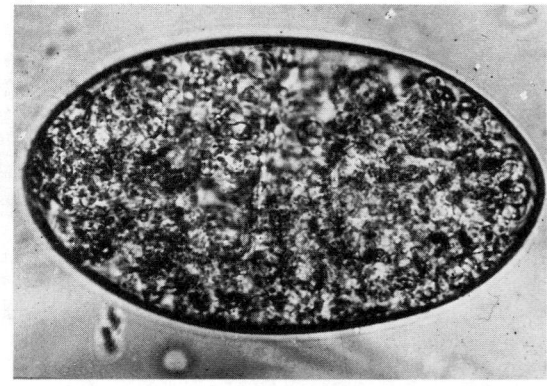

Figure III.2   Egg of *Fasciola hepatica*. (Courtesy of WTIM.)

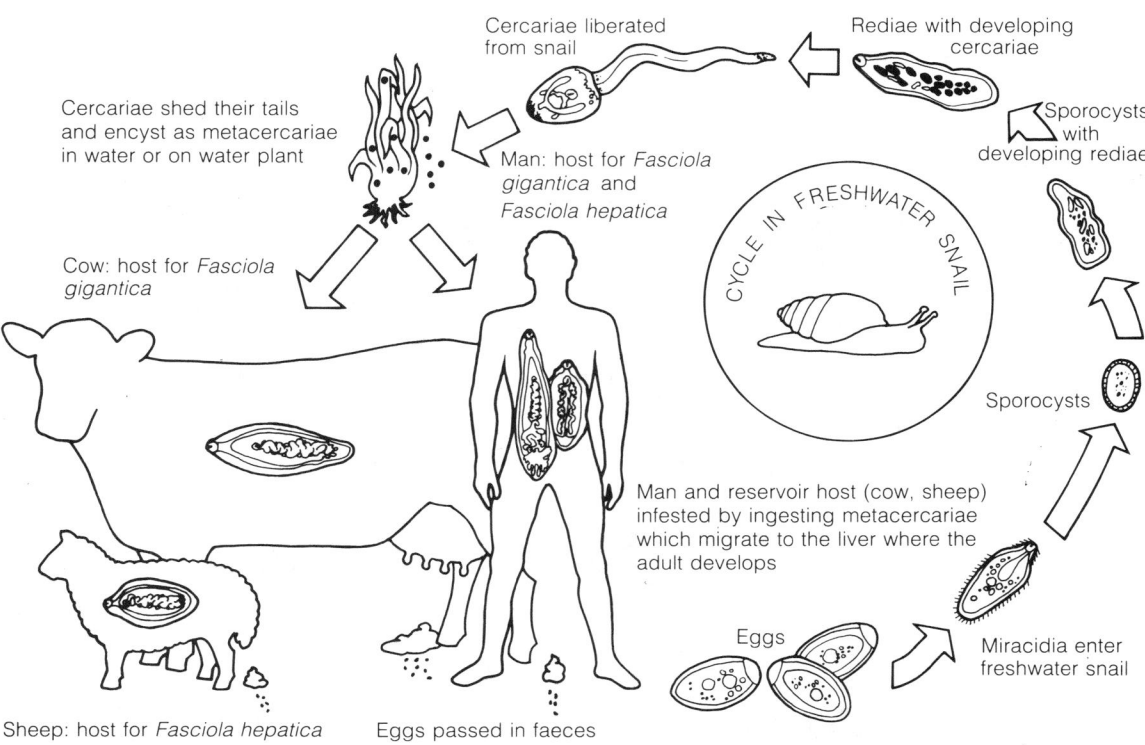

Figure III.3   Life cycle of *Fasciola hepatica* and *F. gigantica*. (Courtesy of WTIM.)

L. bulimoides, *L. humilis* (North America), *L. columella* (Africa, also occasionally North and South America, Australia), *L. cubensis* (Caribbean) and *L. tomentosa* (Australasia). *L. columella* is a proven host for both *F. hepatica* and *F. gigantica* and, in recent years, *L. columella* has become established in South Africa, Australia, New Zealand and Hawaii. In these it becomes a sporocyst, giving rise to rediae (named after the Italian zoologist Redi) and cercariae. Development takes 2 months. The cercaria is blunt tailed and settles in grass or on bark where it secretes mucus to form a cyst containing the metacercaria. Then it is eaten by the mammalian host. Metacercariae excyst in the duodenum and migrate through the intestinal wall into the body cavity, then to the biliary passages where they grow to maturity.

F. gigantica, a liver fluke, similar but larger, is now known to cause human infections in the CIS, Indo-China, West Africa and Hawaii. It develops in fully aquatic lymnaeid snails.

FASCIOLOPSIS BUSKI
(LANKESTER, 1857) (ODHNER, 1902)

Fasciolopsis buski (Figure III.4) is a parasite of the pig and dog; they constitute a reservoir for man.

PARASITOLOGY

F. buski inhabits the small intestine, rarely the stomach; only a small number of those infected show symptoms. This is the

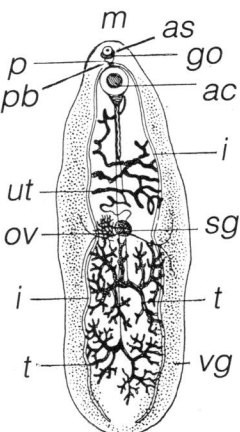

Figure III.4   *Fasciolopsis buski*. The following key is used for the terminology of the anatomy of the trematodes in this and subsequent illustrations.

ac	acetabulum or	ov	ovary
	ventral sucker	ovd	oviduct
as	oral sucker	p	pharynx
exp	excretory pore	pb	pharyngeal bulb
go	genital opening	rs	receptaculum seminalis
gp	genital pore	sg	shell gland
i	intestine	t	testis
ic	branch intestine	ut	uterus
lc	Laurer's canal	va	vagina
m	mouth	vd	vas deferens
nc	nerve cord	vg	vitelline glands
oes	oesophagus	vs	vesicula seminalis
oo	ootype		

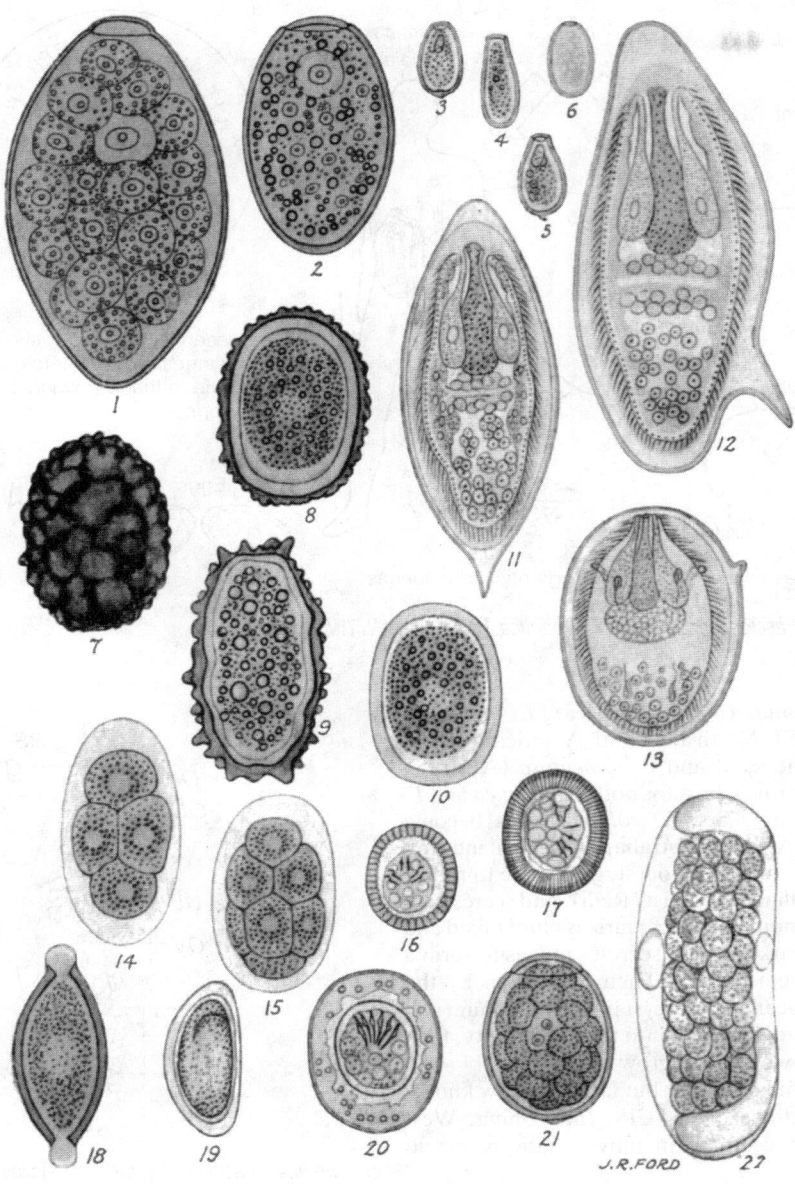

Figure III.5   1, *Fasciolopsis buski*. 2, *Paragonimus westermani*. 3, *Heterophyes heterophyes*. 4, *Opisthorchis felineus*. 5, *Clonorchis sinensis*. 6, *Metagonimus yokogawai*. 7, 8, *Ascaris lumbricoides*, external aspect. 9, *Ascaris lumbricoides*, unfertilized egg. 10, *Ascaris lumbricoides*, decorticated egg. 11, *Schistosoma haematobium*. 12, *Schistosoma mansoni*. 13, *Schistosoma japonicum*. 14, *Ancylostoma duodenale*. 15, *Trichostrongylus colubriformis*. 16, *Taenia solium*. 17, *Taenia saginata*. 18, *Trichuris trichiura*. 19, *Enterobius vermicularis*. 20, *Vampirolepis nana*. 21, *Diphyllobothrium latum*. 22, *Heterodera radicicola*, non-parasitic, ingested with vegetables.

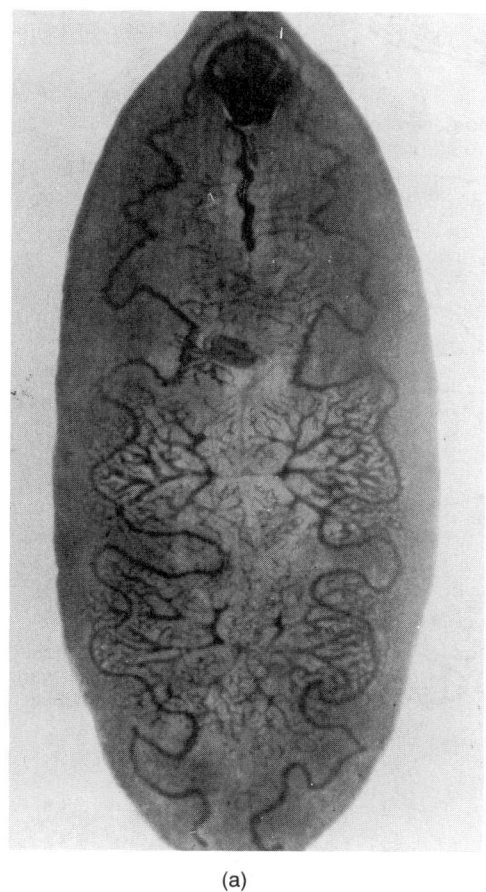

(a)

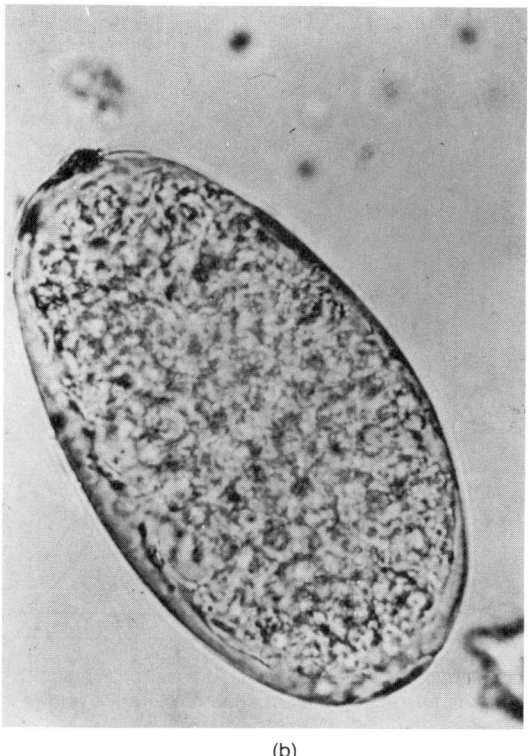

(b)

Figure III.6 (a) Adult *Fasciolopsis buski*. (b) Egg of *F. buski*. (Courtesy of WTIM.)

largest human trematode, measuring 3 cm × 12 mm and 2 mm thick. It is flesh coloured, elongated and oval, with transverse rows of spines, especially numerous near the ventral sucker. The oral sucker is subterminal but ventral in position and is only a quarter of the size of the ventral which is placed close to the oral, and prolonged into the cavity dorsally and backwards, a feature peculiar to this species. (For details of the anatomy see Figure III.4.) The intestinal caeca are simple with two characteristic curves towards the midline. The genital pore is median, placed anterior to the ventral sucker. Branched testes are found in the posterior half of the body; there is a branched ovary and a fine, tortuous, Laurer's canal.

Development in the freshwater snail resembles that of *F. hepatica*.

The egg is operculated and yellow, measuring 130–140 × 80–85 μm (Figures III.5,1 and III.6b). Eggs are found in large numbers in the faeces, the egg capacity of each fluke being about 25 000/day.

LIFE CYCLE (Figure III.7)

After 3–7 weeks in water the eggs hatch a ciliated miracidium which develops in freshwater snails—*Segmentina hemi-*

sphaerula, *Hippeutis umbilicalis* (Far East), *Hippeutis cantori* (Far East) and *Segmentina trochoidens* (India) (Figure III.8). A sporocyst is formed in 3 days, followed by the rediae and daughter rediae, which eventually produce cercariae (the whole cycle takes 2 months).

The cercariae, resembling those of *F. hepatica*, are oval, short lived and lophocercous and measure 0.7 mm; they have a well-developed digestive tract with a muscular bladder and collecting tubules. They encyst, as *metacercariae*, on freshwater plants especially the outer cuticle of the water calthrop, *Trapa* (*Salvinia*) *natans* in China, *T. bicornis* in India, *T. bisponosa* in Taiwan. As many as 20 encysted metacercariae may be found on a single leaf. In south China the most important plant is the water chestnut, *Eliocharis tuberosa*, and water bamboo, *Zigania aquatica*, in Chekiang and Canton, and the water hyacinth, *Eichornia crassipes*, in Taiwan. The outer layers of the plants are torn off by the teeth. All the plants are grown in ponds in China and fertilized by human faeces, thus affording an opportunity for infection; *F. buski* is therefore limited in distribution to that of these plants. The cysts when taken into the mouth pass through the stomach, excyst in the duodenum and become attached to the intestinal wall.

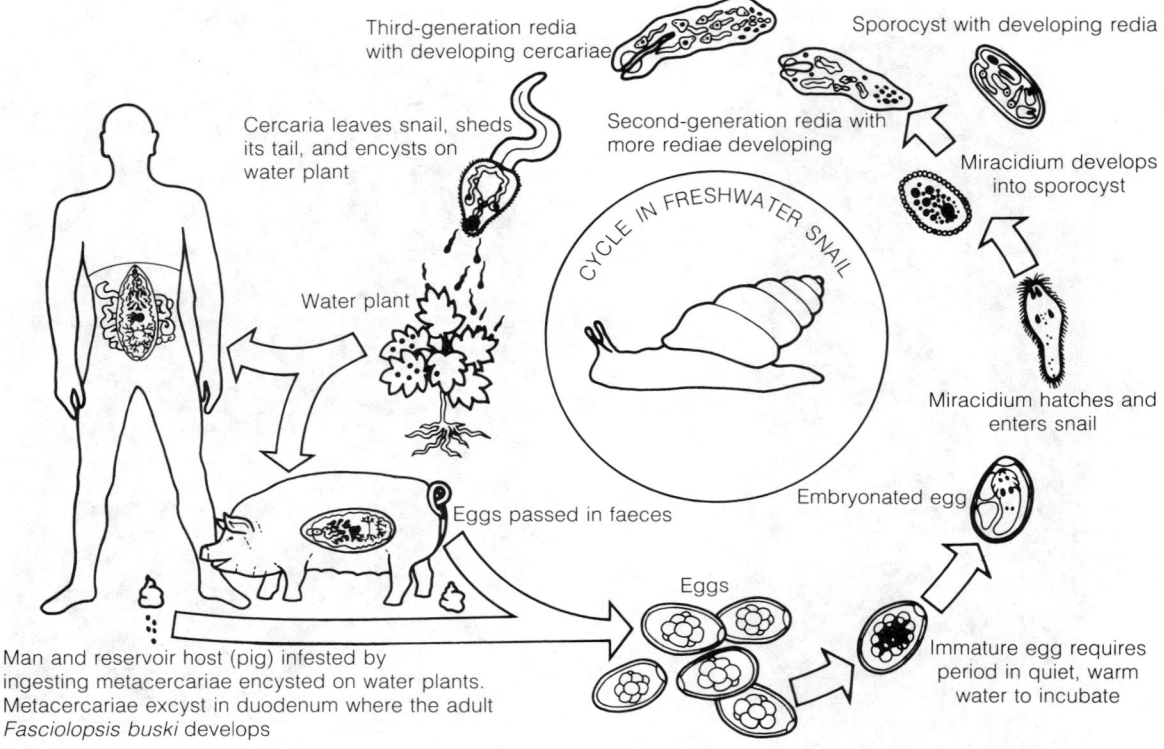

Third-generation redia
with developing cercariae

Sporocyst with developing redia

Cercaria leaves snail, sheds
its tail, and encysts on
water plant

Second-generation redia with
more rediae developing

Miracidium develops
into sporocyst

Water plant

CYCLE IN FRESHWATER SNAIL

Miracidium hatches and
enters snail

Eggs passed in faeces

Embryonated egg

Eggs

Immature egg requires
period in quiet, warm
water to incubate

Man and reservoir host (pig) infested by
ingesting metacercariae encysted on water plants.
Metacercariae excyst in duodenum where the adult
Fasciolopsis buski develops

Figure III.7   Life cycle of *Fasciolopsis buski*. (Courtesy of WTIM.)

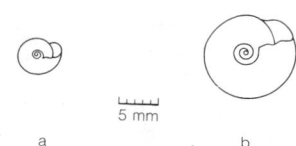

a   b

Figure III.8   Molluscan hosts of *Fasciolopsis buski*. (a) *Segmentina hemisphaerula*. (b) *Hippeutis cantori*.

SUPERFAMILY: OPISTHORCHIOIDEA

GENUS: *CLONORCHIS*

CLONORCHIS SINENSIS (Figures III.9 and III.10)

DISTRIBUTION

Far East, especially China (Kwangtung province in south China, Indo-China and Okayama, Japan).

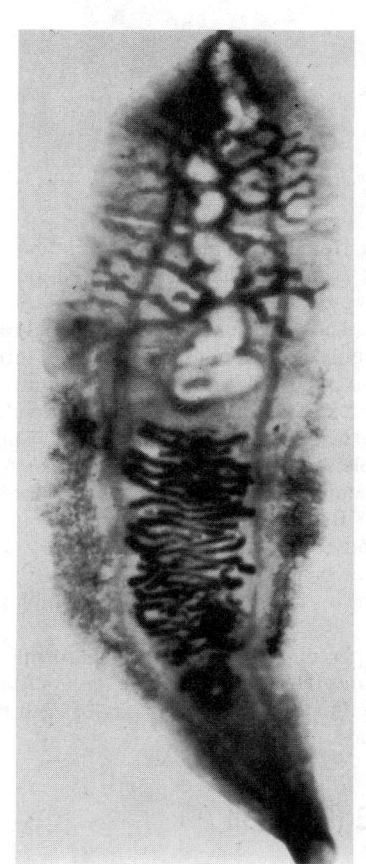

Figure III.9   Adult *Clonorchis sinensis*.

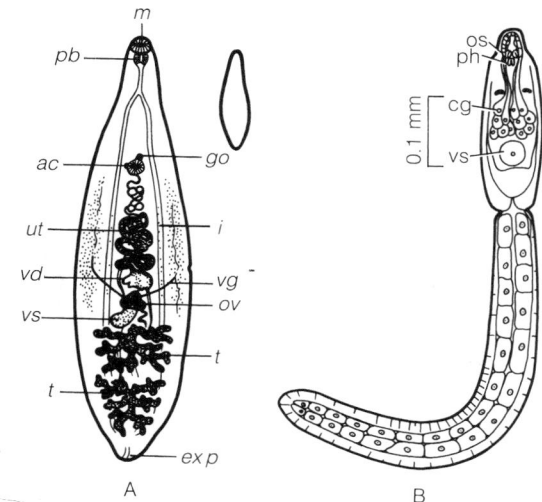

Figure III.10   A, *Clonorchis sinensis*, magnified and natural size.
B, Cercaria of *C. sinensis*.

cg   cephalic secretory gland
os   oral sucker
ph   pharynx
vs   ventral sucker

PARASITOLOGY

This is a common parasite of man and also of the biliary passages of the dog, cat, pig, rat, mouse, camel and badger, etc. It is found rarely in the gallbladder of man but often in the bile ducts, pancreas, pancreatic ducts and duodenum. It is spatulate, tapering anteriorly, reddish, semitransparent and measures 10–25 × 2–5 mm. The tegument is smooth; the oral sucker is larger than the ventral; the intestinal caeca are simple.

The genital pore is median and placed anterior to the ventral sucker. The testes are branched and situated posteriorly one behind the other. The ovary is trilobate with coils anterior to the genital glands. Vitelline glands are moderately developed in the mid-third of the body. Cross-fertilization occurs; the spermatozoa develop before the ova; the sperms enter the female genital pore, pass into the immature uterus and thence to the *spermatheca* (Figure III.10) where they are stored; the ova are fertilized in the spermatheca and then pass on.

The egg measures 20–30 × 14–17 μm; it is operculated, yellow-brown and one of the smallest trematode eggs found in man (Figures III.5,5 and III.11). It is fully embryonated

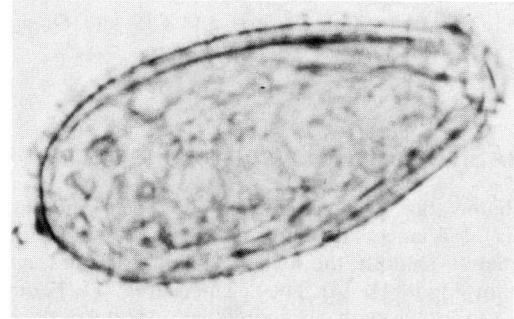

Figure III.11   Egg of *Clonorchis sinensis*.

when discharged. It resembles an electric light bulb with the knob at the bottom. It withstands desiccation but not decomposition.

LIFE CYCLE (Figure III.12)

The egg can remain viable in water for 5 weeks and is ingested by the snail before the escape of the miracidium which has a life span of 20 minutes. Development continues in bythinid snails. The miracidium pierces the oesophagus of the mollusc, casts its cilia and soon becomes a sporocyst; later, the elongated rediae grow within the sporocysts and burst into the perioesophageal sinus and move tailwards into the liver, the whole process taking 3–4 weeks.

The cercariae (Figure III.10B), 450–550 × 100–120 μm, escape from the rediae from the birthpore; they have two pigmented eyespots and a lophocercous blunt-ending tail, and burst through the space between the upper body surface and the shell, emerging into water. Within 24–48 hours they encyst as metacercariae in the muscles and underscales of freshwater fish of families Cyprinidae and Anabantidae. Cercarial glands excrete a hystolytic substance which dissolves the skin of the fish, thus admitting percolating water. The metacercariae secrete a viscous fluid which forms an inner true cyst which in turn is encapsulated by a fibrous layer formed by the tissues of the fish. These are eaten half raw, or pickled in soy sauce by the Chinese. The adolescercaria, the fully developed cyst, possesses a capsule protective against the gastric juice. In some species of fish—*Carassius auratus* (golden carp)—the parasite is found under the scales; in others it is in the flesh so that domestic animals which eat the offal may become heavily infected while man escapes. The cysts withstand a temperature of 50–70°C for 15 minutes. The cyst wall is digested by the succus entericus in the duodenum near the ampulla of Vater and the adolescercariae escape and attach themselves to the mucosa. The young distomes at first have spines but these are soon lost. They attain maturity in 26 days. Attracted by positive chemotaxis a small proportion of them reach the bile ducts but 95% are digested and destroyed. The size of the resulting fluke is determined by the calibre of the bile duct. Egg production is very large; in the cat 2400 eggs are produced daily but fewer in dogs. As many as 9400 adults have been found at autopsy. Life span is 12 years. Adult men are infected more than women.

The following is a list of the molluscs and fishes which may be intermediaries.

HOSTS

First intermediate hosts (molluscs) (Figure III.13)

The most important first intermediate (snail) hosts are: *Parafossarulus manchouricus* and *Bulimus fuchsiana*. Additional first intermediate hosts are *Bythinia longicornis*, *Assiminea lutea* and *Melanoides tuberculatus*.

Second intermediate hosts (fish)

More than 80 species of fish have been incriminated: 71 species of Cyprinidae; two species of Eleotridae; one species

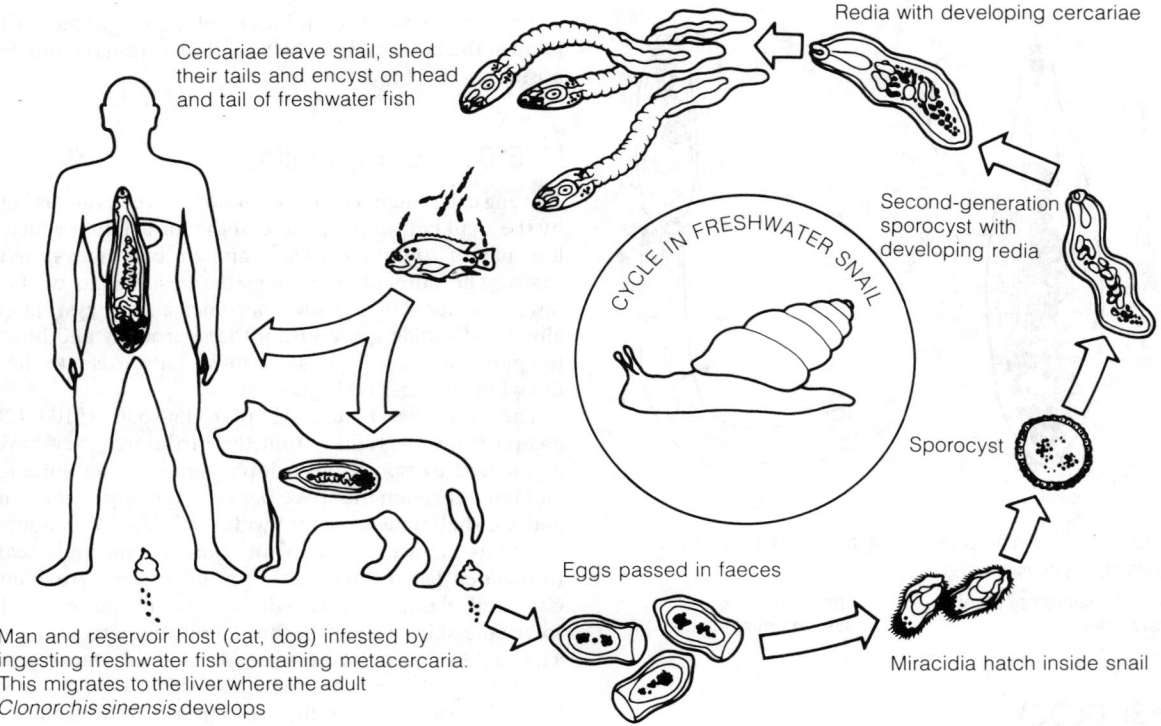

Redia with developing cercariae

Cercariae leave snail, shed their tails and encyst on head and tail of freshwater fish

CYCLE IN FRESHWATER SNAIL

Second-generation sporocyst with developing redia

Sporocyst

Eggs passed in faeces

Miracidia hatch inside snail

Man and reservoir host (cat, dog) infested by ingesting freshwater fish containing metacercaria. This migrates to the liver where the adult *Clonorchis sinensis* develops

Figure III.12   Life cycle of *Clonorchis sinensis*. (Courtesy of WTIM.)

each of Bagridae, Cyprinodontidae, Clupeidae, Osmeripae, Cichlidae, Ophiocephalidae and Gobiidae. The most important cyprinoid fish are *Mylopharyngodon aethiops*, *Ctenopharyngodon idella* (Canton), *Cultur recurviceps* (Peking) and *Carassius auratus* (golden carp).

Major additional fish hosts are *Tribolodon hakonensis*, *Hemibarbus labes*, *Acanthorhodeus asmussi*, *Pungtungia herzi*, *Pseudogobio esocinus*, *Gnathopogon atromaculatus*, *Cultriculus kneri*, *Macropodus chinensis* and *Opsariichthydis bidens*.

In addition in Fukien, China, freshwater shrimps (*Caridinia nilotica*, *Macrobrachium superboum*, *Palaeomonetes sinensis*) are incriminated as sources of infection in children.

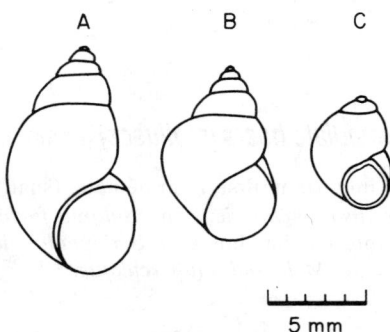

Figure III.13   Molluscan hosts of *Clonorchis sinensis*.
A, *Parafossarulus manchouricus*. B, *Bythinia fuschiana*.
C, *Bythinia longicornis*.

Other fish hosts are *Hemicultur leucisculus*, *H. b. leekeri*, *Acanthorhodeus chankaensis*, *A. gracilis*, *Abbotina rivularis*, *Pseudorasbora parva*, *Hyspeleotris swinhoensis*, *Philypus potamophilus*, *Rhodeus sinensis*, *Sarcocheilichthys nigripennis*, *S. sinensis*, *S. variegatus*, *Macropodus opercularis*, *Biwia zezera*, *Xenocypris davidi*, *Pseudiperilampus typus*, *Abbotina psegma*, *Paraleucogobio strigatus*, *Acheilognathus rhombea*, *A. lanceolata*, *A. limbata*, *A. cyanostigma*, *Lakeo jordani* and *Hypophalmichthys nobilis*.

GENUS: *OPISTHORCHIS* (CAT LIVER FLUKE)

There are two species of cat liver fluke: *Opisthorchis felineus* (Rivolta 1884), eastern Europe and CIS and *O. viverrini* (Poirier 1886) north-east Thailand, Laos.

PARASITOLOGY (*Opisthorchis felineus*)

It inhabits the liver, pancreas, bile ducts and lungs (in Russia). It is lanceolate and measures $8–11 \times 1.5–2$ mm. The tegument is smooth, the suckers equal in size and separated by 2 mm (Figure III.14). The egg measures $30 \times 12\,\mu m$ and is yellowish-brown with an operculum. At the posterior end there is a minute tubercular thickening (Figure III.5,4).

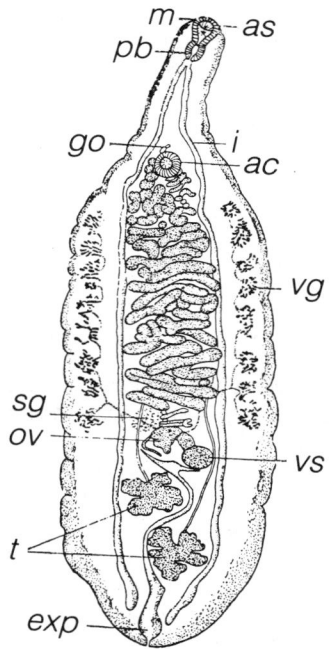

Figure III.14   Opisthorchis felineus. (9×.)

LIFE CYCLE (similar to *C. sinensis*, Figure III.12)

The definitive hosts are man and wild and domestic felines. The first intermediary host is a snail, usually *Bythinia leachi* (Figure III.15); an additional snail host is *Bythinia tentaculata*. The miracidium is fully formed in the egg and hatches in the snail, forming a sporocyst in the intestine measuring 1.2–1.85 mm. Rediae are formed in 1 month and then cercariae which mature in 4 months.

Cercariae, 430–670 × 40–50 μm, which leave the snail in daylight, are phototactic and stimulated by agitation.

The second intermediary hosts are fish—the tench (*Tinca tinca*), the ide (*Leuciscus idus*), the barbel (*Barbus barbus*) and the roach (*Rutilus rutilus*). Additional second intermediary hosts are *Idus melanotus*, *Abramis brama*, *A. sapa*, *Cyprinus carpio*, *Blicca bjorkna*, *Alburnus lucidus*, *Aspilus aspilus*, *Scardinus erythrophthalmus*. The cercariae penetrate in 15 minutes and grow to three or four times their original size forming metacercariae 220 × 160 μm. When ingested by man they pass through the stomach, are freed by

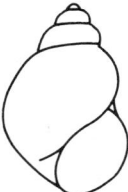

Figure III.15   Bythinia leachi, the molluscan host of *Opisthorchis felineus*.

the succus entericus, attracted by the bile and travel up the bile duct in 5 hours. Infection is therefore contracted by eating raw fish. The entire life cycle requires a minimum of 4 months. This fluke is not specially pathogenic, although 200 or more have been found in the body at autopsies.

Opisthorchis viverrini is the other species and is of importance in Thailand and India. It is morphologically similar.

LIFE CYCLE OF *O. VIVERRINI* (similar to *C. sinensis*, Figure III.12)

The normal definitive hosts are the dog and civet cat. First intermediate hosts are snails. *Bythinia funiculata*, *B. siamensis*, *B. goniomphales* and *B. laevis*. Second intermediate hosts are fish, *Cyclocheilichthys siaja*, *Hampala dispar*, *Puntius orphoides*, *P. gonionotus*, *P. poctozyron*, *Labiobarbus lineatus* and *Osteochilus* sp.

GENUS: *HETEROPHYES*

HETEROPHYES HETEROPHYES (SIEBOLD, 1852)

DISTRIBUTION

Egypt, China, Japan, Brazil, Korea, Spain, France and Greece.

CHARACTERS

Heterophyes heterophyes (Figures III.16 and III.17) inhabits the small intestine of man in large numbers and also that of the rat, fox, dog, wolf, jackal and cat; also in the black kite (*Milvus migrans aegyptius*) and a bat (*Rhinolophus divosus*

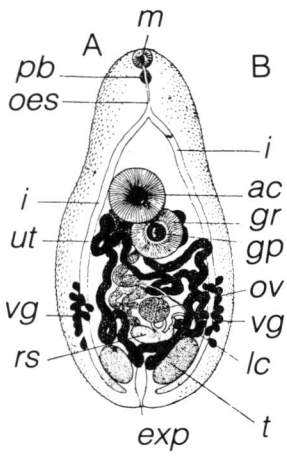

Figure III.16   Heterophyes heterophyes, greatly magnified (A).

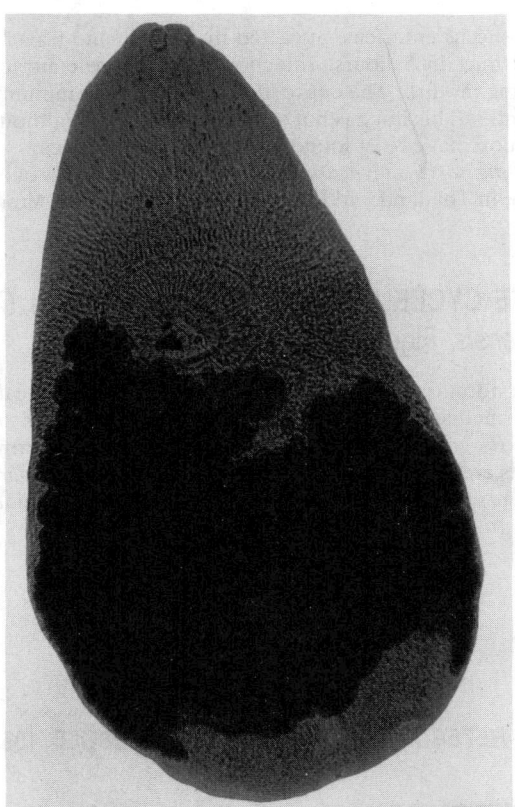

Figure III.17 Adult *Heterophyes heterophyes*. Cuticle covered by fine spines and oral sucker less conspicuous than ventral sucker. (Courtesy of WTIM.)

acrotis) in the Yemen. It imparts a coffee grounds appearance to the intestinal wall. It is pyriform, grey and very small, measuring 1–1.7 × 0.3–0.7 mm. The uterus forms a brown patch in the centre. The oral sucker is subterminal and the ventral sucker is three times the size of the oral sucker. The tegument is thickly set with quadrate scales measuring 5 × 4 μm. There is a short prepharynx and long oesophagus. The intestinal caeca extend to the posterior extremity, converging close to the excretory vesicle. The vitelline glands are posterior, situated in two clumps; the genital pore is posterolateral in the vicinity of the ventral sucker and consists of a muscular ring armed with 70 chitinous cuticular teeth. The testes are oval and posterior, the ovary globular and median. There is a receptaculum seminis as large as the ovary; uterine coils are not numerous. A seminal vesicle and Laurer's canal are present.

The egg measures 20–30 × 15–17 μm, being the same size as that of *C. sinensis* (Figure III.5,3). Its greatest breadth is across the centre. There is no special ring to the operculum, which is light-brown and contains a ciliated miracidium when deposited. It hatches after ingestion by the appropriate snail.

LIFE CYCLE

H. heterophyes develops in brackish water snails. The proven hosts are *Pirinella conica* in the Middle East (Figure

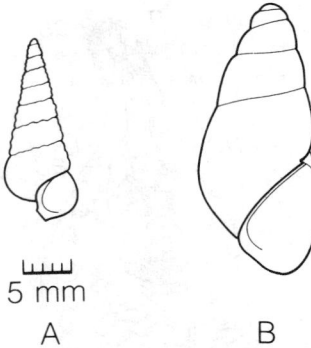

5 mm
A   B

Figure III.18 A, *Pirinella conica*, the molluscan host of *Heterophyes heterophyes*. B, *Semisulcospira libertina*, the molluscan host of *Metagonimus yokogawai*.

III.18A), *Cerithidea cingulata* and *Tympanotomus micropterus* in the Far East. Additional recorded hosts include *Melanoides tuberculata* and *Cleopatra bulimoides*. The cercaria, which is eyed and has a membranous tail, enters the second intermediate host—a freshwater fish the mullet (*Mugil cephalus*) or in Japan a species of *Acanthogobius* in which metacercariae develop and encyst under the scales. Infection is acquired from eating raw fish.

Related species include: *Heterophyes continua*, *Haplorchis pumilio*, *H. vanissimus* and *Procerovum calderon*. In Japan in the vicinity of Kobe a closely related species (or synonym of *Heterophyes heterophyes*), *H. katsuradai*, is recognized which is stouter and has a relatively enormous acetabulum. The eggs are smaller, measuring 25–26 × 14–15 μm.

GENUS: *METAGONIMUS*

METAGONIMUS YOKOGAWAI (KATSURADA, 1912)

DISTRIBUTION

Korea, Taiwan, China, Japan, Philippines and Ukraine. Very common in the Far East.

PARASITOLOGY

Metagonimus yokogawai (Figure III.19) is found in the small intestine of man, higher up than *H. heterophyes*, and also in the cat, dog, pig and fish-eating birds, such as the pelican. It is the smallest fluke parasitic in man with a mean size of 1.4 × 0.6 mm. The tegument is covered with small spines; the ventral sucker is deflected to the right with its long axis in the diagonal phase. There is a genital pore in front; the ovoid testes are posterior; the ovary and receptaculum seminis are situated medially in front of the testes. The yolk glands are found in clumps in the posterior third. The uterus lies between the testes and the ventral sucker and the seminal vesicle in front of the ovary (Figure III.19).

The egg measures 27–28 μm × 16–17 μm and resembles that of *C. sinensis* but is more regularly ovoid (Figure III.5, 6).

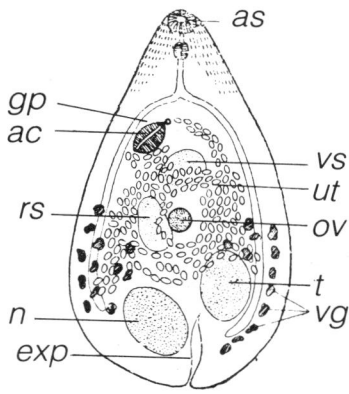

Figure III.19 *Metagonimus yokogawai.* (45×.)

LIFE CYCLE

The first intermediate hosts are molluscs— *Semi-sulcospira libertina* (Figure III.18B) and *S. coreana.* Sporocysts, rediae and cercariae are formed; the last have an anterior end provided with armament. The tail is long and membranous with lateral flutings and is discarded on entering the fish host. *Plecoglossus altivelis* is regarded as the most important source of infection of *M. yokogawai* in Japan. Other freshwater fish hosts recorded include: *Carassius auratus, Cyprinus carpio, Zacco temminckii, Photimus steindachneri, Acheilognathus lanceolata* and *Pseudorasbora parva.* The metacercariae measure about $150 \times 100\,\mu$m and encyst under the scales; infection results from eating raw fish.

SUPERFAMILY: PLAGIORCHIDEA

GENUS: *PARAGONIMUS*

Many species of *Paragonimus* are found in nature and can be divided into four main groups by the nature of the cuticular spines and the ovary.

1. Westermani: *P. westermani, P. pulmonalis.*
2. Compactus: *P. compactus, P. siamensis.*
3. Kellicotti-miyazaki: *P. kellicotti, P. miyazakii, P. heterotremus, P. caliensis, P. amazonicus, P. mexicanus (peruvianus).*
4. Ohirai-ilokstuensis: *P. ohirai, P. ilokstuenensis.*

Other species include: *P. tuanshenensis, P. szechuanensis, P. hueitungensis, P. bangliokensis, P. philippinensis, P. sadoensis, P. shrjabini* and the African species *P. africanus* and *P. uterobilateralis.*

DISTRIBUTION

The Far East from Japan to India, Indonesia, Pacific Islands, West and central Africa and central South America.

PARASITOLOGY

P. westermani measures $8-20 \times 5-9$ mm and is oval (almost round in section), reddish-brown and translucent. The anterior extremity is rounded. The oral sucker is subterminal; the ventral sucker larger and placed anterior to the centre of the body. The pharynx and oesophagus are short and the bifurcation of the intestine is anterior to the ventral sucker (Figures III.20 and III.21). The intestinal caeca run a zigzag

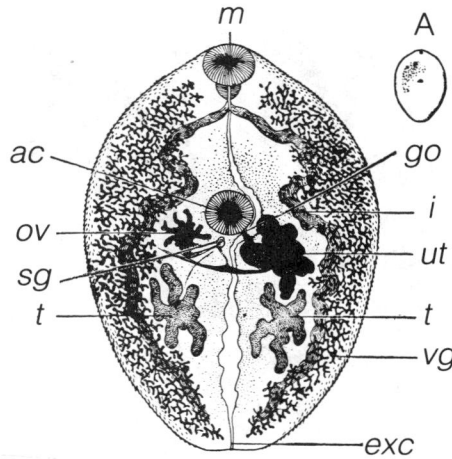

Figure III.20 *Paragonimus westermani* (*ringeri*), natural size (A) and magnified.

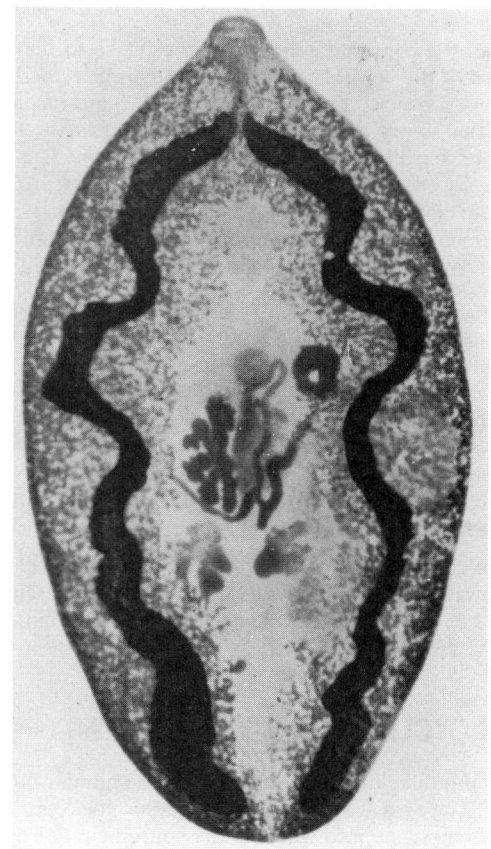

Figure III.21 Adult *Paragonimus westermani.* (Courtesy of WTIM.)

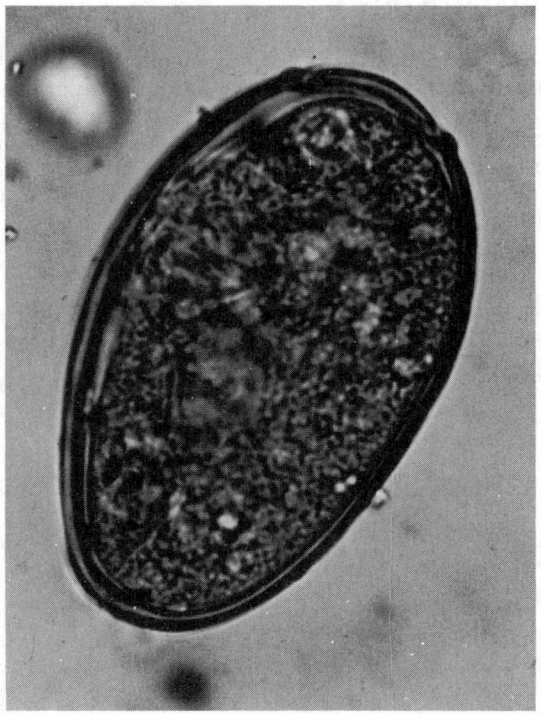

Figure III.22 Egg of *Paragonimus westermani*. (Courtesy of WTIM.)

course; the common genital pore lies close to the posterior margin of the ventral sucker. The body is bisected by a large excretory vesicle. The testes are tubular and racemose; the branched ovary may be to either the right or the left of the midline and posterior to the ventral sucker. The uterus is short, sac-like and lies opposite the ovary. The vitellaria are well developed, extending through the whole body. Laurer's canal and shell gland are present. The cuticle is studded with wedge-shape spines which with the ovary are used to differentiate the four main types:

1. Westermani: cuticular spines singly spaced and ovary simply branched into 4–6 lobes.
2. Compactus: cuticular spines in groups and ovary simply branched into 4–6 lobes.
3. Kellicotti-miyazaki: cuticular spines singly spaced, ovary profusely branched.
4. Ohirai-iloktsuenensis: cuticular spines in groups, ovary profusely branched.

The egg is brown and operculated, measuring $90 \times 55 \mu m$. It shows a thickening at the pole opposite the operculum. The egg of *P. compactus* is smaller, $75 \times 48 \mu m$ (Figures III.5,2 and III.22).

LIFE CYCLE (Figures III.23 and III.24)

The lung fluke can remain viable in the human body for 20 years. The eggs are first voided into cystic pockets in the lungs and then escape into water in the sputum and also in faeces from swallowed sputum. A ciliated miracidium hatches in 16 days to 7 weeks and has distinctive characters. There is a ciliated covering in four rows at the anterior cone. The

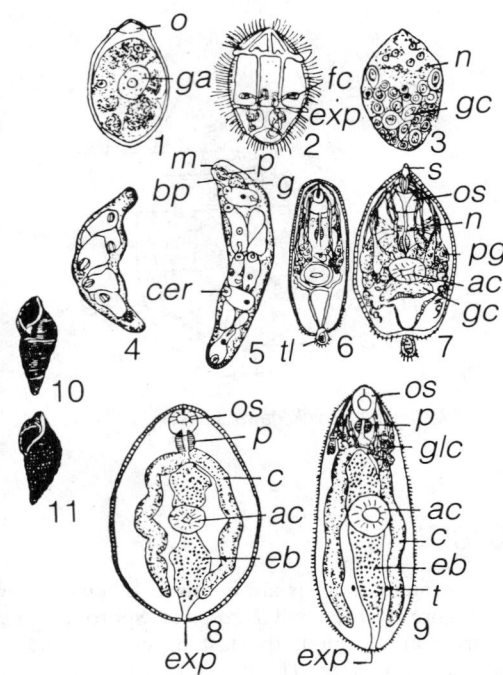

Figure III.23 Life cycle of *Paragonimus westermani* (1–9, 15×; 10 and 11, half natural size). 1, Egg showing yolk cells and germinal area. 2, Miracidium with excretory system and flame cells. 3, Miracidium with ganglionic mass and germ cells. 4, Mature sporocyst in snail containing well-developed first generation rediae. 5, Mature second generation rediae. 6 and 7, Stages of microcercous cercariae after emergence from the snail. 8, Metacercariae from the crab; the cyst wall is not shown. 9, Mature encysted metacercaria. 10, *Semisulcospira libertina*. 11, *Thiara granifera*.

bp	birth pore	n	nervous system
c	caeca	o	operculum
cer	cercaria	os	oral sucker
eb	excretory bladder	p	pharynx
fc	flame cell	pg	periacetabular glands
g	gut	s	stylet
ga	germinal area	tl	tail
gc	genital cells		

excretory pore forms a rosette. It enters the snail hosts (Table III.1). It develops in about 60 days into sporocysts and rediae, each containing 20 cercariae; the latter, ellipsoid and microcercous, have a short knob-like tail and measure $200 \times 70–80 \mu m$ with an anterior stylet and body covered with spines. The cercariae bore into freshwater crabs and become metacercariae in the crabs and crayfish shown in Table III.1.

In the crustacean (the second intermediate) the metacercariae encyst in the liver, muscles and gills. In Japan crabs are eaten but in Korea and Taiwan they are not eaten; the supposition is that the crustacean phase is not always a biological necessity. In Venezuela the appropriate snails and crustacea are present and 30% of dogs are infected but man is not. When the metacercariae enter the stomach of man their cyst wall is digested and the adolescent cercariae emerge, pass through the jejunum, traverse the abdominal cavity, penetrate the diaphragm, pleura and lungs and reach the bronchioles forming cystic cavities.

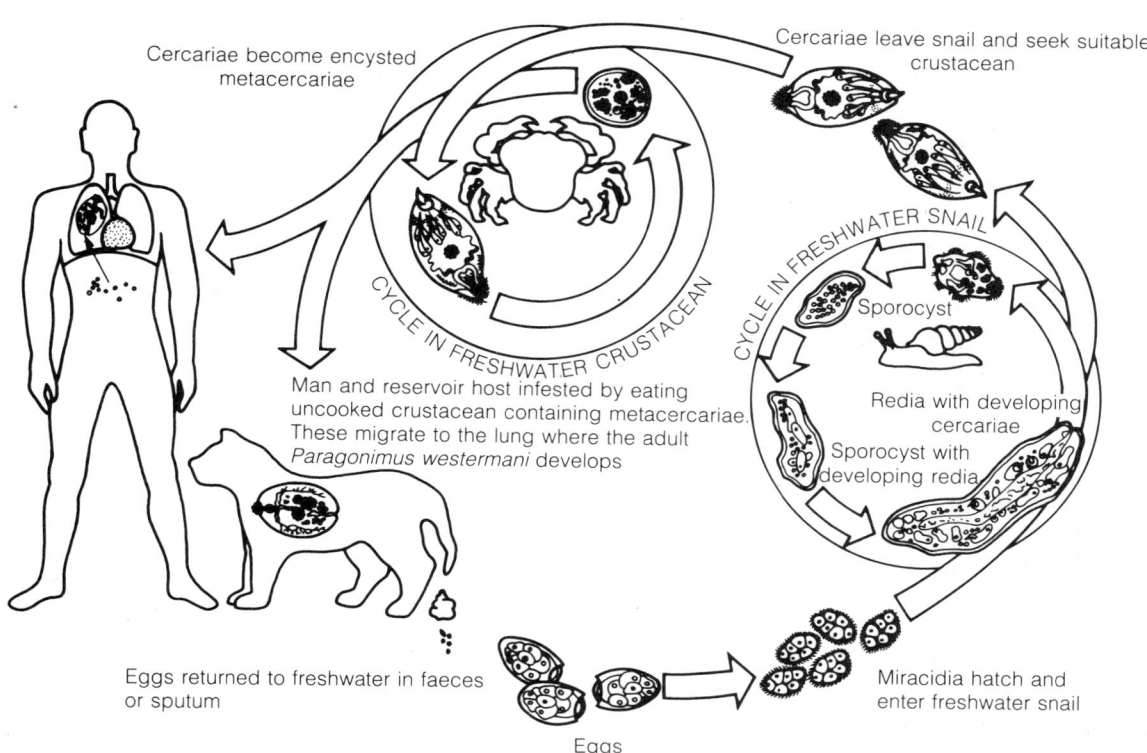

Figure III.24   Life cycle of *Paragonimus westermani*. (Courtesy of WTIM.)

GENUS: *DICROCOELIUM*

Dicrocoeliosis is caused by two species of the genus: *D. dentriticum* and *D. hospes*. *D. dendriticum* is a widely distributed parasite, mainly of ruminants but also of man, occurring in all the European countries, European and Asian parts of the CIS, China, Japan, Indo-Malayan region, USA and Canada, Cuba and parts of South America, e.g. Brazil, Colombia. *D. hospes* has been recorded from many African countries, including Tanzania, Uganda, Sudan, Chad, Ghana and Sierra Leone. The eggs passed in faeces are fully embryonated, resist desiccation and do not hatch in water. They are ingested by land snails. Over 50 species have been recorded as hosts for: *D. dendriticum* including *Theba carthusiana*, *Zebrina detrita*, *Helicella candidula*, *H. itala*, *Cepaea memoralis*, *Helix vulgaris*, *Eulota lantzi*, *E. ruben* and others (Table III.1).

LIFE CYCLE (Figure III.25)

The miracidium is released in the digestive tract of the snail host, penetrates the glandular intestinal epithelium and finally migrates to the hepatopancreas. The mother sporocyst gives rise to daughter sporocysts which in turn give rise to cercariae, the whole process taking 3–5 months. The cercariae leave the sporocyst and migrate to the respiratory chamber of the snail. They leave the host via the respiratory opening in the form of slime balls, cemented by mucus originating from glands located in the posterior region of the cercariae. The slime balls are released from the snails individually or in clusters of 4–16; for the life cycle to continue the slime balls must be eaten fairly quickly by an ant, e.g. *Formica fusca* (17 species have been recorded as secondary intermediate hosts, 14 species belonging to the genus *Formica*, plus *Proformica nasuta*, *Catagliphis bicolor* and *C. aenescens*). Penetration of the intestine occurs and metacercariae are formed in the abdominal cavity. If the infected ant is swallowed by man the cyst wall is disrupted and the young flukes migrate to the bile system and the flukes mature in about 50 days.

SUPERFAMILY: ECHINOSTOMATOIDEA

GENUS: *ECHINOSTOMA*

A trematode of minor importance is *Echinostoma lindoensis*. Until recently it was quite commonly found in man in the environs of Lake Lindoe, Celebes, but not now due to changes in diet. Mice, rats, ducks and pigeons have been experimentally infected. *E. lindoensis* causes diarrhoea, abdominal pains and eosinophilia.

Table III.1 Trematode flukes which can infect man.

Adult fluke	Morphology	Egg	Site	Vertebrate hosts	First intermediate host	Second intermediate host	Geographical distribution	Clinical features
LIVER FLUKES								
Fasciola hepatica (Figure III.1)	Large leaf-shaped, 2–3 × 1.5 cm	130–140 × 63–90 μm (Figure III.2)	Biliary tract	Sheep, cattle, man	Freshwater snails: *Lymnaea truncatula* *L. viridis* *L. viator* *L. bulimoides*, *humilis*, *columella* *Lymnaea tomentosa* Land snail: *Practicoella gresicola* and possibly *Bulinus* sp.	Aquatic vegetation: Watercress	Europe, western Asia, highlands South Africa Far East South America North America Caribbean Australasia	Transient hepatic disturbance with jaundice and fever
Fasciola gigantica	Larger, up to 7.5 cm long	—	Biliary tract	Sheep, cattle, other herbivores and man	Fully aquatic lymnaeid snails	—	Africa and South America	—
Dicrocoelium dendriticum	Small, 1.5 × 2 mm	40 × 25 μm	Biliary tract	Herbivorous animals	Land snails: *Theba carthusiana* *Zebrina detrita* *Hellicella candidula* *H. itala* *Cepaea nemoralis* *Helix vulgaris* *Eulota lantzi* *E. rubens*	Brown ants: *Formica fusca* *F. rufibarbis* *Proformica nasuta* *Catagliphis bicolor* *G. aenescens*	Cosmopolitan in animals. Human cases in Europe, Near East, Africa and China	Dyspepsia and hepatomegaly with eosinophilia
Clonorchis sinensis (Figure III.9)	10–25 × 2.5 mm	20–30 × 15–17 μm (Figure III.11)	Biliary tract	Man, dog, pig, cat, mouse, camel, badger	Freshwater snails: *Byhinia* (*Parafossarulus*) *manchouricus* *B. fuchsiana* Additional: *B. longicornis* *Assiminea lutea* *Melanoides tuberculatus*	Carp species: Most important: Golden carp (*Carassius auratus*) *Ctenopharyngodon idella* *Mylopharyngodon aethiops* *Cultur recurviceps* and more than 80 other species plus some freshwater shrimps (see Appendix III)	China, Taiwan, Indo-China, Korea, Japan — South China	Recurrent cholangitis with jaundice, pancreatitis and cholangiocarcinoma

	Size (worm)	Egg size	Site	Definitive hosts	Intermediate host (snail)	Second intermediate host	Geographical distribution	Clinical features
Opisthorchis tenuicollis (*felineus*)	8–11 × 1.5–2 mm	30 × 12 μm	Biliary tract	Dog, cat, pig, man	*Bythinia leachi.* An additional host is *Bythinia tentaculata*	Freshwater fish: Tench, ide, barbel, roach	Eastern Europe, CIS and India	Recurrent cholangitis
Opisthorchis viverrini	8–11 × 1.5–2 mm	30 × 12 μm	Biliary tract	Civet cat, cat, dog, man	*Bythinia funiculata, B. siamensis, B. goniomphalus, B. laevis*	Freshwater fish: *Cyclochalichthyus siaja, Hampala dispar, Puntius orphoides, P. gonionotus, P. poctozyron, Labiobarbus lineatus, Osteochilus* spp.	North-East Thailand	Recurrent cholangitis

INTESTINAL FLUKES

	Size (worm)	Egg size	Site	Definitive hosts	Intermediate host (snail)	Second intermediate host	Geographical distribution	Clinical features
Fasciolopsis buski (Figure III.6a)	3 cm × 12 cm × 2 mm	130–140 × 80–85 μm (Figure III.6b)	Small intestine	Pig and man	Freshwater snails: *Segmentina hemisphaerula, S. trochoideus, Hippeutis umbilicalis, H. cantori*	Aquatic vegetation: Water calthrop (*Trapa natans*) *T. bicornis, T. bispinosa* Water chestnut (*Eliocharis tuberosa*) Water bamboo (*Zigania aquatica*) Water hyacinth (*Eichornia crassipes*)	China; India and Taiwan, Taiwan, South China; Chekiang and Canton, Taiwan. Also Assam, Malaysia, Borneo and Burma	Chronic diarrhoea, preprandial pain, oedema of face and trunk, malabsorption
Heterophys heterophyes (Figure III.17)	Small 1–1.7 × 0.3–0.7 mm	20–30 × 15–17 μm	Small intestine	Man, rat, fox, dog, wolf, jackal	Brackish water snails: *Pirinella conica, Cerithidea cingulata, Tympanotonus micropterus*	Freshwater fish: Mullet (*Mugil cephalus*), Minnow (*Gambusia affinis*), Goby (*Acanthogobius* sp.), *Tilapia nilotica* and sp. of *Liza, Tridentiga, Glossoglobus* and *Therapon*	Middle East; Far East; Japan; Egypt	Diarrhoea and preprandial pain

continued

Table III.1 (continued)

Adult fluke	Morphology	Egg	Site	Vertebrate hosts	First intermediate host	Second intermediate host	Geographical distribution	Clinical features
Metagonimus yokogawai	Small 1.1 × 0.42–0.7 mm	27 × 16 µm	Small intestine	Man, cat, dog, rat, pig, pelican	Freshwater snails: Semisulcospira liberina Thiara granifera	Freshwater fish: Plecoglossus altivelus (ayu) Carassius auratus (golden carp) Cyprinus carpio (common carp) Zacco temminckii Photinus steindachneri Acheilognathus lanceolata Pseudorasbora parva Tribolodon taczanouski	Korea, Formosa and Japan. Balkan states. Common in Far East	Occasionally temporary abdominal pain and watery diarrhoea
Gastrodiscoides hominis	5–8 × 3–5 mm	150–170 × 60–70 µm	Large intestine	Many herbivores	Freshwater snail: Helicorbis coenosus	Aquatic plants	Assam, Bangladesh, Malaya, Thailand, Philippines, Indonesia	Diarrhoea in heavy infections
Echinostoma lindoensis	1 cm × 1 mm	83–116 × 58–69 µm	Small intestine	Man, rat, pig and other mammals	Freshwater snails: Anisus sarasinorum Gyraulus convexiusculus	Freshwater snail: Vivipara javanica Freshwater mussels: Corbicula lindoensis C. subplanta C. celebensis C. javanica	Japan, Philippines, Indonesia, Malaya	Mostly symptomless. Heavy infections: diarrhoea, abdominal pain and eosinophilia
Echinostoma malayanum	1 cm × 1 mm	83–116 × 58–69 µm (Figure III.26)	Small intestine	Man, rat, pig and other mammals	Freshwater snail: Lymnaea leuteola	Snails: L. leuteola G. convexiusculus Indoplanorbis exustus Fish: Barbus stigma	Malaya, Thailand, India, Sino-Tibetan border	Mostly symptomless. Heavy infections: diarrhoea, abdominal pain and eosinophilia
Euparyphium ilocanum	1 cm × 1 mm	83–116 × 58–69 µm	Small intestine	Man, rat, pig and other mammals	Snails: Gyraulus convexiusculus (Philippines and Indonesia) G. prashadi and Hippeutis umbilicalis (Philippines)	14 Species of snail: G. prashadi Vivipara burranghina Planorbis umbilicatus V. rudipellis	Philippines, Celebes, Indonesia	Mostly symptomless. Heavy infections: diarrhoea, abdominal pain and eosinophilia

LUNG FLUKES								
Paragonimus westermani (Figure III.21)	8–20 × 5–9 mm Cuticular spines singly spaced. Ovary simply branched (4–6 lobes)	90 × 55 μm (Figure III.22)	Cystic cavities in lungs	Wild and domestic felines	Freshwater snails: *Semisulcospira libertina* (optimum host)	Crab: *Eriocheir japonicus* (main host in Japan) Crayfish: *Cambaroides japonicus*	Japan	Pulmonary symptoms, cough and haemoptysis. Cerebral complications. Occasionally eggs in skin
					S. extensa *S. multicincta* *S. nodiperda* *S. cancellata*	Crabs: *Eriocheir sinensis* (main host in China) *Geothelphusa dehaani* *G. obtusipes* *Sinopotamon denticulatus* *Candidopotamon rathbuni* *Sesarma dehaani* *Sesarmops sinensis* Crayfish: *Cambaroides similis* *C. dauricus*, *C. schrenki* *Procambarus clarkii*	China and Korea	Pulmonary symptoms, cough and haemoptysis. Cerebral complications. Occasionally eggs in skin
					Thiara granifera	Crab: *Potamon myazakii*	Taiwan	
					Brotia asperata	Crabs: *Parathelphusa grapsoides* *P. mistio* *Sundathelphusa philippina*	Philippines	
					Melanoides tuberculata	Crabs: *Potamon smithianus* *Parathelphusa degasti* *Parathelphusa* sp.	Thailand	

continued

Table III.1 (continued)

Adult fluke	Morphology	Egg	Site	Vertebrate hosts	First intermediate host	Second intermediate host	Geographical distribution	Clinical features
Paragoninus myazaki	Cuticular spines singly spaced. Ovary profusely branched	—	Lungs	Crab-eating mammals, wild boar and marten as paratenic hosts	—	Crab: Geothelphusa dehaani	Japan	
Paragoninus heterotremus	Cuticular spines singly spaced. Ovary profusely branched	—	Lungs	—	Brotia costula	Crabs: Parathelphusa maculata Potamon cognatus	Thailand, Laos and Malaya	Pulmonary signs. Cerebral involvement and migratory subcutaneous swellings
Paragoninus szechuanensis (skrijabini)	Cuticular spines in groups. Ovary profusely branched	—	Does not develop to maturity. Immature flukes only. No eggs	—	Freshwater snail: Tricula humida	Crabs: Sinopotamon denticulatus	China	Immature flukes only which migrate through body. Subcutaneous swellings (cutaneous larva migrans). Eosinophilic granuloma in brain. Cerebral lesions. Hepatic lesions
Paragoninus hueitungensis	Cuticular spines singly spaced. Ovary profusely branched	—	Does not develop to maturity. Immature flukes only. No eggs	—	Freshwater snail: Tricula cristella	Crabs: Sinopotamon denticulatus S. joshueiense Isopotamon sinense I. papilonaceus	China	Migratory subcutaneous swellings. No ova laid. Pulmonary signs not marked. No cerebral involvement
Paragoninus tuanshenensis	Cuticular spines singly spaced. Ovary profusely branched	—	Lungs	—	Freshwater snail: Oncomelania chiui	Crab: Sinopotamon denticulatus	China	Pulmonary symptoms. No cerebral symptoms or subcutaneous swellings
Paragoninus compactus	Cuticular spines in groups. Ovary simply branched	Smaller, $75 \times 48\,\mu m$	Lungs	—	—		India	Pulmonary symptoms only

Species	Morphology	Size	Location	Reservoir hosts	First intermediate host	Second intermediate host	Distribution	Clinical features
Paragonimus africanus	Cuticular spines in groups. Ovary simply branched	67–113 × 42–56 μm	Lungs	Mongoose (*Crossarchus obscurus*) and *Atilax paludinosus*. Dog, cat and African drill (*Mandrillus leucophaeus*)	Freshwater snail: *Potadoma freethii*	Crabs: *Sudanautes africanus S. ambryi, Liberonautes latidactylus (S. pelii)*	Cameroon and Zaire	Mild pulmonary symptoms. No radiological signs. No cerebral lesions. Retroauricular cysts
Paragonimus uterobilateralis	Double uterus. One on each side	—	Lungs	African civet cat (*Viverra civetta*)	—	*Liberonautes latidactylus*	Nigeria	Pulmonary symptoms only
Paragonimus mexicanus (peruvianus)	—	—	Lungs	Cats	Freshwater snails: *Pomiatopsis lapidaria Aroapyrgus costaricensis*	Crabs: *Pseudothelphusa chilensis Psychophallus tristani Potamocarcinus magnus*	Central and South America	Pulmonary signs and cerebral complications
Paragonimus caliensis Paragonimus ecuadorensis	—	—	Lungs	—	—			

Raw crabs and crayfish

PATHOLOGY

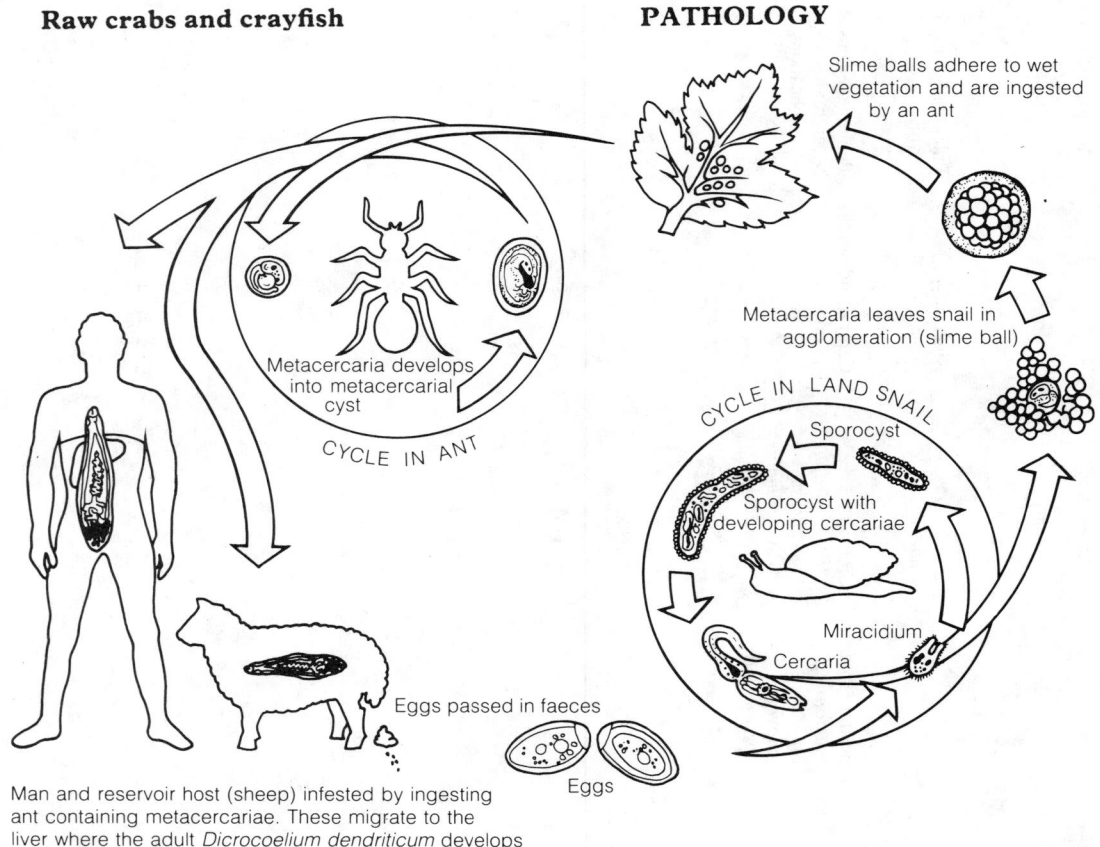

Slime balls adhere to wet vegetation and are ingested by an ant

Metacercaria develops into metacercarial cyst

CYCLE IN ANT

Metacercaria leaves snail in agglomeration (slime ball)

CYCLE IN LAND SNAIL

Sporocyst

Sporocyst with developing cercariae

Miracidium

Cercaria

Eggs passed in faeces

Eggs

Man and reservoir host (sheep) infested by ingesting ant containing metacercariae. These migrate to the liver where the adult *Dicrocoelium dendriticum* develops

Figure III.25   Life cycle of *Dicrocoelium dendriticum*.

LIFE CYCLE

First intermediate: planorbid snails (*Anisus sarasinorum* and *Gyraulus convexiusculus*); second intermediate hosts (metacercariae): snail (*Vivipara javanica rudipellis*) and four species of mussel (*Corbicula lindoensis*, *C. subplanta*, *C. celebensis* and *C. javanica*) (Table III.1). Additional secondary intermediate hosts experimentally are snails and frogs, and *E. lindoensis* has been reported in *Biomphalaria glabrata* in Brazil. The cercariae have simple tails and a body resembling in miniature that of the adult worm. The eggs are straw coloured, operculate and measure 92–124 × 65–76 μm (Figure III.26). Immature when passed in the faeces, they mature in 6–15 days.

Euparyphium ilocanum is found in man in the Philippines, Celebes and Indonesia. The first intermediate hosts are *Gyraulus convexiusculus* in the Philippines and Indonesia, *G. prashadi* and *Hippeutis umbilicalis* in the Philippines. Fourteen species of snail act as second intermediate hosts, e.g. *G. prashadi*, *Vivipara burranghina*, *Planorbis umbilicatus* and *V. rudipellis* (Table III.1). Human cases arise from people eating snails.

Echinostoma malayanum (syn. *Paryphostomum sufrartyfex*) is found in Malaysia, Thailand, India and the Sino-Tibetan border. The natural hosts are pigs and rats. The first intermediate host is the snail *Lymnaea leuteola*. The second intermediate hosts are snails (e.g. *L. leuteola*, *G. convexius-*

culus or *Indoplanorbis exustus*) or the fish (*Barbus stigma*) (Table III.1).

Euparyphium jassyense is found in Romania and has been reported from the USA. The first intermediate host is *Stagnicola emargilatus* and the second intermediate host is a tadpole in Romania and China. Normally the definitive hosts are mink, and trout are the second intermediate hosts.

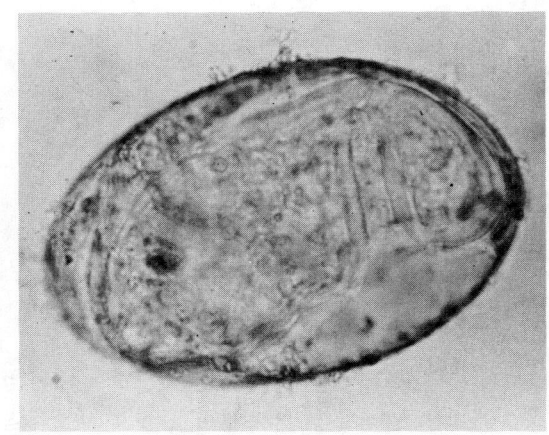

Figure III.26   Egg of *Echinostoma malayanum* containing a fully grown miracidium. (Courtesy of Lie Kan Joe.)

Echinoparyphium recurvatum has been found once in a Japanese who had lived in Taiwan. The natural hosts are ducks, etc.

Echinostoma revolutum is found in man in Thailand. The natural hosts are ducks and geese. At least 14 species of snail are known to act as first intermediate hosts (e.g. *Indoplanorbis exustus*, *Lymnaea rubiginosa* and *L. stagnalis*). Numerous snails of the same species and others (including *Vivipara vivipara*, *Sphaerium corneum* and *Corbizula fluminea*), along with bivalves and tadpoles, are the second intermediate hosts. It is cosmopolitan in distribution in nature and is found in man in Taiwan and Indonesia where human infections result from eating salted or inadequately cooked clams.

Echinostoma hortense: the natural hosts are rats and mice in China, Korea and Japan. About 20 cases have been recorded in man in Japan and Manchuria. The first intermediate hosts are lymnaeid snails (*L. japonica*, *L. pervia* and *L. ollula*). Second intermediate hosts are tadpoles (frogs and newts) and fish (e.g. *Carassius* and *Cyprinus*).

Other human echinostomes are:

E. cinetorchis—in man in Japan (? syn. of *revolutum*);
E. macrorchis—in man in Japan (normally rats, *Capella*);
Echinochasmus perfoliatus—in man in Japan, Taiwan (normally cats, dogs);
E. japonicus—in man in Japan, China, Taiwan (normally birds);
E. jiufoensis—in man in China;
Himasthla muehlensis—a German who had lived 6 years in Columbia picked up this worm, but probably from raw clams (*Vems merceneria*) consumed in New York;
Episthmium caninum—in man in Thailand (normally dogs);
Euparyphium melis—in man in China, Romania;
Hypoderueum conoideum—in man in Thailand, Taiwan (normally birds).

SUPERFAMILY: SCHISTOSOMATOIDEA (STILES & HASSAL, 1926) FAMILY: SCHISTOSOMATIDAE (LOOSS, 1899; POCHE, 1907)

GENUS: *SCHISTOSOMA* (WEINLAND, 1858)

The schistosomes commonly infecting man are:

Schistosoma haematobium (Bilharz, 1852) Weinland, 1858;
Schistosoma mansoni Sambon, 1907;
Schistosoma japonicum Katsurada, 1904;
Schistosoma intercalatum Fisher, 1934;
Schistosoma mekongi Voge, Bruckner & Bruce, 1978.

Differentiation of these five species is shown in Table III.2. Infections of man have also been reported with:

Schistosoma mattheei Veglia & Le Roux, 1929;
Schistosoma bovis (Sonsino, 1876) Blanchard, 1895;
Schistosoma curassoni Brumpt, 1931.

Natural hybrids of *S. haematobium* and *S. intercalatum* and of *S. haematobium* and *S. mattheei* are known to occur in man in Cameroon and South Africa, respectively.[1,2] Although unequivocal evidence exists of *S. mattheei* in man[2] the evidence for *S. bovis* and *S. curassoni* occurring in man is less convincing.

The schistosomes are digenetic trematodes, their life histories consisting of alternating generations, each with its own range of hosts. The adult worms inhabit vertebrates; the larval stages inhabit snails which, in the case of schistosomes pathogenic to man, are freshwater snails.

The schistosomes are dioecious organisms, i.e. the sexes are separate. Adult schistosomes live in the veins of vertebrates; there is an oral cavity but no muscular pharynx; the eggs have no operculum; there is no encysted or metacercarial stage; the cercariae enter the definitive hosts through the skin.

PARASITOLOGY (Figures III.27–III.29)

Like other digenetic trematodes, the schistosomes are equipped with suckers. The *oral sucker* surrounds the mouth and is prehensile; the *ventral sucker* (*acetabulum*) is more posterior, on the ventral surface. With these suckers the worms can attach themselves to the walls of the vessels in which they live. The *mouth* itself is usually near the anterior extremity. The alimentary system consists of an *oral cavity* leading to the *oesophagus* and thence to the *gut* which soon divides into two *caeca* which reunite more posteriorly to form the *single posterior caecum* which ends blindly; there is no anus.

Nutrition is derived from blood in which the worms live; schistosomes consume large amounts of glucose; unused material is rejected through the mouth as adult worms do not possess an anus. Despite having access to relatively unlimited supplies of oxygen, the metabolism is primarily anaerobic with lactate as the major end-product.

The excretory system consists of two longitudinal canals opening posteriorly and fed by collecting tubules. There are flame cells whose function is to fan fluid wastes into the tubules by means of the vibratile cilia with which they are equipped.

There is a rudimentary *nervous system* with an oesophageal ganglion and commissure encircling the oesophagus and two longitudinal nerve cords running to the posterior end and intercommunicating by lateral branches.

The *male reproductive organs* consist of testes dorsal to and posterior to the ventral sucker. Each testis discharges via a *vas efferens*; these unite to form the *vesicula seminalis* at the *genital pore* situated in the midline posterior to the ventral sucker.

The male worm is flat and leaf-like but is folded to form the *gynaecophoric canal*, enfolding the very slender female for almost its entire length (Figure III.27).

The *female reproductive organs* consist of an elongated *ovary* in the posterior half, from which the *oviduct* passes forward, to be joined by the *vitelline duct* from the *vitellaria* (*yolk glands*) to form the *common reproductive duct*. The *common reproductive duct* passes forward, entering the *ootype*, a large egg-shaped chamber which receives the ducts

Table III.2 Differentiation of various species of *Schistosoma*.

Character	S. haematobium	S. mansoni	S. japonicum	S. intercalatum	S. mekongi	S. malayensis
Habitat of adult	Vesical veins; occasionally veins of rectum and portal system	Inferior mesenteric and portal venous system	Superior and inferior mesenteric and portal venous system	Mesenteric and portal venous system	Superior mesenteric and portal veins	—
Adult male	10–15 × 0.75–1.0 mm	6–13 × 1.0 mm	12–20 × 0.5–0.55 mm	11–14 × 0.3–0.4 mm	6–15 mm	4.3–9.2 mm
Tegument	Tubercles and fine spines	Conspicuous tubercle and microscopic tufts of hair	No tubercles; small acuminate spines	Tubercles and fine spines	No tubercles; spined from anterior level of gynaecophoric canal to posterior end of body	—
Oesophagus	Single bulb	Single bulb	Double bulb	Single bulb	Double bulb	—
Caeca	Unite in anterior half; posterior caecum short, one-third of body length	Unite in anterior half; posterior caecum long, two-thirds of body length	Unite in posterior half; posterior caecum medium, one-half of body length	Unite in posterior half; posterior caecum one-fifth to one-quarter of body length	Unite in posterior half; posterior caecum one-fifth of body length	Unite in posterior half of body
Testes	4 or 5	2–14	6–8	4–6	6–7	—
Adult female	20–26 × 0.25 mm	7–17 × 0.25 mm	12–28 × 0.3 mm	10–14 × 0.15–0.18 mm	6–20 mm	6.5–11.3 mm
Tegument	Darker than male, more blood pigment in gut. Transverse striations. Small tubercles at extremity	Darker than male, more blood pigment in gut. Transverse striations. Small tubercles at extremity	Darker than male, more blood pigment in gut. Transverse striations. Minute spines	Darker than male, more blood pigment in gut. Transverse striations, smooth	Darker than male, more blood pigment in gut. Transverse striations	—
Ovary	In posterior third	In anterior half	Central	In posterior half	In anterior 5/8	In anterior half
Uterus	Anterior, long. Holds 10–100 eggs at one time. Produces 20–290 daily	Anterior, short. Holds 1–2 eggs only at one time. Produces 100–300 daily	Anterior, long. Holds 50 or more eggs at one time. Produces 1500–3500 daily	Anterior, long. Holds 5–50 eggs at one time	Anterior, long	Contains many eggs
Eggs	83–187 × 60 μm (Figure III.30,3) Terminal spine	112–175 × 45–70 μm (Figure III.30,1) Lateral spine	70–100 × 50–65 μm (Figure III.30,2) Rudimentary lateral spine	140–240 × 50–85 μm (Figure III.30,4) Long terminal spine	30–55 × 50–65 μm Small lateral knob	52–90 × 33–62 μm Small knob, usually located laterally, occasionally near end of egg
Shell	Pass through bladder wall. Discharged in urine. Non-acid fast with Ziehl–Neelsen stain in tissues	Pass through bowel wall. Discharged in faeces. Acid fast with Ziehl–Neelsen stain in tissues	Pass through bowel wall. Discharged in faeces. Acid fast with Ziehl–Neelsen stain in tissues	Pass through bowel wall. Discharged in faeces. Acid fast with Ziehl–Neelsen stain in tissues	Pass through bowel wall. Discharged in faeces. Acid fast with Ziehl–Neelsen stain in tissues	—
Animal hosts	Occasionally baboons, monkeys, rats, pigs	(Occasional) baboons, rats	Rodents, dogs, cats, cattle, water buffalo, pigs, horses, sheep, goats	?Sheep, goats	Dogs	*Rattus muelleri, R. tiomanicus*

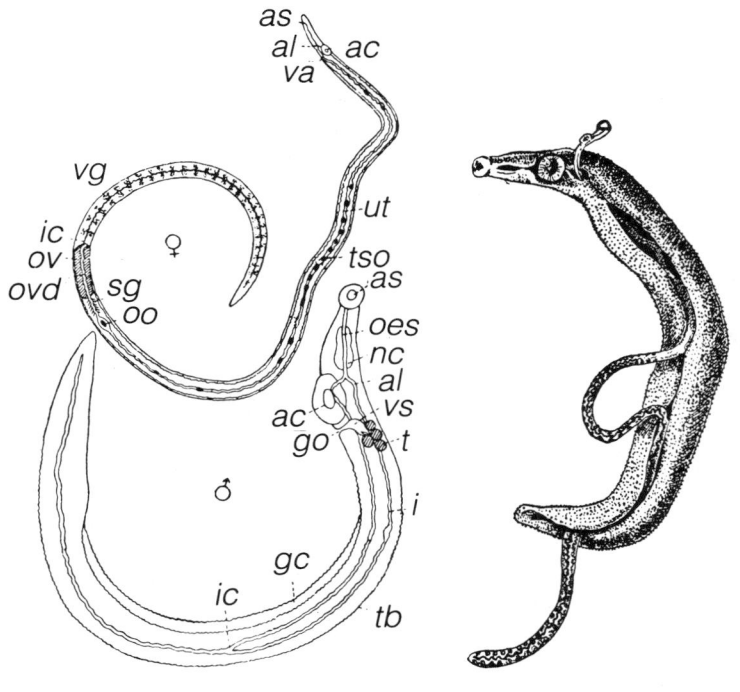

Figure III.27 *Schistosoma haematobium*. (10×.)

al	bifurcation of the alimentary canal
ac	acetabulum
as	oral sucker
gc	gynaecophoric canal
go	gonopore
ic	union of intestinal caeca
nc	nerve cord
oes	oesophagus
oo	ootype
ov	ovary
ovi	oviduct
ps	posterior sucker
sg	shell gland
t	testis
tb	tubercules
tso	terminal spined ovum
ut	uterus
va	vagina
vg	vitelline gland
vs	seminal vesicle

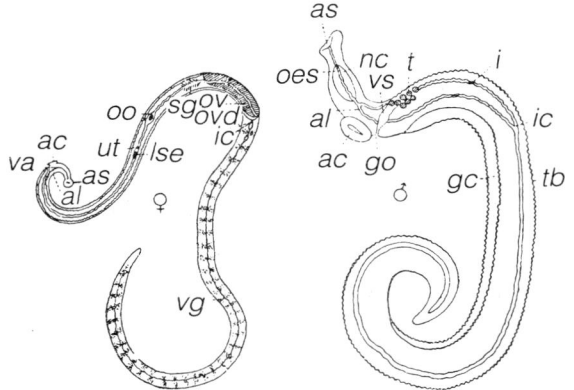

Figure III.28 *Schistosoma mansoni*. (10×.) Key as for Figure III.27. lse, lateral spined egg.

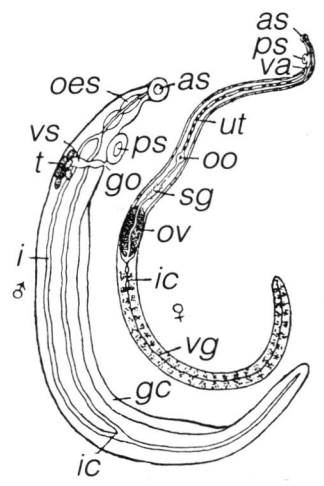

Figure III.29 Male and female *Schistosoma japonicum*. (10×.) Key as for Figure III.27.

of the *Mehlis gland* (*shell gland*), at its posterior end. Anteriorly the *ootype* opens into the uterus which passes forward and opens at the *genital pore* on the median surface posterior to the ventral sucker.

LIFE CYCLE (Figure III.30)

The eggs of the schistosomes are passed by the definitive hosts (vertebrates) in urine (*S. haematobium*) (Figure III.30c) or faeces (*S. mansoni* (Figure III.30a), *S. japonicum* (Figure III.30b), *S. mekongi*, *S. intercalatum* (Figure III.30d)) but this is not an absolute rule since eggs of *S. haematobium* may occasionally be found in faeces and commonly in biopsy specimens of rectal mucosa, and eggs of *S. mansoni* may be found in urine samples, especially in heavy infections. *S. mattheei* (Figure III.30e) is a parasite of sheep and cattle, but *S. mattheei*-shaped eggs have been recorded from the urine of humans in South Africa. Subsequent analyses have demonstrated these eggs to result from *S. haematobium* male × *S. mattheei* female.

Egg-shells of *S. mansoni*, *S. japonicum* and *S. intercalatum* (but not *S. haematobium* or *S. mattheei*) are acid fast when stained by the Ziehl–Neelsen method.

When an egg reaches fresh water it contains a fully embryonated miracidium which hatches within a few minutes, partly as a result of osmosis, partly owing to its own movements. The miracidium swims actively by means of its

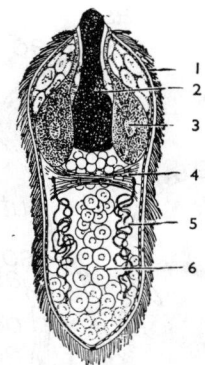

Figure III.31   Miracidium of *Schistosoma haematobium*. 1, Cilia. 2, Apical papilla. 3, Lateral gland. 4, Neural mass. 5, Excretory tubules. 6, Germinal cells.

ciliated epidermis for 8–12 hours, searching for a snail host. Miracidia tend to move to the upper layers of water where many of their snail hosts live but in some circumstances they can infect snails inhabiting the bottom of canals or lakes (e.g. Lake Victoria). These snails, however, frequently move up and down from the depths to the surface of such waters and miracidia have the opportunity of infecting them in the upper reaches.

The miracidium (Figure III.31) has a complex array of sensory receptors which are considered to aid it in locating a snail host. Also the miracidium is endowed with a muscular apical papilla, apical gland and a pair of lateral glands, all of which are considered to play a role in effecting penetration of the snail's epidermis. Miracidia do not appear to discriminate between species of snail and will sometimes enter the incorrect host, thereby preventing further development. However, if a miracidium enters a compatible intermediate host, metamorphosis into the next stage—the mother sporocyst—takes place: the ciliated epidermis is cast off and is replaced by a syncytial tegument with numerous microvilli.

Within the elongated sac of the mother sporocyst germinal cells develop into daughter sporocysts. These leave the mother sporocyst after about 8 days and migrate to the digestive gland (liver) of the snail host, and within them further germinal cells develop into the next stage, the cercaria. Thousands of cercariae may result from one miracidium and all of these will be of the same sex. The cycle from penetration by the miracidium to the production of mature cercariae takes about 3–4 weeks for *S. intercalatum*, about 4–5 weeks for *S. mansoni*, 5–6 weeks for *S. haematobium* and *S. mekongi*, and 7 weeks or more for *S. japonicum*.[3] The snails are damaged in the process and their life span is shortened.

The mature cercaria (Figure III.32) escapes from the daughter sporocyst, migrates through the tissues of the snail and finally emerges to swim free in the water by means of its muscular, bifurcated tail, usually tail first. Its body length is less than 0.5 mm in length, with an oral organ and a smaller ventral sucker, a mouth, oesophagus and a pair of short caeca, and an excretory system of flame cells, tubules and excretory ducts leading into an excretory bladder at the posterior end of the body. It has three types of gland: head glands, four preacetabular and six postacetabular glands. The secretion from the postacetabular glands is thought to help the cercaria attach itself to the skin of the vertebrate

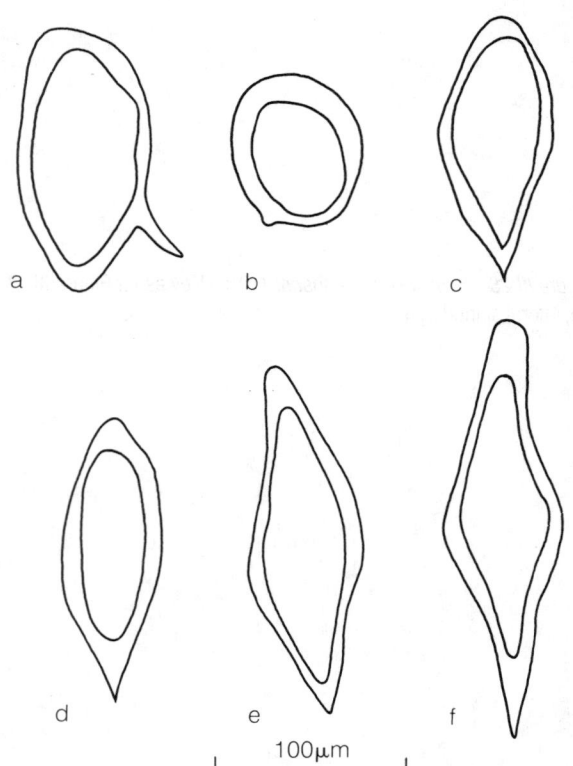

100μm

Figure III.30   Eggs of *Schistosoma* spp. (a) *S. mansoni*. (b) *S. japonicum*. (c) *S. haematobium*. (d) *S. intercalatum*. (e) *S. mattheei*. (f) *S. bovis*.

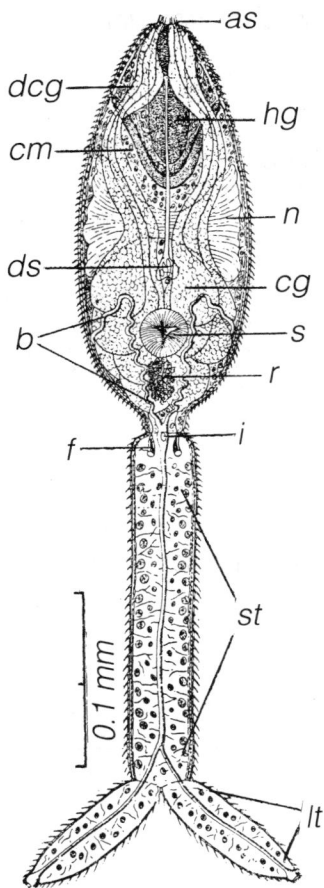

Figure III.32 Cercaria of *Schistosoma japonicum*, ventral view. (240×.)

as	anterior spines	i	island excretory
b	excretory bladder		bladder
cg	cephalic glands	lt	lobe of tail
cm	circular muscles	m	mouth
dcg	ducts of cephalic	n	nervous system
	glands	r	rudimentary genital
ds	digestive system		cells
exp	excretory pore	st	stem of ventral
f	flame cell		sucker
hg	head gland	s	ventral sucker

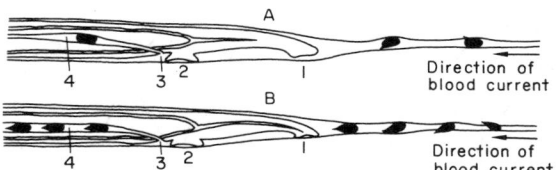

Figure III.33 The deposition of eggs by *Schistosoma mansoni* (A) and *S. haematobium* (B) in the blood vessels and their passage to the exterior. 1, Anterior sucker. 2, Posterior sucker. 3, Vaginal orifice. 4, Uterus containing eggs.

factors, such as turbulence and temperature. In many transmission areas the life span will only be 8–12 hours.

A cercaria can penetrate the skin of a definitive host within a few minutes. In doing so it sheds its tail and in the tissues it becomes a *schistosomulum*. The trilaminate surface of the cercaria is replaced by a multilaminate surface of the schistosomulum and adult. The schistosomulum leaves the skin after about 2–4 days by the venous or lymphatic systems, to be transported to the lungs. In the lungs the schistosomulum becomes longer and thinner and then leaves the lungs via the pulmonary veins and passes through the heart to the systemic circulation. An individual schistosomulum may make several circuits of the pulmonary/systemic circulation before finding its way to the hepatic portal system. Growth takes place in the liver and paired worms may be found after about 26 days. Most worms leave the liver when they are sexually mature and have mated and migrate to the veins of the vesical plexus (*S. haematobium*) or the mesenteric veins (*S. mansoni*, *S. japonicum*, *S. mekongi* and *S. intercalatum*) where they begin to lay eggs. The period between penetration by the cercariae and egg-laying may be 30–50 days or more.

The mated worms move as far as possible towards the fine terminal vessels and the female then leaves the male progressing to the finest vessels where she deposits her eggs, retracting after having done so (Figure III.33). The eggs escape from the venules into the tissues; those of *S. haematobium* largely into the wall of the bladder but occasionally into the wall of the colorectum; those of *S. mansoni*, *S. japonicum*, *S. mekongi* and *S. intercalatum* largely into the wall of the colorectum. Many pass through the mucosa to be excreted in urine or faeces but some remain trapped in the tissues where they give rise to tissue reactions. Some eggs of all species are usually also found in the liver, genital tract, lungs, central nervous system and other organs. Eggs are responsible for most of the pathological effects of the infection (Chapter 72).

INTERMEDIATE HOSTS (SNAILS)

Strains of schistosomes which infect man vary in their ability to infect snail hosts. Usually this variation is associated with geographical area but the subject is complex. The following lists of proved and potential snail hosts have been constructed from Brown[4] and Jordan and Webbe.[3]

host, and the secretion of the preacetabular glands together with that of the postacetabular glands helps to break down the skin barrier.

A snail may shed up to 3000 cercariae per day when in peak production; for example, *Biomphalaria glabrata* shedding *S. mansoni*. However, the number does vary from day to day and some host–parasite relationships are less productive: *Oncomelania hupensis* produces 15–160 cercariae per day of *S. japonicum*. Cercariae tend to swim up to the surface of water, sinking from time to time, and returning. They are influenced by the effect of light, gravity, agitation and touch. They are non-feeding and depend entirely upon their glycogen reserves when free swimming; consequently their life span is short, up to 48 hours, but this depends upon external

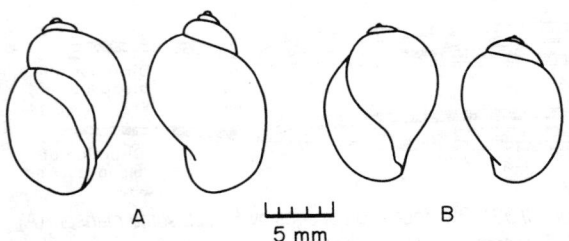

Figure III.34 Molluscan hosts of *Schistosoma haematobium*. A, *Bulinus truncatus*. B, *B. africanus*.

Snail hosts of S. haematobium (Figure III.34)

S. haematobium is a species complex and is, transmitted throughout most of its range by species of the genus *Bulinus*. There is one possible exception: at Gimvi about 250 km south of Bombay, a schistosome considered to be *S. haematobium* is transmitted by *Ferrissia tenuis* but clearly further studies are required on this particular focus. A list of hosts and their distribution is given in Table III.3.

Table III.3   Snail hosts of *S. haematobium*.

Snail species	Locality
Truncatus/tropicus complex	
Bulinus truncatus	Iran, Iraq, Near East, Yemen, North Africa (East Africa, potential), Egypt
B. rohlfsi	West Africa
B. coulboisi (potential)	East Africa
Reticulatus group	
B. reticulatus (potential)	East, central and southern Africa
B. wrighti	Saudi Arabia, South Yemen
Forskalii group	
B. bavayi (potential)	Malagasy Republic
B. beccarii	North and South Yemen, Saudi Arabia
B. camerunensis	Cameroon
B. cernicus	Mauritius
B. senegalensis	Senegal, Gambia, Nigeria
Africanus group	
B. africanus	South and East Africa
B. globosus	Afrotropical region
B. nasutus	East Africa
B. abyssinicus	Ethiopia, Somalia
B. jousseaumei	West Africa
B. obtusispira	Malagasy Republic
B. hightoni (potential)	North-east Kenya
B. umbilicatus	Senegal
Ferrissia tenuis	India

Snail hosts of S. intercalatum

These are shown in Table III.4.

Table III.4   Snail hosts of *S. intercalatum*.

Snail species	Locality
Bulinus globosus	Zaire
B. forskalii	Cameroon, Gabon, São Tomé

Most species of the forskalii and reticulatus groups are capable of acting as hosts for the Cameroon strain of *S. intercalatum* but so far none has been implicated as a natural host.

Snail hosts of S. mansoni (Figure III.35)

These are shown in Table III.5.

Table III.5   Snail hosts of *S. mansoni*.

Snail (Biomphalaria) species	Locality
Biomphalaria pfeifferi	West, East and South Africa, Arabian Peninsula, Malagasy Republic
B. choanomphala	
*B. smithi**	Great Lakes of East Africa
*B. stanleyi**	
B. alexandrina	Egypt
B. angulosa	East and central Africa
B. sudanica	East and central Africa
B. camerunensis	West and central Africa
*B. salinarum**	South-western Africa
B. glabrata	West Indies, Venezuela, Surinam, French Guiana, Brazil
B. tenagophila	Brazil, Bolivia, Peru, Paraguay, Uraguay, Argentina
B. straminea (=*Tropicorbis centimetralis*)	Venezuela, Surinam, French Guiana, Brazil

The following neotropical species have been successfully infected with *S. mansoni* in the laboratory and must, therefore, be regarded as potential hosts.

B. chilensis	Chile
B. havanensis	Antilles, Mexico, Central America, northern South America
B. helphila	Puerto Rico, Cuba, Peru
B. peregrina	Ecuador, Bolivia, Chile, Paraguay, Argentina, Uruguay, Brazil
B. sericea	Ecuador

*Successively infected in the laboratory with *S. mansoni*.

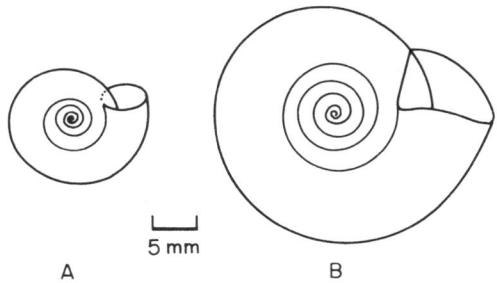

Figure III.35 Molluscan hosts of *Schistosoma mansoni.*
A, *Biomphalaria alexandrina.* B, *B. glabrata.*

Snail hosts of S. japonicum (Figure III.36)

Breeding experiments and detailed cytogenetic and biochemical studies in recent years have indicated that all of the proven hosts for *S. japonicum* should now be regarded as subspecies of a single widespread species, *Oncomelania hupensis.* A distinctive species in Japan, *O. minima*, appears to be resistant to infection. The hosts are listed in Table III.6.

Snail host of S. mekongi

The only recorded host is *Tricula aperta* which is endemic in the Mekong river, Laos and Cambodia. Three races of *T. apeta* are known: alpha, beta and gamma, and the last is considered to be the most important in transmission.

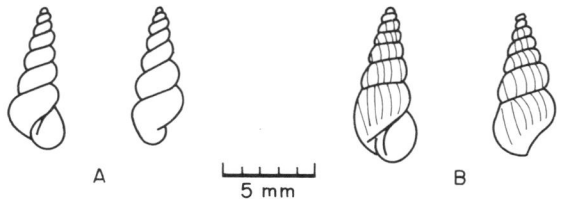

Figure III.36 Molluscan hosts of *Schistosoma japonicum.*
A, *Oncomelania hupensis nosophora.* B, *O. h. hupensis.*

Table III.6 Snail hosts of *S. japonicum.*

Snail species	Locality
Oncomelania hupensis hupensis	China
O. h. formosana	Taiwan*
O. h. chiui	Taiwan
O. h. nosophora	Japan
O. h. quadrasi	Philippines
O. h. lindoensis	Celebes

*The Taiwanese strain is not pathogenic to man.

INTERSPECIFIC ANTAGONISM BETWEEN TREMATODES IN SNAILS

It has been reported[5] that if albino *Biomphalaria glabrata* is infected with *S. mansoni* and also with *Paryphostomum segregatum* (an echinostome from Brazil), the rediae of *P. segregatum* will attack and breach the thin wall of the early mother sporocyst of *S. mansoni* and ingest and destroy the daughter sporocysts within it. They fail, however, to destroy mature daughter sporocysts but can cause degeneration of the schistosome sporocysts by other means. They can ingest whole cercariae. However, the use of echinostomes as a form of biological control for schistosomiasis is not considered practical for field use, since the necessarily high infection rates would not be achieved because of parasite overdispersion. Repeated release of echinostome eggs would be required and the costs of such operations and their evaluation would be high.

SUPERFAMILY: PARAMPHISTOMATOIDEA (*AMPHISTOME TREMATODES*)

GENUS: *GASTRODISCOIDES*
GASTRODISCOIDES HOMINIS
(LEWIS & MCONNELL, 1876; LEIPER, 1913)

DISTRIBUTION

Malaysia, Assam, India, Pakistan, Philippines, Myanmar, South Vietnam, Guyana, CIS. In Kamrup district, Assam, 41% of the population are infected; in Burma 5%. The normal host is the pig or the mouse deer.

CHARACTERS

The fluke is reddish from haemoglobin pigment. When alive it is very expansile and can elongate to 1 cm. Preserved specimens measure 5–7 × 3–4 mm at the widest point. The anterior end is conical, and the posterior discoidal, flattened ventrally to form a concave disc. Prominent genital papillae are seen and the common genital pore is 2.5 mm from the oral sucker. The ventral sucker (acetabulum) is ventrally situated in the caudal portion and measures 2 mm in diameter. The cuticle is smooth. The alimentary canal consists of a pharynx with two pear-shaped pharyngeal pouches. The oesophagus is 1 mm in length and ends in a muscular bulb where the bifurcation of the intestine takes place and caeca run back to the edge of the acetabulum. There are two lobulated testes placed diagonally between the intestinal caeca. A seminal vesicle is present but no cirrus. The ovary lies in the midline, posterior to the testes. An ovoid shell gland is placed near the ovary with a receptaculum seminis anterior to it. The uterus is short. Laurer's canal is present. The vitellaria lie in the mid-third. The ovoid egg measures 152 × 60 μm and has an operculum.

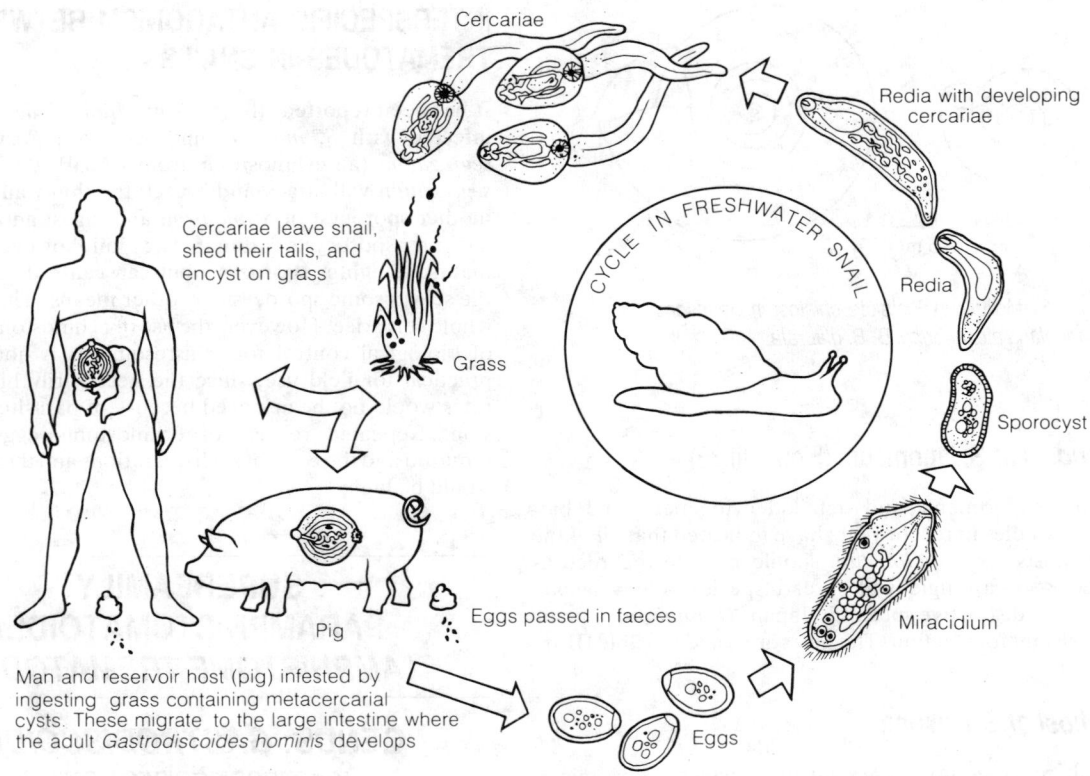

Figure III.37 Life cycle of *Gastrodiscoides hominis*.

LIFE CYCLE (Figure III.37)

The adult lives in the caecum and colon of the definitive host (pig, deer, man). Eggs are passed in the stool which hatch into *Miracidia*. These enter a freshwater snail, *Helicorbis coenosus*, where they develop into sporocysts, and *rediae* forming *cercariae* which leave the snail host to encyst as metacercariae on vegetation which is then eaten by the definitive host.

GENUS: *WATSONIUS*

Watsonius watsoni has been found in large numbers in an African in South-West Africa. Its normal hosts are monkeys of the genera *Cercopithecus* and *Papio* (baboon).

CESTODES (See also Chapters 74–77)
Class: Cestoidea or tapeworms

The name cestode is derived from 'kestos' (Greek = a girdle). There is a head or *scolex*, and the *strobila* or segments have their own musculature which relieves the strain on the head. The worms can live for several years and absorb nutriment through the tegument. They are hermaphroditic normally with male and female in each segment, the male fertilizing the adjacent female (with very few exceptions). Male organs often develop before the female. Human cestodes occur in two orders.

1. Pseudophyllidea with slit-like bothria, oval head (two long grooves with muscular walls), no hooks and the genital orifice on the flat surface.
2. Cyclophyllidea, cup-like or round suckers; genital orifice marginal.

ORDER: PSEUDOPHYLLIDEA

GENUS: *DIPHYLLOBOTHRIUM*

DIPHYLLOBOTHRIUM LATUM (LINNAEUS, 1785)

It is greyish and more translucent and less fleshy than *Taenia* and may attain a length of 3–10 m, lying coiled up in the small intestine. Multiple infections are common. The scolex (3 mm) has no rostellum or hooklets but two slit-like suckers with longitudinal grooves (bothridia). The neck is thin; the

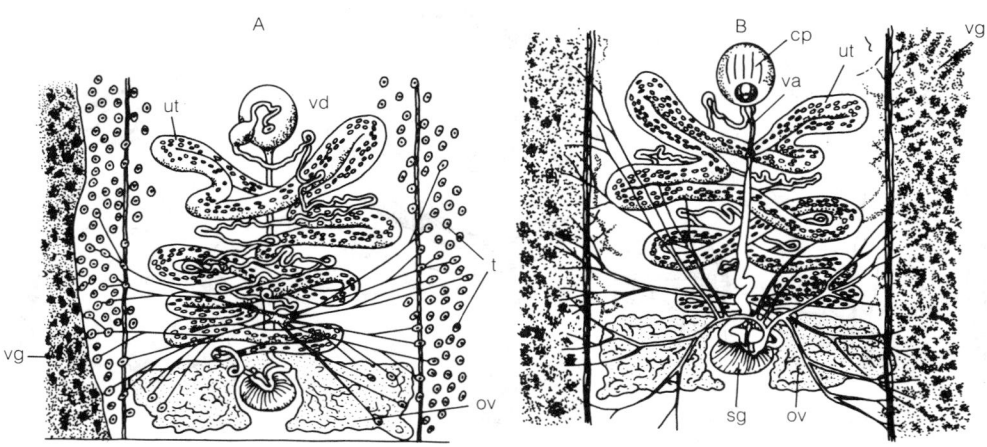

Figure III.38 Mature segment of *Diphyllobothrium latum*. A, Dorsal or male aspect. B, Ventral or female aspect.

cp	cirrus pouch	t	testes	vd	vas deferens
ov	ovary	ut	uterus	vg	vitelline glands
sg	shell gland	va	vagina		

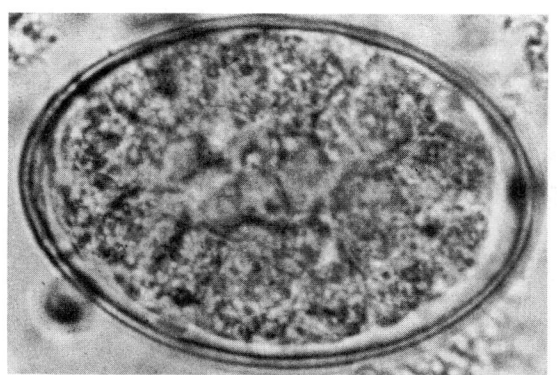

Figure III.39 *Diphyllobothrium latum* (fish tapeworm). Ovum. (Courtesy of D. S. Ridley.)

proglottides number 3000–4000. The number of worms corresponds to the individual plerocercoids swallowed. Mature segments are broader than they are long. A single worm may discharge as many as from 36 000 to a million eggs each day. The worm may be discharged from the bowel naturally without treatment. (For details of anatomy of male and female elements, see Figure III.38.)

The egg is operculated with a brown shell measuring 70 × 45 μm (Figures III.5, and III.39). No segments are passed in faeces (unlike *Taenia*).

LIFE CYCLE (Figures III.40 and III.41)

If the egg is passed in water the operculum is lifted, the ciliated six-hooked coracidium emerges (Figure III.40C); spherical (22.30 μm), it swims by means of its cilia but dies

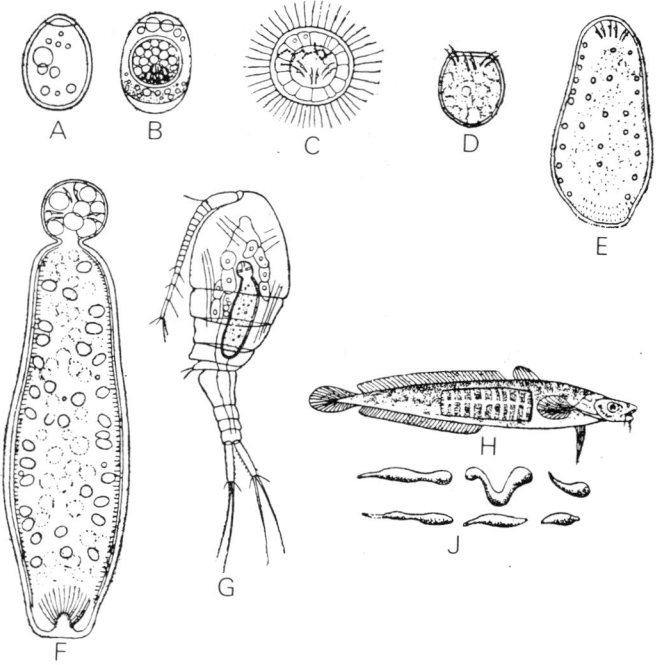

Figure III.40 Life cycle of *Diphyllobothrium latum* (not to scale). A, Egg of *D. latum*. B, Hexacanth embryo. C, Ciliated oncosphere or coracidium. D, E and F, Development of larvae or procercoids in *Cyclops*. G, Procercoid in the body cavity of *Cyclops*. H, Development of plerocercoids in fishes. J, Plerocercoids of different shapes ingested by man, dog or cat.

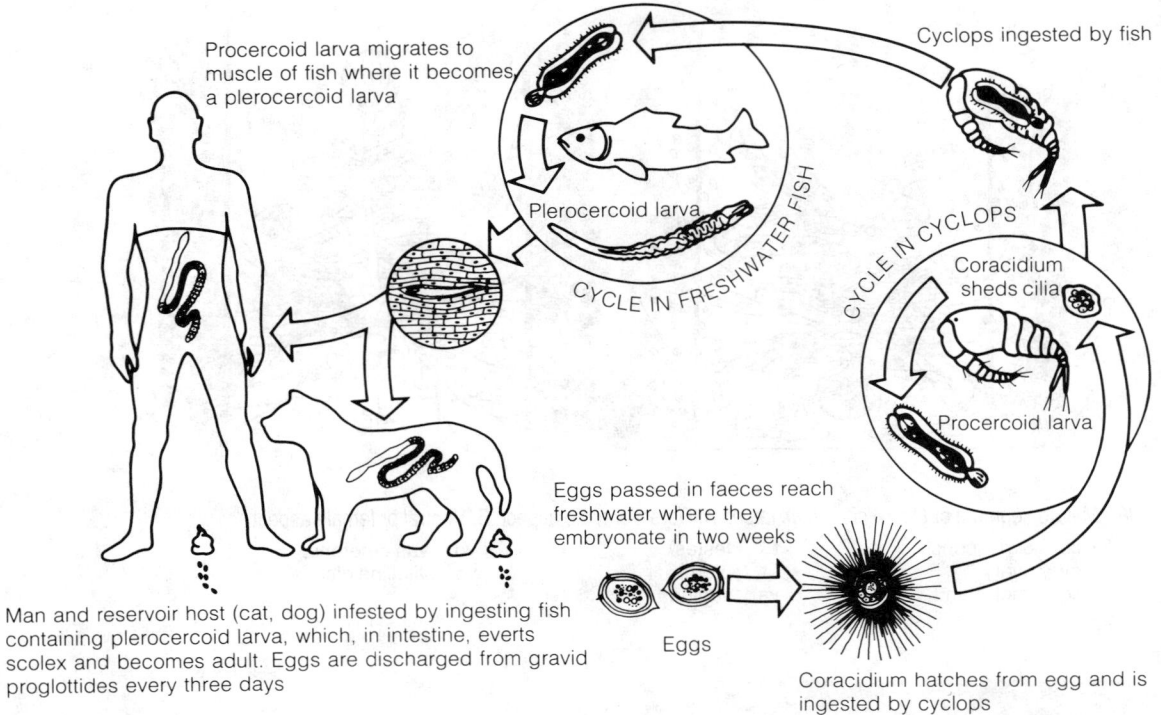

Procercoid larva migrates to muscle of fish where it becomes a plerocercoid larva

Cyclops ingested by fish

Plerocercoid larva

CYCLE IN FRESHWATER FISH

CYCLE IN CYCLOPS

Coracidium sheds cilia

Procercoid larva

Eggs passed in faeces reach freshwater where they embryonate in two weeks

Eggs

Man and reservoir host (cat, dog) infested by ingesting fish containing plerocercoid larva, which, in intestine, everts scolex and becomes adult. Eggs are discharged from gravid proglottides every three days

Coracidium hatches from egg and is ingested by cyclops

Figure III.41   Life cycle of *Diphyllobothrium latum*. (Courtesy of WTIM.)

after 12 hours to 5 days depending on temperature. Normally it is swallowed by fresh water crustacea, the first intermediate host—*Cyclops strenuus*, *Diaptomus gracilis*, *D. graciloides* or *D. oregonensis*, *Cyclops brevisponosus*, and *C. prasenus* in the USA. The outer layer is then digested. The hooks tear a hole in the gut wall; the larva passes into the body cavity and may kill the cyclops. Lying outside the gut wall it becomes the *proceroid larva* (Figure III.40D–G) which is ovoid, 50–60 μm long, with a terminal spherical appendix bearing six hooklets. At most two of these are found in one *Cyclops* which is then swallowed by freshwater fishes of many species—the second intermediate hosts—pike, perch, salmon, trout and grayling. In Africa, the barbel; in the USA the pike, wall-eye and burbot. Reaching the stomach of the fish the procercoid penetrates to the body cavity and after 3–4 days there encysts as a plerocercoid or *Spirometra* larva (6 mm) in the muscular and connective tissues (Figure III.40H). Bothria, nervous and excretory systems are developed. It is then ingested by man with raw roe (caviar) or insufficiently cooked fish and the *plerocercoid* develops in 5–6 weeks into an adult *Diphyllobothrium*.

Freshwater fishes harbour other *Diphyllobothrium* larvae which are difficult to differentiate at this stage. The process of 'kippering' does not kill the plerocercoids and ordinary smoking is ineffectual but brine saturation is effective. The adult tapeworm can live as long as 29 years. *Diphyllobothrium dendriticum* (*minus*) is a small variety found in Lake Baikal and has a similar history. The second intermediate hosts are various species of salmon and grayling which are eaten frozen or salted by Mongolian peoples. *D. alascense* is a species found in Eskimos and can be differentiated by the form of the scolex. The plerocercoids occur in two species of fish—*Pungitus* and *Dallia*.

SPIROMETREA MANSONI (ERINACEI) (*DIPHYLLOBOTHRIUM, DIBOTHRIOCEPHALUS MANSONI*)

PARASITOLOGY

It resembles *D. latum*, is 6–10 m long and has a more delicate structure with a narrower and more ellipsoid egg than *D. latum*.

LIFE CYCLE

The adult stage occurs in the dog and other animals, the plerocercoid (sparganum) under natural conditions in frogs or snakes. The procercoid in *Cyclops leuckarti* shows the same stages as in *D. latum*.

Man is infected by accidentally swallowing a procercoid while drinking, thus becoming a second intermediary. The Chinese custom of applying raw split frogs to sores on the hands or to inflamed eyes may afford entry. The sparganum in man measures 8–36 cm × 0.1–12 mm × 0.5–1.75 mm thick (Figure III.42). Its body is flat and transversely wrinkled with a longitudinal median groove. It is found in many parts of the body: kidneys and iliac fossae, pleural cavities, urethra and subcutaneous tissues.

S. mansonoides (probably = *erinacei*) was formerly thought to be the parent form of *Sparganum proliferum*. It is found in the intestine of the cat in the southern USA and is separable from *D. latum* and *D. cordatum* by the scolex, uterine characteristics and smaller size. Specimens vary from 20 to 60 cm in length but may attain 1 mm × 8 mm. Immature proglottides number 200–300. The egg is pointed, 65 ×

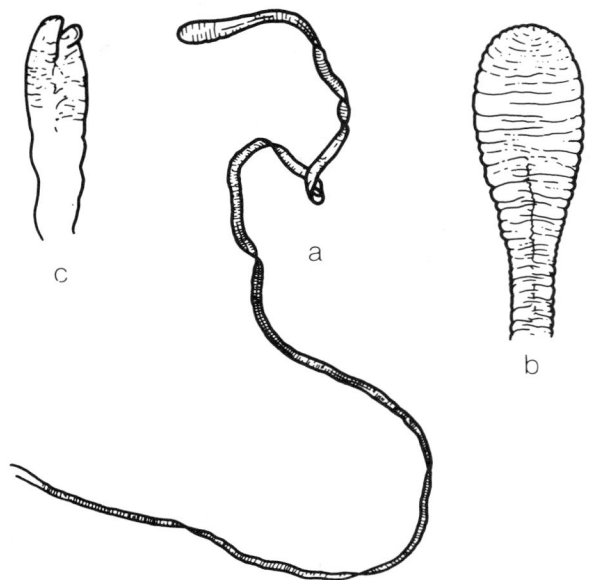

Figure III.42 *Diphyllobothrium mansoni* plerocercoid, extracted from an abscess in a Masai. (a) Natural size. (b) Anterior extremity. (c) Posterior extremity.

$37 \mu m$, with a conical operculum. The life cycle is as in *S. mansoni*.

The plerocercoids (spargana) measure $3-12 \times 2.5 \, mm$ (Figures III.42 and III.43) and are contained in cysts which are found in man in Japan and Florida. The body contains calcareous corpuscles. The cysts may be disseminated throughout the body in subcutaneous tissues, intramuscular fasciae, walls of the alimentary canal, mesentery, kidney, lung, heart and brain. The prognosis in man is grave. Similar plerocercoids have been reproduced in macaque monkeys.

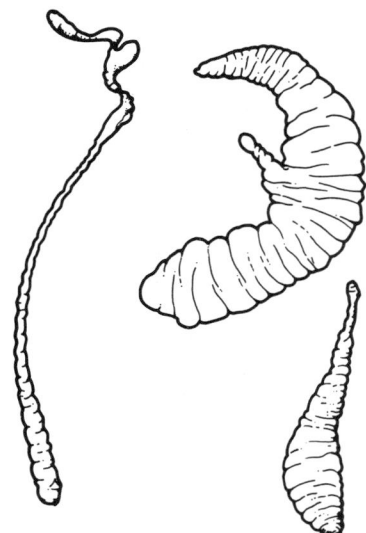

Figure III.43 Different forms of *Sparganum proliferum*.

Sparganosis has been found in Korea and spargana, 23–50 cm in length, were removed from the muscles of the abdomen and chest. All patients had eaten raw snakes—*Dinodon rufozonatum*. It has also been found in abscess(es) of the leg. The adult form is probably *Spirometra erinacei*. Spargana are found near the central African lakes (generally in swellings in the chest) but also in Rwanda and Burundi. The adults are probably *S. theileri* or *S. pretoriensis*.

ORDER: CYCLOPHYLLIDEA

GENUS: *TAENIA*

TAENIA SOLIUM (LINNAEUS, 1758) PORK TAPEWORM

PARASITOLOGY

T. solium (Figure III.44) lives in the upper third of the small intestine. The name 'solium' is derived from the resemblance of the rostellum to the conventional figure of the sun. It attains a length of 2–3 m (exceptionally 8 m), having 800–1000 segments. The head is globular, quadrangular, 1 mm in diameter, and the rostellum short and pigmented, with a double row of 20–50 hooklets (Figure III.45C). The four suckers project slightly and are circular, measuring 0.5 mm in diameter. The anterior proglottides are small, broader than they are long, the more mature ones measuring $12 \times 6 \, mm$. Each proglottis has a marginal genital pore with thick lips; its situation alternates irregularly between the right and left margins. The uterus is median with seven to 13 stout diverticula (Figure III.44A). The testes consist of 150–200 follicles, distributed throughout the dorsal plane. Proglottides number less than 1000. Terminal ripe segments pass out in the faeces and have an independent movement which enables them to migrate outside the anus. Each gravid segment contains 30 000–50 000 eggs.

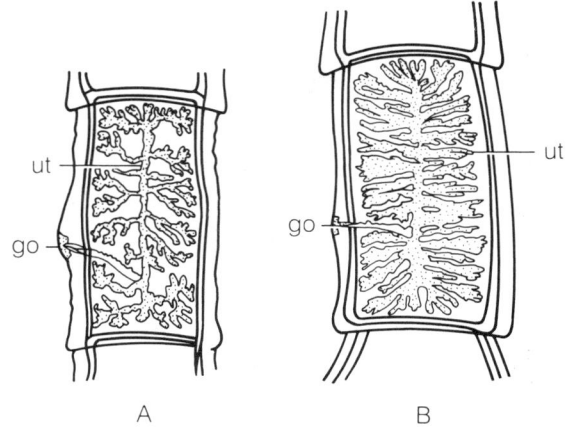

Figure III.44 Segments of tapeworms, showing the characteristic branching of the uterus as seen in mature segments. A, *Taenia solium*. B, *T. saginata*. go, Genital opening; ut, uterus.

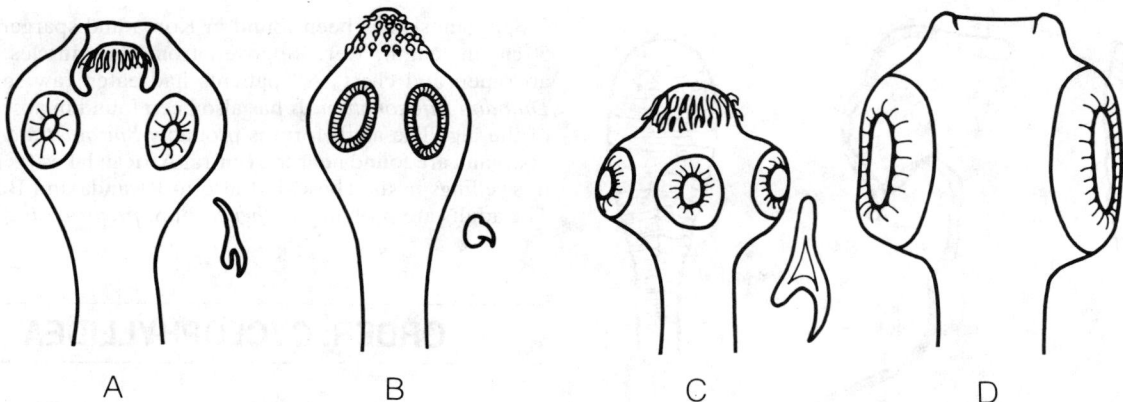

Figure III.45 Heads of human cestodes, showing suckers and, when present, the arrangement of the hooklets. A, *Hymenolepis nana*. B, *Dipylidium caninum*. C, *Taenia solium*. D, *T. saginata*.

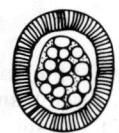 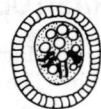

Figure III.46 Eggs of *Taenia saginata* (A) and *T. solium* (B) showing hooklets.

The egg measures 31–56 μm in diameter and is round with no operculum (Figures III.5, and III.46B). It has two radially striated shells, the inner formed by the embryo (thus differing from Pseudophyllidea), and a vitelline membrane when it is in the segment which is lost in the faeces. Small numbers of eggs are found in the faeces when the segments break. They contain the six-hooked oncosphere.

LIFE CYCLE (Figure III.50)

Mature segments are detached and pass out with the faeces; they disintegrate and the eggs are set free and eaten by the

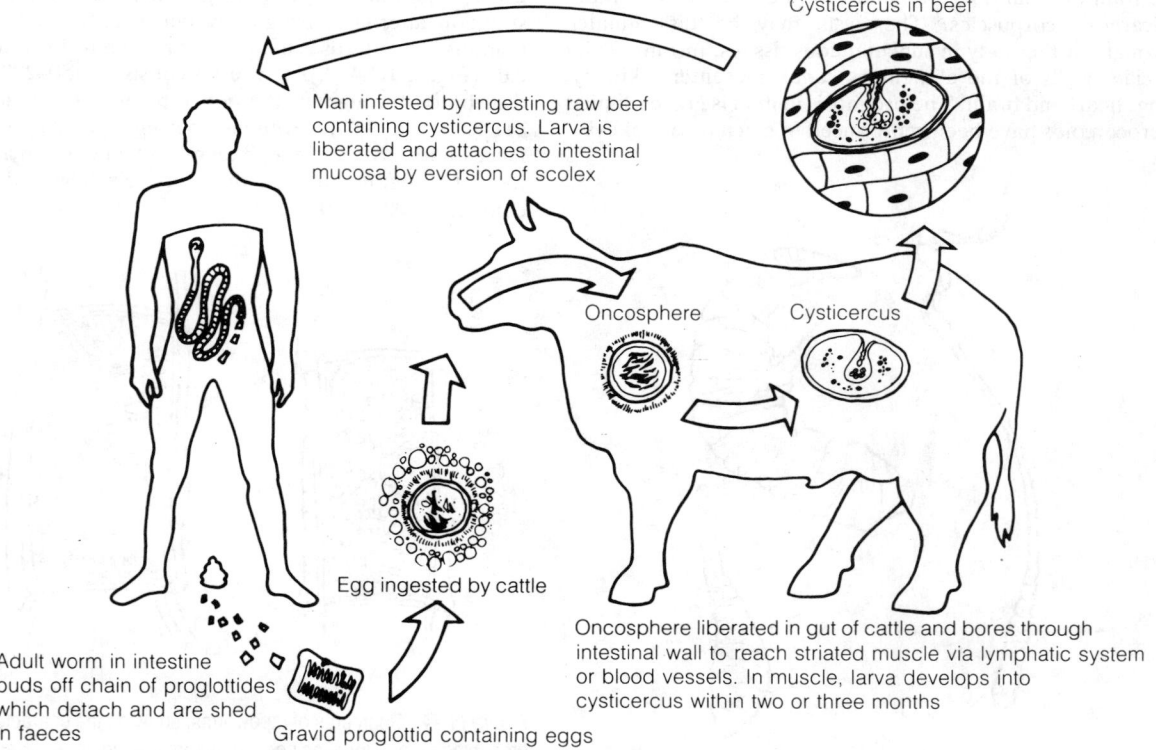

Cysticercus in beef

Man infested by ingesting raw beef containing cysticercus. Larva is liberated and attaches to intestinal mucosa by eversion of scolex

Oncosphere

Cysticercus

Egg ingested by cattle

Oncosphere liberated in gut of cattle and bores through intestinal wall to reach striated muscle via lymphatic system or blood vessels. In muscle, larva develops into cysticercus within two or three months

Adult worm in intestine buds off chain of proglottides which detach and are shed in faeces

Gravid proglottid containing eggs

Figure III.47 Life cycle of *Taenia saginata*. (Courtesy of WTIM.)

intermediate host (the pig). Man is occasionally infected by cysticerci (cysticercosis); so are other primates (macaque monkeys), occasionally sheep or dogs. The oncosphere penetrates the gut wall and enters the bloodstream, settling in the muscles, especially the heart and becomes a *Cysticercus* (5–20 mm) known as cysticercus cellulosae. Infected pork is popularly known as 'measly pork'. At 0°C the cysticerci can persist for 70 days.

In the alimentary tract of man or other definitive host the bladder of the cysticercus is absorbed by the digestive juices; the scolex and head are evaginated and then pass to the small intestine, where the scolex fixes itself to the gut wall and forms proglottides.

TAENIA SAGINATA GOEZE (1782) (BEEF TAPEWORM)

PARASITOLOGY

T. saginata (Figures III.44D, III.45B and III.48) is whitish and semitransparent, measuring 4–10 m; when fully adult it may contain 20–2000 segments. The scolex is pear shaped, cubical and 1–2 mm in diameter, with four lateral suckers but no rostellum or hooks. The suckers and sucker-like organ (Figure III.45D) at the apex are frequently pigmented. The neck is long and half the width of the scolex. The older proglottides are elongated; gravid individuals are three to four times longer than they are broad. The genital pore is single, marginally placed at the hind end of the proglottis, alternating regularly between the right and left margins. There are 20–35 lateral branches on each side of the uterus which may ramify (Figure III.44B). The genital organs in the mature proglottid differ from those of *T. solium* in having about twice the number of testes (300–400) and in lacking the accessory ovarian lobe. Each gravid segment contains about 97 000 eggs. The total output per year is reckoned at 594 million.

T. saginata (like *Enterobius vermicularis*), oviposits on the perianal skin. The ova are expelled when the proglottid has detached itself from the strobila. The gravid uterus carries lateral branches terminating in blind club-shaped sacs. There they form a separate organ resembling a tassel (*thysanus*), which when it disintegrates leaves behind a mass of ova. The thysanus then becomes an aperture for oviposition (*protocostoma*). The stimulus is provided by thousands of eggs compressed within the uterus. The yolk mass which envelops the embryophores of the ova causes them to adhere to the perianal skin.

The egg is globular, 30–40 × 20–30 µm, with a double-shelled striated embryophore, which contains the oncosphere consists of an outer shell, chorionic membrane and two oncospheral membranes (Figures III.5, and III.46A). *T. saginata* embryophores stain well with Ziehl–Neelsen stain, whereas those of *T. solium* do not.[6]

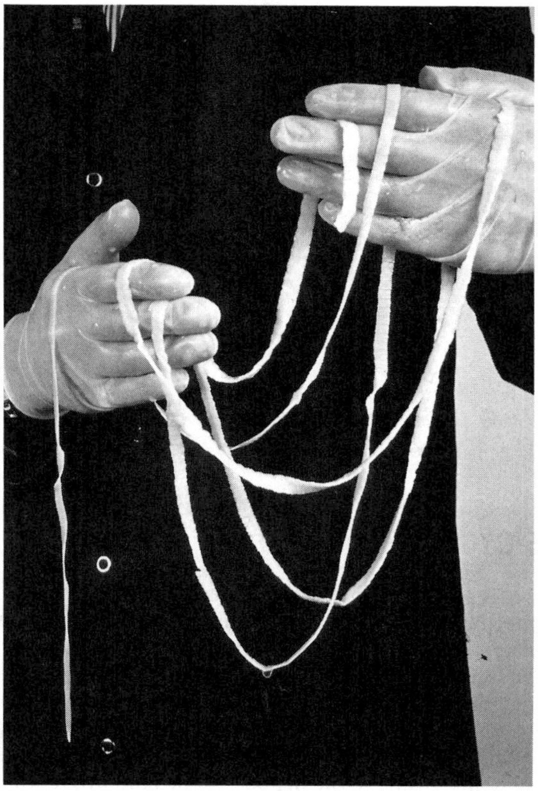

Figure III.48 Adult beef tapeworm (*Taenia saginata*). (Courtesy of G. S. Nelson.)

LIFE CYCLE (Figure III.47)

Gravid proglottides emerge in faeces or pass to the exterior independently; they then creep into grass or herbage, where they disintegrate. When the eggs are eaten by the ox, the oncospheres are set free and pass into the small intestine, where they bore through the wall and are carried to the muscles, especially the pterygoids and the fatty tissues round heart, diaphragm and tongue. Then cysticerci (cysticercus bovis) are formed, measuring 7.5–9 × 5.5 mm. They can be distinguished from other cysticerci by the absence of hooks on the scolices, other cysticerci having large hooks. They live for 8 months in the ox and develop further in man, who constitutes the normal definitive host. The bladder is digested and the liberated scolex, passing to the small intestine, affixes itself by suckers to the gut wall. The cysts die at 48°C. Infected meat is known to inspectors as 'measly beef'. In Egypt and Morocco the camel is the most important intermediate host.

CYSTICERUS

The cysticercus has a small invaginated scolex (and a neck resembling an adult *Taenia*). The external tissue consists of hair-like processes, a peripheral collagenous fibrous layer, two muscle layers, peripheral cells, calcareous corpuscles, flame cells, a duct system embedded in a loose fibrous net and a central band of muscles. The different cestode larvae can be distinguished in human tissues by variations in these structures.[7]

Table III.7 Diagnostic characteristics of cestode larvae found in man.

	Cysticercus cellulosae	Cysticercus bovis	Cysticercus cerebralis	Echinococcus granulosus
Scolex	One	One	Several	Many
Hooks	Present	Absent	Present	Present
Bladder surface	Cuticle	Cuticle	Cuticle	Starified hyaloidine material
Superficial hair-like extensions	Hanging from 1 nm to 2.5 + μm	3–6 μm	1–2 μm	None
Subcuticular groups of muscles	Present	Absent	Absent	Absent
Make-up of wall	Wart-like processes	Rugae	Smooth and rugose	Smooth
Base of superficial protuberances	27–38 μm	50–70 μm	28–46 μm	None
Height of superficial protuberances	15–27 μm	23–27 μm	15–22 μm	None

After Slais.[7]

GENUS: *ECHINOCOCCUS* (See also Chapter 75)

ECHINOCOCCUS GRANULOSUS (BATSCH, 1786)
E. MULTILOCULARIS (LEUCKART, 1863) (VOGEL, 1955)
E. OLOGARTHRUS (DIESING, 1863)
E. VOGELI (RAUSCH & BERNSTEIN, 1972)
(TAENIA ECHINOCOCCUS OR HYDATID)

PARASITOLOGY

E. granulosus is very small, 3–8.5 mm long, with a pyriform scolex, 0.3 mm in diameter, provided at the apex with a projecting rostellum, four suckers and two circular rows of hooks, varying in size and number (Figure III.49). The neck is short and thick; the proglottides usually four in number. The last one is the longest (2–3 mm); only one is sexually mature and this contains up to 5000 eggs. The genital apertures are marginal, one to each proglottis, in an alternating arrangement. The testes are spherical and numerous. The cirrus pouch is large and pear shaped. The uterus is tubular and median with short unbranched lateral diverticula. The adult is difficult to remove from the small intestine of the dog without breaking its head. Eggs appear in dog faeces. Sometimes the fourth segment also comes away. Man is probably not a suitable intermediate host but is, of course, quite susceptible to hydatid infection.

The egg is spherical, 32–38 × 21–30 μm, and is double-shelled, the inner shell being thick. The egg is so similar to those of other tapeworms that it cannot be distinguished from them. The oncosphere contains three pairs of embryonal hooklets.

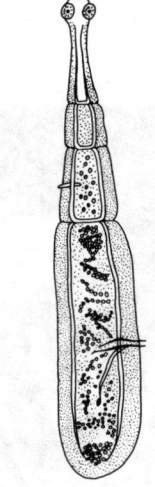

Figure III.49 Echinococcus granulosis. (15×.)

LIFE CYCLE (Figure III.50)

The egg is passed out in the dog's faeces until it is ingested by the intermediate host (sheep or man) either by eating contaminated grass or contaminated food. In the stomach the shell of the egg is digested and the oncosphere escapes. After 8 hours embryos can be found in the portal vein and liver whence they are filtered out. The next filter is the lung where a small number lodge. In 3 weeks the larval worm becomes vesicular and visible to the naked eye; in 3 months it attains a diameter of 5 cm and 5 weeks later has doubled that size. The hydatid cyst wall is composed of a fibrous laminated layer

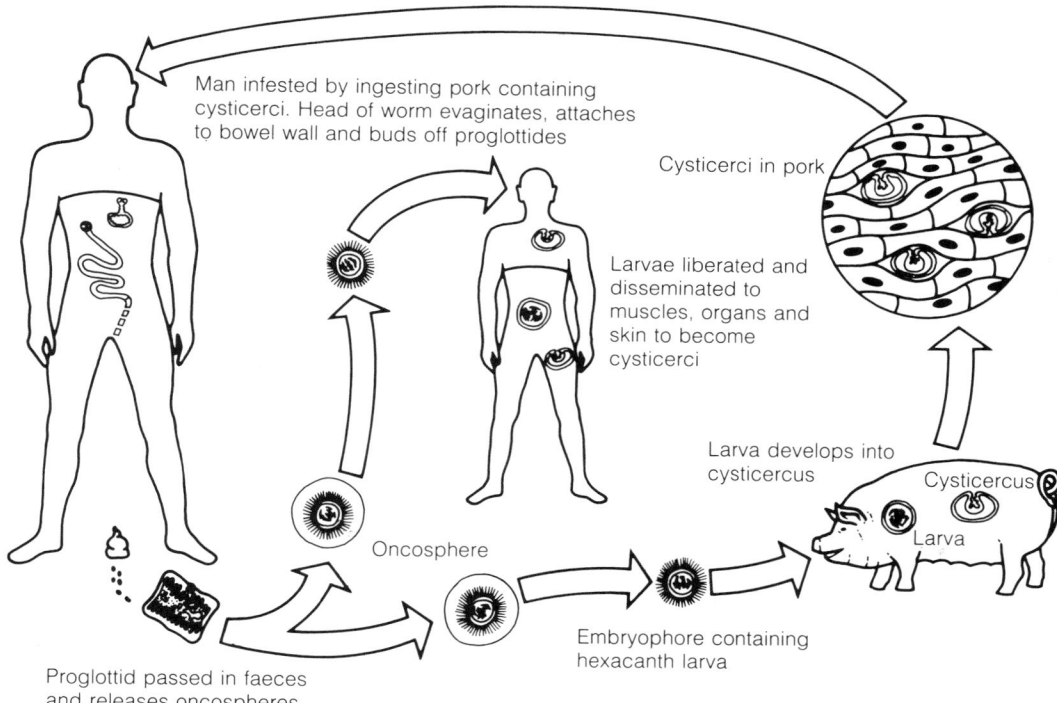

Man infested by ingesting pork containing cysticerci. Head of worm evaginates, attaches to bowel wall and buds off proglottides

Cysticerci in pork

Larvae liberated and disseminated to muscles, organs and skin to become cysticerci

Larva develops into cysticercus

Cysticercus

Larva

Oncosphere

Embryophore containing hexacanth larva

Proglottid passed in faeces and releases oncospheres

Figure III.50   Life cycle of *Taenia solium*. (Courtesy of WTIM.)

formed by the host, a thick median striated layer secreted by the cyst and an inner 'germinal' layer from which the brood capsules and daughter cysts arise. There are two types of proliferation: endogenous and exogenous. In the former, proliferation is inwards towards the cyst cavity; in the latter it is outwards. The varieties of hydatid are so striking that alveolar hydatid (*E. multilocularis*) has now been recognized as a distinct entity which has a limited geographical distribution (see Chapter 75).

The brood capsules are formed from small nuclear masses of the parenchymatous germinal layer; later, they become vacuolated to form vesicles. Larval scolices arise from a local thickening of the wall of the brood capsule; the wall evaginates to form a protective cup for the growing scolex. Near the head end the cuticle thickens and a circle of hooklets develops. The contractile part of the body of the scolex is capable of invaginating the head so that in the typical resting position the scolex has the hooklets inside. These hooklets may be strongly acid fast, a characteristic which can be recognized in histological sections and reveal that the structure is a dead hydatid cyst. Free brood capsules and free scolices in the hydatid cyst cavity are known as 'hydatid sand'. In other cysts the brood capsules never produce scolices and are known as acephalocysts.

Daughter cysts may be produced by injury or by mechanical interference with the mother cyst, inside which they arise from the detached germinal layer and also from the brood-capsule cells; rarely by vesicular changes from the detached scolices. In the liver the daughter cysts are bile stained. Intramuscular injection of scolices causes formation of new cysts and this accounts for the dissemination of hydatid cysts

throughout the body which sometimes occurs after operation.

Exogenous daughter cysts in the omentum and bones are secondary, caused by herniation or rupture of both germinal and laminated layers through weakened parts of the adventitia from intracystic pressure. By final exclusion of these herniations new cysts form.

ALVEOLAR HYDATID (*Echinococcus multilocularis*) (See Chapter 75)

In the adult worm the differences are the position of the genital pore in front of the middle of the proglottis. The number of testes is 21–29 (as against 45–65). These lie behind the posterior end of the proglottis in the region of the cirrus sac. The uterus has no lateral branches. The length of the mature worm is 1.4–3.4 mm (as against 5–8 mm). The alveolar cyst grows by exogenous proliferation which invades the surrounding tissues and metastasizes. The cyst is solid with small irregular vesicles containing fluid and very rarely scolices.

LIFE CYCLE

The definitive hosts of *E. multilocularis* are dogs and foxes and the intermediate hosts rodents.

E. oligarthrus and *E. vogeli* are about half the size of the other echinococci and the rostellar hooks are a means of identification of the protoscolices.

GENUS: *MULTICEPS*

Multiceps multiceps. The adult worm is 40–60 cm in length and has a pyriform scolex about 1 mm in diameter with four suckers and a rostellum armed with a double rank of 22–32 large and small hooks.

Multiceps brauni. The adult worm has a scolex armed with 30 rostellar hooks. The coenurus differs from that of *M. multiceps* in its larger hooks.

LIFE CYCLE

The definitive hosts of *Multiceps* are canines and the intermediate hosts sheep and other herbivorous animals.

GENUS: *VAMPIROLEPIS*

VAMPIROLEPIS NANA (SIEBOLD, 1852)
(HYMENOLEPIS NANA, TAENIA NANA, H. MURINA, DWARF TAPEWORM)

DISTRIBUTION

It is found more commonly in warm countries: Egypt, Sudan, Thailand, India, Japan, South America (Brazil, Argentina and especially Cuba), south Europe (Portugal, Spain and Sicily, where it affects 10% of the children). It lives in the small intestine (Figure III.51).

PARASITOLOGY

H. nana is 25–45 mm long by 0.5–0.9 mm and has 100–200 proglottides. The scolex measures 139–480 μm, is subglobular with a well-developed rostellum, a single crown with 20–30 hooks (14–18 μm) and four globular suckers (80–150 μm) (Figures III.45A and III.51). The neck is long, the proglottides short anteriorly but the posterior ones increase in size and are broader than they are long. The genital pores are marginal and placed near the anterior border. There are three testes. The vas deferens widens into the seminal vesicle and the gravid uterus occupies the entire segment.

The egg is oval and there are up to 180 in each segment. It has two membranes—outer (vitelline), 40–60 μm and inner, 20–30 μm. There is a conspicuous mammillate projection at each pole, enclosing an oncosphere with three pairs of hooklets.

The segments when freed are partially digested and the eggs, set free in the faeces, are easily detected.

LIFE CYCLE (Figure III.52)

This worm forms an exception to other members of the group and does not necessarily have an intermediate host; the larva enters the villus of the intestine to become a

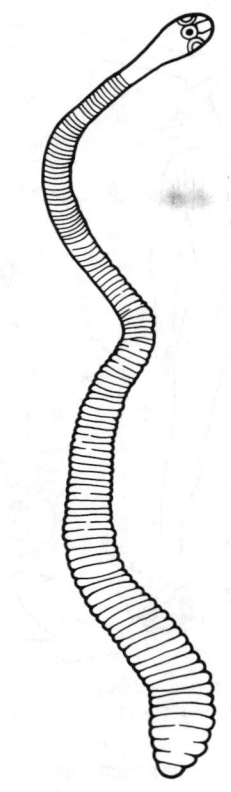

Figure III.51   Hymenolepis nana. Magnified.

cerocyst. In 40–70 hours after infestation the scolex appears; in 80–90 hours the rostellum has hooklets and then passes into the lumen of the intestine attached to the epithelium of the villus by a short neck. The rapidity of development varies greatly. Strobilization is rapid; the proglottides mature in 10–12 days and after 30 days eggs appear in the faeces to be ingested by another human host. *H. fraterna* of the rat is morphologically identical but its intermediate hosts are beetles and fleas (*Nosopsyllus fasciatus* and *Xenopsylla*).

GENUS: *HYMENOLEPIS*

HYMENOLEPIS DIMINUTA (RUDOLPHI, 1819)

This is a parasite of rats (*Rattus norvegicus* (*decumanus*), *R. alexandrinus*) and mice (*Mus musculus* and *Apodemus sylvaticus*); it is found in man throughout the world.

It measures 20–60 mm × 3.5 mm. The head is small and cuboidal. At the apex is a rudimentary rostellum with four small, unarmed suckers. The neck is shorter than the head. The proglottides increase in size as the tail is approached and are broader than they are long.

The egg is circular or ovoid, measuring 60–80 μm. Its outer shell is yellowish and thickened with indistinct radiations and contains a hexanth oncosphere.

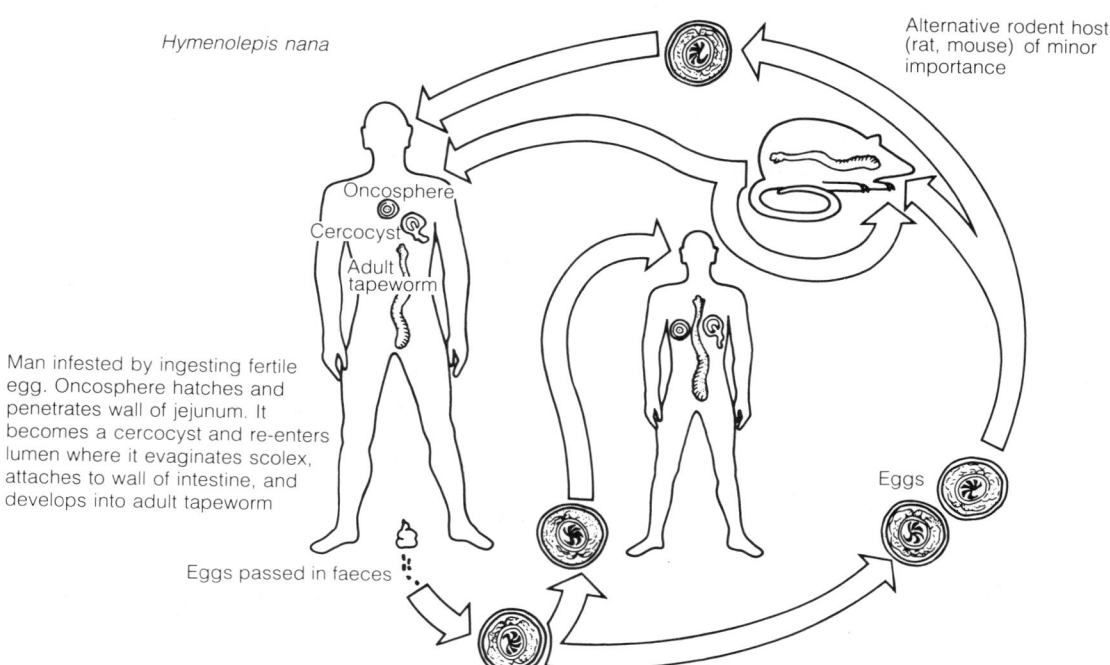

Hymenolepis nana

Alternative rodent host (rat, mouse) of minor importance

Oncosphere

Cercocyst

Adult tapeworm

Man infested by ingesting fertile egg. Oncosphere hatches and penetrates wall of jejunum. It becomes a cercocyst and re-enters lumen where it evaginates scolex, attaches to wall of intestine, and develops into adult tapeworm

Eggs

Eggs passed in faeces

Figure III.52   Life cycle of *Hymenolepis nana*.

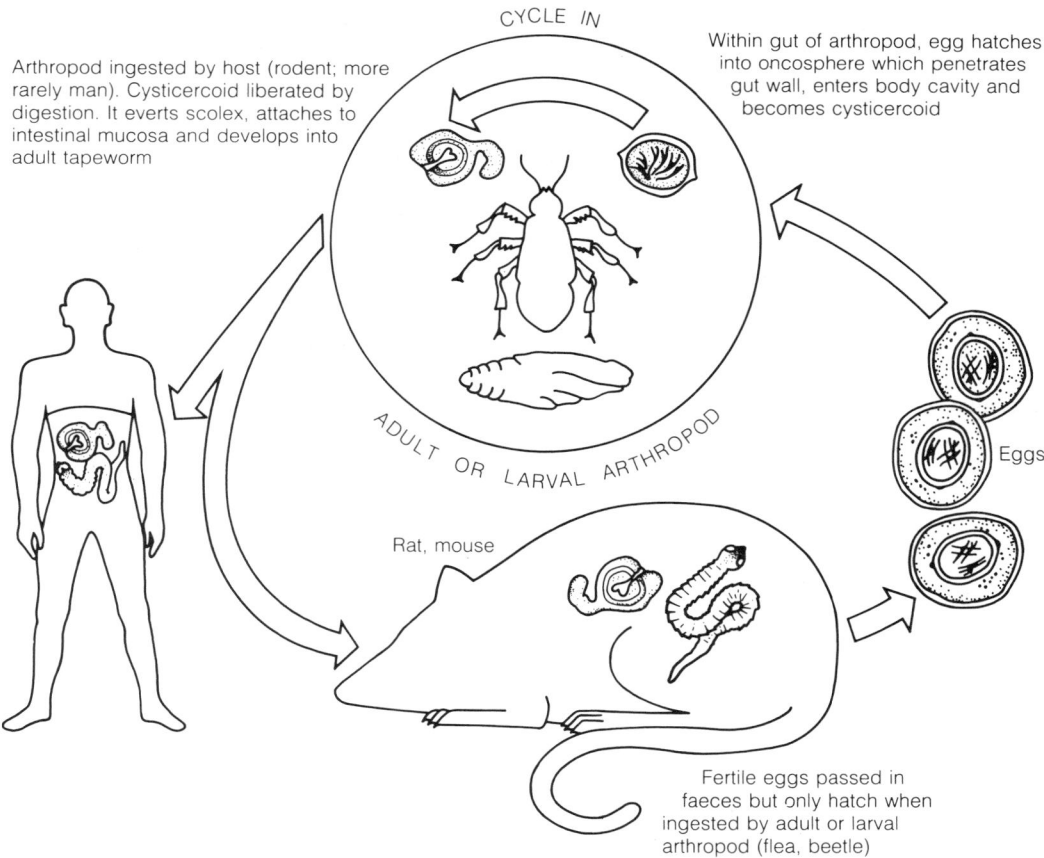

CYCLE IN

Arthropod ingested by host (rodent; more rarely man). Cysticercoid liberated by digestion. It everts scolex, attaches to intestinal mucosa and develops into adult tapeworm

Within gut of arthropod, egg hatches into oncosphere which penetrates gut wall, enters body cavity and becomes cysticercoid

ADULT OR LARVAL ARTHROPOD

Eggs

Rat, mouse

Fertile eggs passed in faeces but only hatch when ingested by adult or larval arthropod (flea, beetle)

Figure III.53   Life cycle of *Hymenolepis diminuta*.

LIFE CYCLE (Figure III.53)

The cysticercus stages occur in the body cavity of insects and fleas during their larval stages: *Nosopsyllus* (*Ceratophyllus*) *fasciatus*; *Xenopsylla cheopis*; *Leptopsylla segnis* (mouse flea); *Pulex irritans*; in coleoptera and lepidoptera such as *Asopia farinalis*, *Anisolabis annulipes*, *Tinea pellionella*, *Akis spinosa* and *Scaurus striatus*; also in South America, in *Dermestes vulpinus*, *D. peruvianus*, *Ulosonia parvicornis* and *Embia argentina* (etc.).

The rat becomes parasitized by eating infected fleas or other insects. The cysticercoids, when ingested by the definitive host, become adult in 17 days.

GENUS: *DIPYLIDIUM*

DIPYLIDIUM CANINUM (LINNAEUS, 1758)

This is a common parasite of the dog, cat and jackal. There are many records of its occurrence in man worldwide, especially in children in European countries.

It lives in the small intestine and measures 15–40 cm × 2–3 mm. The scolex is small and globular, 0.55 mm in diameter. The rostellum has three or four circles consisting of 28–30 hooks (14–18 μm) of 'rose-thorn' shape and four elliptical suckers (Figure III.45B). The proglottides are narrow and there are 200 or more of them. The segments measure 6–7 × 2.3 mm. Two sets of genital apparatus are found in each segment; the genital pores are placed symmetrically at the lateral margins. The uterine cavities contain egg nests, each consisting of 8–15 eggs. Mature proglottides leave the intestine. The egg is round, 35–40 μm across.

The cysticercoid stage is passed through in the dog louse (*Trichodectes canis*), dog flea (*Ctenocephalides canis*), cat flea (*C. felis*) and human flea (*Pulex irritans*). Eggs are eaten by the larval flea and the hexacanth embryo develops in the adipose tissue and muscles, first appearing as a procercoid and later as a cysticercoid larva. Infection of man is accidental due to swallowing infected fleas.

GENUS: *RAILLIETINA*

R. MADAGASCARIENSIS (FORMERLY *TAENIA MADAGASCARIENSIS*), R. DEMERARIENSIS, R. CELEBENSIS, ETC.

These worms are found in Asia, Oceania and South America and *R. demerariensis* has been reported in Ecuador and in Australia from *Rattus fuscipes*. Two cases were reported from Thailand as *R. siviragi*. They are characterized by numerous hooks of 'coal-hammer' shape on the suckers and rostellum and by unilateral genital pores on the proglottides. Ripe segments contain egg capsules. The ovoid eggs possess conspicuously large hooklets. Usually they are parasites of birds, more rarely of rats. Their intermediate hosts are probably flies.

GENUS: *BERTIELLA*

Bertiella studeri has often been found in man and cases of infection with *Bertiella mucronata*, a tapeworm of monkeys, in Central and South America have been reported.[8]

GENUS: *INERMICAPSIFER*

This genus closely resembles the foregoing and cannot be distinguished from it by the ripe proglottides, and, like *Bertiella*, the scolex and suckers are unarmed. *I. arvicanthidis*, a parasite normally of the field rat, was found in a European child from Kenya; since then others have been reported in Ruanda-Buruudi and in Arusha, Tanzania. It is suggested that it is more common than has been supposed. No fewer than 12 species of *Inermicapsifer* are parasites of hyraxes and rodents in Africa. *I. cubensis* appears to be common in Cuba where 76 cases in man have been described. It is identical with the foregoing; *I. madagascariensis* is also identical.

NEMATODES
Phylum: Nemathelminthes
Class: Nematoda or roundworms

The sexes of these worms are separate. They are cylindrical, non-segmented and taper at both ends. They are white or yellow, sometimes semitransparent and their eggs are characteristic.

SUPERFAMILY: ASCARIDOIDEA

GENUS: *ASCARIS*

ASCARIS LUMBRICOIDES (LINNAEUS, 1758)
(ROUNDWORM)

CHARACTERS

Ascaris lumbricoides inhabits the intestine of man, and allied species are found in the pig, cat, dog and horse.

The adult female worm measures 20–35 cm × 3–6 mm, the male 15–31 cm × 2–4 mm (Figure 70.8). Both are pale and brown with whitish longitudinal lines and round tapering ends. The mouth is at the anterior end and is guarded by thin lips with finely denticulated ridges (Figure III.54). The anus is subterminal. In the female the vulva is anterior to the middle of the body. The vagina is directed backward and there are paired genital tubes each containing the uterus, receptaculum seminis, oviduct and ovary. The tubules and ducts attain a length of 12 cm and the capacity at any one time is 27 million eggs, the average daily output being 200 000. The male tail is conical without caudal alae and is curved in a semicircle with two rows of tactile papillae, mostly preanal but a few postanal. There are two chitinous spicules. The adults have a life span of 10–12 months.

The egg measures 50–70 × 40–50 μm and is elliptical, encased in a rough albuminous coat giving it a mamillated appearance. It is usually stained by faecal pigments (Figure III.5).

LIFE CYCLE

When the eggs are passed in the faeces there is no segmentation or differentiated embryo. In water or in moist earth at 36–40°C within 2–4 months the embryo is seen coiled up and moving inside the eggshell. The larva undergoes a moult before hatching and must be transformed into a second stage larva of the 'rhabditoid' type before it is infective. The embryo does not emerge from the egg until it is swallowed. The eggshell is then softened by the digestive juice and hatches in the small intestine. The rhabditiform larva penetrates the mucous membrane, enters the blood via the heart and lungs and reaches the alveolar capillaries where it has a 'blood bath'. As the larvae cannot pass through they burrow through the wall of the alveolus and enter the respiratory tree, finally being carried up the trachea by ciliary action. Eventually, on reaching the vocal cords, the majority of the larvae are swallowed for the second time and reach the small intestine. The second invasion is often accompanied by severe allergic phenomena, urticarial reactions and fall in blood pressure. The whole process occupies 10–14 days. During this time the larva moults twice (once after 5 or 6 days and the second time after the tenth day). The larvae measure 1.3–2 mm on the tenth day (Figure III.55) and 1.75–2.37 mm on the fifteenth. Larvae may reach the intestine as early as the fifth day. The fourth ecdysis takes place in the intestine between days 25 and 29. In man the incubation period (to time of first oviposition) occupies a period of 60–70 days. The diameter of the migrating larvae from the pulmonary capillaries to the terminal air spaces is considerably larger than that of the capillaries.

ASCARIS SUUM (GOEZE, 1782)

Ascaris suum of the pig is almost morphologically identical with *A. lumbricoides* except that the denticular ridges in the mouth are larger and have straight edges but these differences are not constant.

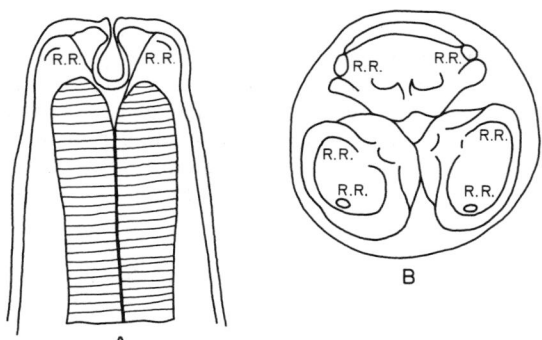

Figure III.54 Head of *Ascaris lumbricoides*. A, Ventral view. B, Anterior view, showing the oral labia.

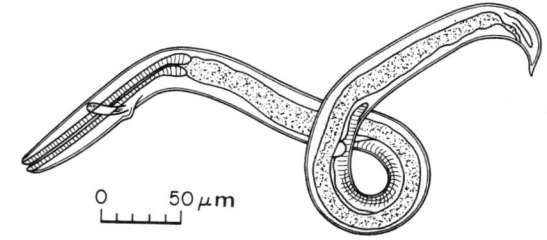

Figure III.55 Larva of *Ascaris lumbricoides* recovered from the trachea of a rat 8 days after ingestion of the eggs.

GENUS: *TOXOCARA*

TOXOCARA CANIS (WERNER, 1782)

Toxocara canis (the dog ascarid) is a cosmopolitan infection of dogs. The morphology is similar to that of *Ascaris*. The male worms are 4–6 cm long and the females 6.5–10 cm. In addition to the three characteristic lips of ascarids there are distinct cervical alae or wings which are much longer than they are broad and extend some distance from the anterior extremity along the lateral margins. The perianal papillae of the male worms are characteristic. The ova are pitted superficially and measure $85 \times 75 \mu$m. They are dark or greyish brown and unembryonated when passed.

The life cycle is similar to that of *A. lumbricoides* with four larval stages. In pregnant bitches the pups are infected transplacentally and are born infected with adult worms laying eggs. They may die within the first few weeks of life, but if they survive acquire some immunity. Puppies are the main source of infection for children who develop toxocariasis.

TOXOCARA CATI (SHRANK, 1788)

This worm is the common ascarid of the domestic cat and some of its wild relatives. The male worms are 4–6 cm long and the females 4–12 cm. The anterior end has characteristic ascarid lips and is provided with a pair of broad lateral cervical alae or wings which give a pyriform outline to the anterior end of the body. The eggs are similar to those of *T. canis*, as is the life cycle.

GENUS: *LAGOCHILASCARIS*

LAGOCHILASCARIS MINOR (LEIPER, 1909)

The usual host of *Lagochilascaris minor* is unresolved. Adult males measure 5–17 mm × 0.19–0.6 mm, females measure 20–60 mm × 0.2–0.81 mm. They are ascarid in morphology but the lips bear no denticles and they have a keel-like cuticular ledge along the entire extent of the lateral line. The eggs are spherical or slightly ovoid and measure $50 \times 65 \mu$m.

LIFE CYCLE

Adult worms live in cavities in the submucosa of the small intestine of the opossum and eggs are passed out in the stool containing infective larvae, which wait until they are ingested by mice and other small mammals when they hatch in the intestine and migrate to skeletal muscle to wait until the definitive host eats its prey.

SUPERFAMILY: SPIRUDOIDEA

GENUS: *GNATHOSTOMA*

GNATHOSTOMA SPINIGERUM (OWEN, 1838)

The adult worms are parasites of both wild and domestic felines and canines. Cats and dogs are important reservoirs.

PARASITOLOGY

The adult worms in the feline host vary in length from 11 to 25 mm for males and 25 to 54 mm for females. They are stout, reddish-coloured, slightly transparent nematodes with a subglobose cephalic swelling separated from the remainder of the worm by a cervical constriction. The anterior half of the nematode is covered with leaf-like spines which are broader and tridented just behind the cervix and narrower and singly pointed more equatorially. These spines are species characteristic.

The cephalic portion of the body is covered with 4–8 transverse rows of sharp recurved hooks. Four conspicuous cervical glands, arranged symmetrically around the oesophagus, fuse in pairs and open through two ducts which perforate the lips. The male has a pseudobursa which is provided with four pairs of perianal papillae. The copulatory spicules are chitinoid rods measuring 1.1 mm and 0.4 mm respectively. The vulva of the female is slightly postequatorial in position. The vagina is long and is anteriorly directed. The other genital tubes are paired.

The eggs (Figure III.56) are ovoid and 65–70 × 38–40 μm in size. They are transparent, superficially pitted, have a mucoid plug at one end and are unembryonated when laid.

The adult lives in tumours in the stomach wall of felines and dogs. Eggs are extruded from lesions and evacuated via the faeces into water where they embryonate and hatch.

A motile first-stage larva, measuring 223–275 × 13.4–17.4 μm and having a rounded anterior end provided with spines, emerges from the shell and actively enters a species of *Cyclops*, bores its way into the haemocoele and metamorphoses in 10–14 days into a second-stage larva (350–450 × 60–65 μm), which is provided with a head bulb armed with four rings of spines and two pairs of cervical glands.

The *third-stage larva* (Figure III.56) develops in a second intermediate host which can be a snake (rock python, cobra in India), freshwater fish (Philippines) or frog (Thailand), crayfish, crabs, amphibia, reptiles, mammals and chickens (Thailand) as well as man, in whom complete maturation does not take place, the larva wandering around the body causing pathological damage. Complete maturation to the adult stage occurs only in the stomach of dogs, cats and other felines in about 6.5 months.

Four species of *Cyclops* can act as the first intermediate host and 28 species of fish and vertebrates as the second intermediate host: two species of freshwater fish, three species of amphibian, five species of reptile, three species of fowl, two species of crab and 13 species of rodents and monkeys.

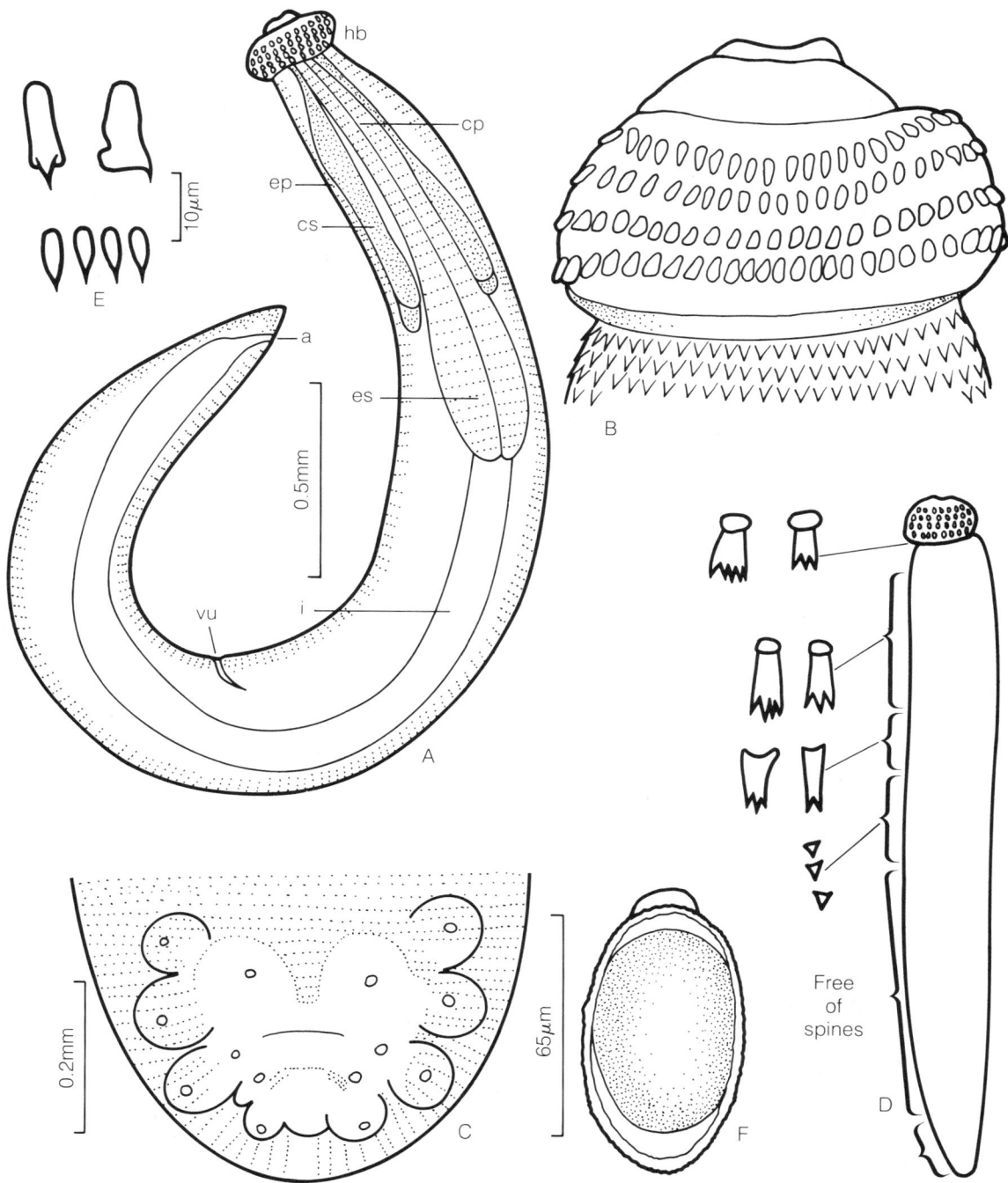

Figure III.56 *Gnathostoma spinigerum.* A, Lateral view of third-stage larva. B, Head bulb of third-stage larva with four rows of hooklets. C, Posterior end of male, ventral view, with minute cuticular spines omitted. D, Diagram of the types of spines at different levels of the body. E, Detail of the spines on the head bulb. F, Fertilized egg.

a	anus		es	oesophagus
cp	cervical papilla		hb	head bulb
cs	cervical sac (gland?)		i	intestine
ep	excretory pore		vu	vulva

GENUS: *PHYSALOPTERA*

PHYSALOPTERA CAUCASICA (LINSTOW, 1902)
(*P. MORDENS*) (LEIPER, 1907)

Normal hosts are monkeys. In man it has been found in central Africa, Mozambique, Uganda and Malawi. It lives in the oesophagus, stomach, small intestine and occasionally the liver.

The female (2.4–10 cm × 1.14–2.8 mm) has a posterior end tapering to a sharp point, two ovaries, a single uterine tube, and a vulva in the anterior part of the body. The male (1.4–5 cm × 0.7–1 mm) has two lateral alae on the tail, formed by expansion of the cuticle, four pairs of pedunculated papillae—six pairs sessile—one unpaired postanal papilla, and two spicules of unequal length. In both sexes the mouth is guarded by two large lips, armed with two papillae and rows of teeth, which serve to grip the mucous membrane (Figure III.57).

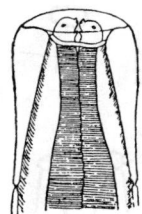

Figure III.57   The head of *Physaloptera caucasica*.

The egg (45 × 35 μm) has a double contour, smooth, thick, colourless shell.

The life cycle is unknown; insects possibly act as intermediaries. The clinical symptoms are indeterminate. The worms live with heads embedded in the digestive tract from the oesophagus to the ileum.

GENUS: *ANISAKIS*

ANISAKIS (*SIMPLEX*) (RUDOLPHI, 1809)

This is an ascarid parasite of herrings and marine animals. Its larval stages have caused symptoms in man.

The adult form inhabits the intestine of sea mammals (whales, dolphins and porpoises) and the larval stages are found in a variety of fish (haddock, mackerel, cod, pike, herring, bonito, salmon and Alaskan pollack) and squid.

The infective larva, as seen in the infective stage, is slender and thread-like, measuring 1.5–2.6 cm long and 0.1 cm in diameter. Its outer surface is somewhat striated and there is a ventriculus between the oesophagus and the intestine, with the latter two structures meeting on an oblique plane. There is an excretory pore in the anterior part of the head, ventral to a small larval tooth, and there are three anal glands near the rectum. Transverse section shows the lateral cords arranged

in a Y-shaped structure along the upper intestine or oesophagus or intestine. The cuticle consists of three layers and shows no alae.

GENUS: *GONGLYONEMA*

GONGLYONEMA PULCHRUM (MOLIN, 1857)

This is a spirurate nematode of a genus in which there are six species. It is a rare infection in man and pig but all ruminants are optimum hosts.

The worm lives most commonly in the upper portion of the digestive tract where it forms sinuous galleries in the mucosa and submucosa of the oesophagus, buccal cavity and tongue.

The male is 62 × 0.15–0.3 mm and the female much larger, 145 × 0.2–0.5 mm. The anterior extremity is covered with a variable number of bosses or scutes arranged in eight longitudinal series.

The transparent thick-shelled oval eggs are embryonated when laid and are 50–70 μm in length by 25–37 μm. Development takes place in dung beetles of genera *Apodius* and *Onthophagus*, as well as in a small cockroach.

SUPERFAMILY: STRONGYLOIDEA

GENUS: *ANCYLOSTOMA*

ANCYLOSTOMA DUODENALE (DUBINI, 1843)
(OLD WORLD HOOKWORM, MINER'S WORM)
(Figure III.58)

Both sexes are cylindrical, white, grey or reddish-brown (from ingested blood). The female (1–1.3 cm × 0.6 mm), is cylindrical and slightly expanded posteriorly. The vagina is in the posterior third. The body cavity is occupied by the ovary and coiled uterine tubes packed with eggs. The maximum egg output occurs 15–18 months after infection. The male (0.8–1.1 cm × 0.4–0.5 mm) has a copulatory bursa consisting of an umbrella-like expansion of the cuticle; the dorsal ray is divided towards the distal end into smaller rays, which again divide into three unequal portions (Figure III.59). There are two long delicate spicules. The genital papillae are tactile, finger-like projections near the anogenital opening. Owing to the situation of the genital openings in both sexes the worms in copulation assume a Y-shaped figure.

Two well-marked cephalic glands occupy the anterior third in both sexes and secrete an anticoagulating ferment. The mouth end is bent dorsally. The excretory pore is ventral, placed at the level of the oesophagus. The buccal capsule is lined with chitin and contains two pairs of sharp teeth on its ventral aspect (Figure III.60). The worm lives mostly in the jejunum and to a lesser extent in the duodenum but not in the

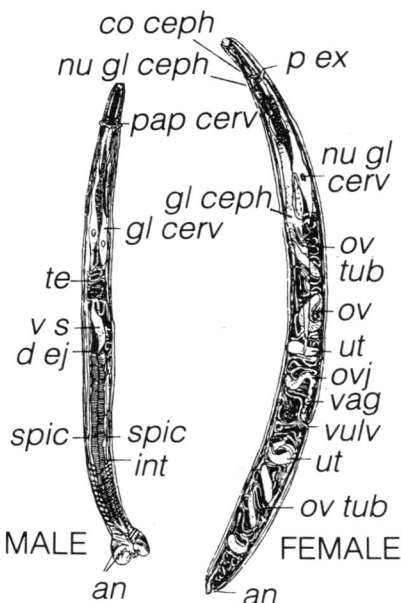

Figure III.58   Male and female *Ancylostoma duodenale*. (14×.)

an	anus
co ceph	cephalic nerve commissure
d ej	ejaculatory duct
gl	cervical gland
int	intestine
nu gl cerv	nucleus of cervical gland
ov	ovary
ovj	ovejector
ov tub	ovarian tubules
p ex	excretory pore
pap cerv	cervical papilla
spic	spicules
te	testes
ut	uterus
vag	vagina
vs	vesicula seminalis
vulv	vaginal opening

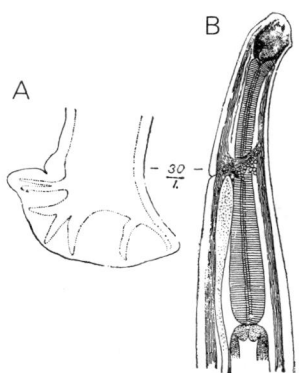

Figure III.59   Bursa (A) and head (B) of male *Ancylostoma duodenale*.

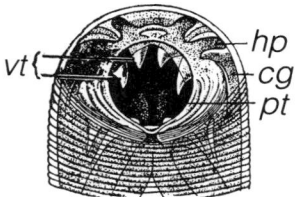

Figure III.60   Head of *Ancylostoma duodenale*, showing the hook-like teeth. (50×.)

cg	cephalic gland	pt	pharyngeal teeth
hp	head papillae	vt	ventral teeth

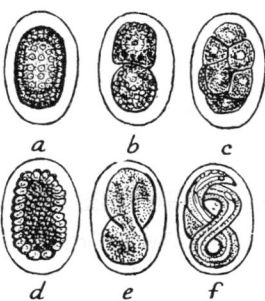

Figure III.61   Development stages of *Ancylostoma duodenale* of the larva in eggs; (a)–(c) are seen in fresh stools, and (d)–(f) when the stools are stale. (300×.)

ileum. The egg is ovoid (Figures III.5,14 and III.61) measuring $60 \times 40\,\mu$m, the shell is thin and hyaline and is passed in the early cleavage stage (Figure III.61a–c). Outside the body it rapidly develops to the morula stage (Figure III.61d) and hatches in 1–2 days.

At autopsy 500–1000 or more worms may be found. They have a life span of 4–7 years. The interval between active infection and the final disappearance of eggs from the faeces may be 76 months. The female produces 25 000–35 000 eggs each day and some 18–54 million eggs during its lifetime.

ANCYLOSTOMA BRAZILIENSE (DE FARIA, 1910)

It is found in dogs and cats in Brazil. In Sri Lanka *A. ceylanicum*, a closely related form from the civet cat, is reported.

It is rarely found in the small intestine and then is part of a mixed hookworm infection in man in India, Malaysia and Thailand. It is smaller than *A. duodenale* and the internal pair of ventral teeth are smaller than the corresponding teeth of that species. The female is 1 cm long and the male 8.5 mm. The rays in the copulatory bursa differ (Figure III.62) from those of *A. duodenale* and are distinctive.

The egg is indistinguishable from that of *A. duodenale*.

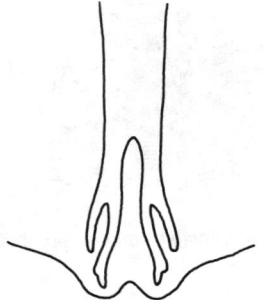

Figure III.62 Dorsal ray of *Ancylostoma braziliense*.

The life cycle is the same as *A. duodenale*. Man is apparently an unsuitable host. The larva does not penetrate into the bloodstream easily but wanders under the skin causing irritation (larva migrans, see Chapter 11).

GENUS: *NECATOR*

NECATOR AMERICANUS (STILES, 1902), NEW WORLD HOOKWORM (Figure III.63)

It is found in the small intestine of man and also of the gorilla, patas monkey, rhinoceros, pangolin and a rodent (*Caendu villosus*) and develops also in puppies. On the whole, *N. americanus* is a shorter and more slender worm than *A. duodenale*. The female (0.9–1.1 cm × 0.4 mm) has the vulva placed slightly in front of the middle of the body so that it copulates at a Y-shaped angle, as in *A. duodenale*. The male (7–9 × 0.3 mm) has the copulatory bursa closed and blunt and a short dorsomedian lobe which appears as if divided.

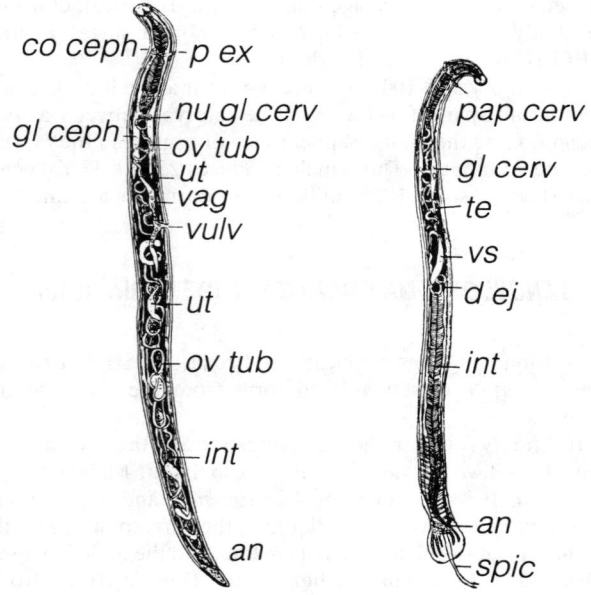

Figure III.63 *Necator americanus*. (12×.) Key as for Figure III.58.

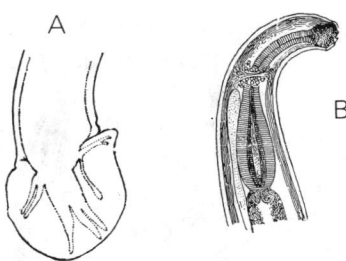

Figure III.64 Bursa (A) and head (B) of *Necator americanus*.

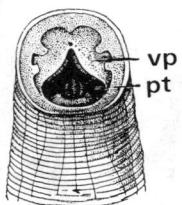

Figure III.65 The head of *Necator americanus*, showing the pharyngeal teeth (pt) and ventral plates (vp). (50×.)

The dorsal ray branches at the base into divergent arms with bipartite tips (tridigitate in *A. duodenale*). The base of the dorsal and dorsolateral rays is short (Figure III.64). Two separate spicules unite to form a single terminal 'fish-hook' barb. The living worms are greyish-yellow, at times reddish.

The sudden dorsal bend of the head, especially in the female, is distinctive (Figure III.64B). The buccal capsule is smaller than in *A. duodenale*, with an irregular border. In place of four hook-like teeth there is a ventral pair of cutting plates (Figure III.65). The first pair of dorsal teeth are represented by chitinous plates, The outlet of the dorsal gland constitutes a 'dorsal rib' or tooth which projects into the oral cavity. Deeply placed in the capsule are one pair of dorsal and one pair of submedian lancets.

The egg is slightly larger than that of *A. duodenale* (64–75 × 36–40 μm) but otherwise similar. The infective (third stage) larva can be differentiated from that of *Strongyloides stercoralis* by the larger buccal vestibule and the intervening space between the oesophagus and midgut and from *A. duodenale* as shown in Table III.73. The presence of 44 eggs per gram of faeces is reckoned to represent one female worm. The female lays from 6000–20 000 eggs/day. The estimated duration of life is about 5 years.

The life cycle is identical with that of *A. duodenale* except that *Necator* infective larvae enter through the skin only, whereas *Ancylostoma* can enter through the buccal mucous membrane as well, and that the migrating larvae of *Necator* grow and develop in the lungs in contrast to those of *Ancylostoma*.

LIFE CYCLE OF HOOKWORMS

The eggs are deposited in the lumen of the intestine with two, four or eight blastomeres. They develop and hatch after

Table III.8 Differentiation of third-stage larvae of *Necator* and *Ancylostoma*.

	Necator	Ancylostoma
Oral capsule	Sharply defined; visible dorsally and ventrally	Hardly visible; more marked dorsally than ventrally
Tail	Rather blunt	Pointed
Zone of closing cells	Leaves only small space between oesophagus and intestine	Leaves considerable space

expulsion in the faeces if they are deposited in damp, shaded soil.

The embryo moves about inside the shell and alters its shape, then escapes and gives rise to the rhabditiform larva which burrows into the faeces and feeds especially on bacteria . At first it has a double-bulbous oesophagus (Figure III.66b). Feeding voraciously, it stores oil globules in its intestinal wall. It moults on the third day; on the fifth the oesophageal bulb disappears and the larva becomes elongated and fully developed at 20–30°C; the larva on the third day is 400 μm and on the fifth it is 500–700 μm long. It then moves away from the faeces into the earth, moults again and becomes the infective filariform, or third-stage larva, with a well-developed mouth capsule, a simple muscular oesophagus and protective sheath, the walls of which are seen as two bright lines in the living specimen. It moves towards the oxygen supply but cannot swim in water. The larvae are most numerous in the upper 2.5 cm of the soil. They can ascend from deeper layers but lateral movements are limited. Attracted by warmth, the larva is quiescent in the cold; it moves along a thin film of water as well as in the earth. Enabled by the sheath to withstand a certain degree of desiccation, it can live in warm damp soil under optimum conditions for 2 years. This is the infective stage (Figure III.66a). Direct sunlight, drying, flooding or salt water are fatal.

On penetrating the skin of the host, the sheath is left behind and the larva then enters the lymphatics, then the bloodstream and reaches the lungs on the third day. If pyogenic bacteria enter the skin with the larvae an open lesion may develop, producing 'ground itch'. *A. duodenale* can infect via the mucous membrane of the mouth, as well as the skin, whereas *N. americanus* infects via the skin. Breaking through the alveoli of the lungs, it enters the bronchioles and travels via trachea and oesophagus to the stomach. During this migration the third moult takes place and the buccal capsule is formed. Migrating larvae of *Necator* grow and develop in the lungs whereas those of *Ancylostoma* do not. On arrival in the intestine on the seventh day it undergoes its fourth moult; the terminal buccal capsule is changed into the 'provisional buccal capsule' with the mouth opening directed dorsally, as in the adult, but without teeth. On the fifteenth day the 'provisional buccal capsule' is cast off and it then assumes the adult form with adult buccal capsule and bursa in the male. In 3–5 weeks it becomes sexually mature, copulates and produces fertile eggs. Adult worms live for 1–9 years and a female *Necator* lays 9000 eggs per day and *Ancylostoma* 30 000.

HYPOBIOSIS

A phenomenon known as hypobiosis has been observed[9] in which there is arrested development of migrating *A. duodenale* larvae, which migrate to the mammary gland, are secreted in milk and infect the child. This is similar to that seen in *A. caninum* which infects puppies in the same way.

CULTIVATION OF HOOKWORM LARVAE

A small portion of faeces is rubbed over a Petri dish with warm water, making a uniform layer like pea soup. Inside the cover is placed a circle of wet blotting paper. This is kept

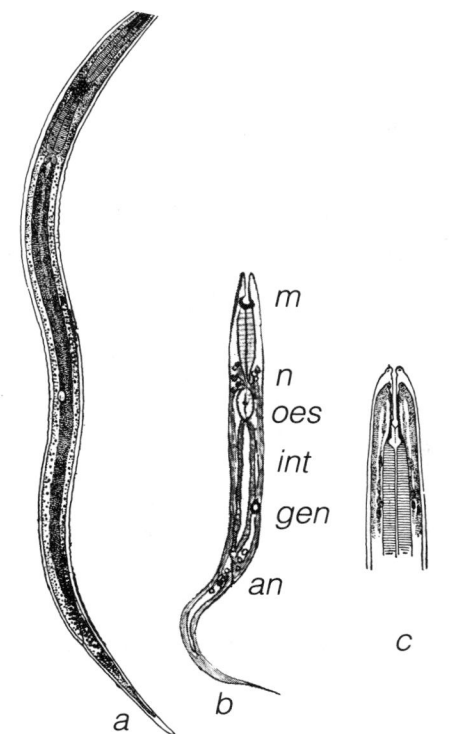

Figure III.66 Ancylostoma duodenale. (a) Mature infective larva. (b) Rhabditiform larva. (120×.) (c) Head of larva.

moist and incubated at 23.9°C under a shade. If there is too much water the eggs will not develop. The larvae climb up the sides of the dish on to the blotting paper where they can be studied.

DIFFERENTIATION OF HOOKWORMS

The striation of the sheath is indistinct in *A. duodenale* but very clear in *A. braziliense*. Rhabditiform ancylostome larvae are similar to those of *S. stercoralis* but are slightly more attenuated posteriorly and possess a much longer buccal vestibule. Infective (third-stage) *A. duodenale* larvae are differentiated from *Necator* by the oesophageal shears, which are unequal in thickness in *Ancylostoma* but equal in *Necator*, and by the features shown in Table III.73.

GENUS: *OESOPHAGOSTOMUM*

OESOPHAGOSTOMUM APIOSTOMUM (WILLACH, 1891)

The female (1 cm × 0.325 mm) terminates posteriorly in a sharp point and has a vulva in its anterior half. The male (0.8–1 cm × 0.35 mm) has a copulatory bursa with a dorsal ray bifurcating into branches and forming a horseshoe-shaped structure, each limb giving off a short lateral horn near its base (Figure III.67).

The egg (60 × 40 μm) closely resembles that of *Ancylostoma* but is passed in an advanced stage of development.

The larvae hatch from the eggs in the soil. When mature, they are unsheathed. The rhabditiform stage is swallowed and passes through the stomach and intestine. Then it invades the wall of the caecum where it forms nodules and, on occasions, may penetrate the intestine and form intraperitoneal abscesses. The immature worms break out into the lumen, attach themselves to mucosa and become adult.

OESOPHAGOSTOMUM STEPHANOSTOMUM (RAILLIET & HENRY, 1909)

This is a common parasite of monkeys (*Cercopithecus callitrichus*) and gorillas. The first case reported in man was in Brazil; the patient died of dysenteric symptoms and peritonitis. It has also been reported in French Guiana and in northern Nigeria.

The morphology resembles that of *O. apiostomum* but both sexes are larger and it is distinguished by a corona radiata with 38 leaf-like spines.

The eggs in the faeces resemble those of *Ancylostoma*.

The life history is probably similar to that of *O. apiostomum*.

GENUS: *TERNIDENS*

TERNIDENS DIMINUTUS (RAILLIET & HENRY, 1905)

The female (14–16 × 0.73 mm) has a genital orifice posterior and subterminal and a short vagina opening into two uterine tubes (Figure III.68). The male (9.5 × 0.56 mm) has the dorsal ray of the copulatory bursa dividing into two distal extremities and each branch bifurcates again (Figure III.69).

The worm resembles a female ancylostome; its anterior extremity is not bent and the mouth capsule is terminal with a corona of setae. At the base of the cup-like buccal capsule three serrated teeth guard the entrance to the oesophagus; this is characteristic of the genus *Ternidens* (Figure III.68).

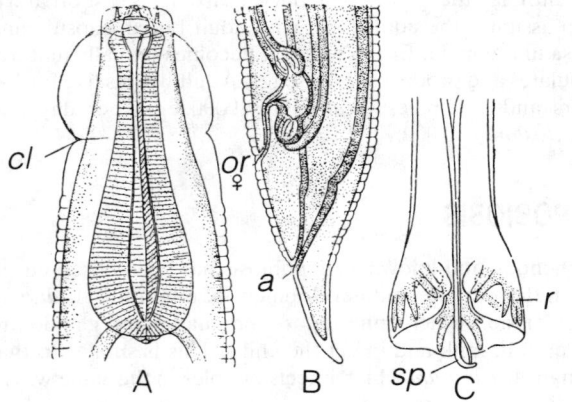

Figure III.67 *Oesophagostomum apiostomum* (*brumpti*). A, Head, showing cuticular expansion and the oral vestibule. B, Tail of the female. C, Tail of the male, showing copulatory bursa.

a	anus	r	characteristic rays
cl	ventral cleft		of bursa
or	vaginal orifice	sp	spicule

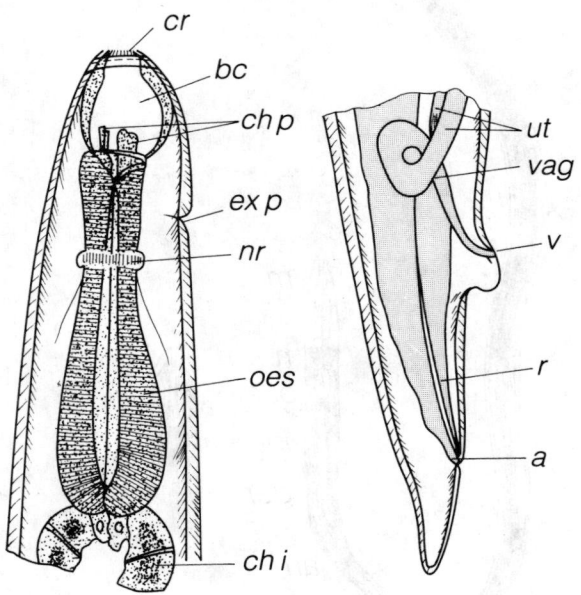

Figure III.68 Female *Ternidens diminutus*. 1, Anterior extremity. 2, Posterior extremity.

a	anus	oes	oesophagus
bc	buccal cavity	r	rectum
ch i	chyle intestine	ut	uterus
ch p	chitinous plates	v	vaginal opening
cr	corona radiata	vag	vagina

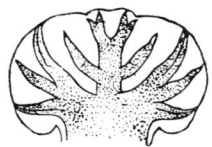

Figure III.69 Bursa of male *Ternidens diminutus*.

The egg (84 × 40 μm) is delicate and transparent and in an advanced stage of segmentation resembles that of an ancylostome.

The rhabditiform larva (0.3 mm) with flagellar tail, hatches from the egg in soil, becomes sheathed and the infective filariform larva (0.6–0.7 mm) is formed. These can survive desiccation, reviving in water; thus they withstand drought.

The filariform infective larvae fail to penetrate human skin but gain entrance through the stomach and intestinal tract after the eggs are swallowed with soil-contaminated food or water.

SUPERFAMILY: METASTRONGYLIDAE

GENUS: *PARASTRONGYLUS*

PARASTRONGYLUS CANTONENSIS (CHEN, 1935)
(*ANGIOSTRONGYLUS CANTONENSIS*)

The male is 15.5–22.0 mm in length × 0.25–0.35 mm in breadth. It is transparent and smooth with faint transverse striae. The head is smoothly rounded and the mouth is without lips. There are four pairs of minute, submedian papillae which are sometimes visible *en face* and two clearly defined minute triangular teeth present at the base of the oral cavity. There may possibly be a third which is difficult to define. The oesophagus is 0.29–0.33 mm long by 0.05 mm at maximum breadth at the posterior end. The intestine is a wide thin-walled tube. The excretory pore opens just posterior to the oesophageal-intestinal junction. The spicules are unequal, flexible and striated rods 1.2 mm in length. The bursa is well developed but the gubernaculum is absent and there is one pair of large adanal papillae.

The female is 18.5–33 mm long × 0.28–0.5 mm in maximum breadth. Cuticle, head, papillae, oesophagus and intestines are as in the male. In life, the spirally wound, milky white uterine tubules and the blood-filled intestine can be seen through the transparent cuticle and form a striking 'barber's pole' pattern. The uterine tubules unite about 2 mm from the posterior end to form the thin-walled vagina. The vulva is a transverse slit. The tail is obliquely truncated. The anus is 0.06 mm and the vulva 0.25–0.28 mm from the tip of the tail which bears a minute terminal projection. The male:female ratio is usually 2:3.

The eggs are ovoid with a thin hyaline shell measuring 46–48 × 68–74 μm. They are passed unembryonated.

The adult *A. cantonensis* lives in the pulmonary arteries of rats. Unsegmented ova are discharged into the bloodstream and lodge as emboli in the smaller vessels. The first-stage larvae which hatch from these eggs break through the respiratory tract, migrate up the trachea and eventually pass out of the body in the faeces. In Hawaii the land snail *Achatina fulica*, the slug *Veronicella leydigi* and the land planarian *Geoplana septemlineata* have been found naturally infected.

Slugs (*Agriolimax laevis*) act as intermediary hosts. Two moults occur in the slug about the seventeenth day. The slugs are then eaten by rats (*R. rattus*) and the larvae remain in their cast skins until freed in the stomach of the rat by digestion. They then pass quickly along the gut as far as the ileum where they enter the bloodstream and congregate in the central nervous system some 17 hours after ingestion. The anterior part of the cerebrum is the favourite site and there the third moult takes place on the sixth or seventh days and the final one on the eleventh to thirteenth. Young adults emerge on the surface of the brain from the twelfth to fourteenth days and spread during the next 2 weeks on the arachnoid surface. From the twenty-eighth to thirty-first days they migrate to the lungs via the venous system, passing through the right side of the heart to their definitive site in the pulmonary arteries. The prepatent period in the rat usually lies between the forty-second and forty-fifth days.

PARASTRONGYLUS COSTARICENSIS (MORENA & CESPEDES, 1971)
(*ANGIOSTRONGYLUS COSTARICENSIS*)

Angiostrongylus costaricensis is larger than *A. cantonensis*. The male measures 22 mm × 140 μm and the female 42 mm × 350 μm and the morphology is similar. The eggs are ovoid and measure 90 μm with a thin hyaline shell and are passed unembryonated.

SUPERFAMILY: TRICHOSTRONGYLOIDEA

GENUS: *TRICHOSTRONGYLUS*

TRICHOSTRONGYLUS COLUBRIFORMIS (GILES, 1892)
AND ALLIED SPECIES

Normally this is a parasite of the upper small intestine of the sheep and goat; it is not infrequently found in the duodenum and upper jejunum of man in agricultural districts of India, central Africa, Egypt, Java, Australia, Japan, Korea and especially in Abadan (Iran) where 70% of inhabitants are infected. It has been found in Java in scrapings from the duodenum where the adults live with head embedded in the mucosa. By a flotation technique the eggs of this species can be found in the faeces, together with ancylostomes, fairly frequently in India and Assam.

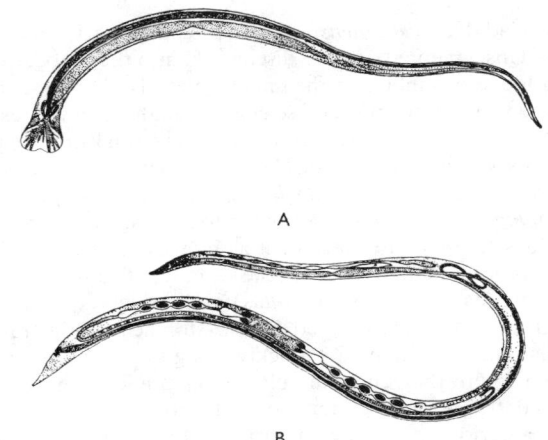

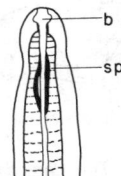

Figure III.71   *Strongyloides stercoralis*. Anterior end of the parasitic male. b, Buccal chamber; sp, buccal spears.

Figure III.70   *Trichostrongylus colubriformis*. A, Female. B, Male. (25×.)

The females (4–6.5 mm) (Figure III.70A) usually outnumber the males. They are very slender and pink with an attenuated anterior extremity and the vulva in the posterior quarter. The males (4–5 × 0.07 mm) have a bilobed copulatory bursa and two spicules (Figure III.70B). These parasites are found a third to a half buried in mucus. When scraped on to a slide they appear as delicate red streaks. When the slide is shaken in saline in a Petri dish they can be seen against a dark background. The adult worms are never found in faeces. The mouth is unarmed.

The egg (85 × 115 μm) is relatively large, oval, thin shelled and contains a morula when deposited. It is apt to be mistaken for that of *Ancylostoma duodenale*, is longer and narrower with more pointed ends.

The eggs hatch outside the body; the rhabditiform larvae metamorphose into infective filariform in 6 days at 22–25°C and can be distinguished from similar stages in *Strongyloides* and *Ancylostoma* by the bead-like swelling at the tip of the tail. The semifilariform third-stage larvae are very resistant to desiccation. These enter the body via the skin or mouth, undergoing two ecdyses.

An eastern form has been separated in Japan (*T. orientalis*). *T. probolurus* (Railliet, 1896) is rarely seen in man; it is a natural infection of the gazelle and camel. *T. orientalis* is common in people who look after donkeys and goats.

SUPERFAMILY: RHABDITOIDEA

GENUS: *STRONGYLOIDES*

STRONGYLOIDES STERCORALIS (BAVAY, 1876)

PARASITOLOGY

Formerly it was thought that embryos were produced by a parasitic, parthenogenetic female, in the absence of a male,

but it is now known that a parasitic male exists, shorter and broader than the female. The oesophagus is characteristic, with a club-shaped anterior part and a postcentral constriction and a posterior bulb (Figure III.71). Later, two copulatory spicules and a gubernaculum are said to become apparent and when developed, the adult male resembles the free-living form (Figure III.72,3). Parasitic males are found in experimentally infected dogs but not in human infections owing to the fact that they do not invade the intestinal wall and so are eliminated from the intestine soon after the females begin to oviposit. Although adolescent parasitic females may be inseminated, probably the majority are

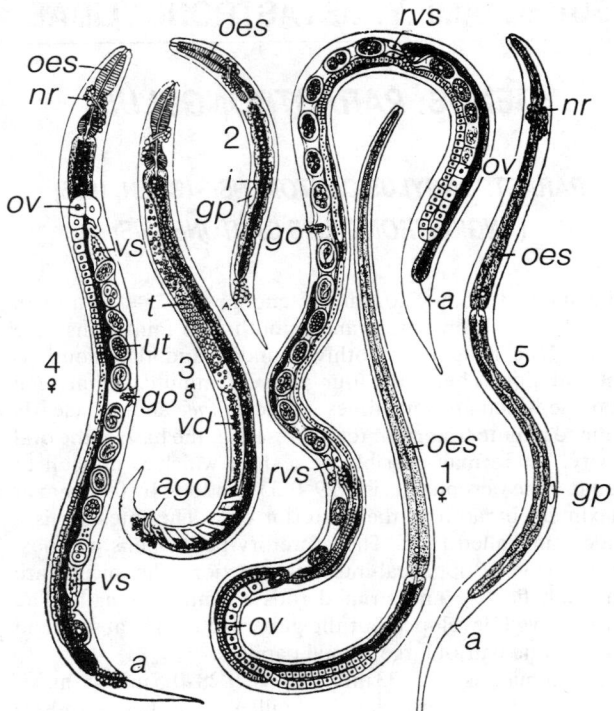

Figure III.72   Life history of *Strongyloides stercoralis*. 1, Parasitic female. 2, Rhabditiform larva. 3, Fully grown male. 4, Fully grown female. 5, Fully developed filariform larva. (30×.) (After Looss.)

a	anus	oes	oesophagus
ago	combined anus and genital pore	ov	ovary
		rvs	rudimentary vesicula seminalis
go	genital opening		
gp	primitive genital organs	t	testes
		ut	uterus
i	intestine	vd	vas deferens
nr	nerve ring	vs	vesicula seminalis

parthenogenetic. This is a process of *reversive metamorphosis*, in which it loses the ability of penetrating tissues and remains a lumen parasite.

The female (2.5 × 0.034 mm) (Figure III.72,4) tapers anteriorly and ends in a conical tail. The mouth has three small lips and leads to an oesophagus occupying a quarter of the length of the body. The vulva lies in the posterior third. There is a prominent uterus containing 50 eggs (50–58 × 30–34 μm) which are laid in the lumen of the bowel in an advanced stage of development and may occasionally be found in the faeces. They hatch immediately to embryos (0.2–0.3 × 0.013 mm), which have a double-bulb oesophagus, apt to be confused with the rhabditiform stage of *Ancylostoma* and *Necator* (Figure III.66b and c). They are passed active in faeces and in 3–5 days are converted into free-living male and female forms, both of which have a rhabditiform, double-bulb muscular oesophagus (Figure III.72,2). The male is a free-living form (0.7 × 0.035 mm) (Figure III.73) with the tail curved ventrally, two spicules and

an accessory piece. The free-living form of the female measures 1 × 0.05 mm. The vulva lies behind the middle of the body. The uterus contains thin-shelled eggs, measuring 70 × 40 μm (Figure III.72,4).

Copulation between the sexes takes place in faeces. The rhabditoid larvae produced are indistinguishable from those derived from the parasitic female. After 3 or 4 days they develop into host-feeding, mature filariform larvae, which are the infective stage, and re-enter the definitive host via the skin or buccal mucosa, as in *Ancylostoma* or *Necator*, but remain alive in the soil for many weeks. The distinguishing feature is that the oesophagus in filariform larvae is half the length of the body (Figure III.72,5); in *Ancylostoma* and *Necator* it occupies about a quarter. Filariform larvae find their way into the small intestine and develop into female parasitic forms. Under unsuitable climatic conditions the sexual phase in the faeces may be omitted and rhabditiform embryos produced by the parasitic female may develop directly into filariform larvae capable of infecting the defini-

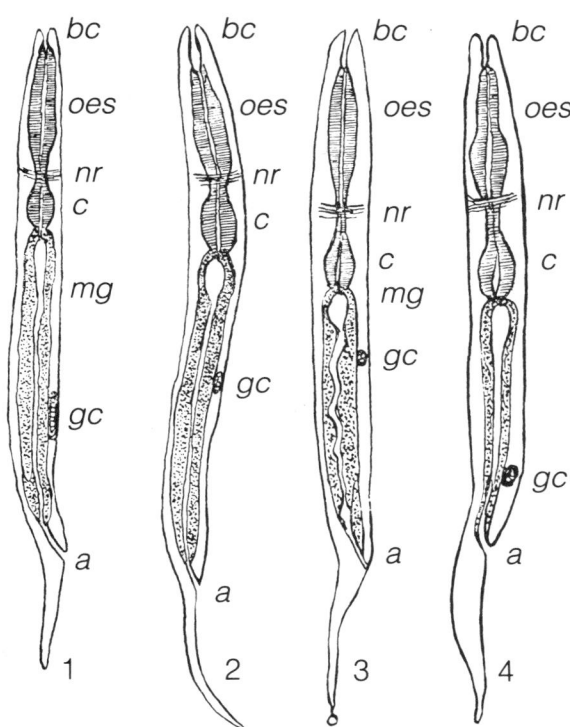

Figure III.73 Distinguishing features of nematode larvae in the faeces. 1, *Strongyloides stercoralis*. 2, *Ancylostoma duodenale*. 3, *Trichostrongylus colubriformis*. 4, *Rhabditis hominis*.

a anus	bc buccal cavity	c cardiac oesophageal bulb	cg genital cells
mg midgut	nr nerve ring	oes oesophagus	

Characters	*Strongyloides*	*Ancylostoma*	*Trichostrongylus*	*Rhabditis*
Average size	225 × 16 μm	275 × 17 μm	275 × 15 μm	240 × 12 μm
Posterior tip	Blunt	Sharp	Sharp with bead-like swelling	Sharp
Buccal chamber	Shorter than width at tip of head	Longer than width at tip of head	Longer than width at tip of head	Longer than width at tip of head
Genital primordia	Fairly large	Small	Very small	Very small

tive host (Figure III.72,5). The larvae of *S. stercoralis* may be confused with those of *Rhabditis hominis*, a free-living worm which may gain entry by accident to the digestive tract of man. These larvae measure 240–360 µm in length × 12 µm in diameter and resemble the parent worm in shape and structure of the oesophagus and filariform larvae of *Ancylostoma duodenale*. The distinguishing features are given in Figure III.73.

LIFE CYCLE

There are two stages: parasitic and free-living in soil.

Parasitic stage

1. *Filariform* (infective) larvae from infective soil penetrate exposed skin or the mouth.
2. They may travel to the lungs via the intestine and copulate as male and female. Filariform larvae enter man by penetrating the skin or through the mouth, and migrate through the lungs to the oesophagus; on arrival in the pulmonary capillaries the larvae produce haemorrhages which form the avenue of escape into the alveoli; followed by cellular infiltration into the respiration passages with output of eosinophil cells. The changes result in *Strongyloides* pneumonitis. These develop in 2 weeks.
3. Females, with or without males, enter the mucosa (especially of the duodenum) and lay eggs.
4. Eggs hatch and larvae escape into the intestine. They may either (a) pass down and be evacuated or (b) become filariform larvae (infective) and re-enter the mucosa or perianal skin (autoinfection) and pass to the organs (e.g. lungs).

Free-living stage

Larvae from faeces in soil are either rhabditoid or filariform (infective). Rhabditoid larvae can either become filariform and invade exposed skin or become male and female and produce rhabditoid larvae which continue the cycle indefintely.

STRONGYLOIDES FÜLLEBORNI (VON LINSTOW, 1905)

S. fülleborni is a common parasite of monkeys and apes widely spread in human populations in tropical Africa, common in the rain forest and sporadic in the savanna, and a similar form is found in Papua New Guinea. It may be identified by prominent vulvar lips and narrowing behind the vulva in the free-living females. The prominent oesophagus in the free-living stages is also characteristic. The eggs are passed in the stools, in contrast to *S. stercoralis*, and resemble hookworm ova, for which they are commonly mistaken.

SUPERFAMILY: OXYUROIDEA

GENUS: *ENTEROBIUS*

ENTEROBIUS VERMICULARIS (LINNAEUS, 1758) (THREADWORM OR PINWORM, *OXYURIS VERMICULARIS*)

This is the only nematode of man with a double-bulb oesophagus in the adult. It is small and white, its mouth surrounded by a cuticular expansion, and its skin transversely striated. The male is seldom seen and does not migrate like the female. Much smaller than the female (2.5 mm), its posterior third is curved spirally and its caudal extremity blunt, with six sensory papillae and a single spicule, 70 µm (Figure III.74B,C). The female (9–12 mm) has a long pointed tail, the anus 2 mm from the posterior extremity, and a transverse, slit-like vulva in the anterior fourth of the body (Figure III.74A). The gravid female lays eggs in a stream of 10 000–15 000 in a few minutes and dies when egg-laying is completed.

The egg (50–54 × 20–27 µm) (Figure III.5) has a characteristic shape, flattened on one side, and is almost colourless, with a bean-shaped double-contour shell, which contains a more or less fully formed embryo.

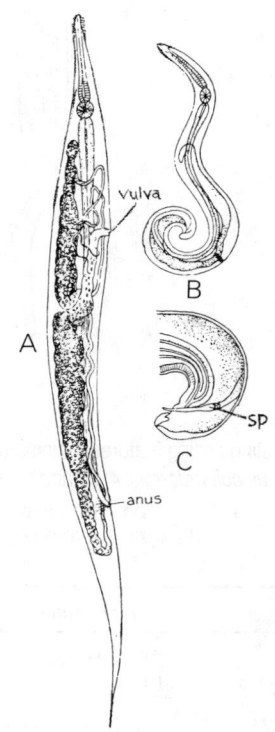

Figure III.74 Enterobius vermicularis. A, Female. B, Male, C, Caudal extremity of male. (12×.)

LIFE CYCLE (Figure III.75)

There is no multiplication of worms inside the body. The egg-shell is weakened by the digestive juices and the larva breaks out of the shell. Soon afterwards it invades the glandular crypts and penetrates into the glands and stroma, where it coils up, causing some liquefaction of the tissues, but no cellular reaction.

The life span of *E. vermicularis* ranges from 37 to 93 days. As soon as the ovary becomes packed with eggs the female worm loosens her hold on the intestinal wall and lies passive in the faecal stream. The fertilized female migrates out of the anus to deposit her eggs in the perianal skin and perineum.

The crawling of the gravid females produces intense pruritus. After a few hours the embryo develops rapidly and attains a length of 140–150 μm. The egg is ingested, generally as a result of deposits of faeces under the fingernails, conveyed to the mouth, and hatches in the digestive juices. Liberated larvae after two moults pass from the small into the large intestine, where they become mature. The whole cycle takes 2–4 weeks. Eggs can be inhaled through the nose from infected garments at some distance, and embryonated eggs have been found in dust. Damp conditions with minimal ventilation are necessary for survival. The eggs require a 6-hour exposure to air before they can hatch.

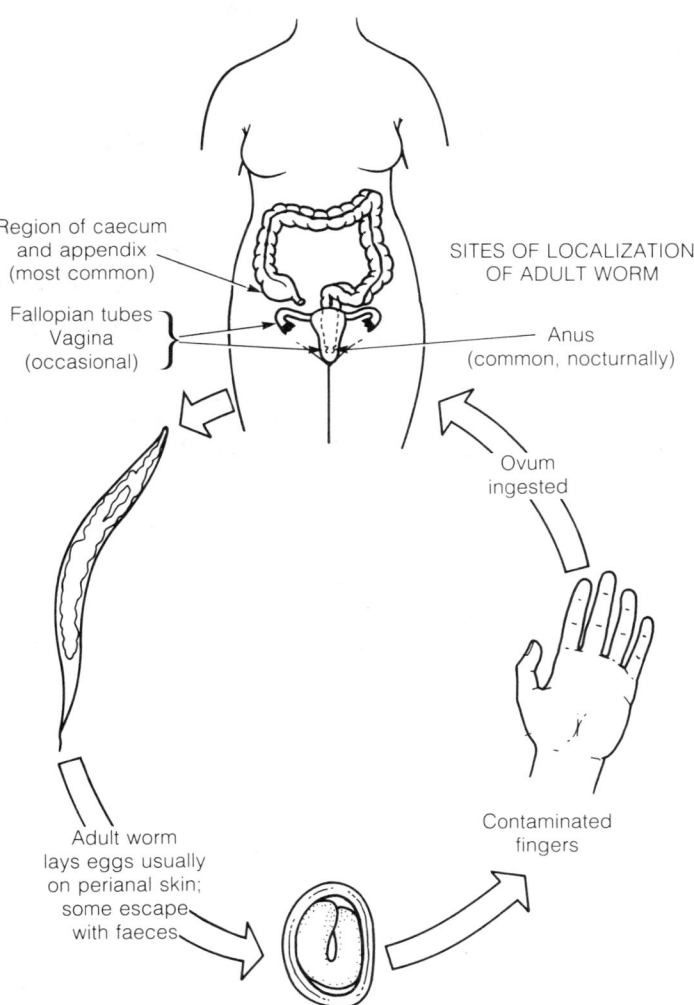

Enterobius (oxyuris) vermicularis
(Pinworm)

Region of caecum and appendix (most common)

Fallopian tubes
Vagina
(occasional)

SITES OF LOCALIZATION OF ADULT WORM

Anus (common, nocturnally)

Ovum ingested

Contaminated fingers

Adult worm lays eggs usually on perianal skin; some escape with faeces

Figure III.75 Life cycle of *Enterobius vermicularis*.

SUPERFAMILY: TRICHINELLOIDEA

GENUS: *TRICHURIS*

TRICHURIS TRICHIURA (LINNAEUS, 1771)
(*TRICHOCEPHALUS DISPAR*, WHIPWORM)

The male (30–45 mm) (Figure III.76,1) has an anterior attenuated portion, containing the cellular oesophagus, which is half as long again as the thicker posterior portion. The caudal extremity is curved ventrally through 360° and there is a single spicule in the sheath, studded with spines (Figure III.76,3).

The female (30–35 mm) (Figure III.76,2) has an anterior attenuated portion, twice as long as the posterior half, which is occupied by a stout uterus, tightly packed with eggs. A sacculate tubular ovary runs forward from the posterior end for over half the thick part of the body. Females preponderate over males in a proportion of over 400 to 1.

The egg (50 × 22 μm) is brown and has a characteristic barrel shape and a single shell with a plug at each end. It contains an unsegmented embryo (Figure III.5).

The worm is greyish-white or slightly pink and lives in the caecum where it maintains its position by transfixing a superficial fold of mucuous membrane with its slender neck, and lying embedded in mucus between the intestinal villi.

LIFE CYCLE (Figure III.77)

Infection is spread chiefly by stale faeces. The egg is unsegmented; embryonation takes at least 21 days. It can withstand a low temperature owing to its thick shell. Moisture is necessary and it cannot withstand desication. Development is direct. The embryo hatches only when the egg is swallowed: the eggshell is digested by the digestive juices, the larva emerges in the small intestine, penetrates the villi where it develops for a week and re-enters the lumen. It then passes to the caecum or colorectum, where it attaches itself to the mucosa and becomes adult.

Trichuris suis of the pig, whose eggs are indistinguishable from those of *T. trichiura*, has been transmitted to man in an experiment in which 1000 infective eggs were swallowed. The volunteer had no symptoms, but eggs appeared in the faeces in about 60 days and continued to be excreted for at least 10 weeks after maturation. *T. suis* may therefore be a cause of trichuriasis in man, especially if in contact with pigs.[10]

GENUS: *CALODIUM*

CALODIUM HEPATICUM (BANCROFT, 1893)
(*CAPILLARIA HEPATICA*, *TRICHOCEPHALUS HEPATICUS*, *HEPATICOLA HEPATICA*)

Calodium hepaticum is a parasite of the liver of the rat. The adult worms are very similar to *Trichuris*; the female measures 2 mm × 10 mm, the male being half as long. The eggs resemble those of *T. trichiura* but have an outer shell distinctly pitted and measuring 51–67.5 × 30–35 μm. It has a direct life cycle like that of *Trichuris*.

GENUS: *AONCHOTHECA*

AONCHOTHECA PHILIPPINENSIS (CHITWOOD, VELASQUEZ & SALAZAR, 1968)
(*CAPILLARIA PHILIPPINENSIS*)

The adult worms resemble *C. hepatica*. The male worm measures 2.1–3.7 mm in length and the female worm 2.6–4.9 mm. The eggs measure 45 × 21 μm and are of two types: one typical bioperculate, with a thick shell resembling a

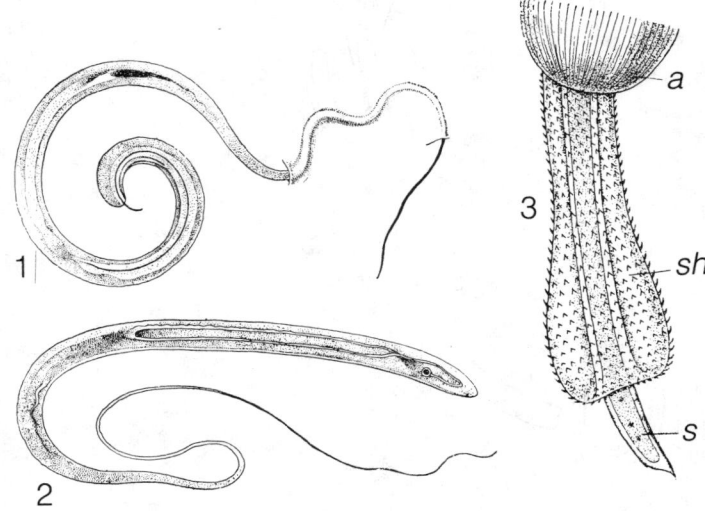

Figure III.76   *Trichuris trichiura*. 1, Male partly embedded in the mucous membrane of the intestine. 2, Female. 3, Copulatory apparatus, greatly magnified. (3×). a, Posterior extremity of body; s, spicule; sh, sheath.

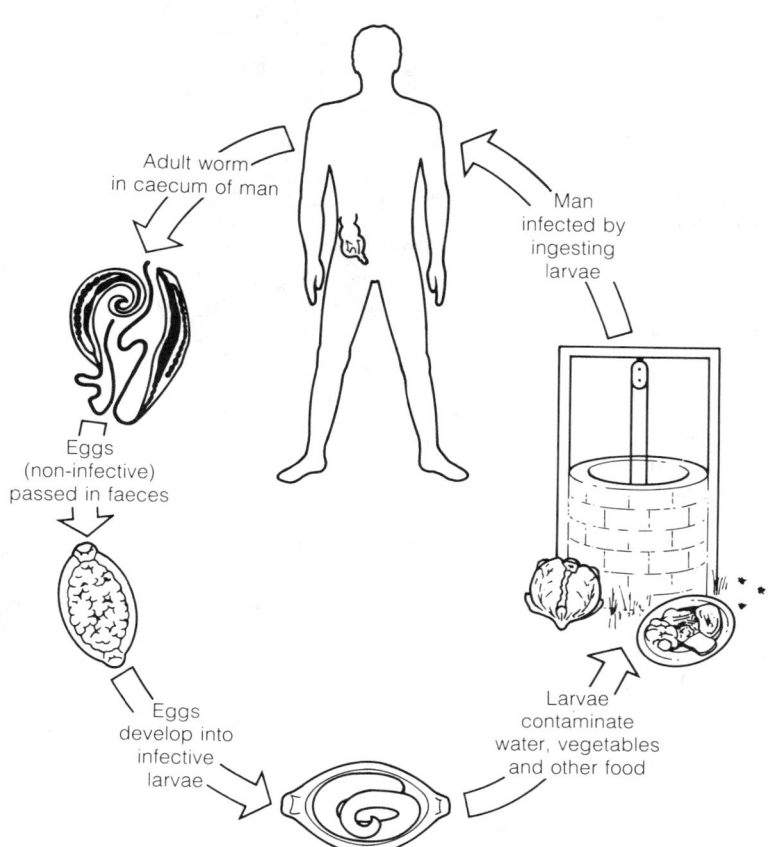

Trichuris trichiura
(Whipworm)

Figure III.77   Life cycle of *Trichuris trichiura*.

Adult worm
in caecum of man

Man
infected by
ingesting
larvae

Eggs
(non-infective)
passed in faeces

Eggs
develop into
infective
larvae

Larvae
contaminate
water, vegetables
and other food

Trichuris ovum which is passed out in the stool unembryonated, and the other atypical, with a thin shell and embryonated resembling a *Strongyloides* ovum.

LIFE CYCLE

The typical eggs pass out in the stool where they are taken up by an intermediate host (small fish) in which they hatch and localize in the mucosa of the small intestine. The atypical eggs hatch in the host's intestine and the larvae reinvade the intestine giving rise to intestinal autoinfection.

GENUS: *TRICHINELLA*

TRICHINELLA SPIRALIS (OWEN, 1835)

Trichinella spiralis (Figure III.78) is a white worm, just visible to the naked eye, which inhabits the small intestine.

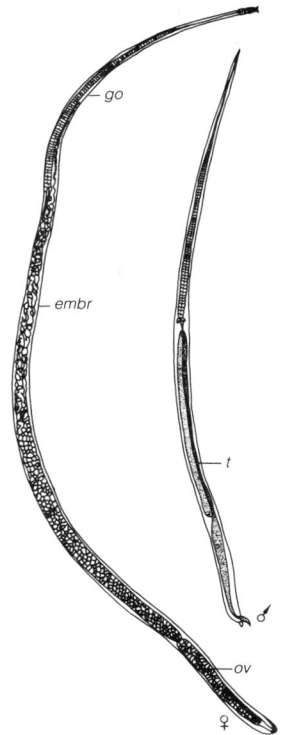

Figure III.78   Female and male *Trichinella spiralis*. (45×.)

embr	embryos	ov	ovary
go	genital opening	t	testes

The male (1.6 × 0.04 mm) has a cloaca situated posteriorly between two caudal appendages and two pairs of papillae. The female (3–4 × 0.06 mm) has a vulva in the anterior fifth, an ovary in the posterior half and an anterior portion occupied by a coiled uterine tube. The anus is terminal. Normally the female lives for 30 days and produces 1500 or more larvae which measure 100 × 6 μm.

LIFE CYCLE (Figure III.79)

The egg (20 μm in diameter) lies in the upper uterus but the embryo soon breaks out from the shell and lives free in the uterine cavity.

The larvae are shed mainly into the lymphatics and bloodstream, reaching all parts of the body and encysting.

The cyst (Figure III.80) is formed by a larva encapsulated by the host tissues. The capsule is an adventitious ellipsoidal sheath with blunt ends which results from round cell and eosinophilic infiltration round the tightly coiled larva. The long axis parallels that of the muscle fibres. Host amino acids can be transferred into the cyst and converted into larval protein so that an encysted larva remains viable for many years.

When consumed by a carnivorous host the cysts are digested in the stomach and, after excysting, the larvae invade the duodenal and jejunal mucosa and develop through four ecdyses into adult males and females, which then enter the lumen of the bowel. Later they re-enter the mucosa and penetrate the villi, even reaching the mesenteric glands. Larviposition takes place over a period of from 4 to 16 weeks or more. The larvae are carried through the right heart and lungs to the arterial circulation which they reach between the

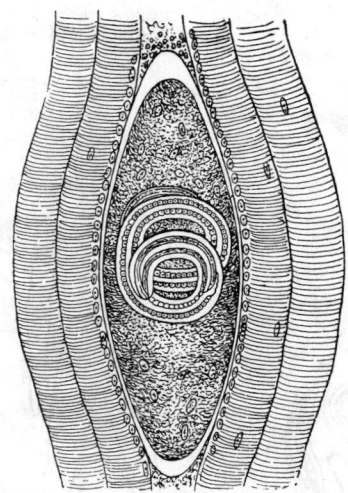

Figure III.80　Encysted larva of *Trichinella spiralis* 15 days after entering muscle. (300×.)

ninth and thirteenth day, finally reaching the striated muscles where they encyst.

There are three biological types (now often considered distinct species) of *Trichinella spiralis*, distinguished by geography and ecology.

1. *T. s. spiralis*: cosmopolitan; involving wild and domestic pigs and predators—domestic dog, cat, also bear and racoon.

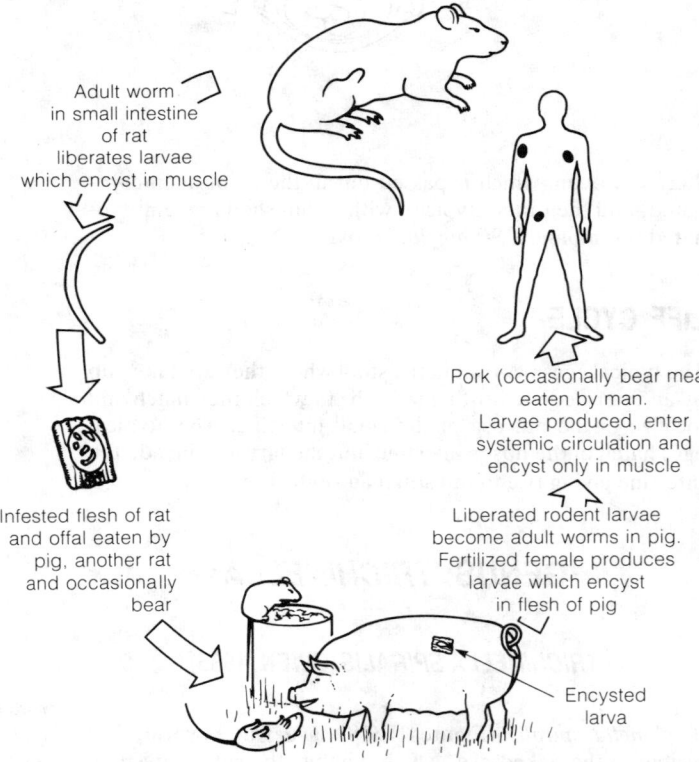

Adult worm
in small intestine
of rat
liberates larvae
which encyst in muscle

Infested flesh of rat
and offal eaten by
pig, another rat
and occasionally
bear

Pork (occasionally bear meat)
eaten by man.
Larvae produced, enter
systemic circulation and
encyst only in muscle

Liberated rodent larvae
become adult worms in pig.
Fertilized female produces
larvae which encyst
in flesh of pig

Encysted
larva

Figure III.79　Life cycle of *Trichinella spiralis*.

2. *T. S. nelsoni*: Europe and Africa; involving pig, bush-pig, wart-hog and predators—dog, fox, wolf, hyena, leopard, lion.

3. *T. s. nativa*: Arctic and subarctic America; probably involving fish and predators—walrus, seal, polar bear, fox.

SUPERFAMILY: FILARIOIDEA

This group includes spirurate filiform nematodes adapted to inhabit the deeper tissues, such as the circulatory, lymphatic and connective tissue layers. Some insect intermediary is necessary to complete their development.

GENUS: *WUCHERERIA*

WUCHERERIA BANCROFTI (COBBOLD, 1877; SEURAT, 1921) (*FILARIA BANCROFTI*)

PARASITOLOGY

Adult filaria

It is a thread-like white worm found in lymphatic vessels and glands. The sexes are coiled together and can be separated with difficulty. The cuticle is adorned with small cuticular bosses.

The male (4 mm × 0.1 mm) is coiled with a corkscrew-like tail and two spicules, the larger of which measures 500 μm. The smaller (300 μm) is grooved on its ventral aspect. There is a short, thick proximal and a whip-like distal portion, ending in a hook, and 15 pairs of minute sensory caudal papillae (Figure III.81a,b). A saddle-shaped thickening of the cuticle on the posterior wall of the cloaca forms a shield, and there is an accessory piece peculiar to *W. bancrofti*. There are 12 pairs of circumanal papillae of which eight are preanal and four postanal in position. There are also two pairs of large sessile papillae and at the tail a solitary pair of minute size. The female (6.5 cm × 0.2–2.8 mm) has a taper-ing anterior end with a rounded swelling (Figure III.82).

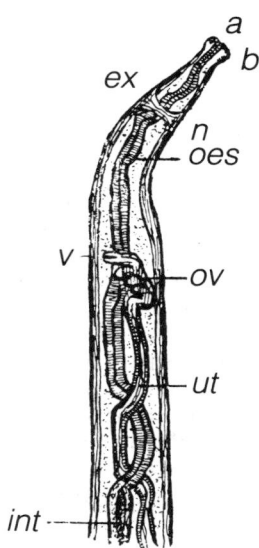

Figure III.82 The head of *Wuchereria bancrofti*, female. (50×.)

a	mouth	oes	oesophagus
b	circumoral papillae	ov	oviduct
ex	excretory pore	ut	uterus
int	intestine	v	vulva
n	nerve ring		

There are sessile papillae on the head and an oral aperture leading to a cylindrical oesophagus. The mid-intestinal tube is one-third to one-fifth of the total diameter and opens into the rectum posteriorly. The caudal extremity is narrow and abruptly rounded (Figure III.81c). The vulva is 0.8 mm behind the anterior extremity. A swollen vagina (0.25 mm in length) leads into the uterus which divides into two tubuli, which are much coiled, occupying the greater portion of the body with a diameter three times that of the mid-intestine (Figure III.82). Two ovaries and ducts extend to within 1 mm of the tail.

The eggs lie in the upper uterus enclosed in a chorionic membrane which becomes a sheath to the living embryos (microfilariae) (Figure III.83). They are emitted by the viviparous female and travel via the lymphatics into the bloodstream, whence they are abstracted by various species of mosquito. Their size in the distal part of the uterus is 38 × 25 μm, but as they are pushed to the vagina they become more elongated. The microfilaria develops from an oval egg

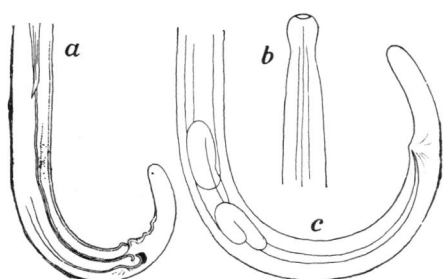

Figure III.81 *Wuchereria bancrofti*. Magnified. (a) Tail of male. (b) Head and neck. (c) Tail of female.

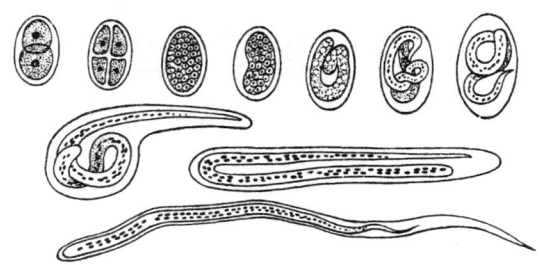

Figure III.83 Evolution of sheathed microfilaria from the ovum in the uterus of the parent worm. The later stages may occasionally take place after emission from the vagina.

and measures at first 216 μm. The embryo often lies curled up in its shell which becomes lobed, resembling a Dutch twist or pretzel.

Microfilaria

The microfilaria (280 × 7 μm) (Figures III.84, III.85 and III.93) in the living state appears structureless. With higher magnification the entire microfilaria is seen to be enclosed in a sheath which is longer than the enclosed microfilaria and stains pale mauve with Giemsa, in contrast to microfilaria of *Loa loa*, the sheath of which does not stain with Giemsa. In this sheath it can move backwards and forwards and the collapsed portion trails after the head or tail. The sheath has been the subject of controversy. It is generally held to be the outstretched vitelline membrane but in the microfilariae of *Litomosoides carinii* of the cotton rat it has been found that a true larval sheath is developed during its sojourn in the blood. In the middle third is some granular material or primitive gut (*Innenkörper*). There is transverse striation of the muscular layer throughout. At one-seventh of the length from the head there is a break which denotes the nerve ring (nr) and at one-fifth of the length there is a triangular V-shaped patch, demonstrated by light staining with dilute haematoxylin, known as 'anterior V-spot', or the excretory pore and excretory cell (ep and ec). A short distance from the tail a second pore represents the anus, cloaca or terminal part of the primitive alimentary canal and is known as the 'posterior V-spot'. Deeply staining cells are known as genital cells (g¹–g⁴) (Figure III.85). When stained, the body of the embryo is seen to be composed of closely packed cells and, by focusing when the movements of the living microfilaria have subsided, the head appears to be covered by a delicate prepuce. A short fang is from time to time shot out from the uncovered cephalic end and suddenly retracted.

Microfilariae pass with difficulty through the peripheral capillaries and they are less active in day than in night blood. They are capable of movement and of transit from place to place.

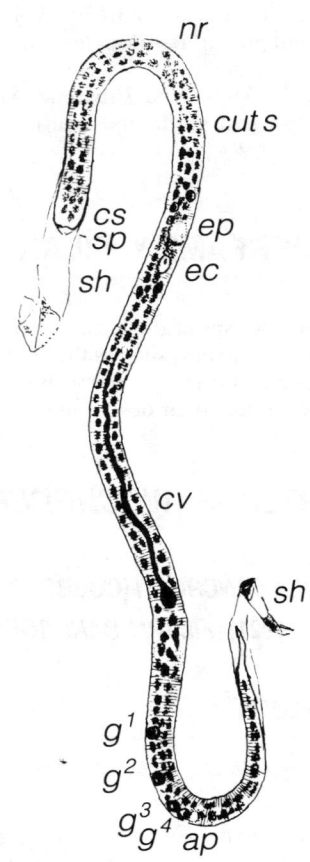

Figure III.85   Morphology of microfilaria of *Wuchereria bancrofti*.

ap	anal pore	g¹–g⁴	'genital cells' of
cs	cephalic space		Rodenwaldt
cuts	cuticular striations	nr	nerve ring
cv	central viscus	sh	sheath
ec	excretory cell	sp	spicule and prepuce
ep	excretory pore		

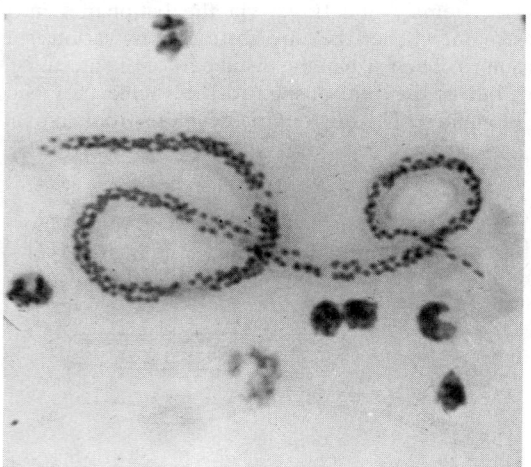

Figure III.84 Sheathed microfilaria of *Wuchereria bancrofti* in a blood film. (Courtesy of W. O'Connor.)

PERIODICITY (Figure III.86)

Microfilariae of *W. bancrofti* exhibit a nocturnal periodicity in certain parts of the world—in the West Indies, South America, North, West and East Africa, China, Indonesia, Papua New Guinea and Melanesia, i.e. they are present in peripheral blood in larger numbers during the night than during the day. The maximum concentration is from 22.00 to 02.00 hours. It occurred to Manson that this nocturnal periodicity was an adaptation to the habits of night-biting mosquitoes—*Culex quinquefasciatus*, *C. pipiens* and certain Anophelines. The numbers of the microfilariae are influenced by sleeping and respond to waking and bodily activity. By reversing the hours of sleeping and waking the periodicity is disturbed for 3 days and then reversed to diurnal periodicity. Periodicity can be easily converted by a change in the rhythm of day and night and was found in emigrants from Okinawa (127° 40'E, 28° 30'N) to Bolivia (63° 30'W, 17° 50'S) to take 116 days.[11] Observations on microfilariae of animals (*Dirofilaria repens* of dog, filaria of

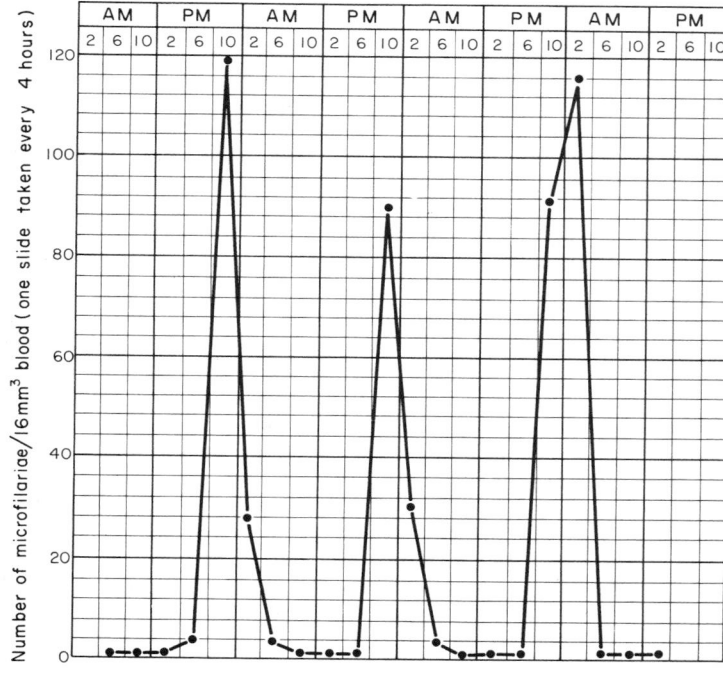

Figure III.86 Filariasis due to *Wuchereria bancrofti*, showing nocturnal periodicity.

American crow and that of Malayan monkey, *Macaca speciosa*) show that they also maintain nocturnal periodicity and reversal is easily established. Periodicity is probably a quality inherent in the microfilaria itself and persists unchanged in transfused blood. This was demonstrated in a patient injected with blood containing microfilariae and in whom a nocturnal periodicity was maintained for 14 days.

In 1897, Manson had an opportunity of ascertaining that during their diurnal absence from the peripheral circulation the microfilariae retire principally to the larger arteries and to the lungs where, during the daytime, they may be found in enormous numbers. Two mechanisms for periodicity have been suggested: alteration in oxygen tension of the blood and phototaxis on the part of the microfilariae.

Considerable light has been shed upon the mechanism of periodicity in general by the discovery of a non-sheathed microfilaria in a monkey (*Macaca speciosa*). In animal, as in man, the curve of microfilarial density in the venous blood follows closely that of the capillary blood. An increase of microfilariae in the blood at night is due to the periodic liberation from accumulations in the small blood vessels of the lungs.

McFadzean and Hawking[12] proved that the microfilariae of *W. bancrofti* are affected by the oxygen concentration in inspired air and by muscular exercise. The periodicity of *W. bancrofti* and *Brugia malayi* may depend on changes in the difference of oxygen tension between venous and arterial blood by day and night. During the daytime the microfilariae accumulate in the lungs where the oxygen tension is high. They manage to hold themselves in the pulmonary capillaries by some force which is increased by the rise in the oxygen tension and decreased by its fall. This force seems to be switched on and off every 12 hours by an unknown mechanism inside the microfilariae.[13] A curious agglutinative phenomenon has been described on the injection of anti-

coagulant (heparin) to the drawn blood. Intravenous injection of this substance during daytime releases microfilariae of *W. bancrofti* into the peripheral blood for a short period. It is presumed that microfilariae gather together in the capillaries and other vessels of the lung during their absence from the peripheral blood by the power of agglutination and thigmotaxis. A different mechanism for periodicity has been suggested,[11] in which the microfilariae possess a photosensitive substance containing a vitamin-A-like carotenoid, similar to visual pigments in fluorescent granules in the epidermis, which causes them to leave the peripheral circulation in daylight and collect in the lungs. Periodic microfilariae possess numerous granules, in contrast to subperiodic and aperiodic forms which have few or none.

A general anaesthetic does not affect the periodicity of *W. bancrofti* but markedly reduces the numbers of *L. loa* microfilariae in the peripheral blood.[13]

Formerly it was thought that nocturnal periodicity was uniformly observed by the microfilariae of *W. bancrofti* the world over but in 1896 it was demonstrated that in Tonga and Fiji the microfilariae were abundant in the blood both by day and by night; those in the western Pacific, the Solomon Islands, Papua New Guinea and Bismarck Archipelago are nocturnally periodic but in New Caledonia the microfilariae are non-periodic. The demarcating line between the two (Buxton's line) lies in longitude 170°E and this also coincides with the distribution of malaria. On the west of this line there are *Anopheles* and malaria, on the east there is neither. It was originally demonstrated that in Indian and Solomon Island immigrants in Fiji these microfilariae maintain their nocturnal periodicity amongst the non-periodic Fijians but, if they and the Europeans also contract the infection in Fiji, the microfilariae are non-periodic. An attempt was made to explain this anomaly by the day-biting habits of the mosquito intermediaries, *Aedes scutellans pseudoscutellaris* and *Ae. s.*

polynesiensis, which have a regional distribution in the Pacific corresponding to that of the non-periodic filariae. As the microfilariae remain true to type after transfusion it was suggested that they are the progeny of a parent distinct from *W. bancrofti*: this has been named *W. bancrofti* var. *pacifica*. The microfilariae of both varieties are morphologically indistinguishable. The non-periodic Pacific type in Fiji differs from that of periodic African *W. bancrofti* in that increased oxygen content of the blood brings about a *slight rise* of the microfilarial counts.

Periodicity is a biological rhythm inherent in the microfilariae but influenced by the rhythm of the host, which itself is influenced by the changes in body temperature which occur every 24 hours.

The two forms of *B. malayi* from Malaysia exhibit different periodicities which correspond with the biting habits of their chief vectors. Therefore attempts have been made to see whether it is possible to change periodicity by feeding mosquitoes by day on a nocturnal periodic infection and transmitting the few filarial larvae which develop in them to experimental animals. Thus when a human infection was transmitted to a cat it was found that the nocturnally periodic microfilariae became semiperiodic. By altering the feeding time and selective breeding of mosquitoes, successive transmission experiments have shown that it is possible to change the periodicity of the mosquito–filarial complex in a relatively small number of generations.

LIFE CYCLE (Figure III.87)

The life cycle was first worked out by Manson in *Culex quinquefasciatus* in China in 1878. Within 1 hour of entering the mosquito's stomach the microfilariae cast the sheaths and bore through the stomach wall. At this stage the microfilariae may be damaged by the buccopharyngeal armature of the mosquito which may explain the differing infection rates of these vectors.[14] At the end of an infective feed the embryos collect at the anterior end of the stomach and then enter the anterior cylindrical portion of the midgut. Forward transportation is effected by reversed peristalsis until they are distributed over the whole of this cylinder. At the end of 16 hours they form a writhing mass behind the valve which prevents their progress into the foregut. The proboscis of the mosquito exerts positive chemotaxis upon microfilariae. Therefore vector female mosquitoes can abstract more embryos than would be present in a similar quantity of circulating blood. The mosquito abstracts 1 mm^3 of blood at each feed and, in so doing, concentrates the embryos tenfold. They next enter the thorax where they lie between the muscular fibres of the indirect or fibrillar flight muscle of the thorax and pharyngeal muscle of the head of the mosquito[15] (Figure III.88). Within 2 days they increase in girth, the 'posterior V-spot' (or anal pore) enlarges and the excretory vesicle becomes more prominent. By rapid nuclear proliferation the larval filaria now assumes a squat 'sausage' form, the tail shrinks and is then absorbed (Figure III.89). Mouth and oesophagus are apparent from the fifth day onwards. The g^2 and g^3 cells (Figure III.85) divide several times and give rise to a column of cells which form the mid-intestine (large gut). The posterior intestine (rectum) is formed from four cells derived from the g^4 cell. The genital primordium is formed from the g^1 cell.

When the larva is 0.5 mm in length a bulbar oesophagus appears at the first and second fourths of the alimentary canal. Now elongated and worm-like the larva moves sluggishly about. Three caudal papillae develop which function in progression and facilitate penetration of human skin (Figure III.90). About the tenth day (in favourable circumstances) the larval filaria, 1.4 mm long, travels forward into the head of the mosquito where it coils up and enters the proboscis sheath (Figure III.91), but occasionally it may penetrate into the abdominal cavity and legs. Two or more ecdyses take place. At high temperatures and in moisture the complete cycle occupies 10–14 days but it is retarded to 6 weeks by cold. Sometimes the larvae die in the thoracic muscles and

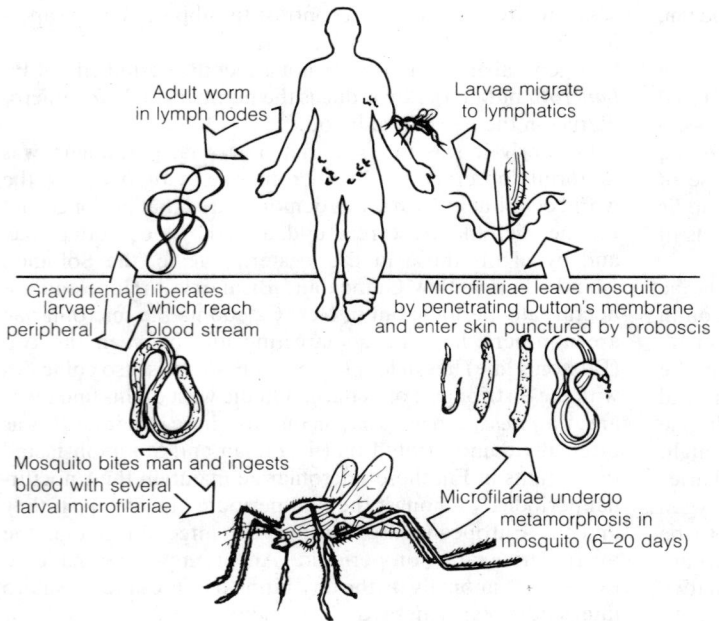

Adult worm in lymph nodes

Larvae migrate to lymphatics

Gravid female liberates larvae which reach peripheral blood stream

Microfilariae leave mosquito by penetrating Dutton's membrane and enter skin punctured by proboscis

Mosquito bites man and ingests blood with several larval microfilariae

Microfilariae undergo metamorphosis in mosquito (6–20 days)

Figure III.87 Life cycle of lymphatic filariasis (*Wuchereria bancrofti*).

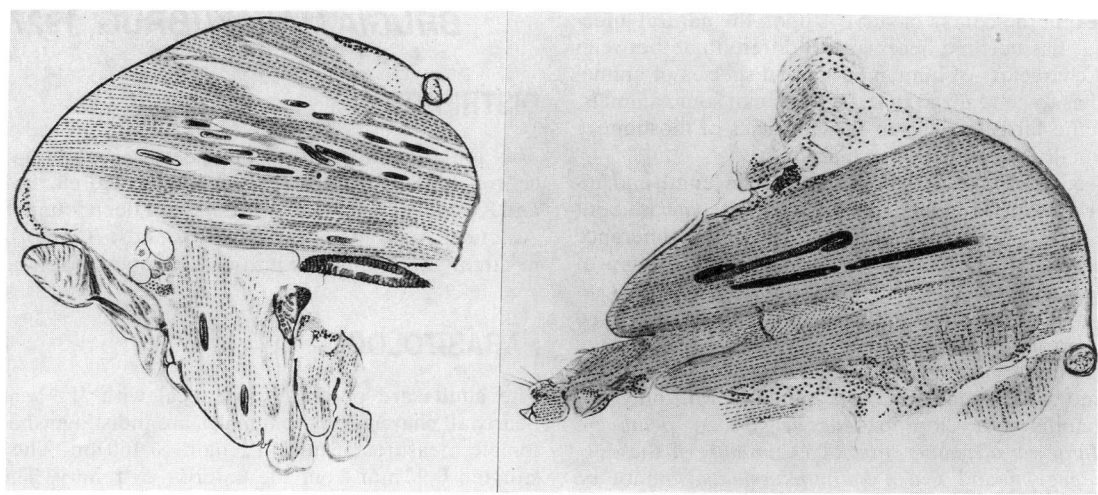

Figure III.88 Section of the thoracic muscles of *Aedes pseudoscutellaris*. Left, The second day after feeding on a filaraemic patient. Right, The second week after feeding on a filaraemic patient.

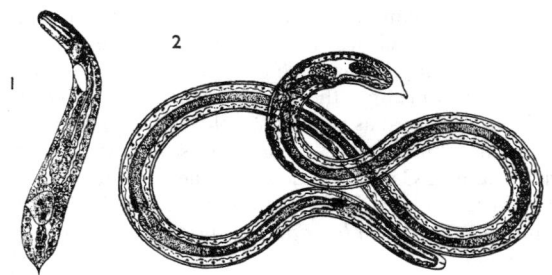

Figure III.89 Stages of the larval forms of *Wuchereria bancrofti* from the thoracic muscles of *Culex quinquefasciatus*. (150×.)

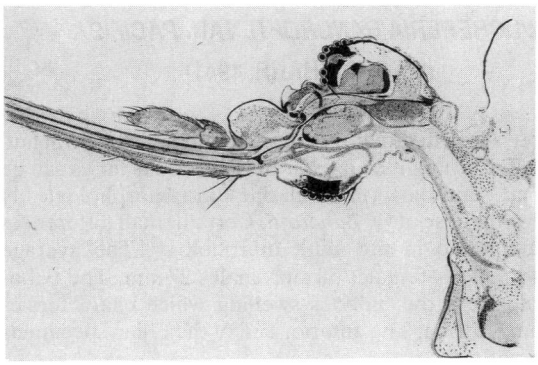

Figure III.91 *Wuchereria bancrofti* in the head and proboscis of the mosquito.

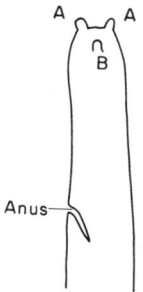

Figure III.90 Larval filaria from the proboscis sheath of *Aedes pseudoscutellaris*. A, Terminal papilla. B, Postanal papilla.

are enclosed in chitin, producing a curious mummy-like structure. When an infected mosquito bites man, the larvae, attracted by warmth, break through the terminal portion of the proboscis sheath in the ligula at the central point of 'Dutton's membrane', wriggle out on to the skin, which they penetrate near the seat of the puncture caused by the stylets of the mosquito. A list of vectors is given in Appendix IV.

In the human host the infective larvae pass through the peripheral blood vessels to the lymphatics where they become mature in an estimated period of 3 months to 1 year. Man is the only known definitive host.

In view of the fact that considerable confusion has been generated by the discovery of larval filariae in wild-caught mosquitoes, in the course of surveys upon the natural infection rate, it has become necessary to differentiate between the larval characters of human and allied species of animal origin. It has to be realized that the filariae of some animals, fruit bats and birds develop in those species of mosquitoes which normally transmit human filariasis.

The infective larva of *B. malayi* is 1–2 mm in length and has three poorly defined caudal papillae; that of *B. patei* is about the same length and has a marked dorsal protuberance resembling a dog's head, in lateral position. The larva of *Dirofilaria corynodes* of monkeys (*Cercopithecus* and *Colobus*) from *Aedes pembaensis* has the typical cigar-shaped tail but less pronounced narrowing between the anus and the extremity, with three small papillae. The larva of *D. repens* of the dog and cat resembles the foregoing but with only one terminal papilla: it develops in *Aedes aegypti*, *Ae. pembaensis* and *Mansonia africanus*; that of *D. immitis* of the dog, from *Ae. aegypti* and *Culex quinquefasciatus*, cannot be distinguished from that of *D. repens*. The larva of *Setaria equina* of the horse, mule and donkey in *Ae. aegypti*, *Ae. pembaensis* and *Culex quinquefasciatus* is about the same length but can easily be distinguished by one large terminal papilla and two subterminal ones, looking like little ears. Distinguishing features are illustrated in a key by Nelson.[16]

WUCHERERIA BANCROFTI, VAR. PACIFICA
(MANSON-BAHR, 1941)

It has been suggested that the filaria found in the central and southern Pacific might be a separate species. As far as can be ascertained, embryos (microfilariae) are morphologically identical with those of *W. bancrofti*. Certain small differences have been noted in the adult morphology. The average length is smaller—females 58 mm, males 27 mm. The tail of the female lacks the bulbous swelling which characterizes those from Guyana. The anterior end of the Fijian specimens is oval in outline.

Microfilariae in polynesians (Fiji, Samoa, Tonga, Cook Islands, New Caledonia) are non-periodic. In these islands as well as in Tokelau, Wallis, Ellice, Gilberts, Marquesas and those beyond 'Buxton's line' (longitude 170° east) they do not exhibit nocturnal periodicity but occur in equal numbers in the blood by day and night. Development of this filaria is confined to mosquitoes indigenous to the South Pacific islands of the *Aedes kochi*, *Ae. vigilax* and *Ae. scutellaris* groups which are adapted to coconut palms and bite by day (see Appendix IV). The non-periodic microfilaria does not develop readily in *C. quinquefasciatus* which is the optimum host for the nocturnally periodic *W. bancrofti*.

GENUS: *BRUGIA* (BUCKLEY, 1959)

The genus *Brugia* contains nine representatives: *B. malayi*, *B. pahangi*, *B. patei*, *B. beaveri*, *B. buckleyi*, *B. ceylonensis*, *B. guyanensis*, *B. tupiae* and *B. timori*.[17]

BRUGIA MALAYI (BRUG, 1927)

DISTRIBUTION

This is the common form in Malaysia, Indonesia, Timor, central India, Sri Lanka, south China, Korea, Indo-China and Koshima Island (Japan). It has not been found in Africa, America, Australia or the Pacific Islands. *B. timori* is found in Timor and islands in south-east Indonesia (Sunda group).

PARASITOLOGY

The adults are practically identical with *W. bancrofti* in nearly all characters; the females are indistinguishable. The female measures 55 mm in length × 160 μm. The vulva is situated 0.92 mm from the anterior extremity. The caudal end is bluntly rounded. The male is 22–23 mm in length by 88 μm in diameter. The posterior extremity has about three turns and the anus is 0.1–0.14 mm from the tip of the tail. One pair of large papillae are just in front of the cloaca and one behind. There are also two smaller pairs. There is a small naviculate gubernaculum and two spicules which are unlike in size and structure: the longer is 0.34–0.36 mm: the shorter 0.11–0.12 mm in length. There are morphological differences in the microfilariae and the mosquito intermediary is distinct—*Mansonia annulifera*. It is identical with the microfilaria of the 'kra' monkey (*Macaca irus*) which is transmitted by the same mosquitoes. It is common in domestic dogs and cats in Malaysia and has been found also in the slow loris (*Nycticebus coucang*), the banded leaf monkey (*Presbytis melalophos*) as well as in the pangolin (*Manis javanica*).

The microfilaria of *B. malayi* was first discovered by Lichtenstein in Celebes and was studied further by Brug in 1927. Brug and de Rook found natural infection in the mosquitoes *Mansonia longipalpis* (also known as *dives*) and *M. annulata*.

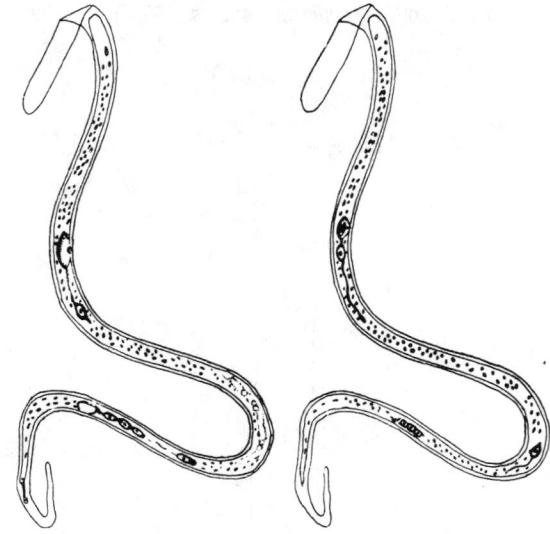

Figure III.92 Comparative morphology of the microfilariae of *Wuchereria bancrofti* (right) and *Brugia malayi* (left).

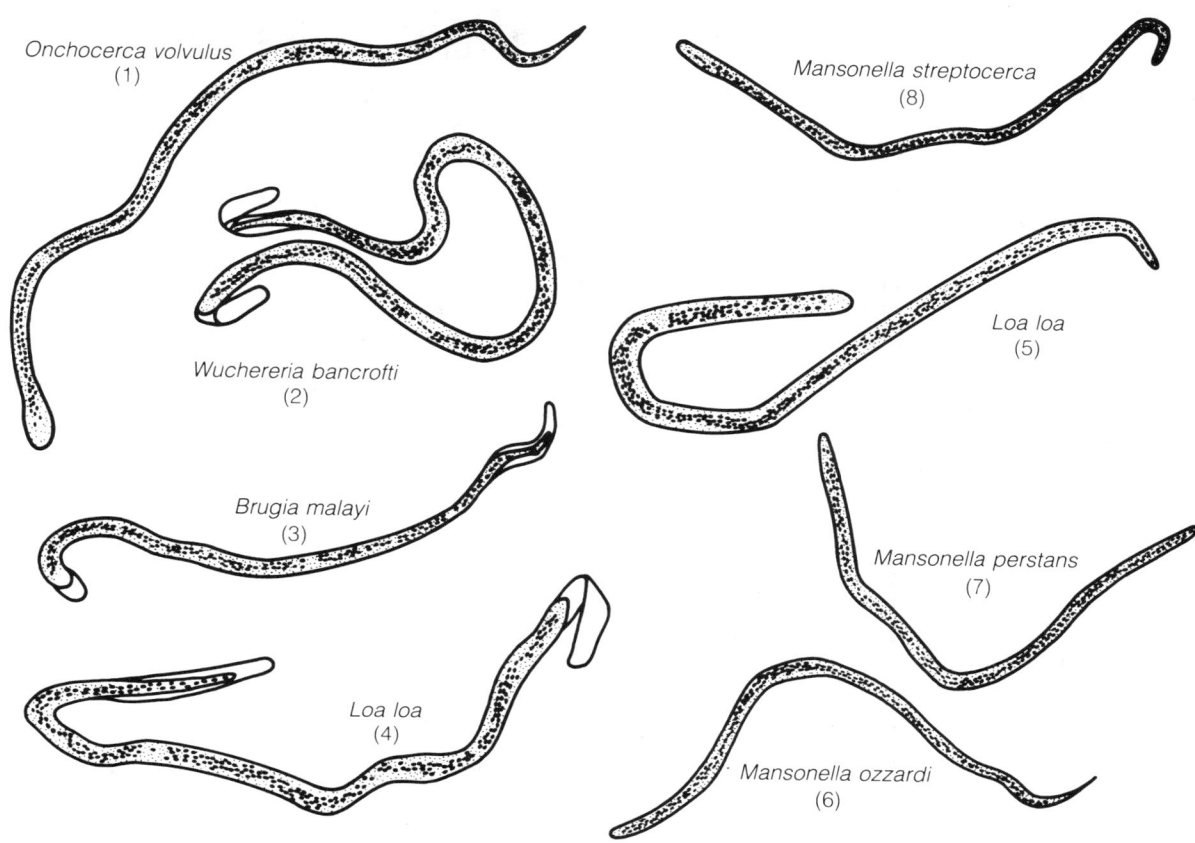

Figure III.93 Microfilariae of medical importance. (Courtesy of D. A. Denham.)

Key to microfilariae found in human blood

Method 1. After staining with Mayer's haemalum

1(a) Sheath present — *W. bancrofti*
 (b) Sheath absent — *Loa loa* (5)
2(a) Nuclei to tip of tail — *B. malayi*
 (a) Nuclei not in tip of tail — *W. bancrofti*

3(a) Two isolated nuclei in tail — *B. malayi*
 (b) Solid column of nuclei in tail — *Loa loa* (4)
4(a) Sheath loosely applied, worm over 250 μm long — *Loa loa* (4)
 (b) Sheath very small, worm under 250 μm long — *Meningonema peruzzi*
5(a) More than 275 μm in length — *M. ozzardi*
 (b) Less than 250 μm in length — *M. perstans*

6(a) Cephalic space longer than twice width of body — *O. volvulus*
 (b) Cephalic space about width of body — *W. bancrofti* (with no sheath)
7(a) Nuclei to tip of tail — *M. streptocerca*
 (b) Nuclei not to tip of tail — *M. ozzardi*
8(a) Tail straight with prominent terminal nucleus — *Dipetalonema perstans*
 (b) Tail bent into crook shape — *Dipetalonema streptocerca*

Method 2. After staining with Giemsa

1(a) Sheath present — *W. bancrofti*
 (b) Sheath absent — *B. malayi*
2(a) Sheath stained red, nuclei in tip of tail — *Brugia* spp.
 (b) Sheath stained pale mauve, no nuclei in tip of tail — *W. bancrofti*
3(a) Nuclei not extending to tip of tail — *Loa loa* (4)
 (b) Nuclei to tip of tail — *M. ozzardi*
4(a) Microfilariae about 300 μm long — *Loa loa* (5)
 (b) Microfilariae 200–225 μm long — *M. ozzardi*
5(a) Cephalic space more than 1½ times diameter of head — *O. volvulus*
 (b) Cephalic space less than or equal to diameter of head — *W. bancrofti* (with no sheath)
6(a) Microfilariae at least 260 μm long — *M. perstans*
 (b) Microfilariae 200–225 μm long — *M. streptocerca*
7(a) Tail with complete column of microfilariae — *Loa loa*
 (b) Tail with two isolated nuclei — *Brugia* (with no sheath)
8(a) Tail with prominent nucleus — *Dipetalonema perstans*
 (b) Tail with crook-shaped bend — *Dipetalonema streptocerca*

Notes 1 The sheath of *Loa loa* does not stain with Giemsa.
2 While *O. volvulus* is normally in the skin appreciable numbers can be detected in the blood.
3 *B. malayi* periodic strain usually loses its sheath in blood smears.
4 Any sheathed microfilaria may lose its sheath.
5 The part of the tail of *M. ozzardi* which is free of nuclei is very fine and may not stain but there is no terminal nucleus as in *D. perstans*.

Although the human form of *B. malayi* is common in dogs and cats in Malaysia and Indonesia, there is a species, *B. pahangi*, which is confined to these animals and which has distinctive morphological characters.

The human form of *B. malayi* can be transmitted to cats by the bite of *Mansonia longipalpis*, The period of full development of the adult filaria in this animal is about 65 days before microfilariae appear in the blood. The adult forms recovered from the cat correspond to the descriptions of *B. malayi* in man. *B. patei* microfilariae have been found in cats in Orissa, India, and in dogs and genet cats in Pate Island, Kenya. The nocturnal periodic form in Malaysia does not develop well in cats and is transmitted by species of *Anopheles* and *Mansonia*. A semiperiodic form occurs in man and commonly in cats, in freshwater swamps and forest. It is transmitted by *Mansonia annulata* and *M. uniformis*.

Microfilaria *B. malayi* has a nocturnal periodicity like that of *W. bancrofti* or may be semiperiodic . It is nocturnal on the west coast of the Malaysia peninsula but non-periodic in the Huantan district on the east coast. It measures 200–250 × 5–6 μm. Its chief points of distinction are the elongated nucleus at the top of the tail and the absence of nuclei in the cephalic space (Figures III.92 and III.93).

Table III.9 summarizes the main points of distinction between the microfilariae of *B. malayi* and *W. bancrofti* and Figure III.93 (with key) shows the differences in the microfilariae of medical importance.

LIFE CYCLE

The most favoured mosquito intermediaries belong to the genus *Mansonia* which are crepuscular or nocturnal feeders.

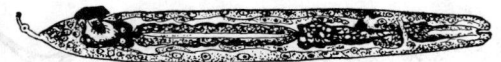

Figure III.94 Developmental stage of *Brugia malayi* showing the terminal nucleus in the tail.

Development in the mosquito is similar to that of *W. bancrofti* but more rapid, in 6–8½ days. Difficulties have been encountered in Malaysia in distinguishing larval forms of ornithofilariae of birds from those of human *B. malayi* in the routine dissection of mosquitoes.

The larval forms of *B. malayi* in *Mansonia* undergo two ecdyses. The buccal cavity is formed from the cephalic space; the oesophagus from the nuclei of the anterior part of the nuclear column; the rectum and anus from the four G cells of Rodenwaldt and the anal pore. The premature genital pore mass is derived from the nuclei of *Innenkörper* and the muscles of the body wall from the 'subcuticular cells' of Rodenwaldt. The tail of the microfilaria, with its two nuclei (terminal nucleus in the tail—Figure III.94), is shed with the first moult. As in the case of *W. bancrofti*, the larva, when in the thoracic muscles, feeds by absorbing food through the cuticle. It does not feed at the expense of these muscles as has been stated.

BRUGIA TIMORI (PARTONO, PURNOMO, DENNIS, ATMOSOEDJONO, OEMIJATI & CROSS, 1977)

The adult male *B. timori* differs from other *Brugia* spp. (except *B. malayi*) in having a spicular ratio of 3:1; it differs

Table III.9 Differentiation between microfilariae of *B. malayi* and *W. bancrofti*.

	Microfilaria malayi	*Microfilaria bancrofti*
General	Often found closely folded with head close to tail, and iregularly disposed for, besides major curves, minor angulations are typical	Usually seen lying with head and tail well separated, and commonly shows three or four major curves of graceful appearance
Nuclei	Blurred and intermingled so that they cannot be easily counted	Well defined and spaced and can easily be counted
Tail	Tapers to a fine point; continues as a fine thread. *Typically* one nucleus at the extremity of the tapered portion and two in the terminal thread	Tapers to a point and the terminal portion contains no nuclei
Cephalic space	Twice as long as broad	As long as broad
Excretory pore and cell	Separated	Close together. A thread of protoplasm runs posteriorly from the latter
Anal pore	Clear space about 40 μm from the tail end	
Sheath	Well stained	Hardly visible

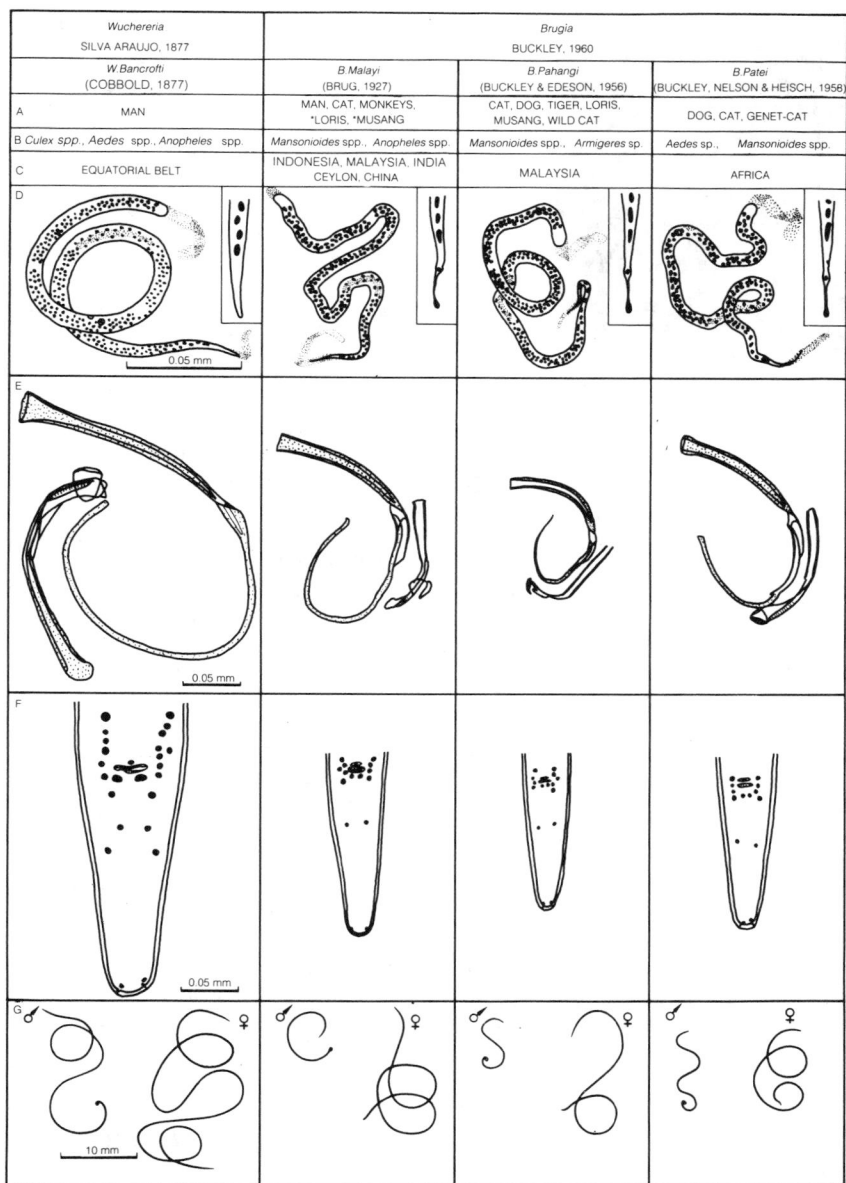

Wuchereria		*Brugia*		
SILVA ARAUJO, 1877		BUCKLEY, 1960		
W. Bancrofti	*B. Malayi*	*B. Pahangi*	*B. Patei*
(COBBOLD, 1877)	(BRUG. 1927)	(BUCKLEY & EDESON, 1956)	(BUCKLEY, NELSON & HEISCH, 1958)
A MAN	MAN, CAT, MONKEYS, *LORIS, *MUSANG	CAT, DOG, TIGER, LORIS, MUSANG, WILD CAT	DOG, CAT, GENET-CAT
B *Culex* spp., *Aedes* spp., *Anopheles* spp.	*Mansonioides* spp., *Anopheles* spp.	*Mansonioides* spp., *Armigeres* sp.	*Aedes* sp., *Mansonioides* spp.
C EQUATORIAL BELT	INDONESIA, MALAYSIA, INDIA CEYLON, CHINA	MALAYSIA	AFRICA

Figure III.95 The morphological distinctions between the genera *Wuchereria* and *Brugia*. A, Definitive hosts. B, Intermediate hosts. C, Geographical distribution. D, Microfilariae and (inset) tail nuclei of microfilariae. E, Spicules of male, lateral view. F, Tails of males, ventral view. G, Adult worms, actual size. *Indicates experimental infection only. (After Bradley; by permission of *Annals of Tropical Medicine and Parasitology.*)

from *B. malayi* in having greater numbers of subventral adanal papillae (up to five on each side) that are loosely spaced and irregularly positioned about the cloaca, a greater diameter of the capitulum of the left spicule and greater length of the proximal section of the right spicule. The adult female has an ovejector of greater length and width than that of *B. malayi*. Microfilariae typical of the *B. timor* have a greater length than other *Brugia* spp., length to width cephalic space ratio of 3:1 and a sheath which does not stain bright pink with Giemsa.[18] The vector is *Anopheles barbirostris*.

Figure III.95 shows the differences between *Wuchereria* and *Brugia* forms of filaria.

GENUS: *ONCHOCERCA*

ONCHOCERCA VOLVULUS (LEUCKART, 1893)

PARASITOLOGY

The body is white and filiform, tapering at both ends. The head is rounded. The cuticle is marked by transverse ridges and raised with prominent angular and oblique thickenings, more distinct posteriorly. It is usually found in nodules but

Male   Female

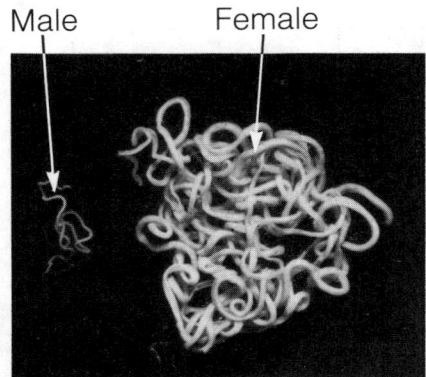

Figure III.96 Adult *Onchocerca volvulus*: male on left, female on right.

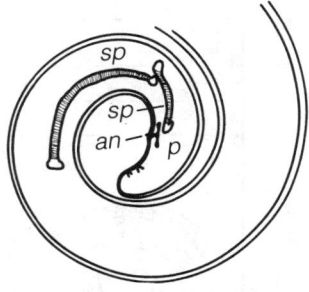

Figure III.97 The caudal extremity of a male *Onchocerca volvulus*. an, anus; p, papillae; sp, spicules.

can reproduce outside them (Figure III.96). The male (2–4 cm × 0.2 mm) has a straight alimentary canal ending in a subterminal anus. The tail ends in a slight spiral and is bulbous at the tip. There are two pairs of preanal, two postanal, an intermediate large papilla, and two unequal spicules (82 μm, 77 μm) protruding from the cloaca (Figure III.97); the former has a fluted end and the latter a narrow neck and knob. The female normally measures 60–70 cm × 0.4 mm but is often smaller, 35–40 cm. The head is round and truncated (0.04 mm), the vulva 0.85 mm from the anterior extremity and the tail curved. Cuticular striations are not so marked as in the male and the presence of two striae in the inner layer of the cuticle is a distinguishing feature of *Onchocerca* in tissue sections.[19] Usually males outnumber females by two to one (four males and two females in each tumour). The female is ovoviviparous and the egg has a striated shell with a pointed process at each pole (like an orange wrapped in tissue paper) measuring 30–50 μm in diameter. The microfilariae (300 × 8 μm) are sheathless and are found in the fluid of the nodule cavity and in the surrounding skin. The body tapers from the last fifth and ends in a sharply pointed, recurved tail (Figure III.93,1). In the anterior fifth is a marked anterior 'V-spot'. The cephalic cone is thickened at the commencement of the nuclear column. This microfilaria is non-periodic; it is found in skin in the femoral, inguinal and cervical lymph glands and in the expressed juice of 'tumours' but sometimes in blood (2%) and also in urine. It is also present in the skin of widely separated portions of the body in apparently healthy people, without producing any nodules or tumours. Microfilariae are easily demonstrated in the skin by biopsy. They are often associated with eye symptoms in the absence of tumours and, by aid of the slit lamp, may be seen in the cornea.

LIFE CYCLE

This was worked out in Sierra Leone. Development takes place in a 'black fly' or 'buffalo gnat' *Simulium damnosum* (*sensulatum*) in Africa and others in South and Central America (see Appendix IV). The fly abstracts microfilariae from the deeper layers of the skin; they then enter the stomach, pierce its walls and pass to the thoracic muscles where they undergo further development. During growth two moults take place. At the seventh day the larva measures

0.65 mm. Development has been traced to the tenth day when the larva escapes from the proboscis; *Simulium* is a day-biting fly (06.00 to 18.00 hours) and 2.6% may be naturally infected. They probably attract and then abstract microfilariae by scraping the skin with their prestomal teeth.

In the South American form, development is similar to that of the central African but occurs in *Simulium metallicum* (*avidum*), *S. ochraceum* and *S. callidum* (*mooseri*), which are common in endemic areas in Central America and other vectors in South American foci. Developing larvae are frequently found in the abdomen and malpighian tubules of these flies. Two caudal papillae are seen in fully developed larvae, which measure 0.45–1.14 mm. In Guatemala 11% of *Simulium* are naturally infected. Non-human filariae can occur in *Simulium*, and a key to their identification and distinction from human *Onchocerca* is given by Nelson and Pester.[20]

Although there are no morphological differences in the various geographical forms of *Onchocerca* there are at least six different *Onchocerca–Simulium* complexes which have their own clinical and biological attributes. Enzyme staining for the presence of acid phosphatase was found to show four distinct patterns in microfilariae from West Africa suggesting that a number of biological strains did exist in West Africa.[21]

ONCHOCERCA GUTTUROSA

O. gutturosa is a parasite of cattle and has occasionally been shown to cause skin nodules in man.[22]

GENUS: *MANSONELLA*

MANSONELLA OZZARDI (MANSON, 1897)
(*TETRAPETALONEMA OZZARDI, FILARIA OZZARDI*)

MORPHOLOGY[23]

The male is 24–28.4 mm long × 0.07–0.08 mm in diameter. It is coiled in one and a half to two turns and has two spicules and caudal alae. The female is twice as long, 32.2–61.5 mm × 0.13–0.16 mm in diameter and has a vulva 0.76 mm from the caudal extremity. The vagina leads to paired uteri filling the body cavity with highly coiled ovaries in the posterior part of the body. The adult worms live in body cavities embedded in adipose tissues and in the mesentery. The microfilariae, which are unsheathed, are 207–232 μm long × 3–4 μm in diameter. The anterior end is round and they have an attenuated tail resembling *M. perstans* but pointed and ending in a hook (Figure III.93,6).

Transfusion experiments have shown that they can live in the blood of the recipient for more than 2 years.

LIFE CYCLE

There are two forms of *M. ozzardi*, one in the Caribbean and the other in Brazil and Venezuela. The insect vectors are a midge and a simulium. Microfilariae are ingested with blood from a blood meal and the larvae migrate within 24 hours to the muscles of the thorax where two ecdyses occur, and the third stage infective larva, measuring 0.7 mm in length, migrates forward to the head to emerge from the proboscis in 8 days from the time of the infective blood meal.

In the Caribbean

Culicoides furens is a vector in St Vincent and Haiti, *C. paraensis* in Antigua and northern Argentina, and *C. phlebotomus* in Trinidad.

In Brazil

The main vector is *Simulium amazonicum* but *Culicoides insinuatus* may also play a part.

MICROFILARIA BOLIVARENSIS[24]

Microfilaria of *M. bolivarensis* has been described in the blood of Amerindians in Bolivar state in Venezuela. The microfilaria measures 256–300 × 7–8 μm and differs from *M. ozzardi*. It superficially resembles microfilaria volvulus but has a greater diameter and a straighter tail.

MANSONELLA (ESSLINGERIA) PERSTANS
(MANSON, 1891)
(*DIPETALONEMA PERSTANS, FILARIA PERSTANS,*
ACANTHOCHEILONEMA PERSTANS,
TETRAPETALONEMA PERSTANS)

PARASITOLOGY

It has a long cylindrical, smooth body and a simple, unarmed mouth. The tail in both sexes is characteristic: incurvated, with a chitinous covering at the extreme tip split into two minute appendages, giving a mitred appearance. The female possesses four cuticular appendages at the posterior ex-

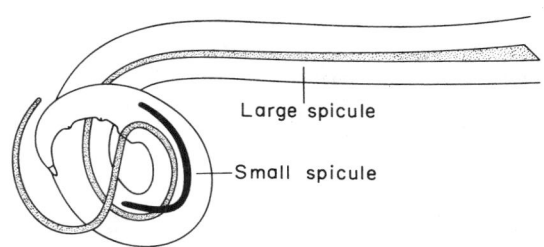

Figure III.98   The tail of *Mansonella perstans*, showing two unequal spicules and papillae. (After Leiper.)

tremity, not two as hitherto believed. The male (4.5 cm × 0.06 mm) is smaller than the female. The head is 0.04 mm in diameter and the cloaca has four pairs of preanal and one pair of postanal papillae, and two unequal spicules (Figure III.98). The female (7–8 cm × 0.12 mm) has a club-shaped head 0.07 mm in diameter, and a vulva situated 1.2 mm from the head. The anus opens at the apex of a papilla in the concavity of the curve formed by the tail; its diameter is 0.02 mm.

The microfilaria (200 × 4.5 μm) is unsheathed (Figure III.93,7). It possesses in a remarkable degree the power of elongation and contraction. Therefore the measurements vary considerably. Long and short forms (90–110 × 4 μm) have been described. It is smaller than that of *W. bancrofti* or *L. loa* and its caudal end is truncated and abruptly rounded (Figure III.99). The tapering tail extends two-thirds of the entire length. The anterior 'V-spot' is 30 μm from the anterior extremity. There is no marked tail spot, no central granular mass, and no cephalic prepuce. It moves freely in the blood.

The embryos occur in equal numbers both by day and night; according to the self-inflicted experiment of Gönnert, this embryo can persist in the recipient 3 years after blood transfusion.

LIFE CYCLE

The insect vectors are species of *Culicoides*. Microfilariae are ingested and the larvae penetrate the stomach to develop in the thoracic muscles. Within 6–9 days third-stage infective larvae 0.7 mm long emerge from the proboscis. Prior to emerging they cause a globular expansion of the labrum

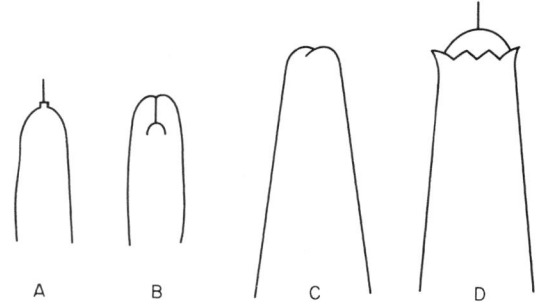

Figure III.99   Structure of the head of microfilaria perstans (A, B) and microfilaria bancrofti (C, D).

which then collapses, allowing the larvae to escape. There is confusion over the identity of the vector in Africa; originally it was described as *C. austeni* but it is more likely that *C. inornatipennis* and possibly *C. grahami* are the vectors. Transmission takes place at night.

MANSONELLA (ESSLINGERIA) STREPTOCERCA (MACFIE & CORSON, 1922) (DIPETALONEMA STREPTOCERCA, AGAMOFILARIA STREPTOCERCA, ACANTHOCHEILONEMA STREPTOCERCA)

This sheathless microfilaria is found commonly in the corium of the skin but not in the blood of people in Ghana (22 out of 50 in Accra). It has a wide distribution especially in Cameroon and other West African countries.

The microfilaria (Figures III.93,8 and III.100) is 215 μm in length and is distinguished by the 'walking stick handle' of the tail extremity and an arrangement of nuclei in the head, and four prominent ones in the tail which has a bifid end[25] which distinguishes it from the microfilariae of *O. volvulus* and *M. perstans*.

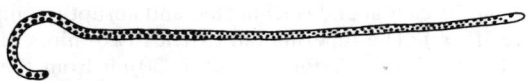

Figure III.100   Microfilaria of *Mansonella streptocerca*, showing the characteristic curvature of the tail. (200×.)

LIFE CYCLE

The vector is *C. grahami* in which development takes place similar to that in *M. perstans*. Transmission takes place during the day.

Microfilariae were found in the skin of six of 11 chimpanzees (*Pan paniscus* and *P. satyrus*) in Zaire. Two adult female worms found in the connective tissue were very similar to *M. perstans*. The microfilariae of this species, *D. vanhoofi*, closely resemble those of the latter. The incubation period of *D. streptocerca* is 3–4 months.

TETRAPETALONEMA BERGHEI (CHARDOME & PEEL, 1951)

This is found in Zaire together with *M. streptocerca*. It is a white nematode, 60.9 × 0.271 mm, with almost imperceptible striations. The head is hemispherical and a relatively large genital opening is situated anteriorly. The uterus divides into two branches. Microfilariae at all stages are visible in the uterus. There are several enlargements of the body at intervals. The caudal extremity narrows rapidly showing four excrescences. The tail is recurved. The microfilaria which is found in the skin resembles that of a small microfilaria

perstans and measures 179 × 3.55 μm. The adult form may turn out to be similar to *M. perstans*.

MENINGONEMA PERUZZII (ORIHEL & ESSLINGER, 1972)

Adults are found in the subarachnoid space of *Cercopithecus* monkeys trapped in equatorial Guinea. The microfilariae resemble those of *M. perstans* but have an inconspicuous sheath. This worm is the same as that described by Peruzzi in 1928 in monkeys in Uganda and causes cerebral filariasis in Zimbabwe.

GENUS: *LOA* (EYE WORM)

LOA LOA (COBBOLD, 1864)

Adult *Loa loa* worms inhabit the subcutaneous connective tissues. Diurnal periodic sheathed microfilariae are shed into the peripheral blood.

PARASITOLOGY

The body is filiform, cylindrical, whitish and semitransparent with numerous round, smooth, translucent protuberances of the cuticle, 12–16 μm in diameter, and 9–11 μm above the surface. These chitinous bosses are more numerous in females. Their distribution is irregular. In the male they are absent at the extremities; in the female they extend to the tail and also the cephalic end. The mouth is unarmed and destitute of papillae; there is no distinct neck but a shoulder 0.15 mm from the mouth where there are two papillae, one dorsal, the other ventral. The alimentary canal commences at a funnel-shaped mouth as a slender straight oesophagus, going on to an intestine 65 μm wide and a short attenuated rectum. The male (3–3.4 cm × 0.35–0.43 mm) (Figure III.101) has its maximum breadth anteriorly; posteriorly it

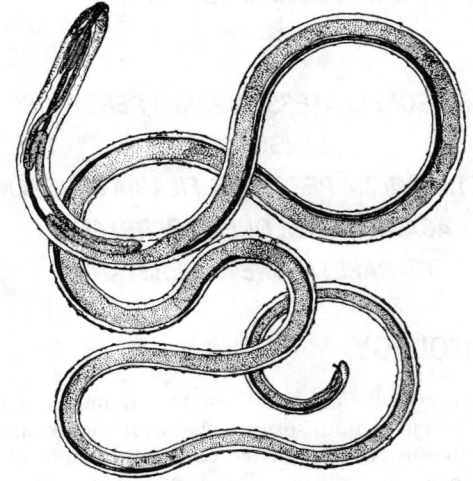

Figure III.101   Male *Loa loa*. (10×.)

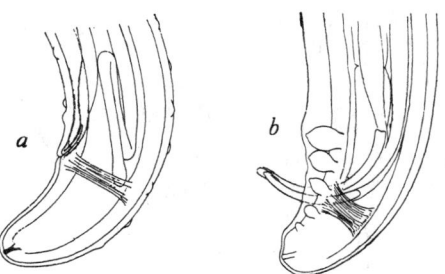

Figure III.102   Posterior extremity of *Loa loa*. a, Female. b, Male.

tapers to a tail which is curved ventrally with two lateral expansions of the cuticle (0.7 × 0.029 mm) (Figure III.102b). In the middle, 0.08 mm from the tail-tip, is the opening of the anogenital orifice with two unequal spicules (123–176 µm and 88–113 µm) surrounded by thick labia. There are four large globular, pedunculated papillae, decreasing in size antero-posteriorly, and a fifth pair of small postanal papillae. The female (5–7 cm × 0.5 mm) (Figure III.103) has a straight, attenuated, broadly rounded posterior extremity and a vulva 2.5 mm from the anterior extremity placed on a small eminence (Figure III.102a). The vagina, 9 mm long, branches off into long uterine tubes extending through the length of the body. At the narrow end are the ovaries with eggs at all stages. Reproduction is ovoviviparous; the embryos develop within the egg envelope, and uncoil themselves on expulsion from the vagina. When dead the adult worm often becomes calcified.

The microfilaria (Figure III.93,4 and 5) is similar in size (298 × 7.5 µm) and structure to that of *W. bancrofti* but its sheath does not stain with Giemsa. In fresh blood it may be impossible to distinguish them. In dried stained films it assumes a stiff angular attitude, the tail end is disposed in a series of sharp flexures, giving it a corkscrew appearance, with the extreme tip flexed, the nuclei of the central column of cells of microfilaria *L. loa* are larger and less deeply stained and the cephalic end of the column is more abruptly terminated (Figure III.93,2 and 4). By special staining methods a large genital cell at the beginning of the posterior third constitutes a marked feature. Microfilaria *L. loa* takes up methylene blue (1 in 5000) in 10 minutes. In microfilaria of *W. bancrofti*, absorption it is much slower but it shows up the excretory pore. Microfilaria of *L. loa* may not be found in the peripheral blood early after infection. It is strictly diurnal, from 08.00 to 20.00 hours—the reverse of microfilaria of *W. bancrofti*. Inversion of periodicity takes place very gradually as, for instance, when daily observations are made on a voyage round the world. The periodicity of microfilaria of *L. loa* is under circadian control by temperature and not by oxygen tension as in periodic *W. bancrofti*.

LIFE CYCLE

There are two parallel and sympatric but ecologically separate cycles of *Loa loa* transmission in the West African rain forest. One cycle is that of human *Loa loa* (*L. loa loa*) which is slightly smaller than the simian *L. loa* and has strictly diurnally periodic microfilariae with day-biting vectors (*Chrysops silacea* and *C. dimidiata*). The slightly larger simian parasite of drills *L. loa papionis* has nocturnally periodic microfilariae with tree-top *Chrysops* (*C. langi* and *C. centurionis*) vectors which feed early in the night.

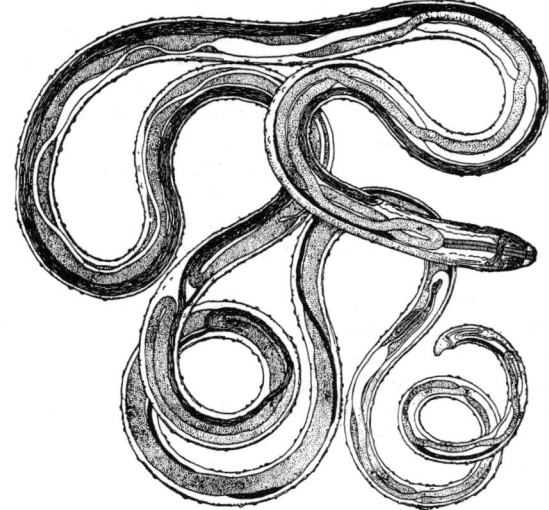

Figure III.103   Female *Loa loa*. (10×.)

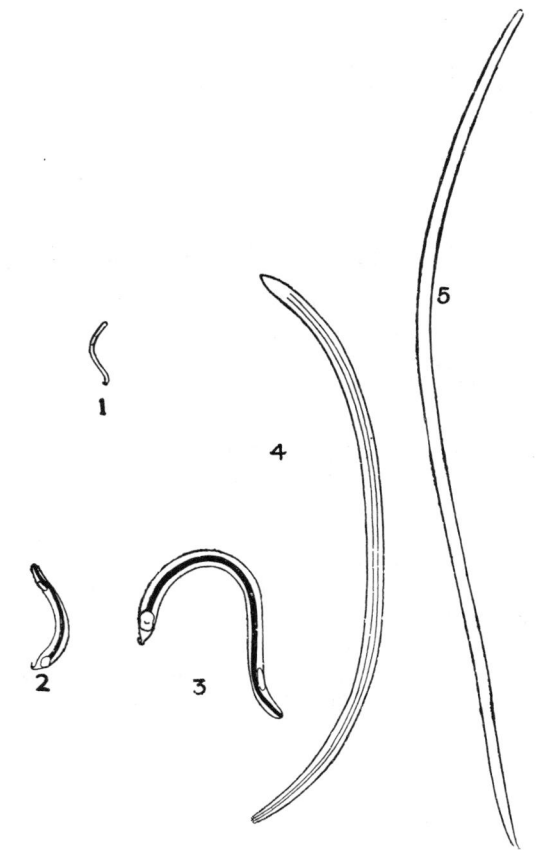

Figure III.104   Development of *Loa loa* in *Chrysops*. (30×.) 1, Larva, 24 hours old. 2, Fourth day, length 390 µm. 3, Fifth day. 4, Seventh day. 5, Tenth day, third-stage infective larva (2 × 0.025 mm).

DEVELOPMENT IN *CHRYSOPS* (Figure III.104)

Microfilariae are taken up with the blood meal and on entering the stomach the microfilaria casts its sheath in 3 hours and, piercing the stomach wall, enters the thoracic muscles and fat body of the thorax, but principally that of the abdomen. Development is complete in 10 days. In 3 days it becomes broad and torpedo-shaped; on the fourth and fifth days the squat form lengthens to 0.8–1 mm; on the sixth day the corkscrew-like appearance is replaced by gentle curves. Then occurs the first ecdysis and the sharp tail is replaced by a rounded, trilobed extremity. By the tenth day it measures 2 × 0.025 mm, and two moults have occurred, and infective third-stage forms migrate forward into the head where they accumulate in large numbers, the majority at the root of the proboscis. At the next feed they break out of the labium and make their way on to the surface of the skin which they penetrate, and migrate along the interfascial planes.

Development of *L. loa* in *Chrysops* generally takes 10–12 days from the original infecting feed. *Chrysops* feeds to repletion once every 14 days and the gestation period is 12 days. It is a pool feeder, straining the blood from the subcutaneous haemorrhages caused by its bite.

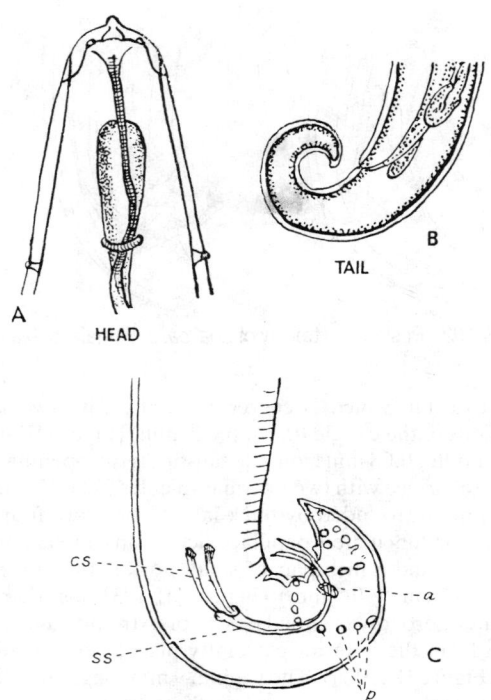

Figure III.106   *Dracunculus medinensis.* A, Anterior end of female. B, Tail of female. C, Posterior end of male. Ventrolateral aspects. (10×.)

a	anus	p	preanal and postanal
cs	copulatory spicules		papillae
		ss	spicular sheath

SUPERFAMILY: DRACUNCULOIDEA

GENUS: *DRACUNCULUS*

DRACUNCULUS MEDINENSIS (LINNAEUS 1758)
(GUINEA-WORM)

PARASITOLOGY

The female is the thickness of a knitting needle and usually 60 cm in length (60 cm × 1.5–1.7 mm; 90 cm is probably exceptional but 120 cm has been recorded). It lives in connective tissue and does not harm its host until about to produce its young when it exhibits 'geotropism', i.e. it is drawn towards earth, towards the limbs—to the fingers, if in the arms; to the scrotum or penis, if in the abdomen; to the breasts in the female, though 90% migrate to the legs and feet, especially behind the outer malleolus.

The body is cylindrical, white and smooth (Figure III.105). The tip of the tail is pointed forming a blunt hook which was

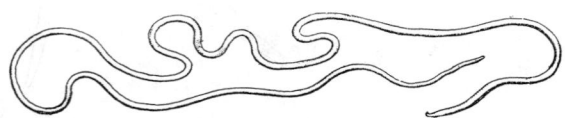

Figure III.105   Female *Dracunculus medinensis.* One-third natural size.

formerly thought to be used for holding firm in tissues, but this is not correct. The head is rounded, terminating in a thickened cuticle cap or 'cephalic shield'. The mouth is triangular, small and surrounded by six papillae and an outer circle of four double papillae. A lateral pair of cervical papillae is situated behind the nerve ring (Figure III.106A). There is a single-bulb oesophagus. The secretion from the head glands is very irritating and histiolytic. The alimentary canal is small and is thrust to one side by the branched uterus. There is no definite anus. The vulva is difficult to see and has been only recently discovered as a very small tube in the centre of the worm. The whole worm is occupied by the double uterus packed with embryos (Figure III.107). The coiled uteri, distended by three million larvae, fill the body. There is a double ovary and double oviducts at the posterior extremity (Figure III.106B,C). When douched with water, waves of contraction force the uterine contents forward, the thickened cuticle gives way and the 'cap' is blown off. The uterus is extruded up to a length of 1.25 cm; this also bursts and the contained embryos are shed into the water. The worm dies when its nervous system is destroyed. The sinus containing the dead worm easily becomes septic, but it may coil itself round tendons and, if pulled upon, may break. It often becomes calcified and can then be demonstrated on radiography.

The male is known from a single specimen in man, 40 mm in length, but was discovered by Moorthy[26] in experimental dogs. It measures 1.2–2.9 cm × 0.4 mm, has subequal spic-

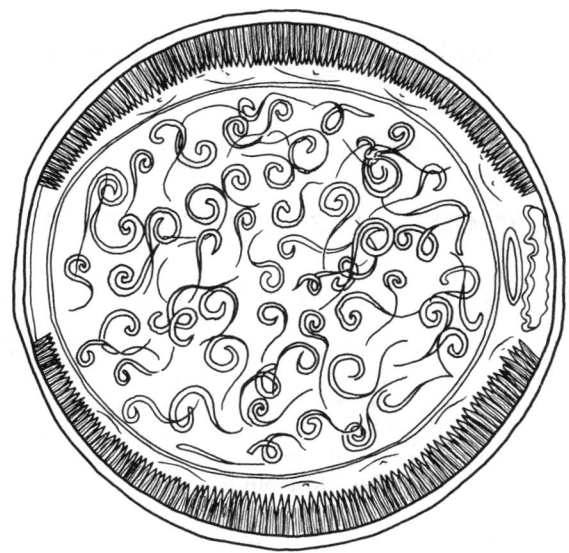

Figure III.107 Transverse section of *Dracunculus medinensis*, showing the contained embryos.

ules (490–730 μm) and a gubernaculum (200 μm). The posterior end is coiled on itself one or more times. There are 10 pairs of caudal papillae, of which four are preanal and six postanal. The copulatory spicules are subequal, 490–730 μm in length. After copulation it dies and is absorbed. It lives in between the muscles of the groin. Copulation probably takes place in the deeper tissues.

The embryo (Figure III.108) measures 500–750 × 17 μm and shows transverse striations of the cuticle. It is flattened, not cylindrical, with a long, slender tail and a rounded head. The alimentary canal has a rudimentary anus and a bulbous oesophagus. There are two glands at the root of the tail. In water the embryos cannot swim but sink and coil up and release again, moving by side-to-side lashing of the tail and tadpole-like movement of the body. Abnormal embryos, with prominences on the dorsal and ventral caudal surfaces, are not uncommon, but do not survive long.

LIFE CYCLE (Figure III.109)

In water they live for 6 days; in muddy water or moist earth for 2 or 3 weeks. If slowly desiccated they can be revived by water. They are swallowed by *Cyclops* (*Cyclops* has a very small mouth). The efficient intermediaries are *Cyclops quadricornis* or allied species (*C. strenuus*, *C. viridis*, *C. coronatus*, *C. bicuspidatus*, *Mesocyclops leuckarti* and *M. hyalinus*) but, in the true tropics, *Tropocyclops multicolor* and other species; in south Nigeria it is *Thermocyclops nigerianus*. Jerky movements of the embryos attract *Cyclops* as a trout is attracted by a fly. As many as 20 may be found in one crustacean but usually they die out when there are more than

Figure III.108 Embryo of *Dracunculus medinensis*. (a) Side view. (b) Front view.

al	alimentary canal	nr	nerve ring
blb	bulb	oes	oesophagus
gl	glands		

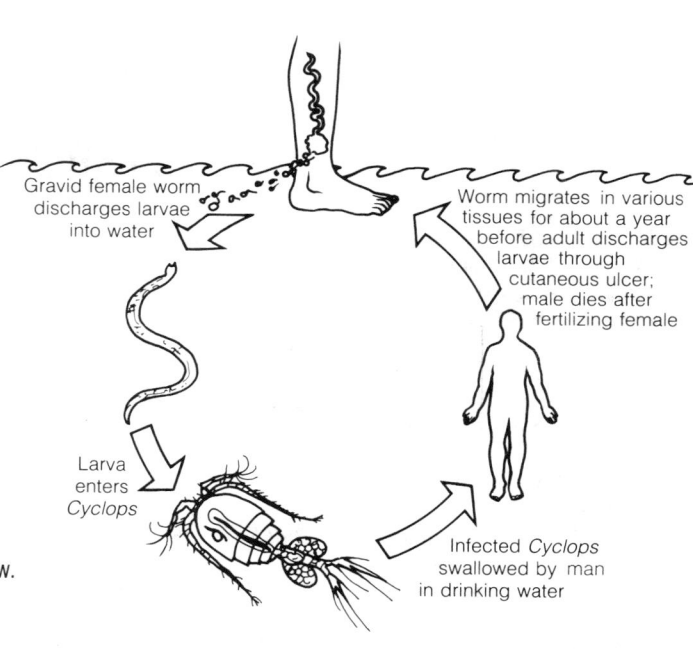

Figure III.109 Life cycle of *Dracunculus medinensis*.

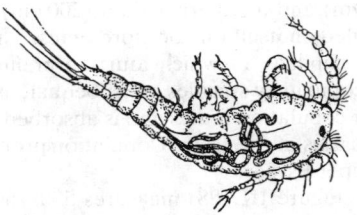

Figure III.110 Larvae of *Dracunculus medinensis* in the body cavity of *Cyclops*.

four (Figure III.110). The pointed tail penetrates the gut wall; they then migrate into the body cavity and feed on the ovary or testes of the cyclops. There is no growth in size but two to three ecdyses take place. The tail is absorbed and they become cylindrical and the posterior extremity trilobed. Development takes 4–6 weeks but the larva may survive for 4 months. When 1 mm in length they acquire a simple muscular oesophagus (Figure III.108) and the tail is truncated. This distinguishes the infective stage.

Cyclops is swallowed by man; in the gastric juice the body of the cyclops is dissolved and the larvae become active and burst out. The migration of the early stages in the mammalian host has been clarified.[27] It takes 3–4 months for the full development of both sexes. Immature stages were recovered 43–48 days while undergoing the fourth ecdysis. The route of the larvae from the alimentary canal to the subcutaneous tissues of the mammalian host takes place via the lymphatic system. The worms reach the subcutaneous tissues by the forty-third day. In this situation the sexes live in equal numbers and sexual differentiation is distinct, though the males have not developed spicules. The final ecdysis takes place in the subcutaneous tissues. The adult worm takes exactly 1 year to develop.

SUPERFAMILY: SPIRUROIDEA

GENUS: *THELAZIA*

THELAZIA CALLIPAEDA (ORIENTAL EYE WORM)

This nematode is a parasite of the conjunctiva of the dog, rabbit and man in India, Myanmar and parts of China.

The adult is a white thread-like worm (males 4.5–13 mm × 0.25–0.75 mm; females 6.2–17 mm × 0.3–0.85 mm). The oral end has a chitinized capsule with two circles of sessile papillae. The male has a recurved posterior end. The vulva of the female opens ventrally in the anterior half of the body. There is a single uterus which bifurcates into two ovaries.

The egg is ovoidal and measures 60 × 34–37 μm, is hyaline, thin-shelled and laid fully embryonated.

LIFE CYCLE

Little is known of the life history but an insect intermediate host is probable since related species have *Musca* spp. as intermediate hosts and *Famina* spp. have been shown to be susceptible larval hosts.[28]

THELAZIA CALIFORNIENSIS

T. californiensis has been found in man in California, the intermediate hosts of which include *Fannia benjamini* and *Musca autumnalis*.

REFERENCES

1 Southgate V R, Van Wijk H B & Wright C A. *Feitschr Parasitol* 1976; 49:145–159.

2 Wright C A & Ross G C. *Trans R Soc Trop Med Hyg* 1980; 74:326–332.

3 Jordan P & Webbe G. *Human Schistosomiasis*, 2nd edn. London: Heinemann, 1982.

4 Brown D S. *Freshwater Snails of Africa and Their Medical Importance*. London: Taylor & Francis, 1980.

5 Kian Joe Lie, Basch P W, Heynemann D et al. *Trans R Soc Trop Med Hyg* 1968; 62:299.

6 Brygoo E R & Randrimalala J C. *Bull Soc Path Exot* 1959; 52:26.

7 Slais J, cited in Dawes, B. *Advances in Parasitology*. London: Academic Press, 1972.

8 Dismuke J C Jun & Routh C F. *Am J Trop Med Hyg* 1963; 12:73.

9 Schad G A et al. *Science* 1973; 180:502.

10 Beer R J S. *BMJ* 1971; ii:44.

11 Masuya T. *Jpn J Parasitol* 1976; 25:283.

12 McFadzean J S & Hawking F. *Trans R Soc Trop Med Hyg* 1956; 50:543.

13 Hawking F. *Trans R Soc Trop Med Hyg* 1956; 50: 397.

14 Bryan J H, Oothman P, Andrews B J et al. *Trans R Soc Trop Med Hyg* 1974; 68:14.

15 Laurence B R. *Trans R Soc Trop Med Hyg* 1985; 79: 690–699.

16 Nelson G S. *J Helminthol* 1959; 33:233.

17 David L & Edeson J F B. *Ann Trop Med Parasitol* 1964; 59:103.

18 Partono F, Purnomo A S & Dennis D T. *J Parasitol* 1977; 63:540.

19 Beaver P C, Horner G S & Bilos J Z. *Am J Trop Med Hyg* 1974; 23:595.

20 Nelson G S & Pester F N R. *Bull World Health Organ* 1962; 27:473.
21 Braun-Munziger R A & Southgate B A. *Bull World Health Organ* 1977; 55:569.
22 Collins R C. *J Parasitol* 1973; 59:1016.
23 Orihel T C & Eberhard M L. *Am J Trop Med Hyg* 1982; 31:1142–1147.
24 Godoy G A, Godoy G, Oriheltic C & Volcan G S. *Am J Trop Med Hyg* 1980; 29:545–547.
25 Orihel T C. *Am J Trop Med Hyg* 1984; 33:1278.
26 Moorthy U N. *J Parasitol* 1937; 23:220.
27 Onobamiro S D. *Ann Trop Med Parasitol* 1956; 50:157.
28 Burnett H S, Warren E P & Lee R D. *J Parasitol* 1957; 43:433.

MEDICAL ACAROLOGY AND ENTOMOLOGY

Edited by G. B. White

Most types of zoological organisms (more than 90% of all known species) belong to the Phylum Arthropoda, having an exoskeleton. Arthropods of medical interest belong to three Classes: Arachnida (ticks, mites, scorpions and spiders, see below); Crustacea (crabs, crayfish, copepods, etc.); and especially the Insecta (insects), characterized by having the body subdivided as head (with antennae), thorax with legs and segmented abdomen.

TICKS AND MITES
M. G. R. Varma

CLASS: ARACHNIDA

The arachnids differ from insects by lacking antennae and wings, and in having an unsegmented body. During the life cycle they undergo incomplete metamorphosis; the eggs hatch into six-legged larvae which develop through the nymphal stage to adults. The nymphs and adults have four pairs of legs.

SUBCLASS: ACARI; ORDER: ACARINA (TICKS AND MITES)

The acarine body is typically composed of an anterior gnathosoma or capitulum and a posterior idiosoma. The gnathosoma represents the head of a generalized arthropod and carries the paired palps, which are sensory in function, the paired chelicerae and the single ventrally situated hypostome, which together make up the cutting and bloodsucking apparatus. The idiosoma carries the paired legs.

There are about 30 000 species of acarines belonging to more than 2000 genera. The mites are usually much smaller than ticks. Of over 200 families of mite that have been described; only a few contain species that affect man.

FAMILY: SARCOPTIDAE

SARCOPTES SCABIEI (ITCH MITE, SCABIES MITE)

Sarcoptes scabiei causes scabies in man and mange in a variety of wild and domestic animals. Scabies mites of dogs and horses, which differ physiologically rather than morphologically from human scabies mites, can establish themselves briefly on humans and cause skin problems similar to scabies. Such infestations are usually mild and cure spontaneously. Increased incidence of human scabies tends to occur in 15–20-year cycles and the cycling is most probably due to changing levels of immunity in the human population. Scabies is widespread in the tropics, although by no means confined there. It may disappear from one area for many years, only to reappear. It is thought that the recent resurgence in scabies is due to large population movements, insufficient or incorrect diagnosis by the medical profession and an altered life style among younger persons in the developed Western countries, resulting in close personal contact. Infestation levels are highest in poorer communities and in children. Even in developed countries, infestation in schoolchildren can reach 5%.

The female *S. scabiei* (0.3–0.4 mm) is bigger than the male (0.2 mm) (Figure IV.1).[1] The first and second pairs of legs of the female and the first, second and fourth pairs of legs of the male carry suckers. The surface of the female is covered with fine transverse striations and the dorsal surface bears a number of specialized spines and conical setae.

Both males and females make short burrows but it is only the fertilized females which make permanent winding burrows in the horny layers of the skin, with the female at the end

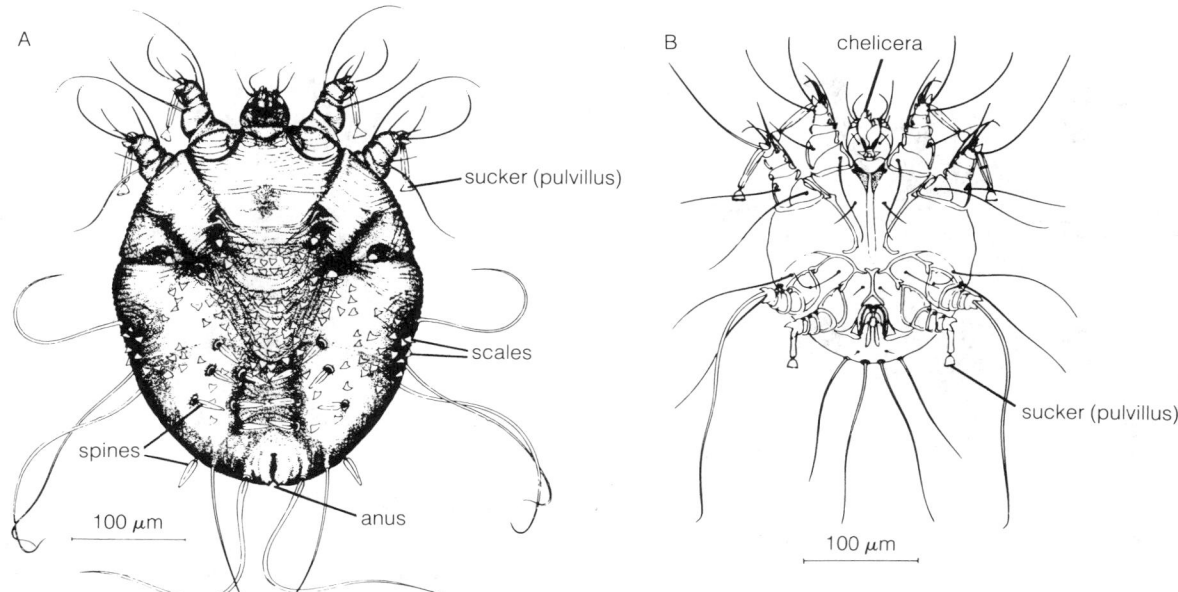

Figure IV.1   A, Dorsal view of female *Sarcoptes scabiei*; B, ventral view of *Sarcoptes scabiei*. (Reproduced from Kettle[1].)

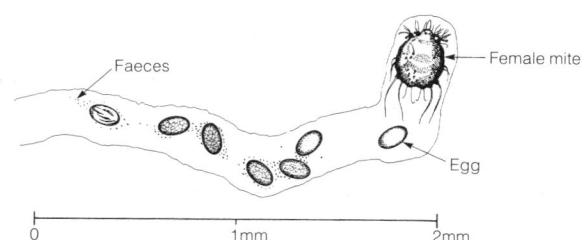

Figure IV.2   Burrow of *Sarcoptes scabiei* with female mite and eggs.

(Figure IV.2). The burrows contain faeces and relatively large eggs. The majority of mite burrows are found in the interdigital skin, bends of the knees and elbows, the penis and breasts. The eggs hatch into larvae which find shelter and presumably food in the follicles. The larval stage is followed by two nymphal stages before the adult stage is reached. The whole life cycle from egg to egg takes about 10–14 days, during which there may be a mortality of about 90%. (For clinical features and treatment see Chapter 11.)

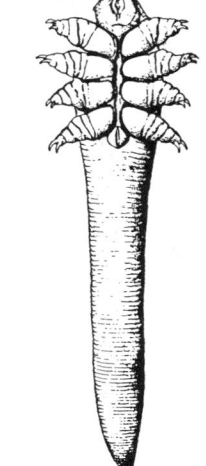

Figure IV.3   *Demodex folliculorum* the follicle mite. Ventral view. (Reproduced from Kettle[1].)

FAMILY: DEMODICIDAE

DEMODEX (FOLLICLE MITES)

These extremely small mites, 0.1–0.4 mm long (Figure IV.3), have a worm-like transversely striated body with four pairs of stubby legs anteriorly. They infest a wide variety of mammalian hosts but are highly host-specific. More than one species may occur on the same host but in different tissues.

For example, *D. folliculorum* lives in the hair follicles of man and the stubby *D. brevis* is found in the sebaceous glands. The entire life cycle occurs in the follicles. In man infestations occur mainly in the region of the eyelids, nose and facial area. Infestations are usually higher in aged persons, in whom they may reach 100%. Diagnosis is by expressing sebum and examining it for mites. Infestations are usually benign, but dry erythema with follicular scaling, particularly in the region of the eyelids, may give rise to blepharitis. In the facial area there may be granulomatous acne. Gammexane (gamma benzene hexachloride) 0.5% in vanishing cream is effective.

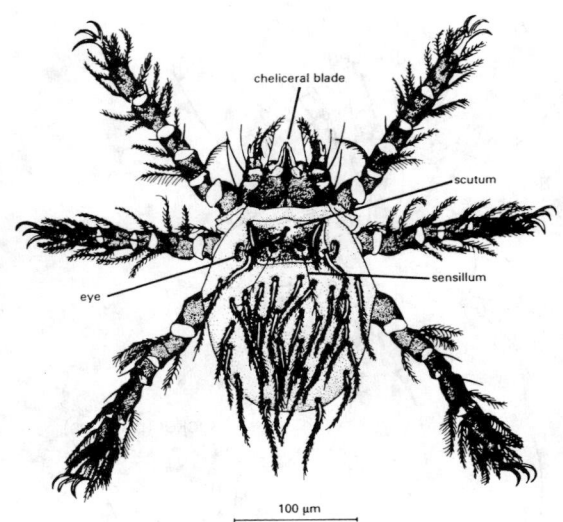

Figure IV.4   Dorsal view of *Leptotrombidium deliense*. (Reproduced from Kettle[1].)

FAMILY: TROMBICULIDAE

Of more than 1200 described species of trombiculid mite, only about 50 are known to attack humans or livestock. Only the larvae, popularly known as chiggers, are parasitic on vertebrates. They are widely distributed and in many countries cause a dermatitis in man, although not all chiggers cause an itchy reaction.

Trombiculid larvae (Figures IV.4 and IV.5) normally parasitize rodents and birds but, given the opportunity, will feed readily on man. The non-parasitic female lays eggs in damp but well-drained soil. Typical breeding places are cultivated alluvial river banks in Japan, scrub jungle, grassy fields or untended gardens with a rank growth of grass and other vegetation.

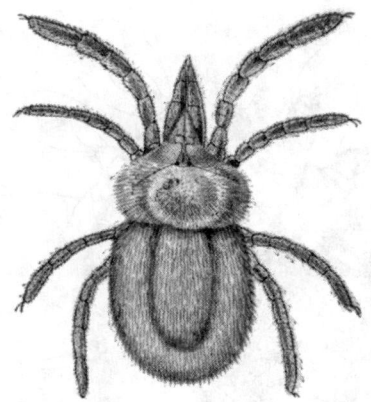

Figure IV.5   Fully grown imago of *Leptotrombidium akamushi*.

LIFE CYCLE (Figure IV.6)

On hatching, the six-legged larvae, which are creamy-white to bright red in colour and 0.25 mm long, ascend grass stems or the tips of fallen leaves and wait in clusters until carbon dioxide from a passing host activates them. The round or oval-shaped larvae have a prominent gnathosoma at the anterior end. The paired toothed chelicerae are flanked by stout palps. The penultimate segment of the palp has a claw which can be apposed to the last segment. Posterior to the gnathosoma on the dorsal side is a chitinized plate or scutum. The shape of the scutum and the shape and disposition of the setae (usually seven) are important characters in the generic and specific identification of the larvae.

The larvae attach in clusters and start feeding on the host's tissues by partially digesting them with saliva and sucking it up. The continual feeding leads to the formation of a feeding tube or stylostome at the point of attachment. The most common sites of attachment are inside the ears of rodents and around the eyes of birds. On man they tend to attach where clothing is tight, i.e. around the waist and on the scrotum. The larvae do not burrow into the skin, nor do they feed on

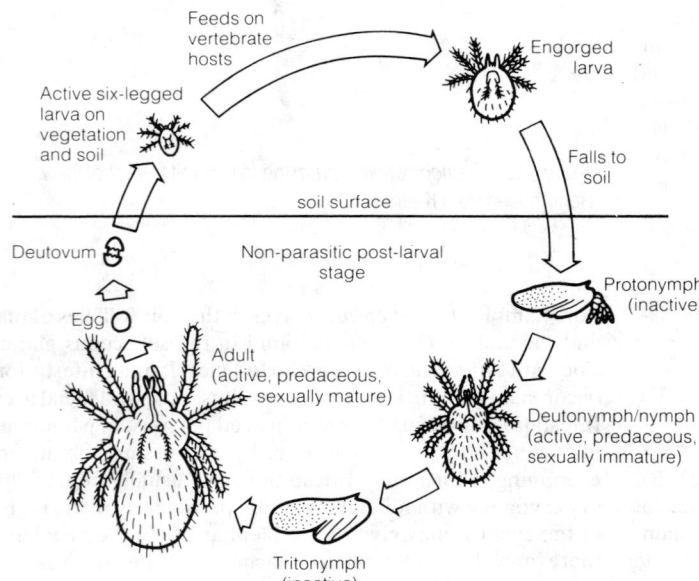

Figure IV.6   Summarized life cycle of trombiculid mites.

blood, although a few blood cells may be ingested. After feeding for several days (minimum 3 days), the larvae fall from the host and enter a quiescent stage before moulting into nymphs. The eight-legged nymphs have a figure-of-eight shape and a dense covering of red hairs which gives them a velvety appearance and the name 'velvet mites'. They are non-parasitic predators and feed on insect eggs or small inactive soil invertebrates. The nymph enters a further quiescent phase from which the adult moults. The adults are larger (about 1 mm long) than nymphs but resemble them in shape and habits. The males deposit stalked spermatophores containing sperms on the substrate and the females are inseminated by walking over them. In tropical regions the life cycle may take about 40 days and breeding occurs continuously throughout the year. In temperate regions there is usually only one generation per year and the chiggers are seasonal, during summer and early autumn.

CHIGGERS AND DERMATITIS

In parts of the world where the mites are present, persons who have been walking in vegetated areas may suffer from a severe itchy dermatitis consisting of pustules and wheals, 3–6 hours after exposure. The sudden appearance of these lesions should suggest attack by chiggers.

Neotrombicula autumnalis is the harvest mite, *'aoutat'* or *'lepte autumnal'* of Europe. The larvae normally parasitize voles, rabbits and hares as well as a ground-frequenting birds and are active in summer and early autumn; hence the name 'harvest mite'.

Eutrombicula alfreddugesi, the common American chigger, feeds readily on man and is also known as *'thalzahuatl'* and *'bicho colorado'*. It extends from continental USA to South America and is most abundant in second growth, cut-over areas. Man is frequently attacked although the usual hosts are domestic and wild animals and birds.

Eutrombicula batatas ranges from the warmer southern states of the USA to Central and South America. It is not a serious pest of man in the USA but commonly attacks man in Panama and other tropical areas of its distribution.

CHIGGERS AND SCRUB TYPHUS

The vectors of scrub typhus (caused by *Rickettsia tsutsugamushi*) are trombiculid mites. The larvae usually infest rodents (*Rattus* spp.) and insectivores which are the vertebrate reservoirs of the rickettsiae. The distribution of the mites on the ground is dependent on the home range of the hosts and, since the home ranges do not usually overlap, mite colonies have a restricted distribution and tend to be isolated from each other in the form of 'mite islands'. Man gets infected by intrusion into a rodent–mite cycle in infected 'mite islands'. Bird hosts of the larval mites can, however, disperse the mites into new areas where a fresh colony could be established.

The habits and life cycle of scrub typhus vectors are similar to that of other trombiculid mites. The parasitic larvae attack man but seldom produce any noticeable itching or skin reaction; but the bite of an infected larva can produce a lesion—the *eschar*. Since only the larvae are parasitic and feed only once, only this stage can acquire and transmit the infection. This means that trans-stadial (stage to stage, i.e. from larva to nymph to adult) and transovarial (through eggs to next generation larvae) transmission are obligatory for maintenance of the infection in nature. Trombiculid mites therefore are the main reservoirs of scrub typhus rickettsiae. In the mites, the rickettsiae eventually localize in the larval salivary glands and transmission is by bite. All the important scrub typhus vectors belong to the genus *Leptotrombidium*, although the genus *Ascoschoengastia* may be involved in transmission among rodents.

L. akamushi is the vector in the classical areas of the disease (tsutsugamushi disease) in Japan. It is found in the cultivated flood plains of rivers.

L. deliense is the main—or an important—vector over most of the distribution of the disease, from coastal Queensland in the south east through Papua New Guinea, Philippines, China, South-East Asia, Sri Lanka and India to Pakistan in the west. Over most of its range, *L. deliense* and the disease are associated with ecologically disturbed vegetation, such as secondary scrub and grass, the result of slash-and-burn cultivation of virgin forest. In South-East Asia and tropical Queensland the coarse fire-resistant kunai grass (*Imperata cylindrica*) is the typical habitat of the mite and its rodent hosts. The mites and the disease are also more likely to occur at the fringes of forests or scrub.

L. fletcheri is an important vector in Malaysia, Borneo, New Guinea and the Philippines.

Other important vectors are *L. arenicola* on sandy beaches in Malaysia, *L. pallidum* in limited areas of Japan, Korea and the Primorye region of Russia; *L. pavlovskyi* in Siberia and the Primorye region of Russia and *L. scutellare* in the Mount Fuji area of Japan.

PROTECTION AGAINST CHIGGER MITES

Personal protection is the best method of preventing attack by the mite larvae. If one has to go into mite-infested areas, impregnation of socks and trouser legs with a repellent, such as permethrin, benzyl benzoate, dimethyl phthalate (DPM) or diethyltoluamide (DEET) will prevent mite attack.

OTHER MITES OF MEDICAL IMPORTANCE

House dust mites, e.g. Dermatophagoides pteronyssinus (Family Pyroglyphidae) (Figure IV.7)

Many mite species are commonly found in house dust, in the tropics and temperate regions. These mites can, in sensitized individuals, cause bronchial asthma, as well as extensive dermatitis. In house dust they feed mainly on desquamated skin scales. The mites become airborne during bed-making and could then be inhaled; not only the living mites but also dead ones and mite faeces contain potent allergens. The best method of controlling the mites would appear to be treatment of carpets, beds and settees with insecticides, followed by thorough vacuum cleaning to remove dead mites and faeces, as these cause symptoms.

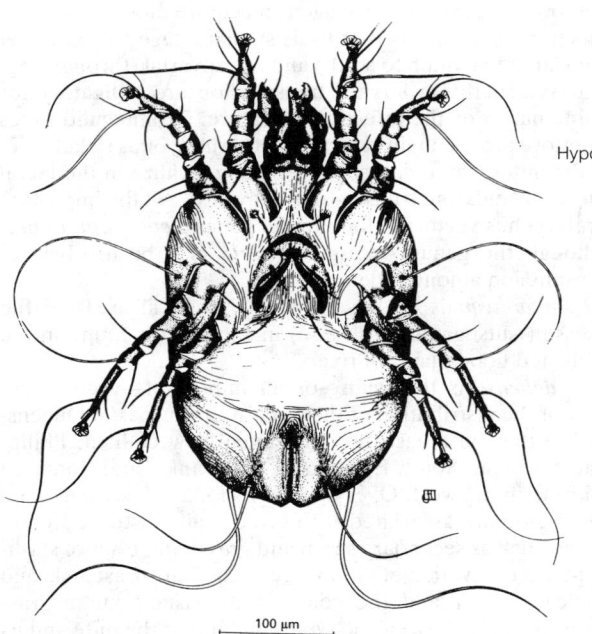

Figure IV.7   *Dermatophagoides pteronyssinus* the house dust mite. Ventral view. (Reproduced from Kettle[1].)

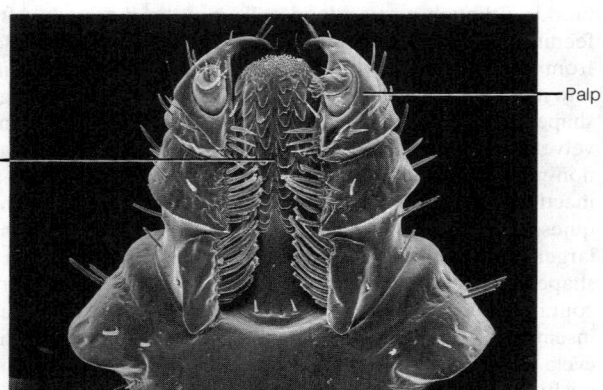

Figure IV.8   Electron micrograph view of ventral capitulum of ixodid tick. (Courtesy of M. Nawar.)

Domestic mites causing dermatosis: Dermanyssus gallinae (*chicken mite*), (*Dermanyssidae*); Ornithonyssus bacoti (*tropical rat mite*), O. sylviarum (*bird mite*) and O. bursa (*tropical poultry mite*) (*Macronyssidae*)

These blood-sucking mites can cause dermatitis in man. In the absence of their natural hosts they will readily attack man. Rat mites are associated with groceries and warehouses. Bird mites are often found in the eaves of houses and in air-conditioning ducts and may be blown into houses when the air-conditioning is switched on.

Forage mites, e.g. Tyrophagus (*Acaridae*)

These are pests of stored food products such as cheese, copra, vanilla pods, flour and macaroni. Persons handling such materials may be bitten or suffer from simple contact allergy, and various names, such as grocers' itch, copra itch and bakers' itch, indicate the occupational nature of these dermatoses. Some forage mites may be swallowed or inhaled and can cause gastric disturbances or respiratory symptoms. The mites do not breed in the body but may be recovered from faeces or sputum (see acarine dermatosis, Chapter 22).

SUBORDER: IXODIDA
SUPERFAMILY: IXODOIDEA (TICKS)

Ticks are larger (adult body length 3–20 mm) and lack the prominent hairs found on mites. All species are obligate blood-sucking ectoparasites of vertebrates. Originally parasites of reptiles, ticks adapted over the last 200 million years to the newly evolving warm-blooded bird and mammals; but some ticks have retained a predilection for cold-blooded vertebrates. The gnathosoma or capitulum is well developed and the prominent ventrally situated median hypostome bears on its underside rows of backwardly directed teeth which help the tick in attaching firmly to the host and prevent it from being easily dislodged by the grooming activities of the host (Figure IV.8).

There are two basic types of ticks: the soft ticks (Family Argasidae) and the hard ticks (Family Ixodidae). Most people are familiar with the slow-feeding ixodid ticks found on dogs, cattle and other domestic animals and which remain attached for several days. The argasids are rapid feeders, usually at night, returning quickly to their hiding places. Primarily parasites of wild animals, about 10% of tick species feed on domestic animals and many will feed opportunistically on man. The soft tick *Ornithodoros moubata* of East, Central and South Africa is probably the only true man-biting tick; it is found in huts and feeds readily on man and chickens. Ticks parasitize a wide range of wild and domestic hosts and many appear to have a preferred host, although this apparent preference may be due to availability rather than choice. Both male and female adult ticks ingest considerable quantities of blood: a fully engorged female ixodid may reach a length of over 20 mm and weigh 2.0 g or more. Because of this, they threaten the health of domestic livestock with very heavy infestations. Control of veterinary pest species with insecticides is being superseded by the development of anti-tick vaccines. Apart from causing blood loss, ticks transmit a variety of pathogens among animals and are therefore important in veterinary medicine. However, because of their indiscriminate feeding habits, ticks acquire infection from animals and transmit it to man during the next blood feed.

Movement of tick-infested animals, particularly of domestic livestock, has resulted in the introduction and establishment of exotic tick species in new areas. The cosmopolitan dog tick *Rhipicephalus sanguineus* is a carnivore parasite from Africa, now a worldwide parasite found in kennels and households. Many tick-borne diseases exist as silent foci where the pathogen, vertebrate host (usually a wild animal) and the tick have evolved to form a balanced relationship. Human population increase and economic pressure have led to ecological changes brought about by clearance of forests

Table IV.1 Differences between argasid ticks and ixodid ticks.

	Argasidae	*Ixodidae*
Morphology		
Scutum	Absent	Present; anterior in larva, nymph and female, covering dorsal side in male
Capitulum	Ventral, not visible from above	Anterior, visible from above
Palps	Long, movable	Short, rigid
Life cycle	Several nymphal stages	One nymphal stage
	Multiple batches of eggs: 100–200 per blood meal	One batch of eggs (several 1000)
Habits	Rapid feeders, usually nocturnal; male and female feed repeatedly	Slow feeders, day and night, several days; only females feed once
	Restricted habitat, burrows or nests of hosts	Diffuse habitat, pasture, etc., where hosts forage

for cultivation, or the growing of cash crops. The intrusion of man into such tick-infested areas and suburban encroachment into tick habitats with silent foci of infection have resulted in closer tick–man contact and an increase in the incidence of tick-transmitted diseases such as Rocky Mountain spotted fever in the eastern USA, tick-borne encephalitis in Europe, and the emergence of apparently 'new' diseases in man such as Kyasanur Forest disease in India and Lyme disease in the USA and Europe.

There are several factors which make ticks efficient vectors of pathogenic organisms. Firm attachment to the host prevents them from being easily dislodged. The slow feeding of ixodids not only gives them ample time to ingest large numbers of pathogens from an infected host and ample time to transmit them to a new host, but also allows dispersal of infected ticks into new areas while still attached to a host. The multiple blood feeds during the life cycle and the wide host range ensure more opportunities to acquire and transmit infections, and makes a blood meal more certain. Many ixodids have a high reproductive potential, laying several thousands of eggs, but this is to offset the very considerable mortality during the life cycle. Some argasids can live for many years and starve for prolonged periods. This is of great survival value and gives them more opportunities to acquire and transmit pathogens during their long life. Transovarial transmission of many pathogens in ticks makes them true reservoirs of infection and some tick-borne infections can be maintained in nature in the absence of vertebrate hosts by transovarial passage through several generations of ticks.

The Argasidae has about 150 species in three genera, of which *Argas* and *Ornithodoros* are the most important. The Ixodidae has about 800 species in 13 genera, of which *Ixodes*, *Amblyomma*, *Hyalomma*, *Haemaphysalis*, *Dermacentor* and *Rhipicephalus* transmit diseases to man, and *Boophilus* cattle ticks are important ectoparasites of domestic livestock. Morphological and biological differences which distinguish the two families are summarized in Table IV.1.

FAMILY: ARGASIDAE

Tough, leathery ticks, with the females ranging in size from small (4 mm) to large (15 mm); the males are smaller but otherwise very similar. In nymphs and adults the capitulum is ventral and not visible from above; in larvae, the capitulum projects anteriorly. The jointed palps are long and movable and in some species may be mistaken for an extra pair of legs. The surface of the integument is covered with mammillae or radially arranged depressions and discs, but the dorsal plate or scutum, characteristic of the Ixodidae is absent (Figure IV.9); hence the name 'soft ticks'. Eyes, when present, are simple and situated laterally. Spiracles or breaching holes are present ventrally between the first segments (coxae) of the third and fourth pairs of legs. The genital opening is anterior and ventral, behind the capitulum, and the anal opening median and about a third of the distance from the posterior margin. Between the first and second pairs of legs are the external openings of the coxal glands which help to concentrate the blood meal by filtering off fluid from the blood and excreting it as two drops of coxal fluid. In many *Ornithodoros* vectors of relapsing fever and arboviruses the coxal glands are infected. Coxal fluid is excreted just before termination of a feed and pathogens in the fluid enter the bite wound. The glands therefore have an important role in disease transmission (Figures IV.10 and IV.11).

Argasids are rapid feeders, the larvae of some species taking only 2–3 minutes to engorge, those of the genus *Argas* remaining attached to their hosts for several days. The six-legged larvae feed once; larvae of *Ornithodoros* do not feed but moult straight into nymphs. Soft ticks are usually nocturnal feeders and the house-haunting *O. moubata* are not unlike bed bugs in their feeding and sheltering habits. Habitats of other Argasids include cracks and crevices in wood, stone or mud, nesting or resting places of the host animals, birds' nests in trees or on the ground, caves, burrows, deer beds, huts, log cabins, chicken coops, pigeon lofts, sheds and pig sties. Access to a blood meal is therefore easy and the hazards in host finding considerably reduced. There are 2–5 or more nymphal stages; each stage feeds once and moults to the next stage. Adults mate off the host. Both males and females feed repeatedly, the females ovipositing after each

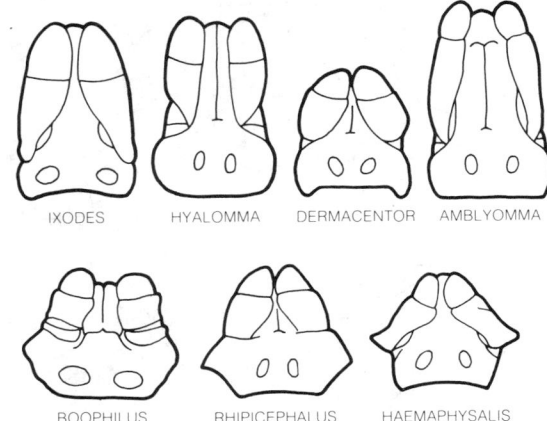

Figure IV.9 Dorsal view of capitulum of Ixodidae, showing characteristics of seven genera.

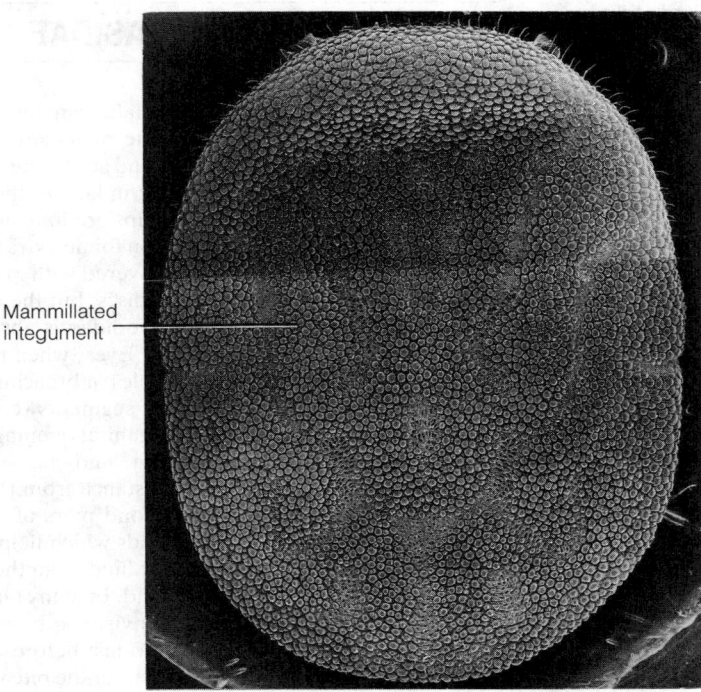

Figure IV.10 Dorsal view of adult female
Ornithodoros moubata.
(Courtesy of M. Nawar.)

blood meal, laying a batch of 100–200 eggs (Figure IV.12). The genera *Argas* and *Ornithodoros* can be separated by the distinct flattened lateral margin of the body in *Argas*, which is evident even when the tick is fully fed.

Argas spp. feed on birds or bats and may attack man, causing painful bites. *Ornithodoros* spp. transmit *Borrelia* spp. spirochaetes causing relapsing fever in man (Table IV.2 and see Chapter 55). Foci of infection are usually restricted in caves, animal shelters, huts or resort cabins. There is a high rate of trans-stadial and transovarial transmission of *Borrelia* among ticks; this and the longevity and ability of the vector to starve for long periods lead to the perpetuation of natural foci

in the absence of vertebrate hosts. Ticks are the main reservoirs of infection, while other animals, such as rodents, probably serve only as amplifiers of infection. Following an infecting feed, the ticks have a disseminated infection of practically all the internal organs. Transmission is usually through salivary secretion containing *Borrelia* and/or contamination of the bite wound through infective coxal fluid.

Ornithodoros moubata, the 'eyeless' tampan tick, transmits relapsing fever (*Borrelia duttoni*) in tropical Africa. The integument is mamillated and greenish-brown. The absence of eyes distinguishes this species from the closely related and widely distributed sand tampan, *O. savignyi*, which has two pairs of eyes on the sides of the body. Both species are night feeders. *O. moubata* inhabits the floor of huts, animal shelters and the burrows of wart-hogs. There are two subspecies: *O. moubata moubata* feeds predominantly on man and

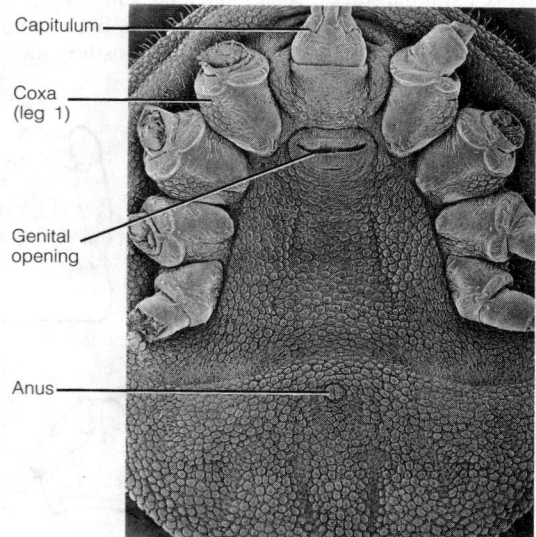

Figure IV.11 Ventral view of adult female *Ornithodoros moubata.*
(Courtesy of M. Nawar.)

A

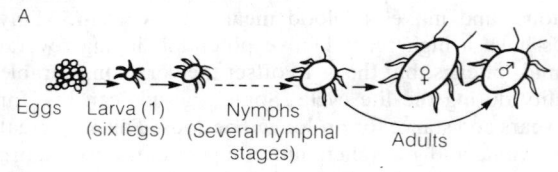

B

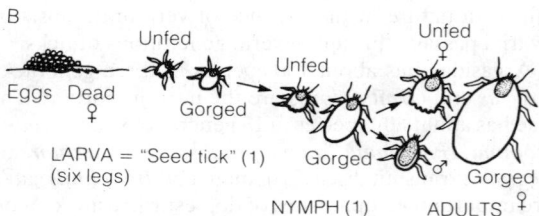

Figure IV.12 Tick life cycles: A, Argasidae; B, Ixodidae.

Table IV.2 Human tick-borne relapsing fever: *Borrelia* spirochaetes and the *Ornithodoros* vectors which transmit them.

Tick vector	Spirochaete	Locality
O. moubata	B. duttoni	E., C. & S. Africa
O. erraticus	B. hispanica	W. Mediterranean, North Africa
O. tholozani	B. persica	E. Mediterranean eastwards through central Asia to western China
O. turicata	B. turicatae	USA, Mexico
O. parkeri	B. parkeri	N., C. & S.
O. hermsi	B. hermsii	America
O. rudis	B. venezuelensis	
O. talajae		
O. turicata		

chickens; *O. m. porcinus* on wart-hogs, antbears and porcupines. In the cool wet habitats of the Kenya highlands and north-west Tanzania, 94% of *O. m. moubata* feed on man and 2% on chickens, but in hot moist habitats these percentages are reversed. Both subspecies have domestic and wild populations and it is the domestic populations which are important in disease transmission; no infected ticks have been found in wild populations. *O. moubata* is common on travel routes and may be carried long distances in mats and bed rolls. Rest houses are usually infested. To prevent the risk of infection with relapsing fever old camping sites and mud houses should be avoided and it is advisable not to sleep on the floor. Since the ticks find shelter in cracks and crevices in mud walls and floors, better housing and the use of concrete and plaster in buildings will help to control the ticks. They can also be controlled by treating the floors and walls of huts with insecticidal powder or spray.

O. savignyi, the eyed or sand tampan, is widely distributed in arid and semi-arid areas from Sri Lanka westwards through India, Arabia, and Africa, where the distributions of *O. savignyi* and *O. moubata* overlap. It is an outdoor tick found near the soil surface in the resting places of cattle, camels and other livestock in the shade of trees and stone fences. It will attack man—given the opportunity, and can transmit relapsing fever in the laboratory.

O. erraticus occurs in north-west Africa, Spain and Portugal. It usually lives in burrows feeding on rodents but considerable populations exist in pig sties where they feed on pigs. It is an important vector of relapsing fever (*B. hispanica*) in north-west Africa and Spain.

O. tholozani (=*O. papillipes*) has a widespread distribution: Libya, north-east Africa, the Mediterranean islands, northern Arabia, south-eastern Europe, southern CIS, northern India and western provinces of China. It is an important vector of relapsing fever (*B. persica*). Typical habitats are caves and large burrows but the tick has successfully adapted to stables and rest houses. *O. tholozani* feeds on domestic livestock, birds and man.

O. lahorensis occurs in Tibet, southern CIS Republics, Pakistan, Turkey, Greece, the Balkans and Bulgaria. It is found in stables and human habitations and is suspected of transmitting relapsing fever.

O. talaje is a South and Central American species extending northwards to the southern states of the USA. It feeds on wild rodents and domestic livestock as well as man, inflicts a very painful bite and transmits relapsing fever in Guatemala, Panama and Colombia.

O. rudis (=*O. venezuelensis*) transmits *B. venezuelensis* in Panama, Colombia, Venezuela and Ecuador. It usually lives in the walls of huts and will feed avidly on man.

O. hermsi is widespread in the Rocky Mountain and Pacific coast states of the USA. It is essentially a rodent parasite. It shelters in summer cabins at higher elevations and transmits relapsing fever (*B. hermsi*) to people occupying the cabins.

O. parkeri and *O. turicata* have similar distributions in the western USA and the range of *O. turicata* extends southwards into Mexico. They feed primarily on rodents and are vectors of relapsing fever (*B. parkeri* and *B. turicatae* respectively) to man.

O. coriaceus extends from California to Mexico. Known as the 'tlaaja' and the 'pajaroello' it is a large argasid, notorious for attacking humans, cattle and deer in their bedding areas. The bites are painful, but it is not a natural vector of relapsing fever.

O. rostratus, the 'quanco', occurs in southern Brazil, Bolivia, Paraguay and north-eastern Argentina. It is an avid biter of man, domestic animals and wild animals, particularly peccaries. The bites are painful and pruritus and inflammation follow, which may become secondarily infected. It is not a natural vector of relapsing fever.

O. muesebecki is associated with marine birds on islands in the Arabian Gulf. The tick eagerly attacks humans and some dexterity is required to avoid being bitten. The bites may be numerous, and irritant bullae develop at the bite sites with intense pruritus, headache and fever. Zirqa virus (Bunyaviridae, Nairovirus) isolated from *O. muesebecki* may be the cause of the illness associated with the bites.

FAMILY: IXODIDAE

Hard ticks are readily distinguished from soft ticks by the presence of the prominent capitulum, projecting anteriorly, visible from above in all stages (Figure IV.13a). The mouthparts of some (*Ixodes* and *Amblyomma*) are long and can produce deep penetrating wounds in animals and man (Figure IV.13b). The shape of the basal plate of the capitulum is an important character in generic identification (see Figure IV.9). The hard shiny scutum is present in all stages, small and restricted to the anterior dorsum in larvae, nymphs and adults, but large and covering the entire dorsal surface in males. The scutum of some ixodids, e.g. *Amblyomma* spp., has a colourful pattern: such ticks are called *ornate* ticks; those in which the scutum is not ornamented are called *inornate* ticks. Paired eyes, when present, are situated on either side of the scutum. Coxal glands are absent in ixodid ticks and the ingested blood is concentrated during the slow feeding by passage of fluid from the stomach into the body cavity, from where it is processed through the salivary glands back into the host. During their slow feeding, ixodid ticks remain attached for several days, anchoring themselves firmly with the chelicerae and hypostome, helped by 'cement' from the salivary glands. Once attached, great care should be taken in removing a tick because the mouthparts may be left

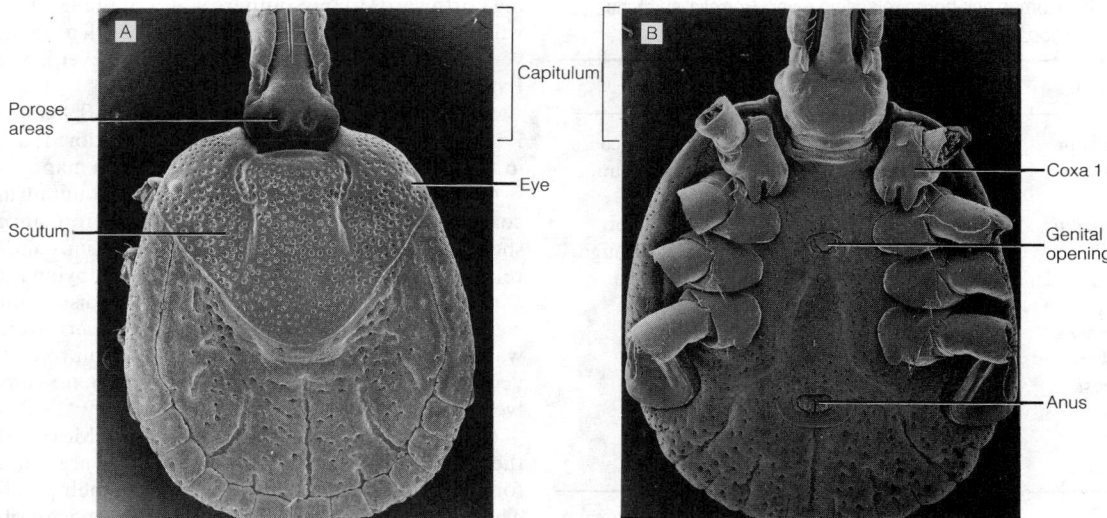

Figure IV.13 Dorsal (A) and ventral (B) views of *Amblyomma variegatum*. (Courtesy of M. Nawar.)

behind in the host tissue and may become a source of irritation and secondary infection.

A few ticks (e.g. *Boophilus* cattle ticks) are host-specific, but most utilize a wide range of hosts. Adult ixodids usually parasitize large mammals, while the immature stages (larvae and nymphs) feed on smaller mammals such as rodents and ground frequenting birds. Man is seldom bitten by the adult ticks, but the larvae or 'seed ticks' of some ixodids feed avidly on man and are a bothersome nuisance in some outdoor areas in America and Africa.

The life cycle of Ixodidae has four stages (see Figure IV.12): the egg, followed by three mobile stage larva, nymph and adult. The fertilized and engorged female drops off the host on to the ground and lays a mass of several thousand eggs. The female dies after oviposition. The six-legged larvae after hatching climb to the tips of leaves, blades of grass or other vegetation to certain heights and gather in clusters questing for a host. They climb on to a passing host, feed for 4–6 days, drop to the ground and moult to the nymphal stage. Unlike the argasid ticks, ixodids have only one nymphal stage. The unfed nymphs quest for hosts like the larvae and after a blood meal (5–8 days) drop to the ground and moult into adults. Adults quest usually at a height greater than that of larvae and nymphs. Mating takes place on the host and the engorged female, after feeding for 6–12 days, drops off to lay a single batch of eggs.

The males may remain attached to the host for many weeks or months, mating with several females. The whole life cycle may take only 2–4 months in warm climates, with continuous breeding throughout the year. In cold or temperate climates the life cycle may take 3–5 years, the ticks being active or developing only in the warmer months. During the colder months and winter, one or more stages enter a diapause of several weeks or months. The parasitic feeding period of the different stages lasts from 4 to 12 days. Most ixodid ticks (e.g. *Amblyomma*, *Dermacentor*, *Ixodes* have a three-host cycle in which each active stage (larva, nymph, adult) parasitizes a different animal of the same or different species. *Boophilus* cattle ticks have only a one-host cycle. A few species of *Hyalomma* and *Rhipicephalus* have a two-host cycle: the fed larva moults on the host (not on the ground) becoming a

nymph which drops to the ground, moults to adulthood and then seeks a second host for a blood meal.

Ixodes scapularis (=*I. dammini*) (American deer tick) is widely distributed in the USA and adjacent Canada; the range appears to be extending, probably due to proliferation of deer, hosts of the adult ticks. Larvae and nymphs parasitize rodents (particularly the white-footed mouse) as well as man. The adult ticks mostly feed on white-tailed deer, or occasionally on man. *I. scapularis* is the vector of human babesiosis (*Babesia microti*) and of Lyme disease (a spirochaetal infection caused by *Borrelia burgdorferi*) in the eastern USA.

I. ricinus (European sheep tick or castor bean tick) is widely distributed in rough pasture and woodland across Europe to the Caspian Sea and northern Iran. *I. ricinus* is the vector of three human flaviviruses: louping ill (primarily of sheep and cattle but affecting man also) in the British Isles (see Chapter 38), tick-borne viral encephalitis (TBE) in central Europe, and Lyme disease (*Borrelia burgdorferi*) (see Chapter 55), which is becoming increasingly widespread in areas with deer populations as hosts for adult *I. ricinus*. Immature ticks are found on rodents and birds; adults attack deer, sheep, cattle and also man. The life cycle takes 2–4 years to complete.

I. persulcatus (the taiga tick) is widepread from the Baltic to Japan, its distribution overlapping with *I. ricinus*. It is more cold-hardy than *I. ricinus*. In Russia, *I. persulcatus* is associated with the taiga forest. The life cycle extends over 2–4 years. It is the chief vector of Russian spring–summer encephalitis (flavivirus). Transovarial transmission occurs but the rate is variable.

I. holocyclus occurs in the humid densely vegetated coastal areas of Queensland and New South Wales in Australia where it infests a variety of mammalian hosts. Its bites may cause tick paralysis in dogs and man. It is the vector of Queensland tick typhus (*Rickettsia australis*).

Haemaphysalis spinigera occurs in Sri Lanka and south India, most abundantly where cattle have been introduced into cleared forests. It is the chief vector of Kyasanur Forest disease (flavivirus). Immatures feed on small forest rodents, monkeys and man. Exposure of humans to the ticks and risk of infection are highest in the dry premonsoon period when villagers go into the forest to gather firewood. Transmission of infection to man is by bite by infected nymphs. There is no transovarial transmission in vector ticks.

H. leachi is widespread on carnivores. In South Africa urban cases of boutonneuse fever (*Rickettsia conori*) are associated with contamination of skin or of eyes from infected ticks crushed while de-ticking dogs.

Rhipicephalus appendiculatus parasitizes cattle and wild game animals in wooded and shrubby grassland from southern Sudan to South Africa but is absent from West Africa. In east Africa it is the vector of the protozoan disease East Coast fever (babesiosis) in cattle. In the South African veld it is the chief vector of African tick typhus (*Rickettsia*) and an avid man biter.

R. sanguineus is a carnivore tick originating from Africa but now a cosmopolitan tick of dogs. In the Mediterranean basin it is the chief vector of boutonneuse fever to man.

Dermacentor andersoni (Rocky Mountain wood tick) is widespread in the western USA and Canada, where it transmits Rocky Mountain spotted fever (*Rickettsia rickettsi*). Larvae and nymphs feed on practically every rodent; adults parasitize wild and domestic herbivores and eagerly bite man. Transmission of the rickettsiae is by bite, and trans-stadial and transovarial transmission occur. There may be an interval of some hours or a day before the attached tick can transmit the rickettsiae. If the tick is removed within a few hours the risk of infection is considerably reduced. This tick also transmits Colorado tick fever virus to man.

D. variabilis (American dog tick) occurs from Mexico to Canada, being particularly abundant along the east coast of the USA. Immatures feed on rodents, adults on wild and domestic carnivores, including dogs and also man. It is the vector of Rocky Mountain spotted fever in the eastern USA. Infestation of dogs with *D. variabilis* brings the disease close to homes and infections occur among women and children.

D. marginatus, *D. silvarum* and *D. nuttalli* are the chief vectors of Siberian tick typhus (*Rickettsia sibirica*). *D. margi-natus* is found in shrubby areas and lowland forests from northern Kazakstan to central Europe. *D. silvarum* extends from the eastern limits of *D. marginatus* to western Siberia. *D. nuttalli* is widely distributed in central and eastern Siberia, Mongolia and China southwards to central Asia and Tibet. *R. sibirica* can survive for long periods in the ticks. Transmission is by bite and both trans-stadial and transovarial transmission have been demonstrated.

D. pictus has the same distribution as *D. marginatus* in mixed and deciduous forests. Omsk haemorrhagic fever arbovirus has been isolated from it, but transmission to man is believed to be by contact with, or drinking water infected with, the urine and faeces of musk-rats.

Amblyomma hebraeum (the South African bont tick) extends from South Africa and Zimbabwe and Mozambique. It is the vector of boutonneuse fever in the South African veld where immatures swarm and feed avidly on humans. *Rickettsia conori* can be maintained for several generations in *A. hebraeum* by hereditary transmission. Apart from man, immature stages feed on birds and small and large mammals, while adults feed on large wild and domestic mammals.

A. americanum (lone-star tick) is widely distributed from South America into central and eastern USA. All stages attack man. It is the vector of Rocky Mountain spotted fever in the USA. The attached feeding ticks are difficult to remove because of the long mouth-parts. Application of 0.6% pyrethrin in methyl benzoate or of camphorated phenol to the skin makes detachment easier.

A. cajennense (Cayenne tick) extends from South America and the Caribbean to southern Texas. Immatures attack man. It is the vector of Rocky Mountain spotted fever to man in Mexico, Panama, Colombia and Brazil.

Hyalomma marginatum is a hardy tick adapted to living under arid or semi-arid conditions in Eurasia. Birds are important hosts of the immature stages and the ticks have been carried to many parts of Europe and Africa by migrating birds. It is the vector of Crimean–Congo haemorrhagic fever arbovirus.

PENTASTOMIDS
J. Riley

Pentastomids, sometimes called linguatulids or 'tongue worms', possess arthropod-like characters and there is evidence to suggest that they may be highly specialized endoparasitic crustaceans.[2] Four species, belonging to two genera, may affect man as dead-end infections: *Linguatula*, which normally infects other mammals, and *Armillifer*, which infects snakes and mammals as intermediate hosts.

FAMILY: LINGUATULIDAE

Linguatula serrata is found worldwide. The adults live in the nasal passages of dogs, foxes and wolves (family Canidae) which are the definitive hosts. Eggs are expelled by sneezing or in nasal discharges, or via the intestine where some premature hatching may occur. Eggs are infective to mammal intermediate hosts, including rodents and domestic animals such as sheep and goats. Primary larvae emerge, penetrate the gut wall and migrate to the viscera, particularly to the mesenteric lymph nodes, where they become encapsulated by host tissue. Within the cyst several moults eventually lead to the formation of an infective larva or nymph. Infection of the definitive host occurs when viscera containing the encysted infective stage are eaten. The epidemiology of *L. serrata* infections is complex, because both eggs and infective larvae can become established in man. When eggs are consumed, primary larvae encyst in the viscera, producing visceral linguatulosis, whereas ingested infective larvae attempt to migrate to the nasal passages producing nasopharyngeal linguatulosis or halzoun (Chapter 73).

The body of adult *Linguatula* (Figure IV.14) is club-shaped, flattened ventrally, convex dorsally and transversely

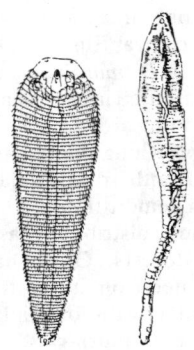

Figure IV.14 Linguatula serrata. Left, Nymph (6×). Right, Adult (natural size).

striated into about 90 superficial annulations. The cephalothorax bears the quadrangular mouth, which is flanked by two pairs of simple retractile hooks. Females are 80–130 mm in length, tapering from 8–10 mm anteriorly to 2 mm posteriorly. The uterine coils, full of reddish-brown eggs, occupy the median line of the body and the translucent flared lateral extensions of the anterior abdomen mould to the contours of the nasal sinuses. Living males are transparent in life but become white when fixed, measure 18–27 mm long and 3 mm broad anteriorly to 0.5 mm posteriorly. The oval eggs, measuring $70 \times 100\,\mu m$ are loosely enveloped by a thin hyaline outer capsule and contain mature primary larvae which have an anterior penetration stylet and four stumpy legs terminating in double claws. Infective nymphs (Figure IV.14) are worm-like, flattened and 4–6 mm in length; the posterior edge of each body annulus carries a row of prominent backward pointing spines which are sufficient to distinguish *Linguatula* spp. in tissue section.

Clinical effects (halzoun; marrara syndrome)
(see Chapter 73)

Encysted infective nymphs are well tolerated and are frequently encountered in the mesenteric glands of domestic animals, as well as in rabbits and hares. Data on human infections arise only from incidental findings during autopsy and in the few instances where sample sizes were large nymphs were not uncommon.[3] Nymphs developing on visceral organs cause no symptoms but occasionally they penetrate the anterior chamber of the eye, causing monocular uveitis. Following surgical removal of these parasites patients recover fully.

In tissue sections, infective larvae of *Linguatula* are enclosed within a thin fibrotic capsule lined by the preceding cast nymphal cuticle. The spinous cuticle is distinctive and the spacious body cavity contains an obvious intestinal tract flanked by a pair of prominent glands composed of large individual gland cells. These characteristics will serve to distinguish them from sparganum (Appendix III).

FAMILY: ARMILLIFERIDAE

Armillifer armillatus infects humans in tropical Africa. In Oriental regions *A. moniliformis* is the usual cause of human infection, which has been recorded from Malaysia, Java, Manila, Sumatra and China.

Adult parasites inhabit the lungs of pythons, and in Africa large vipers; the larval forms encyst in the tissues of many mammal species, including monkeys and man. The parasite is cylindrical, vermiform, yellowish and translucent with conspicuous opaque annulated rings around the body, 1–2 mm apart (Figure IV.15). In females the uterine coils, filled with white or yellowish eggs, are easily visible through the cuticle. The female of *A. armillatus* is 70–140 mm long and 5–9 mm wide, the male 30–50 mm long and 3–4 mm wide: females possess up to 22 annuli and males up to 24. Both sexes of *A. moniliformis* are more slender and have more annuli (26 and above) than *A. armillatus*. The nymphs lie coiled within their cysts in a flat spiral, with the ventral surface corresponding to the convexity of the curve. In shape and structure they resemble the adult. A third species of *Armillifer* (*A. grandis*) has been reported from man in central Africa where nymphs are smaller (9–15 mm long) than those of *A. armillatus* (13–23 mm long): *A. moniliformis* nymphs are intermediate in size (12–20 mm).

The life-history of *Armillifer* is broadly similar to that of *Linguatula*, although man can act only as an intermediate host. Eggs remain viable on soil for at least 3 months and, when ingested, hatch in the intestine and the larvae immediately bore through the intestinal wall to lodge in any tissue. At least six moults occur over a period of 6 months to a year to form infective nymphs. Man acquires the infection by eating poorly cooked snake meat, or by drinking water contaminated by snake faeces. In man the infection comes to a dead end and the nymphs commonly encyst in or on the liver, intestinal tract and lungs.

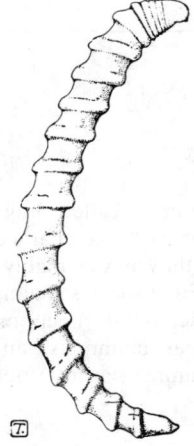

Figure IV.15 Armillifer armillatus (natural size).

FLIES CAUSING MYIASIS
G. B. White

CLASS: INSECTA; ORDER: DIPTERA (TWO-WINGED FLIES)

Myiasis covers a variety of associations between dipterous larvae and mammals. The most comprehensive definition is 'the infestation of live human and vertebrate animals with dipterous larvae which, at least for a certain period, feed on the host's dead or living tissue, liquid body-substance, or ingested food'.[111] Such associations vary from complete endoparasitism, via casual or accidental myiasis, to the bizarre predation on human blood by free-living larvae. A wide range of families of flies are involved, mostly 'higher flies' (Cyclorrhapha) of which the larvae are either specialized endoparasites in other mammals or are scavengers and carrion feeders.

Myiasis can be classified on the basis of either clinical or parasitological criteria. From a medical standpoint the clinical classification is more important as it aids diagnosis and identification of the species responsible. Parasitological classification, based on the host–parasite relationship, assists in understanding the biological background and hence possible methods of prevention or control. Whilst a single incident can be remedied (e.g. by surgical removal) and the larva identified, prevention of further attacks relies on a knowledge of the insects' biology.

Myiasis in man concerns a few common flies (e.g. *Cordylobia*, *Dermatobia*, *Chrysomya*) and a large number of uncommon or rare examples. Numerous cases of myiasis have been published in which the identification of the larva responsible is doubtful.

Clinically, myiasis-producing larvae attack three main parts of the body.

1 Cutaneous tissue, usually invading wounds or sores, producing furuncles, roving swellings or creeping myiasis. 'Sanguinivorous larvae' of the Congo floor maggot (*A. luteola*) are free-living (see Chapter 79).
2 Body cavities such as the nasopharynx, eyes and auditory canal.
3 Organs of the body, principally the gut lumen and urogenital system.

Parasitologically, myiasis producers can be divided into three other categories.

1 Obligate parasites: larvae develop in living tissue; they are unable to develop elsewhere. Larvae are endoparasitic, avoiding the host's immune system. The adults do not normally feed.
2 Facultative myiasis producers, whose larvae usually develop on carrion but may invade wounds. Primary flies initiate myiasis (e.g. *Cochliomyia hominivorax*); secondary flies enter the body only when an animal has prior infestation (e.g. *Cochliomyia macellaria*); tertiary flies become involved at a late stage of necrosis (e.g. many carrion-breeding blowflies).[1]
3 Accidental myiasis producers, whose eggs or larvae are accidentally ingested and are not killed in the intestine.

Larvae causing myiasis are essentially hydrostatic bags against which the muscles work to produce movement. The cephalopharyngeal skeleton has a pair of mouth-hooks to tear at the host's tissues, and a structure to anchor the muscles operating the mouth-hooks. They do not have a recognizable head capsule (except *Psychoda*). The overall shape of the larvae varies from the wedge shape of blow flies (*Calliphora*, *Lucilia*, etc.), through the ovoid tumbu fly (*Cordylobia anthropophaga*) to the pyriform *Dermatobia hominis*. There is often a change of shape during larval development. Some species possess rows of hooks or spines to prevent their expulsion from the host. The distribution and shape of such spines, together with details of the spiracles and cephalopharyngeal skeleton, are used to identify the different species.

MYIASIS OF CUTANEOUS TISSUE
(see Chapter 79)

1 Larvae living in the skin and producing furuncles

These are usually specially adapted endoparasites and are the most commonly encountered by clinicians. Antibiotic prophylaxis is advisable before attempting to remove myiasis larvae from their lesions.

Cordylobia anthropophaga (Figure IV.16) (the African tumbu fly, mango fly or ver du cayor) is a large, robust, yellow-brown fly, 7–12 mm long. Adults of *C. anthropophaga* are difficult to distinguish from numerous other species of the family Calliphoridae, where the larva can be identified by its posterior spiracles (Figure IV.17B).[112]

C. anthropophaga is an obligate parasite found throughout Africa south of the Sahara, although some areas are free from the fly. As a result of air travel, people infested with *C. anthropophaga* arrive in many parts of the world. Recently this species was recorded from a patient in southern Spain who had never visited Africa, thus indicating that it might be possible for *C. anthropophaga* to establish foci outside endemic areas. Adults are active early morning and late afternoon and can be found resting in dark places—huts etc.

The white, banana-shaped eggs of *C. anthropophaga* are

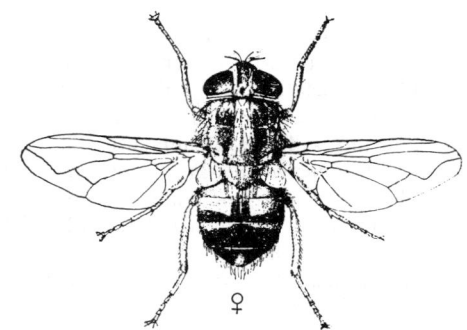

Figure IV.16   Cordylobia anthropophaga (twice natural size).

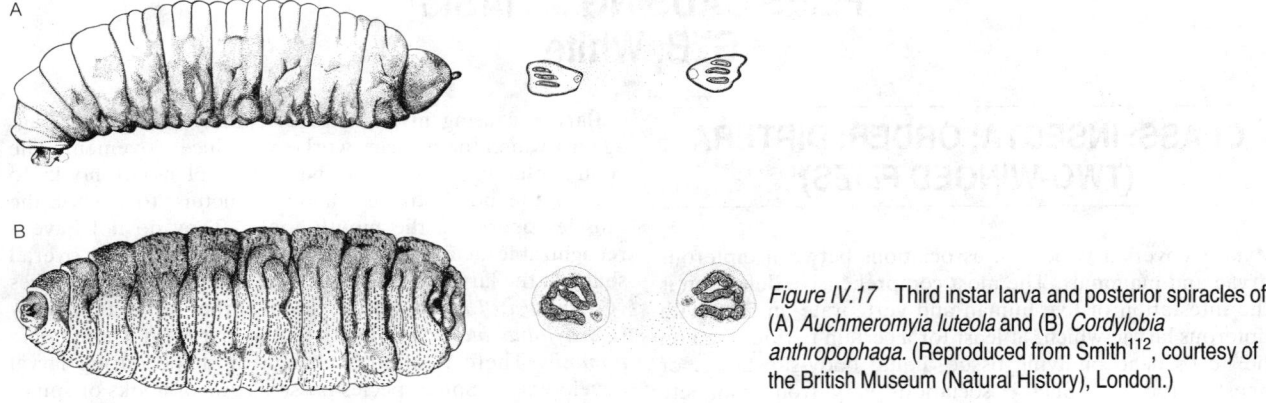

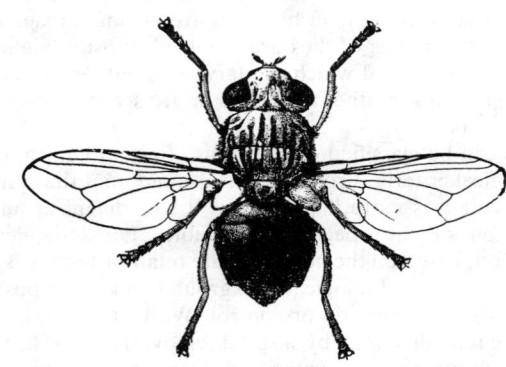

Figure IV.17   Third instar larva and posterior spiracles of (A) *Auchmeromyia luteola* and (B) *Cordylobia anthropophaga*. (Reproduced from Smith[112], courtesy of the British Museum (Natural History), London.)

laid in two batches of 100–300. The female preferentially oviposits on sandy ground, particularly if contaminated with urine or faeces, but can also lay on clothing if similarly contaminated (although such clothing may appear clean to the human eye). Clothing laid on the ground to dry may be affected, but not clothes hanging in bright sunlight since the eggs are laid only in shaded areas. Eggs are not laid directly on to skin, hairs or vegetation. On hatching, the minute first instar larvae hold themselves erect, while waving the anterior part in search of a host, and can remain alive without food for about 9 days. Larvae are sensitive to both heat and vibration and, once they become attached to a host, immediately begin to penetrate the unbroken skin, taking approximately 1 minute. Penetration is usually painless and may involve any part of the body, particularly the back, neck and head of man. Larvae are acquired from lying on the ground or from clothing. They are more common in children. *Cordylobia* breeds all the year round but human cases are more common in the wet season.

Initially, the small papule containing the larva of *C. anthropophaga* may be itchy or pricking at intervals. As the papule increases in size the symptoms recur and may be painful enough to interfere with sleep. Serous fluid may be exuded and gland enlargement may occur, or even febrile reactions and malaise. The larvae are usually noticed when the third stage has been reached. During the time the larva is in the host (which lasts 8–12 days) it has its posterior segment, bearing the respiratory spiracles, protruding from the aperture which can be withdrawn when touched. The cavity containing the larva breaks down to form a swelling, resembling a boil, which bursts without much inflammation. Larvae emerge from the swellings, fall to the ground and pupate within 24 hours. Pupal cases are commonly found in holes of black or brown rats which, together with dogs, are the principal hosts other than man. The adult fly hatches 10–20 days (according to temperature) after pupation.

Larvae can be extracted by manipulation, if mature, or by inducing them to exit of their own accord by covering their respiratory aperture with petroleum jelly. The larvae die when covered with adhesive dressing. To prevent infestation, clothes should be ironed on both sides before wearing and should be hung indoors for drying with the windows closed or screened to exclude the adult flies.

Dermatobia hominis (the American human bot fly, ver macaque, Berne, el tórsalo, beefworm) (Figure IV.18) is widely distributed in the Americas, from Mexico to Argentina and Chile. It attacks a wide range of hosts, including

Figure IV.18   Female *Dermatobia hominis* (twice natural size).

fowls, and is a devastating pest of livestock in some areas. The adult is a large bluish-grey fly, 1.5 cm long with a strong flight. *D. hominis* is primarily found on the edge of tropical forests, particularly hilly areas of secondary forest 160–3000 m above sea level.

D. hominis is remarkable for the unique manner of delivering eggs to a new host, by using other insects as carriers. The adult female *Dermatobia* catches and firmly holds a day-flying mosquito or muscoid fly and attaches up to 30 eggs on to its abdomen (Figure IV.19). The larva remains in the egg shell until it senses proximity to a warm-blooded host, whereupon it rapidly 'hatches' and penetrates the host's skin in 5–10 minutes, remaining at the site of penetration. Each larva penetrates individually and a small nodule develops around it with a central pore through which the larva breathes. Close examination of a lesion containing a larva will reveal its posterior end bearing two small dark brown spots which are the spiracles. The first instar is subcylindrical with circlets of small spines. The second stage (Figure IV.20) is pyriform, with stronger, stout spines on the globular portion and none on the narrow posterior part, which acts like a respiratory siphon. At this stage the larva is difficult to dislodge by virtue of its shape and the numerous concentric rows of backward projecting spines. During larval life the wound continually oozes serous fluid or pus but bacteriostatic activity in the gut of the larva seems to prevent undesirable overgrowth of pyogenic bacteria in its environment,[113] although in some cases secondary infection does occur.

The duration of larval development of *D. hominis* in man is 6–12 weeks, during which it grows slowly, feeding on tissue

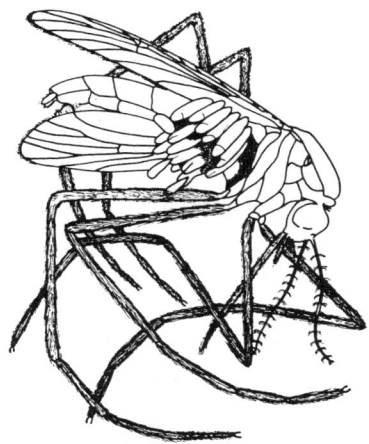

Figure IV.19 The mosquito *Psorophora lutzi* carrying eggs of *Dermatobia hominis*.

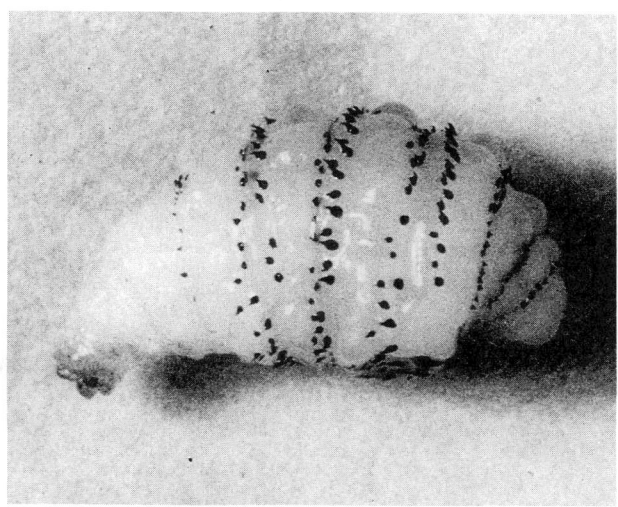

Figure IV.21 Third stage instar of *Dermatobia hominis*.

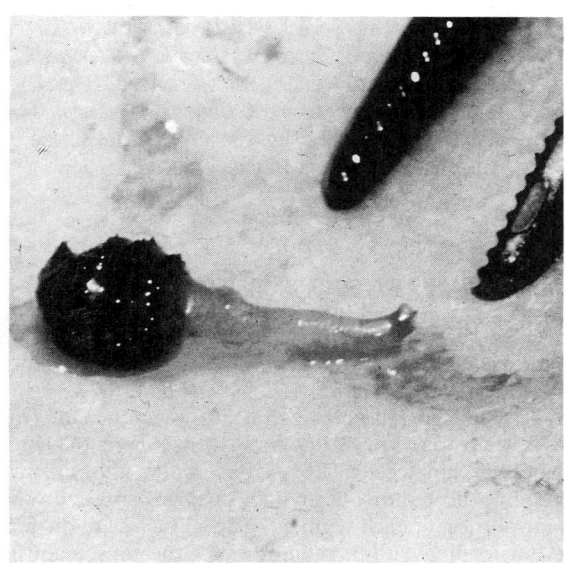

Figure IV.20 Second stage instar of *Dermatobia hominis*.

exudate. The mature larva (Figure IV.21) leaves the host and burrows into the soil to pupate, emerging after 4–11 weeks. The adults live 8–9 days, never feed and are sexually mature about 3 hours after emergence.

Cutaneous swellings harbouring larvae usually occur on exposed areas, although larvae can penetrate clothing and therefore can be found on any part of the body. They are often single, but up to 12 have been reported on one individual. It is a common cause of ocular myiasis in Colombia (see Chapter 10). Rarely, serious complications occur, such as fatal cerebral myiasis in children. Most infestations by *Dermatobia* are painful, so larvae are removed in the first or second stages by the methods described for *Cordylobia* or surgically via a cruciate incision, taking care not to course the central hole as this may result in damage to the larva and give rise to septicaemia.

2 Creeping myiasis and roving swellings
(see Chapter 79)

Species causing this syndrome are usually specialized endo-parasites of other animals which are unable to develop fully in man. It is important to distinguish them from *Ancylostoma* (nematodes) which produce similar effects.

Hypoderma bovis and *H. lineatum* cause creeping swellings and eruptions, especially in persons associated with cattle. On hatching, the larvae penetrate into the subcutaneous tissues, more deeply than *Gastrophilus*, producing an inflamed swelling resembling a boil, which is painful. They migrate sometimes for considerable distances and may invade the nervous system. The larva can be extracted through a cruciform incision.

Gastrophilus spp. are common parasites of horses and occasionally affect man. The larvae penetrate the skin but do not develop beyond the first instar, causing a swelling and a wandering tunnel in the lower epidermis, in which they may progress for long periods.

3 Larvae attacking wounds and sores
(see Chapter 79)

Larvae of flies usually associated with carrion (*Galliphora, Lucilia, Phormia, Musca, Fannia* (Figure IV.22)) have been found in wounds and gangrenous tissue, where they act as facultative parasites feeding on necrotic tissue and occasionally they may attack healthy tissue. Pre-existing lesions may also serve as entry points for larvae of the obligate myiasis flies *C. anthropophaga* in Africa and *D. hominis* in the Americas, as described above. Occasionally, larvae are found living in soiled folds of the skin. Species which are usually found infesting soiled areas around the anus or genitalia may exceptionally enter the rectum or vagina to become internal parasites. At one time it was practice to use larvae of carefully cultivated *Lucilia* (sheep blowflies) to clean septic wounds by removal of infected tissue but this practice has now been abandoned.

Cochliomyia (=*Callitroga*) *hominivorax* (New World

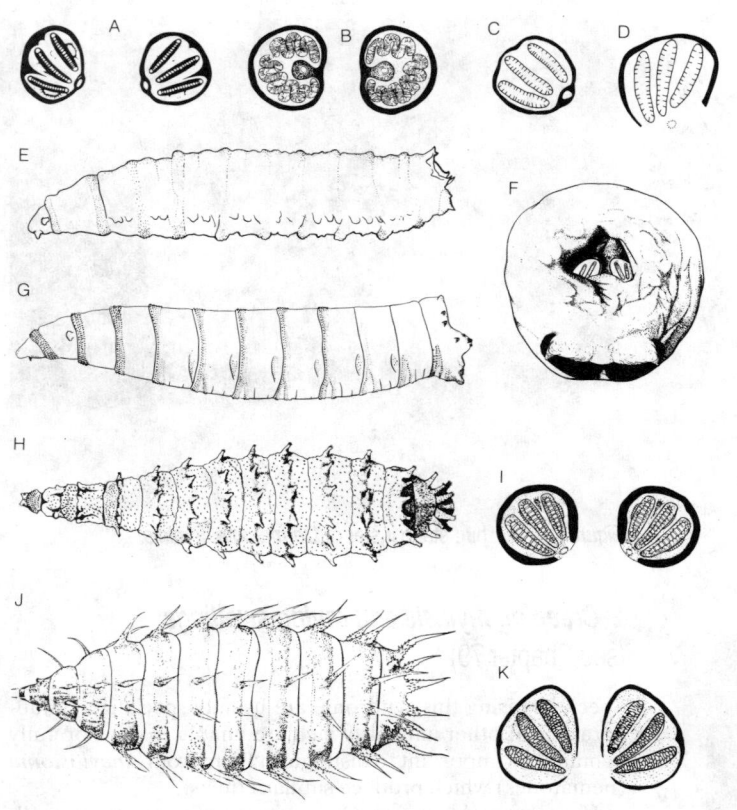

Figure IV.22 General views of mature (third instar) larvae of myiasis-causing flies (Diptera) to show range in form and posterior spiracles used in identification. A, *Lucilia serricata*; B, *Musca domestica*; C, *Calliphora* sp.; D, *Wohlfahrtia* sp.; E and F, *Sarcophaga* spp.; G and I, *Callitroga macellaria*: H and K, *Chrysomyia albiceps*; J, *Fannia* sp. (Reproduced from Smith[112], courtesy of the British Museum (Natural History) London.)

screw-worm fly) is an obligate parasite in the Americas, mainly affecting cattle but also causing serious cases of human myiasis. Clean wounds are attacked, sometimes the smallest abrasions: even a scratch or stubbed toenail can become affected. The fly lays eggs on dry skin and the larvae subsequently invade the wound and feed rapaciously on healthy tissue, usually in groups to produce characteristic pocket-like injuries. Eggs may be deposited in the ears and nasal passages, and even in the vulva and vagina. Larvae grow rapidly and reach maturity in 4–8 days. A case mortality rate of 8% has been reported, and people in close contact with infested cattle are particularly at risk. This species gained recognition for its efficient control in North America by the release of radiation-sterilized males. A related American species, *C. macellaria*, is a facultative parasite responsible for the secondary invasion of wounds as well as scavenging on dead tissues.

Wohlfahrtia magnifica (Old World flesh fly) occurs in the warmer parts of Eurasia where it deposits its larvae in skin lesions, nasal sinuses, ears, sore eyes and vagina, producing serious disfigurement. Like the larvae of *W. vigil* and *Chrysomyia bezziana*, these larvae rely on living tissue for development and do not feed on carrion or excreta.

Wohlfahrtia vigil (Nearctic flesh fly) in North America deposits its larvae in lesions of the skin or mucous membranes, or even on uninjured skin. It is attracted by foul odours from secretions of the ear, eye or nose and possibly from the soiled nappies of babies. Young children are particularly attractive to the flies. The flies do not enter houses. Other species of *Wohlfahrtia* causing cutaneous myiasis are widespread in the northern hemisphere.

4 *Sanguinivorous larvae* (see Chapter 79)

The larvae of several fly genera are obligatory parasites living free in nests of birds and mammals, feeding on the blood of their hosts. Only *Auchmeromyia luteola* (Figure IV.23) (the Congo floor-maggot) has been reported attacking man. This species is widely distributed in Africa, from Nigeria to Natal, in wet and dry climates. The larva is dirty white, about 15 mm long and has three short, fleshy lobes bearing spines on the posterior portion of each segment. The spiracles are distinctive. After feeding with its mouth-hooks, the conspicuously red larva (see Figure IV.17A) retreats to cracks in the floor. Larvae of *A. luteola* are frequently found under sleeping mats and in the earth to a depth of 7.5 cm. They feed mainly

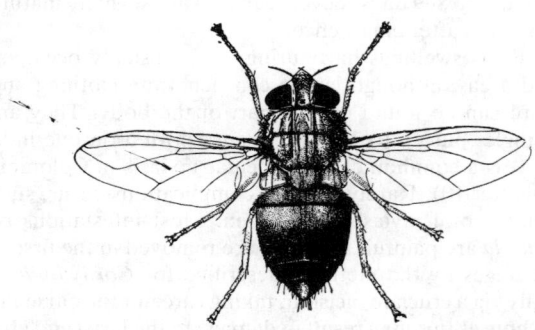

Figure IV.23 Female *Auchmeromyia luteola* (twice natural size).

at night and drop off immediately they are disturbed. The yellowish adults can be found resting in dark areas of huts.

MYIASIS OF BODY CAVITIES (see Chapter 79)

Several species which attack wounds and sores (discussed above) are also involved with myiasis of the eye, orbit, nasal cavities and ear canal. In nasal myiasis the initial symptoms are tickling pain and nasal obstruction. Epistaxis is common, but the discharge soon becomes purulent and fetid. Inhalation of chloroform or packing with chloroform gauze, or the careful local use of weak carbolic acid and turpentine have been advocated but the nasal sinuses may need to be opened.

Chrysomya bezziana (Old World screw-worm) is a large metallic-blue fly with a bright green thorax, found throughout Asia and Africa south of the Sahara. Unlike other species of this genus, it is an obligate parasite. Several other species of *Chrysomyia* have been incriminated as facultative myiasis agents, usually in wounds, but their identification in both the larval and adult stage is difficult.

The females of *C. bezziana* lay numerous eggs in the nasal cavities, especially where there is chronic nasal discharge, or in ulcers or skin wounds (for instance in leprosy), or even in the gums, conjunctiva, ears or vagina. The larvae require living tissue in which to develop, they hatch in a few hours and burrow into the tissues, even to the bones of the nose, producing foul, infected, discharging and disfiguring lesions. These can be treated with a douche of 15% chloroform in light vegetable oil. A few drops of the mixture applied to an infested wound will cause the larvae to appear, and they can be removed with sinus forceps.

Ophthalmomyiasis is the presence of larvae in the orbit, and accessory glands of eye and eyeball. Infections may be quite common (10 per 100 000 population[114]) in some parts of Asia and North Africa, involving obligatory or facultative parasite species. The most common cause of ophthalmomyiasis is first stage larvae of the sheep nasal bot fly (*Oestrus ovis*) (Figure IV.24) which drop their eggs into the orbit, and rarely the mouth or outer ear. Typically patients report being struck in the eye by an insect or foreign object. Within a few hours painful inflammation occurs, which may last for a few days as the larvae cannot develop any further in man. Occasionally larvae reach the nasal cavities (its natural habitat in sheep and goats), where they cause swelling and pain as well as frontal headache, but do not live longer than 10 days. Other obligatory parasites of domestic animals, such as the horse bot fly (*Rhinoestrus purpureus* in Europe, Near East and North Africa), cattle warble fly (*Hypoderma*) and in parts of tropical Africa *Gedoelstia*, may affect man by invading the orbit and (especially in *Hypoderma*) penetrating the eyeball. Rarely, carcass-breeding species such as *Lucilia serricata* (sheep blowfly) cause myiasis of the eye, but only

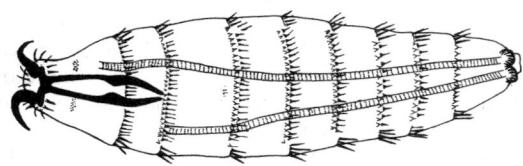

Figure IV.24 First instar larva of *Oestrus ovis*—a common cause of ophthalmomyiasis in North Africa.

when a pre-existing putrefying wound exists near the orbit, and this is therefore typical wound myiasis.

MYIASIS OF ORGAN SYSTEMS (see Chapter 79)

In the majority of cases this is due to accidental 'parasitism'.

INTESTINAL MYIASIS

This type of myiasis is usually diagnosed from the presence of larvae in vomit or faeces. Obligatory gut parasites of animals will not develop in man and therefore species which cause intestinal myiasis are facultative or accidental parasites. About 50 species have been recorded, many cases of suspected gut myiasis have in fact resulted from contamination of samples after collection, as some species (e.g. *Sarcophaga* spp.) can develop to the third larval stage in 24 hours, and others will lay larvae (larviposition) on faeces as they are being deposited. Occasionally previously contaminated collection vessels have been responsible for some mistaken reports.

Larvae may be swallowed in contaminated food and pass through the intestine unaffected by the extreme environment, e.g. *Piophila* (cheese skipper). However, this is unusual as most ingested larvae die and may be passed dead or, exceptionally, live if there is a concurrent intestine infection. Even under these circumstances, larvae may cause intestinal lesions, damage to mucuous membranes or haemorrhagic infiltrations—demonstrated by severe gastrointestinal disturbances (vomiting, diarrhoea, nausea). Reports of larvae developing in the anterior and median gut in man, and even becoming paedogenic, are highly doubtful.[115]

Flies which are normally attracted to faeces may, under particularly poor standards of hygiene, deposit their eggs on or near the anus and the larvae then penetrate into the posterior part of the rectum. Several authentic cases caused by *Eristalis* (Syrphidae), which commonly lives in sewage, have been reported.

UROGENITAL MYIASIS

Larvae of facultative parasites may be excreted in the urine or found in the vagina. The flies concerned are usually of the families Psychodidae, Muscidae, Calliphoridae and Sarcophagidae. A mistaken diagnosis of urinary myiasis due to a larva from a contaminated vessel in which urine has been collected, or introduced into the urine after it has been passed, is not uncommon, but there have been cases in which the larvae have been undoubtedly passed via the urethra from the bladder. If the vulva or vagina is infested there are obvious opportunities for larvae to enter the bladder.

COLLECTION AND PRESERVATION OF LARVAE

After removal of myiasis larvae from the host by irrigation, manipulation or surgery the larvae should be killed in hot water to retain their overall shape. The posterior respiratory spiracles are an important means of identification. The spiracles can be seen under a high-power dissecting microscope, but it may be necessary to remove, macerate and slide mount them for detailed examination. Larvae should be preserved in 80% alcohol. Identification of accidental or facultative parasites is often difficult, as many species can be involved. In contrast, the identification of obligate parasites is easier as fewer species are involved, although the superficial similarity of flies of widely separated genera makes it necessary to submit specimens for identification by a specialist whenever a precise identification is required. Identification is facilitated if larvae are reared to adults on small pieces of meat. Smith[112] gives details for identification.

PHLEBOTOMINE SANDFLIES
R. P. Lane

FAMILY: PSYCHODIDAE; SUBFAMILY: PHLEBOTOMINAE

IMPORTANT GENERA: *PHLEBOTOMUS* (OLD WORLD) AND *LUTZOMYIA* (NEW WORLD)

Phlebotomine sandflies are small, delicate, hairy flies (1.5–3.5 mm) with long, slender legs and filamentous antennae. Both sexes of adult sandflies feed frequently on nectar and other juices from plants. Female sandflies are also haematophagous, i.e. feed regularly on the blood of vertebrates to obtain nutrition for egg production. Of the 700 species found throughout the tropics and subtropics, only a small proportion (*c.* 70 species) are thought to be involved in the transmission of disease to man.

Sandflies are easily distinguished from other small Diptera when alive by the characteristic manner in which they hold their pointed wings above their body (like a vertical V; Figure IV.25). In other blood-sucking Diptera the wings are held flat over the abdomen, either one on top of the other (Culicidae, Simuliidae, *Culicoides*) or outspread (Glossinides, Tabanidae). It is important to differentiate phlebotomine sandflies from other small flies known locally as 'sandflies', i.e. midges of the genus *Culicoides* and blackflies of the family Simuliidae.

There is relatively little morphological difference between sandfly males and females, except that the males have elaborate external genitalia terminalia (see Figure IV.26). Man-biting (anthropophagous) species of sandflies belong to two genera: *Phlebotomus* in the Old World and *Lutzomyia* in the New World. In Africa, some species of the genus *Sergentomyia*, which feed principally on reptiles, occasionally bite man also but are not regarded as vectors of any human or zoonotic pathogen(s).

Phlebotomine sandflies are vectors of visceral leishmaniasis (VL: kala-azar; see Chapter 65), the various forms of cutaneous leishmaniasis (CL: oriental sore, espundia, etc.; see Chapter 65), bartonellosis (Oroya fever, Carrión's disease; see Chapter 46) and sandfly fever (papataci or papatasi fever, 3-day fever, etc.; see Chapter 30). Transmission of pathogens takes place during blood feeding.

Sandflies are not easy to study in relation to disease, as the adults are small and unobtrusive, while finding larvae is almost impossible. This has made the incrimination of vectors during epidemiological studies particularly difficult and, therefore, the vector status of many species remains uncertain.[4] (See also section on epidemiology of leishmaniasis Chapter 65.) Compared with other vector groups (e.g. Culicidae and Simuliidae), the biology of sandflies is poorly known. However, a thorough understanding of the natural history of sandflies is essential, since the epidemiology of the diseases they transmit is largely determined by the ecology and behaviour of the vectors.

DISTRIBUTION AND ECOLOGY

Sandflies are found mainly in the tropics and subtropics, with a few species penetrating into temperate regions in both the northern (to 50°N) and southern hemispheres (to about 40°S). The distribution of leishmaniasis is not as extensive as that of sandflies, for reasons that are not entirely known: e.g. no human leishmaniasis has been recorded from South-East Asia and Australasia, although several potential vectors are present.

In the Old World, man-biting sandflies are confined to the subtropics, there being very few anthropophilic species in tropical Africa. Even in foci of visceral leishmaniasis (e.g. in Kenya) man-biters are not conspicuous. In contrast, the transmission of leishmaniasis in the New World is principally in the tropics.

Sandflies occur in a very wide range of habitats, from sea level (a major focus of leishmaniasis around the Dead Sea is below sea level!) to altitudes of 2800 m or more in the Andes and Ethiopia, and from hot dry deserts, through savannas and open woodland to dense tropical rain forest. Each species of sandfly has rather distinct ecological requirements. If these encompass the conditions in and around the dwellings of man or his domestic animals, the species becomes peridomestic. The majority of peridomestic sandfly species are vectors of infections to man. The highly focal nature of many leishmaniases is undoubtedly a result of ecological constraints on the vectors and probably, to a lesser extent, on the mammalian reservoirs. In central Asia, sandflies are localized, restricted to the natural foci of gerbil colonies and by soil texture and moisture. Even in tropical rain forests, sandflies are not uniformly distributed.

In the Old World most foci of cutaneous leishmaniasis are in dry, semiarid areas, in contrast to the New World where

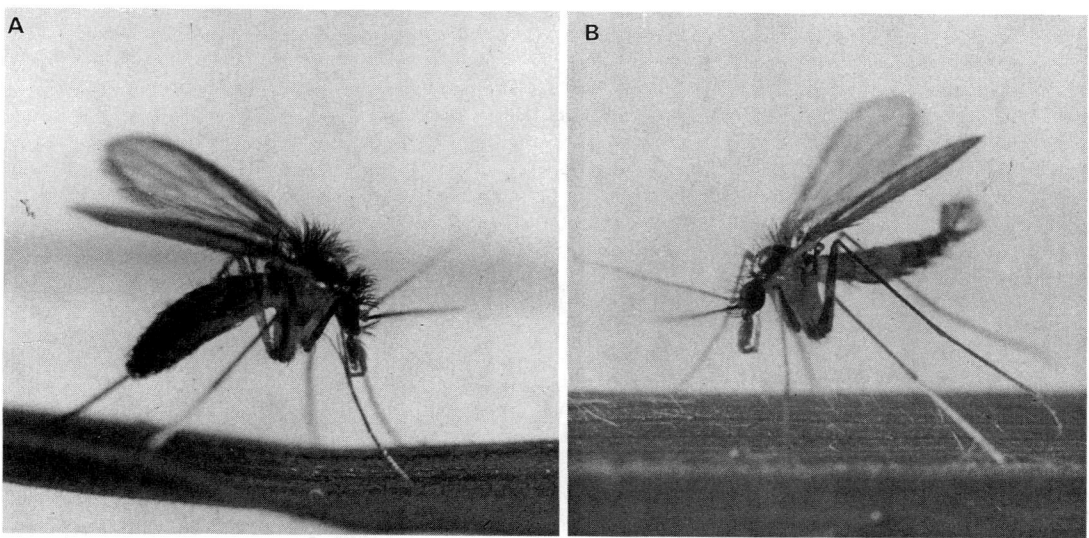

Figure IV.25   Living female (left) and male (right) phlebotomine sandflies (*Lutzomyia longipalpis*), showing the hairy body and wings, the generally mosquito-like stance and appearance except for the characteristic position of the wings, held in a V over the back. (Courtesy of C. J. Webb.)

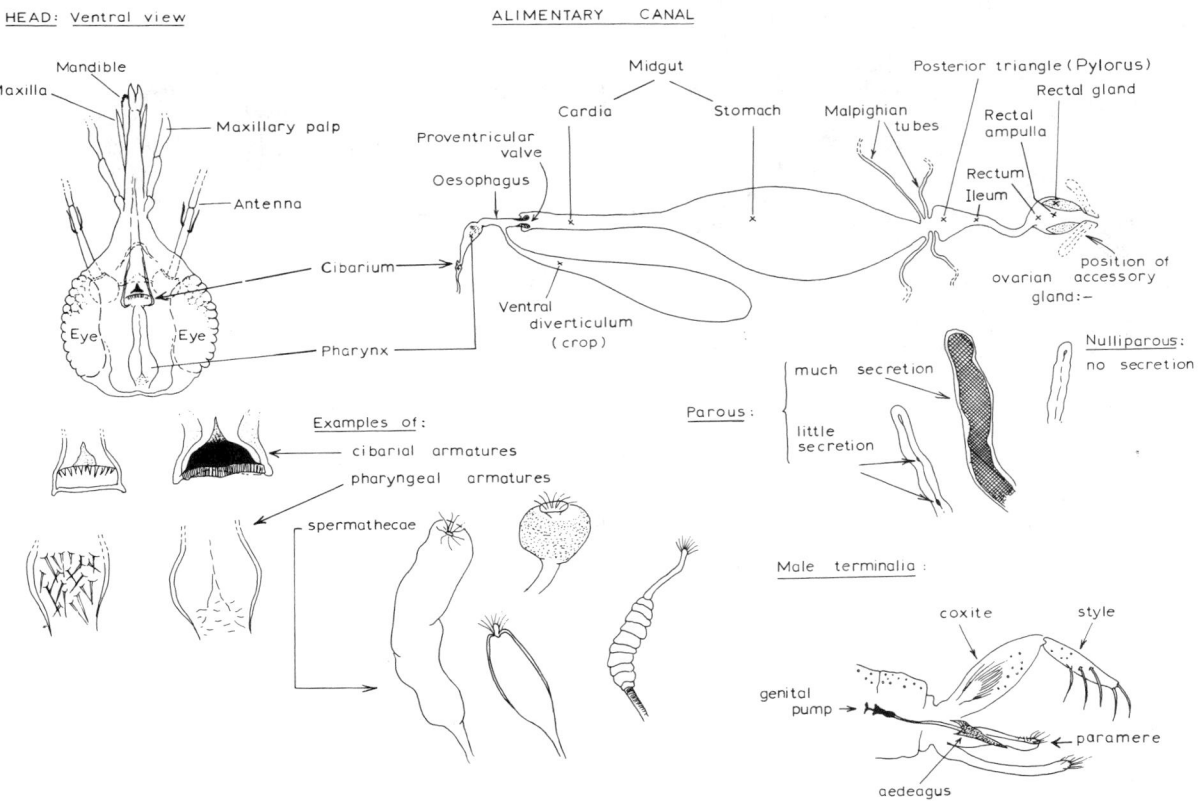

Figure IV.26   The anatomy of the alimentary canal of sandflies, showing the ovarian glands and features of taxonomic importance.

CL is mainly transmitted in forests (Figure IV.27). Hence occupational differences exist between those acquiring infections. Cutaneous disease in Central and South America is primarily associated with working in or modifying the forest environment, whereas in the Old World the disease affects those in rural savanna and urban areas. The open nature of the savanna and steppe environments and the patchy distribution of suitable microclimates for sandflies, has prompted the application of landscape epidemiology in the investigation of many Old World foci of cutaneous leishmaniasis.

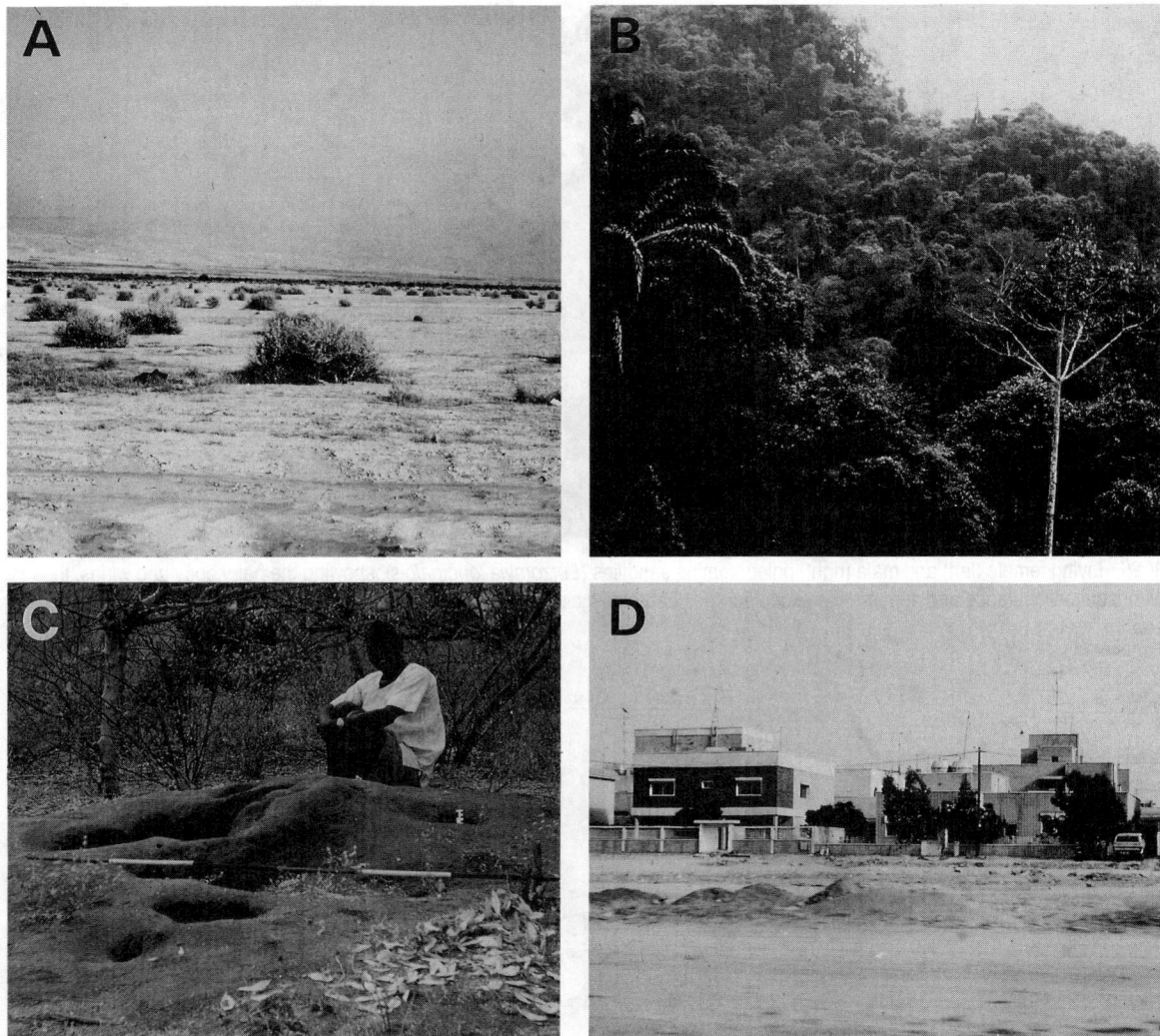

Figure IV.27   A, A typical arid habitat of *Phlebotomus papatasi* (Jordan Valley), where this species transmits *L. (L.) major* from the fat sand rat (*Psammomys obesus*) to man and causes cutaneous leishmaniasis. B, Cutaneous leishmaniasis due to *L (L.) mexicana* is transmitted from tree rats to man by *Lutzomyia olmeca olmeca* in wet forests of Central America (Belize). C, Eroded termite hills are the preferred resting sites of the visceral leishmaniasis vector *Phlebotomus martini* in some areas of East Africa. (Courtesy of D. M. Minter.) D, Occupants of modern housing developments around expanding towns may become infected with visceral leishmaniasis by the bites of peridomestic sandflies, e.g. in Brazil and the Middle East.

The distribution and abundance of sandflies can alter with changing land use. Deforestation in the New World has led to a marked reduction in cutaneous leishmaniasis (after the initial increase in disease during land clearance). Such areas provide opportunities for the extension in the range of the VL vector *Lutzomyia longipalpis* and subsequent transmission of visceral leishmaniasis which has become more prevalent in urban areas of Brazil in recent years, resembling the urban foci of VL with dogs as the reservoir of *Leishmania infantum* in the Old World. By raising the water table, irrigation projects considerably increase the breeding of some vector species, e.g. *Phlebotomus papatasi* but, in some circumstances at least, this may also discourage the rodent reservoir, e.g. the deeply burrowing *Rhombomys opimus* in the steppes of southern Eurasia. In the Middle East there has been a marked increase in cutaneous leishmaniasis due to *L. major* associated with development programmes.

When they are not active, sandflies seek out cool and relatively humid (but not wet) dark niches. Resting sites such as caves, tree holes, tree trunks, cavities between boulders, fissures in the ground, buildings, termite hills and animal burrows are commonly used. By withdrawing to these daytime sites, sandflies are able to survive in very hot and dry climates, in conditions which would otherwise rapidly kill them, emerging at night when the ambient temperature drops and the humidity rises. Such resting sites are very important in the study of sandflies, as their availability determines the ecological distribution of different species: various traps are used to intercept sandflies moving to and from such places.

BEHAVIOUR OF SANDFLIES

Sandflies usually have a short hopping flight, especially when close to prospective hosts. Little is known of their long range movements (e.g. dispersal from breeding sites), although they can fly up to 2.2 km over a period of a few days in open habitats. They only fly at night and in a single night they may fly several hundred metres, in their search for a host and subsequent resting and breeding sites. Climatic factors affect activity markedly; biting does not usually take place below 20°C in tropical species; *P. papatasi* is active between 45 and 60% relative humidity, whereas other species require 75–85% relative humidity, and the flight range of some species (e.g. *P. sergenti*) is greater in humid than in dry climates. Although slight air movement aids the detection of hosts along odour plumes, wind speeds of greater than 1.5 m/s inhibit flight, which ceases altogether in light winds of 4–5 m/s. Forest sandflies, such as the Amazonian *Lutzomyia umbratilis*, often exhibit regular vertical movements in addition to horizontal patterns. The flies rest in the tree buttresses during the day, migrating to the canopy in search of a host at night. Furthermore, within a forest, there is often a marked vertical zonation in which different species of sandflies are active, so that some species remain close to the ground, feeding on ground-dwelling rodents (e.g. the South American vectors *Luzomyia flaviscutellata* and *Lutzomyia olmeca* feeding on the rodents *Proechimys* and *Oryzomys*). For these reasons, the transmission of some parasites between the normal animal hosts is predominantly at ground level (e.g. *L. amazonensis*) and some in the canopy (e.g. *L. panamensis*), although man usually acquires infection at ground level.

SEASONAL DISTRIBUTION

Several abiotic factors affect sandfly numbers, but temperature and rainfall are the most important. Some species in temperate regions may only have one generation per year, and consequently a single peak of activity and transmission. However, such species may have two or three generations per year in climatically more favourable areas. In tropical countries, species react more to rainfall cycles and may be more prevalent in either the wet or dry season. Several anthropophilic species may be present, each with its own annual cycle of activity and potential for transmission.

BLOOD FEEDING

Sandfly females feed on blood, using the nutrients to develop eggs. Feeding takes place on exposed parts of the body by thrusting the tiny mouthparts (0.15–0.57 mm) into the skin and, using minutely serated mandibles in a scissor-like manner, to create a small pool from which the blood is sucked. Blood taken in this manner is directed into the midgut. Liquids taken by other means (e.g. sugar feeding) are directed to the crop for sterilization and then to the midgut; infection of the sandfly gut with bacteria or yeasts appears to depress *Leishmania* development. Both males and females feed on sugars, which they obtain as honeydew or from plants, either passively (extrafloral nectaries, fallen fruits, etc.) or by actively piercing leaves or stems. The presence of sugars is essential for the full development of *Leishmania*

(see section on invertebrate life-cycles of *Leishmania*, Chapter 65).

The site of a bite determines the situation of primary lesions in cutaneous leishmaniasis, and may be influenced as much by the presence of clothes as by the intrinsic preferences of a vector. Consequently, sleeping outside in hot weather without bed-nets, or working in forests during the day without suitable clothing, increases the risk of acquiring an infection.

Sandflies are crepuscular; biting takes place at different times of the night according to the species. When disturbed, sandflies in dense forests, caves or buildings, may bite during the day. Only a few species are endophilic; these are mostly peridomestic species, such as *P. papatasi*, *P. chinensis*, *P. sergenti* and *Lutzomyia longipalpis*, the majority preferring to bite outside, often near their probable breeding and resting sites. It is a relatively small ecological step from rodent burrows and caves to human dwellings. The distinction between peridomestic and 'wild' species has little meaning in sparsely populated areas, where the buildings themselves are made of local materials, perhaps without solid walls. Equally, no species is entirely domestic.

The biting rates of sandflies vary greatly, up to a maximum of about 1000/h. Most species probably have a narrow range of preferred hosts. Species of *Sergentomyia* feed predominantly on reptiles, as do some species of *Lutzomyia* and *Phlebotomus*, but the latter genera feed mainly on mammals. Several peridomestic, mammal-feeding sandflies (*P. papatasi*, *P. sergenti*, and *Lutzomyia longipalpis*), feed readily on poultry also; chicken coops may be a source of biting sandflies.

Most species are gonotrophically concordant, taking one blood meal for each batch of eggs matured. However, autogeny, the ability to lay eggs without a blood meal, is a feature of some man-biting species. Sandflies may feed more than once per ovarian cycle, thus increasing man–fly contact. Oviposition usually takes place 5–10 days after a blood meal. The proportion of parous females within a population (i.e. those which have laid eggs and by inference have had a blood meal, with the concomitant risk of acquiring an infection) indicates the epidemiological potential of the population. The highest parous rates occur in populations towards the end of the 'sandfly season', when sandfly infection rates are maximal and subsequent transmission most likely.

LIFE HISTORY

Relatively little is known about the immature stages of sandflies and their breeding sites, which are terrestrial, in striking contrast to other nematocerous flies such as Culicidae, Simuliidae, Ceratopogonidae and Chironomidae. Breeding and resting often takes place in the same microhabitat—such as the soil accumulated in cracks in walls or among rocks, in animal burrows and shelters, caves, or in damp leaf litter in forests. The main requirements for breeding sites are moisture and the presence of organic detritus, etc., on which the larvae can feed.

Eggs of sandflies (less than 0.7 mm in length) are elliptical with a fine chorionic pattern. Up to 70 eggs are scattered about the potential breeding site by the ovipositing female. Hatching occurs one to two weeks later. The larvae are caterpillar-like and have a distinct dark head-capsule and the pale, cream-coloured body is sparsely covered with characteristic club-shaped hairs ('match-stick' hairs). There are four instars, the first with a single pair, and the remaining instars with two pairs, of long, highly characteristic, caudal bristles on the anal segment. The caudal bristles are almost as long as the body. Diapause occurs during the fourth instar of several species in areas where there are cool winters (e.g. the Mediterranean basin). The pupa is inactive and usually hatches within 5–10 days. The duration of the larval instars varies greatly, both between and within species (in the laboratory at least), as it is regulated mainly by temperature. The period from oviposition to adult eclosion takes between 20 days and several months (in temperate or diapausing species and those living at high altitudes in the tropics, e.g. *P. longipes*).

Emergence takes place during the hours of darkness, often just before dawn. Males usually emerge first. Little is known of mating in sandflies. Although swarming does not generally take place, males may congregate on and around prospective hosts and mate with females there. Pheromones and auditory signals from wing beats are also probably involved. The life of adult flies is unlikely to exceed a few weeks in nature. Once the female becomes infected, perhaps at the first blood meal, parasites can be transmitted to new hosts at intervals throughout the rest of her life.

TRANSMISSION OF DISEASE ORGANISMS

Sandflies transmit viruses, bacteria and protozoa (*Leishmania*), but not nematodes, to vertebrates.

Leishmania

Phlebotomine sandflies are the only vectors of *Leishmania* species to man. Certain species are common vectors of parasites (often peridomestic species) or secondary vectors, while most sandflies rarely if ever come into contact with man. A species may transmit a particular parasite in one area, but not in another: no two areas or foci are the same. The degree of human involvement in leishmaniasis is very variable; many cycles are of reservoir–fly–reservoir, with occasional, almost chance infections; others cause regular zoonotic infections, and some anthroponotic cycles are thought to involve only flies and man. It is important to understand natural transmission cycles for two reasons. Enzootic cycles may pose an unknown threat in remote areas being developed (mining, agriculture, etc.) and, secondly, transmission may be maintained by several species, only one of which transmits the infection to man, e.g. in southern Eurasia *L. major* infections are maintained among rodents by *P. mongolensis*, *P. caucasicus* and *P. andrejevi*, but only *P. papatasi* transmits the parasite to man.

Incrimination of a sandfly species as a vector is difficult, as many criteria have to be satisfied before a species can be unambiguously implicated. These criteria are based on the discovery of natural infections in wild-caught flies, experimental transmission studies, evidence of contact between the sandfly and man, contact between the sandfly and the reservoir host (where known), and the life cycle of the parasite in the fly. As there is often no sharp distinction between important and minor or occasional vectors, it is impossible to draw up a definitive list of vectors. Table IV.3 gives a synopsis of the 'proven' vectors of *Leishmania*; further de-

tails of suspected vectors are given in the section on the epidemiology of leishmaniaisis (see Chapter 65).

Within the genus *Phlebotomus* the majority of subgenera contain vectors or suspected vectors. Species of *Phlebotomus* (*sensu stricto*) are associated with *L. major* transmission in arid environments of East Africa, the Middle East and the former USSR. The subgenus *Paraphlebotomus* contains many species living in rodent burrows in central Asia and transmitting *L. major* between rodents and occasionally to man. One species, the peridomestic *P. sergenti*, is a vector of *L. tropica* in western Asia and the Middle East. Vectors of visceral leishmaniasis in the Old World are distributed through several subgenera: *Larroussius* (Mediterranean basin and Sahel); *Synphlebotomus* (East Africa); *Euphlebotomus* (India); and *Adlerius* (Near East, northern China). The genus *Lutzomyia* is much more diverse than its Old World counterpart; some subgenera contain several vector species (e.g. *Nyssomyia* and *Psychodopygus*), whereas many other subgenera and species groups contain only one or two species which are involved in the transmission of *Leishmania* spp.

Leishmania in the sandfly

After ingestion, the parasites in an infected blood meal undergo metamorphosis to the promastigote form and multiply within the sandfly gut before they become infective. The site in which this development takes place varies between different groups of *Leishmania* and is related to the micromorphology and biochemistry of the sandfly gut. The attachment mechanisms of *Leishmania* are adapted to the surface structure (chitinous or membranous) of the section of the gut to which they adhere. Enzyme activity in the midgut, following blood meals from different hosts, will differentially affect the survival of *Leishmania*.

The location of the parasites in the gut during their development (relative to the pylorus—the sphincter between the mid- and hindgut), has been used in parasite classification (Figure IV.28).[5] This subject is discussed in detail in the section on the genus *Leishmania* (see Appendix III) and may be briefly summarized as follows:

1 Peripylarian ('both sides of the gate') development takes place in the hindgut and then the parasites migrate forward before transmission by bite. Mainly parasites of New World mammals (members of the subgenus *L. (Viannia)*: *L. braziliensis*, *guyanensis*, *panamensis* and *peruviana*). Some parasites of Old World reptiles (e.g. the former *L. adleri*), whose taxonomic status (as '*Sauroleishmania*'; see Appendix III) is presently in doubt, also have a peripylarian form of development in sandflies.
2 Suprapylarian ('above the gate') development is entirely within the midgut prior to anterior migration and transmission by bite. Parasites of New and Old World mammals (members of the subgenus *Leishmania* (*sensu stricto*): *L. donovani* group, *L. mexicana* group, *L. hertigi* group and *L. major* group).

The term hypopylarian ('under the gate') development was used for parasites of some Old World Lizards formerly included in the genus *Leishmania*, but which are currently referred to as *Sauroleishmania* species (of uncertain status), e.g. the former *L. agamae* and *L. ceramodactyli*. Hypopylarian development is confined to the hindgut and transmission is by ingestion or crushing of the infected fly, when fed upon by lizards or other insectivorous vertebrates.

Although transmission occurs through the bite of a sandfly, the exact mechanism by which parasites are taken up or deposited in the skin of a new host is unclear (see: section on vector–parasite interactions, below). Infection with parasites changes the behaviour of a sandfly; a heavily infected fly probes much more frequently than an uninfected fly, in a manner analogous to a flea with *Yersinia*. *Leishmania* can be readily transmitted during each probe, which may only last a few seconds, and this is probably the origin of the multiple lesions seen in some patients (particularly those with *L. major* infections). Infection does not alter the dispersal of sandflies appreciably.

Vector–parasite specificity of sandflies and the *Leishmania* spp. they transmit is affected by several factors, including behaviour (e.g. propensity of a vector to bite a particular species of reservoir host), ecological factors and biochemical factors (e.g. enzyme activity) operating in the sandfly gut. Natural infection rates in wild flies are usually very low

(below 1%), but may be exceptionally high in some foci (e.g. up to 20% in the Jordan Valley).

Viruses

Sandfly fever (papataci or papatasi fever, 3-day fever) is caused by two distinct virus serotypes (Naples and Sicilian) and results in an acute febrile illness in man, lasting 2–4 days, although incapacitation may extend for much longer periods.[6] It is common during the summer months throughout the Mediterranean basin, the Middle East, Pakistan and parts of India and Central America. The disease is of considerable military importance because up to 75% of non-immune individuals arriving in an endemic area may be affected. In Mediterranean areas where the disease is endemic, most of the population is thought to be infected during childhood, possibly suffering only a mild illness (see Chapter 30).

Phlebotomus papatasi was incriminated as the vector in

Table IV.3   Synopsis of proven vectors of leishmaniasis (see also Chapter 65).

Parasite	Vector	Animal reservoir	Principal areas
L. (Leishmania) donovani	*P. (Euphlebotomus) argentipes*	? Man	India
L. (L.) infantum	*P. (Larroussius) ariasi*	Fox, dog	Southern France
	P. (Larroussius) longicuspis	Dog	North Africa
	P. (Larroussius) major syracus	Dog	Eastern Mediterranean
	P. (Larroussius) orientalis	Rodents and carnivores	Sudan
	P. (Larroussius) perfiliewi	Fox; *Rattus* spp.	Italy; former Yugoslavia
	P. (Larroussius) perniciosus	Dog	Western Mediterranean
	P. (Larroussius) smirnovi	Wolves; jackals	Former USSR
	P. (Larroussius) tobbi	Dog	Eastern Mediterranean
	P. (Paraphlebotomus) alexandri	? Man	North-west China: Sinkiang (Xinjiang)
	P. (Adlerius) sichuanensis	?	South-west China: Szechwan (Sichuan)
	P. (Adlerius) chinensis	Dog; racoon dog	China
	P. (Adlerius) longiductus	Dog; jackal	Former USSR
	P. (Synphlebotomus) martini	Dog; man	East Africa
L. (L.) chagasi	*Lutzomyia (Lutzomyia) longipalpis*	Dog; foxes (*Lycalopex, Cerdocyon*)	Brazil
L. (L.) tropica	*P. (Paraphlebotomus) sergenti*	? Man	Middle East to Indus basin
L. (L.) major	*P. (Phlebotomus) papatasi*	Burrowing rodents	North Africa, Middle East: former USSR, north-west India
	P. (Phlebotomus) duboscqi	Rodents	African Sahel (Senegal to East Africa)
	P. (Phlebotomus) salehi	Rodents	North-west India
L. (L.) aethiopica	*P. (Larroussius) pedifer*	Hyrax	Ethiopia, Kenya
L. (L.) maxicana	*Lutzomyia (Nyssomyia) olmeca olmeca*	Forest rodents	Central America
L. (L.) amazonensis	*Lutzomyia (Nyssomyia) flaviscutellata*	Forest rodents; agouti, opossum	Amazon basin (Brazil)
L. (Viannia) braziliensis	*Lutzomyia (Psychodopygus) wellcomei*	?	Brazil
L. (V.) panamensis	*Lutzomyia (Nyssomyia) trapidoi*	Sloth (*Choloepus hoffmani*)	Panama
L. (V.) guyanensis	*Lutzomyia (Nyssomyia) umbratilis*	Sloth (*Choloepus didactylus*)	Northern Brazil, Guyanas
L. (V.) peruviana	?	? (Dog; as secondary host)	Western Andes (South America)

For further details, and for numerous species incriminated, but not conclusively proved as vectors, see also section on epidemiology of the leishmaniases, Chapter 65).

Section of a Phlebotomine sandfly to show the different regions of the alimentary canal

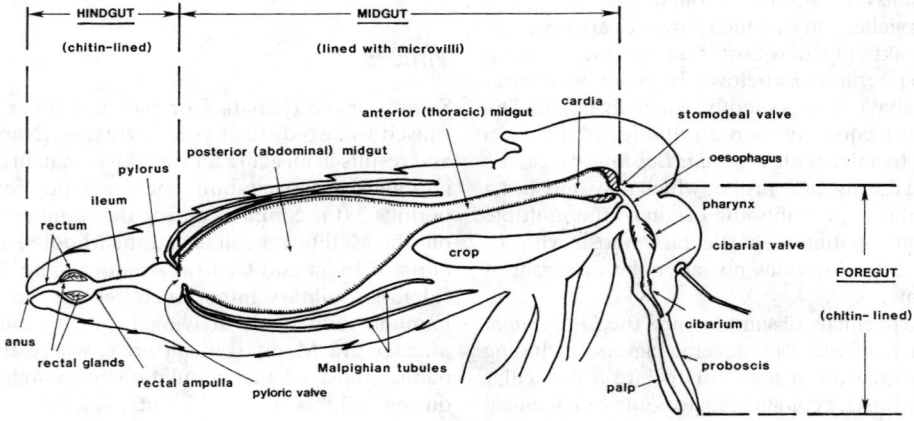

Section SUPRAPYLARIA ("above the gate")

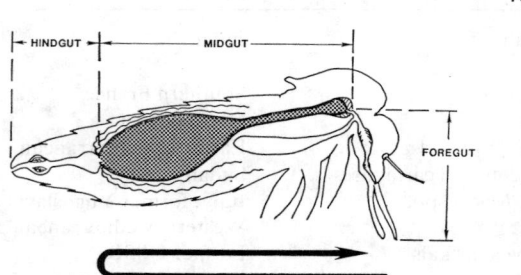

Development in midgut only (no hindgut development). Transmission by bite

Parasites of Old and New World mammals: subgenus Leishmania:

1. Old & New World VL: L. (L.) donovani & L. (L.) infantum (OW)

L. (L.) chagasi (NW)

2. Old World CL: L. (L.) tropica, L. (L.) major, & L. (L.) aethiopica

3. New World CL (members of L. (L.) mexicana complex):

L. (L.) mexicana, L. (L.) amazonensis, L. (L.) pifanoi, L.(L.) garnhami,

L. (L.) enriettii, L. (L.) aristedesi, L. (L.) hertigi, L. (L.) deanei

Section PERIPYLARIA ("on all sides of the gate")

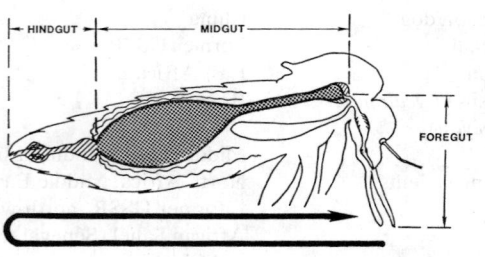

Initial phase of development in hindgut, with subsequent forward migration to

anterior station.   Transmission by bite.

Parasites of New World mammals: subgenus Viannia:

L. (V.) braziliensis, L. (V.) guyanensis, L. (V.) panamensis, L. (V.) peruviana

Note also the former Section HYPOPYLARIA ("under the gate"):

Development in hindgut only: no anterior migration. Transmission by ingestion

of infected insect. Parasites of Old World reptiles:

subgenus Sauroleishmania: (★)   L. (S.) agamae, L. (S.) ceramodactyli

(★ organisms currently of uncertain status and affinity: some may be trypanosomes)

Figure IV.28   Classification of the *Leishmania* species based on their site of development in the phlebotomine host. (After Lanson and Shaw[5].)

Egypt and is generally thought to transmit sandfly fever throughout the Old World range of the disease (i.e. except Central America). Natural infection rates of sandflies are between 0.015 and 0.5%. No natural vertebrate reservoir is known, although infected humans can infect flies, and thus have some amplifying effect during epidemics. It is most likely that the principal maintenance mechanism is by transovarial transmission along genetically susceptible lines of the vector.

Sandflies transmit several other phleboviruses; *Phlebotomus perniciosus* transmits Toscana virus in the northern Mediterranean and in the New World *Lutzomyia trapidoi* and *Lutzomyia ylephiletor* transmit Chagres and Punta Toro viruses. Viruses have been isolated from several other species.

Bacteria

Infections due to *Bartonella bacilliformis* (Oroya fever, verruga peruana) are found only in the central Andean Cordilleras of Peru, Colombia and Ecuador. The disease is endemic in valleys between 750 and 2700 m in altitude apparently restricted by the ecological requirements of the vectors. Little detail is known of the transmission cycle; there are no known animal reservoirs; the sandfly vector acquires the pathogen from an infected human. The lack of a development cycle of *B. bacilliformis* in the vector (it occurs in the gut and on the mouthparts) suggests that transmission may be mechanical. In Peru, *Lutzomyia verrucarum* is considered the vector, although the disease exists in the absence of this species. The closely related *Lutzomyia colombiana* is thought to transmit the disease in Colombia.

REACTION TO SANDFLY BITES

Persons newly exposed to the bites of *P. papatasi* and other species in parts of the Middle East often experience a severe urticarial reaction to sandfly bites after a variable time. This period of sensitization may later be followed by desensitization. Such a reaction may also occur elsewhere in the world.

CONTROL OF SANDFLIES

There is no general method of control for several reasons: the diversity of the habitats in which the diseases occur, behaviour of the vectors, and the public health importance of the disease they transmit. Several different strategies are used, principally aimed at reducing man–fly contact. Control of larvae is often impossible, as the breeding sites of many vectors are either unknown or inaccessible. However, in the former USSR considerable success was achieved by a combined method of pumping insecticides into rodent burrows (breeding and resting sites) with destruction of the rodent reservoirs (*Rhombomys opimus*).

Personal protection

Sandflies are able to penetrate the standard insect screens used in windows of houses and for normal bed-nets, and therefore fine sandfly bed-nets have to be used, which are uncomfortable to sleep under in humid tropical climates. Chemical repellents (deet, DMP) applied to clothing and bed-nets are effective but when applied to the skin are rapidly lost through perspiration. This is especially so when manual work is undertaken (agricultural labour, road building or military operations).

Insecticide control

Leishmaniasis control has occurred in some countries (e.g. India, Mediterranean) as a by-product of antimalarial spraying, with renewed outbreaks after cessation of such spraying. Sandflies are susceptible to insecticides (only one instance of resistance to DDT has been reported) which are applied to resting and breeding sites. Control programmes based on house-spraying with residual insecticides have been directed specifically at sandflies in Egypt, China, CIS, Peru and Saudi Arabia. The use of pyrethroid-treated bed-nets and curtains against sandflies is under evaluation.

Insecticide control of adults is only feasible where peridomestic transmission occurs in discrete and well-populated communities. Where sandflies are exophilic, or bite away from human habitations, insecticide control may not be effective: e.g. there has been little success with attempts to control forest sandflies in the 'neotropics' by barrier spraying.

Environmental modification

This has been effective in some areas, e.g. moving temporary buildings and camps away from microfoci, and ploughing up breeding sties. Often, changing land use affects transmission in an unpredictable way. Sandflies in dense forest will rarely cross a clearing made around isolated houses or villages.

COLLECTION OF SANDFLIES

The diverse biology of sandflies and their habitats means that special methods have to be used to catch then. Most methods rely on an understanding of sandfly behaviour, since they involve catching resting flies, attracting sandflies to a trap, or intercepting them during their nocturnal movements, and thus collecting efficiency will vary between methods and individuals.

The simplest method is to collect flies during the day from their resting sites, either catching them directly with an aspirator or with a fine-mesh net. This is useful for peridomestic flies and for forest flies resting on tree trunks and buttresses. Battery-operated aspirators avoid the risk of histoplasmosis (see Chapter 59). A tent-like device (Damasceno trap) can be put over animal burrows or tree buttresses to catch resting sandflies. The most widely used method of collecting sandflies, at least in the Old World where sandflies live in relatively drier habitats, is setting sticky traps. These are sheets of paper (usually 10 × 17 cm) thinly coated in castor oil and fixed to sticks which are then placed near resting sites. Traps are set before sunset and collected the following morning. The adhering flies are removed with a needle, cleaned in dilute detergent and stored in 70% alcohol. Sticky traps are not usually effective in areas of high humidity. Several types of light traps can be used, although they are less effective in open habitats, such as deserts, than in woodland or forests. Similarly, a range of animal-baited traps have been devised for collecting sandflies. These traps are useful in areas where man-biting species are seldom caught by other means. Baiting such traps with a known reservoir host will help determine potential vector species. Light- and animal-bait methods are combined in the Shannon trap, a rectangular cloth trap with a central wall and an inverted box-like roof.

Man-biting catches provide an accurate method of finding which species are anthropophilic and assessing the extent of man–fly contact. The ethics of collectors being exposed to potential risks of leishmaniasis transmission may be considered acceptable if local residents are employed without substantially increasing their risks. Collecting larvae is enormously time consuming and only rarely productive.

PREPARATION AND PRESERVATION OF SPECIMENS

Because many microscopic characters are used to differentiate species of sandflies, correct preparation of specimens is of paramount importance. Flies can be cleaned in dilute detergent solutions to remove any adherent oil from sticky traps, rinsed in distilled water and mounted in Berlese medium. Other, more permanent, methods of clearing and mounting flies are also used. To display the diagnostic features most clearly, the head should be detached and mounted ventral side uppermost and the remainder of the body mounted laterally. Care must be taken in ringing such mounts to ensure they are permanent. Other mounting media based on Canada balsam are used, but do not show the spermathecae and antennal sensilla very clearly.

In the absence of proper equipment and facilities, sandflies can be preserved in a dry condition, in wisps of paper tissue (not cotton wool), loosely packed in small tubes. Specimens stored dry are, naturally, rather brittle and are easily damaged.

CLASSIFICATION AND IDENTIFICATION OF SANDFLIES

Among the Phlebotominae there is no universal agreement on the ranking of taxa above the species level, although the proposals of Lewis et al,[7] are generally accepted. Different taxonomic opinions can cause confusion, especially when they concern vector species, e.g. the South American *Psychodopygus* is treated as a genus by some, but as a subgenus of *Lutzomyia* by others. Of the five genera of Phlebotominae, only two contain vector species: *Phlebotomus* (Old World) and *Lutzomyia* (New World). The remaining genera, *Sergentomyia* (Old World), *Brumptomyia* and *Warileya* (both New World), rarely feed on man. There is a loose association between the subgenera of sandflies and the affinities of the parasites they transmit, so that deducing potential vectors from their taxonomic relationships with known vector species is important in the initial stages of an epidemiological study.

Identification of sandflies to species is difficult and requires specialist training. Species are differentiated by minute characters, many internal, such as details (teeth- or scale-like processes) of the cibarium and pharynx, and the structure of the spermatheca. External features of the male genitalia and the antennal sensilla are also used. There is often considerable variation within species, making it difficult to determine the limits of particular taxa and to identify some vector species. Cryptic species and complexes of sibling ones make it difficult to separate many species of sandflies. Several new techniques (morphometrics, isoenzyme electrophoresis, DNA probes) are being used to differentiate some members of taxonomically intransigent species groups or complexes of sandflies.

MOSQUITOES
G. B. White

FAMILY: CULICIDAE

Mosquitoes are not confined to tropical regions; the main genera *Anopheles*, *Aedes* and *Culex* are distributed worldwide, even within the Arctic Circle. Approximately 3300 species of Culicidae have been described, more being recognized each year. They are classified in three subfamilies and 35 genera, as shown opposite.

Adult mosquitoes of both sexes feed on nectar and other fluids. Anopheline and culicine females also suck the blood of mammals, birds, frogs, etc., each species of mosquito tending to have particular host preferences. For blood-feeding, the proboscis stylets (Figure IV.29) are pushed into a blood capillary of the hosts' skin. Localized sensitivity to saliva from the mosquito is what causes dermal reactions popularly known as 'mosquito bites'. Each blood meal generally provides enough nutrition for the female mosquito to produce a batch of eggs, 30–150 in number. Anophelines

Subfamily	Tribe	Principal genera
Anophelinae	—	*Anopheles*
Culicinae	Aedini	*Aedes*
		Armigeres
		Eretmapodites
		Haemagogus
		Heizmannia
	Culicini	*Culex*
	Culisetini	*Culiseta*
	Mansoniini	*Coquillettidia*
		Mansonia
	Sabethini	*Limatus*
		Sabethes
		Trichoprosopon
		Tripteroides
		Wyeomyia
Toxorhynchitinae	—	*Toxorhynchites*

show the most regular cycles of blood-feeding and egg-laying. *Toxorhynchites* and some culicines produce eggs autogenously, i.e. without having fed on blood. Male and female mosquitoes may well live for several weeks, feeding repeatedly, under natural conditions. Through their regular attacks on man, female mosquitoes of certain species are important carriers of human diseases. All the vectors of human malaria belong to the genus *Anopheles* (Table IV.4). The main morphological differences between anophelines and culicines are portrayed in Figure IV.30. Various anophelines and especially culicines transmit arboviruses and filariasis of man (Tables IV.5 and IV.6). Mosquitoes also serve as the vectors of enzootic infections (i.e. restricted to animals or birds) and some zoonotic diseases due to pathogens transmitted from animals to man, e.g. yellow fever and subperiodic Brugian filariasis.

Breeding places of mosquitoes are always in water. Eggs may be deposited on damp soil or vegetation, in moist tree-holes or containers, and sometimes directly on to water. It is the choice of specific oviposition sites by female mosquitoes that determines the breeding places of each species. Eggs of the Aedini usually diapause, withstanding drought or winter, whereas other kinds of mosquito eggs hatch within a few days of being laid. Flooding and decreasing oxygen concentration trigger the hatching of eggs that have undergone diapause.

Larval development takes about a week for most tropical mosquitoes, but many temperate species over-winter as larvae. The fourth stage larva moults to the pupal stage, from which the adult mosquito emerges after a few days. Larvae breathe air via a pair of posterior dorsal spiracles mounted on a characteristic 'siphon' (Figure IV.30) which is not developed in anophelines. Pupae breathe via a pair of 'trumpets' on the thorax (Figure IV.31). Although some species have predacious larvae (e.g. *Toxorhynchites*, *Aedes* subgenus *Mucidus*, *Culex* subgenus *Lutzia*), the majority of mosquito larvae have mouthparts adapted for filter-feeding. Maxillary and palatal brushes sweep small food particles from the water, or from the substrate, and pass them to mandibles flanking the larval mouth. The diet of most mosquito larvae comprises micro-organisms and detritus. Rates of mosquito larval growth are influenced by such environmental factors as

temperature, photoperiod, food supply and the degree of crowding. Aquatic predators, pathogenic fungi (e.g. *Coelomomyces*, *Lagenidium*) and protozoa (gregarines, microsporidians), viruses and bacteria, together with water effects such as flushing or drying out, combine to take a heavy toll of immature stages of mosquito. These natural agencies can be manipulated for mosquito control purposes.

Larvae and pupae of mosquitoes are sometimes called 'wrigglers' and 'tumblers' respectively, terms which express their vigorous movements in the water. When undisturbed, the pupa rests beneath the surface preparing for metamorphosis. Pupae do not feed. Eventually the pupal case splits along the back and the adult mosquito works its way out on to the water surface. Wings and legs become extended and the body cuticle begins to harden within half an hour of eclosion. The adult mosquito then flies to shelter and rests for several hours. Males are not able to copulate until their terminalia (external genitalia) have turned upside down, a process known as hypopygial circumversion, taking about one day for completion. Thereafter the males form swarms with specific characteristics at certain times daily. Female mosquitoes flying into or near a swarm are set upon by the males and copulation ensues. Once inseminated, a female mosquito carries in her spermathecae sufficient sperms for fertilization of all the eggs she may produce. Through the action of matrone, a hormone from male accessory glands, mated female mosquitoes normally become unwilling to accept sperm from additional males. Hibernation of mated females is a common way of overwintering among temperate species of mosquito, e.g. *Culex pipiens*, *Culiseta annulata*, *Anopheles maculipennis* complex. Seasonal changes in the duration of daylight govern the onset and end of hibernation. Tropical mosquito adults are generally incapable of long-term quiescence.

When foraging, blood-thirsty female mosquitoes fly upwind searching for the scent trail of an attractive host. Sensilla on the palps and antennae serve to detect the host; eyes of the mosquito help to monitor ground speed, altitude, flight direction and details of host location. Intermittent downwind flights are also a feature of normal activity. The majority of mosquitoes hunt and feed at night, though many aedine mansoniine and sabethine species do so by day. Each

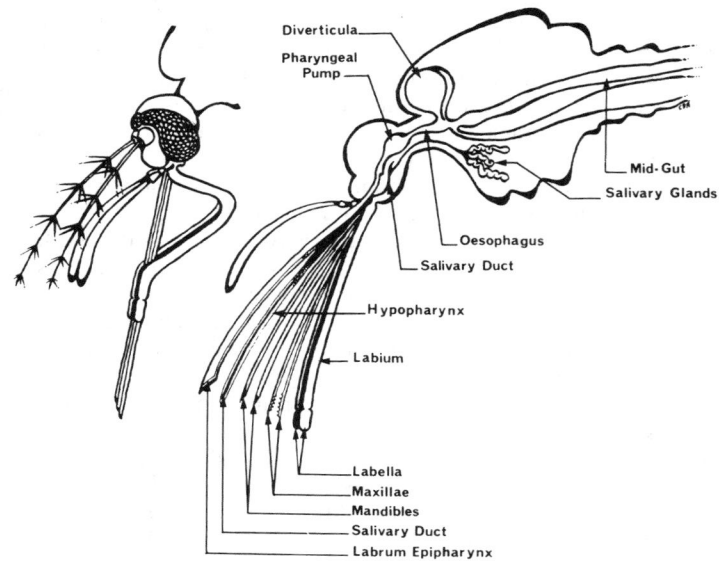

Diverticula
Pharyngeal Pump
Mid-Gut
Salivary Glands
Oesophagus
Salivary Duct
Hypopharynx
Labium
Labella
Maxillae
Mandibles
Salivary Duct
Labrum Epipharynx

Figure IV.29 Anatomy of the proboscis of the female *Anopheles*.

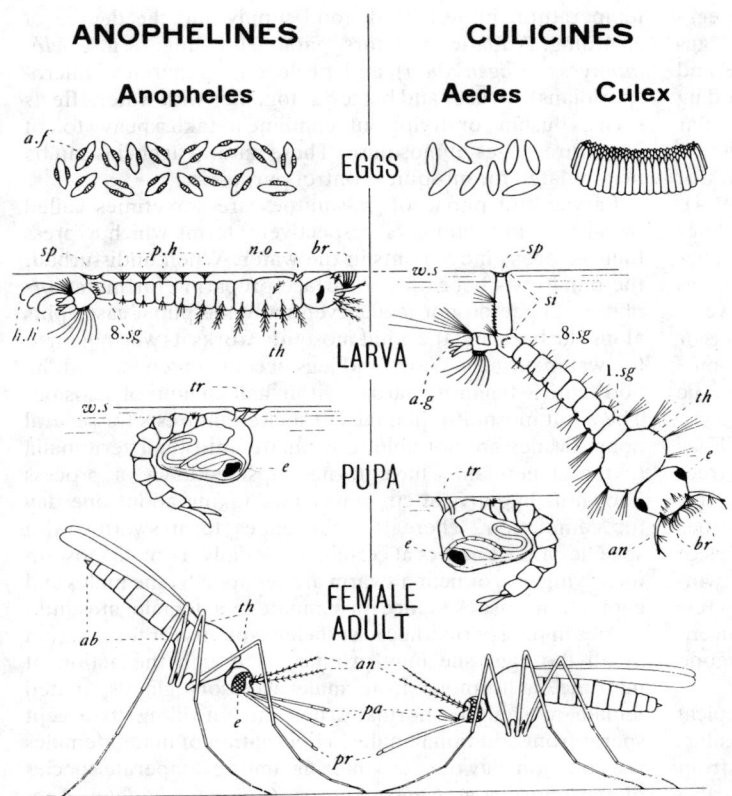

ANOPHELINES | CULICINES

Anopheles | Aedes Culex

EGGS

LARVA

PUPA

FEMALE ADULT

Figure IV.30 Chief distinguishing features of anophelines and culicines. *a.f.*, air floats; *a.g.*, anal gills; *ab*, abdomen; *an*, antenna; *br*, mouth brushes; *e*, eye; *h.h.*, hooked hairs or caudal setae; *n.o.*, notched organ; *pa*, palps (maxillary palpi); *p.h.*, palmate hairs or float hairs; *pr*, proboscis; 1.*sg*, first abdominal segment; 8.*sg*, eighth abdominal segment; *si*, siphon; sp, spiracles; *th*, thorax; *tr*, respiratory trumpets.

species has a well-defined activity cycle: some attack at dusk, others around midnight or at other hours. Species showing strong attraction to man are said to be anthropophilic, or more strictly anthropophagic when man is bitten, as opposed to zoophilic or zoophagic species which attack other creatures. Endophilic mosquitoes are those which favour houses or animal sheds for resting indoors, whereas exophilic species prefer to remain outdoors. Outdoor biting behaviour is termed exophagy, as opposed to the endophagy of mosquitoes which enter dwellings to bite people or animals. It is important to realize that mosquitoes may rest outdoors after feeding indoors or vice versa. Male mosquitoes tend to be less endophilic than females of the same species, while many man-biting species seldom go indoors at all. Few species of mosquito have man as their principal host. In order to quantify amounts of man–mosquito contact for epidemiological purposes it is necessary to estimate (1) the number of bites per person per 24 hours, (2) the percentage of mosquito blood meals obtained from man, versus other animals and (3) the feeding interval, expressed as the mean number of days between times when successive blood meals are taken by a given species of mosquito. These data can be combined with the probability of mosquito daily survival, estimated from the proportion of parous females, in order to calculate an index of vectorial capacity.[9]

Male and female mosquitoes are good fliers and sometimes disperse over many kilometres. However, most kinds of mosquito remain in rather restricted habitats. Those breeding in saltmarshes include some notorious migrants, notably *Aedes taeniorhynchus* along the American east coast. It has been suggested that *Anopheles pharoensis* occasionally travels almost 300 km over desert in the Middle East. Adult mosquitoes can be accidentally transported alive overseas in ships and aeroplanes. For instance, at least six introduced species of mosquito have recently become established on the remote Pacific island of Guam. A survey of planes arriving at Nairobi during the mid-1960s revealed mosquitoes imported from several other countries, *Culex quinquefasciatus* being most frequently encountered, and one African *Anopheles* was found returning on a flight from India. It seems that *Aedes aegypti*, *Anopheles gambiae* and possibly *C. quinquefasciatus* have been inadvertently taken by man from the Old World to the New World, where these mosquitoes have caused inestimable trouble. *A. gambiae* was wiped out again in the 1930s before it had spread from the primary focus in Brazil, but introduced populations of *Aedes aegypti* and *C. quinquefasciatus* are continually spreading throughout the tropics. Fortunately, not many species of mosquito readily become established in fresh situations.

Identification and taxonomy of mosquitoes are matters for specialists. The morphology of hairs, scales and other body structures must be studied in precise detail on adults of both sexes and on all the immature stages. This requires specimens in perfect condition as a basis for conventional identification. Where possible the larval and pupal skins should be preserved with the adult that emerges, so that the taxonomic characteristics of all life stages can be checked. Adult mosquito specimens should be kept on micropins, larvae and skins can be preserved in 60% alcohol or permanently mounted on a microscopic slide in chloral gum or Canada balsam for examination. Many species of mosquito show few points of distinction, although the characteristics of genera and subgenera can be recognized more easily. Most medically important species of mosquito have close similarities to

Table IV.4   Epidemiological zones and vectors of human malaria (see also Chapter 61).

1. North American
   - *A. (A.) freeborni*
   - *A. (A.) quadrimaculatus*
   - *(A. (N.) albimanus)*

2. Central American
   - *(A. (A.) aztecus)*
   - *(A. (A.) punctimacula)*
   - *A. (N.) albimanus*
   - *A. (N.) albitarsis*
   - *A. (N.) aquasalis*
   - *A. (N.) argyritarsis*
   - *A. (N.) darlingi*

3. South American
   - *A. (A.) pseudopunctipennis*
   - *A. (A.) punctimacula*
   - *(A. (K.) bellator)*
   - *(A. (K.) cruzii)*
   - *(A. (K.) neivai*
   - *A. (N.) albimanus*
   - *A. (N.) albitarsis*
   - *A. (N.) aquasalis*
   - *A. (N.) argyritarsis*
   - *A. (N.) darlingi*
   - *(A. (N.) numeztovari)*
   - *(A. (N.) oswaldoi)*
   - *(A. (N.) rangeli)*
   - *(A. (N.) triannulatus)*
   - *(A. (N.) trinkae)*

4. North Eurasian
   - *A. (A.) atroparvus*
   - *(A. (A.) messeae)*
   - *(A. (A.) sacharovi)*
   - *(A. (A.) sinensis)*
   - *(A. (C.) pattoni)*

5. Mediterranean
   - *A. (A.) atroparvus*
   - *A. (A.) claviger*
   - *A. (A.) labranchiae*
   - *(A. (A.) messeae)*
   - *A. (A.) sacharovi*
   - *(A. (C.) hispaniola)*
   - *(A. (C) pattoni)*

6. Afro-Arabian
   - *(A. (C.) hispaniola)*
   - *(A. (C.) multicolor)*
   - *A. (C.) pharoensis*
   - *(A. (C.) sergentii*

7. Afrotropical
   - *A. (C.) arabiensis*
   - *A. (C.) funestus*
   - *A. (C.) gambiae*
   - *(A. (C.) mascarensis)*
   - *(A. (C.) melas)*
   - *(A. (C.) merus)*
   - *(A. (C.) moucheti)*
   - *(A. (C.) nili)*
   - *(A. (C.) pharoensis)*

8. Indo-Iranian
   - *(A. (A.) sacharovi)*
   - *(A. (C.) annularis)*
   - *A. (C.) culicifacies*
   - *A. (C.) fluviatilis*
   - *(A. (C.) pulcherrimus)*
   - *(A. (C.) stephensi)*
   - *(A. (C.) superpictus)*
   - *(A. (C.) tessellatus)*

9. Indo-Chinese Hills
   - *(A. (A.) nigerrimus)*
   - *(A. (C.) annularis)*
   - *(A. (C.) culicifacies)*
   - *A. (C.) dirus*
   - *A. (C.) fluviatilis*
   - *(A. (C.) kunmingensis)*
   - *(A. (C.) maculatus)*
   - *A. (C.) minimus*

10. Malaysian
    - *A. (A.) campestris*
    - *A. (A.) donaldi*
    - *A. (A.) letifer*
    - *A. (A.) nigerrimus*
    - *(A. (A.) whartoni)*
    - *A. (C.) aconitus*
    - *A. (C.) balabacensis*
    - *A. (C.) dirus*
    - *A. (C.) flavirostris*
    - *A. (C.) leucosphyrus*
    - *A. (C.) ludlowae*
    - *A. (C.) maculatus*
    - *A. (C.) minimus*
    - *(A. (C.) philippinensis)*
    - *A. (C.) pseudowillmori*
    - *A. (C.) subpictus*
    - *A. (C.) sundaicus*

11. Chinese
    - *A. (A.) anthropophagus*
    - *A. (A.) sinensis*

12. Australasian
    - *(A. (A.) bancroftii)*
    - *A. (C.) farauti* type 1
    - *A. (C.) farauti* type 2
    - *(A. (C.) hilli)*
    - *(A. (C.) karwari)*
    - *A. (C.) koliensis*
    - *A. (C) punctulatus*
    - *(A. (C.) subpictus)*

Zonation according to the geographical distribution of the main vector species of *Anopheles*. In each zone (cf. map below) behaviour and ecology of *Anopheles* spp. governs transmission characteristics, e.g. indoor or outdoor transmission. *A, Anopheles; C, Celia; K, Kerteszia; N, Nyssorhynchus*. Names in parentheses are those of local or secondary vectors.

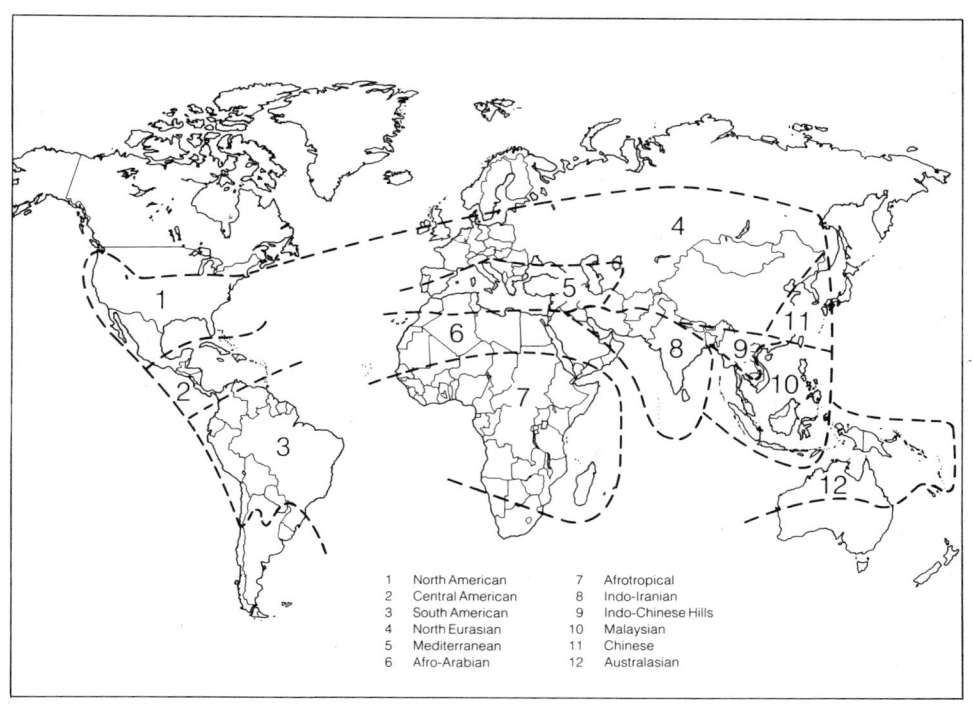

1	North American	7	Afrotropical
2	Central American	8	Indo-Iranian
3	South American	9	Indo-Chinese Hills
4	North Eurasian	10	Malaysian
5	Mediterranean	11	Chinese
6	Afro-Arabian	12	Australasian

Table IV.5 The mosquito vectors of human filariasis (see also Chapter 70).

Mosquito groups and their general distribution	Vector species and places where incriminated	W. bancrofti np	ns	ds	B. malayi np	ns	B. timori np
ANOPHELINAE							
Anopheles (Anopheles)							
bancroftii group: Australian/Papuan areas	*bancroftii* e.g. Papua New Guinea	+					
barbirostris group: Oriental region	*barbirostris*, e.g. Malaysia;	−			+	−	
	Sulawesi, Thailand; Flores				+		+
	campestris Malaysia	−			+	−	
	donaldi, e.g. Malaysia, Sarawak	−			+	−	
	anthropophagus, e.g. China	+			+		
	kewiyangensis, e.g. China				+		
hycanus group: Oriental and Palaearctic regions	*nigerrimus*, e.g. India, Sri Lanka, Thailand	+			+		
	sinensis complex, e.g. China, Korea, Malaysia, Thailand	+			+ −	−	
umbrosus group: Indomalaysian area	*letifer*, e.g. Malaysia	+					
	whartoni, e.g. Malaysia	+			?		
Anopheles (Cellia)							
funestus-minimus group: Afrotropical and Oriental regions	*aconitus*, Flores	+					
	flavirostris, Philippines	+					
	funestus, e.g. Ghana, Kenya, Liberia, Malagasy, Nigeria, Senegal, Sierra Leone, Tanzania, Burkino Faso, Zaire						
	minimus, Hong Kong	+					
gambiae complex: Afrotropical region	*arabiensis*, e.g. Burkino Faso, Kenya, Malagasy, Nigeria, Tanzania	+					
	bwambae, Uganda	+					
	gambiae, e.g. Ivory Coast, Kenya, Malagasy, Nigeria, Tanzania, Zaire	+					
	melas, e.g. Gambia, Guinea, Ivory Coast, Liberia, Sierra Leone	+ +					
	merus, e.g. Tanzania						
jeyporiensis: Oriental region	*candidiensis*, e.g. China	+					
leucosphyrus group: Oriental region	*balabacensis*, e.g. Indonesia	+					
	leucosphyrus, e.g. Malaysia	+					
maculatus: Oriental region	*maculatus*, e.g. Malaysia	+					
nili: Afrotropical region	*nili*, e.g. Liberia	+					
pauliani: Madagascar	*pauliani*, Madagascar	+					
philippinensis: Oriental region	*philippinensis*, e.g. India	+					
punctulatus complex: Papuan area and western Pacific	*farauti*, e.g. Solomon Islands	+					
	koliensis, e.g. Papua New Guinea	+					
	punctulatus, eg. Papua New Guinea	+					
subpictus group: Oriental region and Papuan area	*subpictus*, Flores	+					
tessellatus: Oriental region and Papuan area	*tessellatus*, e.g. Maldives	?					
vagus: Oriental region	*vagus*, e.g. Flores	+					
Anopheles (Kerteszia)							
bellator: South America	*bellator*, e.g. Brazil	+					

Table IV.5 Continued.

Mosquito groups and their general distribution	Vector species and places where incriminated	W. bancrofti np	ns	ds	B. malayi np	ns	B. timori np
Anopheles (Nyssorhynchus)							
albimanus group:	*albimanus*, Caribbean	?					
C. & S. America	*darlingi*, e.g. Brazil, Guyana	+					
argyritarsis group:							
Neotropical region	*aquasalis*, e.g. Brazil, Guyana	+					
CULICINAE							
Aedes (Finlaya)							
kochi group:	*fijiensis*, Fiji		+				
Indomalaysian, Papuan,	*oceanicus*, e.g. Samoa, Tonga			+	+		+
North Australia and	*poicilius*, Philippines	+					
South Pacific	*samoanus*, Samoa		+				+
	tutuilae, Samoa						?
niveus group:	*niveus*, e.g. Philippines	+					
Oriental region	*harinasutai*, Thailand		+				
togoi: East and S.E. Asia	*togoi*, e.g. China, Japan, Korea	+				+	
Aedes (Ochlerotatus)	*scapularis*, e.g. Brazil	+					
scapularis: Neotropical region							
taeniorhynchus group: USA and Neotropical region	*taeniorhynchus*, e.g. Virgin Islands	?					
vigilax group: East Africa, Australian, Indomalaysian, Papuan and South Pacific areas	*vigilax*, e.g. New Caledonia		+				
Aedes (Stegomyia)							
aegypti group: cosmotropical	*aegypti*, filaria susceptible genotypes occur at low frequency, especially in East Africa	−		−	−		
scutellaris group: North Australian,	*cooki*, Niue Islands		?				
	futunae, Horne Islands		+				
Indomalaysian,	*kesseli*, Tonga		?				
Papuan and Pacific areas	*polynesiensis*, central and eastern Polynesia, e.g. Fiji, Samoa, Tahiti, Tuamotu		+				
	pseudoscutellaris, Fiji		+				
	rotumae, Rotuma Island		?				
	tabu, Haapai Tongatapu Island		+				
	tongae, Haapai Islands, Vavau Island		+				
	upolensis, Samoa		+				
Culex (Culex)	*pipiens*, biotype *molestus*, e.g. Egypt, Turkey	+					
pipiens group: cosmopolitan	*pipiens*, form *pallens*, e.g. China, Japan	+					
	quinquefasciatus, tropical Africa, Asia, Caribbean and South America	+					
sitiens group:	*annulirostris*, e.g. West Irian	+					
Afrotropical, Australian and Oriental regions	*bitaeniorhynchus*, e.g. India, West Irian	+					
	gelidus, e.g. India	?					
	sitiens complex, e.g. India, Maldive Islands						
	tritaeniorhynchus, e.g. Bangladesh, India	?					
	vishnui complex, e.g. Bangladesh, India	?			?		
Mansonia (Mansonia)							
titillans: Neotropical region	*titillans*, e.g. Guyana	+					

Table IV.5 Continued.

Mosquito groups and their general distribution	Vector species and places where incriminated	W. bancrofti np	W. bancrofti ns	W. bancrofti ds	B. malayi np	B. malayi ns	B. timori np
Forms of filariasis							
Mansonia (Mansonioides)							
dives group:	*bonneae*, e.g. Malaysia;				−	+	
Oriental region and	Thailand				+		
Papua area	*dives*, e.g. Malaysia, Sumatra, Palawan				+	+	
uniformis group:	*annulata*, e.g. Kalimantan, Malaysia, Sri Lanka	−			+		
Afrotropical,	Sumatra, Thailand						
Australian and	*annulifera*, e.g. India, Kalimantan, Sri Lanka*,				+		
Oriental regions	Thailand						
	indiana, e.g. India, Java, Sri Lanka*, Malaysia,				+		
	Thailand						
	uniformis, e.g. Africa;	−					
	India, Kalimantan, Malaysia, Sri Lanka*;	−		+	+		
	West Irian	+					

np, Nocturnally periodic; *ns*, nocturnally subperiodic or non-periodic; *ds*, diurnally subperiodic; +, proven vector, infective filarial larvae found repeatedly in wild mosquito female; −, non-vector: filarial larvae usually fail to develop; no entry, vector status undetermined or form of filariasis absent.
*Brugia malayi now virtually eradicated from Sri Lanka.

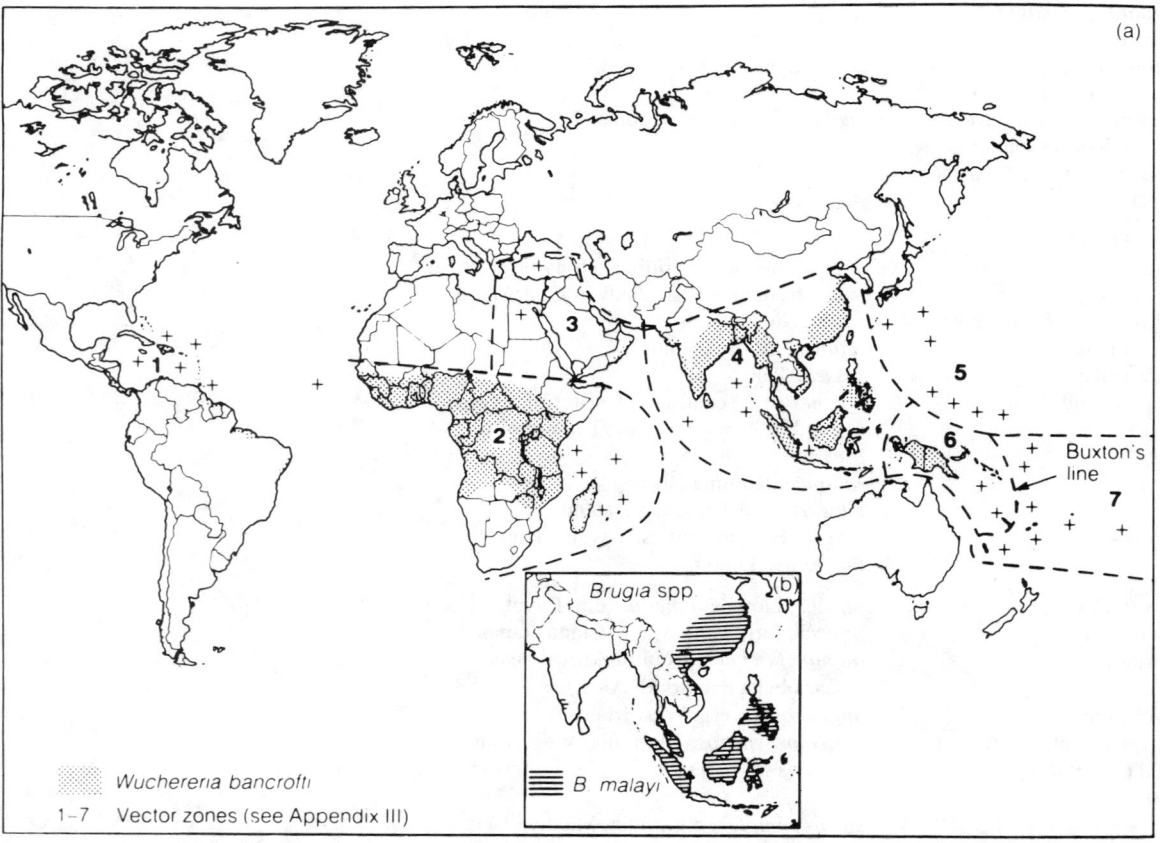

Zone 1: Neotropical: *Anopheles albimanus, aquasalis, bellator, darlingi; Aedes scapularis, taeniorhynchus; Culex quinquefasciatus; Mansonia titillans.*
Zone 2: Afrotropical: *Anopheles funestus, arabiensis, gambiae, melas, merus; Culex quinquefasciatus, sitiens.*
Zone 3: Middle Eastern: *Culex pipiens, molestus.*
Zone 4: Oriental: *Anopheles barbirostris, campestris, donaldi, nigerrimus, sinensis* complex, *letifer, whartoni, aconitus, flavirostris, minimus, candidiensis, maculatus, philippinensis, subpictus, tesselatus; Aedes niveus, harinasutai, togoi, poicilius; Culex bitaeniorhynchus, gelidus, sitiens* complex, *tritaeniorhynchus, vishnui* complex; *Mansonia uniformis, bonneae, annulata, annulifera, indiana.*
Zone 5: Western Pacific: *Culex pipiens; Aedes togoi.*
Zone 6: Papuan: *Anopheles bancrofti, punctulatus, farauti, koliensis, subpictus, tesselatus.*
Zone 7: South Pacific: *Aedes kochi* group *fijiensis, oceanicus, samoanus, tutuilae; Aedes scutellaris* group *cooki, futanae, kesseli, polynesiensis, pseudoscutellaris, rotumae, tabu, tongae, upolensis; Aedes vigilax.*

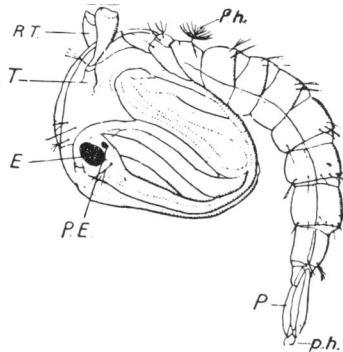

Figure IV.31 Pupa of *Anopheles maculipennis*. E, Eye of developing adult; P, paddle of pupa; PE, pupal eye; RT, respiratory trumpet; T, trachea leading to anterior thoracic spindle.

other species which do not bite man. Specific identification may depend on minute features of the male, the larva or even the egg, often making it unreliable to identify individual female specimens. For some species of mosquito it may be necessary to look at their chromosomal or DNA characteristics, proteins or behaviour in order to distinguish between species which are morphologically identical, or nearly so. Groups of such closely related species are known as 'sibling species complexes'. Genetic evidence shows that these biologically distinct species do not normally interbreed in nature. The significance of species complexes is that some of the species are pests and vectors of disease while others are not.

ANATOMY (Figures IV.29–IV.36)

The body of an adult mosquito consists of three recognizable divisions: head, thorax and abdomen. The head is rounded and attached to the thorax by a slender neck. It is provided with large eyes, antennae and mouthparts. The antennae (Figures IV.34 and IV.35) are composed of 15 segments. Each segment bears a whorl of hairs in the female, but in the male the hairs are profuse, giving a bristly or bottle-brush appearance. The mouthparts in the female consist of a proboscis fitted for piercing and sucking. The labium encloses the other mouthparts (Figure IV.29), except the maxillary palps, and ends distally in two pointed labella lobes clothed with scales and hairs. In the act of biting, the labellae part and are applied to the surface of the skin, forming a sheath for the delicate piercing stylets, and do not enter the wound made for obtaining blood. Within is the labrum-epipharynx, forming a V-shaped channel open on the ventral surface. This extends along the whole length of the labium and ends in a sharp point. Lying directly beneath the labrum-epipharynx, closing the ventral slit, is the hypopharynx, consisting of a thin chitinous lamella, fitting closely to the ventral surface of the labrum-epipharynx, thus forming a tube through which the blood is sucked. In the longitudinal chitinous thickening runs a very fine channel extending from the base to the tip of the hypopharynx; through this the salivary secretion is poured into the wound (Figure IV.29). The mandibles form delicate chitinous stylets at the side of the hypopharynx. The labium buckles in the act of biting and

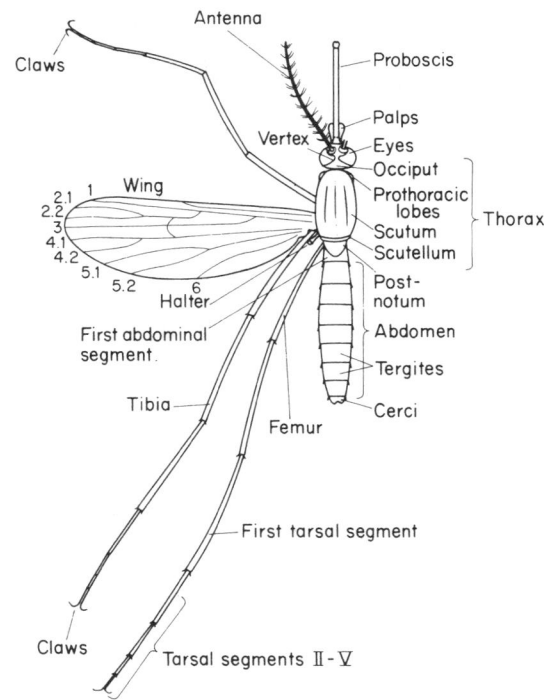

Figure IV.32 The anatomy of the female mosquito, showing wing veins 1–6.

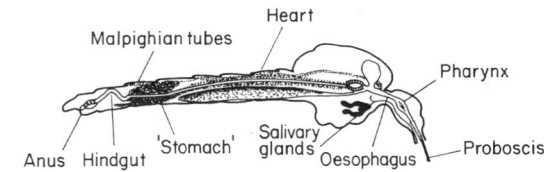

Figure IV.33 Longitudinal section of a female mosquito showing its anatomy.

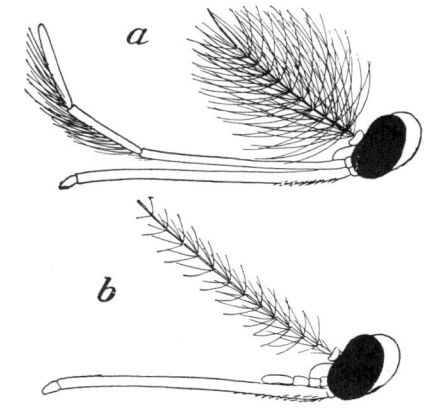

Figure IV.34 Heads of (a) male and (b) female culicine.

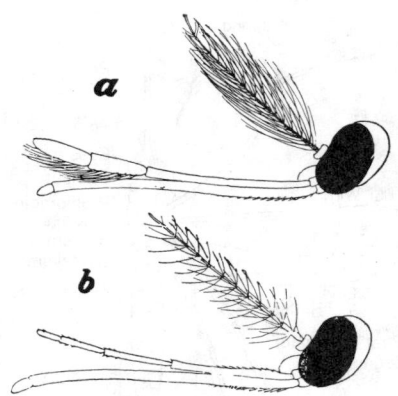

Figure IV.35   Heads of (a) male and (b) female anopheline.

the stylets emerge. Each of these tapers slightly, ending in a sharp point. The maxillary stylets are more robustly constructed, but have the same general form; the tip is generally supplied with a row of backwardly pointing teeth. The maxillary palps consist of five partially fused segments. In the male the mouthparts are not adapted for biting. The maxillary palps are elongated, extending above the proboscis, but the mandibles and maxillae are greatly reduced and may be lacking altogether.

In female anophelines the palps are as long as the proboscis and usually closely applied, but in female culicines the palps are short. In male mosquitoes, both culicine and anopheline, the palps are as long as the proboscis. The palps of the male culicines are bushy and the two terminal segments tend to turn upwards in *Culex*, downward in *Aedes*. Those of the male anophelines are rather club-shaped.

The thorax is wedge-shaped in side view; the sides form the pleura, with scale patches. The various sclerites composing the side of the thorax bear stiff setae or hairs, arranged in definite groups. The scutellum is separated by a transverse suture from the mesonotum. In all genera except *Anopheles*, it is trilobate and each lobe bears a group of stiff setae. In anophelines the scutellum is rounded and reduced. The region behind the scutellum is known as the postnotum and is generally nude. The wings are long and narrow, with venation; the scales are characteristic. Situated immediately posterior to the base of the wings is a pair of halteres or balancers, which have gyroscopic functions during flight.

The legs are long and slender, composed of coxa, trochanter, femur and tibia, as well as a tarsus of five long and slender tarsomeres. The last tarsomere bears a pair of claws (ungues), which vary greatly in size and shape; those of the hind legs are generally smaller than those of others. The abdomen is nearly cylindrical, narrow and elongated, consisting of 10 segments, the last two modified for sexual purposes. The terminal segment in the female is tapered. The ninth is reduced and in the intersegmental area between it and the eighth lies the opening of the reproductive organs. The tenth segment is greatly reduced and bears the anal opening and paired cerci. The abdomen of the male is slightly longer than that of the female. The terminal segments are greatly modified and bear paired claspers, between which lies the aedeagus, a complex organ for use in reproduction. Specific characteristics of these terminalia are the basis of much taxonomy (Figure IV.36).

SUBFAMILY: TOXORHYNCHITINAE

As they are larger than other mosquitoes, it is fortunate that *Toxorhynchites* cannot suck blood. The proboscis is strongly down-curved and suited only for imbibing nectar from plants or free fluids. About 60 species are known, all classified in a single genus. *Toxorhynchites* occur in all warmer regions of the world, between 35°N and 35°S approximately. Breeding places are flooded tree-holes, rock-holes and artificial containers such as buckets and discarded tyres. Female *Toxorhynchites* scatter their rounded buoyant eggs on to water while flying. Larvae soon hatch and become rapacious predators with mouth brushes composed of six to ten strong recurved teeth on each side for grasping prey. When the chance arises cannibalism occurs. A relatively short, dark, strongly chitinous respiratory siphon is present at the abdominal tip, as for larval Culicinae. Populations of some dangerous container-breeding Culicinae, notably *Aedes aegypti*, can be significantly reduced through larval predation by *Toxorhynchites*. This subfamily of mosquitoes should therefore be regarded as beneficial. Adult *Toxorhynchites* are colourful due to their iridescent and metallic scale patterns, with patches of purple, red, orange and green ornamentation on particular species. The lateral abdominal tail tufts and large size (up to 18 mm head to tail; wing span 12–24 mm) are distinctive. *Toxorhynchites* adults are diurnally active and sometimes venture into houses, where they may be found when trying to escape from windows.

SUBFAMILY: ANOPHELINAE

The palps in both sexes are as long, or nearly as long, as the proboscis. The scutellum is rounded. Wings of nearly all species have characteristic patterns of pale and dark spots of scales (Figure IV.37). The subfamily Anophelinae was divided by Edwards into three genera: *Chagasia* (scutellum slightly trilobed), *Bironella* (scutellum evenly rounded, wing with stem of median fork wavy) and *Anopheles* (scutellum evenly rounded, wing with stem of median fork straight). The genus includes over 400 species. When settled, most *Anopheles* stand with the proboscis, head and abdomen in almost a straight line, usually resting on an upright surface at an angle of about 45°; exceptionally, as in *A. culicifacies*, the resting position adopted is more *Culex*-like (Figure IV.38). In flight the hum produced by *Anopheles* is low-pitched, almost inaudible unless close to the ear. Most species require large spaces for mating flights, rendering it difficult to propagate them in captivity. Over-wintering females are fertilized before diapausing, but the males of temperate species cannot overwinter. For tropical species, both sexes are likely to live for several weeks, feeding intermittently. At 25–30°C tropical female *Anopheles* can be expected to suck blood and then lay eggs regularly at intervals of 2 or 3 days. The boat-shaped eggs (Figure IV.39) have an investing membrane inflated laterally to form a pair of floats. These represent air-filled spaces between the exo-chorion and the endo-chorion of the egg shell to resist submersion. Anopheline eggs are 1 mm in length. They are white when freshly laid, but tan to dull brown or black within a few hours. They are laid singly on the

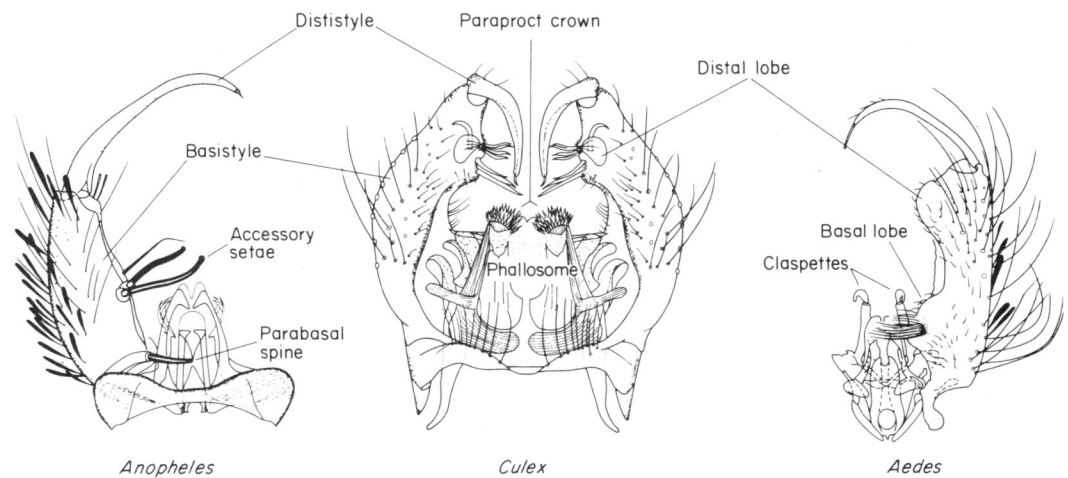

Figure IV.36   Male terminalia (external genitalia) of *Aedes*, *Anopheles* and *Culex* in ventral view, showing the main generic characteristics. These features show specific modifications that are useful for taxonomy and identification of species and genera.

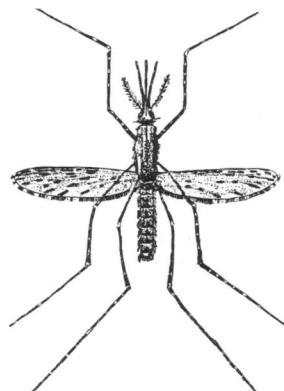

Figure IV.37   Anopheles gambiae. One of a series of drawings made by the late Philip Manson-Bahr, showing the wing markings characteristic of *Anopheles* (6×).

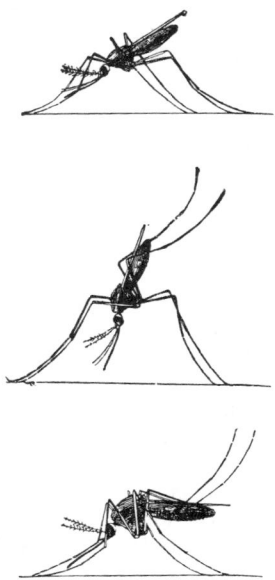

Figure IV.38   The resting positions of *Culex quinquefasciatus* (below), *Anopheles sinensis* (centre) and *Anopheles gambiae* (above).

surface of the water, arrange themselves in a distinct pattern at that site, and hatch in 2 or 3 days. The larva feeds on small floating particles swept into its mouth by feeding brushes which can be folded under its head. When *Anopheles* larvae lie beneath the surface, the dorsal aspects of the thorax and abdomen face upward, but the head is rotated 180° so that its ventral surface lies upward. Food consists of living organisms, bacteria and protozoa obtained beneath the surface, as well as particles of floating food such as dead insect fragments. The head of the larva is complex; the central portion is known as the clypeus, the anterior plaque as the preclypus. It has a pair of short antennae, eyes, a pair of feeding brushes and preclypeal and clypeal hairs. The respiratory opening is composed of two dorsally placed spiracles on the eighth abdominal segment. From the spiracles, the tracheae run the length of the body, conducting air to all regions for respiration.

The larva maintains itself under the surface film in a horizontal position by a row of dorsoabdominal plaques and a series of palmate hairs, known as float hairs. The terminal segment is provided with four anal papillae (gills), which

have respiratory and excretory functions, but are mainly to absorb mineral salts. Above and below the anal gills are dorsal and ventral swimming-brushes (Figure IV.40). The eighth segment has a chitinous plate lying between the two openings of the spiracles; just below it there is a row of teeth arising from a chitinized base, known as the pecten. Small glands secrete a waxy substance around the spiracles, which therefore cannot be wetted. (It is important to note this fact when oiling water to kill larvae.) Respiration also takes place through the cuticle but the oxygen intake from the water is not sufficient to maintain life, except when the temperature is low and metabolism reduced.

The capabilities of any particular species of *Amopheles* to transmit malaria are regulated by a number of factors, such as the numbers present, the degree of anthropophily (human blood index), the probability of survival to a potentially infective age and whether the parasites of malaria can complete their development in the mosquito. A species proved to be a natural carrier in one situation does not necessarily play an important part somewhere else. There is a striking correlation between the incidence of malaria and of *Anopheles* as seen in the case of *A. punctulatus* complex, which occurs on some islands in the South Pacific, but not others. Where these species occur there is malaria; where they do not, there is none. Malaria vector *Anopheles* spp. of the world are listed in Table IV.4.

Mosquito nomenclature is a vexed question. A great many species have been renamed in recent years. In case of doubt recourse should be made to Knight and Stone.[10]

In making a malaria survey an attempt should be made to identify female anophelines; they should be collected and dissected to find out which species are infective. It is necessary to dissect at least several hundred insects and to examine the gut for oocysts and salivary glands for sporozoites. Molecular and immunological detection techniques (e.g. ELISA) are also now available for sporozoite detection. Infectivity rates are generally below 0.1%, though higher rates are often recorded, especially with *A. funestus* and the *A. gambiae* complex in Africa. Adults and larvae should be identified to determine whether known vector species are present. Any locality should be studied for at least a complete year. Seasonal transmission is important; one species may be responsible in spring and another during the autumn.

Identification of the many diverse species of *Anopheles* is specialized work. The following points are of specific importance: size, general colouration, colour of erect scales on the head, pattern of pale scales on the generally dark legs, wings and so on. The distal half of the proboscis may be pale, the palps may be smooth or shaggy, depending on the scales. The palps may be entirely dark or there may be pale bands. The general colouration of the thorax and scales on the mesonotum is helpful. These features are too intricate to be explained in detail here, and identification depends upon characters listed in the published keys.

The distribution and importance of some species of *Anopheles* have been changed in recent years as a result of malaria control or eradication programmes in which residual insecticides have been used. Formerly DDT was the insecticide of choice but, to offset DDT resistance, some more potent pyrethroids and other insecticides (e.g. carbamates, organophosphates) are increasingly being utilized for house spraying (see Table IV.13).

Some species are less responsive than others to insecticides

sprayed indoors because either they tend to leave buildings after feeding, without resting on treated walls, or they tend to bite and rest in the open and therefore do not come into contact with residual insecticides.

Much success has been achieved in eradication programmes in subtropical areas and in some parts of the tropics, but even where eradication has been almost complete, there have been renewed outbreaks of malaria, as in Sri Lanka, India and Guyana. Such outbreaks can occur if surveillance is insufficient, and mosquitoes are allowed to multiply enormously if conditions change so as to stimulate breeding.

In most parts of tropical Africa malaria transmission has hardly changed. Where intensive insecticide spraying has been carried out, *A. funestus* has been eliminated, though it could re-enter the area from the periphery when spraying is discontinued. The main vectors, members of the *A. gambiae* complex (*A. gambiae*, *A. arabiensis*, *A. melas*) breed so prolifically in so many collections of water, and bite man so voraciously indoors and in the open, that control by insecticides is extremely difficult.

In addition to malaria, *Anopheles* spp. transmit *Wuchereria bancrofti*, many of the malaria-carrying species being implicated (Table IV.5). The now recognized Timor filaria parasite of man, *Brugia timori*, has *A. barbirostris* as the only known vector, at least in the island of Flores.[11] *Anopheles* also transmit several arboviruses, for instance eastern equine encephalitis, western equine encephalitis, Venezuelan equine encephalitis, onyong-nyong, tataguine, and others listed in Table IV.6.

Adult anopheline mosquitoes are active only at night when the females seek avidly to feed on the blood of vertebrates. Medically important anthropophilic species belong to the subgenera: *Anopheles*, *Cellia*, *Kerteszia* and *Nyssorhynchus* of the genus *Anopheles*. Neither of the other two anopheline genera, *Bironella* and *Chagasia*, nor the *Anopheles* subgenera *Lophopodomyia* and *Stethomyia* are of any applied interest. Taxonomic separation of *Anopheles* subgenera is based upon the numbers and positions of certain spines on the male basistyle (see Figure IV.36), together with other features summarized by Reid.[12]

Subgenus *Anopheles* predominates in the northern hemisphere, extending southwards with a few species found in Australia and through Africa. These mosquitoes are generally more robust and larger (wing span 8–12 mm) than those belonging to other anopheline subgenera. Taxonomists recognize six series of species within the subgenus *Anopheles*. Vectors of human diseases belong to the *Myzorhynchus* series as well as series *Anopheles* (*sensu stricto*).

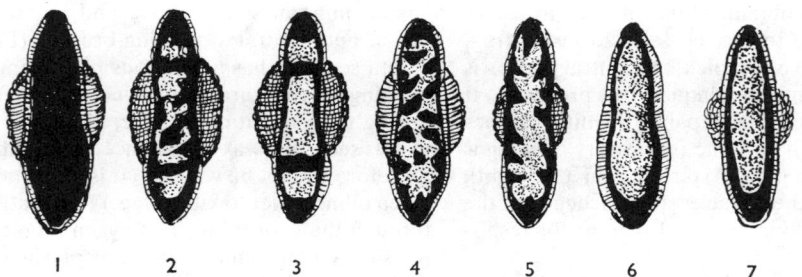

Figure IV.39 Eggs of the *Anopheles maculipennis* complex. 1, *melanoon*; 2, *messeae*; 3, *beklemishevi* or *maculipennis* (*sensu stricto*); 4, *atroparvus*; 5, *labranchiae*; 6, *sacharovi* (summer); 7, *sacharovi* (winter). Species identification is based on the pattern on the deck (upper surface of egg) and the form of floats, i.e. size, number of ribs and striations.

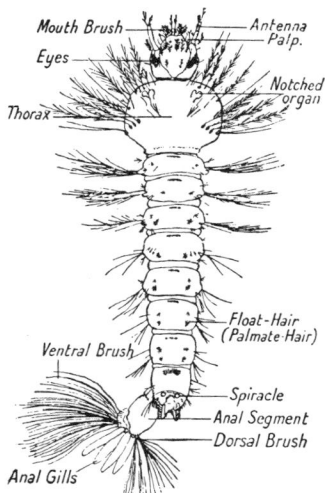

Figure IV.40 Larva of an anopheline (*A. maculipennis*) seen from above. The anal segment is twisted round to display the dorsal and ventral brushes.

Series *Myzorhynchus* occurs mainly in the Oriental region, the following species groups being involved in human disease transmission. *A. hyrcanus* group, mostly zoophilic species, but including *A. sinensis* the main vector of malaria in China, also implicated as a vector of rural filariasis (both *B. malayi* and *W. bancrofti*) in parts of South-East Asia; it thrives where paddy provides suitable breeding places. The closely related *A. nigerrimus*, which breeds in more permanent ponds, also contributes to malaria and filariasis transmission in South-East Asia (see Tables IV.4 and IV.5). *A. barbirostris* group of blackish species with shaggy palps includes two important Malaysian vectors of malaria: darker *A. campestris* associated with clay but not sandy soils, especially alluvial coastal areas, where the larvae occur in lightly shaded deep waters, and paler *A. donaldi* which breeds in swampy forests. These and other members of the *A. barbirostris* group are important vectors of periodic *B. malayi*, but not of the subperiodic form or of *W. bancrofti* to which they are mostly refractory, although *A. donaldi* appears to transmit *W. bancrofti* in Borneo. The only known vector of Timor filariasis (*B. timori*) is said to be *A. barbirostris*,[11] but this mosquito might be the atypical form of *A. barbirostris (sensu lato)* regarded as a local vector of bancroftian filariasis in Sulawesi and perhaps other parts of Indonesia. In the closely related *A. bancroftii* group, the typical species transmits malaria and periodic bancroftian filariasis in Papua New Guinea and Indonesia, and formerly in Australia. Finally in this series the *A. umbrosus* group, having larvae with reduced float hairs, includes two vectors of bancroftian filariasis and malaria in Malaysia: *A. letifer* and *A. whartoni*, both of which breed in partially shaded, acidic stagnant water. Much caution should be exercised in vector studies on mosquitoes belonging to the series *Myzorhynchus*, since they are frequently infected with zoonotic parasites (e.g. monkey malarias) and the taxonomic distinctions between many of the species require expert attention.

Series *Anopheles* includes the notorious *A. maculipennis* complex of a dozen species in the northern hemisphere.[13] Specific patterns on the eggs (Figure IV.39) are the best means of distinguishing these sibling species (i.e. morphologically similar species) which have distinctive biological characteristics despite their anatomical similarities. Differences of the chromosomes and protein electromorphs are also useful for specific identification. Typical *A. maculipennis(sensu stricto)* seldom attacks man, so probably was never a malaria vector, although most malaria transmission in Europe was formerly due to *A. maculipennis sensu lato*, meaning all species combined in the complex. The most widespread member of the *A. maculipennis* complex is *A. messeae*, which is also mainly zoophilic. Arboviruses transmitted by the *A. maculipennis* complex (Table IV.6) are usually associated with *A. messeae*. *A. labranchiae* and *A. sacharovi* around the Mediterranean, and *A. atroparvus* in other parts of Europe were vectors of malaria, and still are in a few places. These three species tend to breed in brackish water, although they are not confined to coastal localities. Because *A. atroparvus* females spend the winter resting indoors, periodically biting people or livestock but not producing eggs until spring, they were responsible for the phenomenon of 'winter malaria' transmission in bygone days. The disappearance of malaria from Europe has been mainly due to the decline of these mosquitoes resulting from housing improvements, draining of marshes, breeding site pollution (soaps and detergents infiltrate the larval tracheae, causing them to drown) and through the application of chemical pesticides. Former malaria vectors in North America belonging to this group are the freshwater-breeding species *A. freeborni* and the more distinctive species *A. quadrimaculatus*.[14] One more medically important species belonging to this series is *A. claviger* which over-winters as larvae and breeds in weedy ponds throughout Europe and the Middle East, where it still transmits some malaria. *A. claviger* may also be involved with myxomatosis transmission among rabbits. Several arboviruses have been isolated from *Anopheles* spp. in Europe and North America (Table IV.6) but it is doubtful if transmission depends upon these vectors in any case.

Subgenus *Cellia* has the majority of species in the genus *Anopheles*, with many complexes of sibling species including disease vectors that are extremely difficult to identify. The taxonomic literature is very inadequate, except for the excellent monographs by Reid[12] covering Malaysian species and by Gillies and De Meillon[15] for African species. *Cellia* species are found almost exclusively in the Old World tropics, being classified into six series: *Cellia, Myzomyia, Neocellia, Neomyzomyia, Paramyzomyia* and *Pyretophorus*, according to the forms of pharyngeal teeth in females. Many *Cellia* spp. are attracted to man for blood meals and representatives of all six series have been implicated as vectors of human diseases.

Series *Cellia* is a group of about ten distinctive savanna species in Africa and the Middle East. Adults differ from most other anophelines through having abdominal scales, those at the sides forming segmental tufts. The thorax and palps are unusually scaly also, the latter appearing shaggy. *A. pharoensis* is the dominant species especially in Egypt where it is the main malaria vector. It also carries arbovirus and helminth infections to animals. The closely related *A. squamosus* is an incidental malaria vector in various parts of Africa.

Series *Myzomyia* includes the *A. funestus–minimus* complex, numbering about a score of small and delicate species with varied host preferences and breeding sites. Three of the

Table IV.6   Mosquitoes implicated as hosts involved in transmission of arboviruses affecting man (see also Chapter 30).

Arbovirus and endemic area	Natural vector (*indicates principal species)
Togaviridae ALPHAVIRUS (=GROUP A) *Barmah Forest Virus (BFV)*	
Australia	*Aedes (Ochlerotatus) vigilax* *Culex (Culex) annulirostris*
Chikungunya (CHIK)	
Africa	*Aedes (Diceromyia) furcifer* *Aedes (Stegomyia) aegypti* *Aedes (Stegomyia) africanus* *Coquillettidia (Coquillettidia) fuscopennata* *Culex (Culex) quinquefasciatus* *Mansonia (Mansonioides) africana* *Mansonia (Mansonioides) uniformis*
South-East Asia	*Aedes (Stegomyia) aegypti* *Aedes (Stegomyia) albopictus?* *Culex (Culex) gelidus* *Culex (Culex) quinquefasciatus* *Culex (Culex) tritaeniorhynchus*
Eastern equine encephalitis (EEE)	
North America	*Aedes (Aedimorphus) vexans* *Aedes (Ochlerotatus) atlanticus* *Aedes (Ochlerotatus) fulvus* *Aedes (Ochlerotatus) mitchellae* *Aedes (Ochlerotatus) sollicitans* *Aedes (Ochlerotatus) sticticus* *Aedes (Ochlerotatus) taeniorhynchus* *Anopheles (Anopheles) crucians* *Coquillettidia (Coquillettidia) perturbans* *Culex (Culex) nigripalpus* *Culex (Culex) quinquefasciatus* *Culex (Culex) restuans* *Culex (Culex) salinarius* *Culiseta (Climacura) melanura* *Culiseta (Culicella) morsitans*
South America	*Aedes (Ochlerotatus) taeniorhynchus* *Culux (Culex) nigripalpus* *Culex (Melanoconion) caudelli* *Culex (Melanoconion) spissipes* *Culex (Melanoconion) taeniopus*
Europe	*Culex (Culex) pipiens*
Everglades (EVE)	
Florida	*Aedes (Ochlerotatus) atlanticus* *Aedes (Ochlerotatus) taeniorhynchus* *Anopheles (Anopheles) crucians* *Culex (Culex) nigripalpus* *Culex (Melanoconion) spp.*

Arbovirus and endemic area	Natural vector (*indicates principal species)
Mayaro (MAY)	
South and Central America	*Culex* spp. *Haemagogus* spp. *Coquillettidia (Rhynchotaemia) venezuelensis* *Psorophora (Janthinosoma) ferox* *Sabethini* spp.
Mucambo (MUC)	
South America	*Aedes* spp. *Aedes (Ochlerotatus) serratus* *Culex* spp. *Culex (Melanoconion) portesi* *Haemagogus* spp. *Sabethini* spp. *Wyeomyia* spp.
O'nong-nyong (ONN)	
Africa	*Anopheles (Cellia) funestus* *Anopheles (Cellia) gambiae (sensu lato)*
Ross River (RR)	
Australasia	*Aedes (Ochlerotatus) vigilax* *Culex (Culex) annulirostris*
Semliki Forest (SF)	
Africa	*Aedes (Aedimorphus) abnormalis* group *Aedes (Aedimorphus) argenteopunctatus* *Aedes (Aedimorphus) denatus* *Aedes (Neomelaniconion) palpalis* *Anopheles (Cellia) funestus* *Eretmapodites grahamii*
Sindbis (SIN)	
Africa	*Aedes (Aedimorphus) cumminsi* *Aedes (Neomelaniconion) circumluteolus* *Anopheles (Celia) pharoensis* *Coquillettidia (Coquillettidia) fuscopennata* *Culex (Culex) antennatus* *Culex (Culex) perexiguus* *Culex (Culex) pipiens (sensu lato)* *Culex (Culex) univittatus* *Mansonia (Mansonioides) africana*
Australasia	*Aedes (Ochlerotatus) normanensis* *Aedes (Ochlerotatus) vigilax* *Culex (Culex) annulirostris* *Mansonia (Mansonioides) septempunctata*
Orient	*Culex (Culex) bitaeniorhynchus* *Culex (Culex) pseudovishnui* *Culex (Culex) tritaeniorhynchus*

Table IV.6 Continued

Arbovirus and endemic area	Natural vector (*indicates principal species)
Venezuelan equine encephalitis (VEE)	
Tropical Americas	about 40 species implicated, including:
	Aedes (Ochlerotatus) angustivittatus
	Aedes (Ochlerotatus) scapularis
	*Aedes (Ochlerotatus) serratus
	Aedes (Ochlerotatus) sollicitans
	*Aedes (Ochlerotatus) taeniorhynchus
	Aedes (Ochlerotatus) thelcter
	Aedes (Stegomyia) aegypti
	Anopheles (Anopheles) aquasalis
	Anopheles (Anopheles) crucians
	Anopheles (Anopheles) neomaculipalpus
	Anopheles (Anopheles) pseudopunctipennis
	Anopheles (Anopheles) punctimacula
	Culex (Culex) corniger
	Culex (Culex) coronator
	Culex (Culex) nigripalpus
	Cilex (Culex) tarsalis
	*Culex (Melanoconion) spp.
	Culex (Melanoconion) iolambdis
	Culex (Melanoconion) ocossa/panocossa
	Culex (Melanoconion) portesi
	Culex (Melanoconion) taeniopus
	Culex (Melanoconion) vomerifer
	Deinocerites pseudes
	Haemagogus spp.
	Limatus flavisetosus
	Mansonia (Mansonia) indubitans
	Mansonia (Mansonia) titillans
	*Psorophora (Grabhamia) confinnis
	Psorophora (Grabhamia) discolor
	Psorophora (Janthinosoma) albipes
	Psorophora (Janthinosoma) cyanescens
	*Psorophora (Janthinosoma) ferox
	Psorophora (Psorophora) ciliata
	Psorophora (Psorophora) cilipes
	Sabethes spp.
	Wyeomyia spp.
Western equine encephalitis (WEE)	
North and South America	mainly *Culex (Culex) tarsalis* in western USA *Culiseta (Climacura) melanura* in eastern USA occasionally *Aedes, Anopheles, Culex, Culiseta* and *Psorophora* spp.
FLAVIVIRUS (=GROUP B)	
Banzi (BAN)	
Africa	*Culex (Culex) nakuruensis*
	*Culex (Eumelanomyia) rubinotus
	Mansonia (Mansonioides) africana
Bussuquara (BSQ)	
South and Central America	*Coquillettidia (Rhynchotaenia) venezuelensis*
	*Culex (Melanoconion) spp.
	Culex (Melanoconion) epanatasis (=crybda)
	Culex (Melanoconion) taeniopus
	Culex (Melanoconion) vomerifer
	Mansonia (Mansonia) titillans
	Trichoprosopon sp.

Arbovirus and endemic area	Natural vector (*indicates principal species)
Dengue (DEN) types 1–4	
between 40°N and 40°S	*Aedes (Finlaya) niveus* group
	Aedes (Stegomyia) spp.
	*Aedes (Stegomyia) aegypti
	Aedes (Stegomyia) albopictus
	Aedes (Stegomyia) polynesiensis
	Aedes (Stegomyia) scutellaris
Ilheus (ILH)	
South and Central America	*Aedes (Ochlerotatus) angustivittatus*
	Aedes (Ochlerotatus) fulvus
	Aedes (Ochlerotatus) scapularis
	Aedes (Ochlerotatus) serratus
	Aedes (Stegomyia) aegypti
	Coquillettidia spp.
	Culex (Culex) nigripalpus
	Culex (Culex) quinquefasciatus
	Culex (Melanoconion) spp.
	Culex (Melanoconion) caudelli
	Culex (Melanoconion) spissipes
	Culex (Melanoconion) taeniopus
	Haemagogus (Conopostegus) leucocelaenus
	Haemagogus (Haemagogus) janthinomys (=falco)
	Psorophora (Janthinosoma) albipes
	*Psorophora (Janthinosoma) ferox
	Psorophora (Janthinosoma) lutzii
	Sabethes (Sabethoides) chloropterus
	Trichoprosopon sp.
	Wyeomyia sp.
Japanese encephalitis (JE)	
South-East Asia to India and Japan and former USSR	*Aedes (Aedimorphus) vexans*
	Aedes (Cancraedes) curtipes
	Aedes (Finlaya) koreicus
	Aedes (Finlaya) togoi
	Anopheles (Anopheles) barbirostris group
	Anopheles (Anopheles) hyrcanus group
	Culex (Culex) bitaeniorhynchus group
	Culex (Culex) epidesmus
	Culex (Culex) gelidus
	Culex (Culex) pipiens group
	Culex (Culex) pseudovishnui
	*Culex (Culex) tritaeniorhynchus
	Culex (Culex) vishnui (=annulus)
	Culex (Culex) whitmorei
Kunjin (KUN)	
Borneo, Australia	**Culex (Culex) annulirostris*
	Culex (Culex) pseudovishnui
	Culex (Culex) squamosus
Murray Valley encephalitis (MVE)	
Australasia	*Aedes (Ochlerotatus) normanensis*
	*Culex (Culex) annulirostris
	Culex (Culex) bitaeniorhynchus
Septik (SEP)	
Australasia	*Armigeres sp.*
	Mansonia (Mansonioides) septempunctata
	Mimomyia (Mimomyia) flavens

Table IV.6   Continued

Arbovirus and endemic area	Natural vector (*indicates principal species)
Spondweni (SPO)	
Africa	Aedes (Aedimorphus) cumminsi
	Aedes (Aedimorphus) fowleri?
	*Aedes (Neomelaniconion) circumluteolus
	Aedes (Ochlerotatus) fryeri?
	Culex (Culex) univittatus
	Eretmapodites spp.
	Eretmapodites silvestris
	Mansonia (Mansonioides) africana
	Mansonia (Mansonioides) uniformis
St Louis encephalitis (SLE)	
North America	Aedes (Ochlerotatus) dorsalis/melanimon
	Aedes (Ochlerotatus) scapularis
	Aedes (Ochlerotatus) serratus
	Anopheles (Anopheles) crucians
	*Culex (Culex) nigripalpus
	Culex (Culex) peus
	*Culex (Culex) pipiens
	*Culex (Culex) quinquefasciatus
	Culex (Culex) restuans
	Culex (Culex) salinarius
	Culex (Culex) tarsalis
South America	Culex (Culex) coronator
	Culex (Culex) declarator (as virgultus)
	Culex (Culex) nigripalpus
	Culex (Melanoconion) caudelli
	Culex (Melanoconion) spissipes
	Culex (Melanoconion) taeniopus
	Psorophora (Janthinosoma) ferox
	Sabethes (Sabethes) belisarioi
	Sabethes (Sabethoides) chloropterus
	Trichoprosopon sp.
	Wyeomyia sp.
Wesselsbron (WSL)	
Africa	Aedes (Aedimorphus) hisutus
	Aedes (Aedimorphus) minutus
	Aedes (Aedimorphus) tarsalis group
	Aedes (Neomelaniconion) spp.
	Aedes (Neomelaniconion) circumluteolus
	Aedes (Neomelaniconion) lineatopennis
	Aedes (Ochlerotatus) caballus
	Anopheles (Cellia) gambiae (sensu lato)
	Anopheles (Cellia) pharoensis
	Culex (Culex) telesilla
	Culex (Culex) univittatus
	Mansonia (Mansonioides) uniformis
Thailand	Aedes (Aedimorphus) mediolineatus
	Aedes (Neomelaniconion) lineatopennis
West Nile (WN)	
Africa	Coquillettidia (Coquillettidia) metallica
	Culex (Culex) theileri
	*Culex (Culex) univittatus
	Culex (Culex) weschei
Europe	Culex (Barraudius) modestus

Arbovirus and endemic area	Natural vector (*indicates principal species)
Middle East	Anopheles (Anopheles) coustani
	Culex (Culex) antennatus
	Culex (Culex) perexiguus (as univittatus)
	Culex (Culex) pipiens group
Asia	Anopheles (Cellia) subpictus
	Culex (Culex) quinquefasciatus
	Culex (Culex) tritaeniorhynchus
	Culex (Culex) vishnui group
Yellow fever (YF)	
Africa	Aedes (Aedimorphus) vittatus
	Aedes (Diceromyia) taylori
	*Aedes (Stegomyia) aegypti
	*Aedes (Stegomyia) africanus
	Aedes (Stegomyia) luteocephalus
	Aedes (Stegomyia) metallicus
	*Aedes (Stegomyia) simpsoni
South and Central America	*Aedes (Stegomyia) aegypti
	Haemagogus (Conopostegus) leucocelaenus
	Haemagogus (Haemagogus) janthinomys (=falco)
	*Haemagogus (Haemagogus) spegazzinii
	Sabethes (Sabethoides) chloropterus
Zika (ZIKA)	
Africa	*Aedes (Stegomyia) africanus
	Aedes (Stegomyia) luteocephalus
Malaysia	Aedes (Stegomyia) aegypti
Bunyaviridae (Bunyavirus)	
BUNYAMWERA GROUP	
Bunyamwera (BUN)	
Africa	*Aedes (Neomelaniconion) circumluteolus
	Aedes (Skusea) pembaensis
	Culex sp.
	Mansonia (Mansonioides) africana
	Mansonia (Mansonioides) uniformis
Calovo (CVO)	
Europe	Anopheles (Anopheles) maculipennis (sensu lato)
	Coquillettidia (Coquillettidia) richiardii
Germiston (GER)	
Africa	Aedes (Neomelaniconion) circumluteolus
	Anopheles (Cellia) arabiensis
	Anopheles (Cellia) funestus
	Culex (Culex) theileri?
	*Culex (Eumelanomyia) rubinotus
Guaroa (GRO)	
South America	Anopheles (Kerteszia) neivai
Ilesha (ILE)	
Africa	Anopheles (Cellia) gambiae (sensu lato)
	Mansonia (Mansonioides) uniformis

Table IV.6 Continued

Arbovirus and endemic area	Natural vector (*indicates principal species)
Tensaw (TEN) South-east USA	*Aedes (Ochlerotatus) atlanticus* *Aedes (Ochlerotatus) infirmatus* *Aedes (Ochlerotatus) mitchellae* **Anopheles (Anopheles) crucians* *Anopheles (Anopheles) punctipennis* *Anopheles (Anopheles) quadrimaculatus* *Coquillettidia (Coquillettidia) perturbans* *Culex (Culex) nigripalpus* *Culex (Culex) salinarius*
Wyeomyia (WYO) South and Central America	*Aedes (Howardina) septemstriatus* *Aedes (Howardina) sexlineatus* *Aedes (Ochlerotatus) fulvus* *Aedes (Ochlerotatus) scapularis* *Aedes (Ochlerotatus) serratus* *Aedes (Protomacleaya) argyrothorax* *Anopheles* spp. *Anopheles (Stethomyia) nimbus* *Coquillettidia (Rhynchotaemia) arribalzagae* *Culex (Aedinus) amazonensis* *Culex (Culex) nigripalpus* *Haemagogous (Conopostegus) leucocelaenus* *Limatus durhamii* *Limatus flavisetosus* *Psorophora (Grabhamia) cingulata* *Psorophora (Janthinosoma) albipes* *Psorophora (Janthinosoma) ferox* *Trichoprosopon (Runchomyia) leucopus* *Trichoprosopon (Runchomyia) longipes* *Trichoprosopon (Trichoprosopon) digitatum* *Wyeomyia (Dendromyia) aporonoma* *Wyeomyia (Dendromyia) complosa* *Wyeomyia (Dendromyia) melanocephala*
BWAMBA GROUP	
Bwamba (BWA) Africa	*Anopheles (Cellia) funestus* *Anopheles (Cellia) gambiae (sensu lato)*
C GROUP	
Apeu (APEU) Brazil	*Aedes (Howardina) arborealis* *Aedes (Howardina) septemstriatus* *Aedes (Ochlerotatus) serratus* *Culex (Melanoconion) acossa/panocossa (=aikenii)*
Caraparu (CAR) South America	*Culex (Melanoconion)* spp. *Culex (Melanoconion) caudelli* **Culex (Melanoconion) portesi* *Culex (Melanoconion) spissipes* *Culex (Melanoconion) vomerifer* *Limatus durhamii* *Wyeomyia* sp.

Arbovirus and endemic area	Natural vector (*indicates principal species)
Itaqui (ITQ) Brazil	*Culex (Melanoconion)* spp. *Culex (Melanoconion) portesi* *Culex (Melanoconion) vomerifer*
Madrid (MAD) Panama	*Culex (Melanoconion) vomerifer*
Marituba (MTB) Brazil	*Culex (Melanoconion) ocossa/panocossa (=aikenii)* *Culex (Melanoconion) portesi*
Murutucu (MUR) South America	*Coquillettidia (Rhychotaenia) venezuelensis* *Culex (Melanoconion) ocossa/panocossa (=aikenii)* *Culex (Melanoconion) portesi* other *Culex* spp. and *Sabethini*
Oriboca (ORI) South America	*Aedes* spp. *Aedes (Ochlerotatus) taeniorhynchus* *Culex* spp. *Culex (Melanoconion) portesi* *Mansonia* sp. *Psorophora (Janthinosoma) ferox* *Sabethini*
Ossa (OSSA) Panama	*Culex (Melanoconion) taeniopus* *Culex (Melanoconion) vomerifer*
Restan (RES) South America	*Culex (Melanoconion) portesi*
CALIFORNIA GROUP	
California encephalitis (CE) South-western USA	*Aedes (Aedimorphus) vexans* **Aedes (Ochlerotatus) dorsalis* **Aedes (Ochlerotatus) melanimon* *Aedes (Ochlerotatus) nigromaculis* *Anopheles (Anopheles) pseudopunctipennis* *Culex (Culex) tarsalis* *Culiseta (Culiseta) inornata* *Psorophora (Grabhamia) signipennis*
Inkoo (INK) Finland	*Aedes (Ochlerotatus) communis/punctor*
La Crosse (LAC) USA	*Aedes (Ochlerotatus) canadensis* *Aedes (Ochlerotatus) communis* *Aedes (Ochlerotatus) trivittatus* **Aedes (Protomacleaya) triseriatus* *Culex (Culex) pipiens*
Melao (MEL) South America	*Aedes (Ochlerotatus) scapularis* *Aedes (Ochlerotatus) serratus* *Psorophora (Janthinosoma) ferox*

Table IV.6   Continued

Arbovirus and endemic area	Natural vector (*indicates principal species)
Tahyna (TAH)	
Africa	*Aedes (Skusea) pembaensis*
Europe	*Aedes (Aedimorphus) vexans*
	Aedes (Ochlerotatus) cantans
	Aedes (Ochlerotatus) caspius
	Aedes (Ochlerotatus) cinereus
	Anopheles (Anopheles) hyrcanus (sensu lato)
	Anopheles (Anopheles) maculipennis (sensu lato)
	Culex (Barraudius) modestus
	Culex (Culex) pipiens (sensu lato)
	Caliseta (Culiseta) annulata

GUAMA GROUP
Catu (CATU)

South America	*Anopheles (Stethomyia) nimbus*
	Coquillettidia (Rhynchotaemia) venezuelensis
	Culex (Aedinus) mojuensis
	Culex (Culex) declarator (=virgultus)
	Culex (Melanoconion) portesi
	Culex (Melanoconion) vomerifer

Guama (GMA)

South and Central America	*Aedes (Howardina) sexlineatus*
	Coquillettidia (Rhynchotaenia) venezuelensis
	Culex (Aedinus) mojuensis
	Culex (Melanoconion) spp.
	Culex (Melanoconion) epanatasis (=crybda)
	Culex (Melanoconion) portesi
	Culex (Melanoconion) spissipes
	Culex (Melanoconion) taeniopus
	Culex (Melanoconion) vomerifer
	Culex (Tinolestes) sp.
	Limatus durhamii
	Wyeomyia sp.

NYANDO GROUP
Nyando (NDO)

Africa	*Anopheles (Cellia) funestus*

SIMBU GROUP
Oropouche (ORO)

South America	Mainly Ceratopogonidae
	Aedes (Ochlerotatus) serratus
	Coquillettidia (Rhynchotaenia) venezuelensis
	Culex (Culex) quinquefasciatus

Shuni (SHU)

South Africa	*Culex (Culex) theileri*

PHLEBOTOMUS FEVER GROUP
Chagres (CHG)

Panama	*Sabethes (Sabethoides) chloropterus* and phlebotomine sandflies

Arbovirus and endemic area	Natural vector (*indicates principal species)
Rift Valley fever (RVF)	
Africa	*Aedes (Aedimorphus) dentatus*
	Aedes (Aedimorphus) tarsalis
	Aedes (Aedimorphus) triseriatus
	Aedes (Neomelaniconion) circumluteolus
	Aedes (Neomelaniconion) lineatopennis
	Aedes (Ochlerotatus) caballus
	Aedes (Ochlerotatus) juppi
	Aedes (Stegomyia) deboeri
	Aedes (Stegomyia) aegypti
	Aedes (Stegomyia) africanus
	Aedes (Stegomyia) dendrophilus
	Anopheles (Anopheles) coustani
	Coquillettidia (Coquillettidia) fuscopennata
	Coquillettidia (Coquillettidia) microbannulata
	Coquillettidia (Coquillettidia) versicolor
	Culex (Culex) neavei
	Culex (Culex) pipiens (sensu lato)
	Culex (Culex) theileri
	Culex (Culex) univattatus
	Culex (Culex) zombaensis
	Eretmapodites chrysogaster group
	Mansonia (Mansonioides) africana
	Mansonia (Mansonioides) uniformis?

GANJAM GROUP
Gamjam (GAN)

India	*Culex (Culex) vishnui* group and ticks (Ixodidae)

ANOPHELES A GROUP
Tataguine (TAT)

Africa	*Anopheles (Cellia) funestus*
	Anopheles (Cellia) gambiae (sensu lato)

UNGROUPED
Zinga (ZGA)

Africa	*Aedes (Neomelaniconion) palpalis* group
	Mansonia (Mansonioides) africana

Poxviridae
Cotia (COT)

South America	*Aedes (Ochlerotatus) serratus*
	Coquillettidia (Rhynchotaenia) venezuelensis
	Culex (Melanoconion) portesi
	Limatus pseudomethysticus
	Psorophora (Janthinosoma) ferox

most efficient malaria vectors in the world are *A. funestus*, which breeds in African swamps and mature paddy, *A. minimus* , which breeds in streams of South-East Asia from the Himalayas to Hong Kong, with *A. flavirostris* doing likewise in the Philippines. These species are also important vectors of bancroftian filariasis. They are extremely endophilic in most areas, so usually respond well to control campaigns with residual insecticides sprayed inside houses. However, exophilic and insecticide-resistant populations of *A. minimus* are an intractable problem in Thailand. *A. fluviatilis* is another important exophilic member of this complex breeding in streams of southern Asia. *A. fluviatilis* maintains highly endemic malaria in localities where *A. minimus* has been eliminated. There is little evidence that these mosquitoes transmit arboviruses, although *A. funestus* has been involved with epidemic o'nyong-nyong fever in East Africa; *A. funestus* is also the type-host of Tanga virus. *A. aconitus* is closely related to the *A. funestus–minimus* complex, probably forming another complex of species in itself. It transmits malaria and possibly filariasis in Indonesia but not in Malaysia. Identification of all these species presents the utmost difficulty, but is vital if effort is not to be wasted in vain attempts to control the exophilic non-vector species in the complex.

A. culicifacies also belongs to series *Myzomyia*, being an opportunistic breeder in temporary pools, wells and other clean water sites from Arabia to China. It is not an efficient malaria vector, but is the only species implicated in Sri Lanka and is clearly of importance in most parts of its range. Exophily makes control difficult and there is good evidence that several sibling species have been confused in what must therefore be regarded as the *A. culicifacies* complex. Similarly in the arid belt of North Africa and the Middle East, *A. sergentii* is an important but inefficient malaria vector, variations of which suggest that it comprises several taxonomic species.

Series *Neocellia* includes a number of oriental malaria vectors, mostly having speckled legs and hind tarsi with white tips. *A. annularis* breeds abundantly in swamps of the kind covered with *Eichornia* weed (cf. *Mansonia*) and in mature paddy, being a widespread and mainly zoophilic mosquito from India to the Philippines. In some situations *A. annularis* is a significant though inefficient malaria vector, often showing multiple resistance to insecticides. *A. karwari* is strongly zoophilic in South-East Asia, where it breeds in trickles of seepage water, but it has been reported to transmit human malaria in West Irian to where it was accidentally introduced. *A. maculatus* is an unusually variable species which also breeds commonly in seepages from Pakistan to Sri Lanka, China and the Philippines. Despite being mainly exophilic and zoophilic it serves as an important vector of malaria and contributes to *W. bancrofti* transmission in some places, especially where hilly countryside is being developed so that breeding sites for *A. maculatus* become plentiful. The African savanna species *A. rufipes* also belongs to this series and was previously regarded as a secondary vector of malaria, because sporozoite infections are frequent, but it is now known that *A. rufipes* more often transmits antelope malaria.[16] Other local vectors of malaria to be mentioned here are *A. pattoni* in China, *A. pulcherrimus* in Afghanistan and *A. superpictus* in the eastern Mediterranean area (see Table IV.4). Finally in this series, *A. stephensi* is essentially a rural cattle-biting species in the Indian subcontinent. However, some populations have adapted to urban conditions in

northern India and Pakistan, where they breed in wells and subsist largely on human blood, becoming important local vectors of urban malaria.[17]

Series *Neomyzomyia* has numerous species in Africa, Asia and Australasia, most of which are either dark and cave-dwelling or heavily spotted and forest-dwelling. *A. nili* breeds in African rivers and streams, being rather seasonal and locally important as an efficient vector of both malaria and bancroftian filariasis. *A. tessellatus* is widespread and usually zoophilic in South-East Asia, breeding in stagnant water. It transmits malaria and filariasis in the Maldive Islands, where it is the only anopheline present. The *A. leucosphyrus* group extends from India to China and the Philippines, comprising at least 12 species, several of which transmit monkey malarias (*P. cynomolgi, P, inui, P. knowlesi* etc.) and sometimes infect man with these zoonotic parasites. *A. leucosphyrus* (*sensu stricto*) is also a regular vector of human malaria in Malaysia and Indonesia. The most important component of the *A. leucosphyrus* group is the *A. balabacensis* complex, which has not yet been analysed satisfactorily. The most widespread form in South-East Asia has been named *A. dirus*, but this seems to consist of four genetic species. In forests from Assam to Indonesia and China, '*A. dirus*' (formerly known as *A. balabacensis*, or simply as *A. leucosphyrus*) is an important vector of human malaria, including chloroquine-resistant *P. falciparum*, and of monkey malarias. True *A. balabacensis* is equally a vector where it occurs in Palawan and northern Borneo. Members of the *A. balabacensis* complex breed in fresh jungle pools; the adults are exophilic and elusive, but not difficult to control by home-spraying with insecticides or by means of forest clearance. Their possible involvement in transmission of arboviruses and filariae remains to be studied.

Also in series *Neomyzomyia*, the *A. punctulatus* complex comprises at least five sibling species which are vectors of malaria and nocturnally periodic bancroftian filariasis from the Moluccas, through Papua New Guinea to the Solomon Islands and formerly in northern Australia. The true *A. punctulatus* is widespread, occurring together with *A. koliensis* and *A. farauti* in some islands. *A. farauti* itself comprises three or more genetic species in Australia and Melanesia. Like the *A. balabacensis* complex, these vectors tend to rest among vegetation and to breed in small fresh pools, making it costly and difficult to attempt their control. However, house spraying with DDT has interrupted filariasis transmission in the Solomons, but malaria persists.[18]

Series *Paramyzomyia* has only four or five species, of which *A. hispaniola* and *A. multicolor* are regarded as malaria vectors in North Africa, although the evidence is equivocal. The latter species can tolerate strong salinity in its breeding places.

Series *Pyretophorus* also has several species adapted to brackish water breeding sites; the adults are characterized by banded tarsi and extensively pale wing markings. *A. sundaicus* is a mainly coastal and locally important vector of malaria in Indonesia, closely related to *A. litoralis* and *A. ludlowae* in the Philippines; the latter species extends to coastal Sulawesi where it joins in malaria transmission. *A. subpictus* ranges from the Middle East to Papua New Guinea, tending to be more anthropophilic and associated with coastal salt-water habitats eastwards; it is a secondary vector of malaria and contributes to *W. bancrofti* transmission locally in Indonesia.

Of the greatest medical importance in Africa and Southern

Arabia is the *A. gambiae* complex, comprising two salt-water adapted species: *A. melas* in West Africa and *A. merus* in East Africa, *A. bwambae* restricted to mineral spring-water sites in the Rift Valley between Uganda and Zaire, and three widespread freshwater breeding species: *A. gambiae* (*sensu stricto*) (species A), *A. arabiensis* (species B) and *A. quadriannulatus* (species C). The last is essentially zoophilic, so not a vector, but the other five species transmit both malaria and bancroftian filariasis.[19] High rates of female mosquito longevity, coupled with marked preferences for human blood, give very high vectorial capacities to *A. arabiensis*, *A. gambiae* and to some extent *A. melas*. Wherever these species are found, malaria is highly endemic. House-spraying with residual insecticides has not reduced malaria transmission to the expected degree, since members of the *A. gambiae* complex are capable of behavioural avoidance of the sprayed surfaces. Resistance to organochlorine and organophosphate insecticides is also spreading in populations of *A. arabiensis* and *A. gambiae*. Control of the salt-water species, *A. melas* and *A. merus*, can be partially achieved by means of drainage and prevention of pool formation in coastal areas, through construction of dikes and bunds. Unfortunately, most breeding of *A. arabiensis* and *A. gambiae* occurs in temporary fresh rainwater pools, or irrigated furrows, which are impossible to prevent or treat adequately with larvicides. Separation of the six sibling species belonging to the *A. gambiae* complex depends upon the examination of chromosomal or protein characters. Adult females of *A. gambiae* (*sensu lato*) have the appearance shown in Figure IV.37, but could easily be confused with various other species in subgenus *Cellia*.

Subgenus *Kerteszia* is restricted to the American tropics, with about ten species that breed exclusively in flooded axils of bromeliad plants or broken bamboos. Since they are found only in the forests of Central and South America, their medical importance is limited, although several species are sometimes abundant and strongly attracted to man. *A. cruzii* and *A. bellator* are significant vectors of malaria, and the latter sometimes contributes to filariasis transmission.[20]

Subgenus *Nyssorhynchus* forms the dominant anopheline fauna of the Neotropical region. Faran[21] has clarified the difficult taxonomy of the *A. albimanus* section, with species having small dark lateral scale tufts on each abdominal segment, including several vectors of disease. *A. albimanus* itself is the main malaria vector in humid lowlands from southern USA to northern South America and in Caribbean islands. It breeds in stagnant water and the adults lack scale tufts on the first full abdominal segment. *A. albimanus* is insufficiently endophilic to be readily controlled by means of house spraying and has become widely resistant to all groups of insecticides. It may contribute to filariasis transmission and has been involved with epidemics of encephalitis and perhaps other arboviruses (Table IV.6). Other malaria vectors closely related to *A. albimanus* are *A. aquasalis*, which also transmits Venezuelan equine encephalitis virus, and is mainly of importance in Trinidad, Tobago, the Guianas and coastal Brazil, usually breeding in brackish water; also *A. nuneztovari* is a primary malaria vector in parts of Colombia and Venezuela, probably comprising a complex of vector and non-vector species. Another section of subgenus *Nyssorhynchus* includes the malaria vectors *A. argyritarsis* and *A. darlingi*. The latter was eradicated from coastal Guyana, but remains of major importance in places from Brazil to Mexico. Infective larvae of *W. bancrofti* have occasionally been found

in *A. darlingi* and *A. aquasalis*, suggesting that these species may contribute to periodic filariasis transmission.

SUBFAMILY: CULICINAE

This large and heterogeneous subfamily of mosquitoes contains over 2500 species and some 30 genera. The scutellum is trilobed, each lobe bearing bristles. The abdomen is blunt and completely clothed with broad flat scales. The eighth segment of the larva bears a patch of comb teeth on each side, used for cleaning the mouth brushes, and is drawn out into a respiratory siphon, with well-developed pecten teeth in a row on each side. There are no abdominal palmate hairs (cf. *Anopheles*). Below the siphon the anal segment of the larva bears a chitinous saddle, four gills, caudal setae and the ventral brush for swimming. Culicine pupae are similar to those of *Anopheles*, but the respiratory trumpets are not so flared distally.

The following are the main characteristics of culicines which distinguish them from anophelines (see Figure IV.30).

1 The eggs are not provided with air floats and are either laid separately (Aedini, Sabethini) or stacked in a floating raft (Culicini, Culisetini) or in a mass on floating vegetation (Mansoniini).
2 The larval spiracles are situated at the tip of a tail-like siphon, projecting dorsally from the eighth abdominal segment. Except for *Mansonia* and some other unimportant genera, which have larvae with the siphon modified for plugging into the air vessels of plants, the larvae hang head downwards from the water surface, supported by the capillary action of five hinged valves surrounding the tip of the siphon. They sweep suspended particles of food with mouth brushes below surface level (see Figure IV.30) or else dive and scavenge at the bottom.
3 The adult has an abdomen densely covered with scales. The female has short and slender palps, from one-fifth to one-half as long as the proboscis. As a rule, the male has long hairy palps which have a plume-like appearance. These mosquitoes usually rest with proboscis and abdomen more or less parallel with the supporting surface (see Figure IV.30.).

TRIBE: AEDINI

GENUS: *AEDES*

Throughout the world, especially in temperate countries, a high proportion of mosquitoes belong to the genus *Aedes* in which there are more than 1000 species, classified as 40 subgenera. Many *Aedes* are vectors of arboviruses, including several of the most important mosquito-borne human diseases (see Chapter 30, Table IV.6). The genus is difficult to define precisely in morphological terms, although adults always possess bristles on the postspiracular area (Figure IV.41) and the tip of the female abdomen is retractable.

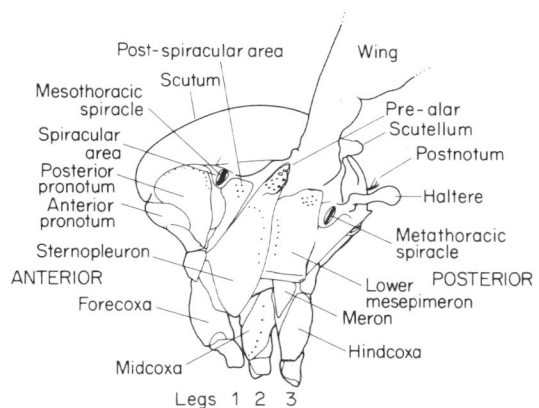

Figure IV.41 Mosquito thorax in side view, showing named components and sites of setae (bristles) referred to in the identification key (Table IV.7).

Separation from other genera in the tribe Aedini depends on characters given in Table IV.7. *Aedes* larvae are characterized by having only a single pair of siphonal hairs, usually branched, in addition to pecten teeth. Many of the medically important *Aedes* spp. are active during daytime, although nocturnal activity is normal for most other species.

Aedes eggs are especially capable of withstanding desiccation. They are laid on damp surfaces, such as soil or around the rim of water in a hole, in situations likely to be flooded causing the eggs to hatch after adequate rainfall. Most species of *Aedes* therefore breed seasonally in swamps and pools, with some significant groups adapted to smaller containers of water such as rock-holes, rot-holes in trees, cut bamboo stumps, old snail shells, buckets and other artificial containers. Almost any kind of water can harbour some sort of *Aedes*—from sea water to melted snow. It is to be expected that, after drought or winter, rainy seasons will cause the hatching of *Aedes* broods so that blood-thirsty females of these species become prevalent early in the season.

In an increasing number of cases, it has been demonstrated that arboviruses can be passed transovarially in *Aedes*, i.e. from mother to progeny via the egg. This is common with California group viruses[22] and has also been reported for yellow fever.[23] This phenomenon, a form of vertical transmission, is of great significance in epidemiology, as it can lead to long-term dormancy and reappearance of virus activity.

Representatives of three subgenera of *Aedes* are natural vectors of *Brugia malayi* and *Wuchereria bancrofti* causing human disease. Where transmission is due to nocturnally active *Aedes* and other mosquitoes, the microfilariae are normally nocturnally periodic in the human bloodstream. In Polynesia, Melanesia and a few areas in South-East Asia (parts of Thailand, Nicobar Islands) there are diurnally active *Aedes* which transmit strains of *W. bancrofti* that are subperiodic so that microfilariae circulate in the human bloodstream during the daytime, enabling their uptake by female mosquitoes which feed by day.

The majority of taxonomic subgenera of *Aedes* have few species and no medical or veterinary significance. Subgenera *Aedes* (*sensu stricto*), *Aedimorphus*, *Mucidus*, *Neomelaniconion*, *Ochlerotatus* and *Verrallina* have numerous species which breed commonly in ground water, with many arbovirus vectors included (see Table IV.6). The habit of breeding in water-filled containers, holes and plant axils is a feature of the important subgenera *Diceromyia*, *Howardina*, *Protomacleaya*, *Finlaya* and *Stegomyia*; arboviruses are transmitted by all five of these subgenera and the last two include filariasis vectors (see Table IV.5).

Subgenus *Stegomyia* is probably of the greatest medical interest. More than 100 species have been described, all diurnally active and having beautiful specific patterns of black and white scales, especially noticeable on the scutum and banded tarsi. They are generally exophilic species which seldom shelter indoors. The *Ae. scutellaris* group numbers approximately 35 species in South-East Asia and the Pacific, including the main vectors of subperiodic *W. bancrofti* in Polynesia: *Ae. pseudoscutellaris* in Fiji, *Ae. cooki*, *Ae. kesseli* and *Ae. tongae* in Tonga, *Ae. upolensis* in Samoa and *Ae. polynesiensis* generally. Adults of the *Ae. scutellaris* group are characterized by having a single white line longitudinally on the middle of the scutum. They also transmit epidemic dengue viruses on many Pacific Islands and in parts of South-East Asia. However, the true *Ae. scutellaris* (*sensu stricto*) is confined to Seram and Papua New Guinea, where it is zoophilic and not a vector. Breeding places of the *Ae. scutellaris* group are in coconut shells, crab holes, holes in trees and coral, axils of plants such as *Pandanus* and bananas, tyres, tins and other artificial containers. All species so far mentioned have complete stripes of broad scales along each side of the thorax, ending above the wing base. This distinguishes the *Ae. scutellaris* subgroup from the *Ae. albopictus* subgroup of species having an incomplete supra-alar stripe, with only narrow scales over the wing base. Species in the latter group are widespread vectors of dengue viruses, notably dengue haemorrhagic fever in the Philippines and South-East Asian countries, but they are apparently refractory to filarial infection. These and other Pacific mosquitoes have been the subject of a monograph by Belkin[24] and a pictorial key provided by Huang.[25] A revision of Tongan species by Huang and Hitchcock[26] gives much information on bionomics and vector functions; vector genetics and speciation of *Ae. scutellaris* group were reviewed by Macdonald.[27]

Aedes (*Stegomyia*) *aegypti* is the most widespread and dangerous species in this subgenus.[28] In African forests, non-anthropophilic populations known as *Ae. aegypti formosus* are distinguished by their lack of pale scales on the abdominal tergites (i.e. the top of the abdomen is entirely dark). Presumably from this ancestral stock, man-biting populations have adapted to domestic breeding sites and become spread throughout the tropics within the 20°C isotherms, i.e. roughly between 35°N and 35°S. The general pattern on adult *Ae. aegypti* is depicted in Fig. IV.42, showing the unique lyre-shaped pattern on the scutum, with narrow longitudinal lines flanked by curved silvery-white markings. *Ae. aegypti aegypti* has some white scales on all abdominal tergites, with *Ae. aegypti* var. *queenslandensis* having the abdomen mainly pale-scaled dorsally.[29] Populations of *Ae. aegypti* breeding indoors in water pots, especially in eastern Africa, usually have the appearance of var. *queenslandensis*, whereas peridomestic populations are mainly of the type form. Evolutionary relationships among various kinds of *Ae. aegypti* (*sensu lato*) are still the subject of much study and debate.[30] This is relevant to the fact that *Ae. aegypti* is the principal vector of chikungunya and dengue viruses in almost every outbreak. Urban yellow fever is also mainly transmitted by *Ae. aegypti* in Central and South America and in West Africa. *Ae.*

Table IV.7   Identification key to the genera of adult mosquitoes likely to be encountered indoors or attacking man.

1	Large iridescent mosquitoes (wing span 12–24 mm); abdominal segments VI–VIII (but not I–V) with distinctive lateral tufts of scales; proboscis curved downwards approx. 90° in middle; feeds on nectar not blood; distribution 40°N to 35°S	*Toxorhynchites*
	Typical mosquitoes of various sizes (wing span 5–16 mm); abdomen usually without distinctive lateral scale-tufts; proboscis usually straight, or curved through no more than 40° downwards or upwards; females often suck blood	2
2	Female palps as long as proboscis; male palps club-shaped (Figure IV.35); wing vein scales usually forming a conspicuous pattern of spots due to *either* clusters of scales at junctions of some veins *or* patches of pale scales and patches of dark scales alternating along some veins; scutellum evenly rounded posteriorly and lacking lateral lobes; abdomen usually not scale-covered, although some narrow scales may be mixed with the covering of fine hairs; worldwide distribution	*Anopheles*
	Female with short palps (Figure IV.34b), usually one-third to one-fifth as long as proboscis; male palps not clubbed, although often apically thickened; wing vein scales usually not forming a distinct pattern of spots or pale and dark patches, although speckling may be due to mixtures of pale and dark scales on some veins; scutellum trilobed, i.e. with large mid-lobe and smaller lateral lobes; abdomen clothed with broad scales (powdery when rubbed) above and below (Culicinae)	3
3	Female with tip of abdomen rounded, terminal segment non-retractable, cerci not conspicuous; postspiracular bristles absent (present in *Mansonia*, see no. 7)	4
	Female with tip of abdomen pointed, ending with a pair of prominent cerci, terminal abdominal segment retractable; postspiracular bristles present (Figure IV.41)	8
4	Pre-alar bristles (Figure IV.41) usually numerous and at least one lower mesepimeral bristle present; postnotum normally without apical tuft; anterior pronotal lobes small; meron well developed, so that upper edge is dorsal to the base of hind coxa	5
	Pre-alar bristles usually absent, no more than four present; no lower mesepimeral bristles; postnotum usually with an apical tuft of small setae; anterior pronotal lobes large and conspicuously ornamented with scales; meron small, so that upper edge is in line with base of hind coxa or ventral to it; essentially sylvatic mosquitoes, i.e. found in jungle	12
5	Tarsi with pulvilli (Figure IV.44) appearing as a pair of pale pads below the claws when examined at 50× magnification or more; worldwide distribution	*Culex*
	Tarsi without pulvilli	6
6	Bristles on spiracular area (Figure IV.41) i.e. setae with roots in a vertical row just in front of the respiratory aperture on side of thorax (mesothoracic spiracle); worldwide distribution	*Culiseta*
	Spiracular bristles absent	7
7	Bristles on spiracular area (Figure IV.41); wing vein scales very broad and forming a mottled pattern on all or most veins; ornamentation without any yellow scales; worldwide distribution	*Mansonia*
	Postspiracle bristles absent; wing vein scales narrow not forming a mottled pattern on most veins; ornamentation mostly yellow, or with at least some bright yellow scales somewhere on body; worldwide distribution	*Coquillettidia*
8	Scutum covered with broad, flat, metallic green scales; legs generally dark; anterior pronotal lobes very large, almost meeting anteriorly; small species (wing span 6–9 mm) active in daytime; Caribbean, South and Central America	*Haemagogus*
	Scutum not covered with shiny green scales; legs often with pale bands, especially on tarsi; anterior pronotal lobes not strongly developed; various sizes (wing span 6–16 mm), diurnal or nocturnal	9
9	Broad silver scales on back of head, sides of thorax and hind corners of abdominal tergites; thoracic cuticle orange or reddish-brown; tropical Africa only	*Eretmapodites*
	Not with silvery scales in the places specified; although some of these areas bear white scales; thoracic cuticle pale or dark, but not orange or reddish; temperate or tropical regions worldwide	10

Table IV.7 Continued

10	Spiracular bristles present (Figure IV.41), i.e. setae with roots in a vertical row just in front of the respiratory aperture on side of thorax (mesothoracic spiracle); New World only	*Psorophora*
	Spiracular bristles absent	
11	Abdomen more than 2 × length of thorax; normally one lower mesepimeral bristle present (Figure IV.41); scales on top of head all broad, flat and decumbent; abdominal segment VIII partially retractile; distributed throughout southern Asia, from India to Japan, Philippines, Indonesia and Melanesia	*Armigeres*
	Abdomen not more than 2 × length of thorax; lower mesepimeral bristle usually absent; top of head with erect scales, seen best in side-view, forming a posterior tuft or more extensive 'crew cut' appearance (easily rubbed off), plus a layer of decumbent scales which are often curved and narrow along the midline but always broad and flat laterally; abdominal segment VIII almost completely retractile; worldwide distribution	*Aedes*
12	Spiracular area bare, i.e. no scales or bristles on the small membranous area between the posterior pronotum and the main thoracic spiracle; South-East Asia only	*Heizmannia*
	Spiracular area with scales and/or at least one bristle	13
13	Australasian or South-East Asian mosquitoes	*Tripteroides*
	New World mosquitoes	14
14	Spiracular area with broad scales only, no bristles; proboscis shorter than fore-femur, thorax with some shiny golden scales; hind tarsi with single claw	*Limatus*
	Spiracular area with at least one spiracular bristle; thoracic scales various, none golden; proboscis longer than or equal to forefemur; each hind tarsus with two claws	15
15	Scutum covered with broad, flat, shiny metallic scales; some tarsi with 'paddles' formed by inner and outer rows of long, mostly dark scales; some tarsi with 'paddles' formed by inner and outer rows of long, mostly dark scales; Central and South America	*Sabethes*
	Scutal scales usually not shiny; tarsi without paddles	16
16	Top of head often with erect scales; pronotal lobes widely separated anteriorly; membrane at wing base (squama) fringed with small setae; bristles on clypeus, i.e. bulbous area of the face between bases of antennae and palps; Central and South America	*Trichoprosopon*
	Top of head without erect scales; pronotal lobes very large and almost meeting anteriorly; membrane at wing base (squama) with no more than three small fringe setae; clypeal area of the face without bristles, although scales may be present; North and South America	*Wyeomyia*

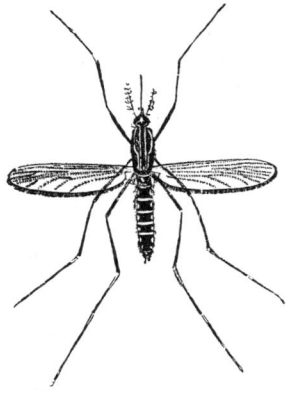

Figure IV.42 Female *Aedes aegypti* (4×).

aegypti formosus is probably involved in the sylvatic cycle of yellow fever in Africa. However, other *Stegomyia* spp. have more often been implicated as vectors of African enzootic yellow fever, especially *Ae. africanus* which also transmits Zika virus. In nature, these arboviruses affect monkeys in the jungle, being transmitted by mosquito species which seldom come into contact with man. At the forest edge, monkeys are likely to be bitten by *Aedes* (*Stegomyia*) *simpsoni* which breeds predominantly in water-filled axils of certain strains of banana plant, or rot holes in stems of paw-paw and candelabra *Euphorbia* (e.g. in Ethiopia). People working and living among such plantations in Africa are especially likely to become infected with yellow fever and other viruses transmitted from monkeys via *Ae. simpsoni*, some populations of which are strongly attracted to man. Man-to-man transmission may then be continued by *Ae. aegypti*. Thus the epidemiology of yellow fever in Africa conforms to the systems shown in Figure IV.43, depending on which species of *Stegomyia* and other mosquitoes are involved. Embryonated eggs of *Stegomyia* spp. can remain dormant for as long

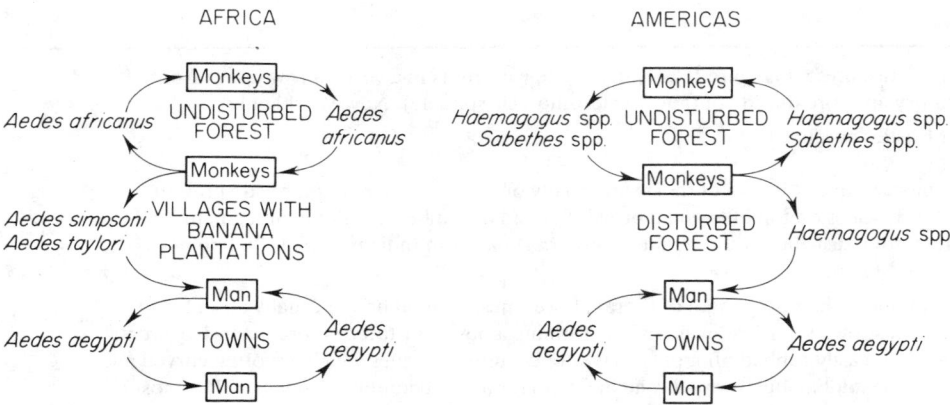

Figure IV.43   Yellow fever ecosystems in Africa and the Americas.

as a year and still hatch when flooded. The fact that *Ae. aegypti* eggs may be laid in portable containers allows this species to be inadvertently spread far and wide; continuously breeding populations often occur in water barrels on board ships and dhows.

Control of *Stegomyia* spp. presents great problems the world over, since breeding sites are small, scattered and usually inaccessible. In emergencies, as when an arbovirus epidemic is under way, periodic insecticidal space-spraying and perifocal applications (see Table IV.13) can be helpful in the vicinity of dwellings. Screening of houses and elimination of mosquito breeding places are desirable preventive measures.

Subgenus *Finlaya* has females with a conspicuous ventral scale tuft on the posterior abdomen; in both sexes the wings are usually spotted. The *Ae. (F.) kochi* group includes several local vectors of periodic *W. bancrofti*. *Ae. poicilius* is the most widespread, in Malaysia, Indonesia and the Philippines, breeding in axils of *Colocasia*, *Pandanus* and bananas (*Musa sapientum*). In parts of the Philippines, where *Musa textiles* (abaca or hemp) is intensively cultivated, *Ae. poicilius* is an important rural filariasis vector. Likewise in Fiji and Samoa, bancroftian filariasis is or was transmitted by several members of the *Ae. kochi* group (see Table IV.5) which breed in plant axils. Around the coasts of South-East Asia, the large, dark-winged species *Ae. (F.) togoi* often breeds in brackish water and contributes to transmission of periodic *B. malayi* and *W. bancrofti*. Finally in this subgenus, members of the *Ae. (F.) niveus* group transmit both periodic and subperiodic strains of *W. bancrofti* locally (see Table IV.5), but are probably of wider importance as vectors of jungle dengue and perhaps other arboviruses.

Subgenus *Diceromyia* of tree-hole breeding species resembling *Stegomyia* but having dark tarsi, includes the African *A. furcifer-taylori* group of species which have been occasionally implicated as vectors of yellow fever and chikungunya.[31]

Subgenus *Protomacleaya* has similarities in the New World, with *Ae. triseriatus* breeding in tree-holes of the eastern USA and being an important vector of California group encephalitides, with evidence of transovarial virus transmission. The closely related *Ae. hendersoni*, which may breed in the same tree-holes, is apparently incapable of virus transmission.

Subgenus *Neomelaniconion* is widespread in the Old World tropics and includes some commonly implicated vectors of arboviruses. These species are recognizable from yellowish stripes edging the scutum and some pale-scaled veins on the wings. They breed prolifically in temporary flood pans in savannas and the adults shelter among grass. About 20 arboviruses have been isolated from *Neomelaniconion* spp., the most important to man being Rift Valley fever transmitted by *Ae. circumluteolus* and *Ae. lineatopennis* in southern Africa and probably elsewhere.

Subgenus *Ochlerotatus* is the dominant component of *Aedes* in terms of numbers of species and their distribution. They are ground pool breeders, mostly in temperate countries. Generally they bite mammals. In North America, *Ae. atlanticus* is an important vector of *D. immitis*, a filarial parasite affecting dogs and capable of causing dog heartworm disease in man. Rift Valley fever virus is commonly transmitted to livestock by *Ae. caballus* in southern Africa, although few *Ochlerotatus* spp. occur in Africa. *Ae. caspius* is widespread in Europe and North Africa, a fairly large speckled species that breeds commonly in brackish water, usually the vector of Inkoo virus in Scandinavia. Various North American *Ochlerotatus* spp. contribute sporadically to the transmission of encephalitides; they are beyond the reach of economical control programmes. Species such as the saltwater-breeding *Ae. detritus* in Europe and *Ae. sollicitans* and *Ae. taeniorhynchus* in America are intolerable pests, and the latter has been implicated in *W. bancrofti* transmission. *Ae. (O.) vigilax* is another salt-water-breeding species locally responsible for periodic bancroftian filariasis transmission in New Caledonia (see Table IV.5) and for Ross River virus in Australia (see Table IV.6). This species and the closely related *Ae. fryeri* are so vicious and prolific as to make many islands uninhabitable in the Indian and Pacific Oceans.

Subgenus *Aedimorphus* and other subgenera of *Aedes* also include some species which are pests and vectors of arboviruses. In particular, *Ae. vexans* is probably the second or third most widespread mosquito in the world (after *C. pipiens* and perhaps *Ae. aegypti*). Seasonal breeding in grassland follows flooding and egg-hatching of broods which are immensely troublesome when the adult females attack; they bite both day and night, being especially numerous in late spring in northern latitudes.

GENUS: *ARMIGERES*

Widespread and common in the Australasian and Oriental regions, this genus is difficult to distinguish from *Aedes*, to which it is closely related. Development always occurs in small containers of water and the larvae grow very rapidly. *Armigeres subalbatus* (=*obturbans*) is a semidomestic species that breeds commonly in foul water, including latrines. This and several other species attack man during night and day. It has been suggested that they may transmit *W. bancrofti* and the encephalitis virus Sepik has been isolated from *Armigeres*.

GENUS: *HAEMAGOGUS*

This genus of forest mosquito is also closely related to *Aedes*. It occurs in Central and South America, breeding in flooded tree-holes. Adults are metallic blue and green due to their covering of scales on thorax and abdomen. Several species are vectors of sylvatic (jungle) yellow fever: *Haemagogus equinus*, *H. janthinomys*, *H. leucocelaenus*, *H. mesodentatus*, *H. spegazzinii* and *H. capricornii*. They are separable only on the characters of the male genitalia and not at all as larvae and pupae. The larvae of these vector species are 'hairy' and are thus distinguishable from some other species of *Haemogogus* which are not vectors. Adult females of *Haemogogus* seldom leave the forest and they attack man mainly during jungle clearance activities. Taxonomy of the genus has been revised by Arnell.[32]

GENUS: *PSOROPHORA*

Three subgenera and almost 50 species are recognized, many of them vicious man-biters. Generic characters are the presence of spiracular *and* postspiracular bristles, plus the retractable postabdomen as in other Aedini. Larvae of the typical subgenus are predacious. Eggs normally diapause before hatching and the breeding places are always in pools and marshes on the ground, not containers as used by some allied genera. Apart from their considerable significance as pests, *Psorophora* spp. are of widespread importance as vectors of arboviruses (see Table IV.6), especially Venezuelan equine encephalitis transmitted by *P. ferox* and *P. confinnis*, the latter being known as the dark rice-field mosquito. Taxonomy of this genus remains unsatisfactory, but Belkin et al[33] and Carpenter and La Casse[14] give summaries.

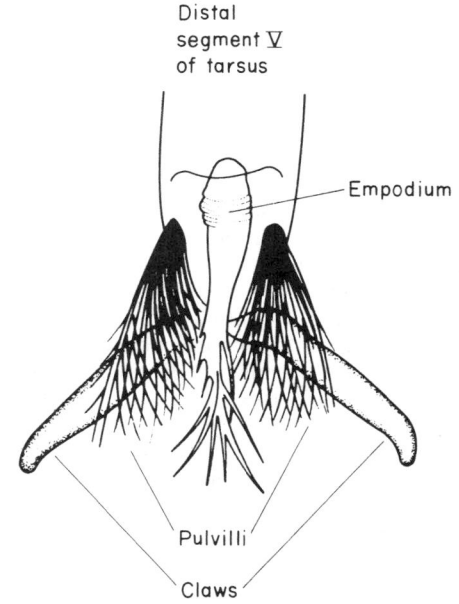

Distal segment $\underline{V}$ of tarsus

Empodium

Pulvilli

Claws

Figure IV.44 Tip of tarsus of *Culex*, showing paired pulvilli below the claws. In life these pulvilli appear as pale pads, more conspicuous than the empodium which is present also in other mosquito genera.

TRIBE: CULICINI

GENUS: *CULEX*

About 800 species of *Culex* are known, being classified in 21 subgenera, with many species acting as the vectors of enzootic arboviruses, protozoa and filariae. They bite at night and some species have much medical significance; many species can be pests when abundant. Generic characteristics are that eggs always form a raft (see Figure IV.30), larvae have several pairs of hair tufts on the siphon, and the adults possess tarsal pulvilli (Figure IV.44) and lack postspiracular bristles, with the tip of the female abdomen being bluntly rounded. Male palps are strongly curved upwards (see Figure IV.34a). General body colouration of the adults is usually brown, with wings plain and vein scales dark. Unlike Aedini, the eggs cannot diapause, so *Culex* breeding is continuous, except when fertilized females hibernate as the overwintering mechanism for species found in temperate countries.

The typical subgenus *Culex* contains the majority of species, usually with a banded proboscis and/or basal pale bands on abdominal tergites. Japanese encephalitis virus is transmitted mainly by *Culex* spp. in the Oriental region (for identification keys see Bram,[34] Sirivanakarn[35]), especially by the following species which breed prolifically in paddy and swamps: *C. tritaeniorhynchus*, *C. gelidus* and *C. vishnui*. Because they are abundant around villages wherever rice is grown in South-East Asia, and the adult females of these species attack various mammals by preference, they readily transfer Japanese encephalitis virus to man from pigs and other amplification hosts. *C. theileri* in southern Africa and members of the *C. pipiens* complex in Egypt are important vectors of Rift Valley fever virus from livestock to man. In Australia, *C. annulirostris* plays a similar role in the epidemiology of Murray Valley encephalitis, but the source of Murray Valley encephalitis virus remains a mystery. Like most other *Culex* spp., *C. annulirostris* feeds to some extent on birds and these may be responsible for virus dissemination. Eastern and Western Equine and St Louis encephalitis viruses in America are mainly found in birds (sparrows and pigeons), being transmitted by *C. nigripalpus*, *C. pipiens*, *C. restuans*, *C. salinarius*, *C. tarsalis* and other mosquitoes which occasionally pass infection to man and other mammals which serve as dead-end hosts. *C. pipiens* serves the same function for Eastern Equine encephalitis virus in Europe. West Nile virus has a similar epidemiology in Africa, being transmitted from birds to man by members of the *C. univittatus* complex.

Culex-borne arboviruses can be carried through the winter in hibernating female mosquitoes, although the ecological importance of this remains uncertain. The arrival of virus in migratory birds may set off seasonal transmission if it coincides with high densities of bird-biting mosquitoes. Investigations of arbovirus epidemiology are frequently hampered by difficulties of distinguishing and identifying the females of *Culex* spp., taxonomy of which is based on the morphology of male terminalia in many cases.

The *Culex pipiens* complex comprises several species, subspecies and forms, with representatives in all parts of the world. Typical *C. pipiens* occurs in temperate countries of the northern hemisphere, spreading through temperate highlands to southern Africa. Closely related species or subspecies are present in temperate parts of Australia and South America, but they seldom attack man in temperate countries. Whenever a man-biting infection occurs to the north of the Mediterranean or equivalent latitude, it is likely to be a form usually known as *molestus* (*autogenicus*). This mosquito causes severe infections due to prolific breeding indoors where circumstances are suitable. Although the females are autogenous (laying one egg batch without having fed on blood) they attack man viciously. Indoor infections of *C. p. molestus*, or autogenous *C. pipiens*, occur as far north as Moscow. It seems that incapacity to hibernate is what keeps these mosquitoes indoors, breeding in flooded basements, cess pits, etc. Southwards especially in North Africa, such populations are more often found breeding freely outdoors and it is unclear to what extent they may interbreed with anautogenous *C. pipiens*. In Egypt, the *C. pipiens* complex is responsible for bancroftian filariasis transmission[36] and has been implicated as the main vector in outbreaks of Rift Valley fever.

C. quinquefasciatus (=*C. p. fatigans*) is the main man-biting tropical member of the *C. pipiens* complex, distributed up to 38°N in USA, 30°N in Asia, but only 24°N in Africa. In the New World it interbreeds with *C. pipiens* (*sensu stricto*), but they can generally be regarded as distinct species. Bancroftian filariasis is largely maintained in tropical villages and towns by *C. quinquefasciatus* alone, although West African strains of *W. bancrofti* do not develop in this species of mosquito. Elsewhere, *C. quinquefasciatus* is an efficient vector of *W. bancrofti* but refractory to *B. malayi*.

C. quinquefasciatus (Figure IV.45) is confined to domestic habitats, breeding abundantly in heavily polluted waters occurring in ditches, village ponds, soakage pits, cess pits and the like. Since these sites are inevitably associated with towns

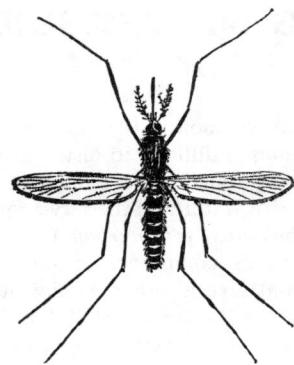

Figure IV.45   Culex quinquefasciatus (4×). The name refers to the way that, when viewed from above with the naked eye, the abdomen seems to have five broad dark bands separated by pale ones (but so do many other species). The alternative name *Culex fatigans* (the mosquito that tends to make one fatigued) has been widely used, although *quinquefasciatus* has priority and is therefore correct.

and urban development, *C. quinquefasciatus* thrives as a tropical pest in developing countries. Some breeding also occurs in rock holes, tree-holes and artificial containers such as tins, buckets and car tyres, where larvae of *Ae. aegypti* commonly mingle with those of *C. quinquefasciatus*. Control of both is best done by elimination of breeding sites, putting covers on water pots, covering soakage pits and taking all possible precautions to prevent there being places where the female mosquitoes can lay their eggs on exposed water containing organic nutrients for the larvae. Larvicidal oils and insecticides have been widely employed, but they are increasingly uneconomical and in many countries *C. quinquefasciatus* has become resistant to both organochlorines and organophosphates. Larger breeding places can be treated (see Table IV.13), with emulsions of organophosphates or to employ costly biocides or insect growth regulators (IGRs) (e.g. diflubenzuron or methoprene), activity of which may be much reduced in polluted water. Application of a floating carpet of expanded polystyrene beads gives the most durable control of *Culex* larvae in enclosed breeding sites such as pit latrines.

As the bites of *C. quinquefasciatus* are painful, whether or not disease is likely to be transmitted, it is advisable to screen houses (plastic mesh, at least six strands per centimetre) and especially bedrooms, making them mosquito proof. Cracks around ceilings and doors should be sealed. The use of bednets is highly desirable wherever *C. quinquefasciatus* occurs. Although several arboviruses have been reported from *C. quinquefasciatus*, it seems that this species is not usually an important vector of such infections. Adult males and females rest both indoors and outdoors during daytime; they are naturally quite tolerant of residual insecticides.

In the Far East, *C. pipiens pallens* seems to be biologically intermediate between *C. pipiens* and *C. quinquefasciatus*. It may be a distinct species or a hybrid. Formerly a filariasis vector in Japan[37] and still a pest there, the importance and distribution of *C. p. pallens* in South-East Asian countries is not well understood.

Taxonomy of the *C. pipiens* complex is a matter of uncertainty and disagreement. Separation of species is traditionally based upon the morphology of male terminalia, as expressed by the ratio of distances between tips of the dorsal

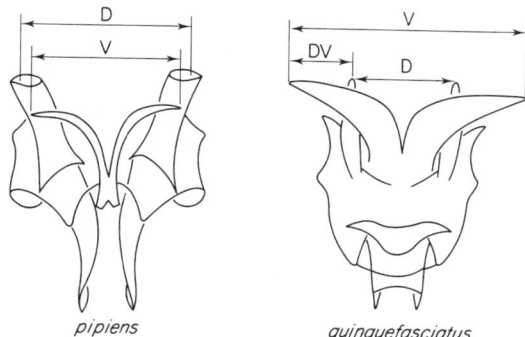

Figure IV.46 Male phallosomes of the *Culex pipiens* complex, ventral views. The shape and spread of the ventral arms is much wider in *C. quinquefasciatus* (= *C. p. fatigans*) than in typical *C. pipiens*. The ratio D/V can be used to express this contrast, sometimes given as DV/V. Members of the *C. pipiens* complex generally have the following values of D/V: *quinquefasciatus* 0.3; *pallens* 0.3–1.0; *pipiens* 0.8–1.0; *molestus* (= *autogenicus*) 0.8–1.2.

and ventral arms of the phallosome (D/V ratio) or the difference between these dimensions (D/DV ratio), as shown in Figure IV.46. General recognition of the *C. pipiens* complex depends upon the following combination of characters: proboscis dark, not banded, paler below in middle; abdominal tergites with transverse pale bands basally and pale spots on hind corners; abdomen pale below, usually with median dark spots in a row; thorax reddish-brown dorsally, straw/pale brown coloured laterally without dark pleural markings, with dark bristles on scutum and whitish scales in patches on pleurae (sides) but without spiracular or postspiracular scales; usually one lower mesepimeral bristle; wings with dark scales on all veins; tarsi entirely dark; mid femur dark anteriorly, without narrow longitudinal pale stripe as in some closely related species (which may also have spiracular or postspiracular scale patches).

Apart from the species already mentioned, which all belong to subgenus *Culex*, some medically important species belong to subgenus *Melanoconion*. These small species are potent vectors of arboviruses in the American tropics (see Table IV.6). As distinct from subgenus *Culex* having narrow scales, species in subgenus *Melanconion* have a rim of broad scales above the eyes, and wing veins one and two with broader scales distally. It is difficult to identify females of *Melanaconion* specifically and breeding places are not easy to find. Usually the larvae occupy large, quiet, non-polluted pools, often sheltering under vegetation. Control is therefore impracticable without environmental damage. Adults of *Melanoconion* spp. shelter among vegetation and their attacks may be locally reduced by insecticidal fogging during the evening flight period. They prefer to feed upon a wide range of wild creatures, but man is often bitten. Taxonomic studies by Sirivanakarn[38] should pave the way to improved understanding of the vectorial significance of the various species.

GENUS: *CULISETA*

Distinctive features of this genus are the presence of spiracular bristles; the wing often has one or two dark spots in the middle (at base of vein three and sometimes vein two); the siphonal tuft is large, at the extreme base of the larval siphon; eggs are usually laid as a raft which is less well formed than in *Culex*. Approximately 35 species are classified in seven subgenera, some of which are given generic status by Maslov.[39] Most are harmless and found only in temperate countries. A few species are pests, notably *C. longiareolata* around the Mediterranean. This species inhabits arid terrain, breeding in wells and rock pools, whereas most other *Culiseta* spp. favour weedy ponds and marshes. In North America, both Eastern and Western Equine encephalitis circulate among birds through *C. inornata*, *C. melanura* and *C. morsitans*. The latter may also be involved as a vector in Old World situations. *Culiseta* spp. breed continuously throughout the year, females of some species (e.g. *C. annulata*) sheltering indoors and feeding intermittently during winter in temperate countries.

TRIBE: MANSONIINI

GENUS: *COQUILLETTIDIA*

Most of these species are mostly yellow, quite large and voracious biters, attacking by day and night. They lay egg masses on the surface of stagnant water or weedy ponds. Larvae and pupae have the respiratory siphon and trumpets pointed and strengthened for plugging into the air ducts of plant stems. The genus occurs in all continents; among 55 known species *C. perturbans* in North America and *C. venezuelensis* in South America are some of the most important pests, and the latter has been implicated as a vector of several arboviruses (see Table IV.6).

GENUS: *MANSONIA*

This genus differs from the preceding one by characters given in the key (Table IV.7) and because egg masses are deposited under floating leaves of certain aquatic plants. Like *Coquillettidia*, larvae and pupae of *Mansonia* breathe air from plant stems and have their respiratory appendages modified accordingly (Figures IV.47 and IV.48). Subgenus *Mansonia* has only a dozen American species, notably the widespread pest *M. titillans* which breeds in swamps and marshes with floating water lettuce (*Pistia*) and water hyacinth (*Eichornia*) or rooted *Pontederia* and other plants favoured by the immature stages. *M. titillans* is an important vector of Venezuelan equine encephalitis and may contribute to transmission of *W. bancrofti*. As with other troublesome *Mansonia* and some *Coquillettidia*, *M. titillans* disperses far from the breeding sites in search of hosts to bite.

Subgenus *Mansonioides* also has a dozen species, endemic to the Old World tropics, being pests arising from breeding sites in water with plenty of *Eichornia*, *Pistia*, rooted *Isachne* (swamp grass), *Zuzania* and other suitable vegetation. When such well-aerated plants are removed, *Mansonioides* disappears. In parts of southern India (Kerala), Sri Lanka and

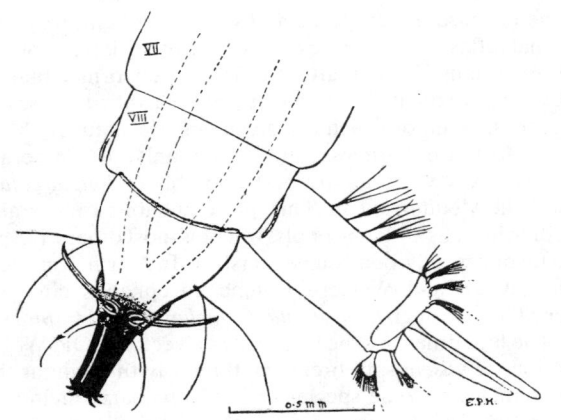

Figure IV.47   Respiratory siphon and terminal segment of the larva of *Mansonioides* (lateral view).

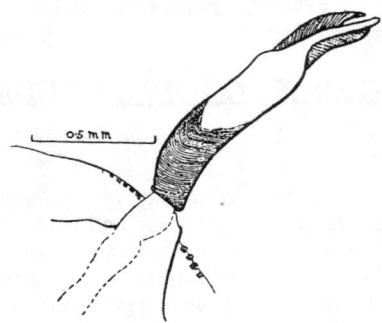

Figure IV.48   Respiratory horn of the pupa *Mansonioides*.

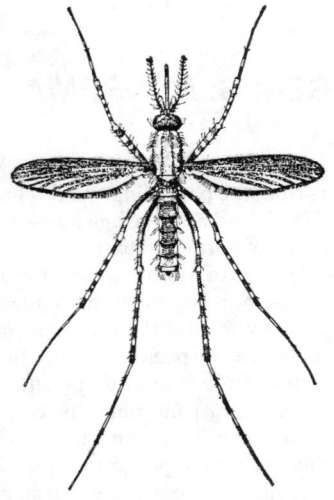

Figure IV.49   Female *Mansonia* (*Mansonioides*) *annulifera* (4×).

elsewhere, *Mansonioides* populations thrive where flooded pits for soakage of coconut husks, from which rope is made, are allowed to provide breeding sites rich in organic food for the larvae. In some areas this problem has now been controlled by keeping the water free of floating plants.

Adult *Mansonioides* are strikingly marked (Figure IV.49),

with banded legs and speckled wings having very broad scales on the veins. The tip of the female abdomen is curiously boat-shaped, to facilitate oviposition under floating leaves. Some arboviruses are transmitted by *Mansonioides* spp., but these species of mosquito are generally refractory to *W. bancrofti*.

In forested localities, or when weather is overcast, the females feed by day; they attack mainly at night outdoors, coming freely into houses, but not resting indoors during the daytime. The bites are more painful than with most other mosquitoes. *Mansonioides* spp. are of particular parasitological interest because, together with *Anopheles* (*Anopheles*) spp., they are the vectors of brugian filariasis (see Table IV.5). In South-East Asia, according to the work of Wharton[40] in Malaysia, swamp-forest populations of *M. annulata*, *M. uniformis* and especially the sibling species *M. bonneae* and *M. dives* share the transmission of zoonotic subperiodic *B. malayi*, which they transmit to man from leaf monkeys and other wild animals. At the same time, *M. annulata*, *M. dives* and other *Mansonioides* spp. are vectors of *B. pahangi* from animal to animal, but rarely to man. Continuous biting activity, with peaks of attack at dusk and dawn, helps to make *Mansonioides* spp. in the forest suitable as vectors of these subperiodic parasites. In areas of paddy on the coastal plains, *M. uniformis* and *Anopheles* spp. are the principal vectors of periodic *B. malayi*, with some involvement of *M. annulata* and *M. dives*. However, *M. bonneae* is apparently refractory to the periodic strains of the parasite. In India and other parts of southern Asia, periodic *B. malayi* is or was generally transmitted by *M. annulata*, *M. annulifera*, *M. indiana* and *M. uniformis*. In eastern Africa, where *B. malayi* is absent, *M. africana* and *M. uniformis* transmit *B. patei* among dogs and cats but rarely to people.

TRIBE: SABETHINI

GENUS: *SABETHES*

These are forest mosquitoes that transmit jungle yellow fever and other arboviruses (see Table IV.6) in South America. *S. chloropterus* is one of the most frequently involved vector species. About 30 species are known. This genus is very distinctive; its characters are given in Table IV.7. The adults have a metallic lustre. The scales of all parts of the body are flat. There is a very large pair of procumbent bristles projecting from the crown of the head and a tuft of setae on the mesonotum. The antennae are similar in both sexes; the palps are short in the female and usually also in the male. The larvae are generally predaceous and live in the water which collects in the axils and bracts of leaves, in tree-holes, or which is secreted by pitchers or other modified parts of plants. They are usually rather hairy and have smooth or stumpy antennae. A siphon is present and a single row of scales on the side of the eighth abdominal segments. The pupae are characterized by the conspicuous fan of bristles at the posterolateral angles of the eighth and ninth abdominal segments and by the small tail-fins. *Sabethes* taxonomy is unsatisfactory and their control is impractical.

LITERATURE ON MOSQUITOES

Information on the many species of mosquito is voluminous, with about five or six publications on Culicidae appearing daily. Much of the literature on mosquito biology and identification is now obsolete, due to advances in knowledge. Some general references to be recommended are: Bates,[41] Gillett,[42] Harbach and Knight,[43] Harwood and James,[44] Horsfall,[45] Mattingly,[46] Service[47] and World Health Organization.[9]

For the identification of mosquito genera and species in each part of the world, the following publications contain the most up-to-date keys and/or other information on medically important species:

Africa: Anophelinae: Gillies and De Meillon.[15]Culicinae: Edwards;[48] Hopkins;[49] Mattingly;[50] Gerberg and Van Someren;[51] Cordellier et al.[52]
Americas: Lane;[53] Forrattini;[54,55] Belkin et al.;[33] Carpenter and LaCasse;[14] Wood et al.;[56] Faran;[21] Darsie and Ward;[57] Sirivanakarn.[38]
Arabia: Mattingly and Knight.[58]
Australia: Lee;[59] Lee and Woodhill;[60] Dobrotworsky;[61] Marks.[62]
Cape Verde Islands: Ribeiro et al.[63]

Europe: Dahl and White.[64]
India: Anophelinae: Christophers;[65] Bhatia et al.[66] Culicinae: Barraud;[67] see also Oriental region.
Jamaica: Belkin et al.[33]
Japan: Tanaka et al.[68]
Madagascar: Grjebine;[69] Ravaonjanahary.[70]
Mediterranean: Rioux;[21] Senevet and Andarelli.[72]
Papua New Guinea: Van den Assem and Bonne-Wepster.[73]
New Zealand: Belkin.[74]
Oriental region: Anophelinae: Bonne-Wepster and Swellengrebel;[75] Reid;[12] Harrison and Scanlon;[76] Culicinae: Mattingly;[77] Bram;[34] Mattingly;[78] Reinert;[79] Sirivanakarn;[75] Huang.[80]
Pacific: Belkin;[24] Huang.[25]
Philippines: Delfinado;[81] Basio.[82]
Russia: Gutsevich et al.[82]
Seychelles: Mattingly and Brown.[84]
World: Foote and Cook;[85] Mattingly;[86] Knight and Stone.[80]

Most recent advances in mosquito control are mentioned in the two volumes edited by Laird and Miles (1983, 1985).[87]

MOSQUITO PHYSIOLOGY AND CONTROL

This subject is becoming more relevant to medical entomology. Some of the newer larvicides for mosquito control act as 'growth regulators'. One mode of action is to impair cuticle formation in the successive larval instars, the pupa and the adult through the application of chitin inhibitors (e.g. diflubenzuron). Another approach is to treat mosquito breeding places with compounds having activity like the juvenile hormones of insects; these 'juvenoids' (e.g. methoprene) prevent successful metamorphosis and maturation of the mosquito. So far there are no practical problems of resistance to these chemicals and there should be little cross-resistance with conventional pesticides.

As for all other insects, the mosquito body is encased in an exoskeleton made of cuticle. Insecticides which act on the nervous system (i.e. organochlorines, organophosphates, carbamates or pyrethroids) must be readily absorbed through insect cuticle, but not through human skin. Cuticular hardness depends on the degree of chitinization. Mosquito larvae have a hard head capsule, siphon and many rigid bristles or setae and spines, but the thorax and abdomen are mostly covered by a more flexible cuticle. Mosquito adults have strong and rigid cuticular plates forming the head, thorax and abdomen, with flexible joints between them, where necessary for articulation of limbs and segments. Respiratory spiracles on the larval siphon, pupal trumpets and on the adult sides (pairs on the mesothorax, metathorax and each abdominal segment) allow air to reach all internal organs via a network of tubes called tracheae. The use of larvicidal oils is intended to drown mosquito larvae by preventing them from reaching air when they try to open their spiracles at the water surface. However, Reiter,[88] working with monomolecular layers for anopheline control,

has found that there may be sufficient dissolved oxygen for larval survival during much of the day and all night without access to free air. Oiling will therefore be most effective when an insecticide is included.

The body cavity or haemocoel of mosquitoes and other insects is filled with colourless haemolymph carrying haemocytes having some of the functions of blood corpuscles. There is an open circulatory system, with a dorsal aorta and heart in the abdomen. The mosquito brain is in the head, with neurosecretory ganglia and *corpus cardiacum* for hormone production. Other important sources of hormones controlling mosquito life processes are the ovaries and the thoracic *corpora allata*. A ventral nerve cord has segmental ganglia and paired lateral branches.

The mosquito gut (Figure IV.50) passes from the proboscis to the pharynx in the head, the oesophagus in the thorax, the midgut or stomach in the abdomen and finally the rectum, where fluids are absorbed before defecation occurs through the anus below the tip of the abdomen. Within the foregut, especially of female anophelines, cuticular teeth protrude into the lumen of the gut; these are thought to have a primary function of rupturing blood corpuscles and they also inflict lethal damage on many ingested microfilariae. A large crop is formed by an oesophageal diverticulum; water and nectar are taken into the crop for digestion of sugars. Excretion is by means of a series of long white malpighian tubules in the abdomen, behind the stomach, with their ducts discharging into the midgut lumen.

When freshly engorged after biting, the abdomen of a female mosquito is swollen and reddened by the blood meal within the stomach. Paired ovaries, each with about 100 follicles for egg production, are situated posteriorly in the

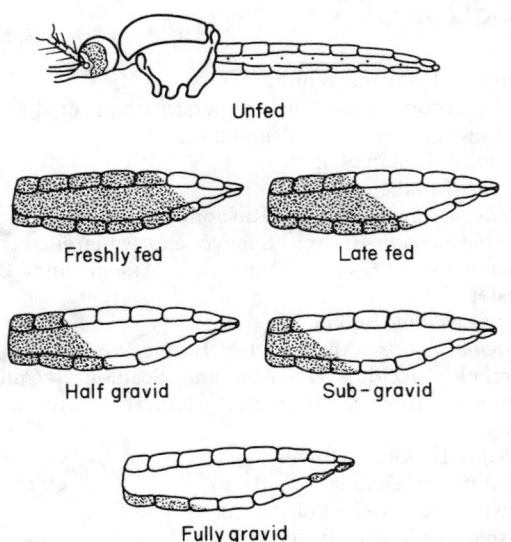

Unfed

Freshly fed   Late fed

Half gravid   Sub-gravid

Fully gravid

Figure IV.50   Classification in the abdominal conditions of female mosquitoes. The dark basal area of the abdomen contains the blood meal in the stomach, decreasing as digestion proceeds. The pale posterior part of the abdomen contains the developing ovaries, increasing as the gonotrophic cycle proceeds. Unfed, fed and gravid female mosquitoes may be either nulliparous or parous.

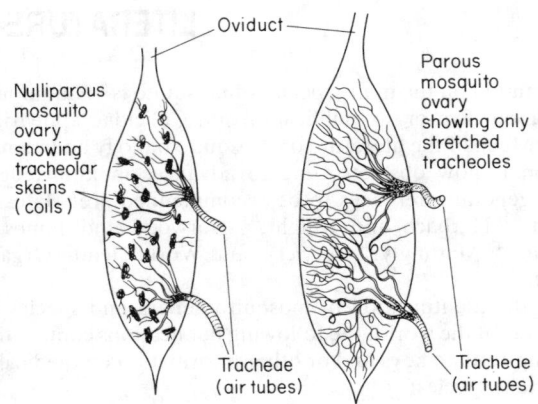

Figure IV.52   Mosquito ovaries, showing how the nulliparous female has coiled tracheolar 'skeins' in the ovary (left); tracheoles become permanently stretched in the parous ovary (right) due to previous growth of eggs. These features of the air tubes can only be seen in mosquito females with 'unfed' abdominal condition.

abdomen. In the terminal abdominal segment of females are spermathecae (three in culicines; one in anophelines) which receive and store sperms from males, so that mature oöcytes can be fertilized as eggs are laid.

As the blood meal becomes digested during the days after blood-feeding, the ovaries develop and fill the rear abdomen with whitish eggs. Figure IV.50 shows how the changes in abdominal condition can be classified as: (1) unfed, (2) freshly fed, (3) one-third gravid or late stage fed, (4) half gravid, (5) two-thirds gravid or sub-gravid, (6) fully gravid.

In parallel with these abdominal stages, it is customary to assess the progress of oögenesis by classifying the development of ovarian follicles. After emergence from the pupa, the follicles pass from stage I to stage II, which is the resting stage. After blood-feeding, yolk is deposited around the oöcyte nucleus, and stage III passes to stage IV when the clear nucleus is no longer visible when examined in saline. Finally stage V represents formation of the full-sized egg, containing the unfertilized oöcyte. These categories of ovarian development in mosquitoes are generally known as 'Christophers' stages' (Figure IV.51).

At tropical temperatures, the eggs of mosquitoes become ready to lay (laying is termed oviposition) 2 or 3 days after ingestion of the blood meal. Blood-feeding and egg-laying are the first and last steps in what is called the gonotrophic cycle. Soon after having laid a batch of eggs, the female mosquito tries to feed again on blood. Thus there are regular and usually continuous gonotrophic cycles. The feeding

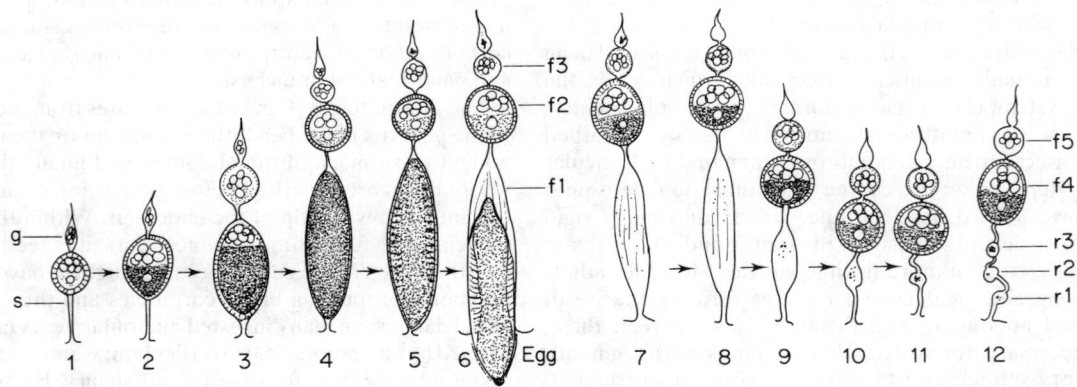

Figure IV.51   Christophers' stages of ovarian follicular development in mosquitoes. Each ovary contains approximately 100 ovarioles. Each ovariole consists of a hollow stalk (s), developing follicles (f1, f2, etc.) and a terminal germarium (g) from which successive follicles arise. Stages I–V of development of the first follicle are shown (1–5). The mature egg then passes from the stalk (6) to the common oviduct. A sac-like swelling of the ovariolar stalk contracts (7–10) to form a small persistent dilatation or follicular relic, which is slightly pigmented (11). Successive eggs formed in each ovariole leave a series of distinct relics (r1, r2, etc.) in the parous mosquito (12), from which the mosquito's age may be estimated in terms of the number of gonotrophic cycles.

interval, or the duration of the gonotrophic cycle, measured in days, is an important factor affecting vectorial capacity. The more often a mosquito feeds on blood, the more likely it is to pick up infections and transmit them. Conversely, at cooler temperatures, the gonotrophic cycle takes longer—maybe 4 or 5 days, reducing the chances of transmission because: (1) occasions when parasites can be acquired or transmitted are less frequent for each female mosquito, (2) the speed of development of parasites to the infective stage in the vectors is proportional to temperature, and (3) mosquitoes are more likely to die before becoming infective. Clearly, if mosquito longevity is less than the time required for completion of parasite development, there is no likelihood of disease transmission. The aim of spraying houses with residual insecticides is to kill the majority of adult female mosquitoes before they reach the age of infectivity, and not to eliminate mosquitoes altogether. Table IV.13 summarizes the insecticidal applications used for mosquito control (see under each type of mosquito for more details on their control).

One way to monitor the age composition and life expectancy of adult mosquito populations is to determine the proportion of females that are parous, i.e. have laid eggs at least once. This involves examination of the ovaries to see whether tracheal skeins are present implying nulliparity, or if follicular relics are present implying parity (Figure IV.52). It may be possible to count the number of relics on each follicular stalk in order to calculate the mosquito's age in terms of the number of gonotrophic cycles it has experienced.[9,89]

More general information on mosquito physiology has been reviewed by Clements.[90] Reviews of mosquito control methods are given by Laird and Miles.[87]

MIDGES
R. P. Lane

FAMILY: CERATOPOGONIDAE (BITING MIDGES)

GENERA: *CULICOIDES, LEPTOCONOPS* AND *FORCIPOMYIA* (SUBGENUS *LASIOHELEA*)

Biting midges are very small flies (1–4 mm long) called 'no-see-ums' in some parts of the world or, confusingly, sandflies in others such as the southern USA and Caribbean. They occur worldwide in habitats ranging from tropical forests and savannas to agricultural districts, coastal and desert areas. The adults are compact, usually dark-brown or black flies, with the wings held flat over the back at rest. Only the females suck blood and often attack in huge numbers, their bites are painful and often elicit a prolonged reaction in sensitive individuals. The males, which can be distinguished by their plumrose antennae, feed only on plant sugars. The larvae are small and worm-like, swimming in a sinusoidal manner through wet or moist habitats such as fresh or brackish water or mud, decomposing vegetation and wet bovine droppings.

The Ceratopogonidae (biting midges) are a large family of over 4000 species in 60 genera but only three contain species of medical significance: *Culicoides, Leptoconops* and *Forcipomyia* (subgenus *Lasiohelea*).[91] Their principal impact on man is as biting pests but species of *Culicoides* transmit filarial nematodes and are also of veterinary importance as virus and nematode vectors.

Leptoconops
Some species are serious pests, biting during the day. The flies are shiny black with milky white wings. Species of the subgenus *Styloconops* breed in sandy beaches surrounding the India Ocean (*L. spinosifrons; L. holoconops*), and are coastal pests in south-east USA, eastern Central America and the Caribbean (*L. becquarti*); *Leptoconops* (*sensu stricto*) breed in fine silt soils inland in south-east USA (*L. torrens*).

A few species of *Forcipomyia* subgenus *Lasiohelea* are serious pests: *F.* (*L.*) *siberica* in central Asia, *F.* (*L.*) *taiwana* in Japan and China and *F.* (*L.*) *townsvillensis* in Australia.

Culicoides
These have a wing length of 2 mm; those of tropical species may be only 1 mm, and usually the wings are patterned (Figure IV.53). Of the 1000 species in this genus, many are biting pests in temperate and tropical countries and may have a significant effect on tourist-based economies. Biting rates of 200–400 per hour are commonly recorded with a maximum of 3000 per hour on a single exposed limb! Attacks may cause severe discomfort, e.g. biting on the eyelids may induce sufficient swelling to prevent their opening for several days. New arrivals to tropical areas often suffer (or are worried) more than locals and subsequent scratching may produce deeply eroding secondary infections to the extent that skin grafting has been used. Dermatitis caused by *Culicoides* has been reported several times, e.g. *C. paraensis* in Bahia, Brazil.

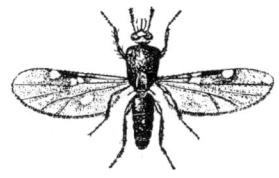

Figure IV.53 Female *Culicoides grahami* (50×).

In the Caribbean and eastern Central America *Mansonella ozzardi* is transmitted by several species of *Culicoides: C. furens* in St Vincent, Haiti;[92] *C. phlebotomus* in Trinidad[93] and *C. paraensis* in Antigua and northern Argentina. Both *C. furens* and *C. phlebotomus* are coastal species the former breeding in mangrove swamps and the latter in streams crossing beaches. *C. paraensis* is a peridomestic species breeding in decaying fruits such as calabash or cacao pods. In the Brazilian and Colombian Amazon regions *M. ozzardi* is primarily transmitted by *Simulium*, but *C. insinuatus* may also play a role.

Culicoides are also vectors of *M. perstans* in Africa and believed to be the vector in the New World. There is considerable confusion over the identity of the species incriminated as the vector of *M. perstans* in West Africa. It was originally recorded as *C. austeni* (and later *C. milnei*), but it is more likely that *C. inornatipennis* (and possibly *C. grahami*) are responsible. The vectors breed in small pools of water in cut stems of bananas and plantains and therefore the incidence of the disease is highest in and around plantations. Transmission takes place at night. In contrast, the transmission of *M. streptocerca* takes place during the day when the vector, *C. grahami*, bites man.

Culicoides paraensis, a domestic pest in many parts of Brazil, has been incriminated as the vector of Oropouche virus, which causes a febrile illness in Amazonian Brazil. Several other viruses have been isolated from ceratopogonids: Japanese B encephalitis (*F.* (*L.*) *taiwana*); Eastern equine encephalitis (pooled *Culicoides* in USA); Rift Valley fever (*Culicoides* in Kenya, Nigeria); and Congo and Dugbe viruses (several pools of *Culicoides* in Nigeria). Although it is most unlikely that midges transmit these viruses, the question does remain open.

Control of ceratopogonids involves the use of insecticides for larviciding or space-spraying, repellents and land management (draining and flooding).[94]

BLACKFLIES, BUFFALO GNATS, TURKEY GNATS (See also Chapter 70)
G. B. White

FAMILY: SIMULIIDAE

GENUS: *SIMULIUM*

The Simuliidae, usually known as blackflies, are small, robust flies (1–5 mm long) (Figure IV.54); the females suck blood and have blade-like mouthparts; in the males these are more or less rudimentary. The flies have a characteristic humped thorax caused by the strong development of the scutum. The antennae are short and similar in both sexes. Most of what is known about blackfly biology and control has been summarized by Crosskey.[124]

Blackflies occur in enormous numbers in favourable localities during late spring and early summer in northern countries and are abundant in the north temperate and subarctic zones. They are also abundant in the tropics where man-biting species transmit *Onchocerca volvulus*. In addition to their role as transmitters of *Onchocerca*, they also act as intermediate hosts of other filariae and blood-borne protozoa of birds and mammals, and are a severe biting nuisance when the flies are numerous. The females attack viciously in the open during the day but do not enter houses. Biting activity is known to be influenced by weather conditions and older (infected) flies may differ in their behaviour from newly emerged, unfed flies.

The females lay their triangular eggs in running (and therefore oxygenated) water, in masses of 300–500, which are attached to rocks, grass and other objects by a gelatinous fluid. The eggs hatch in 1–2 days and the emerging larvae attach themselves by the posterior end to a pad of silk spun from the salivary glands, on to submerged leaves and stones. The larvae and pupae of most species have specialized aquatic niches on stones, twigs or other substrates. Those of the *S. neavei* complex in tropical Africa always occur on freshwater arthropods, mainly crabs, prawns or mayfly nymphs. The larvae feed by straining fine particles from the water through fan-shaped mouth brushes. There are 6–8 larval instars, ending in 1–2 weeks or more. Before pupation, the larva spins a tent-like, silken coccoon which protects the pupa inside it. The pupal period is 2–10 days and both larvae and pupae can be found in large numbers in breeding places.

The following species are actual or potential vectors of *O. volvulus* in man.

Africa

The *Simulium damnosum* and *S. neavei* complexes are groups with sibling species which have been separated into a number of different species by biological and chromosome studies. These species differ in their ecology and feeding preferences which affect their importance as vectors of human onchocerciasis. The *S. damnosum* complex (jinja fly) (see Chapter 70) contains at least 40 sibling species (identified chiefly by the pattern of chromosome banding), including forms that are found in the forest zone or in the savanna zone which are vectors only of the *O. volvulus* strain endemic to their own zones. Clinical manifestations of onchocerciasis in the savanna area are associated with lower biting densities and infection rates in the flies (annual transmission potential) compared to those found in the forest area. Different mem-

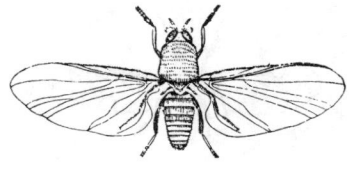

Figure IV.54   Simulium damnosum (10×).

bers of the complex breed in large or small rivers and in the outflow of dams, the larvae attaching to vegetation and stones in the river bed. Females are capable of long flights. In the vast Onchocerciasis Control Programme covering endemic countries of West Africa, involving regular larviciding of all waterways for 20 years, reinvasion of the controlled area was found over distances of 200–400 km due to influx of vector females from far afield.

The *S. neavei* complex is confined to small streams in hilly forest; its flight range is limited. The larvae and pupae are found attached to crabs of the genus *Potamonautes*. The chief vector species are *S. ethiopiense* in Ethiopia, *S. neavei* in Zaire and *S. woodi* in Tanzania. Eradication of *S. neavei* and the interruption of transmission from man to man was achieved in highland foci in Kenya by larviciding and clearance of riverine vegetation.

Central and South America

The *S. ochraceum* complex (orange/yellow species, unusual for a blackfly) are the main vectors in Mexico and Guate-mala. They breed in minute trickles of water, often under leaves, and in innumerable streams in rugged country with heavy vegetational cover; hence these species are difficult to control. They also breed close to villages in irrigated coffee plantations between 500 and 1200 m.

S. metallicum, *S. callidum* and *S. exiguum* are considered to be minor vectors in Central America but *S. exiguum* is the only anthropophilic species and therefore the principal vector in the endemic focus on the western slopes of the Andes in Colombia. *S. metallicum* is the main vector in Venezuela—breeding in small streams, and biting man avidly. In Mexico and Guatemala, however, this species does not feed on man so readily and is associated with larger streams.

In recently discovered foci of onchocerciasis in Amazonia (Brazil and Venezuela) the disease is transmitted by *S. guyanense*, *S. limbatum* and *S. oyapockense* (formerly reported as *S. amazonicum*). The latter also transmits non-pathogenic *Mansonella ozzardi* in South America.

For control of Simuliidae, and onchocerciasis, see Chapter 70.

HORSE FLIES, CLEGS, DEER FLIES
D. M. Minter

SUBORDER: BRACHYCERA
FAMILY: TABANIDAE

GENERA: *TABANUS, HAEMATOPOTA* AND *CHRYSOPS*

The family Tabanidae includes the largest blood-sucking flies known; some have a wing span of over 60 mm. Most species are stoutly built and robust insects, often brightly coloured in life, with large eyes and a body length from 5 to 25 mm. Viewed from above (Figure IV.55a), the eyes of females are widely separated (dichoptic), whilst the eyes of males are contiguous (holoptic). In life, the eyes of both sexes are often shot with species-specific iridescent bands, chevrons or spots of brilliant colours: these colours fade soon after death.

Tabanid antennae have three segments (known as the scape, pedicel and flagellum) that differ in size and proportions in the three main genera, *Tabanus*, *Chrysops* and *Haematopota* (Figure IV.55b). The palps are short and consist of one or two segments only. The wing venation of tabanids is characteristic (Figure IV.55c), particularly the enclosed, almost central, hexagonal discal cell and the open branch of the radial vein which encloses, in a submarginal cell, the wing tip of most species. There is also a second open submarginal cell anterior to the wing tip and five open posterior cells along the hind margin of the wing. The pattern of pigmentation of the wing, or its absence, is a useful feature for identification of the three genera of medical importance, in conjunction with the shape and proportion of the antennal segments (Figure IV.55b,c). Only females bite; because of their large size they take a large blood meal, from 20 to 200 mg. The mouthparts are short and stout; they project downwards below the head and inflict a painful bite.

There are four subfamilies of Tabanidae (Scepsidinae, Pangoniinae, Chrysopsinae and Tabaninae). Medically important species are found only among the Chrysopsinae and Tabaninae. The Tabaninae is subdivided into three tribes (Haematopotini, Tabanini and Diachlorini), of which only the Haematopotini and Tabanini contain species which normally bite man. There are about 3000 species of Tabanidae, in numerous genera, but medically important species occur only in the genera *Tabanus*, *Haematopota* (subfamily Tabaninae) and *Chrysops* (subfamily Chrysopsinae).

The Tabanidae are cosmopolitan; species of *Tabanus*, *Chrysops* and *Haematopota* occur in tropical, subtropical and temperate regions, but species of the genus *Haematopota*, although abundant in Africa, are absent from Australia and South America and are uncommon in North America.

The 'blue-tailed fly', celebrated in the well-known American ballad, is believed to be the widespread *Tabanus atratus* of eastern North America; the species is actually a uniform black colour, but there is a distinctly bluish tinge when the flies are covered with pollen or dust.

Other members of the suborder Brachycera are sometimes a severe biting nuisance, particularly in coastal and mountain regions of western North America. (They have a painful bite and are occasionally the cause of severe allergic manifestations.) These belong to the families Rhagionidae ('snipe-flies') and the closely related Athericidae. Although these

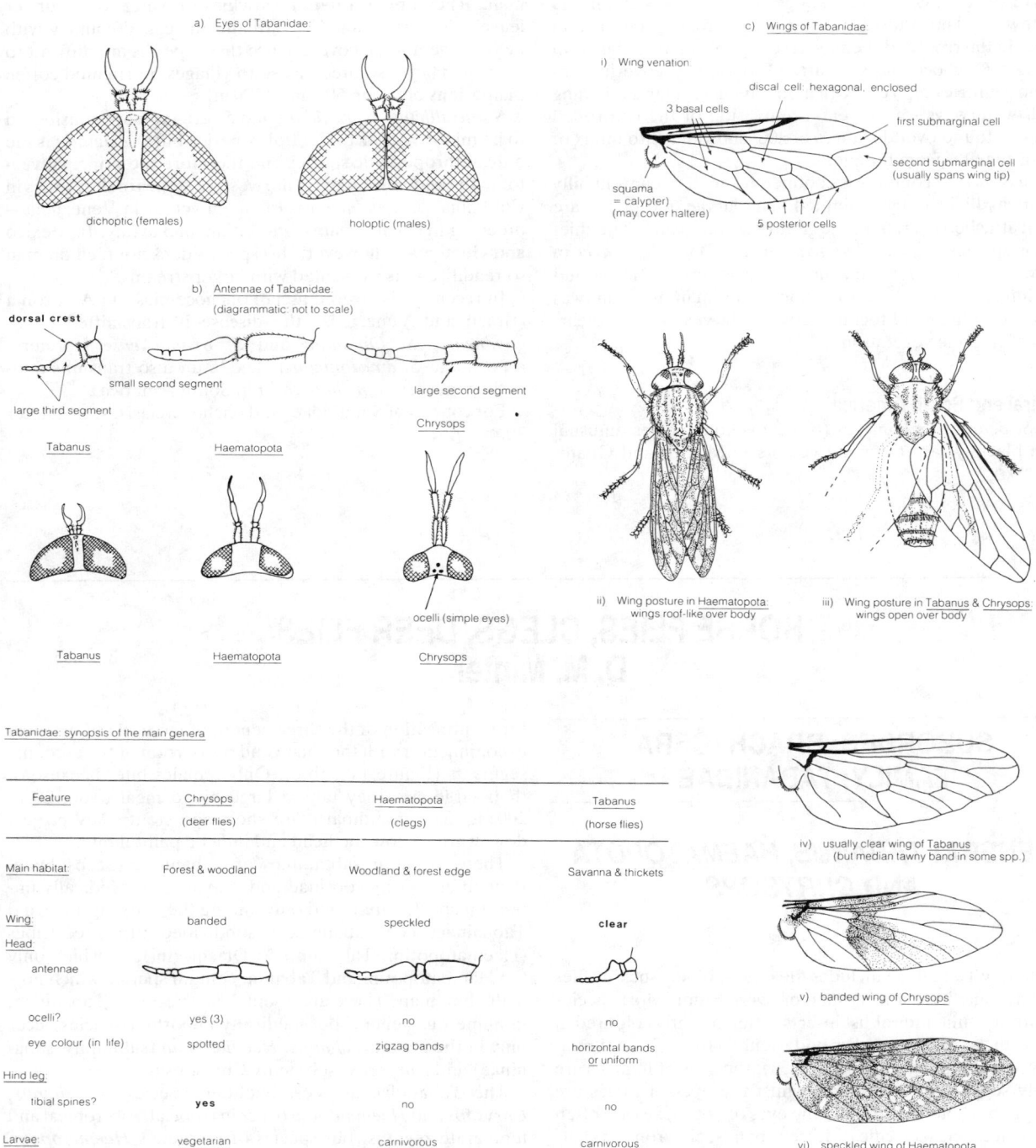

Figure IV.55 Characteristic features of the Tabanidae. (a) Holoptic and dichoptic condition of the head in male and female Tabanidae.
(b) Antennae of adult Tabanidae: antennal features in the genera *Tabanus* (horse flies), *Chrysops* (deer flies) and *Haematopota* (clegs).
(c) Wings of Tabanidae: (i) wing venation of Tabanidae; (ii) wing posture in *Haematopota* sp.; (ii) wing posture in *Tabanus* and *Chrysops* spp.;
(iv) clear wing of *Tabanus* sp; (v) banded wing of *Chrysops* sp.; (vi) speckled wing of *Haematopota* sp.

two families contain blood-sucking species, none has yet been associated with the transmission of pathogens. The rhagionid genus *Symphoromyia* is a vicious biter in the western USA; in Australia, members of the genera *Spaniop-* *sis* and *Austroleptis* are troublesome pests. Since they are of no known medical (or veterinary) importance, these two families are not considered further.

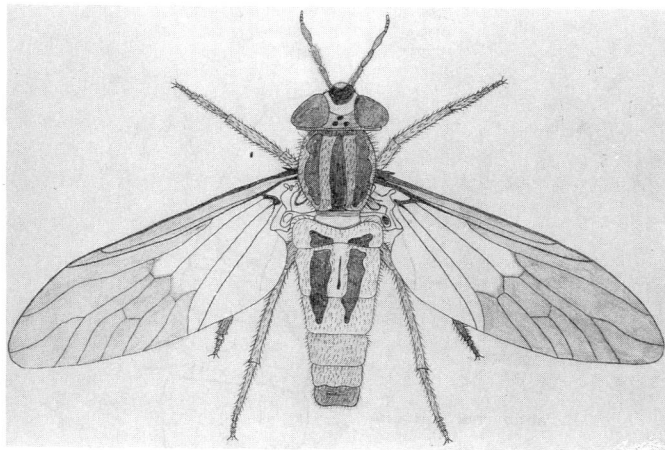

Figure IV.56   Female *Chrysops dimidiatus*. (Courtesy of D. B. Thomas.)

RECOGNITION OF THE GENERA: *CHRYSOPS, TABANUS* AND *HAEMATOPOTA*

Chrysops (deer flies, greenheads, mango flies, mangrove flies) (Figure IV.56)

Medium size, 6–10 mm long. Wings held apart over the body, like a half-open pair of scissors. Wings usually with one or two brownish transverse bands. Antennae (see Figure IV.55b) longer than those of *Tabanus* and *Haematopota*; the three segments are of similar length and project well in front of the head. Three spot-like, light-sensitive ocelli (simple eyes) present on the top of the head, behind the compound eyes. Tibia of hind legs spurred, with paired small distal spines, as well as the more prominent pair on the tibia of the middle legs (the latter found in all three genera). Eyes in life of iridescent colour, often of a golden hue. Mainly found in forest and woodlands, but often also common in marshy scrub and swampy woodlands.

Tabanus (horse flies, gad flies)

Medium to large flies, 9–25 mm long, wings usually clear, held over back like a pair of half-open scissors (as in *Chrysops*). Antennae short (see Figure IV.55b); first two segments small, the third segment long, with a pronounced dorsal 'hump' and an upturned tip. No ocelli. No spines on hind tibia. In life, eyes either of uniform colour or in a series of horizontal coloured bands. Mainly found in more open habitats, such as savanna and thicket vegetation.

Haematopota (clegs, stouts)

Medium size, 6–10 mm long, wings folded over the back in a roof-like manner; in almost all species the wings have a complex mottled dark grey or brown pattern. Antennae (see Figure IV.55b) with first and third segments markedly longer than the short second segment; third segment without dorsal 'hump' or upturned end. No ocelli. No spines on hind tibia. When alive, eyes have zigzag bands of iridescent colour. Mainly flies of woodlands and forest edges.

BIOLOGY AND LIFE CYCLE

The family Tabanidae is believed to have evolved in close association with the ungulates, upon which they mostly feed. Other mammals are also attacked, but seldom birds or reptiles. Most species are diurnal and hunt by sight; they are most active in bright sunlight; *Tabanus paradoxus* of central and southern Europe is unusual in that it is a nocturnal species.

Most tabanids inhabit woodland and forest; many species of *Chrysops* are found in waterlogged scrub and marshy woodlands: other species occupy more open areas of savanna woodland and grassland. Only females feed on blood; both sexes feed on sugary plant secretions. Because the female mouthparts are large and coarse, the bite is deep and painful; blood often continues to ooze from the wound for some time afterwards. Due to the painful bite, females are often forced, by defensive reactions of the human or animal host, to interrupt feeding and later resume on the same individual, or another, in order to feed to repletion. This behaviour considerably increases their efficiency as mechanical vectors of pathogens. Some individuals develop a severe allergic reaction to the large quantity of anticoagulant saliva pumped into the bite wound as the flies feed. With the exception of *Chrysops silaceus*, which will bite indoors, it is rare for tabanids to enter houses, although some species enter by accident and can be seen on windows, in an apparent attempt to escape.

The relatively short-lived adults are strictly seasonal in temperate climates, with biting confined to the warmest summer months. In tropical areas breeding is continuous, but biting activity of different species is very dependent on the rainy or dry season. The natural adult life-span of the important tropical species *Chrysops silaceus* is thought to be about 3–4 weeks.

In this respect rather like tsetse, tabanids are attracted to large, slow-moving dark objects including vehicles; they may enter the windows to bite the occupants, or attack the warm tyres of stationary cars and trucks.

Gravid females are selective of particular plant species or other specific oviposition sites. Females lay lozenge-shaped egg masses, firmly cemented to the underside of grasses, other vegetation, rocks or stones, where these overhang suitable larval breeding places; either shallow water, mud or damp soil (even in tree-holes high above the ground). Egg batches consist of a few dozen, or more than a thousand slender, cigar-shaped eggs—each 1–2.5 mm long (Figure IV.57). The egg batches are coated with a waterproof layer; eggs are commonly off-white in colour, sometimes grey, brownish-black, or even orange. Eggs hatch after 1–2 weeks; the cream-coloured, grub-like larvae drop on to the water, mud or damp soil and soon begin to feed. Larvae of *Chrysops* feed on vegetable detritus, while those of most *Tabanus* and *Haematopota* are carnivorous; they feed on other invertebrates, including members of their own species.

Compared with the relatively short life of adults, the duration of larval life is long, for both tropical and temperate species. For most tropical species, 4–5 months is usual; 1–2 years is not uncommon, and some species in cooler climates may spend up to 3 years as larvae. When mature, after up to eight moults, larvae of different species measure from 10 to 60 mm in length.

Larval habitats differ between the genera and species, but

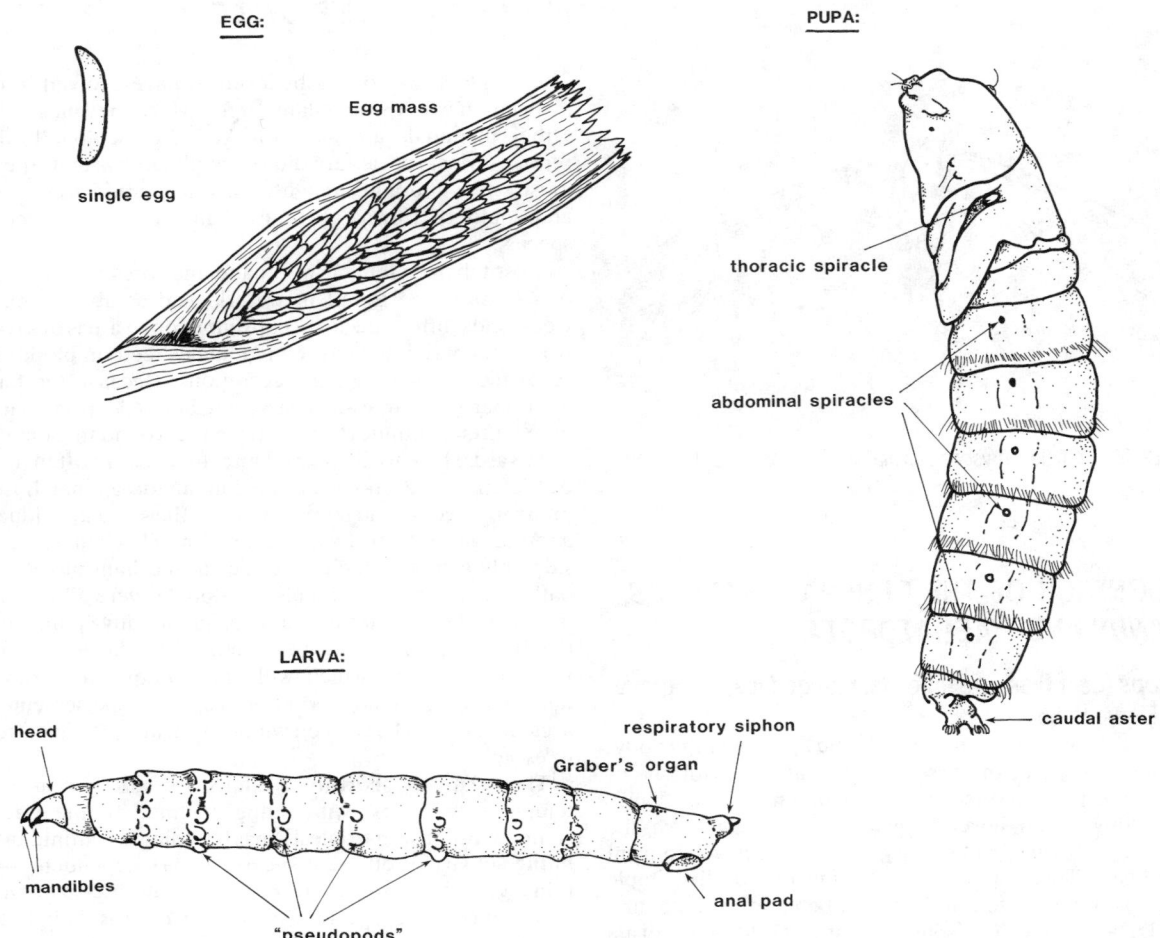

Figure IV.57   Egg, larvae and pupa of Tabanidae.

they are predominantly aquatic or semiaquatic. *Chrysops* larvae generally live in the wettest places, such as the muddy margins of marshes (and salt-marshes), *Tabanus* spp. usually inhabit shallow seasonal pools, mud or wet soil near water, while *Haematopota* are most often found in drier habitats, such as damp soil.

Larvae are easy to recognize (Figure IV.57). They are cylindrical, with rather pointed extremities; at one end is the small head, which can be retracted into the thorax (the head has mouth-hooks like those of the Muscidae). At the other end of the body is the slightly upturned, conical, posterior respiratory siphon. There are tyre-like rings around the body, at the leading edge of each segment, most of which have a number of ventrolateral locomotory protuberances, known as 'pseudopods'.

Graber's organ is a structure unique to larval Tabanidae and of unknown function, possibly sensory or glandular. Visible in life through the integument on the dorsal side, near the base of the respiratory siphon, are a paired row of black, rounded structures (the number of which evidently is increased in older larvae). Together with an internal pyriform sac, which opens via a narrow tube to the exterior between the last two segments, these are the principal parts of Graber's organ that can be seen with a hand-lens or low-power microscope.

Population occurs in drier parts of the habitat: the brown-coloured pupae, 7–40 mm long (Figure IV.57), look rather similar to those of butterflies, but are partly buried, in an upright position, in soil or mud. Some *Tabanus* species whose larvae inhabit seasonal pools, protect the future pupa from exposure to predators or desiccation; the mature larva excavates a vertical spiral burrow to delimit a cylinder of mud, into the centre of which it then burrows before pupation takes place. When the mud of the pool finally dries out, the cylinder cracks free from the surrounding mud and the pupa is securely housed within. The adult eventually emerges, after the pupa has partly rasped away the top of the cylinder. The pupae are provided with rings of spines on each abdominal segment, and a spiny caudal pad (known as an aster); the spines and aster facilitate limited vertical movement, whether in the substrate or in the mud cylinder. The pupal period lasts between 1 and 3 weeks until adult emergence.

CONTROL OF TABANIDAE

There are, in most instances, few or no practicable methods of control for tabanid flies. Drainage of marshy areas would probably limit available breeding places, although this would seldom be justifiable on a cost–benefit basis.

Table IV.8 Diseases transmitted to man by Tabanidae (see also Chapters 30, 38 and 70).

Agent	Disease	Principal hosts	Transmission	Distribution
Loa loa	Loaiasis; Calabar swelling	Man, Drill (*Papio leucophaeus*)	Cyclical: *Chrysops* spp.	West and Central Africa
Bacillus anthracis	Anthrax	Domestic livestock (man)*	Non-cyclic: mechanical	Cosmopolitan
Francisella tularensis	Tularaemia	Lagomorphs, rodents, man	Non-cyclic: mechanical (esp. *Chrysops* and *Tabanus* spp.: *also* ticks)	Cosmopolitan
Borrelia burgdorferi	Lyme disease	Deer, lagomorphs, (man)*	Non-cyclic: mechanical (main vectors: Ixodid ticks)	North temperate zone (Europe, North America) and Australia
Vesicular stomatitis virus (VSV)	Sore mouth (of cattle; horses)	Equines, bovines, pigs, (man)*	Non-cyclic mechanical	North, central and South America
Western equine encephalitis (WEE) virus		Amphibia, reptiles, birds, (man)*	Non-cyclic: mechanical	North and South America
Californian encephalitis virus (CEV) group:				
La Crosse (LAC) virus	—	Rodents, lagomorphs, etc., (man)*	Non-cyclic: mechanical (*also* mosquitoes)	North America (USA)
Jamestown Canyon (JC) virus	—	White-tailed deer [*Odocoileus virginianus*], (man)*	Non-cyclic: mechanical (*Chrysops*, *Tabanus* and *Hybomitra* spp.; *also* mosquitoes)	North America (Alaska, Canada, USA)

*Man an accidental host.

Similarly, the use of insecticides to control likely breeding places would be difficult to justify and would be equally difficult (if not impossible) to carry out effectively, due to the practical difficulty of ensuring adequate contact of insecticide with larval or pupal stages, often buried in wet soil or mud. Tabanid breeding places are in any event generally extensive and diffuse, difficult to delimit, and would be expensive to treat with insecticides. Insecticide-impregnated plastic collars and ear-tags have been developed to protect livestock from the attacks of ticks and various Diptera; they probably help also to reduce biting of tabanids.

Some success in reducing adult numbers of pest species of *Haematopota* has been achieved by the use of dark-coloured plates (about half a metre square) coated with a sticky adhesive, placed in open habitats where the flies are troublesome and the plates visible to the flies for some distance.

The wearing of open-mesh jackets impregnated with a synthetic pyrethroid insecticide (e.g. permethrin) or a repellent such as deet (diethyltoluamide), would afford some personal protection from the attack of tabanids in areas where they are sufficiently troublesome to warrant the inconvenience and expense of an additional garment.

DISEASE RELATIONSHIPS OF THE TABANIDAE (Tables IV.8 and IV.9)

Tabanidae can be a severe biting nuisance to people and livestock, to the extent that their attacks prevent all normal outdoor activities, affect the migration patterns of nomadic herdsmen and prevent the normal use of seasonal pastures by livestock (as in Sudan and parts of North America). In addition to the attacks of the adult flies, ricefield workers in Japan are sometimes attacked by the carnivorous aquatic larvae of *Tabanus* and *Chrysops*, which pierce feet or hands below the water surface; a severe oedematous reaction may ensue from the painful bites of the larvae.

More exceptionally, there are instances where bites of tabanid flies have resulted in the mechanical transmission of anthrax bacilli (*Bacillus anthracis*) to man, but this evidently occurs only under very unusual circumstances, and must surely be a rare event. However, it is very probable that tabanids do play a significant role in the maintenance of anthrax epizootics.

Tularaemia (See Chapter 47)

Of the two principal human diseases transmitted by tabanids, tularaemia is of lesser importance. Tularaemia is a zoonotic bacterial infection widespread in the northern hemisphere and caused by *Francisella tularensis*. In the Old World the disease occurs in most European countries, the former USSR, Iran, Turkey, Tunisia, China and Japan. Ticks are thought to be the major vectors in most affected regions, but infection is contracted also in other ways: mechanically by the bite of various arthropods, directly through the conjunctiva and via abrasions of the skin, and by the consumption of infected meat or contaminated water.

Table IV.9   Animal diseases transmitted by Tabanidae which rarely or never affect man.

Agent	Disease	Principal hosts	Transmission	Distribution
Elaeophora schneideri	Arterial worm disease (sheep)	Sheep, deer, elk, moose (asymptomatic in deer)	Cyclical (*Tabanus* and *Hybomitra* spp.)	West and South-west USA; Italy
Dilofilaria roemeri	—	Wallaroo (*Macropus robustus*)	Cyclical (*Dasybasis hebes*)	Australia
Haemoproteus metchnikovi	—	Turtles	Cyclical (*Chrysops callidus*)	USA
Besnoitia besnoiti	Bovine besnoitiosis	Cattle (intermediate) Cat (definitive host)	Non-cyclic: mechanical (other mechanical vectors are *Glossina* and *Stomoxys*)	Africa, South America, Europe, former USSR, Asia
Anaplasma marginale	Anaplasmosis	Bovines	Non-cyclic: mechanical (esp. *Tabanus* spp.)	Cosmopolitan
Trypanosoma (*Trypanozoon*) *evansi*	Surra (Old World) Derrangadera, Murina (New World)	Bovines, equines, camels, dogs	Non-cyclic: mechanical	Cosmopolitan; tropics and subtropics
Trypanosoma (*Trypanozoon*) *equinum*	Mal de Caderas	Equines, bovines	Non-cyclic: mechanical	South America
Trypanosoma (*Duttonella*) *vivax*	Souma	Bovines, sheep, goats, equines, dogs	Non-cyclic: mechanical	Mauritius, Antilles and South America
Trypanosoma (*Megatrypanum*) *theileri*	—	Bovines, antelopes	Cyclical (?)	Cosmopolitan
Equine infectious anaemia (EIA) virus	Swamp fever	Equines, pheasants	Non-cyclic: mechanical	Cosmopolitan
Hog cholera virus (HCV)	—	Pigs	Non-cyclic: mechanical	North America
Rinderpest virus	—	Ungulates	Non-cyclic (Tabanids are unproved, but potential mechanical vectors)	Cosmopolitan

Tularaemia occurs also in Canada, the USA and Mexico, where it is mainly transmitted between rabbits, rodents, sheep, horses and man, by any of the routes above, including mechanical transmission by biting arthropods, notably ticks. However, in some areas, particularly the western USA, the disease occurs in summer outbreaks (with about 200 cases annually) in circumstances where rabbits are the most important reservoir of infection, and *Chrysops discalis* is certainly implicated as a mechanical vector of infection to man; the human disease is known locally as 'deer-fly fever'. *F. tularensis* bacteria have also been recovered from *C. fulvaster* and *C. aestuans*, but these species appear to play no part in the dissemination of tularaemia to man. (See also Chapter 47.)

Loaiasis

The principal human disease transmitted by tabanids is loaiasis, or Calabar swelling, caused by the filarial nematode *Loa loa*, and transmitted by species of *Chrysops*, notably by *C. silaceus* and *C. dimidiatus* (Bombe form), in which the worms undergo cyclical development. The disease is common and widespread in the rain-forest zones of West Africa, particularly Cameroon, and occurs sporadically across central Africa to the southern Sudan, Ethiopia and western Uganda. There are features of the epidemiology of loaiasis which resemble the sylvatic cycles of yellow fever transmission.

Adult *L. loa* worms inhabit subcutaneous connective tissues; diurnal periodic sheathed microfilariae are shed into the peripheral blood, particularly during the morning hours, and are ingested by day-biting *Chrysops*. When infected people are bitten by *Chrysops*, particularly by *C. silaceus* and *C. dimidiatus* (which may enter houses to feed), a proportion of the exsheathed microfilariae survive digestion in the insect gut, penetrate into the haemocoel, invade the abdominal and thoracic fat-bodies—where they grow, moult twice and develop into infective third stage forms; these migrate forward into the head. Here the infective stages accumulate until the fly next feeds, when they break out of the labium into the mouthparts and infect a new host via the skin. Development of *L. loa* in *Chrysops* generally takes 10–12 days from the original infecting feed.

There are two parallel and sympatric, but ecologically separate, cycles of *L. loa* transmission in the west African

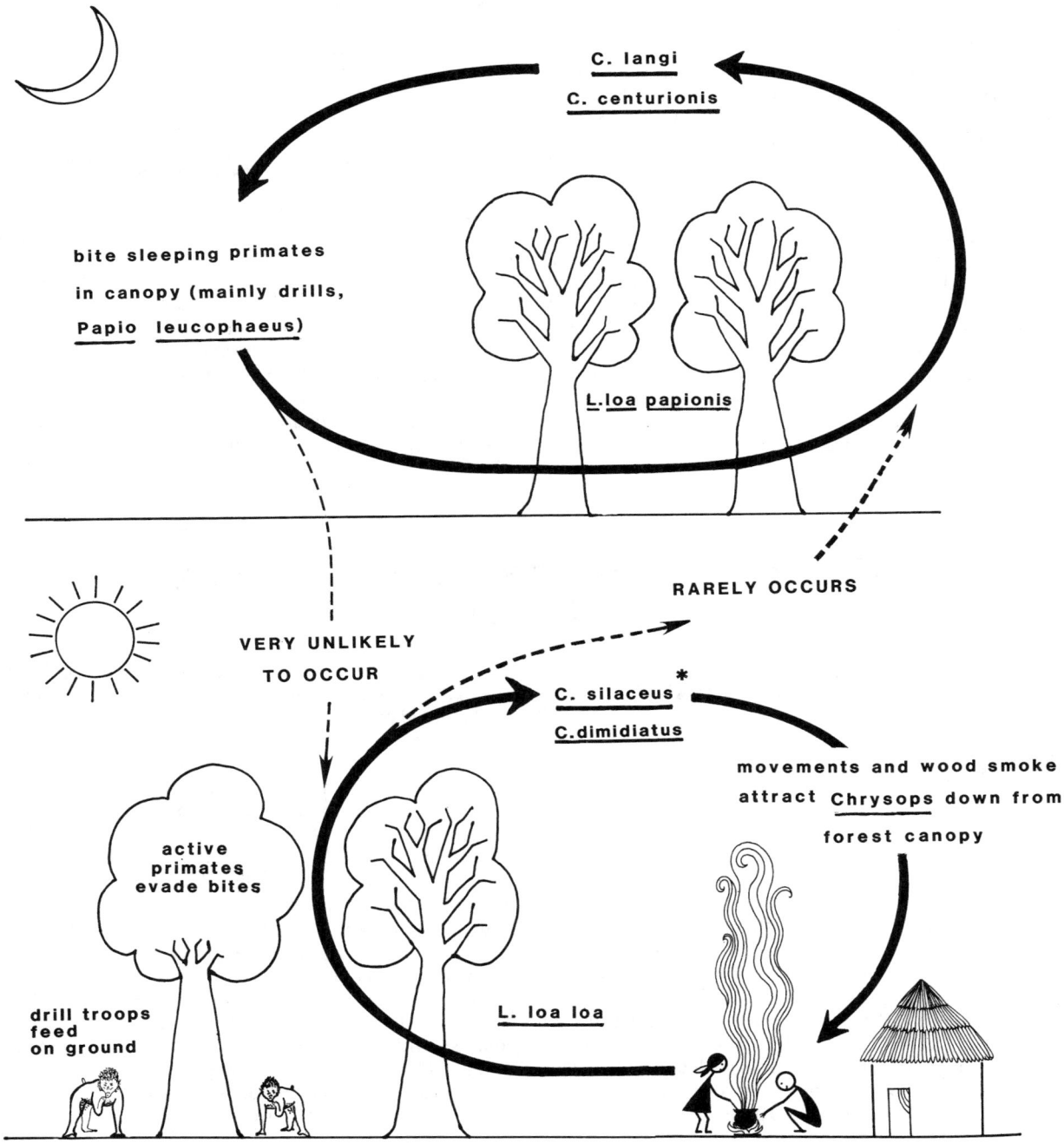

Figure IV.58   Diagram of transmission cycles in *Loa loa* to drills and to man in West African rain-forest.

rain-forests (Figure IV.58). One cycle is that of the slightly smaller human parasite, often given subspecific status as *L. loa loa*. This has a strictly diurnal microfilarial periodicity and day-biting *Chrysops* vectors (*C. silaceus* and *C. dimidiatus*, Bombe form). The other cycle involves the slightly larger simian parasite, *L. l. papionis*, which infects only monkeys. *L. l. papionis* is a nocturnally periodic filarial parasite of drills (forest baboons), *Papio* (=*Mandrillus*) *leucophaeus* (infection rates of 96% and mean adult worm burdens of 17 are recorded in drills). *L. l. papionis* will also naturally infect at

least two cercopithecine monkeys found in the same rain-forests, the putty-nosed guenon and the mona monkey, but the simian worm seems less well adapted to these two hosts. (Infection rates and mean adult worm burdens of 24%/6.3 and 12%/2.4, respectively.)

The vectors of the simian parasite (*L. l. papionis*) are two tree-top *Chrysops* species, both of which are active early in the night and feed on sleeping drills and other monkeys; these are *C. langi* and *C. centurionis*. The vectors of human *Loa* (*C. silaceus* and *C. dimidiatus*) will bite both at canopy level and on the forest floor, but only in daylight hours, when they are seldom able to evade the vigorous response of the monkeys (Figure IV.58).

The obviously closely related parasites of man and monkeys are behaviourally and ecologically distinct; additionally, they are reproductively isolated, although experimental hybrids can be produced. There is evidence which indicates that the simian *Loa* is not transmissible to man, although drills are susceptible to experimental infection with human *Loa*, and occasional natural infections of drills with this infection are known.

The day-biting vectors of human *Loa* are active in the forest canopy, but they are especially attracted to descend to ground level both by some unknown component of woodsmoke (e.g. from cooking-fires) and by human movements. Thus human activities in general, and the scent of wood-fires in particular, combine to draw these canopy-dwellers to ground level and especially into houses in the forest, in order that the females obtain a blood meal (Figure IV.58). These species will also emerge from the natural forest and enter teak or rubber plantations nearby, where there is also a high canopy.

There is at present no practicable method to reduce transmission of loaiasis by means of vector control.

OTHER VECTORS OF HUMAN LOAIASIS

In the grassland and forest mosaic of the highland zone in the west of Cameroon, *C. zahrai* is implicated as a natural vector of local importance.

Chrysops distinctipennis and *C. longicornis* are believed to be vectors of human loaiasis in southern Sudan, beyond the eastern limits of *C. silaceus* and *C. dimidiatus*. The widespread species *C. distinctipennis* may possibly be an occasional vector elsewhere in central Africa, since the range of all three main vectors shows considerable overlap. *C. streptobalius* is the probable vector of the infections reported from Ethiopia. (See also Chapter 70.)

TSETSE FLIES (*Glossina*) (See also Chapter 63)
D. M. Minter

FAMILY: GLOSSINIDAE

GENUS: *GLOSSINA* (WIEDEMANN 1830)

The unique viviparous genus *Glossina* contains some 30 species and subspecies of tsetse, confined to tropical Africa between latitudes 15°N and 30°S, where about $10.4 \times 10^6 \, \text{km}^2$ are infected, roughly half of the surface of the continent.

The tsetse flies are large, brown to greyish, narrow-bodied flies, 6–15 mm long, with a stout proboscis projecting forward well in front of the head (Figure IV.59). The proboscis is adjoined laterally, except during the act of biting, by the paired labial palps. The mouthparts consist of a horny labrum, a slender hypopharynx (through which an anticoagulant saliva is injected into the bite wound) and a stout ventral labium (Figure IV.59). These three parts enclose a space, the food canal, through which blood is sucked by muscular action into the alimentary canal of the fly. During feeding the mouthparts, but not the palps, are lowered some 90° from the line of the body axis. Male and female tsetse feed exclusively on the blood of vertebrates.

Characteristic features which distinguish *Glossina* species (Figure IV.60) from other large biting flies, such as *Stomoxys*, *Haematobia*, *Lyperosia*, *Haematopota*, *Tabanus* and *Chrysops*, include a long straight proboscis with a basal bulb, the presence of branched hairs on the arista (Figure IV.61) (the prominent bristle on the largest, distal, segment of the antenna) and the length of the labial palps (as long as the proboscis in *Glossina*). The manner in which the wings are folded, scissor-like, over the back of the resting fly is also a very characteristic feature. The presence of the 'hatchet' or 'cleaver' cell, enclosed between the fourth and fifth longitudinal wing veins, is diagnostic of *Glossina* (Figure IV.62). This cell is clearly seen in the central area of the wings and contrasts with the triangular shape of the corresponding cell of related flies (e.g. *Stomoxys* (Figure IV.63)).

The genus *Glossina* is usually divided by modern taxonomists into three species groups (Table IV.10) (sometimes given subgeneric status) as follows:

1 The *fusca* group (subgenus *Austenina*).
2 The *palpalis* group (subgenus *Nemorhina*).
3 The *morsitans* group (subgenus *Glossina*).

This taxonomic separation is reflected in the ecological requirements and distribution of the species included in each group: characteristically, flies of the *fusca* group are associated with dense humid tropical forest or forest edges; members of the *palpalis* group are basically dependent on more or less dense riverine or lacustrine vegetation but their distribution extends into savanna zones well away from forested, or formerly forested, areas. Species of the *morsitans* group are the least hygrophilic and occupy vast areas of bushland and thicket vegetation often far from lakes and rivers.

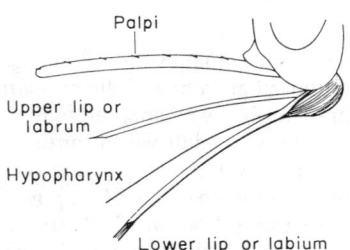

Figure IV.59 Mouth parts of *Glossina*.

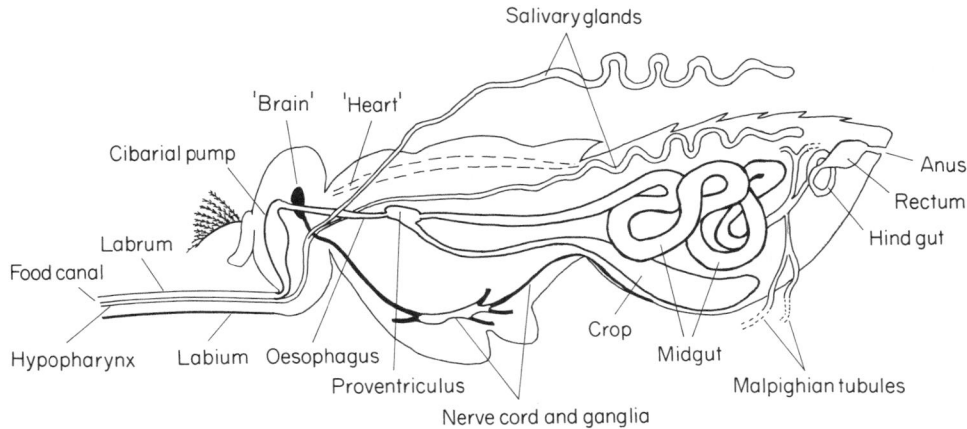

Figure IV.60 Schematic longitudinal section of *Glossina*, showing main features of the internal anatomy.

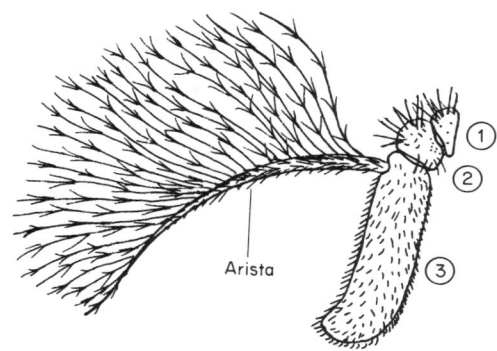

Figure IV.61 Antenna of *Glossina*, showing the dorsal arista with branched hairs, which arises from the third antennal segment. In other flies the hairs of the arista are unbranched.

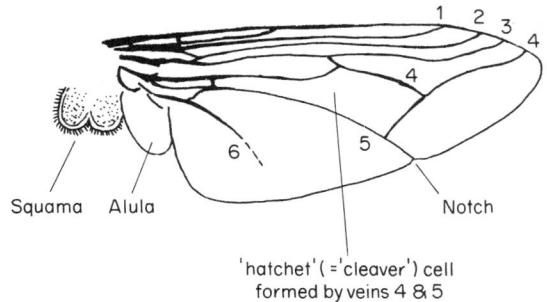

Figure IV.62 Wing of *Glossina*, showing venation and the 'hatchet' (= 'cleaver') cell enclosed between veins 4 and 5. The shape of the 'hatchet' cell is unique to *Glossina*; in all other flies the corresponding cell is triangular. *Glossina* is also unusual among higher flies in that the wings are held scissor-like over the back at rest.

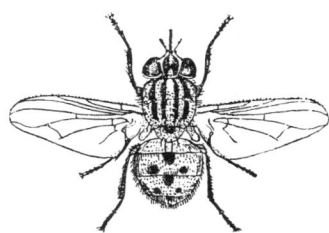

Figure IV.63 *Stomoxys calcitrans* (3×).

Strangely, however, one of the least hygrophilic species, occupying arid and semidesert area, is *G. longipennis*, a member of the *fusca* group. *G. brevipalpis*, also a *fusca* group species, has a distribution which also extends into dry savanna zones. Though flies of the *fusca* group include important vectors of trypanosomes pathogenic to livestock, especially species of the *Trypanosoma vivax* (subgenus *Duttonella*) and *T. congolense* groups (subgenus *Nannomonas*), they have never been associated with the transmission of trypanosomiasis to man and will not be considered further in this section. Figure IV.64 indicates the distribution of the groups of main medical importance and Figure IV.65 shows the general characteristics of some *Glossina* species. Mulligan[98] and Ford[99] summarize current views on the taxonomy and distribution of species and subspecies included in the *fusca*, *palpalis* and *morsitans* groups. Potts[100] gives a detailed key for the identification of all members of the genus and Pollock[101] gives simple regional keys.

LIFE HISTORY

Tsetse flies, in common with a very few other Diptera, have a method of viviparous reproduction uncommon among the higher insects, by which a single larva is produced at a time and is retained and nourished within the body of the female fly. Associated with the production of single offspring is a reduction in the number of ovarioles in the two ovaries to a single pair in each: four ovarioles in all, from which fertilized eggs pass into the uterus in regular rotation. Female flies are normally fertilized only once, shortly after emergence, and store sufficient viable sperm from this single mating to last

Table IV.10 Biotype, distribution and medical importance of Glossina.

Species group/subgenus	Habitat type	Distribution	Species of medical importance
fusca group (*Austenina*)	Mainly rain forest areas	Chiefly forest areas of West and Central Africa, Relict species in dry areas of East Africa	None. But several vectors of livestock trypanosomiasis
palpalis group (*Nemorhina*)	Mainly linear: shores of lakes and rivers in forested or formerly forested areas	15°N to 12°S, approx. 17°W to 15°E, approx.	*G. palpalis*, vector of *T. brucei gambiense* in West Africa
		10°N to 12°S, approx. 10°E to 40°E, approx.	*G. fuscipes* (and subspecies), vectors of *T. brucei gambiense* (West Africa, Central Africa) and *T. brucei rhodesiense* (East Africa)
		12°N to 4°N, approx. 12°W to 40°E, approx.	*G. tachinoides*, vector of *T. b. gambiense* in West Africa and of *T. b. rhodesiense* in South-west Ethiopia
morsitans group (*Glossina*)	'Game' tsetse of the savanna zones; open woodland ('miombo'), bushland and thicket	15°N to 20°S, approx. 17°W to 45°E, approx.	*G. morsitans* (and subspecies), vectors of *T. b. rhodesiense* in East and South-east Africa
		8°N to 20°S, approx. 25°E to 48°E approx.	*G. pallidipes*, vector of *T. b. rhodesiense* in East Africa
		Limited area south-east of Lake Victoria; mainly in Tanzania	*G. swynnertoni*, vector of *T. b. rhodesiense*

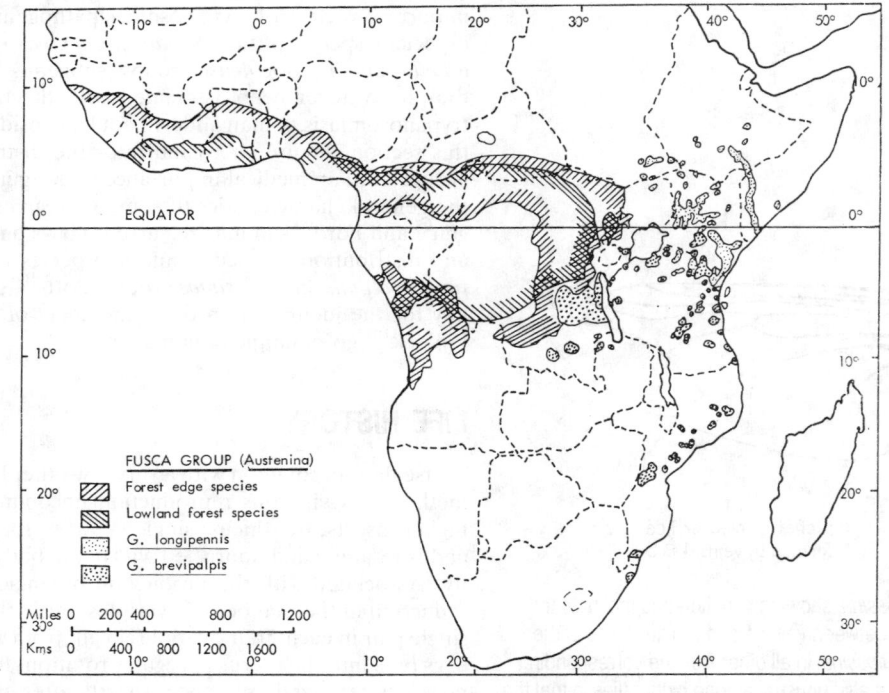

Figure IV.64 Distribution of the important species of *Glossina*. A, *fusca* group; B, *palpalis* group; C, *morsitans* group (see also Chapter 63).

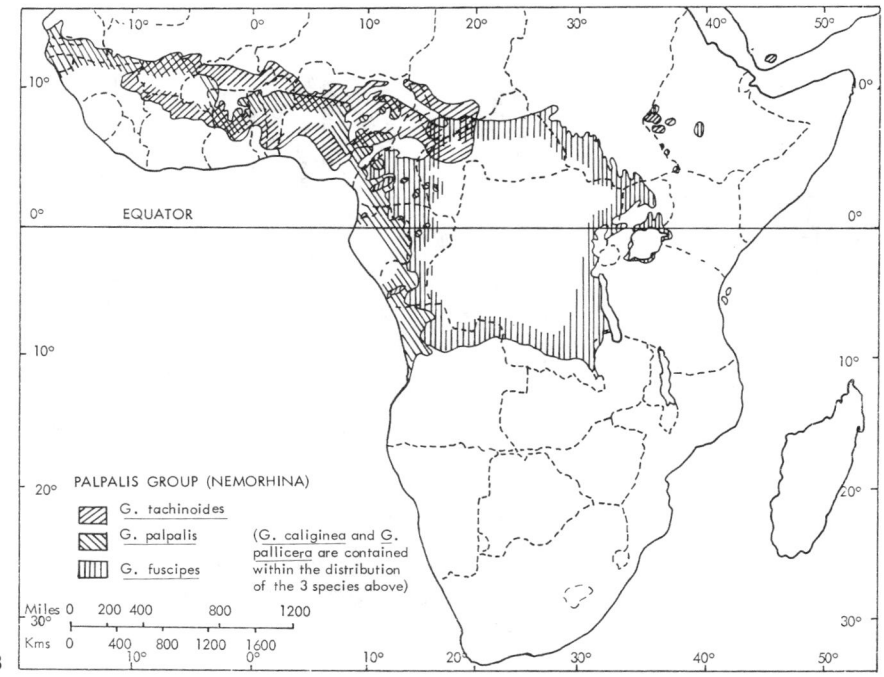

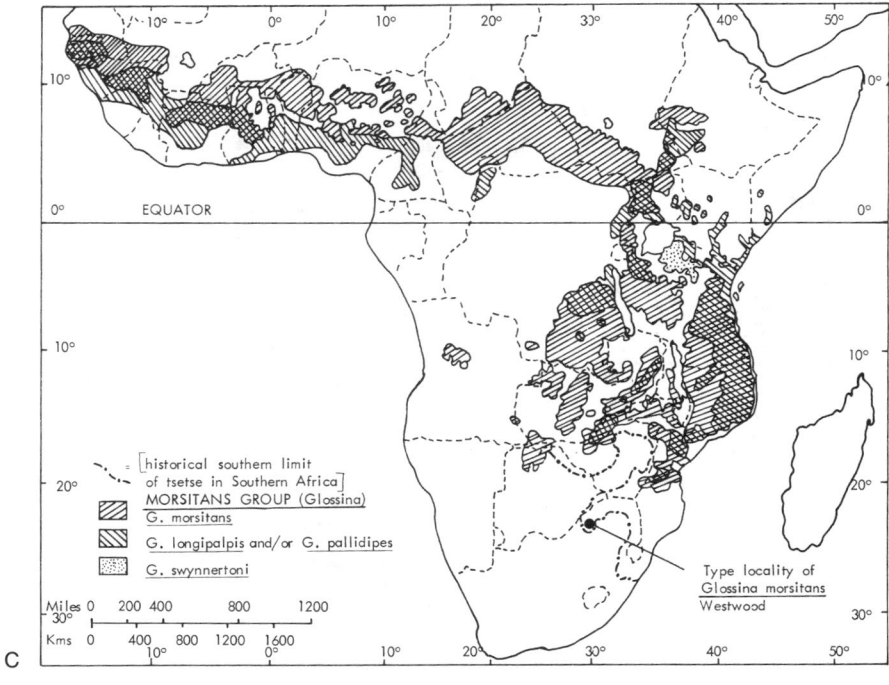

Figure IV.64 Continued

throughout life, during which, under favourable conditions, they may produce, at intervals of about 11 days, some 20 individual larvae.

Each successive fertilized egg (1.5 mm long) passes from the oviduct into the uterus where it hatches into a small, white, grub-like larva. The young larva obtains nutriment solely from the secretion of the uterine (or 'milk') glands of the mother, in which it is bathed. The larva grows, and twice moults, during the 8–12 days of intrauterine development. The mature larva, by now in the third instar, is finally extruded by the mother (by breech delivery) while she is perched on the ground, or on vegetation a few centimetres above it, in a site selected for its shady situation and suitable soil texture. The newly deposited larva, creamy white in

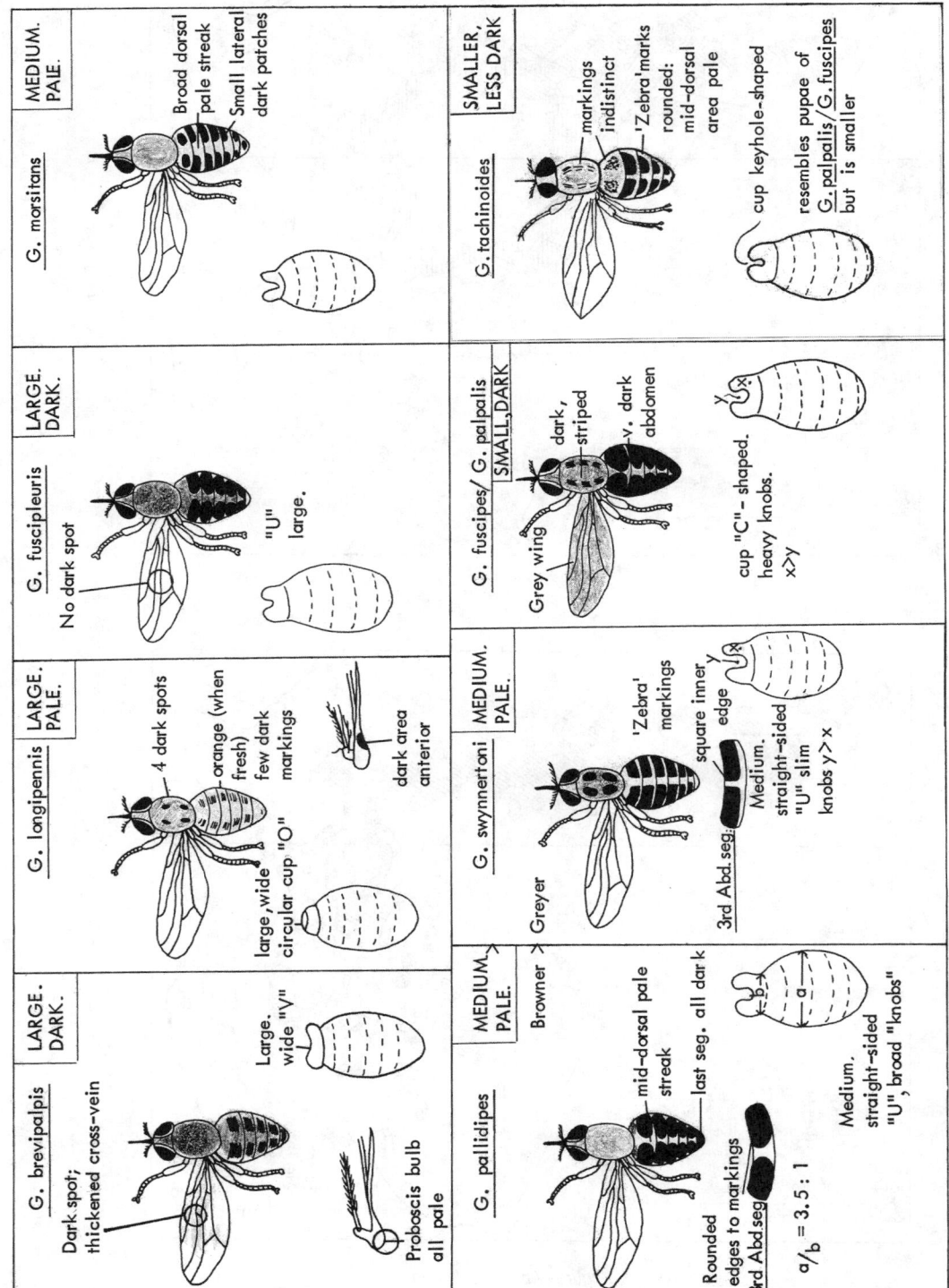

Figure IV.65 Outline guide to the identification of adults and pupae of some *Glossina* species, based on general characteristics visible to the naked eye or with the use of a simple hand-lens. The species illustrated are arranged in order of decreasing size, from top left to bottom right.

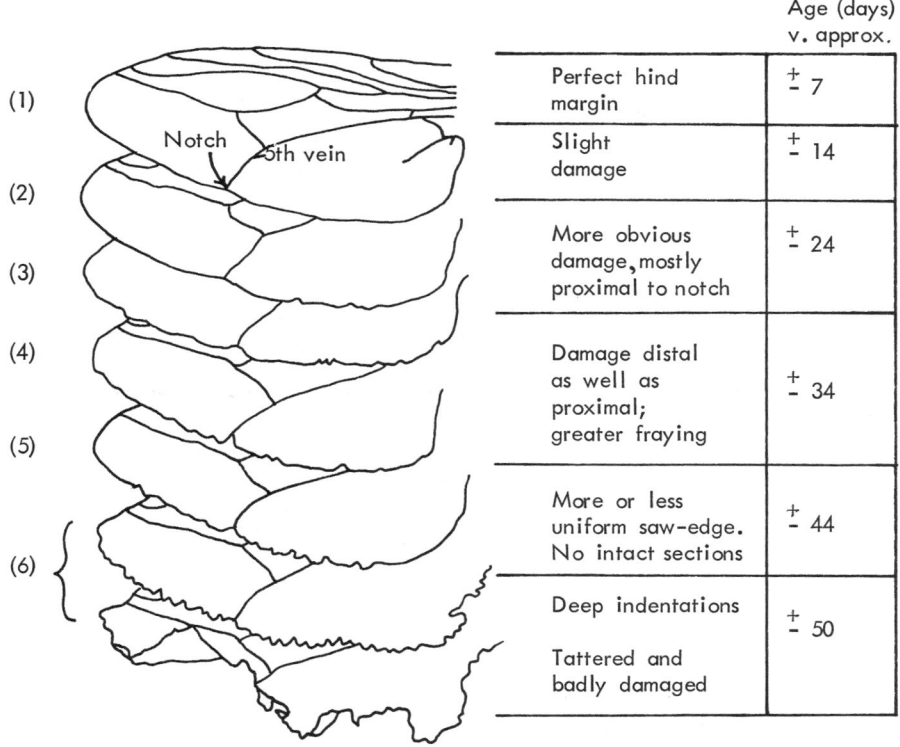

		Age (days) v. approx.
(1)	Perfect hind margin	$\pm$ 7
(2)	Slight damage	$\pm$ 14
(3)	More obvious damage, mostly proximal to notch	$\pm$ 24
(4)	Damage distal as well as proximal; greater fraying	$\pm$ 34
(5)	More or less uniform saw-edge. No intact sections	$\pm$ 44
(6)	Deep indentations Tattered and badly damaged	$\pm$ 50

Notes:
(1) Female wings wear less rapidly
(2) The method is properly applied to find <u>mean</u> age for a <u>group</u> of males
(3) In some species (most) the wings change colour with increasing age, from a smoky brown-grey to a tawny yellow-brown.

Figure IV.66 Age estimation of *Glossina* using a wing fray chart for male flies. Wings of females wear less rapidly, but the degree of female wing fray may be used (in flies of ovarian categories IV to VII in Figure IV.67) to estimate whether flies are in an early or late stage. (Based on Jackson[102] for *G. morsitans*.)

colour, with shiny black posterior polyneustic lobes through which it breathes, actively burrows below the surface soil to a depth of a few millimetres, using vigorous peristaltic movements. Having reached a point below the surface where conditions are suitable, it becomes immobile and begins to pupariate, still within the third larval skin, darkens and hardens. During emergence from the puparium, and in reaching the soil surface, the young fly is aided by an eversible bladder extruded from the front of the head and known as the *ptilinum*. During the first few days of life, this bladder can still be everted, while the body is still soft and 'soapy' in texture—if the young fly is carefully pressed between the fingers. Flies in this stage, so far unfed, are referred to as *teneral* flies: older flies as *non-teneral*, in which the head and body are hardened and horny and the ptilinum can no longer be everted. After the quiescent period, the young teneral flies seek their first blood meal. Flies of each sex normally feed at intervals of 3–4 days, sometimes less, and die of starvation if deprived of a blood meal for 10–12 days. The average life span of female *Glossina* is 2–3 months: exceptionally, up to 6–7 months. Male flies have a much shorter life span.

Male flies exhibit a progressive fraying of the trailing edge of the wings; this can be used to estimate the average age of *groups* of males from the same population. The wings of females also fray with age, usually less rapidly than those of males. With females, however, careful examination of the four ovarioles enables an estimation of the age of *individual* females to be made on a physiological basis. This method of 'ovarian ageing' is accurate to within a few days up to an age of about 40 days; with older flies there is a greater margin of possible error. For a fuller discussion of ageing methods, the reader is referred to Mulligan.[98] Figure IV.66 may be used to assess the degree of wing fray[102] and Figure IV.67 the age of individual females by examination of the ovarioles.[103,104] A new method to estimate age of *Glossina* (of both sexes) is suitable for laboratory automation, but requires sophisticated equipment. This method is based on the quantitative measurement of pteridine eye pigment deposition, which is correlated with age.

Female *G. fuscipes* in the field mate soon after emergence: female *G. pallidipes* are frequently fertilized near the host while seeking the first blood meal. Copulation may last from 2 to 24 hours and, at least in the laboratory, older males (about 14 days) are more potent than younger males.

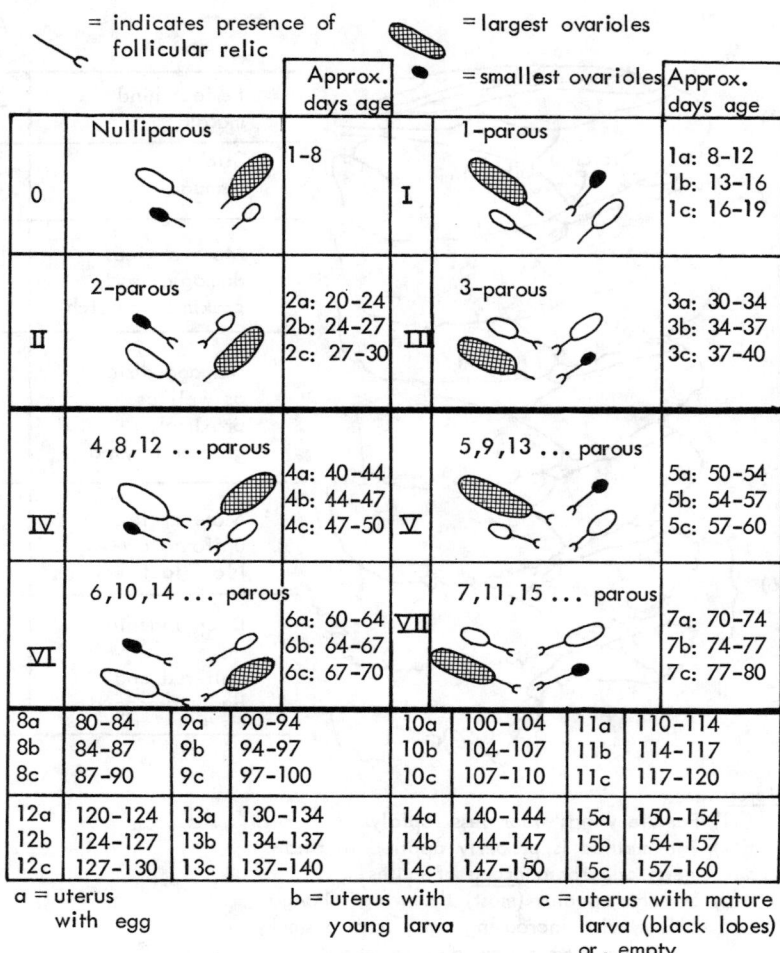

Figure IV.67 Ovarian age grading chart for female *Glossina* as seen in dorsal view. From cycles 0 to III an accurate estimation is possible; from cycles IV to VII (between the heavy lines in the figures) the estimate is subject to error since the same configuration is found in flies of different ages (e.g. 4, 8, 12 parous; 5, 9, 13 parous). The degree of wing fray (see Figure IV.66) is often a useful guide as to which possible physiological age is the most probable. (Modified from Saunders[103] and Challier[104].)

PALPALIS AND *MORSITANS* GROUPS: BIONOMICS AND ECOLOGY IN RELATION TO SLEEPING SICKNESS

Species of these two groups are active only during daylight hours: flight and feeding activities decrease markedly even during dull and overcast weather; few species show evidence of purposive behaviour after dusk. Tsetse flies hunt their prey partly by sight, although scent becomes increasingly important at close range; the flies are often aware of movements at a considerable distance and will fly to investigate any large moving object in their environment. Such objects can include cars, trains, canoes and lake steamers as well as animals and man.

When not actively seeking food, the flies normally rest on woody elements of vegetation. Horizontal or inclined branches, 2–5 cm thick and 1–3 mm from the ground, are favoured resting sites during the day for most species. Resting flies are most numerous where such perches provide a good field of view, as along the edge of thickets or the margins of lakes and streams. Flies in the course of digesting a meal and females seeking to deposit larvae are found in more sheltered places. By night, both sexes of those species so far investigated change from their daytime resting sites on the larger woody elements, to spend the hours of darkness on leaves and small twigs, the change-over takes place very rapidly, during the last few moments of twilight, and a reverse movement occurs at first light in the morning. The change of resting sites has, perhaps, the function of protecting the flies from the activities of nocturnal predators. Challier[105] gives a valuable review of the ecology of tsetse; salient aspects are also dealt with by Molyneux and Ashford.[106]

SLEEPING SICKNESS VECTORS

G. palpalis, G. fuscipes and *G. tachinoides*

Until the closing years of the 1950s it was generally considered, firstly, that flies of the *palpalis* group were limited to, and dependent upon, the woody vegetation along streams and lake shores, and that the flies could not maintain themselves elsewhere except during limited sorties at favourable times of the year. Secondly, flies of the *palpalis* group were considered to be solely responsible for the transmission of Gambian sleeping sickness; while flies of the *morsitans* group transmitted only the acute, Rhodesian, type of disease. These distinctions are no longer completely tenable, though they remain as useful generalizations that apply under most circumstances. However, not only have *G. fuscipes* and *G. tachinoides* been implicated in epidemic outbreaks of the Rhodesian type of disease (*G. fuscipes* in Kenya and Uganda; *G. tachinoides* in Ethiopia) but the same two species have been found (in Kenya and Nigeria) sometimes to live and breed in peridomestic environments far from water. It is now realized that neither species is quite so dependent upon particular vegetational associations as was formerly thought. Many instances of tsetse behaviour once labelled as atypical are now known to be quite commonplace: present-day views of the factors which influence tsetse ecology and behaviour, especially in relation to different types of vegetation, are now less rigid than was once the case.

Peridomestic pigs, sheep and dogs in West and Central Africa harbour *T. brucei* trypanosomes apparently identical to *T. b. gambiense* (on biochemical grounds, particularly isoenzymes) and appear to be significant reservoirs of the disease. Domestic pigs, moreover, are attractive to tsetse and can act as maintenance hosts for *palpalis* group flies. West African chickens are also reported naturally infected with *Trypanozoon* trypanosomes, but their importance (or otherwise) as reservoirs of man-infective organisms is unclear. In Burkina Faso (formerly Upper Volta) both hartebeest (*Alcelaphus* spp.) and kob, *Kobus* (*Adenota*) spp., harbour trypanosomes which are indistinguishable from *T. b. gambiense* by biochemical criteria. These game animals, and possibly other species, are now believed to be natural reservoirs of *T. b. gambiense* in West Africa. These recent observations, with both domestic livestock and game animals, call for a reassessment of the long-held view that there are no animal reservoirs of Gambian sleeping sickness; the evidence to the contrary is now incontrovertible and has obvious epidemiological implications.

In natural circumstances, where there is no close contact with man and domestic animals, flies of the *palpalis* groups show a preference for feeding on large reptiles, such as monitor lizards and crocodiles. Reptiles form more than half of the feeds of wild flies in these conditions; bushbuck (*Tragelaphus scriptus*) account for about a quarter and other animals the remainder. Where man and domestic animals are available, they too are attacked readily by species of the *palpalis* group. In circumstances where man, domestic animals and flies of the *palpalis* group come into close proximity (such as at river-crossings, water-holes, etc.) people and their livestock become a major source of food for the flies, and sharp outbreaks of sleeping sickness are likely to occur, especially in the dry seasons when man, cattle and small populations of flies are likely to depend upon the same limited water sources.

G. morsitans, *G. pallidipes* and *G. swynnertoni*—the 'game' tsetse

Unlike flies of the *palpalis* group which commonly occupy waterside habitats of an essentially linear type, often intersected by patterns of human activity that may lead to close and personal contact, species of the *morsitans* group occupy vast areas of xerophytic woodland, dry bushland and thicket vegetation, particularly in the eastern parts of Africa. Under these conditions contact between man, his livestock and the wild fly populations is seldom close and intense. Species of the *morsitans* group obtain most of their blood meals from the wild game animals, especially Bovidae and Suidae, that roam the savannas and 'miombo' woodlands, and amongst which trypanosomes of the *T. brucei* subgroup are circulated and maintained as a zoonosis. Some of the zoonotic strains are infective to man and give rise to symptoms, characteristically, of the acute, Rhodesian type of disease. Human infections are, however, comparatively rare because of the infrequent and mainly accidental contact between the *morsitans* group and man. The number of cases of Rhodesian sleeping sickness contracted in eastern Africa is very small in comparison with the number of mainly Gambian cases in West Africa and the Congo basin, where man is a principal reservoir of infection, but almost certainly not the only one.

Exposure to *T. rhodesiense* strains is largely occupational: hunters, honey-gatherers, pole-cutters and charcoal burners are among groups likely to enter fly-infested bush. In recent years the rapid growth of the tourist 'package' industry in East Africa has put another large group of itinerants at risk: the tourists themselves. Although species of the *morsitans* group are relatively little interested in man as a source of food if game animals are locally abundant, they often attack in sufficient numbers to be a considerable nuisance. Flies of the *morsitans* group are likely to acquire strains pathogenic to man from prior feeds on bushbuck (the main proved reservoir) or other ungulates. In this latter catgegory must be included domestic cattle; stocks of parasites which caused acute human disease in volunteers were first isolated during a localized outbreak in Kenya (Alego) some years ago. More recently, cattle isolates in Uganda (Busoga) were found to be indistinguishable from man-infective *T. b. rhodesiense* circulating in the human population during an epidemic outbreak, by isoenzymes and other intrinsic criteria. Cattle obviously act as a temporary reservoir, at any rate, under circumstances of human epidemic disease when challenge from animal trypanosomes is sufficiently low to permit survival of the animals. Movement of cattle under these circumstances might also result in the dissemination of man-infective trypanosomes to new foci. Cattle can seldom be kept long in the presence of heavy or moderate fly infestations, however, owing to the damaging incidence of infections with *T. vivax* and *T. congolense*.

NATURAL INFECTION RATES AND METHODS OF FLY DISSECTION

Infective metacyclic trypanosomes of the *T. brucei* subgroup (subgenus *Trypanozoon*) are found in the salivary glands of the tsetse fly. To reach their final station in the glands they undergo a complex migration in the fly that takes nearly 3 weeks to complete; hence it follows that only flies more than 3 weeks old can be infected with trypanosomes infective to man. Even among older flies, infection rates with the *T. brucei* subgroup are always low (commonly 0.1% or less: rarely more than 1%), especially when compared with infection rates with the *T. vivax* (=*Duttonella*) and *T. congolense* (=*Nannomonas*) groups in the same flies. The *T. vivax* group have a short and simple life cycle in the fly: infection rates

Table IV.11   Location of trypanosomes in tsetse flies.

Trypanosome species or group (subgenus)	Approx. time of development in Glossina	Usual range of infection rates in fly	Organs infected		
			Mouth parts	Salivary glands	Gut
T. vivax (*Duttonella*)	4–5 days	75–85%	+	–	–
T. congolense (*Nannomonas*)	8–10 days	18–25%	+	–	+
T. brucei subgroup* (*Trypanozoon*)	15–30 days	0.1–1.5%	+	+	+

*Includes the following parasites:
   T. brucei brucei—not infective to man.
   T. brucei gambiense—cause of Gambian sleeping sickness in man (chronic).
   T. brucei rhodesiense—cause of Rhodesian sleeping sickness in man (acute).

may reach 75% or more. The *T. congolense* group have a longer and slightly more complex cycle in the fly: infection rates may reach 18–25%.

The full dissection of a tsetse involves the removal and microscopic examination of the elongate salivary glands, the midgut and the mouthparts. There are several possible methods of dissection, but given some practice there is probably little to choose between them. The method preferred by the writer is as follows.

1 The fly is killed (with ether, chloroform or by judicious finger pressure against the sides of the thorax), wings and legs may be removed at this stage, or left.
2 The fly is placed on a slide in a *small* amount of physiological saline (or 5% glucose solution).
3 The tough, membranous connection between head and thorax is 'frayed' carefully with the point of a needle to weaken it.
4 The proboscis is held (under a needle or with forceps) by the basal bulb and drawn slowly away from the head. With practice, the proboscis comes away from the head still attached to the salivary glands; continued slow, careful traction enables these to be pulled gradually clear of the body. If the glands break at this stage they can be recovered later.
5 The labrum, hypopharynx and labium are preferably separated with needles and examined in saline under a coverslip. Or the intact semitransparent proboscis can be examined without separating the parts.
6 If removed with the mouthparts, the salivary glands are separated from the former and mounted in a small drop of saline under a coverslip.
7 If the salivary glands were broken during stage 4, the fly is now turned so that its abdomen lies flat on the slide, dorsal side uppermost. The thorax is pulled off and discarded and needles are inserted through the two anterolateral corners of the abdomen, at a point roughly halfway from the

corners towards the long axis of the abdomen, with sufficient pressure to pierce well below the dorsal integument. Firm traction in the direction of the forward corners of the abdomen, to tear them open, will usually result in the recovery of the glands at this state: they may be recognized by their glass-like, refractile appearance. Continued needle traction will normally pull the glands clear of the abdomen, for examination in a separate drop of fresh saline under a coverslip.
8 With a needle or scalpel the sides of the posterior tip of the abdomen are cut and the gut is extracted; the covering of fat-body is stripped off with a needle and the gut is placed in a drop of saline, teased open and examined under a coverslip for the presence of trypanosomes.

Trypanosome infections of tsetse are identified, in the organs dissected, by reference to their location and morphology. Infections of the mouthparts only are likely to be by the *T. vivax* group; infections in the mouthparts and gut only are likely to be *T. congolense* or a mixed infection of *T. vivax* and *T. congolense* groups. Infections involving the salivary glands, gut and mouthparts certainly include the *T. brucei* subgroup but may also be complicated by the presence of *T. vivax*, *T. congolense*, or both. Gut and mouthparts infections could also include immature infections with *T. brucei* subgroup (Table IV.11).

CONTROL OF TSETSE FLIES

The subject of tsetse control is large and complex, beyond the scope of this section. The interested reader is referred to Molyneux[107] for a useful discussion of tsetse control in relation to prevention and control of sleeping sickness generally, to Allsopp[108] for an account of insecticidal control methods, to Jordan[109] for a review of noninsecticidal methods of tsetse control, and also to Jordan.[110]

CIMICID AND TRIATOMINE BUGS (See also Chapter 64)
D. M. Minter

ORDER: HEMIPTERA
SUBORDER: HETEROPTERA
FAMILY: CIMICIDAE

GENUS: *CIMEX*

Bed bugs (Cimicidae) have a worldwide distribution with well over 70 species; all are wingless and dorsoventrally flattened. The species parasitic on man are: *Cimex lectularius* (Figure IV.68), the cosmopolitan bed bug, and *C. hemipterus* (=*rotundatus*), the common bed bug of the tropics, which is distinguished by its elongated narrow abdomen and the shape and proportion of the thorax (Figure IV.68). In West Africa a species of another genus, *Leptocimex boueti*, attacks man. The body of *C. lectularius* is broad and flat, the head short and broad, attached to the thorax, the antennae four-jointed and the eyes present but reduced in size. The mouth-parts consist externally of a segmented rostrum (proboscis) and are normally folded back under the head. The maxillae are serrated at the tip. On the thorax of the adults are short padlike hemielytra, which are vestigial forewings. Both sexes of *Cimex* feed only on blood and can resist starvation well.

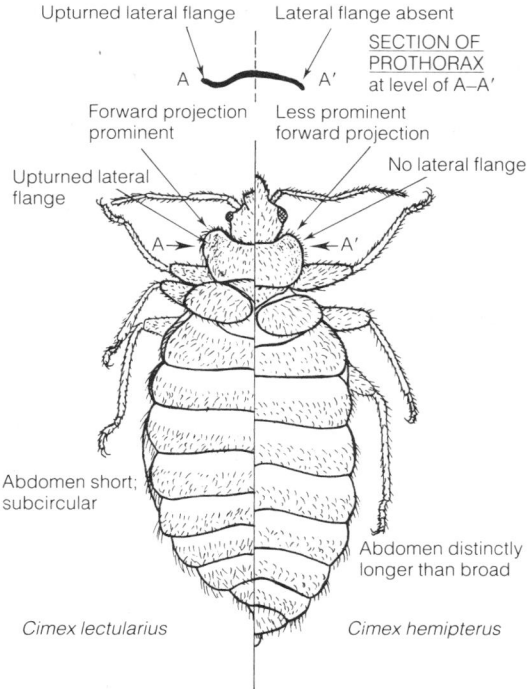

Figure IV.68 Comparison between *Cimex lectularius* (the common bed bug) (left) and *C. hemipterus* (the tropical bed bug) (right) when viewed from above.

The labium does not pierce the skin, but buckles up during feeding like that of a mosquito. The bodies of bugs give out a nasty pungent odour. Bed bugs are nocturnal in their feeding habits, hiding in crevices during the daytime. The eggs are ovoid and operculated and are cemented on to the surfaces of the crevices of woodwork in houses, beds, mattresses, behind pictures and in nail holes. Aggregations of bugs can be located by finding the black faeces round holes.

The females deposit eggs in daily batches from 10 to 50, totalling 200–500. They are large, about 1 mm in diameter, yellowish-white and easily visible to the naked eye. The five successive nymphal stages resemble adults, but have no hemielytra; they mature in about 6 weeks if fed at each stage, but can resist starvation for up to 2 months. Under less favourable conditions, development may be protracted for 6 months or more. Adults may live for many months. Bed bugs are sensitive to high temperatures: even 37.8°C with a fairly high humidity will kill many. A cheap and effective control method is fumigation with sulphur. The dosage necessary varies from 0.34 to 0.74 kg/28 m^3, with an exposure time of at least 6 hours. Sulphur dioxide is cheap and, owing to its smell, free from hazard(s). It kills the active stage of the bug, but a few eggs may escape, and complete combustion must be assured.

Hydrocyanic acid fumigation is very effective, but danger-ous, and has been largely superseded by the use of insecti-cides: 5% DDT emulsion, 2% malathion, 0.5% diazinon or 0.5% dichlorvos or 0.1–0.2% pyrethroids which act as an irritant and cause bugs to leave their hiding places.

Though bed bugs can cause a great deal of irritation by their bites, it has not actually been proved that they dissemi-nate disease, with the possible exception of viral hepatitis (see Chapter 31).

FAMILY: REDUVIIDAE
SUBFAMILY: TRIATOMINAE

Triatomine bugs are also known as 'cone-nose', 'kissing' or, erroneously, 'assassin' bugs; they have many local names in America, including chinchas (Mexico), chipo (Venezuela), barbeiro (Brazil) and vinchucha (Argentina). The group includes more than 100 species, divided into five tribes and 14 genera (Table IV.12). Both sexes and the five nymphal stages feed solely on vertebrate blood. The triatomine bugs are one of more than 20 subfamilies of the family Reduviidae; all the other subfamilies are predators of other insects and are the true 'assassin' bugs. Many species of the predatory Reduvii-dae are, however, capable of inflicting a painful bite, usually in self-defence, but they do not feed on blood. Many superfi-cially resemble the haematophagous Triatominae but can be distinguished by the presence of a rostrum that is frequently curved and is always rigid and inflexible. The triatomines have a three-segmented rostrum that is always both straight and flexible; at rest it lies closely applied to the ventral aspect

Table IV.12 Haematophagous Reduviidae: tribes and genera of the subfamily Triatominae (Jeannel, 1919), with numbers of the 114 species in each genus: the most important genera are shown in bold.

Tribe	Genus	Number of species	Tribe	Genus	Number of species
Alberproseniini	*Alberprosenia*	1	Rhodniini	*Psammolestes*	3
				Rhodnius	**12**
Bolboderini	*Belminus*	4			
	Bolbodera	1	Triatomini	*Dipetalogaster*	1
	Parabelminus	2		*Eratyrus*	2
	Microtriatoma	2		*Linshcosteus*	5
				Panstrongylus	**13**
Cavernicolini	*Cavernicola*	1		*Paratriatoma*	1
				Triatoma	**66**

of the head and more or less parallel to it. Its extreme tip normally lies in a finely ridged stridulatory groove in the anteroventral part of the thorax. (The triatomine genera *Linshcosteus*, and *Cavernicola* are unusual in that they lack this sound-producing stridulatory mechanism, in which the tip of the rostrum acts as a plectrum.)

The outer and visible part of the rostrum is the modified labium, which forms a protective sheath for the paired stylet-like mandibles and maxillae. During the act of feeding the rostrum is swung forward (about 120°) in front of the head and is neither flexed nor telescoped; the tip of the labium rests on the surface of the skin and the apically serrate mandibles penetrate the epidermis and anchor the mouthparts in place. The smooth lanceolate maxillary stylets then penetrate deeply and perforate small blood capillaries. The maxillae enclose the salivary duct and the food canal and form the functional mouth. The bite of triatomines is generally painless but by no means always. This explains why sleeping people are seldom wakened by the bite of bugs and can be bitten repeatedly in the course of the night.

In common with other Heteroptera, the adult triatomines have two pairs of functional wings; the forewings are hardened basally (the corium and clavus) and membranous distally. Thus they are referred to as hemielytra. The posterior wings are membranous throughout and lie beneath the hemielytra at rest. The wings are folded scissor-like over the back of the bug and the lateral margins of the abdominal tergites are visible; these are often colour banded and are a useful taxonomic feature. Female bugs, viewed from above have a broad ovate abdomen which is generally pointed posteriorly; males have a more slender abdomen with a fully rounded posterior end. The plate-like male external genitalia can easily be seen in lateral and ventral view. Female bugs are generally rather larger than males.

The visible dorsal part of the thorax consists of a large trapezoidal pronotum, usually rigid and provided with tubercles. Behind the pronotum and visible between the sclerotized bases of the hemielytra, is a triangular scutellum— strongly pointed posteriorly. The ground colour of the triatomines is usually brownish or black, often relieved with flashes of colour (mainly shades of red, yellow or orange) on thorax and abdomen. Eyes are usually black, but white- or pink-eyed mutants are not uncommon. Adults, unlike all nymphal stages, have paired dorsal ocelli posterior to the prominent compound eyes.

The proportions of the head in lateral view are useful to

separate the three genera of main medical importance (Figure IV.69). The head of *Rhodnius* is elongated with long four-jointed antennae arising close to its apical portion. In *Triatoma* the head is shorter and the antennae are inserted midway between the eye and the forward tip of the head. In the genus *Panstrongylus* the head is stouter and shorter, with the antennae arising close to the eye. See also Figures IV.70–72.

The five nymphal stages are essentially miniatures of the adult but lack wings; in the fifth nymphal stage the 'wing pads' are prominent on either side of the scutellum. Triatomines are generally quite large insects, usually between 20 and 28 mm long in the adult female. Some genera contain species that are only about 5 mm long as adults and the Mexican *Dipetalogaster maxima* is the giant of the triatomines, attaining a length of nearly 4.5 cm. Lent and Wygodzinsky[18] give comprehensive keys to genera and species.

REPRODUCTION AND LIFE CYCLE

Female triatomines commence egg laying 10–30 days after copulation; eggs are laid singly or in small groups, either unattached or cemented to the substrate, depending on species. The ovoid, operculate fresh eggs are whitish; in some species they later turn through pink to cherry-red; in other species the original colour is maintained. The number of eggs laid in life by a female depends upon species and external factors but about 500 is normal and 1000 not uncommon. Virgin females will also lay eggs but these are few in number and infertile. Eggs hatch after 10–30 days; the emerging first stage nymph is at first pink and soft-bodied but hardens sufficiently to take its first blood meal within 48–72 hours of leaving the egg. At least one full blood meal is required by each nymphal stage, sometimes more, before the moult to the next stage can be initiated.

All triatomines have a long life cycle, even in hot climates; the average is about 300 days from egg to adult, though some species may take up to 2 years. *Rhodnius* spp. develop more rapidly than *Triatoma* and *Panstrongylus* and can reach maturity in 3–4 months.

GEOGRAPHICAL DISTRIBUTION

The five tribes occur in tropical and subtropical areas of the neotropical region. Members of one tribe, the Triatomini,

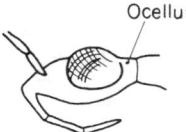

Ocellus

Insect-predatory reduviid
Proboscis curved (mainly)
and rigid

Haematophagous members (Triatominae):
Proboscis straight and flexible

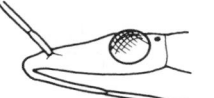

Rhodnius

Head long
Antennae forward
Examples: R. prolixus,
R. pallescens

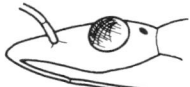

Triatoma

Head medium length
Antennae median
Examples: T. infestans,
T. dimidiata

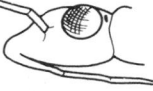

Panstrongylus

Head short
Antennae close to eye
Example: P. megistus

Figure IV.69 Lateral view of the head of an insect-predatory reduviid (top) with usually *curved* and always *inflexible* proboscis which serves to distinguish it from the haematophagous genera of the subfamily Triatominae, all of which have a proboscis which is *straight* and *flexible* (bottom row). The proportions of the head and the site of insertion of the antennae serve to separate members of the triatomine genera *Rhodnius*, *Triatoma* and *Panstrongylus*.

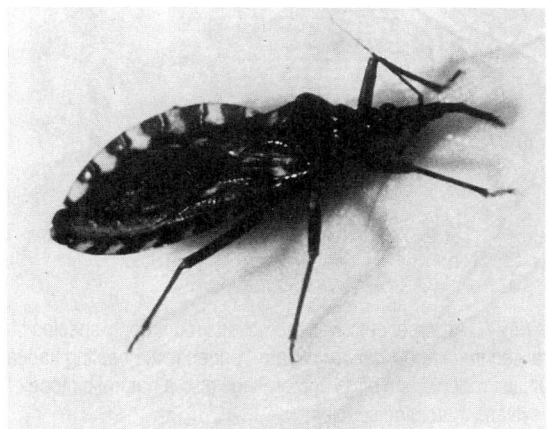

Figure IV.70 Genus *Triatoma*. Head of intermediate length, with antennae set midway between eyes and front of head. The specimen illustrated is a female *Triatoma infestans,* with its proboscis directed forwards whilst feeding. The ground colour is black with yellowish markings on the lateral edge of the abdomen, legs and hemielytra. Males are 21–26 mm long; females 26–29 mm. Nymphal stages lack the coloration seen in the adult. (Courtesy of T. V. Barrett.)

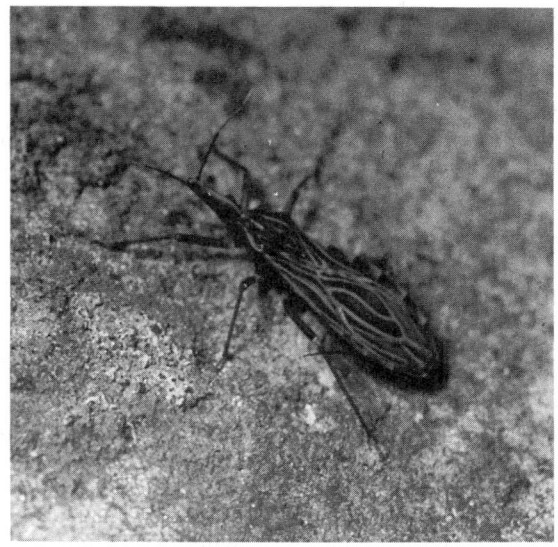

Figure IV.71 Genus *Rhodnius*. Head long, antennae set well forward. The specimen shown is an adult male *Rhodnius prolixus*; males are generally less then 20 mm in length, females up to 21.5 mm. General colour pale brown; lighter markings on thorax and forewings give the overall impression of longitudinal stripes. Nymphal stages have less obvious 'pepper and salt' markings. (Courtesy of C. J. Webb.)

have species which are also found in the oriental region. The Triatomini also marginally enter the Australasian region. The subfamily is entirely absent from the Palaearctic and Afrotropical (=Ethiopian) regions but *T. rubrofasciata* has been spread to all the major tropical ports by human agency. This species is always closely associated with *Rattus* spp., among which it transmits the rat trypanosome *Trypanosoma* (*Megatrypanum*) *conorhini*. Other endemic, and purely sylvatic, species of the tribe Triatomini (members of the *T. rubrofasciata* group) occur in south China, Malaysia, Indonesia, Papua New Guinea and the extreme north-east of Aus-

tralia. The other group of Oriental Triatomini is the genus *Linshcosteus* (six closely related species) which occurs only in India.

The bulk of the Triatominae (four of the five tribes) occur exclusively in the neotropical region: the Rhodniini (the important genus *Rhodnius* and the genus *Psammolestes*) are found from Central America to Argentina; the neotropical species of Triatomini, principally the members of the genus

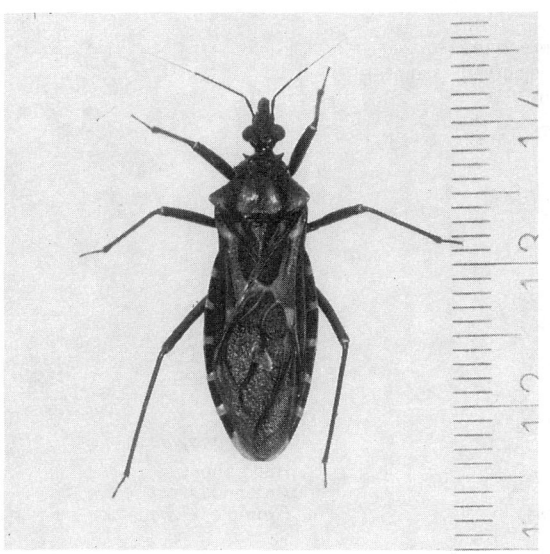

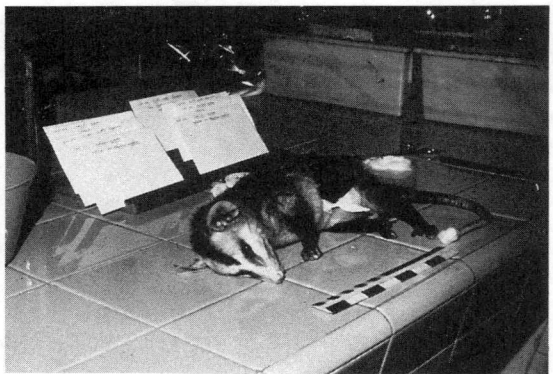

Figure IV.73   The common opossum, *Didelphis* sp., the cat-sized sylvatic marsupial most frequently naturally infected with *Trypanosoma cruzi* throughout the Americas. The animal shown is *D. albiventris* (= *D. azarae*) from Brazil and is anaesthetized whilst undergoing xenodiagnosis and collection of tail blood for microscopic and serological investigation.

Figure IV.72   Genus *Panstrongylus*. Head short, with antennae set close to the eye. The male *Panstrongylus megistus* illustrated is black in overall colour with red, or reddish-brown, markings on the lateral margins of the abdomen, the thoracic pronotum, and scutellum and the hemielytra (forewings). The nymphal stages lack the prominent coloration of the adults. The specimen shown measures 25 mm; females are slightly larger.

Triatoma, range from the northern USA to Patagonia. The genus *Panstrongylus*, the second largest in the Triatomini, with 13 species, extends from Central America to Argentina.

HABITAT OF NEOTROPICAL TRIATOMINES

All triatomines are dependent on the blood of vertebrates (principally mammals and birds, occasionally reptiles) for survival, development and reproduction. The primary habitat of triatomines is thus in or near the shelters, roosts, burrows and nests of a variety of wild animals, prominent amongst which are marsupials (e.g. *Didelphis* (Figure IV.73), *Marmosa*), edentates (e.g. *Dasypus*), rodents (*Rattus*, *Neotoma*), carnivores, bats and birds. Many of the animals and birds find their main shelter in palm fronds or in arboreal epiphytic bromeliads (Figure IV.74), under fallen logs or in hollow trees. Triatomines also occur under rocks, under loose bark and in stone walls and feed on the local rodents or lizards.

A number of triatomine species have the ability to colonize the artificial habitats created by man. Some species seldom penetrate further than the peri-domestic area: stables, cattle enclosures, chicken houses, pig sties, etc., which provide a rich food source. A relatively few species are able to colonize the extensive crevice habitat which is provided by the simple homes of the Latin American peasant majority. These houses are usually constructed of mud and wattle or unplastered adobe brick and roofed with palm fronds (Figure IV.75). More sophisticated houses with smooth plastered walls and roofs of tile or corrugated sheet are less readily and heavily colonized, often being very lightly infested or not at all. The more traditional and basic peasant house, made of local

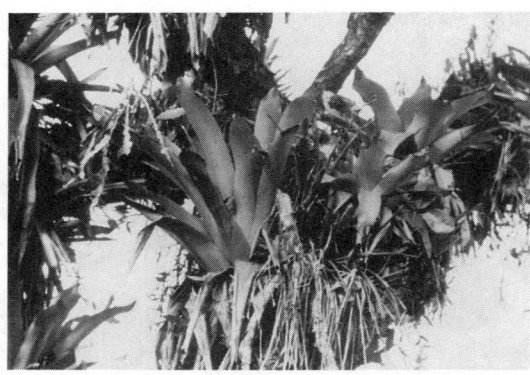

Figure IV.74   Arboreal epiphytic bromeliads (commonly species of the genera *Aechmea* and *Holmbergia*) are frequently the nesting habitat of marsupials, rodents and birds and are thus also a natural biotope of many sylvatic triatomine species.

materials, may support a triatomine population that can run into thousands, particularly of *Rhodnius prolixus* or *Triatoma infestans*.

Although probably all triatomines will support the development of *Trypanosoma cruzi* (well over half the species have been found infected in the wild), it is only relatively few species that have the capacity to colonize human dwellings which are of overriding medical importance as the domiciliary vectors of Chagas' disease to man. By virtue of their wide geographical distribution and large domiciliary populations, together with the large human population in the areas they occupy, the three species *Rhodnius: prolixus*, *Triatoma infestans* and *Panstrongylus megistus* are of prime importance. Other species of the same three genera (particularly *Triatoma* spp. and especially *T. dimidiata*) are of considerable importance on a lesser geographical scale (e.g. *T. dimidiata*, *T. barberi*, *T. brasiliensis*, *T. pallidipennis*, *T. phyllosoma*, *R. pallescens* and *R. ecuadorensis*).

It is possible to divide the triatomines into convenient

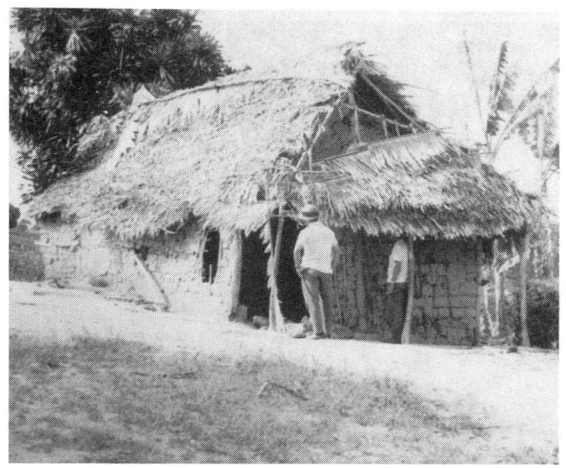

Figure IV.75 A characteristic palm-thatched, mud-and-wattle Latin American peasant house of the type often infested with domiciliary triatomine species. The deep cracks in the mud walls provide ideal harbourage for large populations of *Rhodnius*, *Triatoma* or *Panstrongylus*.

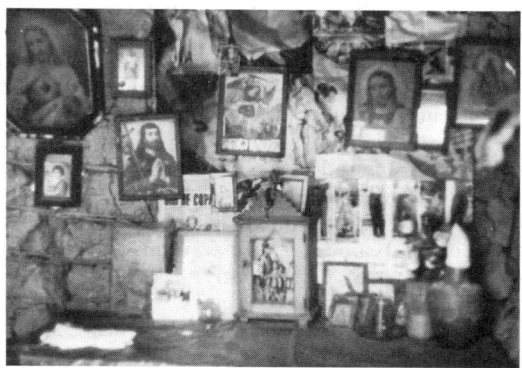

Figure IV.76 Many peasant homes incorporate a domestic shrine such as that shown here; a central case houses the family saints and the walls nearby are covered with pictures, both sacred and profane. Sites such as these are often the principal hiding places for bugs not located in the bedroom walls and furniture.

groups based on their association, or lack of it, with human dwellings.

Most species are fully sylvatic, a few species as flying adults are attracted by light and enter houses (when they may occasionally bite) but seem unable to colonize: an example is the geographically widespread *Panstrongylus geniculatus*, normally closely associated with the burrows of its usual host, the armadillo (*Dasypus* spp.). Others, such as *T. brasiliensis*, are attracted by lights into houses and may establish small domiciliary or peridomestic populations. Species such as the Central American *T. dimidiata* live normally in hollow trees but are often passively transported to houses (in firewood) and form large colonies. *T. sordida* is found naturally in a variety of habitats in the central and southern parts of South America, including crevices among tree bark; it readily adapts to fence-posts and timber outbuildings but never forms large domiciliary populations. This may be because it is regularly found in houses together with heavy infestations of *T. infestans*; in Venezuela and elsewhere in northern South America, *T. maculata* is in a somewhat similar situation when small populations are established in houses among heavy infestations of *R. prolixus*. Both *T. sordida* and *T. maculata* may have the potential to form epidemiologically significant domiciliary populations if and when the major domiciliary species are controlled or eradicated by insecticidal treatment. Much the same happened in southern Brazil when *T. infestans* was controlled by insecticides and within a few years large numbers of *Panstrongylus megistus* (until then a purely sylvatic species in that area) had replaced it as the domiciliary vector of *Trypanosoma cruzi*.

Within human habitations, triatomines prefer to hide during the day in dark and moist places; the extensive crevice habitat provided by unplastered cracked walls of mud or mud-brick can support large populations. Smaller numbers are found among furniture, boxes and, particularly, beds and bedding. Others occur among clothes hanging from pegs in the walls, or behind pictures (Figure IV.76). Some species also readily colonize palm roofs (e.g. *R. prolixus*). Other species are rarely found in the roof (e.g. *P. megistus*).

Most frequently, bugs are found by day close to the areas in which they will encounter sleeping hosts at night—bedrooms are normally the most heavily infested parts of the house. As a rule, feeding behaviour of domiciliary triatomines is governed more by proximity to a suitable host than by specific host preference.

Some entirely or essentially sylvatic species, however, are normally associated with particular hosts: *Cavernicola pilosa* is always associated with bats and all three species of *Psammolestes*, *T. platensis* and *T. delpontei* are found only in the nests of birds. *P. geniculatus* has a close link with burrows of armadillos: *Paratriatoma hirsuta* and species of the *T. protracta* group prey exclusively on *Neotoma* spp., the wood rat (although adults not infrequently fly into houses, attracted by lights, they never colonize; perhaps this is in some way connected with their dependence on wood rats).

All stages of triatomines, in particular the larger nymphal stages, have a remarkable ability to endure long periods of starvation (up to several months). The adults are in general poor fliers and probably take flight only when their nutritional status is poor and their weight lowest, to disperse at random to seek new habitats with new hosts on which to feed. For domiciliary species in particular, passive transport by human agency is probably responsible for nearly all house-to-house dispersal, on or in domestic goods including furniture and clothes. Triatomines of various species have been recovered from the baggage of passengers on long-distance buses and lorries and occasionally even in aircraft. Some species of *Rhodnius* may be transported long distances as young nymphs, or as eggs, in the feathers of large migratory birds (*Jabiru mycteria* (jabiru) and *Mycteria americana* (American wood ibis)) when these leave their nests, in which bugs live and breed, on seasonal migration.

ROLE OF TRIATOMINES AS VECTORS OF *TRYPANOSOMA CRUZI* AND *TRYPANOSOMA RANGELI*

Other blood-sucking arthropods can be experimentally infected with *Trypanosoma cruzi* but only triatomines are important in the epizootiology and epidemiology of Chagas' disease (and of the less important apathogenic trypanosome affecting man in the Neotropical regions, *Trypanosoma* (*Herpetosoma*) *rangeli*). Chagas' disease is a zoonosis and probably all triatomines are potential vectors of *Trypanosoma cruzi*, but *Trypanosoma rangeli* is naturally infective only to species of the genus *Rhodnius* (mainly *R. prolixus*, but also *R. pallescens* and *R. ecuadorensis*); although species of *Triatoma* can be experimentally infected with *Trypanosoma rangeli*, they are rarely infected in the wild. So far as the importance of triatomine species in transmission of *Trypanosoma cruzi* to man is concerned, only a relatively few species of bugs are actual and effective vectors.

Because of the contaminative (and hence inefficient) method of transmission of *Trypanosoma cruzi* in the faeces of the invertebrate, only those bug species which defecate whilst feeding on the human host are able to be effective vectors. Further, only in those species which are capable of colonizing houses in large numbers and feeding predominantly from man, and to a lesser extent his household animals (cats, dogs, chickens, etc.), is contaminative transmission sufficiently intense to lead to a high probability of successful infection among householders, given a high infection rate among the triatomine population. For a domiciliary vector to be of major epidemiological importance, it is also necessary for it to have a wide geographical range.

Of the relatively few triatomine species which fulfil the above criteria, *T. infestans* is the outstanding example in view of its wide occurrence in South America (from 10°N to 40°S and from Atlantic to Pacific coasts). In this extensive area it is almost exclusively a domiciliary species and the geographical range has often been extended by passive movement due to human agency. It is an aggressive and active species with a relatively short life cycle, which helps it to compete successfully with other longer-lived species (such as *P. megistus*) that are also domiciliary and which *T. infestans* tends to displace if accidentally introduced.

There are no domiciliary triatomine species in the broad expanse of the Amazon basin but to the north of this area *R. prolixus* is the main species of epidemiological importance; it is found predominantly from about 3°N (Colombia, Venezuela, the Gyanas) from sea level to an altitude of over 2000 m, and ranges to about 20°N in Mexico. It is the major domiciliary vector of Chagas' disease in Colombia and Venezuela and is one of several important species in Central America. Throughout its range it is also the main vector of *Trypanosoma rangeli* to wild and domestic animals as well as to man. Unlike *T. infestans*, it has an extensive extradomiciliary biotope; particularly important is its frequent occurrence in species of palm trees (where it is found in the nests of mammals and birds) that are frequently used as roofing materials for houses. Among the palms infested the genera *Attalea* and *Acrocomia* are widespread and numerous (Figure IV.77). *R. prolixus* also occurs in the palms *Copernica* and *Leopoldina*.

In the densely populated areas of the eastern seaboard of Brazil, *Panstrongylus megistus* is the important domiciliary triatomine; in the southern part of its range it also occurs in sylvatic foci, but further north it is confined to houses, perhaps because the almost total destruction of the original coastal forest vegetation in this area, over the past four centuries, has rendered conditions unsuitable for its survival in the wild. Alternatively, *P. megistus* may have been passively transported from south to north by human agency, but for various reasons this explanation seems less likely.

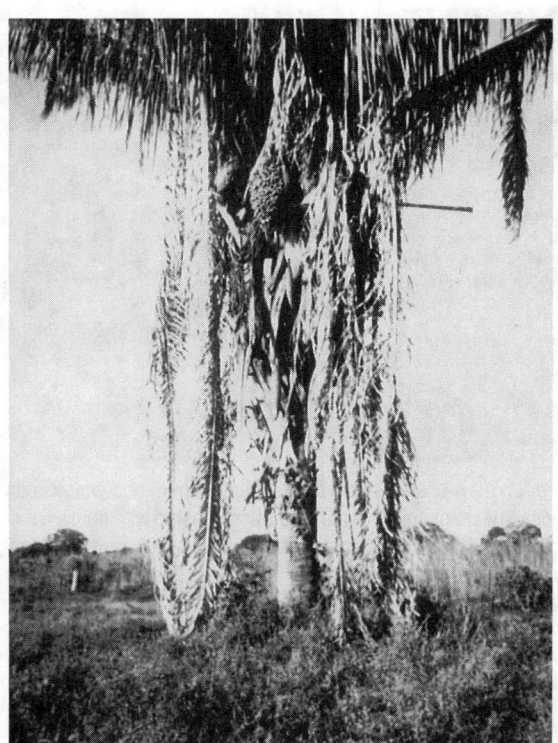

Figure IV.77   Palm tree (*Attalea humboldtiana*), sylvatic habitat of *Rhodnius prolixus* in Venezuela. Several genera and species of palm tree are a principal habitat of many triatomine species throughout Latin America, associated with the nests of various mammals and birds which inhabit the crowns and dependent fronds.

T. dimidiata is a highly variable species in coloration, etc. and was until recently divided into three subspecies (*T. d. dimidiata*, *T. d. maculipennis* and *T. d. capitata*) which are no longer recognized. The species is an important domiciliary vector in Ecuador, Peru and Central America as far as 22°N in Mexico.

The northern limit of domiciliated triatomines, and hence essentially that of human Chagas' disease, is to all intents and purposes the tropic of Cancer: isolated cases have occurred in Texas and elsewhere in the southern USA, but none of the several sylvatic triatomines present have become domiciliated, although some are natural vectors of *Trypanosoma cruzi* in wood rat colonies. Housing standards in the areas of the USA where bugs naturally occur are such that colonization by triatomines is in any event unlikely.

FEEDING BEHAVIOUR OF TRIATOMINES

All triatomines take large blood meals relative to their own body weight; the actual quantity varies greatly from stage to stage and from species to species; the larger bugs obviously take larger quantities.

The first stage nymphs at their first feed take up ten times their own body weight; successive stages take progressively less in terms of body weight, but more in actual quantity. In volumetric terms the fifth stage nymphs take the largest feed; this represents about three to four times their body weight. Adult bugs of both sexes take less blood than the fifth stage, but feed more often; on each occasion about two or three times their own body weight.

Blood meal identifications have been made by precipitin tests and other methods for many species of bugs in different geographical areas and variously from sylvatic, peridomestic and domestic ecotopes. In general terms, the results show that sylvatic species in the wild feed primarily on marsupials (especially the common opossum, *Didelphis* spp.), rodents, birds and edentates (e.g. armadillos, *Dasypus* spp.), bats and occasionally reptiles and amphibians.

Domiciliary bug populations, however, always feed predominantly upon man. Often, the domestic host fed upon most frequently after man is the epidemiologically unimportant chicken (birds are not susceptible to *Trypanosoma cruzi* infection).

Different species of important domiciliary vector may either feed frequently on cats and/or dogs (e.g. *T. infestans*, *T. dimidiata*) or feed infrequently from these hosts (e.g. *R. prolixus*, *P. megistus*). In the case of *T. infestans* and *T. dimidiata*, cats and/or dogs are important domestic reservoirs for Chagas' disease, since infected animals are a perpetual source of *Trypanosoma cruzi* and bugs become infected by feeding on them. Neither *R. prolixus* nor *P. megistus* in houses feed on cats or dogs to any significant extent and these animals, even if infected, thus provide little or no feedback of trypanosomes into the domestic bug population and are thus an epidemiological dead end.

The species of domiciliary bugs so far investigated differ in the frequency with which blood from different hosts can be detected in the same individual triatomine. Since blood proteins are detectable in bugs for up to 100–120 days, the occurrence of many individual meals of mixed origin in a bug population suggests that the bugs are frequently changing from one type of host to the other; a low frequency of multiple blood meals indicates that individuals are feeding repeatedly from the same host species. A high rate of feeds on man, combined with a low rate of feeds from other sources, especially of mixed feeds, clearly indicates that bug-mediated transmission occurs from man to man, rather than from animal to man. This is the situation found with domiciliary *R. prolixus* and *P. megistus*, in Venezuela and Brazil respectively. Domestic populations of *T. maculata* (in Venezuela) and *T. sordida* (in Brazil) feed predominantly from the uninfectable chicken; these species are therefore of very little epidemiological importance in the domestic transmission cycle.

Triatomines can become infected with *Trypanosoma cruzi* (and/or *Trypanosoma rangeli*) at any stage in their life from their first feed onward. Once infected with *Trypanosoma cruzi*, the infection probably almost always persists for life; infection rates found in different stages rise from a small percentage in the first stage nymphs to levels approaching or exceeding 90% among fifth stage nymphs and adults. Bugs appear in no way adversely affected by infection with *Trypanosoma cruzi*. Unlike *Trypanosoma cruzi*, however, *Trypanosoma rangeli* is pathogenic to its invertebrate hosts and causes a disturbance in the moulting mechanism, such that the moult is delayed and mortality during moulting is significantly increased. In adult bugs infected with *Trypanosoma rangeli*, there is also a reduction in the number of eggs laid by females and a decrease in egg viability.

Since, particularly where *R. prolixus* is the domiciliary vector, mixed infections of bugs, animals and man by *Trypanosoma cruzi* and *Trypanosoma rangeli* are common, it is frequently necessary to distinguish the two parasites, in both vertebrate and invertebrate hosts. The bloodstream stages are easily separable by their distinctive morphology; the stages in the bug can be less readily distinguished, except when trypomastigotes occur in the haemolymph and salivary glands (always *Trypanosoma rangeli*). Infective forms of *Trypanosoma rangeli* and *Trypanosoma cruzi* in the recta of bugs are difficult to separate without recourse to animal inoculation and study of the bloodstream stages. *Trypanosoma rangeli* can certainly be transmitted to vertebrates and man by the inoculative route when trypomastigotes occur in the salivary glands. There is controversy, however, as to whether contaminative infection by *Trypanosoma rangeli* (via trypomastigote forms shed in the faeces) occurs to any significant extent, or at all (see also Chapter 64).

TRANSMISSION CYCLES OF *TRYPANOSOMA CRUZI*

The possible cycles and their interrelationship, in bug-mediated *Trypanosoma cruzi* infections of animals and man are summarized in Fig. IV.78. Zoonotic cycles involve the majority of the 114 triatomine species currently recognized and some 120 species and subspecies of mammals. Foremost among the mammal hosts closely associated with sylvatic triatomines, and therefore frequently infected with *Trypanosoma cruzi*, are the marsupials of several genera, particularly *Didelphis* spp., which occupy a range that is more than coextensive with that of *Trypanosoma cruzi*: *Didelphis* spp. play a role in the epizootiology and epidemiology of *Trypanosoma cruzi* that is in some respects reminiscent of that of the bushbuck in the case of *Trypanozoon* trypanosomes in eastern Africa. The cat-sized *Didelphis* (Figure IV.73) are carnivorous and nocturnal and are among the last wild animals to be disturbed by human activities. They frequently enter houses and outbuildings to search for food, steal eggs, etc. and often roost in the roofs of houses or in trees near by. They are thus well placed to introduce sylvatic *Trypanosoma cruzi* strains into the peridomestic and domestic environments. Sylvatic triatomines, already infected with *Trypanosoma cruzi*, may fly into houses or be carried in on palm fronds for roofing or among firewood. Strains of *Trypanosoma cruzi* circulated in houses by domiciliary species are probably most frequently transferred between houses passively, either by passive transfer of infected bugs or by movement of infected people from house to house and from place to place.

Infected sylvatic rodents frequently visit outbuildings to feed on stored grain and other foodstuffs and can introduce new parasites from the wild into the peridomestic area. *Rattus* spp. and *Mus musculus* in houses are not infrequently infected with *Trypanosoma cruzi*, but they probably become infected by ingesting bugs, rather than by being fed upon. In turn, rats and mice form a sources of infection for cats and dogs by the oral route and no doubt hunting dogs and foraging cats frequently eat infected sylvatic animals. It should again be emphasized, however, that neither sylvatic nor domestic birds are ever a source of *Trypanosoma cruzi*, since they are totally insusceptible to infection, possibly owing in part to their higher body temperature, among other factors. The role of cats and dogs within the domestic cycle has been discussed earlier in relation to the feeding behav-

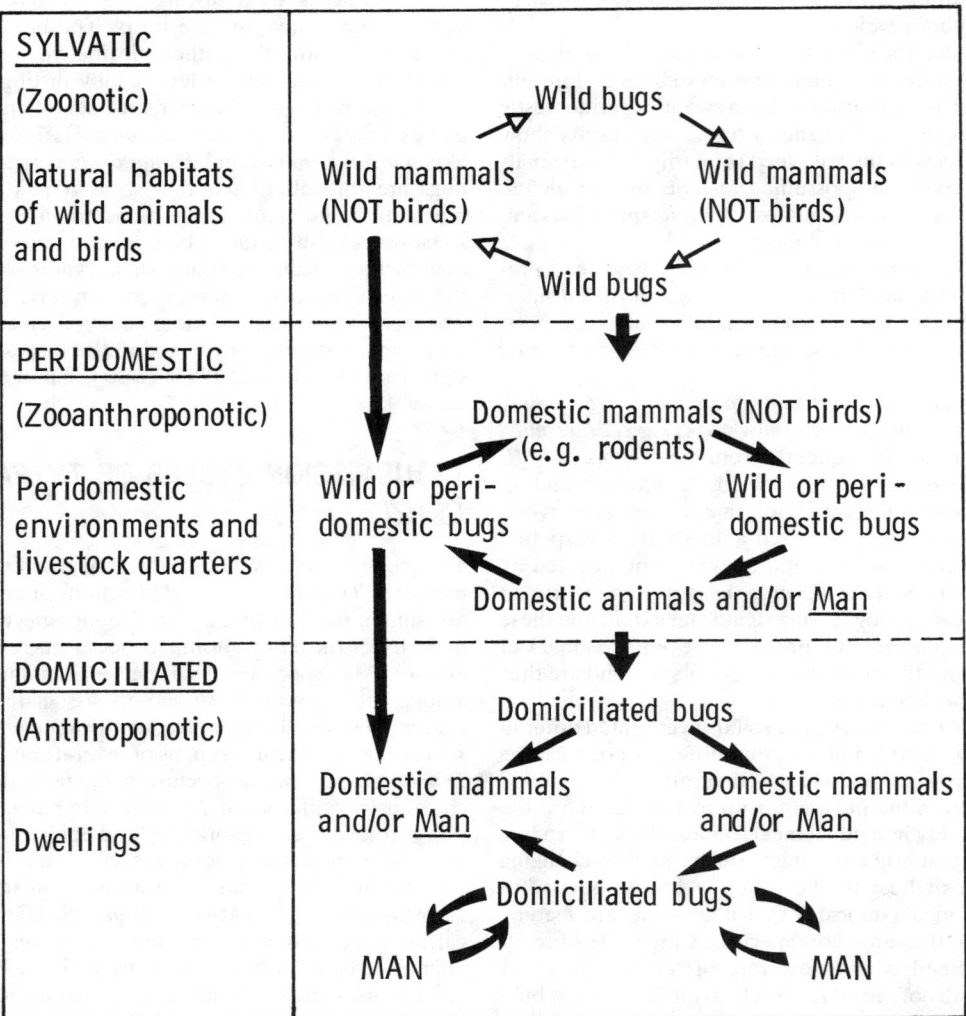

Figure IV.78 Transmission cycles of bug-mediated *Trypanosoma cruzi* infection.

iour of domiciliary triatomines. The role of infected rats and mice in houses can be assessed in a similar way and, from available evidence, it would seem that they are rarely of direct importance in the household epidemiology of Chagas' disease. Although the larger domestic animals, such as pigs, are susceptible to *Trypanosoma cruzi* and are sometimes fed upon by peridomestic/domestic triatomines (e.g. *T. infestans*, *P. megistus*, *T, dimidiata*), it is noteworthy that natural infections have been found only very rarely in pigs, rabbits and other larger domestic animals, which thus appear to play no significant role in the transmission of the parasite or in its transfer from sylvatic to peridomestic circumstances.

Once domiciliary transmission is established in the presence of large bug populations, transmission of *Trypanosoma cruzi* is chiefly man–bug–man and new human infections can occur among uninfected family members at a relatively high rate; among two families (20 persons) living in bug-infected premises in Brazil followed by serology and xenodiagnosis for 4 years, four new parasitologically confirmed infections occurred (a rate of 4% per annum); if two individuals with conversion to positive serology (but negative to xenodiagno-

sis on a single occasion) were included, the annual rate of new infections was 7.5%.

Because the contaminative method of transmission of *Trypanosoma cruzi* by bugs is inherently an inefficient mechanism, a heavy trypanosome challenge over a long period from biting and defaecating bugs is probably necessary for infection to occur. This is probably linked with the fact that young children are seldom infected (except congenitally or via maternal milk) until they are between 2 and 3 years of age, even under conditions of heavy challenge. Rates of infection among children are already high, however, among 5–10 year-olds and rise further in older age groups.

XENODIAGNOSIS AND EPIDEMIOLOGY

The parasitological diagnosis of *Trypanosoma cruzi* infection suggestive of present or future chagasic symptomatology can be made by conventional blood film microscopy only in the initial febrile stage of acute infection, which many infected individuals fail to experience. In the later chronic indeterminate stage of the disease, parasitological diagnosis becomes increasingly difficult, since the parasitaemia falls below the level at which it can be detected by routine methods, including standard concentration techniques. It has been shown that haemoculture is a sensitive diagnostic technique but since only immotile amastigote stages may develop in cultures initially, much skill and experience are required to detect positive cultures in the first weeks, sometimes months, for which they need to be examined until the motile stages appear in sufficient number. The method of haemoculture is also difficult to use in the field.

If triatomine bugs are grown in laboratory culture under conditions which preclude the possibility of their infection with pathogenic organisms (in Latin America this is usually ensured by feeding them on pigeons or chickens), then allowed to feed in sufficient numbers on individuals suspected to be infected with *Trypanosoma cruzi*, kept for several weeks (usually about four) and then examined for the presence of *Trypanosoma cruzi* in their recta, this will often result in the unequivocal detection of parasites and is the process termed xenodiagnosis; the triatomines act as a 'living culture' for the trypanosomes. This technique is expensive, unaesthetic and time consuming, but it is effective and has the great advantage that it can be used under field conditions. Technical details (number of bugs, species and stage) vary from one laboratory or hospital to another, as does the method of examination of the bugs used (expression of a faecal drop, dissection and examination of the entire rectal contents of the individual or pooling and maceration of batches of bugs) and there is much need for increased standardization. There is clear evidence from several sources that local 'strains' of vector are generally most susceptible to infection by the local parasite and that microscopical examination of the rectal contents of individual bugs is more sensitive than the expressed faecal drop or pooling methods; the latter, however, are often adopted for routine purposes because they save time and effort. Whenever possible it is advantageous to use fifth stage nymphs in xenodiagnosis, since these take the largest feed and increase the possibility that a low parasitaemia can be detected. In practice, a minimum number of bugs to use would be five fifth stage nymphs allowed to feed in the dark for about 30 minutes in a secure gauze-covered container; 10 or 20 bugs would be preferable but not always possible for logistic reasons. Repeated xenodiagnosis on several occasions also increases the number of successful diagnoses. On an experimental basis, the 'smaller' instars of the very large *Dipetalogaster maxima* gave results comparable with those with fifth stage nymphs of the main 'standard' xenodiagnosis species (*R. prolixus* and *T. infestans*), with a saving of time and expense on colony maintenance. Artificial xenodiagnosis' is now widely used in Venezuela, in which bugs feed through a membrane on venous blood drawn from the patient. This is claimed to be more acceptable and equally successful as conventional xenodiagnosis.

Xenodiagnosis clearly has many disadvantages and a better and more effective method of parasitological diagnosis is obviously desirable, as a back-up for the increasingly improved serological tests now available. Serological tests, by their nature, detect antibodies to parasite antigen rather than the parasites themselves.

Not only are triatomines the principal means by which people become infected with *Trypanosoma cruzi* (and *Trypanosoma rangeli*), but bugs build up large domiciliary popu-

lations and these are a significant source of blood loss in many households. Calculations show that, in houses in Venezuela with heavy infestations of *R. prolixus*, monthly blood loss was in the order of 100cm^3 per person per month. Occasionally individuals become sensitized to bug bites and may suffer severe allergic reactions as a result. This phenomenon may also be a complicating factor in xenodiagnosis.

Roughly the same number of people, about 250 million in each case, live in countries affected by African trypanosomiasis and in areas of Latin America affected by Chagas' disease. In Africa there are often fewer than 5000 new (treatable) infections annually. In Latin America, for diagnostic and logistic reasons, the number of new (and essentially incurable) cases each year is unknown, but crude estimates suggest up to 850 000 new infections per annum. At any one time, about 24 million people are seropositive for *Trypanosoma cruzi* and a further 65 million at risk in endemic areas. Serological surveys in various countries indicate that between 5 and 10% of national populations are infected.

The magnitude of the problem which such figures suggest, is immense. Unlike sleeping sickness, there is no safe and effective chemotherapy, and diagnosis of Chagas' disease is more difficult; early case detection and treatment are therefore of little value. Ultimately may come the development of an effective vaccine; meanwhile, improvements in standards of new and existing houses (in the latter case, particularly by individual or community-based self-help measures), and increased public health awareness in general, would help to diminish transmission levels to a considerable degree, but alone are probably insufficient to achieve interruption of disease transmission.

CONTROL OF CHAGAS' DISEASE VECTORS

Triatomine control on a large scale must rely on house-spraying using residual insecticides (see Table IV.13). Nowadays pyrethroids such as deltamethrin, cyfluthrin and lambda-cyhalothrin have become the most economical and effective products of choice, but their effects may be negated by active or passive reinvasion. Insecticide resistance has occurred (with dieldrin in Venezuela) but has not become a widespread or serious problem, although it remains a daunting threat everywhere. It is undoubtedly because of the long generation time of triatomines that resistance has yet to become a practical difficulty.

Improved cost-effectiveness of insecticidal treatments can be achieved with slow-release formulations, including paints and mastics applied to wall surfaces.

Simple and cheap methods to improve existing rural houses offer an attractive alternative to the regular use of insecticides, particularly if householders are encouraged, possibly even subsidized, to undertake the work themselves. The plastering of mud walls and/or the replacement of palm-thatched roofs by corrugated metal or plastic sheets, or locally-made tiles, drastically reduces the crevice habitat available to the various domiciliary triatomine species, and hence the level of infestation. A durable and crack-resistant wall plaster can be made from sand, cattle-dung, earth and lime. Lime can often be prepared cheaply from local limestone, by firing it overnight in a suitable kiln fuelled by wood or charcoal.

The mud used to build new mud-and-wattle houses can be

Table IV.13 Insecticides for vector control (based on WHO[126]). Application rates vary according to circumstances, as per local registration authority and manufacturer's instructions.

| Insecticide* | Residual application | | | Space-spray | Larvicide |
	Indoors	Perifocal	Bed-nets		
Organochlorine					
DDT	+	–	–	–	–
Organophosphate					
Temephos	–	–	–	–	+
Malathion	+	+	–	+	+
Fenitrothion	+	+	–	+	+
Pirimiphos-methyl	+	+	+	+	+
Carbamate					
Bendiocarb	+	+	+	+	–
Propoxur	+	+	–	–	–
Pyrethroid					
Bioresmethrin	+	–	–	+	–
Permethrin	+	+	+	+	–
Deltamethrin	+	+	+	+	–
Lambda-cyhalothrin	+	+	+	+	–
Cyfluthrin	+	–	+	–	–
Others					
IGRs	–	–	+	–	+
Bacterials	–	–	–	–	+

*Application rates vary according to circumstance, as per local registration authority and manufacturer's instructions.

stabilized to resist erosion, shrinkage and cracks; this can be done by adding lime, cement or bitumen (to make 'asfadobe'). Hand-operated hydraulic and mechanical rams are available which produce compressed, stabilized soil building blocks with properties similar to fire bricks. The initial capital investment is relatively high (about $US2000), but the machines are rugged and durable; each family which uses the press can produce enough blocks to build a house within a week, by their own unskilled labour and for the cost only of the small amount of lime or cement necessary to stabilize the local soil. The machines can be adapted readily to produce roof and floor tiles, or liners for pit-latrines. Allied with an energetic campaign of health education, and measures to encourage community participation, much could be achieved by the application of simple house improvement measures on a wide scale, particularly were this integrated with the use of insecticides, especially at the start. For further information see Schofield.[125]

FLEAS (See also Chapter 50)
G. B. White

ORDER: SIPHONAPTERA

Fleas are small (length 1–4 mm) and wingless, with laterally compressed bodies composed of a blunt head, compact thorax and a relatively large rounded abdomen (Figure IV.79). In colour they are usually dark brown as adults. Eyes and antennae are small, the latter being modified in males for clasping the female from below during copulation. When not extended, each antenna lies in a groove on the side of the head. This groove may be extended as a strengthening bar within the head from eye to eye (e.g. in *Pulex*). Ventrally the head bears a series of appendages for sensory and feeding functions: paired maxillary palps at the front, slender epipharynx and paired maxillary laciniae form the proboscis, with basal stipes and paired labial palps posteriorly.

Within the thorax, the oesophagus leads to a crop or proventriculus with a constriction before the capacious stomach in the abdomen. Patches of strongly barbed spines protrude into the proventricular lumen so that blood corpuscles may be ruptured as they pass towards the stomach for digestion. Plague vectors, such as *Xenopsylla* spp., have large proventricular spines on which plague bacilli accumulate and multiply, tending to promote thrombus formation and blocking of the proventriculus. Bacilli may then be regurgitated when the flea next tries to feed, so that transmission to another host occurs.

The bodies of adult fleas bear many characteristic setae and spines. The lower margin (gena) of the head and the hind edge of the prothorax are sometimes modified to form cuticular teeth or combs (ctenidia). The size and positions of combs, spines and setae are important in relation to the taxonomy and identification of genera and species of flea. All three pairs of legs are strongly developed, the hindlegs being longest and the forelegs shortest. At the base of each midleg the mesopleuron is usually strengthened with a vertical rod of cuticle internally. Many species of flea can jump to a height of several metres for purposes of reaching hosts or escaping capture. Flea jumps are powered by a mechanism involving energy storage in the thoracic arch, which consists of cuticles impregnated with resilin, a rubbery protein. Tension is built up by the thoracic muscles and released to kick the hindlegs.[119] General information on the anatomy and biology of fleas is summarized by Smit[120] and by Traub and Starcke.[121]

Adult fleas of all species are obligate, temporary ectoparasites of birds (6%) or of mammals (94% of flea species). More than 2000 species of flea have been described and are classified into some 200 genera. They are moderately host-specific, meaning that each kind of flea tends to infest only one or a few kinds of host. Man is frequently attacked by fleas from domestic or wild animals, as well as by the human flea *Pulex irritans*. Development takes place in the nests of particular hosts, including human dwellings. For some flea species (e.g. the European rabbit flea *Spilopsyllus cuniculi*, but not the human flea, cat flea or dog flea) host hormone levels may influence reproductive cycles of the associated fleas so that flea breeding coincides with host nesting.[119] The period of development from egg to pupa is 2 weeks or more, depending on temperature. The active white larvae (Figure IV.80B) have sparse hairs and a small but strong head capsule. Development takes place among dust and litter in the nest of the host, or indoors among fabrics or between floorboards. Larvae feed on organic debris and may require nutrient fragments of dried blood defaecated by adult fleas. There are two larval instars before the pupal stage.

Flea pupae are encased in a cocoon, loosely spun by the

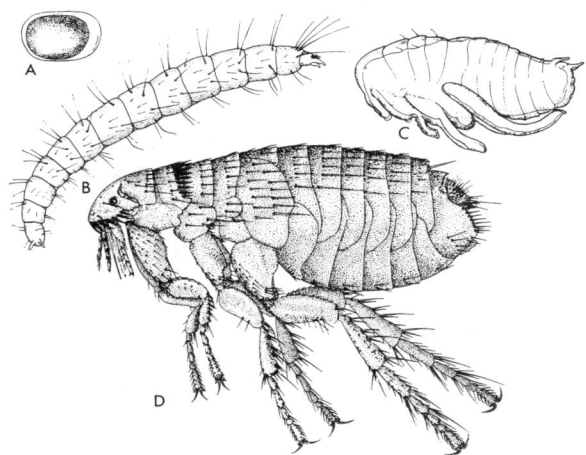

Figure IV.80 Life stages of a flea. A, Egg; B, larva; C, pupa; D, adult female.

larva around itself. Hatching of the adult may be delayed for months until the proximity of a host (vibration, warmth) stimulates emergence. Adult fleas can survive actively and away from the host for many weeks, provided that the climate is not too harsh. In general fleas thrive at temperatures of 20–30°C and humidities of 60–90%. Host temperatures (i.e. 35–42°C) actually inhibit egg hatching and larval development, which is why breeding on the host does not normally occur. Below about 8°C development ceases, and adult fleas become lethargic.

Female fleas tend to be larger than males of the same species. Both sexes feed regularly on blood and so become liable to transmit pathogens from host to host. Recognition of the female depends on presence of the spermatheca within the posterior abdomen (see Figures IV.79 and IV.81), whereas the male abdomen includes a conspicuous, curved phallosome for eventration during copulation.

Relatively large, sticky white eggs are produced by female fleas at a rate of 10–25 per day, being dropped indiscriminately among host fur or feathers or on the floor. In warm situations the eggs hatch within 2 or 3 days.

Identification keys for important genera and species of fleas in all parts of the world have been provided by Smit.[120] Specimens for identification should first be soaked for one or two days in 10% caustic soda to clear them before being washed and slide-mounted. Non-specialists should be cautious in trying to identify fleas, since many species are confusingly alike; The following guidelines may help to distinguish the genera which attack man most frequently.

1 Head rounded; combs absent: *Pulex* or *Xenopsylla*. Mesopleural rod present: *Xenopsylla*; absent: *Pulex*. Cephalic bar present above eyes: *Pulex*; absent: *Xenopsylla*.
2 Head biangular anteriorly, combs absent: *Echidnophaga*.
3 Head sharply pointed anteriorly, combs absent, postabdomen with large spiracles: *Tunga*.
4 Head and prothorax with combs: *Ctenocephalides*.
5 Head without comb, prothorax with comb: *Nosopsyllus*.
6 Head with comb and with two spines anteriorly, eyes absent: *Leptopsylla*.

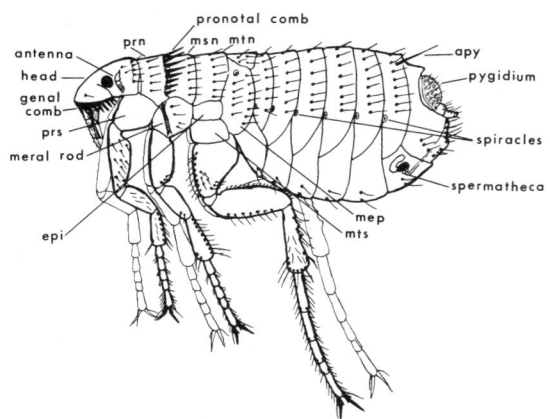

Figure IV.79 Lateral view of an adult female flea showing some of the principal taxonomic features. apy, Antepygidial bristle; epi, episternum; prn, pronotum; prs, prosternum; mep, metepimeron; msn, mesonotum; mtn, metanotum; mts, metepisternum. The meral rod (mesopleural rod) or vertical bar is present in most genera but absent from *Pulex*, the human flea.

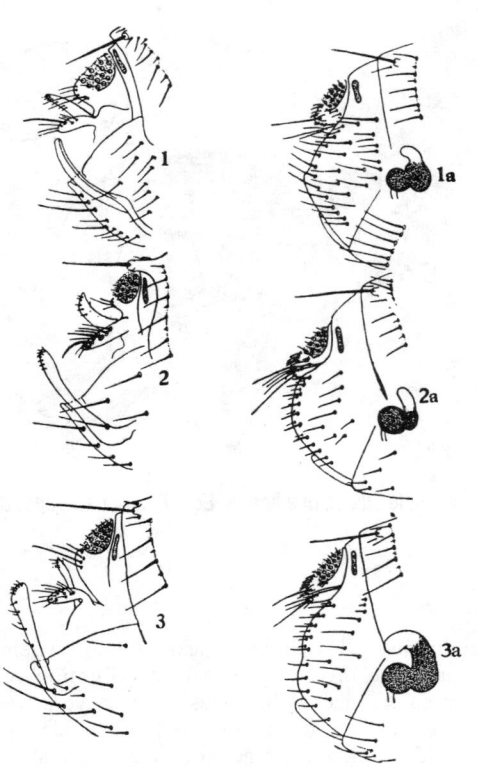

Figure IV.81   Diagnostic characters of the three widespread species of *Xenopsylla* rat fleas. 1, *X. astia*, male terminalia. 1a, *X. astia,* female terminalia with spermatheca. 2, *X. brasiliensis*, male terminalia. 2a, *X. brasiliensis*, female terminalia with spermatheca. 3, *X. cheopis*, male terminalia. 3a, *X. cheopis*, female terminalia with spermatheca. These species all possess the generic characteristics of a strong mesopleural rod, but no combs on head or pronotum.

FAMILY: PULICIDAE

The members of this family, being fleas without ctenidia (combs), include several species of medical importance both as pests and as disease vectors.

Pulex irritans, the human flea, is an ubiquitous pest of man, prevailing in many temperate and tropical situations. It is also commonly associated with various other coarse-coated mammals, both wild and domestic, especially dogs and pigs. Occasionally suspected of bubonic plague transmission from man to man, *P. irritans* is more certainly the vector responsible for vesicular and tonsillar plage outbreaks in Ecuador. Five other *Pulex* spp. are known, of which *P. simulans* also attacks man sometimes in North and South America and is distinguished by laciniae longer than those in *P. irritans*. Like many other fleas found in houses, *P. irritans* occasionally acts as an intermediate host of the dog tapeworm *Dipylidium caninum* which may infect man and is usually transmitted via *Ctenocephalides* fleas.

Xenopsylla cheopis, the oriental or black rat flea, normally infests *Rattus rattus* in urban situations throughout the world, but is scarce in parts of the northern temperature zone. It frequently attacks man in rat-infested buildings, and is the classical vector of epidemic plaque (*Yersinia pestis*) and of

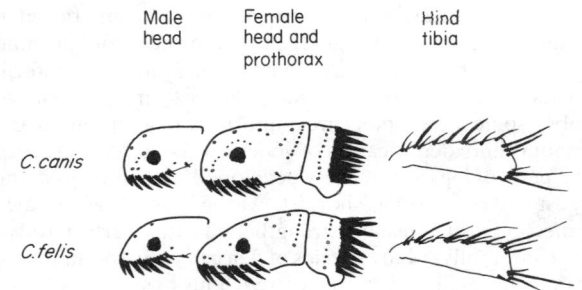

Figure IV.82   *Ctenocephalides* fleas possess rows of comb teeth (ctenidia) below the head and posteriorly on the prothorax. *C. felis*, the cat flea, has a relatively longer and more pointed head than *C. canis*, the dog flea. On the hind tibia, the number of posterior notches bearing strong setae is eight in *C. canis* and six in *C. felis*.

murine typhus (*Rickettsia mooseri*) from rat to rat and from rat to man. Other *Xenopsylla* spp. fulfil similar roles regionally, notably *X. brasiliensis* in tropical Africa where it thrives in wattle huts; the species has spread to parts of India and South America (hence its name). The equivalent endemic Indian flea is *X. astia*. Diagnostic differences between these three common species of *Xenopsylla* are depicted in Figure IV.81. The rat tapeworm *Hymenolepis diminuta* produces eggs which may be ingested by *Xenopsylla* larvae. Intestinal infection of rodents and sometimes children results from eating adult fleas in which cysticercoids have formed. Some strains of *H. nana*, the dwarf tapeworm of man, may also be transmitted from rat to rat via *Xenopsylla* spp.

Echidnophaga gallinacea, the sticktight flea of poultry, sometimes also infests dogs, cats, rabbits and other animals and can be a nuisance to people. Unlike most other fleas they stay attached to the host for prolonged periods and may copulate while feeding. *E. gallinacea* tends to cluster on the head of chickens, which scratch and injure themselves to such an extent that blindness may ensue. Ulceration of the host is often caused by sticktight fleas, and the females are said to oviposit deliberately into such wounds. Usually however, development takes place in the litter of poultry-houses.

Ctenocephalides is a small genus of nine species found mainly on carnivores in Africa and Eurasia, with two species that have become generally distributed: *C. canis* and *C. felis*, the dog and cat flea respectively. Actually, each of these species infests both cats and dogs interchangeably and *C. felis* tends to be more often found on both kinds of host. In modern centrally heated homes in temperate countries, *C. canis* and *C. felis* often thrive, sometimes in the temporary absence of cats and dogs. Recurrent infestations of these species may be more of a nuisance to man than is *P. irritans*, especially in developed countries where intermittent domestic control cannot eliminate *Ctenocephalides* spp. Cat and dog fleas are characterized by pronounced ctenidial combs on the gena (ventral edge of head) and posteriorly on the prothorax. Figure IV.82 shows how *C. felis* has a relatively longer head than *C. canis*. The dog tapeworm *Dipylidium caninum* produces eggs which may be ingested by *Ctenocephalides* larvae. Intestinal infection of cats, dogs and sometimes of man results from eating adult fleas carrying cysticercoids. A similar life cycle involving *Ctenocephalides* is sometimes followed by strains of *Hymenolepis nana*, the human dwarf tapeworm, which usually does not have an intermediate host.

FAMILY: LEPTOPSYLLIDAE

Leptopsylla segnis, the European mouse flea, is frequently found indoors in various parts of the world. It also infests rats and sometimes transmits enzootic plague, but seldom bites man.

FAMILY: CERATOPHYLLIDAE

Ceratophyllus gallinae, the European chicken flea, has spread to many parts of the world, has a wide range of bird hosts and occasionally invades houses and attacks people. It is a particularly large flea with a painful bite. Unlike *Echidnophaga*, it drops off the host directly after feeding. An equivalent North American species is *C. niger*, the western chicken flea. Numerous comb teeth on the pronotum facilitate the identification of *Ceratophyllus* spp.

Nosopsyllus fasciatus, the brown rat flea, has also become widespread with its main host *Rattus norvegicus*; it also infests *R. rattus* and many other small mammals and often attacks man, but is seldom involved in plague transmission. Like *Ctenocephalides*, *N. fasciatus* serves as an intermediate host of the dog tapeworm *D. caninum* which may infect man if infective fleas are eaten.

FAMILY: TUNGIDAE

Tunga penetrans, the sand flea or jigger (chigoe, chique), has females adapted for intracutaneous permanent attachment on the host. *T. penetrans* regularly infects man, pigs, poultry and other creatures in Central America, West and East Africa and parts of the Indian subcontinent. As for other fleas, the larvae are free-living, dusty or sandy soil being best for *T. penetrans*. Adults are also free-living at first, when copulation occurs. The fertilized female then finds a suitable host and tries to penetrate crevices in the skin, such as cracks in the soles of the feet (Chapter 11), between the toes and especially around the toenails. Any part of the human anatomy can be affected. By means of the mouthparts, the female *Tunga* becomes firmly attached and soon swells to the size and shape of a small white pea. Somehow the host skin envelops the jigger, which lies below the stratum corneum but above the stratum granulosum, leaving only the posterior spiracles exposed to the air. Only when the jigger is almost mature and distended, after 8–12 days, does the infection begin to irritate. Severe inflammation and ulceration ensues, so that scratching helps to expel large numbers of white eggs from the jigger. With skill and care it is possible to remove the whole insect, using a needle or forceps, but often the soft abdomen ruptures leaving the head attached in the lesion.

The jigger seldom attacks the leg above the dorsum of the foot, but no part of the body is immune. The soles (Chapter 11), the skin between the toes and that at the roots of the nails are favourite situations. Usually only one or two jiggers are found at a time, but occasionally they are present in hundreds, the small pits left after extraction or expulsion being sometimes so closely set that parts of the surface may look like honeycomb. During her gestation the jigger causes a considerable amount of irritation. In consequence of this pus may form around her distended abdomen which now raises the integument into a pea-like elevation. After the eggs are laid the superjacent skin ulcerates and the jigger is expelled, leaving a small sore which may become infected sometimes causing phagedaena or even tetanus. Ulceration is common and may follow removal of the jigger or natural extrusion of the egg sac. The ulcer commences as a tiny pit and as it extends the sloping edge may develop into a septic ulcer. It remains more or less circular in outline, except under the nail or nail margin, where the outline is more irregular and a pocket of pus forms beneath it. Chronic absorption of pus may lead to thrombophlebitis.

MEDICAL IMPORTANCE AND CONTROL OF FLEAS

More than 50 genera and numerous species of fleas have been implicated as vectors of enzootic plague in various parts of the world (Chapter 50), meaning that they maintain the transmission of *Yersinia pestis* bacilli among rodents. Man is seldom infected primarily through the bites of such zoophilic fleas, except when infected *Xenopsylla* move on to man after plague-stricken rats have died. Rarely are conditions conducive for man-to-man transmission by *Pulex* or *Ctenocephalides* to reach epidemic proportions. Over-wintering of plague bacilli may occur in hibernating fleas.

Various flea species may also be involved in the transmission cycles of murine typhus, tularaemia, pseudotuberculosis, melioidosis, brucellosis, lymphocytic choriomeningitis and possibly other diseases.[122] Only the first depends on fleas, as well as parasitic mites and lice, as vectors. Thus the agent of murine typhus, *Rickettsia typhi* (=*R. mooseri*), is commonly transmitted by *X. brasiliensis*, *X. cheopis*, and possibly *N. fasciatus* or *L. segnis*, with a similar epidemiological picture to that of plague.[123]

As mentioned previously, some fleas serve as the intermediate hosts for tapeworms usually found in animals: *Dipylidium caninum* of dogs and cats; *Hymenolepis diminuta* of rodents; *H. nana* strains endemic in rodents. These occasionally cause diarrhoea in humans, especially children who may happen to become infected by eating infective fleas.

People suffer localized dermal reactions to flea bites, which can be soothed with antihistamines. Generalized allergic sensitization is not uncommon and should be overcome by means of flea control in preference to desensitization treatment of the patient. The irritation and nuisance caused by fleas crawling on the body surface and the pain of their frequent probing and biting always justify control measures.

Simple hygienic measures of keeping houses well swept

and floors washed and clean are beneficial and the regular use of a vacuum suction cleaner is highly effective for gathering up fleas, their eggs and larvae. When flea-infested premises are re-entered after a period of disuse, newly emerged fleas may become activated and attack people in surprising numbers. Temporary relief may be gained through the use of insect repellent creams or lotions based on dimethyl phthalate, diethyltoluamide, indalone and proprietary brands. Floors can be treated with a solution of naphthalenes in benzene, or simply with detergents. Synthetic chemical insecticides should be sprayed or dusted into corners, cracks and fabrics where flea larvae may be expected to occur. The value of DDT for such purposes has become diminished by the problem of insecticide resistance in many areas. Various organophosphates, carbamates and pyrethroids are ample substitutes, but compounds with high mammalian toxicity should not be used indoors. Flea-ridden domestic animals may themselves be washed thoroughly with carbolic soap, dusted with pyrethroid powder, treated with insecticidal lotion or shampoo (e.g. malathion) or fitted with a 'flea-collar' made of plastic impregnated with dichlorvos which has a prolonged, localized vapour action within the fur. For direct killing of fleas it is convenient to employ spray-canisters giving aerosols of synergized pyrethrins or similar quick-acting insecticides.

The particular personal problems caused by sand fleas or jiggers (*T. penetrans*) have already been mentioned. Affected areas of soil may be burnt off in an effort to kill them, and their breeding on livestock and pets should not be allowed. Since female jiggers are not good jumpers, human infestation is normally confined to the feet. Daily inspection of the interdigital clefts, roots of nails and soles of feet should cause freshly burrowing female jiggers to be detected and removed before they have grown significantly. To prevent their attack, good shoes should be worn at all times. An old deterrent is to rub the feet with lysol or creosol in paraffin oil; modern repellents may be better.

In locations where *T. penetrans* is common, the local people become quite skilful at removing them with sharp instruments. The characteristic, circular, open lesions should be dressed antiseptically and protected until healed. Often they become ulcerated and secondarily infected; local pus production may occur, and be complicated by thrombophlebitis or gangrene. Timely use of antibiotics is therefore advisable and the affected limb should be rested.

REFERENCES

1 Kettle D S. *Medical and Veterinary Entomology*. London: Croom Helm, 1984.

2 Riley J. *Adv Parasit* 1986; 15:46–128.

3 Khalil G M. *F Egyptian Publ Hlth Ass* 1972; 47:363–369.

4 World Health Organization. *Wld Hlth Org Tech Rep Ser* 1984; 701:140.

5 Lanson R & Shaw J J. The role of animals in the epidemiology of South American leishmaniasis. In Lumsen W H R & Evans D A (eds) *Biology of the Kinetoplastida*, vol. II. New York and London: Academic Press, 1979: 1.

6 Peters C J & LeDuc J W. Bunyaviruses, Phleboviruses and related viruses. In Belshe R B (ed.) *Textbook of Human Virology*. Littletton, Mass: PSG Publishing, 1985: 547–598.

7 Lewis D J, Young D H, Fairchild G B et al. *Syst Entomol* 1977; 2:319–332.

8 Lane R P. *Insect Sci Applic* 1986; 7:225–230.

9 World Health Organization. *Manual on Practical Entomology in Malaria*. Geneva: World Heath Organization, 1975.

10 Knight L L & Stone A. *A Catalog of the Mosquitoes of the World*. The Thomas Say Foundation, Vol. VI. College Park: Entomological Society of America, 1977 (Supplement 1978).

11 Dennis P T, Partomo F, Durnomo A A et al. *Am J Trop Med Hyg* 1976; 25:797.

12 Reid J A. *Anopheline Mosquitoes of Malaya and Borneo*. Studies from the Institute for Medical Research, Malaysia, No. 31. Kuala Lumpur: Government of Malaysia, 1968.

13 White G B. *Mosquito System* 1968; 10:13.

14 Carpenter S J & La Casse W J. *Mosquitoes of North America*. Berkeley & Loss Angeles: University of Californaia Press, 1974.

15 Gillies M T & de Meillon B. *The Anophelinae of Africa South of the Sahara*. Johannesburg: South African Institute for Medical Research, 1968.

16 Garnham P C C. *Malaria Parasites and Other Haemosporidia*. Oxford: Blackwell Scientific Publications, 1966.

17 Kalra S L. *J Communic Dis* 1978; 10:1.

18 Webber R H. *Trans R Soc Trop Med Hyg,* 1979; 73:722.

19 White G B. *Trans R Soc Trop Med Hyg* 1974; 68:278.

20 Zavortink T J. *Contr Am Ent Inst* 1973; 9:1.

21 Faran M E. *Contr Am Ent Inst* 1980; 15:1.

22 Le Duc J W. *J Med Ent* 1979; 16:1.

23 Dutary B E & Le Duc J W. *Trans R Soc Trop Med Hyg* 1981; 75:128.

24 Belkin J N. *Mosquitoes of the South Pacific*. Berkeley & Los Angeles: California University Press, 1962.

25 Huang Y M. *Mosquito System* 1977; 9:289 (also Document WHO/VBC/76. 654, WHO/FIL/76.143).

26 Huang Y M & Hitchcock J C. *Contr Am Ent Inst* 1980; 17:1.

27 MacDonald W W. Mosquito genetics in relation to filaria infections. *Symp Br Soc Parasit* 1967; 14:1.

28 Christophers S R. *Aedes aegypti (L.), the Yellow Fever Mosquito*. London: Cambridge University Press, 1960.

29 McClelland G A H. *Trans R Ent Soc Lond* 1974; 126:239.

30 Powell J R, Tabachnik W J & Arnold J. *Science, NY* 1980; 208:1385.

31 McIntosh B M. *Mosquitoes as Vectors of Viruses in*

South Africa. Entomology Memoir No. 43, Pretoria: Department of Agricultural and Technical Services, 1975.

32 Arnell J H. *Contr Am Ent Inst* 1973; 10:1

33 Belkin J N, Heinemann S L & Page W A. *Contr Am Ent Inst* 1970; 6:1.

34 Bram R A. *Contr Am Ent Inst* 1967; 2:1.

35 Sirivanakarn S. *Contr Am Ent Inst* 1976; 12:1.

36 Southgate B A. *Trop Dis Bull* 1979; 76:1045.

37 Sasa M. *Human Filariasis.* University of Tokyo Press, 1976.

38 Sirivanakarn S. *Contr Am Ent Inst*, in press, 1982.

39 Maslov A V. *Ent Obozrenie* 1967; 43:193 (English trans. *Ent Rev, Wash*, 43:97.)

40 Wharton R H. *Bulletin No 11.* Institute for Medical Research, Federation of Malaya, 1962.

41 Bates M. *The Natural History of Mosquitoes.* New York: Macmillan, 1949.

42 Gillett J D. *Mosquitoes.* London: Weidenfeld & Nicholson, 1971.

43 Harbach R E & Knight K L. *Taxonomists' Glossary of Mosquito Anatomy.* Marlton, New Jersey: Plexus Publishing, 1980.

44 Harwood R T & James M T. *Entomology in Human and Animal Health.* New York, Toronto & London: Macmillan, 1979.

45 Horsfall, W R. *Mosquitoes—Their Bionomics and Relation to Disease.* New York: Ronald Press, 1955.

46 Mattingly P F. *The Biology of Mosquito-borne Disease.* Science of Biology Series, No. 1. London: Allen & Unwin, 1969.

47 Service M W. *Mosquito Ecology: Field Sampling Methods.* London: Applied Science Publishers, 1976.

48 Edwards F W. *Mosquitoes of the Ethiopian Region. III.—Culicine Adults and Pupae.* London: British Museum (Natural History), 1941.

49 Hopkins G H E. *Mosquitoes of the Ethiopian Region. I.—Larval Bionomics of Mosquitoes and Taxonomy of Culicine Larvae.* London: British Museum (Natural History), 1952.

50 Mattingly, P F. *Bull Br Mus (Nat Hist) (B)* 1952–3; 2:233; 3:1.

51 Gerberg E J & van Someren, E C C. Document WHO/VBC/70.236, 1970.

52 Cordellier R, Germain M, Hervy J P et al. *Guide Pratique pour L'Etude des Vecteurs de Fièvre Jaune en Afrique et Méthode de Lutte.* Initiations, Documentations Techniques, No. 33. Paris: Office de la Recherche Scientifique et Technique Oure-Mer, 1977.

53 Lane J. *Neotropical Culicidae*, Vols 1 and 2. University of São Paulo, 1953.

54 Forratini O P. *Entomologia Médica*, Vol. 1. *Anophelini.* E Blucher and University of São Paulo, 1962.

55 Forratini O P. *Entomologia Médica*, Vol. 2. *Culicini: Culex, Aedes e Psorophora.* E Blucher and University of São Paulo, 1965.

56 Wood D M, Dang P T & Ellis R A. *The Mosquitoes of Canada. The Insects and Arachnids of Canada, Part 6.* Hill, Quebec: Agriculture Canada, 1980.

57 Darsie R F & Ward R A. *Identification and Geographical Distribution of the Mosquitoes of North America.* Fresno, California: American Mosquito Control Association, 1981.

58 Mattingly P F & Knight K L. *Bull Br Mus (Nat Hist) (B)* 1956; 4:89.

59 Lee D J. *An Atlas of the Mosquito Larvae of the Australasian Region. Tribes Megorhinini and Culicini.* Australian Military Forces, 1944.

60 Lee D J & Woodhill A R. *The Anopheline Mosquitoes of the Australasian Region.* Department of Zoology, University of Sydney, Monograph 2, 1944.

61 Dobrotworsky N V. *The Mosquitoes of Victoria.* Melbourne: Melbourne University Press, 1965.

62 Marks E N. *An Atlas of Common Queensland Mosquitoes.* St Lucia: University of Queensland, 1973.

63 Ribeiro H, Ramos H C, Capela R A et al. *Estudios, Ensaios e Documentos No 135.* Lisbon: Junta de Investigacoes Cientificås do Ultramar, 1980.

64 Dahl C & White G B. In Illies J (ed.) *Limnofauna Europaea.* 1978: 390–395.

65 Christophers S R. *Fauna Br India* 1933; 4:1.

66 Bhatia M L, Kalra N L, Rao V V et al. *Vectors of Malaria in India.* Delhi: National Society of India for Malaria and Other Mosquito-Borne Diseases, 1961.

67 Barraud P J. *Fauna Br India* 1934; 5:1.

68 Tanaka K, Mizusawa K & Saugstad E S. *Contr Am Ent Inst* 1979; 16:987.

69 Grjebine A. *Faune de Nadagascar, XXII. Insectes Diptères Culicidae Anophelinae.* Paris: Lahure, 1966.

70 Ravaon Janahary C. *Trav Doc Off Rech Sci Tech Outre-Mer* 1978; 87.

71 Rioux J A. *Encycl Ent B* 1958; 35:1.

72 Senevet G & Andarelli L. *Encycl Ent A* 1959; 37:1.

73 Van den Assem J & Bonne-Wepster J. *Zool Bijdr* 1964; 6:1.

74 Belkin J N. *Contr Am Ent Inst* 1968; 3:1.

75 Bonne-Wepster J & Swellengrebel N H. *The Anopheline Mosquitoes of the Indo-Australian Region.* Amsterdam: de Bussy, 1953.

76 Harrison B A & Scanlon J E. *Contr Am Ent Inst* 1975; 12:1.

77 Mattingly P F. Part I (1957) *Ficalbia*; part II (1957) *Heizmannia*; part III *Aedes (Paraedes)* and *(Cancraedes)*; part IV *Aedes (Skusea)*, *(Diceromyia)* *(Geoskusea)* and *(Christophersiomyia)*; part V *Aedes (Mucidus)*, *(Ochlerotatus)*, and *(Neomelaniconion)*; part VI *Aedes (Stegomyia)*. London: British Museum (Natural History), 1957–65.

78 Mattingly P F. *Contr Am Ent Inst* 1970; 5:1.

79 Reinert J F. *Contr Am Ent Inst* 1973; 9:1.

80 Huang Y M. *Contr Am Ent Inst* 1979; 15:1.

81 Delfinado M D. *Mem Am Ent Inst* 1966; 7:1.

82 Basio R G. *Nat Mus Philipp Monogr* 1971; 4.

83 Gutsevich A V, Monchadsky A S & Stackelberg A A. *Fauna SSSR. VII (4). Family Culicidae.* Leningrad: Akad, Nauk SSSR Zool Inst (English translation (1974) Jerusalem: Keter Press), 1970.

84 Mattingly P F & Brown E S. *Bull Ent Res* 1955; 46:69.

85 Foote R H & Cook D R. *Mosquitoes of Medical Importance.* United States Department of Agriculture, Agricultural Handbook, 1959; 152:1–158.

86 Mattingly P F. *Contr Am Ent Inst* 1971; 7:1. (Reproduced in Smith K G V (1973) *Insects and Other Arthropods of Medical Importance.* London: British Museum (Natural History).)

87 Laird M & Miles J W (eds). *Integrated Mosquito Control Methodologies*, 2 vols. London: Academic Press, 1983, 1985.
88 Reiter P. *Ann Trop Med Parasit* 1980; 74:541.
89 Detinova T S. *Age-grouping Methods in Diptera of Medical Importance*. WHO Monograph Series No 417, 1962.
90 Clements A N. *The Physiology of Mosquitoes*. Oxford: Pergamon Press, 1963.
91 Linley J R, Hoch A L & Pinheiro F P. *J Med Ent* 1983; 20:347–364.
92 Raccurt C, Lowrie R C & McNeeley D F. *Am J Trop Med Hyg* 1980; 29:803–808.
93 Nathan M B. *Bull Ent Res* 1981; 71:97–105.
94 Linley J R & Davies J B. *J Econ Ent* 1971; 64:264–278.
95 Stanek G. *Microb Sci* 1985; 2:231–234.
96 Schmid G P. *Rev Infect Dis* 1985; 7:41–50.
97 Magnarelli L A, Anderson J F & Barbour A G. *J Infect Dis* 1986; 154:355–358.
98 Mulligan H W. *The African Trypanosomiases*. London: George Allen & Unwin, 1970.
99 Ford J. *The Role of the Trypanosomiases in African Ecology: A Study of the Tsetse Fly Problem*. Oxford: Clarendon Press, 1971.
100 Potts.
101 Pollock J N. *Training Manual for Tsetse Control Personnel*, 3 vols. Rome: FAO, 1982.
102 Jackson C H N. *Bull Ent Res* 1946; 37:291.
103 Saunders 1962.
104 Challier 1965.
105 Challier A. *Insect Sci Applic* 1982; 3:97–143.
106 Molyneux D H & Ashford R W. *The Biology of Trypansoma and Leishmania, Parasites of Man and Domestic Animals*. London: Taylor and Francis, 1983.
107 Molyneux D H. *Rev Infect Dis* 1983; 5:945–956.
108 Allsopp R. *Bull Ent Res* 1984; 74:1–23.
109 Jordan A M. *Br Med Bull* 1985; 41:181–186.
110 Jordan A M. *Trypanosomiasis Control and African Rural Development*. Harlow (UK): Longman, 1986.
111 Zumpt, F. *Myiasis in Animals and Man in the Old World*. London, 1965.
112 Smith K G V (ed.). *Insects and Other Arthropods of Medical Importance*. London: British Museum (Natural History), 1973.
113 Landi 1960.
114 Dar M S, Ben Amer M, Dar E K et al. *Trans R Soc Trop Med Hyg* 1980; 74:303.
115 Zumpt F. *SA Med J* 1963; 37:305–307.
116 Clay T. *Bull Br Mus Nat His (Ent)* 1970; 25:73.
117 Scholt L L. *The Epidemiology of Human Pediculosis*, p. 150. Florida: Navy Disease Vector Ecology and Control Centre, 1979.
118 Lent H & Wygodzinsky P. *Bull Am Mus Nat Hist* 1979; 163:123.
119 Rothschild M. *A Rev Ent* 1975; 20:241.
120 Smit F G A M. Siphonaptera (fleas). In Smith K G V (ed.) *Insects and other Arthropods of Medical Importance*. London: British Museum (Natural History), 1973: 325.
121 Traub R & Starcke H. *Fleas*. Rotterdam: Balkema, 1980.
122 Bibikova V A. *A Rev Ent* 1977; 22:1.
123 Traub R, Wisseman C L & Farhang-Azad A. *Trop Dis Bull* 1978; 75:237.
124 Crosskey R W. *The Biology of Blackflies*, 1993.
125 Schofield C J. *Triatominae: Biology and Control*, 1993.
126 WHO. *Chemical Methods for the Control of Arthropod Vectors and Pests of Public Health Importance*, 1984.

LABORATORY DIAGNOSIS

A. H. Moody

HEALTH AND SAFETY

Laboratories are potentially dangerous places in which to work and it is essential that in planning a laboratory great attention is paid to safety.

- Technical staff Gshould be well trained or supervised. They should be aware of the risks of infection in the laboratory and know how to handle the specimens they are examining. Written instructions on how to deal with breakages or spillage involving specimens should be clearly available and a disinfection procedure followed.

- The laboratory should be constructed with adequate benching and lighting. Protective clothing should be supplied and hand-washing facilities should be available.
- Apparatus used in the laboratory should have written instructions for its proper use and maintenance.
- Provision for disinfection and disposal of specimens by incineration is necessary.
- A procedure for disposing of needles and other 'sharps' into a suitable pot should be implemented.

DIAGNOSTIC METHODS

The laboratory diagnosis of tropical diseases is primarily an observer science. Parasitic organisms are recognized by their size, colour and morphological appearance, often with the assistance of stains and after concentration to increase the numbers of parasite stages present in the case of scanty infections. In chronic infections, active stages of a parasite may not be easily found and diagnosis may be more appropriately made by serological means. In a few cases the diagnosis may only be made by histology.

The parasitology laboratory differs from a microbiology laboratory and certain additional pieces of equipment are essential for differentiation and speciation:

- A microscope, equipped with a binocular head and 10× eyepieces is preferred. The microscope should have a good quality substage Abbe condenser with a diaphragm to control the entry of light.
- A calibrated graticule should be available for one of the eyepieces; the graticule can be left in situ or inserted as required. It should be calibrated, using a slide micrometer, for each power objective (see below).
- A filter, which can be nylon or wire gauze, with pore size no more than $600 \mu m$, is required for the faecal concentration method (see below). A vortex mixer and electric or battery powered centrifuge capable of receiving 15 cm centrifuge tubes and operating at $2500 g$ is also required for the faecal concentration method.
- A Swinnex-type holder and Nuclepore membranes, pore size $5 \mu m$, for the filtration of microfilariae (see p. 1745).

Other pieces of apparatus required are commonly available in most laboratories.

CALIBRATION OF EYEPIECE GRATICULE

- Calibration slide: a slide on which is etched a line of 1 cm divided into 100 divisions of *10 μm each*.
- Eyepiece graticule: a circular piece of glass on which is etched a line of variable length with 100 divisions. The graticule fits inside one of the eyepieces.

Calibration

Place the calibrated slide on to the stage of the microscope. Using the 10× objective initially, bring the calibration line into focus. Align the lines of the eyepiece graticule with those of the calibration slide and note the number of lines of each. From these values the micrometre value of each division of the graticule can be calculated.

Example

- If each slide calibration = $10 \mu m$ then if 10 slide divisions = 10 graticule divisions, $100 \mu m$ = 10 graticule divisions and each graticule division will equal $10 \mu m$. Repeat this procedure for the 40× and 100× objectives:
- 40×: if 10 slide divisions = 40 graticule divisions, $100 \mu m$ = 40 graticule divisions and each graticule division will equal $2.5 \mu m$;
- 100×: if 10 slide divisions = 100 graticule divisions then 1 graticule division will equal $1 \mu m$.

USES OF MEASUREMENT

To measure any object the graticule is placed over the object and the number of graticule divisions that exactly cover the object is noted. When this number is multiplied by the number of micrometres calculated for the objective used, the size of the object can be determined.

Measurement enables separation of morphologically similar parasites to be made.

INVESTIGATION OF THE CAUSES OF DIARRHOEA (Figure V.1)

DIRECT EXAMINATION OF FAECES

Direct examination of a suspension of faeces in warm saline enables the presence of motile trophozoites of protozoa to be seen. It will also show cysts and helminth ova present in sufficient numbers. Concentration methods are necessary when cysts and ova are present in low numbers; they do not show motile trophozoites (Figures V.3–V.10).

PREPARATION OF DIRECT FAECAL SMEAR

Materials
- Physiological saline (0.9% sodium chloride)
- Lugol's iodine.

Method
1. Take a microscope slide and label one end with the patient's name.
2. Place a drop of saline at each end of the slide.
3. Using an applicator stick, select a piece of faecal material approximately the size of a small pea and emulsify the faeces into the two drops of saline on the slide. If the faeces contains any blood or mucus, prepare a separate slide for this. Add a drop of iodine solution to the right-hand suspension.
4. Place a 22 mm coverslip on to each preparation and view the slide using the 10× and 40× objectives.

FAECAL CONCENTRATION METHOD

FORMOL–ETHER CONCENTRATION METHOD FOR OVA AND CYSTS

Materials
- 10% formalin (100 ml formaldehyde + 900 ml distilled water)
- Ether or ethyl acetate

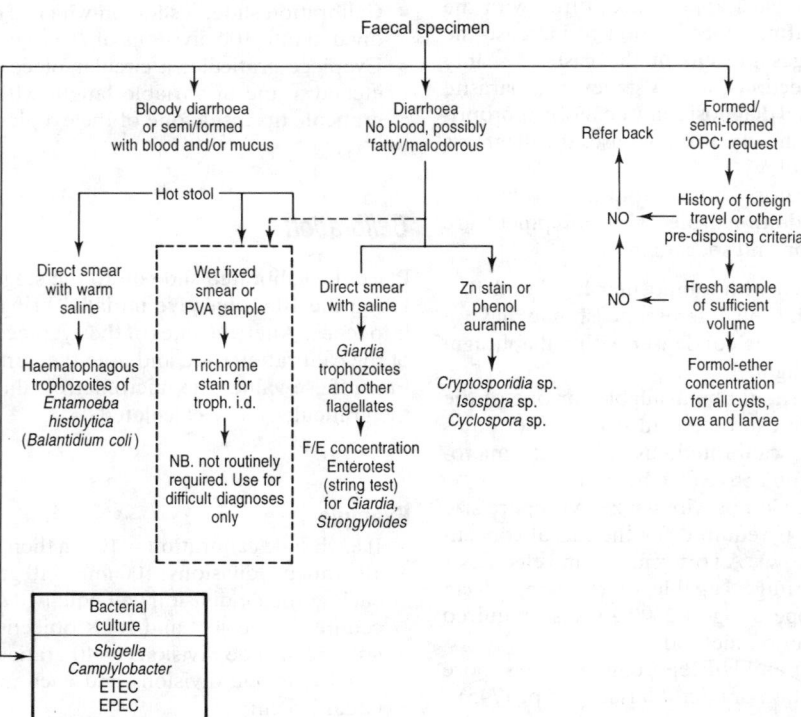

Figure V.1   Investigations of causes of diarrhoea, OCP, ova, cysts, parasites; Zn, Ziehl Neelsen; Troph, trophozoite; i.d., identification.

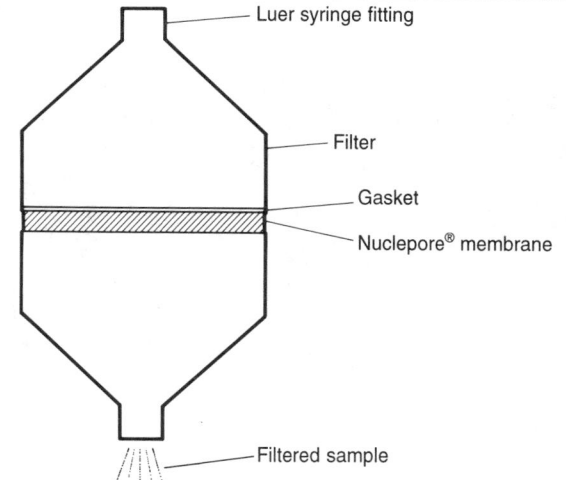

Figure V.2   Swinnex filter for membrane filtration.

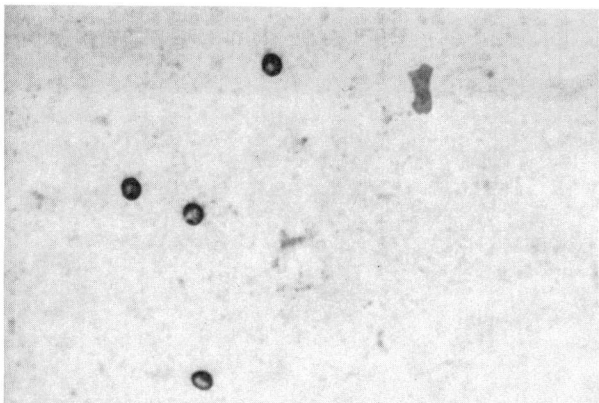

Figure V.3   Oocysts of *Cryptosporidium parvum*.

- 40 Mesh (425 μm) brass wire filter, 3 inch (7.5 cm) in diameter, or a nylon coffee strainer
- Small 3 inch (7.5 cm) dish or beaker.

Method
1. Using applicator sticks, select a quantity of faeces (approximately 1 g) to include external and internal portions.
2. Place in a centrifuge tube containing 7 ml of 10% formalin.
3. Emulsify the faeces in the formalin and filter through the brass/plastic filter into the dish.
4. Wash the filter and discard any lumpy residue.
5. Transfer the filtrate to a boiling tube; add 3 ml of ether and mix well on a vortex mixer for 15 seconds or by hand for 1 minute.
6. Transfer back to the centrifuge tube and centrifuge at 3000 r.p.m. for 1 minute.
7. Loosen the fatty plug with an orange stick and pour the supernatant away by quickly inverting the tube.
8. Allow the fluid on the side of the tube to drain on to the deposit; mix well and transfer a drop to a slide for examination under a coverslip.
9. Use the 10× and 40× objectives to examine the *whole* of the deposit for ova and cysts.

SATURATION SALT FLOTATION METHOD
Method
1. Boil coarse granular NaCl in excess in water to produce a saturated solution which, when cooled, has a specific gravity of 10.18–10.20.
2. Half fill a wide-mouthed flat-bottomed container with the saturated salt solution.
3. Emulsify 1 g of faeces in the solution and remove the larger debris from the surface.
4. Fill the container to the top with saturated salt solution until a convex meniscus forms.
5. Lay a glass slide or coverslip over the top, making sure that no bubbles are trapped.
6. Leave for 20 minutes before quickly inverting the slide.
7. Cover with a coverslip/slide and scan for ova using the 10× objective.

This is a cheap preparation using simple apparatus. Ideally suitable for field work. It concentrates nematode ova well but it does not concentrate cysts.

THE STRING TEST 'ENTEROTEST'

This procedure utilizes a length of thread in a weighted gelatin capsule. The end of the string is taped to the patient's

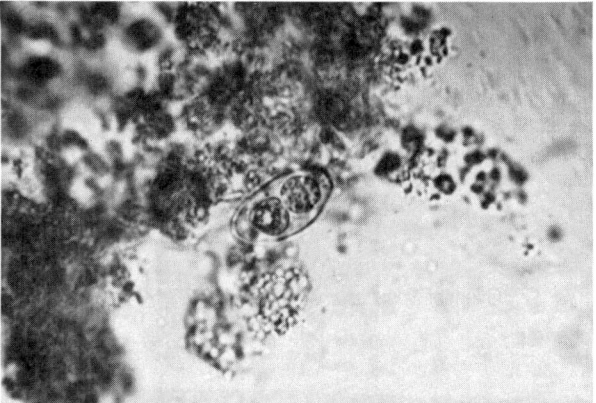

Figure V.4   Oocyst of *Isospora belli*.

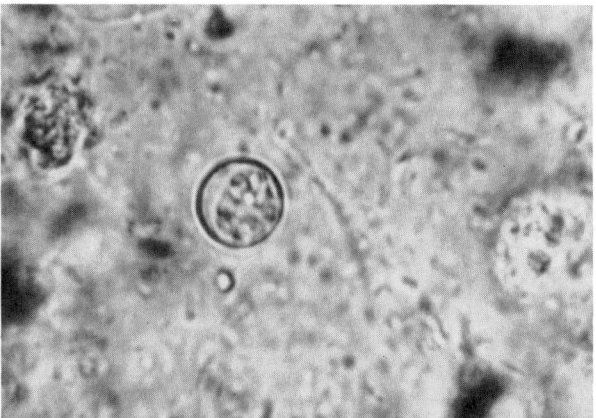

Figure V.5   Oocyst of *Cyclospora cayatenensis*.

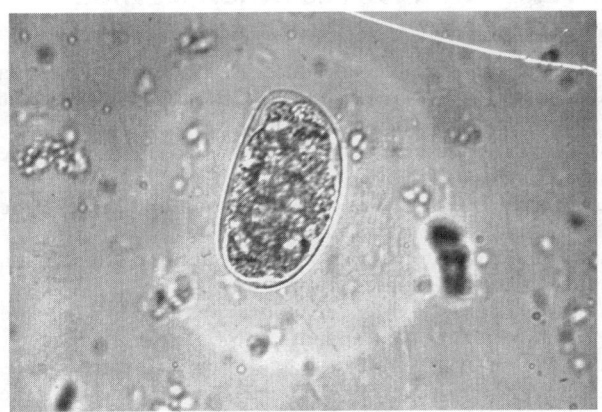

Figure V.6 Ovum of hookworm.

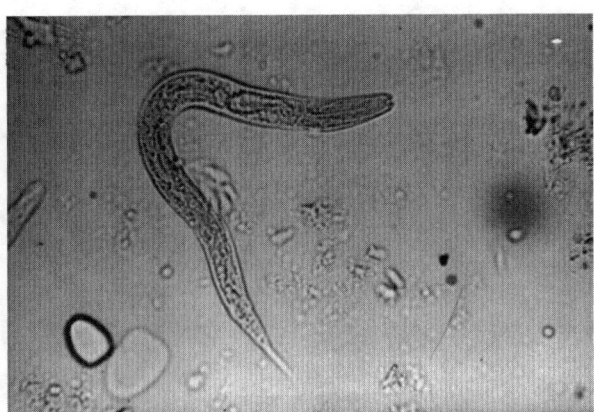

Figure V.9 Larva of *Strongyloides stercoralis*.

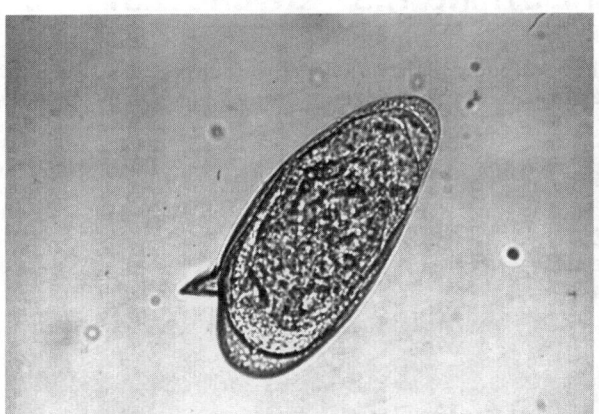

Figure V.7 Ovum of *Schistosoma mansoni*.

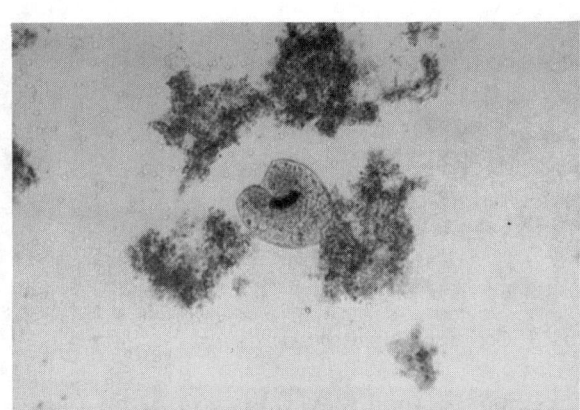

Figure V.10 Protoscoli of *Echinococcus granulosus*.

face and the capsule is swallowed. The patient lies on the right side so that the capsule will travel to the duodenum. After 4 hours the string is pulled up (the weight is passed out in the faeces). The string will be stained yellow with bile and mucus where it has been in the duodenum. If no part of the string is yellow the test should be repeated. The string is placed in a pot and covered with 5 ml of saline.

Method

1. Agitate the string and saline, preferably using a whirli-mixer, to remove jejunal mucus from the string.
2. Wind the string around an applicator stick, pressing it against the side of the container to remove jejunal mucus and excess saline, and then discard it.
3. Centrifuge the saline at 2000 r.p.m. for 2 minutes.
4. Discard the supernatant and transfer the deposit to a microscope slide and examine using the 10× and 40× objectives for trophozoites of *Giardia* and active larvae of *Strongyloides*. Ova from trematodes of the biliary tract may also be found.

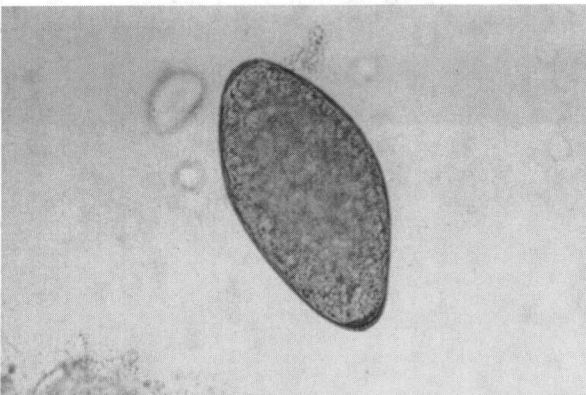

Figure V.8 Ovum of *Fasciola hepatica*.

STAINING METHODS FOR INTESTINAL PROTOZOA

Table V.1 lists the identifying features of common protozoal cysts.

TEMPORARY STAINS

Stains for wet preparations following concentration by the formol–ether method.

LUGOL'S IODINE SOLUTION (DOUBLE STRENGTH)

Reagent 1
- Potassium iodide   20 g
- Iodine   10 g
- Distilled water   100 ml

Add potassium iodide to the distilled water; when dissolved, add the iodine crystals. Store in a brown bottle. Remains stable for many weeks.

Reagent 2
- 25% glacial acetic acid

Method
Mix equal parts of reagents 1 and 2 for use.

Results
Iodine stains glycogen brown and the nuclear chromatin of amoebic cysts brown/black.

BURROWS STAIN

- Thionin   20 mg
- Acetic acid   3 ml
- Ethanol   3 ml
- Distilled water   94 ml

Method
Add an equal volume of the stain to the faecal concentrate and allow to stand for 12–18 hours.

Results
Chromidial bars stain deep blue.

PERMANENT STAINS

TRICHROME STAIN

The trichrome method for staining protozoa is especially recommended for identifying features of amoebic cysts and trophozoites.

Solution A: Schaudinn's fixative
- 95% Ethanol   33.3 ml
- Mercuric chloride 66.6 ml (saturated aqueous solution approximately 14 g/100 ml)

Just prior to use, add 5 ml glacial acetic acid/100 ml of solution.

Table V.1   Identification of cysts of common protozoa.

Protozoan cyst	Size	Nuclear pattern	Inclusions
Entamoeba histolytica	1–4 Nuclei, 9–14 μm	Fine chromatin, central karyosome	Diffuse glycogen, chromidial body
Entamoeba hartmanni	1–4 Nuclei, 7–9 μm	Fine chromatin, central karyosome	Diffuse glycogen, chromidial body
Entamoeba coli	1–8 Nuclei, 14–30 μm	Fine chromatin, eccentric karyosome	Diffuse glycogen, chromidial body rare
Iodamoeba bütschlii	1 Nucleus, 9–15 μm	Coarse chromatin, no karyosome	Compact glycogen vacuole
Endolimax nana	3–4 Nuclei, 6–9 μm	3–4 Granules forming	Nil
Giardia lamblia	Oval, 4 nuclei (not obvious unless stained), 8–12 μm	No diagnostic significance	Refractile axoneme and flagellar remnants
Chilomastix mesnilii	Lemon-shaped, 1 nucleus, 5–6 μm	Fine chromatin	Refractile axoneme

Horen's fixative (alternative to Schaudinn's fixative)
- Cupric sulphate 2% 100 ml
- Ethanol 50 ml
- Glacial acetic acid 7.5 ml

Mix all ingredients together. Fix prepared slides for 30 minutes before they are completely dry.

This fixative does not use the potentially harmful mercuric chloride.

Solution B: iodine alcohol
- To prepare *stock solution* add enough iodine crystals to 70% ethanol to make a dark concentrated solution.
- To prepare *working solution* dilute stock solution by adding 70% ethanol. The exact concentration is unimportant.

Solution C: acid ethanol
- Glacial acetic acid 0.5 ml
- 90% Ethanol 100 ml

Method
1. Make a thin smear of the faecal material on a glass slide.
2. While the smear is still wet, immediately place the slide in a Coplin jar containing Schaudinn's fixative (solution A) for 5 minutes at 50°C or 1 hour at room temperature.

Staining:
3. Iodine alcohol (solution B) 10 minutes
4. 70% Ethanol 3–5 minutes
5. 80% Ethanol 3–5 minutes
6. Parapak trichrome 10 minutes
7. Acid alcohol (solution C) 2–3 seconds
8. 95% Ethanol dip twice
9. 95% Ethanol 5 minutes
10. 95% Ethanol 5 minutes
11. 100% Ethanol 3 minutes
12. Xylene 5 minutes
13. Mount with coverslip using DPX—do not allow the xylene to dry on the slide.

Results
Nuclei, chromidial bars, chromatin, red cells and bacteria stain red. Cytoplasm stains blue-green. Background and yeasts stain green.

INVESTIGATION OF BLOOD/TISSUE PARASITES

- *Plasmodium* spp. (Table V.2)
- *Trypanosoma* spp.
- Spirochaetes
- *Babesia* spp.
- *Leishmania* complex.

Blood parasites can be identified from peripheral blood, bone marrow aspirate, splenic aspirate, gland aspirate or cerebrospinal fluid or from biopsy material. Procedures for identification include (Figures V.11–V.14):

- Direct staining of blood or impression smears
- Culture of appropriate sample
- Concentration methods
- Detection by using DNA recognition methods.

Table V.2 Identification of malaria parasites.

	Plasmodium falciparum	Plasmodium vivax	Plasmodium ovale	Plasmodium malariae
Red blood cells	Normal size and shape	Enlarged	Enlarged, fimbriate, oval	Small, older
Inclusions	Maurer's clefts in mature trophozoite	Schüffner's dots, fine stippling	James' dots, coarse stippling	Ziemann's dots, not seen unless overstained
Trophozoite	Delicate fine rings, accolé forms	Larger, thicker rings	Thick compact rings	Small compact rings
Developing trophozoites	Compact ring, cytoplasm vacuolated	Large amoeboid with central vacuole	Slightly amoeboid but smaller than *P. vivax*	Sometimes seen as a band across cell
Schizont	2–24 merozoites; single, large pigment clump	12–24 Merozoites almost filling red blood cell	8–12 Merozoites fill three-quarters of red blood cell	6–12 Merozoites around central pigment mass
Gametocyte	Crescent-shaped aggregated chromatin and pigment in centre	Large, round, almost fills red blood cell	Smaller, round, fills half red blood cell	Round, may fill between one-half and two-thirds of red blood cell
Pigment	Single clump in schizont	Several fine clumps from late trophozoites	Coarse granules from late trophozoites	Dark fine granules at all stages

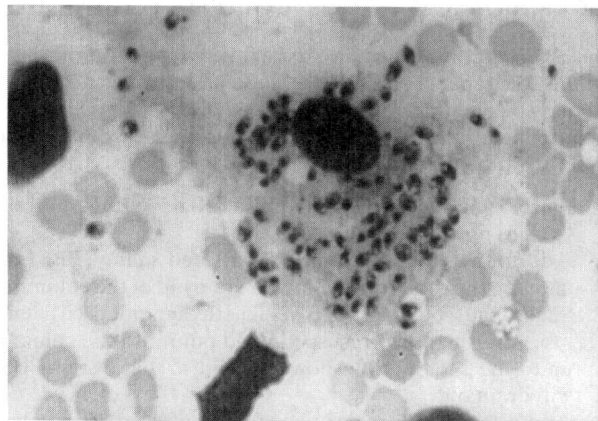

Figure V.11 Amastigotes of *Leishmania* in the bone marrow aspirate.

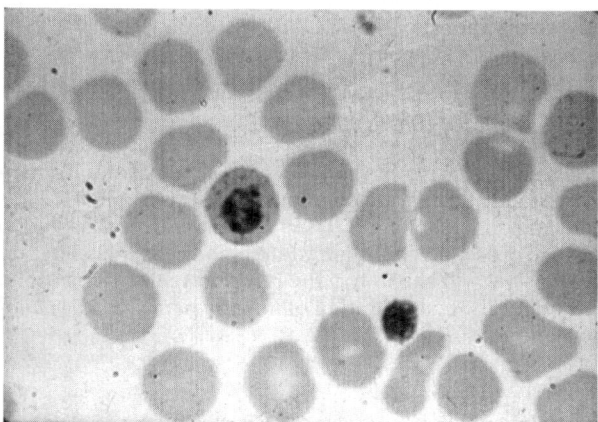

Figure V.12 Schizont of *Plasmodium falciparum* in peripheral blood.

STAINING BLOOD FILMS

GIEMSA STAIN

Giemsa stain is a Romanovsky stain and will stain chromatin material red and cytoplasm blue. Inclusion bodies within the cell will stain red or blue according to their origin.

Materials
- Giemsa stain; a good quality stain is necessary (e.g. Gurr's R66, E. Merck, Poole, Dorset, UK)
- Solvent methanol
- Buffered water pH 6.8 and pH 7.2; tablets are available for the preparation of 1-litre volumes.

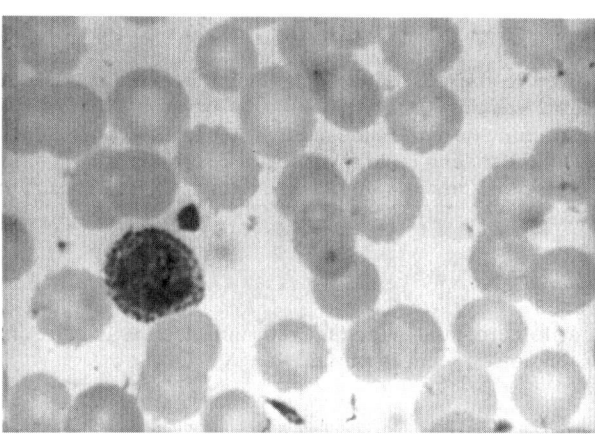

Figure V.13 Gametocyte of *Plasmodium vivax*.

Method
Allow smears prepared from blood, aspirates or CSF deposits to dry thoroughly before staining.

1. Flood the smear with solvent methanol and allow to fix for 1 minute.
2. Tip off the alcohol.
3. Prepare a 1 in 10 dilution of Giemsa stain using 5 drops of stain and 45 drops of appropriate buffered water. Use buffered water pH 7.2 for staining for malaria and pH 6.8 for the other blood parasites.
4. Flood the fixed slide with diluted stain and allow to stain for 30 minutes.
5. At the end of this time, rinse the stain from the slide with buffered water and allow to drain dry.

Results
Parasite chromatin stains red, cytoplasm stains blue and cellular inclusions red. Red cell nuclear remnants (Howell–Jolly bodies) stain deep blue.

CONCENTRATION OF PARASITES FROM BLOOD

Parasites that are scanty can be concentrated before staining by several methods. These include:

- *Thick blood film*: suitable for concentrating malaria parasites, trypomastigotes and spirochaetes.
- *'Buffy coat'*: suitable for concentrating malaria parasites, trypomastigotes and spirochaetes.
- *Mini anion exchange column*: suitable for concentrating trypomastigotes.

THICK BLOOD FILMS

Preparation

Using an applicator stick or directly from a finger prick, place 2 or 3 drops of blood on to one end of a slide. Using the applicator stick spread the blood over an area of $1\,cm^2$ and allow to dry thoroughly.

Field's stain for thick blood films

Field's stain consists of the two components of the Romanovsky stains in separate solutions. These are called Field's stain A and Field's stain B. Used to stain *unfixed* thick blood films the procedure will stain white blood cells, platelets and parasites but will haemolyse the red blood cells. It is a useful method for the concentration of malaria parasites, *Trypanosoma* and *Borrelia* spp.

Materials
- Field's stain A solution (purchased as a prepared stain or prepared as 2.5 g% in distilled or filtered water from the powder form).
- Field's stain B solution (prepared as for Field's stain A).

Method
1. Dip the unfixed, dried, thick blood film in Field's stain A for 3 seconds.
2. Carefully rinse the slide in tap water for 3 seconds.
3. Dip the slide in Field's stain B for 3 seconds.
4. Rinse the slide in water again and then stand vertically to dry.

Results
Parasite chromatin will stain red and cytoplasm blue; inclusion dots, if seen, stain red.

BUFFY COAT EXAMINATION

Method
1. Collect peripheral blood into capillary tubes containing EDTA anticoagulant, filling the tube three-quarters full with blood and rotating to mix the anticoagulant. Seal the end with plasticine and place the tube in the microhaematocrit centrifuge with a corresponding balance tube opposite.
2. Secure the lid and centrifuge the blood at 10 000 r.p.m. for 5 minutes.
3. Remove the tube and using an ampoule blade or a diamond marker score the tube just below the layer of white cells and platelets (buffy coat) at the junction of the plasma layer. Break the tube at this point and expel the buffy coat by tapping on to the end of several slides; push the blood to prepare a thin slide. When dry, fix the slide in methyl alcohol for 5 minutes and stain by Giemsa stain, diluted 1 in 10 with buffered water pH 6.8, for 20 minutes.

Results
The buffy coat will contain malaria parasites, spirochaetes and trypanosomes and may demonstrate parasites when none can be seen in the thick or thin film.

MINI ANION EXCHANGE COLUMN TECHNIQUE

This is a useful concentration technique where other investigations for trypanosomes in the blood have proved negative. Blood is passed through a column of cellulose. Erythrocytes are retained in the column and trypanosomes pass out into a collecting tube.

1. Place a piece of dry sponge into a 2 ml syringe barrel. (This is now termed the column.)
2. Add four drops of phosphate buffered saline (PBS) to dampen the sponge and allow to drain out of the column.
3. Shake the cellulose (DE 52—diethylaminoethyl cellulose) thoroughly to resuspend and pour into the column up to the 2 ml mark. Allow to stand so that excess PBS will drain out.
4. Add a few millilitres of phosphate buffered saline plus glucose (PBSG) to the top of the column and allow it to drain through.
5. Take 150–200 μl of blood (from a finger prick) and drop on to the top of the column. Allow the blood to soak into the column. Attach a collecting pipette to the base of the column.
6. Pipette a few drops of PBSG on top of the blood and *immediately* attach the reservoir and fill with PBSG (approximately 1.5 ml). This will drip slowly on to the column.
7. Leave until all the PBSG has washed through the column. (This should take approximately 4 minutes.)
8. The collecting pipette will now be full of PBSG plus any trypanosomes that were present in the blood.
9. Centrifuge the collecting pipette (in its plastic cover) at 2000 r.p.m. for 10 minutes.
10. Place the pipette on a slide or viewing chamber and, using the 20× objective, examine its tip within 20 minutes for motile trypanosomes.

LABORATORY DIAGNOSIS OF THE FILARIA PARASITES

Filariasis is diagnosed either serologically or by finding the L3 larvae, or microfilariae, in peripheral blood, urine, hydrocele fluid or skin snips. Occasionally adult worms can be removed as they cross the eye (*Loa loa*) or from a subcutaneous nodule (*Onchocerca volvulus*).

Because of the periodic appearance of microfilariae, the peripheral blood sample is collected between 10.00 and 14.00 (day blood) and between 22.00 and 02.00 (night blood). An early morning sample of urine is most suitable.

Urine may show a milky appearance, called chyluria, if filariasis is present.

EXAMINATION OF BLOOD FOR MICROFILARIAE

Filtration method
1. Collect 20 ml of blood into sodium citrate anticoagulant at the appropriate time.
2. Draw the blood up into a syringe and connect it to the

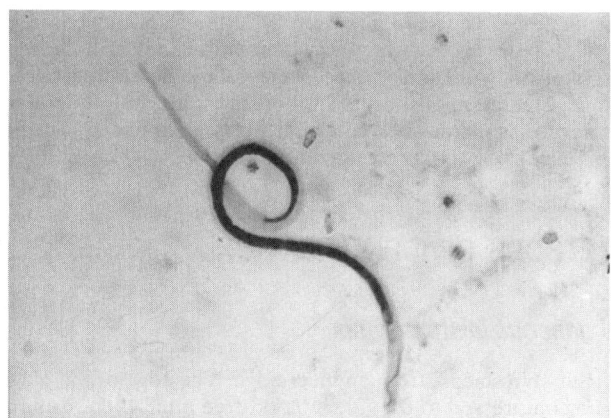

Figure V.14 Microfilaria of *Loa loa*.

Swinnex holder containing the 5 μm pore size Nuclepore membrane.
3. Gently push the blood through the membrane, collecting the filtrate into a container of disinfectant.
4. Draw up 10 ml of normal saline into the syringe and push this through the membrane in a similar manner.
5. Draw several millilitres of air into the syringe and push this through to clear the membrane.
6. Carefully dismantle the holder and, using forceps, remove the membrane and place it on to a slide.
7. Add a drop of normal saline to the membrane and cover with a coverslip.
8. Scan the whole area of the coverslip using the 10× objective to search for the motile microfilariae.
9. Closer inspection using the 40× objective and by allowing a drop of 1% methylene blue dye to run under the coverslip will help to show if the microfilariae has a sheath.

Modification of Knott's method for examining blood for microfilariae

1. Collect 20 ml of blood into sodium citrate anticoagulant, as described above.
2. Add the blood to an equal volume of 1% saponin in saline (or 2% formalin if saponin is not available).
3. Mix well and allow to stand for 15 minutes before transferring to centrifuge tubes and centrifuging for 20 minutes at 2000 r.p.m.
4. Pour off the supernatant into a container of disinfectant and mix the deposit well before transferring a drop to a

slide, covering with a coverslip, and scanning for microfilariae. The saponin preparation will show actively moving larvae; those in the formalin preparation will not be moving.

EXAMINATION OF URINE AND HYDROCELE FLUID

1. Urine and hydrocele fluid can be filtered in a similar manner to blood to show any microfilariae present.
2. Alternatively they can be put into a clean centrifuge tube and centrifuged at 2000 r.p.m. for 5 minutes, the supernatant discarded and a drop of the deposit transferred to a slide. Cover with a coverslip and examine in the same way as for blood.

IDENTIFICATION OF MICROFILARIAE (Table V.3)

Staining

Reagents
• Giemsa stain
• Delafield's haematoxylin

If sufficient microfilariae are present, films prepared directly from peripheral blood can be used to stain them. If not, the blood can be prepared as a thick film or microfilariae can be washed from the membrane filter by placing it into a small pot of saline and agitating. The saline can then be centrifuged at 2000 r.p.m. for 5 minutes and the deposit pipetted on to a slide and dried.

Method
1. Fix the thin blood film or the film prepared from the deposit with methyl alcohol for 5 minutes. If a thick blood film is used it is necessary first to haemolyse the dried slide by placing it vertically in water for 5 minutes. Dry the slide well and fix in methyl alcohol for 5 minutes.
2. Stain the slides with Giemsa stain diluted 1 in 10 with buffered water pH 6.8 for 20 minutes.
3. Wash the stain from the slide with the buffered water, then 'differentiate' the stain by leaving the water on the slide for 5 minutes. At the end of this period look at the slide to see if the nuclei of the microfilariae are clear and

Table V.3 Identification of microfilariae.

Microfilariae	Sheath	Tail	Other features
Loa Loa	Yes, stains pale blue	Blunt, nuclei to tip	Large nuclei
Wuchereria bancrofti	Yes, stains pink	Pointed, nuclei stop short of tail	Nuclei small, discrete; lies in gentle curves
Brugia malayi	Yes, stains deep pink	Blunt, with two discrete nuclei in tail	Nuclei large; lies in sharp angles
Mansonella perstans	No	Blunt	One large nucleus in tail
Mansonella ozzardi	No	Pointed, nuclei stop short of tail	—

discrete. If not, repeat the process, reducing the time of 'differentiation' until nuclei are clearly seen.

4. Tip the buffer from the slide and flood the slide with Delafield's haematoxylin for 15 minutes.
5. Wash the stain from the slide with buffered water and allow the slide to sit in the water for 5 minutes to reach the maximum intensity of staining (called 'blueing' the slide).

Results

Giemsa stain will stain the nuclei of the microfilariae and the haematoxylin will stain the sheath, if present.

Examination of skin snips for microfilariae of Onchocerca volvulus

Filaria worms of *Onchocerca volvulus* live in subcutaneous tissue nodules, and discharge their microfilariae into the tissue. They are identified by examining small pieces of skin taken from various parts of the body.

Method

1. Collect small pieces of skin and subcutaneous tissue, using a corneal punch, to a depth of 1 mm. Alternatively use a needle point to lift the skin and cut it using a scalpel blade.
2. Place the skin snips into a microtitre tray containing a few drops of saline. Alternatively, place them individually on to a slide with a drop of saline and cover with a coverslip.
3. Leave the snips in the saline for at least 4 hours and examine under the low power (10×) objective, or by using an inversion or dissecting microscope, looking for microfilariae which swim out from the snips.
4. An estimate of the number of microfilariae per milligram of tissue can be made by preweighing the fresh snip and counting all the microfilariae released.
5. Areas of the body that can be 'snipped' are usually the back, buttocks and calves of the legs, but any area exhibiting urticaria or itching should be included.

LABORATORY DIAGNOSIS OF LEISHMANIASIS

The leishmanial organisms are a broad complex of species responsible for a wide variety of clinical responses. Laboratory diagnosis is made by identifying the organism in tissue or from the reticuloendothelial system.

Culture is an important diagnostic aid; culture media are varied but NNN media, a rabbit blood-agar base using a salt-based overlay (e.g. Locke's solution) and a liquid tissue culture medium (e.g. Schneider's drosophila medium) with added fetal calf serum, are useful. Cultures are incubated at 20°C for up to 28 days. On examination they will show a conversion from amastigote stage to motile promastigote stage. Detection of specific antibodies is only really useful in visceral leishmaniasis when high titres of antibody can be detected using the direct agglutination test.

METHODS OF IDENTIFICATION

Cutaneous leishmaniasis

- Slit-skin smears from an ulcer edge. The edge of the ulcer is compressed to provide a blood-free area, then, using a fine point (no. 15) scalpel blade, a slit is made into the subcutaneous tissue and the base is gently scraped. The tissue juice and cells are transferred to a slide and smeared over an area of 1 cm^2. The preparation is allowed to dry before being fixed in methyl alcohol and stained with Giemsa stain (see above).
- Needle aspiration using a small syringe to inject saline around the lesion, and then reaspirating it to prepare slides and cultures, can also be used.

  Cultures can also be made from the slit-skin smear.
- Biopsy. Biopsies of the ulcer edge are taken and divided into two parts. One part is fixed in buffered formalin for histopathology. The second piece is aseptically cut into small pieces for culture and to make impression smears.

  Impression smears are made by dabbing the tissue several times on to a slide to deposit the cells. These are then dried and fixed in methyl alcohol before staining with Giemsa stain.

Visceral leishmaniasis

- Bone marrow, splenic aspirate and lymph node aspiration are the tissues used to demonstrate *Leishmania* spp. in this clinical form. Peripheral blood buffy coat may yield parasites in the immunocompromised host.
- Smears are made and stained with Giemsa stain.
- Cultures are also made into NNN and Schneider's media.

IDENTIFICATION OF SPECIES OF *LEISHMANIA*

Identification of specific species of *Leishmania* can be made using two principal techniques.

1. Zymodeme: using the isoenzyme pattern.
2. Polymerase chain reaction (PCR).

EXAMINATION OF CEREBROSPINAL FLUID

Cerebrospinal fluid (CSF) can be used to search for parasites causing cerebral malaria or trypanosomiasis or to demonstrate bacteria causing meningitis.

CSF is collected into two clean sterile containers: one sample is sent for bacteriological culture; the second sample is used for (a) cell count, (b) examination of stained deposit after centrifugation, and (c) biochemical tests on the supernatant, if possible.

METHOD

1. Examine the CSF visually and report one of the following appearances:
   (a) Clear.
   (b) Opalescent or cloudy; this specimen is likely to have a raised cell count.
   (c) Blood-stained. Red blood cells that have disintegrated due to age may give a yellow tinge to the fluid, known as xanthochromia.
2. Note any fibrin clot that may form on standing.
3. Remove the clot carefully using a small wire loop and spread it over a small area of a slide. Allow to dry and, after fixation, stain the slide by the Ziehl–Neelsen method for mycobacteria.
4. Transfer the CSF to a centrifuge tube and centrifuge at 2000 r.p.m. for 5 minutes.
5. Carefully tip off the supernatant into a second tube for biochemical analysis (glucose, protein).
6. Mix the deposit well by tapping the tube and use a clean Pasteur pipette to transfer a drop to each of three slides.
7. Spread the drops over a small area and allow the slides to dry well.

STAINING

Stain one slide with Giemsa stain in order to differentiate any blood cells present. Stain the second with Gram stain to detect any micro-organisms present. Stain the third with Ziehl–Neelsen stain for *Mycobacterium tuberculosis*.

Giemsa stain (see p. 1743)

Result

Normally the CSF has no more than five white blood cells per microlitre and these are usually lymphocytes. Increased white blood cells are seen in bacterial infections. Pyogenic meningitis will give an increase in polymorphonuclear cells, and tubercular meningitis gives an increase in lymphocytes. Red blood cells are not a normal finding and indicate an accidental traumatic tap or bleeding into the subarachnoid space.

Gram stain

Materials

- Gram stain: 1 g gentian or crystal violet dissolved in 100 ml distilled water
- Lugol's iodine
  Reagent 1: Potassium iodide   20 g
              Iodide   10 g
              Distilled water   100 ml
  Add potassium iodide to the distilled water; when dissolved add the iodine crystals. Store in a brown bottle.
- Acetone or methylated spirit
- Neutral red: 0.5 g neutral red dissolved in 100 ml distilled water.

Method

1. Fix the slide by passing it quickly through the flame of a spirit lamp.
2. Place the slide on a rack and flood with Gram stain for 1 minute.
3. Wash the stain from the slide.
4. Flood the slide with Lugol's iodine for 1 minute.
5. Tilt the slide and pour on acetone or alcohol to decolorize; allow the decolorizing agent to stay on the slide for a short time only (5–10 seconds) before washing off with tap water.
6. Flood the slide with the neutral red counterstain for 30 seconds.
7. Wash the stain from the slide with water and stand the slide vertically to dry.

Results

Although almost any group of bacteria can be responsible for meningitis there are some which are seen more commonly: pneumococci—Gram-positive cocci in pairs (diplococci); *Haemophilus influenzae*—small slender Gram-negative bacilli; meningococci—Gram-negative intracellular diplococci seen inside the polymorphonuclear cells). Other bacteria will vary in morphological shape and Gram-stained appearance. *Cryptococcus neoformans* (fungus) may also be visualized.

Ziehl–Neelsen stain

Materials

- Carbol fuchsin stain
- 1% Acid alcohol   1 ml concentrated hydrochloric acid
                      99 ml methylated spirit
- 0.5% Malachite green   0.5 g malachite green dissolved in 100 ml distilled water

Method

1. Fix the smear by passing it through the flame of a spirit lamp.
2. Flood the slide with carbol fuchsin and, using the spirit lamp, gently warm the slide until the surface begins to steam.
3. Stain for 15 minutes.
4. Wash the slide with water.
5. Flood the slide with 1% acid alcohol and gently rock until no more colour will come out.
6. Wash the slide with water.
7. Flood the slide with malachite green counterstain for 1 minute.
8. Wash the slide with water and drain dry.

Results

Mycobacteria are acid-fast bacilli and will stain as red bacilli against a green background.

EXAMINATION OF SPUTUM

Sputum is commonly examined for parasites of the respiratory tract and for bacteria causing pulmonary infections such as tuberculosis or pneumonia. Sputum is usually described by its appearance as:

- Salivary—frothy, white and watery.
- Purulent—thicker consistency, often with a greenish colour.
- Mucopurulent—thick, sticky consistency, containing pus, may be blood-stained.

EXAMINATION FOR PARASITES

Paragonimus spp.

Paragonimus westermani and other *Paragonimus* species discharge ova with the sputum and usually cause a 'rusty', blood-stained sputum.

Ova can be recovered after dissolving mucus in the sputum by mixing a portion with an equal portion of 10% potassium hydroxide and, after mixing thoroughly, standing for 15 minutes before centrifuging for 5 minutes. The deposit is examined for ova using the 10× objective.

The sputum can also be concentrated, after dissolving the mucus, using the formol–ether method.

PNEUMOCYSTIS CARINII

Although now reclassified as a fungal organism, demonstration of this parasitic organism of the immunocompromised host requires specialized laboratory techniques. In sputum the method used is a fluorescent monoclonal antibody stain on a specially prepared concentrate. Kits for this are available from several commercial sources.

EXAMINATION FOR BACTERIA

Two thin smears of sputum are made using a wire loop that can be sterilized in a flame afterwards, or an applicator stick that can be burned. The smears can then be fixed when dry by passing the back of the slide through a flame twice.

One smear is stained for acid-fast bacilli using the Ziehl–Neelsen method (see above). The second is stained for other bacteria using the Gram stain (see above).

Sputum should be sent for routine culture if available, and for culture for *Mycobacterium tuberculosis* if required.

EXAMINATION OF BLOOD FILMS FOR HAEMATOLOGICAL ASSESSMENT

Haematological values are necessary in the diagnosis of infection or anaemia. The most useful criteria include:

- Total white cell count
- Differential white blood cell count
- Haemoglobin
- Haematocrit
- Mean corpuscular haemoglobin
- Platelet count
- Examination of the blood picture.

The *blood picture* can give much useful information even when other parameters are not available.

Method

1. Fix thin blood films in methyl alcohol and stain with Giemsa stain (see p. 1743).
2. Examine the slide using the oil immersion objective (100×).

Observations

Red blood cells

- Note the *size*: a normal erythrocyte measures 7 μm in diameter. The cell may be enlarged (macrocyte), or appear smaller (microcyte).
- Note the *colour*: in a normal erythrocyte the haemoglobin is stained pink with a small area of pallor in the centre. An enlarged area of central pallor (hypochromia) indicates an iron deficiency.
- Note the presence of any *abnormal* erythrocytes. Target cells or sickle cells may indicate an abnormal haemoglobin type.
- Note any *inclusions* of the erythrocytes; basophilic stippling and nucleated cells or spherocytes may indicate a haemolytic process.
- Note any intracellular or extracellular *parasites* which may be present (malaria, *Trypanosoma*, *Babesia*, *Borrelia*, microfilariae).

White blood cells

An impression of the *number* of white cells present can be gained from the thin blood film, an average of 1–2 cells in each field is normally seen. A differential count will indicate the *types* of cells present.

Note the *morphological appearance* of the cells. Neutrophils may show a shift to the left or to the right. Mononuclear cells may be 'atypical', and any primitive cells must be recorded.

Platelets

These are normally seen in every field, either singly or in small clumps. A decrease in platelets is noted when they are scanty, seen in every 3–5 fields only.

FURTHER READING

Fleck S L & Moody A H. *Diagnostic Techniques in Medical Parasitology*. London: Wright, 1988: 135.

RADIOLOGY AND IMAGING SERVICES IN THE TROPICS

W. Peter Cockshott

In many parts of the tropics the provision of diagnostic imaging facilities is undoubtedly deficient when related to Western models. This appendix will present some of the problems and suggest policies that may help to improve the service provided. There are no universal answers since the needs, priorities and possibilities differ so immensely from place to place. What may be applicable to an oil-rich affluent state has little relevance to most of the less fortunate countries that are economically deprived and also lack a trained infrastructure. Even within a country, distortions in levels of radiological health care arise from the competing demands of capital cities and the requirements of provincial and rural centres.

Radiology is often perceived as a luxury, a costly service that devours resources at an alarming rate. The role of radiology in the diagnosis of tropical infectious diseases is limited because laboratory investigations are usually far more effective and useful. Further tension is vented by the relative financial demands of curative and preventive medicine in maximizing effective use of the health budget. However, without entering into these legitimate concerns, I shall assume here that some level of diagnostic imaging is to be provided and that the nature, level and staffing of the service will be as cost effective as possible. There are many factors that militate against such an outcome: utilization, suitability of facilities and equipment, and availability of trained personnel. It becomes obvious that the models of radiological services that have arisen and evolved in industrialized countries are inappropriate for much of the world.

UTILIZATION OF RADIOLOGY

There are considerable variations in the utilization of radiography in Western countries, with annual rates ranging from close to 1000 examinations per 1000 population in the USA and Finland to levels around 500–700 for the European Union. By contrast, for much of Africa the figures are around 20–30 per 1000 population.[1] The number of examinations is a crude index as it does not reflect complexity, but this is of little moment because most studies in the less developed world are simple. This 30-times lower utilization is supported by data on film use—square metres per 1000 population per annum. For the industrialized world the figure is around 130, whereas for equatorial countries of Africa it is below five and figures for South-East Asia are around 28. These are 1977 figures and although there are likely to have been slight changes since then the order of magnitude of the difference is probably little altered. Finally, to indicate the same trend for more complex contrast studies using barium sulphate as a marker, more than 80% of world 'medicinal' barium is consumed by North America, Japan and Europe—the remaining 11% by the rest of the world.[1]

There is no optimal utilization and undoubtedly there is inappropriate overuse in many communities. If guidelines such as those contained in the World Health Organization (WHO) publication *A Rational Approach to Radiodiagnostic Investigations*[2] were applied, utilization would be considerably less in certain countries. The Royal College of Radiologists' guidelines of good practice have been shown to reduce utilization of X-ray services by general practitioners.[3]

In recent years the advent of new modalities, particularly ultrasonography, has led to a reduction in the use of X-ray studies because they have been replaced by non-ionizing techniques, which are often less costly. The high technology imaging modalities of nuclear medicine, computerized tomography and nuclear resonance have an impact on the affluent countries as the proportion of such relatively costly studies rises, but as yet this is a limited problem in the tropics in the government sector.

In the context of the less affluent parts of the tropical world we must ask: What are the main clinical demands for imaging services? The most numerous probably relate to trauma—the ability to detect skeletal injuries resulting from motor, agricultural and industrial accidents. The next clinical need is chest radiography in children and adults to detect pneumonia and tuberculosis. Ultrasonographic pregnancy monitoring and detection of placental site in those with bleeding would probably be next in the list of priorities. Plain abdominal radiographs to deal with acute abdominal conditions and calculi would be the next priority. All these demands can be met with relatively simple radiographic and ultrasonographic apparatus. Fluoroscopic facilities, which are considerably more complex and expensive and require a trained physician, are largely for contrast studies. These are of low volume and, because of the capital investment needed, costly. Thus, ordering and ranking of clinical needs for a particular situation indicates the type and complexity of equipment required.

EQUIPMENT

Throughout the tropics there is a numerical deficiency of equipment, exacerbated by much being obsolete, broken and lacking spare parts and so ineffective. Lack of maintenance facilities, long delayed replacement of equipment because of shortage of capital funds and lack of standardization all contribute to this sorry state. In developed countries there is often about one X-ray unit to every 2000–3000 population, whereas in much of the less developed world the figure is closer to one per 100 000 population.[1] The situation is even worse when it is realized that the capital city plus a few other major cities may contain 80% of the equipment, serving perhaps 15–20% of the population. This type of maldistribution is of course matched by the siting of radiologists and radiographers—rural areas are generally ill served.

All too often there is a mixture of equipment of widely different vintages, made by different firms—a maintenance nightmare. The equipment has been obtained episodically without any planning for standardization and suitability. Radiologists wish to emulate the state of the art in equipment available elsewhere if they can, but the complexity and cost of such a policy is not always wise. Donated equipment is often unsuitable. Too often little attention is paid to the characteristics of the local electrical power supply and the availability of spares and manufacturers' repair facilities. All these considerations point towards the desirability of rationalization and simplification. The equivalent of a Volkswagen can be as effective in transportation as a Rolls Royce, at much less cost. Reliability is related to complexity: the possibility of a malfunction increases according to the product of the number of components and not their sum. In this context the WHO Basic Radiology System BRS needs to be promoted as a solution as it can be the basis of a most efficient X-ray service.

As the name implies, the WHO BRS is a system of hardware (the X-ray unit) and software (manuals for technicians and physicians). Here we shall consider the equipment that has evolved from various manufacturers under WHO guidelines. Incidentally, beware: several makers have used the BRS designation for models that bear little relation to WHO specification. The basic form of the unit is illustrated in Figure VI.1. There is a vertical stand with an X-ray tube and film holder at a fixed distance that can pivot from vertical to horizontal. The patient lies on a wheeled trolley. The power supply can be from special mains or, in some models, operate from conventional wall outlets, the power being stored in batteries and thus enabling the provision of power independently of outside lines for a period. Even solar panels can be used. The X-ray generator has adequate power (12 kW), thanks to solid-state high frequency invertor technology, so that its output is equivalent to that of much more expensive and elaborate hospital units. BRS controls have been rationally simplified for easy operation. The images produced are of the highest quality and proven to be fully comparable with the best that can be obtained with the most sophisticated hospital units. The BRS unit is mechanically simple and there

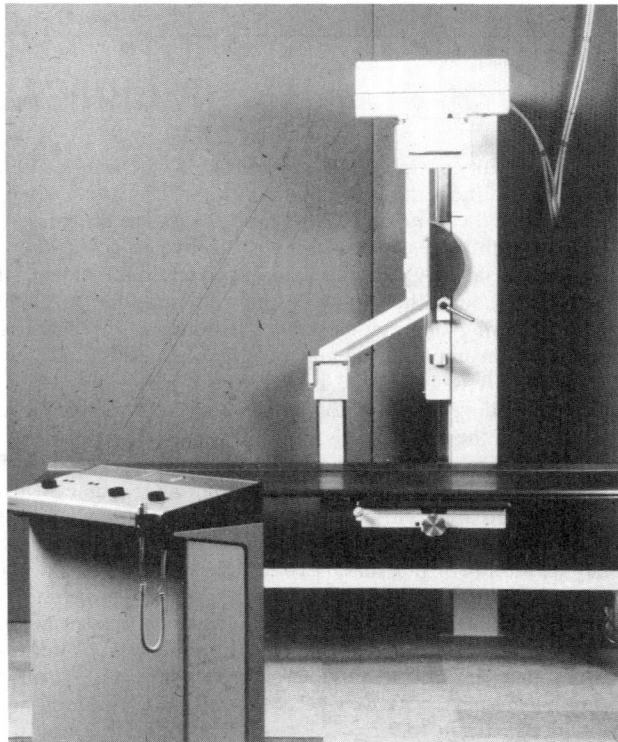

Figure VI.1 Example of a BRS X-ray unit with the swinging tube/receptor arm vertical over the mobile trolley. Note the simplicity of the console with its on/off control, kV selector and mAs control.

is very little to go wrong. In practice the reliability, throughput and freedom from breakdown have been remarkable.

Why has such a paragon taken so long to be adopted? Manufacturers have been reluctant to produce an inexpensive model because it could impede sales of more sophisticated units. Further, the market was considered to be small, limited to the less developed world. However, the adoption of most of the basic BRS concept by 'military units' of Western armies and by Swedish trauma services indicates much wider acceptance. Now several excellent units are available (advice can be obtained from the WHO Section of Radiation Medicine, Geneva).

The BRS unit does not provide fluoroscopy. It is suitable for all levels of hospital, and indeed can probably carry out 80% of the work of a tertiary referral hospital with no loss of quality and usually at a lower radiation dose than that of a standard hospital model.

For fluoroscopy and angiography more elaborate equipment is needed. Once again, if several units are to be purchased, some standardization is an advantage for maintenance purposes. Adequacy of power lines must be ensured as more complex apparatus can be very demanding. Air conditioning may also be essential for newer units with computer controls.

For many applications ultrasonography serves excellently and may obviate the need for fluoroscopy. Apart from obvious diagnostic applications in obstetrics and gynaecology and liver and renal disorders, many interventional studies can be guided by ultrasonography. The cost of ultrasonographic units again varies with complexity. For most situations relatively simple units are the most cost effective and reliable. A WHO Working Party has produced recommendations on appropriate equipment and a manual of interpretation.[4]

TECHNICAL PERSONNEL

The availability of trained staff to operate X-ray units is often a problem. Individuals trained to the certificate level of industrialized countries for 2 or more years are scarce, can demand high wages, and often wish to live in cities where there are what they consider suitable educational and social facilities. Though there may be one radiographer per 3000 population in some industrialized countries, in much of Africa, for example, there may be only one per million.

So what is to be done? Firstly, the highly trained professional radiographer is not usually required outside large hospitals as the workload is small, the equipment is simple and the range of studies limited. This may lead to career dissatisfaction (it is as though a photographer trained with sophisticated apparatus is given an instamatic camera). As a result *ad hoc* on the job training is provided to someone who may divide his or her time between X-ray duties and other tasks. If indeed some training has been given and there is supervision, a workable scheme may develop, sacrificing somewhat on image quality and radiation safety. An alternative approach is to copy the military and some former colonial medical systems where short training periods are provided centrally to form a cadre of X-ray operators who are appropriately skilled. Candidates should preferably be recruited from the locale where they will work so that language is not a problem and the workers will be willing to remain in their community rather than gravitate to the capital when trained.

Once again, the BRS manual for radiographers and the BRS darkroom manual, available from WHO in several languages, are excellent training instruments and indispensable handbooks.[5,6]

The manual for radiographers is designed so that facing pages show how the apparatus is to be arranged and set for a particular study, what size film to use, how to position the patient and the appearance of the final image desired (Figures VI.2 and VI.3). No attempt is made to teach the theory of radiography but notes on radiation safety and patient care are provided. Though initially designed for the primary care level, the text is suitable for use even in tertiary care institutions.

This text has been successfully used in training primary school learners to operate BRS units in Latin America and Africa with periods of training as short as 3 weeks. Occasional follow-up on site by more highly trained supervisory personnel is, of course, desirable to maintain standards, remedy problems and provide encouragement. Organized radiography societies in several developing countries have objected to this training of operators on various professional grounds. Basically they fear loss of status, and wages, as a lower tier of assistant radiographers develops. Instead they should regard it as a challenge to improve their own careers. The scheme provides operators where they are needed at a level that is appropriate for the needs, so relieving highly trained personnel from reiterative simple tasks.

Fully trained radiographers are mobile and subject to the brain drain to better themselves. Jamaica has lost half of its trained radiographers in the last few years due to migration. Assistant radiographers are not subject to the same market forces, as the level of training would only be recognized locally.

Both levels of staffing are needed for major hospitals, where the 2-year radiographer can be fully employed in doing the more complicated radiography and carrying out managerial and supervisory duties.

FILM INTERPRETATION

The majority of medical schools in the world provide relatively little training in diagnostic imaging. Many physicians incidentally obtain further experience during their internship but non-specialists' knowledge in this field is generally limited. Yet perforce such doctors usually find themselves in the role of being the film interpreter because there are no radiologists readily available. In much of Africa and Asia there is less than one radiologist per million population, compared with more than one per 20000 in industrialized countries where radiologists represent about 4% of all physicians. In the less developed world this figure is under 1%.

Consequently, local physicians have to deal with the majority of interpretations with little guidance beyond that acquired from experience. They obviously need to recognize life-threatening emergencies such as tension pneumothorax, pulmonary oedema and acute obstruction. Most become skilled in recognizing fractures. However, there are often perplexing images which give rise to many questions. Is this a

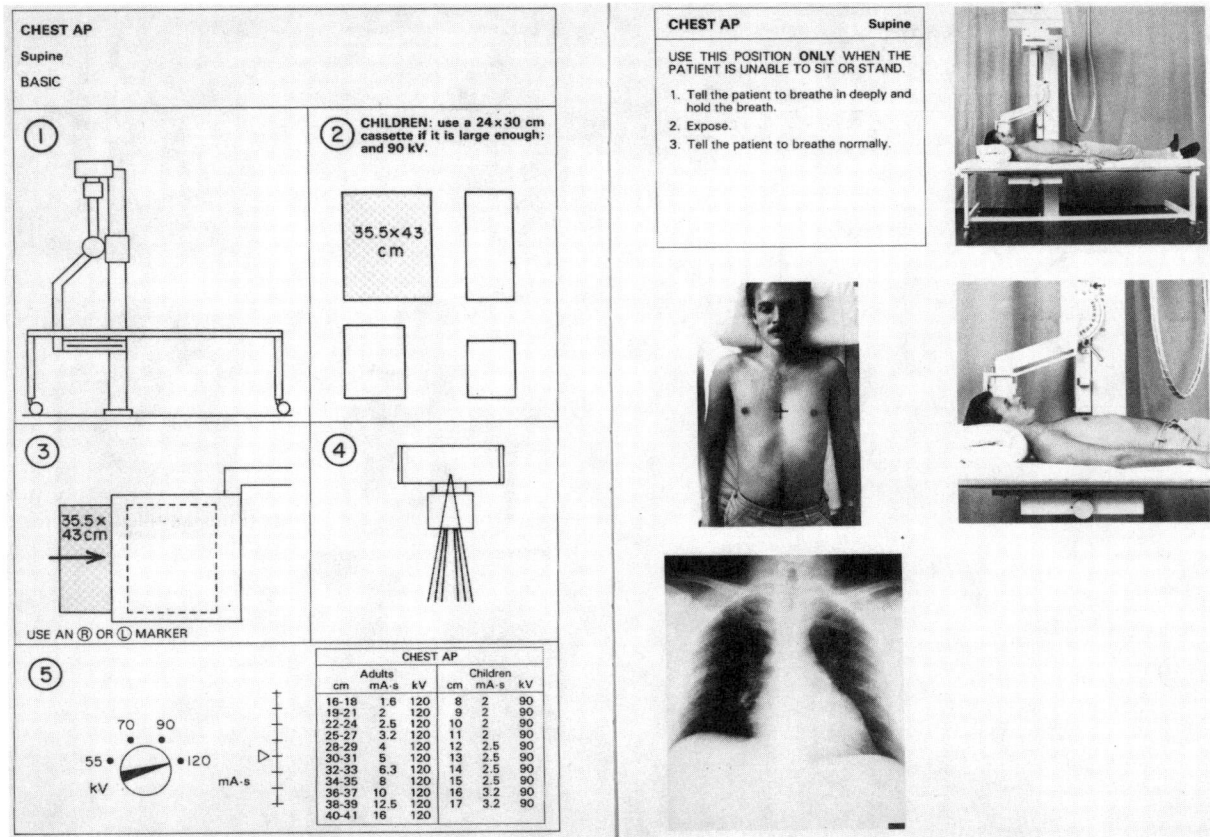

Figure VI.2 Two facing pages from the WHO BRS technique manual showing the position for supine chest AP, which cassette to select, how to collimate and choose the technique, with illustrations of centring and how the finished product should appear.

case that requires further work-up that may be costly or entail a long journey over bad roads? Can I send a film for an opinion or do I have to send the patient as well? No small unit can be expected to possess a comprehensive reference library. There is no easy solution but the BRS *Manual of Radiographic Interpretation for General Practitioners* may be of assistance, together with its companion work on ultrasonographic interpretation.[4,7] Obviously such a work is not comprehensive but concentrates on the most common diagnostic problems that can be managed at the primary care level as well as those conditions that necessitate referral. There are obvious limitations to such an approach but the type of guidance provided has proved to be of value in the short term.

Obviously the provision of trained radiologists is a long-term objective. Where should they be trained? Where possible the source of training should be in the country or region, if there is a local medical school that offers residency training,

so that trainees become familiar with local disorders and with the type of facilities that are available. This is not to say that such training is entirely restricted to local training because exposure to foreign institutions with more modern state-of-the-art equipment and more specialized teachers is obviously valuable. However, entirely foreign training has disadvantages because, on returning to the homeland, a radiologist may suffer severe disappointment at the facilities available and emigrate to find a place elsewhere. A balance has to be sought. Training schemes pioneered in the Caribbean at the University of West Indies, where radiologists spend 3 of their 4 years training in the West Indies, with mainland exposure elsewhere for 1 year, have proved to be highly successful. Similarly the multinational training programme based at the University of Nairobi under the cosponsorship of WHO and the ISR reaches trainees from anglophone East and Central Africa.

GENERAL CONCLUSIONS

In much of the world there is a shortage of trained radiographers and radiologists and they have limited imaging facili-

ties, too often not the most suitable, available to them. The basic economic realities mean that progress will be slow.

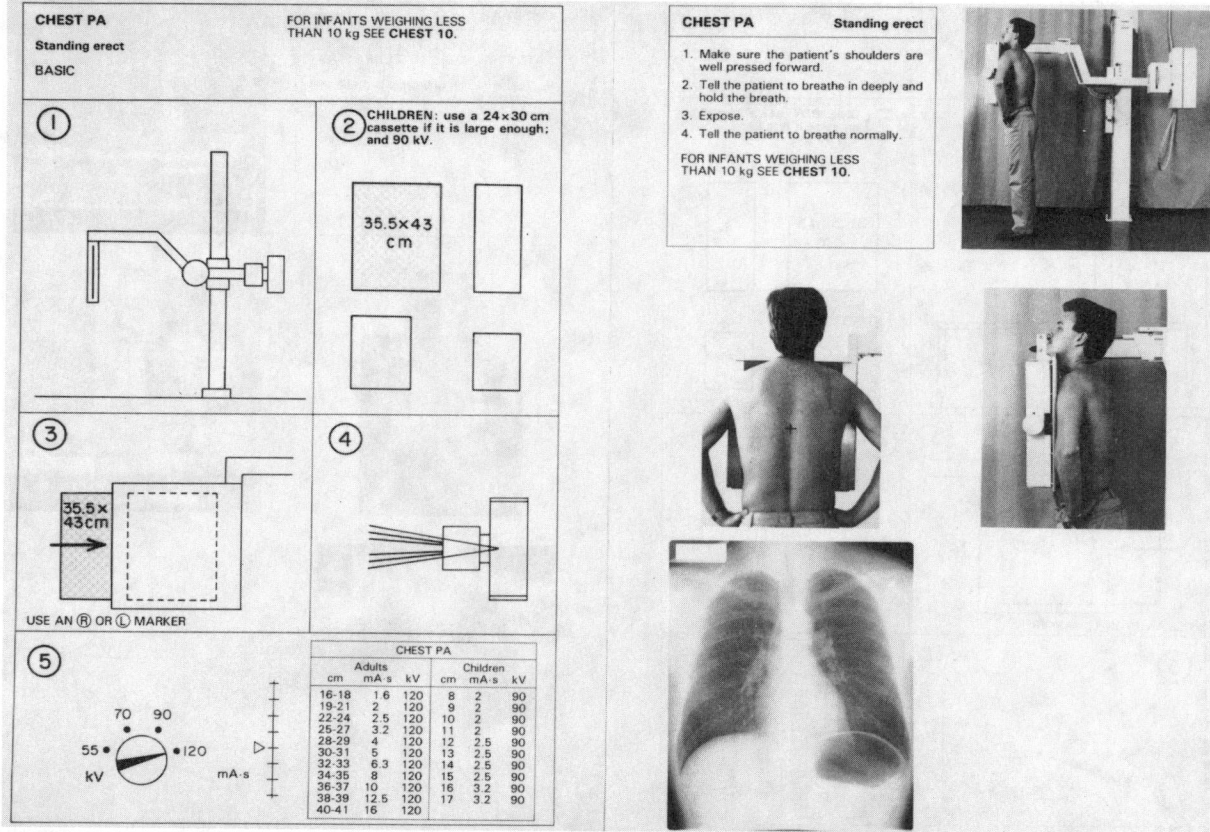

Figure VI.3   BRS set-up for standard PA chest. Note the numbering of the sequences to obtain the correct set-up.

There must be a willingness to use non-traditional approaches so that clinical needs can be met with available funds. Rational simplification of equipment with greater use of staff locally trained to an appropriate level must be considered. This is not to advocate 'barefoot' radiographers and radiologists, but there is no need for all to wear city shoes. Sandals and boots are not amiss if a comprehensive service is to be provided.

REFERENCES

1 Cockshott W P. Diagnostic Radiology: geography of a high technology. *AJR* 1979; 132:339–344.
2 World Health Organization. A rational approach to radiodiagnostic investigations. *WHO Tech Rep Ser* 1983; 689.
3 Royal College of Radiologists Working Party. Influence of Royal College of Radiologists' guidelines on referral from general practice. *BMJ* 1993; 306:110–111.
4 Palmer P E S (ed.). *Manual of Diagnostic Ultrasound.* Geneva: World Federation of Ultrasound, 1993.
5 Palmer P E S. *Manual of Darkroom Technique—WHO Basic Radiological System.* Geneva: WHO, 1985.
6 Holm T, Palmer P E S & Lehtinen E. *Manual of Radiographic Technique.* Geneva: WHO, 1986.
7 Palmer P E S, Cockshott W P, Hegedus V & Samuel E. *Manual of Radiographic Interpretation for General Practitioners.* Geneva: WHO, 1985.

INDEX